D0848649

PEDIATRIC CRITICAL CARE

PEDIATRIC CRITICAL CARE

Third Edition

BRADLEY P. FUHRMAN, MD
Professor of Pediatrics and Anesthesiology
Chief, Pediatric Critical Care Medicine
Children's Hospital of Buffalo
Buffalo, New York

JERRY J. ZIMMERMAN, MD, PHD
Professor of Pediatrics and Anesthesiology
Director, Critical Care Medicine
Children's Hospital and Regional Medical Center
Seattle, Washington

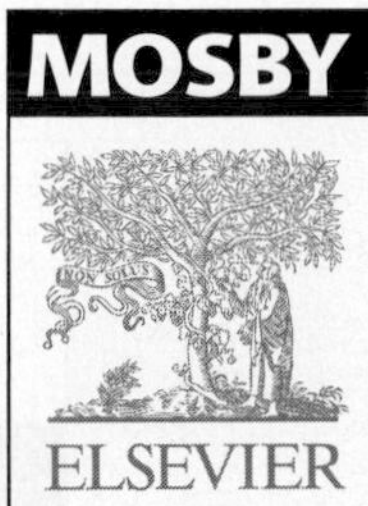

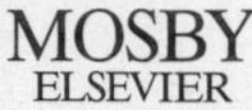

MOSBY
ELSEVIER

1600 John F. Kennedy Boulevard
Suite 1800
Philadelphia, PA 19103-2899

PEDIATRIC CRITICAL CARE
Third Edition
ISBN-13: 978-0-323-01808-1
ISBN-10: 0-323-01808-4

Notice

Knowledge and best practice in this field are constantly changing. As new research and experience broaden our knowledge, changes in practice, treatment and drug therapy may become necessary or appropriate. Readers are advised to check the most current information provided (i) on procedures featured or (ii) by the manufacturer of each product to be administered, to verify the recommended dose or formula, the method and duration of administration, and contraindications. It is the responsibility of the practitioner, relying on his or her own experience and knowledge of the patient, to make diagnoses, to determine dosages and the best treatment for each individual patient, and to take all appropriate safety precautions. To the fullest extent of the law, neither the Publisher nor the Editors assume any liability for any injury and/or damage to persons or property arising out or related to any use of the material contained in this book.

The Publisher

Previous editions copyrighted 1998, 1992.

ISBN 13: 978-0-323-01808-1
ISBN 10: 0-323-01808-4

Publisher: Natasha Andjelkovic
Developmental Editor: Joanne Husovski
Project Manager: Cecelia Bayruns
Design Direction: Ellen Zanolle
Marketing Mananger: Emily Christie

Printed in the United States of America.

Last digit is the print number: 9 8 7 6 5 4

Although in debt to many,
we are especially grateful to our families, friends, and colleagues,
who have been ever so patient, and to the many authors and
counselors who have contributed to this text.

Contributors

P. David Adelson, MD, FACS, FAAP
Professor of Neurosurgery and Vice Chairman of Research
Department of Neurosurgery
Director, Pediatric Neurotrama
Children's Hospital of Pittsburgh
Director, Surgical Epilepsy Center
Director, Brachial Plexus and Peripheral Nerve Center and Clinic
Pittsburgh, Pennsylvania

David B. Allen, MD
Professor of Pediatrics
Director of Endocrinology and Residency Training
University of Wisconsin Children's Hospital
Madison, Wisconsin

Estella M. Alonso, MD
Professor of Pediatrics
Northwestern University Feinberg School of Medicine
Director, Hepatology and Liver Transplantation Program
Children's Memorial Hospital
Chicago, Illinois

Gülay Pinar Alper, MD
Assistant Professor
Division of Child Neurology
Department of Pediatrics
University of Pittsburgh School of Medicine
Children's Hospital of Pittsburgh
Pittsburgh, Pennsylvania

Derek C. Angus, MD, MPH
Associate Professor of Critical Care Medicine and Health Services Administration
Vice-Chair of Research
Department of Critical Care Medicine
University of Pittsburgh School of Medicine
Pittsburgh, Pennsylvania

Sidney Anthone, MD
Clinical Professor Emeritus
Department of Surgery
State University of New York at Buffalo School of Medicine and Biological Sciences
Medical Director; Upstate New York Transplant Services, Inc.
Buffalo, New York

Andrew Argent, MD
Head, Critical Care and Children's Heart Disease
Red Cross War Memorial Children's Hospital
Cape Town, South Africa

John H. Arnold, MD
Associate Professor of Anesthesia
Harvard Medical School
Medical Director, Division of Respiratory Diseases
Senior Associate in Perioperative Anesthesia
Senior Associate in Critical Care Medicine
Children's Hospital Boston
Boston, Massachusetts

Barbara Bambach, MD
Assistant Professor of Hematology/Oncology
Assistant Professor of Pediatrics
State University of New York at Buffalo School of Medicine and Biomedical Sciences
Clinician II, Cancer Research Pediatrician
Attending Physician, Department of Pediatrics
Roswell Park Cancer Institute
Assistant Attending Physician
Children's Hospital of Buffalo
Buffalo, New York

Hülya Bayir, MD
Assistant Professor
Department of Critical Care Medicine
Safar Center for Resuscitation Research
University of Pittsbugh School of Medicine
Pittsburgh, Pennsylvania

Pierre Beaulieu, MD, PhD, FRCA
Assistant Professor of Anesthesiology and Pharmacology
University of Montreal Faculty of Medicine
Centre Hospitalier de l'Université de Montréal–Hôtel-Dieu
Montréal, Quebec, Canada

Laurie O. Beitz, MD
Assistant Professor, Division of Rheumatology
University of Washington School of Medicine
Children's Hospital and Regional Medical Center
Seattle, Washington

Jorge R. Beltrán, MD
Department of Pediatric Surgical Services
Children's Hospital of Buffalo
Buffalo, New York

Wade W. Benton, PharmD
Research Pharmacist, Investigational Drug Service
Children's Hospital and Regional Medical Center
Seattle, Washington

Robert A. Berg, MD
Department of Pediatrics
University of Arizona College of Medicine
Tucson, Arizona

Ira Bergman, MD, PhD
Professor of Pediatrics and Neurology
Department of Pediatrics
University of Pittsburgh School of Medicine
Division of Child Neurology
Children's Hospital of Pittsburgh
Pittsburgh, Pennsylvania

Julie Blatt, MD
Professor and Chief
Division of Pediatric Hematology-Oncology
Department of Pediatrics
University of North Carolina at Chapel School of Medicine
University of North Carolina Hospitals
Chapel Hill, North Carolina

Douglas L. Blowey, MD
Associate Professor of Pediatrics and Pharmacology
Divisions of Pediatric Nephrology and Clinical Pharmacology
University of Missouri–Kansas City School of Medicine
Children's Mercy Hospitals and Clinic
Kansas City, Missouri

Jeffrey L. Blumer, MD, PhD
Professor of Pediatrics and Pharmcology
Case Western Reserve University School of Medicine
Chief, Pediatric Pharmacology and Critical Care
Department of Pediatrics
Rainbow Babies and Children's Hospital
Cleveland, Ohio

John S. Bradley, MD
Director, Division of Infectious Diseases
Children's Hospital and Health Center
San Diego, California

Barbara W. Brandom, MD
Professor, Department of Anesthesiology
University of Pittsburgh Medical Center
Attending Anesthesiologist
Children's Hospital of Pittsburgh
Director, North American Malignant Hyperthermia Registry of Malignant Hyperthermia Association of the United States
Pittsburgh, Pennsylvania

Martin L. Brecher, MD
Associate Professor of Pediatrics
State University of New York at Buffalo School of Medicine and Biomedical Sciences
Chairman, Department of Pediatrics
Roswell Park Cancer Institute
Division Chief, Hematology/Oncology
Children's Hospital of Buffalo
Buffalo, New York

Richard J. Brilli, MD, FAAP, FCCM
Professor, Department of Pediatrics
Associate Chief of Staff
Clinical Director, Pediatric Intensive Care Unit
Medical Director, Patient Transport Services
Cincinnati Children's Hospital Medical Center
Cincinnati, Ohio

Guy F. Brisseau, MD
Department of Pediatric Surgery
Women and Children's Hospital
Buffalo, New York

Thomas V. Brogan, MD
Assistant Professor of Pediatrics and Anesthesia
Division of Pediatric Critical Care Medicine
Department of Pediatrics
University of Washington School of Medicine
Children's Hospital and Regional Medical Center
Seattle, Washington

Timothy E. Bunchman, MD
Adjunct Professor of Pediatrics and Human Development
Michigan State University College of Human Medicine
Department of Pediatric Nephrology, Dialysis, and Transplantation
DeVos Children's Hospital at Spectrum Health
Grand Rapids, Michigan

Sean P. Bush, MD, FACEP
Associate Professor, Department of Emergency Medicine
Loma Linda University School of Medicine
Loma Linda, California

Joseph Carcillo, MD
Associate Professor of Critical Care Medicine and Pediatrics
Department of Critical Care Medicine
University of Pittsburgh School of Medicine
Children's Hospital of Pittsburgh
Pittsburgh, Pennsylvania

Aaron L. Carrel, MD
Assistant Professor of Pediatrics
Division of Endocrinology
University of Wisconsin Children's Hospital
Madison, Wisconsin

Hector Carrillo-Lopez, MD
Professor of Pediatric Critical Care
Universidad Nacional Autonóma de México
Head, Critical Care Division
Hospital Infantil de Mexico
Mexico City, Mexico

Victoria Cartwright, MD, MS
Chief, Pediatric Rheumatology
Department of Pediatrics
Madigan Army Medical Center
Tacoma Washington
Clinical Instructor, Division of Rheumatology
Children's Hospital and Regional Medical Center
Seattle, Washington

Hugo F. Carvajal, MD
Program Director, Department of Pediatrics
Medical Director, Pediatric Critical Care
Baptist Health System
San Antonio, Texas

Leticia Castillo, MD
Boston Children's Hospital
Boston, Massachusetts

Michael G. Caty, MD
Associate Professor of Surgery and Pediatrics
State University of New York at Buffalo School of Medicine and Biomedical Sciences
Surgeon-in-Chief, Department of Pediatric Surgical Services
Women and Children's Hospital of Buffalo
Buffalo, New York

Pelin Cengiz, MD
Division of Critical Care Medicine
Children's Hospital and Regional Medical Center
Seattle, Washington

Anthony C. Chang, MD, MBA
Associate Professor and Chief, Critical Care Cardiology
The Lillie Frank Abercrombie Section of Cardiology
Department of Pediatrics
Baylor College of Medicine
Director, Pediatric Cardiac Intensive Care Unit
Texas Children's Hospital
Houston, Texas

John R. Charpie, MD, PhD
Clinical Associate Professor
Michigan Congenital Heart Center/Pediatric Cardiology
C.S. Mott Children's Hospital
Ann Arbor, Michigan

Adrián Chávez, MD
Chief of Pediatric Intensive Care Department
Hospital Infantil de México
Associate Professor of Pediatric Critical Care
Universidad Nacional Autónoma de México
Mexico City, Mexico

Russell W. Chesney, MD
Professor and Chair, Department of Pediatrics
University of Tennessee Health Science Center
Vice President of Academic Affairs
Le Bonheur Children's Medical Center
Memphis, Tennessee

Michael A. Cimino, MD
Clinical Assistant Professor
Department of Pediatrics
State University of New York at Buffalo School of Medicine and Biomedical Sciences

State University of New York at Buffalo
School of Pharmacy and
Pharmaceutical Sciences
Clinical Pharmacy Services Manager
The Women and Children's Hospital of
Buffalo–Kaleida Health
Buffalo, New York

Robert S.B. Clark, MD
Associate Director, Safar Center for
Resuscitation Research
Pediatric Neuroscience and Molecular
Biology
University of Pittsburgh Medical Center
Pittsburgh, Pennsylvania

Jacqueline J. Coalson, PhD
Professor of Pathology
University of Texas Health Science Center
at San Antonio
San Antonio, Texas

D. Ryan Cook, MD
Professor of Anesthesiology
Division of Pediatric Anesthesia and
Critical Care Medicine
Duke University Medical Center
Durham, North Carolina

Craig M. Coopersmith, MD
Associate Professor of Surgery and
Anesthesiology
Washington University School of
Medicine
Barnes-Jewish Hospital
Saint Louis, Missouri

Christopher P. Coppola, MD
Judson G. Randolph Fellow
Department of Pediatric Surgery
Children's National Medical Center
Washington, District of Columbia

Seth J. Corey, MD, MPH
Associate Professor of Pediatrics
University of Texas at Houston Medical
School
Section Chief, Pediatric
Leukemia/Lymphoma
Division of Pediatrics
MD Anderson Cancer Center
Houston, Texas

Peter N. Cox, MBChB, FRCPC
Associate Professor of Anaesthesia and
Paediatrics
University of Toronto Faculty of
Medicine
Associate Chief and Clinical Director
Department of Critical Care
Hospital for Sick Children
Toronto, Ontario, Canada

Kathleen Culver, RN, MS, CPNP
Nurse Practitioner, Critical Care
Department of Pediatrics
University Hospital and Medical Center
Stony Brook, New York

James J. Cummings, MD
Professor of Pediatrics and Physiology
Brody School of Medicine at East
Carolina University
Section Head, Department of
Neonatology
Children's Hospital of Eastern Carolina
Greenville, North Carolina

Martha A.Q. Curley, RN, PhD, FAAN
Assistant Professor
Department of Anesthesia
Harvard Medical School
Director of Critical Care and
Cardiovascular Nursing Research
Children's Hospital Boston
Boston, Massachusetts

Marek Czosnyka, PhD
Department of Neurosurgery
Cambridge University
Cambridge, England

Heidi J. Dalton, MD
Medical Director
Pediatric Intensive Care Unit
Children's Hospital National Medical
Center
Washington, District of Columbia

Stéphane Dauger, MD
Service de Pédiatrie-Réanimation
Hôpital Robert Debré
Paris, France

Peter J. Davis, MD
Professor of Anesthesia and Pediatrics
Department of Anesthesiology
University of Pittsburgh School of
Medicine
Anesthesiologist in Chief
Children's Hospital of Pittsburgh
Pittsburgh, Pennsylvania

Jenina Deshler, MSW
Practicum Instructor
University of Washington School of Social
Work
Clinical Social Worker, Pediatric Intensive
Care Unit
Senior Social Worker, Department of
Social Work
Children's Hospital
Private practice-psychotherapy
Seattle, Washington

Sonny Dhanani, BSc(pharm), MD, FRCPC
Clinical Fellow
Department of Critical Care Medicine
Hospital for Sick Children
Toronto, Ontario, Canada

Rhonda M. Dick, MD
Associate Professor, Department of Pediatrics
University of Arkansas for Medical Sciences
Medical Director, Emergency Department
Arkansas Children's Hospital
Little Rock, Arkansas

Emily L. Dobyns, MD
Associate Professor of Pediatrics
Section of Critical Care Medicine
University of Colorado Health Sciences Center
The Children's Hospital
Denver, Colorado

Elizabeth J. Donner, MD, FRCP(C)
Assistant Professor of Pediatrics
University of Toronto Faculty of Medicine
Staff Neurologist
Division of Neurology
Department of Pediatrics
Hospital for Sick Children
Toronto, Ontario, Canada

Didier Dreyfuss, MD
Professor of Critical Care
Faculte Xavier Bichat
Paris, France
Chairman of Critical Care Department
Service de Reanimation Medicale
Hôpital Louis Mourier (Assistance Publique–Hopitaux de Paris)
Colombes, France

Philippe Durand, MD
Service de Réanimation Pédiatrique
Hôpital de Bicêtre
Le Kremlin-Bicêtre, France

Susan Duthie, MD
Pediatric Intesivist
Pediatric Critical Care
Children's Hospital and Health Center
San Diego, California

Richard G. Ellenbogen, MD
Chief of Neurosurgery
Children's Hospital and Regional Medical Center
Seattle, Washington

Jacqueline Evans, MD
Department of Anesthesiology and Critical Care Medicine
Children's Hospital Los Angeles
Los Angeles, California

James C. Fackler, MD
Associate Professor of Anesthesiology and Critical Care Medicine
Johns Hopkins Medical School
Johns Hopkins Hospital
Baltimore, Maryland

Kathryn Felmet, MD
Assistant Professor, Critical Care Medicine
University of Pittsburgh School of Medicine
Children's Hospital of Pittsburgh
Pittsburgh, Pennsylvania

Jeffrey R. Fineman, MD
Professor of Pediatrics
Associate Investigator, Cardiology Research Institute
University of California, San Francisco, School of Medicine
San Francisco, California

Debra H. Fiser, MD
Professor and Chair, Department of Pediatrics
University of Arkansas for Medical Sciences
Chief of Pediatrics
Arkansas Children's Hospital
Little Rock, Arkansas

Frank A. Fish, MD
Associate Professor of Pediatrics and Medicine
Division of Pediatric Cardiology
Vanderbilt University School of Medicine
Nashville, Tennessee

James E. Fletcher, MB BS, MRCP, FRCA
Associate Professor of Anesthesiology
University of North Carolina at Chapel Hill School of Medicine
Chapel Hill, North Carolina

J. Julio Pérez Fontán, MD
Alumni Endowed Professor of Pediatrics
Washington University School of Medicine
St. Louis, Missouri

Michael L. Forbes, MD
Assistant Professor of Pediatrics
Drexel University College of Medicine
Philadelphia, Pennsylvania

Norman Fost, MD
Professor of Pediatrics
University of Wisconsin Medical School
Department of Pediatrics
Children's Hospital Clinical Sciences Center
Madison, Wisconsin

Joel E. Frader, MD
Professor of Pediatrics and Professor of Medical Humanities and Bioethics
Feinberg School of Medicine
Northwestern University Medical School
Chief, General Academic Pediatrics
Children's Memorial Hospital
Chicago, Illinois

Deborah Franzon, MD
Pediatric Intensivist
Department of Critical Care
Children's Hospital and Health Center
San Diego, California

F. Jay Fricker, MD
Professor of Pediatrics
University of Florida College of Medicine
Shands Univiversity Medical Center
Gainesville, Florida

Aaron L. Friedman, MD
Sylvia K. Hassenfeld Professor and Chair
Department of Pediatrics
Brown Medical School
Department of Pediatrics
Hasbro Children's Hospital
Providence, Rhode Island

Bradley P. Fuhrman, MD
Professor of Pediatrics and Anesthesiology
Chief, Pediatric Critical Care Medicine
Children's Hospital of Buffalo
Buffalo, New York

France Gauvin, MD, FRCPC, MSc
Assistant Clinical Professor
Department of Pediatrics
Université de Montréal Faculty of Medicine
Hospital Sainte-Justine
Montréal, Quebec, Canada

Eli Gilad, MD
Pediatric Intensive Care Unit
Wolfson Medical Center
Holon, Israel

James C. Gilbert, MD, FACS, FAAP
Assistant Professor of Surgery and Pediatrics
George Washington University Medical Center
Director of Renal Transplantation, Pediatric Surgery
Children's National Medical Center
Washington, District of Columbia

Brett P. Giroir, MD
Kathryne and Gene Bishop Distinguished Chair in Pediatric Care
The University of Texas Southwestern Medical Center at Dallas
Chief Medical Officer, Department of Administration
Children's Medical Center of Dallas
Dallas, Texas

Stuart L. Goldstein, MD
Associate Professor of Pediatrics
Baylor College of Medicine
Medical Director, Renal Dialysis Unit
Texas Children's Hospital
Houston, Texas

James Graham, MD
Associate Professor, Department of Pediatrics
University of Arkansas for Medical Sciences
Associate Medical Director
Emergency Department
Arkansas Children's Hospital
Little Rock, Arkansas

Jerril W. Green, MD
Assistant Professor, Department of Pediatrics
University of Arkansas for Medical Sciences
Assistant Professor, Pediatric Critical Care Medicine
Arkansas Children's Hospital
Little Rock, Arkansas

Thomas P. Green, MD
Woman's Board Centennial Professor and Chairman of Pediatrics
Northwestern University Feinberg School of Medicine
Physician-in-Chief
Children's Memorial Hospital
Chicago, Illinois

Stephanie Greene, MD
Boston Neurosurgical Foundation
Boston, Massachusetts

James A. Griffith, MD
Department of Pediatrics
John A. Burns School of Medicine
University of Hawaii at Manoa
Honolulu, Hawaii

Mauro Grossi, MD
Clinical Associate Professor of Pediatrics
State University of New York at Buffalo School of Medicine and Biomedical Sciences
Hematology/Oncology Division
Children's Hospital of Buffalo
Buffalo, New York

Björn Gunnarsson, MD
Division of Pediatric Critical Care
Children's Hospital of Buffalo
Buffalo, New York

Scott A. Hagen, MD
Assistant Professor of Pediatrics
Division of Critical Care
University of Wisconsin Children's Hospital
Madison, Wisconsin

Cecil D. Hahn, MD
Department of Neurology
Harvard Medical School
Children's Hospital of Boston
Boston, Massachusetts

Craig Hallstrom, MD
Department of Critical Care
Children's Hospital Medical Center
Cincinnati, Ohio

Yong Y. Han, MD
Clinical Instructor of Critical Care Medicine
University of Pittsburgh School of Medicine
Associate Director, Pediatric Intensive Care Unit
Pediatric Critical Care Medicine
Children's Hospital of Pittsburgh
Pittsburgh, Pennsylvania

Cary O. Harding, MD
Division of Metabolism
Departments of Pediatrics and Molecular and Medical Genetics
Oregon Health and Science University
Portland, Oregon

William G. Harmon, MD
Division of Pediatric Critical Care
Department of Pediatrics
University of Rochester Medical Center
Rochester, New York

Eric Harry, MD
Pediatric Critical Care Fellow
Children's Hospital and Regional Medical Center
University of Washington School of Medicine
Seattle, Washington

Mary E. Hartman, MD
Fellow, Deptartment of Critical Care Medicine
University of Pittsburgh Medical Center
Pittsburgh, Pennsylvania

Christopher Heard, MBChB
Clinical Associate Professor of Anesthesiology and Pediatric Critical Care
State University of New York at Buffalo School of Medicine and Biomedical Sciences
Women's and Children's Hospital of Buffalo
Buffalo, New York

Lynn Hernan, MD
Associate Professor of Pediatrics and Anesthesiology
State University of New York at Buffalo School of Medicine and Biomedical Sciences
Director, Pediatric Intensive Care Unit
Children's Hospital of Buffalo
Buffalo, New York

Mark J. Heulitt, MD
Professor of Pediatrics, Physiology and Biophysics
University of Arkansas for Medical Sciences
Pediatric Intensivist
Arkansas Children's Hospital
Little Rock, Arkansas

Robert W. Hickey, MD
Department of Pediatrics
University of Pittsburgh School of Medicine
Pittsburgh, Pennsylvania

Julien I.E. Hoffman, MD, FRCP
Professor of Pediatrics, Emeritus
Senior Member, Cardiovascular Research Institute
Department of Pediatrics and CVR
University of California, San Francisco, School of Medicine
San Francisco, California

Karen T. Hofmann, RN, BSN
Clinical Manger, Pediatric Intensive Care Unit
Children's Hospital and Regional Medical Center
Seattle, Washington

Gregory A. Hollman, MD
Head, Pediatric Critical Care Medicine
University of Wisconsin Children's Hospital
University of Wisconsin Hospitals and Clinics
Madison, Wisconsin

James C. Huhta, MD
Daicoff-Andrews Chair in Perinatal Cardiology
Professor of Pediatrics and Obstetrics and Gynecology
University of South Florida College of Medicine
St. Petersburg, Florida

Hector E. James, MD
Pediatric Neurosurgery
Jacksonville, Florida

David Jardine, MD
Associate Professor of Pediatrics and Anesthesia
Division of Pediatric Critical Care Medicine
Department of Pediatrics
Children's Hospital and Regional Medical Center
Seattle, Washington

Alberto Jarillo, MD
Assistant Professor of Pediatric Critical Care
Universidad Nacional Autónoma de México
Attending Physician, Pediatric Critical Care Unit
Hospital Infantil de México
Mexico City, Mexico

Etienne Javouey, MD
Service de Réanimation et d'Urgences Pédiatriques
Hôpital Edouard Herriot
Lyon, France

James A. Johns, MD
Associate Professor of Pediatrics
Division of Pediatric Cardiology
Vanderbilt University School of Medicine
Nashville, Tennessee

Kristin K. Johnson, BSPharm, PharmD, BCPS
Clinical Pharmacy Instructor
State University of New York at Buffalo School of Medicine and Biomedical Sciences
Clinical Pharmacy Coordinator
Women and Children's Hospital of Buffalo–Kaleida Health
Buffalo, New York

Michael V. Johnston, MD
Professor of Neurology and Pediatrics
Johns Hopkins University School of Medicine
Chief Medical Officer
Kennedy Krieger Institute
Baltimore, Maryland

Deborah P. Jones, MD
Department of Pediatrics
University of Tennessee Health Science Center
Memphis, Tennessee

Prashant Joshi, MD
Medical Director
Western New York Regional Poison Control Center
Buffalo, New York

Prince J. Kannankeril, MD, MSCI
Assistant Professor of Pediatrics
Division of Pediatric Cardiology
Vanderbilt University School of Medicine
Nashville, Tennessee

Robert K. Kanter, MD
Professor of Pediatrics
Director, Critical Care and Inpatient Pediatrics
SUNY Upstate Medical University
Syracuse, New York

John A. Kellum, MD
Associate Professor of Critical Care Medicine
University of Pittsburgh School of Medicine
Pittsburgh, Pennsylvania

Michael Kelly, MD
Pediatric Critical Care Section
Department of Pediatrics
Robert Wood Johnson Medical School
University of Medicine and Dentristry of New Jersey
Newark, New Jersey

Patrick M. Kochanek, MD, FCCM
Professor and Vice Chairman
Department of Critical Care Medicine
Director, Safar Center for Resuscitation Research
University of Pittsburgh School of Medicine
Children's Hospital of Pittsburgh
Pittsburgh, Pennsylvania

Samuel A. Kocoshis, MD
Professor of Pediatrics
Children's Hospital Medical Center
Cincinnati, Ohio

Thomas J. Kulik, MD
Professor of Pediatrics
University of Michigan Hospitals
Ann Arbor, Michigan

Vasanth H. Kumar, MD
Clinical Assistant Professor of Pediatrics
Division of Neonatology
State University of New York at Buffalo School of Medicine and Biomedical Sciences
The Women and Children's Hospital of Buffalo
Buffalo, New York

Jacques Lacroix, MD, FRCPC
Professor of Pediatrics
Université de Montréal
Pediatric Intensive Care Unit
Hôpital Sainte-Justine
Montreal, Quebec, Canada

Yichen Lai, MD
Research Associate
Department of Critical Care Medicine
University of Pittsburgh School of Medicine
Pittsburgh, Pennsylvania

Joanne M. Langley, MD, MSc, FRCPC
Associate Professor of Pediatrics
Community Health and Epidemiology, Clinical Trials Research Center
Dalhousie University Faculty of Medicine
Halifax, Nova Scotia, Canada

Stanley T. Lau, MD
Research Instructor
Department of Pediatric Surgery
State University of New York at Buffalo
Buffalo, New York

Peter Laussen, MB, BS
Associate Professor of Anesthesia
Department of Aneshtesia
Harvard Medical School
Director, Cardiac Intensive Care
Department of Cardiology
Children's Hospital
Boston, Massachusetts

Yi-Horng Lee, MD
Chief Resident
Department of Pediatric Surgery
Women and Children's Hospital of Buffalo
Buffalo, New York

Mary W. Lieh-Lai, MD
Associate Professor of Pediatrics
Director, Intensive Care Unit and Critical Care Medicine Fellowship
Carman and Ann Adams Department of Pediatrics
Children's Hospital of Michigan
Wayne State University School of Medicine
Detroit, Michigan

D. Michael Lindsay, PharmD, BCPS
Pharmacist
Swedish Medical Center
Seattle, Washington

Catherine Litalien, MD, FRCPC
Assistant Clinical Professor of Pediatrics
University of Montreal
Saint-Justine Hospital
Montreal, Quebec, Canada

Naomi L.C. Luban, MD
Chairman, Laboratory Medicine and Pathology
Professor, Pediatrics and Pathology
Laboratory Medicine Department
Children's National Medical Center
Washington, District of Columbia

Robert E. Lynch, MD
Professor and Director
Pediatric Critical Care
St. Louis University School of Medicine
Cardinal Glennon Children's Hospital
St. Louis, Missouri

Frank Maffei, MD
Division of Pediatric Critical Care
Strong Children's Research Center
University of Rochester
Rochester, New York

James P. Marcin, MD, MPH
Associate Professor of Pediatrics and Critical Care Medicine
University of California, Davis, School of Medicine
Sacramento, California

Mary Michele Mariscalco, MD
Assistant Professor of Pediatrics
Baylor College of Medicine
Houston, Texas

Barry P. Markovitz, MD
Associate Professor, Department of Anesthesiology and Pediatrics
Washington University School of Medicine
Attending Physician, Department of Pediatric Intensive Care
Children's Hospital of St. Louis
St. Louis, Missouri

Lynn D. Martin, MD
Professor of Anesthesiology and Pediatrics (adjunct)
University of Washington School of Medicine
Director, Department of Anesthesiology and Pain Management
Children's Hospital and Regional Medical Center
Seattle, Washington

Anne G. Matlow, MD, FRCPC
Associate Professor
University of Toronto Faculty of Medicine
Director, Infection Prevention and Control
Physician Liaison, Patient Safety
The Hospital for Sick Children
Toronto, Ontario, Canada

John E. Mayer, Jr., MD
Department of Cardiac Surgery
Children's Hospital
Boston, Massachusetts

Paula Mazur, MD
Associate Professor of Clinical Pediatrics and Emergency Medicine
State University of New York at Buffalo School of Medicine and Biomedical Sciences
Attending Physician
Department of Pediatrics and Emergency Medicine
Children's Hospital of Buffalo
Buffalo, New York

E. Dean McKenzie, MD
Assistant Professor, Department of Surgery
Baylor College of Medicine
Associate Surgeon, Congenital Heart Surgery
Surgical Director, Heart and Lung Transplant Program
Texas Children's Hospital
Houston, TX

Gwenn E. McLaughlin, MD
Division of Critical Care Medicine
Department of Pediatrics
University of Miami School of Medicine
Miami, Florida

Nilesh Mehta, MD
Medical Surgical Intensive Care Unit
Children's Hospital, Boston
Boston, Massachusetts

Renuka Mehta, MBBS, MRCP, DcH
Assistant Professor of Pediatric Critical Care Medicine
Medical College of Georgia
Children's Medical Center
Augusta, Georgia

Ann J. Melvin, MD, MPH
Assistant Professor
Department of Pediatrics
University of Washington School of Medicine
Division of Infectious Diseases
Department of Pediatrics
Children's Hospital and Regional Medical Center
Seattle, Washington

Jean-Christophe Mercier, MD
Service de Réanimation Pédiatrique
Hôpital Robert Debré
Paris, France

Kelly Michelson, MD, MPH
Assistant Professor of Pediatrics
Northwestern University
Feinberg School of Medicine
Pediatric Critical Care Medicine
Children's Memorial Hospital
Chicago, Illinois

Kelly A. Michienzi, PharmD
Clinical Pharmacy Instructor
The University at Buffalo School of Pharmacy and Pharmaceutical Sciences
Clinical Pharmacy Coordinator
The Women and Children's Hospital at Buffalo–Kaleida Health
Buffalo, New York

Patricia A. Moloney-Harmon, RN, MS, CCNS, CCRN, FAAN
Advanced Practice Nurse/Clinical Nurse Specialist
Children's Services
Sinai Hospital of Baltimore
Baltimore, Maryland

Frederick C. Morin III, MD
Chair, Department of Pediatrics
State University of New York at Buffalo School of Medicine and Biomedical Sciences
Chairman, Department of Pediatrics and Pediatrician-in-Chief
Children's Hospital of Buffalo
Buffalo, New York

Michele Moss, MD
Professor of Pediatrics
Department of Cardiology and Critical Care
University of Arkansas for Medical Sciences
Little Rock, Arkansas

Vinay Nadkarni, MD
Director, Pediatric Critical Care Fellowship Program
Department of Anesthesia and Critical Care
Children's Hospital of Philadelphia
Philadelphia, Pennsylvania

Carol E. Nicholson, MD, MS, FAAP
Program Director
Pediatric Critical Care Medicine and Pediatric Rehabilitation Research
National Institutes of Health/NICHD
Bethesda, Maryland

Victoria F. Norwood, MD
Associate Professor of Pediatrics
Chief, Pediatric Nephrology

Universty of Virginia Children's Medical Center
Charlottesville, Virginia

Daniel Notterman, MD
Professor and Chairman
Department of Pediatrics
Robert Wood Johnson Medical School
University of Medicine and Dentistry of New Jersey
New Brunswick, New Jersey

Alan Nugent, MD
Instructor of Pediatrics
Department of Pediatrics
Harvard Medical School
Assistant Director Cardiac Catheterization Laboratory
Department of Cardiology
Children's Hospital
Boston, Massachusetts

Peter Oishi, MD
Adjunct Clinical Instructor
Department of Pediatrics
University of California, San Francisco
San Francisco, California

Victor Olivar, MD
Assistant Professor of Pediatric Critical Care
Universidad Nacional Autónoma de México
Attending Physician
Pediatric Critical Care Unit
Hospital Infantil de México
Mexico City, Mexico

Richard A. Orr, MD
Associate Professor of Critical Care Medicine and Pediatrics
University of Pittsburgh School of Medicine
Medical Director, Pediatric Transport
Associate Director, Pediatric Intensive Care Unit
Pediatric Critical Care Medicine
Children's Hospital of Pittsburgh
Pittsburgh, Pennsylvania

Yves Ouellette, MD, PhD
Assistant Professor of Pediatrics
Mayo Clinic
Rochester, Minnesota

Daiva Parakininkas, MD
Associate Professor, Department of Pediatrics
Medical College of Wisconsin
Pediatric Pulmonologist/Intensivist
Assistant Medical Director
Pediatric Intensive Care Unit
Pulmonary/Critical Care Division
Children's Hospital of Wisconsin
Milwaukee, Wisconsin
Pediatric Critical Care Staff
St. Vincent's Hospital
Green Bay, Wisconsin

Margaret M. Parker, MD, FCCM
Professor
Department of Pediatrics
Stony Brook University
Director, Pediatric Intensive Care Unit
Stony Brook University Hospital
Stony Brook, New York

Anthony L. Pearson-Shaver, MD, MHSA
Chief, Pediatric Critical Care Medicine
Department of Pediatrics
Medical College of Georgia
Medical Director, Pediatric Intensive Care Unit
Medical College of Georgia Children's Medical Center
Augusta, Georgia

Mary Jane F. Petruzzi, MD
Assistant Professor of Pediatrics
State University of New York at Buffalo
Pediatric Co-Medical Director
Hemophilia Center of Western New York
Children's Hospital of Buffalo
Attending Physician, Roswell Park Cancer Institute
Buffalo, New York

Maury N. Pinsk, MD
Assistant Professor
Division of Pediatric Nephrology
University of Alberta Faculty of Medicine
Walter C MacKenzie Health Sciences Centre
Edmonton, Alberta, Canada

Murray M. Pollack, MD, MBA
Professor of Pediatrics
George Washington University School of Medicine
Executive Director, Center for Hospital-Based Specialties
Chief, Critical Care Medicine
Children's National Medical Center
Washington, District of Columbia

Steven Pon, MD
Associate Professor of Clinical Pediatrics
Department of Pediatrics
Joan and Sanford I. Weill Medical College of Cornell University
Associate Director, Pediatric Intensive Care Unit
Weill Cornell Medical Center
New York-Presbyterian Hospital
New York, New York

Alice Pong, MD
Division of Infectious Diseases
Children's Hospital and Health Center
San Diego, California

Lara Primak, MD
Staff Pediatrics
Dubois Regional Medical Center
Dubois Regional Medical Group
Dubois, Pennsylvania

Audra Prince, MD
Assistant Professor of Pediatrics
University of Arkansas for Medical Sciences
Little Rock, Arkansas

Jean-Damien Ricard, MD, PhD
Associate Professor of Intensive Care Medicine
Service de Reanimation Medicale
Hopital Louis Mourier, Assistance Publique-Hopitaux de Paris, Colombes
Colombes, France
Faculte de Medecine Xavier Bichat
Paris, France

Tom B. Rice, MD
Professor of Pediatrics
Medical College of Wisconsin
Chief, Pediatric Pulmonary/Critical Care Department
Children's Hospital of Wisconsin
Milwaukee, Wisconsin

Gail E. Richards, MD, MM
Professor of Pediatrics
University of Washington School of Medicine
Head, Division of Endocrinology
Children's Hospital and Regional Medical Center
Seattle, Washington

Debra Ann Ridling, RN, MS
Clinical Nurse Manager
Pediatric Intensive Care Unit
Children's Hospital and Regional Medical Center
Seattle, Washington

Joan Roberts, MD
Assistant Professor of Pediatrics and Anesthesiology
University of Washington School of Medicine
Children's Hospital and Regional Medical Center
Seattle, Washington

Kimberly Roth, MD
Fellow, Pediatric Emergency Medicine
Emergency Medicine
Children's Hospital of Pittsburgh
Pittsburgh, Pennsylvania

Alexandre T. Rotta, MD
Department of Anesthesia
Driscoll Children's Hospital
Corpus Christi, Texas

Daniel Rubens, MD
Assistant Professor of Anesthesiology
Children's Hospital and Regional Medical Center
University of Washington
Seattle, Washington

Jeffrey S. Rubenstein, MD
Director, Critical Care Center
University of Rochester Medical Center
Rochester, New York

Christopher M. Rubino, PharmD, BCPS
Assistant Director of Pharmacy–Ambulatory Services
Department of Pharmacy
Roswell Park Cancer Institute
Buffalo, New York

Randall Ruppel, MD
Assistant Professor of Pediatrics
Pediatrics and Critical Care Medicine
Carmel Children's Indianapolis
Saint Vincent Hospital

Peter J. Safar, MD[†]
Safar Center for Resuscitation Research
University of Pittsburgh
Pittsburgh, Pennsylvania

Ashok P. Sarnaik, MD
Professor of Pediatrics
Chief, Division of Critical Care Medicine
Carman and Ann Adams Department of Pediatrics
Children's Hospital of Michigan
Wayne State University School of Medicine
Detroit, Michigan

Joel B. Sarner, MD
Visiting Clinical Associate Professor
Department of Anesthesiology
University of Pittsburgh School of Medicine
Children's Hopital of Pittsburgh
Department of Anesthesiology
Shadyside Hospital
Pittsburgh, Pennsylvania

Georges Saumon, MD
Service de Réanimation Medicale
Hôpital Louis Mouriér
Colombes, France

[†]Deceased

Matthew C. Scanlon, MD
Assistant Professor of Pediatrics
Medical College of Wisconsin
Patient Safety Officer
Children's Hospital of Wisconsin
Milwaukee, Wisconsin

Kenneth Schenkman, MD, PhD
Associate Professor of Pediatrics and Anesthesia
Adjunct Associate Professor of Biomedical Engineering
Director of Pediatric Critical Care Research
University of Washington School of Medicine
Division of Pediatric Critical Care Medicine
Children' s Hospital and Regional Medical Center
Seattle, Washington

Stephen M. Schexnayder, MD
Betty A. Lowe Chair in Pediatric Education
Associate Professor, Department of Pediatrics and Internal Medicine
University of Arkansas for Medical Sciences
Chief, Pediatric Critical Care Medicine
Arkansas Children's Hospital
Little Rock, Arkansas

Charles L. Schleien, MD
Professor of Clinical Pediatrics and Anesthesiology
Director, Pediatric Critical Care Medicine
Children's Hospital of New York
New York, New York

Timothy A. Sentongo, MD
Associate Professor of Pediatrics
The Children's Memorial Hospital
Chicago, Illinois

Thomas P. Shanley, MD
Department of Critical Care
Children's Hospital Medical Center
Cincinnati, Ohio

Frank Shann, MD, FRACP, FJFICM
Department of Pediatrics
University of Melbourne Faculty of Medicine, Dentistry, and Health Sciences
Director, Pediatric Intensive Care
Royal Children's Hospital
Melbourne, Australia

Dennis W.W. Shaw, MD
Professor, Department of Radiology
University of Washington School of Medicine
Division Chief, Interventional Radiology
Pediatric Interventional Neuroradiologist
Children's Hospital and Regional Medical Center
Seattle, Washington

Sam D. Shemie, MD
Associate Professor of Pediatrics
McGill University Faculty of Medicine
Division of Pediatric Critical Care
Montreal Children's Hospital
Montreal, Quebec, Canada

Peter Skippen, MD
Division of Critical Care
Department of Pediatrics
British Columbia Children's Hospital
Vancouver, British Columbia, Canada

Anthony D. Slonim, MD, MPH
Assistant Professor of Medicine and Pediatrics
George Washington University School of Medicine
Medical Director, Performance Improvement and Patient Safety
Children's National Medical Center
Attending Physician, Critical Care Medicine
Washington, District of Columbia

Laurie Smith, MD
Division of Metabolism
Departments of Pediatrics and Molecular and Medical Genetics
Oregon Health and Science University
Portland, Oregon

Lincoln Smith, MD
Division of Critical Care Medicine
Department of Pediatrics
Children's Hospital and Regional Medical Center
Seattle, Washington

David M. Steinhorn, MD
Associate Professor of Pediatrics
Northwestern University Feinberg School of Medicine
Children's Memorial Hospital
Chicago, Illinois

Waldemar E. Storm, MD
Pediatric Critical Care Medicine
MeritCare Children's Hospital
Fargo, North Dakota

Marc Sturgill, PharmD
Associate Professor
Department of Pharmacy Practice and Administration
Ernest Mario School of Pharmacy at Rutgers University

Piscataway, New Jersey
Adjunct Assistant Professor
Division of Pediatric Pharmacology and Toxicology
University of Medicine and Dentistry of New Jersey
Robert Wood Johnson Medical School
New Brunswick, New Jersey

Marianne T. Sweetser, MD, PhD
Acting Assistant Professor
Department of Pediatrics
University of Washington School of Medicine
Seattle, Washington

Jordan M. Symons, MD
Assistant Professor of Pediatrics
University of Washington School of Medicine
Attending Nephrologist
Children's Hospital and Regional Medical Center
Seattle, Washington

Robert C. Tasker, MD
Consultant University Lecturer
Pediatric Intensive Care
Addenbrooke's Hospital
Cambridge, England, United Kingdom

Ann E. Thompson, MD
Professor of Anesthesiology, Critical Care Medicine and Pediatrics
University of Pittsburgh School of Medicine
Director, Pediatric Critical Care Medicine
Children's Hospital of Pittsburgh
Pittsburgh, Pennsylvania

Ann Henderson Tilton, MD
Professor of Pediatrics and Neurology
Louisiana State University Health Science Center
Co-Director, The Rehabilitation Center
Children's Hospital of New Orleans
New Orleans, Louisiana

Nicole H. Tobin, MD
Acting Instructor
Division of Infectious Diseases
Department of Pediatrics
University of Washington School of Medicine
Attending Physician
Children's Hospital and Regional Medical Center
Seattle, Washington

I. David Todres, MD
Professor of Pediatrics
Harvard Medical School
Chief, Pediatrics Ethics Unit
Massachusetts General Hospital
Boston, Massachusetts

Peter Trinkaus, MD
Clinical Associate Professor
Pediatric Intensive Care Unit
Lucile Packard Children's Hospital at Stanford
Palo Alto, California

David J. Vaughan, MBBS
Consultant Respiratory Pediatrician
Department of Pediatrics
Our Lady of Lourdes Hospital
Drogheda, Ireland

Shekhar T. Venkataraman, MD
Associate Professor of Critical Care Medicine and Pediatrics
University of Pittsburgh School of Medicine
Associate Director, Pediatric Intensive Care Unit
Medical Director, Respiratory Care
Children's Hospital of Pittsburgh
Pittsburgh, Pennsylvania

Rapheus C.Q. Villanueva, PharmD
Clinical Pharmacist
Children's Hospital and Regional Medical Center
Seattle, Washington

Patricia C. Wankum, MD
Fellow, Department of Pediatrics
University of Arkansas for Medical Sciences
Fellow, Pediatric Critical Care Medicine
Arkansas Children's Hospital
Little Rock, Arkansas

R. Scott Watson, MD, MPH
Assistant Professor of Critical Care Medicine and Pediatrics
Core Faculty, Clinical Research, Investigation, and Systems Modeling of Acute Illness (CRISMA) Laboratory
University of Pittsburgh School of Medicine
Associate Director, Pediatric Intensive Care Unit
Children's Hospital of Pittsburgh
Pittsburgh, Pennsylvania

Wayne R. Waz, MD
Associate Professor of Clinical Pediatrics
State University of New York at Buffalo School of Medicine and Biomedical Sciences
Chief, Division of Pediatric Nephrology
Women and Children's Hospital of Buffalo
Buffalo, New York

Carl G.M. Weigle, MD, FAAP
Associate Professor of Pediatrics
Medical College of Wisconsin
Associate Director, Pediatric Intensive Care Unit
Medical Director of Information Services
Children's Hospital of Wisconsin
Milwaukee, Wisconsin

Maria B. Weimer, MD
Assistant Professor of Clinical Neurology
Louisiana State University Health Science Center
New Orleans, Louisiana

Ed Weinberger, MD
Children's Hospital and Regional Medical Center
Seattle, Washington

David L. Wessel, MD
Professor of Pediatrics (Anesthesia)
Harvard Medical School
Department of Cardiology
Children's Hospital Boston
Boston, Massachusetts

William T. West, MD
Clinical Instructor
Department of Neonatology
Brody School of Medicine East Carolina University
Greenville, North Carolina

Randall C. Wetzel, MD
Professor of Pediatrics and Anesthesiology
Chair, Anesthesiology Critical Care Medicine
University of Southern California Keck School of Medicine
The Anne O'M. Wilson Professor of Critical Care Medicine
Director, Laura P. and Leland K. Whittier Virtual Pediatric Intensive Care Unit
Children's Hospital Los Angeles
Los Angeles, California

Dale Whitby, PharmD
Pediatric Pharmacy Residency Program Director
Shands at the University of Florida
Gainesville, Florida

Hector R. Wong, MD
Associate Professor of Pediatrics
Director, Division of Critical Care Medicine
Cincinnati Children's Hospital Medical Center
Cincinnati, Ohio

Ellen G. Wood, MD
Professor and Director, Department of Nephrology
St. Louis University
Cardinal Glennon Children's Hospital
St. Louis, Missouri

Alan D. Woolf, MD, MPH
Associate Professor of Pediatrics
Harvard Medical School
Director, Program in Environmental Medicine
Division of General Pediatrics
Children's Hospital
Boston, Massachusetts

James Woytash, MD, DDS, MS
Chief Medical Examiner, Erie County Medical Examiner Office
Director, Department of Pathology
Erie County Medical Center
Staff Pathologist, Buffalo General Hospital
Buffalo, New York

Ofer Yanay, MD
Pediatric Intensive Care Unit
Wolfson Medical Center
Holon, Israel

Arno Zaritsky, MD
Director, Pediatric Critical Care Medicine
Department of Pediatrics
Gainseville, Florida

Danielle M. Zerr, MD, MPH
Assistant Professor
Division of Infectious Diseases
Department of Pediatrics
University of Washington School of Medicine
Attending Physician
Children's Hospital and Regional Medical Center
Seattle, Washington

Jerry J. Zimmerman, MD, PhD
Professor of Pediatrics and Anesthesiology
Director, Critical Care Medicine
Children's Hospital and Regional Medical Center
University of Washington
Seattle, Washington

Preface

This third edition of *Pediatric Critical Care* does not merely update the factual material of previous editions, but revisits that material in the context of current practice. Growth of the field has necessitated extensive revision, reorganization, and rewriting. We believe that this third edition provides a more detailed and complete understanding of the scientific basis of critical care than existed when the first edition published. From that foundation has been constructed a tighter integration of science and practice. In this text we strive to better integrate clinical and scientific issues. Moreover, we try to do so in such a way that clinicians who refer, follow, or consult on patients in the pediatric ICU, but who do not choose to specialize in critical care, can use the text to better appreciate the interdisciplinary aspects of pediatric critical care. We hope to help the subspecialist to see organ failure in the context of holistic critical care, and the referring physician to see critical care in the context of treating the whole child.

Clinical discussions are supplemented by clinical "pearls" and scientific detail is better assimilated into the whole. In this way, we hope the text will prove more useful to the students, residents, fellows, and practitioners for whom it is written.

Bradley P. Fuhrman, MD

Jerry J. Zimmerman, MD, PhD

Contents

Color Plates follow the Contents.

PEDIATRIC CRITICAL CARE

COLOR PLATES

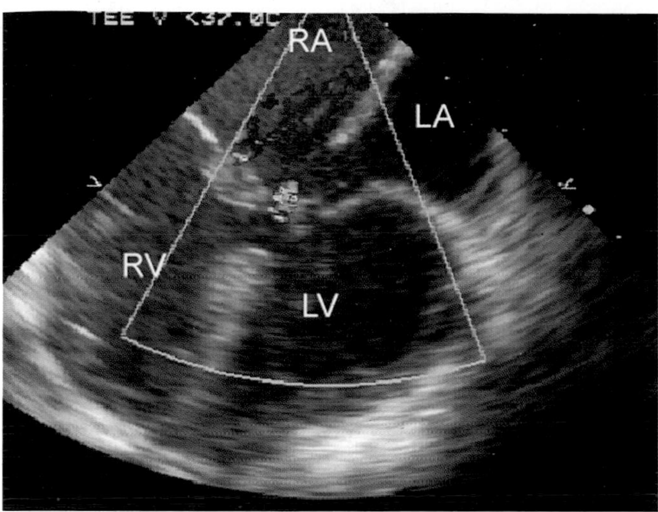

COLOR PLATE 1 • Atrioventricular canal defect with dextrocardia. A large primum atrial septal defect and ventricular septal defect are present. Note the mitral and tricuspid valves are at the same level. *LA,* Left atrium; *LV,* left ventricle; *RA,* right atrium; *RV,* right ventricle. (See also Color Plates.)

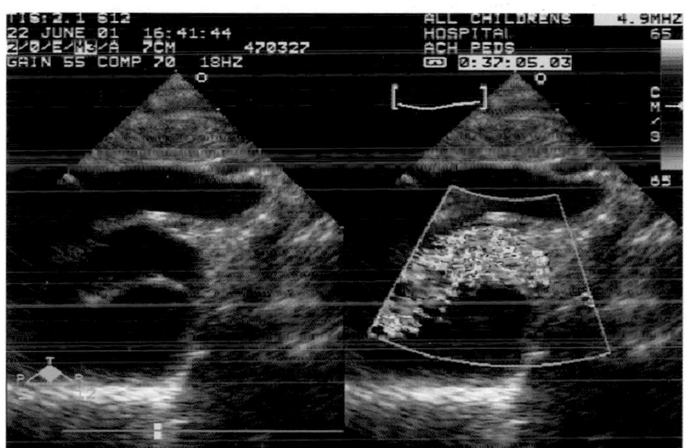

COLOR PLATE 2 • Transposition of the great arteries (discordant ventriculoarterial connection). Note the parallel exit of the anterior aorta and posterior pulmonary artery. (See also Color Plates.)

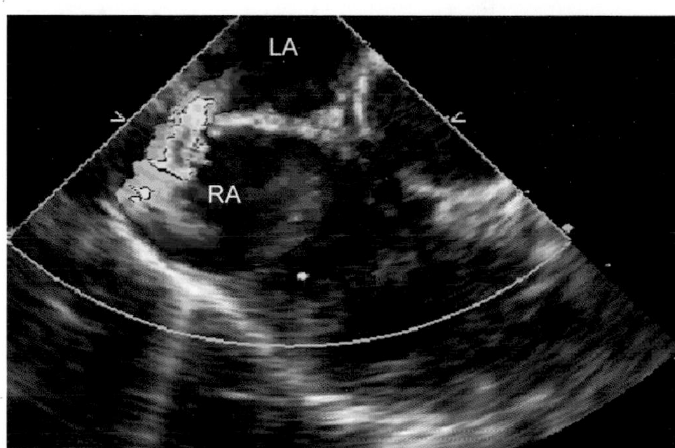

COLOR PLATE 3 • High sinus venosus atrial septal defect between the left atrium *(LA)* and right atrium *(RA).* Left to right shunting is seen by color Doppler (*blue* flow away from the transducer with aliasing). (See also Color Plates.)

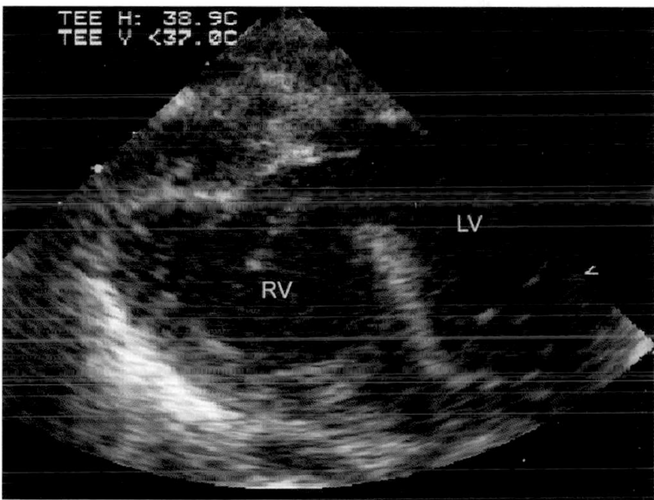

COLOR PLATE 4 • Ventricular septal defect between the left ventricle *(LV)* and right ventricle *(RV).* The defect is in continuity with the tricuspid valve and therefore is a perimembranous defect. (See also Color Plates.)

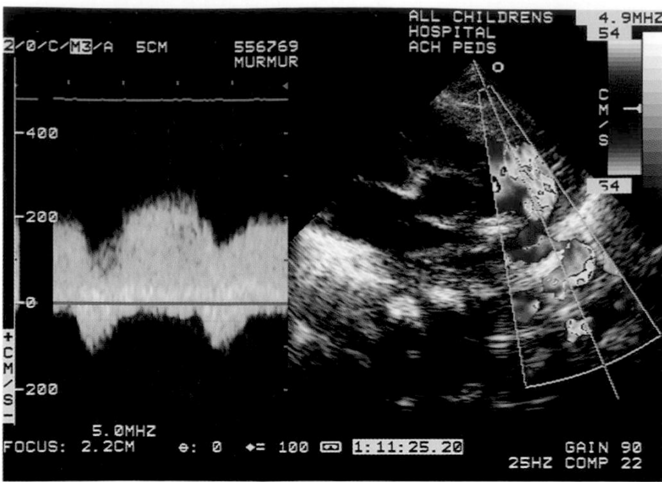

COLOR PLATE 5 • Patent ductus arteriosus in a neonate with a heart murmur. **Right,** Left-to-right shunt into the pulmonary artery is seen by color Doppler. **Left,** Left-to-right shunt velocity is measured by continuous-wave Doppler as a peak of 2.3 m/s. (See also Color Plates.)

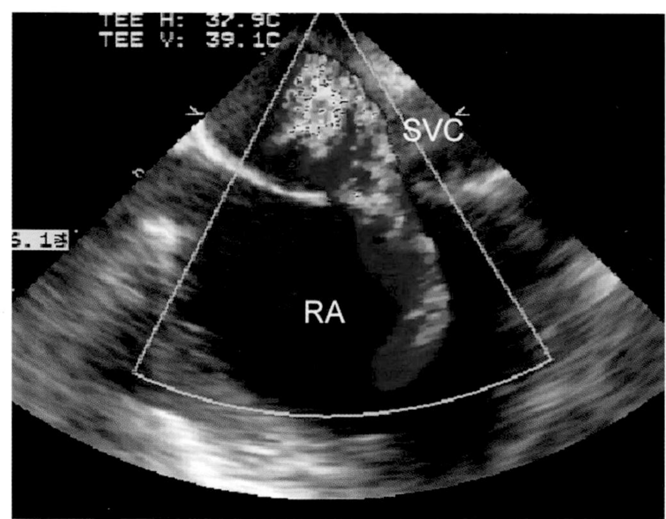

COLOR PLATE 6 • Sinus venosus atrial septal defect on sagittal scan by TEE with left-to-right shunting by color Doppler. *RA,* Right atrium; *SVC,* superior vena cava. (See also Color Plates.)

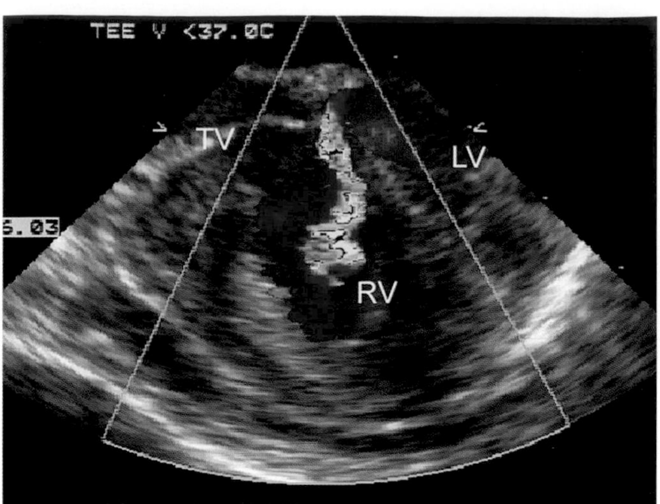

COLOR PLATE 7 • Color Doppler of shunt TEE from the left ventricle *(LV)* to the right ventricle *(RV)* through a ventricular septal defect (VSD). The VSD is perimembranous because of its proximity to the tricuspid valve *(TV).* (See also Color Plates.)

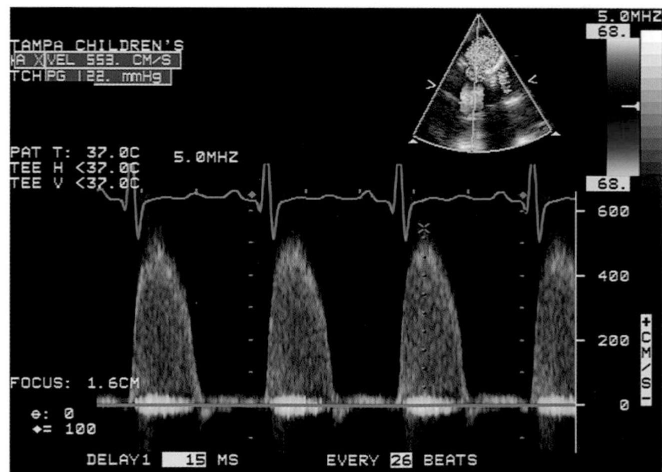

COLOR PLATE 8 • **Right,** Mitral regurgitation from an apical view with alignment of the continuous-wave Doppler cursor. **Left,** The rate of upstroke of mitral regurgitation is quantified by measuring the time from the 1 to the 3 m/s points on the waveform, in this example 15 ms. $dP/dt = 32 \div 15 \text{ ms} \times 1000 = 2133$ mmHg/s, which is normal. (See also Color Plates.)

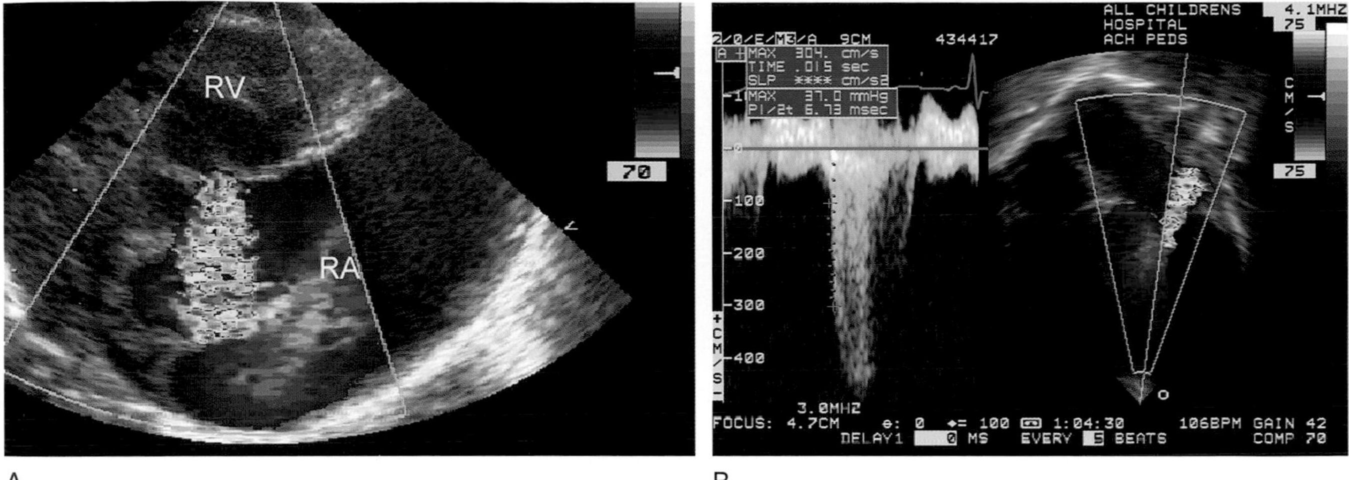

A B

COLOR PLATE 9 • **A,** Tricuspid valve regurgitation in a neonate with pulmonary atresia with intact septum. Note enlargement of the right atrium *(RA)*. *RV,* Right ventricle. **B,** Continuous-wave Doppler shows a very high predicted pressure in the hypoplastic right ventricle. (See also Color Plates.)

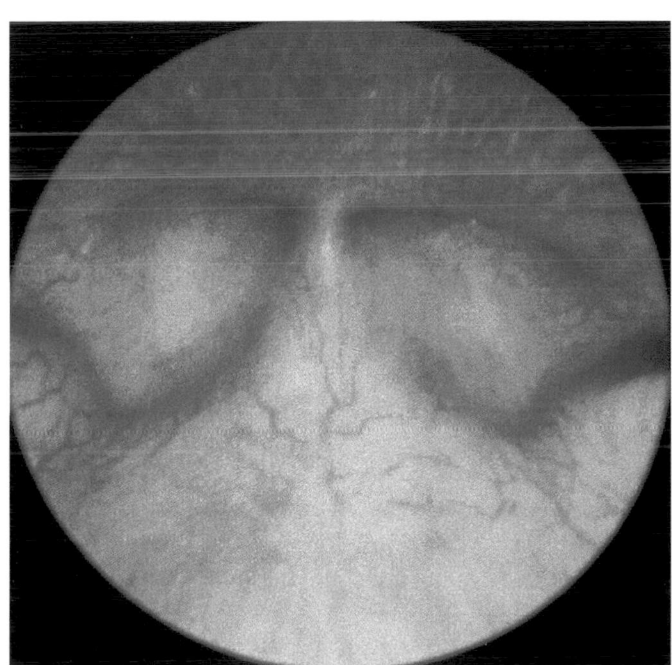

COLOR PLATE 10 • Choanal atresia before repair. View of choanal atresia from posterior nasopharynx. There is complete absence of choanae. (Courtesy Andrew F. Inglis, Jr.)

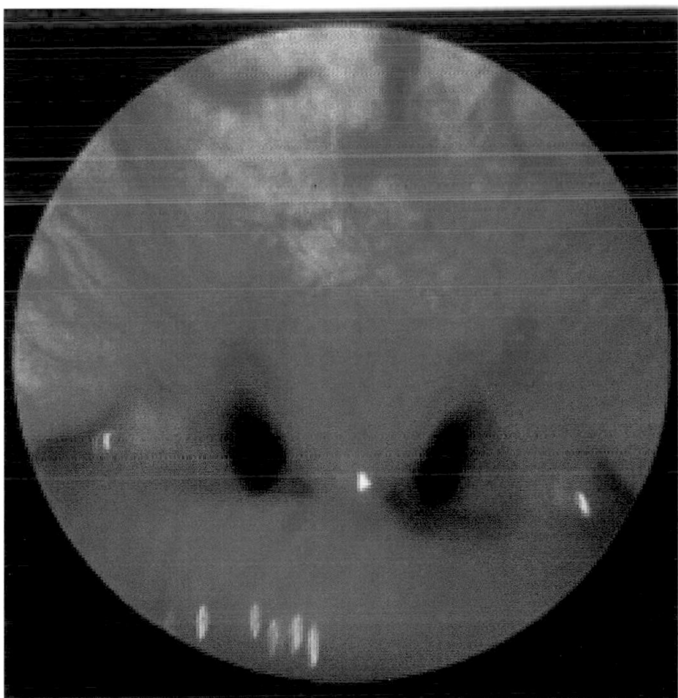

COLOR PLATE 11 • Choanal atresia after repair. View from the posterior of nasopharynx showing patency of choanae after surgery. (Courtesy Andrew F. Inglis, Jr.)

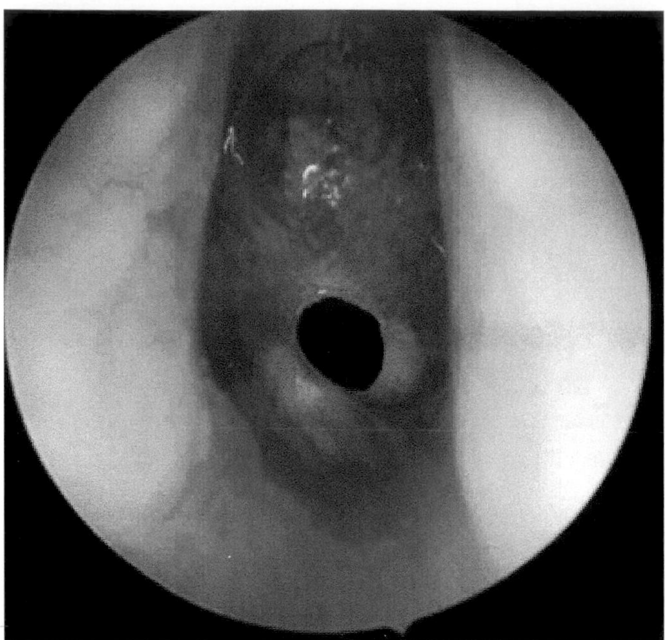

COLOR PLATE 12 • A laryngeal web occludes most of the tracheal lumen in this patient. This web, which is a thin membrane of soft tissue at the level of the glottis, has many of the features that are typical of this class of lesions. (Courtesy Andrew F. Inglis, Jr.)

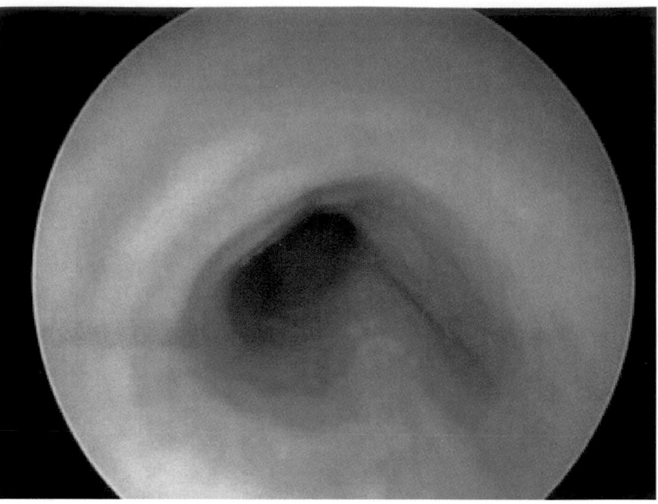

COLOR PLATE 14 • The lateral portion of the tracheal lumen is severely compressed by the impingement of the vascular ring. (Courtesy Andrew F. Inglis, Jr.)

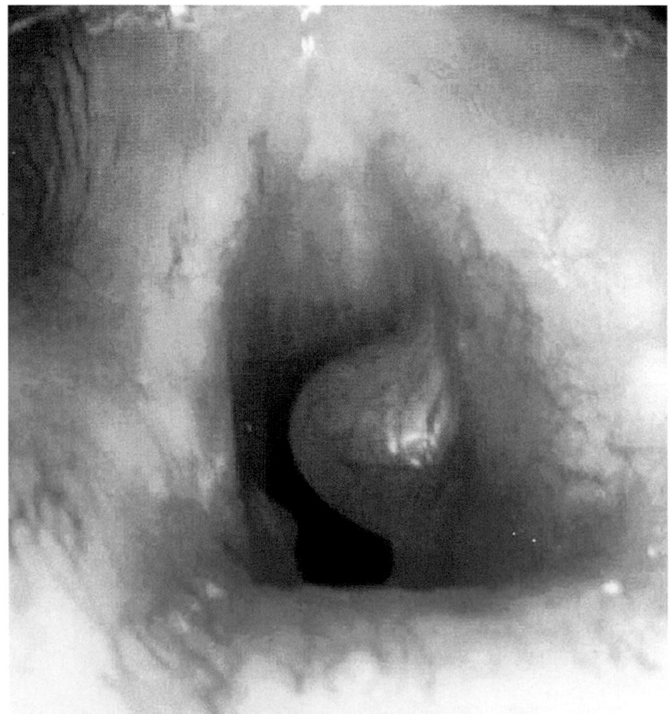

COLOR PLATE 13 • A large laryngeal cyst protrudes from the lateral wall of the trachea, just below the level of the glottis. (Courtesy Andrew F. Inglis, Jr.)

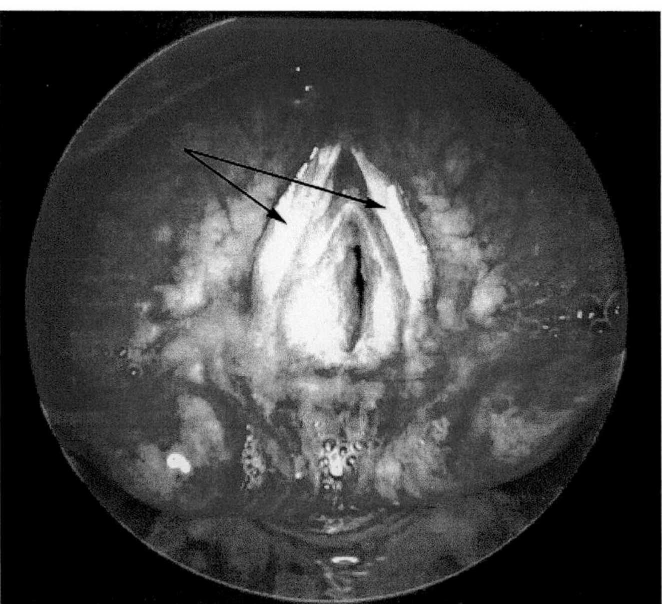

COLOR PLATE 15 • Laryngotracheobronchitis. Below the level of the vocal cords the trachea appears swollen and the tracheal walls are covered with purulent material (vocal cords are indicated by *arrows*). (Courtesy Bruce Benjamin, MD.)

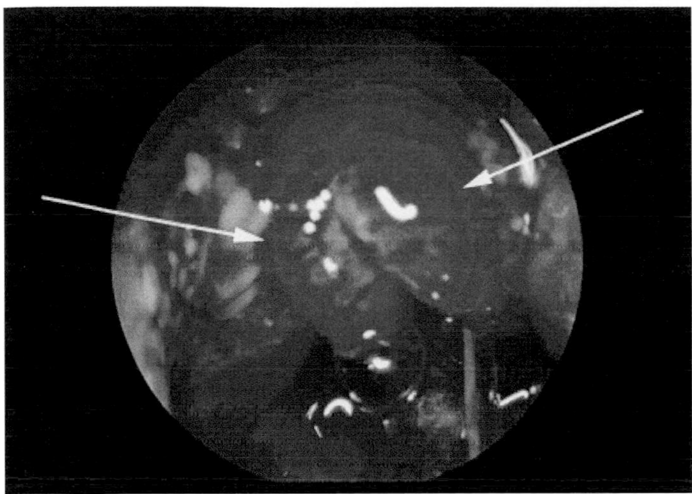

COLOR PLATE 16 • Epiglottitis causing a severely swollen epiglottis (between the *arrows*). In the lower portion of the picture, the endotracheal tube can be seen. (Courtesy Andrew F. Inglis, Jr.)

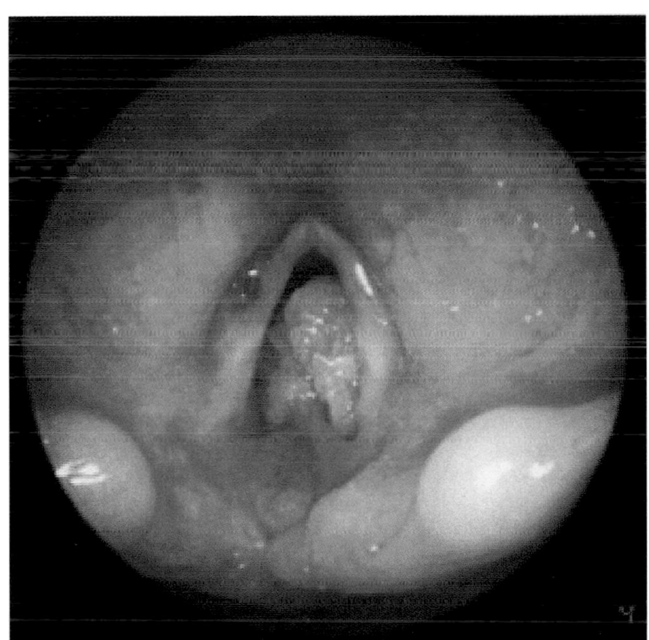

COLOR PLATE 17 • Large, pedunculated papilloma is seen just below the vocal cords. These papillomas almost completely occluded the tracheal lumen and produced marked respiratory distress. (Courtesy Andrew F. Inglis, Jr.)

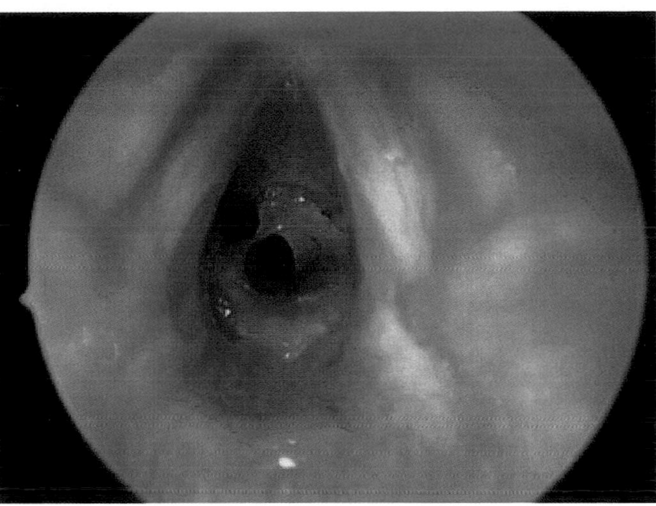

COLOR PLATE 18 • A cicatricial ring is shown just below the glottis. This was caused by trauma from prolonged endotracheal intubation. (Courtesy Andrew F. Inglis, Jr.)

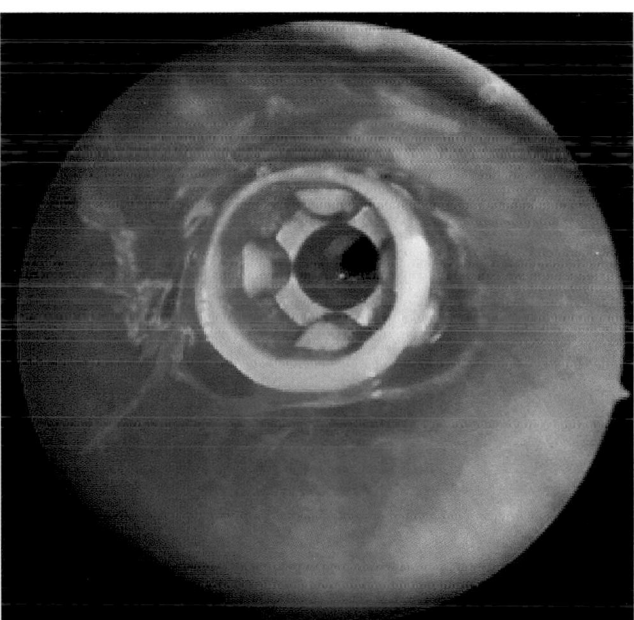

COLOR PLATE 19 • Hollow plastic foreign body in patient's trachea. Because the lumen of the foreign body was aligned with the tracheal lumen, severe respiratory embarrassment did not occur. (Courtesy Andrew F. Inglis, Jr.)

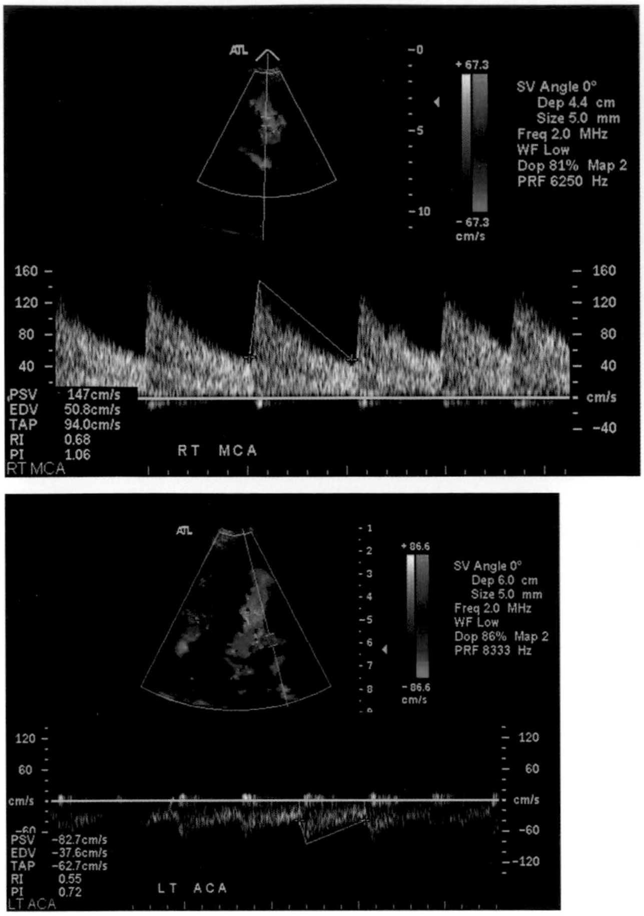

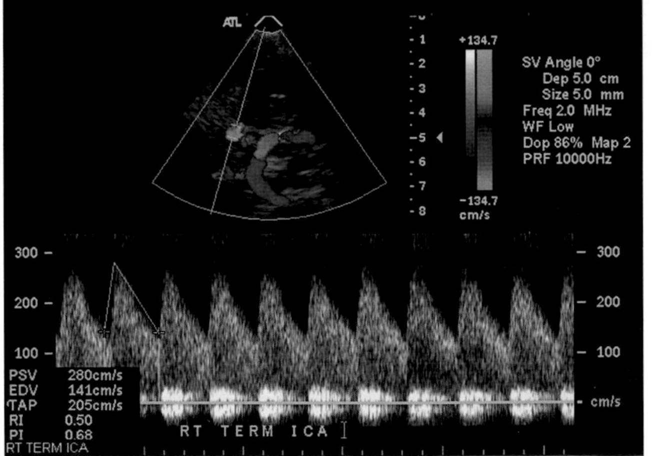

COLOR PLATE 20 • Transcranial Doppler ultrasound images. Color and pulse Doppler waveforms from middle **(A)**, anterior **(B)** and posterior. **(C)** Cerebral arteries are shown. Abnormal middle cerebral (**D**) and terminal carotid. (**E**) Waveforms in another patient with sickle cell disease. See color insert.

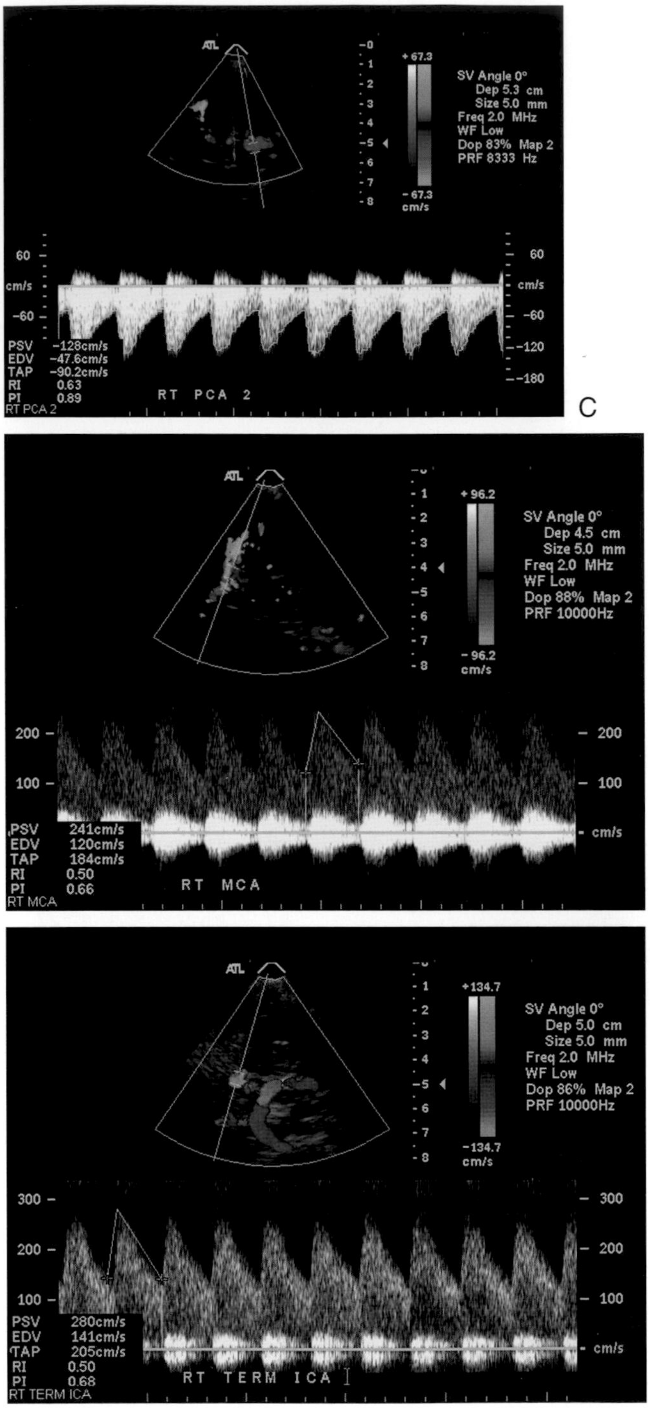

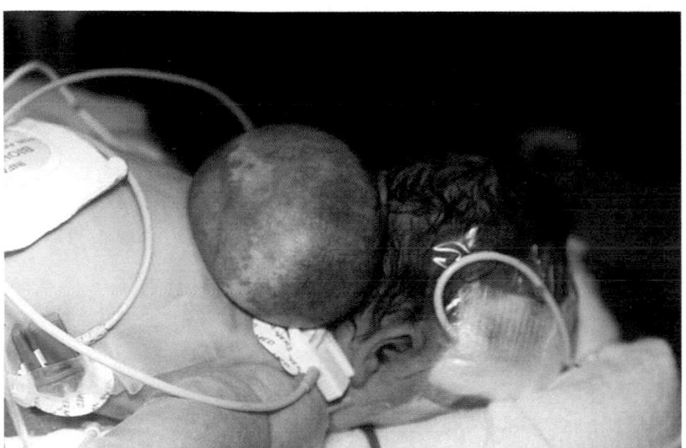

COLOR PLATE 21 • Occipital encephalocele. Used with permission from eMedicine.com, Inc., 2004.

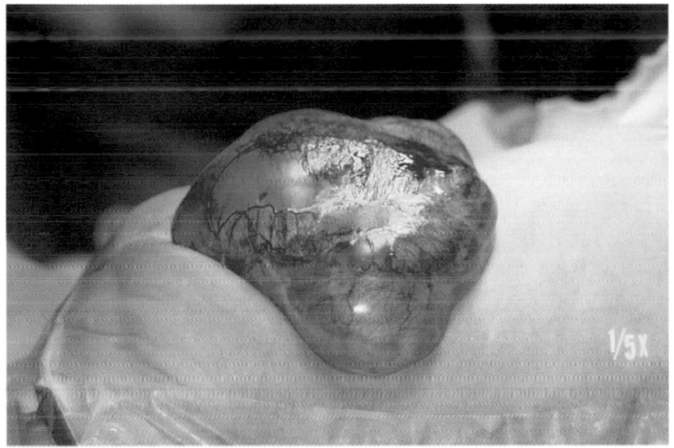

COLOR PLATE 22 • Myelomeningocele. Note the sac of cerebrospinal fluid surrounding the neural placode on the dorsal surface and the area medullovasculosa. Used with permission from eMedicine.com, Inc., 2004.

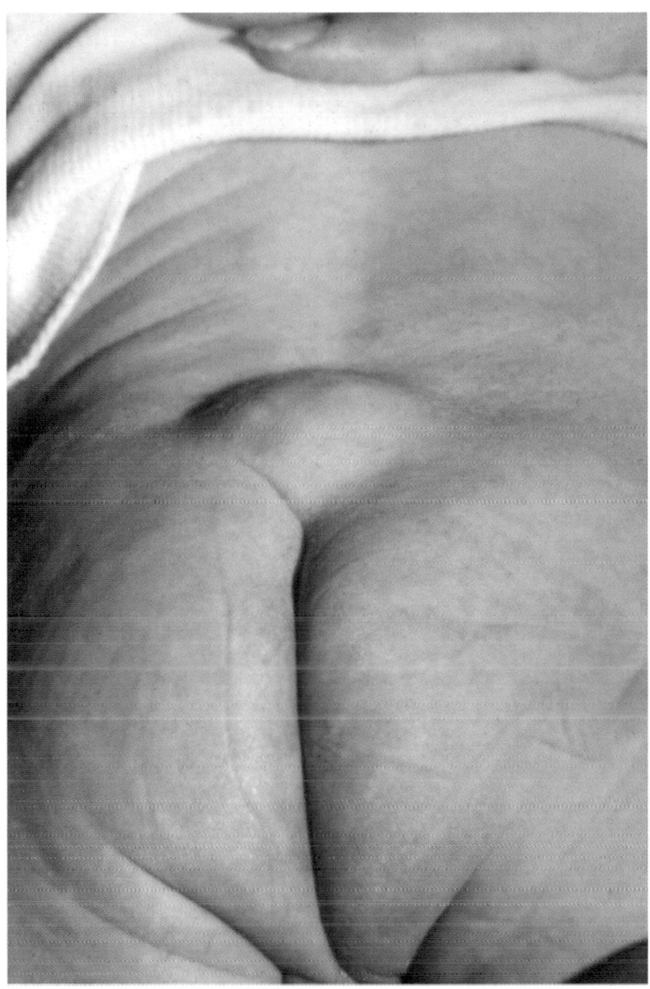

COLOR PLATE 24 • Lipomyelomeningocele. The lesion on the left is pedunculated; the one on the right has a more typical appearance of a lipomyelomeningocele. Used with permission from eMedicine.com, Inc., 2004.

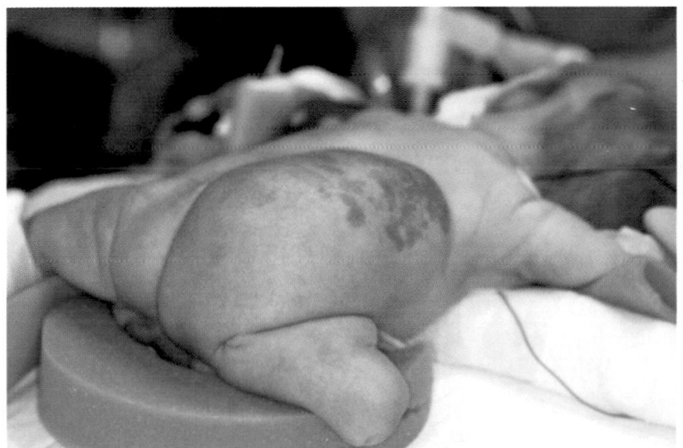

A

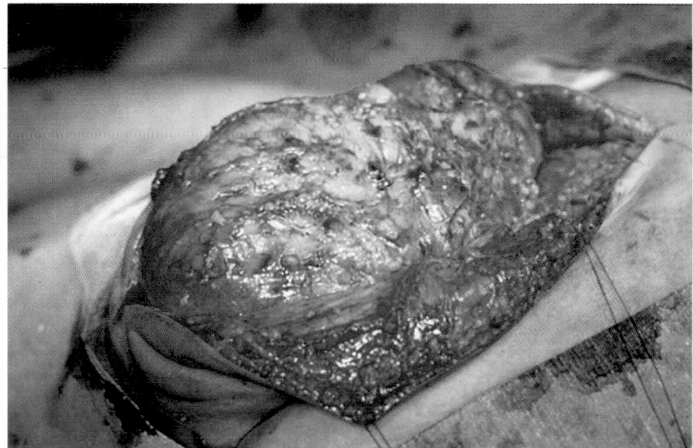

B

COLOR PLATE 23 • Terminal myelocystocele. Note the extremity anomaly. **B**, Figure shows the lipoma commonly seen within the cyst (photo courtesy of Anthony Avellino, MD).

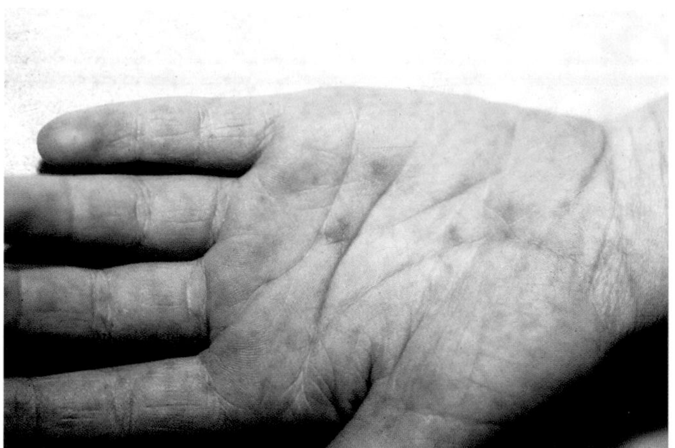

COLOR PLATE 25 • Palmar rash associated with Rocky Mountain spotted fever. (See also Color Insert.) (From Walker DH, Raoult D: Rickettsia rickettsii and other spotted fever group rickettsiae (Rocky Mountain spotted fever and other spotted fevers). In Mandell GL, Bennett JE, Dolin R, editors: *Mandell: principles and practice of infectious diseases,* ed 5, New York, 2000, Churchill Livingstone.)

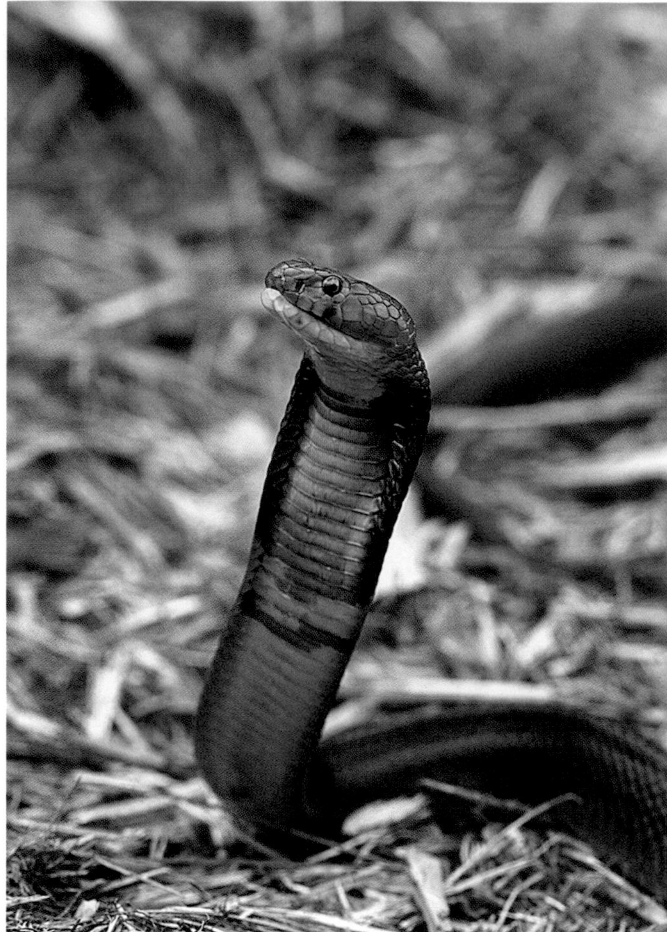

COLOR PLATE 27 • Red spitting cobra (*Naja pallida*). Photo by Mike Cardwell.

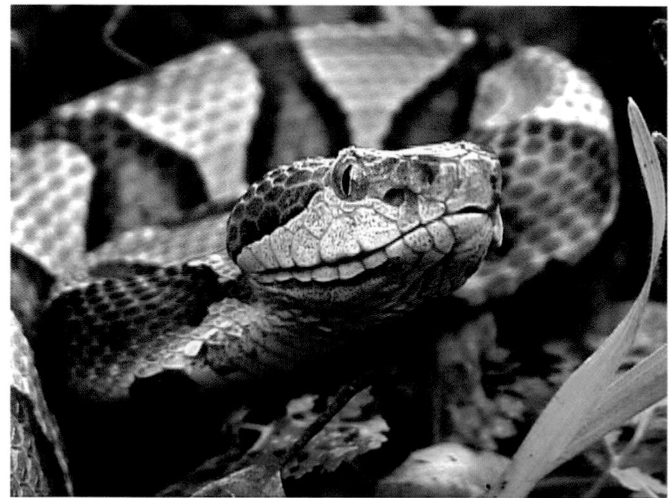

COLOR PLATE 26 • Copperhead (*Agkistrodon contortrix*). (Photo by Sean Bush, MD.)

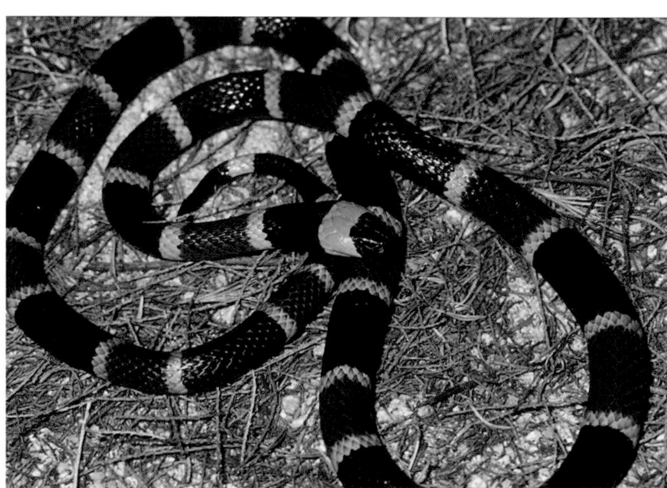

COLOR PLATE 28 • Eastern coral snake (*Micrurus fulvius*). Photo by Mike Cardwell.

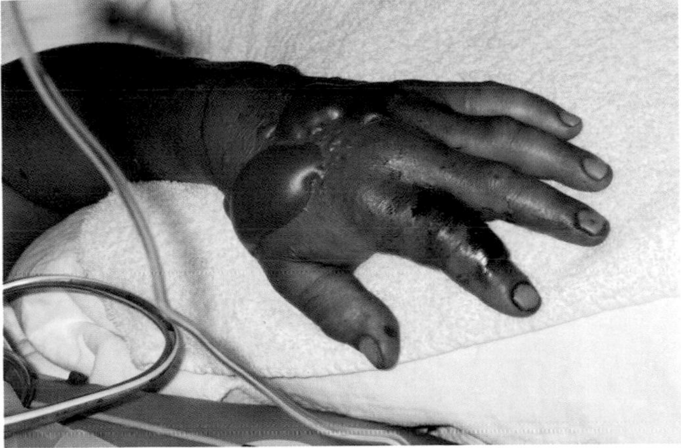

COLOR PLATE 29 • Southern Pacific rattlesnake (*Crotalus helleri*) bite wounds.
Photo by Sean Bush, MD.

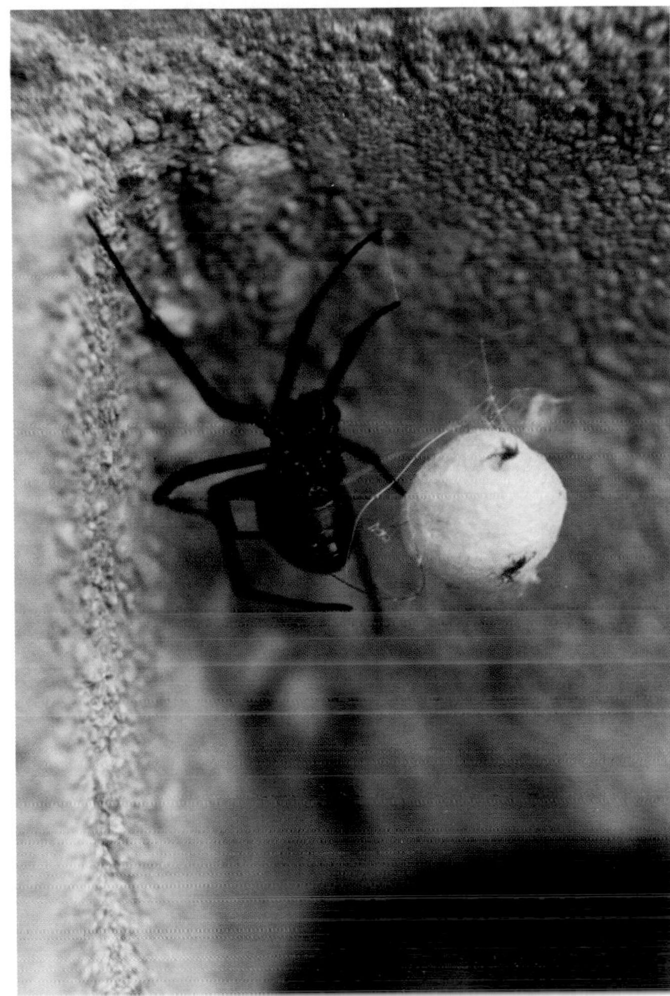

COLOR PLATE 31 • Black widow spider (*Latrodectus hesperus*).
Photo by Sean Bush, MD.

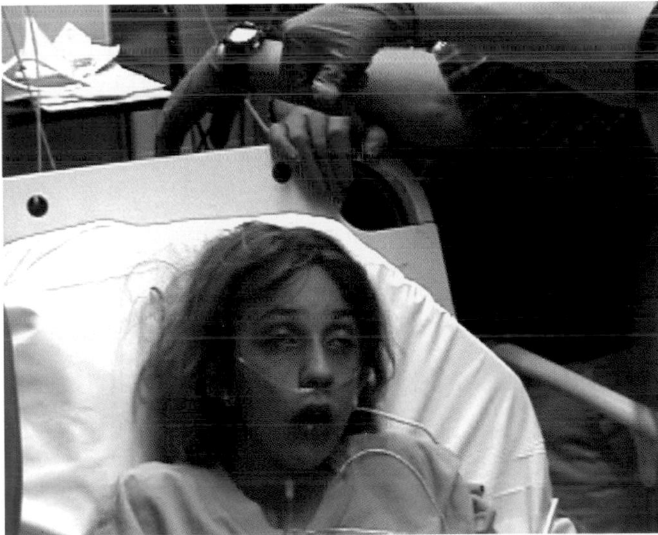

COLOR PLATE 30 • Ptosis after Mohave rattlesnake (*Crotalus scutulatus*) envenomation.
Photo by Sean Bush, MD.

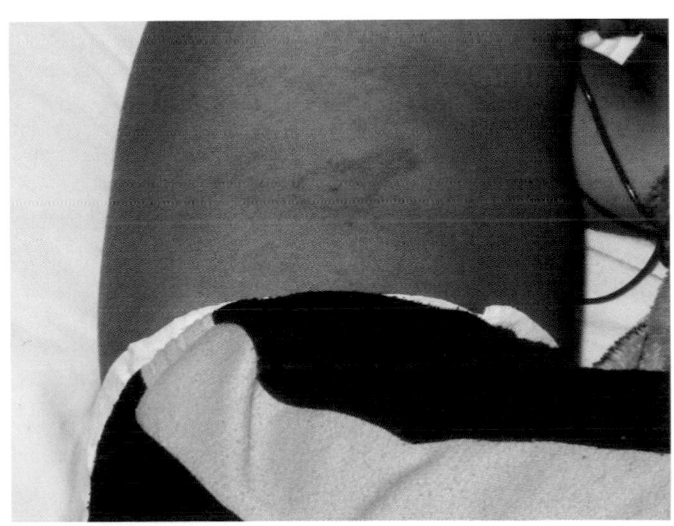

COLOR PLATE 32 • Black widow spider bite site.
Photo by Sean Bush, MD.

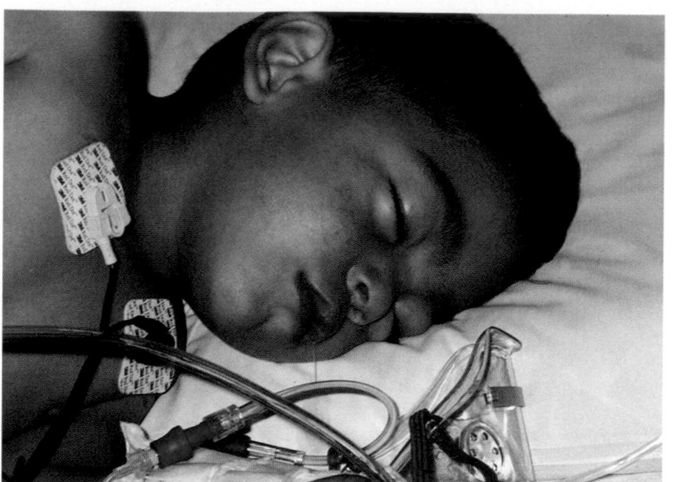

COLOR PLATE 33 • *Latrodectus* facies.
Photo by Sean Bush, MD.

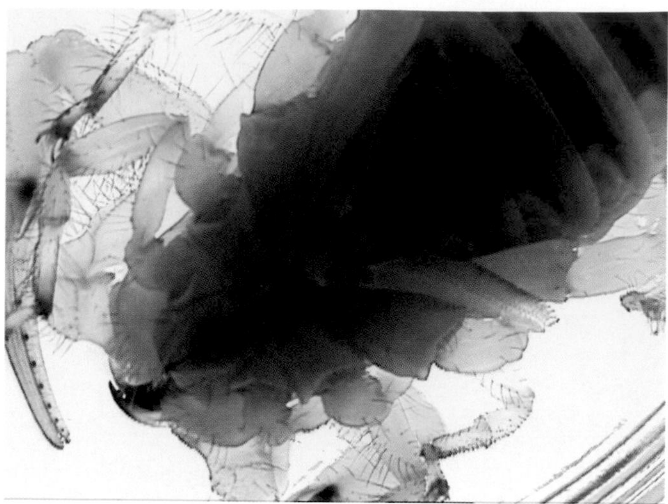

COLOR PLATE 35 • Most scorpions have a pentagonal sternal plate.
Photo by Sean Bush, MD.

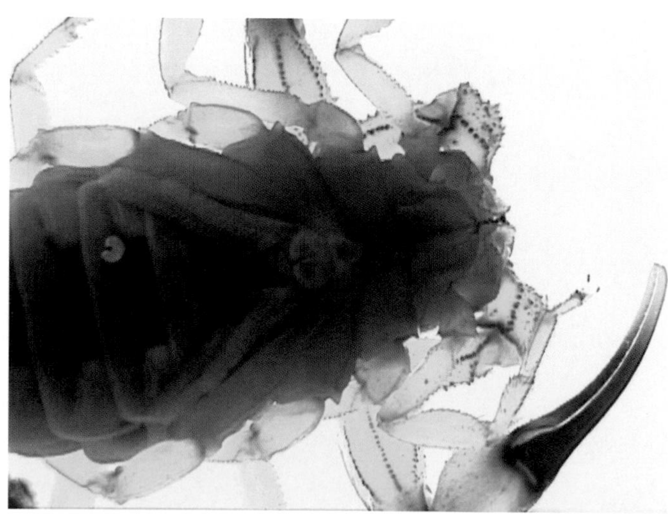

COLOR PLATE 34 • A triangular sternal plate helps distinguish Buthidae from other scorpion families.
Photo by Sean Bush, MD.

PART

I

THE DISCIPLINE

CHAPTER 1

Multidisciplinary Critical Care and the Role of the Subspecialist in the Pediatric Intensive Care Unit

Margaret M. Parker, Richard J. Brilli, and Kathleen Culver

PEARLS

- Coordination of care is essential for optimal care of the critically ill child.
- Communication and collaboration among the members of the health care team improves quality and efficiency of patient care.
- Everyone has an important role in the team, but there must be a "captain of the ship."

Over the past 30 years, the complexity of intensive care unit (ICU) medical care has increased dramatically. The challenge of managing and delivering high-quality care to the critically ill also has increased. Over this same time period, with the maturation of the medical specialty of critical care medicine, it has become apparent that an organized intensive care service, provided by qualified critical care personnel, has many benefits for critically ill patients. These benefits may include improved survival, fewer complications, shortened length of stay, and reduced cost of care.[1–3] Many factors associated with an organized intensive care service may contribute to these benefits, including the composition and leadership of the intensive care team, the timely availability of critical team members, and the ICU administrative structure. The ICU administrative structure includes, but is not limited to, performance improvement activities, data analysis, and use of guidelines to facilitate care with less variability. Another important factor in an organized critical care service may include the interaction among the intensive care specialist, referring physicians, and other medical or surgical specialists. The complexity of the critically ill patient often requires input and expertise from multiple specialists; however, recommendations from one specialist may conflict with recommendations from another. These potentially conflicting recommendations must be evaluated and integrated into a consistent and coordinated care plan for optimal patient care. The ideal model of care in the ICU must be able to integrate and coordinate the recommendations of multiple health care providers into a unified and cohesive plan of action. The Society of Critical Care Medicine and others have suggested that the optimal model of care for delivering organized intensive care services is a multidisciplinary, multiprofessional, intensivist-led model of care.[4] This organizational structure accommodates the various viewpoints of contributing specialists to the care of the critically ill patient as discussed in more detail in this chapter.

Intensive Care Unit Organizational Structure, the Team, and Outcome

A systematic review by Carmel et al.[5] described eight organizational categories that may contribute to patient outcome in the ICU. These factors include staffing, teamwork, patient volume and pressure of work, protocols, admission to intensive care, technology, structure, and error. Physician staffing has received increased attention in the medical literature because some have suggested that the presence of an intensivist in the ICU reduces mortality.[1,6] The active presence of a clinical pharmacist during ICU rounds can significantly improve outcome by reducing medication errors.[7] Appropriate nurse-to-patient ratios also can significantly improve outcome.[1,8] The ubiquitous presence of the nurse at the patient's bedside results in many opportunities to interact in depth with the family, subspecialist consultants, and other members of the health care team. The critical care nurse often plays a pivotal role in helping to coordinate the care plan. The presence of an intensivist dedicated to the ICU facilitates this coordination and reduces the risk that the nurse will need to juggle or negotiate conflicting orders or initiate emergent therapy without a physician order.[9]

Effective multidisciplinary care requires developing a teamwork model in the ICU. True teamwork recognizes the importance of the role of each member of the team and requires respect and trust for the other professions represented on the team.[10] Effective communication among all members of the health care team and the patient/family cannot be overemphasized. A collaborative partnership with shared responsibility for maintaining communication and accountability for patient care includes the recognition that no single provider can perform all parts of patient care; the whole team is much more effective than each member of the team alone. True teamwork is a complementary relationship of interdependence.[10]

Numerous nonrandomized trials report lower mortality and shortened ICU or hospital length of stay in units with an intensivist.[4] In a systematic review of the literature, Pronovost et al.[6] reported that high-intensity ICU physician staffing was associated with reduced hospital and ICU mortality and length of stay compared to low-intensity ICU physician staffing. In summary, organizational structure, intensivist presence, and team composition may contribute to improved care in the ICU; however, little is known about the impact of the nonintensivist specialist's role in care in the ICU.

Most pediatric intensive care units (PICUs) operate using an organizational structure with an intensivist-directed multiprofessional team model of care.[11] In a national survey, Pollack[11] reported that 80% of hospitals with PICUs had a full-time ICU medical director present. In 64% of the PICUs, an intensivist was involved in the care of more than 90% of the patients. Size of the ICU correlated directly with the presence of a pediatric intensivist. In contrast, adult ICUs may have multiple organizational structures.[12] These administrative structures include a full-time intensivist-directed model, a consultant intensivist model, a model using multiple consultants without a designated intensivist, and a model in which the primary care physician provides all ICU care. The relative frequency of these organizational structures depends on the size of the hospital and the type of ICU (medical, surgical, specialty, or general).

Role of the Intensivist and Other Specialists in the Intensive Care Unit

The presence of an intensivist may improve efficiency and coordination of care; however, the patient's primary care physician or nonintensivist subspecialist may be threatened by the presence of an intensivist in the ICU. These other specialists may be concerned about loss of patient control or management, loss of continuity of care, and potentially loss of income; yet collaboration between the intensivist and these other physicians is essential for optimizing ICU care. This collaboration with the patient's primary care physician is particularly important. The primary care physician can help the family develop trust in the intensivist and can provide needed past medical information about the family and the critically ill patient. In addition, the primary care physician likely will provide long-term care for the patient after ICU discharge and thus will be a valuable resource to the family in the future. As a result, the primary care physician must have a good understanding of what transpires in the ICU, even if he/she is not the attending physician of record. In addition to the patient's primary care physician, it is essential to seek the involvement of subspecialists who have medical expertise in specific areas beyond that of the intensivist.[13] The nonintensivist specialist may offer additional clinical expertise or technical skills that the intensivist does not possess. The intensivist must establish rapport and working relationships with multiple medical and surgical specialists and must learn to evaluate, coordinate, and integrate the recommendations of multiple specialists into the patient's plan of care. The intensivist, both by training and by physical presence in the ICU, is in an ideal position to synthesize the recommendations and prioritize the steps of the plan.

There are many barriers to this integration, including patient control issues, personal egos, and reimbursement concerns. However, there are strategies that can lessen the barriers and enhance collaboration. Key among these strategies is coordinating care such that all members of the ICU staff, including the nonintensivist, work as a team.[14] In 1981, the National Joint Practice Commission suggested guidelines and elements to enhance collaboration between nurses and physicians in providing hospital care.[15] These elements included effective communication, respect for individual competence, accountability for care provided, mutual trust, and hospital administrative support for collaboration. Although these parameters focused on collaboration between nurse and physician, they certainly can and should be extrapolated to enhance collaborative care between intensivist and nonintensivist in the ICU environment. Some specific examples that can enhance collaboration include (1) inviting the nonintensivist physician to join morning ICU rounds—this can apply to the patient's primary care physician or the nonintensivist subspecialist; (2) ensuring that the ICU rounding team fully understands the important role of the nonintensivist in the care of the patient; (3) ensuring frequent telephone communication to the specialist or primary care provider to provide medical updates when direct participation during rounds is not possible; (4) inviting the nonintensivist physician to participate in family conferences, especially those that pertain to long-term prognosis or end-of-life decisions; (5) providing written follow-up with either letters or discharge summary information to facilitate continuity of care; (6) inviting or facilitating multispecialty morbidity and mortality conferences or grand rounds wherein the ICU care can be examined from multiple perspectives, including those of the nonintensivist specialist; and (7) working collaboratively with nonintensivist specialists to develop and use clinical pathways that may standardize many facets of patient care. The use of clinical pathways improves efficiency of care and decreases resource utilization and, when developed with input from all members of the ICU team, may enhance the working relationship between intensivist and nonintensivist.[16] Optimally, such clinical pathways should be developed through collaboration among the intensivist, relevant subspecialists, and other members of the ICU team.

Another strategy that further incorporates the nonintensivist physician into the management of the patient includes formalizing multidisciplinary patient care conferences. These conferences often are needed to develop the most appropriate therapeutic direction for the patient. Emphasis must be placed on deciding what is best for the patient, putting individual concerns aside. The team must focus on "what is right," not "who is right." In a prospective, observational study, Bracco et al.[17] reported that human errors were common in treatment of ICU patients. Errors with significant consequences were most commonly related to planning. Careful consideration of all of the diagnostic and therapeutic options, with the development of a treatment plan that is communicated to all members of the health care team, can help prevent many of these errors.

Although multidisciplinary care conferences can enhance communication, the need for effective communication between the intensivist and all other involved health care workers remains paramount. The family must receive one message that is unambiguous, and the intensivist must ensure the integrity of that message. Mixed and/or confusing information greatly increases stress for the family and may result in conflict and mistrust between the family and the health care team. This conflict can be magnified when multiple specialists are involved in the same patient's care. Although the confusion may stem from the family's misinterpretation of the same message being delivered by multiple practitioners, emphasis on a clear and concise message must remain. The subspecialist often has been consulted to answer a specific question, but the intensivist must consider all aspects of the patient's care. The frequency of mixed messages can be reduced if the subspecialist speaks directly with the intensivist before speaking with the family, when possible, or clearly documents in the chart his/her opinion and what has been said to the family. Direct communication among the physician specialists can help prevent errors and minimize confusion and stress for the family.

Financial issues remain a threat to some nonintensivist specialists who traditionally have worked in the intensive care environment, particularly pulmonologists, cardiologists, and nephrologists. The impact of financial issues can be lessened if consultations are obtained where appropriate. In addition, the consultant subspecialist still may receive payment for services as long as the intensivist ensures appropriate consultative paperwork that includes, but is not limited to, formal orders for consultations and formal acknowledgments of the results of the consultations in the intensivist progress note.

A rapidly growing field in medicine is that of the hospitalist. The role of the hospitalist in the ICU remains controversial. Furthermore, the role of the hospitalist may vary among institutions and with the amount of critical care training completed by the hospitalist. In some institutions, the hospitalist cares for his/her own patients in the ICU despite having no specific training in critical care,[18] with the intensivist serving as a consultant. In this model of care, collaboration between the hospitalist and the intensivist is necessary to provide the team with the leadership and coordination of care that is required for optimal patient management. A study by Tenner, Dibrell, and Taylor[19] compared PICU physician coverage using a combination of intensivist-directed care and a hospitalist in hospital when the intensivist was unavailable versus pediatric resident coverage when the intensivist was not in hospital.[19] Their report concluded that the intensivist–hospitalist model was associated with improved survival and shorter length of stay. An ICU model of care that incorporates both intensivists and hospitalists may be both an effective method for optimizing care and an acceptable alternative to the use of pediatric residents as intensivist extenders, especially given the limitations in intensivist manpower. It remains important for each institution to define the role of all health care professionals working in the intensive care environment.

Summary

Critically ill patients have many and varied needs. No single individual can meet all the health care needs of these patients. Close collaboration among all members of the health care team, with overall direction by the intensivist, provides the framework for the most efficient and effective patient care. By weighing the input from all the involved health care professionals, including the nonintensivist physician, the intensivist can and must develop a coordinated plan, even in the face of conflicting recommendations. A single coordinated plan that incorporates input from a variety of sources can improve efficiency, decrease errors, and ultimately improve patient outcome. A variety of administrative models have been implemented in ICUs. The intensivist-directed model, the most common in PICUs, has been associated with improved outcomes. This model works only when communication among all members of the team is effectively coordinated such that there is seamless integration of the multiple perspectives that often must be incorporated into the management of the critically ill child.

REFERENCES

1. Pronovost PJ, Jenckes MW, Dorman T, et al: Organizational characteristics of intensive care units related to outcomes of abdominal aortic surgery. *JAMA* 281:1310-1317, 1999.
2. Hanson CW, Deutschman CS, Anderson HL, et al: Effects of an organized critical care service on outcomes and resource utilization: a cohort study. *Crit Care Med* 27:270-274, 1999.
3. Dimick JB, Pronovost P, Heitmiller R, et al: Intensive care unit physician staffing is associated with decreased length of stay, hospital cost, and complications after esophageal resection. *Crit Care Med* 29:753-758, 2001.
4. Brilli RJ, Spevetz A, Branson RD, et al: Critical care delivery in the intensive care unit: defining clinical roles and the best practice model. *Crit Care Med* 29:2007-2019, 2001.
5. Carmel S, Rowan K: Variation in intensive care unit outcomes: a search for the evidence on organizational factors. *Curr Opin Crit Care* 7:284-296, 2001.
6. Pronovost PJ, Angus DC, Dorman T, et al: Physician staffing patterns and clinical outcomes in critically ill patients. *JAMA* 288:2151-2162, 2002.
7. Leape LL, Cullen DJ, Demspey Clapp M, et al: Pharmacist participation on physician rounds and adverse drug events in the intensive care unit. *JAMA* 282:267-270, 1999.
8. Aiken LH, Clarke S, Sloane D, et al: Hospital nurse staffing and patient mortality, nurse burnout, and job dissatisfaction. *JAMA* 288:1987-1993, 2002.
9. Harvey MA: Invisible excellence. *Crit Care Med* 10:373-374, 2001.
10. Sherwood G, Thomas E, Bennett DS, et al: A teamwork model to promote patient safety in critical care. *Crit Care Nurs Clin North Am* 14:333-340, 2002.
11. Pollack MM, Cuerdon TC, Getson PR, et al: Pediatric intensive care units: results of a national survey. *Crit Care Med* 21:607-614, 1993.
12. Angus DC, Kelley MA, Schmitz RJ, et al: Current and projected workforce requirements for care of the critically ill and patients with pulmonary disease: can we meet the requirements of an aging population? *JAMA* 284:2762-2770, 2000.
13. Charytan C, Kapplan AA, Paganini EP, et al: Role of the nephrologist in the intensive care unit. *Am J Kidney Dis* 38:426-429, 2001.
14. Green TP: What is best for patients is best for the intensive care unit. *Crit Care Med* 29:2038-2039, 2001.
15. National Joint Practice Commission (NJPC): *Guidelines for establishing joint or collaborative practice in hospitals.* Chicago, 1981, NJPC.
16. Holcomb BW, Wheeler AP, Ely EW: New ways to reduce unnecessary variation and improve outcomes in the intensive care unit. *Curr Opin Crit Care* 7:304-311, 2001.
17. Bracco D, Favre J-B, Bissonnette B, et al: Human errors in a multidisciplinary intensive care unit: a 1-year prospective study. *Intensive Care Med* 27:137-145, 2001.
18. Wachter RM, Goldman L: The hospitalist movement 5 years later. *JAMA* 287:487-494, 2002.
19. Tenner PA, Dibrell H, Taylor RP: Improved survival with hospitalists in a pediatric intensive care unit. *Crit Care Med* 31:847-852, 2003.

CHAPTER

2

History of Pediatric Critical Care

I. David Todres

PEARLS

- The history of pediatric intensive care has witnessed remarkable achievements in our ability to understand and treat critical illness in children.
- Neonatal intensive care units in the early 1960s followed a mode not organized along traditional organ system models but instead grouped children according to age and severity of illness.
- New modes of respiratory support and pharmacologic support of the cardiovascular system were major advances in optimizing outcomes of critical illness.
- Introduction of extracorporeal membrane oxygenation followed by nitric oxide inhalation for treatment of pulmonary hypertension were dramatic advances in reducing mortality and morbidity of pediatric critical care patients.
- Nutritional support has evolved as a crucial factor in the patient's recovery in the pediatric intensive care unit.
- A major advance in pediatric intensive care was the development of the intensive care unit laboratory to provide data on blood gases, electrolytes, blood sugar, and, later, measurements of therapeutic drug levels.
- Development of sophisticated interhospital transfer services was significant in reducing mortality and morbidity of critically ill children.
- Better and increasing technology has advanced the care of critically ill children but also has created a greater need for creating a humane, caring environment for the child and family.

"The past matters more than we realize... We walk on its ground, and if we don't know the soil we are lost."

William Carlos Williams

The key to understanding the present practice of intensive care for children lies with its history. Although the history of pediatric intensive care is relatively short, it has witnessed remarkable achievements in our ability to understand and treat critical illness in children. Pediatric intensive care is now a well-established discipline recognized by the professional community and the public at large.

Modern pediatric critical care has its roots in the development of adult intensive care and neonatal intensive care. A landmark in its evolution was the ability to effectively treat respiratory failure resulting from poliomyelitis. The first survivor of respiratory failure requiring artificial respiration was a 9-year-old child who rapidly went into respiratory failure because of polio. The child's survival resulted from use of the tank respirator. The individual credited for this device is Philip Drinker of Boston, who introduced the tank respirator ("iron lung").[1,2] The success of this case was instrumental in establishing the value of the device. One distinguished physician at that time stated:

"I was rather doubtful about the machine at first. It looked cumbersome, it was noisy, and it looked more like a torture chamber than anything else, but certainly the boy I saw getting well in it entirely convinced me as to the practical value of this method of giving artificial respiration."

Intensive care took a quantum leap with the experience gained in the epidemic of poliomyelitis in Copenhagen in 1952. Lassen[3] describes this experience, in which the mortality of the disease, especially the bulbar variety, decreased from 90% to 25%. Instrumental in the dramatic success story was the involvement of Björn Ibsen,[4] an anesthesiologist who applied the principles of effective ventilation for the "paralyzed patient" in the operating room to the care of these patients. Lassen, who was chief of the hospital at the time, described the unusual and dramatic step:

"At this point we consulted our anesthetist colleague, Dr. B. Ibsen, and on August 27th the first patient was treated with the method which soon became our method of choice in patients with impairment of swallowing and reduced ventilation—namely, tracheotomy just below the larynx, with insertion of a rubber-cuff tube into the trachea, and manual positive-pressure ventilation from a rubber bag..."

The ventilation was performed by medical students "bagging" the patient via a tracheostomy with a cuffed tracheal tube (i.e., airway was protected). It was appreciated that ineffective ventilation in the past was responsible for the high incidence of deaths and that periodic monitoring of CO_2 would help guide ventilation for prolonged periods. The director of the laboratory where the patients were managed was Poul Astrup, who proceeded to work with the Radiometer company and introduced practical methods of blood gas analysis.[5,6]

Whereas adult care focused primarily on failure of an organ system (the respiratory system), neonatal intensive care units (NICUs) at various centers in the early 1960s followed with a different mode. These NICUs established a new model for pediatric care. This specialty was not organized along traditional organ system models but instead grouped children according to age and severity of illness with disorders that included respiratory disease, cardiac disease, gastrointestinal problems, infectious disease, and metabolic abnormalities. The neonatologist became the specialized generalist and the leader of a team that used the consultation and advice of a large number of pediatric specialists.

Pediatric intensive care units (PICUs) followed this model. In the 1960s and early 1970s, pediatric anesthesiologists played a major role in developing the early units by extending their activities outside the operating room and into the recovery room phase of care. This process was an adaptation to the operating room experience in which unconscious (anesthetized) and muscle-relaxed (paralyzed), mechanically ventilated children were managed. During surgical procedures, strict attention was paid to adequacy of oxygenation, ventilation, and perfusion. With major blood loss during surgery, infusion of fluids and blood became an important part of the maintenance of adequate perfusion to all major organ systems. The operating room experience was an exercise in applied physiology, especially of the cardiopulmonary system, and in applied pharmacology (see Chapter 30). In many instances, this experience resembled situations encountered when treating critically ill children, for example, multiple trauma including head injuries, septic shock, and near-drowning. Further advances in technology occurred in adult intensive care. For example, Swan-Ganz catheter placement allowed bedside measurement of pulmonary artery pressure and cardiac output so that rational therapeutic decisions could be made. Introduction of these devices in children required therapeutic trials and assessment of the data. Introduction of invasive technology inevitably leads to iatrogenic complications, leading to a situation where the physician is "treating the treatment." Thus the benefits of these devices had to be weighed against their risks. Emphasis was placed on developing noninvasive devices to prevent iatrogenic complications (see Chapter 39). Excellent examples of these devices are end-tidal CO_2 and pulse oximetry for monitoring oxygen saturation. In addition, computerized axial tomography and magnetic resonance imaging have enabled the intensivist to make more precise diagnoses (see Chapter 50). The introduction of echocardiography at the bedside of the critically ill patient provided important practical guidance on cardiovascular status and effects of therapy, thus allowing invasive procedures such as Swan-Ganz catheterization to be performed on a much less frequent basis (see Chapter 21). Pediatric intensive care had moved from clinical evaluation of signs and symptoms of disease to measurement of organ dysfunction, particularly the cardiopulmonary system. Evaluation of the critically ill child now rested on a sound pathophysiologic framework from which rational therapeutic decisions could be made.

The next technologic frontier to be explored was measurement of intracranial pressure (ICP) in the critically ill child (see Chapter 53). This need became apparent as pediatric intensivists succeeded in reversing cardiac and respiratory failure only to see the patient die of cerebral complications. Clinical signs of increased ICP were helpful, but objective measurements of early compromise were needed. The Reye syndrome epidemics of the 1970s and early 1980s demanded both a multisystem approach to pediatric intensive care and experience in ICP monitoring to predict life-threatening increases in ICP before clinical manifestations appeared. This concept was applied to other causes of encephalopathy, such as near-drowning or following cardiac arrest.

Introduction of extracorporeal membrane oxygenation followed by nitric oxide inhalation for treatment of pulmonary hypertension were dramatic advances that reduced mortality and morbidity in pediatric critical care patients (see Chapter 48). Nutritional support has evolved as a crucial factor in the patient's recovery in the PICU (see Chapter 69).

Children in the PICU often suffered multiorgan system failure, which required the expertise of different consulting groups to optimize care. Intensive care needed a "conductor," the pediatric intensivist, with an "orchestra" composed of physicians, nurses, respiratory therapists, social workers, chaplains, and others, all working in harmony to heal the critically ill child. Parents are integral to good care, particularly for pediatric patients. Therefore a great deal of emphasis goes to ensuring that the critical care experience for all involved—the child, family, and health care team—occurs in an environment of humane and compassionate care.

In some areas of the world, rapid development of PICUs occurred over the next few decades. In other areas, rapidity of progress was limited by cost and extent of experience and skill available. The following description of the development of PICUs records some of the landmark steps in development in North America, Europe, Australia and New Zealand, Africa, Asia, and South America. What follows is a brief history. A more comprehensive review would be required in order to include other significant contributions to the development of this specialty.

North America

United States

The first PICU in the United States was established in 1967 at the Children's Hospital of Philadelphia under the direction of John Downes.[7] His experience as an anesthesiologist contributed to the successful innovation of techniques to support critically ill children in respiratory failure and especially status asthmaticus. This contribution opened the door for pediatricians to recognize the worth of the anesthesiologist in caring for the patient with respiratory failure. It is interesting to note that adult intensive care units (ICUs) were more readily attuned to having the anesthesiologist care for the critically ill than were the pediatric units. Downes' contribution to the development of equipment and safety standards for ventilator management of children was crucial in the successful treatment of critically ill children. Downes also recognized early on (1977) the need for developing a home care program for infants and children suffering from severe chronic respiratory failure and requiring mechanical ventilation for survival. This program helped to promote the nurturing of these patients in a more normal home environment.

In 1973, the first child discharged home from a PICU on a mechanical ventilator was a patient under the care of Shannon and Todres at Massachusetts General Hospital. The infant was suffering from congenital central hypoventilation (Ondine curse). As a trial anticipating the child's discharge home, the infant (who was to return home supported in an iron lung, probably for life) was placed on the therapy in the hospital prior to discharge. However, the device malfunctioned, and the infant suffered a cardiac arrest. A check of the patient's blood gas demonstrated a $P{CO_2}$ of 250 mmHg and pH of 6.6. The child was successfully resuscitated and returned home, this time supported with a positive-pressure respirator of the kind used in the PICU. The child went on to make a full recovery with no neurologic deficit. To our knowledge, this was the first child treated at home on a ventilator! I subsequently visited the patient's home to adjust the ventilator as the mother related that the infant had blue lips during sleep. As I made the adjustments to the ventilator, I found the family cat playfully pawing at the respirator tubing! This home visit left me with a new appreciation for the love and dedication of the parents who provided "intensive care" at home without any electronic monitoring or support of ICU staff.

In the early 1970s, as increasing numbers of PICUs were developed, physicians with a pediatric medicine background became active in the PICUs. Between 1968 and 1971, units were developed in other parts of the country. Among these units were those developed by Shannon and Todres at Massachusetts General Hospital, Conn at the Hospital for Sick Children in Toronto, and Gilman at Yale New Haven Hospital. By extending their activities to patient care outside the operating room, pediatric anesthesiologists played a major role in developing the early units. In 1969, Levin, a pediatric cardiologist, impressed by the success of the postoperative PICUs, opened a four-bed PICU at St. Luke's Hospital in Chicago. In some ways this unit was the vanguard for the nonanesthesiologist pediatric intensivist (a term not used until the early 1980s). Kampschulte developed a PICU at the Pittsburgh Children's Hospital in 1971. At the same time units were developed at the Long Island Jewish Hospital by Holzman, a pediatric pulmonologist, and at Montefiore Hospital in New York, with Richard Kravath, a pulmonologist, as director.

An important area of concern to the pediatric intensivist became the care of the child who, on discharge from the ICU, required a "step-down" type of intensive care often referred to as *intermediate intensive care*. Such a unit was developed at the Massachusetts General Hospital under the directorships of Shannon and Todres in 1971. In this setting, it was possible to mechanically ventilate the chronically ill child and monitor the child requiring a lesser degree of intensive care. Focus in this area allowed concentration on the important rehabilitative processes in the child's recovery. Nursing staff and physicians with special interest in this area dedicated their care to such children. Similar areas developed by Downes, Kittrick, and Goldberg in Philadelphia helped stimulate general interest in this important area. Observation of these chronic care patients led to an understanding of how the children and their families coped with illness so that physicians could more appropriately advise and treat those with chronic critical illness. Step-down facilities have been developed in many places and have prompted the development of progressive care facilities so that families of chronically ill children can become increasingly involved in their children's care, ultimately taking over the care themselves and even providing the care at home.

Canada

At The Hospital for Sick Children in Toronto, Alan Conn, anesthetist-in-chief, had the vision of developing an ICU utilizing his anesthesiology skills. In 1970 he took on the position of full-time director of critical care and initiated a flourishing clinical and research program. Conn was followed by Geoffrey Barker, who continued to promote the unit as one of the leading pediatric critical care units in the world. Barker's vision of the need to bring together intensive care from many parts of the world led to his directorship of the World Federation of Pediatric Intensive and Critical Care Societies, which has done much to foster the development of pediatric critical care in countries around the world and to bring the skills and experience so vital in this practice to the benefit of multiple countries.

Africa

Pat Smythe, a pediatrician working with Arthur Bull, an anesthesiologist in Cape Town, South Africa, at the Red Cross Children's War Memorial Hospital, brilliantly conceived a therapeutic plan to treat infants afflicted with tetanus from infected umbilical cord stumps.[8] As a resident in pediatrics in 1959 working in this unit, I administered curare intramuscularly and mechanically ventilated the infants with an early modified Radcliffe respirator via a tracheostomy for 10 days. This method proved to be highly successful. A dedicated group of nursing aides caring for these infants played a crucial role in their survival. Monitoring of these infants depended on close observation of chest movement and visualization of cyanosis. Routine blood gas analyses had not yet entered the scene. The Severinghaus electrode ($P\text{CO}_2$) appeared in 1959 and the Clark electrode ($P\text{O}_2$) in 1961. However, using the Van Slyke method on a sample of end-tidal gas provided a measure of $P\text{CO}_2$ (reflecting venous $P\text{CO}_2$ and, by extrapolation, arterial $P\text{CO}_2$). This labor-intensive method performed by the pediatric resident was applied somewhat infrequently! From this experience the logical step was to apply these principles of ventilator-supported care to the other critically ill infants and children, which followed later with the designation of a special unit for critically ill children with a primary intensivist. Max Klein assumed this role with distinction. Klein's background in pulmonary medicine was an invaluable asset, and his astute clinical observational skill was a model for younger physicians who were quick to resort to sophisticated technology to monitor these patients. Klein's commitment to psychosocial issues in the care of patients was exemplary. His vision went beyond the ICU. In an excellent home-care tracheostomy program of 60 to 70 children, he was successful in ensuring the care of these children despite dreadful home conditions. In talking with him about the program, I recall his enthusiasm for the need to have these children nurtured away from the hospital, and his staff provided these children with visits to the public gardens!

Asia

Japan

In the 1960s Seizo Iwai was the first physician to introduce long-term mechanical ventilation and arterial blood gas analysis of critically ill infants. At that time he was Chief of Anesthesia at the National Children's Hospital in Tokyo. He organized a symposium on respiratory distress in infants at the World Congress of Anesthesiology in Kyoto in 1972. He was a strong force in developing a close relationship with other Asian countries and invited trainees from those countries to promote the teaching and development of pediatric critical care. His close working relationship with Conn and Baker at the Hospital for Sick Children in Toronto, Canada, paved the way for Katsuyuki Miyasaka to study in their highly developed PICU. Miyasaka returned to Japan to stimulate and foster the development of a new generation of pediatric intensivists and continues to play a major role in facilitating this process.

India

Pediatric intensive care followed the establishment of neonatal care, which was started in Delhi in 1961, and its evolution resembles that of the United States'. Pediatricians with other subspecialties, such as anesthesiologists, cardiologists, and surgeons, have attended to this concern with the support of the India Academy of Pediatrics. Intensivists outside the country have been active in establishing teaching programs in various parts of the country. Economics limits the development of ICUs, with their needs for sophisticated technology, ventilators, monitoring equipment, and drugs. However, with support from private hospitals, high-level intensive care comparable with western medicine has been attained. It is recognized that models of intensive care in India must be adapted and developed to meet the needs of the community.

Australia and New Zealand

PICUs started forming in Australia in the early 1960s, arising out of postoperative recovery wards with congenital heart surgery. In 1963 John Stocks and Ian McDonald in Melbourne introduced postoperative respiratory support with prolonged nasal intubation. Other units followed in Adelaide, Perth, Sydney, and Brisbane.

An important contribution to the development of intensive care was the use of plastic endotracheal tubes for prolonged intubation and ventilation. Bernard Brandstater, an Australian working in Lebanon, reported prolonged intubation as an alternate to the tracheosty at the First European Congress in Anesthesia in 1962. In 1963, Allen and Steven in Adelaide introduced this method into practice in Perth and Ian McDonald in Melbourne. The first report of prolonged intubation in 50 patients was described in the *British Journal of Anesthesia* in 1965 by McDonald and Stocks. Pediatric critical care is regionalized in tertiary university services.

To provide such care for critically ill children in remote areas at some distance from major centers led to the development of sophisticated transport service, including fixed wing aircraft.

Until 1991 all critically ill children in New Zealand received care in adult ICUs. The first PICU opened in December 1991 at the Starship Children's Hospital in Auckland.

Europe

In Europe, pediatric intensive care followed shortly after the poliomyelitis epidemic in Denmark in 1952. Even in the early years, it was recognized that children had a higher mortality than adults in these poliomyelitis respiratory units; thus separate PICUs were developed in Uppsala and Stockholm in the 1950s. In 1955 Joran Haglund, an anesthesiologist, established the first PICU for infants and children at the Children's Hospital in Goteburg in Sweden. In 1961 Hans Feychting, a pediatric anesthesiologist, established the first PICU in Stockholm, Sweden, and became recognized as a pioneer in the development of pediatric intensive care in Europe. He introduced many of the skills developed for the operating room and later applied to pediatric intensive care.

In France in July 1963, a newborn presented with tetanus and was admitted to "l'hopital des Enfants Malades" of Paris. Shortly afterward, Gilbert Hualt, a pediatrician trained in pediatrics and adult intensive care, treated a child with respiratory paralysis resulting from polio. In 1964 Hualt opened the first multidisciplinary PICU in Saint Vincent de Paul Hospital. This unit was the first pediatrician-directed PICU in Europe and soon became a major influence on the development of ICUs in which Francois Beaufils and Denis DeVictor were to play an important role in the further development of critical care practice in pediatrics.

In Britain in 1964 the first PICU was opened by G. Jackson Rees, an anesthesiologist, at the Alder Hey Children's Hospital in Liverpool. Other units soon followed. In practice they were postoperative recovering rooms that continued to provide intensive care beyond regular postoperative care and in which children often were mechanically ventilated and closely monitored, particularly their cardiovascular status. The patients were most often postoperative cardiac surgery patients who might require prolonged tracheal intubation, tracheotomy, and mechanical ventilation. I worked in such a unit at the Hospital for Sick Children, Great Ormond Street, London, in 1966. Although not designated "a pediatric ICU," in essence it was a unit that was functionally operating in this manner. This experience formed the foundation of intensive care practice that followed with primary attention to conditions that led to failure of ventilation and circulation. Here David Hatch was instrumental in developing a PICU that provided outstanding clinical care and research.

The first PICUs in the Netherlands were established in the late 1970s and early 1980s at the Sophia Children's Hospital in Rotterdam, the Wilhelmina Children's Hospital in Utrecht, and the Emma's Children's Hospital at the Academic Medical Center in Amsterdam. In 1995 a section on Pediatric Intensive Care Medicine was founded by the Dutch Paediatric Association, which certifies the training of nearly all Dutch pediatric intensivists in fellowship programs. The PICUs are multidisciplinary and manage a variety of childhood diseases, including seizures, hepatic dysfunction, and immunologic and infectious diseases. By 2004 the number of PICUs in the Netherlands had grown to eight, all of which are part of university teaching hospitals and are separate from NICUs. A nationwide transport system to connect this centralized care system of pediatric critical care currently is under development. Albert Bos in Amsterdam and Ed van der Voort in Rotterdam continue to foster the highest standards of pediatric critical care.

Latin America

In Argentina the origin of pediatric intensive care was based on the interests of the general pediatrician. The first PICU was established in Children's Hospital "Dr. R. Gutierrez" in Buenos Aires in 1969 as part of a general surgery ward. In 1972 Jorge Sasbon became the first staff director of the PICU. In 1972 a PICU was set up in Children's Hospital "Pedro Elizalde" under the guidance of Clara Bonno, and the unit has been a pillar of the specialty in Argentina.

Marked progress occurred, and the first liver transplant in a pediatric patient was performed in 1987. With the introduction of international fellowships, physicians were able to travel abroad for further training in units in Toronto, Pittsburgh, Madrid, and London. The pediatric hospital "Dr. J. P. Garraba" was inaugurated as a tertiary center in 1987 and has developed a sophisticated PICU under the direction of Jorge Sasbon.

In Brazil in the 1970s, epidemics of polio and meningococcal disease with high mortality led to the creation of small units for care of patients attended to by personnel with skills and technical resources (although they were scarce). These units were the precursors of PICUs established later in Sao Paolo, Rio de Janeiro, and Porto Allegre. At the same time, neonatal intensive care was developing, and the model of the NICU was transferred to the care of critically ill children in the 1980s.

In 1984 the first Brazilian Pediatric Intensive Care Congress in Sao Paolo took place. These congresses continue annually. At the three major tertiary centers in Sao Paolo, Rio de Janeiro, and Porto Allegre, government agencies are supporting research programs. Pediatric intensivists in the Brazilian Pediatric Society and the Brazilian Critical Care Society worked together to establish the subspecialty, with examination certification commencing in 1990. Brazil's intensivists also are active in cooperative efforts with other Latin American countries, and in 2004 the Sixth Latin American Congress on Pediatric Intensive Care was held.

One of the pioneers of development of pediatric critical care in Latin America was Mauricio Gajer, a dedicated physician from Uruguay. Gajer, with the stimulus of

Professor Ramon Guerra, created the first PICU in Uruguay in 1975. He traveled to France, where he worked with Professors Huault and Beaufils. After returning to Uruguay he created the first private ICU in Uruguay. With his enthusiasm to bring all Latin American pediatricians together in the cause of critical care, he organized the first Latin American Pediatric Intensive Care Congress in Uruguay in 1993, which led to development of the Pediatric Intensive Care Society.

World Federation of Pediatric Intensive and Critical Care Societies

The mission of this federation is exclusively educational, scientific, and charitable in nature. It exists to disseminate and to make available the high standards of pediatric intensive and critical care to all children of the world, with a vision of distributing knowledge across international borders. It was founded in Paris in 1997 and has set up the series of World Congresses of Pediatric and Critical Care. The board of directors recognized individuals who made significant contributions to their field within their country. Each international pioneer was given a gold medal at the World Congress in Montreal in 2000 by the president, Geoff Barker. They include Alan Conn, Canada; Jack Downes, United States; Hans Feychting, Stockholm; Mauricio Gajer, Uruguay; Gilbert Huault, France; Seizo Iwai, Japan; Max Klein, South Africa; and John Stocks, Australia.

Additional Services

Respiratory Therapy

An important development that contributed to pediatric intensive care was respiratory therapy. With the expertise of the respiratory therapist at the bedside, particularly with mechanical ventilation and advances in aerosol treatment, innovative and sophisticated therapies were implemented to benefit critically ill children. Respiratory therapists also participated in interhospital transfer of patients ensuring safety and support of the patient.

Intensive Care Unit Laboratory

A major advance in pediatric intensive care was the development of the ICU laboratory to provide data on blood gases, electrolytes, blood sugar, and, later, measurements of therapeutic drug levels. When pioneer pediatric intensivists first began treating newborns with neonatal tetanus and mechanical ventilation in the late 1950s, adequacy of oxygenation and ventilation was assessed using clinical parameters such as chest movements and skin color. Objective assessment of ventilation was ascertained by obtaining expired alveolar gas and analyzing it for P_{CO_2}, using the Van Slyke manometric apparatus.

The process was tedious, and only one or two assessments per day could be made. The Severinghaus CO_2 electrode appeared in 1957 and the Clark O_2 electrode in 1961; however, the large sample size limited blood gas analysis in children. Ultramicrotechnology for pH and P_{CO_2} analysis was developed in Denmark by Astrup in the mid-1950s and imported to the United States by James at Columbia Medical Center in the late 1950s. Miniaturization of P_{O_2} electrodes and combination with the Astrup system provided a complete blood gas analysis system using less than 1 ml of blood. A commercial system became available in 1965 and gained wide acceptance by 1970.

Transportation of Pediatric Patients

The development of sophisticated interhospital transfer services was significant in reducing mortality and morbidity of critically ill children. This process came out of the recognition that "intensive care" of the patient starts outside of the PICU facility to ensure safe transport and optimal outcome for the patient (see Chapter 14).[9,10]

Human Face of Pediatric Critical Care

The journey of intensive care for children has moved from triumph to triumph. However, in the process the public has perceived that although medicine has succeeded on the technical level, it has lost much of its human touch, becoming more impersonal and forbidding (Figures 2–1 and 2–2). Some have stated that medicine has lost its way. My sense is that we have started to reclaim this lost heritage of caring and compassion. This has been particularly true in end-of-life care and the convening of the expertise of intensivists and palliative caregivers. Pediatric intensivists have come to the realization that caring for critically ill children requires the gathering of information along two parallel lines. One is the disease framework, which includes the symptoms, signs, investigations, and clinical management. The other is the illness framework, which is the patient's and family's agenda of concerns, expectations, feelings, and thoughts that are unique to each individual and family (see Chapter 10). An intensivist acts to bring about a positive good or benefit to the patient; however, experience in the PICU has

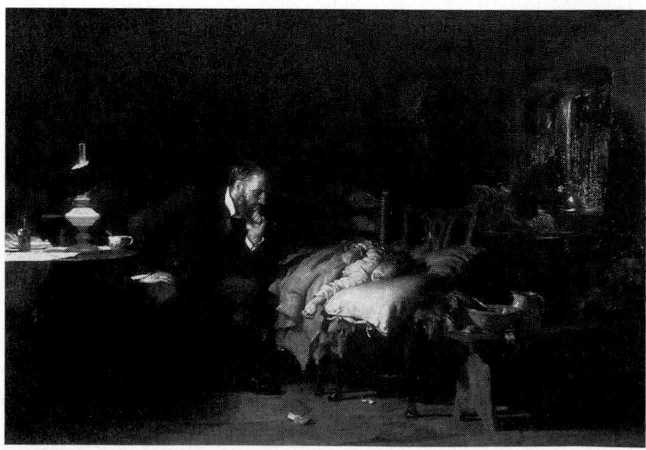

FIGURE 2–1 • "The Doctor," painted by Sir Luke Fildes (1891), shows the concern and compassion, but also the helplessness, of a physician caring for a critically ill child. (Courtesy the Tate Gallery, London, United Kingdom.)

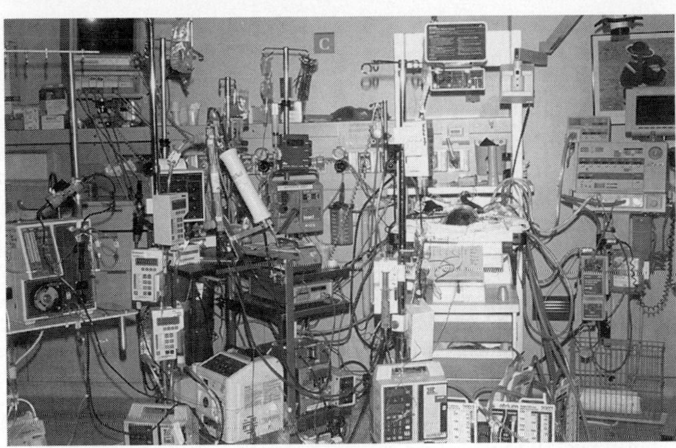

FIGURE 2–2 • Pediatric intensive care unit at Massachusetts General Hospital (2002). In stark contrast to the nineteenth-century view of a sick child, in this picture a critically ill infant is surrounded by sophisticated technology but is isolated from the family and the health care team.

shown that conflicts arise when the presumption to save life (a good) requires interventions that may cause undue suffering. The more aggressive the efforts to reverse illness, often the more suffering is inflicted on the patient. This leads to a situation where the physician begins to question how far to pursue these procedures. These ethical dilemmas are increasingly receiving the attention of intensivists. The establishment of ethics committees has been helpful in providing the health care team with important perspectives in approaching these difficult issues (see Chapter 11 and Chapter 12).

In many units an increasingly diverse patient population has sensitized intensivists to the need to understand and respect individual cultural differences.[11] Stereotyping a particular culture fails to respect individual differences. Increasingly, care is centered on the patient and family in recognition of the effects of personal spiritual/religious, cultural, and family values on patients' illness and recovery and in coping with end of life.[12,13] In many PICUs chaplains are brought to the bedside and become part of the intensive care team.

Addition of child psychiatrists and social workers to the PICU consulting team has helped families and children cope with the severe and devastating effects of critical illness. For the health care team, the long hours of stressful work and the occasional feelings of despair and frustration that all the hard work is not making a difference lead to emotional distress and a sense of loss of fulfillment in their professional life. Understanding this problem and helping the team to realize they are making an important difference and are valued will reduce burnout and enhance staff morale. To illustrate the importance of knowing that one's effort does make a difference in people's lives, the following letter received by one of my nursing staff after a visit to the family at home stated,

"In the almost three weeks that we were in the pediatric ICU (PICU), we witnessed two deaths besides our son's... We know that death is part of your job and therefore must be dealt with as each sees fit... It seems funny that we'd be so happy to see people we barely know but your visit and the effort it took to come signifies a great deal. It meant that you DID care about our baby...and the solace received from your caring was—and is—immense. A special thanks for that... Please do not feel that your encouragement helped to give us false hope. Hope is what got us through those three weeks. Despair could wait."[14]

Rehabilitation

Survival in the PICU often comes at a price. Individuals frequently have significant loss of functional capabilities in addition to organ failure. The skills of the rehabilitation physician now are appreciated as being integrated into the total care of the patient, not only to preserve life but also to assist in restoring or improving physical function and psychological recovery.

Assessment

Evaluation of various treatments and comparison to outcomes must continue so that care is based on science. Following the pioneering work of Cullen in Boston and Knaus in Washington in adult populations, Pollack applied severity scoring in children so that interventions in various diseases can be evaluated on the basis of the common denominator of illness severity. He has continued to develop this system[15] (see Chapter 7). Children who receive care in PICUs as opposed to adult ICUs have a significantly lower mortality rate, especially the most seriously ill children.[16,17]

Summary

Models for pediatric intensive care developed from those established in adult intensive care and neonatal intensive care. The management of the poliomyelitis epidemic in Denmark in 1952 was a major impetus to the development of adult intensive care, which initially focused on treating failure of one organ system (the respiratory system). The respiratory units treated patients with polio, myasthenia gravis, Guillain-Barré syndrome, intoxications, and tetanus. With their experience it was natural to extend management to involvement of other organ systems, especially the cardiac system. Pediatric experience in postoperative recovery rooms with patients following cardiac surgery set the stage for the development of discrete ICUs. Anesthesiologists, by virtue of their operating room experience with patients, played a vital part in the development of these units. In many centers they continue to do so, with the pediatrician taking on an important cooperative or primary role in management of these patients. The development of intensive care technology and facilities also evolved as a progression from the anesthesiologist's work in the operating room and extended recovery room care to multidisciplinary pediatric care units managed by dedicated specialists in pediatric critical care.

In its relatively short history, pediatric critical care has accomplished much for gravely ill infants and children. In the future, pediatric intensivists must continue to strive toward improving morbidity and mortality and helping families cope with these potentially overwhelming times. With increasing technologic advances, every effort must be made to ensure that the critical care experience for the child, family, and health care team is fostered in a humane, caring environment.

There has been increasing awareness of the patients' and families' experience of illness, recognizing each child's uniqueness, human spirit, fear, hope, and desire for comfort and reassurance. In addition, attention to the needs of the health care "family" has become an important and necessary focus to ensure the optimal care of all involved.

Acknowledgments

I express my appreciation to Lucien de Nicola for the significant contributions to this chapter stemming from his coauthorship with me in two previous editions of this text. I also express my appreciation to Geoff Barker, Albert Bos, Denis DeVictor, John Downes, Jonathan Gillis, Katsuyuki Miyasaka, Jefferson Piva, and Jorge Sasbon for their contributions, which provided an international perspective on this history.

REFERENCES

1. Drinker P, Shaughnessy TJ, Murphy DP: The Drinker respirator. Analysis of case reports of patients with respiratory failure treated from October 1928 to June 1930. *JAMA* 95:1249-1253, 1930.
2. Drinker P: Prolonged administration of artificial respiration. *Lancet* 1:1186, 1931.
3. Lassen HCA: A preliminary report on the 1952 epidemic of poliomyelitis in Copenhagen. With special reference to the treatment of acute respiratory insufficiency. Lancet 37-41, 1953.
4. Ibsen B: From anaesthesia to anaesthesiology. Personal experiences in Copenhagen during the past 25 years. *Acta Anaesthsiol Scand Suppl* 61:1-69, 1975.
5. Astrup P: A simple electrometric technique for the determination of carbon dioxide tension in blood and plasma, total content of carbon dioxide in plasma, and bicarbonate content in separated plasma at a fixed carbon dioxide tension (40 mm Hg). *Scand J Clin Lab Invest* 8:33-43, 1956.
6. Severinghaus JW, Astrup PB: History of blood gas analysis. *Int Anesth Clin* 25:1, 1987.
7. Downes JJ: The historical evolution, current status, and prospective development of pediatric critical care. *Crit Care Clin North Am* 8:5, 1992.
8. Smythe PM, Bull A: Treatment of tetanus neonatorum with intermittent positive-pressure respiration. *BMJ* 2:107, 1959.
9. Bergeson PS, Bushore M, Cravens JH, et al: Guidelines for air and ground transportation of pediatric patients. *Pediatrics* 78:943, 1986.
10. Britto J, Nadel S, Machonochie I, et al: Morbidity and severity of illness during interhospital transfer: impact of a specialized paediatric retrieval team. *BMJ* 311:836-839, 1995.
11. Flores G: Culture and the patient-physician relationship: achieving cultural competency in health care. *J Pediatr* 136:14-23, 2000.
12. Mueller PS, Plevak DJ, Rummans TA: Religious involvement, spirituality, and medicine: Implications for clinical practice. *Mayo Clin Proc* 76:1225-1235, 2001.
13. Thoreson CE, Harris MS: Spirituality and health: what's the evidence and what's needed? *Ann Behav Med* 24:3-13, 2002.
14. Todres ID, Armstrong A, Lally P, Cassem EH: Negotiating end-of-life issues. *New Horiz* 6:374-382, 1998.
15. Pollack MM, Rittimann UE, Getson PR: The pediatric risk of mortality (PRISM) score. *Crit Care Med* 16:100, 1988.
16. Pollack MM, Alexander Sr, Clarke N, et al: Improved outcomes from tertiary center pediatric intensive care: a statewide comparison of tertiary and non-tertiary care facilities. *Crit Care* Med 19:150-159, 1991.
17. Hall JR, Reyes HM, Meller JL et al: The outcome for children with blunt trauma is best at a pediatric trauma center. *J Pediatr Surg* 31:72-77, 1996.

CHAPTER

3

Pediatric Critical Care and the Intensivist in the New Hospital Environment

Thomas P. Green

PEARLS

- Intensive care unit costs account for 20% to 28% of hospital costs.
- Multidisciplinary participation in a critical care team appears to be associated with improved patient outcome.
- The Child Health Corporation of America estimates that there will be a need for 27% more pediatric intensivists before 2006.

The past 2 decades have produced many changes in medicine. Advances in the scientific understanding of human biology and the pathophysiology of disease have continued to accelerate and have produced new diagnostic techniques and treatments. For example, in just 20 years, solid organ transplantation has evolved from an experimental concept to an accepted, commonly applied procedure, largely because of scientific discoveries in basic immunology. Technologic breakthroughs have been prominent. New medical equipment and pharmaceutical agents have appeared continuously and impacted all facets of medicine. A notable example is the continuous stream of newly developed antibiotics that has kept ahead of emerging bacterial resistance to older agents.

However, for these and other reasons, the cost of medical care has spiraled upward at the same time these medical breakthroughs have offered promise of better outcomes. Total health care costs now approach 14% of the gross national product.[1] Medical insurance companies, federal and state governments, business leaders, and even the public at large have called for controls on total costs together with accountability for outcomes. Care in intensive care units has been at the center of this attention because intensive care units account for 20% to 28% of hospital costs but only 5% of hospital beds.[2] The costs for intensive care services touch all aspects of hospital operations (Figure 3–1).

Although changes in pediatric care have mirrored many of the developments in medical care for adults, there have been some important differences. Overall costs of children's care have risen more slowly than costs for adults, primarily related to the lower costs of the preventive care prevalent in children contrasted with disease-based care in adults. However, publicly supported care for children is funded through the Medicaid system at rates that generally are substantially below those in the Medicare system, which finances health care for the elderly. Finally, systems of pediatric care, particularly in the critical care units, are more centralized and coordinated than is the case for adult care. The relatively smaller numbers of seriously ill children have resulted in more regionalized care and, perhaps, more collaborative interaction among medical and surgical specialists. Pediatric intensivists typically have been involved in the care, both medical and surgical, of all critically ill children in their institution and coordinate all aspects of

Cost Center	Mean ± SD			Median
Room	52.1%	±	14.9%	52.0%
Laboratory	18.3%	±	11.5%	16.7%
Pharmacy	8.4%	±	7.2%	6.7%
Radiology	7.6%	±	8.7%	5.2%
Respiratory Therapy	5.7%	±	4.4%	4.8%
Medical/Surgical Supply	3.4%	±	2.3%	3.1%
Miscellaneous	4.6%	±	8.2%	1.0%

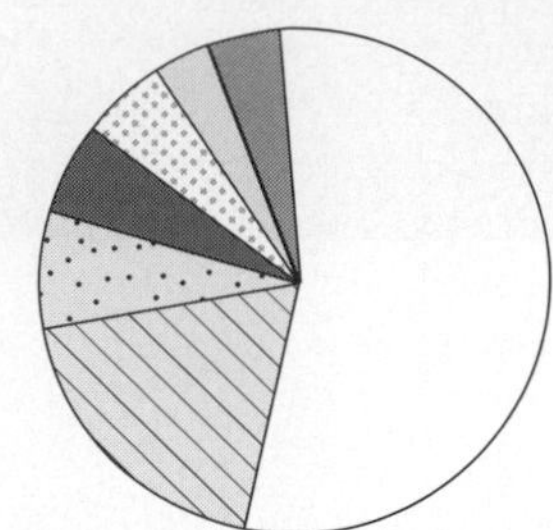

FIGURE 3–1 • Cost distribution (as percentage of each patient admission's total cost) among major cost centers. Mean ± SD and median values are listed, and the pie graph illustrates the distribution for all pediatric intensive care unit care. Miscellaneous includes special diagnostic studies and other services. (From Chalom R, Raphealy RC, Costarino AT: *Crit Care Med* 27:2079-2085, 1999.)

their care. In contrast, intensivists caring for adult patients may focus their attention on one or more critical problems, such as respiratory or cardiac failure.

As a consequence, the pediatric intensive care unit and its multidisciplinary team are major components of hospital planning and operations. In larger hospital systems and networks, the pediatric intensive care unit at the central hospital operates a resource for an entire health system. The leaders of the pediatric intensive care unit are charged with coordinating effective and efficient care with other specialists and primary care providers.

This chapter documents the evolution of this responsibility and role, characterizes some of the essential components, and outlines some of the apparent challenges ahead.

Evolution of Pediatric Critical Care

Critical care units are a relatively recent feature of hospital care. The earliest forerunners of modern intensive care units probably were the special wards, organized in a few hospitals in the early twentieth century, to care for prematurely born infants. Present-day intensive care specialists would recognize the major steps forward made during World War II when separate wards with isolated rooms were reserved for the resuscitation of trauma victims and for the care of surgical patients. During the 1950s, outbreaks of poliomyelitis with respiratory failure led to the formation of respiratory intensive care units. Here the nursing and medical personnel could efficiently care for larger numbers of patients with similar medical problems and common technologic applications. By 1958, 25% of hospitals reported they had an intensive care unit. In the early 1960s, the number of coronary care units increased sharply as the result of reports of improved outcome in patients with myocardial infarction who were closely monitored by personnel trained to intervene acutely. By the late 1960s, most hospitals reported they had organized and were operating one or more intensive care units. In general, workforce and economic issues, rather than technology, were the driving forces in coalescing patients into intensive care units.[3]

The development of pediatric intensive care units evolved more slowly. Advances in mechanical ventilation were applied to the care of prematurely born infants, and neonatal intensive care units were organized in the 1960s and 1970s. For many years after the widespread development of intensive care units for adult patients, nonneonatal pediatric patients with critical illness continued to receive care in adult critical care units, on general medical/surgical wards, and occasionally as exceptional patients in neonatal intensive care units. The lack of a single, high-volume disease, such as hyaline membrane disease in newborns or myocardial infarction in adults, probably contributed to the delayed formation of pediatric intensive care units. However, advances in medical and surgical intensive care and insightful recognition that these developments should be applied to a wide variety of critical problems in children finally resulted in a sharp rise in the organization of pediatric intensive care units in the 1970s and early 1980s.

In 1986 the American Board of Medical Specialists approved certification of specialties in critical care, organized under the auspices of Boards of Anesthesiology, Pediatrics, Medicine, and Surgery. Shortly thereafter, the Residency Review Committee of the American Council on Graduate Medical Education began the review and accreditation of specialty training programs in these disciplines. Beginning with the first certifying examination in 1987 through 2000, the American Board of Pediatrics has certified 994 individuals in Pediatric Critical Care Medicine.

Pediatric intensive care units still vary significantly with regard to size and scope of care provided. A survey by Pollack et al.[4] in 1989 found that 40% of units had four to six beds and only 6% of units had more than 18 beds. Although a similar survey has not been repeated, the promulgation of standards of pediatric critical care practice, outlined by the American College of Critical Care Medicine and the American Academy of Pediatrics, has promoted the organization of regionalized units, staffed by specialized, multidisciplinary teams, led by Board-certified pediatric critical care specialists.[5,6] Notably, the state of Ohio has recognized the value of multidisciplinary pediatric critical care.[7]

Outcomes of Intensive Care

A substantial number of studies now document that the involvement of an intensivist in the care of critically ill patients improves patient outcome. Most of the studies have used historical controls and documented that the involvement of an intensivist was associated with improved patient outcome.[8] However, later cross-sectional surveys have shown that the presence of critical care physicians correlated with better patient outcomes.[9] Further analysis of this dataset suggested that the presence of a critical care training program further enhanced favorable outcomes.[10] Data from adult studies are informative because of the larger numbers of patients, often with more homogeneous diseases such as myocardial infarction or abdominal aortic aneurysm, who can be studied. The involvement of intensivists has been associated with shorter lengths of stay, utilization of fewer resources, fewer complications, and lower overall charges.[11] Outcomes are improved. One investigator summarized that "Daily rounds by an ICU [intensive care unit] physician may be as important as the experience performing a high-risk operation."[12]

Multidisciplinary Intensive Care Team and Role of the Intensivist

The role of the pediatric intensivist has changed considerably in the short time since intensivist involvement has been widespread, although the precise changes and rates of change have been institutionally dependent. In general, pediatric intensive care specialists initially provided consultation on selected patients, often restricting their attention to specific issues, such as management of mechanical ventilation. Gradually at some institutions but more rapidly at others, intensivists assumed all aspects of care for defined groups of patients or even all patients in the intensive care unit.

The models of care in intensive care units continue to vary among institutions. For example, some units operate as a so called *open unit,* contrasted with a *closed unit* approach elsewhere. Typically, in a closed unit all admissions to the intensive care unit are transferred to the care of an intensivist, who manages all aspects of care, with consultative assistance as needed. Other units have varying degrees of "openness," ranging from shared attending responsibilities between intensivists and other specialists on individual patients to open admitting privileges for nonintensivists. Although no controlled trials exist at present, data in the literature suggest that closed units operate with more efficiency[13] and patients have improved mortality and fewer complications.[14]

The most important role of the intensivist is as the leader of the multidisciplinary intensive care team. This team is composed of nursing leadership and staff, pharmacists, respiratory therapists, hospital administrators, social workers, and other medical specialists. Each component of the team contributes a unique expertise directed toward improvement of patient care outcomes, improving efficiency and effectiveness of care and controlling costs.

Interaction among team members is responsible for many of the breakthrough system improvements in critical care. For example, development of protocols for weaning patients from mechanical ventilation have required collaborative development among physicians, nurses, and respiratory therapists. Implementation of these protocols has reduced mechanical ventilation time, reduced intensive care unit length of stay, and thereby reduced hospital costs without affecting outcome.[15] Hospital costs have increased substantially because of rising drug costs. The integral involvement of critical care pharmacists has improved the education of physicians and nurses and improved utilization of cost-effective alternatives.[16] A study has credited the central role for intensive care unit pharmacists in limiting the emergence of antibiotic-resistant strains of bacteria in the intensive care unit.[17] The application of quality improvement methodology has been applicable to intensive care unit procedures and, when implemented with the full multidisciplinary team, results in better outcomes and decreased costs.[18]

The evolution of these many roles for the intensivist has required an increased involvement in both patient care and administrative activities on a daily basis. One of the essential elements of intensive care unit operation is that the responsible intensivist must have no competing clinical responsibilities that would distract him/her from immediate availability to the care of an individual patient or attention to a unit issue. On many units, a pediatric intensivist is present 24 hours per day. This constant availability provides needed expertise in critical situations and appropriate supervision of students and trainees, as required. Current numbers of appropriately qualified pediatric intensivists are insufficient to provide this level of attending coverage in all pediatric critical care units. However, should further investigation demonstrate that continuous intensivist presence improves outcomes in a cost-effective manner, regionalization of units could reduce the redundancy in the health care system.

Opportunities and Challenges

As the role of the pediatric intensivist in the new hospital environment evolves to meet the needs of critically ill patients in a changing social, economic, and medical background, challenges exist for the specialty of pediatric critical care itself. How specialists and their leadership respond to these changes may prominently affect the ability to achieve the continued improvements that have been seen to date.

Intensive care units in neonatology, pediatrics, and adult specialties all began with substantial involvement of trainees in ongoing patient management. A number of factors will decrease the role that students and residents play in pediatric critical care units. To begin, as the specialty has matured, the technical expertise required in bedside decisions has increased, substantially increasing the involvement of fellows and attending physicians directly in care on an ongoing basis. Second, the training curriculum for pediatric residents has expanded substantially in the past decade, increasing the breadth of skills and knowledge that must be acquired and thereby decreasing the amount of time available for critical care.

In addition to changing the manpower mix in the intensive care unit, this change in training focus is having a downstream effect on the skill mix of the pediatric workforce. With less exposure to neonatology and critical care during training, pediatricians are less skilled in the recognition of critical illness and in the initial stabilization and treatment of critically ill and injured children. These factors should be important in organizing health care networks for children's care so that strong support systems are available to pediatricians in primary care practice.

The availability of pediatric critical care specialists will be important to achieve the increasingly prominent role for this specialty. The Child Health Corporation of America has estimated that there will be a need for 27% more pediatric intensivists before 2006, a demand that is equaled by few other specialties in pediatrics.[19] These needs exist in all regions of the country but are most prominent in the north central and southern regions. A survey of member hospitals of the National Association of Children's Hospitals and Related Institutions (NACHRI)[20] revealed that 15.1% of positions in pediatric critical care were vacant.

Many factors have been cited to explain the shortage of critical care specialists, including a reduced interest in residents in specialty careers, compensation issues, and better opportunities in nonspecialty practice. Whether an increased demand for critical care specialists has aggravated this shortage is unclear.

A number of factors appear to contribute to the declining interest of residents in pediatric subspecialty training in general and critical care in particular.[21] Demographic characteristics of residents who tend to choose primary care rather than specialty training include female gender, underrepresented minorities, and U.S. medical school graduates (as opposed to graduates of international medical schools). Each of these groups represents an increasing fraction of residents in training. Those choosing specialty training are more likely to be men, have single marital status, have no children, and have lower total educational debt.

The recruitment of pediatric residents into specialty fellowships may be importantly determined by which medical students chose pediatrics in the first place. As exposure of pediatrics to medical students emphasizes primary care practice, those students who chose pediatrics as residents may already be predestined for careers in primary care. The individuals who would be attracted to specialty pediatrics, with its higher acuity, complexity of care, degree of specialization, and intimate interaction with research and teaching, may be choosing medicine or surgery rather than pediatrics.

Some observers have suggested that educational debt may be among the most prominent determinants of career choice after residency. Not uncommonly, residents accumulate $100,000 or more of educational debt that must be repaid immediately following residency. Compensation differentials between primary care and specialty pediatric practice usually are insufficient to justify the deferment of repayment on economic reasons alone.

The stress of critical care practice, however, may be just as important in determining the recruitment of trainees.[22] Critical care physicians demonstrate the endocrinologic signs of significant physiologic stress during their work hours. The majority of individuals did not perceive stress at the time cortisol levels were increased, and experience did not attenuate this response. However, stress probably is perceptible to trainees and may be especially important to trainees with current or anticipated responsibilities outside of work, such as a family. No data exist on the longevity of careers in pediatric critical care because of the relative newness of the specialty. However, anecdotal information suggests that pediatric intensivists may be leaving direct patient care sooner and in larger numbers than other pediatric subspecialists for administrative positions, careers outside medicine, or retirement.

Unless the organization and systems of care are examined in the context of creating attractive, enduring careers in the specialty, personnel shortages likely will remain a problem or may even worsen.

The interaction of critical care specialists and hospitalists may offer considerable promise for meeting some of the challenges in the changing hospital environment. Beginning with care for adult patients, physicians whose full-time responsibilities were the care of inpatients have been shown to lower length of stay, improve total hospital costs, and preserve or improve patient satisfaction.[23] Increasingly, pediatric units and children's hospitals have recruited physicians for this role. The interface between full-time hospitalists and intensivists is sometimes gray, but frequent situations exist where intensivists or hospitalists practice without the other. In some hospitals, intensivists function as hospitalists during their work time when they are not assigned to the intensive care unit.

Further integration of hospitalist and intensivist roles promises to further improve care along the spectrum of pediatric inpatient medicine. Critical care facilities are expensive to staff and maintain, so timely, appropriate discharge from the pediatric intensive care unit can save costs. Prompt recognition of medical deterioration and intervention can reduce complications and prevent morbidity.

REFERENCES

1. Chalom R, Raphealy RC, Costarino AT: Hospital costs of pediatric intensive care. *Crit Care Med* 27:2079-2085, 1999.
2. Calvin JE, Habet K, Parrillo JE: Critical care in the United States: who are we and how did we get here *Crit Care Clin* 13:363-376, 1997.
3. Fairman J, Kagan S: Creating critical care: the case of the hospital of the University of Pennsylvania, 1950-1965. *ANS Adv Nurs Sci* 22:63-77, 1999.
4. Pollack MM, Cuerdon TC, Getson PR: Pediatric intensive care units: results of a national survey. *Crit Care Med* 21:607-614, 1993.
5. Society of Critical Care Medicine: Guidelines and levels of care for pediatric intensive care units. *Crit Care Med* 21:1077-1086, 1993.
6. Society of Critical Care Medicine: Critical care services and personnel: recommendations based on a system of categorization into two levels of care. *Crit Care Med* 27:422-426, 1999.
7. Ohio Department of Health: Quality assurance: guidelines for pediatric intensive care units, 1996.
8. Pollack MM, Katz RW, Ruttiman UW, et al: Improving the outcome and efficiency of intensive care: the impact of an intensivist. *Crit Care Med* 16:11, 1988.
9. Pollack MM, Cuerdon TT, Patel KM, et al: Impact of quality of care factors on pediatric intensive care mortality. *JAMA* 272: 941-946, 1994.
10. Pollack MM, Patel KM, Ruttiman UE: Pediatric critical care training programs have a positive effect on pediatric intensive care mortality. *Crit Care Med* 25:1637-1642, 1997.
11. Hanson WC, Deutschman CS, Anderson HL, et al: Effects of an organized critical care service on outcomes and resource utilization: a cohort study. *Crit Care Med* 27:270-274, 1999.
12. Pronovost PJ, Jenckes MW, Dorman T, et al. Organizational characteristics of intensive care units related to outcomes of abdominal aortic surgery. *JAMA* 281:1310-1317, 1999.
13. Multz AS, Chalfin DB, Samson IM, et al. A "closed" medical intensive care unit (MICU) improves resource utilization when compared with an "open" MICU. *Am J Respir Crit Care Med* 157:1468-1473, 1998.

14. Ghorra S, Reinert SE, Cioffi W, et al: Analysis of the effect of conversion from open to closed surgical intensive care unit. *Ann Surg* 229:163-171, 1999.
15. Kollef MH, Shapiro SD, Silver P, et al. A randomized, controlled trial of protocol-directed versus physician-directed weaning from mechanical ventilation. *Crit Care Med* 25:567-574, 1997.
16. Montazeri M, Cook DJ: Impact of a clinical pharmacist in a multidisciplinary intensive care unit. *Crit Care Med* 22:1044-108, 1994.
17. Ibrahim KH, Gunderson B, Rotschafer JC: Intensive care unit antimicrobial resistance and the role of the pharmacist. *Crit Care Med* N108-N113, 2001.
18. Clemmer TP, Spuhler VJ, Oniki TA, et al: Results of a collaborative quality improvement program on outcomes and costs in a tertiary critical care unit. *Crit Care Med* 27:1768-1774, 1999.
19. Child Health Corporation of America: *Vital signs: meeting tomorrow's need for pediatric subspecialists.* Shawnee Mission, KS 2001, Child Health Corporation of America.
20. O'Leary K, Katz G, Hollander F: The shortage of pediatric subspecialists. *Children's Hospitals Today* Winter:p 21-23, 2002.
21. Pan RJ, Cull WL, Brotherton SE: Pediatric residents' career intentions: data from the leading edge of the pediatrician workforce. *Pediatrics* 109:182-188, 2002.
22. Fisher J, Calame A, Dettling AC, Zeier H, Fanconi S: Experience and endocrine stress in neonatal and pediatric nurses and physicians. *Crit Care Med* 28:3281-3288, 2000.
23. Wachter RE, Goldman L: The hospitalist movement 5 years later. *JAMA* 287:487-494, 2002.

CHAPTER

4

The Nurse in Pediatric Critical Care

Martha A.Q. Curley and Patricia A. Moloney-Harmon

PEARLS

- *Caring practices* are a constellation of nursing activities that are responsive to the uniqueness of the patient/family and create a compassionate and therapeutic environment with the aim of promoting comfort and preventing suffering.
- Nursing's unique contribution to patients within the health care environment, the one that encompasses all nursing's competencies, is that nurses create safe passage for patients and families.
- Nurses coordinate the patient's and family's experiences by their continuous attention to the person underneath all the high technology.
- Building a humanistic environment that endorses parents as unique individuals capable of providing essential elements of care to their children lays the foundation for family-centered care.
- Excellence in a pediatric critical care unit is achieved through a combination of many factors and is highly dependent on effective leadership.
- Studies have demonstrated that improving manager leadership behaviors is more likely than any other intervention to improve retention of hospital nurses.
- A successful critical care unit–based professional advancement program recognizes varying levels of staff nurse knowledge and expertise and fosters advancement through a wide range of clinical learning and professional development experiences.
- Technical training alone no longer is sufficient to meet the care delivery needs of the nurse in the critical care environment.

Pediatric critical care nursing has evolved tremendously over the past years. The nurse is the singular person in the pediatric critical care unit who creates an environment in which critically unstable, highly vulnerable infants and children benefit from attentive care and who coordinates the actions of a highly skilled team of patient-focused health care professionals. Pediatric critical care nursing practice encompasses the staff nurse providing direct patient care, nursing leadership facilitating an environment of excellence, and professional staff development that assures continued nursing competence and professional growth. This chapter provides the reader with a discussion of the essential components of pediatric critical care nursing practice.

Describing What Nurses Do: The Synergy Model

The *synergy model* describes nursing practice based on the needs and characteristics of patients and their families.[1] The fundamental premise of this model is that patient characteristics drive nurse competencies. When patient characteristics and nurse competencies match and synergize, optimal patient outcomes result. The major components of the synergy model encompass patient characteristics of concern to nurses, nurse competencies important to the patient, and patient outcomes that result when patient characteristics and nurse competencies are in synergy.

Patient Characteristics of Concern to Nurses

Every patient and family member brings unique characteristics to the pediatric intensive care experience. These characteristics—stability, complexity, predictability, resiliency, vulnerability, participation in decision making, participation in care, and resource availability—span the continuum of health and illness. Each is operationally defined as follows. *Stability* refers to the person's ability to maintain a steady state. *Complexity* is the intricate entanglement of two or more systems (e.g., physiologic, family, therapeutic). *Predictability* is a summative patient characteristic that allows the nurse to expect a certain trajectory of illness. *Resiliency* is the patient's capacity to return to a restorative level of functioning using compensatory and coping mechanisms. *Vulnerability* refers to an individual's susceptibility to actual or potential stressors that may adversely affect outcomes. *Participation in decision making and participation in care* are the extents to which the patient and family engage in decision making and in aspects of care, respectively. *Resource availability* refers to resources the patient/family/community bring to a care situation. Resources include personal, psychological, social, technical, and fiscal.

These eight continua apply to patients in all health care settings. This classification allows nursing to have a common language to describe patients that is meaningful to all care areas. For example, a critically ill infant in multisystem organ failure can be described as an individual who is (a) unstable, (b) highly complex, (c) unpredictable, (d) highly resilient, (e) vulnerable, (f) whose family is able to become involved in decision making and care, but (g) has inadequate resource availability.

Individuals fluctuate at different points along these eight continua. For example, in the case of the critically ill infant in multisystem organ failure, stability can range from a high to low, complexity from atypical to typical, predictability from uncertain to certain, resiliency from minimal to strong reserves, vulnerability from susceptible to safe, family participation in decision making and care from no to full capacity, and resource availability from minimal to extensive. When compared to existing patient classification systems, these eight dimensions better describe the needs of patients of concern to nurses.

Nurse Competencies Important to Patients and Families

Nursing competencies, derived from the needs of patients, also are described in terms of essential continua: clinical judgment, advocacy/moral agency, caring practices, facilitation of learning, collaboration, systems thinking, response to diversity, and clinical inquiry. *Clinical judgment* is clinical reasoning that includes clinical decision making, critical thinking, and a global grasp of the situation coupled with nursing skills acquired through a process of integrating formal and experiential knowledge. *Clinical inquiry* is the ongoing process of questioning and evaluating practice, providing informed practice on the basis of available data, and innovating through research and experiential leaning. The nurse engages in clinical knowledge development to promote the best patient outcomes. *Caring practices* are a constellation of nursing activities that are responsive to the uniqueness of the patient/family and create a compassionate and therapeutic environment with the aim of promoting comfort and preventing suffering. Caring behaviors include, but are not limited to, vigilance, engagement, and responsiveness. *Response to diversity* is the sensitivity to recognize, appreciate, and incorporate differences into the provision of care. Differences may include, but are not limited to, individuality, cultural practices, spiritual beliefs, gender, race, ethnicity, disability, family configuration, lifestyle, socioeconomic status, age, values, and alternative care practices involving patients/families and members of the health care team. *Advocacy/moral agency* is defined as working on another's behalf and representing the concerns of the patient/family/community. The nurse serves as a moral agent when assuming a leadership role in identifying and helping to resolve ethical and clinical concerns within the clinical setting. *Facilitation of learning* is the ability to use the self to facilitate patient learning. *Collaboration* is working with others (patients, families, health care providers) in a way that promotes/encourages each person's contributions toward achieving optimal/realistic patient goals. Collaboration involves intradisciplinary and interdisciplinary work with colleagues. *Systems thinking* is appreciating the care environment from a perspective that recognizes the holistic interrelationships that exist within and across health care systems.

These competencies illustrate a dynamic integration of knowledge, skills, experience, and attitudes needed to meet patients' needs and optimize patient outcomes. Nurses become competent within each continuum at a level that best meets the fluctuating needs of their patient population. Logically, more compromised patients have more severe or complex needs; this in turn requires the nurse to possess a higher level of knowledge and skill in an associated continuum. For example, if a patient is stable but unpredictable, minimally resilient, and vulnerable, primary competencies of the nurse center on clinical judgment and caring practices (which include vigilance). If a patient is vulnerable, unable to participate in decision making and care, and has inadequate resource availability, the primary competencies of the nurse focus on advocacy/moral agency, collaboration, and systems thinking. Although all the eight competencies are essential for contemporary nursing practice, each assumes more or less importance depending on a patient's characteristics. Synergy results when there is a match between patient needs/characteristics and nurse competencies.

Clinical Judgment

Clinical judgment, that is, skilled clinical knowledge, use of discretionary judgment, and the ability to integrate complex multisystem data and understand the expected trajectory of illness and human response to critical illness, defines competent nursing practice. In critical care, the novice nurse focuses on individual aspects of the patient and the environment. As expertise develops, the nurse develops a global understanding of the situation. The expert nurse anticipates the needs of patients, predicts the patient's trajectory of illness, and forecasts the patient's level of recovery. Evolving clinical expertise creates *safe passage* for patients. The very best nursing care often is invisible, as it should be, because untoward effects and complications are prevented. Nursing's unique contribution to patients within the health care environment, the one that encompasses all nursing's competencies, is that nurses create safe passage for patients and families. Safe passage may include helping the patient and family move toward a greater level of self-awareness, knowledge, or health; transition through the acute care environment or stressful events; and/or a peaceful death.

Clinical Inquiry

Clinical inquiry optimizes the potential that patients will receive evidenced-based care. Studying the clinical effectiveness of care and how it affects patient outcomes provides information that will help balance cost and quality. Quality improvement methods include multidisciplinary teams working together to help systems operate in the best interests of patient care.[2] Collaborative practice groups working with clinical practice guidelines (CPGs) provide the opportunity to provide evidence-based interventions.

CPGs—patient-centered multidisciplinary multidimensional plans of care—help the team provide evidence-based practice and improve the process of care delivery. CPGs assure practitioner accountability, encourage coordinated care, decrease unnecessary variation in practice patterns, improve quality and cost-effective services, and provide a means to systematically evaluate the quality and effectiveness of practice in moving patients toward desired outcomes. Effective CPGs are driven by patient needs and help provide evidence linking interventions to patient outcomes. CPGs help guide the appropriate use of resources limiting interventions. Interventions that do not benefit patients probably are not worth implementing.

Caring Practices

Caring practices bring clinical judgment to view. Caring practices are activities that are meaningful to the patient and family and help them *feel well cared for.*[3] Families equate caring behaviors with competent behaviors. Families trust that nurses will be vigilant. Vigilance, which includes alert and constant watchfulness, attentiveness, and reassuring presence, is essential to limit the complications associated with a patient's vulnerabilities.[1]

Nurses coordinate the patient's and family's experiences by their continuous attention to the person underneath all the high technology. The unique significance of what nurses do is in making a difference for patients, helping so that patients and their families can better tolerate the experience of critical illness. This aspect of practice, our *presence* with patients, is unique to the profession of nursing.[1] For example, in working with patients with head injuries, caring nurses acknowledge the person by surrounding them with their possessions—family pictures, cards from friends, and their music. They talk with their unresponsive patients, orienting them and telling them what is going on, which preserves the patient's "humanness." Occasionally a response is received from the patient by increasing heart rate or blood pressure or dropping intracranial pressure, sometimes by just shedding a tear. Nurses take this level of communication one step further by teaching this process to family members so that they also can interact with their critically ill loved one.

Pediatric critical care nurses, more than any other intensive care unit (ICU) nursing subspecialty, have made significant progress in integrating family-centered care into the practice of critical care. Building a humanistic environment that endorses parents as unique individuals capable of providing essential elements of care to their children lays the foundation for family-centered care. Family-centered care is more than just unlimited parent access to their children.[4,5]

Nursing research provides the foundation for this change in practice. Based on nursing research, we know that parents have the need for hope, information, and proximity; to believe that their loved one is receiving the best care possible; to be helpful; to be recognized as important; and to talk with other parents with similar issues. Pediatric critical care nurses have gone beyond the identification of family needs to illustrating interventions patients and families find helpful.[4–6] We provide families with what they need to help their child. Parents feel the most important contribution pediatric critical care nurses make is serving as the "interpreter" of their critically ill child's responses and of the pediatric ICU environment.[4]

Response to Diversity

Response to diversity honors the differences that exist in the people we are and in the individuals we care for. At a minimum, it requires that care be delivered in a nonjudgmental, nondiscriminatory manner. Effective communication with patients and families at their level of understanding may require customizing the health care culture to meet the diverse needs and strengths of families. Nurses foresee differences and beliefs within the team and negotiate consensus in the best interest of the patient and family.

Advocacy/Moral Agency

Moral agency acknowledges the particular trust inherent within nurse–patient relationships, a trust gained from nursing's long history of speaking on the patient's behalf in an effort to preserve a patient's "lifeworld" (Hooper, Personal Communication, 1996). The holistic view of the patient that nurses often possess is a reflection of moral awareness.

When cure is no longer possible, nurses turn their focus to secure death with dignity and comfort. Nurses "orchestrate" death, supporting parents and family members through the worst experience in the world, the death of a loved one. Nurses often coordinate the experience for patients and families when death is imminent. This most intimate aspect of care is nursing's most profound contribution to mankind.[7]

Facilitator of Learning

Nurses facilitate learning so that patients and their families become knowledgeable about the health care system and can make informed choices. Teaching is an almost continuous process—helping the patient and the family to understand the critical care environment and therapies contained within it. Also essential is reinforcement of the patient's experience and how, most likely, the infant or child will cope with the ICU experience. This education provides patients with the capacity to help themselves and their infants and children.

Collaboration

Collaboration requires commitment by the entire multidisciplinary team. Knaus et al.[8] found an inverse relationship between actual and predicted patient mortality and the degree of interaction and coordination of multidisciplinary intensive care teams. Hospitals with good collaboration and a lower mortality had a comprehensive nursing educational support program that included a clinical nurse specialist and clinical protocols in which staff nurses were independently responsible. The American Association of Critical-Care Nurses (AACN) Demonstration Project also documented a low mortality ratio, low complication rate, and high patient satisfaction in a unit that had a high perceived level of nurse–physician collaboration, highly rated objective nursing performance, positive organizational climate, and job satisfaction and morale.[9]

Systems Thinking

Today, nurses design, implement, and evaluate whole programs of care, manage units in which care is provided, monitor whether the health care system as a whole is meeting patient needs, and play a role in ethical decision making around caregiving.[10] These vital components require a patient-centered culture that stresses strong leadership, coordination of activities, continuous multidisciplinary communication, open collaborative problem solving, and conflict management.[11] Nurses have learned to manipulate the system to work for the patients; however, systems thinking,[12] the ability to understand the interrelationships and patterns involved in complex problem solving, is a new but necessary skill in taking overall responsibility for the environment in which caregiving occurs.

Managing complex systems is essential to creating a safe environment. Schumacher and Meleis[13] gave evidence supporting "transitions" as a principal concept in nursing. Nurse–patient relationships commonly occur around transitional periods of instability brought about by the demands of the health care situation. Helping with transitions health care system boundaries, for example, into and out of the community, requires systems knowledge and intradisciplinary collaboration.

Optimal Patient Outcomes

According to the synergy model, optimal patient outcomes result when patient characteristics and nurse competencies synergize. Many patient outcome measures are appropriate to study, including physiologic, psychological, functional, behavioral, symptom control, quality of life, family strain, goal attainment, utilization of services, safety, problem resolution, and patient satisfaction.[14] *"Nurse-sensitive" outcome,* a term first coined by Johnson and McCloskey,[15] defines a dynamic patient or family caregiver state, condition, or perception that is responsive to nursing interventions. Brooten and Naylor[16] note: "The current search for 'nurse-sensitive patient outcomes' should be tempered in the reality that nurses do not care for patients in isolation and patients do not exist in isolation" (p. 98). Outcomes have been described at three levels: patient, provider, and system.

Patient Level Outcomes

Major patient level outcomes of concern to pediatric critical care nurses include physiologic changes and the presence or absence of complications. Outcomes related to limiting iatrogenic injury and complications to therapy demonstrate the potential hazards present in illness and in the critical care environment. Patient/family satisfaction and ratings are subjective measures of health and/or quality of health services. Patient satisfaction measures involving nursing typically include technical/professional factors, trusting relationships, and education experiences.[17] Patient-perceived functional change and quality of life are multidisciplinary outcome measures. Linking patient satisfaction, functional status, and quality of life is important because the three factors often are related.

Provider Level Outcomes

Provider level outcomes include the extent to which care/treatment objectives are attained within the predicted time period. Nurses coordinate the day-to-day efforts of the entire multidisciplinary team. The nurse's role as the coordinator of numerous services is essential for optimal patient outcomes and shorter lengths of stay. As discussed, nurse–physician collaboration and positive interaction is associated with lower mortality rates, high patient satisfaction with care, and low nosocomial complications.[8,9]

System Level Outcomes

Critical care units must manage resources *and* maintain quality collaboratively defined by both users and providers in the system. The goal is high-quality care at moderate cost for the greatest number of people. Important patient-system outcome data include recidivism and costs/resource utilization. Recidivism, that is, *re*hospitalization and *re*admission, is rework that adds to the personal and financial burden of providing care. In addition to patient and system factors, nurses can decrease the patient's length of stay through coordination of care, prevention of complications, timely discharge planning, and appropriate referral to community resources. Reducing length of stay and tracking ED visits and rehospitalization assure that cost shifting is not occurring.

Leadership

Excellence in a pediatric critical care unit is achieved through a combination of many factors and is highly dependent on effective leadership.[18] Numerous studies have demonstrated the importance of leadership in creating an environment where both nurses and patients can flourish. Effective leaders help diverse groups work together in harmony.[19]

Current Challenges

The 1990s presented an era of health care reengineering to survive managed care. Organizations were forced to merge and/or reorganize and reengineer to restrain cost in the face of declining reimbursement. In addition, the management structure flattened such that multiple nursing units were managed by one individual. At the same time, management support was reduced and the number of unlicensed assistive personnel was increased while the number of bedside registered nurses (RNs) was decreased through attrition and layoffs.

These significant cuts produced serious questions about quality of care in hospitals. A New York State Nurses Association study found that 52% of the nurses responding stated that patient care was either barely safe or not safe at all. States are attempting to or have passed legislation creating mandatory nursing staff ratios. Many nurses are looking to unions for protection from unsafe working conditions. Overall, stress levels for nurses are high and morale low. One study ranked posttraumatic stress disorder (PTSD) symptomatology across disciplines and found ICU nurses had the highest rate of all groups studied, ahead of Israeli soldiers and Vietnam veterans with PTSD.[20]

A major nursing shortage challenges health care. Vacancies are especially evident in areas that are highly specialized, such as pediatric critical care. The average age of a nurse today is 44 years, and large numbers of RNs will be leaving the profession in the coming years. Compounding this trend, enrollment in nursing schools has decreased, which further jeopardizes the supply of nurses for the future. Couple these facts with the Bureau of Labors projection that more nurses will be needed in the future and the nursing situation looks very challenging. The nursing shortage is geometrically magnified by the ever-increasing ratio of inexperienced to experienced nurses, the number of float and agency nurses, and inadequate support services.

Studies have demonstrated that improving manager leadership behaviors is more likely than any other intervention to improve retention of hospital nurses.[21] In 1994, Shortell et al.[22] studied 42 ICUs to determine whether there was a relationship between performance and managerial and organizational practices. Their study demonstrated that at the unit level, culture, leadership, coordination, communication, and conflict management are significantly associated with lower risk-adjusted length of stay and RN turnover. In 1999, Boyle et al.[21] studied 255 ICU staff nurses working in four urban hospitals. They examined the direct and indirect effects of nurse managers' characteristics of power, influence, and leadership style on critical care nurses' intent to stay within the organization. In many studies, intent to stay had the strongest direct relationship to retention. The study concluded that the nurse manager is the key to understanding why nurses want to stay or leave. The leadership characteristics of nurse managers affect the work environment of critical care nurses, and the environment in turn affects job stress, job satisfaction, and staff members' intent to stay in the unit or hospital.

Effective Leadership

Warren Bennis,[23] a leading expert on leadership, believes we cannot function without leaders. He states that leaders are important for three basic reasons. Leaders are responsible for the overall effectiveness of an organization. The success or failure of all organizations, whether hospitals, football teams, or large corporations such as Microsoft, rests with the perceived quality at the top. Even stock market prices rise and fall according to the public perception of how good the leader is. Leaders give direction through vision and strategic planning. Bennis states that leaders are needed because the change and upheaval of the past has left us with a need for anchors in our lives. Leaders fill that need. Leaders are needed because there is a pervasive, national concern about the integrity of our institutions. Leaders are needed who will act with integrity because how others view a leader or an organizations' integrity will determine the level of trust placed in you or your hospital.

Leadership incorporates core characteristics, which include vision, competence, trust, and constancy. These core characteristics should be integrated into the leader's daily work.

Vision

The first core characteristic is developing a vision for the team. A *vision* is a realistic, credible, attractive future for the organization. It attracts people toward it. Leaders facilitate the process of implementing a shared vision. Effective leaders have the ability to clearly articulate a picture of the future. The picture they present and the values they project are so powerful and meaningful that they bring strong commitment by others.[18]

Competence

The second core characteristic required for leadership is competence. *Competence* refers to having the necessary skills and expertise to lead an organization. Because managers and leaders may not have the same high level of clinical expertise as their staff, they must possess sufficient knowledge to address organizational needs. Competence around leadership skills, such as building relationships, the ability to make decisions, role modeling, team building, mentoring, and accountability, is required to meet those needs.

Relationship building and team building skills are essential to meeting the health care challenges of the future. Teams can develop more creative solutions, make decisions, and take action that will yield more powerful outcomes for the organization. Creating and leading successful teams requires skill and finesse on the part of the leader. Building an environment conducive to maximum team functioning is not a one-time event; rather, it is an ongoing effort and process on the part of both the leader and the team.

High-performance teams are critical to an effective workplace. Certain characteristics make these groups unique. These characteristics include participative leadership that empowers members, a shared commitment for outcomes, clearly defined group goals, effective communication demonstrating mutual trust and respect, a focus on the task to be done and on the future, a celebration of creative thinking, and a tendency for expeditious responses.[18]

Effective leaders promote teamwork by supporting collaboration among all members. These leaders recognize the important contribution that each team member makes to a successful outcome. It is not the skill of one superstar but the level of collaboration among the entire team that promotes success.[18] In addition to relationship and team building, the leader functions as a role model and a mentor to staff. Role modeling and mentoring encourage empowerment, collaboration, and shared accountability for outcomes.

Kerfoot[19] discusses how a leader can use the synergy model as a basis for professional practice. A leader has to work through others to accomplish goals; however, the leader is only as good as the people providing the care. A leader must create the environment in which good people provide optimal care.

Trust

The third core characteristic required leadership is *trust*. Without trust, the leader's vision becomes just words on a document, relationships never reach their potential, and decisions are made without critical information and staff input. Staff must trust their leader, but the leader also must trust his/her staff. If trust is mutual, then trust will lead to team growth, even if mistakes are made.

The foundation of trust is integrity. *Integrity* involves the inherent knowledge of right and wrong and the willingness to stand up for what is right. Integrity includes trusting staff, showing fairness and candor in discussions, and displaying consistency between words and actions. Following through on commitments is an essential component of building integrity and trust.

Constancy

The fourth core characteristic of leadership is *constancy*. In our current health care environment, it is vital that leaders steer a clear and consistent course. Leaders acknowledge uncertainties and deal effectively with the present, while simultaneously anticipating and responding to the future. The leader endlessly expresses, explains, extends, expands, and when necessary revises the units' goals. Because the leader is constantly communicating, seeking feedback, and walking the talk, staff are not waiting for the "other shoe to drop." They know where they are going, and there are no surprises.

Constancy involves putting first things first. Covey[24] states that putting first things first means organizing and executing around priorities and purpose. Leaders focus on what matters most.

Effective leaders create an environment where nurses and patients live beautifully together as part of the organizational structure. By living the core characteristics, effective leaders help to eliminate the chaos often found in patient care and paint a compelling picture of a place where nurses can make their optimal contribution to patients and families.[19]

Professional Development

A critical aspect of development for the nurse is the ability to advance and be recognized professionally. Each pediatric critical care unit should provide a means to meet this professional need. A successful critical care unit–based professional advancement program recognizes varying levels of staff nurse knowledge and expertise and fosters advancement through a wide range of clinical learning and professional development experiences. Essential components of this program include an orientation program, a continuing education plan, inservice education, and an array of other opportunities for clinical and professional development. Unit-based advancement programs are most effective when they are linked to the nursing department's professional advancement program.

A professional advancement program for the recognition and reward of evolving expertise contains elements of both clinical and professional development strategies. The synergy model's ability to describe a patient–nurse relationship that optimizes patient and family outcomes illuminates the various dimensions of critical care nursing practice that require attention from a development perspective.[1,25] The impact of these contributions can be measured based on the nurse's level of expertise, and professional development strategies can be focused to impact patient care.

By combining the nurse competencies identified in the synergy model and the behaviors identified in Benner's levels of practice,[26] a continuum of expertise can be described that matches behavior with practice levels. It focuses recognition and reward on clinical practice. The impact of expert nurses on patient outcomes is presented in quantitative and financial parameters that can be understood throughout the health care system. The model links clinical competencies to patient outcomes.

Nurses require a broad body of knowledge to meet patient and organizational needs. This requirement necessitates a lifelong process of professional development targeted to specific levels of clinical practice. Nurses can choose from many learning options, such as academic education, continuing education, participation in research, collaborative learning, case studies, and simulations. Nurses view the presence of continuing education, both as learning in the unit and inservice education, as very important.[27]

Staff Development

The goal of nursing staff development programs is safe, competent practice. Comprehensive programs provide the critical resources to support and promote practice. In addition, professional nursing standards of practice, health care laws, regulations, and accreditation requirements focus on the components of competent patient care to protect the health care consumer. The establishment of a staff development program that is linked to clinical practice is key to the success of professional nurse development.

Critical care staff development programs can be designed to educate staff nurses within the competencies of the synergy model.[1] The program builds on the nurse's prior education and professional nursing experience, which facilitates attainment and maintenance of competence. Concepts intrinsic to the educational process and to critical care nursing are used as a framework around which professional development opportunities are organized. Once defined based upon a unit's patient population, the organizing framework serves as the structure within which all critical care nursing staff development programs are designed.

Technical training alone is no longer sufficient to meet the care delivery needs of the nurse in the critical care environment. Critical care nurses require broad knowledge and proficiency in areas such as communication, critical thinking, and collaboration.[2] They need to attain the diverse skills necessary to meet the complex needs of their patients and families.

The theory and science required to meet the synergy competencies includes topics such as disease processes, nursing procedures, cultural differences, moral and ethical principles and reasoning, research principles, and educational learning theories. This information can be presented in a variety of methods, including lecture, written information, poster, self–studies, or computer-based technology. However, it is essential that the information is related to realistic clinical situations. Clinical scenarios, case studies, and simulations that represent the dynamic and ambiguous clinical situations nurses encounter daily are most effective.[28]

Bedside teaching is particularly helpful in the development of clinical judgment and caring practice skills. Expert nurses are role models for many of the competencies delineated by the synergy model. Novice nurses learn by watching these expert nurses and emulating behaviors. Clinical teaching also enables the novice practitioner to gain experience with unfamiliar interventions in a safe and protected environment. Communicating and validating clinical knowledge focuses learning, positively affects patient outcomes, and adds to the total body of nursing knowledge.[28]

Information about research and research utilization builds clinical inquiry and system thinking skills. Demystifying research, outcome, and quality processes contributes to the development of these key skills. Use of journal club formats and supporting staff involvement in research develop clinical inquiry skills. Building knowledge in the areas of health care trends and political action expand system thinking skills. Development of critical thinking skills and problem solving skills also assists with development of system thinking.

Nurses acquire facilitation of learning skills by incorporating communication development into their professional development plan. Presenting clinical teaching strategies and assisting staff to determine learner readiness and assess understanding are included in the development of facilitation of learning. The importance of developing patience, flexibility, and a nonconfrontational style is reinforced.

Negotiation, conflict resolution, time management, communication, and team building are components of collaboration skills. Role playing, role modeling, and clinical narratives are methodologies that have been used to develop collaboration skills.

Nurses learn technical skills and scientific knowledge in many ways, but caring practices and advocacy are developed only through relationships that evolve over time.[29] Nurturing professional relationships with experienced staff promote the novice's integration into practice.[30] Expert nurses who share their clinical knowledge and coach other nurses have a tremendous impact on novice nurses.[16] Nurses who coach are in their roles because they are able to clinically persuade and guide situations. They demonstrate expert skills and expedite the ongoing clinical development of others.

A variety of staff development programs exist, but most fall into three general categories: orientation, inservice education, and continuing education programs.

Orientation

Orientation programs help acclimate new staff to unit-based policies, procedures, services, physical facilities, and role expectations in a work setting.[31] A specific type of orientation program that has developed in response to the nursing shortage is the critical care internship program. These types of programs have been developed as a mechanism to recruit and train entry-level nurses. These programs are designed to integrate nurses with little or no nursing experience into the complex critical care environment. They provide extended clinical support for novice nurses and introduce new knowledge more deliberately than traditional orientation programs. Basic information and skill acquisition are the core features of these programs. This foundation builds on the knowledge and skills that these nurses previously acquired in their nursing school programs. Teaching usually is under the direction of a hospital educator and usually involves the less senior staff as preceptors. Typically, the novice nurse starts with providing care to the least complex patients. The program establishes a foundation on which the novice can develop into a competent clinician.[28]

Inservice Education

Inservice education programs are the most frequent type of staff development activity, which involves learning experiences provided in the workplace to assist staff in the performance of assigned functions and maintenance of competency.[32] These programs usually are informal and narrow in scope. They often are spontaneous sessions resulting from new situations on the unit in settings such as patient rounds or staff meetings. Examples of planned inservices are demonstrations of new equipment, procedure reviews, and patient care conferences.

TABLE 4–1

Percentage of Time Caring for Patients with Alterations in Body Systems

System Dysfunction	Pediatric Practice	Neonatal Practice	Adult Practice
Pulmonary	28%	39%	22%
Cardiovascular	24%	15%	39%
Neurologic	15%	6%	8%
Multisystem	12%	22%	10%
Hematology/immunology	7%	5%	4%
Renal	5%	3%	5%
Gastrointestinal	5%	7%	8%
Endocrine	4%	3%	4%

Data from *Role delineation study.* Laguna Niguel, CA, 1990, Certification Corporation, American Association of Critical-Care Nurses.

Continuing Education

Legislation, regulations, professional standards, and expectations of health care consumers help determine the need for continuing education. Continuing nursing education includes planned, organized learning experiences designed to expand knowledge and skills beyond the level of basic education.[33] The focus is on knowledge and skills that are not specific to one institution and build upon previously acquired knowledge and skills. Examples of continuing education programs include formal conferences, seminars, workshops, and courses.

Certification in Pediatric Critical Care Nursing

In 1975 the AACN Certification Corporation was established to formally recognize the professional competence of critical care nurses. The mission of the AACN Certification Corporation is to certify and promote critical care nursing practice that optimally contributes to desired patient outcomes. The program establishes the body of knowledge necessary for CCRN certification, tests the common body of knowledge needed to function effectively within the critical care setting, recognizes professional competence by granting CCRN status to successful certification candidates, and assists and promotes the continual professional development of critical care nurses.

Before 1992, content and construct validity of the CCRN examination were established for critical care nurses who primarily care for adult patients. Pediatric critical care nurses who sat for the CCRN examination were tested on content that did not reflect their practice. In 1989 AACN Certification Corporation conducted a new role delineation study. Major differences among neonatal, pediatric, and adult critical care nursing practice were identified in the types of patient care problems for which direct bedside care is provided and in the amount of time spent caring for patients with specific problems (Table 4–1). The results, for the first time, described the practice of pediatric critical care nursing and justified the need for separate pediatric, neonatal, and adult CCRN examinations.

TABLE 4–2

Pediatric CCNS Examination Blueprint

Dimension	Percentage of Examination Questions
Clinical judgment	25%
Facilitator of learning	18%
Collaboration	14%
Clinical inquiry	13%
Caring practices	10%
Systems thinking	8%
Advocacy/agency	7%
Response to diversity	5%

Data from *CCNS exam blueprint.* Aliso Viejo, CA, 2000, Certification Corporation, American Association of Critical-Care Nurses.

In 1997 the unique competencies of pediatric, neonatal, and adult critical care nurses were rearticulated using the synergy model[1] as a conceptual framework. Again, differences across the lifespan were described, and three separate CCRN programs still exist (Table 4–2). To date more than 1200 pediatric critical care nurses hold CCRN–Pediatric certification.

Summary

Pediatric critical care nursing has evolved into a specialty in its own right. Pediatric critical care nurses make significant and unique contributions to the health care of children. A pediatric critical care nurse requires knowledge and skills in both the art and science of nursing. A supportive, empowered environment and support for professional advancement are essential to the development of knowledge and skills.

REFERENCES

1. Curley MAQ: Patient-nurse synergy: optimizing patients' outcomes. *Am J Crit Care* 7:64-72, 1998.
2. Dickerson P: A CQI approach to evaluating continuing education. *J Nurses Staff Dev* 16:34-40, 2000.

3. Brown L: The experience of care: patient perspectives. *Topics Clin Nurs* 8:56-62, 1986.
4. Curley MAQ: Effects of the nursing mutual participation model of care and parental stress in the pediatric intensive care unit. Unpublished master's thesis. New Haven, CT, 1987, Yale University School of Nursing.
5. Curley MAQ: Effects of the nursing mutual participation model of care and parental stress in the pediatric intensive care unit. *Heart Lung* 17:682-688, 1988.
6. Curley MAQ, Wallace J: Effects of the nursing mutual participation model of care on parental stress in the pediatric intensive care unit—a replication. *J Pediatr Nurs* 7:377-385, 1992.
7. Curley MAQ: The essence of pediatric critical care nursing. In Curley MAQ, Moloney-Harmon PA, editors: *Critical care nursing of infants and children.* Philadelphia, 2001, WB Saunders.
8. Knaus WA, Draper EA, Wagner DP, Zimmermann JE: An evaluation of the outcome from intensive care in major medical centers. *Ann Intern Med* 104:410-418, 1985.
9. Mitchell PH, Armstrong S, Simpson TF, Lentz M: American Association of Critical-Care Nurses Demonstration Project: profile of excellence in critical care nursing. *Heart Lung* 18:219-237, 1989.
10. McBride AB: How nursing looks today. *Indiana Univ Alumni Magazine* Jan-Feb:64, 1994.
11. Zimmerman JE, Shortell SM, Rousseau DM, Duffy J, Gillies RR, Knaus WA, Devers K, Wagner DP, Draper EA: Improving intensive care: observations based on organizational case studies in nine intensive care units: a prospective, multicenter study. *Crit Care Med* 21:1443-1451, 1993.
12. Senge PM: *The fifth discipline: the art and practice of the learning organization.* New York, 1990, Doubleday.
13. Schumacher KL, Meleis AI: Transitions: a central concept in nursing. *Image* 26:119-127, 1994.
14. Lang NM, Marek KD: Outcomes that reflect clinical practice. In: *National Institutes of Health. Patient outcomes research: examining the effectiveness of nursing practice.* Department of Health and Human Services, NIH Publication No. 93-3411, 27-38, 1992.
15. Johnson M, McCloskey JC: Quality in the nineties. In: *Series on nursing administration: volume III. Delivery of quality health care.* St. Louis, 1992, Mosby Year Book.
16. Brooten D, Naylor MD: Nurses' effect on changing patient outcomes. *Image* 7:95-99, 1995.
17. Hinshaw AS, Atwood JR: A patient satisfaction instrument: precision by replication. *Nurs Res* 31:170-175, 1982.
18. Fagan MJ: Leadership in pediatric critical care. In Curley MAQ, Moloney-Harmon PA, editors: *Critical care nursing of infants and children.* Philadelphia, 2001, WB Saunders.
19. Kerfoot K: The leader as synergist. *Crit Care Nurse* 22:126-127, 2002.
20. Allen JJ: *Intensive care nurses: post traumatic stress disorder-like symptomatology.* Dissertation. Loma Linda, 1999, Loma Linda University.
21. Boyle DK, Bott MJ, Hansen HE, Woods CC, Taunton RL: Managers' leadership and critical care nurses intent to stay. *Am J Crit Care* 8:361-371, 1999.
22. Shortell SM, Zimmerman JE, Rousseau DM, Gillies RR, Wagner DP, Draper EA, Knaus WA, Duffy J: The performance of intensive care units: does good management make a difference? *Med Care* 32:508-525, 1994.
23. Bennis W: *On becoming a leader.* Reading, MA, 1989, Addison-Wesley Publishing.
24. Covey SR: *Living the 7 habits.* New York, 1999, Simon and Schuster.
25. Villaire M: The synergy model of certified practice: creating safe passage for patients. *Crit Care Nurse* 16:95-99, 1996.
26. Benner P, Tanner C, Cheslea C: *Expertise in nursing practice: caring, clinical judgment, and ethics.* New York, 1996, Springer Publishing.
27. Darvis JA, Hawkins LG: What makes a good intensive care unit: a nursing perspective. *Aust Crit Care* 15:77-82, 2002.
28. Czerwinski SJ, Martin ED: Facilitation of learning. In Curley MAQ, Moloney-Harmon PA, editors: *Critical care nursing of infants and children.* Philadelphia: 2001, WB Saunders.
29. Chamberlain S, Stengrevics S, Alpert H: Mentorship: A relationship for professional development. In Clifford J, Horvath K, editors: *Advancing professional nursing practice.* New York, 1990, Springer Publishing.
30. Trossman S: Mentoring leads to meaningful relationships, professional growth. *Am Nurse* at *http://www.ana.org/tan/98marapr/feature3.htm.* Accessed 1998.
31. American Nurses Association: *Guidelines for staff development.* Kansas City, 1978, American Nurses Association.
32. American Nurses Association: *Standards for nursing staff development.* Kansas City, 1990, American Nurses Association.
33. American Nurses Association: *Standards for nursing professional development: continuing education and staff development.* Washington DC, 1994, American Nurses Association.

CHAPTER 5

Research in Pediatric Critical Care

Carol E. Nicholson and Randall C. Wetzel

PEARLS

- Research is the right thing to do for critically ill children, their families, and our profession. Whether or not it is supported at your institution does not alter this fact, nor does it relieve you of your scholarly responsibilities as a physician.
- Make inquiry, comparison, and analysis a permanent part of your critical care practice. Keep a follow-up card as a lifelong habit in the practice of medicine. Go to postmortems, and keep looking through the microscope.
- Before you accept dogmatic teaching from anyone, make a habit of analyzing its basis. Keep a "reading" section on your follow up card.
- Rest, don't quit, rest, don't quit!

"A fool is a man who never tried an experiment in his life."

Erasmus Darwin, 1792

Among the factors that define a medical specialty is the recognition of a clearly defined body of knowledge that is intrinsic and unique to that specialty. This body of knowledge is determined by the disease processes that the specialists treat, comprehensive knowledge about the disease processes, and, most importantly, the academic and intellectual constructs that allow the advancement of medical knowledge not only narrowly in the specialty but also in general. Endeavors directed at increasing the specialty's knowledge base are the research interests of that specialty. Thus a recognized medical specialty has a clearly defined patient population, clearly defined disease processes, and clearly defined areas of research interest. Medical specialties frequently have associated societies, professional organizations, and national institutes, all of which facilitate funding, sharing of important research information, and advancing the cutting edge of knowledge in the specialty.

Because organ system classification of specialties is fairly obvious, it is a most common base of specialization. The specialists who treat diseases of the lungs are familiar with the wide spectrum of pulmonary diseases, their pathogenesis, and treatment. There exists a large body of research-derived knowledge and a great deal of ongoing related research activity. This activity is presented at national meetings, such as the annual American Thoracic Society meeting. There is a network of extensive funding sources available to this specialty, such as the American Lung Association; the American Heart Association; and the National Heart, Lung, and Blood Institute (NHLBI). Taken together, these diseases form the clearly defined specialty of pulmonary medicine. Not all specialties are organ specific; for example, infectious disease and immunology are specialties that are concerned with diseases that affect the entire patient. These specialties have managed to clearly define a body of knowledge that is both intrinsic and unique, as well as crucial, to the specialty.

How does critical care medicine compare with this standard? Is attaining this standard desirable for pediatric critical care medicine? Have we succeeded in defining disease processes, patient populations, and research efforts that are unique to critical care medicine? What are these areas? Is it necessary for intensivists to "sub-sub-specialize" in some area other than critical care medicine for their academic and research involvement, as has frequently been the practice in critical care over its first decades? Commonly, physicians whose clinical practice is critical care are involved in research integrated into multiple other specialty areas. To define critical care medicine as a medical specialty able to stand on its own, not only must we define our clinical practice and the pathophysiology of the unique disease entities we manage, we also must make a unique contribution to understanding and treating the pathophysiologic conditions that affect the children we treat. Unless we define a body of research that is unique to critical care medicine, the certainty of the specialty's future will continue to be in question. With this thought in mind, this chapter focuses on the research aspects of our practice and opportunities that may develop into unique research areas for intensivists. A further goal is to provide some insight into scientific process and the rationale behind it.

Research Areas

There are clearly pathophysiologic processes that appear to be unique to critical care medicine. Probably the most clearcut of these processes is acute respiratory distress syndrome (ARDS)[52,62] (see Chapter 40), although this is only one manifestation of a systemic process. The syndrome appears to develop in critically ill patients whose initial injury arises from a wide variety of organ-specific insults. Although the lungs appear to be the primary target organ, all organs are affected by the same, complex underlying pathophysiologic process. This process causes widespread endothelial injury involving many organ systems.[21] This results in tissue edema, decreased organ perfusion, ischemia, and multiple organ failure (see Chapter 97). This pansystemic disease is familiar to the intensivist and is one of the most extensive areas of unique research interest in critical care today. Understanding this systemic inflammatory response is central to understanding critical care.

Another major area that clearly provides a clinical scenario with which critical care physicians are intimately familiar is shock (see Chapter 27). Shock, whether it be hypovolemic, septic, or of some other etiology, by its very nature is a multisystem, nonorgan-specific, acute, life-threatening process.[70,72] Another natural area for critical care research would be specifically aimed at preventing and/or ameliorating the multisystem insults that occur because of the body-wide activation of potentially lethal mediators of the systemic inflammatory response. The spectrum of research opportunities in this area ranges from molecular biologic to large-scale clinical trials and has grown exponentially in the past few years.[11]

Organ system interaction also provides an area of primary interest in critical care. In particular, cardiorespiratory interaction has immediate, everyday application in ventilatory management, cardiopulmonary resuscitation, and cardiac support. The physiology of how changes in the pleural pressure affect cardiac function during either spontaneous or positive pressure ventilation is an area of constant relevance to the intensivist.[60] In a broader sense, cardiorespiratory interaction extends beyond this arena (see Chapter 24). How changes in cardiac function alter ventilation, airway resistance, and lung compliance is an integral part of critical care. The pulmonary endothelial synthesis, release, and degradation of multiple mediators, ranging from myocardial depressant factors to systemic vasoactive substances, that may alter cardiovascular function can be considered cardiorespiratory interaction and are of unique interest to the intensivist.[60] This area also encompasses a broad spectrum of possible approaches from molecular biology to cell physiology to integrated physiology.

An area of research that is particularly important to critical care medicine is cell biology. All organ system failure can be described in terms of cellular failure. For example, the general effects of superoxide radicals produced by leukocytes on other cell functions are legion and clearly of interest to intensivists[70,73] (see Chapter 97). Extending the argument of cellular specialization is possible for other cell types. An argument could be made to consider the endothelium the specialty organ of intensivists.[64] All organs that fail in critically ill children contain large areas of biochemically active endothelium. This endothelium is important because it elaborates hormones and autocoids that have systemic and local effects. These effects include alteration of coagulation and blood viscosity, superoxide generation and tissue damage, smooth muscle regulation, metabolism of circulating vasoactive substances, and interaction with the immunologic system.[16,34] All generalized stressors (e.g., sepsis, hypoxia, hypovolemia) can be expected to alter endothelial cell function. One way of looking at multiple organ system failure is to view it as an "endotheliopathy" (see Chapter 97). This endotheliopathy gives rise to widespread organ-specific damage, such as renal failure, ARDS, myocardial depression, and alterations in the blood-brain barrier, with subsequent cerebral edema. Endothelial cell function undergoes developmental aspects and may be specifically affected by disease processes particularly prevalent in children, such as the infectious vasculitides.[58] This sort of theoretical construct could serve as an organizational basis for research efforts in pediatric critical care and offer new insights into our understanding of critical illness in children.

Because of the astonishing success of the human genome project, the development of gene chips, and the potential of proteomics, understanding the genetic nature of critical illness no longer seems beyond our reach. Understanding the genotype of individuals who physiotypically display fatal responses to meningococcal disease while their classmate remains asymptomatic, albeit colonized by the same serotype organism, holds the promise of prospectively tailoring therapy to each patient individually. It is gratifying to see projects developing within pediatric critical care to help our understanding of the genetic bases of critical illness.

An area unique to critical care is that of caring for children and their families who must cope with acute critical and sometimes fatal illness (see Chapters 10 and 11). No other physicians deal with death and dying more frequently than intensivists. This role is especially important in the care of children. Supporting the family implications of acute, unexpected, critical illness and death of a child requires masterly physician interpersonal skills that are important in attenuating family problems long after the child's death. The entire area of the psychosocial impact of critical illness has been explored very little, and we need to know more. Such issues are intrinsic to critical care medicine, and it is imperative that intensivists become responsible for the research in this area. Potential avenues for the intensivist-investigator include epidemiologic study, such as family bereavement patterns and sibling bereavement, and randomized therapeutic interventions, such as the effect of frequent postmortem follow-up on the high incidence of divorce among couples who have lost a child.

Finally, and not least importantly, the burgeoning area of medical informatics holds the promise of enabling us to understand complex, critical, but rare disease processes previously impossible to study.[25] Understanding knowledge discovery in databases and building national and international collaborative partnerships to understand the scope of pediatric critical care have come within our reach.[35] Informatics research with national funding may provide real-time guidance for management of the rarest critical illnesses.

These examples indicate the wide spectrum of research opportunities in pediatric critical care medicine. There are many more, including the new National Collaborative Pediatric Critical Care Research Network (see *http://grants1.nih.gov/grants/guide/rfa-files/RFA-HD-04-004.html)* funded by the National Institute of Child Health and Human Development (NICHD), one of the National Institutes of Health. Constant sensitivity to identifying the questions (incorrectly answered, unanswered, and unasked) is the character trait required in the academic intensivist if our specialty is to continue to grow. Constantly identifying areas unique to critical care medicine provides the knowledge base for the specialty necessary for its growth and for our patients' well-being. Given the many unique areas of interest in critical care, how do we uncover them and encourage research in the subspecialty?

Wellsprings of Research

Collective Needs

Why must critical care collectively, as a specialty, support research in pediatric critical care? The arguments mentioned previously suggest that without the academic, intellectual, and scientific pursuit of areas that are specifically unique and relevant to critical care, we have no specialty. In this broad sense, research establishes a collegial respect for physicians who practice critical care and engenders the support the specialty deserves. Our colleagues outside intensive care wonder what we do. This concern is real and, in part, justified. If all we do is provide clinical care for dying children—and clinical care that other physicians do not understand by virtue of their not being dedicated to it—their questions are understandable. The frequent challenge of "what do intensivists do?" should only in part be answered by "spend long hours with children who are critically ill and their families." This question also addresses a deeper issue: Are intensivists contributing to the further understanding of critical illness? Are intensivists contributing to the intellectual advancement of medicine and the rich intellectual and academic milieu in the universities in which they find themselves? Are intensivists obtaining extramural funding for university-wide interactive and collaborative research efforts? Are intensivists training future generations of physician-scientists? Until we can affirmatively answer these questions from a uniquely critical care point of view, we should not be surprised that physicians in other subspecialties do not value our labors as highly as do we. This justification—to ensure the viability and respectability of a specialty whose primary concern is treating the critically ill—is a major reason we must encourage and support research. Failure to do so is a failure to critically ill children.

A further reason for the commitment to research by the critical care medicine community is to allow young investigators ample introduction to research. They must

- Discover what research is
- Be provided with the tools and techniques to answer the outstanding questions in the field
- Eventually make contributions both scientifically and educationally

This contribution will occur only if sufficient foresight is exercised to ensure that the facilities and resources are available. One of the chief rewards of developing this integrated structure will be the creation of a true specialty that is able to improve patient care. There are other rewards from this organized research endeavor and the education it provides. If the investigator returns to clinical medicine, never to darken the doorstep of a basic science laboratory again or to organize even one clinical trial, this physician will at least be sensitive to the critical questions in patient care and be able to read and apply the scientific literature with a far better understanding. Many otherwise perfectly adequate young physicians are unable to critically evaluate the medical literature as a tool to improve the management of their patients until they have been involved in contributing to it. It is impossible to teach didactically the rigorous effort required to achieve an article published in a first-class journal. It requires arduous, practical mentoring and doing; however, once done, the emerging clinician is better able to understand and critically review the contributions of her/his colleagues.

There is a further benefit from encouraging our fellows to research. The research effort provides excellent opportunities to observe how modulation of biochemistry, biology, and physiology alters the status of living beings. The practical knowledge gained in learning how to accurately measure the aortic/systemic and pulmonary artery pressures in animal models, determining the growth requirements of endothelial cells, maintaining sterile tissue cultures, and measuring pharmacokinetics provides insights into daily clinical practice unobtainable in any other way but is applicable to every critically ill child. For this reason, it is nearly impossible to become a well-rounded clinician without having learned the basics involved in, and completed the exercise of, addressing a research question. The spinoffs of how to do cutdowns, insert catheters, start arterial lines, measure tidal volumes and pressures, manipulate ventilators, care for cultures, bioassay eicosanoids, perform chromatographic separation of bioactive lipids, and sequence the messenger RNA for endothelin immediately improve the bedside care of children, both intellectually and practically. All of this organized effort would be of no avail, however, without individuals motivated toward research. Without these individuals, the organized support would be purposeless.

Individual Motivation

Research is difficult, expensive, and time consuming. It removes the clinician from patient care, frequently is thankless, often is difficult to plan and organize, and is difficult to execute. Even when excellently done, it may be hard to present and possibly not well received. Why then should any physician dedicated to the critical care of children be even slightly interested in becoming involved in research? Surely the desire to be promoted in the academic setting, see your name in prestigious journals, and impress your family, friends, and colleagues is insufficient motivation to contribute vast amounts of time, exhaust your intellectual and physical energy, and reduce your availability for patient care and family life. Although these aspects may be some of the benefits of a research career, they are merely some of the lesser fruits of research. They are inadequate to provide the primary motivation for being involved in research. They, by and of themselves, are inadequate to support the investigator in long exhausting hours of labor seemingly without reward.

Why should an individual be committed to this arduous task? Personal motivations for research are many, and there are *numerous real rewards.* One of the most obvious is that being an attending physician in a pediatric intensive care unit 12 months of the year is not something that either can or should be done by any physician, no matter how much physical and emotional stamina that individual may have (or think she/he has). Diversion from clinical and administrative responsibilities and refreshment and renewal are some simple rewards of being involved in research. This benefit, prevention of burnout, is not achieved merely by avoiding clinical work. Rather, the invigoration that comes from involvement in, and a commitment to, improving patient care and a long-range commitment to ensure the survival of the specialty and the investigator are the source of the benefits. In turn, active involvement in research provides a broader perspective of our specialty that allows the intensivist to understand the grueling hours of clinical care in their proper perspective.

Of course, research can (and should) be fun. If it is not fun, *if the investigator does not look forward to being involved* in the understanding, development, design, execution, analysis, preparation, and presentation of the research, then *it is not worthwhile for that individual investigator to remain involved.* You must like what you are doing, or the dedication and commitment required for Edison's "99% perspiration for each 1% inspiration" will be lacking. Personal motivation is the necessary starting point, but from where does that motivation come? The noble goal of adding to the knowledge base of the field is excellent; however, it is unlikely that many clinicians wake up in the morning and say, "Aha! I will add to the knowledge base of critical care today." Rather, we are continually challenged by questions that arise from providing critical care for children, by questions about patient management, and by uncertainties and confusion. It is the role of all preceptors and instructors in critical care to make certain that the trainee is aware that these questions are there and that they are asked. *To teach critical care as if it were dogma is destructive to these goals.* To point out and demonstrate constantly where there are failures and conflicts in our understanding and where matters of style, rather than matters of substance, determine our clinical practice is to uncover fertile areas for research. Unless the young intensivist senses these exciting challenges, the personal enthusiasm toward research will not be discovered. There is another motivating factor. Many of our young investigators ask, "What is research?" The great shibboleth of research has been held up before American medical students and our pediatric residents for years. Nevertheless, most young physicians have no idea what research is. They may have seen a fragment of a clinical trial, but they likely did not participate in a basic research experience. All too frequently they do not have the faintest idea about the real application of the scientific method or statistical analysis. Curiosity for what research is should be recognized, fanned, and fed. *The inquisitive clinician must not be lost because of a poor understanding of the research* or a feeling that it is an elitist club. For this reason, our fellowship programs must provide valid scientific research experience guided by seasoned investigators. Not until our junior physicians realize that *they can* acquire the skills to answer the questions that arise clinically, in a rigorous and scientific fashion, can we expect them to do so.

The previously mentioned personally motivating factors, which include personal aggrandizement such as fame, fortune, job security, avoidance of burnout, fun, ability, education, and training, still are not, however, sufficient. All of these possible motivations do not provide the major essential driving force. Individual curiosity, a tireless need to question, and the restless search for answers must be the source of the entire endeavor. Curiosity? Is this the crucial concept? Sir Peter Medawar calls it a "nursery word"—a motive too inadequate.[47] Everyone possesses curiosity, and yet not everyone makes a commitment to seek solutions, occasionally at great personal cost. So it must be more than mere curiosity. Medawar calls this driving compulsion the "exploratory impulsion"; Kant called it "restless endeavor."[47] It is not merely curiosity but surrender to the urge, often sacrificially, to seek the answer that motivates the investigator. This urge must be strong because it will require a great deal of time and energy in training before the question that originally piqued the clinician's curiosity can be addressed. This innate motivation of the individual is the main force driving all medical investigation.

Where the collective needs of the specialty and the individual's needs come together is that both have a genuine, deep-rooted desire to understand better how to help critically ill patients. This symbiosis of specialty needs and individual motivation forms the essential chemistry of discovery. In a fascinating address to the American Society for Clinical Investigation, JL Goldstein[29] presented the formula:

$$\text{Clinical stimulus} \times \text{Basic scientific training} \leftrightarrows \text{Fundamental discovery.}$$

The individual, when clinically stimulated, can make a fundamental contribution only with appropriate training. The specialty can best meet the needs mentioned previously by providing that training. The collective combination of financial and intellectual resources and the individual's blood, sweat, and tears is critical. Resources will be provided only if the physicians involved in critical care are committed to providing, for individual intensivists who have the curiosity and desire, the means to find answers to *their* individual questions. No matter how well organized, the specialty organizations can encourage individuals to labor toward solutions for only the problems that interest them. Selection of these trainees is critical. Erasmus Darwin said in 1792: "A fool is a man who never tried an experiment in his life." Let us not train too many fools. Constantly striving to recruit the seeker, doubter, questioner—and when they are recruited, to support them—is the responsibility of all physicians involved in critical care. Without them, critical care research will be nonexistent. Significant advance in our specialty can grow only from shouldering this responsibility. Without this commitment to encourage and train, critical care medicine will continue to lose promising young clinician-scientists to other specialty areas, because it will be only there that they will be able to seek answers to their questions. We cannot overemphasize this crucial issue and its centrality to the growth of our specialty. The training also must be thorough. This takes time, but without the commitment to train young investigators to think like basic scientists, they will be unable to apply the tools of basic science and will end up paralyzed and lost to the specialty of pediatric critical care.[29]

Doing Research

"Gentlemen, do not think! Try and be patient. Have you performed the experiment?"

John Hunter

The myriad variations in study populations, techniques of data gathering, study designs, questions asked, answers required, and types of analyses and whether the question should be addressed clinically or by a basic science approach (and, if basic science, whether by cellular, physiologic, biochemical, or biophysical experiments) all can be very confusing. Then there is statistics. To understand how to address a given question, familiarity with the basic process of research is necessary. For example, the simple question "Should I give my patients with septic shock sodium bicarbonate?" could be addressed in many ways (and indeed has been)! The options range from experiments to discern the subcellular effect of changes in pH on mitochondrial function all the way to prospective, randomized, double-blind, multicenter clinical trials to determine whether bicarbonate therapy improves survival in septic shock. All of these factors have a part in answering what may first appear to be a simple question. Many factors influence how the researcher goes about answering any question, not the least of which are the researcher's background and training. The availability of resources in the researcher's institution and previous research relevant to the question being asked also are important.

So, what is research? Research is scientific investigation. If the motivation to do research can be matched by the commitment of the specialty to support research, is that sufficient? How is the bedside problem answered? If a keen investigator with a good question has a willing pediatric intensive care unit director with money, or at least one who is willing to help find resources, what next? How is research done? What is the scientific process?

Over the past 200 years, the scientific method has been developed by learning how to test our guesses about the universe.[5] The key factors involved are

- Observation
- Intuition
- Formulation of hypotheses
- Experimentation
- Development of scientific laws, theories, or axioms
- Testing these new theories

Bacon provided one of the first common-sense answers to the question, "How is research done?" The answer was "by observation and experimentation." Which observations and data should be collected may seem fairly obvious at first, but deciding what should be observed and recorded are *the* crucial research questions. Approaches that may be useful in determining whether bicarbonate helps a critically ill child include observing and recording every physiologic parameter and every biochemical response, as well as measuring every enzyme's activity and looking at urinary metabolic products. It is evident that these are not necessarily the best, most direct ways to answer the underlying question. Merely compiling a mountain of data without scientific reasons behind each observation (fishing) is risky, time consuming, inefficient, and often futile. One of the main tasks of the investigator is to decide which observations in the whole set of possible observations are crucial. Lack of critical thinking may result in missing important observations and fruitless experimentation. Similarly, determination of what type of experiment should be performed is equally crucial.

What is an experiment? The original meaning of the term *experiment* was "a test made to demonstrate a known truth." It served as a means of proof for an already "known" truth. This sort of experiment was not designed to generate new knowledge. This Aristotelian concept of experimentation, involving classical deductive logic, has limited application in modern medicine, other than perhaps that of pedantry and teaching high school chemistry. The essential concept of experimentation that has a more contemporary meaning entails an uncertain or unknown outcome. To the present-day researcher, the purpose of performing an experiment is to discriminate between possibilities. How experiments are designed to discriminate between possibilities depends on the underlying assumptions. Understanding the logic that underlies how an experiment is performed is useful in avoiding multiple traps, not only in reviewing the data but also in applying experimental results to real patients. Bacon[6] noted: "If a man begins with certainties, he shall end in doubts, but if he will be content to begin with doubts, he shall end in certainties." This is obviously the starting point, but how do we start? How do we get along?

Many experiments are still designed—*contrived* may be a better word—to demonstrate the validity of preconceived ideas. This reasoning from preconceived ideas or premises to the specific situation is known as the process of *deductive logic.* Deductive logic is reasoning from the general to the specific. A clinical example of such deductive logic is the following syllogism:

Major: Penicillin is an effective treatment for pneumococcal pneumonia.

Minor: My patient has pneumococcal pneumonia.

Inference: I will treat my patient with penicillin.

The experiment performed in this case, treating a patient with penicillin, will have a certain outcome only inasmuch as the deductive logic is correct and the underlying primary assumption (major premise) and diagnostic result (minor premise) are true. In a general way, all specific conclusions that rest on authoritative statements of truth are deductive in origin. By their very nature, although they guide our clinical activity, they do not expand our medical knowledge. The hallmark of deductive logic is complete reliance on the certainty of known or revealed facts. Some 300 years after the modern scientific revolution and the birth of true scientific thought, modern experimental medicine remains beset with this type of logic. Aristotelian experimentation is the process of clinical practice. We reason from general principles and accepted facts to specific interventions and treatments. The entire evidence-based practice movement is based on deducing therapy from sound premises. The difficulty comes when the dogmatic assumptions that underlie our clinical practice, and deductively lead to our therapies, are incorrect. Aristotelian experimentation provides no way to approach outcomes in medicine that are exceptional, yet these are the very occurrences that may be enlightening. Charles Darwin has exhorted us never to allow these exceptions to go unnoticed.[50] Deductive logic is unable to assist in the discovery of new knowledge and therefore general principles. This was clearly noted by Sir Francis Bacon,[4] who stated in 1620:

> *"The syllogism consists of propositions, propositions consist of words, words are symbols of notions. Therefore if the notions themselves (which is the root of the matter) are confused and over-hastily abstracted from the facts, there can be no firmness in the superstructure. Our only hope therefore lies in a true* induction."

The great revolution in scientific and philosophic writing in the 1600s was typified by Bacon's absolute refutation of the concept that any new truths could be discovered merely by a deductive act of the mind[4]:

> *"The discoveries which have hitherto been made in the sciences are such as lie close to vulgar notions, scarcely beneath the surface. In order to penetrate into the inner and further recesses of nature, it is necessary that both notions and axioms be derived from things by a more sure and guarded way; and that a method of intellectual operation be introduced altogether better and more certain."*

The Baconian revolution in scientific thought was dependent on observation and experimentation. The underlying premise was that the general could be determined, inferred, and understood from observing the specific. This led to the realization that by the use of thoughtful inductive logic, linked to observation and understanding, specific discovery of new generalized truths was possible. A clinical example of this sort of contribution to modern medicine is the well-known example of vaccination. Jenner's recurrent observation of the specific immunity to smallpox of patients who had been infected by cowpox led to experimentation with observation and a series of inductive steps that ultimately led not only to the eradication of smallpox in the world but also to generalization of the concept of vaccination to other infectious processes and vast discoveries in the area of immunology. It is impossible to conceive how Aristotelian deductive logic could have led to these discoveries. Bacon's contribution was to realize that observations of the specifics in nature would lead, through application of the intellect, to the discovery of new truths. Bacon did realize that we were unable to rely on "the casual felicity of particular events"[47] to provide us with all the specific information required to discover scientific truths, even if we spent an entire lifetime observing nature. He thus realized the necessity to devise experiences and contrive occurrences to collect factual information by which we would understand the natural world. This is Baconian *experimentation.* However, this still was not true experimentation as we know it today.

True experimentation, as commonly thought of today, is more accurately described as Galilean experimentation.[47,50] The Galilean experiment discriminates between possibilities and, in so doing, confirms a preconceived notion by supplying facts that support the inductive process leading to a sound conclusion. The essence of an experiment as proposed by Galileo was a true test, a trial, or an *ordeal* of a hypothesis. This constructive experimentation more accurately reflects what we think of today when we want to further our understanding of critical illness. As Stephen Hawking[33] put it in *A Brief History of Time:*

> *"Our present ideas about the motion of bodies date back to Galileo and Newton. Before them people believed Aristotle, who said that the*

natural state of a body was to be at rest and that it moved only if driven by a force or impulse. It followed that a heavy body should fall faster than a light one, because it would have a greater pull toward earth."

The Aristotelian tradition also held that you could work out all the laws governing the universe by pure thought: it was not necessary to check by observation. So no one until Galileo bothered to see whether bodies of different weight did, in fact, fall at different speeds. Mythology reports that Galileo demonstrated that Aristotle's belief was false by dropping weights from the leaning tower of Pisa. The story almost certainly is untrue, but Galileo did do something equivalent: he rolled balls of different weights down a smooth slope. The situation is similar to that of heavy bodies falling vertically, but it is easier to observe because the speeds are smaller. Galileo's measurements indicated that each body increased its speed at the same rate, no matter what its weight.

In Galileo's experiment, the hypothesis tested was that objects of different mass fall at different velocities. The "control" group could have been a group of spheres with mass = x. The experimental group (or groups) would have been $x + 1$ kg (or $x + 1$ kg, $x + 2$ kg, and so forth). Because all objects fall at the same velocity, his data failed to support the hypothesis, and it was irrevocably disproved and destroyed, instantly. The old system was dead. The deductively logical syllogism of Aristotle's day was as follows:

Major: The velocity of a falling object is determined by the object's mass.

Minor: These two objects are of different mass.

Inference: They will fall at different rates

This syllogism was disproved by a *single* observation that the conclusion was incorrect. Therefore if the minor premise was true, the major premise had to be false. A new intellectual universe became possible. Every preconceived notion was testable by experiment. All that is required is a testable hypothesis. The routine function of medical experimentation, the purpose of all medical science and the major *modus vivendi* of all the national institutes, is the testing of hypotheses. Although gathering facts and cataloging their relationships as in Aristotelian and Baconian experimentation remains of some value, testing hypotheses is our strongest research tool. Galilean experimentation provided the constant capability of revising our hypotheses and avoiding unnecessary persistence in theoretical structures based on hypothetical errors that lead to no more than a house of cards.

The generation of scientific hypotheses that can be critically tested is the basis of scientific discovery. Discovery has its beginnings in imaginative preconception, which is the creative act of mind that gives rise to a hypothesis.[50] Asking the question or conceiving the question is only the beginning of the scientific process. Casting the question in the form of testable, verifiable, scientific hypotheses is where the creative work of research really begins. The brilliant guess, the falling of scales from the eyes, the eureka moment—these scientific insights are the sources of these hypotheses. The hypothesis is a mark to be attained, a suggestion of the probable, a provisional proposal of the underlying truth, or some specific facet of it. The hypothesis has but one purpose, to be tested. A word of warning here—a hypothesis, no matter how interesting, can never be proven. Absolute proof of a hypothesis is not, by the very nature of inductive logic and Galilean experimentation, ever possible because all possibilities cannot possibly ever be tested. Again, according to Stephen Hawking[33]:

"Any physical theory is always provisional, in the sense that it is only a hypothesis: you can never prove it. No matter how many times the results of experiments agree with some theory, you can never be sure that the next time the result will not contradict the theory. On the other hand, you can disprove a theory by finding even a single observation that disagrees with the predictions of the theory. As philosopher of science Karl Popper has emphasized, a good theory is characterized by the fact that it makes a number of predictions that could in principle be disproved or falsified by observation. Each time new experiments are observed to agree with the predictions the theory survives, and our confidence in it is increased; but if ever a new observation is found to disagree, we have to abandon or modify the theory."

Whereas a theory is an organized system of knowledge used to analyze or explain nature or behavior, a hypothesis has no such value. Theories may be built up from facts learned by testing hypotheses and may even contain partially substantiated hypotheses that are useful in predicting events, but hypotheses are useful only insofar as their testing acts as a focus for the discovery of truths. Without a doubt, hypotheses are the most important instruments in research. Developing a hypothesis is the initial phase of research and scientific investigation. It generates the plan for the research. Nevertheless, it is "a means, not an end," as Thomas Huxley cautioned.[50] The ultimate goal of research is not to hunt blindly for unrelated facts but to test related hypotheses.

If we accept the fact that the purpose of experimentation is to test hypotheses, then it is clear that a necessity for research is to formulate appropriate hypotheses. The hypothesis must be focused, with a limited number of possible outcomes and limited number of implications that lead logically to further investigational steps. This eliminates futile activity. A hypothesis that accommodates all possible phenomena or outcomes is totally uninformative. The more restrictive it is, the more focused it is, the more instructive it is. One final warning about hypotheses—although they are the driving force of research, they must be kept in their place. Accepting unproved hypotheses can clearly lead you down a rabbit hole, often a time-consuming, expensive, and disastrous one. Failure to give up unsubstantiated hypotheses can lead to a futile cycle of experimentation. Although scientists require hypotheses, find them attractive, and may not be able to live without them, they must not fall in love with them.[47,50] The basic fact of science, that hypotheses are never proven and that they are only as good as the results they generate, must never be forgotten. Likewise, the physician-scientist as observer of nature must be encouraged to use quantitative and qualitative descriptive tools in order to develop the platform for meaningful hypothesis generation.

The Null Hypothesis

Galileo's revolutionary experiment proved nothing! Rather, it disproved the accepted dogma by a single observation. When deductive logic is correctly performed and the major and minor premises are correct, the inference is absolutely, positively true. This is not true in the other direction. Reasoning from the inferences is unreliable. The arrival of two objects at the ground at different times does not assure us that the objects are of different mass or that objects of different mass fall at different rates. In the penicillin case, the fact that our patient improved with penicillin proves neither that he had pneumococcal infection nor that penicillin is effective against pneumococcus. He could have just had erysipelas. Then again, if the objects of different mass arrive simultaneously—that is, the inference is wrong—then something also is very wrong with one or both of the premises. If penicillin does not reliably, reproducibly treat pneumococcal pneumonia, then something is wrong with the diagnosis or with the efficacy of penicillin against pneumococcus. Yes, an astute clinician sees all sorts of problems in this statement, but the problems only emphasize the importance of rigid control of nuisance variables (discussed later). Nevertheless, that inference is asymmetrical demonstrates that falsification—the disproving of a hypothesis— is logically a stronger, surer process than the so-called (and impossible) proving of a hypothesis. As Hawking explained, absolute proof is not possible. Instead, to support scientific hypothesis we generally attempt to disprove the *opposite* hypothesis, that is, we try to "refute the null hypothesis." For example, Galileo said:

"All objects, irrespective of mass, fall at the same velocity."

The null hypothesis is that objects of different mass fall at different velocities or, as previously asserted, mass determines velocity. Galileo absolutely refuted this null hypothesis; thus his data were consistent with his own hypothesis. Even so, they did not prove it.

As a clinical example, if the hypothesis is "steroids improve morbidity in shock," then the null hypothesis is that they do not. To refute this null hypothesis, the investigator merely has to demonstrate a difference between steroid-treated and nontreated patients in an adequately randomized and powered trial. If so, the null hypothesis is rejected and the hypothesis survives this test—this time. Statistics are applied to determine the certainty of the rejection of the null hypothesis and actually are performed to demonstrate that the null hypothesis has been rejected with a degree of certainty. For example, if $p = 0.05$, then it is 95% certain that the null hypothesis is incorrect and that the results are consistent with the scientific hypothesis.

It is this *asymmetry* of inference that allows us to disprove major premises by demonstrating the untenability of the inference. This is how we support scientific hypotheses. This refutation of the null hypothesis is generally taken to affirm that the very opposite is true. This is done because falsification of the inference and/or minor premises proving the falseness of the major premise is such a potent tool. Proving the major premise true is, in fact, impossible. Thus the basic tool used to demonstrate that a hypothesis is true is that of proving that the null hypothesis is false. The scientist's experimental goal is to reject the null hypothesis rather than to prove the actual scientific hypothesis. Because refuting the null hypothesis is such a potent tool, good scientific hypotheses must be of such a nature that their null hypothesis (or, indeed, many of their null hypotheses, because several may stem from one hypothesis) can be tested. This test is virtually always a statistical one.

Medical Research

"It is incident to physicians, I am afraid, to mistake subsequence for consequence."

Samuel Johnson

The first great divide in medical research is between clinical and laboratory research. Many consider such a division arbitrary, and the bench to bedside to bench translational models that have enabled modern physician-scientists to bring breakthrough understanding to the care of critical illness mandate that effective pediatric critical care researchers have "feet" in both domains. Still, in this classical distinction, clinical research is carried out in patients. It is an extension of previous experience in patients or of results obtained from laboratory research. Clinical research can occur in any medical arena. Laboratory research clearly does not involve patients; rather, it relies on the results in animals or tissue-derived "subjects."

Clinical research can be either retrospective or prospective. Retrospectively, epidemiologic studies, demographic studies, and studies of disease processes and outcomes of management regimens can provide useful information in directing future therapy. Certainly the great wealth of data now available in patient records can continue to provide worthwhile insights to aid our patients. Unfortunately, retrospective trials cannot convincingly answer therapeutic questions; rather, their utility is in hypothesis generation. Their solution requires true Galilean experimentation. Baconian studies such as these prospective trials require as much planning as possible before the patient actually is observed for the results of a therapeutic intervention, but this has started to change. Learning from reliable observations is the basis of physical science, and applying these research principles to data obtained from human subjects is useful in reliably suggesting a general theory if large enough numbers of observations are collected and analyzed. In medical informatics, this is the basis for knowledge discovery in databases. Thus with a sufficient number of observations (controlled, defined, verified data) we may learn how to manage our patients by applying analytical techniques to retrospective events. The information revolution may be driving knowledge discovery once again toward some reliance on inductive logic.[25]

The principles that guide all medical research, including clinical trials, are in place to minimize the possibility of an incorrect conclusion. A major cause of error is bias, either by the observer or the subject. A further cause of incorrect conclusions results from inadequate study design that may prevent accurate statistical analysis of the information obtained.

The other overwhelming principle that guides clinical research is to preserve the rights, autonomy, and safety of the individual subject.[10,42,56] This is of particular importance in clinical research involving children. The issues of risk, informed consent, and the potential to benefit the patient are particularly finely focused in pediatrics. The spectrum of opinion runs from believing that research in children is not allowable to believing that child subjects should be treated exactly the same as adult experimental subjects. Any researcher who proposes doing clinical research in critically ill children must be familiar with all aspects of these arguments and realize the sensitivity of the issues involved in this area[15,49,64] (see Chapter 11).

Research Design

In the simplest of all experiments, two observable populations, the *experimental* and the *control,* are observed for discrete occurrences. The results of the experiment are that the two observable sets of data from these populations are or are not different. Performance of a critical Galilean experiment that is clearly designed and meticulously executed will unambiguously answer this question. Any experiment that does not contain a control is not truly Galilean. The control group contains subjects as identical as possible to the experimental group. The observations made are the same before and after the introduction of the independent variable.

Designing an experiment involves attention to three separate areas: (1) independent variables, (2) subject selection, and (3) dependent variables. Essentially, an experiment involves controlling or altering independent variables while observing in the subject changes in dependent variables. In short, the scientific method can be reduced to "if I do A, then what happens to B?" An example in early pediatric experimentation is provided by the first demonstration of adrenaline. Sir Henry Dale injected ground-up cow adrenal gland (independent variable) into his small son (subject) and determined the effect on his son's blood pressure (dependent variable). The closer study designs are to this simple algorithm, the more likely they will yield clearly understandable, unambiguous, and true results. Unfortunately, this is rarely possible except in highly controlled settings.

The *independent variable* is that which is under the control of the experimenter. The *dependent variable* is that which reflects the effects associated with altering the independent variable.

Independent Variable

The selection of the independent variable in any experimental design is crucial. Not only can this be a treatment variable but also the level at which treatment is delivered (dose). The independent variable must be one that can be manipulated and rigidly controlled. For example, to determine the effect of light on bilirubin in jaundiced babies, the independent variable is light. This variable can be fluorescent, incandescent, or solar. The duration of exposure and the efficacy of various light wavelengths could be—and indeed have been—experimentally determined by changing the independent variable and measuring the effect on the dependent variable (bilirubin concentration). In most therapeutic trials, the independent variables are either treatment or no treatment. For example, you test the therapeutic efficacy of a drug or the comparison of two or more treatment interventions for a disease, such as acyclovir versus cyclosporine for treatment of herpes encephalitis. A recurrent trial design relevant to critical care is provided by multiple studies on the use of one of many steroids in septic shock. These include steroid versus no steroids as the independent variable and multiple dosing levels of steroids.

The definition of the independent variable must be as precise as possible. Independent variables can be qualitative or quantitative. From the phototherapy example, a qualitative independent variable applies to the type of radiation. The radiation could be solar or incandescent light, and there will be a difference in the response of the dependent variable. There are many different kinds of treatment. Quantitative differences in the independent variable, by contrast, result from the same treatment given at different levels. The simplest of these is comparison of zero (no therapy) to a known dose of therapy, for example, 0 mg of steroids versus 30 mg/kg steroids. In addition, multiple doses can be given for a comparison of dose ranges. The exact selection of the independent variable and the quantitative nature of it ideally should be dictated by the specific hypothesis being tested.

Dependent Variable

Both practical and theoretical considerations are necessary in determining which dependent variables to observe. Clearly the dependent variables will be determined by the expected outcome, as indicated by the hypotheses. In large-scale clinical trials, the dependent variable can be as simple as mortality or as complex as altered hemodynamic function described by a broad spectrum of hemodynamic parameters. The potential for dependent variables is enormous; however, some rules guide selection.

Most statistical analyses limit themselves to assessment of one dependent variable at a time. Selection of the dependent variable is determined by its distribution within the population, how reliably it can be measured, how sensitive and specific it will be to the independent variable, and how practical it is to measure. Clearly, maximum sensitivity and reliability are preferable. The more sensitive and reliable the selected dependent variables, the more likely the time and effort invested, number of subjects required, and cost of investigating the hypothesis will be minimized. With regard to distribution, it is generally assumed that the dependent variables in the study population will undergo a normal (gaussian, bell-shaped curve) distribution. When abnormal distribution occurs, it must be specifically addressed statistically. It also is possible, in some instances, to transform an abnormal distribution to a normal distribution for the purposes of analysis. Unfortunately, a single dependent variable rarely approximates the clinical situation, where a single independent variable intervention may have a series of effects on a host of dependent variables. Therefore it frequently is necessary to evaluate two or more dependent variables at any given time. This process requires advanced study design and analysis that takes requirement into account; for example, multivariant analysis may be required.

Nuisance Variables

Anyone who has ever attempted any form of scientific experimentation is familiar with nuisance variables. *Nuisance variables* are best defined as *undesired causes of variation in the observed or dependent variable.* These variables are of no interest to the investigator but may significantly alter the outcome of the experiment. For example, nuisance variables may include factors such as patient age, gender, disease process, previous therapy, socioeconomic background, nutritional status, and presence or absence of infectious disease processes. The list is long, even infinitely so, and this is a problem for scientists. Unless these nuisance variables are controlled, outcome is uncertain. For example, an epidemiologic experiment to determine whether fatality is more common in lower socioeconomic groups following road traffic accidents could miss the effects of underlying nutritional status, distance from the hospital, and previous disease process and thus arrive at an erroneous conclusion.

One way to control nuisance variables is to ensure that they are both constant and equivalent for all subjects for the entire duration of the experiment. For example, male sheep exactly 6 months old, weighing 30 pounds, and of a specific breed and diet would provide better control for nuisance variables than a population of sheep of any age, weight, gender, size, or breed. In clinical trials it is generally impossible to obtain ideally matched controls. *It must be assumed that some nuisance variables will always escape control.*

The second broad approach to controlling nuisance variables is to assign subjects to experimental groups *randomly*. The principle of randomization rests on the supposition that the study population contains normally distributed nuisance variables and that these nuisance variables will be equally and normally distributed in the experimental subgroups (discussed later). This assumption can be *true only if the experimental groups are of sufficient size to assure normal distribution.* This is one of the major factors determining sample size. Randomization is the most powerful and most commonly used tool for controlling nuisance variables. A third method for eliminating the effect of nuisance variables is merely to include them in the experimental design and thus study their effect on dependent variables. A final, nonexperimental method of controlling nuisance variables is statistical control. *Analysis of covariance* is a method of statistical control that removes the effects of nuisance variables through the use of multiple regression analysis. This is a complex statistical manipulation that should be prospectively designed into any trial when eliminating anticipated (or even reveal unanticipated) effects of nuisance variables is necessary.

Both independent and nuisance variables can be caused by the subject's innate characteristics, such as gender, weight, age, and previous illness, or to external environmental influences. These environmental influences may include temperature, humidity, presence or absence of other caregivers, a variety of pharmacologic interventions, socioeconomic group, diet, and various other factors. Task-related variables also may affect the dependent variable. These factors may be inadvertently introduced into the experiment study design, and they must be rigorously sought and avoided. For example, the experimental design or the particular sequence of observations made may alter the dependent variable in such a fashion as to confound the effects of the independent variable.

Design Efficacy

The problem facing the investigator who wishes to address a medically related question is to design a study (or a series of experiments) that can answer the question as validly and efficiently as possible while taking into consideration the research situation available to the investigator. Efficiency of research design can be accounted for in several ways. Cost can be one of these determinants, and the cost per observation or the cost per experiment can be compared to the amount of information obtained. Alternatively, time can determine efficiency: the maximum useful data in the shortest period of time. In fact, careful stewardship of resources for biomedical research is an underappreciated principle. Every emerging researcher in pediatric critical care must commit herself/himself to incorporating such stewardship as an underlying value. These factors are inherently determined by the amount of variance in the dependent variable that can be attributed to extraneous or nuisance variables.

This situation gives rise to the concept of experimental error variance. A major source of this error is the variability inherent to subjects. A further cause is the lack of precise uniformity in experimental conduct. When comparing two groups it is important to ensure that observations are made at the point where differences between the groups are the greatest. It is possible that the effects of two drugs are equal at higher doses, but significant differences could exist at a lower dose range. Observations at the former would yield negative results but at the latter point reveal a beneficial effect with less drug. Clearly, information about efficacy (dose response) is necessary before a comparison trial. Federer[26] formulated a method for evaluating the efficiency of experimental design that takes into account the number of subjects at each treatment level, the cost of collecting data per subject, the degrees of freedom, and an estimate of error variance per observation.[25] These are the factors the investigator must consider when designing any experiment.

The basic technique of experimental design is that of replication of observations in two or more subjects under identical experimental conditions. The number of replications or the sample size depends on the following five factors[38]:

1. Number of treatment levels
2. Minimum treatment effects to be detected
3. Error variance of the study population
4. Necessary power (probability of rejecting the null hypothesis)
5. Probability of making a type I error

There are two common ways of increasing the power of an experimental design. The first method is to design experiments that provide precise estimates of the desired treatment effects while minimizing error effects. The second method is to increase sample size.

Randomization

All statistical theory is based on the supposition that at some stage during the experiment, a process of random selection is performed. Conclusions based on these statistical studies are valid only inasmuch as the randomization process is understood and observed. A random procedure has at least two possible outcomes, and the probabilities of all possible outcomes are specified prior to the randomization procedure.[51] It is important to note the frequent errors practiced in the name of randomization. First among these is the naive belief that the number of subjects in an experiment is related to randomness. Although the principle of safety in numbers may be reassuring, it is unwarranted. Experiments usually are performed in only a small sample of a normally distributed population. If this sample is truly representative, then the size of the population sample does not matter. By contrast, if the sample of the population is not representative (e.g., it is drawn from patients at one end of the normal distribution), then no matter how large the sample, randomness will not be possible. For example, to determine the case fatality ratio in children with meningitis, it would be just as useless to study 10,000 as 10 autopsies.

It is important to note the difference between a random sample and a haphazard sample. A haphazard sample indicates the investigator has no idea from where the data came. The more a given sample can be constructed wherein as many biases as possible are appreciated, the more likely the results will be truly randomized and known as opposed to haphazard. It is crucial to know that the investigator's *ignorance of the characteristics of the sample population is not the same as randomization.* Similarly, ignorance of associations within a sample population does not make the sample random and provides another serious source for potential bias. Simple inability to show any clear biases in selection does not assure randomization. Another error made in randomization is to confuse the source of bias by mixing populations of unknown bias. Finally, the absence of a clear plan for randomization does not ensure randomization; rather, haphazard sampling leads to haphazard results.

So how do we ensure that randomization takes place? Obviously, with an adequate sample of the best-designed and most homogenous population, randomization can be optimized. In any experiment requiring randomization, the study population must be as explicitly defined as possible before randomization occurs. This is relatively simple if all subjects are prospectively chosen (e.g., 10 patients with sickle cell disease). It is less clear when the subjects can be drawn from a large population (e.g., the next 10 children with ARDS). Second, the system for selection must be prospectively described. Steps should be taken to ensure equal numbers of, for example, boys and girls, age distribution, race, and operative procedure. Once the subjects have been defined and selected, a means of randomizing them, with a representation in the randomization procedure for each subject, must be made (e.g., even or odd numbers, a randomization table, or something as simple as drawing names out of a hat).[51] This process is only as useful as the prerandomization population is homogeneous. Of course, with human experimentation, subjects frequently differ. It also is necessary to describe the action to be taken following randomization; for example, all odd numbers get no therapy, and all even numbers get steroids or prostacyclin. Finally, the subjects are randomized, and nothing is allowed to alter the outcome. A large host of confounding factors in randomization will occur. Other randomizations, such as randomized block design and Latin square design, are potential approaches for solving these problems.[38]

Validity

Evaluating an experimental design requires taking into account those factors that ensure the validity of the results. First of all, the overall field of research must be known so that experimental observations can be made that provide the opportunity for comparison of findings with other investigators. In addition, accepted practices and procedures in the research area should be followed wherever possible. Next it is necessary to decide if the data collection method produces reliable results and that the data obtained are accurate. It also is necessary that the design of the experiment permits the experimenter to determine which effects are caused by experimental error and which results are caused by manipulation of the independent variable. In addition, some attention is necessary to optimizing the efficiency of the experiment and understanding the experimental constraints. Finally, to justify doing any experiments at all, the design should be of sufficient power to be certain that an adequate test of the statistical hypothesis is made.[38]

It is essential to ensure that valid conclusions concerning the effects of the independent variable on the dependent variable can be drawn from the experiment.[17] In general, this is satisfied by statistical analysis. In addition, in the medical setting, generalizations of these results to populations and settings of medical interest are necessary. This requires *probability theory.*[51] It is important to realize that statistical theory and probability theory are not the same.

The purpose of ensuring the validity of the statistical conclusion is to ensure that incorrect data resulting from errors in randomization and inappropriate statistical analyses are not made.[38] There are several threats to the validity of inference from the data.[17] Clearly, the statistical analysis must be correct, but in addition it is necessary to assess the internal validity of the experiment. "Internal validity" deals with the assumption that the relationship between observed variations in the dependent variable is resulting from variations in the independent variable. "Construct validity" of causes or effects deals with the potential that alterations in the independent variable and observations in the dependent variable result from and are construed in terms of other variables. Finally, "external validity" of the results indicates the extent to which the results of a particular experiment can be generalized to populations and subjects. This concerns comparison with existing results and the probability of extending the results of a given experiment to a wider population and ultimately to treatment decisions.[51]

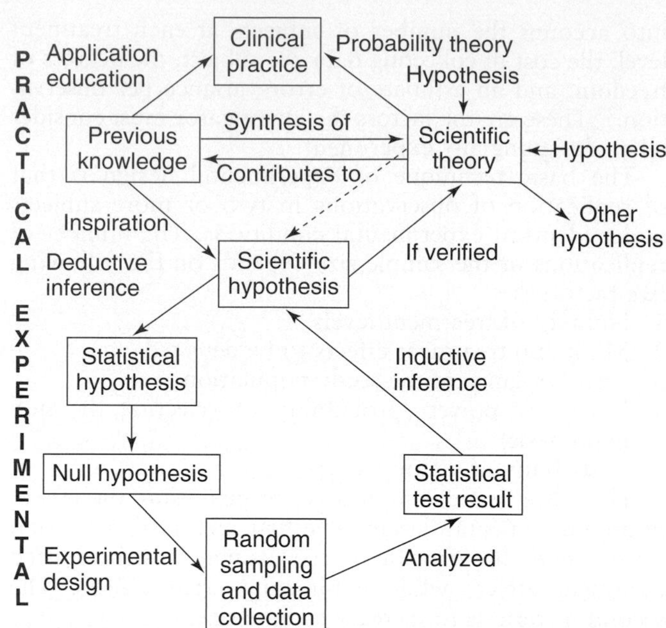

FIGURE 5–1 • General schema of the relationship between clinical practice and medical research. Note the central position of the scientific hypothesis and the steps necessary for verifying it. Also note that the statistical analysis of experimental data does not apply to the application of medical scientific theory (built up of multiple hypotheses) to clinical practice.

Statistics: A Word

This section is not intended to be a primer on statistics or to serve as a catalog of how to do a *t*-test or analysis of variance. Numerous textbooks and computer programs exist for those purposes. Rather, this section emphasizes the common—and most frequently violated—principles that underlie the statistical analysis of experimental data. They are the source of rejection of articles and of grant applications and a great deal of wasted effort—not to mention the potential for misguided therapy. Every study, every paper, every grant, and ultimately the validity of every therapy rests on these principles.

Statistical analysis of the data yields the likelihood of certainty from the experiment at hand.[38] Probability theory deals with the predictive statements based on the outcomes of an experiment.[51] In medicine, both diagnosis and prognosis rely heavily on probability theory. When analyzing experimental data, we generally think in statistical terms. Although statistical analysis of data frequently is used to apply results to the clinical situation, it really is valid only for testing hypotheses and estimating outcomes. Statistical approaches are concerned with the concept of a scientific hypothesis, not with medical treatment. Scientific experimentation is based on testing formulated hypotheses. Therefore a scientific hypothesis must be testable and requires, by its mere formulation, verification. Hypotheses should be reasonable, informed, and intelligent guesses about the phenomena observed in nature. They should be stated as far as possible in the "if A occurs, then B occurs" format. They should be testable. The common technique for assessing the plausibility of a scientific hypothesis is by constructing the hypothesis that manipulation of the independent variable (a treatment) has no effect. This is the so-called *null hypothesis* (as discussed previously). The objective of the experimental scientist is to demonstrate that the null hypothesis is untenable and therefore the hypothesis is supported by default (i.e., variation of the independent variable has some effect on the dependent variable).

For this purpose, the scientific hypothesis must be formulated as a statistical hypothesis by deductive inference, which then can be tested by random sampling and estimation from a population and subjected to a specific statistical test (Figure 5–1). The statistical test will determine whether the null hypothesis is tenable or untenable, and this result, by inductive inference, will be applied to the scientific hypothesis under question. This sequence of demonstrating a scientific hypothesis is the basis of experimental medicine. You should not, however, infer that each scientific hypothesis has a specific and pertinent null hypothesis. Multiple null hypotheses may be compatible with the scientific hypothesis tested, and several may need to be tested to give a broad basis of acceptance to the scientific hypothesis. For example, if the scientific theory is "Mortality can be decreased by steroid use in septic shock," a potentially testable statistical hypothesis might be: "Steroids do not alter pH within 24 hours in patients in septic shock." Although the theory would be statistically difficult to demonstrate (and indeed has been) in a patient population by prospective controlled experiment with all other independent variables held constant, this particular null hypothesis could be tested. There are obviously assumptions between the relationship of pH and outcome. A more useful null hypothesis is that survival at 72 hours is not improved by steroids. This is a testable hypothesis, and with the appropriate study design and statistics it can be tested. Obviously, many other statistical hypotheses bearing on the scientific hypothesis can be designed. It is up to the investigator (and the evaluator of the investigation) to understand the relationship between the statistical hypothesis being presented and the scientific hypothesis being tested.

Type I and Type II Errors

The aim of testing the null hypothesis is to either accept or reject it and thus to refute or support the hypothesis.

Statistical decision		TRUTH: Null true	TRUTH: Null false
	Fails to reject null	Correct acceptance $p = 1 - \alpha$	Type II $p = \beta$
	Rejects null	Type I $p = \alpha$	Correct rejection $1 - \beta$

p = probability of choice

α = level of significance (p value)

β = probability of type II error

FIGURE 5–2 • Difference between type I and type II errors in statistical analysis. *Null* refers to the null hypothesis derived from the scientific hypotheses. Note that the likelihood of a type I error, rejection of a true null hypothesis and therefore acceptance of the statistical/scientific hypothesis, is generally equal to the *p* value of the analysis. Thus, when $p = 0.01$ there is only a 1% chance of a type I error. A type II error is more subtle and requires determination of β (see text) to understand the likelihood of falsely rejecting a true hypothesis.

This decision will be either correct or incorrect. *An incorrect decision that leads to invalid conclusions can be made in two different ways.* The first is *rejection of a null hypothesis that is, in fact, true.* This is a *type I error.* Second, a *false null hypothesis may not be rejected* when in fact it ought to be rejected. This is a *type II error.* The difference between these two arises, in part, from the asymmetry of proof described previously. Support for a null hypothesis does not necessarily disprove the hypothesis. There are also two choices of how a correct decision can be made. If there is a true null hypothesis and the experimenter does not reject it, this is correct acceptance of the null hypothesis. If there is a false null hypothesis that is rejected, then a correct rejection has also been made. These choices are summarized in Figure 5–2.

In general, the likelihood of making a *type I error is determined when the level of significance is specified.* The probability of making a type I error is 0.05, when α equals 0.05. This is the probability of rejecting a true null hypothesis. The determination of α also determines the likelihood of the correct acceptance of a true null hypothesis (1 – α). The *probability of making a type II error is symbolized by β.* Thus the probability of correctly rejecting a false null hypothesis equals 1 – β. Alternative terms for these errors are α errors (type I) and β errors (type II) for obvious reasons. β is determined by a number of factors, including sample size, standard deviation of the population in general, difference between the mean of the sample size and the mean of the overall population, whether a one- or a two-tailed test is used, and level of significance selected. The power of a statistical test is defined as the probability of making a correct rejection (1 – β). Because the mean of the overall population size from which the study population is selected is generally unknown, an estimate of it must be made or a value selected that would be of interest. Statistical techniques are available that determine the sample size and population characteristics necessary for the experimental circumstances.[38]

The investigator must determine whether a type I or type II error is more costly. As an example, with regard to steroids and shock research, experiments are generally designed to test the null hypothesis that steroids are not effective as a therapy for shock. A type I error (rejection of the null hypothesis, when it is in fact true) could result in confirming the effectiveness of steroids and lead to their use. The consequences of this decision would be steroid therapy for septic shock. As long as this did not supplant another useful therapy or carry with it complications of its own, the consequences of this error would not be so severe. In contrast, falsely deciding that steroids were not effective, a type II error, would prevent the use of steroids in septic shock. However, further research might be stimulated that ultimately leads to an effective steroid regimen or alternate therapy. In this case, the long-term consequences of a type II error would be less than those of a type I error. A detailed understanding of the importance of accepting or rejecting the null hypothesis for each scientific hypothesis determines at what level type I and type II errors are acceptable. This is necessary information before designing an experiment. *In general, making a type I error is more serious than making a type II error.* For this reason, α frequently is set at 0.05 or 0.01. If a type I error could be very serious, then $p = 0.001$ may be necessary. Unfortunately, as α decreases, β tends to increase.

There are multiple threats to the statistical validity of experimental design. Some of the threats that increase the likelihood of type II errors are

- Unreliability in measurement of the dependent variable that inflates the error variance
- Unreliable treatment, administration, and implementation
- Heterogeneity in the sample population because of idiosyncratic characteristics of subjects inflates the estimate of error variance
- Presence of nuisance variables

To avoid making invalid conclusions or inferences from the data, you must realize that there are certain assumptions in statistical testing. For example, whenever multiple comparisons are made, there is the possibility of an error rate problem. That is, the likelihood of making an erroneous conclusion increases as the number of comparisons on the same set of data increases. To avoid these major errors in statistical design, multiple comparison tests and the definition of which tests are essential will determine which statistical tests are valid.

This introduction to statistical theory forms the essential basis of all experimental statistical testing. Although simple statistics and analysis of variance are by far the most commonly used statistical tests in medicine, the frequency with which they are inappropriately applied is staggering.[43] Study design must be simplified, and the statistical analysis that is to be used should be determined before the experiments are performed. Haphazardly searching for a statistical test to make the data significant is an all too common error that can be seriously misleading. Thus *a priori* decisions are necessary to ensure the validity of the inferences made from statistical tests.

This point cannot be too strongly emphasized. It is the reason the experimental scientist must be familiar with statistics. Employing a mathematical statistician who does not understand the experimental and medical implications of the study to give some magical statistical analysis is inappropriate, especially if attempted *post hoc.* The more the statistician understands the medical setting of the experiment and the more the experimenter understands statistical theory, the more likely the results will be applicable to the children initially intended to benefit from the research.[26,41]

Research Funding

Obtaining Financial Support

Research takes time and costs money. Investigators must have financial support and support to pay for research materials. It is generally incumbent on the investigator with the idea and the enthusiasm for performing the research to acquire financial support. Less experienced scientists must never be told that their ideas are not of sufficient value to consider supporting them. It is necessary for any investigator with extramural funding to support the broader research effort, especially on behalf of young investigators. Without this commitment, the resources necessary for research will never be available. All investigators are aware of the difficulty of obtaining—and the increased competitiveness for—extramural research support. Despite the prophecies of doom and gloom, myriad funding sources remain available.

Since World War II, the prosperity of the United States has enabled the National Institutes of Health (NIH) to become preeminent as a resource supplier for medical research by conscious governmental effort. Although this system has funded the tremendous surge in medical research that contributed to the growth of medical schools, university faculties, and hospitals and a research effort second to none in the world, it also has rendered this establishment dependent on federal dollars. This dependence has made the politicization of medical research difficult to avoid.[54] Some in the research community may express the opinion that these national funding programs have become less supportive of the ideas of individual investigators and more directive of national medical research priorities. Nevertheless, approximately 80% of overall NIH funding still supports investigator-initiated research. The experienced or emerging investigator is left with the need to be familiar with diverse sources of funding and how to access them.

Sources of Research Funding

From the perspective of the investigator, sources of research funding can be broadly divided into *intramural* and *extramural sources. Intramural funding* is that available from *within the investigator's institution.* The source of funds for this research is private endowments, grants, donations and gifts to the university, and clinical funds directed to research support via individual clinical departments. In addition, universities may receive training grants from federal organizations or other granting agencies (so that the source of these funds is *extramural*) to facilitate training, education, and research endeavors by their faculty, fellows, and staff.

Intramural Funding

The first line of funding for the junior investigator generally is intramural funding. Although intramural funding typically is a first source, *securing it should not delay the investigator's exploration of extramural funding possibilities.* Scientific productivity is the first concern for the new investigator, but being productive financially is always an asset. Intramural funds are developed and administered by individual research directors, division and department chiefs, and dean's offices. Donations from patients, private individuals, and corporations and funds generated by the clinical activity of individual faculty members support innovative entrepreneurial "start-up" research projects that serve as pilot and preliminary studies to ultimately obtain extramural funding.

Providing funds for junior investigators is the responsibility of senior physicians with long-term commitments to critical care medicine. Without this "seed" money, new ideas may never get far enough to generate extramural funding and bear the fruit of complete investigation and experimentation. A commitment to research as a vital part of clinical practice, as well as seeking and dispersing gifts and donations, is crucial to ensure vital funding for the research endeavor in critical care medicine. The percentage of research funded from clinical resources, external donations, and extramural research funding varies widely.

Extramural Funding

Extramural funding comes from numerous private and public sources to which the investigator can apply either independently or through the sponsorship and direction of the institution. Federal funding accounts for a large proportion of available extramural support in U.S. universities performing biomedical research. Much of this funding comes from the NIH, and valuable insight into the agency and the process of obtaining funding can be obtained by bookmarking the NIH web site *http://www.nih.gov/.* In this section, we discuss some of the funding opportunities available through the NIH. A subsequent section discusses the NIH structure and operation as a major part of the "research landscape" in the United States.

Extramural sources include

- Private philanthropy
- Industrial grants
- Private grants and contracts
- Government grants and contracts

Exhaustive lists of granting organizations should be available in the deans' offices and offices of sponsored research and research administration. The staffs in these offices may be an underutilized resource at many institutions, and critical care investigators should identify and contact them. The American Association for the Advancement of Science (AAAS) has made several resources in this case to emerging investigators. The *Science* magazine web site *(http://www.sciencemag.org/)* has many useful links, among them the "Next Wave," which is specifically designed for emerging biomedical researchers. For funding questions that seem perplexing, contact the Grant Doctor (e-mail: grantdoctor@aaas.org). A popular search engine for matching biomedical researchers with funding sources is available at *http://www.grantsnet.org*. Another obvious source of funding opportunities comes from within the specialty's collegial network. Conversations with colleagues within the university, professional organizations such as the Society for Critical Care Medicine and the American Academy of Pediatrics, and personal research contacts frequently provide useful information on the current funding available from various sources. In addition, numerous research publications in this field may be found in the medical school or university library or at the dean's office:

- Annual Register of Grant Support
- Catalog of Federal Domestic Assistance
- Commerce Business Daily
- Federal Register
- Foundation Directory
- Foundation Grant Index
- NIH Extramural Programs
- NIH Guide to Grants and Contracts: The table of contents of new scientific funding initiatives is published weekly by the NIH every Friday afternoon. You can review it by going to *http://grants1.nih.gov/grants/guide/index.html.*
- National Science Foundation Guide to Programs
- Research Awards Index

These publications provide an exemplary, but not exhaustive, list of potential resources for research allocation. They provide an excellent starting point. Additionally, most universities have control of career development awards and institutional granting organizations that can provide interim, emergency, and seed support for research projects with the promise of obtaining extramural funding. Again, reference to the local university offices is suggested.

In recent years, the NIH budget has been aggressively increased by Congress, although increases likely will not continue to that degree. The largest segment of the NIH budget goes to funding *extramural* (that is, the research is conducted outside the NIH) investigator-initiated projects, as summarized in Figure 5–3. *Because of the recent budget growth, it is crucial that those with ongoing research interests develop an understanding of the NIH, our federal government's principal agency for the support of biomedical research.*

Although obtaining funding through the NIH can seem daunting, it is best to begin any such endeavor by understanding some of the basic funding mechanisms because this may ultimately assure successful choices. Funding may take several forms. The most common form is direct *grants,* which are reasonably unrestrictive and awarded to institutions in response to specific applications by investigators. These grants provide the major basis of federal funding. Under most circumstances, institutions receive substantial indirect funds from NIH-funded research: an additional 30% to 50% is added to

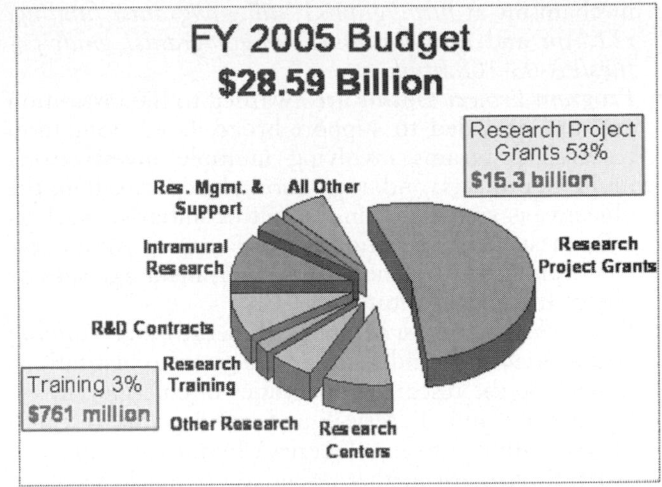

FIGURE 5–3 • National Institutes of Health (NIH) budget for fiscal year 2002. More than 80% of NIH funds support investigator-initiated science outside of the NIH.

the grant amount, supplying the institution with substantial support for facilities and administration (also known as "F and A" or *indirect* costs). There are many types of NIH grants: the investigator should peruse all of them at *http://grants1.nih.gov/grants/index.cfm.* The following brief discussion of a few of these mechanisms is introductory only.

- *Research Project Grants (R01s)* are awarded to an institution on behalf of a principal investigator who has requested support for a specific research project in an area in which he/she is competent and interested. This funding mechanism is widely considered to be the vehicle for successful scientific support and the goal of the investigator with serious research aspirations.

  A characteristic of the R01 from the NIH is that it usually is investigator initiated. (Occasionally there are scientific initiatives published soliciting R01 applications). Most NIH funding goes to investigator- initiated proposals, and the R01 is the most commonly used mechanism. The research plan focuses on a specific set of research aims, and the plan to achieve these aims typically is hypothesis driven. The level of support varies; the budget (direct costs) of an R01 typically is $150,000 to $250,000 per year, with 3 to 5 years of support requested. The award is renewable, in a competitive renewal process.
- *Small Grants and Exploratory/Developmental Grants:* The R03 is a small grant mechanism that offers $50- (direct costs) as a level of support for 2 years. Although not all institutes offer this funding mechanism, it is often used as a first independent funding mechanism by new or emerging investigators. It may be especially useful for obtaining pilot data to answer scientific questions or provide direction for future larger studies. The R21 or exploratory/developmental grant provides 2 years of support for planning research or for exploration of scientific questions, particularly innovative approaches. This funding mechanism is available on an investigator-initiated basis at the NICHD. Pediatric critical care researchers may want to investigate these

mechanisms at *http://grants1. nih.gov/grants/ funding/ r21.htm* and *http://grants1. nih.gov/grants/ guide/pa-files/PA-03-108.html.*

- *Program Project Grants* are awarded to the institution and are provided to support broad-based, long-term research programs involving multiple investigators, multiple projects, and a common objective. Often, the objective is announced in a scientific initiative, such as a Request for Applications, or a Program Announcement, published by one of the government agencies or one of the NIH institutes.
- *Research Career Development* (K series) and *Training Grant Awards* (F and T series) are given to institutions to develop the research capabilities of emerging investigators (F and T series) and to develop research careers with mentoring (K series). In our emerging specialty, these merit further discussion (see below).

  At the junior faculty level, career development awards are available for those wishing to enhance their emerging research careers through work with an experienced mentor. Every junior faculty member with research as a substantial interest should visit the "K Kiosk" at *http://grants1.nih.gov/training/careerdevelopmentawards.htm* and "Career Development Wizard" at *http://grants1.nih.gov/training/kwizard/index.htm* on the NIH web site. These are salary support grants that provide mentored research time for individual emerging investigators. Typically, 75% salary support is provided. This NIH award series has been expanded in recent years. Some of the specific career development and fellowship awards of significance to critical care investigators are listed below. The usefulness of the links to the K Kiosk and Career Development Wizard cannot be overemphasized.

  The K series (K01, K08, K23, and several others) provide mentored investigator funding opportunities from the NIH and often are used as a first funding mechanism. Choice of mentors is *crucial,* and this choice should be made with the emerging investigator's interests foremost. An exciting new development for emerging scientists in pediatric critical care is the Pediatric Critical Care Scientist Development program, established in 2004. The program director is available at Mike.Dean@hsc. utah.edu. A directory of mentors, application materials, and other assistance also is available through Dr. Dean.
- *Institutional Training Grants (T32):* These awards are made to institutions for support of graduate research training, postdoctoral research training, and research fellowships in clinical and basic science investigation.

Another funding source is *contracts.* These formal agreements are made either with the federal government (often the NIH but many other federal agencies also issue research contracts) industry or with private foundations for specific research projects designed by the grantor of the contract. Research contracts can be divided broadly into (1) contracts that provide reimbursement for the cost of investigations and experiments, and (2) fixed-price contracts that basically are awarded to achieve a specific goal at a fixed cost to the grantor of the research contract. *Cooperative agreements* ("U series" funding mechanisms) are becoming increasingly important, especially in research networks. The government agency enters into an agreement with the investigator(s) to manage the project cooperatively, for example, the new National Collaborative Pediatric Critical Care Research Network (see link in research areas section). These awards are made after application for specific funding opportunities published by the NIH. The specific collaborative terms are spelled out between the investigator and the funding organization. It generally is wise that the university office of research administration is intimately involved in establishing these terms. One well-known successful example of a cooperative agreement used to support research is the Collaborative Neonatal Research Network funded since 1986, used as the framework for the National Pediatric Critical Care Collaborative Research Network established in 2005.

Industry is providing a greater portion of research resources. In 1980, 30% of health research was funded by industry compared with 59% by the federal government. By 1990 industry was funding 45% compared with government funding 40%. Such trends likely will continue. Industry supports research in two ways: first by funding foundations that support research and second by contracting with researchers to perform specific, directed product development, such as drug trials, clinical studies, and product evaluation. Information about these programs is available from the sources listed earlier and from the Food and Drug Administration (FDA). In addition, investigators are directly contacted by industry representatives.

Awareness that industry (pharmaceutical agencies, insurance companies, medical equipment companies) has the money to fund their research priorities and wants to carry out such studies should motivate all in pediatric critical care to extend contacts and increase awareness of these opportunities. In addition to direct business contacts, the critical care investigator should become familiar with the Small Business Innovation Research and Technology Transfer (SBIR/STTR) Programs at *http://grants1.nih.gov/grants/funding/sbir.htm.* The NIH SBIR/STTR program is an important source of research funding, and companies seeking professional research consulting are listed on the SBIR/STTR site.

Foundations may be *merely philanthropic* (funding good ideas) or they may be *directive* (addressing issues of specific interest to the foundation).[66] They can bring investigators together, fund research, and disseminate ideas. Foundations are a source of research "venture capital" and as such often take greater risks than federal funding agencies.[66] Accepting research support from *industry* (whether through a foundation or more direct corporate source) has ethical implications.[61] Research and clinical decisions should be guided by data, not funding sources. Private funding for research, especially if lavish, may raise questions regarding the integrity of the researcher; for this reason prospective ethical guidelines are essential. Clear declaration of all potential or even seemingly potential conflicts of interest must be made.[45] Although absolute ethical integrity is the cornerstone of research (see below), it is nowhere more critical or more readily corrupted than when dealing with profit-motivated industry.

National Institutes of Health

The NIH is the federal government's agency for funding biomedical research. It is an agency of the Department of Health and Human Services (DHHS). The DHHS has overall responsibility for many agencies, including the Centers for Disease Control and Prevention, the FDA, the Substance Abuse and Mental Health Services Administration (SAMSHA), Health Resources and Services Administration (HRSA), Agency for Healthcare Research and Quality (AHRQ), and the NIH. Many of these agencies (and other federal agencies) have research funding programs in addition to that of the NIH. The NIH is made up of 27 institutes and centers. Its structure is summarized in Figure 5–4.

Most of these individual NIH institutes and centers have programs that provide both intramural (internal to the NIH) and extramural (outside the NIH) funding support for research. The institutes with only extramural funding programs are shown in black in Figure 5–4. Some of the NIH institutes that may be supportive of critical care research and therefore are familiar are

- National Institute of Child Health and Human Development (NICHD)
- National Heart, Lung and Blood Institute (NHLBI)
- National Cancer Institute (NCI)
- National Institute of Diabetes, Digestive and Kidney Disease (NIDDK)
- National Institute of General Medical Sciences (NIGMS)

Both NICHD and NIGMS have formal programs that are specifically supportive of critical care research. Both institutes offer career development, institutional and individual training awards, and investigator initiated awards. Program staff contacts for each are

NIGMS: Scott Somers, PhD, e-mail: *somerss@mail.nih.gov*

NICHD: Carol E. Nicholson, MD, MS, e-mail: *nicholca@mail.nih.gov*

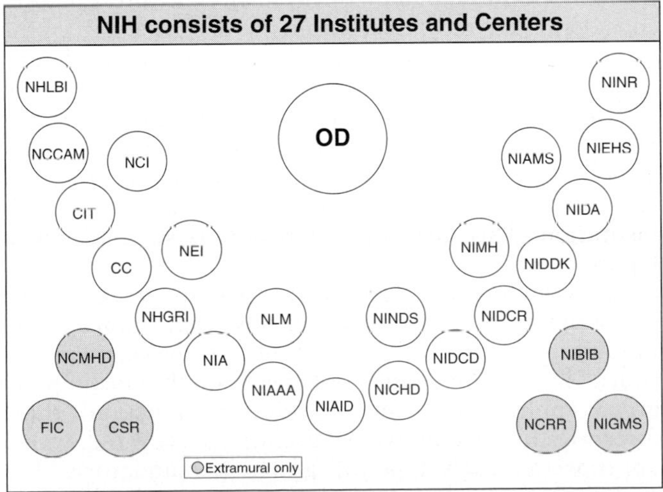

FIGURE 5–4 • The 27 institutes and centers at the National Institutes of Health (NIH). Those shown in *white* support both intramural (at the NIH) and extramural science. Those with *gray backgrounds* support only extramural science.

The NIH extramural programs are divided into grants, contracts, and cooperative agreements. The role of the NIH in each of these programs is, respectively: (1) patron, as granting agency (grants), to provide assistance and encouragement; (2) purchaser (contracts), to provide procurement of necessary resources; and (3) partner (cooperative agreements), an assistance mechanism (rather than an "acquisition" mechanism) in which substantial NIH scientific and/or programmatic involvement with the awardee is anticipated during performance of the activity. *The major type of extramural funding continues to be support for individual investigator-initiated proposals through the grant mechanism.*

The NIH publishes *The NIH Guide for Grants and Contracts*, which announces NIH scientific initiatives and provides NIH policy and administrative information. The guide publishes notices, program announcements (PAs), requests for applications (RFAs), and requests for proposals (RFPs). It is important for investigators to understand the basic differences in these scientific initiatives. Checking the guide weekly (subscribe at *http://grants1.nih. gov/grants/guide/listserv.htm*) provides access to the latest funding initiatives at the NIH. PAs have no specific funds set aside but indicate broad areas of ongoing research interest within the NIH. RFAs are formal announcements describing an institute's initiative in a specified scientific area. *They serve as invitations to investigators in the field to submit research grant applications for a one-time competitive assessment. They are very important funding opportunities, as RFAs have funds already set aside for a certain number of awards in the area requested.*

Following is a general scheme of how an NIH grant application is processed. This scheme serves as the model for grant applications discussed in the following section (Figure 5–5). The investigator initiates a research idea and, in conjunction with the school or other research center, submits an application to the NIH. Applications initially go to the NIH Office of Receipt and Referral, officially part of the Center for Scientific Review (CSR), where the application is assigned to the appropriate study section and institute. The study section, as the peer review groups are widely known, evaluates the study for scientific and technical merit and assigns a priority score. The grant application is evaluated for programmatic relevance by the NIH staff of the individual institutes and submitted to the Advisory Council, which officially recommends funding action to the director of the institute. The responsibility of each component of this review system for grant applications is outlined in Figure 5–6. The first-level peer review provides the initial scientific review of grant applications for scientific merit and assigns them a competitive score, using the criteria in Appendix 5–A. The instructions to reviewers are reproduced here for investigator convenience but can be downloaded from the Center for Scientific Review web site ("Guide for Assigned Reviewers' Preliminary Comments on Research Grant Applications [R01]." Note that different funding mechanisms may have different review criteria. The criteria for each funding mechanism are available at *http://www.csr.nih.gov/guidelines/guidelines.htm.*)

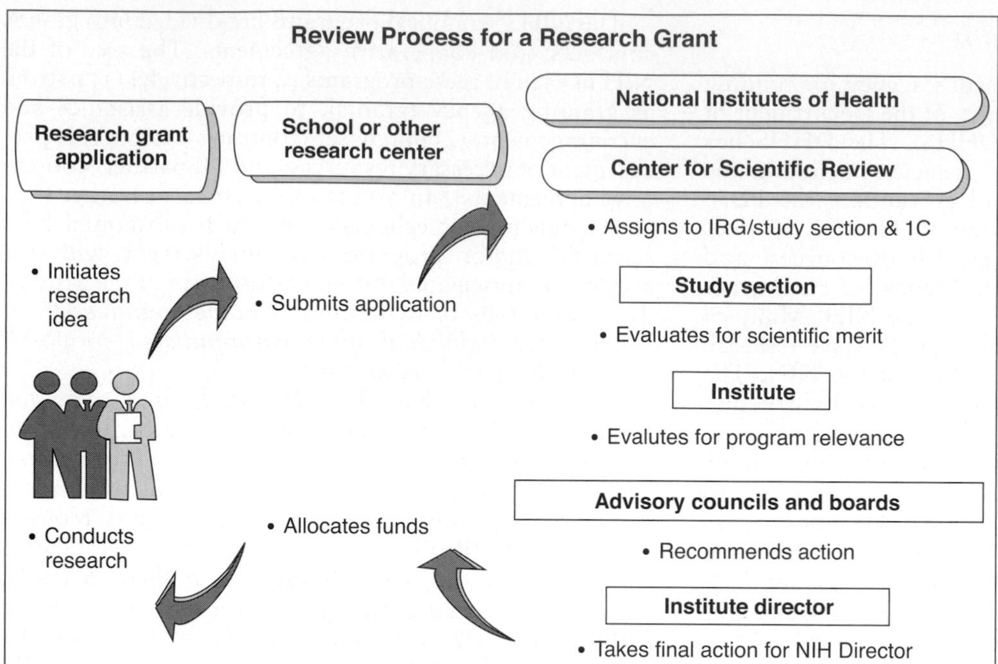

FIGURE 5–5 • Schematic representation of the course a National Institutes of Health grant application follows in the review process. (Courtesy Office of Extramural Research, Office of the Director, National Institutes of Health, Bethesda, MD.)

This first-level review, known as *peer review* (*study section* is often used to describe the first-level review group), does not set program priorities or make funding decisions. Study sections now can triage noncompetitive (those proposals in the bottom 50% of those being reviewed at a given session) submissions.[44] This is called *streamlined review. These proposals are still exhaustively reviewed by the same number of study section members, but the proposal is not scored, and the merits and limitations are not discussed in the study sections.* The reasoning is that these proposals are not presently fundable, and what is really needed is a thorough critique that conveys to the applicant-investigator (1) the level of overall enthusiasm among the reviewers for the proposed research and (2) specific, helpful feedback to the investigators. Sometimes, specific actions required to make the proposal more competitive are suggested. All proposals, scored and unscored, receive this feedback.

After scientific merit review in the study section, the scored proposals go to the second level of review, which is the Advisory Council. The Advisory Council is a national-level group composed of distinguished scientists and community members who advise the director of the institute on policy and funding decisions. Here, the quality of the study review group's assessment of the grant application is evaluated, and the council makes recommendations for funding to the institute's director after considering the recommendations of program staff of the institute. At this second level of review, the council evaluates program priorities and relevance by recommending funding and advises on policy. The institute's director takes final action to allocate funds. When funds are allocated, the individual researcher conducts the research using the allocated funds granted to the investigator's institution. This dual level of review is summarized in Figure 5–6.

Granting organizations have gone to great trouble to prepare extensive instructions that explain the funding procedure and instructions for making applications. Instructions and policies usually accompany grant application forms. Specific reference to these directions for each individual granting agency and, where appropriate, each type of grant is mandatory. The investigator should exhaustively study and adhere to these guidelines and recommendations. Most funding agencies have identified research program staff to assist investigators.

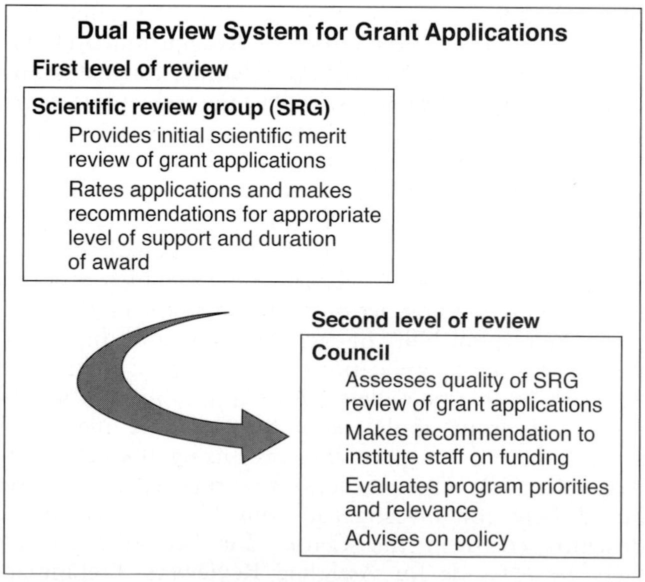

Dual Review System for Grant Applications

First level of review

Scientific review group (SRG)
Provides initial scientific merit review of grant applications
Rates applications and makes recommendations for appropriate level of support and duration of award

Second level of review

Council
Assesses quality of SRG review of grant applications
Makes recommendation to institute staff on funding
Evaluates program priorities and relevance
Advises on policy

FIGURE 5–6 • All National Institutes of Health grant applications undergo two levels of review. Of note is that the study group does not make funding decisions. It can, however, review and advise on the appropriateness of the proposal budget. (Courtesy of Office of Extramural Research, Office of the Director, National Institutes of Health, Bethesda, MD.)

Writing the Grant Application

In making grant applications, particular attention should be paid to the due dates and instructions for application. Although the following guidelines are specifically intended for NIH grant applications, they serve as general guidelines for any granting organization. It seems superfluous to say that no matter how brilliant the idea, it must be presented to the granting organization in a readily accessible, understandable, clear, and concise fashion. Tens of thousands of grants are reviewed annually by the NIH. Those that clearly, concisely, and quickly present their plan are most readily funded. Six simple guidelines follow:

1. Read and study the instructions
2. Present a well-organized, precise, lucid explanation of all points
3. Never assume the reviewers will know what you mean
4. Explicitly and clearly state the rationale of the proposed investigation
5. Refer thoroughly to, and demonstrate thoughtful familiarity with, the literature
6. Use well-designed tables and figures; a picture is worth a thousand words

Remember that your peers who will be reviewing the grants are at the top of the scientific community pyramid (Figure 5–7). They are active and productive researchers who have been through the process themselves. They are both sympathetic and critical. There are no guarantees that they are interested in the individual investigator's area of expertise, that they are uniformly knowledgeable about it, or that they are committed to funding it. As a matter of fact, NIH reviewers are specifically admonished to make no evaluation or recommendation about funding. Rather, the reviewers' judgment of scientific merit is to be precise and thorough. *Most reviewers want to act as advocates for individual research proposals;* it is the investigator's responsibility to *provide the reviewer with the ammunition necessary to support the research proposal accurately and effectively to the study section as a whole.* Reviewers are particularly interested in the following areas:

- Significance and originality of the scientific and technical approach of the proposal
- Qualifications and experience of the principal investigator and staff, not only by previous productivity but also as demonstrated in the body of the proposal
- Likelihood for success by the methodology specifically applied in the proposal
- Availability of resources to complete the research in the proposal
- Reasonableness of the budget and time allocated for the investigation
- Other factors such as the use of human subjects, animal welfare and care provisions, biohazards, and risks within the proposal
- Research career development plan specifics for younger investigators, especially the choice and quality of mentor

When writing a grant, it is essential that the same care and consideration, if not more, for the development of ideas and presentation of concepts be used as in the final publication of the research. The review process of a research grant application will be every bit as critical and rigorous as the review for publication of articles. To allow an ongoing contribution to the research effort in the field, success with grant applications is always a necessary step. The following section serves only as a quick overview of how a grant should be written. Basic concepts that underlie all successful grant applications are that they present a good idea backed up with good science and presented in a well-written format. When writing a grant, bear in mind the advice of the U.S. Public Health Service

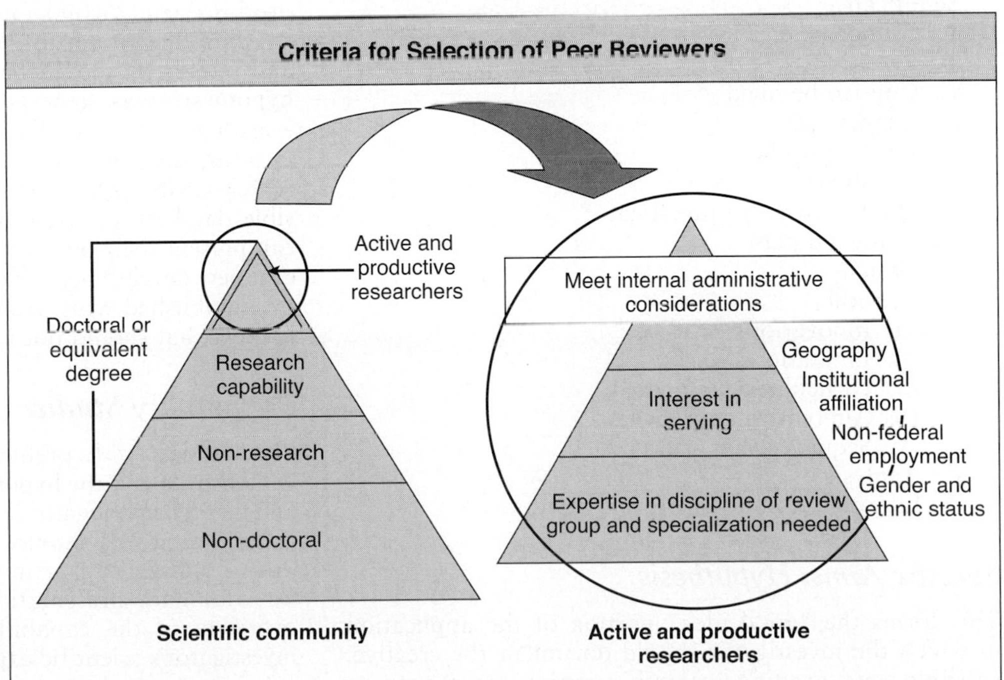

FIGURE 5–7 • Reviewers are chosen from the peak of the scientific community's active researchers. (Courtesy of Office of Extramural Research, Office of the Director, National Institutes of Health, Bethesda, MD.)

application form for grants. Four questions must be approached:

1. What do you intend to do? (specific aims)
2. Why is it important? (significance)
3. What has already been done? (preliminary studies, other investigations)
4. How are you going to do it? (experimental plan)

Writing a grant proposal can be an intimidating and confusing pastime; however, lucidly presenting these simple points not only makes a grant easier to present but also easier to award. As George Eaves pointed out, it is important that even beginning investigators realize they are assessed on the quality of the grant and not just on their track record[22]:

"If you are a beginning investigator submitting your first application and worried because you do not have a professional reputation, remember that you will have already impressed the reviewers in the literature section by your familiarity with the field, and your capability for keen and wise discrimination between the significant and the banal, the valid and the presumed..."

The research grant application provides numerous opportunities to demonstrate qualifications and scholarly attributes; however, it also readily reveals faulty thinking, hasty preparation, superficiality, and inexperience. A "seven steps" process that has been helpful to many investigators is given in Appendix 5–B.

Eaves[22] has expanded the four sections of the Public Health Service Grant as outlined in the following:

1. Aims
   A. Hypothesis
   B. Objectives
2. Significance
   A. Background
   B. Literature
   C. Gaps to be filled
   D. Importance
3. Preliminary studies
   A. Feasibility
   B. Qualifications of investigator
4. Experimental plan
   A. Design
   B. Methods
      I. Innovations
      II. Limitations
      III. Difficulties anticipated
      IV. Alternative approaches
      V. Sequence
   C. Analysis of data
   D. Interpretation of anticipated results

Specific Aims: Hypothesis

This forms the "good idea" portion of the application in which the investigator should document the creative, valuable, and exciting research questions that need to be answered. It justifies the rest of the proposal. Research is generated from this basic hypothesis. In general, the hypothesis should be aimed at delineating, explaining, understanding, or defining mechanisms of action. This is in distinction to those where the goals are merely observational, empirical, or data-gathering exercises. Frequently this is a matter of correctly stating the research endeavor. For example, an investigation to determine whether there are gender differences in hypoxic pulmonary vasoreactivity (HPV) could be justified on a descriptive basis, or it could be justified based on using the differences between male and female responses to investigate the estrogen-modulated endothelial release of prostacyclin, which in turn modifies HPV and provides a mechanistic answer.[68,69] A hypothesis directed at determining the mechanisms modulating HPV is of more interest than merely empirically demonstrating a gender difference in response.[71] The specific research proposal should have specific, achievable, well-defined goals that are neither overly ambitious nor superficial. For NIH proposals, *these research aims should be conveyed, via e-mail, to the program staff of the institute that is the contemplated recipient of the proposals.* Criticism, tightening, and delineation of hypotheses should be completed and reconveyed to the investigator. Then, biostatistical assistance, including power analysis, can be obtained and a detailed research plan generated.

Although the specific proposal should have specific aims, it also is important to present how these research aims fit the broader picture. Relate the research aims and hypotheses of the grant to long-term scientific objectives and integrate them into the overall field relevant to the proposal. All of the problems in an area of research cannot be solved by one research proposal.[31]

Significance

Although the literature supports the significance of the proposed study, you should present a thorough familiarity with the literature, its deficiencies, contradictions, and pitfalls. It should be clear to the reviewer how the hypothesis was generated from the current field of knowledge and exactly how the present proposal fits into that area readily and concisely. Investigators should search CRISP *(http://crisp.cit.nih.gov/)*, a publicly accessible database of federally funded studies, so that they can present their own work as innovative and an important new development of the science in the field. Inclusion of unpublished work from other colleagues, if available, is useful but should not be overused.

Preliminary Studies

Pilot studies with preliminary results are necessary to demonstrate that the hypothesis is testable and supportable and that the investigator has the capabilities of pursuing the research goals. Reference to abstracts and papers previously published by the investigator and preliminary studies with data presentation should provide a complete overview of the capabilities of the investigators. The investigator's scientific capabilities must be evident in the presentation of the proposal.[22,31]

Experimental Plan

The methodology should be appropriate, available, well worked out, and well supported. In addition, it should be specifically targeted and precisely capable of addressing the questions raised in the specific aims. Methodology must be described in sufficient length so that the reviewers can be assured that valid results will be achieved. If the investigator has published results using the methods described in the grant, they should be referenced and perhaps included in the appendix to the grant proposal. If new methodology is being proposed, extensive detail is necessary to assure the reviewers of the applicability of new methodology, as is inclusion of preliminary results demonstrating the likelihood of success of the experiments.[22,31,32]

When assessing the research potential, it is essential to demonstrate a critical awareness of the shortcomings and strengths of the proposal. As clear a statement as possible of the underlying assumptions and their validity and of the limitations and applicability of the proposed research plan should be presented. Investigators applying for career development awards (K awards) should be aware that although the science they propose will be reviewed, the most rigorous analysis will be applied by the reviewers to the career development plan as outlined. The mentor's commitment to the emerging investigator must be specific, and the mentor must be well qualified for the task. Specific discussion must be provided as to how the requested support will result in the development of the scientist who is capable of achieving the aims of the proposal. Formal course work and specifically mentored laboratory work may be two crucial elements in this plan.

Specific attention must be paid to how the data will be evaluated, analyzed, and statistically approached. An expert statistician's input before submission of the proposal, with an estimate of statistical power and the appropriate number and type of experiments to be performed, is of great value in strengthening any research proposal. At the end of reading the method section of the proposal, the reviewer should be sure that the investigator understands and intends to use good scientific method to address specific aims in a logical, clear, focused, and precise manner. The investigator should demonstrate an overall familiarity with the area, with a critical review not only of other researchers but also of his/her own capabilities and potential for actually accomplishing the desired research goals and properly analyzing them.

Presentation

The final necessity for a research proposal is that it be well presented. Although the overall number of grants have not decreased over the years, the competition for them has become greater. Visually attractive, well-presented, easy-to-follow, clearly delineated research proposals will clearly stand out from the herd. Although showmanship will not make up for poor substance, *sloppy applications may obscure good science.* The first rule is strict adherence to the guidelines in the research application with regard to page number, layout, content, and other details. A clear, simple, lucid, grammatically correct, and typographically perfect presentation is essential; leave nothing to assumption and guesswork. Seek as much help as possible. Senior department members, deans, review offices, research administrations, English teachers, spouses, lay people, and other investigators all may have valuable contributions to make to the clarity of a research proposal. Frequently, it is worthwhile to have a grant proposal read by an outside, independent, unbiased assessor before it is submitted to the NIH. Review by a successful investigator who is neither familiar with nor involved in the research area can be invaluable.

It is necessary to demonstrate familiarity with and commitment to the guidelines and recommendations for both human and animal experimentation. Obtaining institutional review board (IRB) approval of research proposals before submission to the NIH is not mandatory. Be aware, however, that the proposal will not be funded until this clearance is officially verified. The internal review process of the institution may be of benefit in establishing and clarifying research proposals. Finally, budget preparation must be meticulous. As a general rule, everything should be justified briefly and concisely. *Although nothing in excess should be asked for, the investigator must request sufficient resources to achieve the specific aims.* Availability of other resources, such as capital equipment, research space, and collaborative resources, to complete the work should be demonstrated. Frequently, preparation of the budget for the proposal is a very time-consuming process. The investigator should not be intimidated by this process. The investigator should first determine precisely what is needed to perform the experiments and what the technical and personnel needs are, then in conjunction with the university determine fair costs for these items, supported with documentation where necessary. Reviewers are most concerned with completeness of budgetary considerations. A grant that has insufficient resources to achieve its goals is a waste of time, money, and effort on behalf of the NIH and the investigator.

These suggestions serve only as guidelines for grant applications. In addition, we (the authors of this chapter) can be contacted for assistance in identifying resources by intensivists serious about research. A "seven steps" guide developed by one of the authors has been helpful to many and is given in Appendix 5–B.

In closing, it is perhaps worthwhile to note why grants fare poorly, as proposed by Cuca and McLoughlin[18] in an eight-point system for describing the shortcomings:

1. *Research Problem:* Hypothesis: ill-defined, lacking, faulty, diffuse, unwarranted
2. *Research Problem:* Significance: unimportant, unimaginative, unlikely to provide new information
3. *Experimental Design:* Study Group or Control: inappropriate, composition, number, characteristic
4. *Experimental Design:* Technical Methodology: questionable, unsuited, defective
5. *Experimental Design:* Data Collection Procedures: confused design, inappropriate instrumentation, timing, or conditions
6. *Experimental Design:* Data Management and Analysis: vague, unsophisticated, not likely to provide accurate and clearcut results

7. *Investigator:* Inadequate expertise or familiarity with literature in the research area, poor past performance or productivity on an NIH grant, insufficient time to be devoted to the project
8. *Resources:* Inadequate institutional setting, support staff, laboratory facilities, equipment, or personnel; restricted access to patient populations; insufficient involvement or collaboration of colleagues or coinvestigators

Before finally submitting a grant application, investigators should look critically at this list and make sure that none of these deficiencies can be found in the application. If deficiencies are determined, then collaboration and help from outside the institution or obtaining further experience and consultation from other investigators is strongly recommended.

Your Chances: Money

Anyone who is in the remotest way connected with the biomedical research effort in the United States is aware that there is never sufficient money to fund all of the worthy ideas. Whether this money crunch arises from the desire to cure acquired immunodeficiency syndrome or map the entire human genome (both laudable goals), budget deficits, or shifting priorities, a competitive system will be necessary for the foreseeable future. The concern for the continued existence of medical research has led to some pretty horrific statements. An optimistic note is that the NIH "has more money, awards more grants and supports more research than ever before."[24] More dollars go to research than at any previous time, and more awards are made. In addition, young researchers appear to have a higher success rate than older researchers as seen by looking at R01s awarded in fiscal 1989.[46] The success rate for principal investigators younger than 36 years was 23% and for those older than 50 years was merely 13%. These facts continue to impress researchers and politicians.

Despite this finding, we all wonder "how we can look so rich and feel so poor."[24] Warnings are sounded throughout the academic world. As the president of the Federation of American Societies and Experimental Biology (FASEB) told the Senate[46]: "The scientists are deeply concerned that without the assurance of sufficient number of new awards for research, promising young investigators are now turning to other careers, depriving the nation of future scientific leadership and economic competitiveness." An article published in *Science* titled "Young Investigators at Risk" concluded that even the best and brightest young scientists are struggling to make it in academic science.[55] The fear remains that "we are going to turn off an entire generation of new biomedical scientists, just at the time when we need them most."[55]

What does this all mean? Here are some facts relative to biomedical research funding:

1. Over the past several years, the NIH budget has doubled, with completion of this process by 2002. Such expansions likely will not be forthcoming again in the foreseeable future. Nevertheless, the Congress has made its intentions quite clear: the desire is for an expanded, rather than contracted, biomedical research effort.
2. The percentage of applications funded varies by institute, budgetary availability, and national priorities. All of these factors have sustained major changes in recent times. It is likely that considerable variation and change will remain in the system for the foreseeable future.
3. In 1993, 4121 of 19,072 R01s were funded.
4. The average period for which grants are funded was 4.3 years in 1990, with 50% of funded grants for more than 5 years.
5. Research project grants undergo an average 12% budget cut after award.
6. Increasingly more people are submitting grants; that is, the competition is getting tougher.

This last fact is one for which we should be grateful. More people are involved in medical research now than at any previous time in our history, and more funding is going toward it. Priorities for biomedical research shift with national priorities, economic change, technologic and business developments, and political interest. Total reliance upon funding from the federal government is unjustified. This is why we must be aware of all available sources of extramural funding. It is necessary for us to continue to encourage industrial and private support for research endeavors in pediatric critical care and to provide clinical income to support this research. The perception of "tight funding" is *not* an excuse to discontinue pursuing the data upon which future grant applications will depend and from which future improvements in pediatric critical care will come.

Your Chances: Cultures in Conflict

By training, philosophy, motivation and research style, doctors and scientists might as well be from different phyla.

New York Times, April 24, 1992

The competition is not merely other pediatric intensivists. Researchers in pediatric critical care must be involved with, collaborate with, and be familiar with the work of investigators from other areas of medicine who are not only clinical researchers but also basic scientists. As pediatric intensivists, our goals are to improve the care of our patients. As basic scientists, our goals are to understand all the issues involved with our hypothesis, regardless of its impact on patient care.

A *JAMA* editorial titled "The Two Cultures of Biomedicine: Can There Be a Consensus?" crystallizes the problem.[30] A researcher-developer stated, "For medicine to advance, you have to be willing to have your patient die on the operating table," whereas a typical clinician said, "The more important thing when you are starting, is to finish with a live patient." These two approaches must be made compatible, and both are essential for our patients' well-being. The practical, goal-oriented, patient-concerned physician must apply the results of biomedical science *and* work in close collaboration with the basic researcher to maintain the appropriate focus. Pure scientists are concerned with studying the underlying abstract mechanisms of diseases, which, to them, may be abstract entities.[2] Frequently conflicts arise when physicians view researchers as detached and cold and pursuing irrelevant goals. The researchers view physicians as poor researchers. This is expressed in the *New York Times* by a research director: "I go through medically oriented publications and see they don't have enough controls and they ignore relevant interpretations of their data. You can get the idea that doctors are too free and easy with science."[2]

The fact that two cultures in biomedical research exist is clear. This is recognized not only by teaching hospitals, where they tend to exist side by side, but also by the community and clearly by the NIH. This division cannot be allowed to develop as a polarized dichotomy. The two sides need each other. Physician-researchers are classically viewed as the pinnacle of academic success, but only inasmuch as they are true researchers who understand patients' needs. The fact that they are so well respected supports the notion that they also are quite rare. Cooperation between these two cultures of biomedical research is the only hope for clinical and basic biomedical science, and neither can exist without the other, contrary to what either may wish. As Tom Stossel said[67]:

"Modern medicine is an increasingly complex and troubled profession, but most will agree that science is at its heart. People know this and demand technical and scientific excellence as well as caring from their physicians. Consumers' wishes aside, the constant evaluation and reevaluation of the knowledge base in medicine—pathogenesis, diagnosis and therapy—is a medical categorical imperative. Physical, biologic and behavioral sciences underpin medicine, but the science that is unique to medicine is clinical investigation."

Competition for limited resources will remain intense. There should, however, be no competition over turf. There need be no competition over areas of interest, and indeed there can be no competition from nonphysicians in the unique science of medicine/clinical investigation. Allocation of resources will be in the direction where collaboration, cooperation, and cross-fertilization between the two cultures of biomedical science are the most fertile. There is no need for competition for ideas. As Stossel concluded: "All kinds of research are needed. The fund of medical knowledge seems vast indeed, but the reservoir of ignorance is even greater."[67]

Ethics in Research

"There is no vice that doth so cover a man with shame as to be found false and perfidious."

Francis Bacon, 1578

A comprehensive presentation of the ethical issues that face investigators in pediatric critical care is beyond the scope of this chapter. Each clinical investigator must be thoroughly aware of the ethics of human investigation before committing children to the necessary uncertainties of research.[39] Issues of information, understanding and consent, risk to patient and investigator, privacy, Health Insurance Portability and Accountability Act (HIPAA; see *http://www.hhs.gov/ocr/hipaa/*) concerns, and the welfare of patients participating in research have been thoroughly discussed in many publications. All of these issues require the investigator's attention. There is, however, more. It cannot be too strongly stressed that intrinsic to these issues is the necessity for well-designed studies that are likely to yield useful results and to be of future benefit either to the patients enrolled in a given trial or to future patients. As Nelson[53] has stated:

"The prospective, randomized, double-blind, controlled, multicenter clinical trial requires a pre-contract among investigator, physician and informed patient that the rigorous rules of statistical mathematics will be enforced...."

Performing shoddy or slipshod science is the single, most unethical action possible for any investigator, experienced or naive, to commit. For those investigators involved in animal research, rigid adherence to standards of ethical animal treatment is necessary.[27,57] These standards should be as stringently maintained as in human trials. One animal sacrificed in a poorly designed study that yields useless results is one too many. These sort of experiments lend credence to the animal rightist's bumper sticker: "Animal research = Scientific fraud." All investigators should adhere to the rules and procedures of their local institution, their state governments, and the NIH when dealing with animals in a humane fashion.[1,12] Constantly reviewing how subjects—children and animals—are treated and the value of any trial or experiment is a mandatory part of professional scientific practice.

Nothing is more important in the practice of medical investigation than absolutely rigid, scrupulous adherence to the truth. The goal of research is to discover true results upon which to base sound conclusions. This goal is threatened in two major ways. The first is poor science, sloppy techniques, and "honest errors." The second is fraud. Both must be avoided. As CP Snow[65] has said:

"The only ethical principle which has made science possible is that the truth shall be told all the time. If we do not penalize false

statements made in error, we open up the way, don't you see, for false statements by intention. And, of course, a false statement of fact, made deliberately, is the most serious crime a scientist can commit."

False statements made intentionally or in error cannot be tolerated. This is important not only during the final summation and reporting of results but also at every step along the way. *The least suggestion of fudging or poor study design, the least bit of misrepresentation of results at any stage, is merely the first step on the slippery slope that ultimately leads to out-and-out fraud.* Advice given by Samuel Johnson[37] in 1778 is valuable for all of us who are concerned with scientific observation and reporting, whether supervising or performing research at any level:

"Accustom your children constantly to this: If a thing happened at one window and they, when relating it, say that it happened in another window, do not let it pass, but instantly check them; you do not know where deviation from the truth will end."

Several threats to the truth occur during the course of medical research. As in all things, recognizing the potential errors is the first step in preventing them. From the very conceptualization of the hypothesis, when there is a risk for plagiarism, through the indifference of senior investigators, to the final analysis of data, the truth is challenged. Charles Babbage, the nineteenth-century mathematical genius remembered as the prophet of the electronic computer, gave us three interesting definitions nearly 150 years ago*:

"Trimming: the smoothing of irregularities to make the data look extremely accurate and precise.
Cooking: analyzing only those results that fit the theory and disregarding others.
Forging: inventing some or all the research data reported, or reporting experiments to obtain those data which were not performed."

Every investigator at every level must incessantly resist these temptations. Meticulously resisting overzealous curve fitting, data smoothing, data elimination, and data insertion is necessary. All forms of unacceptable behavior stem from one or more of these three cases, or from carelessness or plagiarism. Although we may not be certain where the slightest "deviation from the truth will end,"[37] we can be certain that, in time, these deviations will be discovered. As Shakespeare says[63]:

"Time's glory is to calm contending kings,
To unmask falsehood and bring truth to light."

Scientific fraud will be discovered in the long run. An interesting, if extreme, example is that involving the Nobel prize-winning physicist Robert A. Millikan. Not until 1978 was research he published in 1913 discovered to be based on cooked data.[48] Millikan represented his results as being from an unselected, consecutive group of drops, which he examined for electrical charge. As it turns out, the group was highly selected. Although 65 years elapsed before the truth emerged, the certainty of Shakespeare's dictum was supported. Generally the discovery of fraud is not so protracted. This is a good thing; otherwise, the errors resulting from subsequent work based on false data could be quite serious. Adding fraudulent bricks to the edifice of medical knowledge undermines the entire structure and may add to suffering of critically ill children and their families.

In addition to the certainty of discovery aspect of Millikan's error, another lesson is evident. This particular case demonstrates that even the great are not immune to the temptations of dishonestly interfering with results. Perhaps our conviction and love for our hypotheses, which may lead to "honest errors," also occasionally lead to serious and unacceptable overenthusiasm. AJ Balfour,[9] in a letter to a friend in 1918, was well aware of this risk of enthusiasm: "It is unfortunate considering that enthusiasm moves the world, that so few enthusiasts can be trusted to tell the truth."

Perhaps this particular skepticism is what we all must have, most importantly for our own work and not only for the work of others. Although tremendous energy and enthusiasm are necessary to do research, skepticism is necessary to present it. Biased enthusiasm leading to nondeliberate alterations of results and frank dishonesty clutters the history of science.[13] Such alterations not only lead to the dishonor of individuals involved but also contribute to a lack of faith in the entire enterprise, no matter how well intentioned. Perhaps even worse than this, fraud in medical science misleads one's colleague and can lead to years of fruitless investigation and dangerous therapies.[13] *Straightforward honesty is the basis of honor in science.* As Bacon[7] pointed out in his essay *On Truth*: "Clear and sound dealing is the honor of man's nature."

It seems a shame, and no doubt a bit unnecessary to some, to focus on this topic so strongly; however, it has become increasingly clear that we cannot be too cautious.[13,59] Anything less opens the door for the sort of embarrassment that Brunwald and American medicine suffered at the hands of Darsee and continue to suffer by finding research based upon that fraudulent data.[59] Science is a cooperative enterprise. Involvement at every level is necessary for all who participate. Continual questioning of oneself and each colleague and continuous sifting and analysis are necessary. This provides the excellence referred to in a 1983 editorial in *Nature*[23]:

"A research laboratory jealous of its reputation has to develop less formal, more intimate ways of forming a corporate judgment of the work its people do. The best laboratories in university departments are well known for their searching, mutual questioning."

Scrupulous attention to honesty is crucially important because of an inherent characteristic of the scientific method. As discussed earlier, we can support theories only by disproving the null hypotheses. We can never absolutely prove them. Because we can never prove a theory, science is inherently based on uncertainties. The risk of basing our knowledge on uncertainties is obvious. When uncertainties become dishonesties, the entire structure and process of scientific thought are distorted.[23]

This potential for uncertainty is even greater if we apply scientific theories or hypotheses to other inappropriate areas, such as medical therapeutics, sociology, and psychology, where they may not apply. Perhaps the most astonishing example is the widespread application of the theory of evolution.[3,19,35] Although this or any other theory conceivably may be useful to stimulate further research, the far-reaching acceptance of this theory (it is not an incontrovertible fact) is inappropriate.[19,40] The presence of fraudulent data, such as the Piltdown man, and squabbles between experts, such as between Johanson and the Leakeys,[36] undermine the certainty of the entire system.

Add to our communal necessity for rigorous truthfulness and accuracy the fact that many of us are unable to thoroughly and completely understand data generated in areas even closely related to our own, and the situation is even more concerning. We frequently are asked to accept on faith the statistics, results, research techniques, and conclusions based on theories and hypotheses with which we are unfamiliar and certainly unable to test ourselves. In addition, ideas spring into our minds; whether the sources are a paper recently refereed, a research grant recently reviewed, or an idea that occurred to us from our own data is sometimes difficult to ascertain. The potential for chaos and error is great.[23] In this milieu, the presence of police officers, watchdogs, and whistle blowers is too rare and, for the sake of productive research, somewhat undesirable. Journal reviewers should determine whether the results are of sufficient importance to justify publication. Reviewers cannot reliably "police the data." The best source of check and countercheck is at the bench level, where researchers work together.[23,28] The price to be paid by failure and/or fraud at this personal level is far too great. The words of Jacob Bronowski[14] in *Science and Human Values* again demonstrate the overwhelming imperative of honesty:

> *"All our knowledge has been built communally; there would be no astrophysics, there would be no history, there would not even be language, if man were a solitary animal. What follows? It follows that we must be able to rely on other people; we must be able to trust their word. That is, it follows that there is a principle, which binds society together because without it the individual would be helpless to tell the truth from the false. This principle is truthfulness."*

REFERENCES

1. American Psychological Association: *Guidelines for ethical conduct in the care and use of animals,* Washington, DC, 1985, American Psychological Association.
2. Angier N: Cultures in conflict: M.D.'s and Ph.D.'s. *New York Times,* C1, April 24, 1990.
3. Ayala F: Nothing in biology makes sense except in the light of evolution: Theodosus Dobzhansky 1900-1975. *J Hered* 68:3, 1977.
4. Bacon F: Novum Organum, article XIV and article XVIII. In Commins S, Linscott RN, editors: *Man and the universe: the philosophies of science.* New York, 1947, Random House.
5. Bacon F: Novum Organum, book I. In Commins S, Linscott RN, editors: *Man and the universe: the philosophies of science.* New York, 1947, Random House.
6. Bacon F: Advancement of learning, book I, chapter 1. In: *The Oxford dictionary of quotations,* ed 3. New York, 1980, Oxford University.
7. Bacon F: On truth. In: *The essays.* Norwalk, CT, 1980, Eaton Press.
8. Bacon F: On counsels civil and moral. In: *The essays.* Norwalk, CT, 1980, Eaton Press.
9. Balfour AJ: Letter to Mrs. Drew, 1918. In: *The Oxford dictionary of quotations,* ed 3, New York, 1980, Oxford University.
10. Beecher HK: Experimentation in man. *JAMA* 169:109, 461, 478, 1959.
11. Bond RF, Adams HR, Chaudry IH, editors: *Perspectives in shock research.* New York, 1988, Alan R Liss.
12. Breazile JE, Kitchell RL: Euthanasia for laboratory animals. *Fed Proc* 28:1577, 1969.
13. Broad W, Wade N: *Betrayers of the truth.* New York, 1982, Simon & Schuster (original source: Hunt M: A fraud that shook the world of science. *New York Times Magazine,* 42-75, November 1, 1981).
14. Bronowski J: *Science and human values.* New York, 1956, Messner.
15. Campbell AGM: Infants, children, and informed consent. *Br Med J* 3:334, 1974.
16. Chand N, Altura BM: Acetylcholine and bradykinin relax intrapulmonary arteries by acting on endothelial cells: role in lung vascular diseases. *Science* 213:1376, 1981.
17. Cook TD, Campbell DT: *Quasi-experimentation, design and analysis issues for field settings.* Chicago, 1979, Rand McNally.
18. Cuca JM, McLoughlin WJ: Why clinical research grant applications fare poorly in review and how to recover. *Cancer Invest* 5:155, 1987.
19. Denton M: *Evolution: a theory in crisis.* London, 1985, Burnett Books.
20. Diener D, Crandall R: *Ethics in social and behavioral research.* Chicago, 1978, University of Chicago Press.
21. Dorinsky PM, Gadek JE: Clinical implications of basic research mechanisms of multiple nonpulmonary organ failure in ARDS. *Chest* 96:885, 1989.
22. Eaves GN: Preparation of the research-grant application: opportunities and pitfalls. *Grants Magazine* 7:151, 1984.
23. Editorial, Is science really a pack of lies? *Nature* 303:361, 1983.
24. Editorial, Salvation—it's just around the corner! *Physiologist* 33:141, 1990.
25. Fackler JC, Wetzel RC: Critical care for rare diseases. *Pediatr Crit Care Medicine,* 3:1, 2002.
26. Federer WT: *Experimental design: theory and application.* New York, 1955, Macmillan.
27. Feinstein AR: Clinical biostatistics: hard science, soft data, and the challenges of choosing clinical variables in research. *Clin Pharmacol Ther* 22:485, 1977.
28. Foundation for Biomedical Research: *The biomedical investigator's handbook for researchers using animal models.* Washington, DC, 1987, Foundation for Biomedical Research.
29. Glass B: The ethical basis of science. *Science* 150:1257, 1965.
30. Goldstein JL: On the origin and prevention of PAIDS (paralyzed academic investigator's disease syndrome). *J Clin Invest* 78:848, 1986.
31. Greer AL: The two cultures of biomedicine: can there be consensus? *JAMA* 258:2739, 1987.
32. Gordon SL: Obtaining grant funding for clinical research. In Fitzgerald R Jr, editor: *Non-cemented total hip arthroplasty.* New York, 1988, Raven.
33. Gordon SL: Ingredients of a successful grant application to the National Institutes of Health. *J Orthop Res* 7:138, 1989.

34. Hawking SW: *A brief history of time.* New York, 1989, Bantam Books.
35. Hill NS, Fanburg BL: Clinical correlates of endothelial dysfunction. In Ryan US, editor: *Pulmonary endothelium in health and disease.* New York, 1987, Marcel Dekker.
36. Holstead LB: Museum of errors. *Nature* 288:208, 1980.
37. Imhoff M, Webb A, Goldschmidt A: Health Informatics. *Intensive Care Med* 27:179, 2001.
38. Johanson DC, White TD: On the status of Austrophithicus Afarensis. *Science* 207:1104, 1980.
39. Johnson S: In *The Oxford dictionary of quotations.* ed 3, New York, 1980, Oxford University.
40. Kirk RE, editor: *Experimental design: procedures for the behavioral sciences.* ed 2, Pacific Grove, CA, 1982, Brooks/Cole.
41. Lantos JD, Frader J: Extracorporeal membrane oxygenation and the ethics of clinical research in pediatrics. *N Engl J Med* 323:409, 1990.
42. Lewin R: Evolutionary theory under fire. *Science* 210:883, 1980.
43. Lionel NDW, Herxheimer A: Assessing reports of therapeutic trials. *BMJ* 3:637, 1970.
44. Lond CBE: The clinical evaluation of remedies. *Lancet* 2:1085, 1954.
45. Mainland D: The use and misuse of statistics in medical publications. *Clin Pharmacol Ther* 1:411, 1960.
46. Marshall E: NIH tunes up peer review. *Science* 263:1212, 1994.
47. Marwick C: NIH expects conflict-of-interest rule revisions to take at least 6 months. *JAMA* 263:1183, 1990.
48. Mazzaschi A: Young investigators: good news, bad news. *Public Affairs* 4:2953, 1990.
49. Medawar PB: *Advice to a young scientist.* New York, 1979, Harper & Row.
50. Millikan RA: On the elementary electrical charge and the Avogadro constant. *Phys Rev* 2:109, 1913. In Holton G: Subelectrons, presuppositions and the Millikan-Ehrenhaft dispute. *Historical Studies in the Physical Sciences* 9:161, 1978.
51. Mitchell RG: The child and experimental medicine. *BMJ* 1:721, 1964.
52. Muirhead EE: The art of precepts for investigators. *News Physiol Sci* 5:133, 1990.
53. Murphy EA, editor: *Probability in medicine.* Baltimore, 1979, Johns Hopkins University.
54. Murray JF, Matthay MA, Luce JM, Flick MR: Pulmonary perspective: an expanded definition of the adult respiratory distress syndrome. *Am Rev Respir Dis* 138:720, 1988.
55. Nelson NM: On hummingbirds, extracorporeal membrane oxygenation, and IBM. *Pediatrics* 85:374, 1990.
56. Nicholson RS: Congressional pork versus peer review. *Science* 256:1497, 1992.
57. Palca J: Young investigators at risk. *Science* 249:351, 1990.
58. Pickering GW: Section of experimental medicine and therapeutics: the place of the experimental method in medicine. *Proc R Soc Med* 42:229, 1948.
59. Prentice EE, Zucker LH, Jameton A: Ethics of animal welfare in research: the institution's attempt to achieve appropriate social balance. *Physiologist* 28:19, 1986.
60. Rabinovitch M: Endothelial changes associated with high pulmonary blood flow and pressure. In Ryan US, editor: *Endothelial cells,* vol 3, Boca Raton, FL, 1988, CRC.
61. Relman AS: Lessons from the Darsee affair. *N Engl J Med* 308:1415, 1983.
62. Robotham JL, Peters J, Takata M, Wetzel RC: Cardiorespiratory interactions. In Rogers MC, editor: *Pediatric intensive care.* Baltimore, 1991, Williams & Wilkins.
63. Rosner F: Ethical relationships between drug companies and the medical profession. *Chest* 102:266, 1992.
64. Said SI, Foda HD: State of the art: pharmacologic modulation of lung injury. *Am Rev Respir Dis* 139:1553, 1989.
65. Shakespeare W: *The rape of Lucrece.* Line 939.
66. Skegg PDG: English law relating to experimentation on children. *Lancet* 2:754, 1977.
67. Snow CP: *The search,* rev ed. New York, 1959, Charles Scribner's Sons.
68. Stocking B: Using evidence: the role of foundations. *Ann N Y Acad Sci* 703:291, 1993.
69. Stossel TP: Clinical investigation and JAMA. *JAMA* 258:3298, 1987.
70. Sylvester JT, Gordon JB, Malamet RL, Wetzel RC: Prostaglandins and estradiol-induced attenuation of hypoxic pulmonary vasoconstriction. *Chest* 88:252S, 1985.
71. Wetzel RC: The intensivist's system. *Crit Care Med* 21:S341, 1993.
72. Wetzel RC, Tobin J: Shock. In Rogers MC, editor: *Pediatric intensive care.* Baltimore, 1991, Williams & Wilkins.
73. Wetzel RC, Zacur HA, Sylvester JT: Effect of puberty and estradiol on hypoxic vasomotor response in isolated sheep lungs. *J Appl Physiol* 56:1199, 1984.
74. Zimmerman JJ, Dietrich KA: Current perspectives on septic shock. *Pediatr Clin North Am* 34:131, 1987.
75. Zimmerman JJ, Millard JR, Farrin-Rusk C: Septic plasma suppresses superoxide anion synthesis by normal homologous polymorphonuclear leukocytes. *Crit Care Med* 17:1241, 1989.
76. References 10, 15, 20, 42, 49, 56, 64: These definitions are taken from an article in *Awake!* 65:10, 1984, p 7.
77. Boguski MS, McIntosh MW: Biomedical informatics for proteomics. *Nature* 422:233, 2003.
78. Bui AA, Weinger GS, Barretta SJ, et al: An XML gateway to patient data for medical research applications. *Ann N Y Acad Sci* 980:236, 2002.
79. Liebman MN: Biomedical informatics: the future for drug development. *Drug Discov Today* 7(20 suppl):S197, 2002.
80. Leatherman ST, Hibbard JH, McGlynn EA: A research agenda to advance quality measurement and improvement. *Med Care* 41(1 suppl):I80, 2003.

Appendix 5–A

GUIDE FOR ASSIGNED REVIEWERS' PRELIMINARY COMMENTS ON RESEARCH GRANT APPLICATIONS (R01)

Downloaded from *http://www.csr.nih.gov/guidelines/guidelines.htm*

Please use the following guidelines when preparing written comments on research grant applications assigned to you for review. The goals of NIH-supported research are to advance our understanding of biological systems, improve the control of disease, and enhance health. In your written review, you should comment on the following aspects of the application in order to judge the likelihood that the proposed research will have a substantial impact on the pursuit of these goals. **NOTE: Your written reviews should not bear personal identifiers because unaltered comments will be sent to the investigator.**

DESCRIPTION: The NIH now scans the abstract on page 2 of an application for use in the Description section of the summary statement. However, as a reviewer you must be prepared to present a summary of the goals of the application to the Study Section so that all members can follow the critiques and discussion. Thus, any description you write (in prose or in bullet form) is for your use in making this presentation.

CRITIQUE: Include as little descriptive information in this section as possible. Please address, in five individual sections, each criterion listed below. In addition: for competing continuation (renewal) applications, include an evaluation of progress over the past project period; for amended applications, address progress, changes, and responses to the critiques in the summary statement from the previous review, indicating whether the application is improved, the same as, or worse than the previous submission. Comments on progress and response to the previous review should be provided in a separate paragraph and/or under the appropriate criteria.

1. **Significance** Does this study address an important problem? If the aims of the application are achieved, how will scientific knowledge be advanced? What will be the effect of these studies on the concepts or methods that drive this field?
2. **Approach** Are the conceptual framework, design (including composition of study population), methods, and analyses adequately developed, well-integrated, and appropriate to the aims of the project? Does the applicant acknowledge potential problem areas and consider alternative tactics?
3. **Innovation** Does the project employ novel concepts, approaches or methods? Are the aims original and innovative? Does the project challenge existing paradigms or develop new methodologies or technologies?
4. **Investigator** Is the investigator appropriately trained and well suited to carry out this work? Is the work proposed appropriate to the experience level of the principal investigator and other researchers (if any)? PLEASE DO NOT INCLUDE descriptive biographical information unless important to the evaluation of merit.
5. **Environment** Does the scientific environment in which the work will be done contribute to the probability of success? Do the proposed experiments take advantage of unique features of the scientific environment or employ useful collaborative arrangements? Is there evidence of institutional support? PLEASE DO NOT INCLUDE description of available facilities or equipment unless important to the evaluation of merit.

OVERALL EVALUATION: In one paragraph, briefly summarize the most important points of the Critique, addressing the strengths and weaknesses of the application in terms of the five review criteria. Recommend a score reflecting the overall impact of the project on the field, weighing the review criteria, as you feel appropriate for each application. An application does not need to be strong in all categories to be judged likely to have a major scientific impact and, thus, deserve a high merit rating. For example, an investigator may propose to carry out important work that by its nature is not innovative, but is essential to move a field forward.

PROTECTION OF HUMAN SUBJECTS FROM RESEARCH RISKS: Evaluate the application with reference to the following criteria: risk to subjects, adequacy of protection against risks, potential benefit to the subjects and to others, importance of the knowledge to be gained. (If the applicant fails to address **all** of these elements, notify the SRA immediately to determine if the application should be withdrawn.) If all of the criteria are adequately addressed, and there are no concerns write "Acceptable Risks and/or Adequate Protections." A brief explanation is advisable. If one or more criteria are inadequately addressed, write, "Unacceptable Risks and/or Inadequate Protections" and document the actual or potential issues that create the human subjects concern. If the application indicates that the proposed human subjects research is exempt from coverage by the regulations, determine if adequate justification is provided. If the claimed exemption is not justified, indicate "Unacceptable" and explain why you reached this conclusion. Also, if a clinical trial is proposed, evaluate the Data and Safety Monitoring Plan. (If the plan is absent, notify the SRA immediately to determine if the application should be withdrawn.) Indicate if the plan is "Acceptable" or "Unacceptable," and, if unacceptable, explain why it is unacceptable.

GENDER, MINORITY, AND CHILDREN SUBJECTS: Public Law 103-43 requires that women and minorities must be included in all NIH-supported clinical research projects involving human subjects unless a clear and compelling rationale establishes that inclusion is inappropriate with respect to the health of the subjects or the purpose of the research. NIH requires that children (individuals under the age of 21) of all ages be involved in all human subjects research supported by the NIH unless there are scientific or ethical reasons for excluding them. Each project involving human subjects must be assigned a code using the categories "1" to "5" below. Category 5 for minority representation in the project means that only foreign subjects are in the study population (no U.S. subjects). If the study uses both then use codes 1 thru 4. Examine whether the minority and gender characteristics of the sample are scientifically acceptable, consistent with the aims of the project, and comply with NIH policy. For each category, determine if the proposed subject recruitment targets are "A" (acceptable) or "U" (unacceptable). If you rate the sample as "U", consider this feature a weakness in the research design and reflect it in the overall score. Explain the reasons for the recommended codes; this is particularly critical for any item coded "U".

Category
Gender (G)
Minority (M)
Children (C)

1
Both genders
Minority and nonminority
Children and adults

2
Only women
Only minority
Only children

3
Only men
Only nonminority
No children included

4
Gender unknown
Minority representation unknown
Representation of children unknown

5
Only foreign subjects

NOTE: To the degree that acceptability or unacceptability affects the investigator's approach to the proposed research, such comments should appear under "Approach" in the five major review criteria described earlier, and should be factored into the score as appropriate.

ANIMAL WELFARE: Express any comments or concerns about the appropriateness of the responses to the five required points, especially whether the procedures will be limited to those that are unavoidable in the conduct of scientifically sound research.

BIOHAZARDS: Note any materials or procedures that are potentially hazardous to research personnel and indicate whether the protection proposed will be adequate.

BUDGET: Evaluate the direct costs only. Do not focus on detail. Determine whether the total budget is appropriate for the project proposed. Provide a rationale for suggested modification in amount or duration of support.

OTHER CONSIDERATIONS (for Administrative Notes in the Summary Statement): These comments are useful to NIH but should not influence your overall score.

FOREIGN: If the applicant organization is foreign, comment on any special talents, resources, populations, or environmental conditions that are not readily available in the United States or that provide augmentation of existing U.S. resources. In addition, indicate whether similar research is being performed in the U.S. and whether there is a need for such additional research. These aspects do not apply to applications from U.S. organizations for projects containing a significant foreign component.

Appendix 5–B

SEVEN STEPS

Carol E. Nicholson

This is a step-wise process that I use to help investigators approach the NIH for the first time. So far it is working pretty well.

Step I

A. Download forms and instructions and make a notebook with table of contents and dividers.

Here is the link!!!

ftp://ftp.grants.nih.gov/forms/phs398.pdf

You will need all 116 pages and the table of contents. I think it is useful to keep a blank PHS form in the front pocket of the notebook and to download the FAQs as well and keep them there. When you have questions that you need to ask someone besides me, you can call the grants info staff at 301-435-0714 or e-mail them at *GrantsInfo@nih.gov.* They are very friendly, and when you have questions about submission, mailing, labels, copies, FEDEX, etc., they are always there to help. Of course, I really love to hear from the investigators as well!

When you get to steps IV and V, it is helpful to keep handy the material at *http://nextwave.sciencemag.org/cgi/content/full/2001/09/27/1?.*

If you pay special attention to the instructions for reviewers that you can access at *http://www.drg.nih.gov/guidelines/r01.htm,* I think it will be helpful.

Before you start, though, let me review your step II "three things."

So, that is it for today. Now, take a day to think about what you are going to send me. Let me know if you need more help with this very important step!

B. Identify NIH program staff who will advise you. If not sure, contact me and I will help. If you and/or your research do not fit into my program, together we will find an NIH home for your proposal. Please do not worry about that at this stage.

C. Make a time line for the following six steps, working backward from your identified due date.

Step II

A. E-mail the three things you would accomplish for medicine, science, and children with serious illnesses and/or disabilities to your identified program staff (or me).

B. These three things will be criticized and tightened up, hypotheses and null hypotheses suggested where appropriate, and e-mailed back to you. The programmatic appropriateness of these three research aims will be evaluated.

Step III

A. Obtain formal professional biostatistical help, giving the biostatistician the research aims. Ask for a power analysis and a synopsis of the biostatistical modeling/analysis to be used. Make sure you understand the concepts well so that it will be easier to formulate a research plan.

B. Read and reread the world's literature, especially paying attention to studies similar to yours, and search CRISP.

Step IV

A. Make a very ***detailed*** (what species of rats or pigs, what reagents, how many human subjects over what period of time, exclusion, inclusion criteria) outline of your research plans. This step takes about 4 weeks.

B. Give the above three things, power analysis, and detailed outline to an R01-funded researcher(s) at your institution who is not politically connected to you in any way. Ask for a harsh criticism and for any suggestions. Give the researcher a full 3 weeks to do it. The reason is that although all of the reviewers in the study group who evaluate and score your work will be accomplished scientists, many likely will not be in your field. You would be surprised how many things that are patently apparent to a person from one discipline are obscure to those from another field.

C. While IVB is being done, get the IRB forms together on your desk and line up letters of support. Start writing the Introduction, Aims, Background, and Significance and Research plan, following the directions in your notebook very carefully. Call program staff for any clarifications or questions. As you begin to write, keep in mind the purpose of the published RFA or PA (if any) and the NIH evaluation/scoring criteria, which you should have memorized by now.

Step V

A. When the critiqued outline is available, make a grant out of it. Complete a draft of the entire proposal, including the budget. You should allow 8 full weeks for this process. At the end of this time, your proposal should look like a grant. Follow the instructions carefully; adhere to page limits.

B. After at least a 5-day break, look at the grant again, and tune and tweak. Get your institutional and departmental signoffs.

C. Chip away at your IRB submission so that it is ready to turn in the week before you send the grant (or sooner).

Step VI

A. Compose the cover letter. It is very important to contact program staff for editing assistance with this; you probably will back-and-forth it a couple of times. You will use it to request assignment and review. If you are responding to an RFA, the RFA label is necessary for your grant. You *cannot* submit without it, so get help finding it on the web site if you need it.

Step VII

A. FEDEX (overnight) to the NIH 10 days before the due date.
  ** If sending FEDEX, replace last line with Rockville, MD 20852

B. Five days later, make sure the package has arrived.

C. Put it in a drawer for a while, but keep attending to the world literature and to CRISP.

D. Find out who the SRA is for your review.

E. After review, it is important for you to go over your summary statement in detail with program staff, who will be able to give you guidance regarding the likelihood of funding at this point. If you have to do rewrites, wait until you have read and digested the summary statement. Ask the R01 level researcher to review the summary statement with you.
Don't quit, rest, don't quit!

CHAPTER

6

Proving the Point: Evidence-Based Medicine in Pediatric Critical Care

R. Scott Watson, Mary E. Hartman, John A. Kellum, and Derek C. Angus

PEARLS

- The evidence base for critical care is growing rapidly.
- Intensivists have an ethical obligation to use the best available evidence whenever applicable.
- Practicing evidence-based medicine is straightforward, and keeping up with relevant evidence is becoming easier and less time consuming.
- PubMed now includes research methodology filters (found under the "Clinical Queries" heading) that enhance the efficiency of searching the literature.
- Multiple evidence-based medicine–related resources can also be found on the Internet.

"Not all clinicians need to appraise evidence from scratch but all need some skills."[1]

What is evidence-based medicine (EBM)? How is it different from what we have always done? EBM is simply the integration of the best available evidence with individual clinical expertise and patient preferences.[2] The definition is not complicated, and you could easily make the incorrect assumption that its practice is, and always has been, ubiquitous. However, proven interventions are often misapplied, and striking variations in clinical practice (not attributable to patient differences) occur even when high-quality evidence is available.[3–8] Practicing EBM in critical care in general and pediatric critical care in particular poses unique challenges. Decisions, which can have profound implications for a child and his/her family, must be made quickly and, until recently, with little good external evidence. However, our field and EBM both have matured to the point that EBM is an indispensable and realistic component of the practice of pediatric critical care medicine.

Despite 2 decades of international support and growth, the practice of EBM continues to be hindered by misconceptions. It is not "cookbook medicine" that suppresses the individual freedom of practitioners.[9] (To the contrary, EBM relies on individual clinicians to accurately identify clinical situations to which external evidence can be applied.) It is not a cost-cutting tool. (Treatments found to be effective may be more expensive than the previous standard of care.) It is not unrealistic to think that physicians in the "real world" can practice it. (Criticisms that EBM is too difficult and time consuming may have been valid in the past, but advances in literature search engines and the increasing availability of EBM resources make it accessible and applicable for busy clinicians.)

In this chapter, we provide an overview of the steps in practicing EBM, including a summary of common study types, information about many excellent EBM-related resources, and definitions of selected terms used in EBM (Appendix 6–A). EBM is here to stay, and the field of critical care is amidst a groundswell of outstanding clinical research that is improving the outcome of critically ill patients. Our goal is to demystify the process of EBM so that pediatric intensivists can keep up with these changes, understand EBM, and incorporate it as a fundamental element in their practice.

The Evidence-based Medicine Process

The steps in the EBM process are straightforward: (1) define the problem, (2) search for relevant evidence, (3) evaluate the evidence, and (4) apply the evidence.

1. Define the problem.
   EBM starts with a well built clinical question that is constructed to facilitate an efficient literature search (see *www.cebm.net*).[10] The question needs to clearly state the patient population; the intervention(s), event(s), or exposure(s); and the outcome of interest. These steps were codified by Doig and Simpson[10] in the simple mnemonic PICO: Population, Intervention, Comparison, and Outcome. Focusing the question is key, as it enables identification of relevant search terms (described below).
2. Search for relevant evidence.
   Keeping up with the basic pediatric literature alone would require reading at least five articles per day 365 days per year.[11] The objective of searching the literature is to find the answer to the clinical question as quickly and efficiently as possible amidst the 20,000 medical journals and more than 2 million articles published annually.[12] To hone in on relevant articles, a search strategy should take advantage of Medical Subject Headings (MeSH) and incorporate new and useful filters that have been developed. Taking advantage of specific combinations of MeSH terms have been found to increase the speed and effectiveness of searches.[13]
   MeSH are descriptive terms assigned to each bibliographic reference in Medline by the National Library of Medicine. There are 22,568 terms organized into a hierarchical structure. At the most general level are very broad headings such as "Diseases" or "Organisms." More specific headings are found at more narrow levels of the 11-level hierarchy, such as "Sepsis" and "Neisseria meningitidis." There are also thousands of cross-references that assist in finding the most appropriate MeSH (e.g., MODS *see* Multiple Organ Failure).
   So that clinicians need not memorize complicated combinations of search terms, search engines have incorporated many of these terms into easy-to-use research methodology filters for clinicians. These filters are combinations of search terms that can increase searching efficiency. PubMed, for example, allows searchers to select filters for studies of etiology, diagnosis, therapy, and prognosis. Similar filters can be found in Ovid Technologies' search engine, in addition to filters on clinical prediction guides, qualitative studies, costs, and economics. In both, the choices are presented under the "Clinical Queries" heading. Searchers can choose among highly sensitive searches to produce comprehensive retrievals (particularly useful for subjects in which little work has been done), highly specific searches to retrieve only the most rigorous studies and little nonrelevant material (for subjects in which much work has been published), or optimized searches to maximize the tradeoff between sensitivity and specificity.
   In addition to Medline, multiple other specialized databases and Internet-based resources are available that can yield relevant results quickly. Table 6–1 lists a sample of these resources. One of the best known is the Cochrane Library, which contains a large collection of peer-reviewed systematic reviews on a wide variety of health care interventions.[14] It is thoroughly indexed and easily searched. ACP (American College of Physicians) Journal Club and Evidence-Based Medicine are EBM-related journals that are linked for searching through Evidence-Based Medicine Reviews (EBMR) from Ovid Technologies. The British Medical Journal publishes Clinical Evidence, an annual compilation in book and CD-ROM format of the best available evidence on the effects of common medical interventions. In addition, the PedsCCM Evidence-Based Journal Club posts critical reviews of studies related to pediatric critical care.
3. Evaluate the evidence.
   After a search yields potentially useful evidence, the clinician must evaluate the evidence and determine its scientific validity and clinical utility. For a piece of evidence to be useful, it must be valid, have clinically important findings, and be applicable to the particular patient. Guides for assessment of validity, such as those shown in Box 6–1, exist for different types of studies. Worksheets to determine whether a study is valid are available from a number of sources, including the Centre for Evidence-Based Medicine and a number of the web sites listed in Table 6–1.

Study Types

The type of clinical question determines what kinds of studies are most relevant. For example, questions about therapy usually are best answered with a randomized controlled trial (RCT) or systematic review. On the other hand, to determine the prevalence of a disease or risk factors for its development, observational studies are needed.

Interventional Studies

Interventional studies are clinical experiments, the strongest of which is the RCT. RCTs are the "gold standard" in the assessment of the efficacy of an intervention.[15,16] Randomization minimizes the risk of an unequal distribution of known and unknown factors (confounders) that may influence patient outcome. The presence of a control group helps to distinguish changes in outcome that result from the therapy in question from

TABLE 6–1

Partial List of EBM Resources on the Internet

EBM WEB SITES	
Centre for EBM, Oxford	*www.cebm.net//*
Unit for Evidence-Based Practice and Policy, University College London	*www.ucl.ac.uk/openlearning/uebpp/uebpp.htm*
EBM Toolkit, University of Alberta	*www.med.ualberta.ca/ebm/ebm.htm*
User's Guide to Evidence-Based Practice, Centre for Health Evidence	*http://www.cche.net/usersguides/main.asp*
University of Washington EBM internet resources	*http://healthlinks.washington.edu/ebp*
HealthWeb: Evidence Based Health Care	*http://healthweb.org/browse.cfm?subjectid=39*
Netting the Evidence: Database of EBM web sites	*http://www.sheffield.ac.uk/~scharr/ir/netting/*
Health Information Research Unit, McMaster University	*http://hiru.mcmaster.ca*
MEDLINE SEARCHES	
PubMed	*www.pubmed.org*
SYSTEMATIC REVIEWS	
Cochrane Collaboration	*http://www.cochrane.org/*
AHRQ Evidence-Based Practice	*http://www.ahrq.gov/clinic/epcix.htm*
National Guideline Clearinghouse (AHRQ)	*http://www.guidelines.gov/*
Clinical Evidence (from the *British Medical Journal)*	*http://www.clinicalevidence.com/ceweb/conditions/index.jsp*
Best Evidence Topics	*http://www.bestbets.org/index.html*
Centre for Reviews and Dissemination, University of York	*http://www.york.ac.uk/inst/crd*
CRITICAL CARE JOURNAL CLUBS	
PedsCCM Evidence-Based Journal Club	*http://pedsccm.wustl.edu/ebjournal_club.html*
American Thoracic Society, Critical Care Journal Club	*http://www.thoracic.org/assemblies/cc/ccjcframe.html*
ON-LINE EBM JOURNALS	
ACP Journal Club	*http://www.acpjc.org/*
Bandolier	*http://www.jr2.ox.ac.uk/bandolier/*
Evidence-Based Medicine	*http://ebm.bmjjournals.com/*
JOURNALS	
Pediatric Critical Care Medicine	*http://www.pccmjournal.com*
Critical Care Medicine	*http://www.ccmjournal.com*
Critical Care Forum	*http://ccforum.com/*
Pediatrics	*http://pediatrics.aappublications.org/*
Journal of Pediatrics	*http://www.sciencedirect.com/science/journal/00223476*
Archives of Pediatrics and Adolescent Medicine	*http://archpedi.ama-assn.org/*
JAMA	*http://www.jama.com*
New England Journal of Medicine	*http://www.nejm.com*
British Medical Journal	*http://www.bmj.com*
The Lancet	*http://www.thelancet.com/journal*

changes that otherwise would have occurred. Because of their high cost, RCTs usually are designed to maximize the likelihood of finding a positive effect. Therefore they tend to be efficacy studies, with highly selected patient populations treated by experienced providers. The effectiveness of a therapy as used in general practice often requires additional study, usually through subsequent observational studies.[17] In addition, many questions cannot be answered, either ethically or practically, by an RCT.

Observational Studies

The principal alternative to interventional studies involves observation rather than experimentation. Observational studies are powerful tools for addressing many questions that RCTs cannot and for generating hypotheses that can be tested in interventional trials. For example, they can elucidate epidemiologic characteristics and prognosis of diseases or effects of organizational characteristics on outcome. They can inform on a treatment's effectiveness (as opposed to efficacy) and determine cost effectiveness. They have become increasingly sophisticated in design and execution, but, as with all study types, they have limitations. Confounding may be difficult to control, and, even if known confounders are well controlled, unknown or unmeasured confounders may influence study results. Selection of an appropriate control group is crucial but can be difficult. All retrospective studies are subject to recall and selection bias.

BOX 6–1

Critical Appraisal of a Study of Therapy

Are the results of the study valid?
- Were patients effectively randomized?
- Were all the patients accounted for?
- Was follow-up complete?
- Were patients analyzed according to how they were randomized (i.e., intention to treat)?
- Were all people involved in the study blinded?
- Were the groups similar at the start?
- Were the groups treated equally apart from the experimental intervention?

Are the results clinically useful?
- How large was the treatment effect?
- How precise was the estimate of the treatment effect?
- Are the patients similar to the "norm"?
- Were all clinically important outcomes considered?
- Was a cost-to-benefit analysis performed?

Adapted from Sackett DL, Straus SE, Richardson WS, et al: *Evidence-based medicine: how to practice and teach EBM.* London, 2000, Harcourt Publishers Limited.

Different kinds of observational studies are designed to address different types of questions. These include case-control, cross-sectional surveys, and cohort studies.

In case-control studies, researchers compare subjects with a particular outcome (the cases) to subjects who do not have the outcome (controls). Ideally, the cases and controls are identical except for (1) the outcome of interest and (2) the risk factor or exposure that leads to the outcome of interest. With such a study, risk factors or exposures that are responsible for the outcome (e.g., smoking as a risk factor for lung cancer) can be identified. Of course, finding groups of patients that are so identical is impossible. However, well-done case-control studies, with rigorously selected cases and controls, can be extremely informative. They often are the only feasible study method for uncommon outcomes or when the lag time between an exposure and outcome is very long.

Cross-sectional studies provide a snapshot of a population at one point in time. They can identify the prevalence, or frequency, of a condition, such as the frequency of sepsis among intensive care unit patients. They are relatively inexpensive and can be conducted in a short time. Cross-sectional studies usually establish only association, not causality.

In cohort studies, researchers follow a group of subjects through time, recording exposures and development of outcomes. Cohort studies have a number of strengths, including the ability to establish the timing and sequence of events and provide population-based results. The best cohort studies measure exposures and outcomes in a blinded, objective manner, have long and complete follow-up, and identify known confounders. One of the most famous and successful cohort studies in the United States is the Framingham Heart Study, which fashioned the current medical view of atherosclerotic disease.

Case reports may be the only available information in support of a therapeutic strategy, especially for extremely rare or fatal conditions. In addition, some therapies evolved into the standard of care based on case reports and anecdotes prior to the use of randomized trials. The difficulty generalizing from case reports makes them among the weakest forms of clinical evidence.

Research Summaries

Research summaries that provide a standardized, thorough critique of studies are particularly valuable for busy clinicians. Formal summaries of research are becoming increasingly well done and common. Single studies can be presented in a format called a *critically appraised topic* (CAT), which addresses issues of validity and clinical utility in a standardized manner.[18]

Multiple studies of a single topic can be summarized in several different ways. Narrative reviews include traditional review articles and textbooks. A knowledgeable author reviews the literature, formulates an opinion, and disseminates this opinion along with references to support it. Narrative reviews provide a detailed qualitative discussion that usually is easy to comprehend. Unfortunately, the literature is rarely searched and evaluated in an organized, reproducible manner. Textbooks are well organized and synthesize tremendous amounts of information. However, because of the inherent lag in publishing times, they can be an unreliable source of current information. There is no way to ensure that the evidence is complete nor that it receives an unbiased critique. For example, in 1988, pooled data from nearly 9000 patients in 15 studies on the use of prophylactic lidocaine in acute myocardial infarction showed that the practice was useless at best. Nonetheless, in 1990, narrative review articles and textbooks still contained more recommendations for the use of prophylactic lidocaine than against it.[19]

A systematic review combines the results of multiple studies through the systematic search, assembly, and appraisal of primary research. Systematic reviews are an exhaustive effort to find all related information in a given area. Criteria for reviews to be systematic, as opposed to narrative, are explicit. Search criteria, including the inclusion and exclusion criteria for individual studies, are predefined. The methods section provides search terms and key words to establish reproducibility. They can provide an excellent summary of the literature up to the date of the review. The main disadvantage of systematic reviews is that they are only as good as the studies they include. However, even when the studies are weak, systematic reviews can be an important means by which to identify gaps in evidence and thus outline a research agenda.

In a meta-analysis, data are combined from multiple studies to yield a quantitative summary. If the combined studies use similar methodology and are of high quality, meta-analyses can increase the power to find an effect. However, difficulties in interpretation of summary statistics arise when meta-analyses combine studies that vary in quality, population, or intervention.

Levels of Evidence

One of the most widely used taxonomies for classifying evidence and clinical recommendations comes from the

Oxford Centre for Evidence-Based Medicine (Appendix 6–B). Each study can be assigned a level of evidence based on its design and quality. For a given topic, the quality of the entire body of evidence forms the basis for the strength (or grade) of a clinical recommendation. The best studies are level 1a evidence (systematic reviews of studies using similar methods), and the worst studies are level 5 evidence (expert opinion). Clinical recommendations then are graded from A (consistent level 1 evidence) to D (level 5 evidence or troublingly inconsistent or inconclusive studies).

Apply the Evidence

The strongest evidence is useless unless it is effectively applied. Bedside decision making has been the traditional focus of EBM. Clinicians must use their knowledge and experience to understand how the results of studies can be applied to individual patients. With evidence in hand, a clinician practicing EBM will place it in the context of the specific clinical circumstances and the patient's preferences.[20] Patient characteristics or preferences may be sufficiently unique to render even good evidence inapplicable.

EBM can be implemented on a larger scale through clinical practice guidelines and clinical pathways. They can disseminate and promote best practice at institutional, regional, or national levels. They are especially useful for common illnesses and procedures, and they allow implementation of EBM even when individual physicians are unable to incorporate evidence by themselves because of a lack of either time or expertise. The most compelling guidelines contain a summary of the evidence both for and against the guideline and how to apply the recommendations to specific clinical situations.[18]

Challenges to Evidence-Based Medicine

It is impossible to practice EBM without evidence. Until recently, a paucity of strong evidence existed in support of particular care paradigms in the critically ill and even less evidence related to critically ill children. A growing number of studies now offers guidance on a wide set of critical care problems.[21–26] However, much of our care remains largely empiric. A basic tenet of EBM is that a lack of evidence that an intervention is effective is not proof that an intervention is ineffective (i.e., "Absence of evidence is not evidence of absence."[27]). This issue is particularly relevant to pediatric critical care where numerous therapies are used without proven efficacy, and the evidence base for many other therapies comes from studies of adults. Whether unproven therapies should be used depends on (1) whether proven alternatives are available, (2) the likelihood and magnitude of potential harm from the therapy, (3) the natural history of the disease or condition being treated, (4) in the case of prophylaxis, the risk of developing disease, and (5) the cost of treatment (as well as the cost of not treating).

Even for therapies proven to be effective, clinicians must weigh the potential risks and benefits for a given patient. Evidence-based guidelines can be useful in helping clinicians and patients make these decisions, but they cannot take the place of clinical judgment. Treatments that are proven to be useless or harmful should be avoided. However, restrictions on existing therapy solely on the grounds that the therapy is unproven are generally inappropriate.

In the absence of practice guidelines and clinical pathways, EBM relies on individual clinician skill and initiative. Unfortunately, each step of EBM practice can be challenging, particularly for clinicians with little EBM experience. Generating specific, patient-centered questions is difficult. Because of the relative paucity of available evidence, searching for the right article can be akin to searching for a needle in a haystack. Fortunately, electronic databases are increasingly user friendly and efficient. The culture of medicine and the methodology of EBM are changing to put applicable, understandable evidence at the fingertips of clinicians.

Conclusion

The practice of critical care is changing constantly, but studies documenting remarkable practice variation suggest that the change is much too inconsistent. Intensivists tend to be resourceful, creative, and efficient, comfortable with applying clinical skills to desperate circumstances amidst a paucity of evidence. Although critical care physicians often have both the predilection and facility for making important decisions quickly and independently, that same temperament may impede the acquisition and application of a growing body of evidence related to critical illness and critical care. However, time constraints and urgency faced by intensivists are not substantially different than those faced by physicians in other fields.

All physicians have an ethical responsibility for applying EBM. Meticulously designed and executed clinical research is expensive and difficult to perform. Society expends scarce resources on it. Subjects in clinical trials face significant personal risks in hopes of a better outcome and for the advancement of knowledge. Our responsibility extends beyond individual patients, for whom the benefits of using the best available treatment usually are clear. We owe it to subjects of prior trials, researchers who carried out the trials, and the society that supported them to use and build on the knowledge gained. The unique vulnerability of critically ill patients, with their significant risk of death or long-term morbidity, creates perhaps a stronger ethical imperative for intensivists to use evidence whenever it is available. When evidence is inadequate, we are left to do our best with our clinical expertise for our current patient and to generate the evidence needed for future patients.

REFERENCES

1. Guyatt GH, Meade MO, Jaeschke RZ, et al: Practitioners of evidence based care. Not all clinicians need to appraise evidence from scratch but all need some skills. *BMJ* 320:954, 2000.
2. Sackett DL, Rosenberg WM, Gray JA, et al: Evidence based medicine: what it is and what it isn't. *BMJ* 312:71, 1996.
3. Bungard TJ, McAlister FA, Johnson JA, et al: Underutilisation of ACE inhibitors in patients with congestive heart failure. *Drugs* 61:2021, 2001.

4. Bungard TJ, Ghali WA, Teo KK, et al: Why do patients with atrial fibrillation not receive warfarin? *Arch Intern Med* 160:41, 2000.
5. Sim I, Cummings SR: A new framework for describing and quantifying the gap between proof and practice. *Med Care* 41:874, 2003.
6. Bickell NA, McEvoy MD: Physicians' reasons for failing to deliver effective breast cancer care: a framework for underuse. *Med Care* 41:442, 2003.
7. McAlister FA, Teo KK, Lewanczuk RZ, et al: Contemporary practice patterns in the management of newly diagnosed hypertension. *Can Med Assoc J* 157:23, 1997.
8. Eisenberg MJ, Califf RM, Cohen EA, et al: Use of evidence-based medical therapy in patients undergoing percutaneous coronary revascularization in the United States, Europe, and Canada. Coronary Angioplasty Versus Excisional Atherectomy Trial (CAVEAT-I) and Canadian Coronary Atherectomy Trial (CCAT) investigators. *Am J Cardiol* 79:867, 1997.
9. Reinertsen JL: Zen and the art of physician autonomy maintenance. *Ann Intern Med* 138:992, 2003.
10. Doig GS, Simpson F: Efficient literature searching: a core skill for the practice of evidence-based medicine. *Intensive Care Med* 29:2119, 2003.
11. Davidoff F, Haynes B, Sackett D, et al: Evidence based medicine. *BMJ* 310:1085, 1995.
12. Evidence-Based Medicine Working Group: Evidence-based medicine. A new approach to teaching the practice of medicine. *JAMA* 268:2420, 1992.
13. Haynes RB, Wilczynski NL: Optimal search strategies for retrieving scientifically strong studies of diagnosis from Medline: analytical survey. *BMJ* 328:1040, 2004.
14. Sackett DL, Straus SE, Richardson WS, et al: *Evidence-based medicine: how to practice and teach EBM,* ed 2. London, 2000, Harcourt Publishers Limited.
15. Ware JH, Antman EM: Equivalence trials. *N Engl J Med* 337:1159, 1997.
16. Lamas GA, Pfeffer MA, Hamm P, et al: Do the results of randomized clinical trials of cardiovascular drugs influence medical practice? The SAVE Investigators. *N Engl J Med* 327:241, 1992.
17. Rubenfeld GD, Angus DC, Pinsky MR, et al: Outcomes research in critical care: Results of the American Thoracic Society Critical Care Assembly Workshop on Outcomes Research. *Am J Respir Crit Care Med* 160:358, 1999.
18. Sackett DL, Haynes RB, Tugwell P: *Clinical epidemiology: a basic science for clinical medicine.* Boston, 1985, Little, Brown & Co.
19. Mulrow CD: Rationale for systematic reviews. In Chalmers I, Altman DG, editors: *Systematic reviews,* ed 1, London, 1995, BMJ Publishing Group.
20. Cook DJ, Hebert PC, Heyland DK, et al: How to use an article on therapy or prevention: pneumonia prevention using subglottic secretion drainage. *Crit Care Med* 25:1502, 1997.
21. Rivers E, Nguyen B, Havstad S, et al: Early goal-directed therapy in the treatment of severe sepsis and septic shock. *N Engl J Med* 345:1368, 2001.

Appendix 6–A

SELECTED EBM DEFINITIONS AND EQUATIONS

Two-by-Two Table

		Disease or Outcome	
		Present	Absent
Test or Exposure	Positive	a	b
	Negative	c	d

Absolute Risk Reduction (ARR): The difference in event rates in the treated compared with control patients. Note the order is reversed compared with the attributable risk (see below).

$$ARR = [c/(c + d)] - [a/(a + b)]$$

Attributable Risk (AR): The effect of an exposure on the risk of disease in those exposed compared with those unexposed.

$$\begin{aligned} AR &= (\text{Frequency in exposed group}) \\ &\quad - (\text{Frequency in unexposed group}) \\ &= [a/(a + b)] - [c/(c + d)] \end{aligned}$$

Confidence Interval (CI): The range of values likely to include the true value for the entire population. The standard is 95%, in which 95% of such intervals will contain the true population mean.

Intention-to-Treat Analysis: Data are analyzed according to the groups to which subject were assigned, regardless of what treatment subjects actually received ("analyzed as randomized").

Negative Predictive Value: Proportion of people with a negative test who are free of disease: d/(c + d)

Number Needed to Treat (NNT): Number of patients needed to treat to achieve one outcome. It is the inverse of ARR (1/ARR):

$$NNT = 1/[c/(c + d) - a/(a + b)]$$

Odds: Ratio of events to nonevents.

Odds Ratio (OR): The odds of an event in a treated versus the odds in a control patient. For case-control studies, RR cannot be calculated because subjects are selected on the basis of outcome, not exposure. For rare outcomes (e.g., <10% of the population), RR can be estimated by OR.

$$OR = \frac{a/c}{b/d} = \frac{ad}{bc}$$

Positive Predictive Value: Proportion of people with a positive test who have the disease: a/(a + b)

Sensitivity: Proportion of people with disease who have a positive test: a/(a + c)

Specificity: Proportion of people free of a disease who have a negative test: d/(b + d)

Relative Risk (RR): The risk of development of disease in the exposed group relative to those who were not exposed (also called *risk ratio*).

$$RR = \frac{\text{Prevalence in exposed group}}{\text{Prevalence in unexposed group}} = \frac{a/(a + b)}{c/(c + d)}$$

Relative Risk Reduction (RRR): Percent reduction in events in treated versus untreated groups.

$$RRR = (1 - [a/(a + b)]/[c/(c + d)]) \times 100\%$$

Type I Error (alpha): A difference between treated and control groups studied is found when, in reality, there is no difference.

Type II Error (beta): No difference between treated and control groups studied is found when, in reality, there is a difference.

Power (1 − β): Statistical power is the ability of an experiment to find a significant difference between groups when a difference exists.

Appendix 6–B

LEVELS OF EVIDENCE FOR STUDY OF THERAPY OR PREVENTION FROM THE OXFORD CENTRE FOR EVIDENCE-BASED MEDICINE[28]

Level*		Description
1	1a	Systematic review (with homogeneity†) of RCTs
	1b	Individual RCT (with narrow confidence interval)
	1c	All or none‡
2	2a	Systematic review (with homogeneity†) of cohort studies
	2b	Individual cohort study, or low-quality RCT (e.g., <80% follow-up)
	2c	Ecologic studies
3	3a	Systematic review (with homogeneity†) of case-control studies
	3b	Individual case-control study
4		Case series (and poor-quality cohort and case-control studies)
5		Expert opinion without explicit critical appraisal or based on physiology or bench research

RCT = randomized controlled trial.

*A minus sign can be added to denote that evidence fails to provide a conclusive answer because of *either* a single result with a wide confidence interval *or* a systematic review with troublesome (or statistically significant) heterogeneity.

†Homogeneity denotes a systematic review that is free of concerning variations (heterogeneity) in the directions and degrees of results between individual studies.

‡Met when *all* patients died before the treatment became available but some now survive with it *or* when some patients died before the treatment became available but now *none* die with it.

GRADES OF RECOMMENDATION

A	Consistent level 1 studies
B	Consistent level 2 or 3 studies *or* extrapolations from level 1 studies
C	Level 4 studies *or* extrapolations from level 2 or 3 studies
D	Level 5 evidence *or* troublingly inconsistent or inconclusive studies of any level

CHAPTER

7

Outcome Prediction in Pediatric Critical Care

Anthony D. Slonim, James P. Marcin, and Murray M. Pollack

PEARLS

- Prediction of patient outcome by physicians in the intensive care unit (ICU) is subjective and highly variable; therefore more reliable and unbiased measures are needed for accurate prognostication.
- Comparison of practitioner and ICU or institution performance to best practices is known as *benchmarking*. This process helps maintain quality control and improve quality in medicine; however, quality comparisons can be performed only after adjustment for differences in case mix and severity of illness.
- Scoring systems have a variety of uses in clinical medicine and health services research, but their strengths are highly dependent on the quality, reliability, and validity of the data that are collected and on the methodologies used in developing the scores.
- Scoring systems have a number of limitations. They require recalibration as medical care in the ICU changes, they often lack practitioner input, and they have limited utility in prognosticating for individual patients.

Introduction

Physicians, patients, payers, and regulators are interested in risk assessment and quality of care. Risk assessment is fundamental to the practice of medicine and is required for therapeutic decision making and for patient and family counseling. Clinical decisions often are based upon subjective and/or objective predictions of diagnoses, physiologic instability, and prognoses. Physicians often are asked by patients and their families to quantify outcomes from a given illness or clinical event.[1–8]

Physicians often are left to their own subjective assessments of a patient's prognosis. These assessments may be biased, highly variable among practitioners, and inaccurate in providing a true estimate of outcome. There are a number of reasons for this situation. First, physician estimates of outcome may be overly biased by recent events. A tendency exists to overly weight recent experience, especially when experience with a specific condition is limited. Second, there is a "human" limitation to the number of variables that can be processed simultaneously. Integrating the numerous objective data elements that are both available and important in predicting outcome is beyond most of our abilities.[9] The amount of information available to clinicians is expanding exponentially beyond the ability of many practitioners to remain current. Finally, there are differences in a physician's ability to accurately predict outcome based upon the stage of the practitioner's career.[9–16]

The prediction of disease progression and outcome remains a critical component of clinical medicine. This chapter reviews the evolution of outcome prediction, also known as *prognostication,* and its relevance to clinical practice in the pediatric intensive care unit (PICU).

The Past: A Historical Perspective on Prognostication

An emphasis on quality improvement, escalating health care costs, a technology revolution, and important changes in health care reimbursement have propelled the science of prognostication. The past several decades have provided a range of public health events that have impacted the development of reimbursement and the current state of outcome prediction in medicine (Table 7–1).

Fee-for-service care was first seriously evaluated in the 1960s as increased federalism turned its attention on social issues and the health care safety net, in particular. The Medicare and Medicaid programs arose out of the government's attention to social disadvantage to allow improved access to health care services regardless of one's ability to pay.[17] Increased utilization of health care goods and services in the 1970s quickly followed the altruistic gestures of the public health programs of the 1960s.[17] Increased health care costs led to government efforts to modulate costs with attention to hospital and provider behavior.[18] The American Hospital Association introduced a prospective reimbursement system that provided incentives for hospitals that were efficient in the provision of care.[19] "High-tech care," such as dialysis, and the concept of patient entitlements set the stage for the emerging specialty of critical care medicine.[20] The problems of utilization and cost provided a social impetus for the field of prognostication.

Exploding health care costs, inflation, a federal Prospective Payment System (PPS), Diagnostic Related Groupings (DRGs), and the technology revolution enabled researchers to begin to evaluate the quality of care based on different payment systems. Better prognostication methods that adjusted for case mix became increasingly in demand.[21–23] Other social issues, including debates on the utility of care at the end of life, futility, the supply and demand of ICU beds, and objective measures of quality continued to focus on a need for better prognostication methods. Intensive care was, and remains, at the center of many of these issues.[24–39] Thus it is natural for prognostication methods to be a focus for intensivists.

Critical care medicine was prepared for this emphasis on prognostication. The Glasgow Coma Scale and Apgar score are two early examples of how critical care embraced scoring clinical states of disease and prepared the way for current scoring systems.[40,41] The Acute Physiology and Chronic Health Evaluations (APACHE) score, the Therapeutic Intervention Scoring System (TISS), the Pediatric Risk of Mortality (PRISM) score, and the Physiologic Stability Index (PSI) are some of the scores that developed in the 1970s and 1980s, encouraged by

TABLE 7–1

Political, Economic, and Public Health Forces Implicated in the Development of Critical Care and Outcome Analysis

	Pre-1950s	1960s	1970s	1980s	1990s	2000 and beyond
Public health issue	Self-pay No insurance Patients and families bear the burden of health care expenses	Government as safety net Medicare and Medicaid	Runaway expenses health care Economic Stabilization Program (PPS)	HCFA PPS report cards HFCA case mix Adjustment methods questioned	Universal access, resource limits	Quality and safety emerge as major themes Leapfrog group-consumers dictating quality in health care
Development in critical care	No ICUs	First ICUs develop	ICUs and training programs continue to emerge "High-tech" era in health care begins	Questioning the "value" of critical care Who should benefit and how can this be determined? Triage issues become prominent	Variation in ICU care is demonstrated Methods available for quality improvement and benchmarking	Attention to additional outcomes: morbidity, adverse occurrences, nosocomial infection, quality of life, cost effectiveness, benefit
Prognostication and outcome determination	Primarily clinical determinations Lack of scientific foundation (e.g., Apgar)	Remains clinical	Based upon resource use (TISS) and some disease-specific scores	Adult and pediatric severity of illness methods develop (APACHE, MPM, SAPS, PRISM)	Second-generation scores develop and are recalibrated Large datasets emerge Physiologic determinations available for all age groups	Recalibration, Bayesian analysis, computer-based decision support

APACHE, Acute Physiology and Chronic Health Evaluations; *HCFA,* Health Care Financing Administration; *ICU,* intensive care unit; *MPM,* Mortality Probability Models (score); *PPS,* Prospective Payment System; *PRISM,* Pediatric Risk of Mortality (score); *SAPS,* Simplified Acute Physiology Score; *TISS,* Therapeutic Intervention Scoring System.

both the social issues and the intensivists' acceptance of numeric summaries.[27,32,42–45]

The Present: The Current State of Prognostication

Relevant and Reliable Outcomes

Outcome variables must be objective and clearly defined.[30] The three major categories of outcomes that have been used in ICU scoring systems are vitality outcomes, economic outcomes, and quality outcomes.

Vitality Outcomes

Survival and death have been the primary outcome measures used in ICU prognostication. They occur with sufficient frequency in ICU settings, are well defined, and are clearly important. There has been concern that the focus on death may miss other important outcome measures, such as disability.[46] However, it appears that other outcomes, such as morbidity and disability, correlate well with the changes that affect mortality.[46]

Economic Outcomes

Economic outcome indicators are popular in the medical literature because they are widely available and useful when evaluating expensive or resource intensive therapies.[32,35] Several resource outcomes are commonly measured. These include length of stay (LOS), costs (typically estimated as charges), and use of critical care therapies, such as mechanical ventilation or vasoactive infusions.[24,28,30,35,37] Although this emphasis has some immediate appeal, the utility of economic indicators in pediatric patients may be different than in adults for several reasons. First, far fewer children require intensive care services than do adults. Second, children are more likely to live longer than adults after their ICU course and consume resources throughout their period of disability.[30,35] Therefore the total costs associated with the care of children with chronic conditions are likely to be larger than for adults.[30] Third, the delivery of intensive care services for children is more regionalized than for adults. Fourth, the decision to restrict resource allocation in children is highly controversial and subject to a variety of personal and societal values. Hence, policy changes for children have been relatively resistant to the effects of economic outcomes.[30]

Quality Outcomes

Outcomes that relate to the performance or process of care are referred to as *quality outcomes*. These outcomes include adverse events such as nosocomial infection, surgical complications, and outcomes regarding functionality and health status, including disability.[30] Measurement of serious disability has been a difficult problem in pediatrics because it is difficult to define, and there is wide variability in physician estimates of disability. One important effort to quantify disability has been the Pediatric Overall Performance Category (POPC) and Pediatric Cerebral Performance Category (PCPC) scores.[47,48] These scores are global assessments that quantify overall morbidity and cognitive impairment specifically for children.[47,48] Care providers make qualitative assessments based on very general descriptions of POPC and PCPC. Face and content validity for the POPC and PCPC scales have been evaluated. Differences between baseline and discharge POPC and PCPC scores have been associated with several other indicators of morbidity, including length of PICU stay, total hospital charges, discharge care needs, and summary measures of severity of illness.[47–49] Unfortunately, even though POPC and PCPC are statistically correlated with neuropsychological tests, correlation of POPC and PCPC with these tests is not sufficiently precise for use in individual patients. Individuals with the same neuropsychological measure might fall into very different POPC and PCPC groups based on the qualitative assessment of the care giver's assessment of functioning.

Data Issues

Predictor Variables

Data elements should be collected *a priori* to minimize bias associated with the model's development. Generally speaking, the model that is statistically accurate and uses the fewest number of variables in predicting the outcome of interest is best. Variables used for the prediction of the outcome states include physiologic status, diagnoses, physiologic reserve, response to therapy, and intensity of interventions.[30] The ICU exists primarily to monitor and treat alterations in physiology. Hence, physiologic variables make sense in predicting outcomes from ICU care. Diagnostic groupings provide a label for the patient's presentation but may relate only minimally to the degree of physiologic dysfunction, particularly in pediatric patients. Physiologic reserve is a variable that represents the health status of the patient. Age, comorbid conditions, and dependence on a health care technology all may affect the patient's ability to compensate for a given episode of critical illness. The patient's response to a given intervention may provide a useful method for judging illness severity and prognosticating; however, assessing the individual effects of an intervention while multiple diagnoses coexist and several therapies are ongoing is difficult. Finally, the degree of therapeutic intervention (e.g., need for mechanical ventilation) has been used as a variable to measure severity of illness and predict outcome states. Medical interventions, however, often are physician controlled and applied unpredictably, depending upon local practice patterns.

Reliability

A number of considerations with respect to data quality for outcome prediction models need attention prior to the use of these models to predict outcome.[30,50] The reliability of the model must be assured so that the score is consistent in providing the same outcome with a given set of criteria. This begins with clear and concise definitions and timing for the collection of each variable.

Standardized training of data collectors is an important component of this process. Once collected, another opportunity for error occurs during data coding. The measure of reliability can be tested either within or between observers.[30,50] This is necessary to assure consistency in the observations over time and between sites. Failure to perform reliability testing can lead to an inability of a model to perform as designed. Data reliability can be assured by resampling data and evaluating the measure of agreement. Depending on the data type, reliability can be measured by the κ statistic (dichotomous data), the weighted κ statistic (ordinal data), or the intraclass correlation coefficient (interval data). The κ statistic is a measure of agreement scaled from 0 to 1, with 0 representing chance and 1 representing perfect agreement.[30,46,50]

Validity

The validity of the score must be assured to determine if the score measures what it is intended to measure and performs accurately and precisely in the population of interest. Several types of validity have relevance to severity of illness scoring systems.[51] *Face validity* refers to the extent to which a score appears to be related to the outcome of interest. For example, physiologic dysfunction and mortality appear to be related concepts. *Content validity* refers to the extent to which the particular parameters included in a score are representative of the outcome of interest. Vital signs, for example, represent commonly measured physiologic parameters that help determine whether the outcome will be survival or death. Finally, *construct validity* refers to the extent to which the scoring system is able to predict a higher order construct, such as mortality.

The score can be validated internally in the population in which the score was derived or externally by applying the score to a different population and assessing its performance.[30,33] Internal validation can be accomplished by one of three standardized techniques. In *data splitting,* the dataset is split into random subsets known as the *training and validation sets* and validity is tested from one set to the next. In *cross-validation,* multiple training and validation subsets are created and tested. *Bootstrapping* refers to testing the model's performance on a large number of randomly drawn samples from the original dataset.[50]

Two essential and objective measures of model performance are discrimination and calibration.[30] *Discrimination* refers to the ability of a model to distinguish *between* outcome groups. That is, a model with good measures of discrimination is able to differentiate individuals with a low outcome risk from those with a high outcome risk. The area under the receiver operating characteristic (ROC) curve, which affords a measure of the model's accuracy, assesses discrimination.[52] *Calibration* measures the correlation between the predicted outcomes and actual outcome over the entire range of risk prediction. The most accepted methods for assessing calibration are the goodness-of-fit statistic proposed by Lemeshow and Hosmer and the absence of systematic prediction error across predefined or arbitrary deciles.[33,52–55]

Model Development

Individual variables are first typically tested separately for statistical association to the outcome of interest *(univariate analysis).* The set of variables associated with the outcome in univariate analysis then is subjected to *multivariate analysis,* the standard methodology for score development.[30,33] *Multivariate logistic regression* is one of the more common tests and is used when the outcome is dichotomous (e.g., survival/death). It allows the user to predict the probability of a particular outcome based upon a logistic equation and allows for the development of a score, similarly associated with the outcome. Polychotomous and ordinal logistic regressions enable prediction of more than two outcome states but require much larger sample sizes than dichotomous logistic regression.[33,50] For example, these methods could be used to predict the trichotomous discharge outcomes of death, coma, or noncoma.[34] *Linear* and *nonlinear multivariate regression* is most often used for continuous variables (e.g., length of stay), and *multivariate linear* or *quadratic discriminate function analysis* is most often used to predict categorical outcomes (e.g., diagnoses).[50]

Other methods have been proposed for outcome prediction. For example, neural networks are designed to mimic the processes used by the human brain and can be used to predict both categorical and continuous outcomes. Although many involve aspects of artificial intelligence and have been shown in several comparisons to perform as well as standard methods, none has consistently performed better than standard statistical methods when applied to prognostication.[9]

Types

Scoring systems are a means of quantitating clinical states that are difficult to summarize by other subjective or objective means. The three major categories of outcome prediction instruments are dependent upon the variables that predict outcome and include intervention-specific instruments, disease- or condition-specific instruments, and physiology-specific instruments[30] (Box 7–1).

Intervention-Specific Scoring Systems

Prognostic scores may rely on the number of interventions provided to patients. The TISS score is a well-recognized score of this genre and has been applied to pediatric patients.[42] TISS categorizes 76 different therapeutic and monitoring interventions on a scale from 1 to 4 based upon complexity and invasiveness. TISS scores correlate well with resource utilization (and therefore costs) and with mortality risk because as illness severity increases, more therapeutic and monitoring interventions are provided. However, physicians practice and use interventions differently, which affects the score independent of the patient's physiology.

Disease- or Condition-Specific Scoring Systems

Disease- or condition-specific systems represent the severity of a given condition based upon patient characteristics

BOX 7–1

Major Categories and Examples of Outcome Prediction Models

- Intervention-specific instruments
  - Therapeutic Intervention Scoring System (TISS)
- Disease- or condition-specific instruments
  - Apgar score
  - Croup score
  - Meningococcemia score
  - Multiple organ dysfunction score
- Physiology-specific instruments
  - Neonatal
    - Clinical Risk Index for Babies (CRIB)
    - Score for Neonatal Acute Physiology (SNAP)
  - Pediatric
    - Pediatric Risk of Mortality (PRISM) score
    - Pediatric Index of Mortality (PIM)
  - Adult
    - Acute Physiology and Chronic Health Evaluation (APACHE)
    - Mortality Probability Models (MPM)
    - Simplified Acute Physiology Score (SAPS)

that are specific to that disease process or condition. There are many examples of these scoring systems. The Apgar score is a crude measure of newborn vigor that is credited with being one of the original scoring systems. The score comprises five easily graded clinical parameters, each on a scale from 0 to 2.[40] Although the score and its variables were developed solely by the author rather than by statistical methods, its use is widespread in obstetrical suites, delivery rooms, and nurseries. Its utility is derived from its ease of use and its continued relevance in the prediction of neonatal survival.[56] It is only slightly limited by the degree of variation associated with assigning scores among and between providers.[56]

A number of other condition-specific scores are available for general use in pediatrics and in the PICU.[57–70] Examples include the asthma and croup scores.[58,60] The scores are used to assess the severity of the respective disease. These scores use subjective parameters, limiting their reliability.

Two examples of disease-specific scores that have associated objective criteria included in their models are the respiratory failure and meningococcemia scores.[57,59] Both of these scores have found application in the ICU setting.[57,59] The value of these scores is derived from their basis on easily quantifiable disease-specific outcomes that have face validity. However, their ability to perform outside of the setting in which they were constructed reduces their value in other ICUs.

Physiology-Based Scoring Systems

Neonatal Intensive Care Unit Mortality Scores. The Clinical Risk Index for Babies (CRIB) and the Score for Neonatal Acute Physiology (SNAP) are two physiology-based mortality scores for neonates.[61–64] CRIB was developed in the United Kingdom, before the widespread use of antenatal steroids and surfactant, for infants weighing less than 1500 g. It is composed of six commonly measured variables collected within the first 12 hours of birth.[61] CRIB is subject to alterations in physician practice that may not affect the infant's physiology.

SNAP II is a physiology-based score for neonatal severity of illness developed from large samples from United States and Canada.[62–64] SNAP II has also been modified for use as a mortality prediction model (SNAPPE II) by the addition of variables including birth weight, small for gestational age, and low Apgar scores.[62]

Pediatric Intensive Care Unit Mortality Scores. The two most commonly used severity of illness scores in pediatrics are PRISM and the Pediatric Index of Mortality (PIM).[45,65] PRISM is now a third-generation score (PRISM III) developed from more than 11,000 patients in 32 PICUs.[46,65] It has been recalibrated on more than 20,000 patients.[66] Mortality predictions can be made using the first 12 hours (PRISM III-12) or 24 hours (PRISM III-24) of physiologic variables and laboratory and diagnostic data. PRISM III has been used for four national studies and is routinely used in more than 50 PICUs nationally.

PIM was developed on 5695 patients from seven Australian PICUs and one British PICU.[67,68] PIM was developed using physiologic and laboratory data available upon presentation of the patient. This was intended to eliminate the theoretical concern of lead-time bias, the concept that therapies initiated prior to the stabilization of the patient would alter a severity score that used physiologic measures obtained within the first 12 or 24 hours.[68] Thus models such as PRISM III that use data collected over the first 12 or 24 hours after admission might be affected by the quality of the initial pre-PICU management and thus affect the predicted mortality. The PIM score uses data collected from the time the ICU team first contacts the patient (e.g., in the emergency department or in transport) and through the first hours of PICU care. Although PRISM has been externally validated by other national and international PICUs, the performance of PIM has been tested in one published report from the United Kingdom, which failed to demonstrate acceptable calibration.[67]

Adult Intensive Care Unit Mortality Scores. The three most common adult ICU mortality scores are APACHE, the Mortality Probability Models (MPM) score, and the Simplified Acute Physiology score (SAPS).[24,43,44,69–73] APACHE's most recently published version (APACHE III) was derived from more than 17,000 adult ICU patients in 40 institutions.[43,69] The now proprietary model is frequently recalibrated but does not include pediatric, burn, or coronary artery bypass patients. The probability of death is derived from the APACHE III score, which is calculated from physiologic data from the first 24 hours of ICU care.[69,70]

The MPM calculates a probability of death using data obtained from the time of admission (MPM-0) or from the first 24 hours of ICU care (MPM-24).[72,73] MPM-0 is able to assign a probability before ICU interventions begin, thereby theoretically eliminating therapeutic bias. The model was developed on a sample of more than 12,000 patients and excludes pediatric, burn, and cardiac surgery patients.[27]

SAPS is an adult physiology score based upon 17 variables derived from the APACHE score and collected within the first 24 hours of ICU care.[71,72] Data were collected at more than 130 ICUs in North America and Europe. SAPS does not apply to pediatric, burn, or cardiac surgery patients.

Applications

Quality

The compilation of large datasets is useful in gathering significant amounts of patient level data on care characteristics, resource use, and outcome. The datasets also allow the opportunity to compare ICUs within the dataset and with ICUs not included in the dataset. This process is known as *benchmarking*.[74] An example of internal benchmarking is practitioners comparing their performance and outcomes to those of colleagues in order to improve individual performance. The analyses provide the objective feedback that may allow physicians to alter their practice. The scores also can be used to provide an external comparison across other similar ICUs for differences in care or outcome,[74] thereby suggesting best practices or value rating between ICUs of similar structure and organization (Figure 7–1).

The standardized mortality ratio (SMR) is a ratio of observed to predicted mortality based upon a comparison population. The SMR allows comparison between groups of patients after adjustment for severity of illness and case mix.[30,37] The SMR can be used for internal benchmarking, that is, comparison of an ICU's performance over time, or it can be used to determine whether an ICU has a mortality rate that is above or below that of similar external ICUs (external benchmarking).[30,37,75] It often is used as a measure of an ICU's performance and as an index of quality of care.[30,75] The standardized length of stay ratio (SLOSR) is the ratio of observed to predicted LOS and is an indicator of resource use that is adjusted for severity.[75] The SLOSR can be used to compare a particular unit over time on this element of resource use, but it also can be used to determine if a particular ICU's resource use is above or below that of similar ICUs (see Figure 7–1).

Quality outcomes that are related to the performance or process of care are important to consider if an ICU consistently performs beyond the range of its comparison group. For these instances, fundamental process redesign may be necessary to reduce unwanted variability in quality outcomes.[74]

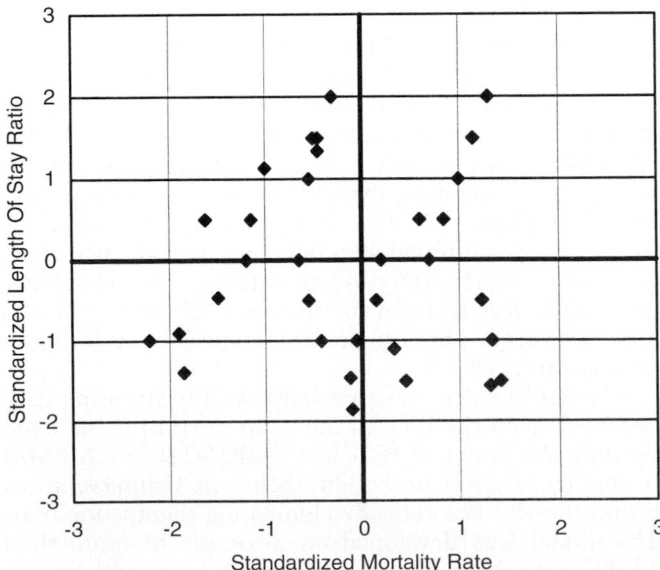

FIGURE 7–1 •

Research

Clinical Trials. Case mix adjustment may be useful for stratifying patients by risk category who may not be able to be randomized prior to their inclusion in clinical studies.[50,76] To determine the efficacy of new or emerging therapies, patients must be compared based upon the type of illness and its severity. Objective scoring systems can convert the clinical characteristics to a summary measure such as probability of death.[76,77] An assessment of the probabilities of death in the study and control groups can assist with determining a therapy's efficacy.

Limitations and Future Needs

There are limitations to the use of scoring systems for outcome prediction in the ICU setting.

First, the degree to which a particular scoring system is able to predict outcome depends significantly on the data quality. Assuring data quality is important to allow determination of the outcomes of interest with appropriate confidence.

Second, scoring systems are suboptimal if the outcome that is being predicted is rare within the dataset. The general rule is that 10 outcomes are needed for each dependent variable, which implies that very large databases are required to develop reliable predictors of rare events.

Third, current technology, experience (database size), and inability to effectively incorporate physician input into these models limit their use for individual patient prognostication. A health care provider's input might enhance the model performance and improve applicability to individual patients and acceptance by physicians for this purpose. Physicians often are better at identifying unique clinical characteristics that are predictors of mortality. Bayesian statistical algorithms have been proposed as a means of combining subjective and objective probabilities and possibly improving both performance and acceptability.[77,78] Bayesian statistics adjust predetermined probability estimate (prior probability) with new data and thereby create a new "updated" probability (posterior probability). These methods have been applied to current prediction methods but have not had substantial impact on either performance or user acceptance.

Finally, the practice of medicine remains a dynamic process. Not only do providers change their practice over time and with experience, but new technologies are developed to improve the practice of medicine. The datasets that support prognostication activities need to keep pace with the changes in medical practice. New patients who represent the new practices and technologies need to be included. Should older patients be excluded because the current practices no longer exist, or do they represent an ongoing source of experience? Regardless of the answers to these questions, the scores that predict the outcomes need to be recalibrated with time to keep pace with the changing medical environment.

Conclusion

Severity of illness scoring systems have achieved broad acceptance for their ability to predict outcomes in populations of critically ill patients, compare across ICUs for quality and resource use, and adjust for case mix differences between groups in clinical research studies. Implicit in this acceptance is an expectation that the models are created from reliable data, are valid, and have the potential to discriminate between the outcomes of interest. Future iterations of these models ideally would allow for practitioner input, dynamic modeling of mortality risk, and applicability at the bedside of individual patients.

REFERENCES

1. Dawes RM, Faust D, Meehl PE: Clinical versus actuarial judgment. *Science* 243:1668-1674, 1989.
2. Kruse JA, Thill-Baharozian MC, Carlson RW: Comparison of clinical assessment with APACHE II for predicting mortality risk in patients admitted to a medical intensive care unit. *JAMA* 260:1739-1742, 1988.
3. Knaus WA, Wagner DP, Lynn J: Short-term mortality predictions for critically ill hospitalized adults: Science and ethics. *Science* 254: 389-394, 1991.
4. McClish DK, Powell SH: How well can physicians estimate mortality in a medical intensive care unit? *Med Decis Making* 9:125-132, 1989.
5. Perkins HS, Jonsen AR, Epstein WV: Providers as predictors: using outcome predictions in intensive care. *Crit Care Med* 14:105-110, 1986.
6. Poses RM, Bekes C, Copare FJ, et al: The answer to "What are my chances, doctor?" depends on whom is asked: prognostic disagreement and inaccuracy for critically ill patients. *Crit Care Med* 17: 827-833, 1989.
7. Poses RM, Bekes C, Winkler RL, et al: Are two (inexperienced) heads better than one (experienced) head? Averaging house officers' prognostic judgments for critically ill patients. 150:1874-1878, 1990.
8. Stevens SM, Richardson DK, Gray JE, et al: Estimating neonatal mortality risk: an analysis of clinicians' judgments. *Pediatrics* 93:945-950, 1994.
9. Morris AH: Developing and implementing computerized protocols for standardization of clinical decisions. *Ann Intern Med* 132: 373-383, 2000.
10. Hanson CW, Marshall BE: Artificial intelligence applications in the intensive care unit. *Crit Care Med* 29:427-435, 2001.
11. Iberti TJ, Fischer EP, Leibowitz AB, et al: A multicenter study of physicians? Knowledge of the pulmonary artery catheter. *JAMA* 264:2928-2932, 1990.
12. Jennings D, Amabile T, Ross L: Informal covariation assessment: data-based versus theory-based judgments. In Kahneman D, Slovic P, Tversky A, editors: *Judgment under uncertainty: heuristics and biases.* New York, 1982, Cambridge University Press.
13. Levetown M, Pollack MM, Cuerdon TT, et al: Limitations and withdrawals of medical intervention in pediatric critical care. *JAMA* 272:1271-1275, 1994.
14. Marcin JP, Pollack MM, Patel KM, Sprague BM, Ruttimann UE: Prognostication and certainty in the pediatric intensive care unit. *Pediatrics* 104:868-873, 1999.
15. Miller G: The magical number seven plus or minus two: some limits on our capacity for processing information. *Psychol Rev* 63:81-97, 1956.
16. Tversky A, Kahneman D: Availability. A heuristic for judging frequency and probability. In Kahneman D, Slovic P, Tversky A, editors: *Judgment under uncertainty: heuristics and biases.* New York, 1982, Cambridge University Press.
17. Litman TJ, Robins LS: *Health politics and policy,* ed 3. New York, 1997, Delmar Publishing.
18. Altman SH, Ostby EK: Paying for hospital care: the impact on federal policy. In Ginzberg E, editor: *Health services research key to health policy.* Boston, 1993, Harvard University Press.
19. Lave J, Lave L, Silverman L: A proposal for incentive reimbursement for hospitals. *Med Care* 11:79-90, 1973.
20. Plough A: *Borrowed time: artificial organs and the politics of extending lives.* Philadelphia, 1986, Temple University Press.
21. Green J, Wintfeld N, Sharkey P, Passman LJ: The importance of severity of illness in assessing hospital mortality. *JAMA* 263: 241-246, 1990.
22. Horn S, Chachich B, Clopton C: Measuring severity of illness: a reliability study. *Med Care* 21:705-714, 1983.
23. Jencks SF, Daley J, Draper D, et al: Interpreting hospital mortality data: the role of clinical risk adjustment. *JAMA* 260:3611-3616, 1988.
24. Berenson RA: *Intensive Care Units (ICUs): Clinical Outcomes, Costs and Decision Making OTA-HCS-28.* Washington DC, 1984, Office of Technology Assessment, US Government Printing Office.
25. Groeger JS, Guntupalli KK, Strosberg M, et al: Descriptive analysis of critical care units in the United States: patient characteristics and intensive care unit utilization. *Crit Care Med* 21:279, 1994.
26. Knaus W, Draper E, Wagner DP: The use of intensive care: new research initiatives and their implications for national health policy. *Milbank Mem Fund Q* 61:561-570, 1983.
27. Lemeshow S, Le Gall JR: Modeling the severity of illness of ICU patients: A systems update. *JAMA* 272:1049-1055, 1994.
28. Miller DH: The rationing of intensive care. *Crit Care Clin* 10: 135-143, 1994.
29. Parrillo JE, Ayres SM: National Institutes of Health: consensus development conference statement on critical care medicine In: *Major issues in critical care medicine.* Baltimore, Williams and Wilkins, 1984.
30. Pollack MM: Prediction of outcome. In Fuhrman BP, Zimmerman JJ, editors: *Pediatric critical care,* ed 2. St. Louis, 1998, Mosby.
31. Pollack MM, Cuerdon TC, Getson PR: Pediatric intensive care units results of a national study. *Crit Care Med* 21:607, 1993.
32. Rappaport J, Teres D, Lemeshow S: Can futility be defined numerically? *Crit Care Med* 26:1781-1782, 1998.
33. Ruttimann UE: Statistical approaches to the development and validation of predictive instruments. *Crit Care Clin* 10:19-37, 1994.
34. Ruttimann UE, Pollack MM, Fiser DH: Prediction of three outcome states from pediatric intensive care. *Crit Care Med* 24:78-85, 1996.
35. Sachdeva, RC, Jefferson, LS, Coss-Bu J, et al: Resource consumption and the extent of futile care among patients in a pediatric intensive care unit setting. *J Pediatr* 128:742-747, 1996.
36. Strosber MA: Intensive care units in the triage mode: an organizational perspective. *Crit Care Clin* 9:415-424, 1993.
37. Teres D, Lemeshow S: Using severity measures to describe high performance intensive care units. *Crit Care Clin* 9:543-574, 1993.
38. Thivault GE, Mulley AG, Barnett GO: Medical intensive care: Indications, interventions, and outcome. *N Engl J Med* 302: 938-945, 1980.
39. Turnbull AD, Goldiner P, Silverman D, et al: The role of an intensive care unit in a cancer center. *Cancer* 37:82, 1976.
40. Apgar V: A proposal for a new method of evaluation of the newborn infant. *Anesth Analg* 32:260-267, 1953.
41. Jennett B, Bond M: Assessment of outcome after severe brain damage. *Lancet* 1:480-484, 1975.
42. Cullen DJ, Civetta JM, Briggs BA, Ferrara LC: Therapeutic intervention scoring system: a method for quantitative comparison of patient care. *Crit Care Med* 2:57-60, 1974.
43. Knaus WA, Draper EA, Wagner DP, et al: APACHE: Acute physiology and chronic health evaluation: A physiologically based classification system. *Crit Care Med* 9:591-595, 1981.
44. Knaus WA, Draper EA, Wagner DP, et al: A severity of disease classification system. *Crit Care Med* 13:818, 1985.
45. Pollack MM, Ruttimann UE, Getson PR: Pediatric risk of mortality (PRISM) score. *Crit Care Med* 16:1110-1116, 1988.

46. Pollack MM: *Prognostication scores.* 2003, Washington, DC, National Academy Press.
47. Fiser DH: Assessing the outcome of pediatric intensive care. *J Pediatr* 121:69-74, 1992.
48. Fiser DH, Long N, Roberson PK, et al: Relationship of Pediatric Overall Performance Category and Pediatric Cerebral Performance Category scores at pediatric intensive care unit discharge with outcome measures collected at hospital discharge and 1- and 6-month follow-up assessments. *Crit Care Med* 28:2616-2620, 2000.
49. Fiser DH, Tilford JM, Roberson PK: Relationship of illness severity and length of stay to functional outcomes in the pediatric intensive care unit: a multi-institutional study. *Crit Care Med* 28:1173-1179, 2000.
50. Marcin JP, Pollack MM: Review of the methodologies and applications of scoring systems in neonatal and pediatric intensive care. *Pediatr Crit Care Med* 1:20-27, 2000.
51. Hulley SB, Cummings SR: *Designing clinical research: an epidemiologic approach.* Baltimore, 2001, Williams & Wilkins.
52. Hosmer DW, Lemeshow S: *Applied logistic regression.* New York, 1989, John Wiley and Sons.
53. Bertolini G, D'Amico R, Nardi D, et al: One model, several results: the paradox of the Hosmer-Lemeshow goodness-of-fit test for the logistic regression model. *J Epidemiol Biostat* 5:251-253, 2000.
54. Hosmer DW, Hosmer T, Le Cessie S, Lemeshow S: A comparison of goodness-of-fit tests for the logistic regression model. *Stat Med* 16:965-980, 1997.
55. Pulkstenis E, Robinson TJ: Two goodness-of-fit tests for logistic regression models with continuous covariates. *Stat Med* 21:79-93, 2002.
56. Casey BM, McIntire DD, Leveno KJ: The continuing value of the Apgar score for the assessment of newborn infants. *N Engl J Med* 344:467-471, 2001.
57. Hachimi-Idrissi S, Corne L, Ramet J: Evaluation of scoring systems in acute meningococcaemia. *Eur J Emerg Med* 5:225-230, 1998.
58. Jacobs S, Shortland G, Warner J, et al: Validation of a croup score and its use in triaging children with croup. *Anaesthesia* 49: 903-906, 1994.
59. Timmons OD, Havens PL, Fackler JC: Predicting death in pediatric patient with acute respiratory failure. Pediatric Critical Care Study Group. Extracorporeal Life Support Organization. *Chest* 108: 789-797, 1995.
60. Wood DW, Downes JJ, Lecks HI: A clinical scoring system for the diagnosis of respiratory failure. Preliminary report on childhood status asthmaticus. *Am J Dis Child* 123:227-228, 1972.
61. The International Neonatal Network: The CRIB (clinical risk index for babies) score: a tool for assessing initial neonatal risk and comparing performance of neonatal intensive care units. *Lancet* 342:193-198, 1993.
62. Richardson DK, Corcoran JD, Escobar GJ, Lee SK: SNAP-II and SNAPPE-II: Simplified newborn illness severity and mortality risk scores. *J Pediatr* 138:92-100, 2001.
63. Richardson DK, Gray JE, McCormick MC, et al: Score for Neonatal Acute Physiology: a physiologic severity index for neonatal intensive care. *Pediatrics* 91:617-623, 1993.
64. Richardson DK, Corcoran JD, Escobar GJ, Lee SK: SNAP-II and SNAPPE-II: simplified newborn illness severity and mortality risk scores. *J Pediatr* 138:92-100, 2001.
65. Pollack MM, Patel KM, Ruttimann UE: PRISM III: an updated Pediatric Risk of Mortality score. *Crit Care Med* 24:743-752, 1996.
66. Pediatric Intensive Care Unit Evaluations. Available at *www.picues.org.* Accessed November 8, 2005.
67. Pearson GA, Stickley J, Shann F: Calibration of the pediatric index of mortality in UK paediatric intensive care units. *Arch Dis Child* 84:125-128, 2001.
68. Shann F, Pearson G, Slater A, et al: Paediatric index of mortality (PIM): a mortality prediction model for children in intensive care. *Intensive Care Med* 23:201-207, 1997.
69. APACHE III Equation Update (version i). Description of the updated predictive equations in the APACHE? Critical Care Series Products 1999.
70. Knaus WA, Wagner DP, Draper EA, et al: The APACHE III Prognostic System. Risk prediction of hospital mortality for critically ill hospitalized adults. Chest 100:1619-1636, 1991.
71. Le Gall JR, Lemeshow S, Saulnier F: A new simplified Acute Physiology Score (SAPS II) based on a European/North American multicenter study. 270:2957-2963, 1993.
72. Le Gall JR, Loirat P, Alperovitch A, et al: A simplified acute physiology score for ICU patients. *Crit Care Med* 12:975-977, 1984.
73. Lemeshow S, Klar J, Teres D, et al: Mortality probability models for patients in the intensive care unit for 48 or 72 hours: A prospective, multicenter study. *Crit Care Med* 22:1351-1358, 1994.
74. Zimmerman JE, Seneff MG: Benchmarking and clinical reengineering in the intensive care unit. In Shoemaker WC, Ayres SM, Grenvik A, Holbrook PR, editors: *Textbook of critical care,* ed 4. Philadelphia, 2000, WB Saunders.
75. Teres D, Lemeshow S: Severity of illness modeling and potential applications. In Rippe JM, Irwin RS, Fink MP, Cerra FB, editors: *Intensive care medicine,* ed 3. Boston, 1996, Little Brown and Company.
76. Knaus WA, Harrell Fem Fisher CJ, et al: The value of measuring severity of disease in clinical research on acutely ill patients. *J Chronic Dis* 37:455-463, 1984.
77. Brannen AL, Godfrey LJ, Goetter WE: Prediction of outcome from critical illness. A comparison of clinical judgment with a prediction rule. *Arch Intern Med* 149:1083-1086, 1989.
78. Hunt DL, Hayes HR, Hanna SE, Smith K: Effects of computer-based clinical decision support systems on physician performance and patient outcomes: a systematic review. *JAMA* 280:1339-1346, 1998.

CHAPTER 8

Safety and Quality Assessment in the Pediatric Intensive Care Unit

Matthew C. Scanlon

PEARLS

- Safety is a prerequisite to achieving quality; however, safety alone does not create quality.
- Understanding systems thinking as it applies to health care is integral to improving safety and quality.
- Data, in the context of both safety and quality, require an appreciation for variation and trends over time.
- In almost all processes, there is normal variation; reacting with interventions to normal variation in a process results in amplified and undesired variation.
- There almost never is a single "root cause" for an event. Belief in a single root cause suggests a fundamentally flawed understanding of the circumstances contributing to the event.
- Quality measures and indicators can be used for improvement, accountability, or both.
- Human errors are endemic and inevitable. Focusing on changing humans to avert errors is shortsighted.
- Reported events (either voluntary or mandatory) do *not* represent measurement that has value as a true rate of events.
- To learn from events, both errors and injuries should be studied.
- Human factors engineering is the science of understanding how humans and systems or processes interact.
- Safe care, economic constraints, and workload are intimately related. Actions that influence one likely impact the others, potentially resulting in less safe care.
- To improve safety and quality in health care, an understanding of how work is done is necessary. Only then can thoughtful design or redesign lead to meaningful improvement.
- All three components of the pediatric medication process (prescription, dispensing, and administration) have unique hazards compared with the adult situation.

Introduction

Both quality improvement (QI) and patient safety have gained increasing recognition of their relevance and importance to health care. An understanding and application of safety and quality principles extends to the pediatric intensive care unit (PICU). Unfortunately, both QI and patient safety draws on knowledge and concepts that are neither part of traditional medical education nor are intuitive. This chapter explores important concepts of safety and quality, with an emphasis on pediatric critical care.

to achieve true quality without improving safety. Others who argue that attention to other aspects of quality beyond safety is critical have confirmed this observation.[2] For the pediatric critical care provider, the important point is that safety is a necessary prerequisite for quality, but improving safety is insufficient to achieve quality.

Systems Thinking

To understand patient safety and quality in health care, you first must recognize the importance of systems in the way care is delivered. The Institute of Medicine, drawing from James Reason's studies of error, defines a system as "a set of interdependent elements interacting to achieve a common aim."[3] The interdependent elements represent both people and technology or equipment. This definition fits with prevailing concepts of systems in the human factors literature.[4] For any given process (e.g., safe administration of a medication, successful endotracheal intubation of a patient, transfer of a patient from a referring hospital), there is a sequence of parts (including people) and actions that must occur to accomplish the desired goal. Understanding the role of systems in the work done in an ICU is crucial to improving efficiency or reducing error.

Although not necessarily intuitive, the concept of interdependent elements interacting with one another is not foreign to pediatric intensivists. Physicians are taught about individual organ systems, such as the pulmonary or circulatory system. However, it is not a forgone conclusion that all health care providers understand the interaction between individual systems in the context of the larger system of an individual patient. Cardiopulmonary interactions are witnessed daily in a PICU, with interventions to one system often leading to predictable (and sometimes unpredictable) changes in the next. The interconnectedness of elements in a system, whether physiologic or process related, is recurrent in health care and central to patient safety and quality efforts.

An understanding of the individual systems in health care is necessary but not sufficient. Before efforts can effectively be made to improve safety or quality, you need to appreciate the importance of interactions between systems. Numerous systems and subsystems exist in health care. A group of physicians, nurses, and respiratory therapists working to resuscitate a child in the PICU can be viewed as one system. This system may interact with other systems (laboratory, radiology) and impact other systems (patient care units asked to take emergent transfers to create bed spaces, the hospital itself). The patient care room in which the resuscitation is occurring resides in the larger system of the PICU itself. PICU-specific issues, including staffing, location of resuscitation carts and medications, and other patients' conditions, all influence the care in the room. Finally, hospital issues, as a larger system, interact with the PICU.

Only by recognizing how almost everything done in the PICU environment can be viewed as part of a system or process can you begin to think about safety and quality.

The fact that we are dealing with complex adaptive systems in the PICU environment has leadership implications that are beyond the scope of this chapter. Interested readers are directed to other works comparing complex adaptive systems with the mechanistic systems that are less common in health care.[5]

As an appreciation of the ubiquitous presence of systems in health care develops, an understanding of the inherent complexity of many systems should follow. Health care has been compared with other systems, such as nuclear energy and aviation. These other industries have been described as *tightly coupled*.[6] A tightly coupled system has events that must occur sequentially; it does not tolerate variation in supplies or inputs without creating delays and may tolerate failures less well than systems with slack designed in them. An example of a complex, tightly coupled system in health care is illustrated in Figure 8–1, a high-level overview of the ordering and dispensing processes of a one-time, first dose of a parenteral medication in a system using computerized physician order entry (CPOE). Of importance is that this flow diagram does not capture details of the process, nor does it include the administration portion of medication delivery. In this process, failure at any step leads to delay, the steps allow for little variation in process, and the majority of steps must occur sequentially. These features of complex, tightly coupled systems are endemic in health care settings.

Quality Improvement

Quality Defined

Quality has been defined as "the degree to which health services for individuals and populations increase the likelihood of desired health outcomes and are consistent with current professional knowledge."[7] This definition, which comes from the Institute of Medicine (IOM), draws from the work of Donabedian.[8] In his work, quality was defined in the context of structure, process, and outcomes.[8] In other words, to measure quality, you should consider the structure or capacities of health care, the process or interactions between patients and care providers, and the outcomes or evidence of changes in a patient's health condition. Ideally, considerations of quality should consider all three components.

More recently, the IOM has identified six key areas for achieving quality.[1] These areas include safety, effectiveness, patient centeredness, timeliness, efficiency, and equity. Based on these and Donabedian's components of quality, efforts to improve quality should consider improvement of process, structure, and/or outcome focused on one of the six areas identified by the IOM.

Quality Assurance

QI grew out of early efforts at quality assurance (QA). In the case of QA, the focus was on identifying "poor performers" and removing them. For a given process (e.g., physician productivity in a group clinic practice measured as number of patients seen per hour), the worst performers were identified and told to improve or find work elsewhere. This approach had at least three limitations. First, if the threshold of unacceptable performance was the bottom 10%, as these providers are removed, the bottom 10% shifts along the curve to the right to now include previously "acceptable providers." Over time, the entire clinic staff would be vulnerable to shrinking the area under the curve by repeatedly removing the bottom 10%.

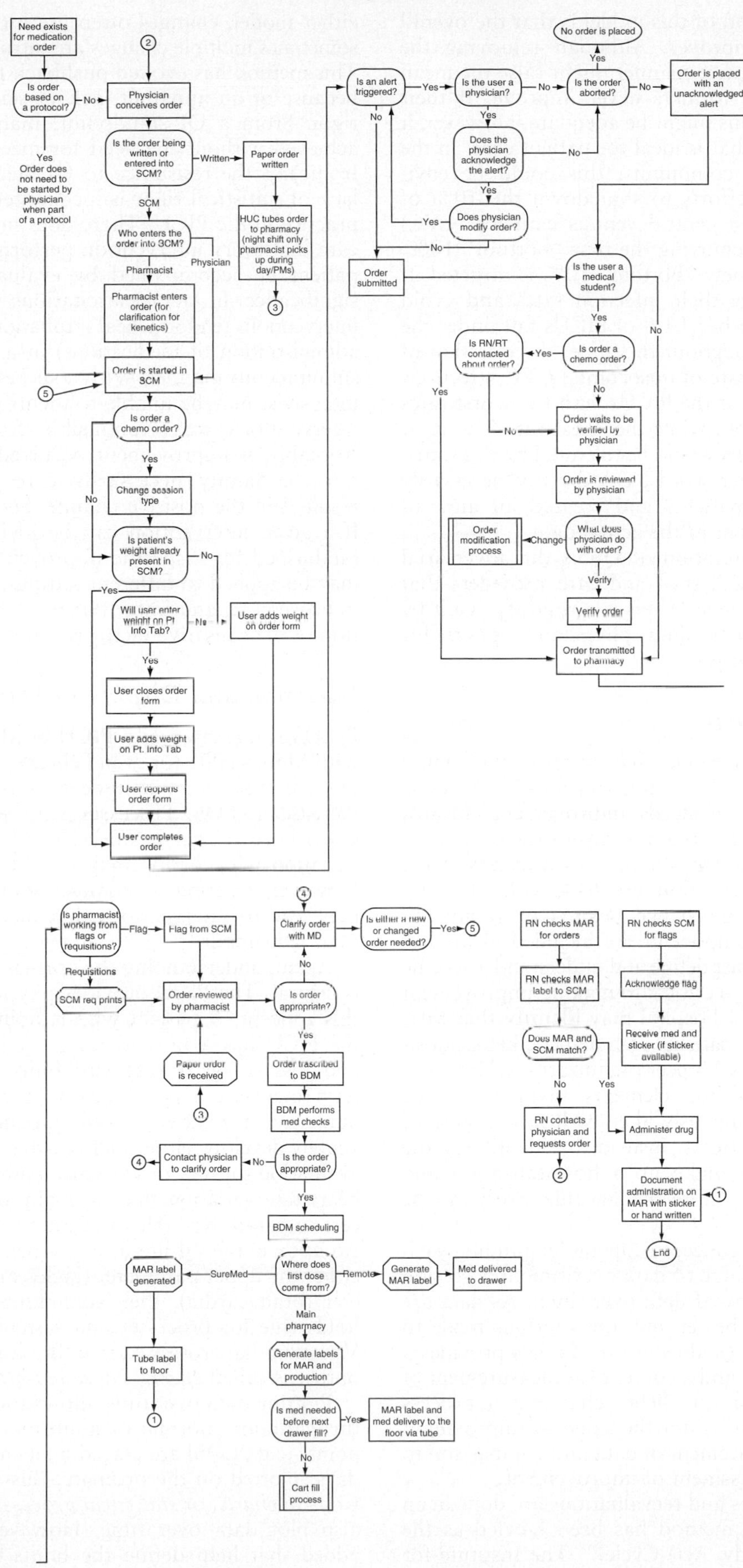

FIGURE 8–1 • Process flow diagram of first order of single parenteral medication using computer order entry from conception through dispensing.

The second limitation of this model is that the overall performance never improves. Although removing the bottom 10% in an iterative manner might raise the mean over time, the top performers never improve. If their performance is ideal, this might be adequate. However, it begs the question of what is ideal for patient care. In the pediatric critical care community, this could be envisioned by regulatory efforts to shut down the 10% of PICUs with the highest central venous catheter (CVC) infection rates. After removing the first "bottom" 10%, the curve shifts and a new "bottom" 10% is targeted. If they manage to reduce their infection rates and avoid punitive measures, another 10% of PICUs fall under the eye of regulators. Throughout this time, the question of what is an acceptable rate of nosocomial CVC infections (if such a thing exists). If the PICUs with the worst rates (say, 50%) were targeted while the "best rates" were at 20%, countless infections would be tolerated by this statistical aberration. In other words, QA did not necessarily improve the care of patients and created an aura of acceptability independent of the actual data.

Finally, the third limitation of QA is the adversarial relationship between QA staff and care providers that developed. The importance of this is a residual "guilt by association," which may limit physician support for efforts to improve quality.

Quality Improvement

In contrast, QI seeks to do just that: improve the quality of care. In order to improve care, you must first define the process of care that needs improvement. Ideally, a goal is set of what is desired in terms of the outputs of the process. Then data are obtained to understand the process, and finally interventions are made with follow-up measurement to assess the change, positive or negative.[9]

Several important components are included in the last paragraph. First, you must define and understand a specific process or system. This is critical to making improvement feasible. For example, a hospital may identify that their length of stay (LOS) for patients with diabetic ketoacidosis is prolonged compared with peer organizations. However, efforts to improve all the elements involved in the hospital course simultaneously likely will fail because of the magnitude of the efforts. Instead, by identifying the components that both make up a hospitalization and contribute to the LOS, more manageable work can be achieved.

A second important concept is the understanding variation of data and the value of data over time (see section on variation and display of data over time). As data are understood, goals can be set and interventions made to assess any change. The establishment of goals provides a target for interventions and a context for measurement of data. To paraphrase a QI cliché, changing a process through an intervention is not the same as improving a process. Instead, measurement of data and comparison to set goals allow for assessment of improvement.

Ideally, these changes and reevaluations are done in an iterative manner. This method has been labeled as the "PDSA (Plan, Do, Study, Act) Cycle."[9] The Institute for Healthcare Improvement *(www.IHI.org)* has advocated use of a PDSA method over a short period of time to create what they call "rapid cycle improvement." With either model, changes often are introduced quickly, and sometimes multiple changes are introduced simultaneously. This method has evoked pushback from some physicians because of an apparent lack of scientific and statistical rigor. From a QI standpoint, many improvements are achieved without the need for meeting a given p value. Ironically, the resistance to QI methodology because of lack of statistical rigor is inconsistent with much clinical practice in the PICU. There does not exist a standard of care that every intervention performed in resuscitating a patient be accompanied by evaluation for statistically significance. In fact, resuscitations may involve multiple interventions (endotracheal intubation, chest compressions, administration of medications) in a rapidly sequential or simultaneous manner. With a successful resuscitation, an intensivist may be unable to identify which of numerous interventions was responsible for the improvement. Arguably, if improvement occurred, neither the patient nor the family necessarily cares which intervention resulted in the positive change. Such is the QI mindset. If a given intervention can be identified and causation established for a specific improvement, this information may be applied to different settings. However, the goal is improvement, and improvement without clear identification of the causative factor remains an improvement.

Variation and Display of Data over Time

If LOS is increased in a PICU in March 2004 compared with March 2003 (or even February 2003), it is a dangerous assumption to assume that there is a meaningful increase in LOS. Processes vary within certain ranges under normal circumstances. The range within which the variation is occurring may be outside the desired goal. However, reacting to changes within normal variation may lead to interventions that increase variation rather than reducing it.[10]

Again, understanding the normal variation in a process is critical. The PICU provides physiologic illustrations of this concept. A patient who is doing reasonably well in the PICU has a normal range of heart rate variability, and loss of heart rate variability has been associated with increased risk of death in certain populations.[11] Similarly, a relatively well patient in the PICU who acutely develops either tachycardia or bradycardia merits evaluation for new or worsened pathology. In this case, the heart rate variation that normally occurs does so within certain parameters. This variation is called *common cause variation* in the QI literature. When the variation crosses either the upper parameter (tachycardia) or lower parameter (bradycardia), then something is amiss. The same holds true for processes and systems within health care. Variation that crosses certain thresholds or is an abnormal outlier is called *special cause variation.*

Plotting data over time allows for an understanding of this variation, normal or abnormal, in data. When data points (e.g., LOS) are placed on a chart with time (e.g., in days) plotted on the ordinate, this is called a *run chart. Control charts,* or *statistical process control charts* (SPC), also plot data over time. However, control limits are added that help define the limits of normal variation. Control limits, described by Walter Shewart in the 1920s, are calculated in a variety of statistical manners, in part depending on the type of control chart. The type and distribution of data determine the choice of control charts,[12] and methods for choosing a control chart are beyond the scope of this chapter. At the most basic limit, control levels are set at three times the standard deviation of the data, around the line of central tendency.

In general, when data exist within the control limits, a process is said to be *in control*. Data that either extend beyond the control limits or demonstrate one of several patterns suggest either an unstable process or a process that is responding to a change. This change may be intentional efforts to alter a process or may represent the effect of an unknown cause. Returning to the heart rate analogy, a patient who becomes bradycardic from hypoxia would demonstrate deviation of the normal heart rate variation in response to the special cause (hypoxia). Correction of the hypoxia ideally returns the heart rate (process) to its normal range of variation. An example of a control chart is displayed in Figure 8–2.

Other Quality Improvement Tools

Interested readers are directed to one of the numerous QI primers available for a thorough discussion of tools used in QI. However, several of these tools bear at least some mention.

A *Pareto chart* is simply a histogram used to identify the major contributors to a problem or variation. For example, if PICU LOS is of concern, it may be beneficial to identify which, if any, diagnosis categories contribute to the prolonged LOS. By plotting LOS in days on the abscissa against diagnosis on the ordinate, those diagnoses that contribute to the greatest portion of the length of hospitalization might be identified. This work is based on the work of Vilfredo Pareto, an Italian economist who mathematically described that 80% of the country's wealth was in the hands of 20% of the population. The *Pareto principle,* also called the *80:20 rule,* suggests that roughly 20% of possible variables account for 80% of the problems or variation. This distribution has been observed in a number of settings and is the basis for targeting where to invest improvement efforts.

Root cause analysis (RCA) is another tool used to attempt to identify the root cause for an event or problem. In its simplest form, RCA is performed by asking the question "why?" five times. Often used in conjunction with a *cause-and-effect* or *Ishikawa diagram,* the process of root cause investigation seeks to identify what caused a failure in a process (safety related or quality related) by defining the contributing factors (Figure 8–3). From each of the five categorical branches, smaller branches are added that answer the question "why?," and in turn the same question of "why?" is asked again. The resultant diagram often is described as a fishbone, explaining the third name for this diagram: a *fishbone diagram.*

By asking the question "why?" repeatedly, the belief is that the root cause of a problem can be identified. This leads to three limitations of RCA. First, there is great danger of introducing hindsight bias. The investigators' beliefs of what happen may lead them to identify only those things on the cause-and effect diagram.[13,14] A second, related limitation is that RCAs may restrict problem solving and brainstorming to only those factors that are known. As you only know what you know and, similarly, you don't know what you don't know, there is the potential for missing important factors.[15]

Finally, the most important limitation of RCA as a tool is the suggestion that there is a single root cause. This is a dangerous belief. Usually there are multiple causes of events. To limit thinking to one or two causes oversimplifies the situation and may preclude meaningful improvement. Use of RCA should be tempered with the knowledge of these limitations and the potential for drawing incorrect conclusions.

Implications of Quality Improvement for Care in the Pediatric Intensive Care Unit

QI has great potential for effecting beneficial change in the PICU. An illustration of this is work that led to improved communication of goals in an adult ICU setting.[16] Identifying an intervention, tracking changes, and modifying the interventions based on feedback, the authors were able to improve understanding of daily patient care goals and reduce ICU LOS. Unlike a rigorous controlled trial, the project was limited in that the authors could not exclude the effect of other confounders. However, the ICU LOS reduction remains significant. This is just one of many published examples of applications of QI methods to ICU care.

There are other implications for the impact of QI in the PICU. First, as many units share the same belief that "our patients are sicker," comparisons between units for either benchmarking or improvement require some adjustment for severity of illness (SOI). Specific tools include Pediatric Risk of Mortality,[17] Pediatric Logistic Organ Dysfunction,[18] and Paediatric Index of Mortality[19] (see Chapter 7). Although a discussion of SOI adjustment is outside the scope of this chapter, comparisons of data without consideration of relative differences in SOI of patients likely will meet significant and appropriate skepticism.

The focus on quality has taken on greater importance nationally with attention from various groups, including

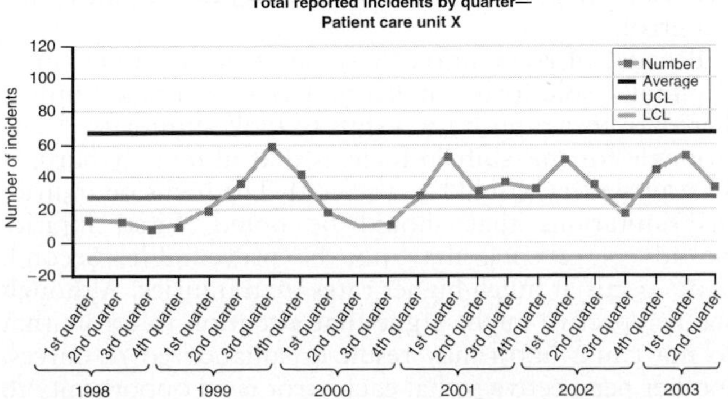

FIGURE 8–2 • Control chart demonstrating normal variation of reported events over time.

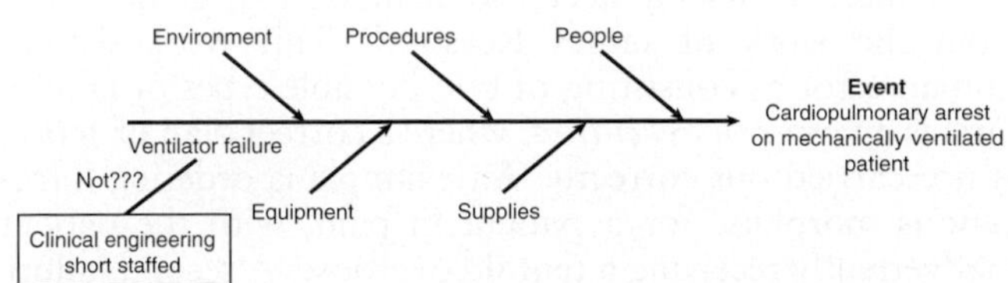

FIGURE 8–3 • Sample cause-and-effect diagram with partial completion to demonstrate structure.

the Joint Commission on Accreditation of Healthcare Organizations (JCAHO; *www.jacho.org*) and the National Quality Forum (NQF; *http://www.qualityforum.org/*). Both groups have pushed health care providers to create or identify quality measures or indicators. Such measures have two potential uses. First, measures of quality can be used strictly for improvement work. By comparing performance on certain measures, an organization then can work to identify causes for any differences. The second application of quality measures is for accountability. In this setting, regulatory bodies, such as JCAHO, use the measures for reporting and evaluations. This process may result in punitive consequences to organizations, which are measured to perform poorly. Current efforts are under way to develop possible PICU-specific measures that might be appropriately used as accountability measures.[20,21] Included in the development of any measures is consideration of the need for risk or SOI adjustment.[22]

Sources of Data for National Pediatric Intensive Care Unit Quality Efforts

A number of administrative databases exist for quality efforts, including HCUPnet *(http://hcup.ahrq.gov/HCUPNet.asp)*. However, two databases specific to PICUs exist that bear mention. First is PICUEs *(http://www.dcchildrens.com/picues/home.aspx)*. This database, which was developed by the team pioneering the Pediatric Risk of Mortality (PRISM) SOI instrument, allows comparisons with other participating institutions. The software has a varying cost structure, although the PRISM III algorithms are available free for research purposes.

The second clinical database is the VPICU Performance System (VPS),[23] a joint product of the Virtual Pediatric Intensive Care Unit (VPICU; *http://www.VPICU.org)* and the National Association of Children's Hospital and Related Institutions (NACHRI). The VPS allows both internal and peer comparisons (with the latter requiring varying fee) and provides a framework for multiinstitutional studies.

Of note, collaboration between PICUEs and VPS allows sharing of common data elements between the two databases. Both systems offer SOI adjustment capabilities and offer potential for health services research related to PICUs.

Patient Safety

Terminology of Patient Safety and Medical Errors

Like many disciplines, the patient safety field is prone to jargon and an evolving lexicon. Any discussion of safety and errors requires a set of definitions with which to work. *Patient safety* is the freedom from preventable injury, an adaptation of the definition used by the Institute of Medicine.[24] A widely accepted definition of error draws from the work of James Reason.[25] This work defines human error as consisting of two possible types of failure. First is an *error of execution,* where a correct plan of action is not carried out correctly. An example is ordering intravenous morphine for a patient in pain, with the patient inadvertently receiving a tenfold overdose. A second failure is an *error of planning*. In this case, the action taken is incorrect. An example is treating a patient with respiratory distress with beta-agonists when he/she is experiencing a pneumothorax. The execution of the action was correct, if the patient's problem was reactive airway disease.

Another definition of medical error considers an error any *overuse, misuse,* or *underuse* of medical care. In this setting, overusing antibiotics for viral illnesses, misuse of analgesics when sedatives are indicated, and underutilization of immunizations all are considered medical errors.

In addition to errors, there are *adverse events.* An adverse event is an undesired outcome of medical care. Adverse events, by definition, are unwanted. However, they are not necessarily the result of an error. Idiosyncratic drug reactions are an example of an undesirable event that is both unpredictable and unpreventable.

Errors and Injuries

There is a disproportionately large focus on errors in the medical literature and regulatory legislative worlds at this time.[26] As a result, there has been a push for mandatory reporting of errors.[27] This emphasis on error reporting may be short sighted based on other observations. First, reported errors do not represent measured data that can be meaningfully interpreted over time.[28] Additionally, simply reporting errors is inadequate. Reported events represent learning opportunities. However, a large influx of reported errors creates a burden for meaningful analysis. An error reporting project in a PICU yielded 1811 errors, of which 1067 were categorized as harmful or potentially harmful.[29] When early findings had previously been presented, the lead researched conceded the challenge of systematically analyzing these reports. Any reporting system "will prove futile in the absence of a strong, well designed system for analysis and response."[30]

Not all errors lead to harm. Many errors are either *near-miss events,* which are errors that are caught before they reach the patient, or *no harm events,* which reach the patient without causing significant harm. Studies of near-miss reports in other industries have identified events that did not reach the point of harm as a rich source of information.[31]

Errors also tend to focus discussion on the people who make them. Unfortunately, humans make errors. Work by Park[32] describes the varied rates of errors in different human endeavors. Focusing on humans rarely creates effective improvement in safety but does create barriers to future reporting and an environment of intimidation. A survey by the Institute for Safe Medication Practice reveals significant concerns of intimidation of staff by physicians that might lead to the execution of an incorrect error.[33]

Because of recognition by some of the safety community that a sole focus on errors may have limited utility, there has been a push for a shift to look at injuries.[34] The rationale for this shift in focus is that ultimately harm is what providers would like to avoid. The focus on injuries has limitations that should be noted. First, injuries (or adverse events) may not be preventable. Second, errors occur at much higher rates than injuries. Although one perspective might argue that attention to errors that do not cause harm may result in squandered resources, another perspective is that each error is an opportunity to learn and prevent injuries. Finally, to learn from an injury, a patient must, by definition, first be harmed. This creates an inherent conflict: patients must first be harmed in order to learn from the event to prevent more harm.

It is more likely that this "either/or" perspective of medical errors and injuries can best be addressed by a "both/and" approach. There is information to be learned from both to ultimately limit errors and, when errors do occur, mitigate harm.

Systems Thinking, Patient Safety, and a "Just Culture"

Perrow[35] identified characteristics of systems that make them more prone to errors. As discussed in section 8.3, the first factor that increases the likelihood of a system failing is its complexity. Not surprisingly, the more complex the system, the more likely a significant failure will occur. The second factor identified by Perrow is the degree to which a system is coupled. As discussed, tightly coupled systems are less forgiving when an error occurs, whereas loosely coupled systems are more forgiving, allowing for time delays and multiples routes for completing work. Most work in a PICU setting can be viewed as tightly coupled. For instance, the steps in dosing a medication (i.e., prescription, preparation and dispensing, administration) follow one another and, in the PICU, often leave no room for delay.

There are several reasons why it is important to understand systems thinking when addressing patient safety challenges. Without understanding systems, you likely will not understand the reasons for failures and, potentially, introduce "solutions" that will increase the likelihood of future failures. Additionally, systems thinking refocuses the discussion from a person who may or may not have committed an error to a flawed system.

As attention is shifted from individuals to systems, inevitably the issue of accountability is raised. Concerns center on whether focusing on systems rather than individuals somehow absolves health care providers from responsibility. In part, this concern arises from a well-intended effort to move from a punitive culture in health care to a "blame-free" environment. The intention was not to create systems deplete of individual accountability but to avoid blaming individuals for situations beyond their control or which resulted from genuine human error.

One solution that represents a system focus is what has been described as a "just culture."[36] Under this model, systems problems and human error are considered. The model promotes efforts to learn from errors without punishing individuals involved. Systems problems that create situations in which individuals are "set up" to make errors also are treated as learning opportunities. When individuals violate policies, often because of "normalization of deviance," the response again is not punitive but instead focused on making it easier to do the right thing. In the PICU, this can be seen when workload constraints make performing required double checks on pump programming unrealistic. The failure to perform double checks may occur daily without event, and no action is taken to stop the behavior. When a neglected double check leads to an error or harm, the traditional mindset is to punish the involved parties, despite a systematic acceptance of this behavior. In a just culture model, rather than punish the individual, efforts are made to again make it easier or more desirable to "do the right thing."

Systems thinking and a just culture are consistent with punishment. This may occur in the face of willful or reckless behaviors that place patients at risk. A physician who provides patient care while intoxicated is an example of reckless behavior that would be unacceptable in a just culture. When behaviors show a pattern of violations that individually may not represent reckless behavior but collectively demonstrate a high-risk pattern, the just culture model proposes two considerations.[36] First, the person may work in a high-risk situation where such patterns are inevitable. Alternatively, the person involved may have individual characteristics, such as marital stress or deteriorating physical abilities, which would require removing the person from that situation in a nonpunitive manner.

A focus on systems provides a rationale for understanding why events happen, suggests tools for investigating flawed systems (see section on risk identification in the pediatric intensive care unit environment), and is consistent with a culture that supports learning from errors and injuries without punishing staff unjustly.

Epidemiology of Pediatric Patient Safety

Pediatric patient safety shares many commonalities with patient safety efforts focused on adult health care. There remains a dearth of fundamental "basic science" research, particularly related to pediatrics[37] (see Chapter 5). Issues of culture change, communication, leadership, reporting, error identification and reduction, and human factors are important to both adult and pediatric safety work. However, many of the same unique characteristics of children, which led to separate medical specialties of pediatrics and pediatric critical care, support the need for separate considerations in patient safety. Unfortunately, little of the work done in the field of medical errors, harm, and pediatrics has centered on the PICU. This section explores what is known about pediatric patient safety, with special attention to where the context of care in the PICU may have added importance.

There have been few systematic investigations of the scope of pediatrics errors and injuries. A study of the utilization of medical care by children referenced finding 0.8% of pediatric discharges associated with a complication.[38] One study using administrative data to assess the risk to hospitalized children found 1.81 to 2.96 medical errors per 100 discharges.[39] This work used ICD-9 coding of medical errors to identify medical errors. The authors identify many of the limitations of using such administrative data, including underreporting, identifying cause and effect related to variables such as LOS, and a lack of clinical and physiological data. These findings are comparable to other published work, which estimated the rate of adverse events in children younger than 5 years at 2.7 per 100 discharges.[40]

A second study applied the Agency for Healthcare Research and Quality's (AHRQ) patient safety indicators (PSIs) to administrative pediatric hospitalization data.[41] This work found rates of patient safety events identified using the AHRQ tool comparable to that of adults. Aside from the previously discussed issues of using administrative datasets, the research is constrained by a limitation of the AHRQ tool. The PSIs, with the exception of birth trauma, were not designed for pediatrics, and the risk adjustment and empirical analyses were done using a dataset containing patients of all ages. AHRQ is working to overcome this limitation by funding the development of indicators specific to the pediatric population. These new indicators will include several focused on patient safety and will provide a new resource for evaluating patient safety events in pediatrics.[42]

Epidemiology of Medication Errors

Of all the possible medical errors that occur in children, the most is known about medication errors. A study of medication errors in children found that the rate of preventable adverse drug events (ADEs) was similar to adult studies.[43] However, the rate of potential adverse drug events (errors that occurred but did not reach the patient) was three times higher. These potential ADEs were most common in neonatal intensive care units (NICUs), a finding consistent with previous work demonstrating a higher number of medication errors in NICUs and PICUs.[44,45]

The provision of medications depends on three main steps: medication prescription, medication dispensing, and medication administration. Each of these steps is associated with errors; in pediatrics each step has additional risks unique to delivering medications for children.

Correct prescribing is the first step to safe medication delivery. A major factor in pediatric prescription errors is the fact that medication dosing is weight based. Prescribing medication requires correct identification of the patient's weight. An incorrect weight can lead to miscalculation of medication dosing. Similarly, confusing the units of weight, pounds, and kilograms can lead to 2× overdosing or underdosing. Identification of accurate weight takes on added importance because patients often experience changes in weight over time. A single weight used as if it were a constant value can lead to dosing errors. Additional factors that have an adverse impact on pediatric medication prescriptions include decimal place errors and computational errors. Because of the weight-based calculation, which may involve small weights, decimals take on added importance. Misplacing a decimal by one place in either direction can lead to a tenfold underdose or overdose. Research reveals that pediatric resident physicians are prone to making computational errors when prescribing medications.[45,47] In the emergency department, another complex care environment that shares some similarities with the PICU, a study of 1532 pediatric emergency department records found 10.1% of the charts reflected a prescribing error.[48] The net effect is that pediatric patients are at increased risk for prescription errors. Kaushal's previously cited work found nearly 80% of potential ADEs occurred at the ordering phase.

Medication dispensing creates another set of challenges. Unit doses can rarely be used for medications because of the weight-based nature of dosing. Consequently, pharmacists and nurses are required to draw up correct amounts from standard vials or containers of medication. Drawing up nonstandard doses manually introduces a new step during which errors can occur. Potential safeguards built into manufacturer's packaging (bar coding or otherwise) are lost when a medication is drawn up into a separate container. Another dispensing hazard occurs because the medication can be administered in both an enteral and a parenteral route. Repackaging or drawing up medications may result in using the wrong syringe, leading, for example, to parenteral administration of an enteral medication. Finally, repackaging in the dispensing phase creates a potential for mislabeling a medication, resulting in the wrong patient receiving the medication.

Administering medications is a source of errors in pediatrics. The potential for mixing up patients or routes of administration can occur. Additionally, pumps designed primarily for adults must be used in pediatrics. Many of these devices are not designed for the volumes or doses that are used in the pediatric population, and they create hazards through features that seem inconsequential in the relatively standardized adult patient population for which they are designed. The majority of pediatric patients are unable to recognize and intervene if they are about to receive a wrong medication or dose. Whereas adults may be able to prevent an error by asking "Why am I getting a red pill? Mine are normally blue," most pediatric patients are unable cognitively and verbally to protect themselves. In PICU patients who are sedated or impaired because of their underlying disease process, any pretense of self-protection from administration errors is lost.

Regardless of where in the medication process a failure occurs, children remain at greater risk for harm. The weight-based nature of dosing increases the likelihood of factor errors and thus larger overdoses or underdoses than an adult might experience. Children are considered to have less physiologic reserve than most adults; a given medication error in a child may yield worse consequences than a proportionately equivalent error in adults. This lower reserve reflects both less physiologic tolerance to stress and a limited ability to "buffer" the effect.

Technology and Medication Errors

The challenges of delivering medications to children are many and, unfortunately, not readily aided by technologic solutions available. Few, if any, CPOE systems provide "off the shelf" rules for pediatric dosing, much less safety checks. Instead, institutions must provide this customization locally, creating another opportunity for error. The true utility of CPOE for the prevention of medical errors and harm is largely undetermined. Reviews of existing literature revealed little evidence to support the claim that CPOE reduces harm.[49,50] These reviews also indicated that the evidence for error reduction with CPOE is in the setting of "homegrown" systems and not in commercially available products.[51] The lack of evidence for the benefit of CPOE may be the result of studies underpowered to identify small differences. In addition, it may be compounded by the potential lack of applications of human factors techniques to the design of this technology.

Reports allude to the potential of harm or other unintended consequences from the introduction of CPOE.[52–54] Although challenges such as selection of incorrect patient for order entry, faulty decision support, and workload implications are identified, there is no mention of the potential impact from a human factors perspective (see sections on human factors engineering in the pediatric intensive care unit and importance of design in patient safety in the pediatric intensive care unit).

Similarly, bar coding technology has added challenges of creating bar codes that fit the wide range of patient sizes that can be encountered in pediatrics. For instance, many wristbands that are marked with bar codes may be "unreadable" to bar code scanning devices because of dressings or curvature of bands because of small extremities.[55] Also, repackaging medications for pediatric use often circumvents safeguards offered by pharmaceutical company bar coding. The need to repackage doses and thus relabel with bar codes introduces yet another source of potential errors. These multiple challenges and their limited technologic solutions create an environment of increased risk to pediatric patients. In the PICU, where baseline use of technology is even greater than in care areas, the potential for both improvement and harm is even greater from the introduction of new technology targeted at improving patient safety.

Risk Identification in the Pediatric Intensive Care Unit Environment

Based on the known epidemiology of pediatric errors and harm, there is a need to identify risk in both new and existing systems. One method, RCA, was discussed in the context of QI. Two other methods worth discussing are sociotechnical probabilistic risk assessment (ST-PRA)[56] and Failure Modes and Effects Analysis (FMEA).[57] Although both methods have limitations, ST-PRA focuses on an undesirable outcome as a starting point, whereas FMEA focuses on a process. The former tool, although not yet widely applied in health care, addresses the importance of interaction between failures at different points, which may not be reflected in risk evaluation with FMEA. The "conditional probabilities"[56] reflected in ST-PRA might better address the marked complexity in health care. A familiarity with one or both of these tools is recommended for analyzing either processes or undesired outcomes in the PICU.

Human Factors Engineering and the Pediatric Intensive Care Unit

One critical topic that has been repeatedly identified in work on patient safety is the need for attention to human factors.[58,59] Human factors engineering (HFE), or *ergonomics,* is the study of the interaction between humans and the systems and tools they use. HFE reflects issues of human cognition, use of the senses, issues of physiology, and the consequences of stress, including fatigue. Additionally, HFE seeks to understand communication between humans and how it is influenced. Research from team building in aviation has been extended to consider the applications for health care.[60]

The true application of HFE to the PICU is largely unknown. However, as a large focus of HFE is on the interaction between humans and technology, the applications quickly become apparent. PICUs are laden with technology: mechanical ventilators, monitoring systems (invasive and noninvasive), and advanced health care information technology such as electronic health records (EHR) and CPOE. The ability of care providers to interact effectively with these technologies ultimately will determine their true benefit in aiding patient care. Conversely, how technologies affect the end users also becomes important. Information from the interaction of human factors in pediatric cardiac surgery supports the value of HFE in the PICU.[61]

Poor design of devices and technology may impair safe application and might facilitate or cause errors.[62–64] The science of usability, a subset of human factors, looks at evaluating the design of products or devices to improve the use. Work by researchers at the Mayo Clinic's usability laboratory led them to observe "if you can't use it... it doesn't work," and "if the system requires training, the system is defective."[65] This mindset of devices being intuitive and simple to use is antithetical to the majority of technology in the PICU. Only by better understanding how devices and technology interact and function (or do not function) in the PICU can we begin to design better, and thus safer, products.

Importance of Design in Patient Safety in the Pediatric Intensive Care Unit

The discussion of patient safety in the PICU has moved from errors and injuries, through systems thinking, to the topic of design. The subject of design may seem far removed from the world of patient care and the PICU. However, work by Rasmussen[66] defined how the design of work is essential to patient safety.

Figure 8–4 illustrates Rasmussen's observations related to safety. This figure has been described as "perhaps the single most important figure we have to guide our research on safety."[67] In this diagram, there is an area bounded by essentially three curves. The area within the curve represents safe practice, with the left-sided border being the *boundary of functionally acceptable practice.* This boundary represents a difficult-to-see and often moving threshold that, when crossed, results in a potentially unsafe practice. This boundary moves based on multiple factors, including the influence of fatigue (tired practitioners are less likely to recognize unsafe care), distractions from the environment, and experience and training. Work focused on errors attempts to influence this boundary, either by creating more tolerance for actions by increasing the "error margin" between normal practice and the boundary of acceptable practice or by making the boundary easier to view. However, efforts to implement well-intended safety efforts that negatively impact the other two boundaries may result in a net negative impact on the safety of patients.

The upper right boundary in Figure 8–4 represents *economic failure.* As financial constraints affect an organization, management increases efficiency demands with a resultant shift in safe practice toward the boundary of acceptable practice. Unfortunately, in today's business environment, health care providers likely will not see increasing reimbursement for their work. Thus economic failure remains a continued factor that will negatively affect patient safety.

The third boundary, *unacceptable workload,* acts similarly to and is intertwined with economic constraints. A common illustration of importance of this boundary to safety is the impact of a sick call on a nursing shift in the PICU. The loss of one or two nurses on a shift increases workload on the remaining nurses. As a result, these nurses have less time for behaviors that may maximize safety, taking shortcuts and violating policies or procedures. Additionally, the added workload and the associated stress serve as distractions that may make the ability to see the boundary of acceptable performance more difficult. The consequence of unacceptable workload is a less safe workplace.

The importance of the interactions of these boundaries cannot be overemphasized. Efforts to improve patient safety should be based on a thorough understanding of the impact of proposed interventions on both the boundaries

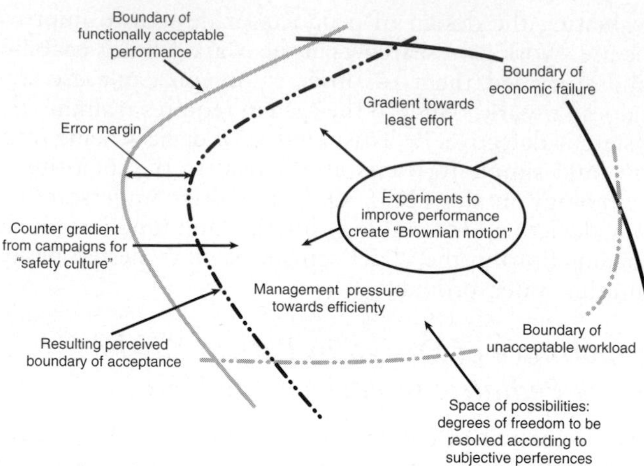

FIGURE 8–4 • Under the presence of strong gradients, behaviors likely migrate toward the boundary of acceptable performance. (Redrawn from Rasmussen J: *Safety Sci* 27:183-213, 1997.)

of economic failures and unacceptable workload. An example of how well-intended safety efforts might negatively impact a unit or hospital can be drawn from proposed National Patient Safety Goals (NPSG) for 2005 that have been suggested by the JCAHO. As part of ongoing, well-intended efforts to regulate health care organizations into safer practice, JCAHO has created a set of safety goals. Failure to comply with the goals may lead to citation by JCAHO and a loss of reimbursement from payers.

Among the proposed goals for 2005 was an expectation regarding nurses performing independent double checks of infusion pumps. Goal 5b states a nurse should "Perform an independent double-check whenever programming or reprogramming infusion pumps."[68] Practically speaking, after a nurse programs an infusion pump, he/she is expected to seek out a second nurse who will independently check the programming. Independent of literature suggesting that the base error rate in which a "monitor or inspector fails to recognize the initial error by the operator" is 10%,[69] there are significant workload implications for complying with this goal.

Internal data at a 220-bed freestanding children's hospital[70] reveals conservative estimates of 339 new infusions in the PICU and 480 new infusions in the NICU in a 30-day period. An additional 1271 modifications to infusions (primarily catecholamines and TPN) occurred during this time period. Assuming an independent double check conservatively took 1 minute to find a person to double check (a gross underestimation) and 1 minute to perform a double check (again, likely an underestimation), for the more than 2000 known changes these units would be required to conservatively devote 4000 minutes or more than 66 hours of nursing time each month for just two of many patient care units. Using conservative estimates for the entire hospital, the numbers of new and modified orders (again excluding changes to intravenous fluid rates) is approximately 8475 per month, requiring (conservatively) more than 282 additional hours of nursing time per month, if the double check process required only 2 minutes.

Practically speaking, in an environment where both economic constraints and the availability of nurses in many markets make the hiring of additional nursing staff unrealistic, this well-intended safety effort (universal double check of infusion pump programming) will add more than 280 hours of nursing work per month for a 220-bed hospital.

In the context of Rasmussen's diagram (see Figure 8–4), the implications for worsened patient safety are dramatic.

The take-home message, based on the work of Rasmussen and findings of both FMEA and ST-PRA, is that understanding work and redesigning work for safety, along with designing new processes in the context of existing work, are essential for improving patient safety. The same concepts apply to considering the implications of quality efforts, whether in the PICU or throughout a hospital.

Safety and Quality Assessment in the Pediatric Intensive Care Unit

There have been relatively few studies of QI or safety efforts in PICUs. Literature and conventional wisdom suggest that children in PICUs are at some of the greatest risk for errors and harm. The opportunities for improvement in safety and quality are great. However, a lack of understanding of the complex environment of the PICU and the work done there lead to undesired harm with either quality or safety efforts.

Organizations, including the Agency for Healthcare Research and Quality, the Society for Critical Care Medicine, and the National Patient Safety Foundation, have demonstrated increased funding for patient safety and QI research over the past 5 years. There are significant opportunities for important, groundbreaking research that can yield genuine improvement in the care of PICU patients.

REFERENCES

1. Committee on Quality of Health Care in America: *Crossing the quality chasm: a new health system for the 21st century.* Washington, DC, 2001, National Academy Press.
2. Woolf SH: Patient safety is not enough: targeting quality improvements to optimize the health of a population. *Ann Intern Med* 140:33-36, 2004.
3. Kohn LT, Corrigan JM, Donaldson MS: Why do errors happen? In Kohn LT, Corrigan JM, Donaldson MS, editors. *To err is human: building a safer health system.* Washington, DC, 1999, National Academy Press.
4. Czaja SJ: Systems design and evaluation. In Salvendy G, editor: *Handbook of human factors and ergonomics,* ed 2. New York, 1997, John Wiley and Sons.
5. Zimmerman B, Lindberg C, Plsek P: *Edgeware: insights from complexity science for health care leaders.* Irving, TX, 1988, VHA Inc.
6. Perrow C: *Normal accidents: living with high-risk technologies,* ed 2. New York, 1984, Basic Books.
7. Lohr KN, editor: *Medicare: a strategy for quality assurance.* Washington, DC, 1990, National Academy Press.
8. Donabedian A: *Explorations in quality assessment and monitoring, volume 1: the definition of quality and approaches to its assessment.* Ann Arbor, MI, 1980, Health Administration Press.
9. Langley GJ, Nolan KM, Nolan TW, et al: *The improvement guide: a practical approach to enhancing organizational performance.* San Francisco, CA, 1996, Jossey-Bass Publishers.
10. Wheeler DJ: *Understanding variation: the key to managing chaos.* Knoxville, TN, 1993, SPC Press.
11. Stein PK. Kleiger RE: Insights from the study of heart rate variability. *Annu Rev Med* 50:249-261, 1999.
12. Kelley DL: *How to use control charts for healthcare.* Milwaukee, WI, 1999, ASQ Quality Press.
13. Reason JT: *Human error.* New York, 1990, Cambridge University Press.
14. Caplan RA, Postner KL, Cheyney FW: Effect of outcome on physician judgments of appropriateness of care. *JAMA* 265:1957-1960, 1991.

15. Runciman WB, Sellen A, Webb RK, et al: The Australian Incident Monitoring Study. Errors, incidents and accidents in anaesthetic practice. *Anaesth Intensive Care* 21:506-519, 1993.
16. Pronovost P, Berebholtz S, Dorman T, et al: Improving communication in the ICU using daily goals. *J Crit Care* 18:17-75, 2003.
17. Pollack MM, Patel KM, Ruttiman UE: PRISM III: an updated Pediatric Risk of Mortality Score. *Crit Care Med* 24:743-752, 1996.
18. Leteurtre S, Martinot A. Duhamel A, et al: Validation of the paediatric logistic organ dysfunction (PELOD) score: prospective, observational, multicentre study. *Lancet* 362:192-197, 2003.
19. Slater A, Shann F, Pearson G: PIM 2: a revised version of the Paediatric Index of Mortality. *Intensive Care Med* 29:278-285, 2003.
20. Scanlon M: Presentation of PICU Quality Indicators. National Association of Children's Hospitals and Related Institutions PICU FOCUS Group Meeting, Alexandria, VA, 2003.
21. Throop C: Personal communication, 2004.
22. Kuhlthau K, Ferris TGG, Iezzoni LI: Risk adjustment for pediatric quality indicators. *Pediatrics* 113:210-216, 2004.
23. Wetzel R, Pon S, Frongello G, et al: Creating a common pediatric critical care Database—A collaboration between the VPICU and NACHRI. *Clin Intensive Care* 10:147, 1999.
24. Kohn LT, Corrigan JM, Donaldson MS: Creating safety systems in health care organizations. In Kohn LT, Corrigan JM, Donaldson MS, editors. *To err is human: building a safer health system.* Washington, DC, 1999, National Academy Press.
25. Reason JT: *Human error.* New York, 1990, Cambridge University Press.
26. McNutt RA, Abrams R, Aron DC: Patient safety efforts should focus on medical errors. *JAMA* 287:1997-2001, 2002.
27. Tokarski C: *Reporting requirements cloud consensus on curbing medical errors.* Rockville, MD, 2000, Agency for Healthcare Research and Quality. Available at *http://www.ahrq.gov/news/ medscap1.htm.*
28. Berwick DM: Communication between health care staff and patients/families. Presented at 3rd Annenberg Conference of Patient Safety, St. Paul, MN, 2001. Available at *http://www.npsf.org/congress archive/2001/summary_thursday.html.*
29. Levy FH: A new error reporting tool in a pediatric intensive care unit. Presented at the Society of Critical Care Medicine's 32nd Critical Care Congress, San Antonio, TX, 2003.
30. Cohen MR: Why error reporting systems should be voluntary. *BMJ* 320:728-729, 2000.
31. Barach P, Small SD: Reporting and preventing medical mishaps: lessons from non-medical near miss reporting systems. *BMJ* 320:759-763, 2000.
32. Park KS: Human error. In Salvendy G, editor: *Handbook of human factors and ergonomics,* ed 2. New York, 1997, John Wiley and Sons.
33. Institute for Safe Medication Practice: Results from ISMP survey on workplace intimidation. 2004. Available at *http://www.ismp.org/Survey0311.htm.*
34. Layde PM, Maas LA, Teret SP, et al: Patient safety efforts should focus on medical injuries. *JAMA* 287:1993-1997, 2002.
35. Perrow C: *Normal accidents: living with high-risk technologies,* ed 2. New York, 1984, Basic Books.
36. Marx DA: Patient safety and a "just culture": a primer for health care executives. Prepared by David Marx, JD, for Columbia University under a grant provided by the National Heart, Lung, and Blood Institute, 2001. Available at *http://www.mers-tm.net/support/Marx_Primer.pdf.*
37. Perrin JM, Bloom SR: Promoting safety in child and adolescent heath care: conference overview. *Ambul Pediatr* 4:43-46, 2004.
38. McCormick MC, Kass B, Elixhauser A, et al: Annual report on access to and utilization of health care for children and youth in the United States—1999. *Pediatrics* 105:219-230, 2000.
39. Slonim AD, LaFleur BJ, Ahmed W, et al: Hospital-reported medical errors in children. *Pediatrics* 111:617-621, 2003.
40. Brennan TA, Leape LL, Laird NM, et al: Incidence of adverse events and negligence in hospitalized patietnes. *N Engl J Med* 324:370-376, 1991.
41. Miller MR, Elixhauser A, Zhan C: Patient safety events during pediatric hospitalizations. *Pediatrics* 111:1358-1366, 2003.
42. Remus D: Personal communication, 2004.
43. Kaushal R, Bates DW, Landrigan C, et al: Medication errors and adverse drug events in pediatric inpatients. *JAMA* 285:2114-2120, 2001.
44. Folli HL, Poole RL, Benitz WE, et al: Medication error prevention by clinical pharmacists in two children's hospitals. *Pediatrics* 79:718-722, 1987.
45. Raju TNK, Kecskes S, Thornton JP, et al: Medication errors in neonatal and paediatric intensive-care units. *Lancet* 2:374-376, 1989.
46. Potts MJ, Phelan KW: Deficiencies in calculation and applied mathematics skills in pediatrics among primary care interns. *Arch Pediatr Adolesc Med* 150:748-752, 1996.
47. Rowe C, Koren T, Koren G: Errors by paediatric residents in calculating drug doses. *Arch Dis Child* 79:56-58, 1998.
48. Kozer E, Scolnik D, Macpherson A, et al: Variables associated with medication errors in pediatric emergency medicine. *Pediatrics* 110:737-742, 2002.
49. Kaushal R, Shojania KG, Bates DW: Effects of computerized physician order entry and clinical decision support on medication safety: a systematic review. *Arch Intern Med* 163:1409-1416, 2003.
50. Oren E, Shaffer ER, Guglielmo BJ: Impact of emerging technologies on medication errors and adverse drug events. *Am J Health Syst Pharm* 60:1447-1458, 2003.
51. Kaushal R, Bates DW: Computerized Physician Order Entry (CPOE with Clinical Decision Support Systems [CDSSs]). In Wachter RM, editor: Making health care safer: a critical analysis of patient safety practices, 2001. Available at *http://www.ahcpr.gov/clinic/ptsafety/chap6.htm.*
52. Kaushal R, Bates DW: Computerized Physician Order Entry (CPOE with Clinical Decision Support Systems [CDSSs]). In Wachter RM, editor: Making health care safer: a critical analysis of patient safety practices, 2001. Available at *http://www.ahcpr.gov/clinic/ptsafety/chap6.htm.*
53. Kuperman GJ, Gibson RF: Computer physician order entry: benefits, costs, and issues. *Ann Intern Med* 139:31-39, 2003.
54. Scanlon M: Computer physician order entry and the real world: we're only human. *Joint Commission Quality Safety* 30:342-346, 2004.
55. Piehl S: Personal communication, 2003.
56. Marx DA, Slonim AD: Assessing patient safety risk before the injury occurs: an introduction to sociotechnical probabilistic risk modelling in health care. *Qual Saf Health Care* 12(suppl 2): ii33-ii38, 2003.
57. FMEA Info Centre: 2004. Available at *http://www.fmeainfocentre.com/.*
58. Murff HJ, Gosbee JW, Bates DW: Human factors and medical devices. In Wachter RM, editor. Making health care safer: a critical analysis of patient safety practices. Available at *http://www.ahrq.gov/clinic/ptsafety/chap41a.htm* (last accessed March 12, 2004).
59. Kohn LT, Corrigan JM, Donaldson MS: Why do errors happen? In: Kohn LT, Corrigan JM, Donaldson MS, editors. *To err is human: building a safer health system.* Washington, DC, 1999, National Academy Press.
60. Sexton JB, Thomas EJ, Helmreich RL: Error, stress and teamwork in medicine and aviation: cross sectional surveys. *BMJ* 320:745-749, 2000.
61. Carthey J, de Leval MR, Reason JT. Human factor in cardiac surgery: errors and near misses in a high technology medical domain. *Ann Thorac Surg* 72:300-305, 2001.
62. Cook RI, Woods DD, Howie MB, Horrow JC, Gaba DM: Case 2-1992. Unintentional delivery of vasoactive drugs with an electromechanical infusion device. *J Cardiothorac Vasc Anesth* 6:238-244, 1992.
63. Scanlon M: Computer physician order entry and the real world: we're only human. *Joint Commission Quality Safety* 30:342-346, 2004.
64. Render ML: Research and redesign are safer than warnings and rules. *Crit Care Med* 32:1074-1075, 2004.
65. Claus PL, Gibbons PS, Kaihoi BH, et al: Usability lab. a new tool for process analysis. Proceedings of 1997 Annual HIMSS Conference, 2:149-159, 1997.
66. Rasmussen J: Risk management in a dynamic society: a modeling problem. *Safety Sci* 1;27:183-213, 1997.
67. Cook RI: Lessons from the war on cancer: the need for basic research on safety. Testimony submitted for the AHRQ sponsored 2nd National Summit on Patient Safety Research, 7 November 2003, Arlington, VA. This document is copyright © 2003 by Richard I. Cook. Contact information: ricook@uchicago.edu, 773-702-4890. Available at *www.ctlab.org.*
68. Joint Commission on Accreditation of Healthcare Organizations. Proposed National Patient Safety Goals, 2004. Available at *www.jcaho.org.*
69. Park KS: Human error. In Salvendy G, editor: *Handbook of human factors and ergonomics,* ed 2. New York, 1997, John Wiley and Sons.
70. Faust T: Estimate of new infusions and infusion order changes. Personal communication, 2004.

CHAPTER

9

Information Technology in Critical Care

Steven Pon, Barry P. Markovitz, and Carl G.M. Weigle

PEARLS

- Information technology promises many benefits but is not without its limitations and pitfalls. Physicians must learn about these technologies to develop realistic expectations, maximize benefit, ensure patient safety, and avoid potentially catastrophic perils.
- Administrators and nurses drive the advancement of various information technologies in most institutions. Physicians, especially intensivists, must become involved in the selection and development of these technologies if their needs and concerns are to be adequately addressed.
- Organizations must ensure the security and confidentiality of personally identifiable health information. They must understand the legislated privacy rules and safeguard the security and confidentiality of patient data.
- All computer users should understand the threats to security and privacy and make informed decisions about the measures required to safeguard them that are commensurate with the task at hand.

Introduction

By one analysis, medicine is an information service. Its practitioners tirelessly gather and assimilate information while adding to the collective body of knowledge. Clinical information is meticulously compiled and interpreted for each patient, the disorders that afflict them, and the therapies to treat them. Efforts to automate medicine do not place patients on conveyor belts to be serially and automatically poked and prodded. Automation efforts are directed at managing the flow of information. Medical information is wielded to protect life and to shepherd death. Compassion, judgment, and technical skill distinguish excellence in the discipline, but information defines medicine.

The volume of medical information, expanding at fantastic rates, threatens to drown even the most conscientious practitioner who devotes every waking hour of every day to collect, catalogue, and assimilate it. Advances in information technology (IT) can both fuel the information explosion and contain it. Computers connected to one another and to large data repositories give practitioners immediate access to vast knowledge and data while streamlining the tedious chores of searching and collating that information. IT has changed the way we practice.

Demonstrations of the potential of IT typically inspire awe and admiration. However, when the technology migrates from demonstration to actual use, awe and admiration sometimes give way to disappointment and disgust. The novel features that users think they need are either impossible to achieve or require significant reengineering of the original product. The lure of the idealized technology suffers from its real limitations. Knowing the limitations helps users to avoid falling victim to them. This understanding can help the clinician focus on what can be accomplished readily while awaiting "the next upgrade."

Programs and Applications

IT has clearly changed our world. The typewriter has disappeared from the office milieu, conspicuously replaced by computers and word processors on every desktop. Lectures are given without slides and overhead projectors, substituted by presentation programs and digital light projectors. Appointment books have given way to personal digital assistants (PDAs) (Box 9–1).

In just over 25 years, the computer industry has sold 1 billion personal computers.[15] The reason those computers are purchased is to run the basic applications: electronic mail (e-mail), web browsers, word processing, and other office productivity programs. Every business card brandishes an e-mail address and a web site address in addition to the name and telephone number. Although embraced by the business world since the torrid 1990s, IT in medicine has achieved only variable penetration.

Calculators, Simulators, and Other Programs

Most of the programs and applications used by physicians are not specifically medically related. They include the ubiquitous word processor and occasionally spreadsheet, database, and presentation programs. Statistics software has liberated us all from the analysis of data by tedious hand calculations while significantly improving accuracy.

The first medical applications of IT came as specialized computer programs that performed ritualized computations. Examples of these were programs that performed

BOX 9–1

A Day with IT in the PICU

ROUNDS

The automatic doors swing open on the thin, bespectacled man in a white coat. His eyes flash brightly but betray a faint weariness not seen in the picture on his identification badge. "Dr. W," it says. He walks briskly to the nearest computer terminal and, with a few taps of the keyboard, logs into the computer-based patient record (CPR) to review the census in the PICU. With a few clicks of the mouse, he requests a printed list of the patients and logs off. The list includes age, height, weight, length of stay, allergies, problems, and a space for scribbled notes. Twenty-four patients on six pages. "A full unit," he muses as he taps impatiently on the printer. He then locates a wireless, mobile, computer cart and wheels it down the corridor to begin rounds with the team.

CPR AND HIPAA

At each bedside, the resident presents a summary of the patient's hospital course. Logged into the CPR, Dr. W follows along, scanning recent orders, reading laboratory results, and searching for trends. The data are displayed in a format configured into his personal profile. Trends in values are evaluated with a plot of values over time. Laboratory data are juxtaposed with clinical data and blood gases with ventilator parameters, and he quickly understands how well this patient is weaning from the ventilator. He asks, almost rhetorically, what the baseline arterial partial pressure of carbon dioxide is for this child with chronic lung disease. He scrolls back in time and reports the answer to the team. Ever mindful of the HIPAA privacy regulations, he is careful to suspend his CPR session when he parks the cart in the hall to walk into the room to examine the patient and speak with the parents. Returning to the cart, he retypes his password, and the chart opens exactly where he left it. He socratically probes the resident for her plan and her reasons for it. Another resident enters orders for changes in mechanical ventilation on the bedside workstation as decisions are made. He suggests that the resident search for an old electrocardiogram to compare to the current one. For this chronic patient, there should be several in the scanned archives of the medical record. The medical records department continues to scan reams of paper into this electronic information warehouse, which is stored on optical disk. Although these records are much more efficient and accessible than paper or microfiche, searching them is still too time consuming to do during rounds. He wishes the two versions of the CPR were more integrated.

Internet References and Calculators

The fellow, expressing concern about the respiratory quotient, asks about the fat content of the tube feeding. Dr. W switches from the CPR to the Internet web browser. Using his favorite search engine, he quickly locates a reliable resource listing the components of a variety of formulas. The formula is changed to one with a more desirable composition. He instructs the resident to estimate the caloric needs of the child and calculate how well the needs are satisfied with the new formula. The fellow whispers to her that the online nutrition calculator does this easily and accurately *(http://info.med.yale.edu/pediat/critcare/nutricalc.htm)*. They move on to the next patient.

The bone marrow transplant patient always presents a challenge, particularly with regard to trying to juggle all the medications. Rather than asking "What was the creatinine yesterday and the day before?," Dr. W answers his own question quickly with two clicks of his mouse. He can see the falling urine output despite the increasing doses of furosemide. Of course, this process frees up time on rounds for more meaningful questions and exchanges between team members, actually synthesizing information rather than simply regurgitating it.

PDA and Web References

He is concerned about the rising creatinine and the need to adjust the medications. The fellow unholsters her PDA and consults a drug reference. The cidofovir must be renally adjusted but not the caspofungin, she reports. A urine collection to measure creatinine clearance is ordered, but a good-natured race ensues to calculate an estimated creatinine clearance. The PDA calculator wins over the web-based calculator only because the network is a bit slow today. Dr. W then uses the web browser to access the hospital formulary database via the hospital's Intranet. This resource uniquely integrates the hospital formulary, hospital policies, and a drug reference database into a single web-enabled database. The cidofovir dose is adjusted pending the measured

Continued on Following Page

BOX 9–1

A Day with IT in the PICU (Continued)

creatinine clearance. The formulary also informs Dr. W that ganciclovir remains in short supply, satisfying his curiosity as to why this more familiar drug was not being used. He asks about drug interactions and assigns the fellow to review all of the medications for this patient, as he thinks of this unfulfilled promise of computerized physician order entry in its current iteration.

Web Paging

The resident is instructed to consult the nephrologist on call about the impending renal failure and the likely need for dialysis. While rounds proceed, he opens the locally developed OnCall system and identifies which nephrologist is on call. The application reveals that at this time of day, this particular physician prefers to be paged rather than called. The resident then goes to the WWW-based paging site and sends a brief text message regarding the consult and requests a call back. Concerned for patient privacy, the resident ensures that the page identifies the resident by name but the patient only by room number.

EBJC

Dr. W notes that the patient's oxygenation had not changed significantly for more than 1 week and the ventilator settings continue to hover around the same. A glance of his printout reveals a 2-week length of stay. "What about steroids for her ARDS?" he inquires. In response to the puzzled look on the resident's face, the fellow again draws out her PDA and opens a copy of the evidence-based journal club appraisal of one of the better clinical trials. Their heads nearly bump as they huddle around the little device. A discussion ensues about the applicability to this patient with a bone marrow transplant and the concerns over treating such a patient with steroids.

THE REMAINS OF THE DAY

Picture Archiving and Communication System

Having completed work rounds, Dr. W leads the team to view the day's radiographs on the picture archiving and communication system (PACS). All radiographic studies—filmless plain radiographs, computerized tomography scans, and magnetic resonance images—are stored on central servers and downloaded to the workstations in clinical areas. Files also are sent to an Internet-based archive that allows viewing from any networked computer, although at a lower resolution than at the dedicated workstations.

The two vertically oriented monitors for the PACS workstation in the PICU have one third the resolution of those used by the radiologists, but Dr. W finds them adequate for his competent ability to read a radiograph. He can magnify, "bright light," and even invert the colors to look for a subtle pneumothorax. He is able to read the radiologist's interpretations and compare them with the actual images. By far his favorite feature is being able to place a single computerized tomography image on the screen and scroll through all of the images in place. He can follow organs or masses through several images without having to reorient himself as he switches from picture to picture. He also can get a three-dimensional reconstruction from a magnetic resonance angiogram and simulate turning the head. After teaching the residents some practical anatomy, Dr. W dismisses the team.

Notes and Billing

After speaking to two consultants and several sets of parents, Dr. W settles into the attending on-service office to write his notes. It was not as much of a struggle to get all the physicians documenting online as he had once feared. It was more like converting to the metric system: laying down the law was a bit painful at first, particularly for the poor typists, but once everyone got accustomed to it, they all recognized it was better even if only for the improved legibility and accessibility. The documentation is better as well, but the notes became profoundly verbose because earlier notes can be copied and pasted into the current note. Some clinicians clamored for voice recognition software or transcription services, but available solutions did not work well with their practice style or were too expensive. He wished that the system could help him write compliant notes, particularly when using the in-patient evaluation and management codes. His greatest wish is to convert the text within the progress notes into real data that can be queried systematically. There are specialized note-writing programs that might accomplish that, but none of those is compatible with their current CPR. He is lost in thought when his PDA starts beeping. With a glance at his watch and a deep sigh, he gets up to go to conference.

Conference: Virtual PICU

At the afternoon research conference, discussion centers on the plans to participate actively in the Virtual PICU (VPICU) project. The initial involvement consisted of assisting with testing the VPICU database tool being codeveloped by the National Association of Children's Hospitals and Related Institutions (NACHRI, *http://www.childrenshospitals.net/*) and the VPICU group *(http://www.picu.org/)*. The section enthusiastically supports the plan of contributing to an effort to contribute to a national database of PICU patient data by adopting a common tool for data collection. It is hoped that interfacing with the clinical information system can facilitate some data collection, even simply for basic patient demographics. The potential for useful interinstitutional benchmarking, as well as internal quality improvement purposes, is a close fit with his section's aims and goals. In the long term, the VPICU group plans to support collection of a highly granular dataset, including frequently sampled physiologic measurements. The section hopes that local information technology developments will allow them to contribute meaningfully to that effort as well.

Consultation

As he emerges from conference, the resident informs Dr. W of a child with status asthmaticus and an increasing oxygen requirement on the general pediatric ward. They want to transfer the patient to the PICU. With the fellow extubating a patient and the unit full, Dr. W goes to see the patient himself. The patient is tachypneic and tachycardic on oxygen via a partial nonrebreather mask. There is minimal wheezing even on forced exhalation. At a nearby workstation, the resident reviews the chart with Dr. W, who notes the frequent, high-dose, nebulized albuterol. "He was requiring more and more oxygen, so we increased the frequency of the albuterol," responded the resident when asked about the reason for the dosing scheme. Dr. W begins his favorite lecture about ventilation-perfusion mismatch and overcoming hypoxemic vasoconstriction with β-agonists. The resident is left with instructions to drastically decrease the albuterol dosing and to call back to the PICU with hourly progress reports. Dr. W writes a quick note in the patient's chart, and he enters into a special physician coding program on his PDA the medical record number, diagnosis,

Continued on Following Page

BOX 9–1

A Day with IT in the PICU (Continued)

and procedure code. He points his PDA toward the infrared (IrDA) port of a nearby printer and prints the information for the billing department. He returns to writing notes for the PICU patients, confident that he has deflected an unnecessary PICU admission.

PICU List

After finishing his notes and ensuring that the asthmatic patient on the pediatric ward is improving, Dr. W searches the Internet but finds almost nothing related to Joint Commission on Accreditation of Healthcare Organizations (JCAHO) guidelines for physical restraints in PICUs. The JCAHO (*http://www.jcaho.org/*) and Centers for Medicare and Medicaid Services (CMS, formerly HCFA, *http://www.cms.hhs.gov*) web sites make it clear that these guidelines were developed originally for elderly residents of nursing homes and appear to have been quite hastily extended to pediatrics. However, the hospital administration, concerned about the risk of a JCAHO citation, developed stringent guidelines that require daily reordering of physical restraints. Clearly, this applies to the vast majority of patients in the PICU, making compliance difficult and strict compliance potentially dangerous. He decides to query the 2000 or so members of the PICU e-mail discussion group (*piculist@vpicu.org or www.picu.net/piculist/*) about their experience with these guidelines. He wants to know how many are trying to comply with the guidelines and how. He is curious if there have been any bad outcomes attributable to compliance with the rules. Being away from his office computer, Dr. W pulls out his new wireless PDA and clicks the tiny keys on the little sheath-like keyboard attachment.

ON CALL

Remote Access

Just before he leaves for home, Dr. W directly supervises the insertion of a central venous catheter by the senior resident while the fellow is tending to other duties. It goes smoothly, and he checks with the fellow before going home. During his ride home, the light on his wireless PDA flashes red, indicating an incoming e-mail. When he pulls into his driveway, he reads a message from the fellow asking Dr. W to look at the follow-up radiograph from the central line insertion. He goes inside, turns on his computer, and connects to the hospital by a VPN. Using a web browser, he logs into the Internet-based PACS. Although not as sophisticated as, and with lower resolution than, the PACS in the PICU, the images are compressed, speeding file transfer. He finds the image and magnifies it, then calls the ICU and tells the fellow to pull the catheter back 5 cm and out of the lumbar vein. He opens a session of the CPR remotely and satisfies himself that there is no interval change in the sickest patients. He then visits each of his children and spouse to bid them goodnight before they go to sleep.

Virtual Care

In the middle of eating his rewarmed dinner, the fellow calls. She had received a telephone call from an intensivist covering the "electronic ICU." Dr. W knows this intensivist who electronically covers a number of adult intensive care units in the hospital network system from a remote command center. With an increased awareness of the role of intensivists on the quality of care in the ICU but with limited numbers of available personnel, the hospital had contracted for a sophisticated system of networked computers and monitors with analytic software and teleconferencing capabilities for each ICU bed. The remote intensivist had been asked to "consult" on a 10 year-old patient in the medical ICU of a community hospital. He reviewed the electronic data over the network and turned on the video cameras and microphones in the patient's room. After a protracted discussion with the bedside nurse and the physician's assistant caring for the patient, he recommended transferring the patient to the pediatric ICU at the children's hospital. Hence the telephone call. Dr. W told the fellow to dispatch the transport team as soon as they got the request directly from the community hospital. As he goes to bed on a full stomach, he wistfully thinks about having the remote, electronic ICU set up in his own home, one with robotics so he could insert a thoracostomy tube from home. Of course, he is dreaming.

CONCLUSION

Although these scenarios are fictional, they represent the experiences of several intensivists and accurately reflect how technology has changed the way many of us practice intensive care. All the technologies described exist today, although few of us have the full range of them. In this case, there is nothing more certain than change.

---

statistical analysis of data, formulated complex parenteral nutrition, calculated hemodynamic and oxygen transport parameters from thermodilution cardiac output measurements, and created tables of emergency medication doses. Other useful but more complex applications have been created and include pharmacokinetics and mechanical ventilation simulators. These programs continue to exist in one form or another. Some have migrated to different platforms on which they run. Many have migrated from mainframe computers to personal computers to networked computers and now to PDAs.

Another important development is that these applications can be written by persons with little or no programming experience in a wide range of programming languages, democratizing advanced computer use that once was reserved for persons with pocket protectors and holstered calculators.

Some of these programs now can be found in a variety of devices not traditionally considered computers but that operate on integrated circuit computer chips. Intravenous pumps, in addition to their standard function, can calculate the dosing of medicated infusions based on the concentration and fluid infusion rate. Although admittedly pedestrian, these peripheral devices in large arrays can feed clinical databases with important information when interfaced properly. Other, more complex devices, such as ventilators, can perform much more sophisticated tasks, sometimes adjusting ventilator settings based on changes in lung compliance or in patient effort, and can feed their data to other devices more accessible to clinicians for interpretation and analysis.

Voice Recognition

Continuous speech recognition has achieved high degrees of accuracy in current iterations. Although this technology results in a 95% accuracy and higher, it is still unclear whether practitioners are ready to use it in their daily practice. Most of the current commercial products are relatively inexpensive but should be complemented by high-quality microphones and a medical lexicon. Without adding prepackaged medical terminology, users may need to add several hundred words manually to achieve 98% accuracy. Some of the more specialized systems made for radiology or pathology have even higher accuracy rates because they do better with jargon-laden text than plain English. Correcting errors further improves accuracy as the voice recognition software learns from its mistakes. Careful editing is still required, lest the benign "The patient was evaluated" becomes the alarming "The patient was violated."

A fast processor, plenty of random access memory (RAM), and a "speech quality" sound card are absolute essentials for speech recognition. Each user typically maintains his/her own voice profile that is continually modified as it is used. Each profile is several megabytes in size, making it impractical to move from machine to machine or to use the profile across a local area network. It is possible to use a high-quality digital microphone to record the dictation to be downloaded later for conversion to text, but most users dictate directly into computers dedicated for this purpose.

As the demands for detailed physician documentation increase with increasing medical, legal, and billing compliance pressures, some physicians are turning to voice recognition. Though it can work for specific types of practices, its role in critical care is not clear.

Medical Knowledgebases

Some physicians and programmers looked to IT to manage complex knowledgebases. Computerized formularies with readily accessible pharmacologic information were developed, and some of them included information about potential drug interactions when they were provided with a list of medications to which a patient was exposed. Other programs were designed with some form of artificial intelligence or codification of the complex process of winnowing down a differential diagnosis. Less technologically impressive but still important is the electronic publication of well-known textbooks and other digital-only textbooks. However, the medical knowledgebase in constant demand is that of the world's burgeoning medical periodic literature.

Intelligent Searching

Gone are the days of pouring over the *Index Medicus* and the *Science Citation Index* to compile lists of journal references and of spending hours in the library stacks and copy room gathering articles. The National Library of Medicine embraced IT long before many of us knew what it was and translated their catalogues of medical literature into electronically searchable databases. Once only available on mainframe computers connected by slow and costly modem connections, Medline databases became available on personal computers via compact disks and eventually the Internet. The Medline interfaces were awkward but have become increasingly easy to use, with graphical user interfaces, hypertext links, and efficient search algorithms.

Resources

Once an online search was executed, access to the full text of the articles necessitated a visit to the library stacks. Some publishers produced electronic versions of their journals on compact disk, but an increasing number are making their journals available on the Internet. A number of publishers require a subscription fee for access to the online journals. Many of them offer access free. Although the revenue may decrease from fewer subscriptions, their not insignificant printing and mailing costs also decrease. The business models continue to be reworked as publishers figure out how to remain competitive in an evolving marketplace.

The knowledgebases available have come to include fully searchable online reference books. Many of these books are electronic versions of established medical textbooks, but some exist only in electronic form. Other knowledgebases include evidenced-based medicine reviews and practice guidelines from various medical societies and agencies. These searchable documents also exist as standalone products for nonnetworked computers and for handheld devices.

Educational software is yet another IT application that is becoming increasingly available. Combined with a network or Internet connection, this becomes a cornucopia of distance learning.

Treasure or Trash?

Ascertaining the veracity and overall quality of medical information obtained from a web site can be difficult, particularly for lay persons. A Harris poll in 2001 concluded that nearly 100 million Americans regularly seek health care information online. A range of organizations have developed methods to evaluate and rate the more than 100,000 web sites offering health-related information.[25] These methods include (1) self-policing by adherence to codes of conduct, (2) user guides to facilitate critical assessment of sites and their information, (3) lists of "quality" filtered sites, (4) quality labels applied to reviewed sites that satisfy quality criteria, and (5) third-party certification or accreditation. Each of these methods has obvious problems, not the least of which is the often absent description of how "quality" is determined and whether it is objective or reproducible.

Perhaps, as in the paper world, reputation should count the most. Health care information from respectable medical organizations or journals should rank high on any list. On the web, one measure of reputation is the number of inbound links to a particular site. If relevant and reputable, other sites will forge hyperlinks to that site. One search engine *(google.com)* ranks web sites partly by this measure.

It is important for practitioners to have some knowledge of what information their patients and families are consuming. Physicians also should be able to direct their patients and families to reputable, high-quality sites with reliable information (Box 9–2).

Evidence-Based Medicine and the Internet

What evidence is best? How do we find it? How do we appraise its validity and results? How do we apply it to our patients? Moreover, perhaps most crucial of all to intensive care unit (ICU) practice: how do we practice evidence-based medicine (EBM) in real time in our units? Every practitioner endeavors to maintain currency with the best evidence to provide optimal care for his/her patients. "Evidence based medicine is the conscientious, explicit, and judicious use of current best evidence in making decisions about the care of individual patients."[19] Its tool set, based upon rules of clinical epidemiology, can help with these questions when properly applied (see Chapter 6).

No longer are sound pathophysiologic reasoning and personal experience sufficient to provide appropriate medical care. Traditional skills now must be supplemented with the results from the burgeoning outcomes-oriented

BOX 9–2

Top-Ten List of Web Sites Relevant to Pediatric Critical Care Medicine

1. PedsCCM: Pediatric Critical Care Medicine web site *(http://PedsCCM.org/)*
   From the feedback received and indirect evidence, this is the headquarters for pediatric critical care medicine on the web. It represents a multidisciplinary educational and practical resource, with announcements, reports, opportunities (including fellowship listings and physician and nursing jobs databases), organized links to original educational material and research reports, and the PedsCCM Evidence-based Journal Club (see Box 9–3).
2. American Academy of Pediatrics *(http://www.aap.org/)*
   The Section on Critical Care of the American Academy of Pediatrics (AAP) is very active in promoting the interests of critically ill children and pediatric intensivists within the Academy. The Academy is the prime advocate for children's health care in the United States. For AAP members, the Members Only channel contains timely announcements relevant to all pediatricians. The AAP Policy Statements and Practice Guidelines are available on this site.
3. Society of Critical Care Medicine *(http://www.sccm.org/)*
   As a prime supporter of the intensivist-directed multidisciplinary critical care team, the Society of Critical Care Medicine (SCCM) plays an important role in education and advocacy. The SCCM's educational and research programs, including the American College of Critical Care's guidelines and practice parameters, are on this site. The organization has launched an online "digital community workplace" with chat rooms, threaded discussion groups, file sharing, and calendar functions. There are designated "e-rooms" for every section, chapter, and committee of the SCCM.
4. Pediatric Critical Care Education *(http://www. picucourse.org/)*
   The product of the Resident Education Committee of the Pediatric Section of the SCCM, this site contains a cornucopia of downloadable lectures (as Microsoft PowerPoint files) on pediatric critical care topics geared toward residents rotating through the PICU. A self-evaluation program is included.
5. *Pediatric Critical Care Medicine* Journal *(http://www. pccmjournal.org/)*
   The subspecialty's first peer-reviewed original journal is online, with full-text available for subscribers.
6. Emedicine Pediatrics *(http://www.emedicine.com/ped/)*
   A well-organized and succinct textbook of pediatrics on the web and freely accessible. Although the critical care section is sparse, it is an excellent resource for many other relevant topics in cardiology, infectious disease, and endocrinology.
7. Calculators on the Web and Handheld Devices
   Several sites maintain online interactive calculators to enable diverse calculations from Yale's (Dr. Michael Apkon) nutritional support page *(http://info.med.yale.edu/pediat/ critcare/nutricalc.htm)* to Cornell's (Dr. Steve Pon) multifunction medical calculators *(http://cornellpicu.org/)*. PICUTools is a downloadable suite of such tools for your Palm OS PDA (Dr. Michael Verive at *http://www. mverive.com/*) Finally, the Harriet Lane Handbook now is available in PDA format *(http://www.skyscape.com/)*.
8. Networking
   The Virtual PICU *(http://www.picu.net)* joins dozens of PICUs learning how to track outcomes, measure quality, and engage in benchmarking. The VPS (VPICU Performance System) is available through the VPICU, as is information on distance learning, pediatric critical care telemedicine, and more. The VPICU also hosts our specialty's premier discussion forum (email and/or web-based), the PICU list.
9. Drug References
   Few resources benefit more from the rapid accessibility and searching capability than drug databases and references. Many exist, from the venerable Physicians Drug Reference *(http://www.pdr.net)* to the well-established Drug Information Handbook from Lexi-Comp *(http://www. lexi.com/)*. PDA versions of several drug databases also are available and rapidly becoming indispensable to junior and experienced clinicians.
10. Subscription-Based Sites
    Many institutions subscribe to Ovid *(http://www.ovid. com/)*, which includes access to several biomedical bibliographic databases, such as Medline and EMBASE, full-text to many biomedical journals, and new interactive diagnostic (MedWeaver) and management (Clineguide) tools. MDConsult *(http://www.mdconsult.com/)* offers a wide range of resources, from contemporary primary clinical research summaries to full-text electronic textbooks.

The URLs listed in this chapter are current and accurate as of the time of publication. For the most up-to-date information, consult the resources linked from the PedsCCMM website *(http://PedsCCM.org)*.

clinical research. No longer is it good enough to know that a new drug will raise the arterial oxygen tension by 10%. Does this agent improve survival, reduce the need for mechanical ventilation, or minimize other significant morbidity? Increasingly, practitioners and their patients now require proof of an improved quality of life as well.

EBM and the Internet are natural partners; they developed contemporaneously but share more than age. The Internet includes a number of excellent resources for learning more about EBM and is a prime source of both primary and preappraised evidence (Box 9–3).

Several excellent resources on the web allow users to explore EBM and many of its current incarnations. The Health Informatics Research Unit web site of McMaster University, the Netting the Evidence web site, and the PedsCCM web site include "meta-sites" or annotated bibliographies with hyperlinks to many other quality resources. Duke University and the University of North Carolina offer web-based tutorials that lead the student through each step of EBM: asking a well-designed clinical question, searching for the evidence, critically appraising the evidence, and learning how to apply the evidence to your own patient. The entire series of Users' Guides to the Medical Literature, originally published in *JAMA,* is available on the Canadian Centre for Health Evidence web site. An interactive version is available by subscription.

The web can provide users with primary evidence. Medline, the bibliographic database maintained by the National Library of Medicine, has an excellent free interface at the PubMed web site. Particularly useful for the evidence-based practitioner is its "clinical queries" tool (on the left side bar of the main search page). This tool automatically applies filters to search terms, enabling focused searching for studies dealing with articles on therapy, diagnosis, prognosis, or etiology. Increasingly useful is PubMed's LinkOut feature, which enables one-click direct access to the full-text article if it is available on the web. In almost all cases, the individual or the institution must own a subscription to the journal to read the text. Some popular third-party interfaces to Medline offer additional features, including full-text articles of many journals.

Searching for and then appraising original clinical research studies can be time consuming and potentially problematic if the evidence is scarce or conflicting. Rather than relying on narrative and potentially biased subjective topical reviews, EBM calls for increasing reliance on preappraised sources of evidence, such as critical appraisals of original trials, systematic reviews (including meta-analyses), and evidence-based guidelines. The web has all three.

Critical appraisals of original clinical research studies are available at numerous "journal clubs" on the web. The Department of Pediatrics at the University of Michigan maintains an excellent collection of pediatric "CATs" (critically appraised topics). These are concise summaries of original research designed around answering specific clinical questions. Perhaps most pertinent to pediatric critical care, the PedsCCM web site includes an evidence-based journal club, where structured appraisals are submitted, peer reviewed, and posted as a resource for our field. More than 250 reviews cover topics from the use of surfactant in pediatric respiratory failure to the role of hypothermia after head injury.

As the body of original clinical research grows, the role of systematic reviews increases. The Cochrane

BOX 9–3

EBM Web Sites

Learning about EBM
- Health Informatics Research Unit, McMaster University
  http://hiru.mcmaster.ca/
- Netting the Evidence
  http://www.nettingtheevidence.org.uk/
- Introduction to Evidence-Based Medicine, Duke University and University of North Carolina
  http://www.hsl.unc.edu/services/tutorials/ebm/index.htm
- PedsCCM
  http://PedsCCM.org/
- Users' Guides to the Medical Literature, Canadian Centre for Health Evidence
  http://www.cche.net/usersguides/main.asp
  http://www.userguides.org/ (interactive version available by subscription)

Primary Sources of Evidence
- PubMed, version of Medline, United States National Library of Medicine
  http://www.pubmed.gov/
- Ovid, version of Medline
  http://www.ovid.com/
- MDConsult
  http://www.mdconsult.com/

Preappraised Sources of Evidence

Critically Appraised Topics
- Department of Pediatrics, University of Michigan
  http://www.med.umich.edu/pediatrics/ebm/
- PedsCCM
  http://PedsCCM.org/

Systematic Reviews
- The Cochrane Library
  http://www.cochrane.org/

Evidence-Based Guidelines
- NIH Guideline Clearinghouse
  http://www.guideline.gov/
- American College of Critical Care Medicine guidelines
  http://www.sccm.org/
- American Academy of Pediatrics
  http://www.aap.org/
- Canadian Pediatric Society
  http://www.cps.ca/

Collaboration is an international organization dedicated to developing, disseminating, and maintaining systematic reviews of virtually all aspects of health care. The Cochrane Library is available on the web by subscription; increasingly more institutions are subscribing to this essential resource. You can easily locate systematic reviews on PubMed with the unique filter button under "clinical queries."

The logical progression of EBM's approach to preappraised evidence involves synthesizing it into evidence-based guidelines for the management of specific conditions. The ultimate guideline resource on the web is the NIH's Guideline Clearinghouse. Specific to critical care is the American College of Critical Care Medicine's list of guidelines and practice parameters. The American Academy of Pediatrics and the Canadian Pediatric Society also maintain a set of such guidelines.

Research Databases

Few areas of clinical or laboratory research do not generate volumes of information that require analysis. All but the simplest studies involve entry of data into an electronic database. Perhaps the most common types of databases involve single flat tables of variables and measured values. In fact, many researchers use spreadsheet programs, not database programs, to perform most of their analyses. As data are acquired and complex relationships among the data are built into the data models, their structure becomes more intricate and better suited to true database programs. Most of these are relational database programs that run on personal computers or on mainframes. Both the characteristics of the data and the nature of the desired output affect the design of the data models and database structure.

There are new areas of research where the sheer volume of information can overwhelm any single program or computer system. The solution to which increasingly more researchers are turning met enormous success in fields such as astronomy, astrophysics, and genetics. That solution is *internetworking* (see Chapter 5).

The new field of *bioinformatics* occupies the intersection between biogenetics and IT. The volume of biologic data being collected cannot be digested without some way of processing it. The data include not only DNA sequencing, but also polymorphisms, cross-species comparisons, levels of mRNA expression, protein–protein interactions and enzyme kinetics, location of gene products within the cell, and the three-dimensional structure of the macromolecular gene products and their ligands. Linking these databases with clinical databases represents additional challenges, but ones that are being met. The Online Mendelian Inheritance in Man database of inherited human disorders is a successful example. Linking genetic variation and clinical response to drugs with the goal of adjusting therapeutic regimens according to genetic profiles represents the challenge of pharmacogenomics.[1,7] Many other areas of research are amenable to this approach, including an initiative on brain research.[17]

The problem of integrating data from multiple, disparate databases is difficult. The separate databases could be consolidated into one large database, but both the data and the data model can easily become asynchronous with the contributing databases. The other approach is *federation,* where the original databases exist on their own but are linked together, some of which are bound by data standards. These include standard, regulated vocabularies, and a standard syntax to govern the form of the data. Rather than adopting a particular platform (Unix or Windows) and a particular program, *eXtensible Markup Language* (XML) has emerged as the standard syntax because of its flexibility. It also allows these databases to be freely available on the Internet, open to query by researchers worldwide. Specialized data that require further characterization are governed by additional specifications such as Biopolymer Markup Language (BIOML) and MicroArray Markup Language (MAML) for microarray data (see Chapter 92).

Ethics and patient privacy and confidentiality represent key issues for some of these research efforts. Biogenetic information about individuals could lead to discrimination, particularly for insurance, employment, or even marriage. Simply removing patient identifiers is not adequate because it is still possible to bring together information from a variety of sources to reconstruct, either exactly or probabilistically, the identity of patients. Fortunately, there are means for adequately protecting confidentiality, including mediation and scrubbing. *Mediation* programs on a database limit the kinds of queries and responses based on specified rules and requester privilege. *Scrubbing* blurs the data by decreasing precision or reporting ranks rather than actual values. It also limits queries to those resulting in more than a specified "bin" size. Queries that violate preset rules would not yield results. Although the privacy and confidentiality issues may be soluble with judicious application of technology, the ethical issues may be more intractable and will require careful study and action.

The methods used in bioinformatics have fundamentally changed the way research is done for an increasing segment of biology and medicine. Rather than first going to the laboratory, researchers move first to the database, and experiments are planned only after the available data are evaluated. One author predicts that "the clinical research teams that will be most successful in the coming decades will be those that can switch effortlessly between the laboratory bench, clinical practice, and the use of these sophisticated computational tools."[2]

Given the direction of this evolving technology, it is conceivable that clinical data from multiple institutions could be linked in similar ways. Detailed analysis for patterns in large volumes of clinical data can serve as a springboard to novel clinical studies. This kind of analysis is known as *data mining* in some disciplines but is referred derogatorily as *data torturing* by some. The true value of this approach cannot yet be predicted, but there can be no argument that the limitation of most studies in pediatric critical care is currently the paucity of data from individual institutions. In aggregate, who knows what we may learn?

Clinical Databases

The *computer-based patient record* (CPR) or *electronic medical record* (EMR) is defined as a comprehensive database of personal, health-related information that is accessed and updated across a health care network. Its potential and real benefits include the following:

- *Improved quality of care* through more timely, more complete, and better organized information delivery to the health care provider, with decision support and clinical pathways
- *Cost savings* through elimination of duplicate testing, shorter lengths of stay, and more efficient data collection and review
- *Higher productivity* by structuring patient care tasks to improve continuity of care and reduce practice variation, by facilitating the creation of more consistent and more comprehensive content, and by making the medical records more readily accessible to more users simultaneously
- *Facilitated research, education, quality improvement, outcomes assessment, and strategic planning*

Although not fully implemented anywhere to date, there is some consensus regarding the content and scope of the CPR. The three principal functions of such a database, like any database, are data acquisition, data access, and data storage.

Data Acquisition

The complete CPR acquires data from a variety of sources, including hospital registration, nursing and physician input, laboratory services, radiology and other test interpretations, therapist and nutrition services, monitoring devices, and physicians' orders. The most important system that feeds the database is the "enterprise-wide master patient index," which ensures that each patient is identified properly and uniquely. All other systems must have the correct identifier in order to deliver their data to the correct patient record. A multimedia database can include images such as radiographs, electrocardiograms, fetal monitoring, sonography, magnetic resonance images, computerized tomograms, and even paper-based documents such as consent forms, questionnaires, and sometimes handwritten notes and hand-drawn diagrams. Data acquisition is organized in a manner that minimizes duplicative effort and maximizes data consistency.

One of the significant challenges to any implementation of a CPR is engineering the various interfaces between it and the host of systems that feed it data. Some of the feeder systems, such as laboratory services, have their own, established, validation protocols that are applied before transmission to the CPR. Other systems, such as bedside data entry, require new validation protocols. These new protocols can include defining error range or acceptable value checks of the input data. The challenge is more daunting when it involves two-way interfaces, as in computerized physician order entry.

Considering that a data element passes from one of several feeder systems through different computers with possible transformations of that data element along the way and considering the possibilities of lost transmissions, computer down times, and network interruptions, consistent error-free data feeding would seem a virtual miracle. In a high-volume environment, a centralized interface engine that routes and converts transaction messages from disparate feeder systems can solve many of the interface issues efficiently and in a timely fashion.

The capture of textual information, such as progress notes, nursing assessments, or even radiology reports, presents particular challenges for several reasons. For the most part, text is entered via a keyboard, but alternatives include voice recognition, handwriting recognition, or hand-held and wireless devices (see section on voice recognition). Many other technologies have failed in practice to date. Semi-automated text entry with menu systems feeding structured and unstructured forms have met with some success. Although these solutions do not have the same expressivity of free text, they lend themselves to the capture of text as data. Collecting data better allows for future analysis, but despite this significant advantage over collecting bland text, it tends to be rigid, can make the unusual impossible, generally requires more time to collect, and may be a significant source of frustration for the clinician. The decision to pursue data rather than text requires an institutional commitment to the philosophy that data are more valuable and are worth the difficulties they can present.

Data Access

The computerized patient record serves as the focal point for most health care professionals. It might be accessed at inpatient sites, but also in emergency departments, nursing facilities, continuing care centers, physician offices, clinics, laboratory facilities, treatment centers, and, in the case of home health services, the patient's home. An ideal computerized patient record should be available when and where it is needed. However, databases with sensitive information must be controlled to prevent unauthorized use or alteration. These systems must satisfy five requirements:

1. *Access control:* Only authorized persons are allowed access for authorized uses.
2. *Authentication:* Some confirmation that a person granted access is, in fact, who they purport to be (see section on Authentication).
3. *Confidentiality:* No unauthorized disclosure of information is allowed (see Health Insurance Portability and Accountability Act).
4. *Integrity:* Information content is unalterable except under authorized circumstances.
5. *Attribution/nonrepudiation:* Actions taken (access, data entry, and data modification) are reliably traceable.

Much has been written about the interface through which most health care providers interact with the computerized patient record. It should be user friendly and intuitive. Most clinicians have little time or patience to sit through tedious training sessions, and, once trained, few clinicians will recall more than a minimum required to complete their immediate, routine tasks.

The system should be capable of providing a full, seamless view of the patient over time and across points of care. Views should be configurable so that a given user's information needs and workflow can be accommodated. Both detailed and summary views that juxtapose relevant data allow the clinician to acquire the information required to optimize expedient decision making. Displays should be configured to highlight key information while suppressing clutter but making all pertinent data readily accessible. Dynamic linkages should exist between the computerized patient record and supporting functions such as expert systems, clinical pathways, protocols, policies, reference material, and the medical literature.

Response times must be sufficiently speedy and workstations should be conveniently accessible to the point of care. Mobile connections would be a bonus. Access of patient data via wireless connections with portable devices or via PDAs are attractive alternatives for users but must overcome usability and security hurdles before they can be fully implemented (see section on wireless networks).

The patient database also supports many areas of research, education, decision support, and external reporting. Thus data in aggregate can be accessed by administration, finance, quality assurance, and research areas.

The critical issues of patient information confidentiality are discussed in the sections on the Health Insurance Portability and Accountability Act (HIPAA) regulations and on privacy (see sections on Health Insurance Portability and Accountability Act and on Privacy). The security of the database includes physical security, prevention of unauthorized access, and protection from malicious software (see section on Security).

Data Storage

The multimedia data of the comprehensive CPR are stored on media that allow for long-term storage while allowing searches and rapid retrieval of enormous volumes of data. The specific type of medium is not as important as the ready availability of the data. The database must be updated in a way that ensures that it is current, complete, and consistent. Data, once entered, should be modifiable only in accordance with strict rules that assure data integrity.

The architecture of the database can be centralized or distributed, replicated or not. A *centralized database* is stored at a single site, whereas a distributed database is a single logical database with segments that are spread across multiple locations connected by a network. A *replicated database* has the advantage over a nonreplicated database by having at least one copy of all records in case the primary copy is inaccessible because of computer or network failure. The challenge of replication is maintaining consistency among all the copies, requiring timely, automatic synchronization of the original database and its replicas.

Even nonreplicated databases must be backed up periodically to ensure against data loss. The strategy for doing so as seamlessly as possible and for establishing a clear and workable recovery strategy is imperative with a CPR.

Once stored, the data should have a time stamp. Although the data can be modified, both the original and the revised versions should be maintained with appropriate time stamping. Appropriate safeguards must ensure database integrity so that its pieces do not lose their links and that the data are not subject to unauthorized modification. Supplanting the paper record with the CPR as the official medical record requires thoughtful consideration of the limitations of paper copies to reflect accurately the electronic record. Sanctioned hard copies of the patient record will be necessary for sharing with other health care institutions or with the legal system.

Whereas a clinical data repository is a database optimized to retrieve data on individual patients, a data warehouse is a database designed to support data analysis across individuals. This function can be distinguished from a simple archival function. The warehouse structure is designed to support a variety of analyses, including elaborate queries on large amounts of data. The data are generally static and updated intermittently in batches rather than continuously.

Hospitals can use data warehouses to perform financial analyses or quality assessments. With decision support tools they can be useful in negotiating managed care contracts or distributing resources to clinical or ancillary services. Subsets of a data warehouse that are structured to support a single department or function are "data marts." These subsets are designed to perform periodic analyses or to produce standard reports run repeatedly, such as monthly financial statements or quality measures. Online analytical processing (OLAP) is decision support on databases that are partially digested for analysis and thus are more rapid. In finance and administration, they can assist in strategic planning, predicting the impact of decisions before they are made. In medicine, it can take the form of a clinical database to support evidence-based decisions. Data mining applications can sift through mountains of data in the warehouse and run complex algorithms to find obscure patterns. However, as with any database, the questions must be defined as precisely as possible and the database designed accordingly if meaningful results are to be expected.

Decision Support

Decision support systems are an integrated set of programs and databases that provide users with the ability to interrogate those databases and analyze information, retrieving data from external sources, if necessary, to assist in decision making.

Most medical decision support systems are designed to improve the process and the outcome of clinical decision making. They can yield most of the benefit of clinical information systems, for example, shorten inpatient length of stay, decrease adverse drug interactions, improve the consistency and content of medical records, improve continuity of care and follow-up, and reduce practice variation.

Retrospective decision support tools can be applied to aggregate patient data to find historical patterns. Real-time decision support systems can be passive or active. *Passive systems* are activated when clinicians request help. Such assistance can come as reference material, automated calculations, or data review. *Active systems* include alerts and reminders that are triggered by preprogrammed rules governing specific circumstances. An order for penicillin in a patient who is allergic to it can cause a warning to display.

An effective decision support system must have accurate data, a user-friendly interface, a reliable knowledgebase, and a good inferencing mechanism. The knowledgebase can include information regarding risks, costs, disease states, clinical and laboratory findings, and clinical guidelines. The inference engine determines how and when to apply the appropriate knowledge.

Safety

Patient safety concerns should remain paramount in any hospital system, including clinical information systems (see Chapter 8).

To the extent possible, redundant systems should be in place to minimize the effect of the failure of a single component. Robust down-time contingency plans must be developed should the clinical information systems cease normal function in either planned or unplanned situations. These contingency plans must account for continued data acquisition and retrieval and provide for mechanisms for communication among health care providers and services. Users should be informed about recovery procedures and what they mean to the clinical database. Do backlogged data generated during the down time ever enter the system? How are they timed? Or is there a gap in the clinical information that the clinicians must fill in for themselves if they want the whole picture?

Many anomalous circumstances related to the EMR can threaten patient safety. Data, such as a laboratory value or a physician order, can be entered into the wrong patient record and prompt the clinician to respond appropriately but on the wrong patient. Similarly, data can be displayed in ways that are so confusing that they are interpreted incorrectly.

Default behaviors of portions of the computerized patient record should be designed carefully because busy or distracted clinicians may accept the default without understanding what they are accepting or considering the consequences. Consider the implications of an order where the default frequency for lorazepam is "every 3 hours" rather than "once."

As some processes are automated, additional sources of error can be introduced.

Human–Automation Interactions

Intelligent, automated systems can support and enhance human performance, but the sources of potential errors include those originating from the human, from the automated system, and at the interface between the two. "The challenge is to develop automated systems that support, rather than confound, the human user."[4]

Although autonomous action of computerized systems in the health care arena remains rare, many kinds of anomalies can induce significant errors. Sources of human–automation interface errors include display-related, data entry, and setup errors. *Display-related errors* can occur when the display of information is incomplete or ambiguous. Consider a laboratory result that reports the test name, the test result, and the normal value: "Acid-fast bacillus seen not seen." Imagine a carriage return before or after "not" and consider the proximity of that word to the name of the test.

Automated systems are particularly prone to *data entry errors*. Results can differ significantly from what is intended with a typographic error or a missed mouse click. Consider other data entry modalities such as voice recognition, and the error rate soars.

Setup errors usually occur remote from the actual error. A data entry error regarding the weight of a patient upon admission is a kind of setup error that will result in a medication error if the dose is calculated based on that weight. A more common type of setup error is a software configuration error that leads to a problem when put into clinical use, such as using an incorrect dose as the default for a drug.

Automation sometimes reduces the human's "situation awareness." The most poignant and spectacular examples of human–automation systems failures come from aerospace, but the lessons are applicable to medicine. Pilots manning a modern, automated cockpit often report that they often are surprised by the actions taken by the automated systems. Inadequate feedback from the automated systems is one of the potential sources of this problem. Because the operator does not understand how the automation functions and is unable to determine what the machine is doing and why, he/she often loses track of what is happening, making it more difficult to reengage in the task if a problem ensues.

Proponents often posit workload reduction as a major benefit of automation. It seems that automation actually has a negative impact on workload, reducing it at times of lower activity, but increasing the human workload burden at times of higher activity.[5] Although automation has other benefits, workload reduction should not be the driving force for automation.

Implementation

Implementation of a computerized patient record requires an investment of additional staff, hardware, software, and an expanded communications infrastructure or network. For large hospital networks, the costs can be exorbitant.

Developing a CPR requires careful planning with implementation in phases. The specific needs of the institution must be examined, particularly with regard to the existing technology and practices. The process should be viewed as an opportunity to enhance care rather than simply to replace the paper and requires reassessment of existing practices and reengineering of health care delivery. As each incremental phase of implementation is approached, there should be a focus on overcoming specific barriers to care rather than the nebulous goal of "creating a paperless process."

The first phase generally provides a patient-centric repository of clinical test results, including laboratory, radiology, pathology, and other textual data. A subsequent phase can include capture of paper document images, radiology images, and other nontextual data. A key phase is the capture of clinical data at the point of care, including vital signs, intake and output, nursing documentation, and physician notes. Implementation of a physician order entry system that satisfies the promises of IT in health care is another key phase that requires careful coordination among services and interdigitating systems. Different classes of orders also can be implemented in phases to ensure the proper function of the required interfaces; however, at the point of care, implementation of all orders at once seems most desirable.

Ensuring that the CPR satisfies required needs involves considerable planning, designing, and testing. Even well-designed, off-the-shelf CPR systems can satisfy only 80% of the complex requirements of any multipractitioner organization. The remainder must be either adapted from other content or created from scratch. Substantial "expert" direction from teams of physicians, nurses, other allied health care providers, medical records, and financial staff is required to assist in developing the design and implementation of all CPRs. If clinicians abdicate their responsibility in participating in this tedious process, they are virtually ensuring that the resulting system will fail to satisfy their needs. Physician acceptance and participation can be enhanced by acknowledging the importance of physicians in the process, training them early and often, frequently and routinely eliciting their feedback, and demonstrating responsiveness to their needs and concerns.

Clinical IT specialists interpret the requests from clinicians for configuration of the information systems. A dedicated technical staff also must ensure instantaneous access to and constant availability of patient information. As the size and variety of information systems increases, enterprises will find it necessary to implement a "help desk" service.

The Promise of IT

The Institute of Medicine, in its report, *Crossing the quality chasm: a new health system for the 21st century,*[6] stated that health care should be safe, effective, patient centered, timely, efficient, and equitable. The Institute further noted that these goals could be more easily reached through judicious application of IT. Automated order entry systems can improve *safety.* Use of automated reminders based on clinical practice guidelines, computer-assisted diagnosis or management, and EBM can improve the *effectiveness* of medical care. IT can enhance *patient-centered* care that is respectful of and responsive to patient preferences, needs, and values by recording them and appropriately reminding the health care professional. It can facilitate access to clinical knowledge through web sites and online support groups. Clinical decision support systems can be used to tailor information and disease management messages based on the patient's individual needs. *Timeliness* can be improved by e-mail, telemedicine, and direct and immediate access to diagnostic test results and other clinical information. IT can improve *efficiency* by using clinical decision support systems to reduce redundant and unnecessary tests and procedures, by improving communication among multiple providers of care to individual patients, and by supplying data for performance and outcome measures. Enhancing *equity* among patients and across socioeconomic, geographic, race, and ethnic lines can be achieved if IT can improve access to clinicians and clinical knowledge, although it would depend upon equitable access to the technology infrastructure. IT is playing the starring role in the current drive to improve the quality of health care today, and the Institute called for a national commitment to build the information infrastructure to support health care.

Health Insurance Portability and Accountability Act

Although the intention of the HIPAA is to protect health insurance coverage for workers and their families when they change or lose their jobs, a portion of the HIPAA[8] attempts to decrease the administrative burdens of health care delivery by standardizing electronic data interchange among health care entities. These provisions for Administrative Simplification standardize patient health, administrative, and financial data and allow it to be transmitted electronically, but these improvements and innovations raise other issues.

The portability and accessibility of patient data and increasing availability of that data in electronic form introduces new vulnerabilities of security and confidentiality of patient data. The Security Standards attempts to provide a uniform level of protection of all health information pertaining to an individual that is housed or transmitted electronically. These standards mandate safeguards for physical storage and maintenance of patient data. They require limiting access to this information. It also specifies a standard for electronic signatures but only where they are used. The implementation of electronic signatures must ensure message integrity, user authentication, and nonrepudiation. This means the recipient can be sure that the message was the one sent by the signatory, that the sender was in fact the signatory, and that the signature is legally binding (see section on electronic signatures).

Protecting confidentiality and privacy of patient information is the purpose of the Standards for Privacy of Individually Identifiable Health Information. Also known as the Privacy Rule, it has far-reaching implications. It affects who has the right to access personally identifiable information whether or not in electronic form. Specifically, the Privacy Rule (1) limits the nonconsensual use and release of private health information, (2) gives patients new rights to access their medical records and to know who accessed them, (3) restricts most disclosures of health information to the minimum needed for the intended purpose, (4) establishes new criminal and civil sanctions for improper use or disclosure, and (5) establishes new requirements for access to records by researchers and others.

The method of implementation in an institution is based on the circumstances within each organization. Hospitals with computer networks must have security measures to permit appropriate access. Whether the security implementation is user based, role based, or context based may depend on the circumstances of the particular institution or the specific resource being accessed. Regardless of the specifics, institutional policies must be established and followed. In the past, violations of such policies, including sharing personal passwords or accessing information to which employees had no right to access, were punishable by official reprimand or, at worse, dismissal. With the new rules, violators may face criminal or civil penalties as well.

The Privacy Rule will also have a significant impact on research as it relates to (1) consent paperwork that safeguards the privacy of patients participating in research, (2) simplified guidelines regarding the limited circumstances where patient health information can be used for research purposes without authorization by the research subject, and (3) clarifying methods by which protected patient health information can be de-identified so that such information can be disclosed freely.

The implications of HIPAA are significant and extend beyond the electronic realm and into the paper world. How difficult and onerous the implementations will be are not yet known. How newer technologies can help safeguard the data and secure patient privacy also remains to be seen.

Security

The security of a networked system involves at least three components: physical security, prevention of unauthorized access, and protection from malicious software.

Physical access to sensitive portions of the system must be secure. Servers should be in locked rooms with controlled access. Networking closets with wiring and hubs should be locked. Sensitive equipment must be protected from extreme temperatures, fire, and water damage. Backup power sources are required. Workstations, wherever possible, should be in open areas where their use can be monitored, but not so open that unauthorized persons can peer over a user's shoulder to steal a user name and password or see sensitive information. Physical security also involves ensuring that the data on storage media are backed up and readily accessible whenever they are needed.

Preventing unauthorized electronic access involves blocking attacks from the outside and authenticating legitimate users before allowing them access. Wireless networks must be configured to minimize the risk of intruders tapping into the system.

Systems can be attacked by malicious software, loosely labeled as *viruses*. Securing systems from these threats is becoming increasingly challenging.

Firewalls

Any computer or network with connections to the outside world, such as the Internet, is vulnerable to attack. These attacks can come in the form of a hacker gaining access to confidential data or another causing data loss or corruption. The first measure of security against such threats is a *firewall*. In the parlance of architects and builders, a firewall isolates part of a building from fire in another part. A network firewall protects the resources of one network from users of other networks. For example, most enterprises have private networks for communication among their workers but have web servers for their public web sites on that network. They also allow their workers access to the Internet. Typically, a firewall isolates the private network from the internetwork traffic, although there are personal firewalls that protect an individual computer from certain kinds of network traffic.

The simplest firewalls are *packet filters*. Information is sent across a network in packets wrapped in layers of protocols with a header that includes Internet protocol (IP) addresses and port numbers. Packet filters examine the headers and, based on a set of rules configured into them, allow or deny passage of each packet. Routers can be configured as packet filters, becoming screening routers. However, not all packets are what they appear to be, and packet filters do not examine their contents. Readily available hacking tools can create normal-appearing packets that can take advantage of well-known security flaws in network applications.

Proxy servers provide the next level of firewall protection. They intercept requests for data from network users and forward them using the proxy address (hiding the requester's internal network address). The reply from the Internet returns to the proxy server, which evaluates it to ensure that the contents contain an expected response. If the commands or data are suspicious, the packet is discarded. Legitimate packets are forwarded to the requester but only after they are repacked in a new packet. No packets ever cross directly from the network to the Internet or from the Internet to the network. The proxy server is always between them, evaluating each packet trying to make its way through.

Software on the user's computer or on a computer that serves as a gateway to other networks can function as a firewall. In fact, home computers constantly connected to the Internet via a broadband connection (e.g., cable modem, digital subscriber line [DSL], or integrated services digital network [ISDN]) should have personal firewall software to protect them from attack. A dedicated "firewall appliance" also can do the job.

Even with a firewall to protect the perimeter of a networked environment, many vulnerabilities remain. For example, any computer on the network connected via modem to any outside system effectively bypasses network firewalls. This security flaw can be plugged with properly configured firewall software. Effective security solutions include network and Internet gateway monitoring, intrusion detection, firewall software for vulnerable nodes, antivirus software, and periodic penetration testing. Firewalls are only one bulwark against attack.

Wireless Networks

Wireless networking allows freedom from the tether of network wiring. In a large intensive care unit with multiple patient rooms and shifting isolation precautions, untethered workstations allow efficient access to information systems during rounds, making it an integral part of the information exchange rather than relegating it to the corner.

Most hospital networks do not provide for wireless technology, citing the lack of security provided by the current products. In fact, most wireless implementations allow the equivalent of the wiring closet completely open for intruders to enter and plug directly into the network because the basic security measures have not been taken. The Institute of Electrical and Electronics Engineers (IEEE) 802.11b standard on which these networks are based includes a provision for encryption called *wireless equivalent privacy* (WEP). This encryption can be either 64-bit or 128-bit. The former is considered insecure, but the latter is not secure either. Because the encryption key does not change, it is possible to crack the key by listening to the network traffic. Surprisingly, most implementations of wireless networks do not use *any* encryption method. Many network administrators do not even bother changing the factory default security settings, including passwords.

Wireless technology is inherently less secure than wired networks because it cannot be locked in an electrical closet. However, it is not impossible to boost its security sufficiently, even for sensitive applications. WEP and all other security features must be configured appropriately. The range of most networking hardware is generally about 100 feet, but with signal-boosting antennae network traffic can be detected much beyond this range. By locating the access points in the center of the building, inadvertent transmission beyond the desired boundaries can be limited. The connections also can be limited in number and by media access control (MAC) address, which identifies each node on a network. The most effective strategy is to place the wireless access points behind a firewall and have the wireless users gain access to the network by using a virtual private network (VPN).

Virtual Private Network

A VPN is a private network set up within a larger public network. It can provide a secure private connection from home or remote office, over the Internet (through an Internet service provider [ISP] by either dial-up connection or high-speed broadband access of digital cable or DSL) or other unsecured network (e.g., wireless), to the hospital's local area network for access to the clinical information system and other applications. With a combination of secure authentication, encryption, and "tunneling," the remote user can have access to the same applications as if he/she were on site. *Authentication* ensures that only authorized persons gain access to the VPN. *Encryption* prevents the data from being read if intercepted. *Tunneling* allows the data to traverse the Internet and get past the firewalls and gain access to the network. (Figure 9–1.)

Network traffic travels in *packets*. Each packet is encapsulated by several layers of protocol codes with addresses. Each layer pertains to different components of networking, from the hardware of the network in the outermost layer to the software application in the innermost layer. Tunneling adds more protocol layers beneath the other layers, and a VPN server does the translation between the internal network and the external network or Internet (Figure 9–2). A user with VPN software connects to a VPN server on the hospital network via the Internet. The VPN server forwards user requests to the specified hospital system server. The packets of data containing the request are enveloped in the tunneling layers and in the standard protocol layers required to traverse the Internet. Once the packets reach the VPN server, the tunneling layers are stripped off and the packet is sent off across the internal network to the clinical information server. Servers on the internal network are unaware that the user is outside of the network, and their response packets undergo the reverse transformation of protocols.

Before implementation of a VPN, the only access to most hospital networks and their applications was through a slow, dial-up access over the telephone (plain old telephone service [POTS] and directly to a host computer on the network. (Figure 9–3). Although not considered extremely secure, direct dial-up is more secure than going through the Internet. However, direct dial-up can be slow and expensive, particularly over long distance. The telephone lines themselves are not necessarily secure.

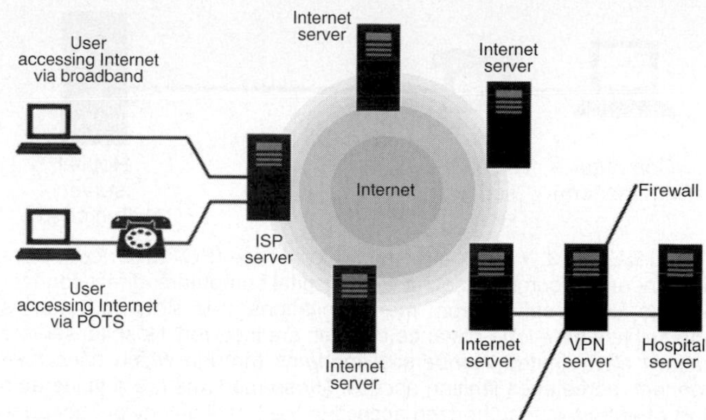

FIGURE 9–1 • Virtual private network (VPN) connection. The user gains access to the Internet through any means, usually an Internet service provider (ISP) while running VPN software. Data are directed at the hospital VPN server by "tunneling" through the public Internet by encryption and special packaging. Once the data stream reaches the hospital's VPN server, the data are unencrypted and sent through the firewall to the hospital server that receives the data, the latter oblivious to the fact that the data came from outside the hospital network. The reply to the user follows the same path through the VPN server that encrypts and packages it to traverse the public Internet. POTS is plain old telephone service.

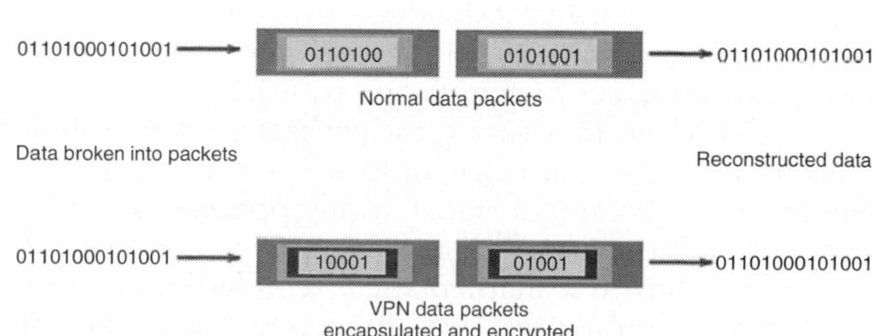

FIGURE 9–2 • Virtual private network (VPN) data transmission. Data streams are prepared to traverse any network by being broken into pieces that are enveloped by as many as seven layers of protocols and address information. Once the packets reach their destination, the protocol layers are peeled off and the data stream is reconstructed. VPN software first encrypts the data, then envelops it in a tunneling layer before adding the standard protocol and address layers. Reconstruction reverses this process.

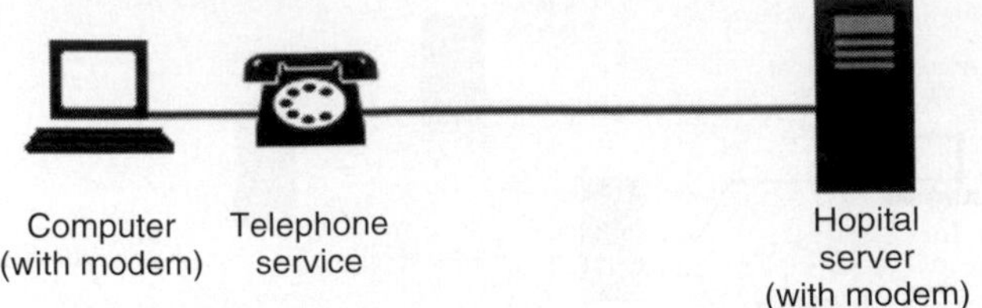

FIGURE 9–3 • Plain old telephone service (POTS). Once a standard means of communicating with hospital computers, direct connection via POTS suffers from many limitations. It is slow and often is unfeasible where long-distance charges are incurred. Hospital servers usually have limited numbers of modems through which users can connect, sometimes limiting access. These modems are a vulnerable port of entry for unauthorized access to the hospital network because they usually are behind the protective firewall.

Access may be limited by the number of modems on the hospital servers relative to the number of users attempting connection. These modems also open vulnerable ports of entry for unauthorized users to the hospital network, particularly as the servers may not be shielded by hospital firewalls.

Remote access to patient data is one of the major issues where physicians and IT administrators clash. Physicians demand it, but the administrators are reluctant to implement it, especially in view of the HIPAA security regulations. The security of a VPN is a function of how tightly authentication, encryption, and access controls are connected. A VPN with a desktop firewall solution and appropriate audit trails is a compromise that is workable in many institutions.

Authentication

Authentication is the process of establishing the identity of a user to a computer or system with some degree of certainty. Most often it is used to grant access. The most common method of authentication uses passwords. Most passwords have personal meaning (a child's nickname, a pet's name, or social security number), making them easier to remember but also easier for others to guess.

"Smart cards" with magnetic strips or barcodes are another method of authentication. Their problems relate to loss or theft if not duplication or forgery.

Biometrics identifies individuals by fingerprints, faces, voices, irises, retinas, signatures, or other physical attributes using some combination of hardware and software. Although the specifics varies, the general process includes collection of the biometric information by a scanner (fingerprints), a camera (face), a microphone (voice), or some other modality. This information is converted by some algorithm to a mathematical template that can be compared with a database of authorized users. The data often are encrypted to prevent intercepted information from being used as keys. Biometric devices are not bulletproof and can be fooled or bypassed. However, as the technology matures, the problems may diminish.

Most security experts agree that the only way to protect any computer system effectively is to layer complementary technologies, hence the adage, "Something you know. Something you carry. Something you are." Items known to the user include passwords and other personal information. Items carried by the user can include keys or identification cards with barcodes or magnetic strips designed to make forgery difficult. Authentication based on an individual's physical characteristics using biometrics composes the last category. Biometric technologies are improving and becoming increasingly more cost effective. A multilayered approach may be necessary to protect super-secret government agencies, but the requirements for most medical information are less stringent. Although some zealous individuals may equate patient privacy with national security, multilayered security systems may be difficult to implement,[16] particularly in an environment where slow or unreliable access may compromise a patient's well-being.

The authentication system widely used remains the combination of user ID and password. These systems are only as secure as the least compliant user. Although there are recommendations regarding choosing and maintaining passwords (Box 9–4), many users ignore these guidelines, making the entire system vulnerable to unauthorized access.

Poorly designed passwords are vulnerable to cracking by any of a number of commercial software programs or by any enterprising programmer. In general, passwords should not be single words. They should be some combination of small words and numbers, and they should be changed with some frequency. They should never be written down, let alone posted to the side of the monitor. Passwords should never be shared. Most hospitals have policies that forbid sharing or borrowing user names and passwords. Dismissal is generally the result for these kinds of violations.

Users should always log out of all systems before stepping away from a workstation to prevent giving others unauthorized access on their login. Because users do not

BOX 9–4

Guidelines for Creating Passwords

1. Passwords should be at least six to eight characters in length. The longer the better.
2. Passwords should include uppercase letters, lowercase letters, and numbers. Non-alphanumeric symbols (e.g., #, @, !, &) can often be used, depending on the system.
3. Passwords should be easy to remember and easy to type.
4. Do not use any readily accessible information as any part of a password. This includes your user name, full name, address, birth date, or social security number.
5. Do not use single words or simple word combinations. Dictionary attacks can test millions of words or word combinations per second, including foreign words.
6. Do not record passwords on any unsecured medium, such as notes beside the computer, on an identification badge, or in a book.
7. Change your password every 4 to 6 weeks.
8. Do not recycle old passwords or use the same password for several different applications.

always remember to do so, there should be a mechanism for automatic logout or lockdown if there is no activity over a specified period. Workstations that have "timed out" should still be available for use after the user has been reauthenticated or when another user is authenticated.

Electronic Signatures

For the bulk of medical applications, electronic signatures are simply an extension of the authentication process. An individual who is authenticated is generally allowed to sign for any changes to the EMR without any additional burden of electronic signature technology. The interest in electronic signatures generally relates to their use on legal documents such as contracts, where the benefits outweigh the additional technical burden. Although it is unlikely that highly secure electronic signatures worthy of million-dollar contracts will become the accepted standard for commonplace electronic documents such as e-mail, some of the principles may be applicable to physicians' signatures on medical documents.

The Electronic Signatures Act (E-Sign) was signed into law in 2000, giving electronic signatures the same legal validity as their handwritten counterparts. The act does not mandate the specific implementation of technology, but it governs the circumstances under which electronic signatures can be used and the standards that must be satisfied for them to be valid.[3]

First invented in the 1970s, digital signatures promised to be better than a handwritten signature because they were unforgeable and uncopyable. It generally involves the creation of two keys that are asymmetric but mathematically related. The individual who owns the keys guards one privately but allows the other to be published publicly (see public key infrastructure discussed in section on electronic mail, security.) When signing a document, the individual creates a digest of the document and encrypts the digest with his/her private key (Figure 9–4). This encrypted digest is permanently attached to the document as the signature. Anyone wishing to verify the signature obtains the public key for the signatory. The signed document is decrypted with the public key. Because keys are related, the verifying calculation proves that the signature is authentic. It also proves that the document had not been altered because such alteration would result in a different digest.

Other similar technologies offer variations on this theme, including electronic signatures embedded in images of a physical signature. All of these technologies are cumbersome and difficult to implement. Newer technologies promise to remove the burden of creating the keys and managing valid public keys, but one of the major problems of electronic signatures is that the computer on which signatures are created may be compromised or coopted to create a false signature or to compromise the privacy of the private key. Their use in medical systems currently is very limited.

Viruses or Malware

All kinds of malicious software have come to be referred to generically as *viruses*. The term *malware* has been coined to be more technically correct. The taxonomy of malware includes viruses, worms, and Trojan horses. With innovative approaches to exploiting security holes in common software, the distinctions are blurring among these methods of wreaking havoc.

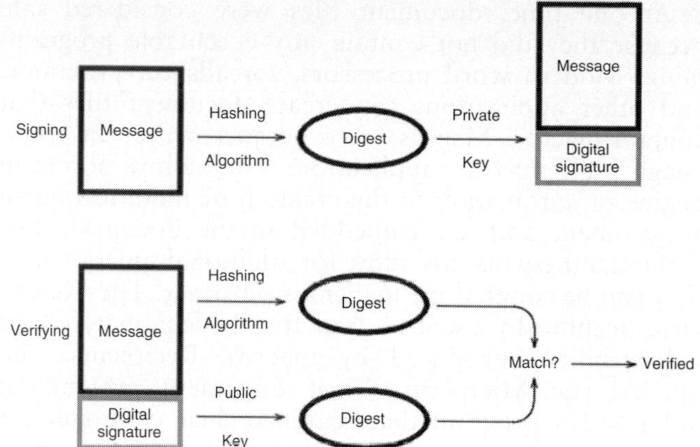

FIGURE 9–4 • Electronic signatures. Among the more common schemes for electronic signatures, this method uses the public key infrastructure. For each user, two keys are created that are not symmetric but are related mathematically. One key is kept private; the other is made publicly available. When a document is signed, a hashing algorithm generates a digest. Minor changes to the document result in a different digest, thus identifying forgeries. The private key is applied to the digest, creating a digital signature that is permanently attached to the document. To verify the signature, the signatory's public key is applied to the digital signature, almost reversing the last step of the signing process. The result is compared to the result of hashing the document again. If the results match, the signature is verified.

Computer viruses are malicious programs attached to executable files or programs. They technically require human intervention to spread from machine to machine, as when users share files on a floppy disk, across a network, or via e-mail. The hidden files on a disk associated with the operating system (boot sector or partition sector) can be infected, as can any program or executable file. Once on a system, the damage occurs when the program is executed and the virus replicates, sometimes replacing or deleting legitimate files, reformatting the hard drive, or corrupting the filing system.

Worms differ from viruses by the method they are transmitted from system to system. No longer limited by human intervention, worms can replicate and spread wildly within a system and across networks, sometimes by hijacking an e-mail program. The damage occurs when the program is executed and replication occurs unchecked throughout the hard disk and/or RAM, using up the computer's resources and eventually overwhelming the system. *Trojan horse programs,* as the name implies, are disguised as, or are embedded in, programs that appear legitimate but perform some illicit activity when they are run. They typically do not replicate themselves or infect other files, but they often dupe users into executing them with the promise of a free game or utility or a clever joke. Some Trojans are written to cause the loss or theft of data, sometimes password information. Others make the system vulnerable to takeover by another computer. Still others simply destroy programs or data on the hard disk.

At one time, document files were considered safe because they did not contain any executable programming. Modern word processors, spreadsheet programs, and other applications can create document files that contain macros. Macros are programs written in a language built into an application. They allow a certain degree of automation in the creation or modification of a document and are embedded in the document file. Although these macros allow for additional functionality, they can be coopted for malicious purposes. The Melissa virus (technically a worm) dramatically demonstrated the vulnerability introduced by macros. Recipients who opened the Microsoft Word document attachment unleashed a program that searched their computer for e-mail addresses and sent copies of itself to those addresses. In 1999, the Melissa virus clogged up thousands of e-mail servers worldwide and caused widespread havoc. Obviously, not all macros are viruses, but if a file contains a macro, it would be wise to consult the author as to its legitimacy and whether it can be disabled without compromising the document. Other types of document files, including Joint Photographic Experts Group (JPG) graphic files, have been shown in laboratories to be capable of carrying viruses, but none have yet surfaced "in the wild."

The increasingly common and dangerous *blended threats* combine features of different kinds of traditional malware while attempting to exploit multiple vulnerabilities on both single-user computers and network servers. By using several different techniques targeting different weaknesses, blended threats can spread rapidly and cause widespread damage before they can be detected and neutralized. Combating blended threats requires an integrated solution at all levels of a network, including web servers, e-mail servers, and client computers to protect every vulnerability.

Hoaxes or *phantom viruses,* although not technically malware, prey on the naïveté of most computer users. Although they generally amount to no more than an e-mail chain letter, they sometimes advise users to delete a needed file, adding that the "virus" cannot be detected by any antivirus software. Most of these false warnings urge users to "forward this to everyone you know" in an effort to perpetuate the hoax. If there is ever any question regarding a legitimate threat or a hoax, users should consult the web pages of any of the antivirus program distributors or perform a simple web search.

Safe computing practices should be used at all times and by all users within a system (Box 9–5). Although some viruses can be intercepted by network administrators who protect their mail servers with antivirus software, there are other means by which malware can infiltrate a system. Sharing files through instant messaging or downloading files via web sites, newsgroups, or file-transfers (file transfer protocol [FTP]) are among the many sources of security breaches.

Antivirus software programs rely on virus *signatures,* strings of bits that uniquely identify each virus. It is

BOX 9–5

Safe Computing Practices

- **Back Up Your Data.** Safe computing practices can decrease the risk to your data but cannot eliminate it altogether.
- **Antivirus Software.** Use real-time virus protection at all times. Scan all files obtained across network or Internet connections, including from e-mail, web sites, instant messaging, or other sources. Scan all floppy disks, zip disks, or CDs that are given you. Scan all software before you install it. (There are verified reports of brand-new, shrink-wrapped retail software that contained viruses.) Periodically scan all hard drives on your computer. Maintain the most up-to-date virus definitions.
- **E-mail Attachments.** Be suspicious of all e-mails, but especially those that are unexpected or out of character. Do not leave infected e-mail attachments or any unwanted attachments on your system. Do not set the e-mail program to automatically open attachments. If the e-mail program can render HTML messages, set it to disallow all executables (ActiveX, Java, JavaScript).
- **Floppy Disks.** Remove all floppy disks before shutdown or start up. Write-protect floppy disks after you finish writing to them.
- **Do Not Share.** File sharing and printer sharing should be disabled if these functions are not needed. If they are needed, limit access to your network. Never allow anonymous sharing of your system. Turn off unneeded services, such as hypertext transfer protocol (HTTP), FTP, Telnet, and personal web servers. Be wary of any files given to you, particularly those with the file extensions *exe, com, bat, pif,* and *vbs.*
- **Firewall.** Use a hardware or software firewall. Files attempting access to the Internet or Internet servers attempting to access your computer should be investigated before they are granted access in the firewall configuration. Know the range of IP addresses used in your network so that intruders can be more easily detected. Test your vulnerabilities with freely available utilities (e.g., Gibson Research's ShieldsUP!).
- **Protect Passwords.** Follow accepted guidelines for creating strong passwords. Do not record passwords in any unsecure documents. Disable password management in the web browser.
- **Security Updates.** Obtain and install all software security updates, particularly for operating systems, e-mail clients, and web browsers.
- **Browser Security.** Consider setting the browser security setting on "high" to prevent ActiveX or Java programs from running. This configuration may degrade your web experience, depending on the web sites that are frequented. Consider obtaining and using software to manage cookies and to warn you of web bugs.
- **Macro Virus Protection.** Offered by some programs, notably Microsoft Office, macro virus protection identifies files that contain any macro before they are opened. It cannot determine if these macros are viruses or legitimate macros.

imperative that these virus definitions be up to date to afford protection from the most recently identified threats.

Some experts view the current reactive paradigm insufficient to secure legitimate users from the threat of increasingly sophisticated, malicious, and destructive attacks we likely will see in the future. Some security developers are turning to more proactive approaches to detect and neutralize yet unknown threats. One approach has distributed attack sensors on servers throughout the Internet to provide early warning. Another approach is heuristic analysis, where abnormal behaviors propagated by files identify and isolate potential threats.

Privacy

The Privacy Rules outlined by HIPAA regulate access to patient information. Most of the requirements can be met with enterprise-wide security measures and changes of behavior supplemented by limiting access by electronic means. However, the privacy of the computer user, related to patient information or not, is vulnerable on many other fronts.

Spyware

Various technologies to spy on computer users exist, and new classes continue to be developed. *Spying software* can log every keystroke, raise flags when key phrases are typed, capture and store periodic screen shots, record e-mail and chat sessions, and report suspicious activities by e-mail. Use of this kind of software in the workplace is becoming more commonplace as employers seek to recoup lost productivity from their workers engaging in non–work-related activities. Some computer viruses or other malicious software (see section on viruses or malware) include spyware that can snoop on and even commandeer the victim's computer. Other spywares attempt to capture passwords or credit card information and forward them via e-mail or Internet relay chat.

Hardware key loggers are inconspicuous devices that can capture every keystroke typed on a keyboard en route to the computer. Hidden in the keyboard or the computer case and completely undetectable by software, they can store up to about 2 MB of data, enough memory to capture a year's worth of typing.

Network sniffers can effectively perform a wiretap on a network or over the Internet by intercepting and recording packets of raw data to and from the victim's computer. Most of the data, particularly e-mail, that traverses networks is not encrypted and therefore is highly vulnerable. Wireless networks (802.11b protocol) are even more accessible (see section on wireless networks).

A computer stores a wide range of backup data and cache information to speed performance and help recovery in the event of system crashes. Even files that you thought you had deleted may continue to exist on your hard drive and may be recoverable by *forensic software.* Web browsers also store a history, cookies, and cache that usually enhance a user's experience on the web, but they also can be a font of information to an investigator. Furthermore, as some White House staffers once discovered to their dismay, e-mail deleted from their own computers was not necessarily removed from their e-mail host server.

Countermeasures require that users be aware of the potential threats. Installing and frequently updating antivirus software is only the beginning. Spying software can take up significant disk space, cause unexpected disk activity, or produce unusual network traffic. Personal firewall software can warn the user that his/her computer is sending information without authorization.

Protecting Privacy

For many of the threats to security and privacy in the electronic world, particularly on the Internet, there are software solutions of varying degrees of effectiveness. These solutions are wide ranging, and some are bundled together to provide integrated control.

Some e-mail services can make the sender anonymous; others provide secure, encrypted mail, saving only one copy to be retrieved by the user. Other software can filter out spam—unsolicited e-mail advertisements—although many standard e-mail agents can perform similar filter functions. Several antispam software packages include antivirus scanning of all incoming mail and some firewall capabilities. It is possible to prevent your IP address from being discovered, even by web bugs, and to encrypt all web page requests. Still other products can block, sort, or clean up cookies. Advertisements can be blocked, as can any site with potentially objectionable material.

The amount of personal information disclosed over the web intentionally or inadvertently can be disturbing to persons concerned about privacy, but every web surfer can take certain steps. Primarily, users should not disclose any information they do not want to share. If personal information is required, as in a financial transaction, make sure the information is transmitted over a secure connection. Avoid answering questions such as your annual income, your mother's maiden name, or your social security number. If some information is "required," you should feel free to make up an answer. In addition, unless you are fond of junk e-mail, you should opt out of getting "special offers."

Your web browser can reveal volumes about you, including your computer's IP address, the web sites recently visited, and the contents of your browser memory cache. Users should routinely purge their browser cache, their browsing history, and the location bar memory. Cookies should be reviewed periodically with one of the available utilities. Those that contain sensitive information or belong to undesirable sites should be deleted. Some advertising networks allow users to opt out of their systems by going to the *http://www.networkadvertising.org* web site. Special applications or services can be used to block web bugs or to surf anonymously through a web proxy server.

It takes a fair amount of effort to protect your privacy. Cookie sorting can take as much as a half-hour per week, but even sporadic use of online commerce requires cookies. Constructing an impervious wall of privacy is not a practical goal. There will be tradeoffs between the services provided by web sites and the personal information you are willing to surrender, but there are abundant wares available that can help keep your business your own.

Initiatives by software manufacturers are under way that, on the surface, appear to help users manage in one location their personal information (such as passwords and e-mail accounts), but there are significant privacy implications. Some privacy groups are concerned that the services that store the data may not use the data appropriately or may not keep the data private and secure. The ultimate fate of these schemes bears watching.

Internet Applications

The Internet continues to evolve. Its dominant applications once were file transfer programs, newsgroups, and e-mail. Today web browsing, instant messaging, and e-mail define the Internet.

Web Browsing

In 1991 Tim Berners-Lee, working at the European Organization for Nuclear Research (CERN), released tools to the public, which allowed them to take part in using a new worldwide hypertext information resource, the world wide web (WWW). This text-based program reached a very small audience. Two years later, Marc Andreesen, working at the National Center for Supercomputing Applications (NCSA) in the United States, released the first version of the WWW browser called *Mosaic*. This browser with a graphical user interface that could accommodate images was the forerunner of *Netscape*. By 1994, the load on the first WWW server *(info.cern.ch)* was one thousand times what it had been in 1991, and the world was changed, propelled by this new information medium.

Cookies

Web pages are considered "stateless," that is, they have no way to remember user preferences from page to page, to know what items are in the electronic shopping cart, or to even remember who the user is. In order to improve the experience, *cookies* were developed. Cookies are data created by a web server, stored on the user's computer, and later read by the originating web server. A cookie includes the address of the web site that sent it. Web browsers will allow a web site to read only those cookies originating from that site and no others. Cookies also include a date after which that cookie is set to expire and to be removed from the user's computer. They can track where on the site the user has been and how often. They can remember user IDs and passwords, and they can remember user preferences so that content can be tailored to the user's interests. Although they can "improve your experience," they also can offer a wealth of information for marketers and others.

Cookies are stored in a file on the hard disk usually named *cookies.txt*. The web browser can be set to accept all cookies, reject all cookies, or notify you if a cookie is being set. The ubiquity and importance of cookies make the latter two choices virtually untenable; however, there are software utilities that are designed to more selectively reject cookies and to allow editing of your cookie file to eliminate any information you would not want sent back to web sites on future visits. Newer versions of popular browsers also provide some of this advanced functionality.

Most reputable web sites mention the use of cookies in their privacy policies. Although these policies often are unread, they are not binding and often are subject to change without notice.

Web Bugs

Information about web traffic and about the persons who visit certain web sites is extremely valuable to commercial web sites, advertisers, and others. Web bugs exploit the way browsers handle web pages to surreptitiously collect limited but important information. These "bugs" (as in clandestine listening devices, not insects or programming errors) also are known by euphemisms such as "web beacons," "clear GIFs," "1-by-1 GIFs," "invisible GIFs," and "beacon GIFs."

A *web bug* is a graphic on a web page designed to feed information back to the owner. The size of these images typically is 1 × 1 pixel; some are not just small but also are invisible. They often are in the graphical interchange format (GIF) file format (Figure 9–5).

The information that can be sent back to the server includes the IP address of the user's computer, the uniform resource locator (URL) of the web page, the URL of the web bug image, the time the web bug was viewed, the kind of web browser used, and any cookies previously set for that server. It can provide an independent accounting of the number of persons visiting a particular web site or the popularity of a particular web browser. Furthermore, anything entered on a web page, whether a zip code, birth date, or even search strings, can be shared among

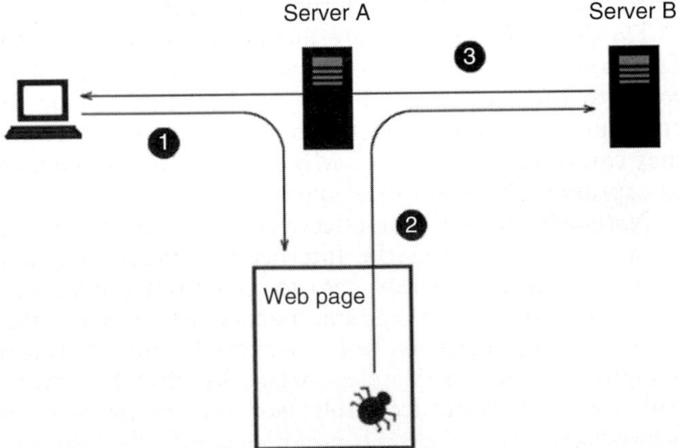

FIGURE 9–5 • Web bugs. **1,** A user requests a web page from server A. **2,** A web bug on the requested page points to an image on server B. That server can record the information that is relayed to it, including the Internet protocol (IP) address of the requesting computer and the uniform resource locator (URL) of the web page containing the web bug. **3,** Server B can send a cookie directly to the requesting computer. If the user visits another site with a server B web bug, that cookie will tell it where else the user had been.

web sites. All these data, including other publicly available data, can be cleverly pieced together by advertising networks, generating a detailed personal profile. This profile can be used to specify the banner ads displayed, and the web bugs can correlate the display frequency of a particular banner ad with what was purchased. Because multiple individuals may be using a computer with a particular IP address, those individuals may remain anonymous. But their collective browsing habits are still disclosed, so it is small solace for this collective invasion of privacy.

Software is available that serves as bug repellant, but its use can make it difficult to navigate certain sites without a barrage of warnings. Most web sites make their privacy policies available. The reputable sites mention the use of web bugs, although they often use one of the euphemisms listed.

Malicious Programs

Similarly, early web documents contained only textual information, graphics, and rudimentary formatting. The wish for enhanced functionality to augment the modern web experience led to the creation of new programming languages. ActiveX and Java programs embedded in a web page can generate eye-popping special effects and can greatly increase the interactive nature of web encounters, but they also can be used as a vehicle to attack computer systems. Web browsers configured with "high" security settings prevent ActiveX and Java programs from executing. Unfortunately, this configuration also can significantly degrade the web experience, and there is no way to selectively block out malicious programs while allowing others to run.

Profiles and Privacy Policies

Reading privacy policies posted on Internet sites can be fairly revealing and can precipitate significant paranoia. These disclosures often admit to using a variety of methods of tracking user patterns, although they are nonbinding and subject to change without notification. The methods of user tracking are not limited to those outlined here. For example, one popular drug information PDA software company admits to tracking the number of times a drug is looked up and the screens viewed. These data are sent back during synchronization and are stored in aggregate and as personally identifiable information. Furthermore, the profiles are supplemented by public information about users from sources such as the American Medical Association.

Although much of these data are collected to "improve customer satisfaction," we should not assume that the intentions of all collectors are to benefit the users. Some may have nefarious intent. Regardless of their intent, creators of certain software or web sites leave few alternatives to these invasions of privacy besides total abstinence.

Electronic Mail

At one time, the Internet consisted of three applications and the medium through which they operated. The three applications were File transfer protocol (FTP), newsgroups, and e-mail. E-mail was the "killer" application, the application that everyone needed. As such, it spurred the rapid development and deployment of computer networks and eventually the interconnection of those networks, or "inter-net."

Once limited to the confines of a local network, e-mail significantly broadened its utility by internetwork connections. The standards adopted for internetworking communications and e-mail protocols made this service nearly universal.

It is possible to send copies of the same message to multiple recipients. Systems known as *list servers* were developed to replicate postings to a set of recipients. In 1994, the pediatric ICU (PICU) e-mail discussion group was started, linking approximately 2000 pediatric intensivists worldwide and heralding a new era of interinstitutional and international sharing and collaboration.

Some users might be tempted to use e-mail as they use the postal service, perhaps corresponding about a patient referred for consultation. However, all e-mail is extremely vulnerable to prying eyes.

Using a mail user agent (MUA) to compose e-mail usually results in a text file that is sent to a mail transfer agent (MTA), a host computer somewhere on the Internet. The MTA sends the message to another MTA using the simple message transfer protocol (SMTP). MTAs use SMTP to move e-mail messages, skipping across the Internet from computer system to computer system, eventually reaching the host of the mail recipient (Figure 9–6), where it is stored. When the intended recipient checks for e-mail, the MUA fetches the message from the host computer, completing the last leg of the journey.

One writer likens e-mail to sending a postcard written in pencil.[18] Just like a postcard that passes through many hands between writer and reader, e-mail can be read by anyone who can view the message as it passes by their electronic eyes either on an MTA or on the network. Not only can the message be read, but it also can be "revised."

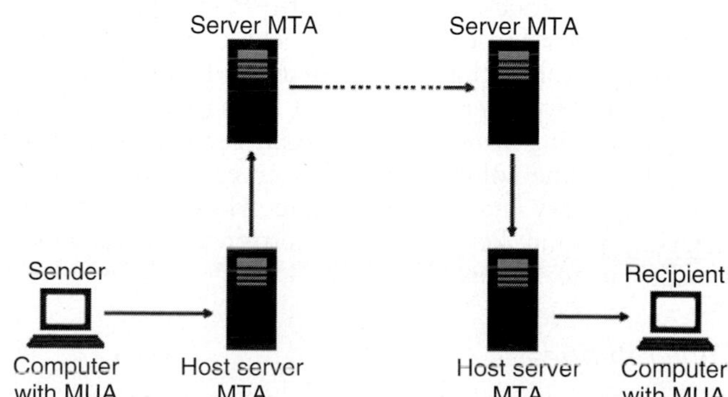

FIGURE 9–6 • Electronic mail (e-mail). A mail user agent (MUA) on a computer is used to compose and send an e-mail message. The message is uploaded to the user's host server, a mail transfer agent (MTA). If the recipient uses the same host server, the message waits for the recipient to pick it up. If a different host server is the target, the message bounces through the Internet until it reaches the recipient's host server. Each MTA will have a copy of the e-mail message and the transaction trail up until the message reached it. How long the messages are kept and who is allowed access to them are locally controlled.

Security

There are methods to protect sensitive information and to ensure that a message had not been altered on the way from the signatory. The primary methods are encryption and digital signatures, but the major obstacle in their implementation is their complexity (see section on electronic signatures).

Encryption generally uses a "key" to scramble a message into incomprehensible strings of data. Simple encryption uses the same key to unscramble the message so that it can be read. The obvious problem arises in getting the key that encoded the message from the sender to the recipient so that the latter can decode the message. Such a security system was as effective as leaving a house key under the doormat.

Public key infrastructure (PKI) cleverly uses a pair of keys that are asymmetric but algorithmically related. A message encoded by one key can be decoded only by the other and not by itself. One of these keys is designated the public key; the other is the private key. Only the user knows the private key, but the public key is posted for anyone to use. Someone wishing to send encrypted mail to the owner of those keys obtains the publicly available key and uses it to encode their message. When the recipient receives the mail, he/she applies the private key and decodes the message. At every point common e-mail is vulnerable to prying eyes, the encrypted mail remains unreadable.

The *pretty good privacy* (PGP) standard was developed because the traditional PKI encryption is slow. It first compresses the message, encrypts it with a one-time key, and then encrypts that key with the recipient's PKI key. The now-encrypted one-time key then is sent to the recipient with the message.

Public keys are available online. Proof that they are authentic, that they actually belong to the person they are supposed to, is offered via *digital certificates* ("certs"). Certificates contain a number of items and can include your user ID, a digital signature made with your private key, your public key, and one or more digital signatures of others that vouch for your identity. Certifying authorities require proof to verify identity. These authorities often are the signatories that vouch for an individual on these certificates. However, the task of managing certificates and determining which are still valid requires significant user effort. The solution may be server-based programs that keep every message encrypted while updating and verifying public keys, making certificate management transparent to the user.[13]

Vulnerabilities

E-mail originally was developed to deliver only plain text (American Standard Code for Information Interchange [ASCII]). Sending anything other than plain text required that the data be "attached" to an e-mail message. Attaching files requires that they be coded for transmission and decoded once received. The most common method in use today is multipurpose Internet mail extensions (MIME) (see Glossary.) Sending files as attachments to e-mail allows users to share documents, photographs, and computer programs, but also viruses (see section on viruses or malware).

The bane of most e-mail users is "spam" or unsolicited advertisements. They are the junk mail and the telemarketers of the Internet. The authors of spam usually purchase your name and e-mail address from a marketing agency or directly from web sites you visited (see section on web bugs).

Other than limiting yourself to web sites that do not collect your e-mail address and refusing to disclose your e-mail address altogether, there are some things you can be do to reduce spam. Some spammers offer opportunities for users to "unsubscribe" from their mailing list. Although these offers sometimes are legitimate, a response often only serves to identify the user's e-mail address as "live" or valid. Addresses that are known to be valid often are subjected to more vigorous spam campaigns. Some users prefer to maintain more than one e-mail address, reserving one for work, one for personal use, and yet another for use in public areas such as web sites that require an e-mail address. Most e-mail software programs offer methods of filtering messages and applying a variety of automatic actions. Users can create filters to automatically delete messages from senders of spam. These messages should be deleted from both the user's computer and the mail server.

If these measures fail to adequately control spam, some software packages are designed specifically for this purpose. This software filters content for common phrases used by spammers. Content filtering can be expanded to eliminate other inappropriate messages, such as sexually explicit language or racial epithets. Many corporations use content filtering on their mail servers, blocking or tracking inappropriate language, corporate secrets, and even viruses.

Although standard e-mail messages are pure text, some e-mail software can view messages that are composed like a web page in hypertext markup language (HTML). This web browsing feature requests images and other components to be downloaded and renders the HTML with fancy text, tables, images, and hyperlinks. Although this capability improves user experience, it also opens new vulnerabilities, particularly the web bug method (see section on web bugs). The most readily accessible information by this method is the user's IP address. Reading this kind of e-mail can synchronize the IP address to an e-mail address, a threat to anonymity that exposes users to an explosion of junk e-mail.

HTML mail opens additional vulnerabilities through exploits of programming languages such as ActiveX, Java, and JavaScript. Users should configure their e-mail client software to disallow the execution of these programs.

Newsgroups, Internet Relay Chat, and Instant Messaging

Newsgroups were first developed in the earlier days of the Internet. They can be likened to a public bulletin board about a particular topic and are hosted by anyone who wants to provide this service to the Internet community; collectively they are known as *Usenet*. Users subscribe to a newsgroup and access a log of previous postings. Users then can post their own messages.

Newsgroups contributed to the early sense of community among Internet users, particularly as they developed around particular areas of interest. Some observers consider it a collective consciousness and a valuable repository of knowledge, although enthusiasm for newsgroups can be dampened by self-serving or insulting postings. Newsgroups differ from e-mail list servers by the way the messages are accessed and by the fact that the histories of the discussion remain intact on newsgroups, at least for some defined period.

Internet relay chat (IRC) provides a way for real-time conferencing over the Internet. IRC servers host one or more "channels." Users join channels and receive all the postings from other members of the channel as they are sent. These channels, otherwise known as *chat rooms,* are accessed by logging into a server and viewing its list of channels.

Instant messaging (IM) provides another way for real-time conferencing over the Internet; however, rather than joining a channel, users create a list of other users with whom they might want to send messages. When one of the users on the list logs into the IM network, the user who created the list is "instantly" notified. An interactive chat session then can be initiated. Because users must share their user names to be included on their friends' lists, users usually are known to one another. Instant messaging has been banned in many business environments because of the loss of employee productivity; however, it can be used to determine if a person is available at their desk for contact by telephone. Some proponents envision the merging of instant messaging and Internet telephone calls, providing seamless transitions from chat to voice-to-chat.

The ability to share files through instant messaging programs opens another portal through which malware can enter a system. Some antivirus programs do not scan files shared this way and can leave their users vulnerable.

Internet2

The effort of nearly 200 universities in collaboration with industry partners and federal agencies, *Internet2* is a closed network of very-high-capacity connections. It consists of a pair of high-performance backbone networks called *Abilene* and *vBNS+* (Very-high-speed Backbone Network Service, plus) connecting high-capacity networking centers known as *gigaPoPs* (very large Points of Presence). This network can achieve a throughput of 2.4 gigabits per second, roughly 43,000 times more data than can flow through a standard 56K modem.

The applications being developed include everything we once dreamed the Internet would be and more. Rather than the small, jerky, low-quality video images we currently know as Internet video, it is possible to be totally immersed in three-dimensional video and audio across thousands of miles with Internet2. The applications being developed are only beginning to tap the potential power, but teleconferencing someday may become virtual reality, or robotic surgery someday may become truly remote.

REFERENCES

1. Altman RB, Klein TE: Challenges for biomedical informatics and pharmacogenomics. *Annu Rev Pharmacol Toxicol* 42:113-133, 2002.
2. Bayat A: Bioinformatics. *BMJ* 324:1018-1022, 2002.
3. Canter S: Electronic signatures. *PC Magazine* 20:102-105, January 2, 2001.
4. Carter JH: Electronic medical records: a guide for clinicians and administrators. American College of Physicians, March 2001.
5. Connors MM: Teaming humans and automated systems in safely engineered environments. *Life Support Biosph Sci* 5:453-460, 1998.
6. Committee on Quality of Health Care in America, Institute of Medicine: *Crossing the quality chasm: a new health system for the 21st century.* Washington, DC, 2001, National Academy Press.
7. Davis A, Long R: Pharmacogenetics research network and knowledge base: 1st annual scientific meeting. *Pharmacogenomics* 2:285-289, 2001.
8. Department of Health and Human Services (HHS): HIPAA, the official government site for HIPAA's Administrative Simplification rules. Available at *http://aspe.os.dhhs.gov/admnsimp.* Accessed September 2, 2002.
9. Gagliardi A, Jadad AR: Examination of instruments used to rate quality of health information on the internet: chronicle of a voyage with an unclear destination. *BMJ* 324:569-573, 2002.
10. Glass B: Are you being watched? *PC Magazine* 21:54-56, April 23, 2002.
11. Hashizume M, Kouzou K, Tsutsumi N, et al: A new era of robotic surgery assisted by a computer-enhanced surgical system. *Surgery* 131:S330-S333, 2002.
12. Hoc JM: From human-machine interaction to human-machine cooperation. *Ergonomics* 43:833, 2000.
13. Karagiannis K: Securing your e-mail. *PC Magazine*, December 24, 2002. Available at *http://www.pcmag.com/article2/0,4149,715713,00.asp.* Accessed January 16, 2003.
14. Masys DR: Electronic medical records: promise and pitfalls, May, 2001. Available at *http://medicine.ucsd.edu/faculty/masys/ASCO_EMR_overview.ppt.* Accessed June 28, 2002.
15. Miller MJ: Forward thinking. *PC Magazine* 21:7, September 3, 2002.
16. Morrissey J: Access denied: Mayo Clinic is a believer in using biometrics to protect medical data, but technological flaws shut doctors out, shut system down. *Mod Healthc* 32:22-30, November 25, 2002.
17. National Institute of Mental Health: Neuroinformatics: the human brain project. Available at *http://www.nimh.nih.gov/neuroinformatics/index.cfm.* Accessed September 2, 2002.
18. Rogers LR: Email: a postcard written in pencil. CERT Coordination Center, Software Engineering Institute, Carnegie Mellon University, 2001. Available at *http://www.cert.org/homeusers/email_postcard.html.* Accessed June 12, 2002.
19. Sackett DL, Rosenberg WM, Gray JA, Haynes RB, Richardson WS: Evidence based medicine: what it is and what it isn't. *BMJ* 312:71-72, 1996.
20. Seltzer L: Password crackers. *PC Magazine*, December 13, 2001. Available at *http://www.pcmag.com/article2/0,4149,696,00.asp.* Accessed January 16, 2003.
21. Society of Critical Care Medicine: CPOE (Computerized Provider Order Entry) System Requirements for Intensive Care Unit Use. Available at http://www.sccm.org/corporate_resources/coalition_for_critical_care_excellence/Documents/cpoe.pdf. Accessed December 14, 2004.
22. Society of Critical Care Medicine: CPOF (Computerized Provider Order Fulfillment) System Requirements for Intensive Care Unit Use. Available at http://www.sccm.org/corporate_resource/coalition_for_critical_care_excellence/Documents/CPOFSystem Requirements_000.pdf. Accessed December 14, 2004.
23. Terry N: Education and debate: regulating health information: a US perspective. *BMJ* 324:602-606, 2002.
24. Weigle CG, Markovitz BP, Pon S: The Internet, the electronic medical record, the pediatric intensive care unit, and everything. *Crit Care Med* 29(8 suppl):N166-N176, 2001.
25. Wilson P: How to find the good and avoid the bad or ugly: a short guide to tools for rating quality of health information on the internet. *BMJ* 324:598-602, 2002.

CHAPTER

10

Family-Centered Care in the Pediatric Intensive Care Unit

Debra Ann Ridling, Karen T. Hofmann, and Jenina Deshler

PEARLS

- Using family-centered care principles to establish the parents as partners with the health care team encourages trust and cooperation, reduces fear and anxiety in both patient and family, and creates an environment of mutual respect.
- Access to their critically ill child is reported by parents to be a high priority. Benefits have been clearly demonstrated when changes in pediatric intensive care unit policies support parent presence in the unit at all times, including those periods that traditionally have been closed to them, such as change of shift and during admissions.
- Access to information provides parents full partnership with the health care team. Participation in rounds, access to their child's medical chart, and daily communication with a care provider result in more accurate exchange of data, fewer errors in communication, and greater patient/family satisfaction.
- Pediatric intensive care unit staff can facilitate parents' participation in the daily care of their child, thereby supporting the parental role, demonstrating appreciation for the parent–child bond, and mitigating the impact on both patient and family of traumatic events, such as procedures and resuscitation.

Introduction

Admission to the pediatric intensive care unit (PICU) constitutes a crisis both for the patient and family. This crisis is amplified by the stress felt by the parents in the ICU environment. In this chapter, the term *parents* is used for the primary caregivers of the child, whether they are biologic, adoptive, legal, or other. The main contributors to the stress are the disruption of the parents' role and the parents' separation from their child. Additionally, the environment, appearance of the child, procedures performed on the child, uncertain outcome, and staff interactions all contribute to stress.[14,15,29,35,36,43,54,59,82] Crisis is an emotionally destabilizing change when a person's normal and usual methods of coping and problem solving are not effective.[65] Reestablishing the parental role in partnership with health care providers as early as possible mitigates the fear and frustration experienced by most families. Establishing this partnership is the core of the family-centered care philosophy, and it requires respectful attention at every level.

Defining the Family

Care teams can spend a great deal of time determining who is "the family" or "the immediate family." Traditionally, visiting and involvement in care have been defined and limited by the preferences of the health care team.

Extended family and important friends often were excluded. The definition of family had been based on the 1950s model of two biologic parents being the primary care givers and the main support being the grandparents.[31,46,82] These assumptions are no longer valid.

The team should ask the parents to define their family so that caregivers are clear on who can receive information, be present, and be integrated into the care team. It is important to understand the legal, as well as the informal, arrangements of the family so that information is communicated to the appropriate members and consenting and other legal requirements are maintained. The health care team should focus on the needs of the child and set policy based on logistical realities of the individual unit rather than defining who may be present. Listening to parents and supporting them is respectful and fosters a collaborative relationship.

Family-Centered Care Principles

Family-centered care is based on the assumption that the family is a child's primary source of strength and support. Family-centered care is characterized by four principles:

1. People are treated with dignity and respect.
2. Health care providers communicate and share complete and unbiased information with patients and families in ways that are affirming and useful.
3. Patients and family members build on their strengths by participating in experiences that enhance control and independence.
4. Patients, family members, and providers collaborate in policy and program development, professional education, and delivery of care.[38]

Some general considerations described by the Institute for Family-Centered Care include a shift in attitudes and the development of new language. Some themes to be considered when developing guidelines around principles of family-centered care should include these concepts (Table 10–1).[1,2,37,38,62,67,79]

Exceptions

Although the majority of families are able to adjust during this crisis, some are overwhelmed to the point of dysfunction. Like any other traumatic situation, there is a small percentage of families for whom the crisis is sufficient to collapse an already overloaded family system.[82] The family who lacks the financial, physical, emotional, or psychological resources to cope with the crisis of a hospitalized child deserves special consideration. All available resources should be directed to the family to assist them in their ability to support their ill child. When appropriate, a referral to a chaplain, social worker, or financial advisor may assist the family in resolving the concerns distracting them from the care of their child. It is helpful to designate one health care provider with whom the family can speak daily for medical updates and to reduce the opportunity for confusion or contradiction among caregivers. If the family is still unable to provide a calm, nurturing atmosphere for their child after provision of these additional practical, psychological, and spiritual supports, it may become necessary to structure or limit the family's participation.

Culturally Sensitive Care

As population trends become more diverse, so do the patients cared for in PICUs. Because individual clinicians cannot be knowledgeable about all cultures or even the major groups of organized religion, the unit should develop principles of cultural competency.[4,20,84] Although a number of resources can be provided, including social workers, chaplains, special interest groups, and written information, each patient/family should be considered unique. In addition to these resources, one of the most effective ways to understand the needs of an individual family is to ask them. Often the spokesperson for the family can provide the team with the necessary information that will assist in the care of the critically ill child.

Personalizing Care

Creating an opportunity where the individual characteristics of the child can be expressed when the child is unable promotes humanization in the PICU setting. Individualizing the environment to include photos, favorite toys and blankets, music, and audio recordings of siblings and family members are effective techniques. It also can be therapeutic for the family to create a collage or poster about their child and family. One such example is the "All About Me©" poster (Figure 10–1), which is well received by families and clinicians alike. Mementos from home draw providers to the bedside and provide a glimpse of the child when he/she was well.[49]

Professional Boundaries

Although family-centered care principles require a shift in professional practices and a change of culture within the hospital, professional roles still must be clearly defined and respectfully maintained. When entering the child's room, clinicians should introduce themselves to the family and explain their role on the care team. Respect toward other members of the health care team should be demonstrated at all times, because parents are observant of such interactions. Providing services beyond the scope of your professional role undermines the health care team partnership, no matter how well intended.

Communication

The highly technical PICU environment with multiple caregivers, paired with parental stress, creates a complex situation where the potential for miscommunication is great. The stressed family is less able to take in, comprehend, and retain information,[28,39,62,77] so explanations must be clear, concise, and repeated. Special attention must be focused on avoiding medical jargon and abbreviations. It may be helpful to advise parents to maintain a bedside journal or log in which they can note information given and list questions to be addressed later.

TABLE 10–1

Family-Centered Care Concepts

Traditional	Contemporary	Concepts
Deficit	Strength	Highly involved parents who require detailed information and continual presence with their child have often been considered a distraction to the delivery of care because of the time and energy required by the health care team to attend to the parents. Sometimes, the parents have been thought of as a nuisance. The paternalistic model of desiring parents to be passive observers of care is now called into question. A family-centered care approach considers the involved parents to be a strength to the child and multidisciplinary team. Appropriately incorporated into the delivery of care to the child, the parents can be an important asset.
Control	Collaboration	Traditionally, the health care team has controlled the degree of involvement parents had in their child's care. This control has included all aspects of care, including access to the child, information, and even the care being delivered. The contemporary approach of collaboration incorporates the parents into all aspects of care and supports the parents as an equal team member for the optimal delivery of care to their ill child.[59]
Expert	Partnership	In the oldest and outdated model of critical care, the delivery of care was driven by the medical physician, without input from other disciplines. As critical care has become more complex and progressed over the years, most intensivists value the contributions of a number of experts from a variety of disciplines such as nursing, respiratory care, social work, pharmacy, and others. Partnerships have been established with a variety of experts to deliver comprehensive critical care. Partnering with parents places value on what the parents bring to the team, such as continuity, history, and how the child responds to illness and treatment.
Information gatekeeper	Information sharing	Health care team members and institutions have desired to control information. This control of information has been thought to be related to the parents' lack of ability to understand medical concepts and/or health care provider's fear of litigation. Information sharing actually decreases the risk of litigation and gives parents the necessary tools to make complex informed decisions.
Rules	Guidelines	Historically, administrators and managers have set rules for how family members should behave while in the hospital. The connotation of the word "rule" is considered harsh and not congruent with the approaches of family-centered care. Using guidelines for behavior is more respectful language and demonstrates an attitude of flexibility and collegiality.
Visitors	Parents	In some of the older models of critical care, parents had strict restrictions on how much time they were permitted to stay with their child. For example, in some settings, only weekly visits were allowed. More recently, visitation has been liberalized, but some units still limit visitors to certain hours of the day or specific time increments. Parents should be exempt from most rules of visitation. Parents should be considered an extension of the child and should have full access. The most respectful language is not to call the parents visitors at all but to use that term for casual acquaintances of the child or family, such as a school friend or teacher.
Rigid	Flexibility	Some units still approach unit standards by rigid rules, setting policy in the strictest sense. In this traditional model of strict adherence to policy, the individual needs of the patient and family are not respected. Some units set policy based upon experience with the worst circumstances. Families ask that policies be created to meet most families' needs with room for flexibility and be dependent upon the needs of the child.

Respectful Language

All written and verbal communication should be respectful in tone and content; it also should be concise and consistent.[39,57] It is helpful to have information communicated in a variety of formats.[4] Information should include an explanation for why some restrictions are necessary (e.g., safety, sterile environment, isolation) and some behaviors prohibited (e.g., smoking, alcohol consumption). Most families respond positively to guidelines that protect their child, especially when the guidelines are presented with rationale. Staff should be reminded that most parents have never had experience in an ICU and do not arrive understanding expected behaviors.

For families for whom English is not a first language, it is an unreasonable expectation that they conduct difficult conversations without a professional interpreter. Even families who speak "pretty good English" will have more difficulty processing new information during this time of crisis. Use of another family member as interpreter is not advised because it puts undue pressure on that person. In addition, the interpretation may be inaccurate, creating additional stress. When an interpreter is not readily available in person, use of telephone services is preferable.

Access to Information

Second only to their need to be with their child, parents need easy access to information.[26,39,40,50,64,68] In addition to conversations with the health care team, parents should be supported with regard to access to their child's medical record. Access to the same information available

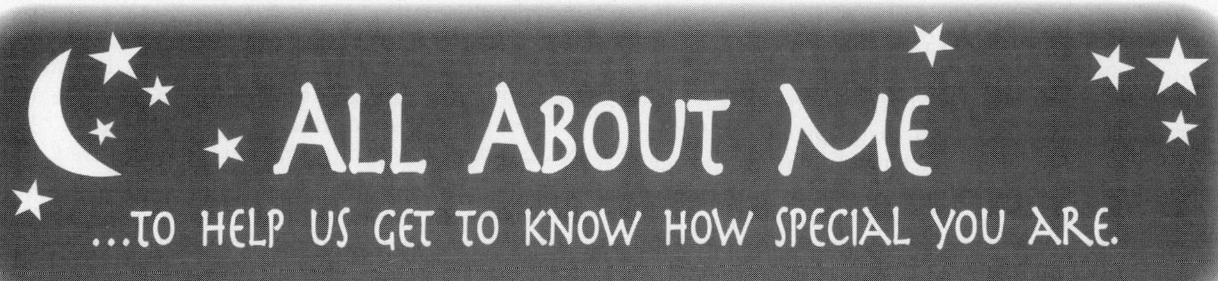

ALL ABOUT ME
...TO HELP US GET TO KNOW HOW SPECIAL YOU ARE.

NAME (AND NICKNAME)
Philip— "Flipper"

BIRTHDAY/AGE...
I'm almost 5

FAMILY...
(INCLUDE YOUR PETS!)
My Mommy
My Daddy
Big Sister, Kira
my cat, Scaredy

HOME...
seattle, WA.

FAVORITE ACTIVITIES...
playing games
helping to cook

FAVORITE TV SHOWS...
Zoboomafoo, Arthur

FAVORITE THINGS...
my scooter, my cat

FAVORITE BOOKS...
"I SPY" books

FAVORITE PLACES...
the playroom, the beach

FAVORITE SONGS...
Wheels on the bus go round...

FAVORITE MOVIES...
Willy Wonka, Scooby Doo

FAVORITE FRIENDS...
Joey, Sammy, Emily, Olivia

FAVORITE FOODS...
grapes, Satsumas
cheese, pasta

SPECIAL INFORMATION...
I like to do things for myself!

FAVORITE GAMES/SPORTS...
Flashlight Hide and Seek

FIGURE 10–1 • "All About Me©" poster.

to the other health care team members in the same format encourages trust and cooperation. Having a health care professional available for clarification as needed may be helpful but is not mandatory. Requiring parents to go through administrative or legal protocols to gain access to this information is destructive to the partnership of care. In that environment, ultimately, no matter how conscientiously delivered, the care of the child suffers.[5]

Rounds

Family-centered care can be effectively enhanced by inviting parents to attend and participate in multidisciplinary rounds. To ask parents to leave when the multidisciplinary team is focused on their child fosters mistrust and decreases efficiency. As a general practice, parents have not been invited to participate in rounds and have been intentionally excluded from the process, or they have been allowed to stay but not encouraged to contribute. Clinicians have feared that parents may misinterpret information, become concerned about staff competence, or delay rounds by asking too many questions. Except for some rare instances, such as legal cases of abuse, parents' participation in rounds works well, improving parental satisfaction and teamwork.[47]

Family participation in rounds provides an opportunity for open communication in clear and supportive language for families, patients, and the entire health care team. All team members should be encouraged to contribute information and ask questions. Parents often are excellent historians and can fill in missing information. They also have experience related to how their child responds to illness and treatment and can provide needed continuity.[39] When this model is fostered by all staff every day, parents recognize this open exchange, which fosters optimal care for their child. It is important to orient the parents to the purpose and system for rounds. If this is to be the primary contact for the day, the parents need to be informed so that they are prepared to ask questions and to ensure they understand the care being delivered. The team should provide adequate time to conduct rounds if this is the model developed. If the model does not provide time for questions from parents, this should be communicated to the parents early on so that they understand their role and do not become disappointed or frustrated by incomplete communication during rounds. In this case, the attending physician needs to ensure time later in the day to meet with the parents.

Shift Report

Traditionally, parents have been asked to leave during nurses' shift report. The same concerns and benefits related to rounds are applicable here. When there are concerns about confidentiality or legal issues, staff can accommodate by relocating report. Other than legal issues of abuse or neglect, parents have a right to know the details of their child's care, so information communicated through the report should already be available to the parents, including unplanned events.[82]

Disclosing Medical Errors

Disclosing errors or unplanned events demonstrates the principle of communicating complete and unbiased information in ways that are affirming and useful. "Building a relationship in which the patient feels respected, supported, and trusting is critical to patient and family satisfaction and malpractice risk reduction."[44] The person delivering these messages needs to follow the same principles as when conveying any other difficult news: Tell the parents as soon as feasible in a private setting. Communicate without blame how the error occurred, let them know what to expect, and help them to understand the implication of the error and its effect on their child. Elicit and acknowledge their responses. Parents should be reassured that everything will be done to prevent reoccurrence. Clearly communicate any plans for follow-up, including an identified contact person.

Daily Communication

To reduce confusion or contradiction among the caregiver's messages, it is helpful to designate one health care provider with whom the family can speak daily. Ideally, this should be the attending physician.[4,78] The content of the communication should include the status of the child, results of any tests, procedures or consultations, and the plan of care. Daily contact should allow sufficient time for questions and support. Consultants should communicate directly with the attending physician who is coordinating the care before talking with the family. Parents can become confused and overwhelmed when they receive different portions of information from a variety of providers.

Multidisciplinary Team

A variety of disciplines are needed in the care of any critically ill child. The components of the team are dependent on the needs of the child, although a physician and nurse are always included. The assignment of a consistent physician and nurse has been shown to decrease parental stress.[77] In the course of a child's stay in the PICU, the family will meet many team members. It is important for the caregivers to understand that any of these team members can become the family's primary source of support.

Social Worker

All parents should have access to a social worker.[20] This individual may be a member of the PICU team or part of a continuity team based on a specialty, such as cardiology, oncology, or organ transplantation. The social worker can provide crisis intervention, supportive care, orientation to the unit, bereavement care, and resources for basic needs. The social worker can liaison with community resources, child protective agencies, and law enforcement when necessary.

Chaplain/Spiritual Care

The chaplain offers spiritual and emotional support to patients and their loved ones and to staff and volunteers.

Provision of spiritual care may take place through conversation and listening, rituals, prayer, help in ethical decision making, and spiritual exploration. They can provide connection with a local or hometown faith group or group representative.

Child Life Specialist

A child life specialist (CLS) should be available to all critically ill children.[20] The CLS can provide support, as well as direct care to the child in several ways, which might include the use of dolls to demonstrate treatments and procedures in preparation for the actual treatment. In addition, the CLS can teach coping techniques, such as distraction, guided imagery, and story telling, as a means to reduce pain and anxiety.[3] Bedside activities can be provided to support a child's need to play. A CLS can work with community resources, schools, and in-home care personnel.

Pet Therapist

In general, there are two main approaches to pet therapy in the ICU. The first is the incorporation of the family pet; the second is that of professional or therapy dog. Incorporating the family pet integrates well with the concepts of family-centered care supporting the family to define the important individuals who will be involved in their child's care, despite biologic relationships. Pets have a significant effect on humans by lowering stress, stabilizing heart rate, and improving mood. Pets have been shown to prevent depression.[17,30,61,80] Many cases of critically ill patients responding to pets in a positive way, such as becoming more interactive and willing to participate in their own care and recovery, have been reported.

It may not always be feasible for a child's pet to visit because of distance, the animal's temperament, or other logistical realities. An alternative to the patient's own pet is the presence of a professional or therapeutic animal. Although the tie to the therapeutic animal will not be present, similar benefits can be observed as with the patient's personal pet.

Parent Advisory Council/Family as Consultant

One of the principles of family-centered care is the collaboration of providers with patients and families.[38] As expert "consumers," families bring an experiential perspective and creative solutions that help advance the best possible care.[34,67] Some hospitals have family advisory councils where consumers can provide recommendations and feedback on policy and organizational changes that affect the family experience. Family "consultants" can be used at the unit level for a variety of activities (Box 10–1).

BOX 10–1

Family Consultant Activities

- Teacher/orienter of new nursing or medical staff by sharing stories and answering questions about the experience as a parent in the PICU
- Author and analyst of satisfaction surveys
- Member of focus groups that are considering changes in service delivery
- Coleader of a parent support group
- Consultant on orientation materials for families
- Consultant for PICU remodel or redesign team
- Committee member for relevant topics, such as ethics or quality improvement

Parent Support Group

While their child is in the PICU, parents naturally seek the understanding of other parents in similar circumstances. Availability of parent support groups can meet this need.[32,37,70] These groups may be led by a trained parent volunteer and/or a professional. Participation can help to normalize the hospital experience by shared stories told in a supportive environment. Other more structured parent support groups and sibling groups meet regularly and usually are convened around a specific population, such as organ transplant, cancer, or bereavement.

Volunteers

Volunteers play an important role in normalizing activities for ill children. They can provide distraction and quiet play, such as reading or watching a movie, or more active play, such as games and crafts.[28] Volunteers can be trained to perform more advanced activities. One example is volunteers who receive training in crisis intervention and then staff the waiting room. Another example occurs at Children's Hospital in Seattle, Washington, where an "Aunties/Uncles" program provides volunteers who develop and maintain an emotional, nurturing bond with a specific hospitalized infant or child when the parents are unable to provide that time at the bedside. This more mature group of individuals must be able to commit to 5 to 6 days per week for a minimum of 6 months. Parents give their permission for this surrogate

Financial Services

Although paying the bill usually is not the concern of the health care team, it may be a serious stressor for a parent in the PICU. This added stress can impact the parent's ability to make careful decisions. In some cases, parents may worry their child will not receive the best care because of their limited financial resources. Providing a financial counselor who can coordinate care with insurance carriers and identify alternative sources for payment can greatly reduce the anxiety of the parents.

Ethicist

Ethical dilemmas are inherent in modern medical practice and are frequently identified in the PICU. Having an ethicist as part of the core multidisciplinary team can foster open discussion and resolution of difficult issues for the entire team, which includes the family.[19] Whenever possible, it is most beneficial to have an ethicist present on a regular basis rather than only during a crisis. Because ethical concerns are recurrent, it is supportive to staff and to families to have a familiar person with whom to consult.

Palliative Care

Palliative care services should be available in the PICU, although these services usually are reserved for patients with a life-limiting condition.[48,77] Palliative care resources should not be misunderstood as simply hospice care because their services are broader in focus and not limited to end-of-life issues. The trained palliative care expert can facilitate discussions between the medical team and the family that takes into consideration the preferences and values of the family, medical indications (benefits and risks), quality of life, and contextual issues such as cultural, spiritual, and community supports. This discussion is coordinated with health providers and family, resulting in the completion of a comprehensive decision-making tool. This tool sets the care plan, which follows the patient through their illness to home[16] (Figure 10–2). Revised as needed, this document allows for earlier coordination in the hospital and within the community, resulting in more consistent and compassionate care on all levels.

Access Concepts

Access to their child is probably the single most important issue for a family with a hospitalized child.[14,29,36,39–41,82] For the child, the family provides a reassuring constant in the unfamiliar PICU environment. To mitigate the anxiety experienced by families in crisis and the displacement of parental roles, access should be supported 24 hours per day, with clear communication related to the importance of parental involvement. Parents should be viewed as partners in care rather than visitors.

Admission Process

The admission process can be frightening for the parents and child, especially for emergent or unplanned admissions.[83] Every effort should be extended to help the parents acclimate to the new environment with compassion, courtesy, and time. Parents report a loss of control, which can be unbearable when separated from their ill child. To support the child and the parents, caregivers should invite the parents to be part of the admission process and support them in remaining with their child.[14,18,22,39,62,83]

If parents cannot be directly at the bedside because of space limitations or caregiving tasks, a space should be provided for the parents where they can see their child. They usually are understanding of the need to be away from the bedside in this instance and, with a brief explanation and a dedicated space near their child, usually are tolerant. As soon as feasible, a caregiver should provide the parents some initial brief information. Anxiety greatly affects short-term memory, so it often is difficult for stressed parents to take in detailed information early on. Once the child is stabilized and caregivers have more

Length of visit: ____________ Prepared by: ____________ ☐ First DMT
Physician of record: ____________ Present: ____________ ☐ Update
Care coordinator: ____________

History of Present Illness	
Medical Indications	**Patient Preferences**
Quality of Life	**Contextual Issues**
Discussion	
Plan	

Action: ____________ Who will do: ____________ By what date: ____________

Physician signature ____________ Date ____________

FIGURE 10–2 • Decision-making tool for palliative care.

time to devote to the parents, they can sit down with the parents either at the bedside or in another confidential space to provide more information.

The initial information given to parents should include the condition of the child, what has been done so far, and the plan of care. Parents often request prognosis as well. The decision to talk at the bedside versus a remote space depends upon the level of consciousness and developmental level of the child, the type of information to be communicated, and the desires of the family. It is crucial to be respectful of the family's preferences based on their cultural and religious backgrounds. Generally, in the case of a conscious adolescent or older, mature school-age child, it may be most appropriate and respectful to include the patient in the conversations rather than excluding them. Alternatively, initial conversations may be conducted away from the bedside and then duplicated at the bedside of the awake, more mature child.

This initial contact should provide adequate time for parents to ask necessary questions and understand the information that is being conveyed. When done well, this discussion is a predictor of later comprehension of what is communicated by the health care team.[4] Once the child is stabilized and the parents have spoken with the physician, cues can be taken as to when the parents are ready for a general orientation to the unit (Box 10–2). For a scheduled stay in the PICU, this orientation can most effectively be done prior to the admission.[55]

Sibling Participation

Sibling presence at the bedside should be supported based on the needs of the patient, parents, and sibling.[42,45,57,75,76,82] Siblings have not always been welcome in the PICU, although the concern that young siblings pose a greater infectious risk to the patient than do adults was disproved in the 1980s. Some fear the siblings will become frightened by what they see. However, the siblings often appear to accept the environment better than some adults. Often the sibling's imagination about an ill brother or sister is much worse than the reality.

During an initial visit by siblings, time should be spent preparing them, the parents, and the patient.[42] Any trained team member can prepare the family, but the preparation might be most effectively done by a social worker or CLS. It often is helpful to show the siblings a photo of the patient and the room and discuss what will be seen. This helps prepare siblings for what they will see. Siblings should be allowed and prepared to visit, but they should always be asked and respected if they change their mind and decline a face-to-face contact. During the visit, a clinician should be available to support the siblings and answer questions. Following a visit, a short debriefing is helpful to answer additional questions and support siblings in expressing their feelings. Providing materials for the child to prepare a memento, such as a card or drawing, to be left at the bedside can be therapeutic for the entire family.

BOX 10–2

General Orientation to the Unit

- Access to the unit
- Communications within the unit (telephone, pager, computer)[56,81]
- Bedside accommodation of family members
- Hand-washing protocols
- Isolation protocols
- Sibling visitation guideline
- Sleep accommodations
- Eating/drinking possibilities at the bedside and within the hospital
- Clinical team member identification and roles
- Multidisciplinary rounds orientation
- Registration paperwork

Family Space

Family-centered care principles can be demonstrated by the physical setting.[64,73,77] The patient bedside should include dedicated space for families. If possible, the space should include a sleep area for parents to stay overnight if they wish, storage, individualized lighting, and phone with voice mail and computer access. Additional support space can include sleep facilities in close proximity to the PICU. Parents should have access to shower, laundry facilities, cafeteria, and transportation.[37]

Participation in Care

Parents are better able to cope when their role as caregiver is maintained.[14,18,43,54,57,60,62,64] Staff are accustomed to providing all care to their patients and often feel parents expect this care. Yet for some parents, such care can be alienating because they may feel incompetent to care for their own child. Staff can help parents provide care for their child, promoting the parent child bond and improving the self-esteem of the stressed parent.[51] Staff, especially nurses, can help delineate the kind of care the parents can provide. Parents may feel frightened by their child's appearance or overwhelmed by the technology, and they require assistance in developing their new role as parents of a critically ill child. The clinician can be most effective by clearly communicating safe and appropriate care for the individual patient and modeling the behavior. This may be as simple as holding the child's hand and helping the parent to do the same. Parents can participate more actively as well. They can be given options, such as assisting with bathing, positioning, or massage.

Procedures

Clinicians may have concerns about parents' presence during procedures, but a growing body of evidence demonstrates parents want to be present, and this approach works well.[6–10,23,51,53,71] In academic hospitals where junior staff are learning procedures on patients, clinicians may feel uncomfortable with parents observing. Because the teaching process will occur whether or not the parents are present, it is honest to support the parents' presence if that is their preference.[23,82] As with any event, the parents should be prepared for what to expect. In addition, parents should be told who will be performing the procedure, any teaching that will take place, how the parent can support the child, and where in the room they can safely remain.

When the parents choose not to stay or cannot be present, they should be provided a comfortable place to wait close to the PICU. There should be a plan for communicating with the parents during the procedure and at its conclusion. If the child will be sedated for the procedure, the parents should be allowed to stay with the child until he/she has been sedated and then brought back to the bedside at the conclusion of the intervention.

Resuscitation

Clinicians have expressed a number of concerns related to parental presence during their child's resuscitation (Box 10–3). However, there is increasing evidence and a wealth of clinical experience supporting the parents' presence.[12,21,23–25,31,33,51–53,58,66,71,72,74] Assisting parents for their presence during resuscitations in the intensive care unit works well. One of the primary benefits is that the parents can see that all efforts were made to save their child. Often when parents are not allowed to be present, their imagination of what is happening behind closed doors is worse than the reality. They may come to mistrust the team and begin to question what really happened in their absence. Additionally, parents may believe their presence gives their child strength and that it is important that they be with them spiritually. Parents come to trust the health care team more because they witness the team working together in a common effort to save their child. Even in cases where resuscitation fails, the partnership developed between the parents and health care providers previous to and during the resuscitation can be helpful for the parent's acceptance of the child's death.[27,63]

It is important that parents be given a choice of whether or not to be present. In all cases, a staff member should be assigned to the parents to explain the care being given to their child. Ideally the parents should be familiar with this caregiver, but this may not be possible nor is it essential. The caregiver should give brief explanations of what is occurring, answer questions, and act as a liaison between the resuscitation team and the parents. This individual should be focused on the parents and not be directly involved in the resuscitation. Because most units have preassigned roles for resuscitations, one should be designated for parental support. Finally, families should be offered the opportunity to be alone should they feel the need.

In some units, the parents of other patients are asked to leave the area if a resuscitation is occurring. This should not be the routine practice unless space is extremely limited and the parents would interfere with the ability of the team to deliver the care. Parents should stay with their own child so that they can comfort them through what is happening around them. It can be frightening when a child is separated from a parent and is left behind, unsupported during a crisis. Parents can be helpful by staying with their child if staff are pulled to another bedside to assist with an emergency. Parents also can share in the experience with their child and provide ongoing and future support related to the event.

Transferring Out of the Pediatric Intensive Care Unit

Transfer from the PICU can be a time of anxiety and uncertainty. Families experience loss when they leave relationships developed during crises. Among the fears reported by patients and families is not knowing what to expect from unknown caregivers. Additionally, they report anxiety related to the higher patient-to-nurse ratios and leaving an area where every patient physiologic event is closely monitored. The family can benefit from a variety of approaches to allay their anxiety, all geared toward providing encouragement, information, and inclusion in the process.[11,13,69]

If the child has been in the PICU for an extended period of time or the parents are particularly anxious, a care conference can be arranged with staff from the receiving unit to delineate who will be caring for the child when the child is transferred, discuss the goals of care, and answer any questions the parents may have. PICU staff would be careful to speak positively about staff in other areas of the hospital and reassure families about their competence in handling emergencies.[69] Written information about the transfer has been shown to significantly reduce parental anxiety about imminent transfer from the PICU.[11] Other potential interventions for improving the transition for families, especially those with long ICU stays, are noted in Box 10–4.

BOX 10–3

Clinicians' Cited Concerns/Fears Regarding Parents' Presence During Resuscitations

- Interference with the resuscitation
- Misinterpretation of the team's performance
- Liability risk
- Team competence questions
- Familial emotional injury
- Staff uncomfortable with grieving family members present
- Distraction, lack of concentration by medical team

BOX 10–4

Activities to Prepare for Transfer

- Initiate transfer process early
- Remove monitor well before transfer if the patient will be off a monitor in the receiving unit
- Identify a primary nurse prior to transfer who will meet with the family to help them plan their involvement in the patient's care
- Conduct a tour of the receiving unit
- Provide written information prior to transfer, including descriptions about the receiving unit and its staff
- Assign a PICU liaison check-in with the family after the transfer

REFERENCES

1. Ahmann E: Family-centered care: shifting orientation. *Pediatr Nurs* 20:113, 1994.
2. Ahmann E: Family-centered care: the time has come. *Pediatr Nurs* 20:52, 1994.
3. American Academy of Pediatrics: Policy statement. Child life services. *Pediatrics* 106:1156, 2000.
4. Azoulay E, Chevret S, Leleu G, et al: Half the families of intensive care unit patients experience inadequate communication with physicians. *Crit Care Med* 28:3044, 2000.
5. Azoulay E, Pochard F, Chevret S, et al: Impact of family information leaflet on effectiveness of information provided to family members of intensive care unit patients. A multicenter, prospective, randomized, controlled trial. *Am J Respir Crit Care Med* 165:438, 2002.
6. Bauchner H, Vinci R, Bak S, et al: Parents and procedures: a randomized controlled trial. *Pediatrics* 98:861, 1996.
7. Bauchner H, Waning C, Vinci R: Pediatric procedures: do parents want to watch? *Pediatrics* 84:907, 1989.
8. Bauchner H, Vinci R, Waning C: Parental presence during procedures in an emergency room: results from 50 observations. *Pediatrics* 87:544, 1991.
9. Boie ET, Moore GP, Brummett C, et al: Do parents want to be present during invasive procedures performed on their children in the emergency department? A survey of 400 parents. *Ann Emerg Med* 35:70, 1999.
10. Boudreaux ED, Francis JL, Loyacano, T: Family presence during invasive procedures and resuscitations in the emergency department: a critical review and suggestions for future research. *Ann Emerg Med* 40:193, 2002.
11. Bouvé LR, Rozmus CL, Giordano P: Preparing parents for their child's transfer from the PICU to the pediatric floor. *Appl Nurs Res* 12:114, 1999.
12. Brown JR. Legally it makes good sense. *Nursing* 89:46, 1989.
13. Cagan J: Weaning parents from intensive care unit care. *Am J Matern Child Nurs* 13:275, 1988.
14. Carter MC, Miles MS, Buford TH, et al: Parental environmental stress in pediatric intensive care units. *Dimens Crit Care Nurs* 4: 181, 1985.
15. Craft MJ: Effect of visitation upon siblings of hospitalized children. *MCN* 15:47, 1986.
16. Children's Hospital, Seattle Palliative Care Program: Decision-making communication tool, adapted from an ethical decision-making model. In: *Clinical ethics*. New York, 2003, McGraw Hill.
17. Cullen L: Family and pet visitation in the critical care unit. *Crit Care Nurse* 19:84, 1999.
18. Curley MA, Wallace J: Effects of the nursing mutual participation model of care on parental stress in the pediatric intensive care unit: A replication. *J Pediatr Nurs* 7:377, 1992.
19. Day LJ, Stannard D: Developing trust and connection with patients and their families. *Crit Care Nurse* 19:66, 1999.
20. Desai PP, Ng JB, Bryant SG: Care of children and families in the CICU: a focus on their developmental, psychosocial, and spiritual needs. *Crit Care Nurs Q* 25:88, 2002.
21. Doyl CH, Post H, Burney RE, et al: Family participation during resuscitation: an option. *Ann Emerg Med* 6:107, 1985.
22. Eberly TW, Miles MS, Carter MC, et al: Parental stress after the unexpected admission of a child to the intensive care unit. *Crit Care Q* 8:57, 1985.
23. Emergency Nurses Association Position Statement: Family presence at the bedside during invasive procedures and/or resuscitation. *J Emerg Nurs* 21:26A, 1994.
24. Eichorn DJ, Meyers TA, Guzetta CE: Letting the family say goodbye during CPR. *Am J Nurs* 95:60, 1995.
25. Eichhorn DJ, Meyers TA, Mitchell TG, et al: Opening the doors: family presence during resuscitation. *J Cardiovasc Nurs* 10:59, 1996.
26. Farrell MF, Frost C: The most important needs of parents of critically ill children: parents' perceptions. *Intens Crit Care Nurs* 8:130, 1992.
27. Fina DK: A chance to say good-bye. *Am J Nurs* May:42, 1995.
28. Gavaghan SR, Carroll DL: Families of critically ill patients and the effect of nursing interventions. *Dimens Crit Care Nurs* 21:64, 2002.
29. Giganti AW: Families in the pediatric critical care: the best option. *Pediatr Nurs* 24:261, 1998.
30. Giuliano KK, Bloniasz E, Bell J: Implementation of pet visitation in critical care. *Crit Care Nurs* 19:43, 1999.
31. Goldsworth JE, Bailey M. Where's the family? *Crit Care Choices* 33, 1999.
32. Halm MA: Effect of family support groups on anxiety of family members during critical illness. *Heart Lung* 19:62, 1990.
33. Hanson C, Strawser D: Family presence during cardiopulmonary resuscitation: Foote hospital emergency department's nine-year perspective. *J Emerg Nurs* 18:104, 1992.
34. Heller R, McKlindon D: Families as "faculty": parents educating caregivers about family-centered care. *Pediatr Nurs* 22:428, 1996.
35. Hickey M: What are the needs of families of critically ill patients? A review of the literature since 1976. *Heart Lung* 19:401, 1990.
36. Hickey PA, Rykerson S: Caring for parents of critically ill infants and children. *Crit Care Nurs Clin North Am* 4:565, 1992.
37. Hostler SL: Family-centered care. *Pediatr Clin North Am* 38:1545, 1991.
38. Institute for Family-Centered Care. Bethesda, Maryland.
39. Jay SS, Youngblut JM: Parent stress associated with pediatric critical care nursing: linking research and practice. *AACN Clin Issues* 2:276, 1991.
40. Kasper JW, Nyamathi AM: Parents of children in the pediatric intensive care unit: what are their needs. *Heart Lung* 17:574, 1988.
41. Kirschbaum MS: Needs of parents of critically ill children. *Dimens Crit Care Nurs* 9:344, 1990.
42. Kleiber C: Information needs of siblings of critically ill children. *Child Health Care* 24:47, 1995.
43. LaMontagne LL, Pawlak R: Stress and coping of parents of children in a pediatric intensive care unit. *Heart Lung* 19:416, 1990.
44. Levinson W: Doctor patient communication and medical malpractice: implications for pediatricians. *Pediatr Ann* 26:186, 1997.
45. Lewandowski LA: Needs of children during the critical illness of a parent or sibling. *Crit Care Nurs Clin North Am* 4:573, 1992.
46. Lewandowski LA: Nursing grand rounds. *J Cardiovasc Nurs* 9:54, 1994.
47. Li JT, Hofmann K, Ridling DA, et al: Family centered care improves parental satisfaction in pediatric intensive care. 2003.
48. Lilly CM, DeMao DL, Sonna LA, et al: An intensive communication intervention for the critically ill. *Am J Med* 109:469, 2000.
49. Mcfall-Bloodworth L: All About Me©. Sparta, NC, 1996, Design for Life.
50. Medland JJ, Ferrans CE: Effectivess of a structured communication program for family members of patients in an ICU. *Am J Crit Care* 7:24, 1998.
51. Meyers A: Family presence during invasive procedures and resuscitation. *Am J Crit Care* 100:32, 2000.
52. Meyers TA, Eichhorn DJ, Guzetta CE: Do families want to be present during CPR? A retrospective survey. *J Emerg Nurs* 24:400, 1998.
53. Meyers TA, Eichorn DJ, Guzetta CE, et al: Family presence during invasive procedures and resuscitation. Experience of family members, nurses, and physicians. *Am J Nurs* 100:32, 2000.
54. Miles MS, Carter MC, Hennessey J, et al: Testing a theoretical model: correlates of parental stress responses in pediatric intensive care unit. *Matern Child Nurs J* 3:207, 1989.
55. Miles MS, Mathew M: Preparation of parents for the ICU experience: what are we missing? CHC 20:132, 1991.
56. Morehead KA, Hunt DM: Using beepers to keep family members involved in the patient's care. *J Healthcare Q* 19:32, 1997.
57. Page NE, Boeing NM: Visitation in the pediatric intensive care unit: controversy and compromise. *AACN Clin Issues Crit Care Nurs* 5:289, 1994.
58. Post H: Letting the family in during a code. *Nursing* 89:43, 1989.
59. Powers PH, Goldstein C, Plank G, et al: The value of patient-and family-centered care. *Am J Nurs* 100:84, 2000.
60. Proctor DL: Relationship between visitation policy in a pediatric intensive unit and parental anxiety. *Child Health Care* 16:13, 1987.
61. Proulx D. Animal assisted therapy. *Crit Care Nurse* 19:43, 1999.
62. Rennick J: Reestablishing the parental role in a pediatric intensive care unit. *J Pediatr Nurs* 1:40, 1986.
63. Reynolds D: Death as a shared experience: families in the resuscitation room. *Emerg Department Manage* December:177, 1992.
64. Riddle II, Hennessey J, Eberly TW, et al: Stresses in pediatric intensive care unit as perceived by mothers and fathers. *Matern Child Nurs J* 18:221, 1989.

65. Roberts AR, editor: *Crisis intervention handbook: assessment, treatment, and research.* Belmont, CA, 1990, Wadsworth.
66. Robinson SM: Psychological effect of witnessed resuscitation on bereaved relatives. *Lancet* 352:614, 1998.
67. Rushton CH: Family-centered care in the critical care setting: myth or reality? *Child Health Care* 19:68, 1990.
68. Rushton CH: Strategies for family-centered care in the critical care setting. *Pediatr Nurs* 16:195, 1990.
69. Saarmann L: Transfer out of critical care: freedom or fear? *Crit Care Nurs Q* 16:78, 1993.
70. Sabo KA: ICU family support group sessions: family members' perceived benefits. *Appl Nurs Res* 2:82, 1989.
71. Sacchetti A, Lichenstein R, Carraccio CA, et al: Family member presence during pediatric emergency department procedures. *Pediatr Emerg Care* 12:268, 1996.
72. Sacchetti A, Caraccio C, Leva E, et al: Acceptance of family member presence during pediatric resuscitations in the emergency department: effects of personal experience. *Pediatr Emerg Care* 16:85, 2000.
73. SCCM, AIA, AACN: video. PICU Design Award, Children's Hospital, Seattle, Washington 2002.
74. Shaner K, Eckle N: Implementing a program to support the option of family presence during resuscitation. *ACCH Advoc* 3:5, 1997.
75. Shea-McAleavey CE, Janusz HB: Sibling visitation. A plan for change. *Dimens Crit Care Nurs* 10:218, 1991.
76. Shonkwiler MA: Sibling visits in the pediatric intensive care unit. *Crit Care Q* 8:67, 1985.
77. Spatt L, Ganus E, Hying S, et al: Informational needs of families of intensive care patients. *Q Rev Bull* 12:16, 1986.
78. Sweeney MM: The value of family-centered approach in the NICU and PICU: one family's perspective. *Pediatr Nurs* 23:297, 1997.
79. Titler MG: Developing family-focused care. *Crit Care Nurs Clin North Am* 7:375, 1995.
80. Titler MA, Drahazol R: Family pet visiting, animal assisted activities, and animal assisted therapies in critical care. In Chulay M, Moltner N, editors: *Protocols for practice. Creating a Healing Environment Series.* Aliso Viejo, California, 1997, American Association of Critical-Care Nurses.
81. Topp R: Can providing paging devices relieve waiting room anxiety? *AORN J* 67:852, 1998.
82. Wincek JM: Promoting family-centered visitation makes a difference. *AACN Clin Issues* 2:293, 1992.
83. Youngblut JM, Jay SS: Emergent admission to the pediatric intensive care unit. Parental concerns. *AACN Clin Issues Crit Care Nurs* 2:276, 1991.
84. Zoucha R: The keys to culturally sensitive care. *Am J Nurs* 100:24GG, 2000.

CHAPTER 11

Ethics in Pediatric Intensive Care

Joel E. Frader and Kelly Michelson

PEARLS

Major Principles of Medical Ethics
- Beneficence: Provide care that benefits patients
- Nonmaleficence: Avoid harming patients
- Autonomy: Individuals should decide what constitutes their own best interests
- Justice: Provide service fairly without bias from factors irrelevant to the medical situation

Informed Consent
- Patients or surrogates must have adequate decision-making capacity (competency)
- Have ability to understand and communicate about the medical situation
- Have ability to manipulate information and deliberate about nature and consequences of alternatives
- Have ability to make a choice among alternatives based on relevant values
- Decision maker should have adequate, comprehensible information
- Professional should assess decision maker's understanding of situation and alternatives
- Valid choices require freedom from undue pressure (coercion)

Decision Standards
- Substituted judgment: surrogates decide based on knowledge of patient's views of situation or, if unavailable, the patient's general beliefs and lifestyle
- Best interests: surrogates decide based on information about the patient's situation, alternatives, and overall judgment about which course best serves the patient

Introduction

Intensivists struggle with value questions all the time, regardless of whether they explicitly label the process *ethical decision making*. This chapter addresses some of the common and more important moral questions arising in pediatric intensive care units (PICUs). It aims to clarify how the values of patients, families, health care professionals, and those of the wider society do and should influence the practice of pediatric intensive care. The goal of the chapter—helping intensivists to help patients and families better—although practical, is best served if the reader appreciates a small amount of the theory that supports much of contemporary medical ethics.

Moral Theory

Medical ethics does not constitute a completely independent field. Most think of medical ethics as an applied discipline of the wider branch of philosophy that is ethics. Like most other intellectual pursuits, ethics has developed according to several theoretical traditions. In western ethics, two particular ways of thinking have dominated for some time. Because these approaches may yield rather different perspectives on some questions, they deserve mention.

Consequentialism

One tradition, known as *consequentialism,* examines the correctness of an action according to what effects the act likely will have on the real world. Good actions produce the most favorable ratio of happiness, pleasure, or some similar value to unhappiness or similarly disvalued result. The utilitarian philosophers Bentham and Mill enjoined us to seek the greatest happiness for the greatest number of individuals possible. These theories emphasize the *social* nature of human moral action, requiring calculation of the consequences of an act. Only after determining the impact of an action for those directly and remotely involved can a person pronounce ethical judgment.

Deontology

The other main approach to moral theory proceeds from different premises. *Deontology* (from the Greek word for *duty)* holds that some actions have intrinsic moral worth. Many religious moral rules conform to this view. Hence the Ten Commandments pronounce that we should not kill. Other approaches, such as Kant's categorical imperative, also proclaim universal truths and rules that persons should honor irrespective of the consequences.

A consequentialist might claim that removal of organs from persons in a persistent vegetative state (PVS) does not harm the individuals because they can no longer experience meaningful life, or even hunger or thirst. The consequentialist also might assert that harvesting the organs best serves the class of PVS patients because, overall, transplantation fosters the well-being (and by implication, happiness) of humans who can actually benefit from continued treatment. Some deontologists, however, surely would argue that the killing that necessarily results from the removal of vital organs, no matter what the intent, undermines human dignity and is morally impermissible.

Prevailing Principles

Despite the "opposing" traditions of ethics, most in *medical* ethics agree on a small number of important principles that should guide medical behavior. The reader should note, however, that narrow adherence to these notions encourages an oversimplified approach. Medical ethics neither begins with nor ends with the principles named here. A more nuanced view includes many more considerations and a clear sense of how different ideas interact, especially how some moral duties conflict with others. Nevertheless, a few guideposts may help intensivists understand that medical ethics, like clinical medicine, uses formal logic and has a recognizable structure.

Beneficence

The first principle, *beneficence,* demands that physicians provide care that benefits the patient. This may seem self-evident until you remember that many potential conflicts of interest can influence medical decisions. For example, parents of children may face tragic choices about the support of a sick child whose survival could endanger the economic or psychological integrity of the rest of their family. Other conflicts may involve doctors, especially those in a fee-for-service system, who benefit financially from providing services that promise only marginal, if any, additional benefit.

Nonmaleficence

Beneficence contrasts with *nonmaleficence.* According to this notion, doctors have a duty to avoid harming patients. Again, the idea may seem obvious, but the practical application involves considerable complexity. For example, when deciding whether to use extracorporeal membrane oxygenation (ECMO) for a desperately ill infant with a diaphragmatic hernia, you must consider the possibility that the technology will extend the life of the baby only by several days, that is, no long-term benefit will accrue. Similar reasoning might apply to cases of malignancy for which chemotherapy and other treatments have no or little likelihood of producing a cure or substantial life prolongation, whereas the treatments impose burdens, such as nausea, itching, extreme fatigue, and high risk of infection. The principle of nonmaleficence reminds us to take potential pain and suffering seriously before recommending no-holds-barred medical intervention.

Autonomy

When considering which medical treatments will best help a patient and what harms to avoid, a natural question arises: whose perspective should we use? The principle of *autonomy* suggests that we must respect individual human differences. To the extent possible, persons should decide for themselves what is in their own best interests. In pediatrics, respecting autonomy can present difficult questions about when children develop the capacity and independence to accept or refuse recommended treatment. The autonomy principle reminds us that individuals or their families often have different values and goals from those of their physicians. Medical decisions usually should be in accordance with the patient's or family's perspective.

Justice

The fourth principle, *justice,* provides some of the most pressing and challenging dilemmas for modern medical care. Put simply, this principle exhorts us to use our services fairly, to avoid decisions that accept or reject candidates for treatment based on factors, such as poverty, that are irrelevant to their medical situation. The application of the justice principle runs into two major obstacles today. First, members of our society seem to have a great deal of difficulty agreeing on what constitutes just or fair allocation of medical resources. Second, we have not yet decided exactly how considerations of justice should affect the medical care *system*.

Medical goods can be distributed, assuming not everyone can have everything, according to a number of different schemes: based on the likelihood of success; by some definition of need (urgency, desperation); as a reward (for past achievement, for waiting the longest, for future contribution); by equal shares; by random assignment until the goods run out; or, as we often do in our society, by ability to pay. Different philosophical and political traditions support each of these approaches, and we seem far from agreeing on which is best.

With respect to the second issue, some urge physicians to ignore financial constraints in order to do everything "medically indicated" for patients, regardless of the economic consequences.[1] The argument goes that at least for individual patient decisions, physicians discharge their fiduciary responsibility only by advocating the best, even if most expensive, care. Macroeconomic concerns, regional and institutional issues, and microeconomics challenge this view.

From a macroeconomic perspective, our society resists increasing medical spending as an ever-increasing proportion of total social expenditure (such as percent of gross domestic product [GDP]). Most western industrial countries spend 7% to 10% of GDP on health care. Does the United States get incrementally better outcomes for its 14% or larger outlay? By many measures of public health (e.g., infant mortality and longevity), the well-being of the U.S. population does not reflect our high medical expenses. Similarly, does the way we spend our health care dollar make the most sense? Should we spend great sums of money on expensive intensive care at the end of life for patients with little likelihood of benefit? In pediatrics, we have reason to believe that preventive measures (immunization, accident prevention) reduce morbidity and mortality[2–4] and, in some cases, save money.[2,3]

Regional and institutional economic questions involve matters such as consolidation of care to increase economic efficiency and medical efficacy. However, political and psychosocial factors often lead to duplication of services and diffusion of experience. Certain programs may even create conflicts of interest. For instance, a hospital could offer a particularly scarce and expensive service (e.g., ECMO or pediatric organ transplantation). The costs of the service might be so high that just a few patients treated "free," that is, without charge to the family, might threaten the economic stability of the enterprise. Such fiscal concerns surely help shape what services institutions offer and the way those services become available (are "marketed") to those in need.

With respect to microallocation, intensivists frequently engage in decisions about the distribution of specific services to particular patients, sometimes with clear awareness that competition exists under conditions of scarcity. With a nearly full ICU and a large demand for postoperative care for the cases on the next day's operating room schedule, intensivists often must negotiate and juggle, trying to meet varying claims about who should occupy scarce beds and receive nursing attention. Even the decision to use one vasoactive drug or antibiotic instead of far more or less expensive agents requires an attempt to balance expected benefit against drains on resources. It seems inappropriate to demand that physicians ignore such actual conflicts. Intensivists, like other practitioners, rarely enjoy the luxury of having a single duty to a single patient with an unlimited ability to pay for services. Although doctors might prefer to leave economic considerations to policymakers and the marketplace, justice issues do find their way into ICU routines.

The challenge for the pediatric intensivist involves applying the various ethical principles and perspectives to individual cases and to policies that affect how the unit operates. The following sections focus on a few topics where ethical concerns arise frequently.

Consent

A major shift in doctor–patient–family relations occurred in the last half of the twentieth century. Doctors now have less freedom to make paternalistic decisions about how to treat patients according to their own beliefs and feelings than they did in the 1950s. With a wider range of technical options, with social trends emphasizing individual liberty and consumer preferences, and with the weakening of traditional authority and trust in professionals, legal and moral arguments at the beginning of the twenty-first century emphasize patient/personal choice in directing medical decisions.

These trends have become embodied in the *doctrine of informed consent*. Backed by philosophical arguments concerning the importance of individual and family autonomy, ethicists, legal scholars, and judges have advanced the notion that patients or their valid surrogates have the right to or should, if they wish, determine which of available medical alternatives to follow. The right, in the law, of a "reasonable person" to accept or refuse offered medical treatment, however, involves some important qualifications. The legal reasonable person standard assumes a *competent* patient or surrogate. To make a valid choice, the patient or surrogate needs comprehensible *information* about the medical situation so that any choice reflects the range of alternatives and their consequences. Simply having the information does not suffice; the decision maker must actually exhibit an *understanding* of what he/she has learned. Finally, choices of individuals or surrogates should occur *voluntarily*, that is, free of any undue pressure, especially from health care providers.

Competency

In most circumstances, minors are legally incompetent; that is, state statutes determine the age at which children become legally entitled to make binding decisions, including those about medical care. In general, children have no legal right to make medical decisions for themselves until age 18 years. As a consequence, like other legally incompetent patients, surrogates must authorize medical treatment for children. Usually, parents serve as the valid surrogates for their children, with certain legal and ethical exceptions.

Almost all states have statutory provisions for children to obtain treatment for sexually transmitted diseases without parental or other surrogate consent. In many states, similar laws apply to children seeking contraception, care for pregnancy-related matters, and sometimes abortion. Children may achieve legal status to make their own medical decisions when "emancipated." Depending on the jurisdiction, this may mean graduation from high school, joining the armed forces, living separately from and economically independent of parents, or being pregnant or being a parent. Thus under some circumstances a critically ill minor may be legally entitled to consent to or refuse treatment, even over and against parental wishes.

In addition to specific legislative rights for some children to consent for themselves, another legal notion may apply. Courts have used the theory of the "mature minor" in judging whether a child has the capacity and maturity to decide what is best for herself/himself. Such cases typically involve chronic or long-standing medical conditions where the minor has had an opportunity to observe the implications of the disorder, to experience the effects of the disease, and to reflect on the religious, moral, and factual matters relevant to medical decisions. Examples of such situations include adolescents with cystic fibrosis, end-stage renal disease, and muscular dystrophies. The mature minor doctrine allows that, in selected cases, the child may accept or decline life-sustaining treatment, such as dialysis, mechanical ventilation, and transplantation, with or without agreement from the family. Other situations might include those where long-standing and well-thought-out beliefs, such as those held by adolescent Jehovah's Witnesses, would lead the child to refuse blood transfusions that otherwise might be essential for appropriate medical care. These cases require careful individual determinations about the actual capacities of the patient and the issues involved, and prudence may suggest judicial review. (This discussion does not imply that legal entitlement equals the best moral solution to dilemmas or disputes. However, the law recognizes that some children have legitimate independent claims regarding their medical care that may differ from the expressed wishes of their parents or guardians. This legal recognition suggests that, at times, professionals should support admittedly divisive stances that minor patients take.)

Legal entitlement does not mean the proposed decision maker actually is competent, whether referring to the child, a parent, or other guardian. More accurately, we should regard competency as a legal determination, and physicians must assess the decision-making *capacity* of the patient or surrogate. This capacity has several features and elements. First, capacity to make medical decisions involves specific determinations for each "significant" decision. A patient or surrogate may have appropriate capacity to accept, generally, medical efforts to prevent death from fulminant hepatic failure. However, the patient's agreement to accept intensive care does not provide a warrant for the doctors to proceed directly to liver transplantation. The proposal of the latter treatment should trigger a separate exploration of the decision-maker's capacity to agree to transplant surgery. Similarly, decisional capacity refers to specific kinds of decisions. Because a parent cannot balance his/her checkbook or pay medical bills on time (because of a lack of understanding of what is involved, rather than a lack of funds), it does not follow that such a parent cannot rationally refuse mechanical ventilation for a son or daughter with a degenerative neuromuscular disease. Further, disagreement with a medical opinion does not, in and of itself, constitute grounds for declaring a patient or surrogate incapable of making sound choices. Rejection of medical recommendations may trigger concern about competency, but such disagreement does not establish the case that the decision maker lacks decision-making capacity.

Although not everyone agrees on how to define *medical decisional capacity,* most accept the notion that it involves (1) an ability to understand and communicate about the medical situation at hand, (2) an ability to manipulate information about the situation and deliberate about the nature and consequences of alternatives, and (3) an ability to make a choice among the alternatives, preferably based on relevant values.

Information

Assuming a patient or surrogate has appropriate decision-making capacity, the decision maker needs information about the patient's condition, prognosis, and alternative treatments. Clinicians should provide details without jargon and abbreviations. Frightened and dependent patients or surrogates may nod or respond as if they understand, but some empirical evidence and common sense suggest otherwise.[5,6] Ethical and legal considerations require that the information be understandable to the decision maker.

In addition to the actual content of any information provided, doctors must consider the timing of decisions and the state of mind of the decision maker. Even the best-prepared patients or surrogates may need complex material presented repeatedly (hence the value of written or audiovisual aids) and may need time to absorb and reflect on what he/she has learned. A common problem here is the assumption by health care professionals that consent (or refusal) occurs at some magic instant in time, usually associated with a signature on a form. Lidz, Appelbaum, and Meisel[6] suggested a superior conception of consent as a process that occurs over time in the context of a relationship among doctors, patients, and surrogates. Although intensivists may object that the nature of their patients' problems and the hectic critical care environment make evolving, deliberative, and relational consent unrealistic, truly emergent treatment decisions remain relatively rare and, in any case, are exempt from legal consent requirements. Most important decisions can occur with adequate time for reflection and with time for relationships to develop. Also, physicians should not consider decisions immutable. Just as medical situations change and require reconsideration, so may the goals of treatment and the acceptable means of reaching those ends remain fluid. The concept of "time-limited trials" may help health care professionals and patients or surrogates remember the value of reassessing courses of action periodically.[7,8]

Understanding

For the capacitated decision maker who has received sufficient understandable information, you can and should ask if he/she actually comprehends the facts and issues. Experts disagree on what criteria to use in assessing understanding. Some accept the decision makers repeating a summary of the facts and concerns (which demonstrates recall, rather than understanding), whereas others have health care providers ask detailed questions probing the matter. Still others permit the assumption of understanding in the absence of questions from the decision maker. Clearly, a "yes" answer to the question "Do you understand what I have just said to you?" demonstrates very little. Research suggests that physicians routinely overestimate what patients and family members understand.[5] Some might say that life-and-death treatment in the ICU is so complicated that parents cannot possibly understand it anyway. Although we should perhaps seriously consider this challenge to the value and importance of informed consent and patient or surrogate autonomy, these concepts remain the legal standard of care and deserve attention on that account.

Voluntariness

The final aspect of informed consent requiring discussion involves whether the patient or surrogate has given permission for treatment or diagnostic tests freely or voluntarily. Permission obtained under duress generally cannot be considered valid consent. Here, as with other aspects of consent, we may encounter difficulty agreeing on how to determine what constitutes freely given acceptance of medical plans or recommendations.

The usual model of informed consent applies most directly to situations where all parties have considerable *time* to reflect on the available options. Although in some cases we need not invoke the notion of emergency, patients or parents may not have many hours or days to consider alternatives. Do time limitations themselves constitute so coercive an influence as to invalidate full consent? Surely the *nature of the patient's situation* can prevent ideal, deliberative decision making. Having to make decisions that may affect life and death may leave parents feeling, "If we don't accept this doctor's plan, we may be harming our child." Undoubtedly, telling parents faced with a life-and-death matter that they must accept their doctor's favored approach when several valid medical alternatives exist cannot be tolerated. ("If you don't do *x*" where *a*, *b*, and *c* might well work, too, "you're killing your child.")

To the extent that parents must make rapid decisions about grave matters in tertiary care settings totally unfamiliar to the patient and family and without benefit of an established, trusting relationship with their doctor, we must worry that parental permission cannot possibly live up to ethical and legal ideals of informed consent.

Surrogate Decision Making: Parental Rights and Obligations

Theorists and courts have agreed that autonomous individuals can accept or reject medical treatment for almost any reason.[9] Doctors have had to defer to adult patients' whims, isolated false beliefs, and strongly held opinions about medical matters to satisfy our society's insistence on respecting individual liberty. (The need, in the end, to accept reluctantly what a person believes to be an inappropriate course of action does not relieve the physician from the burden of trying to dissuade the patient from his/her view.) Parents and others with responsibility for surrogate decision making, however, must adhere to different standards. In the cases of individuals who have had an opportunity to express beliefs about desired or unwanted medical care, surrogates usually must use a standard known as "substituted judgment." In these situations, surrogates attempt, based on their knowledge of the patient's views, to decide what the particular patient would want under the specific circumstances. Written documents (such as "living wills"), oral discussions of particulars (such as the patient's feelings about long-term mechanical ventilation following severe head injury), or a general understanding of the patient's preferences and lifestyle all may form the basis of legally valid surrogate decisions.[10] To the degree that young patients with sufficient decision-making capacity, such as adolescents with sickle cell disease at risk for cerebral hemorrhage or those with muscular dystrophy at risk for cardiac or respiratory failure, have expressed views about possible treatments before becoming unable to express their wishes, the notion of substituted judgment also should prevail in pediatrics.

Far more commonly, however, substituted judgment makes no sense in pediatrics. It only can be a flight of the most fanciful imagination: just how might a toddler with a high spinal cord transection from a motor vehicle accident "think" about what he/she would want (death or a life on a ventilator)? Accordingly, most scholars in ethics and most courts have attempted to apply a different standard for making decisions for children, that of "best interests." The standard enjoins the surrogate to take into account all relevant information about the patient's condition, the alternative treatments (including, presumably, the resources available to obtain and maintain care), and decide, all things considered, what course to follow.[11]

One term used by many, *quality of life*, has received considerable attention in these decisions. The phrase has been used to convey two substantially different concepts. Some reject quality-of-life considerations because they believe parents, doctors, or others use it to make judgments about the social worth of the patient, that is, for some, quality of life implies something about the potential of the patient to contribute to the general social welfare (hold a job, pay taxes, or simply consume resources). Those who fear that social worth will equal quality of life strongly oppose taking quality-of-life evaluations into account in surrogate decisions.

Most commentators mean something different. For them, quality-of-life considerations involve overall prognosis, including pain and/or suffering associated with the patient's condition(s) and treatment(s); the practical likelihood of overcoming barriers to effective treatment, including the financial, social, and psychological resources available to the patient and family; and other nontechnical matters.

Aside from confusion about what meaning to assign to the phrase *quality of life*, it seems quite reasonable to weigh factors beyond simply what technical approaches can affect the child's medical condition(s). Although fears about inappropriate discrimination against the handicapped have a legitimate basis, history raises at least equivalent, if not overriding, concerns about excessive and inhumane treatment, whether in obeisance to the technologic imperative or in pursuit of a vitalist belief.[12]

Arriving at an adequate, practically useful definition of *best interest* has eluded the efforts of many in the pediatric, social work, legal, and ethics communities. Without a clear notion of what constitutes the best interests of the child, it has been difficult to establish readily applicable limits on surrogate decision making. A lively debate continues about the acceptability of including "third party" or parent/family considerations in decisions for or about children, especially life-and-death decisions.

The difficulty for the pediatric intensivist lies in knowing when parental or other surrogate decisions fall outside some socially or morally adequate range. These difficulties involve medical uncertainty about diagnosis and prognosis, varying community standards regarding many different practices (especially the existence of state laws on religious exemptions from child abuse and neglect laws), and changing social attitudes about lifestyle. Concrete examples of these problems illustrate the dilemmas.

Consider a critically ill child with intestinal failure. Over the past few years, several treatments have been offered to children with short bowel syndrome (SBS) and some severe motility disorders who approach exhaustion of their options for total parental nutrition. Controversy exists about the effectiveness of enteral feeding,[13,14] operations for improving intestinal function,[15] and small bowel transplantation.[16]

For each of these approaches, we know little about the long-term outcomes. No one has attempted a straight-on comparative trial of these radically divergent treatment methods, in part because of strong beliefs about which intervention works best. Unfortunately, these convictions have little or no basis in scientifically valid research. Some intensivists caring for a patient with SBS believe that because neither surgical approach nor intensive medical treatment has proven long-term benefit, parents should remain free to accept or reject each intervention and accept palliative/hospice care. Others believe it necessary to challenge parental refusal in court.

Resolving such a dilemma requires consideration of the general question of how much physicians need to know about any therapy, especially of the therapies they recommend, before justifiably attempting to impose treatment, through judicial means, on reluctant patients and families. A helpful question might be the following: what would the doctor choose for her/his own family? A study of neonatologists, pediatric cardiologists, and pediatric cardiac surgeons noted considerable discrepancy between what the physicians recommended to parents of newborns with hypoplastic left heart syndrome and what they would want for their own child.[17] A significantly greater proportion of the physicians accepted nonsurgery—and the inevitability of death—for themselves than they recommended to families.

With regard to community standards of care, we note that the majority of states have laws limiting the application of child abuse and neglect standards where parents invoked religious practices as the reason for delays in, or refusal of, medical care for their children. The manner in which religious exemption laws have been used, either in decisions not to intervene (order treatment, prosecute criminal cases when a child has been harmed) or as a primary defense in court, has varied greatly across jurisdictions. Most agree that parental religious beliefs should not prevent children from receiving clearly beneficial treatment that would permit children to accept or reject their parents' faith when the children become more mature.[18] The difficulty comes in deciding what conditions warrant intervention and what treatments confer obvious benefits.

Criminal prosecutions in California, Massachusetts, Arizona, Florida, and elsewhere remind the pediatric community that certain religious convictions, in these cases Christian Science, favor prayer over antibiotics for meningitis, over surgery for bowel obstruction, and over other standard medical treatments.[19] Assuming timely diagnosis and intervention, deaths of children could have been prevented, and the likely medical outcome would have been excellent. Yet, in some cases that may involve pediatric intensive care, the need for treatment and its benefits leave room for doubt.

Some pediatric cardiothoracic surgeons have taken on the challenge of correcting congenital heart defects using cardiopulmonary bypass without supplemental blood. At the request of families believing in the teachings of the Jehovah's Witnesses, these surgeons agree to operate using saline in the bypass circuitry. Their success has long been available in the peer-reviewed medical literature.[20] Witnesses believe that doctors can frequently provide adequate treatment without using the blood or blood products that their faith cannot accept. In other circumstances, pediatricians may request and receive court permission to transfuse sick children when routine use of blood relies on tradition and not scientifically established need. For example, premature infants may receive packed red cells when blood drawing and inherently slow erythropoiesis drop the hematocrit to between 30% and 40%. Few data support a clear medical need for this intervention: "…no uniformly accepted criteria exist for the transfusion of premature or term infants."[21] In that and other circumstances involving the children of Jehovah's Witnesses, you might think twice before seeking court orders to perform transfusion.

Although understandable, psychosocial factors that lead physicians, anxious to protect their patients, to assert professional control do not constitute an ethical justification for action. In light of the importance of religious freedom in our nation's history and political system, intensive care professionals should consider giving great deference to personal beliefs, especially in medically marginal or uncertain circumstances.

If there is debate about the proper role of parental religious views in determining medical care for children, we have utter confusion about the role of so-called *third party considerations*, such as the impact of a child's disease and treatment on the parents and other family members. Some authors have suggested that when substantial uncertainty exists about the benefits of treatment, when the burdens of treatment seem weighty (e.g., multiple operations, long-term hospitalization, or toxic drugs), or when the ability of the patient to experience human pleasures will be seriously compromised, parents can and should consider the impact of the child's treatment on the family as a whole.[22] Such concerns might include temporal, fiscal, and psychological resources that the sick child will consume and that might otherwise be available to siblings or other dependents.

These matters can become quite confusing, as the following case suggests. A 6-month-old child was referred to a distant center for consideration of organ transplantation. The message to the family at the referring hospital had been heard by the parents as ambivalent, that is, the parents believed the doctors in their hometown were not entirely convinced of the value or likelihood of success of transplantation. The transplantation physicians believed the child was an excellent candidate for the procedure and had a favorable (65% or better 1-year survival, at the time) prognosis. The parents hesitated to accept treatment, stating that transplantation would mean that the mother's recent reentry into her career would be derailed, that they did not want the (considerable) expense of chronic immunosuppressive medication, and that, all things considered, transplantation seemed more of a burden to the family than they thought they could tolerate.

The situation caused considerable distress among the staff at the referral center. Had the parents said, "No, thank you, we'd rather take the money we'll have to spend on antirejection drugs and buy a sailboat," the staff would not have hesitated to challenge their decision-making authority. However, the parents stated coherent and serious concerns. Given the nontrivial risk of complications and the actual burdens of treatment (e.g., lifelong immunosuppression with possible serious infection, malignancy, and toxic injury from medications), their refusal of the "standard of care" (not experimental treatment) seemed difficult to accept but sufficient to prevent an attempt to obtain court intervention. No doubt some other centers would have reacted differently.

With regard to unorthodox parental preferences concerning treatment, courts have not always acted to support mainstream physicians. In one older but still important New York State case, *Matter of Hofbauer,* the courts supported the parents' choice of a licensed physician who agreed to treat the child's Hodgkin's disease with "nutritional or metabolic therapy, including injections of Laetrile."[23] The Court of Appeals of New York decided it could not and should not choose among treatments, each of which was supported by physicians legally practicing within the state. Following that view, parents only need to find a licensed practitioner to endorse their preferred approach to prevail in court. Doubtless the limits on parental or other surrogate decisions will continue to be debated by those concerned with pediatric ethics, laws, and medicine. For the time being, only a rough consensus exists that the best interests of the child should remain the guiding principle in most cases. When doctors and parents experience serious difficulty in defining or predicting what action will best serve the child's interests, other considerations become more important. Other legitimate concerns include the family's religious views or moral commitments, the family's resources, and the ordinary and reasonable plans and projects of family members.[24] Adherence only to narrow technical goals of treatment has little place in the provision of advanced pediatric intensive care.

Pediatric Intensive Care Unit and "Experimentation"

Experimentation has two rather common meanings. In the first sense of the term, *experimentation* refers to research, that is, the scholarly pursuit of generalizable knowledge. Many children receiving intensive care become "subjects" of research when their care follows protocols designed to assess the value of some element of the treatment. Sometimes the research element of the child's care is incidental, possibly even trivial, such as whether one brand of monitoring equipment speeds the jobs of the health care professionals more than another. To the extent that the research determines essential aspects of patient care and may affect outcome, however, doctors must approach such experimentation somewhat differently from their usual practice, that is, experimental treatments (or diagnostic procedures) require greater attention to parental authorization. As noted previously, children may receive *treatment* by court approval, over and against parental wishes, when the therapy constitutes the standard of care. By contrast, parents may, under regulations governing the use of federal research funds, refuse to enter children into research protocols and may withdraw their children from such projects at any time.[25] Under some circumstances, permission for experimental treatment requires written "consent" from both parents, whereas treatment can go forward with permission from only one parent under most circumstances.

The other meaning of experimentation concerns the "use" of the patient for the learning and practice of trainees. When and under what circumstances subjecting critically ill children to additional risk or discomfort related to education can be justified poses a number of difficult questions. First, the patients and their families represent a captive population. The majority of pediatric intensive care takes place in training institutions. Only rarely do parents have an opportunity to express a meaningful preference about which PICU should provide care for their child, given the relative scarcity of units, the relationship of any particular unit to other persons or facilities that parents have chosen (e.g., surgeon, oncologist, or hospital setting), and emergency situations in which legal, bureaucratic, triage, or other considerations leave little room for parental wishes. Unlike the wider "health care market," parents have few substantive choices about their child's ICU.

Second, training must occur. New generations of pediatricians, pediatric nurses, pediatric intensivists, and other specialists need to accrue experience so that they learn to care competently for subsequent critically ill children. Even with use of modern instructional aids, including realistic artificial models, animal laboratory experience, and intellectual preparation, the novice medical professional must perform her/his first intubation, pulmonary artery wedge catheter insertion, and other relatively risky procedures.

The intensivist faces an uncomfortable dilemma: Parental choice is severely constrained yet the education must continue. Whether parental permission, even in the somewhat unlikely event of full disclosure and understanding, could be given freely can easily be questioned.

The institutions of medicine (i.e., the practitioners and the organizations that provide the care and the training) must do a better job of telling patients and surrogates that we continually need to teach people how to provide lifesaving care. Greater efforts at public education would at least help to convince many of the long-term benefits of medical education. More importantly, the profession and the organizations need to promise and actually provide adequate supervision of trainee practice. It is one thing for a new ICU fellow to accomplish her/his first rapid sequence intubation in a trauma victim with a faculty mentor at her/his side, ready to advise or take over as needed, and quite another for the trainee to be thrown into the thick of the action with only telephone connection, if any, to experienced consultation. The dual responsibilities of better education of patients and families and sufficient supervision need more attention from the intensive care community.

What should happen if parents know about and refuse involvement of trainees, despite realistic assurances of adequate supervision? Administrators may suggest holding fast to prevent the establishment of undesirable precedents. Although the worry is legitimate, one wonders if expending the time and energy involved in such a battle results in unreasonable delays in needed patient care, alienates the parties, and undermines the trust needed to facilitate treatment. Flexibility and interpersonal skill might accomplish more than rigid bureaucratic responses. Moreover, parental protest of this sort may reflect underlying anxiety about what is happening to their child or their role in whatever troubles have afflicted the patient. Direct inquiry regarding the parents' fears and guilt may provide greater benefit for all concerned than a confrontation over the educational mission of the unit.

Finally, the matter of practice on insensate or (newly) dead patients deserves mention, if not resolution. In these situations, doctors legitimately claim that the patient or former patient cannot "appreciate" any harm, and substantial benefit may derive from such "harmless" practice. Two problems arise, however. First, in our society we generally hold that dying patients, permanently unconscious individuals, or even dead bodies have interests. Religious and secular laws specify, often in great detail, what constitutes dignified treatment of bodies. In addition, formerly competent individuals have the legal right to specify how they wish to be treated should they become incompetent or die (e.g., via living wills, donor cards, and declarations about funeral arrangements, such as the desire to be buried or cremated). Thus how you construe harm to the body may vary, depending on your perspective, and there is no guarantee that the patient or family will see things the same way as the doctors. The second problem derives from the first. Because most hold that former persons and bodies have interests, you need to determine the interests and obtain permission for the proposed action (assuming a coincidence of interests). Most doctors and other health care professionals do not want to ask permission to use bodies for practice. They fear a premorbid request will trigger unwarranted concern that the physicians will not do everything possible to prevent death and that a postmortem request will only add to family grief, not to mention the guilt and discomfort of the staff. Although this discussion may seem abstract or even absurd, picture a scene where a resident is attempting a difficult intubation on a recently dead patient and a parent unknowingly slips into the room or through the closed curtain. Without proper prior authorization, it seems likely the discovery would produce an unwelcome response.

Again, a clear solution eludes us. Greater public education may help here, as with the problem of training generally. However, the various feelings and rituals that surround death may overpower rationality about the matter. Perhaps the best approach involves finding ever better substitutes (e.g., plastic models and the like) for teaching the skills our trainees need.

REFERENCES

1. Levinsky NG: The doctor's master. *N Engl J Med* 311:1573, 1984.
2. Schoenbaum SC, Hyde JN Jr Bartoshesky L, Crampton K: Benefit-cost analysis of rubella vaccination policy. *N Engl J Med* 294:306, 1976.
3. Matlin NM: The cost of child health supervision services: real concern or red herring? *Child Health Financing Report* II:4, 1985.
4. Nixon J, Clacher R, Pearn J, Corcoran A: Bicycle accidents in childhood. *Br Med J* 294:1267, 1987.
5. Meisel A, Roth LH: What we do and do not know about informed consent. *JAMA* 246:2473, 1981.
6. Lidz CW, Appelbaum PS, Meisel A: Two models of implementing informed consent. *Arch Intern Med* 148:1385, 1988.
7. President's Commission for the Study of Ethical Problems in Medicine and Biomedical and Behavioral Research: *Deciding to forgo life-sustaining treatment: ethical, medical, and legal issues in treatment decisions.* Washington, DC, 1983, US Government Printing Office.
8. *Guidelines on the termination of life-sustaining treatment and the care of the dying.* Briarcliff Manor, NY, 1987, The Hastings Center.
9. Armstrong CJ: Judicial involvement in treatment decisions the emerging consensus. In Civetta J, Taylor RW, Kirby RR, editors: *Critical care.* Philadelphia, 1988, JB Lippincott.
10. *Matter of Conroy.* 98 NJ 321, 1985.
11. Macklin R: Return to the best interests of the child. In Gaylin W, Macklin R, editors: *Who speaks for the child: the problems of proxy consent.* New York, 1982, Plenum Press.
12. Kopelman LM, Irons TG, Kopelman AE: Neonatologists judge the "Baby Doe" regulations. *N Engl J Med* 318:677, 1988.
13. Gambarara M, Ferretti F, Papadatou V, et al: Intestinal adaptation in short bowel syndrome. *Transplant Proc* 29:1862, 1997
14. Gambarara M, Goulet O, Bagolan P, et al: Long-term parenteral nutrition in the management of extremely short bowel syndrome. *Transplant Proc* 30:2539, 1998.
15. Thompson JS: Surgical aspects of the short-bowel syndrome. *Am J Surg* 222:532, 1995.
16. Iyer KR. Srinath C. Horslen S, et al: Late graft loss and long-term outcome after isolated intestinal transplantation in children. *J Pediatr Surg* 37:151, 2002 .
17. Kon AA, Ackerson L, Lo B: Choices physicians would make if they were the parents of a child with hypoplastic left heart syndrome. *Am J Cardiol* 91:1506, A9, 2003.
18. American Academy of Pediatrics, Committee on Bioethics: Religious exemptions from child abuse statutes. *Pediatrics* 81:169, 1988.
19. Margolick D: Death and faith, law and Christian Science. *New York Times,* p. 1, August 6, 1990.
20. Ott DA, Cooley DA: Cardiovascular surgery in Jehovah's Witnesses: report of 542 operations without blood transfusion. *JAMA* 238:1256, 1977.
21. Warkentin PI: The blood and hemopoietic system, part two, blood component therapy for the neonate. In Fanaroff AA, Martin RJ, editors: *Neonatal-perinatal medicine: diseases of the fetus and infant.* ed 4, St. Louis, 1987, Mosby.

22. Strong C: The neonatologist's duty to patient and parents. *Hastings Cent Rep* 14:10, 1984.
23. *Matter of Hofbauer.* 47 NY 2d 648, 1979.
24. Hardwig J: What about the family? *Hastings Cent Rep* 20:5, 1990.
25. Department of Health and Human Services: Additional protections for children involved as subjects in research. *Federal Register* 48:9814, March 8 1983 (also known as 45 CFR [code of federal regulations] part 46).

SUGGESTED READINGS

- American Academy of Pediatrics, Committee on Bioethics: Guidelines on forgoing life-sustaining medical treatment. *Pediatrics* 93:532, 1994.
- American Academy of Pediatrics, Committee on Bioethics: Informed consent, parental permission, and assent in pediatric practice. *Pediatrics* 95:314, 1995.
- American Academy of Pediatrics, Committee on Bioethics: Ethics and the care of critically ill infants and children. *Pediatrics* 98:149, 1996.
- Beauchamp TL, Childress JF: *Principles of biomedical ethics,* ed 5. New York, 2001, Oxford University Press.
- Cooper R, Koch KA: Medical ethics: neonatal and pediatric critical care. *Crit Care Clin* 12:149, 1996.
- Fleischman AR, Cassidy RC, editors. *Pediatric ethics: from principles to practice.* Amsterdam, Netherlands, 1996, Harwood Academic Publishers.
- Frader J, Thompson A: Ethical issues in the pediatric intensive care unit. *Pediatr Clin North Am* 41:6, 1994.
- Orlowski JP, Kanoti GA, editors: *Ethical moments in critical care medicine. Critical Care Clinics,* vol 2. Philadelphia, 1986, WB Saunders.
- Youngner SJ, editor: *Human values in critical care medicine.* New York, 1986, Praeger Publications.

CHAPTER 12

Ethical Issues in Death and Dying

Norman Fost

PEARLS

- There comes a point in every life when continued existence does not serve the interests of the patient, usually because the burdens outweigh the benefits. This point is most clear when the patient has no apparent interests.
- It is not only permissible to discontinue treatments that are not serving the patient's interest, it is obligatory.
- Empiric fact is that, in the United States, no physician has ever been found to have civil or criminal liability for withholding or withdrawing life-sustaining treatment from any patient.
- "Limited codes" or "partial codes" should not generally be tolerated if their only purpose is to treat the sensitivities of medical and nursing staff. One hazard of partial resuscitation is that it may succeed in keeping the patient alive but result in additional damage to the patient because of inadequate oxygenation or perfusion.

Critical care, perhaps more than any other medical specialty, is devoted to saving lives. The intensive care unit (ICU) epitomizes the successes of medical technology in averting or delaying death. But it also is the focal point of claims that sometimes technology goes too far and that we should not always do what we can do. This chapter summarizes the ethical and legal issues involved in death and dying in the pediatric intensive care unit (PICU) and identifies areas of consensus.

Withholding and Withdrawing Life Support

A general ethical and legal presumption in the United States is that life is preferable to death. The medical profession is generally expected to preserve life and to maximize the patient's opportunities to experience and enjoy the benefits of life. Nonetheless, there comes a point in every life when continued existence does not serve the interests of the patient, usually because the burdens outweigh the benefits. This point is most clear when the patient has no apparent interests, such as an infant with anencephaly, who is incapable of experiencing any of the pleasures of biologic existence. Similarly, patients in perpetual coma seem to have no interests. Even the conservative "Baby Doe" regulations,[1] supported by many groups with a strong "right-to-life" orientation, concede that medically beneficial treatment need not be provided to a patient who is irreversibly comatose. The debate is not about whether medically beneficial treatment can be withheld. The challenge is to define acceptable principles that can help identify those patients who should no longer be treated and determine who should decide.

Withholding versus Withdrawing Life-Sustaining Treatment

There is strong consensus in ethics and law that there is no meaningful distinction between withholding and withdrawing life-sustaining treatment. The President's Commission on Ethical Problems in Medicine concluded that contrary to widespread *feelings* on the matter, withdrawing treatment was preferable to withholding for two reasons.[2] First, withdrawing treatment implies there has been more time for assessment of prognosis and the likelihood of a successful outcome. It comes after a clinical trial. Good ethics starts with good facts, and a decision to withhold treatment generally is made with less data than the decision to withdraw after treatment has been tried. Second, a tradition of reluctance to withdraw treatment often led to inappropriate withholding of support from patients who, in retrospect, possibly had a good chance for meaningful long-term survival. One common setting was the delivery room, where high-risk infants sometimes were not resuscitated because of the fear that treatment would succeed in the medical sense but that the infant's prognosis for meaningful survival would vanish without any means of reversing the decision to treat. Allowing treatment to be stopped allows all patients to enjoy the potential benefits of initial intervention and the possibility of success. The central ethical issue is whether treatment is serving the interests of the patient. If it is not, whether it is being considered or has already been tried is irrelevant.

Two types of errors can occur. A *type I error* is one in which a patient lives who in retrospect would have been better off had he/she died much earlier. A *type II error* is one in which a patient dies who in retrospect probably would have enjoyed life. There is consensus that the latter is generally more serious than the former for two reasons: first, because life is valued so highly and most people would prefer even a handicapped life or existence with suffering over death; and second, because a type I error usually is reversible whereas a type II error by definition is not. Particularly in the intensive care setting, prolonged survivors who are better off dead usually are dependent on some technology that can be discontinued to allow a natural death to occur. The increasing ethical and legal acceptance of discontinuing nutrition and hydration makes it theoretically possible to reverse any decision that in retrospect was not in the patient's interest.

A corollary of these observations is that uncertainty generally should be resolved by maintaining the patient's life, because resuscitation that on reflection may not have been indicated usually can be reversed, whereas failure to keep the patient alive cannot be corrected.

Active versus Passive Euthanasia

Once a decision has been made that treatment is no longer serving the patient's interest, it would seem to follow that a quick and painless death would be preferred to a long dying process, with associated discomfort for the patient or his/her family. *Active euthanasia* can be defined as a physical act that causes the death of a patient and was intended to be in the patient's interest. *Passive euthanasia* is generally understood to include withholding or withdrawing treatment, with the intent and expectation that death will occur sooner rather than later, based on the belief that an early death is in the patient's interest. Both practices have the intent and usually the consequence that death will occur sooner rather than later. Active euthanasia is nearly universally prohibited, and passive euthanasia is widely tolerated. The major reason for the distinction is based primarily on concern for future patients, not the patient at hand. Indeed, active euthanasia often seems more merciful from the patient's perspective, precisely because the suffering is reduced. This concern is less relevant when suffering can be relieved with sedation and analgesia.

The major objection to active euthanasia is based on the concern that physicians and others will slide down a "slippery slope," meaning they will become progressively less sensitive and careful about who is a suitable candidate for euthanasia. The claim is made that if the traditional barrier against killing is lowered, doctors will give in to pressures and temptations to end suffering, including that of family, nurses, and the physician, by taking advantage of the quick release that killing provides.

There is some evidence for this view in studies of the two modern societies in which active euthanasia has been widely practiced and tolerated by the state. Lifton's interviews with physicians who worked in Germany in the 1930s and 1940s demonstrate a progression from killing patients with terminal or severely disabling conditions to the slaughter of healthy people in the death camps.[3] Physicians who were directly involved and responsible for the executions reported that they believed at the time that there was no moral distinction between the two types of killings. They justified and defended their involvement in the death camps primarily as an example of their duty as physicians to relieve suffering.

In contemporary Holland, active euthanasia is widely practiced and tolerated by state policy. Public policy limits the practice to clearly competent patients, but cases of children incapable of consenting who were killed at parental request have been reported.

The prohibition of active euthanasia based on slippery slope concerns implies that present patients' interests may be sacrificed to those of future patients. However, if suffering can be eliminated with medications, there should be few, if any, patients whose interests will be harmed by prohibiting active killing. In fact, the vast majority of patients in the contemporary ICU depend on technologies whose discontinuation usually will not result in a long dying process. The major exception is patients who depend only on nutrition and hydration, whose death can take 1 week or longer but for whom sedation can reduce concern for patient suffering.

Withholding Food and Water

Once the judgment has been made that continued existence no longer serves the patient's interest, it should not matter, from the patient's perspective, what treatment is being used to keep him/her alive. The only exception would be treatments that serve to keep the patient comfortable during the dying process. However, if the patient is incapable of experiencing discomfort, whether because of his/her condition or treatments that render him/her unconscious, then any treatment that keeps the patient alive contrary to his/her interests not only may be discontinued but also should be discontinued. It is not only permissible to discontinue treatments that are not serving the patient's interest, it is obligatory.

For these reasons, treatments that provide nutrition and hydration have come to be seen as analogous to other treatments that keep patients alive. In addition to the President's Commission,[2] the American Medical Association, numerous state courts, and the U.S. Supreme

Court have ruled that food and water can be discontinued when other requirements for withdrawing life-sustaining treatment have been met.

It is understandable that discontinuing food and water is psychologically more distressing, particularly to nursing personnel, than withdrawing other forms of treatment, in part because feeding is such an innate human instinct, unlike transfusing, resuscitating, or providing oxygen. Therefore decisions to discontinue food and water often require more discussion and staff support.

One aspect of withholding or withdrawing food and water that distinguishes it from withholding other medical treatments is the extent of the opportunity for abuse. Because every patient requires nutrition and hydration, the power to withhold it gives the physician a power that is almost indistinguishable from active euthanasia. This is not to say opportunities to discontinue other forms of technology, such as mechanical ventilators or surgery, are not subject to abuse. The concern about abuse arises not so much in the ICU, where almost all patients are utterly dependent on some technology, but elsewhere in or out of the hospital where food and water may be the only "treatment" keeping a seriously ill or handicapped patient alive.[4]

Competence, Incompetence, and Baby Doe

Autonomy is a central principle in American medical ethics. It implies that a competent person has a nearly absolute right to decide what shall be done to his/her body. Courts have consistently upheld the right of competent patients to refuse life-saving treatment, even if it appears foolish or unwise to others, whether for religious or secular reasons or for no reason at all.

The definition of *competence* is itself controversial,[5] but many adolescent patients meet the standard. The most common definition relies on the ability of the patient to understand the consequences of his/her decision. Physicians therefore should be sensitive to distinctions between the wants and interests of pediatric patients, which may conflict with the interests of their parents.

The vast majority of PICU patients, regardless of age, are incompetent because of developmental status, disease, or as a consequence of medication. Traditionally, parents had nearly complete discretion to make decisions on behalf of their children. This practice came under intense criticism in the 1970s and 1980s upon disclosure of many cases in which handicapped and critically ill infants who appeared to have good prospects for long, meaningful life were allowed to die.[6,7] These cases most commonly involved infants with Down syndrome or spina bifida. In some instances, infants with Down syndrome and duodenal atresia were allowed to die of dehydration. In one center, more than 50% of infants with spina bifida had standard treatment withheld with the intention that they would die.[8] This pattern of inappropriate undertreatment has been called the *Baby Doe problem,* named after a celebrated case involving a newborn with Down syndrome and esophageal atresia who was allowed to die without surgery.[9]

The response of pediatricians and state courts was generally to respect the wishes of parents, even when decisions appeared to be contrary to the interests of the child.[10,11] In 1982 the federal government promulgated regulations, requiring reports to a hotline and investigations by "Baby Doe squads" of alleged withholding of medically beneficial treatment based on handicap. These regulations were found unconstitutional but were reinstated pursuant to amendments to a child abuse statute that provided funds to the states for implementation of child abuse and neglect programs.[1] The most controversial aspect of these regulations is their apparent prohibition of withholding or withdrawing medically beneficial treatment from any infant based on handicap or prognosis for quality of life. The three exceptions allowed are (1) if the infant is permanently comatose, (2) if the infant is imminently dying, or (3) if the treatment would be "inhumane." The legal significance of these regulations and the role of the law in these cases in general have been the sources of continuing confusion and controversy.

Legal Implications of Withholding or Withdrawing Life Support

Involvement of state and federal legislatures and courts in decisions involving treatment of dying patients is rapidly evolving and varies among jurisdictions.[12,13] Generalizations are difficult, and the law varies among states. Nonetheless, some legal aspects are reasonably clear.

The most widespread source of confusion is the failure to recognize the difference between the law in theory and the law in practice. Although a variety of statutes, court decisions, and regulations have been interpreted as prohibiting discontinuation of treatment in many cases, the empiric fact is that, in the United States, no physician has ever been found to have civil or criminal liability for withholding or withdrawing life-sustaining treatment from any patient. The law in practice has been remarkably deferential to physician discretion.[6]

Even on theoretical grounds, there are reasons to believe that the Baby Doe regulations do not regulate decisions by physicians, parents, or hospitals. Although the substantive standards appear very restrictive, the implementation standards and sanctions defer to the states. All that is necessary for states to be in compliance with the law is to provide assurances to the federal government that reports of alleged medical neglect will be handled in a prescribed way. States are not required to initiate investigations but are permitted to rely on reports, in accordance with traditional regulations involving child abuse and neglect. A study by the U.S. Office of the Inspector General found all states were in compliance with the Baby Doe regulations, although the federal Civil Rights Commission argued that more restrictive legislation is needed.[14]

In 1990, the U.S. Supreme Court issued its first opinion on the specific issue of discontinuing treatment of an incompetent patient. The case involved Nancy Cruzan, a young adult who had been in a persistent vegetative state for 8 years and was being kept alive with nasogastric feedings. Her parents had requested that the feeding be discontinued and that she be allowed to die. The Court upheld a Missouri statute that required "clear and convincing" evidence that a patient had expressed her wish that she would want to die in that specific circumstance. It is unclear whether the decision has any relevance for children, even in Missouri, and it is important to realize that the decision has little or no relevance for decisions in the majority of states that do not have statutes as restrictive as those in Missouri. New York has a similar standard. The central finding in the Court's opinion was that states are free to make their own laws in this area. The majority of states at present defer to physician judgment in theory and virtually all defer in practice. Even in Wisconsin, where an appellate court decision held that parents may never consent to withholding of life-saving treatment of a child unless he/she is in a persistent vegetative state,[15] physicians and hospitals routinely ignore the decision, and there have been no prosecutions.

The difficulty of sustaining a legal challenge against decisions to discontinue treatment was dramatized in an Illinois case involving a 2-year-old child, Sammy Linares, who was in a persistent vegetative state and ventilator dependent for 8 months. The hospital refused the parents' request to discontinue the ventilator, based on the hospital attorney's claim that to do so would be illegal. The father held the medical staff at gunpoint while he discontinued the ventilator until his son died. Despite committing at least two prima facie felonies involving illegal possession and use of a deadly weapon, the district attorney could not convince a grand jury to indict the father. Despite the clear illegality of his action in theory, in practice the legal system was typically sympathetic and supportive of the decision because it appeared to violate no interests of the child.[16] In a similar case, a federal appellate court upheld the right of a hospital to discontinue life support, over parental objection, for a child with profound brain injury.[17]

Despite the nearly universal legal deference to physician judgment, many physicians overtreat infants because they either misunderstand the law or have an exaggerated fear of liability. A survey of neonatologists found that 30% to 50% would continue treatment even when they thought it was not indicated, based on their belief that the Baby Doe regulations required such treatment.[18] Another survey of a group of California neonatologists before and after the Baby Doe regulations also found a trend toward overtreatment.[19]

In a Virginia case, an anencephalic infant known as Baby K was kept alive for 2.5 years, including intermittent ventilator support, at the request of the mother. A federal court ruled that resuscitation was required under a federal statute known as the EMTALA Act, a law that was intended to prevent dumping of patients from emergency rooms. Although the ruling has not been followed in other districts, it is important to note that the courts generally rule only when asked. Nor does the ruling prove that there would have been liability if the doctors had refused to treat the infant. In a related case, a jury acquitted a doctor at the Massachusetts General Hospital who discontinued life-sustaining treatment for a woman in a persistent vegetative state, over the objection of the family. The contrast with the Baby K case is that court opinion was not sought.[20]

Hospital Ethics Committees

With the difficulty in reaching a consensus on substantive standards for decisions to discontinue life support, interest grew in procedural guidelines. The conceptual basis for the guidelines is the general notion that because one can never know whether a decision actually is right, the question of whether or not a decision is morally defensible depends on the process by which the decision is made. The process is similar to other areas of decision making, including the judicial process, in which the legal correctness of a decision resides almost completely in the process by which it is made; in the scientific method, which concedes the impossibility of ultimately knowing the truth but accepts successive approximations if they withstand scrutiny of the process by which they are made; and judgments about the quality of medical care, which ultimately depend less on outcomes than on the process.

One of several procedural theories of ethical decision making is called *ideal observer theory*.[20] The theory argued that a decision is morally right if it could receive approval from an ideal ethical observer with the following characteristics: (1) *omniscient,* meaning access to the relevant and available facts; (2) *omnipercipient,* meaning the ability to empathize, to vividly imagine how others feel, or to put one's self in another's shoes; (3) *disinterested,* having no vested interest in the outcome; (4) *dispassionate,* not being overwhelmed with emotion at the time critical decisions must be made; and (5) *consistent,* meaning that similar cases will be decided similarly.

In retrospect, decisions that appeared to be indefensible could be analyzed in this framework. In most cases, the failure to appreciate readily available facts appeared to be at the center of controversial decisions. Erroneous assumptions about prognosis, the availability of alternative care arrangements, or misunderstandings about the law are common examples. Because no single person can have the godlike qualities of an ideal ethical observer, interest arose in a process that might better emulate the model than traditional doctor–parent decisions. This was the theoretical basis of hospital ethics committees.

The federal Baby Doe regulations recommended but did not require such committees, which they referred to as "Infant Care Review Committees." Since 1994, the Joint Commission on Accreditation of Hospitals has required ethics committees or some other mechanism for resolving disputes about terminal care, and they have become a standard method for resolving controversial decisions.[21] These committees typically are interdisciplinary groups of 10 to 20 people, including hospital-based professionals and community members, which advise and recommend but do not typically decide on treatment plans. Some hospitals have ethics consultants who work independently of an institutional ethics committee. Studies of their activities are limited,[22,23] but their growth has been accompanied by an apparent disappearance of the problem of undertreatment. That problem has been replaced by an apparent growth in overtreatment, which may be aggravated by the influence of hospital attorneys or risk managers on committees.[24] Consultation with committees usually is voluntary.

Ethics committees often serve other functions besides ethical consensus development. They have been used to protect decision makers from liability. Malpractice charges require a finding of negligence, which means the physician failed to take adequate care in how a decision was made. Review and approval by an ethics committee may not only be helpful in defending against such a charge but may deter initiation of a suit. Similarly, a district attorney or judge considering legal charges may be less likely to pursue a case in which there was a special effort to obtain consultation and in which there was broad consensus beyond the family and attending physician. Committees have also served a therapeutic role, helping to manage tensions among medical staff, particularly nurses, when they do not necessarily disagree with a decision but appreciate the opportunity to review it in a broader forum than can be found within the ICU.[25]

Caring for the Terminally Ill

Once a decision has been made that continued treatment is no longer in the patient's interest, attention can turn to implementing the decision in a way that minimizes suffering for the patient, family, medical staff, and other patients.

Decisions to terminate care should be well documented in the chart and in the order book. With regard to legal liability, inadequate documentation is more likely to create vulnerability than the opposite. Because the decision to terminate care should have the support of all involved, there should be no reason to conceal the decision or the reasons for it. Any consultation with an ethics committee should be documented, either by the attending physician or by a representative of the committee.

If a judgment has been made that the patient would be better off dead, there is rarely a reason to continue some treatments while stopping others. The common practice of discontinuing one life-prolonging measure—resuscitation—while maintaining other life-supporting treatments may be illogical. These seemingly contradictory measures are sometimes motivated by concerns for the feelings of family or staff. As long as the patient is not suffering from continued treatment, this practice may be justified for a brief period, but prolonged treatment while waiting and hoping that a patient will die despite the treatment at some point becomes a misuse of limited resources, whether of personnel or an ICU bed.

Similarly, "limited codes" or "partial codes" generally should not be tolerated if their only purpose is to treat the sensitivities of medical and nursing staff. One hazard of partial resuscitation is that it may succeed in keeping the patient alive but result in additional damage to the patient because of inadequate oxygenation or perfusion. In summary, if a decision has been properly made that a patient is better off dead, it usually is best to effect that decision as soon as possible by discontinuing all measures that might prolong the patient's life.

Definition of Death and Organ Retrieval

Determining that a patient is dead is of special interest because of its implications for organ retrieval (see Chapter 13). Death traditionally has been considered a necessary condition for organ retrieval from critically ill patients, although there are increasing challenges to this assumption.

Brain Death

All states now support *brain death* as the legal standard for determination of death, although there is growing controversy about the moral and clinical relevance of the concept.[26] This standard requires irreversible cessation of all brain activity, including the brainstem. The criteria for determining that brain death has occurred are medical criteria not established by statutes or court cases. They change as new technology and research evolves; therefore it is incumbent on the physician to keep abreast of developments in this area. One study showed considerable ignorance and confusion on the subject.[24] The clinical criteria promulgated by a Harvard committee 20 years ago have generally withstood the test of time.[27,28] In ambiguous cases, studies of brain perfusion may be helpful.

Guidelines have been developed for applying these standards to children,[29] with the exception of newborns younger than 7 days. Because of errors in the diagnosis of brain death in this age group, the traditional criteria cannot be relied upon with certainty. At worst, this practice may require maintaining such an infant for 7 days if organ retrieval is desired. It should not generally interfere with decisions to discontinue life support, because such decisions do not depend upon a determination that brain death has occurred.

Infants born alive with *anencephaly* typically have brainstem function and therefore do not meet any current definition of brain death.[22] A controversial protocol at an institution in Loma Linda, California, involved maintaining such infants for 7 days with the expectation that whole brain death might occur. The program did not succeed for various reasons and was suspended by the program's proponents.

The controversy regarding infants with anencephaly has stimulated interest in reexamining the concept of whole brain death as the essential criterion for defining death of the person. Specifically, some have advocated *cortical death* as the critical feature because the brainstem is not associated with functions that are important to most notions of personhood.[30] It has also become clear that patients who meet standard criteria for whole brain death may have residual function of parts of the brain, such as the hypothalamus, as evidenced by normal regulation of antidiuretic hormone release. This observation raises questions about the medical validity of the diagnosis of whole brain death.

Organ Retrieval

There is a wide gap between the number of patients who could benefit from organ transplantation and the supply of organs. There also is a gap between the number of people who say they are willing to donate their own organs or those of family members when death has occurred and the number who actually do donate. These observations led to a national "required request" law, which requires hospitals to inform relatives in appropriate cases that organ donation is an option. The law has not resulted in a substantial increase in organ supply for a variety of reasons. Nonetheless, the ICU staff not only has a legal duty to ask but also should realize that organ donation is generally perceived as a benefit to those who consent to it, not as a burden.

Because the term *donation* implies the giving of a gift, some have objected to its use when pediatric or other nonconsenting patients are involved, who cannot or have not been involved in making such a donation. A person cannot make a gift on behalf of another. For this reason, some have suggested the term *organ source,* as a reminder that the dying pediatric patient is not actually a donor.

Questions may arise regarding who should ask and when. It is a longstanding principle that those involved with the care of potential recipients, such as members of the transplant team, should not be in contact with the family of the potential source of the organ because of the obvious conflicts of interest. It is important to coordinate such decisions to maximize the efficiency and effectiveness of the transplantation; therefore it is appropriate that those caring for the "donor" communicate with the transplant team. It also may be appropriate for members of the transplant team to meet with the family of the "donor" after the decision has been made to answer questions.

The shortage of organs has stimulated new efforts to remove organs more efficiently from patients who are not brain dead and who die by traditional criteria of cessation of heart and lung function. Protocols have been established for discontinuing ventilator support in the operating room so that organs can be removed promptly after death is declared and before organ viability is threatened by warm ischemia[31] (see Chapter 13).

REFERENCES

1. Child Abuse and Neglect Prevention and Treatment Program: Final rule, model guidelines for health care providers to establish infant care review committees. *Federal Register*, DHHS, Office of Human Development Services, 45 CFR Part 1340, Notice 50:14878, 1985.
2. President's Commission for the Study of Ethical Problems in Medicine and Biomedical and Behavioral Research: *Deciding to forego life-sustaining treatment.* Washington, DC, 1981, US Government Printing Office.
3. Lifton RJ: *The Nazi doctors: medical killing and the psychology of genocide.* New York, 1986, Basic Books.
4. Lynn J, editor: *By no extraordinary means: the choice to forego life-sustaining food and water.* Bloomington, 1989, Indiana University Press.
5. Fost N: Ten bad reasons for not treating Baby K. *Trends Health Care Law Ethics* 9:17-18, 22, 1994.
6. Fost N: Treatment of seriously ill and handicapped newborns. *Crit Care Clin* 2:149, 1986.
7. Weir R: *Selective treatment of handicapped newborns.* New York, 1984, Oxford.
8. Gross RH, Cox A, Tatyrek R, Pollay M, Barnes WA: Early management and decision making for the treatment of myelomeningocoele. *Pediatrics* 72:450, 1983.
9. Pless JE: The story of Baby Doe. *N Engl J Med* 309:664, 1983 (case reports, letter).
10. Shaw A, Randolph JG, Manard B: Ethical issues in pediatric surgery: a nationwide survey of pediatricians and pediatric surgeons. *Pediatrics* 60:588, 1977.
11. Todres ID, Krane D, Howell MC, Shannon DC: Pediatrician's attitudes affecting decision making in defective newborns. *Pediatrics* 60:197, 1977.
12. Luce JM, Alpers A: Legal aspects of withholding and withdrawing life support from critically ill patients in the United States and providing palliative care to them. *Am J Respir Crit Care Med* 162:2029-2032, 2000.
13. Holder A: Parents, courts and refusal of treatment. *J Pediatr* 103:515, 1983.
14. United States Commission on Civil Rights: *Medical discrimination against children with disabilities.* Washington, DC, 1989, The Commission.
15. Nancy Montalvo vs Terre Borkovec, 2002 WI App 147 (May 29, 2002), 256 Wis. 2d 472, 647 NW.2d 413
16. Fost N: Do the right thing: Samuel Linares and defensive law. *Law Med Health Care* 17:330, 1989.
17. In Re K.I., B.I. and D.M., Appellants, No. 98-Fs-1683 and 98-Fs-1767 District of Columbia Court of Appeals, 735 A.2d 448; 1999 DC App.
18. Kopelman LM, Irons TG, Kopelman AE: Neonatologists judge the "Baby Doe" regulation. *N Engl J Med* 318:677, 1988.
19. Pomerance JJ, Yu T, Brown SJ: Changing attitudes of neonatologists toward ventilator support. *J Perinatol* 8:232, 1988.
20. Firth R: Ethical absolutism and the ideal observer. *Philos Phenomenol Res* 12:317, 1952.
21. Fost N: Infant care review committees in the aftermath of Baby Doe. In Caplan A, Blank R, Merrick, editors: *Compelled compassion: public policy and the care of handicapped newborns.* 1992, Humana Press.
22. Mahowald MB: Baby Doe committees: a critical evaluation. *Clin Perinatol* 15:789, 1988.
23. Schneiderman LJ, Gilmer T, Teetzel HD, et al: Effect of ethics consultations on nonbeneficial life-sustaining treatments in the intensive care setting: a randomized controlled trial. *JAMA* 290: 1166-1172, 2003.
24. Youngner SJ, Landefeld CS, Coulton CJ, et al: 1989. "Brain death" and organ retrieval. A cross sectional survey of knowledge and concepts among health professionals. *JAMA* 261:2205-2210, 1989.
25. Fost N: What can a hospital ethics committee do for you? *Contemp Pediatr* February:119, 1986.
26. Youngner SJ, Arnold RM, Schapiro R, editors: *The definition of death: contemporary controversies.* Baltimore, 1999, Johns Hopkins Press.
27. A definition of irreversible coma: report of the Ad Hoc Committee of the Harvard Medical School to examine the definition of brain death. *JAMA* 205:337, 1968.
28. President's Commission for the Study of Ethical Problems in Medicine and Biomedical and Behavioral Research: *Defining death: medical, legal and ethical issues in the determination of death.* Washington, DC, 1981, US Government Printing Office.
29. Banasiak KJ, Lister G: Brain death in children. *Curr Opin Pediatr* 15:288-293, 2003.
30. Green MB, Wikler D: Brain death and personal identity. *Philos Public Affairs* 9:105, 1980.
31. Committee on Non-Heart-Beating Transplantation II: *The scientific and ethical basis for practice and protocols.* Washington, DC, 2000, Institute of Medicine, National Academy Press.

CHAPTER

13

Pediatric Transplantation and Organ Donation

Sidney Anthone

PEARLS

- First pediatric kidney transplant occurred in 1952 in Paris, France.
- Preferential use of living donors has become the source of kidneys for pediatric transplant recipients.
- In children younger than 1 year, the most common indication for heart transplantation is congenital heart disease. The quality of life of surviving patients reportedly is normal.
- Brains of infants and young children have increased resistance to brain damage and may recover substantial function after exhibiting unresponsiveness for long periods.
- The physiologic consequences of brain death play a considerable role in affecting multiorgan dysfunction.

Pediatric organ transplantation has proved to be a therapeutic alternative for children with end-stage renal disease, uncorrectable congenital cardiac disease, and liver and intestinal failure.

The history of transplantation is marked by many important events in immunology and transplantation.[1,2] The intent of this chapter is not to review all the events but to point out the landmark events that led up to the present success in transplantation, especially as it relates to pediatric patients.[3] In 1954 Joseph Murray and colleagues[4] performed the first successful kidney transplant between identical twins, thus bypassing the problem of allograft rejection. The first attempted pediatric kidney transplant actually was performed in 1952 in Paris, France, between a 16-year-old boy and his ABO-compatible mother.[5] Although the kidney excreted urine immediately and appeared to be a successful transplant, on postoperative day 21 the kidney abruptly rejected, with subsequent death of the child. In those early years of attempted renal transplantation, the immunologic barrier prevented success between individuals other than identical twins.

The first method of immunosuppression used was total body irradiation, which was used between 1959 and 1962. In 1962 Schwartz and Dameshek[6] suggested that the anticancer drug 6-mercptopurine (6-MP) might be a good immunosuppressive agent as an alternative to irradiation. A derivative of 6-MP, known as *azathioprine* (Imuran), was introduced and subsequently proved to be more effective in controlling rejection.[7] This new drug made it possible for Starzl and colleagues[8] in 1962 to perform the first successful nontwin, living-related donor pediatric kidney transplant. Total body irradiation, azathioprine (Imuran), and prednisone constituted the immunosuppressive regimen used. Imuran and prednisone subsequently became the standard regimen for immunosuppression in the 1960s and early 1970s. In the late1970s, human leukocyte antigen (HLA)-DR matching became refined and added to the long-term success of transplantation.[9]

Following the introduction of Imuran, perhaps the next most significant addition to the pharmacologic armamentarium of the transplant physician was the introduction of cyclosporine (CsA), discovered by Borel,[10] in 1979. As a result of the introduction of this calcineurin inhibitor by Calne[11,12] in 1978 and 1979, there was an unprecedented improvement in the outcome of renal transplantation in both adults and children. This new immunosuppressive agent reduced the need for high-dose steroids, thus avoiding some of the negative growth effects of the steroids in pediatric patients.

Although the introduction of CsA resulted in reduced acute rejection rates and improvement in 1-year graft survival, no substantial improvement was observed in graft survival after 1 year. Some improvement in the long-term results of transplantation was made possible by the addition of monoclonal and polyclonal antibodies used not only for induction therapy but also for reversing acute rejection.[13,14] Tacrolimus (FK506) with similar immunosuppressive activity to CsA was first introduced in 1989 for clinical treatment of pediatric kidney recipients.[15,16]

Several other new immunosuppressive agents have enhanced the success of pediatric transplantation and at the same time reduced the untoward effects of the previous immunosuppressive agents. Mycophenolate mofetil (a substitute for Imuran) and Neoral (the microemulsion formulation of CsA) are now preferred agents to their predecessors.[17,18] New monoclonal antibodies, such as daclizumab and basilsxmab,[19,20] and the new immunosuppressive agent sirolimus[21] are being studied for their effectiveness in controlling acute graft rejection. Prevention of acute rejection remains an important factor for long-term transplant success.

Concerns

The optimal age for transplantation of children with end-stage renal disease once was controversial. Many centers had adopted a policy of waiting until such children reached a certain age or weight, maintaining them on chronic dialysis until the criteria were met. The increased risk of graft thrombosis among the youngest transplant recipients was more apparent when the donor–recipient age difference was highest. More current literature, however, suggests that with proper donor selection and recipient care, no minimum age for infants and children undergoing kidney transplants is required.[22,23]

Of equal concern is the statistics compiled by the North American Pediatric Renal Transplant Cooperative Study (NAPRTCS) showing an increased risk of graft loss, late acute rejection, and incomplete rejection reversal in the adolescent age group.[24,25] Lack of compliance with the immunosuppressive regimen is believed to be a contributing factor to the poor results, although other immunologic factors play a role in the chronic rejection process. NAPRTCS further revealed that 57% of the children who were prepubertal at the time of transplant and were followed to presumed final adult height had suboptimal posttransplant growth.[26] Poor allograft function and corticosteroids are two significant factors responsible for the retarded growth.

Given the improved results of transplantation, the procurement of organs has become a dominant issue. The ever-expanding yearly list of potential recipients combined with the flat number of cadaveric (deceased) donors have led to increasing use of living related and nonrelated donors. This situation has been particularly evident in pediatric transplantation. The NAPRTCS data for the year 2001 reveal a 1-year *graft* survival rate of 91% for living donor (LD) transplants and 83% for deceased donor transplants. The rates decline and differ significantly at 5 years to 80% and 65% for the LD and deceased donor groups, respectively. Hence preferential use of living donors has become the source of kidneys for most pediatric transplant recipients in recent years. The exception may be patients with high risk of recurrent disease, such as rapid progressive focal segmental glomerular sclerosis, in which case a deceased donor may be preferred.

Approximately 3% of recipients on waiting lists are children from birth to 17 years. Kidney allocation policies of the United Network for Organ Sharing (UNOS) give additional points to children on the kidney transplant waiting list. As pointed out in the preceding sections, because of the acute shortage of deceased (cadaver) donors, use of living-related and nonrelated donors has increased, especially in the pediatric age group.

Extrarenal Organ Transplantation

Many centers now report remarkable success with pediatric heart transplantation, and it now is the treatment of choice for infants and children with end-stage heart failure or inoperable congenital heart defects.[27–30] By far, the most common indication for heart transplantation is congenital heart disease in children younger than 1 year. The quality of life in the surviving children reportedly is normal. Somatic growth within the low–normal range has been reported in infants; however, linear growth arrest occurs in adolescent recipients. Long-term patient survival rates continue to improve and are reported to be approximately 75% at 1 year and 65% at 5 years. Over time, accelerated coronary artery disease and rejection account for the slow but constant reduced survival rate.

Significant progress with liver transplantation has been made, including transplantation in the pediatric age group[31–34] (see Chapter 81). Use of living-related and split liver transplantation has reduced the waiting period for children, resulting in improved long-term survival. Similarly, progress has been made with intestinal transplantation.[35–38] The majority of recipients have been children. Refinement in the surgical technique and use of a combination of the newer immunosuppressive agents have resulted in improved survival in children. In some instances the combined use of liver and intestinal transplantation is necessary. Early identification and referral of the potential recipient before the development of TPN-induced cholestatic liver disease can decrease the likelihood of requiring combined liver-intestinal transplantation.

Pediatric Organ Donation

In 1998 the administrator of the Health Care Financing Administration issued a directive requiring that all hospitals participating in Medicare and Medicaid programs refer all potential organ donors to their local organ procurement organization (OPO).[39] The directive further mandates that the family of each potential donor be informed of its options to donate organs, tissues, or eyes. Legislation requires the hospital to appoint a designated requester to discuss organ donation with the family.

Pediatric organ donation requires the coordinated effort of the pediatric medical and nursing staff, the OPO coordinators and family services coordinators, the social service department of the hospital, the clergy, and the medical examiner's office.[40]

The potential deceased pediatric donor must have met the requirements for brain death declaration prior to becoming an organ donor. *Brain death* is defined as the irreversible cessation of all functions of the entire brain, including the brainstem (see Chapter 12). Guidelines have been developed to assist physicians in making such a determination. The hospitals in New York state have adopted the guidelines developed by a task force of the Department of Health. Two sets of guidelines were published, one for children older than 1 year and the other

BOX 13–1

GUIDELINES FOR DETERMINATION OF DEATH BY IRREVERSIBLE CESSATION OF ALL FUNCTIONS OF THE ENTIRE BRAIN, INCLUDING THE BRAIN STEM (AGE OLDER THAN 1 YEAR)

NOTE: All 9 items must be answered YES to declare brain death. — Yes / No

1. Have reasonable efforts been made to notify the patients' next-of-kin or other person closest to the individual that a determination of death based on cessation of brain function will soon be completed? ___ ___
2. Is the cause of the coma known and sufficient to account for the irreversible loss of all brain function? ___ ___
   NOTE: Coma of unknown cause (e.g., no evidence of brain trauma, stroke, hypoxic/hypotensive injury) requires a diligent search for the cause of coma before brain death determination. Similarly, the magnitude of the brain injury must be commensurate with irreversible cessation of all brain function.
3. Are CNS depressant drugs, hypothermia (<32 degrees C) and hypotension (MAP <55 mm Hg) excluded as reversible causes of brain failure and has any effect of neuromuscular blocking agents been excluded as contributing to the results of the neurologic exam? ___ ___
   NOTE:
   - Specific levels of CNS depressants or neuromuscular blocking drugs are left to clinical judgment.
   - Brain death cannot be declared in the setting of hypothermia (<32.2°C).
   - Shock, as defined as a mean arterial blood pressure less than 55 mm Hg, prohibits the declaration of brain death. Pressors to support arterial blood pressure may be used (mean BP = (2 * BP diastolic + BP systolic) / 3).
   - If levels of CNS depressants or neuromuscular blocking agents cannot be excluded as contributing to poor neurologic status but cerebral angiography demonstrates there is no intracranial blood flow, then proceed to item #4.
4. Is all movement attributable to spinal cord function (i.e., there are no other spontaneous movements or motor responses)? ___ ___
   NOTE: Posturing and shivering in the absence of neuromuscular blockade or learned movements in response to pain in any extremity or the head preclude the diagnosis of brain death. Deep tendon reflexes including stereotypic triple flexor responses in the lower extremities are compatible with brain death. These include spontaneous slow movements of an arm or leg. Bizarre movements of entirely spinal origin may sometimes occur in brain dead patients. Also, coordinated movements can occur with shoulder elevation and adduction, back arching and the appearance of intercostal muscle contraction without detectable tidal volumes.

   Finally, in few patients, the "Lazarus sign" may develop when the ventilator is permanently disconnected; the head and torso may flex and for a few seconds rise from the bed with arms outstretched, then falls back and the dead body remains permanently flaccid in the supine position.
5. Absent cough and/or pharyngeal reflexes? ___ ___
6. Absent corneal and pupillary light responses? ___ ___
7. Absent caloric responses to iced water after visual examination of the tympanic membranes? ___ ___
8. Has an apnea test of a minimum 5 minutes duration showed no respiratory movements with a documented PCO_2 greater than 55 mm Hg with a pH of less than 7.40? ___ ___
   NOTE: Extreme caution should be exercised in the performance of the apnea test. The apnea test should be conducted only after all other evaluations are completed. An apnea test should be performed in such a manner as to minimize the risk of hypoxia or hypotension. Delivering a high concentration of oxygen to the airway (4 L/min) before and during the apnea test reduces the risk of hypoxic complications. If mean arterial blood pressure falls significantly during the performance of an apnea test, it should be discontinued with an arterial blood sample drawn to determine whether $PaCO_2$ has either risen above 55 mm Hg or increased by more than 20 mm Hg from the level immediately prior to the test. If so, this validates the clinical diagnosis of brain death.
9. Have one of the following four criteria (A,B,C, or D) been established? ___ ___
   A. Items 2 to 7 have been confirmed by two examinations separated by at least 6 hours, and item 8, the apnea test, validates the clinical diagnosis of death. ___ ___
   B. ___ ___
      1. Items 2 to 7 have been confirmed as YES.
      2. An EEG shows electrocortical silence.
      3. A second exam at least 2 hours after the first, confirms items 2 to 7 as YES, and the apnea test validates the clinical diagnosis of death.
   C. ___ ___
      1. Items 2 to 7 have been confirmed as YES.
      2. No intracranial blood flow is evident.
      3. A second exam at least 2 hours after the first, confirms items 2 to 7 as YES, and the apnea test validates the clinical diagnosis of death.
   D. In the event that any of the items 2 to 7 cannot be determined because the injury or condition prohibits evaluation, (e.g. extensive facial injury precluding caloric testing), then the following criteria apply: ___ ___
      1. ALL items which are assessable are YES.
      2. No intracranial blood flow is evident.
      3. A second exam at least 2 hours after the first confirms all assessable items as YES, and the apnea test validates the clinical diagnosis of death.

BOX 13–1 *(Continued)*

Having considered all the above, I hereby certify the death of:

______________________________ Date: ____________________

Time: __________

Certifier: ______________________________________ M.D.

Printed: ______________________________________

Contemplation of Organ Donation

When organ donation is contemplated, the time of death must be certified by a second physician. Neither the physician who determines brain death nor the second physician who certifies the time of death can participate in the procedure for removing or transplanting the organ.

Second certifier: ________________________________ M.D.

Printed: ______________________________________

for children younger than 1 year (Boxes 13–1 and 13–2). In general, two examinations separated by a defined period of time should be made to confirm brain death but, in some instances of obvious irreparable brain injury, one examination may suffice. Many institutions require that two attending physicians (one a neurologist or neurosurgeon) agree on the brain death determination. In the diagnosis of brain death, it is important to establish the cause of the coma and to rule out reversible causes of unconsciousness, such as depressant drugs, neuromuscular blockade, shock, and hypothermia. The process consists of a physical examination to rule out cortical activity and apnea testing to rule out respiratory activity. Additional studies may be helpful to confirm brain death. These tests are confirmatory and are not required procedures. Electroencephalography is valuable but is not considered a definitive diagnostic tool for determination of brain death. However, cerebral radionucleotide angiography does confirm cerebral death by demonstrating the lack of cerebral blood flow.

Physicians should be particularly cautious when applying neurologic criteria to determine death in children younger than 1 year. The brains of infants and young children have increased resistance to brain damage and may recover substantial function after exhibiting unresponsiveness for longer periods compared with adults. The recommended period of observation depends upon the age of the patient. For infants age 7 days to 2 months, the recommendation is for performance of two examinations and electroencephalograms (EEGs) separated by at least 48 hours prior to brain death declaration. For children age 2 months to 1 year, the recommendation is for performance of two examinations and EEGs separated by at least 24 hours. Repeat examination and EEG are not necessary if a concomitant radionucleotide angiographic study demonstrates no visualization of cerebral flow.

Once brain death has been declared, individuals trained in the social and medical aspects of organ donation should approach the potential donor family in a systematic manner. It has been shown that using OPO staff or a member of the hospital staff specifically trained as a designated requester for organ, tissue, and eye donation, along with the consultation or presence of the child's physician, can increase the rate of family consent to donate. The OPO has family support counselors who provide family support during the donation process and during long-term follow-up of the donor family. Involvement of the child's primary care physician and any subspecialist during organ management and interaction with the family is beneficial.

Medical and forensic investigation of the death of a child attributed to trauma (unintentional or resulting from abuse), sudden death syndrome, and poisoning presents unique issues related to organ procurement.[41] Close cooperation among the forensic personnel, organ recovery team, treating physicians, and the OPO allows for joint evaluation that in most cases leads to successful organ procurement. Cooperation ensures that the evidence will not be destroyed and that any injuries noted during the organ recovery procedure will be documented and reported. If the potential donor's history, surgical and autopsy findings, and laboratory studies are cooperatively examined, most individuals whose death requires investigation can be donors.

Since the 1970s, organs have primarily been recovered from deceased (donors who have been declared "brain dead"). Because of the significant shortage of organs for transplantation, a second type of donor called the *non–heart-beating donor,* recently renamed the *donation after cardiac death,* has been initiated. These are individuals who do not quite meet the criteria of brain death but are maintained on mechanical support measures and for whom a medical and family decision has been made to terminate the support. Death in this situation is determined by the cessation of heart and respiratory function. The decision to withdraw life-sustaining treatment is made independently of and prior to any staff-initiated discussion of organ and tissue donation. This category of organ donation has been thoroughly studied by the Institute of Medicine, which has examined the ethical issues and has endorsed this type of donation.[42,43]

The cost of organ donation is borne entirely by the recipient(s). From the moment consent is obtained, all hospital and professional charges pertaining to the

BOX 13–2

DETERMINATION OF DEATH IN CHILDREN YOUNGER THAN 1 YEAR OF AGE

1. General Statement Policy

The brains of infants and young children have increased resistance to damage and may recover substantial functions even after exhibiting unresponsiveness on neurological examination for longer periods as compared with adults. Physicians should be particularly cautious when applying neurological criteria to determine death in children younger than 1 year.

2. Clinical History and Examination*

*(Taken from Task Force for the Determination of Brain Death in Children 1987 Report)

The critical initial assessment is the clinical history and examination. The most important factor is determination of the proximate cause of coma to ensure absence of remediable or reversible conditions. Most difficulties with the determination of death on the basis of neurological criteria have resulted from overlooking this basic fact. Especially important are detection of toxic and metabolic disorder, sedative-hypnotic drug, paralytic agents, hypothermia, hypotension, and surgically remediable conditions. The physical examination is necessary to determine the failure of brain function.

3. Physical Examination Criteria

a. Coma and apnea must coexist. The patient must exhibit complete loss of consciousness, vocalization, and volitional activity.

b. Absence of brainstem function as defined by:

1. Midposition or fully dilated pupils which do not respond to light. Drugs may influence and invalidate pupillary assessment.

2. Absence of spontaneous eye movements and those induced by occulocephalic and caloric (oculovestibular) testing.

3. Absence of movement of bulbar musculature including facial and oropharyngeal muscles. The corneal, gag, cough, suckling, and rooting reflexes are absent.

4. Respiratory movements are absent with the patient off the respirator. Apnea testing using standardized methods can be performed, but is done after other criteria are met.

c. The patient must not be significantly hypothermic or hypotensive for age.

d. Flaccid tone and absence of spontaneous or induced movements, excluding spinal cord events such as reflex withdrawal or spinal myoclonus, should exist.

e. The examination should remain consistent with brain death throughout the observation and testing period.

4. Observation Periods According to Age

The recommended observation period depends on the age of the patient and the laboratory tests utilized.

Seven days to two months - Two examinations and electroencephalograms (EEGs) separated by at least 48 hours.

Two months to one year - Two examinations and EEGs separated by at least 24 hours. A repeat examination and EEG are not necessary if a concomitant radionuclude angiographic (CRAG) study demonstrates no visualization of cerebral arteries.

5. Laboratory Testing

Electroencephalography—Electroencephalography to document electrocerebral silence should, if performed, be done over a 30-minute period using standardized techniques for brain death determinations. In small children it may not be possible to meet the standard requirement for 10-cm electrode separation. The inter-electrode distance should be decreased in proportion to the patient's head size. Drug concentrations should be insufficient to suppress EEG activity.

Angiography—A cerebral radionucleotide angiogram (CRAG) confirms cerebral death by demonstrating the lack of visualization of the cerebral circulation. A technically satisfactory CRAG that demonstrates arrest of carotid circulation at the base of the skull and absence of intracranial arterial circulation can be considered confirmatory of brain death, even though there may be some visualization of the intracranial venous sinuses. The value of this study in infants younger than 2 months is under investigation. Contrast angiography can document lack of effective blood flow to the brain.

BOX 13–3

Critical Pathway for the Pediatric Organ Donor

Patient name: ______________________________

UNOS ID number: ______________________________

Collaborative Practice	Phase I Identification and Referral	Phase II Declaration of Brain Death and Consent	Phase III Donor Management	Phase III Donor Evaluation	Phase IV Comprehensive Evaluation and Donor Management
The following professionals may be involved to enhance the donation process. *Check all that apply.* O Physician/Intensivist O Primary Care Physician O Critical care RN O Nurse Supervisor O Organ Procurement Organization (OPO) O OPO Coordinator (OPC) O OPO Family Services Coor. O Medical Examiner O Respiratory Therapy O Laboratory O Radiology O Anesthesiology O OR/Surgery Staff O Clergy O Social Worker O Pharmacist O Child Life Specialist	O Identify all patients who may be potential organ and/or tissue donors. O Initial call to OPO to notify of potential donor with devastating neurological injury (organ donor) or patient with grave prognosis (tissue donor) after consultation with treating physician. O Formal contact and referral to OPO when first brain death exam anticipated. O OPC on site and begins evaluation. O Notify charge nurse and intensivist/attending MD of presence on unit. Time______ Date______ Ht ______ Wt ______ ABO confirmed by blood bank ______ O Identify legal guardian/next-of-kin (NOK). O Notify ME/Coroner's office of impending death. O OPC determines suitability of donor following chart review. *Stop Pathway–If not suitable for organ and tissue donation.*	O Brain death documented per hospital protocol. Time______ Date______ O Complete appropriate forms (death cerificate, release of remains, etc.). O If patient does not meet brain death criteria, reevaluate after observation interval. O If withdrawal of life support is anticipated, consider donation after cardiac death (DCD) protocol. In all cases consider tissue donation. O Collaborative plan for family approach with ICU and OPO staff. O Identify/offer support services for family (primary physician, clergy, social worker, etc). O MD notifies family of death. O OPO/hospital staff talks to family about donation. O NOK consents to donation O OPO staff obtains signed consent and medical/social history. Time______ Date______ O ME/Coroner formal notification. O ME/Coroner releases body for donation. O *Family/ME/Coroner denies donation-Stop pathway-initiate post-mortem protocol-support family*	O New orders written in collaboration with intensivists and OPO staff O Begin organ allocation O OPC sets tentative OR time O Ensure adequate IV/arterial access for support and procurement	O Obtain blood/lymph nodes for tissue typing and cross-match O Obtain pre/post transfusion blood for serology testing per OPO protocol and communicate results when available. O Notify the following of pending case: • OR/anesthesiology • Procurement surgeons • House supervisor • Tissue typing labs O Cardiology/pulmonary and other specialty consults as requested by OPC O Lung measurements per CXR by OPC O Organ recovery process discontinued if donor organs unsuitable for transplantation after evaluation	O Notification of OR for needed equipment, time, and organs to be recovered O Pre-op checklist O Communicate appropriate test results to recipient centers O Collaborate with accepting recipient centers on OR time O Procurement supplies present in OR O Prepare patient for transport to OR and maintain ______IV ______O2 ______PEEP ______Pumps O Transport to OR Time______ Date______ O OR nurse confirms completion of all required documentation to include consent and brain death documentation. O OR nurse checks patient identification.
Labs/Diagnostics	O Per ICU protocol	O Review lab results O Review hemodynamics	O Determine need and write orders for ongoing lab testing O Same as adult except for CBC after transfusion, if necessary	O Blood chemistry O CBC with diff O UA O Urine for C&S O PT, PTT O ABO O A Subtype O Liver function tests O Blood culture × 2 obtained 15 minutes to 1 hour apart, different sites O Sputum Gram stain and C&S O Type and cross-match ___# units PRBCs O CXR O ABGs O EKG O Echo O Bedside diagnostic/ therapeutic bronchoscopy	O Labs drawn in OR as per surgeon or OPC request O Communicate with pathology - arrange for pathology testing O BX liver and/or kidneys as indicated
Cardiopulmonary Care	O Pt maintained on ventilator →	→	O Optimize ventilator settings to achieve SaO_2 $> 95\%$ O O_2 challenge for lung placement PEEP = 5cm, FiO_2 @ 100% 20 min, obtain ABG O ABGs as ordered O VS PRN O Pulmonary toilet (bronchial drainage, percussion, turning and suctioning, vest when appropriate)	O Monitor and maintain the following age-specific parameters ______BP ______HR ______CVP ______PaO_2 ______SaO_2 $> 95\%$ ______pH 7.35-7.45	O Portable O_2 @100% FiO_2 for transport to OR O Ambu bag and PEEP valve O Move to OR
Treatments/ Ongoing Care	O ICU staff responsible for maintaining normal hemodynamic parameters, normothermia, and ventilatory support as per ICU protocol →	→	O NG tube placed and functioning O Maintain temperature $>36.5°C$ and $<38°C$ O Eye care		O Set OR temp as directed by OPC O Bronchoscopy as per lung recovery team O Post-mortem care

BOX 13–3 *(Continued)*

Medications	O Continue as per ICU protocol/care plan →	→	O DC former meds except pressors and antibiotics O Initiate broad-spectrum antibiotic if not previously administered O Maintain age-specific parameters for: BP, HR, urine output, electrolytes, glucose, temperature, PT/PTT, CBC O See age-specific donor management recommendations O Medication as requested by OPC		O Management of antidiuretics, diuretics, and heparin per transplant surgeon
Optimal Outcomes	Potential donor is identified, and a referral is made to OPO	Family offered the option of organ/tissue donation, and their decision is supported	Optimize organ function	The donor is evaluated and found to be suitable for donation	All suitable, consented organs are recovered for transplant

For more information about Critical Pathway please contact UNOS Professional Services.

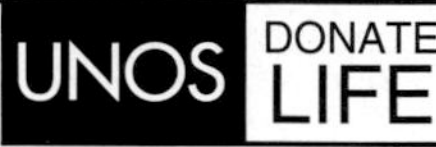

donation process are billed to the OPO, which in turn bills the recipient center(s).

Management of Potential Donors

An aggressive approach to medical management of the potential pediatric donor will help increase the number of medically acceptable transplantable organs. UNOS has developed a protocol called the *Critical Pathway for the Organ Donor* and more recently the *Critical Pathway for the Pediatric Organ Donor* (Box 13–3).[44] The Critical Pathway promotes a cooperative approach by the organ procurement coordinator (OPC), critical care staff, and members of the various disciplines involved with the care of the potential donor. As a standard of care of the donor, the Critical Pathway maximizes the recovery and use of organs for transplantation. The pathway has seen the addition of a protocol for *Cardio-Thoracic Donor Management* (Box 13–4). Studies have shown a significantly increased number of organs recovered and transplanted when these pathway algorithms are followed.[45,46]

The Critical Pathway for the Pediatric Organ Donor consists of four phases:

- Phase I: identification and referral
- Phase II: declaration of brain death and consent
- Phase III: donor management and donor evaluation
- Phase IV: comprehensive evaluation and donor management

Phase I outlines the referral process that essentially is the referral of the potential donor with severe brain insult to the OPC of the local OPO. Once notified, the OPC appears on site and begins evaluation to determine the acceptability of the potential donor as an organ donor.

Phase II consists of the declaration of brain death by a physician and notification of the family of the death. The family is offered the option of donation, a function primarily of the OPC or designated requester. It is helpful if the primary pediatrician and the involved critical care nurse are present.

Phase III of the pathway deals with the major aspects of donor evaluation and management. The physiologic consequences of brain death play a considerable role in affecting multiorgan dysfunction.[47,48] The "catecholamine storm" that results from brain death leads to a diffuse vascular regulatory injury and a diffuse metabolic cellular injury. Once initiated, profound pathophysiologic changes that occur may make the organs unsuitable before they can be recovered. Aggressive donor management can transform a significant number of these donors into acceptable multiorgan donors.

The two parts of phase III provide the OPC with a mechanism necessary to evaluate the functional status of the kidneys, liver, pancreas, heart, and lungs and to proceed with the management steps necessary to optimize the performance of these organs. Once brain death is declared, treatment may be contrary to that which was initiated upon the child's admission. Maintaining ventilatory and homodynamic stability is important. Vigorous fluid resuscitation may be necessary to maintain perfusion of the transplantable organs. It is important to monitor and maintain age-specific parameters, such as blood pressure, heart rate, central venous pressure, PaO_2, SaO_2 greater than 95%, pH 7.35 to 7.45, and urine output. Once adequate fluid volume is restored, vasopressors, such as dopamine, can be used to maintain blood pressure. It now is recommended that hormonal resuscitation be part of the comprehensive donor management protocol, especially to increase the use of extrarenal organs for transplantation[46,49] (see Box 13–4). Hormonal resuscitation consists of administration of T_3 or T_4, arginine, vasopressin, methylprednisolone, and insulin. This "cocktail" has been most beneficial in salvaging the cardiothoracic organs for transplantation.

Phase IV deals with the recovery phase. The ultimate outcome is ensuring that all potentially suitable organs for which consent has been obtained are recovered for transplantation.

The pediatric patient declared brain dead is a potential source of multiple transplantable organs.[50] In 2001, pediatric donors constituted 16% of all deceased (cadaveric) kidney donors. In addition to being a source of kidneys, the pediatric donor is much more likely to be a pancreas, intestine, or heart donor than is an adult donor.

BOX 13–4

Cardio-Thoracic Donor Management

1. **Early echocardiogram for all donors – Insert pulmonary artery catheter (PAC) to monitor patient management (placement of the PAC is particularly relevant in patients with an EF < 45% or on high dose inotropes.)**
   - o Use aggressive donor resuscitation as outlined below
2. **Electrolytes**
   - o Maintain Na < 150 meq/dl
   - o Maintain K+ > 4.0
   - o Correct acidosis with Na Bicarbonate and mild to moderate hyperventilation (pCO_2 30-35 mm Hg)
3. **Ventilation – Maintain tidal volume 10-15 ml/kg**
   - o Keep peak airway pressures < 30 mm Hg
   - o Maintain a mild respiratory alkalosis (pCO_2 30-35 mm Hg)
4. **Recommend use of hormonal resuscitation as part of a comprehensive donor management protocol – Key elements**
   - o Tri-iodothyronine (T3): 4 mcg bolus; 3 mcg/hr continuous infusion
   - o Arginine Vasopressin: 1 unit bolus: 0.5 - 4.0 unit/hour drip (titrate SVR 800-1200 using a PA catheter)
   - o Methylprednisolone: 15 mg/kg bolus (Repeat q 24° PRN)
   - o Insulin: drip at a minimum rate of 1 unit/hour (titrate blood glucose to 120-180 mg/dl)
   - o Ventilator: (see above)
   - o Volume Resuscitation: use of colloid and avoidance of anemia are important in preventing pulmonary edema
     - o albumin if PT and PTT are normal
     - o fresh frozen plasma if PT and PTT abnormal (value ≥ 1.5 × control)
     - o packed red blood cells to maintain a PCWP of 8-12 mm Hg and Hgb > 10.0 mg/dl
5. **When patient is stabilized/optimized repeat echocardiogram. (An unstable donor has not met 2 or more of the following criteria.)**
   - o Mean Arterial Pressure ≥ 60
   - o CVP ≤ 12 mm Hg
   - o PCWP ≤ 12 mm Hg
   - o SVR 800-1200 dyne/sec/cm^5
   - o Cardiac Index ≥ 2.5 l/min/M^2
   - o Left Ventricular Stroke Work Index > 15
   - o Dopamine dosage < 10 mcg/kg/min

HIV = human immunodeficiency virus; VDRL = Venereal Disease Research Laboratory; CMV = cytomegalovirus; CVP = central venous pressure; CXR = chest x-ray; CBC = complete blood count; UA = urinalysis; C & S = culture and sensitivity; PT = prothrombin time; PTT = partial thromboplastin time; RBCs = packed red blood cells; ABGs = arterial blood gases; H & H = hemoglobin and hematocrit; BUN = blood urea nitrogen; Rx = prescription: Bx = biopsy; FIO_2 = fraction of inspired oxygen; PCO_2 = partial pressure of carbon dioxide; NG = nasogastric tube; ECG = electrocardiogram; SaO_2 = arterial oxygen saturation; PEEP = positive end-expiratory pressure; VS = vital signs; BP = blood pressure; HR = heart rate; PaO_2 = partial arterial oxygen pressure; DC = discontinue.

REFERENCES

1. Hamilton D: A history of transplantation. In Morris PJ, editor: *Tissue transplantation,* ed 2. Edinburgh, 1982, Churchill Livingstone.
2. Starzl TE: The birth of clinical organ transplantation. *J Am Coll Surg* 192:431-446, 2001.
3. Papalois VE, Najarian JS: Pediatric kidney transplantation: historic hallmarks and personal perspective. *Pediatr Transplant* 5:239-245, 2001.
4. Murray JE, Merrill JP, Harrison JH: Kidney transplantation between seven pairs of identical twins. *Ann Surg* 148:343, 1958.
5. Michon I, Hamburger J, Oeconomos N, et al: Une tentative de transplantation renale chez l'homme: aspects medicaux et biologique. *Presse Med* 61:1419-1923, 1953.
6. Schwartz R, Dameshek W: Drug-induced immunological tolerance. *Nature* 183:1682, 1959.
7. Calne RY, Alenandre GPJ, Murray JE: The development of immunosuppressive therapy. *Ann N Y Acad Sci* 99:743, 1962.
8. Starzl TE, Marchioro TL, Porter KA, Tanous DF, Carey TA: The role of organ transplantation in pediatrics. *Pediatr Clin North Am* 13:381-422, 1966.
9. Kissmeyer-Nielsen F, Olsen S, Peterson VP, Fjeldborg O: Hyperacute rejection of kidney allografts. *Lancet* 2:662, 1966.
10. Borel JF: Comparative study of in-vitro and in-vivo drug effects on cell-mediated cytotoxicity. *Immunology* 31:631-641, 1976.
11. Calne RY, White DJG, Thiru S, et al: Cyclosporin A in patients receiving renal allografts from cadaver donors. *Lancet* 2:1323-1327, 1978.
12. Calne RY, Rolles K, White DJG, et al: Cyclosporin A initially as the only immunosuppressant in 34 recipients of cadaveric organs: 32 kidneys, 2 pancreases, and 2 livers. *Lancet* 2:1033-1036, 1979.
13. Goldstein G, Barnes L, Hirsch RL: OKT3 monoclonal antibody reversal of renal and hepatic rejection in pediatric patients. *J Pediatr* 111:1046-1050, 1987.
14. Leone MR, Alexander SR, Barry JM, et al: OKT3 monoclonal antibody in pediatric kidney recipients with recurrent and resistant allograft rejection. *J Pediatr* 111:45-50, 1987.
15. Starzl TE, Fung J, Jordan M, et al: Kidney transplantation under FK506. *JAMA* 264:63-67, 1990.
16. Jensen CWB, Jordan ML, Shneck FX, et al: Pediatric renal transplantation under FK506 immunosuppression. *Transplant Proc* 23:3075-3077, 1991.
17. Sollinger HW: Mycophenolate mofetil for the prevention of acute rejection in primary cadaveric renal allograft recipients. *Transplantation* 60:225-232, 1995.
18. Wahlberg J, Wilczek HE, Fauchald P, et al: Consistent absorption of cyclosporine from microemulsion formulation assessed in stable renal transplant recipients over a one-year study period. *Transplantation* 60:648-652, 1995.
19. Vincenti F, Kirkman R, Light S, et al: Interleukin-2 receptor blockade with Daclizumab to prevent acute rejection in renal transplantation. Daclizumab Triple Therapy Study Group. *N Engl J Med* 338:161-165, 1998.
20. Nashan B, Moore R, Amlot P, Schmidt AG, et al: Randomized trial of basiliximab versus placebo for control of acute cellular rejection in renal allograft recipients. CHIB 201 International Study Group. *Lancet* 350:1193-1198, 1997.
21. Sindhi R. Sirolimus in pediatric transplant recipients. *Transplant Proc* 35(suppl 3A):113S-114S, 2003.
22. Humar A, Arrazola L, Mauer M, Matas AJ, Najarian JS: Kidney transplantation in young children: should there be a minimum age? *Pediatr Nephrol* 16:941-945, 2001.
23. Salvatierra O Jr, Alexander SR, Krensky AM: Pediatric kidney transplantation at Stanford. *Pediatr Transplant* 2:165-176, 1998.
24. Seikaly M, Ho PL, Emmett L, Tejani A: 12th Annual Report of the North American Pediatric Renal Transplant Cooperative Study: renal transplantation from 1987 through 1998. *Pediatr Transplant* 5:215, 2001.
25. Watson AR: Non-compliance and transfer from paediatric to adult transplant unit. *Pediatr Nephrol* 14:469, 2000.
26. Fine RN, Ho M, Tejni A: The contribution of renal transplantation to final adult height: a report of the North American Pediatric Renal Transplant Cooperative Study (NAPRTCS). *Pediatr Nephrol* 16:951-956, 2001.
27. Hosenpud JD, Bennett LE, Keck BM, et al: The Registry of the International Society for Heart and Lung Transplantation: eighteenth official report-2001. *J Heart Lung Transplant* 20:805-815, 2001.
28. Webber SA: 15 years of pediatric heart transplantation at the University of Pittsburgh: lessons learned and future prospects. *Pediatr Transplant* 1:8-21, 1997.
29. Boucek RJ, Boucek MM: Pediatric heart transplantation. *Curr Opin Pediatr* 14:611-619, 2002.
30. Suddaby EC: The state of pediatric heart transplantation. *AACN Clin Issues* 10:202-216, 1999.
31. SPLIT Research Group: Studies of pediatric liver transplantation (SPLIT): year 2000 outcomes. *Transplantation* 72:463-476, 2001.
32. Ghobrial RM, Farmer DG, Amersi F, Busuttil RW: Advances in pediatric liver and intestinal transplantation. *Am J Surg* 180: 328-334, 2000.
33. Sindhi R, Rosendale J, Mundy D, et al: Impact of segmental grafts on pediatric transplantation: a review of the United Network for

Organ Sharing Scientific Registry data (1990-1996). *J Pediatr Surg* 34:107-111, 1999.
34. Burdelski M, Nolkemper D, Ganschow R, et al: Liver transplantation in children: long term outcome and quality of life. *Eur J Pediatr* 158:34-42, 1999.
35. Reyes J, Mazariegos CV, Bond GM, et al: Pediatric intestinal transplantation: historical notes, principles and controversies. *Pediatr Transplant* 6:193-207, 2002.
36. Iyer KR, Srinath C, Horslen S, et al: Late graft loss and long-term outcome after isolated intestinal transplantation in children. *J Pediatr Surg* 37:151-154, 2002.
37. Iyer KR, Horslen S, Iverson A, et al: Nutritional outcome and growth of children after intestinal transplantation. *J Pediatr Surg* 37:464-466, 2002.
38. Farmer DG, McDiarmid SV, Yersiz H, et al: Outcome after intestinal transplantation: results from one center's experience. *Arch Surg* 136:1027-1032, 2001.
39. 1998 HCFA Directive on Organ/Tissue Donation Committee on Hospital Care and Section on Surgery, American Academy of Pediatrics: Pediatric organ donation and transplantation. *Pediatrics* 109:982-984, 2002.
40. Graham M: The role of the medical examiner in fatal child abuse: organ and tissue transplantation issues. In Monteleone JA, Brodeur AE, editors: *Child maltreatment: a clinical guide and reference.* St Louis, 1994, GW Medical Publishing.
41. Institute of Medicine: *Non-heart-beating organ transplantation: medical and ethical issues in procurement.* Washington, DC, 1997, National Academy Press.
42. Institute of Medicine: *Non-heart-beating organ transplantation: practice and protocols.* Washington, DC, 2000, National Academy Press.
43. Holmquist M, Chabalewski F, Blount T, et al: A critical pathway: guiding care for organ donors. *Crit Care Nurse* 19:84-98, 1999.
44. Rosendale J, Chabalewski F, McBride M, et al: Increased transplanted organs from the use of a standardized donor management protocol. *Am J Transplant* 2:761-768, 2002.
45. Rosendale J, Kauffman H, McBride M, et al: Aggressive pharmacologic donor management results in more transplanted organs. *Transplantation* 75:482-487, 2003.
46. Mackersie R, Bronsther O, Shackford S: Organ procurement in patients with fatal head injuries. The fate of the potential donor. *Ann Surg* 212:143-150, 1991.
47. Power B, Van Heerden P: The physiological changes associated with brain death: current concepts and implications for treatment of the brain dead organ donor. *Anaesth Intensive Care* 23:26-36,1995.
48. Novitzky D, Cooper D, Human P, et al: Triiodothyronine therapy for heart donor and recipient. *J Heart Transplant* 7:370-376, 1988.
49. Colombani PM, Dunn SP, Harmon WE, et al: Pediatric transplantation. *Am J Transplant* 3(suppl 4):53-63, 2003.

CHAPTER 14

Pediatric Transport: Shifting the Paradigm to Improve Patient Outcome

Richard A. Orr, Yong Y. Han, and Kimberly Roth

PEARLS

- Patients often are subjected to a high-risk moving environment with limited resources and few monitoring capabilities. The goal during transport should be to provide the same or better quality care than the patient had before transport.
- A retrieval system has a responsibility to the referral community to provide accessible tertiary care. The components include a communication center, administrative staff, appropriately trained team members, reliable equipment, and education and safety programs.
- A hospital should not transfer a patient until the patient has been appropriately stabilized, the patient consents to transfer after being informed of the risks of transfer, and the referring physician certifies that the medical benefits expected from the transfer outweigh the risks. The transferring hospital must provide care and stabilization within its ability; copies of the medical records and imaging studies must accompany the patient; the receiving facility must have available space and qualified personnel and agree to accept the patient; and the transport must be made by *qualified* personnel.
- Underutilization of an acquired skill often leads to fear on the part of the provider and an aversion to performing an intervention during a time of crisis. A busy emergency medical services system with 50 active advanced life support providers is expected to have one pediatric bag-valve-mask case every 1.7 years, one pediatric intubation every 3.3 years, and one intraosseus cannulation every 6.7 years!
- The current paradigm of transport must shift if we are to realize improved outcomes in the critically ill who require transport to a critical care center. We must abandon the current paradigm of "scoop and run" through a disjointed system as a means to initiating care. We must adopt a system whereby goal-directed therapy begins in the prehospital arena and continues throughout the critical care continuum.

Along with the regionalization of pediatric emergency and critical care centers has come the growth of interfacility transport programs, allowing geographic expansion of tertiary medical care. Critically ill infants and children often are taken to the nearest local emergency department (ED) by the emergency medical services (EMS) provider or by their parents, where their conditions are assessed to determine the extent of their illnesses or injuries so that initial stabilization can be provided. Many community hospitals do not have the personnel, space, or facilities to provide critical care to infants or children beyond the period of initial stabilization, necessitating their transfer to a tertiary facility. Despite numerous advances in pediatrics, transport of the critically ill child continues to be a problem area in critical care. Children often are subjected to a high-risk environment with limited resources and few monitoring capabilities. Major decisions with regard to the mode of travel and staffing of pediatric transports are made daily, yet little research supports the validity of this decision-making process. The goal during transport should be to provide care commensurate with the degree of illness severity in a safe and effective manner, thereby minimizing the risk of deterioration and unplanned events before and during the en route phase of transport.

Despite significant advancements in potentially lifesaving technologies that continue to shape the practice of pediatric intensive care, we believe that actual improvements in patient outcome will not occur until there is a fundamental shift in the paradigm of how pediatric transport operates in the critical care continuum. We must first understand the problems and strongholds that have stifled progress and improvement in outcomes for children before we can devise a solution. This chapter is not intended to be a "typical" discourse on pediatric transport, complete with illustrations on vehicles, drug lists, backpacks, and safety. This information is more appropriately summarized in the American Academy of Pediatrics (AAP) Guidelines for Air and Ground Transport of Neonatal and Pediatric Patients.[1] Rather, this chapter is designed to challenge the pediatric intensivist, whose patient population is derived from transport, with the notion that a pediatric critical care transport system is much more likely to have a positive impact on patient outcome in the short term than any other area of research in which we currently are involved.

The Problem

Unique Aspects of Pediatric Emergency Medical Services

Epidemiology of Emergency Medical Services

The majority of children are transported by EMS providers who have variable educational backgrounds and experience. EMS includes all aspects of basic life support (BLS), advanced life support (ALS), and critical care transport in which emergency medical personnel are used. EMS encompasses prehospital and interfacility components of transport, including hospital-based specialized teams. A critically ill child in a rural setting might receive care from a basic emergency medical technician (EMT) and an ambulance driver but in a more organized system might have the benefit of a transport team specializing in pediatric critical care. Currently, EMS has no national regulations as they relate to children. Only two states require all the pediatric equipment recommended for BLS ambulances, and only five states require all essential pediatric equipment for ALS ambulances. Pediatric guidelines for EMS are just beginning to evolve from the various national organizations that represent children.[2]

Fewer than 10% of all EMS runs nationwide are for infants and children; 12% of the runs involve ALS and even fewer provide critical care.[3,4] Overall, this number translates into three pediatric patients per month for 60% of the nation's paramedics, and fewer than 3% of the nation's paramedics see 15 or more children per month!

Seidel et al.[3] first described these deficiencies and found that 41% of EMT training programs offered only 10 hours or less in both didactic and clinical pediatric training, 24% did not carry a complete set of pediatric blood pressure cuffs, and 79% of providers were not equipped with a complete set of pediatric ventilation masks! Children were twice as likely to die of trauma in the field compared with adults, attributed to the lack of pediatric training.[3,5,6] Glaeser et al.[4] performed a survey of nationally registered EMS providers and found that NREMT-Ps (National Registry of Emergency Medical Technicians-Paramedics) receive a median of 16 hours of pediatric didactic instruction of a total 358 hours, but they are not required to take pediatric continuing medical education (CME) training. However, 76% of the providers supported a mandate for continuing education in pediatrics.[4] Ramenofsky et al.[7] believed that one consequence of this lack of training was a high incidence of secondary insults and potentially avoidable deaths among children. They determined that 53 of 100 deceased pediatric trauma victims in their study could have been salvaged given an optimally functioning emergency medical system. They also concluded that in 79% of the potentially salvageable cases, mortality was associated with prehospital iatrogenic or secondary insults, again attributed to lack of specialized pediatric training.[7]

Skill Maintenance and Provider Confidence

The logical outcome of limited provider exposure to critically ill children is the problem of maintaining pediatric assessment and interventional skills. Babl et al.[8] demonstrated that in a program with 50 active ALS providers in the current milieu of EMS, each provider is expected to have one pediatric bag-valve-mask (BVM) case every 1.7 years, one pediatric intubation every 3.3 years, and one intraosseus cannulation every 6.7 years! Underutilization of an acquired skill often leads to fear on the part of the provider and an aversion to performing an intervention during a time of crisis, especially in infants and children.

Reluctance to provide advanced airway management is a good example. Aijian et al.[9] examined a population of pediatric patients who had suffered a prehospital cardiopulmonary arrest and determined that endotracheal intubation was attempted only 68% of the time, with a success rate of only 64%. In patients younger than 1 year, endotracheal intubation was attempted only 38% of the time, with a success rate of only 50%.[9] Losek et al.[10] reviewed a series of 1467 children in the prehospital setting and determined that only 78% of endotracheal attempts were successful. For patients who were pulseless and not breathing at the scene, 93% were successfully intubated. For patients who were judged to be in impending respiratory failure, only 48% were successfully intubated.[10]

With any given scenario in the EMS setting, adult patients are more likely to receive an appropriate intervention compared with a child having the same problem. Scribano et al.[11] studied 203 children in the field with respiratory distress and found that 44% received inappropriate interventions. Oxygen and medications were underutilized, but vascular access was overutilized, a procedure that paramedics do frequently. Gausche et al.[12] found that children in the field younger than 14 years were more likely to receive undertreatment compared with adults (33% vs. 3%) but discordant overtreatment with placement of intravenous catheters, again a procedure with which paramedics are more comfortable.

Emergency providers often call upon air medical services to transport children because of their presumed expertise and training in pediatric care compared with local prehospital EMS providers. Air medical services usually are hospital based or near major medical centers where providers are provided the opportunity to rotate through pediatric units and receive hands-on experience in the care of critically ill children. However, the literature suggests that airway management in children remains a problem even among these "more experienced" providers. Mishark et al.[13] found only a 67% success rate of intubation in children compared with an 87% overall success rate in their system. Boswell et al.[14] found unsuccessful intubation attempts in 34% of children compared with 9.8% of adults, where inclusion criteria were trauma patients whose Glasgow Coma Score was ≤8. Doran et al.[15] quoted an overall success rate of only 88% in their series and identified increased level of consciousness, technical problems (identifying airway anatomy, visualization, secretions), access problems (clenched teeth, combativeness), and mechanical problems (patient position, equipment failure) as factors associated with decreased success for pediatric intubation. Each of these air medical studies concluded that additional training in airway management in children and use of medications (neuromuscular blockade) to facilitate intubation probably would result in a higher success rate.

Despite the time and effort given toward training of EMS personnel, cognitive and interventional skills deteriorate over time, especially given the few encounters with children in the field. Su et al.[16] demonstrated through a randomized controlled trial that the knowledge a paramedic attains through education courses deteriorates rapidly over a 6-month period. Henderson[17] also demonstrated that the ability of a provider to intubate or provide BVM ventilation for a child deteriorates significantly over 6 months. The issue of more concern in this study was that 95% of the paramedics who failed both BVM and endotracheal intubation attempts reported confidence and lack of anxiety in their ability to provide these life-saving procedures in the field![17]

Finally, referring hospitals often are not equipped to care for critically ill and injured children. Seidel et al.[3,5,6] demonstrated that many EDs were ill prepared to care for children and suggested that hospital facilities should be designated for pediatric emergency care. Esposito et al.[18] found that frequent errors occur in ED management of pediatric trauma, leading to approximately 9% preventable mortality. In addition, they reported a 64% error rate in the management of children, including gross violations of basic trauma care.[18] Athey et al.[19] found that a significant number of critically ill infants and children still are being admitted to hospitals lacking pediatric specialty facilities or expertise. They reported that nearly 10% of all U.S. hospitals without pediatric intensive care facilities admit critically ill and injured children and that 7% of these hospitals routinely admit these children to adult intensive care units rather than transferring the children to a more appropriate facility. Of the facilities that keep children, few have protocols for obtaining pediatric consultation for emergencies, and most did not have appropriate-size equipment to care for children.[19] Consequently, there are two extremes in handling referrals from these hospitals. The first protocol consists of a "scoop and run" approach with minimal initial care from the ED, using inexperienced personnel en route to the tertiary center "to save time." Harrison et al.[20] found that children were likely to be transferred significantly more quickly from referring hospitals than were adults with injury of equal severity. In the second protocol, the critically ill child is kept in the adult intensive care unit too long until irreparable damage to major organ systems occurs, at which point a transfer is requested.

Unappreciated Differences Between Adults and Children

Airway and respiratory difficulties are the most likely causes of pediatric cardiopulmonary arrest[21,22] and account for more than 50% of intensive care admissions for children.[23] The caregiver on transport should recognize the anatomic and physiologic differences in the respiratory system of a child compared with the system of an adult (see Chapters 32 and 33). Earlier intervention often is required to correct a respiratory problem in a child compared with an adult patient with a similar respiratory derangement because of these differences. Airway interventions should be planned carefully and performed early in the course of respiratory failure to avoid having to deal with a respiratory crisis during the en route phase of transport.

First, adults differ from children with regard to the site of the major contribution to the total airflow resistance. The upper airway, particularly the nose, accounts for the major portion of total resistance in the adult. Conversely, the peripheral airway resistance in children younger than 5 years is approximately four times higher than in adults or older children.[24] This observation explains the high incidence of lower airway obstructive disease in young children. Respiratory distress in an adult patient often can be ameliorated by performing a few simple upper airway maneuvers during transport, obviating the need for intubation and positive pressure breathing, at least until the patient arrives at the receiving facility. This approach will not work in an infant or child, and a delay in performing advanced airway management in an effort to save time can lead to progression of respiratory failure and cardiopulmonary arrest.

Second, infants and small children have more compliant chest walls and weak cartilaginous support compared with older children and adults, leading to several clinical implications.[25] The very low elastic recoil pressure of the newborn chest wall increases the risk of lung collapse. Most tidal volume breathing in infants occurs in the range of the closing capacity of the lung. Children younger than 6 years and adults older than 40 years have a closing capacity greater than functional residual capacity when they are in the supine position.[26] The relatively high closing capacity results from reduced elastic recoil of the lung, raising the subatmospheric pressure in the intrapleural space. This situation leads to early airway closure in the dependent regions of the lung, particularly when disease is present. In addition, the highly compliant chest wall is at a mechanical disadvantage during breathing because the infant must generate greater pressure and perform more work to move the same tidal volume. A portion of the force of contraction of the diaphragm is wasted in distorting the rib cage, giving rise to the clinical observation of retractions.[27] When infants are confronted with the need to increase their work of breathing because of lung disease, a certain percentage of them fatigue and stop breathing.[28] Therefore aggressive airway intervention and positive pressure breathing early in the transport process stop the progression of atelectasis and respiratory failure. In addition, because tidal volume breathing is much more dependent on diaphragmatic function in the infant and small child, a nasogastric tube should always be inserted for patients who are intubated and for those with impending respiratory failure to prevent gastric distension.

Third, the alveolar diameter in an infant is half the adult size, predisposing the infant and small child to alveolar collapse much earlier in the course of respiratory failure.[29] In addition, the adult lung contains anatomic channels that allow ventilation distal to an obstructed airway, also known as *collateral ventilation.*[30] Without these pathways for collateral ventilation, the infant and young child presumably are at increased risk for atelectasis and emphysematous changes and consequent ventilation/perfusion mismatching.

Fourth, the diffusing capacity across the alveolar-capillary membrane in a child is only about one third that of an adult, making gas exchange less efficient.[31]

Finally, infants and children have a higher metabolic rate than adults. Therefore hypoxia progresses more quickly during the course of respiratory failure. In addition, toxic byproducts from an ingestion can be produced more quickly.

Cardiorespiratory compensatory mechanisms are more pronounced in children.[32] For infants and children, blood pressure is preserved during the course of shock, through increases in systemic vascular resistance. In our experience, goal-directed therapy for shock is either delayed or minimized because caregivers in the transport environment often use blood pressure as a guide to therapy, something they are more accustomed to doing with adult patients.

Strongholds

Misguided Concept of the Golden Hour

EMS and regional flight teams are essentially focused on the adult population and have been developed to deal primarily with myocardial infarction and trauma, the major causes of morbidity and mortality in adults.[3] They are designed for rapid response and are expected to minimize time at the scene. EMS personnel often are taught that they are working against a clock (the "golden hour") that begins ticking at the onset of the illness or injury, and for every minute spent away from the critical care center, the probability of survival diminishes. This "golden hour" is the driving force for clinical decision making and usually translates into providing minimal care and moving quickly (Figure 14–1). The concept of the "golden hour" often is described as having its origin from an article by Cowley et al.,[33] who reported that survival of patients with traumatic injuries markedly improved when they reached the shock trauma center within 1 hour of injury or illness. The article was not a study on the outcome of trauma victims but rather a surgical commentary on the success of implementing a helicopter-based program for trauma. In fact, the term *golden hour* never appeared in this article! However, the article by Cowley et al. does contain the following quote taken from *Modern Hospital:* "it has been recorded that for every 30 minutes that elapse between the accident and the time the patient gets to definitive care, the mortality rate can be expected to increase threefold."[34] The truth of the matter is that, at the time of the article by Cowley et al., definitive care rarely occurred until the patient arrived at the shock trauma unit. Prehospital care at that time consisted of providing supplemental oxygen, a fast-moving vehicle, and minimal resuscitation. Intuitively, under these circumstances, a worse outcome was expected as prehospital time increased. Interestingly, even during this era, experience suggested improved survival when stabilization occurred in the field. Military medical experience showed that stabilization in the field markedly improved survival of trauma victims.[35] Field stabilization also improved the outcome of victims requiring cardiopulmonary life support.[36,37] Despite these observations and the modernization of EMS as we know it today, with improved equipment, training, and skills, "scoop and run" and the "golden hour" remain the prevailing philosophies in the transport of infants and children, for whom the speed of transport alone benefits few.

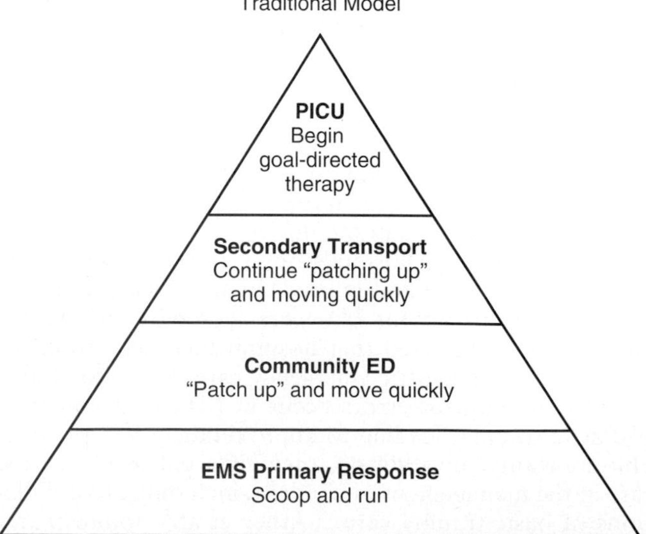

FIGURE 14–1 • Traditional model of emergency care based on the concept of the "golden hour." *ED,* Emergency department; *EMS,* emergency medical services; *PICU,* pediatric intensive care unit.

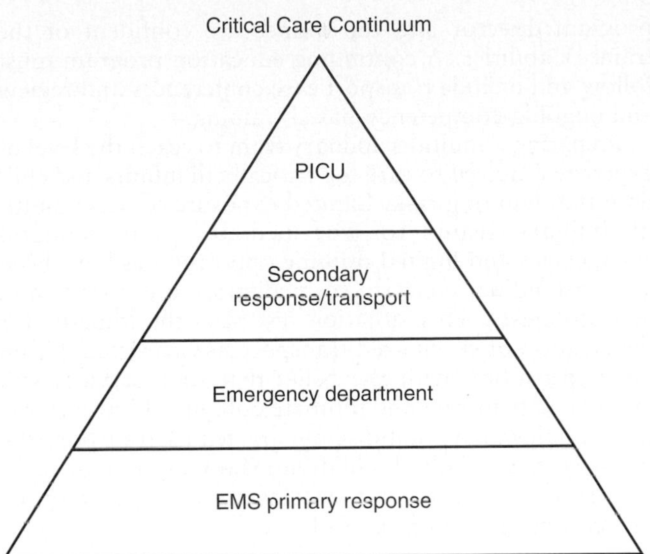

FIGURE 14–2 • Pediatric transport as part of the critical care continuum. *EMS,* emergency medical services; *PICU,* pediatric intensive care unit.

Territorial Issues and Isolation

Pediatric transport is part of a critical care continuum that includes EMS, the referring ED, secondary transfer, and the receiving critical care facility, which could include the receiving pediatric ED and the intensive care unit (Figure 14–2). Ideally, physicians and other caregivers from emergency medicine, neonatology, surgery, and intensive care all take an active role in designing each segment of the continuum and maintaining quality assurance if optimal care is to be provided. The critically ill child ultimately will be the responsibility of the pediatric intensivist, so it behooves him/her to have significant input into system design and protocols. In our experience, the continuum often is fragmented, primarily by territorial issues, resulting in poor communication, isolation, and lack of continuity of care (Figure 14–3). Transport often is considered "someone else's problem" when issues arise. This fragmentation halts the educational process and appropriate quality management that should occur when the segments operate interdependently.

The fact that only 10% of all EMS calls involve children and the differences in size, anatomy, physiology, and psychosocial aspects unique to children will continually challenge the EMS provider. The self-fulfilling prophecy is a system that focuses primarily on the adult population, where training and equipment deficiencies will always be a threat during the transport of infants and children. Caregivers in the current system could conclude that they may never be adept in the care of infants and children and that things will never change. Should we marvel, then, at a quote from an article by Applebaum[38] on pediatric transport outcome: "children are less likely to require or benefit from advanced levels of prehospital care compared to the adult population. When resources for advanced care are limited, priority should be given to adult emergencies!"[38] Is there a solution?

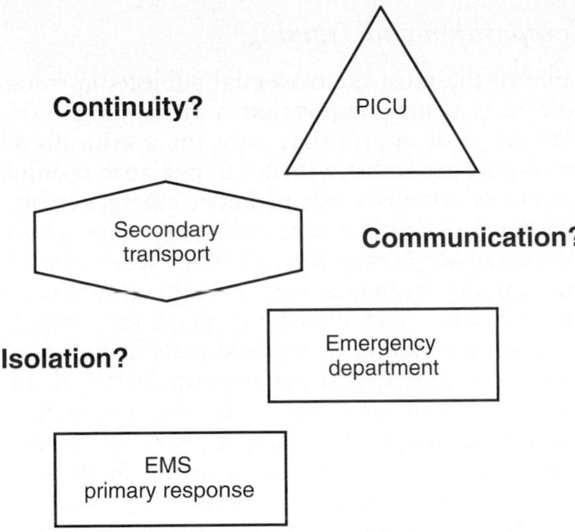

FIGURE 14–3 • Authors' depiction of fragmented critical care continuum within a disjointed system. *EMS,* emergency medical services; *PICU,* pediatric intensive care unit.

The Solution

Retrieval System Focused on Improving Outcome and Not Rapid Movement

The current paradigm of pediatric transport must shift if we are to realize improved outcomes in critically ill infants and children who require transfer to a pediatric critical care center. We must abandon the current paradigm of "scoop and run" through a disjointed system (see Figure 14–3) as a means to initiating definitive care upon arrival to the critical care center. We must adopt a system whereby goal-directed therapy begins in the prehospital arena and continues throughout the critical care continuum (Figure 14–4).

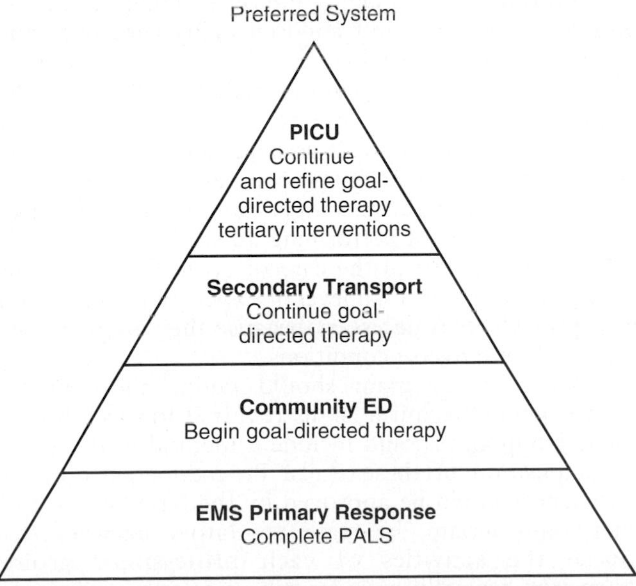

FIGURE 14–4 • Authors' depiction of preferred system of goal-directed care model. *ED,* Emergency department; *EMS,* emergency medical services; *PALS,* pediatric advanced life support; *PICU,* pediatric intensive care unit.

Team Composition and Training

Perhaps one of the most controversial subjects in transport medicine is team composition and training. Who will render the most appropriate care for a critically ill child, a transport generalist with some pediatric training who occasionally attends a true pediatric emergency or a specialized pediatric critical care transport team whose focus and experience is only for children? Team composition and training strategies vary considerably among transport programs. The choice of personnel usually depends on the availability of professionals in the sponsoring facility, the anticipated patient population, financial support for the program, and other practical considerations. Techniques for training personnel depend on the role of a specific professional group in the care of transported patients, their experience in neonatal and pediatric health care, and their familiarity with the transport environment.

Many dedicated pediatric transport teams include a physician, although little objective evidence indicates this configuration results in improved outcome compared with nonphysician teams. Physician attendance is particularly controversial when the role is filled by physicians-in-training. With the exception of advanced trainees (residents in emergency medicine or critical care), most lack the knowledge and experience needed in the transport environment.

Selection of team members is critical to the success of a transport program. Members should be selected based on their experience and competence in the care of children in the inpatient setting. Although the specific requirements of training depend on the professional background of the team members, their experience, and their roles in inpatient care, the goals and general content of training are the same, regardless of the type of personnel. The team transporting a critically ill pediatric patient should include at least one member who is experienced in diagnosing and managing life-threatening illnesses or injuries in neonates and children. This caregiver must understand pathophysiology and the usual clinical course and complications of common pediatric illnesses. This person must understand how to use appropriate laboratory and radiographic tests as diagnostic aids and must have experience in managing neonates and children who require intensive pharmacologic intervention. The team should be capable of performing all standard emergency procedures required in the care of critically ill neonates and children. A very high level of expertise in performing these procedures is necessary because they often are performed under adverse conditions.

A transport program should define the cognitive knowledge and technical skills required for each professional group and should include a method to document the acquisition of these skills. Procedure performance proficiency should be approved by the base facility and, where appropriate, by state regulatory agencies that govern the activities of each professional group. Instruction typically includes didactic sessions designed to assist personnel to acquire cognitive knowledge, a skill development and maintenance program, and a supervised orientation period. The latter should end when the training program director and the trainee are confident of the trainee's abilities. A continuing education program must follow and include transport case conferences and review and ongoing competency-based training.

Preparing a multidisciplinary team to reach the level of expertise required to care for critically ill infants and children is a daunting task. Limited exposure of these multidisciplinary teams to true pediatric and neonatal emergencies and limited training opportunities have been a longstanding concern to pediatric intensivists and neonatologists. This situation has been the impetus for the creation of specialized transport services from within these specialties, with the belief that such services will improve patient care and ultimate outcome. However, the fact remains that multidisciplinary teams transport the majority of crucially ill children. Many argue that pediatric specialized transport systems are not necessary for the reasons given in Box 14–1.

Do Specialized Teams Improve Outcome?

What does the evidence show? In 1978, Chance et al.[39] demonstrated that mortality was significantly reduced when a specialized team transported neonates who weighed less than 1.5 kg compared with transportation by alternative means. Infants were significantly warmer, less hypotensive, and less acidotic on admission to the neonatal intensive care unit when they were transported by a physician and nurse who were trained in neonatal care.[39] Macnab[40] showed that inadequate stabilization and preventable insults were reduced when transport team members received specialized pediatric training. In his study, 72% of all transport preventable insults occurred in the presence of emergency medical attendants (EMAs) who had no formalized pediatric training: 20% with EMAs who had undergone an intensive 18-month pediatric training module but only 8% with transport by a pediatric intensive care team.[40] Edge et al.[41] demonstrated that patients who were transported by nonspecialized teams had a tenfold increase in transport-related adverse events (e.g., loss of an endotracheal tube en route) compared with specialized teams, after adjusting for

BOX 14–1

Arguments Against Use of Specialized Transport Systems

- Expensive and resource intensive
- Limitations of the transport environment—what more can a specialist do?
- ABCs (airway, breathing, circulation) are no different for children
- Specialized teams spend too much time on the scene; no appreciation for what is time critical
- The patient is already packaged to go—what else is there to do?
- Not available in many settings
- Requires two-way transport; takes longer to get to the critical care center

severity of illness (Pediatric Risk of Mortality [PRISM]) and number of interventions (Therapeutic Intervention Scoring System [TISS]). In the United Kingdom, Bellingan et al.[42] compared a specialized retrieval team with current United Kingdom transport practice for adults and found that patients who were transported by the specialized service had improved acid–base balance upon arrival, were hemodynamically more stable, and had fewer deaths. In a later study, Macnab et al.[43] performed a case-control study of head-injured children and calculated the costs associated with secondary adverse events during transport, using the Glasgow Coma Score for case adjustment. They found more preventable insults among the patients transported by untrained escorts compared with trained escorts, and the majority of the insults in the untrained escort group resulted from hypoxia. They determined that the additional cost of care resulting from secondary adverse events occurring during transport by untrained escorts was $135,952! In a prospective risk assessment of 1085 children transported to a children's hospital, Orr et al.[44] found that patients who were transported by nonspecialized transport teams were more likely to suffer from an unplanned event (odds ratio 22.2) and in-hospital death (odds ratio 2.4) compared with children transported by a specialized team, after adjusting for severity of illness, age, and diagnosis. Mobilization time, scene time, and total transport time did not predict unplanned events or death![44]

Goal-Directed Therapies Improve Outcome

In a landmark article, Rivers et al.[45] demonstrated that initiation of goal-directed therapy in the ED setting improved survival in adults with severe sepsis and septic shock. Patients assigned to the early goal-directed therapeutic group also had improved central venous oxygen saturations, lower base deficits, and a lower incidence of multisystem organ dysfunction versus those who had "standard therapy" (minimal resuscitation before arrival to the intensive care unit). Han et al.[46] reported similar results in a pediatric transport study. When community physicians successfully achieved shock reversal through aggressive resuscitation before a transport team arrived, patients had a ninefold increase in their odds of survival. Overall, resuscitation practice was consistent with American College of Critical Care Medicine-Pediatric Advanced Life Support (ACCM-PALS) guidelines in only 30% of children who presented with septic shock in a community ED.[46] This reluctance to treat is typical of the current paradigm of EMS where the "scoop and run" mentality prevails. Caregivers who provide stabilization before the patient arrives to a critical care unit often are criticized for their efforts because of the popular notion that out-of-hospital stabilization "wastes time" and "delays" definitive therapy that should be rendered at the receiving facility.

Responsibility of the Retrieval System

The retrieval system has a responsibility to the referral community to provide accessible tertiary care, including transport. This responsibility begins with a commitment to a formal structure. Optimally, this structure is designed to begin providing intensive care, when necessary, to the patient at the referring institution and to continue appropriate care while en route. Care en route should be similar to the care given in the intensive care unit. The referring community's expectations of the regional center's response to transport requests vary according to the standard of care and topography for that region. Regardless of its origin, a retrieval system should include a communications center, administrative staff, appropriately trained team members, reliable equipment, and a safety program.

Communications

The communications center for the retrieval system should be easily accessible to both the referring physician and the transport team.[47,48] It should be staffed round-the-clock by full-time communication specialists who are trained in handling emergency calls and who have no other distracting duties that would delay a response. The communication specialist should follow a prescribed protocol to minimize the number of calls necessary to organize efforts, notify the appropriate personnel, and arrange all aspects of the transport so that the referring physician can direct his/her attention to patient care rather than waste valuable time on the telephone. A detailed log of transport requests, including time, demographic data, diagnosis, and vehicle availability, is kept for both administrative review and medical-legal documentation. Equipment for direct communication with the center should be available in every transport vehicle. The receiving physician who is responsible for the transport maintains contact with the communications center and with the referring physician. The receiving physician should obtain a brief history of the patient's present illness and a summary of interventions and should give recommendations tailored to the capabilities of the referring hospital and pertinent to the current problem. This information should be documented on a log that remains a part of the patient's medical record. Also suggested is that the referring physician have a copy of the patient's record and radiographs to accompany the transport team.

Staffing a Retrieval System

The administrative staff of a retrieval system should include, at a minimum, a program director, medical director, transport coordinator, and medical command.[47,48] The *program director* is responsible for the structure, activities, and organization of the transport system and assumes overall program responsibilities; acts as a liaison between the team and hospital administration; and develops and implements quality management.

The *medical director* should be a specialist in critical care or emergency medicine. He/she might have training in a surgical subspecialty (trauma) or in pediatrics (neonatology). He/she is a licensed physician who is responsible for supervising and evaluating the quality of medical care provided by the transport team and must have educational experience in the areas of medicine that are commensurate with the mission of the retrieval service.

The medical director should be experienced in both air and ground transport (as appropriate), should understand patient care capabilities and limitations in the transport environment, and should be educated in infection control, stress recognition and management, and altitude physiology and stressors in the flight environment. The medical director must be actively involved in quality management, administrative decisions affecting medical care, and the hiring, training, and continuing education of all transport personnel. He/she must orient physicians who provide on-line medical direction to the policies, procedures, and patient care protocols and should act as a liaison to the referral community for teaching and outreach.[47,48]

The *transport coordinator,* usually a nurse or paramedic, collaborates with the medical director with regard to training, protocols, scheduling, data collection, quality management, and marketing. The medical director and transport coordinator should participate in patient transport, whenever possible, to maintain skill and perspective.

A *command physician* should oversee every transport and provide advice to the referring physician and transport team as necessary. The command physician must be experienced in handling transport calls and offering management suggestions for the period before arrival of the transport team. He/she should be knowledgeable about the availability of resources, have authority to accept transferred patients without further consultation, perform triage, and activate backup systems when necessary. Medical control usually is accomplished in one of two ways: online or offline.[49] Online medical control is direct real-time voice communication (radio, telephone, cellular telephone, or satellite phone) between the medical control physician and the transport team. The transport team must always know who the command physician is throughout the transport process. Responsibility for medical control varies based on local practices and the policies of the transport service. Medical control physicians must be experienced in critical care transports to ensure the crews provide appropriate care. For specialized transports, the transport service should have a mechanism in place for medical control physicians to have timely consultation with subspecialists or the receiving physician. Alternatively, the critical care transport team should have the ability to consult with the receiving physician and to provide updates to the receiving facility. During offline medical control, patient management by the transport team is driven by written protocols or standing orders. There is no direct communication between the team and the medical control physician. The medical director is responsible for developing transport protocols and procedures used for offline medical control.

Transport crew members should be experienced in the care of critically ill patients and be able to deal with complex environments with limited resources. They must be highly skilled in airway management, resuscitation, and vascular access. They should have a fundamental knowledge of field priorities and be able to make decisions independently. All team members should have specific training in transport medicine, which includes methods of functioning in a moving environment, aeromedical physiology, and troubleshooting for equipment-related problems.

Equipment

Equipment taken on transport should be complete and adequate to provide continuing intensive care throughout the trip. Oxygen reserve should be calculated for each patient transported and should be at least twice the amount needed for the expected duration of the trip, in case of delays or equipment malfunction. Portable, compartmentalized equipment packs must be designed for easy access and must be able to withstand the stress of the transport environment. For air medical transport, weight and space restrictions must be considered when selecting equipment and range of medications. Transport monitors should have battery power that will last beyond the expected duration of transport because of the possibility of unexpected delays or vehicle breakdowns and should be free of movement artifact. Most important, the transport team should be self-sufficient and not dependent on the referring hospital for supplies. All equipment should be routinely checked and maintained after transport by a team member dedicated to that task.

Safety

Safety should be a high priority in any transport program. Emergency vehicle operation carries substantial risks, not only to the crew and the patient but also to others in its vicinity. The medical director is responsible for thoroughly researching vendors of air or ground transport services in the areas of maintenance, safety records, experience of drivers and pilots, and reliability of equipment. Written contracts between the institution and the vendor should include specific insurance details. Ambulance drivers should be discouraged from exceeding the speed limit because no evidence indicates that "red-balling" has any positive effect on patient outcome.

Aeromedical transport involves a unique set of safety issues. The four leading causes of accidents are weather, engine failure, collision with an obstacle, and loss of control. Pressure on pilots to fly, competition among aeromedical services within a region, and failure to observe minimal weather standards are among the components contributing to these accidents. In order for pilots to make sound decisions based on the flight conditions, they must be isolated from patient care issues. In regions with competing aeromedical services, the services should act jointly to establish regional safety guidelines, minimum weather standards, and a quality assurance program that examines compliance.

Transport team members must have a good understanding of aviation medicine and of how the aeromedical environment affects both them and the patient. Barometric pressure changes that occur with increasing cabin altitude lower alveolar oxygen tension and increase the volume of any entrapped gas (e.g., in the bowel, sinuses, pneumothorax, and endotracheal tube cuffs) and may affect intravenous infusion rates. The results of poor eating habits (hypoglycemia), sleep deprivation, and drugs (e.g., alcohol, marijuana, antihistamines) are potentiated by increasing altitude. Vibration can produce fatigue, and accelerating and decelerating forces can produce vertigo. Night vision is decreased at cabin altitudes above 5000 feet. The transport team should be adept at survival techniques for their region and should always be prepared to deal with an off-airport landing. Regular sessions to review safety and emergency procedures for each transport mode should be provided for the transport team members.

Referring Hospital Responsibilities

Transfer of patients from one institution to another is regulated by federal statute. The legislation that created the patient stabilization and transfer requirements for hospitals and physicians was the Consolidated Omnibus Budget Reconciliation Act (COBRA) of 1986, also known as the "antidumping law," and its amendment, the Omnibus Reconciliation Act of 1989.[50,51] This is the current legal standard. One of the main objectives of this resolution was to guarantee equal access to emergency treatment to all citizens regardless of their ability to pay. COBRA attributes responsibility for the patient's transfer to the referring hospital and physician. Violations can result in a number of penalties, including termination of Medicare privileges for the physician and hospital. A hospital can be fined between $25,000 and $50,000 per violation, and a physician can be fined $50,000 per violation. A patient can sue the hospital for personal injury in civil court. The Emergency Medical Treatment and Labor Act (EMTALA) established by the COBRA legislation governs how patients can be transferred from one hospital to another. Hospitals cannot transfer patients unless the transfer is "appropriate," the patient consents to transfer after being informed of the risks of transfer, and the referring physician certifies that the medical benefits expected from the transfer outweigh the risks. Appropriate transfers must meet the following criteria: (1) the transferring hospital must provide care and stabilization within its ability; (2) copies of medical records and imaging studies must accompany the patient; (3) the receiving facility must have available space and qualified personnel and agree to accept the transfer; and (4) the interfacility transport must be made by qualified personnel with the necessary equipment.

Emergent interfacility transport should occur after initial stabilization and determination by the referring facility that the patient's needs for definite care are beyond the scope of local capabilities. Transfer of the critically ill patient occurs with the expectation that appropriate care will continue en route to the receiving facility and that complications will be identified and treated. These goals frequently require specialized personnel and equipment. Coordination between referring and receiving institutions and medical direction during transport are fundamental to guarantee continuation of care and maximal utilization of resources. Interfacility transport can be performed by a transport team from the referring facility, the receiving facility, or a third party. It is the responsibility of the referring physician in consultation with the receiving physician to decide the best mode of transportation (air vs. ground) and to ensure that the transporting personnel have the necessary expertise and equipment to deal with the patient's condition and possible complications. For example, some out-of-hospital based personnel may not be trained in the use of certain hospital equipment (drug infusion pumps or other devices).

Complete documentation of all patient care records must be sent. This documentation includes results of all therapeutic and diagnostic interventions, copies of all imaging studies performed, and patient consent for transfer. Teleradiology has a role in allowing receiving centers to review a patient's studies prior to arrival. It is essential that the transport team establish direct communication with both referring and accepting physicians. Communication with the referring physician must detail the following information: (1) identification of the patient and medical history; (2) interventions performed during initial stabilization and patient's response; (3) pertinent physical examination findings; (4) ongoing therapy; and (5) potential complications that may occur during transport.

Conclusion

The current paradigm of transport must shift if we are to realize improved outcomes in the critically ill who require transport to a critical care center. We must abandon the current paradigm of "scoop and run" through a disjointed system as a means to initiating care upon arrival to the critical care center. We must adopt a system whereby goal-directed therapy begins in the prehospital arena and continues throughout the critical care continuum.

REFERENCES

1. Task Force on Interhospital Transport: *Guidelines for air and ground transport of neonatal and pediatric patients.* Elk Grove Village, IL, 1999, American Academy of Pediatrics.
2. Guidelines for pediatric equipment and supplies for emergency departments. Committee on pediatric equipment and supplies for emergency. *Ann Emerg Med* 31:54-57, 1998.
3. Seidel JS, Hornbein M, Yoshiyama K, et al: Emergency medical services and the pediatric patient: are the needs being met? *Pediatrics* 73:769-772, 1984.
4. Glaeser PW, Linzer J, Tunik MG, et al: Survey of nationally registered emergency medical services providers: pediatric education. *Ann Emerg Med* 36:33-38, 2000.
5. Seidel JS: A needs assessment of advanced life support and emergency medical services in the pediatric patient: state of the art. *Circulation* 74:129-173, 1986.
6. Seidel JS: Emergency medical services and the pediatric patient: are the needs being met? I. Training and equipping emergency medical services providers for pediatric emergencies. *Pediatrics* 78:808-812, 1986.
7. Ramenofsky ML, Luterman A, Quindlen E, et al: Maximum survival in pediatric trauma: the ideal system. *J Trauma* 24:818, 1984.
8. Babl FE, Vinci RJ, Bauchner H, et al: Pediatric prehospital advanced life support care in an urban setting. *Pediatr Emerg Care* 17:36-37, 2001.
9. Aijian P, Tsai A, Knopp R, et al: Endotracheal intubation of pediatric patients by paramedics. *Ann Emerg Med* 18:489-494, 1989.
10. Losek JD, Bonadio WA, Walsh-Kelly C, et al: Prehospital endotracheal intubation performance review. *Pediatr Emerg Care* 5:1, 1989.
11. Scribano PV, Baker MD, Holmes J, et al: Use of out-of-hospital interventions for the pediatric patient in an urban emergency medical services system. *Acad Emerg Med* 7:745-750, 2000.

12. Gausche M, Tadeo RE, Zane MC, et al: Out-of-hospital intravenous access: unnecessary procedures and excessive cost. *Acad Emerg Med* 5:878-882, 1998.
13. Mishark KJ, Vukov LF, Gudgell SF: Airway management and air medical transport. *J Air Med Transport* 11:7-9, 1992.
14. Boswell WC, McElveen N, Sharp M, et al: Analysis of prehospital pediatric and adult intubation. *Air Med J* 14:125-127, 1995
15. Doran JV, Tortella BJ, Drivet WJ, et al: Factors influencing successful intubation in the prehospital setting. *Prehosp Disaster Med* 10:259-264, 1995.
16. Su E, Schmidt TA, Mann NC, et al: A randomized controlled trial to assess decay in acquired knowledge among paramedics completing a pediatric resuscitation course. *Acad Emerg Med* 7:779-786, 2000.
17. Henderson DP: Education of paramedics in pediatric airway management effects of different retaining methods on self-efficacy and skill retention. *Acad Emerg Med* 171:429, 1998. (abstract).
18. Esposito TJ, Sanddal ND, Dean JM, et al: Analysis of preventable pediatric trauma deaths and inappropriate trauma. *J Trauma* 47:243-251, 1999.
19. Athey J, Dean JM, Ball J, et al: Ability of hospitals to care for pediatric emergency patients. *Pediatr Emerg Care* 17:170-174, 2001.
20. Harrison T, Thomas SH, Wedel SK: Interhospital aeromedical transports: air medical activation intervals in adult and pediatric trauma patients. *Am J Emerg Med* 15:122-124, 1997.
21. Lewis JK, Minter MG, Eshelman SJ, et al: Outcome of pediatric resuscitation. *Ann Emerg Med* 12:297-299, 1983.
22. Eisenburg M, Bergner L, Hallstrom A: Epidemiology of cardiac arrest and resuscitation in children. *Ann Emerg Med* 12:672-674, 1983.
23. Gregory GA: Respiratory care of the child. *Crit Care Med* 8: 582-587, 1980.
24. Hogg JC, Williams J, Richardson JB, et al: Age as factor in the distribution of lower airway conductance and in the pathologic anatomy of obstructive lung disease. *N Engl J Med* 282: 1283-1287, 1970.
25. Agostini E: Volume-pressure relationships of the thorax and lung in the newborn. *J Appl Physiol* 14:909-913, 1959.
26. Mansell A, Bryan C, Levison H: Airway closure in children. *J Appl Physiol* 33:711, 1972.
27. Guslits BG, Gaston SE, Bryan MH, et al: Diaphragmatic work of breathing in premature human infants. *J Appl Physiol* 62: 1410-1415, 1987.
28. Muller N, Volgyesi G, Bryan MH, et al: The consequences of diaphragmatic muscle fatigue in the newborn infant. *J Pediatr* 95:793-797, 1979.
29. Dunnill MS: The problem of lung growth. *Thorax* 37:561-563, 1968.
30. Macklem PT: Airway obstruction and collateral ventilation. *Physiol Rev* 51:368-436, 1971.
31. Bucci G, Cook C, Barrie H: Studies of respiratory physiology in children. *J Pediatr* 58:820, 1961.
32. *Pediatric advanced life support provider manual.* Dallas, 2002, American Heart Association.
33. Cowley RA, Hudson F, Scanlan E, et al: An economical and proved helicopter program for transporting the emergency critically ill and injured patient in Maryland. *J Trauma Injury Infect Crit Care* 13:1029-1038, 1973.
34. Quote. *Modern Hospital* 112:79-82, 1969.
35. National Academy of Sciences, National Research Council: Accidental death and dismemberment: the neglected disease of modern society. Washington, DC, 1966, The Council.
36. Eisenberg MS, Hallstrom AP, Copass MK, et al: Treatment of ventricular fibrillation: emergency medical technical defibrillation and paramedic services. *JAMA* 251:1723-1726, 1984.
37. Weaver WD, Copass MK, Bufi D, et al: Improved neurologic recovery and survival of early defibrillation. *Circulation* 69: 943-948, 1984.
38. Applebaum D: Advanced prehospital care for pediatric emergencies. *Ann Emerg Med* 14:656-659, 1985.
39. Chance GW, Matthew JD, Gash J, et al: Neonatal transport: a controlled study of skilled assistance. *J Pediatr* 93:662-666, 1978.
40. Macnab AJ: Optimal escort for interhospital transport of pediatric emergencies. *J Trauma* 31:205-209, 1991.
41. Edge WE, Kanter RK, Weigle CG, et al: Reduction of morbidity in interhospital transport by specialized pediatric staff. *Crit Care Med* 22:1186-1191, 1994
42. Bellingan G, Olivier T, Batson S, et al: Comparison of a specialist retrieval team with current United Kingdom practice for the transport of critically ill patients. *Intensive Care Med* 26:740-744, 2000.
43. Macnab AJ, Wensley DF, Sun C: Cost-benefit of trained transport teams: estimates for head-injured children. *Prehosp Emerg Care* 5:1-5, 2001.
44. Orr R, Venkataraman S, Seidberg N, et al: Pediatric specialty care teams are associated with reduced morbidity during pediatric interfacility transport. *Crit Care Med* 27:A30, 1999.
45. Rivers E, Nguyen B, Havstad S, et al: Early goal-directed therapy in the treatment of severe sepsis and septic shock. *N Engl J Med* 345:1368-1377, 2001.
46. Han YY, Carcillo JA, Dragotta MA, et al: Early reversal of pediatric-neonatal septic shock by community physicians is associated with improved outcome. *Pediatrics* 12:793-799, 2003.
47. Ehrenwerth J, Hackel A: Air-to-ground communication: a valuable aid in the transport of critically ill patients. *Crit Care Med* 14: 543-547, 1986.
48. *Accreditation standards of the Commission on Accreditation of Air Medical Services,* ed 5. Anderson SC, 2001, Commission on Accreditation of Air Medical Services.
49. Blumen IJ, Rodenberg H, editors: *Air medical physician handbook.* 1996, Air Medical Physician Association (AMPA).
50. Fell MJ: The Emergency Medical Treatment and Active Labor Act of 1986: providing protection from discrimination in access to emergency medical care. *Specialty Law Digest Health Care Law* 9-42, 1996.
51. Omnibus Budget Reconciliation Act of 1989, sec. 6018 42 USC 1395cc (West Supp. 1990).

CHAPTER 15

Pediatric Vascular Access and Centeses

Debra H. Fiser, James Graham, Jerril W. Green, Michele Moss, Patricia C. Wankum, Mark J. Heulitt, Audra Prince, Stephen M. Schexnayder, and Rhonda M. Dick

PEARLS

Intraosseous Infusion

- Intraosseous infusion is a convenient means of emergency vascular access, but efforts to obtain alternate means of vascular access should be pursued as soon as possible.
- A definite "give" is felt when the needle passes through the cortex of the bone, indicating passage of the needle into the marrow space. Usually, marrow can be aspirated when the needle is properly placed, but occasionally marrow is not aspirated even with proper placement.
- Vigilant observation of the needle insertion site is necessary to recognize extravasation. If extravasation occurs, the infusion must be discontinued.

Central Venous Line Placement

- The relative risk and benefit of catheter placement should be carefully considered prior to each procedure.
- The risk of infection is decreased by use of antibiotic-impregnated catheters, full barrier precautions at the time of placement, and careful aseptic technique when the line is accessed.
- Pneumothorax is less likely with careful patient positioning and attention to anatomic landmarks as the introducer needle is advanced.

Pulmonary Arterial Catheterization

- Pulmonary arterial (PA) catheters are placed either percutaneously or under direct surgical vision for direct measurement of pulmonary arterial pressure. A Swan-Ganz–type PA catheter also allows for direct measurement of the mixed venous oxygen saturation, cardiac output, right atrial or central venous pressure, and pulmonary capillary wedge pressure. Additionally, calculated values for oxygen delivery and vascular resistances can be made.
- Clinical indications for placement of a PA catheter include known or suspected pulmonary hypertension, shock that is unresponsive to standard therapy, and severe respiratory failure with hemodynamic compromise. The catheters can be placed and maintained safely in pediatric patients using the internal jugular, subclavian, or femoral veins for access. Complications have been reported but are relatively infrequent. Despite no outcome studies performed in pediatric patients showing improved outcome with PA catheter use, they are believed to be clinically useful in the situations defined.

Arterial Catheterization

- By allowing access to arterial blood for blood gas analysis and direct, continuous measurement of blood pressure, a transduced arterial catheter allows for immediate assessment of response to therapy directed at oxygen delivery and optimizing perfusion.

- Indications for placement of an arterial catheter are the following: need for frequent measurement of blood pressure, need for frequent sampling of arterial blood for laboratory analysis, need for monitoring of cerebral perfusion pressure, and need for rapid withdrawal of blood for therapeutic procedures.
- Contraindications to placement of an arterial catheter are the following: disruption of the integrity of the skin or evidence of infection at the site of insertion, inadequate collateral circulation, and compromised perfusion at the insertion site.
- Thromboembolic and ischemic complications frequently occur with endovascular procedures. Heparin decreases the risk of these adverse events. Hemorrhage and infection are other possible complications.
- After placement, arterial catheters should always be visible so that any bleeding can be immediately observed in addition to the catheters providing other routine maintenance.

Umbilical Arterial Catheter and Umbilical Venous Catheter Placement

- Infusion of fluids or medications may be warranted when an umbilical arterial catheter (UAC) is present, but placement of UAC is not indicated for infusions alone.
- UACs are commonly used in the care of severely ill neonates. They can serve as extremely valuable tools for the assessment and management of these infants, but their use is not without problems.
- The umbilical vein is catheterized for emergency fluid or medication administration.
- Umbilical venous catheters are more likely to cause complications if they are left in place for prolonged periods or if they are incorrectly positioned.

Pericardiocentesis

- Pericardiocentesis is drainage of fluid or air from the pericardial sac most commonly performed because of cardiac tamponade or for diagnosis of a pericardial effusion. A simple tap may be done, but for large or symptomatic effusions a catheter can be placed by Seldinger technique and left in place for continuous drainage.
- A subxiphoid approach is the most common. Guidance using echocardiography or fluoroscopy results in a safer, more successful procedure. Complications include cardiac perforation, coronary laceration, hemothorax or pneumothorax, and hemoperitoneum or pneumoperitoneum. Studies have shown that the procedure can be safely performed in pediatric patients.
- Causes of effusion include trauma, idiopathic pericarditis, infectious pericarditis, autoimmune pericarditis, and postpericardiotomy syndrome. Laboratory evaluation of the fluid can help determine the etiology.

Thoracentesis

- Ultrasound may facilitate loculated fluid localization.
- Thoracentesis risk is inversely related to the amount of fluid present.
- Uncooperative patients and mechanically ventilated patients increase the risk of pneumothorax.

Tube Thoracostomy

- Tube thoracostomy is required for ongoing removal of fluid or air.
- The fourth intercostal space is the usual location for tube thoracostomy.
- Liberal local anesthesia can reduce sedation and analgesic requirements.
- Needle-dilator systems allow placement of the tube with less dissection of the chest wall.
- Tubes can be safely removed when an air leak has resolved (for pneumothorax) or tube drainage is less than 3 ml/kg/day for freely flowing effusions.

Diagnostic Paracentesis

- Paracentesis is a relatively safe procedure that is a useful diagnostic tool in the evaluation of the patient with ascites.
- Ultrasound guidance may improve the safety and efficacy of paracentesis because ultrasonography can detect small amounts of fluid and differentiate free from loculated fluid.
- Use of the Z-track method of needle insertion is recommended to avoid a direct linear needle track and to minimize persistent leakage of ascitic fluid following paracentesis.
- Laboratory analysis of ascitic fluid should be guided by clinical assessment to identify the most likely diagnosis.

Intraosseous Access

Venous access in critically ill infants and children can be one of the most challenging aspects of their care. Peripheral veins in infants can be particularly difficult to cannulate, particularly in the event of shock with shunting of blood away from the periphery and collapse of small veins. Because of these challenges, intraosseous infusion has become widely accepted as a quick, reliable means to establish short-term, emergency venous access.

Intraosseous infusion was first described in 1922[11] and became widely used in the 1930s and 1940s.[21,51] With the development of disposable needles and catheters, use of intraosseous infusion fell out of favor. It was not commonly used again until the mid 1980s, when a series of publications demonstrated the utility of the technique for rapid venous access in critically ill children.[3,34,52,53]

The marrow space provides a noncollapsible access point to the vascular system. Marrow sinusoids drain into medullary venous channels that empty into the systemic circulatory system. Because of the noncollapsible nature of the marrow space and the direct connection to the venous circulation, fluids and medications infused into the marrow space are distributed rapidly through the venous circulation.

Indications

Intraosseous infusion is indicated in situations requiring the rapid acquisition of intravenous (IV) access in which the establishment of conventional peripheral access is difficult or impossible. The situations in which it is used most often include cardiopulmonary arrest, shock, burns, and status epilepticus. In these situations, one or two attempts at standard peripheral access usually are made prior to placing an intraosseous needle. In addition to its use in the hospital, intraosseous access has been successful in the prehospital setting.[1,18,44,46,48]

The success rate with the technique is high, greater than 95% with experienced practitioners.[33] Most fluids and medications that can be given through a conventional IV line can be given via an intraosseous infusion with comparable results. In the event of cardiac arrest or severe shock, intraosseous access is at least as effective as peripheral venous access in providing fluids and medications to the central circulation.[4,12,17,23,24,27,32,33,36,45,49,50] Studies have shown that commonly used resuscitation, antiepileptic, and antibiotic drugs all can be given effectively through an intraosseous line.[4,12,17,24,27,32,36,45,49,50] Three antibiotics produce subtherapeutic levels when given via an intraosseus line at standard IV doses: chloramphenicol, vancomycin, and tobramycin.[24]

In addition to the administration of fluids and medications, intraosseous access can be used for certain clinical laboratory studies. No significant differences were found when comparing electrolytes, chemistries, pH, pCO_2, or hemoglobin from intraosseous marrow specimen with either arterial or venous blood samples.[28,37] A marrow specimen can be cultured in lieu of a blood culture.[37] Finally, the marrow can be used for blood type and cross-matching.[7]

Contraindications

Intraosseous infusion has few absolute contraindications. A fractured or previously punctured bone should not be used because infused fluid will extravasate and possibly cause compartment syndrome. Alternate sites in other bones can be used in such situations. Bone diseases such as osteogenesis imperfecta and osteopetrosis have been suggested as contraindications to intraosseous infusion,[22,14] but a case of successful intraosseous access in a patient with osteogenesis imperfecta has been reported.[33] Placing the needle into an area of cellulitis or burn could cause osteomyelitis or other infectious complications and is a relative contraindication.

Supplies and Equipment

Access to the bone marrow space is accomplished with one of several different types of needles. Conventional bone marrow needles (Jamshidi, Illinois) work well. Needles made specifically for intraosseous infusion use are available, including a straight needle (Cook) or a needle with a threaded screw device (SurFast). Usually a 15- or 18-gauge needle is chosen. The smaller 18-gauge should be used in infants. Studies have shown no significant differences in time required to insert the needle, success rate, or extravasation rates between standard and threaded intraosseous needles.[20,25,30] If bone marrow or intraosseous needles are not available, standard lumbar puncture needles can be used,[33] although they are prone to bending without the plastic sheath present on standard bone marrow needles. In neonates, even a 19- or 21-gauge butterfly needle can be used.[10,33] Needles with a stylet are preferred to prevent clogging of the needle by bone.

Other equipment required for intraosseous placement includes a towel or sandbag, syringes with saline or heparinized saline flush solution, IV fluid and tubing, a T-connector or stopcock, and antiseptic prep solution (iodine). Optional supplies include a pressure bag and materials for local anesthesia (syringe with 25-gauge needle and 1% lidocaine).

Technique

The intraosseous needle can be placed into the bone marrow at one of several sites, including the proximal tibia, distal femur, distal tibia, iliac crest, and sternum. The proximal tibia is the site most commonly chosen. The sternum has been used in adults but should be avoided in children because of the possibility of perforating the pediatric chest cavity.[40,41] In addition, placing the needle in the sternum can interfere with airway and circulatory resuscitative efforts.

When the needle is placed in the proximal tibia, the insertion site is located by palpation on the flat anterior tibial surface 1 to 3 cm (two fingers breadth) distal to the tibial tuberosity (Figure 15–1). This site is chosen to avoid the proximal growth plate. The midshaft should not be used because of increased risk for fracture. Placing a towel or sandbag under the child's leg helps stabilize the leg and makes insertion easier. The skin overlying the area should be prepped with antiseptic solution.

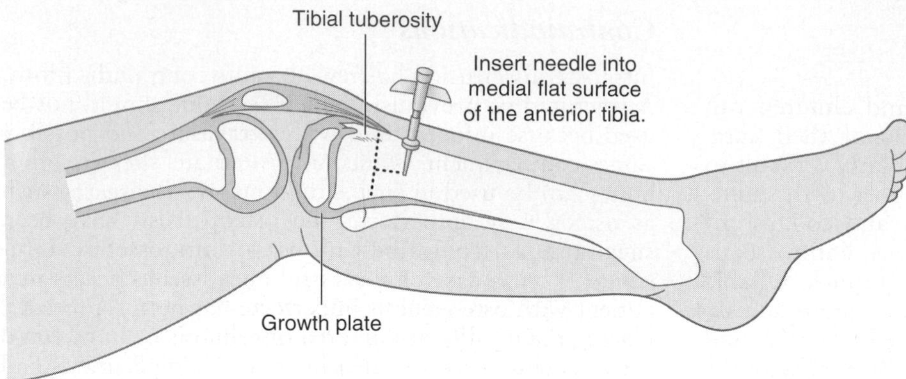

FIGURE 15–1 • Insertion of the intraosseous needle into the anterior tibia.

Because intraosseous lines usually are placed in obtunded patients, local anesthetic often is not necessary. Local anesthesia by infiltration with 1% lidocaine can be performed if the patient is awake. If a needle with a plastic sheath is being used, adjust the sheath so that an adequate length of needle protrudes beyond the sheath. Some authors have suggested inserting the needle at a 60- to 75-degree angle away from the tibial growth plate, but others recommend using a perpendicular or 90-degree angle. The perpendicular angle helps prevent the needle from sliding along the bone. The needle is advanced using firm pressure and a twisting or rotary motion until a "give" or loss of resistance is felt, indicating entry into the marrow space. The force needed to penetrate the bony cortex is considerable; the twisting motion helps significantly in needle insertion. One disadvantage of using a threaded needle is that the "give" or loss of resistance that occurs when the needle enters the marrow space may not be felt, but the needle may be more secure in the bone once the needle is placed.[25] The stylet is removed and a syringe is attached to the needle to attempt to aspirate marrow. Correct placement of the needle should be confirmed to avoid extravasation. Aspiration of bloody fluid into the syringe confirms that the needle is correctly placed. Additional evidence of correct needle placement includes the observation that the needle stands upright in the bone without support and lack of resistance when flush solution is infused into the needle with the syringe. Sometimes, marrow cannot be aspirated even if the needle is correctly placed. If the "give" is felt on insertion and the needle stands alone in the bone but marrow cannot be aspirated, infusion of a small amount of fluid with the syringe can be attempted. Fluid should infuse easily with little pressure and without noticeable swelling of the soft tissues or extravasation of fluid.

When the needle is placed in the distal femur, it should be placed approximately 2 to 3 cm proximal to the patella in the midline. In the distal tibia, the needle is placed 1 cm proximal to the medial malleolus in the midline posterior to the saphenous vein. The proximal tibia usually is selected in children younger than 4 years, but the distal tibia has been recommended in older children in whom the proximal tibial cortex is thicker.

Maintenance

Once correct placement of the needle is confirmed, fluids and medication can be administered with a syringe via a stopcock or T-connector, or a standard IV infusion set can be connected to the needle. The needle is secured using gauze pads and tape. Some have suggested taping a clear plastic cup over the needle to help prevent dislodgment.[33] The site should be observed carefully visually and by palpation for signs of extravasation, both immediately after placement and frequently (every 5–10 minutes) during use. If evidence of extravasation is seen, the needle should be removed to avoid compartment syndrome. If needle placement is attempted at one site and the cortex is penetrated but the line cannot be used because of extravasation, another bone must be chosen for subsequent attempts.

Intraosseous access is intended only for short-term use in emergency resuscitative situations; long-term use increases the risk of extravasation, compartment syndrome, and infection.[2,38,43] Therefore once intraosseous access is secured, efforts should be directed toward obtaining conventional IV access. Once alternate access is obtained, the intraosseous needle should be removed, manual pressure applied for 5 minutes, and a dressing applied to the site. Some authors have suggested administering a course of antistaphylococcal antibiotics to patients who have an intraosseous line.[13]

Complications

Complications of intraosseous infusion are rare. The most common complication is extravasation of fluid. The causes of extravasation include incomplete penetration of the bony cortex, movement of the needle such that the hole is larger than the needle, dislodgment of the needle, penetration of the posterior cortex, and leakage of fluid through another hole in the bone, such as a previous IO site or fracture. Extravasation of small amounts of fluid usually is not problematic, but compartment syndrome may result after extravasation.[9,16,19,31,41,47,54,55] One report documented a compartment syndrome after infusion of only 35 ml of fluid via the intraosseous line.[41] Use of the intraosseous line for prolonged periods and use of the intraosseous line with pressure infusion appear to be risk factors for compartment syndrome. Compartment syndrome associated with intraosseous infusion can result in the need for fasciotomy and amputation. Careful frequent observation of the intraosseous site is necessary to detect extravasation and to prevent compartment syndrome. If extravasation occurs, the needle should be removed and the extremity observed for signs of compartment syndrome.

Other rare complications include infection and bone fracture. Osteomyelitis, cellulitis, and sepsis have been reported in conjunction with intraosseous infusion.[2,38,43] Risk for infection is increased when intraosseous access is used in a bacteremic patient and when the line is used for a prolonged period. The risk of osteomyelitis is small (<1%).[38] Although intraosseous access usually is obtained in emergency situations, precautions to prevent infection should be taken, including use of sterile gloves and equipment and preparation of the skin with antiseptic solution (iodine or alcohol). Fracture of the bone has been reported.[29,35] One report of fracture associated with intraosseous infusion is the case of a 3-month-old in whom a 15-gauge needle was used; smaller needle size (18 gauge) should be used in small infants.

There are some theoretical complications that probably are not significant in clinical practice. Fat embolism occurs with infusion into the bone marrow space. An animal study found fat emboli in the lung with intraosseous infusion, but no changes were seen in oxygen saturation or intrapulmonary shunt.[35] Another animal study in a cardiac arrest model found fat emboli in the lungs in pigs that underwent cardiopulmonary resuscitation, but use of an intraosseous line did not increase the magnitude of fat embolization.[13] There are no reports of clinical fat embolization associated with intraosseous infusion in humans in the English literature. Because of the risk of fat embolization, children with a right-to-left shunt may be at increased risk for cerebral emboli with intraosseous infusion.[33]

The physical effects of infusion on the growing bone seem to be self-limited. Both animal studies and human follow-up studies of the bone and bone marrow show only short-term, minor changes and no long-term changes in bone structure, growth, or bone marrow.[5,6,8,15,39]

Closing Remarks

Intraosseous infusion is a valuable means of obtaining temporary, emergency vascular access in the critically ill infant or child. It has a high success rate and is associated with rare complications. Complications usually can be prevented by using appropriate technique and vigilantly monitoring the site for extravasation.

Central Venous Line Placement

Central venous catheters are among the most important and frequently used tools in the pediatric intensive care unit (PICU). Intensivists must be expert in their placement and use. The need for central access should be anticipated so that circumstances surrounding the procedure, such as sterile technique and the patient's safety and comfort, can be optimized.

Indications and Contraindications

Indications for central venous lines (CVLs) include the need for reliable and durable venous access for administration of vasoactive infusions, TPN, and other medications requiring central vascular access. Frequent blood sampling and measurement of central venous pressure are common indications. Central venous access is required for emergency hemodialysis, continuous venovenous hemofiltration, and plasmapheresis. Central venous catheters also reduce the need for repeated attempts at peripheral venous access.

Contraindications to central access are not absolute and are primarily related to specific sites of catheter placement. In the presence of increased bleeding risk, sites where bleeding may be difficult to control, such as the subclavian, should be avoided if possible. In patients with significant intraabdominal or pelvic trauma, femoral catheters may pose increased risk. Bacteremia present at the time of catheter placement likely will colonize to central venous catheters. Catheters should not be inserted through obviously infected skin. The relative risk and benefit of catheter placement should be carefully considered before each procedure.[58,59]

Technique

Critically ill pediatric patients vary greatly in size. Appropriate catheters for CVL placement in all of these patients should be readily available. In acutely ill patients requiring central access for a relatively short period (days to weeks), plastic polymer catheters are commonly used. These catheters are available in a variety of diameters, lumen number, and length. They can be packaged with appropriate-size introducer needles, guidewires, and vessel dilators, along with other needed equipment such as local anesthetic, skin cleanser, drapes, and suture for securing the catheter. Currently available antibiotic-impregnated catheters may decrease the risk of catheter-related bloodstream infection.[56]

Adequate sedation and analgesia not only provide patient comfort during the procedure but also make the procedure easier and safer with less patient movement (see Chapter 116). Agents with rapid onset and short duration of action, such as midazolam, propofol, and ketamine, are ideal. Even with sedation, local anesthesia should be used to reduce pain and the depth of sedation needed for a patient to be comfortable and still.

Full barrier precautions should be used whenever a CVL is placed in the PICU and should include hair cover, mask, careful handwashing, sterile gown and gloves, a large area of skin prepped with antiseptic solution, and a draped sterile field large enough to eliminate the possibility of inadvertent contamination of equipment and sterile surfaces. This technique, when properly applied, has been shown to decrease the risk of catheter-related infection.[60]

The majority of CVLs placed in the PICU are placed using the Seldinger technique.[63] This technique is essentially the same regardless of the site used. An introducer needle is placed in the desired vein while aspirating with a syringe. When the lumen of the needle is fully within the lumen of the vein, blood flows freely into the syringe. The needle should be held in place with one hand while the syringe is disconnected with the other hand. The rate at which blood passively flows from the open needle hub is dependent upon the gauge of the needle and the venous pressure; however, it should not be obviously pulsatile. A J-tipped guidewire is inserted into the open hub of the needle and advanced into the vein (Figure 15–2, *A*). The wire should meet little or no resistance as it is advanced. If resistance is met, attempts to advance the wire should cease. The position of the needle should be adjusted, by either advancing or withdrawing slightly or changing the angle of entry. The wire can be carefully withdrawn and the syringe reattached to the needle in order to reidentify the lumen of the vein. If resistance is met while withdrawing the wire, the needle and wire should be withdrawn as a unit rather than risk breaking or cutting the wire. Once the guidewire is well within the lumen of the vein, a small incision is made adjacent to the needle to enlarge the puncture site to more easily accommodate the dilator and catheter. Next, the introducer needle is carefully withdrawn along the wire holding the wire completely stationary. A dilator of appropriate size is advanced along the wire into the puncture far enough to dilate all tissue planes into the lumen of the vein. The dilator is withdrawn, and the desired catheter is advanced into position along the wire (Figure 15–2, *B*). The guidewire is removed, leaving the catheter in place. Blood should be easily aspirated from all lumens. Each lumen should be filled with sterile saline or heparinized saline to prevent thrombosis.

Several systems for securing catheters are commercially available. The most common technique uses silk suture. A large loop of suture should be placed in the skin, attached through the wings of the catheter hub, and tied tightly enough to prevent catheter movement but not so tightly as to cause necrosis of the skin within the loop of suture material (Figure 15–2, *C*).

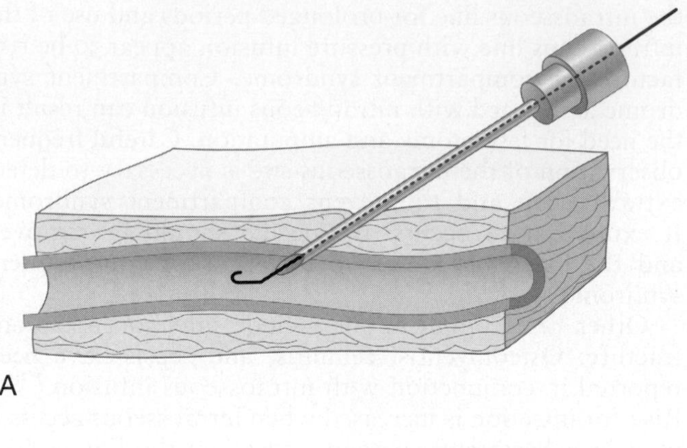

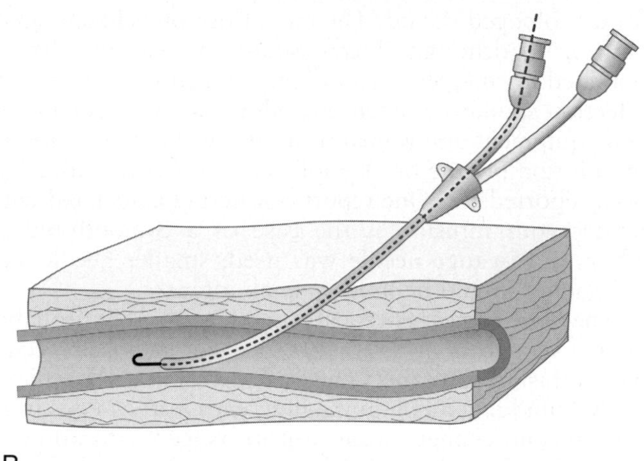

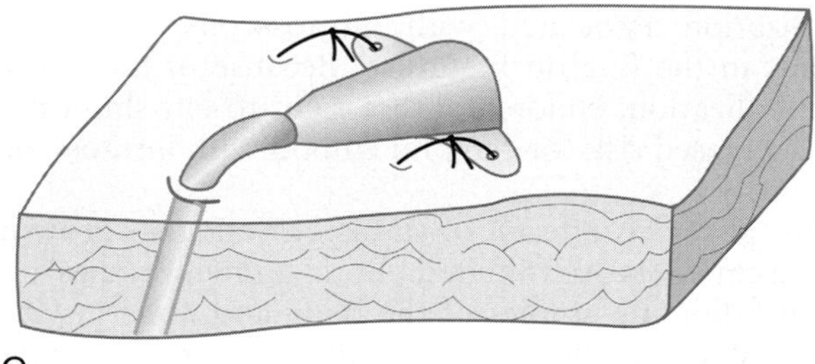

FIGURE 15–2 • **A,** Guidewire is placed through the introducer needle into the lumen of the vein. **B,** Catheter is advanced into the vein lumen along the guidewire. **C,** Hub of the catheter is secured to the skin with suture.

Internal Jugular Vein Cannulation

Multiple approaches can be used to cannulate the internal jugular vein. For each of these approaches, the patient is supine in slight Trendelenburg position, with a roll of bed linen under the shoulders to extend the neck and the face turned to the contralateral side. The middle or low approach is most commonly used (Figure 15–3, *A*). The introducer needle enters the skin at the apex of the triangle formed by the clavicle and the heads of the sternocleidomastoid muscle at a 30-degree angle to the skin directed toward the ipsilateral nipple. For the anterior approach, the introducer needle enters the skin along the anterior margin of the sternocleidomastoid halfway between the mastoid process and the sternum and is directed at the ipsilateral nipple (Figure 15–3, *B*). Using the posterior approach, the needle enters the skin along the posterior border of the sternocleidomastoid halfway between the mastoid process and the clavicle and is directed toward the sternal notch[57] (Figure 15–3, *C*).

Subclavian Vein Cannulation

Place the patient supine in a slight Trendelenburg position. A narrow roll of bed linen is placed beneath the patient between the shoulders. The introducer needle enters the skin inferior to the junction of the middle and lateral third of the clavicle and is directed toward the suprasternal notch. The needle passes slightly inferior to the clavicle and enters the subclavian vein[57] (Figure 15–4).

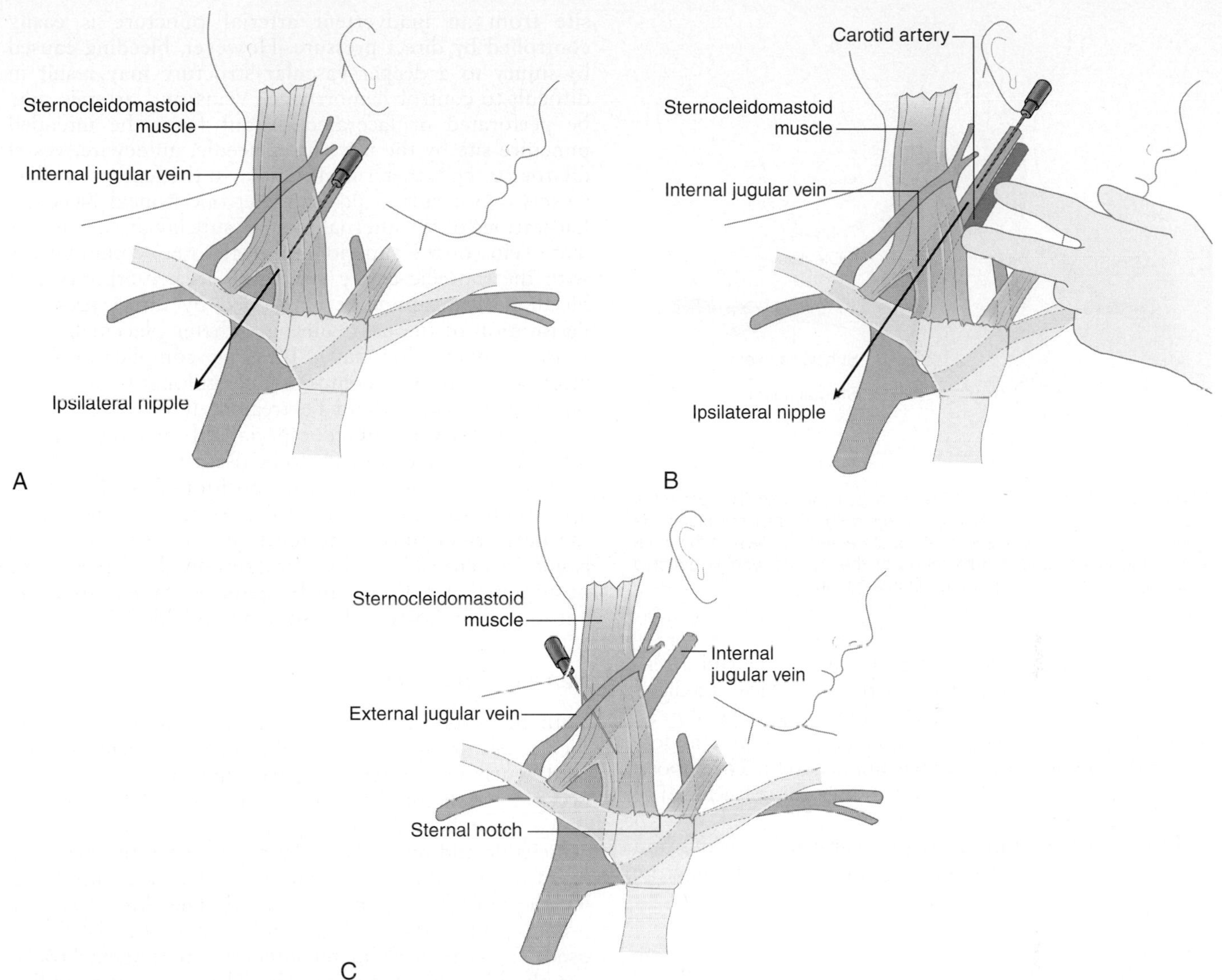

FIGURE 15–3 • Approaches to the internal jugular vein. The patient is supine, in slight Trendelenburg position, with the neck extended over a shoulder roll and the head rotated away from the side of the approach. **A,** Middle approach. The introducer needle enters at the apex of the triangle formed by the heads of the sternocleidomastoid muscle and the clavicle and is directed toward the ipsilateral nipple at an angle of approximately 30 degrees with the skin. **B,** Anterior approach. The carotid pulse is palpated and may be slightly retracted medially. The introducer needle enters along the anterior margin of the sternocleidomastoid about halfway between the sternal notch and the mastoid process and is directed toward the ipsilateral nipple. **C,** Posterior approach. The introducer needle enters at the point where the external jugular vein crosses the posterior margin of the sternocleidomastoid and is directed under its heads toward the sternal notch.

Femoral Vein Cannulation

The patient is placed in a supine position either flat or in slight reverse Trendelenburg position. A pad of bed linen is placed under the hips to slightly raise them off the bed surface. The leg on the side of catheter placement is slightly abducted and externally rotated. The femoral artery pulse is palpated just distal to the inguinal ligament about halfway between the anterior iliac crest and the pubic symphysis. The femoral vein is approximately 5 mm medial to the femoral artery in infants and toddlers and approximately 10 mm in adolescents and adults. The introducer needle enters the skin 1 to 2 cm distal to the inguinal ligament at an approximately 30-degree angle with the skin surface and in line with the course of the vein, approximately parallel to the axis of the thigh[57] (Figure 15–5).

Complications

The risk of bloodstream infection is significantly increased by the presence of a central venous catheter. The increased risk is true for all catheter locations and increases with the total number of catheter days. Routine changing of uninfected catheters either over a guidewire or to a different anatomic site does not change the risk. Coagulase-negative staphylococci, *Enterococcus* species, *Staphylococcus aureus, Enterobacter* species, and *Candida* species account for the majority of infections. The risk of infection is decreased by use of antibiotic-impregnated catheters, full barrier precautions at the time of placement, and careful aseptic technique when the line is accessed.[56,60]

Pneumothorax may result if the lung is punctured during internal jugular or subclavian placement. This complication

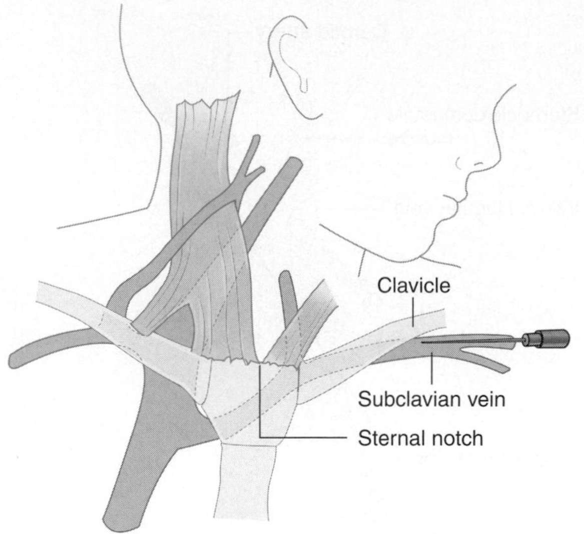

FIGURE 15–4 • Approach to the subclavian vein. The patient is supine, in slight Trendelenburg position, with a small roll along the spine between the shoulders. The needle enters the skin at the junction of the lateral and middle thirds of the clavicle and is directed toward the sternal notch in the horizontal plane.

is less likely with careful patient positioning and attention to anatomic landmarks as the introducer needle is advanced. Chest radiography should be performed after an internal jugular or subclavian catheter is attempted to document that a pneumothorax has not occurred. Thrombosis may occur in the vessel surrounding the catheter. The catheter lumen may become thrombosed.

Bleeding at the time of placement can be serious and potentially life threatening. Bleeding at the skin puncture site from an inadvertent arterial puncture is easily controlled by direct pressure. However, bleeding caused by injury to a deeper vascular structure may result in difficult-to-control hemorrhage. Veins and arteries may be perforated or lacerated distant from the intended puncture site by the introducer needle, guidewire, vessel dilator, or the catheter itself. Injury to the femoral or iliac vessels may result in pelvic or retroperitoneal bleeding. Lacerations of the internal jugular, subclavian, or innominate veins or the superior vena cava may communicate with the thoracic cavity and result in hemothorax and bleeding that cannot be controlled by direct pressure. Perforation of the heart during catheter placement may cause cardiac tamponade. Bleeding complications are more severe in the presence of a coagulopathy or thrombocytopenia and should be treated, if possible, before central access is attempted, especially if the internal jugular and subclavian sites are to be used.[62,65]

A central venous catheter positioned such that it applies pressure to the wall of the vessel or to the wall of the heart risks causing perforation. This situation may result in acute blood loss or tamponade. Undesirable positioning of a CVL can be detected radiographically and should be corrected as soon as possible.[62,65]

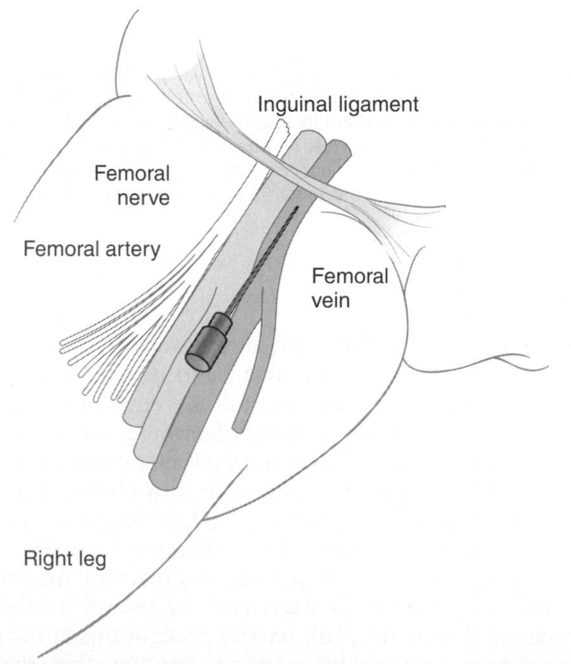

FIGURE 15–5 • Approach to the femoral vein. The patient is flat and supine, with the thigh slightly abducted and externally rotated. The introducer needle enters the skin 2 to 3 cm distal to the inguinal ligament and 0.5 to 1 cm medial to the pulse of the femoral artery.

Venous Cutdown

With the widespread use of central venous access and the use of intraosseous access during emergencies, venous cutdown is less commonly performed. However, it is a necessary skill for the pediatric intensivist. Venous cutdown is indicated when percutaneous access is not achievable and the need for IV access warrants the more invasive procedure. Materials needed depend upon the technique of vein cannulation used. The skin should be prepped and draped, and sterile technique should be used. The skin overlying the intended site is opened transversely with respect to the vein. The tissue surrounding the vein is bluntly dissected to completely expose the vein. Ligatures are passed around the vein distal and proximal to the intended site of cannulation. A small venotomy is created and, using the ligatures to control the vein, a catheter is directly passed into the lumen of the vein. The distal ligature can be tightened to control bleeding and the proximal ligature to help secure the catheter (Figure 15–6). Alternatively, an over-the-needle IV catheter can be directly introduced into the exposed vein without creating the venotomy or using ligatures. An introducer needle and then a guidewire can be inserted into the lumen of the vein for Seldinger technique placement. The latter approach is particularly useful for femoral venous cutdown. After the catheter is in place, it is secured with suture material and the wound is closed around the catheter.

The complications of venous cutdown are similar to the complications of other venous access techniques. The risk of bleeding from the open wound should be considered, especially in patients with increased risk for bleeding (anticoagulation or other coagulopathy). The open wound also increases the risk of infection. Injury to adjacent structures, such as arteries and nerves, during incision and blunt dissection is a risk with cutdown.[57,61,64]

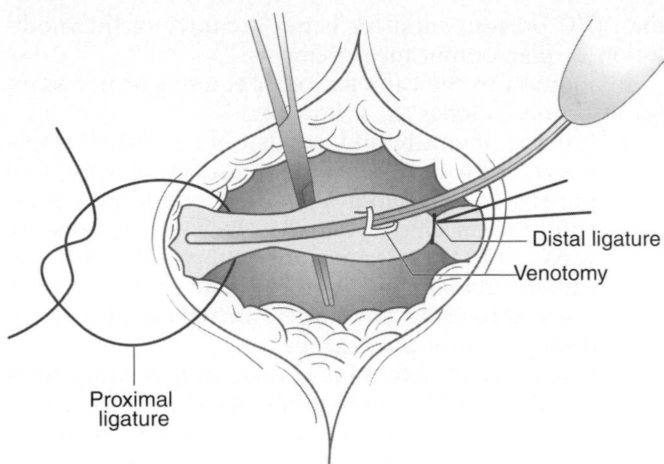

FIGURE 15–6 • Venous cutdown.

Pulmonary Arterial Catheterization

Measurement of pulmonary arterial (PA) pressure at the bedside can be performed using either a single lumen catheter placed directly into the pulmonary artery at the time of cardiac surgery or a balloon-tipped, flow-directed catheter that can be placed at the bedside. Both techniques are used in pediatric patients, but the single-lumen catheter is especially used because of the frequency of pulmonary hypertension complicating the postoperative management of pediatric cardiac patients. The flow-directed, balloon-tipped catheter introduced by Swan and Ganz in the early 1970s has found utilization in pediatric patients but is not as widespread as in adult patients.[77,79,81]

The PA catheter has evolved over the years from the original flexible construction, single-lumen, 6F balloon-tipped catheter to one that houses at least two lumens, often more, with ports for pressure monitoring or delivery of fluids and a thermistor at the tip. It may contain fiberoptic spectrophotometry for continuous measurement of mixed venous oxygen saturation. The basic PA catheter with a thermistor is available as small as 5F for pediatric patients. The catheter diameter, catheter length, and distance between monitoring ports may vary. When in proper position with the tip in the pulmonary artery, the catheter allows direct measurement of PA pressure, right atrial or central venous pressure, and pulmonary arterial occlusion pressure (PAOP), often called the *pulmonary capillary wedge pressure.* Catheters with thermistors allow for direct measurement of cardiac output using the thermodilution technique. From these measurements, multiple calculations pertaining to oxygen delivery and vascular resistance can be made (see Chapter 19).

Indications

Routinely accepted indications for placement of a PA catheter in pediatric patients are (1) pulmonary hypertension, either primary or secondary, including potential pulmonary hypertension in postoperative congenital cardiac patients; (2) severe shock unresponsive to fluid resuscitation and low-dose vasoactive infusions; and (3) severe respiratory failure requiring high positive airway pressure with associated hemodynamic compromise.[15] However, no studies of pediatric patients are available showing improved outcomes when a PA catheter, single-lumen, or Swan-Ganz type was used.

Use of PA catheters in patients with known or potential pulmonary hypertension probably is the most common indication because of the prevalence of pulmonary hypertension in various congenital heart defects, such as truncus arteriosus and complete atrioventricular canal defects. Postoperatively these patients are prone to wide swings in PA pressures associated with variations in oxygenation, ventilation, and even sedation.[71,73,76,83] Additionally, when nitric oxide is used for management of postoperative pulmonary hypertension, direct measurement of PA pressure helps guide therapy.[66]

In shock states, especially septic shock, the hemodynamic profile can be variable and not consistent with the physical examination. Use of a PA catheter in such situations helps to better define the hemodynamic profile, thus allowing more specific therapy. One study by Carcillo et al.[69] showed that patients in septic shock with insufficient fluid resuscitation measured having PAOP less than 8 mmHg. Reynolds et al.[78] also noted in pediatric burn patients with shock that information obtained from a PA catheter contributed to changes in therapy because left ventricular dysfunction was recognized.[78]

With severe respiratory failure, use of high ventilatory pressures can compromise cardiac output. PA catheters have helped to diagnose the cause of low cardiac output in this group of patients and helped to direct therapy. When oxygen delivery in these patients is significantly limited because of hypoxemia, low cardiac output, or both, measurement of oxygen delivery using variables derived from information provided by the catheter may be useful.[72] No studies in pediatric patients have demonstrated better outcomes with the use of the PA catheter.

Contraindications

There are no specific known contraindications to placement of a Swan-Ganz catheter, but there are several relative contraindications, including (1) bleeding diathesis, which makes percutaneous catheter placement risky; (2) severe tricuspid or pulmonary insufficiency, which can make bedside catheter placement prohibitively difficult; and (3) cardiac arrhythmias that are unstable and easily triggered by catheter manipulation. Catheter placement for measurement of cardiac output using the thermodilution technique is contraindicated when in the presence of intracardiac shunts, tricuspid insufficiency, or pulmonary insufficiency. These conditions make the thermodilution measurement inaccurate.

Procedure

Placement of the Swan-Ganz–type PA catheter can be performed percutaneously at the bedside without fluoroscopy. Single-lumen PA catheters are most commonly placed by the surgeon at the time of cardiac surgery in the operating room.

Equipment

Choosing the most appropriate size and type catheter often is difficult because a variety of balloon-tipped, flow-directed catheters are available on the market. At least three major catheter companies make multiple variations of the catheter. Catheters are available with two diameters, 5F and 7F. The 5F-diameter catheter is most appropriate for patients weighing less than 15 kg, and the 7F-diameter catheter is best for patients weighing more than 15 kg. The 5F catheter is available with four channels: (1) proximal "injectate" lumen, which also is used for monitoring right atrial or central venous pressure; (2) distal lumen for measuring PA pressure and PAOP; (3) distal thermistor for cardiac output measurement; and (4) lumen for inflating the balloon for flow direction and occlusion of distal pulmonary arteries. The 7F catheters are available with the same four channels but can additionally have a fifth channel for other uses: (1) a second right atrial port to use as an additional infusion port, (2) fiberoptic oxygen saturation sensor for continuous measurement of mixed venous oxygen saturation, (3) electrodes for measuring right ventricular and PA intracardiac R waves to measure beat-to-beat blood temperature changes, and (4) ventricular endocardial pacing electrode.

The distance between the proximal and distal ports is variable, depending on the catheter. The standards are 10, 15, 20, and 30 cm. This distance can be customized for pediatric patients. In 1986 Borland[68] determined the distance between the right atrium and the pulmonary artery in 61 pediatric patients. These data can be used as a reasonable estimate of the appropriate distance when determining which size catheter to use (Figure 15–7). Using the correct distance is crucial in order to monitor the appropriate pressure, for example, right atrial rather than IVC pressure, and for better accuracy of thermodilution cardiac output measurements.

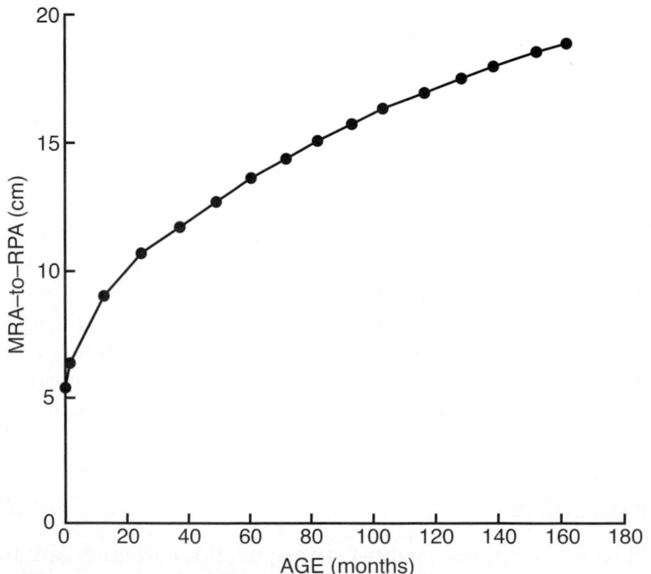

FIGURE 15–7 • MRA-to-RPA (cm) = 1.504 + 0.156 × length − 0.117 × SSSP, where MRA = mid right atrium, RPA = right pulmonary artery, and SSSP = suprasternal to suprapubic distance. (From Borland LM: *Crit Care Med* 14:974-976, 1986.)

In addition to the catheter, other equipment necessary for insertion includes the following:

1. Cardiac monitor and compatible pressure transducers with the ability to transduce at least two pressures. This setup allows for continuous pressure measurement and assessment of pressure waves during insertion and afterward while the catheter remains in place. Cardiac rhythm can be assessed to detect any cardiac arrhythmias occurring during or after placement.
2. Computer to determine cardiac output using thermodilution. Most commonly, the computer is contained as part of the cardiac monitor, but it can also be a freestanding device.
3. Percutaneous introducer sheath with bleedback device to prevent bleeding around the catheter. The introducer can be placed in a vein using the Seldinger technique, then the catheter can be passed through the introducer sheath.
4. Equipment for placing the introducer sheath including povidone-iodine or chlorhexidine for skin preparation, 1% lidocaine for local analgesia with appropriate-size needles and syringes for injection, sterile drapes, introducer needle, guidewire, no. 11 scalpel, slip-tip syringe, sheath dilator, hemostasis valve with side port (depending on brand and size may be part of introducer sheath), catheter sleeve, silk suture, and dressing material. This equipment may be part of an introducer sheath kit or can be assembled separately. All of the equipment must be sterile. The sizes of the introducer needle and guidewire must be appropriate for the size of the patient and the size of the end hole of the sheath dilator. If the equipment is not part of a kit, the wires, needle, and dilator should be checked prior to accessing the vein to ensure they are compatible.
5. Fluid to flush the introducer sheath, catheter, and transducer system. Usually this fluid is normal saline with 1 U heparin added per milliliter of fluid.
6. Optional equipment includes carbon dioxide to inflate the balloon to minimize the risk of air embolization and ability to cool the fluid to be used for injectate. Most commonly room air is used to inflate the balloon.

Technique

The site of access to the vein is determined by the size and medical condition of the patient, the accessibility of the vein, and the skill of the operator. The most commonly used sites are femoral veins, internal jugular veins, and subclavian veins. Any of these sites allows passage of the catheter from the venous system into the right atrium, right ventricle, and ultimately the pulmonary artery. Catheter manipulation is minimized when using the right femoral vein, right internal jugular vein, or left subclavian vein. Although the other veins at these locations can be used, more manipulation of the catheter is necessary and may prolong the procedure.

The site is sterilely prepared with povidone-iodine or chlorhexidine solution and draped with sterile towels and sheets. A wide area of the bed should be barrier draped because of the length of the catheter and sterile pressure tubing. The area surrounding the vein is infiltrated with 1% lidocaine. The vein is accessed using the Seldinger technique, and the introducer sheath is placed in the vein. The sheath has a device with a diaphragm to prevent bleeding back from the sheath and a side port to allow continuous fluid infusion to prevent clot formation. This device may be attached to the sheath or it may be separate. Once the sheath is in place, both the sheath and the side port are aspirated and flushed with fluid to remove air bubbles and clots. Fluid then can be infused through the side port.

The PA catheter is prepared for insertion by flushing all fluid lumens with heparin-containing fluid and inflating the balloon to detect leakage or breakage of the balloon. The thermistor should be tested by connecting it to the computer module that will record a room temperature reading. The length of the catheter from the insertion site to the right atrium can be estimated by laying the catheter on the patient along the course of the vein to the right atrium. The catheter then is ready for insertion. A sterile sleeve is placed on the end of the sheath and the catheter is passed through the sleeve, through the diaphragm and into the sheath. The distal port of the catheter is connected by high-pressure tubing and a pressure transducer to the pressure monitor so that a continuous readout of the pressure contour is visible on the cardiac monitor. The transducer should be "zero" calibrated and then placed at the level of the left atrium at the phlebostatic axis. The proximal lumen also can be connected to a transducer and that pressure monitored during insertion. Once in the vein, all lumens of the catheter are again aspirated and flushed with heparin-containing fluid. Any ports not being monitored during insertion must be closed off with a syringe or stopcock.

The catheter is advanced into the right atrium as determined by the pressure trace and the previous estimate of length. The atrial trace has respiratory variation that helps confirm catheter position in the thorax (Figure 15–8). Once in the right atrium, the balloon is inflated and the catheter advanced until a right ventricular trace is seen. A right ventricular pressure trace is characterized by a rapid upstroke in early systole with an equally rapid downstroke at the end of systole. During diastole the pressure is relatively low and gradually increases until the beginning of systole. Turning the catheter with a clockwise motion usually aids in passing the catheter. Once in the right ventricle, the catheter is further advanced with clockwise motion until a PA trace is noted. The PA trace has the same peak systolic pressure of right ventricular (assuming no anatomic right ventricular outflow tract obstruction.) As systole ends, the trace shows a slower fall that continues through diastole. The diastolic pressure is generally higher than the ventricular diastolic pressure. Once in the pulmonary artery, the catheter can be advanced slightly until a pulmonary capillary wedge trace is seen. This trace is similar in appearance to the right atrial trace, although usually with a higher pressure.

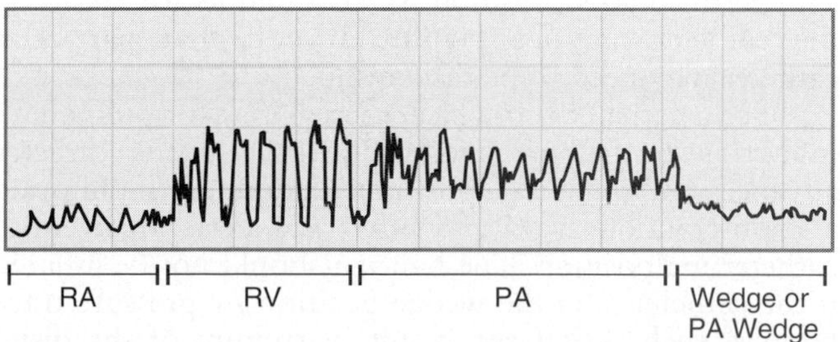

FIGURE 15–8 • Pressure tracing during placement of a pulmonary arterial catheter showing pressures from the right atrium (RA), right ventricle (RV), and pulmonary artery (PA), then pulmonary capillary wedge pressure. (From Adatia I, Cos P: Invasive and noninvasive monitoring. In Chang AC, editor: *Pediatric cardiac intensive care.* Baltimore, 1998, Lippincott, Williams, & Wilkins.)

Once the wedge pressure trace is seen, the balloon is deflated. The PA trace should then return. If the trace is still that of the wedge pressure, the catheter should be retracted until the PA trace is again seen. The balloon should be reinflated just enough to ensure the catheter still floats into the wedge position. The catheter should not be left in the wedge position because of the risk of pulmonary infarction. The catheter is appropriately positioned when the PA pressure trace is present when the balloon is not inflated and the pulmonary capillary wedge trace is present when the balloon is inflated. Catheter position should be confirmed by chest radiography and then secured inside the sleeve and taped or sutured to the patient. The introducer sheath should be sutured in place. Then a sterile occlusive dressing is applied.

Information Acquisition (see Chapter 19)

Much hemodynamic and oxygen delivery information can be obtained from the Swan-Ganz–type PA catheter. Systemic venous oxygen saturation (SvO_2) can be determined directly and continuously with a catheter containing the fiberoptic oximeter. In the absence of the oximeter, intermittent blood sampling from the distal port when in place in the pulmonary artery allows for SvO_2 measurement. Multiple hemodynamic pressures can be obtained, including right atrial pressure, PA pressure, and PAOP. Right atrial pressure is useful for determining preload of the right ventricle. PA pressure is useful for determining the presence of pulmonary hypertension both at baseline and with manipulation of oxygenation, ventilation, ventilator pressures, nitric oxide, and other procedures.

PAOP, also called *pulmonary capillary wedge pressure,* reflects left ventricular preload. In most patients with normal cardiac function and anatomy, right atrial or central venous pressure adequately reflects left ventricular preload as well. However, in the presence of certain congenital heart defects, with significant ventricular dysfunction, or with high mechanical ventilatory pressures, a significant discrepancy may exist between right and left ventricular preload. In such circumstances, measurement of PAOP is useful for guiding fluid and inotropic therapy. PAOP is obtained when the balloon is inflated and the catheter floats into the wedge position. Because the catheter floats to an area of greatest blood flow in the lung, it most likely will be in an area consistent with

West zone III. Zone III is an area where arterial pressure is higher than both venous and alveolar pressure. The transducer should be placed at the level of the left atrium, about the fourth intercostal space, midaxillary line with the patient supine. Measurement of PAOP is best done at end-expiration to minimize the effect of changes in pleural pressure.

The thermistor at the tip of the catheter allows for measurement of cardiac output using the thermodilution method. This method uses the Fick principle, based on the law of conservation of thermal energy. A specific amount of cold fluid is injected in the proximal port (upstream), and the temperature change downstream (at the thermistor) is recorded. The change in temperature over time allows for measurement of blood flow, in this case cardiac output. According to Jansen,[75] this measure of cardiac output is accurate if the following conditions are met: (1) no loss of cold occurs between the injection site and the thermistor, (2) mixing of the cold injectate (indicator using Fick terms) and the blood is complete, and (3) the temperature change caused by the injection of cold fluid is sufficient to be detected by the thermistor.

To perform thermodilution cardiac output measurements, the catheter must be connected to the thermodilution computer, either freestanding or part of the cardiac monitor. A specific volume of injectate, either room temperature or iced, is injected rapidly into the proximal port of the catheter. The temperature difference over time that is detected at the thermistor is recorded as a curve. Some computers have a readout of the curve that allows examination of the quality of the curve. The computer then integrates the area under the curve, which is inversely proportional to the cardiac output. The cardiac output is calculated and projected. For pediatric patients, this number should be divided by their surface area in meters,[77] giving the cardiac index.

The injectate can be either iced or room temperature. The disadvantages to iced injectate include risk of hypothermia in a small patient requiring frequent cardiac output measurements, the poor accuracy of the first injection because of warmer fluid in the catheter, and a greater signal-to-noise ratio. Room temperature injectate prevents these problems and yet is accurate when cardiac output is stable. However, in conditions of extremely high or low cardiac output, less variance occurs with iced injectate compared with room temperature injectate. However, for convenience and safety of pediatric patients, room temperature injectate is recommended.

Other errors in the measurement can be introduced by faulty technique or patient-related issues. Injecting variable volumes or injecting with variable rates can result in inaccurate measures. Multiple injections and averaging of the results can overcome these problems. Usually three to five injections yield adequate results. The presence of tricuspid or pulmonary insufficiency can lead to overestimation of cardiac output. Echocardiography may be necessary to rule out the presence of valvular insufficiency. Intracardiac shunts, such as a ventricular septal defect, result in false values for cardiac output. Mechanical ventilation has been shown to alter stroke volume, which can result in variable measures of cardiac output. Therefore the recommendation is to perform the injection at the same place in the ventilator cycle to standardize the cardiac output measurements.

Maintenance

Care for the catheter is similar to that for any central venous catheter. Pressure transduction of the distal (PA) and proximal (right atrial) ports and continuous electrocardiographic (ECG) monitoring are mandatory. This setup confirms continually proper placement of the catheter. Arrhythmias as noted earlier can occur, particularly if the catheter becomes dislodged. A chest radiogram should be assessed daily for catheter position. The catheter and sheath should be dressed sterilely at all times and the dressing changed according to protocol. The catheter is housed in a sterile sleeve that allows for aseptic technique if further manipulation is necessary. Whenever the balloon is inflated to determine PAOP, allow the balloon to deflate passively by opening the balloon port and removing the syringe. This step helps prevent balloon rupture. Balloon rupture should be suspected if blood is obtained when aspirating the balloon port. In this situation, remove and then replace the catheter if still clinically indicated.

Complications

Complications can result from the initial access to the vein, during catheter passage, or during prolonged catheter use. Depending on the site of venous access, pneumothorax or bleeding may occur during venous access. During passage of the catheter, arrhythmias are frequently seen but generally are transient and benign. Because of the risk of cardiac arrhythmias during insertion, someone other than the operator should observe the ECG monitor for the presence of arrhythmias. When the catheter is in the right atrium, ectopic atrial beats commonly occur. Occasionally, the catheter touches the wall of the atrium, triggering a supraventricular tachycardia. When the catheter is being manipulated through the right ventricle, premature ventricular beats or even ventricular tachycardia may occur. Generally the arrhythmias cease when the catheter is secure in the pulmonary artery. Occasionally pharmacologic or electrical therapy of the arrhythmia may be needed; accordingly, a defibrillator and lidocaine/amiodarone should be readily available. Ventricular ectopy may be excessive even with the catheter is in good position. If so, attempts to reposition the catheter may be helpful; if not, that particular catheter may need to be discontinued.

Once a catheter is in place, there is risk for pulmonary infarction or hemorrhage, particularly if the catheter advances into the wedge position. Continuous monitoring and observation of the pressure trace alert caregivers to catheter malposition. The balloon should not be inflated if the catheter is in the wedge position by pressure trace because such action can result in rupture of the distal pulmonary artery. As with all CVLs, there is a risk of infection that can result in sepsis or endocarditis.[70] Thrombosis in the vein can be seen and may be more frequent in children than adults because of the large catheter-to-vein ratio. To minimize complications, the catheter should be removed as soon as the patient stabilizes and frequent sampling of information is no longer necessary.

Interpretation

A discussion of the use of the hemodynamic data is given in Chapters 14, 19, 20, and 22. Accurate interpretation of the measured hemodynamic data and the derived data is crucial for therapeutic decision making. Multiple studies of physicians and nurses have shown a variable understanding of the data measured and derived from the Swan-Ganz–type catheter.[74,82] A survey that included an examination by the Society of Critical Care Medicine was sent to attending physician members of the Society of Critical Care Medicine (SCCM). The examination contained questions regarding insertion technique, cardiac physiology, interpretation of waveforms, and data related to patient management. This study was believed to show significant deficits by physicians on the basics of PA catheter use, including waveform recognition and data interpretation and application. Previous studies of physician knowledge included as much as 60% trainee participation, whereas this study was performed with 95% of the participants being attending physicians. Based on this study and previous data, the Pulmonary Artery Catheter Consensus Conference concluded that current training and credentialing of practitioners on use of the PA catheter must be reevaluated.[67] No studies evaluating the knowledge of pediatric practitioners on use of the PA catheter have been published. Clearly before large studies can be developed to evaluate the outcome of patients in whom the PA catheter has been used to guide therapy, better understanding and more consistent knowledge of the data by practitioners must occur.

Summary

The PA catheter, either single-lumen or balloon-tipped, flow-directed multiple lumen, is clinically useful in pediatric patients, especially those with known or potential pulmonary hypertension and those whose cardiac output is diminished with an unknown hemodynamic profile. Accurate knowledge of the data obtained from these catheters, either directly measured or derived data, is paramount for making appropriate therapeutic decisions. Currently, there are no studies evaluating the outcome of pediatric patients whose therapy has been guided by use of a PA catheter. The risk of catheter complications is fairly low, but review of the risks and benefits is warranted prior to insertion.

Arterial Access

The cornerstone of medical care of critically ill patients is achieving adequate oxygen delivery and optimizing perfusion. By allowing access to arterial blood for blood gas analysis and direct, continuous measurement of blood pressure, a transduced arterial catheter allows for immediate assessment of response to therapy directed at these goals. Because of the nature of the underlying disease processes and the often rapidly evolving clinical status of the critically ill patient, continuous measurement of blood pressure is essential for timely therapeutic interventions. Other clinical indicators of perfusion, such as capillary refill and skin temperature, often are unreliable. Other indicators, such as urinary output, may require time for measurement and may delay necessary intervention. Indicators such as mentation cannot be assessed in deeply sedated, paralyzed, or comatose patients. Therefore blood pressure measurements become essential.

Access to arterial blood is mandatory to accurately assess oxygenation, ventilation, and acid-base status. For these reasons, use of chronic indwelling arterial catheters became more routine in the 1970s and has since been incorporated into the routine care of critically ill children in whom they are being used with increased frequency.[87,106] Placement of an arterial catheter allows for continuous measurement of systolic, diastolic, and mean blood pressure. It provides a visible pressure waveform that may contribute additional diagnostic information. An arterial catheter also provides direct access to arterial blood for frequent, painless sampling. Hence the ability to place an arterial catheter is a necessary skill in pediatric intensive care medicine.

Indications

Indications for an arterial catheter are as follows:

1. Need for frequent measurement of blood pressure to assess the patient's hemodynamic status and allow for appropriate, timely administration of fluids and titration of inotropes, afterload reduction agents, and antihypertensive infusions. The transduced arterial waveform provides additional clinical information. A patient supported with vasopressors or vasodilators is a candidate to receive an arterial catheter for monitoring.
2. Need for frequent sampling of arterial blood for laboratory analysis. Access to arterial blood through an indwelling catheter increases the ease in painlessly obtaining blood samples for analysis, unskewed by physiologic changes caused by patients' increased respirations with crying or by localized poor perfusion or tourniquet use. A neonatal study showed a significant drop in $Paco_2$ of 6 mmHg and a fall in Pao_2 of 17 mmHg in arterial specimens obtained before and during venipuncture.[94] Another study comparing measurement of pH, $Paco_2$, and Pao_2 between capillary blood gases (CBGs) and arterial blood gases (ABGs) in neonates showed that CBGs did not accurately predict arterial values, suggesting the need for extreme caution in making management decisions based upon CBG results.[88] Differences in pH and $Paco_2$ measured simultaneously with venous blood gases and ABGs have been noted to be greater as cardiac function deteriorates.[84] More accurate measurement of the patient's acid-base status can be obtained with ABGs. Arterial blood allows for meaningful measurement of Pao_2, which cannot be assessed with venous or capillary blood. Indwelling arterial lines permit use of in vivo and ex vivo blood gas monitors, which are capable of continuously measuring blood gases without interrupting the integrity of the arterial catheter

and tubing system.[100] In addition, repeat sampling from an arterial catheter allows for conservation of peripheral veins. Reliable blood cultures can be drawn from indwelling lines. One study comparing blood cultures drawn from an arterial catheter to those drawn from venipuncture revealed 83% equivalent results.[96]

3. Need for continuous monitoring of cerebral perfusion pressure in patients with head injury. Cerebral perfusion pressure is equal to mean arterial pressure minus intracranial pressure (see Chapter 53).
4. Need for arterial access during therapeutic procedures, such as exchange transfusions and continuous arteriovenous hemodialysis.

Contraindications

The skin at the site of arterial access must be intact prior to insertion of a catheter. Any evidence of infection of the skin or underlying structures is a contraindication to catheter placement at this site. Other disruptions in skin integrity, such as burns, are a contraindication.

Evidence of adequate collateral circulation is required prior to placement of an arterial catheter. Twelve percent of the population has either poor collateral flow in their hand or an incomplete palmar arch.[97] Also, 12% of patients have congenital bilateral absence of their dorsalis pedis artery.[97] Collateral circulation can be assessed using the Allen test, in which blood flow to the distal extremity is obstructed by direct pressure over the arteries. The arteries are compressed until the distal extremity is blanched. Pressure over one artery then is released. Capillary refill should return to the distal extremity in less than 5 seconds. The test then is repeated by unblocking the other contributing artery after the distal extremity becomes blanched. Because of time constraints, an arterial catheter is placed without assessing collateral circulation in emergent circumstances. For patients in a shock state, the Allen test becomes less reliable.[97] Some practitioners never perform the Allen test because a normal test result does not guarantee adequate collateral circulation, nor does an abnormal test necessarily indicate possible complications.[108] A catheter should not be placed in an extremity with compromised perfusion.

Severe coagulopathy and systemic heparinization are relative contraindications to arterial catheter placement. The risk of significant bleeding must be weighed when considering this procedure.

Procedure

Box 15–1 lists the supplies and equipment required for arterial catheterization.

BOX 15–1

Supplies and Equipment for Arterial Catheterization

1. Appropriate-size catheter (24-gauge for infants, 22-gauge for toddlers and older)
2. Sterile gloves
3. 10% povidone-iodine or chlorhexidine solution
4. Sterile towels
5. Syringe with 1% lidocaine and 25-gauge needle for local infiltration
6. EMLA
7. Luer-Lok connector with heparinized flush
8. 3-0 silk suture
9. Instrument tray with needle holder and scissors
10. Cloth tape
11. Plastic, nonocclusive dressing
12. Connecting tubing
13. Transducer
14. Fluids containing heparin (1 U/ml) and papaverine

Technique

The initial step in placing an arterial catheter is site selection. If collateral blood flow is sufficient, the radial, posterior tibial, and dorsalis pedis arteries are optimal sites. Catheters also can be placed in the axillary or femoral arteries if no peripheral sites are suitable. Infection rates between femoral and radial catheters are similar.[90] In a study that randomly allocated the placement of 186 catheters between femoral and radial sites, rates of local infection and positive catheter tip cultures were similar between the two sites. Femoral catheters were easier to insert, and blood specimens are easier to obtain via femoral catheters.[110] However, line placement in distal arteries of the extremities is preferred for site observation and hemorrhage control with direct pressure. Preductal placement in the right radial artery is preferred in infants with ductal-dependent heart lesions. Because of the potential complications associated with umbilical arterial catheters (UACs), peripheral arterial lines are being placed in neonates with increasing frequency.[95] Brachial arteries should not be used because of the lack of collateral blood flow. The superficial temporal arteries also should not be used because of poor collateral flow, and retrograde flow from a catheter placed in this artery could result in showering of emboli into the cerebral circulation. Historically, femoral vessel catheterization in neonates has not been used because of complication concerns. A review of complications related to placement of 23 femoral arterial catheters in neonates with gestational age ranging from 23 to 40 weeks revealed that 17% developed transient ischemia of the distal limb.[112] In another series, 158 peripheral arterial lines were placed in 115 neonates. With a complication rate of 1.27% (related to infection), peripheral artery cannulation was demonstrated to be a safe alternative to umbilical artery catheterization.[104]

The selected site must be properly immobilized prior to placement of the indwelling catheter. The wrist is hyperextended 30 degrees to develop a straighter course and bring the radial artery more superficial. Inserting the catheter more than 3 cm proximal to the radiocarpal joint resulted in a greater than four times increased risk of nonpatency.[93]

The site is prepared with a povidone-iodine or chlorhexidine solution and draped with sterile towels.

Lidocaine is infiltrated locally. In addition, lidocaine/prilocaine (EMLA) can be used as a local anesthetic. Systemic narcotics or anxiolytics can be used cautiously.

Percutaneous placement of the catheter can be accomplished using one of several techniques. The first method uses a catheter over a needle. The needle is inserted through the prepped skin at a 30-degree angle (bevel up or down). When a flashback of blood is obtained in the hub, the catheter is advanced another 1 to 2 mm. While holding the needle stable, the catheter is advanced over the needle into the lumen of the vessel in the same manner as placing a peripheral IV line. Blood should be flowing continuously into the catheter hub prior to attempting to advance the catheter. Once the catheter is inserted through the skin to the hub, a flushed Luer-Lok connector is attached to the hub while pressure is applied over the cannulated artery. Correct placement of the catheter is verified by aspirating blood into a syringe attached to the connector. The catheter is flushed and securely sutured and taped into position with DuoDERM dressing placed under the Luer-Lok to protect against skin breakdown, and a plastic dressing, such as Tegaderm, is placed over the catheter and tape as a protective barrier.

Transfixation, the second percutaneous technique, involves inserting a catheter over a needle as described earlier. However, when a flashback of blood is seen in the hub, the needle and catheter are further advanced until the needle and catheter pierce the posterior wall of the artery and transfix this wall to the underlying structures. The needle is pulled out, leaving the catheter in place. The catheter is slowly withdrawn until the tip is again intraluminal, with blood flowing back into the hub. The catheter is advanced. Advancement can be facilitated by attaching a syringe filled with flush to a connecter and gently flushing as the catheter is advanced. The position of the catheter is confirmed, and the catheter secured as described earlier.

The final percutaneous method for catheter placement uses the Seldinger technique. A needle is used to pierce the anterior wall of the artery. A guidewire is placed through the needle and advanced into the lumen of the artery. The needle is removed, and a catheter is advanced over the guidewire into the lumen of the vessel. This method also can be used with a catheter over a needle. Confirmation of correct positioning and securing the catheter completes the procedure. Placement using the Seldinger technique is the preferred method when cannulating larger vessels such as the femoral artery. In addition, some evidence indicates that the Seldinger technique is quicker and requires fewer punctures to obtain access compared with the direct puncture technique.[85] When cannulating a central artery, a longer catheter (e.g., 2.5F–3F, 5-cm line) should be used. This procedure can be accomplished using the Seldinger technique. Commercially made kits are available for arterial access.

If attempts at percutaneous cannulation of an artery are unsuccessful, a cutdown is an alternative to obtain arterial access. A superficial cut is made perpendicular to the artery through the skin. The subcutaneous tissues are bluntly dissected parallel to the vessel using mosquito hemostats. When the artery is identified, the posterior wall is gently dissected away from the adjacent structures. Two loops are placed around the vessel: one proximal and one distal. These loops are used to elevate the artery during the cannulation process; they should never be used to tie off the vessel. After dissection is completed and the loops are in place, the artery is cannulated under direct visualization using the needle over the catheter method. The catheter is secured with a suture through the skin, and the wound is closed with interrupted stitches. If excessive bleeding persists, the proximal loop is pulled gently in an attempt to control the hemorrhage.[97]

Maintenance

Thromboembolic and ischemic complications frequently occur with endovascular procedures secondary to arterial wall injury, thrombogenic characteristics of arterial catheters, contrast media, and implanted devices. Heparin decreases the risk of these adverse events by indirectly blocking thrombin activation.[101] To prolong patency of an arterial catheter, 0.9% NaCl containing heparin 1 U per milliliter[105,113] is infused at 3 ml/hour. Presently, adult protocols are used for children in the absence of more definitive studies in children.[90,109] Comparison of normal saline to D_5W, both with heparin, revealed that infusion of saline resulted in longer catheter life.[103] Use of sodium citrate is not recommended as an anticoagulant for arterial lines because contamination of blood specimens with this additive mimics severe hypocalcemia, metabolic acidosis, and mild hyperglycemia despite wasting an adequate volume of blood before sampling.[86,101] Direct thrombin inhibitors and antibodies to platelet glycoprotein IIb/IIIa may be more effective than conventional anticoagulation and antiplatelet therapies[101] but are not routinely used. Slower infusion rates occasionally are used with caution in small, fluid-restricted infants. By decreasing vasospasm, papaverine added to the infused fluids increases catheter longevity.[92] Papaverine at the routinely used concentration of 60 mg per 500 ml should not have any systemic effects but is contraindicated in patients with head injury.

The catheter should always be visible so that any bleeding is immediately observed. Routine maintenance of an arterial catheter requires changing the fluids and connecting tubing every 72 hours. A study that investigated increasing the change interval from 48 to 72 hours showed no increased risk for catheter-associated infection.[99] The overlying dressing also is changed on a scheduled basis.

CVLs, PA catheters, and arterial lines should be changed only when clinically indicated.[101,107] There is no difference in infection risk whether catheters (CVL, PA, AL) are changed to a new site weekly, changed over a guidewire at the same site weekly, or changed to a new site when clinically indicated.[89]

Inability to draw blood from a catheter or flattening of the waveform on the monitor is suggestive of either a kinked catheter or thrombus formation at the end of the catheter. If no evidence of compromised perfusion related to the catheter is present, changing the catheter over a guidewire is indicated. Vascular insufficiency followed by bleeding is the most common vascular complication after changing a catheter using a guidewire.[90]

Complications

Complications related to arterial catheters include hemorrhage, thrombus formation, emboli and distal ischemia, and infection. In a review of 2119 critically ill adult patients in a medical intensive care unit and a surgical intensive care unit, the most common complication was vascular insufficiency (3.4% in the medical intensive care unit and 4.6% in the surgical intensive care unit), followed by bleeding (1.8% and 2.6%, respectively) and infection (0.4% and 0.7%, respectively).[90,105]

To minimize the complications associated with arterial catheters, close surveillance of the site is required. Inadvertent disconnection of tubing interfaced with the catheter can quickly result in excessive blood loss leading to hemodynamic compromise. Therefore the site of arterial catheterization must always be visible and never covered by clothing or blankets so that any disconnection is quickly noted and acted upon. Suturing the catheter in place and using a Luer-Lok connector decrease the possibility of accidental detachment.

The site of catheter insertion should be closely monitored for any signs of infection or compromised perfusion related to catheter placement. Mottling of the skin proximal and/or distal to the catheter is indicative of intraarterial thrombus formation resulting from initial damage. Discoloration of fingers or toes distal to a catheter may result from emboli. The catheter must be removed if any of these complications are observed.

Catheter-related infections can be local or the focus for systemic sepsis. One study examining infection rates of arterial catheters showed that use of 10% povidone-iodine for cutaneous antisepsis was associated with an incidence of local catheter-related infection of 9.3 per 100 catheters and catheter-related bacteremia of 2.6 per 100 catheters.[98] Duration of placement was an independent risk factor for infection after controlling for white count, antibiotic therapy, and presence of central venous catheters. The cumulative risk of an oncology patient developing a catheter infection increases after 6 days of peripheral arterial catheter placement, from 7% to 17%. Some have advocated routine changing of sites every 4 to 6 days based on these data[102]; however, a review of data collected in the pediatric population indicated different results. Of 340 arterial catheters, only 5% were contaminated (defined as <10 colony-forming units [CFUs] on semiquantitative culture) and 3% were infected (8/340 locally infected defined as ≥10 CFUs; 2/340 associated with a possible catheter-related sepsis). There was almost no risk of infection in the first 48 hours after catheter placement. Subsequently the risk was 6.2%, but this finding did not correlate with duration of catheter placement. Because the incidence of infection related to arterial catheterization is very low in children, the practice of routine catheter reinsertion is not justified.[91] Comparison of blood cultures obtained from arterial catheters prior to removal and catheter tip cultures showed that blood cultures are neither sensitive nor highly predictive of positive catheter tip cultures.[111]

Summary

Transduced arterial lines have become a routine part of the monitoring of many critically ill patients. The additional information gained by catheter use often is integral in the management of the patient. Therefore the ability to place an arterial catheter is a necessary skill when caring for critically ill patients. Prior to placement, however, the risks and benefits must be carefully considered because the complications related to the catheter may be significant.

Umbilical Arterial Catheter and Umbilical Venous Catheter Placement

In newborns, the umbilical vessels are readily accessible for catheterization. They have even been called "the gift to the neonatologist." Even so, catheterization of the umbilical vessels should not be taken lightly. The decision to place umbilical catheters should be based on the patient's clinical situation, gestational age, and expected duration and severity of illness. The risks associated with placement of umbilical lines should be weighed against the benefits prior to catheter placement. Umbilical catheters can be placed in most neonates up to age 1 week and in some newborns up to age 2 weeks.

Umbilical Artery Cannulation

Indications for UAC placement include the need for frequent ABGs, continuous measurement of blood pressure, and, in some instances, exchange transfusion. Infusion of fluids or medications may be warranted when a UAC is present, but placement of a UAC is not indicated for infusions alone. UAC placement is contraindicated in patients with omphalitis, peritonitis, necrotizing enterocolitis, omphalocele, hypercoagulable states, or known ischemia to the perineum or lower extremities.[128]

Supplies and Equipment

A bed with adequate lighting and a heat source are essential. Prepackaged UAC trays are commercially available and contain different sizes and types of catheters. Umbilical catheters should be radiopaque with rounded tips. A Luer-Lok system is available on some catheters; others need trimming and attachment of a blunt needle to connect them to a three-way stopcock. The appropriate-size catheter is determined by the size of the infant. Babies weighing less than 1500 g need a 3.5F catheter; infants weighing more than 1500 g require a 5F catheter.[130] Other supplies needed include povidone-iodine or chlorhexidine solution, umbilical tape, sterile drapes, gloves, scalpel, scissors, iris forceps, pick-ups, gauze pads, 3-0 silk suture, 10-ml syringes, tape, diapers, and heparin flush (1 U heparin per milliliter of normal saline).

Technique

Prior to UAC placement, gently restrain the baby and determine the catheter insertion distance. Restrain the infant in a supine position by taping a diaper across the groin and thighs to immobilize the legs. Gently restrain the patient's arms at his/her side with tape.

To determine the length of catheter insertion, decide whether to place a "high UAC" or a "low UAC." High or low placement of the catheter is based on the vertebral level at which the catheter resides in the aorta. A low UAC should lie at or below the third lumbar vertebra (caudal to the origins of the renal arteries).[125] A high UAC should have its tip between the sixth and ninth thoracic vertebrae. Institutions vary greatly as to their preference for placement of UACs. Some studies have shown fewer complications with high UAC placement; however, thrombosis and hypertension have been reported with both low and high UACs.[122,138,144] The calculation for insertion length can be determined using various methods, such as birth weight, shoulder-to-umbilicus length, and total body length.[118,131,132,137] A simple method for calculating insertion depth for high placement is as follows: 3 × (weight in kg) + 9 = centimeters of catheter to insert from the umbilical ring.[136]

Next, attach the UAC to a three-way stopcock and fill with heparin flush. Turn the stopcock off to the catheter prior to insertion. Prepare the cord and abdominal wall with antiseptic solution, and drape the baby while allowing for visualization of the cord in a generous sterile field. Encircle the cord with umbilical tape placed snugly but not too tightly. The umbilical tape should be able to apply pressure to the cord in the event of acute hemorrhage but should not be so tight as to hamper introduction of the catheter. Use a scalpel to cut the cord horizontally approximately 1 to 2 cm above the umbilical ring. Grasp the cord securely with toothed forceps. It is better to get a firm hold initially rather than grasping the cord repeatedly, which can thin the Wharton's jelly and make placement of the catheter more difficult. At this point, the larger thin-walled umbilical vein in the 12 o'clock position and two small thick-walled UACs usually can be identified. Use the iris forceps to dilate an arterial lumen by first inserting one prong and then the other prong, finally allowing both prongs to spring open and dilate the lumen. Holding the catheter with the iris forceps, introduce the catheter into the artery, taking care to ensure that the catheter is in the lumen of the vessel. Insert the catheter approximately 0.5 cm and pull the umbilical cord toward the infant's head before attempting to advance the catheter. Aspirate blood and flush the catheter once it has been advanced to the desired length. If the catheter meets resistance, apply gentle steady pressure for approximately 30 seconds to determine if the catheter will advance. Do not force the catheter. If the catheter will not advance or no blood return is seen, a false passage may have been created. A double-catheter technique can be attempted in this situation.[134] Leave the catheter that is meeting resistance in place and advance a second catheter beside it to the appropriate distance. If the double-catheter technique fails, the second umbilical artery can be cannulated. Suture the catheter in place using a pursestring stitch cinched tightly to provide hemostasis. Tie a square knot 1 cm above the umbilical stump and loop the catheter one time before tying off. A tape bridge is used to further secure the line. Finally, remove the umbilical tape. Anteroposterior and lateral x-ray films of the abdomen are needed to confirm proper positioning of the catheter. A catheter position that is suboptimal should be adjusted (Table 15–1).

Maintenance

A continuous infusion is needed to keep the lumen of the catheter clear, and catheters should be flushed after blood draws to keep the catheters free of clot. The infusion usually consists of 38 MEq/L NaCl with heparin 1 U/ml, running 0.5 ml/hour for a 3.5F catheter or 1 ml/hour in a 5F catheter. Infants can be placed in the supine position or on their sides; prone positioning usually is not used. Daily changing of the tubing that connects to the UAC may decrease the risk of infection. A dressing should not be applied to the umbilicus so that the catheter insertion site and cord can be easily inspected. The UAC should be removed when continuous blood pressure monitoring and frequent blood gases are no longer needed. To remove the UAC, withdraw it slowly in increments of 1 to 2 cm over a few minutes. This process should allow the artery to spasm and provide hemostasis. If bleeding occurs, apply pressure to the cord. The sutures should be removed at the time of catheter removal.

Complications

A variety of complications are associated with UACs. The most common complication is blanching of the legs or buttocks secondary to vasospasm, which may resolve by applying heat to the contralateral leg.[115,117,119,143] If blanching does not improve, catheter removal is warranted to prevent severe ischemic complication. Thrombotic and embolic complications resulting from fibrin deposition on the catheter are clinically significant in fewer than 10% of patients, but thrombosis of the aorta or its major branches can be devastating. Accidental catheterization of the branches of the internal iliac artery can lead to gross disfigurement of the child.[116,119,127,140] Acute hemorrhage is an infrequent complication that can result in significant morbidity and mortality. Blood loss can occur secondary to accidental withdrawal of the catheter or disconnection from the blunt needle. Close monitoring and proper securing of the catheter can prevent most of these problems. Hypertension secondary to UAC placement has been frequently reported.[138] Catheter-related sepsis occurs in approximately 5% of neonates possessing UACs, with coagulase-negative *Staphylococcus* the most commonly identified pathogen.[120,123] Some complications

TABLE 15–1

Adjustment of Umbilical Artery Catheters

Catheter Position	Adjustment Needed
Too high on x-ray film	Pull back to desired length
Too low on x-ray film	Never advance the catheter once the sterile field has been broken; the catheter should be replaced
In vessel other than aorta	Remove the catheter

infrequently associated with UACs are development of aneurysmal dilatation of the aorta, peritoneal perforation, and umbilical artery rupture.[124,133,141] Death associated with UAC complication is rare.[139]

Summary

UACs are commonly used in the care of severely ill neonates. They can be extremely valuable tools for assessment and management of these infants, but their use is not without problem. Because of the clinical significance of complications associated with UACs, alternative noninvasive tools for patient monitoring have been developed.

Umbilical Vein Cannulation

The umbilical vein is catheterized for emergency fluid or medication administration. The umbilical vein is much easier to cannulate than the umbilical arteries for central access. In addition to resuscitation, the umbilical vein can be catheterized for prolonged parenteral nutrition administration in severely ill neonates. Other indications include exchange transfusion and monitoring of central venous pressure.

Equipment

The materials required for umbilical venous catheter (UVC) placement are identical to the materials required for UAC placement. Three sizes of UVCs are commonly used, based on infant weight (Table 15–2). Double-lumen UVCs are commercially available and are preferred unless the catheter is being placed for exchange transfusion.

Technique

UVC placement requires the same preparation as described for umbilical artery cannulation. The umbilical vein is larger and is not constricted when compared with the umbilical arteries and does not require dilation prior to introduction of the catheter. Another difference with UVC placement compared with UAC placement is that the cord should be gently pulled toward the infant's feet. when attempting to advance the catheter.

When placing the UVC, resistance and bouncing of the line can be encountered when the catheter reaches 4 to 5 cm and usually indicates the catheter has entered the portal vein. If this type of resistance is encountered, the catheter should be pulled back and then gently advanced while the line is flushed. A catheter should never be forcefully advanced when resistance is met. Catheter position should be confirmed radiographically. Length of catheter insertion is determined by the size of the infant and by the indication for placement. In emergency situations (resuscitation) and exchange transfusion, the catheter should be placed only to a depth where rapid blood return is achieved, which is 3 to 5 cm in most infants. When placing a UVC for prolonged central venous access, the line must reside at the junction of the inferior vena cava and right atrium. This distance can be estimated using the formula ([3(wt in kg) + 9]/2) + 1.[136] Other calculation methods include measurement of the shoulder to umbilicus distance or sternal notch to umbilicus measurement multiplied by 0.6.[118,127] The catheter should be sutured using a pursestring stitch and secured with a tape bridge, as described for the UAC.

TABLE 15–2

Umbilical Venous Catheter Selection

Catheter Size (French)	Infant Weight (kg)
8	>3.5
5	1–3.5
3.5	<1

Maintenance

The UVC should be maintained as part of a closed system to prevent air embolism. Infants normally are not placed prone while the UVC is in place, and careful observation of the umbilicus for signs of infection is warranted. Sterile technique should be used to minimize the risk of infection, and a malpositioned catheter should never be advanced. If placed for exchange transfusion, the catheter should be removed immediately after the exchange. If the UVC was placed for central venous access, it should be removed when its clinical utility is no longer indicated. Generally, UVCs should be discontinued within 10 days to 2 weeks after placement to decrease the likelihood of complications.[123] UVCs should be removed in the manner described for UACs.

Complications

The complication rate for UVCs is greater than the rate for UACs, but usually the complications are less severe.[127] The most common complication associated with UVC placement is infection, with increased risk when the line is left in place for prolonged periods.[114,123] Thrombosis is another reported complication of UVC placement and can lead to portal hypertension when it occurs in the portal venous system.[126] Associated hepatic necrosis and necrotizing enterocolitis have been documented in the literature.[129,135] Liver necrosis occurs more frequently when hypertonic solutions are delivered through the UVC. As mentioned previously, air embolus is a potentially deadly complication of UVCs, as are pericardial tamponade, pulmonary embolus, endocarditis, and certain arrhythmias.[121,142]

Closing Remarks

UVCs provide emergency access during resuscitation of a severely ill neonate. In low-birth-weight infants, UVCs can be the initial route for providing valuable high-calorie nutrition. Complications from UVCs are more likely if the catheters are left in place for prolonged periods or are incorrectly positioned. Preferably CVPs are removed within 7 days and inferior vena cava placement confirmed radiographically.

Pericardiocentesis

Pericardiocentesis is the aspiration of fluid or air from the pericardial space. The most compelling indication for the procedure is relief of cardiac tamponade, but it also can be performed to diagnose the cause of a pericardial effusion. Pericardiocentesis can be performed emergently without guidance techniques but should be reserved for dire circumstances because of the risk of the procedure and the higher failure rate when no guidance is used.

Indications

Drainage of a pericardial effusion of any cause is absolutely indicated when cardiac tamponade is present. Often drainage is recommended if the effusion is large, even in the absence of tamponade. In pediatric patients, pericardial effusions most commonly occur with postviral or idiopathic pericarditis, but they also are seen with postpericardiotomy syndrome, collagen vascular disease, oncologic disease, and rarely uremia. Purulent pericarditis resulting from *S. aureus* or *Streptococcus pneumoniae* infection can be seen with concomitant pneumonia with empyema. Although rare, tuberculous pericarditis can occur. Drainage of purulent pericarditis is indicated for relief of tamponade, prevention of constrictive pericarditis, diagnosis, and drainage of infection. Traumatic pericardial effusions secondary to penetrating trauma often require drainage of the blood because tamponade is common (see Chapter 108). Pneumopericardium secondary to pulmonary air leaks in mechanically ventilated patients usually is well tolerated hemodynamically but may require drainage, especially in small infants because of the development of tamponade.

Contraindications

When acute tamponade is present, pericardiocentesis is absolutely indicated. However, when elective or diagnostic pericardiocentesis is to be performed, the presence of a bleeding diathesis is considered a contraindication. Lack of experience with the procedure is a relative contraindication for elective pericardiocentesis. Open drainage is preferred to closed drainage when the patient has traumatic tamponade and is in cardiac arrest.[145] With purulent pericarditis, open drainage may be more effective because of the difficulty in draining thick pus. When the effusion is loculated in a location not easily reached using the subxiphoid approach, needle pericardiocentesis is contraindicated because the risk of complications increases and the possibility of drainage becomes remote.

Procedure

Drainage of a pericardial effusion can be performed either by simple needle aspiration or by insertion of a drainage catheter. If the procedure is for diagnosis only and the effusion is small, then needle drainage is adequate. However, if tamponade is present, the effusion is sizable, or effusion likely will continue, insertion of a catheter for continuous drainage is indicated.

Equipment

1. *Needle for drainage.* The size of the needle ranges from 14 to 20 gauge, depending on the type of fluid and the size of the patient. For thicker fluids, such as pus or blood, a larger-bore needle is used. A steel needle, such as a vascular introducer needle or a spinal needle, can be used, but often an IV catheter is more effective because once the fluid is reached, the steel inner needle can be removed from the IV catheter, leaving the softer, needleless catheter in place while the fluid is aspirated. This process decreases the risk of cardiac puncture.
2. *Syringes, three-way stopcock, and short extension tubing* are assembled for aspiration. A 5- or 10-ml slip-tip syringe is used when accessing the pericardium for easier manipulation. A larger 20- to 30-ml syringe may be needed for fluid drainage, depending on the predicted volume. The stopcock and short tubing are useful when draining large amounts of fluid.
3. *Equipment for insertion* includes povidone-iodine or chlorhexidine solution, sterile gloves and drapes, and 1% lidocaine for local analgesia.
4. Appropriate *sterile sample tubes* should be available for collection of fluid for chemical, cellular, and microbiologic analysis.
5. *Cardiac monitor* is essential for determination of arrhythmias during the procedure.
6. *Catheter, dilator, and flexible* J-*wire* are necessary when the catheter will be left in place. Placement in the pericardial sac of a 5F to 8F pigtail catheter with multiple side holes is recommended. The size of the catheter is determined by the size of the patient and the viscosity of the fluid. If the fluid is fibrinous in appearance by echocardiography, then a larger-bore catheter should be placed. Several pigtail catheters are manufactured specifically for fluid drainage, often available as kits that also contain an appropriate-size dilator and J-wire guide. If a kit is not available, then a venous dilator of appropriate size with a separate J-wire can be used. A J-wire is used to prevent another puncture of the pericardium or heart using a straight wire. Before the needle is inserted, the wire, dilator, and catheter must be checked to ensure their sizes are compatible.

Technique

Needle aspiration can be performed blindly in the event of a true emergency such as traumatic tamponade; however, the technique has a higher complication and failure rate. Fluoroscopy has been useful but is cumbersome because it requires patient transport to a radiologic or catheterization suite in the absence of portable fluoroscopy.

Echocardiographic guidance is recommended for most pericardiocenteses. The most common technique uses transthoracic scanning, which can easily visualize the effusion. Echocardiographic scanning is indicated prior to needle drainage or catheter insertion for any reason except tamponade with cardiac arrest. Pericardial fluid can be identified by computed tomography or magnetic resonance imaging. Because these techniques are cumbersome and time consuming, they should not be used in acute tamponade because echocardiography often is more readily available at the bedside and usually is fast in skilled hands. The echocardiogram can show the size of the effusion, its distribution around the heart including any loculations, presence of fibrin or clots, and evidence of tamponade.[146] Tamponade can be diagnosed using two-dimensional imaging when the right atrium collapses during late diastole. Normally the right atrial free wall is concave throughout the cardiac cycle. With tamponade, the pericardial pressure exceeds the right atrial pressure at end-diastole and causes the right atrial free wall to collapse toward the center of the right atrium. The worse the tamponade, the longer into systole the collapse occurs.[147]

After the fluid has been echocardiographically evaluated, the patient is placed supine with the head elevated approximately 30 degrees. The subxiphoid approach is the safest and most common approach, although other approaches have been described. The subxiphoid and lower costal margin are prepared with povidone-iodine or chlorhexidine. The area is sterilely draped. Lidocaine local analgesia is infiltrated at the junction of the xiphoid and the left costal margin. The needle is inserted at a 30- to 45-degree angle with the needle directed toward the left clavicle (Figure 15–9). The slip-tip syringe is attached and aspirated continually while the needle is inserted (Figure 15–10). Needle advancement is halted when air or fluid is aspirated. If blood is obtained, analysis is necessary to determine if the blood is of pericardial or intracardiac origin. Several techniques are helpful for this determination. The hematocrit of pericardial fluid will be lower than that of intracardiac blood, which will be equal to the patient's hematocrit. Dropping a few milliliters of the fluid on gauze sponges determines if the fluid will clot. Fluid that does not clot is pericardial; fluid that does clot most likely is intracardiac blood.[148] Another technique involves injection of small amounts of saline microbubble contrast (saline in a syringe that has been agitated) through the introducer needle while imaging with echocardiography.[149] If contrast bubbles are seen in the heart, then the tip of the needle is intracardiac. If bubbles appear in the pericardial sac, then the needle is appropriately placed in the pericardium.

During insertion the needle is guided using two-dimensional echocardiography. The echocardiographic probe is placed on the chest where the fluid is best seen. The needle tip is identified and followed as the needle is advanced.[150] Another technique involves mounting the needle on the echocardiographic probe, which has been placed in a sterile sleeve. The needle is advanced while the operator also handles the probe. This technique allows the use of different locations for insertion of the introducer needle other than the subxiphoid approach, with the potential for better fluid visualization.[151]

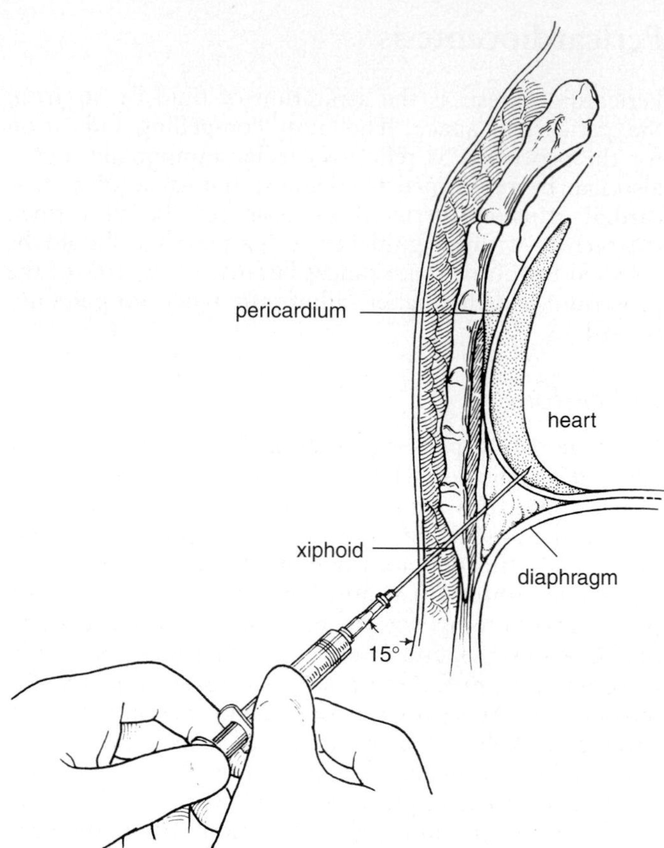

FIGURE 15–10 • In pericardiocentesis, the needle is inserted slowly under continuous aspiration toward the heart at a 15-degree angle to the skin. (From Brundage SI, et al: Pericardiocentesis and pericardial window. In Shoemaker WC, Velmahos GC, Demetriades D, editors: *Procedures and monitoring for the critically ill.* Philadelphia, 2002, WB Saunders.)

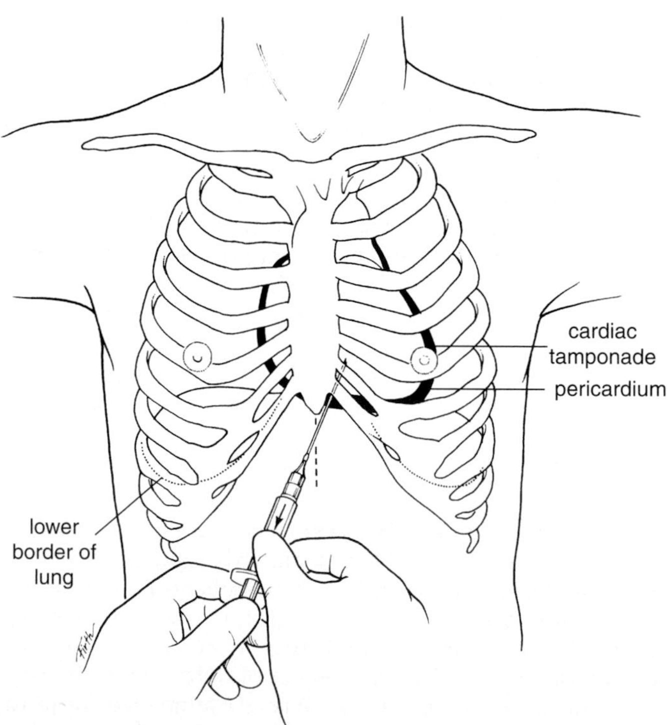

FIGURE 15–9 • Insertion of needle for pericardiocentesis at the junction of the xiphoid and the left costal margin, aiming toward the left shoulder. (From Brundage SI, et al: Pericardiocentesis and pericardial window. In Shoemaker WC, Velmahos GC, Demetriades D, editors: *Procedures and monitoring for the critically ill.* Philadelphia, 2002, WB Saunders.)

Previously the most common guidance technique used electrocardiography to guide the needle. Alligator clamps were placed on the steel insertion needle and connected to an ECG monitor. The ECG complexes were visualized while the needle was inserted. If an injury pattern was noted in the ST segment, then the heart presumably was touched by the needle. The needle was pulled back into the pericardial sac, and the ECG trace would return to normal. Although this technique is simple to perform, echocardiographic guidance offers more specific information about needle position and fluid location, allowing for a safer procedure.

Once the needle is determined to be well positioned in the pericardiac sac, if a catheter is to be inserted, then the J-wire can be passed through the needle as with standard Seldinger technique. The needle is removed, and the dilator is passed over the wire to open the tissues outside the pericardium and enlarge the puncture in the pericardium. The dilator is removed, taking care to leave the J-wire in good position. The catheter is passed over the wire into the pericardial sac. Its position can be viewed echocardiographically. The wire is removed. The connecting tubing and three-way stopcock are connected and the fluid aspirated. The tubing can be connected to a drainage bag for removal of fluid that continues to accumulate. A sample of the aspirated fluid should be sent to the laboratory for appropriate analysis. The catheter is secured with suture and covered with an occlusive dressing. A chest radiogram should be taken at the end of the procedure and daily to confirm the catheter position.

Maintenance

The catheter is simple to maintain. The dressing should be changed according to the ICU protocol for CVLs. The fluid in the drainage bag should be measured and the amount recorded on a regular schedule. If fluid is no longer draining, then a small amount (1–2 ml) of heparinized saline can be infused into the pericardium through the stopcock after preparation with antiseptic solution. This process can release any fibrinous material occluding the catheter. If no fluid is forthcoming, then echocardiography can be performed to determine if residual pericardial fluid remains. If more fluid is present, flush the catheter again in an attempt to open up the catheter. If no fluid remains, the catheter can be removed depending on the patient's condition and the underlying cause of fluid development.

Complications

Cardiac puncture is not an uncommon complication of the procedure. If the ventricle is entered and the needle quickly withdrawn, then the injury is minor and of no clinical consequence. Coronary laceration occurs rarely, resulting in acute ischemia, and has been associated with death from the procedure.[152] The pleural space can be entered with the insertion needle or the catheter, resulting in a hemothorax or pneumothorax. Hemoperitoneum and pneumoperitoneum can occur. Injury to the diaphragm, intestines, and stomach have been reported. Infection of the indwelling catheter can occur but is rare because the catheter usually is not in place for more than 3 to 4 days. Cardiac arrest and death have been reported during pericardiocentesis.[153,154] In a retrospective study of pericardial drainage catheters in pediatric patients, Zahn et al.[155] noted only five complications in a total of 43 procedures. Four of the complications were considered minor and included myocardial perforation with no hemodynamic alteration, pneumopericardium, and ST-segment elevation. One critically ill neonate who had suffered a myocardial perforation during cardiac catheterization died.[155] The results of the study indicated that pericardial catheter placement in pediatric patients is a relatively safe procedure. Most complications of pericardiocentesis with or without catheter placement can be prevented by careful guidance of the needle with echocardiography and greater experience of the practitioner.

Interpretation

Laboratory analysis of pericardial fluid includes cell count and differential, microbiologic evaluation, cytology, and blood chemistry workup, which may include protein, glucose, pH, lactate dehydrogenase (LDH) and triglycerides. Normally pericardial fluid is clear and straw colored. Cloudiness may indicate purulence resulting from infection or chyle if the patient's status is post chest or cardiac surgery. Serosanguinous fluid can be seen with multiple diagnoses, including trauma, postpericardiotomy syndrome, collagen vascular disease, infection, and neoplastic disease.

The presence of white blood cells with a predominance of polymorphonuclear cells greater than 1000 per milliliter is indicative of bacterial infection. When the predominant cell type is lymphocytic, then tuberculous pericarditis should be suspected. In idiopathic or postviral pericarditis, the fluid contains fewer than 1000 cells per milliliter, and the cells are mostly monocytic or lymphocytic. Occasionally the fluid is hemorrhagic with a preponderance of red blood cells. Neoplastic effusions may contain neoplastic cells, which may be missed on routine cell count but will be notable by cytologic examination. With purulent pericarditis the protein level is high and the glucose level and pH are low. LDH is elevated with neoplastic effusions. With purulent effusions the ratio of LDH in the fluid to the blood is increased to greater than 0.6. With chylous effusions, the fluid has an increased triglyceride level.

With acute nonpurulent pericarditis the fluid should be evaluated for viruses, with Coxsackie viruses the most common causes. Viral culture can be performed, although the yield is generally low. Polymerase chain reaction has been used successfully to diagnose the microbial cause, but its use is not yet widespread.[156,157] For purulent pericarditis, Gram stains and acid-fast bacilli stains should be performed, as should appropriate bacterial (both aerobic and anaerobic) and fungal cultures (see Chapter 28).

Closing Remarks

Pericardiocentesis with or without catheter placement is a straightforward procedure that is indicated for relief of cardiac tamponade and for diagnosis of certain pericardial effusions. It is a lifesaving technique for patients with tamponade. Used in conjunction with guidance techniques such as echocardiography or electrocardiography, pericardiocentesis can be performed safely in patients of all ages.

Thoracentesis and Tube Thoracostomy

Thoracentesis

Introduction

Thoracentesis is most often performed as a diagnostic test, but it can be used for relief of respiratory distress caused by large pleural effusions. In pediatric patients, effusions most commonly result from acute pulmonary infections, but they also are seen with many other conditions (Box 15–2). In pediatric critical care, pleural effusions are commonly found in patients with capillary leak, syndromes such as sepsis, and in postoperative cardiac patients.

Indications

Thoracentesis is performed to remove air or fluid from the pleural space. It can be used either to obtain fluid for diagnostic studies or to relieve distress in patients with large effusions. If ongoing evacuation of air or fluid is required, tube thoracostomy should be performed. In the presence of an apparent infectious process, ultrasound can be useful for distinguishing fluid from atelectasis with complete opacification of the hemithorax, detecting loculations, and defining the character of the fluid.[158] Ultrasound guidance may facilitate aspiration of small amounts of fluids, particularly with loculation.[159]

Contraindications

Thoracentesis has no absolute contraindications, but several relative contraindications exist. If a very small volume of fluid is present, the risk of pneumothorax is great, making the procedure relatively contraindicated. Overlying skin infection makes likely the possibility of introduction of microorganisms into the pleural space. An uncorrected coagulopathy is a relative contraindication, but generally thoracentesis can be safely performed in this situation using a small needle and careful technique. An uncooperative patient greatly increases the risks to underlying thoracic structures, making sedation and analgesia a frequent necessity in pediatric patients. Positive pressure ventilation increases the risk of pneumothorax and subsequent tension pneumothorax.

Preparation

Sedation and analgesia frequently are necessary to perform thoracentesis safely in pediatric patients. Appropriate monitoring for these patients, as well as medication choices, are discussed in Chapter 116. Topical agents, such as lidocaine/prilocaine (EMLA) or liposomal lidocaine (LMX-4), may reduce the discomfort of local anesthesia.[160–162] A thick layer of these agents should be applied under an occlusive dressing. Buffering the lidocaine with sodium bicarbonate may reduce the discomfort associated with injecting the lidocaine.[163–165]

BOX 15–2

Causes of Pleural Effusion

- Infection (exudates)
  - Bacterial
  - Viral
  - Fungal
  - Mycobacterial
  - Mycoplasma
- Cardiovascular
  - Congestive heart failure
  - Constrictive pericarditis
  - Superior vena cava obstruction
- Pulmonary
  - Pulmonary infarction
  - Atelectasis
  - Asbestos exposure
  - Drug-induced pleuritis
- Intraabdominal disease
  - Abdominal surgery
  - Pancreatitis
  - Hepatitis
  - Peritonitis
  - Subdiaphragmatic abscess
  - Intrahepatic abscess
  - Meigs syndrome
  - Cirrhosis with ascites
- Iatrogenic
  - Extravascular central venous catheter placement
- Collagen vascular disease
  - Rheumatoid arthritis
  - Systemic lupus erythematosus
  - Sjögren syndrome
  - Wegener granulomatosis
- Neoplastic
  - Lymphoma/leukemia
  - Mesothelioma
  - Chest wall tumors
  - Metastatic carcinoma
  - Bronchogenic carcinoma
- Renal
  - Uremia
  - Urinary tract obstruction
  - Nephrotic syndrome
  - Peritoneal dialysis
- Miscellaneous
  - Esophageal rupture
  - Hemothorax
  - Chylothorax
  - Lymphedema
  - Hypoalbuminemia
  - Myxedema
  - Sarcoidosis
  - Radiation therapy
  - Immunoblastic lymphadenopathy
  - Familial Mediterranean fever

Procedure

Box 15–3 lists the supplies and equipment required for thoracentesis.

BOX 15-3

Supplies and Equipment for Thoracentesis

- Pillows or towels for positioning patient
- Sterile gloves
- Povidone-iodine or chlorhexidine solution
- Commercial thoracentesis tray (for older children and adolescents)
- Or assemble the following items:
  Sterile gauze sponges
  Sterile towels or drapes
  3- to 5-ml syringe for local anesthetic; 27- to 30-gauge needle for skin infiltration
  1% lidocaine; consider sodium bicarbonate to buffer lidocaine
  Over-the-needle catheter: 14- to 20-gauge depending on the size of the patient
  10- or 20-ml syringes for fluid collection
  Three-way stopcock or tubing extension set with clamp
  Sterile dressing
  Tape to secure dressing

Technique

Position the patient in an upright, seated position, if possible. We frequently ask the patient to lean over a bedside tray table that has been padded with a pillow or blanket. An infant or young child can be held in the burping position by an assistant, or the child can be placed in the lateral decubitus position. In this position, the arm on the affected side should be abducted and positioned above the child's head.

If thoracentesis is being performed for a pneumothorax, position the patient supine and perform the aspiration from the second or third intercostal space in the midclavicular line. The usual site for thoracentesis performed to obtain fluid is the posterior axillary line near the tip of the scapula. This site is the seventh intercostal space during full inspiration.

If the area was prepared with a topical anesthetic, remove the cream and occlusive dressing. The site for thoracentesis is prepared with multiple applications of antiseptic solution and then draped with sterile towels. The superior border of the rib is identified and infiltrated with local anesthetic by first creating a skin wheal with a 27- to 30-gauge needle. After allowing time for onset of local anesthesia in the wheal, the same needle is introduced perpendicular to the skin. Lidocaine is injected slowly as the needle is advanced. If the needle is not long enough to reach the rib, the lidocaine is injected as the needle is being withdrawn. A longer 22- to 25-gauge needle is attached to the anesthetic syringe and reintroduced through the anesthetized area. Additional anesthetic is injected until the superior border of the rib is reached and the periosteum infiltrated. Subsequently, the needle is advanced into the pleural space with continuous aspiration until pleural fluid is obtained. The depth of the needle where fluid is obtained should be noted. Applying a hemostat to the needle before the needle is withdrawn may facilitate the process. An over-the-needle catheter is attached to the larger syringe for fluid collection, ensuring the unit is of sufficient length to reach the effusion by comparing it with the previously marked anesthetic needle. If infection is suspected, using a larger (16- to 18-gauge) needle facilitates aspiration of a viscous exudate. Finally, the over-the-needle catheter is advanced through the previously anesthetized tract.

Once pleural fluid is obtained, aspiration is continued until a quantity of fluid sufficient for diagnostic studies is obtained. A three-way stopcock or tubing extension with clamp can be attached at this point. Alternatively, the catheter is advanced until the hub reaches the skin. The inner needle is removed and the needle hub covered with a finger until the stopcock or tubing is attached following connection of the larger syringe to the tubing. If the thoracentesis is being performed for relief of respiratory distress, fluid aspiration is continued until flow ceases. The fluid can be emptied into a basin and measured. The catheter is withdrawn and covered with a sterile dressing.

Complications

Pneumothorax is the most common complication of thoracentesis. For this reason, a chest radiograph should always be obtained following thoracentesis and repeated if respiratory distress develops despite the absence of a pneumothorax on the initial postprocedure radiogram. Some adult data suggest routine chest radiography after thoracentesis is unnecessary unless respiratory distress develops.

Hemothorax may occur, particularly in patients with a coagulopathy. Ideally, the platelet count should be greater than 50,000 and the coagulation times near normal to avoid hemorrhage. If thrombocytopenia is present, platelets can be infused during the procedure. Carefully entering the pleural space over the superior rib border avoids the neurovascular bundle found on the inferior border of the rib. Significant bleeding may require tube thoracostomy. Infection of the skin, soft tissue, and pleural space can be greatly diminished with careful attention to sterile technique.

Pulmonary edema may result if a large volume of fluid is removed, but this complication has not been described in children. It is generally seen in adults from whom more than 1 L of fluid is removed. A "safe" amount of pleural effusion removal in children has not been established.

Interpretation

Evaluation of pleural fluid is largely based on the adult work of Light.[166] Effusions are separated into exudates and transudates, and the causes of each are listed in Box 15–2. Box 15–4 lists the general diagnostic tests for pleural fluid. Box 15–5 lists the differentiating characteristics of transudates versus exudates. If the red blood cell count of the fluid is greater than 100,000, trauma, neoplasm, or pulmonary infarction is likely.[167] A pleural fluid pH less than 7.2, glucose level less than 40 mg/dl, or a Gram-positive stain of the fluid suggests a complicated parapneumonic effusion that requires drainage.[168,169] A consensus statement of the American College of Chest Physicians has stratified the risk of parapneumonic

BOX 15–4

Diagnostic Tests for Pleural Fluid

- pH (by arterial blood gas machine)
- Glucose
- LDH, total protein
- Cell count and differential
- Amylase
- Cytology for malignant cells
- Stains (Gram, fungal, acid-fast bacilli)
- Triglycerides
- Cultures (aerobic/anaerobic, mycobacterial, fungal, viral)
- Polymerase chain reaction for mycobacteria

effusions in adults and has recommended interventions other than simple thoracentesis or tube thoracostomy for drainage of effusions when the effusion is large or loculated, has a positive culture or Gram stain, or has a pH less than 7.20.[170] If mycobacterial disease is suspected, acid-fast staining and mycobacteria culture of the pleural fluid likely will not be diagnostic; rather, polymerase chain reaction analysis of the pleural fluid should be considered.[171]

An elevated amylase level in the pleural fluid suggests pancreatitis or esophageal rupture.[172] When the triglyceride level is more than 110% of the serum value and lymphocytes predominate, chylothorax is likely.[166]

Closing Remarks

Thoracentesis is frequently required in the care of critically ill infants and children. This relatively simple procedure can yield valuable diagnostic information with minimal risk to the patient.

Tube Thoracostomy

Introductory Remarks

Tube thoracostomy is frequently required in the critical care setting. Hippocrates described using a metal tube to drain the chest of "evil humors."[173] Small catheter drainage systems and a wire-guided technique using a series of progressive dilators now have added to the armamentarium of choices for chest drainage.

Indications

Tube thoracostomy is frequently required for pulmonary air leaks in the presence of acute lung injury or acute respiratory distress syndrome and in patients who require ongoing drainage of parapneumonic effusions or empyema. In the pediatric trauma patient with hemothorax or hemopneumothorax, tube thoracostomy is generally required. In the postoperative cardiac patient, tube thoracostomy may be required for treatment of chylothorax.

BOX 15–5

Interpretation of Pleural Fluid

Characteristics of exudative effusions

- Pleural to serum protein ratio >0.5
- Pleural to serum LDH ratio >0.6
- Pleural fluid LDH more than twice the upper limit of the normal serum value

Contraindications

Tube thoracostomy has no absolute contraindications. In patients with a coagulopathy, attempts should be made to correct the coagulopathy, if possible, prior to tube thoracostomy, but the risk of delayed drainage must be compared against the risk of further hemorrhage. Other relative contraindications include hemothorax prior to adequate volume resuscitation, as the hemothorax may tamponade the hemorrhage. If the patient requires thoracotomy, chest tubes can be placed at this time unless they are required in preoperative stabilization.

Supplies and Equipment

Most institutions have a specially designated chest tube tray. Typical contents include sterile gauze sponges, sterile towels for draping, syringes and needles for local anesthesia, a scalpel and blade, curved Kelly clamps of various sizes, needle driver, suture, and suture scissors. Other materials required are the appropriate-size chest tube (Table 15–3), povidone-iodine or chlorhexidine solution, sterile gloves, a drainage apparatus (such as Pleur-Evac), local anesthetic, and tape.

Technique

Tube thoracostomy is a painful procedure. Although the pain can be significantly reduced by generous local anesthesia, sedation and analgesia are frequently required in pediatric patients. Pain of local anesthetic injection can be reduced by buffering with sodium bicarbonate, as discussed in the thoracentesis section.

The patient is positioned in the supine position. The preferred site of entry is either the fourth or fifth intercostal space. Prior to breast development, the nipple overlies the fourth intercostal space. After breast development, the lower border of the breast generally overlies the fourth intercostal space. The area should be prepared

TABLE 15–3

Chest Tube Sizes

Age	Approximate Weight (kg)	Sizes (French)*
Neonate	2–3	8–12
Infant	4–10	10–16
1–2 years	10–15	12–24
3–5 years	15–20	16–28
6–10 years	20–30	16–32
≥10 years	>30	20–40

*Use the tubes on the lower end of the range for evacuating air or suspected transudates. Use a larger tube for viscous fluids such as blood and exudates.

with antiseptic and draped in sterile fashion. It is helpful to either mark the skin with a permanent marker prior to skin preparation or include the nipple area in a younger infant (or the inferior border of the breast after breast development) in the exposed sterile field in order to maintain landmarks.

The area of incision should be infiltrated liberally with lidocaine, including the subcutaneous tissue, intercostal muscles, and entry point into the pleural space. Up to 0.5 ml/kg of 1% lidocaine (5 mg/kg) or 0.7 ml/kg of 1% lidocaine with epinephrine (7 mg/kg) can be used. Generally, the skin incision is one interspace below the chest cavity entry point to generate a skin flap that potentially reduces air leaks.

An incision of appropriate length is made to allow passage of the tube in the midaxillary line parallel to the axis of the rib. A curved Kelly clamp is inserted and the subcutaneous and muscle tissue bluntly dissected until the superior border of the next most superior rib is reached. The clamp with the end closed is inserted and then gently opened to create the tract. Once the superior border of the rib is reached, the clamp is forced through the pleura with pressure, taking care not to deeply drive the clamp into the chest when the pleura is penetrated.

If the child's size permits, a finger can be inserted through the tract into the pleural space to ensure that the tract extends through the pleura. Any adhesions that are felt can be manually disrupted. The end of the tube is side clamped and another clamp placed near the distal end of the tube to prevent free flow of fluid through the tube once the pleural space is entered. The side clamped tube is advanced through the tract. Once the clamp enters the pleural space, the clamp is opened and the tube advanced. The tube should be inserted to a sufficient depth so that the most distal side hole is within the chest cavity to prevent pneumothorax.

While the tube is held securely in place, the distal end of the tube is attached to an appropriate pleural drainage system. Once the system is attached, the clamp on the distal end of the tube is removed to allow chest drainage.

Many techniques for suturing the chest tube in place are available. The most important aspect of the choice of anchoring method is that the operator removing the tube knows how the tube was secured. Some operators prefer a horizontal mattress suture on both sides of the tube; others prefer to place a "pursestring" that can be pulled together after the tube is removed. If the latter technique is used, no knot is placed at the skin level, but extra suture is wrapped around the body of the tube and then tied to the tube itself. Upon removal, the extra suture serves as skin suture for the wound. Rarely, a suture is inadvertently placed through the tube while the device is anchored. In this event, a technique for cutting the suture using endoscopic scissors has been described.[174] "Needleless" anchoring devices for anchoring tubes without suture (Statlock Multipurpose, Venetec International, San Diego, CA, USA) have been developed.

Petroleum gel gauze can be placed around the tube but generally is not necessary when the tube is adequately secured. Tape is applied to the tube to further secure it to the thorax.

A variation tube thoracostomy that is useful for draining air or thin fluid is the pigtail catheter.[175,176] Catheters are available in sizes ranging from 5F to 9F. With this technique, a needle is introduced into the pleural space after anesthesia, as described in the thoracentesis section. After aspiration of air or fluid, the syringe is removed and a guidewire is introduced into the pleural space. The needle is removed, and a small skin incision is made to facilitate passage of a dilator over the wire. Following (successive) dilation, a catheter with multiple side holes is introduced over the wire into the pleural space. The catheter is attached to a standard chest drainage system and sutured in place. Advantages of this technique are that it is much less traumatic than blunt dissection through the chest wall and it is better tolerated. However, blood or viscous fluid may not drain adequately with this technique.

Another variation on traditional tube thoracostomy is the needle-wire-dilator technique.[177] With this technique, a needle and wire are introduced, as described for the pigtail catheter. A series of progressively larger dilators are passed into the pleural space, taking care to insert the dilators only a length sufficient to extend into the pleural space. Placing a stiff dilator far into the chest greatly increases the potential for injury to organs and vasculature. After passage of the largest dilator, the thoracostomy tube is introduced. An inner cannula in the tube facilitates passage of the relatively larger tube over a small wire. The inner cannula is removed, and the chest tube is connected to the suction apparatus. Disadvantages of this technique are that the tube may take slightly longer to place and some of the commercially available tubes are less rigid than traditional thoracostomy tubes, which may predispose the tubes to kinking.[178]

Maintenance

Once the tube has been placed, some authorities suggest "stripping" or "milking" the tube if blood is present. This step results in increased negative pressure within the tube during the procedure, sometimes facilitating drainage, although little data supporting this practice are available.[179,180] Surgeons frequently prescribe prophylactic antibiotics while a tube thoracostomy is in place, especially in trauma patients, but data supporting this practice are mixed.[181,182]

Tubes should be evaluated for ongoing air leaks by observing the leak chamber of the drainage apparatus for air bubbles. If an air leak is noted after the first few minutes, all connections should be checked to ensure air is not being entrained through a loose connection. A chest radiogram is obtained to verify the position of the tube and observe resolution of the pneumothorax or pleural effusion. Persistent pneumothorax and ongoing air leak despite a functional chest tube suggest a bronchopleural fistula or injury to an airway.

Timing of tube removal depends on the indication for tube placement. If a tube was placed for pneumothorax and active air leak has resolved, a trial of water seal drainage to allow accumulation of air over several hours should be considered. If a tube was placed for fluid drainage, the drainage should decrease to 2 to 3 ml/kg over the 24 hours prior to tube removal.

Removal of the thoracostomy tube is painful. Systemic analgesics are frequently used, and topical anesthesia with lidocaine/prilocaine cream reduced the pain of removal when a tube was left in place for 3 hours.[183] Another study found intrapleural bupivacaine was ineffective in reducing the pain of tube removal.[177] One study of adult patients found no difference in the risk of pneumothorax when tubes were removed at the end of inspiration or expiration.[184]

Complications

Many complications can arise from chest tube placement. Any structure in the chest can be penetrated by undue force. For this reason, trocars should not be used. The underlying lung can be penetrated, leading to a persistent bronchopleural fistula. Intraabdominal organs may be injured if tube placement is too caudal. Placement of a tube too far into the pleural space may result in mediastinal perforation.[185] Vascular injuries may result to the great vessels, and the thoracic duct may be injured with left-sided placement. Injury to the long thoracic nerve may result in winging of the scapula, and intercostal nerve injury can cause intercostal neuralgia. Computed tomography of the chest can help identify the exact location of the chest tube in the thorax.[186]

Placement high in the thorax can result in obstruction of the subclavian artery.[187] Development of new subcutaneous emphysema after tube thoracostomy suggests one of the side ports migrated outside the thoracic cavity.[188] Some adult data suggest the risk of recurrent pneumothorax is reduced by a trial of water seal with repeat chest radiography prior to tube removal.[189,190]

Summary

Tube thoracostomy is required frequently in pediatric critical care and can be accomplished safely with careful attention to detail. Newer techniques of drainage using smaller catheters and needle-wire-dilator systems offer additional choices and safety in carefully selected patients.

Diagnostic Paracentesis

Paracentesis is the percutaneous sampling of peritoneal fluid by needle aspiration through the abdominal wall. It is a relatively safe procedure and is useful as a diagnostic tool in the evaluation of patients with ascites. Analysis of ascitic fluid, combined with history and physical examination, frequently confirm the cause of ascites.

Indications

Paracentesis is indicated in any patient with new-onset ascites, patients with chronic ascites and clinical deterioration, and cases of suspected bacterial peritonitis.[197] Paracentesis is not recommended for diagnosis of traumatic hemoperitoneum because of high false-negative rates.[193]

Contraindications

Paracentesis in patients with ascites has no absolute contraindications. Coagulopathy is not a contraindication to paracentesis, although caution should be used in patients with moderate-to-severe coagulopathies.[200–204] Some investigators propose that prophylactic transfusion of fresh-frozen plasma, platelets, or other clotting factors prior to paracentesis in patients with coagulopathy is not necessary.[197,203]

Pregnancy is a relative contraindication to the procedure, but pregnant patients can undergo paracentesis with the site of needle insertion above the umbilicus and lateral to the midline.[193] Paracentesis should not be performed through an area of cellulitis.[193]

Procedure

Presence of ascites must be confirmed prior to paracentesis. Physical examination findings supporting the presence of ascites include flank dullness, shifting dullness, and fluid waves.[191] Although the presence of ascites may be obvious in patients with massive ascites, physical examination alone often is not sufficient. Many clinicians believe that unless ascites is unquestionably present, ultrasound should be performed before proceeding with paracentesis.[199] Ultrasonography is more sensitive than physical examination in diagnosing ascites, can detect small amounts of fluid, and can differentiate free from loculated fluid.[194] Ultrasound guidance may improve the safety and efficacy of paracentesis.[195]

Supplies

Box 15–6 lists the supplies required for diagnostic paracentesis.

Technique

The patient is positioned in the sitting, semisupine, or lateral decubitus position.[198,201] The bladder should be emptied by voiding or catheterization. The site of needle

BOX 15–6

Supplies for Diagnostic Paracentesis

- Antiseptic solution
- Alcohol preps
- Sterile gauze
- Sterile drapes
- Sterile gloves
- 1% lidocaine with or without epinephrine
- 3- to 10-ml syringe with small-gauge needle for local anesthesia
- 22- to 16-gauge spinal needle or intravenous catheter (22- to 20-gauge needle for small children, 16- to 20-gauge needle for larger children)
- 20-ml (or larger) syringe
- Specimen vials

insertion is selected by physical examination or ultrasound location of ascitic fluid, with the preferred site midline, 2 cm below the umbilicus in the area of the avascular linea alba. A lateral approach can be used in the right or left lower quadrant a few centimeters above the inguinal ligament and lateral to the rectus abdominus muscle.[198,200] Needle insertion in pregnant patients should be above the umbilicus and lateral to the midline. Puncture sites in the area of surgical scars or any area of cellulites should be avoided.[193]

The entry site is prepared with antiseptic solution, followed by 70% alcohol and application of sterile drapes. Infiltration of the skin and peritoneum is achieved with 1% lidocaine using a small-gauge needle. After attaching a syringe to a needle or catheter appropriate for the patient's age, the needle is inserted through the site of infiltration while traction is applied to the skin in a caudal direction. Use of this Z-track method of insertion is recommended to prevent a direct linear needle track, which could result in a fluid leak after the procedure is completed. The needle is advanced slowly using negative pressure on the syringe until a "pop" is felt as the needle passes through the peritoneum and free flow of fluid into the syringe is noted. A spinal needle, if used, can be secured in place with a free hand or hemostat. An over-the-needle catheter, if used, is advanced into the peritoneal cavity, the needle is removed, and the syringe is replaced. Approximately 20 to 40 ml of fluid is collected for diagnostic evaluation. If fluid return stops or is sluggish, changing the patient's position may be helpful. Following removal of the needle or catheter, direct pressure is applied to the insertion site and then a sterile pressure dressing is applied.[198,200,201]

Complications

Potential complications of paracentesis are few but may include persistent leakage of ascitic fluid, bladder or intestinal perforation, introduction of infection with resultant peritonitis, subcutaneous abdominal wall hematoma, and bleeding.[198,200,204] Persistent leakage of ascitic fluid can be minimized by using the Z-track method for needle insertion. Bladder emptying decreases the risk of bladder perforation.[198] Risk of intestinal perforation with subsequent complications is minimal but is increased in patients with previous abdominal surgical procedures and adhesions. This risk can be minimized by not using abdominal surgical scars as the needle insertion site.[200,204] Risk of intestinal perforation can be increased if the bowel is markedly distended (as in bowel obstruction), so decompression should be considered prior to paracentesis in these cases.[200] Appropriate selection of the needle insertion site minimizes the risk of bleeding. Visible collateral venous channels on the abdominal wall should be avoided.[200] Strict adherence to sterile technique and avoidance of areas of skin or soft tissue infection decrease the risk of infection. Scrotal edema following paracentesis has been described, typically in patients with massive ascites. Use of small needles is proposed as a method to prevent this occurrence.[192]

Interpretation

Analysis of ascitic fluid may not yield a definitive diagnosis but is useful in the evaluation of ascites. Clinical assessment identifies the most likely diagnosis, helps determine which tests which should be ordered, and influences interpretation of results.[197,203]

Studies that should be obtained include total protein, glucose, albumin, LDH, cell count with differential, Gram stain, and aerobic and anaerobic cultures. Other studies to consider are pH, amylase, triglycerides, bilirubin, creatinine, electrolytes, cytology, and cultures and stains for tuberculosis.[191,197] Corresponding serum chemistries should be obtained for comparison.

Fluid obtained for cultures should be directly inoculated into blood culture bottles at the bedside.[205] Gram stain should be performed on the cell pellet generated from centrifuged fluid.[197] These measures increase the likelihood of recovering or identifying organisms from infected fluid.

Analysis of the serum–ascites albumin gradient (SA gradient) is useful for differentiating between ascites caused by portal hypertension and ascites resulting from other causes. The SA gradient is calculated by subtracting the albumin concentration of the ascitic fluid from the albumin concentration of the serum. An SA gradient of 1.1 g/dl or higher correlates with portal hypertension with 97% accuracy.[197]

Characteristics of ascitic fluid in various conditions are as follows.

Portal hypertension. The ascitic fluid typically is clear or straw colored, with a total protein of less than 2.5 to 3 g/dl. Leukocyte count is generally less than 250 to 500 cells per milliliter, and fewer than one third of cells are neutrophils. Gram stain and culture reveal no organisms.[191]

Bacterial peritonitis. The ascitic fluid generally appears cloudy or turbid, with an absolute neutrophil count of greater than 250 cells per milliliter.[197] In spontaneous bacterial peritonitis, total protein generally is less than 1 g/dl, and LDH and glucose levels are similar to serum levels. A single organism may be identified by Gram stain or culture, although Gram stain is only about 10% specific in detecting bacteria in early spontaneous peritonitis and cultures may be negative.[197,203] Spontaneous bacterial peritonitis occasionally is present without a significant increase in the ascitic fluid neutrophil count. In these cases, low ascitic fluid pH has been proposed as an indicator of peritonitis, but Runyon[202] demonstrated that the pH of ascitic fluid is not consistently decreased in spontaneous bacterial peritonitis without increased neutrophil count. In secondary bacterial peritonitis, the total protein may be greater than 3 g/dl.[191,197] LDH is higher than serum LDH, and the glucose level may be less than 50 mg/dl.[203] Multiple organisms may be identified by Gram stain or culture. It has been reported that the SA gradient typically is 1.1 g/dl or higher in spontaneous peritonitis but less than 1.1 g/dl in secondary peritonitis.[197]

Chylous ascites. The fluid appears milky but may appear clear or yellowish if the patient has not recently ingested fat. Leukocyte count is 1000 to 5000 cells/ml3, and the majority of the cells are lymphocytes.[191] Triglyceride levels are markedly higher than serum levels and may be greater than 1500 g/dl. Total protein concentration generally is less than 3 g/dl.

Pancreatic ascites. The fluid generally is turbid but may be tea colored or bloody. Leukocyte count and total protein level are elevated. Amylase and lipase levels in ascitic fluid are greater than serum levels. In infants younger than 4 to 6 months, amylase levels may be low, and lipase levels should be used to evaluate the ascitic fluid.[191]

Urinary ascites. Protein levels are less than 1 g/dl.[201] Creatinine levels are higher than serum levels.[191]

Malignant ascites. Malignant ascites are rare in children. The ascitic fluid may appear bloody, with elevated protein and LDH levels. Glucose level may be low, and the SA gradient is less than 1.1 g/dl in 93% of affected patients.[191]

Nephrotic syndrome. The fluid is similar to the fluid in portal hypertension, appearing straw colored with a total protein less than 2.5 g/dl.[191]

Biliary ascites. Fluid is bile stained. Bilirubin levels are greater than serum levels and may be 100 to 400 mg/ml.[206]

Tuberculous ascites. The fluid may be bloody or yellow, or it may exhibit fibrin clots. Total protein typically is greater than 2.5 g/dl. Leukocyte count is elevated to greater than 1000 cells per milliliter, and the cells are primarily lymphocytic.[193] The glucose level may be less than 30 mg/dl.[196]

Closing Remarks

Needle aspiration of ascitic fluid is a relatively safe procedure when performed with appropriate precautionary measures. Analysis of ascitic fluid obtained by paracentesis is useful in the evaluation of patients with new-onset ascites, chronic ascites with clinical deterioration, or suspected bacterial peritonitis.

REFERENCES

Intraosseous Access

1. Anderson TE, Arthur K, Kleinman M, et al: Intraosseous infusion: success of a standardized regional training program for prehospital advanced life support providers. *Ann Emerg Med* 23:52-55, 1994.
2. Barron BJ, Tran HD, Lamki LM, et al: Scintigraphic findings of osteomyelitis after intraosseous infusion in a child. *Clin Nucl Med* 19:307-308, 1994.
3. Berg RA: Emergency infusion of catecholamines into bone marrow. *Am J Dis Child* 138:810-811, 1984.
2. Biello JF, O'Hair KC, Kirby WC, et al: Intraosseous infusion of dobutamine and isoproterenol. *Am J Dis Child* 145:165-167, 1991.
3. Bielski RJ, Bassett GS, Fideler B, et al: Intraosseous infusions: effects on the immature physis: an experimental model in rabbits. *J Pediatr Orthop* 13:511-515, 1993.
4. Brickman K, Rega P, Koltz M, et al: Analysis of growth plate abnormalities following intraosseous infusions through the proximal tibial epiphysis in pigs. *Ann Emerg Med* 17:121-123, 1988.
5. Brickman KR, Krupp K, Ruga P, et al: Typing and screening of blood from intraosseous access. *Ann Emerg Med* 19:1207, 1990.
6. Brickman KR, Rega P, Schoolfield L, et al: Investigation of bone developmental and histopathologic changes from intraosseous infusion. *Ann Emerg Med* 28:430-435, 1996.
7. Burke T, Kehl DK: Intraosseous infusion in infants: case report of a complication. *J Bone Joint Surg* 75:428-429, 1993.
8. Daga SR, Gosavi DG, Verma B: Intraosseous access using butterfly needle. *Trop Doct* 29:142-144, 1999.
9. Drinker CK, Drinker KR, Lund CC: The circulation in mammalian bone marrow. *Am J Physiol* 62:1-92, 1922.
10. Dubeck MA, Pfeiffer JW, Clifford CD, et al: Comparison of intraosseous and intravenous delivery of hypertonic saline/dextran in anesthetized, euvolemic pigs. *Ann Emerg Med* 21:498-503, 1992.
11. Fiallos M, Kissoon N, Abdelmoneim T, et al: Fat embolism with the use of intraosseous infusion during cardiopulmonary resuscitation. *Am J Med Sci* 314:73-79, 1997.
14. Fiser DH: Intraosseous infusion. *N Engl J Med* 32:1579-1581, 1990.
15. Fiser RT, Walker WM, Seibert JJ, et al: Tibial length following intraosseous infusion: a prospective, radiographic analysis. *Pediatr Emerg Care* 13:186-188, 1997.
16. Galpin RD, Kronick JB, Willis RB, et al: Bilateral lower extremity compartment syndromes secondary to intraosseous fluid resuscitation. *J Pediatr Orthop* 11:773-776, 1991.
17. Getschman SJ, Dietrich AM, Franklin WH, et al: Intraosseous adenosine. As effective as peripheral or central venous administration? *Arch Pediatr Adolesc Med* 148:616-619, 1994.
18. Glaeser PW, Hellmich TR, Szewczuga D, et al: Five-year experience in pediatric intraosseous infusions in children and adults. *Ann Emerg Med* 22:1119-1124, 1993.
19. Gunal I, Kose N, Gurer D: Compartment syndrome after intraosseous infusion: an experimental study in dogs. *J Pediatr Surg* 31:1491-1493, 1996.
20. Halm B, Yamamoto LG: Comparing ease of intraosseous needle placement: Jamshidi versus Cook. *Am J Emerg Med* 16:420-421, 1998.
21. Heinild S, Sondergaard T, Tudvad F: Bone marrow infusion in childhood: experiences from a thousand infusions. *J Pediatr* 30:400-412, 1947.
22. Hodge D: Intraosseous infusions: a review. *Pediatr Emerg Care* 1:215-218, 1985.
23. Hodge D III, Delgado-Paredes C, Fleisher G: Intraosseous infusion flow rates in hypovolemic "pediatric" dogs. *Ann Emerg Med* 16:305-307, 1987.
24. Jaimovich DG, Kumar A, Francom S: Evaluation of intraosseous versus intravenous antibiotic levels in a porcine model. *Am J Dis Child* 145:946-949, 1991.
25. Jun H, Hanuyama AZ, Chang KS, et al: Comparison of a new screw-tipped intraosseous needle versus a standard bone marrow aspiration needle for infusion. *Am J Emerg Med* 18:135-139, 2000.
26. Katz DS, Wojtowzcz AR: Tibial fracture: a complication of intraosseous infusion. Am J Emerg Med 12:258-259, 1994.
27. Kentner R, Haas T, Gervais H, et al: Pharmacokinetics and pharmacodynamics of hydroxyethyl starch in hypovolemic pigs: a comparison of peripheral and intraosseous infusion. *Resuscitation* 40:37-44, 1999.
28. Kissoon N, Rosenberg H, Gloor J, et al: Comparison of the acid-base status of blood obtained from intraosseous and central venous sites during steady and low flow states. *Crit Care Med* 21:1765-1769, 1993.
29. LaFleche FR, Slepin MJ, Vargas J, et al: Iatrogenic bilateral tibial fractures after intraosseous infusion attempts in a 3-month-old infant. *Ann Emerg Med* 18:1099-1101, 1989.
30. LaSpada J, Kissoon N, Melker R, et al: Extravasation rates and complications of intraosseous needles during gravity and pressure infusion. *Crit Care Med* 23:2023-2028, 1995.
31. Moscanti R, Moore GP: Compartment syndrome with resultant amputation following intraosseous infusion. *Am J Emerg Med* 8:470-471, 1990.
32. Neufeld JD, Marx JA, Moore EE, et al: Comparison of intraosseous, central, and peripheral routes of crystalloid infusion for resuscitation of hemorrhagic shock in a swine model. *J Trauma Injury Infect Crit Care* 34:422-428, 1993.
33. Orlowski JP: Emergency alternatives to intravenous access: intraosseous, intratracheal, sublingual, and other site drug administration. *Pediatr Clin North Am* 41:1183-1200, 1994.
34. Orlowski JP: My kingdom for an intravenous line. *Am J Dis Child* 138:803, 1984.
35. Orlowski JP, Julius CJ, Petras RE, et al: The safety of intraosseous infusions: risks of fat and bone marrow emboli to the lungs. *Ann Emerg Med* 18:1062-1067, 1989.
36. Orlowski JP, Porembka DT, Gallagher JM, et al: Comparison study of intraosseous, central intravenous, and peripheral intravenous infusions of emergency drugs. *Am J Dis Child* 144:112-117, 1990.

37. Orlowski JP, Porembka DT, Gallagher JM, et al: The bone marrow as a source of laboratory studies. *Ann Emerg Med* 18:1348-1351, 1989.
38. Platt SL, Notterman DA, Winchester P: Fungal osteomyelitis and sepsis from intraosseous infusion. *Pediatr Emerg Care* 9:149-150, 1993.
39. Plewa MC, King RW, Fenn-Buderer N, et al: Hematologic safety of intraosseous blood transfusion in a swine model of pediatric hemorrhagic hypovolemia. *Acad Emerg Med* 2:799-809, 1995.
40. Ravitch MM: Suppurative anterior medistinitis in an infant following intrasternal blood transfusions. *Arch Surg* 47:250-257, 1943.
41. Ribeiro JA, Price CT, Knapp DR: Compartment syndrome of the lower extremity after intraosseous infusion of fluid: a report of two cases. *J Bone Joint Surg* 75:430-433, 1993.
42. Rosetti VA, Thompson RM, Miller J, et al: Intraosseous infusion: an alternative route of pediatric intravascular access. *Ann Emerg Med* 14:885-888, 1985.
43. Rosovsky M, Fitzpatrick M, Goldfarb CR, et al: Bilateral osteomyelitis due to intraosseous infusion: case report and review of the English literature. *Pediatr Radiol* 24:72-73, 1994.
44. Salassi-Scotter M, Fiser DH: Adoption of intraosseous infusion technigque for prehospital pediatric mergency care. *Pediatr Emerg Care* 6:263-265, 1990.
45. Sapien R, Stein H, Padbury JF, et al: Intraosseous versus intravenous epinephrine infusions in lambs: pharmacokinetics and pharmacodynamics. *Pediatr Emerg Care* 8:179-183, 1992.
46. Seigler RS: Intraosseous infusion performed in the prehospital setting: South Carolina's six-year experience. *J South Carolina Med Assoc* 93:209-215, 1997.
47. Simmons CM, Johnson NE, Perkin RM, et al: Intraosseous extravasation complication reports. *Ann Emerg Med* 23:363-366, 1994.
48. Smith RJ, Keseg DP, Manley LK, et al: Intraosseous infusions by prehospital personnel in critically ill pediatric patients. *Ann Emerg Med* 17:491-495, 1988.
49. Spivey WH, Malone D, Unger HD, et al: Comparison of intraosseous, central, and peripheral routes of administration of sodium bicarbonate during CPR in pigs. *Ann Emerg Med* 14:1135-1140, 1985.
50. Tobias JD, Nichols DG: Intraosseous succinylcholine for orotracheal intubation. *Pediatr Emerg Care* 6:108-109, 1990.
51. Tocantins LM, O'Neill JF, Jones HW: Infusions of blood and other fluids via the bone marrow: application in pediatrics. *JAMA* 117:1229-1234, 1941.
52. Turkel H: Intraosseous infusion. *Am J Dis Child* 137:706, 1983.
53. Valdes MM: Intraosseous fluid administration in emergencies. *Lancet* 1:1235-1236, 1977.
54. Vidal R, Kissoon N, Gayle M: Compartment syndrome following intraosseous infusion. *Pediatrics* 91:1201-1202, 1993.
55. Wright R, Reynolds SL, Nachtsheim B. Compartment syndrome secondary to prolonged intraosseous infusion. *Pediatr Emerg Care* 10:157-159, 1994.

Central Venous Line Placement

56. Darouiche RO, Raad II, Heard SO, et al: A comparison of two antimicrobial-impregnated central venous catheters. Catheter Study Group. *N Engl J Med* 340:1-8, 1999.
57. Dieckman RA, Fiser DH, Selbst SM: *Pediatric emergency and critical care procedures.* St. Louis, 1997, Mosby.
58. Fuhrman BP, Zimmerman JJ: *Pediatric critical care*, ed 2, St. Louis, 1998, Mosby.
59. Olson ME, Lam K, Bodey GP, et al: Evaluation of strategies for central venous catheter placement. *Crit Care Med* 20:797-804, 1992.
60. Raad II, Hohn DC, Gilbreath BJ, et al: Prevention of central venous catheter related infections by using maximal barrier precautions during insertion. *Infect Control Hosp Epidemiol* 15:231-238, 1994.
61. Randolph J: Technique for insertion of a plastic catheter into the saphenous vein. *Pediatrics* 631-35, 1959.
62. Scott WL: Complications associated with central venous catheters. A survey. *Chest* 94:1221-24, 1988.
63. Seldinger SI: Catheter replacement of the needle in percutaneous arteriography. *Acta Radiol* 39:368, 1953.
64. Simon RR, Hoffman JR, Smith M: Modified new approaches for rapid intravenous access. *Ann Emerg Med* 16:44-49, 1987.
65. Smith-Wright DL, Green TP, Lock JE, et al: Complications of vascular catheterization in critically ill children. *Crit Care Med* 12:1015-1017, 1984.

Pulmonary Arterial Catheterization

66. Adatia I, Atz AM, Jonas RA, et al: Diagnostic use of inhaled nitric oxide after neonatal cardiac operations. *J Thorac Cardiovasc Surg* 112:1403-1405, 1996.
67. Anonymous: Pulmonary Artery Catheter Consensus Conference: Consensus Statement. *New Horizons* 5:175-193, 1997.
68. Borland LM: Allometric determination of the distance from the central venouns pressure port to wedge position of balloon-tip catheters in pediatric patients. *Crit Care Med* 14:974-976, 1986.
69. Carcillo JA, Davis AL, Zaritsky A: Role of early fluid resuscitation in pediatric septic shock. *JAMA* 266:1242-1245, 1991.
70. Damen J, Van der Tweel I: Positive tip cultures and related risk factors associated with intravascular catheterization in pediatric cardiac patients. *Crit Care Med* 16:221-228, 1988.
71. Damon J, Wever JEAT: The use of balloon-tipped pulmonary artery catheters in children undergoing cardiac surgery. *Intensive Care Med* 13:266-272, 1987.
72. DeBruin W, Notterman DA, Magid M, et al: Acute hypoxemic respiratory failure in infants and children: clinical and pathologic characteristics. *Crit Care Med* 20:1223-1234, 1992.
73. Hopkins RA, Bull C, Hawaorth SG, et al: Pulmonary hypertensive crises following surgery for congenital heart defects in young children. *Eur J Cardiothorac Surg* 5:628-634, 1991.
74. Iberti TJ, Fischer EP, Leibowitz AB, et al: A multicenter study of physician's knowledge of the pulmonary artery catheter. *JAMA* 264:2928-2932, 1990.
75. Jansen JRC: The thermodilution method for the clinical assessment of cardiac output. *Intensive Care Med* 21:691-697, 1995.
76. Morray JP, Lynn AM, Mansfield PB: Effect of pH and PCO_2 on pulmonary and systemic hemodynamics after surgery in children with congenital heart disease and pulmonary hypertension. *J Pediatr* 113:474-479, 1988.
77. Pollock MM, Reed TP, Holbrook PR, et al: Bedside pulmonary artery catheterization in pediatrics. *J Pediatr* 96:274-278, 1980.
78. Reynolds EM, Ryan CP, Sheridan RL, et al: Left ventricular failure complicating severe pediatric burn injuries. *J Pediatr* 30:264-270, 1995.
79. Swan HJC, Ganz W, Forester J, et al: Catheterization of the heart in man with use of a flow-directed balloon-tipped catheter. *N Engl J Med* 283:447-450, 1970.
80. Thompson AE: Pulmonary artery catheterization in children. *New Horizons* 5:244-249, 1997.
81. Todres ID, Crone RK, Rogers MC, et al: Swan-Ganz catheterization in the critically ill newborn. *Crit Care Med* 7:330-334, 1979.
82. Trottier SJ, Taylor RW: Physicians' attitudes toward and knowledge of the pulmonary artery catheter. Society of Critical Care Medicine Membership Survey. *New Horizons* 5:201-206, 1997.
83. Wheedon D, Shore DF, Lincoln C: Continuous monitoring of pulmonary artery pressure after cardiac surgery in infants and children. *J Cardiovasc Surg* 22:307-311, 1981.

Arterial Access

84. Adrogue HJ, Rashad MN, Gorin AB: Assessing acid-base status in circulatory failure. Differences between arterial and central venous blood. *N Engl J Med* 18:1312-1316, 1989.
85. Beards SC, Doedens L, Jackson A, et al: A comparison of arterial lines and insertion techniques in critically ill patients. *Anaesthesia* 49:968-973, 1994.
86. Cardinal P, Allan J, Pham B, et al: The effect of sodium citrate in arterial catheters on acid-base and electrolyte measurements. *Crit Care Med* 28:1388-1392, 2000.
87. Cilley RE: Arterial access in infants and children. *Semin Pediatr Surg* 1:174-180, 1992.
88. Courtney SE, Weber KR, Breakie LA, et al: Capillary blood gases in the neonate. A reassessment and review of the literature. *Am J Dis Child* 144:168-172, 1990.
89. Eyer S, Brummitt C, Crossley K, et al: Catheter-related sepsis: prospective, randomized study of three methods of long-term catheter maintenance. *Crit Care Med* 18:1073-1079, 1990.
90. Frezza EE, Mezghebe H: Indications and complications of arterial catheter use in surgical or medical intensive care units: analysis of 4932 patients. *Am Surg* 64:127-131, 1998.

91. Furfaro S, Gauthier M, Lacroix J, et al: Arterial catheter-related infections in children. A 1-year cohort analysis. *Am J Dis Child* 145:1037-1043, 1991.
92. Heulitt MJ, Farrington EA, O'Shea TM, et al: Double-blind, randomized, controlled trial of papaverine-containing infusions to prevent failure of arterial catheters in pediatric patients. *Crit Care Med* 21:825-829, 1993.
93. Kaye J, Heald GR, Morton J, et al: Patency of radial arterial catheters. *Am J Crit Care* 10:104-111, 2001.
94. Kim EH, Cohen RS, Ramachandran P: Effect of vascular puncture on blood gases in the newborn. *Pediatr Pulmonol* 10:287-290, 1991.
95. Lemke RP, al-Saedi SA, Belik J, et al: Use of tolazoline to counteract vasospasm in peripheral arterial catheters in neonates. *Acta Paediatr* 85:1497-1498, 1996.
96. Levin PD, Hersch M, Rudensky B, et al: The use of the arterial line as a source for blood cultures. *Intensive Care Med* 26:1350-1354, 2000.
97. Lual, Gonzales M, Guzzetta PC, Toro-Figueroa LO. Arterial access and catheters. In Levin DL, Morriss FC, editors: *Essentials of pediatric intensive care,* ed 2. 1997, Quality Medical Publishing.
98. Maki DG, Ringer M, Alvarado CJ: Prospective randomised trial of povidone-iodine, alcohol, and chlorhexidine for prevention of infection associated with central venous and arterial catheters. *Lancet* 338:339-343, 1991.
99. McLane C, Morris L, Holm K: A comparison of intravascular pressure monitoring system contamination and patient bacteremia with use of 48- and 72-hour system change intervals. *Heart Lung* 27:200-208, 1998.
100. Peruzzi WT, Shapiro BA: Blood gas monitors. *Respir Care Clin North Am* 1:143-156, 1995.
101. Qureshi AI, Luft AR, Sharma M, et al: Prevention and treatment of thromboembolic and ischemic complications associated with endovascular procedures: Part I—pathophysiological and pharmacological features. *Neurosurgery* 46:1344-1359, 2000.
102. Raad I, Umphrey J, Khan A, et al: The duration of placement as a predictor of peripheral and pulmonary arterial catheter infections. *J Hosp Infect* 23:17-26, 1993.
103. Rais-Bahrami K, Karna P, Dolanski EA: Effect of fluids on life span of peripheral arterial lines. *Am J Perinatol* 7:122-124, 1990.
104. Randel SN, Tsang BH, Wung JT, et al: Experience with percutaneous indwelling peripheral arterial catheterization in neonates. *Am J Dis Child* 141:848-851, 1987.
105. Randolph AG, Cook DJ, Gonzales CA, et al: Benefit of heparin in peripheral venous and arterial catheters: systematic review and meta-analysis of randomised controlled trials. *BMJ* 316:969-975, 1998.
106. Ruble K, Long C, Connor K: Pharmacologic treatment of catheter-related thrombus in pediatrics. *Pediatr Nurs* 20:553-557, 1994.
107. Saint S, Matthay MA: Risk reduction in the intensive care unit. *Am J Med* 105:515-523, 1998.
108. Steinhart CM. Arterial catheterization. In Diechmann RA, Fisher DH, Selbst SM, editors: *Illustrated textbook of pediatric and critical care procedures.* St. Louis, 1997, Mosby.
109. Sutor AH, Massicotte P, Leaker M, et al: Heparin therapy in pediatric patients. *Semin Thromb Hemost* 23:303-319, 1997.
110. Thomas F, Burke JP, Parker J, et al: The risk of infection related to radial vs femoral sites for arterial catheterization. *Crit Care Med* 11:807-812, 1983.
111. Thomas F, Orme JF Jr, Clemmer TP, et al: A prospective comparison of arterial catheter blood and catheter-tip cultures in critically ill patients. *Crit Care Med* 12:860-862, 1984.
112. Wardle SP, Kelsall AW, Yoxall CW, et al: Percutaneous femoral arterial and venous catheterization during neonatal intensive care. *Arch Dis Child Fetal Neonatal Ed* 85:F119-F122, 2001.
113. Zevola DR, Dioso J, Moggio R: Comparison of heparinized and nonheparinized solutions for maintaining patency of arterial and pulmonary artery catheters. *Am J Crit Care* 6:52-55, 1997.

Umbilical Arterial Catheter and Umbilical Venous Catheter Placement

114. Anagnostakis D, Kamba A, Petrochilou V, et al: Risk of infection associated with umbilical vein catheterization: a prospective study in 75 newborn infants. *J Pediatr* 86:759, 1975.
115. Cole ARF, Rogin SH: A technique for rapid catheterization of the umbilical artery. *Anesthesiology* 53:254, 1980.
116. Cumming WA, Burchfield DJ: Accidental catheterization of internal iliac artery branches: a serious complication of umbilical artery catheterization. *J Perinatol* XIV:304-309, 1994.
117. Dorand RD, Cook LN, Andrew BF: Umbilical vessel catheterization: the low incidence of complications in a series of 200 newborn infants. *Clin Pediatr* 16:569, 1977.
118. Dunn PM: Localization of the umbilical catheter by postmortem measurement. *Arch Dis Child* 41:69, 1966.
119. Gupta JM, Roberton NRC, Wigglesworth JS: Umbilical artery catheterization in the newborn. *Arch Dis Child* 43:382, 1968.
120. Hodson WA, Truog WE: Principles of management of respiratory problems. In Avery GB, Fletcher MA, MacDonald MG, editors: *Neonatology, pathophysiology and management of the newborn.* Philadelphia, 1994, JB Lipponcott.
121. Johns AW, Kitchen WH, Leslie DW: Complications of umbilical vessel catheters. *Med J Aust* 2:810, 1972.
122. Kempley ST, Bennett S, Loftus BG, et al: Randomized trial of umbilical arterial catheter position: clinical outcome. *Acta Paediatr* 82:173-176, 1993.
123. Landers S, Moise AA, Fraley JK, et al: Factors associated with umbilical catheter-related sepsis in neonates. *Am J Dis Child* 145:675, 1991.
124. Malloy MH, Nicholas MM: False abdominal aortic aneurism: an unusual complication of umbilical arterial catheterization for exchange transfusion. *J Pediatr* 90:285, 1977.
125. Oppenheimer D, Carroll B, Garth K: Ultrasonic detection of complications following umbilical arterial catheterization in the neonate. *Radiology* 145:667, 1982.
126. Oski FA, Allen DM, Diamond LK: Portal hypertension-a complication of umbilical vein catheterization. Pediatrics 31:297, 1963.
127. Pierce JR, Turner BS: Physiologic monitoring. In Merenstein GB, Gardner SL, editors: *Handbook of neonatal intensive care.* St. Louis, 1998, Mosby-Yearbook.
128. Raval NC: Umbilical vessel vcatheterization. In Spitzer AR, editor: *Intensive care of the fetus and neonate.* St. Louis, 1996, Mosby-Year Book.
129. Rejjal AR, Galal MO, Nazar HM, et al: Complications of parenteral nutrition via umbilical vein catheter. *Eur J Pediatr* 152:624, 1993.
130. Rodriguez RJ: Umbilical vessel catheterization. In Klaus MH, Fanaroff AA, editors: *Care of the high-risk neonate.* Philadelphia, 2001, WB Saunders.
131. Rosenfeld W, Biagtan J, Schaeffer H, et al: A new graph for insertion of umbilical artery catheters. *J Pediatr* 96:735, 1980.
132. Rosenfeld W, Estrada R, Jhaveri R, et al: Evaluation of graphs for insertion of umbilical artery catheters below the diaphragm. *J Pediatr* 98:627, 1981.
133. Sasidhanan P: Umbilical artery rupture: a major complication of catheterization. *Indiana Med* 78:34, 1985.
134. Schreiber MD, Perez CA, Kitterman JA: A double-catheter technique for caudally misdirected umbilical artery catheter. *J Pediatr* 104:768, 1984.
135. Shah KJ, Corkery JJ: Necrotizing enterocolitis following umbilical vein catheterization. *Clin Radiol* 29:295, 1978.
136. Shukla H, Ferrara A: Rapid estimation of insertional length of umbilical catheters in newborns. *Am J Dis Child* 140:786, 1986.
137. Simpson JS: Misdiagnosis complicating umbilical vessel catheterization. *Clin Pediatr* 16:569, 1977.
138. Stork E, Carlo W, Kliegman R, et al: Neonatal hypertension appears unrelated to aortic catheter position. *Pediatr Res* 18:321A, 1984.
139. Umbilical Artery Catheter Trial Study Group: Relationship of intraventricular hemorrhage or death with the level of umbilical artery placement: a multicenter randomized trial. *Pediatrics* 90:881, 1992.
140. Vailas GN, Brouilette RT, Scott JP, et al: Neonatal aortic thrombosis r: recent experience. *J Pediatr* 109:101, 1986.
141. Van Leeuwen G, Patney M: Complications of umbilical artery catheterizations: peritoneal perforation. *Pediatrics* 44:1028, 1969.
142. Walker D, Pellet JR: Pericardial temponade secondary to umbilical vein catheters. *J Pediatr Surg* 7:79, 1972.
143. Weber AL, Deluce S, Shannon DL: Normal and abnormal position of umbilical artery and venous catheter on the roentgenogram and review of complications. *AJR Am J Roentgenol* 20:361, 1974.

144. Wesstrom G, Finnstrom O, Stenport G: Umbilical artery catheterization in newborns: thrombosis in relation to catheter type and position. *Acta Paediatr Scand* 68:575, 1979.

Pericardiocentesis

143. Armstrong G, Cardon L, Vikomerson D, et al: Localization of needle tip with color doppler during pericardiocentesis: in vitro validation and initial clinical application. *J Am Soc Echocardiogr* 14:29-37, 2001.
144. Chandraratna PA, Reid CL, Nimalasuriya A, et al: Application of 2-dimentional contrast studies during pericardiocentesis. *Am J Cardiol* 52:1120-1122, 1983.
145. Duvernoy O, Borowiec J, Helmius G, et al: Complication of percutaneous pericardiocentesis under fluoroscopic guidance. *Acta Radiol* 33:309, 1992.
146. Guberman BA, Fowler N, Engel PJ, et al: Cardiac tamponade in medical patients. *Circulation* 64:633, 1981.
147. Inkelis SH: Pericardiocentesis. In Dieckman RA, Fiser DH, Selbst SM, editors: *Pediatric emergency and critical care procedures.* St. Louis, 1997, Mosby-Year Book.
148. Maggiolini S, Bozzano A, Russo P, et al: Echocardiography-guided pericardiocentesis with probe-mounted needle: report of 53 cases. *J Am Soc Echocardiogr* 14:821-824, 2001.
149. Satoh T: Demonstration of the Epstein-Barr genome by the polymerase chain reaction and in situ hybridization in a patient with viral pericarditis. *Br Heart J* 69:563-564, 1993.
150. Silverman NH: Postoperative evaluation. In Silverman NH, editor: *Pediatric echocardiography.* Baltimore, 1993, Williams & Wilkins.
151. Snider AR, Serwer GA: Echocardiographic evaluation of the postoperative patient. In Snider AR, Serwer GA, editors: *Echocardiography in pediatric heart disease.* St. Louis, 1990, Mosby-Year Book.
152. Sobol SM, Thomas JM, Jr. Evans RW: Myocardial laceration not demonstrated by continuous electrocardiographic monitoring occurring during pericardiocentesis. *N Engl J Med* 292:1222, 1975.
153. Szymanski M, Petric M, Saunders FE, et al: Mycoplasma pneumoniae pericarditis demonstrated by polymerase chain reaction and electron microscopy. *Clin Infect Dis* 34:16-17, 2002.
154. Van Heeckeren DW, Moss MM: Pericardiocentesis and pericardial tube insertion. In Blumer JL, editor: *A practical guide to pediatric intensive care.* St. Louis, 1990, Mosby-Year Book.
155. Zahn EM, Houde C, Benson L, et al. Percutaneous pericardial catheter drainage in childhood. *Am J Cardiol* 70:678-680, 1992.

Thoracentesis and Tube Thoracostomy

156. Ahmed MY, Silver P, Nimkoff L, et al: The needle-wire-dilator technique for the insertion of chest tubes in pediatric patients. *Pediatr Emerg Care* 11:252-254, 1995.
157. Bartfield JM, Crisafulli KM, Raccio-Robak N, et al: The effects of warming and buffering on pain of infiltration of lidocaine. *Acad Emerg Med* 2:254-258, 1995.
158. Bell RL, Ovadia P, Abdullah F, et al: Chest tube removal: end-inspiration or end-expiration. *J Trauma* 50:674-677, 2001.
159. Bucalo BD, Mirikitani EJ, Moy RL: Comparison of skin anesthetic effect of liposomal lidocaine, nonliposomal lidocaine, and EMLA using 30-minute application time. *Dermatol Surg* 24:537-541, 1998.
160. Buckley MM, Benfield P: Eutectic lidocaine/prilocaine cream: a review of the topical anaesthetic/analgesic efficacy of a eutectic mixture of local anaesthetics (EMLA). *Drugs* 46:126-151, 1993.
161. Cerfolio RJ, Bass C, Katholi CR: Prospective randomized trial compares suction versus water seal for air leaks. *Ann Thorac Surg* 71:1613-1617, 2001.
162. Colice GL, Curtis A, Deslauriers J, et al: Medical and surgical treatment of parapneumonic effusions: an evidence-based guideline. *Chest* 118:1158-1171, 2000.
163. Duncan C, Erickson R: Pressures associated with chest tube stripping. *Heart Lung* 11:166-71, 1982.
164. Freimanis AS: Ultrasound and thoracentesis. *JAMA* 238:1631, 1977.
165. Gammie JS, Banks MC, Fuhrman CR, et al: The pigtail catheter for pleural drainage: a less invasive alternative to tube thoracostomy. *J Soc Laparoendosc Surg* 3:57-61, 1999.
166. Gayer G, Rozenman J, Hoffmann C, et al: CT diagnosis of malpositioned chest tubes. *Br J Radiol* 73:786-790, 2000.
167. Gonzalez RP, Holevar MR: Role of prophylactic antibiotics for tube thoracostomy in chest trauma. *Am Surg* 64:617, 1998; discussion 620-621.
168. Hippocrates: Writings. In RM H, editor: *Great books of the western world.* Chicago, 1952, Encyclopedia Brittanica.
169. Houston MC: Pleural fluid pH: diagnostic, therapeutic, and prognostic value. *Am J Surg* 154:333-337, 1987.
170. Jetty P, Mehran RJ: Inadvertent suture through the chest tube: a simple solution to a frustrating problem. *Ann Thorac Surg* 69:261-262, 2000.
171. Jones PM, Hewer RD, Wolfenden HD, et al: Subcutaneous emphysema associated with chest tube drainage. *Respirology* 6:87-89, 2001.
172. Keske U: Ultrasound-aided thoracentesis in intensive care patients. *Intensive Care Med* 25:896-897, 1999.
173. Lander J, Hodgins M, Nazarali S, et al: Determinants of success and failure of EMLA. *Pain* 64:89-97, 1996.
174. Light RW, Erozan YS, Ball WC Jr: Cells in pleural fluid: their value in differential diagnosis. *Arch Intern Med* 132:854-860, 1973.
175. Light RW, Girard WM, Jenkinson SG, et al: Parapneumonic effusions. *Am J Med* 69:507-512, 1980.
176. Light RW, Macgregor MI, Luchsinger PC, et al: Pleural effusions: the diagnostic separation of transudates and exudates. *Ann Intern Med* 77:507-513, 1972.
177. Light RW: Pleural effusions. *Med Clin North Am* 61:1339-1352, 1977.
178. Martino K, Merrit S, Boyakye K, et al: Prospective randomized trial of thoracostomy removal alogrithms. *J Trauma* 46:369-371, 1999; discussion 372-373.
179. Meyer G, Henneman PL, Fu P: Buffered lidocaine. *Ann Emerg Med* 20:218-219, 1991.
180. Moskal TL, Liscum KR, Mattox KL: Subclavian artery obstruction by tube thoracostomy algorithms. *J Trauma* 43:368-369, 1997; discussion 372-373.
181. Nagesh BS, Sehgal S, Jindal SK, et al: Evaluation of polymerase chain reaction for detection of Mycobacterium tuberculosis in pleural fluid. *Chest* 119:1737-1741, 2001.
182. Pierce JD, Piazza D, Naftel DC: Effects of two chest tube clearance protocols on drainage in patients after myocardial revascularization surgery. *Heart Lung* 20:125-130, 1991.
183. Puntillo KA: Effects of interpleural bupivacaine on pleural chest tube removal pain: a randomized controlled trial. *Am J Crit Care* 5:102-108, 1996.
184. Rashid MA, Wikstrom T, Ortenwall P: Mediastinal perforation and contralateral hemothorax by a chest tube. *Thorac Cardiovasc Surg* 46:375-376, 1998.
185. Roberts JS, Bratton SL, Brogan TV: Efficacy and complications of percutaneous pigtail catheters for thoracostomy in pediatric patients. *Chest* 114:1116-1121, 1998.
186. Rosen DA, Morris JL, Rosen KR, et al: Analgesia for pediatric thoracostomy tube removal. *Anesth Analg* 90:1025-1028, 2000.
187. Scarfone RJ, Jasani M, Gracely EJ: Pain of local anesthetics: rate of administration and buffering. *Ann Emerg Med* 31:36-40, 1998.
188. Wilson RF, Nichols RL: The EAST practice management guidelines for prophylactic antibiotic use in tube thoracostomy for trraumatic hemopneumothorax: a commentary: Eastern Association for Trauma. *J Trauma* 48:758-759, 2000.

Diagnostic Paracentesis

189. Cochran WJ: Ascites. In McMillan JA, DeAngelis CD, Feigin RD, Warshaw JB, editors: *Oski's pediatrics: principles and practice.* Philadelphia, 1999, Lippincott, Williams & Wilkins.
190. Conn H: Sudden scrotal edema in cirrhosis: a postparacentesis syndrome. *Ann Intern Med* 74:943-945, 1971.
191. Glauser JM: Paracentesis. In Roberts JR, Hedges JR, editors: *Clinical procedures in emergency medicine.* Philadelphia, 1991, WB Saunders.
192. Goldberg BB, Goodman GA, Clearfield HR: Evaluation of ascites by ultrasound. *Radiology* 96:15-22, 1970.
193. Heller M, Jehle D: *Ultrasound in emergency medicine.* Philadelphia, 1995, WB Saunders.
194. Hickerson SL, Cross JT, Schutze GE, et al: Diagnostic procedures. In Dieckmann RA, Fiser DH, Selbst SM, editors: *Pediatric emergency and critical care procedures.* St. Louis, 1997, Mosby-Year Book.
195. Hoefs JC, Jonas GM: Diagnositic paracentesis. *Adv Intern Med* 37:391-409, 1992.

196. Huges WT, Buescher ES: *Pediatric procedures*. Philadelphia, 1995, WB Saunders.
197. Kandel G, Diamant NE: A clinical view of recent advances in ascites. *J Clin Gastroenterol* 8:85-99, 1986.
198. Mallory A, Schaefer JW: Complications of diagnostic paracentesis in patients with liver disease. *JAMA* 239:628-630, 1978.
199. McCoy J, Wolma FJ: Abdominal tap: indication, technic and results. *Am J Surg* 122:693-695, 1971.
200. Runyon BA, Antillon MR: Ascitic fluid pH and lactate: insensitive and nonspecific tests in detecting ascitic fluid infection. *Hepatology* 13:929-935, 1991.
201. Runyon BA: Care of patients with ascites. *N Engl J Med* 330:337-342, 1994.
202. Runyon BA: Paracentesis of ascitic fluid: a safe proecedure. *Arch Intern Med* 146:2259-2261, 1986.
203. Runyon BA, Umland ET, Merlin T: Inoculation of blood culture bottles with ascitic fluid: improved detection of spontaneous bacterial peritonitis. *Arch Intern Med* 147:73-75, 1987.
204. Smith SD, Vazquez WD: Ascites. In O'Neill JA, Rowe MI, Grosfield JL, Fonkalsrud EW, Coran AG, editors: *Pediatric surgery*. St. Louis, 1998, Mosby Year-Book.
205. Unger SW, Chandler JG: Chylous ascites in infants and children. *Surgery* 93:455-461, 1983.

CHAPTER

16

Pediatric Intensive Care in Developing Countries

Frank Shann and Andrew Argent

PEARLS

- In the 52 high-income countries, annual expenditure on health averages US $2702 per capita, which is *128 times* the amount available in the 66 poorest countries.
- Overseas development aid from members of the Organisation of Economic Co-operation and Development (OECD) has fallen to 0.25% of gross domestic product, which is well short of the United Nations' target of 0.70%.
- More than 99% of all child deaths occur in developing countries, and 10.1 million of the 10.9 million deaths in children younger than 5 years are preventable.
- Pneumonia is the most common cause of death in children. It causes 2.1 million deaths per year in children younger than 5 years. It also contributes to many of the 1.1 million deaths each year from measles.
- Gastroenteritis is the second most common cause of child mortality. It causes 2 million child deaths every year.
- The diagnosis of tuberculosis may be difficult in children because of the paucity of organisms in sputum and other body fluids. Often treatment for tuberculosis must be started without bacteriologic confirmation of the diagnosis.
- Malnutrition contributes to 56% of child deaths, and 83% of this effect is associated with mild-to-moderate rather than severe malnutrition.
- When treating severe malnutrition, sodium and water intake should be limited, protein intake restricted initially, intravenous albumin avoided, and calorie intake increased gradually.
- Ideally, every child in the world should have access to an intensive care unit with facilities for endotracheal intubation and mechanical ventilation. No ethical justification exists for providing these treatments to children in rich countries while denying them to children in poor countries.
- Providing intensive care is not in the interests of a child if the prognosis is very poor because such care simply prolongs suffering, and it is not in the interests of the health services if such care results in poor utilization of limited resources.
- When mortality in children younger than 5 years is greater than 30 per 1000, many deaths are caused by infections. A high proportion of the deaths can be prevented by immunization and primary health care, which are far less expensive than intensive care.
- When resources are limited, admitting to the intensive care unit only children who have a good chance of long-term survival is important. If intensive care unit mortality rates are greater than 10%, patient selection probably is inappropriate.

In the year 2000, 132 million children were born in the world. Of these children, 10.9 million died before age 5 years, with 99.4% of the deaths occurring in developing countries.[113] If the whole world had a under 5-year mortality rate equal to that of the developed world, only 0.8 million deaths in children under 5 deaths would occur each year. Therefore of the 10.9 million deaths in children under 5 years that occur each year, 10.1 million are preventable.

Why Lower Child Mortality?

If too many people already exist in the world, is it sensible to try to reduce child mortality? First, this question is always asked about other people's children. Second, reducing child mortality rates is important both for humanitarian reasons and to enable lower birth rates.[53] Governments of poor countries are not able to provide old-age or sickness benefits, so surviving children are crucially important to provide security. To increase their chances of having surviving children when mortality rates are high, people need to have many children. A vicious circle is created because high birth rates perpetuate poverty so that governments cannot provide social security, people need surviving children, and birth rates remain high. Reducing child mortality is, therefore, a necessary (but not sufficient) condition for reducing birth rates and slowing the growth of the world's population.

Expenditure on Health

In 1999, 40% of the world's population lived in the 66 poorest countries (with an annual gross national income of less than US $746 per capita).[116] In 1990 to 1998, the total annual expenditure on health in these countries averaged only US $21 per capita.[117] In the 52 high-income countries, annual expenditure on health averaged US $2702 per capita, which is 128 times the amount available in low-income countries.

Child Mortality, Infections, and Intensive Care

Most of the unnecessary child deaths in developing countries are caused by infectious diseases, and most of these deaths can be prevented by immunization and basic primary health care. Figure 16–1 shows the relationship between the under 5-year mortality rate and the percentage of deaths caused by infection in different regions of the world.[59] When the under 5-year mortality rate is less than 20 per thousand live births, few deaths are caused by infections, and intensive care can make an important contribution to further reduce mortality from noninfectious causes such as congenital heart disease, trauma, and asthma. As under 5-year mortality increases from 20 to 30 per 1000, the proportion of deaths caused by infections increases rapidly, and the role of intensive care becomes less clear. When under 5-year mortality is greater than 30 per 1000, many deaths are caused by infections, and a high proportion of these deaths can be prevented by immunization and primary health care, which are far less expensive than intensive care.

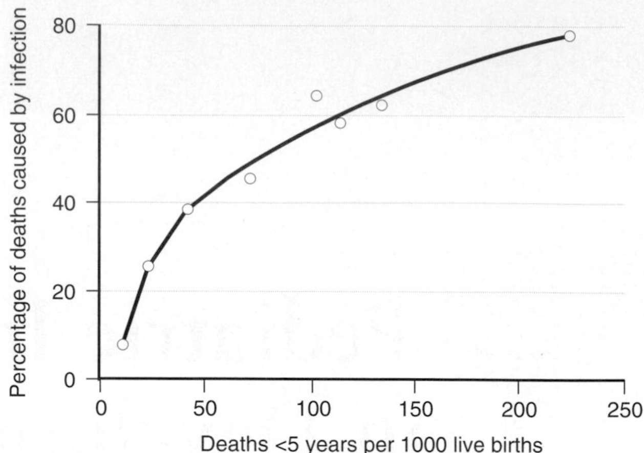

FIGURE 16–1 • Under 5-year mortality rates and percentage of deaths caused by infection in different regions of the world.[59]

Role of Intensive Care

Optimal use must be made of the limited resources available to treat critically ill children in developing countries. Many lives can be saved with effective use of relatively inexpensive therapies, such as intravenous (IV) fluids, oxygen, antibiotics, thermal control, and good nutrition. However, if we define intensive care as endotracheal intubation with the capacity for mechanical ventilation, publicly funded pediatric intensive care in communities with under 5-year mortality rates greater than 30 per 1000 live births probably have little place. In communities with intermediate under 5-year mortality rates of approximately 20 to 30 per 1000, use of intubation and ventilation for carefully selected patients using basic equipment may have a limited role. When resources are limited, admitting only children who have a good chance of long-term survival is important. If intensive care unit (ICU) mortality rates are greater than 10%, patient selection probably is inappropriate.

The main argument in favor of providing endotracheal intubation and ventilation to children in developing countries is that every child in the world should have access to these therapies. No ethical justification exists for providing intensive care to children in developed countries while denying it to children in poor countries. In addition, educated families in developing countries reasonably demand that their children have access to intensive care.

The main argument against providing intensive care in high-mortality areas is that intensive care diverts scarce resources away from far more effective low-cost interventions such as immunization and primary health care. Skilled staff, in particular, are in short supply in many developing countries; if they are used to provide curative services in urban hospitals, the rural poor are at grave risk of being neglected. Strong arguments exist for providing basic public and primary health care to all children rather than intensive care to a small proportion of children.[58] In addition, intubation and ventilation are difficult to do well. Done poorly, they may actually increase mortality. For example, a study in six pediatric ICUs in Mexico and Ecuador found that endotracheal intubation and central venous cannulation were associated with increased mortality in low-risk admissions.[24]

Ethical Dilemma

An ethical dilemma exists. Children in rich countries have access to intensive care. In poor countries, we can either deny intensive care to children (and perhaps increase the probability they will be immunized and receive primary health care) or provide intensive care (often at the expense of immunization and primary health care).

This dilemma cannot be resolved while extreme poverty persists in developing countries. Unfortunately, the rich countries are doing even less to help now than in the past. Overseas development aid from members of the Organisation of Economic Co-operation and Development (OECD) has fallen to 0.25% of gross domestic product, which is well short of the United Nations' target of 0.70%.[92] Even worse, OECD countries now spend more than US $1 billion every day on farm subsidies, which is more than six times the amount given in aid and seriously undermines primary producers in developing countries. If developing countries could increase their export share by just 5%, it would generate US $350 billion per year, seven times more than the total amount they receive in aid.[36,67]

Causes of Death

Greater than 99% of all child deaths occur in developing countries, and 10.1 million of the 10.9 million deaths in children younger than 5 years are preventable. Table 16–1 shows that most of the deaths are caused by infectious diseases, particularly pneumonia, diarrhea, and measles, with malnutrition an important contributing factor.[73,96] Table 16–2 shows that the major pathogens are *Streptococcus pneumoniae*, measles, *Haemophilus influenzae*, rotavirus, malaria, human immunodeficiency virus (HIV) and respiratory syncytial virus (RSV).[96] Unfortunately, the number of deaths caused by HIV is increasing rapidly. The following sections discuss individual diseases that are common causes of mortality in children in developing countries, starting with the diseases that cause the most deaths (see Table 16–1). On rare occasions, children with these diseases require intensive care in developed countries. The suggested treatments assume that the child is in a hospital that can deliver a high standard of intensive care. Other hospitals should follow the World Health Organization (WHO) guidelines for care at the first-referral level in developing countries.[122]

Pneumonia

Pneumonia is the most common cause of death in children. It causes 2.1 million deaths each year in children younger than 5 years. It also contributes to many of the 1.1 million deaths each year from measles.[88] A total of 165 million episodes of acute lower respiratory tract infection occur in children each year, 11 to 20 million of which are severe enough to require hospital admission.[83]

Fatal pneumonia in children usually is caused by *S. pneumoniae* or *H. influenzae*. The etiology of pneumonia can be determined accurately only by culture of lung aspirates from children with no antibiotic activity

TABLE 16–1

Causes of Death in Children Younger than 5 Years in 1995

Cause	No. of Deaths (in Millions)
Pneumonia	2.1
Diarrhea	2.0
Measles	1.1
Prematurity	1.0
Birth asphyxia	0.9
Malaria	0.7
Acquired immunodeficiency syndrome	0.5
Congenital abnormalities	0.5
Pertussis	0.4
Neonatal tetanus	0.4
Other	1.3
Total	10.9

From World Health Organization: *The world health report 1998.* Geneva, 1998, World Health Organization.[120]

TABLE 16–2

Approximate Annual Number of Deaths in Children Younger than 5 Years Caused by Individual Pathogens

Pathogen	No. of Deaths (in Millions)
Pneumococcus	1.2
Measles	1.1
Haemophilus (a, b, c, d, e, f, nonserotypable)	0.9
Rotavirus	0.8
Malaria	0.7
Human immunodeficiency virus	0.5
Respiratory syncytial virus	0.5
Pertussis	0.4
Tetanus	0.4
Tuberculosis	0.1
Hepatitis B	<0.1
Influenza virus	<0.1
Meningococcus	<0.1
Parainfluenza virus	<0.1
Varicella	<0.1
Total	6.7

From Shann F, Steinhoff MC: Vaccines for children in rich and poor countries. *Lancet* 354(suppl II):7, 1999.[96]

detectable in serum or urine.[91] Most cases of pneumonia in children are caused by aspiration of bacteria from the nasopharynx, and mixed infections with *S. pneumoniae*, *H. influenzae*, and *Moraxella catarrhalis* are common.[95] *H. influenzae* pneumonia often is caused by nonserotypable strains, as well as by type b and the other serotypes (a, c, d, e, f).[90]

In children who do not respond to penicillin and gentamicin, consider staphylococcal pneumonia (give cloxacillin and gentamicin), HIV infection, chlamydia or mycoplasma (give clarithromycin), and tuberculosis (see section on tuberculosis).

Antibiotic Treatment

Children with pneumonia who are sick enough to require hospitalization usually should be treated with benzyl penicillin and gentamicin given intravenously.[122] This combination of antibiotics has synergistic activity against many strains of *S. pneumoniae* and *H. influenzae*. It usually is effective even for pneumonia caused by strains of *S. pneumoniae* that have reduced sensitivity to penicillin. However, if meningitis caused by a partially resistant strain also is present, vancomycin or a third-generation cephalosporin (e.g., cefotaxime or ceftriaxone) should be used if available.

Staphylococcal pneumonia is suggested by a poor response to penicillin and gentamicin, pneumatoceles, pneumothorax, empyema, or associated soft tissue or joint infection. Cloxacillin (or oxacillin, flucloxacillin, or dicloxacillin) and gentamicin given intravenously are appropriate treatment.

Oxygen and Ventilation

Oxygen therapy may be lifesaving in patients with severe pneumonia.[118] The most efficient means of administration is 1 to 2 L/min of humidified oxygen via an 8F nasopharyngeal catheter inserted 1 cm less than the distance from the side of the nose to the front of the ear. As well as providing oxygen, this method delivers low levels of continuous positive airway pressure (CPAP).[25] Care should be taken to remove and clean the catheter every 12 hours, to verify that the catheter is not inserted too far (to avoid delivering oxygen into the esophagus), and to limit the flow to a maximum of 2 L/min (to avoid distending the stomach). A special low-flow oxygen flowmeter with a scale of 0–2 or 0–3 L/m should be used.

If mechanical ventilation is not available, oxygenation and ventilation can be improved using mask or nasopharyngeal CPAP up to 12 cm H_2O pressure. If endotracheal intubation and mechanical ventilation are available, a sensible plan is to start with low tidal volumes of 6 to 8 ml/kg, positive end-expiratory pressure 8 to 10 cm, inspiratory time 1 second with a rate of 20 to 30 per minute in an infant (assuming no bronchiolitis or asthma is present), and peak pressure less than 30 cm to minimize ventilator-associated lung injury (see Chapters 45 and Chapter 46). Right ventricular failure may occur secondary to pulmonary hypertension.[89] Nitric oxide 5 to 10 ppm and high-frequency oscillatory ventilation may be helpful and should be administered if available.

Fluid Therapy

Patients with pneumonia often have increased secretion of antidiuretic hormone (syndrome of inappropriate antidiuretic hormone secretion),[18,97] so children with pneumonia should not be given too much water. Hyponatremia usually is caused by excess water rather than sodium deficiency and should be treated by fluid restriction rather than administration of hypertonic saline. A small proportion of children with pneumonia have septic shock with hypovolemia, which may be exacerbated by positive pressure ventilation (causing severe hypoxemia). A helpful procedure in these children may be to insert a central venous catheter and give 10 ml/kg boluses of 0.9% saline to achieve a central venous pressure of 10 to 12 mmHg (see Chapters 22 and 99). Large amounts of fluid may be needed to restore the intravascular volume, but thereafter fluid requirements often are only 30% to 40% of normal because the child may have high antidiuretic hormone concentrations.

Feeding

The blood glucose level should be monitored closely and the glucose infusion rate adjusted to prevent hypoglycemia. If necessary, 50% dextrose can be infused via the central venous catheter. Small amounts of continuous nasogastric feeds should be started from the time of admission as long as no cardiovascular compromise is evident. Full enteral feeds usually can be achieved within 24 to 48 hours. If gastric feeds are not tolerated, nasojejunal feeding may be successful if a nasojejunal tube can be placed (see Chapter 69).

Gastroenteritis

Gastroenteritis is the second most common cause of child mortality. It causes 2 million child deaths every year (see Table 16–1). Particular problems include shock, acid-base abnormalities, electrolyte abnormalities, and secondary bacterial infection. Diarrhea may be a symptom of other disease processes, including sepsis and metabolic abnormalities, so it should not be assumed to be caused by gastroenteritis.

The consequences of fluid loss depend on the rate and the amount of loss. In gastroenteritis, fluid moves from the intravascular space into the gut lumen. Depending on the relative rates of fluid loss and fluid replacement from the extracellular fluid space, patients may be in shock with no clinical signs of dehydration, dehydrated with no features of shock, or dehydrated and in shock. Loss of only 20 ml/kg from the intravascular space causes shock, but clinical signs of dehydration occur only when approximately 30 to 40 ml/kg of fluid is lost from the body (i.e., 3%–4% dehydration).[51]

Shock requires immediate and vigorous replacement with IV fluids. Dehydration can be corrected over 2 or 3 days and usually can be adequately treated with oral fluids. The management of dehydration is complicated by the relative inaccuracy of the clinical signs of dehydration (particularly in malnourished or obese children)[51] and by the variable amount of ongoing stool losses (see Chapter 29). During rehydration, the patient's body weight and serum sodium concentration should be measured every 4 hours and the rate of fluid and sodium administration adjusted accordingly.

Shock

Shock in gastroenteritis usually is caused by hypovolemia secondary to fluid loss. However, a high incidence of bacterial sepsis also is observed in patients with severe gastroenteritis. The initial therapy for shock should include provision of oxygen and rapid IV administration of fluid with an electrolyte content similar to plasma (e.g., 0.9% sodium chloride, Plasmalyte, or Ringer's lactate). Shock should be corrected rapidly over 10 to 15 minutes with continuous or frequent assessment of the response. Intraosseous vascular access may be the most appropriate route of administration if venous access is difficult.

Evidence indicates that Ringer's lactate may be preferable to sodium chloride because high chloride intake may aggravate metabolic acidosis.[98] However, lactate-containing solutions should not be given to patients with metabolic alkalosis caused by excessive vomiting. Additional aliquots of fluid should be given under close observation until the patient is normovolemic. Once the patient is normovolemic, inotropic support will be required if the patient still exhibits shock. Patients who are hypovolemic from gastroenteritis do not require colloid as volume replacement.

Fluid and Electrolyte Abnormalities

Once intravascular volume has been restored, attention should be paid to the management of the sodium derangements and dehydration (see Chapter 62). Normal hydration should be achieved over 48 to 72 hours. If renal function is normal, the kidneys will resolve most of the electrolyte abnormalities given adequate treatment of shock and gradual replacement of fluid and electrolyte deficits.

Calculation of fluid therapy is more difficult in the presence of ongoing diarrhea, which may amount to 300 ml/kg in 24 hours. Fluid therapy is best monitored using a combination of serial weighing and electrolyte measurement. If any doubt exists about urine output, insert a urinary catheter to help distinguish between renal losses and diarrhea. A metabolic bed may be used so that both stool and urine output can be measured separately. Oliguric renal failure is common, but polyuric renal failure may occur, particularly in children with severe hypokalemia or hyperglycemia.

Sodium Abnormalities

Hypernatremia may result from excessive water loss, excessive salt intake (usually in poorly constituted rehydration solutions), or a combination of both. It is associated with significant morbidity (especially of the central nervous system) and mortality. Hypernatremia is more common in infancy than later life and may be associated with use of formula feeds.[3]

Once shock has been treated, the goal of therapy is to reduce the sodium concentration no faster than 0.5 mmol/L/hour. Once hypovolemia has been corrected, the remaining fluid deficit should be replaced over 48 to 72 hours using a solution containing approximately 70 mEq/L of sodium.

Hyponatremia may be related to errors of measurement, excessive fluid intake, or excessive sodium loss. Pseudohyponatremia occasionally is seen secondary to hyperlipidemia or hyperproteinemia. Fictitious hyponatremia is seen in the context of hyperglycemia or mannitol infusions. Measured sodium levels decrease by approximately 1.6 mmol/L for every 100 mg/dl (approximately 5.5 mmol/L) increase in glucose concentration. This factor must be taken into account when calculating fluid management. Hyponatremia should be treated with sodium intake that will increase the sodium concentration by not more than 0.5 mmol/L/hour. This rate is ideally monitored with measurement of sodium levels every 4 hours.

Hypokalemia

Hypokalemia is common in patients with severe gastroenteritis, particularly if rehydration solutions without potassium are used. In the face of bradycardia secondary to severe hypokalemia that is causing poor cardiac output, rapid replacement of potassium may be required to establish a heart rate that is appropriate to the circulatory status of the child. In all other situations, potassium supplementation should not exceed 0.5 mmol/kg/hour IV. If polyuria occurs, a safe approach is to provide maintenance fluids and replace urinary losses greater than 2 ml/kg/hour with fluid with an electrolyte content similar to that of the urine.

Hypophosphatemia

Hypophosphatemia is similarly common in patients with severe gastroenteritis and should be treated with IV potassium or sodium phosphate if the child is symptomatic. Joules' solution can be provided enterally but may exacerbate diarrhea. Phosphate concentrations less than 0.3 mmol/L usually are associated with severe symptoms and should be treated, but phosphate supplementation is not required with concentrations greater than 0.6 mmol/L unless other symptoms are associated.

Metabolic Acidosis

Metabolic acidosis is common in children admitted to the ICU with gastroenteritis. It may be related to hypoperfusion (usually elevated serum lactate levels), renal dysfunction with renal tubular acidosis, or ingestion of medication (e.g., salicylates or toxins such as Mpilo toxin). Many "traditional" medications given to children in developing countries can exacerbate the metabolic acidosis. Mpilo toxin is a plant toxin that causes severe renal and hepatic damage that usually manifests as severe metabolic acidosis.

If acidosis persists despite correction of hypovolemia, consider measuring serum lactate and urine ketone levels, excluding the ingestion of toxins such as salicylates and iron, and screening for metabolic disease. Inborn errors of metabolism may present following the stress of an illness such as acute gastroenteritis.

If acidosis is related to excessive loss of bicarbonate via stool or urine, bicarbonate administration may be appropriate. To prevent sodium overload, try using a solution of 5% dextrose containing 50 to 70 mmol/L of sodium bicarbonate, with potassium added according to requirements.

Hyperglycemia

Severe hyperglycemia may occur with severe gastroenteritis and is thought to be a consequence of a severe stress reaction.[79] Treatment of shock and ongoing fluid replacement lead to resolution of hyperglycemia. Insulin therapy is required occasionally but should be used cautiously at a dose of 0.025 U/kg/hour because these children often are extremely sensitive to insulin and may become hypoglycemic very rapidly. The dose can be cautiously increased if no response is seen.

Measles

Despite the effectiveness of measles immunization, more than 1 million children still die every year as a result of measles (see Table 16–1). It is a devastating viral infection with a case fatality rate up to 30%, particularly in malnourished children. Measles is highly infectious, and its course frequently is complicated by secondary infection with adenovirus or bacteria.[21,88]

Diagnosis

Measles has a 3- to 5-day prodromal period consisting of coryzal symptoms, fever, cough, and conjunctivitis. Koplik spots develop in the mouth from days 2 to 4. They are seen on the inner surface of the cheeks and have the appearance of salt granules on a red background. A maculopapular rash appears from day 4. The rash starts on the head and neck, and it spreads to the trunk and the rest of the body over several days. The rash darkens 5 to 6 days after it appears. The skin may peel and have a scaly appearance. Diarrhea is common throughout the early phase of the disease. Upper respiratory tract symptoms may progress to involve the larynx with croup and the rest of the respiratory system with severe bronchopneumonia.

Persistence of fever after the rash, apparent for 3 days, usually is caused by secondary infection, often involving the respiratory system. Measles may precipitate features of acute malnutrition. Vitamin A deficiency may interact with the illness to produce acute xerophthalmia with blindness. An acute allergic encephalitis with demyelination may occur, typically during the second week of the illness as the rash is clearing. Acute measles inclusion body encephalitis may occur and is more common in immunocompromised children. Subacute sclerosing panencephalitis presents some years after the acute infection. Bronchiectasis may be a complication of severe measles pneumonia with secondary infection.

Infection Control

Children are infectious before the rash appears and for up to 7 days after the first symptoms appear. The incubation period is 10 to 12 days. Ensure that all children who possibly came into contact with the infected child have been immunized with measles vaccine. In children older than 4 months, immediate immunization at the time of exposure protects against infection. Younger infants usually are protected by maternal antibodies; however, in communities where maternal antibody levels likely are low, every effort should be made to ensure that young infants are not exposed to measles patients, and immunoglobulin should be administered to contacts if possible.

General Measures

The common complications of measles are pneumonia, diarrhea, croup, conjunctivitis, keratitis, xerophthalmia, malnutrition, otitis media, stomatitis, and nosocomial infection.[21,43] Practical treatment of the acutely ill child includes ensuring adequate oxygenation, obtaining cultures and providing cloxacillin and gentamicin as needed, and initiating mechanical ventilation. Fluid therapy should be closely tailored to the clinical situation, taking into account factors such as diarrhea and fever. Hydration status may be difficult to assess clinically, so regular weighing facilitates fluid balance assessment. Vitamin A 200,000 IU/day should be administered orally for 2 days to reduce mortality and prevent xerophthalmia.[19] Whether immunoglobulin has a role in treatment of severe measles is not clear.[21] Measles may exacerbate tuberculosis and malnutrition.

Low Birth Weight

Babies born weighing less than 2500 g are said to have a low birth weight. Approximately 1 million low-birth-weight infants die each year (see Table 16–1 and Chapter 42). Small-for-gestational-age births are relatively more common in developing countries than in developed countries. The decision on whether a low-birth-weight baby is premature, small for gestational age, or both is important. Problems associated with prematurity (babies younger than 37 weeks of gestation) include respiratory distress syndrome, apnea, poor feeding, intraventricular hemorrhage, jaundice, infection, and hypothermia. Problems associated with small-for-gestational-age status are intrauterine hypoxia, birth asphyxia, meconium aspiration, hypoglycemia, and infection.

Only the general principles of management are outlined in this chapter; more detailed information is available elsewhere.[93,124] Vitamin K 1 mg intramuscularly (IM) is administered after birth. The baby should be kept warm (well wrapped up in a room 27°–30°C, which is crucially important) and handled as little as possible. Apnea monitors should be used for babies younger than 32 weeks of gestation and aminophylline provided if apnea occurs. Cultures are obtained and penicillin and gentamicin administered if any signs of infection, including respiratory distress, appear. Use of breast milk and strict handwashing procedures help prevent cross-infection in the nursery. Desaturation can be treated with nasopharyngeal CPAP. Facilities for intubation and mechanical ventilation, if available, may be indicated, but nasal CPAP is much safer and often is just as effective.

Kangaroo care is defined as skin-to-skin contact between mother and baby with frequent and exclusive or nearly exclusive breast-feeding and early discharge from hospital. Many of the controlled trials of kangaroo care are of poor quality. A Cochrane Review concluded that kangaroo care appears to reduce morbidity, but more well-designed trials are needed.[11]

Breast-feeding on demand is preferred if the baby is active and sucks well. If the baby does not feed well, feeding expressed breast milk with a cup and spoon (not a bottle) is appropriate. If the baby is too weak to feed with a cup and spoon, nasogastric tube feeds are indicated. Close attention to serum glucose is warranted with IV and/or enteral glucose administration as needed to provide 5 to 10 mg/kg/min.

Poliomyelitis, bacille Calmette-Guérin (BCG), and hepatitis B vaccines should be administered before discharge at a time when the baby is fully breast-fed and gaining weight. A solution of ferrous sulfate (to be given at a dose of 2 mg/kg/day of elemental iron) should be provided to the infant's mother and follow-up scheduled.

Neonatal Asphyxia

Approximately 900,000 infants die every year from asphyxia. In many cases, the cause is an hypoxic-ischemic insult during labor, but it also may be caused by fetal abnormalities that were present before labor. Asphyxia is more common in small-for-gestational-age babies and carries a grave prognosis in low-birth-weight babies. Even if the baby improves during the first few hours after delivery, observe the baby closely for at least 24 hours because rapid deterioration may occur at 6 to 24 hours as cerebral edema develops.

Oxygen is provided as required to maintain an oxygen saturation greater than 90%. Intubation and mechanical ventilation should be used in the event of airway or breathing compromise and should not be discontinued too early because deterioration may occur 6–24 hours after delivery.

Poor cardiac output is common with severe asphyxia because of hypovolemia from capillary leak and impaired myocardial contractility. Cardiac echocardiography may help distinguish among hypovolemia (small left atrium), poor ventricular contractility, and pulmonary hypertension (treat with nitric oxide, if available). After correction of hypovolemia, the total fluid intake initially should be limited to 30 to 40 ml/kg/day.

The baby's temperature should be kept at 36° to 37°C. Controlled trials assessing the role of hypothermia are in progress.[31] The blood glucose should be kept in the normal range.

Close infection surveillance should be undertaken for neonatal sepsis, which can present as asphyxia. Treatment with penicillin and gentamicin is appropriate, but cefotaxime or ceftriaxone also may be indicated if evidence of meningitis is present. Convulsions should be treated with phenobarbital 20 mg/kg IV over 60 minutes. One small study reported phenobarbital 40 mg/kg administered intravenously to all babies with asphyxia was beneficial,[33] but it may cause dangerous sedation unless the infant is ventilated.

Hypocalcemia is treated with 10% calcium gluconate 0.5 ml/kg IV over 10 minutes. Empiric corticosteroids are not indicated. Coagulopathy should be treated with fresh-frozen plasma, if available. Vitamin K should be given to all babies. Paralytic ileus and necrotizing enterocolitis are common after severe asphyxia; accordingly, enteral feeds should not be started until bowel sounds are present and the baby passes meconium. Renal failure and hyperkalemia may require treatment with glucose and insulin, an ion-exchange resin enema, or peritoneal dialysis. Babies who do not start to breathe within 48 hours rarely make a good recovery. It is important not to continue treatment given no realistic chance of intact survival.

Malaria

Severe malaria is caused by *Plasmodium falciparum*, which is the only species of malaria that causes parasitized erythrocytes to adhere to endothelial cells and produce microvascular disease. At any one time, more than 1 billion people are infected with malaria, and the disease causes 0.5 to 3 million deaths each year.[30]

Malaria starts with fever, with possible coughing and vomiting. Especially in nonimmune patients, the illness may progress very rapidly over 1 to 2 days, with coma (cerebral malaria), shock, convulsions, anemia, hypovolemia, hypoglycemia, jaundice, respiratory distress, renal failure, and coagulopathy.

Diagnosis

The diagnosis is made by examination of thick and thin blood smears (false-negative results may occur with inexperienced staff) or by detection of *P. falciparum* antigen using enzyme-linked immunosorbent assay, polymerase chain reaction (PCR), or immunoassay for parasite lactate dehydrogenase. Commercially available rapid blood tests use a dipstick or test strip with monoclonal antibodies directed against a parasite antigen.[30] They have a sensitivity and specificity greater than 90% for *P. falciparum*.

Severe malaria is present if severe anemia (hemoglobin <6 g/dl) or hypoglycemia (blood glucose <2.5 mmol/L) is evident. In nonimmune patients, severe malaria is present if hyperparasitemia (>250,000 parasites/µl or >5% parasitemia) is evident, but partially immune patients may have greater than 5% parasitized erythrocytes without evidence of clinical illness.

Initial Treatment

Patients with coma or shock should be intubated and ventilated. Insertion of a central venous line to allow monitoring of central venous pressure and infusion of drugs should be considered. Hypovolemia should be corrected with 10 ml/kg boluses of 0.9% saline. If poor perfusion persists despite an adequate central venous pressure, echocardiography may aid in assessing intravascular volume and ventricular contractility (see Chapter 23). Hypoglycemia is common in small children, and the blood glucose concentration should be monitored closely. Convulsions are treated with phenobarbital 20 mg/kg IV over 1 hour, then 5 mg/kg daily.

Routine phenobarbital may increase mortality in unventilated patients but likely does not in ventilated patients.[56]

Antimalarial Drugs

The choice of antimalarial drug depends on which drugs are available and local drug resistance patterns. The best choice usually is either quinine or artesunate. Evidence suggests that artesunate clears parasites faster than quinine and increases survival rates.[55] Patients with severe malaria are infected by a large number of parasites and should always be treated with two antimalarial drugs to reduce the risk of selecting resistant strains with recrudescence of disease.[64]

Artesunate is given in an initial dose of 2.5 mg/kg IV, then 1.2 mg/kg/day after 12 to 24 hours for 6 days.[49,122] When the child can swallow, artesunate should be administered orally. After 7 days of artesunate, mefloquine 15 mg/kg orally then 10 mg/kg 12 hours later should be given.

Quinine sulfate (or quinine dihydrochloride) is given in an initial dose of 20 mg/kg IV over 4 hours, then 10 mg/kg IV over 2 hours every 12 hours for 7 days.[122] Quinine can be given orally when the child can tolerate it. After 7 days of quinine, mefloquine 15 mg/kg orally then 10 mg/kg 12 hours later should be provided.

Quinidine can be used if artesunate and quinine are not available, but quinidine is more likely to cause cardiac toxicity than quinine.[122] Following a loading dose of 15 mg/kg quinidine IV over 4 hours, the drug is dosed 7.5 mg/kg over 4 hours, every 8 hours, for 7 days. After 7 days of quinidine, mefloquine 15 mg/kg orally then 10 mg/kg 12 hours later should be given.

Other Treatment

Bacterial infection is common in children with clinical findings suggestive of cerebral malaria. Following a blood culture, cefotaxime (or penicillin if cefotaxime is not available) and gentamicin are appropriate empirical treatments. Lumbar puncture should be deferred until the child recovers consciousness. Antibiotics are discontinued after 48 to 72 hours if the blood culture is negative and lumbar puncture is normal.

Children with a hemoglobin level of 4 g/dl or less require urgent transfusion with packed erythrocytes. Children with a hemoglobin level of 4 to 6 g/dl should be transfused if they have coma, shock, or more than 10% parasitized erythrocytes.[57,122] Transfusion should occur slowly over 6 hours to a hemoglobin level of 10 g/dl, taking care to avoid fluid overload in children with severe malnutrition. Furosemide is not indicated unless evidence of fluid overload (pulmonary edema with a high central venous pressure) is seen. Exchange transfusion, if it can be performed safely, may be beneficial in patients with coma, renal failure, adult respiratory distress syndrome, or a parasitemia of 10% or more.[77]

No evidence supports the use of corticosteroids,[78] cyclosporin, dextran, heparin, iron chelating agents,[99] or prostacyclin. The patient should be turned every 2 hours, hypoglycemia prevented, and vital signs and fluid balance monitored carefully. Acidosis may be associated with severe hyperkalemia initially, but total body potassium often is low and hypokalemia may occur in the recovery phase.

Human Immunodeficiecny Virus

The vast majority of HIV-infected children are located in the developing world (see Chapter 88). Despite advances in antiretroviral therapy, no evidence indicates a decrease in the number of children born with HIV infection each year. As a result, the spectrum of disease seen in pediatric wards in the developing world over the past 10 years has changed dramatically, with a marked increase in HIV-related disease.[129]

HIV disease has produced an effect on pediatric ICUs in developing countries.[126] Patients with HIV admitted to these units are predominantly infants who have severe pneumonia or respiratory symptoms.[44,126] Initially, children admitted to the ICU with respiratory disease had a very high mortality, but the rate has improved gradually with time.[126] Much of the improvement probably came from the recognition that *Pneumocystis jeroveci* is a major pathogen in these children.[46] Other studies have highlighted the importance of cytomegalovirus,[45] tuberculosis,[45,126] and bacterial infections, particularly *Staphylococcus aureus*.[126]

Little information is available on the long-term outcome of HIV-infected children requiring intensive care in the developing world. However, the impression is that, in the absence of antiretroviral therapy, the majority of these children die within months of being admitted to the ICU. A decision about whether to admit a child to the ICU should be influenced by the medium- to long-term prognosis and not just survival in intensive care.[13] It is not in the interests of a child to provide intensive care if the prognosis is very poor because such care simply prolongs suffering, and it is not in the interests of the health services if such care results in poor utilization of limited resources.

In the absence of antiretroviral therapy, admitting infants with severe infection to the ICU appears to be of limited benefit. However, one consequence of programs directed at reducing maternal-to-child transmission of HIV (using nevirapine or zidovudine [AZT]) is that the diagnosis of HIV infection in the infant is more complex. Thus there is a place for admitting HIV-exposed (and possibly HIV-infected) infants with severe infection to the ICU while the diagnosis is being established. There is little or no place for prolonged intensive care when the diagnosis of HIV infection is established but antiretroviral therapy is not available. As antiretroviral therapy becomes more generally available in the developing world, the role of intensive care in the management of HIV-infected children will require review.

Pertussis

Pertussis syndrome is caused by *Bordetella pertussis* or *Bordetella parapertussis*. WHO estimates that 400,000 children die from pertussis each year, but PCR testing has shown that pertussis is much more common than previously thought,[16] so the total number of deaths may be much higher.

The illness starts with rhinorrhea, fever, and a cough that comes in spasms for approximately 10 days until the whoop starts. The cough may last for up to 3 months and recur with subsequent respiratory infections. A large amount of very thick sputum is produced, which causes the child to cough so many times that he or she becomes cyanotic. The child then inspires so strongly that a loud stridor, or whoop, is heard. The cough may be accompanied by expectoration of tenacious mucus or vomiting. Young infants may have no whoop and may present with apnea.

In endemic areas, encephalopathy is common in patients with severe pertussis, and up to one third of infants may present with coma or seizures.[68] Mortality is high in infants with severe pertussis if the total white cell count is greater than 40,000/µl, they have encephalopathy, or they need mechanical ventilation for pneumonia. Severe pulmonary hypertension may occur, particularly in children with a white cell count greater than 100,000/µl.[74]

Diagnosis

In developing countries, the diagnosis usually must be made on clinical grounds. Pertussis likely is present in children with typical clinical findings who have a lymphocyte count greater than 10,000/µl. Children with lower respiratory infection and a total white cell count of 40,000/µl or more have a high mortality rate, and many of these children probably have pertussis even if they do not have typical symptoms.[94]

Culture of *B. pertussis* is difficult, and the sensitivity is low even if the test is performed correctly. Immunofluorescent antibodies are present in approximately 80% of cases if the specimen is obtained within 2 weeks of the onset of the cough and erythromycin or chloramphenicol has not been given. PCR for pertussis is sensitive and specific,[16] but the test is difficult to perform and is expensive. In one study, 33% of children with pertussis also had RSV infection.[16]

Treatment

Antibiotics probably do not alter the course of the illness unless they are given before the paroxysmal cough develops, but they do render the patient noninfectious. In developing countries, chloramphenicol usually is the antibiotic of choice. Chloramphenicol is active against *B. pertussis* and most of the bacteria that cause secondary pneumonia. Erythromycin also is active, but erythromycin stearate is less effective than the estolate and must be given in high doses for 14 days.[7,39] Clarithromycin and azithromycin are highly effective, but they are expensive.[39]

Severe paroxysms should be treated with oxygen and gentle suction. Convulsions can be treated with diazepam, followed by phenobarbital as prophylaxis. The available evidence does not support the use of diphenhydramine, pertussis immunoglobulin, or salbutamol.[75] Four controlled trials of steroid use for pertussis all suggested benefit from the use of systemic steroids, but the studies were not well designed.[10,82,112,128] Inhaled steroids appeared to be helpful in one report.[115]

Nasal mask or prong CPAP may be helpful in infants with apnea as an alternative to mechanical ventilation.[109] The prognosis is poor if mechanical ventilation is required for pneumonia in children with pertussis.[27] Exchange transfusion should be considered if the total white cell count is more than 100×10^9/L or severe pulmonary hypertension is present.[74]

Tetanus

Tetanus is responsible for 400,000 child deaths each year (see Table 16–1). Most of the deaths result from neonatal tetanus caused by lack of maternal immunization and poor umbilical cord hygiene. Tetanus has occurred occasionally in older children with infected wounds but has decreased substantially since the institution of adequate immunization practices. Tetanus toxins affect most body organs and not just the central nervous system. The prognosis depends on age (with higher mortality rates in newborn babies and elderly adults), the source of infection, and delay in treatment.[84] Children with tetanus present with difficulty feeding; trismus; muscle spasms; hypertonicity; convulsions; and autonomic, cardiac, and respiratory instability.

Treatment

If spasms are severe, oxygen should be provided until adequate sedation is achieved with diazepam and chlorpromazine. Diazepam at a dose of 0.5 mg/kg is administered slowly intravenously every 15 to 30 minutes until severe spasms are controlled and then 0.5 mg/kg is given every 12 hours by nasogastric tube. Diazepam given intravenously should be diluted 1:20 with 0.9% saline and injected slowly over 5 minutes. Diazepam should not be given intramuscularly. After spasms have been controlled with IV diazepam, maintenance doses can be given orally or by nasogastric tube; up to 40 mg/kg/day may be needed as tolerance develops. In addition to diazepam or midazolam, chlorpromazine 5 mg/kg every 12 hours intramuscularly or by nasogastric tube is useful. Tracheostomy should be performed in older children with severe tetanus. Paralysis and mechanical ventilation will be needed if severe spasms persist despite heavy sedation.

Autonomic instability may cause large and sudden variations in blood pressure and pulse rate. In ventilated patients, morphine 20 to 40 µg/kg/hour may be a helpful addition to diazepam and chlorpromazine. Atropine, clonidine, and magnesium have been used[12] but have not been demonstrated to be superior to careful use of large doses of chlorpromazine, diazepam, and morphine. Beta-blockers should not be given.[12]

If IV human tetanus immunoglobulin is available, a total dose of 4000 U is recommended, although some centers now use only 500 U. The entire dose can be infused intravenously over 1 hour. Alternatively, 1.5 ml (≈100 U) can be administered intrathecally, 1.5 ml infiltrated around the umbilicus in neonatal tetanus (after cleaning the stump with hydrogen peroxide), and the remainder infused intravenously. If immunoglobulin is given intrathecally, dexamethasone 4 mg (2 mg in neonates) every 12 hours intramuscularly should be administered for 5 days. The role of intrathecal administration of tetanus immunoglobulin is unclear,[2] but it may reduce mortality if corticosteroids are given as well.[87] If IV human tetanus immunoglobulin is not available, 750 U (three ampoules) of IM human or horse tetanus immunoglobulin on the first day and 500 U on the next 2 days should be given. IM preparations should not be administered by intrathecal injection.

After the site of infection is identified, any necrotic tissue is removed, and benzyl penicillin 50 mg/kg intravenously every 6 hours is given. A full course of immunization with tetanus toxoid should be given during convalescence (usually three doses at 2-month intervals).

Tuberculosis

Tuberculosis is common in the developing world. In association with the HIV pandemic, there has been an increase in the incidence of tuberculosis and multidrug-resistant tuberculosis. Most children with tuberculosis do not require intensive care. However, tuberculosis may be an unexpected additional finding during an ICU admission, or it may be the cause of an ICU admission. In a report from a pediatric ICU, tuberculosis was not initially considered as a diagnosis in 30% of eventually confirmed cases.[38] In general, the sputum of children does not contain a large number of *Mycobacterium tuberculosis* organisms, so children are rarely a source of infection. However, in the ICU, children who have *M. tuberculosis* in the sputum may constitute a risk to staff because sputum is aerosolized from an endotracheal tube during suctioning. In the case of young children, the risk of either parent being infected is high. In one series of infants younger than 3 months with tuberculosis, 42% of the index cases identified by history were parents, and 30% of the mothers had previously unsuspected pulmonary tuberculosis.[85] Patients' relatives may be a source of infection for staff and other hospital patients.[61] If a child presents with tuberculosis, the public health authorities must be informed, the source of infection investigated, and appropriate therapy instituted. Children are rarely the source of infection, whereas adults with tuberculosis are highly infectious.

Pathophysiology

In children, tuberculosis usually results from primary infection with *M. tuberculosis* inhaled into the lungs. The organism spreads into the lymphatic system and the mediastinal lymph nodes (setting up the primary focus) and then via the thoracic duct into the bloodstream, with hematologic dissemination throughout the lungs (miliary tuberculosis). Spread to the rest of the body may occur from erosion of the pulmonary vessels and subsequent dissemination via the systemic circulation.

Diagnosis

The diagnosis of tuberculosis may be difficult in children because of the paucity of organisms in sputum and other body fluids. Often treatment for tuberculosis must be started without bacteriologic confirmation of the diagnosis. However, particularly when resistant tuberculosis is possible, every effort should be made to isolate the organisms from sputum, body fluids, tissue biopsy, or culture of the suspected sources of infection. Gastric lavage has been shown to be superior to BAL,[1] and evidence suggests that induced sputum may be superior to gastric lavage.[127] Table 16–3 summarizes the diagnostic approaches to tuberculosis.

Chest x-ray films showing a miliary pattern, a typical Ghon focus with associated lymphadenopathy, or more diffuse consolidation are strongly suggestive of tuberculosis. Pleural effusions are common, especially in older children. Computerized tomography scan of the chest demonstrates typical lymph nodes with rim enhancement after contrast administration.

Tuberculin tests can be used to ascertain infection. False-negative results frequently occur in children with malnutrition, immune compromise, overwhelming disease, or recent significant illness. Induration of more than 10 mm at the site of tuberculin administration indicates infection in children who have not received BCG vaccination, whereas induration of more than 15 mm indicates infection in children who have received BCG vaccination.

Presentation to the Intensive Care Unit

Children with tuberculosis who require intensive care usually have infection of the respiratory tract; however, central nervous system disease or abdominal complications also may cause critical illness. In areas where tuberculosis commonly occurs, the diagnosis should be considered in any child with acute pneumonia that does not respond to therapy as expected. Radiologic changes in the lung may be surprisingly extensive for the severity of lung disease in patients with tuberculous bronchopneumonia.

Acute respiratory distress syndrome is a well-recognized complication of miliary and bronchogenic tuberculosis in adults but is less common in children.[22,23,42,52,60,66,76] Some reports have suggested that steroid therapy may be useful for acute respiratory distress syndrome with miliary tuberculosis, whereas other reports suggest the outcome is worse. No randomized trials have been performed.

Lower Airway Obstruction

Intrathoracic lymph node tuberculosis may cause severe airway obstruction. Airway obstruction may be a consequence of external compression of the airways by

TABLE 16–3

Investigation for Tuberculosis in Children

Investigation	Technique	Problems and Possible Benefits
Gastric lavage	Lavage of the stomach with a variable volume of 0.9% saline	Should be performed when the patient has been NPO for several hours to avoid contamination of specimen with food; not applicable once patient has been intubated because theoretically the sputum will be removed by suction and will not be swallowed; relatively noninvasive
Induced sputum	Aspirate of the nasopharyngeal secretions following nebulization with 5% saline; generally, patients should be given salbutamol prior to nebulization to decrease the risks of bronchospasm related to the hypertonic saline	Potential risk to staff because organisms can be nebulized to environment with coughing; better yield than gastric lavage
Bronchoalveolar lavage	Bronchoalveolar lavage of affected areas of the lung	Patient requires general anesthesia; technically difficult and requires expensive equipment if a particular area of the lung is lavaged; can be conducted nonbronchoscopically, but a particular area of the lung cannot then be lavaged; yield not as good as with gastric lavage

circumferential lymph nodes, erosion of the bronchial wall with extrusion of caseous material into the bronchial lumen, or a combination of both. Clinical presentation of airway compression by lymph nodes includes features of lower airway obstruction and a "klaxon cough." Typically a wheeze that is worse on expiration, particularly with forced expiration, is heard. Air trapping is less than expected based upon the severity of the wheeze.

Acute obstruction may be temporarily relieved by use of inhaled epinephrine, and administration of steroids may ameliorate the symptoms.[111] If the airway obstruction does not resolve with steroid therapy or if the obstruction is so severe that supportive ventilation is required, relief may be achieved by surgical intervention.[37,62,69,125] Surgery should be preceded by bronchoscopy to define the site of compression and remove endobronchial material that may be contributing to the obstruction. If the lymph nodes are compressing the trachea or major bronchi, surgical decompression may dramatically relieve symptoms; however, if segmental bronchi are being compressed, surgery is less likely to relieve the symptoms. Surgery usually is effective if the nodes are filled with fluid material. Relieving obstruction caused by hard caseous nodes with extensive surrounding fibrosis often is difficult.

Bronchoesophageal Fistula

An acquired bronchoesophageal fistula can be caused by erosion of peribronchial lymph nodes into both the esophagus and a bronchus.[26,50] The fistula may present either with features of bronchial aspiration of swallowed material and associated coughing and other symptoms or with respiratory failure. Ventilation in this situation is complicated by the constant leak of air from the bronchus into the esophagus and gastrointestinal tract. Fistulas from the esophagus into the pleural space have been described.

Laryngeal Tuberculosis

Tuberculosis may cause laryngeal airway obstruction, particularly in the setting of HIV infection.[44] In one study, laryngeal tuberculosis accounted for 15.8% of episodes of laryngeal obstruction in HIV-infected children admitted to the ICU.[20] Clinical features include hoarseness and laryngeal obstruction.

Tuberculous Meningitis

Children with tuberculous meningitis usually present to the ICU with a depressed level of consciousness or status epilepticus (see Chapter 59). Lumbar puncture should not be performed on a child who has a depressed level of consciousness, but a computerized tomography scan should be performed to determine if hydrocephalus, cerebral edema, or a mass lesion is present. The typical cerebrospinal fluid features include an increased cell count (usually >500 per microliter, predominantly lymphocytes, although neutrophils may predominate early in the disease); absence of other bacteria; and high protein, relatively low sugar, and low chloride levels. Hyponatremia is common because of increased secretion of antidiuretic hormone (71% of cases in one study).[14] Therapy should be started with high-dose antituberculous therapy and steroids.[86] Of note, antituberculous drugs such as rifampicin may accelerate the metabolism of steroids, and a high dose may be required.

Tuberculous Pericarditis

Tuberculous pericarditis is an uncommon complication. Few children present with features of shock. The most common presentation consists of long-standing symptoms of illness with some features of pericardial tamponade.[41] Tuberculous pericarditis requires urgent drainage only in cases of significant symptoms or diagnostic concerns. Antituberculous therapy should be started early, and steroids should be given to patients at risk of developing constrictive pericarditis.[102,103]

Miliary and Abdominal Tuberculosis

Miliary tuberculosis is relatively rare in the ICU but may be associated with tuberculous meningitis and development of ARDS. Abdominal tuberculosis is characterized by marked abdominal lymphadenopathy, with associated malabsorption, gut obstruction, or protein-losing enteropathy.

Treatment Regimens

For drug-susceptible tuberculosis, the usual treatment starts with isoniazid, pyrazinamide, and rifampicin,[4] but starting with just isoniazid and rifampicin is acceptable if pyrazinamide is contraindicated. If drug resistance is likely, ethambutol or streptomycin should be added. Children diagnosed with tuberculosis during an intensive care admission usually are started on a daily treatment regimen, although later treatment may be given only two or three times per week. One (non-ICU) study showed that three-drug therapy administered two times per week from the start was as effective as daily therapy.[108]

Many drugs interact with antituberculous therapy, and great care must be taken with all other medications given. In particular, anticonvulsant, theophylline, paracetamol, antiretroviral, and steroid dosing may require adjustment for patients receiving tuberculosis therapy.[54]

Metronidazole is not a first-line antituberculous agent; however, it has a marked effect against dormant *M. tuberculosis* under anaerobic conditions. One report from India showed significant improvement in clinical outcome when metronidazole was added to conventional therapy for adults with pulmonary tuberculosis.[17] Steroids may be useful in tuberculous meningitis and when intrathoracic airways are compressed by tuberculous lymph nodes. Table 16–4 summarizes tuberculosis antimicrobial drugs.

Poor absorption of drugs from the gastrointestinal tract may occur in critically ill children, especially those with abdominal tuberculosis. Given concerns about the absorption of medication from the gut, rifampicin and isoniazid should be administered intravenously. Liver toxicity may occur, with side effects ranging from mild elevation of transaminases to acute severe hepatic failure and death. All the first-line antituberculous drugs have a marked postantibiotic effect, and daily administration is not essential.

Diphtheria

Diphtheria is an acute infectious disease caused by toxigenic strains of *Corynebacterium diphtheriae.* Since the introduction of immunization, the incidence of diphtheria has decreased dramatically; however, the disease still caused 4000 deaths in 1999.[123] Frequently, colonization

TABLE 16–4

Drugs Used to Treat Tuberculosis in Children

Drug	Usual Daily Dose	Comment
FIRST-LINE THERAPY		
Isoniazid	10–15 mg/kg orally (max 300 mg), IV, or IM	Part of usual three-drug regimen; has marked effect on rapidly dividing cells
Rifampicin	10–15 mg/kg (max 600 mg) orally or IV over 3 hours	Part of usual three-drug regimen; has significant postantibiotic effect
Rifabutin	Dosing for children not established	
Rifapentine	Dosing for children not established	
Pyrazinamide	15–30 mg/kg (max 2 g) orally	
Ethambutol	25 mg/kg orally (max 2.5 g); give 80% of oral dose if given IV	Can be used in young children if resistant organisms suspected; older children should undergo regular visual testing during therapy
SECOND-LINE THERAPY		
Cycloserine	10–15 mg/kg orally (max 1 g)	
Ethionamide	15–20 mg/kg orally (max 1 g)	
Streptomycin	20–40 mg/kg (max 1g) IM	
Amikacin or kanamycin	15–30 mg/kg (max 1 g) IM or IV daily; drug level monitoring essential	
p-Aminosalicylic acid (PAS)	200–300 mg/kg (max 10 g) in 2–4 divided doses orally	

IM = intramuscular; IV = intravenous.

of chronic skin sores by *C. diphtheriae* often induces immunity. As standards of hygiene improve and chronic skin sores become rare, clinical diphtheria becomes more common unless it is prevented by immunization.

The organisms are transmitted by contact or droplet spread. After an incubation period of 2 to 4 days, the organisms invade the pharynx in 90% of pediatric cases, but they may infect the nose, mouth, or skin. Satellite lesions may occur in the stomach, esophagus, or lower airways.[32] Bronchial involvement mimicking bacterial tracheitis has been described.[105]

First week: Nasal diphtheria initially may be indistinguishable from the common cold but later may be characterized by a serosanguinous nasal discharge, white patches on the septal mucosa, and erosions on the upper lip. Toxemia usually is mild. Pharyngeal diphtheria is characterized by the development of a pseudomembrane composed of sloughed mucosa plus an inflammatory exudate of neutrophils, fibrin, and bacterial colonies. The membrane typically forms over one or both tonsils and may extend throughout the nasopharynx, oropharynx, and soft palate and down into the larynx. The pseudomembrane initially is white and changes to a dirty gray over time. It is associated with intense underlying inflammation, and attempts to remove the pseudomembrane cause bleeding. The intense inflammation may obstruct the airway, and occasionally the entire pseudomembrane sloughs off and causes airway obstruction.[32] Pharyngeal diphtheria usually is associated with severe toxemia and the development of enlarged cervical lymph nodes with associated edema (bullneck).

Laryngeal and tracheobronchial diphtheria can be primary infections or extensions of pharyngeal lesions. These lesions are relatively rare but can cause severe airway compromise and are associated with severe toxicity.[32] Oral lesions in adults have been described but are rare in children. Skin involvement with formation of slough may occur at any site; toxicity, if present, is mild.

During the initial phase of the illness, systemic features such as pyrexia and toxemia are caused by absorption of toxin from the inflammation site. Disseminated intravascular coagulation, acute renal damage, and acute cardiac failure may occur.[34,35,114] Fever and toxemia usually resolve after approximately 1 week.

Subsequent course: During the second or third week of the illness, myocarditis and neurologic problems may occur if the toxin has not been inactivated by administration of antiserum. Myocarditis has been described in 10% to 20% of patients presenting with oropharyngitis. Mortality associated with diphtheritic myocarditis ranges from 14% to 60%.[40] Clinical features include rapid onset of cardiac failure with cardiac gallop, muffled heart sounds, and apical murmurs; rhythm disturbances including sinoatrial node dysfunction, extrasystoles, atrial flutter, atrial fibrillation, nodal rhythm, and ventricular tachycardia; and conduction abnormalities with bundle branch and atrioventricular block. Conduction abnormalities on electrocardiogram were a marker of severe myocardial damage and poor prognosis in one study.[101] A wide range of electrocardiographic changes is seen in myocarditis, ranging from ST-segment changes to extensive infarctlike patterns.[47] On echocardiography, left ventricular dilatation with poor function but retained muscle mass has been described. Biochemical features of myocarditis include increased serum myoglobin, lactic dehydrogenase, and creatine phosphokinase.

Neurologic complications usually occur between 10 days and 3 months after onset of oropharyngeal disease. Palatal palsies with difficulty swallowing are a common complication during the first 3 weeks of illness. Paralysis of the diaphragm, eye muscles, and skeletal muscles may occur up to 3 months after onset of disease. Examination of affected nerves has shown degeneration of the myelin sheaths and axon cylinders.[32]

Diagnosis

Early diagnosis and treatment are important for limiting the effects of toxin and minimizing the severity of illness. Initial symptoms are those of upper respiratory tract infection, but the presence of toxemia with a membrane on the pharyngeal surface in an unimmunized child (or a child immunized in a program where the refrigeration chain may not have been maintained) should alert the clinician. The organisms can be cultured from a portion of the membrane or from a swab taken from under it. The presence of diphtheroids on Gram stain is not sufficient evidence of infection; complete cultures should be performed. Presence of an antibody titer to diphtheria toxin may help confirm the diagnosis.

Antibiotics

Penicillin 50 mg/kg intravenously every 4 hours is a first-line therapy. Once the toxemia settles, a change to IM procaine penicillin 25,000 to 50,000 U/kg/day or oral phenoxymethylpenicillin 12.5 mg/kg every 6 hours is appropriate.[15] Erythromycin is an alternative for patients allergic to penicillin, but some strains of the organism are resistant.[70]

Antitoxin

Antitoxin should be administered as soon as the condition is suspected. Evidence is clear that mortality is higher in children who receive antitoxin late. The antitoxin is made in horses, and a test dose should be given to assess for possible allergy. Diphtheria antitoxin may be difficult to obtain. In the United States, the antitoxin is available only through the Centers for Disease Control and Prevention (CDC). In some other countries, less purified antitoxin is available but cannot be given intravenously. The dose of antitoxin is not related to the patient's size but to the severity of the disease:

Mild disease (nasal and tonsillar)	20,000 U IM
Moderate disease (laryngeal with symptoms)	40,000 U IM or IV
Moderately severe (nasopharyngeal with symptoms)	60,000–100,000 U IV
Malignant disease (combined sites or delayed diagnosis)	60,000–100,000 U IV

Supportive Care

Oxygen by face mask or nasal prong should be provided if the child has an oxygen saturation less than 92% in room air. Nasal or nasopharyngeal catheters are not advisable because they may precipitate airway obstruction. Endotracheal intubation or tracheostomy may be indicated if increasing obstruction is evident. Endotracheal intubation may be difficult if marked tissue swelling and distortion of the pharyngeal and laryngeal anatomy occur. Intubation is ideally performed following gas induction, and great care must be taken not to dislodge pieces of the membrane into the trachea and obstruct the airway. Dexamethasone may help decrease airway edema and relieve obstruction,[35] but it does not reduce the incidence of cardiac and neurologic complications.[110] Maintaining the airway using a tracheostomy may be easier if the inflammation extends down through the larynx into the trachea. Patients may develop palatal palsies that make swallowing difficult, and nasogastric tube feeding may be needed for some time. Patients must be regularly monitored for 3 months after the acute illness because neurologic problems may persist during this time.

Cardiac

Carnitine may have a role in the therapy of diphtheria carditis. Animal data and a randomized controlled trial showed a decreased incidence of myocarditis and complications.[80,81] Cardiac support may dictate use of inotropes and optimization of preload with diuretics or intravenous fluid. Ventricular pacing may improve the outcome in children with diphtheritic myocarditis and associated heart block, although one study reported that all patients with third-degree heart block died despite use of a pacemaker.[101] Prolonged cardiac follow-up may be indicated because of possible considerable delay between onset of symptoms and development of cardiac dysfunction.[29] Recovery from myocarditis may require more time than previously appreciated.[8]

Prevention of Spread

All hospital staff in contact with the patient should be fully immunized. When possible, the child with diphtheria should be isolated. Alternatively, only fully immunized children should be housed in the same area of the ward. All patients' contacts require investigation for diphtheria by obtaining throat swabs and checking immunization status. Patients who have recovered from diphtheria should be immunized with diphtheria toxoid, with dose dependent on age and immunization status.[6]

Dengue

Dengue is an acute febrile illness caused by four different dengue viruses transmitted by Aedes mosquitos (principally *Aedes aegypti*). Dengue symptoms include fever, myalgia, arthralgia, rash, leukopenia, and lymphodenopathy.[121] Dengue usually causes a nonspecific febrile illness. However, it also causes dengue hemorrhagic fever and dengue shock syndrome, the latter characterized by increased vascular permeability.[121] Associated thrombocytopenia, spontaneous bleeding, and intravascular coagulation are common. Severe dengue is one of the most common causes of pediatric admission to hospitals in Asia, with up to 500,000 cases reported annually to the WHO.[121] Dengue shock syndrome usually occurs between the days 3 and 5 of the illness. Mortality is highest when the pulse pressure is 10 mmHg or less at the time of presentation.[63]

Fluid Therapy

The main treatment for dengue shock syndrome is prompt, vigorous fluid therapy. Boluses of 20 ml/kg of 0.9% saline should be given every 15 minutes until the pulse pressure is at least 30 mmHg. After resuscitation, normal maintenance fluid is initiated, with extra boluses of 10 ml/kg if the pulse pressure falls below 30 mmHg. A randomized controlled trial of four different types of fluid in 230 children in Vietnam concluded that 0.9% saline was the crystalloid fluid of choice for the majority of patients with dengue shock syndrome.[63] Lactated Ringer's solution was not as effective as the other solutions, and allergic reactions occurred in 5 of the 56 children given 3% gelatin. Children given dextran 70 recovered more quickly, but they had not been as ill as the children in the other treatment groups. None of the 230 children with dengue shock syndrome died, even though 51 children had a pulse pressure of 10 mmHg or less at the time of presentation.

Other Treatment

Because of severe capillary leak, pleural effusion and ascites are common in patients with severe dengue. However, because of the risk of bleeding, centesis should not be undertaken unless fluid accumulations are causing severe respiratory or circulatory embarrassment.[100] Similarly, the risks of central venous line insertion usually are greater than the benefits. Corticosteroids and carbazochrome should not be used routinely.[104,106,107] A report of a single case from Tahiti has suggested that desmopressin may reduce capillary leak in patients with severe dengue.[72]

A small proportion of children do not respond to aggressive fluid therapy. Respiratory distress may require oxygen and nasal CPAP or mechanical ventilation. If shock persists despite vigorous fluid therapy, a central venous catheter should be inserted if possible. The risk of bleeding can be reduced by using a femoral venous line. Central venous pressure should be maintained at 10 to 12 cm H_2O. However, if severe lung disease is causing right ventricular failure, central venous pressure may be normal or high even though the child is hypovolemic. In these circumstances, echocardiography should be performed to assess left atrial size (as a measure of intravascular volume) and to locate evidence of impaired ventricular contractility. Hypovolemia should be corrected, and dobutamine 5 to 15 μg/kg/min given if ventricular contractility is poor. Bleeding can be severe and often is associated with platelet dysfunction and intravascular coagulation; low-dose heparin 10 to 15 U/kg/hour and fresh-frozen plasma may be helpful. Platelets should be transfused only if the count is less than 20,000/mm^3 or less than 40,000/mm^3 with significant bleeding. IV administration of immunoglobulin 500 mg/kg/day for 5 days may decrease bleeding and increase the platelet count. Renal failure may require hemofiltration or peritoneal dialysis. Coma usually results from hypoxic-ischemic injury, cerebral edema, intracranial hemorrhage, or intravascular coagulation but occasionally is caused by dengue encephalitis.

Malnutrition

Malnutrition contributes to 56% of child deaths, and 83% of this effect is associated with mild-to-moderate rather than severe malnutrition.[73] WHO has published detailed guidelines on the management of severe malnutrition for physicians and health workers at first-referral level,[119,122] and useful summaries of the management of malnutrition have been published.[5,9]

Severe malnutrition is defined as nutritional edema (kwashiorkor), severe wasting with weight-for-height more than three standard deviations below the median (marasmus), or severe stunting with height-for-age more than three standard deviations below the median.[119] Although improvements in the management of severe malnutrition have lowered the mortality from greater than 50%, it remains high even with intensive management. Kwashiorkor now appears not to be caused by protein deficiency but rather by antioxidant deficiency.[28]

Diagnostic workup for malnutrition should include a blood glucose level, blood film for malaria, hemoglobin, microscopy and culture of urine, microscopy of feces (blood suggests dysentery; *Giardia lamblia* cysts or trophozoites may be present), chest x-ray film, and a Mantoux test. Measurement of serum proteins and electrolytes rarely is helpful and may lead to inappropriate therapy. Testing for HIV depends on local circumstances.

Malnutrition mimics many of the clinical signs of dehydration (sunken eyes, poor skin turgor, apathy). Malnourished children often have excess body water and sodium, and giving too much fluid is dangerous. On the other hand, severe sepsis in a malnourished child may be present with remarkably few clinical signs. In particular, no fever may be present, and mortality is high in afebrile patients with malnutrition and sepsis. If the child exhibits shock, hypovolemia should be corrected with 10 ml/kg boluses of 0.9% saline (not albumin). Once hypovolemia is corrected, care should be taken not to administer excess sodium and water intravenously. Nasogastric feeding should be used whenever possible; IV fluids should be avoided.[122] Benzyl penicillin and gentamicin should be given parenterally after taking cultures. The child should be maintained normothermic. Blood glucose level initially should be measured every 4 hours and hypoglycemia treated promptly. Diuretics should not be given for treatment of edema.

Total body sodium is high in malnutrition, even in the presence of hyponatremia, so sodium intake should be restricted. Deficiencies of potassium, magnesium, zinc, copper, selenium, iodine, vitamin A, and folic acid must be corrected immediately. Usually, this is best accomplished with oral or nasogastric administration of electrolyte solution.[9,122] Iron supplements should be given orally only when the child starts to recover (after the first week of treatment).

After initial correction of hypovolemia and replacement of any continuing losses, water intake should be limited to 100 to 130 ml/kg/day. Hypoosmolar feeds should be given initially, with a moderate calorie intake of 80 to 100 kcal/kg/day and protein intake restricted to 1 to 1.5 g/kg/day.[9,119,122] Albumin should not be given intravenously for treatment of hypoalbuminemia. Feeds usually are given every 2 hours for the first 2 days, every 3 hours on days 3 to 5, and every 4 hours thereafter. Appetite usually returns after the first 5 to 7 days. The strength of the feeds then can be gradually increased to 150 to 220 kcal/kg/day and protein to 4 to 5 g/kg/day, but fluids still are limited to 130 ml/kg/day.

During treatment of severe malnutrition, sodium and water intake should be limited, protein intake restricted initially, IV albumin avoided, and calorie intake increased gradually. Deficiencies of potassium and magnesium should be corrected early, with empiric antibiotic therapy given and care taken to prevent hypoglycemia and hypothermia.

Conclusion

Ideally, every child in the world should have access to an ICU with facilities for endotracheal intubation and mechanical ventilation. No ethical justification exists for providing these treatments to children in rich countries while denying them to children in poor countries. However, attempting to make intensive care available to all children while many extremely poor countries have so little money to spend on health care is not helpful.

In countries where the mortality rate in the first 5 years of life is greater than 30 per 1000 live births, most deaths are caused by infections. Using government funding to provide intensive care actually might increase mortality if such care diverts resources away from immunization and primary health care. When the under 5-year mortality rate is between 20 and 30 per 1000, limited use of intubation and ventilation for carefully selected indications may have a role. When the under 5-year mortality rate is less than 20 per 1000, fewer deaths can be prevented by immunization and primary health care, and intensive care can make an important contribution to further reducing child mortality.

REFERENCES

1. Abadco DL, Steiner P: Gastric lavage is better than bronchoalveolar lavage for isolation of Mycobacterium tuberculosis in childhood pulmonary tuberculosis. *Pediatr Infect Dis J* 11:735, 1992.
2. Abrutyn E, Berlin JA: Intrathecal therapy in tetanus, a meta-analysis. *JAMA* 266:2262, 1991.
3. Abu-Ekteish F, Zahraa J: Hypernatraemic dehydration and acute gastro-enteritis in children. *Ann Trop Paediatr* 22:245, 2002.
4. American Thoracic Society, Centers for Disease Control and Prevention, Infectious Diseases Society of America: Treatment of tuberculosis. *Am J Respir Crit Care Med* 167:603, 2003.

5. Ashworth A: Treatment of severe malnutrition. *J Pediatr Gastroenterol Nutr* 32:516, 2001.
6. Atkinson W, Wolfe C, Humiston S, et al: *Epidemiology and prevention of vaccine-preventable diseases,* ed 6. Atlanta, 2000, Centers for Disease Control.
7. Bass JW: Erythromycin for treatment and prevention of pertussis. *Pediatr Infect Dis* 5:154, 1986.
8. Bethell DB, Nguyen MD, Ha Thi Loan, et al: Prognostic value of electrocardiographic monitoring of patients with severe diphtheria. *Clin Infect Dis* 20:1259, 1995.
9. Bhan MK, Bhandari N, Bahl R: Management of the severely malnourished child: perspective from developing countries. *BMJ* 326:146, 2003.
10. Chandra H, Rao CS, Karan S, Mathur YC: Evaluation of betamethasone and isoniazid along with chloramphenicol in the management of whooping cough. *Indian Pediatr* 9:70, 1972.
11. Conde-Agudelo A, Diaz-Rossello JL, Belizan JM: Kangaroo mother care to reduce morbidity and mortality in low birthweight infants (Cochrane Review). In: *The Cochrane Library,* Issue 4, Chichester, 2003, John Wiley & Sons.
12. Cook TM, Protheroe RT, Handel JM: Tetanus: a review of the literature. *Br J Anaesth* 87:477, 2001.
13. Coovadia HM, McNally LM, Jeena PM: The etiology and outcome of pneumonia in HIV-infected children admitted to intensive care in a developing country: a commentary. *Pediatr Crit Care Med* 2:280, 2001.
14. Cotton MF, Donald PR, Schoeman JF, et al: Plasma arginine vasopressin and the syndrome of inappropriate antidiuretic hormone secretion in tuberculous meningitis. *Pediatr Infect Dis J* 10:837, 1991.
15. Coulter B: Diphtheria. In Southall D, et al: *International child health care: a practical manual for hospitals worldwide.* London, 2001, BMJ Books.
16. Crowcroft NS, Booy R, Harrison T, et al: Severe and unrecognised: pertussis in UK infants. *Arch Dis Child* 88:802, 2003.
17. Desai CR, Heera S, Patel A, et al: Role of metronidazole in improving response and specific drug sensitivity in advanced pulmonary tuberculosis. *J Assoc Physicians India* 37:694, 1989.
18. Dreyfuss D, Leviel F, Paillard M, et al: Acute infectious pneumonia is accompanied by a latent vasopressin-dependent impairment of renal water excretion. *Am Rev Respir Dis* 138:583, 1988.
19. D'Souza RM, D'Souza R: Vitamin A for the treatment of children with measles—a systematic review. *J Trop Pediatr* 48:323, 2002.
20. Du Plessis A, Hussey G: Laryngeal tuberculosis in childhood. *Pediatr Infect Dis J* 6:678, 1987.
21. Duke T, Mgone CS: Measles: not just another exanthem. *Lancet* 361:763, 2003.
22. Dyer RA, Potgieter PD: The adult respiratory distress syndrome bronchogenic pulmonary tuberculosis. *Thorax* 39:383, 1984.
23. Dyer RA, Chappell WA, Potgieter PD: Adult respiratory distress syndrome associated with miliary tuberculosis. *Crit Care Med* 13:12, 1985.
24. Earle M, Natera OM, Zaslavsky A, et al: Outcome of pediatric intensive care at six centers in Mexico and Ecuador. *Crit Care Med* 25:1462, 1997.
25. Frey B, Shann F: Oxygen administration in infants. *Arch Dis Child Fetal Neonatal Ed* 88:F84, 2003.
26. Gie RP, Kling S, Schaaf HS, et al: Tuberculous broncho-esophageal fistula in children: a description of two cases. *Pediatr Pulmonol* 25:285, 1998.
27. Gillis J, Grattan-Smith T, Kilham H: Artificial ventilation in severe pertussis. *Arch Dis Child* 63:364, 1988.
28. Golden MHN: Oedematous malnutrition. *Br Med Bull* 54:433, 1998.
29. Groundstroem KW, Molnar G, Lumio J: Echocardiographic follow-up of diphtheric myocarditis. *Cardiology* 87:79, 1996.
30. Guerin PJ, Olliaro P, Nostin F, et al: Malaria: current status of control, diagnosis, treatment, and a proposed agenda for research and development. *Lancet Infect Dis* 2:564, 2002.
31. Gunn AJ, Gluckman PD, Gunn TR: Selective head cooling in newborn infants after perinatal asphyxia: a safety study. *Pediatrics* 102:885, 1998.
32. Hadfield TL, McEvoy P, Polotsky Y, et al: The pathology of diphtheria. *J Infect Dis* 181:S116, 2000.
33. Hall RT, Hall FK, Daily DK: High-dose phenobarbital therapy in term newborn infants with severe perinatal asphyxia: a randomized, prospective study with three-year follow-up. *J Pediatr* 132:345, 1998.
34. Havaldar PV, Patil VD, Siddibhavi BM: Haemorraghic diphtheria. *Ann Trop Paediatr* 9:178, 1989.
35. Havaldar PV: Dexamethasone in laryngeal diphtheritic croup. *Ann Trop Paediatr* 17:21, 1997.
36. Hewett A: Global blockade. *The Australian* April 17, 2002, page 8.
37. Hewitson JP, Von Oppell UO: Role of thoracic surgery for childhood tuberculosis. *World J Surg* 21:468, 1997.
38. Heyns L, Gie RP, Kling S, et al: Management of children with tuberculosis admitted to a pediatric intensive care unit. *Pediatr Infect Dis J* 17:403, 1998.
39. Hoppe JE: State of art in antibacterial susceptibility of Bordetella pertussis and antibiotic treatment of pertussis. *Infection* 26:242, 1998.
40. Hoyne A, Welford N: Diphtheritic myocarditis, a review of 496 cases. *J Pediatr* 5:642, 1934.
41. Hugo-Hamman CR, Scher H, de Moor MMA: Tuberculous pericarditis in children: a review of 44 cases. *Pediatr Infect Dis J* 13:13, 1994.
42. Huseby JS, Hudson LD: Miliary tuberculosis and adult respiratory distress syndrome. *Ann Intern Med* 85:609, 1976.
43. Hussey GD, Clements CJ: Clinical problems in measles case management. *Ann Trop Paediatr* 16:307, 1996.
44. Jeena PM, Bobat R, Kindra G, et al: The impact of human immunodeficiency virus 1 on laryngeal airway obstruction in children. *Arch Dis Child* 87:212, 2002.
45. Jeena PM, Coovadia HM, Chrystal V: Pneumocystis carinii and cytomegalovirus infections in severely ill, HIV-infected African infants. *Ann Trop Paediatr* 16:361, 1996.
46. Klein M, Zar H: ICU outcome in HIV-associated childhood pneumonia. *S Afr Med J* 88:1483, 1998.
47. Loukoushkina EF, Bobko PV, Kolbasova, EV, et al: The clinical picture and diagnosis of diphtheritic carditis in children. *Eur J Pediatr* 157:528, 1998.
48. Kuppermann N, Inkelis SH, Saladino R: The role of heparin in the prevention of extremity and digit necrosis in meningococcal purpura fulminans. *Pediatr Infect Dis J* 13:867, 1994.
49. Lesi A, Meremikwu M: High first dose quinine regimen for treating severe malaria. In: *The Cochrane Library,* Issue 1, Chichester, 2003, John Wiley & Sons.
50. Lucaya J, Sole S, Badosa J, Manzanares R: Bronchial perforation and bronchoesophageal fistulas: tuberculous origin in children. *AJR Am J Roentgenol* 135:525, 1980.
51. Mackenzie A, Barnes G, Shann F: Clinical signs of dehydration in children. *Lancet* 2:605 and 1529, 1989.
52. Martinez-Azagra A, Serrano A: Adult respiratory distress syndrome in children, associated with miliary tuberculosis. *J Pediatr* 126:678, 1995.
53. Mason KO: Explaining fertility transitions. *Demography* 34:443, 1997.
54. McAllister WA, Thompson PJ, Al-Habet SM, Rogers HJ: Rifampicin reduces effectiveness and bioavailability of prednisolone. *BMJ* 286:923, 1983.
55. McIntosh HM, Olliaro P: Artemisinin derivatives for treating severe malaria (Cochrane Review). In: *The Cochrane Library,* Issue 1, Oxford, 2003, Update Software.
56. Meremikwu M, Marson AG: Routine anticonvulsants for treating cerebral malaria (Cochrane Review). In: *The Cochrane Library,* Issue 1, Oxford, 2003, Update Software.
57. Meremikwu M, Smith JH: Blood transfusion for treating malarial anaemia (Cochrane Review). In: *The Cochrane Library,* Issue 1, Oxford, 2003, Update Software.
58. Morley D: Paediatric priorities in evolving community programmes for developing countries. *Lancet* 2:1012, 1976.
59. Murray CJL, Lopez AD: *Global comparative assessments in the health sector.* Geneva, 1994, World Health Organization.
60. Murray HW, Tuazon CU, Kirmani N, Sheagren JN: The adult respiratory distress syndrome associated with miliary tuberculosis. *Chest* 73:37, 1978.
61. Musher DM: How contagious are common respiratory tract infections. *N Engl J Med* 348:1256, 2003.
62. Nakvi AJ, Nohl-Oser HC: Surgical treatment of bronchial obstruction in primary tuberculosis in children: report of seven cases. *Thorax* 34:464, 1979.

63. Ngo NT, Cao XT, Kneen R, et al: Acute management of dengue shock syndrome: a randomized double-blind comparison of 4 intravenous fluid regimens in the first hour. *Clin Infect Dis* 32:204, 2001.
64. Nosten F, Brasseur P: Combination therapy for malaria the way forward? *Drugs* 62:1315, 2002.
65. Nurnberger W, Kries RV, Bohm O, Gobel U: Systemic meningococcal infection: which children may benefit from adjuvant haemostatic therapy? Results from an observational study. *Eur J Pediatr* 158:S192, 1999.
66. Onwubalili JK, Scott GM, Smith H: Acute respiratory distress related to chemotherapy of advanced pulmonary tuberculosis: a study of two cases and review of the literature. *QJM* 59:599, 1986.
67. Oxfam: Make trade fair. Available at *www.maketradefair.com.* Accessed January 27, 2005.
68. Paine BG: Pertussis in the highlands: a clinical review. *P N G Med J* 16:36, 1973.
69. Papagiannopoulos KA, Linegar AG, Harris DG, Rossouw GJ: Surgical management of airway obstruction in primary tuberculosis in children. *Ann Thorac Surg* 68:1182, 1999.
70. Parry CM, White NJ: Penicillin vs. erythromycin in the treatment of diphtheria. *Clin Infect Dis* 27:845, 1998.
71. Pavesio D, Ponzone A: Salbutamol and pertussis. *Lancet* 1:150, 1977.
72. Pea L, Roda L, Moll F: Desmopressin treatment for a case of dengue hemorrhagic fever/dengue shock syndrome. *Clin Infect Dis* 33:1611, 2001.
73. Pelletier DL, Frongillo EA, Schroeder DG, Habicht JP: The effects of malnutrition on child mortality in developing countries. *Bull World Health Organ* 73:443, 1995.
74. Pierce C, Klein N, Peters M: Is leukocytosis a predictor of mortality in severe pertussis infection? *Intensive Care Med* 26:1512, 2000.
75. Pillay V, Swingler G: Symptomatic treatment of the cough in whooping cough (Cochrane Review). In: *The Cochrane Library,* Issue 4, Chichester, 2003, John Wiley & Sons.
76. Piqueras AR, Marruecos L, Artigas A, Rodriguez C: Miliary tuberculosis and adult respiratory distress syndrome. *Intensive Care Med* 13:175, 1987.
77. Powell VI, Grima K: Exchange transfusion for malaria and Babesia infection. *Transfus Med Rev* 16:239, 2002.
78. Prasad K, Garner P: Steroids for treating cerebral malaria (Cochrane Review). In: *The Cochrane Library,* Issue 1, Oxford, 2003, Update Software.
79. Rabinowitz L, Joffe BI, Abkiewicz C, et al: Hyperglycaemia in infantile gastroenteritis. *Arch Dis Child* 59:771, 1984.
80. Ramos AC, Barrucand L, Elias PR, et al: Carnitine supplementation in diphtheria. *Indian Pediatr* 29:1501, 1992.
81. Ramos AC, Elias PR, Barrucand L, Silva JA: The protective effect of carnitine in human diphtheric myocarditis. *Pediatr Res* 18:815, 1984.
82. Roberts I: Randomised controlled trial of steroids in pertussis. *Pediatr Infect Dis J* 11:982, 1992.
83. Rudan I, Tomaskovic L, Boschi-Pinto C, et al: Global estimate of the incidence of clinical pneumonia among children under five years. *Bull World Health Organ,* 82:895, 2004.
84. Sanders RK: The management of tetanus 1996. *Trop Doctor* 26:107, 1996.
85. Schaaf HS, Gie RP, Beyers N, et al: Tuberculosis in infants less than 3 months of age. *Arch Dis Child* 69:371, 1993.
86. Schoeman JF, Van Zyl LE, Laubscher JA, Donald PR: Effect of corticosteroids on intracranial pressure, computed tomographic findings and clinical outcome in young children with tuberculous meningitis. *Pediatrics* 99:226, 1992.
87. Shann F: Intrathecal administration of tetanus antiserum. *Med J Aust* 2:604, 1983.
88. Shann F: Meta analysis of trials of prophylactic antibiotics for children with measles: inadequate evidence. *BMJ* 314:334, 1997.
89. Shann F: Cardiac failure in children with pneumonia in Papua New Guinea. *Pediatr Infect Dis J* 17:1141, 1998.
90. Shann F: Haemophilus influenzae pneumonia: type b or non-type b? *Lancet* 354:1488, 1999.
91. Shann F: Bacterial pneumonia: commoner than perceived. *Lancet* 357:2070, 2001.
92. Shann F: Research in developing countries. *N Engl J Med* 346:627, 2002.
93. Shann F, Biddulph J, Vince J: *Paediatrics for doctors in Papua New Guinea.* Port Moresby, 2003, PNG Department of Health.
94. Shann F, Germer S: Leukaemoid reaction in Eastern Highlands children. *P N G Med J* 22:55, 1979.
95. Shann F, Gratten M, Germer S, et al: Aetiology of pneumonia in children in Goroka Hospital, Papua New Guinea. *Lancet* 2:537, 1984.
96. Shann F, Steinhoff MC: Vaccines for children in rich and poor countries. *Lancet* 354(suppl II):7, 1999.
97. Singhi S, Dhwan A: Frequency and significance of electrolyte abnormalities in pneumonia. *Indian Pediatr* 29:735, 1992.
98. Skellett S, Mayer A, Durward A, et al: Chasing the base deficit: hyperchloraemic alkalosis following 0.9% saline fluid resuscitation. *Arch Dis Child* 83:514, 2000.
99. Smith JH, Meremikwu M: Iron chelating agents for treating malaria (Cochrane Review). In: *The Cochrane Library,* Issue 1, Oxford, 2003, Update Software.
100. Soni A, Chugh K, Sachdev A, Gupta D: Management of dengue fever in ICU. *Indian J Pediatr* 68:1051, 2001.
101. Stockins BA, Lanas FT, Saavedra JG, Opazo JA: Prognosis in patients with diphtheric myocarditis and bradyarrhythmias: assessment of results of ventricular pacing. *Br Heart J* 72:190, 1994.
102. Strang JIG, Gibson DG, Mitchison D, et al: Controlled clinical trial of complete open surgical drainage and of prednisolone in treatment of tuberculous pericardial effusion in Transkei. *Lancet* 2:759, 1988.
103. Strang JIG, Gibson DG, Nunn AJ, et al: Controlled trial of prednisolone as adjuvant in treatment of tuberculous constrictive pericarditis in Transkei. *Lancet* 2:1418, 1987.
104. Sumarmo, Talogo W, Asrin A, et al: Failure of hydrocortisone to affect outcome in dengue shock syndrome. *Pediatrics* 69:45, 1982.
105. Suresh GK, Dhawan A, Kohli V: Tracheal diphtheria mimicking bacterial tracheitis. *Pediatr Infect Dis J* 11:502, 1992.
106. Tassniyom S, Vasanawathana S, Chirawatkul A, et al: Failure of high dose methylprednisolone in established dengue shock syndrome: a placebo controlled double blind study. *Pediatrics* 92:11, 1993.
107. Tassniyom S, Vasanawathana S, Dhiensiri T, et al: Failure of carbazochrome sodium sulfonate (AC-17) to prevent dengue vascular permeability or shock: a randomized, controlled trial. *J Pediatr* 131:525, 1997.
108. Te Water Naude JM, Donald PR, Hussey GD, et al: Twice weekly vs. daily chemotherapy for childhood tuberculosis. *Pediatr Infect Dis J* 19:405, 2000.
109. Theilade D: Nasal continuous positive airway pressure in the treatment of whooping cough. *Anaesthesia* 34:1028, 1979.
110. Thisyakorn U, Wongvanich J, Kumpeng V: Failure of corticosteroid therapy to prevent diphtheritic myocarditis or neuritis. *Pediatr Infect Dis* 3:126, 1984.
111. Toppet M, Derde MP, Toppet V, et al: Corticosteroids in primary tuberculosis with bronchial obstruction. *Arch Dis Child* 65:1222, 1990.
112. Torre D: Treatment with steroids in children with pertussis. *Pediatr Infect Dis J* 12:419, 1993.
113. UNICEF: *The state of the world's children 2002.* New York, 2001, UNICEF.
114. Wesley AG, Pather M, Chrystal V: The haemorrhagic diathesis in diphtheria with special reference to disseminated intravascular coagulation. *Ann Trop Paediatr* 1:51, 1981.
115. Winrow AP: Inhaled steroids in the treatment of pertussis. *Pediatr Infect Dis J* 14:922, 1995.
116. World Bank: Data and statistics: country groups. Available at *http://worldbank.org/data/countryclass/classgroups.htm.* Accessed April 11, 2003.
117. World Bank: Health, nutrition and population statistics: health expenditure, services and use. Available at *http://devdata.worldbank.org/hnpstats/files/Tab2_15.xls.* Accessed April 11, 2003.
118. World Health Organization: *Oxygen therapy for acute respiratory infections in young children in developing countries (WHO/ARI/93.28).* Geneva, 1993, World Health Organization.
119. World Health Organization: *Management of severe malnutrition: a manual for physicians and other senior health workers.* Geneva, 1998, World Health Organization.
120. World Health Organization: The world health report 1998. Geneva, 1998, World Health Organization.

121. World Health Organization: *Prevention and control of dengue and dengue haemorrhagic fever: comprehensive guidelines.* New Delhi, 1999, World Health Organization.
122. World Health Organization: *Management of the child with a serious infection or severe malnutrition: guidelines for care at the first-referral level in developing countries (WHO/FCH/CAH/00.1).* Geneva, 2000, World Health Organization.
123. World Health Organization: *The world health report 2000.* Geneva, 2000, World Health Organization.
124. World Health Organization: *Managing newborn problems: a guide for doctors, nurses and midwives.* Geneva, 2003, World Health Organization.
125. Worthington MG, Brink JG, Odell JA, et al: Surgical relief of acute airway obstruction due to primary tuberculosis. *Ann Thorac Surg* 56:1054, 1993.
126. Zar HJ, Apolles P, Argent A, et al: The etiology and outcome of pneumonia in human immunodeficiency virus-infected children admitted to intensive care in a developing country. *Pediatr Crit Care Med* 2:108, 2001.
127. Zar HJ, Tannenbaum E, Apolles P, et al: Sputum induction for the diagnosis of pulmonary tuberculosis in infants and young children in an urban setting in South Africa. *Arch Dis Child* 82:305, 2000.
128. Zoumboulakis D, Anagnostakis D, Albanis V, Matsaniotis N: Steroids in treatment of pertussis. *Arch Dis Child* 48:51, 1973.
129. Zwi KJ, Pettifor JM, Soderlund N: Paediatric hospital admissions at a South African urban regional hospital: the impact of HIV, 1992-1997. *Ann Trop Paediatr* 19:135, 1999.

PART

II

Organ System Function and Failure

CHAPTER 17

Structure and Function of the Heart

Julien I.E. Hoffman

PEARLS

- The basic form of the human heart and great vessels is complete 8 weeks after conception, after which the structures grow and mature.
- The parietal pericardium is a stiff membrane that surrounds the heart loosely, separated from the heart by a small amount of lubricating pericardial fluid.
- Immediately after birth, there is a large increase in total body oxygen consumption and cardiac output to approximately twice its later values.
- Although large arteries are regarded as conduits and capillaries as vessels allowing transport of substances to and from the tissues, many substances can move across arterial walls.

The Heart

Anatomical Development and Structure

Gross Anatomy

The basic form of the human heart and great vessels is complete 8 weeks after conception, after which the structures grow and mature. The ventricular mass enlarges by cellular hyperplasia and hypertrophy; hyperplasia ceases shortly after birth. Increase of ventricular volumes depends on the increasing flow through each ventricle; diverting flow from a ventricle causes hypoplasia of that ventricle and its associated great artery. Before birth, left and right ventricles have equal wall thickness. After birth, with rise in aortic pressure and decrease in pulmonary arterial pressure, the left ventricle becomes thicker than the right ventricle. Left ventricular wall thickness is proportional to the logarithm of age from conception.[139] The ventricular septum is flat in the fetus. After birth, it bulges into the right ventricle and functions like part of the left ventricle. In the embryo, coronary arteries form in the embryonic epicardial tissue[201] and join the aorta to supply flow to the thickening heart muscle that can no longer get enough blood from sinusoids from the ventricular cavity.

Muscle fibers in the ventricles form a complex helical array. Fibers in the left ventricular midwall are circumferential, parallel to the atrioventricular groove. From this position the fibers twist gradually as they move toward each surface so that at the epicardial surface they are 75 degrees and at the endocardial surface 60 degrees from the circumferential fibers.[241] Some investigators believe that the muscle fiber layers form one continuous sheet that is wrapped around itself like a turban.[257] When the ventricle is dilated, the fiber angles change and become less effective in ejecting blood.[9]

Microscopic Anatomy

The myocardium is a syncytium made of branching fibers, each consisting of bundles of myocytes in series. The myocytes are joined to adjacent myocytes by the intercalated disc, a set of mechanical junctions: adherens junctions with N-cadherin, catenins, and vinculin;

desmosomes with desmin, desmoplakin, desmocollin, and desmoglein; and gap junctions with connexins and N-cadherin.[144,271,289] The gap junctions transmit the electrical impulse from one cell to the next.

Myocyte. The major components of the myocyte are the *sarcomeres,* which contain the myofibrillar contractile apparatus; the *mitochondria,* which contain enzymes for energy production; the *sarcolemma,* which contains the cell envelope and its extensions into the cytoplasm; the *sarcoplasmic reticulum;* and the *cytosol.* The numerous proteins in these structures not only play a role in normal function but, if abnormal for genetic or extraneous reasons, contribute to myocardial dysfunction.[130]

Contractile Apparatus. The functional unit is the *sarcomere,* defined as the structure between two transverse Z lines,[53,222,233] representing discs that contain proteins such as α-actinin and filamin that connect the actin and titin filaments of adjacent myocytes. On each side of the Z line is a light zone, the I (isotropic) band, and in the center of the sarcomere are two dark zones, the A (anisotropic) bands, separated by a light H band in the middle of which is a dark thin M band (Figure 17–1). The I bands contain paired thin filaments of actin coiled in a helix and attached to the Z lines. In humans, cardiac α-actin makes up 80% of the actin in fetuses and neonates, but in adults skeletal α-actin makes up 60% of the total.[24] Two long tropomyosin filaments lie in the grooves between each pair of actin filaments[148] (Figure 17–2, *left*). Every 400 Å, near the crossover points of two actin filaments, is a troponin complex with the following three distinct troponins: (1) troponin T, which binds troponin to tropomyosin; (2) troponin I, which inhibits actin-myosin interaction; and (3) troponin C, which is a high-affinity calcium receptor. The thin actin filaments overlap with thick myosin filaments at the A bands. These myosin filaments are composed of light and heavy chains. The light chains coil around each other to form the long core of the myosin molecule. The heavy chains form globular myosin heads that project from the sides of the thick filament toward the actin molecules (Figure 17–2, *right*). A collar of cardiac myosin binding protein C encircles the thick filaments. Mutations of this protein are a common cause of hypertrophic cardiomyopathy.[175] Between two A bands there is usually a thin lighter band, the H band, which has myosin but no actin filaments.[148,233]

Titin, the largest known molecule (molecular weight 3–3.6 MDa, 1 mm long), is the third most abundant fibrillar protein. It extends from the Z band to the M band, has two isoforms, and is the main protein responsible for the elastic behavior of the myocyte.[119] It is essential for sarcomere assembly and for sensing sarcomere length[160] and, with myomesin, supports the actomyosin filaments.

Myocytes have fewer myofibrils and more water and cytoplasm before birth than after birth, and the myofibrils do not have the uniformly parallel arrays that they will have after birth.[5]

Sarcolemma and Sarcoplasmic Reticulum. The cell membrane contains receptors, ion channels, pumps, and exchangers. It has indentations overlying the Z bands, and from these indentations small tubules termed *T* (for transverse) *tubules* penetrate the cell. Abutting against the T tubules are dilated expansions of the sarcoplasmic reticulum (junctional reticulum or cisternae), which join the free sarcoplasmic reticulum, a network of longitudinal tubules inside the cell that surround the thick (myosin) filaments (see Figure 17–1). These tubular systems modulate the entry of calcium to, or its exclusion from, the cytoplasm.[5,53]

The cisternae contain the calcium-binding protein calsequestrin, whereas the longitudinal tubules contain phospholamban and the adenosine triphosphate (ATP)-dependent calcium pump.[5,178] Phospholamban inhibits the affinity of the sarcoplasmic reticulum Ca^{2+}-ATPase (SERCA) pump for calcium, and phospholamban phosphorylation relieves the inhibition and increases calcium entry with resulting increase in inotropy.[34,55,92,216] In heart failure, phospholamban phosphorylation is decreased by an increase in unphosphorylated calcineurin,[179] leading to decreased SERCA activity.[93,196] A similar decrease in SERCA has been found in sepsis[287] and in some forms of dilated cardiomyopathy.[161] Cisternae store and release

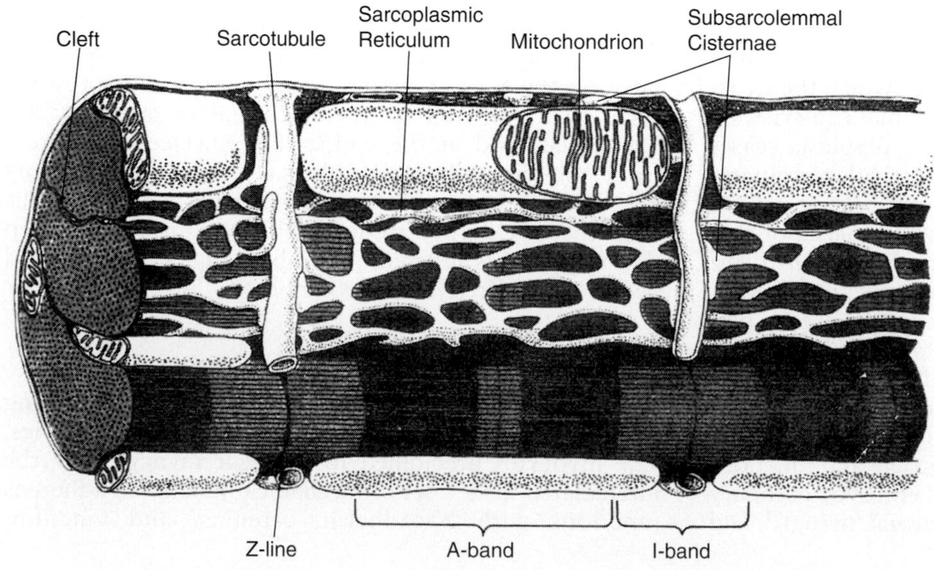

FIGURE 17–1 • Diagram of cardiac muscle unit showing organization of contractile elements and sarcoplasmic reticulum. (Drawn by Bunji Tagawa. From Chidsey CA III: Calcium metabolism in the normal and failing heart. In Braunwald E, editor: *The myocardium: failure and infarction.* New York, 1974, HP Publishing.)

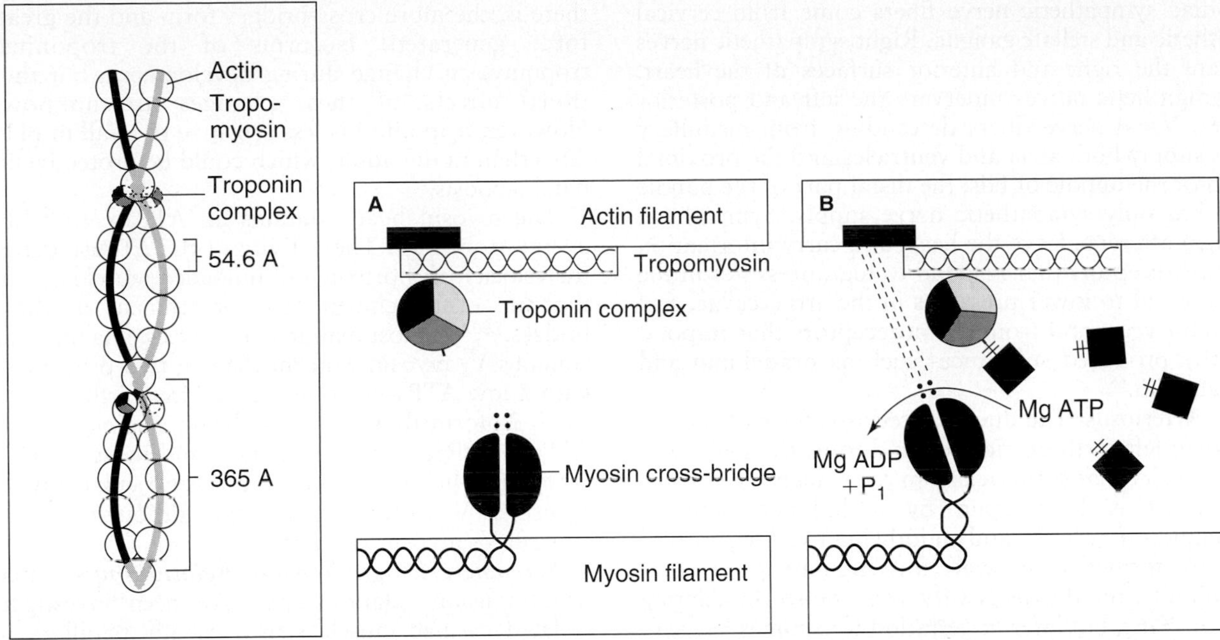

FIGURE 17–2 • **Left,** Diagram of actin and tropomyosin filaments and their relation to the troponin complex. **Right,** Diagram showing the role of troponin in contraction. **A,** In diastole, the interaction between myosin and actin is inhibited. **B,** Calcium *(black squares)* binds to the troponin complex so that myosin and actin can interact. (Original drawing by Gaetano di Palma. Redrawn from Katz A: Contractile proteins in normal and failing myocardium. In Braunwald E, editor: *The myocardium: failure and infarction,* New York, 1974, HP Publishing.)

activator calcium, whereas longitudinal tubules remove calcium from the cytosol. Both T tubules and sarcoplasmic reticulum are sparse, undifferentiated, and disorganized early in gestation but increase and differentiate markedly late in gestation and after birth in mammals. Therefore the immature heart depends mainly on extracellular sources for activator calcium,[5,148] partly explaining its marked calcium sensitivity.

Cytoplasm. During development, the proportion of mitochondria in the myocyte increases, particularly at the time of birth, and mitochondria become larger and develop more complex cristae.[5] In the adult, approximately 30% to 40% of the muscle mass is made up of mitochondria.

The cytosol contains other calcium-binding proteins[5,6] and other major proteins such as tubulin and desmin.

Cytoskeleton and Extracellular Matrix. For contractile proteins to shorten the whole myocyte, they must be linked to the cell wall and the extracellular matrix. Longitudinal connections are made via the Z lines, representing discs that contain proteins such as α-actinin and filamin that connect the actin and titin filaments of adjacent myocytes.[121,236] More lateral connections are made by the extrasarcomeric skeleton. There is an intermyofibrillar cytoskeleton with intermediate filaments, microfilaments, and microtubules.[48,49,121,239] Desmin intermediate filaments provide a three-dimensional scaffold throughout the extrasarcomeric cytoskeleton and connect longitudinally to adjacent Z discs and laterally to subsarcolemmal costameres.[48,239] *Costameres* are subsarcolemmal domains located in a periodic pattern, flanking the Z lines and overlying the I bands on the cytoplasmic side of the sarcolemma.[71,190,191,220,243] They contain the focal adhesion-type complex, the spectrin-based complex, and the dystrophin/dystrophin-associated protein complex. The focal adhesion-type complex, made up of cytoplasmic proteins such as vinculin, ankyrin, and talin, connects with cytoskeletal actin filaments and with transmembrane proteins such as the dystroglycans and the sarcoglycans.[13,17,43] Dystrophin is linked to dystroglycan, laminin, and actin. These proteins help to fix sarcomeres to the lateral sarcolemma, stabilize the T-tubular system, and connect the sarcolemma to the extracellular matrix. Voltage-gated sodium channels colocalize with dystrophin, spectrin, ankyrin, and syntrophins. Potassium channels interact with the Z line and intercalated discs. In many of the genetic dilated cardiomyopathies these proteins are abnormal,[258–260] thereby explaining the abnormal muscle function.

Extracellular collagen plays a major role in cell–cell and cell–vessel interactions and in ventricular stiffness.[25,205,206,292] With maturation, more collagen is type III and less is type I.[168] The relationship between sarcomeres and cytoskeleton changes with maturation, perhaps accounting for maturational differences in the rest sarcomere's mean length in myocytes.[182] In addition, cell adhesion proteins stimulated by growth factors from the myocyte are in greatest amount in the neonate, decrease with postnatal age, but increase again during hypertrophy.[254,255] Other elements in the extracellular matrix (e.g., laminin, fibronectin, and tenascin) play a major role during morphogenesis and during contraction[33] and are important mediators in hypertrophy.

Nerves and Receptors. Adrenergic, muscarinic, and other receptors appear early and are functional even before innervation. Parasympathetic innervation precedes sympathetic innervation in all species.[5,22,97] Innervation is present in the earliest viable human premature infants but may not be fully mature. Innervation is most advanced in species that are most independent immediately after birth.

Cardiac sympathetic nerve fibers come from cervical sympathetic and stellate ganglia. Right sympathetic nerves innervate the right and anterior surfaces of the heart. Left sympathetic nerves innervate the left and posterior surfaces. Vagal nerve fibers descending from medullary centers supply both atria and ventricles and the proximal portion of the bundle of His; the distal part of the bundle of His has only sympathetic nerve supply. Sympathetic and vagal afferents leave the heart and carry information from baroreceptors that respond to high pressures in the ventricles and to lower pressures in the atria, cavae, and pulmonary veins and from chemoreceptors that respond to locally produced substances such as bradykinin and prostaglandin.[68]

Ductus Arteriosus. The ductus arteriosus forms from the embryonic left sixth aortic arch and joins the main pulmonary artery that separates from the truncus arteriosus. The ductus is kept open by a balance between prostaglandin E_2 (PGE_2) and endothelin-1 (ET-1), both of which are formed in its wall and circulate from other sites. Initially, the ductus is very sensitive to the dilating action of PGE_2, but later in gestation it becomes less sensitive to dilator and more sensitive to constrictor prostaglandins.[57–59] After birth, oxygen reacts with a cytochrome P-450 and causes release of ET-1 (the most powerful ductus constrictor).[64] A switch from dilator to constrictor prostaglandins occurs. In addition, oxygen modulates the function of mitochondrial electron chain transport by increasing the generation of H_2O_2, inhibiting voltage-gated potassium channels in ductus smooth muscle, thereby opening voltage-gated L-type Ca^{2+} channels to cause influx of calcium and ductus constriction.[172,202,261] These constrictor effects overpower the dilating effect of nitric oxide that is released from the ductus when oxygen tension rises.[62] The ductus constricts, usually within the first 24 hours and almost invariably within 3 weeks. The lumen then becomes permanently occluded by fibrosis.[59,60]

Physiological Development and Function

Myocardial Mechanics

Cardiac Sarcomere Function

Excitation-Contraction Coupling. When an electrical impulse reaches cardiac muscle, myocyte membranes depolarize. Extracellular calcium in high concentration at the sarcolemmal membrane and the T tubules enters the cell rapidly. Spread of electrical excitation into the myocyte via the T tubules also causes release of intracellular calcium from the sarcoplasmic reticulum.[53,84,158]

Cytosolic calcium increases from a concentration of 10^{-7} M in diastole to 10^{-5} M in systole. When the calcium that entered the cytosol binds to troponin C, the inhibitory effect of troponin I is antagonized, and a conformational change of troponin and tropomyosin exposes the actin-myosin binding sites.[53,84,148,158] These sites interact with the myosin heads to form the cross-bridges (see Figure 17–2, *right*). The myosin heads rotate, generate force, and move the actin filaments, just as oars move a boat through the water. Interaction between actin and myosin pulls the two Z lines toward each other, shortening the muscle and generating force. The more calcium there is, the more cross-bridges form and the greater the force generated. Isoforms of the troponins and tropomyosin change during development, but the functional effects of these changes are unknown.[5,164] However, troponin I is less sensitive to a fall in pH in the fetus than in the adult, which could be protective in perinatal acidosis.

The myosin head contains an ATPase that liberates energy from ATP. The activity of the ATPase determines the velocity of shortening of unloaded muscle by affecting the rate of attachment and detachment of the cross-bridges.[5,232] In most mammalian species, fetal myocardium contains V_3 myosin isoform (having two β heavy chains) with a low ATPase activity rate. After birth this changes to V_1 isoform (having two α heavy chains) with a high ATPase activity rate. In humans and most of the larger mammals, however, almost all ventricular myocardial myosin is V_3 isoform at any age, although human atria contain V_1 myosin isoform.[5]

Sarcomere Length-Tension Relationships. Sarcomere length-tension relationships have been investigated in isolated cardiac muscle strips, usually papillary muscle with its nearly parallel fibers. The muscle strip is placed in a water bath. One end is tied to a lever and the other to a force transducer (Figure 17–3, *A*). Weights attached to the other end of the lever extend the muscle to any desired length before contraction (preload); excessive stretching is prevented by a stop. Other weights added to the lever after initial length is set affect the muscle only after contraction has started and so are termed the *afterload.* The muscle can be stimulated to contract by an electrical impulse. Instruments for measuring muscle length, sarcomere length by laser diffraction, calcium entry by various fluorescence methods, and a host of other specialized functions can be added.[158,192,229]

Stretching relaxed muscle produces an exponential-like increase in passive tension (see Figure 17–3, *B*). This elasticity results mainly from titin.[119,120,229,242] At very low sarcomere lengths, the actin filaments from each Z line overlap each other. As the sarcomere lengthens, the Z lines move farther apart and a gap appears between the two sets of actin filaments. When the sarcomere reaches a length of approximately 2.2 μm, there is a maximal overlap between actin and myosin filaments[158,232,233] (see Figure 17–3, C). At longer muscle and sarcomere lengths, actin and myosin filaments overlap increasingly less. The maximal sarcomere length is 3.0 μm. Further elongation of the muscle occurs by slippage of fibers and not by further sarcomere lengthening.[158,232,233]

Active contraction is studied in two ways[192] (see Figure 17–3, *D*). First, muscle is stimulated to contract at different initial muscle lengths but is not allowed to shorten (isometric contraction). At the shortest lengths no force is generated; the muscle remains slack. As sarcomere lengths increase, force is generated and increases to reach a maximum at sarcomere lengths of approximately 2.2 μm. At longer sarcomere lengths, there may even be a decrease in force.[232]

If, at any length, passive tension is subtracted from the tension generated during isometric contraction, the resulting curve demonstrates active tension as a function of length (see Figure 17–3, *B*).

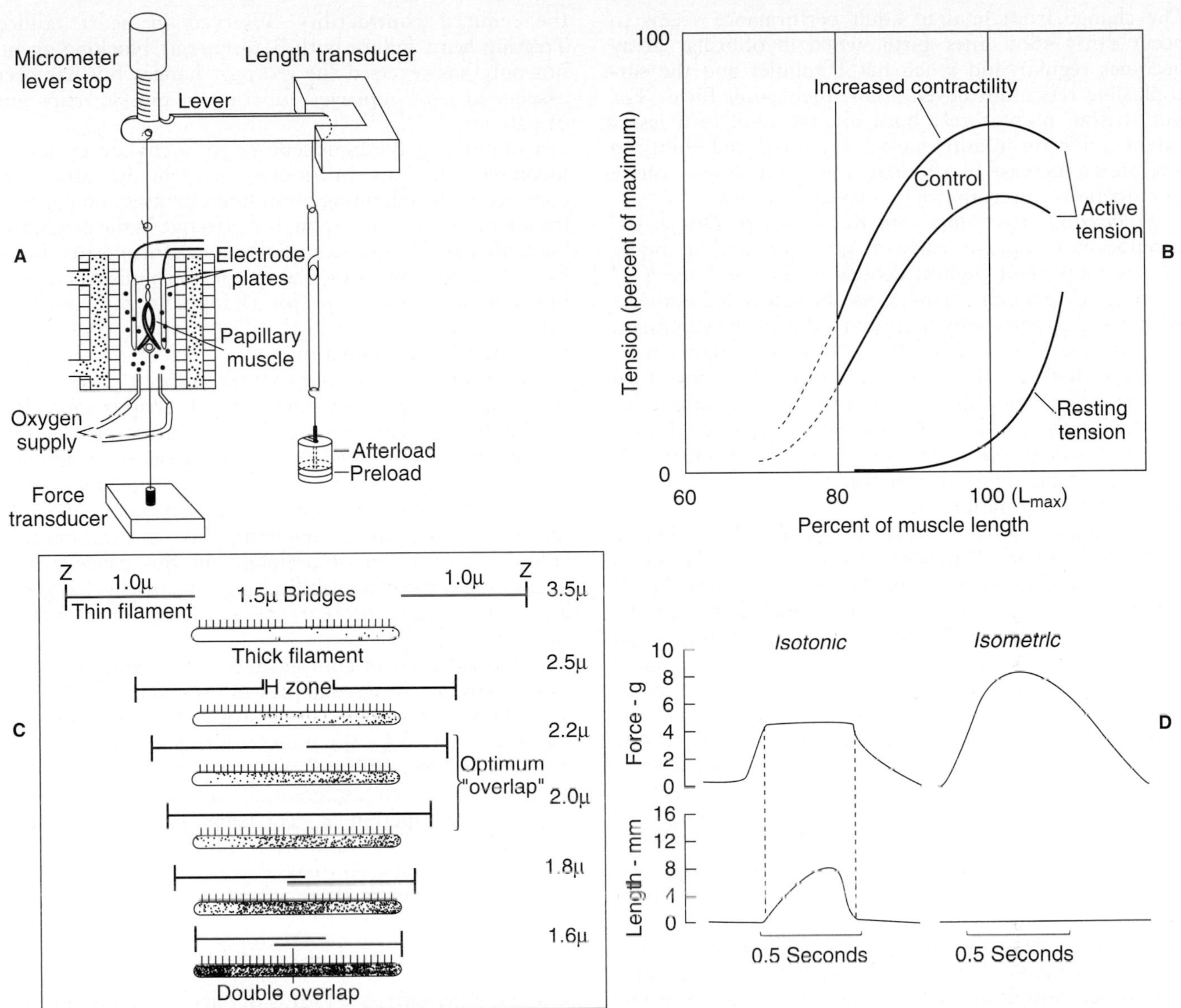

FIGURE 17–3 • **A,** Diagram of isolated muscle strip in a water bath and attached to transducers for measuring force and length. Preload is set by the lever stop. (From Parmley WW, Tyberg JV: Determinants of myocardial oxygen consumption. In Yu PN, Goodwin JF, editors: *Progress in cardiology.* Philadelphia, 1976, Lea & Febiger.) **B,** Relationship between muscle length and resting tension or active tension at three different contractile levels. (Original drawing by Albert Miller. Redrawn from Sonnenblick EH: Myocardial ultrastructure in the normal and failing heart. In Braunwald E, editor: *The myocardium: failure and infarction.* New York, 1974, HP Publishing.) **C,** Diagram showing relationships of sarcomere length, positions of the actin and myosin filaments, and contractile force. (Original drawing by Albert Miller. Redrawn from Sonnenblick EH: Myocardial ultrastructure in the normal and failing heart. In Braunwald E, editor: *The myocardium: failure and infarction.* New York, 1974, HP Publishing.) **D,** Typical length tracings for isotonic **(left)** and isometric **(right)** contractions. The *dashed vertical lines* in the **left tracing** indicate the portion of contraction in which the muscle shortens against a constant force. (Redrawn from Parmley WW, Tyberg JV: Determinants of myocardial oxygen consumption. In Yu PN, Goodwin JF, editors: *Progress in cardiology.* Philadelphia, 1976, Lea & Febiger.)

Second, if afterload is small the contracting muscle generates an appropriate force and then shortens while force remains constant (isotonic contraction). The rate of shortening is fastest at the onset of shortening and from it the velocity of shortening is measured (see Figure 17–3, *D*). The shortening velocity ranges from zero when the load is so heavy that it prevents shortening to a maximum when the external load is zero[158]; however true zero loading is impossible because of internal viscosity and elastic forces.[5,232] Increases in cytosolic calcium increase the force generated during contraction but have little influence on the maximal velocity of shortening.

In fetal lambs, the passive tension of muscle strips is abnormally high. Active tension per mm^2 cross-sectional myocyte area at any given afterload is below adult values but is proportional to the reduced number of myofibrils.[5,6,97] Contractile material accounts for approximately 60% of cardiac muscle in adults but only 30% in fetuses. The extent and velocity of shortening are reduced in fetal heart muscle, but correcting for the amount of contractile machinery suggests the intrinsic performance of fetal and adult actin-myosin filaments is similar. Some of the differences between fetal and adult cardiac muscle may result from the differences in collagen and cytoskeletal composition.[5]

The change from fetal to adult performance seems to occur fairly soon after birth, when myofibrillar array becomes regular and when the T tubules and the sarcoplasmic reticulum develop into their adult form.[5] For this reason, prematurely born infants (and, to a lesser extent, full-term infants) have a much-reduced ability to tolerate an increase in afterload and are unduly sensitive to reductions in serum calcium concentrations.

Myocardial Receptors and Responses to Drugs. α_1-adrenoceptors appear early in gestation and in many species reach their highest density in the neonate.[5,22,169] These developmental changes may be associated with the normal cell hypertrophy that occurs during development. By contrast, β-adrenoceptors increase progressively with age. Both β_1- and β_2-adrenoceptors are present on myocytes.[36,129] In addition, histamine H_2, vasoactive intestinal polypeptide (VIP), adenosine A_1, acetylcholine M_2, and somatostatin receptors have been identified. They act on the myocyte's contractile apparatus through one of two main pathways.

The major pathway involves the membrane-bound receptor–G protein–adenylate cyclase complexes. G proteins include the Gs (stimulatory) and Gi (inhibitory) proteins.[244] In their inactive state, these G proteins include α, β, and γ subunits and guanine diphosphate (GDP). When agonists stimulate β-adrenergic, histamine, or VIP receptors, the G proteins undergo a conformational change. The change induces the Gs protein to exchange its GDP for guanine triphosphate (GTP) and release the β and γ subunits. The Gs–α–GTP complex interacts with adenylate cyclase to convert ATP to cyclic AMP, which activates a variety of protein kinases to phosphorylate proteins, including voltage-dependent calcium channels, phospholamban, and troponin I. Consequently, calcium entry during depolarization and uptake of calcium into the sarcoplasmic reticulum storage pool are increased, thus increasing contractility. The Gs–α–GTP complex has intrinsic GTPase activity that converts GTP to GDP. The β and γ subunits rejoin the complex, which now is available for further activation by the receptor. In this way, as long as receptors are occupied by the agonist, the Gs cycle produces increasingly more cyclic AMP, thereby amplifying the stimulatory signal. The Gi protein complex undergoes a similar cycle when adenosine, acetylcholine, or somatostatin receptors are stimulated, but activating Gi protein reduces cyclic AMP formation and decreases contractility.

Another signal-transducing system in the human heart is the phospholipase C-diacylglycerol-inositol triphosphate pathway, activated by α_1-adrenergic and M_2-muscarinic receptors.[18,19,186] Occupation of the receptors activates phospholipase C, which cleaves phosphatidylinositol triphosphate in the cell membrane to produce diacylglycerol and inositol triphosphate. The former activates protein C kinase in the membrane, which may hinder the effects of cyclic AMP. The latter facilitates calcium release from the sarcoplasmic reticulum. This pathway is important in smooth muscle contraction but is of less importance in heart muscle.

In heart failure, the number of β_1-adrenergic and VIP receptors are down-regulated, and β_2-adrenergic receptors are uncoupled from G proteins.[34–37,129] These changes make the myocardium less responsive to circulating or locally released catecholamines or VIP and play a role in the reduced contractility observed in heart failure. Treating heart failure with β-adrenergic blocking agents not only has reversed the receptor hanges but has been associated with improved function of muscle strips and of patients.[38,89,156,189]

Coupling of β-adrenoceptors to adenylate cyclase is incomplete at birth. Milrinone, an agent that stimulates contractility by inhibiting phosphodiesterases and bypasses the adenylate cyclase system, is ineffective in the newborn.[8] Nevertheless, because contractile mechanisms are almost fully developed at birth, the major mechanisms controlling contractility (except for changes in the source of calcium) are in place at birth.

Integrated Muscle Function

Relationship Between Muscle Strips and Intact Ventricles. Preload stretching a muscle strip is equivalent to end-diastolic fiber length of the intact ventricle. This length can be measured by various devices in animals, but in the intact human ventricle it is best related to end-diastolic diameter or volume. Frequently, end-diastolic pressure has been used interchangeably with end-diastolic volume as an index of preload, but this usage can be misleading if the distensibility of the ventricle changes or if pressure outside the heart (pericardial or intrathoracic) rises.[111,112,262,264]

Afterload is more complicated in the intact ventricle. Commonly, aortic systolic pressure is equated with afterload. However, in the muscle strip, afterload represents the force exerted by the muscle during contraction, and pressure and force are not the same.[210,211,242] It is preferable to calculate circumferential wall stress, which at the midwall is a function of ventricular pressure, diameter, and wall thickness. Both peak systolic and end-systolic wall stress can be used to assess ventricular function.

Calculations of wall stress are based on the Laplace relationship:

$$\text{Wall stress} = \text{Pr}/2\text{h},$$

where P = pressure, r = radius of curvature, and h = wall thickness. Because the left ventricle is not a regular sphere, particularly in systole, the Laplace formula is an oversimplification.[171] A fairly simple and accurate formula was developed by Grossman and colleagues:[122]

$$\text{Wall stress} = 1.35\text{PD}/[4\text{h}(1\text{h}/\text{D})],$$

where P = pressure, D = left ventricular minor axis dimension, and h = wall thickness at the level of the minor axis. This equation can be written as:

$$\frac{Pr}{2h}\left(\frac{1.35}{1+\dfrac{h}{r}}\right)$$

that is, as the Laplace equation modified by the expression in parentheses. Note that if the left ventricle dilates acutely, wall stress rises markedly because r gets bigger and h gets smaller.

The major findings from studies of muscle strips have been confirmed in intact ventricles. Increasing preload increases the pressure generated by an isolated ventricle that is not allowed to eject, as observed in the last century by Otto Frank. If the ventricle is allowed to eject, then increased preload allows the heart to eject the same stroke volume against an increased afterload or else to eject a greater stroke volume against a constant afterload. This is the Starling component of the Frank-Starling law.[114,215] The mechanism of this response is twofold: (1) lengthening the sarcomere narrows it and places the myosin and actin fibrils closer together for stronger interaction, and (2) increased calcium sensitivity is mediated in some way by titin stretching.[160] If an inotropic drug is given, then contractility increases and from a given fiber length greater force of contraction is achieved, which is a phenomenon seen every day in the intensive care unit.

The force-frequency relationship can be determined in intact hearts[4,195] by examining the response of the maximal rate of change of pressure (dP/dt max) in the ventricles after premature beats. The results in intact ventricles and muscle strips are similar. Subsequently, Seed and colleagues[217] applied this technique to humans with normal or abnormal left ventricular function and found an optimal R-R interval of 800 ms. They also examined dP/dt max for two beats given at optimum intervals after the premature stimulus. As expected, the first normal beat after the premature beat was potentiated because the extra calcium introduced into the cytosol by the premature beat was available to potentiate the first beat after the premature stimulus. The second postpremature beat also was potentiated but less so. They used the ratio of the potentiation of these two beats to calculate the fraction of calcium recirculating from one beat to the next. This amount was constant in any one patient but was much less in those with left ventricular dysfunction.

Pressure-Volume Loops. If left ventricular pressure and volume are measured simultaneously, the resulting pressure volume loop gives information about ventricular function and can be used to assess myocardial contractility in the intact heart.

The modern approach to analyzing these loops is based on the elastance concept of Suga and Sagawa.[213,214,215] *Elastance* is the ratio of pressure change to volume change. Consider an isolated ventricle containing a balloon that can be inflated to different volumes. At each volume the ventricle is stimulated to contract and generates a peak systolic pressure (Figure 17–4, *A*). As volumes increase, so do the peak systolic pressures generated, and the relationship is linear (Frank's law). The line joining the peak pressures intercepts the volume axis at a positive value, termed V_0, that indicates the unstressed volume of the ventricle. The equation for this line is as follows:

$$P_{es} = E_{es}(V_{es} - V_0),$$

where P_{es} = end-systolic pressure, E_{es} = slope of the line, V_{es} = end-systolic volume, and V_0 = unstressed volume. If contractility increases (more calcium enters the cells), the ventricle can generate greater pressures at any given volume, thereby generating a steeper pressure-volume line (higher value of E_{es}; dashed line I in Figure 17–4, *A*). If contractility decreases, the ventricle generates lower pressures at any given volume, and the pressure-volume line is less steep (lower value of E_{es}; dotted line D in Figure 17–4, *A*). Es is also termed E_{max}.

If the ventricle is allowed to eject, the typical pressure-volume loop shown in Figure 17–4, *B* is seen.

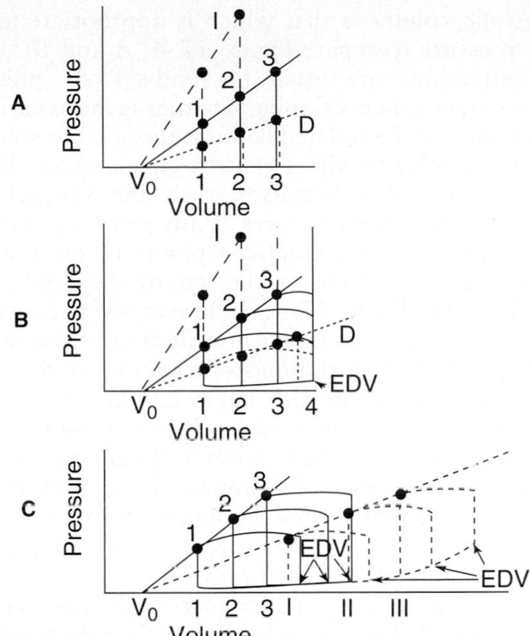

FIGURE 17–4 • Diagrams illustrating the concept of ventricular elastance. **A,** Isolated ventricle contracting at volumes 1, 2, and 3, generating corresponding pressures. *Dashed line I* indicates results at increased contractility. *Dotted line D* indicates results at decreased contractility. V_0, resting (unstressed) volume. **B,** Ventricular pressure-volume loops achieving end-systolic pressures of 1, 2, and 3 at corresponding volumes. *Dashed line I* indicates results at increased contractility, with greater end-systolic pressures at each volume. *Dotted line D* indicates results at decreased contractility. From a given end-diastolic volume, either the same ejection fraction is delivered at a lower end-systolic pressure *(dotted line 1)* or the same end-systolic pressure is achieved but at a much smaller stroke volume and ejection fraction *(line 4)*. **C,** When the ventricular end-diastolic volumes *(EDV)* increase as afterload increases, as is normal, then stroke volume can be maintained, even though ejection fraction decreases. If contractility is decreased *(dotted line)*, then stroke volume can be maintained only with increasing end-diastolic pressures. *1, 2, 3,* End-systolic volumes and pressures at normal contractility. *I, II, III,* End-systolic volumes at decreased contractility.

During diastolic filling, volume increases and diastolic pressure rises slightly because of the increase in passive tension. At the end of diastole, isovolumic systole occurs, and ventricular pressure rises with no change in volume. When ventricular pressure exceeds aortic diastolic pressure, the aortic valve opens, blood is ejected, and ventricular volume decreases. Ejection ends, and pressure falls to diastolic levels as isovolumic relaxation occurs. The pressure and volume reached at the end of systole are those that would have been attained by the isolated ventricle at that same end-systolic volume. In other words, at a given volume, no higher pressure can be generated (loop 1, see Figure 17–4, *B*). The decrease in volume during ejection is the stroke volume which, divided by the end-diastolic volume, gives the ejection fraction; normally, ejection fraction is greater than 65%.

If afterload is suddenly increased by raising aortic pressure, the normal heart responds as shown in Figure 17–4, *B*. In the first beat after the increase, the ventricle has to generate a higher pressure before the valve opens (loop 2). It then ejects but cannot eject a normal stroke volume because that would require higher pressure from the same end-diastolic length (preload). In fact, the end-systolic volume is that which is appropriate for the higher pressure (compare Figure 17–4, *A* and *B*). If different afterloads are used, the end-systolic pressure-volume points define a sloping line that is the same as the line obtained in the isolated heart at those same volumes; this is the line of maximal ventricular elastance. If ventricular contractility increases, then the ventricle can attain higher ejection pressures at any given volume, and the end-systolic pressure-volume points lie on a steeper line that lies above and to the left of the normal line (dashed line I in Figure 17–4, *B*). If ventricular contractility decreases, then the ventricle cannot generate normal pressures at any given end-diastolic volume, and the end-systolic pressure-volume line lies below and to the right of the normal line (dotted line in Figure 17–4, *B*). Note from Figure 17–4, *B* that, from a given end-diastolic volume, the ventricle with impaired contractility can either eject a normal stroke volume at much reduced pressures or eject at a normal pressure only by reducing its stroke volume drastically (loop 4).

In beats that follow a sudden increase in afterload, the ventricles adjust. Because of the reduced stroke volume in the first beat, the end-systolic volume is larger than normal. During diastole, however, a normal stroke volume enters the ventricle so that end-diastolic volume increases (loop 2 in Figure 17–4, C). In normal ventricles, the increased end-diastolic fiber length causes little increase in diastolic pressure. The pressures during ejection and the end-systolic pressure-volume point are unchanged, but stroke volume and ejection fraction increase. After a few more cycles, a new equilibrium is established (loop 3) in which the ventricle ejects a normal stroke volume at the higher afterload. The ejection fraction, however, is subnormal because although the stroke volume is normal, the end-diastolic volume is increased. The ventricle has adapted to the higher afterload by increasing end-diastolic fiber length, a phenomenon described by Starling and discussed by Ross[210,211] under the term *preload reserve.* If the ventricle has decreased contractility (dashed loops), the same pattern of response occurs, but with some important differences. With decreased contractility, the ventricle cannot eject a normal stroke volume from a normal end-diastolic volume. Compensation results in a larger than normal increase in end-diastolic volume even at normal afterloads. Any increase in afterload causes a further increase in end-diastolic volume, and this increase causes diastolic pressures to rise to high values that cause pulmonary congestion. The normal preload reserve has been used up in the attempt to eject a reasonable stroke volume against a modestly increased afterload. In more depressed hearts, even normal afterloads cannot be handled by the ventricle without getting a pathologically raised diastolic pressure in the ventricles or else a drastic decrease in stroke volume. Note that in these hearts, because of the relatively flat slope of the maximal ventricular elastance line, a slight reduction of afterload produces a relatively large increase in stroke volume and a relatively large decrease in ventricular end-diastolic volume and pressure. This is one of the mechanisms for cardiac improvement with afterload reduction.

Assessing Myocardial Contractility. An index of contractility must reflect the ability of the ventricle to perform work independent of changes in preload and afterload. Contractility can perhaps best be defined as the alterations in cardiac function that occur secondary to changes in cytosolic calcium availability or sarcomere sensitivity to calcium. Thus β-adrenergic agonists or phosphodiesterase inhibitors, which increase cytosolic calcium, and thyroxine, which alters myosin ATPase sensitivity to calcium in some species by altering the dominant isoform, are positive inotropic agents. However, quantifying contractility in the intact heart or assessing the contractile effects of an intervention is difficult[192] because all indices of contractility are indices of overall performance and are not independent of the other determinants of performance. For example, cardiac output is an excellent index of the systolic performance of the intact ventricle, but it is not a useful index of contractility because of its high sensitivity to preload, afterload, and heart rate.

It is convenient to divide methods of assessing contractility into those based on early events in the cardiac cycle (isovolumic phase indices) and those that occur later (ejection phase indices).

Isovolumic phase indices. The concept of maximal velocity of contraction against zero load (V_{max}) once was popular, but the complexity of the mechanics of cardiac muscle made it difficult to assess what would have been the true index, namely, V_{max} of the contractile element alone.[91] In practice, too, it is not possible to abolish internal loading of the muscle fiber. Applying this concept to the intact heart was even more difficult.[268]

As a substitute for V_{max}, investigators used dP/dt max (maximal rate of change of ventricular pressure) or dP/dt at a developed ventricular pressure of 40 mmHg. These values usually are achieved before the aortic valve opens and are relatively unaffected by changes in preload. The index is, however, affected markedly by changes in afterload and so must be used with care when afterloads are very different. This method is more useful for measuring acute changes in contractility than for assessing absolute contractility.

Ejection phase indices. The index of contractility most commonly used today is the maximal (end-systolic) ventricular elastance of Suga and Sagawa, which is independent of changes in preload (see previous text). Several different afterloads must be obtained, and either ventricular volumes must be measured or echocardiographic dimensions must be used as substitutes for volumes. The most clear-cut results have been obtained when reflex changes in contractility are prevented, which may explain why the relationship is less well established in conscious than in anesthetized animals.[50,242] Several studies have shown that the maximal elastance line often is alinear and gives a negative intercept on the pressure axis, that is, a negative resting volume.[146,155] To deal with this simply, some investigators use the values of E_{max} in the mid range of pressures.[155]

Ejection fraction and velocity of shortening also provide information about ventricular function. Because these two variables depend on afterload (see Figure 17–4), it is necessary to adjust for changes in afterload. This adjustment has been made in adults and children[26,27,65–67,94] by providing normal data for the relationship between end-systolic wall stress and either velocity of shortening or ejection fraction (Figure 17–5). However, the relationship is not linear,[10] so single-point determinations are of little use.

Ventricular Function Curves. Sarnoff and Mitchell[215] introduced the ventricular function curve. They measured left ventricular diastolic pressure and stroke work, then infused fluids and examined the relationship between the two variables (Figure 17–6, *A*). If contractility increased, the curve shifted up and to the left; at any end-diastolic pressure, a greater stroke work was achieved. If contractility decreased, the curve shifted down and to the right. One problem with this technique, recognized by Sarnoff, was that curvilinearity of the diastolic length-pressure relationship produced an S-shaped curve when relating stroke work to end-diastolic pressure and that techniques for measuring fiber length or ventricular volume were inadequate. In addition, using pressure instead of fiber length or volume may lead to misinterpretations if pericardial or pleural pressures change substantially. Several groups of investigators adapted this function curve to examine the stroke volume to end-diastolic pressure relationship, but this is even less satisfactory because stroke volume is affected by the resulting increases of afterload.

More recently, the relationship of stroke work to end-diastolic fiber length or ventricular volume has been examined in conscious dogs with autonomic blockade.[114] This relationship, termed *preload recruitable stroke work,* was linear and independent of changes in afterload (see Figure 17–6, *B*). The line intercepted the length or volume axis at values close to the unstressed length or volume, that is, at the length or volume that the ventricle has at zero transmural pressure. Calcium infusion increased the slope of the line without changing the intercept on the length axis. Subsequently, the same group extended this analysis to ischemic ventricles.[113] Depression of ventricular function shifted the stroke work to end-diastolic segment length relationship to the right (increased intercept) and decreased the slope. This concept and the ventricular elastance concept have much in common. Both require measurements of wall force, stroke work, ventricular

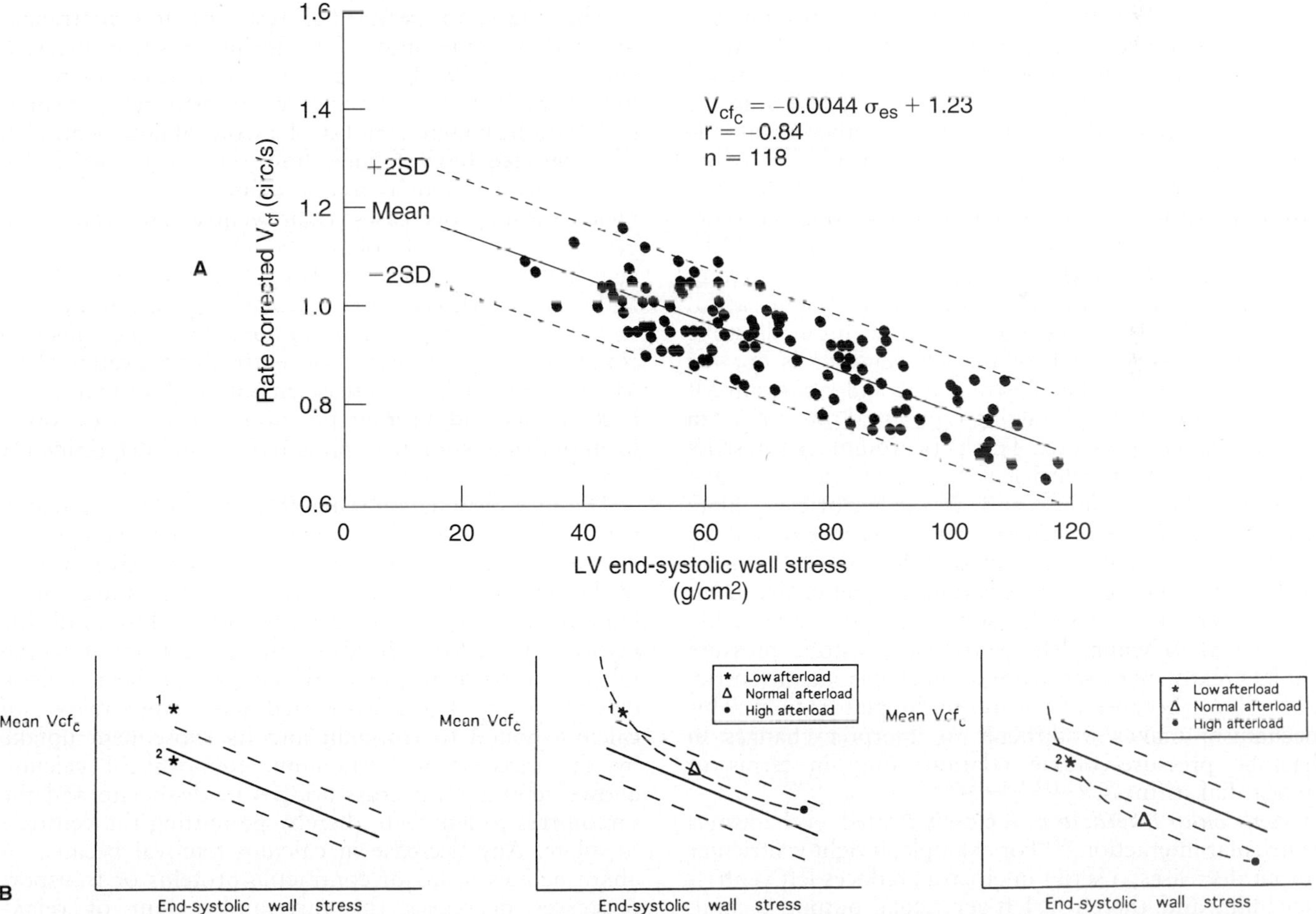

FIGURE 17–5 • **A,** Relationship between rate-corrected mean velocity of fiber shortening *(Vcf)* and left ventricular *(LV)* end-systolic wall stress. (From Colan SD, Borow KM, Neumann A: *J Am Coll Cardiol* 4:715, 1984.) **B,** Possibility of misinterpreting the relationship between mean velocity of fiber shortening and end-systolic wall stress. **Left,** Data point 1 is more than 2 standard deviations *(SD)* above normal relation (taken from left panel), suggesting increased contractility. Data point 2 is within the normal range, suggesting normal contractility. **Middle,** Alternative explanation for point 1 is that contractile state is normal, but points obtained at very low afterloads follow a hyperbolic, not a linear, relationship. **Right,** Alternative explanation for point 2 is that contractility is decreased, but because of the hyperbolic relationship and the low afterload it appears within the "normal" linear range. (From Banerjee A, et al: *J Am Coll Cardiol* 23:514, 1994.)

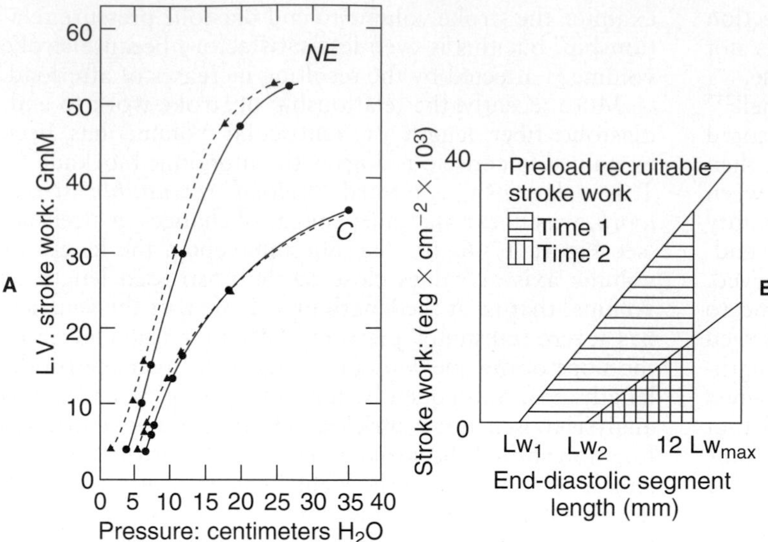

FIGURE 17–6 • Ventricular function curves. **A,** Typical function curve relating left ventricular diastolic pressure to left ventricular (external) stroke work. *C,* Control state; *NE,* increased contractility resulting from norepinephrine infusion. *Solid* and *dashed lines* indicate repeatability of the measurement. (Redrawn from Sarnoff SJ, Mitchell JH: The control of the function of the heart. In Hamilton WF, Dow P, editors: *Handbook of physiology, section 2: circulation,* vol 1. Washington, DC, 1962, American Physiological Society.) **B,** Preload recruitable stroke work area, in which the area under the curve relating end-diastolic segment length to stroke work is indicated for two different contractile states of the ventricle. Lw_1, Lw_2, Intercepts on the x axis; Lw_{max}, maximal value of *Lw* for the whole experiment. For details, see reference. (Redrawn from Glower DD, et al: *Am J Physiol* 255:H85, 1988.)

volume, or minor axis diameter and changing them over a range so that the lines or areas defining these indexes can be obtained.

Pericardial Function. The parietal pericardium is a stiff membrane that surrounds the heart loosely, separated from it by a small amount of lubricating pericardial fluid. Intrapericardial pressure is negative, reflecting the negative intrapleural pressure. On the other hand, the pericardium exerts a surface pressure on the heart that would exist even if all fluid were removed. If the pericardium had holes in it, fluid would leak out and there would be no fluid pressure, but the heart still could be compressed. This surface pressure varies in different regions but in general is similar to right atrial pressure.[262,265] Therefore normally transmural diastolic pressure across the wall of the left ventricle is not the same as left ventricular diastolic ventricular pressure. It can be estimated by subtracting right atrial pressure from left ventricular pressure. The pericardium can restrict dilatation of the left ventricle if there is a tense pericardial effusion (tamponade)[227] and if the ventricles dilate acutely. Thus if the ventricles enlarge because of sudden volume load or sudden myocardial depression, the pericardium becomes tense and restrains further enlargement of the ventricles.[262,264] In some patients with acute myocardial ischemia, left ventricular diastolic pressure can be greatly increased without much change in ventricular volume because of tension in the pericardium. This mechanism makes it difficult to interpret changes in diastolic pressure-volume relations only in terms of myocardial stiffness.[111,112,224,228,265]

Ventricular Interaction. A closely related mechanism is ventricular interaction.[224] For example, if right ventricular output decreases, a series interaction reduces left ventricular filling and, therefore, left ventricular output. Second, a direct interaction occurs because the left and right ventricles share the ventricular septum and are contained within the same relatively rigid pericardium. Consequently, right ventricular distension, as in acute pulmonary embolism or congestive heart failure, pushes the septum to the left, thereby decreasing left ventricular volume and preload. The resulting decrease in cardiac output should not be taken to indicate left ventricular dysfunction.[15,16,262]

The effects of pericardial restraint and ventricular interaction come into play during positive pressure ventilation.[263] With a normal circulation, increased intrathoracic pressure decreases transmural pressures, end-diastolic volumes, and stroke work of both ventricles. In congestive heart failure, however, where pericardial restraint regulates total cardiac volume, increased intrathoracic pressure decreases right ventricular transmural pressure, filling, and volume, resulting in increased left ventricular transmural pressure, end-diastolic volume, and stroke work via the Frank-Starling relationship.

Diastolic Ventricular Function. Diastolic function concerns the rate and extent of ventricular relaxation.[103,112] Many forms of heart disease manifest abnormalities of both systolic and diastolic function, but one or the other form of dysfunction may predominate and determine the type of therapy needed.

Diastolic dysfunction is manifested mainly by increased ventricular diastolic pressure at normal ventricular volume.[103] This can result from increased passive stiffness of the ventricles because of chronic infiltrates (e.g., amyloid), myocardial scars, constrictive pericarditis, or diffuse myocardial fibrosis. It also can result from impaired relaxation. Normally, relaxation of ventricular muscle in diastole is rapid and associated with rapid release of calcium bound to troponin and its subsequent uptake by the sarcoplasmic reticulum. Removal of calcium allows actin-myosin cross-bridges to dissociate and the sarcomeres to lengthen, thereby permitting the ventricle to dilate. Any decrease in calcium removal because of abnormalities in major contractile proteins or transport processes decreases the rate and extent of relaxation.[20,165,229] Ischemia is one major factor that impairs calcium metabolism and diastolic ventricular function, but many other forms of heart disease have similar effects.[90,93,161,195] Clinically, diastolic function is assessed by relating end-diastolic pressure and volume, by observing the rate of ventricular filling by angiography or by

Doppler studies of the mitral valve inflow, by measuring the peak rate of fall of ventricular pressure (–dP/dt max), or by calculating the time constant of the fall in ventricular pressure.

Neural Control of the Heart. The heart can function without any cardiac nerves, for example, after cardiac transplantation. However, the response to exercise in these denervated hearts is slow and due to increases in circulating catecholamines and the rise in body temperature. In intact animals and humans, β-adrenoceptor blockade blunts the heart rate increase with exercise and abolishes the inotropic response, as judged by the increase in dP/dt max.[274]

Studies of the neural control of the heart must consider the basal level of sympathetic and parasympathetic tone.[274] In conscious animals, resting sympathetic tone is low, and resting parasympathetic tone is high. Therefore sympathetic blockade has little effect on heart rate and myocardial contractility, but parasympathetic blockade causes marked tachycardia. On the other hand, many anesthetics depress the sympathetic nervous system, leading to impaired contractility and bradycardia. Postoperatively patients often have high circulating catecholamine concentrations, and the effects on myocardial function depend on the balance of catecholamine concentrations, stimulation of the sympathetic nervous system by pain, and the extent of myocardial depression caused by the drugs used for sedation.

The carotid and aortic baroreceptors respond to changes in arterial blood pressure. If basal sympathetic tone is low, as is normal, then inhibiting sympathetic tone by raising aortic pressure has little effect on myocardial contractility. On the other hand, lowering arterial pressure causes a reflex increase in sympathetic tone, with increases in heart rate and contractility. Baroreceptor sensitivity increases throughout gestation in fetal lambs[221] but may decrease after birth.[23] Also in fetal lambs, denervating the baroreceptors did not alter mean arterial blood pressure or heart rate but increased the variability of pressure and heart rate. Similar increased variability of pressures but not of heart rate occurred in adult sheep.[141] Denervation in the fetuses in the same study also decreased peripheral resistance.

Carotid and aortic chemoreceptors are stimulated by low PO_2, high PCO_2, and low pH, but the changes have to be marked, and even then the increase in myocardial contractility is modest. The fetus seems to be less sensitive than the adult to chemoreceptor stimulation.[1] The bradycardia that accompanies severe hypoxemia results from vagal stimulation.

During exercise and hemorrhage, plasma catecholamines increase markedly, but the inotropic responses are different. With exercise, dP/dt max increases by as much as fourfold, the peripheral vascular bed is dilated, and cardiac output increases, whereas with hemorrhage, dP/dt max increases by only 30% to 50%, cardiac output falls, and most vascular beds vasoconstrict. Thus the pattern of sympathetic neural stimulation rather than the circulating catecholamine concentrations determines how the heart responds to these stimuli.

Vagal effects on the heart are shown most prominently by changes in heart rate, but their effects on myocardial contractility depend on the existing level of sympathetic tone. Vagal stimulation has little effect on myocardial contractility given little sympathetic tone but markedly reduces the inotropic effects of increases in circulating catecholamines or sympathetic nerve stimulation. Conversely, blockade of muscarinic receptors can intensify the myocardial contractile response to sympathetic stimulation.

Cardiac Output. Cardiac output in the fetus is determined mainly by heart rate because of a limited capacity to increase stroke volume. This limitation results partly from decreased diastolic distensibility and partly from positive extracardiac pressures.[118] Consequently, fetal bradycardia is detrimental to blood flow and oxygen delivery. The fetal heart, however, can respond to increased preload (Starling's law) with increased stroke volume, provided there is no concomitant increase in afterload.[127] Usually, infusion of fluid into an animal causes arterial pressure to rise, and the increased afterload tends to inhibit the increase in stroke volume that would otherwise occur.[109,110,127] Immediately after birth, there is a large increase in total body oxygen consumption and cardiac output to about twice its later values (per unit body size).[162] This increase has been related to an increase in adrenergic receptors stimulated by fetal thyroid hormones.[32] In addition, because at birth approximately 80% of the infant's hemoglobin is in the form of fetal hemoglobin, the reduced ability of this hemoglobin to unload oxygen at the tissue level compels the infant to have a higher cardiac output than the infant will have 4 to 6 weeks later.[162] Therefore the neonate has limited cardiac output reserve and the heart has near-maximal contractility.[153,252] These features make the neonate unusually susceptible to diseases that impair cardiac function. The Frank-Starling mechanism, however, is intact at this time.[269] Evidence indicates β-adrenoceptor stimulation helps the neonatal ventricle adapt to volume loads.[61] Thus β-adrenoceptor blockade might be expected to be much more harmful in the neonate than in the older person with minimal sympathetic tone.

Myocardial Metabolism

Normal Myocardial Energy Metabolism

Basic Metabolic Processes. Basal metabolic processes can be studied by measuring oxygen uptake, production of heat, or utilization of high-energy phosphates. In isolated papillary muscle, most of the oxygen consumed is used in generating force (internal work), approximately 15% is used in shortening (external work), approximately 20% is used for basal metabolic processes (protein synthesis, sarcolemmal Na-K transport), and approximately 10% is used for the activity of Na/K-ATPase and Ca-ATPase.[52,79,108] Similar conclusions can be drawn from studies of whole hearts.[136]

The myocardium has a brisk rate of metabolism, consuming approximately 8 to 10 ml oxygen/100 g muscle/min under basal conditions. Potassium-induced cardioplegia can reduce myocardial oxygen consumption, but "resting" cardiac muscle still consumes more than five times as much oxygen as does resting skeletal muscle. During maximal exercise, the myocardium may consume as much as 60 to 80 ml oxygen/100 g muscle/min.[151]

Cardiac energy is generated by oxidizing substrates to carbon dioxide and water. During this process, energy is both used and stored, and most of the stored energy is in the form of ATP. When needed, ATP breaks down to adenosine diphosphate (ADP) or adenosine monophosphate (AMP) and releases energy for contractile or transport processes.[187] The substrates for energy production can be glucose, lactate, or fatty acids.[188] In a mixture, the fatty acids are preferred over the others, and an increase in plasma fatty acid concentrations, as in fasting or sympathetic stimulation, suppresses oxidation of carbohydrates by the heart.[33,188] Therefore lactate consumption or extraction cannot be used as an accurate guide to cardiac metabolism unless the concentration of the fatty acids is evaluated at the same time.[107]

ATP usually is generated by oxidative phosphorylation. Various transport systems move the substrates into the mitochondria for oxidation by the tricarboxylic cycle. Other transport systems move the ATP out of mitochondria into the cytosol, where they can break down and supply energy. The ATP is replenished by transfer of a high-energy phosphate moiety from creatine phosphate to ADP, mediated by the enzyme creatine kinase.[75,187] When oxygen supply is restricted, ATP can be generated by anaerobic glycolysis, an inefficient but useful temporary pathway. Furthermore, products of glycolysis, if they accumulate, inhibit key enzymes and interfere with further ATP production. Therefore the myocardium is unable to build an oxygen debt without further depressing energy production and, hence, contractility. Oxidative metabolism is so important to the heart that more than 30% of the mass of the myocardium is mitochondria.[52]

Fetal lamb ventricles have the same oxygen consumption per unit mass as the adult left ventricle. Because fetal oxygen content is lower than that in the adult, however, myocardial blood flow per unit mass is about twice as high in the fetus as in the adult.[86,87] Oxidative capacity is relatively lower, and glycogen stores and glycolytic flux are relatively higher in the fetal heart. This condition may explain why the immature heart is more resistant to hypoxemia than is the adult heart, provided an adequate supply of glucose is available for glycolysis. The main substrates used by the fetal heart are glucose, lactate, and pyruvate, although ketones, amino acids, and short- and medium-chain fatty acids also can provide energy.[56] After birth, long-chain fatty acids become the predominant substrates. For these reasons, prolonged severe hypoglycemia can seriously depress cardiac function in the neonate but is unlikely to do so in the older person.

L-Carnitine is essential for fatty acid transport across the mitochondrial membrane. Most of the body's carnitine is produced endogenously when protein degradation releases trimethyl-lysine, which is transformed into carnitine. Carnitine is present in red meats and dairy products (including breast milk), but only small amounts are present in vegetable products. It can be absorbed by the intestine, is not broken down in the body, and is excreted by the kidney.

In all except young infants, the preferential source of energy for myocardial function comes from the β-oxidation of long-chain fatty acids. After fatty acids enter the cell, they are activated to fatty acid (or acyl) coenzyme A (CoA) compounds by palmitoyl-CoA synthetase, then linked by carnitine palmitoyl transferase I to carnitine to form acylcarnitines, thus releasing CoA. The acylcarnitines cross the mitochondrial membrane, and at the inner surface of the membrane another enzyme, carnitine palmitoyl transferase II, transfers the fatty acids back to CoA. The fatty acids now can undergo β-oxidation with the production of ATP. These enzymes also help transport acylcarnitine esters of CoA out of the mitochondria. These esters are toxic in high concentrations. Fetuses and neonates have decreased activity of carnitine palmitoyl transferase and palmitoyl-CoA synthetase, so glucose, lactate, and short-chain fatty acids are the preferred myocardial energy substrates at this age.[5,200]

Endogenous carnitine production usually is sufficient for growth, but plasma (and tissue) carnitine concentrations may decrease after 1 month of parenteral nutrition without carnitine supplements. Energy demands increase when renal excretion of carnitine increases in conditions of burns, sepsis, starvation or after surgery; with excess excretion in Fanconi syndrome; with drugs such as valproic acid, pivampicillin, and pivmecillinam, which bind to carnitine and are excreted; with decreased production during chronic hemodialysis (see Chapter 76); and with cirrhosis of the liver.[73,77] Carnitine concentrations may be low in very premature infants.[199] Ischemia of heart or skeletal muscle depletes carnitine in the affected tissues, as does chronic congestive heart failure.[204,231] Most cases of severe carnitine deficiency in children, however, result from inherited defects in intermediary metabolism.[208]

Carnitine deficiency may produce acute or chronic syndromes, including a Reye syndrome–like encephalopathy, hypoglycemia, myopathy, cardiomyopathy, and failure to thrive. Once the diagnosis is established, treatment is with a diet high in carbohydrates and short-chain fatty acids, plus carnitine supplements by mouth (25–300 mg/kg/day) or even intravenously if needed. Patients with congestive heart failure who do not show overt evidence of carnitine deficiency may improve after taking carnitine supplements.[231]

Determinants of Myocardial Oxygen Consumption. In 1958, Sarnoff and Mitchell[215] reported that pressure work by the heart consumed more oxygen than did volume work and found a good correlation between the area under the left ventricular pressure curve in systole (termed the *tension time index)* and left ventricular oxygen consumption. Subsequently, others found that peak wall tension (or stress) was a better predictor of left ventricular oxygen consumption.[170,193,240,251] It is important to take account of wall thickness and ventricular dimensions in estimating myocardial oxygen consumption, which is why the tension time index, which ignores wall stress, is not a good predictor. Increases of contractility or heart rate also increase myocardial oxygen consumption, but because they decrease ventricular size and thus wall stress, increased oxygen consumption is not as great as would be expected from studies in muscle strips.[117]

Stroke volume is an added predictor of myocardial oxygen consumption.[209,222,277,280,281] The approaches used include examining the area within the pressure-flow loop. This approach has been extended by Suga and colleagues,[125,126,245–249] who concluded that the best predictor of left ventricular oxygen consumption was the area in the pressure-volume loop plus the area representing end-systolic pressure energy (Figure 17–7). By subtracting the contributions of basal myocardial metabolism, they were able to show that the oxygen consumption-pressure volume area (PVA) relationship was independent of contractile state. Further studies by these investigators showed that PVA-independent oxygen consumption was a function of contractility, defined by E_{max}. Certain interventions, for example, acidosis, made the slope of this relation between PVA-independent V_{O_2} to E_{max} steeper, that is, they decreased the efficiency of the system.

Because oxidizing fats uses up more oxygen than does oxidizing carbohydrates, theoretically more oxygen should be used per unit of work when burning fatty acids.[75] This situation has not always been found, but there are few good studies of this phenomenon.

Myocardial Oxygen Demand-Supply Relationship. One way of assessing myocardial oxygen demand is to note that it is roughly proportional to the ventricular systolic pressure generated and the duration of systole, that is, to the area under the real-time pressure curve of the ventricle in systole: the systolic pressure time index (SPTI).[135,137] SPTI is dramatically influenced by cardiac afterload; for instance, aortic stenosis raises SPTI (at constant stroke volume). The correlation between SPTI and myocardial oxygen demand is imperfect because it does not take into account wall stress, which involves radius and wall thickness, or contractility.[134]

Because left ventricular myocardial perfusion is restricted to diastole (see Chapter 18), myocardial oxygen supply is proportional to both duration of diastole and myocardial perfusion pressure in diastole. In general, diastolic myocardial perfusion pressure can be represented graphically as the difference between superimposed aortic and left ventricular pressure curves. The area between these curves, from the instant of aortic valve closure in diastole to reopening of the aortic valve in systole, has been termed the *diastolic pressure time index* (DPTI) and is proportional to subendocardial blood flow. When multiplied by arterial oxygen content, this index correlates with subendocardial oxygen supply.[31]

(DPTI × arterial oxygen content)/SPTI (Figure 17–8) is a fair indicator of myocardial oxygen balance. At critical levels, subendocardial ischemia occurs.[135,137] This ratio is worsened by tachycardia, which shortens diastole and the duration of myocardial perfusion; by elevation of end-diastolic pressures in the ventricles; or by elevation of coronary sinus pressure. It is adversely affected by low aortic diastolic pressure (as in shock, aortic valve insufficiency, or other large diastolic runoff lesions) and by elevated ventricular systolic pressure (as in aortic stenosis,

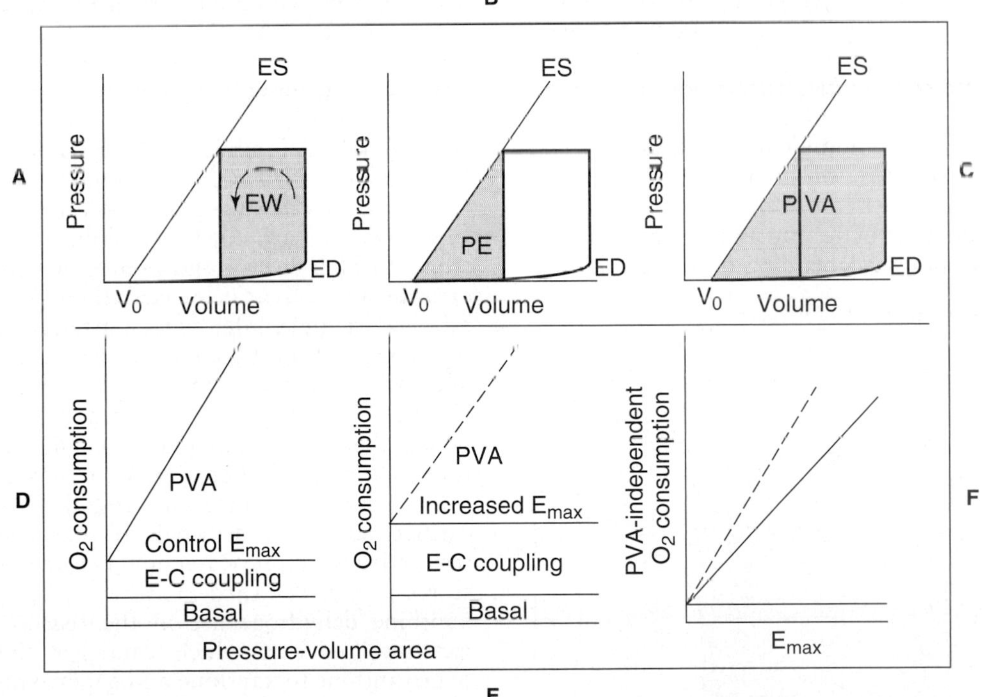

FIGURE 17–7 • Relationship of myocardial oxygen consumption to the pressure volume area (PVA). **A,** Ventricular pressure-volume loop with pressure plotted on the ordinate and volume on the abscissa. *Arrow* shows the direction of inscription of the loop. *ED,* End-diastolic pressure-volume line; *ES,* line of end-systolic pressure-volume points (end-systolic elastance); *EW,* area representing external mechanical work; V_0, unstressed ventricular volume. **B,** *Shaded area* to the left of the pressure-volume loop in the pressure-volume diagram represents potential energy (PE). **C,** Total area (PVA = EW + PE) between the end-systolic and end-diastolic lines is shown. This area is proportional to myocardial oxygen consumption. **D,** PVA is linearly proportional to oxygen consumption, but some oxygen consumption is independent of PVA. The PVA-independent oxygen consumption shown below the *upper horizontal line* results from excitation-contraction (E-C) coupling and basal oxygen consumption. **E,** When contractility is increased, as indicated by the increased value for E_{max}, the relationship between PVA and oxygen consumption is unchanged, but PVA-independent oxygen consumption increases. **F,** Relationship between E_{max} and PVA-independent oxygen consumption is linear. With myocardial depression, the slope of this relationship is steeper *(dashed line).* Thus for any value of E_{max}, PVA-independent oxygen consumption is increased so that myocardial efficiency is reduced. (Data from references 61, 62, 125–127.)

systemic hypertension, or pulmonary hypertension). The ratio is favorably affected by balloon aortic counterpulsation, which elevates aortic diastolic pressure and reduces systolic afterload. Given the imperfect nature of this ratio, too much emphasis should not be placed on any given value, but two points are clear: (1) a fall in the ratio in any patient moves them toward a supply:demand imbalance and (2) any ratio less than 0.45 that typifies normal subjects likely indicates myocardial ischemia.[12]

Effects of Myocardial Ischemia on Cardiac Function and Metabolism. Ischemia indicates a flow that is inadequate to supply the demand for oxygen by an organ or tissue; it also implies reduced clearance of metabolites.[128,203] The second part of the definition is what distinguishes ischemia from hypoxemia, in which there is a normal flow with a decreased oxygen delivery. Because the heart cannot sustain an oxygen debt, inadequate oxygen supply rapidly decreases the energy supply to the muscle cells, which cease to contract normally. If a branch of the left coronary artery is severely narrowed or occluded acutely, within 5 to 15 seconds the myocardium supplied by that branch stops contracting, turns blue, and bulges and thins during each systole. If the acute ischemia is global, that is, all coronary arteries have similar reductions in oxygen supply, then the subendocardial muscle becomes ischemic first because this muscle has the lowest coronary flow reserve. Subendocardial function is selectively decreased.[46,104,273] Global cardiac contractility decreases. Cardiac pump function is impaired, but survival is possible. More extensive global ischemia leads to death. Chronic imbalance of oxygen supply and demand leads to death of the affected muscle cells, producing either a localized infarct or diffuse, perhaps patchy, subendocardial fibrosis as occurs commonly with severe aortic stenosis, cyanotic heart disease, or dilated cardiomyopathy (see Chapter 18).

Temporary imbalance of supply and demand leads to two patterns of response, depending on the duration of the ischemia. If a branch coronary artery is occluded for 15 to 30 minutes and then the occlusion is removed, flow returns to normal rapidly, but the muscle may not contract normally for many hours. Some biochemical changes that occurred take many hours to reverse. This phenomenon is known as *reperfusion injury* or *stunning*.[69,150,152,163] It should be distinguished from the "no reflow" phenomenon in which, after a longer occlusion, release of the occlusion is followed by incomplete restoration of flow because of myocardial edema, cell swelling, plugging by neutrophils, and endothelial damage. Stunning may occur after prolonged cardiopulmonary bypass surgery and may account for some of the cardiac depression that often is observed in the early recovery period.[147,253]

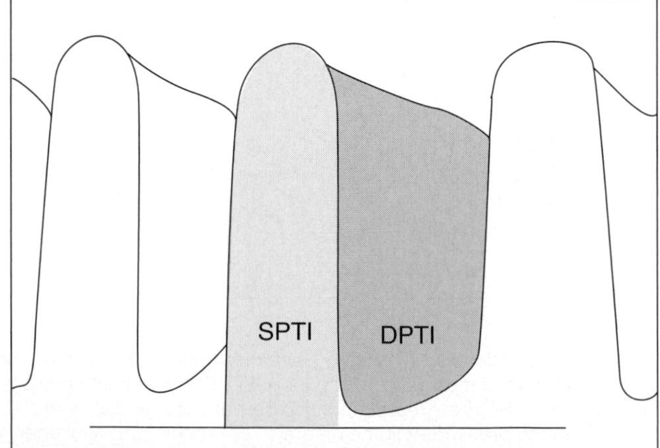

FIGURE 17–8 • Systolic pressure time index (SPTI) reflects myocardial work and oxygen demand. Diastolic pressure time index (DPTI) reflects myocardial blood flow. (Redrawn from Fuhrman BP: Regional circulation. In Fuhrman BP, Shoemaker WC, editors: *Critical care: state of the art,* vol 10. Fullerton, CA, 1989, Society of Critical Care Medicine.)

Chronic ischemia of moderate severity causes myocardial hibernation, an adaptive response that leads to metabolic down-regulation and reduction of flow without extensive cell death.[47,132,133,166] Regional function is reduced, but restoration of flow leads to functional recovery. This phenomenon is best known from studies of coronary artery disease but can be present in some children with normal coronary arteries and subendocardial ischemia.

Many biochemical changes occur when the heart becomes ischemic, and which are the primary causes of the dysfunction is not always clear. As soon as oxygen supply is cut off, all components of the mitochondrial electron chain become reduced because of the absence of the final electron acceptor. Nicotinamide adenine dinucleotide (NAD) is reduced to NADH within 2 seconds after the onset of sudden ischemia.[11] Glycogenolysis increases rapidly, thereby helping to supply ATP, but then is progressively inhibited by increasing concentrations of hydrogen ion, NADH, and lactate. (This inhibition is less marked with pure hypoxemia because the associated high flows help to wash out these inhibitory metabolites.) The stores of high-energy phosphates become depleted. First creatine phosphate decreases, then ATP concentrations fall. For example, after sudden arterial occlusion, creatine phosphate is almost completely depleted within 3 minutes, and ATP is reduced to 35% of control concentration within 15 minutes. ATP is degraded to ADP and AMP, which then is deaminated to adenosine. Adenosine in turn is rapidly broken down to inosine and hypoxanthine. Because of these changes, the nucleotide pool of cardiac muscle is depleted so that even after flow is restored, a long time is required before normal high-energy stores are replenished. Furthermore, during ischemia, xanthine dehydrogenase in the tissues is converted to xanthine oxidase, which catalyzes the conversion of hypoxanthine to xanthine and superoxide radicals. These in turn can be converted by superoxide dismutase into hydrogen peroxide, which can be converted by catalase to produce highly reactive hydroxyl radicals. These free radicals can react with lipids in the cell membranes and cause lipid peroxidation, which produces several toxic and arrhythmogenic substances and impairs the functions of the cell membrane.[154] Oxygen-derived free radicals can be introduced by activation of neutrophils by the damaged endothelium and by the formation of peroxynitriles from nitric oxide.

Accompanying these changes are accumulation of hydrogen ions, lactate, and many other catabolites. These entities create an osmotic load within the cells with resultant swelling of the cells and the mitochondria. The cell and mitochondrial membranes become impaired, and myoglobin and enzymes such as creatine kinase leak out of the cell, as do essential ions such as magnesium and potassium. Free calcium may accumulate in the cytosol (because of loss of chelating agents) and the mitochondria, particularly during reperfusion, and this calcium load may be highly detrimental to cell function. Finally, ischemia is associated with decreased myocardial carnitine concentrations, defective transport of long-chain fatty acids into the mitochondria, and accumulation of toxic acylcarnitine esters of CoA. These changes further delay the recovery of energy production and muscle contraction.

Systemic Vasculature

General anatomy. The large arteries are elastic. Their media contain concentric lamellae of perforated elastic tubes cross-linked by transverse collagen (type III) and smooth muscle.[25,286] When smooth muscle contracts, the wall becomes stiffer. Smaller arteries have fewer lamellae. The media is bounded by the external and internal elastic laminae, beyond which are the adventitia with nerves and vasa vasorum and the intima with sparse fibrous tissue and a metabolically active endothelium, respectively. Arterioles have no lamellae and only a thin media with circular or spiral smooth muscle; the only elastic tissue is in the inner and outer elastic laminae. Capillaries are thin walled and nonmuscular, ideal for transport of materials into and from the tissues; however, they contain pericytes that have myosin, actin, and tropomyosin and so might have some contractile function. Veins have medial muscle but thinner walls relative to lumen diameter than do arteries. Their endothelium may have different properties. The numerous extracellular matrix components are reviewed by Buga and Ignarro.[40] The developmental aspects of blood vessels are reviewed by Stenmark and Weisen.[238]

Physiologic Mechanisms

General features. Although large arteries are regarded as conduits and capillaries as vessels allowing transport of substances to and from the tissues, many substances can move across arterial walls. Oxygen and carbon dioxide can diffuse across arteriolar walls, and lipoproteins can penetrate the walls of large arteries. Whether atheromatous deposits form in arteries depends on the balance of the amount of lipoprotein that enters and leaves the arterial wall. This balance depends on the concentration and chemical nature of lipoproteins and the action of components of the wall, such as glycosaminoglycans, in binding altered lipoprotein molecules and preventing their transit through the wall.

Arteriolar tone controls peripheral resistance and, with cardiac output, determines blood pressure and regional flow. Regions of the circulation may differ markedly in their patterns of vascular regulation. A stimulus that potently increases vascular resistance in one region of the circulation may have a different effect in another. For example, during hemorrhagic shock, flow is maintained to heart and brain but is reduced to muscle, kidneys, and gut. Venous and venular tone, together with diuretic and antidiuretic factors, determine blood volume and venous pressure.

The two active components of the systemic circulation are the medial smooth muscle and the endothelium. They both have receptors for innumerable agonists and antagonists that diffuse from autonomic nerve endings, circulate from remote regions, or are produced locally. The smooth muscle is responsible for vasoconstriction or vasodilatation. The endothelium, one of the metabolic powerhouses of the body, has several major functions:

1. Endothelial cells play important roles in the response to injury by causing leukocyte adhesion and extravasation, mediated by cell adhesion molecules such as selectins, cadherins, and integrins.[40,235]
2. They are intimately bound up with coagulation[7,40] by virtue of the production of procoagulant (e.g., platelet activating factor [PAF], von Willebrand factor, fibronectin, and factors V and X) and anticoagulant factors (e.g., heparan, dermatan sulfate, thrombomodulin, and ectonucleotidase) and by the production of nitric oxide and PGI_2, which inhibit platelet aggregation and degranulation.
3. They regulate capillary permeability by producing ET-1 (increase) or PGE_1 (decrease) and respond with increased plasma leakage to substances such as bradykinin, histamine, thrombin, oxygen radicals, and PAF.
4. They regulate smooth muscle contraction in response to shear stress, in keeping with an overriding principle that shear rate must be kept constant within narrow limits to prevent endothelial damage.[96,100] In general, most of the vascular resistance resides in microvessels smaller than 150 μm in diameter,[54,276] which are subject to the controls discussed here.

Any increase in local organ flow resulting from a decrease in resistance in these microvessels increases shear stress in the larger upstream arteries. This increase is sensed by endothelial integrins[223] that set off a cascade of responses that relax smooth muscle by activating Ca^{++}-sensitive K^+ channels and hyperpolarizing the endothelial cell membrane and by releasing acetylcholine, nitric oxide, PGI_2, ATP, and substance P.[40,223] A chronic increase in shear stress activates the nuclear factor-κB transcription complex and induces a number of early response genes.[40,223]

Control of vascular tone. In general, regional circulations regulate their flow so that they obtain required amounts of oxygen and nutrients. Any or all of the mechanisms discussed may be invoked. Vasomotor tone is strongly influenced by several mechanisms: (1) innervation and neural processes, (2) circulating endocrine and neuroendocrine mediators, (3) blood gas composition, (4) local metabolic products, (5) endothelial derived factors, and (6) myogenic processes.

1. Receptors responsive to neural products (norepinephrine, acetylcholine, neuropeptides) are found throughout the circulation. Nevertheless, innervation and receptor distributions are organ specific, which allows rapid, patterned, coordinated redistribution of blood flow and an orchestrated response to hypoxia, changes in posture, and hemorrhage. Although these

receptors respond to circulating agonists (including angiotensin II and adrenal epinephrine) and to those liberated locally, they are generally associated with innervation by autonomic nerves. In general, presynaptic α-adrenergic stimulation causes norepinephrine reuptake, whereas postsynaptic α-adrenergic stimulation causes norepinephrine release and vasoconstriction. β-Adrenergic stimulation generally causes vasodilatation. Cholinergic stimulation (whether sympathetic or parasympathetic) generally causes vasodilatation (see Chapters 29 and 103).

In all organs, sensory and efferent nerve endings contain nonadrenergic, noncholinergic (NANC) peptides, for example, neuropeptide Y, VIP, calcitonin gene-related peptide (CGRP), and substance P.[14,74,91,95,105,123,131,174,185,197,250,278,283] Neuropeptide Y is colocalized and released with norepinephrine[102] and VIP is colocalized with acetylcholine and released upon stimulation of vagal nerve endings. Most of these peptides except neuropeptide Y are vasodilatory, and they help modulate blood pressure and regional flows. Substance P and CGRP are released when sensory nerves are stimulated by capsaicin, thus accounting for the flushing that accompanies the eating of hot peppers. (Many neuropeptides also occur throughout the central nervous system, where they may play roles in cardiovascular regulation.)

2. Humoral regulators of vascular tone and blood volume include angiotensin, adrenomedullin, aldosterone, arginine vasopressin (AVP), bradykinin, histamine, serotonin, thyroxine, natriuretic peptides, and various reproductive hormones. Most of these regulators have both direct effects and secondary effects, which tend to be organ specific or regional. They tend to have altered concentrations in hypertension, congestive heart failure, or shock, and their antagonists are used in therapy. Some agents, such as histamine, serotonin, and thyroxine, probably affect peripheral resistance only in abnormal states and are not physiologic regulators.

Angiotensin plays a special role in the homeostasis of blood pressure. Its concentration increases in hemorrhagic or hypovolemic shock following increased renal production of renin that produces angiotensin I from angiotensinogen. Angiotensin I is converted to active angiotensin II by angiotensin-converting enzyme (ACE) in the endothelium, especially in the pulmonary vessels. However, angiotensin II also is produced locally in the heart and vessel walls by renin that enters from the blood and perhaps by other local proteases.[106,177] It causes generalized vasoconstriction in both systemic and pulmonary circulations, but locally it stimulates the release of vasodilating prostaglandins in lung and kidney. Angiotensin II via angiotensin I receptors plays a role in cardiac and smooth muscle cell hypertrophy. In excess it results in cardiac inflammation, fibrosis, and apoptosis.[42,76,266,267] Adrenomedullin, originally found in pheochromocytomas, is produced in many normal cell types, including endothelium. Among its many actions are long-lasting vasodilatation and diuresis.[82,157] It shares homologous sequences with CGRP, calcitonin, and amylin.[284] Its release may be stimulated by ET-1. It may play a role in treating heart failure.[198]

Aldosterone, known primarily for its effect on sodium excretion and potassium retention, has indirect central effects on blood pressure.[207,212,290] Its concentration increases when renin release is stimulated. In patients with congestive heart failure its decreased breakdown in the liver accounts for very high blood concentrations, which are harmful to the heart and blood vessels. Inhibition of aldosterone by spironolactone may have great clinical value.[212,230,282]

AVP, which is released from the axonal terminals of magnocellular neurons in the hypothalamus, causes vasoconstriction by stimulating VP1 receptors. However, at low concentrations AVP dilates coronary, cerebral, and pulmonary vessels. It is an antidiuretic hormone that acts on VP2 receptors in the renal collecting ducts.[138] Its concentration is low in septic shock,[146] with ventricular arrhythmias and after cardiac surgery[293] but is increased in myocardial and hemorrhagic shock, congestive heart failure, and cirrhosis of the liver.[115,138,275] Selective AVP antagonists promote free water excretion without concomitant electrolyte excretion[218,219,256,275] and are useful in treating fluid overload in patients with congestive heart failure, cirrhosis of the liver, and the syndrome of inappropriate antidiuretic hormone secretion without causing electrolyte imbalance.

Bradykinin is a potent pulmonary and systemic vasodilator released locally by the action of proteolytic enzymes on kallikrein after tissue injury.[45,80,81,145] Bradykinin is metabolized by kininase II, which is the same as ACE, so ACE inhibitors not only reduce angiotensin II production but increase bradykinin concentrations. Bradykinin also causes endothelial cell release of tissue-type plasminogen activator.[285]

Histamine, released by mast cells in response to injury, is a potent vasodilator in most regions of the circulation but causes vasoconstriction in the lung. It also increases endothelial permeability.[270] No evidence indicates histamine plays a part in normal vasoregulation.

The natriuretic peptides are released from the heart when it is distended in congestive heart failure. They cause vasodilatation and increased diuresis. A-natriopeptide (mainly from atria) and B-natriopeptide (from ventricles) are released from myocardial cells, and C-natriopeptide is released from cardiac endothelium.[41,78,124,149] A recombinant B-natriopeptide (nesiritide) is more effective than dobutamine in treating acute severe congestive heart failure.[41,78,124,149] These natriopeptides and the kinins are broken down by neutral endopeptidase. Inhibition of this breakdown combined with inhibition of ACE by vasopeptidase inhibitors (e.g., omapatrilat) greatly augments vasodilatation.[88,159,183]

Serotonin probably acts mainly in the central nervous system, but peripherally it can act on S1 receptors to produce vasodilatation and on S2 receptors to cause vasoconstriction. It also augments the action of other vasoconstrictors.[98,99]

3. Tissue levels of oxygen and carbon dioxide reflect adequacy of perfusion and oxygen delivery. These blood

gases are potent determinants of regional blood flow and have effects that differ among regions of the circulation. They also have a more general effect mediated by carotid chemoreceptors.

4. Local metabolic regulation of vasomotor tone provides an ideal homeostatic mechanism whereby metabolic demand can directly influence perfusion. For instance, adenosine, which accumulates locally when tissue metabolism is high and tissue oxygenation is marginal, causes pronounced vasodilatation in the coronary, striated muscle, splanchnic, and cerebral circulations. Cerebral autoregulation has been suggested to take advantage of local metabolite production as an indicator of adequacy of blood flow. According to the argument, when perfusion pressure falls, cerebral blood flow might decline but for local accumulation of vasodilating metabolites. The perivascular concentration of these metabolites is restored to normal as flow rises, washing out the metabolites. Potassium is released from muscle in response to increased work, ischemia, and hypoxia.[85] Hypokalemia causes vasoconstriction.[28,29] Hyperkalemia, within the physiological range, causes vasodilatation by stimulating K_{Ir} channels.[180,181,237] Many of the agents discussed in section 2 (page 218) are produced locally and are effective as circulating hormones.

   At least four different types of potassium channels are present on arterial smooth muscle cells[237]: voltage-activated channels (K_v), calcium-activated channels (BK_{Ca}), inward rectifiers (K_{Ir}), and ATP-dependent channels (K_{ATP}). These channels are activated by vasodilators. As a result, the cells hyperpolarize, voltage-dependent calcium channels close, intracellular calcium concentrations decrease, and vasodilatation results.[30] Pharmacological vasodilators, such as cromakalim, pinacidil, and diazoxide, directly activate K_{ATP} channels, as do endogenous vasodilators such as CGRP, VIP, prostacyclin, and adenosine.[30] Inhibitors of K_{ATP} channels, such as glibenclamide, cause vasoconstriction.

5. The endothelial lining of blood vessels plays a prominent role in the regulation of vascular tone.[101] In addition to its roles in the elaboration of vasoactive eicosanoids[234] and in the metabolism of angiotensin, the endothelium secretes several other categories of vasoactive substances, including adrenomedullin (discussed previously), nitric oxide, endothelial cell hyperpolarizing factor, and endothelins.

   Endothelium-derived relaxing factor (EDRF) has been identified as nitric oxide.[140] Nitric oxide is a potent vasodilator released from endothelium after stimulation and accounts for some or all of the activity generally ascribed to other agonists. For instance, acetylcholine causes constriction of vessels stripped of their intima and causes dilatation only in the presence of the vascular endothelium.[101] Adenosine, prostacyclin, and epinephrine dilate vessels stripped of their endothelium. Bradykinin, substance P, thrombin, and potassium cause only endothelium-dependent relaxation. Nitric oxide also is released from endothelium when flow increases, an example of positive feedback. Nitric oxide increases smooth muscle soluble guanylate cyclase activity, raises muscle cyclic GMP, and thereby relaxes vascular smooth muscle (see Chapter 44). In addition to EDRF, an unidentified endothelial cell hyperpolarizing factor dilates vessels.[44]

   The vascular endothelium elaborates the *endothelins* (ET-1, ET-2, ET-3), a family of compounds that are vasoactive, structurally related peptides. ET-1 is the most potent vasoconstrictor known. It also promotes mitogenesis and stimulates the renin-angiotensin-aldosterone system and the release of vasopressin and atrial natriuretic peptide.[3,83,116,194,212] These peptides act on one of two receptor subtypes: ET(A) and ET(B). ET(A) is located mainly on vascular smooth muscle cells and is responsible for mediating vasoconstriction and cell proliferation. ET(B) is present predominantly on endothelial cells and mediates vasorelaxation, as well as ET-1 clearance. Endothelins cause local vasoconstriction or vasodilatation, depending on dose and location in the circulation.[173] Individual endothelins occur in low levels in the plasma, generally below their vasoactive thresholds. This finding suggests they are primarily effective at the local site of release. Even at these levels, however, they may potentiate the effects of other vasoconstrictors such as norepinephrine and serotonin.[288] Endothelin antagonists, such as bosentan, now are being used.[184,279]

6. Myogenic responses of vessels are changes in smooth muscle tone in response to stretch or increased transmural pressure. An increase in inflow pressure causes a rise in vessel wall tension and transmural pressure[143] that causes localized vasoconstriction. The reverse occurs when inflow pressure falls. The mechanisms of this response are complex. There probably is initial sensing by surface integrins,[72] followed by activation of cation channels with calcium entry.[272] In some way, protein kinase C, MAP kinases, and Rho kinase are also involved.[21,167,225]

As expected, a complex interplay exists among myogenic, flow-mediated, and metabolic regulation of vessel tone.[70] The relative importance of these mechanisms likely varies in different vascular beds.

Autoregulation. In all organs, when inflow pressure is suddenly raised or lowered while oxygen consumption remains constant, flow rises or falls transiently but then returns to the earlier value. The phenomenon is termed *autoregulation*. Myogenic tonic response is partly responsible for this phenomenon, but it is not the only mechanism. Some investigators believe tissues have oxygen sensors that respond to transient increases or decreases in oxygen supply.[2,39,51] Others believe the process is mediated by greater or lesser release of nitric oxide carried to the tissues by hemoglobin in the form of S-nitrosohemoglobin or by ATP release by the red blood cell.[45a,51,110a,141a,196a,236a] Carbon monoxide produced by the action of hemoxygenase in endothelium and smooth muscle may play a regulatory role.[63,142,176,291]

REFERENCES

1. Acker H: Chemoreceptor and baroreceptor control of perinatal oxygen supply in different organs. In Jones CT, editor: *Research in perinatal medicine,* vol 7, *Fetal and neonatal development.* Ithaca, NY, 1988, Perinatology Press.

2. Acker H: Cellular oxygen sensors. *Ann N Y Acad Sci* 718:3, 1994.
3. Agapitov AV, Haynes WG: Role of endothelin in cardiovascular disease. *J Renin Angiotensin Aldosterone Syst* 3:1, 2002.
4. Anderson PA, et al: Evaluation of the force-frequency relationship as a descriptor of the inotropic state of canine left ventricular myocardium. *Circ Res* 39:832, 1976.
5. Anderson PAW: Immature myocardium. In Moller JH, Neal WA, editors: *Fetal, neonatal, and infant cardiac disease.* Norwalk, CT, 1992, Appleton & Lange.
6. Anderson PAW: Developmental cardiac physiology and myocardial function. In Moller JH, Hoffman JIE, editors: *Pediatric cardiovascular medicine.* New York, 2000, Churchill Livingstone.
7. Andrews M, Massicotte P: Hemostasis. In Gluckman PD, Heymann MA, editors: *Pediatrics and perinatology. The scientific basis.* London, 1996, Edward Arnold.
8. Artman M, et al: Inotropic responses change during postnatal maturation in rabbit. *Am J Physiol Heart Circ Physiol* 255:H335, 1988.
9. Athanasuleas CL, et al: Optimizing ventricular shape in anterior restoration. *Semin Thorac Cardiovasc Surg* 13:459, 2001.
10. Banerjee A, et al: Nonlinearity of the left ventricular end-systolic wall stress-velocity of fiber shortening relation in young pigs: a potential pitfall in its use as a single-beat index of contractility. *J Am Coll Cardiol* 23:514, 1994.
11. Barlow CH, et al: Evaluation of cardiac ischemia by NADH fluorescence photography. *Ann Surg* 186:737, 1977.
12. Barnard W, et al: Ischemic response to sudden strenuous exercise in healthy men. *Circulation* 48:936, 1973.
13. Barth AI, et al: Cadherins, catenins and APC protein: interplay between cytoskeletal complexes and signaling pathways. *Curr Opin Cell Biol* 9:683, 1997.
14. Beaulieu P, Lambert C: Peptidic regulation of heart rate and interactions with the autonomic nervous system. *Cardiovasc Res* 37:578, 1998.
15. Belenkie I, et al: The importance of pericardial constraint in experimental pulmonary embolism and volume loading. *Am Heart J* 123:733, 1992.
16. Belenkie I, et al: Ventricular interaction: from bench to bedside. *Ann Med* 33:236, 2001.
17. Ben-Ze'ev A, Geiger B: Differential molecular interactions of beta-catenin and plakoglobin in adhesion, signaling and cancer. *Curr Opin Cell Biol* 10:629, 1998.
18. Berridge MJ: Inositol trisphosphate and diacylglycerol: two interacting second messengers. *Annu Rev Biochem* 56:159, 1987.
19. Berridge MJ: The 1996 Massry Prize. Inositol trisphosphate and calcium: two interacting second messengers. *Am J Nephrol* 17:1, 1997.
20. Bers DM: Cardiac excitation-contraction coupling. *Nature* 415:198, 2002.
21. Bevan JAM: Pressure and flow-dependent vascular tone. *FASEB J* 5:2267, 1991.
22. Birk E: Myocardial receptors. In Gluckman PD, Heymann MA. editors: *Pediatrics and perinatology. The scientific basis.* London, 1996, Edward Arnold.
23. Blanco CE, et al: Carotid baroreceptors in fetal and newborn sheep. *Pediatr Res* 24:342, 1988.
24. Boheler KR, et al: Skeletal actin mRNA increases in the human heart during ontogenic development and is the major isoforn of control and failing adult hearts. *J Clin Invest* 88:323, 1991.
25. Borg TK, et al: Structural basis of ventricular stiffness. *Lab Invest* 44:49, 1981.
26. Borow KM, et al: Left ventricular end-systolic stress-shortening and stress-length relations in human. Normal values and sensitivity to inotropic state. *Am J Cardiol* 50:1301, 1982.
27. Borow KM, et al: Sensitivity of end-systolic pressure-dimension and pressure-volume relations to the inotropic state in humans. *Circulation* 65:988, 1982.
28. Brace RA: The course and mechanisms of the acute effects of hypokalemia and hyperkalemia on vascular resistance. *Proc Soc Exp Biol Med* 145:1389, 1974.
29. Brace RA, et al: Local effects of hypokalemia on coronary resistance and myocardial contractile force. *Am J Physiol* 227:590, 1974.
30. Brayden JE: Functional roles of K_{ATP} channels in vascular smooth muscle. *Clin Exp Pharmacol Physiol* 29:312, 2002.
31. Brazier J, et al: The adequacy of subendocardial oxygen delivery: the interaction of determinants of flow, arterial oxygen content and myocardial oxygen need. *Circulation* 49:968, 1974.
32. Breall JA, et al: Role of thyroid hormone in postnatal circulatory and metabolic adjustments. *J Clin Invest* 73:1418, 1984.
33. Bristow JD: Cardiac and myocardial structure and myocardial cellular and molecular function. In: Gluckman PD, Heymann MA, editors: *Pediatrics and perinatology. The scientific basis.* London, 1996, Edward Arnold.
34. Bristow M: Of phospholamban, mice, and humans with heart failure. *Circulation* 103:787, 2001.
35. Bristow MR: Mechanistic and clinical rationales for using beta-blockers in heart failure. *J Card Fail* 6:8, 2000.
36. Bristow MR, et al: Beta 1- and beta 2-adrenergic-receptor subpopulations in nonfailing and failing human ventricular myocardium: coupling of both receptor subtypes to muscle contraction and selective beta 1-receptor down-regulation in heart failure. *Circ Res* 59:297, 1986.
37. Bristow MR, et al: The role of third-generation beta-blocking agents in chronic heart failure. *Clin Cardiol* 21:13, 1998.
38. Bruns LA, Canter CE: Should beta-blockers be used for the treatment of pediatric patients with chronic heart failure? *Paediatr Drugs* 4:771, 2002.
39. Budinger GR, et al: Hibernation during hypoxia in cardiomyocytes. Role of mitochondria as the O_2 sensor. *J Biol Chem* 273:3320, 1998.
40. Buga GM, Ignarro LJ: Vascular endothelium and smooth muscle function. In Gluckman PD, Heymann MA, editors: *Pediatrics and perinatology. The scientific basis.* London, 1996, Edward Arnold.
41. Burger AJ, et al: Effect of nesiritide (B-type natriuretic peptide) and dobutamine on ventricular arrhythmias in the treatment of patients with acutely decompensated congestive heart failure: the PRECEDENT shady. *Am Heart J* 144:1102, 2002.
42. Burlew BS, Weber KT: Connective tissue and the heart. Functional significance and regulatory mechanisms. *Cardiol Clin* 18:435, 2000.
43. Burridge K, Chrzanowska-Wodnicka M: Focal adhesions, contractility, and signaling. *Annu Rev Cell Dev Biol* 12:463, 1996.
44. Busse R, et al: EDHF: bringing the concepts together. *Trends Pharmacol Sci* 23:374, 2002.
45. Campbell DJ: The kallikrein-kinin system in humans. *Clin Exp Pharmacol Physiol* 28:1060, 2001.
45a. Cannon RO III, Schechter AN, Panza JA, et al: Effects of inhaled nitric oxide on regional blood flow are consistent with intravascular nitric oxide delivery. J Clin Invest 108:279, 2001.
46. Canty JM Jr: Coronary pressure-function and steady-state pressure-flow relations during autoregulation in the unanesthetized dog. *Circ Res* 63:821, 1988.
47. Canty JM Jr, Fallavollita JA: Lessons from experimental models of hibernating myocardium. *Coron Artery Dis* 12:371, 2001.
48. Capetanaki Y, Milner DJ: Desmin cytoskeleton in muscle integrity and function. *Subcell Biochem* 31:463, 1998.
49. Capetanaki Y, et al: Desmin in muscle formation and maintenance: knockouts and consequences. *Cell Struct Funct* 22:103, 1997.
50. Carabello BA, Spann JF: The uses and limitations of end-systolic indexes of left ventricular function. *Circulation* 69:1058, 1984.
51. Chandel NS, Schumacker PT: Cellular oxygen sensing by mitochondria: old questions, new insight. *J Appl Physiol* 88:1880, 2000.
52. Chapman JB: Heat production. In Drake-Holland A, Noble MIM, editors: *Cardiac metabolism.* Chichester, England, 1983, John Wiley & Sons.
53. Chidsey CA: Calcium metabolism in the normal and failing heart. In Braunwald E, editor: *The myocardium: failure and infarction.* New York, 1974, HP Publishing.
54. Chilian WM, et al: Redistribution of coronary microvascular resistance produced by dipyridamole. *Am J Physiol* 256:H383, 1989.
55. Chu G, Kranias EG: Functional interplay between dual site phospholamban phosphorylation: insights from genetically altered mouse models. *Basic Res Cardiol* 97(suppl 1):143, 2002.
56. Clark JB, Clark CM Jr: The growth and metabolism of the developing heart. In Jones CT, editor: *The biochemical development of the fetus and neonate.* Amsterdam, 1982, Elsevier Biomedical.
57. Clyman RI: Developmental physiology of the ductus arteriosus. In Polin Long WA, editors: *Fetal and neonatal cardiology.* New York, 1989, WB Saunders.
58. Clyman RI: Medical treatment of the ductus arteriosus in premature infants. In Polin Long WA, editors: *Fetal and neonatal cardiology.* New York, 1989, WB Saunders.
59. Clyman RI: Patent ductus arteriosus in the premature infant. In Avery ME, editor: *Diseases of the newborn.* Philadelphia, 1998, WB Saunders.

60. Clyman RI, et al: Permanent anatomic closure of the ductus arteriosus in newborn baboons: the roles of postnatal constriction, hypoxia, and gestation. *Pediatr Res* 45:19, 1999.
61. Clyman RI, et al: The role of beta-adrenoreceptor stimulation and contractile state in the preterm lamb's response to altered ductus arteriosus patency. *Pediatr Res* 23:316, 1988.
62. Clyman RI, et al: Regulation of ductus arteriosus patency by nitric oxide in fetal lambs: the role of gestation, oxygen tension, and vasa-vasorum. *Pediatr Res* 43:633, 1998.
63. Coceani F: Carbon monoxide in vasoregulation: the promise and the challenge. *Circ Res* 86:1184, 2000.
64. Coceani F, Kelsey L: Endothelin-1 release from lamb ductus arteriosus: relevance to postnatal closure of the vessel. *Can J Physiol Pharmacol* 69:218, 1991.
65. Colan SD, et al: Use of the indirect axillary pulse tracing for noninvasive determination of ejection time, upstroke time, and left ventricular wall stress throughout ejection in infants and young children. *Am J Cardiol* 53:1154, 1984.
66. Colan SD, et al: Left ventricular end-systolic wall stress-velocity of fiber shortening relation: a load-independent index of myocardial contractility. *J Am Coll Cardiol* 4:715, 1984.
67. Colan SD, et al: Use of the calibrated carotid pulse tracing for calculation of left ventricular pressure and wall stress throughout ejection. *Am Heart J* 109:1306, 1985.
68. Coleridge JCG, Coleridge HM: Chemoreflex regulation of the heart. In Berne RM, Sperelakis N, editors: *Handbook of physiology, section 2: the cardiovascular system,* vol 1, *The heart.* Bethesda, Md, 2001, American Physiological Society.
69. Cooper HA, Braunwald E: Clinical importance of stunned and hibernating myocardium. *Coron Artery Dis* 12:387, 2001.
70. Cornelissen AJ, et al: Balance between myogenic, flow-dependent, and metabolic flow control in coronary arterial tree: a model study. *Am J Physiol Heart Circ Physiol* 282:H2224, 2002.
71. Craig SW, Pardo JV: Gamma actin, spectrin, and intermediate filament proteins colocalize with vinculin at costameres, myofibril-to-sarcolemma attachment sites. *Cell Motil* 3:449, 1983.
72. Davis MJ, et al: Integrins and mechanotransduction of the vascular myogenic response. *Am J Physiol Heart Circ Physiol* 280:H1427, 2001.
73. DiPalma JR: Carnitine deficiency. *Am Fam Physician* 38:243, 1988.
74. DiPette DJ, et al: Systemic and regional hemodynamic effects of calcitonin gene-related peptide. *Hypertension* 9:III142, 1987.
75. Drake-Holland AJ: Substrate utilization. In Drake-Holland AJ, Noble MIM, editors: *Cardiac metabolism.* Chichester, England, 1983, John Wiley & Sons.
76. Dzau VJ, et al: Pathophysiologic and therapeutic importance of tissue ACE: a consensus report. *Cardiovasc Drugs Ther* 16:149, 2002.
77. Editorial: Carnitine deficiency. *Lancet* 335:631, 1990.
78. Elkayarn U, et al: Nesiritide: a new drug for the treatment of decompensated heart failure. *J Cardiovasc Pharmacol Ther* 7:181, 2002.
79. Elzinga G: Cardiac oxygen consumption and the production of heat and work. In Drake-Holland AJ, Noble MIM, editors: *Cardiac metabolism.* Chichester, England, 1983, John Wiley & Sons.
80. Erdos EG: Kinins, the long march—a personal view. *Cardiovasc Res* 54:485, 2002.
81. Erdos EG, Deddish PA: The kinin system: suggestions to broaden some prevailing concepts. *Int Immunopharmacol* 2:1741, 2002.
82. Eto T: A review of the biological properties and clinical implications of adrenomedullin and proadrenomedullin N-terminal20 peptide (PAW), hypotensive and vasodilating peptides. *Peptides* 22:1693, 2001.
83. Evans JJ, et al: Effects of endothelin-1 on release of adrenomedullin and C-type natriuretic peptide from individual human vascular endothelial cells. *J Endocrinol* 175:225, 2002.
84. Fabiato A: Calcium release in skinned cardiac cells: variations with species, tissues, and development. *Fed Proc* 41:2238, 1982.
85. Feigl EO: Coronary physiology. *Physiol Rev* 63:1, 1983.
86. Fisher DJ: Cardiac output and regional blood flows during hypoxaemia in unanaesthetized newborn lambs. *J Dev Physiol* 6:485, 1984.
87. Fisher DJ: Increased regional myocardial blood flows and oxygen deliveries during hypoxemia in lambs. *Pediatr Res* 18:602, 1984.
88. Floras JS: Vasopeptidase inhibition: a novel approach to cardiovascular therapy. *Can J Cardiol* 18:177, 2002.
89. Fowler M: Beta-adrenergic blocking drugs in severe heart failure. *Rev Cardiovasc Med.*
90. Frais MA, et al: The dependence of the time constant of left ventricular isovolumic relaxation (tau) on pericardial pressure. *Circulation* 81:1071, 1990.
91. Franco-Cereceda A, et al: Cardiovascular effects of calcitonin gene-related peptides I and II in man. *Circ Res* 60:393, 1987.
92. Frank K, Kranias EG: Phospholamban and cardiac contractility. *Ann Med* 32:572, 2000.
93. Frank KF, et al: Modulation of SERCA: implications for the failing human heart. *Basic Res Cardiol* 97(suppl 1):172, 2002.
94. Franklin RC, et al: Normal values for noninvasive estimation of left ventricular contractile state and afterload in children. *Am J Cardiol* 65:505, 1990.
95. Frase LL, et al: Cardiovascular effects of vasoactive intestinal peptide in healthy subjects. *Am J Cardiol* 60:1356, 1987.
96. Friedman MH, Fry DL: Arterial permeability dynamics and vascular disease. *Atherosclerosis* 104:189, 1993.
97. Friedman WF: The intrinsic physiologic properties of the developing heart. In Friedman WF, et al., editors: *Neonatal heart disease.* New York, 1973, Grune & Stratton.
98. Frishman WH, Grewall P: Serotonin and the heart. *Ann Med* 32:195, 2000.
99. Frishman WH, et al: Serotonin and serotonin antagonism in cardiovascular and noncardiovascular disease. *J Clin Pharmacol* 35:541, 1995.
100. Fry DL: Acute vascular endothelial changes associated with increased blood velocity gradients. *Circ Res* 22:165, 1968.
101. Furchgott RF: Role of endothelium in responses of vascular smooth muscle. *Circ Res* 53:557, 1983.
102. Furness JB, et al: Neuropeptides contained in peripheral cardiovascular nerves. *Clin Exp Hypertens A* 6:91, 1984.
103. Gaasch WH, et al: Diastolic properties of the left ventricle. In Levine HJ, Gaasch WH, editors: *The ventricle:* basic and clinical aspects. Boston, 1985, Martinus Nijhoff.
104. Gallagher KP, et al: Significance of regional wall thickening abnormalities relative to transmural myocardial perfusion in anesthetized dogs. *Circulation* 62:1266, 1980.
105. Gangula PRY, et al: Increased blood pressure in alpha-calcitonin gene-related peptide/calcitonin gene knockout mice. *Hypertension* 35:470, 2000.
106. Ganong WF: Origin of the angiotensin II secreted by cells. *Proc Soc Exp Biol Med* 205:213, 1994.
107. Gertz EW, et al: Myocardial lactate extraction: multi determined metabolic function. *Circulation* 61:256, 1980.
108. Gibbs CJ, Chapman JB: Cardiac energetics. In Berne RM Sperelakis N, editors: *Handbook of physiology, section 2, the cardiovascular system,* vol 1, *the heart.* Bethesda, MD, 2001, American Physiological Society.
109. Gilbert RD: Effects of afterload and baroreceptors on cardiac function in fetal sheep. *J Dev Physiol* 4:299, 1982.
110. Gilbert RD: Control and distribution of cardiac output in the fetus. In Jones CT, editor: *Research in perinatal medicine,* vol 7, *fetal and neonatal development.* Ithaca, NY, 1988, Perinatology Press.
110a. Gladwin MT, Shelhamer JH, Schechter AN, et al: Role of circulating nitrite and S-nitrosohemoglobin in the regulation of regional blood flow in humans. Proc Natl Acad Sci USA 97:11482, 2000.
111. Glantz SA, et al: The pericardium substantially affects the left ventricular diastolic pressure volume relationship in the dog. *Circ Res* 42:433, 1978.
112. Glantz SA, Parmley WW. Factors which affect the diastolic pressure-volume curve. *Circ Res* 42:433, 1978.
113. Glower DD, et al: Quantification of regional myocardial dysfunction after acute ischemic injury. *Am J Physiol* 255:H85, 1988.
114. Glower DD, et al: Linearity of the Frank-Starling relationship in the intact heart: the concept of preload recruitable stroke work. *Circulation* 71:994, 1985.
115. Goldsmith SR: Congestive heart failure: potential role of arginine vasopressin antagonists in the therapy of heart failure. *Congest Heart Fail* 8:251, 2002.
115a. Gonzalez-Alonso J, Olsen DB, Saltin B: Erythrocyte and the regulation of human skeletal muscle blood flow and oxygen delivery: role of circulating ATP. *Circ Res* 91:1046, 2002.
116. Goraca A: New views on the role of endothelin (minireview). *Endocr Regul* 36:161, 2002.
117. Graham TP Jr, et a1: Control of myocardial oxygen consumption: relative influence of contractile state and tension development. *J Clin Invest* 47:375, 1968.

118. Grant DA: Pericardial influence on the left ventricle of the neonatal lamb. In Jones CT, editor: *Research in perinatal medicine*, vol 7, *fetal and neonatal development*. Ithaca, NY, 1988, Perinatology Press.
119. Granzier H, Labeit S: Cardiac titin: an adjustable multi-functional spring. *J Physiol* 541:335, 2002.
120. Granzier HL, Irving TC: Passive tension in cardiac muscle: contribution of collagen, titin, microtubules, and intermediate filaments. *Biophys J* 68:1027, 1995.
121. Gregorio CC, Antin PB: To the heart of myofibril assembly. *Trends Cell Biol* 10:355, 2000.
122. Grossman W, et al: Wall stress and patterns of hypertrophy in the human left ventricle. *J Clin Invest* 56:56, 1975.
123. Hagner S, et al: Calcitonin receptor-like receptor: identification and distribution in human peripheral tissues. *Cell Tissue Res* 310:41, 2002.
124. Hansson M: Natriuretic peptides in relation to the cardiac innervation and conduction system. *Microsc Res Tech* 58:378, 2002.
125. Hata K, et al: Hypercapnic acidosis increases oxygen cost of contractility in the dog left ventricle. *Am J Physiol* 266:H730, 1994.
126. Hata K, et al: Stunned myocardium after rapid correction of acidosis. Increased oxygen cost of contractility and the role of the Na^+H^+ exchange system. *Circ Res* 74:794, 1994.
127. Hawkins J, et al: Effects of increasing afterload on left ventricular output in fetal lambs. *Circ Res* 65:127, 1989.
128. Hearse DJ: Ischaernia definition. *Cardiovasc Res* 28:1737, 1994 (editorial).
129. Heilbrunn SM, et al: Increased beta-receptor density and improved hemodynamic response to catecholamine stimulation during long-term metoprolol therapy in heart failure from dilated cardiomyopathy. *Circulation* 79:483, 1989.
130. Hein S, et al: The role of the cytoskeleton in heart failure. *Cardiovasc Res* 45:273, 2000.
131. Henning RJ, Sawmiller DR: Vasoactive intestinal peptide: cardiovascular effects. *Cardiovasc Res* 49:27, 2001.
132. Heusch G, Schulz R: The biology of myocardial hibernation. *Trends Cardiovasc Med* 10:108, 2000.
133. Heusch G, Schulz R: Hibernating myocardium: new answers, still more questions! *Circ Res* 91:863, 2002.
134. Hoffinan JI, Buckberg GD: The myocardial supply:demand ratio—a critical review. *Am J Cardiol* 41:327, 1978.
135. Hoffman JIE: Transmural myocardial perfusion. *Prog Cardiovasc Dis* 29:429, 1987.
136. Hoffman JIE: Coronary physiology. In Garfield OB, editor: *Current concepts in cardiovascular physiology.* New York, 1990, Academic Press.
137. Hoffinan JIE, Buckberg GD: Transmural variations in myocardial perfusion.
138. Holmes CL, et al: Physiology of vasopressin relevant to management of septic shock. *Chest* 120:989, 2001.
139. Huhta JC, et al: Left ventricular wall thickness in complete transposition of the great arteries. *J Thorac Cardiovasc Surg* 84:97, 1982.
140. Ignarro LJ, et al: Endothelium-derived relaxing factor from pulmonary artery and vein possesses pharmacologic and chemical properties identical to those of nitric oxide radical. *Circ Res* 61:866, 1987.
141. Itskovitz J, et al: Baroreflex control of the circulation in chronically instrumented fetal lambs. *Circ Res* 52:589, 1983.
141a. Jagger JE, Bateman RM, Ellsworth ML, et al: Role of erythrocyte in regulating local O_2 delivery mediated by hemoglobin oxygenation. *Am J Physiol Heart Circ Physiol* 280: H2833, 2001.
142. Johnson FK, et al: Vascular effects of a heme oxygenase inhibitor are enhanced in the absence of nitric oxide. *Am J Hypertens* 15:1074, 2002.
143. Johnson PC: The myogenic response. In Bohr DF, et al., editors: *Handbook of physiology. The cardiovascular system*, vol 2. Bethesda, MD, 2001, American Physiological Society.
144. Kanno S, Saffitz JE: The role of myocardial gap junctions in electrical conduction and arrhythmogenesis. *Cardiovasc Pathol* 10:169, 2001.
145. Kaplan AP, et al: Pathways for bradykinin formation and inflammatory disease. *J Allergy Clin Immunol* 109:195, 2002.
146. Kass DA, et al: Influence of contractile state on curvilinearity of in situ end-systolic pressure-volume relations. *Circulation* 79:167, 1989.
147. Kato R, Foex P: Myocardial protection by anesthetic agents against ischemia-reperfusion injury: an update for anesthesiologists. *Can J Anaesth* 49:777, 2002.
148. Katz AM: Contractile proteins in normal and failing myocardium. In Braunwald E, editor: *The myocardium: failure and infarction.* New York, 1974, HP Publishing.
149. Keating GM, Goa KL: Nesiritide: a review of its use in acute decompensated heart failure. *Drugs* 63:47, 2003.
150. Kern KB: Postresuscitation myocardial dysfunction. *Cardiol Clin* 20:89, 2002.
151. Kitamura K, et al: Hemodynamic correlates of myocardial oxygen consumption during upright exercise. *J Appl Physiol* 32:516, 1972.
152. Kloner RA, et al: Evidence for stunned myocardium in humans: a 2001 update. *Coron Artery Dis* 12:349, 2001.
153. Klopfenstein HS, Rudolph AM: Postnatal changes in the circulation and responses to volume loading in sheep. *Circ Res* 42:839, 1978.
154. Korthuis RJ, Granger DN: Ischemia-reperfuson injury: role of oxygen-derived free radicals. In Taylor AE, et al., editors: *Physiology of oxygen radicals.* Bethesda, MD, 1986, American Physiological Society.
155. Krosl P, Abel FL: Problems with use of the end systolic pressure-volume slope as an indicator of left ventricular contractility: an alternate method. *Shock* 10:285, 1998.
156. Kukin ML: Beta-blockers in chronic heart failure: considerations for selecting an agent. *Mayo Clin Proc* 77:1199, 2002.
157. Lah JJ, Frishman WH: Adrenomedullin: a vasoactive and natriuretic peptide with therapeutic potential. *Heart Dis* 2:259, 2000.
158. Lakatta EG: Length modulation of myocardial performance: Frank-Starling law of the heart. In Fozzard HA, et al., editors: *The heart and cardiovascular system: scientific foundations.* New York, 1991, Raven Press.
159. Lapointe N, Rouleau JL: Cardioprotective effects of vasopeptidase inhibitors. *Can J Cardiol* 18:415, 2002.
160. Le Guennec JY, et al: Is titin the length sensor in cardiac muscle? Physiological and physiopathological perspectives. *Adv Exp Med Biol* 481:337, 2000.
161. Lennon NJ, Ohlendieck K: Impaired Ca2+-sequestration in dilated cardiomyopathy (review). *Int J Mol Med* 7:131, 2001.
162. Lister G, et al: Oxygen delivery in lambs: cardiovascular and hematologic development. *Am J Physiol* 237:H668, 1979.
163. Luss H, et al: Biochemical mechanisms of hibernation and stunning in the human heart. *Cardiovasc Res* 56:411, 2002.
164. Mahony L: Development of myocardial structure and function. In Emmanouilides GC, et al., editors: *Heart disease in infants, children, and adolescents, including the fetus and young adult.* Baltimore, MD, 1998, Williams & Wilkins.
165. Maier LS, Bers DM: Calcium, calmodulin, and calcium-calmodulin kinase 11: heartbeat to heartbeat and beyond. *J Mol Cell Cardiol* 34:919, 2002.
166. Mari C, Strauss WH: Detection and characterization of hibernating myocardium. *Nucl Med Commun* 23:311, 2002.
167. Massett MP, et al: Different roles of PKC and MAP kinases in arteriolar constrictions to pressure and agonists. *Am J Physiol Heart Circ Physiol* 283:H2282, 2002.
168. Mays PK, et al: Age-related changes in the proportion of types I and 111 collagen. *Mech Ageing Dev* 45:203, 1988.
169. McCormack J, et al: In vivo demonstration of maturational changes of the chronotropic response to alpha-adrenergic stimulation. *Pediatr Res* 24:50, 1988.
170. McDonald RH Jr, et al: Measurement of myocardial developed tension and its relation to oxygen consumption. *Am J Physiol* 211:667, 1966.
171. McHale PA, Greenfield JC Jr: Evaluation of several geometric models for estimation of left ventricular circumferential wall stress. *Circ Res* 33:303, 1973.
172. Michelakis ED, et al: O_2 sensing in the human ductus arteriosus: regulation of voltage-gated K+ channels in smooth muscle cells by a mitochondria1 redox sensor. *Circ Res* 91:478, 2002.
173. Minkes RK, Kadowitz PJ: Differential effects of rat endothelin on regional blood flow in the cat. *Eur J Pharmacol* 55:161, 1989.
174. Mione MC, et al: Peptides and vasomotor mechanisms. *Pharmacol Ther* 46:429, 1990.
175. Moolman-Smook J, et al: Identification of novel interactions between domains of myosin binding protein-C that are modulated by hypertrophic cardiomyopathy missense mutations. *Circ Res* 91:704, 2002.

176. Morse D, et al: Carbon monoxide-dependent signaling. *Crit Care Med* 30:S12, 2001.
177. Muller DN, Luft FC: The renin-angiotensin system in the vessel wall. *Basic Res Cardiol* 93:7, 1998.
178. Muller FU, et al: Junctional sarcoplasmic reticulum transmembrane proteins in the heart. *Basic Res Cardiol* 97(suppl 1):152, 2002.
179. Munch G, et al: Evidence for calcineurin-mediated regulation of SERCA 2a activity in human myocardium. *J Mol Cell Cardiol* 34:321, 2002.
180. Murray PA, et al: The role of potassium in the metabolic control of coronary vascular resistance of the dog. *Circ Res* 44:767, 1979.
181. Murray PA, Sparks HV: The mechanism of K+-induced vasodilation of the coronary vascular bed of the dog. *Circ Res* 42:35, 1978.
182. Nassar R, et al: Developmental changes in the ultrastructure and sarcomere shortening of the isolated rabbit ventricular myocyte. *Circ Res* 61:465, 1987.
183. Nawarskas J, et al: Vasopeptidase inhibitors, neutral endopeptidase inhibitors, and dual inhibitors of angiotensin-converting enzyme and neutral endopeptidase. *Heart Dis* 3:378, 2001.
184. Ono K, Matsumori A: Endothelin antagonism with bosentan: current status and future perspectives. *Cardiovasc Drug Rev* 20:1, 2002.
185. Onuoha GN, et al: Distributions of VIP, substance P, neurokinin A and neurotensin in rat heart: an immunocytochemical study. *Neuropeptides* 33:19, 1999.
186. Opie L: Receptors and signal transducers. In: Opie LH, editor: *The heart: physiology and metabolism*. New York, 1991, Raven Press.
187. Opie LH: High energy phosphate compounds. In Drake-Holland AJ, Noble MTM, editors: *Cardiac metabolism*. Chichester, England, 1983, John Wiley & Sons.
188. Opie LH: Fuels: carbohydrates and lipids. In Opie LH, editor: *The heart: physiology and metabolism*. New York, 1991, Raven Press.
189. Packer M, et al: Effect of carvedilol on the morbidity of patients with severe chronic heart failure: results of the carvedilol prospective randomized cumulative survival (COPERNICUS) study. *Circulation* 106:2194, 2002.
190. Pardo JV, et al: Vinculin is a component of an extensive network of myofibril-sarcolemma attachment regions in cardiac muscle fibers. *J Cell Biol* 97:1081, 1983.
191. Pardo JV, et al: A vinculin-containing cortical lattice in skeletal muscle: transverse lattice elements ("costameres") mark sites of attachment between myofibrils and sarcolemma. *Proc Natl Acad Sci U S A* 80:1008, 1983.
192. Parmley WW, et al: Comparative evaluation of the specificity and sensitivity of isometric indices of contractility. *Am J Physiol* 228:506, 1975.
193. Parmley WW, Tyberg JV: Determinants of myocardial oxygen demand. In Yu P, Goodwin JF, editors: *Progress in cardiology*. Philadelphia, 1988, Lea & Febiger.
194. Parris RJ, Webb DJ: The endothelin system in cardiovascular physiology and pathophysiology. *Vasc Med* 2:31, 1997.
195. Pidgeon J, et al: The contractile state of cat and dog heart in relation to the interval between beats. *Circ Res* 47:559, 1980.
196. Pieske B, et al: Sarcoplasmic reticulum Ca2+ load in human heart failure. *Basic Res Cardiol* 97(suppl 1):963, 2002.
196a. Pollack GH: Maximum velocity as an index of contractility in cardiac muscle. A critical evaluation. *Circ Res* 26:111, 1970.
197. Preibisz JJ: Calcitonin gene-related peptide and regulation of human cardiovascular homeostasis. *Am J Hypertens* 6:434, 1993.
198. Rademaker MT, et al: Long-term adrenomedullin administration in experimental heart failure. *Hypertension* 40:667, 2002.
199. Rebouche CJ: Carnitine function and requirements during the life cycle. *FASEB J* 6:3379, 1992.
200. Rebouche CJ, Paulson DJ: Carnitine metabolism and function in humans. *Annu Rev Nutr* 6:41, 1986.
201. Reese DE, et al: Development of the coronary vessel system. *Circ Res* 91:761, 2002.
202. Reeve HL, et al: Redox control of oxygen sensing in the rabbit ductus arteriosus. *J Physiol* 533:253, 2001.
203. Reimer KA, Jennings RB: Myocardial ischemia, hypoxia, and infarction. In Fozzard HA, et al., editors: *The heart and cardiovascular system: scientific foundations*. New York, 1991, Raven Press.
204. Retter AS: Carnitine and its role in cardiovascular disease. *Heart Dis* 1:108, 1999.
205. Robinson TF, et al: Structure and function of connective tissue in cardiac muscle: collagen types I and III in endomysial struts and pericellular fibers. *Scanning Microsc* 2:1005, 1988.
206. Robinson TF, et al: Coiled perimysial fibers of papillary muscle in rat heart: morphology, distribution, and changes in configuration. *Circ Res* 63:577, 1988.
207. Rocha R, Funder JW: The pathophysiology of aldosterone in the cardiovascular system. *Ann N Y Acad Sci* 970:89, 2002.
208. Roe CR, Coates PM: Mitochondrial fatty acid oxidation disorders. In Scriver CL, et al., editors: *The metabolic basis of inherited disease*. New York, 1989, McGraw-Hill.
209. Rooke GA, Feigl EO: Work as a correlate of canine left ventricular oxygen consumption, and the problem of catecholamine oxygen wasting. *Circ Res* 50:273, 1982.
210. Ross J Jr: Afterload mismatch and preload reserve: a conceptual framework for the analysis of ventricular function. *Prog Cardiovasc Dis* 18:255, 1976.
211. Ross J Jr: Mechanisms of cardiac contraction. What roles for preload, afterload and inotropic state in heart failure? *Eur Heart J* 4(suppl A): 19, 1983.
212. Rossi GP, et al: The endothelin-aldosterone axis and cardiovascular diseases. *J Cardiovasc Pharmacol* 38(suppl 2):S49, 2001.
213. Sagawa K: The ventricular pressure-volume diagram revisited. *Circ Res* 43:677, 1978.
214. Sagawa K: The end-systolic pressure-volume relation of the ventricle: definition, modifications and clinical use. *Circulation* 63:1223, 1981.
215. Sarnoff SJ, Mitchell JH: The control of the function of the heart. In Hamilton WE, Dow P, editors: *Handbook of physiology. Section 2: circulation*, vol 1. Washington, DC, 2001, American Physiological Society.
216. Schmidt AG, et al: Phospholamban: a promising therapeutic target in heart failure? *Cardiovasc Drugs Ther* 15:387, 2001.
217. Seed WA, et al: Relationships between beat-to-beat interval and the strength of contraction in the healthy and diseased human heart. *Circulation* 70:799, 1984.
218. Serradeil-Le Gal C: An overview of SRl21463, a selective non-peptide vasopressin V_2 receptor antagonist. *Cardiovasc Drug Rev* 19:201, 2001.
219. Serradeil-Le Gal C, et al: Nonpeptide vasopressin receptor antagonists: development of selective and orally active V1a, V2 and V1b receptor ligands. *Prog Brain Res* 139:197, 2002.
220. Sharp WW, et al: Mechanical forces regulate focal adhesion and costamere assembly in cardiac myocytes. *Am J Physiol* 273:H546, 1997.
221. Shinebourne EA, et al: Development of baroreflex activity in unanesthetized fetal and neonatal lambs. *Circ Res* 31:710, 1972.
222. Shroff SG, et al: Mechanical and energetic behavior of the intact left ventricle. In Fozzard HA, et al., editors: *The heart and cardiovascular system: scientific foundations*. New York, 1991, Raven Press.
223. Shyy JY, Chien S: Role of integrins in endothelial mechanosensing of shear stress. *Circ Res* 91:769, 2002.
224. Slinker BK, Glantz SA: End-systolic and end-diastolic ventricular interaction. *Am J Physiol* 251: H1062, 1986.
225. Slish DF, et al: Diacylglycerol and protein kinase C activate cation channels involved in myogenic tone. *Am J Physiol Heart Circ Physiol* 283:H2196, 2002.
226. Smart EJ, et al: Caveolins, liquid-ordered domains, and signal transduction. *Mol Cell Biol* 19:7289, 1999.
227. Smiseth OA, et al: left and right ventricular diastolic function during acute pericardial tamponade. *Clin Physiol* 11:61, 1991.
228. Smiseth OA, et al: Assessment of pericardial constraint: the relation between right ventricular filling pressure and pericardial pressure measured after pericardiocentesis. *J Am Coll Cardiol* 7:307, 1986.
229. Smith V-E, Zile MR: Relaxation and diastolic properties of the heart. In Fozzard HA, et al., editors: *The heart and cardiovascular system: scientific foundations*. New York, 1991, Raven Press.
230. Soberman J, et al: Aldosterone antagonists in congestive heart failure. *Curr Opin Investig Drugs* 3:1024, 2002.
231. Sole MJ, Jeejeebhoy KN: Conditioned nutritional requirements: therapeutic relevance to heart failure. *Herz* 27:174, 2002.
232. Sonnenblick EH: Myocardial ultrastructure in the normal and the failing heart. In Braunwald E, editor: *The myocardium: failure and infarction*. New York, 1974, HP Publishing.
233. Sonnenblick EH, et al: The ultrastructural basis of Starling's law of the heart. The role of the sarcomere in determining ventricular size and stroke volume. *Am Heart J* 68:336-346, 1964.
234. Sparks HV: Effect of local metabolic factors on vascular smooth muscle. In Bohr DF, et al., editors: *Handbook of physiology*.

The cardiovascular system, vol. 2. Bethesda, MD, 1980, American Physiological Society.
235. Springer TA: Traffic signals on endothelium for lymphocyte recirculation and leukocyte emigration. *Annu Rev Physiol* 57:827, 1995.
236. Squire JM: Architecture and function in the muscle sarcomere. *Curr Opin Struct Biol* 7:247, 1997.
236a. Stamler JS, Jia L, Eu JP, et al: Blood flow regulation by S-nitrosohemoglobin in the physiological oxygen gradient. *Science* 276:2034, 1997.
237. Standen NB, Quayle JM: K+ channel modulation in arterial smooth muscle. *Acta Physiol Scand* 164:549, 1998.
238. Stenmark KR, Weiser MC: Vascular development and function. In Gluckman PD, Heymann MA, editors: *Pediatrics and perinatology. The scientific basis.* London, 1996, Edward Arnold.
239. Stewart M: Intermediate filament structure and assembly. *Curr Opin Cell Biol* 5:3, 1993.
240. Strauer B-E: Myocardial oxygen consumption in chronic heart disease: role of wall stress, hypertrophy and coronary reserve. *Am J Cardiol* 44:730-740, 1979.
241. Streeter DD Jr: Hanna WT: Engineering mechanics for successive states in canine left ventricular myocardium. 11. Fiber angle and sarcomere length. *Circ Res* 33:656, 1973.
242. Strobeck JE, Sonnenblick EH: Myocardial contractile properties and ventricular performance. In Fozzard HA, et al., editors: *The heart and cardiovascular system: scientific foundations.* New York, 1991, Raven Press.
243. Stromer MH: The cytoskeleton in skeletal, cardiac and smooth muscle cells. *Histol Histopathol* 13:283, 1998.
244. Stryer L, Bourne HR: G proteins: a family of signal transducers. *Annu Rev Cell Biol* 2:391, 1986.
245. Suga H: Ventricular energetics. *Physiol Rev* 70:247, 1990.
246. Suga H: Paul Dudley White International Lecture: cardiac performance as viewed through the pressure-volume window. *Jpn Heart J* 35:263, 1994.
247. Suga H, et al: O_2 consumption of dog heart under decreased coronary perfusion and propranolol. *Am J Physiol* 254:H292, 1988.
248. Suga H, et al: Regression of cardiac oxygen consumption on ventricular pressure-volume area in dog. *Am J Physiol* 240:H320, 1981.
249. Suga H, et al: Effect of positive inotropic agents on the relation between oxygen consumption and systolic pressure volume area in canine left ventricle. *Circ Res* 53:306, 1983.
250. Tamburino G, Malatino LS: The vasoactive peptidergic system. *Ann Ital Med Int* 9:88, 1994.
251. Taylor RR: Myocardial oxygen consumption, left ventricular fibre shortening and wall tension. *Cardiovasc Res* 1:219, 1967.
252. Teitel DF, et al: Developmental changes in myocardial contractile reserve in the lamb. *Pediatr Res* 19:948, 1985.
253. Tennyson H, et al: Treatment of post resuscitation myocardial dysfunction: aortic counterpulsation versus dobutamine. *Resuscitation* 54:69, 2002.
254. Terracio L, et al: Expression of collagen adhesion proteins and their association with the cytoskeleton in cardiac myocytes. *Anat Rec* 223:62, 1989.
255. Terracio L, et al: Expression of collagen binding integrins during cardiac development and hypertrophy. *Circ Res* 68:734, 1991.
256. Thibonnier M, et al: Molecular pharmacology and modeling of vasopressin receptors. *Prog Brain Res* 139:179, 2002.
257. Torrent-Guasp F, et al: The structure and function of the helical heart and its buttress wrapping. I. The normal macroscopic structure of the heart. *Semin Thorac Cardiovasc Surg* 13:301, 2001.
258. Towbin JA: The role of cytoskeletal proteins in cardiomyopathies. *Curr Opin Cell Biol* 10:131, 1998.
259. Towbin JA, Bowles NE: Molecular genetics of left ventricular dysfunction. *Curr Mol Med* 1:81, 2001.
260. Towbin JA, Bowles NE: The failing heart. *Nature* 415:227, 2002.
261. Tristani-Firouzi M, et al: Oxygen-induced constriction of rabbit ductus arteriosus occurs via inhibition of a 4-aminopyridine-, voltage-sensitive potassium channel. *J Clin Invest* 98:1959, 1996.
262. Tyberg JV, et al: Ventricular interaction and venous capacitance modulate left ventricular preload. *Can J Cardiol* 12:1058, 1996.
263. Tyberg JV, et al: Effects of positive intrathoracic pressure on pulmonary and systemic hemodynamics. *Respir Physiol* 119:171, 2000.
264. Tyberg JV, et al: A mechanism for shifts in the diastolic, left ventricular, pressure-volume curve: the role of the pericardium. *Eur J Cardiol* 7(suppl):163, 1978.
265. Tyberg JV, et al: The relationship between pericardial pressure and right atrial pressure: an intraoperative study. *Circulation* 73:428, 1986.
266. Unger T: The role of the renin-angiotensin system in the development of cardiovascular disease. *Am J Cardiol* 89:3A, 2002.
267. Usui M, et al: Important role of local angiotensin I1 activity mediated via type 1 receptor in the pathogenesis of cardiovascular inflammatory changes induced by chronic blockade of nitric oxide synthesis in rats. *Circulation* 101:305, 2000.
268. Van den Bos GC, et al: Problems in the use of indices of myocardial contractility. *Cardiovasc Res* 7:834, 1973.
269. Van Hare GF, et al: The effects of increasing mean arterial pressure on left ventricular output in newborn lambs. *Circ Res* 67:78, 1990.
270. van Hinsbergh VW, van Nieuw Arnerongen GP: Intracellular signalling involved in modulating human endothelial barrier function. *J Anat* 200:549, 2002.
271. van Veen AA, et al: Cardiac gap junction channels: modulation of expression and channel properties. *Cardiovasc Res* 51:217, 2001.
272. VanBavel E, et al: Role of T-type calcium channels in myogenic tone of skeletal muscle resistance arteries. *Am J Physiol Heart Circ Physiol* 283:H2239, 2002.
273. Vatner SF: Correlation between acute reductions in myocardial blood flow and function in conscious dogs. *Circ Res* 47:20l, 1980.
274. Vatner SF: Sympathetic mechanisms regulating myocardial contractility in conscious animals. In Fozzard HA, et al., editors: *The heart and cardiovascular system: scientific foundations.* New York, 1991, Raven Press.
275. Verbalis JG: Vasopressin V2 receptor antagonists. *J Mol Endocrinol* 29:1, 2002.
276. Vicaut E: Microcirculation and arterial hypertension. *Drugs* 59:1, 1999.
277. Vinten-Johansen J, et al: Prediction of myocardial O_2 requirements by indirect indices. *Am J Physiol* 243:H862, 1982.
278. Wang BC, et al: Cardiovascular effects of calcitonin gene-related peptide in conscious dogs. *Am J Physiol* 257:R726, 1989.
279. Webb DJ, Strachan FE: Clinical experience with endothelin antagonists. *Am J Hypertens* 11:71S, 1998.
280. Weber KT, Janicki JS: Myocardial oxygen consumption: the role of wall force and shortening. *Am J Physiol* 233:H421, 1977.
281. Weber KT, Janicki JS: Interdependence of cardiac function, coronary flow, and oxygen extraction. *Am J Physiol* 235:H784, 1978.
282. Weber MA: Clinical implications of aldosterone blockade. *Am Heart J* 144:s12, 2002.
283. Wharton J, Gulbenkian S: Peptides in the mammalian cardiovascular system. *Experientia* 43:821, 1987.
284. Wimalawansa SJ: Amylin, calcitonin gene-related peptide, calcitonin, and adrenomedullin: a peptide superfamily. *Crit Rev Neurobiol* 11:167, 1997.
285. Witherow FN, et al: Marked bradykinin-induced tissue plasminogen activator release in patients with heart failure maintained on long-term angiotensin-converting enzyme inhibitor therapy. *J Am Coll Cardiol* 40:961, 2002.
286. Wolinsky H, Glagov S: Comparison of abdominal and thoracic aortic medial structure in mammals. Deviation of man from the usual pattern. *Circ Res* 25:677, 1969.
287. Wu LL, et al: Altered phospholamban-calcium ATPase interaction in cardiac sarcoplasmic reticulum during the progression of sepsis. *Shock* 17:389, 2002.
288. Yang ZH, et al: Threshold concentrations of endothelin-1 potentiate contractions to norepinephrine and serotonin in human arteries. A new mechanism of vasospasm? *Circulation* 82:188, 1990.
289. Yeager M, Nicholson BJ: Structure of gap junction intercellular channels. *Curr Opin Struct Biol* 6:183, 1996.
290. Young MJ, Funder JW: Mineralocorticoid receptors and pathophysiological roles for aldosterone in the cardiovascular system. *J Hypertens* 20:1465, 2002.
291. Zhang F, et al: Vasoregulatory function of the heme-heme oxygenase-carbon monoxide system. *Am J Hypertens* 14:62S, 2001.
292. Zhao MJ, et al: Profound structural alterations of the extracellular collagen matrix in postischemic dysfunctional ("stunned") but viable myocardium. *J Am Coll Cardiol* 10:1322, 1987.
293. Zimmerman MA, et al: Vasopressin in cardiovascular patients: therapeutic implications. *Expert Opin Pharmacother* 3:505, 2002.

CHAPTER

18

Regional Circulation

Peter Oishi, Julien I. Hoffman, Bradley P. Fuhrman, and Jeffrey R. Fineman

PEARLS

- Critical illness tends to focus attention on the unique properties of crucial regions of the circulation.
- Individual regional circulations differ in their response to vasoactive substances, alterations in hemodynamics, and disease.
- When delivering critical care, one must understand the specific properties that characterize the various regional circulations because therapies that benefit one region may be detrimental to another.
- Blood flow to a regional vascular bed is determined by inflow pressure, vascular resistance, and outflow pressure.
- Vasomotor tone is influenced by: (1) innervation and neural processes; (2) circulating endocrine and neuroendocrine mediators; (3) local metabolic products; (4) blood gas composition; (5) endothelial-derived factors; and (6) myogenic processes.
- The transition from the fetal pulmonary circulation to the postnatal pulmonary circulation is marked by a dramatic fall in pulmonary vascular resistance and rise in pulmonary blood flow. A number of neonatal and infant diseases result from a failure to successfully make this transition.
- Under normal conditions, the pulmonary circulation is maintained in a dilated, low-resistance state following the immediate postnatal period.
- Blood flow to the brain is specially regulated to facilitate the myriad of complex functions overseen by the brain.
- An important feature unique to the cerebral circulation is the presence of a blood-brain barrier. As a result, the cerebral vasculature responds differently than other vascular beds to humoral stimuli.
- Regulation of myocardial perfusion is tailored to match regional myocardial oxygen supply to demand over the widest possible range of cardiac workload. Increases in myocardial oxygen demand must be met by increases in myocardial blood flow.
- Critically ill patients are at risk for impaired splanchnic blood flow that can impair the two chief functions of the gastrointestinal system: (1) digestion and absorption of nutrients, and (2) maintenance of a barrier to the translocation of enteric antigens. Splanchnic ischemia is associated with increased morbidity and mortality in critically ill patients.
- Although renal blood flow remains constant over a wide range of renal artery perfusion pressures, urinary flow rate varies as a function of renal perfusion pressure.
- Unsuccessful arbitration among regional circulations may contribute to multiple organ systems failure.

General Features

General Anatomy

Vascular anatomy is generally described as distinct layers. Moving from the innermost layer outward are the metabolically active endothelium, the intima (with nerves and vasa vasorum), the media, and the adventitia. The composition of these layers differs among vessel types (with some vessels consisting of fewer layers), depending on the position and function of the vessel within the circulation.

The large arteries are elastic. Their media contain concentric lamellae of perforated elastic tubes cross-linked by transverse collagen and smooth muscle. When smooth muscle contracts, the wall becomes stiffer. Smaller arteries have fewer lamellae. The media is bounded by the external and internal elastic laminae. Arterioles, which are less elastic, have no lamellae, a thin media with circular or spiral smooth muscle, and inner and outer elastic laminae. Capillaries are thin walled and nonmuscular, ideal for transport of materials into and from the tissues. Veins have medial muscle but have thinner walls relative to lumen diameter than do arteries. The vascular endothelium has important metabolic characteristics, which may differ between vessel types (i.e., arteries vs. veins).

Basic Physiology

Blood flow to a regional vascular bed is determined primarily by inflow pressure, vascular resistance, and outflow pressure. Inflow pressure usually is systemic arterial pressure. Outflow pressure generally approximates venous pressure but at times exceeds venous pressure if vascular tone is great enough to close the circulation above venous pressure or if external pressure impinges on the vasculature.

In a model explaining the relation of arterial pressure to flow, the circulation is represented by two capacitance vessels separated by a resistance. A standpipe full of blood is allowed to discharge its contents into the arterial vasculature (proximal capacitance). Blood flows across the resistance site (microvessels), traverses the venous vasculature (distal capacitance), and drains to a reservoir at some outflow pressure (P_o), taken to be atmospheric in this example (Figure 18–1).

The pressure head of the system (P_i) is generated by the weight of the column of blood in the standpipe and is proportional to its height (P_i = blood column height in cm H_2O). As the standpipe discharges, the height decreases and P_i falls. This in turn reduces the rate of flow (Q) through the vasculature. Q falls almost linearly with P_i until the column is quite low. Ultimately, flow ceases while there is still pressure in the standpipe. The pressure at which flow ceases is the critical closing pressure of the circulation (P_{cc}).[1] Lower P_i is insufficient to maintain vessel patency and permit continued flow (Figure 18–2).

Incremental resistance to flow is generally defined as the change in pressure per unit change in flow (dP_i/dQ). At pressures well above critical closing pressure, incremental resistance is nearly identical to vascular resistance (R) defined clinically as follows:

$$R = (P_i - P_o)/Q.$$

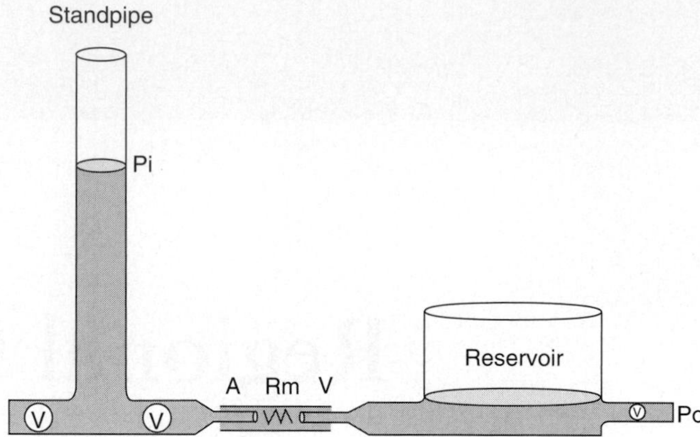

FIGURE 18–1 • Model for facilitating interpretation of vascular pressure-flow relations. When valves (V) are properly positioned, fluid filling the standpipe to height Pi discharges across the circulation to the reservoir at outflow pressure Po. *A,* Artery; *Rm,* microvascular resistance; *V,* vein.

When P_i does not greatly exceed P_{cc} but P_{cc} does greatly exceed P_o, however, incremental resistance can differ substantially from this clinical estimate. Thus an increase in P_{cc} can be confused with a true increase in incremental resistance. For example, when excessive levels of airway pressure are applied to the normal lung (raising P_{cc}), the measured rise in pulmonary artery pressure may not be a result of pulmonary vasoconstriction. Pulmonary hypertension must be interpreted with caution during mechanical ventilation for lung disease.

Venous Return and Cardiac Output

A second model can be used to illustrate the relationship of cardiac output to intrinsic mechanical properties of

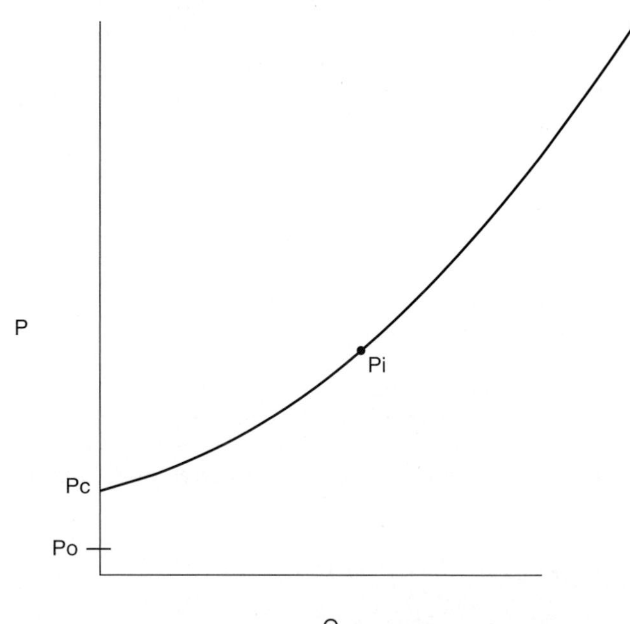

FIGURE 18–2 • As the standpipe in Figure 18–1 discharges, Pi falls. Flow consequently slows and ultimately stops when Pi = Pc, the critical closing pressure of the circulation. Pi only reaches outflow pressure Po if Po ≥ Pc.

the systemic vasculature. In this model, the heart is functionally replaced by a roller pump, creating a circulation much like that achieved during extracorporeal membrane oxygenation (Figure 18–3).

The roller pump displaces blood from the veins to the arteries, where some of it builds up before the resistive barrier of the arterioles. The higher the flow (Q), the more blood resides in the arteries and the less resides in the veins. This complex partitioning of the blood volume depends on arterial capacitance (C_a), venous capacitance (C_v), and arteriolar incremental resistance to flow. At maximal Q, P_i is high and arterial blood volume (Pi × Ca) is high, so much of the vascular blood volume is displaced to the arteries, and venous pressure (P_v) approaches P_{cc}. No further increase in roller pump speed can be sustained because any further increase in P_i would drive venous pressure substantially below venous critical closing pressure, causing vessel collapse and preventing venous return.

As Q is reduced by turning down the roller pump, P_i falls and the volume of blood that resides in the arterial circuit also declines. This process allows more blood to reside in the veins, and venous pressure rises. As Q approaches zero, venous pressure approaches the mean circulatory pressure (P_m) (Figure 18–4). The importance of this model is that it can be used to illustrate the role of venous return as an independent determinant of cardiac output.

In its simplest form, cardiac output and central venous pressure of the intact circulation can be assumed to behave as illustrated in Figure 18–5. An increase in venous pressure distends the heart and elevates cardiac output. This behavior of the heart (see Chapter 17) can be superimposed on pressure flow characteristics of the vasculature. Venous return and cardiac output achieve equilibrium at one theoretical point for any given state of cardiac function (Starling curve) and simultaneous set of vascular characteristics (venous return curve). This imaginary point defines a unique equilibrium relation of cardiac output to venous pressure (Figure 18–5). This venous return curve is dramatically influenced by changes in blood volume, vascular capacitance, and arteriolar vascular resistance.

Transfusion elevates the maximal venous return that can be achieved without venous closure. Phlebotomy has the opposite effect. Because neither transfusion nor phlebotomy directly alters resistance or capacitance, the slope of the curve is not altered (Figure 18–6). The two interventions alter mean circulatory pressure because both interventions change blood volume.

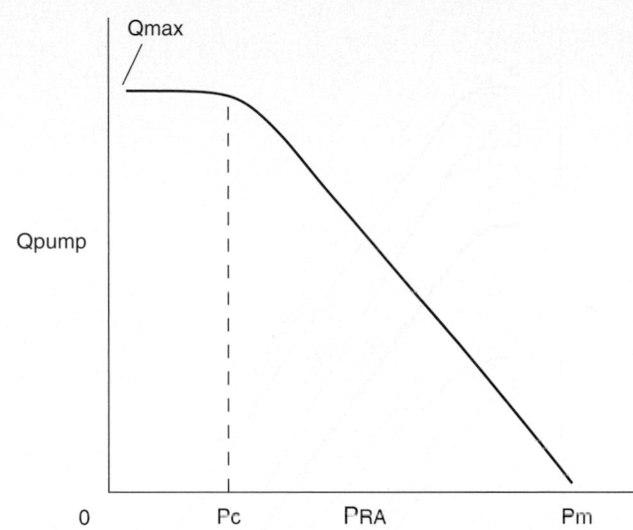

FIGURE 18–4 • Venous return curve. As pump flow *(Qpump)* varies, right atrial pressure *(PRA)* is altered by redistribution of blood between arteries and veins. Qpump cannot be increased above Qmax because PRA would fall below critical closing pressure *(Pc)* of the venous circulation. *Pm,* Mean circulatory pressure of the vasculature at no flow.

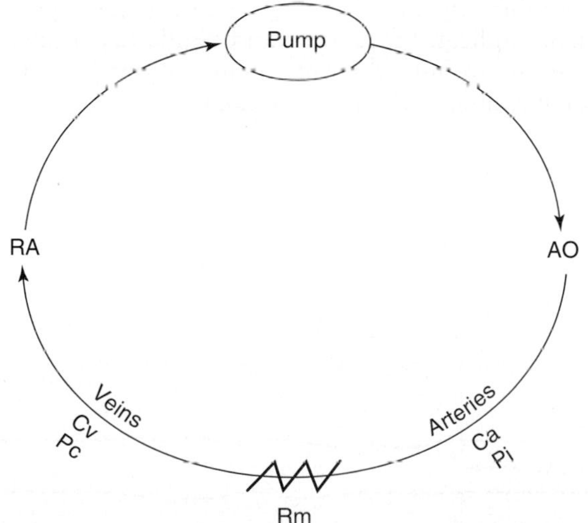

FIGURE 18–3 • Model for facilitating interpretation of the relation of venous return to right atrial pressure. The heart is replaced by a mechanical roller pump. The right atrium *(RA)* is drained by the pump, and blood is infused into the aorta *(AO)*. Blood then traverses the arteries, which have a capacitance *(Ca)* at an inflow pressure *(Pi)* determined by flow rate and microvascular resistance *(Rm)*. Blood then returns through veins having capacitance *(Cv)* and critical closing pressure *(Pc)* to the right atrium.

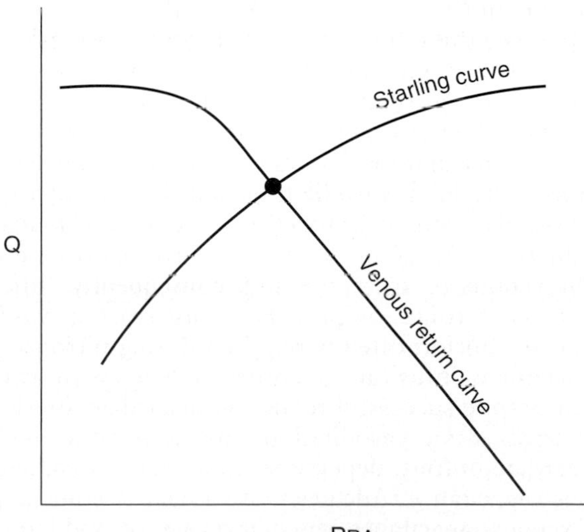

FIGURE 18–5 • Theoretical superimposition of venous return and Starling curves. For any state of the heart and vasculature, these curves intersect at a point that characterizes right atrial pressure *(PRA)* and cardiac output *(Q)*.

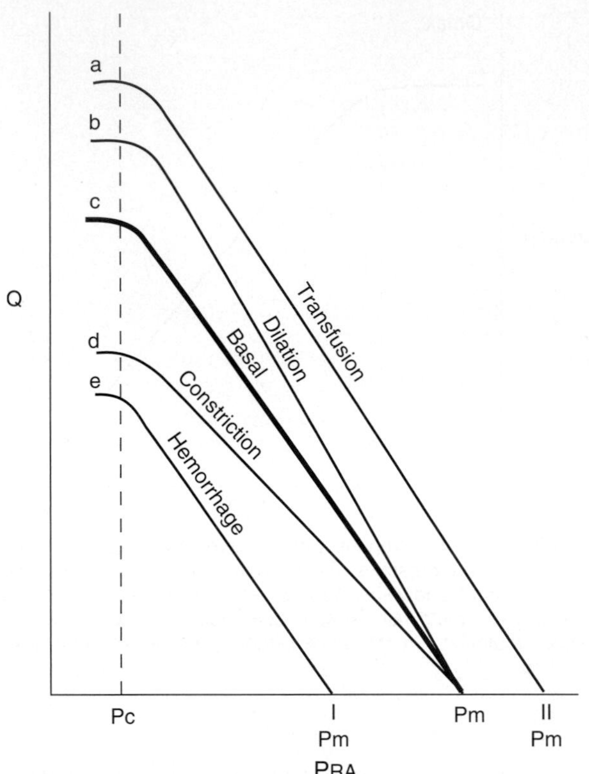

FIGURE 18–6 • Effects of changing blood volume and microvascular resistance on the venous return curve. Curves *a, c,* and *e* are parallel but have different mean circulatory pressure *(Pm)* at zero flow. Curves *b, c,* and *d* are nonparallel but have the same Pm. *Pc,* Critical closing pressure; *PRA,* right atrial pressure.

Acute alterations in vascular capacitance can be expected to have effects similar to transfusion or phlebotomy, but any disparity between the change in C_a and the change in C_v alters the slope of the venous return curve.

Isolated manipulation of incremental resistance alters the maximum venous return attainable without venous collapse yet does not alter mean circulatory pressure. Thus changes in incremental resistance change the shape of the venous return curve (see Figure 18–6).

In clinical practice, the occurrence of any of these changes in vascular mechanics in isolation is unusual. For instance, arteriolar vasodilation and dilation of capacitance vessels often occur together. Arteriolar vasodilation and dilation of capacitance vessels have opposite effects on the venous return curve and, consequently, different effects on cardiac output. For this reason, vascular volume expansion often is required during nitroprusside or tolazoline infusion to ensure adequacy of cardiac output despite successful reduction in cardiac afterload.

In sepsis, toxic vasodilation may cause either high or low cardiac output, depending on associated changes in venous capacitance. Adequacy of vascular volume expansion, venous capacitance, vascular resistance, and inotropic state of the heart can profoundly influence cardiac output in sepsis. Septic shock is warm only if the circulation is adequately filled, cardiac function is sufficient, and incremental resistance is low.

Critical Closing Pressure

In many organs, as inflow pressure is lowered, flow decreases and then ceases at a pressure—the critical closing pressure (P_{cc})—that is higher than venous pressure. The probable mechanism is the vascular waterfall or Starling resistor. In 1910 Jerusalem and Starling[2] described a device that was designed to control afterload to the left ventricle and that made possible the study of cardiac contractility. The device consisted of a collapsible rubber tube traversing a pressurized glass chamber (Figure 18–7). When pressure surrounding the rubber tube exceeded the outflow pressure set by the reservoir, surrounding pressure opposed the flow of blood and became the true outflow pressure of the device. The physiologic counterpart of this process occurs in small vessels surrounded by tissue pressure. In the heart, for example, a Starling resistor effect occurs in extramyocardial coronary veins, although evidence also exists for critical closure of small arterioles. Vessel closure has not been demonstrated directly but may not be necessary. The wall becomes convoluted as small vessels narrow upon compression, and blood cells may become obstructed by the folds even when externally the vessel does not appear to be closed.

Autoregulation

In all organs, when inflow pressure is suddenly raised or lowered while oxygen consumption remains constant, flow rises or falls transiently but then returns to its former value in the phenomenon termed *autoregulation.* Myogenic tonic response is partly responsible for this phenomenon but is not the only mechanism. Some investigators believe tissues have oxygen sensors that respond to transient increases or decreases in oxygen supply; others believe the process is mediated by greater or lesser release of nitric oxide (NO) carried to the tissues by hemoglobin in the form of S-nitrosohemoglobin.[3–5] Evidence indicates that some autoregulatory mechanisms are specific to individual microcirculations (e.g., macula densa signaling in the renal circulation).

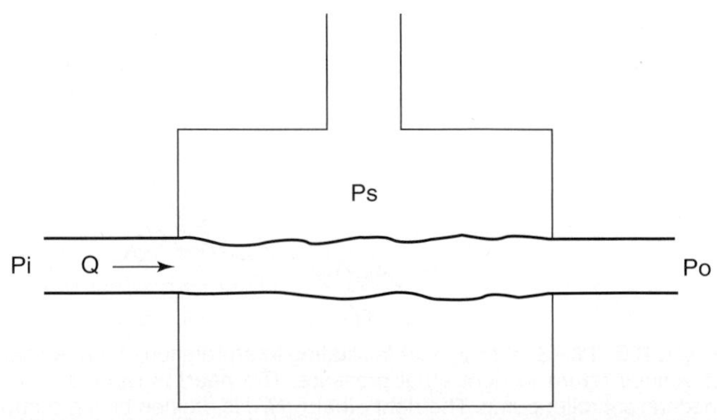

FIGURE 18–7 • Starling resistor is a compressible conduit exposed to surrounding pressure *(Ps).* When Ps is less than outflow pressure *(Po),* Ps does not oppose blood flow. When Ps is between inflow *(Pi)* and outflow pressures, it opposes blood flow. No flow is possible when Ps exceeds Pi.

Distensibility and Compliance

The *distensibility* of a vessel is defined as the change in volume as a proportion of the initial volume for a given change in pressure:

$$\text{Distensibility} = \frac{\Delta V}{\Delta P} \times \frac{1}{V},$$

where V = volume and P = pressure.

Veins are much thinner than arteries, so they are approximately eight times more distensible. Multiplying distensibility by volume yields ΔV/ΔP, which is the definition of compliance. Because venous volume usually is more than three times arterial volume, venous compliance is approximately 20- to 30-fold greater than arterial compliance. As a result, whenever fluids are infused, the bulk of the fluid volume is accommodated in the veins.

Vascular Resistance

Under normal circumstances, vascular resistance is the major regulator of organ flow and can be understood by considering the resistance of a newtonian liquid passing through a rigid tube as defined by the Hagen-Poiseuille equation:

$$R = \left(\frac{8}{\pi}\right)\left(\frac{l}{r^4}\right)\eta$$

where R = resistance, l = tube length, r = internal radius of the tube, and η = fluid viscosity. Applying this equation to the vasculature, the fact that blood is not a newtonian fluid does not have much of an effect on vascular resistance. However, we must account for the fact that vascular beds contain many "tubes" in parallel by adding a factor k to represent the number of vessels. The equation thus becomes

$$R = \left(\frac{8}{\pi}\right)\left(\frac{l}{kr^4}\right)\eta.$$

Because the length and number of vessels and blood viscosity are relatively constant at any one time, change in vessel radius is the major mechanism of changing vascular resistance. Because resistance is related to the fourth power of the radius, small changes in radius cause large changes in resistance. Vessel radius is influenced by vascular elasticity and transmural pressure but is mainly regulated by changes in vessel wall smooth muscle tone.

Vascular Impedance

Resistance is strictly a steady-state concept. In a pulsatile system, the factors affecting the relationship of pressure dissipation to flow are resistance resulting from friction and viscosity, fluid inertia, and vessel wall compliance. These factors combine to produce an *impedance* to flow that varies with frequency. At zero frequency we have the familiar steady-state resistance obtained by taking mean pressure drop and mean flow, but substantial contributions made by the first three harmonics are ignored in our usual calculations.

Local Regulatory Mechanisms

Regions of the circulation may differ markedly in their patterns of vascular regulation. A regulatory stimulus can have multiple effects that differ among locations. An agent that potently regulates vascular resistance in one region of the circulation may have no effect in another region. For example, during hemorrhagic shock, flow is maintained to heart and brain but is reduced to muscle, kidneys, and gut.

Vasomotor tone is strongly influenced by several mechanisms: (1) innervation and neural processes, (2) circulating endocrine and neuroendocrine mediators, (3) local metabolic products, (4) blood gas composition, (5) endothelial-derived factors, and (6) myogenic processes.

Innervation and Neural Processes

Receptors responsive to neural products (norepinephrine, acetylcholine) are found throughout the circulation; nevertheless, innervation and receptor distribution is organ specific. This situation allows rapid, patterned, coordinated redistribution of blood flow and permits an orchestrated response to hypoxia, changes in posture, and hemorrhage. Although these receptors respond to circulating agonists (including adrenal epinephrine) and to those liberated locally, they are generally associated with innervation by autonomic nerves. In general, presynaptic α-adrenergic stimulation causes norepinephrine reuptake, whereas postsynaptic α-adrenergic stimulation causes norepinephrine release and vasoconstriction. β-Adrenergic stimulation generally causes vasodilation. Cholinergic stimulation (whether sympathetic or parasympathetic) generally causes vasodilation (see Chapters 23 and 111).

Circulating Endocrine and Neuroendocrine Mediators

Humoral regulators of vascular tone include angiotensin, arginine vasopressin, bradykinin, histamine, and serotonin. Of less certain significance are aldosterone, thyroxine, antinatriuretic peptide, and various reproductive hormones. Most of these regulators have both direct and secondary effects, which tend to be organ specific or regional in nature. Angiotensin plays a special role in the homeostasis of blood pressure and is produced in hemorrhagic or hypovolemic shock. It causes generalized vasoconstriction in both systemic and pulmonary circulations, but locally it stimulates the release of vasodilating prostaglandins in lung and kidney. Bradykinin is a potent pulmonary and systemic vasodilator released locally by the action of proteolytic enzymes on kallikrein after tissue injury. Histamine, which is released by mast cells in response to injury, is a potent vasodilator in most regions of the circulation but causes vasoconstriction in the lung.

Local Metabolic Products

Local metabolic regulation of vasomotor tone provides an ideal homeostatic mechanism whereby metabolic demand can directly influence perfusion. The precise mechanisms underlying the coupling of blood flow with metabolic activity remain unclear. One theory posits that formation of some vasodilating substance increases as the metabolic rate increases. Thus the regional vasculature relaxes, allowing more oxygen delivery in support of this work. As flow rises, the metabolites are washed out and their concentration is restored to normal. For example, adenosine, which accumulates locally when tissue metabolism is high and tissue oxygenation is marginal, causes pronounced vasodilation in the coronary, striated muscle, splanchnic, and cerebral circulations. Another example is potassium, which is released from muscle in response to increased work, ischemia, and hypoxia.[6] Hypokalemia causes vasoconstriction, and hyperkalemia (within the physiologic range) causes vasodilation.[7,8]

Increasing data demonstrate the importance of the local redox state on regulation of blood flow through the microcirculation. Reactive oxygen species, such as superoxide, hydrogen peroxide, and peroxynitrite, influence normal regulatory processes and participate in the pathophysiology of a wide array of cardiovascular disorders. For example, the rapid reaction of NO with the superoxide anion results in formation of peroxynitrite, a potent oxidant. Under normal conditions peroxynitrite inhibits leukocyte adherence and platelet aggregation without evidence of cellular injury.[9,10] In disease states, however, peroxynitrite can lead to protein nitration and DNA damage. In addition, elevated levels of superoxide may decrease the bioavailabilty of NO, leading to abnormal vasomotion.[11]

Blood Gas Composition

Tissue levels of oxygen and carbon dioxide reflect the adequacy of perfusion and oxygen delivery.[12] These blood gases are potent determinants of regional blood flow and have effects that differ among regions of the circulation. They also have a more general effect mediated by carotid chemoreceptors.

Endothelial-Derived Factors

Vascular endothelial cells are capable of producing a variety of vasoactive substances that participate in the regulation of normal vascular tone. These substances, such as NO and endothelin-1 (ET-1), are capable of producing vascular relaxation and constriction, modulating the propensity of the blood to clot, and inducing and inhibiting smooth muscle migration and replication[13,14] (Figure 18–8). Understanding the role of vascular endothelium in regulating blood flow in health and disease has resulted in several treatment strategies that target the endothelium. Treatments include inhaled NO for pulmonary hypertension, L-arginine supplementation for coronary artery disease and pulmonary vasculopathy of sickle cell disease, phosphodiesterase inhibitors (e.g., sildenafil, which prevents breakdown of cyclic guanosine 3′5′-monophosphate [cGMP]) for pulmonary hypertensive disorders, endothelin receptor antagonists for pulmonary hypertensive disorders and subarachnoid hemorrhage, and NO

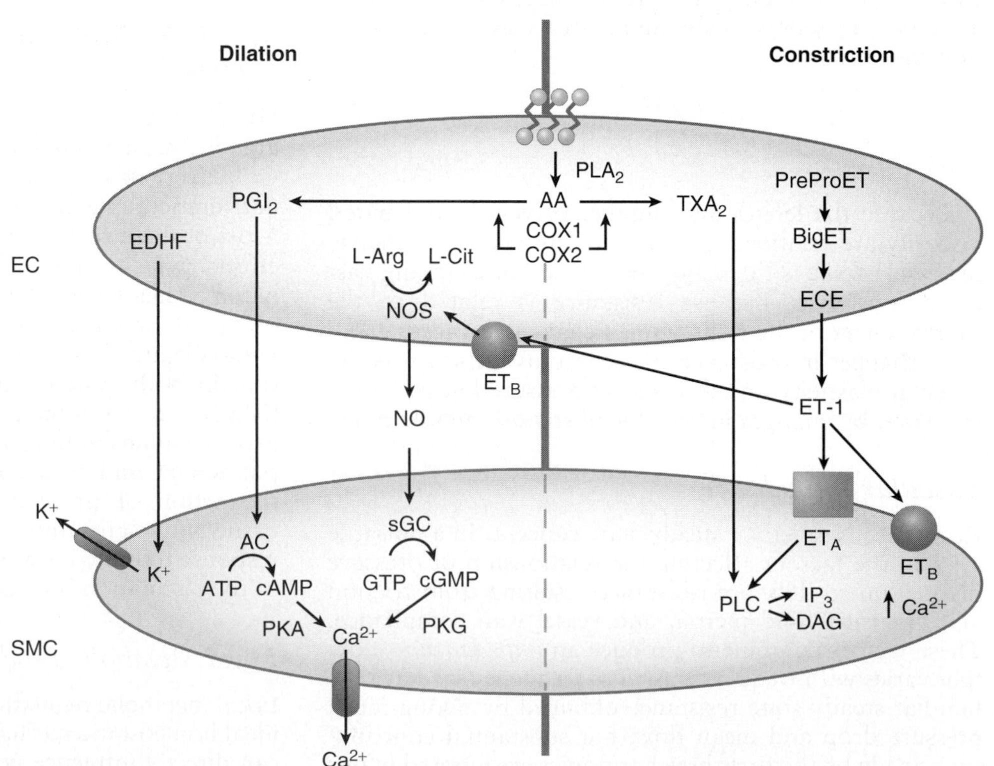

FIGURE 18–8 • Schematic of some endogenous vasoactive agents produced by the vascular endothelium. *AA,* arachidonic acid; *AC,* adenylate cyclase; *ATP,* adenosine triphosphate; *cAMP,* cyclic adenosine monophosphate; *cGMP,* cyclic guanosine monophosphate; *COX,* cyclooxygenase; *DAG,* diacylglycerol; *EC,* endothelial cell; *ECE,* endothelin converting enzyme; *EDHF,* endothelial-derived hyperpolarizing factor; *ET-1,* endothelin-1; *GTP,* guanosine triphosphate; *IP_3,* inositol 1,4,5, triphosphate; *L-arg,* L-arginine; *L-cit,* L-citrulline; *NO,* nitric oxide; *NOS,* nitric oxide synthase; *PGI_2,* prostacyclin; *PKA,* protein kinase A; *PKC,* protein kinase C; *PLA,* phospholipase A_2; *sGC,* soluble guanylate cyclase; *SMC,* smooth muscle cell; *TXA_2,* thromboxane A_2.

inhibitors for refractory hypotension secondary to sepsis. Many older therapies, such as nitrovasodilators, affect endothelial function, a fact that was not appreciated until now.

NO is a labile humoral factor produced by nitric oxide synthase (NOS) from L-arginine in the vascular endothelial cell. NO diffuses into the smooth muscle cell and produces vascular relaxation by increasing concentrations of cGMP, via activation of soluble guanylate cyclase. NO is released in response to a variety of factors, including shear stress (flow) and binding of certain endothelium-dependent vasodilators (such as acetylcholine, adenosine triphosphate [ATP], and bradykinin) to receptors on the endothelial cell. Basal NO release is an important mediator of both resting pulmonary and systemic vascular tone in the fetus, newborn, and adult and of the fall in pulmonary vascular resistance normally occurring at the time of birth.[15–18]

ET-1 is a 21-amino-acid polypeptide also produced by vascular endothelial cells.[19] The vasoactive properties of ET-1 are complex, and studies have shown varying hemodynamic effects on different vascular beds. However, its most striking property is its sustained hypertensive action. ET-1 is the most potent vasoconstricting agent discovered, with a potency 10 times that of angiotensin II. The hemodynamic effects of ET-1 are mediated by at least two distinctive receptor populations: ET_A and ET_B. ET_A receptors are located on vascular smooth muscle cells, and they mediate vasoconstriction. ET_B receptors may be located on endothelial cells, and they mediate both vasodilation and vasoconstriction. Individual endothelins occur in low levels in the plasma, generally below their vasoactive thresholds. This finding suggests endothelins are primarily effective at the local site of release. Even at these levels, they may potentiate the effects of other vasoconstrictors such as norepinephrine and serotonin.[20] The role of endogenous ET-1 in the regulation of normal vascular tone is unclear.[21] Nevertheless, alterations in ET-1 have been implicated in the pathophysiology of a number of disease states.[22]

Endothelial-derived hyperpolarizing factor (EDHF), a diffusible substance that causes vascular relaxation by hyperpolarizing the smooth muscle cell, is another important endothelial factor. EDHF has not yet been identified, but current evidence suggests the action of EDHF is dependent on K^+ channels[23] (see Figure 18–8). Activation of potassium channels in the vascular smooth muscle results in cell membrane hyperpolarization, closure of voltage-dependent calcium channels, and ultimately vasodilation. Potassium channels also are present in endothelial cells. Activation within the endothelium results in changes in calcium flux and may be important in the release of NO, prostacyclin (PGI_2), and EDHF. Potassium channel subtypes include ATP-sensitive K^+ channels, Ca^{2+}-dependent K^+ channels, voltage-dependent K^+ channels, and inward rectifier K^+ channels.[23]

Breakdown of phospholipids within vascular endothelial cells results in production of important byproducts of arachidonic acid, including PGI_2 and thromboxane (TXA_2). PGI_2 activates adenylate cyclase, resulting in increased cAMP production and subsequent vasodilation, whereas TXA_2 results in vasoconstriction via phospholipase C signaling (see Figure 18–8). Other prostaglandins and leukotrienes also have potent vasoactive properties.

In general, regional circulations regulate their flow so that they obtain required amounts of oxygen and nutrients, and all the mechanisms described can be invoked. However, an overriding principle is that shear rate must be kept constant within narrow limits to prevent endothelial damage.[24,25] Any increase in local organ flow is sensed by endothelial integrins that set off a cascade of responses that culminate in NO release.[26]

Myogenic Processes

In 1902 Bayliss[27] described an intrinsic increase in vascular tone in response to elevated intravascular pressure. This myogenic response results in alterations in vascular tone following changes in transmural pressure or stretch.[28] This response is especially important at the arteriolar level and is thought to participate in regional autoregulation. Increases in intravascular pressure and/or stretch result in an increase in arteriolar smooth muscle tone; decreasing pressures have the reverse effect. The precise mechanisms mediating this response are unclear, but a role for dynamic changes in intracellular Ca^{2+} and myosin light-chain phosphorylation has been documented.[29] Later work has focused on the role of tyrosine phosphorylation pathways in this response.[30]

Regional Circulations

Pulmonary Circulation

Maldevelopment and/or maladaptation of the pulmonary vascular bed are important components of several neonatal and infant disease states (e.g., chronic lung disease, persistent pulmonary hypertension of the newborn, congenital heart disease). Therefore an understanding of the fetal and transitional pulmonary circulations is crucial for the critical care physician caring for these infants. In addition, strategies aimed at altering postnatal pulmonary vascular resistance are commonly used in infants and children with congenital heart disease or acute lung injury. Therefore a complete understanding of the regulation of postnatal pulmonary vascular tone also is clinically relevant.

Morphologic development of the pulmonary circulation affects the physiologic changes that occur in the perinatal period. In the fetus and immediate newborn, small pulmonary arteries of all sizes have a thicker muscular coat compared with the external diameter of the vessels than do similar arteries in the adult. This greater muscularity is generally held responsible, at least in part, for the vasoreactivity and high pulmonary vascular resistance found in the fetus, particularly as it draws close to term. In fetal lamb lungs fixed at perfusion pressures similar to those found normally in utero, the medial smooth muscle coat is most prominent in the smallest arteries (fifth- and sixth-generation arteries; external diameter 20–50 μm). During the latter half of gestation, the medial smooth muscle thickness remains constant in relationship to the external diameter of the artery.[31] Similar observations using slightly different techniques have been made in human lungs.[32,33] After birth, particularly within the first several weeks, the medial smooth muscle involutes and the thickness of the media of the small pulmonary arteries decreases rapidly and progressively.[34]

Toward the periphery of the lung, the completely encircling smooth muscle of the media gives way to a region of incomplete muscularization.[33] In these partially muscularized arteries, the smooth muscle is arranged in a spiral or helix. More peripherally, the muscle disappears from arteries that are still larger than capillaries (nonmuscularized small pulmonary arteries). In these nonmuscular small pulmonary arteries, an incomplete pericyte layer is found within the endothelial basement membrane. In the nonmuscular portions of the partially muscular small pulmonary arteries, intermediate cells, that is, cells intermediate in position and structure between pericytes and mature smooth muscle cells, are found.[35] These cells are precursor smooth muscle cells. Under certain conditions, such as hypoxia, they may rapidly differentiate into mature smooth muscle cells.[35]

Small pulmonary arteries (20–50 μm in external diameter) are conveniently identified by their relationship to airways. Preacinar pulmonary arteries lie proximal to or with terminal bronchioli. Intraacinar pulmonary arteries course with respiratory bronchioli or alveolar ductus or within the alveolar walls. In the fetus during the last quarter of gestation, only about half of the pulmonary arteries associated with respiratory bronchioli (precapillary) are muscularized or partially muscularized, and the alveoli are free of muscular arteries.[32] In the adult, complete circumferential muscularization extends peripherally along the intraacinar arteries so that the majority of small pulmonary arteries in relationship to alveoli are completely muscularized. Between birth and the teenage years, the arteries undergo progressive peripheral muscularization. The adult pattern is reached at about the time of puberty.

During fetal growth in lambs, the number of small arteries increase greatly, not only in absolute terms but also per unit volume of lung.[31] In humans, the main preacinar pulmonary arterial branches that accompany the larger airways are developed by 16 weeks.[32] However, development of the intraacinar circulation relates more closely to alveolar development that occurs late in gestation and perhaps even predominantly after birth.[34] As the alveoli multiply, so do the arteries, a process that is generally complete by age 10 years. In early postnatal life (first 2 years in humans), pulmonary arterial growth is more rapid than alveolar growth.[34]

In the lung, extraalveolar vessels course along connective tissue planes that partition the lung into lobes, lobules, and smaller segments, following the airway. These vessels branch and extend into the walls of alveoli (alveolar vessels) or penetrate the "corners" where several alveoli meet. Corner vessels give rise distally to alveolar vessels. Venules and veins, loosely wrapped in connective tissue, follow tissue planes to the hilus of the lung. This intimate anatomic relation of vessels to airspaces provides a structural basis for interactions between circulation and ventilation.

Normal Fetal Circulation

In the fetus, normal gas exchange occurs in the placenta and pulmonary blood flow is low, supplying only nutritional requirements for lung growth and some metabolic functions. Pulmonary blood flow in near-term lambs is about 100 ml/100 g wet lung weight, representing between 8% and 10% of total output of the heart.[36] Pulmonary blood flow is low despite the dominance of the right ventricle, which in the fetus ejects about two thirds of total cardiac output. Most of the right ventricular output is diverted away from the lungs through the widely patent ductus arteriosus to the descending thoracic aorta, from which a large proportion reaches the placenta through the umbilical circulation for oxygenation. In young fetuses (about 0.5 of gestation), pulmonary blood flow is approximately 3% to 4% of the total combined left and right ventricular outputs of the heart (fetal cardiac output). This value increases to approximately 6% at nearly 0.8 gestation, corresponding temporally with the onset of release of surface active material into lung fluid. This step is followed by another progressive slow rise in pulmonary blood flow, reaching approximately 8% to 10% near term.[36] Fetal pulmonary arterial pressure increases with advancing gestation. At term, mean pulmonary arterial pressure is about 50 mm Hg, generally exceeding mean

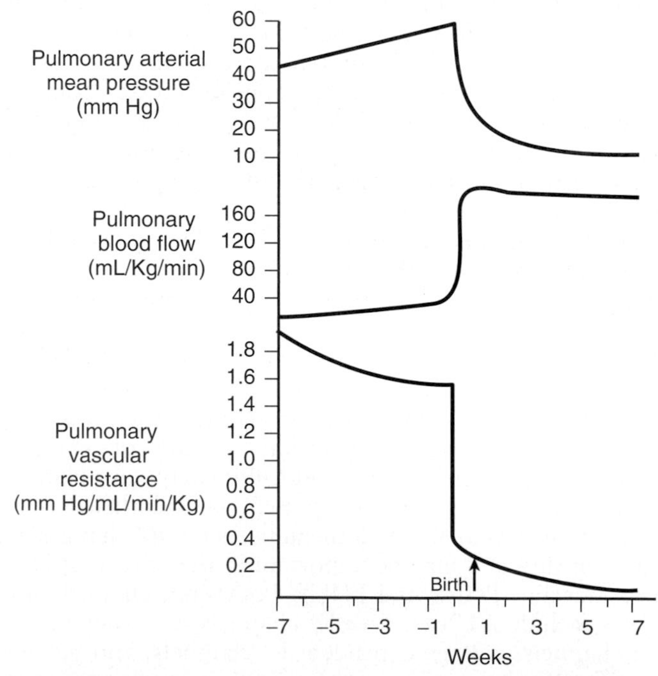

FIGURE 18–9 Changes in mean pulmonary arterial pressure, pulmonary blood flow, and pulmonary vascular resistance at birth. (Data from Morin FC III, Egan E: Pulmonary hemodynamics in fetal lambs during development at normal and increased oxygen tension. *J Appl Physiol* 73:213-218, 1993; Soifer SJ, Morin FC III, Kaslow DC, et al: The developmental effects of prostaglandin D2 on the pulmonary and systemic circulations in the newborn lamb. *J Dev Physiol* 5: 237-250, 1983.)

descending aortic pressure by 1 to 2 mm Hg.[37] Pulmonary vascular resistance early in gestation is extremely high relative to that in the infant and adult, probably because of the low number of small arteries. Pulmonary vascular resistance falls progressively during the last half of gestation, new arteries develop, and cross-sectional area increases. However, baseline pulmonary vascular resistance still is much higher than after birth.[37,38]

Changes in Pulmonary Circulation at Birth

After birth, with initiation of ventilation by the lungs and the subsequent increase in pulmonary and systemic arterial blood O_2 tensions, pulmonary vascular resistance decreases and pulmonary blood flow increases by 8- to 10-fold to match systemic blood flow (300–400 ml/min/kg body weight). This large increase in pulmonary blood flow increases pulmonary venous return to the left atrium, increasing left atrial pressure. The valve of the foramen ovale closes, preventing significant atrial right-to-left shunting of blood. In addition, the ductus arteriosus constricts and closes functionally within several hours after birth, effectively separating the pulmonary and systemic circulations. Mean pulmonary arterial pressure decreases and, by age 24 hours, is approximately 50% of mean systemic arterial pressure. Adult values are reached 2 to 6 weeks after birth[39,40] (Figure 18–9).

The decrease in pulmonary vascular resistance with ventilation and oxygenation at birth is regulated by a complex and incompletely understood interplay between metabolic and mechanical factors, which in turn are triggered by the ventilatory and circulatory changes that occur at birth. Physical expansion of the fetal lamb lung without changing O_2 tension increases fetal pulmonary blood flow and decreases pulmonary vascular resistance, but not to newborn values.[41] A small proportion of this decrease is related to replacement of fluid in the alveoli with gas, which allows unkinking of the small pulmonary arteries, and to changes in alveolar surface tension, which exert a negative dilating pressure on the small pulmonary arteries, maintaining their patency.[42] Physical expansion of the lung releases vasoactive substances such as PGI_2, which increases pulmonary blood flow and decreases pulmonary vascular resistance in the fetal goat and lamb.[43] Net production of PGI_2 by the lung occurs with initiation of ventilation at birth.[43] In addition, inhibitors of prostaglandin synthesis (such as indomethacin and meclofenamic acid) not only block PGI_2 production but also attenuate the increase in pulmonary blood flow and decrease in pulmonary vascular resistance that occur with physical expansion of the fetal lung, although not the changes that occur with oxygenation.[44] Therefore PGI_2, or perhaps (but less likely) another metabolite of arachidonic acid, plays an important role in the increase in pulmonary blood flow and decrease in pulmonary vascular resistance that occur in association with the mechanical component (stretch) of ventilation at birth.

Ventilation of the fetus without oxygenation produces partial pulmonary vasodilatation, whereas ventilation with air or oxygen produces complete pulmonary vasodilatation. The exact mechanisms of oxygen-induced pulmonary vasodilation during the transitional circulation remain unclear. The increase in alveolar or arterial O_2 tension may decrease pulmonary vascular resistance either directly by dilating the small pulmonary arteries or indirectly by stimulating production of vasodilator substances such as PGI_2 or NO. In particular, NO has been implicated as an important mediator of the decrease in pulmonary vascular resistance at birth associated with increased oxygenation.[45–50] However, the immediate decrease in pulmonary vascular resistance minutes after birth is not attenuated by NO inhibition. Therefore the decrease in pulmonary vascular resistance with initiation of ventilation and oxygenation consists of at least two components. First is partial pulmonary vasodilatation caused by physical expansion of the lung and the production of prostaglandins (PGI_2 and PGD_2). This process probably is independent of fetal oxygenation and results in a modest increase in pulmonary blood flow and decrease in pulmonary vascular resistance. Second is a further maximal pulmonary vasodilatation associated with fetal oxygenation, which is not necessarily dependent on prostaglandin production. This process results in an increase in pulmonary blood flow and a decrease in pulmonary vascular resistance to newborn values. The latter pulmonary vasodilatation likely is caused by synthesis of NO. Both components are necessary for successful transition to extrauterine life. An additional mechanism by which vasodilatation occurs is related to the stimulation by increased shear forces of endothelial cells to produce both NO and PGI_2. It is possible that after the initial decrease in pulmonary vascular resistance because of another mechanism, this particular mechanism acts to maintain pulmonary vasodilatation.

Control of perinatal pulmonary circulation probably reflects a balance between factors producing pulmonary vasoconstriction (low O_2, leukotrienes, other vasoconstricting substances) and those producing pulmonary vasodilatation (high O_2, PGI_2, NO, other vasodilating substances). The dramatic increase in pulmonary blood flow with initiation of ventilation and oxygenation at birth reflects a shift from active pulmonary vasoconstriction in the fetus to active pulmonary vasodilatation in the newborn.

Failure of the pulmonary circulation to undergo this normal fall in pulmonary vascular resistance at birth (persistent pulmonary hypertension of the newborn) is associated with a variety of conditions, including aspiration syndromes, sepsis, in utero stress events, and certain congenital heart defects (e.g., obstruction of pulmonary venous drainage, hypoplastic left heart syndrome with restrictive atrial septum).

Regulation of Postnatal Pulmonary Vascular Resistance

As stated earlier, mean pulmonary arterial pressure decreases to approximately 50% of mean systemic arterial pressure by age 24 hours. Adult values are reached 2 to 6 weeks after birth.[39,40] Therefore after the immediate postnatal state, the pulmonary circulation is maintained in a dilated, low-resistance state.

Because the inflow pressure of the pulmonary circulation is low, a vertical gradation to the distribution of

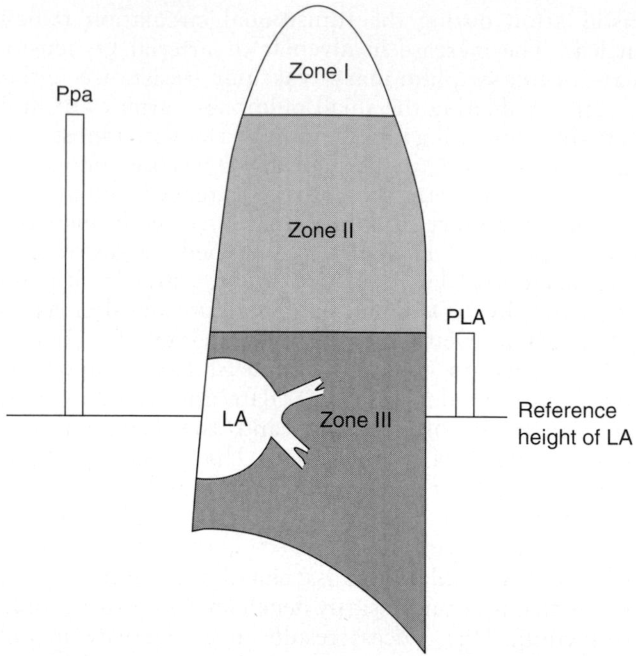

FIGURE 18–10 • The lung is divided vertically into three regions. Zone I alveolar capillary units are unperfused because they see no functional inflow pressure. Zone II units are perfused in proportion to their height above the left atrium *(LA)*. Zone III vasculature is more uniformly perfused because gravity has comparable effects on inflow and outflow pressures. (Redrawn from Fuhrman BP: Regional circulation. In Fuhrman BP, Shoemaker WC, editors: *Critical care: state of the art,* vol 10, Fullerton, CA, 1989, Society of Critical Care Medicine.)

blood flow in the lung occurs. Hydrostatic pressure must be adjusted for vertical height above the left atrium, both at the inflow and at the outflow of every alveolar capillary unit. For example, given a pulmonary artery mean pressure of 20 cm H_2O (zeroed at the level of the left atrium), an alveolar capillary unit 12 cm above the left atrium faces an inflow pressure of only 8 cm H_2O. A left atrial pressure of 5 cm H_2O generates no opposing outflow pressure to alveolar capillary units more than 5 cm above the left atrium. Critical closing pressure of postcapillary vessels therefore sets outflow pressure for a unit 10 cm above the left atrium. Were intrinsic vascular resistance identical throughout the lung, flow at any vertical height would be determined by hydrostatic driving pressure (inflow-outflow) and would be greatest at the base and least at the apex of the lung. West, Dollery, and Naimark[51] reported that this phenomenon partitions the lung into three vertical regions (Figure 18–10). Zone I vessels are higher above the left atrium than pulmonary artery pressure (expressed in cm H_2O) and are not perfused by the pulmonary artery. Zone II vessels lie above the height defined by the hydrostatic left atrial pressure but below the height of pulmonary artery pressure. These units are perfused in proportion to the driving pressure across them, which is approximately pulmonary artery pressure less vertical height (or critical closing pressure, whichever is higher). Zone III vessels lie at a vertical height less than outflow pressure expressed in cm H_2O. Driving pressure across these units is independent of height because inflow and outflow pressures are comparably influenced by gravity.

Again, because of the intimate relation of small pulmonary vessels to alveoli, airway pressure modulates pulmonary blood flow. Alveolar capillary unit now is known to have similar properties.[52] Alveolar pressure can be loosely translated into surrounding pressure for alveolar vessels. Positive airway pressure applied to the lung can impinge on alveolar vessels whenever alveolar pressure exceeds the other determinants of outflow pressure. During positive pressure ventilation, outflow pressure of the pulmonary circulation can be determined predominantly by the mechanics of ventilation. The lung is partitioned into zones, but the distribution of flow becomes a complex function of alveolar pressure and of left atrial and critical closing pressures.

To further complicate this view of the pulmonary circulation, lung volume and alveolar pressure both change over the respiratory cycle during positive pressure ventilation. In inspiration, extraalveolar and corner vessels are dilated by radial traction, reducing their resistance to flow, whereas alveolar vessels narrow and elongate.[53] During lung inflation, alveolar surface tension rises, diminishing the transmission of alveolar pressure to alveolar vessels.[54] Evidence also indicates that, in the infant lamb, lung stretch may directly augment pulmonary vascular tone in a manner that is dependent on calcium flux and subject to calcium channel blockade using verapamil.[55] Mechanical ventilation can have profound direct effects on the intact pulmonary circulation that depend on the waveform of airway pressure applied and not on mean airway pressure alone.[56,57]

In nonuniform lung disease, application of positive airway pressure can modulate and redistribute blood flow away from ventilated regions and toward unventilated regions of the lung by directly elevating the pulmonary vascular resistance of lung segments exposed to elevated airway pressure, that is, segments not protected by consolidation or airway obstruction.[44]

Evidence suggests that basal release of NO and the subsequent increase in smooth muscle cell concentrations of cGMP partly mediate the low resting pulmonary vascular resistance of the newborn.[17,58] Other vasoactive substances, including histamine, 5-hydroxytryptamine, bradykinin, and metabolites of arachidonic acid by the cyclooxygenase and lipoxygenase pathways, have been implicated in mediation of postnatal pulmonary vascular tone. However, their roles, if any, are not well elucidated. Two of the most important factors affecting pulmonary vascular resistance in the postnatal period are oxygen concentration and pH. Decreasing oxygen tension and decreases in pH elicit pulmonary vasoconstriction of the resting pulmonary circulation.[59] Alveolar hypoxia constricts pulmonary arterioles, diverting blood flow away from hypoxic lung segments and toward well-oxygenated segments.[60] This process enhances ventilation/perfusion matching and prevents wasting of blood flow on diseased lung. This is an unusual response to hypoxia, which probably is greater in the younger animal than in the adult.[61] In most vascular beds (i.e., cerebral vasculature), alveolar hypoxia is a potent vasodilator. The mechanism of alveolar hypoxic pulmonary vasoconstriction remains to be defined and is the subject of several extensive reviews.[62] Acidosis potentiates hypoxic pulmonary vasoconstriction, and alkalosis reduces it.[59] The exact mechanism of pH-mediated pulmonary vasoactive responses is incompletely understood but appears to be independent of Pa_{CO_2}.[63] Alveolar hyperoxia and alkalosis often are used to relax pulmonary vascular tone because they generally relieve pulmonary vasoconstriction but have little apparent effect on the systemic circulation as a whole. However, detrimental effects of hypocarbia or respiratory alkalosis on cerebral and myocardial blood flow may occur.[64]

The lung is innervated, but neural effects on pulmonary vascular resistance appear to be of little consequence to basal tone. However, pulmonary neurohumoral receptors are sensitive to α-adrenergic, β-adrenergic, and dopaminergic agonists. Therefore vasoactive agents that stimulate these receptors affect the vascular tone of both the pulmonary and systemic circulations. The degree of pulmonary versus systemic alterations induced by these agents is variable and often dictated by the relative tone of each vascular bed at a given time. The response of these agents is difficult to predict in an individual critically ill patient.

A selective pulmonary vasodilator for treatment of pulmonary hypertension has long been sought. However, with the exception of oxygen, the response of the pulmonary circulation to humoral vasoactive agents is generally similar to that of the systemic circulation as a whole. Inhaled NO may prove to be the long-sought selective pulmonary vasodilator. Of note, its selectivity is not based on a differential effect in the pulmonary and systemic circulations. When NO is delivered as a free gas via the inhalational route, it is rapidly bound to hemoglobin after uptake in the circulation and therefore is not delivered to the systemic circulation. To take advantage of this pharmacologic selectivity, other agents with rapid metabolism delivered via inhalational routes are being studied (i.e., inhaled prostacyclin).

Cerebral Circulation

Although the general principles governing circulation certainly hold true for the cerebral circulation, blood flow to the brain is specially regulated to facilitate the myriad of complex functions overseen by the brain.

The brain makes up 2% of body mass, receiving approximately 14% of the cardiac output, but accounts for close to 20% of the body's O_2 consumption. Other organ systems receive a larger percentage of the total cardiac output (e.g., the lung) and use larger amounts of oxygen (e.g., skeletal muscle), but the brain is unique in its intolerance for diminished blood flow. Unconsciousness occurs in seconds and irreversible damage and death within minutes of circulatory arrest under normal conditions.[65–68]

Blood is supplied to the brain by the carotid and vertebral arteries. The common carotid artery bifurcates, forming the internal carotid artery (ICA) and external carotid artery. The ICA gives rise to its major branches, the posterior communicating, anterior cerebral, middle cerebral, and anterior choroidal arteries, which compose the *anterior circulation*. The vertebral arteries give rise to the anterior spinal and posterior inferior cerebellar arteries before merging to form the basilar artery, which in turn gives rise to the anterior inferior cerebellar, superior cerebellar, and posterior cerebral arteries. These vessels compose the *posterior circulation*. Venous drainage from the superficial and deep cerebral veins enters the dural sinuses and exits the cranium mostly via the internal jugular vein, although the vertebral veins are an important secondary pathway available for venous outflow.[69]

The cranium has three compartments: tissue, cerebral spinal fluid, and blood. The Monro-Kellie doctrine states that these compartments occupy a relatively fixed space and that an increase in one compartment can occur only at the expense of another. For example, with brain swelling, cerebrospinal fluid and cerebral venous blood must be displaced if intracranial pressure (ICP) is to remain unchanged. As the limits of cerebrospinal fluid and blood evacuation are approached, ICP rises. Raised ICP and/or venous obstruction can impede cerebral blood flow (CBF). Therefore cerebral perfusion pressure (CPP), generally defined as the difference between the MAP and ICP, is a more accurate descriptor of the pressure causing flow to the brain. This observation has important implications with respect to autoregulation because CPP and not simply MAP modulates autoregulation.[70] CBF declines when CPP falls below the lower limit of the autoregulatory curve. In the setting of raised ICP or venous hypertension, this process occurs even in the face of elevated systemic arterial pressures.

At rest, CBF is approximately 50 ml/100 g tissue/min.[71] Cerebral oxygen consumption is surprisingly high, averaging 3.2 ml/100 g tissue/min. Glucose is the primary energy substrate, although ketones can be used during

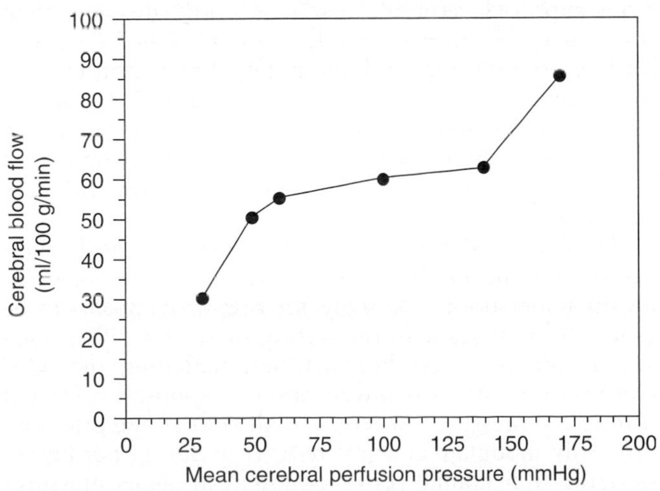

FIGURE 18–11 • Cerebral blood flow *(CBF)* autoregulates at perfusion pressures between 50 and 160 mmHg. Below 50 mmHg, CBF falls. Above 160 mmHg, CBF rises. (Redrawn from Fuhrman BP: Regional circulation. In Fuhrman BP, Shoemaker WC, editors: *Critical care: state of the art,* vol 10, Fullerton, CA, 1989, Society of Critical Care Medicine.)

periods of starvation. The brain has no functional capacity to store energy. It is completely dependent on a steady supply of O_2 as up to 92% of its ATP production results from the oxidative metabolism of glucose.[65–68]

An important feature unique to the cerebral circulation is the presence of a blood-brain barrier (BBB). The vascular endothelium of brain capillaries forms a continuous sheet, with adjacent cells joined by tight junctions. Unlike the endothelium of nonneural capillaries, vascular endothelium does not contain intercellular clefts through which water-soluble particles can traverse, and pinocytosis is markedly diminished. Lipid-soluble substances, CO_2, and O_2, however, can freely diffuse across the endothelium. Metabolically important components, such as glucose, lactate, and amino acids, depend upon specific carrier proteins to facilitate their diffusion into the brain. Furthermore, the BBB has a biochemical component, with high levels of degradative enzymes that protect the vascular smooth muscle and extracellular fluid from the effects of circulating vasoactive substances, such as catecholamines.[72] As a result of the BBB, the cerebral vasculature responds differently than other vascular beds to humoral stimuli. However, humoral stimuli can significantly alter the vascular tone of large cerebral arteries and can affect blood flow to parts of the brain lacking a complete BBB, such as the choroid plexus, median eminence, and area postrema.[73,74]

For more than 60 years it has been recognized that CBF remains constant over a wide range of mean systemic arterial pressures (60–150 mmHg)[75] (Figure 18–11). Constant CBF is maintained in the face of increasing inflow pressures by compensatory vasoconstriction. Conversely, in the setting of low systemic arterial pressures (i.e., low inflow pressures), the cerebral vasculature dilates in order to maintain steady CBF. At systemic arterial pressures outside the autoregulatory range, further dilation or constriction can no longer regulate blood flow. At pressures greater than 150 mmHg, disruption of the BBB ensues with subsequent edema and even hemorrhage from ruptured cerebral vessels. At pressures less than 60 mmHg, CBF begins to fall, with continued decreases leading to ischemia and ultimately brain death.[66,76–78] Importantly, normal cerebral autoregulation can be impaired in the setting of disease. Traumatic brain injury, subarachnoid hemorrhage, and stroke, for example, all can abolish or impair the normal autoregulatory response.[79–82]

The brain's ability to autoregulate flow is well established, but the mechanisms underlying it are not completely understood.[78] A *myogenic response* appears to be especially important in the setting of raised CPP. Large- and medium-size cerebral arteries, including the ICA, constrict both *in vitro* and *in vivo* in response to elevated transmural pressures. Whereas small arteries and arterioles primarily modulate cerebral resistance during normotension, the large cranial vessels dominate at higher pressures (>110 mmHg). Thus at high perfusion pressures, smaller more delicate vessels are protected by changes in upstream resistance.[70,78]

In marked contrast to other vascular beds, neural stimuli have relatively little effect on basal CBF. Cerebral vessels display extensive perivascular innervation, especially by the sympathetic nerves arising from the superior cervical sympathetic ganglia, but the brain is well protected from circulating catecholamines by the BBB. Thus many of the vasoactive agents used in the critical care setting (α- and β-adrenergic agonists) have minimal effects on resting cerebral vascular tone. Mild-to-moderate electrical stimulation, as well as surgical resection of both the sympathetic and parasympathetic nervous system, does not alter cerebral vascular tone under resting conditions. However, vigorous sympathetic stimulation, as occurs with strenuous exercise or hypertension, does result in vasoconstriction of large- and medium-size cerebral vessels.[68] Thus a neurogenic mechanism may not mediate cerebral vascular resistance under normal conditions, but it does provide protection at times of stress.[70,83,84] Patients with chronic hypertension have shown a rightward shift of the autoregulatory curve.[68,78]

With the advent of sophisticated methods for detecting and measuring CBF, such as radioactive xenon, intracerebral regional circulatory variations could be mapped and were found to correlate with local central nervous system activation.[71,85,86] Blood flow to the occipital cortex increases with visual stimulation.[87] Motor activity augments flow to the motor strip and speech enhances flow to Broca's area.[88,89] CBF decreases during deep sleep but returns to normal awake levels during rapid eye movement sleep.[90]

As in other vascular beds, CBF appears to be linked or "coupled" to changes in metabolism.[91–93] For example, hypothermia decreases the cerebral metabolic rate of oxygen ($CMRO_2$), and therefore CBF, in both animal and human studies.[94–97] Seizure activity and fever both increase $CMRO_2$ and CBF, which explains the deleterious consequences of the two conditions for patients with raised ICP.[98] The mechanisms underlying this coupling of blood flow and metabolism are unclear. A number of substances affect cerebrovascular tone, including carbon dioxide,

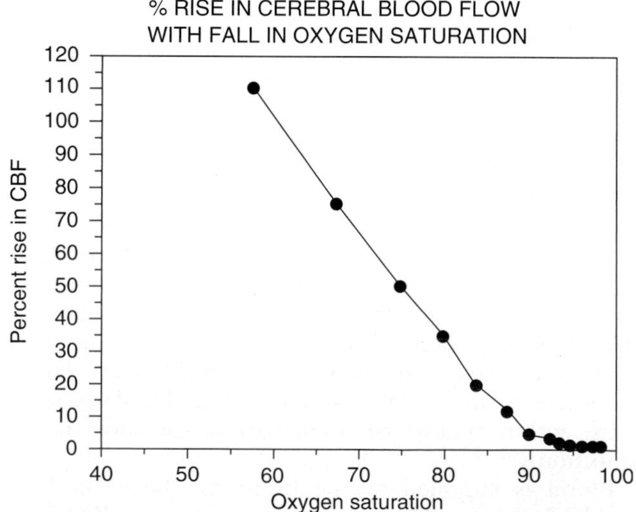

FIGURE 18–12 • Arterial hypoxia dilates cerebral vessels and maintains cerebral oxygen delivery. *CBF,* Cerebral blood flow. (Redrawn from Fuhrman BP: Regional circulation. In Fuhrman BP, Shoemaker WC, editors: *Critical care: state of the art,* vol 10, Fullerton, CA, 1989, Society of Critical Care Medicine.)

oxygen, hydrogen ions, lactic acid, histamine, potassium ions, prostaglandin, ET-1, NO, and adenosine.[66,68]

Carbon dioxide plays a critical role in regulation of CBF. A linear increase in CBF is seen with increasing $PaCO_2$, making CO_2 one of the most potent known cerebral vasodilators.[99,100] Carbon dioxide exerts its effect via reduction of perivascular pH. Arterial H^+ cannot cross the BBB, but CO_2 can easily diffuse into the brain. Carbonic anhydrase facilitates the reaction between CO_2 and H_2O, forming carbonic acid with subsequent dissociation producing H^+ ions. Perivascular acidosis dilates the cerebral vasculature, whereas alkalosis leads to vasoconstriction.[101,102] In this way the cerebral vasculature is distinct in that respiratory acidosis and alkalosis alter tone and CBF, whereas metabolic acidosis and alkalosis do not.[100,103] Although CO_2 predominates in affecting transient changes in the extracellular pH, other metabolic byproducts, such as lactate and pyruvate, also can have an effect and contribute to changes in regional blood flow.

Several workers demonstrated that the cerebral vasculature adapts to chronically elevated $PaCO_2$, with changes in the pH of the brain extracellular fluid.[104] This finding has obvious implications for the clinician attempting to treat raised ICP with chronic hyperventilation. Interestingly, abnormal CO_2 reactivity has been associated with several disease processes, including traumatic brain injury, subarachnoid hemorrhage, stroke, carotid stenosis, and congestive heart failure.[79–81] Abnormal CO_2 vasoreactivity has been used as a means to prognosticate in some disease states.[81,82]

Arterial oxygen tension (PaO_2) also participates in regulation of CBF. Arterial hypoxia dilates cerebral vessels at PaO_2 less than 40 to 50 mmHg (Figure 18–12).[99] The relation between CBF and arterial oxygen content is almost linear, and cerebral oxygen delivery can be maintained unless arterial oxygen content falls below 4 vol%. However, hyperoxia does not appear to be a highly potent stimulus for vasoconstriction.[99,105] Hypoxic vasodilation is not limited to the cerebral circulation. Efforts to fully elucidate this phenomenon continue, but adenosine and both Ca^{2+} activated and ATP activated potassium channels are known to be particularly important. Adenosine, which leads to vasodilation through an increase in cAMP, increases more than fivefold with hypoxia.[106–109] Adenosine also is critical in autoregulation. Experimental data reveal a sixfold rise in brain adenosine levels as MAP falls from 135 to 45 mmHg.[110]

A large body of evidence from both animals and humans implicates NO in a number of important processes within the cerebral circulation.[105,111–116] NO antagonists mitigate the normal increase in CBF resulting from neuronal activation.[113,117,118] Multiple lines of evidence suggest NO has a role in maintenance of basal cerebrovascular tone.[119] Exogenously administered inhibitors of NOS constrict cerebral vessels and decrease CBF in the basal state of several species, including humans.[118,120–123] Interestingly, ADMA, an endogenous and potent inhibitor of NOS that has been implicated in a number of vascular disorders, is produced in the brain, but its precise role in regulating CBF is not clear.[124,125] Vascular reactivity to CO_2 also is strongly influenced by NO.[126] One study of humans found decreased MCA flow in response to hypercapnia following NOS inhibition.[105] Similar results have been confirmed by others and documented in animal studies as well.[112,122,126] CO_2 reactivity is not completely ablated, however, suggesting that other factors also contribute. Further, in a neuronal-NOS-knockout mouse model, CO_2 reactivity remained intact, again suggesting redundant systems underlying the response.[126–128] Of note clinically, nitroprusside and other NO donor compounds can dilate cerebral vessels.[129] This process greatly complicates the management of hypertension in patients with increased ICP. In such patients, nitroprusside may reduce arterial pressure but raise both CBF and blood volume, thereby causing herniation.

Vasodilation in response to acetylcholine, oxytocin, substance P, histamine, ET-1, ADP, ATP, and prostaglandin all have been shown to be NO dependent.[23] In some studies, NOS inhibition blunted the increase in blood flow in response to hypoxia.[111] A role for NO in other disease states also has been demonstrated. Treatment with L-arginine, the substrate for NOS, and tetrahydrobiopterin, an important cofactor for NOS, reverse impaired endothelial function resulting from acute hypertension, hypercholesterolemia, and atherosclerosis.[130–132] In addition, impaired NO signaling is important in the pathophysiology of subarachnoid hemorrhage in which endothelial dysfunction has been well documented, leading to the important clinical problem of vasospasm. A number of mechanisms have been proposed, including decreased endothelial NOS activity, alterations in soluble guanylate cyclase activation and cGMP production, inactivation of NO by hemoglobin, and increased superoxide anion production.[133–137] Furthermore, alterations in vascular tone in response to shear force are mediated, at least in part, by NO.[23] Beyond its effects on vascular tone, NO is protective in the cerebral circulation by its inhibition of platelet aggregation and leukocyte adherence.[138]

Prostacyclin, a metabolite of arachidonic acid, is another important dilator of the cerebral vasculature. The cyclooxygenase enzymes COX-1 and COX-2 appear to be involved in basal cerebral vascular tone and in the vasodilation associated with various stimuli, such as inflammation and hypoxia, depending on the species investigated.[23,67,68]

ET-1 is another important mediator of cerebrovascular tone.[139] Both ET_A and ET_B receptors have been identified in the cerebral vasculature.[140] ET-1 given in high concentrations constricts cerebral vessels, probably via ET_A receptor activation.[141] However, ET-1 given in low concentrations relaxes cerebral vessels via endothelial cell ET_B receptor activation, a response that is NO dependent. Sarafotoxin 6c (a selective ET_B agonist) causes cerebral vasodilation.[140] However, ET_A and combined receptor antagonists do not alter basal cerebrovascular tone.[23] ET-1 has been identified as an important mediator of vasospasm following subarachnoid hemorrhage.[141,142] ET-1 levels are increased following subarachnoid hemorrhage. In association with the increase in ET-1 levels are increases in ET_A receptor levels, smooth muscle cell ET_B receptor levels (which mediate vasoconstriction), and endothelin-converting enzyme activity.[143] The potential clinical use of ET receptor antagonists following subarachnoid hemorrhage is under investigation.

Reactive oxygen species, especially superoxide, participate in regulation of cerebral vascular tone. Production of superoxide anion has been associated with acute hypertension, seizures, head injury, meningitis, and cerebral ischemia.[144–148]

Coronary Circulation

Right and left coronary arteries arise from the sinuses of Valsalva and course over the surface of the heart. Nutrient branches penetrate the myocardium to supply both superficial (epicardial) and deep (subendocardial) layers of the muscle. Venous blood drains primarily to the coronary sinus, although some blood returns via anterior coronary veins to the right atrium or sinusoids directly to the ventricles.

Because life itself is blood flow dependent, myocardial work load (which sets myocardial oxygen demand) is determined not only by the needs of the heart but also by the demands of the body. Furthermore, the heart is required to generate its own perfusion pressure. Accordingly, regulation of myocardial perfusion is tailored to match regional myocardial oxygen supply to demand over the widest possible range of cardiac workload and under conditions fashioned not so much for maximal cardiac efficiency but rather for benefit of the body.

Myocardial perfusion normally is approximately the same per gram of tissue in the outer (subepicardial), mid, and inner (subendocardial) layers of the left ventricle, but the dynamics during the cardiac cycle are complicated.[6] At the end of diastole, when the ventricle is relaxed and tissue pressures probably are less than 10 mmHg in any layer of the left ventricle, pressures in the intramural arteries probably are similar to each other and to aortic pressure. At the beginning of systole, tissue pressure rises to equal intracavitary pressure in the subendocardium but then falls off linearly across the wall to approximately 10 mmHg in the subepicardium.[149] These pressures are for an instant added to those inside the vessels because the vessels walls are not rigid. As a result, intravascular pressures in subendocardial arteries exceed aortic pressures, but aortic pressures are higher than pressures in subepicardial arteries.[150] These pressure gradients and the greater shortening of subendocardial than subepicardial muscle fibers during systole compress the subendocardial vessels and squeeze blood out of them both forward into the coronary sinus and backward toward the epicardium.[151–153] Narrowing of the subendocardial vessels facilitates thickening and shortening of the myocytes.[154] This backflow enters the subepicardial arteries to supply their systolic flow.[150] In systole, some forward flow occurs into the orifices of the coronary arteries but does not perfuse the myocardium; it merely fills the extramyocardial arteries.[6,150,155] In fact, often reverse flow occurs in the epicardial coronary arteries.[156] In early diastole, blood flows first into the subepicardial vessels that have not been compressed but takes longer to refill the narrowed subendocardial vessels. Given enough time and perfusing pressure, all the myocardium will be perfused, but if diastole is too short or perfusion pressure too low, subendocardial ischemia occurs. On the other

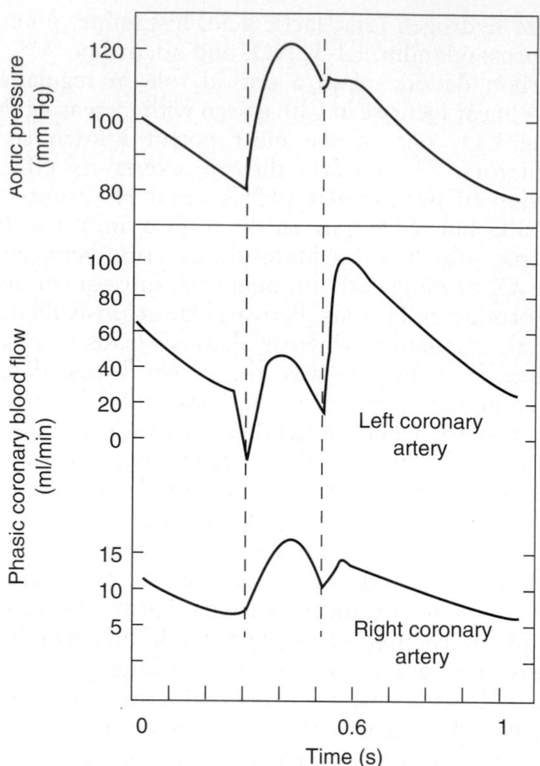

FIGURE 18–13 • Myocardial blood flow is modulated by ventricular wall tension. Most of the perfusion of the left ventricular myocardium occurs in diastole. (Adapted from Berne RM, Levy MN: *Cardiovascular physiology*, ed 7, St. Louis, 1997, Mosby.)

hand, right ventricular myocardium normally is perfused in both systole and diastole (Figure 18–13) because of lower tissue pressures.[157,158] We expect perfusion of the hypertrophied right ventricle of severe pulmonic stenosis or tetralogy of Fallot to resemble that of the left ventricle.[159]

Myocardial Oxygen Demand-Supply Relationship

The left ventricle extracts most of the oxygen from the blood passing through the myocardium; coronary sinus oxygen saturation normally is approximately 30%. Therefore increases in myocardial oxygen demand must be met by increases in myocardial blood flow. At rest, left ventricular myocardial blood flow is approximately 80 to 100 ml/100 g/min. With maximal exertion, left ventricular oxygen consumption increases about fourfold, as does left ventricular blood flow in normal people and animals.[160] If coronary perfusion pressure does not change during exertion, the increased flow must be achieved by a decrease in coronary vascular resistance; the response is termed *metabolic regulation.*

Coronary vascular resistance has three components: a basal low resistance in the arrested heart with maximally dilated vessels, an added resistance when vessels have tone, and a phasic resistance added whenever the ventricle contracts.[161,162] In the beating heart with vessels maximally dilated by a pharmacologic dilator, the second

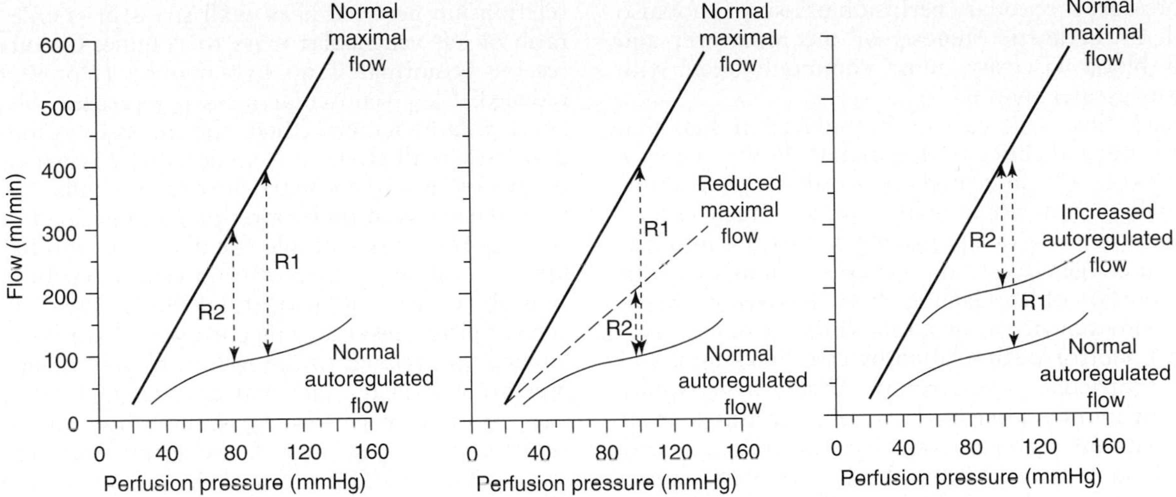

FIGURE 18–14 • **A,** Normal pressure-flow relations in the left coronary artery during normal autoregulated flow and during maximal vasodilation. Values are appropriate for a left ventricle weighing approximately 100 g. *R1, R2,* coronary flow reserve measurements at two different coronary perfusing pressures. *B1,* pressure at which autoregulation fails. **B,** Effect on coronary flow reserve of a reduced maximal flow. At the same coronary perfusing pressure, flow reserve is reduced from the normal R1 to R2. *B1, B2,* pressures at which autoregulation fails. **C,** Effect on coronary flow reserve of an increased autoregulated flow. Reserve is reduced from R1 to R2. *B1, B2,* pressures at which autoregulation fails. In panels **B** and **C,** the *dashed lines* and *white arrowheads* indicate abnormal flows and pressures.

of these resistances is absent. Perfusion of the left ventricular myocardium then produces a steep pressure-flow relation that is linear at higher flows but usually curvilinear at low pressures and flows (Figure 18–14, *A*). Because the vessels are maximally dilated, flow is uncoupled from metabolism and depends only on driving pressure and resistance. If heart rate is increased, maximal flow at any perfusion pressure decreases because the heart is in a relaxed state for a smaller proportion of each minute.

If tone is allowed to return to the coronary vessels, then the pressure-flow relationship can be assessed at different perfusion pressures after the left coronary artery is cannulated. This step is necessary because when cardiac metabolism and blood flow are coupled, increasing aortic blood pressure increases coronary flow not only by increasing perfusion pressure but also by increasing myocardial oxygen demand. Under normal conditions, coronary blood flow is autoregulated. If perfusion pressure is raised or lowered from its normal value, a range exists over which almost no change in flow occurred; a rise in pressure caused vasoconstriction, and a fall in pressure caused vasodilatation.[163] At perfusion pressures above some upper limit, flow increases, probably because the pressure overcomes the constriction. More importantly, at pressures less than approximately 40 mmHg (but varying, as discussed later) flow decreases (see Figure 18–14, *A*), indicating that some vessels have reached maximal vasodilatation and can no longer decrease resistance to compensate for the decreased perfusion pressure. If this pressure dependency occurs, then further decrease in perfusion pressure decreases local blood flow below its required amount, or if myocardial oxygen demands increase at the same low perfusion pressure (as occurs if the ventricle becomes dilated), the requisite increase in flow does not occur. These two conditions cause ischemia.

At any given pressure, the difference between autoregulated and maximal flows is termed *coronary flow reserve*.[164–166] (Coronary flow reserve can be measured in units of ml/min but also can be assessed by a dimensionless flow reserve ratio derived by dividing maximal flow by resting flow.) Flow reserve depends on perfusion pressure because of the steepness of the pressure-flow relation in maximally dilated vessels. Coronary flow reserve indicates how much extra flow the myocardium can receive at a given pressure to meet increased demands for oxygen. If reserve is much reduced, then flow cannot increase sufficiently to meet demands and myocardial ischemia occurs. What the figure does not show is that coronary flow reserve normally is lower in the subendocardium than in the subepicardium, and that decreases in coronary flow reserve are always more profound in the subendocardium than in the subepicardium.

If autoregulated flow is normal but maximal flow is decreased, as indicated by the decreased slope of the pressure-flow relation during maximal dilatation (Figure 18–14, *B*), then coronary flow reserve will be reduced. Such a change can occur with marked tachycardia; decrease in the number of coronary vessels because of small-vessel disease, as in some collagen vascular diseases, especially systemic lupus erythematosus; increased resistance to flow in one or more large coronary vessels because of embolism, thrombosis, atheroma, or spasm; impaired myocardial relaxation because of ischemia; myocardial edema; marked increase in left ventricular diastolic pressure; marked increase in left ventricular systolic pressure if coronary perfusion pressure is not also increased, as in aortic stenosis or incompetence; and increased blood viscosity, most commonly seen with hematocrits greater than 65%.

Coronary flow reserve can be reduced if maximal flows are normal but autoregulated flows increase (Figure 18–14, *C*). Increased myocardial flows above normal values can occur with exercise, tachycardia, anemia, carbon monoxide poisoning, leftward shift of the hemoglobin oxygen dissociation curve (as in infants with a high proportion of fetal hemoglobin), hypoxemia, thyrotoxicosis, acute ventricular dilatation (because of increased wall stress), inotropic stimulation by catecholamines, and acquired ventricular hypertrophy. When hypertrophy occurs a few months after birth, ventricular muscle mass increases without a concomitant increase in conducting coronary blood vessels. Ventricular hypertrophy returns wall stress to normal, and myocardial flow per minute per gram of muscle is approximately normal. Therefore total left ventricular flow is increased in proportion to ventricular mass, but because maximal flow per ventricle usually is unchanged, the coronary flow reserve is diminished. Often autoregulated flow is increased and maximal flows are reduced at the same time, for example, with severe tachycardia or cyanotic heart disease with hypoxemia, ventricular hypertrophy, and polycythemia. Under these circumstances, coronary flow reserve can be drastically reduced. A third mechanism that reduces coronary flow reserve is a shift to the right of the pressure-flow line. If with maximally dilated vessels diastolic coronary flow is measured at different mean diastolic perfusion pressures, a pressure-flow line is obtained that is linear at higher pressures but curved in the low pressure-flow region.[167,168] Zero flow occurs at a pressure of approximately 8 to 12 mmHg; this is the critical closing pressure that is above right atrial pressure.[169,170] The whole pressure-flow line can be shifted to the right by several factors, most important of which are pericardial tamponade, a rise in right or left ventricular diastolic pressures, and α-adrenergic stimulation. Such a rightward shift decreases flow reserve (Figure 18–14, *D*). Of note, because the line of maximal pressure-flow relations slopes up and to the right, any decrease in that slope (see Figure 18–14, *B*), any increase in autoregulated flow (see Figure 18–14, *C*), or any rightward shift of the slope (see Figure 18–14, *D*) raises the pressure at which autoregulation fails to compensate for decreased perfusing pressure. Also important to reemphasize is that any decrease in coronary flow reserve affects the subendocardium predominantly so that autoregulation fails first and ischemia occurs in the subendocardium before these changes occur in the subepicardium.[171] The predominant reduction in subendocardial flow and reserve is particularly marked when left ventricular diastolic pressure is very high.

The interactions between myocardial blood flow and ventricular function are of particular importance in the presence of ventricular hypertrophy. Myocardial wall stress is regulated within a fairly narrow range, with or without myocardial hypertrophy. Consequently, myocardial blood flow per unit mass is fairly constant at approximately 1 ml/min/g of left ventricle at rest.[172–177] Strauer and colleagues[173,175,178,179] showed a close relationship between peak wall stress in systole and the ratio of left ventricular mass to volume. Coronary flow reserve is normal if no hypertrophy is present but is reduced if left ventricular mass is increased. Should the heart dilate acutely, then the mass-to-volume ratio decreases, wall stress and myocardial oxygen consumption increase, and coronary flow reserve falls. Decreasing ventricular dilatation by afterload and preload reduction reverses these unfavorable events and is another reason for the resulting improvement in ventricular function.

Right ventricular myocardial blood flow follows the general principles regarding coronary blood flow, but differences are related to the low right ventricular systolic pressure and to the fact that changes in aortic pressure alter coronary perfusing pressure without altering right ventricular pressure work. If the normal right ventricle is acutely distended, for example, by pulmonary embolism, eventually right ventricular failure occurs. The increased wall stress increases oxygen consumption, but the raised systolic pressure reduces coronary flow, so when supply cannot match demand right ventricular myocardial ischemia occurs.[180] Raising aortic perfusing pressure mechanically or with α-adrenergic agonists increases right ventricular myocardial blood flow, relieves ischemia, and restores right ventricular function to normal. Improved coronary flow is not the only mechanism of this improvement; increased left ventricular afterload moves the ventricular septum toward the right ventricle and improves left ventricular performance.[181] If right ventricular pressure is chronically elevated so that right ventricular hypertrophy occurs, as in pulmonic stenosis, many forms of cyanotic congenital heart disease, and some chronic lung diseases, then right ventricular myocardial blood flow behaves in the same way as left ventricular blood flow, with one exception.[182–184] If aortic pressure is lowered, left ventricular pressure also decreases, as does left ventricular work and oxygen consumption. In the right ventricle, however, the workload may not be reduced (if no ventricular septal defect is present), so an imbalance between myocardial oxygen supply and demand may occur. The worst imbalance occurs when aortic systolic pressure is maintained but coronary perfusing pressure decreases, which can occur in a child with tetralogy of Fallot who has too large an aortopulmonary anastomosis. The high aortic and left ventricular systolic pressures mandate an equally high right ventricular systolic pressure, but the low diastolic aortic pressure reduces coronary perfusion pressure in diastole and can cause both left and right ventricular ischemia and failure.[185]

Gastrointestinal Circulation

Maintenance of adequate splanchnic blood flow in critically ill patients is important. In a globally compromised circulation, the gastrointestinal system is particularly prone to injury that impairs its two chief functions: (1) digestion and absorption of nutrients and (2) maintenance of a barrier to the translocation of enteric antigens.[186–191] Moreover, splanchnic ischemia has been associated with multiple organ failure and increased morbidity and mortality in these patients.[192–195]

The three major arteries supplying blood to the gastrointestinal circulation arise directly from the aorta. The celiac artery supplies blood to the stomach, liver, and spleen. The superior mesenteric artery supplies the small intestine, pancreas, and proximal colon. The inferior mesenteric artery supplies the remaining middle and distal colon. There is extensive collateral blood flow.[69] Total flow accounts for 20% to 25% of the cardiac output in the resting unfed state.[196]

The gastrointestinal circulation has multiple levels of regulation that can be broadly divided into intrinsic and extrinsic mechanisms. Intrinsic mechanisms include local metabolic processes, locally produced vasoactive substances, and myogenic reflexes. Extrinsic factors include circulating vasoactive substances, neural innervation, and general hemodynamic forces.[196,197] Neural input arising from the medulla oblongata through preganglionic fibers of the intermediolateral area of the spinal cord participates in regulation of large blood vessels (>50 μm), largely through sympathetic α-adrenergic control.[198,199] Blood flow to the intestinal circulation, like other vascular beds, is autoregulated such that oxygen delivery remains fairly constant, with inflow pressures varying from 30 to 120 mmHg.[197,200–202] Oxygen, carbon dioxide, H^+ ions, and adenosine are important local metabolic mediators of this process.[203–209] Other important vasoactive mediators of intestinal blood flow include serotonin, histamine, bradykinin, and prostaglandin, although their role in autoregulation is unclear.[210–214] Finally, various gastrointestinal hormones and peptides released from the intestinal mucosa and intestinal glands, including gastrin, vasoactive intestinal polypeptide, cholecystokinin, secretin, glucagon, enkephalins, somatostatin, and kallidin, have vasoactive properties.[196,215]

A phenomenon unique to the gastrointestinal circulation is the increase in flow following consumption of nutrients.[216] This *postprandial intestinal hyperemia* appears to involve multiple factors. However, the composition of the chyme is particularly important.[217] Luminal distension, mechanical stimulation, and extrinsic neural stimulation are not necessary for the response to occur.[196,218–220] Lipids in combination with bile salts are the most potent triggers for postprandial hyperemia.[221–223] Glucose is the most potent single stimulus for this response.[224] Blood flow to skin and skeletal muscle decreases and cardiac output increases during postprandial hyperemia.[216] Furthermore, nutrients that induce the largest increase in blood flow illicit the largest oxygen debt within the intestinal villi.[225–230]

Interestingly, postprandial hyperemia may be protective in some instances of low blood flow to the intestinal mucosa. Glucose ameliorates mucosal ischemia in models of septic and hemorrhagic shock, and early enteral feeding has been advocated in human studies.[231–233] Conversely, enteral feeding has been associated with bowel ischemia and injury in some patients, such as premature infants, thus complicating decisions regarding enteral feeding during or after low-flow states.[234–236]

Increasing data demonstrate a large role for NO in the regulation of gastrointestinal blood flow. Endothelial nitric oxide synthase (eNOS) is expressed throughout the gastrointestinal vasculature, including the liver and pancreas.[237] A number of stimuli, such as shear stress, adenosine, bradykinin, and serotonin, activate eNOS production of NO.[238] NO at least partly mediates basal mesenteric and hepatic blood flow. Inhibitors of NOS decrease splanchnic blood flow and increase hepatic pressure.[239,240] A number of studies implicate endothelial dysfunction, particularly aberrations in NO signaling, in portal hypertension and cirrhosis.[241–243] NO also participates in maintenance of the mucosal barrier function and is further protective by virtue of its inhibitory effect on platelet and leukocyte adhesion.[244] Furthermore, postprandial hyperemia involves adenosine-mediated NO release.[245,246] Finally, neuronal nitric oxide synthase (nNOS) and inducible nitric oxide synthase (iNOS) are important in both normal and abnormal gastrointestinal motility and gastrointestinal inflammatory disorders, respectively.[247–252]

Although NO is integral to gastrointestinal health and disease, therapies for gastrointestinal disorders that use the NO signaling cascade are sparse. Inhibition and potentiation of NOS activity have been studied for treatment of portal hypertension, with mixed results.[244,253,254] NO donor agents have been investigated as therapy for diseases with impaired mucosal barrier function, such as gastric ulcerative disease. These therapies also have been of limited success.[255,256]

ET-1 is another important mediator of intestinal blood flow. The intestinal vasculature displays increased vasoconstriction in response to ET-1 compared with other vascular beds.[257–259] This finding has particular importance for gastrointestinal blood flow in critically ill patients, as ET-1 levels have been found to be elevated following surgery and in association with a number of disease states, including hypoxia, pancreatitis, and sepsis.[260–266] ET-receptor antagonism ameliorates ischemic injury to the bowel in several models of low flow states.[267,268] Interestingly, as in the pulmonary circulation, there appear to be developmental changes in the activity of ET-1.[269] Infusion of ET-1, however, results in sustained vasoconstriction of intestinal vessels across age groups.[202]

Finally, drugs used to augment systolic blood pressure and/or to enhance cardiac output can have various effects on the gastrointestinal circulation. Fenoldopam, a dopamine-1 receptor agonist, improves intestinal perfusion during hemorrhage.[270] Results with more common agents, such as norepinephrine, dopamine, and vasopressin, have been mixed, depending on the doses used and the models or clinical situations studied.[271–275] Thus investigations aimed at determining the optimum strategy to improve overall cardiac output and oxygen delivery without compromising flow to specific organs, such as the bowel, continue.

Renal Circulation

Blood flow to the kidneys greatly exceeds the metabolic needs of the organs themselves. In a 70-kg adult, combined renal blood flow is approximately 1200 ml/min, accounting for more than 20% of total cardiac output supplying organs that represent less than 0.5% of total body weight.[276] This high renal blood flow is necessary to support glomerular filtration, such that solute and fluid homeostasis are maintained.

Blood is supplied to the kidneys by the renal arteries, which branch to form the interlobar, arcuate, and interlobular arteries. Interlobular arteries progress to form the afferent arterioles, which lead to the glomerular capillaries within the glomerulus, the site of fluid and solute filtration. The distal glomerular capillaries re-form into the efferent arterioles, which then lead to a second capillary system, the peritubular capillaries. An elevated hydrostatic pressure within the glomerular capillaries supports filtration, whereas a much lower pressure within the peritubular capillary system supports absorption.[276] Alterations in the resistances of the afferent and efferent arterioles regulate these pressures and allow for dynamic changes in renal function in response to overall fluid and solute needs.[277] The venous system branches in a similar fashion as the arterial supply, with blood eventually entering the inferior vena cava from the renal veins.

Renal blood flow is determined by the difference between renal artery pressure (which is generally equivalent to systemic arterial pressure) and renal vein pressure, over the renal vascular resistance. In general, three vascular segments limit renal vascular resistance: interlobular arteries, afferent arterioles, and efferent arterioles.[278–280] Regulation of renal vascular resistance can be broadly divided into extrinsic mechanisms and intrinsic mechanisms. Extrinsic mechanisms, which include the sympathoadrenal system, atrial natriuretic system, and renin-angiotensin-aldosterone axis, modulate renal blood flow by alterations in intrarenal vascular tone, mesangial tone, intravascular volume, and systemic vascular resistance.[276] Intrinsic mechanisms, which primarily alter afferent arteriolar resistance, are responsible for autoregulation of renal blood flow in response to changes in renal perfusion pressure.[281]

The juxtaglomerular apparatus, which is composed of the afferent and efferent arterioles, macula densa, and glomerular mesangium, is an important site involved in the regulation of renal perfusion and glomerular filtration. Glomerular filtration is largely a function of glomerular filtration pressure, which in turn depends on renal perfusion pressure and, importantly, the balance between afferent arteriolar and efferent arteriolar tone. Increased efferent arteriolar tone increases glomerular filtration by increasing glomerular pressure, whereas increased afferent arteriolar tone has the opposite effect.

Endogenous epinephrine and norepinephrine derived from sympathetic neural input have various effects on renal perfusion and glomerular filtration. Mild sympathetic output preferentially constricts the efferent arterioles, thereby increasing glomerular pressure and filtration.[282] However, intense sympathetic discharge results in afferent arteriolar constriction, which decreases glomerular filtration.[283] Furthermore, sympathetic stimulation of afferent arterioles results in renin release, which leads to increased sodium reabsorption and fluid retention. Sympathetic stimulation can affect renal blood flow more generally by alterations in systemic arterial pressure. Clinically norepinephrine increased renal perfusion and renal function (measured by changes in creatinine clearance) in patients with septic shock.[284]

Angiotensin II, which is produced by cleavage of angiotensin I by the enzyme angiotensin-converting enzyme (ACE), has important effects on renal perfusion. Like catecholamine stimulation, the effects of angiotensin II are dose related. Angiotensin II at low levels results in efferent arteriolar constriction, whereas angiotensin II at high levels results in both afferent and efferent arteriolar constriction.[282,285] Angiotensin II alters renal blood flow further by changing intravascular volume through aldosterone and arginine vasopressin and by increasing systemic vascular resistance.

Arginine vasopressin (AVP) is synthesized in the anterior hypothalamus and released from the posterior pituitary gland. It plays a critical role in maintaining serum osmolality within a narrow range. Both V_1 and V_2 receptors have been indentified.[286,287] V_2 receptors are located on the renal collecting ducts. Stimulation of V_2 receptors results in increased reabsorption of water.[288,289] Activation of V_1 receptors on systemic vessels results in vasoconstriction. Interestingly, V_1-receptor activation in the pulmonary vasculature results in vasodilation, at least in part via NO production.[290] Triggers for AVP release include changes in serum osmolality, hypovolemia, and hypotension. Patients with septic shock have decreased levels of AVP, which has led to clinical use of AVP supplementation.[291] Unlike catecholamines and angiotensin II, high levels of AVP appear to preferentially constrict efferent arterioles, which preserves glomerular filtration.[292]

ET-1 has diverse effects on the kidney.[293] In general, endothelin results in vasoconstriction, decreased renal perfusion, and decreased glomerular filtration. ET-1 constricts both afferent and efferent arterioles.[294] ET-1 also stimulates cell proliferation within the kidney. Conversely, ET-1 may promote natriuresis through ET_B-receptor activation.[295] Furthermore, alterations in ET-1 signaling have been implicated in a host of renal diseases, including acute and chronic renal failure, essential hypertension, glomerulonephritis, renal fibrosis, and renal transplant rejection.[293,296–301]

Important vasodilators within the renal circulation include prostaglandins and atrial natriuretic peptide (ANP). The vasodilating prostaglandins (D_2, E_2, and I_2) are synthesized from arachidonic acid by the enzyme phospholipase A_2.[302–304] Most of the important vasoconstricting factors, such as catecholamines, angiotensin II, and AVP, stimulate the release of prostaglandins, promoting increased renal perfusion and glomerular filtration.[305] ANP is produced within the atrial myocytes and is released in response to increased atrial stretch. Through cGMP signaling, ANP results in afferent arteriolar dilation and increased renal perfusion and glomerular filtration. ANP also antagonizes the actions of endogenous catecholamines, angiotensin II, and AVP.

Like other organ systems, renal blood flow is autoregulated via mechanisms intrinsic to the renal vasculature.[276] Early studies demonstrated that renal blood flow and glomerular filtration remain constant at renal artery perfusion pressures between 80 and 180 mm Hg.[281,306] Importantly, urinary flow rate is not constant within the autoregulatory range but changes as a function of renal perfusion pressure. The precise mechanisms for this autoregulation are unclear. Alterations in vascular tone in response to changes in intravascular pressure (myogenic mechanism) may participate. However, other evidence suggests that signaling at the macula densa in response to tubular electrolyte concentrations also is important.[276]

Increasing data suggest that NO plays an important role in normal renal function and that alterations in NO signaling mediate renal pathophysiology.[307–311] Techniques that use intrarenal NO antagonism decrease renal blood flow and increase systemic arterial pressure. Intramedullary administration of NO inhibitors increases afferent arteriolar tone with lesser effects on the efferent arterioles.[307] Various experiments demonstrate that NO signaling modulates angiotensin II-mediated vasoconstriction. Furthermore, NO appears to modulate salt and water reabsorption within the nephron independent of changes in glomerular filtration or renal blood flow.[309] Chronic NO antagonism increases systemic arterial pressure, decreases medullary blood flow, and results in a positive sodium balance. Administration of L-arginine, the substrate for NO production, abrogates the development of hypertension to salt in salt-sensitive rats and decreases blood pressure in spontaneously hypertensive rats.[308,311]

Reactive oxygen species also participate in the regulation of renal blood flow, largely by altering the bioavailability of NO.[312,313] Superoxide dismutase attenuates the development of hypertension in spontaneously hypertensive rats.[313–315] Furthermore, superoxide dismutase diminishes angiotensin II-induced vasoconstriction and increases renal medullary blood flow.[313,316]

A number of disease states that affect critically ill patients result in loss of renal autoregulation. Acute tubular necrosis, septic shock, hepatic failure, and cardiopulmonary bypass all have been associated with renal dysfunction and loss of renal autoregulation.[317–320]

Conflicting Needs of Regional Circulations

Individual regional circulations respond to threats to homeostasis both independently and in concert. This response is natural because individual organs have their own separate needs. Yet each region also has a responsibility to the body as a whole. At times individual need and responsibility conflict. Life-threatening illness accentuates these "conflicts of interest." An example follows.

Pulmonary vascular resistance is pathologically elevated in persistent pulmonary hypertension of the newborn and idiopathic pulmonary hypertension and in certain patients with congenital cardiac disease, chronic pulmonary disease, or acquired cardiac disease. Often this problem is managed acutely by hyperventilation, which is easily induced and requires no sodium or osmotic load. However, hypocarbic alkalosis is a vasoconstrictor in brain and myocardium, whereas metabolic alkalosis has little acute effect on cerebral circulation. A good understanding of the regulation of regional circulations is necessary to adequately arbitrate this conflict. Treatment of elevated pulmonary vascular resistance following cavopulmonary anastomosis for single-ventricle physiology is an excellent example of this conflict. In this postoperative setting, mild elevations of pulmonary vascular resistance may decrease pulmonary blood flow and venous return. With this anatomy, pulmonary blood flow depends upon superior vena cava venous return. If hyperventilation is used to decrease pulmonary vascular resistance, hypocarbic alkalosis decreases CBF and subsequent superior vena cava return. This process may result in a net decrease in pulmonary blood flow and desaturation.

Another example occurs in the daily treatment of acute lung injury. The lung is responsible for gas exchange for the entire body. When the lung fails or becomes frankly inefficient as a result of disease, other organs may be subjected to hypoxia, hypercarbia, and acidosis. Positive pressure ventilation may be essential to life. Yet mechanical ventilation can impede cardiac output (see Chapter 24), and increasing ventilator pressures with high inspired oxygen concentrations may induce further lung injury. The need for positive pressure ventilation may impose a trade: good peripheral perfusion with desaturated blood for less perfusion, better arterial oxygen content, and lower risk of iatrogenic lung injury. Decisions based on optimal oxygen delivery are generally global. Bowel and brain vascular beds autoregulate to blood pressure, but cerebral vessels dilate to hypoxia, whereas mesenteric vessels constrict. The bowel might benefit from a different combination of PO_2, cardiac output, and blood pressure than the brain, although any of several combinations of these parameters may be associated with the same net oxygen delivery.

Unsuccessful arbitration among regional circulations may contribute to the genesis of the syndrome of multiple organ systems failure (see Chapter 97). A greater understanding of the mechanisms that regulate regional, microcirculatory blood flow will lead to new and improved treatments that optimize blood flow and allow the intensivist to successfully arbitrate the regional blood flow "conflict of interests" that will best serve the short- and long-term interests of the critically ill patient.

REFERENCES

1. Sylvester JT, Gilbert RD, Traystman RJ, Permutt S: Effects of hypoxia on the closing pressure of the canine systemic arterial circulation. Circ Res 49:980-987, 1981.
2. Jerusalem E, Starling EH: On the significance of carbon dioxide for the heart beat. J Physiol 40:279, 1910.
3. Stamler JS, Jia L, Eu JP, et al: Blood flow regulation by S-nitrosohemoglobin in the physiological oxygen gradient. Science 276:2034-2037, 1997.
4. Gladwin MT, Shelhamer JH, Schechter AN, et al: Role of circulating nitrite and S-nitrosohemoglobin in the regulation of regional blood flow in humans. Proc Natl Acad Sci U S A 97:11482-11487, 2000.
5. Cannon RO III, Schechter AN, Panza JA, et al: Effects of inhaled nitric oxide on regional blood flow are consistent with intravascular nitric oxide delivery. J Clin Invest 108:279-287, 2001.
6. Feigl EO: Coronary physiology. Physiol Rev 63:1-205, 1983.
7. Brace RA, Anderson DK, Chen WT, et al: Local effects of hypokalemia on coronary resistance and myocardial contractile force. Am J Physiol 227:590-597, 1974.

8. Murray PA, Sparks HV: The mechanism of K+-induced vasodilation of the coronary vascular bed of the dog. *Circ Res* 42:35-42, 1978.
9. Beckman JS, Koppenol WH: Nitric oxide, superoxide, and peroxynitrite: the good, the bad, and ugly. *Am J Physiol* 271:C1424-C1437, 1996.
10. Beckman JS: The double-edged role of nitric oxide in brain function and superoxide-mediated injury. *J Dev Physiol* 15:53-59, 1991.
11. Cai H, Harrison DG: Endothelial dysfunction in cardiovascular diseases: the role of oxidant stress. *Circ Res* 87:840-844, 2000.
12. Sparks HV: Effect of local metabolic factors on vascular smooth muscle. In Bohr DF, Somlyo AP, Sparks HV, editors: *Handbook of physiology. The cardiovascular system.* Bethesda, MD, 1980, Amercian Physiological Society.
13. Moncada S, Higgs A: The L-arginine-nitric oxide pathway. *N Engl J Med* 329:2002-2012, 1993.
14. Dinh-Xuan AT: Endothelial modulation of pulmonary vascular tone. *Eur Respir J* 5:757-762, 1992.
15. Palmer RM, Ashton DS, Moncada S: Vascular endothelial cells synthesize nitric oxide from L-arginine. *Nature* 333:664-666, 1988.
16. Rubanyi GM, Romero JC, Vanhoutte PM: Flow-induced release of endothelium-derived relaxing factor. *Am J Physiol* 250: H1145-H1149, 1986.
17. Fineman JR, Heymann MA, Soifer SJ: N omega-nitro-L-arginine attenuates endothelium-dependent pulmonary vasodilation in lambs. *Am J Physiol* 260:H1299-H1306, 1991.
18. Abman SH, Chatfield BA, Hall SL, McMurtry IF: Role of endothelium-derived relaxing factor during transition of pulmonary circulation at birth. *Am J Physiol* 259:H1921-H1927, 1990.
19. Yanagisawa M, Kurihara H, Kimura S, et al: A novel potent vasoconstrictor peptide produced by vascular endothelial cells. *Nature* 332:411-415, 1988.
20. Yang ZH, Richard V, von Segesser L, et al: Threshold concentrations of endothelin-1 potentiate contractions to norepinephrine and serotonin in human arteries. A new mechanism of vasospasm? *Circulation* 82:188-195, 1990.
21. Rubanyi GM, editor: *Endothelin.* New York, 1992, Oxford University Press for the American Physiological Society.
22. Vane JR, Anggard EE, Botting RM: Regulatory functions of the vascular endothelium. *N Engl J Med* 323:27-36, 1990.
23. Faraci FM, Heistad DD: Regulation of the cerebral circulation: role of endothelium and potassium channels. *Physiol Rev* 78:53-97, 1998.
24. Ling SC, Atabek HB, Fry DL, et al: Application of heated-film velocity and shear probes to hemodynamic studies. *Circ Res* 23:789-801, 1968.
25. Friedman MH, Fry DL: Arterial permeability dynamics and vascular disease. *Atherosclerosis* 104:189-194, 1993.
26. Shyy JY, Chien S: Role of integrins in endothelial mechanosensing of shear stress. *Circ Res* 91:769-775, 2002.
27. Bayliss W: On the local reactions of the arterial wall to changes of internal pressure. *J Physiol* 28:220-231, 1902.
28. Johnson PC: The myogenic response. In Bohr DF, Somlyo AP, Sparks HV, editors: *Handbook of physiology. The cardiovascular system.* Bethesda, MD, 1980, American Physiologic Society.
29. Davis MJ, Hill MA: Signaling mechanisms underlying the vascular myogenic response. *Physiol Rev* 79:387-423, 1999.
30. Murphy TV, Spurrell BE, Hill MA: Cellular signalling in arteriolar myogenic constriction: involvement of tyrosine phosphorylation pathways. *Clin Exp Pharmacol Physiol* 29:612-619, 2002.
31. Levin DL, Rudolph AM, Heymann MA, Phibbs RH: Morphological development of the pulmonary vascular bed in fetal lambs. *Circulation* 53:144-151, 1976.
32. Hislop A, Reid L: Intra-pulmonary arterial development during fetal life-branching pattern and structure. *J Anat* 113:35-48, 1972.
33. Reid LM: Structure and function in pulmonary hypertension. New perceptions. *Chest* 89:279-288, 1986.
34. Hislop A, Reid L: Pulmonary arterial development during childhood: branching pattern and structure. *Thorax* 28:129-135, 1973.
35. Meyrick B, Reid L: The effect of continued hypoxia on rat pulmonary arterial circulation. An ultrastructural study. *Lab Invest* 38:188-200, 1978.
36. Rudolph AM, Heymann MA: Circulatory changes during growth in the fetal lamb. *Circ Res* 26:289-299, 1970.
37. Rudolph AM: Fetal and neonatal pulmonary circulation. *Annu Rev Physiol* 41:383-395, 1979.
38. Heyman MA, Soifer S: Control of the fetal and neonatal pulmonary circulation. In Weir EK, Reeves JT, editors: *Pulmonary vascular physiology and pathophysiology.* New York, 1989, Marcel Dekker.
39. Iwamoto HS, Teitel D, Rudolph AM: Effects of birth-related events on blood flow distribution. *Pediatr Res* 22:634-640, 1987.
40. Rudolph AM: Distribution and regulation of blood flow in the fetal and neonatal lamb. *Circ Res* 57:811-821, 1985.
41. Dawes GS, Mott JC, Widdicombe JG, Wyatt DG: Changes in the lungs of the new-born lamb. *J Physiol* 121:141-162, 1953.
42. Enhorning G, Adams FH, Norman A: Effect of lung expansion on the fetal lamb circulation. *Acta Paediatr Scand* 55:441-451, 1966.
43. Leffler CW, Hessler JR, Green RS: The onset of breathing at birth stimulates pulmonary vascular prostacyclin synthesis. *Pediatr Res* 18:938-942, 1984.
44. Velvis H, Moore P, Heymann MA: Prostaglandin inhibition prevents the fall in pulmonary vascular resistance as a result of rhythmic distension of the lungs in fetal lambs. *Pediatr Res* 30: 62-68, 1991.
45. Tiktinsky MH, Morin FC III: Increasing oxygen tension dilates fetal pulmonary circulation via endothelium-derived relaxing factor. *Am J Physiol* 265:H376-H380, 1993.
46. Shaul PW, Farrar MA, Zellers TM: Oxygen modulates endothelium-derived relaxing factor production in fetal pulmonary arteries. *Am J Physiol* 262:H355-H364, 1992.
47. Shaul PW, Farrar MA, Magness RR: Pulmonary endothelial nitric oxide production is developmentally regulated in the fetus and newborn. *Am J Physiol* 265:H1056-H1063, 1993.
48. Cornfield DN, Chatfield BA, McQueston JA, et al: Effects of birth-related stimuli on L-arginine-dependent pulmonary vasodilation in ovine fetus. *Am J Physiol* 262:H1474-H1481, 1992.
49. Black SM, Johengen MJ, Ma ZD, et al: Ventilation and oxygenation induce endothelial nitric oxide synthase gene expression in the lungs of fetal lambs. *J Clin Invest* 100:1448-1458, 1997.
50. Fineman JR, Wong J, Morin FC III, et al: Chronic nitric oxide inhibition in utero produces persistent pulmonary hypertension in newborn lambs. *J Clin Invest* 93:2675-2683, 1994.
51. West JB, Dollery CT, Naimark A: Distribution of blood flow in isolated lung; relation to vascular and alveolar pressures. *J Appl Physiol* 19:713-724, 1964.
52. Lopez-Muniz R, Stephens NL, Bromberger-Barnea B, et al: Critical closure of pulmonary vessels analyzed in terms of Starling resistor model. *J Appl Physiol* 24:625-635, 1968.
53. Riley RL: Effects of lung inflation on the pulmonary vascular bed. In Adams WW, Veith I, editors: *Pulmonary circulation.* New York, 1959, Grune & Stratton.
54. Sun RY, Nieman GF, Hakim TS, Chang HK: Effects of lung volume and alveolar surface tension on pulmonary vascular resistance. *J Appl Physiol* 62:1622-1626, 1987.
55. Fuhrman BP, Smith-Wright DL, Venkataraman S, Howland DF: Pulmonary vascular resistance after cessation of positive end-expiratory pressure. *J Appl Physiol* 66:660-668, 1989.
56. Fuhrman BP, Everitt J, Lock JE: Cardiopulmonary effects of unilateral airway pressure changes in intact infant lambs. *J Appl Physiol* 56:1439-1448, 1984.
57. Fuhrman BP, Smith-Wright DL, Kulik TJ, Lock JE: Effects of static and fluctuating airway pressure on intact pulmonary circulation. *J Appl Physiol* 60:114-122, 1986.
58. Braner DA, Fineman JR, Chang R, Soifer SJ: M&B 22948, a cGMP phosphodiesterase inhibitor, is a pulmonary vasodilator in lambs. *Am J Physiol* 264:H252-H258, 1993.
59. Rudolph AM, Yuan S: Response of the pulmonary vasculature to hypoxia and H+ ion concentration changes. *J Clin Invest* 45: 399-411, 1966.
60. Marshall C, Marshall B: Site and sensitivity for stimulation of hypoxic pulmonary vasoconstriction. *J Appl Physiol* 55:711-716, 1983.
61. Custer JR, Hales CA: Influence of alveolar oxygen on pulmonary vasoconstriction in newborn lambs versus sheep. *Am Rev Respir Dis* 132:326-331, 1983.

62. Cutaia M, Rounds S: Hypoxic pulmonary vasoconstriction. Physiologic significance, mechanism, and clinical relevance. *Chest* 97:706-718, 1990.
63. Schreiber MD, Heymann MA, Soifer SJ: Increased arterial pH, not decreased $PaCO_2$, attenuates hypoxia-induced pulmonary vasoconstriction in newborn lambs. *Pediatr Res* 20:113-117, 1986.
64. Cartwright D, Gregory GA, Lou H, Heyman MA: The effect of hypocarbia on the cardiovascular system of puppies. *Pediatr Res* 18:685-690, 1984.
65. Harper AM, Jennett B, Miller D, editors: *Blood flow and metabolism in the brain. Proceedings of the 7th international symposium on cerebral blood flow and metabolism.* New York, 1975, Churchill Livingstone.
66. Mchedlishvili G, Purves M, Kovach A, editors: *Regulation of cerebral blood flow.* Budapest, 1979, Akademiaikiado.
67. Vavilala MS, Lee LA, Lam AM: Cerebral blood flow and vascular physiology. *Anesthesiol Clin North Am* 20:247-264, v, 2002.
68. Zijlstra W: Physiology of the cerebral circulation. In Minderhoud J, editor: *Cerebral blood flow: basic knowledge and clinical implications.* Princeton, 1981, Princeton Press.
69. Williams P, Warwick R, Dyson M: Angiology. In *Gray's anatomy.* New York, 1989, Churchill Livingstone.
70. Sadoshima S, Thames M, Heistad D: Cerebral blood flow during elevation of intracranial pressure: role of sympathetic nerves. *Am J Physiol* 241:H78-H84, 1981.
71. Kety S, Schmidt JF: The determination of cerebral blood flow in man by the use of nitrous oxide in low concentrations. *Am J Physiol* 143:53-66, 1981.
72. Hardebo JE, Owman C: Barrier mechanisms for neurotransmitter monoamines and their precursors at the blood-brain interface. *Ann Neurol* 8:1-31, 1980.
73. Rapoport S: *Blood-brain barrier in physiology and medicine.* New York, 1976, Raven Press.
74. Paulson OB: Blood-brain barrier, brain metabolism and cerebral blood flow. *Eur Neuropsychopharmacol* 12:495-501, 2002.
75. Fog M: Cerebral circulation. The reaction of pial arteries to a fall of blood pressure. *Arch Neurol Psychiat* 37:351-364, 1937.
76. Panerai RB, Dawson SL, Eames PJ, Potter JF: Cerebral blood flow velocity response to induced and spontaneous sudden changes in arterial blood pressure. *Am J Physiol Heart Circ Physiol* 280:H2162-H2174, 2001.
77. Strandgaard S, Paulson OB: Cerebral autoregulation. *Stroke* 15:413-416, 1984.
78. Strandgaard S, Paulson OB: Regulation of cerebral blood flow in health and disease. *J Cardiovasc Pharmacol* 19(suppl 6):S89-S93, 1992.
79. Dernbach PD, Little JR, Jones SC, Ebrahim ZY: Altered cerebral autoregulation and CO_2 reactivity after aneurysmal subarachnoid hemorrhage. *Neurosurgery* 22:822-826, 1988.
80. Georgiadis D, Sievert M, Cencetti S, et al: Cerebrovascular reactivity is impaired in patients with cardiac failure. *Eur Heart J* 21: 407-413, 2000.
81. Lam JM, Smielewski P, al-Rawi P, et al: Prediction of cerebral ischaemia during carotid endarterectomy with preoperative CO_2-reactivity studies and angiography. *Br J Neurosurg* 14:441-448, 2000.
82. Schalen W, Messeter K, Nordstrom CH: Cerebral vasoreactivity and the prediction of outcome in severe traumatic brain lesions. *Acta Anaesthesiol Scand* 35:113-122, 1991.
83. Faraci FM, Heistad DD: Regulation of large cerebral arteries and cerebral microvascular pressure. *Circ Res* 66:8-17, 1990.
84. Heistad DD, Marcus ML: Effect of sympathetic stimulation on permeability of the blood-brain barrier to albumin during acute hypertension in cats. *Circ Res* 45:331-338, 1979.
85. Lassen NA, Ingvar DH, Skinhoj E: Brain function and blood flow. *Sci Am* 239:62-71, 1978.
86. Madsen PL, Holm S, Herning M, Lassen NA: Average blood flow and oxygen uptake in the human brain during resting wakefulness: a critical appraisal of the Kety-Schmidt technique. *J Cereb Blood Flow Metab* 13:646-655, 1993.
87. Kato M, Ueno H, Black P: Regional cerebral blood flow of the main visual pathways during photic stimulation of the retina in intact and split-brain monkeys. *Exp Neurol* 42:65-77, 1974.
88. Olesen J: Contralateral focal increase of cerebral blood flow in man during arm work. *Brain* 94:635-646, 1971.
89. Wallesch CW, Henriksen L, Kornhuber HH, Paulson OB: Observations on regional cerebral blood flow in cortical and subcortical structures during language production in normal man. *Brain Lang* 25:224-233, 1985.
90. Madsen PL, Schmidt JF, Wildschiodtz G, et al: Cerebral O_2 metabolism and cerebral blood flow in humans during deep and rapid-eye-movement sleep. *J Appl Physiol* 70:2597-601, 1991.
91. Bryan RM Jr, Hollinger BR, Keefer KA, Page RB. Regional cerebral and neural lobe blood flow during insulin-induced hypoglycemia in unanesthetized rats. *J Cereb Blood Flow Metab* 7:96-102, 1987.
92. Fox PT, Raichle ME: Focal physiological uncoupling of cerebral blood flow and oxidative metabolism during somatosensory stimulation in human subjects. *Proc Natl Acad Sci U S A* 83: 1140-1144, 1986.
93. Mintun MA, Lundstrom BN, Snyder AZ, et al: Blood flow and oxygen delivery to human brain during functional activity: theoretical modeling and experimental data. *Proc Natl Acad Sci U S A* 98:6859-6864, 2001.
94. Ehrlich MP, McCullough JN, Zhang N, et al: Effect of hypothermia on cerebral blood flow and metabolism in the pig. *Ann Thorac Surg* 73:191-197, 2002.
95. McCullough JN, Zhang N, Reich DL, et al: Cerebral metabolic suppression during hypothermic circulatory arrest in humans. *Ann Thorac Surg* 67:1895-1899, 1999; discussion 1919-1921.
96. Cheng W, Hartmann JF, Cameron DE, et al: Cerebral blood flow during cardiopulmonary bypass: influence of temperature and pH management strategy. *Ann Thorac Surg* 59:880-886, 1995.
97. Greeley WJ, Kern FH, Ungerleider RM, et al: The effect of hypothermic cardiopulmonary bypass and total circulatory arrest on cerebral metabolism in neonates, infants, and children. *J Thorac Cardiovasc Surg* 101:783-794, 1991.
98. Brodersen P, Paulson OB, Bolwig TG, et al: Cerebral hyperemia in electrically induced epileptic seizures. *Arch Neurol* 28:334-338, 1973.
99. Ellingsen I, Hauge A, Nicolaysen G, et al: Changes in human cerebral blood flow due to step changes in PAO_2 and $PACO_2$. *Acta Physiol Scand* 129:157-163, 1987.
100. Severinghaus JW, et al: Step hypocapnia to separate arterial from tissue PCO_2 in the regulation of cerebral blood flow. *Circ Res* 20:272-278, 1967.
101. Harper AM, Bell RA: The effect of metabolic acidosis and alkalosis on the blood flow through the cerebral cortex. *J Neurol Neurosurg Psychiatry* 26:341-344, 1963.
102. Peng HL, Ivarsen A, Nilsson H, Aalkjaer C: On the cellular mechanism for the effect of acidosis on vascular tone. *Acta Physiol Scand* 164:517-525, 1998.
103. Kontos HA, Raper AJ, Patterson JL: Analysis of vasoactivity of local pH, PCO_2 and bicarbonate on pial vessels. *Stroke* 8:358-360, 1977.
104. Muizelaar JP, van der Poel HG, Li ZC, et al: Pial arteriolar vessel diameter and CO_2 reactivity during prolonged hyperventilation in the rabbit. *J Neurosurg* 69:923-927, 1988.
105. Schmetterer L, Findl O, Strenn K, et al: Role of NO in the O_2 and CO_2 responsiveness of cerebral and ocular circulation in humans. *Am J Physiol* 273:R2005-R2012, 1997.
106. DiGeronimo RJ, Gegg CA, Zuckerman SL: Adenosine depletion alters postictal hypoxic cerebral vasodilation in the newborn pig. *Am J Physiol* 274:H1495-H1501, 1998.
107. Ko KR, Ngai AC, Winn HR: Role of adenosine in regulation of regional cerebral blood flow in sensory cortex. *Am J Physiol* 259:H1703-H178, 1990.
108. Morii S, Ngai AC, Ko KR, Winn HR: Role of adenosine in regulation of cerebral blood flow: effects of theophylline during normoxia and hypoxia. *Am J Physiol* 253:H165-H175, 1987.
109. Winn HR, Rubio R, Berne RM: Brain adenosine concentration during hypoxia in rats. *Am J Physiol* 241:H235-H242, 1981.
110. Winn HR, Welsh JE, Rubio R, Berne RM: Brain adenosine production in rat during sustained alteration in systemic blood pressure. *Am J Physiol* 239:H636-H641, 1980.
111. Berger C, von Kummer R: Does NO regulate the cerebral blood flow response in hypoxia? *Acta Neurol Scand* 97:118-125, 1998.
112. Buchanan JE, Phillis JW: The role of nitric oxide in the regulation of cerebral blood flow. *Brain Res* 610:248-255, 1993.
113. Dirnagl U, Niwa K, Lindauer U, Villringer A: Coupling of cerebral blood flow to neuronal activation: role of adenosine and nitric oxide. *Am J Physiol* 267:H296-H301, 1994.

114. Iadecola C, Pelligrino DA, Moskowitz MA, Lassen NA: Nitric oxide synthase inhibition and cerebrovascular regulation. *J Cereb Blood Flow Metab* 14:175-192, 1994.
115. Lavi S, Egbarya R, Lavi R, Jacob G: Role of nitric oxide in the regulation of cerebral blood flow in humans: chemoregulation versus mechanoregulation. *Circulation* 107:1901-1905, 2003.
116. Lindauer U, Megow D, Matsuda H, Dirnagl U: Nitric oxide: a modulator, but not a mediator, of neurovascular coupling in rat somatosensory cortex. *Am J Physiol* 277:H799-H811, 1999.
117. Irikura K, Maynard KI, Moskowitz MA: Importance of nitric oxide synthase inhibition to the attenuated vascular responses induced by topical L-nitroarginine during vibrissal stimulation. *J Cereb Blood Flow Metab* 14:45-48, 1994.
118. White RP, Hindley C, Bloomfield PM, et al: The effect of the nitric oxide synthase inhibitor L-NMMA on basal CBF and vasoneuronal coupling in man: a PET study. *J Cereb Blood Flow Metab* 19:673-678, 1999.
119. Thompson BG, Pluta RM, Girton ME, Oldfield EH: Nitric oxide mediation of chemoregulation but not autoregulation of cerebral blood flow in primates. *J Neurosurg* 84:71-78, 1996.
120. Cholet N, Seylaz J, Lacombe P, Bonvento G: Local uncoupling of the cerebrovascular and metabolic responses to somatosensory stimulation after neuronal nitric oxide synthase inhibition. *J Cereb Blood Flow Metab* 17:1191-1201, 1997.
121. Cholet N, Bonvento G, Seylaz J: Effect of neuronal NO synthase inhibition on the cerebral vasodilatory response to somatosensory stimulation. *Brain Res* 708:197-200, 1996.
122. Joshi S, Young WL, Duong DH, et al: Intracarotid infusion of the nitric oxide synthase inhibitor, L-NMMA, modestly decreases cerebral blood flow in human subjects. *Anesthesiology* 93: 699-707, 2000.
123. Niwa K, Lindauer U, Villringer A, Dirnagl U: Blockade of nitric oxide synthesis in rats strongly attenuates the CBF response to extracellular acidosis. *J Cereb Blood Flow Metab* 13:535-539, 1993.
124. Kotani K, Ueno S, Sano A, Kakimoto Y: Isolation and identification of methylarginines from bovine brain. *J Neurochem* 58:1127-1129, 1992.
125. Xiong Y, Li YJ, Yu XJ, et al: Endogenous inhibitors of nitric oxide synthesis and lipid peroxidation in hyperlipidemic rabbits. *Zhongguo Yao Li Xue Bao* 17:149-152, 1996.
126. McPherson RW, Kirsch JR, Ghaly RF, Traystman RJ: Effect of nitric oxide synthase inhibition on the cerebral vascular response to hypercapnia in primates. *Stroke* 26:682-687, 1995.
127. Irikura K, Huang PL, Ma J, et al: Cerebrovascular alterations in mice lacking neuronal nitric oxide synthase gene expression. *Proc Natl Acad Sci U S A* 92:6823-6827, 1995.
128. Wang Q, Kjaer T, Jorgensen MB, et al: Nitric oxide does not act as a mediator coupling cerebral blood flow to neural activity following somatosensory stimuli in rats. *Neurol Res* 15:33-36, 1993.
129. Ivankovich AD, Miletich DJ, Albrecht RF, Zahed B: Sodium nitroprusside and cerebral blood flow in the anesthetized and unanesthetized goat. *Anesthesiology* 44:21-26, 1976.
130. Clarkson P, Adams MR, Powe AJ, et al: Oral L-arginine improves endothelium-dependent dilation in hypercholesterolemic young adults. *J Clin Invest* 97:1989-1994, 1996.
131. Rossitch E Jr, Alexander E 3rd, Black PM, Cooke JP: L-arginine normalizes endothelial function in cerebral vessels from hypercholesterolemic rabbits. *J Clin Invest* 87:1295-1299, 1991.
132. Stroes E, Kastelein J, Cosentino F, et al: Tetrahydrobiopterin restores endothelial function in hypercholesterolemia. *J Clin Invest* 99:41-46, 1997.
133. Hino A, Tokuyama Y, Weir B, et al: Changes in endothelial nitric oxide synthase mRNA during vasospasm after subarachnoid hemorrhage in monkeys. *Neurosurgery* 39:562-567, 1996; discussion 567-568.
134. Kajita Y, Suzuki Y, Oyama H, et al: Combined effect of L-arginine and superoxide dismutase on the spastic basilar artery after subarachnoid hemorrhage in dogs. *J Neurosurg* 80:476-483, 1994.
135. Kim P, Schini VB, Sundt TM Jr, Vanhoutte PM: Reduced production of cGMP underlies the loss of endothelium-dependent relaxations in the canine basilar artery after subarachnoid hemorrhage. *Circ Res* 70:248-256, 1992.
136. Macdonald RL, Weir BK: A review of hemoglobin and the pathogenesis of cerebral vasospasm. *Stroke* 22:971-982, 1991.
137. Nishizawa S, Yamamoto S, Yokoyama T, et al: Chronological changes of arterial diameter, cGMP, and protein kinase C in the development of vasospasm. *Stroke* 26:1916-1920, 1995; discussion 1920-1921.
138. Lindauer U, Dreier J, Angstwurm K, et al: Role of nitric oxide synthase inhibition in leukocyte-endothelium interaction in the rat pial microvasculature. *J Cereb Blood Flow Metab* 16:1143-1152, 1996.
139. Yoshimoto S, Ishizaki Y, Kurihara H, et al: Cerebral microvessel endothelium is producing endothelin. *Brain Res* 508:283-285, 1990.
140. Nilsson T, Cantera L, Adner M, Edvinsson L: Presence of contractile endothelin-A and dilatory endothelin-B receptors in human cerebral arteries. *Neurosurgery* 40:346-351, 1997; discussion 351-353.
141. Kobayashi H, Hayashi M, Kobayashi S, et al: Cerebral vasospasm and vasoconstriction caused by endothelin. *Neurosurgery* 28: 673-678, 1991; discussion 678-679.
142. Roux S, Loffler BM, Gray GA, et al: The role of endothelin in experimental cerebral vasospasm. *Neurosurgery* 37:78-85, 1995; discussion 85-86.
143. Hino A, Tokuyama Y, Kobayashi M, et al: Increased expression of endothelin B receptor mRNA following subarachnoid hemorrhage in monkeys. *J Cereb Blood Flow Metab* 16:688-697, 1996.
144. Armstead WM, Mirro R, Leffler CW, Busija DW: Cerebral superoxide anion generation during seizures in newborn pigs. *J Cereb Blood Flow Metab* 9:175-179, 1989.
145. Armstead WM, Mirro R, Busija DW, Leffler CW: Postischemic generation of superoxide anion by newborn pig brain. *Am J Physiol* 255:H401-H403, 1988.
146. Kasemsri T, Armstead WM: Endothelin production links superoxide generation to altered opioid-induced pial artery vasodilation after brain injury in pigs. *Stroke* 28:190-196, 1997; discussion 197.
147. Leib SL, Kim YS, Chow LL, et al: Reactive oxygen intermediates contribute to necrotic and apoptotic neuronal injury in an infant rat model of bacterial meningitis due to group B streptococci. *J Clin Invest* 98:2632-2639, 1996.
148. Pourcyrous M, Leffler CW, Mirro R, Busija DW: Brain superoxide anion generation during asphyxia and reventilation in newborn pigs. *Pediatr Res* 28:618-621, 1990.
149. Heineman FW, Grayson J: Transmural distribution of intramyocardial pressure measured by micropipette technique. *Am J Physiol* 249:H1216-H1223, 1985.
150. Flynn AE, Coggins DL, Goto M, et al: Does systolic subepicardial perfusion come from retrograde subendocardial flow? *Am J Physiol (Heart Circ Physiol)* 262:H1759-H1769, 1992.
151. Goto M, Flynn AE, Doucette JW, et al: Cardiac contraction affects deep myocardial vessels predominantly. *Am. J. Physiol* 261: H1417-H1429, 1991.
152. Hiramatsu O, Goto M, Yada T, et al: In vivo observations of the intramural arterioles and venules in beating canine hearts. *J Physiol* 509:619-628, 1998.
153. Kajiya F, Goto M: Integrative physiology of coronary microcirculation. *Jpn J Physiol* 49:229-241, 1999.
154. Willemsen MJ, Duncker DJ, Krams R, et al: Decrease in coronary vascular volume in systole augments cardiac contraction. *Am J Physiol Heart Circ Physiol* 281:H731-H737, 2001.
155. Gregg DE, Khouri EM, Rayford CR: Systemic and coronary energetics in the resting unanesthetized dog. *Circ Res* 16:102-113, 1965.
156. Kajiya F, Tomonaga G, Tsujioka K, et al: Evaluation of local blood flow velocity in proximal and distal coronary arteries by laser Doppler method. *J Biomech Eng* 107:10-15, 1985.
157. Berne RM, Levy MN: Coronary circulation. In Berne RM, editor: *Cardiovascular physiology*. Toronto, 1986, Mosby.
158. Berne RM, Rubio R. Coronary circulation. In Berne RM, Sperelakis N, editors: *Handbook of physiology, section 2: the cardiovascular system.* Bethesda, 1979, American Physiological Society.

159. Lowensohn HS, Khouri EM, Gregg DE, et al: Phasic right coronary artery flow in conscious dogs with normal and elevated right ventricular pressures. *Circ Res* 39:760-766, 1976.
160. Kitamura K, Jorgensen CR, Gobel FL, et al: Hemodynamic correlates of myocardial oxygen consumption during upright exercise. *J Appl Physiol* 32:516-522, 1972.
161. Dole WP, Yamada N, Bishop VS, Olsson RA: Role of adenosine in coronary blood flow regulation after reductions in perfusing pressure. *Circ Res* 56:517-524, 1985.
162. Klocke FJ: Coronary blood flow in man. *Prog Cardiovasc Dis* 19:117-166, 1976.
163. Hoffman JIE: Transmural myocardial perfusion. *Prog Cardiovasc Dis* 29:429-464, 1987.
164. Hoffman JIE: Maximal coronary flow and the concept of coronary vascular reserve. *Circulation* 70:153-159, 1984.
165. Hoffman JIE: A critical view of coronary reserve. *Circulation* 75(suppl I):6-11, 1987.
166. Hoffman JI: Problems of coronary flow reserve. *Ann Biomed Eng* 28:884-896, 2000.
167. Bellamy RF: Diastolic coronary pressure-flow relations in the dog. *Circ Res* 43:92-101, 1978.
168. Hoffman JIE, Spaan JAE: Pressure-flow relations in coronary circulation. *Physiol Rev* 70:331-390, 1990.
169. Scharf SM, Bromberger-Barnea B, Permutt S: Distribution of coronary venous flow. *J Appl Physiol* 30:657-662, 1971.
170. Uhlig PN, Baer RW, Vlahakes GJ, et al: Arterial and venous coronary pressure-flow relations in anesthetized dogs. Evidence for a vascular waterfall in epicardial coronary veins. *Circ Res* 55:238-248, 1984.
171. Coggins DL, Flynn AE, Austin RE Jr, et al: Nonuniform loss of regional flow reserve during myocardial ischemia in dogs. *Circulation Res* 67:253-264, 1990.
172. Strauer BE: Left ventricular hypertrophy, myocardial blood flow and coronary flow reserve. *Cardiology* 81:274-282, 1992.
173. Strauer B-E: Ventricular function and coronary hemodynamics in hypertensive heart disease. *Am J Cardiol* 44:999-1006, 1979.
174. Strauer B-E: Myocardial oxygen consumption in chronic heart disease: role of wall stress, hypertrophy and coronary reserve. *Am J Cardiol* 44:730-740, 1979.
175. Strauer B-E: The coronary circulation in hypertensive heart disease. *Hypertension* 6(suppl III):74-80, 1984.
176. Strauer BE: The significance of coronary reserve in clinical heart disease. *J Am Coll Cardiol* 15:775-783, 1990.
177. Hoffman JIE, Grattan MT, Hanley FL, Messina LM: Total and transmural perfusion of the hypertrophied heart. In ter Keurs HEDJ, Schipperheyn JJ, editors: *Cardiac left ventricular hypertrophy.* Boston, 1983, Martinus Nijhoff.
178. Vogt M, Motz W, Strauer BE: Coronary haemodynamics in hypertensive heart disease. *Eur Heart J* 13(suppl D):44-49, 1992.
179. Strauer BE: Significance of coronary circulation in hypertensive heart disease for development and prevention of heart failure. *Am J Cardiol* 65:34G-41G, 1990.
180. Vlahakes GJ, Turley K, Hoffman JIE: The pathophysiology of failure in acute right ventricular hypertension: hemodynamic and biochemical correlations. *Circulation* 63:87-95, 1981.
181. Belenkie I, Horne SG, Dani R, et al: Effects of aortic constriction during experimental acute right ventricular pressure loading. Further insights into diastolic and systolic ventricular interaction. *Circulation* 92:546-554, 1995.
182. Archie JP, Brown R: Effect of preload on the transmural distribution of diastolic coronary blood flow. *J Surg Res* 16: 215-223, 1974.
183. Manohar M, Bisgard GE, Bullard V, Rankin JHG: Blood flow in the hypertrophied right ventricular myocardium of unanesthetized ponies. *Am J Physiol Heart Circ Physiol* 240:H881-H888, 1981.
184. Murray PA, Vatner SF: Carotid sinus baroreceptor control of right coronary circulation in normal, hypertrophied, and failing right ventricles of conscious dogs. *Circ Res* 49:1339-1349, 1981.
185. Cooper N, Brazier J, Buckberg G: Effects of systemic-pulmonary shunts on regional myocardial blood flow in experimental pulmonary stenosis. *J Thorac Cardiovasc Surg* 70:166-176, 1975.
186. Mayers I, Johnson D: The nonspecific inflammatory response to injury. *Can J Anaesth* 45:871-879, 1998.
187. Vallet B, Lund N, Curtis SE, et al: Gut and muscle tissue PO_2 in endotoxemic dogs during shock and resuscitation. *J Appl Physiol* 76:793-800, 1994.
188. Swank GM, Deitch EA: Role of the gut in multiple organ failure: bacterial translocation and permeability changes. *World J Surg* 20:411-417, 1996.
189. Baker JW, Deitch EA, Li M, et al: Hemorrhagic shock induces bacterial translocation from the gut. *J Trauma* 28:896-906, 1988.
190. Riddington DW, Venkatesh B, Boivin CM, et al: Intestinal permeability, gastric intramucosal pH, and systemic endotoxemia in patients undergoing cardiopulmonary bypass. *JAMA* 275: 1007-1012, 1996.
191. Ohri SK, Bowles CW, Mathie RT, et al: Effect of cardiopulmonary bypass perfusion protocols on gut tissue oxygenation and blood flow. *Ann Thorac Surg* 64:163-170, 1997.
192. Moore FA, Moore EE: Evolving concepts in the pathogenesis of postinjury multiple organ failure. *Surg Clin North Am* 75: 257-277, 1995.
193. Moore FA, Sauaia A, Moore EE, et al: Postinjury multiple organ failure: a bimodal phenomenon. *J Trauma* 40:501-510, 1996; discussion 510-512.
194. Kirton OC, Windsor J, Wedderburn R, et al: Failure of splanchnic resuscitation in the acutely injured trauma patient correlates with multiple organ system failure and length of stay in the ICU. *Chest* 113:1064-1069, 1998.
195. Doglio GR, Pusajo JF, Egurrola MA, et al: Gastric mucosal pH as a prognostic index of mortality in critically ill patients. *Crit Care Med* 19:1037-1040, 1991.
196. Matheson P, Wilson M, Garrison R: Regulation of intestinal blood flow. *J Surg Res* 93:182-196, 2000.
197. Lundgren O: Autoregulation of intestinal blood flow: physiology and pathophysiology. *J Hypertens* 7:S79-S84, 1989.
198. Donald DE, Shepherd JT: Autonomic regulation of the peripheral circulation. *Annu Rev Physiol* 42:429-439, 1980.
199. Hilton SM, Spyer KM: Central nervous regulation of vascular resistance. *Annu Rev Physiol* 42:399-411, 1980.
200. Bohlen HG: Na+-induced intestinal interstitial hyperosmolality and vascular responses during absorptive hyperemia. *Am J Physiol* 242:H785-H789, 1982.
201. Granger DN, Granger HJ: Systems analysis of intestinal hemodynamics and oxygenation. *Am J Physiol* 245:G786-G796, 1983.
202. Matheson PJ, Wilson MA, Garrison RN: Regulation of intestinal blood flow. *J Surg Res* 93:182-196, 2000.
203. Pawlik WW, Fondacaro JD, Jacobson ED: Metabolic hyperemia in canine gut. *Am J Physiol* 239:G12-G17, 1980.
204. Shepherd AP: Intestinal capillary blood flow during metabolic hyperemia. *Am J Physiol* 237:E548-E554, 1979.
205. Granger DN, Granger JP, Brace RA, et al: Analysis of the permeability characteristics of cat intestinal capillaries. *Circ Res* 44:335-344, 1979.
206. Sawmiller DR, Chou CC: Role of adenosine in postprandial and reactive hyperemia in canine jejunum. *Am J Physiol* 263: G487-G493, 1992.
207. Sawmiller DR, Chou CC: Adenosine plays a role in food-induced jejunal hyperemia. *Am J Physiol* 255:G168-G174, 1988.
208. Sawmiller DR, Chou CC: Jejunal adenosine increases during food-induced jejunal hyperemia. *Am J Physiol* 258:G370-G376, 1990.
209. Sawmiller DR, Chou CC: Adenosine is a vasodilator in the intestinal mucosa. *Am J Physiol* 261:G9-15, 1991.
210. Meyer T, Brinck U: Differential distribution of serotonin and tryptophan hydroxylase in the human gastrointestinal tract. *Digestion* 60:63-68, 1999.
211. Fan L, Iseki S: Immunohistochemical localization of vascular endothelial growth factor in the globule leukocyte/mucosal mast cell of the rat respiratory and digestive tracts. *Histochem Cell Biol* 111:13-21, 1999.
212. Rothschild AM, Gomes EL, Fortunato IC: Bradykinin release from high molecular weight kininogen and increase in plasma kallikrein-like activity following sensory stimulation by food in the rat. *Naunyn Schmiedebergs Arch Pharmacol* 358:483-488, 1998.
213. Alemayehu A, Chou CC: Thromboxane plays a role in postprandial jejunal oxygen uptake and capillary exchange. *Am J Physiol* 259:G430-G435, 1990.

214. Gallavan RH Jr, Chou CC: Prostaglandin synthesis inhibition and postprandial intestinal hyperemia. *Am J Physiol* 242:G140-G146, 1982.
215. Gallavan RH Jr, Chen MH, Joffe SN, Jacobson ED: Vasoactive intestinal polypeptide, cholecystokinin, glucagon, and bile-oleate-induced jejunal hyperemia. *Am J Physiol* 248:G208-G215, 1985.
216. Chou CC: Splanchnic and overall cardiovascular hemodynamics during eating and digestion. *Fed Proc* 42:1658-1661, 1983.
217. Gallavan RH Jr, Chou CC: Possible mechanisms for the initiation and maintenance of postprandial intestinal hyperemia. *Am J Physiol* 249:G301-G308, 1985.
218. Nyhof RA, Chou CC: Evidence against local neural mechanism for intestinal postprandial hyperemia. *Am J Physiol* 245: H437-H446, 1983.
219. Nyhof RA, Ingold-Wilcox D, Chou CC: Effect of atropine on digested food-induced intestinal hyperemia. *Am J Physiol* 249:G685-G690, 1985.
220. Chou CC, Alemayehu A, Mangino MJ: Prostanoids in regulation of postprandial jejunal hyperemia and oxygen uptake. *Am J Physiol* 257:G798-G808, 1989.
221. Kvietys PR, Gallavan RH, Chou CC: Contribution of bile to postprandial intestinal hyperemia. *Am J Physiol* 238:G284-G288, 1980.
222. Kvietys PR, McLendon JM, Granger DN: Postprandial intestinal hyperemia: role of bile salts in the ileum. *Am J Physiol* 241: G469-G477, 1981.
223. Chou CC, Nyhof RA, Kvietys PR, et al: Regulation of jejunal blood flow and oxygenation during glucose and oleic acid absorption. *Am J Physiol* 249:G691-G701, 1985.
224. Chou CC, Burns TD, Hsieh CP, Dabney JM: Mechanisms of local vasodilation with hypertonic glucose in the jejunum. *Surgery* 71:380-387, 1972.
225. Bohlen HG: Intestinal tissue PO_2 and microvascular responses during glucose exposure. *Am J Physiol* 238:H164-H171, 1980.
226. Bohlen HG: Intestinal mucosal oxygenation influences absorptive hyperemia. *Am J Physiol* 239:H489-H493, 1980.
227. Kvietys PR, Perry MA, Granger DN: Intestinal capillary exchange capacity and oxygen delivery-to-demand ratio. *Am J Physiol* 245:G635-G640, 1983.
228. Kvietys PR, Wilborn WH, Granger DN: Effect of atropine on bile-oleic acid-induced alterations in dog jejunal hemodynamics, oxygenation, and net transmucosal water movement. *Gastroenterology* 80:31-38, 1981.
229. Sit SP, Chou CC: Time course of jejunal blood flow, O_2 uptake, and O_2 extraction during nutrient absorption. *Am J Physiol* 247:H395-H402, 1984.
230. Tso P, Fujimoto K: The absorption and transport of lipids by the small intestine. *Brain Res Bull* 27:477-482, 1991.
231. Flynn WJ Jr, Gosche JR, Garrison RN: Intestinal blood flow is restored with glutamine or glucose suffusion after hemorrhage. *J Surg Res* 52:499-504, 1992.
232. Gosche JR, Garrison RN, Harris PD, Cryer HG: Absorptive hyperemia restores intestinal blood flow during Escherichia coli sepsis in the rat. *Arch Surg* 125:1573-1576, 1990.
233. Revelly JP, Tappy L, Berger MM, et al: Early metabolic and splanchnic responses to enteral nutrition in postoperative cardiac surgery patients with circulatory compromise. *Intensive Care Med* 27:540-547, 2001.
234. Kliegman RM, Pittard WB, Fanaroff AA: Necrotizing enterocolitis in neonates fed human milk. *J Pediatr* 95:450-453, 2001.
235. Lucas A, Cole TJ: Breast milk and neonatal necrotising enterocolitis. *Lancet* 336:1519-1523, 1990.
236. Stoll BJ: Epidemiology of necrotizing enterocolitis. *Clin Perinatol* 21:205-218, 1994.
237. Fischer H, Becker JC, Boknik P, et al: Expression of constitutive nitric oxide synthase in rat and human gastrointestinal tract. *Biochim Biophys Acta* 1450:414-422, 1999.
238. Shah V, Haddad FG, Garcia-Cardena G, et al: Liver sinusoidal endothelial cells are responsible for nitric oxide modulation of resistance in the hepatic sinusoids. *J Clin Invest* 100:2923-2930, 1997.
239. Kusayama T, Yamazaki J, Nagao T: Flow dependence of nitric oxide-mediated pressure change in rat mesenteric beds with different tonus. *Eur J Pharmacol* 312:301-307, 1996.
240. Mittal MK, Gupta TK, Lee FY, et al: Nitric oxide modulates hepatic vascular tone in normal rat liver. *Am J Physiol* 267: G416-G422, 1994.
241. Cahill P, Redmond E, Sitzmann JV: Endothelial dysfunction in cirrhosis and portal hypertension. *Pharmacol Ther* 89: 273-293, 2001.
242. Pannen BH, Bauer M, Noldge-Schomburg GF, et al: Regulation of hepatic blood flow during resuscitation from hemorrhagic shock: role of NO and endothelins. *Am J Physiol* 272:H2736-H2745, 1997.
243. Clemens MG: Nitric oxide in liver injury. *Hepatology* 30:1-5, 1999.
244. Shah V, Lyford G, Gores G, Farrugia G: Nitric oxide in gastrointestinal health and disease. *Gastroenterology* 126: 903-913, 2004.
245. Matheson PJ, Wilson MA, Spain DA, et al: Glucose-induced intestinal hyperemia is mediated by nitric oxide. *J Surg Res* 72:146-154, 1997.
246. Matheson PJ, Spain DA, Harris PD, et al: Glucose and glutamine gavage increase portal vein nitric oxide metabolite levels via adenosine A2b activation. *J Surg Res* 84:57-63, 1999.
247. Watkins CC, Sawa A, Jaffrey S, et al: Insulin restores neuronal nitric oxide synthase expression and function that is lost in diabetic gastropathy. *J Clin Invest* 106:373-384, 2000.
248. Russo A, Fraser R, Adachi K, et al: Evidence that nitric oxide mechanisms regulate small intestinal motility in humans. *Gut* 44: 72-76, 1999.
249. Boughton-Smith NK, Evans SM, Hawkey CJ, et al: Nitric oxide synthase activity in ulcerative colitis and Crohn's disease. *Lancet* 342:338-340, 1993.
250. Perner A, Andresen L, Normark M, et al: Expression of nitric oxide synthases and effects of L-arginine and L-NMMA on nitric oxide production and fluid transport in collagenous colitis. *Gut* 49:387-394, 2001.
251. Middleton SJ, Shorthouse M, Hunter JO: Increased nitric oxide synthesis in ulcerative colitis. *Lancet* 341:465-466, 1993.
252. Lundberg JO, Hellstrom PM, Lundberg JM, Alving K: Greatly increased luminal nitric oxide in ulcerative colitis. *Lancet* 344:1673-1674, 1994.
253. Shah V, Chen AF, Cao S, et al: Gene transfer of recombinant endothelial nitric oxide synthase to liver in vivo and in vitro. *Am J Physiol Gastrointest Liver Physiol* 279:G1023-G1030, 2000.
254. Fiorucci S, Antonelli E, Morelli O, et al: NCX-1000, a NO-releasing derivative of ursodeoxycholic acid, selectively delivers NO to the liver and protects against development of portal hypertension. *Proc Natl Acad Sci U S A* 98:8897-902, 2001.
255. Lanas A, Bajador E, Serrano P, et al: Nitrovasodilators, low-dose aspirin, other nonsteroidal antiinflammatory drugs, and the risk of upper gastrointestinal bleeding. *N Engl J Med* 343:834-839, 2000.
256. Fiorucci S, Antonelli E, Santucci L, et al: Gastrointestinal safety of nitric oxide-derived aspirin is related to inhibition of ICE-like cysteine proteases in rats. *Gastroenterology* 116:1089-1106, 1999.
257. Clozel M, Clozel JP: Effects of endothelin on regional blood flows in squirrel monkeys. *J Pharmacol Exp Ther* 250:1125-1131, 1989.
258. Minkes RK, Kadowitz PJ: Influence of endothelin on systemic arterial pressure and regional blood flow in the cat. *Eur J Pharmacol* 163:163-166, 1989.
259. MacLean MR, Randall MD, Hiley CR: Effects of moderate hypoxia, hypercapnia and acidosis on haemodynamic changes induced by endothelin-1 in the pithed rat. *Br J Pharmacol* 98:1055-1065, 1989.
260. Cargill RI, Kiely DG, Clark RA, Lipworth BJ: Hypoxaemia and release of endothelin-1. *Thorax* 50:1308-1310, 1995.
261. Chou MC, Wilson MA, Spain DA, et al: Endothelin-1 expression in the small intestine during chronic peritonitis. *Shock* 4:411-414, 1995.
262. Ferri C, Bellini C, De Angelis C, et al: Circulating endothelin-1 concentrations in patients with chronic hypoxia. *J Clin Pathol* 48:519-524, 1995.
263. Fukuda S, Taga K, Tanaka T, et al: Relationship between tissue ischemia and venous endothelin-1 during abdominal aortic aneurysm surgery. *J Cardiothorac Vasc Anesth* 9:510-514, 1995.

264. te Velthuis H, Jansen PG, Oudemans-van Straaten HM, et al: Circulating endothelin in cardiac operations: influence of blood pressure and endotoxin. *Ann Thorac Surg* 61:904-908, 1996.
265. Miura S, Fukumura D, Kurose I, et al: Roles of ET-1 in endotoxin-induced microcirculatory disturbance in rat small intestine. *Am J Physiol* 271:G461-G469, 1996.
266. Wilson MA, Steeb GD, Garrison RN: Endothelins mediate intestinal hypoperfusion during bacteremia. *J Surg Res* 55:168-175, 1993.
267. Burgener D, Laesser M, Treggiari-Venzi M, et al: Endothelin-1 blockade corrects mesenteric hypoperfusion in a porcine low cardiac output model. *Crit Care Med* 29:1615-1620, 2001.
268. Ozel SK, Yuksel M, Haklar G, et al: Nitric oxide and endothelin relationship in intestinal ischemia/reperfusion injury (II). *Prostaglandins Leukot Essent Fatty Acids* 64:253-257, 2001.
269. Nankervis CA, Reber KM, Nowicki PT: Age-dependent changes in the postnatal intestinal microcirculation. *Microcirculation* 8:377-387, 2001.
270. Guzman JA, Rosado AE, Kruse JA: Dopamine-1 receptor stimulation attenuates the vasoconstrictive response to gut ischemia. *J Appl Physiol* 91:596-602, 2001.
271. Jakob SM, Ruokonen E, Takala J: Effects of dopamine on systemic and regional blood flow and metabolism in septic and cardiac surgery patients. *Shock* 18:8-13, 2002.
272. Clemmesen JO, Galatius S, Skak C, et al: The effect of increasing blood pressure with dopamine on systemic, splanchnic, and lower extremity hemodynamics in patients with acute liver failure. *Scand J Gastroenterol* 34:921-927, 1999.
273. LeDoux D, Astiz ME, Carpati CM, Rackow EC: Effects of perfusion pressure on tissue perfusion in septic shock. *Crit Care Med* 28:2729-2732, 2000.
274. Lindner KH, Brinkmann A, Pfenninger EG, et al: Effect of vasopressin on hemodynamic variables, organ blood flow, and acid-base status in a pig model of cardiopulmonary resuscitation. *Anesth Analg* 77:427-435, 1993.
275. Prengel AW, Lindner KH, Wenzel V, et al: Splanchnic and renal blood flow after cardiopulmonary resuscitation with epinephrine and vasopressin in pigs. *Resuscitation* 38:19-24, 1998.
276. Dworkin LD, Sun AM, Brenner BM: The renal circulations. In Brenner BM, editor: *The kidney*, ed 6. Philadelphia, 2000, WB Saunders.
277. Arendshorst WJ, Navar LG: Renal circulation and glomerular hemodynamics. In Schirer RW, Gottschalk CW, editors: *Diseases of the kidney*, ed 5. Boston, 1993, Brown.
278. Kallskog O, Lindbrom LO, Ulfendahl HR, Wolgast M: Hydrostatic pressures within the vascular structures of the rat kidney. *Pflugers Arch* 363:205-210, 1976.
279. Fretschner M, Endlich K, Fester C, et al: A narrow segment of the efferent arteriole controls efferent resistance in the hydronephrotic rat kidney. *Kidney Int* 37:1227-1239, 1990.
280. Mulvany MJ, Aalkjaer C: Structure and function of small arteries. *Physiol Rev* 70:921-961, 1990.
281. Gilmore JP, Cornish KG, Rogers SD, Joyner WL: Direct evidence for myogenic autoregulation of the renal microcirculation in the hamster. *Circ Res* 47:226-230, 1980.
282. Myers BD, Deen WM, Brenner BM: Effects of norepinephrine and angiotensin II on the determinants of glomerular ultrafiltration and proximal tubule fluid reabsorption in the rat. *Circ Res* 37:101-110, 1975.
283. Edwards RM: Segmental effects of norepinephrine and angiotensin II on isolated renal microvessels. *Am J Physiol* 244:F526-F534, 1983.
284. Desjars P, Pinaud M, Bugnon D, Tasseau F: Norepinephrine therapy has no deleterious renal effects in human septic shock. *Crit Care Med* 17:426-429, 1989.
285. Steinhausen M, Sterzel RB, Fleming JT, et al: Acute and chronic effects of angiotensin II on the vessels of the split hydronephrotic kidney. *Kidney Int Suppl* 20:S64-S73, 1987.
286. Jard S, Lombard C, Marie J, Devilliers G: Vasopressin receptors from cultured mesangial cells resemble V1a type. *Am J Physiol* 253:F41-F49, 1987.
287. Naitoh M, Suzuki H, Murakami M, et al: Arginine vasopressin produces renal vasodilation via V2 receptors in conscious dogs. *Am J Physiol* 265:R934-R942, 1993.
288. Gellai M, Silverstein JH, Hwang JC, et al: Influence of vasopressin on renal hemodynamics in conscious Brattleboro rats. *Am J Physiol* 246:F819-F827, 1984.
289. Azzawi SA, Shirley DG: The effect of vasopressin on renal blood flow and its distribution in the rat. *J Physiol* 341:233-244, 1983.
290. Russ RD, Walker BR: Role of nitric oxide in vasopressinergic pulmonary vasodilatation. *Am J Physiol* 262:H743-H747, 1992.
291. Landry DW, Levin HR, Gallant EM, et al: Vasopressin deficiency contributes to the vasodilation of septic shock. *Circulation* 95:1122-1125, 1997.
292. Edwards RM, Trizna W, Kinter LB: Renal microvascular effects of vasopressin and vasopressin antagonists. *Am J Physiol* 256: F274-F278, 1989.
293. Naicker S, Bhoola KD: Endothelins: Vasoactive modulators of renal function in health and disease. *Pharmacol Ther* 90:61-88, 2001.
294. Takabatake T, Ise T, Ohta K, Kobayashi K: Effects of endothelin on renal hemodynamics and tubuloglomerular feedback. *Am J Physiol* 263:F103-F108, 1992.
295. Tomita K, Nonoguchi H, Marumo F: Regulation of NaCl transport by endothelin in renal tubules. *Semin Nephrol* 12:30-36, 1992.
296. Yoshimura A, Iwasaki S, Inui K, et al: Endothelin-1 and endothelin B type receptor are induced in mesangial proliferative nephritis in the rat. *Kidney Int* 48:1290-1297, 1995.
297. Simonson MS, Emancipator SN, Knauss T, Hricik DE: Elevated neointimal endothelin-1 in transplantation-associated arteriosclerosis of renal allograft recipients. *Kidney Int* 54: 960-971, 1998.
298. Shichiri M, Hirata Y, Ando K, et al: Plasma endothelin levels in hypertension and chronic renal failure. *Hypertension* 15:493-496, 1990.
299. Roccatello D, Mosso R, Ferro M, et al: Urinary endothelin in glomerulonephritis patients with normal renal function. *Clin Nephrol* 41:323-330, 1994.
300. Krum H, Viskoper RJ, Lacourciere Y, et al: The effect of an endothelin-receptor antagonist, bosentan, on blood pressure in patients with essential hypertension. Bosentan Hypertension Investigators. *N Engl J Med* 338:784-790, 1998.
301. Firth JD, Ratcliffe PJ: Organ distribution of the three rat endothelin messenger RNAs and the effects of ischemia on renal gene expression. *J Clin Invest* 90:1023-1031, 1992.
302. Laragh JH: Atrial natriuretic hormone, the renin-aldosterone axis, and blood pressure-electrolyte homeostasis. *N Engl J Med* 313:1330-1340, 1985.
303. de Bold AJ, Borenstein HB, Veress AT, Sonnenberg H: A rapid and potent natriuretic response to intravenous injection of atrial myocardial extract in rats. *Life Sci* 28:89-94, 1981.
304. Levenson DJ, Simmons CE Jr, Brenner BM: Arachidonic acid metabolism, prostaglandins and the kidney. *Am J Med* 72: 354-374, 1982.
305. Gerber JG, Olson RD, Nies AS: Interrelationship between prostaglandins and renin release. *Kidney Int* 19:816-821, 1981.
306. Shipley RE, Study RS: Changes in renal blood flow, extraction of inulin, glomerular filtration rate, tissue pressure and urine flow with acute alterations of renal artery blood pressure. *Am J Physiol* 167:676-688, 1951.
307. Nakanishi K, Mattson DL, Cowley AW Jr: Role of renal medullary blood flow in the development of L-NAME hypertension in rats. *Am J Physiol* 268:R317-R323, 1995.
308. Miyata N, Cowley AW Jr: Renal intramedullary infusion of L-arginine prevents reduction of medullary blood flow and hypertension in Dahl salt-sensitive rats. *Hypertension* 33: 446-450, 1999.
309. Mattson DL, Roman RJ, Cowley AW Jr: Role of nitric oxide in renal papillary blood flow and sodium excretion. *Hypertension* 19:766-769, 1992.
310. Mattson DL, Lu S, Nakanishi K, et al: Effect of chronic renal medullary nitric oxide inhibition on blood pressure. *Am J Physiol* 266:H1918-H1926, 1994.
311. Larson TS, Lockhart JC: Restoration of vasa recta hemodynamics and pressure natriuresis in SHR by L-arginine. *Am J Physiol* 268:F907-F912, 1995.
312. Oury TD, Day BJ, Crapo JD: Extracellular superoxide dismutase: a regulator of nitric oxide bioavailability. *Lab Invest* 75:617-636, 1996.

313. Zou AP, Li N, Cowley AW Jr: Production and actions of superoxide in the renal medulla. *Hypertension* 37:547-553, 2001.
314. Schnackenberg CG, Wilcox CS: The SOD mimetic tempol restores vasodilation in afferent arterioles of experimental diabetes. *Kidney Int* 59:1859-1864, 2001.
315. Schnackenberg CG, Welch WJ, Wilcox CS: TP receptor-mediated vasoconstriction in microperfused afferent arterioles: roles of O(2)(-) and NO. *Am J Physiol Renal Physiol* 279:F302-F308, 2000.
316. Rhinehart KL, Pallone TL: Nitric oxide generation by isolated descending vasa recta. *Am J Physiol Heart Circ Physiol* 281:H316-H324, 2001.
317. Kelleher SP, Robinette JB, Miller F, Conger JD: Effect of hemorrhagic reduction in blood pressure on recovery from acute renal failure. *Kidney Int* 31:725-730, 1987.
318. Conger JD, Hammond WS: Renal vasculature and ischemic injury. *Ren Fail* 14:307-310, 1992.
319. Cumming AD, Driedger AA, McDonald JW, et al: Vasoactive hormones in the renal response to systemic sepsis. *Am J Kidney Dis* 11:23-32, 1988.
320. Mackay JH, Feerick AE, Woodson LC, et al: Increasing organ blood flow during cardiopulmonary bypass in pigs: comparison of dopamine and perfusion pressure. *Crit Care Med* 23:1090-1098, 1995.

CHAPTER 19

Principles of Invasive Monitoring

Jacqueline M. Evans, Eric D. Harry, and Kenneth A. Schenkman

PEARLS

- *Hemodynamic monitoring* refers to measurement of the functional characteristics of the heart and the circulatory system that affect the perfusion of tissues with oxygenated blood.
- Hemodynamic monitoring can be performed invasively or noninvasively and can be used for diagnosis, surveillance, or titration of therapy.
- The central venous waveform is composed of three waves (a, c, and v) and two descents (x and y).
- The arterial waveform has three components: rapid upstroke, dicrotic notch, and runoff.
- Changes in the central venous or arterial waveform can be seen with certain pathologic conditions.
- Cardiac output can be calculated using the Fick method or measured directly via thermodilution.
- A pulmonary artery catheter can be used to directly measure cardiac output and indices of oxygen delivery and extraction.

Role of Invasive Hemodynamic Monitoring

Since William Harvey's early observation that the heart pumps blood in a continuous circuit, the function of the circulatory system has been the subject of intense scrutiny from a variety of perspectives. *Hemodynamic monitoring* refers to measurement of the functional characteristics of the heart and the circulatory system that affect the perfusion of tissues with oxygenated blood in order to maintain homeostasis and to remove byproducts of metabolism. Several different types of invasive hemodynamic monitoring can be used concurrently to guide management. *The goal of hemodynamic monitoring* is to provide more accurate diagnoses and to institute additional interventions in order to deliver improved care to the critically ill patient in the intensive care unit.

In his 1733 report, "*Statical essays: containing haemastaticks; or, an account of some hydraulick and hydrostatical experiments made on the blood and blood-vessels of animals,*" Hales[1] described early experiments in horses in which he was the first to measure central venous pressure (CVP). Figure 19–1 depicts Hales and an assistant in the process of these early experiments.

Clinical hemodynamic measurements at the bedside begin with noninvasive measurements such as heart rate (HR), blood pressure, urine output, and peripheral perfusion. Other noninvasive studies that may contribute to assessment of hemodynamic status include electrocardiograms, chest x-ray films, and echocardiography. Frequently, in the pediatric intensive care unit these measurements are supplemented by invasive hemodynamic measures that require entrance into the intravascular space. Such invasive hemodynamic measurements include placement of central venous catheters to assess right atrial filling pressures, arterial catheters to assess arterial blood pressure, and pulmonary artery catheters to assess left-sided pressures, cardiac output (CO), and vascular resistances. Although invasive hemodynamic monitoring

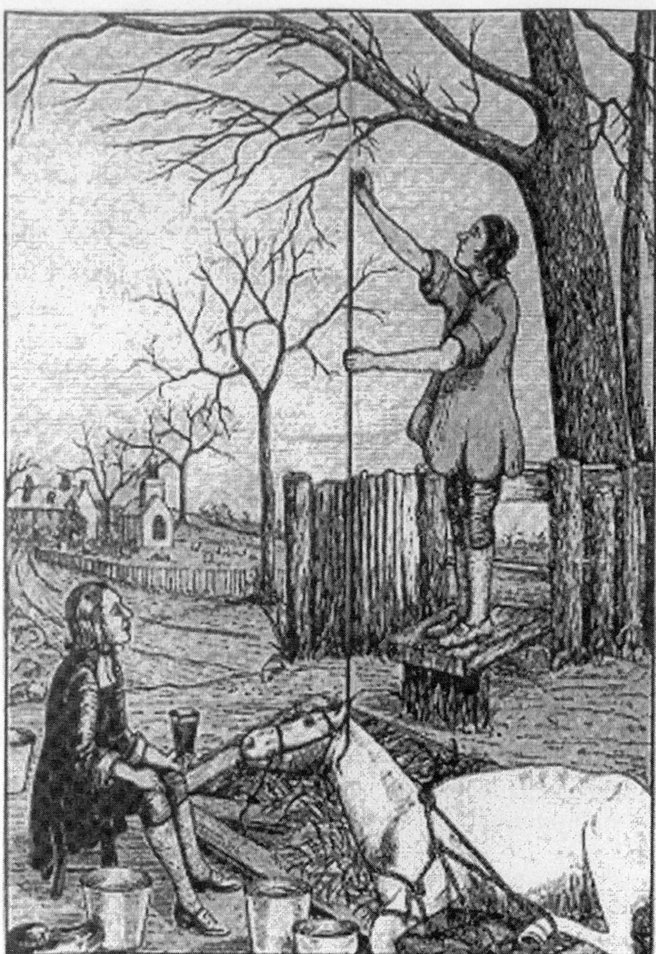

FIGURE 19–1 • Stephen Hales and an assistant measuring the blood pressure of a horse. (From Pickering G: Systemic arterial hypertension. In Fishman AP, Dickinson WR, editors: *Circulation of the blood: men and ideas.* New York, 1964, Oxford University Press.)

can provide the skilled intensivist with a plethora of valuable information, it is not meant to take the place of or minimize the extensive amount of information that can be gained by less invasive measures. Successful use of invasive hemodynamic measurements necessitates that the clinician possesses the requisite skills to obtain these measures safely and with utmost attention to the multiple potential risks imposed upon the patient. Furthermore, for invasive hemodynamic measurements to be useful, the clinician must be able to successfully interpret the information provided by the measurements. Finally, as with any technology, the use of invasive hemodynamic monitoring is in evolution, and it is incumbent upon the clinician to be familiar with developments as they arise and with current controversies regarding these procedures.

This chapter aims to be a practical guide on the use of hemodynamic monitoring in the pediatric intensive care unit. The chapter reviews general principles of measurement and then discusses the three main types of invasive hemodynamic monitoring: central venous catheter, arterial catheter, and pulmonary artery catheter. Indications and controversies, sites of insertion, interpretation of waveforms, and potential complications are addressed. CO monitoring and calculation of oxygen consumption and delivery are reviewed. Chapter 15 discusses the specific techniques for gaining access in order to make these measurements.

Indications for Invasive Hemodynamic Measurements

The three main indications for invasive hemodynamic monitoring are diagnosis, surveillance, and titration of therapy. *Diagnosis* may include the differentiation of septic shock (through assessment of factors such as diminished right heart filling pressures or preload and decreased systemic vascular resistance) from cardiogenic shock (which is characterized by elevated left heart pressures and afterload). *Surveillance* implies observation over time. The purpose of surveillance may be to assess the stability of a patient at risk for adverse changes or to determine the response to therapy. Invasive measurements performed for diagnostic purposes often are continued for surveillance purposes. *Titration of therapy* often is based on information gleaned from invasive measurements.

Principles of Measurement

Intensive care clinicians rely on a wide variety of measurement systems to assess patient clinical status or response to therapy. However, not all clinicians have a good understanding of how physiologic variables are measured and thus may not be able to troubleshoot monitoring systems or recognize when information presented is inaccurate. A detailed discussion of monitoring is beyond the scope of this chapter and may be impractical for the busy clinician to study, but a basic understanding of the principles of measurement is helpful in deciding which measurements to trust and how to assess a monitoring system for accuracy. Detailed descriptions of monitoring systems are given elsewhere.[2–4]

Signal Analysis

Measurements generally are made directly by comparison with known standards or indirectly by use of a calibration system. Determination of length or weight usually is made by direct comparison with a standard ruler or standard mass. Most invasive measurements in the intensive care unit are made indirectly, therefore requiring use of a calibration system. Thus understanding the basis for calibration of a system is important to determine the validity of the measurement.

Measurement systems detect and transform signals so that they can be presented in an interpretable way to the user. Signals can be characterized as static or dynamic. Slowly changing signals, such as body temperature, can be thought of as static. Hemodynamic measurements change from moment to moment and thus are dynamic. Physiologic signals may be periodic, for example, arterial pressure, which varies with the cardiac cycle.

Complex periodic signals, such as an arterial pressure waveform, can be described mathematically as the sum of a series of simpler waveforms called a *Fourier series.*

Alternatively, the arterial tracing can be thought of as a sum of simpler waveforms, sine waves, and cosine waves. Figure 19–2 depicts an arterial pressure waveform as the sum of the first six terms in the Fourier series. The sum of the first six terms in the series forms a waveform similar to the original tracing. Adding additional terms from the Fourier series, or *higher harmonics,* results in an increasingly better representation of the actual waveform. In general, to reproduce a pressure tracing without loss of significant characteristics for clinical use, the measurement system must have an accurate frequency response to approximately 10 times the fundamental frequency (first 10 harmonics).

The sampling rate of a measurement system determines how often a physiologic value is measured. For body temperature, sampling every few minutes might be sufficient, but for arterial pressure measurement a higher rate is needed. This principle may seem obvious, but as an example of the importance of sampling rate, consider the number of points needed to define a circle. If we place three equidistant points on a circle, we describe a triangle, not a circle. Similarly, four points describe a square. If we increase the number of points (sampling rate), we can describe the circle more completely. For a sine wave, the minimum frequency of sampling needed to preserve the waveform is twice the frequency. This mathematical minimum is known as the *Nyquist frequency.*[2] For complex waveforms such as arterial pressure tracings, the sampling rate must be at least twice the highest frequency component in the waveform.

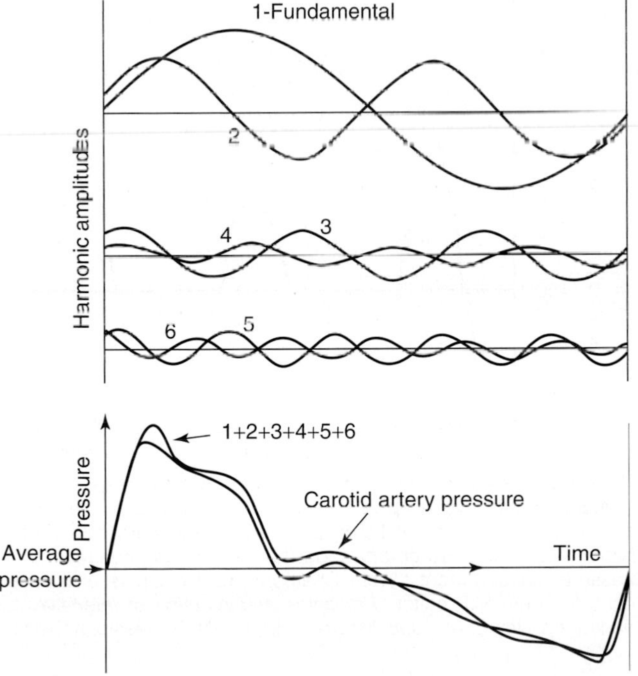

FIGURE 19–2 • Fourier series representation of an arterial pressure tracing. **Bottom,** High-fidelity carotid artery pressure tracing and the sum of the first six harmonics of its Fourier series representation. Despite the few terms used in the synthesis, the close fit of the two curves is evident. **Top,** Individual harmonic components labeled with their harmonic number. (Redrawn from *RSC: Transducers for biomedical measurements: principles and applications.* New York, 1974, John Wiley & Sons, from Hansen AT: *Acta Physiol Scand* 19[suppl 68]:1, 1949.) (From Perloff WH: Invasive measurements in the PICU. In Fuhrman BP, Zimmerman JJ, editors: *Pediatric critical care,* ed 2. St. Louis, 1998, Mosby.)

Measurement Systems

Hemodynamic monitoring in the clinical setting usually uses a fluid-coupled system where changes in pressure are transmitted via a column of (uncompressible) fluid in a (ideally incompressible) tube to a mechanical transducer. The mechanical transducer, usually a displaceable screen diaphragm, converts a change in pressure to an electrical signal, which can be processed and displayed. In laboratory settings, vascular pressures can be measured by a transducer at the point of interest rather than remotely as in the clinical setting. Measuring pressure at the point of interest, in the aorta directly, for example, decreases loss of signal integrity because of the measurement system. Most clinical pressure measuring systems have sufficient fidelity for clinical purposes. However, compliance, resistance, or impedance in the pressure tubing can result in damping or alteration of the recorded signal. The presence of bubbles in the fluid can further damp the recorded signal.

Errors in Measurement

The ideal measurement system determines the actual or "true" value for the measured variable. However, determination of a true value may be difficult. Every measurement system is subject to various errors. Errors in measurement can be classified as either *systematic* or *random.* Systematic errors occur in a predictable manner and are reproduced with repeated measures. *Bias* in a measurement system, for example, a baseline offset, results in a systematic error. Random errors are unpredictable and do not recur predictably with repeated measures.

Accuracy of a measurement is defined by the difference between the measured and true values, divided by the true value. *Precision* is defined by the reproducibility of the measurement; thus a more precise system yields more similar values for repeated measures under the same conditions than does a less precise system. *Imprecision* can be thought of as a representation of random errors, whereas *bias* can be thought of as a representation of systematic errors.

Calibration

Many measurement systems are *linear,* that is, based upon an assumption that the relationship between the inputs and outputs from a measurement device can be fitted to a straight line. This assumption allows a system to be calibrated under two conditions, with the rest of the values falling on the line defined by those two points. Actual nonlinearity of the system adversely affects the measurements.

Calibration is a process in which the reading, or output of a device, is adjusted to match a known input value. For example, an electronic pressure transducer may be calibrated against a mercury manometer. If the input to the device is zero, the output should be adjusted so that the reading also is set to zero. This *zeroing* reduces any baseline offset, thus reducing systematic errors in subsequent readings. The system then is calibrated to a nonzero value, for example, 100 mmHg pressure, and the system *gain* is adjusted to read this value as well.

Frequency Response

The ability of a measurement system to accurately measure an oscillating signal, such as arterial blood pressure, is dependent upon the system's *frequency response*. The system can either overestimate or underestimate the true amplitude of a signal. If the system is *overdamped*, the value reported underestimates the amplitude, and waveform characteristics may be lost. *Resonance* in the system may result in overestimation of the amplitude. Measurement of arterial systolic pressure—the amplitude of the arterial waveform—may be inaccurate because of overdamping, and important waveform characteristics may be lost if the frequency response of the measurement system is poor. Figure 19–3 illustrates the effects of damping on measurement of blood pressure.

Impedance

Impedance is the ratio of the change in blood flow along a vessel to the change in the pressure in the vessel. Impedance has both resistive and reactive components. In a pulsatile system such as the cardiovascular system, resistance alone does not fully describe the impediment or *impedance* to forward flow of blood. The caliber, length, and arrangement of the blood vessels and the mechanical properties of the blood determine resistance in the blood vessels. Reactance includes compliance of the vessels and inertia of the blood and thus is a dynamic component of impedance. This is important because the pulsatile nature of the cardiovascular system is dynamic.

When blood is propelled through a vessel at a branch point, a reflected pressure wave back toward the heart increases the impedance of the system. The major sites of wave reflection from vessel branching are from vessels approximately 1 mm in diameter (Tobin[3], p. 96). Thus these small vessels contribute significantly to overall impedance. Figure 19–4 shows the relationships between pressure and flow velocity with distance along the length of the aorta. Because blood pressure increases with distance from the heart and flow velocity decreases with distance, the impedance increases toward the peripheral vasculature. Hemodynamic measuring systems are essentially physical extensions of the vascular system; thus the configuration and characteristics of the tubing and transducer system can alter the overall effect of impedance.

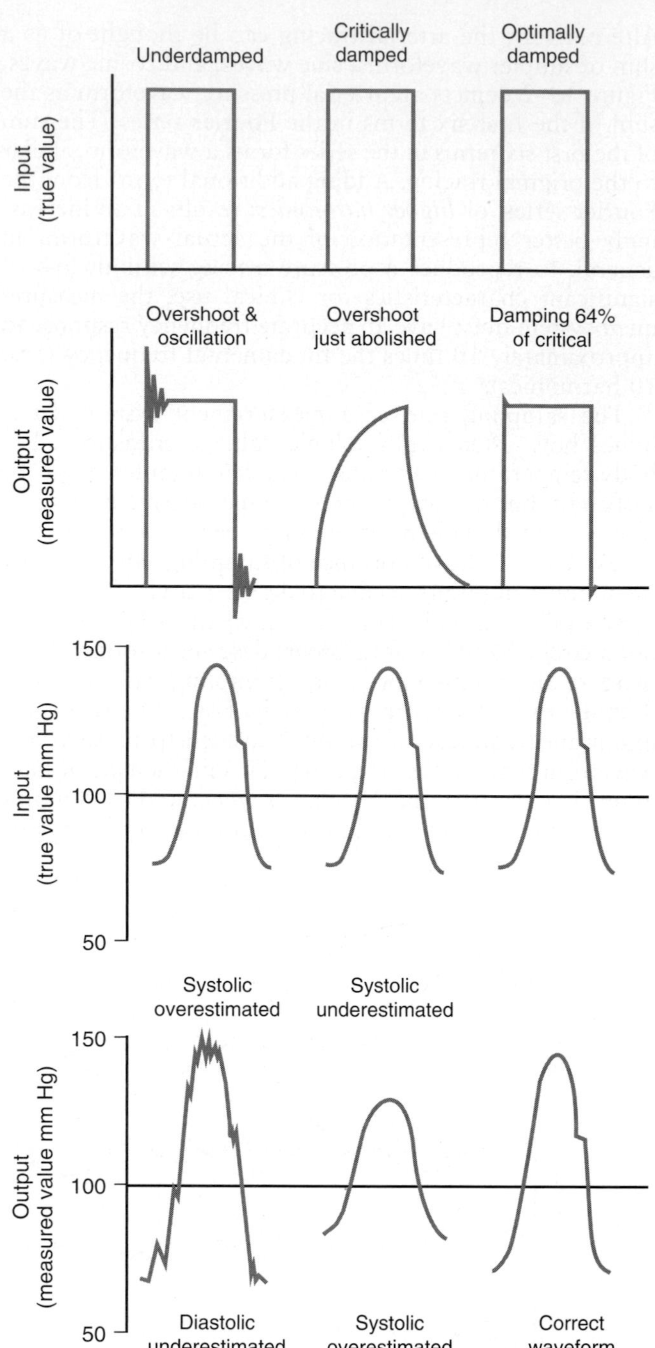

FIGURE 19–3 • Effects of dampening on blood pressure measurement. **Upper two graphs** depict the response to a square-wave input from three different blood pressure transducers with different dampening. *Lower two graphs* show the effect of dampening on blood pressure measurement. (From Chatburn RL: Principles of measurement. In Tobin MJ, editor: *Principles and practice of intensive care monitoring,* New York, 1998, McGraw-Hill, Health Professions Division.)

Invasive Techniques

Central Venous Pressure Catheters

Indications

Indications for CVP catheter placement in pediatric patients include assessment of right heart filling pressure (CVP), monitoring of large fluid shifts from the intravascular to the extravascular space and vice versa, infusion of vasoactive substances, and infusion of hyperosmolar fluids and/or irritants.[5,6] For these types of fluids to be infused into a peripheral vein, they would need to be diluted to such a large extent so as to potentially cause fluid overload.[5]

Interpretation of Waveforms

CVP is a measure of right atrial pressure, although it may be measured in the inferior or superior vena cava. It is a

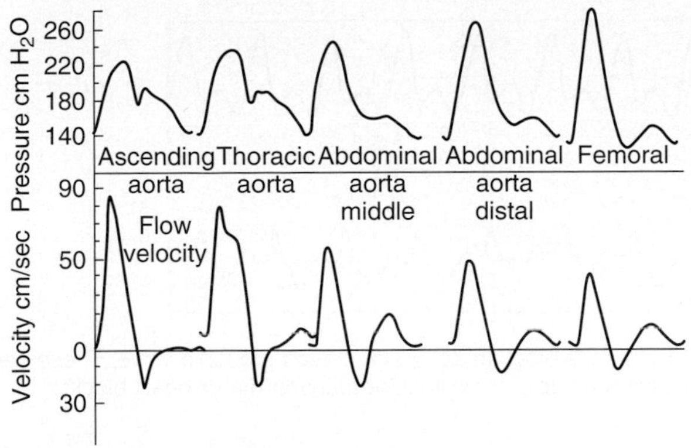

FIGURE 19–4 • Pressure pulses and flow velocity at various points in the systemic arterial circulation. Data were obtained from dogs and are similar to measurements made in humans. The data indicate that both peak and pulse pressure increase with distance from the heart, whereas oscillation in flow velocity shows a progressive decrease. Consequently *impedance* (discussed in the text) must increase toward the periphery. (From Perloff WH: Invasive measurements in the PICU. In Fuhrman BP, Zimmerman JJ, editors: *Pediatric critical care,* ed 2. St. Louis, 1998, Mosby.)

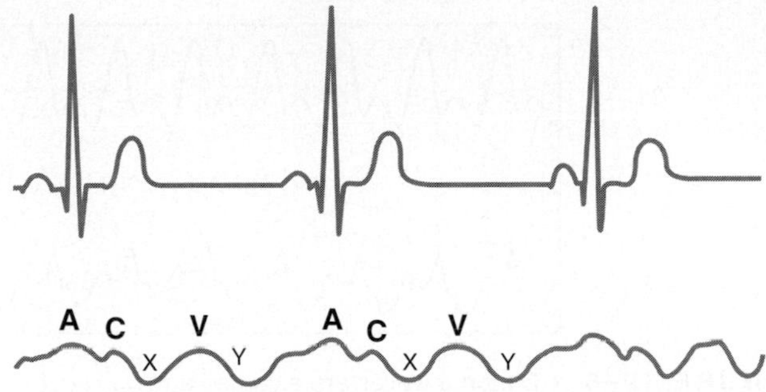

FIGURE 19–5 • Central venous pressure (A) tracing with corresponding electrocardiogram (ECG). The *a wave* is produced by atrial contraction and occurs after the P wave of the ECG during the PR interval. The *c wave* (C) is produced by closure of the tricuspid valve and takes place early in systole at the end of the QRS complex in the RST junction. The *v wave* (V) is caused by rapid filling of the right atrium late in systole prior to opening of the tricuspid valve and is seen between the T and P waves of the ECG. The *x descent* (X) reflects the decrease in pressure in the right atrium after the *a wave* as the tricuspid valve is pulled away from the right atrium by the right ventricle as the ventricle contracts during systole. The *y descent* (Y) is the decrease in right atrial pressure that occurs after the *v wave* as the tricuspid valve opens and blood moves from the right atrium into the right ventricle. (From O'Rourke RA: The measurement of systemic blood pressure: normal and abnormal pulsations of the arteries and veins. In Hurst JW, editor: *The heart,* New York, 1990, McGraw-Hill.)

measure of preload—the force or load on the right ventricle during relaxation or filling. CVP is measured at the end of diastole, just prior to ejection. Final filling of the right ventricle occurs at the end of atrial contraction. When the tricuspid valve is open during diastole, the right atrium and right ventricle form a continuous column; therefore right atrial pressure reflects right ventricular end-diastolic pressure (RVEDP). CVP is used to measure filling pressure or preload and as such is an indicator of volume status. It is commonly used in patients with hypovolemic or septic shock in whom volume resuscitation is desirable prior to institution of vasopressor therapy. In patients with decreased right ventricular function or pulmonary hypertension, an increased CVP well beyond normal limits may be observed, and further fluid resuscitation may promote the development of congestive failure. Increases in the positive end-expiratory pressure (PEEP) can decrease preload despite a paradoxically increased CVP. Finally, increases in extrathoracic pressure, such as that caused by increased abdominal girth, can increase CVP (see Chapter 24).

The CVP waveform is divided into three components: *a, c,* and *v* waves (Figure 19–5). Each component can be correlated with a specific portion of the electrocardiogram tracing. The *a wave* occurs with atrial contraction and is seen after the P wave of the electrocardiogram during the PR interval. Thus the mean value of the *a wave* approximates RVEDP. *Canon a waves* (Figure 19–6), which are enlarged *a waves* seen when the right atrium is ejecting against a closed tricuspid valve, may be seen when atrioventricular discordance occurs (i.e., during an ectopic junctional or ventricular tachycardia or heart block). The *c wave* occurs in early systole with closure of the tricuspid valve and is seen at the end of the QRS complex in the RST junction. The *v wave* occurs during filling of the right atrium in late systole prior to opening of the tricuspid valve and is seen between the T and P waves of the ECG. The v wave is increased in the setting of tricuspid regurgitation. The *x descent* is the decrease in pressure after the *a wave.* The *y descent* is the decrease in pressure that occurs after the *v wave* as the tricuspid valve opens.

Arterial Pressure Catheters

Indications

The transition to direct monitoring of arterial blood pressure dates back to the mid 1950s when two separate studies compared invasive arterial measurements to noninvasive or cuff measurements in healthy adults.[7,8] Van Bergen and co-workers[8] noted a frequent difference between direct and indirect measurements, with indirect measurements increasingly lower than direct measurements as the systemic blood pressure increased. The greatest disparity was found in the young, hypertensive patient. Similarly, Cohn and Luria[9] observed that invasive arterial pressures were significantly greater than cuff pressures and emphasized the importance of direct measurements of systemic arterial pressure in the care of patients with hypotension and shock. Continuous direct monitoring of arterial blood pressure should be considered when treating patients requiring more than minimal vasopressor therapy.

Indications for arterial catheterization include continuous monitoring of systemic arterial blood pressure, frequent blood sampling, and withdrawal of blood during exchange transfusions.[10] In addition to the value of the measurements themselves, these measurements provide components of derived measures of CO and oxygen delivery.

Interpretation of Waveforms

Systolic blood pressure (SBP) in children varies greatly with age and gender. Similar to the CVP waveform, the arterial waveform can be correlated with specific parts

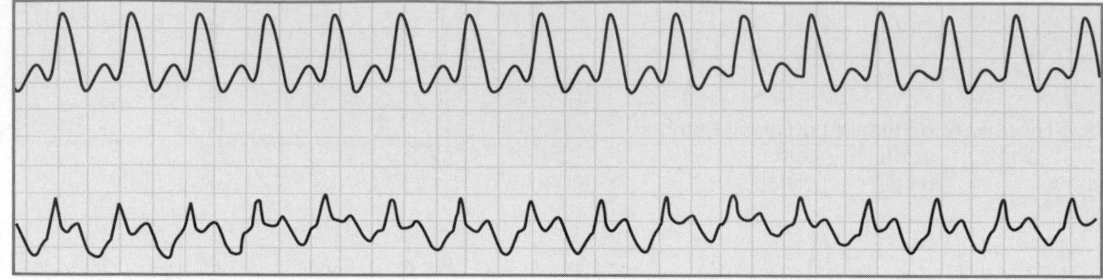

FIGURE 19–6 • Canon a waves are enlarged a waves seen when the right atrium is ejecting against a closed tricuspid valve. These waves are typically seen when atrioventricular discordance occurs, such as during junctional ectopic or ventricular tachycardia or heart block.

of the cardiac cycle. The arterial waveform has three main components (Figure 19–7): (1) rapid upstroke and downslope that correlates with systolic ejection, (2) dicrotic notch that correlates with closure of the aortic valve, and (3) a smooth runoff that correlates with diastole. The dicrotic notch or incisura is decreased in situations of hyperdynamic CO in which left ventricular output and stroke volume (SV) are increased, pulse pressure is widened, and diastolic blood pressure (DBP) is increased (e.g., surgical systemic-to-pulmonary shunts, patent ductus arteriosus, aortic regurgitation, anemia, fever, sepsis, hypovolemia, exercise).[11] Conversely, cardiac tamponade and severe aortic stenosis can narrow the pulse pressure and are associated with a deflection (anacrotic notch) on the ascending limb of the waveform.[11]

Systolic pressures measured in the periphery typically are greater than those measured more centrally because of pulse amplification of pressure waves reflected back from arterial branch points[11,12] (see Figure 19–4). More peripheral sites, such as the radial artery, have greater SBP and lower DBP than more central sites and thus taller and narrower waveforms with greater pulse pressures (difference between SBP and DBP). Important to note is that the mean arterial pressure (MAP in Equation 1) represents the area under the waveform curve, and the overall magnitude of the reading remains the same regardless of the location of the tracing.

$$MAP = DBP + (SBP - DBP)/3. \quad (1)$$

Pulmonary Artery Catheters

History and Controversy

In 1847 Claude Bernard, a French researcher with widespread interests in experimentation, described a method for recording intracardiac pressures in animals by inserting a glass tube in the heart.[13] However, the true pioneers of cardiac catheterization were two other Frenchman: Jean Baptiste Auguste Chaveau, at that time a veterinarian interested in the relationship between the dynamic motion of the heart and heart sounds, and Etienne-Jules Marey, a physician interested in the physiology of the circulation. In the early 1860s, using techniques adapted from Bernard's work, Chaveau and Marey inserted a double-lumen catheter into the right atrium of a horse to record phasic changes in intracardiac pressures as they simultaneously recorded the apical impulse.[13–16]

Right heart catheterization was not considered a safe practice in humans until the early twentieth century. In 1929 Werner Forssman, a German surgeon, secretly performed a right heart catheterization on himself. Forssman had been interested in the work of Bernard, Chaveau, and Marey and wanted to advance their techniques in order to apply them to humans. In direct contradiction to his supervisor's instructions, Forssman inserted a urinary catheter into his own left antecubital vein and then advanced it approximately 1 foot to the head of his humerus. He then went to the radiology department and asked a nurse to hold up a mirror while he advanced the catheter the remainder of the way to his right atrium under fluoroscopic guidance. At this point, Forssman was forced to wrestle with a colleague who

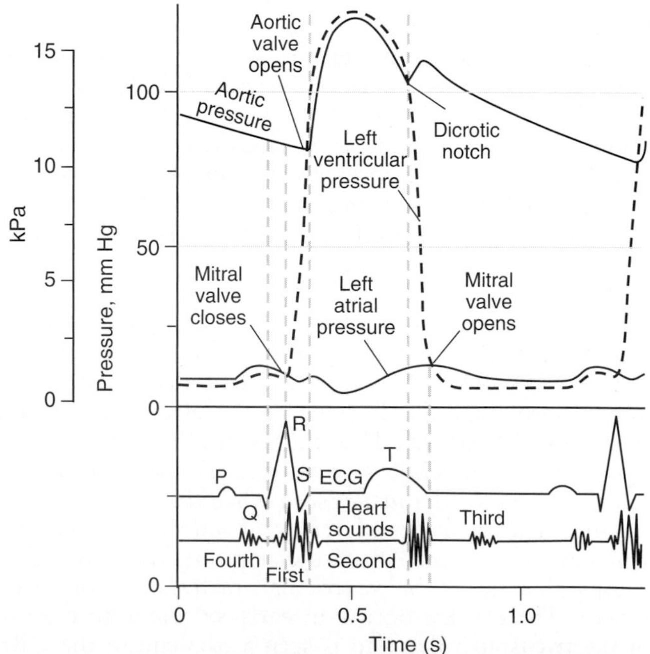

FIGURE 19–7 • Aortic, left ventricular, and left atrial pressure waveforms as they correspond to the electrocardiogram (ECG), opening and closing of the aortic and mitral valves, and heart sounds. Note the presence of the dicrotic notch on the descending limb of the aortic waveform. (From Peura RA: Blood pressure and sound. In Webster JG, editor: *Medical instrumentation: application and design,* Boston, 1978, Houghton Mifflin Company.)

burst into the room and attempted to stop Forssman from completing the final stages of the procedure. Forssman performed right heart catheterizations on himself a total of nine additional times without adverse consequences and expanded his findings by demonstrating the feasibility of injecting contrast dye during the procedure.[17,18]

In the early 1940s Andres Cournand and Dickinson Richards, working at Bellevue Hospital in New York City, continued Forssman's work. They performed right heart catheterization in healthy humans and in those with cardiac failure.[18–21] In 1956 Forssman, Cournand, and Richards won the Nobel Prize for Physiology–Medicine for their work in developing cardiac catheterization. In his Nobel lecture entitled "The Role of Heart Catheterization and Angiography in the Development of Modern Medicine," Forssman remarked[18]:

One may compare the art of healing with a work of art, which from different standpoints and under different lighting reveals ever new and surprising beauty.

Lewis Dexter, at the Peter Bent Brigham Hospital in Boston, was the first to describe the pathophysiologic abnormalities in many forms of congenital heart disease (CHD). Dexter's group studied patients with atrial and ventricular septal defects, patent ductus arteriosus, tetralogy of Fallot, and pulmonic stenosis. In addition, they carefully assessed the pathophysiology of pulmonary embolism, valvular heart disease, right and left ventricular dysfunction, and pulmonary hypertension. They were the first investigators to measure pulmonary capillary wedge pressures using cardiac catheterization.[22,23]

Dexter initially was interested in renal physiology. On December 7, 1944 Dexter was in the process of catheterizing the renal vein of a hypertensive patient when his catheter inadvertently passed into the pulmonary circulation, an event that led Dexter to change his field of interest to cardiology.[23]

...I decided to wander around the heart which I understood was above the diaphragm somewhere. Suddenly, this catheter came clear out into the lung field and I was sure I [had] perforated the heart. I didn't have any idea of what to do and ... I turned on the overhead lights and said, "Mr. S___, how are you?" He said, "I feel a hell of a lot better than you look." Then I was pretty sure that, having perforated the heart, it just sort of sealed itself off and [I] wondered what would happen when I pulled it back. So I closed my eyes and then pulled the catheter back and nothing happened. And then I went and looked up the anatomy of the chest and I figured I had gone into the pulmonary artery.

In 1953 Michael Lategola and Hermann Rahn,[24] two pulmonary physiologists from Rochester, New York, performed experiments in dogs in which they were the first to use a self-guiding balloon-tipped catheter to measure pressures in the pulmonary circulation. Seventeen years later, Swan, Ganz, and coworkers[25] at the University of California, Los Angeles, used this technique to assess right heart pressures in humans and in doing so brought this methodology to the bedside where it is commonly used today.

The past 2 decades have seen much debate over the safety and efficacy of PACs in critically ill adults,[26–31] with multiple calls for a moratorium on PAC usage.[32,33] The data regarding the use of PACs in clinical and research settings were carefully reviewed.[34–36] Because scarce high-level objective evidence supports the use of PACs,[36] the recommendations were based primarily on expert opinion. These reviews found no basis for a moratorium on PACs and called for standardization and monitoring of the education of nurses and physicians with regard to PAC use and future clinical trials.[34,35] A randomized, controlled clinical trial underscores the lack of evidence supporting a benefit to therapy directed by PACs compared with standard care.[31] The basis for the difficulties in interpreting the efficacy of PACs may not be caused by inherent problems with the tool itself but rather differences in physicians' abilities to insert the PAC correctly and to interpret the information it provides. Studies have revealed a significant lack of knowledge and expertise on the part of physicians using PACs.[37,38]

With regard to pediatric patients, the Pulmonary Artery Catheter Consensus Conference, based on a consensus of expert opinions, concluded that the PAC was useful for clarifying cardiopulmonary physiology in critically ill infants and children with pulmonary hypertension, shock refractory to fluid resuscitation and/or low-to-moderate doses of vasoactive medications, severe respiratory failure requiring high mean airway pressures, and on rare occasions multiple organ failure.[34] They found no data indicating that PAC use increases mortality in children; however, they also failed to find any controlled trials that proved benefit. The panel recommended PAC use for selected patients and called for randomized, controlled trials, a registry of PAC use, and studies to assess the impact of PAC use on cost and duration of ICU/hospital stay.[34]

Indications

Indications for PAC use in children include patients with septic shock unresponsive to fluid resuscitation and low-dose vasopressor support,[39–41] refractory shock following severe burn injuries,[42] children with CHD,[41] multiple organ failure,[43] and respiratory failure requiring high mean airway pressures.[41,44]

Capabilities of PACs include determination of CVP, pulmonary artery pressure (PAP), and pulmonary artery occlusion pressure (PAOP), also referred to as *pulmonary capillary wedge pressure* (Pw). PAOP is a measurement of left atrial pressure and left ventricular end-diastolic pressure (when the mitral valve is open). PACs also are used to assess CO, tissue oxygenation (Svo_2), oxygen delivery

(DO_2) and consumption (VO_2), and pulmonary vascular resistance (PVR) and systemic vascular resistance (SVR). A fundamental application of the PAC is to examine the function of the right and left ventricles separately. PACs are used to establish diagnoses, guide response to therapy, and assess the determinants of oxygen delivery. PACs are especially helpful in cases of discordant ventricular function.

One of the most common uses of the PAC in infants and children is monitoring pulmonary pressures during and after repair of CHD. In addition to flow-directed balloon-tipped PACs, transthoracic left atrial catheters are often used in these patients.[45] Use of PACs has altered the management of children with CHD by identifying residual anatomic defects and diagnosing pulmonary hypertensive crisis.[46,47] The ability to monitor PAP provides the means to titrate response to inhaled nitric oxide (iNO) and other pulmonary vasodilators.[48,49] The lack of response to iNO may suggest a residual structural anomaly in postoperative patients and indicate the need for repeat cardiac catheterization and/or repair.[49] In addition to monitoring for pulmonary hypertensive crisis, PACs can be used to assess the effects of changes in concentration of inspired CO_2 on mean pulmonary artery pressure (MPAP), pulmonary vascular resistance index (PVRI), and cardiac index (CI).[50]

Catheter Ports

PACs contain the following ports (see Figure 19–7). The *proximal port* is located 15 cm from the tip in 5F catheters and 30 cm from the tip in larger catheters. It opens into or near the right atrium. The proximal port provides access for infusion of fluid or drugs, injection of cold saline as indicator (thermodilution method), CVP monitoring, and blood sampling. In infants or small children, PAC placement via the internal jugular or subclavian vein may result in the improper location of the proximal port before the right atrium such that the port lies inside the sheath or outside the body. Therefore it is essential to verify not only the placement of the distal tip in the pulmonary artery but also the location of the proximal port in the right atrium.

The *distal port* opens at the tip of the catheter. It is used for monitoring PAP and PAOP, for blood sampling of mixed venous blood gases, and for infusion of fluids. By monitoring pressure continuously through this port during catheter placement, the location of the tip can be determined from the characteristic pressure tracings shown in Figure 19–7. After placement, PAP should be monitored continuously in order to identify inadvertent migration into the pulmonary capillary bed or "wedged" position. It is important to allow the catheter tip to "float" into the wedged position only when actively measuring PAOP in order to minimize risk of pulmonary artery infarct or rupture.

The *balloon inflation port* inflates the balloon, which is located 1 cm proximal to the catheter tip. The balloon is inflated for flow-directed catheter placement and for PAOP monitoring.

The *thermistor* is located just proximal to the balloon and connects to a bedside computer in order to measure changes in the temperature of pulmonary artery blood.

The *oximeter* uses a fiberoptic-based sensor to continuously measure the mixed venous oxygen saturation (SvO_2).

Larger catheters may also have cardiac pacing ports. An adult-size catheter is available for "continuous" CO determination when coupled to an appropriate bedside computer (Figure 19–8).

Measurement of Cardiac Output

CO is the volume of blood pumped by the heart or SV multiplied by the number of ejections per minute or heart rate (CO = HR × SV) and often is expressed as CI, which is CO divided by the body surface area (BSA) in m^2. The normal range for infants and children is approximately 3.3 to 6 L/min/m^2.[51,52] Two methods for calculating CO are discussed here: the Fick method and thermodilution.

Fick Method

In 1870 Adolph Fick, a brilliant mathematician, was the first to study the relationship between blood flow and gas exchange in the lungs using a mathematical model.[53] Fick hypothesized that the amount of oxygen extracted by the body from the blood must equal the amount of oxygen taken up by the lungs during breathing. Fick also reasoned that the flow of blood through the lungs must equal the CO to the remainder of the body in the absence of a shunt. If the amount of oxygen consumed by the body and the amount of oxygen extracted by the body from the blood can be determined, then the CO can be determined. In Fick's time, oxygen consumption was measured using a basal metabolism spirometer, and the oxygen content in arterial and venous blood was measured using a rudimentary method. In his *Compendium der Physiologie des Menschen*, Fick reported that the CO of the resting adult was 4.6 L/min.[53] This value is consistent with values obtained from healthy patients using modern methods. Although Fick's method remains the gold standard, it is rarely used in the intensive care unit because it is less practical than the more commonly used thermodilution method described in the next section. However, Fick's method is commonly used in the cardiac catheterization laboratory because the required data are readily available in this setting, although oxygen consumption typically is estimated.

$$\text{Amount of oxygen extracted by the body from the blood} = \text{Amount of oxygen taken up from the lungs during breathing}$$

As noted previously, Fick's equation is based on the assumption that the amount of oxygen extracted by the body from the blood equals the amount of oxygen taken up from the lungs during breathing. The amount of oxygen extracted by the body from the blood equals the difference in oxygen content of arterial (CaO_2) and venous blood (CvO_2) in ml/L, also referred to as

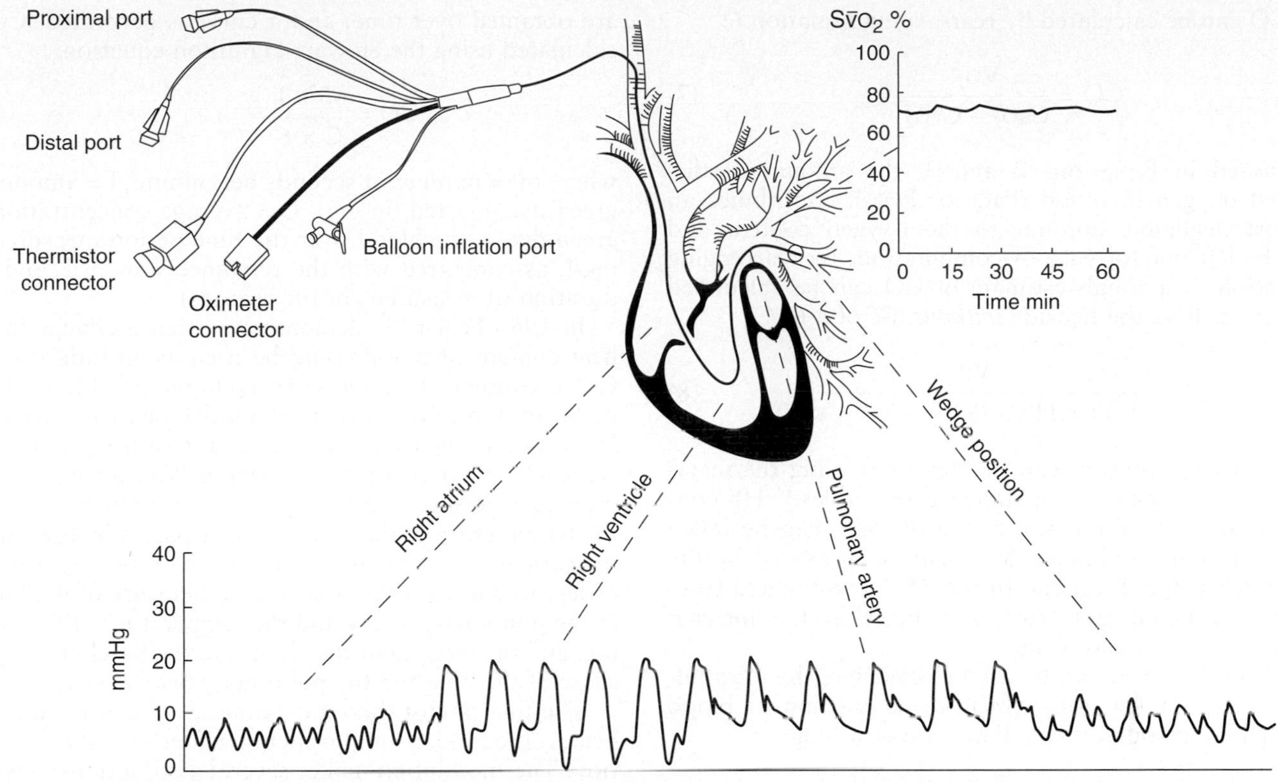

FIGURE 19–8 • Components and functional features of a thermodilution flow-directed pulmonary artery catheter. The flexible multilumen catheter with the balloon at the distal tip inflated is in the wedge position. The proximal ends of the five lumens are labeled. The distal port is connected to a pressure measurement system for catheter insertion and subsequent monitoring. When the distal tip is within the central venous circulation, the balloon is inflated to enhance flow direction of the tip through the right atrium into the right ventricle and then to the pulmonary artery. Recorded pressures **(lower panel)** correspond to these locations, confirming the course of the catheter. The **last tracing on the right** corresponds to the "wedge" position, commonly reflecting pressure transmitted from the left atrium via the pulmonary veins and capillaries. **Upper right panel** shows an example of a continuous $Sv\text{O}_2$ tracing from the fiberoptic monitor available on adult-size catheters. (Redrawn from Daily EK, Tilkian AG: Hemodynamic monitoring. In Tilkian AG, Daily EK, editors: *Cardiovascular procedures, diagnostic techniques and therapeutic procedures.* St. Louis, 1986, Mosby). (From Perloff WH: Invasive measurements in the PICU. In Fuhrman BP, Zimmerman JJ, editors: *Pediatric critical care, 2nd edition,* p. 79, St. Louis, 1998, Mosby.)

arterial-mixed venous oxygen content difference ($avD\text{O}_2$), multiplied by the total amount of blood pumped through the lungs body (CO).

The oxygen content of the blood is a function of the hemoglobin (Hb) concentration of blood in g/dl, the systemic or venous oxygen saturation ($Sa\text{O}_2$ or $Sv\text{O}_2$) expressed in decimal form, and the partial pressure of arterial oxygen ($Pa\text{O}_2$) in mmHg. The oxygen carrying capacity of adult Hb is 1.34 ml O_2 per gram Hb and the Bunsen solubility coefficient of O_2 in plasma at 37° C equals 0.003. A true $Sv\text{O}_2$ is measured in the pulmonary artery; however, in the presence of an intracardiac shunt, $Sv\text{O}_2$ should be measured in the superior vena cava.

$$Ca\text{O}_2 = (1.34 \times 10 \times Hb \times Sa\text{O}_2) + (Pa\text{O}_2 \times 0.003) \quad (2)$$

$$Cv\text{O}_2 = (1.34 \times 10 \times Hb \times Sv\text{O}_2) + (Pv\text{O}_2 \times 0.003). \quad (3)$$

Note that the units for oxygen content in this chapter are milliliters of oxygen per *liter* of blood rather than milliliters of oxygen per deciliter of blood, as is in many other sources. (Thus the values for $Ca\text{O}_2$ and $Cv\text{O}_2$ must be converted to ml/L by multiplying in a correction factor of 10 dl/L.) Expressing oxygen content in these units allows for easy computation of CO, which is expressed as liters per minute.

The arterial-mixed venous oxygen content difference ($avD\text{O}_2$) is the difference between $Ca\text{O}_2$ and $Cv\text{O}_2$ and normally ranges from 20 to 78 ml/L.[52]

$$avD\text{O}_2 = Ca\text{O}_2 - Cv\text{O}_2. \quad (4)$$

As noted earlier, the amount of oxygen extracted by the body from the blood equals $avD\text{O}_2$ multiplied by the amount of blood that flows through the lungs (Q_P). Assuming Q_P equals the flow of blood through the systemic circulation (Q_S), then Q_P is a measure of CO. (Note pulmonary and systemic blood flows cannot be assumed to be identical in children with CHD with single-ventricle physiology or with shunts).

$$O_2 \text{ extraction} = (Ca\text{O}_2 - Cv\text{O}_2) \times CO. \quad (5)$$

The amount of oxygen taken up by the lungs equals the amount of oxygen consumed by the body. According to Fick, the amount of oxygen extracted by the body from the blood (Equation 5) equals oxygen consumption ($V\text{O}_2$).

$$(Ca\text{O}_2 - Cv\text{O}_2) \times CO = V\text{O}_2. \quad (6)$$

CO can be calculated by rearranging Equation 6:

$$CO = \frac{V_{O_2}}{Ca_{O_2} - Cv_{O_2}}. \quad (7)$$

As noted in Equations 2 and 3, the amount of dissolved oxygen in blood (Pa_{O_2} or Pv_{O_2}), contributes an almost negligible amount to the oxygen content and can be left out for ease of computation. By rearranging Equation 7, a rough estimate of CO can be calculated rather easily at the bedside *without* use of a PAC:

$$CO = \frac{V_{O_2}}{1.34 \times Hb \times (Sa_{O_2} - Sv_{O_2}) \times 10}. \quad (8)$$

Oxygen consumption can be measured using the metabolic cart or taken from standardized tables.[11] Hb concentration can be measured directly. Sa_{O_2} can be taken from the pulse oximeter. Sv_{O_2} can be measured by the oximeter at the distal end of the PAC or estimated from a venous blood gas from a catheter in the internal jugular or subclavian vein.

These data also can be used to calculate the intrapulmonary shunt fraction, which is the fraction of blood that passes through unventilated areas of lung:

$$Qs = \frac{(Cpv_{O_2} - Ca_{O_2})}{Qt\ (Cpv_{O_2} - Cv_{O_2})}, \quad (9)$$

where Ca_{O_2} = systemic arterial oxygen content and Cv_{O_2} = mixed venous oxygen content.

Cpv_{O_2} is the oxygen content in the pulmonary vein and can be calculated using the alveolar gas equation:

$$Cpv_{O_2} = PA_{O_2}\ (P_{atm} - P_{wp}) - Pa_{CO_2}/R, \quad (10)$$

where PA_{O_2} = alveolar partial pressure of oxygen, P_{atm} = barometric pressure, P_{wp} = vapor pressure of water (47 mmHg at 37° C), Pa_{CO_2} = arterial CO_2, and R = respiratory quotient, which is normally assumed to be 0.8.

The normal shunt fraction is 3% to 7%.

Thermodilution Method

In 1921 Stewart[54] first described an indicator-dilution method for measuring CO. Flow was calculated by measuring the change in concentration of an indicator over time. The "ideal" indicator is "stable, nontoxic, uniformly distributed, and [does] not leave the system between sites of injection and detection. However, it should be rapidly cleared in a single circulation time to prevent recirculation interfering with measurement."[55] Initially indocyanine green was used as an indicator, but recirculation was problematic because the dye is unstable and accumulates. A known amount of green dye, usually 5 mg, is injected into the pulmonary artery or elsewhere in the venous system and then a continuous stream of blood is withdrawn from the femoral artery. The optical density of the arterial blood is measured and compared with a known standard. Multiple readings are obtained over time, and a curve is generated. CO is calculated using the Stewart-Hamilton equation:

$$CO = \frac{60 \times I}{C \times t}, \quad (11)$$

where 60 = number of seconds per minute, I = amount of green dye injected (in mg), C = average concentration of green dye in the blood over the time period measured in mg/L as compared with the reference standard, and t = duration of measurement (in seconds).

In 1953 Fegler[56,57] demonstrated that a change in the heat content of blood could be used as an indicator for CO measurement. A bolus of cold liquid of a known temperature, typically normal saline, 5% dextrose, Ringer's lactate, or sterile water, is injected into or proximal to the right atrium. A thermistor near the PAC tip in the pulmonary artery or a pulmonary artery branch measures the temperature of the injectate as it passes by the end of the catheter. A computer calculates the ratio between the difference between the baseline temperature of the blood in the pulmonary artery and the temperature of the injectate and the integral of the change in the baseline temperature of the blood in the pulmonary artery over time.

The first law of thermodynamics, the conservation of heat, is the fundamental principle underlying thermodilution. Thermodilution makes several assumptions: physiologic conditions must remain constant during the period of observation, all heat exchange occurs between the indicator and the blood without heat loss to the surrounding tissues, mixing of the injectate and blood is complete upstream of the temperature measurement, and the temperature sensor is sufficiently sensitive, accurate, and rapidly responsive to depict accurately the change in temperature over time.

Measurement of CO using the thermodilution method can be understood by examining a modified version of the Stewart-Hamilton equation.[55] V_1 = injectate volume (in ml), Tb = temperature of the pulmonary artery at baseline (in °C), Ti = temperature of the injectate (in °C), K^1 = density factor that equals the specific heat of the injectate multiplied by the specific gravity of the injectate, divided by the product of the specific heat and specific gravity of blood, and K^2 = constant that figures in the dead space of the catheter and the loss of heat from the injectate as it moves through the catheter. The denominator of the equation is the integral of the change in the temperature of the blood (Tb) over time (t) (adapted from reference 55):

$$CO = \frac{V_1(Tb - Ti)\ K^1K^2}{\int \Delta Tb(t)dt}. \quad (12)$$

The computer generates a CO curve the height of which varies *inversely* with the magnitude of the CO. In settings of low CO, less warm blood flows with the injectate, and the injectate stays cooler. A smaller change in baseline pulmonary artery temperature occurs over time, the difference between the injectate temperature and that of the blood remains large, and the CO curve has a high domed shape. In contrast, in situations of high CO, pulmonary artery blood flow with the injectate increases and the temperature of the injectate approaches or equals that of the blood. In these situations because the difference between the final temperature of the injectate and that of the blood is small, the CO curve is flattened and the CO may be impossible to measure. In extreme low-flow states, the change in temperature of the injectate resulting from handling alone, before the injectate even enters the catheter from the proximal port, may be greater than the change caused by warming of the injectate by the flow of blood.

A correction factor is added to the equation to account for warming of the injectate because of handling alone; however, the correction factor may be inaccurate if the injection is too slow or the syringe is held in the injector's hands for too long. Therefore CO readings should be made as quickly as possible and should be repeated until three successive readings are within 15% of each other. Other sources of error include a falsely elevated CO because of inadvertent warming of the thermistor when it is up against the wall of the pulmonary artery, but this usually is not a concern as long as the catheter is not in the wedged position. The thermodilution method generally should not be used in patients with an intracardiac shunt; however, if the shunt fraction is less than 10%, the error likely is negligible.[11]

The thermodilution method is preferable to the dye dilution method for several reasons. Much less concern exists about recirculation and mixing because the cold injectate is quickly warmed by the warmer temperature of the blood and mixes better with the blood than does green dye. This method does not necessitate withdrawal of blood in order to measure dye concentration because temperature is calculated by the thermistor at the distal end of the PAC. The indicators are safe, inexpensive, and readily available. Rapid sequence readings can be performed in order to accumulate successive measurements.

Calculation of Oxygen Delivery and Consumption

Metabolic derangements, such as fever, sepsis, and shock, interfere with oxygen delivery (DO_2) to and consumption by (VO_2) the tissues. The mixed venous oxygen saturation (SvO_2) is a measure of the oxygenation of blood returning to the heart. SvO_2 is measured continuously by the fiberoptic oximeter (see description of PAC ports in the catheter ports section) and normally ranges from 65% to 75%. The oxygen extraction ratio (ERO_2) is $avDO_2$ (see Equation 4) divided by CaO_2 (Equation 2) and usually is approximately 25%[51,52]:

$$ERO_2 = \frac{avDO_2}{CaO_2}. \quad (13)$$

DO_2 also can be expressed as the product of CI and CaO_2 and VO_2 as the product of CI and $avDO_2$. The normal value for DO_2 is 620 ± 50 ml/min/m², whereas VO_2 typically ranges from 120 to 200 ml/min/m².[51,52]

$$DO_2 = CI \times CaO_2 \quad (14)$$

$$VO_2 = CI \times avDO_2. \quad (15)$$

Chapter 99 provides a complete discussion of oxygen demand, delivery, and consumption.

Interpretation of Waveforms

The waveforms corresponding to the right atrium and the systemic arterial blood pressure were discussed in previous sections. The pressure in the RA ranges from approximately 3 to 12 mmHg. As the catheter passes into the right ventricle, the diastolic pressure drops to 0 to 10 mmHg and the systolic pressure increases to 13 to 42 mmHg.[11] As the catheter enters the pulmonary artery, the diastolic pressure increases to 3 to 21 mmHg while the systolic pressure remains relatively similar to that of the right ventricle, 11 to 36 mmHg.[11] Once the catheter tip advances into the pulmonary capillary bed and the pulmonary artery is occluded by the inflated balloon, the measured pressure decreases to 2 to 14 mmHg.[11] By recognizing the changes in the various tracings, the movement of the catheter tip can be followed through the chambers of the right heart and into the pulmonary circulation, without simultaneous imaging.

The waveforms are affected by the components of the respiratory cycle. As expected, the effects of respiration differ during spontaneous breathing (negative pressure) versus mechanical ventilation (positive pressure). During spontaneous ventilation, pulmonary artery pressures decrease during inhalation and increase during exhalation. In contrast, during mechanical ventilation, pressure increases during inhalation and pressure decreases during exhalation. The cyclical changes induced by the respiratory cycle cause the tracings to take on a sinusoidal pattern once the tip of the catheter enters the thorax. By measuring pressures at the *end* of expiration, when pleural pressures are closest to zero, the effects of respiration on PAC determinations can be minimized.

Because CVP is a measure of preload or filling of the right ventricle, it reflects changes in volume status, right ventricular function, and pulmonary vascular tone. Similarly, PAOP (Pw) measures filling pressures of the left atrium and ventricle. When the pulmonary artery is occluded, the pressure from the left atrium is transmitted back to the catheter tip. During diastole, when the mitral valve is open and the aortic valve is closed, a continuous fluid-filled column is formed from the catheter tip to the aortic valve, and PAOP is equivalent to the left ventricular end-diastolic pressure. PAOP usually is approximately equivalent to the pulmonary artery end-diastolic pressure (PAEDP). PAEDP may provide a safer means for monitoring left ventricular filling.

In patients with cardiogenic shock, an elevated PAOP may reflect decreased function of the left ventricle. Rather than provide further fluid resuscitation or preload, increasing contractility or decreasing afterload may be preferable. *Afterload* is the load that the heart must eject blood against and is inversely related to SV (volume of blood ejected by the heart with each beat) and CO. It is determined by the impedance of the vasculature, ejection pressure, preload, and ventricular wall stress.

According to Laplace's law, ventricular wall stress (T) is proportional to ventricular transluminal pressure (P) (intraluminal pressure − extraluminal pressure) and radius (r) and is inversely related to twice the wall thickness (t):

$$T = \frac{P \times r}{2t}. \quad (16)$$

For a given pressure, wall stress is increased by an increase in radius (ventricular dilation); therefore volume administration may increase ventricular diameter and consequently wall stress. Thus afterload is preload dependent. Similarly, during spontaneous breathing the transluminal pressure and consequently the wall stress increase, whereas during mechanical ventilation (positive pressure) the transluminal pressure and wall stress both decrease. Ventricular hypertrophy increases wall thickness and therefore decreases wall stress.

Resistance

To understand resistance, returning to Ohm's law is helpful: voltage (V) varies directly with resistance (R) and current (I):

$$V = IR. \quad (17)$$

Rearranging Equation 17 by substituting pressure for voltage and flow for current gives Equation 18:

$$R = \frac{Pin - Pout}{Q}, \quad (18)$$

where R = resistance, Pin = pressure going into a vessel, Pout = pressure exiting the vessel, and Q = flow. According to Poiseuille's law, the resistance of flow through a tube varies directly with the viscosity of the fluid and the length of the tube and is inversely proportional to the radius to the fourth power multiplied by pi (π):

$$R = \frac{8\eta l}{\pi r^4}, \quad (19)$$

where η = viscosity, l = length, and r = radius. Unfortunately, Poiseuille's law assumes uniform viscosity, length, and radius, none of which holds true in the case of the pulmonary or systemic circulation; however, the principles behind the law are valuable in understanding the major determinants of resistance.

By substituting the appropriate values into Equation 16, the formulas for systemic vascular resistance (SVR) and pulmonary vascular resistance (PVR) can be derived. CO is substituted for Qs and Qp in the absence of a right-to-left or left-to-right shunt or single-ventricle physiology. In the case of the equation for PVR (21), PAOP is substituted for pulmonary vein pressure in determining Pout:

$$SVR = \frac{MAP - CVP}{CO} \quad (20)$$

$$PVR = \frac{MPAP - PAOP}{CO}. \quad (21)$$

SVR and PVR are measured in mmHg $\times$ minute $\times$ L^{-1} (or mmHg/L/min). These units also are referred to as *hybrid resistance units* (HBUs) or Wood units after the cardiologist Paul Wood.[11] By multiplying by 80, HBUs or Wood units can be converted to the centimeter-gram-seconds (cgs) system, where resistance is measured as dynes $\times$ seconds $\times$ cm^{-5}, also known as *absolute resistance units* (ARUs).

PVR and SVR often are indexed for BSA (in m^2). The systemic vascular resistance index (SVRI) and PVRI are measured as dyne-s/cm^5/m^2:

$$SVRI = \frac{MAP - CVP}{CI} \times 80 \quad (22)$$

$$PVRI = \frac{MPAP - PAOP}{CI} \times 80. \quad (23)$$

SVRI usually is 800 to 1600 dyne-s/cm^5/m^2 in children[51,52] and 2180 ± 210 in adults.[58]

Calculation of Intracardiac Shunt

If the oxygen saturations throughout the cardiopulmonary circulation are known, derivation of the values for the ratio of pulmonary to systemic blood flow or intracardiac shunt (Qp/Qs) is possible:

$$Qp = \frac{Vo_2}{1.34 \times 10 \times Hb\,(Spvo_2 - Spao_2)} \quad (24)$$

$$Qs = \frac{Vo_2}{1.34 \times 10 \times Hb\,(Sao_2 - Svo_2)} \quad (25)$$

$$\frac{Qp}{Qs} = \frac{Sao_2 - Svo_2}{Spvo_2 - Spao_2}, \quad (26)$$

where $Spvo_2$ = oxygen saturation in the pulmonary vein and $Spao_2$ = oxygen saturation in the pulmonary artery. In the absence of severe intrapulmonary shunt, $Spvo_2$ approaches 98% to 100%. In a complete mixing lesion, $Spao_2$ and Sao_2 should be equal by definition, enabling Sao_2 to be substituted for $Spao_2$.

Directly and Indirectly Measured Variables

Measurements of CO include directly and indirectly measured or derived variables. Directly measured variables include CVP, MAP, MPAP, PAOP, CO, Sao_2, and Svo_2. Derived parameters include CI, PVR, SVR, PVRI, and SVRI (as noted earlier), as well as SV (in ml/L) and stroke volume index (SVI; in ml/L/m^2). SI normally is 30 to 60 ml/m^2.[51,52]

$$SV = CO/HR \quad (27)$$

$$SVI = SV/BSA \quad (28)$$

$$SI = SVI \times 1000. \quad (29)$$

Left ventricular stroke work index (LVSWI) and right ventricular stroke work index (RVSWI) normally are 56 ± 6 and 0.5 ± 0.06 gm-m/m^2, respectively.[51,52] Note all values are for pediatric patients unless otherwise indicated.

$$LVSWI = SI \times MAP \times 0.0136 \quad (30)$$

$$RVSWI = SI \times MPAP \times 0.0136. \quad (31)$$

REFERENCES

1. Hales S: *Statical essays: containing haemastaticks; or, an account of some hydraulick and hydrostatical experiments made on the blood and blood-vessels of animals*. London, 1733, Innys, Manby, and Woodward.
2. Bronzino JD, editor: *The biomedical engineering handbook*. Boca Raton, 1995, CRC Press.
3. Tobin MJ, editor: *Principles and practice of intensive care monitoring*. New York, 1998, McGraw-Hill.
4. Webster JG, editor: *Medical instrumentation*. Boston, 1978, Houghton Mifflin Company.
5. Lowrie L, Difiore J, Martin R: Monitoring in the pediatric and neonatal intensive care units. In Martin J, Tobin M, editors: *Principles and practice of intensive care monitoring*. San Francisco, 1998, McGraw-Hill.
6. Heitmiller E, Wetzel R: Hemodynamic monitoring considerations in pediatric critical care. In Rogers M, editor: *Textbook of pediatric intensive care*. Baltimore, 1996, William & Wilkins.
7. Roberts L, Smiley J: A comparison of direct and indirect blood pressure determinations. *Circulation* 8:232-242, 1953.
8. Van Bergen F, Weatherhead S, Treloar A, et al: Comparison of indirect and direct methods of measuring blood pressure. *Circulation* 10:481-490, 1954.
9. Cohn J, Luria M: Studies in clinical shock and hypotension. *JAMA* 190:113-118, 1964.
10. Kaye W: Invasive monitoring techniques: arterial cannulation, bedside pulmonary artery catheterization, and arterial puncture. *Heart Lung* 12:395-427, 1983.
11. Vargo T: Cardiac catheterization: hemodynamic measurements. In Garson A, Bricker J, Fisher D, Neish S, editors: *The science and practice of pediatric cardiology*, ed 2. Baltimore, MD, 1998, Williams & Wilkins.
12. Murgo J, Westerhof N, Giolma J, Altobelli S: Aortic input impedance in normal man: relationship to pressure waveforms. *Circulation* 62:105-116, 1980.
13. Fye WB: Profiles in cardiology: Jean-Baptiste Auguste Chaveau. *Clin Cardiol* 26:351-353, 2003.
14. Chaveau J, EJ M: Determination graphique des rappats de la pulsation cardiaque avec les mouvements de l'oriellette et du ventrucule, obtenu au moyen d'un appareil enregisteeur. *CR Mear Soc Biol* 3:3-11, 1861.
15. Chaveau J, EJ M: De la force deployeu par la contraction des differentes cavites du coeur. *CR Soc Biol* 3:151-154, 1862.
16. Chaveau A, Marey E: *Appareils at Experiences Cardiographiques Demonstration Nouvelle du Mechanisme des Mouvements du Coeur par l'Emploi des Instruments Enregistreurs a Indications Continuees*. Paris, 1863, JB Balliere.
17. Forssman W: Die Sondierung des rechten herzens. *Klin Wochenschr* 8:2085-2087, 1929.
18. Fontenot C, O'Leary J: Dr. Werner Forssman's self-experimentation. *Am Surg* 62:514-515, 1996.
19. Cournand A, Ranges H: Catheterization of the right auricle in man. *Proc Soc Exp Biol Med* 46:462-466, 1941.
20. Richards D, Cournand A, Darling R, et al: Pressure of blood in the right auricle in animals and man: under normal conditions and in right heart failure. *Am J Physiol* 136:115-123, 1942.
21. Cournand A: Measurement of the cardiac output in man using the right heart catheterization. *Fed Proc* 4:207-212, 1945.
22. Hellems H, Haynes F, Dexter L, Kinney T: Pulmonary capillary pressure in animals estimated by venous and arterial catheterization. *Am J Physiol* 155:98-105, 1948.
23. Mukhopadhyay M: A biographical sketch of Lewis Dexter. *Texas Heart Inst J* 28:133-138, 2001.
24. Lategola M, Rahn H: A self-guiding catheter for cardiac and pulmonary artery catheterization and occlusion. *Proc Soc Exp Biol Med* 84:667-668, 1953.
25. Swan H, Ganz W, Forrester J, et al: Catheterization of the heart in man with use of a flow-directed balloon-tipped catheter. *N Engl J Med* 283:447-451, 1970.
26. Gore J, Goldberg R, Spodick D, et al: A community-wide assessment of the use of the use of pulmonary artery catheters in patients with acute myocardial infarction. *Chest* 92:721-727, 1987.
27. Connors A, Speroff T, Dawson N, et al: The effectiveness of right heart catheterization in the initial care of critically ill patients. SUPPORT investigators. *JAMA* 276:889-897, 1996.
28. Zion M, Balkin J, Rosenmann D, et al: Use of pulmonary artery catheters in patients with acute myocardial infarction: analysis of experience in 5841 patients in the SPRINT registry. *Chest* 98: 1331-1335, 1990.
29. Williams G, Grounds M, Rhodes A: Pulmonary artery catheter. *Curr Opin Crit Care* 8:251-256, 2002.
30. Vincent J-L, Dhainaut J-F, Perret C, Suter P: Is the pulmonary artery catheter misused? A European view. *Crit Care Med* 26: 1283-1287, 1998.
31. Sandham J, Hull R, Brant R, et al: A randomized, controlled trial of the use of pulmonary-artery catheters in high-risk surgical patients. *N Engl J Med* 348:5-14, 2003.
32. Robin E: Death by pulmonary artery flow-directed catheter. Time for a moratorium? *Chest* 92:727-731, 1987.
33. Dalen J, Bone R: Is it time to pull the pulmonary artery catheter? *JAMA* 276:916-918, 1996.
34. Pulmonary Artery Catheter Consensus conference: consensus statement. *Crit Care Med* 25:910-925, 1997.
35. Bernard G, Sopko G, Cerra F, et al: Pulmonary artery catheterization and clinical outcomes: National Heart, Lung, and Blood Institute and Food and Drug Administration workshop report. Consensus statement. *JAMA* 283:2568-2572, 2000.
36. Cooper AB, Doig GS, Sibbald WJ: Pulmonary artery catheters in the critically ill. An overview using the methodology of evidence-based medicine. *Crit Care Clin* 12:777-794, 1996.
37. Iberti T, Fischer E, Leibowitz A, et al: A multicenter study of physicians' knowledge of the pulmonary artery catheter. Pulmonary Artery Catheter Study Group. *JAMA* 264:2928-2932, 1990.
38. Gnaegi A, Feihl F, Perret C: Intensive care physicians' insufficient knowledge of right heart catheterization at the bedside: time to act? *Crit Care Med* 25:213-220, 1997.
39. Carcillo J, Davis A, Zaritsky A: Role of early fluid resuscitation in pediatric septic shock. *JAMA* 266:1242-1245, 1991.
40. Mercier J, Beaufils F, Hartmann J, Azema D: Hemodynamic patterns of meningococcal shock in children. *Crit Care Med* 16: 27-33, 1988.
41. Pollack M, Reed TP, Holbrook P, Fields A: Bedside pulmonary artery catheterization in pediatrics. *J Pediatr* 96:274-276, 1980.
42. Reynolds E, Ryan D, Sheridan R, Doody D: Left ventricular failure complicating severe pediatric burn injuries. *J Pediatr Surg* 30: 264-270, 1995.
43. Thompson A: Pulmonary artery catheterization in children. *New Horiz* 5:244-250, 1997.
44. DeBruin W, Notterman D, Magid M, et al: Acute hypoxemic respiratory failure in infants and children. *Crit Care Med* 20:1223-1234, 1992.
45. Wheedon D, Shore D, Lincoln C: Continuous monitoring of pulmonary artery pressure after cardiac surgery in infants and children. *J Cardiovasc Surg* 22:307-311, 1981.
46. Damen J, Weaver J: The use balloon-tipped pulmonary artery catheters in children undergoing cardiac surgery. *Intensive Care Med* 13:266-272, 1987.
47. Hopkins R, Bull C, Haworth S, et al: Pulmonary hypertensive crisis following cardiac surgery in infants and children. *Eur J Cardiothorac Surg* 5:628-634, 1991.
48. Atz A, Adatia I, Jonas R, Wessel D: Inhaled nitric oxide in children with pulmonary hypertension and congenital mitral stenosis. *Am J Cardiol* 77:316-319, 1996.
49. Adatia I, Atz A, Jonas R, Wessel D: Diagnostic use of inhaled nitric oxide after neonatal cardiac operations. *J Thorac Cardiovasc Surg* 112:1403-1405, 1996.
50. Morray J, Lynn A, Mansfield P: Effect of pH and PCO_2 on pulmonary and systemic hemodynamics after surgery in children with congenital heart disease and pulmonary hypertension. *J Pediatr* 113:474-479, 1988.
51. Cayler G, Rudolph A, Nadas A: Systemic blood flow in infants and children with and without heart disease. *Pediatrics* 32:186, 1963.
52. Krovetz L, McLoughlin T, Mitchell M, Schiebler G: Hemodynamic findings in normal children. *Pediatr Res* 1:122-130, 1967.
53. Gottschall CAM: The greatest medical discovery of the millennium (fundamental steps to the understanding of cardiac performance). *Arq Bras Cardiol* 73:320-330, 1999.

54. Stewart G: The output of the heart in dogs. *Am J Physiol* 57:27-50, 1921.
55. Moise S, Sinclair C, Scott D: Pulmonary artery blood temperature and the measurement of cardiac output by thermodilution. *Anaesthesia* 57:562-566, 2002.
56. Fegler G: A thermocouple method of determination of heart output in anaesthetized dogs. In: Nineteenth International Physiological Congress, Montreal, Canada, 1953:341.
57. Fegler G: Measurement of cardiac output in anesthetized animals by a thermodilution method. *Q J Exp Physiol* 39:153-164, 1954.
58. Shoemaker W, Chang P, Bland R, et al: Cardiorespiratory monitoring in postoperative patients. II. Quantitative therapeutic indices as a guide to therapy. *Crit Care Med* 7:243, 1979.

CHAPTER 20

Assessment of Cardiovascular Function

John R. Charpie and Thomas J. Kulik

PEARLS

- Cardiovascular assessment and monitoring in the pediatric intensive care unit requires careful integration of physical findings, laboratory studies, and electronic data in order to make appropriate therapeutic decisions.
- The four primary determinants of cardiac function are preload, end-systolic wall stress, myocardial contractility, and heart rate. These determinants can be altered by many factors in the intensive care unit.
- Noninvasive monitoring includes physical examination, chest radiography, echocardiography, blood pressure monitoring, and pulse oximetry. Invasive monitoring includes intravascular pressure monitoring, cardiac output measurements (thermodilution or Fick method), and laboratory studies.
- Management of the neonate with hypoplastic left heart syndrome poses several unique challenges to the cardiac intensivist, including optimization of pulmonary-to-systemic blood flow ratios and preservation of myocardial function.

Introduction

Cardiovascular assessment and monitoring in the pediatric intensive care setting involves both invasive and noninvasive techniques. Multiple studies have investigated the predictive value and use of surrogate indicators of cardiovascular function, but in practice it is the clinician who integrates all of the relevant physiologic parameters, accurately diagnoses cardiovascular dysfunction, and makes appropriate therapeutic decisions for an individual patient. One study evaluated the ability of pediatric intensive care physicians to estimate cardiac index in ventilated children based on physical examination, clinical data, and bedside laboratory data.[1] Overall, a poor correlation between measured cardiac index (by thermodilution) and the clinicians' categorical and numerical estimate was observed. Thus overreliance on physical findings, laboratory studies, or raw electronic data, with their inherent errors, may compromise the safe and efficient care of patients. These findings support the need for safe, accurate, repeatable techniques for monitoring cardiovascular function in children who are critically ill. This chapter briefly reviews determinants of myocardial function and discusses the various noninvasive and invasive methods that are commonly used to assess and monitor the cardiovascular system in the pediatric intensive care unit. The applicability of these methods for assessing cardiovascular function are highlighted in a particularly unique and challenging patient population, namely, pediatric patients with single-ventricle physiology.

Myocardial Function

The function of the heart and vasculature is to deliver oxygen and other nutrients to various tissues in order to meet the metabolic demands of the organism. Mild-to-moderate depression of oxygen delivery (DO_2) normally is compensated by augmented oxygen extraction at the tissue level, thereby maintaining a stable level of oxygen consumption ($\dot{V}O_2$). When DO_2 falls below some critical level, this compensatory mechanism fails and a state of oxygen supply dependency exists,[2] such that any further drop in DO_2 leads to a parallel fall in $\dot{V}O_2$.[3–5] Under a state of supply-dependent oxygen consumption, affected tissues and organs maintain homeostasis partly through anaerobic metabolism. Left unchecked, inadequate tissue oxygenation may be reflected in abnormal specific end-organ function. The effect of inadequate oxygen delivery on the heart may manifest as depressed systolic or diastolic ventricular function, hypotension, and delayed capillary refill.

Cardiac output is the product of stroke volume (quantity of blood ejected per beat) and heart rate. The four primary determinants of cardiac function are preload (which determines the precontractile lengths of the myofibrils), end-systolic wall stress (function of the pressure and physical characteristics of the arterial system, ventricular wall thickness, and chamber dimension), myocardial contractility, and heart rate. Although the separate roles of these factors have been studied extensively in isolated myocardial strips and intact hearts, data suggest these parameters are interrelated and may influence both systolic and diastolic ventricular function *in vivo*. Furthermore, the four determinants of ventricular function can be altered by many factors in the intensive care setting. Preload, or end-diastolic volume, is affected by ventricular compliance (rate and extent of cardiomyocyte relaxation, and cardiac connective tissue), intravascular volume status, and intrathoracic pressure. Expansion of the heart resulting from transmural filling pressure, rather than the left atrial pressure per se, determines the force of contraction. Therefore intrathoracic (or intrapericardial) pressure is a key determinant of preload. Thus ventricular hypertrophy, vasodilator and diuretic therapies, and positive pressure mechanical ventilation all may have an adverse effect on preload. Similarly, cardiac function is inversely related to afterload, or end-systolic wall stress. Anatomic obstructions and systemic or pulmonary hypertension may negatively impact ventricular systolic and diastolic function, particularly in the critically ill patient. Heart rate and normal atrioventricular conduction are other important determinants of cardiac output. Excessively fast or slow heart rates and inappropriately timed atrial contraction (relative to ventricular systole) may negatively affect ventricular function. Tachyarrhythmias are associated with a shorter diastole leading to impaired diastolic filling (decreased preload) and decreased coronary perfusion, both of which limit ventricular performance. When a compensatory increase in stroke volume is not possible, extreme bradyarrhythmias also decrease ventricular function. Finally, myocardial contractility is often affected in the intensive care setting. Hypoxemia, acidosis, hypomagnesemia, hypocalcemia, hypoglycemia, hyperkalemia, cardiac surgery, sepsis, and cardiomyopathies impair the function of cardiac contractile proteins in forming cross-bridges and developing tension. The remainder of the chapter addresses the techniques used to assess and monitor the determinants of cardiovascular function.

Noninvasive Monitoring

Physical Examination

The physical examination often is the initial and perhaps most common technique used to assess and monitor cardiovascular function. Significantly diminished cardiac output may manifest as diminished peripheral pulses, cool or mottled extremities, and delayed capillary refill. However, certain clinical signs of low cardiac output may be unreliable depending on the particular diagnosis. For example, in the context of cardiac lesions associated with a large arterial pulse pressure (e.g., severe aortic insufficiency and aortopulmonary shunts), peripheral pulses may be increased despite low cardiac output and reduced systemic DO_2. In septic shock, patients often are peripherally vasodilated and warm despite hypotension, diminished pulses, and reduced DO_2 (at the tissue level). Dependent edema, a physical finding most often associated with chronic low cardiac output, may be influenced by a number of additional factors (e.g., hypoalbuminemia, capillary leak syndrome) that may render it a less helpful sign.

Impaired oxygenation may present as cyanosis of the skin, lips, and/or nail beds. Central cyanosis, from either cardiac or respiratory causes, results from arterial oxygen desaturation. In contrast, peripheral cyanosis results from vasoconstriction and low blood flow at the microcirculatory level. In some patients, cyanosis is a relatively subtle physical finding, particularly if the patient has a dark complexion or is anemic.

Hydration status can be assessed by skin turgor, dryness of mucous membranes, and fullness of the anterior fontanel (in infants). It is important to note that these manifestations of hydration status, which relate mostly to interstitial fluid, may poorly reflect intravascular volume, which must be directly measured.

Cardiac auscultation for abnormal heart sounds, including valve clicks, rubs, gallops, and murmurs, may provide the first clue to the presence of a significant functional or structural cardiac abnormality. Unfortunately, the lack of a heart murmur, especially with low cardiac output, does not necessarily rule out a significant residual cardiac lesion.

The presence of pulmonary rales, particularly in the older pediatric patient, may signify pulmonary edema perhaps associated with congestive heart failure. However, pulmonary rales are nonspecific and may be caused by lung disease (e.g., pneumonia), fluid overload, or a disorder of cardiac structure or function.

Finally, jugular venous distension and hepatomegaly often are indicative of high right-sided filling pressures often associated with right ventricular dysfunction.

Chest Radiography

The chest radiograph may be helpful for assessment and monitoring of cardiovascular status in the critically ill pediatric patient. If the chest film is technically adequate, the clinician can assess heart size, contour, and configuration; pulmonary vascularity; pleural effusions; lung parenchyma; and abdominal situs. Some of these findings, when abnormal, may help determine the etiology of cardiovascular dysfunction, and several of these findings are useful for monitoring response to therapy. Nonetheless, the chest radiograph is insensitive with regard to revealing cardiac status.

Increased pulmonary arterial vasculature may be indicated by enlarged pulmonary arteries in the hila that radiate toward the periphery of the lung. Conditions that increase pulmonary blood flow at least twice normal increase the size of the pulmonary arteries. Increased pulmonary capillary pressure may be indicated by the presence of pulmonary edema. The edema may present as a "fluffy" hilum, but in neonates it may appear as diffuse granularity throughout both lung fields. Pleural effusions may accompany pulmonary edema, particularly in conditions associated with poorly compensated congestive heart failure. Increased pulmonary venous markings are indicative of elevated pulmonary venous pressures of any cause, although usually from decreased left ventricular compliance or obstruction in the pulmonary veins or left atrium. Rarely, pulmonary venous hypertension is seen as enlargement of the more horizontally positioned pulmonary veins and is commonly accompanied by pulmonary edema.

In conditions of cardiovascular compromise, cardiac size is frequently enlarged. The cardiothoracic ratio gives a quantitative estimate of cardiac size. The size is obtained by dividing the transverse diameter of the heart in the posteroanterior view by the width of the thoracic cavity. Cardiomegaly is present if the cardiothoracic ratio is greater than 0.5 in adults and 0.6 in infants. Although useful for assessing left ventricular enlargement, the cardiothoracic ratio is not as sensitive to right ventricular enlargement. Right ventricular enlargement results in lateral and upward displacement of the cardiac apex on the posteroanterior view and filling of the retrosternal space on the lateral view.

Significant cardiac problems, such as constrictive pericarditis, restrictive myocarditis, and obstructed total anomalous pulmonary venous return, may be associated with a normal-size heart on chest radiograph.

In the early postoperative period, the most important information obtained from the chest radiograph is (1) the positions of the endotracheal tube, chest tubes, and intracardiac lines; (2) the presence of extrapulmonary fluid or air; and (3) the presence of pulmonary edema.

Blood Pressure Monitoring

The auscultatory method of blood pressure measurement with cuff and pressure gauge is difficult if access to the patient is limited, the patient is small or uncooperative, and when frequent recordings are required. Therefore two techniques—Doppler and oscillometric measurements—have been developed. The Doppler technique uses a Doppler ultrasound probe that is applied to the radial or brachial artery. A cuff wrapped around the upper arm is inflated until the audible Doppler signal is obliterated and then deflated until the signal first becomes audible again (systolic blood pressure). This method has been validated in low-flow states and in small children.[6] The oscillometric method has the advantage of being readily automated. The Dinamap (Device for Indirect Noninvasive Mean Arterial Pressure) is based on the principle that blood flow through a vessel produces oscillation of the arterial wall that may be transmitted to an inflatable cuff encircling the extremity. As cuff pressure decreases, a characteristic change occurs in the magnitude of oscillation at the levels at which systolic, diastolic, and mean pressures are registered. Accuracy of Dinamap blood pressures has been validated in children, and it correlates well with direct intravascular radial artery pressures.[7]

The accuracy of these two techniques relates to the cuff size. If the cuff is too narrow, the pressure recorded may be erroneously high; if the cuff is too wide, the pressure recorded may be too low. Both techniques are unreliable and inadequate in patients with low cardiac output, hypotension, dysrhythmias, significant edema, and/or systemic vasoconstriction.

Pulse Oximetry

Pulse oximetry measures the quantity of hemoglobin saturated with oxygen in arterial blood. It depends on two principles: (1) oxygenated and reduced hemoglobin have different absorption spectra; and (2) at constant light intensity and hemoglobin concentration, oxygen saturation of hemoglobin is a logarithmic function of the intensity of transmitted light (Beer Lambert law). Two wavelengths of light, which have different absorption spectra for reduced hemoglobin and oxyhemoglobin, are transmitted from the light-emitting diodes through the arterial bed. Light absorption at the two wavelengths is compared, yielding the ratio of oxyhemoglobin to reduced hemoglobin, or the oxygen saturation. Pulse oximeters have a high potential for error at saturations below 80%.[8] Furthermore, the oxygen dissociation curve flattens out at the high range so that at saturations greater than 90% to 95%, large changes in PaO_2 accompany small changes in saturation. This principle is important in preventing hyperoxia in premature infants and in patients with univentricular hearts and shunt-dependent pulmonary blood flow.

Invasive Monitoring

Intravascular pressure monitoring often is essential in the management of critically ill neonates and infants in an intensive care unit. Pressures also can be measured in the cardiac chambers or in the pulmonary vasculature. However, the necessity for intravascular or intracardiac lines always should be considered carefully, and they should be removed as soon as the clinical condition permits. The risk of thrombosis and systemic thromboembolism is constant, particularly with relatively large catheters in small vessels for prolonged periods.

Typically, an end-hole catheter is inserted into a vessel or cardiac chamber and connected to a pressure transducer by a coupling system composed of fluid-filled extension tubing, a stopcock for withdrawing blood and balancing the transducer to atmospheric pressure, and a continuous infusion device to flush out blood and air. The transducer translates pressure into an electrical signal that can be processed through a preamplifier into a waveform or numerical display on a monitor. The pressure transducer must be properly calibrated, dampened, and positioned (at midchest level). Inaccurate measurements can occur for a variety of reasons. A thorough review of the physics of invasive pressure monitoring is presented in Chapter 19.

Central venous access affords the opportunity to measure central venous pressure (CVP), deliver drugs or high osmolarity nutritional solutions, and repeatedly sample blood to monitor venous oxygen saturations and for other laboratory studies. Intraarterial lines offer the opportunity to continuously monitor arterial pressure and for intermittent blood gas analysis.

Intravascular pressures provide information about ventricular preload and afterload. Right ventricular preload is assessed by CVP. The CVP is determined by a variety of factors, including patient age, preoperative status (i.e., patient with right ventricular hypertrophy and increased right atrial pressure), cardiac performance, intrathoracic pressure, blood volume, vasopressor therapy, and status of the pericardium. The CVP "a wave" reflects atrial contraction and the "v wave" reflects atrial filling. Serial measurements of CVP are frequently used to evaluate the response to fluid administration. Right ventricular afterload can be assessed using a pulmonary arterial catheter. This catheter is particularly important for monitoring pulmonary artery pressure and therapeutic response to vasodilators in patients with elevated pulmonary vascular resistance. The pulmonary arterial wedge pressure reflects left atrial pressure (in the absence of pulmonary vein stenosis). In the postoperative cardiac patient, a direct left atrial line can be placed in order to directly assess left ventricular preload. Left ventricular afterload is assessed by measurement of systemic arterial pressure, provided no left ventricular outflow tract obstruction is present. In the pediatric population, blood pressure is age dependent and is a relatively insensitive marker of systemic blood flow and DO_2. Blood pressure is the product of cardiac output and systemic vascular resistance. Therefore, hypotension may result from diminished cardiac output and/or decreased systemic vascular resistance.[9] Because the treatment options are different, differentiating low cardiac output from low systemic vascular resistance is important.

When catheters are placed in more distal arteries, be aware of pulse wave amplification. The exact causes of pulse wave amplification are unknown but may be related to reflected waves from the periphery, the resonant frequency of arterial walls, distortion of particular waveforms by the arterial wall, or conversion of kinetic energy to hydrostatic energy. Characteristically, pulse wave amplification results in a higher systolic pressure, a lower diastolic pressure, but a constant mean arterial pressure.

Cardiac Output

Cardiac output can be measured by a variety of techniques, including the Fick method, the thermodilution technique, the dye dilution technique, Doppler echocardiography (see section of Doppler echocardiography), and magnetic resonance imaging. Each of the first three methods applies a similar principle of dilution of an indicator: oxygen, cold, or indocyanine green dye, respectively. According to the principle, the change in concentration of a substance is proportional to the volume of blood in which it is being diluted. In general, the thermodilution technique is the method most widely used in the intensive care setting. However, for conditions of low cardiac output, the Fick method is more reliable than the thermodilution or dye dilution technique. Conversely, the Fick method is less accurate in conditions of high cardiac output because of difficulty in measuring narrow arteriovenous oxygen differences in the blood.

Thermodilution Technique

The thermodilution technique for measuring cardiac output requires use of a specialized pulmonary arterial catheter. Cardiac output is calculated by injecting a known volume of ice water or saline into the right atrium (proximal catheter port) and measuring the temperature change at the catheter tip in the pulmonary artery. Cardiac output (CO) is calculated by the following equation:

$$CO = 1.08 \times V_i \, (T_b - T_i) / \int_0 T_b(t)dt,$$

where V_i = injectate volume (ml), T_b = temperature of blood (°C), T_i = injectate temperature (°C), and $T_b(t)dt$ = area under the curve. In general, thermodilution cardiac outputs are performed using a completely automated system, and the calculations are performed by a computer. This method (as with any indicator dilution method) requires complete mixing and thus is most accurate in situations where a mixing chamber is located proximal to the thermistor. It is generally used only in patients who do not have intracardiac or great vessel-level shunts or an insufficient valve between the injection site and the sampling site. The injection must be made rapidly because a slow injection gives a falsely elevated cardiac output.

Possible sources of error with this method include inaccurate measurement of the volume of injectate or of the temperature of the blood or injectate, close approximation of the thermistor to a vessel wall, and inadequate mixing, as sometimes seen in venous systems with low flow.

Fick Method

According to the Fick principle, cardiac output equals oxygen consumption divided by the arteriovenous oxygen content difference. Measurement of oxygen consumption in an intensive care unit is difficult and cumbersome but has been accomplished by analysis of expired gases. Because measuring $\dot{V}O_2$ in the intensive care setting is difficult, the arteriovenous oxygen difference is often used as an indirect measure of cardiac output. A wide arteriovenous oxygen difference generally reflects a low cardiac output and indicates a large oxygen extraction by the tissues, whereas a narrow arteriovenous oxygen difference usually reflects a high cardiac output. Particular care must be taken to select the appropriate sampling site for a true mixed venous blood sample. Under most circumstances, the best site to obtain a mixed venous sample is within the pulmonary artery. If a left-to-right shunt is present, however, the mixed venous site should be the cardiac chamber proximal to the site of the shunt. When a site other than the pulmonary artery is used for the mixed venous site, the resultant value for arteriovenous oxygen difference is a less reliable reflection of the absolute cardiac output, but it can be used for serial observations and for monitoring response to therapy. Unfortunately, studies suggest $\dot{V}O_2$ is quite variable for any individual patient in an intensive care setting.[10] Furthermore, mixed venous oxygen saturation (and hence arteriovenous oxygen difference) may be misleading in patients with decreased tissue O_2 extraction.[11,12]

Laboratory Studies

When systemic oxygen transport (product of cardiac output and arterial oxygen content) is reduced below a critical level, oxygen uptake (product of cardiac output and arteriovenous oxygen content difference) declines with further reductions in oxygen delivery. Tissue hypoxia then occurs, and affected tissues and organs resort, in part, to anaerobic metabolism, which leads to increased production of lactate, CO_2, and hydrogen ions. Alterations in hydrogen ion concentration cause the clinical problems of acid-base disorders. Severe acidosis (pH <7.2) depresses myocardial contractility, sensitizes the heart to arrhythmias, and causes arteriolar dilatation and hypotension. Alterations in hydrogen ion concentration are resisted by a complex defense system that includes extracellular and intracellular chemical buffers and respiratory compensation by the lungs or metabolic compensation by the kidneys. Extracellular buffers, including serum bicarbonate and proteins, are the first line of defense, rapidly titrating the increased hydrogen ion concentration. Extracellular fluid buffering is handled primarily by the bicarbonate-carbonic acid system, which can be assessed clinically by measuring blood gas pH and PCO_2 and serum bicarbonate concentration or total CO_2 content. When a primary decrease in extracellular bicarbonate concentration causes a fall in pH below 7.35, metabolic acidosis occurs. A laboratory clue to the cause of metabolic acidosis is the anion gap, the difference in unmeasured serum anions and unmeasured serum cations. If the anion gap is normal (8–16 mEq/L), loss of bicarbonate has occurred, usually via the kidneys or gastrointestinal tract, or rapid dilution of the extracellular fluid has occurred. Treatment consists of sodium bicarbonate replacement. If the anion gap is increased, strong acids may have been added to the system either by retention of endogenous acids produced in excess, such as lactic acidosis, or by addition of exogenous acids. Treatment ultimately consists of correcting the underlying disorder, but acute therapy with sodium bicarbonate may be necessary if the pH is dangerously low.

End-tidal PCO_2, determined noninvasively by capnography, accurately identifies the critical point for systemic oxygen transport; however, further work is necessary to determine whether this method has clinical applicability.[13] Other indirect methods include gastric tonometry to assess gut intramucosal pH or PCO_2[14,15] and measurement of blood lactate concentration.[16,17] These two methods are readily available for use in clinical practice, but both techniques have limitations. With advancements in blood gas analyzer technology, blood lactate measurements now are rapid, simple, accurate, and relatively inexpensive and thus may hold promise for clinical monitoring and evaluating response to therapy. We observed that initial absolute blood lactate levels were less important than the temporal trend in lactate concentrations for predicting mortality in postoperative cardiac patients.[18] Unfortunately, the specificity of blood lactate is imperfect and may lack sensitivity for detecting supply-dependent oxygen consumption, particularly if it is only regional. In addition, blood lactate depends on hepatic metabolism and the rate of production. In these respects, gastric tonometry may have an advantage in that it can uncover regional hypoxia and hypoperfusion involving the gut and can be adapted for continuous online measurement.[15] Nonetheless, this technique assumes that a critical reduction in oxygen transport manifests in the splanchnic circulation before it can be detected systemically (probably a reasonable assumption), and tonometric methods are not entirely noninvasive.

Urine output generally reflects adequate systemic blood flow, but oliguria may occur in the context of good systemic blood flow with or without hypotension, particularly in the postoperative congenital heart disease patient. Patients who return to the intensive care unit following surgery with cardiopulmonary bypass frequently have significant total body water and salt overload from dilution of blood with crystalloid pump priming solution. In the first 2 to 4 hours following admission, most patients who have undergone bypass produce more than 1 ml/kg/hour of urine. After this initial period of adequate urine output, the rate often decreases to less than 1 ml/kg/hour and continues at a lower rate for up to 48 hours. Increased abdominal pressure, most often associated with ascites, may contribute to decreased renal blood flow and hence oliguria.

Near-infrared spectroscopy (NIRS) is a newer noninvasive technique that has been applied to assess systemic and regional oxygen transport in several clinical and laboratory studies.[19–27] In an experimental setting in which DO_2 is controlled, NIRS has been used to correlate cytochrome aa_3 (terminal link in the electron transport chain responsible for mitochondrial respiration), $\dot{V}O_2$, and lactate flux.[24] Thus NIRS has the potential to identify a regional critical reduction in oxygen transport at the cellular level.

Several studies suggest the initial metabolic response to hypoxemia differs between the newborn and older ages. In adults at rest, DO_2 is in great excess of $\dot{V}O_2$. This "oxygen surplus" means moderate reductions of oxygen transport are generally well tolerated without compromise of $\dot{V}O_2$. In contrast to the metabolism of the adult, the metabolism of the newborn may be particularly susceptible to modest alterations in oxygen transport because of the high resting demands for oxygen, the ease with which these demands can be increased by small environmental changes, and the apparently limited reserve for augmenting cardiac output or oxygen extraction acutely.[28,29]

Echocardiography

Echocardiography has emerged as an invaluable method for assessing cardiac function. The noninvasive nature of echocardiography allows for serial measurements of systolic and diastolic ventricular function. Unfortunately, the continually and rapidly changing hemodynamic status of patients in an intensive care setting may limit use of this imaging modality. Nonetheless, echocardiography provides a simple means for assessing global ventricular function through implementation of M-mode, two-dimensional, and Doppler techniques.

M-Mode Echocardiography

M-mode echocardiography provides a single line of information at a higher frame rate than can be obtained by two-dimensional echocardiography. This technique enhances accurate determination of linear dimensions and improves quantitation of chamber size and wall thickness. M-mode measurements have been used extensively to evaluate left ventricular function, but they are not as useful in assessing function in ventricles of irregular shapes (e.g., right ventricles or single ventricles) or in the presence of segmental wall-motion abnormalities. M-mode measurements of function include the fractional shortening (diastolic dimension minus systolic dimension divided by diastolic dimension; normal 28% to 40%), mean rate of circumferential fiber shortening (fractional shortening divided by ejection time), and mitral E-point septal separation (distance between most anterior excursion of the mitral valve and most posterior excursion of ventricular septum). When corrected for left ventricular end-diastolic volume, mitral E-point septal separation provides a good index of systolic function but is rarely used as a clinical measure.

Two-Dimensional Echocardiography

In two-dimensional echocardiography, various tomographic views of the heart and great vessels are obtained along different axes. These views allow detailed analysis of the anatomy and function of the cardiac structures, obviating the need for cardiac catheterization in many infants and children. In addition, in most patients, ventricular masses and volumes can be accurately measured, and an ejection fraction can be calculated (usually by the Simpson rule). In the setting of a critically ill child, the two-dimensional echocardiogram may prove invaluable for assessing the extent and pattern of left ventricular contraction, for detecting the presence of pericardial effusions, and for detecting intracardiac thrombi or vegetations. Unfortunately, echocardiography has several limitations, including inadequate determination of ventricular function in the univentricular heart and imprecise assessment of diastolic function.

Doppler Echocardiography

Doppler echocardiography has emerged as an important noninvasive procedure to determine hemodynamic information. Doppler imaging is based on the principle that the frequency of the reflected echocardiographic wave provides information on the location, direction, and velocity of the blood flowing through the structures being interrogated. Doppler blood flow velocities can provide estimates of intracardiac and intrapulmonary pressures by using the simplified Bernoulli equation:

$$P_1 - P_2 = 4V^2,$$

where V = measured velocity (cm/s), P_1 = pressure proximal to measured velocity, and P_2 = pressure distal to measured velocity.

Doppler flow velocities have been used to assess right ventricular systolic pressure and pulmonary artery systolic, diastolic, and mean pressures. Because pulmonary artery and right ventricular systolic pressures are nearly equal in the absence of disease of the right ventricular outflow tract, pulmonary valve, or supravalvular region, pulmonary artery systolic pressure is commonly estimated by techniques that measure right ventricular systolic pressure. In the method most commonly used, the peak velocity of the tricuspid regurgitation jet is used to calculate the right ventricular–right atrial pressure gradient using the Bernoulli equation. In patients with a ventricular septal defect, right ventricular systolic pressure can be estimated using a Doppler recording of the peak velocity across the septum and the systolic blood pressure (assuming no left ventricular outflow tract obstruction). In patients with pulmonary regurgitation, quantification of diastolic velocities is helpful in calculating pulmonary artery end-diastolic pressure. In the presence of mild pulmonary regurgitation, normal right ventricular end-diastolic pressure, and low pulmonary artery diastolic pressure, pulmonic regurgitation Doppler velocities return to the baseline at end-diastole. In patients with elevated pulmonary artery systolic and diastolic pressures, the velocity of the pulmonary regurgitation jet is high at the end of diastole, and can be calculated from the Bernoulli equation.[30] Masuyama and colleagues[30] showed that the peak of the pulmonary regurgitation flow velocity in early diastole correlates well with the mean pulmonary artery pressure using the regression equation:

$$4V^2 = 0.70\ (\text{MPAP}) - 2,$$

where $4V^2$ = peak of all pulmonary artery-to-right ventricular diastolic pressure gradients, and MPAP = mean pulmonary artery pressure.

Doppler technique also can be used to measure cardiac output. Cardiac output equals the mean velocity of systolic flow, the heart rate at the time of measurement, and the cross-sectional area of the artery in which measurements are being made (usually the ascending aorta):

$$\text{CO} = \text{A} \times \text{V} \times \text{HR},$$

where A = area of the orifice, V = integrated flow velocity, and HR = heart rate. To determine the integrated flow velocity, the area under the Doppler curve must be measured. The area of the aortic orifice is commonly obtained by measuring the aortic diameter from the two-dimensional image, where $A = 0.785 \times d^2$.

Another technique for assessing left ventricular function by Doppler echocardiography is interrogating Doppler flow in patients with mitral regurgitation. The rate at which left ventricular pressure rises (dP/dt) is a measure of left ventricular contractility and is reflected by the rate at which blood moves from left ventricle to left atrium in mitral regurgitation. By taking two points along the slope of the mitral regurgitation jet, the pressure gradient at each point can be calculated and the pressure difference between the two points obtained. Dividing by the time between the two points provides the dP/dt (normal LV dP/dt = 1800 mmHg/s). When dP/dt is used to assess ventricular systolic function, remember that dP/dt, like any ejection phase index, is influenced by preload, afterload, and inotropic state of the heart.

Single-Ventricle Physiology

With advances in surgical techniques and preoperative and postoperative care, survival of children with single-ventricle physiology continues to improve. Therefore these patients may represent an ever-increasing population in pediatric and pediatric cardiothoracic intensive care units. In many ways, these patients are distinct from children with two functioning ventricles, so they pose several unique challenges to the pediatric intensivist.

For many single-ventricle patients, initial palliation in infancy often involves placement of an aortopulmonary (e.g., modified Blalock-Taussig) shunt that provides a source of (limited) pulmonary blood flow. Following this operation, the total cardiac output of the single ventricle represents the sum of the pulmonary (Q_p) and systemic (Q_s) blood flows. The relative percentage of blood flow to the pulmonary and systemic circulations depends on the total resistance in each vascular bed. Because pulmonary vascular resistance usually is substantially less than systemic vascular resistance soon after birth, the size (diameter, length, and vessel of origin) of the aortopulmonary shunt is a major contributor to total pulmonary vascular resistance and hence an important determinant of Q_p/Q_s. Therefore in shunt-dependent single-ventricle patients with complete admixture, arterial oxygen saturation is influenced not only by lung function (e.g., pulmonary venous saturation) but also by pulmonary blood flow and myocardial function (which influences systemic blood flow and hence mixed venous saturation). Computer modeling of shunt-dependent single ventricle physiology[31] suggests $Q_p/Q_s \ll 1.0$ is ideal for optimizing systemic oxygen availability for a given pulmonary venous saturation, cardiac output, and $\dot{V}O_2$. However, pulmonary venous saturation,[32] cardiac output, and $\dot{V}O_2$ are variable, particularly in the immediate postoperative period; thus the "ideal" Q_p/Q_s remains unclear. In addition, an accurate mixed venous saturation may be difficult to obtain because it requires placement of a catheter in the proximal superior vena cava (vs. distal superior vena cava, right atrium, or inferior vena cava that may be contaminated by highly saturated pulmonary venous blood) and because PCO_2 may influence cerebral blood flow and hence mixed venous O_2.

In vivo data from our institution and others highlight the impracticality and difficulty of accurately measuring Q_p/Q_s in a postoperative single-ventricle patient.[33] Thus some investigators have proposed surrogate indices of inadequate systemic oxygen delivery. In our patients following single-ventricle palliation, a progressive decline in the serum lactate concentration (regardless of the initial postoperative concentration) is a sensitive and specific marker for early survival. In contrast, rising lactate is an accurate predictor of early postoperative cardiovascular collapse.[18]

After total cavopulmonary anastomosis (Fontan palliation), single-ventricle patients again demonstrate unique physiology that may require special cardiovascular monitoring. For instance, right atrial and left atrial catheters placed intraoperatively are extremely useful for measuring the transpulmonary gradient. An elevated right atrial (or central venous) pressure with a normal left atrial pressure often reflects pulmonary hypertension secondary to elevated pulmonary vascular resistance (branch pulmonary artery stenoses or elevated arteriolar resistance). In contrast, elevated right and left atrial pressures (with a normal transpulmonary gradient) usually signify elevated ventricular end-diastolic pressures. In the presence of a Fontan baffle fenestration, elevated right atrial (central venous) pressures are associated with increased right-to-left shunting and decreased arterial oxygen saturations. Further evaluation and treatment options would be very different depending on the particular clinical scenario as described above.

REFERENCES

1. Tibby SM, Hatherhill M, Marsh MJ, et al: Clinicians' abilities to estimate cardiac index in ventilated children and infants. *Arch Dis Child* 77:516-518, 1997.
2. Schlictig R: Oxygen delivery and consumption in critical illness. In Civetta JM, Taylor RW, Kirby RR, editors: *Critical care,* ed 2, Philadelphia, 1997, Lippincott-Raven.
3. Adams RP, Dieleman LA, Cain SM: A critical value for O_2 transport in the rat. *J Appl Physiol* 53:660-664, 1982.
4. Cain SM: Oxygen delivery and uptake in dogs during anemic and hypoxic hypoxia. *J Appl Physiol* 42:228-234, 1977.
5. Schwarz S, Frantz RA, Shoemaker WC: Sequential hemodynamic and oxygen transport responses in hypovolemia, anemia and hypoxia. *Am J Physiol* 241:H864-H871, 1981.
6. Waltemath C, Preuss D: Determination of blood pressure in low-flow states by the Doppler technique. *Anesthesiology* 34:77-79, 1971.
7. Park M, Menard S: Accuracy of blood pressure measurement by the Dinamap monitor in infants and children. *Pediatrics* 79:907-914, 1987.
8. Webb R, Ralston A, Runciman W: Potential errors in pulse oximetry. II. Effects of changes in saturation and signal quality. *Anaesthesia* 46:207-212, 1991.
9. Argenziano M, Chen JM, Choudhri AF, et al: Management of vasodilatory shock after cardiac surgery: identification of predisposing factors and use of a novel pressor agent. *J Thorac Cardiovasc Surg* 116:973-980, 1998.
10. Jain A, Shroff SG, Janicki JS, et al: Relation between mixed venous oxygen saturation and cardiac index: nonlinearity and normalization for oxygen uptake and hemoglobin. *Chest* 99:1303-1409, 1991.
11. Scheinman MM, Brown MA, Rapaport E: Critical assessment of use of central venous oxygen saturation as a mirror of mixed venous oxygen in severely ill cardiac patients. *Circulation* 40:165-172, 1969.
12. Chang AC, Kulik TJ, Hickey PR, et al: Real-time gas-exchange measurement of oxygen consumption in neonates and infants after cardiac surgery. *Crit Care Med* 21:1369-1375, 1993.
13. Guzman JA, Lacoma FJ, Najar A, et al: End tidal PCO_2 as a noninvasive indicator of systemic oxygen supply-dependency during hemorrhagic shock and resuscitation. *Shock* 8:427-431, 1997.
14. Guzman JA, Lacoma FJ, Kruse JA: Relationship between systemic oxygen supply dependency and gastric intramucosal PCO_2 during progressive hemorrhage. *Trauma* 44:696-700, 1998.
15. Guzman JA, Kruse JA: Development and validation of a technique for continuous monitoring of gastric intramucosal pH. *Am J Respir Crit Care Med* 153:694-700, 1996.
16. Kruse JA: Blood lactate and oxygen transport. *Intensive Care World* 4:121-125, 1987.

17. Kruse JA, Haupt MT, Puri VK, et al: Lactate levels predict the relationship between oxygen delivery and consumption in patients with the adult respiratory distress syndrome. *Chest* 98:959-962, 1990.
18. Charpie JR, Dekeon MK, Goldberg CS, et al: Serial blood lactate measurements predict early outcome after neonatal repair or palliation for complex congenital heart disease. *J Thorac Cardiovasc Surg* 120:73-80, 2000.
19. Slavin KV, Dujovny M, Ausman JI, et al: Clinical experience with transcranial cerebral oximetry. *Surg Neurol* 42:531-541, 1994.
20. Wyatt JS, Cope M, Delpy DT, et al: Quantitation of cerebral blood volume in human infants by near-infrared spectroscopy. *J Appl Physiol* 68:1086-1091, 1990.
21. Edwards AD, Wyatt JS, Richardson C, et al: Cotside measurement of cerebral blood flow in ill newborn infants by near-infrared spectroscopy. *Lancet* 2:770-771, 1988.
22. Tateishi A, Maekawa T, Soejima Y, et al: Qualitative comparison of carbon dioxide-induced change in cerebral near-infrared spectroscopy versus jugular venous oxygen saturation in adults with acute brain disease. *Crit Care Med* 23:1734-1738, 1995.
23. Lewis SB, Myburgh JA, Thornoton EL, et al: Cerebral oxygenation monitoring by near-infrared spectroscopy is not clinically useful in patients with severe closed-head injury: a comparison with jugular venous bulb oximetry. *Crit Care Med* 24:1334-1338, 1996.
24. Guery BPH, Mangalaboyi J, Menager P, et al: Redox status of cytochrome a,a_3: a noninvasive indicator of dysoxia in regional hypoxic or ischemic hypoxia. *Crit Care Med* 27:576-582, 1999.
25. Hampson NB, Piantadosi CA: Near-infrared monitoring of human skeletal muscle oxygenation during forearm ischemia. *J Appl Physiol* 64:2449-2457, 1988.
26. Tashiro H, Suzuki S, Kaneshiro M, et al: A new method for determining graft function after liver transplantation by near-infrared spectroscopy. *Transplantation* 56:1261-1263, 1993.
27. Noriyuki T, Ohdan H, Yoshioka S, et al: Near-infrared spectroscopic method for assessing the tissue oxygenation of living lung. *Am J Respir Crit Care Med* 156:1656-1661, 1997.
28. Lister G, Walter TK, Versmold HT, et al: Oxygen delivery in lambs: cardiovascular and hematologic development. *Am J Physiol* 237: H668-H675, 1979.
29. Klopfenstein HS, Rudolph AM: Postnatal changes in the circulation and responses to volume loading in sheep. *Circ Res* 42:839-845, 1978.
30. Masuyama T, Kodama K, Kitabatake A, et al: Continuous-wave Doppler echocardiographic detection of pulmonary regurgitation and its application to noninvasive estimation of pulmonary artery pressure. *Circulation* 74:484-492, 1986.
31. Barnea O, Austin EH, Richman B, et al: Balancing the circulation: theoretic optimization of pulmonary/systemic flow ratio in hypoplastic left heart syndrome. *J Am Coll Cardiol* 24:1376-1381, 1994.
32. Taeed R, Schwartz SM, Pearl JM, et al: Unrecognized pulmonary venous desaturation early after Norwood palliation confounds Q_p:Q_s assessment and compromises oxygen delivery, *Circulation* 103:2699-2704, 2001.
33. Charpie JR, Dekeon M, Goldberg CS, et al: Postoperative hemodynamics after Norwood palliation for hypoplastic left heart syndrome. *Am J Cardiol* 87:198-202, 2001.

CHAPTER

21

Echocardiography and Noninvasive Diagnosis

James C. Huhta

PEARLS

- When congenital heart disease or myocardial dysfunction is suspected during the management of a neonate or child in the intensive care unit, echocardiography is the noninvasive diagnostic tool of choice.
- Difficulty in oxygenation may lead to a noninvasive study. The goals are to (1) confirm normal intracardiac anatomy, (2) assess intracardiac shunting as a cause of cyanosis, (3) assess left and right ventricular function, (4) assess right-sided heart pressures, (5) assess valve competence, and (6) look for pleural or pericardial effusion.
- In neonatal patients, it is important to assess the status of the ductus arteriosus and to measure the aorta-to-pulmonary artery pressure difference.
- In the postoperative period, information about the pulmonary-to-systemic flow ratio facilitates manipulation of pulmonary vascular resistance.
- All postoperative patients should undergo assessment of diaphragm function bilaterally.

Since the early 1980s, echocardiography (also known as *ultrasonic imaging of the heart and cardiovascular system*) has been at the forefront of advances in pediatric cardiology. This technology allows imaging of anatomy, assessment of ventricular function, and determination of peripheral blood flow velocities in both arteries and veins. This noninvasive technique has enhanced the assessment of fetal and neonatal congenital heart disease and facilitated the management of postoperative and other patients in the pediatric intensive care unit. Early in the history of pediatric cardiology, the electrocardiogram was the dominant tool for exploration of intracardiac anatomy, whereas chest radiography was the screening tool for signs of congestive heart failure and abnormalities of extracardiac anatomy, such as pulmonary artery size and vascularity. Now, complete anatomic and physiologic assessment can be obtained in the neonate and in the fetus at 20 weeks of gestation. Intracardiac and extracardiac anatomy can be defined in most patients, and details of the physiologic state, such as fluid balance, cardiac output, and myocardial contractility, can be determined noninvasively.

The technique of echocardiography and the practice of "echocardiology" have slowly changed the practice of pediatric cardiology by replacing cardiac catheterization for the diagnosis of congenital malformations. Combined with use of prostaglandin for maintaining the patency of the ductus arteriosus, echocardiography has dramatically reduced the need for emergency cardiac catheterization in neonates. Most patients with congenital heart disease detected in the neonatal period can undergo palliative surgery without cardiac catheterization. Most definitive surgical repairs can be performed successfully without the risk of invasive studies. Pulsed, continuous-wave, color, and tissue Doppler have added important capabilities for anatomic and functional assessment. Intraoperative and postoperative management of congenital heart defects has been aided by the addition of transesophageal echocardiography (TEE). This mode can improve resolution in neonates and older patients in whom transthoracic imaging is difficult and greatly aids the surgeon by providing feedback about the quality of the repair prior to separation from the heart-lung machine. Higher-resolution imaging systems continue to evolve. Multielement transducer technology and advances in high-speed computing, three-dimensional real-time imaging, color Doppler, and tissue Doppler have facilitated the assessment of systolic and diastolic function of the myocardium.[1] This chapter focuses on the detection of congenital heart disease in pediatric patients presenting with cardiopulmonary compromise at any age and illustrates the use of TEE for physiologic assessment and management.

Diagnosis of Congenital Heart Disease

Comprehensive analysis of cardiovascular anatomy requires a step-by-step segmental approach. In certain complex congenital malformations, portions of the heart may be absent or malpositioned. Delineation of cardiac anatomy may require that data obtained from several echocardiographic windows be combined. A complete, step-by-step approach to cardiac diagnosis includes the diagnosis of atrial situs diagnosis; identification of the chambers and their interconnections; and systematic assessment of valves, septa, coronaries, systemic and pulmonary veins, and aortic anatomy. Imaging of the thymus and diaphragm is part of the detailed echocardiographic examination.

The segmental approach is based on the principle that all aspects of abnormal cardiovascular morphology can be broken down into discrete, mutually exclusive descriptors, allowing unambiguous description of any complex congenital malformation. The schema must include information on the presence, position, and connection of each cardiac segment. Classically, three segments have been recognized: atria, ventricles, and great arteries. By describing the anatomic segments and indicating the normality or abnormality of each, a complete description of the cardiac anatomy is possible. It now is possible to code cardiac anatomic abnormalities by segmental analysis.[2]

Cardiac Function Assessment

Echocardiography is a tomographic anatomic tool, but it also provides dynamic information about cardiac function and structure. Observations about the cardiac walls, their movement, thickness, and degrees of shortening and thickening can be extremely useful in determining segmental and global cardiac function. In general, the shortening fraction of the left ventricle should be at least 28% (end-diastolic minus end-systolic divided by end-diastolic dimension), and the walls of the left ventricle should move inward symmetrically.

Doppler echocardiography can provide functional information that is not available by any other method. Pulsed Doppler can interrogate a site in the circulation and measure the direction and speed of blood flow in systole and diastole. For example, sampling in the aorta allows comparison of upper and lower body resistances to blood flow by revealing the direction of flow in systole and diastole. The structure and function of the cardiac valves can be determined, perhaps the most powerful application of echocardiography. For example, atrioventricular (AV) valve regurgitation can be diagnosed and its severity, which depends on many technical and physiologic factors, estimated. In addition to visualizing a ventricular septal defect (VSD), the jet of a left-to-right shunt can be detected by pulsed Doppler, the pressure gradient quantified by continuous-wave Doppler (using the simplified Bernoulli equation: Pressure gradient = $4V^2$, where V = peak velocity), and the defect spatially localized by color Doppler. Using the continuity equation and the proximal isovelocity surface area (PISA) concept, flow area and volume can be calculated in left-to-right shunts, and the regurgitant volume and area can be calculated in AV valve regurgitation. Pulmonary artery pressure often can be estimated using the peak velocity of the tricuspid regurgitation jet, and the severity of semilunar stenosis or coarctation can be estimated using the peak and mean gradients. This hemodynamic information can be integrated into the segmental description using the anatomic segment as the finding and the functional aspect as the modifier. For example, the morphologic mitral valve is an anatomic site and location, for which regurgitation might be a modifier. This step-by-step approach to diagnosis answers specific questions about cardiac function and screens for congenital and acquired abnormalities.[3,4]

Structure-Oriented Approach

Adult-oriented, two-dimensional echocardiographic reports usually are based on standard views of the cardiac anatomy that are highly reproducible. The investigators describe the appearance of a given cardiac lesion as seen on a standard parasternal, apical, or subcostal scan. However, this approach can lead to diagnostic errors when applied to congenital heart disease.[5] For example, a scan of an aortopulmonary window from the right ventricular outflow tract can simulate the origin of the aorta from the right ventricle (i.e., transposition of the great arteries). In congenital heart disease, the various views must be integrated, scanning from one echocardiographic window to another to obtain a complete anatomic examination. Although the echocardiographic examiner with experience learns to identify the normal appearances of the heart without congenital defects from various echocardiographic windows, a structure-oriented or anatomic approach always is superior to an approach based on standardized views.

Achieving high sensitivity in the detection of congenital heart disease requires a compulsive approach to locate rare anatomic variations that may be important. For example, coronary artery anomalies such as a coronary originating from the pulmonary artery can be reliably detected using a standardized approach to defining the origins and courses of the coronary branches.[6]

Segmental Analysis—Situs Diagnosis

Determination of cardiac position and atrial-visceral situs is a standard portion of the echocardiographic assessment of congenital heart disease and is the foundation of the segmental approach. Atrial situs and atrial morphology are diagnosed together, and four possibilities exist: solitus (normal), inversus, and heterotaxy that may be right atrial isomerism or left atrial isomerism. For example, for situs solitus, the morphologic right atrium is on the right and the morphologic left atrium is on the left. Abnormal atrial situs and cardiac malposition, such as dextrocardia, frequently are associated. Both can be diagnosed by obtaining a short-axis scan of the abdomen, identifying the spine and the inferior vena cava and the descending aorta. The location of the cardiac apex is important for later scanning from the apex. Subcostal scanning above the diaphragm immediately shows the position of the cardiac apex. From this scan below the diaphragm, the position of the inferior vena cava and aorta usually can be identified, and their location with respect to the spine identifies the situs (Figure 21–1).

The descending aorta and inferior vena cava are oriented symmetrically with respect to one another, with the inferior vena cava to the right in situs solitus and to the left in situs inversus. In right atrial isomerism, the aorta and inferior cava run together on either side of the spine, with the cava anterior. A venous structure that courses behind the aorta and does not enter the heart suggests azygos continuation of the inferior vena cava, which is associated with left atrial isomerism. These patients usually have separate, anomalous hepatic venous connections to the heart. Occasionally, atrial appendage morphology can be identified and the diagnosis of atrial situs confirmed directly. A broad-based atrial appendage usually is a morphologic right one, and a narrow-based appendage is morphologic left. Symmetrical appendages suggest atrial isomerism. Situs diagnosis is important clinically for care of the intensive care patient. Complex congenital malformations occur predictably with right and left isomerism, and asplenia (associated with right atrial isomerism) may place the child at risk for recurrent or persistent infection. Left isomerism is associated with a high rate of gastrointestinal obstruction after birth.

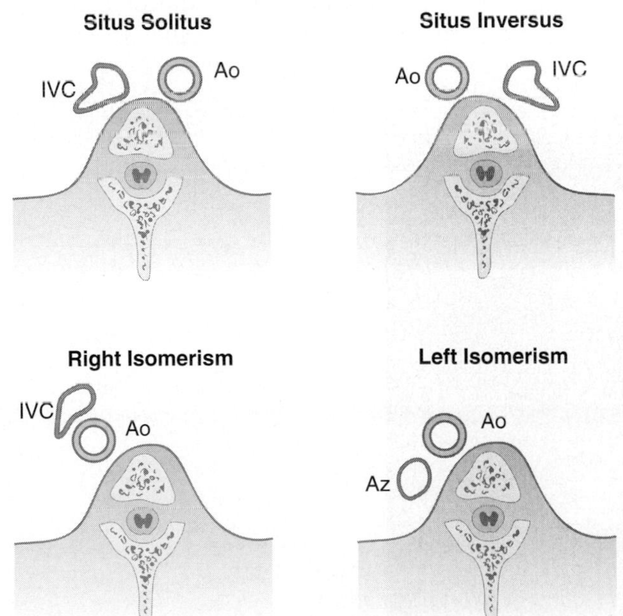

FIGURE 21–1 • Situs by echocardiography. Situs solitus is normal, and the aorta *(Ao)* and inferior vena cava *(IVC)* are symmetrically positioned adjacent to the spine. In situs inversus, there is a mirror image relationship. In right atrial isomerism, the IVC and Ao run together on either side of the spine. In left isomerism, there is azygos continuation of the IVC(Az) located retroperitoneally with the Ao.

Segmental Analysis—Atrioventricular Connection

Description of the connection of the atria and ventricles (i.e., AV connection) requires knowledge of both atrial and ventricular morphology. The echocardiographic criteria for a morphologic left ventricle include insertion of the mitral valve at the crux of the heart farther from the cardiac apex than that of the tricuspid valve, two normally placed left ventricular papillary muscles, mitral semilunar continuity, a typical elliptical, smooth septal wall, and a fishmouth appearance of a mitral valve having two commissures. In the absence of typical offsetting of the AV valves and with cardiac malposition, the trabecular pattern of the ventricles sometimes can be recognized: a smooth wall pattern of the left ventricle and coarser, more heavily trabeculated pattern of the right ventricle. The appearance of the ventricular outflow tracts may aid in ventricular morphologic diagnosis and should be observed as part of the segmental approach. Normally, there is continuity between the mitral valve of the left ventricle and the aortic valve, but muscle of the right ventricular outflow tract separates the tricuspid and pulmonary valves. The most reliable criterion for identifying the morphologic right ventricle is tricuspid valve chordal attachments to the septum. With an atrial septal defect of the primum type, the AV valves are at the same level (Figure 21–2).

Four patterns of AV connection exist: concordant (i.e., normal); discordant; univentricular through a single inlet

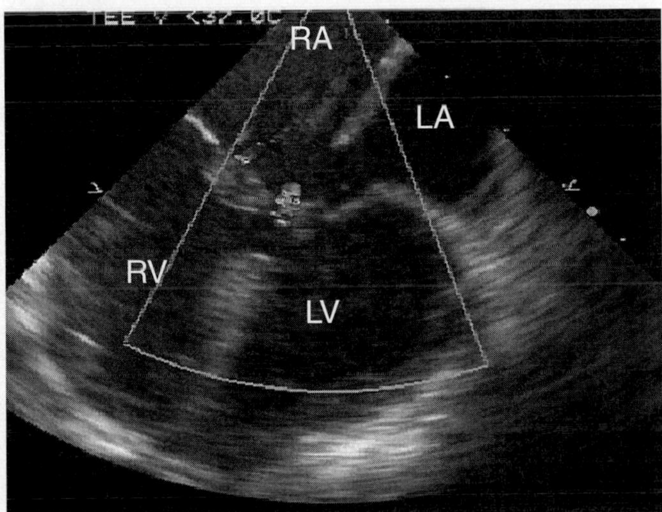

FIGURE 21–2 • Atrioventricular canal defect with dextrocardia. A large primum atrial septal defect and ventricular septal defect are present. Note the mitral and tricuspid valves are at the same level. *LA,* Left atrium; *LV,* left ventricle; *RA,* right atrium; *RV,* right ventricle. (See also Color Plates.)

(i.e., tricuspid or mitral atresia), double inlet, or common inlet; and ambiguous (i.e., two ventricles with atrial isomerism). When the morphologic right atrium connects normally to the morphologic right ventricle and the left atrium connects to the left ventricle, AV concordance is present. When this connection is reversed and the morphologic right atrium connects to the morphologic left ventricle, AV connection is discordant and sometimes is referred to as *ventricular inversion*. Patients with these abnormalities have "corrected transposition" and may present with complete heart block and have a high incidence of associated congenital cardiac malformations, such as VSD and pulmonary stenosis. They usually also have ventriculoarterial discordance. Atrioventricular discordance occurs rarely, whereas the ventriculoarterial connection is normal.

If most of the AV connection is to one ventricle, the connection is univentricular through one valve (i.e., single inlet with atresia of the other valve), double inlet (i.e., two AV valves), or common inlet (i.e., common AV valve). A common inlet ventricle is part of the spectrum of AV septal defect (i.e., AV canal) in which hypoplasia of one of the ventricular chambers occurs and the AV connection is predominant to the other.

The accuracy of echocardiographic imaging in the diagnosis of AV connection is unsurpassed by other modalities. Occasionally, an inexperienced observer confuses a common inlet with a common (four-leaflet) valve with a single inlet, but this should not be a problem after experience is gained with imaging the variations of AV septal defect. Identification of the lower atrial septum unequivocally identifies the crux of the heart and points to a single inlet with atresia of the other valve. The general consensus is that echocardiography in experienced hands is the best method for assessing AV connection and abnormalities of the cardiac valves.

Segmental Analysis—Ventriculoarterial Connection

Ventriculoarterial connection is the manner in which the great arteries and semilunar valves connect to the ventricular outflow tracts. Normally, the morphologic right ventricle connects to the pulmonary valve and the morphologic left ventricle connects to the aortic valve. Four possibilities exist: concordant (i.e., normal); discordant (i.e., right ventricle to the aorta and left ventricle to the pulmonary trunk); double outlet (usually the right ventricle); and single outlet (i.e., aortic or pulmonary atresia or truncus arteriosus).

The most common type of abnormality of ventriculoarterial connection is transposition of the great arteries, in which the morphologic right ventricle gives rise to the aorta and the morphologic left ventricle gives rise to the pulmonary trunk (i.e., ventriculoarterial discordance) (Figure 21–3). To diagnose this abnormality, the great vessels must be identified. The pulmonary artery is identified by its branching pattern into left and right pulmonary arteries and ductus arteriosus, and the aorta is identified by the coronary, carotid, and subclavian arteries. Both great vessels may originate from one ventricle (usually the morphologic right ventricle), creating a double-outlet right ventricle. If the aortic or pulmonary valve is atretic, a single-outlet ventricle is the result. Another example of a single outlet is truncus arteriosus, in which a single truncal valve originates from the ventricular mass but overrides the ventricular septum. The ventriculoarterial connection is designated as a single outlet with an overriding truncal valve. In complex malformations, including right atrial isomerism with the asplenia syndrome, the AV septal defect often is associated with a double-outlet right ventricle. In cases of tetralogy of Fallot, overriding of the aortic valve is often present so that almost half of the

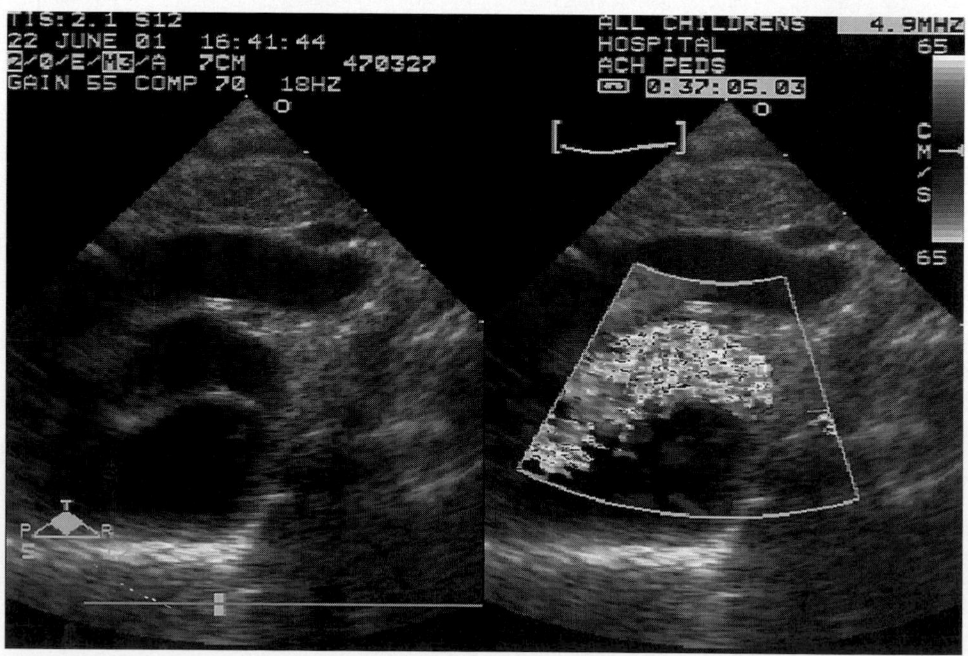

FIGURE 21–3 • Transposition of the great arteries (discordant ventriculoarterial connection). Note the parallel exit of the anterior aorta and posterior pulmonary artery. (See also Color Plates.)

valve annulus appears to arise from the right ventricle. Mitral aortic continuity is present and, except for the rare circumstance in which more than 50% overriding of the aortic valve occurs, the ventriculoarterial connection in tetralogy of Fallot is concordant.

Reports of neonates with abnormalities of ventriculoarterial connection and children with transposition of the great arteries show that echocardiography can accurately detect these abnormalities. A newborn with cyanosis caused by transposition can be diagnosed without catheterization, and most neonates now undergo surgery without catheterization.

Ventricular and Atrial Septa

Atrial Septum

Before birth, the atrial septum usually bows toward the morphologic left atrium because of the significant blood flow to the left side of the heart through the fossa ovalis. After birth, aneurysmal bowing of the atrial septum may be a clue to right-to-left or left-to-right intertrial shunting. Color Doppler studies have confirmed that left-to-right shunting through a patent foramen ovale is a normal finding soon after birth, particularly if the ductus arteriosus has not closed. After the infant reaches age 6 weeks, persistent shunting at the atrial level is considered abnormal if the color diameter of the shunt is greater than 4 mm.

Results of echocardiographic imaging of atrial septal defects are good. Detailed analysis of the venous connections is needed to exclude partial anomalous pulmonary venous return, for example. The triage of patients with an atrial defect requires detailed measurements of the rims of the defect to determine whether the patient is a candidate for device closure of the defect in the catheterization laboratory. The popular Amplatzer device straddles the hole, effectively closing it permanently. Another practical application of echocardiography is evaluation of the atrial defect created by balloon atrial septostomy or blade and balloon techniques.

A thin strand of tissue in what appears to be a common atrium suggests right atrial isomerism. The upper atrial septum where a sinus venosus defect may occur can be difficult to evaluate in an older child, but color flow mapping has improved the accuracy of diagnosis in all forms of atrial septal defect (Figure 21–4; see Figure 21–9).

Ventricular Septum

Defects of the ventricular septum can be analyzed using multiple tomographic imaging approaches, and defects can be separated into perimembranous, muscular, and subarterial. An inlet perimembranous defect (i.e., AV canal-type defect) can be differentiated from complete AV canal by the presence of the central fibrous body at the internal crux of the heart (Figure 21–5). Small muscular VSDs and even a significant defect in the perimembranous region may be missed by imaging alone, but color Doppler has improved substantially the sensitivity of echocardiography in detecting muscular defects. Color may be crucial for detection of multiple VSDs. The details of complicated interventricular communications in the trabecular septum may be aided by angiography or a detailed evaluation using TEE. TEE with color Doppler appears adequate for evaluation of these patients, especially when they are older. Three-dimensional echocardiography offers the promise of improved spatial orientation and delineation of the defect(s).

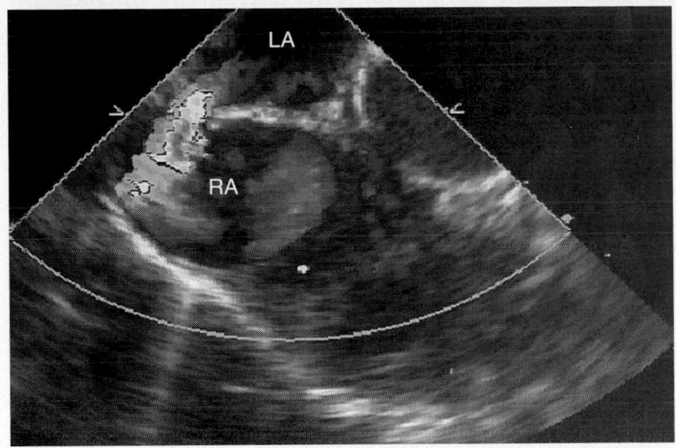

FIGURE 21–4 • High sinus venosus atrial septal defect between the left atrium *(LA)* and right atrium *(RA)*. Left-to-right shunting is seen by color Doppler (*blue* flow away from the transducer with aliasing). (See also Color Plates.)

Segmental Analysis—Valves

Atrioventricular Valves

A wide variety of malformations may involve the left or right AV valves. The mitral or tricuspid valve may be abnormally positioned, stenotic, regurgitant, or hypoplastic, or the valve may have a cleft or exhibit prolapse, straddling,

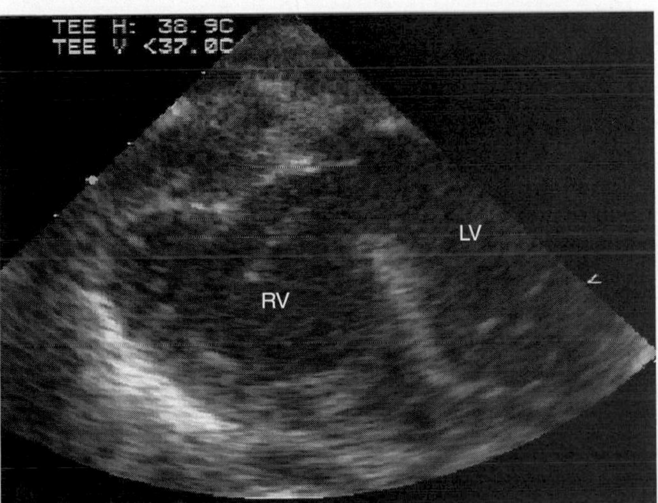

FIGURE 21–5 • Ventricular septal defect between the left ventricle *(LV)* and right ventricle *(RV)*. The defect is in continuity with the tricuspid valve and therefore is a perimembranous defect. (See also Color Plates.)

or Ebstein malformation. The pattern of opening on real-time imaging is augmented by Doppler or M-mode functional assessment. Almost all forms of congenital abnormalities of the mitral valve can be recognized immediately by imaging alone, with the possible exception of supravalvar mitral ring, in which the ring may adhere to the valve tissue. The normal papillary muscles in this disorder differentiate it from most other congenital forms of mitral stenosis. Color flow mapping and continuous-wave Doppler more effectively evaluate the hemodynamics of AV valve stenosis than do invasive techniques. Regurgitation of AV valves can be detected with excellent sensitivity, and color Doppler can be used to grade the severity of regurgitation of the AV and semilunar valves (Figure 21–6).

Semilunar Valves

Semilunar valves (either pulmonary or aortic) are described by their age-adjusted size, cusp morphology, and pattern of opening. Because the size of a valve annulus reflects the flow through it, hypoplasia of the valve annulus usually is associated with severe stenosis. Echocardiographic imaging may detect this condition, doming of a stenotic valve, or muscular hypertrophy of infundibular stenosis. Abnormal coaptation of the semilunar valve cusps also correlates with regurgitation of the valve. Because of flow variability through a stenotic valve, a flow-independent method, known as the *continuity equation,* may be useful. The ratio of mean velocity at the valve to velocity below the valve is used to estimate the ratio of effective subvalvar to valvar area. As a rule of thumb, a peak velocity of stenosis that is four times the velocity below the valve is predictive of critical narrowing of functional valve area. Prosthetic valves may be present in the pediatric population and require a combination of transthoracic and transesophageal echocardiographic assessment.

Segmental Analysis—Veins

Systemic Venous Connections

Segmental diagnosis of systemic venous connection is possible by echocardiography before and after birth. Systemic venous return may be typical of the atrial situs (e.g., azygos continuation with left atrial isomerism). Systemic venous return that is abnormal in situs solitus may be normal if the situs is not solitus. Normal inferior and superior venae cavae connecting to the right atrium indicate a normal systemic venous connection to the morphologic right atrium. Imaging the inferior vena cava connecting to the heart and its extensions into the abdomen is important so that hepatic veins connecting separately to the atrium are not mistaken for it. Each of the systemic venous segments, including the right superior vena cava, left superior vena cava, inferior vena cava, coronary sinus, and hepatic veins, should be examined individually.

Systemic Venous Anomalies

A persistent left superior vena cava is present in up to 10% of patients with congenital heart disease and can be detected by echocardiography and confirmed by contrast studies. Persistent left superior vena cava is the most common venous defect and is present in 0.5% of patients without congenital cardiac defects. Rarely does this minor defect require attention, except to document its presence in case surgical management is needed for other forms of congenital heart disease. If the persistent left superior vena cava appears to be connected to the left atrium or drains to this site because of unroofing of the coronary sinus, cyanosis results. Echocardiographic contrast injection in the left arm shows immediate opacification of the left atrium. A sinus venosus atrial septal defect can direct superior vena caval drainage to the left atrium, causing mild cyanosis in an otherwise normal child.

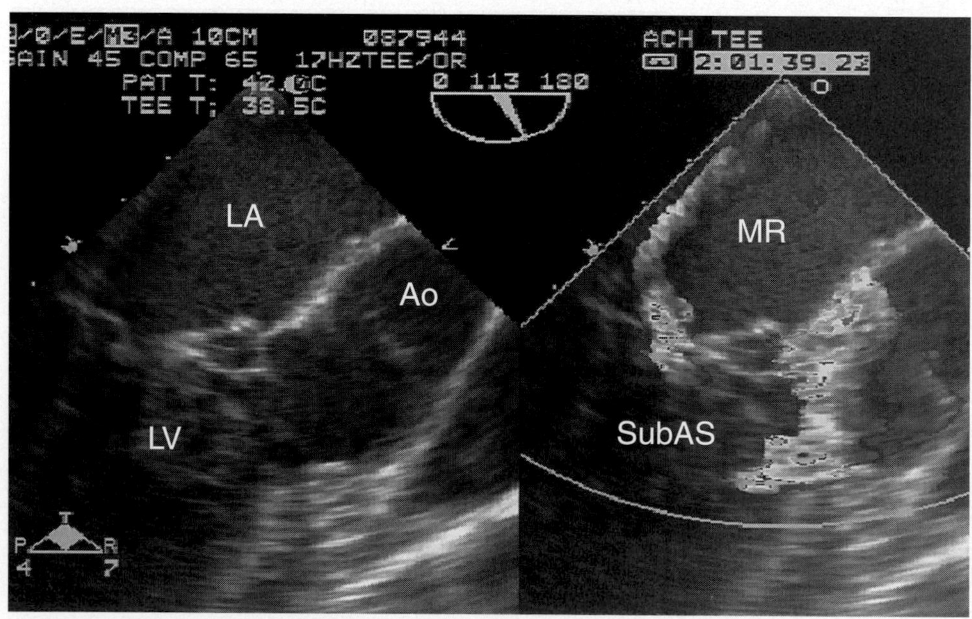

FIGURE 21–6 • Mitral regurgitation *(MR)* between the left ventricle *(LV)* and the left atrium *(LA)* created by a subaortic membrane causing subaortic stenosis *(SubAS)*. *Ao,* Aorta.

Pulmonary Veins

Each pulmonary vein connecting to the morphologic left atrium must be imaged in a sequential fashion. A four-chamber view often reveals at least two pulmonary veins connecting to the left-sided morphologic left atrium. The suprasternal scan may demonstrate all four pulmonary veins connecting to the left atrium. Total anomalous pulmonary venous connection can be detected with high sensitivity, depending on the experience of the examiner. Although accurate diagnosis of isolated total anomalous pulmonary venous connection can be made in neonates and infants, the ability of any noninvasive tool to exclude an isolated partial anomalous connection of one vein has not been tested. Color Doppler can confirm pulmonary venous flow in the location where the vein is thought to be connecting. Detection of variations of pulmonary venous obstruction depends on Doppler imaging. Direct visualization of all four pulmonary veins is mandatory before corrective surgery for any defect, especially for atrial septal defect or anomalous pulmonary venous connection. Any deviation from the usual anatomy should prompt a complete angiographic study or a detailed study by magnetic resonance imaging, which in experienced hands can clarify the defect. Severely cyanotic neonates with atrial isomerism usually have abnormalities of pulmonary venous connection and may require angiography prior to palliative surgery.

Segmental Analysis—Coronary Arteries

The coronary arteries are examined in a sequential fashion to detect abnormalities. One approach is summarized in Box 21–1. The two proximal coronary arteries are identified, the proximal branching of the left is visualized, the distal course of the right and left coronaries is imaged in the AV valve grooves, and the distal anterior and posterior descending branchs are imaged. If intracardiac repair is contemplated, the origin of the coronary vessels and their courses must be visualized using a segmental approach. Any coronary passing between the two semilunar valve annuli is abnormal. With the exception of aneurysm detection in Kawasaki disease or the abnormal origin of the common left or right coronary artery, the ability of ultrasonography to define abnormalities of the coronary circulation is limited. Use of TEE can significantly improve diagnosis of the intramural course of coronary arteries. In the case of fistulae, enlargement of one of the coronaries usually can be detected, and pulmonary atresia with a significant fistula can be diagnosed. In our experience, an isolated coronary fistula can be repaired without bypass, and the entry site can be defined by color Doppler.

Anomalous origin of one or both coronaries from the pulmonary trunk can be detected with high specificity using high-frequency two-dimensional/color Doppler and a low peak repetition frequency. Any electrocardiographic evidence of coronary insufficiency should prompt immediate coronary angiography if surgical intervention is contemplated. Imaging studies of the coronary artery anatomy in tetralogy of Fallot and transposition should be successful with experience. All patients with tetralogy should undergo assessment of the coronaries to define the origin of the left anterior descending branch before a right ventriculotomy is performed.

BOX 21–1

Coronary Artery Segmental Analysis

- Define both proximal arteries from the aorta
- Image the bifurcation of the left coronary
- Exclude coronary passing between the aortic and pulmonary arteries
- Confirm normal direction of flow in the left coronary
- Examine the distal courses of the coronaries

Segmental Analysis—Aorta

Segmental analysis of the aorta and congenital abnormalities that affect it includes assessment of the (1) ascending aorta, (2) aortic arch branching, (3) aortic isthmus, and (4) descending aorta. Echocardiography is highly accurate for diagnosing abnormalities of the aorta in neonates, infants, and children. Each segment of the aorta is located in a slightly different tomographic plane, requiring a sequential, segmental approach. Normal branching of the right innominate artery indicates a left aortic arch with normal branching. Branching to the left indicates a right aortic arch with mirror-image branching. A left-sided patent ductus arteriosus is the most common abnormality of the aorta. Color and continuous-wave Doppler echocardiography are indicated in every study to detect ductal shunting (Figure 21–7).

Coarctation of the aorta, which in the neonatal period has a typical appearance that includes hypoplasia of the transverse aortic arch and right ventricular enlargement, can be diagnosed by echocardiography. The typical Doppler pattern confirms the diagnosis if the ductus has closed. The presence of a posterior ledge and a transverse arch that is similar in size to the left subclavian artery makes the diagnosis. With an open ductus, the flow pattern may be mildly turbulent without gradient. In patients with a large VSD, the status of the aorta always should be investigated to exclude coarctation. In hypoplastic left heart syndrome with aortic atresia, the patent ductus arteriosus has bidirectional shunting similar to that seen in interrupted aortic arch. In hypoplastic left heart syndrome, the ascending aorta is small, with reversed flow in the arch (Figure 21–8).

In adults, the segmental analysis of the aorta is less reliable, but Doppler techniques have significantly improved the detection of aortic obstruction in cases where imaging had been poor. TEE allows identification and measurement of internal mammary branches.

Systemic Arteriovenous Fistulas

Systemic arteriovenous fistulas cause enlargement of the artery feeding the fistula and generalized enlargement of the aorta. Sequestration and hepatic and cerebral fistulas are most common. Sequestration of the lung and other

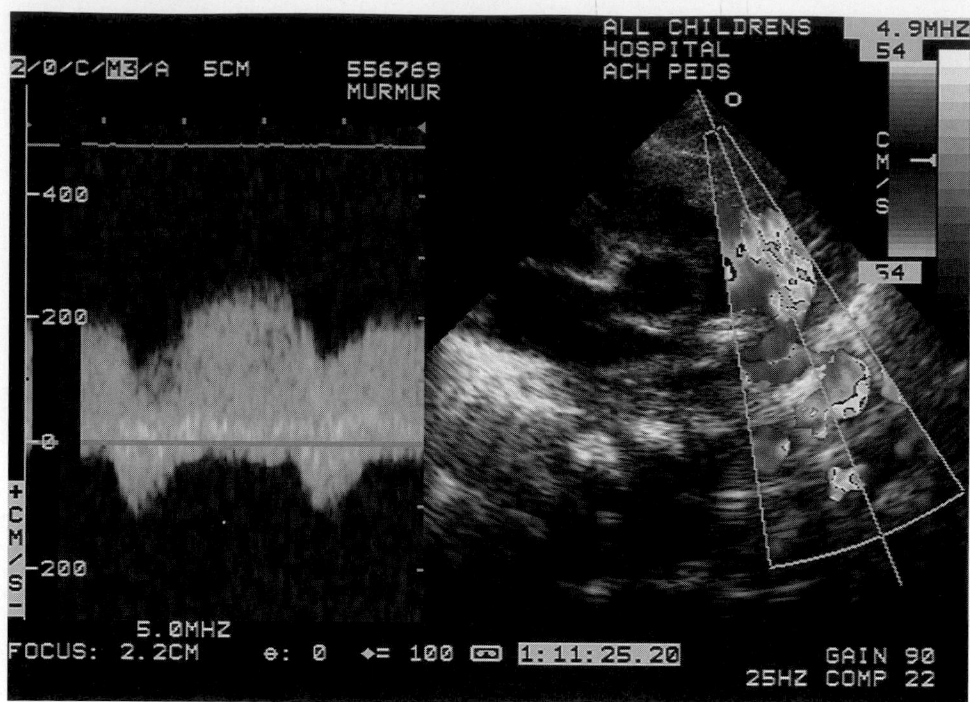

FIGURE 21–7 • Patent ductus arteriosus in a neonate with a heart murmur. **Right,** Left-to-right shunt into the pulmonary artery is seen by color Doppler. **Left,** Left-to-right shunt velocity is measured by continuous-wave Doppler as a peak of 2.3 m/s. (See also Color Plates.)

fistulas causing an obligatory shunt can be detected but require careful technique. The defect known as a *vein of Galen aneurysm* may simulate coarctation of aorta because of the aortic isthmus morphology created by branching of the ductal flow to the upper and lower body. Cerebral angiography is required for definition of small-vessel anatomy preoperatively.

Pulmonary Arteries

The most common abnormality of the pulmonary arteries indicating congenital heart disease is hypoplasia. The pulmonary arteries normally are confluent in the midline, and this detail of anatomy is important when planning a palliative approach to cyanotic congenital heart disease. Abnormalities of the origin or size of the pulmonary arteries may occur. In severe right ventricular outflow tract obstruction in neonates, pulmonary artery hypoplasia is associated with a reciprocal increase in the size of the aorta, and the ratio of size of the pulmonary arteries to the aorta may be useful in diagnosing the abnormality and making surgical decisions where the ability of the pulmonary vascular bed to carry the total combined cardiac output is questionable. Assessment of the details of the distal arteries requires angiography or magnetic resonance imaging. A pulmonary arteriovenous fistula presents with cyanosis and enlargement of the pulmonary arteries and veins on echocardiography and should be confirmed by angiography and pulmonary venous oxygen saturation measurements.

Tetralogy with pulmonary atresia and major aortopulmonary artery collaterals may be difficult to evaluate. The neonate with this condition can be differentiated from a neonate with ductal-dependent pulmonary supply by the oxygen saturation off of prostaglandin and by imaging the ductus and poorly developed confluent pulmonary arteries. All patients with collateral arteries and multifocal pulmonary supply must undergo complete angiographic evaluation prior to surgery. Comparison of the sum of the diameters of the right and left pulmonary arteries with the diameter of the descending aorta can be useful in planning surgery.

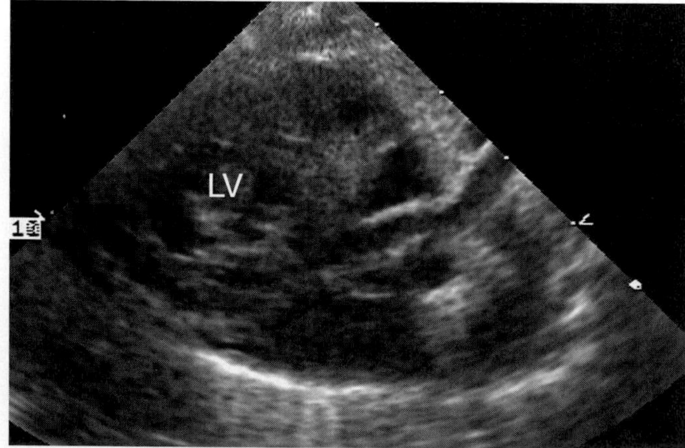

FIGURE 21–8 • Small ascending aorta in a neonate with aortic atresia (hypoplastic left heart syndrome). Note the large remnant of left ventricle *(LV)*.

Ventricular Function Assessment and Hemodynamics

Temporal resolution of two-dimensional echocardiography is limited by the scanning rate limits of the equipment.

M-mode techniques, on the other hand, interrogate the heart at a much higher rate (800–1500 times per second) and allow tracking of the ventricular wall and valves at rapid rates of movement. The most useful application of M-mode echocardiography is the measurement of absolute cardiac chamber dimensions and wall thicknesses and their dynamic changes. Normal values for the systolic and diastolic dimensions of the left atrium and ventricle increase with age and body size, and comparison of right and left heart measurements to normal ranges should be part of every echocardiogram. M-mode parameters from the left ventricle can be used to estimate the wall stress of the left ventricle and its dynamic changes and the rate of relaxation. Systolic function can be estimated by measuring shortening fraction: SF = (end-diastolic dimension – systolic dimension)/end-diastolic dimension. In normovolemic patients, dimensional shortening of the left ventricular endocardial cavity can be used to estimate stroke volume.

Diastolic function can be assessed using tissue Doppler techniques and may be useful in the diagnosis of cardiac transplant rejection. Tissue Doppler is a technique by which low-velocity, high-intensity signals from the valve annuli and cardiac walls are examined to assess contraction and relaxation of the myocardium. New advances in the calculation of segmental wall strain are being studied. An easily obtained nongeometric parameter that is useful for assessment of right and left ventricular performance is the *myocardial performance index*. The so-called *Tei index* is the ratio of the isovolemic contraction time to the ejection time of the ventricle. This nongeometric index is useful for detecting systolic or diastolic function abnormalities when ventricular shape is not ideal, as in the morphologic right ventricle.

Valvular regurgitation allows estimation of the first derivative over time of the pressure change in the ventricle using the continuous-wave Doppler waveform. Practically, this can be calculated by measuring the time (in seconds) from the waveform at the 1 and 3 m/s points and dividing it into 32, which yields dP/dt (in mmHg/s).

Contrast Echocardiography

An ultrasonic contrast agent is a substance that stabilizes microbubbles in solution, which are large enough to reflect ultrasound but small enough that they disappear rapidly and are physiologically safe. The agent may be as simple as an injection of saline into the circulation during two-dimensional echocardiographic imaging or as complex as precision-engineered microbubbles of polysaccharide that dissolve in the circulation after injection. Advances in bubble technology allow imaging of myocardial capillary perfusion. Contrast also can be useful in defining the identity of an imaged structure. For example, a structure under the aortic arch may be confusing but can be confirmed to be the innominate vein by echocardiographic contrast injection in a left arm vein. In congenital heart disease, the major application of contrast echocardiography is in the postoperative patient with residual shunts or as a means to exclude congenital heart disease. Systemic venous injection of contrast fills the right side of the heart sequentially, and the site of residual right-to-left shunting can be defined. In the neonatal or pediatric intensive care unit, contrast injections using agitated saline can detect right-to-left interatrial shunting in cases of persistent pulmonary hypertension with difficulty oxygenating the patient.

Transesophageal Echocardiography

The indications for TEE in patients with congenital heart disease are expanding because TEE greatly aids intracardiac imaging. TEE is a technique that pediatric cardiologists cannot be without in a surgical practice or in the critically ill neonate or child. As with any new technique, there has been a learning curve, but the methods are now well developed and useful.[7] Use of training guidelines and frequent continuing education is desirable.[8] Biplane probes now come in many sizes so that even in neonates weighing 2.5 to 5 kg, a biplane probe can be passed safely in the operating room under general anesthesia with minimal hemodynamic compromise. Multiplane probes for pediatric patients are improving slowly. Current technology allows use of a multiplane probe in patients weighing as little as 5 kg.

The reproducibility of quantitative measurements with TEE is good, that is, reproducible to within 5% for multiple examiners. TEE has special value in pediatric practice, particularly in left ventricular outflow obstruction and assessment of AV and semilunar valves. Assessment of mitral regurgitation is important after repair and re-repair of AV canal defects. TEE can identify the type and severity of mitral regurgitation and is superior to transthoracic echocardiography or cineangiography.[9,10]

Complications of TEE are more common in smaller patients. Failure to pass the probe occurs in approximately 0.8% of children with congenital heart disease, and airway obstruction occurs in approximately 1%.[11]

Echocardiography can be used during transcatheter closure for precise positioning of a device or coil. TEE also is useful during ductal closure. Intraoperatively, ductal patency can be monitored during minimally invasive procedures.[12] For example, in neonates with critical aortic stenosis, balloon positioning can be monitored using TEE. Guidance of radiofrequency ablation catheters can be facilitated with TEE, particularly where single-ventricle anatomy is present.

Cardiac output can be estimated by TEE from the minute distance (time-velocity integral) measured in the descending aorta. Assessment of ventricular function using Doppler to estimate the first derivative of pressure in the left ventricle (dP/dt) is useful for identifying patients in need of inotropic support.[13]

Both pre-TEE and postoperative use are increasing in the intensive care unit. Critically ill infants and children and those on assisted circulatory devices can be optimally evaluated this way. The average duration for performance of TEE includes approximately 42 minutes of technician time and 32 minutes of physician time.

Adults with congenital heart disease are best studied by TEE. Reviews of TEE use in pediatric patients suggest the technique will be increasingly utilized in the future[14,15] (Box 21–2).

BOX 21–2

Transesophageal Echocardiographic Scans and Structures Visualized

TRANSVERSE SCANS

1. Inferior vena cava
2. Right atrium
3. Atrial septum
4. Right and left pulmonary veins
5. Left atrium
6. Superior vena cava
7. Ventricular inlets: tricuspid and mitral valves
8. Left ventricular outflow tract
9. Aortic valve
10. Coronary arteries

SAGITTAL SCANS

1. Right superior vena cava
2. Right atrium and appendage
3. Atrial septum
4. Ascending aorta
5. Right ventricular outflow tract
6. Pulmonary valve
7. Pulmonary arteries
8. Aortic arch/ductus arteriosus

Specific Lesions

Shunts

Shunting lesions are well seen from the multiple-view possibilities offered by TEE. Shunts at the atrial level, for example, are most accurately defined by TEE. Defects at the fossa ovalis can be quantitated with regard to size and shunt. Sinus venosus defect can be readily seen, and the associated anomalies of pulmonary venous drainage detailed (Figure 21–9).

VSDs can be studied in detail, and multiple coexisting VSDs can be distinguished. The most common VSD is perimembranous VSD, which often is partially closed by tricuspid valve tissue. The larger defects in this position may extend into either the inlet or the outlet septum. With experience, both size and position can be determined (Figure 21–10). Shunt is defined by color Doppler. Shunting through the patent ductus arteriosus can be observed from high probe positions.

Complex Heart Defects

Evaluation of complex congenital heart defects requires a segmental approach, exactly as with transthoracic imaging. For example, with a single AV valve, the situs, AV connection, and ventriculoarterial connection must be defined. With hypoplastic left heart syndrome, the function of the tricuspid valve is important, and the atrial septum should be assessed at each preoperative examination because of the possibility of late constriction. The details of AV canal defect can be defined, and the commitment of the valves and valvular function can be analyzed. With pulmonary artery atresia, a high-velocity jet from the right ventricle to right atrium is seen (Figure 21–11).

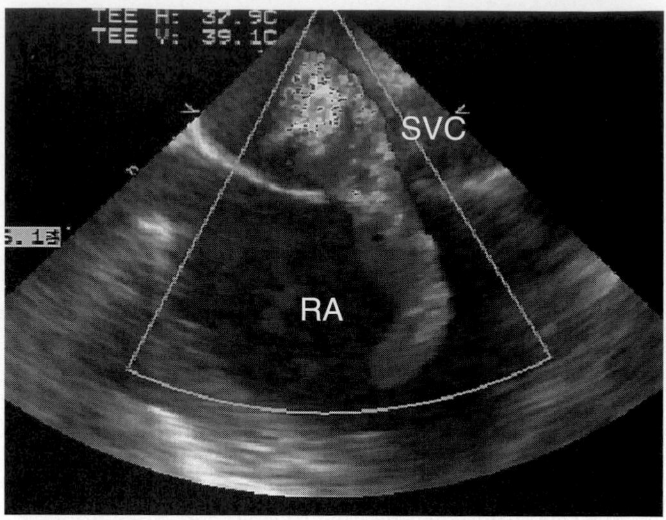

FIGURE 21–9 • Sinus venosus atrial septal defect on sagittal scan by TEE with left-to-right shunting by color Doppler. *RA,* Right atrium; *SVC,* superior vena cava. (See also Color Plates.)

Left Heart Lesions

TEE can define left ventricular outflow obstruction with great accuracy. Details of the aortic valve, subvalvar region, and mitral valve can be easily seen. Three-dimensional imaging now is possible in real time, but with low resolution in the infant and child. This situation is expected to improve significantly in the future. TEE can precisely define the structure and function of the aortic valve and subaortic area. No other imaging tool performs as well in examining the fine structure of the cusps and the presence of regurgitation. After the Ross procedure, in which the pulmonary valve is transplanted into the left ventricular outflow tract, neoaortic valve function can be evaluated without difficulty.

Regurgitation of the mitral valve can be diagnosed, but assessment of the valve requires information about

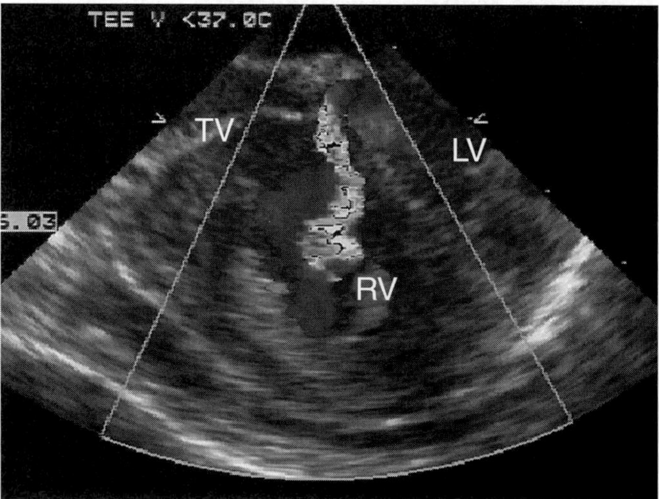

FIGURE 21–10 • Color Doppler of shunt TEE from the left ventricle *(LV)* to the right ventricle *(RV)* through a ventricular septal defect (VSD). The VSD is perimembranous because of its proximity to the tricuspid valve *(TV)*. (See also Color Plates.)

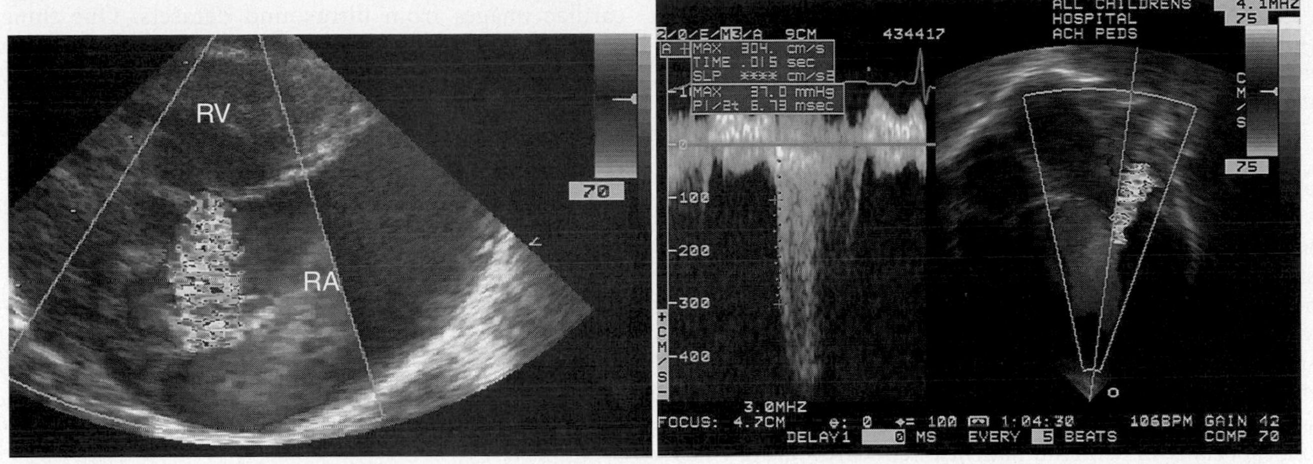

FIGURE 21–11 • **A,** Tricuspid valve regurgitation in a neonate with pulmonary atresia with intact septum. Note enlargement of the right atrium *(RA)*. *RV,* Right ventricle. **B,** Continuous-wave Doppler shows a very high predicted pressure in the hypoplastic right ventricle. (See also Color Plates.)

the mechanism of the regurgitation. A posteriorly directed jet is consistent with mitral valve prolapse. Doppler can be used to assess the hemodynamics, including dP/dt[13] (Figure 21–12).

Right Heart Lesions

In general, the right ventricular outflow tract is more difficult to evaluate by TEE because it is farther away from the transducer. Nonetheless, the details of tetralogy of Fallot can be seen and communicated to the surgeon in the operating room. The presence of complicating lesions can be defined. Accurate assessment of tetralogy of Fallot can be accomplished before and after surgery. The right ventricle to pulmonary artery gradient can be

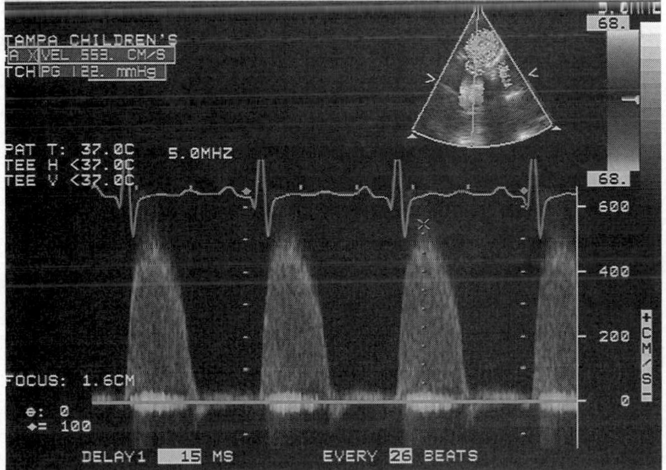

FIGURE 21–12 • **Right,** Mitral regurgitation from an apical view with alignment of the continuous-wave Doppler cursor. **Left,** The rate of upstroke of mitral regurgitation is quantified by measuring the time from the 1 to the 3 m/s points on the waveform, in this example 15 ms. dP/dt = 32 ÷ 15 ms × 1000 = 2133 mmHg/s, which is normal. (See also Color Plates.)

assessed using continuous-wave Doppler. The tricuspid valve can be seen well, and the details of its leaflets, chordal attachments, and function can be assessed. This observation is particularly important in infants with pulmonary atresia, intact septum, and hypoplasia of the valve. More than absolute measurements, diastolic and systolic function and structure of the valve best predict its potential for growth.

Special Considerations After Chest Trauma

Trauma to the chest can result in dissection or transection of the aorta. TEE imaging is the best technique for examining the ascending and descending portions of the aorta.

Myocardial contusion can be recognized after edema develops in the myocardial wall but may be suspected when cardiac enzyme elevations are disproportionate to the degree of myocardial dysfunction. Air in the chest may make transthoracic echocardiography difficult but often does not hamper a transesophageal approach.

Safety of Ultrasound

Significant adverse effects of ultrasound imaging, M-mode, or Doppler evaluation have not been reported. The potentially negative bioeffects of ultrasound can be classified as those caused by either cavitation or heating. *Cavitation* refers to the development of tiny, gas-filled bubbles that resonate at the ultrasonic frequency and induce neighboring particles of liquid to vibrate, potentially damaging the ultrasound-transmitting medium. Practically, the sound intensities used for echocardiography (typically 10 W/cm^2) are almost an order of magnitude less than those known to produce cavitation. *Thermal effects* may result from heat generated in the tissue. To reach the thermal threshold for damage using modern ultrasonic intensities, an average intensity of 1000 W/cm^2 must be applied for hours.

Higher intensities with pulsed Doppler have the potential to cause cavitation, and concerns regarding Doppler use for first-trimester fetal assessment are being investigated.

Costs and Benefits

One major reason for the rapid proliferation of ultrasound use in pediatric practice is that the technique is noninvasive and generally painless. Ultrasound equipment is less expensive than radiographic equipment. Indications for cardiac catheterization are being reassessed. The development of echocardiography as an extension of the clinician's other assessment skills has decreased the need for catheterization, especially in neonatal patients. Echocardiography has the potential to decrease the cost of medical care for these patients.

For the most effective cardiovascular use of ultrasound, the physician should be involved in the study and its interpretation. A more physician-intensive diagnostic process may benefit the patient but may be more expensive than comparable tests performed by technicians.

Trends

Technology is changing so rapidly that predicting which technique will be optimal for a given lesion in 5 years is difficult. The rapid development of nuclear magnetic resonance for imaging and spectroscopy is beginning to show potential. Rapid computed tomography has potential to create high-quality, three-dimensional images in pediatric patients. These two modalities will become indispensable for assessment of extracardiac anatomy and the coronary arteries. Positron emission tomography can be used to assess myocardial perfusion, although it is rarely used in pediatric patients at this time. Emerging areas in echocardiography include the development of contrast agents, some of which allow myocardial blood flow assessment by ultrasonography; tissue characterization techniques; automated cardiac function assessment; three-dimensional real-time imaging and color Doppler display; invasive imaging probes for intracardiac imaging; transesophageal imaging in neonates for intraoperative functional assessment; and offline three-dimensional reconstruction of cardiac images from ultrasound datasets. One thing is certain, the roles of the various noninvasive diagnostic modalities used in assessing congenital heart disease will require continued reevaluation.

REFERENCES

1. Frommelt MA, Frommelt PC: Advances in echocardiographic diagnostic modalities for the pediatrician. *Pediatr Clin North Am* 46: 427-39, xi, 1999.
2. Lacour-Gayet F, Clarke D, Jacobs J, et al: The Aristotle score for congenital heart surgery. *Semin Thorac Cardiovasc Surg Pediatr Card Surg Annu* 7:185-191, 2004.
3. Phoon CK, Divekar A, Rutkowski M: Pediatric echocardiography: applications and limitations. *Curr Probl Pediatr* 29:157-185, 1999.
4. Rice MJ, McDonald RW, Reller MD, Sahn DJ: Pediatric echocardiography: current role and a review of technical advances. *J Pediatr* 128:1-14, 1996.
5. Stanger P, Silverman NH, Foster E: Diagnostic accuracy of pediatric echocardiograms performed in adult laboratories. *Am J Cardiol* 83:908-914, 1999.
6. Frommelt PC, Berger S, Pelech AN, et al: Prospective identification of anomalous origin of left coronary artery from the right sinus of Valsalva using transthoracic echocardiography: importance of color Doppler flow mapping. *Pediatr Cardiol* 22:327-332, 2001.
7. Smallhorn JF: Intraoperative transesophageal echocardiography in congenital heart disease. *Echocardiography* 19:709-723, 2002.
8. Aronson S: Adherence to physician training guidelines for pediatric transesophageal echocardiography affects the outcome of patients undergoing repair of congenital cardiac defects. *J Am Soc Echocardiogr* 12:1008, 1999.
9. Singh GK, Shiota T, Cobanoglu A, et al: Diagnostic accuracy and role of intraoperative biplane transesophageal echocardiography in pediatric patients with left ventricle outflow tract lesions. *J Am Soc Echocardiogr* 11:47-56, 1998.
10. Kececioglu D, Kehl HG, Schmid C, et al: Morphologic characterization and assessment of mitral regurgitation after repair of atrioventricular defects in children. *Thorac Cardiovasc Surg* 45:70-74, 1997.
11. Stevenson JG: Incidence of complications in pediatric transesophageal echocardiography: experience in 1650 cases. *J Am Soc Echocardiogr* 12:527-532, 1999.
12. Hijazi Z, Wang Z, Cao Q, et al: Transcatheter closure of atrial septal defects and patent foramen ovale under intracardiac echocardiographic guidance: feasibility and comparison with transesophageal echocardiography. *Catheter Cardiovasc Interv* 52:194-199, 2001.
13. Rhodes J, Marx GR, Tardif JC, et al: Evaluation of ventricular dP/dt before and after open heart surgery using transesophageal echocardiography. *Echocardiography* 14:15-22, 1997.
14. Tibby SM, Hatherill M, Murdoch LA: Use of transesophageal Doppler ultrasonography in ventilated pediatric patients: derivation of cardiac output. *Crit Care Med* 28:2045-2050, 2000.
15. Wolfe LT, Rossi A, Ritter SB: Transesophageal echocardiography in infants and children: use and importance in the cardiac intensive care unit. *J Am Soc Echocardiogr* 6(3 pt 1):286-289, 1993.

CHAPTER 22

Diagnostic and Therapeutic Cardiac Catheterization

Peter Laussen and Alan Nugent

PEARLS

- The cardiac catheterization laboratory plays important diagnostic and therapeutic roles in the management of children in the pediatric intensive care unit.
- For patients with cardiac disease whose critical care course is not progressing as expected, the diagnosis of unsuspected or residual defects by cardiac catheterization often improves outcomes.
- To derive the maximum benefit from hemodynamic, angiographic, and interventional procedures, effective communication between the intensive care physician and the interventional cardiologist before, during, and after the procedure is essential.

Introduction

The cardiac catheterization laboratory plays an important diagnostic and therapeutic role in the management of children in the critical care environment. Invasive intravascular monitoring often is not possible because of restrictions in patient size, vascular access, or underlying anatomy in the case of patients with complex congenital heart disease. Obtaining comprehensive hemodynamic data in the catheterization laboratory helps formulate and tailor management strategies. The diagnosis of unsuspected or residual cardiac anatomic defects using hemodynamic data and angiography obtained during cardiac catheterization may enable therapeutic surgical or catheter-directed interventions to improve a patient's outcome. Numerous interventions can be performed during cardiac catheterization, such as balloon dilation of stenotic blood vessels, atrioventricular, and semilunar valves, device closure of intracardiac and extracardiac shunts, and radiofrequency ablation of an arrhythmic focus. The pediatric critical team must be aware of the possible benefits and limitations of catheterization procedures, and effective communication between the intensive care physician and the physician performing the procedure is crucial.

Catheterization Laboratory Environment

Cardiac catheterization laboratories usually are remote from the intensive care unit and rarely are configured to accommodate critical care personnel and equipment. Relative to patient size, the lateral and anteroposterior cameras used for imaging are in close proximity to the patient's head and neck, limiting access to the airway. A mechanical ventilator and monitors around the patient further confine the space in which the critical care team works and limit access to the patient during a procedure. In addition, the environment is darkened to facilitate viewing of images, and full monitoring, either invasive or noninvasive, must be established before the procedure begins. Because of limited access to the patient and airway, end-tidal capnography and pulse oximetry are mandatory to ensure adequate ventilation and oxygenation during the procedure and to provide immediate detection of disconnection or dislodgment of the endotracheal tube and mechanical ventilator that could inadvertently occur during movement of the catheterization table and cameras. The environment is cooler because of computer and x-ray equipment, and children may become hypothermic from conductive and convective heat loss; this is a particular problem in neonates and infants. In addition, frequent flushing of the catheters and sheaths to prevent clotting or air embolism may contribute to hypothermia. Unnecessary exposure of the child must be prevented, and convective warming blankets used where possible. Care must be taken when positioning a patient on the catheterization table because of the risk to pressure areas and of nerve traction injury. In particular, brachial plexus injury may occur when the patient's arms are positioned above the head for prolonged periods to enable better exposure for the lateral camera. To facilitate femoral vein and arterial access, the pelvis is commonly elevated from the catheterization table. This position may displace abdominal contents cephalad, restricting diaphragm excursion and increasing the risk for respiratory depression in a sedated patient.

Safe transportation of a critically ill child from the intensive care unit to the catheterization laboratory can be a significant challenge but should not be a deciding factor as to whether or not the procedure should be performed. Safe transport requires planning and multidisciplinary coordination. This process includes physician and nursing staff accompanying the patient with complete monitoring and resuscitation equipment, respiratory therapy staff to assist with ventilation and establishing mechanical ventilation in the catheterization laboratory if indicated, coordinating timing with the catheter laboratory staff to prevent needless delays, assistance with establishing adequate space for equipment and patient access in the laboratory, and correct positioning on the catheterization table to enable access for both the catheterizer and intensive care staff as necessary.

Adequate sedation and anesthesia during cardiac catheterization are essential to facilitate acquisition of meaningful hemodynamic data and to assist during interventional procedures. For the most part, hemodynamic or diagnostic catheterization procedures can be performed with the patient under sedation in all age groups.[1] For many interventional procedures, sedation may be appropriate; however, for procedures that are associated with significant hemodynamic compromise or are prolonged, general anesthesia is preferable. Whatever technique is used, hemodynamic data must be attained in conditions as close to normal as possible. For accurate calculation of the intracardiac shunt, reducing the inspired oxygen concentration to room air may be necessary, although this step requires close collaboration with the catheterizer because lowering FiO_2 may be inadvisable in patients with significant desaturation and lung injury.

Hemodynamic and Oxygen Saturation Data

Hemodynamic cardiac catheterization is not necessary when echocardiographic analysis with Doppler measurements and color flow mapping is complete and unambiguous. However, in patients with complex cardiac anatomy, severe low cardiac output state, pulmonary hypertension, severe lung injury of uncertain etiology, or with concerns for important residual problems after cardiac surgery, physiologic data from catheterization may provide important information.[2] Catheterization allows description of the direction, magnitude, and approximate location of intracardiac and intrapulmonary shunts. Intracardiac and intravascular pressures are measured to determine the presence of obstructions and whether shunt orifices are restrictive or nonrestrictive. Pressure gradients across sites of obstruction must be considered in light of estimated cardiac output. A small pressure gradient measured at a time of low cardiac output is misleading.

Normally, no significant change in oxygen saturation from venae cavae to pulmonary artery is observed. In the child with congenital heart disease, the superior vena cava provides the simplest mixed venous oxygen saturation. A greater than 5% increase in oxygen saturation from the superior vena cava through to the pulmonary artery suggests the presence of a left-to-right shunt at the level of the right atrium with an atrial septal defect (ASD), in the right ventricle (RV) with a ventricular septal defect (VSD), and in the pulmonary artery with a patent ductus arteriosus (PDA).[3] The magnitude of the left-to-right shunt can be calculated by applying the Fick equation to the pulmonary and systemic vascular beds separately (assuming O_2 uptake and consumption are equal):

$$Q_p = VO_2/(SpvO_2 - SpaO_2)(Hb)(1.36)(10) \quad (1)$$

$$Q_s = VO_2/(SaO_2 - SsvcO_2)(Hb)(1.36)(10), \quad (2)$$

where Q_p = pulmonary blood flow, Q_s = systemic blood flow, VO_2 = oxygen consumption, $SpvO_2$ = pulmonary vein saturation, which can be assumed to be 0.98 in the absence of significant pulmonary disease, $SpaO_2$ = pulmonary artery saturation, SaO_2 = arterial oxygen saturation, $SsvcO_2$ = superior vena cava oxygen saturation, and Hb = hemoglobin. (Note that saturation data in the equations is expressed as a decimal number and not as a percentage, e.g., 98% saturation = 0.98.)

In pediatric patients, the pulmonary and systemic flows usually are indexed to body surface area:

$$CI = Q_s/BSA, \quad (3)$$

where CI = cardiac index, and BSA = body surface area.

Thermodilution can be used to calculate the cardiac output in pediatric patients, although it is confounded by the presence of intracardiac or extracardiac shunts.[4] Although measurement of oxygen consumption is preferable[5] because assumed values are unreliable in patients with critical illness and in those requiring substantial hemodynamic support, the practical reality is that the majority of catheterization laboratories tend to assume oxygen consumption from tables.[6] The inherent error of all calculations should always be considered, particularly with respect to flow and resistance calculations.

The pulmonary to systemic blood flow ratio (Q_p/Q_s) can be derived simply from the measured oxygen saturation values because all other variables cancel out (from Equations 1 and 2):

$$Q_p/Q_s = (SaO_2 - SsvcO_2)/(SpvO_2 - SpaO_2). \quad (4)$$

The patient whose aortic blood is fully saturated can be assumed to have no significant right-to-left intracardiac shunt. However, when a right-to-left shunt is present, oxygen saturations also should be obtained from the pulmonary veins, left atrium, and left ventricle to determine the source of desaturated blood. Pulmonary venous desaturation implies a primary pulmonary source of venous admixture (e.g., pneumonia, atelectasis, or other pulmonary disease).

Vascular resistance is calculated by the change in pressure divided by the flow ($\Delta p/Q$):

$$\text{Pulmonary vascular resistance (PVR)} = (\text{Mean PAP} - \text{Mean LAP})/Q_p \quad (5)$$

$$\text{Systemic vascular resistance (SVR)} = (\text{Mean AOp} - \text{Mean SVCP})/Q_s, \quad (6)$$

where PAP = pulmonary artery pressure, LAP = left atrial pressure, AOP = aortic pressure, SVCP = superior vena cava pressure, Q_p = pulmonary blood flow, and Q_s = systemic blood flow.

Once again for pediatric patients, the vascular resistance usually is indexed to body surface area and expressed as Wood units:

$$\text{PVR} = (\text{Mean PAP} - \text{Mean LAP})(\text{BSA})/Q_p \quad (7)$$

$$\text{SVR} = (\text{Mean AOP} - \text{Mean SVCP})(\text{BSA})/Q_s \quad (8)$$

Assessment of Critical Illness

The cardiac catheterization laboratory can be useful in a number of situations during the management of critically ill infants and children who have structurally normal hearts (Table 22–1) or with congenital heart disease. Fluoroscopy can be used to assist with placing difficult central venous or pulmonary artery lines, performing pericardiocentesis and pleurocentesis, and assessing diaphragm function.

Patients with pulmonary hypertension can benefit from investigation in the catheterization laboratory. Catheterization may help diagnose or rule out structural disease involving the pulmonary arteries or pulmonary veins, as in cases of multiple thromboembolic disease or undiagnosed pulmonary vein stenosis. Data obtained during catheterization are important for evaluation of the response of pulmonary vasculature to vasodilator treatment, for example, with increased FiO_2 or inhaled nitric oxide.[7] Such evaluation and measurement of a specific response are important for longer-term management strategies of patients with pulmonary hypertension. In the presence of a left-to-right shunt and elevated PVR, pressure and saturation measurements often are repeated with the patient breathing 100% oxygen to assess both the reactivity of the pulmonary vascular bed and any contribution of ventilation/perfusion abnormalities to hypoxemia. If breathing 100% oxygen and inhaled nitric oxide increases pulmonary blood flow and dramatically increases Q_p/Q_s (with a fall in PVR), potentially reversible processes such as hypoxic pulmonary vasoconstriction may be contributing to the elevated PVR. The patient with a high, unresponsive PVR and a small left-to-right shunt may have extensive pulmonary vascular damage from the underlying lung injury or irreversible obstructive pulmonary vascular disease.

The reactivity of the pulmonary vascular bed and change in PVR are important components to the assessment of patients potentially listed for cardiac transplantation. An elevated PVR is a risk factor for cardiac transplantation. PVR likely is elevated in patients with heart failure associated with left atrial hypertension. However, if PVR decreases with nitric oxide when these patients are tested during pretransplant catheterization, they still may be suitable candidates for cardiac transplantation.

Patients who present with severe cardiac failure because of myocarditis or idiopathic dilated cardiomyopathy or intractable dysrhythmias often require cardiac catheterization not only for hemodynamic assessment but also for endomyocardial biopsy. Biopsies in these circumstances

TABLE 22–1

Indications for Cardiac Catheterization or Management in the Catheterization Laboratory of Pediatric Intensive Care Patients with Noncongenital Heart Disease

Diagnostic	Hemodynamic evaluation of pressures and oxygen saturations
	Cardiac output measurement
	Pulmonary hypertension assessment and reactivity
	Fluoroscopy:
	Central venous catheter position
	Diaphragm movement
	Myocardial biopsy
Therapeutic	Pericardiocentesis
	Pleurocentesis
	Radiofrequency catheter ablation

can be associated with significant morbidity, and treatment should not be delayed until catheterization is performed.[8,9] The risk of myocardial perforation is particularly increased in infants with thin-walled ventricles, and biopsy should be reconsidered in infants with a very dilated and poorly functioning left ventricle. Patients who have a low cardiac output state associated with fulminant myocarditis are at risk for dysrhythmias during catheterization, and resuscitation resources must be immediately available, including mechanical support. The catheterization study and desire for a biopsy in an effort to establish a diagnosis must not take priority over efforts to support the circulation and maintain cardiac output.

Transcatheter Radiofrequency Ablation

Pediatric patients undergoing radiofrequency catheter ablation (RFCA) vary in age and diagnosis.[10] Ablation may be necessary in newborns or infants with persistent reentrant tachycardia or ectopic atrial tachycardia[11] and in older children with ectopic foci but otherwise structurally normal hearts that are refractory to or poorly controlled by conventional antiarrhythmic drugs. If an incessant dysrhythmia, particularly a supraventricular tachycardia such as ectopic atrial tachycardia or permanent junctional reciprocating tachycardia, is the primary cause of a dilated poorly contracting heart at the time of presentation, electrophysiologic study and mapping of the dysrhythmia focus may be important diagnostic steps performed in the catheterization laboratory. Successful RFCA in this circumstance may enable recovery of ventricular function.[12]

An increasing population of patients undergoing ablation consists of those with previous surgical repair of congenital heart defects. Patients with persistent volume or pressure load on the right atrium and those who required an extensive incision and suture lines within the right atrium, such as following a Mustard, Senning, or Fontan procedure, may be at increased risk for supraventricular tachyarrhythmia (SVT) such as atrial flutter and fibrillation.[13,14] Ventricular tachyarrhythmias may develop late after repair of certain congenital heart defects, such as right ventricular outflow tract reconstruction for tetralogy of Fallot.[15]

RFCA procedures can be lengthy. Because children find it difficult to lie still for prolonged procedures, endotracheal general anesthesia is preferred. In addition, patients must remain immobile to prevent catheter movement at the time of ablation because sudden patient movement may result in creation of a radiofrequency lesion at an incorrect site. For instance, if the focus is close to the AV node, inadvertent movement might displace the catheter and cause permanent AV conduction blockade. On occasion, holding ventilation in either inspiration or expiration may be necessary to ensure adequate contact of the ablation catheter with the arrhythmic focus. For the most part, RFCA procedures are hemodynamically well tolerated and blood loss is minimal. During mapping, the focus is stimulated and the tachyarrhythmia induced. This situation may result in hypotension but usually is short lived and can be readily converted via intracardiac pacing. If hypotension is prolonged and intracardiac conversion is unsuccessful, transthoracic cardioversion may be necessary; therefore a defibrillator should be immediately available.

Congenital Heart Disease

Although most congenital heart defects can be evaluated noninvasively by echocardiography or, more recently, by magnetic resonance imaging, further evaluation by angiography is essential in some instances. Rarely is hemodynamic assessment required in newborns with congenital heart disease, perhaps except for Ebstein anomaly where hemodynamic evaluation, including balloon occlusion of the atrial septum, may assist in decision making with regard to medical or operative management.[16]

Patients with pulmonary atresia and intact ventricular septum require careful examination of the coronary anatomy prior to decompressing the RV either surgically or with catheterization techniques because of the possible presence of fistulas from the RV to the coronary artery circulation.[17,18] RV to coronary artery fistulas can be seen on echocardiography, but selective right ventricular angiography and aortography, or even selective coronary angiography if necessary, are important to determine any associated coronary stenoses or atresia (RV-dependent coronary circulation).[19] At another end of this spectrum, patients with tetralogy of Fallot and pulmonary atresia often have diminutive native pulmonary arteries. Aortopulmonary collaterals may contribute greatly to pulmonary blood flow. Angiography can delineate the exact location and anatomy of these collaterals and, if indicated, may be followed by coil occlusion of aortopulmonary collaterals that provide dual supply to the native pulmonary arteries.

Therapeutic Interventions in the Newborn

Interventional cardiac catheterization has matured. Many specific anatomic defects can be treated in the catheterization laboratory to alleviate the need for surgical intervention.

Atrial Communication Procedures

The first therapeutic procedure performed in the catheterization laboratory for congenital heart disease was balloon atrial septostomy in newborns diagnosed with transposition of the great arteries (TGA) with intact ventricular septum.[20] A balloon atrial septostomy usually is needed in newborns with TGA to facilitate mixing of systemic and pulmonary venous return at the atrial level prior to the arterial switch operation. This procedure can be performed by echocardiographic guidance[21] (Figure 22–1) or in the cardiac catheterization laboratory if additional diagnostic information is required or there are potential vascular access problems. Via either the femoral or umbilical vein, a balloon catheter is advanced across the atrial defect from right atrium to left atrium (Figure 22–2, *A*) and position confirmed by echocardiographic or fluoroscopic guidance. The balloon is inflated to the desired volume and jerked back to the right atrium to tear the septum primum (Figure 22–2, *B*).

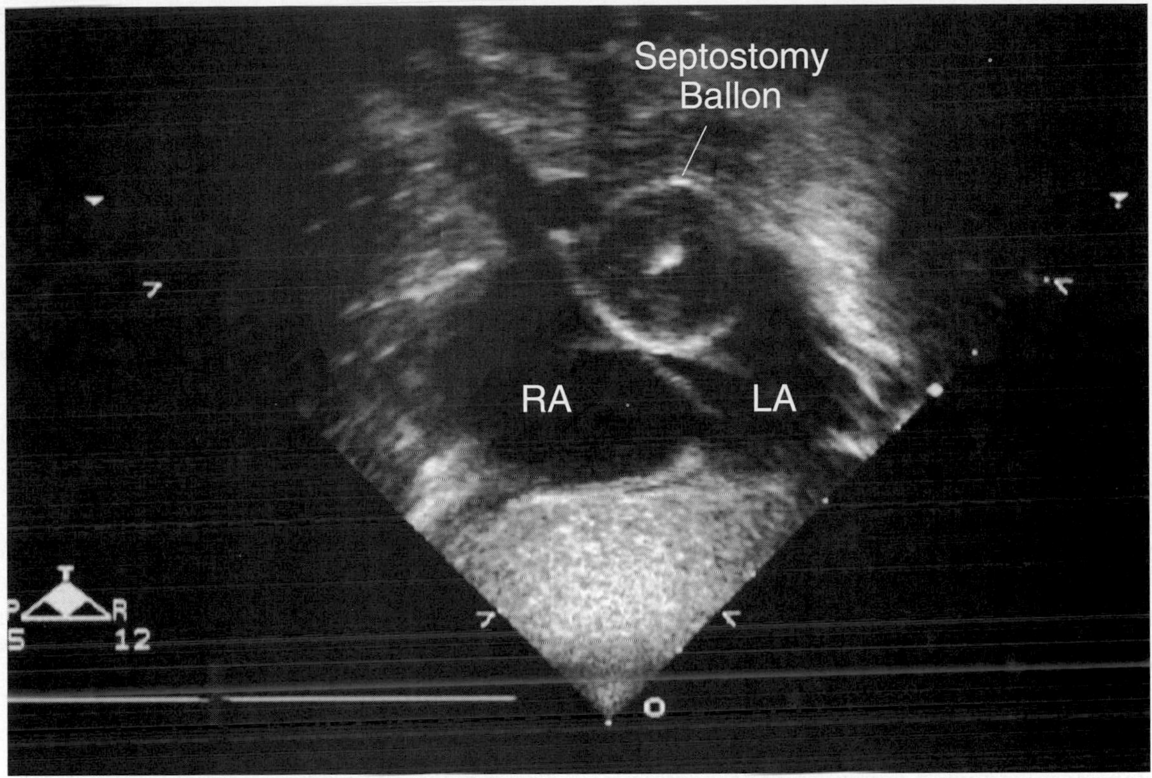

FIGURE 22–1 • Echocardiography-guided balloon atrial septostomy. From the subcostal view, the septostomy balloon is easily seen as it inflates in the left atrium *(LA)*. *RA,* Right atrium.

In some patients with a single-ventricle lesion, such as mitral atresia or hypoplastic left heart syndrome, and who also have a restrictive or near intact atrial septum, the left atrial pressure may be very high at birth, causing pulmonary edema and pulmonary artery hypertension. The physiology in this circumstance is identical to that of patients with obstructed totally anomalous pulmonary venous drainage. Patients usually are cyanotic with a low cardiac output state, and urgent dilation of the atrial septum to lower the atrial pressure and improve mixing can be lifesaving.[22,23] It also allows the pulmonary artery pressure to decrease and pulmonary edema to resolve

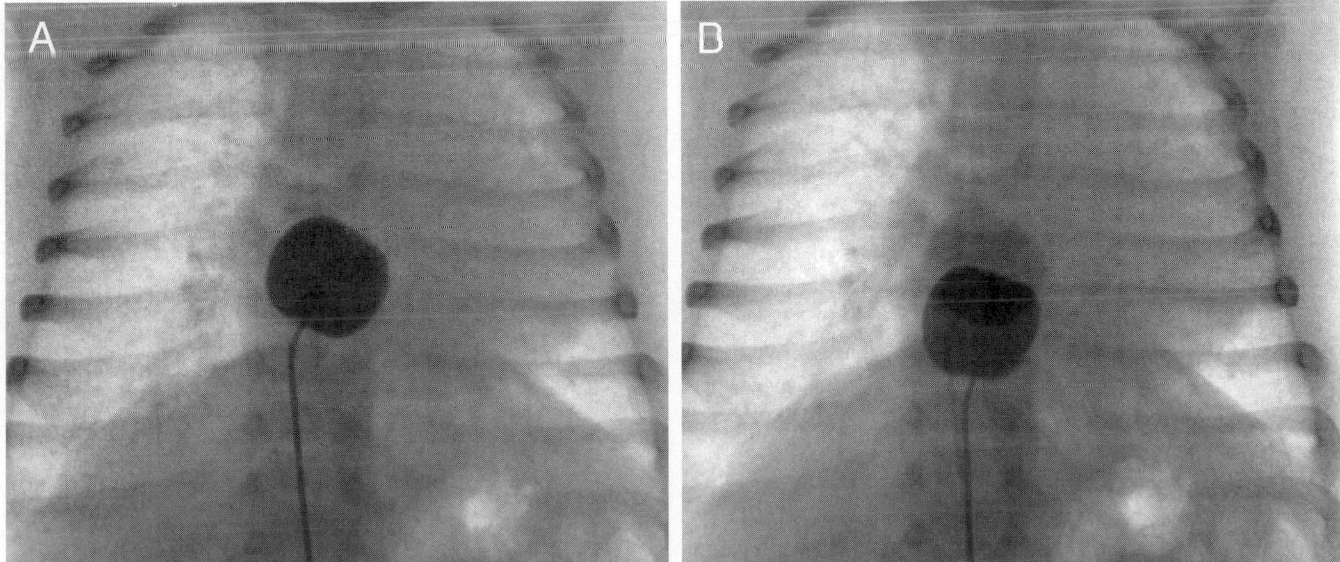

FIGURE 22–2 • Fluoroscopy-guided balloon atrial septostomy. **A,** The balloon is inflated with diluted contrast and positioned in the left atrium. **B,** The balloon is rapidly "jerked" across the atrial septum, resulting in a tear in the septum primum and enabling complete mixing of blood in the atria.

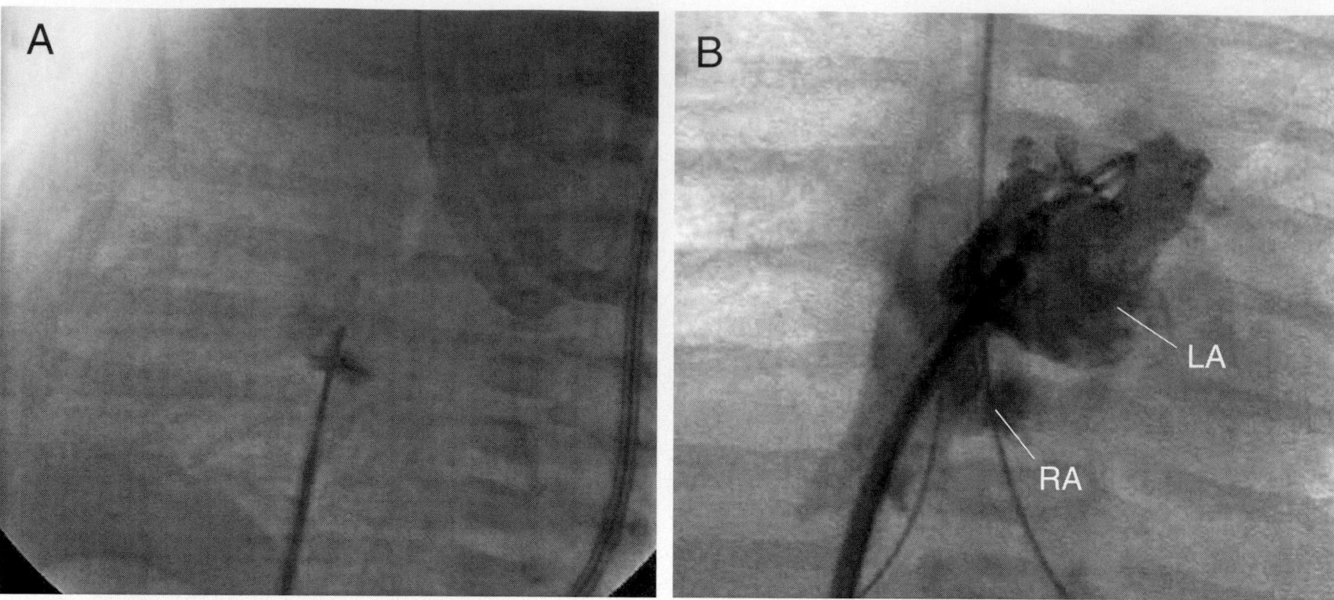

FIGURE 22–3 • Atrial septoplasty in a newborn with restrictive atrial septum and hypoplastic left heart syndrome. **A,** Lateral view of a Brockenbrough transseptal needle introduced across the thickened atrial septum and contrast injected into the small left atrium. **B,** Anteroposterior view following stent placement across the thickened atrial septum. Contrast is seen equally in both the left atrium *(LA)* and the right atrium *(RA).*

prior to stage 1 palliation. It is important to appreciate that the atrial septum often is thickened in these patients, which is quite different than the thin-walled restrictive foramen ovale of patients with TGA. Because of its thickness, disruption of the septum using a balloon atrial septostomy technique usually is not possible. In addition to the thickened atrial septum, atrial cavity size usually is small, so inflating a balloon in the left atrium without causing myocardial injury or tearing a pulmonary vein may be difficult. Instead, decompression of the pulmonary atrium can be achieved with a Brockenbrough transseptal puncture (Figure 22–3, *A*), followed by an atrial septoplasty involving balloon dilation of the thickened or restrictive atrial septum and possible stent placement across the defect to maintain a gradient across the septum of 4 to 6 mmHg (Figure 22–3, *B*). Because of the degree of cyanosis and low cardiac output state, concurrent resuscitation with volume replacement, inotrope support, and mechanical ventilation usually are necessary during this procedure until adequate mixing is established and pulmonary veins are decompressed.

Pulmonary Balloon Valvotomy

Congenital pulmonary valve stenosis may present as a murmur heard in the newborn period. If the obstruction is mild, intervention with balloon dilation can be deferred. Newborns with critical pulmonary valve stenosis or pulmonary valve atresia have severe restriction or absence of antegrade flow across the right ventricular outflow and, as a result, have ductus arteriosus-dependent pulmonary blood flow. Balloon dilation in the catheterization laboratory is the therapeutic procedure of choice (Figure 22–4).[24,25] A balloon catheter is passed over a guidewire antegrade across the pulmonary valve, and balloon dilation usually up to 120% size of the pulmonary valve annulus is performed. Heart block and ventricular ectopy may occur with wire manipulation in the RV but usually are transient. Antegrade flow across the pulmonary valve may not increase significantly after balloon dilation until right ventricular compliance improves, and continuation of prostaglandin E_1 (PGE_1) infusion to maintain patency of the ductus arteriosus for several days following balloon dilation may be necessary. Perforation of the relatively thin right ventricular

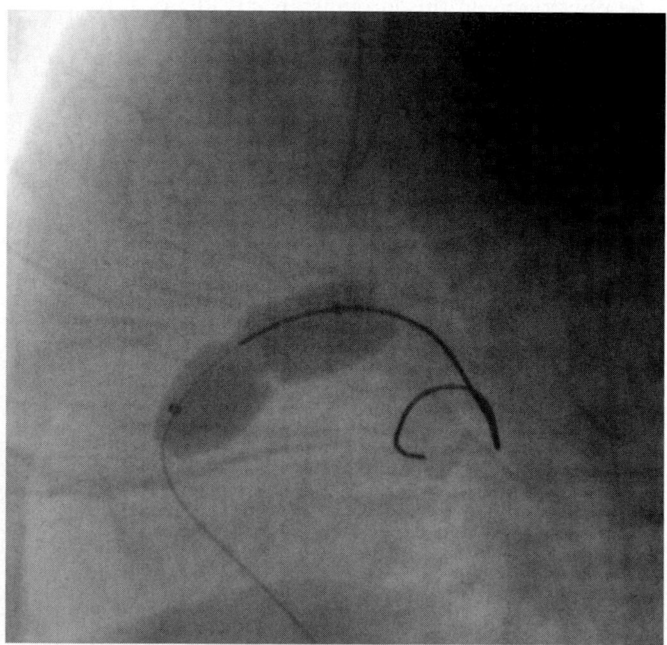

FIGURE 22–4 • Pulmonary valvuloplasty in a newborn with severe pulmonary valve stenosis. Lateral view with balloon catheter centered across a stenotic pulmonary valve. As the balloon is inflated, a "waist" representing the stenotic valve is seen.

outflow tract with the guidewire is a potential complication, particularly in low-birth-weight and premature newborns. Tamponade occurs immediately, and urgent pericardiocentesis or surgical exploration may be necessary.

Aortic Balloon Valvotomy

The newborn with critical valvar aortic stenosis who develops hypotension and acidosis as the ductus arteriosus closes requires resuscitation with PGE_1 to restore aortic flow plus mechanical ventilation and inotropic support to achieve stabilization before an intervention is performed. Balloon dilation of the stenotic aortic valve during cardiac catheterization is the preferred intervention (Figure 22–5),[26] although surgical valvotomy under direct vision using cardiopulmonary bypass (CPB) is the surgical alternative. At catheterization, a guidewire is passed either retrograde (via femoral artery) or antegrade (via femoral vein) across the aortic valve. A balloon catheter is passed over the wire and serial dilations performed up to 90% to 100% size of the aortic valve annulus. The pressure gradient across the aortic valve is remeasured after each dilation, and an ascending aortogram is obtained to evaluate aortic valve regurgitation. Because of the initial minimal flow across the valve, balloon dilation of critical neonatal aortic stenosis usually is well tolerated. Despite the successful relief of obstruction, antegrade flow across the valve may not increase significantly until left ventricular compliance and function improve; therefore continuation of PGE_1 infusion, mechanical ventilation, and vasoactive drugs following dilation for some days may be necessary. Until flow across the valve increases, the residual gradient across the aortic valve will be underestimated by echocardiography, and serial studies usually are necessary to track the evolving gradient and left ventricular function. Other complications include possible mitral valve damage from a relatively stiff guidewire if an antegrade approach is used for dilation and possibly ventricular fibrillation and an acute low cardiac output state secondary to coronary ischemia in patients with a hypertrophied ventricle.

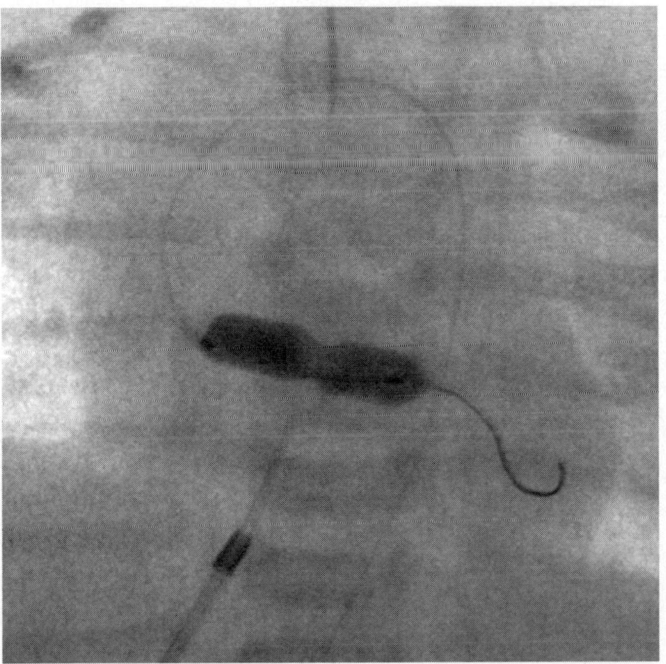

FIGURE 22–5 • Aortic valvuloplasty in a newborn with critical aortic stenosis. Anteroposterior view with retrograde catheter course from the femoral artery. The balloon, also with the waist apparent, is seen being inflated across the aortic valve.

Perioperative Interventional Procedures

A thorough understanding of the anatomy and morphology of complex congenital heart defects is essential for successful management of patients with complex congenital heart disease. This is particularly critical when establishing a diagnosis and planning surgical intervention. Important for the successful perioperative management in the intensive care unit is a thorough understanding of the pathophysiology of various defects. This understanding includes not only the preoperative pathophysiology associated with defects but also the potential alteration in pathophysiology related to surgical repair and/or development of complications in the postoperative period. As a general guide, if patients are not progressing as expected and low cardiac output persists, cardiac catheterization should be performed to investigate and exclude the possibility of undiagnosed or residual structural defects.

Transcatheter treatment of congenital cardiac defects continues to evolve and expand and in some circumstances is effectively replacing the need for conventional intraoperative surgical procedures.[27] This experience has a significant impact on the severity and complexity of illness seen in the operating room and interventional laboratory. In addition to the procedures described, other interventions now routinely performed in the catheterization laboratory include angioplasty often combined with transcatheter placement of endovascular stents for treatment of systemic and pulmonary arterial and venous stenoses, and device occlusion or embolization of systemic-to-pulmonary arterial communications, venous channels, fistulas, muscular VSDs, ASDs, and PDA.

Risks and Complications

Placement of catheters in and through the heart increases the risk for dysrhythmias, perforation of the myocardium, damage to valve leaflets and chordae, cerebral vascular accidents, and air embolism. Use of radiopaque contrast material may cause an acute allergic reaction (rare in children with non-ionic contrast media), pulmonary hypertension, renal impairment, and myocardial depression. Blood loss may be sudden and unexpected when large-bore catheters are used or vessels are ruptured. More insidious blood loss may occur over several hours in heparinized small children or neonates because of bleeding around the catheter site or multiple aspirations and flushes of catheters. Transfusion requirements and appropriate vascular access should be continually assessed.

Arrhythmias, albeit transient, may be recurrent and fatal if not promptly treated. Arrhythmias include catheter-induced SVTs, ventricular tachycardia, ventricular fibrillation, and occasionally complete heart block requiring temporary transvenous pacing support. On most occasions, removing the wire or catheter resolves the arrhythmia, but full resuscitation and cardioversion equipment must be available in case the arrhythmia does not resolve.

Complications of various interventional procedures are related in part to the type of procedure, but all share the risks associated with percutaneous vascular access with large catheters that course through the heart and vessels.[28–31] Table 22–2 lists the specific problems that can occur during various transcatheter procedures. Although the underlying cardiac status or American Society of Anesthesiologists (ASA) classification of a patient may increase his or her risk of adverse events during catheterization, in many circumstances complications are sudden, occur without warning, and reflect the inherent risk for specific procedure. Many complications are potentially life threatening, and successful treatment of complications depends on prompt action by critical care physicians and/or anesthesiologists cooperating closely with the interventional cardiologists who are manipulating the catheters.

Inadvertent release or detachment of embolic and closure devices results in systemic and pulmonary arterial embolization. Embolization usually occurs immediately after placement. Devices often can be retrieved using a variety of retrieval catheters, but in a small minority of cases surgical removal is required. If the device is lodged in the heart or a great vessel, CPB may be required for removal. Device embolization usually does not cause extreme hemodynamic instability or cardiovascular decompensation requiring emergency surgical removal, but an unscheduled surgical procedure still is required. Even after successful transcatheter retrieval, femoral artery and vein reconstruction during anesthesia occasionally is necessary when embolized devices or large dilation balloons are removed through these vessels.

TABLE 22–2

Potential Complications in the Catheterization Laboratory

Procedure	Representative Lesion	Complications
Hemodynamic evaluation	Congenital heart disease	Blood loss requiring transfusion
	Pulmonary hypertension	Air embolism
	Postoperative course: progress not as expected, persistent low cardiac output state, inability to wean from mechanical ventilation, persistent chylous effusions, evaluate residual intracardiac shunt or outflow tract obstruction	Vascular access: trauma, dissection, occlusion, perforation Myocardial perforation and tamponade Arrhythmias: ventricular and supraventricular tachycardia, ventricular fibrillation, complete heart block
Coil embolization	Aortopulmonary collaterals	Fevers
	Systemic-to-pulmonary shunts	Excessive hypoxemia
		Systemic embolization
Transcatheter device closure	Patent ductus arteriosus	Air or device embolization
	Atrial septal defect	Interference with atrioventricular valve function
	Ventricular septal defect	Ventricular arrhythmias, complete heart block
	Baffle leak	Ventricular arrhythmias, complete heart block
Balloon and stent dilations	Pulmonary artery stenosis	Pulmonary artery tear and hemorrhage
		Pulmonary edema: high flow
		False aneurysm
		Right ventricle ischemia
	Pulmonary valve stenosis	Right ventricle perforation
		Pulmonary valve regurgitation
	Aortic valve stenosis	Aortic regurgitation, mitral valve trauma
		Left ventricle ischemia
		Ventricular fibrillation
	Mitral valve stenosis	Mitral insufficiency
		Pulmonary hypertension
	Coarctation of the aorta	Aortic dissection
		Hypertension
	Right ventricular conduit	False aneurysms
		Stent embolization
Atrial septostomy	Transposition of the great arteries	Air embolus, mitral valve or pulmonary vein trauma
Atrial septoplasty	Mitral stenosis (atresia), restrictive atrial septum	Air embolus, mitral valve or pulmonary vein trauma, atrial perforation and tamponade

Balloon Dilation of Pulmonary Arteries

Pulmonary artery balloon dilation and stent placement to relieve stenosis is a common procedure performed in the catheterization laboratory.[32] Pulmonary artery stenoses may be congenital or acquired lesions. They may be discrete involving the main or branch pulmonary arteries or multiple involving distal segmental vessels. The increase in pulmonary artery pressure and fixed resistance to antegrade pulmonary blood flow may have related and deleterious consequences, which include the following:

1. An increase in the afterload on the RV, which in turn causes right ventricular hypertension. The RV can cope with a significant pressure load for some time. However, as right ventricular end-diastolic pressure increases and tricuspid regurgitation possibly develops, right atrial pressure increases and manifests as hepatomegaly, ascites, and persistent or recurrent pleural effusions.
2. Reduced antegrade flow across the pulmonary outflow, which in turn reduces preload to the left ventricle and contributes to a low cardiac output state. Further, the hypertrophy of the ventricular septum reduces the compliance of the left ventricle and increases left ventricular end-diastolic pressure.
3. An increase in right ventricular pressure and ventricular hypertrophy may compromise coronary blood flow. Hypotension or tachycardia with altered coronary filling time may cause myocardial ischemia, with the subendocardium at particular risk.
4. If the pulmonary valve is incompetent, for example, following right ventricular outflow reconstruction for repair of tetralogy of Fallot with or without pulmonary atresia, a considerable amount of pulmonary regurgitation may occur that causes an additional volume load on the RV, leading to right ventricular dilation and systolic failure. In addition, the increased pulsatility to the branch pulmonary arteries may cause extrinsic compression of the main stem bronchi.

Patients with persistent signs of right ventricular failure, such as low cardiac output state, hepatomegaly, ascites, recurrent pleural effusions (particularly if chylous in nature), and inability to wean from mechanical ventilation, should be considered for catheterization. Although echocardiography may help determine a specific problem, catheterization provides quantitative data that can direct vasoactive support and enable interventions such as pulmonary artery dilation, coiling of collateral vessels, and creation of an atrial communication that allows an atrial level right-to-left shunt.

The function of the RV is critical, and often the cause of complication is related to pulmonary artery dilation. At the time of balloon dilation, cardiac output may decrease significantly, causing hypotension, bradycardia, arterial oxygen desaturation, and a fall in end-tidal CO_2. Because the balloon is inflated for only a few seconds and provided preload is maintained, the procedure usually is well tolerated and the circulation usually recovers spontaneously. Patients who have a hypertrophied, poorly compliant RV with intraventricular pressures at systemic or suprasystemic levels may not tolerate the sudden increase in afterload associated with balloon dilation, even for a short period. In particular, myocardial ischemia and arrhythmias may occur, causing severe acute right ventricular failure and loss of cardiac output. General anesthesia and controlled ventilation are recommended prior to intervention in this at-risk group of patients.

Pulmonary artery disruption is signaled by local extravasation of contrast in the lung parenchyma, sudden hemodynamic deterioration from cardiac tamponade or acute hemothorax, or sudden onset of hemoptysis.[33] The tear in the pulmonary artery may be confined (Figure 22–6, *A*) and therefore controlled, or unconfined, resulting in hemodynamic collapse and possible need for immediate surgical intervention. The potential for pulmonary artery disruption is increased because of the high atmospheric pressure used to inflate the balloon and maintain tension on the vessel wall to tear the intima and media. The risk for pulmonary artery disruption may be increased in early postcardiac

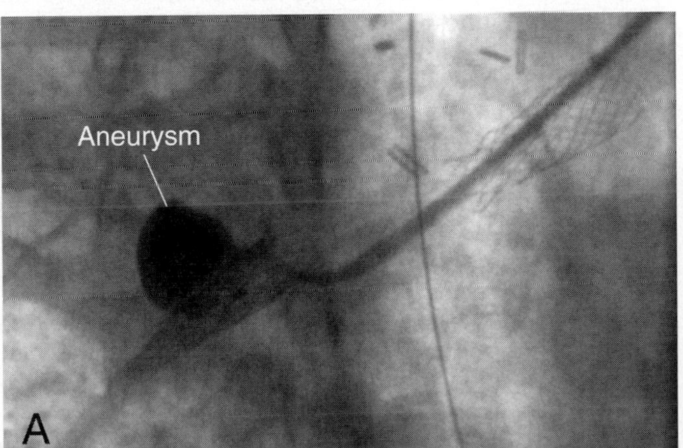

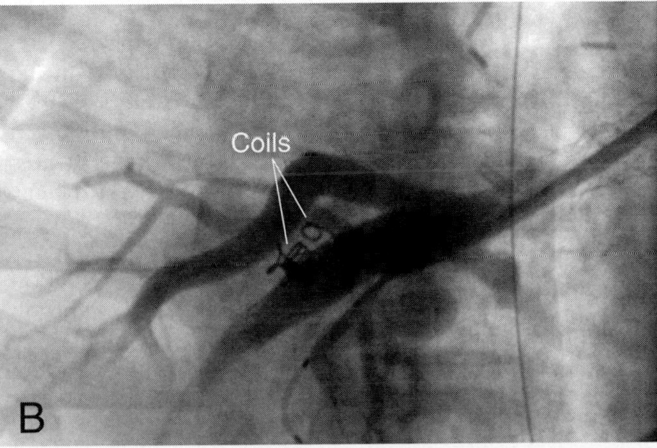

FIGURE 22–6 • Pulmonary artery trauma in a patient with multiple peripheral pulmonary artery stenoses. **A,** Pulmonary artery aneurysm following balloon dilation. Note that a stent has been placed but the aneurysm is still present. **B,** Resolution after coils are placed in the neck of the aneurysm.

surgery patients if the dilation is performed across a recent pulmonary artery anastomosis. The safe time frame to wait for the anastomosis to heal before attempting balloon dilation has not been determined. If the patient is stable without signs of right ventricular failure or low cardiac output state, we prefer to wait 6 weeks after surgery before proceeding with balloon dilation. However, early balloon dilation may be necessary in the immediate postoperative period, particularly if the patient has severe right ventricular failure, low cardiac output state, or inability to wean from mechanical ventilation. Provided the dilation is performed cautiously with all resuscitation facilities immediately available, successful balloon dilation can be achieved in the immediate postcardiac surgery period.[34] Cutting balloons have been added to the options available for achieving successful balloon dilation.[35] The relative safety between a cutting balloon and high pressure dilations is unknown, but a high index of suspicion should be maintained in patients with peripheral pulmonary artery stenosis treated with a cutting balloon. In the presence of substantial hemoptysis, immediate endotracheal intubation is indicated for airway control and ventilation. Hypertension and further airway stimulation should be prevented, the addition of positive end-expiratory pressure may be useful, and instillation of 1 ml of 1:100,000 epinephrine via the endotracheal tube may help reduce immediate bleeding by causing vasoconstriction of mucosal vessels. An immediate intervention by the catheterizer to tamponade the disrupted branch pulmonary artery with a balloon catheter may be lifesaving. Occlusion of the vessel permanently with a coil (Figure 22-6, *B*) or covered stent may be necessary to prevent further hemorrhage.

Transient unilateral or unilobar pulmonary edema is also seen in the setting of pulmonary artery dilation. This finding is related to sudden large increases in pulmonary blood flow and distal pulmonary artery pressure after dilation in a previously underperfused pulmonary vascular bed. Pulmonary edema after dilation usually occurs immediately following balloon dilation but can be delayed for up to 24 hours. Pulmonary edema and disruption of a pulmonary artery can occur abruptly, in isolation, or together, during pulmonary artery dilation procedures. Both can cause the appearance in the airway of frank blood or blood-tinged edema fluid in substantial quantities.

Patients who have a dilated RV secondary to a long-standing volume load, such as chronic pulmonary regurgitation, are at risk for arrhythmias and low output during catheter manipulations and interventions. As noted earlier, on most occasions the changes in rhythm are short lived and settle once the catheters are withdrawn. Nevertheless, anesthesia and airway control are recommended if the circulation is compromised, and a defibrillator and transvenous pacing must be immediately available.

Potential movement at the time of critical balloon dilation or stent placement must be prevented. Dilation of pulmonary arteries is painful and often causes patients to waken from sedation and move. In addition, dilation of the pulmonary arteries may induce coughing. The coughing usually is not a problem for isolated pulmonary artery dilation, but if the patient moves during stent placement, lobar or segmental branch pulmonary arteries may be obstructed inadvertently by the stent. Therefore the patient must be immobile, and additional sedation should be considered immediately prior to stent placement.

Occlusion Device Insertion

Although device closures of PDA and ASD are commonly performed interventions in the catheterization laboratory, they are relatively uncommon procedures in pediatric intensive care patients. A persistent *left-to-right* shunt at the atrial level contributing to right ventricular volume overload, increased pulmonary blood flow, and inability to wean from mechanical ventilation may be one indication, although often the ASD must be of considerable size to cause these symptoms and may be too large for safe deployment of the device. Conversely, a large *right-to-left* shunt across an ASD may result in significant cyanosis and increase the risk for paradoxical embolism and cerebral vascular accident. A similar circumstance exists in patients who have undergone a fenestrated Fontan operation. Placement of a PDA or ASD device usually is associated with minimal hemodynamic disturbance. Although placement can be performed in most patients using sedation techniques,[36] endotracheal tube placement for airway protection may be necessary if transesophageal echocardiography is used to guide device placement.

Indications for VSD device placement include closure of a residual or recurrent septal defect, preoperative closure of defects that may be difficult to reach surgically while on CPB (Figure 22–7, *A*), and closure of acquired defects such as postmyocardial infarction or trauma.[37] A residual VSD may cause considerable volume load to the ventricles and result in a low cardiac output state and congestive heart failure requiring prolonged mechanical ventilation and inotropic or vasoactive support. In contrast to our experience with closure of PDAs or ASDs, transcatheter VSD device closures are prolonged procedures that often are associated with profound hemodynamic instability and blood loss.[38] Although the clinical condition of patients undergoing VSD device placement may vary considerably, the preoperative clinical condition or ASA status is not a sole predictor of hemodynamic disturbance during device placement. Rather, it is the technique necessary for deploying the occlusion device that results in significant hemodynamic compromise; therefore all patients are susceptible. Factors contributing to hemodynamic instability include blood loss, arrhythmias from catheter manipulation in the ventricles and across the septum, atrioventricular or aortic valve regurgitation from stenting open of valve leaflets by stiff wire/catheters, and device-related factors such as malposition of the umbrella with arms impinging on valve leaflets or dislodgment from the ventricular septum.

Because of the large sheath required for positioning of the delivery pod and device (Figure 22–7, *B* and *C*) and the need for frequent catheter changes through the sheath, considerable blood loss may occur (often concealed by drapes) and the risk for air embolism is increased. In patients with intracardiac shunts, air embolization may be life threatening and can be diagnosed by fluoroscopy. When unoccupied by the device carrier system and collapsed device, the large delivery sheath represents a potential

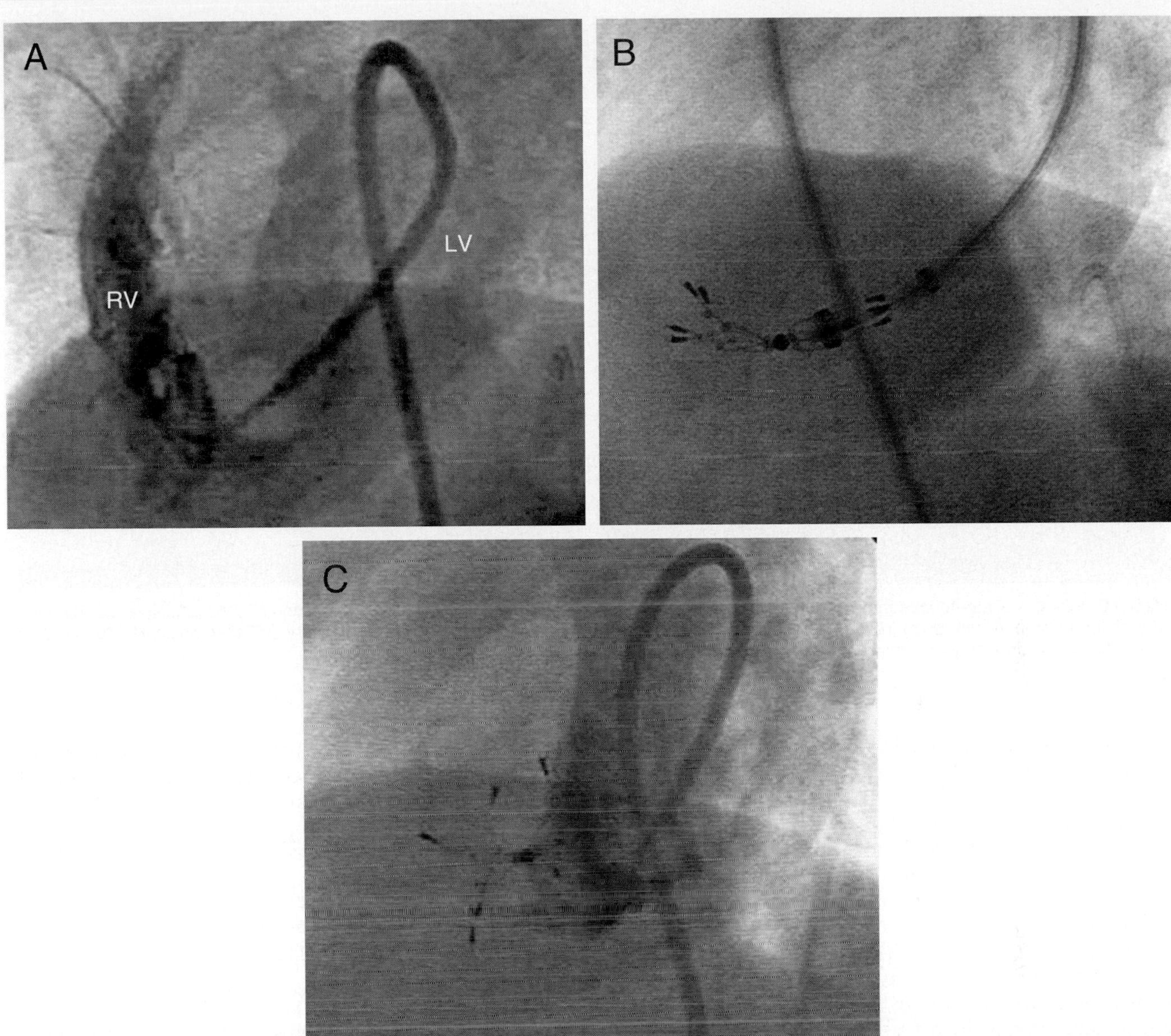

FIGURE 22-7 • Ventricular septal defect closure using the CardioSEAL™ device. **A,** Long axial oblique view of the interventricular septum reveals an apical muscular defect. The catheter course is from inferior vena cava, right atrium, across atrial septum to left atrium, and across the mitral valve to the left ventricle *(LV)*. **B,** Same projection demonstrates dense delivery. The long sheath has been retracted over the arms positioned in the right ventricle *(RV)* and is still covering the left-sided arms. During this stage of the procedure, hemodynamic instability occurs with the large sheath and delivery system interfering with ventricular contraction and valve function. **C,** Left ventricular angiogram after device release.

space for air accumulation and subsequent delivery into the heart. In addition, when the entry port of the large delivery sheath is open during removal and reinsertion of various catheters and devices, extreme inspiratory efforts may introduce air into the heart air. Air in the right atrium may be shunted across an ASD even in the presence of nominal left-to-right shunting. Left heart air embolization produces ST-segment elevation and often hemodynamic changes as it passes into the aorta. The resultant ST-segment changes, hypotension, arterial desaturation, and bradycardia generally respond to aspiration and then sealing of the entry port, along with administration of atropine and inotropic and pressor support to maintain coronary perfusion. Meticulous purging of air from the catheter system and sealing of open ports should help minimize the incidence of air embolism. Use of controlled positive pressure ventilation through an endotracheal tube in an anesthetized paralyzed patient also may decrease the potential for transcatheter air embolus.

Cardiac Catheterization and Extracorporeal Membrane Oxygenation

Cardiac catheterization may be necessary in patients supported with extracorporeal membrane oxygenation

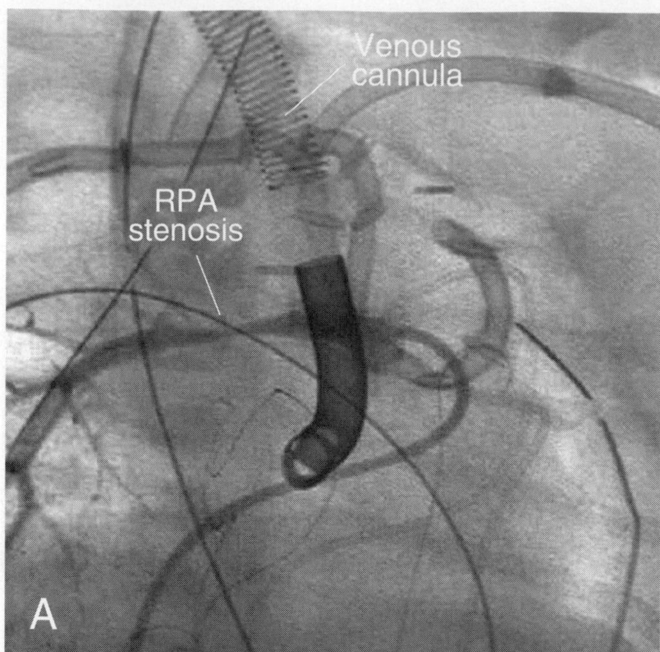

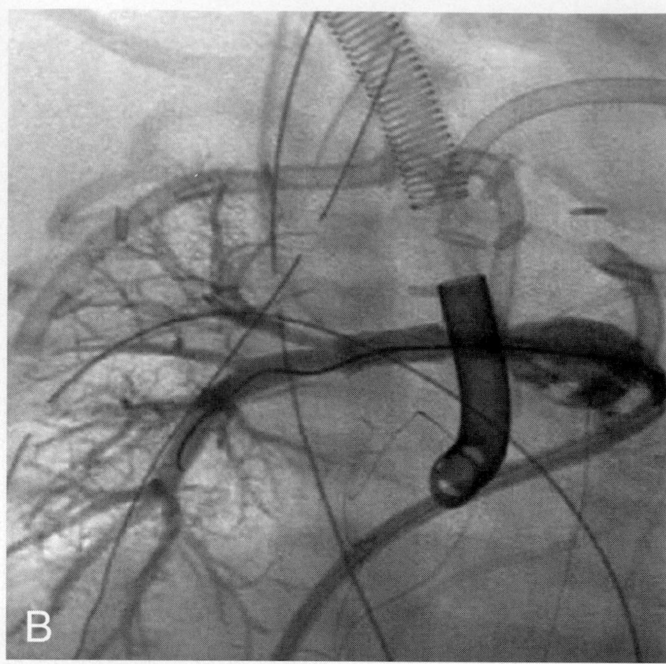

FIGURE 22–8 • Catheterization procedure in a patient undergoing extracorporeal membrane oxygenation (ECMO). **A,** Note ECMO cannula and monitoring lines. A right pulmonary artery angiogram reveals significant proximal right pulmonary artery *(RPA)* stenosis. **B,** Much improved distal right pulmonary artery flow following stent placement across the stenotic area.

(ECMO) for either diagnostic or therapeutic procedures, often to facilitate subsequent weaning and decannulation.[39] Reversible respiratory failure and pulmonary hypertension remain common indications for ECMO, but mechanical support of the failing circulation using ECMO has been increasingly used given indications including refractory low cardiac output state, unexpected cardiac arrest, failure to wean from CPB, severe cyanosis, and refractory arrhythmias.[40]

A small number of published series have described the feasibility and utility of cardiac catheterization of patients supported by ECMO.[34,39,41,42] As the use of ECMO for supporting the circulation after cardiac surgery has increased,[43] so has the potential utility of cardiac catheterization during ECMO. Indications for catheterization have included assessment of surgical repair and interventions to treat residual defects, left heart decompression via a percutaneous transatrial vent in order to prevent overdistension of the left ventricle, hemodynamic assessment and myocardial biopsy in patients with fulminate myocarditis/cardiomyopathy, and catheter-based interventions such as arrhythmia ablation.[44] Despite the high risk, few complications during catheterization were reported in the series, and the complications did not contribute to morbidity or mortality.

It is important to have a high index of suspicion for residual lesions in postoperative cardiac surgery patients who cannot be weaned from ECMO within 72 hours of expected myocardial recovery.[40] Transthoracic echocardiography often is limited in this setting because of less satisfactory windows for standard views and altered hemodynamics during ECMO. Catheterization during the course of ECMO can make possible the diagnosis of residual lesions that could limit successful weaning from ECMO (Figure 22–8, *A* and *B*). Early catheterization and subsequent interventions may facilitate recovery of myocardial function, reduce ECMO duration, and lessen the potential for ECMO-related complications.

REFERENCES

1. Javorski JJ, Hansen DD, Laussen PC, et al: Anesthesia for pediatric cardiac catheterization: innovations. *Can J Anaesth* 42:310-329, 1995.
2. Wilkinson JL: Haemodynamic calculations in the catheter laboratory. *Heart* 85:113-120, 2001.
3. Freed MD, Miettinen OS, Nadas AS: Oximetric detection of intracardiac left to right shunts. *Br Heart J* 42:690-694, 1979.
4. Freed MD, Keane JF: Cardiac output measured by thermodilution in infants and children. *J Pediatr* 92:39-42, 1978.
5. Lundell BPW, Casas ML, Wallgren CG: Oxygen consumption in infants and children during heart catheterization. *Pediatr Cardiol* 17:207-213, 1996.
6. LaFarge CG, Miettinen OS: The estimation of oxygen consumption. *Cardiovasc Res* 4:23-30, 1970.
7. Atz AM, Adatia IA, Lock JE, Wessel DL: Combined effects of nitric oxide and oxygen during acute pulmonary vasodilator testing. *J Am Coll Cardiol* 33:813-819, 1999.
8. Pophel SG, Sigfussen G, Booth KL, et al: Complications of endomyocardial biopsy in children. *J Am Coll Cardiol* 34:2105-2110, 1999.
9. Wu LA, Lapeyre AC, Cooper LT: Current role of endomyocardial biopsy in the management of dilated cardiomyopathy and myocarditis. *Mayo Clin Proc* 76:1030-1038, 2001.
10. Tanel RE, Walsh EP, Triedman JK, et al: Five-year experience with radiofrequency catheter ablation: implications for management of arrhythmias in pediatric and young adult patients. *J Pediatr* 131: 878-887, 1997.
11. Blaufox AD, Felix GL, Saul JP, Pediatric Catheter Ablation Registry: Radiofrequency catheter ablation in infants </= 18 months old: when is it done and how do they fare?: short-term data from the pediatric ablation registry. *Circulation* 104:2803-2808, 2001.
12. De Giovanni JV, Dindar A, Griffith MJ, et al: Recovery pattern of left ventricular dysfunction following radiofrequency ablation of

incessant supraventricular tachycardia in infants and children. *Heart* 79:588-592, 1998.

13. Gelatt M, Hamilton RM, McCrindle BW, et al: Arrhythmia and mortality after the Mustard procedure: a 30 year single center experience. *J Am Coll Cardiol* 29:194-201, 1997.
14. Fishberger SB, Wernovsky G, Gentles TL, et al: Factors that influence the development of atrial flutter after the Fontan operation. *J Thorac Cardiovasc Surg* 113:80-86, 1997.
15. Deanfield JE, McKenna WJ, Presbitero P, et al: Ventricular arrhythmia in unrepaired and repaired tetralogy of fallot. relation to age, timing of repair and hemodynamic status. *Br Heart J* 52:77-81, 1984.
16. Atz AM, Munoz RA, Aditia I, Wessel DL: Diagnostic and therapeutic uses of inhaled nitric oxide in neonatal Ebstein's anomaly. *Am J Cardiol* 91:906-908, 2003.
17. Giglia TM, Mandell VS, Connor AR, et al: Diagnosis and management of right ventricle-dependent coronary circulation in pulmonary atresia with intact ventricular septum. *Circulation* 86:1516-1528, 1992.
18. Justo RN, Nykanen DG, Williams WG, et al: Transcatheter perforation of the right ventricular outflow tract as initial therapy for pulmonary valve atresia and intact ventricular septum in the newborn. *Cathet Cardiovasc Diagn* 40:408-413, 1997.
19. Satou GM, Perry SB, Gauvreau K, Geva T: Echocardiographic predictors of coronary artery pathology in pulmonary atresia with intact ventricular septum. *Am J Cardiol* 85:1319-1324, 2000.
20. Rashkind WJ, Miller WW: Creation of an atrial septal defect without thoracotomy. A palliative approach to complete transposition of the great arteries. *JAMA* 196:991-992, 1966.
21. Steeg CN, Bierman FZ, Hordof AJ, et al. "Bedside" balloon septostomy in infants with transposition of the great arteries: new concepts using two dimensional echocardiographic techniques. *J Pediatr* 107:944-946, 1985.
22. Atz AM, Feinstein JA, Jonas RA, et al: Preoperative management of pulmonary venous hypertension in hypoplastic left heart syndrome with restrictive atrial septal defect. *Am J Cardiol* 83:1224-1228, 1999.
23. Cheatham JP: Intervention in the critically ill neonate and infant with hypoplastic left heart syndrome and intact atrial septum. *J Interv Cardiol* 14:357-366, 2001.
24. Colli AM, Perry SB, Lock JE, Keane JF: Balloon dilation of critical valvar pulmonary stenosis in the first month of life. *Cathet Cardiovasc Diagn* 34:23-28, 1995.
25. Latson LA: Critical pulmonary stenosis. *J Interv Cardiol* 14:345-350, 2001.
26. Egito ES, Moore P, O'Sullivan J, et al: Transvascular balloon dilation for neonatal critical aortic stenosis: early and midterm results. *J Am Coll Cardiol* 29:442-447, 1997.
27. Lock JE, Keane JF, Perry SB: *Diagnostic and interventional catheterization in congenital heart disease.* Norwell, MA, 1999, Kluwer Academic Publishers.
28. Vitiello R, McCrindle BW, Nykanen D, et al: Complications associated with pediatric cardiac catheterization. *J Am Coll Cardiol* 32:1433-1440, 1998.
29. Cassidy SC, Schmidt KG, Van Hare GF, et al: Complications of pediatric cardiac catheterization: a 3-year study. *J Am Coll Cardiol* 19:1285-1293, 1992.
30. Zeevi B, Berant M, Fogelman R, et al: Acute complications in the current era of therapeutic cardiac catheterization for congenital heart disease. *Cardiol Young* 9:266-267, 1999.
31. Schroeder VA, Shim D, Spicer RL, et al: Surgical emergencies during pediatric interventional catheterization. *J Pediatr* 140:570-575, 2002.
32. O'Laughlin MP: Catheterization treatment of stenosis and hypoplasia of pulmonary arteries. *Pediatr Cardiol* 19:48-56, 1998.
33. Baker CM, McGowan FX Jr, Keane JF, Lock JE: Pulmonary artery trauma due to balloon dilation: recognition, avoidance and management. *J Am Coll Cardiol* 36:1684-1690, 2000.
34. Zahn EM, Dobrolet NC, Nykanen DG, et al: Interventional catheterization performed in the early postoperative period after congenital heart surgery in children. *J Am Coll Cardiol* 43: 1264-1269, 2004.
35. Bergersen LJ, Perry SB, Lock JE: Effect of cutting balloon angioplasty on resistant pulmonary artery stenosis. *Am J Cardiol* 91: 185-189, 2003.
36. Wessel DL, Keane JF, Parness I, Lock JE: Outpatient closure of the patent ductus arteriosus. *Circulation* 77:1068-1071, 1988.
37. Bridges ND, Perry SB, Keane JF, et al: Preoperative transcatheter closure of congenital muscular ventricular septal defects. *N Engl J Med* 324:1312-1317, 1991.
38. Laussen PC, Hansen DD, Fox LM, et al. Hemodynamic instability associated with VSD device closure: anesthetic implications. *Anesth Analg* 80:1076 1082, 1995.
39. Booth KL, Roth SJ, Perry SP, et al: Cardiac catheterization of patients supported by extracorporeal membrane oxygenation. *J Am Coll Cardiol* 40:1681-1686, 2002.
40. Duncan BW, Hraska V, Jonas RA, et al: Mechanical circulatory support in children with cardiac disease. *J Thorac Cardiovasc Surg* 117:529-542, 1999.
41. Ettedgui JA, Fricker FJ, Park SC, et al: Cardiac catheterization in children on extracorporeal membrane oxygenation. *Cardiol Young* 6:59-61, 1996.
42. Desjardins SE, Crowley DC, Beekman RH, Lloyd TR: Utility of cardiac catheterization in pediatric cardiac patients on ECMO. *Cathet Cardiovasc Interv* 46: 62-67, 1999.
43. *ECMO registry report.* Ann Arbor, Mich, 2004, Extracorporeal Life Support Organization.
44. Carmichael TB, Walsh EP, Roth SJ: Anticipatory use of venoarterial extracorporeal membrane oxygenation for a high risk interventional cardiac procedure. *Respir Care* 47:1002-1006, 2002.

CHAPTER

23

Pharmacology of the Cardiovascular System

Michael Kelly, Marc Sturgill, and Daniel Notterman

PEARLS

- Clinical acumen is needed to distinguish between the need for an inotropic agent, which is used to increase cardiac contractility, and the need for a vasopressor agent, which is used to increase vascular tone.
- The failing myocardium may require support with an agent that increases contractility and reduces afterload, such as milrinone or dobutamine. Dobutamine should not be used to directly increase blood pressure.
- Multiple polymorphisms discovered in receptors are relevant to the intensivist. Although the clinical importance of these polymorphisms has yet to be determined, physicians must stay abreast of changes in this rapidly expanding area.

In many pediatric critical care units, disorders of the cardiovascular and respiratory systems are the most frequent reasons for admission. Children with these disorders constitute a large group of patients who may require pharmacologic support to maintain adequate end-organ perfusion and oxygenation. The *catecholamines* are the class of drug most often used for this support and remain a mainstay of therapy for the pediatric critical care physician, although the role of other agents has expanded. The *bipyridines,* such as milrinone, have been used in the support of patients with hemodynamic compromise of varying etiologies. The role of *vasopressin* continues to be investigated in the management of the patient with vasodilatory shock or after cardiopulmonary bypass. This chapter examines the clinical pharmacology of the five clinically useful catecholamines, the newer agents, and the venerable cardiac glycosides.

Mechanisms of Response

Pharmacologic manipulation of the cardiovascular system often entails increasing the inotropic state of the myocardium or altering the tone of the systemic vascular tree so as to improve perfusion. The final common mediator for both processes is the concentration of calcium in the cytosol. The pathway by which pharmacologic agents affect this parameter is a function of their specific cell surface receptors.

Adrenergic Receptors

Catecholamines modify cellular physiology by interacting with a specific adrenergic receptor. The classic paradigm of α and β classes of adrenergic receptors remains unchanged, although investigations of new subtypes and sub-subtypes continue. Currently, three subtypes of α_1 and three subtypes of α_2 receptors have been described, and three subtypes of β receptors are recognized.[112] Advances in the biology of the adrenergic receptor have led to a greater understanding of the α receptor's role in the heart, adrenergic receptor regulation of cardiac myocyte apoptosis, and coupling of the β_2 receptor to more than one G protein. The discovery of various polymorphisms for the adrenergic receptors has added even more complexity, but the clinical relevance of many of these polymorphisms has not been elucidated. Despite our increased understanding of the adrenergic receptor, the clinical classification of the catecholamines into α and β agents remains functionally unchanged (Table 23–1).

TABLE 23–1

Adrenergic Receptors: Physiologic Responses, Agonist Potency, and Representative Antagonists

Receptor	G Protein	Physiologic Response	Agonist	Antagonist
α_1	G_q	Increase $InsP_3$, 1,2-DG, and intracellular Ca^{+2}; muscle contraction; vasoconstriction; inhibit insulin secretion	E > NE > D	Prazosin
α_2	G_i	Decrease cAMP; inhibit NE release; vasodilation; negative chronotropy	E > NE	Yohimbine
β_1	G_s	Increase cAMP; inotropy, chronotropy; enhance renin secretion	I > E ≥ D ≥ NE	Propranolol Metoprolol
β_2	G_s	Increase cAMP; smooth muscle relaxation; vasodilation; bronchodilation; enhance glucagon secretion; hypokalemia	I ≥ E > D > NE	Propranolol
D_1	G_s	Increase cAMP; smooth muscle relaxation	D	Haloperidol Metoclopramide
D_2	G_i	Decrease cAMP; inhibit prolactin and β-endorphin	D	Domperidone

$InsP_3$, Inositol 1,4,5-triphosphate; *1,2-DG*, 1,2 diacylglycerol; *E*, epinephrine; *NE*, norepinephrine; *D*, dopamine; *I*, isoproterenol.
Adapted from Notterman DA: *Prob Anesth* 3:288, 1989.

Signal Transduction

Adrenergic receptors mediate their effects through G proteins and as such are classified as G protein–coupled receptors. The adrenergic receptor itself contains seven membrane-spanning α-helical domains, an extracellular N-terminal segment, and a cytosolic C-terminal segment (Figure 23–1). G proteins are heterotrimeric proteins, consisting of α, β, and γ subunits, each of which has multiple subfamilies.[134] There are at least 20 α subunits, 5 β subunits, and 6 γ subunits. The action resulting from a ligand binding to a particular adrenergic receptor is a function of the specific type of subunits compromising the G protein-receptor complex. An evolving concept is spontaneous receptor activation, as described for the β_2-adrenergic receptor.[171,310] In this model, the receptor "toggles" between different conformational states, some of which are active and each of which may be bound to different G proteins. Binding of a ligand may stabilize or invoke a shift to a particular conformation and in doing so promote changes in the expression of second messengers, most commonly protein kinases. Hence the response of ligand binding may depend not only on the ligand involved but also on the state of the receptor at the time of binding.

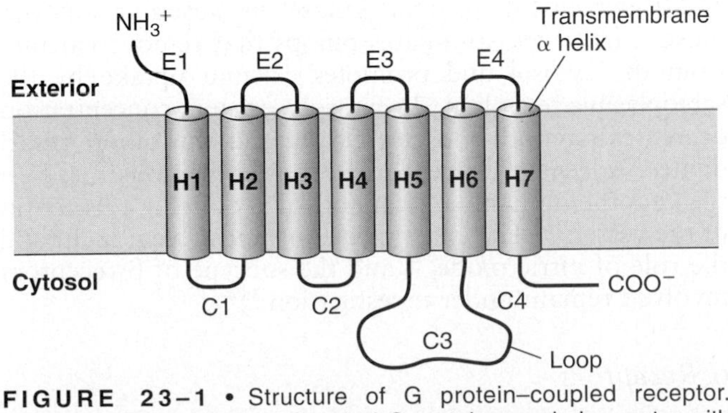

FIGURE 23–1 • Structure of G protein–coupled receptor. Schematic representation of typical G protein–coupled receptor with seven membrane spanning regions (H1–H7), cytoplasmic (C1–C4), and extracellular (E1–E4) loops. (From Lodish H, et al: *Molecular cell biology,* ed 4. New York, 1999, WH Freeman.)

Adrenergic receptors are typically coupled to one of three types of G proteins: G_s, G_i, or G_q. G_s proteins produce an increase in adenylate cyclase activity, whereas G_i proteins promote a decrease in adenylate cyclase activity. G_q protein receptors stimulate phospholipase C to generate diacylglycerol and inositol 1,4,5-triphosphate (IP_3). The nature of the G protein is usually a function of the type of α subunit (α_s, α_I, α_q, $\alpha_{12/13}$).[264] Events involving interaction of G proteins, the receptor protein, and adenylate cyclase are summarized in Figure 23–2. In the example of the G_s protein, ligand binding to the coupled receptor causes a conformational change in the G protein, resulting in GDP disassociating from the G_s α subunit and GTP binding to the α subunit. This GTP-G_α complex then disassociates from the $G_{\beta\gamma}$ subunit and binds to adenylate cyclase, leading to an increase in activity of this enzyme. Adenylate cyclase catalyzes the conversion of adenosine triphosphate (ATP) to cyclic adenosine monophosphate (cAMP), thus increasing cellular levels of cAMP. G_i proteins have a different α subunit. When the $G_{i\alpha}$-GTP complex binds to adenylate cyclase, the enzyme is inactivated. By inhibiting this enzyme, G_i-coupled receptor agonists produce a decrease in the cellular concentration of cAMP. The specific cellular response that follows an alteration in the concentration of cAMP depends on the specialized function of the target cell.[3] Typically, an increase in concentration of cAMP leads to activation of a cAMP-dependent protein kinase. These kinases then phosphorylate and activate other structures and enzymes. Many compounds other than adrenergic agents also increase intracellular levels of cAMP. The question of how different agents produce specific responses through the expression of common second messengers continues to be investigated. One proposed mechanism involves anchoring proteins, such as A kinase anchoring proteins (AKAP). These proteins localize protein kinase A (PKA) to particular cellular locales and may offer binding sites for other regulatory proteins.[144] Similarly, anchoring

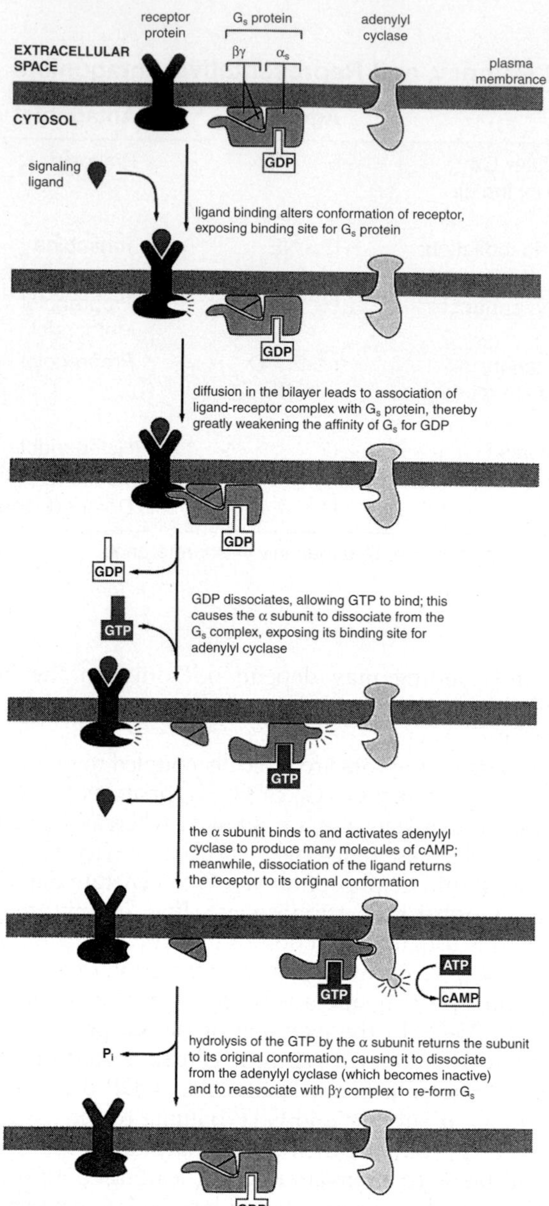

FIGURE 23–2 • Adrenergic receptor complex. When the receptor is engaged by an appropriate ligand (e.g., isoproterenol for a β_1 receptor), the receptor associates with the α_s polypeptide of the G_s protein. This causes the α_s to extrude GDP and incorporate GTP. α_s then associates with and activates the adenylate cyclase. The process is terminated when GTP is hydrolyzed to GDP and α_s dissociates. (From Alberts B et al: Cell signaling. In *Molecular biology of the cell,* ed 3. New York, 1994, Garland Publishing.)

proteins for both the active and inactive forms of protein kinase C (PKC) have been described.[193] Different subtypes of anchoring proteins may create another level of specificity in the effector response for a particular ligand by confining the response to a particular area.

β-*Adrenergic Receptors*

Myocardial β_1-adrenergic receptors are associated with G_s. When this receptor type is engaged by an agonist agent, the result is enhanced activity of adenylate cyclase and a rise in the concentration of cAMP. This activates PKA. PKA in turn phosphorylates voltage-dependent calcium channels, increasing the fraction of channels that can be open and the probability that these channels are open, producing an increase in intracellular calcium concentration (Figure 23–3).[143] Calcium then binds to troponin C, allowing for actin-myosin cross-bridge formation and sarcomere contraction. Also, PKA phosphorylates phospholamban, relieving the disinhibitory effect of the unphosphorylated form on calcium channels in the sarcoplasmic reticulum. The accumulation of calcium by the sarcoplasmic reticulum is enhanced, increasing the rate of sarcomere relaxation (lusitropy) and subsequently increasing the amount of calcium available for the next contraction. This process leads to both enhanced contractility and active diastolic relaxation.

The question of a PKA-independent mechanism by which β-adrenergic receptors can activate calcium channels remains controversial.[301] Experimental evidence indicates β_1 receptors are preferentially coupled to cardiac calcium channels in a cAMP-independent mechanism; however, a binding site on the calcium channel has not been delineated.[148,302] β_2-Adrenergic receptors physically complex with the calcium channel v1.2 in neuronal tissue.[70] Of note, whereas the β_2 receptor once was believed to have little presence and no role in the heart, later evidence suggests just the opposite. β_2 receptors are present in the heart and in fact couple with both G_s and G_i.[149] The response to β_2 activation in the heart remains controversial. β_2 activation is actually more effective at increasing cAMP levels than β_1 activation, but the effect on PKA is localized rather than diffuse, as is the case following β_1 activation. This finding could result from localization of receptor signaling by the G_i component. Evidence supporting this hypothesis is that treatment with pertussis toxin (an inhibitor of G_i) transforms the β_2 signal from a local to a diffuse one.[57] In summary, the role of β_2 receptors in the heart and the signaling processes involved are not fully resolved.[264, 297] Their role in the failing heart and implications for disease also remain to be elucidated.[164,307] To add further complexity, functional β_3 receptors have been demonstrated in the heart and appear to have a negative inotropic effect.[101]

In vascular smooth muscle, both β_1 and β_2 receptors are present although β_2 predominate.[112] The β_2 receptor is coupled to G_s; therefore activation of β_2 receptors promotes formation of cAMP. The resulting activation of cAMP-dependent protein kinase in vascular smooth muscle, however, stimulates pumps that remove calcium from the cytosol and promotes calcium uptake by the sarcoplasmic reticulum. As cytosolic calcium concentration decreases, smooth muscle relaxes and the blood vessel dilates. Adrenergic receptors have been demonstrated on the endothelium and are capable of producing relaxation of the vessel.[282] The exact mechanism involved, including the role of nitric oxide[274] and the subtype of β receptors involved remain under investigation.[112]

α *Receptors*

Vascular smooth muscle contraction is mediated via α_1-adrenergic receptors, of which there are three subtypes: 1A, 1B, and 1D. The individual contributions of each

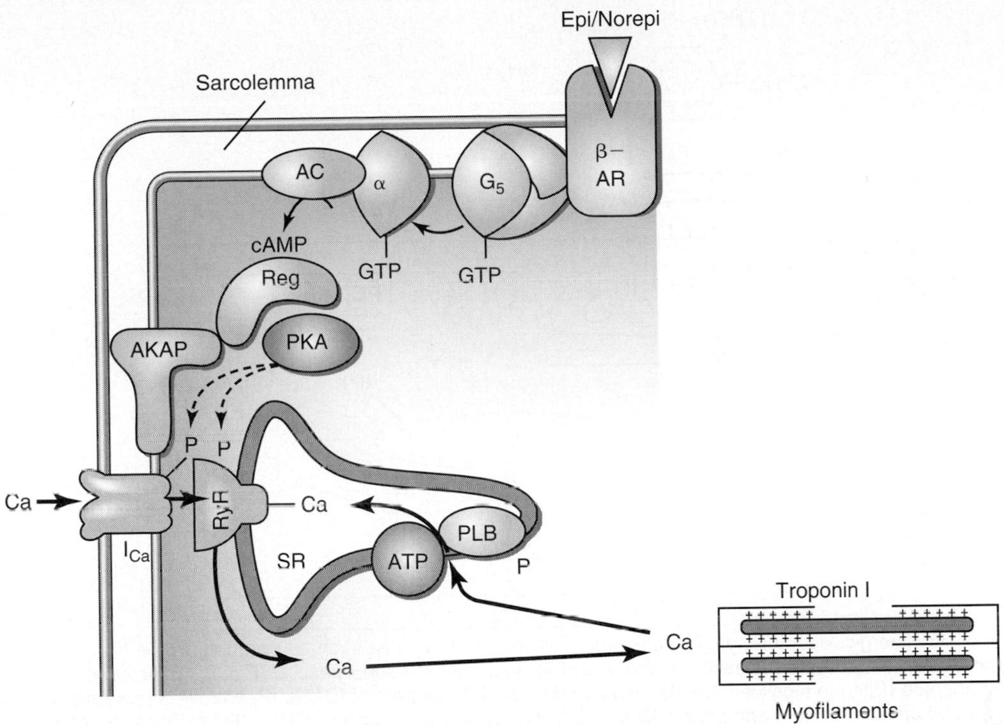

FIGURE 23–3 • β_1-Adrenergic receptor signaling cascade. Agonist (epinephrine/norepinephrine [Epi/Norepi]) to β-adrenergic receptor (β-AR) results in the α subunit binding to GTP, which activates adenylate cyclase (AC). AC then converts ATP to cyclic AMP (cAMP), which binds to regulatory unit (Reg) on protein kinase A (PKA). PKA then promotes an increase in the intracellular concentration of calcium (Ca) by acting on voltage-gated channels (I_{Ca}) and on the sarcoplasmic reticulum (SR). Calcium then promotes sarcomere contraction. See text for further details. *AKAP,* A kinase anchoring protein; *PLB,* phospholamban; *RyR,* ryanodine receptor. (From Bers DM: *Nature* 415:198, 2003.)

subtype to the control of vascular tone remain an active area of investigation. Each subtype may be expressed in all of the vascular beds, but one type is thought to predominate for a particular bed.[214] A mouse knockout model of the α_{1D} receptor showed that α_1 binding in the aorta was lost but preserved in the heart. The knockout model also had lower blood pressures and a decreased response to norepinephrine.[269] α_{1A} and α_{1B} are thought to be involved in both the heart and vasculature.[151] A knockout model of α_{1A} demonstrated decreased blood pressure and response to phenylephrine.[214] An animal model of overexpression of the α_{1A} receptor was associated with marked increase in cardiac contractility without a change in blood pressure or heart rate.[172] In a knockout model of α_{1B} receptors in mice, chronic exposure to norepinephrine did not lead to cardiac hypertrophy or vascular remodeling.[285] Overexpression of a mutant α_{1B} receptor led to increased expression of mitogen-activated protein kinases and decreased responsiveness to isoproterenol in isolated cardiac preparations.[51] Thus although α receptors may have an inotropic effect less than that of β-adrenergic receptors, they do have significant effects in the myocardium. Interestingly, in heart failure, down-regulation of β receptors has been noted but α receptors are preserved.[191] The α_1 receptor is coupled to the family of $G_{q/11}$ proteins, which act independently of cAMP. Signal transduction across this receptor is initiated by the activation of phospholipase C (PLC), which hydrolyzes phosphatidylinositol 4,5-biphosphate (PIP_2) to inositol 1,4,5-triphosphate ($InsP_3$) and 1,2-diacylglycerol (1,2-DG). $InsP_3$ binds to specific receptors on the sarcoplasmic reticulum, causing a release of calcium into the cytosol, and promotes movement of extracellular calcium into the cell. 1,2-DG with calcium activates PKC, which regulates movement of calcium into the cytosol (Figure 23–4). In vascular smooth muscle, medium light-chain kinase is activated as a result and phosphorylates myosin light-chain 2, leading to smooth muscle contraction.[260] A similar mechanism underlies the inotropic effect of the α_1 receptor in the myocardium.[10] The α_{1A} receptor appears to be the most efficiently coupled of the different subtypes.[271] The α_1 receptors also activate calcium influx through voltage-dependent and voltage-independent calcium channels.[192] The α receptors also promote activation of the mitogen-activated kinase family, which is a key regulator of cell growth.

Receptor Down-Regulation

The mechanisms described provide numerous sites at which the activity of the system can be modified, thereby affecting the sensitivity of target cells to both exogenous and endogenous catecholamines. Some of these receptor modifications are clinically important to the critical care physician. The best-documented type of modification involves agonist-mediated receptor desensitization. Exposure of receptors to agonists markedly reduces the sensitivity of the target cell to the agonist. Within seconds

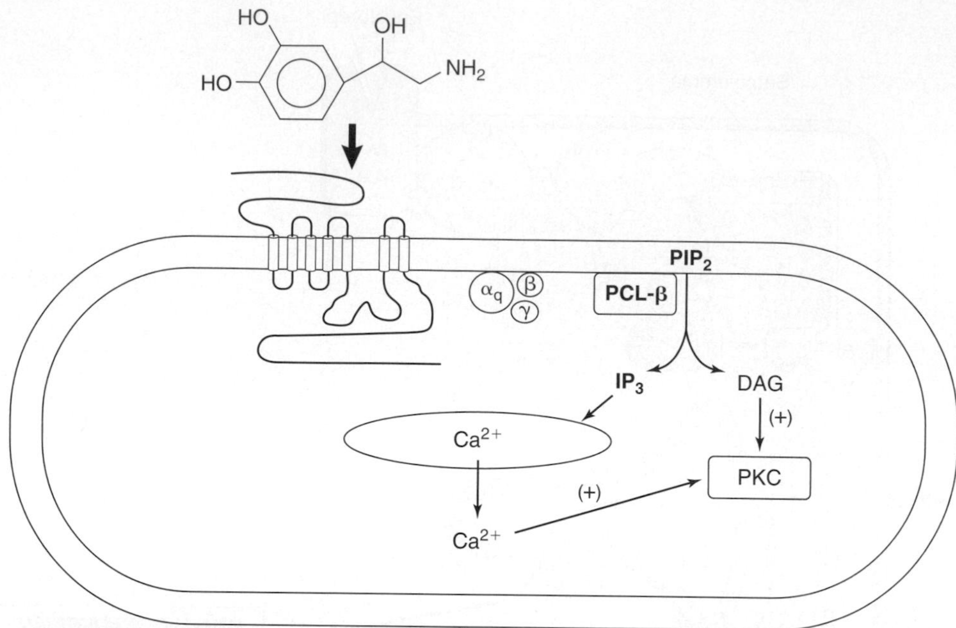

FIGURE 23–4 • α_1-Adrenergic receptor signaling cascade. Binding of an agonist such as norepinephrine to a G protein–coupled receptor activates the $G_{q/11}$ protein, leading to disassociation of the α and $\beta\gamma$ subunits. Phospholipase C (PLCβ-) is activated in turn and cleaves phosphatidylinositol 4,5-biphospate (PIP_2) to inositol 1,4,5-triphosphate (IP_3) and diacylglycerol (DAG). IP_3 and DAG promote an increase in intracellular calcium through the sarcoplasmic reticulum and protein kinase C (PKC). See text for further details. (From Zhong H, Minneman KP: *Eur J Pharm* 375:26, 1999.)

to minutes after agonist binding, the receptor may be uncoupled as a result of receptor phosphorylation. The receptor may be phosphorylated by PKA or PKC or by a member of the family of G receptor kinases (GRKs). These kinases, which include β-adrenergic receptor kinases 1 and 2, phosphorylate only receptors that have bound agonist. Compared with PKA and PKC, phosphorylation by GRKs enhances the ability of β arrestin, a cytosolic protein, or clathrin to bind to the receptor and disrupt further signaling. The role of GRKs has been established for β_1, β_2, and α_2 receptors.[164, 253] Sequestration of receptors within the target cell and degradation of sequestered receptors is another mechanism by which receptors are down-regulated. Desensitization of α_1 receptors has been extensively reviewed.[100] Homologous desensitization is mediated by GRKs, which are activated by soluble $G_{\beta\gamma}$ subunits and phosphatidylinositol biphosphate. As with the other adrenergic receptors, once phosphorylated, the receptors are internalized into vesicles. The α_1 receptors also demonstrate heterologous desensitization, in which a second messenger kinase, generated as a result of ligand binding, inactivates the receptor and prevents further signaling from the receptor. In addition to agonist-mediated desensitization, other stimuli have been implicated in down-regulation, including endotoxin, tumor necrosis factor, and congestive heart failure (CHF).[247] Lymphocyte β-adrenergic receptor density in children with CHF was reduced in proportion to the degree of elevation in plasma norepinephrine concentration.[296] Several pharmacologic agents, such as corticosteroids and ketotifen, are thought to up-regulate β-adrenergic receptors, and evidence indicates both immaturity and senescence are associated with β-adrenergic receptor desensitization.[47]

Polymorphisms

With the rapid advances in molecular biology, knowledge of polymorphisms within the genetic code has increased dramatically. Polymorphisms within the adrenergic receptors (Table 23–2) are reviewed briefly here. The reader is also directed toward a published comprehensive review.[251] Two polymorphisms have been described in the β_1 receptor. At position 49, glycine may be substituted for serine. The frequency of the minor allele gly is approximately 15%. In cell culture studies, the minor allele is associated with enhanced agonist-promoted down-regulation and increased affinity for agonists.[165] Another polymorphism occurs at position 389, where glycine may be substituted for arginine. This position is in the carboxy-terminus, a site involved with binding with the G protein. In a fibroblast cell line, the arginine alleles (wild-type) were observed to have higher levels of adenyl cyclase expression with agonist binding, representing more efficient coupling.[188] In a model using isolated human myocardial tissue, the wild-type allele (Arg389) was associated with enhanced inotropic potency in response to norepinephrine, although maximal force generated did not differ between the two alleles.[231] Another study demonstrated higher resting heart rates and diastolic blood pressure in patients with the Arg389 allele.[132] Three polymorphisms have been demonstrated in the β_2 receptor. Of note, at position 164 isoleucine may be substituted for threonine. This polymorphism is associated with a threefold decrease in affinity for agonist binding.[170] In a transfected cell line, the Ile164 type is associated with decreased basal adenyl cyclase activity and decreased activity after agonist stimulation.[278] Similar results were found in a study of patients heterozygous for the Ile164 allele. These patients had blunting of the

TABLE 23–2

Common Polymorphisms of Adrenergic Receptors

Receptor	Position		Alleles		Clinical Effect*
	Nucleotide	Amino Acid	Major	Minor	
$A_{1A}AR$	1441	492	Cysteine†	Arginine	
$A_{2A}AR$	753	251	Asparagine	Lysine	
$A_{2B}AR$	901-909	301-303		Deletion	
				Glutamic acid-Glutamic acid-Glutamic acid	
$A_{2C}AR$	964-975	322-325		Deletion	Minor allele associated with abnormal vasomotor regulation
				Glycine-Alanine Glycine-Proline	
β_1AR	145	49	Serine	Glycine	Minor allele associated with increased affinity for agonists
	1165	389	Arginine	Glycine	Major allele associated with more efficient coupling
β_2AR	46	16	Glycine	Arginine	
	79	27	Glutamine	Glutamic acid	
	491	164	Threonine	Isoleucine	Minor allele associated with decreased affinity for agonists
β_3AR	190	64	Tryptophan	Arginine	

*See text for details.
†In African Americans, arginine is a major allele.
Adopted from Small KM, McGraw DW, Liggett SB: *Annu Rev Pharmacol Toxicol* 43:381, 2003.

increase in both heart rate and duration of systole during terbutaline infusion with a trend toward lower systolic blood pressure.[46] A single polymorphism has been delineated in the α_1 receptor; it does not appear to have any clinical significance. A restriction fragment length polymorphism was identified in the gene for the α_{2C} receptor.[96] This polymorphism was associated with abnormal vasomotor regulation, sodium excretion, and platelet function. The presence of both the Arg389 β_1-receptor polymorphism and a deletion polymorphism in the α_{2C} receptor in black patients has been shown to increase the risk of heart failure.[252] This study is an example of the difficulty in linking genetic variations to the clinical scenario in that a single polymorphism may not have an effect except in the presence of another polymorphism. None of these particular polymorphisms has yet been shown to have a significant role in the pediatric intensive care unit (PICU), but they no doubt will continue to add in our understanding of the adrenergic pathways.

Vasopressin Receptors

Arginine vasopressin (AVP) is a nonpeptide hormone synthesized in the supraoptic and paraventricular nuclei of the hypothalamus. The three subtypes of vasopressin receptors are known as V_1, V_2, and V_3 (or V_{1b}). V_2 receptors are present in the renal collecting duct; V_1 receptors are located in the vascular bed, kidney, bladder, spleen, and hepatocytes, among other tissues.[129] AVP is released in response to small increases in plasma osmolality or large decreases in blood pressure or blood volume.[136] The plasma osmolality threshold for release of AVP is 280 mOsm/kg; above this level there is a steep linear relation between serum osmolality and AVP levels.[136] Changes of at least 20% in blood volume are needed to effect a change in AVP levels, although levels then may increase by 20- to 30-fold.[136] Hypovolemia also shifts the response curve for AVP to osmolar changes to the left and increases the slope of the curve (Figure 23–5). Vasopressin can produce vasoconstriction through V_1 receptors in the vascular bed (see later), but it also activates V_1 receptors in the central nervous system (CNS), including receptors in the area postrema.[118] This region is responsible for the reflex bradycardia seen with AVP infusion. This reflex attenuates the increase in blood pressure that would result from the vasoconstrictor effects of AVP.[177, 279] In fact, vasopressin causes a greater reduction in heart rate than do other vasoconstrictors.[129] Thus if this feedback loop is abolished, AVP induces a greater vasopressor response than do other agents.[118]

V_1 Receptors

Vasopressin receptors belong to the family of G protein–coupled receptors. V_1 receptors are coupled to G_q, and V_2 receptors are coupled to G_s.[136] When vasopressin binds to the V_1 receptor, PLC is activated with the eventual production of $InsP_3$ and 1,2-DG. These molecules increase the

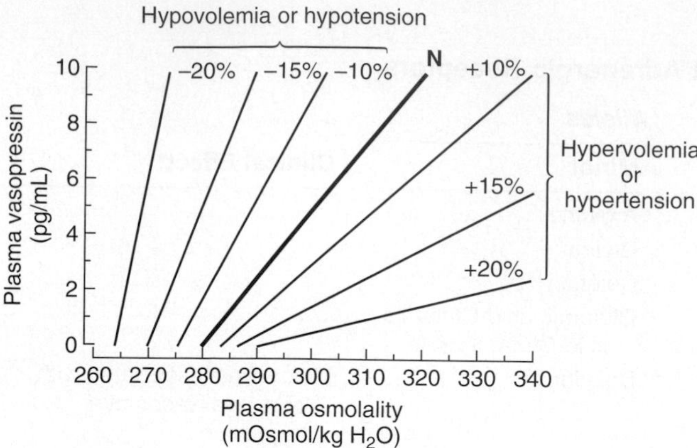

FIGURE 23–5 • Relationship between plasma vasopressin levels and plasma osmolality. As hypovolemia worsens, vasopressin levels increase for any given plasma osmolality. (Adapted from Robertson GL, Athar S, Shelton RL: Osmotic control of vasopressin function. In Androli TE, Grantham JJ, Rector FC Jr, editors: *Disturbances in body fluid osmolality.* Bethesda, MD, 1977, American Physiological Society.)

release of calcium from the endoplasmic reticulum and the entry of calcium through gated channels (Figure 23–6).[199] The increase in intracellular calcium leads to an increase in the activity of myosin light-chain kinase. This kinase acts upon myosin to increase the number of actin-myosin cross-bridges, enhancing contraction of the myocyte. Of note, vasopressin produces vasoconstriction in the skin, skeletal muscle, and fat while producing vasodilatation in the renal, pulmonary, and cerebral vasculature.[95] This effect may be mediated through nitric oxide or may be a function of the isoform of adenyl cyclase with which the receptor is coupled.[290] AVP increases the pressor effects of catecholamines,[24,146] although in two different vascular smooth muscle cell lines, AVP had opposing effects on isoproterenol-induced activation of adenyl cyclase.[290] Other effects of vasopressin binding to V_1 receptors are shown in Figure 23–6.

AVP may increase vascular tone by interacting with so-called ATP-sensitive potassium channels termed K_{ATP}.[288]

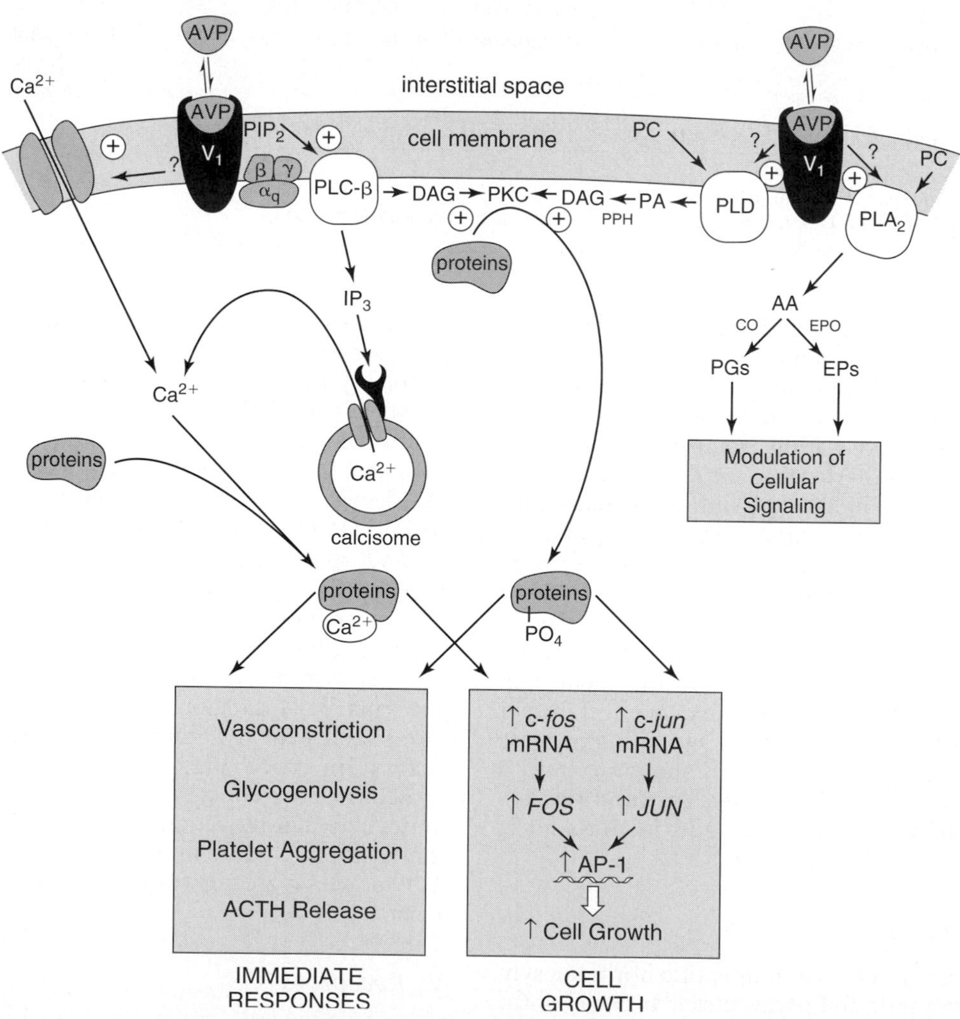

FIGURE 23–6 • V_1 receptor signaling cascade. Binding of arginine vasopressin (AVP) to the V_1 vasopressin receptor (V_1) leads to activation of phospholipase C (PLC-β) via the Gq protein with the production of inositol 1,4,5-triphosphate (IP_3). IP_3 promotes an increase in intracellular calcium, resulting in figure. *AA,* Arachidonic acid; *AP-1,* transcription factor consisting of heterodimer of FOS and JUN; *CO,* cyclooxygenase; *DAG,* diacylglycerol; *EPO,* epoxygense; *EPs,* epoxyeicosatrienoic acids; *PA,* phosphatidic acid; *PC,* phosphatidylcholine; *PGs,* prostaglandins; *PIP_2,* phosphatidylinositol 4,5-biphosphate; *PKC,* protein kinase C; *PLA_2,* phospholipase A_2; *PLD,* phospholipase D; *PPH,* phosphatidate phosphohydrolase. "?" indicates the mechanism of coupling is unclear. (From Jackson EK: Vasopressin and other agents affecting the renal conservation of water. In Hardman JG, Limbird LE, editors: *Goodman and Gilman's the pharmacologic basis of therapeutics,* ed 10. New York, 2001, McGraw Hill.)

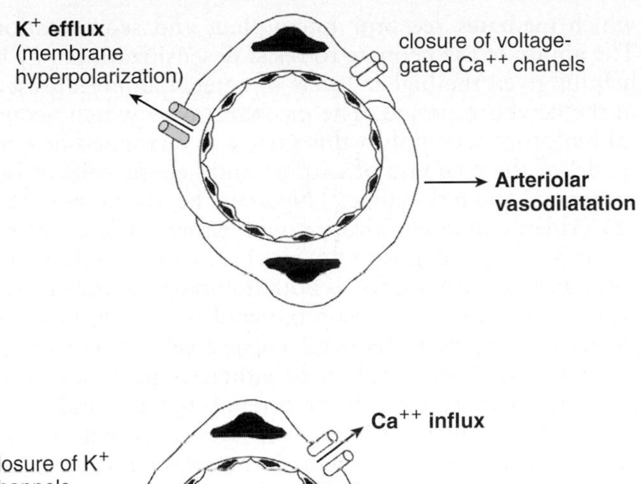

FIGURE 23–7 • K^+ channels vascular tone. Diffusion of K^+ through open K_{ATP} channels in vascular smooth muscle cell results in membrane hyperpolarization, closure of voltage-gated Ca^{2+} channels, and decreased intracellular calcium, resulting in vasodilatation. Closing of K_{ATP} channels has the opposite effects. (From Jackson W: *Hypertension* 35:173, 2000.)

Activation of K_{ATP} channels hyperpolarizes the cell, closes calcium channels, and prevents contraction.[45,157] The result may be protection of the cell.[303] AVP can induce PKC, which in turn inhibits the K_{ATP} channel when the cellular concentration of ATP is low.[276] Inhibition of K_{ATP} channels allows for cell depolarization and calcium entry, resulting in vasoconstriction (Figure 23–7).[137] V_1 receptors also have a weak positive inotropic effect in the heart, although the clinical significance of this finding has not been established.[53]

Receptor Down-Regulation

As with adrenergic receptors, vasopressin receptors undergo down-regulation. AVP promotes the phosphorylation of its own receptor immediately after binding. The receptor is removed from the cell surface within 3 minutes after binding.[36] As with adrenergic receptors, G protein–coupled receptor kinases catalyze phosphorylation of the receptor. PKC also mediates this reaction and may serve as the means by which other agents down-regulate the vasopressin receptor in a heterologous manner.[36]

Polymorphisms

Although numerous mutations in the V_2 receptor exist and result in nephrogenic diabetes insipidus, much less is known about the V_1 receptor. One study established two polymorphisms in the V_1 receptor gene but failed to establish a linkage with hypertension.[272]

Phosphodiesterase Regulation of Cyclic Adenosine Monophosphate

Phosphodiesterases are a class of enzyme that catalyze the hydrolysis of cAMP and cyclic guanosine monophosphate (cGMP) into AMP and GMP, respectively. Therefore, these enzymes can down-regulate the signals transduced by cAMP, such as PKA activity (see earlier). There are several families of this enzyme, each with subtypes. Phosphodiesterase III (PDE3) is present in many cell types, including cardiac myocytes, vascular smooth muscle cells, adipocytes, platelets, and pancreatic islet cells. PDE3 has a much higher V_{max} for cAMP than it does for cGMP and therefore is functionally a cAMP esterase.[81] Different isoforms of PDE3 are present in cardiac (PDE3A1) and vascular smooth muscle cells (PDE3A2) and are localized to different cellular compartments. As such they are able to regulate the function of their target enzymes in response to particular cellular signals.[198] The C-terminus of the enzyme codes for the central catalytic core that is the active binding site and the N-terminus coding region may determine cellular targeting.[198] The bipyridines, such as milrinone, are competitive inhibitors of PDE3,[93,234] that is, they bind to PDE3, preventing the enzyme from binding to cAMP. They appear to bind near the binding site for cAMP, although different PDE3 inhibitors may have different binding sites.[309] Inhibition of PDE3 produces an increase in cAMP. This increase in cAMP results in a positive inotropic effect in the myocardium and vasodilatation in the systemic and pulmonary vasculature.[245] In contrast, methylxanthines such as theophylline, which inhibit all phosphodiesterases, cause cGMP (thought to decrease contractility) and cAMP levels to increase. This dual increase attenuates their inotropic effects. Bipyridines may also enhance contractility by increasing the sensitivity of myofilaments to cytosolic calcium.[56] Milrinone enhances the sarcomere uptake of calcium and thereby augments left ventricular (LV) relaxation (lusitropy).[300] In the peripheral vasculature, PD3 inhibitors may produce vasodilatation via a cGMP mechanism.[150] The bipyridines offer the combination of positive inotropy, lusitropy, and afterload reduction. Long-term exposure to PDE inhibitors has been speculated to result in adrenergic receptor desensitization via heterologous desensitization but has not been demonstrated clinically.[40]

ATPase Inhibition

Membrane-bound sodium/potassium adenosine triphosphatase (Na/K-ATPase) is responsible for maintaining electrochemical gradients across the cellular membrane. It does so by extruding three molecules of sodium from and incorporating two molecules of potassium into the cell, both against their respective concentration gradients. This process occurs at the cost of one molecule of ATP. The enzyme consists of an α and β subunit; there are four α subtypes and three β subunits.[236] The β subunit may be involved in enzyme trafficking.[92] The α subunit contains both the binding site and catalytic site.[236] The isoforms expressed are dependent on the type of tissue.[289] The putative mechanism of action of the cardiac glycosides is inhibition of the Na/K-ATPase pump, which results in increased intracellular sodium. The elevated level of intracellular sodium then effects a decrease in the activity of the sodium/calcium exchange pump (NCX). This pump exchanges three molecules of extracellular sodium for one molecule of intracellular calcium.[15,244] The net result is a rise in intracellular calcium and, in the cardiac myocyte, enhanced contractility. The particular α isoform expressed may affect the function of the enzyme. In a mouse knockout model, animals heterozygous for α_1 ($\alpha_1^{-/+}$) and α_2 ($\alpha_2^{-/+}$) were generated.[139] The cardiac myocytes from α_2 heterozygous animals demonstrated a hypercontractile state compared with controls (similar to that seen with administration of cardiac glycosides). In contrast, the α_1 heterozygous animals had a hypocontractile state. The authors note that this phenotype is similar to that seen with cardiac glycoside toxicity. Although the classic explanation has been described, the precise mechanism for the increase in intracellular calcium with Na/K-ATPase inhibition remains controversial. Some studies have demonstrated a rise in intracellular calcium without the expected, concomitant rise in intracellular sodium,[14,109] suggesting that perhaps the NCX pump was not involved. In contrast, a study of mice lacking the NCX pump demonstrated that ouabain (an Na/K-ATPase inhibitor) did not increase intracellular calcium.[224,283] No evidence suggests the development of tolerance to digoxin with long-term use.[235]

Developmental Issues

It is often stated that the immature myocardium is less sensitive to inotropic agents than the adult heart. The exact nature of the mechanism responsible for these differences represents an area of active investigation. The majority of studies involve animal models or isolated human tissue. As there are inherent differences between intact healthy animal models and the ill child, as well as pharmacokinetic differences between the infant and adult patient,[40] caution must be exercised when extrapolating laboratory data to the bedside. Nonetheless, a brief review of developmental differences is appropriate.

There are age-related differences in the response of the developing myocardium to inotropic agents, receptor regulation, and calcium handling.[15,39] In puppy heart models, the inotropic response to dopamine and isoproterenol increases with increasing age.[83,227] Maximal developed pressure and relaxation velocity in response to isoproterenol were higher in adult rabbit hearts compared with neonatal hearts.[233] However, in a model of rat ventricular myocytes, zinterol (a selective β_2 agonist) increased intracellular calcium gradients and cAMP accumulation and augmented cell shortening in neonatal myocytes at much lower concentrations than in adult myocytes.[153] Sun[267] showed in a rabbit model that isolated adult hearts had a greater increase in systolic function in response to isoproterenol than neonatal hearts but that the response to continuous infusions was less attenuated in the neonatal hearts, suggesting less desensitization. In another study, neonatal rat hearts did not show any evidence of homologous uncoupling in response to isoproterenol.[308] In fact, the receptors demonstrated an enhanced response after prolonged exposure to agonist. This process occurred despite increased activity of β-adrenergic receptor kinase-1, which mediates receptor uncoupling and sequestration. The ability of the neonate to resist desensitization may be helpful given the higher levels of catecholamines present in the newborn period. The mechanism by which neonatal receptors accomplish this goal was examined in a rat model of the response of cardiac and hepatic cells to isoproterenol and terbutaline.[16] Neonatal hearts did not show any evidence of desensitization with either single injections of, or prolonged exposure to, isoproterenol or terbutaline. Adult hearts had evidence of both homologous and heterologous desensitization to isoproterenol but not terbutaline. In marked contrast, neonatal hepatic cells demonstrated homologous desensitization to either single doses of, or prolonged exposure to, isoproterenol and terbutaline. In fact, there was increased sensitivity to agents that increase adenyl cyclase through nonadrenergic mechanisms. These findings suggest the resistance of neonatal myocytes to desensitization is the result of processes downstream from the adrenergic receptor and may involve developmental changes in the expression of adenyl cyclase isoforms or the compartmentalization of PKA activity.

Another area of difference is the handling of intracellular calcium. In the adult heart, the majority of released calcium is derived from the sarcoplasmic reticulum, but this is less so in the neonatal heart.[15] Calcium flux across the sarcolemma is the predominant source of calcium utilized in excitation-contraction coupling. Neonatal rabbit hearts express more NCX protein than do adult hearts. With maturation, expression of NCX decreases, accompanied by enhanced contractility. In addition, differences between neonatal and adult hearts could be demonstrated on the concentration-response curves for ouabain (dP/dt min) and calcium (dP/dt min), but not for isoproterenol.[233] An experimental agent that blocks the NCX did not increase contractility in the neonatal heart, although it did have an inotropic effect on adult myocardium.[233] The role of voltage-gated calcium channels as the source of intracellular calcium in the neonatal myocardium is unclear. Studies suggest these channels are the major source of intracellular calcium[119,176] although their exact role is unclear.[15]

Developmental differences may exist in the expression of PDE isoforms. In a model of rabbit ventricular myocytes, administration of IBMX (a nonselective PDE inhibitor) and rolipram (PDE type IV inhibitor) increased intracellular calcium currents in the neonatal cells both at baseline and in response to isoproterenol but not in the adult cells. In contrast, milrinone (PDE type III inhibitor) increased intracellular calcium currents at baseline and in response to isoproterenol only in the adult cells.[1] Thus it appears that PDE type IV may be the dominant isoenzyme that regulates intracellular calcium currents in the neonatal myocardium.

Developmental changes may involve the peripheral vascular system. In developing swine, Gootman[110] found that the peripheral vascular response to several adrenergic agonists developed at different rates and that complete reflex integration was not present at birth. He predicted that overall responses to stress or to treatment with these agents would be age dependent. Gootman's physiologic studies are complemented by receptor-binding studies indicating developmental changes in the adrenergic receptor content of a variety of organs, although later work indicates lymphocyte β-adrenergic receptors are fully mature and functional at birth.[42,292] There are also structural and ultrastructural differences between immature and mature hearts. These differences include reduced ventricular compliance, greater ventricular interdependence, and a reduction in the ratio of myocardial contractile to noncontractile protein in the immature heart. The net effect is that the immature myocardium neither responds to nor tolerates volume loading as well as the adult heart. In addition to this diminished "preload reserve," the baseline heart rate of infants and children is high. This finding limits the extent to which tachycardia can augment cardiac output before diastolic filling is compromised.

The combination of impaired preload reserve, limited chronotropic reserve, and reduced sensitivity of the heart and peripheral vasculature to adrenergic agents implies that the response of the immature organism to infusion of inotropic and vasopressor agents differs from the pattern noted in adults.[98,213]

Sympathomimetic Amines

Virtually all sympathomimetics currently used to treat hemodynamic problems are catecholamines. This class includes the endogenous compounds epinephrine, norepinephrine, and dopamine and the synthetic products isoproterenol and dobutamine. Catecholamines have a β-phenylethylamine core with hydroxyl (OH) substituents at the 3 and 4 aromatic ring positions (Figure 23–8). Minor differences in molecular substitution about the N-terminus or the α or β carbon produce marked differences in activity. Structure-activity relationships are complex for the catecholamines and have been reviewed.[125] It is possible to generalize by noting that increasing size of the substituent on the amino group enhances β-adrenergic activity, whereas decreasing size is associated with α-adrenergic selectivity. Tyrosine serves as the base compound for catecholamine synthesis. Tyrosine hydroxylase catalyzes the conversion of tyrosine to dopa, which undergoes decarboxylation, producing dopamine. Dopamine β-hydroxylase converts dopamine to norepinephrine. In the adrenal medulla, norepinephrine is converted to epinephrine by N-methyl transferase (Figure 23–9).

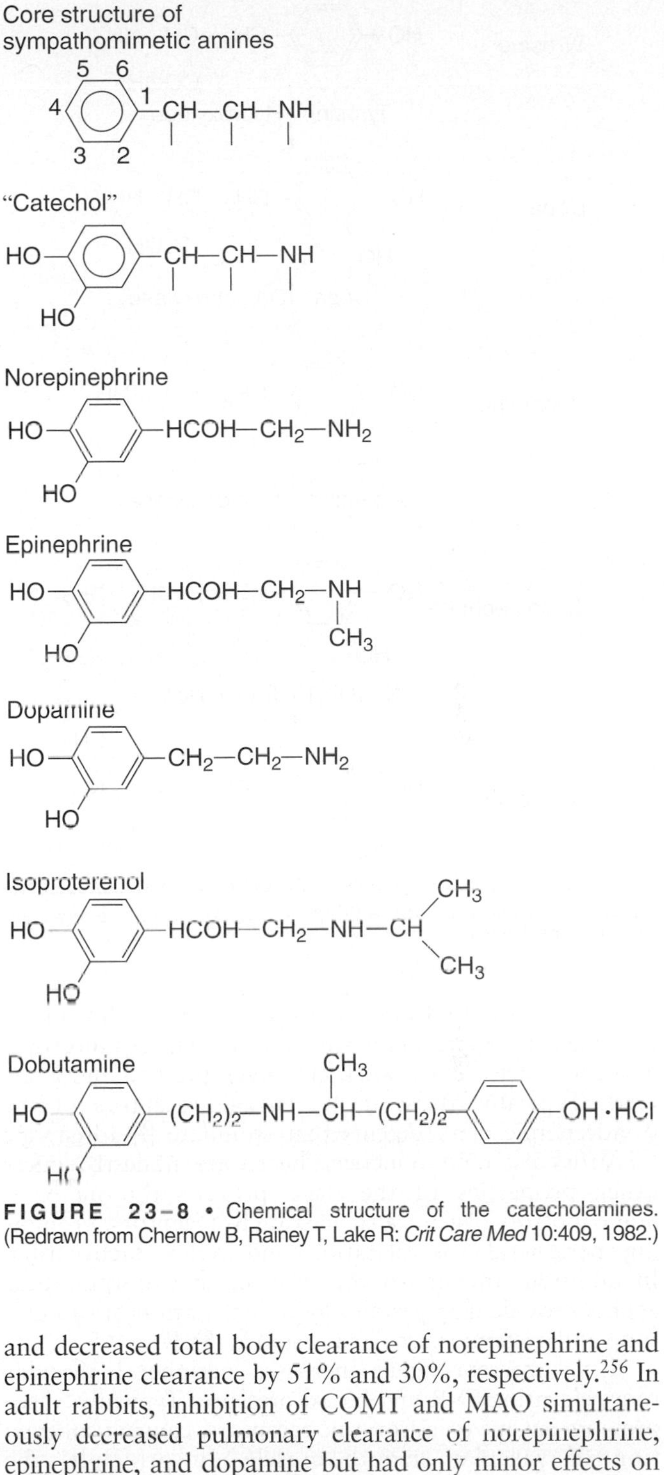

Catecholamines are subject to several different elimination processes.[150] Infused dopamine provides an example in which elimination occurs through a variety of processes. A small proportion is excreted unchanged in the urine. A proportion likely undergoes neuronal reuptake. The principal means of elimination appears to be O-methylation by catechol O-methyltransferase (COMT) to form metanephrines, followed by either sulfoconjugation (by phenolsulfotransferase) or by deamination (by monoamine oxidase [MAO]) to homovanillic acid.[203] Substitution at the α carbon determines the rate of deamination by MAO.[262] The contribution of these pathways to total body clearance of catecholamines varies with age and the particular circulatory bed. In newborn lambs, the lungs accounted for 35% of the total body clearance of norepinephrine and 15% of the clearance of epinephrine. Inhibition of MAO by desipramine decreased pulmonary clearance to near zero

FIGURE 23–8 • Chemical structure of the catecholamines. (Redrawn from Chernow B, Rainey T, Lake R: *Crit Care Med* 10:409, 1982.)

and decreased total body clearance of norepinephrine and epinephrine clearance by 51% and 30%, respectively.[256] In adult rabbits, inhibition of COMT and MAO simultaneously decreased pulmonary clearance of norepinephrine, epinephrine, and dopamine but had only minor effects on total body clearance.[97] Inhibition of COMT did not change extracellular levels of catecholamines in the CNS.[168] Furthermore, individual differences in COMT activity are not well correlated with dopamine clearance.[5] The liver and gut clear between 30% and 52% of the circulating norepinephrine and epinephrine.[61,89] Processes or drugs that disturb these routes of elimination likely decrease the overall metabolic clearance of catecholamines. Organ dysfunction associated with critical illness increases the blood concentration of dopamine during a given infusion rate of the compound. For example, with liver dysfunction the clearance of dopamine is reduced.[203]

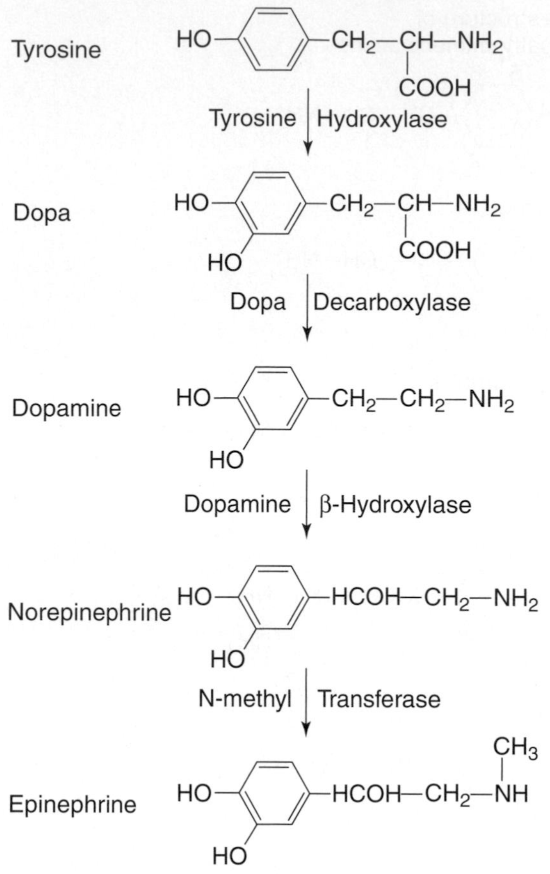

Tyrosine — HO–C_6H_4–CH_2–CH(NH_2)–COOH

Tyrosine Hydroxylase

Dopa — (HO)$_2$$C_6H_3$–$CH_2$–CH($NH_2$)–COOH

Dopa Decarboxylase

Dopamine — (HO)$_2$$C_6H_3$–$CH_2$–$CH_2$–$NH_2$

Dopamine β-Hydroxylase

Norepinephrine — (HO)$_2$$C_6H_3$–HCOH–$CH_2$–$NH_2$

N-methyl Transferase

Epinephrine — (HO)$_2$$C_6H_3$–HCOH–$CH_2$–NH–$CH_3$

FIGURE 23–9 • Biosynthetic pathways of the endogenous catecholamines. (Redrawn from Chernow B, Rainey T, Lake R: *Crit Care Med* 10:409, 1982.)

It is practical to divide the properties of catecholamines into their inotropic and vasopressor effects. An inotropic agent increases stroke work at a given preload and afterload. Typically, these agents engage receptors of the β_1-adrenergic class. Agents that stimulate β_1-adrenergic receptors also tend to increase heart rate modestly, unless other properties of the drug prevent the increase. Some inotropic agents also activate β_2 receptors, promoting peripheral vasodilatation and reflex tachycardia. In addition, the improvement in cardiac output these agents provide may permit a reflex relaxation of vascular tone and systemic vascular resistance (SVR).

A vasopressor agent increases peripheral vascular tone, elevating SVR and blood pressure. Typically, vasopressors engage α_1-adrenergic receptors, causing contraction of vascular smooth muscle. In principle, the physician uses a vasopressor agent to treat peripheral vascular failure and an inotropic agent when the major problem is impaired cardiac contractility. In practice, most available agents display a blend of inotropic, chronotropic, and vasopressor activity. Norepinephrine has both inotropic and vasopressor effects, although it is most commonly used as a vasopressor agent. Phenylephrine (a noncatecholamine) has considerable specificity for the α-adrenergic receptor, so it is almost a pure pressor. Isoproterenol and dobutamine have little α-adrenergic agonist activity but considerable activity at the β receptor; they are used mostly as inotropes. Epinephrine and dopamine have both inotropic and vasopressor activity. At relatively low infusion rates, they enhance myocardial function and increase heart rate (β_1 and β_2). At higher rates, pressor activity (α_1) becomes manifest.

Dopamine

Basic Pharmacology

In the enzymatic pathway leading from tyrosine to epinephrine (see Figure 23–9), decarboxylation transforms L-dopa to dopamine. Dopamine is a central neurotransmitter. It also is found in sympathetic nerve terminals and in the adrenal medulla, where it is the immediate precursor of norepinephrine. In healthy individuals, plasma levels of dopamine range from 50 to 100 pg/ml.

Clinical Pharmacology

Dopamine simulates dopamine (D_1 and D_2) receptors located in the brain and in vascular beds in the kidney, mesentery, and coronary arteries (Table 23–3).[106] It also stimulates α and β receptors, although the compound's affinity for these receptors is lower. D_1 receptors are coupled to G_s and thus enhance adenylate cyclase and produce a rise in cAMP, which evokes vasodilatation. This increases blood flow to these organs and may enhance renal solute and water excretion by the kidney. Dopamine modulates release of aldosterone and prolactin (D_2 receptors), which also may affect renal solute clearance.[281] The physiologic role of dopamine has been extensively reviewed.[125,238]

In healthy adult volunteers, infusion rates between 1 and 10 μg/kg/min increase stroke volume and cardiac output without major effect on heart rate or blood pressure.[28,105,294] These infusion rates are associated with plasma concentrations of 50 to 100 ng/ml. Low infusion rates augment renal sodium excretion; intermediate rates (10 μg/kg/min) produce chronotropic and inotropic effects, and still higher infusion rates increase vascular resistance.[305] Renal blood flow, glomerular filtration rate, and sodium excretion are maintained or even increase during dopamine infusion in patients with poor cardiac output. Work by Gundert-Remy in healthy adults indicated that even at a relatively low infusion rate of 400 μg/min (5–6 μg/kg/min), significant augmentation of heart rate and blood pressure likely plays a role in improved renal function.[113]

Evidence for the view that infants display reduced sensitivity to dopamine is not conclusive. In support of reduced sensitivity, Perez and associates[212] found that in critically ill neonates, infusion rates of 50 μg/kg/min did not cause clinically evident impairment of cutaneous or renal perfusion. Some experimental evidence also indicates diminished sensitivity to dopamine in infants; however, this finding is limited to studies of immature animals. A contrary observation was made by Padbury et al.,[209] who measured cardiac output in a group of infants and found that mean blood pressure increased at doses of 0.5 to 1 μg/kg/min, whereas heart rate increased beyond 2 to 3 μg/kg/min. Cardiac output and stroke volume increased before heart rate, and SVR did not change within the range of dopamine infusion rates (0.5–8 μg/kg/min). The threshold values obtained were 14 ± 3.5 ng/ml for increase in mean blood

TABLE 23–3

Major Hemodynamic Effects of Adrenergic Receptor Activation by Catecholamines

	Receptor			
Agent	α_1	β_1	β_2	D_1
Dopamine*	Vasoconstriction; ↑ SVR, PVR	Inotropy; chronotropy	Vasodilation	Vasodilation (renal)
Norepinephrine	Vasoconstriction; ↑ SVR, PVR	Inotropy (minor)	—	—
Epinephrine†	Vasoconstriction; ↑ SVR, PVR	Inotropy; chronotropy	Vasodilation	—
Isoproterenol	—	Inotropy	Vasodilation	—
Dobutamine	See text	Inotropy	—	—
Amrinone/milrinone	Nonreceptor-mediated inotropy and vasodilation			

D_1, Dopamine receptor; *SVR*, systemic vascular resistance; *PVR*, pulmonary vascular resistance.
*Dose related. At low infusion rates, D_1 receptor effects predominate; at intermediate rates, β_1 and β_2 receptor effects predominate; and at high rates, α receptor effects predominate.
†Dose related. At low infusion rates, β receptor effects predominate; at high rates, α receptor effects predominate.
Adapted from Notterman DA: *Prob Anesth* 3:288, 1989.

pressure, 18 ± 4.5 ng/ml for increase in systolic blood pressure, and 35 ± 5 ng/ml for increase in heart rate. The steady-state concentration at infusion rates between 1 and 2 μg/kg/min was 16.5 ± 3.4 ng/ml. Thus newborns may exhibit clinical response at doses as low as 0.5 to 1 μg/kg/min. Seri et al.[239] demonstrated an increase in blood pressure without a change in heart rate in premature infants. Doses ranged from 2.5 to 7.5 μg/kg/min. Interestingly, in this study, a greater increase in blood pressure was associated with a lower gestational age. The authors attributed this finding to the enhanced α-adrenergic sensitivity of the immature myocardium.

Infused dopamine crosses the blood-brain barrier in preterm neonates but was shown not to increase blood flow velocity in the middle cerebral artery.[239] Dopamine inhibits the release of prolactin, thyrotropin, growth hormone, and the gonadotropins, but the clinical significance of these effects is unclear.[58,226,239] Low infusion rates of dopamine are frequently used to augment renal function during critical illness.[104] Although evidence indicates this method may increase the fractional excretion of sodium and the creatinine clearance,[133] a large, randomized, double-blind placebo control study of low-dose dopamine (2 μg/kg/min) administered to critically ill patients at risk of renal failure did not show any benefits.[27] The study group and the control group did not differ in peak creatinine concentration, need for renal replacement therapy, length of intensive care unit (ICU) or hospital stay, or mortality. Seri et al.[239] demonstrated increased urine output among premature infants associated with increased blood pressure and decreased renal vascular resistance with dopamine, although they did not take into account the role of postnatal physiologic changes in urine volume. Use of low-dose dopamine in pediatric and neonatal ICUs to augment renal function is not uncommon despite the lack of evidence suggesting a beneficial effect.[217]

Pharmacokinetics

Plasma dopamine clearance ranges from 60 to 80 ml/kg/min in normal adults and is lower in patients with renal or hepatic disease.[141,203] In subjects with normal renal function, the elimination half-life of infused dopamine is approximately 2 minutes.[179] Among critically ill children, the elimination half life is 26 ± 14 minutes,[91] and in neonates the elimination half-life is 5 to 11 minutes.[80] Age has a striking effect on clearance of dopamine, and clearance in children younger than 2 years is approximately twice as rapid as the rate in older children (82 vs. 46 ml/kg/min).[203] Wide interindividual variations in the rate of dopamine clearance have been reported in critically ill children[29] as well as in healthy adults.[178] Dopamine clearance also may decrease after 24 hours of continuous infusion.[5] Allen et al.[5] confirmed that during the first 20 months of life, clearance of infused dopamine decreased by almost 50%, with an additional 50% decrease from ages 1 to 12 years. Another study did not show a correlation between age and dopamine clearance, although the patients in this study had a mean age of 37 months.[29] Age-related differences in COMT activity cannot account for the higher dopamine clearance values exhibited in neonates.[5] Banner et al.[21] studied the pharmacokinetics of infused dopamine in 15 patients ranging in age from 3 days to 8 years and noted nonlinear behavior, possibly resulting from saturable plasma protein binding in neonates. Although dopamine clearance correlated significantly with body weight, the authors questioned the utility of evaluating total body clearance in this age group. Differences in the rate of sulfoconjugation[29] as a route of elimination also may contribute to the wide variations in the clearance of dopamine in critically ill children.[5,203] The possible role of concomitantly administered dobutamine on the clearance of dopamine has been suggested by some authors,[91] but an in vitro study showed that although dopamine and dobutamine are competitors for both COMT and MAO, the concentrations achieved under clinical situations are unlikely to produce clinically significant levels of inhibition.[299] A pharmacokinetic difference between children and infants, rather than a difference in receptors or myocardial sensitivity, may account for the observation that infants require and tolerate higher infusion rates. Dopamine crosses the human placenta, but the effect on the fetus is not known. The pharmacokinetics of dopamine and other cardiovascular drugs has been reviewed.[263]

Clinical Role

Clinicians use dopamine to enhance renal function and to exploit its inotropic and vasopressor properties. Dopamine has been shown to be an effective inotropic and vasopressor agent in neonates and infants with a variety of conditions associated with circulatory failure, including hyaline membrane disease, asphyxia, sepsis syndrome, and cyanotic congenital heart disease.[240,306] There are very few trials of pharmacologic therapy for hypotension in the neonate. Osborn et al.[207] found that although dopamine increases blood pressure, dobutamine produced a greater increase in blood flow as judged by superior vena cava flow. Four other trials showed that dopamine was more effective than dobutamine in treating hypotension, but there was no difference in mortality.[265] Fewer data evaluating the efficacy of dopamine in older children are available. However, it remains a mainstay of pharmacologic support for the child with inadequate perfusion. Dopamine is recommended as the first-line agent for children with fluid refractory septic shock[50] and has been recommended for adults as well,[287] but this topic is debated.[241] Dopamine also may be appropriate for children with mild impairment of myocardial function and hypotension after resuscitation from cardiac arrest.[9,280] Severe impairment of vascular tone or cardiac contractility suggest the need for other agents. Children with primary myocardial disease not complicated by frank hypotension will benefit from a more selective inotropic agent such as dobutamine or milrinone. Infusion rates of dopamine needed to improve signs of severe myocardial dysfunction may be associated with troublesome tachycardia or dysrhythmia and may increase myocardial oxygen consumption disproportionately to myocardial perfusion.

Although dopamine is used extensively following cardiac surgery,[291] reports indicate that dopamine is less effective following cardiac surgery in infants than in older children or adults. Lang et al.[158] treated five children with dopamine following cardiac surgery. For the group as a whole, hemodynamic improvement did not occur at infusion rates less than 15 μg/kg/min. Any increase in cardiac output was attributed to an increase in heart rate rather than to improved stroke volume. Another study indicated that following cardiac surgery, dopamine and dobutamine have similar inotropic efficacy but that dopamine was associated with pulmonary vasoconstriction at dosages greater than 7 μg/kg/min in the absence of α-adrenergic blockade.[41] Dopamine 10 μg/kg/min improved right ventricular (RV) function after RV injury in a young swine model.[189] Increased RV ejection fraction with a decrease in end-systolic RV volume was noted in premature hypotensive infants treated with dopamine.[63] To treat shock associated with hypotension, therapy is initiated at an infusion rate of 5 to 10 μg/kg/min. The rate of infusion is increased in steps of 2 to 5 μg/kg/min, guided by evidence of improved blood flow (skin temperature, capillary refill, sensorium, urine output) and by restoration of a blood pressure that is appropriate for age. Infusion rates greater than 25 to 30 μg/kg/min of dopamine are not customary, even if they maintain a "normal" blood pressure. At infusion rates of this magnitude, the effect on blood pressure likely represents an increase in SVR (α-adrenergic activation) rather than cardiac output. A requirement for a dopamine infusion of this magnitude suggests the physician should reexamine the physiologic diagnosis or select a different agent, such as epinephrine or norepinephrine.

Adverse Effects

Dopamine toxicity is mainly cardiovascular: tachycardia, hypertension, and dysrhythmia. Dopamine is less likely to produce severe tachycardia or dysrhythmias than either epinephrine or isoproterenol.[125] With the possible exception of the bipyridines, all inotropes increase myocardial oxygen consumption because they increase myocardial work. If the resulting increase in oxygen consumption is balanced by improved coronary blood flow, the net effect on oxygen balance is beneficial. When shock is caused or complicated by myocardial disease, improved myocardial contractility may reduce preload and afterload, improve coronary perfusion pressure (increase oxygen supply), and prolong diastolic coronary perfusion by reducing heart rate. If the same drug is administered to a patient with normal myocardial contractility, the result may be increased cardiac oxygen consumption without increased oxygen delivery to the myocardium. Tachycardia, by both increasing oxygen consumption and shortening diastole, is a particular burden. Thus the effect of dopamine on myocardial oxygen balance is better than that of isoproterenol, but not as good as dobutamine, amrinone, and milrinone.[20] Dopamine depresses the ventilatory response to hypoxemia and hypercarbia by as much as 60%.[163] Dopamine (and other β agonists) decrease PaO_2 by interfering with hypoxic vasoconstriction.[223] In one study, dopamine increased intrapulmonary shunting in patients with acute respiratory distress syndrome (ARDS) from 27% to 40%.[163] The effect of dopamine on perfusion to the splanchnic bed is widely debated. Evidence suggests that dopamine increases splanchnic blood flow during sepsis[175] and after cardiac surgery,[273] increases gastric pH,[246] and leads to less lactate production than epinephrine.[71] However, dopamine may increase blood flow or oxygen delivery but reduce oxygen consumption in sepsis.[116,138] In infants and children who have undergone cardiac surgery, dopamine may have several endocrinologic effects. Prolactin levels are decreased, the pulsatility of growth hormone is decreased in infants, and thyrotropin levels are decreased.[281] Dopamine can cause or worsen limb ischemia, gangrene of distal parts and entire extremities, and extensive loss of skin.[202] Infusion rates as low as 1.5 μg/kg/min have been associated with limb loss. Because dopamine promotes release of norepinephrine from synaptic terminals (and is also converted to norepinephrine in vivo), it is more often associated with limb ischemia than other adrenergic compounds. Extravasations of dopamine should be treated immediately by local infiltration with a solution of phentolamine (Regitine, 5–10 mg in 10 ml of normal saline) administered with a fine hypodermic needle.[248]

Preparation and Administration

Dopamine hydrochloride is available in 5-ml vials at concentrations of 40, 80, and 160 mg/ml, and as 250-ml or

TABLE 23–4

Method for Preparing Vasoactive Infusions in Pediatric Patients

Drug	Preparation	Infusion Rate	Maximum Concentration	Drug
Isoproterenol Epinephrine Norepinephrine Milrinone	**0.6** mg × body weight (kg), added to diluent to make 100 ml	1 ml/hour delivers **0.1** μg • kg^{-1}• min^{-1}	6.4 mg/100 ml 24 mg/100 ml 12.8 mg/100 ml 40 mg/100 ml	Isoproterenol Epinephrine Norepinephrine Milrinone
Dopamine Dobutamine Amrinone*	**6** mg × body weight (kg), added to diluent to make 100 ml	1 ml/hour delivers **1** μg • kg^{-1}• min^{-1}	1280 mg/100 ml 800 mg/100 ml	Dopamine Dobutamine Amrinone

*Not compatible with dextrose.
Adapted from Zaritsky A, Chernow B. *J Pediatr* 105:341, 1984.

500-ml premixed solutions for infusion at concentrations of 0.8, 1.6, and 3.2 mg/ml in 5% dextrose.[80] Dopamine is administered by central vein to prevent skin injury because of extravasation. In an emergency, dopamine can be administered through an intraosseous needle.[206] Tables 23–4 and 23–5 provide information regarding preparation of infusions and compatibility.[111,201] Dopamine is not compatible with some of the 3:1 solutions used for parenteral nutrition[275] or with sodium bicarbonate. Dopamine is stable in solutions of 5% dextrose or normal saline for 24[211] to 84 hours.[103] At the low infusion volumes often used for infants and children, available infusion pumps may produce cyclic variations in fluid delivery rate. These variations may be of sufficient magnitude to cause oscillations in hemodynamic response. Therefore in infants and small children, dopamine (and other vasoactive compounds) should be administered by a syringe pump.

Interactions

Dopamine is metabolized by MAO, and concurrent use of an MAO inhibitor (e.g., pargyline) potentiates its effect.[125] In this rare circumstance, the initial dosage of dopamine should be reduced to one tenth the usual dosage.[284] Dopamine antagonists such as metoclopramide or haloperidol may attenuate response to dopamine. An increase in infusion rate will overcome the receptor blockade if necessary.

Summary

Dopamine is used to treat mild-to-moderate cardiogenic or distributive (septic, hypoxic-ischemic) shock associated with moderate degrees of hypotension. In the absence of hypotension, acute severe cardiac failure is treated with dobutamine or amrinone. When septic or cardiogenic shock is complicated by severe hypotension, epinephrine

TABLE 23–5

Compatibility of Vasoactive Drugs with Commonly Used Continuous Infusions

DRUG	Aminoph	Cis	Dobut	Dopa	Epi	Fentanyl	Furosemide	Heparin	Lidocaine	Loraz	Midazolam	Milrinone	Norepi	Vec
Aminophylline		C/I	I	C	I		C	C	C				I	C
Cisatracurium	C/I		C	C	C	C	C/I	C/I	C	C	C		C	
Dobutamine	I	C		C	C	C	C/I	C/I	C	C	C	C	C	C
Dopamine	C	C	C		C	C	C/I	C/NS	C	C	C	C	C	C
Epinephrine	I	C	C	C		C	C	C	C	C	C	C	C	C
Fentanyl		C	C	C	C		C	C		C	C	C	C	C
Furosemide	C	C/I	C/I	C/I	C	C		C	C	C	I	I	C	I
Heparin	C	C/I	C/I	C/NS	C	C	C		C	C	C	C	C	C
Lidocaine	C	C	C	C	C		C	C				C		
Lorazepam		C	C	C	C	C	C	C			C	C	C	C
Midazolam		C	C	C	C	C	I	C		C		C	C	C
Milrinone			C	C	C	C	I	C	C	C	C		C	C
Norepinephrine	I	C	C	C	C	C	C	C		C	C	C		C
Vecuronium	C		C	C	C	C	I	C		C	C	C	C	

C, Compatible; C/I, may be unstable at higher concentrations of additives; C/NS, this combination more stable in normal saline (NS) than D_5W because of an exothermic reaction; I, incompatible.
*Norepinephrine ⇒ More stable in D_5W at higher concentrations because of its high acidity (pH 3).
From Trissel LA: *Handbook on injectable drugs,* ed 11. 2001.

TABLE 23–6

Selecting Inotropic and Vasopressor Agents for Specific Hemodynamic Disturbances in Children

Hemodynamic Pattern	Blood Pressure or SVR		
	Normal	**Decreased**	**Elevated**
Septic shock			
Stroke index ↑		Norepinephrine	
Stroke index ↓	Dobutamine or dopamine	Dopamine or epinephrine (or dobutamine and norepinephrine)	Dobutamine plus vasodilator and/or PDIII inhibitor
Cardiogenic shock	Dobutamine or dopamine or PDIII inhibitor	Dopamine or epinephrine	Dobutamine plus vasodilator and/or PDIII inhibitor
Myocardial dysfunction* (complicating critical illness)	Dobutamine or dopamine or PDIII inhibitor	Dopamine or epinephrine	Dobutamine plus vasodilator and/or PDIII inhibitor
Congestive heart failure	Dobutamine or dopamine or PDIII inhibitor		Dobutamine plus vasodilator and/or PDIII inhibitor
Bradycardia		Isoproterenol	

*For example, acute respiratory distress syndrome or anthracycline therapy
PDIII inhibitor: amrinone or milrinone
Adapted from Notterman DA: *Prob Anesth* 3:288, 1989.

or norepinephrine is preferred, depending on hemodynamic measurements (Table 23–6).

Norepinephrine

Basic Pharmacology

Dopamine is hydroxylated at the β carbon to produce norepinephrine, the principal neurotransmitter of the sympathetic nervous system (see Figures 23–8 and 23–9). Because there is no substituent on the N (amino)-terminus, norepinephrine has little β_2 activity and is considerably less potent at that receptor than epinephrine.[125] It is a moderately potent α and β_1 agonist.

Clinical Pharmacology

Infusion in normal subjects elevates SVR because α-adrenergic stimulation is not opposed by β_2 stimulation.[125] Reflex vagal activity reduces the rate of sinus node discharge, thereby blunting the expected β_1 chronotropic effect. In normal subjects renal, splanchnic, and hepatic blood flows decrease. The increase in afterload may augment coronary blood flow. This effect may be enhanced by α-adrenergic receptors located in the coronary arteries, although in coronary arteries from explanted human hearts the vasodilatation in response to norepinephrine was mediated via β_2 receptors.[266] Norepinephrine does have inotropic effects on the heart, mediated via α_1 and β_1 receptors. The proportion of inotropic response related to α_1 stimulation may be affected by the pressure load on the right ventricle.[43] In the failing heart, the relative contribution from each type of adrenergic receptor appears to be equal.[249] In the isolated rat heart, the inotropic effects of norepinephrine are diminished in the presence of a nitric oxide synthetase inhibitor but restored when a nitric oxide donor is present.[102] Interestingly, the contractile effects of norepinephrine in the rat are lost when it is pretreated with peroxynitrite.[268] In healthy volunteers, norepinephrine produces a decrease in creatinine clearance because of the effect on renal blood flow; however, in patients with hypotension the improvement in global perfusion may actually produce an increase in urine output.[76]

Figure 23–10 compares the acute hemodynamic effects of norepinephrine with those of epinephrine and isoproterenol. Experience in critically ill children indicates the hemodynamic responses are not different than those observed in adults.

Pharmacokinetics

Basal plasma levels of norepinephrine are much higher than basal plasma levels of epinephrine (250 to 500 vs. 20 to 60 pg/ml). The minimum concentration at which norepinephrine produces detectable hemodynamic activity is at least 1500 to 2000 pg/ml, suggesting that endogenous plasma norepinephrine simply represents "spillover" from sympathetic activity and that norepinephrine is not a true hormone.[68] The clearance of norepinephrine in healthy adults is 24 to 40 ml/kg/min, with the half-life averaging 2 to 2.5 minutes.[200] The clinical effect of norepinephrine ceases within 2 minutes of the infusion being stopped.[200] Little pharmacokinetic information in children is available. Norepinephrine is inactivated by reuptake into nerve terminals with some elimination occurring by enzymatic degradation in the liver, adrenal glands, and kidney, either by methylation to normetanephrine (by COMT) or by oxidative deamination.[107] Most of the metabolites formed by either MAO or COMT are reduced or oxidized further. 3-Methoxy-4-hydroxymandelic acid is the major metabolite in the urine.[126]

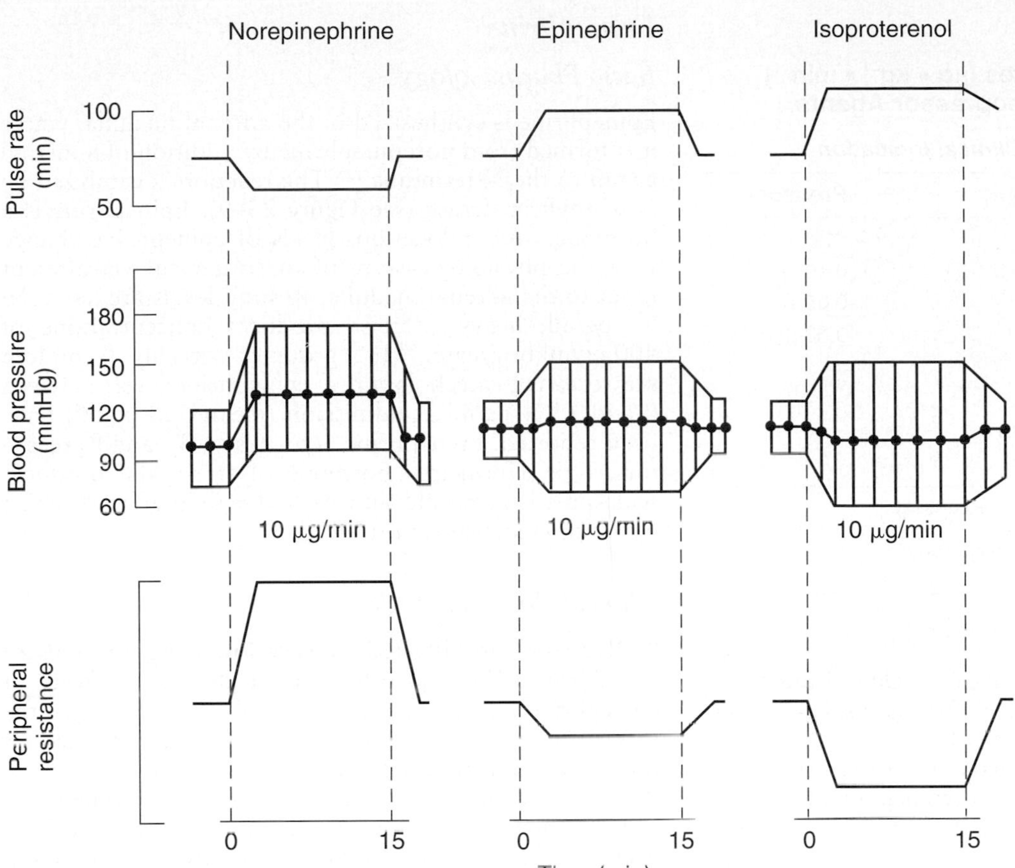

FIGURE 23–10 • Effects of intravenous infusion of norepinephrine, epinephrine, and isoproterenol in adult humans. (Redrawn from Allwood MJ, Cobbold AF, Ginsberg J: *Br Med Bull* 19:132, 1963.)

Clinical Role

Norepinephrine improves perfusion in children with low blood pressure and a normal or elevated cardiac index (CI). Septic shock is the usual context in which norepinephrine is beneficial. Norepinephrine is administered only after intravascular volume repletion and is best guided by estimates of cardiac output and SVR. Little experience on use of norepinephrine for treatment of distributive shock in children has been published; however, publications on adult patients provide a rationale for using this agent in patients with hypotension unresponsive to volume repletion and infusion of dopamine.[75,99,124,184] In children, norepinephrine is the recommended agent for warm shock refractory to fluid loading and dopamine.[50] A prospective, unblinded randomized study (in adults) indicates norepinephrine is superior to dopamine for treating hypotension and other hemodynamic abnormalities associated with hyperdynamic septic shock. In this study, the average infusion rate for norepinephrine was 2.7 μg/kg/min[185] compared with the average dopamine dose of 22 μg/kg/min. Others have reported that somewhat lower average dosages (0.4 μg/kg/min) were effective in adults with sepsis.[221] Coronary and renal blood flow increased in lambs at a dose of 0.4 μg/kg/min while mesenteric blood flow decreased.[77] Thus titration is important and may entail fairly rapid escalation of dosage. Norepinephrine produces increases in SVR, arterial blood pressure, and urine flow. It is most valuable in the context of tachycardia because drug infusion does not produce significant elevation of heart rate and may even lower heart rate through reflex mechanisms. In a study of adults with abdominal sepsis, norepinephrine infusion was associated with increases in systemic blood pressure and SVR. Stroke volume increased as heart rate declined. CI did not change, although creatinine clearance increased substantially.[221] Norepinephrine has been shown to improve RV performance in adults with hyperdynamic septic shock.[185]

The usual starting dosage is an infusion of 0.1 μg/kg/min (Table 23–7), with the goal of elevating perfusion pressure so that flow to vital organs is above the threshold needed to meet metabolic requirements.[8] Arbitrary values of SVR or blood pressure are not appropriate end points for therapy.[73] The lowest infusion rate that improves perfusion as judged by skin color and temperature, mental status, urine flow, and reduction in plasma lactate level should be used.

Other causes of distributive shock (e.g., vasodilator ingestion, intoxication with CNS depressants) should respond to norepinephrine infusion when the predominant hemodynamic problem is low SVR and blood pressure.

Adverse Effects

The increase in afterload that norepinephrine produces should increase myocardial oxygen consumption. However, norepinephrine may reflexively decrease heart rate, which should reduce oxygen consumption and improve diastolic coronary perfusion.[125] Injudicious use of norepinephrine compromises organ blood flow. Norepinephrine infusion may

TABLE 23–7

Suggested Infusion Rates ($\mu g \cdot kg^{-1} \cdot min^{-1}$) for Inotropic and Vasopressor Agents

Agent	Clinical Indication	
	Inotropic	Pressor
Dopamine	2–15	>12
Epinephrine	0.05–0.5	0.10–1
Norepinephrine		0.05–1
Vasopressin		0.02–0.04*
Dobutamine	2.5–20	
Amrinone†	5–10	
Milrinone†	0.25–0.75	
Isoproterenol	0.05–1	

*Units/kg/min (see text for other published doses).
†Loading dose required (see text).
Adapted from Park MK: *J Pediatr* 108:871, 1987.

elevate blood pressure yet not improve clinical indices of perfusion. This type of poor clinical response usually is associated with a low CI, stroke volume, LV stroke work index, and elevated pulmonary capillary wedge pressure.[75,99] Using excessive dosages or using norepinephrine to elevate blood pressure without improving perfusion may produce multiple organ system failure.

Preparation and Administration

Tables 23–4 and 23–5 provide information regarding preparation and compatibility. Norepinephrine bitartrate is available in 4-ml ampules at a concentration of 1 mg/ml.[200] Norepinephrine should be diluted in 5% dextrose or 5% dextrose in 0.9% sodium chloride for preparation of infusions. Norepinephrine is administered only by central venous catheter, except in extreme emergencies. Extravasation of norepinephrine should be treated immediately by local infiltration with a solution of phentolamine (Regitine 5–10 mg in 10 ml of normal saline) administered with a fine hypodermic needle.[200,248] As with dopamine, norepinephrine should be administered by a syringe-type infusion device.

Interactions

Tricyclic antidepressants potentiate the action of norepinephrine by reducing neuronal uptake of the compound.[125] MAO inhibitors do not appear to enhance the activity of infused norepinephrine. α-Adrenergic blocking agents reduce efficacy of norepinephrine.

Summary

Norepinephrine is the agent of choice when the principal hemodynamic disturbance involves hypotension with an abnormally low SVR and a normal or high cardiac output after fluid resuscitation (see Table 23–6). Septic shock is the usual indication and frequently is useful in other diseases associated with distributive shock.

Epinephrine

Basic Pharmacology

Epinephrine is synthesized in the adrenal medulla, where it is formed from norepinephrine by addition of a methyl group to the N-terminus.[125] The reaction is catalyzed by N-methyltransferase (see Figure 23–9). Epinephrine is a hormone, and endogenous levels of epinephrine change with the physiologic state of the organism via afferent input to the adrenal medulla. Resting levels are less than 50 pg/ml; heavy exercise produces concentrations of 400 pg/ml or greater.[68] In a group of critically ill children not receiving catecholamines, epinephrine levels between 0 and 1378 pg/ml at admission (mean 508 pg/ml) have been reported. Epinephrine activates α, β_1, and β_2 receptors. It is a principal hormone of stress and produces widespread metabolic and hemodynamic effects, which have been extensively reviewed.[125]

Clinical Pharmacology

β_1 Receptors are affected by very low concentrations of epinephrine. Consequently, one of the early effects of epinephrine infusion is activation of β_1 receptors in the myocardium and conducting systems. This accelerates phase 4 of the action potential. The rate of sinoatrial node discharge and heart rate increase, and systolic time intervals are shortened. The inotropic state of the myocardium is enhanced, producing an increase in force of contraction and rate of rise of pressure. Evidence indicates myocardial oxygen consumption is out of proportion to the increase in force of contraction, decreasing myocardial efficiency.[125] High concentrations of epinephrine or exposure to the compound when the myocardium is sensitive because of infarction, operation, or myocarditis may produce serious atrial and ventricular dysrhythmias.[125]

Stimulation of peripheral β_2 receptors promotes relaxation of resistance arterioles. SVR decreases and diastolic blood pressure falls (see Figure 23–10). The decrease in SVR enhances the direct chronotropic effect of epinephrine. Higher plasma concentrations are associated with activation of vascular α receptors, and SVR increases. Higher doses are associated with an increase in pulmonary vascular resistance (PVR), from direct effect and secondary to increased venous return to the right side of the heart.[125] The effect of epinephrine on the pulmonary vasculature may vary as a result of the dose used.[189] During infusion of epinephrine, hepatic and splanchnic blood flow increase, while renal blood flow may be reduced.[125]

The thresholds for producing these effects in healthy adults has been examined.[68] Normal basal levels are approximately 40 pg/ml. Heart rate accelerates between 50 and 100 pg/ml; changes in blood pressure (systolic blood pressure increases, diastolic blood pressure decreases) occur between 75 and 100 pg/ml. Various metabolic effects (hyperglycemia, cytogenesis, glycolysis) occur between 150 and 200 pg/ml. Concentrations of this magnitude are achieved during therapeutic infusion of the drug. Other metabolic effects include hypophosphatemia and hypokalemia. Desensitization to elevated levels of epinephrine occurs rapidly and may be present prior to administration of exogenous catecholamines in the ICU.

Pharmacokinetics

In healthy male volunteers, the plasma clearance of epinephrine is 35 to 89 ml/kg/min.[35,64] The elimination half-life is approximately 1 minute.[179] Epinephrine is methylated by COMT to metanephrine in the liver and kidneys or deaminated via the action of MAO.[126] It also may be metabolized by extraneuronal uptake.[107] The resulting catabolites may be conjugated to sulfate or glucuronide and excreted in the urine. A wide interindividual variation in clearance is observed in healthy adults. In critically ill children receiving epinephrine at doses from 0.03 to 0.2 μg/kg/min, plasma concentrations at steady state ranged from 0.67 to 9.4 ng/ml and were linearly related to dose.[94] In this study, clearance ranged from 15 to 79 ml/kg/min, demonstrating wide interindividual variation as with dopamine. Variability between the ordered dose of catecholamines and the measured dose has been noted.[6] Combined with the interindividual variation in clearance, there may be significant differences in serum levels between patients receiving the "same" dose of epinephrine or dopamine.

Clinical Role

Epinephrine is used to treat shock associated with myocardial dysfunction. Thus it may be appropriate for treatment of cardiogenic shock unresponsive to dopamine or following cardiac surgery.[43] In a model of RV injury, epinephrine increased pulmonary artery blood flow and RV power with greater efficiency than dopamine or dobutamine.[189] It also can be used to increase pulmonary flow across left-to-right shunts.[291] The septic patient who does not improve adequately after intravascular volume repletion and treatment with dopamine or dobutamine may benefit from epinephrine infusion. Epinephrine most likely will be useful when hypotension exists in the context of a low CI and stroke index ("cold shock").[50] At modest infusion rates (0.05–0.1 μg/kg/min), SVR decreases slightly; heart rate, cardiac output, and systolic blood pressure increase. At intermediate infusion rates, α_1-adrenergic activation becomes important but is balanced by the improved cardiac output and activation of vascular β_2 receptors. Even though epinephrine constricts renal and cutaneous arterioles, renal function and skin perfusion may improve. Very high infusion rates (>1–2 μg/kg/min) are associated with significant α_1-adrenergic-mediated vasoconstriction. Blood flow to individual organs is compromised, and the associated increase in afterload may further impair myocardial function. The effects of epinephrine on splanchnic blood flow continue to be investigated. Studies have shown decreased splanchnic blood flow, decreased oxygen uptake, and increased lactate[190] with epinephrine compared with norepinephrine despite similar increases in global oxygen delivery. Dopamine led to a decrease in lactate and increase in arterial pH, whereas epinephrine was associated with increases in lactate and metabolic acidosis despite similar increases in CI and oxygen delivery.[71] At a dose of 3.2 μg/kg/min in newborn piglets, epinephrine increased SVR and PVR, with a decrease in hepatic blood flow and oxygen delivery and an increase in lactate.[60] However, these effects may be a result of the dosages used as well as the concomitant catecholamines used. Seguin et al.[237] demonstrated increased gastric blood flow with epinephrine as compared with norepinephrine with dobutamine. They note that the doses of norepinephrine they used were higher than in previous studies. Other studies have shown that the degree of shock also may influence splanchnic blood flow.[72] In a study of adult patients with septic shock, stepwise infusion of epinephrine was associated with linear increases in cardiac rate, mean arterial pressure (MAP), cardiac index, LV stroke work index, oxygen consumption, and oxygen delivery. In that study, neither PVR nor SVR was affected by epinephrine infusion.[197]

Epinephrine has been evaluated for treatment of hypotension in very-low-birth-weight infants.[122] Epinephrine increased blood pressure and heart rate without decreasing urine output in infants with hypotension who did not respond to a dopamine infusion up to 15 μg/kg/min. Urine output tended to increase among infants who had been oliguric.

Bolus injections of epinephrine are used to treat asystole and other nonperfusing rhythms. The recommended initial dosage[9] is 0.01 mg/kg (10 μg/kg or 0.1 ml/kg of the 1:10,000 solution). The recommendation that subsequent doses be 10-fold greater (so-called "high-dose epinephrine") has been deemphasized. Although initial studies using high-dose epinephrine were encouraging, later publications indicate no improvement in return of spontaneous circulation or survival after high-dose epinephrine following out-of-hospital cardiac arrest in children[78] or adults.[48] Epinephrine may be given by endotracheal tube at a dose of 100 μg/kg. Intraosseous administration is appropriate for both bolus and continuous administration of epinephrine. The dosage is the same as for intravenous injection. Epinephrine by infusion is also the agent of choice for hypotension or shock following successful treatment of cardiac arrest. Shock following an episode of hypoxemia or ischemia usually is cardiogenic and may respond to epinephrine infusion.

Preparation and Administration

Epinephrine should be infused by a syringe-type pump into a central vein. Tables 23–4 and 23–5 provide dilution and compatibility information.

Adverse Effects

Central Nervous System. Epinephrine produces CNS excitation manifested as anxiety, dread, nausea, and dyspnea.[125]

Heart. Enhanced automaticity and increased oxygen consumption are the main serious toxicities.[125] Extreme tachycardia carries a substantial oxygen penalty, as does hypertension. A severe imbalance of myocardial oxygen delivery and oxygen consumption produces characteristic ECG changes of ischemia. A subischemic, but persistently unfavorable, ratio of oxygen delivery to consumption may be harmful to the myocardium. This subject has not been adequately examined in the setting of critical illness in children.

Dysrhythmias. Epinephrine produces tachycardia. Increases in infusion rate lead to successively more serious events, including atrial and ventricular extrasystoles, atrial and ventricular tachycardia, and ultimately ventricular fibrillation. Ventricular dysrhythmias in the pediatric age group are not common but may occur in the presence of myocarditis, hypokalemia, or hypoxemia.

Epinephrine overdosage is serious. Several neonates died when they were inadvertently subjected to oral administration of huge amounts of epinephrine.[259] The syndrome mimicked an epidemic of neonatal sepsis with shock and metabolic acidosis. Intraaortic injection in infants (per umbilical artery) produces tachycardia, hypertension, and renal failure. Intravenous overdosage of epinephrine is immediately life threatening. Manifestations include myocardial infarction, ventricular tachycardia, extreme hypertension (up to 400/300 mmHg), cerebral hemorrhage, seizures, renal failure, and pulmonary edema. Bradycardia also has been observed.

Manifestations of acute overdosage are treated symptomatically. β-receptor antagonists such as propranolol are contraindicated. Hypertension is treated with short-acting antihypertensives (e.g., nitroprusside).

Metabolic Effects. Hypokalemia is produced by epinephrine infusion as a result of stimulation of β_2-adrenergic receptors, which are linked to Na/K-ATPase located in skeletal muscle.[49] Infusion of 0.1 μg/kg/min lowered serum potassium by 0.8 mEq/L. Hyperglycemia results from β-adrenergic-mediated suppression of insulin release.

Skin. Epinephrine is an α_1-adrenergic agonist, and infiltration into local tissues or intraarterial injection can produce severe vasospasm and tissue injury.[125] Concurrent activation of β_2 receptors by epinephrine limits vasospasm, and local injury to tissue is less frequent than with either norepinephrine or dopamine.

Interactions

Tricyclic antidepressants potentiate the effects of epinephrine.[125] Use of fluorinated anesthetics may increase the frequency of ventricular dysrhythmia.[140,174,257] Administration of epinephrine with a β-adrenergic antagonist such as propranolol may be dangerous because of residual unopposed α_1 activity. The result can be severe hypertension and bradycardia terminating in asystole.

Summary

Epinephrine is useful for treating shock associated with myocardial dysfunction and hypotension. In pediatric critical care, the most frequent indications for epinephrine infusion are cardiogenic shock, septic shock associated with reduced stroke volume, and shock following severe hypoxemia-ischemia (see Table 23–6).

Isoproterenol

Basic Pharmacology

Isoproterenol is the synthetic N-isopropyl derivative of norepinephrine (see Figure 23–8). The bulky N-terminal substituent confers β (β_1 and β_2)-receptor specificity; the compound does not affect the α-adrenergic receptor. Thus the principal cardiovascular activities of isoproterenol relate to its inotropic, chronotropic, and peripheral vascular vasodilator effects.[125]

Clinical Pharmacology

Isoproterenol enhances cardiac contractility and cardiac rate.[125] Peripheral vasodilatation produces a fall in SVR, augmenting the direct chronotropic action of the drug. Significant tachycardia ensues. Systolic blood pressure increases while mean and diastolic pressures fall (see Figure 23–10). If normal prior to infusion of isoproterenol, mesenteric and renal perfusions fall; however, if the subject was in shock, then the increase in cardiac output associated with isoproterenol administration may result in an increase in blood flow to these tissues.[125] Isoproterenol increases myocardial demand for oxygen and decreases supply by reducing diastolic coronary filling. If the patient is intravascularly fluid depleted, hypotension may complicate initiation of isoproterenol infusion.

Pulmonary bronchial and vascular bed β_2-adrenergic receptors produce bronchodilation and pulmonary vasodilatation, respectively.[125] For this reason, isoproterenol by continuous intravenous infusion was used as adjunctive therapy in children with refractory or rapidly worsening status asthmaticus.[82] At present, continuously nebulized albuterol and intravenous infusion of albuterol or terbutaline have largely supplanted isoproterenol for this indication.

Isoproterenol has few important metabolic effects. Hyperglycemia is not usually observed, although the drug does promote release of free fatty acids. Isoproterenol infusion causes sympathetic neurons to release norepinephrine, producing an increase in plasma levels of norepinephrine. This effect relative to the hemodynamic response to isoproterenol has not been studied.[108]

Pharmacokinetics

Isoproterenol is metabolized by COMT.[125] The plasma elimination half-life of isoproterenol is 1.5 to 4.2 minutes.[66,67] Information about therapeutic isoproterenol concentrations in critically ill patients is not available. In healthy volunteers, tachycardia and increases in stroke volume were observed at 50 pg/ml.[108]

Clinical Role

Isoproterenol was used in the past for a variety of indications, including septic shock and cardiogenic shock associated with myocardial infarction. Newer agents such as dopamine and dobutamine, together with a more subtle understanding of the pathophysiology of shock, have limited the use of this compound to very few specific indications.

Isoproterenol can be used to treat hemodynamically significant bradycardia,[243] but epinephrine infusion probably is preferable.[8] When bradycardia results from heart block, placement of a pacemaker is definitive treatment. Bradycardia resulting from anoxia is treated by administering oxygen and improving gas exchange.

Interactions

Few drug interactions have been documented. Propranolol given before an operation for repair tetralogy of Fallot attenuates the response to isoproterenol postoperatively.[23] Isoproterenol decreases serum theophylline concentrations during concomitant therapy of status asthmaticus. It may be necessary to increase theophylline dosage when isoproterenol therapy is initiated and reduce theophylline dosage when isoproterenol is discontinued.[123]

Summary

Isoproterenol is rarely used to treat children or adults. In the acute setting, it may play a role in the treatment of symptomatic bradycardia. Although it is effective adjunctive therapy for respiratory failure associated with status asthmaticus, more selective β_2 agonists are safer and are preferred.

Dobutamine

Basic Pharmacology

The structure of dobutamine, a synthetic catecholamine, resembles dopamine in that the β carbon is not hydroxylated. Unlike other catecholamines, there is a large aromatic substituent on the N-terminus. Like isoproterenol, dobutamine is administered a racemate. (+) Dobutamine is a strong β agonist and an α antagonist, and (–) dobutamine is an α agonist and a weak β agonist.[230] That dobutamine delivers significant inotropic and usually trivial chronotropic and vasopressor activity has been ascribed to this blend of receptor activities.

Clinical Pharmacology

In adults with CHF, dobutamine increased CI from 2.4 to 2.9 L/min/m, decreased LV end-diastolic volume, and increased LV dP/dt.[4] Although renal function and urine output may improve as the increase in cardiac output fosters relaxation of sympathetic tone and improved perfusion, dobutamine did not improve indices of renal function compared with dopamine in critically ill patients.[133] Dobutamine improved RV systolic function and decreased PVR in piglets with RV injury.[189] In healthy children, dobutamine increased LV systolic function and relaxation.[117] In the newborn piglet, dobutamine increased superior mesenteric and renal artery blood flow after 60 minutes, increased CI, and decreased SVR.[59] A threshold model with a log-linear dose-response relationship above the threshold has been demonstrated in critically ill term and preterm neonates[186] and in children between 2 months and 14 years old.[29] In one small study, dobutamine infusion (10 µg/kg/min) was associated with increases in cardiac output (30%), blood pressure (17%), and heart rate (7%). The thresholds for these increases were 13, 23, and 65 ng/ml, respectively, demonstrating that dobutamine is a relatively selective inotrope with little effect on heart rate at customary infusion rates.[114] Somewhat greater thresholds for improved cardiac output were observed in a second group of children[29] and in infants,[186] but in all studies, dobutamine improved cardiac contractility without substantially altering heart rate unless high infusion rates were used. Dobutamine increases cerebral blood flow velocity but not cerebral oxygen consumption in patients with septic shock.[34]

Pharmacokinetics

The plasma elimination half-life of dobutamine in adults is approximately 2 minutes.[179] CHF increases the volume of distribution. In adults with CHF, the terminal elimination half-life ($t\frac{1}{2}_{\beta}$) of dobutamine has been reported to be 2.37 minutes, with an apparent volume of distribution of 0.2 L/kg and total body clearance of 2.33 L/min/m^2.[162] Reported clearance values in children ranged from 32 to 625 ml/kg/min in one study[22] and from 40 to 130 ml/min/kg in another study.[114] Infusions in the range used clinically yield plasma dobutamine concentrations from approximately 50 to 190 ng/ml in children[114] and adults. The principal route of elimination is methylation by COMT, followed by hepatic glucuronidation and excretion into urine and bile.[125] 3-O-Methyldobutamine also is a major route of elimination for dobutamine, with up to 33% of the infused drug eliminated as the sulfoconjugated compound.[298] Dobutamine also is cleared from the plasma by nonneuronal uptake. Some investigators have reported nonlinear elimination kinetics,[22] but other data suggest that dobutamine's kinetics can be adequately described by a simple first-order (linear) model.[29,114,263]

Clinical Role

In adults, dobutamine produces improvement in a variety of conditions associated with poor myocardial performance, such as cardiomyopathy, atherosclerotic heart disease, and acute myocardial infarction. Dobutamine has been used following surgery for myocardial revascularization, cardiac transplantation, and other procedures associated with postoperative myocardial dysfunction, although undesirable chronotropic effects were recorded with its use after cardiac surgery.[180] Whether septic shock is an appropriate context in which to prescribe dobutamine is not clear, unless the primary disturbance is complicated by myocardial dysfunction. Although impaired myocardial performance can be demonstrated early in septic shock, the main problem relates to regulation of vascular tone. Preferred agents are those that increase SVR. When ventricular dysfunction becomes an important complicating factor, however, dobutamine may be a useful adjunct. In this context, dobutamine alone or in combination with dopamine has produced an increase in cardiac output, LV stroke work, and blood pressure.[235] As indicated in Table 23–6, dobutamine can be combined with norepinephrine to treat the patient with myocardial dysfunction associated with hyperdynamic shock (e.g., a child who received a cardiotoxic agent to treat cancer and subsequently developed septic shock).

Several studies in infants and children[29,114,186] demonstrate that dobutamine improves myocardial function in a variety of settings. Stroke volume and CI improve without a substantial increase in cardiac rate. SVR and PVR may decrease toward normal.[161] Dobutamine has been evaluated in children following cardiac surgery with cardiopulmonary bypass. In a study by Bohn et al.,[37] dobutamine enhanced cardiac output by increasing heart rate; indeed, tachycardia prompted discontinuation of the infusion in several patients. The expected fall in SVR was not observed in children receiving the drug after cardiopulmonary bypass. The authors found no benefit over isoproterenol or dopamine. These differences between adults and children may result from the fact that myocardial dysfunction and CHF are not characteristic of the circulatory status of many children undergoing repair of congenital heart disease. Unlike adults, indication for the operation involves abnormalities in ventricular architecture or abnormal circulatory anatomy. Berner and associates[33] found that children undergoing operations for mitral valve disease responded to dobutamine with an increase in stroke volume; children with tetralogy of Fallot repair did not, and their cardiac output increased only through a higher heart rate. A later report by the same group indicated that, following repair of tetralogy of Fallot, dobutamine enhanced cardiac output when it was combined with atrial pacing to increase heart rate. Isoproterenol without pacing provided a higher cardiac output than either dobutamine alone or dobutamine in combination with pacing.[32] Booker et al.[41] found that dobutamine and dopamine had equivalent inotropic effects in children following cardiac surgery. Specific indications for prescribing dobutamine in the pediatric age group are those associated with low-output CHF and a normal to moderately decreased blood pressure (see Table 23–6). Typical examples include viral myocarditis; cardiomyopathy associated with use of anthracyclines, cyclophosphamide, or hemochromatosis (related to hypertransfusion therapy); or myocardial infarction (Kawasaki disease).

Dobutamine is *not* a first-line agent for treatment of low-output states caused by intracardiac shunt or abnormal cardiac chamber structure. Dobutamine is used following corrective or palliative cardiovascular surgery in the child; however, in this context its use should be limited to occasions with demonstrated or suspected myocardial dysfunction. Dobutamine may be of adjunctive value in treating myocardial dysfunction that complicates a primary condition such as ARDS or septic shock. Rarely, however, will it be appropriate to use dobutamine as the sole agent for treatment of hemodynamic compromise associated with sepsis, ARDS, or shock following an episode of severe hypoxia-ischemia.

Adverse Effects

Dobutamine usually increases myocardial oxygen demand. In subjects with myocardial dysfunction, coronary blood flow and oxygen supply improve with the increase in demand. However, if dobutamine is used when myocardial contractility is normal, oxygen balance is adversely affected.[208] Tachycardia greatly increases oxygen use by the heart and should prompt a reduction in dobutamine dosage or use of an alternate agent.

Although dobutamine is less likely than other catecholamines to induce serious atrial and ventricular dysrhythmias, they may occur in patients receiving dobutamine, particularly in the context of myocarditis, electrolyte imbalance, or high infusion rates.[161] Dobutamine and other inotropes should be administered cautiously to patients with dynamic LV outflow obstruction (hypertrophic aortic stenosis). Prolonged infusion of dobutamine inhibits the second wave of ADP-induced platelet aggregation. A few adult patients have developed petechial bleeding attributed to dobutamine.[254]

Preparation and Administration

Tables 23–4 and 23–5 provide information on dilution and compatibility. Therapy is initiated at a rate of 2.5 to 5 μg/kg/min (see Table 23–7). A change to epinephrine should be considered if no substantial improvement is seen with infusion rates of 20 μg/kg/min.

Interactions

Few drug interactions have been reported. Evidence indicates dobutamine may increase the insulin requirement of diabetic patients,[295] and dobutamine may interfere with measurement of chloramphenicol by high-performance liquid chromatography.[215]

Summary

Dobutamine is a positive inotropic agent that should be reserved for treatment of poor myocardial contractility. Following cardiac surgery, dobutamine can be used when contractility is abnormal. For septic shock and other acute hemodynamic disturbances, dobutamine is an adjunct when the primary problem is complicated by poor myocardial function (see Table 23–6). In this context, concomitant use of a vasopressor such as norepinephrine may be appropriate.

Vasopressin

Basic Pharmacology

Vasopressin is a highly conserved hormone. Vasopressin-like peptides are present in numerous species. Its main function is to preserve fluid balance in the organism. In man, it is released in response to two main stimuli: increases in plasma osmolality and decreases in effective circulating volume or blood pressure. Although vasopressin has long been used for treatment of diabetes insipidus, its name derives from its vasopressor effect. Vasopressin has a number of effects beyond volume regulation. It acts as a neurotransmitter in the CNS, has a role regulating adrenocorticotropin hormone release, and is involved in thermoregulation, platelet aggregation, and smooth muscle contraction in the uterus and gastrointestinal tract.[129,136]

Clinical Pharmacology

As noted previously, the response patterns are different for the two stimuli for vasopressin release. An increase in plasma osmolality above 280 mOsm/kg leads to a dramatic increase in the release of vasopressin from the posterior pituitary, and the hormone exerts its effect by increasing water reabsorption in the renal collecting duct. The dose-response curve is so steep that when osmolality is 290 mOsm/kg, vasopressin levels exceed those that produce maximal urinary concentration. In contrast, the threshold for release in response to hypovolemia or hypotension is much higher, with decreases of greater than 20% required. However, once the threshold is reached, plasma levels rise 20- to 30-fold (far exceeding levels seen with hyperosmolality).[136] Vasopressin exerts its hemodynamic effects via the V_{1a} receptor, which is coupled to G_q. In the peripheral vasculature, intracellular calcium is increased, enhancing contraction and restoring systemic vascular tone. Vasopressin also inhibits potassium channels, further increasing intracellular calcium.[157,225] Baroreceptors in the left atrium, left ventricle, and pulmonary veins sense changes in volume while baroreceptors in the carotid sinus and aorta sense changes in arterial pressure.[136] Decreased pressure leads to a reduced rate of firing and release of the tonic inhibition of vasopressin release.[129]

Vasopressin is a potent vasopressor when present in the plasma at high concentration. At the lower concentrations associated with the vasopressin response to hyperosmolarity rather than hypotension, it does not elevate blood pressure because the resulting decrease in heart rate offsets the increase in SVR. For this reason, vasopressin was not considered a clinically useful agent for treatment of hypotension.[222] Landry et al.[155] measured plasma vasopressin levels in 19 patients with septic shock and 12 patients with cardiogenic shock (all receiving catecholamine support). Surprisingly, plasma levels of vasopressin were not elevated in patients with septic shock (mean 3.1 pg/ml; normal <5 pg/ml). Patients with cardiogenic shock had an expected mean level of 22.7 pg/ml. Vasopressin infusion (0.04 U/min intravenously) in 10 patients with septic shock who were receiving catecholamines produced an increase in SVR and MAP, associated with a decrease in CI. The resulting plasma level of vasopressin was 30 pg/ml, an appropriate concentration considering the level of hypotension. Therefore vasopressin plasma levels are inappropriately low in vasodilatory septic shock, possibly because of impaired baroreflex-mediated secretion. The authors hypothesized that this process contributes to the hypotension of vasodilatory septic shock.

It appears that vasopressin levels are higher than normal in the early stages of septic shock but decrease to either low levels or levels that represent a relative deficiency (normal level in the setting of hypotension) as shock continues.[242] This pattern has also been shown in a model of hemorrhagic shock.[195] In this study, neurohypophysis stores of vasopressin were depleted. In three patients with septic shock and low vasopressin levels, the high intensity signal from the posterior pituitary on T1-weighted magnetic resonance imaging was lost, suggesting depletion of vasopressin.[242] Thus vasopressin deficiency may occur early in vasodilatory shock and contribute to its pathogenesis.

Pharmacokinetics

Vasopressin circulates as a free peptide and does not exhibit any protein binding.[95] It is degraded rapidly in the kidneys and liver, with 5% to 15% of an intravenous dose eliminated unchanged in the urine.[284] Renal failure or hepatic insufficiency can prolong the elimination half-life.[11,258] The normal elimination half-life is 10 to 20 minutes.[284]

Clinical Role

The original report by Landry et al.[155] generated intense investigation into the clinical applications of vasopressin in the setting of vasodilatory shock. The same group prospectively evaluated vasopressin in patients with vasodilatory shock after placement of an LV assist device.[13] At a dose of 0.1 U/min, vasopressin increased MAP and SVR but not CI. Among patients with a high level of endogenous vasopressin, the increase in blood pressure tended to be less. A rapid response to vasopressin was noted in all patients, allowing the dose to be decreased to as low as 0.01 U/min. This group also reported experience with vasopressin in patients with septic shock[156] and children after cardiac surgery.[228] In five patients with septic shock, vasopressin was given at doses ranging from 0.03 to 0.05 U/min. Again, blood pressure and SVR increased, allowing for discontinuation of catecholamine support in four patients. In 11 children, vasopressin was used to treat hypotension following cardiac surgery. At doses ranging from 0.0003 to 0.002 U/kg/min, vasopressin increased blood pressure within 1 hour, and the epinephrine infusion could be decreased in five of eight patients. Two patients who had echocardiographic evidence of poor function died. The remaining nine patients with vasodilatory shock survived to ICU discharge. The authors cautioned against vasopressin use in patients with cardiogenic shock, in view of the potential effect on CI. Vasopressin levels were measured in three patients; two had an absolute deficiency and one had a relative deficiency of vasopressin. In adults, vasopressin deficiency (relative or absolute) was associated with shock following cardiopulmonary bypass. Hemodynamic function improved with vasopressin and the need for other vasopressors decreased.[12] In a small double-blind randomized study, prophylactic vasopressin (0.03 U/min) decreased the need for norepinephrine and ICU length of stay in patients receiving angiotensin-converting enzyme inhibitors who underwent cardiopulmonary bypass.[196] In another small study (N = 10), patients admitted to a trauma unit with the diagnosis of septic shock were randomized to placebo or vasopressin at 0.04 U/min if they remained in shock with catecholamine support.[181] In the treatment group (n = 5), systolic blood pressure and SVR increased. Other vasopressors were discontinued within 24 hours in patients receiving vasopressin; in only one patient in the placebo group was other vasopressor support discontinued. In a larger, prospective, randomized study, the combination of vasopressin and norepinephrine was evaluated versus norepinephrine alone in patients with catecholamine-resistant vasodilatory shock.[86] Vasopressin was given at a dose of 0.06 U/min. The patients in the vasopressin-norepinephrine arm had a lower heart rate and higher blood pressure, SVR, and CI. They also had reduced requirements for norepinephrine. In addition, the norepinephrine group had a higher rate of new-onset dysrhythmias. Gastric perfusion was better preserved in the vasopressin group.

In summary, in several studies of patients with vasodilatory shock, vasopressin improved blood pressure, increased SVR, lessened the need for catecholamines, improved markers of myocardial ischemia, and improved urine output.[84,87,130,277] Published experience in pediatric patients with septic shock is limited. Bojko et al.[38] reported one case in abstract form. At a dose of 0.02 U/min, blood pressure and SVRI increased and urine output improved with subsequent discontinuation of catecholamine therapy. Liedel et al.[169] reported their experience with five patients who ranged in age from 2 weeks (23-week premature infant) to 14 years. Doses used were between 0.0006 and 0.008 U/kg/min (one patient was given 0.06 U/min). In all five patients, blood pressure increased (in one patient blood pressure increased briefly prior to rapid deterioration and death) and catecholamine support could be decreased. In three patients, urine output improved. No formal randomized trial of vasopressin in pediatric patients with septic shock or following cardiac surgery has been published to date. Vasopressin also has been used as a vasopressor in children undergoing evaluation for brain death.[147] At a dose of 0.04 U/kg/hour, blood pressure increased and α-agonist support decreased. No deleterious effect on organ function was noted. Vasopressin has also become part of the Advanced Cardiovascular Life Support (ACLS) protocol for ventricular fibrillation in adults.[9] No recommendations were made for pediatric patients or patients in asystole. Mann et al.[183] reported their experience with vasopressin during CPR in pediatric patients. In six events involving four patients, vasopressin was given at a dose of 0.4 U/kg after conventional therapy had failed to achieve restoration of spontaneous circulation. In all six events, pulseless electrical activity was the initial rhythm. At the time vasopressin was given, four patients were in asystole, one had pulseless ventricular tachycardia, and one had ventricular fibrillation. In four events (three patients), restoration of spontaneous circulation was achieved for more than 60 minutes. Of the two patients who survived for more than 24 hours, one was discharged home in a condition close to her neurologic baseline; care was electively withdrawn in the other patient.

Adverse Effects

Few adverse events have been reported with vasopressin use in the setting of vasodilatory shock. Elevation of liver enzymes and total bilirubin with a decrease in platelet count has been reported.[87] One series noted six cardiac arrests among 50 patients receiving vasopressin for hemodynamic support.[130] All six patients had "severe refractory shock", and five were receiving a vasopressin dose greater than 0.05 U/min. Thirty percent of patients receiving vasopressin developed ischemic skin lesions of the distal limbs, trunk, or tongue. Preexisting peripheral arterial occlusive disease and the presence of septic shock were identified as risk factors.[85] Extravasation of vasopressin from a peripheral intravenous catheter was associated with skin necrosis.[142]

Preparation and Administration

Vasopressin does not demonstrate any significant incompatibilities.

Interactions

No significant drug interactions have been reported for vasopressin.

Summary

Vasopressin is a recent addition to the PICU practitioner's armamentarium for treatment of decreased SVR. Its use may elevate blood pressure and urine output in catecholamine refractory vasodilatory shock. The optimal dose has not been determined, and the pharmacokinetics of the drug in conditions such as septic shock or after cardiopulmonary bypass must be investigated. It may have a role in pediatric advanced life support in the future. Vasopressin should not be used in settings where impaired myocardial function is the principal problem. Controlled trials in the pediatric age group are urgently needed and should be accompanied by appropriate pharmacokinetic measurements.

Bipyridines

Amrinone, milrinone, enoximone, and piroximone are nonsympathomimetic inotropic agents. The structures (not a catecholamine) of amrinone and milrinone are shown in Figure 23–11. Amrinone and milrinone currently are available for intravenous use only. As described previously, the pharmacologic effects of the bipyridines result from selective inhibition of phosphodiesterase III and not from interaction with adrenergic receptors or inhibition of Na/K-ATPase.[234] These agents produce positive inotropic and lusitropic effects on isolated ventricular tissue as well as relaxation of vascular smooth muscle. They are often used to improve myocardial contractility and to decrease ventricular afterload.

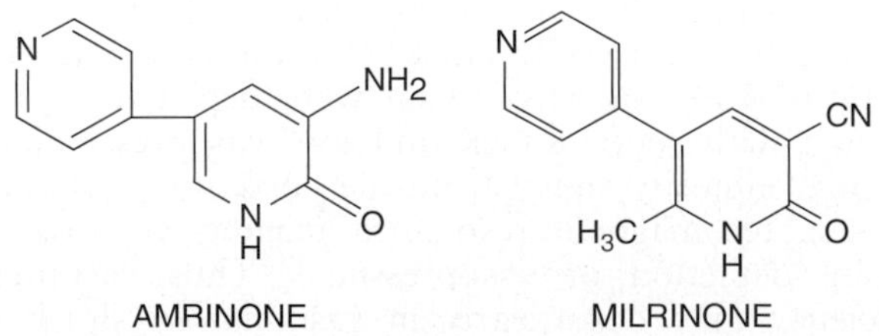

AMRINONE MILRINONE

FIGURE 23–11 • Structure of amrinone plus milrinone.

Amrinone

Clinical Pharmacology

Administration of phosphodiesterase inhibitors to subjects with CHF results in an increase in cardiac output and a reduction of SVR, central venous pressure (CVP), and pulmonary capillary wedge pressure.[44] Heart rate is not affected. Amrinone was shown to be a direct pulmonary vasodilator in a newborn lamb model, and the effect occurred at lower dosages than those causing increased cardiac output.[182] When amrinone is administered to patients who are intravascularly volume depleted or in whom the expected improvement in cardiac output does not occur, hypotension may result.[293] Improvement in cardiac function likely results from a combination of a positive inotropic effect and a direct reduction of preload and afterload.[55,234] In patients with CHF, the amelioration in global hemodynamic function is associated with an improvement in the ratio of myocardial oxygen delivery to consumption.[19] Amrinone may improve contractility in patients who have not responded to catecholamines and may further increase CI even in patients who have responded to dobutamine. Therapeutically effective concentrations range from 2 to 7 μg/ml, and there is a strong correlation between concentration and improvement in hemodynamic function.[159] Amrinone reduces PVR in children with intracardiac left-to-right shunts. In one study, children with elevated PVR exhibited a 47% reduction in PVR on infusion of amrinone.[226] The ratio of PVR to SVR decreased by 45%. In these children, both pulmonary blood flow and left-to-right shunt increased. In children with normal pulmonary pressure, amrinone infusion was associated with a decrease in SVR but not PVR. Amrinone may be undesirable in children with an elevated pulmonary artery pressure associated with a high-flow left-to-right shunt but normal PVR. Conversely, the phosphodiesterase type III inhibitors may be an effective adjunctive therapy in the child with elevated PVR and reduced pulmonary blood flow. Amrinone increases CI and decreases SVR after the Fontan procedure.[261] Whether the inotropic effects of amrinone derive more from its ability to decrease SVR than a positive inotropic effect has been questioned.[31] Bailey et al.[17] compared the effects of nitroprusside and amrinone. Although both agents decreased SVR to a similar extent, amrinone increased CI and produced a greater increase in the ratio of change in CI to change in mean arterial blood pressure. In infants following cardiac surgery, amrinone increased LV fractional shortening and the mean velocity of circumferential fiber shortening and decreased LV end-diastolic wall stress.[270]

In a cell culture line, amrinone decreased the expression of nuclear factor-κB and inducible nitric oxide synthetase in cardiac myocytes exposed to lipopolysaccharide and tumor necrosis factor (TNF)-α. Interleukin (IL)-1β production in response to TNF-α also was decreased, as was intercellular adhesion molecule expression.[52] The authors of the study note that the results imply amrinone is acting downstream at a central point for proinflammatory signaling. The clinical implications of these findings have yet to be explored.

Pharmacokinetics

Amrinone is metabolized by N-acetyltransferase. In addition, up to 40% is eliminated unchanged in the urine.[7] In healthy adults, the half-life of amrinone in "slow acetylators" is 4.4 hours and in "fast acetylators" 2 hours.[115] It is unclear if this difference is clinically important.[154] Protein binding is not extensive. One study of children younger than 1 year following cardiopulmonary bypass found that the half-life was prolonged in those younger than 4 weeks and that volume of distribution (1.7–1.8 L/kg) was threefold greater than others have reported in adults.[159] A second study among children older than 1 month found wide interpatient variability in pharmacokinetic measurements. There was no relation between age and any measured pharmacokinetic parameter. Average clearance was approximately 1.2 ml/kg/min (range 0.4–2.2 ml/kg/min). The mean half-life was 5.5 hours.[6] There was no correlation noted between amrinone pharmacokinetics and hepatic or renal function. In infants younger than 1 month, half-life is increased and clearance decreased.[154] Neonates have a smaller volume of distribution at steady state.[154]

Clinical Role

In adults with CHF, phosphodiesterase type III inhibitors are safe and effective when given intravenously, and their clinical place in short-term management of patients with refractory heart failure is clearly established. Bipyridines are most useful in management of children and adolescents with isolated cardiac dysfunction, particularly when it results from myocardial failure, or in the setting of decreased cardiac output following cardiopulmonary bypass. They provide both inotropic and afterload reduction and may be an alternative to coadministration of dobutamine and an afterload-reducing agent (see Table 23–7). Although amrinone is useful for increasing CI and decreasing SVR in children following cardiac surgery, its role has been largely supplanted by milrinone because of concern over thrombocytopenia induced by amrinone (see later).

Adverse Effects

Amrinone produces reversible dose-dependent thrombocytopenia (incidence 2.4%), which is more common during prolonged therapy. This finding was not seen in the largest published pediatric study,[159] but case reports suggest it occurs in children as well. In one series,[229] 8 of 18 patients developed thrombocytopenia. The plasma concentration of amrinone did not correlate with thrombocytopenia, although N-acetylamrinone levels were increased in the patients with thrombocytopenia. Supraventricular and ventricular dysrhythmias have occurred during infusion of amrinone but may have been related to the patient's underlying condition. Fatal progressive hypotension not responsive to peritoneal dialysis has been reported for amrinone overdose.[160] Too rapid infusion of amrinone or milrinone during the loading dose produces hypotension. This problem is exacerbated in volume-depleted patients.

Preparation and Administration

Amrinone lactate is available in 5 mg/ml vials for injection. Loading doses may be administered undiluted over 2 to 3 minutes. In adults the manufacturer recommends an amrinone loading dose of 0.75 mg/kg, which may be repeated once. This is followed by a continuous infusion of 5 to 10 μg/kg/min. Maintenance infusions should be prepared in 0.45% or 0.9% Sodium Chloride Injection USP at a final concentration of 1 to 3 mg/ml. Amrinone is not compatible with 5% Dextrose USP or furosemide. The dosage in children has not been conclusively established, although the publication previously cited contains a suggestion for a much higher loading dose (children younger than 1 year: initial intravenous amrinone bolus 3.0–4.5 mg/kg in four divided doses followed by a continuous infusion of 10 μg/kg/min; neonates: similar bolus followed by continuous infusion of 3–5 μg/kg/min).[159] These recommendations are supported by a second study in which this regimen was associated with a generally satisfactory plasma concentration of amrinone.[7] As with the catecholamines, significant differences between the ordered concentration and the measured concentration of amrinone have been shown.[7]

Interactions

Significant drug interactions have not been documented.

Milrinone

Clinical Pharmacology

Milrinone, a derivative of amrinone, shares the same mechanism of action and pharmacodynamic profile. The major advantage is that milrinone, unlike amrinone, does not appear to evoke thrombocytopenia. In adults, milrinone acts both as an inotrope and vasodilator. In adults with CHF, milrinone causes a much greater decrease in left and right filling pressures and SVR than does dobutamine, even at equivalent contractility dosing.[145] Compared with dobutamine, milrinone produces a greater reduction in SVR for a given degree of improvement in inotropic state.[65] Blood pressure is well maintained, even in the face of reduced SVR, because of the associated improvement in contractility and stroke volume. Increasing doses of milrinone correlate with increasing mixed venous oxygen saturation (SvO_2).[204] Milrinone has been extensively used following cardiac surgery[166] and in adults with CHF,[245] where it increases CI and reduces SVR, filling pressures, and often systemic blood pressure.[74] When given perioperatively, milrinone attenuated decreases in gastric mucosal pH in patients undergoing coronary artery bypass grafting.[194] Splanchnic oxygenation improved and systemic levels of endotoxin and IL-6 decreased. Although a cell culture study failed to show a decrease (with a possible increase) in proinflammatory markers in response to milrinone,[52] milrinone decreased serum levels of IL-1β and IL-6 following cardiopulmonary bypass.[121] The decrease in IL-6 correlated inversely with cAMP levels.

Several studies evaluated milrinone in children following surgery for congenital heart disease. In one study, a loading dose of 50 μg/kg followed by continuous infusion of 0.5 μg/kg/min was associated with mild tachycardia and a slight decrease in systemic blood pressure.[54] CI increased from 2.1 to approximately 3.1 L/min/m^2, while SVR index and PVR index decreased from approximately 2100 to 1300 and 488 to 360 dyne•sec•/cm^5•m^2, respectively. In a completed double-blind, placebo-controlled trial, high-dose milrinone (75 μg/kg bolus followed by continuous infusion at 0.75 μg/kg/min) was associated with a decreased incidence of low cardiac output syndrome.[127] Length of hospital stay was similar among the treatment groups, but prolonged stay (>15 days) was more common in the placebo arm. Milrinone has been evaluated in children with nonhyperdynamic septic shock (normal-to-low CI, normal-to-elevated SVR). In a double-blind crossover study, milrinone increased CI, stroke volume index, and oxygen delivery while decreasing SVR.[25] No differences in blood pressure or PVR were seen. Milrinone was given at a dose of 0.5 μg/kg/min as a continuous infusion after a bolus dose of 50 μg/kg.

Pharmacokinetics

In contrast to amrinone, milrinone is approximately 70% bound to plasma proteins, with approximately 85% renal elimination.[304] Hepatic glucuronidation accounts for a minor elimination pathway. In healthy adults, milrinone has an apparent volume of distribution of 0.32 ± 0.08 L/kg, clearance of 6.1 ± 1.3 ml/kg/min, and elimination half-life of 0.8 ± 0.22 hours.[304] Both renal dysfunction and CHF affect the elimination profile of milrinone, extending the elimination half-life to approximately 2 hours.[88] In infants and young children undergoing cardiac surgery, the weight-adjusted clearance of milrinone increases with age, ranging from 2.6 ml/kg/min at age 3 months to 5.6 ml/kg/min at age 22 months.[18] In a separate study of milrinone in infants and children (ages 1–13 years) following open heart surgery, milrinone clearance was significantly lower in infants than in children (3.8 ± 1 ml/kg/min vs. 5.9 ± 2 ml/kg/min, respectively).[219] Importantly, the milrinone clearance values for both infants and children were significantly higher than the clearance of milrinone reported in adults following cardiac surgery (2 ± 0.7 ml/kg/min).[69] In the pediatric study, the plasma concentration versus time data fit a two-compartment model.[219] The apparent volume of distribution by area (V_β), which reflects the volume of distribution during the terminal elimination phase, was not significantly different between infants and children (0.9 ± 0.4 L/kg vs. 0.7 ± 0.2 L/kg). However, the value reported for infants differed significantly from the value reported in adults following cardiac surgery (0.3 ± 0.1 L/kg).[69] In children with septic shock, the median half life of milrinone was 1.5 hours.[173] Plasma levels did not correlate with changes in CI or SVR. One patient with acute renal failure had an eightfold increase in the serum milrinone level even though the same dosing regimen was used as in the patients without renal failure.

Clinical Role

Based on its shorter elimination half-life and possibly a lower incidence of thrombocytopenia, milrinone is generally preferred to amrinone for pediatric patients.[18] Milrinone can be used to increase cardiac contractility following cardiac surgery and may have a role in improving perfusion in patients with "cold shock." Its properties as a vasodilator also suggest milrinone may be useful in the setting of pulmonary hypertension.[62]

Adverse Effects

In the largest pediatric study, serial measurements showed no difference in platelet count over time (baseline, 36 hours, 72 hours, discharge) by treatment arm, and there was no difference in the incidence of thrombocytopenia (platelet count <50,000) during the study infusion (7.4% placebo, 8.8% low dose, 2.6% high dose).[127]

Preparation and Administration

Milrinone lactate is available in 10-, 20-, and 50-ml single dose vials, each at a concentration of 1 mg/ml, and in 100- and 200-ml flexible containers at a concentration of 200 μg/ml in 5% dextrose.[216] Loading doses can be drawn from a single-dose vial and administered undiluted over 15 minutes. A loading dose of 50 μg/kg is generally used in children.[18,54] For preparation of maintenance infusions, milrinone should be diluted with 0.45% or 0.9% Sodium Chloride Injection USP or 5% Dextrose Injection USP to a final concentration of 200 μg/ml or less. Maintenance infusion rates are generally initiated at 0.5 μg/kg/min, titrated to clinical response. Based on the higher clearance and volume of distribution values discussed, Ramamoorthy et al.[219] suggested a loading dose and initial maintenance infusion rate of 104 μg/kg and 0.49 μg/kg/min, respectively, in infants and 67 μg/kg and 0.61 μg/kg/min, respectively, in children. In patients not given a loading dose of milrinone, changes in CI and plasma levels of milrinone after 3 hours were similar to those seen in patients given a loading dose.[26] Milrinone is not compatible with furosemide but is compatible with a large number of drugs used in the PICU,[286] including dopamine, epinephrine, fentanyl, and vecuronium.[2]

Summary

The bipyridines offer an attractive combination of positive inotropy with decreased SVR. The bipyridines likely will be effective in the short-term management of infants and children with myocardial disease. Milrinone has an established role in the management of impaired cardiac contractility following cardiopulmonary bypass. Its role in other settings has not been conclusively established by randomized trials.

Digitalis Glycosides

The role of digoxin in the acute care of critically ill children has always been limited by a narrow therapeutic range, slow onset of action, and the potential for life-threatening adverse effects. With the advent of new therapies for both the acute and chronic management of CHF and myocardial dysfunction, its role has been further decreased. A review is offered here because the practitioner in the PICU may still encounter patients taking the drug, particularly for control of dysrhythmias. Digoxin, as do the catecholamines and other drugs discussed in this chapter, exerts its inotropic effects by increasing intracellular calcium.

Basic Pharmacology

The cardiac glycosides consist of a steroid moiety with one to four sugar molecules attached.[205] The number and composition of the associated sugar molecules affect the pharmacokinetics of the specific glycoside. All digitalis glycosides have similar pharmacodynamic properties. Glycosides bind to and inhibit Na/K-ATPase. Binding of digoxin to ATPase is affected by serum potassium. Hyperkalemia depresses digoxin binding, whereas hypokalemia has the opposite effect,[167] accounting in part for potentiation of digoxin-induced dysrhythmias during hypokalemia. As described earlier in this chapter, inhibition of ATPase produces an increase in intracellular calcium and enhances the inotropic state of the myocardium.

Clinical Pharmacology

In patients with CHF, the positive inotropic action of digoxin leads to increased cardiac output and reductions in filling pressures, edema, and sinus node rate. In a study of 10 adult patients with acute myocardial failure, a single 10 μg/kg dose of digoxin produced a 69% increase in LV stroke work index, 25% reduction in wedge pressure, 16% to 28% increase in CI, and 25% increase in stroke index within 2 hours of infusion.[117] Many of the changes occurred within 60 minutes.[218] In infants, digoxin produces changes in echocardiographic measurements that are associated with an improved inotropic state, although detailed invasive hemodynamic measurements have not been made in infants or children.[30,210,232] Demonstrating benefit is more difficult when CHF is caused by obstructive lesions or left-to-right shunts than when CHF is caused by myocardial failure.

In patients with CHF who have a sinus rhythm, administration of digoxin produces a decrease in heart rate, likely secondary to improvement of the inotropic state and withdrawal of compensatory sympathetic activity. In addition, digoxin enhances vagal tone by increasing baroceptor sensitivity and directly stimulating central vagal centers.[167] This process causes direct slowing of heart rate in addition to that permitted by improved function. Another effect of digoxin-mediated enhanced vagal tone is slowed conduction of atrial impulses through the atrioventricular node to the ventricle. This property is exploited with use of digoxin for control or treatment of supraventricular rhythm disturbances such as supraventricular tachycardia and atrial flutter or fibrillation. This aspect of digitalis pharmacology is reviewed in Chapter 25.

Use of digoxin in the PICU is further complicated by the large number of pharmacokinetic and pharmacodynamic interactions between digoxin and other pharmacologic agents used in critical care patients.[79] For example, carvedilol (a beta-blocker) decreases digoxin elimination in children, necessitating a reduction in digoxin dosage.[220] Toxicity is a major limiting factor in administering digitalis glycosides to critically ill patients. The most frequent side effects are gastrointestinal; the most serious are disturbances in cardiac rhythm.[152,205,210] Digitalis toxicity is reviewed in several references.[120,131] In adults and older children, the dominant manifestations of digoxin toxicity are tachydysrhythmias such as ventricular premature contractions, ventricular tachycardia, and ventricular fibrillation. Atrial tachycardia and junctional tachycardia also may be noted. Bradycardia and A-V conduction block are noted with acute, profound intoxication. In infants, enhanced vagal tone and diminished sympathetic activity alter this pattern; the dominant findings are A-V conduction block and sinus bradycardia.

Digitalis toxicity is made more likely by factors that increase myocardial irritability, such as myocarditis, ischemia, hypoxemia, or catecholamine support. Hypokalemia and alkalosis also potentiate digoxin-induced dysrhythmias. Treatment of digoxin toxicity involves supportive treatment and correction of electrolyte disturbances.[135] Specific pharmacologic support (atropine, lidocaine, phenytoin, magnesium sulfate) may be necessary (although frequently unsuccessful). In life-threatening circumstances, treatment with digoxin-specific Fab antibody fragments is indicated.[255]

Pharmacokinetics

The dosage of digoxin prescribed for young children and infants is much higher than that applied to older children and adults. In the past, this method was ascribed to the incorrect belief that developmental immaturity was associated with decreased myocardial sensitivity to digitalis. It now is understood that neonates are not less sensitive to digoxin but eliminate digoxin more rapidly.[210] Clearance is dependent on age, although there is wide interindividual variation during the first year of life.[187] Thus infants may require higher loading ("digitalizing") and maintenance dosages (Table 23–8) to achieve a therapeutically effective plasma concentration of 1 to 2 ng/ml. Distribution of digoxin is relatively slow; therefore plasma levels will be misleadingly elevated if determined sooner than 6 hours after dose administration. At distribution equilibrium, the concentration of digoxin in the heart is 15 to 30 times greater than that in the plasma. In the non-acutely ill child, the half-life of digoxin is 36 hours with a clearance of 8.6 L/hour.[90] Digoxin is eliminated by the kidney through glomerular filtration and renal tubular secretion, through a renal tubular mechanism that includes the efflux pump P-glycoprotein. A polymorphism that decreases the activity of this enzyme was associated with increased serum digoxin levels.[128] Elimination is strongly affected by renal dysfunction, which complicates use of the agent in the critically ill child.

TABLE 23–8

Recommended Intravenous Digoxin Dosage for CHF

Age	Digitalizing Dose (μg/kg)	Maintenance Dose (μg/kg/day)
Premature infant	15	3.75
Term neonate	22	6.0–7.5
Children <2 years	30–35	7.5–9.0
Children >2 years	22–30	6.0–7.5

Adapted from Park MK: *J Pediatr* 108:871, 1987.

Clinical Role

The role of digoxin in the care of the pediatric patient continues to be refined and narrowed. Its role as an inotropic agent has been supplanted by other drugs (e.g., milrinone) with a more favorable pharmacodynamic profile in the acute setting. Use of digoxin to improve cardiac function in children with systemic-to-pulmonary shunts has decreased greatly, and it now is used primarily for control of certain dysrhythmias and for improvement of systolic function in children without structural lesions.[131] Because digoxin does not produce β-adrenergic receptor desensitization and has beneficial effects by virtue of decreased sympathetic activity, it continues to have a clinical role.

Summary

Digitalis glycosides are effective inotropic agents that have the desirable property of slowing rather than accelerating heart rate. As a result of its narrow therapeutic window, long half-life, and the emergence of newer medications, the role of digoxin in the acute setting has diminished.

Conclusion

Our understanding of the mechanisms underlying adrenergic receptor signaling, the control of vascular tone, and the influence of genetic polymorphisms on the pathways involved in these processes continue to grow. Despite our increased understanding, the therapeutic options for supporting the patient with evidence of impaired end-organ perfusion has not changed significantly. The catecholamines remain the mainstay of therapy, with dopamine often the initial drug of choice for either inotropic or vasopressor support. Epinephrine or norepinephrine is used when poor cardiac performance or decreased systemic vascular tone, respectively, is the hemodynamic derangement and perfusion does not improving with dopamine. Milrinone (or amrinone) or dobutamine can be used to increase myocardial contractility if no frank hypotension is present. Milrinone is particularly useful for hemodynamic support after surgery for congenital heart disease. Vasopressin has emerged as an option for vasodilatory shock resistant to catecholamine therapy. Often the clinical picture is mixed, and the patient may require both inotropic and vasopressor support. Careful attention to the clinical signs of end-organ perfusion and an understanding of cardiovascular pharmacology are necessary for the care of these patients.

Acknowledgments

The authors gratefully acknowledge the assistance of Christine Jaderlund, PharmD, with drug preparation and compatibility information and Donna Farrell with manuscript preparation.

REFERENCES

1. Akita T, Joyner RW, Lu C, et al: Developmental changes in modulation of calcium currents of rabbit ventricular cells by phosphodiesterase inhibitors. *Circulation* 90:469, 1994.
2. Akkerman SR, Zhang H, Mullins RE, et al: Stability of milrinone lactate in the presence of 29 critical care drugs and 4 i.v. solutions. *Am J Health Syst Pharm* 56:63, 1999.
3. Alberts B: *Molecular biology of the cell,* ed 3. New York, 1994, Garland Publishing.
4. Al-Hesayen A, Azevedo ER, Newton GE, et al: The effects of dobutamine on cardiac sympathetic activity in patients with congestive heart failure. *J Am Coll Cardiol* 39:1269, 2002.
5. Allen E, Pettigrew A, Frank D, et al: Alterations in dopamine clearance and catechol-O-methyltransferase activity by dopamine infusions in children. *Crit Care Med* 25:181, 1997.
6. Allen EM, Van Boerum DH, Olsen AF, et al: Difference between the measured and ordered dose of catecholamine infusions. *Ann Pharmacother* 29:1095, 1995.
7. Allen-Webb EM, Ross MP, Pappas JB, et al: Age-related amrinone pharmacokinetics in a pediatric population. *Crit Care Med* 22:1016, 1994.
8. American Academy of Pediatrics: Drugs for pediatric emergencies. *Pediatrics* 101:e13, 1998.
9. American Heart Association: Guidelines 2000 for cardiopulmonary resuscitation and emergency cardiovascular care, part 6: Advanced Cardiovascular Life Support: agents to optimize cardiac output and blood pressure. *Circulation* 102:I129, 2000.
10. Anderson GO, Qvigstad E, Schiander I, et al: AR induced positive inotropic response in heart is dependent on myosin light chain phosphorylation. *Am J Physiol Heart Circ Physiol* 283:H1471, 2002.
11. Argent NB, Wilkinson R, Baylis PH: Metabolic clearance rate of arginine vasopressin in severe chronic renal failure. *Clin Sci* 83:583, 1992.
12. Argenziano M, Chen JM, Choudhri AF, et al: Management of vasodilatory shock after cardiac surgery: identification of predisposing factors and use of a novel pressor agent. *J Thorac Cardiovasc Surg* 116:973, 1998.
13. Argenziano M, Choudhri AF, Oz MC, et al: A prospective randomized trial of arginine vasopressin in the treatment of vasodilatory shock after left ventricular assist device placement. *Circulation* 96:II286, 1997.
14. Arnon A, Hamlyn JM, Blaustein MP: Ouabain augments Ca^{2+} transients in arterial smooth muscle without raising cytosolic Na^{+}. *Am J Physiol Heart Circ Physiol* 279:H679, 2000.
15. Artman M, Henry G, Coetzee WA: Cellular basis for age-related differences in cardiac excitation-contraction coupling. *Prog Pediatr Cardiol* 11:185, 2000.
16. Auman JT, Seidler FJ, Tate CA, et al: Are developing beta-adrenoceptors able to desensitize? Acute and chronic effects of beta-agonists in neonatal heart and liver. *Am J Physiol Regul Integr Comp Physiol* 283:R205, 2002.
17. Bailey JM, Miller BE, Kanter KR, et al: A comparison of the hemodynamic effects of amrinone and sodium nitroprusside in infants after cardiac surgery. *Anesth Analg* 84:294, 1997.
18. Bailey JM, Miller BE, Lu W, et al: The pharmacokinetics of milrinone in pediatric patients after cardiac surgery. *Anesthesiology* 90:1012, 1999.
19. Baim DS: Effect of phosphodiesterase inhibition on myocardial oxygen consumption and coronary blood flow. *Am J Cardiol* 63:23A, 1989.
20. Balakuraman K, Hugenholtz PG: Cardiogenic shock. Current concepts in management. *Drugs* 32:372, 1986.
21. Banner W Jr, Vernon DD, Dean JM, et al: Nonlinear dopamine pharmacokinetics in pediatric patients. *J Pharmacol Exp Ther* 249:131, 1989.
22. Banner W Jr, Vernon DD, Minton SD, et al: Nonlinear dobutamine pharmacokinetics in a pediatric population. *Crit Care Med* 19:871, 1991.
23. Barazzone C, Jaccard C, Berner M, et al: Propranolol treatment in children with tetralogy of Fallot alters the response to isoprenaline after surgical repair. *Br Heart J* 60:2, 1988.
24. Bartelstone HJ, Nasmyth PA: Vasopressin potentiation of catecholamine actions in dog, rat, cat, and rat aortic strip. *Am J Physiol* 208:754, 1965.
25. Barton P, Garcia J, Kouatli A, et al: Hemodynamic effects of i.v. milrinone lactate in pediatric patients with septic shock. A prospective, double-blinded, randomized, placebo-controlled, interventional study. *Chest* 109:1302, 1996.
26. Baruch L, Patacsil P, Hameed A, et al: Pharmacodynamic effects of milrinone with and without a bolus loading infusion. *Am Heart J* 141:e6, 2000.
27. Bellomo R, Chapman MJ, Finfer S, et al: Low dose dopamine in patients with early renal dysfunction. ANZICS Clinical Trials Group. *Lancet* 356:2139, 2000.
28. Beregovich J, Bianchi C, Rubler S, et al: Dose-related hemodynamic and renal effects of dopamine in congestive heart failure. *Am Heart J* 87:550, 1974.
29. Berg RA, Padbury JF, Donnerstein RL, et al: Dobutamine pharmacokinetics and pharmacodynamics in normal children and adolescents. *J Pharmacol Exp Ther* 265:1232, 1993.
30. Berman W Jr, Yabek SM, Dillon T, et al: Effects of digoxin in infants with congested circulatory state due to a ventricular septal defect. *N Engl J Med* 308:363, 1983.
31. Berner M, Jaccard C, Oberhansli I, et al: Hemodynamic effects of amrinone in children after cardiac surgery. *Intensive Care Med* 16:85, 1990.
32. Berner M, Oberhansli I, Rouge JC, et al: Chronotropic and inotropic supports are both required to increase cardiac output early after corrective operations for tetralogy of Fallot. *J Thorac Cardiovasc Surg* 97:297, 1989.
33. Berner M, Rouge JC, Friedli B: The hemodynamic effect of phentolamine and dobutamine after open-heart operations in children: influence of the underlying heart defect. *Ann Thorac Surg* 35:643, 1983.
34. Berre J, De Backer D, Moraine JJ, et al: Dobutamine increases cerebral blood flow velocity and jugular bulb hemoglobin saturation in septic patients. *Crit Care Med* 25:392, 1997.
35. Best JD, Halter JB: Release and clearance rates of epinephrine in man: importance of arterial measurements. *J Clin Endocrinol Metab* 55:263, 1982.
36. Birnbaumer M: Vasopressin receptors. *Trends Endocrinol Metab* 11:406, 2000.
37. Bohn DJ, Poirier CS, Edmonds JF, et al: Hemodynamic effects of dobutamine after cardiopulmonary bypass in children. *Crit Care Med* 8:367, 1980.
38. Bojko T, Wirywan B, Saps M, et al: Usefulness of vasopressin in pediatric vasodilatory shock. *Pediatr Crit Care Med* 1S:100, 2000.
39. Booker PD: Myocardial stunning in the neonate. *Br J Anaesth* 80:371, 1998.
40. Booker PD: Pharmacological support for children with myocardial dysfunction. *Paediatr Anaesth* 12:5, 2002.
41. Booker PD, Evans C, Franks R: Comparison of the haemodynamic effects of dopamine and dobutamine in young children undergoing cardiac surgery. *Br J Anaesth* 74:419, 1995.
42. Boreus LO, Hjemdahl P, Lagercrantz H, et al: Beta-adrenoceptor function in white blood cells from newborn infants: no relation to plasma catecholamine levels. *Pediatr Res* 20:1152, 1986.
43. Borthne K, Haga P, Langslet A, et al: Endogenous norepinephrine stimulates both alpha 1- and beta-adrenoceptors in myocardium from children with congenital heart defects. *J Mol Cell Cardiol* 27:693, 1995.
44. Bottorff MB, Rutledge DR, Pieper JA: Evaluation of intravenous amrinone: the first of a new class of positive inotropic agents with vasodilator properties. *Pharmacotherapy* 5:227, 1985.
45. Brayden JE: Functional roles of K_{ATP} channels in vascular smooth muscle. *Clin Exp Pharmacol Physiol* 29:312, 2002.

46. Brodde OE, Buscher R, Tellkamp R, et al: Blunted cardiac responses to receptor activation in subjects with Thr164Ile beta2-adrenoceptors. *Circulation* 103:1048, 2001.
47. Brodde OE, Petrasch S, Bauch HJ, et al: Terbutaline-induced desensitization of beta 2-adrenoceptor in vivo function in humans: attenuation by ketotifen. *J Cardiovasc Pharmacol* 20:434, 1992.
48. Brown CG, Martin DR, Pepe PE, et al: A comparison of standard-dose and high-dose epinephrine in cardiac arrest outside the hospital. The Multicenter High-Dose Epinephrine Study Group. *N Engl J Med* 327:1051, 1992.
49. Brown MJ, Brown DC, Murphy MB: Hypokalemia from beta2-receptor stimulation by circulating epinephrine. *N Engl J Med* 309:1414, 1983.
50. Carcillo JA, Fields AI: Clinical practice parameters for hemodynamic support of pediatric and neonatal patients in septic shock. *Crit Care Med* 30:1365, 2002.
51. Chalothorn D, McCune DF, Edelmann SE, et al: Differential cardiovascular regulatory activities of the alpha 1B- and alpha 1D-adrenoceptor subtypes. *J Pharmacol Exp Ther* 305:1045, 2003.
52. Chanani NK, Cowan DB, Takeuchi K, et al: Differential effects of amrinone and milrinone upon myocardial inflammatory signaling. *Circulation* 106:I284, 2002.
53. Chandrashekhar Y, Prahash AJ, Sen S, et al: The role of arginine vasopressin and its receptors in the normal and failing rat heart. *J Mol Cell Cardiol* 35:495, 2003.
54. Chang AC, Atz AM, Wernovsky G, et al: Milrinone: systemic and pulmonary hemodynamic effects in neonates after cardiac surgery. *Crit Care Med* 23:1907, 1995.
55. Chatterjee K: Phosphodiesterase inhibitors: alterations in systemic and coronary hemodynamics. *Basic Res Cardiol* 84(suppl 1):213, 1989.
56. Chatterjee K: Newer oral inotropic agents: phosphodiesterase inhibitors. *Crit Care Med* 18:S34, 1990.
57. Chen-Izu Y, Xiao RP, Izu LT, et al: Gi-dependent localization of beta2-adrenergic receptor signaling to L-type Ca^{2+} channels. *Biophys J* 79:2547, 2000.
58. Chernow B, Rainey TG, Lake CR: Endogenous and exogenous catecholamines in critical care medicine. *Crit Care Med* 10:409, 1982.
59. Cheung PY, Barrington KJ, Bigam D: The hemodynamic effects of dobutamine infusion in the chronically instrumented newborn piglet. *Crit Care Med* 27:558, 1999.
60. Cheung PY, Barrington KJ, Pearson RJ, et al: Systemic, pulmonary and mesenteric perfusion and oxygenation effects of dopamine and epinephrine. *Am J Respir Crit Care Med* 155:32, 1997.
61. Chu CA, Sindelar DK, Neal DW, et al: Hepatic and gut clearance of catecholamines in the conscious dog. *Metabolism* 48:259, 1999.
62. Chu CC, Lin SM, New SH, et al: Effect of milrinone on postbypass pulmonary hypertension in children after tetralogy of Fallot repair. *Zhonghua Yi Xue Za Zhi (Taipei)* 63:294, 2000.
63. Clark SJ, Yoxall CW, Subhedar NV: Right ventricular performance in hypotensive preterm neonates treated with dopamine. *Pediatr Cardiol* 23:167, 2002.
64. Clutter WE, Bier DM, Shah SD, et al: Epinephrine plasma metabolic clearance rates and physiologic thresholds for metabolic and hemodynamic actions in man. *J Clin Invest* 66:94, 1980.
65. Colucci WS, Wright RF, Braunwald E: New positive inotropic agents in the treatment of congestive heart failure. Mechanisms of action and recent clinical developments. *N Engl J Med* 314:290, 1986.
66. Conolly ME, Davies DS, Dollery CT, et al: Metabolism of isoprenaline in dog and man. *Br J Pharmacol* 46:458, 1972.
67. Conway WD, Minatoya H, Lands AM, et al: Absorption and elimination profile of isoproterenol III. *J Pharm Sci* 57:1135, 1968.
68. Cryer PE: Physiology and pathophysiology of the human sympathoadrenal neuroendocrine system. *N Engl J Med* 303:436, 1980.
69. Das PA, Skoyles JR, Sherry KM, et al: Disposition of milrinone in patients after cardiac surgery. *Br J Anaesth* 72:426, 1994.
70. Davare MA, Avdonin V, Hall DD, et al: A beta2 adrenergic receptor signaling complex assembled with the Ca2+ channel Cav1.2. *Science* 293:98, 2001.
71. Day NP, Phu NH, Bethell DP, et al: The effects of dopamine and adrenaline infusions on acid-base balance and systemic haemodynamics in severe infection. *Lancet* 348:219, 1996.
72. De Backer D, Creteur J, Silva E, et al: Effects of dopamine, norepinephrine and epinephrine on the splanchnic circulation in septic shock. *Crit Care Med* 31:1659, 2003.
73. De Backer D, Vincent JL: Norepinephrine administration in septic shock: how much is enough? *Crit Care Med* 30:1398, 2002.
74. De Hert SG, Moens MM, Jorens PG, et al: Comparison of two different loading doses of milrinone for weaning from cardiopulmonary bypass. *J Cardiothorac Vasc Anesth* 9:264, 1995.
75. Desjars P, Pinaud M, Bugnon D, et al: Norepinephrine therapy has no deleterious renal effects in human septic shock. *Crit Care Med* 17:426, 1989.
76. Desjars P, Pinaud M, Potel G, et al: A reappraisal of norepinephrine therapy in human septic shock. *Crit Care Med* 15:134, 1987.
77. Di Giantomasso D, May CN, Bellomo R: Norepinephrine and vital organ blood flow. *Intensive Care Med* 28:1804, 2002.
78. Dieckmann RA, Vardis R: High-dose epinephrine in pediatric out-of-hospital cardiopulmonary arrest. *Pediatrics* 95:901, 1995.
79. Digoxin. In McEvoy G, editor: *AHFS drug information*. Bethesda, 2003, American Society of Health-System Pharmacists.
80. Dopamine hydrochloride. In McEvoy GK, editor: *AHFS drug information*. Bethesda, MD, 2003, American Society of Health-System Pharmacists.
81. Dousa TP: Cyclic-3′,5′-nucleotide phosphodiesterase isozymes in cell biology and pathophysiology of the kidney. *Kidney Int* 55:29, 1999.
82. Downes JJ, Wood DW, Harwood I, et al: Intravenous isoproterenol infusion in children with severe hypercapnia due to status asthmaticus. *Crit Care Med* 1:63, 1973.
83. Driscoll DJ, Gillette PC, Ezrailson EG, et al: Inotropic response of the neonatal canine myocardium to dopamine. *Pediatr Res* 12:42, 1978.
84. Dunser MW, Mayr AJ, Stallinger A, et al: Cardiac performance during vasopressin infusion in postcardiotomy shock. *Intensive Care Med* 28:746, 2002.
85. Dunser MW, Mayr AJ, Tur A, et al: Ischemic skin lesions as a complication of continuous vasopressin infusion in catecholamine-resistant vasodilatory shock: incidence and risk factors. *Crit Care Med* 31:1394, 2003.
86. Dunser MW, Mayr AJ, Ulmer H, et al: Arginine vasopressin in advanced vasodilatory shock: a prospective, randomized, controlled study. *Circulation* 107:2313, 2003.
87. Dunser MW, Mayr AJ, Ulmer H, et al: The effects of vasopressin on systemic hemodynamics in catecholamine-resistant septic and postcardiotomy shock: a retrospective analysis. *Anesth Analg* 93:7, 2001.
88. Edelson J, Stroshane R, Benziger DP, et al: Pharmacokinetics of the bipyridines amrinone and milrinone. *Circulation* 73:III145, 1986.
89. Eisenhofer G, Rundquist B, Aneman A, et al: Regional release and removal of catecholamines and extraneuronal metabolism to metanephrines. *J Clin Endocrinol Metab* 80:3009, 1995.
90. El Desoky ES, Nagaraja NV, Derendorf H: Population pharmacokinetics of digoxin in Egyptian pediatric patients: impact of one data point utilization. *Am J Ther* 9:492, 2002.
91. Eldadah MK, Schwartz PH, Harrison R, et al: Pharmacokinetics of dopamine in infants and children. *Crit Care Med* 19:1008, 1991.
92. Fambrough DM, Lemas MV, Hamrick M, et al: Analysis of subunit assembly of the Na-K-ATPase. *Am J Physiol* 266:C579, 1994.
93. Farah AE, Frangakis CJ: Studies on the mechanism of action of the bipyridine milrinone on the heart. *Basic Res Cardiol* 84(suppl 1): 85, 1989.
94. Fisher DG, Schwartz PH, Davis AL: Pharmacokinetics of exogenous epinephrine in critically ill children. *Crit Care Med* 21:111, 1993.
95. Forrest P: Vasopressin and shock. *Anaesth Intensive Care* 29:463, 2001.
96. Freeman K, Farrow S, Schmaier A, et al: Genetic polymorphism of the alpha 2-adrenergic receptor is associated with increased platelet aggregation, baroreceptor sensitivity, and salt excretion in normotensive humans. *Am J Hypertens* 8:863, 1995.
97. Friedgen B, Wolfel R, Graefe KH: The contribution by monoamine oxidase and catechol-O-methyltransferase to the total-body and pulmonary plasma clearance of catecholamines. *Naunyn Schmiedebergs Arch Pharmacol* 353:193, 1996.

98. Friedman WF, George BL: New concepts and drugs in the treatment of congestive heart failure. *Pediatr Clin North Am* 31:1197, 1984.
99. Fukuoka T, Nishimura M, Imanaka H, et al: Effects of norepinephrine on renal function in septic patients with normal and elevated serum lactate levels. *Crit Care Med* 17:1104, 1989.
100. Garcia-Sainz JA, Vazquez-Prado J, del Carmen Medina L: Alpha 1-adrenoceptors: function and phosphorylation. *Eur J Pharmacol* 389:1, 2000.
101. Gauthier C, Tavernier G, Charpentier F, et al: Functional beta3-adrenoceptor in the human heart. *J Clin Invest* 98:556, 1996.
102. Geier S, Muller-Strahl G, Zimmer HG: The inotropic response of the isolated, perfused, working rat heart to norepinephrine is attenuated by inhibition of nitric oxide. *Basic Res Cardiol* 97:145, 2002.
103. Ghanayem NS, Yee L, Nelson T, et al: Stability of dopamine and epinephrine solutions up to 84 hours. *Pediatr Crit Care Med* 2:315, 2001.
104. Girardin E, Berner M, Rouge JC, et al: Effect of low dose dopamine on hemodynamic and renal function in children. *Pediatr Res* 26:200, 1989.
105. Goldberg LI: Dopamine—clinical uses of an endogenous catecholamine. *N Engl J Med* 291:707, 1974.
106. Goldberg LI, Rajfer SI: Dopamine receptors: applications in clinical cardiology. *Circulation* 72:245, 1985.
107. Goldstein DS, Eisenhofer G, Kopin IJ: Sources and significance of plasma levels of catechols and their metabolites in humans. *J Pharmacol Exp Ther* 305:800, 2003.
108. Goldstein DS, Zimlichman R, Stull R, et al: Plasma catecholamine and hemodynamic responses during isoproterenol infusions in humans. *Clin Pharmacol Ther* 40:233, 1986.
109. Golovina VA, Song H, James PF, et al: Na+ pump alpha 2-subunit expression modulates Ca2+ signaling. *Am J Physiol Cell Physiol* 284:C475, 2003.
110. Gootman N: Cardiovascular effects of catecholamine infusions in developing swine. In Tumbleson M, editor: *Swine in biomedical research*. New York, 1986, Plenum.
111. Grillo JA, Gonzalez ER, Ramaiya A, et al: Chemical compatibility of inotropic and vasoactive agents delivered via a multiple line infusion system. *Crit Care Med* 23:1061, 1995.
112. Guimaraes S, Moura D: Vascular adrenoceptors: an update. *Pharmacol Rev* 53:319, 2001.
113. Gundert-Remy U, Penzien J, Hildebrandt R, et al: Correlation between the pharmacokinetics and pharmacodynamics of dopamine in healthy subjects. *Eur J Clin Pharmacol* 26:163, 1984.
114. Habib DM, Padbury JF, Anas NG, et al: Dobutamine pharmacokinetics and pharmacodynamics in pediatric intensive care patients. *Crit Care Med* 20:601, 1992.
115. Hamilton RA, Kowalsky SF, Wright EM, et al: Effect of the acetylator phenotype on amrinone pharmacokinetics. *Clin Pharmacol Ther* 40:615, 1986.
116. Hannemann L, Reinhart K, Grenzer O, et al: Comparison of dopamine to dobutamine and norepinephrine for oxygen delivery and uptake in septic shock. *Crit Care Med* 23:1962, 1995.
117. Harada K, Tamura M, Ito T, et al: Effects of low-dose dobutamine on left ventricular diastolic filling in children. *Pediatr Cardiol* 17:220, 1996.
118. Hasser EM, Bishop VS, Hay M: Interactions between vasopressin and baroreflex control of the sympathetic nervous system. *Clin Exp Pharmacol Physiol* 24:102, 1997.
119. Hatem SN, Sweeten T, Vetter V, et al: Evidence for presence of Ca2+ channel-gated Ca2+ stores in neonatal human atrial myocytes. *Am J Physiol* 268:H1195, 1995.
120. Hauptman PJ, Kelly RA: Digitalis. *Circulation* 99:1265, 1999.
121. Hayashida N, Tomoeda H, Oda T, et al: Inhibitory effect of milrinone on cytokine production after cardiopulmonary bypass. *Ann Thorac Surg* 68:1661, 1999.
122. Heckmann M, Trotter A, Pohlandt F, et al: Epinephrine treatment of hypotension in very low birthweight infants. *Acta Paediatr* 91:566, 2002.
123. Hemstreet MP, Miles MV, Rutland RO: Effect of intravenous isoproterenol on theophylline kinetics. *J Allergy Clin Immunol* 69:360, 1982.
124. Hesselvik JF, Brodin B: Low dose norepinephrine in patients with septic shock and oliguria: effects on afterload, urine flow, and oxygen transport. *Crit Care Med* 17:179, 1989.
125. Hoffman BB: Catecholamines, sympathomimetic drugs and adrenergic receptor antagonists. In Hardman JG, Limbird LE, editors: *Goodman & Gilman's the pharmacologic basis of therapeutics*. New York, 2001, McGraw Hill.
126. Hoffman BB, Taylor P: Neurotransmission. In Hardman JG, Limbird LE, editors: *Goodman and Gilman's the pharmacologic basis of therapeutics*. New York, 2001, McGraw Hill.
127. Hoffman TM, Wernovsky G, Atz AM, et al: Efficacy and safety of milrinone in preventing low cardiac output syndrome in infants and children after corrective surgery for congenital heart disease. *Circulation* 107:996, 2003.
128. Hoffmeyer S, Burk O, von Richter O, et al: Functional polymorphisms of the human multidrug-resistance gene: multiple sequence variations and correlation of one allele with P-glycoprotein expression and activity in vivo. *Proc Natl Acad Sci U S A* 97:3473, 2000.
129. Holmes CL, Patel BM, Russell JA, et al: Physiology of vasopressin relevant to management of septic shock. *Chest* 120:989, 2001.
130. Holmes CL, Walley KR, Chittock DR, et al: The effects of vasopressin on hemodynamics and renal function in severe septic shock: a case series. *Intensive Care Med* 27:1416, 2001.
131. Hougen TJ: Digitalis use in children: an uncertain future. *Prog Pediatr Cardiol* 12:37, 2000.
132. Humma LM, Puckett BJ, Richardson HE, et al: Effects of beta1-adrenoceptor genetic polymorphisms on resting hemodynamics in patients undergoing diagnostic testing for ischemia. *Am J Cardiol* 88:1034, 2001.
133. Ichai C, Soubielle J, Carles M, et al: Comparison of the renal effects of low to high doses of dopamine and dobutamine in critically ill patients: a single-blind randomized study. *Crit Care Med* 28:921, 2000.
134. Insel PA: Adrenergic receptors—evolving concepts and clinical implications. *N Engl J Med* 334:580, 1996.
135. Iseri LT, Freed J, Bures AR: Magnesium deficiency and cardiac disorders. *Am J Med* 58:837, 1975.
136. Jackson E: Vasopressin and other agents affecting the renal conservation of water. In Hardman JG, Limbird LE, editors: *Goodman & Gilman's the pharmacologic basis of therapeutics*. New York, 2001, McGraw Hill.
137. Jackson WF: Ion channels and vascular tone. *Hypertension* 35:173, 2000.
138. Jakob SM, Ruokonen E, Takala J: Effects of dopamine on systemic and regional blood flow and metabolism in septic and cardiac surgery patients. *Shock* 18:8, 2002.
139. James PF, Grupp IL, Grupp G, et al: Identification of a specific role for the Na,K-ATPase alpha 2 isoform as a regulator of calcium in the heart. *Mol Cell* 3:555, 1999.
140. Johnston RR, Eger EI II, Wilson C: A comparative interaction of epinephrine with enflurane, isoflurane, and halothane in man. *Anesth Analg* 55:709, 1976.
141. Juste RN, Moran L, Hooper J, et al: Dopamine clearance in critically ill patients. *Intensive Care Med* 24:1217, 1998.
142. Kahn JM, Kress JP, Hall JB: Skin necrosis after extravasation of low-dose vasopressin administered for septic shock. *Crit Care Med* 30:1899, 2002.
143. Kamp TJ, Hell JW: Regulation of cardiac L-type calcium channels by protein kinase A and protein kinase C. *Circ Res* 87:1095, 2000.
144. Kapiloff MS: Contributions of protein kinase A anchoring proteins to compartmentation of cAMP signaling in the heart. *Mol Pharmacol* 62:193, 2002.
145. Karlsberg RP, DeWood MA, DeMaria AN, et al: Comparative efficacy of short-term intravenous infusions of milrinone and dobutamine in acute congestive heart failure following acute myocardial infarction. *Clin Cardiol* 19:21, 1996.
146. Karmazyn M, Manku MS, Horrobin DF: Changes of vascular reactivity induced by low vasopressin concentrations: interactions with cortisol and lithium and possible involvement of prostaglandins. *Endocrinology* 102:1230, 1978.
147. Katz K, Lawler J, Wax J, et al: Vasopressin pressor effects in critically ill children during evaluation for brain death and organ recovery. *Resuscitation* 47:33, 2000.

148. Keef KD, Hume JR, Zhong J: Regulation of cardiac and smooth muscle Ca^{2+} channels Ca(V)1.2a,b by protein kinases. *Am J Physiol Cell Physiol* 281:C1743, 2001.
149. Kilts JD, Gerhardt MA, Richardson MD, et al: Beta2-adrenergic and several other G protein-coupled receptors in human atrial membranes activate both Gs and Gi. *Circ Res* 87:705, 2000.
150. Kopin JJ: Catecholamine metabolism: basic aspects and clinical significance. *Pharmacol Rev* 37:333, 1985.
151. Koshimizu TA, Tanoue A, Hirasawa A, et al: Recent advances in alpha1-adrenoceptor pharmacology. *Pharmacol Ther* 98:235, 2003.
152. Krasula R, Yanagi R, Hastreiter AR, et al: Digoxin intoxication in infants and children: correlation with serum levels. *J Pediatr* 84:265, 1974.
153. Kuznetsov V, Pak E, Robinson RB, et al: Beta 2-adrenergic receptor actions in neonatal and adult rat ventricular myocytes. *Circ Res* 76:40, 1995.
154. Laitinen P, Ahonen J, Olkkola KT, et al: Pharmacokinetics of amrinone in neonates and infants. *J Cardiothorac Vasc Anesth* 14:378, 2000.
155. Landry DW, Levin HR, Gallant EM, et al: Vasopressin deficiency contributes to the vasodilation of septic shock. *Circulation* 95:1122, 1997.
156. Landry DW, Levin HR, Gallant EM, et al: Vasopressin pressor hypersensitivity in vasodilatory septic shock. *Crit Care Med* 25:1279, 1997.
157. Landry DW, Oliver JA: The pathogenesis of vasodilatory shock. *N Engl J Med* 345:588, 2001.
158. Lang P, Williams RG, Norwood WI, et al: The hemodynamic effects of dopamine in infants after corrective cardiac surgery. *J Pediatr* 96:630, 1980.
159. Lawless S, Burckart G, Diven W, et al: Amrinone in neonates and infants after cardiac surgery. *Crit Care Med* 17:751, 1989.
160. Lebovitz DJ, Lawless ST, Weise KL: Fatal amrinone overdose in a pediatric patient. *Crit Care Med* 23:977, 1995.
161. Leier CV, Unverferth DV: Drugs five years later. Dobutamine. *Ann Intern Med* 99:490, 1983.
162. Leier CV, Unverferth DV, Kates RE: The relationship between plasma dobutamine concentrations and cardiovascular responses in cardiac failure. *Am J Med* 66:238, 1979.
163. Lemaire F: Effect of catecholamines on pulmonary right-to-left shunt. *Int Anesthesiol Clin* 21:43, 1983.
164. Leone M, Albanese J, Martin C: Positive inotropic stimulation. *Curr Opin Crit Care* 8:395, 2002.
165. Levin MC, Marullo S, Muntaner O, et al: The myocardium-protective Gly-49 variant of the beta 1-adrenergic receptor exhibits constitutive activity and increased desensitization and down-regulation. *J Biol Chem* 277:30429, 2002.
166. Levy JH, Bailey JM, Deeb GM: Intravenous milrinone in cardiac surgery. *Ann Thorac Surg* 73:325, 2002.
167. Lewis RP: Digitalis: a drug that refuses to die. *Crit Care Med* 18:S5, 1990.
168. Li YH, Wirth T, Huotari M, et al: No change of brain extracellular catecholamine levels after acute catechol-O-methyltransferase inhibition: a microdialysis study in anaesthetized rats. *Eur J Pharmacol* 356:127, 1998.
169. Liedel JL, Meadow W, Nachman J, et al: Use of vasopressin in refractory hypotension in children with vasodilatory shock: five cases and a review of the literature. *Pediatr Crit Care Med* 3:15, 2002.
170. Liggett SB: Beta2-adrenergic receptor pharmacogenetics. *Am J Respir Crit Care Med* 161:S197, 2002.
171. Liggett SB: Update on current concepts of the molecular basis of beta2-adrenergic receptor signaling. *J Allergy Clin Immunol* 110: S223, 2002.
172. Lin F, Owens WA, Chen S, et al: Targeted alpha1A-adrenergic receptor overexpression induces enhanced cardiac contractility but not hypertrophy. *Circ Res* 89:343, 2001.
173. Lindsay CA, Barton P, Lawless S, et al: Pharmacokinetics and pharmacodynamics of milrinone lactate in pediatric patients with septic shock. *J Pediatr* 132:329, 1998.
174. Lippmann M, Reisner LS: Epinephrine injection with enflurane anesthesia: incidence of cardiac arrhythmias. *Anesth Analg* 53: 886, 1974.
175. Lisbon A: Dopexamine, dobutamine, and dopamine increase splanchnic blood flow: what is the evidence? *Chest* 123:460S, 2003.
176. Liu W, Yasui K, Opthof T, et al: Developmental changes of Ca^{2+} handling in mouse ventricular cells from early embryo to adulthood. *Life Sci* 71:1279, 2002.
177. Luk J, Ajaelo I, Wong V, et al: Role of V1 receptors in the action of vasopressin on the baroreflex control of heart rate. *Am J Physiol* 265:R524, 1993.
178. MacGregor DA, Smith TE, Prielipp RC, et al: Pharmacokinetics of dopamine in healthy male subjects. *Anesthesiology* 92:338, 2000.
179. MacLeod CM: Drugs used in the acutely ill patient. *Dis Mon* 39:362, 1993.
180. Majerus TC, Dasta JF, Bauman JL, et al: Dobutamine: ten years later. *Pharmacotherapy* 9:245, 1989.
181. Malay MB, Ashton RC Jr, Landry DW, et al: Low-dose vasopressin in the treatment of vasodilatory septic shock. *J Trauma* 47:699, 1999.
182. Mammel MC, Einzig S, Kulik TJ, et al: Pulmonary vascular effects of amrinone in conscious lambs. *Pediatr Res* 17:720, 1983.
183. Mann K, Berg RA, Nadkarni V: Beneficial effects of vasopressin in prolonged pediatric cardiac arrest: a case series. *Resuscitation* 52:149, 2002.
184. Martin C, Eon B, Saux P, et al: Renal effects of norepinephrine used to treat septic shock patients. *Crit Care Med* 18:282, 1990.
185. Martin C, Viviand X, Leone M, et al: Effect of norepinephrine on the outcome of septic shock. *Crit Care Med* 28:2758, 2000.
186. Martinez AM, Padbury JF, Thio S: Dobutamine pharmacokinetics and cardiovascular responses in critically ill neonates. *Pediatrics* 89:47, 1992.
187. Martin-Suarez A, Falcao AC, Outeda M, et al: Population pharmacokinetics of digoxin in pediatric patients. *Ther Drug Monit* 24:742, 2002.
188. Mason DA, Moore JD, Green SA, et al: A gain-of-function polymorphism in a G-protein coupling domain of the human beta1-adrenergic receptor. *J Biol Chem* 274:12670, 1999.
189. McGovern JJ, Cheifetz IM, Craig DM, et al: Right ventricular injury in young swine: effects of catecholamines on right ventricular function and pulmonary vascular mechanics. *Pediatr Res* 48:763, 2000.
190. Meier-Hellmann A, Reinhart K, Bredle DL, et al: Epinephrine impairs splanchnic perfusion in septic shock. *Crit Care Med* 25:399, 1997.
191. Michelotti GA, Price DT, Schwinn DA: Alpha 1-adrenergic receptor regulation: basic science and clinical implications. *Pharmacol Ther* 88:281, 2000.
192. Minneman KP: Alpha 1-adrenergic receptor subtypes, inositol phosphates, and sources of cell Ca2+. *Pharmacol Rev* 40:87, 1988.
193. Mochly-Rosen D, Gordon AS: Anchoring proteins for protein kinase C: a means for isozyme selectivity. *FASEB J* 12:35, 1998.
194. Mollhoff T, Loick HM, Van Aken H, et al: Milrinone modulates endotoxemia, systemic inflammation, and subsequent acute phase response after cardiopulmonary bypass. *Anesthesiology* 90:72, 1999.
195. Morales D, Madigan J, Cullinane S, et al: Reversal by vasopressin of intractable hypotension in the late phase of hemorrhagic shock. *Circulation* 100:226, 1999.
196. Morales DL, Garrido MJ, Madigan JD, et al: A double-blind randomized trial: prophylactic vasopressin reduces hypotension after cardiopulmonary bypass. *Ann Thorac Surg* 75:926, 2003.
197. Moran JL, O'Fathartaigh MS, Peisach AR, et al: Epinephrine as an inotropic agent in septic shock: a dose-profile analysis. *Crit Care Med* 21:70, 1993.
198. Movsesian MA: PDE3 cyclic nucleotide phosphodiesterases and the compartmentation of cyclic nucleotide-mediated signalling in cardiac myocytes. *Basic Res Cardiol* 97:I83, 2002.
199. Nemenoff RA: Vasopressin signaling pathways in vascular smooth muscle. *Front Biosci* 3:D194, 1998.
200. Norepinephrine bitartrate injection. In: *USP package insert.* Chicago, 1999, Abbott Laboratories.
201. Notterman DA: Pharmacologic support of the failing circulation: an approach for infants and children. *Prob Anesth* 3:288, 1989.

202. Notterman DA: Inotropic agents. Catecholamines, digoxin, amrinone. *Crit Care Clin* 7:583, 1991.
203. Notterman DA, Greenwald BM, Moran F, et al: Dopamine clearance in critically ill infants and children: effect of age and organ system dysfunction. *Clin Pharmacol Ther* 48:138, 1990.
204. Nunez S, Maisel A: Comparison between mixed venous oxygen saturation and thermodilution cardiac output in monitoring patients with severe heart failure treated with milrinone and dobutamine. *Am Heart J* 135:383, 1998.
205. Ooi H, Colucci WS: Pharmacological treatment of heart failure. In Hardman JG, Limbird LE, editors: *Goodman and Gilman's the pharmacologic basis of therapeutics.* New York, 2001, McGraw Hill.
206. Orlowski JP, Porembka DT, Gallagher JM, et al: Comparison study of intraosseous, central intravenous, and peripheral intravenous infusions of emergency drugs. *Am J Dis Child* 144:112, 1990.
207. Osborn D, Evans N, Kluckow M: Randomized trial of dobutamine versus dopamine in preterm infants with low systemic blood flow. *J Pediatr* 140:183, 2002.
208. Pacold I, Kleinman B, Gunnar R, et al: Effects of low dose dobutamine on coronary hemodynamics, myocardial metabolism, and anginal threshold in patients with coronary artery disease. *Circulation* 68:1044, 1983.
209. Padbury JF, Agata Y, Baylen BG, et al: Dopamine pharmacokinetics in critically ill newborn infants. *J Pediatr* 110:293, 1986.
210. Park MK: Use of digoxin in infants and children, with specific emphasis on dosage. *J Pediatr* 108:871, 1986.
211. Peddicord TE, Olsen KM, ZumBrunnen TL, et al: Stability of high-concentration dopamine hydrochloride, norepinephrine bitartrate, epinephrine hydrochloride, and nitroglycerin in 5% dextrose injection. *Am J Health Syst Pharm* 54:1417, 1997.
212. Perez CA, Reimer JM, Schreiber MD, et al: Effect of high-dose dopamine on urine output in newborn infants. *Crit Care Med* 14:1045, 1986.
213. Perloff WA: Cardiovascular problems in pediatric critical care. In Swedlow DB, Raphaely RC, editors: New York, 1986, Churchill Livingston.
214. Piascik MT, Perez DM: Alpha1-adrenergic receptors: new insights and directions. *J Pharmacol Exp Ther* 298:403, 2001.
215. Powel MB, Robinson CA, Furner RL: Interference with high performance liquid chromatographic chloramphenicol assay in a patient receiving dobutamine. *Ther Drug Monit* 7:121, 1985.
216. Primacor. In: *Physician's Desk Reference.* Montvale, NJ, 2003, Thomson.
217. Prins I, Plotz FB, Uiterwaal CS, et al: Low-dose dopamine in neonatal and pediatric intensive care: a systematic review. *Intensive Care Med* 27:206, 2001.
218. Rackow EC, Packman MI, Weil MH: Hemodynamic effects of digoxin during acute cardiac failure: a comparison in patients with and without acute myocardial infarction. *Crit Care Med* 15:1001, 1987.
219. Ramamoorthy C, Anderson GD, Williams GD, et al: Pharmacokinetics and side effects of milrinone in infants and children after open heart surgery. *Anesth Analg* 86:283, 1998.
220. Ratnapalan S, Griffiths K, Costei AM, et al: Digoxin-carvedilol interactions in children. *J Pediatr* 142:572, 2003.
221. Redl-Wenzl EM, Armbruster C, Edelmann G, et al: The effects of norepinephrine on hemodynamics and renal function in severe septic shock states. *Intensive Care Med* 19:151, 1993.
222. Reid IA: Role of vasopressin deficiency in the vasodilation of septic shock. *Circulation* 95:1108, 1997.
223. Rennotte MT, Reynaert M, Clerbaux T, et al: Effects of two inotropic drugs, dopamine and dobutamine, on pulmonary gas exchange in artificially ventilated patients. *Intensive Care Med* 15:160, 1989.
224. Reuter H, Henderson SA, Han T, et al: The Na+-Ca2+ exchanger is essential for the action of cardiac glycosides. *Circ Res* 90:305, 2002.
225. Robin JK, Oliver JA, Landry DW: Vasopressin deficiency in the syndrome of irreversible shock. *J Trauma* 54:S149, 2003.
226. Robinson BW, Gelband H, Mas MS: Selective pulmonary and systemic vasodilator effects of amrinone in children: new therapeutic implications. *J Am Coll Cardiol* 21:1461, 1993.
227. Rockson SG, Homcy CJ, Quinn P, et al: Cellular mechanisms of impaired adrenergic responsiveness in neonatal dogs. *J Clin Invest* 67:319, 1981.
228. Rosenzweig EB, Starc TJ, Chen JM, et al: Intravenous arginine-vasopressin in children with vasodilatory shock after cardiac surgery. *Circulation* 100:II182, 1999.
229. Ross MP, Allen-Webb EM, Pappas JB, et al: Amrinone-associated thrombocytopenia: pharmacokinetic analysis. *Clin Pharmacol Ther* 53:661, 1993.
230. Ruffolo RR Jr, Spradio TA, Pollock GD, et al: Alpha and beta-adrenergic effects of the sterioisomers of dobutamine. *J Pharmacol Exp Ther* 219:447, 1981.
231. Sandilands AJ, O'Shaughnessy KM, Brown MJ: Greater inotropic and cyclic AMP responses evoked by noradrenaline through Arg389 beta 1-adrenoceptors versus Gly389 beta 1-adrenoceptors in isolated human atrial myocardium. *Br J Pharmacol* 138:386, 2003.
232. Sandor GG, Bloom KR, Izukawa T, et al: Noninvasive assessment of left ventricular function related to serum digoxin levels in neonates. *Pediatrics* 65:541, 1980.
233. Schiffmann H, Flesch M, Hauseler C, et al: Effects of different inotropic interventions on myocardial function in the developing rabbit heart. *Basic Res Cardiol* 97:76, 2002.
234. Schlepper M, Thormann J, Kremer P, et al: Present use of positive inotropic drugs in heart failure. *J Cardiovasc Pharmacol* 14(suppl1): S9, 1989.
235. Schmidt TA, Allen PD, Colucci WS, et al: No adaptation to digitalization as evaluated by digitalis receptor (Na,K-ATPase) quantification in explanted hearts from donors without heart disease and from digitalized recipients with end-stage heart failure. *Am J Cardiol* 71:110, 1993.
236. Schwinger RH, Bundgaard H, Muller-Ehmsen J, et al: The Na, K ATPase in the failing human heart. *Cardiovasc Res* 57:913, 2003.
237. Seguin P, Bellissant E, Le Tulzo Y, et al: Effects of epinephrine compared with the combination of dobutamine and norepinephrine on gastric perfusion in septic shock. *Clin Pharmacol Ther* 71:381, 2002.
238. Seri I: Cardiovascular, renal, and endocrine actions of dopamine in neonates and children. *J Pediatr* 126:333, 1995.
239. Seri I, Abbasi S, Wood DC, et al: Regional hemodynamic effects of dopamine in the sick preterm neonate. *J Pediatr* 133:728, 1998.
240. Seri I, Tulassay T, Kiszel J, et al: Cardiovascular response to dopamine in hypotensive preterm neonates with severe hyaline membrane disease. *Eur J Pediatr* 142:3, 1984.
241. Sharma VK, Dellinger RP: The International Sepsis Forum's controversies in sepsis: my initial vasopressor agent in septic shock is norepinephrine rather than dopamine. *Crit Care* 7:3, 2003.
242. Sharshar T, Blanchard A, Paillard M, et al: Circulating vasopressin levels in septic shock. *Crit Care Med* 31:1752, 2003.
243. Shekerdemian L, Reddington A: Cardiovascular pharmacology. In Chang AC, Hanley F, Wernovsky G, Wessel DL, editors: *Pediatric cardiac intensive care.* Baltimore, 1998, Williams & Wilkins.
244. Shigekawa M, Iwamoto T: Cardiac Na(+)-Ca(2+) exchange: molecular and pharmacological aspects. *Circ Res* 88:864, 2001.
245. Shipley JB, Tolman D, Hastillo A, et al: Milrinone: basic and clinical pharmacology and acute and chronic management. *Am J Med Sci* 311:286, 1996.
246. Silva E, DeBacker D, Creteur J, et al: Effects of vasoactive drugs on gastric intramucosal pH. *Crit Care Med* 26:1749, 1998.
247. Singh M, Notterman DA, Metakis L: Tumor necrosis factor produces homologous desensitization of lymphocyte beta 2 adrenergic responses. *Circ Shock* 39:275, 1993.
248. Siwy BK, Sadove AM: Acute management of dopamine infiltration injury with Regitine. *Plast Reconstr Surg* 80:610, 1987.
249. Skomedal T, Borthne K, Aass H, et al: Comparison between alpha-1 adrenoceptor-mediated and beta adrenoceptor-mediated inotropic components elicited by norepinephrine in failing human ventricular muscle. *J Pharmacol Exp Ther* 280:721, 1997.
250. Skoyles JR, Sherry KM: Pharmacology, mechanisms of action and uses of selective phosphodiesterase inhibitors. *Br J Anaesth* 68:293, 1992.
251. Small KM, McGraw DW, Liggett SB: Pharmacology and physiology of human adrenergic receptor polymorphisms. *Annu Rev Pharmacol Toxicol* 43:381, 2003.

252. Small KM, Wagoner LE, Levin AM, et al: Synergistic polymorphisms of beta1- and alpha2C-adrenergic receptors and the risk of congestive heart failure. *N Engl J Med* 347:1135, 2002.
253. Smiley RM, Kwatra MM, Schwinn DA: New developments in cardiovascular adrenergic receptor pharmacology: molecular mechanisms and clinical relevance. *J Cardiothorac Vasc Anesth* 12:80, 1998.
254. Smith RE: Dobutamine-induced inhibition of platelet function. *Int J Clin Pharm Res* 2:89, 1982.
255. Smith TW, Butler VP Jr, Haber E, et al: Treatment of life-threatening digitalis intoxication with digoxin-specific Fab antibody fragments: experience in 26 cases. *N Engl J Med* 307:1357, 1982.
256. Smolich JJ, Cox HS, Esler MD: Contribution of lungs to desipramine-induced changes in whole body catecholamine kinetics in newborn lambs. *Am J Physiol* 276:R243, 1999.
257. Snow JC, Shamsai J, Sakarya I: Effects of epinephrine during halothane anesthesia in mastoidotympanoplastic surgery. *Anesth Analg* 47:252, 1968.
258. Solis-Herruzo JA, Gonzalez-Gamarra A, Castellano G, et al: Metabolic clearance rate of arginine vasopressin in patients with cirrhosis. *Hepatology* 16:974, 1992.
259. Solomon SL, Wallace EM, Ford-Jones EL, et al: Medication errors with inhalant epinephrine mimicking an epidemic of neonatal sepsis. *N Engl J Med* 310:166, 1984.
260. Somlyo AP, Somlyo AV: Signal transduction and regulation in smooth muscle. *Nature* 372:231, 1994.
261. Sorensen GK, Ramamoorthy C, Lynn AM, et al: Hemodynamic effects of amrinone in children after Fontan surgery. *Anesth Analg* 82:241, 1996.
262. Steel A, Bihari D: Choice of catecholamine: does it matter. *Curr Opin Crit Care* 6:347, 2000.
263. Steinberg C, Notterman DA: Pharmacokinetics of cardiovascular drugs in children. Inotropes and vasopressors. *Clin Pharmacokinet* 27:345, 1994.
264. Steinberg SF: The molecular basis for distinct beta-adrenergic receptor subtype actions in cardiomyocytes. *Circ Res* 85:1101, 1999.
265. Subhedar NV, Shaw NJ: Dopamine versus dobutamine for hypotensive preterm infants. *Cochrane Database Syst Rev* CD001242, 2000.
266. Sun D, Huang A, Mital S, et al: Norepinephrine elicits beta2-receptor-mediated dilation of isolated human coronary arterioles. *Circulation* 106:550, 2002.
267. Sun LS: Regulation of myocardial beta-adrenergic receptor function in adult and neonatal rabbits. *Biol Neonate* 76:181, 1999.
268. Takakura K, Xiaohong W, Takeuchi K, et al: Deactivation of norepinephrine by peroxynitrite as a new pathogenesis in the hypotension of septic shock. *Anesthesiology* 98:928, 2003.
269. Tanoue A, Nasa Y, Koshimizu T, et al: The alpha1D-adrenergic receptor directly regulates arterial blood pressure via vasoconstriction. *J Clin Invest* 109:765, 2002.
270. Teshima H, Tobita K, Yamamura H, et al: Cardiovascular effects of a phosphodiesterase III inhibitor, amrinone, in infants: non-invasive echocardiographic evaluation. *Pediatr Int* 44:259, 2002.
271. Theroux TL, Esbenshade TA, Peavy RD, et al: Coupling efficiencies of human alpha 1-adrenergic receptor subtypes: titration of receptor density and responsiveness with inducible and repressible expression vectors. *Mol Pharmacol* 50:1376, 1996.
272. Thibonnier M, Graves MK, Wagner MS, et al: Study of V1-vascular vasopressin receptor gene microsatellite polymorphisms in human essential hypertension. *J Mol Cell Cardiol* 32:557, 2000.
273. Thoren A, Elam M, Ricksten SE: Differential effects of dopamine, dopexamine, and dobutamine on jejunal mucosal perfusion early after cardiac surgery. *Crit Care Med* 28:2338, 2000.
274. Toyoshima H, Nasa Y, Hashizume Y, et al: Modulation of cAMP-mediated vasorelaxation by endothelial nitric oxide and basal cGMP in vascular smooth muscle. *J Cardiovasc Pharmacol* 32: 543, 1998.
275. Trissel LA, Gilbert DL, Martinez JF, et al: Compatibility of medications with 3-in-1 parenteral nutrition admixtures. *JPEN J Parenter Enteral Nutr* 23:67, 1999.
276. Tsuchiya M, Tsuchiya K, Maruyama R, et al: Vasopressin inhibits sarcolemmal ATP-sensitive K+ channels via V1 receptors activation in the guinea pig heart. *Circ J* 66:277, 2002.
277. Tsuneyoshi I, Yamada H, Kakihana Y, et al: Hemodynamic and metabolic effects of low-dose vasopressin infusions in vasodilatory septic shock. *Crit Care Med* 29:487, 2001.
278. Turki J, Lorenz JN, Green SA, et al: Myocardial signaling defects and impaired cardiac function of a human beta 2-adrenergic receptor polymorphism expressed in transgenic mice. *Proc Natl Acad Sci U S A* 93:10483, 1996.
279. Undesser KP, Hasser EM, Haywood JR, et al: Interactions of vasopressin with the area postrema in arterial baroreflex function in conscious rabbits. *Circ Res* 56:410, 1985.
280. Ushay HM, Notterman DA: Pharmacology of pediatric resuscitation. *Pediatr Clin North Am* 44:207, 1997.
281. Van den Berghe G, de Zegher F, Lauwers P: Dopamine suppresses pituitary function in infants and children. *Crit Care Med* 22:1747, 1994.
282. Vanhoutte PM: Endothelial adrenoceptors. *J Cardiovasc Pharmacol* 38:796, 2001.
283. Vasarhelyi B, Ver A, Nobilis A, et al: Functional and structural properties of Na+/K(+)-ATPase enzyme in neonatal erythrocytes. *Eur J Clin Invest* 28:543, 1998.
284. Vasopressin. In McEvoy GK, editor: *AHFS drug dnformation.* Bethesda, 2003, American Society of Health-System Pharmacists.
285. Vecchione C, Fratta L, Rizzoni D, et al: Cardiovascular influences of alpha1b-adrenergic receptor defect in mice. *Circulation* 105:1700, 2002.
286. Veltri MA, Conner KG: Physical compatibility of milrinone lactate injection with intravenous drugs commonly used in the pediatric intensive care unit. *Am J Health Syst Pharm* 59:452, 2002.
287. Vincent JL, de Backer D: The International Sepsis Forum's controversies in sepsis: my initial vasopressor agent in septic shock is dopamine rather than norepinephrine. *Crit Care* 7:6, 2003.
288. Wakatsuki T, Nakaya Y, Inoue I: Vasopressin modulates K^+ channel activities of cultured smooth muscle cells from porcine coronary artery. *Am J Physiol* 263:H491, 1992.
289. Wang J, Schwinger RH, Frank K, et al: Regional expression of sodium pump subunits isoforms and Na+–Ca++ exchanger in the human heart. J Clin Invest 98:1650, 1996.
290. Webb JG, Yates PW, Yang Q, et al: Adenylyl cyclase isoforms and signal integration in models of vascular smooth muscle cells. *Am J Physiol Heart Circ Physiol* 281:H1545, 2001.
291. Wessel DL: Managing low cardiac output syndrome after congenital heart surgery. *Crit Care Med* 29:S220, 2001.
292. Whitsett JA, Noguchi A, Moore JJ: Developmental aspects of alpha- and beta-adrenergic receptors. *Semin Perinatol* 6:125, 1982.
293. Wilmhurst PT, Webb-Peploe MM: Side effects of amrinone therapy. *Br Heart J* 49:447, 1983.
294. Wilson RF, Sibbald WJ, Jaanimagi JL: Hemodynamic effects of dopamine in critically ill septic patients. *J Surg Res* 20:163, 1976.
295. Wood SM, Milne JR, Evans SF, et al: Effect of dobutamine on insulin requirement in diabetic ketoacidosis. *Br Med J (Clin Res Ed)* 282:946, 1981.
296. Wu JR, Chang HR, Huang TY, et al: Reduction in lymphocyte beta-adrenergic receptor density in infants and children with heart failure secondary to congenital heart disease. *Am J Cardiol* 77: 170, 1996.
297. Xiao RP, Cheng H, Zhou YY, et al: Recent advances in cardiac beta2-adrenergic signal transduction. *Circ Res* 85:1092, 1999.
298. Yan M, Webster LT Jr, Blumer JL: 3-O-methyldobutamine, a major metabolite of dobutamine in humans. *Drug Metab Dispos* 30:519, 2002.
299. Yan M, Webster LT Jr, Blumer JL: Kinetic interactions of dopamine and dobutamine with human catechol-O-methyltransferase and monoamine oxidase in vitro. *J Pharmacol Exp Ther* 301:315, 2002.
300. Yano M, Kohno M, Ohkusa T, et al: Effect of milrinone on left ventricular relaxation and Ca^{2+} uptake function of cardiac sarcoplasmic reticulum. *Am J Physiol Heart Circ Physiol* 279:H1898, 2000.
301. Yatani A, Brown AM: Rapid beta-adrenergic modulation of cardiac calcium channel currents by a fast G protein pathway. *Science* 245:71, 1989.
302. Yatani A, Tajima Y, Green SA: Coupling of beta-adrenergic receptors to cardiac L-type Ca2+ channels. *Cell Signal* 11:337, 1999.
303. Yost CS: Potassium channels: basic aspects, functional roles, and medical significance. *Anesthesiology* 90:1186, 1999.

304. Young RA, Ward A: Milrinone. A preliminary review of its pharmacological properties and therapeutic use. *Drugs* 36:158, 1988.
305. Zaritsky A: Essentials of critical care pharmacology. In Chernow B, editor: Baltimore, 1994, Williams & Wilkins.
306. Zaritsky A, Chernow B: Use of catecholamines in pediatrics. *J Pediatr* 105:341, 1984.
307. Zaugg M, Schaub MC, Pasch T, et al: Modulation of beta-adrenergic receptor subtype activities in perioperative medicine: mechanisms and sites of action. *Br J Anaesth* 88:101, 2002.
308. Zeiders JL, Seidler FJ, Iaccarino G, et al: Ontogeny of cardiac beta-adrenoceptor desensitization mechanisms: agonist treatment enhances receptor/G-protein transduction rather than eliciting uncoupling. *J Mol Cell Cardiol* 31:413, 1999.
309. Zhang W, Ke H, Colman RW: Identification of interaction sites of cyclic nucleotide phosphodiesterase type 3A with milrinone and cilostazol using molecular modeling and site-directed mutagenesis. *Mol Pharmacol* 62:514, 2002.
310. Zhou YY, Yang D, Zhu WZ, et al: Spontaneous activation of beta2- but not beta1-adrenoceptors expressed in cardiac myocytes from beta1 beta2 double knockout mice. *Mol Pharmacol* 58:887, 2000.

CHAPTER

24

Cardiopulmonary Interactions

Bradley P. Fuhrman

PEARLS

- Mechanical ventilation can alter right ventricular preload and ejection, pulmonary circulation, left ventricular preload, and left ventricular afterload.
- In patients who are hypovolemic, effects of positive airway pressure on right ventricular preload generally predominate, whereas in patients who have myocardial dysfunction, effects on left ventricular afterload may predominate.
- Respiratory effort imposes critical loads on the heart, and respiratory muscle failure from inadequate circulation is a final common pathway to death in shock and circulatory impairment.

Introduction

Both spontaneous and mechanical ventilation affect the circulation in predictable ways. The cardiovascular system also has important effects on respiration, ventilation, and gas exchange.

Effects of Ventilation on Circulation

For clarity of discussion, wherever the term *positive pressure ventilation* is used in this chapter, the patient is presumed to respond passively, as though subjected to neuromuscular blockade.

As shown by Cournand[1] in his sentinel paper, mechanical ventilation can have important effects on circulation. The magnitude of these effects may be accentuated by factors that compromise cardiovascular adaptability, such as hypovolemia, cardiac dysfunction, or disordered vascular tone.

Mechanical ventilation can alter right ventricular preload and ejection, pulmonary circulation, left ventricular preload, and left ventricular afterload. These interactions may occur simultaneously and yet not act in the same direction on cardiac output. The net effect on cardiac output depends on which interaction predominates over the course of the respiratory cycle.

Right Ventricular Filling and Stroke Volume

The effects of mechanical ventilation on filling of the right heart are the best understood of the various heart–lung interactions and are generally the preponderant effects on cardiac output. They are mediated by changes in intrathoracic pressure and venous return over the respiratory cycle. Spontaneous breathing and positive pressure mechanical ventilation have opposite effects on intrathoracic pressure, which largely explains their different effects on cardiac output.

Venous Return

The mean systemic pressure of the circulation (P_{ms}) is thought to be the inflow pressure driving blood toward the right ventricle.[2] This driving pressure is not measurable in the intact patient, but it can be thought of as the static mean pressure that might exist throughout the circulation if there were no blood flow.[3] P_{ms} approximates the weighted average of pressures in venous reservoirs throughout the body during the circulation of blood. The backpressure that opposes flow toward the right heart is the right atrial pressure (P_{ra}). The impact of these pressures on return of venous blood to the heart is described by the venous return curve (Figure 24–1A). Picture the systemic circulation as compliant arteries and veins separated by high-resistance arterioles and a pump that receives venous return and propels it into the arteries (Figure 24–1B). The faster the pump circulates the blood, the more blood piles up before the arterioles and the higher the arterial pressure will be. In contrast, the faster the pump moves blood from vein to artery, the less blood resides on the venous side of the circuit and the lower the venous pressure will be. As the pump is slowed down, venous pressure rises until flow reaches zero and pressure equilibrates throughout the circulation at P_{ms}. Resistance to venous return (R_{vr}) is the reciprocal of the slope of the linear part of the venous return curve. Simply stated:

$$\text{Venous return} = (P_{ms} - P_{ra})/R_{vr}. \qquad (1)$$

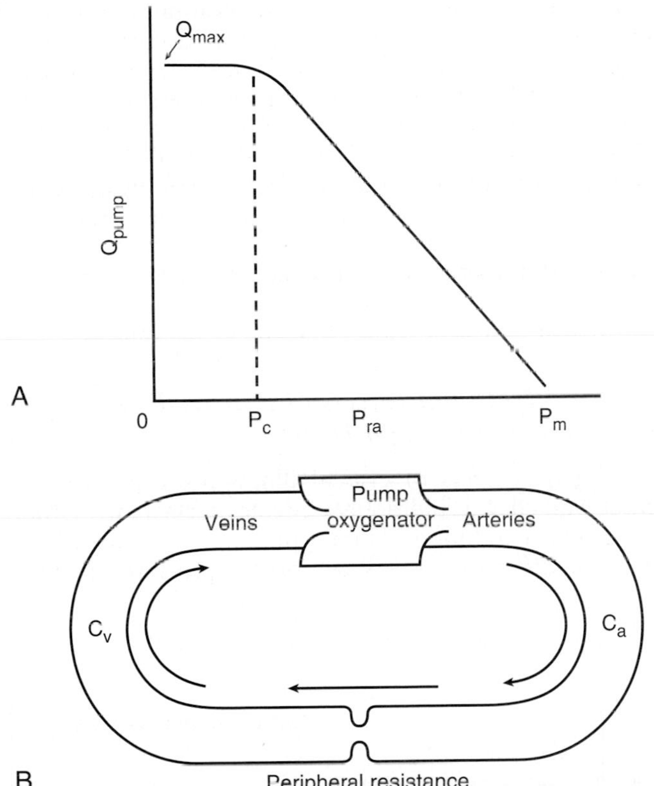

FIGURE 24–1 • **A,** Systemic venous return curve. Flow (Q_{pump}) is plotted on the ordinate but is treated as the independent variable. Right atrial pressure (P_{ra}), the dependent variable, is plotted on the abscissa. **B,** Circulation is treated as though a pump transferred blood from veins to arteries, generating arterial pressure sufficient to overcome peripheral arterial resistance. Arterial compliance (C_a) and venous compliance (C_v) determine the volume of blood distending arteries and veins at any Q_{pump}. When there is no flow, pressure equilibrates throughout the circulation at the mean systemic pressure of the circulation P_{ms}. As pump flow is progressively increased, venous pressure falls and arterial pressure rises because of the net transfer of blood from veins to arteries by the pump and because of the accumulation of blood before the peripheral resistance. When venous pressure falls to P_c, the critical closing pressure of the venous system, no further increase in pump flow is possible. (Adapted from Guyton AC: *Physiol Rev* 35:123, 1955.)

P_{ms} is sensitive to the volume of blood in the circulation and to the capacitance of the venous reservoir. It can be altered by transfusion, volume infusion, hemorrhage, and diuresis. It also is sensitive to changes in venous tone. P_{ms} is an extrathoracic measurement and is less sensitive than P_{ra} to changes in intrathoracic pressure.[4] P_{ra}, in contrast, is quite sensitive to changes in intrathoracic pressure.

At functional residual capacity (FRC), the thorax exerts recoil force, tending to spring outward, while the lung exerts recoil force (mostly as a result of alveolar surface tension), tending to collapse inward. These forces result in subambient pleural pressure. The cardiac fossa, or juxtacardiac space, which surrounds the pericardium and heart, shares in this balance of forces and has slightly negative pressure at apneic FRC. At any right atrial volume, P_{ra} is influenced by juxtacardiac pressure because these two forces act together to oppose the right atrium's balloonlike tendency to recoil inward. Therefore it is not surprising that all of these pressures (pleural, juxtacardiac, and right atrial) are influenced by the respiratory cycle.[5–7]

During spontaneous breathing, lung volume rises from FRC to end-inspiratory volume by expansion of the rib cage and descent of the diaphragm. This reshaping of the thorax stretches the lung, increasing its recoil tension, so pleural pressure and juxtacardiac pressure both become more negative (subambient). At any right atrial volume, this process reduces right atrial pressure. Therefore spontaneous inspiration reduces pleural, juxtacardiac, and right atrial pressures. By the mathematical relationship in Equation 1, this augments venous return.[8] Over the course of passive spontaneous expiration, all three pressures return toward their values at FRC.

Right Ventricular Preload and Stroke Volume

Transmural pressure is the pressure difference across (inside to outside) a hollow structure. This pressure difference and the wall tension of the structure determine its radius. P_{ra} approximates the pressure within the right ventricle during cardiac filling. Juxtacardiac pressure approximates the pressure surrounding the ventricle. During spontaneous inspiration, systemic venous return to the right atrium and ventricle are augmented (Equation 1), and end-diastolic ventricular volume rises. P_{ra} falls, but not as much as juxtacardiac pressure falls. Transmural pressure is, therefore, increased by spontaneous inspiration. Despite the falling P_{ra}, right ventricular stroke volume normally rises during spontaneous inspiration. Hence there is a paradoxical inverse relationship between P_{ra} and right ventricular stroke volume over the spontaneous respiratory cycle (Figure 24–2).[9] If transmural right atrial pressure is plotted against right ventricular stroke volume during various respiratory maneuvers, the expected positive slope is revealed (Figure 24–3).[10]

Positive Pressure Mechanical Ventilation and Right Ventricular Preload

The effects of positive pressure ventilation on pleural, juxtacardiac, and right atrial pressure are opposite those of spontaneous breathing. A common goal in the application of positive end-expiratory pressure (PEEP) is restoration

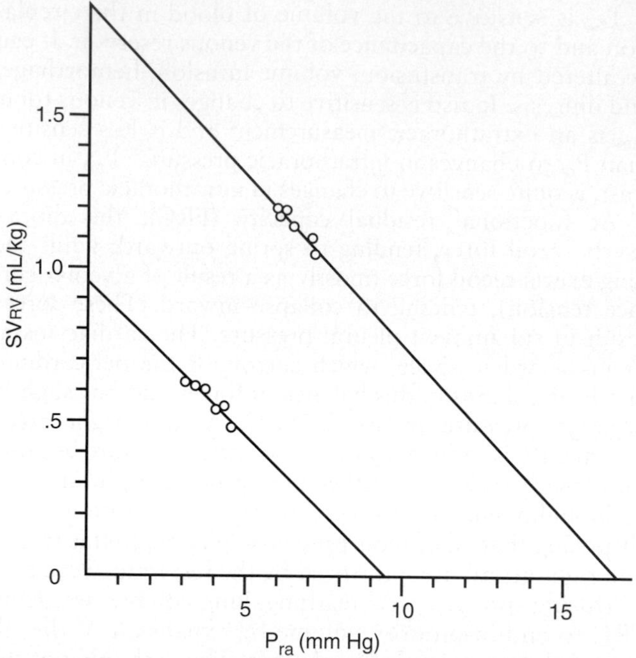

FIGURE 24–2 • During spontaneous inspiration, right atrial pressure (P_{ra}) falls, but this decline is associated with an increase in right ventricular stroke volume (SVRV). Shown at two different mean P_{ra}. (From Pinsky MR: *J Appl Physiol* 56:765, 1984.)

of normal end-expiratory lung volume (normal FRC). All other things being equal, pleural pressure, which opposes thoracic recoil, should be the same at end-expiration whether breathing is spontaneous or mechanical. Pleural pressure is, after all, determined by thoracic volume.

During spontaneous inspiration, active reshaping of the thorax by the respiratory muscles and diaphragm inflates the lungs by reducing pleural pressure. In contrast, throughout positive pressure mechanical inspiration, pleural pressure rises because the passive thorax is pushed outward by the expanding lungs. Passive expiration restores pleural pressure to that of FRC. Averaged over the entire respiratory cycle, pleural pressure is higher during positive pressure breathing than it would be during spontaneous breathing (Figure 24–4). (This elevation of pleural pressure during positive pressure mechanical ventilation is generally called *transmission of airway pressure to the pleural space.*) Positive pressure ventilation, therefore, reverses the effects of spontaneous breathing on venous return[11] and right ventricular transmural pressure.

Positive pressure inspiration impedes venous return by raising P_{ra}. Right ventricular stroke volume declines over positive pressure inspiration because right ventricular transmural pressure is reduced. Averaged over the entire respiratory cycle, P_{ra} is raised and right ventricular stroke volume and cardiac index are reduced by positive airway pressure relative to their expected values during spontaneous breathing (Figure 24–5).

It is easy to argue from these observations that positive pressure ventilation will invariably decrease venous return to the right heart. This is not always the case. PEEP tends to elevate intrathoracic pressure over the entire respiratory cycle and opposes venous return. However, it may also displace blood from the pulmonary circulation and from the abdominal viscera (by descent of the diaphragm), thereby raising P_{ms}. Positive airway pressure may also have favorable effects on left heart function (see the section on left ventricular afterload). In patients whose left heart function improves, both left and right ventricular inflow pressures fall, enhancing venous return.

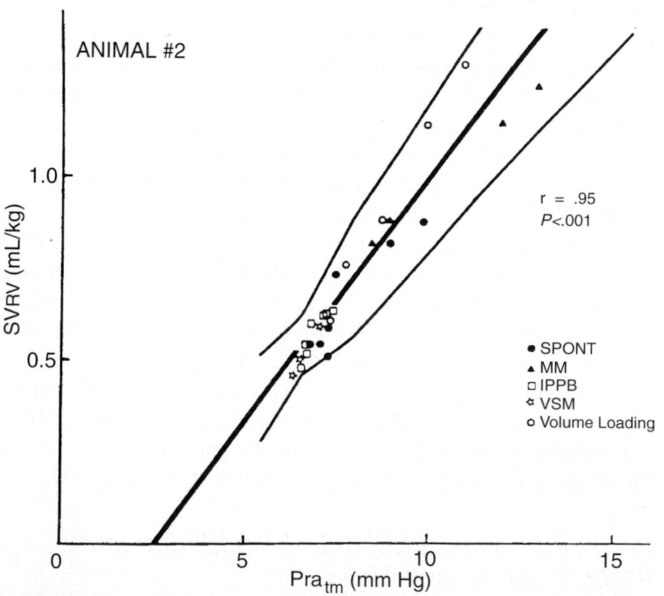

FIGURE 24–3 • Over a wide range of respiratory maneuvers, right ventricular stroke volume (SVRV) varies directly with transmural right atrial pressure (Pra_{tm}). *IPPB,* Intermittent Positive Pressure Breathing; *MM,* Müller Maneuver; *SPONT,* spontaneous breathing; *VSM,* Valsalva Maneuver. (From Pinsky MR: *J Appl Physiol* 56:1237, 1984.)

Critical Illness and Effects of Positive Pressure Breathing on the Right Heart

Among the effects of critical illness are capillary leak, chest wall edema, pulmonary edema, surfactant dysfunction, abnormal blood volume, and abdominal distension. Each modifies the effects of positive pressure breathing on the right heart.

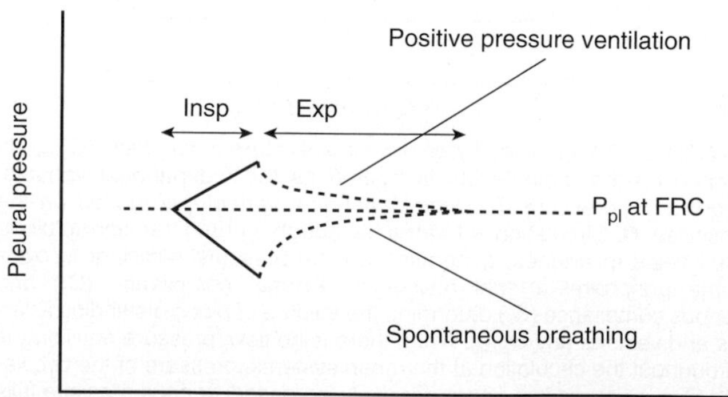

FIGURE 24–4 • Over the course of the respiratory cycle, if spontaneous and positive pressure breaths both begin and end at the same functional residual capacity (FRC), spontaneous breathing takes place at lower pleural pressure than does positive pressure ventilation.

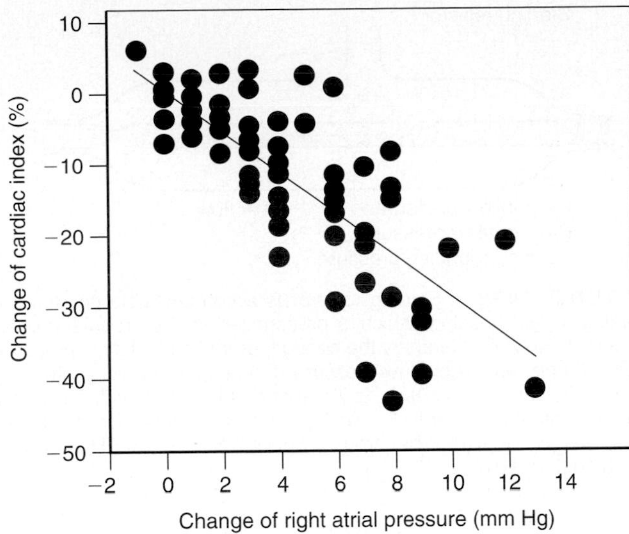

FIGURE 24–5 • Relationship between the percentage change in cardiac index and the percentage change in right atrial pressure that was produced by the application of graded levels of positive airway pressure in adults. (From Jellinek H, Krafft P, Fitzgerald RD, et al: *Crit Care Med* 28:672, 2000.)

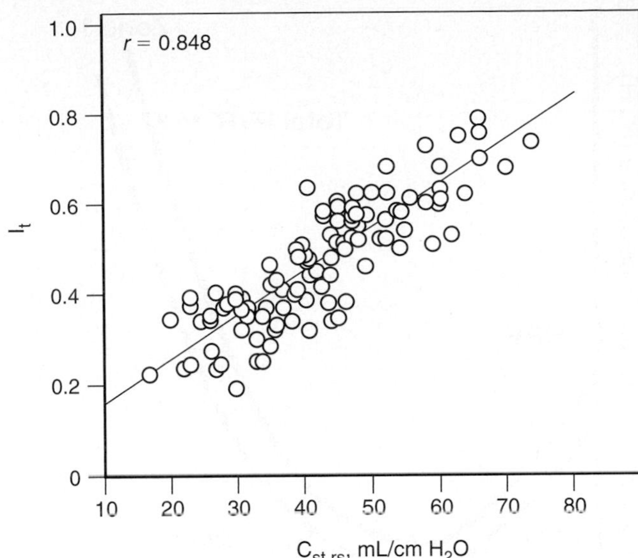

FIGURE 24–6 • Relationship between the static compliance of the respiratory system ($C_{st,rs}$) and the index of transmission (I_t, decimal fraction) of a change in static airway pressure to the pulmonary circulation in adults. I_t values for pleural and juxtacardiac spaces are presumed to be comparable. (From Teboul JL, Pinsky MR, Mercat A, et al: *Crit Care Med* 28:3631, 2000.)

Capillary leak alters the compliance of the atrial and ventricular chambers, modifying the responsiveness of the heart to changes in preload. Sepsis and inflammation decrease cardiac contractility, directly altering the way the heart responds to changes in preload. Chest wall edema, pulmonary edema, surfactant dysfunction, and abdominal distension alter thoracic and pulmonary compliances, which in turn alter pleural and juxtacardiac pressures.

Reduced respiratory system compliance diminishes the transmission of alveolar pressure to the juxtacardiac space.[12] The change in intrathoracic pressure that occurs with a change in static airway pressure is essentially the same as the change observed in pulmonary artery wedge pressure,[13] which is readily measured. Recognizing this relationship in adults has made it possible to estimate percent transmission of airway pressure to the juxtacardiac space by measurement of respiratory system compliance (Figure 24–6).

Both abnormal blood volume and abnormal vascular compliance can change P_{ms} and thereby alter venous return. Vascular hypovolemia can exaggerate the adverse effects of positive pressure ventilation on preload.

Pulmonary Circulation

By modifying pulmonary vascular resistance (PVR), the effects of breathing on pulmonary circulation modify right ventricular afterload. The effects of breathing also can change the distribution of pulmonary blood flow within the lung. Both effects are significant.

Lung Volume

The alveolar septa are highly vascular (Figure 24–7). More than 90% of the alveolar surface makes contact with alveolar capillaries. These vessels can be separated into two categories according to their location or their response to lung inflation. Most alveolar vessels are capillaries and lie in septa, which separate adjacent alveoli. Other alveolar vessels are termed *corner vessels* because they are located at the intersection of alveolar septa.

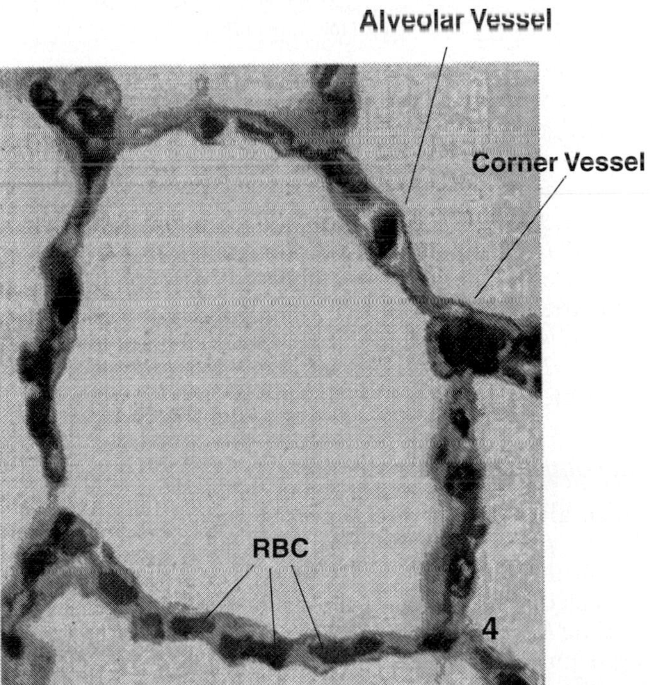

FIGURE 24–7 • Alveolus is encased in a network of capillaries. Alveolar vessels are those that lie between adjacent alveoli. Corner vessels are those that lie at the intersection of alveolar septa. *RBC,* Red blood cell. (Modified from Reith EJ, Ross MH: *Atlas of descriptive histology.* New York, 1965, Harper & Row.)

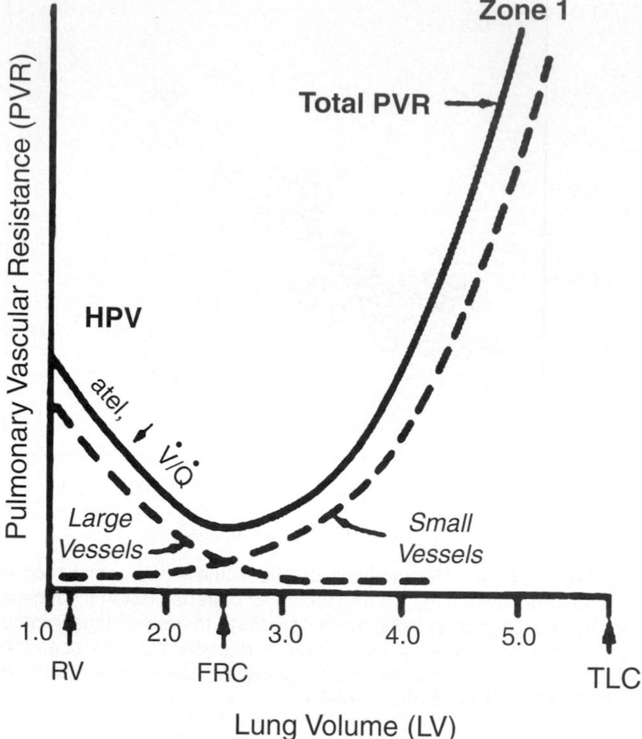

FIGURE 24–8 • Effects of lung volume on pulmonary vascular resistance (PVR). As whole lung is distended from functional residual capacity (FRC) toward total lung capacity (TLC), PVR rises, predominantly by increasing resistance to flow through the small alveolar vessels that course between adjacent alveoli (alveolar vessels). As whole lung is collapsed from FRC toward residual volume, PVR rises, predominantly by effects on corner vessel that traverse the intersection of alveolar septa. (Modified from Cassidy SS, Schwiep F: Cardiovascular effects of positive end-expiratory pressure. In Scharf SM, Cassidy SS, editors: *Heart lung interactions in health and disease,* vol 42, *Lung biology in health and disease.* New York, 1989, Dekker.)

These corner vessels are generally larger and probably divide later in their course to become alveolar capillaries located in septa between adjacent alveoli. When the lung is stretched, either by spontaneous inspiration or by positive pressure distension, corner vessels are pulled open by radial traction, and their resistance to blood flow is reduced. When alveolar septa are stretched, alveolar capillaries thin and restrict flow. The net effect of these factors is a U-shaped relation of PVR to lung volume (Figure 24–8);[14–17] PVR is least at FRC and rises with either atelectasis or overdistension.

Alveolar Pressure

When alveolar pressure is greater than ambient, as it is during positive pressure ventilation, the vessels that course through alveolar septa between adjacent alveoli can be compressed.[18,19] This behavior is akin to that of a Starling resister, a collapsible tube traversing a rigid housing (Figure 24–9). Flow (Q) is propelled through the tube by inflow pressure (P_i) and is opposed by outflow pressure (P_o). The tubing has some intrinsic resistance (R). If the housing is pressurized to a surrounding pressure (P_s), flow through the tube is determined as follows:

$$P_s < P_o < P_i, \quad Q = (P_i - P_o)/R \qquad (2)$$

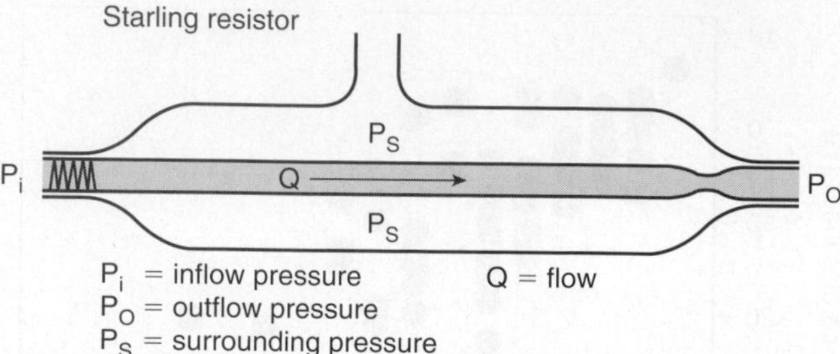

FIGURE 24–9 • Starling resistor is a compressible conduit traversing a rigid housing, which is pressurized to a surrounding pressure (P_s). Flow (Q) traverses the conduit, propelled by inflow pressure (P_i) and opposed by outflow pressure (P_o) such that driving pressure is ($P_i - P_o$) for $P_s < P_o$. As P_s is increased, it begins to influence flow, but only after it exceeds P_o. At $P_s > P_o$, the driving force for flow becomes ($P_i - P_s$). (Modified from Jerusalem E, Starling EH: *J Physiol Lond* 40:279, 1910.)

$$P_o < P_s < P_i, \quad Q = (P_i - P_s)/R \qquad (3)$$

$$P_o < P_i < P_s, \quad Q = 0. \qquad (4)$$

Alveolar pressure, then, appears to modulate local pulmonary blood flow as though it surrounds the pulmonary capillary (Figure 24–10).

From this discussion, the degree to which alveolar pressure (P_s) affects flow is influenced by the magnitude of inflow pressure, which, for the pulmonary capillary, must be adjusted for vertical height. Alveolar pressure causes greater reduction in flow at low pulmonary artery pressure than it does at high pressure.

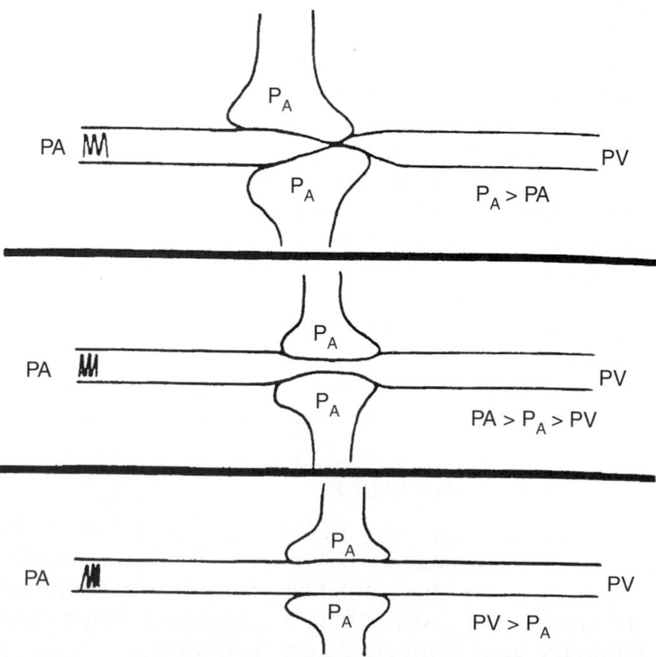

FIGURE 24–10 • Pulmonary capillaries are, in essence, surrounded by gas-filled alveoli. The influence of alveolar pressure (P_A) on regional lung blood flow is similar to the influence of surrounding pressure on flow through a Starling resistor. At ambient values of P_A, pulmonary vein pressure (PV) opposes inflow. As P_A rises, it begins to oppose inflow only after P_A > PV. It modulates inflow until P_A reaches hydrostatic inflow pressure (PA), at which point flow ceases.

Pulmonary hypertension (high P_i) dampens this cardiopulmonary interaction, whereas hypovolemia (low P_o) accentuates it.

Hydrostatic pressure in the lung is a function of vertical height (see Chapter 18).[20] To estimate the hydrostatic inflow pressure of a pulmonary capillary, a pressure equivalent to that exerted by a water column extending from the left atrium to the capillary must be subtracted from the pressure within the main pulmonary artery. The greater the vertical height of the pulmonary capillary, the lower its inflow pressure and the greater the attenuation of flow by alveolar pressure. This can produce areas of no flow, especially at peak inspiration, high in the supine lung. These high V_A/Q alveolar capillary units waste ventilation and can cause hypercarbia (see Chapter 36).

Compression of pulmonary capillaries is a local phenomenon. It can divert pulmonary blood flow away from normal lung segments toward consolidated or atelectatic lung segments whose airways do not effectively transmit airway pressure to the alveolus.[21] By this mechanism, the application of high PEEP in the presence of lobar pneumonia may increase blood flow through unventilated lung and worsen hypoxemia (Figure 24–11). From a more positive perspective, PEEP may relieve atelectasis and improve ventilation, thereby relieving alveolar hypoxic vasoconstriction. Whether PEEP benefits or impairs pulmonary blood flow may depend on the balance of its effect on atelectasis and its effect on alveolar capillaries.

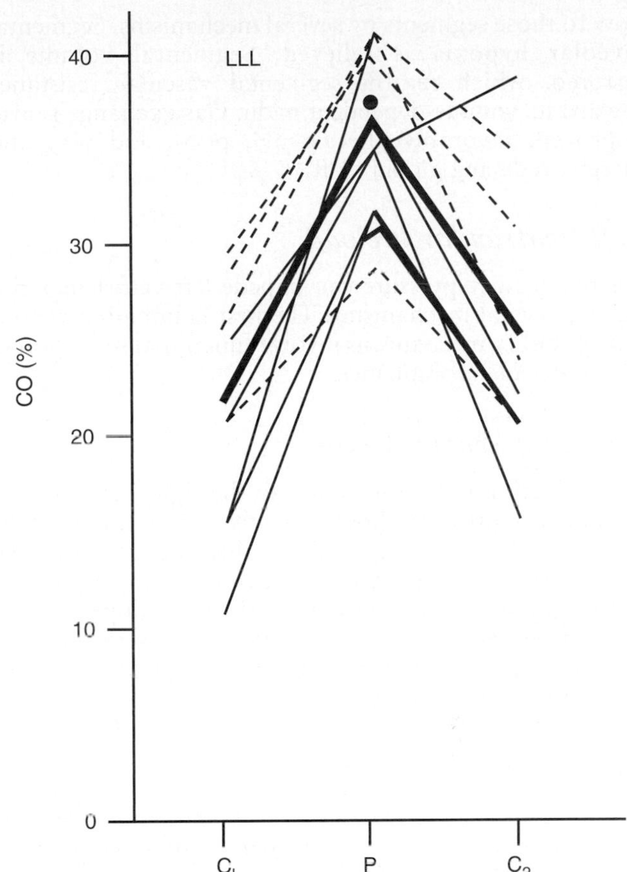

FIGURE 24–11 • Blood flow to the left lower lobes of dogs (LLL) with LLL pneumonia, measured at zero positive end-expiratory pressure (PEEP) (C_1), 6 to 12 cmH_2O PEEP (P), and on cessation of applied PEEP (C_2). PEEP diverted blood flow away from more normal lung toward the consolidated LLL. (From Mink SN, Light RB, Cooligan T, et al: *J Appl Physiol* 50:517, 1981.)

Direct Effects of Airway Pressure on Pulmonary Vascular Tone

Pulmonary vessels are stretched by lung inflation. The lung of infant lambs responds to abrupt changes in airway pressure with changes in vascular tone. Abrupt distension of one lung of the intact infant lamb increases the PVR of that lung alone.[22] The resistance change is sensitive to the waveform of the lung distension[23] and persists after relief of distending pressure and return of lung volume to baseline.[24] This effect is calcium channel dependent[25] and resembles a myogenic reflex whereby direct vessel stretch causes constriction.

Regulation of Pulmonary Vascular Resistance

The resistance to flow through a vessel is described by the following:

$$R = \frac{8\eta l}{\pi r^4}, \tag{5}$$

where η = viscosity, l = length, and r = radius. It follows that PVR can be effectively controlled by active changes in vessel radius. Mechanical ventilation may alter blood pH and alveolar po_2, both of which influence vessel tone and radius (Figure 24–12).[26,27]

Hypoxic pulmonary vasoconstriction is a powerful mechanism for sustaining systemic oxygenation in the face of lung disease.[28–31] Relief of atelectasis and restoration of segmental ventilation not only increase the fraction of the lung that is ventilated but also restore blood

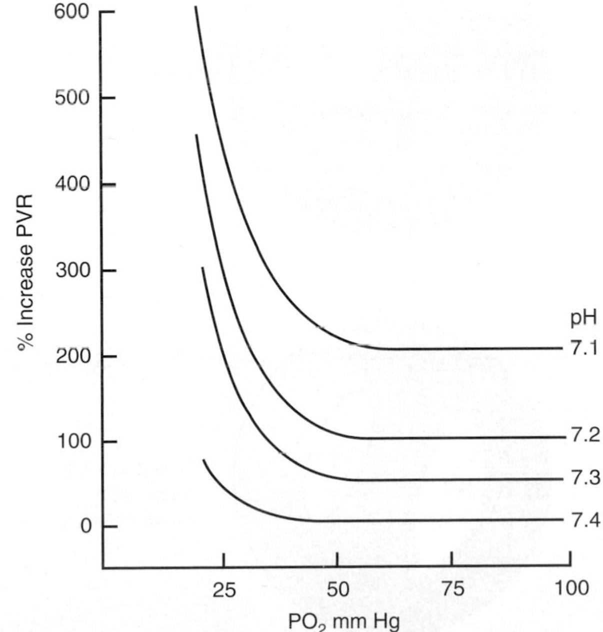

FIGURE 24–12 • Pulmonary vascular resistance (PVR) is a function of both pH and arterial po_2. (From Rudolph AM, Yuan S: *J Clin Invest* 45:399, 1966.)

flow to those segments by several mechanisms. Segmental alveolar hypoxia is relieved. Segmental volume is restored, which returns segmental vascular resistance toward its volume-dependent nadir. Gas exchange is also improved, favorably altering pH, pCO_2, and pO_2, and thereby reducing global PVR.

Left Ventricular Preload

Positive airway pressure can impede left ventricular filling via several mechanisms. The first is impaired venous return. Other mechanisms involve functional reduction in left ventricular compliance.

Decreased Venous Return

The reduction in venous return to the right heart seen at high airway pressure should directly reduce filling of the left heart. But there is a trap in this line of reasoning. Venous return, when averaged over several respiratory cycles, equals cardiac output. If other cardiopulmonary interactions and compensatory mechanisms restore cardiac output to normal, then right and left heart venous return will not be diminished.

Ventricular Interdependence

The right and left ventricles share a common muscle mass and pericardial space. It follows that compliance of either ventricle will be influenced by volume of the other chamber (Figure 24–13). Increased venous return to the right heart, as occurs during spontaneous inspiration and especially during execution of a Muller maneuver, tends to shift the interventricular septum to the left, reducing compliance of the left ventricle.[32] Similarly, excessive compression of the pulmonary circulation by positive airway pressure may impede right ventricular ejection, causing the right ventricle to dilate and encroach on the left.

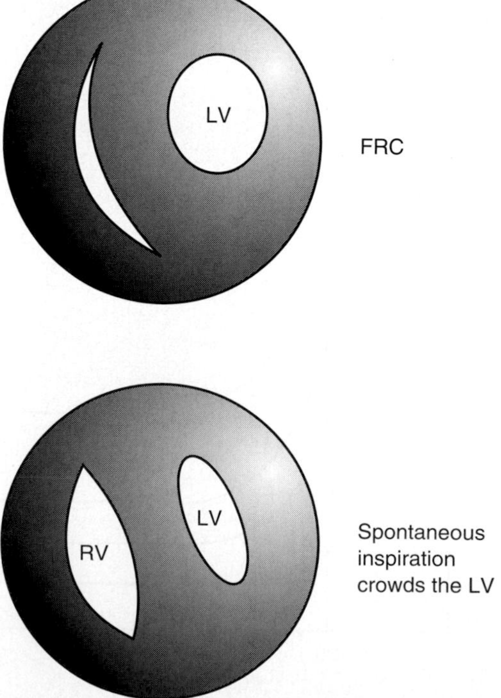

FIGURE 24–13 • Increasing the diastolic volume of the right ventricle reduces compliance of the left ventricle (LV). *FRC,* Functional residual capacity; *RV,* right ventricle.

Cardiac Crowding

Overinflation of the lungs may crowd the cardiac fossa in which the heart resides. To the extent that this creates a mechanical barrier to cardiac filling, it may reduce left ventricular compliance.

Left Ventricular Afterload

The left ventricle ejects blood from within the thorax to the extrathoracic arteries and arterioles. Most of the resistance to this forward flow resides in the arterioles. From a practical point of view, the pressure in the extrathoracic arteries can be described by the following equations:

$$(P_{artery} - P_{ms}) = Q \times R_{arteriole} \quad (6)$$

or

$$P_{artery} = Q \times R_{arteriole} + P_{ms} \quad (7)$$

where Q = cardiac output, P_{artery} = inflow pressure before the arteriole, and P_{ms} = outflow pressure after the arteriole as defined for the venous return curve.

It follows that, at any given blood volume, arterial pressure is determined by forward flow and arteriolar resistance. These two parameters set the afterload opposing left ventricular ejection.

When the left ventricle contracts, it creates internal pressure against the closed aortic valve by generating tension in the myocardium that encircles the ventricular chamber. This "wall" tension causes ventricular pressure to rise until it reaches aortic diastolic pressure, opening the aortic valve and ejecting the stroke volume. Creation of wall tension and subsequent shortening of myocardial fibers perform the external mechanical work of the heart (see Chapter 17)

When the heart squeezes, it creates a pressure difference between the ventricle and the juxtacardiac space. In effect, the myocardium creates a transmural pressure to produce a ventricular pressure sufficient to open the aortic valve. Aortic diastolic pressure and external (juxtacardiac) pressure determine the myocardial wall tension needed to open the aortic valve. Both pressures represent afterloads to left ventricular ejection.[33,34]

An infusion of phenylephrine, by raising $R_{arteriole}$, increases the afterload of the left ventricle (Figure 24–14). It raises the pressure required to open the aortic valve. This increases the wall tension the heart must generate to eject blood.

The Muller maneuver, forced inspiration against a closed glottis, does the same thing. It reduces juxtacardiac pressure, thereby raising the transmural pressure required to open the aortic valve. Thus the Muller maneuver also increases the afterload of the left ventricle.

Positive pressure inspiration or application of PEEP may raise juxtacardiac pressure to such an extent that the

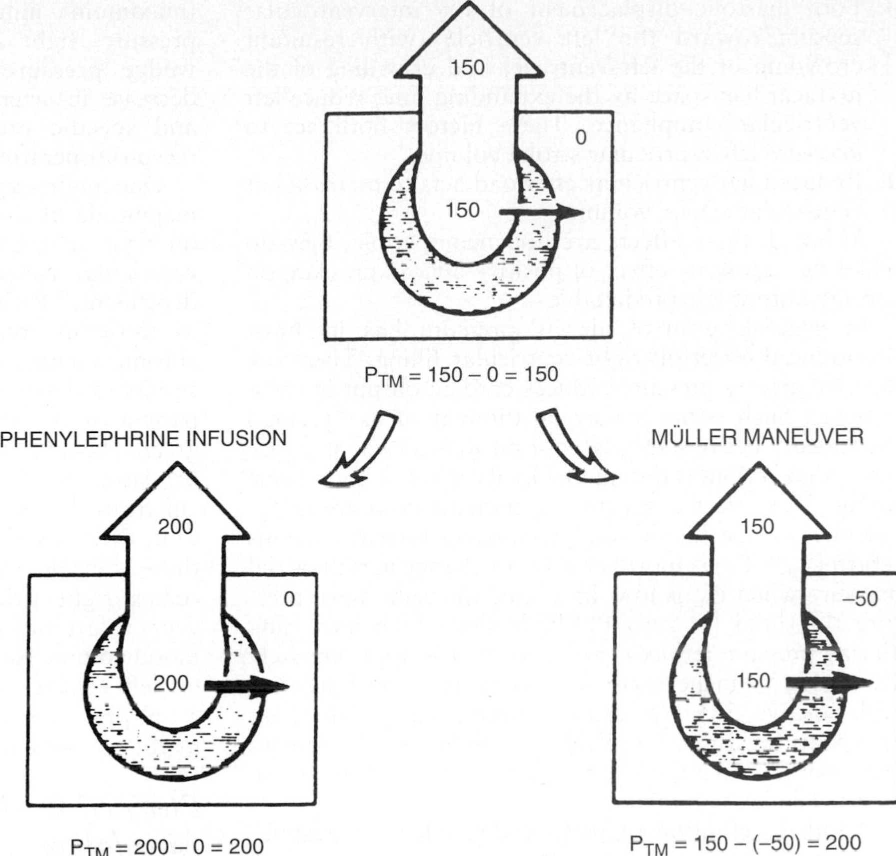

FIGURE 24–14 • Negative pressure in the juxtacardiac space (Muller maneuver) increases the wall tension required to eject blood into the aorta. This respiratory maneuver acts like a phenylephrine infusion to increase left ventricular afterload. (From Buda AJ, Pinsky MR, Ingels NB Jr, et al: *N Engl J Med* 301:453, 1979.)

wall tension required to open the aortic valve is diminished. Mechanical ventilation may, therefore, reduce the afterload of the left ventricle.

The net effect of positive pressure inspiration often is augmentation of left ventricular ejection. Stroke volume may consequently rise, cardiac output increase, and arterial pressure rise. Arterial pressure is commonly observed to rise during positive pressure inspiration, whereas it falls during spontaneous inspiration. These are effects of afterload on stroke volume.

Cardiac Contractility

Studies of the effects of positive airway pressure on left ventricular contractility have yielded conflicting results. Certainly changes in preload and afterload have secondary effects on stroke volume, but independent effects of positive airway pressure on left ventricular contractility have not been consistently demonstrated. Negative inotropic effects modulated by reflexes, mediators, or alterations in coronary blood flow have been described,[35–40] but most animal and human studies fail to show that positive airway pressure has any primary effect on myocardial contractility.[41–44]

It has been suggested that high levels of PEEP may compress coronary vessels, cause myocardial ischemia, and thereby impair ventricular function.[45–47] The left ventricular myocardium is perfused predominantly in diastole. To the extent that juxtacardiac pressure exceeds left ventricular diastolic pressure, such an effect is plausible. This assertion appears more compelling for patients in shock and for those with intrinsic coronary blood flow limitations than for otherwise normal individuals.

Right ventricular myocardial perfusion normally occurs in both systole and diastole.

In systole, right ventricular coronary inflow pressure is aortic systolic pressure, and right ventricular coronary outflow (or surrounding) pressure is right ventricular or pulmonary artery systolic pressure. To the extent that positive pressure ventilation impedes pulmonary blood flow and increases pulmonary artery pressure, it may impede right ventricular systolic myocardial perfusion.

Right ventricular diastolic myocardial perfusion may be subject to modulation by positive airway pressure as described for the left ventricle.

Overall, it does not appear likely that judicious levels of positive airway pressure have much effect on myocardial contractility.

Preload Dependence versus Afterload Dependence

The expected effects of an abrupt rise in airway pressure are as follows:

1. Decreased filling of the right ventricle acts to decrease right ventricular stroke volume.
2. Impaired pulmonary blood flow or increased right ventricular afterload acts to decrease right ventricular stroke volume.

3. Both diastolic displacement of the interventricular septum toward the left ventricle (with resultant crowding of the left ventricle) and crowding of the juxtacardiac space by the expanding lung reduce left ventricular compliance. These factors both act to *decrease* left ventricular stroke volume.
4. Reduced left ventricular afterload acts to *increase* left ventricular stroke volume.

Although these effects are not incompatible, they do make the aggregate effect of positive airway pressure on cardiac output less predictable.

In general, positive airway pressure has its most pronounced effect on right ventricular filling. Therefore positive airway pressure reduces cardiac output in most patients. Such patients may be thought of as "preload dependent" because the effect of positive airway pressure on cardiac output is dominated by its effect on right heart filling. This effect is greatest in patients who are hypovolemic because the driving pressure for systemic venous return ($P_{ms} - P_{ra}$) is more sensitive to change in right atrial pressure when P_{ms} is low. In adults, the right atrial pressure threshold (at zero PEEP) below which increasing airway pressure reduces cardiac output is approximately 12 mmHg.[48] Furthermore, the rise in right atrial pressure with positive airway pressure is mechanical and does not appear to be a function of blood volume, so the percent reduction in driving pressure is exaggerated in the hypovolemic patient.

Another definition of preload dependence is responsiveness to vascular volume infusion. By this definition, when the dominant effect of positive airway pressure is to impede right heart filling, vascular volume infusion raises cardiac output. Four measurable parameters (Figure 24–15) predict responsiveness to vascular volume infusion: variation over the respiratory cycle (maximum – minimum) in pulse pressure, arterial systolic pressure, right atrial pressure, and pulmonary artery wedge pressure.[49] Of these parameters, expiratory decrease in arterial pulse pressure is the most sensitive and specific predictor of "preload dependence" (by receptor operating characteristic curve) (Figure 24–16).[50]

One might expect the converse also to apply. Reduced magnitude of the effects of positive pressure ventilation on right ventricular filling or augmented effects on left ventricular ejection may make the patient "afterload dependent." Patients who have high blood volume, such as those in congestive cardiac failure or those with chronic anemia, should have high P_{ms} and decreased sensitivity to changes in right atrial pressure.[51] Moreover, the patient with poor left ventricular contractility may greatly benefit from the afterload reduction of positive pressure ventilation.[52] If positive airway pressure enhances the ejection of blood into the systemic circulation, this may directly reduce left atrial pressure. From these considerations, better cardiac output may also reduce right atrial pressure by transferring blood from veins to arteries and reducing venous capacitance vessel blood volume (see Figure 24–1B). When favorable effects on left ventricular ejection act to reduce right and left atrial pressures, cardiac output improves. Such a patient might be thought of as "afterload dependent."

Elevated Work of Breathing and the Circulation

During quiet respiration, the heart has no difficulty satisfying the demand of the respiratory muscles for perfusion

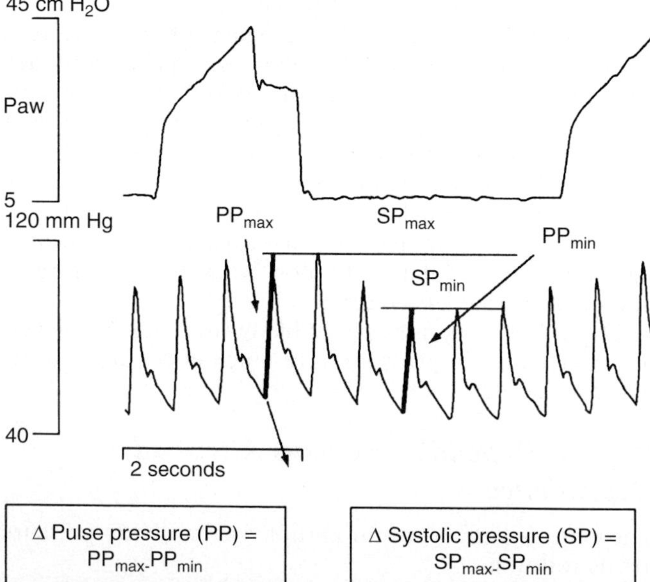

FIGURE 24–15 • Positive pressure inspiration generally raises aortic pulse pressure (PP), systolic pressure (SP), right atrial pressure, and pulmonary artery wedge pressure. (From Michard F, Chemla D, Richard C, et al: *Am J Respir Crit Care Med* 159: 935, 1999.)

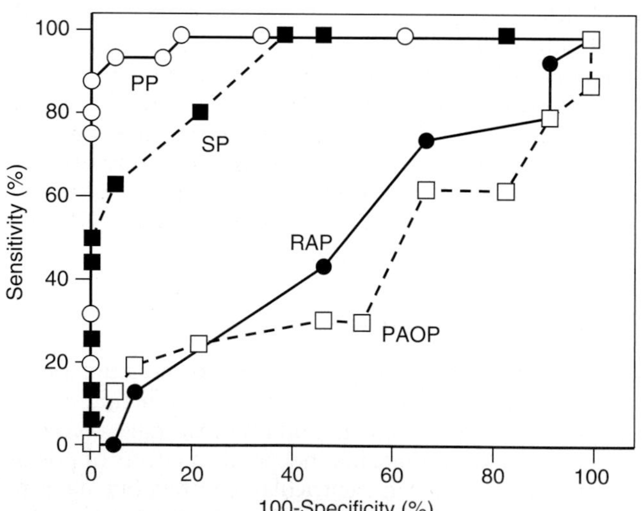

FIGURE 24–16 • Septic patients on positive end-expiratory pressure were challenged by volume infusion. In response to volume loading, some patients had a greater than 15% increase in cardiac index. These responsive patients were deemed preload dependent. The sensitivity and specificity of variation in pulse pressure (PP) across the respiratory cycle as a predictor of responsiveness to volume loading yielded a near-perfect receptor operating characteristic (ROC) curve. Greater than 15% inspiratory rise in PP appears to identify adults with preload dependence during positive pressure ventilation. *PAOP,* pulmonary artery occlusion pressure; *RAP,* right atrial pressure: *SP,* systolic pressure. (From Michard F, Boussat S, Chemla D, et al: *Am J Respir Crit Care Med* 162:134, 2000.)

and muscle oxygen delivery. In respiratory failure, however, respiratory muscle perfusion may not be adequate. The diaphragm and the accessory muscles of respiration all are taxed to the limit by respiratory distress. Unlike cardiac muscle, respiratory muscles can accumulate an oxygen debt, but persistent hypoperfusion may interfere with their ability to perform the requisite work of breathing. In many clinical scenarios, including shock, congestive heart failure, and respiratory disease, the inability of the circulation to maintain adequate respiratory muscle blood flow causes weakness, respiratory muscle fatigue, and ultimate respiratory arrest.[53] Loaded breathing,[54] respiratory muscle failure, and impending respiratory arrest all pose a strain on the circulation, demanding greater cardiac output.

Mechanical ventilation is, therefore, a highly effective if not essential intervention in the patient with cardiac decompensation and respiratory distress.

Pulsus Paradoxicus in Respiratory Distress

Arterial pressure normally falls during spontaneous inspiration, which is best explained as a result of increasing left ventricular afterload at a time in the respiratory cycle when ventricular interdependence restricts left ventricular filling. It is well known that pericardial tamponade causes accentuation of the normal inspiratory decrease in systemic blood pressure, a phenomenon known as *pulsus paradoxus*. This finding has been attributed to accentuation of ventricular interdependence, which favors right over left ventricular filling, at the same time in the respiratory cycle when inspiration is raising left ventricular afterload.

During loaded spontaneous inspiration, as in the Müller maneuver or in the presence of inspiratory airway obstruction (e.g., croup), the inspiratory fall in juxtacardiac pressure is exaggerated, and left ventricular afterload is accentuated. Again, the result is pulsus paradoxicus, an accentuated drop in blood pressure during inspiration.

Blood pressure commonly rises during positive pressure inspiration, which is termed *reverse pulsus paradoxus*. This finding has been attributed to left ventricular afterload reduction by the rise in juxtacardiac pressure that occurs during positive pressure inspiration.[55] Reverse pulsus paradoxicus is a normal finding during positive pressure ventilation but may be accentuated in afterload-dependent states (e.g., left ventricular dysfunction, vascular hypervolemia, and so on, as discussed in the Preload Dependence versus Afterload Dependence section).

Effects of Breathing on Measurement of Hemodynamic Parameters

Because hemodynamic measurements vary with respiration, mechanical ventilation may complicate assessment of cardiac function. Yet it may not be advisable to discontinue PEEP or mechanical ventilation to assess hemodynamics. Measuring vascular pressures at a consistent time in the respiratory cycle usually is sufficient. End-expiratory measurements are generally used because airway pressures are least at that time.

It should be understood that the effects of mechanical ventilation on the circulation are not merely artifactual. They are real. There is no greater accuracy of measurements made off the ventilator. Measurements performed after ventilator disconnect are subject to the effects of respiratory dysfunction and instability.

A special circumstance can occur when a balloon flotation catheter with its tip in zone I lung is used to measure pulmonary artery pressure and when such a catheter with its tip in zone I or II lung is used to measure pulmonary artery wedge pressure.[56] Under such circumstances, airway pressures that exceed vascular pressures may be erroneously reported as vascular pressures.

Effects of Cardiovascular Function on Respiration

Shock States and Respiratory Function

Shock of any cause diminishes perfusion of respiratory muscles and can lead to respiratory failure and respiratory arrest. It also causes metabolic acidosis, which constricts pulmonary vessels and opposes lung blood flow.[57,58] Acidosis is a potent stimulus of respiratory effort and contributes to tachypnea and respiratory distress, which in turn worsen the demand on the heart. Shock is injurious to both heart and lung, and one final common pathway to recovery is the initiation of mechanical ventilation, which benefits both organ systems.

Hypovolemic shock can create extreme preload dependency.[59] In hypovolemic shock, diastolic blood pressure may fall during positive pressure inspiration, impairing coronary perfusion. This may cause myocardial ischemia and worsen cardiac function.

Cardiogenic shock, by reducing oxygen delivery to tissues, elevates tissue oxygen extraction from the blood. The resultant decline in venous oxygen tension has a paradoxical effect. It increases the efficiency of pulmonary blood flow by allowing greater oxygen uptake per unit of pulmonary blood flow. That is, the more desaturated the blood that enters the pulmonary circulation, the more new oxygen it can upload. This process requires that alveolar pO_2 not limit the amount of oxygen available for uptake and is one reason to administer oxygen to patients suffering cardio-respiratory failure.

Congestive Heart Failure

All that has been said about shock is equally true of congestive heart failure (CHF). In fact, there is a continuum from CHF to cardiogenic shock. CHF elicits physiologic responses that restore cardiac output toward normal. As these homeostatic responses are exhausted, cardiac output declines and the patient develops obvious manifestations of cardiogenic shock and respiratory failure.

In addition to the impact of shock on respiratory function and reserve, CHF generally causes fluid retention and pulmonary edema. Treatment of cardiogenic shock by vascular volume expansion may, by augmenting cardiac filling pressures, improve cardiac output at the expense of pulmonary edema. The edematous lung is stiff, may have elevated airway resistance, and can have alveolar flooding, atelectasis, intrapulmonary shunt, and severe ventilation/perfusion mismatch.

Again, mechanical ventilation addresses most of these issues. Furthermore, PEEP improves lung function and supplemental oxygen supports gas exchange. Treatment of CHF can itself dramatically improve lung function.

When a premature infant has a large patent ductus arteriosus, the primary manifestation of cardiac volume overload may be respiratory embarrassment.

Cardiac Disease as a Cause of Blood Gas Abnormalities

Cardiac disease can cause arterial hypoxemia or hypercarbia by several mechanisms. The most obvious cardiac cause of arterial hypoxemia is right-to-left intracardiac shunting of blood as seen in tetralogy of Fallot. This situation allows venous blood to directly reenter the arterial circulation, causing arterial desaturation. In admixture lesions, such as transposition of the great arteries, tricuspid atresia, or total anomalous pulmonary venous connection, there is obligatory mixing of the systemic and pulmonary circulations, which allows desaturated blood to reach the systemic circulation, causing hypoxemia.

Arterial oxygen tension in right-to-left shunt lesions is sensitive to the volumes of systemic and pulmonary venous return that enter the aorta. The greater the ratio of pink to blue blood, the greater the arterial saturation. When oxygen-enriched air is administered after an excessively large aortopulmonary shunt, arterial blood may become fully saturated as a result of oxygen dissolved at high pO_2 in the torrential pulmonary venous return.

In transposition of the great arteries, arterial oxygenation may be inherently limited by the degree of mixing that can occur. Pulmonary blood flow may be enormous, yet little of the pink pulmonary venous return escapes to the systemic circulation. Only the pulmonary venous return that reaches the systemic circulation delivers oxygen to the tissues.

In hypoplastic left heart syndrome, which is an admixture lesion, supplemental oxygen may, by reducing PVR, dramatically divert blood flow to the pulmonary circulation at the expense of systemic blood flow. This can both dramatically drop blood pressure and raise arterial pO_2. In this situation, the rise in pO_2 can be attributed to the fall in cardiac output and to the increase in pulmonary blood flow. These two changes alter the ratio of pink to blue blood that admixes in the atria.

Cardiac disease can cause hypercarbia by several mechanisms.[60] CHF can cause pulmonary edema, which interferes with lung function. As discussed in the Shock States and Respiratory Function section, it can weaken the muscles of respiration and thereby reduce minute ventilation during spontaneous breathing.

Certain cardiac defects (or their treatments) can create large-scale ventilation/perfusion (V/Q) abnormalities, which may include underperfusion of large volumes of lung. An example is branch pulmonary artery stenosis, which may accompany tetralogy of Fallot or follow its surgical repair. Another example is maldistribution of pulmonary blood flow caused by a surgical shunt, which predominantly perfuses only one lung. The resultant high ventilation/perfusion defect functionally wastes ventilation. The airflow to high V/Q (underperfused) segments does not contribute to carbon dioxide clearance (as the scanty perfusion carries little, if any, CO_2 to that region of the lung). This waste of ventilation functionally reduces effective minute alveolar ventilation, causing CO_2 retention. In contrast, the gas exhaled by high V/Q segments mixes with gas from perfused alveoli during expiration, lowering the end-tidal pCO_2. The result is elevated arterial pCO_2 and reduced end-tidal pCO_2, an apparent high arterial-alveolar pCO_2 gradient. This is also called *elevated alveolar dead space.*

One additional mechanism of hypercarbia in cardiac disease is extremely low pulmonary blood flow in the presence of admixture or right-to-left shunting. In this situation, so little blood reaches the lung that the circulation cannot deliver to the alveoli as much carbon dioxide per minute as the body produces until venous pCO_2 becomes quite elevated. This can occur in ductus-dependent cyanotic cardiac defects upon ductus closure and presents the paradoxical findings of clear (underperfused) lung fields and hypercarbia despite adequate ventilation. When there is no right-to-left shunt, elevation of venous (and occasionally arterial) pCO_2 can occur without cyanosis. This commonly occurs during cardiopulmonary resuscitation (or in severe shock) when circulation is inadequate.

Hypercyanotic Spells

One special scenario that warrants discussion is the hypercyanotic spell, often called a *tetrad spell.* In these episodes, pulmonary blood flow is inadequate to take up sufficient oxygen from the lung to meet the mitochondrial demand for oxygen. Mixed venous pO_2 progressively falls. In the presence of admixture or right-to-left shunting, this directly reduces arterial oxygen tension. Sometimes the cause of the spell is abrupt reduction in pulmonary blood flow, as occurs with worsening obstruction of the infundibulum of the right ventricular outflow tract in tetralogy of Fallot or increased right-to-left shunting because of systemic vasodilation. However, pulmonary blood flow need not fall for a hypercyanotic spell to occur. Oxygen demand may rise (as in crying, fever, or exertion), outstripping the capacity of pulmonary blood flow to take up oxygen from alveolar air. Blood loss or acute anemia can cause worsening hypoxia and acidosis in the presence of underlying cyanotic disease. Hypercyanotic spells can occur in any cyanotic heart defect or in the child with lung disease and cyanosis.

The cycle put in place by this abrupt inadequacy of pulmonary oxygen uptake includes acidosis, physical distress, exaggerated skeletal muscle work, respiratory distress, exaggerated respiratory muscle work, and a further increase in muscle oxygen utilization. The cycle can progress to death unless it is interrupted.

Although respiratory distress and tachypnea may suggest a pulmonary cause, the treatment is directed at restoration of pulmonary blood flow (volume expansion, squatting, propranolol, transfusion if there has been blood loss), assurance of adequate alveolar oxygen for uptake (supplemental oxygen), reduction of oxygen demand (calming, sedation, paralysis, intubation, and mechanical ventilation, propranolol), or ductus manipulation (prostaglandin E_1).

Glenn and Fontan Procedures

Hearts that cannot support two separate circulations after repair (univentricular hearts and hearts having one hypoplastic ventricle) often are palliated and then repaired using systemic venous return to directly perfuse the lung (Glenn and Fontan procedures). This procedure frees the one functional ventricle to support the systemic circulation.

After such a procedure, the pressure of venous return drives pulmonary blood flow. At low pulmonary artery driving pressures, gravitational and airway pressure-mediated changes in V/Q matching may be exaggerated. The pressure of alveolar gas impinging on alveolar capillaries mediates this effect during mechanical ventilation. High airway pressure (from high PEEP or high tidal volume) tends to create alveolar dead space and waste ventilation as described in the Alveolar Pressure section. Use of high PEEP and large tidal volumes in Glenn and Fontan patients requires caution and attention to gas exchange, although low levels of PEEP are generally well tolerated.

One additional effect of elevated airway pressure in these patients is impaired venous return. The heart does not compensate for increases in right ventricular afterload following a Fontan procedure. It is predictable that venous filling pressure will rise in proportion to the rise in alveolar pressure, so a 5 cm H_2O rise in PEEP is expected to raise venous pressure by 4 mmHg. This might reduce cardiac output in proportion to the reduction in venous return as described for the normal circulation.

The advisability of PEEP after a Fontan or Glenn procedure must take into account the heart's inability to compensate for any elevation of PVR that may accompany atelectasis or lung disease. After either one of these procedures, the disadvantages of PEEP must be weighed against the risks of low FRC lung dysfunction.

Pulmonary Hypertension

Pulmonary hypertension makes the pulmonary circulation less susceptible to gravitational and airway pressure (Starling resistor)-mediated changes in V/Q matching. In contrast, it raises the tension in pulmonary vessels and invariably leads to smooth muscle hypertrophy and increased vasomotor reactivity. Even the infant with pulmonary hypertension because of a large interventricular communication and large left-to-right shunt (low PVR) may be capable of intense pulmonary vasoconstriction. The lung with pulmonary hypertension must be ventilated with special attention to blood pH, arterial pCO_2, alveolar pO_2, and probably degree of lung stretch, all of which alter PVR.

Pulmonary hypertensive crises can be transparent unless pulmonary artery pressure is monitored. They are only obvious in the presence of a right-to-left shunt. In the absence of such a shunt, an abrupt rise in PVR presents as a fall in cardiac output, sometimes associated with right ventricular ischemia, which may be evident on the electrocardiogram. Cardiovascular deterioration in a patient with underlying pulmonary hypertension should always direct attention to the patient's respiratory status.

There are numerous potential treatments of pulmonary hypertensive crises. Central to these is assurance of normal gas exchange and adequate (but not excessive) lung expansion. Oxygen, inhaled nitric oxide, selective phosphodiesterase inhibitors, calcium channel blockers, and other vasodilators have been used. Treatments that address oxygen demand also are essential.

Vascular Impingement on the Lungs

There are several recognizable cardiovascular syndromes of vascular impingement on airways.[61,62] The respiratory effects of these lesions are predictable from their location. Complete vascular rings may compress the trachea, causing airway narrowing, obstruction, and localized tracheomalacia. A pulmonary artery sling is origin of the left pulmonary artery from the right. The left pulmonary artery then wraps around the right mainstem bronchus to pass between the trachea and esophagus on its course to the left lung. It may impinge on the right mainstem bronchus, often causing right lung air trapping and overdistension. In congenital cardiac defects, pulmonary hypertension and left atrial hypertension often occur together. In this situation, the left atrium may elevate the left mainstem bronchus and trap it against the hypertensive left pulmonary artery.[63] This situation often leads to left lung atelectasis. In tetralogy of Fallot with absent pulmonary valve, massive dilation of the main pulmonary artery may occur with impingement on the bifurcation of the trachea. Tracheobronchial malacia may cause critical respiratory problems in this lesion, even after successful repair of the cardiac defect.

Effect of Initiating Mechanical Ventilation

At the time of initiation of mechanical ventilation, the interactions between breathing and circulation are abruptly altered. Moreover, these changes are superimposed on simultaneous sedation, paralysis, other pharmacologic regimens, and instrumentation of the pharynx and airway. Whereas narcotics, paralytics, atropine, and other drugs have well-defined effects, the effects of initiation of mechanical ventilation on circulation are not as consistent.

In many cases, effects on right ventricular preload predominate. This is generally the case in patients who are hypovolemic, such as asthmatics who have not been drinking, patients who are dehydrated, and septic children who may be hypovolemic because of capillary leak syndrome. Air trapping, as occurs in asthma, may be worsened by positive pressure ventilation, high ventilator rates, or use of long inspiratory times,[64] with consequent amplification of effects on venous return. Vascular volume expansion should accompany intubation in these patients.[65] It is noteworthy that the decrease in stroke volume that is often caused by positive pressure ventilation is not generally accompanied by a compensatory rise in heart rate,[66,67] so hemodynamic embarrassment that occurs upon institution of mechanical ventilation is not generally signaled by tachycardia.

Patients with segmental lung disease may undergo redistribution of blood flow upon initiation of positive pressure ventilation. Patients with lobar pneumonia or large segments of atelectasis may become more hypoxemic upon institution of positive pressure breathing because of diversion of pulmonary blood flow away from normal lung toward low V/Q lung segments. In contrast, application of PEEP may quickly reexpand collapsed areas of lung, improving V/Q matching and enhancing oxygenation.

Patients with pulmonary vascular disease may benefit from restoration of normal blood gases and alveolar gas composition, as alveolar hypoxia, arterial hypercarbia, and acidosis all increase pulmonary vascular tone. Inadvertent overdistension of lung may, in contrast, cause a calcium channel mediated rise in PVR.[68]

Patients in congestive cardiac failure, especially those with elevated filling pressures, may benefit almost immediately from afterload reduction as described in the Left Ventricular Afterload section. Relief of respiratory distress and diminished work of breathing can quickly benefit the circulation. Septic patients with myocardial depression also may show prompt improvement.

REFERENCES

1. Cournand A, Motley HL, Werko L, et al: Physiologic studies of the effects of intermittent positive pressure breathing on cardiac output in man. *Am J Physiol* 152:162-174, 1948.
2. Brengelmann GL: A critical analysis of the view that right atrial pressure determines venous return. *J Appl Physiol* 94:849-859, 2003.
3. Guyton AC: Determination of cardiac output by equating venous return curves with cardiac output curves. *Physiol Rev* 35:123-129, 1955.
4. Fessler HE, Brower RG, Wise RA, Permutt S: Effects of positive end-expiratory pressure on the canine venous return curve. *Am Rev Respir Dis* 146:4-10, 1992.
5. Cassidy SS, Robertson CH Jr, Pierce AK, et al: Cardiovascular effects of positive end-expiratory pressure in dogs. *J Appl Physiol* 44:743-750, 1978
6. Brookhart JM, Boyd TE: Local differences in intrathoracic pressure and their relation to cardiac filling pressure in the dog. *Am J Physiol* 148:434-444, 1947.
7. Marini JJ, O'Quin R, Culver BH, et al: Estimation of transmural cardiac pressure during ventilation with PEEP. *J Appl Physiol* 53:384-391, 1982.
8. Brecher GA, Hubay CA: Pulmonary blood flow and venous return during spontaneous respiration. *Circ Res* 3:210-214, 1955.
9. Pinsky MR: Instantaneous venous return curves in an intact canine preparation. *J Appl Physiol* 56:765-771, 1984.
10. Pinsky MR: Determinants of pulmonary arterial flow variation during respiration. *J Appl Physiol* 56:1237-1245, 1984.
11. Morgan BC, Abel FL, Mullins GL, et al: Flow patterns in cavae, pulmonary artery, pulmonary vein and aorta in intact dogs. *Am J Physiol* 210:297-305, 1969.
12. Teboul JL, Pinsky MR, Mercat A, et al: Estimating cardiac filling pressure in mechanically ventilated patients with hyperinflation. *Crit Care Med* 28:3631-3636, 2000.
13. Pinsky MR: Recent advances in the clinical application of heart-lung interactions. *Curr Opin Crit Care* 8:26-31, 2002.
14. Burton AC, Patel DJ: Effect on pulmonary vascular resistance of inflation of the rabbit lungs. *J Appl Physiol* 12:239-246, 1958.
15. Barer GR, Howard P, McCurrie JR, et al: Changes in the pulmonary circulation after bronchial occlusion in anesthetized dogs and cats. *Circ Res* 25:747-764, 1969.
16. Benumof JL: Mechanism of decreased blood flow to atelectatic lung. *J Appl Physiol* 46:1047-1048, 1979.
17. Whittenberger JL, McGregor M, Berglund E, et al: Influence of state of inflation of the lung on pulmonary vascular resistance. *J Appl Physiol* 15:878-882, 1960.
18. Lopez-Muniz R, Stephens NC, Bromberger-Barnea B, et al: Critical closure of pulmonary vessels analyzed in terms of Starling resistor model. *J Appl Physiol* 24:625-635, 1968.
19. West JB, Dollery CT, Naimark A: Distribution of blood flow in isolated lung: relation to vascular and alveolar pressures. *J Appl Physiol* 19:713-724, 1964.
20. West JB, Dollery CT: Distribution of blood flow and the pressure flow relations of the whole lung. *J Appl Physiol* 20:175-183, 1965.
21. Mink SN, Light RB, Cooligan T, et al: Effect of PEEP on gas exchange and pulmonary perfusion in canine lobar pneumonia. *J Appl Physiol* 50:517-523, 1981.
22. Fuhrman BP, Everitt J, Lock JE: Cardiopulmonary effects of unilateral airway pressure changes in intact infant lambs. *J Appl Physiol* 56:1439-1448, 1984.
23. Fuhrman BP, Smith-Wright DL, Kulik TJ, et al: Effects of static and fluctuating airway pressure on intact pulmonary circulation. *J Appl Physiol* 60:114-122, 1986.
24. Fuhrman BP, Smith-Wright DL, Venkataraman S, Howland DF. Pulmonary vascular resistance after cessation of positive end-expiratory pressure. *J Appl Physiol* 66:660-668, 1989.
25. Venkataraman ST, Fuhrman BP, Howland DF: PEEP-induced calcium channel-mediated rise in PVR in neonatal lambs. *Crit Care Med* 21:1066-1076, 1993.
26. Schreiber MD, Heymann MA, Soifer SJ: Increased arterial pH, not decreased PaCO2 attenuates hypoxia-induced pulmonary vasoconstriction in newborn lambs. *Pediatr Res* 20:113-117, 1986.
27. Rudolph AM, Yuan S: Response of the pulmonary vasculature to hypoxia and H^+ ion concentration changes. *J Clin Invest* 45: 399-411, 1966.
28. Fishman AP: Vasomotor regulation of the pulmonary circulation. *Annu Rev Physiol* 42:211-220, 1980.
29. Doyle JST, Wilson JS, Warren JV: The pulmonary vascular responses to short-term hypoxia in human subjects. *Circulation* 5:263-270, 1952.
30. Wagner WW: Pulmonary circulation: control through hypoxic vasoconstriction. *Semin Respir Med* 7:124-135, 1985.
31. Peake MD, Harabin AL, Brennan NJ, et al: Steady-state vascular responses to graded hypoxia in isolated lungs of five species. *J Appl Physiol* 51:1214-1219, 1981.
32. Taylor RR, Covell JW, Sonnenblick EH, et al: Dependence of ventricular distensibility on filling of the opposite ventricle. *Am J Physiol* 213:711-718, 1967.
33. Buda AJ, Pinsky MR, Ingels NB Jr, et al: Effect of intrathoracic pressure on left ventricular performance. *N Engl J Med* 301: 453-459, 1979.
34. Pinsky MR, Summer WR, Wise RA, et al: Augmentation of cardiac function by elevation of intrathoracic pressure. *J Appl Physiol* 54:950-955, 1983.
35. Patten MT, Liebman PR, Hechtman HB: Humorally mediated decreases in cardiac output associated with positive end expiratory pressure. *Microvasc Res* 13:137-139, 1997.
36. Patten MT, Liebman PR, Manny J, et al: Humorally mediated alterations in cardiac performance as a consequence of positive end-expiratory pressure. *Surgery* 84:201-205, 1978.
37. Grindlinger GA, Manny J, Justice R, et al: Presence of negative inotropic agents in canine plasma during positive end-expiratory pressure. *Circ Res* 45:460-467, 1979.
38. Dunham BM, Grindlinger GA, Utsunomiya T, et al: Role of prostaglandins in positive end-expiratory pressure-induced negative inotropism. *Am J Physiol* 241:783-788, 1981.
39. Manny J, Grindlinger G, Mathe AA, et al: Positive end-expiratory pressure, lung stretch and decreased myocardial contractility. *Surgery* 84:127-133, 1978.
40. Glick G, Wechsler AS, Epstein SE: Reflex cardiovascular depression produced by stimulation of pulmonary stretch receptors in the dog. *J Clin Invest* 48:467-473, 1969.
41. Calvin JE, Driedger AA, Sibbald WJ: Positive end-expiratory pressure (PEEP) does not depress left ventricular function in patients with pulmonary edema. *Am Rev Respir Dis* 124:121-128, 1981.
42. Dhainaut JF, Bricard C, Monsallier FJ, et al: Left ventricular contractility using isovolumic phase indices during PEEP in ARDS patients. *Crit Care Med* 10:631-635, 1982.

43. Johnston WE, Vinten-Johansen I, Santamore WP, et al: Mechanism of reduced cardiac output during positive end-expiratory pressure in the dog. *Am Rev Respir Dis* 140:1257-1264, 1989.
44. Rankin JS, Olsen CO, Arentzen CE, et al: The effects of airway pressure on cardiac function in intact dogs and man. *Circulation* 66:108-120, 1982.
45. Schulman DS, Biondi JW, Matthay RA, et al: Effect of positive end-expiratory pressure on right ventricular performance: importance of baseline right ventricular function. *Am J Med* 84:57-67, 1988.
46. Schulman DS, Biondi JW, Zohgbi S, et al: Coronary flow limits right ventricular performance during positive end-expiratory pressure. *Am Rev Respir Dis* 141:1531-1537, 1990.
47. Fessler HE, Brower RG, Wise R, et al: Positive pleural pressure decreases coronary perfusion. *Am J Physiol* 258:H814-H820, 1990.
48. Jellinek H, Krafft P, Fitzgerald RD, et al: Right atrial pressure predicts hemodynamic response to apneic positive airway pressure. *Crit Care Med* 28:672-678, 2000.
49. Michard F, Chemla D, Richard C, et al: Clinical use of respiratory changes in arterial pulse pressure to monitor the hemodynamic effects of PEEP in patients with acute lung injury. *Am J Respir Crit Care Med* 159:935-939, 1999.
50. Michard F, Boussat S, Chemla D, et al: Relation between respiratory changes in arterial pulse pressure and fluid responsiveness in septic patients with acute circulatory failure. *Am J Respir Crit Care Med* 162:134-138, 2000.
51. Van Den Berg P, Jansen JR, Pinsky MR: Effect of positive pressure on venous return in volume-loaded cardiac surgical patients. *J Appl Physiol* 92:1223-1231, 2002.
52. Pinsky MR, Matuschak GM, Klain M: Determinants of cardiac augmentation by increase in intrathoracic pressure. *J Appl Physiol* 58:1189-1198, 1985.
53. Aubier M, Trippenbach T, Roussos C: Respiratory muscle fatigue during cardiogenic shock. *J Appl Physiol* 51:499-508, 1981.
54. Coast JR, Jensen RA, Cassidy SS, et al: Cardiac output and O2 consumption during inspiratory threshold loaded breathing. *J Appl Physiol* 64:1624-1628, 1988.
55. Abel JG, Salerno TA, Panos A, et al: Cardiovascular effects of positive pressure ventilation in humans. *Ann Thorac Surg* 43:198-206, 1987.
56. Berryhill RE, Benumof JL: PEEP-induced discrepancy between pulmonary arterial wedge pressure and left atrial pressure: the effects of controlled vs spontaneous ventilation and compliant vs noncompliant lungs in the dog. *Anesthesiology* 51:303-308, 1979.
57. Enson Y, Giuntini C, Lewis ML, et al: The influence of hydrogen ion concentration and hypoxia on the pulmonary circulation. *J Clin Invest* 43:1146-1162, 1964.
58. Rudolph AM, Yuan S: Response of the pulmonary vasculature to hypoxia and H^+ ion concentration changes. *J Clin Invest* 45: 339-411, 1966.
59. Pepe PE, Lurie KG, Wigginton JG, et al: Detrimental hemodynamic effects of assisted ventilation in hemorrhagic states. *Crit Care Med* 32(suppl):S414-S420, 2004.
60. Fuhrman BP, Pokora TJ, Bessinger FB Jr, et al: Hypercarbia in the infant with congenital cardiac disease. *Pediatr Cardiol* 2:245-250, 1982.
61. Smith RJ, Smith MC, Glossop LP, et al: Congenital vascular anomalies causing tracheoesophageal compression. *Arch Otolaryngol* 110:82-87, 1984.
62. Berlinger NT, Lucas RV Jr, Foker J: Pulmonary arteriopexy to relieve tracheobronchial compression by dilated pulmonary arteries. *Ann Otol Rhinol Laryngol* 93(5 pt 1):473-476, 1984.
63. Berlinger NT, Long C, Foker J, Lucas RV Jr: Tracheobronchial compression in acyanotic congenital heart disease. *Ann Otol Rhinol Laryngol* 92(4 pt 1):387-390, 1983.
64. Pepe PE, Marini JJ: Occult positive end-expiratory pressure in mechanically ventilated patients with airflow obstruction: the auto-PEEP effect. *Am Rev Respir Dis* 126:166-170, 1982.
65. Morgan BC, Crawford EW, Guntheroth WG: The hemodynamic effects of changes in blood volume during intermittent positive-pressure ventilation. *Anesthesiology* 30:297-305, 1969.
66. Cassidy SS, Eschenbacher WL, Robertson CH Jr, et al: Cardiovascular effects of positive-pressure ventilation in normal subjects. *J Appl Physiol* 47:453-461, 1979.
67. Cassidy SS, Mitchell JH: Effects of positive pressure breathing on right and left ventricular preload and afterload. *Fed Proc* 40: 2178-2181, 1981.
68. Venkataraman ST, Fuhrman BP, Howland DF: Air trapping causes a Ca2 (+) channel mediated increase in pulmonary vascular resistance in neonatal lambs. *Pediatr Res* 29:89-92, 1991.

CHAPTER 25

Myocardial Dysfunction, Extracorporeal Membrane Oxygenation, and Ventricular Assist Devices

Anthony C. Chang and E. Dean McKenzie

PEARLS

- Type and duration of mechanical circulatory support should be individualized to meet the needs of each specific cardiac scenario.
- Time to myocardial recovery in children varies with the indication for support. The myocardium usually recovers from postcardiotomy dysfunction absent residual defect or coronary insufficiency within 72 hours, more rapidly than with fulminant myocarditis or acute respiratory distress syndrome.
- Choosing among specific devices will become more complicated. Factors such as anticipated duration of support, patient size and age, necessity for biventricular support, and spectrum of anticipated device complications will enter into the decision-making process.

Introduction

Low cardiac output from a failing myocardium is often seen in the pediatric cardiac intensive care setting. Catecholamines and new pharmacologic agents such as milrinone[1,2] remain the mainstay of therapy for the failing heart. This form of therapy has obvious limitations, especially in neonates who have age-related differences in sympathetic neurohumoral activity and adrenergic receptor agonism.[3]

Results of mechanical cardiopulmonary support in infants, children, and young adults have steadily improved in the past decade as a result of improved technology.[4–6] Yet such support remains in its nascent stages and is largely limited to extracorporeal membrane oxygenation (ECMO).[7–25] Pediatric mechanical circulatory support has become an essential component of state-of-the-art pediatric cardiac intensive care,[26,27] and additional innovative modalities and extended indications for mechanical cardiopulmonary support are being explored.[28]

General Principles

In both pediatric and adult patients, myocardial failure can be divided into (1) intrinsic failure of the myocardium from general pathophysiologic processes such as myocardial ischemia, myocarditis/cardiomyopathy, graft rejection after transplantation, or injury from prolonged intraoperative course (prolonged cross-clamp time, insufficient myocardial protection, or coronary ischemia) and (2) extrinsic factors such as sepsis or metabolic derangement (e.g., acidosis or hypoxia). There are important differences, however, between pediatric and adult patients with cardiac failure. Pediatric patients with failing hearts often also have right ventricular failure, pulmonary hypertension, profound hypoxemia, or anatomic variations that provide daunting challenges in planning surgical cannulation and support strategy. In addition, mechanical support for pediatric patients with heart disease, particularly those with congenital heart disease, demands even more forethought and individualization than for pediatric patients with respiratory disease with normal intracardiac anatomy.

General Principles of Cardiac Intensive Care in Anticipation of Mechanical Support

As with pediatric cardiac intensive care in general, the care of critically ill patients requires a multidisciplinary team involving the cardiologist; cardiac surgeon; cardiac anesthesiologist; intensivist or neonatologist; support personnel in perfusion, respiratory therapy, pharmacology, and nursing; and other relevant subspecialists such as pulmonologists, nephrologists, hematologists, neurologists, and infectious disease specialists. The present strategy uses mechanical cardiopulmonary support as a bridge to either myocardial recovery or heart transplantation, although the concept that the failing heart needs rest to recover is not entirely novel.[29]

For all patients being considered for mechanical cardiopulmonary support, it is essential to make an accurate diagnosis of the cardiac anatomy and physiology prior to instituting support. One lesion that occasionally is missed is anomalous left coronary artery from the pulmonary artery; these infants often have clinical presentations that mimic myocarditis yet are amenable to surgical correction. Total anomalous pulmonary venous connection often was misdiagnosed as pulmonary disease before the widespread use of color Doppler. Last, both venous and aortic arch anatomy require careful evaluation prior to cannulation, especially when an interrupted aortic arch or coarctation is a consideration. These diagnoses are difficult to exclude in the presence of a patent ductus arteriosus.[30]

It is strategically beneficial to ameliorate ventricular dysfunction by pharmacologic means before surgery to lessen the likelihood of need for postoperative support. Cardiopulmonary bypass induces myocardial inflammation that can cause subsequent myocardial dysfunction. Moreover, the increased myocardial wall stress seen in patients with deteriorating myocardial function before surgery may reduce the safety margin for successful separation from bypass after surgery. For instance, a 3-year-old child with severe mitral regurgitation and shortening fraction of 22% may benefit from 24 to 48 hours of inotropic support before surgery to decrease end-diastolic and end-systolic dimensions and wall stress.

Certain congenital heart defects, such as anomalous left coronary artery from the pulmonary artery or transposition of the great arteries in an older infant, have predicted high risk for postoperative ventricular dysfunction. Anticipation of need for postoperative mechanical support should be heightened.

After cardiac surgery, indications for mechanical support include poor hemodynamic profile, metabolic acidosis, oliguria, poor perfusion, and rising serum lactate level (>0.75 mmol/L/hour)[31] despite escalating inotropic support. Prior to placing a postoperative patient on support, it is prudent to rule out significant postoperative residua (such as residual atrioventricular valve regurgitation/stenosis or left-to-right shunt) or coronary insufficiency as a result of surgical manipulation (such as ostial stenosis or compression by surgical conduit). Such an evaluation may require diagnostic and interventional cardiac catheterization. If the patient's condition is very unstable and warrants immediate support, it is technically feasible to obtain hemodynamic and angiographic data at a later time while the patient is on mechanical support by introducing brief periods of circuit interruptions. The presence of postoperative residua is not a contraindication for support but rather a situation that warrants surgical or catheter intervention to improve the likelihood of eventual survival. Untreated significant postoperative residua that require mechanical cardiopulmonary support confer a very low likelihood of survival.[32]

In general, an anticipatory strategy for early institution of mechanical support is preferable to a resuscitative rescue. For example, for a 6-week-old infant with transposition of the great arteries after an arterial switch operation with left ventricular dysfunction and a left atrial pressure of 22 mmHg who is on inotropic support consisting of epinephrine at 0.4 μg/kg/minute, serious consideration for mechanical support should be discussed prior to reaching the nadir period of cardiac output at 6 to 12 hours postoperatively.[33] Optimal timing of support is subjective yet critical to minimize end-organ ischemia and maximize opportunity for multiorgan recovery. Use of ECMO for postcardiotomy support reported in the literature ranges from 1.5% to 8.3% but is even lower at some institutions (currently <1% at Texas Children's Hospital). Although criteria for postoperative cardiac ECMO support based solely on serum lactate level have been proposed, such an approach may oversimplify a complex decision that should be made on a case-by-case basis. Such criteria can create intellectual limitations that discourage the management flexibility vital in perioperative cardiac intensive care.

The decision for institution of mechanical support should be individualized, taking into consideration hemodynamic instability, low urine output, metabolic acidosis, poor perfusion with decreased capillary refill, and high level of inotropic support. As a guide, an inotropic requirement of epinephrine greater than or equal to 0.2 μg/kg/minute (without evidence for vasodilatory shock as seen in sepsis, in which case norepinephrine or vasopressin is indicated) usually is indicative of severe low cardiac output syndrome and may warrant mechanical support. Irreversible damage to the neonatal myocardium may occur when high epinephrine dosages are used for sustained periods.

Before a final decision for mechanical support is made, a thorough echocardiographic examination should be performed to rule out any reversible mechanical problem (e.g., pericardial tamponade). Acute sternal opening in the intensive care unit setting is an acceptable strategy as a maneuver to improve oxygen delivery[34] prior to mechanical support.

Preparation for mechanical support includes acquisition of packed red blood cells (2 units that are cytomegalovirus-negative irradiated and leukocyte reduced in case the patient becomes a transplant candidate) and fresh-frozen plasma. Baseline hematologic studies including complete blood cell count, prothrombin time, partial thromboplastin time, platelet count, activated clotting time (ACT), plasma hemoglobin, antithrombin 3, fibrinogen, and thromboelastogram also should be obtained. Lastly, both arterial and venous lines and the endotracheal tube should be secured and be accessible during the cannulation process.

Indications and Contraindications for Mechanical Support

Appropriate patient selection and stabilization for mechanical support are of paramount importance to maximize survival and outcome. Among indications for mechanical cardiopulmonary support in children are the following.

Myocardial Dysfunction: Bridge to Recovery

Mechanical support in children with potentially reversible myocardial dysfunction, including postcardiotomy myocardial dysfunction (e.g., anomalous left coronary artery from the pulmonary artery[35,36] or transposition of the great arteries with postoperative left ventricular dysfunction),[37] acute myocarditis, exacerbation of cardiomyopathy, and acute transplant rejection,[38] entails a clinical strategy to create a bridge to eventual myocardial recovery.

Perioperative patients with postcardiotomy syndrome can be further divided into those who fail to separate from cardiopulmonary bypass ("early" postcardiotomy cardiac failure) and those who require mechanical support hours or days after operation because of myocardial dysfunction and low cardiac output ("late" postcardiotomy cardiac failure). There is a higher likelihood of survival if cannulation occurs after an initial period of stability rather than immediately after cardiopulmonary bypass (except for children with anomalous left coronary artery from the pulmonary artery).

Children with acute fulminant myocarditis often succumb to low cardiac output syndrome despite escalating inotropic support and can benefit greatly from mechanical support with eventual myocardial recovery.[39,40] In adult patients with fulminant myocarditis, aggressive hemodynamic support with assist technology has yielded excellent long-term survival.[41] Mechanical support probably is underused in children with this diagnosis. Children should not succumb to myocarditis without an attempt to bridge to myocardial recovery on mechanical support because survival among these patients is excellent.[42] In the absence of a severity of illness score for myocarditis, escalating requirement for inotropic support (particularly use of epinephrine) associated with relentless metabolic acidosis and rising serum lactate level should provide a clinical indication for institution of mechanical support. Children with myocarditis usually require a longer duration of support (>72 hours) than children with myocardial dysfunction after cardiac surgery.

Myocardial Dysfunction: Bridge to Transplantation

Children who are critically ill with primary myocardial failure secondary to dilated cardiomyopathy, end-stage congenital heart disease, or prolonged graft rejection after heart transplantation are candidates for consideration of mechanical cardiopulmonary support as a bridge to transplantation.[43,44] Although these children are less likely to recover myocardial function compared with patients in the former category, nevertheless there is a continuum of recovery and reversibility of myocardial dysfunction. In addition, although ECMO has been the mainstay of therapy for this group of patients with survival of approximately 50%,[45–47] there is a growing need for more longer-term (>2 weeks) mechanical support alternatives for these patients[48–50] because complications can develop during ECMO that preclude transplantation before a donor heart is available.[51] Although extracorporeal life support can be used as a bridge to pediatric cardiac transplantation for at least 2 weeks with acceptable survival,[52] mortality while waiting for heart transplantation in patients on inotropic support, especially infants, is greater than 50% at 6 months.[53]

Cardiopulmonary Resuscitation

Use of mechanical support as a rescue after failed conventional resuscitation was first described by del Nido[55] in pediatric cardiac patients and has been described in adults with acceptable results.[55,56] Such capability for rapid deployment of a mechanical support system is essential for any cardiac intensive care setting and demands an organized team effort. It is essential that such a maneuver be instituted within 20 minutes; thus a crystalloid primed circuit is essential as the initial setup to obviate the need for blood products. The current survival results for such rescue therapy can be 50% or higher as long as resuscitation is effective and cannulation is performed in a timely manner.[57–59]

Preoperative Stabilization

Cardiopulmonary support can be provided to any neonate who presents with profound hypoxemia and/or cardiovascular collapse before definitive intervention is possible.[60] Clinical situations that demand such support among preoperative patients include those with hypercyanotic spells,[61] pulmonary hypertensive crises,[62] or certain diagnoses such as total anomalous pulmonary venous connection,[63,64] common pulmonary vein atresia,[65] or tetralogy of Fallot with absent pulmonary valve.[66] Timely surgical or catheter palliation/repair of these lesions, however, remains an essential part of the management strategy.

Acute Respiratory Distress Syndrome

Parenchymal lung disease is the most common indication for ECMO use in the neonatal population, but good results also have been observed with non-neonatal respiratory failure.[67] A patient with congenital heart disease could develop parenchymal lung disease before or after cardiac surgery and not respond to conventional therapy such as high-frequency ventilation, surfactant administration, or even inhaled nitric oxide. The highest-risk patient populations include children with respiratory syncytial virus,[68,69] bronchopulmonary dysplasia,[70] or unusual associated respiratory diseases such as plastic bronchitis.[71] Duration of necessary support may be weeks rather than days because patients with lung parenchymal disease tend to recover over longer periods. Venovenous ECMO has been used for respiratory disease in children with cardiac diagnoses, including a neonate after a Norwood operation.[72]

Severe Pulmonary Hypertension

A few selected patients with hemodynamic instability because of pulmonary hypertension unresponsive to inhaled nitric oxide have benefited from mechanical support. Such support may be especially useful during the postoperative period when pulmonary vascular resistance may be transiently elevated.[73] However, mechanical support is controversial in any patient with irreversible pulmonary hypertension. For postoperative patients with pulmonary hypertension who undergo mechanical support, postoperative anatomic residua (e.g., residual shunt or pulmonary venous obstruction) must be ruled out by noninvasive imaging or cardiac catheterization while on mechanical support. The advent of inhaled nitric oxide has reduced the need for mechanical support for this indication.[74–76] Elevated right atrial pressure in a Fontan patient, indicating elevated pulmonary vascular resistance, has been treated with ECMO.[77] Although mechanical support provides hemodynamic stability and reduces pulmonary vascular resistance (as a result of less aggressive mechanical ventilation), it potentially can rekindle the inflammatory milieu that leads to pulmonary vasoreactivity.

Malignant Dysrhythmias

Patients who do not respond to aggressive medical therapy for incessant tachydysrhythmias may benefit from a short trial of mechanical support to prevent further myocardial depressant effects of antiarrhythmic agents, especially beta-blockade.

Patients who have benefited under this indication include those with lethal arrhythmias associated with myocardial disease,[78] supraventricular tachycardia,[79] junctional ectopic tachycardia, or ventricular tachycardia after cardiac surgery.[80–82] However, it is imperative to identify etiologic factors such as postoperative residua and/or coronary ischemia. Use of ECMO has been reported for malignant ventricular tachydysrhythmias[83] and for quinidine toxicity with refractory bradydysrhythmias and profound hypotension.[84]

Profound Cyanosis

In patients with severe cyanosis, the underlying anatomic and/or physiologic etiology must be diagnosed and palliated or corrected. Mechanical support for cyanosis should be considered on a case-by-case basis. For example, an infant who is profoundly cyanotic after a bidirectional cavopulmonary anastomosis without an anatomic cause may benefit from inhaled nitric oxide and sternal opening. If these maneuvers fail, mechanical support could be justified to stabilize and resuscitate a patient while diagnostic and possibly interventional catheterizations are performed to delineate the etiologic factors for cyanosis.

Proactive Support

This indication is controversial but may be valid in certain high-risk clinical situations. High-risk interventional catheterizations, such as balloon valvotomy, in a critically ill neonate with aortic stenosis may warrant support on ECMO.[85,86] In addition, certain electrophysiologic procedures can be performed while on ECMO support to minimize end-organ ischemia in the event of cardiac arrest.[87] Last, there is even discussion of using mechanical support in a proactive fashion for children following Norwood palliative repair.[88]

Mechanical Device Selection

Device options for short-term support are limited. They include ECMO in its various technologic forms and centrifugal ventricular assist device (VAD) (Table 25–1). Longer-term support options for the pediatric patient population do not exist.

At present, ECMO is the mainstay support device for all neonates and for children with biventricular dysfunction or hypoxemia. Biventricular assist devices are too large for most children. The decision for specific devices will become more complex as factors such as anticipated duration of support, patient size and age, necessity for biventricular support, and spectrum of anticipated device complications all enter into the decision-making process.

General Principles of Cardiac Intensive Care During Support

Extracorporeal Membrane Oxygenation

It is imperative that the team understands not only the pathophysiology of the failing myocardium but also the circulatory physiology of mechanical support (Figure 25–1 A and B).[89] In addition, confounding issues (e.g., presence of atrial and ventricular septal defects, patent ductus arteriosus) may complicate mechanical support of cardiac patients.

Mechanical cardiovascular support reduces cardiac wall stress, work, and oxygen consumption when the heart is appropriately decompressed. The changes in preload and afterload that occur on initiation of mechanical support are clinically significant. Blood flow becomes nonpulsatile. Central venous pressure usually is lowered as a result of adequate venous drainage and should be maintained low to minimize sequelae from elevated central venous pressure such as pleural effusions, ascites, and deleterious effects on the cerebral, gastrointestinal,

TABLE 25–1

Comparisons of ECMO and Centrifugal VAD for Children with Heart Disease

	ECMO	Centrifugal VAD (Biomedicus)
PEDIATRIC EXPERIENCE	Large (>4,000 since 1989)	Growing (n/a)
EASE OF USE	No	Yes
MEMBRANE OXYGENATOR	Yes	Possible
PERIPHERAL CANNULATION	Yes	No
VENTRICULAR CANNULATION	No	No
ANTICOAGULATION	Yes	Yes (but less than ECMO)
UNIVENTRICULAR SUPPORT	Yes	Yes
BIVENTRICULAR SUPPORT	Yes	Possible (but difficult in infants)
NEED FOR LA DECOMPRESSION	Occasional	No
DURATION OF SUPPORT	Days to weeks	Days to weeks
PATIENT MOBILITY	No	No
COST	High	Low
COMPLICATIONS	Moderate	Low

hepatic, and renal blood flows. Left atrial pressure (which can be noninvasively estimated by echocardiographic examinations of the position of the atrial septum) should be carefully monitored. Inadequate unloading of the left atrium and ventricle with resultant distension can lead to mitral regurgitation and pulmonary edema/hemorrhage and will minimize the likelihood of myocardial recovery. One strategy to decrease left atrial pressure is to increase the ECMO flow as much as 150 ml/kg/minute. If left atrial distension persists, mechanical decompression can be achieved by surgical left atrial venting (with an additional cannula and a Y connector to the venous tubing of the ECMO circuit)[90] or by balloon/blade atrial septostomy/septectomy after transseptal puncture.[91–93] The presence of aortopulmonary collaterals, patent ductus arteriosus, or insufficiency of the aortic valve (occasionally as a result of flow of the arterial cannula directed at the aortic valve) can create a persistently elevated left atrial pressure. If an adequate atrial septal defect is present, as in some patients with congenital heart disease, no intervention should be necessary to decompress the left atrium.

Systolic hypertension and increased systemic vascular resistance[94] associated with ECMO are thought to be related to high plasma renin activity or to result from higher ECMO flows and should be aggressively treated with a vasodilator such as nitroprusside, nitroglycerin, phenoxybenzamine, or milrinone. Adequate afterload reduction decreases the likelihood of elevated left ventricular wall stress,[95,96] surgical bleeding, and intracranial hemorrhage.[97] Mean pressure should be maintained at what is appropriate for body weight (≈30–40 mmHg in neonates and ≈50–75 mmHg in older children depending on size). Other etiologic factors for elevated systemic resistance include hypothermia, seizures, pain, and acidosis. Occasionally, intermittent doses of intravenous hydralazine are necessary for more rapid treatment of elevated systolic blood pressure, although this therapy does not necessarily improve cardiac performance.[98]

Left ventricular ejection, manifested by arterial pulsation, may indicate ventricular recovery. Myocardial stun can be observed in 5% of neonates on ECMO, even in infants without prior myocardial injury, and is manifested by a lack of adequate arterial pulsation.[99] This stun phenomenon, which resembles electromechanical dissociation, usually occurs within the first 6 hours after initiation of flow and can last up to 64 hours.[100] One theory to explain this apparent lack of myocardial function is that the heart is not able to eject antegrade against an excessively elevated afterload. Therefore maneuvers to diminish afterload (by reducing ECMO flow or by pharmacologic afterload reduction) may improve left ventricular ejection.

Mechanical support should decrease myocardial oxygen consumption (less tachycardia and lower wall stress) and increase myocardial perfusion (augmentation of coronary diastolic pressure and concomitant diminution of end-diastolic filling pressure). Low-dose inotropic support can be used to maintain baseline inotropy and renal perfusion. Continuous monitoring of mixed venous saturation is used to maintain vigilance of overall cardiac output. In addition, elevated serum lactate levels and abnormal acid-base status should normalize after initiation of mechanical support and thereby demonstrate adequate oxygen delivery. Overall, the right and left ventricular outputs decrease in proportion to the amount of bypass flow provided.[101]

Hemodynamic compromise can persist or develop during ECMO. Effective troubleshooting may require measurement of right and left atrial pressures and mean arterial pressure. If the arterial pressure and the filling pressures are low, consider (1) hypovolemia and administer volume; (2) excessive bleeding (including occult bleeding) and correct coagulopathy; (3) excessive vasodilation and decrease dose of vasodilators or initiate vasopressors; and (4) excessive runoff into pulmonary circulation (shunts or collaterals such as a large patent ductus arteriosus) and discuss with the cardiovascular surgeon the possibility of obliterating such a runoff. If the arterial pressure is low but the filling pressures are elevated, then consider (1) inadequate venous drainage from cannulas and adjust as necessary; (2) tamponade and perform echocardiography and consider exploring the mediastinum[102]; (3) left atrial distension from ventricular dysfunction and (4) noncardiac issues such as tension pneumothorax or hemothorax.[103] Patients with arrhythmias require special consideration while on mechanical support. Readily reversible issues, such as lowered mean perfusion pressure or metabolic derangements leading to arrhythmias, should be reversed (rather than performing cardiopulmonary resuscitation or countershock). Resuscitation has potential deleterious sequelae, and chest compressions are contraindicated during satisfactory ECMO because the maneuver can easily dislodge the cannulas or injure the myocardium.

Although mechanical support provides a temporary reprieve from the constant threat of cardiac arrest, it remains a good strategy to continue to aggressively pursue any postoperative residua that may be amenable to interventional catheterization. Although transthoracic echocardiography can be limited because of suboptimal acoustic windows, it can be useful for delineating cannula position, intracardiac thrombi, or certain intracardiac anatomic residua.[104] Even transesophageal echocardiography can have inherent limitations for accurate diagnosis given that the loading conditions while on mechanical support make hemodynamic assessment of residual defects using with Doppler studies less likely.

Cardiac catheterizations can be safely performed while on ECMO and can aid in the diagnosis of potential residual lesions. ECMO is not a contraindication to interventional catheterization (balloon dilations, stent implantations, coil placements).[105–107] Failure to correct postoperative residua in the mechanical support population contributes to poor survival.[108,109] Leaving a large interventricular communication after corrective surgery, for instance, reduces the effectiveness of ECMO because right atrial drainage alone usually is inadequate to decompress the left atrium. Moreover, a patent ductus arteriosus may require closure because it can create a large amount of runoff.[110] Transport of these critically ill patients to the catheterization laboratory requires meticulous care during the entire process. Potential complications can be prevented with support equipment that is directly attached to the bed, which may reduce the risk of dislodging cannulas.

In ECMO patients with single ventricles and shunts, optimal management of the shunt (open, partially ligated, or totally ligated) remains controversial. Many options have been described, including the option of pump support without an oxygenator, relying on pulmonary gas exchange with the aortopulmonary shunt as the sole source of pulmonary blood flow.[111,112] One report indicated a higher survival in 10 patients if the shunt remained open.[113] If the shunt is left totally open, adequate alveolar ventilation should be made sufficient to prevent pulmonary interstitial edema from excessive pulmonary blood. In addition, flow from the ECMO circuit may need to be increased to maintain both pulmonary blood flow and adequate systemic perfusion. In certain patients with particularly low pulmonary vascular resistance, such as low-birth-weight neonates, leaving the shunt open may not be a feasible option because pulmonary blood flow may be excessive. In addition, evidence indicates deleterious effects on cerebral oxygenation and hemodynamics when an aortopulmonary communication such as ductus arteriosus is present.[114] In contrast, totally occluding the shunt may lead to extensive pulmonary ischemia and infarction because bronchial flow alone may not be adequate to supply the pulmonary parenchyma. Thus ECMO support for single-ventricle patients requires even more forethought and flexibility than for biventricular patients, but the usual goals of single-ventricle physiology still apply (Q_p and Q_s balance as much as possible).[115]

This clinical scenario is particularly challenging in patients with single ventricle and bidirectional cavopulmonary anastomosis. Cannulation is necessary in both the superior vena cava and the right atrium because jugular venous cannulation alone may not supply sufficient venous return and right atrial cannulation alone may not decompress the cerebral venous system adequately. Cannulation of the common iliac vein may be necessary. Similar considerations may be necessary in Fontan patients to assure adequate venous drainage.[116]

The optimal strategy for ventilator management during extracorporeal support remains controversial. Animal studies show that pulmonary sequelae from prolonged venoarterial bypass are significant and include pulmonary edema with parenchymal necrosis and intraalveolar hemorrhage.[117] Ventilatory support may be necessary to minimize atelectasis and to maximize oxygenation of blood returning to the left atrium (with the theoretical advantage that the coronary blood flow from the left ventricle can receive the highest oxygen tension possible).[118]

Another consideration is possible use of surfactant for lungs with evidence of parenchymal disease. Lung ischemia may cause endothelial dysfunction and surfactant deficiency during ECMO (not dissimilar to that observed with cardiopulmonary bypass).[119] Therefore surfactant therapy may decrease pulmonary dysfunction and duration of ECMO.[120] Excessive fluid overload evidenced by interstitial edema on chest roentgenogram can be addressed by use of hemofiltration via the extracorporeal circuits to remove excessive fluid and to improve gas exchange.[121]

The neurologic system must be assessed after successful resuscitation and cannulation for support. Central nervous system (CNS) evaluation may be hampered by neuromuscular blockade and narcotic analgesia. Neurologic injury is a major category of morbidity in neonates and children on ECMO. Daily head ultrasound examinations should be performed, especially in the first few days of ECMO, which is the highest risk period for CNS bleeding.[122] Cerebrovascular accidents and hemorrhages can occur during resuscitation and during ECMO, so other investigative procedures such as computed tomography may be necessary when feasible. Seizures while on ECMO support are common (manifested occasionally as tachycardia, elevated blood pressure, and pupillary changes) but often go undetected. A study showed that intermittent-discontinuous electroencephalograms did not indicate poor prognosis if normalization of the electroencephalogram occurred within 7 days.[123] Hyperthermia after cardiopulmonary arrest may confer higher likelihood of neurologic recovery.[124] Longer-term neurologic complications include acquired hydrocephalus associated with superior vena cava syndrome.[125]

Optimal renal perfusion during mechanical support is vital. Renal failure with an elevated creatinine is a poor prognostic factor of overall survival of pediatric patients on mechanical support. Low-dose dopamine or new drugs such as the dopamine-agonist fenoldapam[126] may have a role in maintenance of renal perfusion while patients are on mechanical support with nonpulsatile flow. Peritoneal dialysis can be used as a strategy to remove fluid in appropriate patients and may be beneficial for minimizing capillary leak syndrome by removing unwanted inflammatory mediators.[127]

Fluid and electrolyte issues include electrolyte disturbances such as hypercalcemia/hypocalcemia[128,129] or hyperkalemia.[130] Diuresis can be encouraged with intermittent or continuous furosemide infusion. In addition, continuous hemofiltration via a circuit parallel to the oxygenator[131] can be used to maintain optimal fluid balance, because these patients usually have capillary leak and fluid retention secondary to elevated levels of inflammatory mediators but may be limited by flow rates.[132,133] Fluid administration in the form of albumin or lipids should be performed postmembrane to prevent thrombosis.

Significant complications of the gastrointestinal system have been reported in patients on mechanical support, so nutrition probably should be parenteral rather than enteral, especially in the immediate postcannulation period.[134] Because some cardiac diagnoses (such as hypoplastic left heart syndrome and truncus arteriosus) are at higher risk for necrotizing enterocolitis, enteral feeding may need to be avoided in these patients, especially in the presence of low cardiac output. Evidence indicates that gastric tonometry pH is a predictor of survival in children on ECMO.[135] Hepatic function should be monitored closely.

The hematologic system is a vital aspect of ECMO management. Appropriate anticoagulation must be maintained because hematologic abnormalities cause morbidity. This is a particularly challenging aspect in the early postoperative period. Hematocrit is maintained at 40% to 50% for most cardiac patients with leukocyte-reduced cytomegalovirus-negative and irradiated packed red blood cells. The mainstay of anticoagulation therapy has been continuous intravenous infusion of heparin sodium (10–50 units/kg/hour) to maintain whole blood ACT of 180 to 220 seconds. Vigilance is necessary for device-related or mediastinal bleeding and for bleeding in the CNS. Increased risk of hemorrhage and intracranial bleeding is associated with low platelet counts, so appropriate platelet transfusion (given postmembrane with a 50% increase in heparin infusion during transfusion to prevent thrombosis) to maintain a count greater than 100,000/μl is important to minimize bleeding complications.[136,137] Routine echocardiography should be performed to look for intracavitary thrombi, which are especially prevalent in patients on mechanical support with preexisting prosthetic valves, or pericardial fluid/blood collections.

In the presence of persistent significant bleeding (>10 ml/kg/hour), other blood products such as cryoprecipitate or fresh-frozen plasma and even ε-amino caproic acid (Amicar) at 30 mg/kg/hour for up to 72 hours (with a loading dose of 100 mg/kg over 5–10 minutes) or the kinin inhibitor aprotinin at an infusion dose of 10,000 IU/kg/hour for 6 hours following a bolus of 30,000 IU/kg[138,139] can be administered. Serum fibrinogen usually is maintained at greater than 100 mg/dl. Thromboelastogram[140] has been useful for more precise delineation of the bleeding and product profile. Normal maintenance issues during the support period involve clearing the mediastinum and surveillance of tubing for thrombi. In addition, hemolysis is monitored by plasma-free hemoglobin (should be <60 mg/dl). Increase of plasma-free hemoglobin and change of pressure gradient across the oxygenator should raise suspicion for thrombus formation; consider changing the pump head or even the circuit. A difference between ECMO and VAD is that patients on VADs can run ACTs lower (≈140–180 seconds) than those on conventional ECMO.

Sepsis and mediastinitis are especially prevalent in children on ECMO after the first week of support. An open chest is a risk factor for infection.[141] Routine administration of antibiotics should include vancomycin and ceftazidime and nystatin for candida coverage. The risk of life-threatening infection in these patients is compounded by the usual intensive care unit-related infections of ventilated patients with central lines and prolonged usage of parenteral nutrition and antibiotics. The risk is further increased by support device-related access such as the mediastinum and cannulas, not to mention possible immunosuppression from prolonged ECMO support. Antibiotic coverage should be broadened, especially if transsternal cannulation was necessary.

Ventricular Assist Device

Most of the aforementioned principles pertaining to ECMO also apply to VADs with a few key differences.

Although children with myocarditis, acute rejection, and end-stage congenital heart disease have some degree of biventricular dysfunction, left ventricular unloading with the VAD with concomitant physiologic assist of the right ventricle has generally made unnecessary the use of a biventricular VAD. For left VADs, it is essential to appreciate its major inherent difference from ECMO. Cardiac output that is generated from the assist device depends entirely on right ventricular output; in other words, the right ventricular output is the preload to the left VAD. Inadequate filling of the left VAD can result from low intravascular volume, tamponade, improper cannula positioning, right ventricular dysfunction, elevated pulmonary vascular resistance, or dysrhythmias. Thus monitoring of central venous pressure is even more critical compared with ECMO, and frequent echocardiographic assessment of right ventricular function and estimation of right ventricular pressure are mandatory. An elevated central venous pressure indicates right ventricular dysfunction and/or elevated pulmonary vascular resistance, and these issues must be treated in a timely fashion.

As in the management of patients on ECMO, overall management of the VAD depends on both the atrial filling and systemic blood pressures. Low systemic blood pressures with a low left atrial pressure indicate hypovolemia/bleeding, sepsis, or right ventricular failure and should be treated with volume resuscitation or appropriate inotropic agents. A low inlet pressure may be secondary to collapse of atrial wall around the cannula and can be managed by decreasing the revolutions per minute (RPM) temporarily to allow the tissue to be freed from the cannula. On the other hand, low systemic blood pressure with a high left atrial pressure may indicate tamponade or cannula malposition, and both of these possible situations can be checked by noninvasive imaging. High systemic blood pressure with an elevated left atrial pressure may indicate fluid overload and should be treated with diuresis and afterload reduction.

The presence of an atrial septal defect should be evaluated prior to VAD placement to avoid cyanosis (if left atrial pressure falls below right atrial pressure). Other troubleshooting issues for the VAD involve (1) air in the system, which requires immediate attention (patient can be placed in Trendelenburg position), and revision of the system if necessary, and (2) thrombus in the pump head, which requires more aggressive anticoagulation and possible exchange for a new component.

Considerations During the Weaning Process

Before the actual weaning process, both cardiac and pulmonary support should be escalated to accommodate the weaning process.

During the usual weaning process over 6- to 24 hours, flow is slowly reduced in 5% to 10% decrements to 25% flow with unclamping of the bridge between the arterial and venous systems. Modification of the anticoagulation strategy may be necessary during this period, and ECMO flow probably should not be reduced to less than 100 to 200 ml/minute to prevent thrombosis. If the bridge is used, cannulas should be flushed frequently (approximately every 4 hours) to maintain patency. A trial period of 2 to 4 hours off support can be used to assure higher likelihood of a successful decannulation. Some surgeons may prefer a shorter weaning period because any significant decrease in flow, particularly in infants, may be conducive to oxygenator failure. If the patient tolerates the weaning process, the arterial and venous cannulas are clamped.

Although echocardiography[142] and even newer noninvasive ultrasound methodology[143] are useful for assessing myocardial function, interpretation of the results of such studies must take into account the observation that ECMO decreases circumferential fiber shortening and myocardial performance by reducing preload and increasing afterload. Occasionally a patient fails to meet criteria for decannulation and yet surprisingly survives after removal of support. One possible reason is that the relative large size of the venous cannula impedes venous return (especially in a neonate) during low-flow weaning trials.

Types of Mechanical Support

Mechanical support can be divided into several categories as follows:

1. Short-term (<30 days) mechanical support devices
   A. ECMO
   B. VAD
   C. Miscellaneous
2. Long-term (>30 days) mechanical support devices
   A. Pulsatile type
   B. Rotary/axial type

Short-Term Mechanical Support Devices

These devices are used to support the myocardium in the intensive care setting for hours to days but rarely beyond 30 days. Much confusion exists about the lexicon of short-term devices. ECMO and VAD are methodologies of mechanical cardiac support and have little to do with the nature of their pumps (i.e., ECMO can have centrifugal pumps and the BioMedicus VAD can have an oxygenator, so the two support methodologies do have some overlap).

Extracorporeal Membrane Oxygenation

At present, venoarterial ECMO is the most common type of mechanical cardiopulmonary support device used in infants and children.

Use of ECMO in children with cardiac disease initially was reported in the 1970s in patients with concomitant lung disease.[144,145] ECMO support for primary cardiac failure, mainly postcardiotomy syndrome, initially was reported in the 1970s by Bartlett[146] but has been steadily increasing in volume, with a survival range of 42% to 64% and an overall survival rate of approximately 55%[147] (see Table 25-2A for larger reported series for cardiac failure and Table 25-2B for the Extracorporeal Life Support Organization (ELSO) registry data up to July 2002).

ECMO remains the preferred strategy in neonates with biventricular failure and cardiopulmonary failure because other support means have technical and size limitations. ECMO is also a good initial mechanical support strategy for "screening," before use of a VAD.[148,149] Venovenous ECMO possibly can be used in a few selected cases of pediatric cardiac patients.

ECMO uses either a roller pump system with a servoregulatory mechanism for controlling circuit flow or a centrifugal pump that may be more efficient at maintaining flow (Figure 25–1). When using a roller pump, the blood is drained into a compliant bladder and goes through the circuit above at rates of 100 to 150 cm^3/kg/minute in neonates and 75 to 100 cm^3/kg/minute in older infants. The servoregulating bladder turns off the pump if venous return is inadequate. The ECMO circuit consists of the pump that pushes blood to a membrane or hollow fiber oxygenator followed by a heat exchanger. The blood gases can be adjusted by altering the gas sweep rate and composition of the gases passing across the membrane. The oxygenated blood then is returned to the patient via the arterial cannula. A hemofilter can be attached via a circuit parallel to the patient.

Cannulation can be peripheral via the right internal jugular vein and the common carotid artery, but it also can be transsternal via the right atrial appendage and the aorta in the postcardiotomy cardiac surgical patient.

Advantages of ECMO include its relative ease of implementation, rapid potential for stabilization,

TABLE 25–2A

Extracorporeal Membrane Oxygenation for Children with Heart Disease

Author	Year	Patients	Types of Patients	Support Duration Range	Weaned from Support	Survival to Discharge
Kanter et al.	1987 (1982-1985)	13 9 days to 17.6 years (mean 3.8 years)	Postoperative (100%)	12 hours to 9 days (mean 3.4 days)	54%	46%
Rogers et al.	1989 (1981-1987)	10 2 days to 5 years (NA)	Postoperative (100%)	15 hours to 6 days (mean 3.8 days)	80%	70%
Weinhaus et al.	1989 (1985-1988)	13 2 days to 7.4 years (mean 1.4 years)	Postoperative (93%)	6 hours to 11.2 days (mean 3.8 days)	64%	36%
Anderson et al.	1990 (1971-1989)	16 NA	Postoperative (69%)	NA	NA	25%
Klein et al.	1990 (1984-1989)	39 1 day to 7 years (mean 13.6 months)	Postoperative (92%)	6 hours to 9 days (mean 4.4 days)	61%	58%
Meliones et al.	1991 (1981-1990)	189 1 day to 16.8 years (median 7 months)	Postoperative (93%)	NA (mean 4.8 days)	NA	43%
Delius et al.	1992 (1981-1990)	25 1 day to 8 years (median 7 months)	Postoperative (80%)	8 hours to 15.8 days (mean 6.1 days)	52%	40%
Raithel SC et al.	1992 (1982-91)	65 1 day to 14 years (mean 2.4 years)	Postoperative (100%)	12.5 hours to 17.6 days (mean 5.2 days)	68%	35%
Ziomek et al.	1992 (1989-1991)	24 14 hours to 6 years (mean 12.5 months)	Postoperative (100%)	17 hours to 8.3 days (mean 4 days)	75%	54%
Dalton et al.	1993 (1981-1990)	29 2 weeks to 7 years (mean 1.4 years)	Cardiac arrest (59%) Postoperative (93%)	15 hours to 9.2 days (NA)	62%	45%
Black et al.	1995 (1990-1994)	31 NA (mean 1.2 years)	Postoperative (81%) Myocarditis (19%)	NA (mean 5 days)	45%	41%
Walters et al.	1995 (1984-1994)	73 NA (median 7.2 months)	Preoperative (10%) Failure to wean (26%) Postoperative (74%)	NA (mean 4.8 days)	67%	58%
del Nido et al.	1996 (1981-1994)	68 (1 day to 18 years)	NA	NA	NA	38%
Mehta et al.	2000 (1995-1999)	34 1 day to 17.5 years (median 7 months)	Postoperative (53%)	1 day to 58 days (median 6.4 days)	50%	35%
Aharon et al.	2001 (1997-2000)	50 1 day to 11 years (median 40 days)	Postoperative (100%)	1 hour to 15 days (mean 4 days)	60%	50%

TABLE 25–2B

ELSO Registry (data up to July 2002)

Category	Total	% Survived
NEONATE		
Respiratory	17333	86
Cardiac	1685	55
Pediatric		
Repiratory	2324	63
Cardiac	2396	55
ADULT		
Repiratory	777	57
Cardiac	375	44
TOTAL	25201	77

peripheral cannulation, capability for biventricular support, accommodation of neonatal size limitations, effective oxygenation, and large international neonatal and pediatric experience (see Table 25–1 for comparison with VADs). Disadvantages are its large circuit volume and requirement for blood prime, extensive anticoagulation, carotid artery ligation, nonpulsatile flow, decreased pulmonary blood flow, occasional inadequate left atrial decompression, relatively complex circuit that requires higher level of expertise for its use, lack of durability, bleeding tendencies in postoperative patients, and relatively high incidence of neurologic complications.

Centrifugal Ventricular Assist Device

The BioMedicus centrifugal pump (Medtronic BioMedicus, Eden Prairie, MN, USA) can be used for cardiopulmonary bypass, ECMO,[150] or ventricular assistance[151]; therefore this centrifugal pump should not be synonymous with VAD. This nonpulsatile VAD concept has been in existence since the late 1970s[152] but only recently has been used more frequently in children.[153–157] Although the terminology VAD is used, it also can be used to describe other types of devices that support the ventricle and thereby leads to some confusion. The VAD experience in the pediatric patient population in the United States is limited to the nonpulsatile centrifugal type device, described in the following paragraph, but includes other systems elsewhere in the world, particularly Europe.

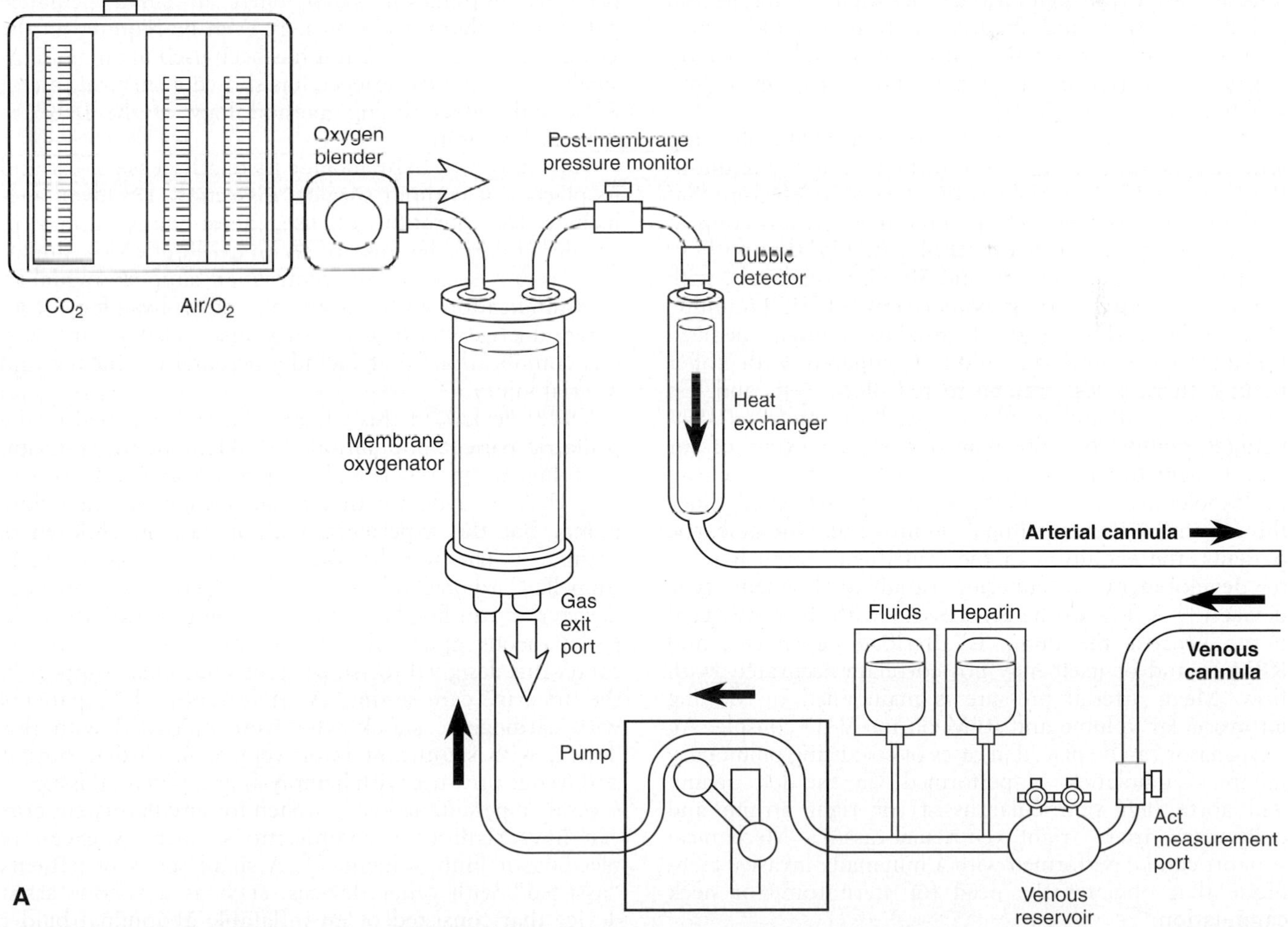

FIGURE 25–1 • **A,** Setup for venoarterial extracorporeal membrane oxygenation via neck cannulation. (From Walker LK: Myocardial assist devices. In Nichols D, editor: *Critical heart disease in infants and children.* Philadelphia, 1995, Mosby.)

(Continued)

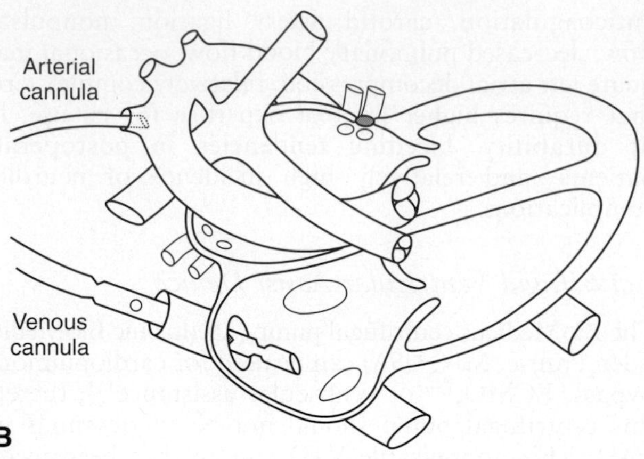

FIGURE 25–1—cont'd • B, Close-up view of cannulation via the neck vessels for support with venoarterial extracorporeal membrane oxygenation. (From del Nido PJ: *Ann Thorac Surg* 61:336-339, 1996.)

This device evolved as the need for a mechanical support device superior to conventional ECMO became necessary, especially for patients with isolated ventricular failure. Common uses for VAD as ventricular support include myocarditis or dilated cardiomyopathy, acute rejection after transplantation, older infants after arterial switch operation, and children after surgery for correction of anomalous coronary artery from the pulmonary artery.[158] Experience with single-ventricle patients is limited but has been positive.[159]

With this VAD, an extracorporeal centrifugal pump with acrylic rotator cones produces a vortex continuous flow (Figure 25–2), which creates a negative pressure that enables blood to move. The pump is magnetically coupled to a driver that controls the RPM. The BP-80 and BP-50 models have volumes of 80 and 50 ml, respectively, with the former capable of maximal flow of 10 L/minute. Heparin-bonded tubing can be used to minimize the need for aggressive anticoagulation. Compared with roller pumps, there is less trauma to red blood cells and less pronounced inflammatory response.[160] In addition, centrifugal pumps are advantageous in the event of air entrainment because the acrylic cones create an air trap (as bubbles accumulate in the middle of the vortex). Since the advent of the centrifugal pump device for pediatric patients, the evolution of the centrifugal pump has led to development of superior rapid deployment type devices.[161] A flow probe is necessary with the centrifugal pump because the pump is afterload dependent, and RPM in and of itself may not correlate accurately with flow. Mean arterial pressure is maintained by varying intravascular volume and RPM on the VAD console. An oxygenator can be placed in cases of coexisting pulmonary failure. Cannulation is performed via the left atrium and aorta (left ventricular assist) or right atrium and pulmonary artery (right ventricular assist). Mechanical support can be performed with a minimally invasive technique that obviates the need for sternotomy or neck cannulation.[162]

Advantages of the VAD include its relative ease of use compared with ECMO, ease of implantation, fast setup time, low priming volume, and low-level anticoagulation because it usually does not have an oxygenator or a heat exchanger. There is purported evidence that myocardial recovery may be superior to ECMO (although this is controversial if the left atrium is decompressed in ECMO support).[163,164] Disadvantages include its shorter duration of usage, occasional thrombus formation in the circuit, and its nonpulsatile flow nature. In addition, the right ventricle must have adequate function because it supplies preload to the left ventricle supported by the VAD. There is a size limitation if biventricular support is necessary.[165]

Miscellaneous

The intraaortic balloon pump (IABP) is a support device with a balloon of 0.75- to 10-ml size mounted on 4F to 5F catheters that works on the following principle. The balloon inflates during diastole (after aortic valve closure) for optimal coronary flow augmentation and then deflates before the next systole for optimal ventricular afterload diminution. The device usually is less effective in smaller children because of their increased compliance of the aorta, size constraints within the aorta, higher heart rates, and difficulty in synchronization.[166] This modality of support has had limited experience in the pediatric population, particularly in small pediatric patients in whom insertion may even be required in the ascending aorta,[167–171] but it has been used in an infant as small as 2 kg.[172] Experience has shown a survival rate of 62% with novel timing methodology of the IABP to echocardiography.[173]

Advantages of IABP include its relative ease of use and its placement without surgical dissection. Disadvantages include less duration of use, questionable utility in smaller children because of technical limitations, limitation as an isolated left ventricular support modality, contraindication with certain anatomy/physiology (e.g., patent ductus arteriosus or aortic insufficiency), and serious complications that include mesenteric ischemia and arterial injury.[174]

Other devices in this category have been used in the pediatric patient population. The Hemopump (Johnson & Johnson Interventional Systems, Rancho Cordova, CA, USA) is a device that is an intraaortic axial flow pump, but the experience with its use in children is limited.[175] The Impella Recover 100 microaxial VAD (Impella Cardiotechnik AG, Aachen, Germany) is an axial device that can be placed in either the femoral artery via percutaneous approach or the aorta by transthoracic route. It is designed for short-term ventricular support in the intensive care setting. A study reported 12 patients with cardiogenic shock who were unloaded with this device, with significant improvement in cardiac output and wedge pressure with hemolysis as a potential issue.[176] Overall, a percutaneous approach for circulatory support can have significant complications, such as excessive bleeding or limb ischemia.[177] A small series of patients "assisted" with other devices, such as a venous assist device that consisted of an inflatable abdominal binder for intermittent external compression of the abdomen in Fontan patients, has been reported.[178]

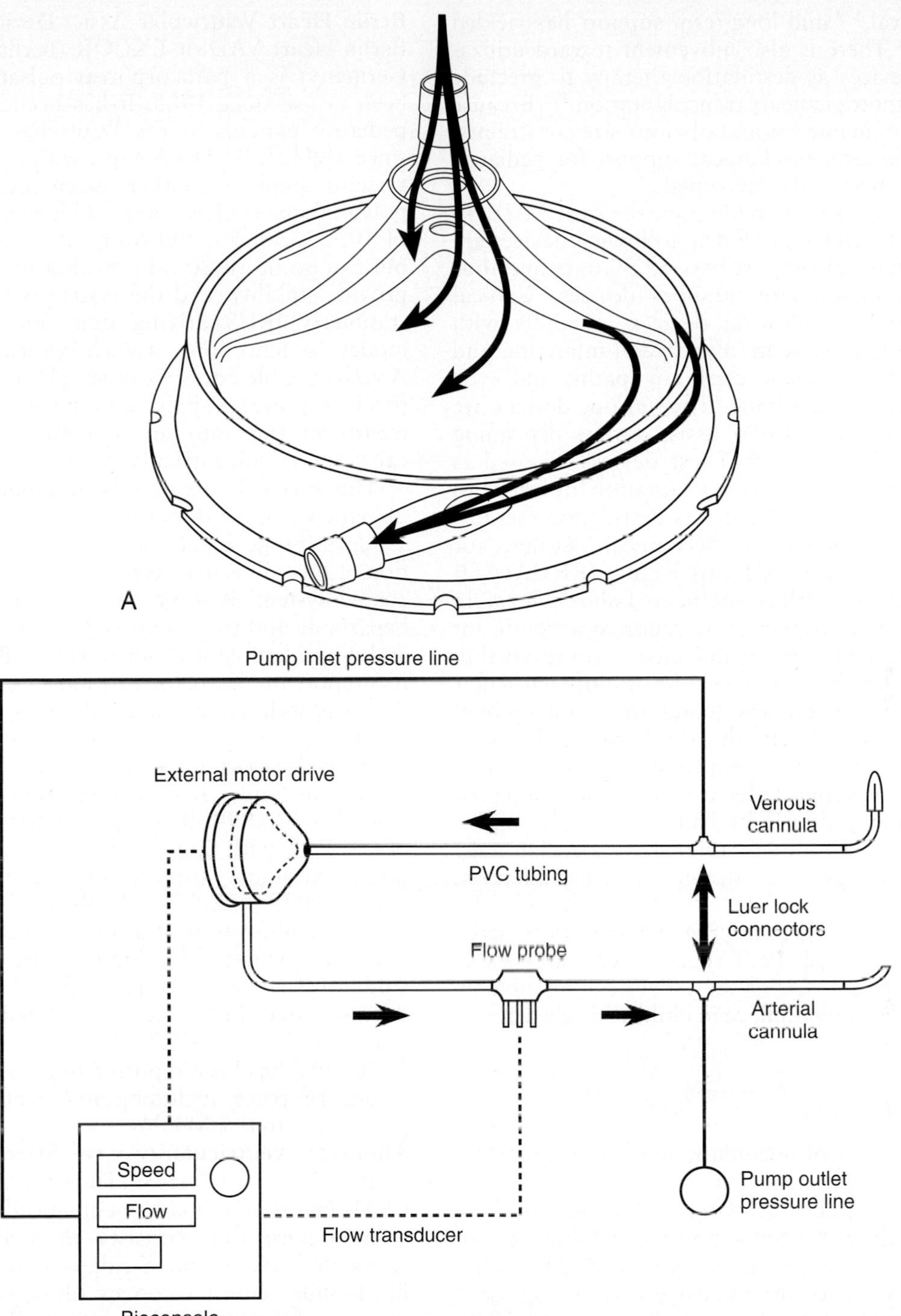

FIGURE 25-2 • **A,** Schematic diagram of the BioMedicus centrifugal pump. Blood enters the cones via the apex of the cone, and the kinetic energy of the spinning cones is transferred to the blood leaving the side port. (From Karl TR, Horton SB: Centrifugal pump ventricular assist device in pediatric cardiac surgery. In Duncan BW, editor: *Mechanical support for cardiac and respiratory failure in pediatric patients.* New York, 2001, Marcel Dekker.) **B,** BioMedicus centrifugal pump setup. (From Karl TR, Horton SB: Centrifugal pump ventricular assist device in pediatric cardiac surgery. In Duncan BW, editor: *Mechanical support for cardiac and respiratory failure in pediatric patients.* New York, 2001, Marcel Dekker.)

Long-Term Mechanical Support Devices

The emergence of better long-term mechanical support devices for adults has made this modality possible for selected pediatric patients. The advent of this newer type of device has provided a better range of equipment for mechanical support in children in the intensive care setting, but longer-term mechanical support devices, especially for neonates and children, still are lacking. An occasional patient requires transition from ECMO or centrifugal VAD to a longer-term device. The adult experience with ECMO to implantable device conversion has reported improved survival,[179] and long-term support has yielded good results.[180] There is also movement toward utilization of these devices as destination therapy to preclude the need for orthotopic heart transplantation.[181] Because of lack of corporate interest and obvious size constraints, this area of long-term mechanical support for pediatric patients has not been fully developed.

Much progress has been made since the early VAD initially described by DeBakey.[182] The following devices are capable of mechanical support beyond 30 days and thus are considered longer-term support devices. Clinical experience with the following devices in adults with postcardiotomy failure, acute myocardial infarction and cardiogenic shock, ischemic cardiomyopathy, and even myocarditis is rapidly growing. The various devices are used as single or biventricular assist devices depending on the device and the patient. These devices are used as bridge to recovery, bridge to transplantation, or bridge to same or other mechanical devices as destination therapy. The Randomized Evaluation of Mechanical Assistance for the Treatment of Congestive Heart Failure (REMATCH) trial in adult patients with severe heart failure who were ineligible for heart transplantation reported a significant improvement in quality of life and short-term survival in patients with severe heart failure with use of ventricular devices as destination therapy (compared with optimal medical management).[183] In the same study, the most common causes of death were infection and device failure.

No longer-term support devices are widely accepted for use in smaller pediatric patients with body surface area less than 1.2 M^2. Implantable left ventricular assist systems have been used for bridge to transplantation, bridge to myocardial recovery, or permanent circulatory support only in larger children. These devices, separated into pulsatile and axial type devices, are briefly discussed here because use of these devices undoubtedly will become more commonplace in children in the coming years.

Pulsatile Type Devices

Since the early report of pneumatic paracorporeal VADs in children,[184] the pediatric experience with long-term pulsatile devices has been growing. Advantages of these devices include their chronic support capability, ease of use, capability for biventricular support without an oxygenator, mobility out of the intensive care setting, need for low-level anticoagulation, and their pulsatile flow nature. Disadvantages include a propensity for thromboembolic complications, difficulty of implantation/explantation, cumulative cost, need for exteriorization of the cannulas, and size limitations, especially with need for biventricular support. Infection is a serious complication, but immobilization of the drive line or cannulas as close to the exit site as possible with a binder can decrease the incidence of infections.

Hypertension while on support can be treated with a myriad of agents, such as milrinone, calcium channel blockers, angiotensin-converting enzyme inhibitors, beta-blockers, alpha-antagonists, nitroprusside, or nitroglycerin. Anticoagulation regimen usually consists of heparin or warfarin with antiplatelet therapy.

Berlin Heart Ventricular Assist Device or EXCOR. The Berlin Heart VAD or EXCOR (Berlin Heart AG, Berlin, Germany) is a paracorporeal pulsatile device that has been in use since 1988. It has been available for use in pediatric patients at the Deutsches Herzzenrum Berlin since 1992.[185,186] The pumps, with its two different valve systems made of either mechanical tilting disks or polyurethane leaflets, have a wide range of stroke volumes of 10, 25, 30, 50, and 60 ml designed for pediatric use but can go up to 80 ml for adult use. Three membranes provide stability, and the system is heparin coated. The stationary IKUS driving unit can operate in various modes (synchronous, asynchronous, and independent). A rechargeable battery can supply up to 5 hours of independent power supply, and its mobile drive unit can transform this into an outpatient device. The device can provide univentricular or biventricular support.

The survival rate has been reported to be 52% in 28 patients ages 6 days to 16 years, for a mean support of 17 days (range 12 hours to 98 days).[187] Early complication of thrombus has been lessened with use of a heparin-coated system. Postoperative care includes initial use of heparin at 400 to 1200 units/kg/day, followed by aspirin and dipyridamole without warfarin. Because of its ability to support the heart for this longer duration of time, the device is well suited for children with myocarditis, with longer recovery periods for even biventricular assist.[188]

MEDOS Ventricular Assist Device. The MEDOS VAD (Medizintechnik, Berlin, Germany) was developed in Germany in 1994. It is a pneumatically driven paracorporeal VAD with three left ventricular sizes (10-, 25-, and 60 ml maximum stroke volume) and three right ventricular sizes (9-, 22.5-, and 54-ml stroke volume).[189–191] A later modification of a three-leaflet blood pump valve improved dynamic blood flow of the pump.[192] An animal study of 3-week-old lambs with right ventricular failure demonstrated the device was successful with a miniaturized pulsatile right VAD.[193]

Survival has been reported to be 36.2% in children up to age 16 years, including an infant with body surface area less than 0.3 M^2.[194]

Thoratec Ventricular Assist System. The Thoratec Ventricular Assist System (Thoratec Corp., Berkeley, CA, USA) (Figure 25–3) is a pneumatically powered pulsatile assist device that consists of a flexible, seam-free, segmented sac within a ridged polycarbonate housing. Bjork-Shiley concave-convex tilting disc valves are present in the inlet and outlet portions. The stroke volume is 65 ml with a maximum output of 7 L/minute. The inlet is cannulation via left atrial or left ventricular apex, and the outlet is to the aorta with both of the cannulas exteriorized. The three modes for this assist system are fixed rate, synchronous (with wean to 1:3), and fill to empty. The device is flexible in terms of usage in smaller-size patients.

The pediatric experience is limited. In a reported series of 101 patients, the survival rate was 68.8%,[195–197] including a child who weighed as little as 17 kg (body surface area 0.7 M^2) who had viral cardiomyopathy and was supported for 22 days.[198] These results in children are similar to results of adult series.[199,200] Neurologic complications in these pediatric patients seem to

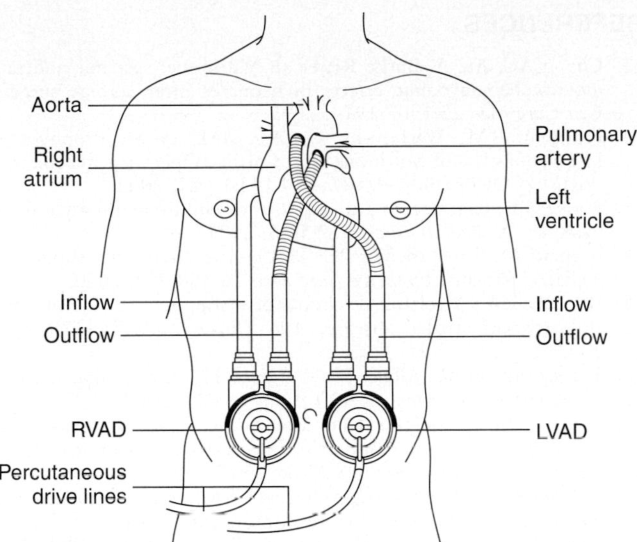

FIGURE 25–3 • Schematic diagram of the Thoratec ventricular assist system for biventricular support. (From Patel H, Pagani FD: Extracorporeal mechanical circulatory assist. *Cardiol Clin* 21:29–41, 2003.)

be higher when cannulation is performed in the left atrium.[201]

Rotary/Axial-Type Devices

Although the pediatric experience with these devices is extremely small and limited to a few adolescents, their smaller size holds promise for future pediatric use. This class of devices consists of relatively small axial pumps that involve an impeller within its housing that are almost entirely implantable (Figure 25–4). Some of these devices can even be implanted without cardiopulmonary bypass. The apex of the left ventricle can be used as the inflow (to maximize flow conditions), and the ascending aorta has been used for the outflow graft because of thrombus formation when the graft was placed in the descending aorta.[202] Adding pulsatility to almost all of these devices is under discussion.

Advantages of such an axial system are their relatively small size, implant/explant procedures that are relatively easy, noiseless system, decreased infection, relatively less cost, and continuous flow that not only provides unloading throughout the cardiac cycle but also minimizes stasis and thrombus formation.[203] Disadvantages include the need for a relatively large-size ventricular apical cannulation and relative size limitation to pediatric patients greater than 1.5 M^2.

MicroMed DeBakey VAD. The MicroMed DeBakey VAD (MicroMed Technology, Houston, TX, USA) is an axial device with inflow from the left ventricle and outflow to the ascending aorta pushing blood at 7500 to 12,500 RPM and up to 10 L/minute (see Figure 25–4). In a collaborative effort between Drs. DeBakey and Noon with NASA engineer David Saucier, computational fluid dynamics were used to build this axial flow pump designed to minimize hemolysis and thrombosis.

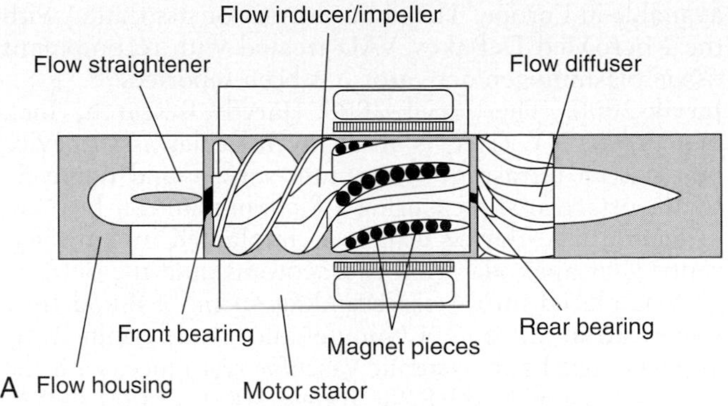

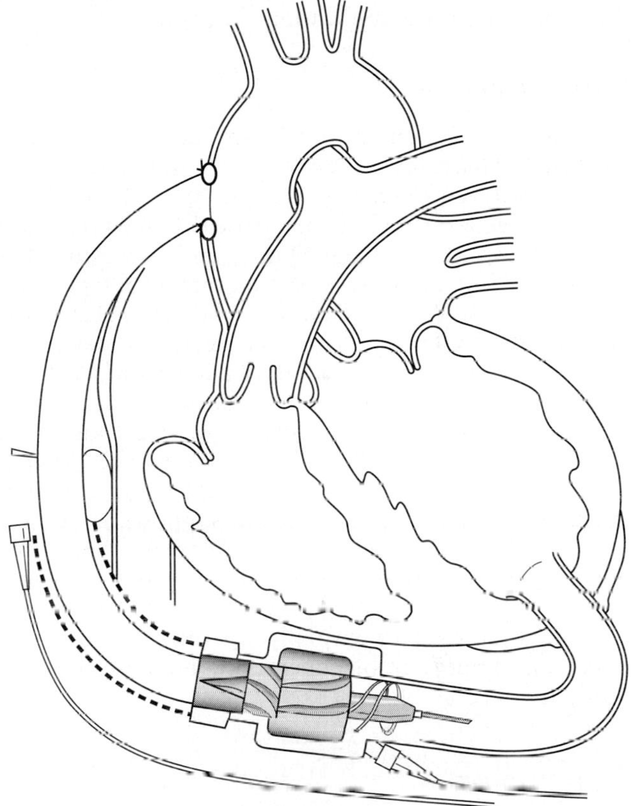

FIGURE 25–4 • **A,** DeBakey ventricular assist device in a cutaway view. (Courtesy MicroMed Technology, Houston, TX, USA.) **B,** DeBakey ventricular assist device with its position next to the heart. (From Kukuy EL, Oz MC, Rose EA, et al: Devices as destination therapy. Cardiol Clin 21:67–73, 2003.)

VAD flow increases and decreases in concert with systole and diastole.

This device was the first long-term axial flow circulatory assist device introduced into clinical trials (November 1998) as a bridge to transplant. It has the largest clinical experience with close to 200 patients worldwide.[204] Because of its relatively small size, it is an attractive potential device for use in children, with the present experience of patients ranging in age from 12 to 76 years and body surface area as low as 1.3 M^2. There have been three successful implantations of the pediatric DeBakey VAD to date. The device has been modified to have a Carmeda coating and now is commercially available in Europe. Thrombus formation associated with the MicroMed DeBakey VAD treated with recombinant tissue plasminogen activator has been reported.[205]

Jarvik-2000. The Jarvik-2000 (Jarvik Research, Inc., New York, NY, USA) is an intraventricular assist device that has an ultrasmooth titanium surface and relatively small surface area measuring 1.8 cm in diameter by 5 cm in length. The device usually is implanted into the left ventricular apex via a left thoracotomy, and the outflow graft is placed into the descending aorta.[206] Blood flow ranges from 2 to 7 L/minute and is determined by impeller speed and systemic vascular resistance, with the usual setting at 9000 RPM (range 8000–12,000 RPM). There has been virtually no pediatric experience, but there may be future applications in children.[207]

Future Devices

One new device under preclinical investigation is the modified HeartSaver VAD, a pulsatile and fully implantable ventricular assist system.[208] There is also the new generation of magnetically levitated axial (HeartQuest from HeartQuest and CorAide from Arrow)[209,210] or similarly levitated centrifugal type devices (HeartMate III from Thoratec and DuraHeart from Terumo Corporation).[211,212] The levitated devices are designed to have virtually no device inner surface contact with their own parts to minimize thrombus formation.

Progress had been rapid toward the ideal mechanical support device. The ideal device would accommodate a large range of patient ages and sizes and expanding indications (including biventricular support). In addition, it would have near-perfect flow dynamics, high durability, reliability with lifetime (more than 10 years) approaching that of a pacemaker, simple design, high biocompatibility with virtually no thromboembolus or infections, imperceptible operation (no noise or vibration), and reasonable cost.

Conclusion

Principles of mechanical circulatory support emphasize the need for an individualized approach. Indications should broaden to include pediatric patients with myocarditis and septic shock. Short-term experience with mechanical devices had been limited to ECMO, but pediatric experience with VADs is growing. The pediatric experience with long-term devices is lacking, but the advent of small axial type devices holds great promise. Long-term biventricular support in neonates and infants remains a daunting challenge. With better clinical management, improved technology, broader use of mechanical support devices, and attention to economic restraints, survival of pediatric patients with severe heart failure will continue to improve.

Acknowledgment

We thank Dr. Stephen Stayer for critical review of the manuscript and the perfusion team at Texas Children's Hospital for assistance.

REFERENCES

1. Chang AC, Atz A, Burke RP, et al: Milrinone: systemic and pulmonary hemodynamic effects in neonates after cardiac surgery. *Crit Care Med* 23:1907-1914, 1995.
2. Hoffman TM, Wernovsky G, Atz AM, et al: Prophylactic Intravenous Use of Milrinone after Cardiac Operation in Pediatrics (PRIMACORP) Study. *Am Heart J* 143:15-21, 2002.
3. Booker PD: Pharmacological support for children with myocardial dysfunction. *Pediatr Anesth* 12:5-25, 2002.
4. Beghetti M, Rimensberger PC: Mechanical circulatory support in pediatric patients. *Intensive Care Med* 26:350-352, 2000.
5. Duncan BW: Mechanical circulatory support for infants and children with cardiac disease. *Ann Thorac Surg* 73:1670-1677, 2002.
6. Throckmorton AL, Allaire PE, Gutgesell HP, et al: Pediatric circulatory support systems. *ASAIO J* 48:216-221, 2002.
7. Kanter KR, Pennington DG, Weber TR, et al: Extracorporeal Membrane oxygenation for postoperative cardiac support in children. *J Thorac Cardiovasc Surg* 93:27-35, 1987.
8. Redmond CR, Graves ED, Falterman KW, et al: Extracorporeal membrane oxygenation for respiratory and cardiac failure in infants and children. *J Thorac Cardiovasc Surg* 93:199-204, 1987.
9. Weinhaus L, Canter C, Noetzel M, et al: Extracorporeal membrane oxygenation for circulatory support after repair of congenital heart defects. *Ann Thorac Surg* 48:206-212, 1989.
11. Rogers AJ, Trento A, Siewers RD, et al: Extracorporeal membrane oxygenation for postoperative cardiogenic shock in children. *Ann Thorac Surg* 47:903-906, 1989.
12. Anderson HL, Attorri RJ, Custer JR, et al: Extracorporeal membrane oxygenation for pediatric cardiopulmonary failure. *J Thorac Cardiovasc Surg* 99:1011-1021, 1990.
13. Klein MD, Shaheen KW, Whittlesey GC, et al: Extracorporeal membrane oxygenation for circulatory support of children after repair of congenital heart disease. *J Thorac Cardiovasc Surg* 100:498-505, 1990.
14. Ferrazzi P, Glauber M, DiDomenico A, et al: Assisted circulation for myocardial recovery after repair of congenital heart disease. *Eur J Cardiothorac Surg* 5:419-423, 1991.
15. Delius RE, Bove EL, Meliones JN, et al: Use of extracorporeal life support in patients with congenital heart disease. *Crit Care Med* 20:1216-1222, 1992.
16. Raithel SC, Pennington DG, Boegner E, et al: Extracorporeal membrane oxygenation in children after cardiac surgery. *Circulation* 86(suppl 2):305-310, 1992.
17. Ziomek S, Harrell JE, Fasules JW, et al: Extracorporeal membrane oxygenation for cardiac failure after congenital heart operation. *Ann Thorac Surg* 54:861-868, 1992.
18. Meliones JN, Custer JR, Snedecor S, et al: Extracorporeal life support for cardiac assist in pediatric patients. Review of ELSO Registry Data. *Circulation* 84(5 suppl):III168-III72, 1991.
19. Dalton HJ, Siewers RD, Fuhrman BP, et al: Extracorporeal membrane oxygenation for cardiac rescue in children with severe myocardial dysfunction. *Crit Care Med* 21:1020-1028, 1993.
20. Pennington DG, Swartz MT: Circulatory support in infants and children. *Ann Thorac Surg* 55:233-237, 1993.
21. Del Nido PJ: Extracorporeal membrane oxygenation for cardiac support in children. *Ann Thorac Surg* 61:336-339, 1996.
22. Walters HL, Hakimi M, Rice MD, et al: Pediatric cardiac surgical ECMO: multivariate analysis of risk factors for hospital death. *Ann Thorac Surg* 60:329-336, 1995.
23. Montgomery VL, Strotman JM, Ross MP: Impact of multiple organ system dysfunction and nosocomial infections on survival of children treated with extracorporeal membrane oxygenation after heart surgery. *Crit Care Med* 28:526-531, 2000.
24. Mehta U, Laks H, Sadeghi A, et al: Extracorporeal membrane oxygenation for cardiac support in pediatric patients. *Am Surg* 66: 879-886, 2000.
25. Aharon AS, Drinkwater DC, Churchwell KB, et al: Extracorporeal membrane oxygenation in children after repair of congenital cardiac lesions. *Ann Thorac Surg* 72:2095-2101, 2001.
26. ECMO Registry Report. Ann Arbor, MI, 2001, Extracorporeal Life Support Organization.
27. Chang AC, Hanley FL, Wernovsky G, Wessel DL: Pediatric cardiac intensive care. Baltimore, 1998, Williams & Wilkins.

28. Chang AC: Pediatric cardiac intensive care: current state of the art and beyond the millennium. *Curr Opin Pediatr* 12:238-246, 2000.
29. Pennington DG, Swartz MT: Circulatory support in infants and children. *Ann Thorac Surg* 55:233-237, 1993.
30. Burch GE: On resting the human heart. *Am Heart J* 71:422-428, 1966.
31. Kahwaji I, Ramaciotti C, Nikaidoh H, et al: Images in cardiovascular medicine. Echocardiographic diagnosis of anomalous drainage of the superior vena cava into the left atrium. *Circulation* 107:1560-1561, 2003.
32. Charpie JR, Dekeon MK, Goldberg CS, et al: Serial blood lactate measurements predict early outcome after neonatal repair or palliation for complex congenital heart disease. *J Thorac Cardiovasc Surg* 120:73-80, 2000.
33. Langley SM, Sheppard SB, Tsang VT, et al: When is extracorporeal life support worthwhile following repair of congenital heart disease in children? *Eur J Cardiothorac Surg* 13:520-525, 1998.
34. Wernovsky G, Chang AC, Wessel DL: Intensive care. In Emmannouilides GC, Riemenschneider TA, Allen HD, et al, editors: Heart disease in infants, children, and adolescents. Baltimore, MD, 2000, Williams & Wilkins.
35. Hakami M, Walters HL, Pinsky WW, et al: Delayed sternal closure after neonatal cardiac operations. *J Thorac Cardiovasc Surg* 107:925-933, 1994.
36. Alexi-Meskishvili V, Hetzer R, Weng Y, et al: Successful extracorporeal circulatory support after aortic reimplantation of anomalous left coronary artery. *Eur J Cardiothorac Surg* 8:533-536, 1994.
37. Del Nido PJ, Duncan BW, Mayer JE Jr, et al: Left ventricular assist device improves survival in children with left ventricular dysfunction after repair of anomalous origin of the left coronary artery from the pulmonary artery. *Ann Thorac Surg* 67:169-172, 1999.
38. Mee RB, Harada Y: Retraining of the left ventricle with a left ventricular assist device (Biomedicus) after the arterial switch operation. *J Thorac Cardiovasc Surg* 101:171-173, 1991.
39. Mitchell MB, Campbell DN, Bielefeld MR, et al: Utility of extracorporeal membrane oxygenation for early graft failure following heart transplantation in infancy. *J Heart Lung Transplant* 19: 834-839, 2000.
40. Grundl PD, Miller SA, del Nido PJ, et al: Successful treatment of myocarditis using extracorporeal membrane oxygenation. *Crit Care Med* 21:302-304, 1993.
41. Duncan BW, Bohn DJ, Atz AM, et al: Mechanical circulatory support for the treatment of children with acute fulminant myocarditis. *J Thorac Cardiovasc Surg* 122:440-448, 2001.
42. Acker MA: Mechanical circulatory support for patients with acute-fulminant myocarditis. *Ann Thorac Surg* 71(3 suppl):S73-S76, 2001.
43. Lee KJ, McCrindle BW, Bohn DJ, et al: Clinical outcomes of acute myocarditis in childhood. *Heart* 82:226-233, 1999.
44. Bohn D: Extracorporeal life support in heart and lung transplantation. *Semin Thorac Cardiovasc Surg Pediatr Card Surg Annu* 4: 94-102, 2001.
45. Levi D, Marelli D, Plunkett M, et al: Use of assist devices and ECMO to bridge pediatric patients with cardiomyopathy to transplantation. *J Heart Lung Transplant* 21:760-770, 2002.
46. Del Nido PJ, Armitage JM, Fricker FJ, et al: Extracorporeal membrane oxygenation support as a bridge to pediatric heart transplantation. *Circulation* 90(5 pt 2):II66-II69, 1994.
47. Hopper AO, Pageau J, Job L, et al: Extracorporeal membrane oxygenation for perioperative support in neonatal and pediatric cardiac transplantation. *Artif Organs* 23:1006-1009, 1999.
48. Ishino K, Weng Y, Alexi-Meskishvili V, et al: Extracorporeal membrane oxygenation as a bridge to cardiac transplantation in children. *Artif Organs* 20:728-732, 1996.
49. Farrar DJ, Hill JD: Univentricular and biventricular Thoratec VAD support as a bridge to transplantation. *Ann Thorac Surg* 55: 276-282, 1991.
50. Warnecke H, Berdjis F, Hennig E, et al: Mechanical left ventricular support as a bridge to cardiac transplantation in childhood. *Eur J Cardiothorac Surg* 5:330-333, 1991.
51. Hetzer R, Loebe M, Weng Y, et al: Pusatile pediatric ventricular assist device: current results for bridge to transplantation. *Semin Thorac Cardiovasc Surg Pediatr Card Surg Annu* 2:157-176, 1999.
52. Delius RE, Zwischenberger JB, Cilley R, et al: Prolonged extracorporeal life support of pediatric and adolescent cardiac transplant patients. *Ann Thorac Surg* 50:791-795, 1990.
53. Gajarski RJ, Mosca RS, Ohye RG, et al: Use of extracorporeal life support as a bridge to pediatric cardiac transplantation. *J Heart Lung Transplant* 22:28-34, 2003.
54. Morrow WR, Naftel D, Chinnock R, et al: Outcome of listing for heart transplantation in infants younger than six months: predictors of death and interval to transplantation. The Pediatric Heart Transplantation Study Group. *J Heart Lung Transplant* 16: 1255-1266, 1997.
55. Del Nido PJ, Dalton HJ, Thompson AE, et al: Extracorporeal membrane oxygenation for cardiac rescue in children with severe myocardial dysfunction. *Crit Care Med* 21:1020-1028, 1993.
56. Kurose M, Okamoto K, Sato T, et al: Extracorporeal life support for patients undergoing prolonged external cardiac massage. *Resuscitation* 25:35-40, 1993.
57. Chen YS, Chao A, Yu HY, et al: Analysis and results of prolonged resuscitation in cardiac arrest patients rescued by extracorporeal membrane oxygenation. *J Am Coll Cardiol* 41:197-203, 2003.
58. Parra DA, Totapally BR, Zahn E, et al: Outcome of cardiopulmonary resuscitation in a pediatric cardiac intensive care unit. *Crit Care Med* 28:3296-3300, 2000.
59. Dembitsky WP, Moreno-Cabral RJ, Adamson RM, et al: Emergency resuscitation using portable extracorporeal membrane oxygenation. *Ann Thorac Surg* 55:304-309, 1993.
60. Duncan BW, Ibrahim AE, Hraska V, et al: Use of rapid deployment extracorporeal membrane oxygenation for the resuscitation of pediatric patients with heart disease after cardiac arrest. *J Thorac Cardiovasc Surg* 116:305-311, 1998.
61. Salzer-Muhar UE, Marx M, Wimmer M: Pediatric cardiac extracorporeal membrane oxygenation in congenital heart disease: the cardiologist's view. *Artif Organs* 23:995-1000, 1999.
62. Hunkeler NM, Canter CE, Donze A, et al: Extracorporeal life support in cyanotic congenital heart disease before cardiovascular operation. *Am J Cardiol* 69:790-793, 1992.
63. McKay VJ, Stewart DL, RobinsonTW, et al: Preoperative versus postoperative extracorporeal life support in neonatal cardiac patients. *Perfusion* 12:179-186, 1997.
64. Lupinetti FM, Kulik TJ, Beekman RH, et al: Correction of total anomalous pulmonary venous connection in infancy. *J Thorac Cardiovasc Surg* 106:880-885, 1993.
65. Stewart DL, Mendoza JC, Winston S, et al: Use of extracorporeal life support in total anomalous pulmonary venous drainage. *J Perinatol* 16(2 pt 1):186-190, 1996.
66. Dudell GG, Evans ML, Krous HF, et al: Common pulmonary vein atresia: the role of extracorporeal membrane oxygenation. *Pediatrics* 91:403-410, 1993.
67. McDonnell BE, Raff GW, Gaynor JW, et al: Outcome after repair of tetralogy of Fallot with absent pulmonary valve. *Ann Thorac Surg* 67:1391-1396, 1999.
68. Adolph V, Heaton J, Steiner R, et al: Extracorporeal membrane oxygenation for nonneonatal respiratory failure. *J Pediatr Surg* 26:326-330, 1991.
69. Khongphatthanayothin A, Wong P, Samara Y, et al: Impact of respiratory syncytial virus infection on surgery for congenital heart disease: postoperative course and outcome. *Crit Care Med* 27:1974-1981, 1999.
70. Moler FW, Palmisano JM, Green TP, et al: Predictors of outcome of severe respiratory syncytial virus-associated respiratory failure treated with extracorporeal membrane oxygenation. *J Pediatr* 23:46-52, 1993.
71. Hibbs A, Evans JR, Gerdes M, et al: Outcome of infants with bronchopulmonary dysplasia who receive extracorporeal membrane oxygenation therapy. *J Pediatr Surg* 36:1479-1484, 2001.
72. Brogan TV, Finn LS, Pyskaty DJ, et al: Plastic bronchitis in children: a case series and review of the medical literature. *Pediatr Pulmonol* 34:482-487, 2002.
73. Boigner H, Trittenwein G, Marx M, et al: Pulmonary failure after Norwood procedure: indication for extracorporeal membrane oxygenation? A case report. *Artif Organs* 23:1036-1037, 1999.
74. Dhillon R, Pearson GA, Firmin RK, et al: Extracorporeal membrane oxygenation and the treatment of critical pulmonary hypertension in congenital heart disease. *Eur J Cardiothorac Surg* 9:553-556, 1995.
75. Chang AC, Wernovsky G, Kulik T, et al: Management of the neonate with transposition of the great arteries and persistent pulmonary hypertension. *Am J Cardiol* 68:1253-1255, 1991.

76. Cullen M, Splittgerber F, Sweezer W, et al: Pulmonary hypertension postventricular septal defect repair treated by extracorporeal membrane oxygenation. *J Pediatr Surg* 21:675-677, 1986.
77. Goldman AP, Delius RE, Deanfield JE, et al: Nitric oxide might reduce the need for extracorporeal membrane support in children with critical postoperative pulmonary hypertension. *Ann Thorac Surg* 62:750-755, 1996.
78. Saito A, Miyamura H, Kanazawa H, et al: Extracorporeal membrane oxygenation for severe heart failure after Fontan operation. *Ann Thorac Surg* 55:153-155, 1993.
79. Thomas JA, Raroque S, Scott WA, et al: Successful treatment of severe dysrhythmias in infants with respiratory syncytial virus infections: two cases and a literature review. *Crit Care Med* 25:880-886, 1997.
80. Walker GM, McLeod K, Brown KL, et al: Extracorporeal life support as a treatment of supraventricular tachycardia in infants. *Pediatr Crit Care Med* 4:52-54, 2003.
81. Azzam FJ, Fiore AC: Postoperative junctional ectopic tachycardia. *Can J Anesth* 45:898-902, 1998.
82. Marino BS, Wernovsky G, Rychik J, et al: Early results of the Ross procedure in simple and complex left heart disease. *Circulation* 100(19 suppl):II62-II66, 1999.
83. Chen RJ, Ko WJ, Lin FY: Successful rescue of sustained ventricular tachycardia/ventricular fibrillation after coronary artery bypass grafting by extracorporeal membrane oxygenation. *J Formos Med Assoc* 101:283-286, 2002.
84. Cohen MI, Gaynor JW, Ramesh V, et al: Extracorporeal membrane oxygenation for patients with refractory ventricular arrhythmias. *J Thorac Cardiovasc Surg* 118:961-963, 1999.
85. Tecklenburg FW, Thomas NJ, Webb SA, et al: Pediatric ECMO for severe quinidine cardiotoxicity. *Pediatr Emerg Care* 13:111-113, 1997.
86. Butler TJ, Yoder BA, Seib P, et al: ECMO for left ventricular assist in a newborn with critical aortic stenosis. *Pediatr Cardiol* 15: 38-40, 1994.
87. Ward CJ, Mullins CE, Barron LJ, et al: Use of extracorporeal membrane oxygenation to maintain oxygenation during pediatric interventional cardiac catheterization. *Am Heart J* 130(3 pt 1): 619-620, 1995.
88. Carmichael TB, Walsh EP, Roth SJ: Anticipatory use of venoarterial extracorporeal membrane oxygenation for a high risk interventional high-risk cardiac procedure. *Respir Care* 47:1002-1006, 2002.
89. Fuhrman BP, Hernan LJ, Rotta AT, et al: Pathophysiology of cardiac extracorporeal membrane oxygenation. *Artif Organs* 23: 966-969, 1999.
90. Del Nido PJ, Armitage JM, Fricker FJ, et al: Extracorporeal membrane oxygenation support as a bridge to pediatric heart transplantation. *Circulation* 90(5 pt 2):II66-II69, 1994.
91. Koenig PR, Ralston MA, Kimball TR, et al: Balloon atrial septostomy for left ventricular decompression in patients receiving extracorporeal membrane oxygenation for myocardial failure. *J Pediatr* 122:S95-S99, 1993.
92. Johnston TA, Jaggers J, McGovern JJ, O'Laughlin MP: Bedside transseptal balloon dilation atrial septostomy for decompression of the left heart during extracorporeal membrane oxygenation. *Catheter Cardiovasc Interv* 46:197-199, 1999.
93. Seib PM, Faulkner SC, Erickson CC, et al: Blade and balloon atrial septostomy for left heart decompression in patients with severe ventricular dysfunction on extracorporeal membrane oxygenation. *Catheter Cardiovasc Interv* 46:179-186, 1999.
94. Edmunds LH. Pulseless cardiopulmonary bypass. *J Thorac Cardiovasc Surg* 84:800-804, 1982.
95. Bavaria JE, Ratcliff MB, Gupta KB, et al: Changes in left ventricular systolic wall stress during biventricular circulatory assistance. *Ann Thorac Surg* 45:526-532, 1988.
96. Martin GR, Short BL: Doppler echocardiographic evaluation of cardiac performance in infants on prolonged extracorporeal membrane oxygenation. *Am J Cardiol* 62:929-934, 1988.
97. Sell LL, Cullen ML, Lerner GR, et al: Hypertension during extracorporeal membrane oxygenation: cause, effect, and management. *Surgery* 102:724-730, 1987.
98. Martin GR, Chauvin L, Short BL: Effects of hydralazine on cardiac performance in infants receiving extracorporeal membrane oxygenation. *J Pediatr* 118:944-948, 1991.
99. Martin GR, Short BL, Abbott C, et al: Cardiac stun in infants undergoing extracorporeal membrane oxygenation. *J Thorac Cardiovasc Surg* 101:607-611, 1991.
100. Rosenberg EM, Cook LN: Electromechanical dissociation in newborns treated with extracorporeal membrane oxygenation: an extreme form of cardiac stun syndrome. *Crit Care Med* 19: 780-784, 1991.
101. Walther FJ, van de Bor M, Gangitano ES, et al: Left and right ventricular output in newborn infants undergoing extracorporeal membrane oxygenation. *Crit Care Med* 18:148-151, 1990.
102. Kurian MS, Reynolds ER, Humes RA, et al: Cardiac tamponade caused by serous pericardial effusion in patients on extracorporeal membrane oxygenation. *J Pediatr Surg* 34:1311-1314, 1999.
103. Zwischenberger JB, Cilley RE, Hirschl RB, et al: Life-threatening intrathoracic complications during treatment with extracorporeal membrane oxygenation. *J Pediatr Surg* 23:599-604, 1988.
104. Kececioglu D, Galal O, Halees Z, et al: Transesophageal echocardiography in children with cardiac assist. *Thorac Cardiovasc Surg* 42:21-24, 1994.
105. Ettedgui JA, Fricker FJ, Park SC, et al: Cardiac catheterization in children on extracorporeal membrane oxygenation. *Cardiol Young* 6:59-61, 1996.
106. desJardins SE, Crowley DC, Beekman RH, et al: Utility of cardiac catheterization in pediatric cardiac patients on ECMO. *Cathet Cardiovasc Interv* 46:62-67, 1999.
107. Booth KL, Roth SJ, Perry SB, et al: Cardiac catheterization of patients supported by extracorporeal membrane oxygenation. *J Am Coll Cardiol* 40:1681-1686, 2002.
108. Black MD, Coles JG, Williams WG, et al: Determinants of success in pediatric cardiac patients undergoing extracorporeal membrane oxygenation. *Ann Thorac Surg* 60:133-138, 1995.
109. Walters HL, Hakimi M, Rice MD, et al: Pediatric cardiac surgical ECMO: multivariate analysis of risk factors for hospital death. *Ann Thorac Surg* 60:329-336, 1995.
110. Brown KL, Shekerdemian LS, Penny DJ: Transcatheter closure of a patent arterial duct in a patient on veno-arterial extracorporeal membrane oxygenation. *Intensive Care Med* 28:501-503, 2002.
111. Hoskote A, Bohn D, VanArsdell G, et al: Extracorporeal life support in functional single ventricle following palliative surgery. *Pediatr Crit Care Med* 4:A119, 2003 (abstract).
112. Darling EM, Kaemmer D, Lawson DS, et al: Use of ECMO without the oxygenator to provide ventricular support after Norwood stage I procedures. *Ann Thorac Surg* 71:735-736, 2001.
113. Jaggers JJ, Forbess JM, Shah AS, et al: Extracorporeal membrane oxygenation for infant postcardiotomy support: significance of shunt management. *Ann Thorac Surg* 69:1476-1483, 2000.
114. Van Heijst AF, van der Staak FH, Hopman JC, et al: Ductus arteriosus with left-to-right shunt during venoarterial extracorporeal membrane oxygenation: effects on cerebral oxygenation and hemodynamics. *Pediatr Crit Care Med* 4:94-99, 2003.
115. Nelson DP, Schwartz S, Chang AC: Single ventricle physiology before and after Norwood operation. *Cardiol Young* 14(suppl 1): 52-60, 2004.
116. Saito A, Miyamura H, Kanazawa H, et al: Extracorporeal membrane oxygenation for severe heart failure after Fontan operation. *Ann Thorac Surg* 55:153-155, 1993.
117. Koul B, Willen H, Sjoberg T, et al: Pulmonary sequelae of prolonged total venoarterial bypass: evaluation with a new experimental model. *Ann Thorac Surg* 51:794-799, 1991.
118. Shen I, Levy FH, Benak AM, et al: Left ventricular dysfunction during extracorporeal membrane oxygenation in a hypoxemic swine model. *Ann Thorac Surg* 71:868-871, 2001.
119. McGowan FX, Ikegami M, del Nido PJ, et al: Cardiopulmonary bypass significantly reduces surfactant activity in children. *J Thorac Cardiovasc Surg* 106:968-977, 1993.
120. Bui KC, Walther FJ, David-Cu R, et al: Phospholipid and surfactant protein A concentration in tracheal aspirates from infants requiring extracorporeal membrane oxygenation. *J Pediatr* 121:271-274, 1992.
121. Coraim FJ, Coraim HP, Ebermann R, et al: Acute respiratory failure after cardiac surgery: clinical experiences with the application of continuous arteriovenous hemofiltration. *Crit Care Med* 14: 714-718, 1986.
122. Biehl DA, Stewart DL, Forti NH, et al: Timing of intracranial hemorrhage during extracorporeal life support. *ASAIO J* 42: 938-941, 1996.
123. Korinthenberg R, Kachel W, Koelfen W, et al: Neurological findings in newborn infants after extracorporeal membrane oxygenation,

with special reference to EEG. *Dev Med Child Neurol* 35: 249-257, 1993.
124. The Hypothermia after Cardiac Arrest Study Group: Mild therapeutic hypothermia to improve the neurologic outcome after cardiac arrest. *N Engl J Med* 346:549-556, 2002.
125. McLaughlin JF, Loeser JD, Roberts TS: Acquired hydrocephalus associated with superior vena cava syndrome in infants. *Childs Nerv Syst* 13:59-63, 1997.
126. Tobias JD: Controlled hypotension in children: a critical review of available agents. *Paediatr Drugs* 4:439-453, 2002.
127. Sorof JM, Stromberg D, Brewer ED, et al: Early initiation of peritoneal dialysis after surgical repair of congenital heart disease. *Pediatr Nephrol* 13:641-645, 1999.
128. Pettignano R, Heard M, Davis R, et al: Total enteral nutrition versus total parenteral nutrition during pediatric extracorporeal membrane oxygenation. *Crit Care Med* 26:358-363, 1998.
129. Duke T, Butt W, South M, et al: The DCO2 measured by gastric tonometry predicts survival in children receiving extracorporeal life support. *Chest* 111:174-179, 1997.
130. Sell LL, Cullen ML, Whittlesey GC, et al: Hemorrhagic complications during extracorporeal membrane oxygenation: prevention and treatment. *J Pediatr Surg* 21:1087-1091, 1986.
131. Dela Cruz TV, Stewart DL, Winston SJ, et al: Risk factors for intracranial hemorrhage in the extracorporeal membrane oxygenation patient. *J Perinatol* 17:18-23, 1997.
132. Horwitz JR, Cofer BR, Warner BW, et al: A multi-center trial of 6-aminocaproic acid (Amicar) in the prevention of bleeding in infants on ECMO. *J Pediatr Surg* 33:1610-1613, 1998.
133. Biswas AK, Lewis L, Sommerauer JF: Aprotinin in the management of life-threatening bleeding during extracorporeal life support. *Perfusion* 15:211-216, 2000.
134. Zavadil DP, Stammers AH, Willett LD, et al: Hematological abnormalities in neonatal patients treated with extracorporeal membrane oxygenation. *J Extra Corpor Technol* 30:83-90, 1998.
135. O'Neill JM, Schutze GE, Heulitt MJ, et al: Nosocomial infections during extracorporeal membrane oxygenation. *Intensive Care Med* 27:1247-1253, 2001.
136. Fridriksson JH, Helmrath MA, Wessel JJ, et al: Hypercalcemia associated with extracorporeal life support in neonates. *J Pediatr Surg* 36:493-497, 2001.
137. Meliones JN, Moler FW, Custer JR, et al: Hemodynamic instability after the initiation of extracorporeal membrane oxygenation: role of ionized calcium. *Crit Care Med* 19:1247-1251, 1991.
138. Bolton DT: Hyperkalemia, donor blood and cardiac arrest associated with ECMO priming. *Anaesthesia* 55:825-826, 2000.
139. Sell LL, Cullen ML, Whittlesey GC, et al: Experience with renal failure during extracorporeal membrane oxygenation: treatment with continuous hemofiltration. *J Pediatr Surg* 22:600-602, 1987.
140. Hirther M, Simoni J, Dickson M: Elevated levels of endotoxin, oxygen-derived free radicals, and cytokines during extracorporeal membrane oxygenation. *J Pediatr Surg* 27:1199-1202, 1992.
141. Heiss KF, Pettit B, Hirschl RB, et al: Renal insufficiency and volume overload in neonatal ECMO managed by continuous ultrafiltration. *ASAIO Trans* 33:557-560, 1987.
142. Marcus B, Atkinson JB, Wong PC, et al: Successful use of transesophageal echocardiography during extracorporeal membrane oxygenation in infants after cardiac operations. *J Thorac Cardiovasc Surg* 109:846-848, 1995.
143. Vermes E, Houel R, Simon M, et al: Doppler tissue imaging to predict myocardial recovery during mechanical circulatory support. *Ann Thorac Surg* 70:2149-2151, 2000.
144. Hill JD, de Leval MR, Fallat RJ, et al: Acute respiratory insufficiency: treatment with prolonged extracorporeal oxygenation. *J Thorac Cardiovasc Surg* 64:551-562, 1972.
145. Soeter JR, Mamiya RT, Sprague AY, et al: Prolonged extracorporeal oxygenation for cardiorespiratory failure after tetralogy correction. *J Thorac Cardiovasc Surg* 66:214-218, 1973.
146. Bartlett RH, Gazzaniga AB, Fong SW, et al: Extracorporeal membrane oxygenator support for cardiopulmonary failure. Experience in 28 cases. *J Thorac Cardiovasc Surg* 73:375-386, 1977.
147. Zwischenberger JB: Personal communication, 2002.
148. Kihara S, Kawai A, Endo M, et al: Extracorporeal membrane oxygenation and left ventricular assist device: a case of double mechanical bridge. *Heart Vessels* 16:164-166, 2002.
149. Wang SS, Ko WJ, Chen YS, et al: Mechanical bridge with extracorporeal membrane oxygenation and ventricular assist device to heart transplantation. *Artif Organs* 25:599-602, 2001.
150. Borowski A, Korb H: Experience with uni (LAVD) and biventricular (ECMO) circulatory support in postcardiotomy pediatric patients. *Int J Artif Organs* 20:695-700, 1997.
151. Noon GP, Lafuente JA, Irwin S: Acute and temporary ventricular support with Biomedicus centrifugal pump. *Ann Thorac Surg* 68:650-654, 1999.
152. Golding LR, Harasaki H, Loop FD, et al: Use of a centrifugal pump for temporary left ventricular assist system. *Trans Am Soc Artif Int Organs* 24:93-97, 1978.
153. Moat NE, Pawade A, Lewis BC, et al: Circulatory support in infants with post-cardiopulmonary bypass left ventricular dysfunction using a left ventricular assist device. *Eur J Cardiothorac Surg* 4:649-652, 1990.
154. Scheinin SA, Radovancevic B, Parnis SM, et al: Mechanical circulatory support in children. *J Cardiovasc Thorac Surg* 8:537-540, 1994.
155. Chang AC, Hanley FL, Weindling SN, et al: Left heart support with a ventricular assist device in an infant with acute myocarditis. *Crit Care Med* 20:712-715, 1992.
156. Karl TR, Sano S, Horton S, et al: Centrifugal pump left heart assist in pediatric cardiac operations. *J Thorac Cardiovasc Surg* 102:624-630, 1991.
157. Thuys CA, Mullaly RJ, Horton SB, et al: Centrifugal ventricular assist in children under 6 kg. *Eur J Cardiothorac Surg* 13: 130-134, 1998.
158. Del Nido PJ, Duncan BW, Mayer JE Jr, et al: Left ventricular assist device improves survival in children with left ventricular dysfunction after repair of anomalous left coronary artery from the pulmonary artery. *Ann Thorac Surg* 67:169-172, 1999.
159. Perko MJ, Sander-Jensen K, Dehnke C, et al: BioMedicus ventricular assist for postcardiotomy heart failure: evaluation of univentricular assistance. *Artif Organs* 19:777-781, 1995.
160. Morgan IS, Codispoti M, Sanger K, et al: Superiority of centrifugal pump over roller pump in pediatric cardiac surgery: prospective randomised trial. *Eur J Cardiothorac Surg* 13:526-532, 1998.
161. Jacobs JP, Ojito JW, McConaghey TW, et al: Rapid cardiopulmonary support for children with complex congenital heart disease. *Ann Thorac Surg* 70:742-750, 2000.
162. Marelli D, Laks H, Meehan DA, et al: Minimally invasive mechanical cardiac support without extracorporeal membrane oxygenation in children awaiting heart transplantation. *Ann Thorac Surg* 68:2320-2323, 1999.
163. Ratcliffe MB, Bavaria JE, Wenger RK, et al: Left ventricular mechanics of ejecting, postischemic hearts during left ventricular circulatory assistance. *J Thorac Cardiovasc Surg* 101:245-255, 1991.
164. Eugene J, Ott RA, McColgan SJ, et al: Vented cardiac assistance: ECMO vs left heart bypass for acute left ventricular failure. *ASAIO Trans* 32:538-541, 1986.
165. Williams MR, Quaegebeur JM, Hsu DT, et al: Biventricular assist device as a bridge to transplantation in a pediatric patient. *Ann Thorac Surg* 62:578-580, 1996.
166. Pantalos GM, Minich LL, Tani LY, et al: Estimation of timing errors for the intraaortic balloon pump use in pediatric patients. *ASAIO J* 45:166-171, 1999.
167. Veasy LG, Blalock RC, Orth JL, et al: Intra-aortic balloon pumping in infants and children. *Circulation* 68:1095-1100, 1983.
168. Pollock JC, Charlton MC, Williams WG, et al: Intraaortic balloon pumping in children. *Ann Thorac Surg* 29:522-528, 1980.
169. Park JK, Hsu DT, Gersony WM: Intraarotic balloon pump management of refractory congestive heart failure in children. *Pediatr Cardiol* 14:19-22, 1993.
170. Pozzi M, Santoro G, Makundan S: Intraaortic balloon pump after treatment of anomalous origin of left coronary artery. *Ann Thorac Surg* 65:555-557, 1998.
171. Akomea-Agyin C, Kejriwal NK, Franks P, et al: Intraaortic balloon pumping in children. *Ann Thorac Surg* 67:1415-1420, 1999.
172. Del Nido PJ, Swan PR, Benson LN, et al: Successful use of intraaortic balloon pumping in a 2-kilogram infant. *Ann Thorac Surg* 46:574-576, 1988.
173. Pinkney KA, Minich LL, Tani LY, et al: Current results with intraaortic balloon pumping in infants and children. *Ann Thorac Surg* 73:887-891, 2002.

174. Spence PA, Peniston CM, Mihic N, et al: A rational approach to the selection of an assist device for the failing right ventricle. *Ann Thorac Surg* 41:606-608, 1986.
175. Scheinin SA, Radovancevic B, Parnis SM, et al: Mechanical circulatory support in children. *Eur J Cardiothorac Surg* 8:537-540, 1994.
176. Meyns B, Dens JO, Sergeant P, et al: First clinical experience with the Impella micropump in patients with cardiogenic shock. In: El-Banayosy A, Korfer R, editors: Proceedings of the Third Mechanical Circulatory Support Meeting: Today's Facts and Future Trends. Bad Oeyenhausen, Germany, December, 2002.
177. Hata M, Shiono M, Orime Y, et al: Strategy of circulatory support with percutaneous cardiopulmonary support. *Artif Organs* 24:636-639, 2000.
178. Milliken JC, Laks H, George B: Use of venous assist device after repair of complex lesions of the right heart. *J Am Coll Cardiol* 8:922-929, 1986.
179. Smedira NG, Blackstone EH: Postcardiotomy mechanical support: risk factors and outcomes. *Ann Thorac Surg* 71(3 suppl): S60-S66, 2001.
180. El-Banayosy A, Minami K, Arusoglu L, et al: Long-term mechanical circulatory support. *Thorac Cardiovasc Surg* 45:127-130, 1997.
181. Goldstein DJ, Oz MC, Rose EA: Implantable left ventricular assist devices. *N Engl J Med* 339:1522-1533, 1998.
182. DeBakey ME: Left ventricular bypass for cardiac assistance: clinical experience. *Am J Cardiol* 27:3-10, 1971.
183. Rose EA, Gelijns AC, Moskowitz AJ, et al: Long-term mechanical left ventricular assistance for end-stage heart failure. *N Engl J Med* 345:1435-1443, 2001.
184. Matsuda H, Taenaka Y, Ohkubo N, et al: Use of paracorporeal pneumatic ventricular assist device for postoperative cardiogenic shock in two children with complex cardiac lesions. *Artif Organs* 12:423-430, 1988.
185. Loebe M, Hennig E, Muller J, et al: Long-term mechanical circulatory support as a bridge to transplantation, for recovery from cardiomyopathy, and for permanent replacement. *Eur J Cardiothorac Surg* 11(suppl):S18-S24, 1997.
186. Ishino K, Loebe M, Uhlemann F, et al: Circulatory support with paracorporeal pneumatic ventricular assist device (VAD) in infants and children. *Eur J Cardiothorac Surg* 11:965-972, 1997.
187. Hetzer R, Loebe M, Potapov EV, et al: Circulatory support with pneumatic paracorporeal ventricular assist device in infants and children. *Ann Thorac Surg* 66:1498-1506, 2000.
188. Stiller B, Dhanert I, Weng YG, et al: Children may survive severe myocarditis with prolonged use of biventricular assist devices. *Heart* 82:237-240, 1999.
189. Herwig V, Severin M, Waldenberger FR, et al: Medos/HIA-Assist System: first experiences with mechanical circulatory assist in infants and children. *Int J Artif Organs* 20:692-694, 1997.
190. Konertz W, Hotz H, Schneider M, et al: Clinical experience with the MEDOS HIA-VAD System in infants and children: a preliminary report. *Ann Thorac Surg* 63:1138-1144, 1997.
191. Busch U, Waldenberger FR, Redlin M, et al: Successful treatment of postoperative right ventricular heart failure with the HA-Medos Assist System in a two year-old girl. *Pediatr Cardiol* 20:161-163, 1999.
192. Reul H: The MEDOS/HIA System: development, results, perspectives. *Thorac Cardiovasc Surg* 47(suppl 2):311-315, 1999.
193. Shum-Tim D, Duncan BW, Hraska V, et al: Evaluation of a pulsatile pediatric ventricular assist device in an acute right heart failure model. *Ann Thorac Surg* 64:1374-1380, 1997.
194. Weyand M, Keceicioglu D, Kehl HG, et al: Neonatal mechanical bridging to total orthotopic heart transplantation. *Ann Thorac Surg* 66:519-522, 1998.
195. Joharchi MS, Neiser U, Lenschow U, et al: Thoratec left ventricular assist device for bridging to recovery in fulminant acute myocarditis. *Ann Thorac Surg* 74:234-235, 2002.
196. Reinhartz O, Keith FM, El-Banayosy A, et al: Multicenter experience with the Thoratec ventricular assist device in children and adolescents. *J Heart Lung Transplant* 20:439-448, 2001.
197. Reinhartz O, Stiller B, Eilers R, et al: Current clinical status of pulsatile pediatric circulatory support. *ASAIO J* 48:455-459, 2002.
198. Copeland JG, Arabia FA, Smith RG: Bridge to transplantation with a Thoratec left ventricular assist device in a 17-kg child. *Ann Thorac Surg* 71:1003-1004, 2001.
199. Farrar DJ, Hill JD, Pennington DG, et al: Preoperative and postoperative comparison of patients with univentricular and biventricular support with the Thoratec ventricular assist device as a bridge to transplantation. *J Thorac Cardiovasc Surg* 113:202-209, 1997.
200. McBride LR, Naunheim KS, Fiore AC, et al: Clinical experience with 111 Thoratec ventricular assist devices. *Ann Thorac Surg* 67:1233-1239, 1999.
201. Reinhartz O, Keith FM, El_Banayosy A, et al: Multicenter experience with the Thoratec ventricular assist device in children and adolescents. *J Heart Lung Transplant* 20:439-448, 2001.
202. Frazier OH: Personal communication, 2004.
203. Frazier OH, Myers TJ, Gregoric ID, et al: Initial clinical experience with the Jarvik 2000 implantable axial flow left ventricular assist system. *Circulation* 105:2855-2860, 2002.
204. Noon GP: Personal communication, 2004.
205. Rothenburger M, Wilhelm MJ, Hammel D, et al: Treatment of thrombus formation associated with the Micromed DeBakey VAD can be treated with recombinant tissue plasminogen activator. *Circulation* 106(suppl I):I-189-I-192, 2002.
206. Raman J, Jeevanadam V: Destination therapy with ventricular assist devices. *Cardiol* 101:104-110, 2004.
207. Kaplon RJ, Oz MC, Kwiatkowski PA, et al: Miniature axial flow pump for ventricular assistance in children and small adults. *J Thorac Cardiovasc Surg* 111:13-18, 1996.
208. Jassawalla JS: Optimized HeartSaver VAD. In: El-Banayosy A, Korfer R, editors: Proceedings of the Third Mechanical Circulatory Support Meeting: Today's Facts and Future Trends. Bad Oeyenhausen, Germany, December, 2002.
209. Golding L: The CorAide left ventricular assist system. In: El-Banayosy A, Korfer R, editors: Proceedings of the Third Mechanical Circulatory Support Meeting: Today's Facts and Future Trends. Bad Oeyenhausen, Germany, December, 2002.
210. Long JW: HeartQuest™ next generation VAD. In: El-Banayosy A, Korfer R, editors: Proceedings of the Third Mechanical Circulatory Support Meeting: Today's Facts and Future Trends. Bad Oeyenhausen, Germany, December, 2002.
211. Bourque K, Gernes DB, Loree HM II, et al: HeartMate III: pump design for a centrifugal LVAD with a magnetically levitated rotor. *ASAIO J* 47:401-405, 2001.
212. Takatani S, Matsuda H, Hanatani A, et al: Mechanical circulatory support devices (MCSD) in Japan: current status and future directions. *J Artif Organs* 8:13-27, 2005.

CHAPTER 26

Disorders of Cardiac Rhythm

Frank A. Fish, Prince J. Kannankeril, and James A. Johns

PEARLS

- Arrhythmias may result from ongoing therapies: ask "What's the DEAL?":
  - *D*rugs and drips
  - *E*lectrolytes
  - *A*irway and acid base
  - *L*ines
- Appropriate diagnosis is key. Always attempt to document arrhythmia in multiple leads before instituting therapy.
- For ventricular fibrillation or pulseless ventricular tachycardia, *begin cardiopulmonary resuscitation and defibrillate immediately.*
- Involve a cardiologist before initiating (chronic) antiarrhythmic drug therapy.
- Whenever possible, use available means to document atrial rate to discern correct ventricular-atrial relationship.
- "Supraventricular tachycardia" is a nonspecific electrocardiographic pattern. There are multiple types, and appropriate therapy depends on appropriate diagnosis.
- Whenever possible, opt for therapies that maintain AV synchrony.

Cardiac rhythm disturbances (arrhythmias) are commonly observed in critically ill pediatric patients.[1] A given arrhythmia may represent the primary disease process, occur secondary to another disorder (e.g., recent cardiac surgery or myocarditis), or represent a complication of management (Table 26–1). Associated metabolic or hemodynamic derangements may confuse the diagnostic process.[2] Furthermore, arrhythmias that, under most circumstances, would be tolerated hemodynamically may be immediately life threatening to the critically ill child. Finally, certain treatment strategies may be available in the critical care unit that might not be normally considered, particularly for serious but transient arrhythmias. Therefore optimal evaluation and management of arrhythmias in the critical care setting should emphasize prompt hemodynamic stabilization of the patient using modalities immediately available at the bedside, along with concurrent identification and correction of predisposing factors. This chapter attempts to emphasize the most common clinical scenarios and treatment approaches encountered in the intensive care setting while providing a broader overview of the array of arrhythmia mechanisms and their associated presentations in pediatric patients.

Classification of Arrhythmias

Arrhythmias are commonly classified according to electrocardiographic (ECG) findings, or they can be grouped according to underlying electrophysiologic mechanisms.

TABLE 26–1

Classification of Arrhythmias by Type and Basis

	Primary	Secondary
Ventricular premature beats and supraventricular premature beats	+++	+++
Sinus bradycardia, sick sinus syndrome	++	++
Incomplete AV block		
Mobitz I	++	+++
Mobitz II		++
Congenital third-degree AV block	+++	++
Acquired third-degree AV Block		++
Paroxysmal SVT (AV reentrant tachycardia, AV nodal reentrant tachycardia)	+++	
Ectopic atrial tachycardia	++	
Atrial flutter and intraatrial reentry	++	+++
Atrial fibrillation	+	+++
Chaotic atrial tachycardia		++
Junctional ectopic tachycardia	+	+++
Monomorphic ventricular tachycardia	++	++
Torsades de pointes	+	+
Ventricular fibrillation	+	++
Bidirectional ventricular tachycardia	++	+

+++, typical; ++, occasional; + = rare.

In the intensive care setting, it is helpful to discern whether an arrhythmia represents a primary versus secondary process (see Table 26–1). Electrocardiographically, arrhythmias can be characterized as bradycardias, tachycardias, or extrasystoles. Bradycardias are further subdivided into sinus node bradycardia or atrioventricular (AV) block. Extrasystoles and tachycardias are categorized as supraventricular or ventricular in origin. Tachycardias can be further attributed to one of three possible mechanisms: reentry, automaticity, and triggered activity. Whereas most treatment algorithms assume a reentrant mechanism, abnormal triggering and automaticity may be particularly important in various disease states. These mechanisms may respond quite differently to given therapies, such as pacing or direct current cardioversion. Yet differentiating between mechanisms may be difficult, particularly when more than one mechanism contributes to a given arrhythmia. However, when initial therapies unexpectedly fail to terminate an arrhythmia, the possibility of an alternative mechanism may require consideration.

Bradycardias

Appropriate versus "Normal Heart Rate"

Normal heart rate ranges vary tremendously during childhood. Although a clear relationship between age and "intrinsic heart rate" can be demonstrated in the presence of "total autonomic blockade," the normal heart rate at any particular moment is predominantly a reflection of relative sympathetic and parasympathetic tone. Thus in a given clinical situation, "appropriate" heart rate is a more useful concept than "normal rate." Most critically ill patients manifest some degree of sinus tachycardia in response to pain, sepsis, shock, fever, or adrenergic agonist infusions. Therefore elevations in sinus rate are expected in most critically ill patients, and the degree of tachycardia serves as a gauge of pain or hemodynamic instability. Under such circumstances, inappropriate absence of sinus tachycardia may be an ominous indicator of severe hemodynamic embarrassment and may require aggressive intervention to reestablish a more appropriate rate.

Sinus Bradycardia and Sinus Pauses

Transient interruptions in the sinus mechanism (sinus pauses) may occur as an exaggeration of vagally mediated sinus arrhythmia or be caused by intrinsic sinus node dysfunction. Intermittent sinus bradycardia or sinus pauses may be caused by intense vagal episodes, such as those occurring during neurocardiogenic syncope. Whereas vagal stimulation may produce profound bradycardia, pauses, or even asystole lasting for several seconds, transient bradycardia should not be construed as an absolute indication for pacing. Prolonged sinus pauses in the setting of persistent bradycardia are attributed to sinus node exit block or sinus arrest and often warrant pacing. It may be important to distinguish apparent sinus bradycardia or pauses from blocked premature atrial depolarizations (where premature P waves may be obscured in the preceding t wave). Primary sinus node dysfunction in childhood is rare but has been described.[3]

Conduction Abnormalities

First-degree atrioventricular (AV) block is characterized by a prolonged PR interval for age and rate while maintaining 1:1 AV conduction. First-degree AV block usually is exaggerated with increasing heart rate except when related to high vagal tone, in which case it resolves as vagal tone is blocked or diminished.

Second-degree block occurs when atrial depolarizations intermittently fail to conduct to the ventricle. Second-degree block can be further characterized as Mobitz type I or Mobitz type II. Mobitz type I, also called *Wenckebach conduction,* displays progressively prolonged PR intervals (and correspondingly shorter RR intervals) prior to a single nonconducted atrial complex. Wenckebach conduction usually represents block in the AV node, is unlikely to progress suddenly to high-grade block, and in some settings may be benign. Mobitz type II, characterized by abrupt failure to conduct without prior lengthening of the PR interval, usually is attributed to block within the His conduction system and may indicate greater potential for sudden progression to complete AV block. As such, type II block may be more ominous and may require more aggressive intervention (i.e., pacing). In attempting to distinguish type I from type II block, it is useful to compare the PR interval of the first conducted beat following block to the last conducted beat prior to block to best appreciate whether PR prolongation preceded block.

Higher grades of second-degree AV block are best characterized by the ratio of atrial to ventricular depolarizations (2:1, 3:1, 4:1, etc.). This ratio of conduction does not imply the level of block or even whether any conduction abnormality exists. Atrial tachyarrhythmias, including atrial flutter, often result in second-degree AV block in those with normal AV nodal function. Likewise, vagally mediated AV block may result in transient high-grade block (although the sinus rate usually slows concurrently).

Complete or *third-degree AV block* represents complete failure of the atrial depolarizations to propagate to the ventricle. As with sinus bradycardias, there may be a junctional or idioventricular rhythm escape rhythm that typically is regular but may be quite slow. Periodic shortening of the RR interval may be the only clue to distinguish complete AV block from high-grade second-degree block with intermittent conduction (Figure 26–1). In complete AV block, ventricular systole may alter the sinus rate (ventriculo-phasic variation).

Bundle branch block patterns occur when impaired conduction in the specialized intraventricular conduction system results in delayed right or left ventricular depolarization, resulting in an aberrant QRS complex. Bundle branch block and AV block sometimes represent normal

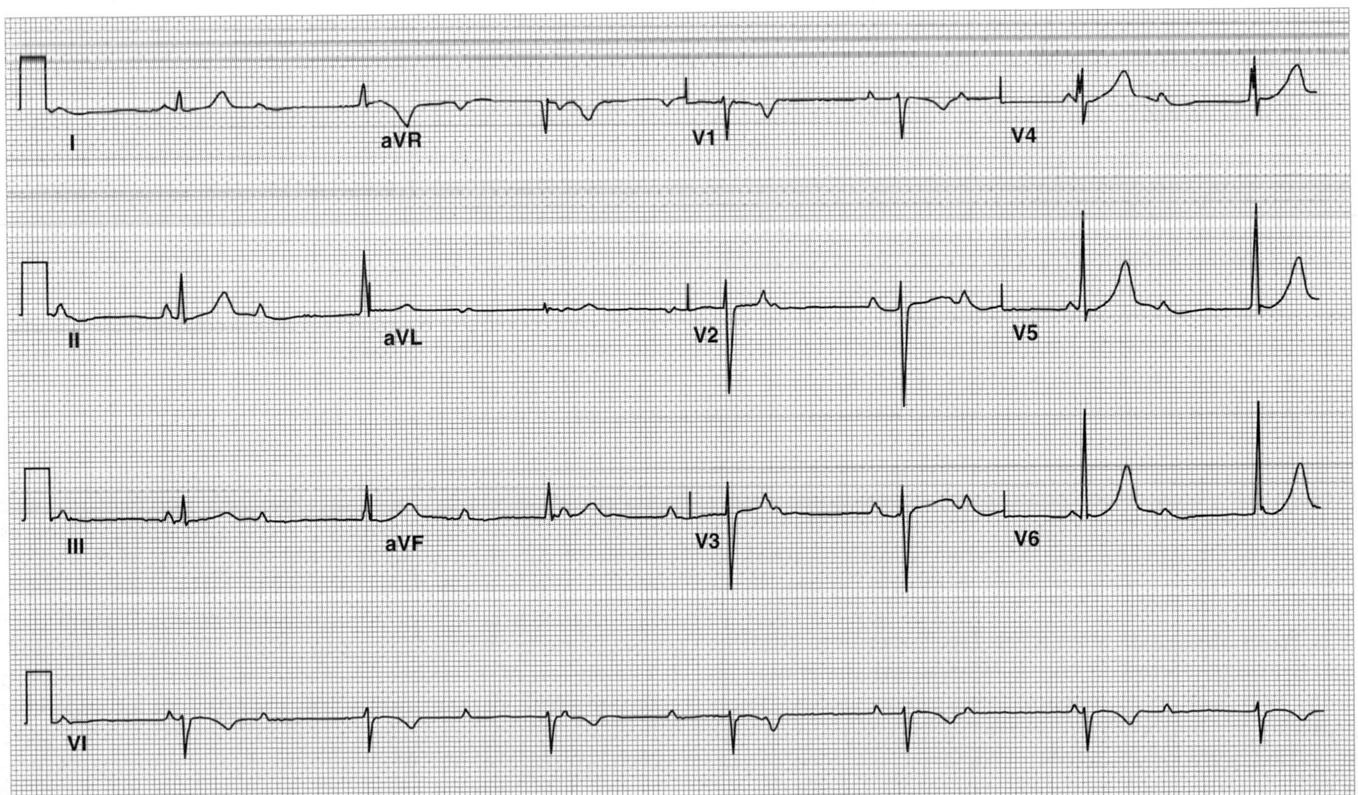

FIGURE 26–1 • Complete AV block, presumably congenital, in an asymptomatic 9 year old with slow resting heart rate. Note the regular RR interval, which confirms complete rather than incomplete (second-degree) AV block.

physiologic responses to shortening of the cycle length (as with premature atrial systoles or tachycardia initiation) or may result from increased vagal tone, pharmacologic effects, or primary disease within the specialized conduction tissue.

Escape Rhythms

AV nodal and Purkinje cell "subsidiary pacemakers" are revealed only as "escape rhythms" when the sinus mechanism is depressed or fails to propagate normally. Transient or sustained escape rhythms may arise from the atrium, AV node, or ventricles, but they usually are slower than the appropriate sinus rate. Sometimes these escape rhythms become accelerated and compete with the sinus focus. It is important to distinguish these accelerated subsidiary rhythms from both pathologic tachycardias and escape rhythms resulting from AV block. Only rarely does an accelerated junctional or ventricular rhythm result in significant symptoms in a healthy child.[4] However, in the critically ill patient, the resultant loss of AV synchrony may compromise cardiac output and warrant efforts to pace the atrium at a slightly faster rate.

Tachycardias

Classification by Mechanism

As discussed earlier, most patients in critical care settings display some degree of sinus tachycardia as an appropriate response to the primary illness. The degree of sinus tachycardia for age may provide important insights into level of sedation, pain, or hemodynamic stress of a given patient. However, exaggerated sinus tachycardia must be distinguished from other tachycardia mechanisms that may appear similar.

Most abnormal tachycardias encountered clinically are caused by abnormal impulse propagation in the form of reentry. This may represent reentry using an accessory AV connection (AV reentry), the AV node and its adjacent tissues (AV nodal reentry), atrial myocardium (intraatrial reentry including atrial flutter and fibrillation), or ventricular myocardium (most ventricular tachycardias). Automatic tachycardias represent abnormal impulse formation arising from either ectopic foci or usual subsidiary pacemaker tissues at a significantly accelerated rate. These also may originate from the atria, from AV nodal or junctional regions, or within the ventricles. They presumably arise when pathologic conditions confer abnormally accelerated depolarization to the usual subsidiary pacemaker tissues or when diseased atrial or ventricular myocardium acquires abnormal spontaneous depolarization. Triggered tachycardias are thought to arise from abnormal secondary depolarizations (afterdepolarizations) following normal myocardial depolarizations, which may propagate to adjacent tissues. These probably are important in several specific situations such as cardiac glycoside toxicity (delayed afterdepolarizations), drug-induced long QT syndromes (early afterdepolarizations), and probably the congenital long QT syndromes (see section on long QT syndromes).

Classification by Site

Although tachycardia behavior and response to therapy may be highly dependent on the mechanisms, in common practice tachycardias usually are grouped primarily according to the site of origin and only secondarily based on specific or presumed mechanism. Most treatment algorithms place primary emphasis on distinguishing supraventricular tachycardias from ventricular tachycardias.

Supraventricular Tachycardias

"Supraventricular tachycardia" (SVT), "paroxysmal atrial tachycardia" (PAT), and "paroxysmal supraventricular tachycardia" (PSVT) are common and descriptive but nonspecific terms often used interchangeably to describe tachycardias with a regular rate (usually in excess of 200–220 bpm), normal QRS morphology, and P waves that either are nondiscernible or follow the QRS complex. This phenotype represents the most common form of SVT seen in otherwise healthy neonates and children and usually can be attributed to AV nodal reentry or AV reentry using an accessory connection (see next section). However, these typical ECG features can be produced by a more diverse array of tachycardia mechanisms.[5] Furthermore, intermittent AV block or QRS prolongation may be observed in certain types of "SVT," such that the ECG distinction of "SVT" from other atrial arrhythmias becomes obscured. Therefore it is most useful to include among SVTs all tachycardias originating from the atrium, the AV node, or both, regardless of whether the ventricles participate primarily (i.e., AV reentry) or merely as a secondary consequence of AV conduction. This broad and inclusive definition appropriately allows inclusion of nonreciprocating mechanisms that need to be included in the differential diagnosis of "SVT" such as intraatrial reentry.[4]

AV Reciprocating Tachycardias

AV reciprocating tachycardias use one or more accessory AV connections to allow a reentrant circuit to develop involving both atrial and ventricular tissues. By definition, they display a fixed 1:1 AV relationship. Orthodromic reciprocating tachycardia (ORT) is the most common AV reentrant tachycardia and in otherwise normal infants also is the most common mechanism of SVT.[5,6] In ORT, antegrade conduction is over the AV node whereas retrograde conduction to the atria occurs via an accessory AV connection. QRS morphology and duration usually are normal, with retrograde P waves often evident following each QRS complex. If the accessory connection conducts antegrade during sinus rhythm, ventricular preexcitation occurs prior to conduction over the AV node (Wolff-Parkinson-White [WPW] syndrome). The fusion of preexcited ventricular depolarization with the normal depolarization of the AV node and His-Purkinje system produces the short PR interval and Δ wave characteristic of WPW syndrome. Many patients experiencing ORT have normal QRS morphology during sinus rhythm and (concealed) accessory connections, which conduct only retrograde. Thus the accessory pathway is clinically evident only during tachycardia or during ventricular pacing.

Antidromic reciprocating tachycardia (ART) is a much less common AV reciprocating tachycardia in which the circuit is reversed. Antegrade conduction during ART occurs exclusively via the accessory connection and results in a "maximally preexcited" QRS. As a result, ART is not readily distinguished from ventricular tachycardia by ECG features alone. Retrograde conduction occurs over the AV node (or commonly a second accessory connection) producing a 1:1 ventricular-atrial (VA) relationship. By definition, patients with ART also have the ECG features of WPW syndrome during sinus rhythm because antegrade conduction over the accessory pathway also should be evident during sinus rhythm. ART should be distinguished from ORT with aberrant conduction.

A specific form of antidromic AV reentry uses Mahaim fibers, which are accessory AV connections with decremental antegrade conduction. Most Mahaim fibers are located on the right ventricular free wall (atriofascicular connections), although some arise from the AV node itself (nodoventricular connections). Tachycardia using a Mahaim fiber should be suspected in a young patient with a regular tachycardia and left bundle branch block QRS pattern. Typically, ART and tachycardia using Mahaim fibers have a 1:1 VA relationship. However, because retrograde conduction in either case may be supported over a second accessory connection, maneuvers typically resulting in AV nodal block may not terminate these tachycardias, further confusing clinical distinction between these wide QRS complex tachycardias and ventricular tachycardia.

Permanent junctional reciprocating tachycardia (PJRT) is a variant of ORT with retrograde conduction over a slowly conducting accessory AV connection that possesses decremental ("AV nodelike") conduction.[7] The relative conduction and refractory properties of the accessory connection and the AV node are such that the PR interval is short or normal and tachycardia is incessant. In a single-lead rhythm strip, PJRT may mimic sinus tachycardia, although a 12-lead electrocardiogram reveals atypical P wave morphology with P-wave inversion in the inferior leads. This tachycardia typically displays repeated spontaneous termination and prompt reinitiation resulting in incessant tachycardia until adequately treated (Figure 26–2).

AV Nodal Reentrant Tachycardia

AV nodal reentrant tachycardia (AVNRT) is the most common cause of SVT in older children and young adults without WPW syndrome or structural heart disease. It is seen less commonly in infants.[5,6] Occasionally, it is precipitated for the first time by a serious illness or by other secondary factors associated with arrhythmias in the intensive care unit (ICU). This tachycardia can be attributed to so-called "dual AV nodal physiology." Conceptually, one functional "limb" of the AV node typically displays slow conduction and a short refractory period, whereas the other limb typically displays more rapid conduction but a longer refractory period. The differential conduction between the two "limbs" of the AV node (slow and fast pathways) provides the functional substrate for reentry. In actuality, these "limbs" represent differential conduction properties of the fibers inputting the AV node from upper and lower approaches of the atrial septum, representing so-called "fast" and "slow" inputs.

Classically, two electrocardiographically distinct forms of AVNRT may occur. In the "typical" form, antegrade conduction during tachycardia is over the slow AV node inputs, and the P waves often are obscured by the preceding QRS complex. In the "atypical" form, antegrade conduction is via the fast inputs of the AV node, and retrograde conduction is over the slow limb. The typical form of AVNRT cannot be reliably distinguished from ORT in which P waves are also often obscured. The atypical form of AVNRT may be indistinguishable from PJRT (see later), although the tachycardia is paroxysmal rather than incessant. Like PJRT, atypical AVNRT must be carefully distinguished from other tachycardias with a normal PR interval, including sinus tachycardia, intraatrial reentry, or ectopic atrial tachycardias (see later). Other atypical forms of AV nodal reentry using "intermediate" pathways can occur but are uncommon in children. Other variations of AVNRT can be characterized during the course of formal intracardiac electrophysiologic study.

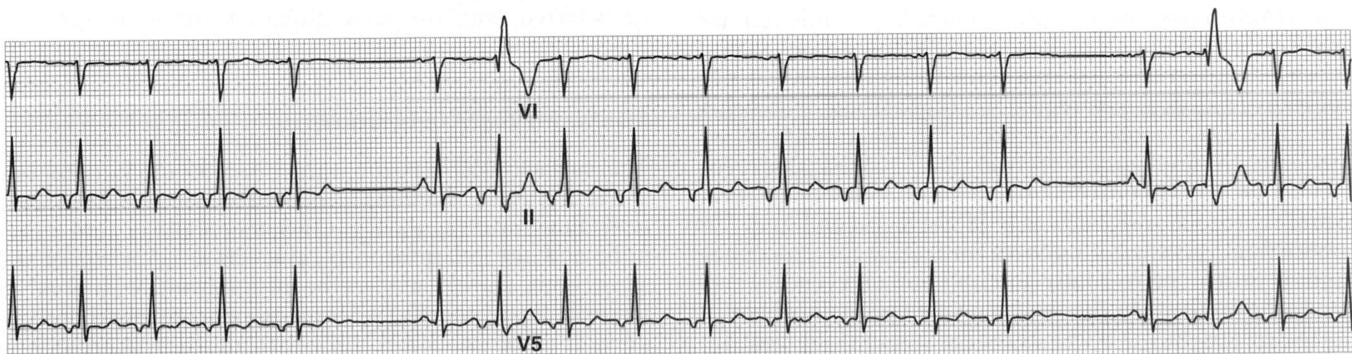

FIGURE 26–2 • Supraventricular tachycardia resulting from the permanent form of junctional reciprocating tachycardia. Note the slow rate, long RP and short PR interval, and inverted P waves in ECG leads II and III. At rest, this rhythm often shows incessantly repetitive termination (with retrograde block), followed by immediate reinitiation (after single, isolated sinus complexes). With exercise, this rhythm often is faster and sustained, rendering it electrocardiographically indistinguishable from the atypical nodal reentry.

Primary Atrial Tachycardias

Primary atrial tachycardias are tachycardias originating solely from atrial tissue. They include tachycardias with discrete P waves (ectopic atrial tachycardia, intraatrial reentry), sawtooth flutter waves (atrial flutter), or disorganized atrial activity (atrial fibrillation, chaotic atrial tachycardia).[8] The ECG appearance alone may not adequately distinguish the underlying mechanism.

In all cases, conduction to the ventricles is over the AV node (except in patients with associated WPW syndrome). The resulting ventricular rate determines the degree of clinical compromise during these tachycardias. If conduction is rapid or occurs over an accessory connection, the QRS morphology may be aberrant and difficult to distinguish from ventricular tachycardias. However, interventions that limit AV nodal conduction usually allow the ongoing and faster atrial rhythm to be revealed. It is useful and often necessary to directly record atrial depolarization (via esophageal, epicardial, or intraatrial recordings) to discern atrial activation. Despite the potential ECG similarities of the various primary atrial tachycardias, the varying mechanisms confer important differences in clinical behavior.

Junctional Ectopic Tachycardia

Junctional ectopic tachycardia (JET) probably arises from an abnormal automatic focus or a protected microreentrant circuit in the region of the AV node or proximal His bundle. Antegrade conduction usually is over the normal His-Purkinje system with a narrow QRS. Retrograde (VA) block or complete VA dissociation with a slower atrial rate aids in the recognition of this mechanism. Variants include a congenital form, the more common postsurgical form, and paroxysmal JET described primarily in adults.[7,9] As in primary atrial tachycardias, atrial depolarization may be obscure, and direct atrial recordings aid the diagnosis. Occasionally JET is associated with 1:1 VA conduction, in which case additional pacing or pharmacologic maneuvers are necessary to distinguish it from other mechanisms of SVT.

Ventricular Tachycardias

Ventricular tachycardias include all tachycardias that arise exclusively within the ventricle(s) and require neither the atrium nor the AV node for perpetuation. Because ventricular depolarization is aberrant, the QRS duration is always prolonged for a given age and heart rate. The QRS morphology may be either uniform or changing (bidirectional, polymorphic). Classically, ventricular tachycardias are associated with VA dissociation (atrial rhythm at a slower rate). However, in children, VA conduction over the AV node (or an accessory connection) may be sufficient to allow intermittent or even 1:1 VA conduction. Thus VA dissociation when present is helpful but when absent (or uncertain) does not exclude ventricular tachycardia as the underlying mechanism. The presence of periodic fusion complexes (QRS morphology intermediate between tachycardia morphology and sinus morphology) is virtually pathognomonic for ventricular tachycardia with VA dissociation.

Although often regarded as a homogeneous group of arrhythmias, ventricular tachycardias actually constitute diverse rhythms representing each of the underlying tachycardia mechanisms (reentry, automaticity, triggered activity) with important therapeutic implications.[10] Likewise, although sometimes lethal, they may range in complexity and severity from benign accelerated ventricular rhythm to rapid polymorphic ventricular tachycardia and ventricular fibrillation. Both the clinical setting and the QRS morphology during ventricular tachycardia may provide important clues to the mechanism and pathogenesis, anatomic origin or tachycardia focus (see incessant ventricular tachycardias), and treatment strategies as discussed later.

Approach to Diagnosis

Monitoring and General Assessment

In the intensive care setting, there may be a tradeoff between precision of diagnosis and urgency of therapy. Even so, appropriate diagnosis remains key to ongoing therapy. When an arrhythmia develops, rapid assessment of hemodynamic stability dictates the extent to which diagnostic studies can be pursued relative to the urgency of treatment. This should include assessment of level of consciousness, ventilation, tissue perfusion, and blood pressure. If time allows, determination of acid-base balance or other indicators of tissue perfusion (e.g., mixed venous oxygen saturation, serum lactate levels) is helpful. Minimal diagnostic evaluation should always include a timely evaluation of available ECG rhythm strips and a rapid review of drugs being administered, potential toxic exposures, respiratory and acid-base status, and known associated illnesses. Electrolyte assessment (potassium, calcium, and possibly magnesium) and drug screening may provide valuable diagnostic clues and should be obtained. The history of surgical procedures for congenital heart disease and trauma (chest and cranial) should be quickly reviewed. Indwelling catheters should be surveyed on radiographs for potential intracardiac position. Concurrent with this brief survey, a differential diagnosis of the rhythm disturbance should be quickly established, followed by the most appropriate emergency therapy. If the patient is sufficiently stable, therapy may be deferred until the arrhythmia can be more precisely characterized.

Surface Electrocardiogram

The surface electrocardiogram remains the cornerstone of arrhythmia diagnosis, providing key information regarding rate, regularity, QRS morphology and duration, and AV relationship (Table 26–2). A strip of the arrhythmia should always be printed and examined in multiple leads (ideally, with calipers) to assess these features (Figure 26–3). A full 12-lead electrocardiogram should be obtained whenever possible because diagnostic details, such as QRS aberrancy, atrial rate, and P-wave morphology, or hidden features, such as "flutter waves," may be evident only in selected leads (Figure 26–4). Most contemporary monitoring systems now have automatic

TABLE 26–2

Electrocardiographic Patterns

AV BLOCK	
Mobitz I	Shortened PR of first conducted beat after block
Mobitz II	No change in PR before/after block
	Periods of high-grade block
Third-degree	Fixed, rather than variable, RR interval
SUPRAVENTRICULAR TACHYCARDIAS	
AV reentrant supraventricular tachycardia	P waves obscured or buried in ST segment
AV nodal reentrant supraventricular tachycardia	P waves obscured by terminal QRS
	"Pseudo" R′ in lead V_1 during tachycardia, not sinus
Junctional ectopic tachycardia	Narrow QRS tachycardia, VA dissociation
	RR periodically shortened because of sinus capture complexes*
Atrial ectopic tachycardia	Monotonous rate, inappropriately fast
	Abnormal P-wave morphology (may be subtle)
Intraatrial reentrant tachycardia	Inappropriately fast rate, discrete P waves, variable AV conduction in postoperative congenital heart disease patient
Atrial flutter	Variable RR interval
	Rapid, sawtooth flutter waves (>280 bpm)
Atrial fibrillation	Irregular ventricular rate
	Coarse baseline with no discernible P waves
Chaotic atrial tachycardia	Three or more P-wave morphologies, irregular atrial rate, variable AV conduction (periods or atrial flutter or fibrillation common)
VENTRICULAR TACHYCARDIAS	
Monomorphic	Wide QRS for age, different from baseline
	Slurred upstroke of QRS
	Variable VA conduction†
	Sinus capture complexes†
Idiopathic types	Left bundle branch block, inferior axis (right ventricular outflow tract origin)
	Right bundle branch block, left superior axis (left ventricular septal origin)
Bidirectional	Alternating QRS axis (beat-to-beat)
Torsades de pointes	Initiation with "short-long-short" sequence
	QT-interval prolongation prior to onset
	"Twisting" of QRS axis

*Junctional ectopic tachycardia may be associated with third-degree AV block.
†Helpful when seen; absent if 1:1 VA relationship.

arrhythmia detection and storage capabilities. Familiarity with the capabilities and limitations of the specific system available is important. "Full-disclosure" capabilities can provide invaluable review of subtle physiologic changes leading up to an otherwise seemingly "sudden" arrhythmia event.

For bradycardias, the surface electrocardiogram usually is sufficient to characterize the arrhythmia and differentiate between an abnormality in sinus nodal function and AV block, based upon the ratio of atrial-to-ventricular rate. The diagnosis of tachycardias may not be feasible from the surface electrocardiogram alone. Nevertheless, a

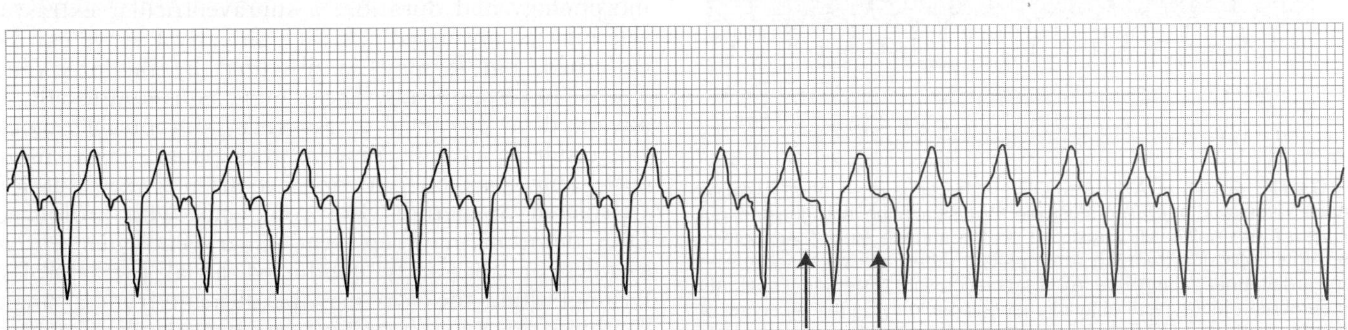

FIGURE 26–3 • Ventricular tachycardia in an 8 year old with previous muscular ventricular septal defect repair. Note transient VA block *(arrows)*, excluding a supraventricular mechanism with aberrant conduction.

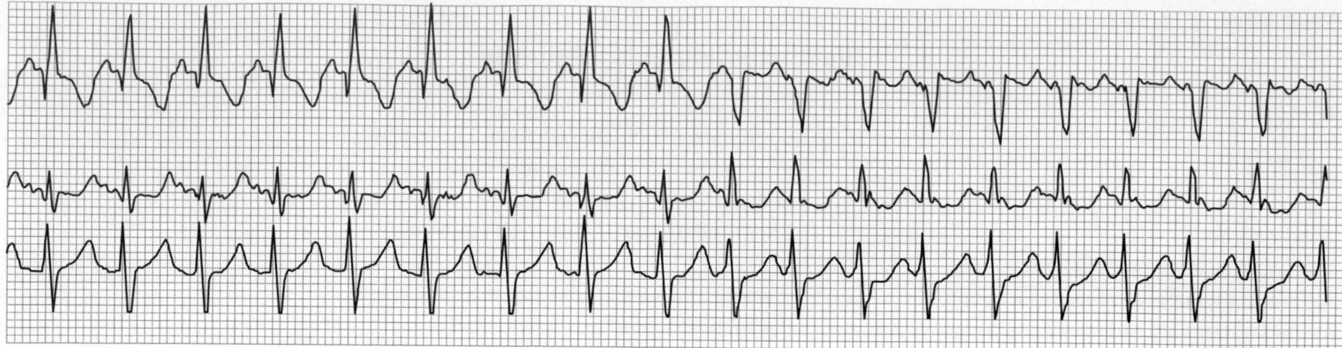

FIGURE 26–4 • Ventricular tachycardia following cardiac surgery. Note similarity between QRS complexes during sinus rhythm and ventricular in two of three recorded leads.

combination of surface electrocardiogram and simple diagnostic maneuvers, sometimes coupled with direct recording of atrial activation, should allow accurate determination of most tachycardias. As with bradycardias, the surface electrocardiogram should be inspected for the ventricular rate and regularity, QRS duration and morphology, and atrial-to-ventricular relationship. Too often the apparent atrial-to-ventricular relationship is not clearly reflected on the surface electrocardiogram, and direct atrial recording, either with temporary atrial pacing wires or an esophageal electrocardiogram, is necessary to facilitate the diagnosis (Figure 26–5).

Bradycardias

In the absence of AV block, bradycardias are characterized by the origin of the initiating impulse as sinus, atrial, junctional, or ventricular. It is important to distinguish junctional or ventricular bradycardia from sinus bradycardia with an underlying junctional or ventricular escape, respectively. Terms such as *nodal rhythm* and *dissociated* are imprecise and demand further characterization. When the atrial rate exceeds the ventricular rate, second-degree or third-degree AV block is present. In complete AV block, the resultant escape rhythm usually is regular; in second-degree AV block, the ventricular intervals vary (see Figure 26–1). Occasionally, sinus node disease and complete AV block coexist, so it is important in the setting of a slow atrial rate to note "sinus capture" complexes when appropriately timed P waves conduct to the ventricle. When atrial pacing is feasible (as in patients with recent cardiac surgery), temporary atrial pacing can be used to demonstrate normal AV conduction, and the maximum rate at which 1:1 conduction can be maintained can be easily determined and followed serially.

The distinction between bradycardia resulting from AV block and sinus nodal dysfunction may have important therapeutic implications. If AV nodal conduction is intact, it usually is most appropriate to pace the atrium only (see AAI mode) rather than perform dual-chamber pacing. In contrast, isolated AV block is best managed by sensing and tracking the intrinsic atrial rate (see DDD mode).

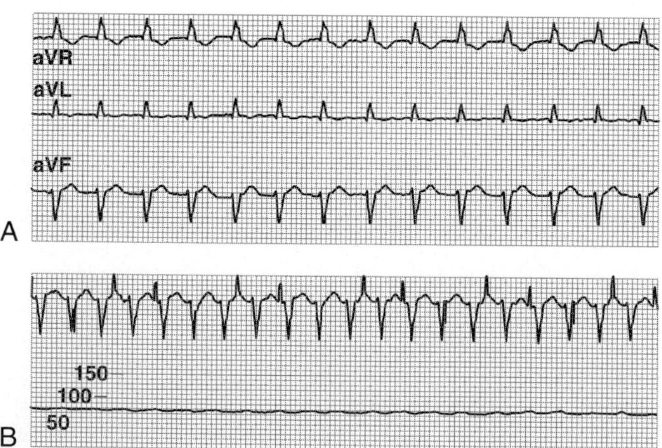

FIGURE 26–5 • **A,** Narrow QRS tachycardia in an infant following stage I Norwood operation. Possible AV dissociation is suggested, but P waves are not easily discerned on the surface electrocardiogram. **B,** Atrial recording from the same patient (after rate increased) using epicardial atrial pacing wire. AV dissociation with faster junctional rate is demonstrated, typical of junctional ectopic tachycardia. Absence of clearly shortened RR intervals because of sinus capture might indicate associated AV block.

Extrasystoles

Extrasystoles, or *premature beats*, usually are defined as supraventricular (supraventricular premature beats or premature atrial complexes) or ventricular (premature ventricular complexes, ventricular premature beats [VPBs]) in origin. True junctional extrasystoles are uncommon. When the extrasystole results in an early QRS with normal morphology and duration, a supraventricular extrasystole may be presumed. Usually, an early P wave can be discerned, but it may be obscured by the preceding T wave in certain leads. The ensuing sinus beat usually is advanced by the atrial extrasystole, but entrance block can result in a "full compensatory pause" (as is more commonly observed following a ventricular extrasystole).

Isolated premature QRS complexes with prolonged QRS duration may represent either ventricular extrasystoles or aberrantly conducted atrial extrasystoles. Distinguishing the two may be difficult from a single rhythm strip. Premature P waves often may be obscured in a particular lead, or the ventricular extrasystole morphology may appear similar to the sinus QRS in one lead (but totally dissimilar in another). The ECG features favoring ventricular extrasystoles over aberrantly conducted atrial extrasystoles include (1) wide QRS morphology, (2) a full compensatory pause, (3) presence of fusion beats, and (4) absence of a discernible premature P wave. In the setting of ventricular preexcitation, variable fusion can occur as a result of exaggerated preexcitation with premature atrial depolarizations. As noted earlier, ventricular extrasystoles usually are followed by a full compensatory pause because the sinus node is not reset by the ventricular depolarization. However, an atrial extrasystole may sometimes fail to reset the sinus node (because of entrance block) or a ventricular extrasystole may occasionally reset the sinus node because of retrograde (VA) conduction. The simultaneous occurrence of both narrow QRS and wide QRS extrasystoles usually favors normally and aberrantly conducted atrial extrasystoles, particularly when the QRS width varies with the degree of prematurity (excluding fusion complexes).

The distinction of atrial versus ventricular extrasystoles may be somewhat academic in otherwise asymptomatic individuals because neither generally warrants therapy. However, either might be a harbinger for underlying myocardial irritability and should prompt a search for underlying causes. Occasionally, measures to suppress ectopy may appear to improve cardiac output by "regularizing" filling time in an otherwise tenuous patient. The relative advantages and risks of any such measure, whether achieved with medications or temporary pacing, need to be considered individually.

Tachycardias with Normal QRS

By definition, all tachycardias with normal QRS represent either sinus tachycardia or a form of SVT. It should be noted that the terms "supraventricular tachycardia" (SVT)," "paroxysmal supraventricular tachycardia" (PSVT), and "paroxysmal atrial tachycardia" (PAT) often are used in reference to tachycardias with normal QRS, a regular rate in excess of 200 bpm, and no readily discernible P waves. In otherwise healthy infants, children, and adolescents, these features usually result from either AV reentrant tachycardia or AVNRT (Figure 26–6). Further distinction between these two mechanisms has little impact on acute management. However, in the ICU setting, primary atrial tachycardias (including sinus tachycardia) and junctional tachycardias also must be considered (particularly following cardiac surgery). Abnormal P-wave morphology (determined by 12-lead electrocardiogram), PR interval greater than 50% of the RR interval, or completely obscured P waves favor a nonsinus mechanism. Finally, the QRS duration may appear normal by adult standards but be significantly prolonged for age.

In young patients, intraatrial reentry, atrial flutter, and atrial fibrillation usually are seen following surgical treatment for congenital heart defects involving the atrium (atrial septal defects, atrial repair of transposition of the great arteries, or the Fontan operation).[11] The sawtooth pattern typical of atrial flutter may be absent in these patients, and the term *intraatrial reentrant tachycardia* (IART) may be more appropriate when discrete P waves

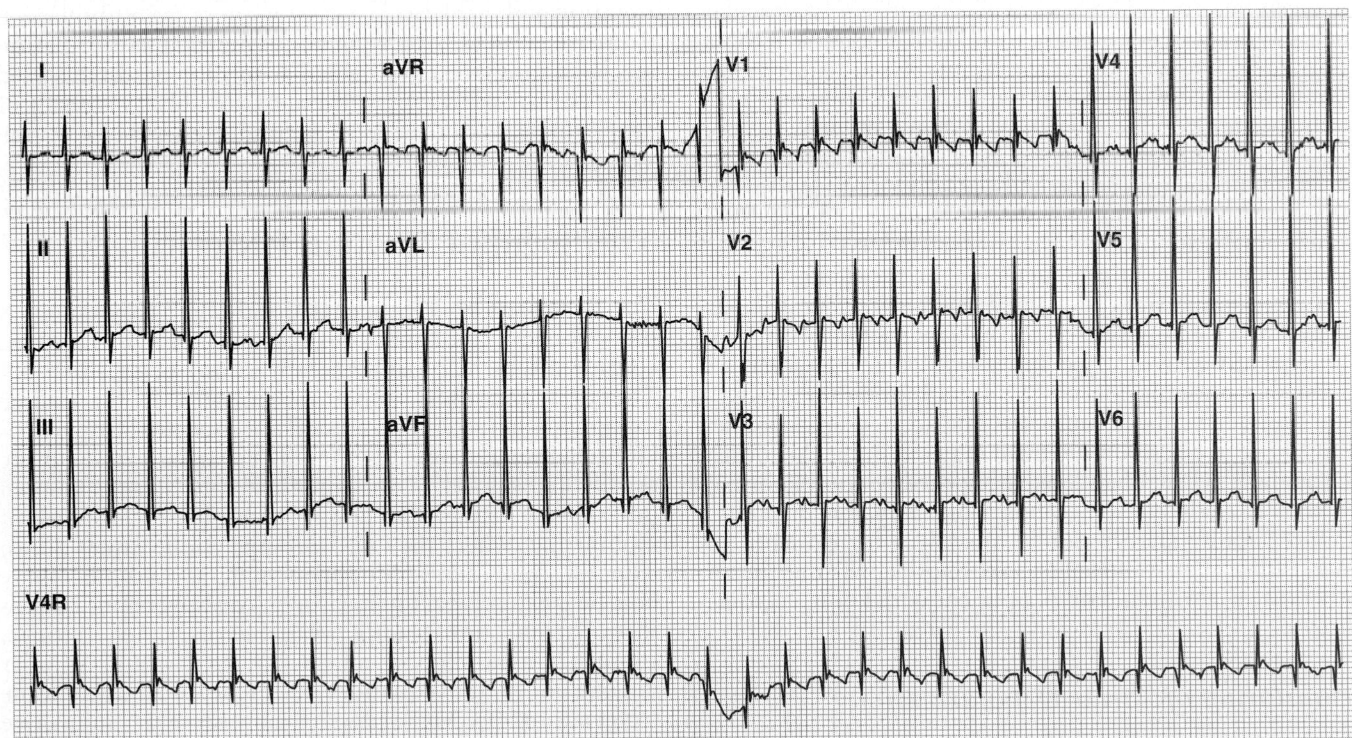

FIGURE 26–6 • Supraventricular tachycardia resulting from AV nodal reentry in an infant. Although considerably less common than orthodromic reciprocating tachycardia in this age group, the P wave on the terminal portion of the QRS complex results in a "pseudo rSr′ pattern." During sinus rhythm, this terminal deflection on the QRS was absent, and the transesophageal recording confirmed the mechanism.

are present. Because the atrial rate often is relatively slow in comparison to "typical" atrial flutter, a high index of suspicion is required. In some cases, the atrial rate is slow enough that consistent 1:1 conduction (with discrete P waves) further obscures the diagnosis by simulating sinus tachycardia. Similarly, with 2:1 conduction, alternate P waves may be obscured by the T wave, giving the impression of sinus rhythm.

Distinguishing sinus tachycardia from various types of SVT may be difficult. The appropriateness and variation of the rate (or lack thereof) may be particularly helpful in differentiating sinus from nonsinus tachycardias. Observing the heart rate response to interventions such as volume expansion, analgesia, antipyretics, and catecholamine infusions often is helpful. Depending on the pattern of atrial activation, P waves may even simulate a normal sinus P-wave morphology during primary atrial tachycardias. In other cases, AV conduction may appear to be 1:1 on the surface electrocardiogram when, in fact, a second P wave is obscured by the QRS complex or T wave. Direct atrial recordings using transesophageal electrocardiography or temporary epicardial atrial pacing wires usually facilitate the diagnosis (see Figure 26–5B). Vagal maneuvers or administration of adenosine to interrupt AV conduction transiently often helps characterize the true AV relationship and determine whether the AV node participates in the tachycardia mechanism.

Tachycardias with Prolonged QRS

Generally, tachycardias with prolonged QRS should be presumed to be ventricular tachycardias until or unless evidence of an alternative diagnosis is demonstrated. VA dissociation, the hallmark ECG feature of ventricular tachycardia, may not be seen in childhood because of rapid retrograde conduction over the AV node (see Figure 26–3). The distinction between ventricular tachycardia and SVT with aberrant conduction can be difficult and may require invasive electrophysiologic study. Prolonged attempts to differentiate the two at the bedside by noninvasive means often are fruitless and may delay treatment. The wrong conclusion may prompt inappropriate and potentially dangerous therapeutic maneuvers. In the acute setting, treatment based on a presumed diagnosis of ventricular tachycardia is rarely deleterious, even when the mechanism subsequently proves to be supraventricular. However, an erroneous presumption of "SVT with aberrant conduction" may have disastrous consequences. When feasible, a full 12-lead electrocardiogram may aid in the diagnosis, particularly when a baseline electrocardiogram in normal rhythm is available for comparison. Apparent hemodynamic stability should not be mistaken for evidence of SVT rather than ventricular tachycardia, whether in an otherwise healthy child or in a patient with known cardiac disease.

Monitoring of Atrial Depolarization

When the AV relationship during a tachycardia is unclear, sometimes it can be inferred indirectly by other available monitoring. Invasive arterial and venous pressure waveforms can help define atrial contractile action in some situations. For example, cannon A waves commonly are noted in patients with atrial flutter or JET.

Direct recording of atrial activity is necessary when the AV relationship cannot be determined from the surface electrocardiogram or otherwise inferred by the means described. Patients recovering from cardiac surgery frequently have temporary atrial epicardial pacing wires in place that can be used to record atrial electrograms directly while simultaneously recording the surface electrocardiogram (see Figure 26–5B). Attachment of the atrial wires to a unipolar precordial lead ("V lead") on the monitor is an easy way to observe atrial activation. Otherwise, atrial activity can be readily recorded with a bipolar esophageal catheter inserted in the esophagus behind the left atrium.

Diagnostic Uses of Adenosine

Although most widely used as an acute therapy for terminating SVT involving the AV node, adenosine administration also may yield important diagnostic clues to the underlying arrhythmia mechanism.[12] By producing transient block in the AV node during tachycardia, it often is possible to distinguish AV reentrant tachycardias and AVNRTs (either of which should terminate) from atrial tachycardias and ventricular tachycardias. However, adenosine's effects are not confined to the AV node. Ectopic (automatic) atrial and junctional tachycardias, intraatrial reentry, and certain ventricular tachycardias also may terminate with adenosine. Extreme caution should be taken when administering adenosine during wide QRS tachycardia. Adenosine produces vasodilatation, which theoretically can result in hemodynamic deterioration and tachycardia acceleration, or even fibrillation, if tachycardia fails to terminate. Ventricular fibrillation has been rarely observed when adenosine is administered in the setting of WPW syndrome, probably as a result of atrial fibrillation that then is conducted rapidly to the ventricles.

Treatment of Rhythm Disturbances

The approach to treatment of cardiac arrhythmias is influenced by the clinical setting, but several important considerations help guide therapy in any given situation. The first and most important concern is the degree of hemodynamic compromise associated with a particular arrhythmia. Minor rhythm disturbances may be more readily recognized in the intensive care setting than in other usual situations simply because of the level of monitoring, where they may prompt undue attention. In contrast, potentially life-threatening arrhythmias may best be treated by acute measures (cardioversion, temporary pacing) not readily available in other settings. Extracorporeal support and assist devices add another dimension to the equation. Extracorporeal membrane oxygenation (ECMO) support may serve as adjunctive therapy for refractory arrhythmias, whereas other modes of support (assist device, balloon pump) may require a regular rhythm for appropriate coordination of the device with spontaneous cardiac activity.

A second important consideration in critically ill patients, particularly those undergoing cardiac surgery, is to favor therapies that maintain appropriate AV synchrony. In the setting of marginal hemodynamics, an otherwise acceptable ventricular rate during arrhythmias such as atrial tachycardias and fibrillation, junctional tachycardia, or AV block may further compromise cardiac output as a result of loss of AV synchrony (see Figure 26–4).

A third facet of the management of arrhythmias in this setting is the recognition that many arrhythmias in the ICU are iatrogenic. Even minor arrhythmias may herald more serious issues, such as electrolyte disturbances, acidosis, subendocardial ischemia, excessive catecholamine infusions, or increased intracranial pressure. It is important to identify and correct any such underlying causes because therapies directed at the rhythm itself may not protect from more serious rhythm decompensation.

Finally, whenever feasible, acute and short-term measures with limited potential to impair hemodynamics should generally be favored over chronic therapies. Thus nonpharmacologic therapies, such as pacing or cardioversion, or ultrashort-acting drugs, such as adenosine and esmolol, may be preferable over chronic antiarrhythmic therapy. Whether chronic therapy is warranted for a given arrhythmia is determined more by its underlying mechanism, clinical setting, and frequency than by the severity of the arrhythmias encountered in the intensive care setting. Before beginning chronic antiarrhythmic therapy, consultation with a cardiologist versed in the spectrum of arrhythmias seen in childhood is advisable. The impact of acute measures on chronic arrhythmia management becomes increasingly crucial with the emergence of amiodarone use in the ICU and the increasing availability of nonpharmacologic therapies such as radiofrequency catheter ablation and implantable defibrillators for a broader spectrum of arrhythmias and patient populations.[13–15]

Bradycardia Therapies

Whenever treatment is instituted for a rhythm disturbance, an underlying cause should be sought. This is especially important in the treatment of bradycardias occurring in the intensive care setting, where airway compromise and respiratory insufficiency probably are the most common causes of acute bradycardias. Increased intracranial pressure, hypothermia, or iatrogenic causes also may produce bradycardias that require specific interventions beyond those outlined here. Emergency interventions for AV nodal and sinus nodal dysfunction are essentially identical.

Pharmacologic Treatment of Bradycardias

After appropriate confirmation or restoration of airway integrity and ventilatory function, initial treatment of symptomatic bradycardias usually is pharmacologic whether the cause is sinus node slowing or AV nodal block. Atropine (0.01–0.04 mg/kg intravenously or, if necessary, intramuscularly or via endotracheal tube) may transiently ameliorate the bradycardic effects of hypoxia (or other vagal stimulants), digoxin, intracranial hypertension, or AV block as a result of Lyme disease. Atropine is less likely to reverse bradycardic effects of beta-blocking agents or other antiarrhythmic drugs, particularly in the setting of underlying sinus node disease. Epinephrine (0.1 μg/kg) can be administered by various routes to accelerate the heart rate. Continuous infusions of epinephrine (0.05–0.5 μg/kg/min) or isoproterenol (0.02–0.2 μg/kg/min) may be instituted. In general, high-dose epinephrine or isoproterenol infusions should be replaced by temporary pacing as soon as feasible. Even if lower doses of these agents prove adequate, temporary pacing should be available as backup. Occasionally, methylxanthines are useful as an alternative to pacing for nonlethal bradycardias.

Temporary and Permanent Pacing for Bradycardias

Pacing is an essential adjunct to medical management of arrhythmias in the ICU. Several reviews of pacing in children are available.[16–18] Pacing can be accomplished using permanently implanted pacemaker and lead systems, temporary leads attached to the heart at the time of cardiac surgery or passed through the venous system to the heart, a lead passed into the esophagus to stimulate the atrium, or transcutaneous patches to stimulate the ventricle. Most pacing is performed for bradyarrhythmias, although temporary pacing may be used to terminate reentrant tachyarrhythmias. Examination of atrial electrograms obtained from epicardial, transvenous, or esophageal pacing leads can be helpful in diagnosing arrhythmias.

Principles of Pacing

All pacing requires a complete circuit with at least one lead on or near each chamber that is to be paced. Often, two leads are placed on each chamber (bipolar leads), although sometimes only the cathode is attached to the heart (unipolar leads), with a subcutaneous electrode acting as the anode. The metal can of a permanent pacemaker also can serve as the anode. The intensity of the pacing stimulus is related to the stimulus duration (pulse width) and its amplitude, which can be expressed either as current (mA) or voltage (V). Energy is proportional to the pulse width and the square of the amplitude. Most temporary pacemakers provide a fixed pulse width, with an adjustable current output (mA). Permanent pacemakers generally have both an adjustable pulse width and an adjustable amplitude.

Sensing of intrinsic activity of the heart is important to prevent pacing at inappropriate times. The sensitivity of permanent and temporary pacers is adjustable. The sensitivity setting (mV) actually refers to a sensing threshold for detection of spontaneous cardiac activity. The spontaneous activity must exceed that threshold to be detected. Thus a lower numeric sensitivity setting makes the pacemaker more sensitive to both spontaneous activity of the atrium or ventricle (appropriate sensing) and other electrical signals (oversensing).

The timing circuits of the pacemaker determine when the pacemaker fires and its response to sensed events.

A simplification of the North American Society of Pacing and Electrophysiology/British Pacing and Electrophysiology Group (NASPE/BPEG) pacing code uses three letters to describe pacing modes.[19] The first two letters refer to the chamber(s) paced and chamber(s) sensed, respectively (A, atrium; V, ventricle; D, dual). The third letter refers to the response to sensed events (I, inhibit; T, trigger; D, dual). Thus a single-chamber atrial or ventricular pacing demand mode is AAI or VVI mode, whereas dual-chamber pacing is generally DDD mode. In evaluating and adjusting pacemakers, it is helpful to think in terms of intervals rather than rates. Because there are 60,000 ms in 1 minute, to convert a rate (bpm) to an interval (ms) you must divide 60,000 by the rate. For example, a rate of 100 bpm corresponds to an interval of 600 ms. Thus for a ventricular demand (VVI) pacemaker programmed to a rate of 100, the pacemaker stimulates the ventricle 600 ms after the previous paced or sensed ventricular beat unless there is another sensed ventricular beat. If there is another sensed ventricular beat, the pacemaker output is inhibited and another interval of 600 ms is started. Similarly, for dual-chamber pacing with an AV interval of 150 ms, the ventricle is paced 150 ms after an atrial paced or sensed beat unless a ventricular sensed beat occurs during that interval.

Temporary Pacing

In the pediatric ICU, temporary pacing is most commonly used in patients after surgical treatment of congenital heart disease. At the time of operation, most surgeons place temporary epicardial pacing wires on the atria and ventricles of patients undergoing open repair of congenital heart disease. These wires can be used to maintain AV synchrony if there is AV block or to pace the atrium if there is sinus nodal dysfunction. Temporarily attaching an atrial wire to one of the leads of the bedside monitor can facilitate observation of atrial activity, which helps in the diagnosis of tachyarrhythmias such as JET. Atrial burst pacing can be used to terminate reentrant supraventricular arrhythmias such as IART, AVNRT, and ORT. Pace termination of ORT is shown in Figure 26–7. Although JET generally cannot be terminated with burst pacing, atrial pacing at a rate faster than the JET rate often improves hemodynamics by allowing AV synchrony until the JET resolves or is pharmacologically controlled (Figure 26–8).

In patients who do not have temporary epicardial pacing wires, transcutaneous pacing can be performed using specially designed pads applied to the chest. In general, transcutaneous pacing is used only for a short time while a temporary transvenous pacing lead is placed. Often the quickest and easiest method is to place a transvenous lead from the internal jugular or subclavian approach, although they also can be placed from a femoral venous approach using fluoroscopy. Temporary pacing leads can be passively positioned with or without fluoroscopy, usually with an inflatable balloon similar to positioning a Swan-Ganz catheter. A temporary active-fixation lead can be placed under direct fluoroscopy, allowing more secure positioning and the choice of pacing the atrium, the ventricle, or both (in dual-chamber mode).

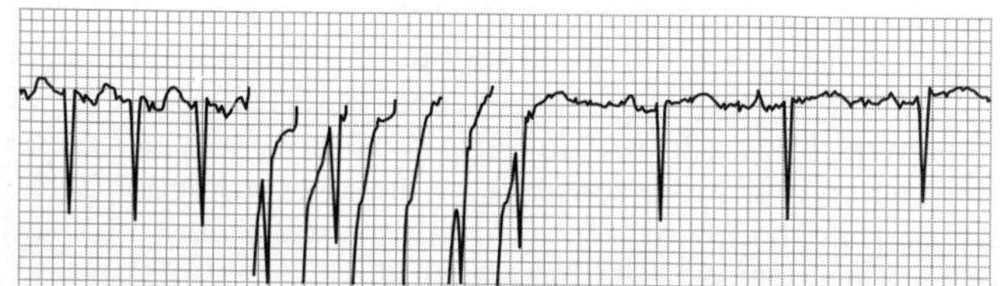

FIGURE 26–7 • Pace termination of orthodromic reciprocating tachycardia with a burst of atrial pacing.

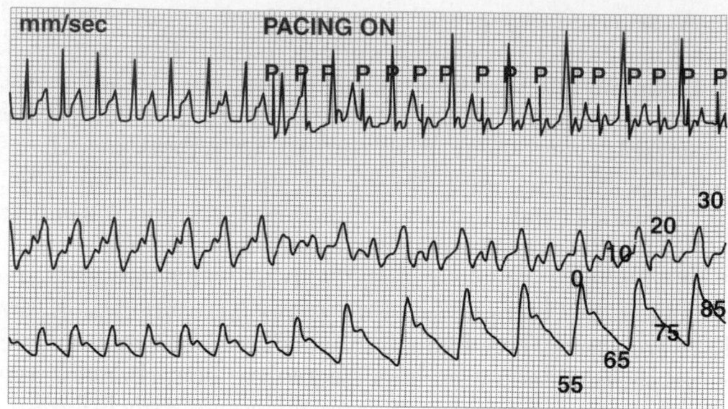

FIGURE 26–8 • Junctional ectopic tachycardia with hypotension immediately improved with faster atrial pacing (in this case, resulting in 2:1 AV block and AV synchrony).

Setting Temporary Pacing Parameters

For single-chamber atrial (AAI) or ventricular (VVI) demand pacing, the pacemaker usually is initially set at a rate higher than the patient's intrinsic atrial or ventricular rate. The pacemaker's output expressed in mA (current) or V (voltage) is gradually reduced until there is loss of capture and then is increased again. The lowest output that captures the chamber being paced is known as the *pacing threshold*. Usually, the output is set at twice the threshold output. The pacemaker rate is lowered to a rate below the intrinsic rate of the chamber being paced, unless the patient is hemodynamically unstable at that rate. The pacemaker should indicate that it is sensing the intrinsic atrial or ventricular activity, usually with a blinking indicator light. The sensitivity of the pacemaker is adjusted to higher numeric settings (less sensitive) until the pacemaker stops sensing the intrinsic activity. The sensitivity then is reduced to a lower numeric value (more sensitive). The highest numeric value at which the pacemaker senses appropriately is known as the *sensing threshold*. Ideally, the sensitivity is set to a numeric value that is half the sensing threshold, but this is not always possible, especially for temporary atrial leads. Failure to sense can result in inappropriate pacing, which can induce tachyarrhythmias. Figure 26–9 shows a single inappropriate atrial stimulus initiating sustained ORT.

Dual-chamber pacing is more complex. The atrial and ventricular sensitivity and output are set using basically the same process described for single-chamber pacing. In addition to setting the low rate of the pacemaker, you

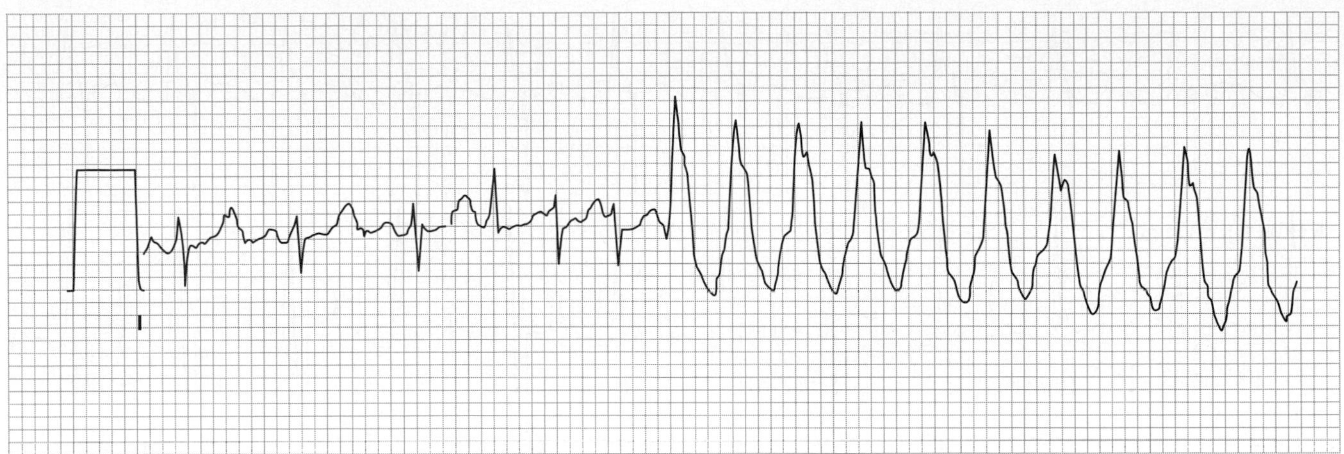

FIGURE 26–9 • Initiation of orthodromic reciprocating tachycardia with a single atrial paced beat that falls at a vulnerable time. After several narrow-complex beats, bundle branch block in tachycardia results in a wide-complex rhythm.

must set several other timing parameters, including the upper tracking limit (UTL), the AV delay, and the postventricular atrial refractory period (PVARP). UTL defines the fastest rate at which the pacemaker will pace the ventricle. PVARP refers to a period after a ventricular paced event during which the pacemaker is refractory to atrial sensed events and ignores any spontaneous atrial beats. The pacemaker is also refractory to spontaneous atrial events during the AV interval. Thus the total atrial refractory period (TARP) includes both the AV interval and the PVARP. Although TARP is not a programmable parameter (it is the sum of the programmed AV interval and the programmed PVARP), it is an important concept for understanding high rate behavior.

If the spontaneous atrial cycle length (60,000 ms/min divided by the spontaneous atrial rate in bpm) is less than the TARP, only half of the spontaneous atrial beats will be sensed, resulting in 2:1 block. The point at which this occurs is known as the *2:1 block rate*. Abrupt 2:1 block is generally an undesirable situation, so most temporary pacemakers will not allow the UTL to be set above the 2:1 block rate. Thus before increasing the UTL, it often is necessary to shorten the AV interval or the PVARP. If the atrial rate exceeds the UTL, the ventricular output will be delayed, producing a rhythm that resembles Wenckebach AV conduction, known as *pacemaker Wenckebach*. It is important to remember that pacemaker Wenckebach is a desirable response to high atrial rates. The alternatives, tracking rapid atrial rates 1:1 and abrupt 2:1 ventricular tracking of the atrium, are more likely to cause hemodynamic compromise. Occasionally appropriate pacemaker Wenckebach is mistaken for failure to sense the atrium or failure to pace the ventricle. Figure 26–10 shows 1:1 conduction, 2:1 block, and pacemaker Wenckebach at different pacemaker settings in a patient with a dual-chamber pacemaker for high-grade AV block.

When initiating dual-chamber pacing, it is important to be sure that the atrial lead senses appropriately and that the rates, intervals, and refractory periods are set appropriately to allow the pacemaker to track the spontaneous atrial rate. If the intrinsic atrial activity is not appropriately sensed and the dual-chamber temporary pacemaker's low rate is lower than the patient's intrinsic atrial rate, you may falsely assume that dual-chamber pacing is occurring when it is not. The presence of cannon A waves on the central venous pressure tracing may provide a clue that AV synchrony is not occurring. Reversing the atrial leads, lowering the numeric atrial sensitivity, or adjusting the AV interval, UTL, or PVARP may remedy this situation. If the atrium still cannot be sensed appropriately, setting the pacemaker's low rate higher than the patient's own atrial rate will allow AV synchrony. In effect, you are pacing in DVI mode, pacing atrium and ventricle, sensing the ventricle, and inhibiting pacemaker output when spontaneous ventricular beats occur. Older temporary dual-chamber pacemakers offered only DVI mode; newer devices allow true DDD pacing as long as atrial sensing can occur.

Occasionally, you may see a reentrant arrhythmia known as *pacemaker-mediated tachycardia* (PMT), in which a DDD pacemaker senses the atrium and paces the ventricle, with the patient's own AV node conducting the impulse up from the ventricle to the atrium and the cycle repeating again. Thus the pacemaker acts as the antegrade limb of the reentrant circuit, while the patient's own AV node acts as the retrograde limb. Usually, you can avoid PMT with careful adjustment of the pacemaker's AV interval and PVARP. Acutely, you usually can terminate PMT by placing a magnet over the pacemaker, which makes the pacemaker pace asynchronously, ignoring any sensed events, thus interrupting the antegrade limb of the reentrant circuit. Figure 26–11 shows initiation of PMT by loss of atrial capture with termination of the tachycardia by a spontaneous ventricular beat.

Permanent Pacing

The two most common indications for permanent pacing are high-grade AV block and sinus nodal dysfunction. AV block may be congenital or acquired, with surgical damage to the conduction system the most common cause of acquired AV block. In patients with surgical AV block, there may be recovery of normal conduction with resolution of edema. In general, permanent pacing is not

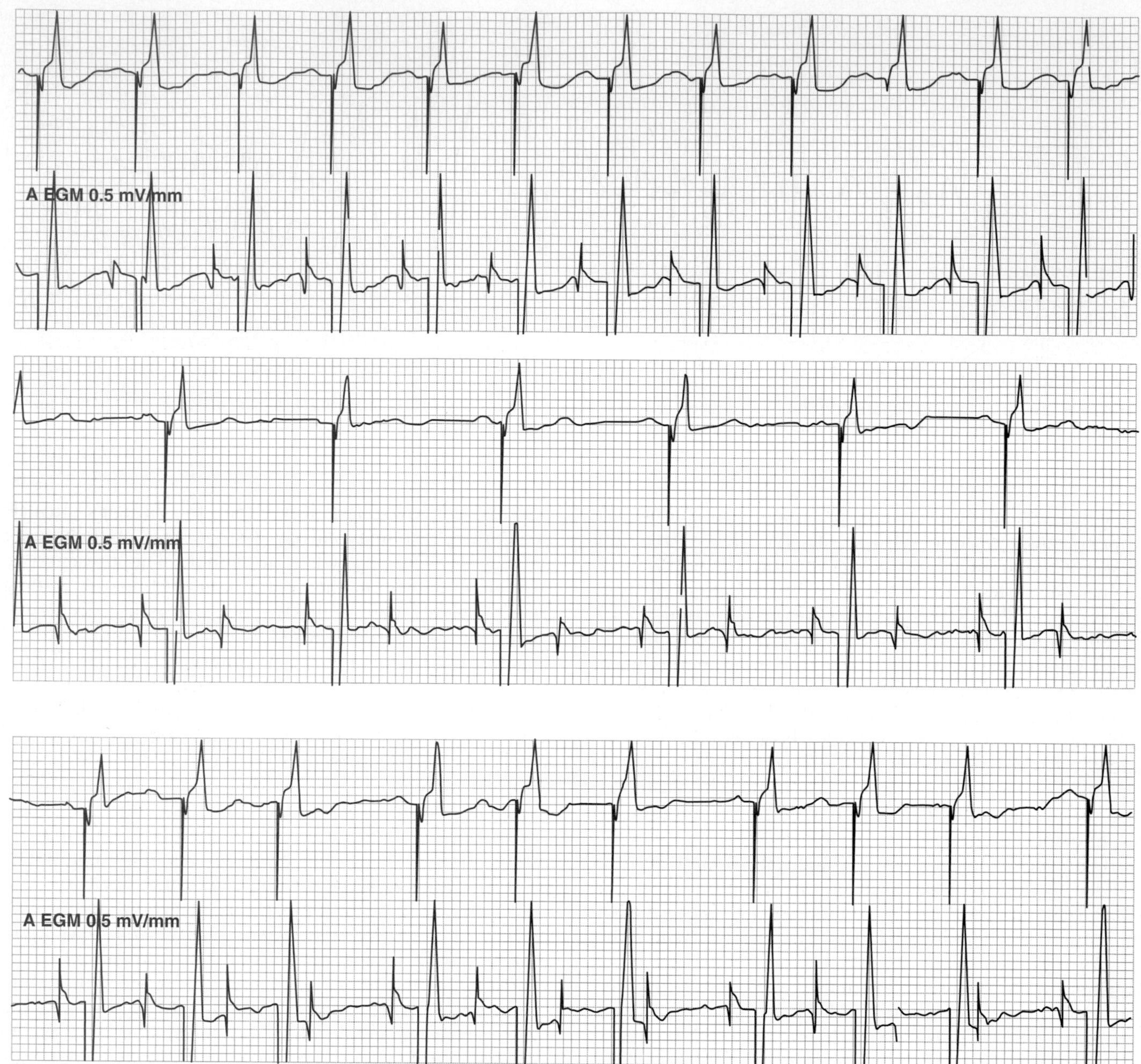

FIGURE 26–10 • Examples of pacemaker high-rate behavior. Each panel shows a surface electrocardiogram with the simultaneous atrial electrogram below. **Top,** 1:1 Atrioventricular conduction. Each sensed atrial event falls outside the total atrial refractory period, resulting in a corresponding paced ventricular event. **Middle,** 2:1 Block occurs when the total atrial refractory period exceeds the spontaneous atrial cycle length. Every other atrial beat falls within the refractory period and fails to trigger a ventricular pacing stimulus. **Bottom,** "Pacemaker Wenckebach" operation occurs when the atrial rate reaches the upper tracking rate. Gradual lengthening of the AV delay ensures that the ventricular pacing does not occur above the upper tracking rate. Eventually, an atrial sensed event falls within the refractory period so that a ventricular pacing stimulus is not triggered. All three recordings were obtained in the same patient over a short period by adjusting the programmable pacemaker parameters. (From Sliz NB Jr, Johns JA. *Cardiol Rev* 8:223-239, 2000.)

recommended unless there has been no recovery for 7 to 14 days.[20] Occasionally, if the surgeon is confident that the conduction system has been permanently damaged or if temporary pacing is not reliable, permanent pacemakers may be implanted before 7 days after the initial injury. Elective pacing for congenital AV block in the first decade of life usually is prompted by symptoms, low ventricular rates, or ventricular ectopy. Elective pacing is commonly recommended in the second decade of life even for asymptomatic patients with congenital heart block, based on studies showing that the first symptom in teenagers and adults may be catastrophic.[21] Pacing for sinus nodal dysfunction is most commonly performed in patients with structural heart disease, usually following extensive atrial surgery such as Fontan operation or atrial repair of transposition of the great arteries.

In older children and adults, transvenous pacing is the preferred route for pacing because of better pacing

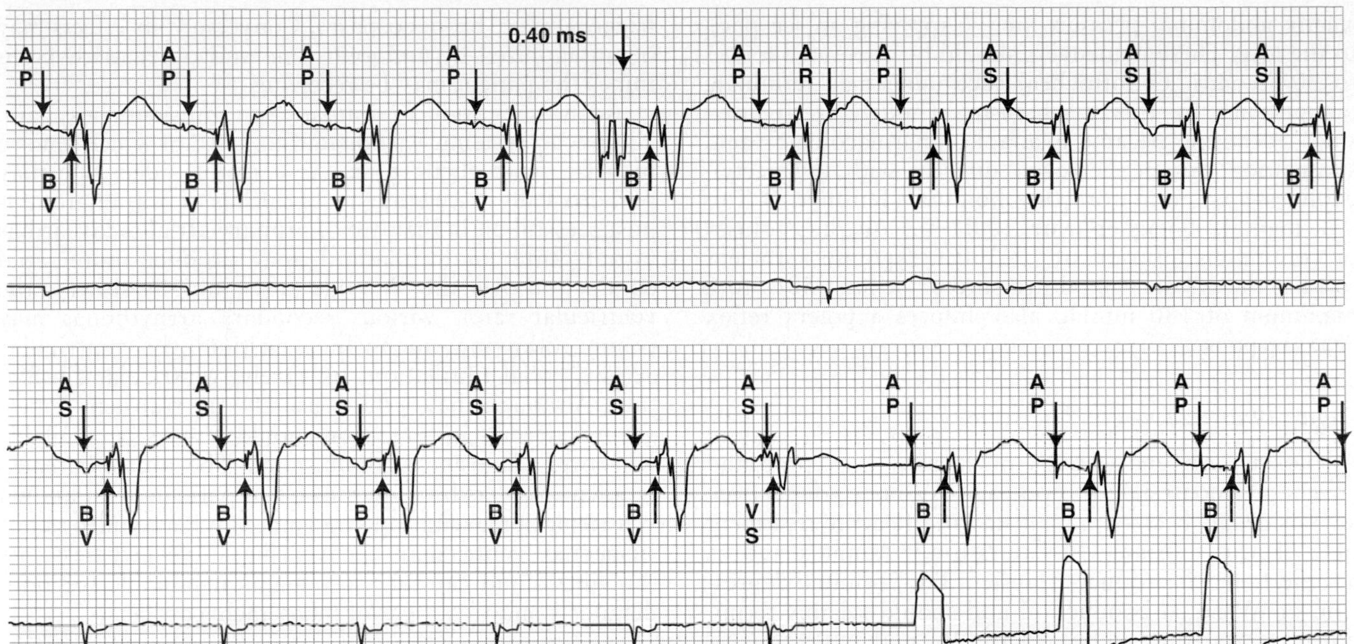

FIGURE 26–11 • Initiation and termination of pacemaker-mediated tachycardia. **Top,** Two atrial pacing stimuli fail to capture, followed by ventriculoatrial conduction of a ventricular paced beat. The resulting atrial beat *(AS)* is sensed and triggers another ventricular beat, and the process repeats. Had the retrograde atrial beat occurred during the postventricular atrial refractory period, it would not have triggered a ventricular paced beat. **Bottom,** Spontaneous ventricular beat inhibits the ventricular pacing, terminating the process. Atrial electrogram tracings are shown at the **bottom** of each panel. *AP,* Atrial pace; *AR,* atrial refractory; *BV,* biventricular pace; *VS,* ventricular sense.

thresholds, easier lead placement, and lower susceptibility to lead fractures than with epicardial leads. In younger children, however, concern about venous occlusion in a patient who will require many decades of pacing often favors placement of epicardial pacemaker leads. The development of epicardial leads that elute a small amount of dexamethasone appears to improve epicardial lead performance,[22] although epicardial lead fractures remain a concerning problem. In patients requiring a lifetime of pacing, various approaches to allow atrial and ventricular pacing are commonly needed (Figure 26–12).

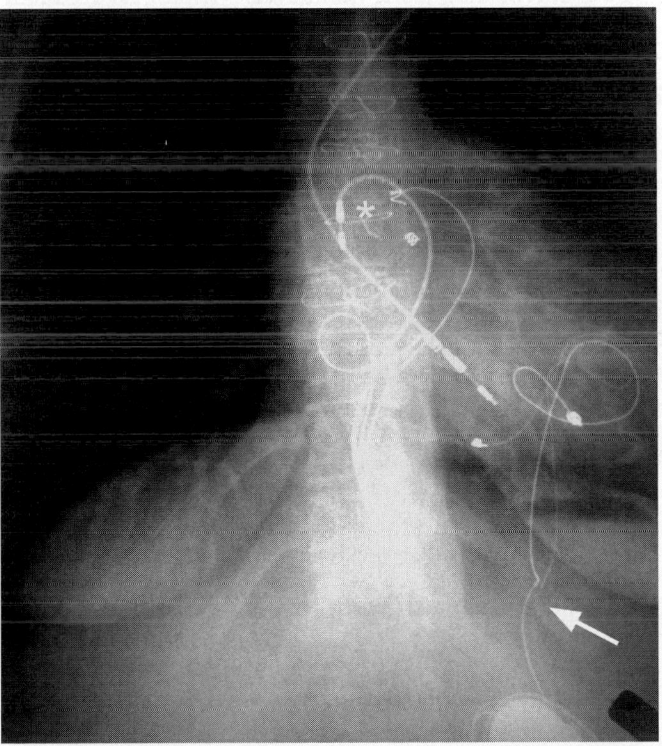

FIGURE 26–12 • Chest x-ray film of a patient with many abandoned pacing leads. There is a bipolar transvenous lead with the tip in the right ventricle. Another bipolar transvenous lead has been used as an epicardial atrial lead *(asterisk).* There are two screw-in epicardial leads, one atrial and one ventricular. The atrial lead has a fractured electrode. There are two other types of epicardial leads more toward the apex, one of which is fractured *(arrow),* and the other of which is kinked. Only the kinked lead is functional. (From Sliz NB Jr, Johns JA. *Cardiol Rev* 8:223-239, 2000.)

Newer Indications for Pacing

Data on adults have suggested that biventricular pacing, with independent stimulation of the right and left ventricles, improves ventricular function in patients with heart failure. Limited data are available in the pediatric population. Ventricular pacing also has been suggested to be helpful in patients with hypertrophic cardiomyopathy.

Tachycardia Therapies

Vagal Maneuvers

"Vagal maneuvers" once were the most commonly used intervention for terminating SVTs. They occasionally terminate ventricular tachycardias as well. Mechanical maneuvers such as the Valsalva maneuver or carotid sinus massage usually produce effective vagal stimulation beyond infancy. In infants, a similar reflex vagal response sometimes can be elicited by applying firm, steady abdominal pressure or by applying an ice pack to the face. These maneuvers should be attempted for 15 to 30 seconds. Endotracheal suctioning may terminate tachycardias by this mechanism. Though rarely used since adenosine became available, pharmacologic vagal stimulation can be achieved directly with the acetylcholinesterase inhibitor edrophonium (Tensilon, 0.1 to 0.2 mg/kg). Phenylephrine (0.01–0.1 mg/kg boluses or continuous infusion of 10–100 μg/kg/min) sufficient to raise the systolic blood pressure by at least 50% to a maximum of 180 mmHg also induces a potent reflex vagal response.

Acute Pharmacologic Therapies

Adenosine. An endogenous nucleoside with profound effects on sinoatrial (SA) node and AV node conduction, adenosine has become a mainstay in the acute treatment of SVT with normal QRS duration.[12] Administered as a rapid bolus, it produces transient but profound depression of AV nodal conduction and should reliably terminate reciprocating tachycardias (AV nodal reentry, AV reentry). Although less commonly recognized, adenosine also may interrupt AV reentry by directly blocking accessory pathway conduction.

Given the prevalence of AV reentry and AV nodal reentry among otherwise healthy young patients, adenosine often is advocated for wide QRS tachycardias as a therapeutic and/or diagnostic maneuver.[21] Its effects are mediated through specific membrane receptors coupled to inhibitory G proteins modulating K channel function. These receptors are found not only in the AV and SA nodes but also on atrial myocytes. It usually causes transient AV block without terminating most primary atrial tachycardias but instead may transiently suppress atrial automatic tachycardias (ectopic atrial or junctional) and occasionally may terminate intraatrial reentrant tachycardias. Certain ventricular tachycardias may be adenosine sensitive, particularly those originating because of abnormal triggering in the right ventricular outflow tract.

Adenosine must be administered rapidly (50–250 μg/kg) because of rapid metabolism by erythrocytes. If tachycardia is not terminated, determination must be made of whether a larger dose is warranted, the dose was given too slowly, or VA or AV conduction was altered without terminating tachycardia (see discussion on diagnosis). Therefore it is important to record an ECG strip during adenosine administration so that important diagnostic or therapeutic clues are not missed. Because of its brief effect (half-life 8–10 seconds), tachycardias sometimes immediately reinitiate following successful termination. If they do, readministration of the same dose should be attempted rather than increasing the dose further.

In addition to effects on the AV node, adenosine can produce sinus arrest, which may be prolonged in the setting of intrinsic SA nodal dysfunction, in the presence of drugs that interfere with its metabolism such as dipyridamole and diazepam, or with drugs that may exaggerate its effects, such as class I, II, or III antiarrhythmic drugs. High doses should not be used indiscriminately in these situations. Its usage in patients with reactive airway disease may be problematic because adenosine occasionally triggers severe bronchospasm. Conversely, its effects may be antagonized by aminophylline and other methylxanthines the patient may be receiving.

Adenosine produces dramatic but transient chest pain, along with systemic vasodilatation, both of which tend to increase sympathetic tone. As a result, adenosine may paradoxically accelerate tachycardias if termination is unsuccessful or, in the case of primary atrial tachycardias (atrial flutter or fibrillation), may produce more rapid conduction over the AV node (after initially slowing the ventricular rate). Various secondary arrhythmias may occur following adenosine, particularly ventricular ectopy, atrial fibrillation, or, rarely, ventricular fibrillation. Although these effects usually are transient, emergency external cardioversion should always be available whenever adenosine is administered. The appropriateness of adenosine has been questioned in patients with known ventricular preexcitation syndromes (WPW syndrome) or suspected ventricular tachycardias. Nevertheless, its thoughtful and careful use remains invaluable for both diagnosis and treatment of many tachycardias.

Antiarrhythmic agents

Selection and Classes of Drug Action. The addition of pharmacologic agents following adenosine administration should be guided by the clinical situation, known or suspected tachycardia mechanism, and response to adenosine administration. In some cases (wide QRS tachycardia or hemodynamically compromised patients), it may be most appropriate to proceed directly to pacing termination or cardioversion if adenosine is unsuccessful in restoring sinus rhythm. In other instances, acute antiarrhythmic drug therapy may be warranted.[23]

Antitachycardia drugs usually are classified according to their surface ECG effects, which often correlate closely with their cellular electrophysiologic effects. The Vaughan Williams classification divides drugs into those that block cardiac sodium channels (class I), block beta-adrenoreceptors (class II), prolong repolarization (class III), and block calcium channels (class IV). Digoxin and adenosine, which are not included in this classification scheme, exert their primary antiarrhythmic effects on the AV node. Magnesium also has depressant effects on the AV node and suppresses early and late afterdepolarizations (triggered activity). Many of the available drugs manifest properties of more than one class, which contribute collectively to their antiarrhythmic action.[24]

In general, class I drugs (particularly IA and IC) slow conduction in atrial, ventricular, or accessory pathway tissue and class III drugs increase refractoriness in these same tissues. Class IA drugs usually accomplish both effects. β-Adrenergic antagonists, calcium channel antagonists, digoxin, and adenosine act primarily by slowing AV nodal conduction or inhibiting abnormal automaticity. Thus the latter group of drugs is primarily used for reciprocating tachycardias using the AV node (ART, ORT, AVNRT) or to induce second-degree AV block during a primary atrial tachycardia. In contrast, class IA, IC, and III drugs may be more effective in terminating or directly suppressing primary atrial tachycardias and may be effective for reciprocating tachycardias.[5,23]

Despite the various antiarrhythmic agents available for chronic therapy, relatively few are suitable (Tables 26–3A and 26–3B) for acute administration to the critically ill patient either because the drugs are not available in intravenous formulation or they have significant negative inotropic effects when administered intravenously. This discussion is limited to agents suitable for acute and short-term parenteral administration.

All antiarrhythmic agents have the potential for producing bradycardia, particularly when administered acutely, and most have negative inotropic and/or hypotensive effects. Careful observation is required during initial administration and subsequent infusion of all intravenous antiarrhythmic agents. Although many are contraindicated in cases of heart failure or hypotension, therapy may be necessary if the arrhythmia is contributing significantly to the patient's hemodynamic compromise.

Procainamide. Procainamide is useful for various SVTs and ventricular tachycardias in the intensive care setting. Its broad electrophysiologic effects include both conduction slowing and increased refractoriness in atrial tissue, ventricular tissue, and accessory AV connections. Unlike quinidine, procainamide can be administered intravenously. Effective plasma concentrations (6–10 μg/dl) can be readily achieved with a total loading dose of 15 mg/kg over

TABLE 26–3A

Treatment of Bradycardias and Supraventricular Tachycardias

	Primary Therapies	Secondary Therapies	Long-Term Therapies
BRADYCARDIAS			
Sinus bradycardia	Atropine 0.01 mg/kg Epinephrine 0.1 mg/kg Transcutaneous pacemaker	Temporary pacemaker Isoproterenol infusion	Permanent pacemaker (AAIR, DDDR)
AV block (high-grade)	Transcutaneous pacemaker	Temporary pacemaker	Permanent pacemaker (DDDR)
SUPRAVENTRICULAR TACHYCARDIAS			
Sinus tachycardia	Identify cause(s)	Sedation, pain control Adjust catecholamines Respiratory support	Beta-blockers, if chronic Consider nonsinus mechanism
Paroxysmal supraventricular tachycardia (AV reentrant tachycardia, AV nodal reentrant tachycardia)	Vagal maneuvers Adenosine Transesophageal termination Procainamide	Esmolol Verapamil Procainamide (IV) Amiodarone (IV) Class I, class III	Beta-blockers, class I, class III Amiodarone Radiofrequency ablation Radiofrequency ablation
AET and other incessant supraventricular tachycardia	Amiodarone Esmolol Avoid cardioversion	Beta-blockers Amiodarone	
Atrial flutter <24 hours	Rate-control (diltiazem IV) Procainamide Pace termination with pacemaker DC cardioversion Ibutilide (transesophageal echocardiography if duration unknown or >24 hours to rule out thrombus)	Pace termination (transesophageal, intracardiac)	Radiofrequency ablation Antitachycardia pacemaker
Atrial fibrillation <24 hours	Same as above, except pace termination not feasible)		
Chaotic atrial tachycardia	Procainamide, amiodarone	Beta-blocker (rate control)	Propafenone, amiodarone

TABLE 26–3B

Treatment of Ventricular Tachycardias

	Primary Therapies	Secondary Therapies	Long-Term Therapies
Monomorphic (conscious, stable)	Procainamide/lidocaine DC cardioversion Pace termination if PM, ICD	Procainamide/lidocaine Amiodarone	Defined by substrate
*Known heart disease	Same	Amiodarone	ICD, Radiofrequency ablation Amiodarone
*Known idiopathic	Consider IV verapamil Avoid cardioversion	Beta-blocker	Ca-channel blocker Beta-blocker Radiofrequency ablation
Pulseless (monomorphic, polymorphic)	DC cardioversion Beta-blocker Amiodarone	Amiodarone (unless long QT) Beta-blocker Magnesium	ICD
Ventricular fibrillation	Defibrillation	Epinephrine Vasopressin	ICD

ICD, implantable cardioverter-defibrillator.

15 minutes (or in small bolus increments at a similar rate). Careful and repeated blood pressure monitoring is required as loading ensues because of potential negative inotropic and direct vasodilator effects. We prefer to administer intravenous procainamide by hand in 1 mg/kg aliquots at 1- to 2-minute intervals, rather than using a continuous infusion on a pump. In a patient not set up for continuous direct arterial blood pressure monitoring, we set the noninvasive blood pressure monitor to measure blood pressure at 1- or 2-minute intervals. An acceptable noninvasive blood pressure measurement is then the cue to give the next aliquot of procainamide. If hypotension results, the administration should be momentarily interrupted until blood pressure returns toward normal. In primary atrial tachycardias, a vagolytic effect may increase the ventricular response over the AV node. Occasionally, atrial tachycardia that is conducting 2:1 to the ventricle slows sufficiently to allow 1:1 conduction, converting a hemodynamically stable rhythm to an unstable rhythm. Thus you should always be prepared to use cardioversion if necessary.

Procainamide, like other class IA and class III drugs, is contraindicated in the congenital or acquired long QT syndromes. Regular monitoring of plasma concentration every 6 to 12 hours is necessary during intravenous administration to maintain levels between 5 and 10 μg/dl. The active metabolite N-acetylprocainamide (NAPA) contributes to the antiarrhythmic action; higher levels of the parent drug may be necessary in patients lacking the enzyme to produce this metabolite.

Lidocaine. Intravenous lidocaine is useful for suppressing and sometimes terminating ventricular tachycardias in children. Although somewhat less likely to acutely terminate ventricular tachycardias than procainamide, bretylium, or amiodarone, lidocaine's lack of significant negative inotropic effect often makes it more attractive for this indication. The usual loading dose is 1 to 2 mg/kg acutely or 3 mg/kg over 20 to 30 minutes, followed by 20 to 50 μg/kg/min infusion. Lidocaine levels should be monitored to prevent central nervous system (CNS) toxicity. With chronic use (4–7 days), accumulation of the metabolite glycine xylide may impair drug efficacy by interfering with the parent drug effect at the sodium channel. Despite traditional recommendations for its use in ventricular fibrillation, lidocaine actually increases defibrillation energy requirements. It probably is superior to phenytoin for ventricular arrhythmias related to digitalis toxicity, but more specific therapies are available (see magnesium, pharmacologic, and toxic arrhythmias).

Beta-Blocking Agents. A limited number of beta-blocking agents are useful for intravenous treatment of tachycardias. Acutely, their role is generally limited to incessant tachycardias, which seem to be dependent on sympathetic tone, and ventricular tachycardias related to myocarditis, ischemia/reperfusion injury, or congenital long QT syndromes. In hemodynamically unstable patients, beta-blocking agents should be used cautiously because of hypotension and potential sinus bradycardia once tachycardia terminates. All may produce bronchospasm, hypotension, or bradycardia or may depress ventricular function.

Esmolol, a short-acting, nonselective beta-blocker with a half-life of 2 to 5 minutes, can be administered as a continuous infusion. A loading dose of 500 μg/kg is followed by an infusion of 50 to 100 μg/kg/min. The infusion can be titrated upward by doubling every 3 to 5 minutes up to 500 μg/kg/min. Repeat loading doses may be useful as the infusion is increased. Its very short half-life is excellent for short-term use, but extended efficacy is limited by tachyphylaxis. For longer-term intravenous administration, propranolol (0.02–0.1 mg/kg) and metoprolol (0.05–0.10 mg/kg) are administered by slow intravenous infusion every 4 to 6 hours, carefully observing for hypotension (or bradycardia). Metoprolol, a selective β_1-blocker, may be preferable for ventricular arrhythmias and in patients with reactive airway disease.

Amiodarone. Amiodarone has only recently become available for intravenous use in the United States. Yet extensive clinical trials in the United States and experience in other countries have indicated amiodarone is highly effective in controlling various tachycardias refractory to other antiarrhythmic agents.[9,23,44] Although typically regarded as a class III agent, its effects are considerably more diverse. It not only prolongs repolarization (by blocking potassium channels), but to varying degrees it blocks some sodium channel (class I effect), calcium channel (class IV effect), and β receptors (class II effect).

Amiodarone is administered as a total loading dose of 5 mg/kg divided into 1 mg/kg aliquots given at 5- to 10-minute intervals. The loading can be truncated if arrhythmia control is achieved. If hypotension ensues, volume expansion or calcium chloride (10–30 mg/kg) should be administered. If arrhythmia control is not achieved, a second loading dose can be administered 30 to 60 minutes later. A continuous infusion of 10 mg/kg over 24 hours can be administered if ongoing therapy is desired.

Because of amiodarone's slow elimination and its potential for significant vasodilatation, its usage usually should be limited to arrhythmias truly refractory to other agents or certain arrhythmias recognized as poorly responsive to conventional therapy. Furthermore, because of its slow elimination, the absence of spontaneous arrhythmias following acute administration may obscure the determination of whether ongoing therapy is warranted for several days or weeks. Similarly, amiodarone may obscure subsequent diagnostic efforts and inhibit induction of arrhythmias at electrophysiologic study for days or weeks after ceasing administration. Cessation of intravenous therapy at the earliest possible opportunity is advisable. When necessary, oral therapy should be deferred until necessary diagnostic issues (sometimes including formal electrophysiologic study) have been addressed.

Calcium Channel-Blocking Agents. Verapamil and, more recently, diltiazem have proved useful for terminating SVT involving the AV node (AV reentry, AV nodal reentry). However, their acute efficacy is no greater than that of adenosine, and both may cause hypotension or cardiovascular collapse in young infants or patients with poor ventricular function.[25] Either can be useful as an alternative to adenosine when tachycardias have repeatedly reinitiated following termination with adenosine.

Both agents may help slow the ventricular response over the AV node during atrial flutter or fibrillation. Verapamil is administered as a bolus of 0.15 mg/kg. Diltiazem can be administered as a bolus of 0.15 to 0.35 mg/kg and can be infused continuously at 0.05 to 0.2 mg/kg/hour if ongoing effect is necessary. In addition to vasodilatation and negative inotropic effects, both can accelerate antegrade conduction over accessory pathways in patients with WPW syndrome. Therefore they are contraindicated for WPW syndrome with atrial fibrillation over the accessory pathway, and generally they should not be administered during uncharacterized wide QRS tachycardias. Likewise, oral calcium channel blockers should generally not be used as maintenance therapy for patients with WPW syndrome. If hemodynamic compromise develops, intravenous calcium gluconate should be administered immediately.

Magnesium Sulfate. Magnesium (administered as 25–50 mg/kg magnesium sulfate) has proved useful in the treatment of certain ventricular and supraventricular arrhythmias. Its actions appear to be mediated through depression of early and late afterdepolarizations; depressant effects on AV nodal conduction; and, at high doses, indirect inhibition of sodium-potassium ATPase. It has proved most effective in the acute treatment of torsades de pointes and as a temporizing measure in the treatment of arrhythmias associated with digoxin toxicity (see page 391).[26] Therapeutic efficacy is not restricted to situations where hypomagnesemia is present (although hypomagnesemia may predispose to afterdepolarization-dependent arrhythmias).

Although magnesium has efficacy comparable to that of adenosine in the acute termination of SVT resulting from AV reentry and AV nodal reentry, it has more severe and lasting side effects. It has little demonstrable effect in the acute treatment of monomorphic ventricular tachycardias or polymorphic ventricular tachycardias not associated with QT prolongation. Although administration of magnesium for various ventricular arrhythmias has become popular, its usage should generally be restricted to the situations described or for cases of documented severe hypomagnesemia.

Digoxin. Digoxin historically has been used for various supraventricular arrhythmias, including AV reentry, AV nodal reentry, and primary atrial tachycardias. Its therapeutic role has been questioned in numerous situations. Digoxin terminates ORT slowly, is associated with a high recurrence rate in infants, and may increase the risk of rapid antegrade conduction during atrial fibrillation in older patients and possibly infants with preexcitation. Its usage is further confounded by potentially dangerous interactions with other medications likely to be administered concurrently including quinidine, verapamil, amiodarone, flecainide, phenytoin, and warfarin. Even with intravenous loading, therapeutic effect on the AV node may be unpredictable in onset and often inadequate. Like calcium channel-blocking agents, it should be avoided altogether in the treatment of patients with ventricular preexcitation (WPW syndrome). At toxic dosages, its direct cellular effects may predispose to dangerous tachycardias and bradycardias. Thus given the availability of an increasing number of preferable alternatives, its appropriate usage as an acute antiarrhythmic agent is limited.

Cardioversion and Defibrillation

Cardiovascular collapse or failure of mechanical and pharmacologic interventions for tachycardias may warrant cardioversion. For tachycardias with discrete QRS complexes, synchronization with the QRS should be confirmed (the default mode for most defibrillators is nonsynchronized, and most revert to nonsynchronized shocks after each shock is delivered). Proper synchronization may require changing the ECG lead configuration to achieve an upright QRS complex.

Several factors may determine the success of cardioversion and defibrillation. Energy requirements may vary from 0.25 to 1 J/kg for SVTs to greater than 2 J/kg for ventricular tachycardias. Newer defibrillators with a "biphasic" rather than "monophasic" waveform have reduced defibrillation energy requirements. Electrode (paddle) location is an important variable. If conversion is not achieved with low or moderate energy levels, consideration should be given to changing electrode position before using higher energy levels. Automatic tachycardias are characteristically refractory to cardioversion and may account for treatment failure. Finally, some antiarrhythmic drugs, particularly sodium channel-blocking drugs (see later), increase defibrillation energy requirements and pacing thresholds, whereas other drugs (QT-prolonging drugs) appear to have a favorable effect.[27]

The availability of automatic external defibrillators injects an additional complexity into the use of external cardioversion and defibrillation. Each ICU should carefully consider how to best configure devices for automatic versus manual defibrillation operation and which electrode system (ECG leads, paddles, and patches) best suits the particular patient population and care team.[28]

Approach to therapy

Extrasystoles

In general, isolated extrasystoles do not require treatment unless they are sufficiently frequent to impair hemodynamics (e.g., incessant bigeminy or trigeminy with pulse deficit) or they serve as frequent initiating events for tachycardias. In otherwise healthy children and adolescents, they may be a benign finding. In other settings, "complex" ventricular extrasystoles may identify patients at increased risk for cardiac arrest. Even in such situations, prophylaxis may not decrease and may actually increase the risk. Effort should instead be directed at identifying possible causes and correcting any predisposing factors, which include ischemia, electrolyte disorders, acidosis, pericarditis, or direct trauma from recent cardiac surgery, blunt or penetrating chest trauma, and intracardiac catheter-induced irritation. Numerous drugs, including digoxin, catecholamines, or drugs associated with the acquired long QT syndrome, may produce extrasystoles. Frequent asystoles occasionally are the sole manifestation of myocarditis.

Sustained Tachycardias

Most sustained tachycardias observed in the intensive care setting warrant immediate attention and intervention. Sinus tachycardia may indicate the need for additional sedation and analgesia or may reflect hemodynamic compromise as a consequence of anemia, hypovolemia, or impaired myocardial function. Sinus tachycardia as a consequence of hyperthermia may be poorly tolerated in children already critically ill, especially following cardiac surgery. Sinus tachycardia may reflect an underlying neuroendocrine process such as hyperthyroidism or pheochromocytoma requiring acute medical intervention (beta-blocker) while instituting therapy for the underlying disorder.

Nonsinus tachycardias in patients with primary rhythm disturbances (rather than as a complication of another problem) may warrant therapy to prevent life-threatening events, prevent the development of myocardial dysfunction as a consequence of chronic (incessant) tachycardia, or simply alleviate acute tachycardia-related symptoms such as chest pain, lightheadedness, and palpitations. The acuity of the situation dictates the approach to therapy. Tachycardias occurring secondary to other abnormalities (structural heart disease, metabolic derangements, drug toxicity) should always be regarded as high risk for serious hemodynamic deterioration.

Unstable Patients

The approach to patients with tachycardia is determined largely by the degree of hemodynamic compromise (see Tables 26–3A and 26–3B). Patients who are hemodynamically unstable or in cardiovascular collapse resulting from sustained tachycardia almost always warrant prompt cardioversion or defibrillation. In these patients, measures that otherwise would be appropriate, such as vagal maneuvers, adenosine administration, or attempts to differentiate SVT from ventricular tachycardia, should be deferred. Delaying prompt termination of tachycardia in the unstable patient may further compromise the hemodynamic status and increase the risk of other end-organ damage. Only when tachycardia is known to be incessant or unresponsive to cardioversion (JET, atrial ectopic tachycardia, chaotic tachycardia, PJRT) should antiarrhythmic medications (and other supportive measures) replace cardioversion in the unstable patient.

Cardiopulmonary resuscitation should always be instituted in the absence of a pulse or blood pressure, as is typically the case for polymorphic ventricular tachycardia and ventricular fibrillation. Although hemodynamic and ventilatory support should be initiated immediately and maintained following tachycardia termination as necessary, cardioversion (with bag and mask ventilation initially) should take precedence over other interventions.[29] Although congestive heart failure may accompany tachycardias (as an infant with SVT of several hours' duration), aggressive diuresis should be avoided; patients may benefit initially from fluid resuscitation. Even mild intravascular volume contraction in the face of subsequent tachycardia recurrences further compromises ventricular filling and results in more severe hypotension. Underlying factors contributing to the tachycardia should be sought, including hypoxia, infection (cardiac or systemic), drug toxicities (see later), and electrolyte derangements.

Once tachycardia is terminated, acute therapies may focus on either suppressing recurrences or terminating them when they recur. In critically ill patients, the latter may be preferable, at least initially. Although antiarrhythmic medications eventually may be necessary to suppress recurrences, most have negative inotropic or vasodilating effects, particularly when administered intravenously. Often it is preferable to delay specific therapy after initial termination until ventricular function improves. Most recurrences of SVTs can be safely treated with temporary pacing or adenosine rather than with repeated cardioversions. In the event of frequent recurrences, a transesophageal catheter may be left in place for this purpose, or a transvenous atrial pacing catheter may be warranted in selected patients. Similarly, temporary ventricular pacing may be useful in some circumstances for recurrent ventricular tachycardia. Although adenosine can be administered repeatedly because of its short half-life, the resulting vasodilatation may be poorly tolerated in patients with tachycardia mechanisms unresponsive to adenosine.

Treatment Errors

When seemingly appropriate electrical and pharmacologic interventions fail to terminate tachycardias, three possibilities should be considered: erroneous diagnosis, unrecognized tachycardia reinitiation, or a technical error in the termination technique.

Errors in Diagnosis

As noted previously, automatic atrial tachycardias, JET, and occasionally chaotic atrial tachycardia might be mistaken for tachycardias with reentrant mechanism (ORT, AVNRT, primary atrial reentry). Each of these conditions usually is refractory to electrical termination (either pace termination or cardioversion), yet the diagnosis may be subtle if atrial activity is obscured.

Confusion between ventricular tachycardias and SVTs with prolonged QRS probably remains the most frequent diagnostic error. Occasionally the presumption of ventricular tachycardia may lead to ineffective treatments. For example, following cardiac surgery, incessant, monomorphic wide QRS tachycardia that is refractory to cardioversion may actually be JET with postsurgical bundle branch block. Brief atrial pacing at a faster rate may be necessary to confirm the diagnosis.

Certain tachycardias such as torsades de pointes related to long QT syndromes (congenital or drug-induced) or bidirectional ventricular tachycardia resulting from digoxin toxicity must be recognized to provide more appropriate and specific therapies to prevent recurrences following cardioversion.

Unrecognized Reinitiation

Unrecognized reinitiation may occur following medical termination, pace termination, or cardioversion. In some tachycardias (as in PJRT or other incessant forms of SVT), reinitiation is expected, but it also may occur inadvertently as the result of continued pacing beyond the point of termination or may be facilitated by sinus pauses, junctional beats, or ectopic beats following adenosine or cardioversion. Again, measures to decrease the factors favoring reinitiation (shorter pacing bursts, antibradycardia pacing, coadministration of an antiarrhythmic drug) should be used rather than further increases in energy or dose of the terminating therapy. With frequent terminations and reinitiations of tachycardia, multiple repeated cardioversions are likely ineffective and may cause myocardial injury.

Errors in Technique

Appropriate administration of adenosine is accomplished through an intravenous catheter (peripheral or central), by rapid push followed immediately with ample flush. Because of rapid metabolism by erythrocytes, arterial administration may be ineffective in terminating tachycardia (yet still produce vasodilatation). Errors in cardioversion or pacing technique are generally attributable to insufficient energy or improper electrode (or paddle) placement.[28] For pace termination, the stimulator must be capable of sufficient output for the pacing modality being used (see section on temporary pacing). Intensive care personnel should be familiar with the defibrillation devices available in the ICU, including adjustment of ECG gain and lead selection to allow synchronous cardioversion when appropriate. However, in ventricular fibrillation or polymorphic tachycardia, asynchronous countershock is necessary. Use of excessive energy may damage the myocardium and, when repeated, may lead to preterminal bradycardias, which are refractory to all pacing modalities and progress to complete electromechanical dissociation if hypoxia and acidosis are not corrected.

Specific Arrhythmias

Primary Arrhythmias

Some arrhythmias require unique therapeutic approaches or are seen with sufficient frequency to warrant a brief review (Box 26–1).

Orthodromic Reciprocating Tachycardia in Infancy

Infants with ORT can present with tachycardia in utero, at birth, or within the first weeks to months of life. Intrauterine tachycardia can result in abnormal hemodynamics resulting from limited ventricular filling times accentuated by atrial systole against closed AV valves. Retrograde systemic venous flow during tachycardias may contribute to low cardiac output, congestive heart failure, and nonimmune hydrops fetalis prenatally.[30] Postnatally, tachycardia sustained beyond a few hours may result in congestive heart failure that may progress to shock, acidosis, and complete cardiovascular collapse.[31] In the latter situation, ORT may be terminated during resuscitation efforts such that its causative role remains unrecognized. Thus SVT should be considered in the differential diagnosis of neonatal shock, along with other conditions such as sepsis, aortic coarctation, and congenital adrenal hyperplasia in which sinus tachycardia associated with cardiovascular collapse would be expected.

BOX 26–1

PRIMARY RHYTHM DISTURBANCES

Paroxysmal supraventricular tachycardias (AV reentrant tachycardia, AVNRT)
Congenital AV block
Congenital long QT syndrome, Brugada syndrome, other genetic arrhythmia syndromes?
Other genetic arrhythmias
Ventricular tachycardias resulting from Purkinje hamartoma
Verapamil-sensitive ventricular tachycardias
Accelerated ventricular rhythm

SECONDARY RHYTHM DISTURBANCES

Early Postoperative Arrhythmias

JET
Postsurgical AV block
Early primary atrial tachycardia

Late Postoperative Arrhythmias

Ventricular arrhythmias (postoperative tetralogy of Fallot)
Sick sinus syndrome

Metabolic Derangements

Electrolyte disturbances
Endocrine derangements (thyroid)
CNS injury
Hypothermia, hyperthermia
Acute hypoxia (newborns)
Acute myocardial infarction

Drug Toxicity, Proarrhythmia

Digoxin
Cocaine
Tricyclic antidepressants
Antiarrhythmic drugs
Quinidine/sotalol
Flecainide/encainide
Organophosphates

Infectious

Lyme disease
Myocarditis, endocarditis

The transesophageal electrophysiologic (TEP) study is useful in determining tachycardia mechanism[32] and especially for assessing drug efficacy. The negative predictive value of TEP (noninducible with no clinical recurrence) is 89% and increases to 96% when stimulation is also performed after administration of proterenol.[33] Long-term drug therapy is not always necessary, because approximately one third of infants have no inducible tachycardia at TEP by age 1 year.[6,34]

Tachycardia-Induced Cardiac Dysfunction

Although most SVTs are paroxysmal or episodic, chronic SVTs pose a unique problem. Many are minimally symptomatic and are recognized only by the inappropriately fast rate. However, with time, varying degrees of congestive heart failure become evident, and ventricular dysfunction may be severe. Even then, the diagnosis may not be immediately evident. As a consequence, chronic tachycardia must be considered in any patient presenting with gradually progressive congestive heart failure. In one series, chronic atrial tachycardia was present in 37% of patients initially diagnosed with "idiopathic" cardiomyopathy and listed for heart transplant.[35]

In patients with structurally normal hearts, the most common incessant SVTs are PJRT and ectopic atrial tachycardia. These conditions may occur throughout infancy, childhood, and adolescence. The rates (often <200 bpm) and normal PR interval during tachycardia may lead to an erroneous diagnosis of sinus tachycardia secondary to the hemodynamic compromise (see Approach to Diagnosis). An abnormal P-wave axis on 12-lead electrocardiogram, determination of the "intrinsic heart rate" following complete autonomic blockade, and Holter monitoring to look for interruptions in the tachycardia with changes in P-wave morphology are helpful. Electrophysiologic study still may be necessary to establish the diagnosis. In infants, incessant ventricular tachycardias and the rare congenital form of JET are also seen.

In each of these entities, it is important first to recognize the primary role of the tachycardia in producing secondary congestive symptoms and to recognize the futility of acute therapies such as adenosine, pace termination, and cardioversion. Most are catecholamine dependent so that inotropic agents may aggravate the situation and compromise the efficacy of antiarrhythmic regimens, whereas beta-blocking agents may be useful despite the presence of heart failure. Once the diagnosis is established, chronic antiarrhythmic therapy is instituted to control or limit the tachycardia. Uncontrolled, severe cardiac symptoms may result, but ventricular dysfunction improves once tachycardia is suppressed medically or treated with catheter ablation.[36] Despite the severity of heart failure, antiarrhythmic medications that depress ventricular function usually are well tolerated.

Congenital AV Block

Congenital heart block is usually the result of either maternal connective tissue disease (45%) or structural congenital heart disease (53%), particularly L-transposition of the great arteries or left atrial isomerism. Mothers with connective tissue disease are frequently asymptomatic but may have detectable anti-Ro/SSA antibodies. In a prospective study of mothers with anti-Ro/SSA antibodies, the risk of congenital AV block was 2%.[37] The L-type calcium channel is the likely target of these autoantibodies.[38]

Rarely, congenital AV block is the initial manifestation of congenital long QT syndrome.[39] Temporary pacing in congenital AV block may be required to treat symptoms or secondary ventricular arrhythmias. A subset of patients may develop ventricular dysfunction despite pacing therapy.[40] Guidelines and indications for permanent pacing have been established.[20]

Chaotic Atrial Tachycardia

Chaotic atrial tachycardia is a primary atrial tachycardia characterized by three or more different P-wave morphologies and irregular, rapid atrial rates (Figure 26–13). Although atrial flutter may be associated with it, episodes usually are self-limited, and cardioversion is neither indicated nor effective. Asymptomatic patients with slow or intermittent tachycardia may require no treatment. Digoxin is occasionally used to limit AV conduction when atrial rates are excessive or to enhance contractility in the setting of tachycardia-induced cardiomyopathy.[41] An association with respiratory syncytial virus has been described in some patients.[42] Various agents have been used in symptomatic cases; amiodarone and propafenone are most effective.[43,44]

Long QT Syndromes

The long QT syndromes are a diverse group of disorders, both congenital and acquired, in which individuals are at risk for torsades de pointes and sudden death because of abnormalities in ventricular repolarization (Figure 26–14). In both congenital and acquired forms, the rate-corrected QT intervals usually exceed 0.46 second, and more typically are greater than 0.48 to 0.50 second. Associated anomalies of T-wave morphology, including T-wave alternans, "bifid" T waves, and prominent U waves, are common. It may be difficult to establish the diagnosis of congenital long QT syndrome because QT prolongation may not be severe. In fact, affected individuals sometimes have a normal QTc.[45] Congenital long QT syndrome should be considered in all patients with QT prolongation and a history of syncope, cardiac arrest, or seizures or a family history of unexplained sudden death. The diagnosis should be strongly considered in any child presenting with syncope or sudden death in whom polymorphic ventricular tachycardia or multiform ventricular premature beats are documented. Long QT syndrome may be familial. Incidental QT prolongation in an asymptomatic child (with negative family history) may warrant further scrutiny and possibly serial Holter monitoring. However, unless the QTc is markedly prolonged (>0.48–0.50 second), the diagnosis should be withheld until or unless further suggestive features are noted. Finally, all infants presenting with second-degree or third-degree AV block should be evaluated for the possibility of long QT syndrome.[46]

Patients with symptoms or arrhythmias associated with QT prolongation require careful evaluation for secondary causes, which include CNS injury, hypocalcemia, hypokalemia, and drugs that prolong the QT interval. The list of drugs that prolong the QT interval is extensive and includes antiarrhythmic and noncardiac drugs, most of which block I_{Kr}, the rapid component of the delayed rectifier potassium current.[47] Updated lists of these drugs are available at *www.torsades.org* and *www.qtdrugs.org*.

Torsades de pointes is the specific arrhythmia associated with long QT syndromes and is responsible for the symptoms. This characteristic arrhythmia is recognized by progressive undulation in the QRS axis, resulting in a "twisting" appearance, and usually is associated with a specific initiation with a VPB following a pause (often following a previous VPB). Many episodes are not sustained, and even prolonged episodes may terminate spontaneously. Torsades de pointes that degenerates to ventricular fibrillation requires defibrillation. As the stress caused by defibrillation may trigger recurrent arrhythmias, defibrillation should be performed in an unconscious or sedated patient. Treatment of immediate recurrence of torsades de pointes is challenging and includes magnesium sulfate, increasing the heart rate with temporary pacing or isoproterenol, and sedation.[48,49] For most acquired long QT syndromes (and some congenital forms), increasing the heart rate using isoproterenol or by pacing shortens the QT interval, but isoproterenol may exacerbate some forms of the congenital long QT syndrome.[50] Therefore isoproterenol should be used only when there is underlying bradycardia and cardiac pacing cannot be started immediately. Correcting hypokalemia,

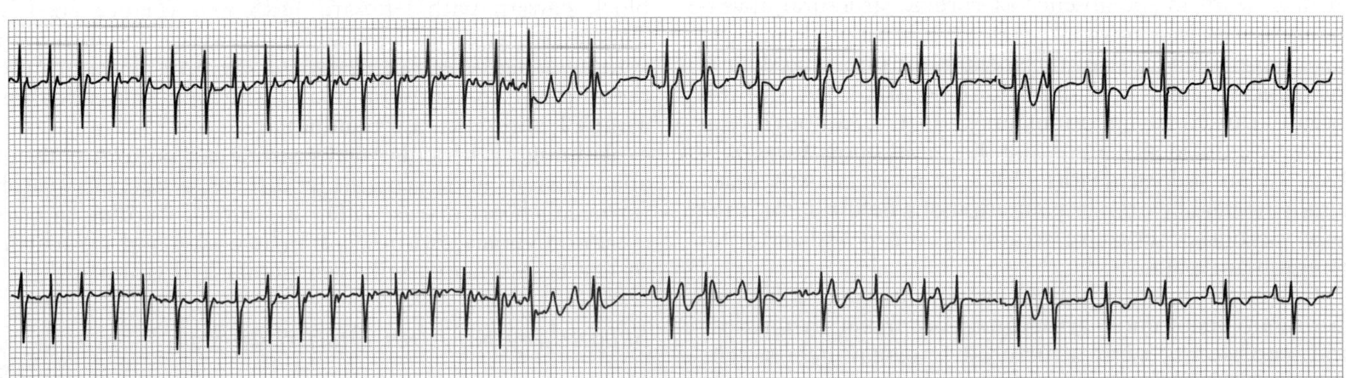

FIGURE 26–13 • Chaotic atrial tachycardia. Note two discrete P-wave morphologies before conversion to sinus.

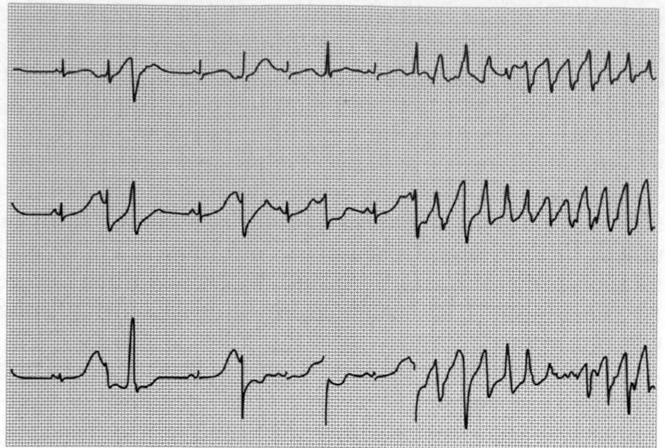

FIGURE 26–14 • Torsades de pointes in a teenage patient with long QT syndrome. This arrhythmia is associated with no pulse and results in syncope. It often terminates spontaneously but otherwise rapidly degenerates to ventricular fibrillation.

hypomagnesemia, or hypocalcemia and removing potentially causative agents may be important in the ICU setting.

The molecular/genetic basis of the congenital long QT syndrome was discovered in the 1990s. To date, more than 150 mutations have been discovered in seven genes.[51] Six of these genes encode channels that regulate potassium *(KCNQ1, KCNH2, KCNE1, KCNE2, KCNJ2)* and sodium *(SCN5A)* currents, and one gene encodes a cytoskeletal protein (ankyrin B) that may affect sodium or calcium channel kinetics. Currently, known mutations in the seven genes account for an estimated 50% of patients affected with long QT syndrome. The type and location of the genetic mutation may determine to some extent the expression of the clinical syndrome, the phenotype. However, as mentioned earlier, this disorder has variable expression of severity (i.e., variable penetrance). This variability in expression in related individuals with the same mutation suggests the influence of environmental factors and/or the presence of other modifier genes.

Genetic Arrhythmias

Other genetic causes of arrhythmias deserve brief mention. Brugada syndrome, the syndrome of ST-segment elevation in the right precordial leads and a high incidence of sudden cardiac death in the absence of cardiac structural abnormalities, was first recognized in 1992.[52] Since then, there has been tremendous advancement in the understanding of the clinical, genetic, cellular, and molecular aspects of this disease, caused by mutations in *SCN5A*.[53] Although relatively rare (incidence 5 per 10,000), it accounts for 4% to 12% of all sudden deaths (20% in patients with structurally normal hearts). Implantation of a defibrillator is the only established effective treatment and is indicated for symptomatic patients.[54]

Catecholaminergic bidirectional ventricular tachycardia is an uncommon arrhythmia occurring in children and adolescents with structurally normal hearts. The characteristic arrhythmia of ventricular tachycardia with beat-to-beat alternation of the QRS axis occurs with physical or emotional stress and can be asymptomatic. Mutations in the cardiac ryanodine receptor gene *(RyR2)* underlie catecholaminergic bidirectional ventricular tachycardia, and patients with the disease are at risk for sudden cardiac death and ventricular fibrillation.[55] Beta-blockers can suppress bidirectional ventricular tachycardia, but data suggest they provide incomplete protection from arrhythmias.[56]

Genetic cardiomyopathies that are associated with sudden death include arrhythmogenic right ventricular dysplasia (ARVD) and hypertrophic cardiomyopathy. ARVD is a disease of autosomal dominant inheritance characterized by fatty replacement of right ventricular myocardium and risk for ventricular tachycardia and sudden death.[57] Linkage analysis has yielded eight different ARVD loci including *RyR2,* and wider genetic heterogeneity cannot be ruled out.[58] Hypertrophic cardiomyopathy is an inherited cardiac muscle disorder disease that affects sarcomeric proteins, resulting in small vessel disease, myocyte and myofibrillar disorganization, and fibrosis with or without myocardial hypertrophy.[59] These features may result in significant cardiac symptoms and are a potential substrate for arrhythmias. Risk stratification for sudden death is an important component in the management of these patients (Table 26–4).

Ventricular Tachycardia in Ostensibly Healthy Patients

Accelerated ventricular rhythm is observed in occasional neonates in the first few days of life at rates only slightly faster than the appropriate sinus rates. The rhythm competes with the sinus mechanism, and alternation between sinus and ventricular rhythm with fusion beats is common. The rhythm is self-limited, does not usually result in hemodynamic compromise, and carries a good prognosis. No specific therapy is necessary unless rates are excessive.[60] A similar rhythm is seen in older children and usually has a similarly benign course.[61] Two other characteristic ventricular tachycardias may be seen in otherwise healthy children and adolescents. One arises from the right ventricular outflow tract, resulting in a left bundle branch block pattern with inferior QRS axis. This pattern may be incessant, in which case the term *repetitive monomorphic ventricular tachycardia* has been used. The other arises from the posterior fascicle of the left-sided conduction system, producing a right bundle branch block pattern with leftward QRS axis (Figure 26–15). This tachycardia has been called *fascicular, Belhassen,* or *verapamil-sensitive ventricular tachycardia.* Interestingly, the response to verapamil may result in misclassification as "SVT with aberrant conduction."

Although ventricular tachycardia can be seen without any apparent underlying heart disease, a rigorous search for occult heart disease often is fruitful. Cardiac tumors (rhabdomyomas, fibromas, hamartomas) and myocarditis can be associated with ventricular arrhythmias.[62]

Secondary Rhythm Disturbances

Certain arrhythmias characteristically follow operative treatment of congenital heart disease. Among those observed in the early postoperative period are complete heart block, JET, and primary atrial tachycardias. Late postoperative arrhythmias include ventricular arrhythmias following tetralogy of Fallot repair and atrial arrhythmias following the Mustard/Senning and Fontan procedures.

Postoperative Arrhythmias

Postsurgical AV Block. Inadvertent damage to the AV conduction system may occur with cardiac surgery, especially after closure of ventricular septal defects (particularly associated with L-loop ventricles), during resection of septal tissue, or after insertion of prosthetic valves in the tricuspid, aortic, or mitral position. Bradycardia from AV block can be initially managed using isoproterenol to accelerate the ventricular rate. When anticipated or recognized in the operating room, temporary pacing wires usually are left in place. Although temporary pacing frequently is necessary for rate support, permanent pacemaker implantation usually should be delayed 7 to 14 days to allow for potential recovery of AV conduction. Most patients who recover AV conduction do so within 9 days of surgery.[63]

Junctional Ectopic Tachycardia. JET immediately following cardiac surgery may be mistaken for third-degree AV block, but on rewarming ventricular rates approach or exceed 200 bpm. Atrial wires or esophageal electrography confirms the key diagnostic features: AV dissociation with normal QRS and the regular ventricular rate faster than the atrial rate. Appropriately timed atrial systoles conducted to the ventricle result in "advancement" of the tachycardia cycle (without a change in QRS morphology or subsequent pause). If the QRS is normal but the RR interval does not shorten with appropriately timed atrial systoles, JET with retrograde (VA) conduction or third-degree AV block with JET as the escape rhythm should be suspected.

Infants with JET usually are severely ill, and β-adrenergic agonists, fever, and endogenous catecholamines accelerate the tachycardia. Initial treatment of postoperative JET includes sedation and analgesia, withdrawal of adrenergic stimulants (to the extent possible), and cooling blankets or cool soaks using an electric fan to foster evaporative cooling. The tachycardia may be suppressed by temporary overdrive (atrial) pacing, by pacing at a rate sufficient to produce 2:1 AV block, or by AVT mode pacing to provide AV synchrony.[64] Intravenous amiodarone has been used with perhaps the greatest efficacy.[66] Although emergency radiofrequency ablation has been performed in rare instances, aggressive temporizing measures, including ECMO, appear warranted given the transient nature of this arrhythmia.

Late Postoperative Arrhythmias

Atrial tachycardia and bradycardia are common late sequelae following the Senning and Mustard operations for D-transposition of the great arteries, atrial septal defect closure, and the Fontan procedure for tricuspid atresia and single ventricle.[66–68] Patients with these arrhythmias appear to be at increased risk for sudden death, although whether death is the result of atrial tachycardia itself, associated bradycardia, degeneration to ventricular tachycardia, or even nondysrhythmic events remains unclear.[69,70]

Likewise, patients with repaired or palliated congenital heart disease may develop ventricular arrhythmias that are associated with risk for sudden death. Long-term data suggest the risk of sustained arrhythmias and sudden death is much lower than previously estimated.[71,72] There seems to be little justification for empirical drug therapy to suppress asymptomatic ventricular arrhythmias in these patients. Earlier repair is believed to decrease the incidence of serious problems. Still, the relative contributions of postoperative hemodynamic abnormalities, natural history of the unrepaired lesions, and surgical technique to the development of late arrhythmias remain uncertain. Similarly, the roles of pacemaker/defibrillator therapy, prospective electrophysiologic study, and antiarrhythmic drug testing are not well established. Because many patients develop both bradycardias and tachycardias, the correlation of symptoms with electrophysiologic abnormality is important in guiding therapy.

TABLE 26–4

Genetic Arrhythmia Syndromes

Phenotype	Gene(s) Affected
Long QT syndromes	*KCNQ1, KCNH2, SCN5A, ANK2, KCNE1,KCNE2*
Brugada syndrome*	*SCN5A*
Short QT syndrome	*KCNH2*
Right ventricular dysplasia†	*RYR2, DSP*
(Naxos disease)	*JUP*
Catecholaminergic polymorphic ventricular tachycardia	*RYR2*
Bidirectional ventricular tachycardia and periodic paralysis (Andersen syndrome)‡	*KCNJ2*
Congenital sinus nodal dysfunction	*SCN5A*

*A second locus on chromosome 3, distinct from *SCN5A,* has been linked to Brugada syndrome.
†At least six other genes on chromosomes 2, 3, 10, and 14 also have been linked to arrhythmogenic right ventricular dysplasia.
‡Andersen syndrome is termed LQT7 by some authors, as a prolonged QT interval can be part of the phenotype. The significant extracardiac manifestations and characteristic bidirectional ventricular tachycardia distinguish it from other forms of long QT syndrome.

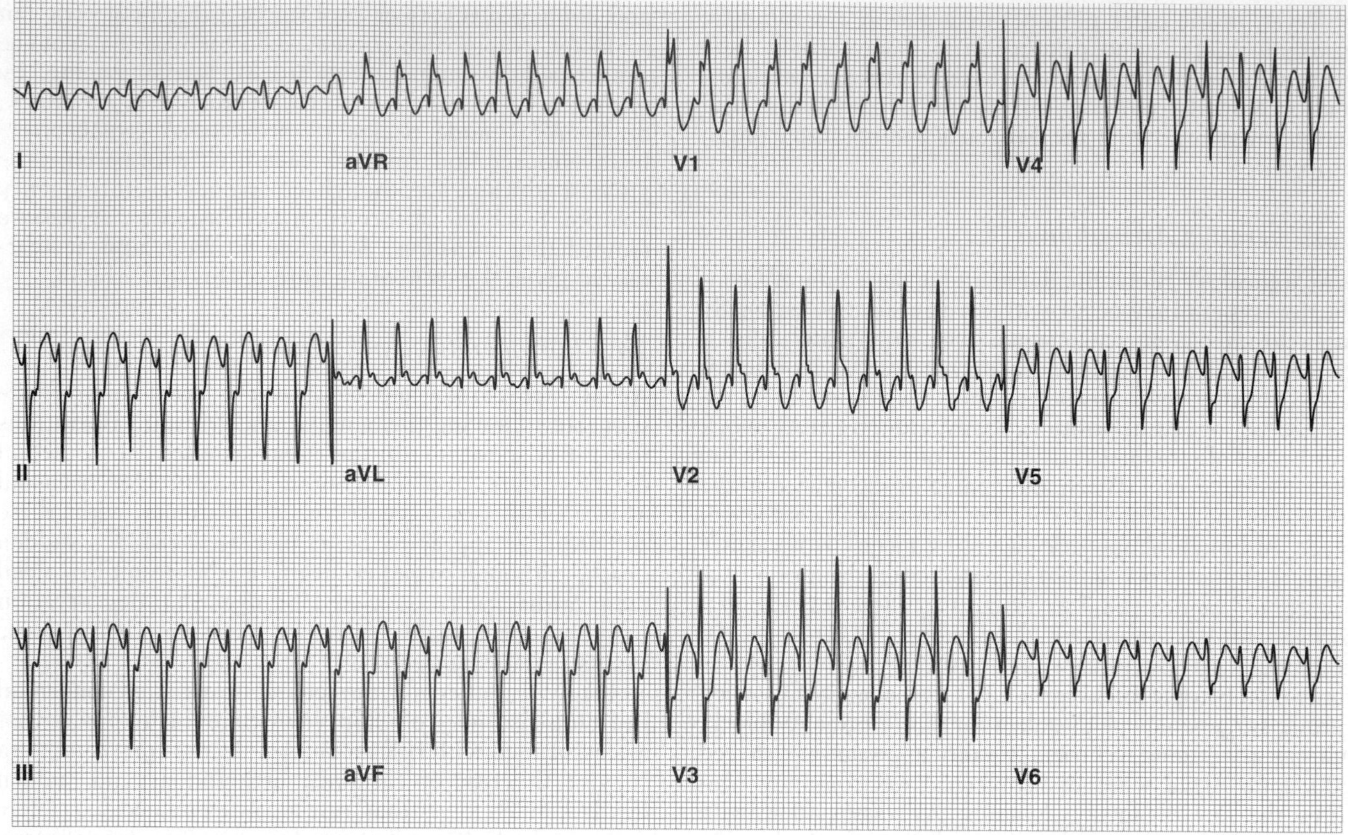

FIGURE 26–15 • Idiopathic ventricular tachycardia in an otherwise healthy 12 year old. Note right bundle branch block pattern with superior axis, typical of origin within the left posterior fascicle region of the left ventricular septum (sometimes called *Belhassen tachycardia).*

Metabolic Derangements

Electrolyte Disturbances. Hyperkalemia causes characteristically tall ("peaked" or "tented") t waves with a narrow base with progressive changes at higher concentrations, including decreased P-wave amplitude, QRS prolongation, SA nodal and AV nodal block, and ultimately ventricular fibrillation. Mild-to-moderate hypokalemia may cause prominent U waves, diminished T-wave amplitude, T-wave inversion, and fusion of the T wave and U wave, along with increased spontaneous ventricular ectopy and inducible ventricular arrhythmias. Arrhythmias caused by hypokalemia are potentiated by catecholamines, and hypokalemia itself potentiates the toxic effects of digoxin and the proarrhythmic effects of drugs associated with drug-induced long QT syndrome.[73] Severe hypokalemia is associated with ventricular fibrillation.

Hypercalcemia produces T-wave inversion and shortens the QT interval. Hypocalcemia prolongs the time to the peak of the T wave (Q-aT) but not the QT interval itself. Isolated calcium abnormalities are uncommon, and arrhythmias caused by such abnormalities are rare, although hypercalcemia may aggravate digitalis toxicity.[2]

Endocrine Disorders (Thyroid). Hyperthyroidism exerts both sympathetic-like and direct cardiovascular actions that produce sinus tachycardia and atrial fibrillation, but ventricular arrhythmias are uncommon. These arrhythmias respond to beta-blockers and resolve when the euthyroid state is restored. Combination treatment with digoxin potentiates AV nodal block while minimizing negative inotropic effects. Hypothyroidism causes sinus bradycardia and AV conduction disturbances; QT interval prolongation is common but rarely associated with torsades de pointes.[74]

Central Nervous System Injury. The most common ECG change associated with CNS trauma and increased intracranial pressure is sinus bradycardia, usually with associated hypertension. These bradycardias appear to be vagally mediated and usually respond to atropine. However, potentially serious arrhythmias may occur within 24 hours following blunt trauma to the head, subdural hematoma, and subarachnoid hemorrhage. QT-interval prolongation is common and, in combination with bradycardia and hypokalemia, may provoke torsades de pointes.

Hypothermia and Hyperthermia. Mild hypothermia can cause a range of reversible ECG changes, including sinus bradycardia; prolongation of the PR, QRS, and QT intervals; and a characteristic secondary deflection on the terminal portion of the QRS (Osborn wave).[75] Severe hypothermia may cause more significant bradycardias, including AV block and asystole or ventricular tachycardias and ventricular fibrillation. In contrast, hyperthermia causes sinus tachycardia and may enhance other tachycardias such as PSVT, ectopic atrial arrhythmias, and especially JET in susceptible patients.

Acute Myocardial Infarction. Acute myocardial infarction is uncommon in young patients but may occur in anomalous origin of the left coronary artery, in perinatal stress, following Kawasaki disease, with blunt chest wall trauma, and following cardiac transplantation and the arterial switch procedure. It can occur after air embolism in cyanotic congenital heart disease or after open heart operations. The diagnosis may be overlooked in infants and children because of the inconsistency of symptoms and relatively poor (60%) clinical recognition by electrocardiography.[76] Nevertheless, acute infarction may result in various rhythm disturbances, including sinus bradycardia (as a result of the Bezold-Jarisch reflex), AV conduction disturbances, intraventricular block, and asystole.

Arrhythmias Resulting from Drug Toxicity

Digoxin. Digoxin toxicity may cause various arrhythmias and should be suspected in any patient who develops a new arrhythmia during digoxin therapy. Likewise, digoxin ingestion should be considered in acute arrhythmias, particularly those associated with CNS and gastrointestinal symptoms (although noncardiac side effects may be absent with acute ingestion). Accelerated junctional rhythm may be the first arrhythmia seen. Progressive AV block is common. Sinus bradycardia resulting from either SA node exit block or sinus arrest may occur, as can atrial fibrillation (but usually not atrial flutter). Ectopic atrial arrhythmias may occur. Nearly any ventricular arrhythmia may occur, including multiform ventricular extrasystoles, bigeminy, ventricular tachycardia (particularly "bidirectional" VT; Figure 26–16), and ventricular fibrillation.[77]

In general, digoxin concentrations less than 2 ng/ml are considered nontoxic. Neonates usually tolerate levels as high as 3.5 ng/ml. Nevertheless, neonates and other intensive care patients may be more susceptible to digoxin toxicity because of renal dysfunction, electrolyte imbalances, and hypoxia. Hypokalemia, excessive calcium infusions, and rapid sinus rates exacerbate digitalis-related arrhythmias.

Purified digoxin-specific Fab antibody fragment, which binds the drug and is eliminated in the urine, is used to treat digoxin toxicity. Prophylactic treatment with this preparation should be gauged according to the quantity ingested, the time since ingestion, and the serum digoxin level. Magnesium sulfate is a useful temporizing treatment while specific antibody treatment is being implemented. Cardioversion should be reserved for life-threatening tachycardias or those unresponsive to these therapies.

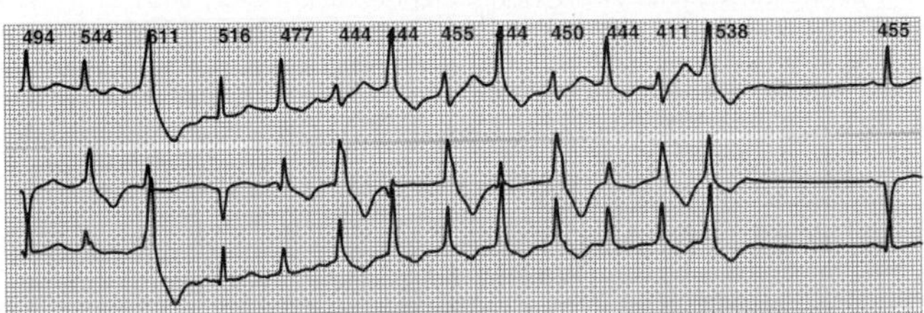

FIGURE 26–16 • Bidirectional ventricular tachycardia in a patient with Andersen syndrome (periodic paralysis and ventricular arrhythmias). The patient is asymptomatic during this arrhythmia, but patients appear to be at risk for polymorphic ventricular tachycardia. This syndrome is sometimes included among the long QT syndromes.

Cocaine. Life-threatening ventricular arrhythmias, cardiac arrest, and myocardial infarction can occur in healthy individuals with normal coronary arteries following cocaine ingestion and in prenatally exposed neonates.[78,79] Cocaine produces myocardial ischemia and infarction by inducing severe local coronary vasoconstriction, increasing myocardial-metabolic demand through its potent chronotropic effects, and increasing afterload. In infarct models, cocaine directly potentiates arrhythmias induced by catecholamines.[80] These factors favor the use of β-adrenergic antagonists as first-line treatment for cocaine-related arrhythmias. Additionally, cocaine blocks fast inward sodium channels, similar to class I antiarrhythmic agents.[81] QT prolongation and torsades de pointes have been observed.[82]

Tricyclic Antidepressants and Phenothiazine. Phenothiazines and tricyclic antidepressants produce electrophysiologic (and potentially antiarrhythmic) effects similar to quinidine and procainamide. They slow conduction velocity in atrial and ventricular tissue, prolong repolarization, and exert anticholinergic effects accounting for the observed ECG changes of conduction disturbances, prolonged QT intervals and QRS duration, and various tachycardias and bradycardias.[83] Sinus tachycardia, atrial and ventricular tachycardias, and AV conduction disturbances distal to the AV node occur occasionally during normal therapeutic administration and may reflect individual susceptibility to QT-prolonging agents. "Unmasking" of the Brugada syndrome has been reported after administration of tricyclic antidepressants.[84]

Arrhythmias commonly follow intentional overdose, resulting in hypotension (due to alpha-blocking effects), severe anticholinergic effects (neuromuscular and mucosal), seizures, and coma. Quinidine and procainamide are contraindicated for tachycardias because of these agents. Patients manifesting early cardiotoxicity may develop arrhythmias 3 to 7 days following ingestion, apparently because of release of tissue stores. Therefore ECG monitoring should be continued for at least 24 to 48 hours after apparent ECG and rhythm normalization and longer if severe arrhythmias are observed.

Infections

Myocarditis may cause atrial and ventricular tachycardias or acquired heart block. Lyme disease may produce high-grade acute AV block. Although AV conduction usually normalizes with appropriate antibiotic therapy, temporary pacing may be required.[85] Antibiotic treatment should be instituted based on the history and ECG findings alone while awaiting confirmatory serology. Bacterial endocarditis can cause AV conduction disturbances, particularly when the aortic valve is involved. Unstable or persisting conduction abnormalities (>7 days) carry a high risk of mortality (43%–80%) and are indications for early valve replacement.[86]

Myocarditis may be responsible for some cases of ventricular tachycardia in otherwise healthy individuals and may range from chronic ventricular ectopy or tachycardia to fulminant and refractory arrhythmias leading to electromechanical dissociation. Chaotic atrial tachycardia may occur in the setting of infection with respiratory syncytial virus, although the cause of this association is unclear. Finally, paroxysmal tachycardias of any etiology may be exacerbated by acute infections that cause fever, dehydration, and increased sympathetic tone. Short-term modifications of chronic therapy may be necessary, particularly when oral administration becomes impractical.

REFERENCES

1. Valsangiacomo E, Schmid ER, Schupbach RW, et al: Early postoperative arrhythmias after cardiac operation in children. *Ann Thorac Surg* 4:792-796, 2002.
2. Ramaswamy K, Hamdan MH: Ischemia, metabolic disturbances, and arrhythmogenesis: mechanisms and management. *Crit Care Med* 28:N151-N157, 2000.
3. Benson DW, Wand DW, Dyment M, et al: Congenital sick sinus syndrome caused by recessive mutation in the cardiac sodium channel gene (SCN5A). *J Clin Invest* 12:1019-1028, 2003.
4. Pfammatter JP, Bauersfeld U: Idiopathic ventricular tachycardias in infants and children. *Cardiac Electrophys Rev* 6:88-92, 2002.
5. Paul T, Bertram H, Bokenkamp R: Supraventricular tachycardia in infants, children and adolescents: diagnosis, and pharmacological and interventional therapy. *Paediatr Drugs* 2:171-181, 2000.
6. Etheridge SP, Judd VE: Supraventricular tachycardia in infancy: evaluation, management, and follow-up. *Arch Pediatr Adolesc Med* 153:267-271, 1999.
7. Wren C: Incessant tachycardias. *Eur Heart J* 19:E32-E36, 1998.
8. Benditt DG, Benson DW Jr, Dunnigan A, et al: Atrial flutter, atrial fibrillation, and other primary atrial tachycardias. *Med Clin North Am* 68:895-918, 1984.
9. Lan Y-T, Lee J CR, Wetzel G: Postoperative arrhythmia. *Curr Opin Cardiol* 18:73-78, 2003.
10. Yabek SM: Ventricular arrhythmias in children with an apparently normal heart. *J Pediatr* 119:1-11, 1991.
11. Kanter RJ, Garson A Jr: Atrial arrhythmias during chronic follow-up of surgery for complex congenital heart disease. *Pacing Clin Electrophysiol* 20:502-511, 1997.
12. Wilbur SL, Marchlinski FE: Adenosine as an antiarrhythmic agent. *Am J Cardiol* 79:30-37, 1997.
13. McKee MR: Amiodarone: an "old" drug with new recommendations. *Curr Opin Pediatr* 15:193-199, 2003.
14. Paul T, Guccione P: New antiarrhythmic drugs in pediatric use: amiodarone. *Pediatr Cardiol* 15:132-138, 1994.
15. Campbell RM, Strieper MJ, Frias PA: The role of radiofrequency ablation for pediatric supraventricular tachycardia. *Minerva Pediatr* 56:63-72, 2004.
16. Walsh EP, Cecchin F: Recent advances in pacemaker and implantable defibrillator therapy for young patients. *Curr Opin Cardiol* 19:91-96, 2004.
17. Cohen MI, Bush DM, Vetter VL, et al: Permanent epicardial pacing in pediatric patients: seventeen years of experience and 1200 outpatient visits. *Circulation* 103:2585-2590, 2001.
18. Sliz NB Jr, Johns JA. Cardiac pacing in infants and children. *Cardiol Rev* 8:223-239, 2000.
19. Bernstein AD, Daubert JC, Fletcher RD, et al: The revised NASPE/BPEG generic code for antibradycardia, adaptive-rate, and multisite pacing. North American Society of Pacing and Electrophysiology/British Pacing and Electrophysiology Group. *Pacing Clin Electrophysiol* 25:260-264, 2002.
20. Gregoratos G, Abrams J, Epstein AE, et al: Guideline Update for Implantation of Cardiac Pacemakers and Antiarrhythmia Devices—summary article: a report of the American College of Cardiology/American Heart Association Task Force on Practice Guidelines (ACC/AHA/NASPE Committee to Update the 1998 Pacemaker Guidelines). *J Am Coll Cardiol* 40:1703-1719, 2002.
21. Michaelsson M, Riesenfeld T, Jonzon A: Natural history of congenital complete atrioventricular block. *Pacing Clin Electrophysiol* 20:2098-2101, 1997.
22. Horenstein MS, Walters H III, Karpawich PP: Chronic performance of steroid-eluting epicardial leads in a growing pediatric population: a 10-year comparison. *Pacing Clin Electrophysiol* 26: 1467-1471, 2003.
23. Bink-Boelkens MT: Pharmacologic management of arrhythmias. *Pediatr Cardiol* 21:508-515, 2000.
24. Roden DM: Antiarrhythmic drugs: from mechanisms to clinical practice. *Br Heart J* 84:339-346, 2000.
25. Weindling SN, Saul JP, Walsh EP: Efficacy and risks of medical therapy for supraventricular tachycardia in neonates and infants. *Am Heart J* 131:66-72, 1996.
26. Gomez MN: Magnesium and cardiovascular disease. *Anesthesiology* 89:222-240, 1998.
27. Fish FA: Ventricular fibrillation: basic concepts. *Pediatr Clin North Am* 51:1211-1221, 2004.
28. Atkins DL, Kenney MA: Automated external defibrillators: safety and efficacy in children and adolescents. *Pediatr Clin North Am* 51:1443-1462, 2004.
29. The American Heart Association in collaboration with the International Liaison Committee on Resuscitation: Guidelines 2000 for Cardiopulmonary Resuscitation and Emergency Cardiovascular Care. Part 10: pediatric advanced life support. *Circulation* 102:I-291-I-342, 2000.
30. Strasburger JF, Duffy CE, Gidding SS: Abnormal systemic venous Doppler flow patterns in atrial tachycardia in infants. *Am J Cardiol* 80:640-643, 1997.
31. Gikonyo BM, Dunnigan A, Benson DW Jr: Cardiovascular collapse in infants: association with paroxysmal atrial tachycardia. *Pediatrics* 76:922-926, 1985.
32. Samson RA, Deal BJ, Strasburger JF, Benson DW, Jr: Comparison of transesophageal and intracardiac electrophysiologic studies in characterization of supraventricular tachycardia in pediatric patients. *J Am Coll Cardiol* 26:159-163, 1995.
33. Rhodes LA, Walsh EP, Saul JP: Programmed atrial stimulation via the esophagus for management of supraventricular arrhythmias in infants and children. *Am J Cardiol* 74:353-356, 1994.
34. Benson DW Jr, Dunnigan A, Benditt DG: Follow-up evaluation of infant paroxysmal atrial tachycardia: transesophageal study. *Circulation* 75:542-549, 1987.
35. Zimmerman FJ, Pahl E, Rocchini A: High incidence of incessant supraventricular tachycardia in pediatric patients referred for cardiac transplantation. *Pacing Clin Electrophysiol* 19:663, 1996.
36. Noe P, Van Driel V, Wittkampf F, Sreeram N: Rapid recovery of cardiac function after catheter ablation of persistent junctional reciprocating tachycardia in children. *Pacing Clin Electrophysiol* 25:191-194, 2002.
37. Brucato A, Frassi M, Franceschini F, et al: Risk of congenital complete heart block in newborns of mothers with anti-Ro/SSA antibodies detected by counterimmunoelectrophoresis: a prospective study of 100 women. *Arthritis Rheum* 44:1832-1835, 2001.
38. Qu Y, Xiao GQ, Chen L, Boutjdir M: Autoantibodies from mothers of children with congenital heart block downregulate cardiac L-type Ca channels. *J Mol Cell Cardiol* 33:1153-1163, 2001.
39. Trippel DL, Parsons MK, Gillette PC: Infants with long-QT syndrome and 2:1 atrioventricular block. *Am Heart J* 130:1130-1134, 1995.
40. Moak JP, Barron KS, Hougen TJ, et al: Congenital heart block: development of late-onset cardiomyopathy, a previously underappreciated sequela. *J Am Coll Cardiol* 37:238-242, 2001.
41. Bradley DJ, Fischbach PS, Law IH, et al: The clinical course of multifocal atrial tachycardia in infants and children. *J Am Coll Cardiol* 38:401-408, 2001.
42. Donnerstein RL, Berg RA, Shehab Z, Ovadia M: Complex atrial tachycardias and respiratory syncytial virus infections in infants. *J Pediatr* 125:23-28, 1994.
43. Dodo H, Gow RM, Hamilton RM, Freedom RM: Chaotic atrial rhythm in children. *Am Heart J* 129:990-995, 1995.
44. Fish FA, Mehta AV, Johns J: Characteristics and management of chaotic atrial tachycardia of infancy. *Am J Cardiol* 78:1052-1055, 1996.
45. Priori SG, Napolitano C, Schwartz P: Low penetrance in the long-QT syndrome: clinical impact. *Circulation* 99:529-533, 1999.
46. Scott WA, Dick M: Two:one atrioventricular block in infants with congenital long QT syndrome. *Am J Cardiol* 60:1409-1410, 1987.

47. Yang T, Snyders D, Roden D: Drug block of I(kr): model systems and relevance to human arrhythmias. *J Cardiovasc Pharmacol* 38:737-744, 2001.
48. Tzivoni D, Banai S, Schuger C, et al: Treatment of torsade de pointes with magnesium sulfate. *Circulation* 77:392-397, 1988.
49. Viskin S: Long QT syndromes and torsade de pointes. *Lancet* 354:1625-1633, 1999.
50. Roden DM, Lazzara R, Rosen M, et al: Multiple mechanisms in the long-QT syndrome. Current knowledge, gaps, and future directions. The SADS Foundation Task Force on LQTS. *Circulation* 94:1996-2012, 1996.
51. Moss AJ: Long QT Syndrome. *JAMA* 289:2041-2044, 2003.
52. Brugada P, Brugada J: Right bundle branch block, persistent ST segment elevation and sudden cardiac death: a distinct clinical and electrocardiographic syndrome. A multicenter report. *J Am Coll Cardiol* 20:1391-1396, 1992.
53. Antzelevitch C, Brugada P, Brugada J: Brugada syndrome: 1992-2002. A historical perspective. *J Am Coll Cardiol* 41: 1665-1671, 2003.
54. Brugada P, Brugada R, Brugada J, Geelen P: Use of the prophylactic implantable cardioverter defibrillator for patients with normal hearts. *Am J Cardiol* 83:98D-100D, 1999.
55. Priori SG, Napolitano C, Tiso N, et al: Mutations in the cardiac ryanodine receptor gene (hRyR2) underlie catecholaminergic polymorphic ventricular tachycardia. *Circulation* 103:196-200, 2001.
56. Priori SG, Napolitano C, Memmi M, et al: Clinical and molecular characterization of patients with catecholaminergic polymorphic ventricular tachycardia. *Circulation* 106:69-74, 2002.
57. Marcus FI: Update of arrhythmogenic right ventricular dysplasia. *Card Electrophysiol Rev* 6:54-56, 2002.
58. Danieli GA, Rampazzo A: Genetics of arrhythmogenic right ventricular cardiomyopathy. *Curr Opin Cardiol* 17:218-221, 2002.
59. McKenna WJ, Behr ER: Hypertrophic cardiomyopathy: management, risk stratification, and prevention of sudden death. *Heart* 87:169-176, 2002.
60. Van Hare GF, Stanger P: Ventricular tachycardia and accelerated ventricular rhythm presenting in the first month of life. *Am J Cardiol* 67:42-45, 1991.
61. Reynolds JL, Pickoff AS. Accelerated ventricular rhythm in children: a review and report of a case with congenital heart disease. *Pediatr Cardiol* 22:23-28, 2001.
62. Alexander ME: Ventricular arrhythmias in children and young adults. In Walsh EP, Saul JP, Triedman JK, editors: *Cardiac arrhythmias in children and young adults with congenital heart disease.* Philadelphia, 2001, Lippincott Williams & Wilkins.
63. Weindling SN, Saul JP, Gamble WJ, et al: Duration of complete atrioventricular block after congenital heart disease surgery. *Am J Cardiol* 82:525-527, 1998.
64. Janousek J, Vojtovic P, Gebauer RA: Use of a modified, commercially available temporary pacemaker for R wave synchronized atrial pacing in postoperative junctional ectopic tachycardia. *Pacing Clin Electrophysiol* 26:579-586, 2003.
65. Laird WP, Snyder CS, Kertesz NJ, et al: Use of intravenous amiodarone for postoperative junctional ectopic tachycardia in children. *Pediatr Cardiol* 24:133-137, 2003.
66. Cohen MI, Rhodes LA: Sinus node dysfunction and atrial tachycardia after the Fontan procedure: the scope of the problem. *Semin Thorac Cardiovasc Surg Pediatr Card Surg Annu* 1:41-52, 1998.
67. Murphy JG, Gersh BJ, McGoon MD, et al: Long-term outcome after surgical repair of isolated atrial septal defect. Follow-up at 27 to 32 years. *N Engl J Med* 323:1645-1650, 1990.
68. Williams WG, Trusler GA, Kirklin JW, et al: Early and late results of a protocol for simple transposition leading to an atrial switch (Mustard) repair. *J Thorac Cardiovasc Surg* 95:717-726, 1988.
69. Silka M, Kron J, McAnulty J: Supraventricular tachyarrhythmias, congenital heart disease, and sudden cardiac death. *Pediatr Cardiol* 13:116-118, 1992.
70. Saul JP, Alexander M: Preventing sudden death after repair of tetralogy of Fallot: complex therapy for complex patients. *J Cardiovasc Electrophysiol* 10:1271-1287, 1999.
71. Nollert G, Fischlein T, Bouterwek S, et al: Long-term survival in patients with repair of tetralogy of Fallot: 36-year follow-up of 490 survivors of the first year after surgical repair. *J Am Coll Cardiol* 30:1374-1383, 1997.
72. Wilson NJ, Clarkson PM, Barratt-Boyes BG, et al: Long-term outcome after the mustard repair for simple transposition of the great arteries. 28-year follow-up. *J Am Coll Cardiol* 32:758-765, 1998.
73. Roden DM, Woosley RL, Primm R: Incidence and clinical features of the quinidine-associated long QT syndrome: implications for patient care. *Am Heart J* 111:1088-1093, 1986.
74. Klein I, Ojamaa K: Thyroid hormone and the cardiovascular system. *N Engl J Med* 344:501-509, 2001.
75. Mattu A, Brady WJ, Perron AD: Electrocardiographic manifestations of hypothermia. *Am J Emerg Med* 20:314-326, 2002.
76. Towbin JA, Bricker JT, Garson A Jr: Electrocardiographic criteria for diagnosis of acute myocardial infarction in childhood. *Am J Cardiol* 69:1545-1548, 1992.
77. Hastreiter AR, van der Horst RL, Chow-Tung E: Digitalis toxicity in infants and children. *Pediatr Cardiol* 5:131-148, 1984.
78. Kloner RA, Rezkalla SH: Cocaine and the heart. *N Engl J Med* 348:487-488, 2003.
79. Frassica JJ, Orav EJ, Walsh EP, Lipshultz SE: Arrhythmias in children prenatally exposed to cocaine. *Arch Pediatr Adolesc Med* 148: 1163-1169, 1994.
80. Inoue H, Zipes DP: Cocaine-induced supersensitivity and arrhythmogenesis. *J Am Coll Cardiol* 11:867-874, 1988.
81. Chakko S: Arrhythmias associated with cocaine abuse. *Card Electrophysiol Rev* 6:168-169, 2002.
82. Chakko S, Sepulveda S, Kessler KM, et al: Frequency and type of electrocardiographic abnormalities in cocaine abusers (electrocardiogram in cocaine abuse). *Am J Cardiol* 74:710-713, 1994.
83. Witchel HJ, Hancox JC, Nutt DJ: Psychotropic drugs, cardiac arrhythmia, and sudden death. *J Clin Psychopharmacol* 23:58-77, 2003.
84. Babaliaros VC, Hurst JW: Tricyclic antidepressants and the Brugada syndrome: an example of Brugada waves appearing after the administration of desipramine. *Clin Cardiol* 25:395-398, 2002.
85. Pinto DS: Cardiac manifestations of Lyme disease. *Med Clin North Am* 86:285-296, 2002.
86. DiNubile MJ, Calderwood SB, Steinhaus DM, Karchmer AW: Cardiac conduction abnormalities complicating native valve active infective endocarditis. *Am J Cardiol* 58:1213-1217, 1986.

CHAPTER

27

Shock States

Lincoln Smith and Lynn Hernan

PEARLS

- Shock can be recognized by the features of tachycardia, tachypnea, and abnormalities of perfusion as evidenced by skin perfusion, quality of pulses, mental status, and other organ system dysfunction.
- Pediatric patients with shock most often present with myocardial dysfunction ("cold" shock), although older children and adolescents may present with the adult picture of vascular dysfunction ("warm" shock).
- Neonates in shock must be treated for both septic shock and cardiogenic shock resulting from ductal-dependent congenital heart disease until an echocardiogram can confirm the cardiac anatomy. These conditions cannot be ruled out by physical examination. Therefore all neonates with shock should be given prostaglandin infusion as part of their resuscitation. Pulmonary hypertension, hypocalcemia, and hypoglycemia frequently complicate shock in neonates.
- Pediatric patients in shock generally have absolute or relative hypovolemia, and the first line of resuscitation should be a fluid bolus of 20 ml/kg. Administration of more fluid should be based on rapid assessment of hemodynamic status.
- Early endotracheal intubations allow advantageous redistribution of the compromised cardiac output, and afterload reduces the left ventricle.
- Promising therapies for treatment of septic shock in children include use of activated protein C, stress dose steroids, extracorporeal membrane oxygenation, and plasma exchange therapy.

The clinical syndrome of shock is one of the most dramatic, dynamic, life-threatening problems faced by the physician in the critical care setting. Although untreated shock is universally lethal, mortality may be considerably reduced with proper recognition, diagnosis, monitoring, and treatment.

Definition and Physiology

Shock is an acute, complex state of circulatory dysfunction that results in failure to deliver sufficient amounts of oxygen and other nutrients to meet tissue metabolic demands. If prolonged, it leads to multiple organ failure and death.[37] Therefore shock states can be viewed as a state of acute cellular oxygen deficiency. Shock can be caused by any serious disease or injury, but whatever the causative factors it is always a problem of inadequate cellular sustenance. It is the final common pathway to death. Delivery of oxygen is a direct function of cardiac output (CO) and arterial oxygen content (Cao_2):

Delivery of Oxygen

$$Do_2 = CO$$

$$CO = \text{Heart rate (HR)} \times \text{Stroke volume (SV)}$$

$$Cao_2 = (Hgb \times 1.34 \times Sao_2) + (0.003 \times Pao_2).$$

Stroke volume is a function of preload, afterload contractility, and diastolic relaxation. Therefore increasing heart rate, improving contractility and diastolic relaxation, and optimizing preload and afterload improves cardiac output. Oxygen carrying capacity can be increased by raising hemoglobin and optimizing its saturation with oxygen. Oxygen delivery can be improved by manipulation of all these factors.[29]

Calculation of oxygen delivery provides a measure of global oxygen delivery and may not reflect regional hypoperfusion and localized ischemia. Inadequate oxygen delivery can result from either limitation or maldistribution of blood flow. Reduced oxygen content (anemia, poor arterial oxygen saturation) necessitates higher cardiac output to maintain oxygen delivery. In certain situations (fever, sepsis, trauma), metabolic demands may exceed normal oxygen delivery. Impairment of the extraction or utilization of oxygen by cells and mitochondria creates a functional arteriovenous shunt and may be the harbinger of multiorgan dysfunction syndrome.[20,42,43,52,115]

When oxygen delivery fails to meet cellular oxygen demands, various compensatory mechanisms are activated. Therefore shock is a dynamic process. The exact cardiorespiratory pattern detected clinically depends on the complex interaction of patient, illness, time elapsed, and treatment provided.

Because of its progressive nature, shock can be divided into phases: compensated, uncompensated, and irreversible. In *compensated shock*, vital organ function is maintained primarily by intrinsic regulatory mechanisms. Previously healthy children can compensate and maintain normal blood pressure during hypoperfusion states. Therefore identification of the early compensated stage of shock is crucial. Diagnosing a patient as having early compensated shock, rather than as mere dehydration, may be the difference between a patient who is appropriately resuscitated and one for whom resuscitative efforts are delayed. As shock progresses, the cardiovascular system's ability to compensate is exceeded, and microvascular perfusion becomes marginal. Cellular function deteriorates, affecting all organ systems. *Terminal* or *irreversible shock* implies damage to key organs of such magnitude that death occurs even if therapy restores cardiovascular function to adequate levels.

The ability to respond to shock states varies with age and depends on developmental aspects of the autonomic nervous, circulatory, respiratory, renal, and immunologic systems,[37] as well as the presence of other medical conditions.

Recognition and Assessment of the Shock State

The early diagnosis of shock requires a high index of suspicion and knowledge of conditions that predispose children to shock. Interviews of the parents, physicians, nurses, and emergency medical services personnel caring for the child provide valuable information. A rapid and focused physical examination of a patient in shock is essential (Box 27–1).

BOX 27–1

Physical Assessment in Shock

1. State of consciousness: restless, anxious, agitated, comatose
2. Skin: temperature, perfusion, moistness, color, turgor, rash
3. Mucous membranes: color, moistness
4. Nail beds: color, capillary refill
5. Central capillary refill
6. Peripheral veins: collapsed or distended
7. Pulse: rate, rhythm, quality
8. Blood pressure: orthostatic changes, pulse pressure
9. Respiration: rate, depth, effort, crackles, adequacy of aeration
10. Urine: concentration, hourly output

Early signs of compensated shock may be subtle and should not be missed. They include tachycardia, tachypnea, mildly prolonged capillary refill, orthostatic hypotension, and mild alteration of mental status (e.g., lethargy, irritability). In patients with sepsis, other signs of early compensated shock are plethora, warm extremities, bounding pulses, and a widened pulse pressure.

The contribution of laboratory tests to the initial evaluation of patients in shock is limited. Blood gases and serum lactate levels may quantify the degree of acidosis and are widely used as markers for the effectiveness of treatment. However, an increased understanding of microcirculatory aberrations and cellular hypoxia has raised awareness of the limitations of tests on pooled venous samples.[115] This has stimulated a search for a minimally invasive means of sampling regional circulations.[100] Gastrictonometry,[2,53] near-infrared spectroscopy,[32,79] rectal tonometry,[27] and sublingual capnography[76,104] are methods currently being investigated to evaluate regional circulation. Their clinical utility is unproved at this time.

Repeated evaluation and monitoring of the patient in shock by a competent observer, with appropriate intervention, remains the most effective and sensitive physiologic monitor available.

Treatment of Shock

General Principles

Shock is a clinical syndrome of inadequate tissue oxygenation. In addition to treatment of the primary underlying process, therapeutic efforts involve optimizing and balancing oxygen delivery and oxygen consumption. Efforts to reduce oxygen requirements at a time when oxygen delivery is compromised are important. Intubation, mechanical ventilation, sedation, paralysis and control of fever are ways to reduce oxygen consumption. Even routine nursing procedures can increase oxygen consumption by up to 20% to 30% in healthy adults.[126]

Intubation and Mechanical Ventilation

Viires et al.[127] studied spontaneously breathing dogs during cardiogenic shock. During a low cardiac output state, blood flow to the diaphragm was substantially increased, while blood flow to the liver, brain, and quadriceps was significantly decreased. Intubation, mechanical ventilation, and paralysis resulted in redistribution of blood flow from the diaphragm to the liver, brain, and quadriceps. A similar study of endotoxic shock in dogs demonstrated that respiratory muscle blood flow rose significantly in spontaneously breathing dogs.[63] During shock states, there is often increased work of breathing and respiratory distress related to capillary leak in the pulmonary bed and acidosis.

Intubation and mechanical ventilation can allow redistribution of cardiac output from the muscles of respiration to vital organs during shock (when cardiac output and oxygen delivery are compromised). Positive pressure ventilation also has the effect of reducing afterload to the left ventricle (thereby allowing improved stroke volume) (see Chapter 24).

Fluid Resuscitation

Regardless of the underlying insult, patients in shock have an absolute or relative hypovolemia. A primary goal of initial therapy must be restoration of effective circulating volume. Early fluid resuscitation is the cornerstone of immediate therapy.[22,23] In a study of pediatric septic shock patients, Carcillo et al.[22] correlated the volume of fluid given in the first hour of presentation and reversal of hypovolemia to outcome. Patients who received the largest volume of fluid in the first hour of resuscitation had the lowest mortality. Persistent hypovolemia was associated with increased mortality. Fluid resuscitation must be guided by repeated evaluation of the patient's hemodynamic status.

Vasoactive Infusions

Vasoactive infusions are commonly used when patients are adequately fluid resuscitated but hemodynamics remain deranged. Infusions of catecholamines (dopamine, dobutamine, epinephrine, norepinephrine), phosphodiesterase inhibitors (inamrinone, milrinone), and vasopressin are most commonly used. The choice of vasoactive infusion is dependent on the physiologic derangement requiring treatment (Table 27–1). Catecholamines work through stimulation of α_1, α_2, β_1, β_2, and dopaminergic receptors to increase intracellular cyclic guanosine monophosphate (cGMP) and cause the appropriate response (Table 27–2). Phosphodiesterase inhibitors increase cGMP by preventing its degradation within the cell (see Chapter 23). Vasopressin causes vasoconstriction by direct stimulation of vascular smooth muscle cells V_1 receptors.[4,59,60] Vasopressin also potentiates systemic adrenergic effects.[7,81,82,122]

Other Therapies

The finding of hypocalcemia in infants who present in shock should raise the suspicion of left ventricular dysfunction. Hypocalcemia has been reported as a cause of left ventricular dysfunction in neonates and is reversible with calcium therapy.[84] Of note, 30% of neonates with DiGeorge syndrome are hypocalcemic. Neonates also have low glycogen stores, and increased metabolic requirements during shock states may quickly develop hypoglycemia.[84]

Shock in neonates is frequently complicated by pulmonary hypertension. Adrenal insufficiency should be suspected in patients with refractory shock resulting from trauma (head or abdominal), history of steroid use within past 6 months, or sepsis. Direct damage to the hypothalamus, anterior pituitary, or adrenals may result in cortisol deficiency. In septic shock, adrenal hemorrhage has been the paradigm of adrenal insufficiency, but increasing evidence indicates transient relative or functional adrenal insufficiency in septic shock (see section on septic shock).

Extracorporeal membrane oxygenation (ECMO) has been used to support patients of all ages with shock. The Extracorporeal Life Support Organization (ELSO) maintains a database of patients treated with ECMO from member institutions around the world. The registry was searched for data on patients treated with ECMO with any mention of the diagnosis of shock (Lynn Hernan, personal communication, 2003). The registry revealed 952 patients who were treated with ECMO for any mention of the diagnosis of shock. The overall mortality was 64%. Fifty-two percent of patients were younger than 1 year. Mortality was 62% to 69% in all age groups (infant, pediatric, adult). In patients younger than 21 years treated with ECMO, the etiology of the shock was septic/hypovolemic (45%), cardiogenic (42.4%), unspecified (8.2%), postsurgical (2.2%), and toxic shock syndrome (2.2%).

TABLE 27–1

Therapies for Hemodynamic Patterns in Shock States

	Blood Pressure or Systemic Vascular Resistance		
Hemodynamic Pattern	**Normal**	**Decreased**	**Elevated**
Septic shock			
Stroke index ↑↔	None, D_1	α_1,V_1	None
Stroke index ↓	β_1	α_1 and β_1	β_1 plus β_2, or PDE
Cardiogenic shock	β_1	α_1 and β_1	β_1 plus β_2, or PDE
Myocardial dysfunction (complicating critical illness)*	β_1 and/or β_2	α_1 and β_1	β_1 plus β_2, or PDE
Congestive heart failure	β_1 and/or β_2	β_1	β_1 plus β_2, or PDE
Bradycardia	None	β_1	None

*For example, acute respiratory distress syndrome or anthracycline therapy.
PDE, phosphodiesterase inhibitor.

TABLE 27–2

Vasoactive Medications

	α_1	β_1	β_2	D_1	V_1
Dopamine*	Vasoconstriction; ↑ SVR, PVR	Inotropy; chronotropy	Vasodilation	Vasodilation (renal)	
Norepinephrine	Vasoconstriction; ↑ SVR, PVR	Inotropy (minor)			
Epinephrine†	Vasoconstriction; ↑ SVR, PVR	Inotropy; chronotropy	Vasodilation		
Dobutamine		Inotropy			
Inamrinone Milrinone	Nonreceptor-mediated inotropy, lusitropy, and vasodilation				
Vasopressin	Potentiates	Potentiates			Vasoconstriction

*Dose related. At low infusion rates, D_1-receptor effects predominate; at intermediate rates, β_1- and β_2- receptor effects predominate; and at high rates, α-receptor effects predominate.
†Dose related. At low infusion rates, β-receptor effects predominate; at high rates, α- receptor effects predominate on peripheral vasculature.
D_1, dopamine receptor; *PVR,* peripheral vascular resistance; *SVR,* systemic vascular resistance.

Multisystem Effects of Shock

Management of the multisystem deterioration that occurs in shock states is as important as treating the underlying condition. Respiratory, gastrointestinal, central nervous system, renal, and hematologic abnormalities in shock must be identified and treated.

Respiratory

Respiratory failure frequently accompanies shock states. It may result from failure of the ventilator pump (i.e., respiratory muscle fatigue) and/or deterioration of lung function (i.e., acute respiratory distress syndrome). For these reasons and for maximizing oxygen delivery, increased inspired oxygen is essential in all children with shock. Early tracheal intubation protects the airway, provides relief from respiratory muscle fatigue, facilitates provision of positive airway pressure, redistributes blood flow from the muscles of respiration to core organs, afterload reduces the left ventricle, and reduces oxygen demands of respiratory muscles. Patients should be ventilated with a lung protective strategy (see Chapter 45).

Renal

Renal failure may develop in association with any of the shock syndromes. Shock-related renal failure is a continuum of acute prerenal azotemia through classic acute tubular necrosis to cortical necrosis. Renal support is essential to prevent prolonged renal shutdown in shock states. Volume augmentation to correct absolute or relative hypovolemia is essential. Low-dose dopamine (3–5 μg/kg/min) improves renal blood flow and may be beneficial in preventing acute renal failure in shock states[46,88]; however, it may inhibit secretion of prolactin, growth hormone, and thyrotropin in critically ill children.[124] Acute anuric renal failure may require treatment with peritoneal dialysis, ultrafiltration, continuous hemofiltration or hemodiafiltration, or hemodialysis (see Chapter 65). High-output renal failure may occur in shock states without previous oliguria. The polyuria associated with this condition may falsely suggest adequate renal perfusion and adequate vascular volume at a time when the patient's intravascular volume is, in fact, depleted.

Although there is a potential drug that is directly renal protective in endotoxic shock,[9] restoration of perfusion pressure remains the standard of care. Populations for whom early renal replacement therapies result in decreased mortality have not been consistently demonstrated.[13,74,99,106] If renal dysfunction exists, all medications and therapies should be adjusted for creatinine clearance.

Coagulation

Coagulation abnormalities (e.g., disseminated intravascular coagulation) probably occur to some extent in all forms of shock. Monitoring of prothrombin time, partial thromboplastin time, and platelet count and observation for abnormal bleeding are essential. Replacement therapies specifically designed to replace absent clotting factors seem to be the most advantageous treatments. Use of vitamin K, fresh-frozen plasma, cryoprecipitate, and platelet transfusions should correct most coagulopathies. If replacement therapy is ineffective and the patient is at risk for purpura fulminans, heparinization[69] or antithrombin III infusions may be of value.[45,47]

Coagulopathy is ubiquitous in all patients with severe sepsis.[50] Recombinant activated protein C has been shown to decrease mortality in adults with severe sepsis (see section on septic shock).

Use of plasmapheresis, plasma exchange, and plasma filtration as therapy for treating sepsis-induced multiple organ system failure and improving outcome remains experimental. Their efficacy is controversial.[19,90,106,114,120]

Hepatic

The degree of hepatic dysfunction may determine a patient's ultimate outcome in severe shock states. Maintaining adequate circulation helps maintain liver function and prevents further hepatocellular damage. Liver function tests should be performed early and followed frequently. If dysfunction exists, drugs requiring hepatic metabolism must be carefully titrated.

Gastrointestinal

Gastrointestinal disturbances after hypoperfusion and stress include bleeding, ileus, and bacterial translocation. Ileus may result from electrolyte abnormalities, administration of narcotic medications, or from shock itself. Abdominal distension from ileus or ascites may cause respiratory compromise, especially in infants. Use of prophylactic medications (H_2 blockers, protein pump inhibitors, sucralfate) to prevent gastrointestinal hemorrhage is unproven.[41] Use of histamine antagonists has been associated with an increased incidence of nosocomial pneumonias.[41,116]

Acute nonocclusive mesenteric ischemia is a devastating condition characterized by intense, prolonged splanchnic vasoconstriction, intestinal mucosal hypoxia, and acidosis. Mesenteric ischemia eventually leads to transmural necrosis of the bowel, bacterial translocation, sepsis, and multisystem organ dysfunction.[38,44,108] Morbidity and mortality for this condition are high because the signs/symptoms are nonspecific, delaying diagnosis. Prevention of gut ischemia through adequate oxygen delivery may prevent bacterial translocation. Some clinicians advocate the use of selective gut decontamination and early enteral nutrition.[26,30,107]

Endocrine

Multiple endocrine problems involving fluid, electrolytes, and mineral balance may arise and complicate the management of children in shock. Severe abnormalities of calcium homeostasis can occur during the course of acute hemodynamic deterioration.

Hypoadrenalism may exacerbate the shock state. Patients who have been administered corticosteroids within 6 months preceding the onset of shock should be considered for stress doses of glucocorticoids.

Patients in shock because of head or abdominal trauma may have disruption of the hypothalamic-anterior pituitary-adrenal axis. Adrenal hemorrhage has been demonstrated as a manifestation of severe sepsis, but more commonly patients may develop a relative or functional adrenal insufficiency (see section on septic shock).

Functional Classification and Common Underlying Etiologies

Shock states can be classified into six functional categories (Box 27–2). Such tidy classifications imply a degree of precision that will be misleading when approaching an individual patient. Vicious cycles play a prominent role in most shock syndromes. Any given patient, over time, may display features of any functional category.[86] Hemodynamic profiles of these categories are summarized in Table 27–1.

BOX 27–2

Shock States

Hypovolemia
Cardiogenic
Obstructive
Distributive
Septic
Endocrine

Courtesy Dr. Mark S. McConnell and Dr. Ronald M. Perkin.

Hypovolemic Shock

Etiology and Pathophysiology

Hypovolemia is the most common cause of shock in infants and children. *Hypovolemic shock* is best defined as a decrease in the intravascular blood volume to such an extent that effective tissue perfusion cannot be maintained. Etiologies include hemorrhage (see Chapters 105 and 109), fluid and electrolyte loss (see Chapter 60), endocrine disease (see Chapter 70), and plasma loss (Box 27–3).

Hypovolemia causes a decrease in preload leading to a decrement of stroke volume and reduction in cardiac output. Activation of peripheral and central baroreceptors produces an outpouring of catecholamines, and the resulting tachycardia and peripheral vasoconstriction are initially adequate to support the blood pressure with little or no evidence of hypotension. Acute losses of 10% to 15% of the circulatory blood volume may be well tolerated and in healthy children are compensated. An acute loss of 25% or more of the circulating blood volume, however, frequently results in a clinically apparent hypovolemic state that requires immediate, aggressive management.

The most reliable indicators of early, compensated hypovolemic shock in children are persistent tachycardia, cutaneous vasoconstriction, and diminution of the pulse pressure. The best clinical evidence of decreased tissue perfusion is skin mottling, prolonged capillary refill, cool extremities, and decreased urine output. Systemic arterial blood pressure is frequently normal, the result of increased systemic vascular resistance, making blood pressure measurement of limited value in managing the patient with compensated hypovolemic shock. Neurologic status is normal or only minimally impaired.

With continued loss of blood volume or with delayed or inadequate blood volume replacement, the intravascular fluid losses surpass the body's compensatory abilities, causing circulatory and organ dysfunction. Stroke volume and cardiac output are decreased. The pronounced systemic vasoconstriction and hypovolemia produce ischemia and hypoxia in the visceral and cutaneous circulations.

BOX 27–3

Etiologies of Hypovolemic Shock

I. Whole blood loss
  A. Absolute loss: hemorrhage
    1. External bleeding
    2. Internal bleeding
      a. Gastrointestinal
      b. Intraabdominal (spleen, liver)
      c. Major vessel injury
      d. Intracranial (in infants)
      e. Fractures
  B. Relative loss
    1. Pharmacologic (barbiturates, vasodilators)
    2. Positive pressure ventilation
    3. Spinal cord injury
    4. Sepsis
    5. Anaphylaxis
II. Plasma loss
  A. Burns
  B. Capillary leak syndromes
    1. Inflammation, sepsis
    2. Anaphylaxis
  C. Protein-losing syndromes
    1. Nephrosis
    2. Intestinal disorders or obstruction
III. Fluid and electrolyte loss
  A. Vomiting and diarrhea
  B. Excessive diuretic use
  C. Endocrine
    1. Adrenal insufficiency
    2. Diabetes insipidus
    3. Diabetic ketoacidosis

Courtesy Dr. Mark S. McConnell and Dr. Ronald M. Perkin.

Altered cellular metabolism and function occur in these areas, resulting in damage to blood vessels, kidneys, liver, pancreas, and bowel. Patients become hypotensive, acidotic, lethargic or comatose, and oliguric or anuric. It is important to emphasize that arterial blood pressure falls only after compensations are exhausted, which may occur long after the precipitating event and only after a severe reduction in cardiac output. Terminal phases of hypovolemic shock are characterized by myocardial dysfunction and widespread cell death.

Therapy

Initial treatment of the child in hypovolemic shock is similar regardless of etiology. Therapy begins with the establishment or assurance of adequate oxygenation and ventilation. Oxygen should always be the first drug administered. Once the airway is ensured or established (may require intubation) and ventilation is adequate, measures to restore an effective circulating blood volume should begin. Placement of an adequate intravenous or intraosseous catheter and rapid volume replacement are the most important therapeutic maneuvers to reestablish the circulation (see Chapter 15). Central venous catheterization is infrequently necessary during initial resuscitation.

The choice of fluid depends on the nature of the loss.[130,131] Early correction of hypovolemia is the major factor preventing the later complications of shock. Crystalloid solutions, which are readily available, safe, and the least expensive, should be used in initial volume resuscitation. The first fluid bolus (20 ml/kg) should be administered as rapidly as possible. Heart rate, pulse pressure, blood pressure, peripheral perfusion, quality of mentation, and volume of urine output should be monitored. Improvement in these measurements should be expected if the blood volume loss is approximately 20%. Under these conditions, a rapid response to resuscitation can be anticipated. Maintenance fluid administration then can be initiated and vital signs monitored. The appropriate maintenance fluid depends on the measurements of serum electrolytes, total protein, and hematocrit.

The endpoint of fluid resuscitation should be normalization of arterial blood pressure, pulse pressure, peripheral perfusion, and heart rate; establishment of adequate urine output; and a decrease in the metabolic acidosis. If shock persists, continued aggressive fluid resuscitation in aliquots of 20 ml/kg should be initiated with rapid assessment of response to therapy. If the patient does not show improvement after several isotonic fluid boluses, more aggressive monitoring and reevaluation of the diagnosis may be required. Causes of ongoing vascular depletion should be sought. Such patients in profound hypovolemic shock will require frequent or continuous monitoring of heart rate, arterial blood pressure, arterial blood gases, central venous pressure (CVP), and urinary output.

Uncomplicated, promptly treated hypovolemic shock usually does not lead to a significant capillary injury and leak. However, severe, prolonged hypovolemic shock, traumatic shock with extensive soft tissue injury, and burn shock may significantly damage the pulmonary and other capillary membranes. Sepsis complicating hypovolemic shock may seriously impair capillary integrity.[58] Therefore once adequate circulation and urine output have been restored, fluid administration may be reduced unless there are demonstrable ongoing fluid losses. Continued assessment of hemodynamic status and vascular volume is essential to guide further therapy.

The amount of fluid necessary to restore effective circulating blood volume depends on the amount lost (deficit) and the rate of ongoing loss. The total amount of fluid given often exceeds the total volume lost because of expanded capacitance of the vascular space and dysfunction of cellular membranes. Ongoing fluid losses from chest tube drains, biliary drains, bowel, or other sources of bodily fluids may dictate the use of solutions other than crystalloid. Enough fluid must be given to provide adequate cardiac filling pressure. Adequate filling pressure only ensures that one determinant of cardiac performance—preload—has improved. It does not ensure adequate contractility, ejection of blood, and perfusion of tissue beds. A child with nonhemorrhagic hypovolemic shock should respond to 40 ml/kg of crystalloid solution. If a child is unresponsive to this amount of fluid resuscitation, the child must be evaluated for complicating factors. Causes of refractory shock include unrecognized pneumothorax or pericardial effusion, intestinal ischemia (volvulus, intussusception, necrotizing enterocolitis), sepsis, myocardial dysfunction, adrenocortical insufficiency, and pulmonary hypertension.

The first approach to further diagnosis of patients in persistent hypovolemic shock is the establishment of a central venous catheter for measurement of CVP. In the hypotensive patient, a CVP of less than 10 mmHg, in the absence of pulmonary edema, should be carefully augmented by fluid infusion until that level of preload is reached. If there is no improvement in blood pressure, peripheral perfusion, or urine output, cardiogenic causes of circulatory failure must be considered. Arterial blood gases, hematocrit, serum electrolytes, glucose, and calcium should be reevaluated. Correction of acidosis, hypoxemia, or metabolic derangements is essential. Blood and other appropriate sites must be cultured and broad-spectrum parenteral antibiotic coverage begun if sepsis is suspected. Shock persisting in the face of a CVP exceeding 10 mmHg may be an indication for placement of a flow-directed thermodilution pulmonary artery catheter and/or an echocardiogram.

Because many factors affect preload measurements, the absolute value of the CVP and pulmonary capillary pressure measurement may be less important than the change in measurement in response to therapeutic interventions. Used this way, these measurements allow detection of limitation in cardiac competence and therefore provide an important guide for volume replacement. Fluid administration should be discontinued when ventricular filling pressure rises without evidence of improvement in cardiovascular performance. At such a time, an inotropic agent may be necessary.

In the case of hemorrhagic hypovolemia, blood must be obtained and transfused if hypotension persists despite early crystalloid infusions. The patient with severe anemia in shock may need emergency transfusion of uncrossed matched blood as part of the initial resuscitation. The hematocrit may be a poor indicator of the severity of hemorrhage because it may not immediately decline in the setting of acute hemorrhagic shock. The possibility of occult intrathoracic or intraabdominal bleeding must be considered. Concomitant with fluid resuscitation of hemorrhagic shock, early surgical intervention may be indicated to control the source of bleeding. In the setting of hemorrhagic shock caused by penetrating trauma in adults, surgical control of the bleeding site may be more important than initial fluid resuscitation in improving patient outcome.[14]

Cardiogenic Shock or Congestive Heart Failure

Etiology and Pathophysiology

Cardiac shock is the pathophysiologic state in which an abnormality of cardiac function is responsible for the failure of the cardiovascular system to meet the metabolic needs of tissues. The common denominator is depressed cardiac output, which in most instances is the result of decreased myocardial contractility.[95] Cardiogenic shock or congestive heart failure (CHF) during infancy and childhood is a diagnostic and therapeutic challenge because of its myriad etiologies[21] (Box 27–4).

BOX 27–4

Etiologies of Cardiogenic Shock

I. Heart rate abnormalities
  A. Supraventricular tachycardia
  B. Ventricular dysrhythmias
  C. Bradycardia
II. Cardiomyopathies/carditis
  A. Hypoxic/ischemic events
    1. Cardiac events
    2. Prolonged shock
    3. Head injury
    4. Anomalous coronary artery
    5. Excessive catecholamine state
    6. Cardiopulmonary bypass
  B. Infectious
    1. Viral
    2. Bacterial
    3. Fungal
    4. Protozoal
    5. Rickettsial
    6. Sepsis
  C. Metabolic
    1. Hypothyroid/hyperthyroid
    2. Hypoglycemia
    3. Pheochromocytoma
    4. Glycogen storage disease
    5. Mucopolysaccharidoses
    6. Carnitine deficiency
    7. Disorders of fatty acid metabolism
    8. Acidosis
    9. Hypothermia
    10. Hypocalcemia
  D. Connective tissue diseases
    1. Systemic lupus erythematosus
    2. Juvenile rheumatoid arthritis
    3. Polyarteritis nodosa
    4. Kawasaki disease
    5. Acute rheumatic fever
  E. Neuromuscular disorders
    1. Duchenne muscular dystrophy
    2. Myotonic dystrophy
    3. Limb girdle (Erb)
    4. Spinal muscular atrophy
    5. Friedreich ataxia
    6. Multiple lentiginosis
  F. Toxic reactions
    1. Sulfonamides
    2. Penicillins
    3. Anthracyclines
  G. Tachydysrhythmias
    1. Supraventricular tachycardia
    2. Atrial flutter
    3. Ventricular tachycardia
  H. Other
    1. Idiopathic dilated cardiomyopathy
    2. Familial dilated cardiomyopathy
III. Congenital heart disease
IV. Trauma

Courtesy Dr. Mark S. McConnell and Dr. Ronald M. Perkin.

Cardiac function can be depressed in patients with shock of noncardiac origin. Myocardial dysfunction is frequently a late manifestation of shock of any etiology. Although the cause of myocardial dysfunction in such patients is not completely understood, the following mechanisms have been proposed: (1) specific toxic substances released during the course of shock that have a direct cardiac depressant effect, (2) myocardial edema, (3) adrenergic receptor dysfunction, (4) impaired sarcolemmic calcium flux, and (5) reduced coronary blood flow resulting in impaired myocardial systolic and diastolic function.[21]

Another form of cardiogenic shock is caused by diastolic dysfunction. Impaired myocardial relaxation changes the pressure-to-volume ratio during diastole and increases ventricular pressure at any volume. This lack of myocardial relaxation is hemodynamically unfavorable because increased left ventricular diastolic pressure is transmitted to the lung and results in pulmonary edema and dyspnea. Elevated left ventricular diastolic pressure also decreases myocardial perfusion pressure and can lead to subendocardial ischemia. Such patients present with "heart failure" but may have normal left ventricular systolic function. Diastolic properties of the ventricle appear to be the first to become abnormal in patients with ischemic heart disease or disorders associated with ventricular hypertrophy.[6,48] Therefore when approaching a patient with cardiogenic shock, it is important to characterize both systolic and diastolic function. Therapy designed to improve systolic function may impair myocardial diastolic function[48] (see Chapter 17).

BOX 27–5

Recognition of Congestive Heart Failure in Infancy

HISTORY

Excessive respiratory effort
Prolonged feeding time
Poor weight gain
Excessive sweating
Frequent respiratory tract infections

PHYSICAL EXAMINATION

Tachycardia, tachypnea
Gallop rhythm
Cold extremities, weak peripheral pulses
Wheezing, rales
Dyspnea, cough
Cyanosis
Diaphoresis
Hepatomegaly
Neck vein distension
Peripheral edema
Hypotension

CHEST X-RAY FILM

Cardiomegaly
Pulmonary venous congestion
Hyperinflation

Courtesy Dr. Mark S. McConnell and Dr. Ronald M. Perkin.

Clinical Assessment

The appropriate management of CHF in infancy is critically dependent upon the specific etiology; accurate and rapid diagnosis is of prime importance. Recognition begins with a careful history and physical examination (Box 27–5) and is supplemented by chest radiography, electrocardiography, and echocardiography.

Two-dimensional and Doppler echocardiographic studies provide important information about the size, thickness, and performance of the heart and delineation of cardiac malformations. Doppler investigation of the diastolic mitral inflow pattern is useful in assessing the presence of diastolic dysfunction.[48]

As opposed to hypovolemic shock, compensatory responses can have deleterious effects in patients with cardiogenic shock. Compensatory responses are nonspecific and imprecise and may contribute to the progression of shock by further depressing cardiac function. As contractility deteriorates and cardiac output decreases, systemic vascular resistance increases, in response to neurohumoral mediators, in order to maintain circulatory stability.[10] However, this increase in afterload adds to the heart's workload and further decreases pump function. Therefore in cardiogenic shock, a vicious cycle is established. Because of the self-perpetuating cycle, compensated phases of cardiogenic shock may not be observed. Patients are tachycardic, hypotensive, diaphoretic, oliguric, acidotic, and poorly perfused. Extremities are cool and mental status is altered. Hepatomegaly, jugular venous distension, rales, and peripheral edema may be observed. Cardiac output is depressed, and elevations in CVP, pulmonary capillary wedge pressure, and systemic vascular resistance are observed.

Therapy

Box 27–6 lists the general supportive and pharmacologic measures used in the treatment of severe CHF or cardiogenic shock. These measures are designed to increase tissue oxygen supply, decrease tissue oxygen requirements, and correct metabolic abnormalities. The initial therapy for cardiogenic shock is to support the heart with supplemental oxygen and mechanical ventilation. Preload should be optimized to allow the patient to take advantage of Starling mechanisms.

Although volume expansion and correction of metabolic derangements (e.g., pH, glucose, calcium, magnesium) may enhance cardiac function, pharmacologic interventions usually are necessary to improve cardiac function. This approach to treatment relies on the use of drugs having the ability to restore or augment myocardial contractility, improve cardiac output, and bring about restoration and maintenance of blood flow. The proper choice of drug(s) requires knowledge of the exact hemodynamic disturbance and of the pharmacology of the drugs (see Tables 27–1 and 27–2 and Chapter 23).

In neonates presenting in shock within the first 2 weeks of life, a lesion with ductal-dependent systemic output should be suspected, and prostaglandin E_1 (PGE)

BOX 27-6

General Principles in the Management of Severe Congestive Heart Failure or Cardiogenic Shock

MINIMIZE MYOCARDIAL OXYGEN DEMANDS

Intubation, mechanical ventilation
Maintain normal core temperature
Provide sedation
Correct anemia

MAXIMIZE MYOCARDIAL PERFORMANCE

- Correct dysrhythmias
- Optimize preload
  - Salt and water restriction
  - Augment preload by fluid challenges
  - Diuretics, venodilators for congestion
- Improve contractility
  - Provide oxygen
  - Guarantee ventilation
  - Correct acidosis and other metabolic abnormalities
  - Inotropic, lusitropic drugs
- Reduce afterload
  - Provide sedation and pain relief
  - Correct hypothermia
  - Appropriate use of vasodilator

EXCLUDE CONGENITAL OR TRAUMATIC HEART DISEASE

EXPLORE SURGICAL OPTIONS

Courtesy Dr. Mark S. McConnell and Dr. Ronald M. Perkin.

(0.05–0.1 μg/kg/min) should be infused emergently until a cardiac echocardiogram can be obtained. This is a lifesaving intervention; opening and maintaining ductal patency is the only intervention that allows systemic cardiac output.

Proper use of the various vasoactive drugs often requires the presence of indwelling arterial and central venous catheters. A pulmonary artery catheter may be helpful if the patient is not responding to therapy and shock is not resolving as expected. The presence of these monitoring devices allows the generation of data that will characterize the hemodynamic state, direct appropriate therapy, and allow for evaluation of the response to therapy. There is no usual drug or dose in shock; instead, therapy must be continually tailored to the patient's response.[94]

Myocardial Contractility: Inotropic Agents. The catecholamines are the most potent positive inotropic agents available; however, effects are not limited to inotropy. The catecholamines also possess chronotropic properties and have complex effects on vascular beds of the various organs of the body. Consequently, the choice of an agent may depend as much on the state of the circulation as it does on the myocardium.[91] The most commonly used catecholamines are norepinephrine, epinephrine, dopamine, and dobutamine.[11] Novel dopamine receptor agonists, such as dopexamine and fenoldopam, are being developed for management of CHF and preservation of renal function but are not yet clinically available in the United States.[87]

The digitalis glycosides may augment myocardial contractility, but because of a narrow therapeutic-to-toxic ratio, long half-life, and dependence of clearance on renal (digoxin) or hepatic function, their use in patients with cardiogenic shock should be avoided. These compounds have the advantage of improving contractility without further increasing the heart rate. They can be used once the shock is resolved.

Inamrinone, milrinone, and enoximone belong to a class of nonglycoside, nonsympathomimetic inotropic agents. They appear to act via potent and selective inhibition of phosphodiesterase.[17,71,91] Intravenous administration of inamrinone or milrinone increases cardiac output and reduces cardiac filling pressures and systemic vascular resistance with minimal effect on the heart rate and systemic blood pressure of adult patients. These drugs are particularly useful in the treatment of cardiogenic shock because they improve diastolic function (lusitropy), increase contractility, and reduce afterload by peripheral vasodilation without a consistent increase in myocardial oxygen consumption. These agents require careful bolus dosing prior to initiating an infusion; a rapid infusion of the bolus dose may cause hypotension.[71] Both of these drugs have relatively long half-lives, and they should be used cautiously in the presence of significant hypotension. Milrinone may be preferred over inamrinone because of inamrinone's tendency to cause thrombocytopenia. Enoximone is currently in phase III clinical trials in the United States, and it has been used in pediatric sepsis.[112]

Afterload Reduction: Vasoactive Drugs. Neurohumoral compensatory mechanisms that initially compensate for a fall in output of the failing heart in time become a major part of the problem.[10] The kidney's response to a decrease in cardiac output leads to expansion of extracellular fluid volume and, potentially, to circulatory congestion and edema. Systemic vasoconstriction raises aortic impedance, which, while tending to maintain perfusion pressure in the face of declining cardiac output, eventually impairs ventricular function. After resuscitation, therapy is directed to counteract these physiologic responses: for example, use of vasodilators to oppose systemic vasoconstriction, angiotensin-converting enzyme inhibitors to block the renin-angiotensin system, and diuretics to prevent or reverse abnormal fluid retention.[1] They should not be used as first-line therapy to reverse shock.

Numerous vasodilators, representing several different pharmacologic classes, improve cardiac performance and lessen clinical symptoms via arterial and venous smooth muscle relaxation.[1,94] Arterial relaxation should increase ejection fraction, increase stroke volume, and decrease end-systolic left ventricular volume. Some evidence suggests some vasodilator drugs increase left ventricular compliance, which should improve diastolic function.[48] Venous relaxation should shift blood into the periphery and reduce right and left ventricular diastolic volume, with attendant beneficial effects on pulmonary and systemic capillary pressure. This, in turn, ought to be reflected in decreased edema, reduced myocardial wall stress, and improved diastolic perfusion of the myocardium.

For treatment of cardiogenic shock, intravenous vasodilators with rapid onsets of action and short half-lives are preferred. Selection of a vasodilator agent should depend on its principal hemodynamic effects and the specific hemodynamic abnormalities in individual patients. Factors that increase systemic resistance, such as hypothermia, acidosis, hypoxia, pain, and anxiety, should be treated before vasodilator drugs are considered.

Use of vasodilators in shock is generally limited to situations in which cardiac dysfunction is associated with elevated ventricular filling pressures, elevated systemic vascular resistance, and normal or near-normal systemic arterial blood pressure. Occasionally, the combination of vasodilator and inotropic therapy results in hemodynamic improvement not attainable with either drug alone.

There is a growing awareness that right ventricular dysfunction plays a pivotal role in some of the most frequently encountered and important cardiopulmonary disorders in children, including congenital heart disease, acute respiratory distress syndrome, bronchopulmonary dysplasia, and other chronic pulmonary disorders. The ability of the right ventricle to respond to increased pulmonary vascular resistance seen in these situations often determines outcome. Therefore measures to decrease pulmonary vascular resistance have become more common in the treatment of many seriously ill pediatric patients. Such measures include supplemental oxygen, hyperventilation, metabolic and respiratory alkalosis, inhaled nitric oxide, prostaglandin E_1, prostacyclin, analgesia, and sedation.[67,93,111]

Surgical Intervention. A number of congenital cardiac defects may present in severe CHF and cardiogenic shock. Diagnosis of these defects is critical because surgery is the definitive therapy. Prostaglandin E_1 infusion allows for resuscitation and stabilization until surgery can be accomplished.

Cardiac function can be supported temporarily by mechanical means, including intraaortic balloon counterpulsation, left ventricular assist device, and ECMO. Cardiac transplantation has become an important tool for treating patients with severe myocardial dysfunction who otherwise would die of their heart disease.

Specific Etiologies

Cardiomyopathy. Patients may present in shock with dilated cardiomyopathy. The etiologies of acute dilated cardiomyopathies are listed in Box 27–4. Myocarditis is one of the more common causes of dilated cardiomyopathy in previously healthy children. The clinical presentation of myocarditis in pediatric patients is varied. Carditis may cause myocardial dysfunction or dysrhythmia, or it may be "clinically silent." Tachycardia (in the absence of fever) and tachypnea are usual presenting symptoms. In acute myocarditis, the history of illness is very short (hours to days). Life-threatening dysrhythmias in patients with acute myocarditis include ventricular tachycardia and supraventricular tachycardia. Initial resuscitation of the patient with myocarditis is the same as for other forms of cardiogenic shock; however, patients with myocarditis and other dilated cardiomyopathies may not respond as well to traditional inotropic therapy.[56,70] In addition, catecholamine infusions may promote the development of dysrhythmias. Once the diagnosis of myocarditis is made, treatment with steroids or intravenous immunoglobulin (IVIg) (1g/kg/day for 2 days) is recommended to modulate the inflammatory response.[80,121] Use of ECMO has been lifesaving in patients with acute myocarditis whose shock does not reverse with conventional therapy or in whom arrhythmias are unremitting. We queried the ELSO registry for cases of myocarditis treated with ECMO through April 2003. There were 124 cases, with a median run time of 6 days. The survival was 57% (Lynn Hernan, personal communication, 2003).

Hypoxic-Ischemic Injury. Shock following a generalized hypoxic ischemic episode (e.g., near-drowning, sudden infant death syndrome) is frequently encountered in infants and children with no preexisting cardiovascular or pulmonary disease. Data have shown that shock following hypoxic-ischemic events is cardiogenic. This shock is characterized by a low cardiac index, elevated right and left heart filling pressures, elevated systemic and pulmonary vascular resistances, decreased oxygen consumption, and elevated oxygen extraction index. In many patients, the mean systemic arterial blood pressure is elevated, which suggests the increase in systemic vascular resistance is exaggerated. Studies have documented progressive systolic and diastolic myocardial dysfunction immediately after successful cardiac resuscitation.[123] All of these observations have important therapeutic implications because the increased vascular resistance and decreased cardiac output may prevent adequate tissue perfusion following anoxic injury.

Cardiac Injury in Trauma. Blunt cardiac injury can cause myocardial contusion, myocardial concussion, aneurysm, septal defects, chamber rupture, valvular rupture, and damage to the pericardium. Each of these entities has separate presentations, although the lesions often are concurrent. Every pediatric trauma patient deserves a careful cardiac evaluation. Of note, both left and right ventricular function may be impaired significantly in children with isolated head injury. The myocardial injury seen in children with head injury appears to be related to high levels of catecholamines with resultant myocardial ischemia.[40]

Obstructive Shock

Etiology and Pathophysiology

Obstructive shock is caused by the inability to produce adequate cardiac output despite normal intravascular volume and myocardial function. Causative factors may be located within the pulmonary or systemic circulation or associated with the heart itself. Examples of obstructive shock include acute pericardial tamponade, tension pneumothorax, pulmonary or systemic hypertension, and congenital or acquired outflow obstructions. Recognition of the characteristic features of these syndromes is essential because most of the causes can be treated provided the diagnosis is made early.

Specific Etiologies

Cardiac Tamponade. Cardiac tamponade is defined as hemodynamically significant cardiac compression resulting from accumulating pericardial contents that evoke and defeat compensatory mechanisms. The pericardium may contain effusion fluid, purulent fluid, blood, or gas.

Clinical manifestations of tamponade may be insidious, especially when it occurs in conditions such as malignancy, connective tissue disorders, renal failure, or pericarditis. In early phases, the symptoms are nonspecific. As cardiac output becomes restricted, the overall picture resembles CHF; however, the lungs usually are clear. Findings on physical examination that suggest cardiac tamponade include pulsus paradoxus, narrowed pulse pressure, pericardial rub, and jugular venous distension. Echocardiography is of particular value in detecting the presence of pericardial effusion and can provide clues about the presence of tamponade. In rapid tamponade caused by hemorrhage, as in trauma, shock dominates the picture. Left untreated, it leads to electromechanical dissociation.

The definitive treatment of cardiac tamponade is removal of pericardial fluid or air by surgical drainage or pericardiocentesis. Removal of even a small volume of fluid can rapidly improve blood pressure and cardiac output. Surgical drainage by either thoracotomy or a subxiphoid limited surgical approach should be considered for traumatic tamponade.

Pericardiocentesis should be performed as soon as possible if the patient is considered in a life-threatening condition. Pericardiocentesis is a blind procedure; introduction of the needle should be monitored by echocardiography whenever possible. The subxiphoid approach is generally preferable in most cases (see Chapter 15).

Medical management is not a substitute for drainage but may avert a catastrophe until pericardiocentesis or surgical drainage can be safely performed. The principles of medical management include (1) blood volume expansion to maintain venoatrial gradients and (2) inotropic agents. In addition, any anticoagulant or thrombolytic therapy should be withheld or discontinued if pericardiocentesis is anticipated. Diuretics, which reduce blood volume, and digoxin or other agents, which slow the heart, are contraindicated in tamponade.

Coarctation/Interrupted Arch. Infants with aortic arch interruption or juxtaductal coarctation of the aorta may depend on patency of the ductus arteriosus to provide adequate lower body perfusion. In many such infants, the ductus arteriosus constricts after birth, resulting in severe heart failure, poor systemic perfusion, and acidemia. Many of the signs and symptoms of coarctation with shock are indistinguishable from shock of other etiologies.[117] A high index of suspicion must be maintained for infants who present in shock between birth and age 4 months. In severely ill infants in whom the diagnosis of coarctation or interruption of the aorta is clinically suspected, it is appropriate and often lifesaving to start a continuous prostaglandin E_1 infusion before diagnostic evaluation is performed.

Distributive Shock

Etiology and Pathophysiology

Distributive shock results from maldistribution of blood flow to the tissue. Abnormalities in distribution of blood flow may result in profound inadequacies in tissue oxygenation, even in the face of a normal or high cardiac output. Such maldistribution of flow generally results from widespread abnormalities in vasomotor tone. Distributive shock may be seen with anaphylaxis, spinal or epidural anesthesia, disruption of the spinal cord, or inappropriate administration of vasodilatory medication.

Treatment generally includes reversal of the underlying etiology and vigorous fluid administration. In severe cases of distributive shock unresponsive to fluids, vasopressor infusions may be necessary.

Septic Shock

The incidence of pediatric septic shock in the United States is approximately 0.56 cases per 1000 population.[132] The incidence is highest in infants (5.16 cases per 1000 population) and falls rapidly after the first year. There are an estimated 42,000 cases per year with a case fatality rate of 10.3% (or ≈4400 deaths per year). The average cost per case of pediatric sepsis in the U.S. is estimated to be greater than $40,000. The estimated national total annual cost is $1.97 billion.[132] Sepsis and septic shock are significant causes of mortality in children and consume a significant amount of U.S. health care dollars.

Etiology and Pathophysiology

Septic shock is the most complex and controversial type of shock and merits independent classification. Septic shock often is a combination of multiple problems, including infection, relative and absolute hypovolemia, maldistribution of blood flow, myocardial depression, and multiple metabolic, endocrine, and hematologic problems. Thus shock in sepsis contains many elements of the other types of shock discussed previously (hypovolemic, cardiogenic, and distributive shock) (see Chapters 84 and 96).[86,113]

Septic shock encompasses a cascade of metabolic, hemodynamic, and clinical changes resulting from invasive infection and the release of microbial toxins in the bloodstream. Correlation of clinical findings with the type of invading microorganism has been attempted. However, the systemic inflammatory response is independent of the type of invading organism (bacterial, virus, fungus, rickettsia) and is a host-dependent response.[15,51,113] Recognizing that etiologies other than bacterial infection cause a similar shock syndrome, researchers at the American College of Chest Physicians—Society of Critical Care Medicine Consensus Conference developed definitions for a variety of septic shock syndromes (Box 27–7).[73]

The pathophysiology of septic shock is incompletely understood. A combination of the direct effects of microbial agents, microbiologic toxins, the patient's inflammatory response to infection, and activation of endogenous mediators results in the cardiovascular instability and

BOX 27–7

*Definitions for Sepsis and Septic Syndromes**

INFECTION

Microbial phenomenon characterized by an inflammatory response to the presence of microorganisms or the invasion of normally sterile host tissue by those organisms

BACTEREMIA

Presence of viable bacteria in the blood

SYSTEMIC INFLAMMATORY RESPONSE SYNDROME (SIRS)

Systemic inflammatory response to a variety of severe clinical insults; indicated by two or more of the following conditions:

- Temperature >38°C or <36°C
- Heart rate >90 bpm (adults)
- Respiratory rate >20 breaths/min (adults) or PA_{CO_2} <32 mmHg
- White blood cell count >12,000 cells/ml^3, <4000 cells/ml^3, or >10% band forms

SEPSIS

Systemic response to infection manifested by two or more of the following conditions as a result of infection:

- Temperature >38°C or <36°C
- Heart rate >90 bpm (adults)
- Respiratory rate >20 breaths/min (adults) or PA_{CO_2} <32 mmHg
- White blood cell count >12,000 cells/ml^3, less than 4000 cells/ml^3, or >10% band forms

SEVERE SEPSIS

Sepsis associated with organ dysfunction, hypoperfusion, or hypotension. Hypoperfusion and other perfusion abnormalities may include, but are not limited to, lactic acidosis, oliguria, or an acute alteration in mental status.

SEPTIC SHOCK

Sepsis with hypotension despite adequate fluid resuscitation along with the presence of perfusion abnormalities that may include, but are not limited to, lactic acidosis, oliguria, or an acute alteration in mental status. Patients who are taking inotropic or vasopressor agents may not be hypotensive at the time that perfusion abnormalities are measured.

HYPOTENSION

Systolic blood pressure <90 mmHg (adults) or a reduction of >40 mmHg from baseline in the absence of other causes for hypotension

MULTIPLE ORGAN DYSFUNCTION SYNDROME

Presence of altered organ function in an acutely ill patient such that homeostasis cannot be maintained without intervention

*Modified from Bone RC, Balk RA, Cerra FB, et al: *Chest* 101:1644, 1992. Courtesy Dr. Mark S. McConnell and Dr. Ronald M. Perkin.

multisystem organ failure.[31,86,113] Septic shock is a constellation of signs and symptoms that reflect multiple organ system derangement at the subcellular level. Mediator release seems to be the final common pathway to the development of this shock state regardless of etiology.[51] Some mediators are cytokines, tumor necrosis factor, interleukin-1, interleukin-6, kinins, eicosanoids, platelet activating factor, and nitric oxide.

The clinical pattern and presentation of septic shock vary greatly and are dependent on the dynamic interplay of the invading organism, time to treatment, and the host response to the infection and treatment. All patients present with an absolute or functional hypovolemia. Several factors may contribute to hypovolemia. Increased microvascular permeability, arteriolar and venular dilation with peripheral pooling of intravascular volume, inappropriate polyuria, and poor oral intake all combine to result in reduced effective blood volume. Volume loss secondary to fever, diarrhea, vomiting, or sequestered third space fluid also contributes to hypovolemia. Abnormal hemodynamic responses constitute a primary hallmark of septic shock.[97,113] The most common presentation (80%) in children is low cardiac index with or without abnormalities of vascular tone.[75] These children present with tachycardia, mental status changes, diminished peripheral pulses, mottled cold extremities, and prolonged capillary refill (>2 seconds). Adults and some children (20%) present in a hyperdynamic state characterized by an elevated cardiac output and decreased systemic vascular resistance. On physical examination, patients appear plethoric with warm extremities. They have tachycardia, bounding pulses, and a widened pulse pressure. High fever, mental confusion, and hyperventilation may be present. At this stage the inexperienced observer may fail to recognize shock. Paradoxically, hypotension may occur in the presence of a normal or elevated cardiac output. In either case, hypotension is not necessary to make the diagnosis of shock.

Progression of sepsis is characterized by a loss of cardiac compensation for diminishing systemic vascular resistance, possibly as a result of inflammatory-mediated capillary leak, vasodilation, and/or toxin-mediated cardiac depression. Some patients die of refractory hypotension as a result of a low systemic vascular resistance.[96,101]

The progression from high to low cardiac output may occur rapidly. As cardiac output decreases, the physical symptoms change to those of a hypoperfused state. The patient has tachypnea, tachycardia, hypotension, weak thready pulses, mottled cold extremities, and delayed capillary refill. As tissue perfusion worsens, anaerobic metabolism ensues and lactic acid accumulates.

Progressive deterioration in oxygen consumption and oxygen extraction portends a poor prognosis. In addition to oxygen, impaired use of other metabolic substrates has been demonstrated in septic shock. Prior to the onset of cellular hypoxia,[20,42,43,52,115] dysregulation of glucose, fat, and amino acids occurs. Changes in glycolysis and gluconeogenesis are possibly the earliest metabolic manifestation of sepsis.[18] Insulin responsiveness,[75] intracellular calcium,[35] glucose distribution,[28] and adrenergic effects[109] all have been implicated.

Although most adults present with hyperdynamic septic shock, most children and especially infants who have limited cardiac reserve present with a low cardiac output state, clinically indistinguishable from cardiogenic shock.[25] Even during the hyperdynamic state seen in adults, myocardial contractility is depressed because of myocardial depressant factor, diffuse myocardial edema, adrenergic receptor dysfunction, and impaired sarcolemmic calcium flux.[68,101] Survival of children in septic shock is related to the speed and adequacy of resuscitation. When resuscitation is delayed or inadequate, cellular hypoxia and multiple system organ failure ensue and are the final common pathway to death.

Therapy

Primary therapeutic goals for the initial treatment of septic shock are identification of the shock state, rapid reversal of cardiovascular dysfunction, and control of the infection.

Removal or control of microorganisms by surgical debridement, drainage, and antibiotic therapy is a crucial component of treatment of septic shock. Antibiotic treatment is appropriate in patients with circulatory shock whenever an infectious etiology is suspected. Although not always possible, blood, urine, and samples from other potential infected sites should be sent for culture and susceptibility testing before broad-spectrum antibiotic therapy is initiated.

Cardiovascular Support. The primary goal in the initial management of septic shock is to restore hemodynamic stability. Increasing oxygen delivery by maximizing cardiac output and arterial oxygen content and minimizing oxygen requirements are fundamentals of management.[22]

Restoration of preload by volume resuscitation is the first therapeutic measure.[23] Early and effective expansion of the circulating blood volume may enhance oxygen delivery and prevent progression of the septic shock state. Patients in septic shock have an enormous fluid requirement caused primarily by peripheral vasodilation and capillary leak. Initial fluid requirements of septic patients frequently exceed the 60 ml/kg discussed by Carcillo and Fields.[23] Patients may require as much as 200 ml/kg. Fluids must be given incrementally, with attention to clinical signs of volume overload, and the administration of pressors may mask hypovolemia.[3] Placement of a thermodilution pulmonary artery catheter may be indicated in children who demonstrate a sluggish response to fluid infusion, show clinical or echocardiographic evidence of myocardial dysfunction, or fail to respond to appropriate cardiovascular support.

There continues to be debate regarding the use of crystalloid or colloid solutions for volume expansion in sepsis.[66] Packed red blood cells may be used if the hematocrit is less than 30% because red blood cell transfusion increases oxygen delivery to the tissues. However, expansion of oxygen-carrying capacity may not improve oxygen consumption.[83]

Whereas some patients respond to fluid resuscitation alone, many patients require therapy with vasoactive infusions (inotropes, pressors, or dilators). Inotropy with catecholamines or phosphodiesterase inhibitors may be effective in reversing myocardial depression and improving contractility. An evidence-based guideline for the management of resuscitation and support of children and neonates with septic shock was issued in 2002.[23] Algorithms for resuscitation for children (Figure 1 in Carcillo and Fields, 2002[23]) and neonates (Figure 2 in Carcillo and Fields, 2002[23]) can help guide management. Early reversal of septic shock with adherence to these guidelines is associated with improved survival in children with septic shock.[54]

A significant advancement in the treatment of severe sepsis has developed from the finding of the close interweaving of the immune/inflammatory cascade and the coagulation pathways.[50,92] Cytokines activate coagulation and inhibit fibrinolysis, and the procoagulant thrombin can activate inflammation. Patients with severe sepsis may be coagulopathic, and several studies have demonstrated acquired protein C deficiency in up to 90% of adult septic patients.[50] This deficiency is associated with poor outcome.[133] Phase III trials of recombinant human activated protein C (rhAPC) demonstrate significant reductions in morbidity[129] and mortality in adults. In the PROWESS study, a randomized, double-blind, placebo-controlled multicenter, multinational study of the use of activated protein C in severe sepsis,[12] 1690 patients with an average age of 60 years were enrolled in a study of the mortality difference between patients who received activated protein C (24 μg/kg/hour for 96 hours) and placebo. Seventy-five percent of patients had at least two organs failing at the time of enrollment. Patients who received placebo had a mortality of 30.8%, whereas patients who received activated protein C had a mortality of 24.7%, for an absolute reduction of 6.1%. Bleeding was more common in patients who received activated protein C (3%) than in those who received placebo (2.5%). The number need to treat to save one life was 16.

A study of 83 pediatric patients with severe sepsis aged newborn to 18 years showed that the pharmacokinetic, pharmacodynamic, effective dose and safety profiles were similar to those reported in the PROWESS study.[8] The mortality of sepsis is significantly lower in children than adults, and there is currently a randomized, placebo-controlled trial of rhAPC use in children.[50]

Nutrition. Septic patients develop protein/caloric malnutrition as a principal manifestation of their metabolic response to sepsis.[16] In patients who were previously malnourished or remained hypermetabolic, this rapidly developing malnutrition is believed to contribute to morbidity and mortality. However, the abnormalities in intermediary metabolism (see the Multisystem Effects of Shock section) make the provision of an adequate level of metabolic support challenging. Parenteral or enteral nutrition should begin as soon as cardiovascular stability is achieved. Many clinicians advocate the early use of enteral feedings to prevent gut mucosal atrophy and bacterial translocation.[85]

Experimental/Unproved Therapies. ECMO has been used to support myocardial and/or pulmonary function during sepsis. We queried the ELSO registry for ECMO use in all (neonatal, pediatric, and adult) patients with sepsis or septic shock. A total of 2194 patients identified: 2031 neonates (93%) and 163 patients older than 1 month (7%). Overall survival was 72%, but there was a significant difference in the survival of neonates versus other patients. Survival in the neonatal group was 74% versus 40% in all other patients.

The presence of adrenal insufficiency in septic shock has been widely studied. Meta-analyses of early studies using a short course of high-dose ("shock") glucocorticoids found no benefit and possibly increased mortality.[34,72]

Subsequent observations of adrenal hemorrhage and cytokine-mediated adrenal insufficiency identify a select group of patients who benefit from glucocorticoid replacement (50 mg intravenously every 6 hours) over a prolonged period (7 days).[5,33] Increased knowledge of the close intertwining of the hypothalamic-pituitary-adrenal axis with inflammatory mediators led to the concepts of "functional adrenal insufficiency" or "relative adrenal insufficiency."[33] In many cases, the insufficiency is temporary.[5,33] A random cortisol level of 25 μg/dl or less in hypotensive septic adult patients is more sensitive and specific than low-dose or high-dose corticotropin stimulation tests at identifying a group of septic patients as steroid responsive. Responsiveness was defined as cessation of the need for pressor support within 24 hours of initiation of steroids (100 mg every 8 hours). Sixty-one percent of adult patients had relative adrenal insufficiency as defined by the random cortisol level or response to steroid therapy.[77]

A randomized, double-blind, crossover study of a continuous infusion of low-dose (100 mg loading dose over 30 minutes followed by 10 mg/hour) hydrocortisone in septic adults showed improved hemodynamics and an antiinflammatory benefit without evidence of immunosuppression.[65]

The incidence of adrenal dysfunction in pediatric sepsis may be as high as 52% and is associated with increased vasopressor requirement and longer duration of shock.[57] These patients may benefit from stress doses of steroids for the duration of the shock.

Many pharmacologic agents and therapies have been evaluated as adjunctive treatments in sepsis and septic shock. They include inhibitors of arachidonic acid metabolism and inhibitors of thromboxane and leukotriene formation; exchange transfusion and plasmapheresis[19,24,90,105]; white blood cell transfusions; passive immunotherapy; toxic oxygen scavengers; inhibitors of myocardial depressant factors; and fibronectin administration.[64,97] Although these therapies have significant potential therapeutic usefulness, further study is required before they can be recommended.

The recognition of sepsis as the systemic inflammatory response to an invading microorganism led to therapies targeted at modulating inflammation, such as the administration of antagonists or antibodies to various cytokines (e.g., tumor necrosis factor).[62,64] In preliminary studies, monoclonal antibodies and therapies directed toward lipid A of endotoxin appeared to favorably affect the outcome of patients with gram-negative sepsis. Further trials demonstrated no improvement in survival in patients given these antibodies.[78] Anticytokine therapies directed at tumor necrosis factor and interleukin-1 similarly demonstrated no benefit or worsened survival in patients with septic shock.[62,89] However, reevaluations of studies using anti-tumor necrosis factor-α may have revealed subpopulations for whom there is a survival benefit.[110] Therapies designed to modulate the immune response,[36,39] inhibit neutrophil function, or inhibit synthesis of nitric oxide (endothelial-derived relaxing factor) have demonstrated no clinical benefit in septic shock.[89] Other areas being explored with regard to the pathophysiology and treatment of septic shock include factors that promote apoptosis,[39,62,102] use of insulin to maintain tight glucose control and normoglycemia,[55,103,125,128] and use of vasopressin[61,98,118,119] in sepsis. These therapies have shown some promise in adults, but little information about their efficacy in children is available.

Summary

Shock is a life-threatening condition that has a myriad of causes. In order to survive shock, recognition of the shock state and resuscitative efforts must be achieved early, the etiology elucidated, and ongoing monitoring and therapy instituted. The astute clinician who recognizes shock, institutes therapy, and continuously assesses response to therapy is the child's best chance for a quality survival.

REFERENCES

1. Effect of enalapril on mortality and the development of heart failure in asymptomatic patients with reduced left ventricular ejection fractions. The SOLVD Investigators. *N Engl J Med* 327:685-691, 1992.
2. Ackland G, Grocott MP, Mythen MG: Understanding gastrointestinal perfusion in critical care: so near, and yet so far. *Crit Care* 4:269-281, 2000.
3. Alston TA: Sepsis and hypovolemia: two bad. *Crit Care Med* 31:991-992, 2003.
4. Altura BM: Altura BT: Vascular smooth muscle and neurohypophyseal hormones. *Fed Proc* 36:1853-1860, 1977.
5. Annane D: Corticosteroids for septic shock. *Crit Care Med* 29 (7 suppl):S117-S120, 2001.
6. Arques S, Ambrosi P, Gelisse R, et al: Prevalence of angiographic coronary artery disease in patients hospitalized for acute diastolic heart failure without clinical and electrocardiographic evidence of myocardial ischemia on admission. *Am J Cardiol* 94:133-135, 2004.
7. Bartelstone HJ, Nasmyth PA: Vasopressin potentiation of catecholamine actions in dog, rat, cat, and rat aortic strip. *Am J Physiol* 208:754-762, 1965.
8. Barton P, Kalil AC, Nadel S, et al: Safety, pharmacokinetics, and pharmacodynamics of drotrecogin alfa (activated) in children with severe sepsis. *Pediatrics* 113(1 pt 1):7-17, 2004.
9. Begany DP, Carcillo JA, Herzer WA, et al: Inhibition of type IV phosphodiesterase by Ro 20-1724 attenuates endotoxin-induced acute renal failure. *J Pharmacol Exp Ther* 278:37-41, 1996.
10. Benedict CR: Neurohumoral aspects of heart failure. *Cardiol Clin* 12:9-23, 1994.
11. Berg RA, Donnerstein RL, Padbury JF: Dobutamine infusions in stable, critically ill children: pharmacokinetics and hemodynamic actions. *Crit Care Med* 21:678-686, 1993.
12. Bernard GR, Vincent JL, Laterre PF, et al: Efficacy and safety of recombinant human activated protein C for severe sepsis. *N Engl J Med* 344:699-709, 2001.
13. Best C, Walsh J, Sinclair J, Beattie J: Early haemo-diafiltration in meningococcal septicaemia. *Lancet* 347:202-201, 1996.
14. Bickell WH, Wall MJ Jr, Pepe PE, et al: Immediate versus delayed fluid resuscitation for hypotensive patients with penetrating torso injuries *N Engl J Med* 331:1105-1109, 1994.
15. Bone RC, Balk RA, Cerra FB, et al: Definitions for sepsis and organ failure and guidelines for the use of innovative therapies in sepsis. The ACCP/SCCM Consensus Conference Committee.

American College of Chest Physicians/Society of Critical Care Medicine. *Chest* 101:1644-1655, 1992.
16. Bower RH: Nutrition during critical illness and sepsis. *New Horiz* 1:348-352, 1993.
17. Brecker SJ, Xiao HB, Mbaissouroum M, Gibson DG: Effects of intravenous milrinone on left ventricular function in ischemic and idiopathic dilated cardiomyopathy. *Am J Cardiol* 71:203-209, 1993.
18. Bruins MJ, Deutz NE, Soeters PB: Aspects of organ protein, amino acid and glucose metabolism in a porcine model of hypermetabolic sepsis. *Clin Sci (Lond)* 104:127-141, 2003.
19. Busund R, Koukline V, Utrobin U, Nedashkovsky EP: Plasmapheresis in severe sepsis and septic shock: a prospective, randomised, controlled trial. *Intensive Care Med* 28:1434-1439, 2002.
20. Cairns CB: Rude unhinging of the machinery of life: metabolic approaches to hemorrhagic shock. *Curr Opin Crit Care* 7:437-443, 2001.
21. Califf RM, Bengtson JR: Cardiogenic shock. *N Engl J Med* 330:1724-1730, 1994.
22. Carcillo JA, Davis AL, Zaritsky A: Role of early fluid resuscitation in pediatric septic shock. *JAMA* 266:1242-1245, 1991.
23. Carcillo JA, Fields AI: Clinical practice parameters for hemodynamic support of pediatric and neonatal patients in septic shock. *J Pediatr (Rio J)* 78:449-466, 2002.
24. Carcillo JA, Kellum JA: Is there a role for plasmapheresis/plasma exchange therapy in septic shock, MODS, and thrombocytopenia-associated multiple organ failure? We still do not know—but perhaps we are closer. *Intensive Care Med* 28:1373-1375, 2002.
25. Ceneviva G, Paschall JA, Maffei F, Carcillo JA: Hemodynamic support in fluid-refractory pediatric septic shock. *Pediatrics* 102: e19-e18, 1998.
26. Cerra FB, Maddaus MA, Dunn DL, et al: Selective gut decontamination reduces nosocomial infections and length of stay but not mortality or organ failure in surgical intensive care unit patients. *Arch Surg* 127:163-167, 1992.
27. Chendrasekhar A, Pillai S, Fagerli JC, et al: Rectal pH measurement in tracking cardiac performance in a hemorrhagic shock model. *J Trauma Injury Infect Crit Care* 40:963-967, 1996.
28. Chinkes D, deMelo E, Zhang XJ, et al: Increased plasma glucose clearance in sepsis is due to increased exchange between plasma and interstitial fluid. *Shock* 4:356-360, 1995.
29. Cilley RE, Scharenberg AM, Bongiorno PF, et al: Low oxygen delivery produced by anemia, hypoxia, and low cardiac output. *J Surg Res* 51:425-433, 1991.
30. Cockerill FR III, Muller SR, Anhalt JP, et al: Prevention of infection in critically ill patients by selective decontamination of the digestive tract. *Ann Intern Med* 117:545-553, 1992.
31. Cohen J: The immunopathogenesis of sepsis. *Nature* 420:885-891, 2002.
32. Cohn SM, Varela JE, Giannotti G, et al: Splanchnic perfusion evaluation during hemorrhage and resuscitation with gastric near-infrared spectroscopy. *J Trauma Injury Infect Crit Care* 50:629-634, discussion 634-635, 2001.
33. Cooper MS, Stewart PM: Corticosteroid insufficiency in acutely ill patients. *N Engl J Med* 348:727-734, 2003.
34. Cronin L, Cook DJ, Carlet J, et al: Corticosteroid treatment for sepsis: a critical appraisal and meta-analysis of the literature. *Crit Care Med* 23:1430-1439, 1995.
35. Crouser ED, Dorinsky PM: Metabolic consequences of sepsis. Correlation with altered intracellular calcium homeostasis. *Clin Chest Med* 17:249-261, 1996.
36. Das UN: Critical advances in septicemia and septic shock. *Crit Care* 4:290-296, 2000.
37. De Bruin WJ, Greenwald BM, Notterman DA: Fluid resuscitation in pediatrics. *Crit Care Clin* 8:423-438, 1992.
38. Deitch EA: The role of intestinal barrier failure and bacterial translocation in the development of systemic infection and multiple organ failure. *Arch Surg* 125:403-404, 1990.
39. Despond O, Proulx F, Carcillo JA, Lacroix J: Pediatric sepsis and multiple organ dysfunction syndrome. *Curr Opin Pediatr* 13: 247-253, 2001.
40. Dujardin KS, McCully RB, Wijdicks EF, et al: Myocardial dysfunction associated with brain death: clinical, echocardiographic, and pathologic features. *J Heart Lung Transplant* 20:350-357, 2001.
41. Fabian TC, Boucher BA, Croce MA, et al: Pneumonia and stress ulceration in severely injured patients. A prospective evaluation of the effects of stress ulcer prophylaxis. *Arch Surg* 128:185-191, 1993.
42. Fink MP: Cytopathic hypoxia. Mitochondrial dysfunction as mechanism contributing to organ dysfunction in sepsis. *Crit Care Clin* 17:219-237, 2001.
43. Fink MP: Cytopathic hypoxia. Is oxygen use impaired in sepsis as a result of an acquired intrinsic derangement in cellular respiration? *Crit Care Clin* 18:165-175, 2002.
44. Fink MP: Gastrointestinal mucosal injury in experimental models of shock, trauma, and sepsis. *Crit Care Med* 19:627-641, 1991.
45. Finney SJ, Evans TW: Emerging therapies in severe sepsis. *Thorax* 57(suppl 2):II8-II14, 2002.
46. Flancbaum L, Choban PS, Dasta JF: Quantitative effects of low-dose dopamine on urine output in oliguric surgical intensive care unit patients. *Crit Care Med* 22:61-68, 1994.
47. Fourrier F, Chopin C, Huart JJ, et al: Double-blind, placebo-controlled trial of antithrombin III concentrates in septic shock with disseminated intravascular coagulation. *Chest* 104:882-888, 1993.
48. Gaasch WH: Diagnosis and treatment of heart failure based on left ventricular systolic or diastolic dysfunction. *JAMA* 271:1276-1280, 1994.
50. Giroir BP: Recombinant human activated protein C for the treatment of severe sepsis: is there a role in pediatrics? *Curr Opin Pediatr* 15:92-96, 2003.
51. Giroir BP: Mediators of septic shock: new approaches for interrupting the endogenous inflammatory cascade. *Crit Care Med* 21:780-789, 1993.
52. Gutierrez G, Lund N, Bryan-Brown CW: Cellular oxygen utilization during multiple organ failure. *Crit Care Clin* 5:271-287, 1989.
53. Hamilton MA, Mythen MG: Gastric tonometry: where do we stand? *Curr Opin Crit Care* 7:122-1227, 2001.
54. Han YY, Carcillo JA, Dragotta MA, et al: Early reversal of pediatric-neonatal septic shock by community physicians is associated with improved outcome. *Pediatrics* 112:793-799, 2003.
55. Hansen TK, Thiel S, Wouters PJ, et al: Intensive insulin therapy exerts antiinflammatory effects in critically ill patients and counteracts the adverse effect of low mannose-binding lectin levels. *J Clin Endocrinol Metab* 88:1082-1088, 2003.
56. Harding SE, MacLeod KT, Jones SM, et al: Contractile responses of myocytes isolated from patients with cardiomyopathy. *Eur Heart J* 12(suppl D):44-48, 1991.
57. Hatherill M, Tibby SM, Hilliard T, et al: Adrenal insufficiency in septic shock. *Arch Dis Child* 80:51-55, 1999.
58. Haupt MT, Kaufman BS, Carlson RW: Fluid resuscitation in patients with increased vascular permeability. *Crit Care Clin*: 341-353, 1992.
59. Holmes CL, Landry DW, Granton JT: Science review: vasopressin and the cardiovascular system part 1—receptor physiology. *Crit Care (Lond)* 7:427-434, 2003.
60. Holmes CL, Landry DW, Granton JT: cience review: vasopressin and the cardiovascular system part 2—clinical physiology. *Crit Care (Lond)* 8:15-23, 2004.
61. Holmes CL, Patel BM, Russell JA, Walley KR: Physiology of vasopressin relevant to management of septic shock. *Chest* 120: 989-1002, 2001.
62. Hotchkiss RS: Karl IE: The pathophysiology and treatment of sepsis. *N Engl J Med* 348:138-150, 2003.
63. Hussain SN, Graham R, Rutledge F, Roussos C: Respiratory muscle energetics during endotoxic shock in dogs. *J Appl Physiol* 60:486-493, 1986.
64. Jafari HS, McCracken GH Jr: Sepsis and septic shock: a review for clinicians. *Pediatr Infect Dis J* 11:739-748, 1992.
65. Keh D, Boehnke T, Weber-Cartens S, et al: Immunologic and hemodynamic effects of "low-dose" hydrocortisone in septic shock: a double-blind, randomized, placebo-controlled, crossover study. *Am J Respir Crit Care Med* 167:512-520, 2003.
66. Khandelwal P, Bohn D, Carcillo JA, Thomas NJ: Pro/con clinical debate: do colloids have advantages over crystalloids in paediatric sepsis? *Crit Care* 6:286-288, 2002.
67. Kinsella JP, Toews WH, Henry D, Abman SH: Selective and sustained pulmonary vasodilation with inhalational nitric oxide

therapy in a child with idiopathic pulmonary hypertension. *J Pediatr* 122(5 pt 1):803-806, 1993.
68. Krishnagopalan S, Kumar A, Parrillo JE, Kumar A: Myocardial dysfunction in the patient with sepsis. *Curr Opin Crit Care* 8: 376-388, 2002.
69. Kuppermann N, Inkelis SH, Saladino R: The role of heparin in the prevention of extremity and digit necrosis in meningococcal purpura fulminans. *Pediatr Infect Dis J* 13:867-873, 1994.
70. Lang R: Medical management of chronic heart failure: inotropic, vasodilator, or inodilator drugs? *Am Heart J* 120(6 pt 2): 1558-1564, 1990.
71. Lawless ST, Zaritsky A, Miles M: The acute pharmacokinetics and pharmacodynamics of amrinone in pediatric patients. *J Clin Pharmacol* 31:800-803, 1991.
72. Lefering R, Neugebauer EA: Steroid controversy in sepsis and septic shock: a meta-analysis. *Crit Care Med* 23:1294-1303, 1995.
73. Levy MM, Fink MP, Marshall JC, et al: 2001 SCCM/ESICM/ACCP/ATS/SIS International Sepsis Definitions Conference. *Crit Care Med* 31:1250-1256, 2003.
74. Lewis MA: Veno-venous haemodiafiltration in meningococcal septicaemia. *Lancet* 347:612-613, 2, 1996.
75. Maitra SR, Wojnar MM, Lang CH: Alterations in tissue glucose uptake during the hyperglycemic and hypoglycemic phases of sepsis. *Shock* 13:379-385, 2000.
76. Marik PE: Sublingual capnography: a clinical validation study. *Chest* 120:923-927, 2001.
77. Marik PE, Zaloga GP: Adrenal insufficiency during septic shock. *Crit Care Med* 31:141-145, 2003.
78. McCloskey RV, Straube RC, Sanders C, et al: Treatment of septic shock with human monoclonal antibody HA-1A. A randomized, double-blind, placebo-controlled trial. CHESS Trial Study Group. *Ann Intern Med* 121:1-5, 1994.
79. McKinley BA, Marvin RG, Cocanour CS, Moore FA: Tissue hemoglobin O2 saturation during resuscitation of traumatic shock monitored using near infrared spectrometry. *J Trauma Injury Infect Crit Care* 48:637-642, 2000.
80. McNamara DM, Holubkov R, Starling RC, et al: Controlled trial of intravenous immune globulin in recent-onset dilated cardiomyopathy. *Circulation* 103:2254-2259, 2001.
81. Medina P, Acuna A, Martinez-Leon JB, et al: Arginine vasopressin enhances sympathetic constriction through the V1 vasopressin receptor in human saphenous vein. *Circulation* 97:865-870, 1998.
82. Medina P, Noguera I, Aldasoro M, et al: Enhancement by vasopressin of adrenergic responses in human mesenteric arteries. *Am J Physiol* 272(3 pt 2):H1087-H1093, 1997.
83. Mink RB, Pollack MM: Effect of blood transfusion on oxygen consumption in pediatric septic shock. *Crit Care Med* 18:1087-1091, 1990.
84. Moller JH, Hoffman JIE: Congestive *heart failure pediatric cardiovascular medicine*. New York, 2000, Churchill Livingstone.
85. Moore FA, Feliciano DV, Andrassy RJ, et al: Early enteral feeding, compared with parenteral, reduces postoperative septic complications. The results of a meta-analysis. *Ann Surg* 216:172-183, 1992.
86. Mouchawar A, Rosenthal M: A pathophysiological approach to the patient in shock. *Int Anesthesiol Clin* 31:1-20, 1993.
87. Murphy MB, Elliott WJ: Dopamine and dopamine receptor agonists in cardiovascular therapy. *Crit Care Med* 18(1 pt 2): S14-S18, 1990.
88. Myles PS, Buckland MR, Schenk NJ, et al: Effect of "renal-dose" dopamine on renal function following cardiac surgery. *Anaesth Intensive Care* 21:56-61, 1993.
89. Natanson C, Hoffman WD, Suffredini AF, et al: Selected treatment strategies for septic shock based on proposed mechanisms of pathogenesis. *Ann Intern Med* 120:771-783, 1994.
90. Nguyen TC, Hall MW, Han YY, et al: A randomized control trial of plasma exchange therapy in pediatric patients with thrombocytopenia associated multiple organ failure. *Soc Pediatr Res* 49:42A, 2001.
91. Om A, Hess ML: Inotropic therapy of the failing myocardium. *Clin Cardiol* 16:5-14, 1993.
92. Opal SM, Esmon CT: Bench-to-bedside review: functional relationships between coagulation and the innate immune response and their respective roles in the pathogenesis of sepsis. *Crit Care* 7:23-38, 2003.
93. Pacher R, Globits S, Wutte M, et al: Beneficial hemodynamic effects of prostaglandin E1 infusion in catecholamine-dependent heart failure: results of a prospective, randomized, controlled study. *Crit Care Med* 22:1084-1090, 1994.
94. Packer M: Treatment of chronic heart failure. *Lancet* 340:92-95, 1992.
95. Packer M: Pathophysiology of chronic heart failure. *Lancet* 340:88-92, 1992.
96. Parker MM, McCarthy KE, Ognibene FP, Parrillo JE: Right ventricular dysfunction and dilatation, similar to left ventricular changes, characterize the cardiac depression of septic shock in humans. *Chest* 97:126-131, 1990.
97. Parrillo JE, Parker MM, Natanson C, et al: Septic shock in humans. Advances in the understanding of pathogenesis, cardiovascular dysfunction, and therapy. *Ann Intern Med* 113:227-242, 1990.
98. Patel BM, Chittock DR, Russell JA, Walley KR: Beneficial effects of short-term vasopressin infusion during severe septic shock. *Anesthesiology* 96:576-582, 2002.
99. Pearson G, Khandelwal PC, Naqvi N: Early filtration and mortality in meningococcal septic shock? *Arch Dis Child* 83:508-509, 2000.
100. Pinsky MR: Beyond global oxygen supply-demand relations: in search of measures of dysoxia. *Intensive Care Med* 20:1-3, 1994.
101. Porembka DT: Cardiovascular abnormalities in sepsis. *New Horiz* 1:324-341, 1993.
102. Power C, Fanning N, Redmond HP: Cellular apoptosis and organ injury in sepsis: a review. *Shock* 18:197-211, 2002.
103. Preiser JC, Devos P, Van den BG: Tight control of glycaemia in critically ill patients. *Curr Opin Clin Nutr Metab Care* 5:533-537, 2002.
104. Rackow EC, O'Neil P, Astiz ME, Carpati CM: Sublingual capnometry and indexes of tissue perfusion in patients with circulatory failure. *Chest* 120:1633-1638, 2001.
105. Reeves JH: A review of plasma exchange in sepsis. *Blood Purif* 20:282-288, 2002.
106. Reeves JH, Butt WW, Shann F, et al: Continuous plasmafiltration in sepsis syndrome. Plasmafiltration in Sepsis Study Group. *Crit Care Med* 27:2096-2104, 1999.
107. Reidy JJ, Ramsay G: Clinical trials of selective decontamination of the digestive tract: review. *Crit Care Med* 18:1449-1456, 1990.
108. Reilly PM, Bulkley GB: Vasoactive mediators and splanchnic perfusion. *Crit Care Med* 21(2 suppl):S55-S68, 1993.
109. Reinelt H, Radermacher P, Fischer G, et al: Effects of a dobutamine-induced increase in splanchnic blood flow on hepatic metabolic activity in patients with septic shock. *Anesthesiology* 86:818-824, 1997.
110. Reinhart K, Karzai W: Anti-tumor necrosis factor therapy in sepsis: update on clinical trials and lessons learned. *Crit Care Med* 29(7 suppl):S121-S125, 2001.
111. Rich GF, Murphy GD Jr, Roos CM, Johns RA: Inhaled nitric oxide. Selective pulmonary vasodilation in cardiac surgical patients. *Anesthesiology* 78:1028-1035, 1993.
112. Ringe HI, Varnholt V, Gaedicke G: Cardiac rescue with enoximone in volume and catecholamine refractory septic shock. *Pediatr Crit Care Med* 4:471-475, 2003.
113. Saez-Llorens X, McCracken GH Jr: Sepsis syndrome and septic shock in pediatrics: current concepts of terminology, pathophysiology, and management. *J Pediatr* 123:497-508, 1993.
114. Schmidt J, Mann S, Mohr VD, et al: Plasmapheresis combined with continuous venovenous hemofiltration in surgical patients with sepsis. *Intensive Care Med* 26:532-537, 2000.
115. Schumacker PT, Samsel RW: Oxygen delivery and uptake by peripheral tissues: physiology and pathophysiology. *Crit Care Clin* 5:255-269, 1989.
116. Schuster DP: Stress ulcer prophylaxis: in whom? With what? *Crit Care Med* 21:4-6, 1993.
117. Schwangel DA, Nichols DG, Cameron DE: Coarctation of the aorta and interrupted aortic arch. In Nichols DG, Cameron DE, Greeley WJ, Lappe DG, Underleider RM, Wetzel RC, editors: *Critical heart disease in infants and children*. St. Louis, 1995, Mosby-Year Book.
118. Sharshar T, Blanchard A, Paillard M, et al: Circulating vasopressin levels in septic shock. *Crit Care Med* 31:1752-1758, 2003.

119. Sharshar T, Carlier R, Blanchard A, et al: Depletion of neurohypophyseal content of vasopressin in septic shock. *Crit Care Med* 30:497-500, 2002.
120. Stegmayr B: Apheresis of plasma compounds as a therapeutic principle in severe sepsis and multiorgan dysfunction syndrome. *Clin Chem Lab Med* 37:327-332, 1999.
121. Stouffer GA, Sheahan RG, Lenihan DJ, et al: The current status of immune modulating therapy for myocarditis: a case of acute parvovirus myocarditis treated with intravenous immunoglobulin. *Am J Med Sci* 326:369-374, 2003.
122. Streefkerk JO, Mathy MJ, Pfaffendorf M, van Zwieten PA: Vasopressin-induced presynaptic facilitation of sympathetic neurotransmission in the pithed rat. *J Hypertens* 20:1175-1180, 2002.
123. Tang W, Weil MH, Sun S, et al: Progressive myocardial dysfunction after cardiac resuscitation. *Crit Care Med* 21:1046-1050, 1993.
124. Van den BG, de ZF, Lauwers P: Dopamine suppresses pituitary function in infants and children. *Crit Care Med* 22:1747-1753, 1994.
125. Van den BG, Wouters P, Weekers F, et al: Intensive insulin therapy in the critically ill patients. *N Engl J Med* 345:1359-1367, 2001.
126. Verderber A, Gallagher KJ: Effects of bathing, passive range-of-motion exercises, and turning on oxygen consumption in healthy men and women. *Am J Crit Care* 3:374-381, 1994.
127. Viires N, Sillye G, Aubier M, et al: Regional blood flow distribution in dog during induced hypotension and low cardiac output. Spontaneous breathing versus artificial ventilation. *J Clin Invest* 72:935-947, 1983.
128. Vincent JL, Abraham E, Annane D, et al: Reducing mortality in sepsis: new directions. *Crit Care* 6(suppl 3):S1-18, 2002.
129. Vincent JL, Angus DC, Artigas A, et al: Effects of drotrecogin alfa (activated) on organ dysfunction in the PROWESS trial. *Crit Care Med* 31:834-840, 2003.
130. Wagner BK, D'Amelio LF: Pharmacologic and clinical considerations in selecting crystalloid, colloidal, and oxygen-carrying resuscitation fluids, part 1. *Clin Pharm* 12:335-346, 1993.
131. Wagner BK, D'Amelio LF: Pharmacologic and clinical considerations in selecting crystalloid, colloidal, and oxygen-carrying resuscitation fluids, part 2. *Clin Pharm* 12:415-428, 1993b.
132. Watson RS, Carcillo JA, Linde-Zwirble WT, et al: The epidemiology of severe sepsis in children in the United States. *Am J Respir Crit Care Med* 167:695-701, 2003.
133. Yan SB, Helterbrand JD, Hartman DL, et al: Low levels of protein C are associated with poor outcome in severe sepsis. *Chest* 120:915-922, 2001.

CHAPTER

28

Cardiopulmonary Bypass for Repair of Congenital Heart Disease in Infants and Children

John E. Mayer, Jr.

PEARLS

- Pulsatile perfusion, in contrast to nonpulsatile perfusion, is associated with better tissue perfusion, lower arterial resistance, and less accumulation of extracellular fluid, but is technically difficult to achieve in small children.
- Cardiopulmonary bypass usually is accompanied by hypothermia, which reduces metabolic rate by about 50% for every 10°C below 37°C. At 20°C oxygen consumption is approximately 20% of its value at 37°C.
- Deep hypothermic circulatory arrest is used to achieve ideal operating conditions for complex intracardiac repairs, especially in infants. Safe circulatory arrest time may be as short as 35 to 40 minutes.

Introduction

The term *cardiopulmonary bypass* is generally used to describe the techniques by which some of the functions of the heart and lungs are temporarily replaced with a mechanical system in order to support the remaining organ systems of the patient during surgical interventions on the cardiovascular and/or pulmonary subsystems. In simplest terms, this apparatus consists of a pumping device to deliver blood to the patient and an oxygenator in which gas exchange occurs. Almost all current systems also incorporate a heat exchanger by which the temperature of the blood in the oxygenator can be altered, thus allowing control of the patient's temperature. Bypass systems for cardiac operations initially were used clinically in the early 1950s, with significant mortality and morbidity. With improvements in materials and bypass techniques, cardiac operations using cardiopulmonary bypass now are performed safely on a daily basis throughout the world. However, cardiopulmonary bypass continues to be an unphysiologic state with nontrivial morbidity and mortality. This chapter outlines the ways in which various techniques of cardiopulmonary bypass can be used for performing intracardiac operations in infants and children and discusses the existing problems and limits of current techniques in this patient population. Because repair of most defects requires that the heart, and often the entire circulatory system, be arrested, techniques of cardioplegia and deep hypothermic circulatory arrest are discussed.

Principles and Mechanics of Cardiopulmonary Bypass

The primary function of cardiopulmonary bypass is to circulate blood of appropriate composition to the body to maintain viability of the patient. This maintenance of viability obviously involves the provision of oxygen and the removal of carbon dioxide, but the constraints imposed by the need to provide optimal operating conditions and by the damaging effects of unmodified cardiopulmonary bypass itself require that a number of other variables, including pH, temperature, hematocrit, oncotic pressure, electrolyte and glucose composition, and the pharmacologic milieu be manipulated. These various manipulations are directed at minimizing the damaging effects of cardiopulmonary bypass and offsetting the deleterious effects of cardiac and/or whole body ischemia required to provide suitable conditions for the conduct of the repair.

Circulation

In order to establish cardiopulmonary bypass, the surgeon must introduce cannulas into the venous system (generally the right atrium and/or vena cavae) through which venous blood is drained from the patient to the pump system. In almost all systems, the venous blood is *siphoned* from the patient into a reservoir by the force of gravity; therefore, the cannulas must be of large caliber to minimize resistance to blood flow. Active suction has been used increasingly in adult cardiac surgical programs, and there is initial experience in pediatric cardiac surgery. However, if significant amounts of air are entrained with the suctioned blood, significantly more blood trauma occurs and hemolysis is possible. Once the blood reaches the reservoir, it passes through the oxygenator where gas exchange occurs and then is pumped back into the patient through a cannula, which has been introduced into the systemic arterial system (usually the ascending aorta). This pumping of blood is generally carried out with a roller pump that compresses the tubing containing the blood in a rotary fashion and thereby "pumps" it back into the patient. The resulting arterial waveform is relatively nonpulsatile with a difference of no more than 5 to 10 mmHg between the highest and lowest pressures. The consequences of this nonpulsatile arterial flow are difficult to totally separate from other effects of cardiopulmonary bypass, but evidence indicates a pulsatile waveform may be associated with better tissue perfusion, lower systemic arterial resistance, and less accumulation of extracellular fluid, particularly after a period of reduced perfusion.[1,2] A reliable system for providing pulsatile flow has become commercially available. The ability to deliver pulsatile flow is particularly limited in neonates and infants because only small arterial cannulas (10–12F) can be placed into the ascending aorta, and in general these cannulas considerably dampen any pulsatile waveform. The advantages of pulsatile flow over nonpulsatile flow in the clinical setting remain a subject of debate.[3] In general, systemic vascular resistance falls during the initial phases of cardiopulmonary bypass and then progressively rises to supernormal levels with time.[3] The renal response to nonpulsatile flow has been well described and includes an increase in renin production that, in turn, contributes to the increase in systemic resistance.[4] A generalized increase in sympathetic tone with release of epinephrine from the adrenal has been documented in adults[5] and to an even greater degree in neonates.[6] Total bypass flow rates nearly equal to the cardiac output of an anesthetized patient are generally attainable, but pump output must not exceed the venous return to the pump because such a situation would result in the pump "running dry" and air being pumped into the patient. One of the functions of the perfusionist is to regulate the arterial output of the pump (by altering the rotation speed of the pump head) to match the rate at which venous blood is returning to the pump oxygenator system. This regulation is accomplished by maintaining a constant level of blood in the reservoir portion of the system, but close communication between the perfusionist and the surgeon is necessary to maintain smooth control of the system. Apparently minor changes in venous cannula position that may significantly alter venous return are detected by the perfusionist as falls in the reservoir level. To compensate for fluid losses during bypass, including urine output and fluid sequestration in the tissues, the perfusionist may be forced to add volume in the form of crystalloid or blood to maintain an adequate level of perfusate in the reservoir.

As a general approach at the Children's Hospital, Boston, perfusion flow rate rather than perfusion pressure is used to set bypass parameters. In infants, flow rates of approximately 150 ml/kg/min are used, and no attempt is made to pharmacologically elevate perfusion pressures. α-Adrenergic blockade with phentolamine is routinely used in an attempt to improve tissue perfusion and to enhance the evenness of cooling prior to the onset of circulatory arrest as described below.

Respiration

The introduction of oxygen and the removal of carbon dioxide occurs in the oxygenator portion of the cardiopulmonary bypass apparatus. This gas exchange must occur across an interface between the gas(es) introduced into the oxygenator and the plasma and erythrocytes that are in the oxygenator at that moment. In early oxygenator systems, this interface was created by direct contact between the blood and the gas source either by spreading the blood into thin films that then were exposed to an oxygen-enriched gas phase (disk oxygenator) or by introducing "bubbles" of oxygen into the blood so that gas exchange occurred across the blood-bubble interface (bubble oxygenator). In more current designs, thin-walled "membranes" are interposed between the gas and blood (membrane oxygenators) in an attempt to reduce the deleterious effects of the direct gas-blood interface on the plasma proteins and the formed elements of the blood. The gas exchange characteristics of oxygenators vary; therefore, familiarity with a particular system is important for the perfusionist to be able to set the gas flow rate and gas composition supplied to the particular type of oxygenator at a given blood flow rate and temperature in order to achieve the appropriate blood gas concentrations in the arterial outflow to the patient. In general, all systems can achieve normal to supernormal levels of oxygen and normal to hypocapnic levels of CO_2 in the blood leaving the oxygenator.

Respiration at the cellular level is dependent on several variables that can be manipulated during bypass. On bypass at normothermic temperatures, total body oxygen consumption is related to blood flow, and bypass flows of at least 2 L/min/m^2 are required to achieve relatively normal O_2 consumption rates for anesthetized patients of 110 to 130 ml/min/m^2. If bypass flow rates are lower than these values, then total body O_2 consumption falls and metabolic acidosis may result.[3] As temperatures are reduced, O_2 consumption falls and bypass flow requirements are likewise reduced with less dependence of total body O_2 consumption on bypass flow rate.[7] To improve operating conditions and the overall tolerance to cardiopulmonary bypass, most congenital heart surgeons now use at least moderate levels of hypothermia with reduced flow rates during cardiac operations on bypass. Deep hypothermia (<20°C) with circulatory arrest is used for many repairs in neonates and infants.

The optimal management of respiration, particularly pH and PCO_2, under hypothermic conditions remains unsettled, although it is our institutional preference to use the pH strategy outlined here. In general, two strategies, termed *pH stat* and *alpha stat,* have been used. In the pH-stat approach, PCO_2 and pH are maintained such that the values are 40 torr and 7.40, respectively, at the given temperature. These values are the "corrected" values that account for the patient's temperature. They are not the values obtained when the sample is introduced into a blood gas analyzer (which brings the temperature of the blood to 37°C prior to analysis). Therefore the actual PCO_2 result from the blood gas analyzer (at 37°C) of a sample collected at a patient temperature of 20°C is approximately 65 torr, yielding a "corrected" value of 40 torr (the actual partial pressure of CO_2 if it was determined at 20°C). Similarly, to achieve a "corrected" pH value of 7.40 for the patient at 20°C, the blood gas analyzer yields a reading of 7.16. Functionally, these blood gas targets are achieved by adding CO_2 to the gases entering the oxygenator as cooling is carried out. With the alpha-stat strategy, PCO_2 is reduced, and consequently pH rises during hypothermia. The target values, as actually measured in the blood gas analyzer, are approximately PCO_2 = 40 torr and pH = 7.40. If the measurements were actually made with the blood at 20°C, the actual PCO_2 is considerably lower (17.6 torr) with an actual pH of almost 7.7. Interestingly, in "natural" situations of hypothermia, both strategies are used in different species. Hibernating mammals use a pH-stat strategy, whereas poikilothermic species (e.g., reptiles, frogs) generally use an alpha-stat strategy[8] and reduce PCO_2 by relative hyperventilation in response to lower temperatures. In man and in many other "homeotherms," temperature variations exist in various parts of the arterial system (and body) under normal conditions, but these variations occur at a relatively constant total CO_2 content.[9] Actual sampling of the arterial and venous blood shows that lower temperatures are associated with lower PCO_2 and higher pH in accordance with values obtained with the alpha-stat strategy.[9] The change in blood pH/°C is approximately −0.0147. It appears from studies in a variety of mammalian and other species that the evolutionary goal of PCO_2 (and consequent pH) regulation is to maintain a constant state of ionization of the intracellular proteins,[9] particularly the enzyme systems. The two ionizing species with a pK in the physiologic pH range (6–8) are the imidazole moiety of histidine and the alpha NH_3^+ terminal group of peptide chains, with the histidine groups being much more numerous. The ratio of nonprotonated (non-ionized) imidazole groups to the total of protonated (NH_3^+) and nonprotonated imidazole groups is denoted by the symbol $alpha_{Im}$. Of note, the pK of $alpha_{Im}$ also varies inversely with temperature. As a result, the ionization state of the imidazole moieties does not change appreciably with temperature if PCO_2 also falls and pH rises.[9] If the ionization state of the intracellular proteins does not change with temperature changes (if these pH and PCO_2 conditions are met), then the enzymatic functions of these proteins will not be impaired by temperature change. Of note, the ionization of water also varies inversely with temperature so that the pH of water rises with a fall in temperature, and the change in pH of water/°C also is −0.0147. Thus it is intuitively attractive to believe that the alpha-stat strategy for regulation of PCO_2 on bypass during hypothermic conditions most likely will preserve the function of important enzyme systems. This strategy was adopted in our unit and a number of other units as the method by which to regulate blood gas tensions and pH. However, studies comparing the alpha-stat and pH-stat strategies on oxygen consumption during bypass procedures in adults have yielded conflicting results.[10,11] The important effect of CO_2 on cerebral blood flow and thus on cerebral protection is a particularly important consideration in the choice of pH management strategy. Ekroth and coworkers[12] noted an inverse correlation between creatine kinase BB levels (a probable marker for neuronal injury) and pH in infants undergoing operations using circulatory arrest. The question of whether the alpha-stat or pH-stat strategy is optimal if the tissue is to be made ischemic (in addition to being made hypothermic) remains to be more definitively answered, although some evidence favors the alpha-stat strategy when myocardial preservation during ischemia is considered.[13] In contrast, a group of patients undergoing deep hypothermia and circulatory arrest managed with a pH-stat strategy appeared to have better developmental scores late after surgery than patients managed with an alpha-stat strategy.[14]

Temperature

As indicated earlier, some degree of hypothermia is used in most cardiac operations. The rationales for use of hypothermia are multiple but are centered around safely providing optimal operating conditions for the conduct of the operation. The protective effects of hypothermia for tissues exposed to periods of reduced or absent blood flow during experimental cardiac surgery were investigated by Bigelow and coworkers[15] in 1950, and the principle of hypothermic protection was used by Lewis and Tauffic[16] in 1953 for a clinical "open heart" operation in which an atrial septal defect was closed during a short period of circulatory arrest at a moderate level of hypothermia without any cardiopulmonary bypass. The mechanism by which hypothermia is protective during ischemia is not completely defined but must involve the reduced metabolic demands of the tissues as a result of the lower temperatures. The effect of temperature on metabolic rate (as reflected by oxygen consumption) is described by the term Q_{10}, which is the ratio of the oxygen consumptions at two different temperatures (10° apart). For man, this value has been estimated to be approximately 1.9; therefore oxygen consumption at 20°C is reduced to about 20% of that at 37°C.[17] It seems likely, however, that hypothermia has protective effects other than the reduction in metabolic rate. If the central nervous system has a safe ischemic period of 5 minutes at normothermia, then a fivefold reduction in metabolic demand would only be expected to increase the "safe" interval of ischemia to 25 minutes. Clinically, it seems that total circulatory arrest times of up to 45 to 60 minutes are well tolerated neurologically in the majority of cases, suggesting that hypothermia has other protective effects.

The technique of deep hypothermia and circulatory arrest provides ideal operating conditions for intracardiac repairs in neonates and infants, including defects such as transposition of the great arteries, total anomalous pulmonary venous connection, complete AV canal, tetralogy of Fallot, hypoplastic left heart syndrome, and truncus arteriosus. At the Children's Hospital in Boston, bypass is established with single aortic and single right atrial cannulas when circulatory arrest is planned for a procedure, and the perfusate is precooled to approximately 25°C. Cooling is carried out predominantly with perfusion (core cooling), although some surface cooling is achieved after the induction of anesthesia by using a cooling blanket and exposing the child to the ambient temperature in the operating room. Cooling on bypass is generally carried out for at least 15 minutes, and the tympanic and rectal temperatures are brought to less than 20°C. Ice is placed around the head, and the cooling blanket remains cold during the period of circulatory arrest. The introduction of metal-tipped, right-angle venous cannulas has enabled direct cannulation of the superior and inferior vena cavae in many, if not most, procedures, thereby allowing continuous low-flow perfusion with intermittent short periods of circulatory arrest as needed. Whether this strategy is preferable to a single, more prolonged period of hypothermic circulatory arrest remains unclear. The ductus arteriosus/ligamentum is ligated to prevent air entry into the aortic arch during the period of circulatory arrest and to prevent spontaneous reopening of the ductus during the postoperative period. After the aorta is clamped and cardioplegia administered, blood is drained to the oxygenator by leaving the venous line open and stopping the arterial inflow to the patient. In situations where two caval cannulas are used, bypass flows can be reduced while perfusion is maintained. The cardiac repair then is carried out. After completion of the parts of the repair in which circulatory arrest is necessary for visualization, the right atrium is closed, and the venous cannula is reinserted. To shorten the circulatory arrest time, low-flow bypass can be restarted using cardiotomy suction for venous return while the atrium is closed. Another technique, developed by Pigula et al.[18] for neonatal operations that include reconstruction of the aortic arch (such as stage I palliation for hypoplastic left heart syndrome), uses selective hypothermic perfusion of the right innominate artery via a prosthetic graft that is subsequently used as a systemic-to-pulmonary artery shunt in this palliative procedure. Once the portions of the procedure requiring circulatory arrest are completed, the circulation can be resumed; generally rewarming is begun once the circulation is reestablished, keeping the temperature of the heat exchanger no more than 10°C above the temperature of the blood returning from the patient in order to prevent dissolved gases from coming out of solution. Rewarming is carried out until a rectal temperature of 35°C to 36°C is reached. Careful attention to the rates of cooling and rewarming of the rectal, esophageal, and tympanic probes may uncover residual anatomic problems, particularly in the aortic arch.

The safe period of circulatory arrest in human neonates and infants has not been established with certainty.[3] We previously thought that periods of 45 to 60 minutes were well tolerated in the vast majority of our patients. However, more current studies suggest the "safe" period of circulatory arrest may be as short as 35 to 40 minutes.[19] O'Connor and coworkers[20] showed that 1 hour of circulatory arrest at 13°C in dogs was associated with neither functional nor anatomic evidence of injury. Tharion et al.[21] reported a low incidence of neurologic problems after circulatory arrest in children. Transient seizure activity has been noted in approximately 5% to 10% of patients,[3] and very occasionally patients develop choreoathetoid movements. Despite these favorable clinical results, however, Greeley and coworkers[22] showed that recovery of cerebral blood flow after a period of deep hypothermic circulatory arrest is remarkably lower than if hypothermic bypass without arrest was used. The interaction of preoperative, intraoperative, and postoperative events on ultimate neurologic outcome makes evaluation of the impact of circulatory arrest alone difficult, but Blackwood et al.[23] showed that developmental outcome was not different between a group of patients undergoing operations using circulatory arrest and a group having repairs on bypass without arrest. Evidence from earlier studies indicates that continuous hypothermic bypass without circulatory arrest can result in severe neurologic injury, particularly if hemodilution is not used,[24,25] but our own studies demonstrated that a short period of circulatory arrest at deeply hypothermic levels with low-flow bypass (50 ml/kg/min) for periods up to 90 minutes was associated with better neurologic and developmental outcomes compared with patients who had periods of circulatory arrest of more than 40 to 45 minutes.[19,26]

One side effect of hypothermia of unknown significance is sequestration of fluid in the tissues. This effect occurs even without bypass and was reported by Chen and coworkers[27] in both animals and humans undergoing surface cooling to 25°C. The explanation for this effect is unknown but may involve changes in capillary permeability and/or sequestration of whole blood and plasma in certain portions of the circulatory bed with hypothermia.

Hematocrit and Oncotic Pressure

Reduction of the hematocrit during the period of cardiopulmonary bypass (hemodilution) appears to be desirable for a number of reasons and is widely used. First, with hypothermia the viscosity of blood increases, which contributes to a rise in the resistance to blood flow, particularly in the microcirculation.[3] When this factor is added to the nonpulsatile nature of bypass flow, significant underperfusion of the microcirculation may occur with resulting tissue ischemia. The importance of hemodilution during hypothermia is highlighted by the early experiences reported by Bjork and Hultquist[24] and Egerton et al.[25] using deep hypothermia with normal hematocrit, in which there was a high incidence of significant neurologic deficits when deep hypothermia without circulatory arrest was used. Of interest, hibernating (hypothermic) mammals become naturally hemodiluted.[28] A second advantage to hemodilution is the reduction in usage of blood products to "prime" the cardiopulmonary bypass circuit with its attendant reduction in transfusion risk. For several years, the "target" hematocrit while on bypass at the Children's Hospital, Boston, was 20% to 25%, and this was achieved by using a balanced crystalloid priming solution (pH 7.4) and adding citrated whole blood to the prime (when necessary) to account for the hematocrit and calculated blood volume of the patient so that the mixed final hematocrit of the patient plus oxygenator circuit was in the desired range. In recent years, experimental and clinical studies have indicated a higher hematocrit may be preferable in terms of cerebral protection under conditions of deep hypothermia and circulatory arrest.[29] The mechanisms by which an increase in hematocrit is beneficial remain speculative, although an increase in the oxygen content in the blood remaining in the capillary bed could result in increased oxygen availability during periods when the circulation is interrupted. Other mechanisms also may be operative. However, based on these studies, the target hematocrit in our center has been raised to between 25% and 30%. However, several centers continue to use more significant degrees of hemodilution without apparent deleterious effects.[30]

Hemodilution with nonblood priming solutions also results in a fall in the protein concentration of the blood, and concerns have been expressed regarding the development of tissue edema as a result of the decreased oncotic pressure.[3] However, Marelli and coworkers[31] were unable to show any significant advantages by the addition of albumin to the priming solution. Most infants undergoing operations on bypass seem to accumulate a considerable amount of extravascular fluid, and some evidence indicates the capillary beds of immature animals are more leaky than those of the mature animal,[32] but the impact of this fluid accumulation on ultimate outcome after cardiac surgery is unclear. An effect of serum protein concentration and oncotic pressure mitigates the effects of hemodilution in experimental studies,[33] and for this reason future studies on the relationship between hematocrit and outcomes after cardiopulmonary bypass and circulatory arrest should include the ability to separate the effect of altering protein concentration from the effect of altering the red cell concentration.

Electrolyte and Glucose Composition

Logic seems to dictate that concentrations of serum electrolytes and glucose should be maintained within normal ranges in order to maintain the normal milieu for the cells of the body. Such a strategy has been used, in general, for most of these constituents, but at least two exceptions are worth noting. Glucose concentrations during bypass have frequently been raised using glucose-containing priming solutions with the goal of inducing an osmotic diuresis during bypass and thereby attempting to minimize the risk of renal failure in the postbypass period.[3] However, evidence suggests that elevated glucose levels may have a deleterious effect on the outcome of central nervous system tissue subjected to ischemia.[34] Ekroth and coworkers[12] showed that levels of creatine kinase BB, which is thought to be specific for central nervous system injury, were highly correlated with elevations of glucose prior to circulatory arrest. Therefore we have used a priming solution for bypass that does not contain glucose, particularly when circulatory arrest is anticipated. Calcium is generally thought to be involved in the ischemia/reperfusion process, and massive increases in intracellular calcium have been noted during reperfusion after lethal periods of ischemia.[35] Rebeyka and colleagues (Personal Communication) at the Hospital for Sick Children in Toronto, Canada, have suggested that hypothermia induces the intracellular accumulation of calcium and recommended that cardioplegic arrest be effected prior to reaching deep hypothermic levels in order to prevent the hypothermia-induced rise in intracellular calcium that will increase the metabolic demands during ischemia. When applied to the whole organism, one might infer that reduced levels of calcium, prior to or immediately following ischemia, reduce ischemic injury, but the advantages of such an approach at this point are hypothetical. At the Children's Hospital, Boston, we have serendipitously arrived at preischemic hypocalcemia, particularly in neonatal patients, because a calcium-free crystalloid priming solution is used and the citrated bank blood that is added to the pump prior to bypass is not supplemented with calcium. Ionized calcium concentrations are generally about 0.3 mM/L during the preischemic phase and are not raised to normocalcemic levels until midway through the postischemic rewarming period near the end of bypass. The advantages of this strategy of calcium management remain highly speculative. All other electrolytes are maintained within the normal ranges.

Pharmacologic Manipulations

As alluded to previously, cardiopulmonary bypass remains an unphysiologic state and results in a number of deleterious effects on the patient, as reviewed by Kirklin and Kirklin.[36] As these effects have become known (and sometimes before the mechanisms of the effects were precisely characterized), a variety of pharmacologic manipulations have been introduced to offset the ill effects of bypass. The most obvious effect of bypass is on the circulating blood. The contact of the blood with the inner surfaces of the bypass tubing and oxygenator results in prompt thrombus formation unless the coagulation system is inhibited. Therefore heparin must be given to the patient before the blood makes contact with any of these surfaces. Heparin acts by enhancing the activity of antithrombin III (heparin cofactor), which inhibits the serine active sites of many of the factors in the coagulation cascade, including thrombin.[37] Because there is a very low incidence of deficiency of this heparin cofactor in the general population,[37] the recommendation is that a prolongation of the clotting time be confirmed after administration of heparin but before initiation of bypass. Clinically significant deficiencies of this cofactor have generally been reported only in adults[37] and can be reversed by administering normal (fresh-frozen) plasma. Platelet function and numbers are impaired by cardiopulmonary bypass,[36,38] and a variety of platelet-inhibiting agents have been used experimentally to reduce these effects.[36,39,40] However, agents such as prostacyclin,[39,40] dipyridamole, and iloprost have potent vasodilatory effects that may lower perfusion pressure quite remarkably on bypass. There is concern that the platelets activated in the bypass circuit may aggregate and lodge in the microcirculation, leading to organ dysfunction.[40] Prevention of this effect theoretically could reduce the morbidity of bypass.

Bypass elicits an inflammatory response from the contact of the blood and plasma with the nonendothelial surfaces of the pump oxygenator,[36] which involves the kallikrein-bradykinin system and complement activation.[36,41] C3a is released in the early phases of bypass and is continually produced throughout the duration of bypass.[36,41,42] Granulocytes also are activated during bypass, with rises in plasma levels of granulocyte myeloperoxidase, lactoferrin, and elastase.[41] The levels of lactoferrin and elastase could be reduced with infusion of nifedipine during bypass, but this agent did not affect the levels of C3a.[41] Oxygen free radicals and hydrogen peroxide are produced by neutrophils during bypass.[42] Experimentally, bypass has been shown to increase microvascular permeability, which appears to result from an increase in the size of large pores in the microvascular bed.[43] Corticosteroids have been used as an ingredient in the bypass prime at the Children's Hospital, Boston, for many years and initially were added based on observations of beneficial effects in patients with low cardiac output following cardiac operations.[44] The multiple antiinflammatory effects of corticosteroids, including the reduction of complement activation during bypass,[45] may be a more rational justification for the use of steroids prior to bypass. Mannitol, which originally was used to induce an osmotic diuresis, has now been shown to be a free radical scavenger and therefore may have significant benefit in reducing free radical injury that occurs during reperfusion after a period of ischemia.[46] To offset the remarkable increases in catecholamines and the consequent effects on systemic vascular resistance, phentolamine is added to the bypass prime in our institution, based initially on the favorable effects noted in postoperative patients.[44] Cardiopulmonary bypass circuits with coatings that appear to cause less activation of the inflammatory response system have become available. Based on animal experiments, these circuits may prove to reduce the amount of inflammation associated with cardiopulmonary bypass.

Myocardial Protection

The subject of myocardial preservation during surgical ischemia has been the subject of hundreds of publications in recent years. Most surgeons now use cardioplegia during periods of myocardial ischemia, although clinical and experimental evidence have not conclusively proved its value, particularly in the immature myocardium.[47,48] Multiple problems are associated with the extrapolation of experimental animal data to the human infant, and significant variations exist among species.[49] The basic components of cardioplegic solutions seem to be potassium (to achieve diastolic arrest) and cold temperatures to reduce the metabolic demands of the heart during ischemia. Magnesium, which is an important component in the St. Thomas solution, probably has a beneficial effect through antagonism of calcium entry.[50,51] Oxygenation of the cardioplegic solution has some benefit experimentally.[52] The addition of free radical scavengers to the cardioplegia solution has been reported to be of benefit experimentally.[46] Substrate modification, particularly by the addition of amino acids such as aspartate and glutamate, has been shown to be of benefit as well.[53–55] Single dose rather than multiple doses seems to provide better protection in immature rabbits,[56] and our clinical observations indicate this also may apply in infants.

Control of reperfusion conditions, particularly with regard to perfusion pressure, seems to have an important impact on recovery of function in the experimental setting.[57,58] We have focused a significant amount of laboratory effort on examining the effects of reperfusion interventions directed at preserving endothelial function. There is relatively good evidence that endothelial function is impaired after ischemia and reperfusion,[59,60] and this impairment likely results from a reduction in the endothelial production of nitric oxide.[59] Subsequent studies have shown that infusion of the nitric oxide precursor L-arginine during reperfusion results in enhanced recovery of ventricular and endothelial function.[61] Administration of nitroglycerine, which causes vasodilation through a nitric oxide mechanism, has similar beneficial effects on the recovery of ventricular function after a period of hypothermic ischemia.[62]

Neutrophil-endothelial interactions seem to have an important role in recovery of the heart after ischemia and reperfusion.[60] Experiments in our laboratory with either leukocyte depletion[60] or antibodies directed against neutrophil adhesion molecules seem to result in significant improvements in ventricular and endothelial function.[63]

Clinically, we currently use dilute oxygenated blood potassium cardioplegia, to which both magnesium and lidocaine are added for almost all neonates and infants at the Children's Hospital, Boston. We also use intravenous nitroglycerine during reperfusion while the patient is still on bypass. In addition, we attempt to maintain the perfusion pressures in the range from 20 to 30 mmHg during the early phases of reperfusion based on the laboratory work described. The value of these interventions is hard to quantify because of the difficulties in obtaining load-independent measures of ventricular function in the clinical situation; myocardial dysfunction and the need for inotropic support seem to be less but have not been totally eliminated.

Summary

Reparative cardiac surgery of all types requires use of cardiopulmonary bypass and periods of myocardial and total body ischemia in order to provide satisfactory surgical conditions for the repair. Despite improved materials and better understanding of the pathophysiology of this form of support, its application remains limited by the morbid effects of bypass and tissue ischemia. Continued efforts are necessary to further reduce the morbidity of tissue ischemia and cardiopulmonary bypass in order to allow safer conduct of reparative operations for congenital heart defects.

REFERENCES

1. Mori F, Ivey TD, Itoh T, et al: Effects of pulsatile reperfusion on postischemic recovery of myocardial function after global hypothermic cardiac arrest. *J Thorac Cardiovasc Surg* 93:719-727, 1987.
2. Bregman D, Marrin CAS, Spotnitz HM: Pulsatile flow in extracorporeal circulation. In Ionescu MI, editor: *Techniques in extracorporeal circulation,* ed 2. London, 1981, Butterworths.
3. Kirklin JW, Barratt-Boyes B: Hypothermia, circulatory arrest, and cardiopulmonary bypass. In Kirklin JW, Barratt-Boyes B, editors: *Cardiac surgery,* ed 1. New York, 1986, John Wiley and Sons.
4. Bartlett RH, Gazzaniga AB: Physiology and pathophysiology of extracorporeal circulation. In Ionescu MI, editor: *Techniques in extracorporeal circulation,* ed 2. London, 1981, Butterworths.
5. Tan CK, Glisson SN, El-Etr AA, Ramakrishnaiah KB: Levels of circulating norepinephrine and epinephrine before, during, and after cardiopulmonary bypass operation in man. *J Thorac Cardiovasc Surg* 71:928-931, 1976.
6. Anand KJ, Hansen DD, Hichkey PR: Hormonal-metabolic stress responses in neonates undergoing cardiac surgery. *Anesthesiology* 73:661, 1990.
7. Hickey RF, Hoar PF: Whole body oxygen consumption during low-flow hypothermic cardiopulmonary bypass. *J Thorac Cardiovasc Surg* 86:903-906, 1983.
8. White FN: A comparative physiological approach to hypothermia. *J Thorac Cardiovasc Surg* 82:821-831, 1981.
9. Reeves RB, Rahn H: Patterns in vertebrate acid-base regulation. In Wood SC, Lenfant C, editors: *Evolution of respiratory processes: a comparative approach,* ed 1. New York, 1979, Marcel Dekker.
10. Alston RP, Singh M, McLaren AD: Systemic oxygen uptake during hypothermic cardiopulmonary bypass: effects of flow rate, flow character, and arterial pH. *J Thorac Cardiovasc Surg* 98:757-768, 1989.
11. Tuppurainen T, Settergren G, Stensved P: The effect of arterial pH on whole body oxygen uptake during hypothermic cardiopulmonary bypass in man. *J Thorac Cardiovasc Surg* 98:769-773, 1989.
12. Ekroth R, Thompson RJ, Lincoln C, et al: Elective deep hypothermia with total circulatory arrest. Changes in plasma creatinine kinase BB, blood glucose, and clinical variables. *J Thorac Cardiovasc Surg* 97:30-35, 1989.
13. Becker H, Vinten-Johansen J, Buckberg GD, et al: Myocardial damage caused by keeping pH 7.40 during systemic deep hypothermia. *J Thorac Cardiovasc Surg* 82:810-820, 1981.
14. Jonas RA, Bellinger DC, Rappaport LA, et al: Relation of pH strategy and developmental outcome after hypothermic circulatory arrest. *J Thorac Cardiovasc Surg* 106:362-368, 1993.
15. Bigelow WG, Callaghan JC, Hopps JA: General hypothermia for experimental intracardiac surgery. *Ann Surg* 132:531-539, 1950.
16. Lewis FJ, Tauffic M: Closure of atrial septal defects with the aid of hypothermia: experimental accomplishments and the report of one successful case. *Surgery* 33:52-58, 1953.
17. Harris EA, Seelye ER, Barratt-Boyes B: Respiratory and metabolic acid-base changes during cardiopulmonary bypass in man. *Br J Anaesth* 42:912, 1970.
18. Pigula FA, Siewers RD, Nemoto EM: Regional perfusion of the brain during neonatal aortic arch reconstruction. *J Thorac Cardiovasc Surg* 117:1023, 1999.
19. Newburger JW, Jonas RA, Wernovsky G, et al: A comparison of the perioperative neurologic effects of hypothermic circulatory arrest versus low flow cardiopulmonary bypass in infant heart surgery. *N Engl J Med* 329:1057-1064, 1993.
20. O'Connor JV, Wilding T, Farmer P, et al: The protective effect of profound hypothermia on the canine central nervous system during one hour of circulatory arrest. *Ann Thorac Surg* 41:255-259, 1986.
21. Tharion J, Johnson DC, Celermajer JM, et al: Profound hypothermia with circulatory arrest: nine years' clinical experience. *J Thorac Cardiovasc Surg* 84:66-72, 1982.
22. Greeley WJ, Ungerleider RM, Smith LR, Reves JG: The effects of deep hypothermic cardiopulmonary bypass and total circulatory arrest on cerebral blood flow in infants and children. *J Thorac Cardiovasc Surg* 97:737-745, 1989.
23. Blackwood MJA, Haka-Ikse K, Steward DJ: Developmental outcome in children undergoing surgery with profound hypothermia. *Anesthesiology* 65:437-440, 1986.
24. Bjork VO, Hultquist G: Contraindications to profound hypothermia in open heart surgery. *J Thorac Cardiovasc Surg* 44:1, 1962.
25. Egerton N, Egerton WS, Kay JH: Neurologic changes following profound hypothermia. *Ann Surg* 157:366-382, 1963.
26. Bellinger DC, Jonas RA, Rappaport LA, et al: Developmental and neurologic status of children after heart surgery with hypothermic circulatory arrest or low flow cardiopulmonary bypass. *N Engl J Med* 332:549-555, 1995.
27. Schubert T, Vetter H, Owen P, et al: Adenosine cardioplegia: adenosine versus potassium cardioplegia: effects on cardiac arrest and postischemic recovery in the isolated rat heart. *J Thorac Cardiovasc Surg* 98:1057-1065, 1989.
28. Kent KM, Popovic V: Cardiovascular responses in hypothermia and hibernation. *Physiologist* 8:318, 1965.
29. Jonas RA, Wypij D, Roth SJ, et al: The influence of hemodilution on outcome after hypothermic cardiopulmonary bypass: results of a randomized trial in infants. *J Thorac Cardiovasc Surg* 126:1765, 2003.
30. Cooper MM, Elliott M: Haemodilution. In Jonas RA, Elliott M, editors: *Cardiopulmonary bypass in neonates, infants, and young children.* Oxford, 1994, Butterworth Heinemann.
31. Marelli D, Paul A, Samson R, et al: Does the addition of albumin to the prime solution in cardiopulmonary bypass affect clinical outcome? *J Thorac Cardiovasc Surg* 98:751-756, 1989.
32. Harake B, Power GC: Thoracic duct lymph flow: a comparative study in newborn and adult sheep. *J Dev Physiol* 8:87-95, 1986.
33. Shin'oka T, Shum-Tim D, Laussen PC, et al: Effects of oncotic pressure and hematocrit on outcome after hypothermic circulatory arrest. *Ann Thorac Surg* 65:155-164, 1998.
34. Siemkowicz I, Gjedde A: Postischemic coma in rat: effect of different preischemia blood glucose levels on cerebral metabolic recovery after ischemia. *Acta Physiol Scand* 110:225-232, 1980.
35. Fitzpatrick D, Karmazyn M: Comparative effects of calcium channel blocking agents and varying extracellular calcium concentration on hypoxia/reoxygenation and ischemia/reperfusion-induced cardiac injury. *J Pharmacol Exp Ther* 84:761-768, 1984.
36. Kirklin JK, Kirklin JW: Cardiopulmonary bypass for cardiac surgery. In Sabiston DC, Spencer FC, editors: *Surgery of the chest,* ed 5. Philadelphia, 1990, WB Saunders.
37. Rosenberg JS, Rosenberg RD: Advances in the understanding of the anticoagulant function of heparin. In Silverglade A, editor: *A heparin symposium,* ed 1. Tenafly, NJ, 1975, Therapeutic Research Press.
38. Addonizio VP, Fisher CA, Jenkin BK, et al: Iloprost (ZK36374), a stable analogue of prostacyclin, preserves platelets during simulated extracorporeal circulation. *J Thorac Cardiovasc Surg* 89:926-933, 1985.
39. DeSesa VJ, Huval W, Leluk S, et al: Disadvantages of prostacyclin infusion during cardiopulmonary bypass: a double-blind study of 50 patients having coronary revascularization. *Ann Thorac Surg* 38:514-519, 1984.
40. Fish KJ, Sarnquist FH, van Steenis C, et al: A prospective, randomized study of the effects of prostacyclin on platelets and blood loss during coronary bypass operations. *J Thorac Cardiovasc Surg* 91:436-442, 1986.
41. Riegel W, Spillner G, Schlosser V, Horl WH: Plasma levels of main granulocyte components during cardiopulmonary bypass. *J Thorac Cardiovasc Surg* 95:1014, 1988.
42. Cavarocchi NC, England MD, Schaff HV, et al: Oxygen free radical generation during cardiopulmonary bypass: correlation with complement activation. *Circulation* 74(suppl III):III-130–III-133, 1986.
43. Smith EJ, Naftel DC, Blackstone EH, Kirklin JW: Microvascular permeability after cardiopulmonary bypass. *J Thorac Cardiovasc Surg* 94:225-233, 1987.
44. Dietzman RH, Ersek RA, Lillehei CW: Low output syndrome, recognition and treatment. *J Thorac Cardiovasc Surg* 57:138, 1969.

45. Cavarocchi NC, Pluth JR, Schaff HV, et al: Complement activation during cardiopulmonary bypass. *J Thorac Cardiovasc Surg* 91:252, 1986.
46. Gardner TJ, Stewart JR, Casale AS, et al: Reduction of myocardial ischemic injury with oxygen-derived free radical scavengers. *Surgery* 94:423-427, 1983.
47. Fujiwara T, Heinle J, Britton L, Mayer JE Jr: Myocardial preservation in neonatal lambs: comparison of hypothermia with crystalloid and blood cardioplegia. *J Thorac Cardiovasc Surg* 101:703-712, 1991.
48. Bull CM, Cooper J, Stark J: Cardioplegic protection of the child's heart. *J Thorac Cardiovasc Surg* 88:287-293, 1984.
49. Baker JE, Boerboom LE, Olinger GN: Is protection of ischemic neonatal myocardium by cardioplegia species dependent? *J Thorac Cardiovasc Surg* 99:280-287, 1990.
50. Reynolds TR, Geffin GA, Titus JS, et al: Myocardial preservation related to magnesium content of hyperkalemic cardioplegic solutions at 8°C. *Ann Thorac Surg* 47:907-913, 1989.
51. Geffin GA, Love TR, Hendren WG, et al: The effects of calcium and magnesium in hyperkalemic cardioplegic solutions on myocardial preservation. *J Thorac Cardiovasc Surg* 98:239-250, 1989.
52. Bodenhamer RM, DeBoer WV, Geffin GA, et al: Enhanced myocardial protection during ischemic arrest. *J Thorac Cardiovasc Surg* 85:769-780, 1983.
53. Rosenkranz ER, Okamoto F, Buckberg GD, et al: Safety of prolonged aortic clamping with blood cardioplegia: III. Aspartate enrichment of glutamate-blood cardioplegia in energy-depleted hearts after ischemic and reperfusion injury. *J Thorac Cardiovasc Surg* 91:428-435, 1986.
54. Rosenkranz ER, Okamoto F, Buckberg GD, et al: Safety of prolonged aortic clamping with blood cardioplegia: II. Glutamate enrichment in energy-depleted hearts. *J Thorac Cardiovasc Surg* 88:402-410, 1984.
55. Robertson JM, Vinten-Johansen J, Buckberg GD, et al: Safety of prolonged aortic clamping with blood cardioplegia. *J Thorac Cardiovasc Surg* 88:395-401, 1984.
56. Kempsford RD, Hearse DJ: Protection of the immature heart. *J Thorac Cardiovasc Surg* 99:269-279, 1990.
57. Fujiwara T, Kurtts T, Silvera M, Mayer JE Jr: Physical and pharmacological manipulation of reperfusion conditions in neonatal myocardial preservation. *Circulation* 78(suppl II):II-444, 1988.
58. Lazar HL, Wei J, Dirbas FM, et al: Controlled reperfusion following regional ischemia. *Ann Thorac Surg* 44:350-355, 1987.
59. Sawatari K, Kadoba K, Bergner KA, et al: Influence of initial reperfusion pressure after hypothermic cardioplegia on endothelial modulation of coronary tone in neonatal lambs: impaired coronary vasodilator response to acetylcholine. *J Thorac Cardiovasc Surg* 101:777-782, 1991.
60. Kawata H, Sawatari K, Mayer JE: Evidence for the role of neutrophils in reperfusion injury after cold cardioplegic ischemia in neonatal lambs. *J Thorac Cardiovasc Surg* 103:908-918, 1992.
61. Hiramatsu T, Forbess JM, Miura T, Mayer JE Jr: Effects of L-arginine and L-nitro-arginine methyl ester on recovery of neonatal lamb hearts after cold ischemia: evidence for an important role of endothelial production of nitric oxide. *J Thorac Cardiovasc Surg* 109:81-87, 1995.
62. Kawata H, Aoki M, Mayer Jr: Nitroglycerin improves functional recovery of neonatal lamb hearts after 2 hours of cold ischemia. *Circulation* 88(suppl II):II-366–II-371, 1993.
63. Kawata H, Aoki M, Hickey PR, Mayer JE Jr: Effect of antibody to leukocyte adhesion molecule cd18 on recovery of neonatal lamb hearts after 2 hours of cold ischemia. *Circulation* 86(suppl II): II-364–II-370, 1992.

CHAPTER

29

Cardiac Intensive Care

David L. Wessel and Peter C. Laussen

Introduction

Among the causes of infant mortality in the United States, congenital anomalies account for the largest diagnostic category.[1,2] Structural heart disease leads the list of congenital malformations. Of the more than 4 million children born each year in the United States, nearly 40,000 have some form of congenital heart disease (CHD). Approximately half of these children appear for therapeutic intervention within the first year of life, and the vast majority of them require critical care expertise. Patients with congenital or acquired heart disease compose a major diagnostic category for admissions in large pediatric intensive care units (ICUs) across the country, representing 30% to 40% or more of ICU admissions in many centers.

Newborn Considerations

Care of the critically ill neonate requires an appreciation of the special structural and functional features of immature organs, the interactions of the "transitional" neonatal circulation, and the secondary effects of the congenital heart lesion on other organ systems.[3–7] The neonate appears to respond more quickly and profoundly to physiologically stressful circumstances, which may be expressed in terms of rapid changes in pH, lactic acid, glucose, and temperature. Neonates have diminished fat and carbohydrate reserves. The higher metabolic rate and oxygen consumption of the neonate account for the rapid appearance of hypoxia when these patients become apneic. Immaturity of the liver and kidney may be associated with reduced protein synthesis and glomerular filtration such that drug metabolism is altered and hepatic synthetic function is reduced. These issues may be compounded by the normal increased total body water of the neonate compared with the older patient, along with the propensity of the capillary system of the neonate to leak fluid from the intravascular space. This is especially prominent in the lung of the neonate in whom the pulmonary vascular bed is nearly fully recruited at rest, and lymphatic recruitment required to handle increased mean capillary pressures associated with increases in pulmonary blood flow may be unavailable.[6,7] The neonatal myocardium is less compliant than that of the older child, is less tolerant of increases in afterload, and is less responsive to increases in preload. Younger age also predisposes the myocardium to the adverse effects of cardiopulmonary bypass (CPB) and hypothermic ischemia implicit in surgical support techniques used for reparative operations. These factors do not preclude intervention in the neonate but simply dictate that extraordinary vigilance be applied to the care of these children and that intensive care management plans emerge to account for the immature physiology.

The observed benefits of neonatal reparative operations in patients with two ventricles are numerous (Table 29–1). They continue to dictate that care of the newborn with complex CHD after CPB be a central feature of cardiac intensive care. Elimination of cyanosis and congestive heart failure (CHF) early in life optimize conditions for normal growth and development. Palliative procedures such as pulmonary artery bands and systemic-to-pulmonary artery shunts may not fully address cyanosis or CHF and may introduce their own set of physiologic and anatomic complications. Some examples of improved outcomes with a single reparative operation rather than staged palliation as a newborn are well known, are supported by published literature, and evoke little controversy. Approaches that have been abandoned include banding the pulmonary arteries in truncus arteriosus,[8] staging repair of type B interrupted aortic arch (IAA),[9] and staging rather than repairing in a single session transposition of the great arteries with IAA.[10] In other conditions (e.g., severely cyanotic newborn with tetralogy of Fallot [TOF]), the risks and benefits of neonatal repair versus a palliative shunt are debated.[11]

Whereas the neonate may be more labile than the older child, there is ample evidence that this age group is more resilient in its response to metabolic or ischemic injury. In fact, the neonate may be particularly capable of coping with some forms of stress. Tolerance of hypoxia in the neonate is characteristic of many species,[12] and the plasticity of the neurologic system in the neonate is well known. Neonates with obstructive left heart lesions often present with profound metabolic acidosis but can be

TABLE 29–1

Advantage of Neonatal Repair

Advantage of Neonatal Repair
Early elimination of cyanosis
Early elimination of congestive heart failure
Optimal circulation for growth and development
Reduced anatomic distortion from palliative procedures
Reduced hospital admissions while awaiting repair
Reduced parental anxiety while awaiting repair

effectively resuscitated without persistent organ system impairment or sequelae as the rule rather than the exception. The pliability and mobility of vascular structures in the neonate improve the technical aspects of surgery. Reparative operations in neonates take best advantage of normal postnatal changes, allowing more normal growth and development in crucial areas such as myocardial muscle, pulmonary parenchyma, and coronary and pulmonary angiogenesis. Neonatal repair may obviate irreversible secondary organ damage arising from unrepaired or palliative approaches. Postoperative pulmonary hypertensive events are more common in the infant who has been exposed to weeks or months of high pulmonary pressure and flow.[8,13] This seems especially true for such lesions as truncus arteriosus, complete atrioventricular (AV) canal defects, and transposition of the great arteries with ventricular septal defects (VSDs). Finally, cognitive and psychomotor abnormalities associated with months of hypoxemia or abnormal hemodynamics may be diminished or eliminated by early repair. However, if early reparative surgery results in more exposures to CPB (e.g., repeated conduit changes) and any associated cognitive or subtle adverse effects on motor function, then the risk-to-benefit assessment needs to be modified accordingly.

Preoperative Care

Optimal preoperative care involves (1) initial stabilization, airway management, and establishment of vascular access; (2) complete and thorough noninvasive delineation of the anatomic defect(s); (3) resuscitation with evaluation and treatment of secondary organ dysfunction, particularly the brain, kidneys, and liver; (4) cardiac catheterization if necessary, typically for (A) physiologic assessment, (B) interventional procedures such as balloon atrial septostomy or valvotomy, or (C) anatomic definition not visible by echocardiography (e.g., coronary artery distribution in pulmonary atresia with intact ventricular septum or delineation of aorticopulmonary collaterals in TOF with pulmonary atresia); and (5) surgical management when cardiac, pulmonary, renal, and central nervous systems are optimized.

Physical Examination and Laboratory Data

A complete history and physical examination are required. When such information is obtained, attention should be directed to the extent of cardiopulmonary impairment, airway abnormalities, and associated extracardiac congenital anomalies.[14,15] Upper and lower airway problems in patients with Down syndrome, calcium and immunologic deficiencies in patients with aortic arch abnormalities, and renal abnormalities in patients with esophageal atresia and CHD are a few of the associated congenital abnormalities with which the anesthesiologist should be familiar. Intercurrent pulmonary infection is a common and significant finding in chronically overcirculated lungs. The presence, degree, and duration of hypoxemia are important details that, in the absence of iron deficiency, are reflected in the hematocrit. The nadir of physiologic anemia during infancy may contribute to left-to-right shunting by decreasing the relative pulmonary vascular resistance (PVR).[16]

Chest radiography shows heart size, pulmonary vascular congestion, airway compression, and areas of consolidation or atelectasis. The electrocardiogram (ECG) may reveal rhythm disturbances and demonstrate ventricular strain patterns (ST and T-wave changes) characteristic of unphysiologic pressure or volume burdens on the ventricles. Electrolyte abnormalities caused by CHF and forced diuresis also must be evaluated preoperatively. Severe hypochloremic metabolic alkalosis may occur in some patients. It is more important to discontinue digoxin preoperatively and to avoid hyperventilation and administration of calcium to these patients during induction of anesthesia. The alkalotic hypokalemic, hypercalcemic, hypotensive, dilated, digoxin-bound myocardium fibrillates with ease.

Echocardiographic and Doppler Assessment

Advances in echocardiographic imaging have had an enormous impact on the diagnosis of CHD.[17] Accurate anatomic diagnosis now is routine in children without the need for cardiac catheterization. Echocardiography is the preferred imaging modality for assessment of intracardiac anatomic features in young children. However, the anesthesiologist should be aware of the current limitations of echocardiographic and Doppler techniques so that alternative diagnoses can be considered when intraoperative or postoperative findings are inconsistent with the working echocardiographic diagnosis.

Skilled echocardiographers accurately interpret the alignment of cardiac chambers and great vessels but cannot always visualize an atrial septal defect (ASD) or VSD, although color flow mapping techniques have vastly improved diagnostic capabilities. An ASD can be indirectly inferred from right ventricular (RV) volume overload and interventricular septal shift. Distal pulmonary artery architecture and conduits between a ventricle and a great artery are poorly imaged by echocardiography, and pressure gradients in these areas are not always measurable with Doppler techniques. Quantification of AV valve regurgitation may be subjective and nonquantitative. Accuracy of echocardiographic diagnosis is limited by an inadequate window for imaging in obese patients, older children, and some postoperative patients. Techniques for three-dimensional echocardiography that may improve diagnostic capabilities, such as defining the mechanism of valve regurgitation, are available, although real-time three-dimensional imaging currently is not readily available.

Doppler measurements add greatly to noninvasive diagnostic capabilities. Measurements of pressure gradients across semilunar valves and other obstructions frequently are accurate but may not always correlate with peak systolic ejection gradients measured at catheterization. As good as echocardiographic diagnosis of anatomic defects and Doppler measurements of pressure gradients and valve function have become, the standard for assessment of physiology when other clinical information is ambiguous or contradictory remains cardiac catheterization.

Cardiac Catheterization

When echocardiographic analysis with Doppler measurements and color flow mapping is complete and unambiguous, preoperative assessment may no longer require cardiac catheterization. Catheterization typically is not performed before infant or neonatal operations for VSDs, complete AV canal defects, TOF, IAA, hypoplastic left heart syndrome (HLHS), or coarctation of the aorta. However, in older patients with complex anatomy, such as a single ventricle, physiologic data from catheterization may be essential. This technique allows description of the direction, magnitude, and approximate location of intracardiac shunts. Intracardiac and intravascular pressures are measured to determine the presence of obstructions and whether shunt orifices are restrictive or nonrestrictive. Pressure gradients across sites of obstruction must be considered in light of simultaneous blood flow; a small pressure gradient measured at a time of low cardiac output is misleading.

Normal intracardiac pressure and saturation values in children are described in Chapter 22. Normally, there is no significant change in oxygen saturation from vena cava to pulmonary artery. In the child with CHD, the superior vena cava (SVC) gives the best indication of true mixed venous oxygen saturation; a 5% or greater step-up in saturation downstream suggests the presence of a left to right shunt.[18] It would occur at the level of the right atrium with an ASD, in the right ventricle with a VSD, and in the pulmonary artery with a patent ductus arteriosus (PDA). The magnitude of the left-to-right shunt can be calculated from the Fick equation. The oxygen consumption of the patient usually is measured, as are the saturation values, but subsequent flow and resistance calculations can be in error. The frequently used term Q_p/Q_s (pulmonary-to-systemic blood flow ratio) can be derived simply from the measured oxygen saturation values.

The patient whose aortic blood is fully saturated can be safely assumed to have no significant right-to-left shunting. However, when a right-to-left shunt is present, aortic blood is hypoxemic. Blood samples should also be obtained from the pulmonary veins, left atrium, and left ventricle for oxygen saturation determination and ascertainment of the source of desaturated blood. Pulmonary venous destruction implies a pulmonary source of venous admixture (e.g., pneumonia, atelectasis, or other pulmonary disease). Intrapulmonary shunting may substantially alter the anesthetic plan and the postoperative ventilatory requirements of the patient.

In the presence of a left-to-right shunt and elevated PVR, pressure and saturation measurements often are repeated, with the patient breathing 100% oxygen to assess both the reactivity of the pulmonary vascular bed and any contribution of ventilation-perfusion abnormalities to hypoxemia. If breathing 100% oxygen increases pulmonary blood flow and dramatically increases Q_p/Q_s (with a fall in PVR), potentially reversible processes such as hypoxic pulmonary vasoconstriction probably are contributing to the elevated PVR. The patient with a high, unresponsive PVR and a small left-to-right shunt despite a large shunt orifice may have extensive pulmonary vascular damage from irreversible obstructive pulmonary vascular disease. If so, surgical repair usually is contraindicated if the child is older than 1 year.[19]

During cardiac catheterization, anatomic abnormalities are identified angiographically. Special angled views provide specific information about the location and extent of congenital defects.[20,21] Ventricular function is assessed angiographically and physiologically (e.g., by pressure measurements). The calculated size of a cardiac chamber may have an important bearing on its ability to support the circulation of a child with hypoplastic ventricles.

Magnetic Resonance Imaging and Angiography

Magnetic resonance imaging (MRI) and magnetic resonance angiography (MRA) have emerged as important diagnostic modalities in the evaluation of the cardiovascular system following the development of ECG-gated MRI. Image acquisition is triggered to the patient's ECG to counter motion artifacts and to acquire cine sequences that allow imaging of cardiac structures and visualization of blood flow throughout the cardiac cycle. In addition to providing excellent anatomical and three-dimensional images, particularly of the pulmonary veins and thoracic aorta, it also is possible with MRA to qualitatively assess valve and ventricular function and to quantify flow, ventricular volume, mass, and ejection fraction.[22,23] Whereas ferromagnetic implants near the region of interest might produce artifact, sternal wires and vascular clips produce relatively minor disturbances; therefore MRI can be performed in patients who have undergone previous cardiac surgery. Contraindications include patients with pacemakers, recently implanted endovascular or intracardiac implants, and aneurysm clips on vessels that will be exposed directly to the magnetic field.

Assessment of Patient Status and Predominant Pathophysiology

Frequently congenital heart defects are complex and can be difficult to categorize or conceptualize. Rather than trying to determine the management for each individual anatomic defect, a physiologic approach can be taken. The following questions should be asked:

1. How does the systemic venous return reach the systemic arterial circulation to maintain cardiac output? What intracardiac mixing, shunting, or outflow obstruction exists?
2. Is the circulation in series or parallel? Are the defects amenable to a two-ventricle or single-ventricle repair?

3. Is pulmonary blood flow increased or decreased?
4. Is there a volume load or pressure load on the ventricles?

Appropriate organization of preoperative patient data, preparation of the patient, and decisions about monitoring, anesthetic agents, and postoperative care are best accomplished by focusing on a few major pathophysiologic problems, beginning with whether the patient is cyanotic, is in CHF, or both. Most pathophysiologic mechanisms in the patient's disease that are pertinent to the perioperative plan and to optimal preparation of the patient focus on one of the following major problems: severe hypoxemia, excessive pulmonary blood flow, CHF, obstruction of blood flow from the left heart, and poor ventricular function. Although some patients with CHD present with only one problem, many have multiple interrelated problems.

Severe Hypoxemia

Many of the cyanotic forms of CHD present in the ICU with severe hypoxemia (Pa_{O_2} <50 mmHg) during the first few days of life, but without respiratory distress. Infusion of prostaglandin E_1 (PGE_1) in patients with decreased pulmonary blood flow maintains or reestablishes pulmonary flow through the ductus arteriosus. This may also improve mixing of venous and arterial blood at the atrial level in patients with transposition of the great arteries.[24] Consequently, neonates rarely require surgery while they are severely hypoxemic. During preoperative preparation with PGE_1, neurologic examination and blood chemistry analysis of renal, hepatic, and hematologic function are necessary to assess the effects of severe hypoxemia during or after birth on end-organ dysfunction.

Cyanotic patients who present for surgery after infancy require adequate preoperative and postoperative hydration to prevent the thrombotic problems caused by their high hematocrit levels. Adequate quantities of blood products for treatment of the coagulopathies also are needed, as outlined earlier. Premedication must be given cautiously so as not to cause hypoventilation in these patients.

PGE_1 dilates the ductus arteriosus of the neonate with life-threatening ductus-dependent cardiac lesions and improves the patient's condition before surgery. PGE_1 can reopen a functionally closed ductus arteriosus for several days after birth, or it can maintain patency of the ductus arteriosus for several months postnatally.[24,25] The common side effects of PGE_1 infusion—apnea, hypotension, fever, central nervous system (CNS) excitation—are easily managed in the neonate when normal therapeutic doses of the drug (0.02–0.05 μg/kg/min) are used.[26] However, PGE_1 is a potent vasodilator, so intravascular volume frequently requires augmentation. Patients with intermittent apnea resulting from administration of PGE_1 may require mechanical ventilation preoperatively.

PGE_1 usually improves the arterial oxygenation of hypoxemic neonates who have poor pulmonary perfusion as a result of obstructed pulmonary flow (critical pulmonic stenosis or pulmonary atresia). By providing pulmonary blood flow from the aorta via the ductus arteriosus, an infusion of PGE_1 improves oxygenation and stabilizes the condition of neonates with these lesions. The improved oxygenation reverses the lactic acidosis that may have developed during episodes of severe hypoxia. PGE_1 administration for 24 hours usually markedly improves the condition of a severely hypoxemic neonate with restricted pulmonary blood flow.[27]

Excessive Pulmonary Blood Flow

Excessive pulmonary blood flow is frequently the primary problem of patients with CHD. The intensivist must carefully evaluate the hemodynamic and respiratory impact of left-to-right shunts and the extent to which it contributes to the perioperative course in the ICU. Children with left-to-right shunts may have chronic low-grade pulmonary infection and congestion that cannot be eliminated despite optimal preoperative preparation. If so, surgery should not be postponed further. Respiratory syncytial viral infections are particularly prevalent in this population, but improvements in intensive care have markedly improved outcome with this and other viral pneumonias.[28]

Aside from the respiratory impairment caused by increased pulmonary blood flow, the left heart must dilate to accept pulmonary venous return that is several times normal. If the body requires more systemic blood flow, the heart responds inefficiently. Most of the increment in cardiac output is recirculated to the lungs. Eventually symptoms of CHF appear.

Children with failing hearts increase endogenous catecholamine production and redistribute cardiac output to favored organs by their increased heart rate and decreased extremity perfusion.[29] In the most severe cases, the evaluation reveals a child whose body weight is below the third percentile for age and who is tachypneic, tachycardic, and dusky in room air. The child may have intercostal and substernal retractions and skin that is cool to the touch. Capillary refill may be prolonged. Expiratory wheezes usually are audible. Medical management with digoxin and diuretics may improve the patient's condition, but the diuretics may induce a profound hypochloremic alkalosis and potassium depletion and may still be abnormal after surgery.

Obstruction of Left Heart Outflow

Patients who require surgery to relieve obstruction to outflow from the left heart are among the most critically ill children for whom the intensivist must care. These lesions include interruption of the aortic arch, coarctation of the aorta, aortic stenosis (AS), and mitral stenosis or atresia as part of the HLHS. These neonates present with inadequate systemic perfusion and profound metabolic acidosis. The initial pH may be below 7 despite a low Pa_{CO_2}. Systemic blood flow is largely or completely dependent on blood flow into the aorta from the ductus arteriosus.

Ductal closure in the neonate with these problems causes dramatic worsening of the patient's condition. The patient becomes critically ill or even moribund and requires PGE_1 infusion (see earlier) for survival. PGE_1 allows blood flow into the aorta from the pulmonary artery because it maintains the patency of the ductus arteriosus.[27,30,31]

In neonates with acidosis, metabolic derangements, and renal failure because of inadequate systemic perfusion, PGE_1 infusion improves perfusion and metabolism, and surgery can be deferred until the patient's condition improves. Ventilatory and inotropic support and correction of metabolic acidosis, along with calcium, glucose, and electrolyte abnormalities, are often indicated preoperatively. The stabilization period also allows assessment of the magnitude of end-organ dysfunction caused by the preceding period of inadequate systemic perfusion. Adequacy of resuscitation, rather than severity of illness at presentation, appears to influence postoperative outcome.[32]

Ventricular Dysfunction

Ideally the intensivists should participate in the presentation of all preoperative patients who have a planned admission to the ICU. Understanding the extent of ventricular dysfunction preoperatively provides considerable insight into intraoperative and postoperative events. Although patients with large shunts may have complete mixing of systemic and venous blood and only mild-to-moderate hypoxemia as a result of their excessive pulmonary blood flow, the price paid for near-normal arterial oxygen saturation is chronic ventricular dilation and dysfunction and pulmonary vascular obstructive disease. Consequently, narrowing the shunt or a staged approach to single-ventricle repair may be indicated before any other elective surgery can be undertaken. Older patients with CHD and poor ventricular function as a result of chronic ventricular volume overload (aortic or mitral valve regurgitation or long-standing pulmonary-to-systemic arterial shunts) present a different problem, amenable to some extent by afterload reduction. However, in all of these circumstances when the heart is dilated and volume overloaded, there is a propensity for ventricular fibrillation during sedation, anesthesia, and/or intubation of the airway.

Assessment should include an estimation of the patient's functional limitation as an indicator of myocardial performance and reserve, quantification of the degree of hypoxia and the amount of pulmonary blood flow, and evaluation of PVR. For patients with increased Q_p/Q_s, systemic blood flow should be optimized without further augmenting pulmonary flow during induction of anesthesia in the ICU or in the operating room. However, during maintenance and emergence from anesthesia, retraction of the lung, positional changes, and abdominal distension may increase the hypoxemia and compromise the function of a dilated, poorly contractile ventricle. If this sequence occurs during surgery, the management must be altered to improve pulmonary blood flow.

In addition, systolic function of the ventricle may be impaired by intrinsic myopathic abnormalities related to drug toxicity (e.g., doxorubicin [Adriamycin]), inborn enzyme deficiencies, or acquired inflammatory or infectious disease. Patients with such dilated cardiomyopathies require optimization of ventricular performance with emphasis on inotropic support and afterload reduction. In many centers, these patients are admitted to the ICU for inotropic support and optimization of hemodynamic state prior to a planned surgical intervention.

Postoperative Care

Assessment

When the clinical course of patients after cardiac surgery deviates from the usual expectation of uncomplicated recovery, our first responsibility is to verify the accuracy of the preoperative diagnosis and the adequacy of surgical repair. For example, a young infant who is acidotic, hypotensive, and cyanotic after surgical repair of TOF may tempt us to ascribe these findings to the vagaries of ischemia/reperfusion injury of CPB or transient, postoperative stiffness of the right ventricle. However, the real culprit may be an additional VSD undetected preoperatively and therefore not closed, a residual VSD around the surgical patch, or residual RV outflow obstruction. Any of these anatomic issues and more can produce serious adverse outcomes. Getting the right postoperative assessment is imperative and treatment follows accordingly. Evaluation of the postoperative patient relies on examination, monitoring, interpretation of vital signs, or other bedside data and imaging (Table 29–2). When the accuracy of the diagnosis and adequacy of the repair are established, then a low cardiac output state can be presumed and treatment optimized. Treating low cardiac output states and preventing cardiovascular collapse often are the central features of pediatric cardiac intensive care and are the focus of this chapter. The details of the specific considerations for each lesion are presented in their respective chapters.

Optimizing preload involves more than just giving volume to a hypotensive patient. There are numerous considerations to fluid balance involving types of isotonic fluid, ultrafiltration in the operating room, optimal hematocrit, and use of furosemide, thiazides, and possibly newer drugs such as fenoldapam or nesiritide. Fluid itself can be detrimental if excess extravascular water results in interstitial edema and end-organ dysfunction of

TABLE 29–2

Ten Intensive Care Strategies to Diagnose and Support Low Cardiac Output States

1. Know in detail the cardiac anatomy and its physiologic consequences
2. Understand the specialized considerations of the newborn and implications of reparative rather than palliative surgery
3. Diversify personnel to include experts in neonatal and adult congenital heart disease
4. Monitor, measure, and image the heart to rule out residual disease as a cause of postoperative hemodynamic instability or low cardiac output
5. Maintain aortic perfusion and improve the contractile state
6. Optimize preload (including atrial shunting)
7. Reduce afterload
8. Control heart rate, rhythm, and synchrony
9. Optimize heart lung interactions
10. Provide mechanical support when needed

vital organs such as the heart, lungs, and brain. Perhaps permitting a right-to-left shunt at the atrial level would optimize preload to the left ventricle in some conditions (see later). Maintaining aortic perfusion after CPB and improving the contractile state of the heart with higher doses of catecholamines are reasonable goals but may have particularly deleterious consequences in the newborn myocardium after hypothermic CPB. The benefits of afterload reduction are well known, but in excess it results in hypotension and cardiovascular collapse or renal or cerebral insufficiency. Pacing the heart can stabilize the rhythm and hemodynamics, but it also may contribute to dyssynchronous, inefficient contraction of the heart or induce other arrhythmias. Mechanical support of the failing myocardium, in the form of extracorporeal membrane oxygenation (ECMO) or ventricular assist devices, although lifesaving in many instances, has its own set of time limitations and morbid complications. Almost every treatment approach has its own set of adverse effects that may be damaging. Supporting cardiac output in the postoperative patient is a balance between the promise and poison of therapy.

The initial assessment following cardiac surgery begins with review of the operative findings. This includes details of the operative repair and CPB, particularly total CPB or myocardial ischemia (aortic cross-clamp) times; concerns about myocardial protection; recovery of myocardial contractility; typical postoperative systemic arterial and central venous pressures; findings from intraoperative transesophageal echocardiography, if performed; and vasoactive medication requirements. This information guides subsequent examination, which should focus on the quality of the repair or palliation plus clinical assessment of cardiac output (Table 29–3). In addition to a complete cardiovascular examination, a routine set of laboratory tests should be obtained, including a chest radiograph, 12- or 15-lead ECG, blood gas analysis, serum electrolytes and glucose, an ionized calcium level, complete blood count, and coagulation profile.

TABLE 29–3

Signs of Heart Failure or Low Cardiac Output States

SIGNS
Cool extremities/poor perfusion
Oliguria and other end-organ failure
Tachycardia
Hypotension
Acidosis
Cardiomegaly
Pleural effusions
MONITOR AND MEASURE
Heart rate, blood pressure, intracardiac pressure
Extremity temperature, central temperature
Urine output
Mixed venous oxygen saturation
Arterial blood gas pH and lactate
Laboratory measures of end-organ function
Echocardiography

Monitoring

Monitoring central venous pressure is routine for many patients following cardiac surgery, except those who undergo the least complex procedures. For example, we do not routinely place a central venous catheter in patients undergoing thoracic procedures, such as coarctation of the aorta, vascular ring, or PDA ligation, or in patients undergoing cardiotomy with a short period of mildly hypothermic CPB, such as an ASD repair. Intracardiac or transthoracic left atrial (LA) catheters are often used to monitor patients after complex reparative procedures. Pulmonary arterial (PA) catheters now are seldom used but may be particularly useful if the postoperative management anticipates a problem such as (1) a residual lesion producing an intracardiac left-to-right shunt (e.g., multiple VSDs); (2) residual RV outflow tract obstruction, as a catheter "pullback" can be performed to measure the RV-to-PA pressure gradient; and (3) pulmonary hypertension, thereby allowing rapid detection of pressure changes and assessment of the response to interventions.

Left atrial catheters are especially helpful in the management of patients with ventricular dysfunction, coronary artery perfusion abnormalities, and mitral valve disease. The mean LA pressure typically is 1 to 2 mmHg greater than mean right atrial (RA) pressure, which generally varies between 1 and 6 mmHg in nonpostoperative pediatric patients undergoing cardiac catheterization. In postoperative patients, mean LA and RA pressures both are often greater than 6 to 8 mmHg. However, they should generally be less than 15 mmHg. The compliance of the right atrium is greater than that of the left atrium except in the newborn, so pressure elevations in the right atrium of older patients with two ventricles typically are less pronounced.

Possible causes of abnormally elevated LA pressure are listed in Table 29–4. In addition to pressure data, intracardiac catheters in the right atrium (or a percutaneously

TABLE 29–4

Common Causes of Elevated Left Atrial Pressure after Cardiopulmonary Bypass

1. Decreased ventricular systolic or diastolic function
Myocardial Ischemia
Dilated cardiomyopathy
Systemic ventricular hypertrophy
2. Left atrioventricular valve disease
3. Large left-to-right intracardiac shunt
4. Chamber hypoplasia
5. Intravascular or ventricular volume overload
6. Cardiac tamponade
7. Arrhythmia
Tachyarrhythmia, junctional rhythm
Complete heart block

TABLE 29–5

Causes of Abnormal Right Atrial, Left Atrial, or Pulmonary Artery Oxygen Saturation

Location	Elevated	Reduced
RA	Atrial level left-to-right shunt Anomalous pulmonary venous return Left ventricular-to-right atrial shunt ↑Dissolved O_2 content ↓O_2 extraction Catheter tip position (e.g., near renal veins)	↑Vo_2 (e.g, low CO, fever) ↓Sao_2 saturation with a normal A-V O_2 difference Anemia Catheter tip position (e.g., near CS)
LA	Does not occur	Atrial level right-to-left shunt ↓Pvo_2 (e.g., parenchymal lung disease)
PA	Significant left-to-right shunt Small left-to-right shunt with incomplete mixing of blood Catheter tip position (e.g., PA "wedge")	↑ O_2 extraction (e.g., low CO, fever) ↓Sao_2 saturation with a normal A-V O_2 difference Anemia

A-V, arteriovenous; *CO,* cardiac output; *CS,* coronary sinus; *LA,* left atrium; *PA,* pulmonary artery; *Pvo_2,* pulmonary vein oxygen tension; *RA,* right atrium; *Sao_2,* arterial oxygen saturation; *Vo_2,* oxygentation consumption.

placed central venous catheter), left atrium, and pulmonary artery can be used to monitor the oxygen saturation of systemic venous or pulmonary venous blood.

Table 29–5 lists the causes of abnormally high or low RA, LA, and PA oxygen saturations, which can be measured at the bedside in the ICU. Following reparative surgery, patients with no intracardiac shunts and adequate cardiac output may have a mild reduction in RA oxygen saturation to approximately 60%. Lower RA oxygen saturation does not necessarily indicate low cardiac output, if a patient has arterial desaturation (common mixing lessons, lung diseases, etc.) the arteriovenous oxygen difference is normal at 25%, there may be appropriate oxygen delivery and extraction. Elevated RA oxygen saturation often is the result of left-to-right shunting at the atrial level (e.g., from the left atrium, anomalous pulmonary vein, or left ventricular [LV]-to-RA shunt). Blood in the left atrium normally is fully saturated with oxygen (i.e., approximately 100%). The two chief causes of reduced LA oxygen saturation are an atrial level right-to-left shunt and pulmonary venous desaturation from abnormal gas exchange.

In the absence of left-to-right shunts, PA oxygen saturation is the best representation of the "true" mixed venous oxygen saturation because all sources of systemic venous blood should be thoroughly combined as they are ejected from the right ventricle. When elevated, this saturation is useful in identifying residual left-to-right shunts following repair of VSD(s). The absolute value of the PA oxygen saturation is a predictor of significant postoperative residual shunt. In patients following TOF or VSD repair, PA oxygen saturation greater than 80% within 48 hours of surgery with supplemental O_2 at a fractional inspired oxygen concentration (FIO_2) less than 0.5 is a sensitive indicator of significant left-to-right shunt (Q_p/Q_s >1.5) 1 year after surgery.[33] Determination of PA oxygen saturation also can be useful in patients with systemic-to-pulmonary artery collaterals because flow from these vessels into the pulmonary arteries can increase oxygen saturation.

Low Cardiac Output Syndrome

Although some causes of low cardiac output after CPB are attributable to residual or undiagnosed structural lesions, progressive low cardiac output states do occur. A number of factors have been implicated in the development of myocardial dysfunction following CPB including (1) the inflammatory response associated with CPB, (2) the effects of myocardial ischemia from aortic cross-clamping, (3) hypothermia, (4) reperfusion injury, (5) inadequate myocardial protection, and (6) ventriculotomy (when performed). The expression and prevention of reperfusion injury after aortic cross-clamping on CPB currently is the subject of intense investigation. We previously showed the typical decrease in cardiac index in newborns following an arterial switch operation (ASO) (Figure 29–1).[34] In this group of 122 newborns, the median maximal decrease in cardiac index that typically occurred 6 to 12 hours after separation from CPB was 32%. One fourth of these newborns reached a nadir of cardiac index that was less than 2 L/min/m² on the first postoperative night. Low cardiac output syndrome (LCOS) does occur in the postoperative patient, but appropriate anticipation and intervention can do much to avert morbidity or the need for mechanical support. Signs of low cardiac output are listed in Table 29–3. Mixed venous oxygen saturation, whole blood pH, and lactate are laboratory measures commonly used to evaluate the adequacy of tissue perfusion and hence cardiac output.

Volume Adjustments

After CPB, the factors that influence cardiac output, such as preload, afterload, myocardial contractility, heart rate, and rhythm, must be assessed and manipulated. Volume therapy (increased preload) is commonly necessary, followed by appropriate use of inotropic and afterload-reducing agents.[3] Atrial pressure and the ventricular response to changes in atrial pressure must be evaluated. Ventricular response is judged by observing systemic arterial pressure

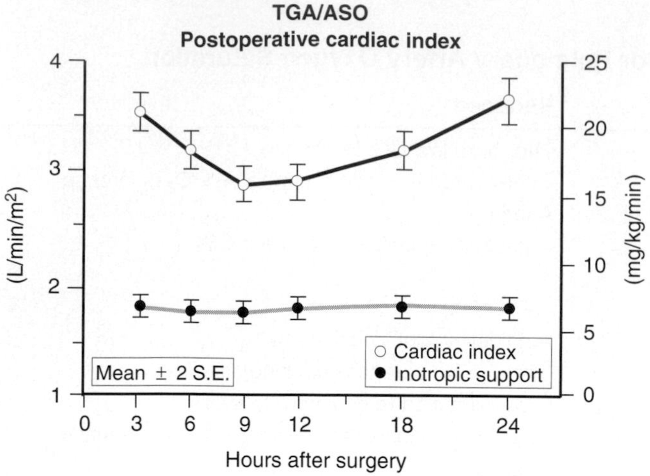

FIGURE 29–1 • Cardiac index **(left axis)** measured in infants following the arterial switch operation declines during the first 12 hours and was not the result of any reduction in inotropic support **(right axis).** One fourth of the patients reach a value less than 2 L/min/m^2. The median reduction in cardiac index the first night is 33%. (From Wernovsky G, Wypij D, Jonas RA, et al: Postoperative course and hemodynamic profile after the arterial switch operation in neonates and infants. A comparison of low-flow cardiopulmonary bypass and circulatory arrest. *Circulation* 92:2226-2235, 1995.)

and waveform, heart rate, skin color, peripheral extremity temperature, peripheral pulse magnitude, urine flow, core body temperature, and acid-base balance.

Preserving and Creating Right-to-Left Shunts

Selected children with low cardiac output may benefit from strategies that allow right-to-left shunting at the atrial level in the face of postoperative RV dysfunction. A typical example is early repair of TOF, when the moderately hypertrophied, noncompliant right ventricle has undergone a ventriculotomy and may be further compromised by an increased volume load from pulmonary regurgitation secondary to a transannular patch on the RV outflow tract. In these children it is very useful to leave the foramen ovale patent to permit right-to-left shunting of blood, thus preserving cardiac output and oxygen delivery despite the attendant transient cyanosis. If the foramen is not patent or is surgically closed, RV dysfunction can lead to reduced LV filling, low cardiac output, and ultimately LV dysfunction. In infants and neonates with repaired truncus arteriosus, the same concerns apply and may even be exaggerated if RV afterload is elevated because of pulmonary artery hypertension.

Right Ventriculotomy and Restrictive Physiology

Right ventricular "restrictive" physiology in infants and children who have undergone congenital cardiac surgery has been demonstrated by echocardiography as persistent antegrade diastolic blood flow into the pulmonary circulation following reconstruction of the RV outflow. This occurs in the setting of elevated RV end-diastolic pressure and RV hypertrophy, and the right ventricle demonstrates diastolic dysfunction with an inability to relax and fill during diastole. The right ventricle usually is not dilated in this circumstance, and pulmonary regurgitation is limited because of the higher diastolic pressure in the right ventricle.[35–37]

The term *restrictive RV physiology* is also commonly used in the immediate postoperative period in patients who have a stiff, poorly compliant, and sometimes hypertrophied right ventricle. The elevated ventricular end-diastolic pressure restricts filling during diastole, and therefore stroke volume and preload to the left ventricle causes an increase in right atrial filling pressure and therefore causes systemic venous hypertension. Because of the phenomenon of ventricular interdependence, changes in RV diastolic function and septal position in turn affect LV compliance and function. Factors contributing to diastolic dysfunction include lung and myocardial edema following CPB, inadequate myocardial protection of the hypertrophied ventricle during aortic cross-clamp, coronary artery injury, residual outflow tract obstruction, volume load on the ventricle from a residual VSD or pulmonary regurgitation, and dysrhythmias.

A low cardiac output state with increased right-sided filling pressure (usually >10 mmHg) is the common feature of neonatal restrictive RV physiology. As a result of the low cardiac output state, patients often have cool extremities, are oliguric, and may have a metabolic acidosis. As a result of the elevated right atrial pressure, hepatic congestion, ascites, increased chest tube losses, and pleural effusions may be evident.

These patients may be tachycardic and hypotensive with a narrow pulse pressure. Preload must be maintained despite elevation of RA pressure. Significant inotropic support often is required (typically dopamine 5–10 μg/kg/min and/or low-dose epinephrine 0.05–0.1 μg/kg/min), and a phosphodiesterase inhibitor, such as milrinone, is beneficial because of its lusitropic properties. Sedation and paralysis often are necessary for the first 24 to 48 hours to minimize the stress response and associated myocardial work.

Patients may be desaturated initially following surgery (75% to 85% range typically) because of this shunting. As RV compliance and function improve (usually within 2–3 postoperative days), the amount of shunt decreases and both antegrade pulmonary blood flow and SaO_2 increase.

Mechanical ventilation may have a significant impact on RV afterload and the amount of pulmonary regurgitation. In addition, an increase in PVR because of hypothermia, acidosis, and either hypoinflation or hyperinflation of the lung also increases afterload on the right ventricle and pulmonary regurgitation. Intermittent positive pressure ventilation with the lowest possible mean airway pressure should be the aim, as discussed previously.

This concept has been extended to older patients with single-ventricle physiology who are at high risk for Fontan operations.[38] The Fontan circulation relies on passive flow of blood through the pulmonary circulation without benefit of a pulmonary ventricle. If an atrial septal communication or fenestration is left at the time of the Fontan procedure, the resulting right-to-left shunt helps to preserve cardiac output. These children have fewer postoperative complications.[39] It is better to shunt blood right to left and accept some decrement in oxygen saturation but maintain ventricular filling and cardiac output rather than have high oxygen saturation but low blood pressure and cardiac output.

Pharmacologic Support

Catecholamines

Preload adjustments often do not provide adequate cardiac output. Use of pharmacologic agents to support cardiac output is common.[40,41] Table 29–6 lists common vasoactive drugs used in the ICU and their actions. Many prefer to use dopamine first in doses of 3 to 10 µg/kg/min. Dosages greater than 15 µg/kg/min are rarely used because of the known vasoconstrictor and chronotropic properties of dopamine at very high doses. However, extreme biologic variability in pharmacokinetics and pharmacodynamics defies placing narrow limits on recommended dosages. Dobutamine's chronotropic and vasodilatory advantages recognized in adults with coronary artery disease have not always proved equally efficacious in clinical studies in children. In fact, dobutamine has fewer, or no, dopaminergic advantages for the kidney.[42] This may be an especially important limitation in infants with excess total body water and interstitial edema. The significant chronotropic effect and increased oxygen consumption induced by isoproterenol have also increasingly limited its use in neonates and infants. Epinephrine is occasionally useful for short-term therapy

TABLE 29–6

Summary of Selected Vasoactive Agents

Agent	Doses (IV)	Peripheral Vascular Effect	Cardiac Effect	Conduction System Effect
NONCATECHOLAMINES				
Digoxin (total digitalizing dose)	20 µg/kg premature 30 µg/kg neonate (0–1 mo) 40 µg/kg infant (< 2yr) 30 µg/kg child (2-5yr) 20 µg/kg child (> 5 yr)	Increase peripheral vascular resistance 1–2+; acts directly on vascular smooth muscle	Inotropic effect 3–4+; acts directly on myocardium	Slows sinus node slightly; decreases AV conduction more
Calcium chloride	10–20 mg/kg/dose (slowly)	Variable; age-dependent; vasoconstrictor	Inotropic effect 3+; depends on ionised Ca^{2+}	Slows sinus node; decreases AV conduction
Gluconate	50–100 mg/kg/dose (slowly)			Reflex tachycardia
Nitroprusside	0.5–5 µg/kg/min	Donates nitric oxide group to relax smooth muscle and dilate pulmonary and systemic vesels	Indirectly increases cardiac output by decreasing afterload	
Nitroglycerin	0.5–10 µg/kg/min	Primarily venodilator, as a nitric oxide donor may cause pulmonary vasodilation and enhance coronary vasoreactivity after aortic cross-clamping	Decreases preload; may decrease afterload; reduces myocardial work related to change in wall stress	Minimal
Milrinone	50–75 µg/kg loading dose 0.25–1.0 µ/kg/min maintenance	Systemic and pulmonary vasodilator Potent vasoconstrictior	Diastolic relaxation (lusitropy); measurable inotopic effect	Minimal tachycardia
Vasopressin	0.003–0.002 µ/kg/min	Mild vasodilator	No direct effect	None known
Thyroid hormone Triiodothyronine (T_3)	0.05–0.10 µ/kg/min	Vasodilation	Positive inotropy	Tachycardia
Natriuretic Peptide (Nesiritide)	0.01–0.03 µ/kg/min	Natriuresis; little experience in children; diuretic effects controversial	Positive inotropy; diastolic relaxation	

		Peripheral Vascular Effect			*Cardiac Effect*		
Agent	**Dose Range**	α	$β_2$	Δ	$β_1$	$β_2$	**Comment**
CATECHOLAMINES							
Phenylephrine	0.1–0.5 µg/kg/min	4+	0	0	0	0	Increases systemic resistance, no inotropy; may cause renal Ischemia; useful for treatment of TOF spells

TABLE 29–6

Summary of Selected Vasoactive Agents *(Continued)*

Agent	Dose Range	α	β_2	ε	β_1	β_2	Comment
Isoproterenol	0.05–0.5 μg/kg/min	0	4+	0	4+	4+	Strong inotropic and chronotropic agent; peripheral vasodilator; reduces preload; pulmonary vasodilator; limited by tachycardia and oxygen consumption
Norepinephrine	0.1–0.5 μg/kg/min	4+	0	0	2+	0	Increases systemic resistance; moderately inotropic; may cause renal ischemia
Epinephrine	0.03–0.1 μg/kg/min 0.2–0.5 μg/kg/min	2+ 4+	1–2+ 0	0 0	2–3+ 4+	2+ 3+	Beta$_2$ effect with lower doses; best for blood pressure in anaphylaxis and drug toxicity
Dopamine	2–4 μg/kg/min 4–8 μg/kg/min >10 μg/kg/min	0 0 2–4+	0 2+ 0	2+ 2+ 0	0 1–2+ 1–2+	0 1+ 2+	Splanchnic and renal vasodilator; may be used with isoproterenol; increasing doses produce increasing α effect
Dobutamine	2–10 μg/kg/min	1+	2+	0	3–4+	1–2+	Less chronotropy and arrhythmias at lower doses; effects vary with dose similar to dopamine; chronotropic advantage compared with dopamine may not be apparent in neonates
Fenoldapam	0.05–1 μg/kg/min (see text; little experience in children)						Powerful D_1 agonist; little chronotropic or inotropic effect but may redistribute flow to renal bed and improve urine output

AV, atrioventricular; *TOF,* tetralogy of fallot.

when high systemic pressures are sought, provided the temporary increase in peripheral vascular resistance can be tolerated. High doses of epinephrine occasionally are necessary to increase pulmonary blood flow across significantly narrowed systemic-to-pulmonary artery shunts when oxygen saturations are low and falling. Arginine vasopressin has been advocated for states of refractory vasodilation associated with low circulating vasopressin levels as may rarely occur after CPB in children.[43] Vasopressin has been used to treat low systemic blood pressure in postoperative pediatric cardiac patients with pulmonary hypertension where it may ameliorate hypoxic pulmonary vasoconstriction and not exacerbate pulmonary hypertension.[44]

In the past, the side effects of inotropic support of the heart with catecholamines seemed a lesser concern in children than in adults with an ischemic, noncompliant heart. Tachycardia, an increased end-diastolic pressure and afterload, and increased myocardial oxygen consumption, despite their undesirable side effects, were tolerated by most children in need of inotropic support after CPB. However, with increasing perioperative experience in neonates and young infants, the adverse effects of vasoactive drugs have become more evident. The less compliant neonatal myocardium, like the ischemic adult heart, may raise its end-diastolic pressure during higher doses of dopamine infusion or may develop even more extreme noncompliance. Actual myocardial necrosis caused by high doses of epinephrine infusions has been identified in neonatal animal models after CPB.[45,46] Although these agents do increase the cardiac output, the concomitant increase in ventricular filling pressure is less well tolerated by the immature myocardium than it is in older children. Many of the complex corrective procedures performed in neonates and small infants are accompanied by transient postoperative arrhythmias that are either induced or exacerbated by catecholamines, which can have a profound adverse effect on the patient's recovery after surgery. Diastolic function is crucial in older patients with single ventricles and can be adversely affected by catecholamines. Nevertheless, the predictable and often significant decrease in cardiac output documented by many investigators after CPB in infants and older children continues to justify the practice of judiciously using catecholamines to support the heart and circulation while weaning them from CPB and during the immediate postoperative period.

Type III Phosphodiesterase Inhibitors

Milrinone has emerged as an important inotropic agent for use in children after open heart surgery.[47–49] It is a nonglycosidic, noncatecholamine inotropic agent with additional vasodilatory and lusitropic properties used extensively in adults for treatment of heart failure and more recently introduced to pediatric practice. This class of drugs exerts its principal effects by inhibiting phosphodiesterase III, the enzyme that metabolizes cyclic adenosine monophosphate (cAMP). By increasing intracellular cAMP, calcium transport into the cell is favored, and the increased intracellular calcium stores enhance the contractile state of the myocyte. In addition, reuptake of calcium is a cAMP-dependent process, and these agents may enhance diastolic relaxation of the myocardium by increasing the rate of calcium reuptake after systole (lusitropy). The drug also appears to work synergistically with low doses of β-agonists and has fewer side effects than other catecholamine vasodilators, such as isoproterenol. In critically ill postoperative newborns, milrinone increases cardiac output, lowers filling pressures, and reduces pulmonary artery pressures.[48]

The Prophylactic Intravenous Use of Milrinone after Cardiac Operation in Pediatrics (PRIMACORP) trial investigated the efficacy and safety of prophylactic milrinone use to prevent LCOS after cardiac surgery in high-risk pediatric patients.[49] The study was a multicenter, randomized, double-blind, placebo-controlled trial using three parallel treatment groups (low-dose: 25 μg/kg bolus over 60 minutes followed by a 0.25 μg/kg/min infusion for 35 hours; high-dose: 75 μg/kg bolus followed by 0.75 μg/kg/min; or placebo). The composite endpoint of death or the development of LCOS was evaluated at 36 hours and at the follow-up visit. Among 238 treated patients, the prophylactic use of high-dose milrinone significantly reduced the risk of death or the development of LCOS relative to placebo with a relative risk reduction of 55% (p = 0.023) in the treated patients. Patients who developed LCOS had a significantly longer cumulative duration of mechanical ventilation and hospital stay in comparison with those who did not develop LCOS. The authors concluded that the prophylactic use of high-dose milrinone following pediatric congenital heart surgery reduces the risk of LCOS. Dopamine and milrinone have emerged as our most commonly used inotropic agents, often used in combination to achieve increased cardiac output, maintain arterial perfusion pressure, and improve diastolic relaxation.

Thyroid Hormone

LCOS typically overlaps with the time that free and total triiodothyronine (T_3) levels are significantly suppressed following surgical reconstruction, namely, during the first 24 to 48 hours postoperatively. This is a significant observation, as T_3 is the predominant form of biologically active thyroid hormone and is known to improve cardiac output by improving the inotropic state of animal and human hearts while decreasing systemic vascular resistance. Limited studies of T_3 supplementation after cardiac surgery have been performed in children. Mainwaring et al.[50] gave two bolus doses of T_3 after the Fontan procedure to 10 children aged 19 to 42 months. Compared with a historical control group, the T_3 patients had a significantly shorter period of mechanical ventilation. Bettendorf et al.[51] randomized 40 children undergoing a wide variety of cardiac procedures to receive bolus dosing of T_3 or placebo. Cardiac output reportedly was higher in the treatment group but was estimated by echocardiography. Chowdhury et al.[52] randomized 28 children aged 0 to 18 years to a 5-day continuous infusion of T_3 (0.05–0.15 μg/kg/hour) or placebo. Among neonates, the T_3 group had lower severity of illness scores and lower inotrope requirements. The T_3 group also had a trend toward higher mixed venous oxygen saturations, fewer days of mechanical ventilation, and a shorter postoperative length of stay. No adverse effects of T_3 administration were recorded in any of these small series.

Thus the current literature demonstrates that infants undergoing cardiac surgery experience significant depression of T_3 levels and that supplementation of T_3 may have an impact on physiologic variables if not other measures of improved outcomes. Larger trials with more rigorous trial designs are under way and may address whether certain subgroups at particular risk for LCOS may benefit from T_3 administration. Preliminary analysis of a blinded trial of T_3 administration to patients after reconstructive surgery for HLHS at Children's Hospital Boston was disappointing, and routine use of T_3 is not supported by the existing literature.[53]

Other Afterload Reducing Agents

When systemic blood pressure is elevated and cardiac output appears low or normal, a primary vasodilator is indicated to normalize blood pressure and to decrease the afterload on the left ventricle. This is especially true for the newborn myocardium, which is particularly sensitive to changes in afterload and tolerates elevated systemic resistances poorly. Although nitroprusside has no known direct inotropic effects, this potent vasodilator has the advantage of being readily titratable and possessing a short biologic half-life. Use of nitroglycerin avoids the toxic metabolites cyanide and thiocyanate associated with nitroprusside use (especially in hepatic and renal insufficiency), but its potency as a vasodilator is less than that of nitroprusside. Inhibitors of angiotensin converting enzyme have proved to be important adjuvants to chronic anticongestive therapy in pediatric patients. Intravenous (IV) forms are available and may be useful in treatment of systemic hypertension immediately after coarctation repair or when afterload reduction with these inhibitors would benefit patients unable to receive oral medications. Sudden hypotension with the IV forms may limit use among infants.

The natriuretic hormone system is an important regulator of neurohumoral activation, vascular tone, diastolic function, and fluid balance. Preliminary data suggest that the endogenous biologic activity of the natriuretic hormone system is decreased following pediatric CPB. In theory, infusions of brain natriuretic peptide could oppose the neurohumoral mechanism associated with vasoconstriction and fluid retention after pediatric CPB. In randomized adult studies following CPB, natriuretic hormone infusions suppress the renin-angiotensin-aldosterone axis and improve cardiac loading conditions, cardiac index, and urine output.[54–57] We have increasing experience with nesiritide infusions in children.

Fenoldapam is a new dopaminergic agent useful in the treatment of systemic hypertension. It may have salutary effects on renal blood flow. It has no known chronotropic or inotropic effects on the heart but reduces afterload and may augment urine output in critically ill newborns after cardiac surgery.

Levosimendan is a calcium sensitizer that enhances the contractile state of the ventricle by increasing myocyte sensitivity to calcium and induces vasodilation. Levosimendan increases cardiac output by increasing stroke volume. It is independent of cAMP pathways that characterize the mechanism of action of both the catecholamines and the type III phosphodiesterase inhibitors. With its positive inotropic effects, levosimendan may be of value as adjunctive therapy to other inotropic drugs in patients who are refractory or tachyphylactic to other forms of inotropic support. Its hemodynamic effect in children is uncertain, but its pharmacokinetic profile seems similar to adults.[58]

Other Strategies

Newer strategies to support low cardiac output associated with cardiac surgery in children include use of atrio-*bi*ventricular pacing for patients with complete heart block or prolonged interventricular conduction delays and asynchronous contraction.[59] Appreciation of the hemodynamic effects of positive and negative pressure ventilation may assist cardiac output. Avoidance of hyperthermia and even induced hypothermia may provide end-organ protection during periods of low cardiac output. Antiinflammatory agents including monoclonal antibodies, competitive receptor blockers, inhibitors of compliment activation, and preoperative preparation with steroids are being actively investigated in an effort to prevent and protect major organs from ischemic injury imposed by CPB and the reperfusion injury associated with the recovery period.

Diastolic Dysfunction

Occasionally there is an alteration of ventricular relaxation, an active energy-dependent process, which reduces ventricular compliance. This is particularly problematic in patients with a hypertrophied ventricle undergoing surgical repair, such as TOF or Fontan surgery, and following CPB in some neonates when myocardial edema may significantly restrict diastolic function (i.e., "restrictive physiology").[36,37] The ventricular cavity size is small, and the stroke volume is decreased. β-Adrenergic antagonists and calcium channel blockers add little to the treatment of this condition. In fact, hypotension or myocardial depression produced by these agents often outweigh any gain from slowing the heart rate. Calcium channel blockers are relatively contraindicated in neonates and small infants because of their dependence on transsarcolemmal flux of calcium to both initiate and sustain contraction.

A gradual increase in intravascular volume to augment ventricular capacity, in addition to the use of low doses of inotropic agents, has proved to be of modest benefit in patients with diastolic dysfunction. Tachycardia must be avoided to optimize diastolic filling time and decrease myocardial oxygen demands. If low cardiac output continues despite treatment, therapy with vasodilators can be carefully attempted to alter systolic wall tension (afterload) and thus decrease the impediment to ventricular ejection. Because the capacity of the vascular bed increases after vasodilation, simultaneous volume replacement is often indicated. Milrinone or enoximone is useful under these circumstances because these agents are noncatecholamine so-called inodilators with vasodilating and lusitropic (improved diastolic state) properties, in contrast with other inotropic agents. Nesiritide also may play a particularly important role in lowering LV filling pressures in patients with heart failure.

Managing Acute Pulmonary Hypertension in the Intensive Care Unit

Children with many forms of CHD are prone to develop perioperative elevations in PVR.[60] This situation may complicate the postoperative course, when transient myocardial dysfunction requires optimal control of RV afterload.[61]

Although postoperative patients with pulmonary hypertension often are presumed to have active and reversible pulmonary vasoconstriction as the source of their pathophysiology, the critical care physician is obligated to explore anatomic causes of mechanical obstruction that impose a barrier to pulmonary blood flow. Elevated LA pressure, pulmonary venous obstruction, branch pulmonary artery stenosis, or surgically induced loss of the vascular tree all raise RV pressure and impose an unnecessary burden on the right heart. Similarly, a residual or undiagnosed left-to-right shunt raises pulmonary artery pressure postoperatively and must be addressed surgically. Extended use of pulmonary vasodilator strategies only augments residual or undiagnosed shunts and increases the volume load on the heart.

Several factors peculiar to CPB may raise PVR: Pulmonary vascular endothelial dysfunction, microemboli, pulmonary leukosequestration, excess thromboxane production, atelectasis, hypoxic pulmonary vasoconstriction, and adrenergic events all have been suggested to play a role in postoperative pulmonary hypertension. Postoperative pulmonary vascular reactivity has been related not only to the presence of preoperative pulmonary hypertension and left-to-right shunts but also to the duration of total CPB. Treatment of postoperative pulmonary hypertensive crises has been partially addressed by surgery at earlier ages, pharmacologic intervention, and other postoperative management strategies (Table 29–7).

Pulmonary Vasodilators

Many IV vasodilators have been used with variable success in patients with pulmonary hypertensive disorders requiring critical care. Older-style vasodilators such as tolazoline, phenoxybenzamine, nitroprusside, or isoproterenol had little biologic basis for selectivity or enhanced activity in the pulmonary vascular bed.[62] However, if myocardial function is depressed and the afterload reducing effect on the left ventricle is beneficial to myocardial function and cardiac output, then these drugs may be of some value. However, in addition to drug-specific side effects, they all have the limitation of potentially profound systemic hypotension, critically lowering right (and left) coronary perfusion pressure and simultaneously increasing intrapulmonary shunt. Even with selective infusions of rapidly metabolized, intravenously administered vasoactive drugs into the pulmonary circulation, systemic drug concentrations and systemic hemodynamic effects can be appreciable.

TABLE 29–7

Critical Care Strategies for Postoperative Treatment of Pulmonary Hypertension

Encourage	Avoid
1. Anatomic investigation	1. Residual anatomic disease
2. Opportunities for right-to-left shunt as "popoff"	2. Intact atrial septum in right heart failure
3. Sedation/anesthesia	3. Agitation/pain
4. Moderate hyperventilation	4. Respiratory acidosis
5. Moderate alkalosis	5. Metabolic acidosis
6. Adequate inspired oxygen	6. Alveolar hypoxia
7. Normal lung volumes	7. Atelectasis or overdistention
8. Optimal hematocrit	8. Excessive hematocrit
9. Inotropic support	9. Low output and coronary perfusion
10. Vasodilators	10. Vasoconstrictors/increased afterload

Prostacyclin appears to have somewhat more selectivity for the pulmonary circulation but at high doses can precipitate a hypotensive crisis in unstable postoperative patients with refractory pulmonary hypertension. It is best suited for chronic outpatient therapy in severe forms of primary pulmonary hypertension.[63–66] Agents that improve ventricular function in addition to reducing afterload (e.g., type III phosphodiesterase inhibitors) are more appealing when cardiac output is low.

As an alternative approach to nonspecific vasodilators, it seems logical to target vasoconstrictors known to be associated with pathologic states or critical events. In this regard, endothelin, a potent vasoconstrictor, is elevated in persistent pulmonary hypertension of the newborn, in children with CHD, and in patients after CPB, and seems a likely candidate for investigation of specific receptor blockers. Petrossian et al.[67] showed promising amelioration of postoperative pulmonary hypertension associated with CPB in animal models of increased pulmonary blood flow (from intracardiac shunts) when pretreated with endothelin-A receptor blockers. Undoubtedly, because the causes of pulmonary hypertension in the intensive care setting frequently are multifactorial, our "best" therapy will be multiply targeted. Adding phosphodiesterase inhibitors to prostacyclin infusions, endothelin blockers, thromboxane inhibitors, and inhaled nitric oxide (NO) all may have individual and combined merit with synergism enhancing efficacy.

Nitric oxide is a selective pulmonary vasodilator that can be breathed as a gas and distributed across the alveoli to the pulmonary vascular smooth muscle.[68,69] It is formed by the endothelium from L-arginine and molecular oxygen in a reaction catalyzed by NO synthase. It then diffuses to the adjacent vascular smooth muscle cells where it induces vasodilation through a cyclic guanosine monophosphate-dependent pathway.[70] Because NO exists as a gas, it can be delivered by inhalation to the alveoli and then to the blood vessels, which lie in close proximity to ventilated lung. Because of its rapid inactivation by hemoglobin, inhaled NO may achieve selective pulmonary vasodilation when pulmonary vasoconstriction exists. It has advantages over intravenously administered vasodilators that cause systemic hypotension and increase intrapulmonary shunting. Inhaled NO lowers pulmonary artery pressure in a number of diseases without the unwanted effect of systemic hypotension. This effect is especially dramatic in children with cardiovascular disorders and postoperative patients with pulmonary hypertensive crises.[61,71–73]

Therapeutic uses of inhaled NO in children with CHD abound in the ICU. For example, newborns with total anomalous pulmonary venous connection (TAPVC) frequently have obstruction of the pulmonary venous pathway as it connects anomalously to the systemic venous circulation. When pulmonary venous return is obstructed preoperatively, pulmonary hypertension is severe and demands urgent surgical relief. Increased neonatal pulmonary vasoreactivity, endothelial injury induced by CPB, and intrauterine anatomic changes in the pulmonary vascular bed in this disease contribute to postoperative pulmonary hypertension. Inhaled NO dramatically reduces pulmonary hypertension without change in heart rate, systemic blood pressure, or vascular resistance.

Patients with TAPVC, congenital mitral stenosis, and other pulmonary venous hypertensive disorders associated with low cardiac output appear to be among the most responsive to NO. These infants are born with significantly increased amounts of smooth muscle in their pulmonary arterioles and veins. Histologic evidence of muscularized pulmonary veins and pulmonary arteries suggests the presence of vascular tone and capacity for change in resistance at both the arterial and venous sites. The increased responsiveness to NO seen in younger patients with pulmonary venous hypertension may result from pulmonary vasorelaxation at a combination of precapillary and postcapillary vessels.

Several groups have reported successful use of inhaled NO in a variety of other congenital heart defects following cardiac surgery. It may be especially helpful when administered during a pulmonary hypertensive crisis.[73] NO use after Fontan procedures,[74] following VSD repair, and with a variety of other anatomic lesions has been described. Prophylactic use of inhaled NO in patients at risk for developing postoperative pulmonary hypertensive crises is thought by some to reduce the duration of mechanical ventilation.[75] Oxygen saturation in response to inhaled NO generally does not improve in very young infants who are excessively cyanotic after a bidirectional Glenn anastomosis. Increasing cardiac output and cerebral blood flow may have much greater impact on arterial oxygenation. Elevated pulmonary vascular tone is seldom the limiting factor in the hypoxemic patient after the bidirectional Glenn operation.[76]

Inhaled NO can be used diagnostically in neonates with RV hypertension after cardiac surgery to discern those with reversible vasoconstriction. Failure of the postoperative newborn with pulmonary hypertension to respond to NO successfully discriminated anatomic obstruction to pulmonary blood flow from pulmonary vasoconstriction. Failure of the postoperative newborn to respond to NO should be regarded as strong evidence of anatomic and possibly surgically remediable obstruction.[77]

If withdrawal of NO is necessary before resolution of the pathologic process, hemodynamic instability can be expected. We previously suggested that the withdrawal response to inhaled NO can be attenuated by pretreatment with the type V phosphodiesterase inhibitor sildenafil (Viagra).[78] Sildenafil inhibits the inactivation of cyclic guanosine monophosphate within the vascular smooth muscle cell and has the potential to augment the effects of endogenous or exogenously administered NO to effect vascular smooth muscle relaxation. Sildenafil can be administered in an oral or IV form and has a somewhat selective pulmonary vasodilating capacity while lowering LA pressure and providing a modest degree of afterload reduction in some postoperative children. Chronic oral administration of sildenafil to adults with primary pulmonary hypertension improves exercise capacity, which suggests an important therapeutic application of the IV preparation in postoperative congenital heart surgery.

Cardiac Tamponade

Chest closure is a time of particular instability after operations for CHD. The small infant's mediastinum makes compression of the heart and cardiac tamponade ever-present possibilities after chest closure despite patent drainage tubes and surgical resection of the anterior pericardium. The warning signs of tamponade frequently are subtle in small children, even minutes before cardiovascular collapse from tamponade. Any significant deterioration in hemodynamics after chest closure first should be attributed to tamponade if ventilation and cardiac rhythm are adequate. The signs of tamponade include tachycardia, hypotension, narrow pulse pressure, and high filling pressures on both the left and right sides of the heart.

Acute myocardial perforation with tamponade occasionally occurs during interventional cardiac catheterization procedures. Prompt support of the circulation with volume infusions and pressor support, along with immediate catheter drainage of the pericardial space, are essential in the event of this complication. Hemopericardium after ventricular puncture usually is self-limited, as the muscular ventricle seals the perforation after the responsible wire or catheter is removed. However, laceration of the more thin-walled atrium may require suture repair under direct vision in the operating room.

Other causes of cardiac tamponade are seen in patients with CHD, and treatment frequently requires the assistance of an intensivist for either pericardiocentesis or sedation and monitoring for that definitive procedure. Postoperative tamponade from bleeding immediately after operation, as discussed earlier, is best handled by facilitation of chest tube drainage or reopening the sternotomy. These patients usually are still anesthetized and mechanically ventilated so that new anesthetic considerations and choices are limited. However, some children develop pericardial effusions during other phases of their illness because of hydrostatic influences (e.g., patients with modified Fontan operations) or postpericardiotomy syndrome. Fluid in the pericardial space may accumulate under considerable pressure, and filling of the heart is impaired. If this problem is left unattended, the transmural pressure in the atria diminishes as intraatrial pressures rise, and diastolic collapse of the atria can be observed echocardiographically. Patients become symptomatic with a narrow pulse pressure, pulsus paradoxus, tachycardia, respiratory distress, abdominal pain progressing to decreased urine output, hyperkalemia, metabolic acidosis, and hypotension with tremendous endogenous catecholamine response.[79–81]

In summary, aggressive identification and treatment of low cardiac output conditions after cardiac surgery is central to the critical care of children with CHD. Successful application of these strategies and thoughtful use of pharmacologic intervention undoubtedly has contributed to the remarkable decline in mortality associated with congenital heart surgery in the past two decades. However, despite these interventions, additional (mechanical) support is sometimes necessary as a bridge to recovery.

Mechanical Support of the Circulation

Despite the expanding options for pharmacologic support, the circulation cannot be adequately supported in some patients in both preoperative and postoperative situations. Mechanical assist devices have an important role in providing short-term circulatory support to enable myocardial recovery and the potential for longer-term support while the patient is awaiting cardiac transplantation. Although a variety of assist devices are available for adult-size patients, ECMO is the predominant mode of support for children.

Currently, more than 300 children per year who receive ECMO for cardiac support are reported to the Extracorporeal Life Support Registry, with the majority of patients placed on ECMO following cardiotomy.[82–84] Although more than 50% of these patients are decannulated from ECMO, the overall survival to discharge has been only 35% to 40% of reported cases over the past decade.

At Children's Hospital Boston, we have used ECMO to support the circulation in more than 200 patients. Neonates comprise 41% of all our cardiac ECMO patients, with a survival rate to discharge of 50%. The pediatric group (infant through 16 years) comprises 55% of our total experience with an improved survival rate to discharge of 59%.

Substantial institutional variability in patient selection for ECMO makes comparison of published experience difficult. Centers with an efficient and well-established ECMO service are more likely to use this form of support in patients with low cardiac output. Furthermore, surgical technique and bypass management are additional confounding factors that make comparisons of the use and indications for ECMO between institutions difficult to interpret. Nevertheless, this form of mechanical support can be demonstrated to be lifesaving, and it can be argued that it should be available when needed for selected patients following congenital heart surgery. ECMO for pediatric resuscitation (rapid deployment during active cardiopulmonary resuscitation [CPR]) in a pulseless circulation remains a controversial issue. A rapid response ECMO system was started at Children's

Hospital Boston in 1996.[85] Of more than 200 cardiac ECMO patients, 50% were cannulated during active CPR (rapid response system), and 55% of these patients have been successfully discharged from the hospital. General indications and contraindications for ECMO support of the circulation in patients with CHD are summarized in Tables 29–8 and 29–9.

Preoperative Stabilization

Extracorporeal membrane oxygenation may be useful for critically ill neonates prior to cardiac surgery, thereby enabling preoperative stabilization and limiting end-organ dysfunction prior to repair. Indications include severe low output state (e.g., critical AS), pulmonary hypertension (e.g., obstructed totally anomalous pulmonary venous return), and severe hypoxemia (e.g., transposition with pulmonary hypertension). These have been rare indications for ECMO at Children's Hospital Boston.

Failure to Wean from Cardiopulmonary Bypass

Patients who fail to wean from CPB may be connected directly to an ECMO circuit in the operating room and brought to the ICU in the hope of recovering myocardial function. These children typically had poorer survival rates for many reasons, including severity and complexity of disease and increased bleeding.[82] A critical decision for using ECMO in this circumstance is whether the patient is a suitable candidate for cardiac transplantation if there is no significant recovery of function. Clearly, patient selection can have an enormous influence on outcomes in this category. As practitioners gained experience with and acceptance of mechanical support, its successful use in the transition from CPB increased.[86]

TABLE 29–8

Typical Indications for ECMO

- I. Inadequate oxygen delivery
  - A. Low cardiac output
    1. Chronic (cardiomyopathy)
    2. Acute (myocarditis)
    3. Weaning from cardiopulmorary bypass
    4. Preoperative stabilization
    5. Progressive postoperative failure
    6. Pulmonary hypertension
    7. Refractory arrhythmias
    8. Cardiac arrest
  - B. Profound cyanosis
    1. Intracardiac shunting and cardiovascular collapse
    2. Acute shunt thrombosis
    3. Acute respiratory failure exaggerated by underlying heart disease
    4. Congestive heart disease complicated by other newborn indications for ECMO, such as meconium aspiration syndrome, PPHN, pneumonia, sepsis, respiratory distress syndrome
- II. Support for intervention during cardiac catheterization

ECMO, Extracorporeal membrane oxygenation.

TABLE 29–9

Relative Contraindications for Extracorporeal Membrane Oxygenation

1. End-stage, irreversible, or inoperable disease
2. Family, patient directives to limit resuscitation
3. Significant neurologic or end-organ impairment
4. Uncontrolled bleeding within major organs
5. Extremes of size and weight
6. Inaccessible vessels during resuscitation

Postcardiotomy

In general, ECMO appears to be most effective as a therapeutic option for patients who have a period of relative stability after reparative cardiac surgery but then develop progressive myocardial or respiratory failure or have a sudden cardiac arrest. This typically occurs during the first 24 hours after surgery, and subsequent survival may be better in this group of patients following a period of myocardial rest and decompression. Our current survival rate for this group at Children's Hospital Boston is 64%.

Bridge to Transplantation

Although ECMO can be used to resuscitate the circulation and prevent end-organ dysfunction while the patient is awaiting potential myocardial recovery, it also can be used as a bridge to transplantation.[87] However, with limitations related to donor availability and the potential complications while the patient is on ECMO, in particular bleeding, end-organ dysfunction, and sepsis, the decision to proceed with listing for transplantation should be made early during the ECMO run. If there is no discernible recovery of myocardial function after 48 to 72 hours on ECMO support, transplant evaluation should be completed for appropriate patients.[88] Our current median waiting time on ECMO after listing for transplantation is 6 days for all patients, and we have been able to successfully bridge 63% of our patients to transplant. However, there are important age and size differences, with older children and adolescents being much more likely to survive a successful ECMO bridge to transplantation.

Resuscitation

The rapid deployment of ECMO during active CPR in a pulseless circulation remains a contentious issue. The underlying premise is that survival following a sudden cardiac arrest and standard resuscitation in children is poor irrespective of the resuscitation setting.[89,90] Therefore a number of pediatric institutions have developed a rapid response system to provide early deployment and cannulation for ECMO.[85,91,92] A rapid response ECMO system was started at Children's Hospital Boston in 1996. Through January 2003, more than 150 patients have been placed on ECMO with an overall survival-to-discharge rate of 57%. Of these patients, 52% were placed on ECMO during active CPR (rapid response system), and 55% of these patients have been successfully discharged from the hospital.

The ability to efficiently and rapidly support the circulation or respiration in patients following cardiac surgery (and in children with cardiac disease in general) has improved our ability to salvage a group of children who previously most likely would have died. This type of support is believed to account for a substantial part of the decline in surgical mortality during the end of the 1990s.

We have used the rapid deployment system during cardiopulmonary arrest and resuscitation at a variety of locations throughout the hospital, including the ICU, cardiac catheterization laboratory, emergency department, and noncardiac operating rooms. Typically, we now wait only moments (i.e., after one or two rounds of resuscitation medications) before determining that return of cardiovascular stability during CPR is unlikely and that ECMO should be deployed. An ECMO circuit is ready and saline primed at all times in the ICU. A neonatal membrane is used in this setup (size 0.8–1.5 M^2; appropriate for patients 2–15 kg). For older children and adults, a fresh circuit with a hollow-fiber membrane is used that takes little time to de-air and can be established within 15 minutes. Once the patient is stable on ECMO, the hollow fiber can be changed out for a conventional membrane if longer-term support is necessary. Blood products are added when they are available (typically after cannulation), and crystalloid is removed by direct withdrawal from the circuit into a syringe or by a volume-matched amount of ultrafiltration. Cardiac surgeons who are trained in cannulation techniques for open chest, groin, or neck routes, ECMO specialists, and cardiac ICU physicians are immediately available in-house 24 hours per day.

Extracorporeal Membrane Oxygenation Cannulation, Stabilization, and Evaluation

Depending on the circumstances of hemodynamic decompensation (impending or actual cardiac arrest; nonoperated or postoperative cardiac patient) and surgeon preference, vascular access is obtained either by transthoracic approach with direct cannulation of the right atrium and aorta or peripherally through the neck or femoral vessels. Medical support and resuscitation (i.e., airway stabilization with hand ventilation, intravascular volume replacement, catecholamine infusions, correction of electrolyte imbalance, sodium bicarbonate administration, arrhythmia suppression, cardiac pacing, core temperature cooling, and cardiac massage) are continued throughout the cannulation procedure and commencement of venoarterial extracorporeal support until a stable circulation is achieved.

The ECMO circuit is a "closed" circuit, which is an important distinction to a CPB circuit in which cardiotomy suction is used during cardiac surgery. There is very limited ability to handle any air in the venous limb of the ECMO circuit, and careful de-airing of both the arterial and venous cannulas is essential when connecting to the ECMO circuit. In our institution, blood flow is driven by a roller pump using a servoregulatory mechanism. This system permits high flow rates with minimal hemolysis and protects against air entrainment. Priming volumes are determined by the surface area of the oxygenator membrane. The circuit is initially vacuumed with carbon dioxide to eliminate nitrogen, which leads to bubble formation after introduction of the saline priming solution. Normosol solution (Abbott Laboratories, Abbott Park, IL, USA) is used to displace the CO_2, and after the system has been de-bubbled, 5% albumin is added to decrease adsorption of fibrinogen to the circuit components during the subsequent blood priming.

Following cannulation, the patient is connected to the ECMO circuit and the roller pump is adjusted to gradually achieve the desired flow rates of 100 to 150 ml/kg depending on the underlying cardiopulmonary physiology. Intracardiac and arterial blood pressures, including waveform characteristics, are noted. Usually, vasopressor infusions are used to maintain mean arterial blood pressure greater than 45 mmHg in neonates and greater than 60 to 70 mmHg in children and adults. A chest radiograph is obtained to check cannulas, line position, endotracheal tube, and lung parenchymal status.

Elevated premembrane pressures (i.e., >350 mmHg) at normal flows without change in postmembrane pressure and evidence of blood-to-gas leak constitute membrane oxygenator dysfunction and may dictate oxygenator replacement. Extensive thrombus or consumptive coagulopathy with hypofibrinogenemia and thrombocytopenia are other indications for circuit replacement. When ECMO flow appears inadequate to meet the needs of the patient and limited venous drainage restricts additional flow, interpretation of arterial and atrial pressures may aid the formulation of a differential diagnosis (Table 29–10). Low flow states and/or significant hypotension require immediate analysis and intervention.

Assessing the adequacy of flow soon after initiation of ECMO is of paramount importance. Answering a checklist of questions assists this assessment.

Is the Systemic Ventricle Adequately Decompressed? Venting the left atrium may be necessary to lower the LA pressure and decrease LV wall stress, thereby minimizing ongoing myocardial injury. Adequate decompression and signs of pulmonary edema can be assessed early by echocardiography. If not decompressed, strategies include (1) placing a vent in the left atrium by direct placement via the atrial appendage or pulmonary veins through an open chest or by a transcatheter approach in the catheterization laboratory[93] and (2) augmenting ventricular ejection by judicious use of inotropic agents.

Are the Perfusion Pressure and Flow Adequate? This determination can be made by assessment of perfusion pressure, patient color and appearance, presence of an acidosis, adequate clearance of lactate, and appropriately sized and positioned cannulas. Hypotension with mean arterial blood pressure less than 30 mmHg in neonates or less than 50 mmHg in larger children and adults requires prompt evaluation and treatment.

Is Hemostasis Achieved? This is not an uncommon problem in the immediate postoperative period. Prompt control of bleeding has a direct influence on subsequent outcome. Tamponade physiology affects venous return, circuit line pressure, and ECMO flows; mediastinal reexploration may be necessary to evacuate clot and control bleeding. In addition to surgical exploration, replacement of coagulation factors and use of antifibrinolytics must

TABLE 29–10

Assessment of Low Flow States During ECMO

Problem	Observations	Treatment Options
Inadequate oxygen delivery and organ perfusion	Tachycardia, mottled skin, cool extremities, poor capillary refill, hypotension, oliguria, metabolic acidosis, hyperlactatemia, rising serum creatinine and liver function tests	Check cannula position Increase ECMO flow Increase native cardiac output
Inadequate ECMO flow: circuit chatters, bladder collapses, inadequate venous return or high postmembrane pressure	Atrial pressures normal	
	Venous cannula malposition	Reposition venous cannula
	Venous cannula too small	Replace or add second venous cannula
	Venous thrombus formation	Surgically remove thrombus or thrombolysis
	Excessive runoff through aortopulmonary shunt	Narrow shunt, embolize collaterals
	Atrial pressures low	
	Bleeding	Surgically explore, administer coagulation factors and blood, administer antifibrinolytics, reduce heparin
	Systemic vasodilation	Treat sepsis, administer vasoconstrictors
	Atrial pressures high	
	Tamponade	Surgically explore, evacuate blood and clot
	Left ventricular overdistension	Place vent in left atrium, support ejection with catecholamine
	Aortic regurgitation	Reposition aortic cannula, assess need for aortic valve replacement
	Membrane pressure high	
	Arterial cannula malposition	Reposition cannula
	Arterial cannula too small	Replace or add second arterial cannula (bifemoral arterial cannulation)

ECMO, Extracorporeal membrane oxygenation.

be considered (e.g., aminocaproic acid bolus 100 mg/kg followed by 30 mg/kg/hour infusion; an alternative for persistent postcardiotomy bleeding may be aprotinin 30,000 IU/kg bolus and 10,000 IU/kg/hour for 6 hours). Initial guidelines include transfusion of packed red blood cells to maintain the hematocrit at greater than 35%, cryoprecipitate to keep the serum fibrinogen level greater than 150 mg/dl, and concentrated platelet transfusions to maintain the platelet count greater than $100,000/mm^3$. A heparin bolus (30 U/kg) usually is given at the time of cannulation, followed by infusion (20–30 U/kg/hour) adjusted to maintain an activated clotting time of 180 to 200 seconds.

Are There Specific Considerations Based on Underlying Pathology? Management of an aortopulmonary shunt is critical in patients with single-ventricle physiology. Systemic and pulmonary flow should be balanced by either partially clipping the shunt or by using high ECMO flows. On ECMO, circuit flows up to 200 ml/kg/min or more usually are necessary to maintain adequate systemic perfusion while accounting for runoff into the pulmonary circulation through the shunt. Although partial temporary narrowing of the shunt may be advisable in some circumstances, it is unwise to completely occlude the only source of pulmonary blood flow to the pulmonary endothelium. It is possible to bypass the membrane oxygenator in patients following the Norwood procedure with a Blalock shunt without lung disease if higher flows are maintained and the shunt is patent.[94] This maneuver simplifies the circuit and may permit less use of heparin. Thus ECMO effectively becomes a ventricular assist device.

Problems related to cannula placement and adequacy of venous drainage must be considered in patients with single-ventricle physiology and complex venous anatomy, such as heterotaxy syndrome or possible vessel occlusion from prior catheterizations, and in patients with a cavopulmonary connection. The site of cannulation is affected by vessel patency, and the underlying physiology might influence the number of venous cannulae used. For example, patients with a superior cavopulmonary anastomosis (bidirectional Glenn shunt [BDG]) as the primary source of pulmonary blood flow often require separate venous drainage of the SVC and inferior vena cava (IVC), unless there is congenital interruption of the infrahepatic IVC with drainage of lower body blood to the azygos vein. In the latter case, a single venous cannula in the SVC might be sufficient. On the other hand, placement of a cannula in the SVC may be detrimental in patients with BDG physiology because of the potential for reduced cerebral venous drainage and therefore decreased cerebral perfusion. This also is a concern for patients with Fontan physiology. Although it may be possible to achieve adequate drainage with a venous cannula placed in the Fontan baffle, in our experience an additional SVC catheter often is necessary to achieve the desired or necessary flows on ECMO.[95]

Is There Adequate End-Organ Perfusion? Once stable flows and perfusion have been achieved, the ventricles have been decompressed, and hemostasis has been secured, potential end-organ injury should be evaluated. For patients who have long-standing cyanotic heart disease, it may be preferable to start ECMO using a lower oxygen concentration (closer to room air) to attenuate the potential ischemia/reperfusion injury and potential for oxygen free radical injury. Neurologic protection must be considered. For patients placed on ECMO during active resuscitation, mild hypothermia (34°C) should be maintained for the first 12 to 24 hours on ECMO to prevent secondary neurologic injury. Assessment with head ultrasound, electroencephalography, or computed tomographic (CT) scan should be considered early. Muscle relaxants should not be given and sedation minimized to allow an appropriate daily clinical assessment. In addition, renal function, liver function, risk for sepsis, and possible gut ischemia should be frequently evaluated.

Residual Cardiac Defects. If a patient fails to wean from ECMO or if there is a delay in anticipated recovery of myocardial function, the possibility of a residual surgical problem must always be considered. This usually is difficult to diagnose by echocardiography alone, and cardiac catheterization (i.e., diagnostic or interventional) should be considered.

Daily Management

The daily management of a patient on ECMO or other forms of extracorporeal life support requires meticulous assessment of cardiorespiratory function, end-organ perfusion and injury, evolving complications such as bleeding or sepsis, and the mechanics of the ECMO circuit.[84] Following ECMO cannulation and initial resuscitation, high flow rates (100–200 cc/kg/min depending on the underlying pathophysiology) are used to "rest" the heart and decompress the ventricle(s). However, in contrast to the concept of "resting the lungs" for patients who are placed on ECMO for respiratory failure and lung injury, it is important that the heart regain contractile function and conduction as soon as possible to maintain a workload and avoid involution of the myocardial mass. For this reason, inotropic support may be reintroduced earlier in cardiac patients compared with those on ECMO purely for respiratory support. Atrioventricular synchrony should be established as soon as possible. This can be achieved with external pacing if necessary. It is very important that dysrhythmias occurring on ECMO be treated promptly. Although it may be possible to maintain adequate systemic perfusion and ECMO flows, the heart may overdistend in the presence of certain dysrhythmias, particularly ventricular fibrillation, and cause irreversible myocardial injury.

Transient endothelial dysfunction is common after ECMO is established, identical to the injury resulting from CPB, and causes an elevated PVR and ventilation/perfusion abnormalities.[96] Permitting or promoting the heart to eject some blood into the pulmonary circulation while on ECMO may help endothelial recovery and prevent pulmonary hypertension when weaning from ECMO. It is important to remember that the pulmonary venous blood entering the left ventricle and ejected into the coronary circulation may be significantly desaturated, which could cause myocardial ischemia or delay myocardial recovery. For this reason, mechanical ventilation is continued on cardiac ECMO to ensure pulmonary venous blood is well saturated. Ventilator settings are adjusted primarily according to lung compliance, which may reflect the degree of preexisting cardiac-related or parenchymal lung disease. Tidal volumes of 7 to 9 ml/kg with peak inspiratory pressures not exceeding 25 to 28 cmH_2O and FiO_2 of 0.3 to 0.4 usually are maintained in patients with normal lung compliance. Changes in ventilator settings are guided by physical examination, assessment of compliance based on hand ventilation and lung volumes, and appearance of the lung fields on daily chest radiographs. Fluid retention and body wall edema are very common in cardiac patients on ECMO because of (1) endothelial dysfunction and capillary leak associated with reperfusion injury and inflammatory response,[97] (2) changes in oncotic pressure depending on the priming solution, and (3) decreased urine output secondary to alterations in perfusion and the influence of antidiuretic hormone, renin-angiotensin, and atrial natriuretic factor production.[98] Diuretic therapy is started early to achieve a negative fluid balance and treat anasarca as soon as possible; fluid overload is one of the most important factors that will determine eventual successful weaning from cardiac ECMO and longer-term survival. Furosemide bolus (1 mg/kg) followed by continuous infusion (0.2–0.3 mg/kg/hour) usually is the first choice to induce a diuresis, provided adequate renal perfusion has been achieved with ECMO flow and no significant or irreversible renal injury occurred prior to starting ECMO. Chlorothiazide (10 mg/kg per dose every 12 hours) is added if the response to furosemide is suboptimal. Modified ultrafiltration is used in the setting of excessive fluid retention despite maximal diuretic therapy and circulatory support. Suspension of ultrafiltration is advisable in the setting of low atrial pressures with hypotension and frequent circuit shutdown because of low volume or pressure sensing within the bladder, at least until hemodynamics stabilize.

Neurologic assessment, although difficult in patients on ECMO, must be performed regularly. Abrupt changes in heart rate, blood pressure, skin perfusion, and pupillary size could indicate seizure activity in paralyzed patients. Findings of concern should be promptly evaluated by cranial ultrasound, head CT scan, or electroencephalography because changes or abnormalities will impact the decision to continue ECMO support. Sedation and analgesia also must be continually reassessed. Muscle relaxation is advisable in unstable patients but can be used intermittently as needed once the patient and ECMO flows are stable enough to allow neurologic evaluation. Parenteral nutritional support should be initiated within 1 to 2 days after establishing ECMO, although it can be deferred if the ECMO course likely will be relatively short (i.e., <4 days), and introduction of enteral nutrition soon after discontinuing ECMO is anticipated. Patients receiving mechanical support are at high risk for nosocomial infection, especially from skin flora with a direct portal of entry through catheters, chest sites, and open or closed sternotomy wounds. Patients with unexplained hemodynamic instability, coagulopathy, and elevated white blood cell count or fever should be pan-cultured and broad-spectrum antibiotic cover initiated.

Weaning from Extracorporeal Membrane Oxygenation

The strategies for weaning from cardiac ECMO often are quite different from those used for weaning patients who are on ECMO for respiratory support. A thorough understanding of the underlying cardiac physiology and cardiorespiratory interactions and an appreciation for the expected range of oxygen saturations is important. Because of the high risk of complications and substantial mortality in cardiac patients associated with duration of mechanical circulatory support beyond 1 week, consideration as to when and how to wean cardiac patients from ECMO should begin soon after cannulation once circulatory stability has been established. The disease process and circumstances resulting in hemodynamic failure or cardiac arrest may influence the expected duration of mechanical support. For example, patients who fail to separate from CPB after cardiac surgery because of severe pulmonary hypertension usually respond to a 24- to 48-hour period on ECMO with inhaled NO therapy and inotropic support of the right heart. Similarly, patients who have a low cardiac output state or suffer cardiac arrest after cardiac surgery may have residual defects that allow rapid weaning and decannulation soon after reoperation. The likelihood of recovery of ventricular function should be decided within the first 48 to 72 hours so that cardiac transplantation status can be ascertained. ECMO instituted for catheter intervention or arrhythmia ablation procedures may be discontinued within hours of patient cannulation.[99] In contrast, patients with severe cardiomyopathies or those awaiting heart transplantation may require mechanical assistance for a much longer period. Patients with severe bronchiolitis as a result of respiratory syncytial virus complicating repair of CHD on CPB typically require 2 to 3 weeks of ECMO support for respiratory failure.

For patients with structurally normal hearts who require ECMO support for respiratory illness, the ability to wean is dependent on resolution of the primary pulmonary process, often with little need for support of the myocardium beyond moderate inotropic support, fluid and electrolyte management, and nutritional support. Once lung compliance and gas exchange have normalized, improvement of the lungs on chest radiograph is apparent, and a stable circulation with sufficient negative fluid balance has been achieved, the patient is sedated, paralyzed, and fully ventilated, and the ECMO circuit is clamped.

Patients requiring cardiovascular support with ECMO are partially weaned within the first 48 hours in order to assess myocardial function by echocardiography and hemodynamic evaluation. An acceptable PaO_2 obtained while the ECMO circuit is clamped varies substantially according to the underlying anatomy and pathophysiology. If transthoracic cannulation was used and bleeding problems occurred during the ECMO run, the mediastinum may require exploration prior to or during the weaning process. If only a short period of reconditioning of the myocardium is anticipated, the patient frequently is sedated and paralyzed, dopamine infusion is increased to 5 to 10 μg/kg/min, intravascular volume status is optimized, and ventilator settings are adjusted according to lung compliance and expected arterial O_2 saturation. ECMO flow is decreased by 25% to 50% over a period of several hours until the circuit is clamped. Volume is infused to achieve appropriate preload. Echocardiographic assessment of ventricular systolic function, valvar function, systemic and pulmonary outflow obstruction, and location and direction of intracardiac shunts is useful prior to weaning and when a change in hemodynamics occurs after the circuit has been clamped. Arterial blood gases, serum lactate levels, and systemic (mixed) venous saturation are important guides to the stability of the circulation, ventilation, and adequacy of perfusion after the circuit has been clamped. Decannulation from ECMO is undertaken once the patient has maintained a stable circulation and acceptable gas exchange for a period of up to 4 hours.

Cardiovascular Interactions with Other Organs

Respiratory Function and Heart–Lung Interaction

Altered respiratory mechanics and positive pressure ventilation may have significant influence on hemodynamics following congenital heart surgery. Therefore the approach to mechanical ventilation not only should be directed at achieving a desired gas exchange but also should be influenced by the potential cardiorespiratory interactions of mechanical ventilation and method of weaning. The mode of ventilation must be matched to the hemodynamic status of each patient in order to achieve adequate cardiac output and gas exchange. Frequent modifications to the mode and pattern of ventilation may be necessary during recovery after surgery, with attention to changes in lung volume and airway pressure. Changes in lung volume have a major effect on PVR, which is lowest at the lung's functional residual capacity (FRC), whereas both hypoinflation or hyperinflation may result in a significant increase in PVR because of altered traction on alveolar septa and extraalveolar vessels.

Positive pressure ventilation influences preload and afterload on the heart (Table 29–11).[100–102] Increased lung volume and intrathoracic pressure decreases preload to both the right and left atria. The afterload on the pulmonary ventricle is increased during a positive pressure breath secondary to the changes in lung volume and increase in mean intrathoracic pressure. If this is significant or there is limited functional reserve, RV stroke volume may be reduced and end-diastolic pressure increased. This in turn may contribute to a low cardiac output state and signs of RV dysfunction, including tricuspid regurgitation, hepatomegaly, ascites, and pleural effusions. In contrast to the right ventricle, the afterload on the systemic ventricle is decreased during a positive pressure breath secondary to a fall in the ventricle transmural pressure. The systemic arteries are under higher pressure and are not exposed to radial traction effects during inflation or deflation of the lungs. Therefore changes in lung volume will affect LV preload, but the effect on afterload is

TABLE 29–11

Cardiorespiratory Interactions of a Positive Pressure Mechanical Breath

	Afterload	Preload
Pulmonary ventricle	Elevated Effect: ↑ RVEDp ↑ RVp ↓ Antegrade PBF ↑ PR and/or TR	Reduced Effect: ↓ RVEDV ↓ RAp
Systemic ventricle	Reduced Effect: ↓ LVEDp ↓ LAp ↓ Pulmonary edema ↑ Increase cardiac output	Reduced Effect: ↓ LVEDV ↓ LAp

LAp, left atrial pressure; *LVEDp,* left ventricular end-diastolic pressure; *LVEDV,* left ventricular end-diastolic volume; *PBF,* pulmonary blood flow; *PR,* pulmonary regurgitation; *RAp,* right atrial pressure *RVEDp,* right ventricular end-diastolic pressure; *RVEDV,* right ventricular end-diastolic volume; *RVp,* right ventricular pressure; *TR,* tricuspid regurgitation.

dependent upon changes in intrathoracic pressure alone rather than changes in lung volume. Therefore positive pressure ventilation and positive end-expiratory pressure (PEEP) may have a significant beneficial effect in patients with LV failure.

Patients with LV dysfunction and increased end-diastolic volume and pressure can have impaired pulmonary mechanics secondary to increased lung water, decreased lung compliance, and increased airway resistance. The work of breathing is increased, and neonates can fatigue early because of limited respiratory reserve. A significant proportion of total body oxygen consumption is directed at the increased work of breathing in neonates and infants with LV dysfunction, contributing to poor feeding and failure to thrive. Therefore positive pressure ventilation has an additional benefit in patients with significant volume overload and systemic ventricular dysfunction by reducing the work of breathing and oxygen demand.

The use of PEEP in patients with CHD has been controversial. It initially was perceived not to have a significant positive impact on gas exchange, and there was concern that the increased airway pressure could have a detrimental effect on hemodynamics and contribute to lung injury and air leak. Nevertheless, PEEP increases FRC, enabling lung recruitment, and redistributes lung water from alveolar septal regions to the more compliant perihilar regions. Both of these actions improve gas exchange and reduce PVR. Therefore PEEP should be used in mechanically ventilated patients following congenital heart surgery. However, excessive levels of PEEP can be detrimental by increasing afterload on the right side of the circulation. This may be especially true in the Fontan circulation. Usually 3 to 5 cmH_2O of PEEP helps maintain FRC and redistribute lung water without causing hemodynamic compromise. Of course the optimal condition for the Fontan circulation occurs when the patient can breathe spontaneously, generating negative pleural and intrathoracic pressures that assist systemic venous return. If lung volume can be maintained and work of breathing minimized without any positive pressure ventilation, then the Fontan circulation is best served. Early transition to a pressure-support mode of breathing and aim to extubation during the first few postoperative hours is our goal.

Special Problems for the Cardiac Patient

Diaphragmatic paresis (reduced motion) or paralysis (paradoxical movement) may precipitate and promote respiratory failure, particularly in the neonate or young infant who relies on diaphragmatic function for breathing more than older infants and children (who can recruit accessory and intercostal muscles if diaphragmatic function proves inadequate). Injury to the phrenic nerve, usually the left, may occur during operations that require dissection of the branch pulmonary arteries well out to the hilum (e.g., TOF, ASO), arch reconstruction from the midline (e.g., Norwood operation), manipulation of the SVC (Glenn shunts), takedown of previous systemic-to-pulmonary shunts, or after percutaneous central venous access. Phrenic injury may occur more frequently at reoperation, when adhesions and scarring may obscure landmarks. Topical cooling with ice during deep hypothermia may also cause transient phrenic palsy. Increased work of breathing on low ventilator settings, increased PCO_2, and a chest radiograph revealing an elevated hemidiaphragm are suggestive of diaphragmatic dysfunction. The chest x-ray film may be misleading, however, if it is taken during peak positive pressure ventilation. Ultrasonography or fluoroscopy is useful for identifying diaphragmatic motion or paradoxical excursion. Recovery of diaphragmatic contraction usually occurs; however, if a patient fails to tolerate repeated extubations despite optimizing cardiovascular and nutritional status and diaphragmatic dysfunction persists with volume loss in the affected lung, then the diaphragm may require surgical plication. Although only a temporary effect is gained, the prevention of collapse and volume loss in the affected lung may provide the critical advantage.

Pulmonary edema, pneumonia, and *atelectasis* are the most common causes of lower airway and alveolar abnormalities that interfere with gas exchange. If a bacterial pathogen is identified, therapy includes antibiotics and pulmonary toilet. If the cause is pulmonary edema, therapy is aimed at lowering the LA pressure through diuresis and pharmacologic means to reduce afterload and improve the lusitropic state of the heart. For infants, fluid restriction frequently is incompatible with adequate nutrition; therefore an aggressive diuretic regimen is preferable to restriction of caloric intake. Adjustment of end-expiratory pressure and mechanical ventilation serve as supportive therapies until the alveoli and pulmonary interstitium are cleared of the fluid that interferes with gas entry.

Pleural effusions and *ascites* may occur in patients after a Fontan operation or reparative procedures requiring a right ventriculotomy (e.g., TOF, truncus arteriosus) with transient RV dysfunction. Especially in young patients, pleural effusions and increased interstitial lung water may be a manifestation of right heart failure. This seems logically related to raised systemic venous pressure impeding lymphatic return to the venous circulation. The lymphatic circuit often is functioning at full capacity in these children. Fluid in the pleural space or peritoneum and intestinal distension compete with intrapulmonary gas for thoracic space. Evacuation of the pleural space or drainage of ascites and decompression of the intestinal lumen allow the intrapulmonary gas volume to increase.

Weaning from Mechanical Ventilation

Early tracheal extubation of children following congenital heart surgery is not a new concept but has received renewed attention with the evolution of "fast track" management for cardiac surgical patients. Early extubation generally refers to tracheal extubation within a few hours (i.e., 4–8 hours) after surgery, although in practice it means the avoidance of routine overnight mechanical ventilation. Factors to consider when planning early extubation are given in Table 29–12. For any patient, a thorough review of the preoperative clinical status and surgical procedure is necessary immediately upon admission to the ICU, followed by a detailed examination and assessment of monitoring and laboratory data. Although procedures vary from patient to patient, carefully constructed postoperative order sheets are useful for directing initial management and planning.

A number of published reports have described successful tracheal extubation in neonates and older children following congenital heart surgery, either in the operating room or soon after in the cardiac ICU.[103,104] This has been possible without significant compromise of patient care, and a low incidence of reintubation or hemodynamic instability has been reported. This fast track strategy has been extended to routine early (within 24 hours of surgery) discharge from hospital. Although overzealous attempts to achieve this goal can have a negative impact on patients and families (e.g., discharge at 24 hours to hotel with chest tube still in place), the practice has streamlined the care of these children and highlights the advances in perioperative care that now permit hospital discharge of infants and older children within 24 hours of repair of congenital heart defects on CPB.[105]

TABLE 29–12

Considerations for Planned Early Extubation after Congenital Heart Surgery

Patient factors	Limited cardiorespiratory reserve of the neonate and infant
	Pathophysiology of specific congenital heart defects
	Timing of surgery and preoperative management
Anesthetic factors	Premedication
	Hemodynamic stability and reserve
	Drug distribution and maintenance of anesthesia on bypass
	Postoperative analgesia
Surgical factors	Extent and complexity of surgery
	Residual defects
	Risks for bleeding and protection of suture lines
Conduct of bypass	Degree of hypothermia
	Level of hemodilution
	Myocardial protection
	Modulation of the inflammatory response and reperfusion injury
Postoperative management	Myocardial function
	Cardiorespiratory interactions
	Neurologic recovery
	Analgesia management

Central Nervous System

The dramatic reduction in surgical mortality in recent decades has been accompanied by a growing recognition of adverse neurologic sequelae in some survivors. Central nervous system abnormalities may be a function of coexisting brain abnormalities or acquired events unrelated to surgical management (e.g., paradoxical embolus, brain infection, effects of chronic cyanosis), but CNS insults appear to occur most frequently during or immediately after surgery. In particular, support techniques used during neonatal and infant cardiac surgery (e.g., CPB, profound hypothermia, circulatory arrest) have been implicated as important causes of brain injury.[106]

During hypothermic CPB, multiple perfusion variables may influence the risk of brain injury. These variables include (but probably are not limited to) (1) the total duration of CPB and the duration and rate of core cooling, (2) pH management during core cooling, (3) duration of circulatory arrest, (4) type of oxygenator, (5) presence of arterial filtration, and (6) depth of hypothermia. Undoubtedly, there is interaction between these various elements, and CNS injury following CPB most likely is multifactorial. Early postoperative studies (in the ICU) revealed a higher incidence of neurologic perturbation in patients undergoing circulatory arrest, including a higher incidence of clinical and electroencephalographic (EEG) seizures, a longer recovery time to the first reappearance of EEG activity, and greater release of the brain isoenzyme of creatine kinase.

Seizures are the most commonly observed neurologic consequence of cardiac surgery with an incidence in older studies of 4% to 25%. Although the incidence of seizures in the ICU has dramatically declined in recent years, when seizures occur we treat them aggressively with benzodiazepines, phenobarbital, or phenytoin. Importantly, we have reduced possible practices that may have been associated with brain injury after CPB: rapid cooling on CPB and use of prolonged hypothermic circulatory arrest, extreme alpha-stat strategy of intraoperative pH management, extreme hemodilution to hematocrits less than 20, applying heat lamps to infants upon arrival in ICU, hypocapnic hyperventilation, and prolonged muscle relaxation (masking seizure observations). We are especially loath to permit hyperthermia to any degree in the early postoperative period.

Intraventricular hemorrhage may occur as a consequence of perinatal events or circulatory collapse in the first few days of life. It is commonly associated with prematurity. Our approach has been to screen all premature infants or asphyxiated babies with a head ultrasound prior to CPB, which involves extensive anticoagulation, hemodynamic perturbation, and risk for bleeding extension. Surgical intervention is delayed for several days if intraventricular bleeding is documented. Our strategy of deferring operations in very premature newborns for several days after birth is associated with a low incidence of intraventricular hemorrhage in these high-risk patients despite use of CPB.[107]

Renal Function and Postoperative Fluid Management

Risk factors for postoperative renal failure include preoperative renal dysfunction, prolonged bypass time, low cardiac output, and cardiac arrest. In addition to relative ischemia and nonpulsatile flow on CPB, angiotensin II-mediated renal vasoconstriction and delayed healing of renal tubular epithelium have been proposed as one mechanism for renal failure. Postoperative sepsis and nephrotoxic drugs may further damage the kidneys.

Because of the inflammatory response to bypass and significant increase in total body water, fluid management in the immediate postoperative period is critical. Capillary leak and interstitial fluid accumulation may continue for the first 24 to 48 hours following surgery, necessitating ongoing volume replacement with colloid or blood products. A fall in cardiac output and increased antidiuretic hormone secretion contribute to delayed water clearance and potential prerenal dysfunction, which could progress to acute tubular necrosis and renal failure if a low cardiac output state persists.

During CPB, optimizing the circuit prime, hematocrit, and oncotic pressure; attenuating the inflammatory response with steroids and protease inhibitors such as aprotinin;[108] and use of modified ultrafiltration techniques have been recommended to limit interstitial fluid accumulation.[109] During the first 24 hours following surgery, maintenance fluids should be restricted to 50% of full maintenance and volume replacement titrated to appropriate filling pressures and hemodynamic response.

Oliguria in the first 24 hours after complex surgery and CPB is common in neonates and infants until cardiac output recovers and neurohumoral mechanisms abate. Although diuretics are commonly prescribed in the immediate postoperative period, the neurohumoral influence on urine output is powerful. Time after CPB and enhancement of cardiac output through volume and pharmacologic adjustments are the most important factors that will promote diuresis.

Peritoneal dialysis, hemodialysis, and continuous venovenous hemofiltration provide alternate renal support in patients with severe oliguria and renal failure.[110] Besides enabling water and solute clearance, maintenance fluids can be increased to ensure adequate nutrition. The indications for renal support vary but include blood urea nitrogen greater than 100 mg/dl, life-threatening electrolyte imbalance such as severe hyperkalemia, ongoing metabolic acidosis, fluid restrictions limiting nutrition, and increased mechanical ventilation requirements secondary to persistent pulmonary edema or ascites.

A peritoneal dialysis catheter can be placed into the peritoneal cavity at the completion of surgery or later in the ICU. Indications in the ICU include the need for renal support or for reducing intraabdominal pressure from ascites that may compromise mechanical ventilation. Drainage may be significant in the immediate postoperative period as third space fluid losses continue, and replacement with albumin and/or fresh-frozen plasma may be necessary to treat hypovolemia and hypoproteinemia.

Gastrointestinal Issues

Following cardiac surgery in neonates and children, adequate nutrition is exceedingly important. These critically ill children often have decreased caloric intake and increased energy demand after surgery; the neonate in particular has limited metabolic and fat reserves. Total parenteral nutrition can provide adequate nutrition in the early hypercatabolic phases of the early postoperative period.

Upper gastrointestinal bleeding and ulcer formation may occur following the stress of cardiac surgery in children and adults. There are limited reports of the efficacy of histamine H_2 antireceptors, sucralfate, or oral antacids in pediatric cardiac patients, although their use is common in many ICUs. Hepatic failure may occur after cardiac surgery (particularly after the Fontan operation and typically is characterized by elevated liver enzymes and coagulopathy).

Necrotizing enterocolitis, although typically a disease of premature infants, is seen with considerable frequency in neonates with CHD. Risk factors include (1) left-sided obstructive lesions, (2) umbilical or femoral arterial catheterization/angiography, (3) hypoxemia, and (4) lesions with wide pulse pressures (e.g., systemic-to-pulmonary shunts, PDA, especially in transposition of the great arteries and severe aortic regurgitation) producing retrograde flow in the mesenteric vessels during diastole. Frequently, multiple risk factors exist in the same patient, making a specific etiology difficult to establish. Treatment includes continuous nasogastric suction, parenteral nutrition, and broad-spectrum antibiotics. Bowel exploration or resection may be necessary in severe cases.

Infection

Low-grade (<38.5°C) fever during the immediate postoperative period is common and may be present for up to 3 to 4 days, even without a demonstrable infectious etiology. However, there are several reports of increased susceptibility to infection after CPB. CPB may activate complement and other mediators of inflammation but also can lead to derangements of the immune system and increase the likelihood of infection. A centrally mediated etiology of fever following CPB has been postulated.

Sepsis and nosocomial infection after cardiac surgery contribute substantially to overall morbidity. Despite the recent increased use of broad-coverage, third-generation cephalosporins, these agents did not seem to be more effective in decreasing postoperative infections. Meticulous catheter insertion and daily care routines, along with early removal of indwelling catheters in the postoperative patient, may reduce the incidence of sepsis.

Mediastinitis occurs in up to 2% of patients undergoing cardiac surgery. Risk factors may include delayed sternal closure, early reexploration for bleeding, or reoperation. Mediastinitis is characterized by persistent fever, purulent drainage from the sternotomy wound, instability of the sternum, and leukocytosis. *Staphylococcus* is the most common offending organism. Treatment usually involves debridement and irrigation with parenteral antibiotic therapy. Duration of therapy seldom exceeds 2 weeks.

Critical Care Management of Specific Lesions

Single-Ventricle Anatomy and Physiology

For a variety of anatomic lesions, the systemic and pulmonary circulations are parallel, with a single ventricle effectively supplying both systemic and pulmonary blood flow (Table 29–13). The relative proportion of ventricular output to either the pulmonary or systemic vascular bed is determined by the relative resistance to flow in the two circuits. The pulmonary arterial and aortic oxygen saturations are equal, with mixing of the systemic and pulmonary venous return within a "common" atrium. Assuming equal mixing, normal cardiac output, and full pulmonary venous saturation, SaO_2 of 80% to 85%, with MvO_2 of 60% to 65%, indicates $Q_p/Q_s \approx 1$ and hence a balance between systemic and pulmonary flow. Although "balanced," the single ventricle still must receive and eject twice the normal amount of blood: one part to the pulmonary circulation and one part to the systemic circulation. $Q_p/Q_s > 1$ implies an intolerable volume burden on the heart. Although there may be specific management issues for certain defects with single-ventricle physiology, nevertheless there are common management considerations to balance flow and augment systemic perfusion.

TABLE 29–13

Factors Contributing to a Lower Than Anticipated Oxygen Saturation in Patients with Common Mixing Lesions

Etiology	Considerations
Low FiO_2	Low delivered oxygen concentration Failure of oxygen delivery device
Pulmonary vein desaturation	**1. Ventilation perfusion defects** Alveolar process, e.g., edema/ infectious/atelectasis Restrictive process, e.g, effusion/ bronchospasm **2. Intrapulmonary shunt** Severe RDS Pulmonary AVM PA-to-PV collateral vessel(s)
↓ Pulmonary blood flow	Anatomic RV outflow obstruction Anatomic pulmonary artery stenosis Increased PVR Atrial level right-to-left shunt Ventricular level right-to-left shunt
↓ Oxygen content	**1. Low mixed venous oxygen level** Increased O_2 extraction: hypermetabolic state Decreased O_2 delivery: low cardiac output state **2. Anemia**

AVM, arteriovenous malforamtion; *FiO_2*, fractional inspired concentration of oxygen; *PA*, pulmonary artery; *PV*, pulmonary vein; *PVR*, pulmonary vascular resistence; *RDS*, respiratory distress syndrome; *RV*, right ventricle.

Preoperative Management

Changes in PVR have a significant impact on systemic perfusion and circulatory stability, especially preoperatively when the ductus arteriosus is widely patent. In preparation for surgery, it is important that systemic and pulmonary blood flow be as well balanced as possible to prevent excessive volume overload and ventricular dysfunction that reduces systemic and end-organ perfusion. For example, a newborn with HLHS who has an arterial oxygen saturation greater than 90%, a wide pulse width, oliguria, cool extremities, hepatomegaly, and metabolic acidosis has severely limited systemic blood flow. Even though ventricular output is increased, the blood flow that is inefficiently partitioned back to the lungs is unavailable to the other vital organs. Immediate interventions are necessary to prevent imminent circulatory collapse and end-organ injury. In this "overcirculated" state, PVR is falling as it should in the normal postnatal state, and the ductus arteriosus is maintained widely patent with prostaglandin infusion to permit unrestricted blood flow from the single right ventricle across the ductus to the systemic bed. Blood flow manipulation of mechanical ventilation and inotrope support may temporarily stabilize the patient (see later), but surgery should not be delayed. Similarly, in a patient with pulmonary atresia and an intact ventricular septum, LV-dependent pulmonary circulation occurs. Ductal patency is necessary for pulmonary blood flow. As PVR falls, pulmonary blood flow will be excessive and eventually will steal from the systemic circulation. Preoperative management should focus on an assessment of the balance between pulmonary (Q_p) and systemic flow (Q_s). This is best achieved by thorough and continuous reevaluation of the clinical examination for cardiac output state and perfusion, an evaluation of chest radiograph for cardiac size and pulmonary congestion, a review of laboratory data for alterations in gas exchange, acid-base status, and end-organ function, and echocardiographic imaging to assess ventricular function and AV valve competence. A central venous line positioned in the proximal superior vena cava (SVC) may be useful to monitor volume status and sample for mixed venous oxygen saturation as a surrogate of cardiac output and oxygen delivery. Central venous lines are not necessary in all circumstances; they may have significant complications in small newborns and do not substitute for clinical examination.

Initial resuscitation involves maintaining patency of the ductus arteriosus with a PGE_1 infusion at a rate of 0.02 to 0.05 μg/kg/min. Intubation and mechanical ventilation are not necessary in all patients. Patients usually are tachypneic, but provided the work of breathing is not excessive and systemic perfusion is maintained without a metabolic acidosis, spontaneous ventilation often is preferable to achieve an adequate systemic perfusion and balance of Q_p and Q_s. A mild metabolic acidosis and low bicarbonate level may be present but may not indicate poor perfusion and a lactic acidosis specifically. If the presentation involved circulatory collapse and end-organ dysfunction, then a period of days may be required to establish stability and allow return of vital organ function prior to surgery.

Patients require intubation and mechanical ventilation because of apnea secondary to PGE_1, presence of a low cardiac output state, or for manipulation of gas exchange to assist balancing pulmonary and systemic flow. SaO_2 greater than 90% indicates pulmonary overcirculation, that is, $Q_p/Q_s > 1$. PVR can be increased with controlled mechanical hypoventilation to induce a respiratory acidosis, often necessitating sedation and neuromuscular blockade, and with a low FiO_2 to induce alveolar hypoxia. Ventilation in room air may suffice, but occasionally a hypoxic gas mixture is necessary. This is achieved by adding nitrogen to the inspired gas mixture, reducing the FiO_2 from 0.17 to 0.19. Although these maneuvers often are successful in increasing PVR and reducing pulmonary blood flow, remember that these patients have a limited oxygen reserve and may desaturate suddenly and precipitously. Controlled hypoventilation in effect reduces FRC and therefore the oxygen reserve, which is further reduced by use of an hypoxic inspired gas mixture. An alternate strategy is to add carbon dioxide to the inspiratory limb of the breathing circuit, which also increases PVR, but because an hypoxic gas mixture is not used, systemic oxygen delivery is maintained.[111,112] Patients who have continued pulmonary overcirculation with high SaO_2 and reduced systemic perfusion despite these maneuvers require early surgical intervention to control pulmonary blood flow. At the time of surgery, a snare can be placed around either branch of the pulmonary artery to effectively limit pulmonary blood flow.

Decreased pulmonary blood flow in preoperative patients with a parallel circulation is reflected by hypoxemia with SaO_2 less than 75%. Preoperatively this may result from restricted flow across a small ductus arteriosus, increased PVR secondary to parenchymal lung disease, or increased pulmonary venous pressure secondary to obstructed pulmonary venous drainage or a restrictive ASD. Sedation, paralysis, and manipulation of mechanical ventilation to maintain an alkalosis may be effective if PVR is elevated. NO as a specific pulmonary vasodilator also may be useful in this situation. Systemic oxygen delivery is maintained by improving cardiac output and maintaining hematocrit >40%. Among some newborns with HLHS, pulmonary blood flow may be insufficient because mitral valve hypoplasia in combination with the occasional finding of a restrictive or nearly intact atrial septum severely restricts pulmonary venous return to the heart. The newborn is intensely cyanotic and has a pulmonary venous congestion pattern on chest radiograph. Urgent interventional cardiac catheterization with balloon septostomy or dilation (or stent placement) of a restrictive ASD may be necessary.[113,114] Immediate surgical intervention and palliation is preferred in some centers.

Systemic perfusion is maintained with the use of volume and vasopressor agents. Inotropic support often is necessary because of ventricular dysfunction secondary to the increased volume load. Systemic afterload reduction with agents such as phosphodiesterase inhibitors may improve systemic perfusion, although they also may decrease PVR and thus not correct the imbalance of pulmonary and systemic flow. Oliguria and a rising serum creatinine level may reflect re-renal insufficiency from a low cardiac output. Necrotizing enterocolitis is a risk secondary to splanchnic hypoperfusion, and we prefer not to enterally feed newborns with a wide pulse width and low diastolic pressure (usually <30 mmHg) prior to surgery. It is important to evaluate end-organ perfusion and function.

Bidirectional Cavopulmonary Anastomosis

In this procedure, also known as a *bidirectional Glenn shunt,* the SVC is transected and connected end-to-side to the right pulmonary artery, but the pulmonary arteries are left in continuity. Therefore flow from the SVC is bidirectional into both left and right pulmonary arteries. This is the only source of pulmonary blood flow, and IVC blood returns to the common atrium. Performed between age 3 to 6 months, the BDG has proved to be an important early staging procedure for patients with single-ventricle physiology because the volume and pressure load is relieved from the systemic ventricle yet effective pulmonary blood flow is maintained. Q_p/Q_s is always less than 1, and the volume load to the single right ventricle is relieved compared with a systemic-to-pulmonary artery shunt. However, it is impractical in the newborn whose pulmonary cross sectional area is inadequate to accommodate sufficient passive pulmonary blood flow for tolerable oxygenation.

The BDG usually is performed on CPB using mild hypothermia with a beating heart. Therefore the complications related to CPB and aortic cross-clamping are minimal, and patients can be weaned and extubated in the early postoperative period.[115] Systemic hypertension is common following a BDG. The etiology remains to be determined, but possible factors include improved contractility and stroke volume after the volume load on the ventricle is removed and brainstem-mediated mechanisms secondary to the increased systemic and cerebral venous pressure. Treatment with vasodilators may be necessary during the immediate postoperative period and during the weaning process.

Following the BDG anastomosis, arterial oxygen saturation should be in the 80% to 85% range. Persistent hypoxemia often is secondary to a low cardiac output state and low SvO_2. Treatment is directed at improving contractility, reducing afterload, and ensuring the patient has a normal rhythm and hematocrit. Increased PVR is an uncommon cause, and inhaled NO is rarely beneficial in these patients. This finding is not surprising because PA pressure and resistance and vascular tone are not high enough following this surgery to see a demonstrable benefit from NO.[76] Persistent profound hypoxemia should be investigated in the catheterization laboratory to evaluate hemodynamics, look for residual anatomic defects limiting pulmonary flow, such as PA stenosis or a restrictive ASD, and coil any significant venous decompressing collaterals, if present.

Fontan Procedure

Since the original description in 1971,[116] the Fontan procedure and subsequent modifications have been successfully used to treat a wide range of simple and complex single-ventricle congenital heart defects.[117] The repair is "physiologic" in that the systemic and pulmonary circulations are in series and cyanosis is corrected. However, given the current long-term outcome data, perhaps the repair should be viewed as palliative rather than curative.[118–120] The mortality and morbidity associated with this surgery have declined substantially over the years, and many patients with stable single-ventricle physiology can lead normal lives.[121] Considerations in managing a cavopulmonary connection are given in Table 29–14. Systemic venous pressure of 10 to 15 mmHg and LA pressure of 5 to 10 mmHg, that is, a transpulmonary gradient of 5 to 10 mmHg, is ideal.

Intravascular volume must be maintained and hypovolemia must be treated promptly. Venous capacitance is increased, and as patients rewarm and vasodilate following surgery, a significant volume requirement of approximately 30 to 40 ml/kg on the first postoperative night is not unusual. Changes in mean intrathoracic pressure and PVR have a significant effect on pulmonary blood flow. Pulmonary blood flow has been shown to be biphasic following the Fontan procedure, and earlier resumption of spontaneous ventilation is recommended to offset the detrimental effects of positive pressure ventilation.[122,123] Using Doppler analysis, it has been demonstrated that pulmonary blood flow predominantly occurs during inspiration in a spontaneously breathing patient, that is, when the mean intrathoracic pressure is subatmospheric. Therefore the method of mechanical ventilation following a Fontan procedure requires close observation. A tidal volume of 10 to 15 ml/kg with the lowest possible mean airway pressure is appropriate. Although it is preferable to wean from positive pressure ventilation in the early postoperative period, hemodynamic responses must be closely monitored.

If appropriate selection criteria are followed, patients undergoing a modified Fontan procedure will have a low PVR without labile pulmonary hypertension. Therefore vigorous hyperventilation and induction of a respiratory and/or metabolic alkalosis often are of little benefit in this group of patients, and the related increase in mechanical ventilation requirements may be detrimental. A normal pH and $Paco_2$ of 40 mmHg should be the goal and, depending on the amount of right-to-left shunt across the fenestration, the arterial oxygen saturation usually is in the 80% to 90% range.

However, PVR may increase following surgery, particularly secondary to an acidosis, hypothermia, atelectasis and hypoventilation, vasoactive drug infusions, and stress response. Any acidosis must be treated promptly. If the cause is respiratory, ventilation must be adjusted. A metabolic acidosis reflects poor cardiac output and treatment directed at the potential causes, including reduced preload to the systemic ventricle, poor contractility, increased afterload, and loss of sinus rhythm.

The use of PEEP continues to be debated. The beneficial effects of an increase in FRC, maintenance of lung volume, and redistribution of lung water need to be balanced against the possible detrimental effect of an increase in mean intrathoracic pressure. A PEEP of 3 to 5 cmH_2O, however, rarely has either hemodynamic consequence or substantial effect on effective pulmonary blood flow.

Alternative methods of mechanical ventilation have been used in these patients. High-frequency ventilation has been used successfully, although the hemodynamic consequences of the raised mean intrathoracic pressure must be continually evaluated.[124] Negative-pressure ventilation can be beneficial by augmenting pulmonary

TABLE 29–14

Management Considerations Following a Modified Fontan Procedure

	Aim	Management
Baffle (right side)		→ or ↑ Preload
pressure 10–15 mmHg	Unobstructed venous return	Low intrathoracic pressure
	PVR <2 Wood units • m^2	Avoid increases in PVR, such as from acidosis,
Pulmonary circulation	Mean Pap <15 mmHg	hypoinflation and hyperinflation of the lung,
	Unobstructed pulmonary vessels	hypothermia, and excess sympathetic stimulation
		Early resumption of spontaneous respiration
Left atrial	Sinus rhythm	Maintain sinus rhythm
pressure 5–10 mmHg	Competent AV valve	→ or ↑ Rate to increase CO
	Ventricle	→ or ↓ Afterload
	Normal diastolic function	→ or ↑ Contractility
	Normal systolic function	
	No outflow obstruction	PDE inhibitors useful because of vasodilatory, inotropic, and lusitropic properties

AV, atrioventricular; *CO*, cardiac output; *Pap*, pulmonary arterial pressure; *PDE*, phosphodiesterase; *PVR*, pulmonary vascular resistance.

blood flow.[125] The development of new negative-pressure ventilators and cuirasses and jackets has increased the interest in this mode of ventilation for this group of patients, but the experience is relatively small and indications are not defined. Application is cumbersome.

Nonspecific pulmonary vasodilators, such as sodium nitroprusside, glycerol trinitrate, PGE_1, and prostacyclin have been used to dilate the pulmonary vasculature in an effort to improve pulmonary blood flow after a Fontan procedure, but the results are variable. Although PVR may fall, pulmonary blood flow also could increase as a result of reduced ventricular end-diastolic pressure following improved ventricular function secondary to the fall in systemic afterload. The response to inhaled NO also is variable, and the improvement may be related to changes in ventilation/perfusion matching rather than a direct fall in PVR.

Afterload stress is poorly tolerated after a modified Fontan procedure because of the increase in myocardial wall tension and end-diastolic pressure. The phosphodiesterase inhibitors milrinone and amrinone are particularly beneficial. Besides being weak inotropes with pulmonary and systemic vasodilating properties, their lusitropic action assists by improving diastolic relaxation and lowering ventricular end-diastolic pressure, thereby improving effective pulmonary blood flow and cardiac output.

Specific Complications after the Fontan Procedure

Pleuropericardial Effusions. The incidence of recurrent pleural effusions and ascites has decreased since the introduction of the fenestrated baffle technique. Nevertheless, for some patients they remain a major problem with associated respiratory compromise, hypovolemia, and possible hypoproteinemia. They usually occur secondary to persistent elevation of systemic venous pressure, and reevaluation with cardiac catheterization may be indicated.

Rhythm Disturbances. Atrial flutter and/or fibrillation; heart block; and, less commonly, ventricular dysrhythmia may have a significant impact on immediate recovery and on long-term outcome.[126,127] Sudden loss of sinus rhythm initially causes an increase in LA and ventricular end-diastolic pressure and a fall in cardiac output. The SVC or PA pressure must be increased, usually with volume replacement, to maintain the transpulmonary gradient. Prompt treatment with antiarrhythmic drugs, pacing, or cardioversion is necessary.

Premature Closure of the Fenestration. Not all patients require a fenestration for a successful, uncomplicated Fontan operation. Those with ideal preoperative hemodynamics often maintain adequate pulmonary blood flow and cardiac output without requiring a right-to-left shunt across the baffle. Similarly, not all Fontan patients who received a fenestration use it for a right-to-left shunt in the immediate postoperative period. These patients are fully saturated following surgery and may have an elevated right-sided filling pressure but nevertheless maintain an adequate cardiac output. The problem is predicting which patients are at risk for low cardiac output after a Fontan procedure, and who will benefit from placement of a fenestration. Even patients with ideal preoperative hemodynamics may manifest a significant low output state after surgery. Because of this possibility, essentially all patients having a Fontan procedure at Children's Hospital, Boston are fenestrated.

Premature closure of the fenestration may occur in the immediate postoperative period, leading to a low cardiac output state with progressive metabolic acidosis and large chest drain losses from high right-sided venous pressures. Patients may respond to volume replacement, inotrope support, and vasodilation; however, if hypotension and acidosis persist, cardiac catheterization and removal of thrombus or dilation of the fenestration may be urgently needed.

Persistent Hypoxemia. Arterial O_2 saturation levels may vary substantially following a modified Fontan procedure. Common causes of persistent arterial O_2 desaturation less than 75% include a poor cardiac output with a low SvO_2, a large right-to-left shunt across the fenestration, or additional "leak" in the baffle pathway producing more shunting. An intrapulmonary shunt and venous admixture from decompressing vessels draining either from the pulmonary artery to the systemic venous circulation or from the systemic vein to the pulmonary venous system are additional causes. Reevaluation with echocardiography and cardiac catheterization may be necessary.

Low Cardiac Output State. An elevated LA pressure after a modified Fontan procedure may reflect poor ventricular function from decreased contractility or increased afterload stress, atrioventricular valve regurgitation, and loss of sinus rhythm (Table 29–15). The right-sided filling pressure must be increased to maintain the transpulmonary gradient and treatment with inotropes and vasodilators initiated. If a severe low output state with acidosis persists, takedown of the Fontan operation and conversion to a BDG anastomosis or other palliative procedure is lifesaving.

Tetralogy of Fallot

Pathophysiology

The four anatomic features of TOF are VSD, RV outflow tract obstruction, overriding of the aorta, and RV hypertrophy. In addition, there may be VSDs of the muscular region of the septum and right-sided obstruction of the pulmonary valve and the main and branch pulmonary arteries.

Resistance to RV outflow forces systemic venous return from right to left across the VSD (complex shunt) and into the aorta, producing arterial desaturation. Pulmonary blood flow is less than systemic flow. The amount of blood that shunts right to left through the VSD varies with the magnitude of the RV outflow tract obstruction and with SVR. Distal PVR is low and has minimal influence on shunting. Systemic vasodilation, in conjunction with increasing dynamic infundibular stenosis, intensifies right-to-left shunting and therefore hypoxemia, producing hypercyanotic "spells." Such spells can occur at any time before surgical correction of the anomalies and can be life threatening. Their treatment is outlined in the following section. Because the morbidity associated with recurrent hypercyanotic spells is significant, many

TABLE 29–15

Etiology and Treatment Strategies for Patients with Low Cardiac Output Immediately Following the Fontan Procedure

Low Cardiac Output	Etiology	Treatment
INCREASED TPG		
Baffle >20 mmHg LAp <10 mmHg ↑ TPG >>10 mmHg	Inadequate pulmonary blood flow and preload to left atrium Increased PVR Pulmonary artery stenosis	Volume replacement Reduce PVR Correct acidosis Inotropic support
Clinical State High Sao_2/low Svo_2 Hypotension/tachycardia Core temperature high Poor peripheral perfusion SVC syndrome with pleural effusions and increased chest tube drainage Ascites/hepatomegaly Metabolic acidosis	Pulmonary vein stenosis Premature fenestration closure	Systemic vasodilation Catheter or surgical intervention
NORMAL TPG		
Baffle >20 mmHg LAp >15 mmHg TPG normal 5–10 mmHg	Ventricular failure Systolic dysfunction Diastolic dysfunction AVV regurgitation and/or stenosis	Maintain preload Inotrope support Systemic vasodilation Establish sinus rhythm or atrioventricular synchrony
Clinical State Low Sao_2/low Svo_2 Hypotension/tachycardia Poor peripheral perfusion Metabolic acidosis	Loss of sinus rhythm ↑ Afterload stress	Correct acidosis Mechanical support Surgical intervention, including takedown to BDG and transplantation

AVV, atrioventricular valve; *BDG,* bidirectional glenn anastomosis; *LAp,* left atrial pressure; *PVR,* pulmonary vascular resistance; *Sao_2,* systemic arterial oxygen saturation; *SVC,* superior vena cava; *Svo_2,* SVC oxygen saturation; *TPG,* transpulmonary gradient.

physicians consider recurrent episodes of hypercyanosis an indication for corrective surgery at any age.

Critical Care Management for the Early Postoperative Course

The surgical approach to TOF may involve either an early or delayed repair. Delayed repair requires early palliation with a systemic-to-pulmonary artery shunt to prevent hypercyanotic episodes, followed by a transatrial and transpulmonary artery repair between ages 12 to 18 months. Excellent outcome has been achieved with this approach, and the need for a transpulmonary valve annulus outflow patch (transannular patch) at the time of surgery is reduced.[128] The risks of cyanosis and complications related to a systemic-to-pulmonary artery shunt argue for early complete repair of TOF. This can be performed in the neonate or young infant depending on the degree of obstruction and arterial oxygen saturation level.[35,129] Complete repair in neonates and young infants may more often require a transventricular approach to close the VSD, with pericardial augmentation of the RV outflow tract. A ventriculotomy is performed in the RV outflow tract and frequently is extended distally through the pulmonary valve annulus and beyond any associated pulmonary artery stenosis. The outflow tract is enlarged with pericardium or synthetic material, and obstructing muscle bundles are resected to relieve the outflow tract obstruction.[130,131] Being smaller and younger, these patients may be at increased risk for complications associated with CPB. Pulmonary regurgitation results after a transannular incision that may compromise ventricular function in the postoperative period. In approximately 8% of patients, abnormalities in the origin and distribution of the coronary arteries preclude placement of the RV outflow patch,[132,133] making it necessary to bypass the stenosis by placing an external conduit from the body of the right ventricle to the pulmonary artery.[134]

Critical care management of these patients should maintain systemic vascular resistance, minimize PVR, and avoid myocardial depression. Hypercyanotic spells in nonanesthetized children are traditionally treated initially with 100% oxygen by face mask, a knee-chest position, and morphine sulfate. This regimen usually causes the dynamic infundibular stenosis to relax while maintaining systemic resistance. Deeply cyanotic and lethargic patients are given IV crystalloid infusions to augment circulating blood volume. Continued severe hypoxemia is treated with a vasopressor (e.g., phenylephrine 1–2 μg/kg) to increase SVR and sometimes with judicious use of IV propranolol or esmolol to slow the heart rate. The latter allows more filling time and relaxes the infundibulum.[135] If a hypercyanotic spell persists despite treatment, immediate surgical correction of the anomaly is indicated. The child can be anesthetized with IV narcotics, and an inhalation agent such as halothane may be beneficial to reduce hyperdynamic outflow tract obstruction. Anesthetic agents that predominantly decrease SVR, such as isoflurane, should be used with caution. The pattern of mechanical ventilation is critical, as excessive inspiratory pressure or short expiratory times increases the mean intrathoracic pressure and further reduces antegrade flow across the RV outflow.

When weaning patients from CPB following tetralogy repair, the aim of therapy is to support RV function and minimize afterload on the right ventricle. This is particularly important following repair in neonates or small infants. Although systolic dysfunction of the right ventricle may occur following neonatal ventriculotomy, more commonly the clinical picture is one of a "restrictive physiology" reflecting reduced RV compliance or diastolic function.[36,37] Factors contributing to diastolic dysfunction include ventriculotomy, lung and myocardial edema following CPB, inadequate myocardial protection of the hypertrophied ventricle during aortic cross-clamp, coronary artery injury, residual outflow tract obstruction, volume load on the ventricle from a residual VSD or pulmonary regurgitation, and arrhythmias.

Patients usually separate from CPB with a satisfactory blood pressure and atrial filling pressures less than 10 mmHg on inotropic support, such as dopamine 5 to 10 μg/kg/min. However, in neonates during the first 6 to 12 hours after surgery, a low cardiac output state with increased right-sided filling pressures from diastolic dysfunction is common following a right ventriculotomy, and continued sedation and paralysis usually are necessary for the first 24 to 48 hours to minimize the stress response and associated myocardial work. Preload must be maintained, despite elevation of RA pressure.

In addition to high right-sided filling pressures, pleural effusions and/or ascites may develop. Significant inotrope support is often required, and a phosphodiesterase inhibitor, such as milrinone, is beneficial because of the lusitropic properties. Because of the restrictive defect, even a relatively small volume load from a residual VSD or pulmonary regurgitation is often poorly tolerated in the early postoperative period, and 2 to 3 days may be required before RV compliance improves following surgery and cardiac output increases. Although the patent foramen ovale or any ASD usually is closed at the time of surgery in older patients, it is beneficial to leave a small atrial communication following neonatal repair. In the face of diastolic dysfunction and increased RV end-diastolic pressure, a right-to-left atrial shunt maintains preload to the left ventricle and therefore cardiac output. Patients may be desaturated initially following surgery because of this shunting. As RV compliance and function improve, the amount of shunt decreases and both antegrade pulmonary blood flow and arterial oxygen saturation increase.

Arrhythmias following repair include heart block, ventricular ectopy, and junctional ectopic tachycardia. It is important to maintain sinus rhythm to prevent additional diastolic dysfunction and an increase in end-diastolic pressure. Atrioventricular pacing may be necessary for heart block. Complete right bundle branch block is typical on the postoperative ECG.

Most patients recover systolic ventricular function postoperatively. However, there is a small group of patients, especially those repaired at older ages, in whom significant ventricular dysfunction remains.[136,137] Pulmonary valve insufficiency may contribute to residual ventricular systolic dysfunction.[138] The most common cause of systolic dysfunction immediately after repair of CHD is a residual or unrecognized additional VSD,[139,140] which causes a volume load on the left ventricle and pressure load on an already stressed right ventricle, leading to RV failure and poor cardiac output. A residual VSD combined with a residual RV outflow obstruction is particularly deleterious.[141]

In some patients the distal pulmonary arteries may be so hypoplastic and stenotic that they cannot be satisfactorily corrected. Suprasystemic pressure develops in the right ventricle, which in some cases can be ameliorated by partially opening the VSD to allow an intracardiac right-to-left ventricular shunt. This shunt unloads the compromised right ventricle at the expense of decreased arterial oxygen saturation.

Critical Care Management for Late Postoperative Care

Reconstruction of the RV outflow tract may lead to significant problems that affect RV function and risk for arrhythmias over time. These patients may return to the ICU months or years after their repair for related or unrelated reasons pertaining to their heart disease. Although most of the long-term outcome data pertain to patients following TOF repair, similar complications and risks are likely for those who have undergone an extensive RV outflow reconstruction, such as placement of a conduit from the right ventricle to the pulmonary artery for correction of pulmonary atresia, truncus arteriosus, and the Rastelli procedure for transposition of the great arteries with pulmonary stenosis.

Complete surgical repair of TOF has been successfully performed for more than 40 years, with studies reporting a 30- to 35-year actuarial survival of approximately 85%.[142,143] Many patients report leading relatively normal lives, but RV dysfunction may progress after repair and may be evident only on exercise stress testing or echocardiography. A spectrum of problems may develop, ranging from a dilated right ventricle with systolic dysfunction to diastolic dysfunction from a poorly compliant right ventricle, and these problems must be thoroughly evaluated preoperatively. In addition, continued evaluation is necessary because of the increased risk for ventricular arrhythmias and late sudden death. Factors that may adversely affect long-term survival include older age at initial repair, initial palliative procedures, and residual chronic pressure and/or volume load as occurs from pulmonary insufficiency or stenosis.

Systolic dysfunction secondary to a residual volume load from pulmonary regurgitation after tetralogy repair is a predictor of late morbidity. It is reflected as cardiomegaly on chest x-ray film, an increase in RV end-diastolic volume by echocardiography,[138] and a reduction in anaerobic threshold, maximal exercise performance, and endurance on exercise testing.[144] Patients who have significant pulmonary regurgitation and reduced RV function are at potential risk for a fall in cardiac output during anesthesia, particularly as positive pressure ventilation may increase the amount of regurgitation. Once again, it is difficult to predict those patients who are more likely to have instability during anesthesia for noncardiac surgery, nor is it possible to formulate a "recipe" for anesthesia that will be suited to all patients. Nevertheless, preoperative exercise testing may provide some insight into hemodynamic reserve.

An important group to distinguish consists of those who have continued restrictive physiology or diastolic dysfunction secondary to reduced ventricular compliance. They usually do not have cardiomegaly, they demonstrate better exercise tolerance, and the risk for ventricular dysrhythmias is possibly decreased. Although the right ventricle is hypertrophied, function is generally well preserved on echocardiography, with minimal pulmonary regurgitation.[46]

The incidence of significant RV outflow obstruction developing over time is low. Residual obstruction contributes to early mortality within the first year after surgery but is well tolerated in the long term. A gradient more than 40 mmHg across the RV outflow is uncommon, and the pressure ratio between the right ventricle and left ventricle usually is less than 0.5. The gradient may become more significant with time, but as the progression usually is slow, RV dysfunction occurs late.

A wide variation in the incidence of ventricular ectopy has been reported in numerous follow-up studies, including up to 15% of patients on routine ECG and up to 75% of patients on Holter monitor. Multiple risk factors, including an older age at repair, residual hemodynamic abnormalities, and duration of follow-up, have all been considered important.[145–147] In common with these factors are probable myocardial injury and fibrosis from chronic pressure and volume overload, as well as cyanosis. Although ventricular ectopy is common in asymptomatic patients during ambulatory ECG Holter monitoring and exercise stress testing, it often is low grade and has not identified those patients at risk for sudden death. Electrophysiologic induction of sustained ventricular tachycardia (VT), especially when monomorphic, is suggestive of the presence of a reentrant arrhythmic pathway. Although dependent on the stimulation protocol used to induce VT, the presence of monomorphic VT in a symptomatic patient with syncope and palpitations is significant and indicates treatment with radiofrequency ablation, surgical cryoablation, antiarrhythmic drugs, or placement of an implantable cardioverter-defibrillator.[148] The risk for ventricular dysrhythmias during anesthesia and ICU care for subsequent hospitalizations is unknown. Although preoperative prophylaxis with antiarrhythmic drugs is not recommended, a means for external defibrillation and pacing must be readily available.

Pulmonary Atresia

Pathophysiology

Atresia of the pulmonary valve or main pulmonary artery forms a spectrum of cardiac defects, the management of which depends on the extent of atresia, size of the right ventricle and tricuspid valve (TV), presence of a VSD and collateral vessels, surface area of the pulmonary vascular bed, and coronary artery anatomy. At birth, pulmonary blood flow is derived from either a PDA or other aortopulmonary collateral blood vessels. These collaterals, which arise from the descending aorta and supply both lungs, may be extensive. The right ventricle usually is hypertrophied, and a restrictive physiology is common during initial postoperative recovery.[149,150]

At one end of the spectrum, critical pulmonary stenosis may exist with a variable degree of hypoplasia of the right ventricle, TV, and pulmonary artery. There is no VSD. With critical pulmonic stenosis, only a pinhole orifice is present in the pulmonic valve, but the right ventricle is generally less hypoplastic than with pulmonary atresia. A fixed obligatory shunt of all systemic venous return occurs from the right to the left atrium, where blood mixes completely with pulmonary venous blood. Some blood may flow into the right ventricle, but because there is no outlet, blood regurgitates back across the TV and eventually reaches the left atrium and left ventricle. Pulmonary blood flow is derived exclusively or predominantly from a PDA. These patients usually do not have extensive aortopulmonary collateral blood flow; consequently, they often become cyanotic when the PDA closes after birth. Critical pulmonary valve stenosis can be effectively treated by balloon dilation in the catheterization laboratory. Antegrade flow across the RV outflow may not improve immediately but may gradually increase over days as RV compliance improves.

Pulmonary valve atresia or short-segment main pulmonary artery atresia, with a VSD and normal-size TV, right ventricle, and branch pulmonary arteries, is completely repaired in the neonate. The procedure usually involves placement of a pericardial patch to reconstruct the outflow tract. If there is long-segment pulmonary artery atresia, a homograft "conduit" is necessary to reconstruct the RV outflow. Conduits may be extrinsically compressed or kinked at the time of sternal closure, causing partial RV outflow obstruction or direct compression of a coronary artery leading to ischemia.

The intracardiac anatomy of TOF with pulmonary atresia is similar to that of simple TOF, but the RV outflow tract is atretic. Because of the atretic RV outflow tract, all systemic venous return courses right to left through the VSD. Therefore complete mixing of pulmonary and systemic venous return occurs in the left ventricle and aorta, producing arterial hypoxemia. Infants with TOF and associated pulmonary atresia regularly exhibit significant systemic-to-pulmonary collateral flow. If antegrade flow is established from the right ventricle into the main pulmonary artery by a reparative procedure, the left-to-right shunt via collateral flow will impose a diastolic load on the left ventricle. Preoperative occlusion of these collateral vessels can be accomplished by interventional techniques in the cardiac catheterization laboratory but may leave the child precariously cyanotic in the hours before operation. The most effective temporizing therapy is to reduce oxygen consumption (e.g., anesthesia, mechanical ventilation) and to increase the systemic perfusion pressure across other systemictopulmonary communications.

Patients with pulmonary atresia, a VSD, but small right ventricle and TV may not tolerate a complete initial repair. The right ventricle may be unable to cope with the entire cardiac output, resulting in a low output state and RV failure (see later). Alternative management strategies therefore include initial palliation with a shunt and/or RV outflow patch to improve pulmonary blood flow, or a repair of the outflow tract with fenestration of the VSD patch to enable a right-to-left shunt at that level. Two-ventricle repair ultimately may be limited by growth of the TV.[149] If the right ventricle subsequently grows, the shunt and the patent foramen ovale ASD and VSD can be closed surgically.

Patients with pulmonary atresia and an intact ventricular septum usually have a small right ventricle and TV, a condition that often makes them unsuitable for a two-ventricle repair in the long term. Initial palliation with an aortopulmonary shunt is necessary. Reconstruction of the RV outflow with a pericardial patch or interventional catheter techniques also may be considered if the right ventricle is a sufficient size such that a two ventricle could be considered. Prior to intervention, the coronary anatomy should be determined, usually by cardiac catheterization. A large conal branch or aberrant left coronary artery across the RV outflow tract may restrict the size of a ventriculotomy and placement of a patch or conduit. Patients with pulmonary atresia, a hypoplastic right ventricle, and intact ventricular septum may have numerous fistulous connections between the small hypertensive RV cavity and the coronary circulation.[150,151] Therefore a significant proportion of the myocardium may depend on coronary perfusion directly from the right ventricle. If, in addition, proximal coronary artery stenoses are restricting coronary perfusion from the aortic root, then decompression of the right ventricle following reconstruction of the RV outflow tract can lead to myocardial infarction.

At the worst end of the spectrum, severe pulmonary atresia may be associated with a hypoplastic right ventricle and diminutive pulmonary arteries that are not suitable for primary repair. A palliative procedure with a Blalock-Taussig or central shunt is usually necessary at first to improve pulmonary blood flow, followed by staged single-ventricle repair (see section on managing Fontan physiology).

Multiple aortopulmonary collateral arteries may be present, supplying some or all segments of the lung. They can be associated with a large left-to-right shunt, contributing to volume overload and pulmonary hypertension. Larger collateral vessels supplying significant portions of the lung can be anastomosed or "unifocalized" to the native pulmonary arteries, with the ultimate aim being to establish full antegrade pulmonary blood flow. Smaller vessels to some segments of lung can be coiled in the cardiac catheterization laboratory, provided there is antegrade flow from the native pulmonary arteries to those lung segments.

When the pulmonary arteries are very diminutive, it is important to establish early antegrade flow from the right ventricle to the pulmonary artery, in an effort to promote growth and establish a pathway to the pulmonary arteries for subsequent balloon dilation. A Blalock-Taussig shunt may be necessary to provide sufficient pulmonary blood flow if the pulmonary arteries and right ventricle are small. Initially, the VSD can be left open, and postoperative management of cyanosis or CHF will be determined by the size of and the resistance offered by the pulmonary circuit. The course in these patients can be dynamic and demanding for even the most experienced practitioners. When collaterals are occluded in the operating room and right ventricle to diminutive pulmonary artery continuity is established, cyanosis may ensue and therapy is aimed at lowering PVR and/or (re)establishing adequate pulmonary blood flow. On the other hand, if the child is fully saturated in the aorta with elevated pulmonary artery oxygen saturation and LA pressure, then a left-to-right shunt through the VSD may be developing, which will produce a volume load on the left ventricle and an unstable postoperative course, dictating VSD closure. When the patient is not fully saturated in the aorta but is suffering from a volume-loaded left ventricle with low cardiac output and high LA pressure postoperatively, excessive systemic-to-pulmonary collaterals may be the culprits, requiring catheterization laboratory investigation and occlusion or immediate reoperation.

Critical Care Management

Critical care management of patients with pulmonary atresia is similar to that for TOF, except that hypercyanotic spells do not occur in the same fashion. Maintaining the patency of the ductus for the perioperative treatment of neonates with pulmonary atresia and critical pulmonary stenosis is essential. If the right ventricle is sufficiently well developed and the main pulmonary artery is present, it may be possible to perform a pulmonary valvotomy and provide adequate pulmonary blood flow without a supplemental systemic-to-pulmonary artery shunt. The goal of therapy is to improve oxygenation and decrease RV afterload. Because the underdeveloped noncompliant right ventricle requires high filling pressures, consequently there may be substantial right-to-left shunting through the foramen ovale, making these infants hypoxemic during the immediate postoperative period. With growth and improved compliance of the right ventricle, the right-to-left shunting diminishes and the infant's oxygenation improves substantially. If hypoxemia persists, a PGE_1 infusion should be started to increase pulmonary blood flow through the ductus arteriosus while arrangements are made to surgically create a pulmonary artery to systemic artery shunt.

In patients with long-segment pulmonary atresia, the need for a conduit to bridge the gap between the right ventricle and the pulmonary artery complicates the repair. Again, RV failure may occur postoperatively, especially when there is a residual VSD or an outflow obstruction. The conduit may obstruct acutely during chest closure, further elevating pressure in the right ventricle.

After the VSD is closed and blood flow is from the right ventricle to the pulmonary arteries, there may be excessive pulmonary blood flow ($Q_p/Q_s > 1$) as a result of the combined flow into the pulmonary arteries from the right ventricle and from aortopulmonary collaterals just described. If this occurs, the patient develops CHF and requires intraoperative inotropic support of the heart and an extended period of postoperative mechanical ventilation.

With large collateral flows, the pulse pressure is large and diastolic pressure low. The patient may require surgery to ligate the collateral vessels or may require embolization.

Critical Care Management for Late Postoperative Care

Patients with TOF and pulmonary atresia are subject to the same late problems and complications as patients with TOF alone. In addition, they may develop progressive conduit obstruction after surgery. Conduit obstruction is accelerated by the presence of a porcine valve in the conduit.[152,153] Consequently, unless the patient has severe pulmonary hypertension, valveless conduits or homografts now are preferred.[134]

Tricuspid Atresia

Pathophysiology

In this condition, an imperforate TV and hypoplasia of the right ventricle are present, often accompanied by a VSD of variable size and by pulmonic stenosis. A fixed obligatory shunt of all systemic venous return occurs from the right atrium through the patent foramen ovale or ASD into the left atrium, where complete mixing takes place. The degree of hypoxemia depends on the amount of pulmonary blood flow, which is regulated by the severity of the pulmonic stenosis. The common presentation is characterized by significant hypoxemia caused by the decreased pulmonary blood flow induced by either a restrictive VSD or a severe pulmonic stenosis.

Critical Care Management

The reparative operation of choice for tricuspid atresia is a modified Fontan procedure, but a palliative procedure may initially be required to improve pulmonary blood flow. A pulmonary artery band may be needed if the pulmonary blood flow is increased, or a shunt may have to be created for the severely hypoxemic child with decreased pulmonary blood flow. The critical care management and complications are those discussed in the sections on shunts, banding, and modified Fontan procedures. Complications of chronic hypoxemia and cyanosis are also present.

Transposition of the Great Arteries

Pathophysiology

With transposition of the great arteries, the right ventricle gives rise to the aorta. Almost 50% of patients with this anomaly have a VSD, and some of them have a variable degree of subpulmonic stenosis. Oxygenated pulmonary venous blood returns to the left atrium and is recirculated to the pulmonary artery without reaching the systemic circulation. Similarly, systemic venous blood returns to the right atrium and ventricle and is ejected into the aorta again. Obviously, this arrangement is compatible with life only for a few circulation times unless there is some mixing of pulmonary and systemic venous blood via a PDA or an opening in the atrial or ventricular septum at birth. The physiologic disturbance in these patients is one of inadequate mixing of pulmonary and systemic blood rather than one of inadequate pulmonary blood flow.

Mixing of blood at the atrial level can be improved by balloon atrial septostomy. If dangerous levels of hypoxemia persist after the septostomy and metabolic acidosis ensues, an infusion of PGE_1 can maintain the patency of ductus arteriosus, increase pulmonary blood flow (by increasing left-to-right shunting across the PDA), and thereby increase the volume of oxygenated blood entering the left atrium. The volume-overloaded left atrium is likely to shunt part of its contents into the right atrium and thereby improve the oxygen saturation of aortic blood. Unlike the kinetics with other lesions, increased shunting of blood during anesthesia improves arterial oxygen saturation before correction of the transposition.

Depending on the particular anatomy and the presence of a VSD or pulmonary stenosis, one of three corrective procedures is used. The intraoperative and postoperative problems encountered differ with each type of procedure.

Atrial Baffle Procedure (Mustard and Senning). An atrial level partition is created with baffling to redirect pulmonary venous blood across the TV to the right ventricle and thus to the aorta.[154–157] Systemic venous return is directed across the atrial septum to the mitral valve, into the left ventricle, and out the pulmonary artery. Although the pulmonary and systemic circuits are then connected serially instead of in parallel, this arrangement leaves the patient with a morphologic right ventricle and TV in continuity with the aorta. Therefore this ventricle must work against systemic arterial pressure and resistance.

One problem with atrial baffles is that they can obstruct systemic and pulmonary venous return.[158] When this occurs, the patient manifests signs and symptoms of systemic venous obstruction, as evidenced by SVC syndrome or other signs of systemic venous hypertension. When the pulmonary venous pathway is obstructed, pulmonary venous hypertension may be manifested by respiratory failure, poor gas exchange, and pulmonary edema (seen on chest radiograph). Severe pulmonary venous obstruction is manifested in the operating room by the presence of copious amounts of bloody fluid in the endotracheal tube, low cardiac output, and frequently poor oxygenation. Residual interatrial shunts also may cause intraoperative or postoperative hypoxemia. Long-term rhythm disturbances and the limitations of ventricular and AV valve function have made this operation nearly obsolete.

Arterial Switch Operation. Because of the complications associated with atrial baffle procedures, Jatene and others explored whether anatomic correction of this lesion, by dividing both great arteries and reattaching them to the opposite anatomically correct ventricle, would improve survival.[159–163] This procedure requires excision and reimplantation of the coronary arteries to the neoaorta (formerly the proximal main pulmonary artery). The success of the arterial switch procedure depends on adequate preparation of the left ventricle and technical proficiency with the coronary transfer. Anatomic correction of transposition of the great vessels is done during the neonatal period when PVR (LV afterload) and LV pressure are high.

Left ventricular mass decreases progressively after birth in this lesion, and if the ability of the left ventricle to tolerate the work required is misjudged, the child may develop severe LV failure postoperatively and require inotropic support and afterload reduction to provide normal cardiac output. Infants with transposition of the great arteries who are older than a few weeks of age and have an intact ventricular septum may have decreased LV pressure and mass. In such cases, the left ventricle may not tolerate the work required to perfuse the systemic vessels. However, if the neonate has a nonrestrictive VSD, the left ventricle is accustomed to high pressure and may tolerate the increased workload at any age. In older patients with an intact ventricular septum, banding the pulmonary artery can prepare the left ventricle to function as a systemic ventricle by increasing its afterload and muscle mass. If the left ventricle is "prepared" by banding the pulmonary artery and augmenting pulmonary blood flow with a modified Blalock-Taussig shunt, then an arterial switch procedure usually can be accomplished 1 week later, after hypertrophy and hyperplasia have occurred.[164] However, during this interval these patients are cyanotic, with a volume-loaded right ventricle and a pressure-loaded left ventricle, and they may require considerable pharmacologic support.[165,166]

In experienced centers, the incidence of mortality after neonatal repair of transposition of the great arteries now is less than 3% and may be less than 2% for most anatomic arrangements of coronary arteries if the aortic arch is normal.[10,106,167–169] Mid-term follow-up of these patients shows excellent outcome. Alternative operations are reserved almost exclusively for patients with particularly difficult coronary anatomy[170,171] or pulmonic (neoaortic) stenosis.

Myocardial ischemia or infarction may occur after mobilization and reimplantation of the coronary arteries, especially if they are stretched or twisted. Inotropic support, maintenance of coronary perfusion pressures, control of heart rate, and treatment with vasodilators may be particularly useful, as in adult patients with myocardial ischemia. Postoperative bleeding and tamponade occur more commonly with this operation because of the presence of multiple arterial anastomoses.

Ventricular Switch (Rastelli Procedure). In patients with a large VSD and severe subpulmonic stenosis, the VSD can be closed obliquely to direct LV flow to the aorta. The pulmonary valve is oversewn and the right ventricle is connected to the pulmonary artery with a conduit.[172]

Complications of the Rastelli procedure include obstruction of LV outflow as a result of narrowing of the subaortic region by the VSD patch. The conduit also may obstruct during or after the immediate postoperative period.[152,153] A small but significant incidence of heart block in these patients can be a difficult postoperative problem.

Critical Care Management

Patients who have both a pulmonary ventricle and a morphologic right ventricle remaining as the systemic ventricle can be regarded as having a physiologic or functional two-ventricle repair. Actuarial survival rates at 15 years have been quoted up to 85%; however, significant long-term functional deterioration is likely with increasing risk for right heart failure, sudden death, and dysrhythmias.[158,173–178] This situation is evidenced by systemic (right) ventricular dysfunction and TV regurgitation long after the repair.[179,180] These patients also are prone to develop significant atrial dysrhythmias, including supraventricular tachyarrhythmias and sick sinus syndrome later in life.[181,182] The arrhythmias may be preceded by RV dysfunction but also may be an isolated finding and is potentially the major cause of sudden death in these patients. A number of large follow-up series have reported the probability of a patient remaining in sinus rhythm after an atrial level repair is 50% at 10 years and 40% at 20 years. Function of the sinus node may be seriously impaired by the atrial manipulations during surgery, and sick sinus syndrome (requiring pacemaker insertion) may occur late in the postoperative period. The atrial baffle provides a functional repair, although despite this, many patients continue to maintain relatively active lives with few subjective symptoms.[183] Objective exercise testing on intermediate and late follow-up may demonstrate limited RV reserve in as many as 50% of patients. Exercise duration, peak heart rate response, and peak minute oxygen consumption have all been reported to be reduced compared with age-matched controls.[184]

One of the major advances in congenital heart surgery over the past 10 to 15 years has been the development of the ASO to correct transportation of the great arteries. In experienced centers, the early hospital mortality is less than 3%, and actuarial analyses indicate a 98% survival rate at 5 to 10 years.[169] Long-term survival data are not available given that the oldest survivors are only in their teenage years, but based on intermediate-term follow-up data the risk for reoperation and complications after ASO remains small.

Virtually all coronary artery patterns are amenable to ASO. No particular pattern has been associated with late death. A report of coronary artery angiography in 366 patients following ASO (median age at follow-up 7.9 years) revealed coronary artery stenosis or occlusion in 3% of patients.[185] The long-term significance of these coronary artery abnormalities has not been determined. Despite the angiographic findings, evaluation with serial ECG, exercise testing, and wall-motion abnormalities on echocardiography rarely demonstrate evidence of ischemia.[186,187]

After repair, the "native" pulmonary valve becomes the "neo-aortic" valve. A 30% incidence of trivial-to-mild aortic regurgitation has been reported on intermediate-term follow-up, without significant hemodynamic changes.[188] Severe regurgitation is unusual.

There appears to be a very low incidence of significant rhythm disturbances after ASO.[189] Supravalvar pulmonary artery stenosis was an early complication but now is less common with surgical techniques that extensively mobilize, augment, and reconstruct the pulmonary arteries. Supravalvar AS may develop but is rare.

Assessment of myocardial performance using echocardiography, cardiac catheterization, and exercise testing following ASO have demonstrated function identical to that in age-matched controls.[190] Based upon the currently available clinical, functional, and hemodynamic data, a patient who has undergone ASO with no evidence of subsequent problems should be treated as any patient with a structurally normal heart when presenting for noncardiac surgery.

Late complications of the Rastelli procedure include progressive conduit obstruction and RV hypertension, residual VSDs, and occasionally subaortic obstruction from diversion of LV outflow across the VSD to the aorta.

Total Anomalous Pulmonary Venous Connection

Pathophysiology

Patients with TAPVC are cyanotic because their pulmonary veins connect to a systemic vein and they have various degrees of pulmonary venous obstruction. The venous connection may be above the level of the heart (e.g., to the SVC, innominate, or azygos vein), directly to the right atrium, or below the level of the heart and the diaphragm (e.g., to the hepatic veins). Patients with this anomaly must have a patent foramen ovale or an ASD that allows blood flow to the left side of the heart.

This anatomic arrangement provides complete mixing of all systemic and pulmonary venous blood in the right atrium. Unless there is significant stenosis of the pulmonary venous connection, most of this right atrial blood passes through the right ventricle into the pulmonary artery, which increases pulmonary blood flow. If pulmonary venous return is significantly inhibited, there is increased pulmonary venous congestion and decreased pulmonary blood flow.

Critical Care Management

These patients may be very ill, with hypoxemia, severe pulmonary edema, and pulmonary artery hypertension. Resuscitation, including mechanical ventilation, PEEP, and inotropic support of the myocardium, is followed by early surgical intervention to relieve the pulmonary venous obstruction. Although patients are hypoxemic, their primary pathology is caused by obstructed venous return from the lungs. Therapy that increases pulmonary blood flow (e.g., PGE_1) must be avoided. Surgical repair of TAPVC requires attachment or redirection of the pulmonary venous confluence to the left atrium.[191]

Intraoperative and postoperative problems often are related to residual or recurrent stenosis of the pulmonary veins. In patients who had severe stenosis and pulmonary venous hypertension preoperatively, the pulmonary vascular bed is highly reactive. This reactivity may produce high pulmonary artery pressures and poor RV function after bypass and during the early postoperative period. Critical care management of these patients after completion of the repair should emphasize inotropic support of the right ventricle, avoidance of myocardial depressant drugs, and minimization of PVR. Early extubation of the trachea usually is not feasible. Mechanical ventilation with hyperventilation and other postoperative therapy to decrease PVR are required. Inhaled NO has been particularly useful in this population.[192]

Critical Care Management for Late Postoperative Care

Other than the potential for late development of recurrent pulmonary venous obstruction, these patients generally do well and have good cardiovascular reserve once recovery from the surgery is complete.[193] The size of the pulmonary veins at birth may be a predictor of late complications with recurrent pulmonary vein stenosis.[194]

Atrial Septal Defect

Pathophysiology

There are three anatomic varieties of ASD. The most common, *ASD secundum*, is a deficit in the septum primum, which ordinarily covers the region of the foramen ovale. *ASD primum* is a deficit of the inferior portion of the atrial septum (endocardial cushion) usually accompanied by a cleft in the anterior leaflet of the mitral valve. *Sinus venous defects* are located near the junction of the right atrium and the SVC or IVC. They frequently are associated with a partial anomalous pulmonary venous connection.

Left-to-right shunting (simple) occurs at the atrial level, causing a low-pressure volume load to the right ventricle. Pulmonary blood flow is increased, but not enough to make these patients symptomatic during early childhood. However, later in life, as the left ventricle becomes less compliant and the LA pressures increase, the left-to-right shunt and volume load increase and symptoms of CHF may occur. In rare patients the long-standing increase in pulmonary blood flow causes pulmonary vascular obstructive disease.[195]

Critical Care Management

The defect can be closed directly with sutures or, if it is sufficiently large, with a synthetic patch. Sinus venosus defects associated with partial anomalous pulmonary venous connection require a more extensive patch that also directs the partial anomalous pulmonary venous return into the left atrium.

These patients are among the healthiest encountered. Their anesthesia can be managed in many ways. Early tracheal extubation is usual. Atrial arrhythmias, including atrial flutter and atrial fibrillation, are rarely seen during the postoperative period. Mitral regurgitation may occur in patients who have undergone repair of an ASD primum. Although transient LV failure has been reported, these patients rarely require inotropic support. Residual ASDs are uncommon, but occasionally failure to recognize partial anomalous pulmonary venous return results in a residual left-to-right shunt. Most patients can be extubated during the immediate postoperative period or in the operating room. With the exceptions mentioned, these patients usually have nearly normal cardiovascular function and reserve after repair.[196]

Ventricular Septal Defect

Pathophysiology

Defects in the ventricular septum occur at several locations in the muscular partition dividing the ventricles. Simple shunting occurs across the ventricular septum. The magnitude of pulmonary blood flow is determined by the size of the VSD and the PVR.[197] With a nonrestrictive defect, high LV flows and pressures are transmitted to the pulmonary artery. Therefore surgical repair is indicated within the first 2 years of life to prevent the progression of pulmonary vascular obstructive disease.[60,198,199] In patients with established pulmonary vascular disease, the pulmonary arteriolar changes may not recede when the defect is closed. In such cases, there may be progressive PVR elevation.[200–202] The growth and development of the pulmonary vascular bed are significant factors in the patient's ability to normalize pulmonary vascular hemodynamics after surgery.[203] When PVR approaches or exceeds systemic vascular resistance, right-to-left shunting occurs through the VSD and the patients develop progressive hypoxemia (Eisenmenger syndrome). Closing the VSD in this circumstance adds the risk for acute right heart failure to that of progressive increases in PVR.

Critical Care Management

The defects are closed during CPB. The most common septal defect, the membranous defect, is often repaired through a right atriotomy and the TV. However, lesions in the inferior apical muscular septum or those high in the ventricular outflow tract may require a left or right ventriculotomy. If so, postoperative ventricular function may be impaired.

Before repair, measures that decrease PVR may appreciably increase left-to-right shunting in patients with a nonrestrictive defect and may increase the degree of CHF. Postoperative right or LV failure may be a manifestation of the preoperative status of the myocardium, a result of the ventriculotomy and CPB, or both. Small infants who fail to thrive, who are malnourished, and who have significant CHF preoperatively may have excessive lung water and may require prolonged mechanical ventilation postoperatively.[204] Such infants may have limited intraoperative tolerance for anesthetics that depress the myocardium or for maneuvers that increase pulmonary blood flow.

Persistent CHF and an audible murmur postoperatively, evidence of low cardiac output, or the need for extensive inotropic support intraoperatively suggests that a residual or previously unrecognized additional VSD is continuing to place a volume and pressure load on the ventricles. When PVR is increased preoperatively, the increase in RV afterload caused by closure of the VSD may be poorly tolerated, leading to the need for inotropic support of the heart and measures to decrease PVR. Occasionally ventricular outflow tract obstruction is caused by placement of the septal patch. Aortic regurgitation caused by prolapse of one of the aortic valve cusps can develop in subaortic or subpulmonic VSDs. In addition, heart block may occur after closure of VSDs with a patch. A pacemaker may be needed to maintain an adequate heart rate and cardiac output.

Critical Care Management for Late Postoperative Care

In the absence of residual VSDs, outflow obstruction, and heart block, most of these patients regain relatively normal myocardial function, especially if the VSD is repaired early.[205] However, a small percentage of patients, especially those in whom a large defect was repaired late in childhood, continue to have some degree of ventricular dysfunction and some pulmonary hypertension.[206–208]

Atrioventricular Canal Defects

Pathophysiology

The endocardial cushion defect, or complete common AV canal, consists of defects in the atrial and ventricular septa and the AV valvular tissue. All four chambers communicate and share a single common AV valve. The atrial and ventricular shunts communicate volume and systemic pressures to the right ventricle and pulmonary artery. The ventricular shunt orifice usually is nonrestrictive (simple shunt); therefore PVR governs the degree of excess pulmonary blood flow. Mitral regurgitation and direct left-ventricular-to-right-atrial shunting may further contribute to atrial hypertension and total left-to-right shunting.

Critical Care Management

Surgical repair of this lesion consists of division of the common AV valve and closure of the ASD and VSD with a single patch.[209] In addition, the mitral valve (and sometimes the TV) requires suture approximation and resuspension of the separated portions.

These patients have large left-to-right shunts. As a result of their high pulmonary blood flows, they have CHF and pulmonary hypertension. Myocardial depressants and therapies that decrease PVR while increasing shunt flow may be poorly tolerated before repair. Some patients, especially older children, may have obstructive pulmonary vascular disease. All of the potential complications of ASD and VSD closures are seen in these patients. In addition, the mitral valve may be severely regurgitant.[210] Inotropic support for the failing heart, afterload reduction for mitral regurgitation, and measures to decrease PVR may be required intraoperatively and postoperatively after repair.

Patients with Down syndrome frequently have an associated complete AV canal. Measures to decrease PVR and the use of prolonged ventilatory support are often necessary because their airways and pulmonary vascular beds are hyperreactive. The large tongues, upper airway obstruction, and difficult vascular access of these patients pose additional problems. The most frequent postoperative problems in patients with Down syndrome are residual VSDs, mitral insufficiency,[211,212] and pulmonary hypertension.[13]

Patent Ductus Arteriosus

Pathophysiology

The ductus arteriosus is a fetal vascular communication between the main pulmonary artery at its bifurcation and the descending aorta below the origin of the left subclavian artery. When patent, it provides a simple shunt between the systemic and pulmonary arteries. The magnitude and direction of flow between the systemic and pulmonary vessels are determined by the relative resistances to flow in the two vascular beds and the diameter (resistance) of the ductus itself. With a large, nonrestrictive ductus and low PVR, the pulmonary blood flow is excessive and the volume load of the left heart is large. Systolic and diastolic flow away from the aorta may steal blood from vital organs (e.g., pulmonary steal) and compromise end-organ function at many sites.[213] In addition, overcirculated lungs and elevated LA pressure increase the work of breathing.[214,215]

Critical Care Management

Although the PDA of premature infants can often be closed medically with indomethacin, contraindications to use of this agent (e.g., intracranial hemorrhage, renal dysfunction, and hyperbilirubinemia) may require surgical closure of the defect.[216] Whereas thoracotomy and surgical ligation of the ductus arteriosus are standard in older infants and children, some centers now occlude the ductus with a percutaneously inserted vascular umbrella[217] or by using video-assisted thoracoscopic surgery (VATS).[218,219] Advantages of VATS compared with open thoracotomy include decreased postoperative pain, shorter hospital stay, and decreased incidence of chest wall deformity.[220]

Healthy asymptomatic patients undergoing surgery can be extubated in the operating room, allowing many options for anesthetic management. However, the fragile premature infant with severe lung disease may require mechanical ventilation for protracted periods after ligation of the ductus arteriosus. Fentanyl, pancuronium, oxygen, and air constitute a common anesthetic regimen for this procedure.[221] Management of the premature infant in the operating room requires special considerations of gas exchange, hemodynamic performance, temperature regulation, metabolism, and drug and oxygen toxicity. Thoracotomy and lung retraction usually decrease lung compliance and increase oxygen and ventilatory requirements. A transient rise in systemic blood pressure with ligation of the ductus arteriosus may increase LV afterload or elevate cerebral perfusion pressure to the detriment of a premature patient. Inadvertent ligation of the left pulmonary artery or descending aorta has occurred because the ductus arteriosus is often the same size as the descending aorta.

The ductus is located near the recurrent laryngeal nerve (RLN), which may be damaged during the procedure. In addition to the close relationship of the RLN to the PDA and descending aorta, the RLN has a variable course that may be difficult to identify during dissection. Prior reports of PDA ligation performed by open thoracotomy indicate that the incidence of RLN injury is 1.2% to 8.8%.[222,223] RLN paralysis causes hoarseness and is not detected until the endotracheal tube is removed. The incidence may be reduced by location of the RLN within the thorax prior to ligation or clip placement using direct intraoperative stimulation of the RLN and evoked electromyogram monitoring.[224]

Ligation of an isolated ductus arteriosus generally results in normal cardiovascular function and reserve several months postoperatively.[225,226]

Truncus Arteriosus

Pathophysiology

With truncus arteriosus the embryonic truncus fails to separate normally into the two great arteries. A single great artery leaves the heart and gives rise to the coronary, pulmonary, and systemic circulations. The truncus straddles a large VSD and receives blood from both ventricles.[227]

Complete mixing of systemic and pulmonary venous blood in the single great artery causes mild hypoxemia. One or two pulmonary arteries may originate from the ascending truncus; the pulmonary artery orifice is seldom restrictive. The resulting shunt (simple) produces excessive pulmonary blood flow early in life as the PVR decreases. This "pulmonary steal" may elevate the arterial oxygen saturation and decrease the systemic blood flow. In such a case, net systemic oxygen transport decreases and lactic acidosis develops. Children with truncus arteriosus are at risk for developing early pulmonary vascular obstructive disease.[228] Regurgitation of blood through the truncal valve may place an additional volume load on the ventricles.

Critical Care Management

Complete repair of this lesion should be performed early, even in the neonate, before the development of irreversible pulmonary vascular changes.[8,229] The VSD is closed with a synthetic patch, and the pulmonary arteries are detached from the truncus. Continuity is established between the right ventricle and the pulmonary arteries with a valved conduit.[230] The truncal valve may require valvuloplasty if a significant amount of blood regurgitates through it.

Critical care management centers around control of pulmonary blood flow and ventricular support. Pulmonary blood flow may increase further with anesthetic agents, hyperventilation, alkalosis, and oxygen administration, resulting in hypotension and acute ventricular failure. If measures for *increasing* PVR do not decrease pulmonary flow, occlusion of one branch of the pulmonary artery with a tourniquet limits pulmonary flow and restores systemic perfusion pressure until CPB can be instituted. Because these patients are often in high-output CHF, myocardial depressants should be used with caution.

Immediately after repair, the combination of persistent pulmonary artery hypertension and RV failure can be fatal. Hence, aggressive measures should be taken to provide normal myocardial function and lower PVR. A residual VSD adds volume and pressure load on the ventricles and may have a devastating impact on the patient's hemodynamics and oxygenation. A VSD should be suspected in patients who are not doing well postoperatively. Any residual VSD should be repaired if feasible. Truncal valve regurgitation or stenosis may induce LV failure early during the postoperative period.

Critical Care Management for Late Postoperative Care

Obstruction of the pulmonary conduit and the accompanying RV hypertension may occur early or late during the postoperative course. Usually the conduit is unable to support flow in the growing child after several postoperative years. Late development of truncal (aortic) valve regurgitation is possible. For patients who underwent repair later in childhood, residual persistent pulmonary hypertension may be a problem.

Left-Sided Obstructive Lesions

Pathophysiology

This category includes valvar, subvalvar, and supravalvar mitral and aortic stenosis (AS), aortic coarctation, and IAA. Although these lesions can occur as isolated defects, they often are accompanied by other congenital cardiac defects. Identification of additional structural defects is necessary for optimal preoperative, surgical, and postoperative treatment.

Patients with LV outflow tract obstruction tend to present as either neonates or young infants with significant LV dysfunction and CHF or later in childhood with LV hypertrophy but few symptoms. The dramatic presentation of a neonate with circulatory collapse typically occurs with lesions that obstruct systemic blood flow so severely that right-to-left shunting at the ductus arteriosus is required to perfuse the body. As the ductus significantly narrows or closes, the left ventricle becomes acutely pressure overloaded and begins to fail, leading to pulmonary edema and respiratory distress. When systemic perfusion becomes inadequate, the patient develops hypotension, weak pulses, metabolic acidosis, and oliguria. Classic examples include severe (or "critical") valvar AS, coarctation of the aorta, and HLHS (see earlier single ventricle discussion).

If the obstruction is less severe, the child can make the transition through ductal closure without notable LV dysfunction and maintain an adequate cardiac output. Over time, however, the pressure overload on the LV stimulates generalized hypertrophy. If untreated and significant, long-term pressure overload can cause LV diastolic dysfunction (compliance falls and end-diastolic pressure rises, causing pulmonary venous hypertension), LV systolic dysfunction, and episodic myocardial ischemia. Clinical manifestations of these changes can include reduced exercise tolerance, exertional chest pain, ventricular dysrhythmias, syncope, and sudden death. Significant LV dilation and/or clinical signs of CHF are ominous findings associated with a poor prognosis and an increased surgical mortality rate.

Aortic Stenosis

Of the three anatomic subtypes of AS, valvar AS occurs more frequently than subvalvar or supravalvar AS. The newborn with critical valvar AS who develops hypotension and acidosis as the ductus arteriosus closes requires resuscitation with PGE_1 to restore aortic flow plus mechanical ventilation and inotropic support to achieve stabilization before an intervention is performed. Currently, balloon dilation of the stenotic aortic valve during cardiac catheterization is the preferred intervention at many centers.[231] A surgical valvotomy under direct vision using CPB is the surgical alternative. Despite successful relief of obstruction, significant LV dysfunction and low cardiac output often persist for days after the procedure and require continued treatment with mechanical ventilation and vasoactive drugs. Until LV function recovers and can support the entire cardiac output, continuation of prostaglandin infusion may be necessary to maintain patency of the ductus arteriosus. Patients should be carefully evaluated after balloon aortic valvuloplasty for residual AS and aortic regurgitation, the chief potential complication of valve dilation, especially if cardiac output does not improve over several days.

Older infants, children, and adolescents with moderate (pressure gradient 50–70 mmHg at catheterization) or severe (pressure gradient >70 mmHg at catheterization) valvar AS also are generally good candidates for balloon aortic valvuloplasty. If more than mild aortic regurgitation coexists with AS, however, a surgical intervention is preferred to balloon valvuloplasty.

The pathophysiology produced by all types of aortic outflow obstruction is similar, that is, the pressure-overloaded LV becomes progressively hypertrophied and develops reduced compliance and an abnormally elevated end-diastolic pressure.

Initial assessment of obstruction relief can occur when the patient is still in the catheterization laboratory or operating room by either direct pressure measurements or echocardiography. Nevertheless, reevaluation for residual obstruction by physical examination and/or echocardiography in the ICU as patients recover from anesthesia and baseline physiology returns is important because outflow gradients can change. A significant residual obstruction should be suspected in any patient with persistent low cardiac output following the intervention. Poor recovery of LV function after surgery can occur secondary to inadequate myocardial protection with cardioplegia in hearts with significant ventricular hypertrophy. Patients with marked hypertrophy are also at greater risk for developing VT and ventricular fibrillation early after surgery.

In patients with preserved LV systolic function who undergo an uncomplicated procedure, such as aortic valvuloplasty or subvalvar membrane resection, myocardial recovery after CPB is typically rapid and inotropic support is usually not required. Systemic hypertension is more common following relief of LV outflow obstruction, especially during emergence from anesthesia and sedation. Antihypertensive therapy in the initial 24 to 48 hours may be necessary to prevent an aortic suture line and reconstructed valve leaflet disruption from excessive stress and to allow adequate hemostasis. Both beta-blockers (e.g., labetalol, propranolol, and esmolol) and vasodilators (e.g., nitroprusside), alone or usually in combination, are effective for lowering blood pressure in these patients.

In addition to assessing aortic valve and LV function, an evaluation for complications specific to each procedure is required. For example, if a myectomy is required as part of the resection of fibromuscular subvalvar AS, the possibility of a new VSD, mitral valve injury, and left bundle branch block should all be assessed. Following the Ross procedure, it is important to assess patients for RV outflow tract and LV outflow tract obstruction, because the RV outflow tract is also reconstructed with a valved conduit.

Coarctation of the Aorta

Coarctation of the aorta is a constriction in the descending aorta located at the level of insertion of the ductus arteriosus. Narrowing of the aortic lumen is asymmetric, with the majority of the obstruction occurring because of posterior tissue infolding, leading to the common description of a posterior aortic "shelf." Depending on the severity of constriction, patients can present as neonates with severe obstruction (a "critical" coarctation of the aorta) during ductal closure, as infants with CHF, or as children/adolescents with no symptoms except for upper body hypertension (especially with exercise).

Neonates presenting with critical coarctation of the aorta can often be distinguished clinically from patients with critical AS by their clearly discrepant upper versus lower body pulses, perfusion, and blood pressures. Other features at presentation, including evidence of CHF and inadequate blood flow to tissues, are similar. Because ductal narrowing or closure is common after hospital discharge, these patients often become critically ill and suffer end-organ damage before the ductus arteriosus can be reopened and resuscitation accomplished. Intestinal and renal ischemia leading to necrotizing enterocolitis and renal failure, respectively, are well-known complications of critical coarctation of the aorta. Echocardiography often reveals additional left-sided defects such as bicuspid aortic valve, valvar AS, aortic arch hypoplasia, and VSD. Preoperative management includes treatment with PGE_1 plus mechanical ventilation, inotropic agents, and diuretic agents, as needed, and adequate time for end-organ recovery before performing an intervention.

Coarctation of the aorta also occurs in association with complex defects such as D-transposition of the great arteries, single ventricle, and complete AV canal defect. If the ductus arteriosus is patent during echocardiographic evaluation of a neonate with suspected CHD, it often is not possible to predict the severity of coarctation of the aorta with confidence. A patient can have an abnormally narrowed aorta just proximal to the site of ductal insertion (i.e., the aortic isthmus) and a posterior shelf but still not develop a severe coarctation of the aorta following ductal closure. Therefore evaluation of the potential severity of coarctation of the aorta in the ICU often involves a strategy of close monitoring for aortic obstruction without PGE_1 to allow the PDA to close, followed by clinical and echocardiographic reassessment. An intervention to reduce aortic obstruction is indicated in any neonate with clinical or echocardiographic evidence of reduced ventricular function or impaired cardiac output. These indications are more important than the systolic blood pressure difference between upper and lower body per se, although differences greater than 30 mmHg often are accompanied by diminished ventricular function.

The postoperative management of patients following surgical repair of coarctation of the aorta can vary depending on age at intervention. However, the key issues for assessment in all patients are adequate relief of obstruction and preservation of spinal cord function. Upper and lower body blood pressures and pulses should be compared serially and the lower extremities monitored closely for the return of sensation and voluntary movement in the early postoperative period. Equal pulses and a reproducible systolic blood pressure difference less than 10 to 12 mmHg between upper and lower extremities indicate an excellent repair. Neonates and young infants typically require 1 to 2 days of mechanical ventilation after repair, and they are more likely to receive inotropic agents, especially if ventricular function was diminished before surgery. Older children and adolescents can frequently be extubated in the operating room and rarely require inotropic support. In fact, these patients are increasingly likely with older age at repair to have significant hypertension,[232] which should be treated aggressively early after surgery to reduce the risk of aortic suture disruption and bleeding. Beta-blockers and vasodilators, along with adequate analgesia and sedation, are effective. Patients with long-standing coarctation of the aorta frequently have persistent systemic hypertension despite an adequate repair; continued treatment with angiotensin-converting enzyme inhibitors is advocated to achieve normal blood pressures.

Four uncommon complications are associated with surgical repair of coarctation of the aorta. Postcoarctectomy syndrome manifests as abdominal pain and/or distension in older patients and is presumed to be caused by mesenteric ischemia from reflex vasoconstriction after restoration of pulsatile aortic flow. Recurrent laryngeal nerve and phrenic nerve trauma can cause vocal cord paralysis and hemidiaphragm paresis or paralysis, respectively, with neonates and infants at highest risk. Disruption of lymphatic vessels or thoracic duct trauma can produce a chylous effusion and chylothorax that may require treatment by drainage and/or dietary modification.

Catheter-directed balloon angioplasty is used to treat both native and residual coarctation of the aorta.[233–235] The results of native coarctation of the aorta dilation after early follow-up appear similar to published surgical results, but aortic aneurysm formation has been reported.[234] Balloon angioplasty of recurrent coarctation of the aorta after surgery is effective and now is generally preferred to reoperation.

Interrupted Aortic Arch

Patients with IAA typically present as neonates with either a loud systolic murmur or circulatory compromise as the ductus arteriosus closes. Therefore patient presentation can be similar to other severe left-sided obstructive lesions such as critical AS, critical coarctation of the aorta, and HLHS. Unlike either critical AS or coarctation of the aorta, however, severe pressure overload on the LV does not occur in the presence of an unrestrictive VSD, which functions as a "pop off" for LV outflow. The approach to resuscitation is similar to that described for the other ductal-dependent left-sided obstructive lesions, with attention to the possibility of pulmonary overcirculation as for HLHS.

Postoperative management issues specific to patients with IAA include assessment of possible residual left-sided obstruction, both in the aortic arch and in the subaortic region, shunting across a residual VSD, hypocalcemia, dysrhythmias, and LV dysfunction with low cardiac output secondary to global effects of CPB and DHCA. Left-lung hyperinflation on postoperative chest radiographs suggests compression of the left mainstem bronchus. This complication tends to occur after difficult arch reconstructions when tension on the aorta causes it to press on the anterior surface of the bronchus, thus producing distal air trapping.

Mitral Stenosis

Hypoplastic Left Heart Syndrome.

Pathophysiology. Among the congenital heart lesions, perhaps the most controversial has been management of HLHS. HLHS is a uniformly fatal disease if left untreated, and debates continue over a staged palliation,[236] versus neonatal transplantation,[237,238] versus comfort care alone.[239] The results of surgical management vary among institutions and are clearly dependent upon expertise and experience,[240] the clinical condition of the neonate at presentation,[241] prematurity, multiple congenital anomalies, presence of an intact atrial septum, later age of presentation,[242] and degree of hypoplasia of left heart structures.[243–246]

This common example of single-ventricle physiology also represents the most severe form of obstructive left heart lesion. An anatomic spectrum of disease is implied for the lesion, but in its most severe and common presentation there is atresia or marked hypoplasia of the aortic and mitral valves with critical underdevelopment of the left atrium, left ventricle, and ascending aorta. A 1- or 2-mm ascending aorta gives rise to the coronary circulation and the head vessels before converging with the ductus arteriosus, where the aorta becomes larger and supplies the circulation to the lower body. Pulmonary venous return arrives in the diminutive left atrium and cannot cross the atretic mitral valve; therefore it is directed to the right atrium and right ventricle, where common mixing occurs with the systemic venous return and all blood is ejected into the pulmonary artery. Systemic blood flow is then supplied from the pulmonary artery, right-to-left, across the PDA. As the PDA constricts in the neonatal period, systemic blood flow decreases and all ventricular output is directed to the lungs. The Q_p/Q_s ratio approaches infinity as Q_s nears zero. Therefore the paradoxical presentation of high Po_2 (70–150 mmHg) in the face of profound metabolic acidosis is seen. When the ductus arteriosus is reopened with PGE_1, systemic perfusion is reestablished, the acidosis resolves, and the Po_2 returns to the range of 40 to 60 mmHg range, representative of a Q_p/Q_s ratio between 1 and 2.

Critical Care Management. Adequate preoperative resuscitation with PGE_1 and correction of metabolic acidosis and end-organ dysfunction are crucial to the preparation and management of patients with this lesion. Further facilitation of resuscitation can be enhanced by judicious use of inotropic agents, which can optimize cardiac output and blood flow to organs such as the kidneys. However, excessive delay in the timing of surgical intervention results in gradual reduction in PVR over days, with excessive pulmonary blood flow and inadequate systemic perfusion. The surgical reconstructive approach to this lesion now commonly entails three operations that ultimately aim to provide a 2- to 5-year-old child with a reconstructed aortic arch and a Fontan-type circulation for single-ventricle physiology.[236,245,247] In the first stage of the reconstruction (Norwood operation),[31] the pulmonary artery is transected at the bifurcation and an anastomosis is performed to the ascending aorta, which has been surgically incised so that the aortic and pulmonary arterial confluence arises together from the single right ventricle as the neoaorta, which is extended into the remaining native aorta using homograft material. Pulmonary blood flow is established with a modified Blalock-Taussig shunt, usually 3.5 mm in diameter. The atrial septum is excised to ensure free flow of pulmonary venous return over to the TV. In addition to HLHS, the Norwood operation is used to repair other complex single-ventricle defects with systemic outflow obstruction or hypoplasia.[248]

The critical care considerations are the same as those outlined for patients with single-ventricle physiology. Perioperative management requires careful manipulation of PVR and SVR and support of ventricular function to provide adequate, but not excessive, pulmonary blood flow and systemic oxygen delivery while maintaining sufficient systemic and coronary artery perfusion.

Postoperative Management.

Evolution of treatment strategies. Common teaching has held that postoperative mortality and hemodynamic lability are attributable to myocardial dysfunction and the physiologic burden imposed by a shunt-dependent pulmonary circulation in parallel with systemic blood flow. Treatment strategies have emphasized factors that may affect the balance between pulmonary and systemic blood flow. Immediately following a Norwood operation, PVR may be transiently elevated but soon decreases. Once PVR falls, treatment is aimed at raising resistance to blood flow through the lungs and redirecting cardiac output to the systemic circulation. High inspired concentration of oxygen, hyperventilation, alkalosis, systemic vasoconstriction, and anemia may cause further pulmonary vasodilation and are avoided. Therapies designed to raise PVR and thereby direct aortic blood flow to the systemic circulation have focused on lowering the Fio_2 or allowing the $Paco_2$ to rise with the pH falling toward 7.3. Further measures, such as ventilation with hypoxic gas mixtures or added carbon dioxide, have been advocated by some centers and have been intermittently embraced and abandoned by others. Validation of the effectiveness of these techniques to balance the pulmonary and systemic circulations has been difficult.

The clinical focus on caring for the newborn who has undergone Norwood palliation for HLHS has evolved in stages over the past 20 years. The early emphasis was on manipulating the PVR by optimizing mechanical ventilation (i.e., mean airway pressure, tidal volume, rate and inspiratory time, Fio_2, and Pco_2). It soon became apparent that the majority of this effort was aimed in the postoperative period to raise PVR and lower pulmonary blood flow while increasing systemic blood flow. Like any therapeutic strategy, manipulating gas exchange and inspired gases had its own set of adverse effects. High FiO_2 has well-defined pulmonary toxicity that may appear in a matter of days or even hours after exposure. Use of low FiO_2 (below room air concentrations) to raise PVR transiently and stabilize patients is both counterintuitive and a relatively uncommon therapy in clinical medicine. Whether iatrogenically induced or as part of a pathologic process, alveolar hypoxia can be life threatening when aggravated by unexpected hypoventilation. A mechanically ventilated and sedated patient on an FiO_2 less than 0.21 has little safety margin for dangerous hypoxemia even in the most intensively monitored environments. Excellent animal models of chronic pulmonary hypertension are produced by relatively brief exposure to hypoxic gas. A newborn breathing hypoxic gas mixtures in the preoperative period of stabilization may have a favorable response by raising PVR and diminishing pulmonary blood flow. However, if this treatment is prolonged during preparation for reconstructive or transplantation surgery, the caretakers may be frustrated by subsequent elevation in PVR that persists during and after weaning from CPB.

In centers where neonates are allowed to awaken and breathe spontaneously during the immediate postoperative period, pulmonary blood flow may become excessive and further stimulate hyperventilation and respiratory alkalosis. Adding carbon dioxide to the inspired gas may reverse this trend toward respiratory alkalosis and stabilize the relative balance of the pulmonary and systemic circulations if the forces that drive minute ventilation are suppressed with agents for sedation or analgesia. However, the metabolic cost of carbon dioxide breathing in an awakening child given little analgesia may discourage widespread application of this technique until the physiologic advantage over conventional means of controlling alveolar ventilation and $PaCO_2$ has been demonstrated. This is especially true in unsedated, preoperative patients where factors controlling respiration during carbon dioxide breathing may permit minimal change of $PaCO_2$ but substantially increase the respiratory rate and work of breathing.

The introduction of a 3.5-mm systemic-to-pulmonary shunt (rather than a 4-mm shunt) and the appreciation of the surgical complexity of an appropriately placed shunt did as much to reduce excessive pulmonary blood flow in the infants as did manipulation of the ventilator. Although the smaller shunts were associated with a rare but real incidence of shunt thrombosis, those involved in postoperative care found patient management with a small shunt substantially easier than struggling with a 4-mm shunt off of an innominate artery. By the late 1980s it was apparent that this palliated circulation was required for only 10 to 12 weeks to reach an adequate patient size for the newly applied second stage of the procedure (bidirectional Glenn) to be performed. Therefore a relative increase in cyanosis (from a smaller shunt) was believed to be a justifiable price for more stable early postoperative hemodynamics. However, mortality rates did not plummet with the recognition of the advantage of smaller shunts and manipulating PVR, although by then many more centers were undertaking a staged reconstructive approach to HLHS. In the early 1990s attention was redirected to the observation that arterial oxygen saturation was only one variable in the assessment of Q_p/Q_s and that a perfectly "acceptable" arterial oxygen saturation of 80% in this disease may represent severe pulmonary overcirculation if the mixed venous oxygen saturation was only 20%. Hence a renewed interest in measuring and monitoring arterial and mixed venous oxygen saturations emerged. Thus in overcirculated patients with a small (3.5-mm) fixed-diameter shunt off of the subclavian artery, there was less emphasis on micromanagement of PVR and more interest in pharmacologically supporting cardiac output while reducing the *systemic* afterload to diminish the driving pressure across the shunt. Use of the alpha-blocker phenoxybenzamine has been advocated by some for blunting systemic vascular reactivity and dilating the peripheral circulation,[249] but its potent, long-lasting effects and associated hypotension can be challenging. The phosphodiesterase inhibitors then enjoyed a new and extensive application in pediatric critical care: lowering SVR, increasing cardiac output, and lowering filling pressures. The new strategy was to monitor (arteriovenous) DO_2, support cardiac output, and reduce SVR.

Later in the decade, the observation of limited coronary reserve, low mixed venous oxygen saturation, rising lactate, and hemodynamic collapse in the first 48 hours helped emphasize the fundamental limitation of myocardial function and cardiac output in the early postoperative period. The morphologic right ventricle and TV seem ill suited to support adequate systemic plus pulmonary blood flow. Several centers then embraced mechanical support of the circulation temporarily for the failing Norwood patient in the early postoperative period.

Specific considerations for the Norwood operation. Management of patients following a Norwood-type operation is complex. Intensive monitoring is essential because the patient's clinical status can change abruptly with rapid deterioration. Persistent or progressive metabolic acidosis is a bad prognostic sign and must be aggressively managed. Considerations in the assessment of the circulation following the Norwood operation are given in Table 29–16.

Ideally the pH should be 7.40, $PaCO_2$ 40 mmHg, and PaO_2 40 mmHg in room air, with a mixed venous O_2 saturation of 60% reflecting a well-balanced circulation. Higher saturations can be achieved if the systemic circulation is well dilated without compromising perfusion pressure. Frequent changes in mechanical ventilation settings and FiO_2 may be necessary in the first few hours after surgery. However, manipulations of FiO_2 in the face of a restrictive 3.5-mm shunt may have less impact on pulmonary blood flow than would systemic vasodilation.[250] Leaving the sternum open after surgery may facilitate lower filling pressures, a balanced circulation, and stable ventilation pattern.

Deep sedation or even muscle paralysis and anesthesia often are continued after surgery to minimize the stress response until the patient has a stable circulation and gas exchange. Inotropic support with dopamine and occasionally low doses of epinephrine usually are required, titrated to systemic pressure and perfusion. Afterload reduction with milrinone as second-line agents is beneficial to reduce myocardial work and improve systemic

TABLE 29–16

Management Considerations for Patients Following a Norwood Procedure

Scenario	Etiology	Management
Sao_2 ~ 80% Svo_2 ~ 60% Normotensive	Balanced Flow $Q_p = Q_s$	No intervention
Sao_2 >90% Hypotension	OVERCIRCULATED $Q_p = Q_s$ Low PVR Large BT shunt Residual arch obstruction	Raise PVR Controlled hypoventilation Low Fio_2 (0.17–0.19) Add CO_2 (3%–5%) Increase systemic perfusion Afterload reduction, vasodilation Inotropic support Surgical shunt revision
Sao_2 <75% Hypertension	UNDERCIRCULATED $Q_p < Q_s$ High PVR Small, kinked, thrombosed BT shunt	Lower PVR Controlled hyperventilation Alkalosis Sedation/paralysis Increase cardiac output Inotropic support Hematocrit >40% Surgical intervention
Sao_2 <75% Hypotension Low Svo_2	Low Cardiac Output Ventricular failure Myocardial ischemia Residual arch obstruction Atrioventricular valve regurgitation	Minimize stress response Inotropic support Surgical revision Consider mechanical support Consider transplantation

BT, Blalock-Taussing; *Fio_2,* inspired oxygen concentration; *PVR,* pulmonary vascular resistance; *Q_p,* pulmonary blood flow; *Q_s,* systemic blood flow; *Sao_2,* arterial oxygen saturation; *Svo_2,* mixed venous oxygen saturation.

perfusion. Monitoring SVC O_2 saturations, as a measure of mixed venous O_2 saturation (Svo_2) and cardiac output, is useful in this assessment.[251] Volume replacement to maintain preload is essential, aiming for a common atrial pressure approximating 10 mmHg.

The type, diameter, length, and position of the shunt affects the balance of pulmonary and systemic flow. Generally, a 3.5-mm Blalock-Taussig shunt from the distal innominate artery provides adequate pulmonary blood flow without excessive steal from the systemic circulation for most full-term neonates. Nevertheless, a shunt resulting in a low diastolic pressure (<30 mmHg) in turn affects perfusion to other vascular beds, particularly the coronary, cerebral, renal, and splanchnic perfusion. This may contribute to a prolonged and difficult postoperative course.

Overcirculation in the immediate postoperative period with an Sao_2 greater than 90% may reflect a low PVR or increased flow across the shunt if the shunt size is too large or the perfusion pressure increased from residual aortic arch obstruction distal to the shunt insertion site. The increased volume load on the systemic ventricle results in congestive cardiac failure and progressive systemic hypoperfusion with cool extremities, oliguria, and possibly metabolic acidosis. Although manipulation of mechanical ventilation and inspired oxygen concentration may help limit pulmonary blood flow, surgical revision to reduce the shunt size may be necessary.

If there is significant systemic steal through a large shunt, coronary perfusion may be reduced and lead to ischemia, low output, and arrhythmias. Rhythm disturbances are uncommon in the immediate postoperative period following a Norwood operation, and a sudden loss of sinus rhythm, and particularly heart block or ventricular fibrillation, should increase the suspicion of myocardial ischemia.

In the immediate postoperative period, mild hypoxemia with a Sao_2 of 70% to 75% and Pao_2 of 30 to 35mmHg is preferable to an overcirculated state with high systemic oxygen saturations and falling mixed venous oxygen saturation. Pulmonary blood flow often increases on the first postoperative day as ventricular function improves and PVR falls during recovery from CPB. Pulmonary venous desaturation from parenchymal lung disease such as atelectasis, pleural effusions, and pneumothorax requires aggressive management.

Persistent desaturation and hypotension reflects a low cardiac output from poor ventricular function, thereby decreasing the perfusion pressure across the shunt. Svo_2 is low (often <40%), and treatment directed first at augmenting contractility with inotropic agents and subsequently reducing afterload with a vasodilator. This is a serious clinical problem with a high mortality after a Norwood operation. The related myocardial ischemia and acidosis further impair myocardial function and systemic perfusion, leading to circulatory collapse.

Atrioventricular valve regurgitation and residual aortic arch obstruction are important causes of persistent low cardiac output and inability to wean from mechanical ventilation. Echocardiography is useful for assessing valve and ventricular function but is less accurate for assessing the degree of residual arch obstruction. Cardiac catheterization is sometimes necessary and will enable fine-tuning of hemodynamic support or balloon dilation of a hypoplastic segment of narrowed aorta. Occasionally, surgical revision of the aortic arch or atrioventricular valve is necessary, although this is seen more commonly in the interval before the bidirectional cavopulmonary shunt.

A more recent modification of the Norwood procedure involves placement of conduit from the right ventricle to the PA confluence (ventriculopulmonary shunt).[252–254] The primary advantage of this procedure in the immediate postoperative period is improved diastolic perfusion without runoff across an aortopulmonary shunt. Ventricular function is less likely to be compromised after surgery because the volume load to the ventricle is reduced from a lower Q_p/Q_s, along with a reduced risk for myocardial ischemia because of improved coronary perfusion. Perfusion to cerebral, renal, and splanchnic circulations also is likely to be improved with the lack of diastolic runoff to the pulmonary circulation, which may enhance postoperative recovery. Because pulmonary blood flow occurs only during ventricular systole across the right ventricle to pulmonary artery conduit, there may be a critical reduction in pulmonary blood flow and excessive hypoxemia, especially during periods of low cardiac output or if there is dynamic obstruction to flow at the ventricular insertion site. Efforts to overcome this limitation by creating a larger RV incision run the longer-term risk of ventricular dysfunction or aneurysm formation. The short-term survival advantage of the Sano modification of the Norwood operation for centers where mortality rate after the Norwood operation already was below 15% will be hard to demonstrate.

Orthotopic heart transplantation has gained acceptance as an alternative treatment for HLHS.[255] Neonatal transplants appear to be well tolerated, and some centers have avoided maintenance steroid therapy while achieving excellent mid-term results using transplantation as the sole therapeutic option for this disease.[255,256] Others have successfully advocated a combined approach using either transplantation or staged reconstruction, depending on the pathophysiologic state of the child and the availability of a donor heart.[257] However, the critical shortage of donor organs places a marked limitation on correction of this common congenital heart lesion.

It is apparent that many children have derived benefit from a completed, staged reconstruction or heart transplantation for this previously fatal illness. They are often able to lead active, productive lives and to develop normally.[258,259] Both survival and developmental outcomes for this disease are improving worldwide. However, the long-term prognosis for this evolving therapy will not be known for several years.

SUMMARY

The cardiac ICU has become the epicenter of activity in large cardiovascular programs. Nowhere are collaborative practices and multidisciplinary skills more valued or necessary. A curriculum in cardiac intensive care is now formally incorporated into cardiology training. Pediatric intensive care training programs have a mandate to include curricula and experience in management of postoperative cardiac patients. Specialists in this field must have in-depth training in cardiology but also be well versed in diagnosis and management of multiorgan system dysfunction, which is so vital to the discipline of intensive care. Increased complexity of disease, advances in technology and applied research, shortened lengths of stay, and improved survival all describe the fast-paced specialized environment that has accompanied the development of this new specialty of pediatric cardiac intensive care. Although the dramatic reduction in mortality has been gratifying in cardiac intensive care and is attributable to many factors, achieving 100% survival with minimal morbidity remains our elusive goal. It will challenge the next generation of practitioners.

REFERENCES

1. Guyer B, Hoyert DL, Martin JA, et al: Annual summary of vital statistics—1998. *Pediatrics* 104:1229-1246, 1999.
2. Arias E, MacDorman MF, Strobino DM, et al: Annual summary of vital statistics—2002. *Pediatrics* 112:1215-1230, 2003.
3. Friedman WF, George BL: Treatment of congestive heart failure by altering loading conditions of the heart. *J Pediatr* 106:697-706, 1985.
4. Friedman WF: The intrinsic physiologic properties of the developing heart. *Prog Cardiovasc Dis* 15:87-111, 1972.
5. Romero TE, Friedman WF: Limited left ventricular response to volume overload in the neonatal period: a comparative study with the adult animal. *Pediatr Res* 13:910-915, 1979.
6. Mills AN, Haworth SG: Greater permeability of the neonatal lung. Postnatal changes in surface charge and biochemistry of porcine pulmonary capillary endothelium. *J Thorac Cardiovasc Surg* 101:909-916, 1991.
7. Feltes TF, Hansen TN: Effects of an aorticopulmonary shunt on lung fluid balance in the young lamb. *Pediatr Res* 26:94-97, 1989.
8. Hanley FL, Heinemann MK, Jonas RA, et al: Repair of truncus arteriosus in the neonate. *J Thorac Cardiovasc Surg* 105:1047-1056, 1993.
9. McCrindle BW, Tchervenkov CI, Konstantinov IE, et al: Risk factors associated with mortality and interventions in 472 neonates with interrupted aortic arch: a Congenital Heart Surgeons Society study. *J Thorac Cardiovasc Surg* 129:343-350, 2005.
10. Planche C, Serraf A, Comas JV, et al: Anatomic repair of transposition of great arteries with ventricular septal defect and aortic arch obstruction. One-stage versus two-stage procedure. *J Thorac Cardiovasc Surg* 105:925-933, 1993.
11. Gladman G, McCrindle BW, Williams WG, et al: The modified Blalock-Taussig shunt: clinical impact and morbidity in Fallot's tetralogy in the current era. *J Thorac Cardiovasc Surg* 114:25-30, 1997.
12. Fisher DJ, Heymann MA, Rudolph AM: Fetal myocardial oxygen and carbohydrate consumption during acutely induced hypoxemia. *Am J Physiol* 242:H657-H661, 1982.
13. Clapp S, Perry BL, Farooki ZQ, et al: Down's syndrome, complete atrioventricular canal, and pulmonary vascular obstructive disease. *J Thorac Cardiovasc Surg* 100:115-121, 1990.
14. Greenwood RD, Rosenthal A, Parisi L: Extracardiac abnormalities in infants with congenital heart disease. *Pediatrics* 55:485, 1975.
15. Greenwood RD: Cardiovascular malformations associated with extracardiac anomalies and malformation syndromes. *Clin Pediatr* 23:145, 1984.
16. Lister G, Hellenbrand WE, Kleinman CS, et al: Physiologic effects of increasing hemoglobin concentration in left-to-right shunting in infants with ventricular septal defects. *N Engl J Med.* 306:502, 1982.
17. Sanders S: Echocardiography and related techniques in the diagnosis of congenital heart defects. *Echocardiography* 1:185, 1984.

18. Freed MD, Miettinen OS, Nadas AS: Oximetric detection of intracardiac left-to-right shunts. *Br Heart J* 42:690-694, 1979.
19. Rabinovitch M: Pulmonary hypertension. In Adams FH, Emmanouilides GC, editors: Moss' heart diseases in infants, children and adolescents. Baltimore, MD, 1983, Williams & Wilkins.
20. Bargeron LMJR, Elliot LP, Soto B: Axial cineangiography of congenital heart disease. *Radiology* 56:1075, 1977.
21. Fellows KE, Keane JF, Freed MD: Angled views in cineangiography of congenital heart disease. *Radiology* 56:485, 1977.
22. Geva T: Introduction: magnetic resonance imaging. *Pediatr Cardiol* 21:3-4, 2000.
23. Chung T: Assessment of cardiovascular anatomy in patients with congenital heart disease by magnetic resonance imaging. *Pediatr Cardiol* 21:18-26, 2000.
24. Freed MA, Heyman MA, Lewis AB: Prostaglandin E1 in infants with ductus arteriosus-dependent congenital heart disease. *Circulation* 64:889, 1981.
25. Yokota M, Muraoka R, Aoshima M, et al: Modified Blalock-Taussig shunt following long-term administration of prostaglandin E1 for ductus-dependent neonates with cyanotic congenital heart disease. *J Thorac Cardiovasc Surg* 90:399-403, 1985.
26. Lewis AB, Freed MA, Heymann MA: Side effects of therapy with prostaglandin E1 in infants with critical congenital heart disease. *Circulation* 64:893, 1981.
27. Donahoo JS, Roland JM, Ken J: Prostaglandin E1 as an adjunct to emergency cardiac operation in neonates. *J Thorac Cardiovasc Surg* 81:227, 1981.
28. Moler FW, Khan AS, Meliones JN, et al: Respiratory syncytial virus morbidity and mortality estimates in congenital heart disease patients: a recent experience. *Crit Care Med* 20:1406-1413, 1992.
29. Talner NS. Heart failure. In: Adams FH, Emmanouilides GC, editors: Moss' heart diseases in infants, children and adolescents. Baltimore, MD, 1983, Williams & Wilkins.
30. Jonas RA, Lang P, Mayer JE, et al: The importance of prostaglandin E1 in resuscitation of the neonate with critical aortic stenosis. *J Thorac Cardiovasc Surg* 89:314, 1985.
31. Norwood WI, Lang P, Hansen DD: Physiologic repair of aortic atresia-hypoplastic left heart syndrome. *N Engl J Med* 308:23, 1983.
32. Jonas RA, Hansen DD, Cook N, et al: Anatomical subtype and survival after reconstructive surgery for hypoplastic left heart syndrome. *J Thorac Cardiovasc Surg* 107:1121-1127, 1994.
33. Lang P, Chipman CW, Siden M: Early assessment of hemodynamic status after repair of tetralogy of Fallot: a comparison of 24 hour and one year postoperative data in 98 patients. *Am J Cardiol* 58: 795-799, 1982.
34. Wernovsky G, Wypij D, Jonas RA, et al: Postoperative course and hemodynamic profile after the arterial switch operation in neonates and infants. A comparison of low-flow cardiopulmonary bypass and circulatory arrest. *Circulation* 92:2226-2235, 1995.
35. Di Donato RM, Jonas RA, Lang P, et al: Neonatal repair of tetralogy of Fallot with and without pulmonary atresia. *J Thorac Cardiovasc Surg* 101:126-137, 1991.
36. Cullen S, Shore D, Redington A: Characterization of right ventricular diastolic performance after complete repair of tetralogy of Fallot. Restrictive physiology predicts slow postoperative recovery. *Circulation* 91:1782-1789, 1995.
37. Redington AN, Penny D, Rigby ML: Antegrade diastolic pulmonary arterial flow as a marker of right ventricular restriction after complete repair of pulmonary atresia with intact ventricular septum and critical pulmonary valve stenosis. *Cardiol Young* 2:382-386, 1992.
38. Bridges ND, Mayer JE Jr, Lock JE, et al: Effect of baffle fenestration on outcome of the modified Fontan operation. *Circulation* 86: 1762-1769, 1992.
39. Lemler MS, Scott WA, Leonard SR, et al: Fenestration improves clinical outcome of the Fontan procedure: a prospective, randomized study. *Circulation* 105:207-212, 2002.
40. Bohn DJ, Poirer CS, Demonds JF: Efficacy of dopamine, dobutamine, and epinephrine during emergence from cardiopulmonary bypass in children. *Crit Care Med* 8:367-373, 1980.
41. Wessel DL: Managing low cardiac output syndrome after congenital heart surgery. *Crit Care Med* 29(10 suppl):S220-S230, 2001.
42. Habib DM, Padbury JF, Anas NG, et al: Dobutamine pharmacokinetics and pharmacodynamics in pediatric intensive care patients. *Crit Care Med* 20:601-608, 1992.
43. Rosenzweig EB, Starc TJ, Chen JM, et al: Intravenous arginine-vasopressin in children with vasodilatory shock after cardiac surgery. *Circulation* 100:II182-II186, 1999.
44. Scheurer MA, Bradley SM, Atz AM: Vasopressin to attenuate pulmonary hypertension and improve systemic blood pressure after correction of obstructed total anomalous pulmonary venous return. *J Thorac Cardiovasc Surg* 129:464-466, 2005.
45. Caspi J, Coles JG, Benson LN, et al: Age-related response to epinephrine-induced myocardial stress. A functional and ultrastructural study. *Circulation* 84(suppl III):III-394-III-399, 1991.
46. Caspi J, Coles JG, Benson LN, et al: Effects of high plasma epinephrine and Ca2+ concentrations on neonatal myocardial function after ischemia. *J Thorac Cardiovasc Surg* 105:59-67, 1993.
47. Bailey JM, Miller BE, Lu W, et al: The pharmacokinetics of milrinone in pediatric patients after cardiac surgery. *Anesthesiology* 90: 1012-1018, 1999.
48. Chang AC, Atz AM, Wernovsky G, et al: Milrinone: systemic and pulmonary hemodynamic effects in neonates after cardiac surgery. *Crit Care Med* 23:1907-1914, 1995.
49. Hoffman TM, Wernovsky G, Atz AM, et al: Efficacy and safety of milrinone in preventing low cardiac output syndrome in infants and children after corrective surgery for congenital heart disease. *Circulation* 107:996-1002, 2003.
50. Mainwaring R, Lamberti J, Nelson J, et al: Effects of tri-iodothyronine supplementation following modified Fontan procedure. *Cardiol Young* 7:194-200, 1997.
51. Bettendorf M, Schmidt KG, Grulich-Henn J, et al: Tri-iodothyronine treatment in children after cardiac surgery: a double-blind, randomised, placebo-controlled study. *Lancet* 356:529-534, 2000.
52. Chowdhury D, Parnell VA, Ojamaa K, et al: Usefulness of tri-iodothyronine (T3) treatment after surgery for complex congenital heart disease in infants and children. *Am J Cardiol* 84:1107-1109, A10, 1999.
53. Dimmick S, Badawi N, Randell T: Thyroid hormone supplementation for the prevention of morbidity and mortality in infants undergoing cardiac surgery. *Cochrane Database Syst Rev* CD004220, 2004.
54. Colucci WS, Elkayam U, Horton DP, et al: Intravenous nesiritide, a natriuretic peptide, in the treatment of decompensated congestive heart failure. Nesiritide Study Group. [published erratum appears in *N Engl J Med* 343:1504, 2000] *N Engl J Med* 343:246-253, 2000.
55. Mills RM, LeJemtel TH, Horton DP, et al: Sustained hemodynamic effects of an infusion of nesiritide (human b-type natriuretic peptide) in heart failure: a randomized, double-blind, placebo-controlled clinical trial. Natrecor Study Group. *J Am Coll Cardiol* 34:155-162, 1999.
56. Publication Committee for the VMAC Investigators (Vasodilatation in the Management of Acute CHF): Intravenous nesiritide vs nitroglycerin for treatment of decompensated congestive heart failure: a randomized controlled trial. [published erratum appears in *JAMA* 288:577, 2002] *JAMA* 287:1531-1540, 2002.
57. Yancy CW, Saltzberg MT, Berkowitz RL, et al: Safety and feasibility of using serial infusions of nesiritide for heart failure in an outpatient setting (from the FUSION I trial). *Am J Cardiol* 94:595-601, 2004.
58. Turanlahti M, Boldt T, Palkama T, et al: Pharmacokinetics of levosimendan in pediatric patients evaluated for cardiac surgery. *Pediatr Crit Care Med* 5:457-462, 2004.
59. Janousek J, Vojtovic P, Hucin B, et al: Resynchronization pacing is a useful adjunct to the management of acute heart failure after surgery for congenital heart defects. *Am J Cardiol* 88:145-152, 2001.
60. Heath D, Edwards JE: The pathology of hypertensive pulmonary vascular disease: a description of six grades of structural changes in the pulmonary arteries with special attention to congenital cardiac septal defects. *Circulation* 18:533-547, 1958.
61. Wessel DL: Current and future strategies in the treatment of childhood pulmonary hypertension. *Prog Pediatr Cardiol* 12:289, 2001.
62. Drummond WH, Gregory GA, Heymann MA, et al: The independent effects of hyperventilation, tolazoline, and dopamine on infants with persistent pulmonary hypertension. *J Pediatr* 98:603-611, 1981.
63. Barst RJ, Rubin LJ, Long WA, et al: A comparison of continuous intravenous epoprostenol (prostacyclin) with conventional therapy for primary pulmonary hypertension. The Primary Pulmonary Hypertension Study Group. *N Engl J Med* 334:296-302, 1996.
64. Palevsky HI, Long W, Crow J, et al: Prostacyclin and acetylcholine as screening agents for acute pulmonary vasodilator responsiveness in primary pulmonary hypertension. *Circulation* 82:2018-2026, 1990.
65. Rosenzweig EB, Kerstein D, Barst RJ: Long-term prostacyclin for pulmonary hypertension with associated congenital heart defects. *Circulation* 99:1858-1865, 1999.

66. Zobel G, Dacar D, Rodl S, et al: Inhaled nitric oxide versus inhaled prostacyclin and intravenous versus inhaled prostacyclin in acute respiratory failure with pulmonary hypertension in piglets. *Pediatr Res* 38:198-204, 1995.
67. Petrossian E, Parry AJ, Reddy VM, et al: Endothelin receptor blockade prevents the rise in pulmonary vascular resistance after cardiopulmonary bypass in lambs with increased pulmonary blood flow. *J Thorac Cardiovasc Surg* 117:314-323, 1999.
68. Frostell CG, Fratacci MD, Wain JC, et al: Inhaled nitric oxide: A selective pulmonary vasodilator reversing hypoxic pulmonary vasoconstriction. *Circulation* 83:2038-2047, 1991.
69. Furchgott RF, Zawadzki JV: The obligatory role of endothelial cells in the relaxation of arterial smooth muscle by acetylcholine. *Nature* 288:373-376, 1980.
70. Ignarro LJ, Buga GM, Wood KS, et al: Endothelium-derived relaxing factor produced and released from artery and vein is nitric oxide. *Proc Natl Acad Sci U S A* 84:9265-9269, 1987.
71. Atz AM, Wessel DL: Inhaled nitric oxide in the neonate with cardiac disease. *Semin Perinatol* 21:441-455, 1997.
71. Wessel DL, Adatia I, Giglia TM, et al: Use of inhaled nitric oxide and acetylcholine in the evaluation of pulmonary hypertension and endothelial function after cardiopulmonary bypass. *Circulation* 88(5 pt 1):2128-2138, 1993.
73. Journois D, Pouard P, Mauriat P, et al: Inhaled nitric oxide as a therapy for pulmonary hypertension after operations for congenital heart defects. *J Thorac Cardiovasc Surg* 107:1129-1135, 1994.
74. Goldman AP, Delius RE, Deanfield JE, et al: Pharmacological control of pulmonary blood flow with inhaled nitric oxide after the fenestrated Fontan operation. *Circulation* 94(9 suppl):II44-II48, 1996.
75. Miller OI, Tang SF, Keech A, et al: Inhaled nitric oxide and prevention of pulmonary hypertension after congenital heart surgery: a randomised double-blind study. *Lancet* 356:1464-1469, 2000.
76. Adatia I, Atz AM, Wessel DL: Inhaled nitric oxide does not improve systemic oxygenation after bidirectional superior cavopulmonary anastomosis. *J Thorac Cardiovasc Surg* 129:217-219, 2005.
77. Adatia I, Atz AM, Jonas RA, et al: Diagnostic use of inhaled nitric oxide after neonatal cardiac operations. *J Thorac Cardiovasc Surg* 112:1403-1405, 1996.
78. Atz AM, Wessel DL: Sildenafil ameliorates effects of inhaled nitric oxide withdrawal. *Anesthesiology* 91:307-310, 1999.
79. Brecker SJ, Xiao HB, Mbaissouroum M, et al: Effects of intravenous milrinone on left ventricular function in ischemic and idiopathic dilated cardiomyopathy. *Am J Cardiol* 71:203-209, 1993.
80. Remme WJ: Inodilator therapy for heart failure. Early, late, or not at all? *Circulation* 87:IV97-IV107, 1993.
81. Vincent JL, Leon M, Berre J, et al: Addition of enoximone to adrenergic agents in the management of severe heart failure. *Crit Care Med* 20:1102-1106, 1992.
82. Duncan BW, Hraska V, Jonas RA, et al: Mechanical circulatory support in children with cardiac disease. *J Thorac Cardiovasc Surg* 117:529-542, 1999.
83. Extracorporeal Life Support Organization: *ECLS Registry Report: International Summary. 2002*. Ann Arbor, MI, 2002, Extracorporeal Life Support Organization.
84. Wessel D, Almodovar M, Laussen P: Intensive care management of cardiac patients on extracorporeal membrane oxygenation. In Dunan B, editor: *Mechanical support for cardiac and respiratory failure*. 2000.
85. Duncan BW, Ibrahim AE, Hraska V, et al: Use of rapid deployment extracorporeal membrane oxygenation for the resuscitation of pediatric patients with heart disease after cardiac arrest. *J Thorac Cardiovasc Surg* 116:305-311, 1998.
86. Chaturvedi RR, Macrae D, Brown KL, et al: Cardiac ECMO for biventricular hearts after paediatric open heart surgery. *Heart* 90:545-551, 2004.
87. Del Nido PJ, Armitage JM, Fricker FJ, et al: Extracorporeal membrane oxygenation support as a bridge to pediatric heart transplantation. *Circulation* 90(5 pt 2):II66-II69, 1994.
88. Ibrahim AE, Duncan BW, Blume ED, et al: Long-term follow-up of pediatric cardiac patients requiring mechanical circulatory support. *Ann Thorac Surg* 69:186-192, 2000.
89. Slonim AD, Patel KM, Ruttimann UE, et al: Cardiopulmonary resuscitation in pediatric intensive care units. *Crit Care Med* 25: 1951-1955, 1997.
90. Schindler MB, Bohn D, Cox PN, et al: Outcome of out-of-hospital cardiac or respiratory arrest in children. *N Engl J Med* 335: 1473-1479, 1996.
91. Chen YS, Chao A, Yu HY, et al: Analysis and results of prolonged resuscitation in cardiac arrest patients rescued by extracorporeal membrane oxygenation. *J Am Coll Cardiol* 41:197-203, 2003.
92. Del Nido PJ, Dalton HJ, Thompson AE, et al: Extracorporeal membrane oxygenator rescue in children during cardiac arrest after cardiac surgery. *Circulation* 86(5 suppl):II300-II304, 1992.
93. Booth KL, Roth SJ, Perry SB, et al: Cardiac catheterization of patients supported by extracorporeal membrane oxygenation. *J Am Coll Cardiol* 40:1681-1686, 2002.
94. Jaggers JJ, Forbess JM, Shah AS, et al: Extracorporeal membrane oxygenation for infant postcardiotomy support: significance of shunt management. *Ann Thorac Surg* 69:1476-1483, 2000.
95. Booth KL, Roth SJ, Thiagarajan RR, et al: Extracorporeal membrane oxygenation support of the Fontan and bidirectional Glenn circulations. *Ann Thorac Surg* 77:1341-1348, 2004.
96. Wessel DL, Adatia I, Giglia TM, et al: Use of inhaled nitric oxide and acetylcholine in the evaluation of pulmonary hypertension and endothelial function after cardiopulmonary bypass. *Circulation* 88:2128-2138, 1993.
97. Burch M, Lum L, Elliott M, et al: Influence of cardiopulmonary bypass on water balance hormones in children. *Br Heart J* 68: 309-312, 1992.
98. Ationu A, Singer DR, Smith A, et al: Studies of cardiopulmonary bypass in children: implications for the regulation of brain natriuretic peptide. *Cardiovasc Res* 27:1538-1541, 1993.
99. Carmichael TB, Walsh EP, Roth SJ: Anticipatory use of venoarterial extracorporeal membrane oxygenation for a high-risk interventional cardiac procedure. *Respir Care* 47:1002-1006, 2002.
100. Jenkins J, Lynn A, Edmonds J, et al: Effects of mechanical ventilation on cardiopulmonary function in children after open-heart surgery. *Crit Care Med* 13:77-80, 1985.
101. Robotham JL, Lixfeld W, Holland L, et al: The effects of positive end-expiratory pressure on right and left ventricular performance. *Am Rev Respir Dis* 121:677-683, 1980.
102. Pinsky MR, Summer WR, Wise RA, et al: Augmentation of cardiac function by elevation of intrathoracic pressure. *J Appl Physiol* 54:950-955, 1983.
103. Barash PG, Lescovich F, Katz JD, et al: Early extubation following pediatric cardiothoracic operation: a viable alternative. *Ann Thorac Surg* 29:228-233, 1980.
104. Schuller JL, Bovill JG, Nijveld A, et al: Early extubation of the trachea after open heart surgery for congenital heart disease. A review of 3 years' experience. *Br J Anaesth* 56:1101-1108, 1984.
105. Vricella LA, Dearani JA, Gundry SR, et al: Ultra fast track in elective congenital cardiac surgery. *Ann Thorac Surg* 69:865-871, 2000.
106. Newburger JW, Jonas RA, Wernovsky G, et al: Perioperative neurologic effects of hypothermic arrest during infant heart surgery. The Boston Circulatory Arrest Study. *N Engl J Med* 329: 1057-1064, 1993.
107. Reddy VM, McElhinney DB, Sagrado T, et al: Results of 102 cases of complete repair of congenital heart defects in patients weighing 700 to 2500 grams. *J Thorac Cardiovasc Surg* 117:324-331, 1999.
108. Costello JM, Backer CL, de Hoyos A, et al: Aprotinin reduces operative closure time and blood product use after pediatric bypass. *Ann Thorac Surg* 75:1261-1266, 2003.
109. Elliott M: Modified ultrafiltration and open heart surgery in children. *Paediatr Anaesth* 9:1-5, 1999.
110. Paret G, Cohen AJ, Bohn DJ, et al: Continuous arteriovenous hemofiltration after cardiac operations in infants and children. *J Thorac Cardiovasc Surg* 104:1225-1230, 1992.
111. Tabbutt S, Ramamoorthy C, Montenegro LM, et al: Impact of inspired gas mixtures on preoperative infants with hypoplastic left heart syndrome during controlled ventilation. *Circulation* 104(12 suppl 1):I159-I164, 2001.
112. Ramamoorthy C, Tabbutt S, Kurth CD, et al: Effects of inspired hypoxic and hypercapnic gas mixtures on cerebral oxygen saturation in neonates with univentricular heart defects. *Anesthesiology* 96:283-288, 2002.
113. Atz AM, Feinstein JA, Jonas RA, et al: Preoperative management of pulmonary venous hypertension in hypoplastic left heart syndrome with restrictive atrial septal defect. *Am J Cardiol* 83: 1224-1228, 1999.
114. Vlahos AP, Lock JE, McElhinney DB, et al: Hypoplastic left heart syndrome with intact or highly restrictive atrial septum: outcome after neonatal transcatheter atrial septostomy. *Circulation* 109: 2326-2330, 2004.

115. Chang AC, Hanley FL, Wernovsky G, et al: Early bidirectional cavopulmonary shunt in young infants: postoperative course and early results. *Circulation* 88(5 pt 2):II149-II158, 1993.
116. Fontan F, Baudet E: Surgical repair of tricuspid atresia. *Thorax* 26:240, 1971.
117. Castaneda AR: From Glenn to Fontan. A continuing evolution. *Circulation* 86:II80-II84, 1992.
118. Fontan F, Kirklin JW, Fernandez G, et al: Outcome after a "perfect" Fontan operation. *Circulation* 81:1520-1536, 1990.
119. Driscoll DJ, Offord KP, Feldt RH, et al: Five- to fifteen-year follow-up after Fontan operation. *Circulation* 85:469-496, 1992.
120. Gentles TL, Mayer JE, Jr., Gauvreau K, et al: Fontan operation in five hundred consecutive patients: factors influencing early and late outcome. *J Thorac Cardiovasc Surg* 114:376-391, 1997.
121. Gentles TL, Gauvreau K, Mayer JE, Jr., et al: Functional outcome after the Fontan operation: factors influencing late morbidity. *J Thorac Cardiovasc Surg* 114:392-403, 1997.
122. Penny DJ, Redington AN: Doppler echocardiographic evaluation of pulmonary blood flow after the Fontan operation: the role of the lungs. *Br Heart J* 66:372-374, 1991.
123. Redington AN, Penny D, Shinebourne EA: Pulmonary blood flow after total cavopulmonary shunt. *Br Heart J* 65:213-217, 1991.
124. Meliones JN, Bove EL, Dekeon MK, et al: High-frequency jet ventilation improves cardiac function after the Fontan procedure. *Circulation* 84:III364-III368, 1991.
125. Shekerdemian LS, Bush A, Shore DF, et al: Cardiopulmonary interactions after Fontan operations: augmentation of cardiac output using negative pressure ventilation. *Circulation* 96:3934-3942, 1997.
126. Gewillig M, Wyse RK, De Leval MR, et al: Early and late arrhythmias after the Fontan operation: predisposing factors and clinical consequences. *Br Heart J* 67:72-79, 1992.
127. Fishberger SB, Wernovsky G, Gentles TL, et al: Factors that influence the development of atrial flutter after the Fontan operation. *J Thorac Cardiovasc Surg* 113:80-86, 1997.
128. Karl TR, Sano S, Pornviliwan S, et al: Tetralogy of Fallot: favorable outcome of nonneonatal transatrial, transpulmonary repair. *Ann Thorac Surg* 54:903-907, 1992.
129. Pigula FA, Khalil PN, Mayer JE, et al: Repair of tetralogy of Fallot in neonates and young infants. *Circulation* 100(19 suppl):II157-II161, 1999.
130. Castaneda AR, Freed MD, Williams RG: Repair of tetralogy of Fallot in infancy. *J Thorac Cardiovasc Surg* 74:372, 1977.
131. Rocchini AP, Rosenthal A, Freed M, et al: Chronic congestive heart failure after repair of tetralogy of Fallot. *Circulation* 56: 305-310, 1977.
132. Fellows KE, Freed MD, Keane JF: Results of preoperative coronary angiography in tetralogy of Fallot. *Circulation* 51:561, 1975.
133. Dabizzi RP, Capriolo G, Aiazzi L: Distribution and anomalies of coronary arteries in tetralogy of Fallot. *Circulation* 61:95, 1980.
134. Shabbo FP, Wain WH, Ross DN: Right ventricular outflow reconstruction with aortic homograft conduit: analysis of the long-term results. *Thorac Cardiovasc Surg* 28:21-25, 1980.
135. Nudel D, Berman N, Talner N: Effects of acutely increasing systemic vascular resistance on arterial oxygen tension in tetralogy of Fallot. *Pediatrics* 58:248, 1976.
136. Borrow KM, Green LH, Castenda AR: Left ventricular function after repair of tetralogy of Fallot and its relationship to age at surgery. *Circulation* 61:1150, 1980.
137. Reduto LA, Berger HJ, Johnstone DE, et al: Radionuclide assessment of right and left ventricular exercise reserve after total correction of tetralogy of Fallot. *Am J Cardiol* 45:1013-1018, 1980.
138. Bove EL, Byrum CJ, Thomas FD: The influence of pulmonary insufficiency on ventricular function following repair of tetralogy of Fallot. *J Thorac Cardiovasc Surg* 85:691, 1983.
139. Lang P, Chipman CW, Siden H: Early assessment of hemodynamic status after 24 hours (intensive care unit) and one year postoperative data in 98 patients. *Am J Cardiol* 49:1733, 1982.
140. Murphy JD, Freed MD, Keane JF: Hemodynamic results after intracardiac repair of tetralogy of Fallot by deep hypothermia and cardiopulmonary and cardiopulmonary bypass. *Circulation* 62:1168, 1980.
141. Guntheroth WG, Kawabori I, Baum D: Tetralogy of Fallot. In Adams FH, Emmanouilides GC, editors: *Moss' heart disease in infants, children, and adolescents.* Baltimore, MD, 1983, Williams & Wilkins.
142. Murphy JG, Gersh BJ, Mair DD, et al: Long-term outcome in patients undergoing surgical repair of tetralogy of Fallot. *N Engl J Med* 329:593-599, 1993.
143. Nollert G, Fischlein T, Bouterwek S, et al: Long-term survival in patients with repair of tetralogy of Fallot: 36-year follow-up of 490 survivors of the first year after surgical repair. *J Am Coll Cardiol* 30:1374-1383, 1997.
144. Carvalho JS, Shinebourne EA, Busst C, et al: Exercise capacity after complete repair of tetralogy of Fallot: deleterious effects of residual pulmonary regurgitation. *Br Heart J* 67:470-473, 1992.
145. Gatzoulis MA, Balaji S, Webber SA, et al: Risk factors for arrhythmia and sudden cardiac death late after repair of tetralogy of Fallot: a multicentre study. *Lancet* 356:975-981, 2000.
146. Chandar JS, Wolff GS, Garson A Jr, et al: Ventricular arrhythmias in postoperative tetralogy of Fallot. *Am J Cardiol* 65:655-661, 1990.
147. Deanfield JE, McKenna WJ, Presbitero P, et al: Ventricular arrhythmia in unrepaired and repaired tetralogy of Fallot. Relation to age, timing of repair, and haemodynamic status. *Br Heart J* 52:77-81, 1984.
148. Marie PY, Marcon F, Brunotte F, et al: Right ventricular overload and induced sustained ventricular tachycardia in operatively "repaired" tetralogy of Fallot. *Am J Cardiol* 69:785-789, 1992.
149. Hanley FL, Sade RM, Blackstone EH, et al: Outcomes in neonatal pulmonary atresia with intact ventricular septum. *J Thorac Cardiovasc Surg* 105:406-427, 1993.
150. Hawkins JA, Thorne JK, Boucek MM, et al: Early and late results in pulmonary atresia and intact ventricular septum. *J Thorac Cardiovasc Surg* 100:492-497, 1990.
151. Giglia TM, Mandell VS, Connor AR, et al: Diagnosis and management of right ventricle-dependent coronary circulation in pulmonary atresia with intact ventricular septum. *Circulation* 86:1516-1528, 1992.
152. Silver MM, Pollock J, Silver MD, et al: Calcification in porcine xenograft valves in children. *Am J Cardiol* 45:685-689, 1980.
153. Heck HA, Schieken RM, Lauer RM, et al: Conduit repair for complex congenital heart disease. *J Thorac Cardiovasc Surg* 75:806, 1978.
154. Otero Coto E, Norwood WI, Lang P: Modified Senning operation for treatment of transposition of the great arteries. *J Thorac Cardiovasc Surg* 78:721, 1979.
155. Quaegebeur JM, Rohmer J, Brom AG: Revival of the Senning operation in the treatment of transposition of the great arteries. Preliminary report on recent experience. *Thorax* 32:517-524, 1977.
156. Senning A: Surgical correction of transposition of the great vessels. *Surgery* 59:334-336, 1966.
157. Senning A: Correction of the transposition of the great arteries. *Ann Surg* 182:287-292, 1975.
158. Hagler DJ, Ritter DG, Mair DD: Clinical, angiographic and hemodynamic assessment of late results after Mustard operation. *Circulation* 57:1214, 1978.
159. Danielson GK, Gale AW, McGraw DC: Great-vessel switch operation without coronary relocation for transposition of great arteries. *Mayo Clin Proc* 53:675, 1978.
160. Yacoub MH: The case for anatomic correction of transposition of the great arteries. *J Thorac Cardiovasc Surg* 78:3-6, 1979.
161. Jatene AD, Fontes VF, Souza LCB: Anatomic correction of transposition of the great arteries. *J Thorac Cardiovasc Surg* 83:20, 1982.
162. Castaneda AR, Norwood WI, Jonas RA: Transposition of the great arteries and intact ventricular septum: anatomical repair in the neonate. *Ann Thorac Surg* 38:438, 1984.
163. Pacifico AD, Stewart RW, Bargeron LM: Repair of transposition of the great arteries with ventricular septal defect by an arterial switch operation. *Circulation* 68(pt II):49, 1983.
164. Di Dontato RM, Fujii AM, Jonas RA, et al: Age-dependent ventricular response to pressure overload. Considerations for the arterial switch operation. *J Thorac Cardiovasc Surg* 104:713-722, 1992.
165. Wernovsky G, Giglia TM, Jonas RA, et al: Course in the intensive care unit after "preparatory" pulmonary artery banding and aortopulmonary shunt placement for transposition of the great arteries with low left ventricular pressure. *Circulation* 86:II133-II139, 1992.
166. Jonas RA, Giglia TM, Sanders SP, et al: Rapid, two-stage arterial switch for transposition of the great arteries and intact ventricular septum beyond the neonatal period. *Circulation* 80(3 pt 1): I203-I208, 1989.

167. Serraf A, Lacour-Gayet F, Bruniaux J, et al: Anatomic correction of transposition of the great arteries in neonates. *J Am Coll Cardiol* 22:193-200, 1993.
168. Kirklin JW, Blackstone EH, Tchervenkov CI, et al: Clinical outcomes after the arterial switch operation for transposition. Patient, support, procedural, and institutional risk factors. Congenital Heart Surgeons Society. *Circulation* 86:1501-1515, 1992.
169. Wernovsky G, Mayer JE Jr, Jonas RA, et al: Factors influencing early and late outcome of the arterial switch operation for transposition of the great arteries. *J Thorac Cardiovasc Surg* 109: 289-301, 1995.
170. Wernovsky G, Sanders SP: Coronary artery anatomy and transposition of the great arteries. *Coron Artery Dis* 4:148-157, 1993.
171. Day RW, Laks H, Drinkwater DC: The influence of coronary anatomy on the arterial switch operation in neonates. *J Thorac Cardiovasc Surg* 104:706-712, 1992.
172. Rastelli GC, McGoon DC, Wallace RB: Anatomic correction of transposition of the great arteries with ventricular septal defect and subpulmonary stenosis. *J Thorac Cardiovasc Surg* 58:545-552, 1969.
173. Mair DD: Long-term follow-up of Mustard operation survivors. *Circulation* 50(pt II):46, 1974.
174. Williams WG, Trusler GA, Kirklin JW, et al: Early and late results of a protocol for simple transposition leading to an atrial switch (Mustard) repair. *J Thorac Cardiovasc Surg* 95:717-726, 1988.
175. Merlo M, de Tommasi SM, Brunelli F, et al: Long-term results after atrial correction of complete transposition of the great arteries. *Ann Thorac Surg* 51:227-231, 1991.
176. Graham TP Jr, Atwood GF, Boucek RJ Jr, et al: Abnormalities of right ventricular function following Mustard's operation for transposition of the great arteries. *Circulation* 52:678-684, 1975.
177. Deanfield J, Camm J, Macartney F, et al: Arrhythmia and late mortality after Mustard and Senning operation for transposition of the great arteries. An eight-year prospective study. *J Thorac Cardiovasc Surg* 96:569-576, 1988.
178. Helbing WA, Hansen B, Ottenkamp J, et al: Long-term results of atrial correction for transposition of the great arteries. Comparison of Mustard and Senning operations. *J Thorac Cardiovasc Surg* 108:363-372, 1994.
179. Parrish MD, Graham TO, Bender HW: Radionuclide angiographic evaluation of right and left ventricular function during exercise after repair of transposition of the great arteries. Comparison with normal subjects and patients with congenitally corrected transposition. *Circulation* 67:178, 1983.
180. Benson LN, Bonet J, McLaughlin P: Assessment of right ventricular function during supine bicycle exercise after Mustard's operation. *Circulation* 65:1052, 1982.
181. Gillette PC, Kugler JD, Garson A: Mechanisms of cardiac arrhythmias after Mustard operation for transposition of the great arteries. *Am J Cardiol* 45:1225, 1980.
182. Gelatt M, Hamilton RM, McCrindle BW, et al: Arrhythmia and mortality after the Mustard procedure: a 30-year single-center experience. *J Am Coll Cardiol* 29:194-201, 1997.
183. Sagin-Saylam G, Somerville J: Palliative Mustard operation for transposition of the great arteries: late results after 15-20 years. *Heart* 75:72-77, 1996.
184. Ramsay JM, Venables AW, Kelly MJ, et al: Right and left ventricular function at rest and with exercise after the Mustard operation for transposition of the great arteries. *Br Heart J* 51:364-370, 1984.
185. Tanel RE, Wernovsky G, Landzberg MJ, et al: Coronary artery abnormalities detected at cardiac catheterization following the arterial switch operation for transposition of the great arteries. *Am J Cardiol* 76:153-157, 1995.
186. Weindling SN, Wernovsky G, Colan SD, et al: Myocardial perfusion, function and exercise tolerance after the arterial switch operation. *J Am Coll Cardiol* 23:424-433, 1994.
187. Massin M, Hovels-Gurich H, Dabritz S, et al: Results of the Bruce treadmill test in children after arterial switch operation for simple transposition of the great arteries. *Am J Cardiol* 81:56-60, 1998.
188. Jenkins KJ, Hanley FL, Colan SD, et al: Function of the anatomic pulmonary valve in the systemic circulation. *Circulation* 84:III173-III179, 1991.
189. Rhodes LA, Wernovsky G, Keane JF, et al: Arrhythmias and intracardiac conduction after the arterial switch operation. *J Thorac Cardiovasc Surg* 109:303-310, 1995.
190. Colan SD, Boutin C, Castaneda AR, et al: Status of the left ventricle after arterial switch operation for transposition of the great arteries. Hemodynamic and echocardiographic evaluation. *J Thorac Cardiovasc Surg* 109:311-321, 1995.
191. Fiser B: Infradiaphragmatic total anomalous pulmonary venous drainage. *J Cardiovasc Surg* 20:69, 1979.
192. Adatia I, Atz AM, Jonas RA, et al: Diagnostic use of inhaled nitric oxide after neonatal cardiac operations. *J Thorac Cardiovasc Surg* 112:1403-1405, 1996.
193. Raisher BD, Grant JW, Martin TC, et al: Complete repair of total anomalous pulmonary venous connection in infancy. *J Thorac Cardiovasc Surg* 104:443-448, 1992.
194. Jenkins KJ, Sanders SP, Orav EJ, et al: Individual pulmonary vein seize and survival in infants with totally anomalous pulmonary venous connection. *J Am Coll Cardiol* 22:201-206, 1993.
195. Haworth SG: Pulmonary vascular disease in secundum atrial septal defect in childhood. *Am J Cardiol* 51:265, 1983.
196. Horvath KA, Burke RP, Collins JJ, et al: Surgical treatment of adult atrial septal defect: early and long term results. *J Am Coll Cardiol* 20:1156-1159, 1992.
197. Collins G: Ventricular septal defect: clinical and hemodynamic changes in the first five years of life. *Am Heart J* 84:695, 1972.
198. Hoffman JIE, Rudolph AM, Heymann MA: Pulmonary vascular disease with congenital heart lesions: pathologic features and causes. *Circulation* 64:873-877, 1981.
199. Hoffman JI: Ventricular septal defect: indications for therapy in infants. *Pediatr Clin North Am* 18:1091, 1971.
200. Rabinovitch M, Haworth SG, Castaneda AR, et al: Lung biopsy in congenital heart disease: a morphometric approach to pulmonary vascular disease. *Circulation* 58:1107-1122, 1978.
201. DuShane JW, Kirklin JW: Late results of the repair of ventricular septal defect on pulmonary vascular disease. In Kirklin JW, editor: *Advances in cardiovascular surgery.* Orlando, FL, 1973, Grune & Stratton.
202. Friedman WF, Heiferman MF: Clinical problems of postoperative pulmonary vascular disease. *Am J Cardiol* 50:631-636, 1982.
203. Haworth SG, Sauer U, Buhlmeyer K, et al: Development of the pulmonary circulation in ventricular septal defect: a quantitative structural study. *Am J Cardiol* 40:781-788, 1977.
204. Vincent RN, Lang P, Elixson EM, et al: Measurement of extravascular lung water in infants and children after cardiac surgery. *Am J Cardiol* 54:161-165, 1984.
205. Cordell D, Graham TP, Atwood GF: Left heart volume characteristics following ventricular septal closure defects in infancy. *Circulation* 54:417, 1976.
206. Jarmakani JM, Graham TP, Canent RV: The effect of corrective surgery on heart volume and mass in children with ventricular septal defect. *Am J Cardiol* 27:254, 1971.
207. Jarmakani JM, Graham TP, Canent RV: Left ventricular contractile state in children with successfully corrected ventricular septal defect. *Circulation* (pt I):102, 45-47, 1972.
208. Jablonsky G, Hilton JD, Liu P: Rest and exercise ventricular function in adults with congenital ventricular septal defects. *Am J Cardiol* 51:293, 1983.
209. Mair DD, McGoon DC: Surgical correction of atrioventricular canal during the first year of life. *Am J Cardiol* 40:66-69, 1977.
210. Studer M, Blackstone EH, Kirklin JW, et al: Determinants of early and late results of repair of atrioventricular septal (canal) defects. *J Thorac Cardiovasc Surg* 84:523-542, 1982.
211. Capouya ER, Laks H, Drinkwater DC, et al: Management of the left atrioventricular valve in the repair of complete atrioventricular septal defects. *J Thorac Cardiovasc Surg* 104:196-203, 1992.
212. Rizzoli G, Mazzucco A, Maizza F, et al: Does Down syndrome affect prognosis of surgically managed atrioventricular canal defects? *J Thorac Cardiovasc Surg* 104:945-953, 1992.
213. Spach MS, Serwer GA, Anderson PA, et al: Pulsatile aortopulmonary pressure-flow dynamics of patent ductus arteriosus in patients with various hemodynamic states. *Circulation* 61:110-122, 1980.
214. Bancalari E, Jesse MJ, Gelband H, et al: Lung mechanics in congenital heart disease with increased and decreased pulmonary blood flow. *J Pediatr* 90:192, 1977.
215. Gerhardt T, Bancalari E: Lung compliance in newborns with patent ductus arteriosus before and after surgical ligation. *Biol Neonate* 38:96, 1980.

216. Mahony L, Carnero V, Brett C: Prophylactic indomethacin therapy for patent ductus arteriosus in very-low-birth-weight infants. *N Engl J Med* 306:506, 1982.
217. Rashkind WJ, Mullins CE, Hellenbrand WE, et al: Nonsurgical closure of patent ductus arteriosus: clinical application of the Rashkind PDA Occluder System. *Circulation* 75:583-592, 1987.
218. Laborde F, Noirhomme P, Karam J, et al: A new video-assisted thorascopic surgical technique for interruption of patent ductus arteriosus in infants and children. *J Thorac Cardiovasc Surg* 105: 278-280, 1993.
219. Burke RP, Chang AC: Video-assisted thoracoscopic division of a vascular ring in an infant. *J Card Surg* 8:537-540, 1993.
220. Burke RP, Wernovsky G, van der Velde M, et al: Video-assisted thoracoscopic surgery for congenital heart disease. *J Thorac Cardiovasc Surg* 109:499-507, 1995.
221. Robinson S, Gregory GA: Fentanyl-air-oxygen anesthesia for ligation of patent ductus arteriosus in preterm infants. *Anesth Analg* 60:331-334, 1981.
222. Zbar RI, Chen AH, Behrendt DM, et al: Incidence of vocal fold paralysis in infants undergoing ligation of patent ductus arteriosus. *Ann Thorac Surg* 61:814-816, 1996.
223. Fan LL, Campbell DN, Clarke DR, et al: Paralyzed left vocal cord associated with ligation of patent ductus arteriosus. *J Thorac Cardiovasc Surg* 98:611-613, 1989.
224. Odegard KC, Kirse DJ, Del Nido PJ, et al: Intraoperative recurrent laryngeal nerve monitoring during video-assisted thoracoscopic surgery for patent ductus arteriosus. *J Cardiothorac Vasc Anesth* 14:562-564, 2000.
225. Baylen B, Meyer RA, Korfhagen J: Left ventricular performance in the critically ill premature infant with patent ductus arteriosus and pulmonary disease. *Circulation* 55:182, 1977.
226. Elliott LP, Anderson RH, Bargeron KM, et al: Single or univentricular heart. In Adams FH, Emmanouilides GC, editors: *Moss' heart disease in infants, children and adolescents*. Baltimore, MD, 1983, Williams & Wilkins.
227. Mair DD, Edwards WD, Fister V: Truncus arteriosus. In Adams FH, Emmanouilides GC, editors: *Moss' heart disease in infants, children, and adolescents*. Baltimore, MD, 1983, Williams & Wilkins.
228. Marcelletti C, McGood DC, Mair DD: The natural history of truncus arteriosus. *Circulation* 54:108, 1976.
229. Bove EL, Lupinetti FM, Pridjian AK, et al: Results of a policy of primary repair of truncus arteriosus in the neonate. *J Thorac Cardiovasc Surg* 105:1057-1066, 1993.
230. Ebert PA, Robinson SJ, Stanger P: Pulmonary artery conduits in infants younger than six months of age. *J Thorac Cardiovasc Surg* 72:351, 1976.
231. Roth S, Keane JF: Balloon aortic valvuloplasty. *Prog Pediatr Cardiol* 3-16, 1992.
232. Anyanwu E, Klemm C, Achatzy R, et al: Surgery of coarctation of the aorta: a nine-year review of 253 patients. *Thorac Cardiovasc Surg* 32:350-357, 1984.
233. Lock JE, Bass JL, Amplatz K, et al: Balloon dilation angioplasty of aortic coarctations in infants and children. *Circulation* 68: 109-116, 1983.
234. Rao PS, Thapar MK, Galal O, et al: Follow-up results of balloon angioplasty of native coarctation in neonates and infants. *Am Heart J* 120:1310-1314, 1990.
235. McCrindle BW, Jones TK, Morrow WR, et al: Acute results of balloon angioplasty of native coarctation versus recurrent aortic obstruction are equivalent. Valvuloplasty and Angioplasty of Congenital Anomalies (VACA) Registry Investigators. *J Am Coll Cardiol* 28:1810-1817, 1996.
236. Jacobs ML, Norwood WI. Hypoplastic left heart syndrome. In Jacobs ML, Norwood WI, editors: *Pediatric cardiac surgery*. Boston, 1992, Butterworth-Heinemann.
237. Jenkins PC, Flanagan MF, Jenkins KJ, et al: Survival analysis and risk factors for mortality in transplantation and staged surgery for hypoplastic left heart syndrome. *J Am Coll Cardiol* 36:1178-1185, 2000.
238. Canter C, Naftel D, Caldwell R, et al: Survival and risk factors for death after cardiac transplantation in infants. A multi-institutional study. The Pediatric Heart Transplant Study. *Circulation* 96:227-231, 1997.
239. Osiovich H, Phillipos E, Byrne P, et al: Hypoplastic left heart syndrome: "to treat or not to treat." *J Perinatol* 363-365, 1920.
240. Ashburn DA, McCrindle BW, Tchervenkov CI, et al: Outcomes after the Norwood operation in neonates with critical aortic stenosis or aortic valve atresia. *J Thorac Cardiovasc Surg* 125: 1070-1082, 2003.
241. Kumar RK, Newburger JW, Gauvreau K, et al: Comparison of outcome when hypoplastic left heart syndrome and transposition of the great arteries are diagnosed prenatally versus when diagnosis of these two conditions is made only postnatally. *Am J Cardiol* 83:1649-1653, 1999.
242. Iannettoni MD, Bove EL, Mosca RS, et al: Improving results with first-stage palliation for hypoplastic left heart syndrome. *J Thorac Cardiovasc Surg* 107:934-940, 1994.
243. Forbess JM, Cook N, Roth SJ, et al: Ten-year institutional experience with palliative surgery for hypoplastic left heart syndrome. Risk factors related to stage I mortality. *Circulation* 92(suppl II): II-262-II-266, 1995.
244. Donner R: Hypoplastic left heart syndrome. *Curr Treat Options Cardiovasc Med* 2:469-480, 2000.
245. Mahle WT, Spray TL, Wernovsky G, et al: Survival after reconstructive surgery for hypoplastic left heart syndrome: a 15-year experience from a single institution. *Circulation* 102(19 suppl 3): III136-III141, 2000.
246. Tchervenkov CI, Jacobs ML, Tahta SA: Congenital Heart Surgery Nomenclature and Database Project: hypoplastic left heart syndrome. *Ann Thorac Surg* 69(4 suppl):S170-S179, 2000.
247. Mosca RS, Kulik TJ, Goldberg CS, et al: Early results of the Fontan procedure in one hundred consecutive patients with hypoplastic left heart syndrome. *J Thorac Cardiovasc Surg* 119: 1110-1118, 2000.
248. Daebritz SH, Nollert GD, Zurakowski D, et al: Results of Norwood stage I operation: comparison of hypoplastic left heart syndrome with other malformations. *J Thorac Cardiovasc Surg* 119:358-367, 2000.
249. Hoffman GM, Tweddell JS, Ghanayem NS, et al: Alteration of the critical arteriovenous oxygen saturation relationship by sustained afterload reduction after the Norwood procedure. *J Thorac Cardiovasc Surg* 127:738-745, 2004.
250. Mosca RS, Bove EL, Crowley DC, et al: Hemodynamic characteristics of neonates following first stage palliation for hypoplastic left heart syndrome. *Circulation* 92(suppl II):II-267-II-271, 1995.
251. Riordan C, Randsbaek F, Storey J: Balancing pulmonary and systemic arterial flows in parallel circulations: the value of monitoring systemic venous oxygen saturations. *Cardiol Young* 7: 74-79, 1997.
252. Maher KO, Pizarro C, Gidding SS, et al: Hemodynamic profile after the Norwood procedure with right ventricle to pulmonary artery conduit. *Circulation* 108:782-784, 2003.
253. Sano S, Ishino K, Kawada M, et al: Right ventricle-pulmonary artery shunt in first-stage palliation of hypoplastic left heart syndrome. *Semin Thorac Cardiovasc Surg Pediatr Card Surg Annu* 7:22-31, 2004.
254. Sano S, Ishino K, Kawada M, et al: Right ventricle-pulmonary artery shunt in first-stage palliation of hypoplastic left heart syndrome. *J Thorac Cardiovasc Surg* 126:504-509, 2003.
255. Bailey LL, Gundry SR, Razzouk AJ, et al: Bless the babies: one hundred fifteen late survivors of heart transplantation during the first year of life. *J Thorac Cardiovasc Surg* 105:805-815, 1993.
256. Armitage JM, Fricker FJ, del Nido P, et al: A decade (1982 to 1992) of pediatric cardiac transplantation and the impact of FK 506 immunosuppression. *J Thorac Cardiovasc Surg* 105:464-473, 1993.
257. Starnes VA, Griffin ML, Pitlick PT, et al: Current approach to hypoplastic left heart syndrome. Palliation, transplantation, or both? *J Thorac Cardiovasc Surg* 104:189-194, 1992.
258. Freedom RM: Neurodevelopmental outcome after the fontan procedure in children with the hypoplastic left heart syndrome and other forms of single ventricle pathology: challenges unresolved. *J Pediatr* 137:602-604, 2000.
259. Wernovsky G, Stiles KM, Gauvreau K, et al: Cognitive development after the Fontan operation. *Circulation* 102:883-889, 2000.

CHAPTER 30

Cardiac Transplantation

F. Jay Fricker

PEARLS

- Indications for transplantation are cardiomyopathy and complex palliated congenital heart disease with severe myopathic ventricular dysfunction.
- Pediatric patients on inotropic support or circulatory support and who have life-threatening arrhythmia receive priority for available donors.
- Selection of the agent to initiate inotropic support has evolved from sympathomimetic agents (dobutamine/dopamine) to the phosphodiesterase inhibitor milrinone.
- Nesiritide, a recombinant B-type natriuretic peptide, now is approved for treatment of acutely decompensated heart failure.
- It is imperative that immune suppression is initiated immediately after heart transplantation.
- The high-risk period for acute allograft rejection is in the first month after transplantation.
- Complications of immune suppression are infection, acute renal failure, and hyperglycemia.

Critical Care after Orthotopic Heart Transplant

It has now been a quarter of a century since the first successful pediatric heart transplant was performed at Stanford University.[2] The introduction of cyclosporine as the primary immune suppressant agent used in solid organ transplantation was a key discovery because it was the first selective immune suppressive agent used in solid organ transplant recipients. It has spared corticosteroid use and has made heart transplantation a cost-effective procedure.[17,48] In the past 25 years, perioperative mortality has become negligible. Advances have occurred in our understanding of the immune system, and improvement in critical care management of both donor and recipient patients has resulted in increased survival benefit. This chapter reviews critical care management of the pediatric patient with cardiopulmonary failure who is evaluated for orthotopic heart transplantation. Donor management, physiology of the transplanted heart, and preoperative and perioperative critical care all play important roles in the successful outcome of critically ill children with no option other than heart replacement surgery.

Indications for transplantation are cardiomyopathy and complex palliated congenital heart disease with severe myopathic ventricular dysfunction. Infants with hypoplastic left heart/aortic atresia and its variants have the option of palliation with the Norwood procedure and subsequent single ventricle approach with atrial to pulmonary connection. Heart transplantation in this group of infants is still an acceptable alternative approach to the Norwood procedure.[3,4]

The Pediatric Heart Transplant Study Group reviewed the causes of death after heart transplantation from a prospective database initiated in 1993. Patients were entered into the database on an "intention to treat" basis.[10,30,31,46] Using parametric data analysis with competing outcomes, death while waiting for transplant has been analyzed for all age groups, pretransplant diagnosis, blood type, and urgency status. Early death after heart transplant has been categorized as primary heart allograft failure. This includes inadequate preservation from long ischemic time and primary right ventricular failure from high pulmonary vascular resistance (PVR). Acute allograft rejection is an exceedingly rare event immediately after implantation. Late death after transplant is the result of posttransplant coronary vasculopathy, malignancy, or nonadherence to immune suppression regimens.[41,50]

The technical complexities of heart transplantation in children with palliated congenital heart disease resulted in perioperative mortality that exceeded 30% in the early experience. Difficulties in estimating PVR, variable pulmonary artery anatomy, and complications from multiple repeat thoracotomy and sternotomy all contributed to early morbidity and mortality.[56] Improvements in preservation techniques, technical experience, and recipient selection have reduced perioperative mortality to levels equivalent to transplantation in the primary cardiomyopathy patient who has not undergone previous operation.[46,56] Primary transplantation in the neonate with hypoplastic left heart syndrome (HLHS) has caused controversy because an acceptable surgical alternative is available and infant donor heart resource is limited.[3,4] In reviews from the Pediatric Heart Transplant Study Group Database, the mortality of infants waiting for donor heart availability exceeds 25%.[10] Currently, death while waiting for transplantation has decreased, but this decrease reflects the smaller number of infants listed and those who have opted for Norwood procedure and single ventricle palliation. The Norwood procedure does not preclude the possibility of future transplantation.

Late death after heart transplantation is related to either accelerated allograft coronary artery disease or primary malignancy.[42,50] The major cause of death in the adolescent heart transplant recipient now is noncompliance with the medical regimen.[13,41] With the decrease in perioperative mortality, we now expect 5-year survival after heart transplantation to exceed 70%. Rehospitalization after the first year is rare, and quality of life has been excellent.[25,41]

Critical Care of the Pediatric Patient Waiting for Heart Transplantation

An inadequate number of good donor hearts are available to satisfy the number of potential adult recipients. Statistics from United Network for Organ Sharing (UNOS) demonstrate this discrepancy between the number of potential recipients for heart and lung transplants and the availability of potential donors.[59] Donor availability for the pediatric patient is not as critical. Pediatric patients usually receive an appropriate donor offer unless they are infants or adolescents of a size that they are competing with critically ill adult patients. Guidelines from UNOS regarding organ distribution have changed to assure that pediatric adolescent donors are available first to potential adolescent and young adult pediatric recipients for both heart and lungs.

For potential heart transplant recipients, urgency criteria have been established for the most critically ill patient. Pediatric patients on inotropic support or circulatory support or who have life-threatening arrhythmia receive priority for available donors (Table 30–1).

Management of the Potential Heart Transplant Recipient

The pre-transplant management of the critically ill patient with end-stage myocardial function can determine the outcome of that patient after transplant. The principles of inotropic support, preservation of end-organ function, and attention to issues of nutrition and infection are the same for all critically ill patients in the pediatric intensive care unit.

Evaluation of the potential heart transplant recipient requires a careful pre-transplant hemodynamic assessment. This information can guide the fluid and inotropic therapy by optimizing preload and afterload while waiting for organ availability. The critical hemodynamic information influencing the function of the donor heart is an assessment of pulmonary artery pressure and PVR of the recipient before implantation. High PVR is associated with increased perioperative transplant mortality and adverse long-term outcome.[1,54] A transpulmonary gradient greater than 15 mmHg (mean pulmonary arterial pressure − mean left atrial pressure) is associated with higher incidence of heart graft dysfunction.[32,33] Preoperative hemodynamic assessment should include measurement of both left and right heart pressures with interventions to manipulate the PVR if elevated. Remeasuring hemodynamics with FiO_2 of 1, nitric oxide, prostacyclin, and aggressive vasodilator therapy to decrease systemic vascular resistance (SVR) can help determine if the patient is a heart transplant candidate or if he or she should be considered for lung or heart and lung transplantation.[21]

TABLE 30–1

Heart Transplantation Justification Pediatric Cardiology Status IA

- Requires assistance with a ventilator
- Requires assistance with a mechanical assist device (e.g., extracorporeal membrane oxygenation, left ventricular assist device)
- Requires assistance with intraaortic balloon pump
- Patient younger than 6 months with congenital or acquired heart disease exhibiting reactive pulmonary hypertension >50% of systemic blood pressure levels
- Requires infusion of a single high-dose inotrope (e.g., dobutamine ≥7.5 μg/kg/minute or milrinone ≥0.5 μg/kg/minute)
- Patient does not meet any of the criteria specified above but has a life expectancy without a heart transplant of <14 days (i.e., refractory arrhythmia)

Inotropic Support

Critically ill children with myopathic ventricular dysfunction severe enough for them to be in the intensive care unit are on inotropic support. These agents increase contractility through a common pathway of increasing intracellular levels of cyclic adenylate monophosphate (cAMP). Increased cytoplasmic levels of cAMP cause increased release of calcium from the sarcoplasmic reticulum and increase contractile force generation. Increases in cAMP occur either by β-adrenergic–mediated stimulation (increase in production) or phosphodiesterase III (PDE III) inhibition (decreased degradation.). Milrinone has proven to be a well-tolerated agent. Intravenous administration of milrinone increases cardiac output and reduces cardiac filling pressures, PVR, and SVR, with minimal effect on heart rate. Milrinone has been well studied in the pediatric population, and the benefit is primarily related to effect on SVR and PVR rather than inotropy.[19,58] Milrinone is initiated at doses of 0.25 μg/kg/min and increased to 1 μg/kg/min without adverse effects. We have not seen the heart acceleration or atrial or ventricular ectopy associated with dobutamine. Neither have we seen rapid tachyphylaxis with this agent. Milrinone has a long half-life and should be used cautiously in patients with hypotension. This drug is primarily excreted in the urine, so concentrations can increase in the presence of renal failure. We have observed severe hypotension and renal dysfunction precipitated by use of an angiotensin-converting enzyme inhibitor in a patient already on milrinone infusion. The addition of low-dose dobutamine (5–10 μg/kg/min) or epinephrine (dose 0.01–0.05 μg/kg/min) can help stabilize the critically ill child who is not responding adequately to milrinone therapy alone.

Nesiritide, a recombinant B-type natriuretic peptide, is now approved for treatment of acutely decompensated heart failure. Endogenous B-type natriuretic peptide is a cardiac hormone produced by the failing heart, and nesiritide is identical to the naturally occurring peptide. Nesiritide reduces preload and afterload, leading to increases in cardiac output/index without reflex tachycardia or direct inotropic effect. In addition, this drug promotes natriuresis, diuresis, and suppresses the renin-angiotensin axis and endogenous catecholamines. Although this drug has not been studied extensively in the pediatric group, in our and others' experiences, it has been found to be a safe and effective adjunctive therapy.[12]

Mechanical Support

Most patients waiting for transplantation who are on inotropic support do not remain hemodynamically stable indefinitely. Progressive end-organ dysfunction ensues, requiring escalation of support that includes multiple inotropic agents, in addition to respiratory and circulatory support. Mechanical circulatory support has become an important addition to the treatment armamentarium for the infant or child with decompensated heart failure and low cardiac output unresponsive to pharmacologic maneuvers. Options include extracorporeal membrane oxygenator (ECMO), intraaortic balloon, and left and right ventricular assist devices. Experience with ECMO as a bridge to heart transplantation has been reported by several pediatric transplant centers.[23,29] ECMO support can be used for 2 to 3 weeks without major complications from bleeding or infection, extending the window for donor organ availability. Isolated ventricular support devices, such as the Thoratec, Berlin heart, and DeBakey centrifugal pump, are now available for children.[40,51] These devices can be used in children as small as 0.7 m^2 or 20 kg. In the past, use of these devices had always been considered extraordinary and usually proposed in patients with severe end-organ dysfunction. Placement of a device in a patient with multisystem organ failure usually results in poor outcome. We propose that these devices be placed early before end-organ dysfunction, which enables rehabilitation of the patient, who then becomes a more optimal candidate for organ transplantation.

Anticoagulation

All patients with severe myocardial dysfunction are at risk for complications of systemic and pulmonary embolus. In our experience, nearly all explanted hearts have mural thrombi in both the left and right ventricles. Pulmonary emboli lead to increased PVR and the potential for lung abscess. The most devastating result of systemic embolus is stroke. All patients waiting for transplantation should be managed with systemic anticoagulation. Heparin is preferred but warfarin is acceptable in a stable patient on inotropic support. We add a word of caution regarding the use of low-molecular-weight heparin for prophylaxis. Enoxaparin cannot be easily reversed in a patient who must go to the operating room emergently because a donor heart has been identified. Cardiovascular surgeons prefer using heparin for prophylactic anticoagulation.

Management of the Potential Heart Donor

Many potential heart donors are lost because of suboptimal management after brain death has occurred. Associated with brain death is a catecholamine surge causing unnatural circulatory physiology that rapidly evolves, making management of the donor difficult. This intense sympathomimetic outflow initially causes vasoconstriction resulting in tachycardia, hypertension, and increased myocardial oxygen demand. The result can be a direct injury to the myocardium in the potentially transplantable heart. Myocardial structural damage is seen and includes myocytolysis, contraction band necrosis, subendocardial hemorrhage, edema formation, and interstitial mononuclear infiltration.[36] This initial sympathetic outflow is followed by a loss of sympathetic tone resulting in marked vasodilatation and hypotension. The hypotension and cardiovascular collapse are related to decreased SVR rather than primary myocardial dysfunction. Large fluid volumes and high-dose inotropic agents at α-adrenergic dosing range are administered, causing volume overload and vasoconstriction that can injure all donor organs. Hearts that are supported on high-dose inotropic agents likely will exhibit myocardial injury. A risk factor that predicts donor heart failure is a history of high-dose dopamine, dobutamine greater than 20 μg/kg/min, and epinephrine greater than 0.1 μg/kg/min.

Hormonal changes occur with brainstem injury and death. Early depletion of antidiuretic hormone causes inappropriate diuresis. Depletion of free triiodothyronine (T_3) has been implicated in myocardial dysfunction. Falling insulin levels lead to decreased intracellular glucose levels. Significant decrease in cortisol levels contribute to cardiovascular instability.[34,35,44]

Our present understanding of the physiology of brain death has resulted in "protocol" development for management of the potential donor.[45] The principles of support include the following:

- Invasive cardiovascular monitoring maintaining a mean arterial blood pressure greater than 60 mmHg and central venous pressure of 6 to 10 mmHg.
- Vasopressin is now the first-line blood pressure support medication because it treats diabetes insipidus in addition to supporting blood pressure. Infusion of less than 2.5 U/hour usually is sufficient to increase mean arterial blood pressure and not cause end-organ injury.
- Respiratory support to maximize oxygen delivery to transplantable organs. Recommended ventilatory strategies are aimed at optimizing oxygenation and preventing lung injury.
- Hormonal support including high-dose corticosteroids in the form of Solu-Medrol, insulin, and possibly infusions of the thyroid hormone T_3 or T_4. The benefits of thyroid hormone replacement in the brain-dead donor are debated, but there are studies supporting their use.[34,35,44] Resuscitation of the "marginal donor heart" is worth the effort given the shortage of available donor organs. Administration of T_3 has been advocated for reversal of myocardial dysfunction induced by the catecholamine surge of brain death.[44]

Critical Care Management of the Orthotopic Heart Transplant Recipient

Intraoperative Considerations

Heart replacement can be accomplished in virtually any congenital heart anomaly because the aorta, pulmonary arteries, and left atrium are in a relatively constant position near the midline. Regardless of malposition or positional relationships of the great arteries, the aorta of the recipient can be mobilized to make anastomosis with the donor aorta possible. The left atrium is a midline structure, and even when anomalies of the pulmonary venous return exist, pulmonary veins usually approach the midline and can be incorporated into the repair.[28]

Techniques of implantation have not changed significantly since the original description.[2,49] The newest innovation is the bicaval anastomosis.[22,55] This technique has the advantage of preserving sinus node function. Implantation techniques require that the pulmonary veins come to the midline. The pulmonary artery and aorta can be malpositioned but add little to the technical difficulty of the procedure. Aortic root size mismatch can, however, cause technical difficulty. Implantation of recipients with complex congenital heart disease usually can be accomplished by harvesting additional donor pulmonary artery, aorta, and caval tissue to replace deficient recipient tissue or to correct malposition of vena cava or great arteries.[11,28]

Donor heart function is related to proper management of the donor and the total ischemic time of the donor heart. The amount of time the aorta is cross-clamped on the donor until the aortic anastomosis is completed on the recipient (total ischemic time) is a major factor in early donor heart function. Nevertheless, donor hearts have been exposed to more than 8 hours of ischemia and recovered function after transplantation.

Early Perioperative Management

The early perioperative management of the recipient is not significantly different from the management of any postcardiac surgical patient. Significant physiologic changes in the newly transplanted heart can alter its response because of denervation. The major changes in the physiology of the transplanted heart related to autonomic denervation include alterations in diastolic dysfunction and exaggerated response to exogenously administered catecholamines. The transplanted heart also must adapt to a new environment related to recipient lung function and elevated PVR.

Autonomic system denervation results in a relatively fixed heart rate without respiratory variation. Heart rates are between 90 and 110 bpm but can be faster related to exogenous catecholamine administration. (Sinus node is transplanted with the donor heart.) Heart rates can be slower with injury to the donor sinus node. Injury to the blood supply of the sinus node in the donor heart is not uncommon, and 10% of recipients require permanent pacemaker therapy after transplant.[9]

Early blood pressure instability is common because of loss of regulation of baroreceptors and dependence of the transplanted heart on catecholamine administration. Hypertension occurs because of a fixed stroke volume into a systemic vascular bed that is abnormal because of longstanding compensatory changes in peripheral resistance arterioles.[61] Size mismatch between donor and recipient can also contribute. The other concern about donor heart/recipient mismatch is "big-heart" or hyperperfusion syndrome. A well-functioning large allograft generates a large stroke volume causing systemic hypertension and high cardiac output in a patient who previously had low cardiac output state. This increase in cerebral blood flow has the potential to cause cerebral vasoconstriction and symptomatic seizures, headache, or changes in mental status.[15,39,53] These symptoms are limited to the first few days after transplantation. There is a gradual adaptation in allograft stroke volume to the needs of the recipient. This adaptation of oversized cardiac allografts in children is part of the "shrink-and grow" phenomenon previously described.[14,18,39] The oversized donor heart eventually undergoes remodeling with regression of hypertrophy. Although this is a rare problem in children, symptomatic hypertension must be treated aggressively early in the perioperative period.

Early myocardial function of the transplanted heart is dependent on catecholamine support. Small infusions of β-adrenergic agents such as isoproterenol for several days often are necessary to maintain optimal heart allograft function.[52]

Hemodynamics of the transplanted heart reflect a significant shift to the left of the pressure/volume curve. Diastolic dysfunction can be demonstrated from the early transplant period. Why this hemodynamic abnormality is present early because of preservation injury is understandable, but diastolic dysfunction persists well into the recovery phase and beyond. Fluid administration of 10 ml/kg to a heart transplant recipient months remote from transplant will uncover an occult restrictive hemodynamic pattern. Pulmonary artery wedge pressure will increase by twofold, and right atrial pressure will increase more than expected.[48,60] In the normal heart, right atrial pressure will not change and left atrial pressure will increase by 1 to 2 mmHg in response to a fluid challenge.

Diastolic dysfunction is a significant impairment to early allograft function, limiting cardiac output. Diastolic dysfunction emphasizes the importance of heart rate and early sinus node function. The capability of temporary pacing in the early perioperative period is mandatory.

Management of Early Heart Allograft Dysfunction

Early heart allograft dysfunction is related to primary failure of the heart allograft because of unsuspected injury to the heart prior to procurement or because of preservation injury. The other major cause of primary allograft failure is elevated PVR in the recipient. Allograft failure is rarely caused by acute antibody-mediated injury. Risk factors associated with donor heart dysfunction, if present, should be factored into the decision of accepting that particular heart for your patient. Obviously the condition of the donor and expected length of survival can require the acceptance of a “marginal heart.”

Risk factors for donor heart dysfunction include “down time of the donor” (length of initial resuscitation), evidence of myocardial injury with elevation of troponin I, and a history of high-dose inotropic support (dopamine/dobutamine >20 μg/kg/min or epinephrine/norepinephrine >0.1 μg/kg/min) in the donor. Objective assessment of donor heart function can be made by obtaining an echocardiogram and electrocardiogram. The echocardiogram assesses donor heart systolic function (shortening fraction or left ventricular ejection fraction), presence of mitral valve regurgitation, and wall-motion abnormalities. The presence of any of these abnormalities makes the donor heart “marginal” for transplantation.

The other major reason for primary donor heart dysfunction is inaccurate measurement of the recipient’s PVR during the initial evaluation. We have known since the early days of heart transplantation that the donor right ventricle will not function when exposed to an abnormal pulmonary circulation. High PVR in the recipient increases perioperative morbidity and mortality and can affect late survival. All potential heart recipients undergo cardiac catheterization prior to heart transplantation to document the anatomy of systemic and pulmonary venous connections, determine pulmonary artery size and distribution, and calculate PVR. The upper limit of PVR associated with successful orthotopic heart transplantation is not known. Criteria developed from the adult heart transplant experience indicate a PVR greater than 6 Wood units or a transpulmonary gradient (pulmonary artery mean pressure − left atrial mean pressure) greater than 15 mmHg is associated with increased perioperative mortality.[1] The transpulmonary gradient is the most useful number for estimating PVR because measurement of cardiac output can be flawed. In children, PVR index (PVRI) determined by dividing transpulmonary gradient by cardiac index is more useful because children come in all sizes. PVRI less than 6 index units is associated with low perioperative mortality. Orthotopic heart transplants have been successful with PVRI greater than 6 and as high as 10 index units but with increased mortality. Diagnosis of high PVR is evident as the patient is weaned from cardiopulmonary bypass. Intraoperative transesophageal echocardiography (TEE) demonstrates dilatation of the right ventricle and small underfilled left heart. Acute management of high PVR and right heart dysfunction includes high FiO_2, and nitric oxide is administered at 20 to 40 ppm. The need for continuous pulmonary vasodilator medications in the immediate perioperative period is unusual, but prostacyclin and sildenafil both have proved effective in this situation.[24]

The sinus node artery from the donor heart is at risk at the time of procurement, and the incidence of sinus node dysfunction causing junctional rhythm or atrial flutter/fibrillation is 10% to 20%. Nearly 5% of children require pacemaker therapy after transplantation because of sinus node dysfunction.[9] All transplant recipients have temporary pacing wires, so bradyarrhythmias are not an issue. If the patient is in atrial flutter/fibrillation, then cardioversion should be performed. Persistent sinus node dysfunction with bradycardia can be problematic because of early diastolic dysfunction of the heart allograft. In the usual scenario, the patient returns from the operating room in an atrial paced rhythm. When the pacemaker is turned off, the underlying rhythm is a junctional rate between 100 and 120 bpm. As inotropic support is discontinued, the junctional rate slows to an unacceptable rate in the 50 to 80 bpm range. Usually an occasional atrial contraction is conducted, but the sinus node has been injured. Initiating theophylline at a dose of 10 mg/kg/day is helpful. Permanent pacing is recommended if sinus or atrial conducted rhythm has not returned within 2 weeks.

Heart Allograft Rejection and Immune Suppression

It is imperative that immune suppression be initiated immediately after heart transplantation. Solid organ transplants transfer antigen-presenting cells (APCs) that are recognized by the recipient’s human leukocyte antigen (HLA) immune system as foreign, which sets up a cascade of lymphocyte stimulation and proliferation. These lymphocytes then migrate to the heart allograft, where they can adhere to myocytes and endothelial receptors and cause tissue destruction. T-cell activation is the prime mover of allograft rejection. The initial signal is T-cell receptor binding of antigen on the surface of an APC. The APC is derived from the donor, a monocyte, or a tissue macrophage. Interaction of the APC and T-cell receptor causes release of interleukin (IL)-1 from the APC, which causes activation of the T cell. Activated T cells secrete IL-2 and other lymphokines that induce proliferation of activated T cells, which migrate to the allograft causing tissue damage.

Initial immune suppression protocols include high-dose corticosteroids, induction with IL-2 receptor blockade, or antithymocyte globulin, followed by introduction of the calcineurin inhibitors cyclosporine or tacrolimus (Table 30–2).

Induction protocols with lympholytic agents OKT3 or antithymocyte globulin are effective in delaying the time until the first allograft rejection episode but do not have a long-term survival benefit.[7] The benefit of induction with IL-2 receptor blockade has not been proven.

Corticosteroids have been part of standard protocols since the early days of solid organ transplantation. High-dose methylprednisolone (5–10 mg/kg) is administered at the time of aortic cross-clamp removal and continued in tapering doses over the first several days after surgery. Corticosteroids have immunosuppressive properties and benefit the allograft because of membrane-stabilizing and antioxidant effects on the graft.

More controversial is the timing of the introduction of calcineurin inhibitors cyclosporine and tacrolimus. A major complication in the early perioperative course is renal dysfunction, to which cyclosporine and tacrolimus are major contributors. The APC and lymphocyte receptor interaction occurs within hours of the transplant; therefore, early introduction of calcineurin inhibitors is important. Because bioavailability of these drugs is so variable, early, continuous intravenous administration of these drugs have been a standard protocol.[43] We continue to experience a group of recipients who develop acute renal failure with intravenous administration of these drugs. Current protocols are based on oral/nasogastric administration of a standard dose of tacrolimus beginning on the day of transplant. Target levels of this drug are reached 3 to 5 days after transplant if subsequent doses are based on the trough level obtained each morning[5] (see Table 30–2).

The high-risk period for acute cellular rejection (ACR) is the first month after transplantation. ACR is a phenomenon that rarely occurs in the first week after transplant. Hyperacute rejection is uncommon but can occur when a heart transplant recipient has preformed HLA antibody that reacts with a donor who has those specific HLA antigens. A positive cross-match will be reported, which means the recipient's serum causes lysis of donor T cells obtained from lymph nodes obtained at the time of organ procurement. Heart transplant recipients at risk for hyperacute rejection are identified by measuring evidence of prior sensitization to HLA antigens as part of the transplant evaluation. Children with palliated congenital heart disease are at particular risk for HLA sensitization because of exposure to blood products at the time of their previous surgical procedures. Rapid institution of plasmapheresis is the optimal way to clear the offending antibody causing heart allograft dysfunction.

The diagnosis of ACR is made by endomyocardial biopsy. Histopathology in cardiac tissue obtained by endomyocardial biopsy remains the gold standard for diagnosis of acute cardiac allograft rejection. The numbers of infiltrating lymphocytes and the presence of myocyte injury are used to grade rejection and to guide allograft rejection therapy. Surveillance endomyocardial biopsies are performed within the first 2 weeks after transplant and then at strategic times depending on the size of the child, access, and the technical difficulty of obtaining tissue.

Clinical recognition of acute allograft rejection can be subtle but obviously important because tissue diagnosis is not always possible, and surveillance techniques using peripheral blood, electrocardiography, and echocardiography have limitations. Acute cellular rejection can be present in the allograft without any symptoms or clinical findings. When ACR has progressed to hemodynamically significant allograft dysfunction, then symptoms of abdominal pain and vomiting are prevalent, and findings of systemic venous congestion, liver enlargement, and low cardiac output dominate. Symptoms of pulmonary venous congestion/pulmonary edema are rare findings. When ACR is suspected, histologic confirmation is always desirable if it can be safely performed. The principles of management are to acutely augment immune suppression with methylprednisolone or a lympholytic agent depending on the histologic and clinical severity of the heart allograft dysfunction. Following acute treatment, increases in maintenance of immune suppression agents are prescribed and follow-up endomyocardial biopsy is scheduled.

Complications of Immune Suppression in Heart Transplant Recipients Occurring in the Pediatric Intensive Care Unit

Infection

Infections are a major cause of mortality and morbidity early after heart transplantation.[16,47] Factors that predispose to infection can be divided into preexisting factors related to the donor and recipient, and factors secondary to events in the intraoperative and postoperative periods. For example, the site of the organ transplanted provides a clue to the site of infection. Renal transplant recipients acquire urinary tract infections, whereas heart transplant recipients are exposed to chest cavity infections. The type and severity of the underlying illness leading to organ failure can increase the risk for rejection. Children with cardiomyopathy can be severely malnourished, require prolonged mechanical respiratory or circulatory support, and have chronic indwelling venous catheters, all of which predispose to infection. The presence of a pretransplant pulmonary infarction is associated with lung abscess in the posttransplant recovery period.[20] Neonates may experience severe sepsis from coagulase-positive staphylococci more often than older children.

TABLE 30–2

Immune Suppression in Intensive Care Unit

Agent	Mechanism of Action	Dose	Monitoring	Major Side Effect(s)
INDUCTION IMMUNE SUPPRESSION				
Corticosteroids	Redistribution of peripheral lymphocytes, inhibit lymphokine IL-2 production, impair macrophage response to lymphocyte signals	2 mg/kg days 1–3 1 mg/kg days 4–7	Glucose	Infection, cushingoid appearance, hypertension, hyperlipidemia, glucose intolerance
Basiliximab	Monoclonal AB binds to IL 2 receptor	20 mg > 35 kg 10 mg < 35 kg, administer days 1, 4	CBC	Anaphylaxis
Antithymocyte globulin	Nonspecific T-cell lysis	1.5 mg/kg/day for 5–7 days	T-lymphocyte subsets	Thrombocytopenia, anaphylaxis, infection, PTLD, localized pain with RATG administration, serum sickness
Cyclosporine	Calcineurin inhibitor, inhibition of T-cell receptor lymphokine production and T-cell proliferation	2.5 mg/kg/ 24 hours IV	Monoclonal whole blood assay 100–400 ng/ml, depending on time since transplantation	Nephrotoxicity, central nervous system seizures, decreased magnesium, hypertension, hirsutism/gingival hyperplasia
Tacrolimus (FK 506)	Calcineurin inhibitor, inhibition of T-cell receptor lymphokine production and T-cell proliferation	IV 0.03 0.05 mg/kg/ 24 hours Oral 1.0 mg bid–increase (Baran), dose based on daily level	5–15 ng/ml, whole blood	Nephrotoxicity, anemia/neutropenia, headache, tremors, insomnia, glucose intolerance
MAINTENANCE IMMUNE SUPPRESSION				
Cyclosporine		5–20 mg/kg bid or tid		
Tacrolimus		0.3 mg/kg/day divided bid		
Sirolimus	Inhibition of T-cell activation and proliferation by preventing translation of mRNA	Loading dose of 3 mg/m^2 PO, then 1 mg/m^2/day given 4 hours after cyclosporine or tacrolimus	Triglycerides, platelets 5–10 mg/ml	Nephrotoxicity, hyperlipidemia, thrombocytopenia, leukopenia, gastrointestinal intolerance
Azathioprine	Antimetabolite inhibits purine and DNA synthesis	1–2 mg/kg/day	WBC <4000, ANC >1500	Bone marrow suppression
Mycophenolate mofetil		30–60 mg/kg/day in divided doses	WBC <4000 ANC >1500	Bone marrow suppression, gastrointestinal intolerance
Prednisone		1–3 mg/kg/day		
ACUTE CELLULAR REJECTION				
Methylprednisolone		10–25 mg/day for 3–4 days		
Antithymocyte globulin		1.5 mg/kg/day for 7–14 days		

ANC, absolute neutrophil count < 1000; *PTLD,* post-transplant lymphoproliferative disease; *RATG,* rabbit anti-thymocyte globulin.

The herpes virus family plays a significant role in infections occurring after transplantation. The clinical expression of cytomegalovirus and Epstein-Barr virus infection in the young patient is more severe because it is often a primary exposure.[8] Clinical infections related to these viruses rarely present before 1 month following organ transplantation and are most common in the first 6 months after heart transplantation.

Antibiotic management of the heart transplant recipient in the intensive care unit can be focused primarily on clinical suspicion, time of infection after transplant, and predisposing factors. Immune suppression is selective and targets T cells. Neutrophil function is normal except for the effect of high-dose corticosteroids. Neutropenia can be a problem occasionally because of bone marrow suppression caused by antimetabolites and tacrolimus. Prophylactic antibiotics in the form of third-generation cephalosporin is used for patients after sternotomy and continued until chest tubes and central lines are removed. The strategy against infection includes initial isolation, routine surveillance cultures, and regular replacement of indwelling catheters. In the early setting after transplantation, temperature elevation should indicate active infection and serious complication. If an infection is suspected, early aggressive investigation is necessary and broad-spectrum antibiotics/antifungal agents initiated until the source of the fever is identified.

Renal Function

Acute renal failure is a major complication following orthotopic heart transplantation. Renal failure is multifactorial in etiology, and the premorbid risk factors of heart transplant recipients cannot necessarily be controlled. We can monitor and control use of calcineurin inhibitor immune suppression agents. Therapeutic strategies include delayed initiation of cyclosporine and tacrolimus by using antithymocyte globulin IL-2 receptor blockade daclizumab for induction of immune suppression. The other option is to use a modified oral/nasogastric protocol for tacrolimus administration. This protocol targets tacrolimus levels to below 6 ng/ml in the first 3 days after transplantation and then aggressively increases dosing and target level over the next 4 days. It is important to avoid early intravenous administration of these agents because they invariably lead to renal afferent arteriolar vasoconstriction and oliguria. If renal dysfunction is complicating posttransplant course, it is still difficult to withdraw calcineurin inhibitors completely, but lowering the target level to less than 6 ng/L and substituting higher doses of mycophenolate mofetil and adding sirolimus are reasonable options.[26] The other means for reversing renal toxicity is to target mechanisms of calcineurin inhibitor toxicity. Renal arteriolar vasoconstriction is an imbalance between vasodilator prostaglandins and vasoconstrictor thromboxaneA_2. Thus prostaglandin E_1 (PGE_1) has been used for promoting renal vasodilatation with some success. Oral PGE_1 analogues have received mixed reviews. Calcium channel antagonists also have been used to prevent renal toxicity. Felodipine has been shown to cause a naturesis and prevent decline in renal hemodynamics produced by angiotensin II. We have not had enough experience using this potentially useful drug in reversing cyclosporine/tacrolimus nephrotoxicity.[27]

Diabetes Mellitus

Hyperglycemia is common after heart transplantation with tacrolimus-based immune suppression. The combination of decreased insulin production from islet cells caused by tacrolimus and decreased peripheral utilization related to high-dose corticosteroids results in nonketotic hyperglycemia. Insulin is initially mandatory in management but often can be discontinued if tacrolimus dose is reduced and the corticosteroid portion of maintenance immune suppression is discontinued.[37]

Future Management Strategies for Critical Care of Infants and Children with Cardiopulmonary Failure

Heart transplantation in children has gained wide acceptance as an important adjunct to treatment of children with end-stage cardiomyopathic function from cardiomyopathy and palliated congenital heart disease. Successful transplantation has produced longer and quality lives for many infants and children. Ten-year survival free of malignancy and coronary vasculopathy is the expected outcome.[6,57]

The future is moving toward fewer transplant procedures in children. Palliation techniques for complex congenital heart disease (i.e., single ventricle Fontan) are improving, and most of these patients will survive well into adulthood before requiring transplantation. Complications of adolescents with transposition of the great arteries who have undergone a Senning procedure and now present with systemic or right ventricular dysfunction will begin to disappear because of success with the arterial switch.

The natural history of cardiomyopathy is changing because of our understanding of the cellular mechanisms of myocardial function. New treatment strategies using angiotensin receptor and β-adrenergic blockade therapy are delaying or replacing the need for heart transplantation.

Circulatory support is being miniaturized by the development of the German heart and the DeBakey centrifugal pump. These devices can cause reversed ventricular modeling, allowing discontinuation of support without heart replacement therapy. The other major benefit of circulatory support is that, if initiated early, it can rehabilitate the child, recover end-organ function, and reduce the risks of heart transplantation surgery.

REFERENCES

1. Addonizio LJ, Gersony WM, Robbins RC, et al: Elevated pulmonary vascular resistance and cardiac transplantation. *Circulation* 76:52, 1987.

2. Baum D, Stinson EB, Shumway NE: The place for heart transplantation in children. In Godman, editor: *Pediatric cardiology,* vol 4. London, 1981, Churchill Livingstone.
3. Bailey LL, Gundry SR, Razzouk AJ, et al: Bless the babies; one hundred fifteen late survivors of heart transplantation during the first year of life. *J Thorac Cardiovasc Surg* 105:805, 1993.
4. Bailey L, Nehlsen-Cannarella S, Doroshow R, et al: Cardiac allotransplantation in newborns as therapy for hypoplastic left heart syndrome. *N Engl J Med* 315:949, 1986.
5. Baran DA, Galin I, Sandle D, et al: Tacrolimus in cardiac transplantation: efficacy and safety of a novel dosing protocol. *Transplantation* 74:1136, 2002.
6. Boucek MM, Edwards LB, Kec BM, et al: Registry for the ISHLT: seventh official pediatric report. *J Heat Lung Transplant* 23:933, 2004.
7. Boucek RJ, Naftel D, Boucek MM, et al: Induction immunotherapy in pediatric heart transplantation recipients: a multicentered study. *J Heart Lung Transplant* 18:460, 1999.
8. Boyle GJ, Michaels MG, Webber SA, et al: Post-transplantation lymphoproliferative disorders in pediatric thoracic organ recipients. *J Pediatr* 131:309, 1997.
9. Bryant RM, Harker K, Fricker FJ, et al: Natural history and treatment of sinus node dysfunction following pediatric heart transplantation. *Pediatrics* 102(suppl):684, 1998.
10. Canter C, Naftel DC, Caldwell R, et al: Survival and risk factors for death after cardiac transplantation in infants: a multi-institutional study. *Circulation* 96:227, 1997.
11. Chartrand C, Guerin R, Kangah M, et al: Pediatric heart transplantation; surgical considerations for congenital heart diseases. *J Heart Transplant* 9:608, 1990.
12. Colucci WS: Nesiritide for the treatment of decompensated heart failure. *J Card Fail* 7:92, 2001.
13. Douglas JF, Hsu DT, Addonizio LJ, et al: Noncompliance in pediatric heart transplant patients. *J Heart Lung Transplant* 111:S92, 1993.
14. Fukushima N, Gundry SR, Razzouk AJ, et al: Growth of oversized grafts in neonatal heart transplantation. *Ann Thorac Surg* 60:1659, 1995.
15. Fullerton DA, Gundry SR, Alonso de Bergma J, et al: The effects of donor-recipient size disparity in infant and pediatric heart transplantation. *J Thorac Cardiovasc Surg* 104:1314, 1992.
16. Green M, Wald E, Fricker FJ: Infections in pediatric heart transplant recipients. *Pediatr Infect Dis J* 8:87, 1989.
17. Griffith BP, Hardesty RL, Bahnson HT: Powerful but limited immunosuppression for cardiac transplantation with cyclosporine and low-dose steroid. *J Thorac Cardiovasc Surg* 87:35, 1984.
18. Hirsch R, Huddleston CB, Mendeloff EN, et al: Infant and donor organ growth after heart transplantation in neonates with hypoplastic left heart syndrome. *J Heart Lung Transplant* 15:1093, 1996.
19. Hoffman TM, Wernovsky G, Atz AM, et al: Prophylactic intravenous of milrinone after cardiac operations in pediatrics (PRIMACORP) study. *Am Heart J* 143:15, 2002.
20. Hsu DT, Addonizio LJ, Hordof AJ, et al: Acute pulmonary embolism in pediatric patients awaiting heart transplantation. *J Am Coll Cardiol* 17:1621, 1991.
21. Kao B, Balzer DT, Huddleston CB, et al: Long term prostacyclin infusion to reduce pulmonary hypertension in pediatric cardiac transplant candidate prior to transplantation. *J Heart Lung Transplant* 20:785, 2001.
22. Kirklin JK, McGriffin DC, Pinderski LJ, et al: Selection of patients and techniques of heart transplantation. *Surg Clin North Am* 84:257, 2004.
23. Kirshborn PM, Bridges ND, Myung RJ, et al: Use of extracorporeal membrane oxygenation in pediatric thoracic organ transplantation. *J Thorac Cardiovasc Surg* 1223:130, 2002.
24. Kulkarni A, Singh TP, Sarniak A, et al: Sildenaphil for pulmonary hypertension after heart transplantation. *J Heart Lung Transplant* 23:1441, 2004.
25. Lawrence KS, Fricker FJ: Pediatric heart transplantation: quality of life. *J Heart Lung Transplant* 6:329, 1987.
26. Lobach NE, Polllock-BarZiv SM, West LJ, et al: Sirolimus immunosuppression in pediatric heart transplant recipients: single-center experience. *J Heart Lung Transplant* 24:184, 2005.
27. Madsen JK, Sorensen SS, Hansen HE, et al: The effect of felodipine on renal function and blood pressure in cyclosporine-treated renal transplant recipients during the first three months after transplant. *Nephrol Dial Transplant* 13:2327, 1998.
28. Mayer JE, Perry S, O'Brien P: Orthotopic heart transplantation for complex congenital heart disease. *J Thorac Cardiovasc Surg* 99: 484, 1990.
29. Mehta U, Laks H, Sadeghi A, et al: Extracorporeal membrane oxygenation for cardiac support in pediatric patients. *Am Surg* 66:879, 2000.
30. McGriffin DC, Naftel DC, Kirklin J, et al: Predicting outcome following listing for cardiac transplantation in children: comparison of Kaplan-Meier and parametric competing risk analysis. *J Heart Lung Transplant* 16:713,1997
31. Morrow WR, Frazier E, Naftel DC: Survival after listing for cardiac transplantation in children. *Prog Pediatr Cardiol* 11:99, 2000.
32. Murali S, Uretsky BF, Armitage JM, et al: Utility of prostaglandin E1 in the pretransplantation evaluation of heart failure patients with significant pulmonary hypertension. *J Heart Lung Transplant* 11:716, 1992.
33. Murali S, Uretsky BF, Reddy PS, et al: Reversibility of pulmonary hypertension in congestive heart failure patients evaluated for car diac transplantation: comparative effects of various pharmacologic agents. *Am Heart J* 122:1375, 1991.
34. Novitzky D, Cooper DKC, Reichart B: Hemodynamic and metabolic responses to hormonal therapy in brain-dead potential organ donors. *Transplantation* 43:852, 1987.
35. Novitzky D, Cooper DKC, Human PA, et al: Triiodothyronine therapy for heart donor and recipient. *J Heart Transplant* 7:370, 1988.
36. Novitzky D: Donor management: state of the art. *Transplant Pro* 29:3773, 1997.
37. Paolillo JA, Boyle GJ, Law YM, et al: Posttransplant diabetes mellitus in pediatric thoracic organ recipients receiving tacrolimus-based immunosuppression. *Transplantation* 71:252, 2001.
39. Razzouk AJ, Johnston JK, Larsen RL, et al: Effect of over-sizing cardiac allografts on survival in pediatric patients with congenital heart disease. *J Heart Lung Transplant* 24:195, 2005.
40. Reinhartz O, Keith FM, EL-Banayosy A, et al: Multicenter experience with the Thoratec ventricular assist device in children and adolescents. *J Heart Lung Transplant* 20:439, 2001.
41. Ringewald JM, Gidding SS, Crawford SE, et al: Non-adherence is associated with late rejection in pediatric heart transplant recipients. *J Pediatr* 139:75, 2001.
42. Robbins RC, Barlow CW, Oyer PE, et al: Thirty years of cardiac transplantation at Stanford University. *J Thorac Cardiovasc Surg* 117:939, 1999.
43. Robinson BC, Boyle GJ, Miller SA, et al: Optimal dosing of intravenous tacrolimus following pediatric heart transplantation. *J Heart Lung Transplant* 18:786, 1999.
44. Rosendale JD, Kaufman HM, McBride MA: Hormonal resuscitation yields more transplanted hearts with improved early function. *Transplantation* 75:1336, 2003.
45. Rosendale JD, Chabalewski FL, McBride MA: Increased transplanted organs from the use of a standardized donor management protocol. *Am J Transplant* 2:761, 2002.
46. Rosenthal DM, Dubin AM, Chin C, et al: Outcome while awaiting heart transplantation in children: a comparison of congenital heart disease and cardiomyopathy. *J Heart Lung Transplant* 19:751, 2000.
47. Schowengerdt K, Naftel D, Selb P, et al: Infections after pediatric heart transplantation: results of a multi-institutional study. The Pediatric Heart Transplant Study Group. *J Heart Lung Transplant* 16:1207, 1997.
48. Schroeder JS, Hunt S: Cardiac transplantation: update 1987. *JAMA* 258:3142, 1987.
49. Shumway NE: Heart transplantation. *J Coll Physicians Surg* 24: 7, 1995.
50. Sigfusson G, Fricker FJ, Bernstein D, et al: Long-term survivors of pediatric heart transplantation: a multi-centered report of sixty-eight children who have survived longer than five years. *J Pediatr* 130:862, 1997.
51. Sidiropoulos A, Hotz H, Konertz W: Pediatric circulatory support. *J Heart Lung Transplant* 17:1172, 1998.

52. Stover EP, Siegel LC: Physiology of the transplanted heart. *Int Anesthesiol Clin* 33:11, 1995.
53. Tamisier D, Vouhe P, LeBidois J, et al: Donor-recipient size matching in pediatric heart transplantation: a word of caution about small grafts. *J Heart Lung Transplant* 15:190, 1996.
54. Tenderich G, Koener MM, Stuettgen B, et al: Pre-existing elevated pulmonary vascular long-term hemodynamic follow-up and outcome of recipients after orthotopic heart transplant. *J Cardiovasc Surg* 41:215, 2000.
55. Tsilimingas NB: Modification of bicaval anastomosis: an alternative technique for orthotopic cardiac transplantation. *Ann Thorac Surg* 75:1333, 2003.
56. Webber SA, Fricker FJ, Michaels M, et al: Orthotopic heart transplantation in children with congenital heart disease. *Ann Thorac Surg* 58:1664,1994.
57. Webber SA: The current state of, and future prospects for, cardiac transplantation in children. *Cardiol Young* 13:64, 2003.
58. Wessel DL: Managing low cardiac output syndrome after congenital heart surgery. *Crit Care Med* 29;S220, 2001.
59. UNOS. United Network for Organ Sharing. Available at www.unos.org.
60. Young JB, Leon CA, Short HD, et al: Evolution of hemodynamics after orthotopic heart and heart–lung transplantation: early restrictive patterns persisting in occult fashion. *Heart Transplant* 6:34, 1987.
61. Zelis R, Longhurst J, Capone RJ, et al: Peripheral circulatory control mechanisms in congestive heart failure. *Am J Cardiol* 32:82, 1973.

CHAPTER 31

Structure of the Respiratory System

Jacqueline J. Coalson

PEARLS

- The site where osseous and cartilaginous portions of the septum converge is frequent site of trauma that results in epistaxis because of the anastomosing vessels in the lamina propria.
- In infants, there is incomplete formation of the turbinate nasal bones, which likely makes nose breathing easier.
- In the nose of a child, there is relatively more mucosa and lymphoid tissue than in the nose of an adult.
- By the time the child reaches age 4 to 7 years old, the airway contains abundant tonsillar and adenoidal tissues.
- The epiglottis in the infant is longer, stiff, and U- or V-shaped and projects over the larynx at a 45-degree angle compared with the adult epiglottis, which is situated closer to the base of the tongue.
- The trachea in a child is smaller and shorter than the adult; this smaller size makes any reduction in the cross-sectional area substantially increase resistance to airflow.
- Lungs increase in volume from about 250 ml at birth to 6000 ml in the adult.
- At birth, the pulmonary artery and aorta are comparable in medial thickness and configuration and are the same size; by age 2 years, elastic tissue decreases in the pulmonary artery and its thickness is only about 60% that of the aorta.
- The diaphragm, the principle muscle of respiration, is essential during deep anesthesia because other muscles of respiration become inactive.

The respiratory system can be divided into several functional parts: conducting, respiratory, and ventilatory portions. The conducting portion of the respiratory system includes the nasal cavity and the associated sinuses, the nasopharynx, larynx, trachea, and bronchial and bronchiolar passages of the lungs. The primary function of this part of the respiratory system is to filter and cleanse the inspired air and then warm and moisten it before it reaches the respiratory level in the lungs. The respiratory portion is designed to facilitate the exchanges of gases between the inspired air and blood. The diaphragm and other respiratory muscles accomplish ventilatory function. This overview includes references to several excellent chapters and pertinent references that should be utilized for additional details.

Upper Respiratory System

Nasal Cavity[1,2,5,19,21,22]

The nasal cavity extends from the nares to the choanae, where it opens into the nasopharynx. In the child, the nares are angled forward and the passageway through the turbinates to the posterior nasopharynx is straighter toward the occiput.[5] It is divided into symmetrical halves by a median cartilaginous and bony septum. The inferior region of each fossa, the vestibule, is located immediately posterior to the external nasal opening and is lined by epidermis (continuous with the facial skin), which contains sebaceous glands and, after preadolescence, vibrissae (hairs). The vestibule serves as the first defensive site to filter large particulates and funnels air posteriorly. At the site where the osseous and cartilaginous portions of the septum converge, the epithelium thins and changes from squamous to respiratory. This is a frequent site of trauma that results in epistaxis because of the anastomosing vessels in the lamina propria. The ciliated respiratory epithelium covers the nasal cavity with a thin layer of mucus that provides immune protection (secretory immunoglobulin [Ig]A, lactoferrin, lysozyme, kallikrein). Seromucous glands are abundant in the mucosa of the nose and sinuses and are found superficially just below the surface epithelium or deeper with the blood vessels. Mucus is moved toward the nasopharynx by the cilia.

The primary nasal chambers are located within the skull. Within the nasal chambers, the wall along the septum is smooth, whereas laterally, turbinated projections (superior, middle, and inferior turbinates) protrude from the underlying ethmoid and inferior turbinate bones. This configuration ensures turbulence and increased surface area that allow for more contact between the inhaled particulate matter and the mucous lining. In infants, there is incomplete formation of the turbinate nasal bones, which likely makes nose breathing easier.

In the nose of a child, there is relatively more mucosa and lymphoid tissue than in the nose of an adult. In most sites, it is closely adherent to the underlying periosteum of the bone so that any swelling, as occurs in an inflammatory response or allergic disease, gives rise to edema or polyps that hamper or occlude the narrow air passages.

The olfactory mucosa in humans is found on the roof of the nasal cavity and the upper portions of the nasal septum. The mucous membranes of the frontal, ethmoid, and sphenoid sinuses are very thin and are closely applied to the underlying periosteal layer. The paranasal sinuses (maxillary, ethmoid, frontal, and sphenoid) are lined by a single layer of pseudostratified ciliated columnar epithelium in continuity with the nasal epithelium. The ethmoid and maxillary sinuses are present at birth, the frontal appears by age 5 to 6 years, and the sphenoid develops before adolescence.

Nasopharynx[1,19,21,22]

The nasopharynx is a continuation of the nasal portion of the respiratory tract and is covered with respiratory epithelium. Its mucosa differs from that of the nose in that large lymphoid aggregates are located beneath the epithelium, so *lymphoepithelium* is an appropriate term. The lymphoid component is particularly prominent in the fossa of Rosenmüller and in the upper posterior wall of the nasopharynx, where it constitutes the adenoids. Although lymphoid aggregates are small at birth, by the time the child reaches age 4 to 7 years, the pediatric airway contains abundant tonsillar and adenoidal tissues. The pharynx extends to the level of the cricoid cartilage. The lowest portion of the pharynx divides into the larynx and the esophagus.

Larynx

The larynx sits on the ring-shaped cricoid cartilage, which abuts on the trachea.[1,5,7,21,22] In the infant, the larynx is situated more cephalad than in the adult. As the neck lengthens with growth, it moves caudad. The supporting structures of the larynx consist of four cartilaginous structures: epiglottic cartilage, thyroid cartilage, arytenoid cartilages, and cricoid cartilage. Internally, the larynx has three pairs of lateral folds: the aryepiglottic, then the ventricular folds or false folds, followed by the true vocal folds. Between the true vocal and ventricular folds, side walls of the larynx recess to form the laryngeal ventricles. The epiglottis projects upward from the interior wall of the larynx and is broad and flat in the adult (Figure 31–1). The epiglottis in the adult is situated closer to the base of the tongue. In the infant, the epiglottis is longer, stiff, and U- or V-shaped and projects over the larynx at a 45-degree angle. The mucosa of the larynx, being continuous with that of the pharynx and trachea, has features of both. Stratified squamous epithelium extends over the aryepiglottic folds, the entire lingual side of the epiglottis, the upper half of the epiglottis' laryngeal aspect, the vocal folds, and the arytenoid cartilages (supraglottic area). Beneath the vocal cords, the larynx is lined by pseudostratified ciliated columnar epithelium, with a transition zone of stratified columnar epithelium. The glands of the larynx are comparable with those in the trachea and bronchi, but they are not present within the

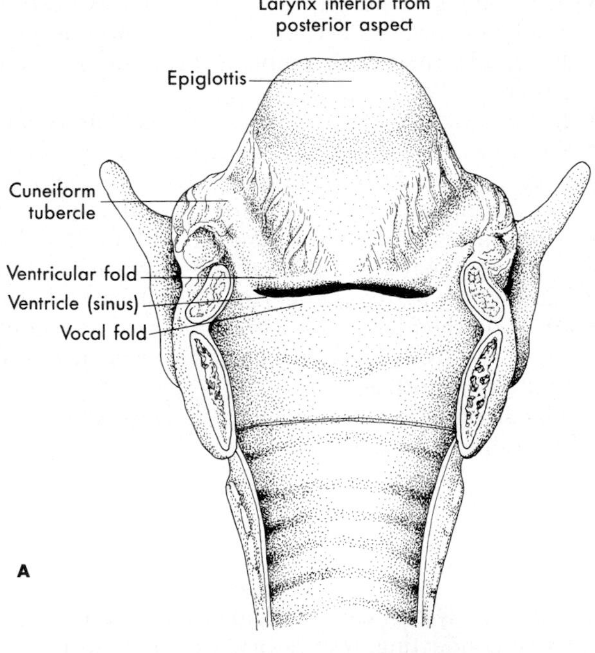

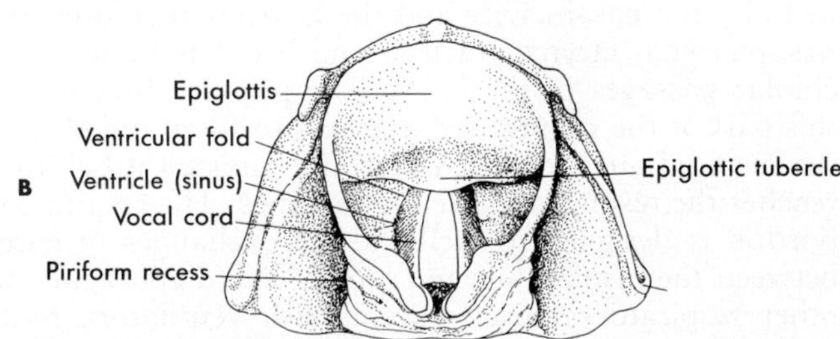

FIGURE 31–1 • **A,** Interior of the larynx, posterior view. **B,** Larynx from above. (Redrawn from Grant JB: *Atlas of anatomy,* ed 4. Baltimore, 1956, Williams & Wilkins.)

true vocal folds. Constriction of the pharyngeal wall and upward movement of the larynx, trachea, and pharynx associated with a depression of the epiglottis are noted during swallowing. Innervation of the larynx represents both sensory and motor cortices, which help to control phonation, cough reflex, and swallowing.

Lower Respiratory System

Trachea[4,8,12,13,19,21]

Originating at the base of the larynx and ending at the carina, the trachea is reinforced by a skeleton of cartilage and conditions the air as it passes to the lungs. In the adult, it is approximately 22 cm long and 2 cm in diameter. Because the trachea is smaller and shorter in the child, any reduction in cross-sectional area substantially increases the resistance to air flow. Its respiratory mucosa contains several cell types, including ciliated columnar, goblet, nonciliated columnar cells (brush cells), and short cells. By electron microscopy, an additional neurosecretory cell type is noted. The C-shaped hyaline cartilages are surrounded by perichondrium that blends into a fibroelastic membrane that intermingles with some muscle in the cartilage-free zone posteriorly. The abundant tubuloalveolar tracheal glands extend into the submucosa and consist of ciliated and collecting duct cells and mixed mucus with serous cell crescents. They open into the tracheal lumen at intervals of at least 1 mm. The primary bronchi of the right and left lungs are extrapulmonary, arising in the mediastinum from the bifurcation of the trachea at the level of T5-6. The left main bronchus is narrower and longer and branches at a greater angle from the trachea than the right bronchus. They differ from the trachea only in their cartilage configuration (less regular) and musculature (more complete muscularis).

The trachea's nervous, vascular, and lymphatic supplies are independent of those to the lungs. The trachea receives its systemic blood through the branches of the inferior thyroid artery (Figure 31–2). Near the carina, the branches anastomose with the bronchial arteries. Tracheal lymphatics drain to the superior deep cervical chain of lymph nodes, along with a few paratracheal nodes. Visceral afferent fibers and sympathetic and parasympathetic efferent fibers constitute the neural supply to the trachea.

Lungs[8,11,12,13,19,20,21,24,25]

Lung weights of children from birth to age 12 years have been published.[4] At birth, the lungs weigh about 40 g and double in weight by 6 months. By age 2 years, when most of the alveolarization process is completed, they weigh about 170 g total. In the normal adult, the lungs weigh approximately 1000 g.[20] Lungs increase in volume from about 250 ml at birth to 6000 ml in the adult. The height of a normal adult lung is 27 cm at total lung capacity, but in the range of normal breathing it is

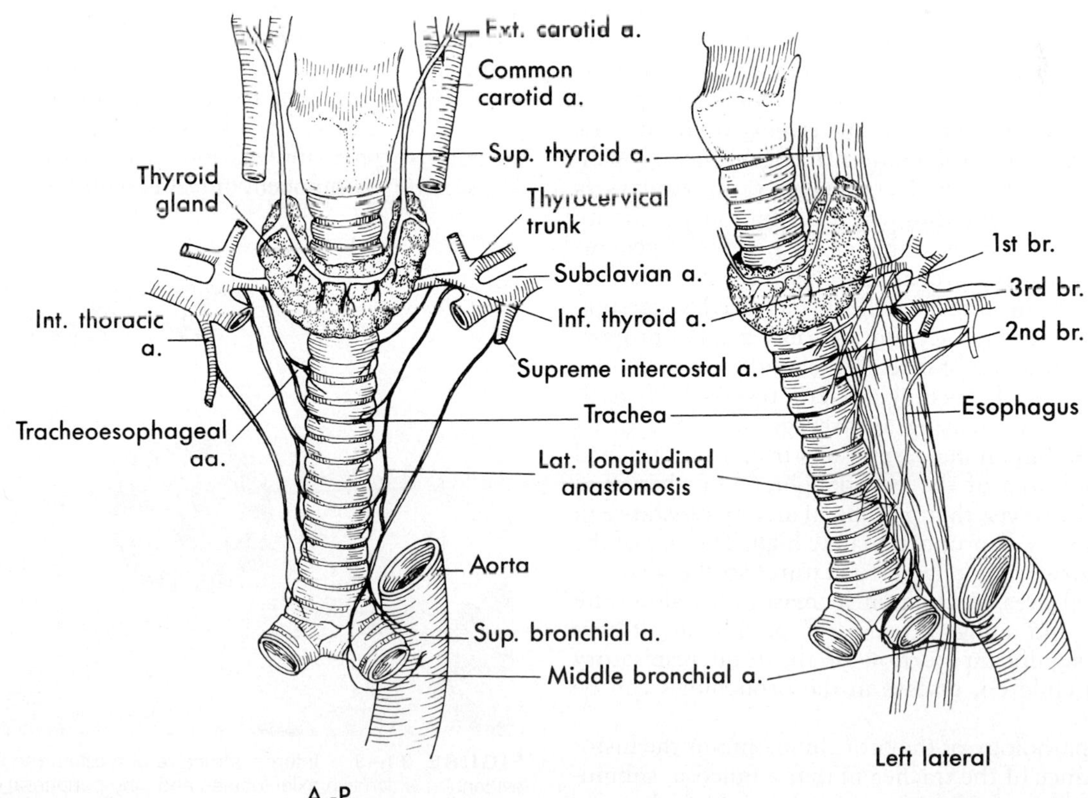

FIGURE 31–2 • Vascular supply of the trachea. (Redrawn from Ravitch MM: *Atlas of general thoracic surgery.* Philadelphia, 1988, WB Saunders.)

approximately 24 cm in height. Externally, the lungs are paired structures that, with the mediastinum, fill the thoracic cavity. The right lung, with its three lobes, and the left, with its two lobes, have hili that receive a primary bronchus, pulmonary artery and veins, bronchial arteries and veins, lymphatics, and nerves. The lobes are subdivided into bronchopulmonary segments, which are demarcated by fissures over the surface of the lung. The visceral pleura covers the surface of, and dips into, the lung to form the interlobular septa. On entering the lung from their short extrapulmonary course, the bronchi and their accompanying pulmonary artery branch into lobar bronchi and then into segmental bronchi that supply the 19 bronchopulmonary segments of the lung. The bronchopulmonary segments are bounded by connective tissue septa that allow surgeons to perform resections. The pulmonary veins do not course with the airway and pulmonary artery dyad; instead they course midway between the dyads and can be readily identified in the septa.

Airways and Bronchus-Associated Lymphoid Tissue[4,8,11,12,16,21,24]

The airway branching pattern in the lung undergoes multiple generations, yielding a total of 27 or 28 divisions when counting begins from the primary bronchus. The bronchi are the larger intrinsic cartilaginous airways and comprise 9 to 12 generations starting with the primary bronchus and terminating in bronchi having a diameter of approximately 1 mm. Bronchioles, sometimes called *membranous bronchioles* or *distal noncartilaginous airways,* are the last of the conducting system. They comprise an additional 12 generations before ending as terminal bronchioles, the last purely conducting structure in the lung. Horsfield and Cumming[11] showed that the course from the trachea to the alveolar level may be as few as 8 or as many as 24 airway branch points. This points out that a particular airway diameter may occur at various points along the distribution of the bronchial wall. Determination of the total cross section of airways is important in understanding the distribution of airway resistance. Weibel[25] showed that as the peripheral generations of the airways are approached, the total cross-sectional area of the lung is markedly increased, suggesting that peripheral airways account for only a small proportion of total airway resistance. In the adult, the asymmetrical dichotomous branching pattern results with each daughter branch decreasing an average of 0.75% of its parent branch, but an increase results from the combined cross-sectional area of the two daughter branches. It is well known, however, that peripheral airway resistance in children's lungs is disproportionately high. The size of the conducting airways is related to stature, so the airways' cross-sectional area in children increases at a slow rate with growth and aging. Because the peripheral airways make up a significant portion of the total respiratory resistance in children, disease in the bronchioles can be serious.

The histopathology of the bronchi maintains the histologic appearance of the trachea in that a mucosa, submucosa, muscularis, and adventitia are present. As the bronchi branch deeper into the lung parenchyma, the cartilage rings become plates and less regular, and the muscularis becomes continuous, being located between the submucosa and the cartilage plates. As the bronchi decrease in diameter, the pseudostratified columnar epithelium becomes lower, and the mucoserous glands become fewer in number. Although the glands wane in number in the more distal parts of the lung, mucous cells persist and are found in very small bronchi and in some of the membranous bronchioles. A rich capillary plexus, a loose network of fibers and cells, and unmyelinated nerves encircle the airways.

The pseudostratified columnar epithelium of the bronchi contains several cell types: ciliated, epithelial mucous, basal, brush, and neuroendocrine. The ciliated cell constitutes more than 90% of the epithelial cell population in the conducting airways, but the proportion and number of cilia per cell decrease from the proximal to distal airways. The 9+2 microtubular structure within the cilia has been shown to be altered in the primary ciliary syndromes (Figure 31–3). In addition to its ciliary beating movement, the ciliated cells regulate the depth of the composition of the periciliary fluid and transports ions across the epithelium. The basal cell, like mucous and Clara cells, has a progenitor cell role; it also functions to adhere the columnar cells to the basement membrane. The brush cell, thought to have a role in fluid absorption and/or chemoreceptor function, is found rarely in the tracheobronchial and alveolar epithelia.

The mucociliary apparatus is the primary defense mechanism in the respiratory system. Although mucous cells secrete mucin, the submucosal glands produce more than 90% of the mucus needed for mucociliary function. The glands contain mucous, serous, myoepithelial cells, collecting duct cells, and occasional neuroendocrine (Kulchitsky) cells. The physical characteristics of the mucous layer reveal that the superficial layer is more viscous than the deeper layer. This difference in consistency of the mucous layer allows the cilia to function properly, allowing a power and recovery stroke mechanism. The secretions include lysozyme, antileukoprotease, lactoferrin, and IgA. The secretory component of IgA is synthesized in bronchial

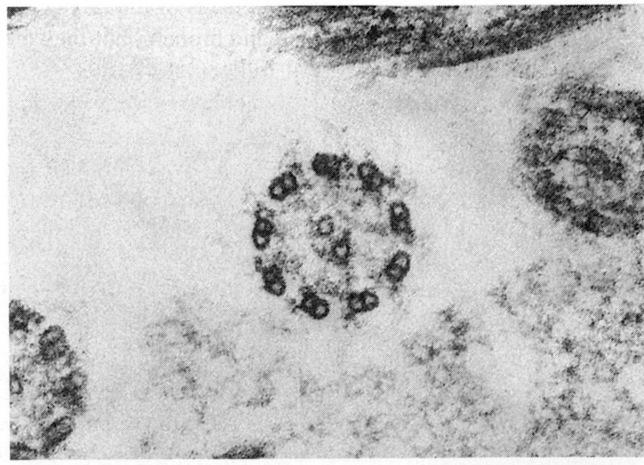

FIGURE 31–3 • Internal structure of a cilium (no cell membrane evident) in which two axial tubules and nine peripheral duplex tubules are seen. Dynein arms are attached to several of the peripheral duplex tubules (magnification ×13,500).

gland cells and expressed on their basolateral cell surfaces to which IgA dimers synthesized by plasma cells bind. The complex is endocytosed by the glandular cell and then is secreted from its luminal surface.

Neuroendocrine cells can be solitary near the basal lamina between columnar cells or in collections called *neuroepithelial bodies* that occur near branch points of bronchi. A number of neural markers are expressed (e.g., 5-hydroxytryptamine, chromogranin A, neuron-specific enolase, synaptophysin) and a number of hormones produced (e.g., endothelin, calcitonin, bombesin [gastrin-releasing peptide]). They are more abundant in the fetus and likely have a role in lung growth or maturation.

Mast cells are an important population of cells found in great abundance in the submucosa and connective tissue in lungs. They contain cytoplasmic granules and produce two neutral proteases: chymase and tryptase. They release lysosomal enzymes (arylsulfatase, B-glucuronidase, myeloperoxidase) and various mediators (e.g., histamine, eosinophil chemotactic factor of anaphylaxis, heparin), and they help mediate important physiologic events, such as IgE-dependent bronchial asthma.

Bronchus-associated lymphoid tissue (BALT) appears as isolated nodules in the connective tissue of the lamina propria of the bronchial tree and produces primarily IgG and secretory IgA. Collections of BALT cells tend to occur at airway bifurcations and are covered by a special epithelium that can pinocytose and transport solutes and particulate antigens. BALT is sparse at birth but starts accumulating thereafter. It is prominent in lungs of children and in diseased lungs of smokers and patients with bronchiectasis. Although more than 50% of the cells are B lymphocytes, T lymphocytes are also found (18%), along with follicular dendritic cells[4]. Sometimes these nodules bulge into the bronchial lumen. Additional lymphoid tissue in the lung is a rich supply of lymph nodes within the lung, at the carina, and along the trachea.

Although originally defined as having a lumen diameter less than 2 mm, the term *small airway* usually refers to a bronchiole. A bronchiole is characterized by columnar epithelium in which the secretory Clara cell replaces the mucous cell, by an increased muscular layer, and by a lack of submucous glands and cartilage. Occasionally referred to as *membranous,* it ends as a terminal bronchiole. The terminal bronchiole branches into two generations of respiratory bronchioles, which through further divisions give rise to additional respiratory bronchioles that have more alveoli in their walls, so-called *second-* and *third-order respiratory bronchioles.* By definition, respiratory bronchioles are alveolated, and they branch into two to three generations of alveolar ducts. The alveolar ducts are defined as those channels from which a series of alveoli open and are histologically characterized by having small clublike ends that contain muscle sphincters and elastic fibers. The ducts open into a final generation of alveolus-lined spaces, the multiloculated cup-shaped alveolar sacs (Figure 31–4).

In the bronchiolar epithelium, a ratio of about three ciliated cells to two nonciliated cells lines the lower intrapulmonary airways. The epithelium contains the Clara cell, which is a dome- or tongue-shaped cell that protrudes into the bronchiolar lumen among the shorter ciliated cells. The Clara cell has varying features according to species but possesses an abundance of agranular reticulum and secretory granules. The Clara cells can synthesize and secrete an antileukoproteinase, a unique 10-kDa protein similar to rabbit uteroglobin, and surfactant-associated proteins A, B and D. Importantly, the Clara cell also is the progenitor cell that differentiates into ciliated cells following injury, and some investigators have shown that the Clara cell can differentiate into a type II epithelial cell.

Definitions of Special Lung Unit and Alveolar Formation[6,13,14,15,18,23]

A *secondary lobule* now is defined as a cluster of three to five terminal bronchioles and their associated respiratory tissue situated at the end of a bronchial pathway. A *primary lobule* constitutes a respiratory bronchiole and its subsidiary divisions. A *terminal respiratory unit* is defined as several alveolar ducts with their accompanying alveoli. The *acinus,* which is approximately spherical in shape and has a diameter of about 7 mm and a length of 0.5 to 1 cm, is the beginning of the gas exchange portion of the lung. The acinus consists of those structures distal to the terminal bronchiole, namely,

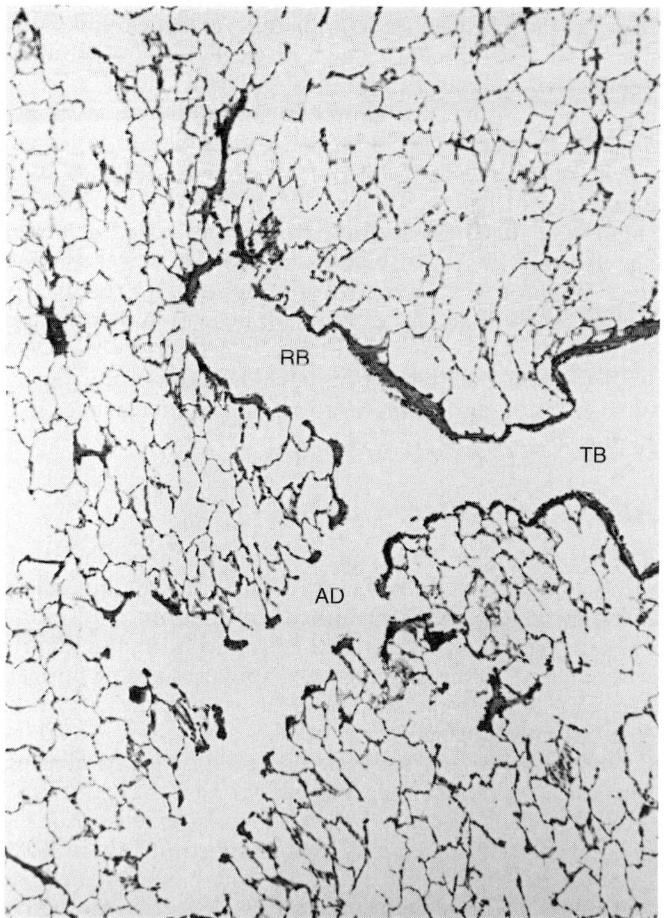

FIGURE 31–4 • Light micrograph shows a terminal bronchiole *(TB)* that branches into respiratory bronchioles *(RB),* which further branch into alveolar ducts *(AD)* (magnification ×30).

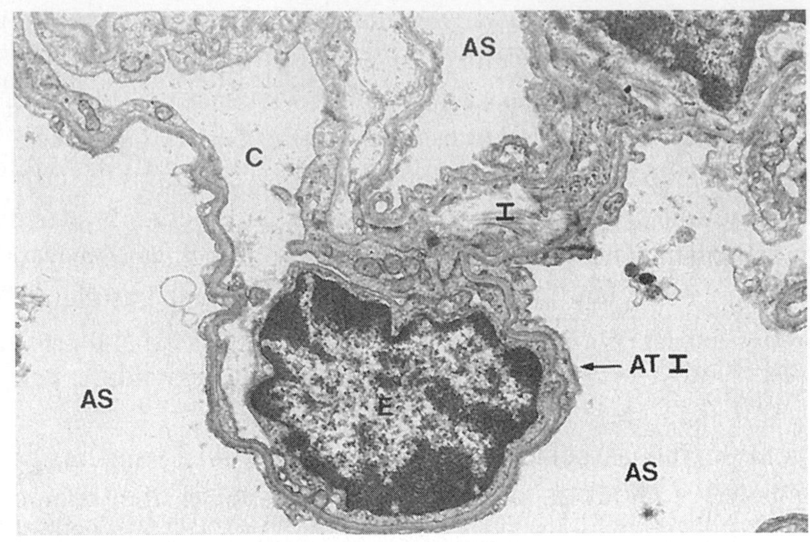

FIGURE 31–5 • Both surfaces of the alveolar wall that separates the alveolar spaces *(AS)* are covered by thin extensions of alveolar type I epithelial cells *(ATI)*. The capillary *(C)* is lined by endothelium *(E)*. The epithelium and endothelium rest on a fused basement membrane on the thin portion of the alveolar wall and are separated by an interstitial space *(I)* in the thick portion of the alveolar wall (magnification ×5500).

several respiratory bronchioles, alveolar ducts, and finally the alveolar sacs, which are entirely lined by alveoli. *Alveoli* are the gas-exchanging structures.

At the alveolar level, many changes occur in the postnatal period. Although there is disparity concerning the time alveolarization is completed, evidence links the postnatal development of alveoli with elastic tissue fiber deposition.[15] At birth, primitive alveoli called *saccules* are evident, but approximately 50 million alveoli are already formed.[14] The number of alveoli in a normal adult can vary from 300 to 500 million, and they have a diameter of 150 to 200 μm. The early work by Dunnell[6] suggesting that new alveolar formation ceased at about age 8 years has been challenged by Thurlbeck,[23] who has shown that alveolarization appears to be nearly complete at about age 2 years. Lung volume correlates with body size, but alveolar surface area correlates with metabolic activity; thus alveoli become more complex in shape during maturation and as increasing O_2 is required.

Alveolar-Capillary Unit[4,8,10,13,19,24]

The alveolar-capillary unit is highly specialized to allow diffusion between the blood and air gases (Figure 31–5). A continuous epithelium consisting of highly specialized epithelial cells covers an abundantly vascularized connective tissue. Capillaries are positioned between two epithelial layers in a gridlike network. The internal surface area of the adult lung is 70 to 80 m^2, of which 90% covers the pulmonary capillaries; thus the air-blood surface available for gas exchange is 60 to 70 m^2. This vascular bed is the most extensive in the body. The endothelial cells, which constitute about 30% of the total lung cells, are thin and have few cellular organelles. A number of adenine nucleotides, vasoactive amines, prostaglandins, vasoactive peptides, and lipoproteins can be metabolized and taken up within the endothelial cells. Importantly, endothelial cells synthesize nitric oxide, the endothelins, prostacylin, tissue plasminogen activator, and thrombomodulin. Other functions include liquid and solid exchange and enzyme activity within the walls of the caveolae. The capillaries are bounded by their basement membrane, which on the thin side of the air-blood barrier fuses with that of the overlying epithelium, the site where gas exchange takes place. On the other side of the alveolar wall, designated the thick portion of the alveolar wall, the alveolar epithelium and capillary endothelium are separated by the interstitial space.

The connective tissue space, or interstitium of the lung at the alveolar level, does not have lymphatics, but it can accumulate fluid that can be absorbed into the lymphatic system, which ends usually at the respiratory bronchiolar level. The interstitial cell population includes resident and migratory cell populations. Normally, the interstitium contains macrophages, pericytes, myofibroblasts, mast cells, infrequent lymphocytes, and a few cells that are best termed *undifferentiated, mesenchymal,* or *pluripotential* because in disease they can differentiate into various cell types, fibroblasts, smooth muscle cells, and others. Greater than 25% of the interstitial cells cannot be identified definitively with the electron microscope, so it is understandable why most of the cells cannot be identified by light microscopy without special cell marker stains.

Two epithelial cell types line the alveoli. Type I cells have thin cytoplasmic extensions and have a very large surface area covering approximately 90% of the total alveolar surface (Figure 31–6). Numerically, they form only about 40% of the epithelial cells, whereas the type II cell, which is cuboidal, constitutes 60% of the total number of epithelial cells but contributes less than 10% of the total alveolar surface area. Type I cells form about 8% and type II cells about 16% of the total cells of the lung. Type I cells are exquisitely well adapted to allow for the rapid exchange of gases, and their micropinocytotic system likely plays a major role in the

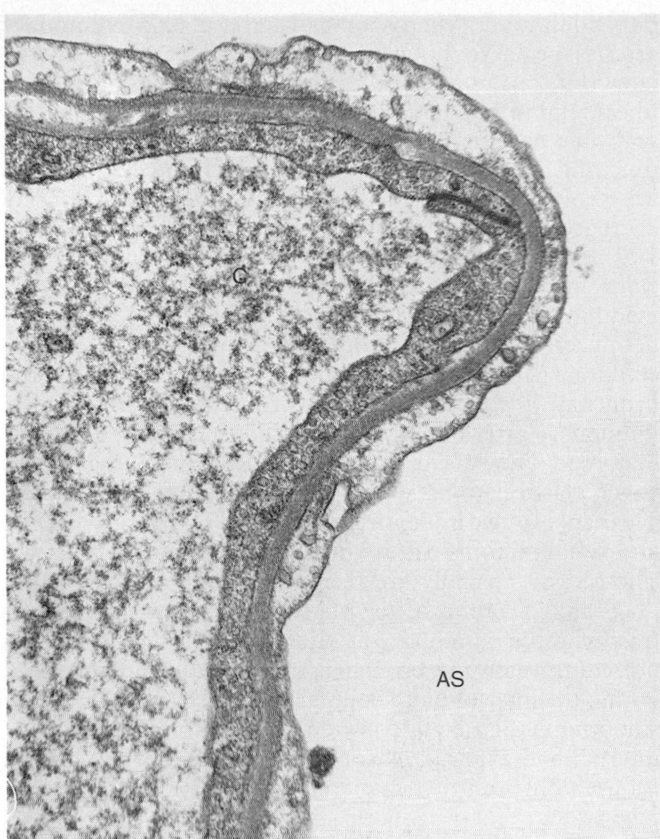

FIGURE 31–6 • Electron micrograph showing the thin side of the air-blood barrier. The thin cytoplasmic extension of the type I epithelium contains only a few vesicles and shares a fused basement membrane with the endothelium that contains many caveolae (magnification ×18,000). *AS,* Alveolar space; *C,* capillary.

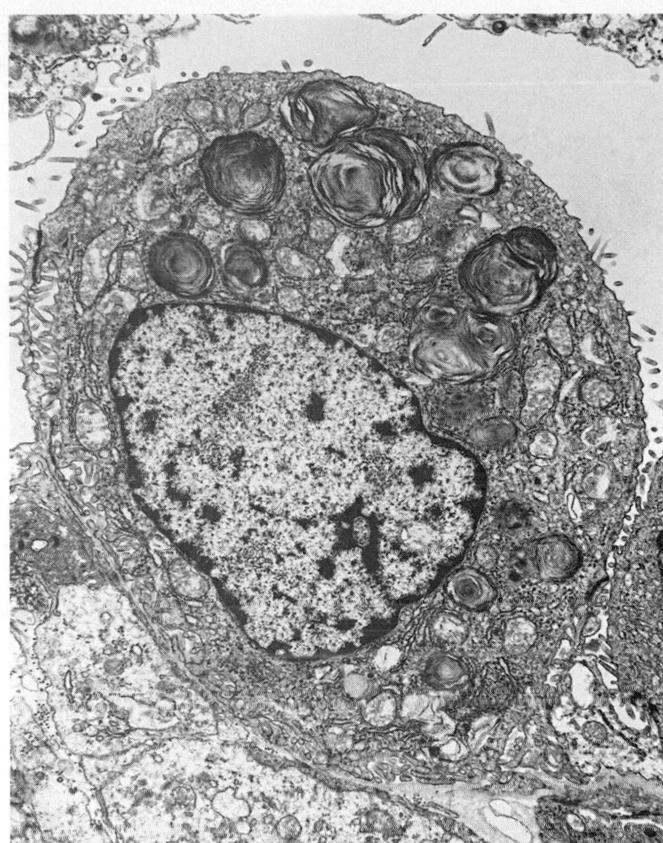

FIGURE 31–7 • Cytoplasm of the alveolar type II cell has abundant lamellar inclusion bodies and surface membrane microvilli (magnification ×7500).

transport of solutes, such as albumin and immunoglobulin, in small quantities. They can be induced to ingest some particulates and can increase their number of pinocytotic vesicles, but they are not active in surfactant uptake.

The type II cell is the regenerative cell of the alveolus. Following injury, it serves as the stem cell for the alveolar surface. It can repopulate the alveolar surface in about 5 days. It is cuboidal in shape and only numbers about one per alveolus. The type II cell has characteristic surface microvilli and cytoplasmic lamellar inclusions, which are the intracellular cytoplasmic storage forms of surfactant (Figure 31–7). The inclusions evolve from multivesicular bodies or lysosomal granules, which progressively acquire the characteristic lamellae. In addition to its roles in the synthesis, secretion, and reuptake of surfactant, the type II cell synthesizes arachidonic acid metabolites, synthesizes and secretes connective tissue components of the basement membrane including fibronectin, synthesizes and secretes components of the complement system, and expresses class II proteins of the major histocompatibility complex among others.

Considerable data clearly demonstrate that there are several populations of macrophages: intraalveolar (PAM), septal (interstitial), pulmonary intravascular (PIM), and airway. Within the alveolar spaces, alveolar macrophages, an important arm of the defense mechanism of the lung, are abundant (Figure 31–8). They number approximately 23×10^9 in the lung (10% of the total cells of the alveolar compartment), and 50 to 100 are estimated per alveolus. They derive from three sources: bone marrow via blood monocyte, the interstitial macrophage pool, and proliferation of macrophages in the alveolar space. They are actively phagocytic and scavenge the surface of the alveoli for respired particulates. Although seen free-floating in alveolar spaces in light microscopic preparations, the alveolar macrophage crawls along the surface of epithelium, adhering with its filopodia. The macrophage has remarkable metabolic activities, has known immune functions, and is involved in lung injury and repair phenomena. More than 100 macrophage-synthesized mediators have been identified, and numerous ligands have been demonstrated. In normal bronchoalveolar lavage fluid, 90% of the cells are alveolar macrophages and 1% to 5% are lymphocytes (T-cell lymphocytes constituting 60%–70% and B cells 5%–10%). Alveolar macrophages also play a role in surfactant uptake, removal, or catabolism.

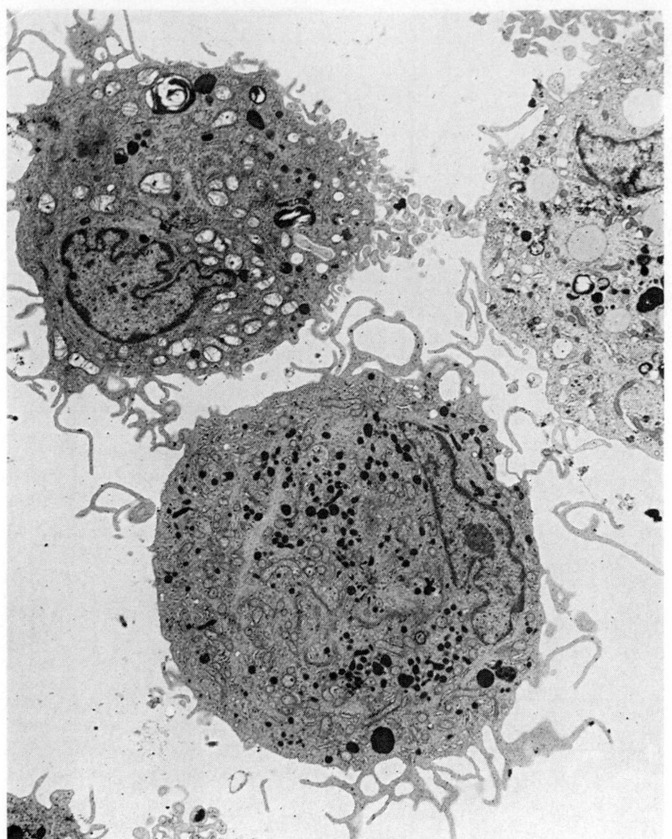

FIGURE 31–8 • Alveolar macrophages recovered from bronchoalveolar lavage fluid contain abundant lysosomes and other cytoplasmic contents, including lipid droplets and surfactant remnants (magnification ×5300).

Lung Circulation

Pulmonary Vascular System[2,4,8,9,13,19,21,24]

The pulmonary circulation is furnished by the pulmonary and the bronchial vascular systems. During gestation, branches of the pulmonary arterial system are thick-walled and contain a medial layer of smooth muscle. At birth, the pulmonary artery and aorta are comparable in medial thickness and configuration and are of the same size. By age 2 years, elastic tissue has decreased in the pulmonary artery and its thickness is only about 60% that of the aorta. Only a few muscular arteries are seen accompanying terminal bronchioles at birth. Following birth, when pulmonary arterial pressures fall to normal levels, the muscle fibers diminish. New vessels without muscle are formed, along with new respiratory units during lung growth. Smooth muscle extends peripherally into small arteries slowly, reaching arterioles at the respiratory bronchiolar level at 4 months, alveolar duct level at 3 years, and some alveoli at age 10 years.

The criteria for recognizing various types of pulmonary vessels were put forth by Brenner[3] in 1935. The pulmonary arteries, which exceed 1000 μm in external diameter, are called *elastic pulmonary arteries* and traverse with the cartilaginous airways. They extend from the hilum to nearly halfway in the bronchial tree of the newborn, a pattern completed by week 16 of gestation and retained into adulthood. Microscopically, the elastic pulmonary arteries begin to undergo maturational changes in the newborn, but until approximately 2 years of age elastic fibers tend to be long, uniform, unbranched, and parallel with one another, similar to those in the aorta. At that time, the adult pattern evolves in which the elastic fibers are short, irregular, and branched and form a loosely arranged network. Pulmonary arteries measure between 100 and 1000 μm in diameter and have a distinct muscular media and internal and external limiting elastic membranes. The muscular arteries of the lung have thinner media than their counterparts in the systemic circulation. Muscular pulmonary arteries branch with the bronchial tree and lie close to bronchi and bronchioles. Pulmonary arterioles are vessels that measure 100 μm in diameter. They have only an endothelial lining and a single elastic lamina with little, if any, muscular media. Their appearance is identical to that of a pulmonary venule, and serial sections are required to differentiate the two. These vessels usually are seen at the level of the alveolar ducts and in certain sites within the alveolar walls. In contrast with the pulmonary arteries, the pulmonary veins do not course with the bronchial tree; instead they are seen within the interlobular septa. Their media is composed of smooth muscle fibers, collagen, and elastin with no clear internal and external elastic lamina. Pulmonary capillaries are nonfenestrated, whereas bronchial capillaries are fenestrated.

Bronchial Vascular System[4,8,9,13,24]

Whereas the pulmonary circulation returns all venous blood to the lung and serves some nutritive function to peripheral capillaries, the bronchial circulation is the primary blood source for the lung. Although two major bronchial arteries for each lung is a common pattern, this is present less than 40% of the time. There usually are two bronchial arteries in the left lung and one in the right lung. Although variable, the left bronchial arteries usually arise from the upper portion of the descending aorta. The right bronchial artery arises from the descending aorta, one of the right intercostal branches, or subclavian or internal thoracic arteries. The bronchial arteries traverse along the dorsal portion of each bronchus. They lose their distinctness along the respiratory bronchioles and drain with the alveolar capillaries into the peribronchiolar venous network. They form a capillary plexus in the bronchi that supplies the submucosa and muscle. The capillary plexus communicates with branches of the pulmonary artery that empty into pulmonary veins. Other bronchial arteries supply the interlobular tissue and the pleura. They drain into the bronchial veins. The diameter of the bronchial artery is much smaller than that of the accompanying pulmonary artery. It has an internal elastic lamina and media but no external elastic lamina.

Pulmonary Lymphatics

Pulmonary lymphatics[17] invariably have less elastic tissue in their walls than either arteries or veins.[17,24] They are lined by endothelium, and valves are present especially near and in the visceral pleura. There are two lymphatic systems in the human lung: a superficial network in the pleura and a deep network around the bronchi and pulmonary arteries and veins and in the connective tissue septa between the secondary lobules. The two separate systems have anastomoses, both in the pleura and near the hilum. Lymphatics can be demonstrated to the level of the septal walls that comprise the atria but are not found at the alveolar level. Lymph flow from both lower lobes drains into the infratracheal lymph nodes. The remaining right and left lung lobes drain into the tracheobronchial lymph nodes on each side of the trachea, respectively. Lymph from the right tracheobronchial nodes drains into the right bronchomediastinal trunk, whereas the left tracheobronchial nodes drain into thoracic duct.

Understanding the lymphatic drainage of the pleura is of clinical value. All lymph from the visceral pleura eventually reaches parabronchial and hilar lymph nodes by flowing either on the surface or in lymphatic trunks that course through the lung. Lymphatic vessels in the parietal pleura are in communication with the pleural space via 2- to 6-mm stomas found on the mediastinal pleura or the intercostal surfaces of the lower thorax. The parasternal nodes in the second and third interspaces receive lymph from a significant portion of the parietal pleura, so biopsy of these nodes may reveal an etiology of the pleural effusion. The portion of lymph that drains caudally from the lower parietal pleural region into retroperitoneal nodes can explain metastases of tumor to adrenals and kidneys.

Diaphragm[10,17]

Although the diaphragm is the principal muscle of respiration, it is not essential for breathing in the awake state. It becomes essential during deep anesthesia because other muscles of respiration become inactive. The diaphragm is a musculotendinous sheet that is the main source of inspiratory muscle force. Anatomically it separates the thoracic from the abdominal cavity. It has two distinct muscular components: the sternocostal portion and the crural. These two portions have distinct embryologic origins and have separate segmental innervations and varying muscle fiber composition. There are changes in fiber composition following birth. The muscle fibers vary morphologically, physiologically, and cytochemically. The diaphragm has three openings near its central portion for the aorta, inferior vena cava, and esophagus. The vagus nerve passes through the esophageal hiatus, whereas the azygos vein and thoracic duct pass through the aortic hiatus. There are small paravertebral perforations for splanchnic nerves. Because of the way the fibers originate from the bones and traverse to the central tendon, triangular areas may result in spaces or clefts in the diaphragm. Anteriorly these are called *Morgagni foramina,* and posteriorly they are known as the *foramina of Bochdalek.* Both are potential sites for hernias. The phrenic nerve innervates the diaphragm.

During contraction in adults, the dome of the diaphragm descends and the lower ribs elevate. In infants, because of their very compliant rib cage, descent opposes elevation of the lower ribs and results in the subcostal retractions. Other muscles of respiration include the intercostals, the majority of which are arranged to enhance inspiration by elevating the lower ribs, and the abdominal muscles, which are powerful muscles of expiration but do not participate in expiration during quiet breathing. Scalenes act to elevate the first two ribs and are active even during quiet breathing. Although the sternocleidomastoid muscles usually are not active in quiet breathing, when inspiratory efforts are marked, they become the most important accessory muscles of inspiration. This is well seen in infants with respiratory distress who elevate the upper portion of their sterna.

REFERENCES

1. Ash JE, Raum M: *An atlas of otolaryngic pathology,* ed 4. Washington, DC, 1956, The American Registry of Pathology and The Armed Forces Institute of Pathology.
2. Baroody FM: Anatomy and physiology. In Naclerio RM, Durham SR, Mygind N, editors: *Rhinitis: mechanisms and management.* New York, 1999, Marcel Dekker.
3. Brenner O: Pathology of the vessels of the pulmonary circulation. *Arch Intern Med* 56:211, 1935.
4. Corrin B: Normal lung structure. In Corrin B, editor: *Pathology of the lungs.* New York, 2000, Churchill Livingstone.
5. Dickison AE: In the normal and abnormal pediatric upper airway, recognition and management of obstruction. *Clin Chest Med* 8:583, 1987.
6. Dunnell MS: Postnatal growth of the lung. *Thorax* 17:329, 1962.
7. Eckenhoff JE: Some anatomic considerations of the infant larynx influencing endotracheal anesthesia. *Anesthesiology* 12:4, 1951.
8. Hasleton PS, Curry A: Anatomy of the lung. In Hasleton PS, editor: *Spencer's pathology of the lung,* ed 5. New York, 1996, McGraw-Hill.
9. Harris P, Heath D. The structure of the normal pulmonary blood vessels after infancy. In Harris P, Heath D: *The human pulmonary circulation,* ed 2. New York, 1977, Churchill Livingstone.
10. Hinshaw HC, Murray JF: Anatomy of the thorax. In Hinshaw HC, Murray JF: *Diseases of the chest,* ed 4. Philadelphia, 1980, WB Saunders.
11. Horsfield K, Cumming G: The morphology of the bronchial tree in man. *Appl Physiol* 24:373, 1968.
12. Jeffrey PK: Microscopic structure of normal lung. In Brewis RAL, Corrin B, Geddes DM, Gibson GJ, editors: *Respiratory medicine.* London, 1995, WB Saunders.
13. Kuhn C: Normal anatomy and histology. In Thurlbeck WM, Churg AM, editors: *Pathology of the lung,* ed 2. New York, 1995, Thieme Medical Publishers.
14. Langston C, Kida K, Reed M, et al: Human lung growth in late gestation and in the neonate. *Am Rev Respir Dis* 129:607, 1984.
15. Loosli CG, Potter EL: Pre- and postnatal development with reference to elastic fibers. *Am Rev Respir Dis* 80(suppl):5, 1959.
16. Matsuba K, Thurlbeck WM: A morphometric study of bronchial and bronchiolar walls in children. *Am Rev Respir Dis* 105:908, 1972.
17. Murray JF: Postnatal growth and development of the lung. In Murray JF, editor: *The normal lung,* ed 2. Philadelphia, 1986, WB Saunders.
18. Reid L, Simon G: The peripheral pattern in the normal bronchogram and its relation to peripheral pulmonary anatomy. *Thorax* 13:103, 1958.
19. Ross MH, Kaye GI, Pawlina W: Respiratory system. In Ross MH, Kaye GI, Pawlina W, editors: *Histology: a text and atlas,* ed 4. Baltimore, 2003, Lippincott Williams & Wilkins.
20. Saphir O: *Autopsy diagnosis and technique,* ed 3. New York, 1951, Paul B Hoeber.
21. Sorokin SP: The respiratory system. In Weiss L, editor: *Cell and tissue biology: a textbook of histology,* ed 6. Baltimore, 1988, Urban and Schwarzenberg.

22. Stocks J, Hislop AA: Structure and function of the respiratory system: developmental aspects and their relevance to aerosol therapy. In Lenfant C, editor: *Drug delivery to the lung*. New York, 2002, Marcel Dekker.
23. Thurlbeck WM: Postnatal human lung growth. *Thorax* 37:564, 1982.
24. Wang N-S: Anatomy. In Dail DH, Hammar SP, editors: *Pulmonary pathology*, ed 2. New York, 1994, Springer-Verlag.
25. Weibel E: *Morphometry of the human lung*. New York, 1963, Academic Press.

CHAPTER

32

Pediatric Airway Management

Ann E. Thompson

PEARLS

- Safe management of the critically ill child's airway requires understanding the anatomic and physiologic changes that occur from birth through adolescence, recognition of congenital and acquired airway abnormalities, appreciation of the pathophysiologic consequences of airway manipulation, and preparation for potentially difficult airways.
- Laryngoscopy and intubation are potent physiologic stimuli that are associated with severe discomfort, profound cardiovascular and cerebrovascular changes, and increased airway reactivity.
- Recognition of, and preparation for, managing a difficult airway are essential for preventing potentially lethal complications of intubation.
- The approach to intubation must be tailored to specific circumstances, such as full stomach, elevated intracranial pressure, cervical spine injury, and upper airway obstruction.
- Alternative approaches to airway management, such as the lighted stylet, laryngeal mask airway, cricothyrotomy, retrograde intubation, and tracheostomy, may be lifesaving.

Accurate assessment and safe management of the critically ill child's airway is the essential first step in providing effective intensive care. It requires understanding of the anatomic and physiologic changes that occur from birth through adolescence, recognition of congenital and acquired airway abnormalities, appreciation of the pathophysiologic consequences of airway manipulation, and preparation for potentially difficult airways.

Anatomic Considerations

The configuration of the child's airway changes dramatically from birth to adulthood (Figure 32–1). The nose is the site of nearly half of the total respiratory resistance to air flow at all ages. The infant's nose is short, soft, and flat with small, nearly circular nares. The nasal valve, the narrowest portion of the nasal airway, approximately 1 cm proximal to the alar rim in newborns, is only about 20 mm^2.[1,2] By 6 months, dimensions of the nares have nearly doubled, but they are still easily occluded by edema, secretions, or external pressure. Although perhaps not as much the obligate nose breather as commonly assumed, the infant frequently develops signs of airway obstruction when the nose is blocked.[3,4]

In infancy, the mandible is small, and the basicranium, which provides the roof of the nasopharynx, is flat, creating a small oral cavity. Over the years of development, the jaw grows primarily down and forward, with the ramus increasing in height and width. The posterior portion of the basicranium develops a progressively more rounded configuration through childhood, which results in a larger nasal airway to meet the need for increased air flow (and provides a chamber for the resonance of adult speech).

Under normal conditions, the genioglossus muscle and other muscles of the pharynx and larynx help maintain airway patency. Both tonic and phasic inspiratory

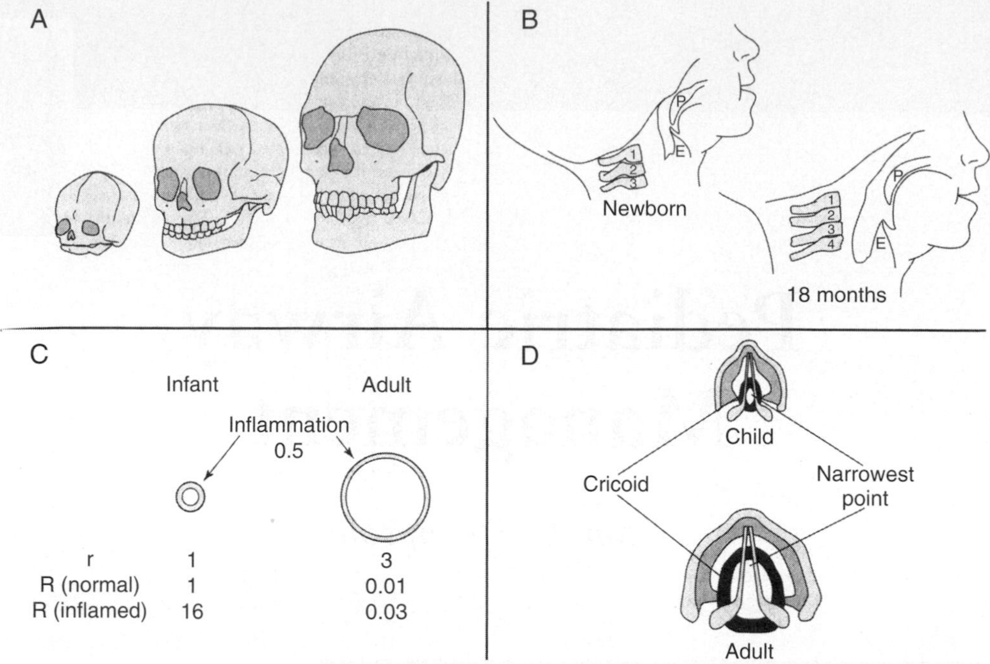

FIGURE 32–1 • Characteristics of the pediatric airway. **A**, Changes in mandibular shape from infancy through adolescence. **B**, The epiglottis is initially cephalad in infancy, then descends throughout childhood. *E*, Epiglottis; *P*, palate. **C**, Edema has a much greater effect on airways resistance in the young child than later in life. *r*, Relative radius of the trachea; *R*, relative airways resistance. **D**, The cricoid is the narrowest portion of the airway until age 8 to 10 years.

activity synchronized with phrenic contraction have been noted in animal and human studies. In particular, the genioglossus increases the dimensions of the pharyngeal airway by displacing the tongue anteriorly.[5] In the infant and young child, the tongue is large relative to the bony structures surrounding it and the cavities they form. Relatively little displacement is possible at any time, and loss of tone during sleep, sedation, or central or peripheral nervous system dysfunction is more likely than in older patients to allow the tongue to relax into the posterior pharynx and cause upper airway obstruction.

The infant larynx is high in the neck at birth, with the epiglottis at the level of the first cervical vertebra and overlapping the soft palate. This approximation of structures, in combination with the relatively large tongue and small mandible, probably contributes to the vulnerability to airway obstruction in infants and young children. By 6 months the epiglottis has moved to about the level of the third cervical vertebra and is separate from the palate. It continues to descend to its adult position at about the fifth or sixth cervical vertebra by early adolescence. The infant epiglottis is soft and omega shaped, in contrast with the more rigid, flatter adult structure, and has greater potential to occlude the airway. The immature larynx is funnel shaped, with the subglottic portion angled posteriorly relative to the supraglottic portion rather than forming a straight vertical column as seen in the adult. It tapers to the cricoid cartilage, the narrowest point in the child's extrathoracic airway.

The internal dimensions of the trachea in the newborn are approximately one third those of the adult, and absolute resistance to air flow is higher than in older children and adults. Because the most important factor determining resistance (R) is the radius (r) of an airway ($R \propto 8\ l/r^4$), small changes in airway diameter in infants or young children as a consequence of edema or secretions have a far greater effect on resistance than similar changes in larger patients (see Figure 32–1).

Basic Airway Management

Airway management depends on a brisk assessment of the patient's breathing and knowledge of the likely progression of the airway problem, that is, deterioration versus improving function. In virtually any setting where respiratory difficulty is suspected, oxygen should be administered until the specific abnormality can be identified and adequately treated. Although extreme hypercarbia usually is well tolerated, hypoxia is routinely catastrophic. From the alveolar air equation, it is obvious that hypercarbia produces hypoxia at low FiO_2. If the patient is breathing spontaneously, attention is directed first to signs of upper airway obstruction, including absence of audible or palpable air flow, stertorous sounds, stridor, or rocking chest and abdominal motion rather than the normal, smooth rise and fall that should occur with inspiration and expiration.

An alert child with normal neuromuscular function usually instinctively assumes a body position that minimizes upper airway obstruction. However, a child with an altered level of consciousness or severe neuromuscular weakness may be unable to maintain a patent airway because of inability to alter his or her position or maintain adequate glossopharyngeal muscle tone.

Nasopharyngeal Airway

A nasopharyngeal airway that extends through nasal passages to the posterior pharynx and beyond the base of the tongue often is adequate to relieve obstruction and is tolerated by most patients, even those who are conscious (Figure 32–2). An appropriate-size airway extends from the nares to the tragus of the ear and is of the largest diameter that passes through nasal passages without causing blanching of the skin surrounding the nares. It should be well lubricated before placement. Risks of nasopharyngeal airways include nasal ulceration, bleeding, laceration of friable lymphoid tissue, rupture of a pharyngeal abscess, laryngospasm, and potential passage through the cribriform plate in patients with basilar skull fractures. Topical vasoconstricting agents reduce, but do not eliminate, the risk of bleeding. Like other nasal tubes, nasal airways increase the risk of sinusitis. Contraindications to their use therefore include severe coagulopathies, cerebrospinal fluid (CSF leaks), and basilar skull fractures.

Oropharyngeal Airways

Oropharyngeal airways displace the base of the tongue from the posterior pharyngeal wall and break contact between the tongue and palate (see Figure 32–2). Size selection is important. An excessively long airway may encroach upon the larynx and cause laryngospasm. An airway that is too short may actually push the tongue posteriorly and exacerbate obstruction. If the airway is held at the side of the face with the flange just anterior to the incisors, the tip should be at or near the angle of the mandible. The airway should be positioned following the curve of the tongue while the tongue is held down and forward with a tongue depressor. Inserting the airway with its concave side facing the palate and then rotating it may traumatize the oral mucosa or damage teeth. Oral airways are poorly tolerated in any patient with a functional gag reflex and may induce vomiting. As a consequence, they are of little more than temporary value in the critically ill child. They may support a patent airway for bag-valve-mask ventilation in preparation for intubation.

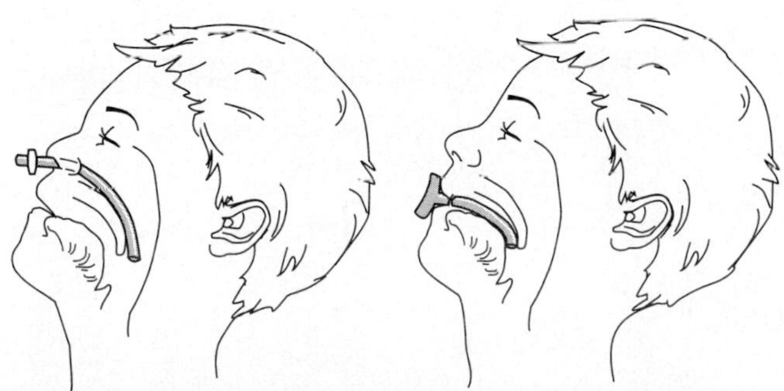

FIGURE 32–2 • Nasopharyngeal and oropharyngeal airways in good position.

Oxygen Delivery Devices

Nasal Cannulas

Nasal cannulas consist of two hollow prongs projecting from a hollow face piece. Humidified oxygen (100%) flows from a standard source, effectively delivering a pharyngeal concentration of 25% to 40% after mixing with variable amounts of room air. The cannulas are easy to use, often readily tolerated, lightweight, economical, and disposable and take advantage of the humidifying properties of the nasopharynx. Their use is limited by the relatively low oxygen concentration that can be delivered. High-flow nasal cannulas can deliver positive distending pressure similar to that provided by nasal continuous positive airway pressure. The pressure generated is dependent on the interaction among the flow rate, patient size, and anatomy of the patient's airway.[6]

Oxygen Hoods

Oxygen hoods are cylinders or boxes that enclose an infant's or small child's head. Oxygen enters through a gas inlet port, and exhaled gas leaves primarily through the opening for the neck. Hoods provide up to 80% to 90% oxygen, good humidification, and controlled temperature. They allow easy access to the child for other care. Tents for older children provide the same environment advantages but allow less ready access to the patient and usually provide only 21% to 50% oxygen. Both have the disadvantage of being very noisy for the patient.

Masks

A variety of masks are available for delivering oxygen. Simple masks fit loosely. The oxygen concentration delivered varies, depending on the patient's inspiratory flow rate and the oxygen flow into the system. Partial rebreathing masks incorporate some sort of reservoir, usually a bag below the chin. Provided flow into the system exceeds the patient's minute ventilation and that the bag does not collapse on inspiration, little carbon dioxide is inhaled, and concentrations of oxygen up to about 60% can be achieved. Nonrebreathing masks must fit snugly. They incorporate a mask, reservoir, and one-way valves that vent expired gas but do not permit inspiration of room air. As a result, they can deliver close to 100% oxygen.

Establishing a Functional Airway

A patient who is apneic or in very severe respiratory distress requires ventilation assisted initially with bag and mask. If the child is too weak or obtunded to maintain pharyngeal tone independently, the head should be placed on a thin cushion to cause slight cervical spine flexion and gentle extension at the atlantooccipital joint. In infants, the large occipitofrontal diameter makes the cushion unnecessary, although a thin pad under the shoulders may be useful. Current recommendations are to avoid overextending the baby's very flexible cervical spine, which may stretch and compress the trachea and potentiate, rather than relieve, obstruction. Studies have questioned the existence of this phenomenon but to date have included a very small number of infants, all with normal airways.[7] Appropriate head tilt separates the tongue from the posterior pharyngeal wall. If airway obstruction persists, the chin can be pulled forward by encircling the mandible behind the lower incisors between thumb and fingers. The most effective means of relieving functional obstruction is the so-called *triple airway maneuver:* With the fingers behind the vertical ramus of the jaw, the mandible is displaced downward, forward, and finally upward again until the mandible and lower incisors are anterior to the maxilla. This action effectively pulls the tongue forward and away from the pharyngeal wall.

In some patients, establishing a functional airway is sufficient to allow resumption of effective spontaneous ventilation. In other patients, steady positive airway pressure is necessary to overcome residual obstruction. If breathing remains inadequate, manual ventilation is necessary. Effective ventilation requires a good mask fit. The mask should sit smoothly on the bridge of the nose and the bony prominence of the chin. It is important to avoid airway occlusion with the mask or hand or pressure on eyes, soft nasal structures, or branches of the trigeminal and facial nerves. A good mask fit is predictably difficult in patients without teeth, very flat or prominent noses, or micrognathia. A nasal or oropharyngeal airway may help maintain an adequate airway. Once a good mask fit is ensured, ventilation may be assisted.

Two types of bags are in general use: self-inflating resuscitation bags and standard anesthesia bags. Self-inflating bags vary substantially, so specific directions for their use must be followed carefully. All incorporate an adapter to connect to a mask or endotracheal tube, a bag, a pressure-relief valve, and a port for fresh gas inflow. Most bags designed for children have pressure-relief valves designed to pop off at 35 to 45 cmH_2O pressure to prevent excessive volume delivery and subsequent barotrauma. In patients with very poor compliance or increased airway resistance, it may be necessary to bypass this valve temporarily to provide effective ventilation.

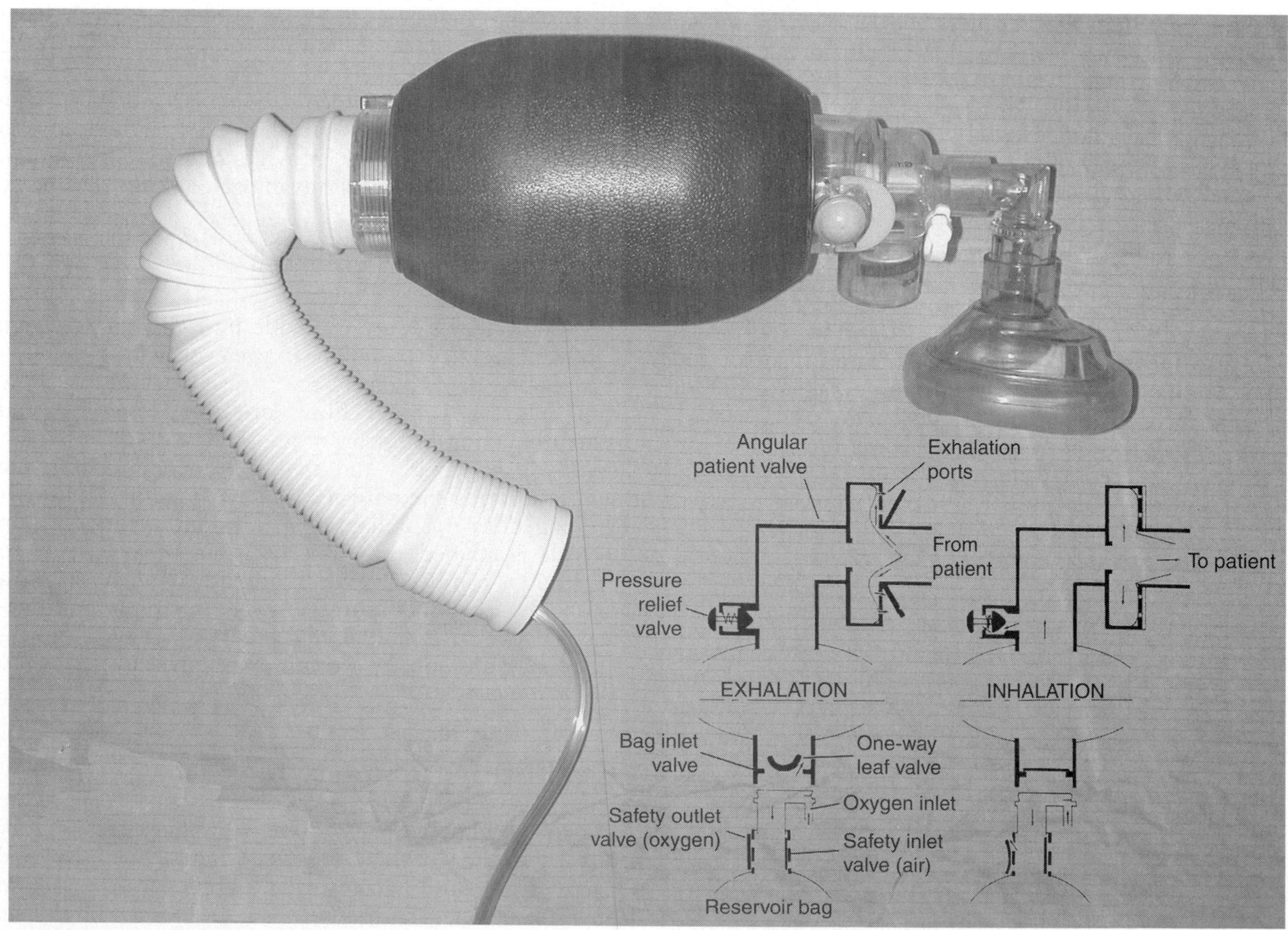

FIGURE 32–3 • Self-inflating manual ventilation bag with tubing as a reservoir. **Inset** shows function of one type of valve, permitting manual positive pressure breathing, or spontaneous breathing, but requiring generation of negative pressure by the patient to open the valve.

Most systems incorporate valves that prevent rebreathing. Fresh gas flows through the valve on spontaneous inspiration (negative pressure) or on creation of positive pressure by squeezing the bag (Figure 32–3). Exhaled gas is vented to the atmosphere. Not all systems allow spontaneous breathing. Those that do demand that the patient generate at least a little negative pressure, so a good mask fit is necessary. Holding the mask *above* the patient's face provides *no* supplemental oxygen. The percentage of oxygen delivered depends on the percentage of oxygen from the source, the fresh gas flow rate, and the respiratory rate, which determines the time available for the bag to refill. Most require some sort of reservoir assembly in addition to the self-inflating bag to prevent entrainment of room air. With a reservoir, 100% oxygen may be delivered; without a reservoir, most deliver less than 50%.

Anesthesia bags require flow from a source of gas under pressure in order to expand. Many variations have been extensively reviewed in the anesthesia literature. These circuits depend on the location of the fresh gas inflow and overflow valves, the rate of fresh gas flow, the respiratory rate, tidal volume, carbon dioxide production, and whether ventilation is spontaneous or controlled. Many intensive care units (ICUs) use the Mapleson D configuration, with the fresh gas source attached just distal to the patient connection. The overflow valve is proximal to the reservoir bag. During expiration, the patient's exhaled tidal volume mixes with fresh gas flowing into the system and accumulates in the tubing and bag. With sufficiently high fresh gas flow, alveolar gas is washed to the overflow valve and eliminated from the circuit. The system requires higher fresh gas flow to avoid rebreathing during spontaneous ventilation than during controlled breathing, but a safe rule of thumb recommends fresh gas flow two to three times the minute ventilation. During controlled ventilation, a minimum of 100 ml/kg/min ensures that carbon dioxide elimination is proportional to minute ventilation.[8,9] At flows less than 90 ml/kg/min, increasing ventilation may only increase CO_2 rebreathing.

Endotracheal Intubation

The pediatric intensivist is frequently called on to intubate critically ill patients when brief ventilation with bag and mask is inadequate to reverse the underlying disorder. Few of these intubations are performed under the optimal conditions commonly attainable in the operating room: relatively healthy children with empty stomachs, previously sedated, and intubated in a controlled environment, with all members of the team experienced in and prepared for airway management. Instead, patients are often critically unstable and require intubation suddenly, often in settings where the procedure is not routine. Intubation is often viewed only as a means to an end, namely, mechanical ventilation. However, it is associated with profound physiologic effects that may dramatically affect the patient. The intensivist's appreciation of these factors and ability to minimize the adverse physiologic consequence of airway manipulation may as decisively determine patient outcome as his/her skill in providing the intensive care that follows.

Indications

Respiratory Failure

Respiratory failure may result from dysfunction at any point along the ventilatory pathway. In order to provide appropriate support and to avoid hazards specific to the individual disorder, airway intervention must be tailored to the underlying cause. Outside the operating room, the need for intubation is most commonly associated with respiratory failure resulting from lower airway or pulmonary parenchymal disorders that require mechanical ventilation. Respiratory failure is defined in terms of either inadequate oxygenation (in the absence of cyanotic congenital heart disease) or carbon dioxide elimination. Box 32–1 contains one set of criteria for intubation.

Hemodynamic Instability

Patients with hemodynamic instability often benefit from assisted ventilation. The need for controlled ventilation as a component of cardiopulmonary resuscitation is obvious. In addition, early intubation in anticipation of impending cardiovascular collapse may prevent catastrophic tissue hypoxia. Redistribution of blood flow away from respiratory muscles, especially the diaphragm, in patients with marginal cardiac output may improve perfusion of other vital organs, including the heart, and help prevent cardiac arrest.[10–14]

Neuromuscular Dysfunction (see Chapter 58)

Neuromuscular dysfunction or severe chest wall instability (or deformity) may cause failure of the bellows apparatus for breathing.[15] Initially, tidal volume remains normal or at least sufficient to maintain normal blood gas tensions, but vital capacity and maximal inspiratory and expiratory pressures decrease. Inability to take a deep breath or cough forcefully risks progressive segmental or

BOX 32–1

Indications for Intubation

1. Pa_{O_2} <60 mmHg with Fi_{O_2} ≥0.6 (in absence of cyanotic congenital heart disease)
2. Pa_{CO_2} >50 mmHg (acute and unresponsive to other intervention)
3. Upper airway obstruction, actual or impending
4. Neuromuscular weakness
   - Maximum negative inspiratory pressure > −20 cmH_2O
   - Vital capacity <12–15 ml/kg
5. Absent protective airway reflexes (cough, gag)
6. Hemodynamic instability (cardiopulmonary resuscitation, shock)
7. Controlled therapeutic (hyper)ventilation
   - Intracranial hypertension
   - Pulmonary hypertension
   - Metabolic acidosis
8. Pulmonary toilet
9. Emergency drug administration

lobar atelectasis, inability to clear secretions, bronchial obstruction, and possible major airway obstruction with sudden severe hypoxia or carbon dioxide retention. Increasing weakness results in progressively smaller tidal volumes, loss of upper airway tone, and, ultimately, inadequate minute ventilation. Bulbar dysfunction may lead to aspiration secondary to impaired swallowing and inadequate cough.

Measurement of ventilatory reserve provides a better assessment of the patient's need for ventilatory assistance than arterial blood gas tensions alone. Maximum negative inspiratory pressure and vital capacity are two simple, commonly used tests for this purpose. A variety of other measures also help assess respiratory "strength," but most are difficult to perform in sick, uncooperative infants and children. Patients with diffuse neuromuscular weakness of any cause, spinal cord dysfunction above the level of T6, or loss of phrenic nerve or diaphragm function are particularly prone to respiratory failure.[16] Because of the extreme compliance of their chest walls and relative ineffectiveness of intercostal muscles, infants younger than approximately 6 months tolerate diaphragmatic paralysis poorly.[17–21]

Many patients with neuromuscular weakness respond well to noninvasive forms of ventilatory support.[15,22] Decisions about the best approach to airway management should be based on the nature and likely progression of the illness, the child's maturity and level of consciousness, and the timing of the onset of respiratory insufficiency. In an emergency, endotracheal intubation is likely to be safest, with transition to noninvasive support when careful planning allows.[22]

Failure of Central Nervous System Regulation of Ventilatory Drive

Failure of central nervous system regulation of ventilatory drive may prompt intubation (see Chapters 54 and 57). Centrally mediated hypoventilation is manifest as CO_2 retention, usually in the absence of increased work of breathing. On occasion the decision to support ventilation may be based on observing abnormal ventilatory patterns in anticipation of neurologic deterioration. Loss of protective airway reflexes, including the cough and gag reflexes, can result from central nervous system depression, cranial nerve abnormalities, or severe motor weakness. In such patients, intubation is indicated to prevent aspiration. Intubation may be appropriate in anticipation of the need to protect the airway and support ventilation during deep sedation for procedures or diagnostic studies.

Other Indications

Intubation is indicated as a step toward therapeutic controlled (hyper)ventilation (e.g., in patients with increased intracranial pressure [ICP] or pulmonary hypertension) or to support spontaneous hyperpnea in patients with metabolic acidosis and other conditions. Patients with profuse, thick, or tenacious secretions may benefit from an artificial airway as a means of providing effective suction (e.g., bacterial pneumonitis, smoke inhalation). Impaired mucociliary clearance occurs in patients exposed to high oxygen concentrations or other airway irritants (including particulate and gaseous components of smoke), those suffering from severe hypoxia or hypercarbia, and, paradoxically, those suffering from airway trauma induced by endotracheal intubation and suction. Endotracheal intubation also provides an effective means of delivering drugs during cardiopulmonary resuscitation when venous access is not available (see Chapter 119)

Physiologic Effects of Intubation

Laryngoscopy is a potent physiologic stimulus[23,24] (Box 32–2). At the very least, laryngoscopy is uncomfortable, causing significant pain and severe anxiety, especially in children who cannot understand or accept the need for it. Laryngoscopy causes an increase in systemic blood pressure and heart rate initiated by pressure on the back of the tongue or lifting of the epiglottis.[25] This effect is augmented by endotracheal intubation and suction.[26] Nodal or ventricular dysrhythmias may occur. Sensory impulses triggering this reflex probably are carried along the vagus nerve supplying the base of the tongue, epiglottis, and trachea. The efferent limb is less well defined but most likely is the product of enhanced sympathetic activity. Infants respond more variably than do older patients. Most develop hypertension, but a few become hypotensive, especially if they are hypoxic.[27] They may demonstrate moderate-to-severe bradycardia rather than tachycardia, perhaps as a consequence of their greater parasympathetic tone. Sedation and light anesthesia decrease but do not obliterate the hypertension and tachycardia; surface anesthesia and deeper general anesthesia are more effective.[28] Children with previous hypertension display an exaggerated vasopressor response. Sedation and neuromuscular blockade during airway manipulation in infants minimizes the associated bradycardia and systemic hypertension.[29–33] The impact of positive pressure ventilation on cardiac performance depends on the underlying disorder (discussed in Chapter 44) but should be carefully considered in preparation for intubation.

BOX 32–2

Potential Physiologic Effects of Laryngoscopy and Intubation

Pain	Tachycardia
Anxiety	Bradycardia
Hypoxia	Systemic hypertension
Hypercarbia	Decreased systemic venous return
Increased intraocular pressure	Decreased jugular venous return
Increased intragastric pressure	Increased intracranial pressure
Laryngospasm	Bronchoconstriction
	Pulmonary hypertension

Laryngoscopy and intubation are potent stimulators of laryngospasm and may cause bronchoconstriction, especially in patients with a history of reactive airways disease. Increased airway resistance probably results from parasympathetic stimulation, with release of acetylcholine and stimulation of muscarinic receptors on airway smooth muscle, especially large central airways.

During intubation, oxygen delivery to the patient is commonly interrupted. Ineffective breathing or apnea increases the likelihood of hypoxia, especially in children, with their relatively low functional residual volume and higher basal metabolic rate. Patients with severe pulmonary disease and abnormally low FRC are at particular risk.[29,32] During apnea, carbon dioxide tension increases at a rate of 3 to 4 mmHg/min in healthy, sedated adults and probably more rapidly in children, particularly those with severe cardiopulmonary disease or increased metabolic rate secondary to fever, sepsis, or pain.[34,35]

ICP rises immediately during laryngoscopy even in patients without intracranial pathology, before changes in blood gas tensions occur.[28,30,36,37] Cerebral metabolic rate and blood flow increase. Hypoxia, hypercarbia, and diminished jugular venous drainage, particularly in struggling patients, contribute further. Although normally very transient, such intracranial hypertension may predispose patients with coagulopathies or vascular malformations to intracranial hemorrhage. Systemic hypertension in patients with impaired autoregulation of the cerebral circulation (e.g., sick infants or patients with a variety of intracranial disorders) and impedance to jugular venous return by jugular compression, pneumothorax, or coughing and struggling stress both the arterial and venous sides of the cerebral circulation. In patients with poor intracranial compliance, this effect is exaggerated and prolonged. In infants without primary central nervous system disease, muscle paralysis (even without sedation or analgesia) effectively blocks the rise in ICP associated with intubation.[32] The systemic hypertensive response is generally unaffected by neuromuscular blocking agents but can be modified by analgesia and sedation or intravenous anesthesia.

Patients with severe pulmonary hypertension are at high risk for adverse effects of laryngoscopy. Decreased oxygenation and progressive hypercarbia lead to elevated pulmonary artery pressure. The noxious stimulus of visualizing the airway, itself, may precipitate life-threatening hypertension.

Recognition of a Difficult Airway

Recognition of a difficult airway is important if potentially lethal surprises in airway management are to be minimized (Box 32–3). A history of difficult intubations in the past or episodes of upper airway obstruction (including snoring or sleep apnea) suggests structural abnormalities that may or may not be evident at the moment. Micrognathia, glossoptosis, facial clefts, midface hypoplasia, prominent upper incisors or maxillary protrusion, facial asymmetry, high arched narrow palate, a small mouth, and a short, muscular neck or morbid obesity are features that can interfere with effective bag-and-mask ventilation or visualization of the larynx.

BOX 32–3

Recognizing the Difficult Airway

HISTORY

Difficult intubation
Upper airway obstruction, current or past, including snoring and sleep apnea

ANATOMIC FEATURES

Gross macrocephaly
Facial asymmetry
Midface hypoplasia
Small mouth
Glossoptosis
Midline clefts or high arched palate
Micrognathia
Limited neck mobility
Laryngotracheal abnormalities (congenital or acquired)
Severe obesity
Facial trauma
Airway bleeding
Oropharyngeal mass
Abnormal soft tissue infiltration
Limited temporomandibular joint mobility
Nasal obstruction

Limited temporomandibular joint or cervical spine mobility may make laryngoscopy and tube placement very difficult. Midface instability or upper airway bleeding, edema, masses, and foreign bodies are additional reasons for concern.[38] Ability to visualize the faucial pillars, soft palate, and uvula usually predicts an uncomplicated intubation but may be difficult to assess in a sick, uncooperative child.[39] Children with severe hypoxia, severe hypovolemia, intracranial hypertension, full stomach, or some combination of these conditions present added difficulties that must be considered.

When airway problems are anticipated, the intensivist should approach intubation with a plan specific to the difficulty noted and with a backup strategy in mind.[40,41] Extra equipment should be on hand, including a variety of laryngoscope blades, forceps, tubes, bronchoscopes, tracheostomy or cricothyrotomy trays, and additional skilled personnel as needed. If sedation is required, agents that can be reversed pharmacologically are desirable and should be titrated slowly to the desired effect. Figure 32–4 shows a modification of the American Society of Anesthesiologist's difficult airway algorithm and provides an approach to managing the difficult airway.[42] A similar plan is necessary at the time of extubation, with serious consideration given to extubation in the operating room or with an airway exchange catheter left in place to facilitate reintubation if necessary.

Process of Intubation

All equipment for intubation must be available prior to the procedure (Figure 32–5). A source of suction and appropriate catheters, oxygen and necessary tubing, ventilation bag, mask, laryngoscope and proper-sized blade with a well-functioning light, endotracheal tubes of the expected size and larger and smaller sizes, airway forceps, stylet, and a means of securing the endotracheal tube should be present at the head of the bed so that the

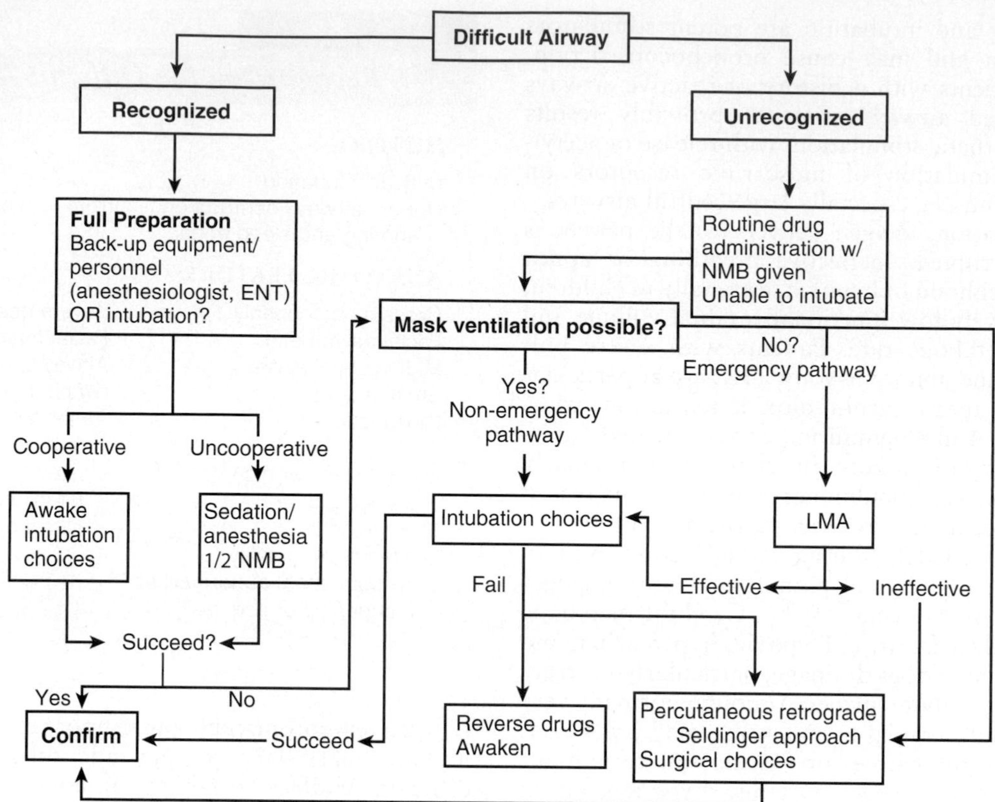

FIGURE 32–4 • Modification of the American Society of Anesthesiologist's difficult airway algorithm. (From *Anesthesiology* 98:1269, 2003.)

intubator does not need to look away from the patient. A functioning intravenous catheter for drug infusion is essential in all but the most extreme emergencies.

Laryngoscope handles are available in standard adult and pediatric sizes. The smaller diameter of the pediatric handle makes it easier to manipulate, particularly when intubating infants and very young children. Blades of many descriptions are available. The most important characteristic is length. Inexperienced operators often select a blade that is too short, making visualization of the larynx difficult. Excessively long blades make it difficult to avoid pressure on the upper lip and teeth. Straight blades provide good exposure in infants and young children. The slightly curved tip of the Miller blade makes visualization of the larynx possible without actually lifting the epiglottis. The broader blade and bore of the Wis-Hipple helps displace soft tissues in the young infant's oropharynx. The Miller no. 2 blade is especially versatile in a broad age group (about 3 to 10 years old). In older children, a curved blade is often best. If a cuffed endotracheal tube is to be used, a curved Macintosh no. 2 or 3 blade is effective in the majority of patients and may provide more room to manipulate a cuff in the oropharynx.

Virtually all endotracheal tubes in use in the United States today are sterile, disposable, implant-tested plastic tubes. Tubes vary with regard to the type of material used, external markings, and other factors, but few data on the relative risk of tracheal injury, propensity to kink, or other characteristics are available. Selecting the proper tube size (diameter) is important, both to achieve effective mechanical ventilation and to prevent tracheal injury. A variety of formulas are in use; the most common is that of Cole: Tube size (inner diameter) = (Age [years]/4) + 4. For infants, no formula is very accurate. Table 32–1 gives reasonable guidelines. Individual differences require that tube size be modified for each child such that the tube passes easily and allows gas to leak around it at roughly 15 to 30 cmH_2O pressure, but fits snugly enough to allow delivery of adequate mechanical breaths at a given chest compliance.

Traditional teaching has held that cuffed endotracheal tubes are not necessary or appropriate in young pediatric patients (younger than 8 years) because the narrow diameter of the trachea at the cricoid ring allows a fairly snug fit without a cuff, and a cuff may make tracheal injury at that level more likely. In addition, the bulk of the cuff usually requires using a tube of 0.5-mm smaller diameter, with the associated increased resistance to gas flow and greater risk of occlusion. Cuffed tubes are routinely recommended for children older than 8 to 10 years because the cricoid ring has been replaced by the triangular opening of the vocal cords as the narrowest point in the airway (see Figure 32–1). In addition, the greater elastic recoil of the lungs and chest wall of older patients may demand higher airway pressures for effective ventilation.

However, cuffed tubes of all sizes are available and may be useful in patients in whom consistent minute ventilation is essential (e.g., in the presence of severely elevated ICP or very reactive pulmonary vasculature) or those requiring relatively high airway pressures. Although data are limited, evidence is growing that cuffed tubes

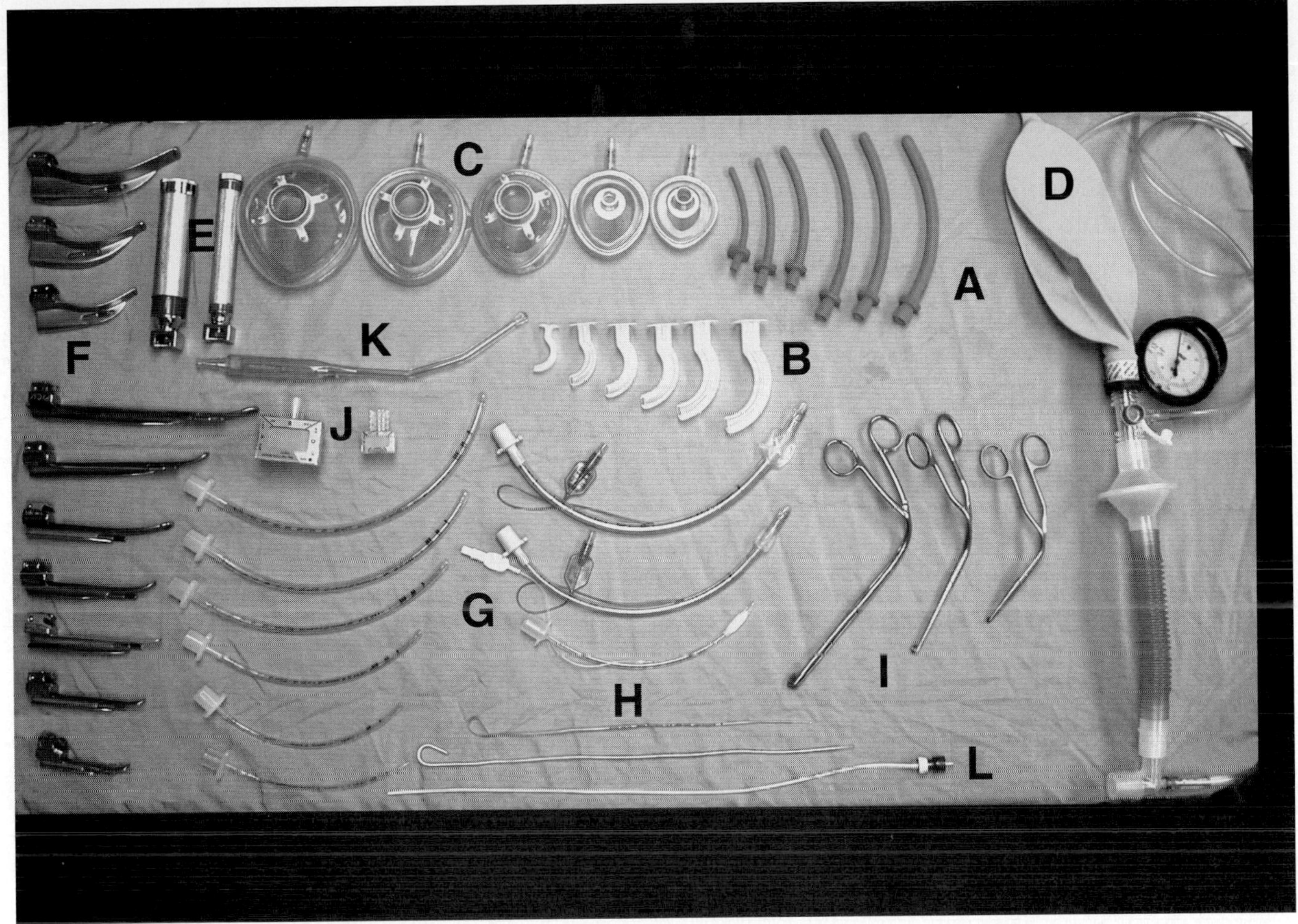

FIGURE 32–5 • Equipment for intubation, showing a variety of sizes available for pediatric patients.

can be used in young children without higher incidence of airway complications.[43–47] The modern low-pressure, high-volume cuff requires a much lower pressure to obtain a seal than did the endotracheal tube cuffs of the past. When a cuffed tube is used, great care should be taken to inflate it with the "minimum occlusive volume," the *minimum* volume required to "just seal" the gas leak around the tube during mechanical inspiration and prevent mucosal ischemia and subsequent tracheal damage. Potential advantages of cuffed tubes include

TABLE 32–1

Guidelines for Endotracheal Tube Diameter in Infants and Children*

Age	Internal Diameter (ID)	Orotracheal Length (cm)	Nasotracheal Length (cm)
Premature	2.0–3.0	6–8	7–9
Newborn	3.0–3.5	9–10	10–11
3–9 mo	3.5–4.0	11–12	11–13
9–18 mo	4.0–4.5	12–13	14–15
1.5–3 yr	4.5–5.0	12–4	16–17
4–5 yr	5.0–5.5	14–16	18–19
6–7 yr	5.5–6.0	16–18	19–20
8–10 yr	6.0–6.5†	17–19	21–23
11–13 yr	6.0–7.0†	18–21	22–25
14–16 yr	7.0–7.5†	20–22	24–25

*Ideal tube size varies according to age, height, weight, specific airway anatomy, and ventilatory requirements of a child. In general, an air leak around the tube at 15–30 cmH_2O pressure is desirable.

†Cuffed tube.

decreased likelihood of multiple intubations to identify the correct size and avoidance of changing the endotracheal tube of a critically unstable patient if lung disease worsens. Ability to occlude the leak also facilitates pulmonary function testing.

Pharmacologic Agents Facilitating Intubation (Table 32–2)

Although intubation often is possible without use of drugs, the physiologic and psychological benefits of their use usually outweigh the disadvantages.[48,49] This is equally true in neonates, in whom sedation and neuromuscular blockade are still commonly not used, with no evidence they are harmful.[50] In neonates the predominance of evidence indicates that use of neuromuscular blockade is associated with a lower risk of intracranial hemorrhage and pulmonary airleak.[51] Excellent technical airway skills are an *absolute* prerequisite, however, because loss of control of the airway invites catastrophe.

Anticholinergic Agents

Anticholinergic agents decrease oral secretions and prevent bradycardia, particularly in young infants. Atropine (0.02 mg/kg) and glycopyrrolate (0.01 mg/kg intravenously) both are effective. Scopolamine provides amnesia, decreases secretions, and prevents bradycardia.

TABLE 32–2

Drugs Facilitating Intubation

	Drugs	Dose	Duration	Comments
Intravenous anesthetics	Thiopental	4–7 mg/kg IV	5–10 min	Anesthesia, apnea, myocardial depression, decreased venous tone, ↓$CMRO_2$, ↓CBF, ↓ICP, ↓IOP
	Etomidate	0.3 mg/kg IV	3–5 min	Anesthesia, minimal CV effect, apnea, ↓$CMRO_2$, ↓CBF, ↓ICP
	Ketamine*	1–2 mg/kg IV 4–6 mg/kg IM	10–15 min	Anesthesia, ↑systemic arterial pressure, ↑HR, ↑ICP, ↑IOP, hallucinations, laryngospasm, bronchodilation
	Propofol	1–3.5 mg/kg IV, then 0.05–0.3 mg/kg/min	10–15 min	↓Systemic arterial pressure, ↓$CMRO_2$, ↓CBF, ↓ICP, metabolic acidosis
Sedatives/analgesics	Fentanyl*	2–5 mcg/kg IV	30–90 min	Analgesia, respiratory depression, cardiovascular stability, occasional bradycardia, or chest wall rigidity
	Remifentanil	1–3 mcg/kg, then 0.25–1 mcg/kg/min		Analgesia, respiratory depression, cardiovascular stability
	Morphine*	0.1–0.2 mg/kg IV	2–4 hr	Analgesia, respiratory depression, ↓systemic arterial and venous tone, ↓systemic blood pressure
	Midazolam*	0.1–0.3 mg/kg IV	1–2 hr	Amnesia, sedation or euphoria, ±cardiovascular stability, occasional respiratory depression
	Lorazepam	0.1–0.3 mg/kg IV	2–4 hr	Sedation, anxiolysis, minimal cardiovascular effect
Neuromuscular blocking agents	Rocuronium*	0.6–1.2 mg/kg IV	15–45 min	Minimal cardiovascular effect, prolonged duration in liver failure
	Vecuronium*	0.1–0.3 mg/kg IV	30–75 min	Minimal cardiovascular effect, prolonged effect in hepatic failure
	Cis-atracurium	0.1 mg/kg, then 1–5 mg/kg/min	20–35 min	Metabolized by plasma hydrolysis, mild histamine release
	Atracurium	0.5 mg/kg	30–40 min	Metabolized by plasma hydrolysis, mild histamine release
	Succinylcholine*	1–4 mg/kg IV	5–10 min	↓HR, K^+ release in neuromuscular disease, trauma or burns, masseter spasm, malignant hyperthermia, myoglobinuria

CBF, cerebral blood flow; *$CMRO_2$*, cerebral metabolic oxygen requirement; *HR*, heart rate; *ICP*, intracranial pressure; *IOP*, intraocular pressure.
Duration of effect is only approximate and varies with age and physiologic state of the patient.
*Agents may be given IM but will have slower onset and more variable duration of effect.

The drying effect commonly requires approximately 15 to 30 minutes and is rarely achieved in emergency intubation.

Sedative and Analgesic Agents

Most patients benefit from some degree of sedation. Drugs commonly used include intravenous anesthetic agents, anxiolytics, and narcotic analgesics. The appropriate choice in a particular patient depends on the child's hemodynamic status, level of anxiety, and underlying disease process.

Thiopental is a short-acting barbiturate that can provide deep anesthesia, obliterating awareness of the intubation process. It decreases cerebral oxygen consumption and thereby sharply lowers cerebral blood flow (CBF) and ICP. However, it is also a potent myocardial depressant; it decreases peripheral vascular resistance and may precipitate cardiovascular collapse in patients with myocardial dysfunction or hypovolemia. At anesthetic doses (4–7 mg/kg), it reliably causes apnea.

Etomidate is another short-acting intravenous anesthetic that causes rapid loss of consciousness (at 0.3 mg/kg) and respiratory depression, although it is less potent than thiopental. It also decreases cerebral oxygen consumption, CBF, and ICP, but without significant detrimental effects on cardiovascular function and with less respiratory depression than thiopental. These characteristics have led to its increased use for emergency intubation.[52,53] It has no analgesic properties and may be best combined with a narcotic analgesic. Side effects include vomiting, myoclonus, and lowering of the seizure threshold. With continuous infusion for sedation, it can cause adrenal insufficiency, making it inappropriate for long-term use in the ICU.[54] Limited evidence suggests it may suppress adrenal function even after a single dose, particularly in patients with sepsis and shock, raising questions about its use in these settings.[55]

Ketamine is another potent nonnarcotic analgesic and anesthetic that has been used safely in children in the critical care setting.[56,57] It increases heart rate, systemic blood pressure, and cardiac output and is a fairly potent bronchodilator. However, myocardial depression may be apparent after administration to patients with catecholamine depletion. Spontaneous ventilation is preserved in most patients, but laryngospasm may occur. It increases cerebral metabolic rate, blood flow, and ICP, making it an inappropriate agent for use in patients with suspected intracranial hypertension. Investigation suggests its use in already sedated patients at risk for intracranial hypertension can be accomplished without adverse effects, but the associated increased CBF makes its use in unmonitored patients unnecessarily risky.[58] Emergence delirium and hallucinations occur frequently and may be prolonged and recurrent, particularly in adolescents. Use of ketamine for a variety of procedures in children has been successful, with little reported difficulty with neuropsychiatric complications, but follow-up in most studies has been short and superficial.[59–62] Whereas the majority of patients do not suffer severe disturbances, those who do may have severe and prolonged distress. Benzodiazepines or barbiturates may decrease the incidence and severity of such side effects and the incidence of vomiting, although the data in children are limited and conflicting.[59,63,64]

Propofol is an ultra-short-acting agent with rapid onset and offset unless given by continuous infusion. It causes respiratory depression, desaturation, and systemic hypotension secondary to its negative inotropic effects and peripheral venous and arterial vasodilation. Its role in airway management of critically ill children is limited because of these effects. It has gained widespread acceptance as an anesthetic agent in children, however, and has been used extensively for procedural sedation.[65,66] Longer use in the ICU remains controversial because of its still unexplained association with deaths among pediatric ICU patients.[67,68]

The *benzodiazepines*, including diazepam and midazolam, relieve anxiety, produce sedation in most children, and provide amnesia for noxious procedures. They do not relieve pain. They have relatively little hemodynamic effect in most patients and rarely interfere with spontaneous breathing at therapeutic doses. Although they decrease cerebral oxygen consumption, their effect on cerebral metabolism is much less pronounced than that of thiopental. They are best combined with a narcotic analgesic when used for intubation in order to decrease the pain associated with laryngoscopy and passage of the tube.

Narcotics commonly used for intensive care include morphine, fentanyl, and some of the ultra-short-acting agents such as remifentanil. They cause respiratory depression in a dose-dependent fashion and increase intracranial blood flow in proportion to the increase in $Pa{CO_2}$. If hypercarbia is prevented, they decrease cerebral metabolic rate and blood flow. In the setting of altered cerebral autoregulation, they may not protect the patient from alterations of CBF.[69,70] Morphine causes histamine release and peripheral vasodilation and may precipitatesystemic hypotension. Fentanyl is approximately 100 times more potent than morphine but does not release histamine and has little hemodynamic effect, even at anesthetic doses. Large doses given rapidly can cause bradycardia or chest wall rigidity. Remifentanil is a rapid-onset, ultra-short-acting opiate, even more potent than fentanyl, which may have potential benefit in intubation for procedures.

Neuromuscular Blocking Agents

Neuromuscular blocking agents cause reversible paralysis, facilitating visualization of the airway and insertion of the endotracheal tube in an atraumatic fashion. Most drugs in use are nondepolarizing relaxants, with very similar action. Differences are primarily in their hemodynamic effects, metabolism, and excretion.[71,72] Vecuronium and rocuronium are the agents most commonly used. Both are amino-steroid agents. Vecuronium has virtually no hemodynamic effect. Its duration of action varies depending on the the patient's age, approximately 70 minutes in infants and 35 minutes in older children. It is metabolized exclusively by the liver. Rocuronium provides good intubating conditions nearly as rapidly as succinylcholine (in about 45–90 seconds)[73–75] without the side effects. Its duration is longer at 15 to 45 minutes (and longer in infants).[76–78] Like vecuronium, it has minimal hemodynamic effect, is metabolized by the liver, and largely is excreted in bile (with a small amount excreted by the kidneys). Atracurium and cis-atracurium, both benzylquinolinium agents, also have minimal hemodynamic effects in most patients but may cause histamine release and hypotension in some. Metabolism occurs by spontaneous plasma hydrolysis; thus neither renal nor hepatic function is necessary for elimination. Its duration of action is short at about 15 to 20 minutes.

The only depolarizing relaxant in clinical use is succinylcholine. Its only advantage is its rapid onset of action (45–60 seconds) and brief duration of action (5–10 minutes). Muscle fasciculations occur at the onset of action in patients older than 4 years and may increase intracranial, intraocular, and intragastric pressure. Defasciculating doses of a nondepolarizing neuromuscular blocker minimize such effects. Massive hyperkalemia may occur following its use in patients with spinal cord injury, severe burns, crush injuries, or neuromuscular disease. It is a known trigger for malignant hyperthermia and frequently causes myoglobinuria in otherwise healthy children. The US Food and Drug Administration (FDA) has issued a warning against its use for routine intubation in children because of these complications. Although it is frequently used for emergency intubations and is widely recommended,[49,79,80] the difference in time to conditions for intubation between succinylcholine and rocuronium is small (~30 seconds), *very rarely* of clinical significance, and inadequate to justify the added risk in the vast majority of cases.

A more extensive discussion of anesthetic agents and their use is given in Chapters 114, 115, and 116.

Orotracheal Intubation

When all equipment is ready, an assistant is assigned to monitor the child's color, heart rate, blood pressure, and oxygen saturation and to administer drugs when ordered. The child is placed supine with the head in the "sniffing" position. The infant's large occipitofrontal diameter naturally results in good position most of the time, but a small pad under the shoulders may be helpful. In older children, a thin pad under the occiput helps establish slight neck flexion (Figure 32–6). The head is extended to align the oral, pharyngeal, and laryngeal axes as much as possible. Spontaneous or manual ventilation with supplemental oxygen is maintained as drugs to facilitate intubation are given. Applying cricoid pressure during manual ventilation helps minimize gastric distension by air (Figure 32–7).[81] After the drugs take effect, the pharynx is suctioned and stomach contents are aspirated. The patient is again briefly oxygenated, and the mask is removed. In a fully relaxed patient in good position, the mouth falls open. It can be opened more widely with caudad pressure on the chin by the intubator's left fifth finger as the laryngoscope is introduced into the right-hand corner of the mouth. In an unsedated patient or when the mouth opens abnormally, it may be necessary to open the jaw with the often recommended scissorslike use of the right thumb and forefinger, but this action places the intubator at risk of both trauma and infection and should be avoided when possible.

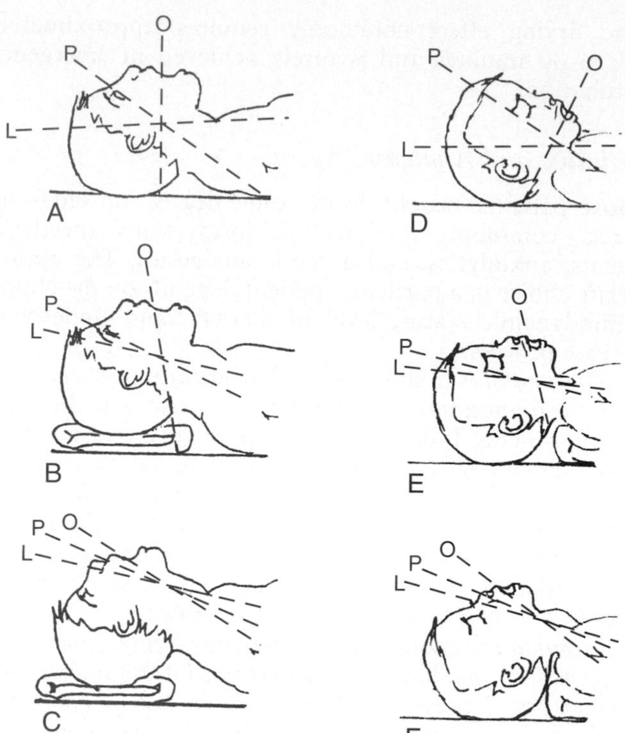

FIGURE 32–6 • Positioning of the young child and infant for laryngoscopy and tracheal intubation. Placing the child's head on a thin pad *(B)* flexes the neck slightly and helps align the pharyngeal and laryngeal axes. Extension of the atlantooccipital joint (into the sniffing position) further aligns the oral axis with the pharyngeal and laryngeal axes. Under the age of approximately 3 years, the child's large frontal occipital diameter makes the pad beneath the head unnecessary, but a small pad under the shoulders may improve alignment of the pharyngeal and laryngeal axes. As with the older child, head extension improves alignment of the oral, pharyngeal, and laryngeal axes. (From McAllister JD, Gnauck KA: *Emerg Med* 46:1255, 1999.)

The laryngoscope is gently advanced into the pharynx and leftward, sweeping the tongue out of the way. Holding the handle at a 45-degree angle to the bed and lifting along the line of the handle to avoid pressure on the lips, teeth, or alveolar ridge, the intubator displaces the mandible until the vocal cords are in view. Application of gentle cricoid pressure by an assistant may be helpful. Once the larynx is clearly visualized, the tube is advanced from the right corner of the mouth into the larynx (not through the blade itself). The nearly universal tendency to plumb the depths of the child's airway with extra centimeters of tube results in mainstem intubation. It can be avoided if the intubator is careful to place the appropriate markings near the tip of the endotracheal tube at the level of the cords. If such markings are absent, careful attention to advancing the tip of the tube only a few centimeters[2–4] beyond the cords prevents mainstem intubation.

With the tube in place, the child again receives manual ventilation with oxygen, and the presence of an appropriate leak is documented. Correct tracheal placement of the tube is suggested by observation of moisture condensing in the tube, good chest excursion, symmetrical breath sounds, and effective oxygenation. The most reliable means of ensuring proper placement, following clear visualization of the tube passing between the vocal cords,

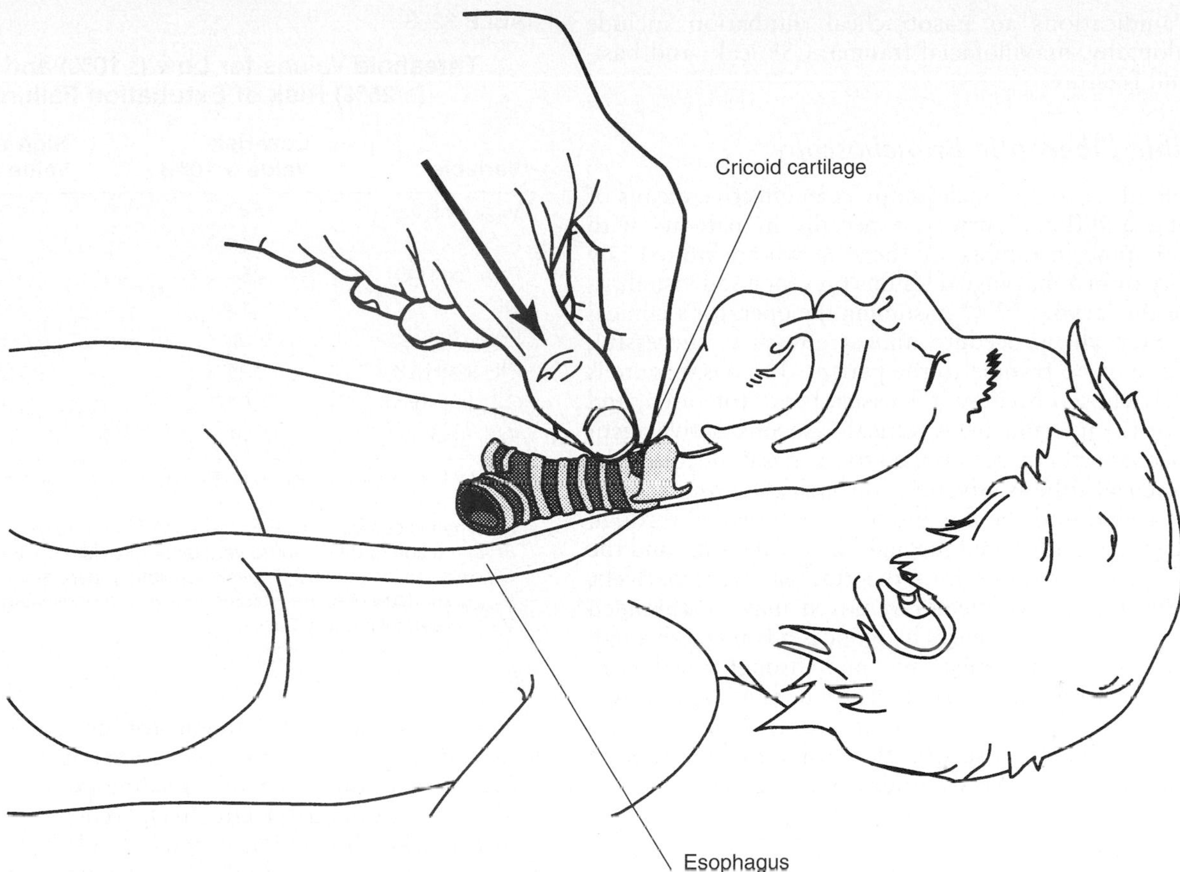

FIGURE 32–7 • Sellick maneuver. Pressure on the cricoid cartilage occludes the esophagus.

is documentation of carbon dioxide in expired gas (by capnometry or a disposable CO_2 detector). Only in the settings of full cardiac arrest or *extremely* low pulmonary blood flow can the endotracheal tube be in the airway without detection of expired carbon dioxide. Under other conditions, malposition of the tube, most commonly in the esophagus, must be assumed. It is important to remember that capnometry does not assure correct positioning within the airway: carbon dioxide will be detected with the tube anywhere from a bronchus to above the vocal cords. Documenting location of the tip of the tube between the thoracic inlet and T4 on chest radiograph is important. An inflated cuff can often be palpated at the sternal notch when quick pressure is applied to the sentinel balloon. The tube is secured, avoiding pressure on the lips, particularly at the angle of the mouth, and keeping the vermilion border of the lip free of tape.

Nasotracheal Intubation

If nasotracheal intubation is preferred, it should generally follow orotracheal intubation so that an assistant can ventilate the child while the somewhat more difficult intubation is accomplished. A topical vasoconstricting agent such as phenylephrine 0.25% or oxymetazoline 0.05%, sprayed into the nasal fossa, minimizes the risk of bleeding. In most children a tube of the same diameter as the oral tube can be gently advanced along the floor of the nasal cavity, essentially directly posteriorly, into the nasopharynx with firm, but not brutal, pressure. With the oral tube in the left-hand corner of the mouth, the laryngoscope is again advanced into the pharynx until the oral tube is visualized passing through the cords and the tip of the nasal tube is seen in the nasopharynx. The nasal tube is advanced until it lies directly above the cords, anterior to the oral tube. Magill forceps may facilitate this maneuver. When the nasal tube is in good position to enter the larynx, the assistant removes the oral tube and helps advance the nasal tube. Difficulty advancing the tube after it has passed the vocal cords may be overcome by rotating the tube or flexing the neck. The tube is secured; pressure on the septum or anterior rim of the nares should be avoided.

Although an orotracheal tube usually is placed more rapidly in emergencies, it often stimulates gagging, makes mouth care difficult, and it is more easily kinked or bitten. Anchoring the tube often is difficult because of saliva, and tongue movement may contribute to palatal or tracheal erosion and increase the likelihood of accidental extubation. Trauma to lips, teeth, tongue, and other oropharyngeal structures may occur. Nasotracheal intubation is more comfortable for most conscious patients, causes less stimulation of the gag reflex, is more easily secured, and prevents the problem of biting in patients with seizures, decerebrate rigidity, or extreme agitation. Bleeding, adenoid injury, sinusitis, and trauma to the nasal turbinates, septum, or nares may occur. The risk of sinusitis is greater than with orotracheal tubes.[82,83]

Contraindications to nasotracheal intubation include coagulopathy, maxillofacial trauma, CSF leak, and basilar skull fracture.

Flexible Fiberoptic Bronchoscopy

Flexible fiberoptic bronchoscopy is an effective means of securing a difficult airway, especially in patients with cervical spine instability or those in whom limited jaw mobility or oropharyngeal lesions prevent good visualization of the larynx.[38,41,84] Assuming the operator's clinical proficiency, the procedure almost always is successful, with little or no trauma to the patient. The nasal route is routinely chosen because it is easier, better tolerated, and safer for the instrument. A topical vasoconstrictive agent and local anesthetic are applied to the nasal mucosa. The endotracheal tube is advanced through the nose into the nasopharynx, and the flexible scope is threaded through it. The scope is advanced through the vocal cords, and the tube is passed over it into the trachea. (Alternatively, the tube with its connector removed may be threaded retrograde over the scope. The scope is advanced through the nose, to the nasopharynx, and through the larynx into the trachea. The endotracheal tube is advanced over the bronchoscope into good position.) The bronchoscopist visualizes and secures the position of the tube in the trachea and carefully withdraws the scope.

Extubation

Extubation is appropriate when the conditions for intubation are no longer present. In general, this means the work of breathing has decreased to a level manageable by the patient. In most cases, this situation occurs when oxygenation is adequate with the administration of 40% oxygen or less, spontaneous tidal volume is greater than 3.5 ml/kg, the patient can sustain a normal $Pa{CO_2}$ without mechanical breaths and without the use of accessory muscles, secretions are manageable, upper airway reflexes are intact, and neuromuscular function is sufficiently good to achieve an adequate vital capacity and maximum inspiratory pressure (Table 32–3).[85] If intubation was for relief of upper airway obstruction, extubation usually is possible when a leak develops around the endotracheal tube or when direct inspection reveals more normal anatomy. In patients with a previously difficult airway, extubation over a tube changer or in the operating room should be considered.

Before extubation, the child is kept NPO (nothing by mouth) for 4 to 6 hours. The tube and pharynx are suctioned thoroughly, and the child is ventilated with 100% oxygen to provide a reservoir of oxygen as a buffer against laryngospasm at extubation. With the lungs fully inflated, the endotracheal tube is removed, and the child is provided with humidified oxygen and observed closely.

Postextubation stridor is common and may range from mild to life threatening. Children younger than 4 years are most frequently affected. Factors contributing to airway edema include a tight endotracheal tube or cuff, traumatic or repeated intubations, excessive movement of the tube (or patient), preexistent airway abnormalities, and airway infection.[86] Cool mist or humidified oxygen is sufficient treatment for children with mild symptoms. Nebulized racemic epinephrine (0.5 ml of a 2.25% solution in 2.5 ml of saline delivered intermittently or continuously) effectively relieves more severe upper airway obstruction in most children, probably by local vasoconstriction. Only the L-isomer in the racemic formulation is biologically active. Epinephrine available for cardiovascular use is as safe, effective, and less expensive if half the racemic dose is used. Following its use, edema may recur, so close observation must continue. The value of corticosteroids is more controversial, in part because most studies do not differentiate multiple causes of croup.[87–89] Dexamethasone (0.3–0.5 mg/kg for 1 or 2 days) is recommended.

The work of breathing through a narrowed upper airway can be decreased by inhalation of a low-density gas mixture. Oxygen in helium is less dense than air or pure oxygen and permits higher inspiratory flow at lower resistance. Helium-oxygen mixtures are commercially available, usually providing 20% oxygen in 80% helium. More oxygen can be added to the mix as needed. Although traditional teaching holds that at least 70% helium is necessary to decrease airway resistance enough to make a clinical difference in the work of breathing, experience demonstrates value at considerably lower concentrations.

If pharmacologic treatment is ineffective, reintubation with a smaller tube for 12 to 24 hours, maintenance of dexamethasone dosing, and sedation to minimize agitation and further trauma to the airway may permit resolution of symptoms. Persistent symptoms are an indication for diagnostic laryngotracheobronchoscopy.

TABLE 32–3

Threshold Values for Low (≤10%) and High (≥ 25%) Risk of Extubation Failure

Variable	Low-risk Value (<10%)	High-risk Value (≥25%)
V_{tspon} (mL/kg)	≥6.5	≤3.5
Fio_2	≤0.30	>0.40
Paw (cmH_2O)	<5	>8.5
OI	≤1.4	>4.5
FrVe (%)	≤20	≥30
PIP (cmH_2O)	≤25	≥30
C_{dyn} (ml/kg/cmH_2O)	≥0.9	<0.4
V_t/T_i (ml/kg/s)	≥14	≤8

From Venkataraman ST, Khan N, Brown A: *Crit Care Med* 28:2991, 2000.

C_{dyn}, dynamic compliance; Fio_2, fraction of inspired oxygen; *FrVe,* fraction of total minute ventilation provided by the ventilator; *OI,* oxygenation index; *PIP,* peak ventilatory inspiratory pressure; V_{tspont}, spontaneous tidal volume indexed to body weight; V_t/T_i, mean inspiratory flow.

Complications of Endotracheal Intubation

Complications of intubation can be divided into those related to placement of the artificial airway, those that occur while the endotracheal tube is in place, and those related to extubation or appearing late (Table 32–4).

TABLE 32–4

Complications of Endotracheal Intubation

	Immediate	Maintenance	Extubation/Late
Physiologic	Hemodynamic instability Dysrhythmias Apnea ↓Pa_{O_2} ↑Pa_{CO_2} Coughing Laryngospasm Gagging, vomiting, regurgitation, aspiration ↑Intracranial pressure ↑Intraocular pressure	Obstruction Sinusitis Otitis (similar to immediate)	Laryngospasm Gagging, vomiting Aspiration Sore throat Dysphonia, aphonia
Traumatic	Nasal septum laceration, perforation Nasal turbinate injury Tooth loss or injury Lip, tongue, palate laceration, hematoma Tonsillar or adenoid avulsion, laceration, hematoma Laryngeal strictures Cervical spine subluxation Esophageal position	Lip, tongue ulceration Nares ulceration Palatal erosion, cleft formation Vocal cord edema, ulceration Laryngeal and tracheal mucosal ischemia, ulceration, necrosis Recurrent laryngeal nerve damage Subglottic edema, ulceration	Laryngeal or tracheal granuloma Vocal cord paralysis Subglottic stenosis
Malposition	Esophageal Mainstem bronchus Intracranial Soft tissue	Mainstem intubation Inadvertent extubation Atelectasis	

Immediate complications usually are related to the underlying disease process, the physiologic effects of laryngoscopy and intubation, or direct trauma to airway structures. The child's general condition, tube size, cuff pressure, movement, airway infection, systemic perfusion, duration of intubation, and attention to meticulous airway care are factors influencing the development of problems during maintenance of the airway.[90] Laryngospasm, aspiration, and failure (or inability) to deflate a cuff cause complications at extubation. Although laryngeal or tracheal injury may be obvious at the time of intubation, symptoms may be delayed 2 to 6 weeks.

Prolonged Intubation

The safe duration of endotracheal intubation in infants and children is not clear. Since the 1950s, the accepted period has increased from less than 12 hours to an undefined, much longer period. Subglottic stenosis is reported to occur in 1% to 8% of infants after prolonged intubation, but a similar incidence has been noted after intubation for less than 1 week.[91] In older infants, children, and adults, it is becoming clear that there is no clear "safe" period. Complications can occur immediately at intubation or may not be seen after many weeks or even months with an endotracheal tube in place.[92] The decision to switch to tracheostomy should not be based on an arbitrary time limit but rather on the relative advantages and disadvantages of one artificial airway over another in each individual patient.

Special Circumstances

Full Stomach

Patients with a full stomach are at high risk for aspiration of gastric contents during airway manipulation, particularly if protective airway reflexes are impaired. Much of the morbidity associated with aspiration can be attributed to the effects of acid aspiration. Aspiration of fluid with a pH below 1.8 is associated with a very high incidence of severe pulmonary dysfunction and death. Aspiration of fluid with a pH between 1.8 and 2.5 produces symptoms of moderate severity. When fluid with pH above 2.5 is aspirated, sequelae are less a consequence of the acid than of other characteristics of the material aspirated.[93] Other risk factors include the volume aspirated, the presence and nature of particulate food particles, contamination by bacterial pathogens, underlying pulmonary or systemic disease, and immunosuppression.[94]

Food particles may physically obstruct small or even large central airways, with the expected alterations in lung volume in segments distal to the obstruction. In addition, certain foods may cause severe local inflammatory changes. Bacterial contamination of the upper gastrointestinal tract secondary to bowel obstruction or even antacid administration greatly increases the risks of respiratory infection following aspiration.

Patients who have eaten shortly before intubation (<6 hours) should be assumed to have a full stomach. In addition, those with bowel obstruction, pharyngeal or upper gastrointestinal bleeding, trauma, or acute onset of illness within 6 hours of eating and those who are pregnant or who have ileus or tense abdominal distension from any cause should be considered to have a full stomach.

Although delaying airway manipulation might be the measure most certain to prevent aspiration, such an approach is not a realistic option in most situations confronting the intensivist. In a conscious child, the volume of gastric contents can be minimized by suction through a relatively large-gauge nasogastric tube, but complete emptying of the stomach, particularly of large food particles and blood clots, is rarely possible. Although H_2 antagonists such as cimetidine and ranitidine effectively decrease both the volume and acid content of gastric secretions, an adequate effect requires 60 to 90 minutes following administration. Neither antacid nor H_2 blockers decrease the volume of gastric contents already present in the stomach. Anticholinergic agents such as atropine or glycopyrrolate also reduce gastric acidity but slowly and less effectively than the H_2 antagonists. They may decrease gastroesophageal sphincter tone. They appear to have no value in preventing the acid aspiration syndrome.

Antacids can effectively neutralize gastric pH. However, when aspirated, particulate antacids (aluminum and magnesium hydroxides) produce inflammatory changes as severe as gastric acid and food particles. Clear antacids, such as sodium citrate or Alka-Seltzer, appear to provide true protection. They effectively increase gastric pH and, when aspirated, appear to produce damage no more severe than that caused by normal saline. However, their use has not become common clinical practice.

Intubation is at once protective of the patient vulnerable to gastric aspiration and itself a risk to the patient. In an alert child with intact protective airway reflexes, it may be appropriate to pass a nasogastric tube to decrease the volume of gastric contents. A clear antacid (e.g., sodium citrate, 10–30 ml) can be administered orally or through the tube, which then is removed. In a child with impaired reflexes, no effort to pass a nasogastric tube should be made because of the risk of inducing vomiting or regurgitation and subsequent aspiration.

The intensivist should examine the patient's airway to be as certain as possible that intubation will not be difficult, as discussed earlier. If intubation likely will be straightforward, a rapid-sequence intubation is indicated (Box 32–4). The goal of this method of intubation is to minimize the likelihood of vomiting or regurgitation and the time between loss of protective reflexes and correct positioning of the endotracheal tube. The sequence consists of preoxygenation, cricoid pressure, administration of an intravenous sedative or anesthetic, pharmacologic paralysis, and endotracheal intubation.

BOX 32–4

Rapid-Sequence Intubation for Full Stomach

INDICATIONS

Food intake <4–6 hours before intubation
Pharyngeal or upper gastrointestinal bleeding
Intestinal obstruction or ileus (includes acute onset of illness)
Tense abdominal distension
Pregnancy

RELATIVE CONTRAINDICATIONS

"Difficult" airway
Profuse hemorrhage obscuring visualization
Upper airway obstruction
Increased intracranial pressure

PROCEDURE

Prepare *all* necessary equipment, including suction devices
Allow patient to breathe 100% oxygen for 3 minutes
Direct assistant to apply cricoid pressure
Rapid intravenous infusion of anesthetic or sedative/analgesic and neuromuscular blocking agents
Allow patient to continue to breathe oxygen until apneic
Avoid manual ventilation to minimize gastric distension
Perform laryngoscopy and orotracheal intubation with stylet in endotracheal tube
Confirm endotracheal tube placement
Release cricoid pressure

Cricoid pressure effectively occludes the esophagus, preventing regurgitation of gastric contents into the trachea, and often improves visualization of the larynx (see Figure 32–7).[81,95,96]

The patient spontaneously breathes 100% oxygen by mask for 3 to 5 minutes before further manipulation. If the child can cooperate, four deep breaths are comparable to 5 minutes of tidal breathing. Once preoxygenation is complete, the anesthetic or sedative is administered by rapid intravenous infusion, cricoid pressure is applied immediately by an assistant, and, as consciousness is lost, a muscle relaxant is given. The mask supplying oxygen is kept in place until the patient becomes apneic, but *no* effort to assist ventilation is made in order to avoid gastric distension and regurgitation. Once the patient is flaccid and apneic, the intensivist performs laryngoscopy and intubates the patient. Using a stylet in the endotracheal tube facilitates rapid intubation. Only after correct tube position is verified and the tube cuff, if present, is inflated should cricoid pressure be relieved and manual ventilation begun. In the case of unexpected difficulty intubating the patient and evidence of progressive hypoxemia, manual ventilation between attempts may be necessary but should be done with continued cricoid pressure.

The "classic" combination of drugs used for rapid sequence induction/intubation is sodium thiopental (4–6 mg/kg) and succinylcholine (1–4 mg/kg) with a prior defasciculating dose of a nondepolarizing muscle relaxant such as vecuronium. In hemodynamically unstable patients, alternative drugs include ketamine, etomidate, or a benzodiazepine alone or in combination with a short-acting narcotic. Succinylcholine has multiple undesirable side effects (as noted previously) that may include increased intragastric pressure. Most of the nondepolarizing relaxants, given in amounts two to three times the usual intubating dose, produce good conditions for intubation nearly as quickly as succinylcholine (60–90 seconds), without adverse side effects but lasting longer. Rocuronium is the current best alternative, with its rapid onset and short duration of action. Table 32–2 lists suggested drugs and doses.

Increased Intracranial Pressure and Neurologic Dysfunction

The intensivist is frequently called upon to intubate children with severe central nervous system dysfunction resulting from infection, hemorrhage, trauma, hydrocephalus, or mass lesions, any of which may be associated with actual or imminent intracranial hypertension and herniation. The pathophysiology of such disorders is discussed in depth in Chapters 52 and 53; a few points merit brief review.

In most circumstances, the intensivist can observe signs of elevated ICP or recognize settings where the likelihood is high, but there is no clinical measure of its severity. Current guidelines recommend intubation for Glasgow coma score of 8 or less.[97] Intubation under these conditions should be undertaken with the recognition that it is a likely stimulus for further and potentially lethal intracranial hypertension. The most immediate means of lowering ICP involves decreasing CBF (volume) through hyperventilation. Unfortunately, the process of intubation likely will decrease minute ventilation and increase cerebral blood volume for this and other reasons, as discussed earlier.

Under normal circumstances, CBF is closely coupled to the cerebral metabolic oxygen requirement ($CMRO_2$). Cerebral oxygen consumption and blood flow increase with increasing body temperature, motor activity, pain or other noxious stimuli, and seizure activity. Blood flow also increases rapidly when PaO_2 falls below 50 to 60 mmHg and linearly as $PaCO_2$ increases over a wide range. With intact autoregulation, blood flow is independent of systemic blood pressure except at very high or low levels, but when autoregulation is impaired, mean arterial pressure may affect CBF over a much broader range. Elevated intrathoracic pressure during struggling, coughing, or Valsalva maneuvers may impede jugular venous drainage and result in intracranial venous congestion.

Laryngoscopy and intubation are powerful noxious stimuli. In the awake unsedated child and even in the severely obtunded patient, laryngoscopy and intubation likely will precipitate vigorous struggle, coughing, pain (anxiety), and marked evidence of autonomic stimulation.[23,36,37,98] In most patients, sympathetic discharge predominates with tachycardia, hypertension, and diaphoresis. In the infant, vagal stimulation often predominates with resulting bradycardia.

Even in the lightly anesthetized patient, laryngoscopy itself and then intubation are associated with hypertension, tachycardia, and increased ICP. As might be predicted, massive surges in ICP are more likely to occur in patients suspected of having borderline or high baseline ICP before intubation than in those with intracranial pathology with well-compensated or previously controlled pressure. Arterial hypertension may precipitate further hemorrhage in the child with a vascular malformation, coagulopathy, or bleeding into a tumor. ICP waves may reduce cerebral perfusion pressure to ischemic levels or cause frank herniation.

Given the risk of life-threatening systemic and intracranial hypertension in these patients, it is clear that laryngoscopy and intubation should be undertaken with every effort to minimize stimulation and associated struggle.[70,99–101] In general, this implies ensuring excellent oxygenation, ventilation, and intubation under protection of profound sedation or anesthesia, with the assistance of neuromuscular blockade (Box 32–5). Neurologists and neurosurgeons are frequently loathe to relinquish the opportunity to examine the patient following intubation, but the risk of life-threatening intracranial hypertension justifies temporarily obscuring the neurologic examination. In most cases, adequate assessment is possible before intubation, and diagnostic studies require deep sedation for a period afterward.

The patient is provided 100% oxygen by bag and mask. An anesthetic or sedative agent in combination with a neuromuscular blocking agent is given, and manual ventilation is initiated to lower ICP as much as possible before airway manipulation. Although extreme hyperventilation may decrease CBF to ischemic levels, current guidelines support ventilation to a $PaCO_2$ of

BOX 32–5

Intubation for Increased Intracranial Pressure

- Prepare equipment. Monitor heart rate, blood pressure, and SaO_2
- Provide 100% oxygen and assisted ventilation as tolerated by patient
- Consider possible difficult airway
- If no airway contraindications, administer anesthetic and neuromuscular blocking agents:
  - Associated cardiovascular compromise or hypovolemia:
    - Etomidate (0.3 mg/kg IV), or midazolam (0.2–0.3 mg/kg IV), and fentanyl (5–10 mcg/kg IV), plus lidocaine (1.0–1.5 mg/kg IV), and rocuronium (0.6–1.2 mg/kg IV) or other relaxant
  - No associated cardiovascular compromise or hypovolemia:
    - Thiopental (4–6 mg/kg IV), plus lidocaine (1.0 mg/kg IV), plus rocuronium (0.6–1.2 mg/kg IV) or other relaxant
- Ventilate patient until drug effect achieved (consider short-term hyperventilation in patients with signs of critically elevated intracranial pressure)
- Perform laryngoscopy and orotracheal intubation

approximately 30 to 35 mmHg for patients with intracranial hypertension.[102]

In the hemodynamically stable patient, thiopental provides relatively deep anesthesia associated with a rapid decline in $CMRO_2$, CBF, and ICP.[99,101] Alternative agents include narcotic analgesics alone or in combination with a benzodiazepine, which has less hemodynamic effect but also less effect on $CMRO_2$ unless given in anesthetic doses.

Etomidate is widely used in patients with suspected intracranial hypertension. Its ability to decrease CBF without apparent detrimental effect on systemic hemodynamic stability makes it a useful agent, although concerns about its effect on adrenal function, perhaps even following a single dose, require caution in the patient with sepsis or shock. Because it lacks analgesic properties, combining it with an intravenous narcotic agent should be considered.

Lidocaine 1 to 1.5 mg/kg decreases $CMRO_2$ and modestly decreases the systemic and intracranial hypertensive response and the cough reflex, as long as a dose below the seizure-producing threshold is used. Effective serum concentrations are obtained more quickly and at lower doses by the intravenous route than when the agent is administered endotracheally. The available literature addresses patients fully premedicated and monitored undergoing neurosurgical procedures or patients already intubated, ventilated, and monitored in the ICU. Studies addressing intubation in the acute setting are lacking and unlikely to be accomplished.[102–106]

Although newer studies suggest that ketamine, given in already sedated patients, may not increase ICP as much as previously thought, it does increase systemic blood pressure and CBF and should be avoided in these patients until further evidence is available.[58,107]

In nearly all patients, orotracheal intubation is preferred because it is accomplished quickly and easily with less risk of prolonged manipulation and interrupted ventilation. Nasotracheal intubation is contraindicated in patients with basilar skull fractures and CSF leaks as a potential source of infection or even perforation of the cribriform plate and intracranial tube placement.

Cervical Spine Instability

Flexion and extension of the head on the neck occur between the atlas (C1) and the basiocciput. Rotation occurs between the atlas and axis (C2), as the thin arch of the atlas pivots around the odontoid process. Below the axis, the cervical vertebrae articulate with each other anteriorly at the intervertebral disks and posteriorly at the facet joints. Further neck flexion and extension occur at these joints. Anterior and posterior ligaments complete the stable spine.

Spinal cord injury generally occurs as a result of bony fracture, compression, or disruption of cervical ligaments. In young children, actual ligamentous disruption or bony fracture is not necessary for severe cord injury, even transection, to occur; extreme stretching, as may occur in acceleration or deceleration injury, is sufficient.[108–110] Instability results from disruption of both the anterior and posterior columns. Congenital or degenerative anatomic abnormalities, penetrating wounds, or expanding mass lesions in the spinal canal may compromise cord integrity.

During routine intubation, the intensivist flexes the neck and extends the head. In children with known or suspected cervical spine injury or instability resulting from other causes (e.g., Down syndrome or rheumatoid arthritis), manipulating the head and neck for intubation risks extending the existing condition or injury and may precipitate new problems. Cervical spine films and knowledge about the nature of the traumatic event help define the precise injury and predict maneuvers most likely to do harm, but such information rarely is complete and may be falsely reassuring.

The ideal approach to intubation in this setting is controversial.[111–114] Although evidence in cadavers, in addition to common sense, indicates typical airway maneuvers can cause anterior or posterior subluxation or widening of the disk space, evidence in patients is lacking.[115] Axial traction increases distraction and even subluxation in some patients[116]; in others traction is helpful. However, information about the appropriate amount of force or the correct plane in which it should be applied is rarely sufficient to make a timely informed decision. Therefore immobilization of the head and neck in the midline without traction is recommended.

Current advanced trauma life support guidelines no longer recommend blind nasotracheal intubation.[117,118] Orotracheal intubation is more reliably accomplished and less time-consuming than blind nasotracheal intubation and is associated with far fewer complications, including tube malposition and bleeding, even in adults.[119] The high anterior location of the pediatric larynx makes nasotracheal intubation even more difficult in young children. As a result, it is rarely a necessary or desirable choice for emergency airway stabilization in children.

Just as manipulation of the airway for intubation may risk additional cord injury, patient movement can cause additional damage. Few children of any age will tolerate awake intubation by any route without violent struggle. Even heavily sedated patients likely will cough upon stimulation of the airway.

Patients with spinal cord injuries are at risk for extreme hyperkalemia and resulting dysrhythmias or cardiac arrest following administration of succinylcholine. This response occurs from approximately 48 hours to 6 to 9 months after injury. Cervical injury often also disrupts sympathetic nervous system outflow and results in unopposed vagal tone and severe bradycardia. For these reasons, in most instances intubation is best accomplished in these patients via the orotracheal route, using an intravenous anesthetic or combination of sedative and analgesic agents, atropine, and a nondepolarizing neuromuscular blocking agent with an assistant immobilizing the head and neck in neutral position with one hand over the ear on either side of the head. If time, equipment, and available expertise permit, fiberoptic bronchoscopy may assist visualization of the larynx and intubation with minimal head or neck movement.[120]

If orotracheal or nasotracheal intubation cannot be accomplished because of associated facial or airway injuries or other technical obstacles, cricothyrotomy or primary tracheotomy may be indicated. However, no data support either the necessity or safety of routinely using a surgical approach before attempting orotracheal intubation.

Upper Airway Obstruction

Upper airway obstruction may result from many disorders (see Chapter 39). When symptoms are related to loss of oropharyngeal muscle tone, changing the patient's position, reversing the effects of a drug, or placing a nasal airway may be sufficient, if the duration of the underlying process likely will be brief. However, where airway structures likely are severely or progressively distorted by edema, inflammation, trauma, or other space-occupying process, an endotracheal airway is necessary.

Patients should be allowed to assume whatever position is most comfortable. Supplemental oxygen is provided at the maximum concentration possible, but a young child's anxiety should not be heightened with an overly aggressive approach with a mask. Contrary to popular fear, breathing *can* be assisted in nearly all cases by application of positive pressure, initially with continuous positive airway pressure and then gradually with assisted breaths.

In general, no action should be taken that compromises the child's ability to breathe spontaneously until the capacity to control ventilation is certain. In particular, use of neuromuscular blocking agents is dangerous and inappropriate until *after* the airway is controlled. Distortion of the airway may be so extreme that recognition of landmarks for intubation is impossible, and loss of pharyngeal tone in such patients may remove the last barrier to complete airway occlusion. However, reducing a child's anxiety with *cautious* sedation (with a reversible agent) may decrease peak inspiratory flow rate and symptoms of obstruction and make it easier to assist breathing and establish an artificial airway. When possible the child is gently lowered to a supine position (or to 30 degrees) and intubated by the orotracheal route. When time and available expertise permit, intubation in the operating room using an inhalational anesthetic in a high oxygen concentration allows spontaneous breathing until the patient is deeply anesthetized and untroubled by airway manipulation. This method may be especially helpful in cases of supraglottitis. In most cases, the proper tube size is 0.5 to 1.0 mm smaller in diameter than predicted for age because of airway inflammation and edema, and no leak will be present. Extubation usually is well tolerated when a leak develops.

Facial and Laryngotracheal Injury

Children with facial injuries present airway problems nearly as varied as the injuries themselves. Appropriate management depends primarily on accurate assessment of airway patency at presentation, the rate of bleeding (if any) into the airway, and the amount of additional swelling and distortion likely to occur later. Evaluation of possible ocular and intracranial injury must proceed simultaneously.

Profuse bleeding, unstable facial fractures, or aspiration of blood, gastric contents, or teeth causes early respiratory distress. Maxillary fractures may result in a free-floating maxilla with occlusion of the nasopharynx and pressure on the tongue. Isolated mandibular fractures often cause trismus but rarely cause airway obstruction or interfere with visualization of the larynx.

Airway management begins with suctioning the mouth and pharynx of blood and debris. If other injuries permit, the child is placed with the head down and turned to the side. The tongue and maxilla are pulled forward manually if necessary. A spontaneously breathing patient receives oxygen by mask and may not require further intervention before surgery. Patients with persistent obstruction may require an immediate artificial airway.

In most cases, orotracheal intubation is accomplished first. If ventilation can be assisted with bag and mask and bleeding is controlled, the patient may be sedated, paralyzed, and intubated with full stomach precautions. If bag-and-mask ventilation exacerbates airway obstruction, awake intubation may be necessary. Uncontrollable bleeding, inability to visualize the larynx, or violent struggle in a child with cervical spine instability or evidence of increased ICP may make primary tracheostomy desirable. Nasotracheal and nasogastric tubes are avoided until the possibility of a basilar skull fracture and CSF leak is eliminated.

Laryngotracheal injuries may be subtle or dramatic. They should be suspected in children with a history of anterior neck trauma and often cause hoarseness, stridor, subcutaneous emphysema, pneumothorax, or pneumomediastinum. Aerosolized epinephrine may temporarily decrease swelling and provide a little extra time to evaluate the airway and plan intervention. Awake intubation, with cautious sedation and topical anesthesia, under direct vision by laryngoscopy or fiberoptic bronchoscopy minimizes the risk of sudden, complete obstruction or creation of a false passage adjacent to the airway.

Open Globe Injury

Children with penetrating eye injuries may require emergency intubation for respiratory failure resulting from associated injuries or other underlying problems. Management in these cases seeks to prevent increased intraocular pressure with subsequent extrusion of the vitreous and permanent blindness. Intraocular pressure can be increased by struggling, crying, coughing, straining, or rubbing the eye. Hypoxia and hypercarbia can increase intraocular pressure. In general, central nervous system depressants lower intraocular pressure, with the possible exception of ketamine. Intubation should be performed smoothly under full muscle relaxation if possible, taking into consideration associated injuries and the risk of a full stomach.

The child should be preoxygenated with 100% oxygen, taking care not to apply pressure to the eye with the mask. Efforts to empty the stomach are delayed until the patient is fully relaxed and intubated. In hemodynamically stable patients, thiopental or other rapidly acting sedative/anesthetics are administered, followed by a nondepolarizing neuromuscular blocking agent if other airway anatomy permits. Succinylcholine, a *depolarizing* relaxant, has been associated with increased intraocular pressure, even in the absence of fasciculations. As in patients with head trauma, a combination of sedative and analgesic agents may replace thiopental if hemodynamic stability is uncertain. Lidocaine supplements the effect of other agents in blunting the rise in intraocular pressure that may occur even during a smooth intubation. Heavy sedation or paralysis should be maintained following intubation until after repair.

Alternative Approaches to the Airway

Lighted Intubation Stylet (Light Wand)-Assisted Intubation

A number of lighted intubation stylets have become available in the last decade. Each uses transillumination of the neck to guide placement of an endotracheal tube. The devices consist of a handle containing the power source and a malleable wand (stylet) with a light at the tip. Pediatric versions accommodate tubes as small as 3.5 mm.

Use of the lighted stylet for intubation is a technique recommended for use in patients with difficult airways. Reported experience in children is limited, but the technique has been successful in the hands of both highly skilled and novice operators.[121–125] The equipment is fairly simple to use and easy to learn. It does not require visualization of the airway, is less stimulating than laryngoscopy, allows nasal or oral intubation, and is portable and relatively inexpensive. Reported series indicate that mucosal and dental injuries are uncommon, and sore throat is less of a problem than following standard laryngoscopy.[126] Because intubation may be accomplished from the patient's side, it may be useful in awkward settings such as emergency transport vehicles.

Potential disadvantages include trauma to the upper airway and larynx. Anything that obscures transmission of light through the anterior neck interferes with its use, including scarring, massive edema, subcutaneous emphysema, or mass lesions. Profuse bleeding or thick airway secretions that obscure the bulb also interfere with effective use.

A lubricated lighted stylet is inserted through an endotracheal tube of desired size until the light is just short of the end of the tube, and the tube is firmly attached. The tube and stylet are bent to approximately 90 degrees, just proximal to the cuff if present. Dimming the room lights improves appreciation of the transillumination. The intubator may stand at the head of the bed or to the side of the patient. The head is extended. A shoulder roll may be useful. The mandible and tongue are pulled forward and upward by the intubator, and the styletted tube is introduced into the patient's mouth in the midline. It is advanced into the pharynx, while the operator observes transillumination of the soft tissues of the neck. Entry into the airway typically is recognized by the presence of a focused glow of light in the midline below the thyroid prominence; more diffuse light suggests esophageal placement. The tube is advanced until the light is at the level of the sternal notch. The lighted stylet is withdrawn and placement confirmed with capnography.

Nasal intubation is possible with the light wand. In this case, the trocar is removed to increase the flexibility of the device. When a glow is noted above the thyroid prominence, the tube is likely in the vallecula. The epiglottis can be moved out of the way with a jaw thrust, allowing further advancement of the tube into the trachea. An alternative is to flex the patient's neck as is sometimes necessary with visualized nasotracheal intubation.

Laryngeal Mask Airway

The laryngeal mask airway (LMA) is a relatively new and fairly safe means of securing a difficult airway in an infant or child.[127–129] It consists of a small mask with an inflatable rim and a tube with a "universal adaptor," which permits attachment to an anesthesia bag or ventilator (Figure 32–8). The insertion technique can be learned quickly by physicians and other providers, including emergency transport personnel, often more quickly than endotracheal intubation. Experience on a manikin appears to be effective training. Once in place, it can serve as a means of ventilating the patient until an alternative airway can be established. It is often used as a means subsequently of facilitating fiberoptic bronchoscopic intubation.

Proper placement is essential but is most uncertain in infants requiring the LMA size 1, most likely because the margin of error for placement in the small pharynx is so small. In general, the risk of downfolding the epiglottis, occluding the trachea, is greater in children than in adults. Successful placement depends on the shape and tone of the pharynx, adequate matching of the cuff, palatopharyngeal curve and shape of the posterior pharynx, the extent to which anterior structures (such as tonsils) obliterate the curve, the position of the head and neck, efficacy of digital manipulation, and the depth of anesthesia/sedation, muscle relaxation, or loss of airway reflexes.[128] Tissue trauma is uncommon, and there is minimal need to manipulate the cervical spine during placement. In most patients the autonomic response to placement is less pronounced than with laryngoscopy and intubation. On the other hand, the device does not fully protect against aspiration in the setting of a full stomach. In addition, it may not be effective in patients with glottic or subglottic pathology.

Although its primary use is in the operating room, growing experience demonstrates it can be lifesaving in a variety of other settings when no other nonsurgical means of maintaining an airway is successful, particularly in patients with anatomically abnormal airways.[130] The ease and rapidity of insertion and decreased gastric air insufflation during resuscitation make it a valuable tool when intubation fails during adult resuscitation.[131] The current Pediatric Advanced Life Support textbook supports the LMA as an effective alternative to intubation during resuscitation when inserted by trained providers.[132] In neonatal resuscitation, when face mask

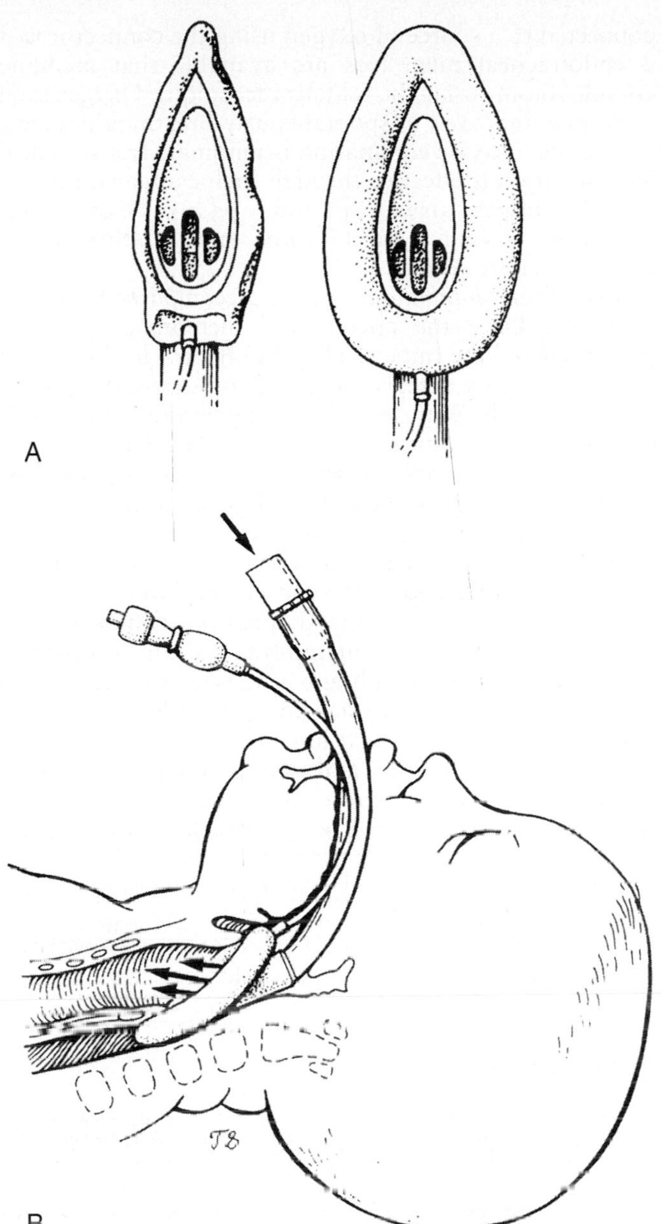

FIGURE 32–8 • Laryngeal mask airway (LMA). **A,** Mask portion of the airway with the rim deflated for insertion **(left)** and inflated **(right). B,** LMA in position, with the rim inflated around the laryngeal inlet. (From Efrat R, Kadari A, Katz S: *J Pediatr Surg* 29:206, 1994.)

ventilation or intubation is not successful, the LMA provides a means of rapidly improving oxygenation and heart rate. It is not, however, effective for aspirating meconium and may be inadequate for infants with severely noncompliant lungs. Use by prehospital personnel has been effective for critically ill adults, but experience in children in the field has not been reported.[133]

It is poorly tolerated by patients with intact protective reflexes, so its use is largely limited to those with severely depressed levels of consciousness or heavy sedation or anesthesia. Lidocaine jelly on the inflatable rim or lidocaine pharyngeal spray may promote tolerance in patients with active airway reflexes.

Choice of LMA size is based on weight: size 1 for patients weighing 2.5 to 6.0 kg, size 2 for 6.0 to 30 kg, and size 3 for patients weighing more than 30 kg.[134,135] With the rim deflated or partially inflated, the mask is placed blindly behind the tongue with the dorsum of the mask facing the palate. It is advanced into the hypopharynx until resistance of the upper esophageal sphincter is encountered. The cuff is filled with air, forming a seal around the laryngeal outlet, and the attached tube is connected to a source of oxygen and positive pressure. Although the seal is somewhat protective, patients with a full stomach remain at risk for aspiration. Positive airway pressure should be minimized as much as possible and a nasogastric tube passed to decrease gastric distension. Cricoid pressure may further decrease the risk of aspiration but also may interfere with proper LMA placement. If desired, an endotracheal tube can be inserted through the mask, either blindly or with fiberoptic bronchoscopy.[136]

Tracheostomy

Indications for tracheostomy include structural abnormalities of the upper airway requiring surgery, laryngeal trauma or complex craniofacial injury, severe facial burns, congenital anomalies lacking surgical treatment, vocal cord paralysis, and iatrogenic injury to the upper airway. Severe chronic neurologic dysfunction with impaired protective reflexes is an additional indication. Even in the absence of evidence of upper airway damage, tracheostomy may be performed to provide a more comfortable airway, which simultaneously allows airway protection, respiratory support, and greater patient mobility so that nutritional, developmental, and psychosocial needs may be met, especially, but not only, in the chronically ventilated patient.[137–140]

Tracheostomy spares laryngeal and subglottic structures from the trauma of an artificial airway, particularly in active or thrashing patients. Tracheostomy tubes are less likely to be inadvertently dislodged or to become obstructed, but if either problem does occur early following tracheostomy, it is more likely to be catastrophic. Because the tube is inserted below the cricoid ring, it often is possible to use a larger tracheostomy tube than endotracheal tube. Nevertheless, a larger leak around the tube may interfere markedly with effective ventilation in patients requiring high airway pressures.

Complications in the early postoperative period include bleeding, subcutaneous air dissection, pneumothorax, pneumomediastinum, injury to the recurrent laryngeal nerve, and death, usually as a consequence of loss of control of the airway intraoperatively or an unrecognized complication from the preceding list. Nearly all pediatric patients can and should be intubated before tracheostomy. Prior intubation decreases the incidence of most technical problems. Exceptions include patients with complex facial or airway injuries or deformities and those in whom no other means of establishing an airway have been successful. Wound colonization occurs rapidly. Bacterial infection may occur, rarely involving major cervical and mediastinal structures. Swallowing difficulty is common and may result from the tube and fixation tapes limiting excursion of the larynx. Aspiration may result from alteration of the laryngeal closure reflex.

Tracheostomy tube obstruction or accidental dislodgment is suspected when the patient becomes agitated and shows signs of increased respiratory distress, a suction catheter no longer passes freely, manual ventilation is ineffective, or, in case of dislodgment, the child is suddenly able to vocalize. The tube should be removed and replaced with a new one. The child is placed supine with the head and neck extended. Oxygen is delivered to the nose, mouth, and tracheal stoma. If manual ventilation is necessary, the stoma can be occluded to allow bag-and-mask ventilation from above. A fresh tracheostomy tube is inserted, initially directly posteriorly and then caudad. Replacement with a smaller tube or endotracheal tube may be necessary if resistance is encountered. Resistance to passage of a suction catheter or ineffective ventilation following replacement of a tracheostomy tube, particularly in the first 7 to 10 days postoperatively, is highly suggestive of creation of a "false passage" in a tissue plane outside the tracheal lumen. Reestablishing tracheal cannulation may require surgical intervention. Life-threatening pneumothorax or pneumomediastinum occurs frequently in such patients.

Late complications include granuloma or stricture formation at the stoma or where the tip of the tube meets the tracheal wall. Persistent posterior wall pressure may cause tracheoesophageal fistula formation. Erosion into the innominate artery is another rare occurrence, usually when the tracheostomy incision is below the third tracheal ring. The importance of an experienced, well-trained staff immediately available to address problems is supported by data demonstrating that mortality related to tracheostomy is significantly lower when performed in a children's hospital and decreases with increasing volume.[141]

Decannulation occurs when the indications for tracheostomy are no longer present. Diagnostic laryngotracheobronchoscopy before a planned decannulation permits identification of problems likely to interfere with effective breathing, including granulation tissue, severely stenotic areas, or vocal cord abnormalities. If none is present, the indwelling tube is replaced with successively smaller tubes until the smallest available is in place and the child is breathing well. If no distress occurs, the tube is removed and the stoma covered.

Cricothyrotomy and Retrograde Intubation

Although airway management by endotracheal intubation is possible and endotracheal intubation is the appropriate first choice in the vast majority of pediatric patients, intubation is not possible or should not be done on certain occasions. Such situations include massive facial trauma, oropharyngeal hemorrhage or foreign body, or severe upper airway obstruction.[142] Cricothyrotomy is an alternative to tracheostomy for rapidly establishing an airway in apneic or severely distressed patients.

The child's head and neck are extended with a roll under the shoulders. The cricothyroid membrane is palpated between the inferior margin of the thyroid cartilage and the superior edge of the cricoid cartilage. With one hand (or an assistant) stabilizing the larynx and trachea, the membrane is punctured in the midline with a large angiocath, the stylet is withdrawn, and the catheter is connected to a source of oxygen using the connector to a 3 endotracheal tube. Kits are available that facilitate cricothyrotomy using the Seldinger technique. Oxygenation is rapidly improved in spontaneously breathing patients, but carbon dioxide elimination is minimal. Transtracheal jet ventilation is effective through such catheters, providing the upper airway permits passive exhalation; otherwise, severe hyperinflation and life-threatening barotrauma are certain.

Retrograde intubation can be accomplished by this approach. Once the cricothyroid membrane has been punctured and the catheter placed in the tracheal lumen, a long wire from a vascular access kit is advanced cephalad into the mouth. With the wire firmly secure, an endotracheal tube may be advanced into the trachea. Once the tube is in the tracheal lumen, the wire is withdrawn and the tube is further advanced into the desired position. If the wire is insufficiently stiff to permit passage of the tube into the trachea, an endotracheal tube exchanger can be advanced over the wire first, followed by the endotracheal tube.

In adults and adolescents, a small horizontal incision over the cricothyroid membrane is an alternative approach. Once the membrane is incised, it is spread vertically, and a standard tracheostomy or endotracheal tube is inserted into the tracheal lumen. This approach is not recommended in infants and young children, except in highly skilled hands because of the potential for grave injury to a small, soft trachea or nearby neurovascular structures.

Complications are similar to those of tracheostomy. Complication rates of 10% to 40% are reported in adults.[142] There is little reported experience in pediatric patients, particularly in younger children.

REFERENCES

1. Buenting JE, Dalston RM, Drake AF: Nasal cavity area in term infants determined by acoustic rhinometry. *Laryngoscope* 104: 1439-45, 1994.
2. Arens R, McDonough JM, Corbin AM, et al: Linear dimensions of the upper airway structure during development: assessment by magnetic resonance imaging. *Am J Respir Crit Care Med* 165: 117-22, 2002.
3. Rodenstein DO, Perlmutter N, Stanescu DC: Infants are not obligatory nose breathers. *Am Rev Respir Dis* 131:343-347,1985.
4. Bergeson PS, Shaw JC: Are infants really obligatory nasal breathers? *Clin Pediatr* 40:567-569, 2001.
5. Onal E, Lopata M, O'Connor TO: Diaphragmatic and genioglossal electromyelogram response to CO_2 rebreathing in humans. *J Appl Physiol* 50:1052, 1981.
6. Sreenan C, Lemke RP, Hudson-Mason A, et al: High-flow nasal cannulae in the management of apnea of prematurity: a comparison with conventional nasal continuous positive airway pressure. *Pediatrics* 107:1081-1083, 2001.
7. Wheeler M, Roth AG, Dunham ME, et al: A bronchoscopic, computer-assisted examination of the changes in dimension of the infant tracheal lumen with changes in head position: implications for emergency airway management. *Anesthesiology* 88:1183-1187, 1998.
8. Rose DK, Froese AB: The regulation of $PaCO_2$ during controlled ventilation of children with a t-piece. *Can Anaesth Soc* J 26:104, 1979.
9. Waters DJ, Mapleson WW: Rebreathing during controlled respiration with various semiclosed anaesthetic systems. *Br J Anaesth* 33:374, 1961.
10. Aubier M, Viires N, Syllie G, et al: Respiratory muscle contribution to lactic acidosis in low cardiac output. *Am Rev Respir Dis* 126: 648, 1982.

11. Field S, Kelly SM, Macklem PT: The oxygen cost of breathing in patients with cardiorespiratory disease. *Am Rev Respir Dis* 126: 9, 1982.
12. Rasanen J: Conventional and high frequency controlled mechanical ventilation in patients with left ventricular dysfunction and pulmonary edema. *Chest* 91:225-229, 1987.
13. Naughton MT, Rahman MA, Hara K, et al: Effect of continuous positive airway pressure on intrathoracic and left ventricular transmural pressures in patients with congestive heart failure. *Circulation* 91:1725-1731, 1995.
14. Kaye DM, Mansfield D, Naughton MT: Continuous positive airway pressure decreases myocardial oxygen consumption in heart failure. *Clin Sci* 106:599-603, 2004.
15. MacDuff A, Grant IS: Critical care management of neuromuscular disease, including long-term ventilation. *Curr Opin Crit Care* 9:106-112, 2003.
16. Robotham JL: A physiological approach to hemidiaphragm paralysis. *Crit Care Med* 7:563, 1979.
17. Muller N, Volgyesi G, Bryan MH, et al: The consequences of diaphragmatic muscle fatigue in the newborn infant. *J Pediatr* 95:793, 1979.
18. Le Souef PN, England SJ, Stogryn HA, et al: Comparison of diaphragmatic fatigue in newborn and older rabbits. *J Appl Physiol* 65:1040-1044, 1988.
19. Watchko JF, Mayock DE, Standaert TA, et al: The ventilatory pump: neonatal and developmental issues. *Adv Pediatr* 38: 109-134, 1991.
20. Gaultier C: Respiratory muscle function in infants. *Eur Respir J* 8:150-153, 1995.
21. de Leeuw M, Williams JM, Freedom RM, et al: Impact of diaphragmatic paralysis after cardiothoracic surgery in children. *J Thorac Cardiovasc Surg* 118:510-517, 1999.
22. Bach JR, Niranjan V, Weaver B: Spinal muscular atrophy type 1: a noninvasive respiratory management approach. *Chest* 117: 1100-1105, 2000.
23. Kaplan JD, Schuster DP: Physiologic consequences of tracheal intubation. *Clin Chest Med* 12:425-432, 1991.
24. Kovac AL: Controlling the hemodynamic response to laryngoscopy and endotracheal intubation. *J Clin Anesth* 8:63-79, 1996.
25. Wicks TC: The pharmacology of rocuronium bromide (ORG 9426). *AANA J* 62:33, 1994.
26. Durand M, Sangha B, Cabal LA, et al: Cardiopulmonary and intracranial pressure changes related to endotracheal suctioning in preterm infants. *Crit Care Med* 17:506, 1989.
27. Marshall TA, Deeder R, Pai S, et al: Physiologic changes associated with endotracheal intubation in preterm infants. *Crit Care Med* 12:501, 1984.
28. Bode H, Ummenhofer W, Frei F: Effects of laryngoscopy and tracheal intubation on cerebral and systemic haemodynamics in children under different protocols of anaesthesia. *Eur J Pediatr* 152:905-908, 1993.
29. Fanconi S, Duc G: Intratracheal suctioning in sick preterm infants: prevention of intracranial hypertension and cerebral hypoperfusion by muscle paralysis. *Pediatrics* 79:538, 1987.
30. Friesen RH, Honda AT, Thieme RE: Changes in anterior fontanel pressure in preterm neonates during tracheal intubation. *Anesth Analg* 66:874, 1987.
31. Ninan A, O'Donnell M, Hamilton K, et al: Physiologic changes induced by endotracheal instillation and suctioning in critically ill preterm infants with and without sedation. *Am J Perinatal* 3:94, 1986.
32. Barrington KJ, Finer NN, Etches PC: Succinylcholine and atropine for premedication of the newborn infant before nasotracheal intubation: a randomized, controlled trial. *Crit Care Med* 17:1293, 1989.
33. DeBoer SL, Peterson LV: Sedation for nonemergent neonatal intubation. *Neonat Netw J Neonat Nurs* 20:19-23, 2001.
34. Gentz BA, Shupak RC, Bhatt SB, et al: Carbon dioxide dynamics during apneic oxygenation: the effects of preceding hypocapnia. *J Clin Anesth* 10:189-194, 1998.
35. Patel R, Lenczyk M, et al: Age and onset of desaturation in apnoeic children. *Can J Anaesth* 41:771-774, 1994.
36. Millar C, Bissonnette B: Awake intubation increases intracranial pressure without affecting cerebral blood flow velocity in infants. *Can J Anaesth* 41:281-287, 1994.
37. Stow PJ, McLeod ME, Burrows FA, et al: Anterior fontanelle pressure responses to tracheal intubation in the awake and anaesthetized infant. *Br J Anaesth* 60:167-170, 1988.
38. Christianson L: Anesthesia for major craniofacial operations. *Int Anesthesiol Clin* 23:117, 1985.
39. Mallampati SR, Gatt SP, Gugino LD, et al: A clinical sign to predict difficult tracheal intubation—a prospective study. *Can J Anaesth* 32:429–434, 1985.
40. Sullivan KJ, Kissoon N: Securing the child's airway in the emergency department. *Pediatr Emerg Care* 18:108-121, 2002.
41. Walker RW: Management of the difficult airway in children. *J R Soc Med* 94:341-344, 2001.
42. Practice guidelines for the management of the difficult airway: an updated report by the American Society of Anesthesiologists Task Force on Management of the Difficult Airway. *Anesthesiology* 98:1269–1277, 2003.
43. Deakers TW, Reynolds G, Stretton M, et al: Cuffed endotracheal tubes in pediatric intensive care. *J Pediatr* 125:57, 1994.
44. Newth CJ, Rachman B, Patel N, et al: The use of cuffed versus uncuffed endotracheal tubes in pediatric intensive care. *J Pediatr* 144:333-337, 2004.
45. Verive M, Reyes G, et al: International survey on the use of cuffed versus uncuffed endotracheal tubes. *Clin Intensive Care* 10, 1999.
46. Fine GF, Borland LM: The future of the cuffed endotracheal tube. *Paediatr Anaesth* 14:38-42, 2004.
47. Mhanna MJ, Zamel YB, Tichy CM, et al: The "air leak" test around the endotracheal tube, as a predictor of postextubation stridor, is age dependent in children. *Crit Care Med* 30:2639-643, 2002.
48. Bledsoe GH, Schexnayder SM: Pediatric rapid sequence intubation: a review. *Pediatr Emerg Care* 20:339-344, 2004.
49. McAllister JD, Gnauck KA: Rapid sequence intubation of the pediatric patient. Fundamentals of practice. *Pediatr Clin North Am* 46:1249-1284, 1999.
50. Whyte S, Birrell G, Wyllie J: Premedication before intubation in UK neonatal units. *Arch Dis Child Fetal Neonatal Ed* 82:F38-41, 2000.
51. Cools F, Offringa M: Neuromuscular paralysis for newborn infants receiving mechanical ventilation. *Cochrane Database Syst Rev* CD002773, 2000.
52. Sokolove PE, Price DD, Okada P: The safety of etomidate for emergency rapid sequence intubation of pediatric patients. *Pediatr Emerg Care* 16:18–21, 2000.
53. Rothermel LK: Newer pharmacologic agents for procedural sedation of children in the emergency department—etomidate and propofol. *Curr Opin Pediatr* 15:200-203, 2003.
54. Wagner RL, White PF, Kan PB, et al: Inhibition of adrenal steroidogenesis by the anesthetic etomidate. *N Engl J Med* 310:1415-1421, 1984.
55. Schenarts CL, Burton JH, Riker RR: Adrenocortical dysfunction following etomidate induction in emergency department patients. *Acad Emerg Med* 8:1-7, 2001.
56. Slonim AD, Ognibene FP: Sedation for pediatric procedures, using ketamine and midazolam, in a primarily adult intensive care unit: a retrospective evaluation. *Crit Care Med* 26:1900-1904, 1998.
57. Green SM, Denmark TK, Cline J, et al: Ketamine sedation for pediatric critical care procedures. *Pediatr Emerg Care* 17:244-248, 2001.
58. Bourgoin A, Albanese J, Wereszczynski N, et al: Safety of sedation with ketamine in severe head injury patients: comparison with sufentanil. *Crit Care Med* 31:711-717, 2003.
59. Kennedy RM, McAllister JD: Midazolam with ketamine: who benefits? *Ann Emerg Med* 35:297-299, 2000.
60. Kennedy RM, Porter FL, Miller JP, et al: Comparison of fentanyl/midazolam with ketamine/midazolam for pediatric orthopedic emergencies. *Pediatrics* 102:956-963, 1998.
61. Parker RI, Mahan RA, Giugliano D, et al: Efficacy and safety of intravenous midazolam and ketamine as sedation for therapeutic and diagnostic procedures in children. *Pediatrics* 99:427-431, 1997.
62. Pena BM, Krauss B: Adverse events of procedural sedation and analgesia in a pediatric emergency department. *Ann Emerg Med* 34:483-491, 1999.
63. Sherwin TS, Green SM, Khan A, et al: Does adjunctive midazolam reduce recovery agitation after ketamine sedation for pediatric procedures? A randomized, double-blind, placebo-controlled trial. *Ann Emerg Med* 35:229-238, 2000.

64. Wathen JE, Roback MG, Mackenzie T, et al: Does midazolam alter the clinical effects of intravenous ketamine sedation in children? A double-blind, randomized, controlled, emergency department trial. *Ann Emerg Med* 36:579-588, 2000.
65. Hertzog JH, Dalton HJ, Anderson BD, et al: Prospective evaluation of propofol anesthesia in the pediatric intensive care unit for elective oncology procedures in ambulatory and hospitalized children. *Pediatrics* 106:742-747, 2000.
66. Wheeler DS, Vaux KK, Ponaman ML, et al: The safe and effective use of propofol sedation in children undergoing diagnostic and therapeutic procedures: experience in a pediatric ICU and a review of the literature. *Pediatr Emerg Care* 19:385-392, 2003.
67. Parke TJ, Stevens JE, Rice AS, et al: Metabolic acidosis and fatal myocardial failure after propofol infusion in children: five case reports. *BMJ* 305:613-616, 1992.
68. Bray RJ: Propofol infusion syndrome in children. *Paediatr Anaesth* 8:491-499, 1998.
69. de Nadal M, Munar F, Poca MA, et al: Cerebral hemodynamic effects of morphine and fentanyl in patients with severe head injury: absence of correlation to cerebral autoregulation. *Anesthesiology* 92:11-19, 2000.
70. Werner C, Kochs E, Bause H, et al: Effects of sufentanil on cerebral hemodynamics and intracranial pressure in patients with brain injury. *Anesthesiology* 83:721-726,1995.
71. Doobinin KA, Nakagawa TA: Emergency department use of neuromuscular blocking agents in children. *Pediatr Emerg Care* 16:441-447, 2000.
72. Sparr HJ, Beaufort TM, Fuchs-Buder T: Newer neuromuscular blocking agents: how do they compare with established agents? *Drugs* 61:919-942, 2001.
73. Stoddart PA, Mather SJ: Onset of neuromuscular blockade and intubating conditions one minute after the administration of rocuronium in children. *Paediatr Anaesth* 8:37-40, 1998.
74. Naguib M, Samarkandi AH, Ammar A, et al: Comparison of suxamethonium and different combinations of rocuronium and mivacurium for rapid tracheal intubation in children. *Br J Anaesth* 79:450-455, 1997.
75. Scheiber G, Ribeiro FC, Marichal A, Bredendiek M, et al: Intubating conditions and onset of action after rocuronium, vecuronium, and atracurium in young children. *Anesth Analg* 83:320-324, 1996.
76. Motsch J, Leuwer M, Pfau M, et al: Time course of action and recovery of rocuronium bromide in children during halothane anaesthesia: a preliminary report, *Eur J Anaesthesiol Suppl* 9:75, 1994.
77. Mazurek AJ, Pae B, Hann S, et al: Rocuronium versus succinylcholine: are they equally effective during rapid sequence induction of anesthesia? *Anesth Analg* 87:1259-1262, 1998.
78. Rapp HJ, Altenmueller CA, Waschke C: Neuromuscular recovery following rocuronium bromide single dose in infants. *Paediatr Anaesth* 14:329-335, 2004.
79. Gerardi MJ, Sacchetti AD, Cantor RM, et al: Rapid-sequence intubation of the pediatric patient. *Ann Emerg Med* 28:55-74, 1996.
80. Robinson AL, Jerwood DC, Stokes MA: Routine suxamethonium in children. A regional survey of current usage. *Anaesthesia* 51:874-878, 1996.
81. Moynihan RJ, Brock-Utne JG, Archer JH, et al: The effect of cricoid pressure on preventing gastric insufflation in infants and children, *Anesthesiology* 78:652, 1993.
82. Bach A, Boehrer H, Schmidt H, Geiss HK: Nosocomial sinusitis in ventilated patients: nasotracheal versus orotracheal intubation. *Anaesthesia* 47:335-339, 1992.
83. Mevio E, Benazzo M, Quaglieri S, et al: Sinus infection in intensive care patients. *Rhinology* 34:232-236, 1996.
84. Niggemann B, Haack M, Machotta A: How to enter the pediatric airway for bronchoscopy. *Pediatr Int* 46:117-121, 2004.
85. Venkataraman ST, Khan N, Brown A: Validation of predictors of extubation success and failure in mechanically ventilated infants and children. *Crit Care Med* 28:2991-2996, 2000.
86. Koka BV, Jean IS, Andre JM, et al: Post-intubation croup in children. *Anesth Analg* 56:501, 1977.
87. Anene O, Meert KL, Uy H, et al: Dexamethasone for the prevention of postextubation airway obstruction: a prospective, randomized, double-blind, placebo-controlled trial. *Crit Care Med* 24: 1666-1669, 1996.
88. Harel Y, Vardi A, Quigley R, et al: Dexamethasone does not prevent post-extubation stridor in pediatric patients who previously failed extubation due to stridor. *Crit Care Med* 23: A186, 1995.
89. Tellez DW, Galvis AG, Storgion SA, et al: Dexamethasone in the prevention of post-extubation stridor in children. *J Pediatr* 118: 289-294 , 1991.
90. Black AE, Hatch DJ, Nauth-Misir N: Complications of nasotracheal intubation in neonates, infants and children: a review of 4 years' experience in a children's hospital. *Br J Anaesth* 65: 461-467, 1990.
Benjamin B: Prolonged intubation injuries of the larynx: endoscopic diagnosis, classification and treatment. *Ann Otol Rhinol Laryngol* 160:1-15, 1993.
91. deSilva OP: Factors influencing acquired upper airway obstruction in newborn infants receiving assisted ventilation because of respiratory failure: an overview. *J Perinatol* 16:272-275,1996.
92. Rivera R, Tibballs J: Complications of endotracheal intubation and mechanical ventilation in infants and children. *Crit Care Med* 20:193-199, 1992.
93. James CF, Modell JH, Gibbs CP, et al: Pulmonary aspiration: effects of volume and pH in the rat. *Anesth Analg* 63:665, 1984.
94. Schwartz DJ, Wynne JW, Gibbs CP, et al: The pulmonary consequences of aspiration of gastric contents at pH values greater than 2.5. *Am Rev Respir Dis* 21:119, 1980.
95. Salem MR, Wong AY, Fizzotti GF: Efficacy of cricoid pressure in preventing aspiration of gastric contents in paediatric patients. *Br J Anaesth* 44:401, 1972.
96. Brock-Utne JG: Is cricoid pressure necessary? *Paediatr Anaesth* 12:1-4, 2002.
97. Adelson PD, Bratton SL, Carney NA, et al: Guidelines for the acute medical management of severe traumatic brain injury in infants, children, and adolescents. Chapter 3. Prehospital airway management. *Pediatric Critical Care Medicine* 4:S9-11, 2003.
98. Belfort M, Kirshon B, Bowen R, et al: The cardiovascular and intracranial effects of laryngoscopy and endotracheal intubation in hypercarbic neonatal piglets. *S Afr Med J* 83:117-121, 1993.
99. Ampel L, Hott KA, Sielaff GW, et al: An approach to airway management in the acutely head-injured patient. *J Emerg Med* 6:1, 1988.
100. Walls RM: Rapid-sequence intubation in head trauma. *Ann Emerg Med* 22:1008-1013, 1993.
101. Bedell E, Prough DS: Anesthetic management of traumatic brain injury. *Anesthesiol Clin North Am* 20:417-439, 2002.
102. Adelson PD, Bratton SL, Carney NA, et al: Guidelines for the acute medical management of severe traumatic brain injury in infants, children, and adolescents. Chapter 12. Use of hyperventilation in the acute management of severe pediatric traumatic brain injury. *Pediatr Crit Care Med* 4:S45-48, 2003.
103. Adelson PD, Bratton SL, Carney NA, et al: Guidelines for the acute medical management of severe traumatic brain injury in infants, children, and adolescents. Chapter 9. Use of sedation and neuromuscular blockade in the treatment of severe pediatric traumatic brain injury. *Pediatric Critical Care Medicine* 4:S34-37, 2003.
104. Lev R, Rosen P: Prophylactic lidocaine use preintubation: a review. *J Emerg Med* 12:499-506, 1994.
105. Butler J, Jackson R: Towards evidence based emergency medicine: best BETs from Manchester Royal Infirmary. Lignocaine premedication before rapid sequence induction in head injuries. *Emerg Med J* 19:554, 2002.
106. Robinson N, Clancy M: In patients with head injury undergoing rapid sequence intubation, does pretreatment with intravenous lignocaine/lidocaine lead to an improved neurological outcome? A review of the literature. *Emerg Med J* 18:453-457, 2001.
107. Albanese J, Arnaud S, Rey M, et al: Ketamine decreases intracranial pressure and electroencephalographic activity in traumatic brain injury patients during propofol sedation. *Anesthesiology* 87:1328-1334, 1997.
108. Pang D, Wilberger JE: Spinal cord injury without radiologic abnormalities in children. *J Neurosurg* 57:114, 1982.
109. Brown RL, Brunn MA, Garcia VF: Cervical spine injuries in children: a review of 103 patients treated consecutively at a level 1 pediatric trauma center. *J Pediatr Surg* 36:1107-1114, 2001.
110. Cirak B, Ziegfeld S, Knight VM, et al: Spinal injuries in children. *J Pediatr Surg* 39:607-612, 2004.

111. Doolan LA, O'Brien JF: Safe intubation in cervical spine injury. *Anaesth Intensive Care* 13:319, 1985.
112. Knopp RK: The safety of orotracheal intubation in patients with suspected cervical-spine injury. *Ann Emerg Med* 19:603, 1990.
113. Rhee KJ, Green W, Holcroft JW, et al: Oral intubation in the multiply injured patient: the risk of exacerbating spinal cord damage. *Ann Emerg Med* 9:511, 1990.
114. Stene JK, Grande CM: General anesthesia: management considerations in the trauma patient. *Crit Care Clin* 6:73, 1990.
115. Bivins HG, Ford S, Bezmalinovic Z, et al: The effect of axial traction during orotracheal intubation of the trauma victim with an unstable cervical spine, *Ann Emerg Med* 17:25, 1988.
116. Joyce SM: Cervical immobilization during orotracheal intubation in trauma victims. *Ann Emerg Med* 17:88, 1988.
117. Suderman VS, Crosby ET, Lui A: Elective oral tracheal intubation in cervical spine-injured adults. *Can J Anaesth* 38:785, 1991.
118. Airway management and ventilation. In: *Advanced trauma life support instructor manual.* 1997.
119. McHale SP, Brydon CW, Wood ML, et al: A survey of nasotracheal intubating skills among Advanced Trauma Life Support course graduates. *Br J Anaesth* 72:195, 1994.
120. Minck EJ Jr, Clinton JE, Plummer D, et al: Fiberoptic intubation in the emergency department. *Ann Emerg Med* 19:359, 1990.
121. Davis L, Cook-Sather S, Schreiner MS: Lighted stylette intubation: a review. *Anesth Analg* 90:745, 2000.
122. Fox DJ, Matson MD: Management of the difficult pediatric airway in an austere environment using the lightwand. *J Clin Anesth* 2:123-125, 1990.
123. Fisher QA, Tunkel DE: Lightwand intubation of infants and children. *J Clin Anesth* 9:275-279, 1997.
124. Holzman RS, Nargozian CD, Florence FB: Lightwand intubation in children with abnormal upper airways. *Anesthesiology* 69:784-787, 1988.
125. Pfitzner L, Cooper MG, Ho D: The Shikani Seeing Stylet for difficult intubation in children: initial experience. *Anaesth Intensive Care* 30:462-466, 2002.
126. Friedman PG, Rosenberg MK, Lebenbom-Mansour M: A comparison of light wand and suspension laryngoscopic intubation techniques in outpatients. *Anesth Analg* 85:578-582,1997.
127. Broennle AM, Cohen DE: Pediatric anesthesia and sedation, *Curr Opin Pediatr* 5:310, 1993.
128. Lopez-Gil M, Brimacombe J, Alvarez M: Safety and efficacy of the laryngeal mask airway. A prospective survey of 1400 children. *Anaesthesia* 51:969-972, 1996.
129. O'Neill B, Templeton JJ, Caramico L, et al: The laryngeal mask airway in pediatric patients: factors affecting ease of use during insertion and emergence. *Anesth Analg* 78:659-662, 1994.
130. Berry AM, Brimacombe JR, Verghese C: The laryngeal mask airway in emergency medicine, neonatal resuscitation, and intensive care medicine. *Int Anesthesiol Clin* 36:91-109, 1998.
131. Dorges V, Ocker H, Wenzel V, et al: Emergency airway management by non-anaesthesia house officers—a comparison of three strategies. *Emerg Med J* 18:90-94, 2001.
132. American Heart Association: Airway, ventilation, and management of respiratory distress and failure. In: *PALS Provider Manual.* 2002.
133. Martin SE, Ochsner MG, Jarman RH, et al: Use of the laryngeal mask airway in air transport when intubation fails. *J Trauma Injury Infect Crit Care* 47:352-357, 1999.
134. Efrat R, Kadari A, Katz S: The laryngeal mask airway in pediatric anesthesia: experience with 120 patients undergoing elective groin surgery, *J Pediatr Surg* 29:206, 1994.
135. Ferrari LR, Goudsouzian NG: The use of the laryngeal mask airway in children with bronchopulmonary dysplasia. *Anesth Analg* 81:310, 1995.
136. Benumof JL: Use of the laryngeal mask to facilitate fiberoptic endoscopy intubation. *Anesthesiology* 74:313, 1992.
137. Carron JD, Derkay CS, Strope GL, et al: Pediatric tracheotomies: changing indications and outcomes. *Laryngoscope* 110:1099-1104, 2000.
138. Arcand P, Granger J: Pediatric tracheostomies: changing trends. *J Otolaryngol* 17:121-124, 1988.
139. Wetmore RF, Marsh RR, Thompson ME, et al: Pediatric tracheostomy: a changing procedure? *Ann Otol Rhinol Laryngol* 108:695-699, 1999.
140. Dutton JM, Palmer PM, McCulloch TM, et al: Mortality in the pediatric patient with tracheotomy. *Head Neck* 17:403-408, 1995.
141. Lewis CW, Carron JD, Perkins JA, et al: Tracheotomy in pediatric patients: a national perspective. *Arch Otolaryngol Head Neck Surg* 129:523-529, 2003.
142. Spaite DW, Maralee J: Prehospital cricothyrotomy: an investigation of indications, technique, complications, and patient outcome, *Ann Emerg Med* 19:279, 1990.

CHAPTER

33

Physiology of the Respiratory System

Mark J. Heulitt

PEARLS

- During childhood, the most important chest diseases have obstructive pictures that are best measured using interrupter and oscillation techniques.
- Wheezing is a sound heard when there is flow limitation in a compliant tube. It is a sign of expiratory flow limitation. The wheezing is caused by a "flutter" of the walls at the site of flow limitation. This is secondary to the conservation of energy in the system because the driving pressure exceeds that which is required to produce $\dot{V}_{max}$ and is dissipated, causing the flutter. However, flow limitation can occur in the absence of wheezing.
- The equation of motion changes when a spontaneously breathing patient is placed on positive pressure mechanical ventilator support. P_{APP} (pressure applied to the airway) equals the sum of pressure generated by the patients muscles (P_{mus}) plus the ventilator pressure (P_{vent}). Thus $P_{mus} + P_{vent} = {}^{1}/_{C}V + RV$.

Physiology of the Respiratory System

Given the increasing emphasis on molecular biology today, many physicians in training have received limited exposure to physiologic principles that are the basis of clinical medicine. There has been a resurgence of interest in translational research with a reemphasis on a path from molecular research to applied animal physiology before these products of research are used in clinical research.[1] In an editorial in the *European Journal of Physiology,* Dr. R. Rossier stated that research is refocusing itself to make a change from the past, when its mantra was "from function to the gene," to the future, when the focus must be on the "gene to function." The focus of this chapter is to expose the reader to the important, basic principles of respiratory physiology and to serve as a primer to other chapters that use these principles.

The main function of the lungs is (rapid) gas exchange. Gas exchange is accomplished by a well-coordinated interaction of the lungs with the central nervous system, the diaphragm and chest wall musculature, and the circulatory system.

Gas exchange occurs in the alveolus, where the thin laminar blood flow and inspired air are separated by only a thin tissue layer. Gas exchange takes 0.25 seconds or one third of the total transit time of a red cell. The entire blood volume of the body passes through the lungs each minute in the resting state, that is, 5 L/min. The total surface area of the lungs is approximately 80 m^2, equivalent to the size of a tennis court. The primary function of the lungs is to supply oxygen (O_2) and to remove carbon dioxide (CO_2) from the tissues of the body. For the lungs to achieve this function, two interrelated processes must occur: *ventilation,* the movement of air between the outside of the body and the alveoli, and *gas exchange,* the transfer of O_2 and CO_2 between the alveolar gas and the mixed venous blood entering the lungs.

Only approximately 10% of the lungs are occupied by solid tissue; the remainder is filled with air and blood.

Supporting structures of the lungs must be delicate enough to allow gas exchange yet strong enough to maintain architectural integrity, that is, to sustain alveolar structure. The functional structure of the lungs can be divided into (1) conducting airways (dead air space) and (2) gas exchange portions. The two plumbing systems are (1) airways for ventilation and (2) the circulatory system for perfusion. Both are under low pressure.

Conducting Airways

The diameter of the lower airways is maintained by a balance of forces. Sympathetic impulses relax and parasympathetic impulses constrict the muscles. Airway dilatation may occur as a result of sympathomimetic agents (e.g., epinephrine or adrenaline). Narrowing forces are bronchial smooth muscle contraction, mediated by efferent autonomic nerve control. Constriction also can occur as a result of irritants (e.g., dust, smoke, or cold), hyperventilation, or vasoactive agents (e.g., acetylcholine, histamine, or bradykinin).

Additional narrowing occurs during forced expiration, when there is dynamic airway compression caused by pleural and peribronchial pressures. This is counteracted by the intraluminal pressure and the tethering action of the surrounding lung. The luminal diameter of a branch is related to the number of alveoli at the end of that branch (axial and lateral pathways). Because the longer airways with more branches and more alveoli usually have a wider lumen that allows greater airflow, newly inspired air reaches all of the alveoli throughout both lungs at the same time and in approximately the same amount, that is, there is an even distribution of inspired air throughout all lobes in a given period of time. There are approximately 23 airway divisions to the level of the alveoli. The divisions include the main bronchi, lobar bronchi, segmental bronchi (to designated bronchopulmonary segments), and so on until the terminal bronchioles, which are the smallest of the divisions; these bronchioles do not have alveoli and are lined completely by bronchial epithelium. Although the base airway diameter decreases with branching, the overall or total cross-sectional diameter increases tremendously so that peripheral airway resistance decreases.

Model of the Respiratory System

The respiratory system can be represented by a collection of physical components interacting with one another and with their environment. Although in vivo analysis demonstrates that the lungs do not function as a single compartment, analyzing the respiratory system in a linear model simplifies the presentation.

A single balloon on a pipe is the simplest model, although this model has its deficiencies because the airway is more complex than a simple pipe. Also, it now appears that the alveolus is more like a cluster of grapes, not a single balloon or group of balloons. The alveoli are not physically independent structures but are interconnected.[2] An excellent review of the structure of the alveoli and the role of surfactant is offered by Gatto et al.[3] However, to lay the groundwork for our understanding of respiratory mechanics, we consider this simple model of a balloon on a pipe.

The relationship at any moment (t) between the pressure applied at the opening of the model [$P(t)$] and the volume in the model [$V(t)$] during emptying of this balloon can be described as a first-order model:

$$P(t) = E \cdot V(t) + R \cdot \dot{V}(t)$$

where E = elastance of the balloon, R = resistance of the pipe, and $\dot{V}$ = flow through the opening. Using regression analysis, E and R can be calculated from $P(t)$, $V(t)$, and $\dot{V}(t)$.

The values of R and E, as applied to the respiratory system, reflect the resistance of the airways and the elastance of the respiratory system, whereas $V(t)$ is the volume increase from functional residual capacity (FRC) when the mouth pressure is zero.

The three important components of this linear model are the time constant (τ), compliance (C) or elastance (E), and resistance (R). The relationship of these components is given by the following equation:

$$\tau = C \cdot R \text{ or } \tau = \frac{R}{E}.$$

Each of these components is discussed separately.

Elastic Properties of the Respiratory System

The respiratory system is composed of a collection of elastic structures. The response to a force applied to the elastic structure of the respiratory system is to resist deformation by producing an opposing force, known as *elastic recoil,* to return the structure to its relaxed state.[4] In the respiratory system, this opposing force produces a pressure known as the *elastic recoil pressure* (P_{EL}). The force required to stretch an elastic structure depends on the volume at which the outward recoil of the chest wall balances the inward recoil, known as the *elastic equilibrium volume* (EEV). The pressure of the elastic recoil or P_{EL} divided by the lung volume (V) gives a measure of the elastic properties of respiratory system and is called *elastance* (E):

$$E = \frac{P_{EL}}{V}.$$

When lung volume is plotted on the ordinate and P_{EL} is plotted on the abscissa, the slope of the static pressure–volume curve is equivalent to the reciprocal of elastance, called *compliance.*

Ventilation of the lungs involves producing the forces necessary to overcome the elasticity, flow-resistance, and inertial properties of the lungs and chest wall to create motion of the respiratory system. Respiratory muscles normally produce these forces.

Overcoming forces to move gas into the airway can be exemplified by moving a block of wood over a surface. The movement of the block is determined by the friction between the block of wood and the surface and how fast the wood is moving. The block's position is irrelevant. Similarly, the pressure required to produce a flow of gas between the atmosphere and the alveoli must overcome the frictional resistance of the airways. This pressure is proportional to flow ($\dot{V}$) (the rate at which volume is changing) as follows:

$$P_{ao} - P_{alv} = P_{fr} \alpha \dot{V},$$

where P_{ao} = pressure at the airway opening (usually atmospheric pressure), P_{alv} = alveolar pressure, and P_{fr} = pressure required to overcome frictional resistance. The pressure required to produce a unit of flow is known as *flow resistance* (R):

$$R = P_{fr} / \dot{V}.$$

If the respiratory system is modeled as a single compartment with a single constant elastance (E) and a single constant resistance (R), then the equation of motion describes the balance of forces acting on the system as follows:

$$P = EV + R\dot{V} + I\dot{V}$$

The inertance (I) usually is negligible and therefore is ignored. Of the pressure produced during tidal respiration, most is required to overcome the elastic forces, and a minimal amount is required to overcome the flow-resistant forces.

Traditionally it was thought that little energy was dissipated by the tissues of the respiratory system, and that the majority of the force developed during breathing was required to move gas through the airways. The lung parenchyma is a complex system consisting of alveolar walls composed of collagen, elastin, and proteoglycan macromolecules; an air–liquid interface of surfactant; and interstitial cells that have the capacity to act in a contractile fashion. The viscoelastic behavior of the pulmonary parenchyma could explain this behavior. In addition, this action is difficult to study because the boundary where the airways end and parenchyma begins is unclear. Airway smooth muscle exists in the terminal bronchioles and alveolar ducts, and the behavior of these structures may influence parenchymal mechanics.

The energy expended while moving the tissue is called the *tissue viscance* or *resistance,* although it is a non-newtonian resistance. In other words, the viscosity depends on the force applied. When measured during inspiration, tissue resistance increases with increasing lung volume, whereas airway resistance falls. Tissue resistance contributes approximately 65% of respiratory system resistance at FRC in mechanically ventilated animals and increases as much as 95% at higher lung volumes.[5] The contribution of tissue resistance to respiratory system resistance in humans under the same circumstances is unknown.

Resistance is expressed as changes in pressure divided by changes in flow:

$$R = \frac{\Delta P}{\Delta \dot{V}}$$

The other part of elastic recoil depends on the surface tension at the alveolar gas–liquid interface (surface forces). Surface tension is produced by the interface between air in the alveolus and the thin film of liquid that covers the alveolar surface. Surface tension in the alveolus is created by interacting water molecules that direct a force inward and could cause the alveoli to collapse. This action is described by the Laplace equation, where the pressure inside a bubble exceeds the pressure outside the bubble by twice the surface tension, divided by the radius. In other words, the smaller a bubble, the more the pressure inside it exceeds the pressure on the outside. The Laplace equation is defined as follows:

$$P = \frac{2T}{r},$$

where P = internal pressure, T = tension in the wall of the structure, and r = radius. Comparing two different alveoli with the same surface tension, the smaller the radius the greater the pressure created by a given surface tension. Air flows from higher pressure (small alveoli) to lower pressure (larger alveoli). Thus smaller alveoli are more likely to collapse. The surface tension of the alveoli is affected by a substance produced in the alveoli called *surfactant.* Surfactant contains a mixture of lipids and proteins, is manufactured by alveolar type II cells, and exists as a monolayer on top of the alveolar subphase. Three surfactant-associated protein groups have been identified.[6] Surfactant lowers surface tension at the alveolar air–liquid interface and thereby decreases elastic recoil of the lungs.[7] Another action of surfactant is to reduce the development of pulmonary edema by diminishing one component of the pressure gradient. In the lung there is a gradient between pulmonary capillary pressure and alveolar pressure. In most of the lung the pulmonary capillary pressure is greater than the alveolar pressure; thus pulmonary edema would develop if not checked by the oncotic pressure of the plasma proteins. By reducing surface tension the surfactant reduces the pressure gradient, but if there is a deficiency of surfactant and thus a rise in surface tension, pulmonary edema may develop.[8] In addition, surfactant has been described as an antiwetting agent keeping the lungs dry.[9] Currently there is agreement on the fact that surfactant plays an essential role in alveolar mechanics, but there is debate on its mechanism. This description outlines the classic discussion on the role of surfactant, but opinions on its true role are diverse. Scapelli[10] described the role of the surfactant foam bubbles within the alveoli as "inner tubes." In contrast, Hills and Scapelli[11,12] propose that surfactant coats the alveolar walls as a "biologic wax." The clinical implications of a deficiency of surfactant was described in a famous editorial by Lachmann entitled "Open up the lung and keep the lung open."[13]

Compliance and Elastance

Compliance is how much a compartment will expand if the pressure in that compartment is changed. A balloon has a high compliance because a small pressure increase inside the balloon will greatly expand the balloon. A rigid tube has a low compliance because a small pressure increase inside the rigid tube will not result in a significant increase in the volume of the rigid tube. Two major forces contribute to lung compliance: tissue elastic forces and surface tension forces. The compliance (C) is determined by the change in elastic recoil pressure (ΔP) produced by a change in volume (ΔV).

$$C = \frac{\Delta V}{\Delta P}.$$

The compliance of the lungs (C_L), chest wall (C_{CW}), and respiratory system (C_{RS}) can be determined by measuring the change in distending pressure and the associated change in volume. The distending pressure represents the pressure change across the structure, where P_{ao}, P_{pl}, and P_{bs} = pressure measured at the airway opening, pleural pressure, and pressure at the body surface (atmospheric pressure), respectively.

$$C_L = \frac{\Delta V}{\Delta(P_{ao} - P_{pl})}$$

$$C_{CW} = \frac{\Delta V}{\Delta(P_{pl} - P_{bs})}$$

$$C_{RS} = \frac{\Delta V}{\Delta(P_{ao} - P_{bs})}.$$

Lung volume and volume–pressure relationships (e.g., compliance) reflect parenchymal (air space) development, whereas airflow and pressure–flow relationships (resistance and conductance) predominantly reflect airway development. The lungs become stiffer (i.e., compliance decreases) at higher lung volumes.

Pulmonary compliance changes with growth and maturation, depending on the number of expanded air spaces, the size and geometry of the air spaces, the characteristics of the surface lining layer, and the properties of the lung parenchyma. This is represented by changes in the shape of the volume–pressure curve. When these curves are corrected by expressing the volumes as a percentage of the maximal observed lung volume, they are more curved in infants than in older children[14] (Figure 33–1). It is important to note that there may be boundaries for dynamic changes in alveolar size and shape during ventilation as a result of the tensile forces of the connective tissue and surface tension supporting the alveoli and alveolar ducts.

The change in shape of the volume–pressure curve represents the immature, rather than the mature, alveoli and hence the differences in the elastin/collagen ratio with age.[14] The lung volume at which airway closure occurs is higher in children younger than 7 years.[15] Pressure–volume relationships are also more curvilinear in infants.[16] Chest wall compliance is 50% greater in infants.

Elastance is defined as the change in distending pressure divided by the associated change in volume:

$$E = \frac{\Delta P}{\Delta V}.$$

Elastance is the reciprocal of compliance; therefore stiff lungs have a high elastance.

Elastic Recoil of the Respiratory System

A series is created between the lungs and the chest wall by the forces within the pleural space. In the intact thorax, the inward recoil of the lungs is opposed by the outward recoil of the chest wall below its resting volume. Both the lungs and the chest wall recoil inwardly when this volume is exceeded.

By having a subject exhale in increments from total lung capacity (TLC) to residual volume, the pressure required to balance the elastic recoil of the lungs, chest wall, and respiratory system (elastic recoil pressure) can be determined. At each volume, the subject relaxes against a fixed obstruction with glottis open, and the pressure difference across the lung, chest wall, and entire respiratory system is recorded. Pressure–volume curves are derived in this way for the respiratory system, and its components are shown in Figure 33–2.[17] The static pressure–volume curves of the respiratory system, lung,

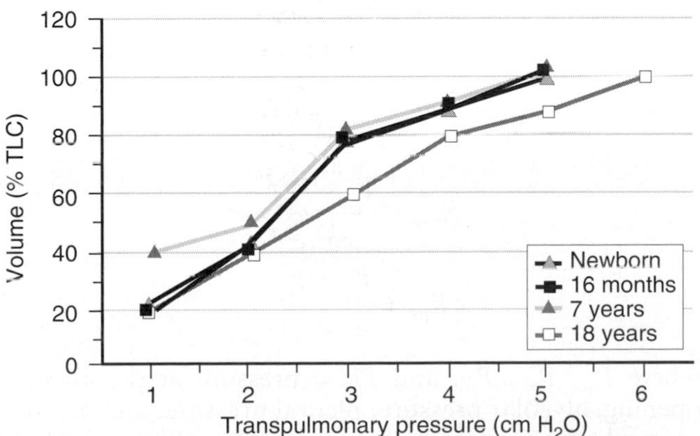

FIGURE 33–1 • Deflation volume-pressure curves of the lung at different ages (obtained from studies on excised lungs).[8] With increasing age up to young adulthood, the curves become straighter and, at a given lung volume, elastic recoil pressure is greater. The curve from elderly individuals resembles that of a 7-year-old respiratory system.

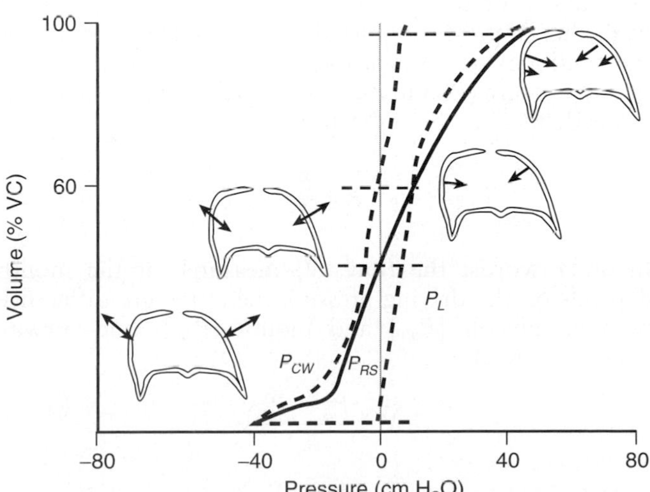

FIGURE 33–2 • Pressure–volume relationship of the lung (P_L), chest wall (P_{CW}), and entire respiratory system (P_{RS}). *Large arrows* represent the elastic recoil of the lungs and the chest wall. (Adapted from Agostoni E, Mead J: Statics of the respiratory system. In Fenn WO, Rahn H, editors: *Handbook of physiology, respiration.* Washington, DC, 1964, American Physiological Society.)

and chest wall are different during inspiration and expiration. Thus lung volumes at a given transpulmonary pressure are higher during deflation than during inflation. The phenomenon is called *hysteresis*. Hysteresis is the failure of a system to follow identical paths of response on application and withdrawal of a forcing agent, as occurs during inspiration and expiration. Hysteresis in the respiratory system depends on viscoelasticity, such as stress adaptation (i.e., rate-dependent phenomenon), and plasticity (i.e., rate-independent phenomenon). In the lungs, hysteresis results mainly from surface properties and alveolar recruitment-derecruitment. In comparison, chest wall hysteresis is related to the action of both muscles and ligaments because both skeletal muscles and elastic fibers exhibit hysteresis. Hysteresis is negligible when volume changes are minimal, as during quiet breathing. This is important because the area of the hysteresis loop represents energy lost from the system.

The resting volume of the respiratory system, FRC, is the volume at which the elastic recoil of the lungs and the chest wall exactly balance. Above and below this equilibrium point, progressively increasing pressure is required to change the volume of the respiratory system. The total pressure required at each volume is the sum of the pressures required to overcome the elastic recoil of the lungs and chest wall.

Flow Resistance of the Respiratory System

The response of the lung to movement is governed by its response to the physical impedance of the respiratory system. Impedance can be categorized into (1) elastic resistance at the alveolar gas–liquid interface and tissue and (2) frictional resistance to gas flow. Under static conditions, pressure is required only to oppose the elastic recoil of the respiratory system. However, when the lungs and chest wall are in motion and air moves into and out of the lungs, pressure must also be provided to overcome the frictional or viscous forces. The ratio of this additional pressure (P) and the rate of airflow that it produces ($\dot{V}$) is defined as the resistance.

$$R = \frac{P}{\dot{V}}.$$

In other words, the flow ($\dot{V}$) measured at the mouth depends on the driving pressure (i.e., pressure difference between alveoli [P_{alv}] and mouth [P_{mo}]) and airway resistance (R_{aw}):

$$\dot{V} = \frac{P_{mo} - P_{alv}}{R_{aw}}.$$

If the mouth pressure is zero (i.e., atmospheric pressure), the driving pressure is the alveolar pressure.

Airway resistance (R_{aw}) is the sum of peripheral airway resistance (peripheral intrathoracic airways <2-mm diameter; R_{awp}), central airway resistance (large intrathoracic airways >2-mm diameter; R_{awc}), and extrathoracic airway resistance (especially glottis; R_{ext}). In healthy people, R_{ext} accounts for 50% of the total R_{aw} and R_{awp} accounts for approximately 15%. R_{awp} and R_{awc} are influenced by lung volume. Higher lung volumes give higher P_{el} and therefore increase airway diameter. With increasing volumes during inspiration, the increased P_{el} is counteracted by P_{pl}, resulting in increased radial distending force. This distending force is the transmural pressure and is the difference between pressure in (P_{in}) and pressure outside (P_{out}) the airway.

At zero airflow the pressure inside the airways (P_{in}) equals atmospheric pressure and transmural pressure (P_{tm}) equals the elastic recoil pressure (P_{el}):

$$P_{in} = P_{mo}, P_{tm} = P_{el}.$$

The total respiratory resistance (R_{RS}) consists of the resistance of the airways (R_{aw}), the resistance of the lung (R_L), and the resistance of the chest wall (R_{CW}):

$$R_{RS} = R_{CW} + R_L + R_{aw}.$$

In older children, R_{CW} and R_L represent only 10% to 20% of R_{RS},[18] but in newborns R_L could be higher.[19]

Airway diameter of the intrathoracic airways approximates a sigmoidal relationship with P_{tm}. This results in volume dependency of R_{aw}. At higher lung volumes R_{awp} decreases. The specific relation between R_{awp} (or its reciprocal conductance G_{aw} [= $1/R_{aw}$]) and volume is mirrored by the specific R_{aw} (sR_{aw}) and specific G_{aw} (sG_{aw}):

$$sR_{aw} = \frac{R_{aw}}{V}, sG_{aw} = \frac{G_{aw}}{V}.$$

The resistance of the airways (R_{AW}), lungs (airway and parenchyma) (R_L), chest wall (R_{CW}), and entire respiratory system (R_{RS}) can be calculated by measuring the rate of airflow and the associated transstructural pressure by subtracting from the total pressure the amount required to overcome elastic recoil:

$$R_{AW} = \frac{P_{ao} - P_{alv}}{\dot{V}}$$

$$R_L = \frac{P_{ao} - P_{pl}}{\dot{V}}$$

$$R_{CW} = \frac{P_{pl} - P_{bs}}{\dot{V}}$$

$$R_{RS} = \frac{P_{ao} - P_{bs}}{\dot{V}},$$

where P_{ao}, P_{alv}, P_{pl}, and P_{bs} = pressure at the airway's opening, alveolar pressure, pleural pressure, and pressure at the body surface, respectively. The resistance of the lung parenchyma can be derived by subtracting airway from total lung resistance.

The relationship between the flow rate and the airway pressure gradient is nonlinear because of the relative contribution of the various components of the respiratory system to the total pressure required to overcome the viscous forces. The viscous forces increase disproportionately as flow rate increases, and airway resistance increases. In contrast, the resistance of the chest wall and lung parenchyma remains constant over a wide range of flow rates.[20] During quiet breathing by mouth, airway resistance accounts for greater than 50% of the total respiratory system resistance.[21] However, as flow rate increases, the contribution of the airways to total resistance progressively increases.

Changing patterns of airflow results in the nonlinear flow-resistance characteristics of the airways. Subsequently, as the flow rate to the airway increases, airflow becomes progressively more turbulent. The more turbulent the flow, the greater the pressure required to overcome the viscous forces. Turbulence occurs at lower flow rates in the upper airway because of the tortuous geometry of the upper (extrathoracic) airway and the narrow glottic aperture than in the lower (intrathoracic) airways. Therefore the upper airway is responsible for most of the increase in airway resistance with increase in flow rate. Studies have shown that the resistance of the lower airways is nearly constant up to flow rates of 2 L/s.[20] For patients who are breathing quietly by mouth, total airway resistance is divided almost equally between the upper and lower airways. As their effort increases, the flow rate increases, and the ratio of upper to lower airway resistance progressively increases as described earlier.

Depending on whether laminar or turbulent flow predominates, resistance to airflow varies inversely with either the fourth or fifth power of airway radius.[22] Thus major changes in airway resistance occur by factors that affect airway diameter.[23] During spontaneous lung inflation, airway diameter increases as airway resistance decreases. This is produced by two mechanisms. First, as lung volume increases, the increasing elastic recoil of the pulmonary parenchyma provides a tethering effect that dilates the intrapulmonary airways. Second, extrapulmonary and large intrapulmonary airways are surrounded by pleural pressure, which becomes increasingly negative during inspiration. This leads to an increasing pressure gradient across the airway wall and therefore to an increasing diameter. The change in airway resistance with lung volume is curvilinear and is illustrated in Figure 33–3.[23] When the reciprocal of airway resistance, airway conductance (G_{AW}), is plotted against lung volume, this relationship is nearly linear.

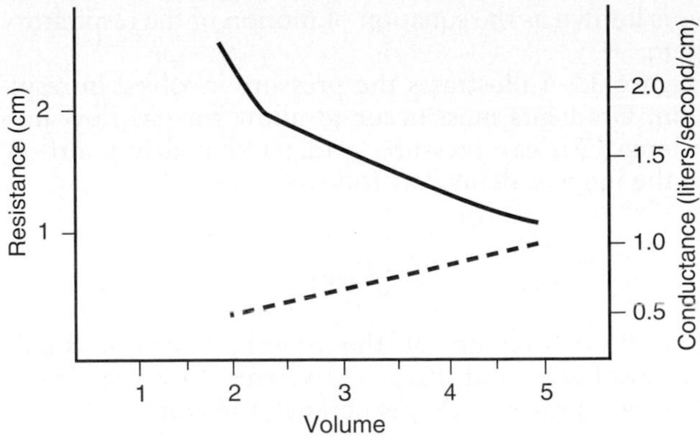

FIGURE 33–3 • Relationship between lung volume and airway resistance *(solid line)* and conductance *(dashed line)*. (Adapted from Briscoe WA, Dubois AB: *J Clin Invest* 37:1280, 1958.)

Dynamic Change in Airway Caliber During Respiration

Airway caliber is partially dependent on transmural pressure. Transmural pressure is the difference between interstitial pressure and atmospheric pressure. The external airway wall for the intrathoracic airways is subjected to the interstitial pressure, which is approximately equal to the pleural pressure. In contrast, the external walls of extrathoracic airways are subjected to the atmospheric pressure. The intraluminal pressure is dependent on the generation of the airway. During inspiration, pleural pressure is negative relative to atmospheric pressure. Alveolar pressure is approximately equal to pleural pressure, and pressure at the mouth is atmospheric. This pressure difference creates a gradient from the mouth to the alveoli. Extrathoracic airways tend to narrow during inspiration because the transmural pressure is positive. In contrast, the intrathoracic airways' transmural pressure is negative, causing a tendency for these airways to dilate during inspiration. The degree of airway caliber change during inspiration depends on both the magnitude of the transmural pressure and the airway wall compliance. At the end of inspiration there is relaxation of the inspiratory muscles; thus the elastic recoil of the respiratory system produces, relative to atmospheric pressure, a positive pleural and alveolar pressure. Because of the dynamic pressure changes described earlier in this section, there is a tendency of intrathoracic airways to narrow and extrathoracic airways to dilate during expiration.

Applied Forces

Ventilation of the lungs involves motion of the respiratory system, which is produced by the forces required to overcome the flow-resistance, inertial, and elastic properties of the lungs and chest wall. Under normal circumstances, these forces are produced by the respiratory muscles.

If ventilation is to occur, opposing forces must be overcome by pressure applied to the respiratory system to create motion. At each instant, the applied pressure (P_{APP}) must equal the sum of the pressure required to balance elastic recoil (P_{ER}) and the pressure lost to viscous forces (P_R).

$$P_{APP} = P_{ER} + P_R.$$

Using previous equations this can be converted to the following:

$$P_{APP} = \frac{1}{C}V + R\dot{V}.$$

This is known as the equation of motion of the respiratory system.

Figure 33–4 illustrates the pressure involved in respiration. Gradients must occur to allow for gas flow into the lungs. Airway pressure gradient that drives airflow into the lungs is defined as follows:

$$P_M - P_{ALV},$$

where P_M = pressure at the mouth, which normally is atmospheric, and P_{ALV} = alveolar pressure. Transpulmonary pressure (P_{TP}) is defined as follows:

$$P_{TP} = P_{ALV} - P_{Pl}$$

where P_{ALV} = alveolar pressure, P_{PL} = intrapleural pressure, and P_{TP} = elastic recoil of the lungs when there is no airflow. P_{TP} increases and decreases with lung volume. Transchest wall pressure (P_{TC}) is defined as follows:

$$P_{TC} = P_{Pl} - P_{bs}$$

where P_{PL} = intrapleural pressure, and P_{bs} = pressure at the body surface, which usually is atmospheric. P_{TC} is equal in magnitude to elastic recoil of the chest when there is no airflow and, like P_{TP}, increases and decreases with lung volume.

Transmural pressure (P_{RS}) is defined as follows:

$$P_{RS} = P_{ALV} - P_{bs}$$

where P_{ALV} = alveolar pressure, P_{bs} = pressure at the body surface, and P_{RS} = transmural pressure across the entire respiratory system, including the lungs and the chest, and is equal to the net passive elastic recoil pressure of the whole respiratory system when airflow is zero.

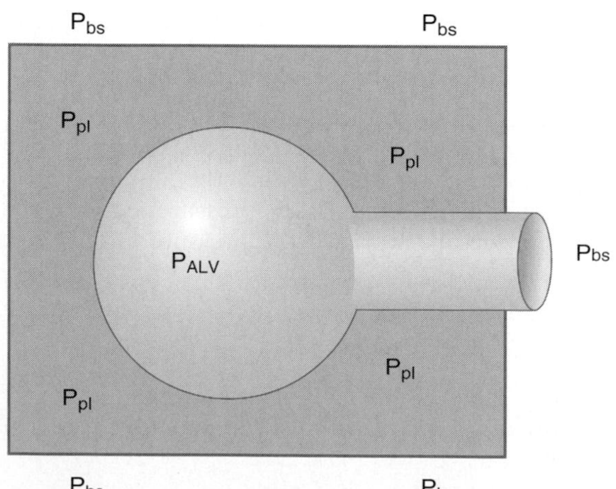

FIGURE 33–4 • Illustration of the pressure involved in respiration. Gradients must occur to allow for gas to flow into the lungs.

TABLE 33–1

Balance of Forces

$P_{RS} + P_{MUS}$	=	$P_L + P_{CW}$
$P_{ALV} - P_{bs} + P_{MUS}$	=	$P_L + P_{CW}$
Inspiratory muscle contraction		Lung, chest wall elastic recoil
Outward acting forces when positive		Inward acting forces when positive

During inspiration the respiratory muscles provide the applied pressure, which expand the chest wall and the lungs causing the alveolar and airway pressure to lower. The net result is that alveolar pressure becomes less than atmospheric pressure. Once alveolar pressure is less than atmospheric pressure, air flows into the lungs along a pressure gradient and the lungs inflate, thus storing potential energy in the elastic structures for expiration. In order for gas flow to occur there must be balance of forces. Table 33–1 describes these forces.

Expiration usually is passive (excluding disease states where the patient actively tries to empty the lungs), that is, the energy stored in the elastic recoil of the lungs and the chest wall produces the positive alveolar pressure and airway pressure needed to overcome flow resistance and air is forced from the lungs.

In order to inflate the lungs, there must be an increase in alveolar pressure, which usually is done with positive pressure ventilation, a decrease in body surface pressure, as in negative pressure ventilation (iron lung), or activation of the respiratory muscles (normal breathing).

Under resting conditions, expiration usually is passive. At times of increased ventilatory requirements, such as during exercise, contraction of the abdominal and internal intercostal muscles can aid expiration.

Interactions between Lungs and Chest Wall

The lungs and the chest wall operate in series, and their compliance adds reciprocally to make total compliance.

$$1/C_T = 1/C_L + 1/C_{CW}.$$

The chest wall is like a spring that can be either compressed or distended. Transthoracic pressure is negative at residual volume and FRC, meaning the chest wall is smaller than its unstressed volume and has a tendency to spring out. Normal tidal breathing is entirely in the negative pressure range for transthoracic pressure. When examining the compliance curve of the chest wall (lung volume vs. transthoracic pressure), pressure is zero at approximately 65% of TLC. Thus the chest is at its unstressed volume and has no tendency to collapse or expand. Transthoracic pressure is positive at volumes greater than 65% TLC. The chest tends to collapse above its unstressed volume.

Time Constant of Emptying

The time for the volume in the respiratory system to be reduced by 63% when the respiratory system is allowed to empty passively and the volume-time profile is measured is known as the time constant (τ) of the respiratory system.[24] If we use a model of the respiratory system with a single compartment, a single constant elastance, and a single constant resistance, the following occurs:

$$\tau = R/E.$$

In a single-compartment model, the volume-time profile can be represented by a single exponential decay.

In healthy adults, the time constant of the passive respiratory system is short, approximately 0.5 seconds. Such a short time constant allows the lungs to empty to the EEV at the end of each expiration. Thus FRC and EEV are equal. Because the respiratory system is relaxed at the end of expiration, inspiration can begin as soon as inspiratory muscle activity is initiated. The expiratory time constant is shorter in children, with values approximating 0.3 seconds reported in infants with normal lungs.[25] Infants with hyaline membrane disease have stiffer than normal lungs with expiratory time constants reported as low as 0.1 seconds. In patients with obstructive airway diseases, such as asthma, resistance is increased, and the expiratory time constant is longer. Therefore a longer time is required for the lungs to empty and return the respiratory system to EEV. Patients with chronic airway obstruction frequently have carbon dioxide retention and an increased respiratory drive. This results in an increased respiratory rate with a shorter respiratory cycle and less time available for expiration. In this situation the respiratory system frequently does not have time to return to EEV before the next inspiration starts. FRC occurs at a volume higher than EEV, not equal to EEV, causing the respiratory system not to be relaxed at the end of expiration. This lack of relaxation of the respiratory system at the end of expiration causes a positive recoil pressure. This pressure is called *intrinsic positive end-expiratory pressure* ($PEEP_i$). Before inspiratory flow can begin, the patient's inspiratory muscle must produce enough force to overcome $PEEP_i$; thus this force is "lost" to produce inspiratory flow and represents a load that must be overcome by the inspiratory muscle. In patients with severe airway obstruction, this pressure can be as high as 15 to 20 cmH_2O.

Gas Exchange

The basic respiratory function of the respiratory system is to supply oxygen to the body and to remove excess carbon dioxide. The following are the essential steps involved in this process:

1. Ventilation, the exchange of gas between the atmosphere and the alveoli
2. Diffusion across the alveolar-capillary membrane
3. Transportion of gases in the blood
4. Diffusion of the gases from the capillaries of the systemic circulation to the cells of the body
5. Use of oxygen and production of carbon dioxide within the cells as a byproduct of metabolism

During the process of ventilation, air is transported back and forth between the outside of the body and the terminal respiratory units of the lungs. In the alveoli, the air is exposed to a thin film of blood. O_2 diffuses across the alveolar-capillary membrane, enters the blood, and combines with hemoglobin. Simultaneously, CO_2 diffuses from the blood and enters the alveolar gas. In this way, the mixed venous blood entering the lungs is altered through the addition of O_2 and the removal of CO_2. This is the process of gas exchange.

The partial pressure of O_2 in the arterial blood (PaO_2) and the partial pressure of CO_2 in the arterial blood ($PaCO_2$), and therefore the adequacy of gas exchange, are dependent on a number of factors. These factors include the composition of the alveolar gas and the extent to which equilibrium is reached between the alveolar gas and the pulmonary capillary blood. The alveolar gas composition in turn is dependent on the content of the inspired air and the mixed venous blood, the quantity of air (ventilation) and blood (perfusion) reaching the alveoli, and the ratio of alveolar ventilation to perfusion ($\dot{V}_A/\dot{Q}$). Of the factors determining the adequacy of gas exchange, structure and function of the lungs primarily influence (1) ventilation/perfusion relationships, (2) alveolar ventilation, and (3) diffusion of O_2 and CO_2.

Ventilation/Perfusion Relationships

In the normal upright lung, both alveolar ventilation and perfusion increase from apex to base because of the effects of gravity. Blood flow increases more rapidly than ventilation; therefore ($\dot{V}_A/\dot{Q}$) ratios are high at the apex and decrease progressively toward the base of the lungs. The regional differences in perfusion are called *West's zone of perfusion.*[26-28] In West's zone I, mean pulmonary arterial pressure is less than or equal to alveolar pressure; therefore no blood flow occurs. In zone I conditions of the lung apices of an upright adult, there is unperfused yet ventilated alveoli and thus dead space ventilation. In zone II, which consists of the mid lung, pulmonary arterial pressure is greater than alveolar pressure. Conditions in this zone are governed by the fact that blood flow is not influenced by venous pressure but by the difference between arterial and alveolar pressures. In zone III or the lower zone of the lung, pressure at the alveolus is exceeded by the pressures in the pulmonary artery and vein. Flow then is a function of both pulmonary arterial and venous pressures. At the very base of the lung, because of higher perivascular pressures and reduced lung expansion, flow again is diminished.[29]

Any disorder affecting the airways or the lung parenchyma will result in an increased imbalance between ventilation and perfusion and therefore a greater than normal range of $\dot{V}_A/\dot{Q}$ ratios. The presence of varying $\dot{V}_A/\dot{Q}$ ratios, whether in the normal or the diseased lung, has several important effects on gas exchange. PO_2 and PCO_2 of an alveolus, and therefore of the capillary blood leaving it, are dependent on the ratio of ventilation to perfusion. As this ratio decreases, PO_2 decreases and PCO_2 increases. The opposite occurs as the $\dot{V}_A/\dot{Q}$ ratio increases. Figure 33–5 demonstrates the relationship between ventilation/perfusion ratios.

Lung units with low $\dot{V}_A/\dot{Q}$ ratios decrease arterial PO_2 and increase arterial PCO_2. In extreme cases where no ventilation reaches a lung unit, $\dot{V}_A/\dot{Q}$ equals zero, and mixed venous blood is added unchanged to the arterial circulation. A right-to-left shunt occurs. The contribution of low $\dot{V}_A/\dot{Q}$ units and shunts to arterial blood can be determined by calculating the venous admixture ($\dot{Q}_S/\dot{Q}_T$):

$$\dot{Q}_S/\dot{Q}_T = \frac{C_C - C_a}{C_c - C_{\bar{V}}},$$

whereas C_c, C_a and $C_{\bar{V}}$ are the O_2 contents of end-capillary, arterial, and mixed venous blood, respectively. This contribution also can be assessed by calculating the difference between alveolar and arterial PO_2 ($AaDO_2$), which varies directly with the extent of venous admixture. Because of difficulties in accurately measuring it, the mean alveolar PO_2 (PAO_2) is calculated from the alveolar air equation:

$$P_AO_2 = P_IO_2 - \frac{PCO_2}{R},$$

where P_IO_2 = PO_2 of inspired air, and R = respiratory exchange quotient, the ratio of CO_2 production to O_2 consumption. In healthy young subjects, $AaDO_2$ averages 8 mmHg.[30]

When ventilation to a lung unit exceeds its perfusion (i.e., $\dot{V}_A/\dot{Q} > 1$), the excess ventilation is considered to be "wasted" because it does not participate in gas exchange. The sum of the excess ventilation contributed by lung units with high $\dot{V}_A/\dot{Q}$ ratios is referred to as the *alveolar dead space.*

The effect of increasing ventilation/perfusion imbalance on gas exchange is that, as the amount of inequality increases, both the ratio of physiologic dead space to tidal volume and venous admixture increase and arterial PO_2 fall rapidly. Arterial PCO_2 changes little at first but then progressively increases. In the diseased lung, ventilation/perfusion imbalance can result in arterial hypercarbia. This is not often observed clinically because the patient usually increases minute ventilation and thereby maintains PCO_2 at a normal level.

Factors other than pulmonary disease can alter the balance between ventilation and perfusion. For example, ventilation can become increasingly uniform between the apex and the base if either the flow rate or the tidal volume is increased by excess effort by the patient. As a result, ventilation/perfusion inequality increases.

Alveolar Ventilation

The volume of air entering the lungs each minute that actually participates in gas exchange is called the *alveolar ventilation* ($\dot{V}_A$). It is the difference between the total volume of air entering the lungs each minute, the minute ventilation ($\dot{V}_E$), and the volume of air entering the lungs that does not participate in gas exchange, the dead space ($\dot{V}_D$).

$$\dot{V}_A = \dot{V}_E - \dot{V}_D.$$

The type of total or physiologic dead space ($\dot{V}_D$) is dependent on the location of the volume not exchanged, either in the anatomic airways or the alveolus. The anatomic dead space is equal to the volume of airways proximal to the terminal respiratory units. Approximately 25% of each tidal volume is lost in these conducting airways. The ultimate volume is dependent on body size and equals approximately 1 ml/lb.[33] This volume is divided almost equally between the upper and lower airways. The alveolar dead space is produced by all alveoli that are overventilated relative to their perfusion. Thus more gas is available than is blood for

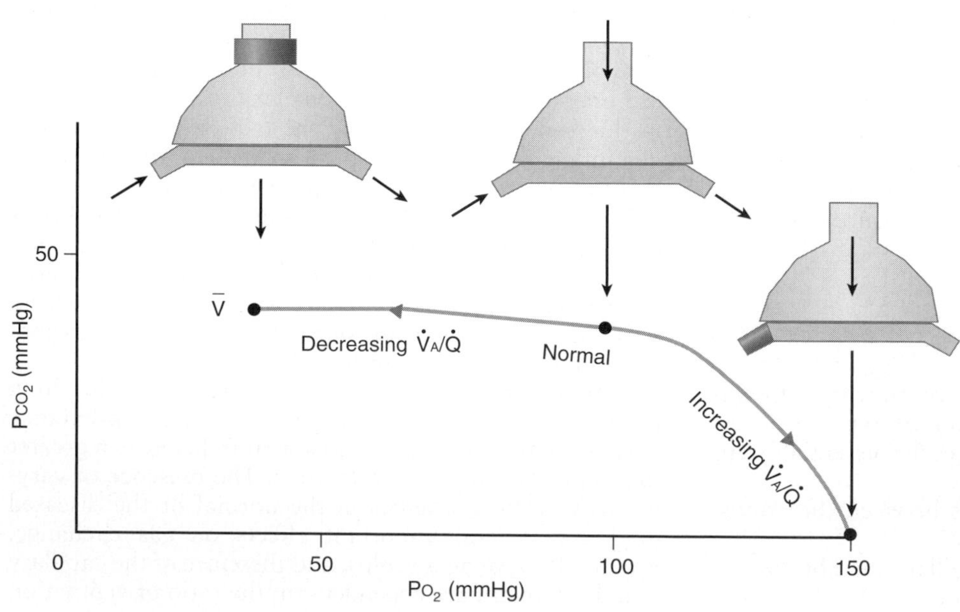

FIGURE 33–5 • Relationship between the ventilation/perfusion ratio ($\dot{V}_A/\dot{Q}$) of an alveolus and the PO_2 and PCO_2 of alveolar gas and end-capillary blood. PO_2 and PCO_2 vary from the mixed venous blood ($\bar{V}$) to inspired air (I) as ($\dot{V}_A/\dot{Q}$) changes from zero to infinity. (Adapted from West JB: *Ventilation blood flow and gas exchange, ed 3.* Oxford, 1977, Blackwell Scientific Publications.)

diffusion. The physiologic dead space usually is expressed as a fraction of the tidal volume ($\dot{V}_D/\dot{V}_T$).

Alveolar ventilation is an important determinant of gas exchange because it, along with the rate at which tissue metabolism produces CO_2 ($\dot{V}CO_2$), determines the PCO_2 of arterial blood.

$$PCO_2 \; \alpha \; \frac{\dot{V}CO_2}{\dot{V}_A}$$

When $\dot{V}CO_2$ is constant, PCO_2 varies inversely with $\dot{V}_A$. At any given minute during ventilation, PCO_2 varies directly with the amount of physiologic dead space. As dead space changes, PCO_2 can be kept constant only by increasing or decreasing $\dot{V}_E$ by an identical amount.

The measurement of dead space has evolved from the original description by Bohr in 1891, when dead space was considered simply the gas from the conducting airways. Today measurement of the physiologic dead space has been modified as follows:

$$V_D/V_T = (Pa_{CO_2} - PE_{CO_2})/Pa_{CO_2}.$$

Diffusion of O_2 and CO_2

Gas must travel through a number of barriers between the alveolus and blood. These barriers include the alveolar epithelial lining, basement membrane, capillary endothelial lining, plasma, and red blood cell. The amount of gas (Q) diffusing through a membrane is directly proportional to the surface area available for diffusion (S), the pressure difference for the gas on either side of the membrane ($p1 - p2$), and a constant (K) that depends on the solubility coefficient of the gas, membrane characteristics, and liquid used. This association is defined by the Fick principle of the diffusion state as follows:

$$Q/\text{min} = Kx(p1 - p2)/d.$$

Q is inversely proportional to the distance it has to diffuse, whereas K is proportional to the solubility of the gas and inversely proportional to the square root of the molecular weight.

In healthy subjects at rest, equilibration of PO_2 and PCO_2 of the alveolar gas and the pulmonary capillary blood is achieved in approximately 0.75 seconds.[32] This is about one third of the time spent by the blood in the capillary network; therefore the rate of blood flow can be increased greatly by impairing equilibration. For this reason, diffusion disequilibrium has been demonstrated in healthy persons only during strenuous exercise at high altitudes.

In the presence of parenchymal disease, diffusion impairment may occur solely as a result of thickening of the alveolar-capillary membrane. Much more commonly, however, diffusion disequilibrium is associated with destruction of the pulmonary capillary bed. This results in greatly increased blood flow velocity in the remaining capillaries that may allow insufficient time for equilibration. Even when parenchymal disease is severe, however, diffusion disequilibrium usually occurs only when cardiac output, and therefore rate of flow, is markedly increased.

REFERENCES

1. Hall JE: The promise of translational physiology. *Am J Physiol Lung Cell Mol Physiol* 283:L235–L236, 2002 (editorial).
2. Fung YC: A model of the lung structure and its validation. *J Appl Physiol* 64:2132–2141, 1988.
3. Gatto LA, Fluck RR, Nieman GF: Alveolar mechanics in the acutely injured lung: role of alveolar instability in the pathogenesis of ventilator induced lung injury. *Respir Care* 49:1045–1055, 2004.
4. Karlinsky JB, Snyder GL, Franzblaw C, et al: In vitro effects of elastase and collagenase on mechanical properties of hamster lungs. *Am Rev Respir Dis* 113:769–777, 1976.
5. Ludwig MS, Dreshaj I, Solway J, et al: Partitioning of the pulmonary resistance during constriction in the dog: effects of volume history. *J Appl Physiol* 62:807–815, 1987.
6. Wright JR, Hawgood S: Pulmonary surfactant metabolism. *Clin Chest Med* 10:83, 1989.
7. Bangham AD: Lung surfactant: how it does and does not work. *Lung* 165:17–25, 1987.
8. Hills BA: What forces keep the air spaces of the lung dry? *Thorax* 37:713–717, 1982.
9. Hills BA: Water repellency induced by pulmonary surfactants. *J Physiol* 325:175–186, 1982.
10. Scapelli EM: The alveoli surface network: a new anatomy and its physiologic significance. *Anat Rec* 251:491–527, 1998.
11. Hills BA: An alternative view of the roles surfactant and the alveolar model. *J Appl Physiol* 87:1567–1583, 1999.
12. Scapelli EM, Hills BA: Opposing views on the alveolar surface, alveolar models, and the role of surfactant. *J Appl Physiol* 89:408–412, 2000 (comment).
13. Lachmann B: Open up the lung and keep the lung open. *Intensive Care Med* 18:319–321, 1992 (editorial).
14. Fagan DG: Post-mortem studies of the semistatic volume-pressure characteristics of infant's lungs. *Thorax* 31:534, 1976.
15. Mansell AL, Bryan C, Levison H: Airway closure in children. *J Appl Physiol* 319:1112, 1988.
16. Thorsteinsson A, Larsson A, Jonmarker C, Werner O: Pressure-volume relations of the respiratory system in healthy children. *Am J Respir Crit Care Med* 150:421, 1994.
17. Rahn H, Otis AB, Chadwick EL, et al: The pressure-volume diagram of the thorax and lung. *Am J Physiol* 146:161–178, 1946.
18. Murray JF, editor: *The normal lung*. Philadelphia, 1986, WB Saunders.
19. Polgar G, String ST: The viscous resistance of the lung tissues in newborn infants. *J Pediatr* 69:787, 1996.
20. Ferris BG, Mead J, Opie LH: Partitioning of respiratory flow resistance in man. *J Appl Physiol* 19:653–658, 1964.
21. Hogg JC, Williams J, Richardson JB, et al: Age as a factor in the distribution in the distribution of lower airway conductance and in the pathologic anatomy of obstructive lung disease. *N Engl J Med* 282:1283, 1970.
22. Dubois AB: Resistance to breathing. In Fenn WO, Rahn H, editors: *Handbook of physiology, respiration*, vol 1.Washington DC, 1964, American Physiological Society.
23. Brisco WA, Dubois AB: The relationship between airway resistance, airway conductance and lung volume in subjects of different age and body size. *J Clin Invest* 37:1279–1285, 1958.
24. Brody AW: Mechanical compliance and resistance of the lung-thorax calculated from the flow during passive expiration. *Am J Physiol* 178:189–196, 1954.
25. Kano A, Lanteri CJ, Pemberton PJ, et al: Fast versus slow ventilation for neonates. *Am Rev Respir Dis* 148:578–584, 1993.
26. West JB: *Ventilation/blood flow and gas exchange*, ed 3. London, 1979, Blackwell Scientific Publications.
27. West JB, Dollery CT: Distribution of blood flow and the pressure-flow relations of the whole lung. *J Appl Physiol* 19:713, 1964.
28. West JB, Dollery CT, Naimark AL: Distribution of blood flow in isolated lung: relation to vascular and alveolar pressure. *J Appl Physiol* 19:713, 1964.

29. Hughes JMB, Glazier JB, Maloney JE, et al: Effect of lung volume on the distribution pulmonary blood flow in man. *Respir Physiol* 4:58, 1968.
30. Mellemgaard K: The alveolar-arterial oxygen difference: its size and components in normal man. *Acta Physiol Scand* 67:10–20, 1966.
31. Radford EP: Ventilation standards for use in artifical respiration. *J Appl Physiol* 61:1560, 1955.
32. Roughton FJ: Average time spent by blood in human lung capillary and its relation to the rates of CD uptake and elimination in man. *Am J Physiol* 143:621, 1945.

CHAPTER

34

Control of Breathing and Acute Respiratory Failure

Robert K. Kanter

PEARLS

- Powerful neural regulation of breathing maintains a constant supply of oxygen to the tissue, despite wide variations of metabolic rate and respiratory system disorders, until an advanced stage of respiratory failure is reached.
- Impaired controls of breathing may interfere with respiratory cycle timing, respiratory effort, or functional patency of the airway. In some cases a disorder of respiratory regulation may be the patient's primary problem. Other patients have secondary impairment of respiratory regulation as a result of acute or chronic systemic illness.
- Sick or injured patients usually hyperventilate in compensation for their stressful disorder. Stressed patients with irregular breathing or inappropriately comfortable effort to breathe have a severely depressed respiratory drive. Immediate ventilatory support usually is warranted.
- Respiratory depression or apnea may be the clue that an underlying systemic illness requires specific treatment.

Powerful neural regulatory processes defend breathing. In the critically ill or injured patient, systemic oxygen requirements are determined by functional needs of stressed tissue and cannot be reduced, even if the supply of oxygen is limited by physiologic derangements. No biologic oxygen reservoir is available. Therefore survival depends on uninterrupted delivery of fresh oxygen to the lungs. Neural responses increase respiratory activity in compensation for increased metabolic demands, airway obstruction, pulmonary parenchymal disorders, and impairment of the respiratory muscles. If respiratory controls are functioning normally, a relatively constant internal chemical environment is maintained until an advanced stage of respiratory failure is reached.

A primary disorder of respiratory regulation may cause respiratory failure. In other cases, chronic disease or acute systemic disorders may cause secondary impairment of central respiratory regulation and prevent the patient from adequately compensating for a respiratory stress. Impaired controls of breathing may interfere with respiratory cycle timing, respiratory effort, or functional patency of the airway.

This chapter summarizes the normal regulatory mechanisms that defend alveolar ventilation. Next, factors that may impair respiratory neural controls are considered.

Normal Regulation of Breathing

Respiratory Control System

The elements of the respiratory control system are shown in Figure 34–1. The breathing pattern is generated by neurons in the brainstem. Microdissection studies of neonatal rat brainstem have revealed that only a limited portion of rostral ventrolateral medulla oblongata is necessary for the generation of rhythmic neural discharges in respiratory motor neurons.[42] Afferent signals from sensors in the brainstem and in peripheral sites modify the intensity and cycle timing of respiratory motor output.

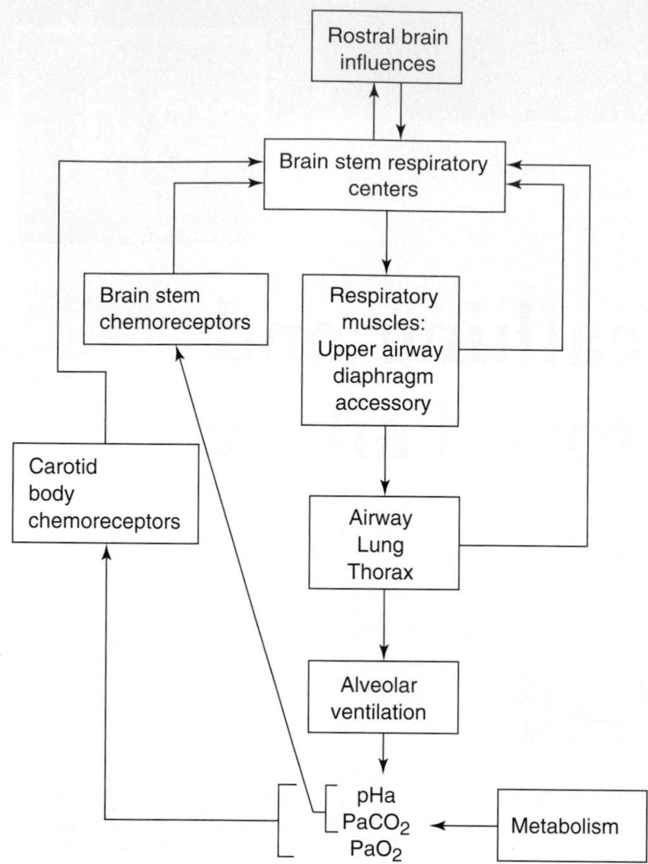

FIGURE 34–1 • Elements of the respiratory control system.

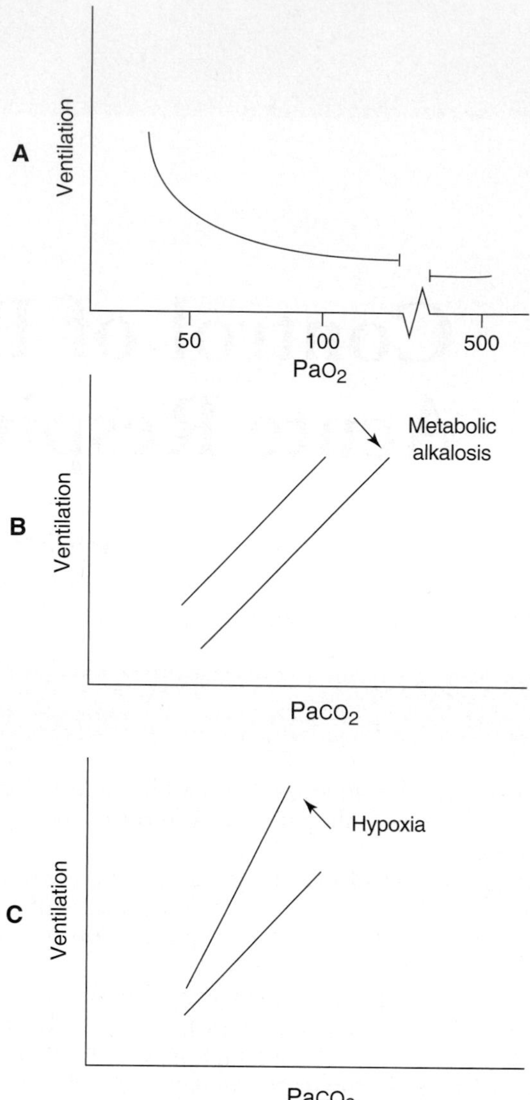

FIGURE 34–2 • Chemoreceptor activity, as reflected by minute ventilation, varies as a function of Pa_{O_2} **(A)**, Pa_{CO_2} **(B)** (superimposed metabolic alkalosis inhibits breathing), and Pa_{CO_2} **(C)** (superimposed hypoxia stimulates breathing).

With high-intensity stimulation, accessory respiratory muscle groups are recruited. Rostral brain influences, including sleep, have an additional powerful influence on respiratory activity. It is notable that the brainstem regions that mediate respiratory control overlap anatomically with areas regulating cardiovascular activity.[28] This is not surprising in view of the coordinated cardiorespiratory functions involved in the transport of oxygen and the clearance of carbon dioxide. For example, afferent impulses from the peripheral chemoreceptor in response to hypoxia[9] and from the baroreceptor in response to hypotension[25] appear to converge to common neuronal populations in medulla oblongata, with sympathoexcitation and hyperventilation resulting from either stimulus.

Chemical Stimuli

Hypoxemia is a powerful stimulus to ventilation mediated by sensory input originating in the carotid body chemoreceptor. Peripheral chemoreceptor activity (reflected in minute ventilation) increases slightly with decrements in Pa_{O_2} below 500 mmHg and rises steeply as Pa_{O_2} falls below 50 mmHg (Figure 34–2, *A*). Low oxygen tension, rather than low oxygen content, is the important ventilatory stimulus. Little carotid body response results from profound anemia. Carotid chemoreceptor response also contributes to arousal from sleep during episodes of hypoxia.[10]

Hydrogen ion concentration and carbon dioxide tension independently activate chemoreceptors in the carotid body and in the brainstem (Figure 34–2, *B*). The simultaneous presence of hypoxia augments the hypercapnic ventilatory response (Figure 34–2, *C*).

Mechanical Loads

Mechanical loads on breathing influence respiratory efforts independent of chemical stimuli. Sensors for load-compensating reflexes are located in respiratory muscles and the chest wall. Reduction in lung volume also is detected by pulmonary stretch receptors. Afferent signals travel via the spinal cord, vagus nerves, and perhaps the phrenic nerves. Both conscious and reflex responses are involved in compensatory increases of effort, including the recruitment of accessory muscles in response to increased respiratory resistance or to a decrease in compliance. Glottic closure at the end of inspiration with braking of expiratory flow maximizes the duration of lung expansion with minimal additional effort. This accounts for the grunting breathing pattern of dyspneic infants. Stimulation to breathe is further augmented by hypercapnia or hypoxia when loaded breathing reduces ventilation.

Upper Airway

Reflexes protecting the patency of the upper airway are vital in health and disease. Important activities include coordination of breathing with swallowing, avoidance of aspiration, and variation of pharyngeal muscle tone with respiratory phase or neck position. Protective upper airway reflexes may be exaggerated in the newborn, with resultant irregular breathing patterns and apnea when fluid is introduced into the pharynx.[33]

Factors Impairing Respiratory Controls

Many factors can blunt neural responses to respiratory stimuli. As a result, deterioration of a sick patient may be accelerated or recovery from respiratory failure prolonged. Recognition of some of these risk factors may allow corrective interventions or, when these disorders cannot be reversed, may enable close monitoring and timely administration of general supportive care, including mechanical ventilation.

Biological Variation in the Normal Population

Familial differences in respiratory chemosensitivity probably account for some of the individual variation in compensations for respiratory disease. The genetic determination of variation in central respiratory sensitivity appears to be greater at younger ages, more important for hypoxic than for hypercapnic chemosensitivity, and less important for perception of dyspnea.[19] Obstructive sleep apnea is partly determined by familial factors.[36] The potential importance of genetic variation is evident in adults with chronic pulmonary disorders. Adults with chronic lung disease can be classified as normocapnic or hypercapnic. Healthy adult offspring of patients with CO_2 retention tend to have lower ventilatory responses to hypoxia and hypercapnia than offspring of patients with normal CO_2 levels. Subclinical individual variation in respiratory controls may be a determinant of some patients' decompensation during acute respiratory disease. Adults studied after recovery from near-fatal asthma episodes had significantly reduced ventilatory responses to hypoxia and blunted perception of dyspnea compared with normal subjects and with asthmatics who had not had near-fatal attacks.[17] Although these asthmatics were not known to have a primary disorder of respiratory control, their insensitivity to hypoxia and poor perception of respiratory mechanical loads impaired the intensity of their respiratory effort, resulting in severe hypercapnia, hypoxia, and need for mechanical ventilation in 8 of 11 patients. These observations suggest that respiratory neural responses at the lower end of the normal intensity range, which are adequate for unstressed breathing, may be insufficient during severe illness. Normal biologic variations in respiratory drive may account for some of the pediatric patients who deteriorate during acute respiratory disease, whereas others tolerate a similar illness.

Immaturity

In the normal adult, hypoxia evokes sustained hyperventilation. However, newborns have a biphasic response to hypoxia. Transient hyperventilation is followed by ventilatory depression to below normoxic levels. This hypoxic depression may greatly exacerbate the adverse impact of transient respiratory compromise in the young infant. The response to hypoxia matures in the first few weeks of life.

Some newborns also have a developmental insensitivity to hypercapnia. Muscular and mechanical factors, as well as immaturity of controls, may contribute to the early limitations in hypercapnic ventilatory response.

An immediate compensation for mechanical loads on breathing is observed in newborns, even in preterm infants. Animal studies reveal small improvements with age in the ability to defend ventilation against experimental loads, but whether this difference is biologically important is not clear.[24] In addition, whether immature control mechanisms are responsible for the differences or whether muscle endurance, compliance of thoracic structures, or metabolic differences are the predominant developmental variables is not clear.

Primary Disorders of Respiratory Control

Congenital or long-standing acquired disorders of the central nervous system may impair respiratory centers, leading to respiratory failure. Acute respiratory insufficiency may accompany progression of a central lesion. A static regulatory impairment may be revealed by its failure to compensate for acute systemic illness. Primary central abnormalities may manifest as ineffective respiratory cycle generation (central apnea), deficient responses to respiratory stimuli (hypoventilation during stress), or inadequate motor control of the vocal cords or pharynx (obstructive apnea). These patterns of regulatory dysfunction may occur individually or in combination. Respiratory compromise usually is the worst during sleep. Medications with central nervous system inhibitory actions may have an exaggerated impact on patients with primary disorders of respiratory controls. Pulmonary hypertension as a result of recurrent hypoxia and aspiration pneumonia associated with impaired airway protective reflexes complicate the clinical situation in some cases. Although comprehensive clinical data are lacking, some consideration should be given to the possibility that the patient with a primary disorder of respiratory controls is potentially at risk for ineffective cardiovascular responses during periods of stress[3] because some of the same neural structures are involved in regulating each of these systems. The reader is referred to the textbook by Mathews[26] for more detailed information on primary disorders of respiratory controls. Although apnea often occurs in the newborn, apnea of prematurity is beyond the scope of this chapter.

Central neurologic causes of airway obstruction must be distinguished from primary anatomic disorders of the airway. Central disorders of respiratory control also may be confused with neuromuscular disorders that present with weakness or pharyngeal airway obstruction on a motor basis.[15] In disorders of motor neurons or myopathy, weak respiratory muscle activity is observed despite intensified respiratory drive.[4]

Recognition of certain structural brain lesions is important because some of the lesions are correctable. In other cases general supportive care is effective. Congenital structural neurologic malformations may manifest as apnea or profound hypoventilation at birth[5] or may be recognized later if respiratory impairment is mild. In particular, patients with Arnold-Chiari malformation often have vocal cord paralysis and airway obstruction. The vocal cord motor dysfunction often is reversed with neurosurgical decompression of the brainstem.[35] Other children with myelodysplasia suffer nonobstructive central hypoventilation, ranging from asymptomatic disordered sleep breathing patterns and reduced ventilatory response to hypercapnia[45] or to life-threatening apnea.[7] Various other structural disorders may interfere with brainstem respiratory regulation, including posterior fossa tumors,[21] vascular malformations,[30] and skeletal disorders.[37]

Nonstructural neurologic disorders with respiratory depression have been recognized. Maternal drug abuse with opiates, cocaine, or phencyclidine during pregnancy results in the birth of infants with sleep breathing pattern abnormalities that persist for months. Rett syndrome[12,14,44] occurs in girls and is characterized by a unique pattern of disorganized breathing while awake and a tendency for breathing to normalize while asleep. Hyperventilation alternates with severe apnea and hypoxia. The cause is unknown, and progressive neurologic deterioration is typical. Children with cerebral palsy occasionally have neurologic deficits of pharyngeal tone, although central drive to breathe usually is intact. Adenotonsillectomy may alleviate the severity of airway obstruction, but tracheostomy is necessary in other patients. Children with congenital central hypoventilation syndrome lack specific anatomic malformations or any obvious cause of the central disturbance.[41,48] These patients may first come to medical attention because of growth failure, neurodevelopmental delay, or cor pulmonale. A diffuse central nervous system disorder, perhaps with a genetic basis, likely is responsible for congenital central hypoventilation syndrome. These patients typically have seizures, deficits in cognition, or impaired motor performance. Radiologic imaging and autopsy findings of atrophy and gliosis suggest a generalized brain disorder. Sleep hypoventilation predominates in congenital central hypoventilation syndrome, although some patients also suffer respiratory insufficiency while awake. The disorder often is fatal without mechanical ventilation. Early mechanical ventilation may reduce the sequela and improve long-term neurodevelopmental outcome.

Sudden infant death syndrome (SIDS) is the leading cause of postneonatal infant mortality in the United States. Clinicians have long speculated that SIDS is caused by a disorder of cardiorespiratory regulation and arousal, a hypothesis that remains unproved. Cardiorespiratory observations have been obtained on thousands of apparently normal infants, some of whom subsequently died of SIDS. The respiratory pattern of the SIDS victims overlapped sufficiently with survivors such that detection of the individual infant at high risk for SIDS based on respiratory observations is impossible. Evidence of an underlying central disorder is suggested by the finding that SIDS victims tended to have reduced variability of heart rate when compared with matched sleep-waking state data of control infants.[38] Decreased muscarinic receptor binding has been noted in the brainstem arcuate nucleus of infants who died of SIDS.[18] Complete investigation of an apparent SIDS death includes an autopsy to rule out an underlying medical disorder or trauma.[2]

In evaluating an acutely ill patient for possible respiratory control disorders, it should be emphasized that apnea may be the most obvious manifestation of various acute systemic illnesses (see section on evaluating controls of breathing during respiratory deterioration). The acute illness must be recognized and treated specifically. It also should be recalled that apnea may be the presenting manifestation of child abuse.[29] Apnea reported in infants older than 12 months (older than typical for SIDS), especially if accompanied by a suspicious history or injury, raises the consideration of abuse.

The first priority in evaluation of the patient with a possible primary disorder of respiratory control is to recognize life-threatening respiratory depression. Severe disorders of respiratory regulation usually result in hypoxia and hypercapnia, especially during sleep. General supportive care is instituted when necessary. When the history and physical examination suggest a central nervous system structural problem, imaging studies of the brainstem are warranted. When an infant has been resuscitated successfully from an apparent life-threatening event, a period of hospital observation should be considered to prevent a dangerous recurrence. A medical evaluation is carried out according to individual features of the history and physical examination. When no specific correctable cause of infant apnea is found, the decision to recommend home monitoring is difficult. Cardiorespiratory monitoring in the home has not decreased the risk of SIDS. Home cardiorespiratory monitoring may be warranted for infants who are technology dependent, have unstable airways, or have rare medical conditions affecting regulation of breathing. Monitors should be equipped with an event recorder. Plans should be made for periodic review and discontinuation of home monitoring.[1]

Chronic Underlying Conditions

In critically ill patients, compensations for respiratory disorders may be limited by chronic underlying conditions that impair respiratory controls. Recognizing these disorders allows identification of patients who may be at higher risk for respiratory failure during acute illness. In addition to the apparent genetic influences that may impair control of breathing, chronic hypercapnia can cause compensatory renal bicarbonate retention in patients with chronic obstructive pulmonary disease. Respiratory drive associated with a given level of CO_2 is opposed by this compensatory rise in pH (Figure 34–2, *B*). Also, some adults with chronic lung disease fail to increase effort when presented with an external respiratory load. The respiratory response elicited by a resistive load may significantly increase after naloxone injection, suggesting that endogenous opioids play a role in respiratory depression of chronic lung disease. A concern regarding supplemental oxygen is sometimes raised in the care of patients with chronic lung disease and acute exacerbations. It is sometimes argued that administration of excessive supplemental oxygen causes respiratory failure in patients with chronic CO_2 insensitivity who might depend on hypoxic drive to breathe. Of greater concern are the adverse effects of hypoxia. Because hypoxic drive to breathe only increases substantially at oxygen tension below 50 mmHg (Figure 34–2, *A*), it is virtually impossible to maintain stable respiratory stimulation with mild and "safe" hypoxia, without risking episodic dangerous hypoxia.[27] If a patient is so poorly compensated that removal of hypoxic drive results in hypoventilation, then mechanical ventilation is the safest management strategy.

Congenital heart disease with high pulmonary blood flow elevates work of breathing and causes ventilation/perfusion mismatch. More subtle is the reversible blunting of hypoxic ventilatory response that occurs in children with cyanotic heart disease. It is not clear how early in infancy blunted hypoxic sensitivity develops in these patients. Resolution occurs over a period of weeks after surgical correction of cyanotic lesions.

In addition to its many other adverse systemic effects, hypothyroidism is associated with reduced ventilatory response to hypoxia and hypercapnia, especially in adult patients with myxedema. There is no evidence regarding hypothyroidism and respiratory regulation in critically ill infants.

Infants born prematurely continue to experience irregularities of respiratory pattern even at postconceptional age older than 40 weeks. This susceptibility is especially exacerbated by anesthesia.[22] Among infants born prematurely and anesthetized for surgery before 60 weeks' postconceptional age, 37% had prolonged postoperative apnea. Apnea was most common in the younger patients. Apneic events occurred within 2 hours of surgery in 72%, but in the remainder respiratory irregularity began as late as 12 hours postoperatively. In some patients, apnea recurred for as long as 48 hours. Both obstructive and central mechanisms of apnea were observed.[23] Continuous monitoring for at least 12 hours after anesthesia is warranted when surgery is required for infants born prematurely who are still younger than 60 weeks' postconceptional age.

Systemic Factors in Acute Illness

The patient with a critical illness or injury generally hyperventilates. At least some of the increased respiratory drive can be attributed to a higher metabolic rate. Stress-related release of catecholamines, glucagon, and cortisol contributes to the hypermetabolic state. Conscious experience of pain, discomfort, and fear also stimulate ventilation. When a stressed patient fails to hyperventilate, incipient respiratory failure should be suspected.

Some common factors in the critically ill patient interfere with regulation of breathing. The normal breathing pattern in the awake state is modified by sleep, and compensation for respiratory illness is most likely to fail during sleep. Ventilatory responses to hypercapnia and, in some subjects, hypoxia are diminished during sleep. Reduced upper airway tone and cough reflexes worsen the risk of obstruction and aspiration. Infants are at greater risk for obstruction and aspiration. Infants also are at greater risk for sleep-associated respiratory compromise than are older patients. In infants whose compliant thorax tends to collapse, lung volume is maintained by thoracic muscle tone and breathing at sufficiently high frequencies that expiration seldom reaches the passive resting lung volume. During sleep the processes that brake expiratory flow, glottic closure, and maintenance of inspiratory muscle tone are attenuated. Respiratory frequency also slows in sleep, with resulting decreases in infants' expiratory lung volume. Infants' compensation for mechanical loads is compromised during the rapid eye movement stage of sleep more than during quiet sleep. Although sleep is a period of high risk for the sick infant, depriving the patient of sleep is counterproductive. Significantly worse obstructive and central apnea occur in healthy infants after sleep deprivation.[6]

Seizures often contribute to respiratory failure, whether the seizure is the patient's primary problem or a complication of a brain injury. The neurologic basis of seizure-induced respiratory depression is multifactorial.

Moderate brain injuries typically are associated with hyperventilation. The hypermetabolic state, lung pathology, and loss of inhibitory cortical influences probably combine to augment ventilation. Even when the brain-injured patient does hyperventilate, airway protective reflexes usually are impaired, seizures may ensue, and subtle progression of the brain lesion may lead to pathologic breathing patterns (Figure 34–3). Each of these problems may lead to abrupt and catastrophic hypoxia.

Iatrogenic depression of respiratory control is common. Some agents inhibit brain function nonselectively, whereas others have specific actions on respiratory regulation without impairing consciousness. Relative effects on upper airway patency and hypoxic, hypercapnic, and loading responses may be dissociated. For example,

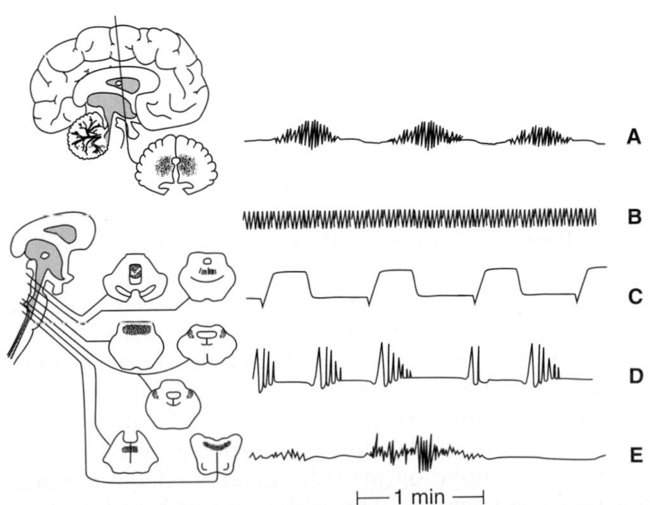

FIGURE 34–3 • Abnormal respiratory patterns associated with lesions *(shaded areas)* at various levels of the brain. Inspiration reads up. **A,** Cheyne-Stokes respiration. **B,** Central neurogenic hyperventilation. **C,** Apneusis. **D,** Cluster breathing. **E,** Ataxic breathing. (From Plum F, Posner JB: *The diagnosis of stupor and coma,* ed 3. Philadelphia, 1980, FA Davis Co.)

chloral hydrate has little effect on chemosensitivity but reduces genioglossus muscle tone and predisposes to obstructive apnea. Concern regarding respiratory depression does not warrant withholding analgesia. Rather, monitoring should be appropriate. In fact, episodic hypoxia during treatment procedures may be reduced when appropriate analgesia is provided.[34] Parenteral sedatives and analgesics usually can be safely administered without endotracheal intubation after considering the patient's underlying medical condition, anatomic or functional risk factors involving the airway, history of past drug reactions, and recent dietary intake. Equipment for suctioning, mask bag ventilation, and intubation should be accessible. Vital signs and oximetry are monitored. Slow intravenous infusion of analgesics is less likely to cause hypoventilation than is bolus administration. After sedation or anesthesia, respiratory depression sometimes appears to worsen after completion of the procedure, as arousing stimulation ceases. Several other pharmacologic mechanisms of delayed respiratory depression after opiates have been hypothesized.[20] Monitoring should continue until the patient is completely awake. It is important to note that respiratory depression can occur after epidural, intrathecal, and intravenous opiates.[32] Low-dose systemic infusion of naloxone may attenuate respiratory depression of epidural opiates, without interfering with analgesia. To better anticipate the duration of respiratory depression after intravenous analgesic administration, it must be recognized that drugs that are rapidly cleared after a single dose may be more slowly cleared after repeated or continuous infusion.[39] Some special considerations are important in infants. For example, newborns have a longer elimination half-life of morphine than do older children and adults. Distinct receptors mediate the respiratory inhibitory and analgesic actions of opioids. It appears that opioid tolerance develops sooner for analgesic effects than does respiratory depression.[40] Therefore effective analgesia may be accompanied by respiratory depression when opioids are necessary over a prolonged course. An important goal of current research is the development of a drug that selectively stimulates opiate receptors to provide analgesia without respiratory depression or other central nervous system toxicity.[8] Opioid-induced respiratory depression can be reliably reversed with naloxone. In patients with cardiovascular compromise (e.g., cardiac surgery), naloxone should be avoided in the immediate postoperative period, as the stress of abruptly eliminating opioid anesthesia would be hazardous. The benzodiazepine antagonist flumazenil reduces respiratory depression resulting from benzodiazepines, but little pediatric experience with this agent has been reported. Flumazenil may lower the threshold for seizures.[11] The duration of action of antagonists may be shorter than the agent depressing breathing. Close monitoring is essential, and repeated doses of antagonists may be necessary. In other cases of drug-induced respiratory depression, mechanical ventilation provides greater safety than pharmacologic antagonists. This is the case with multifactorial central depression or in severely ill patients.

Some pharmacologic agents depress respiration without general central nervous system depression. Although the site of action is unknown, infusions of dopamine even at low doses may depress breathing in patients who are dependent on hypoxic ventilatory drive. Likewise, prostaglandin E_1, given to maintain patency of the ductus arteriosus in infants with cyanotic heart disease, is associated with respiratory depression in 12% of infants.

Respiratory inhibitory action of metabolic alkalosis may account for hypoventilation, with Pa_{CO_2} exceeding 55 mmHg in adult patients.[13] Metabolic alkalosis may be caused by exogenously administered bicarbonate or an endogenous metabolic etiology. The impact of alkalosis on breathing in sick infants has not been systematically studied but may contribute to prolonged dependence on mechanical ventilation in infants receiving bicarbonate and diuretics following cardiac surgery. When metabolic alkalosis accompanies prolonged recovery from respiratory failure, correction of the alkalosis with potassium chloride and occasionally acetazolamide may enable ventilator weaning.

Nutrition has complex effects on respiratory reserve. Muscle strength is diminished and metabolic rate falls in starvation. In addition, ventilatory response to hypoxia is greatly reduced in some otherwise healthy subjects after a 10-day hypocaloric diet. Although important benefits derive from nutritional supplementation in the critically ill patient, the immediate impact is unpredictable. For example, carbohydrate infusions increase production of carbon dioxide exceeding the patient's ventilatory reserve. In healthy subjects, specific augmentation of ventilatory response to CO_2 was seen with branched-chain amino acid infusion.[46] Much remains to be learned about the relationships among nutrition, metabolism, and respiratory homeostasis.

Finally, temperature exerts profound effects on ventilation. Hyperthermia and environmental cold stress induce hyperventilation, but deep accidental hypothermia depresses ventilatory drive. When evaluating blood gas results in patients with extreme variations in temperature, noting the difference between values measured at standard instrument temperature (37°C) versus the patient's body temperature clarifies the interpretation. For example, in a spontaneously breathing patient whose body temperature is 42°C, a Pa_{CO_2} reported as 40 mmHg corresponds to an actual (in vivo) Pa_{CO_2} of 49 mmHg. Thus the patient's tendency to hypoventilate is revealed.

Controls of Breathing in Advanced Respiratory Failure

Initially compensatory, the vigorous respiratory effort of the dyspneic patient may become counterproductive. Agitation increases oxygen consumption, and forced respiratory efforts may cause dynamic obstruction of airways. Large negative intratracheal pressure with forced inspiration worsens upper airway obstruction, whereas positive intrapleural pressure during forced expirations can cause collapse of intrathoracic airways. Dynamic airway obstruction in the dyspneic child may account for rapid progression of respiratory failure in some cases.

As the severely stressed respiratory system decompensates, the labored efforts of the dyspneic patient tend to give way to depressed breathing patterns. Although irregular breathing and apnea have been widely recognized in infants in respiratory failure,[43] observations in adults with near-fatal asthma reveal a similar tendency for respiratory arrest to precede cardiovascular collapse.[31] Slowing of respiratory frequency or reduction of effort appears to be a typical response of the organism on the brink of respiratory failure because of mechanical loads.[16,47,49] Slowing of respiratory frequency occurs in both immature[47] and adult[16,49] experimental models of loaded breathing and precedes muscle fatigue or circulatory collapse. Respiratory depression occurs in hyperoxic experimental models of loaded breathing and does not depend on hypoxemia.[16,47]

Implications for Patient Management

Evaluating Controls of Breathing During Respiratory Deterioration

In the sick, stressed patient, hyperventilation is typical, with increased respiratory frequency and obvious use of accessory muscles of breathing. The clinician should recognize thoracic retraction, grunting respiratory sounds, nasal flaring, head bobbing, and active use of expiratory abdominal muscles as signs of increased respiratory drive.

Controls of upper airway patency and protective reflexes should be assumed to be absent in the comatose patient or the drowsy patient with the snoring sounds of pharyngeal obstruction. Prompt efforts to secure the airway will avert aspiration and obstruction.

If time allows, arterial blood gas (ABG) analysis assists in the evaluation of ventilatory drive in a crisis. If moderate respiratory effort and hypocapnia ($Pa{CO_2}$ <35 mmHg) accompany an acute respiratory disorder, it can be inferred that ventilatory drive is (at least temporarily) sufficient, and alveolar ventilation relative to CO_2 production is satisfactory. If $Pa{CO_2}$ exceeds 40 to 45 mmHg in an acute respiratory disorder, then lung function, the respiratory pump, or drive to breathe is compromised. This may represent a rapidly worsening trend. Close monitoring is essential, and immediate intervention may be warranted. In the sick, stressed patient with irregular breathing or inappropriately comfortable respiratory effort and $Pa{CO_2}$ exceeding 40 to 45 mmHg, respiratory drive is severely impaired. Immediate ventilatory support usually is indicated.

Evaluation of patients during respiratory decompensation often is limited by their rapidly evolving state. Given the safety and effectiveness of conventional measures of respiratory intensive care, endotracheal intubation and mechanical ventilation should be performed promptly when there is substantial suspicion concerning impaired regulation of breathing in the critically ill patient. Apnea may suggest the presence of a systemic disorder requiring specific treatment (Box 34–1).

BOX 34–1

Systemic Causes of Apnea that Require Specific Therapy

Central nervous system
- Head injury, child abuse
- Seizure
- Meningitis, encephalitis
- Hydrocephalus
- Posterior fossa mass

Circulation
- Dysrhythmia
- Congestive heart failure

Infection
- Sepsis

Gastrointestinal
- Gastroesophageal reflux

Metabolic
- Poisons
- Hypoglycemia
- Many inborn errors of metabolism

Evaluating Controls of Breathing During Recovery from Respiratory Failure

Impairment of respiratory controls may contribute to prolonged dependence on mechanical ventilation during recovery from critical illness. In contrast to the limited evaluation of respiratory controls in patients during respiratory emergencies, careful study of specific ventilatory responses is feasible and may be warranted in the patient with slow recovery from respiratory failure.

Coordination of the upper airway is assessed by testing the gag reflex. If the gag reflex is vigorous in the alert patient, upper airway control will seldom be a limiting factor in the patient's recovery.

In attempting to decide whether to discontinue mechanical ventilation and remove an endotracheal tube, a trial of spontaneous breathing with the endotracheal tube still in place provides important insights. Once $Pa{CO_2}$ exceeds the apneic threshold of 30 to 35 mmHg, respiration should become regular and comfortable without apnea. $Pa{CO_2}$ less than 45 mmHg, pH greater than 7.35, and safe oxygenation with a comfortable effort suggest that drive and other components of the respiratory system are adequate to withdraw mechanical ventilation. If the patient becomes tachypneic, breathes laboriously, or complains of dyspnea, pulmonary disease or impaired respiratory muscle capacity probably is a limiting factor. Failure to cough, to at least double resting tidal volume, and to generate peak inspiratory negative pressures of at least 30 cmH_2O all suggest that respiratory muscle strength is inadequate to accomplish the necessary work of breathing. When pulmonary disease and muscle weakness are present, independent evaluation of respiratory drive is difficult without special testing. Finally, some patients fail to increase effort despite hypercapnia and hypoxia during the trial of spontaneous breathing. Others lack a gag response. In these cases, obvious deficiency of neural controls of breathing contributes to persistence of their respiratory insufficiency.

Measuring Respiratory Drive

In the experimental setting, respiratory efferent neural output is most rigorously measured as the phrenic nerve electrical activity or the amplitude of the diaphragm electromyogram. Measurements of mean inspiratory airflow rate (tidal volume/inspiratory time [V_T/T_I]) and the pressure generated at the mouth in the first 0.1 seconds of inspiration against an occluded airway ($P_{0.1}$) parallel direct measures of respiratory center output if respiratory system mechanics and muscle function remain constant. Devices to measure gas flow and pressure at the endotracheal tube are becoming more readily available for routine use in infants. Therefore assessing the response of V_T/T_I, $P_{0.1}$, and minute ventilation to variations in chemical stimuli and determining ventilatory compensation for loads have become feasible methods for noninvasive evaluation of respiratory controls in sick infants. Future application of such techniques in the pediatric critical care setting can advance our understanding of how respiratory controls defend against respiratory failure and how derangements in controls contribute to respiratory insufficiency in infants and children.

Therapy Related to Respiratory Controls

The underlying chronic conditions and systemic derangements acquired in acute illness that are outlined here suggest strategies for managing the critically ill or injured patient. Patients with disorders of respiratory controls should be monitored continuously during periods of severe stress and especially during sleep. Mechanical ventilation should be initiated when hypoventilation poses a substantial threat.

Although theophylline and doxapram have been successful in alleviating apnea of prematurity, there is little evidence for the effectiveness of respiratory-stimulating drugs in other pediatric critical care applications. If a trial of respiratory stimulant therapy is used in a patient with a disorder of respiratory regulation to avert acute respiratory failure, such therapeutic trials should be undertaken with continuous observation in an intensive care setting.

Long-term management of uncorrectable disorders of respiratory controls may include home apnea monitors, positive or negative pressure ventilation, and diaphragm pacing.[26]

REFERENCES

1. AAP Committee on Fetus and Newborn: Apnea, sudden infant death syndrome, and home monitoring. *Pediatrics* 111:914, 2003.
2. AAP Task Force on Infant Sleep Position and Sudden Infant Death Syndrome: changing concepts of sudden infant death syndrome: Implications for infant sleeping environment and sleep position. *Pediatrics* 105:650, 2000.
3. Arcaya J, Cacho J, Del Campo F, et al: Arnold Chiari malformation associated with sleep apnea and central dysregulation of arterial pressure. *Acta Neurol Scand* 88:224, 1993.
4. Baydur A: Respiratory muscle strength and control of ventilation in patients with neuromuscular disease. *Chest* 99:330, 1991.
5. Brazy JE, Kinney HC, Oakes WJ: Central nervous system structural lesions causing apnea at birth. *J Pediatr* 111:163, 1987.
6. Canet E, Gaultier C, D'Allest AM, et al: Effects of sleep deprivation on respiratory events during sleep in healthy infants. *J Appl Physiol* 66:1158, 1989.
7. Cochrane DD, Adderly R, White CP, et al: Apnea in patients with myelomeningocele. *Pediatr Neurosurg* 16:232, 1990–1991.
8. Davies MF, Maguire PA, Chen SW, et al: Separation of analgesia and respiratory depression in an analog of fentanyl. *Soc Neurosci Abstr* 20:750, 1994.
9. Erickson JT, Millhorn DE: Hypoxia and electrical stimulation of the carotid sinus nerve induce fos-like immunoreactivity within catecholaminergic and serotoninergic neurons of the rat brainstem. *J Comp Neurol* 348:161, 1994.
10. Fewell JE, Kondo CS, Dascalu V, et al: Influence of carotid denervation on the arousal and cardiopulmonary response to rapidly developing hypoxemia in lambs. *Pediatr Res* 25:473, 1989.
11. Fine JS, Goldfrank LR: Update in medical toxicology. *Pediatr Clin North Am* 39:1031, 1992.
12. Glaze DG, Frost JD, Zoghbi HY, et al: Rett's syndrome: characterization of respiratory patterns and sleep. *Ann Neurol* 21:377, 1987.
13. Javaheri S, Kazemi H: Metabolic alkalosis and hypoventilation in humans. *Am Rev Respir Dis* 136:1011, 1987.
14. Julu PO, Derr AM, Apartopoulos F, et al: Characterization of breathing and associated central autonomic dysfunction in the Rett disorder. *Arch Dis Child* 85:29, 2001.
15. Kanter RK: Neuromuscular disorders. In Holbrook PR, editor: *Textbook of pediatric critical care*. Philadelphia, 1993, WB Saunders.
16. Kanter RK, Fordyce WE: Central contribution to hypoventilation during severe inspiratory resistive loads. *Crit Care Med* 21:1915, 1993.
17. Kikuchi Y, Okabe S, Tamura G, et al: Chemosensitivity and perception of dyspnea in patients with a history of near-fatal asthma. *N Engl J Med* 330:1329, 1994.
18. Kinney HC, Filiano JJ, Sleeper LA, et al: Decreased muscarinic receptor binding in the arcuate nucleus in sudden infant death syndrome. *Science* 269:1446, 1995.
19. Kobayashi S, Nishimura M, Yamamoto M, et al: Dyspnea sensation and chemical control of breathing in adult twins. *Am Rev Respir Dis* 147:1192, 1993.
20. Krane BD, Kreutz JM, Johnson DL, et al: Alfentanil and delayed respiratory depression: case studies and review. *Anesth Analg* 70: 557, 1990.
21. Kuna ST, Smickly JS, Murchison LC: Hypercarbic periodic breathing during sleep in a child with a central nervous system tumor. *Am Rev Respir Dis* 142:880, 1990.
22. Kurth CD, Spitzer AR, Broennle AM, et al: Postoperative apnea in preterm infants. *Anesthesiology* 66:483, 1987.
23. Kurth CD, LeBard SE: Association of postoperative apnea, airway obstruction, and hypoxia in former premature infants. *Anesthesiology* 75:22, 1991.
24. LaFramboise WA, Standaert TA, Guthrie RD, et al: Developmental changes in the ventilatory response of the newborn to added airway resistance. *Am Rev Respir Dis* 136:1075, 1987.
25. Li YW, Dampney RAL: Expression of fos-like protein in brain following sustained hypertension and hypotension in conscious rabbits. *Neuroscience* 61:613, 1994.
26. Mathews O: *Respiratory controls and disorders in the newborn*. New York, 2003, Marcel Dekker.
27. McEvoy C, Durand M, Hewlett V: Episodes of spontaneous desaturations in infants with chronic lung disease at two different levels of oxygenation. *Pediatr Pulmonol* 15:140, 1993.
28. Millhorn DE, Guyunet P, Kiley JP: Neurobiology of brainstem cardiopulmonary control mechanisms. *J Appl Physiol* 69:1916, 1990.
29. Mitchell I, Brummitt J, DeForest J, et al: Apnea and factitious illness (Munchausen Syndrome) by proxy. *Pediatrics* 92:810, 1993.
30. Miyazaki M, Hashimoto T, Sukarama N, et al: Central sleep apnea and arterial compression of the medulla. *Ann Neurol* 29:564, 1991.
31. Molfino NA, Nannini LJ, Martelli AN, et al: Respiratory arrest in near-fatal asthma. *N Engl J Med* 324:285, 1991.
32. Nichols DG, Yaster M, Lynn AM, et al: Disposition and respiratory effects of intrathecal morphine in children. *Anesthesiology* 79:733, 1993.
33. Pickens DL, Schefft GL, Thach BT: Pharyngeal fluid clearance and aspiration preventive mechanisms in sleeping infants. *J Appl Physiol* 66:1164, 1989.
34. Pokela ML: Pain relief can reduce hypoxemia in distressed neonates during routine treatment procedures. *Pediatrics* 93:379, 1994.
35. Pollack IF, Kinnunen D, Albright AL: The effect of early craniocervical decompression on functional outcome in neonates and young infants with myelodysplasia and symptomatic Chiari II malformation. *Neurosurgery* 38:703, 1996.
36. Redline S, Tosteson T, Tishler PV, et al: Studies in the genetics of obstructive sleep apnea. *Am Rev Respir Dis* 145:440, 1992.
37. Ryken TC, Menezes AH: Cervicomedullary compression in achondroplasia. *J Neurosurg* 81:43, 1994.

38. Schechtman VL, Raetz SL, Harper RK, et al: Dynamic analysis of cardiac R-R intervals in normal infants and in infants who subsequently succumbed to the Sudden Infant Death Syndrome. *Pediatr Res* 31:606, 1992.
39. Shafer SL, Varvel Jr: Pharmacokinetics, pharmacodynamics, and rational opioid selection. *Anesthesiology* 74:53, 1991.
40. Shook JE, Watkins WD, Camporesi EM: Differential roles of opioid receptors in respiration, respiratory disease, and opiate-induced respiratory depression. *Am Rev Respir Dis* 142:895, 1990.
41. Silvestri JM, Chen ML, Weese-Mayer DE, et al: Idiopathic congenital central hypoventilation syndrome: the next generation. *Am J Med Genet* 112:46, 2002.
42. Smith JC, Ellenberger HH, Ballanyi K, et al: Pre-Botzinger complex: a brainstem region that may generate respiratory rhythm in mammals. *Science* 254:726, 1991.
43. Southall DP, Kerr AM, Tirosh E, et al: Hyperventilation in the awake state: potentially treatable component of Rett syndrome. *Arch Dis Child* 63:1039, 1988.
44. Southhall DP, Thomas MG, Lambert HP: Severe hypoxaemia in pertussis. *Arch Dis Child* 63:598, 1988.
45. Swaminathan S, Paton JY, Davidson Ward SL, et al: Abnormal control of ventilation in adolescents with myelodysplasia. *J Pediatr* 115:898, 1989.
46. Takala J, Askanazi J, Weissman C, et al: Changes in respiratory control induced by amino acid infusions. *Crit Care Med* 16:465, 1988.
47. Watchko JF, Standaert TA, Mayock DE, et al: Ventilatory failure during loaded breathing: the role of central neural drive. *J Appl Physiol* 65:249, 1988.
48. Weese-Mayer DE, Silvestri JM, Menzies LJ, et al: Congenital central hypoventilation syndrome: diagnosis, management, and long-term outcome in thirty-two children. *J Pediatr* 120:381, 1992.
49. Yanos J, Keamy M, Leisk L, et al: The mechanism of respiratory arrest in inspiratory loading and hypoxia. *Am Rev Respir Dis* 141: 933, 1990.

CHAPTER 35

Assessment and Monitoring of Respiratory Function

Emily L. Dobyns

PEARLS

- Clinical assessment of respiratory function remains invaluable in the diagnosis and management of patients with respiratory failure. Initial evaluation:
  - Assess child's comfort and activity level.
  - Observe child's body position, respiratory pattern, and body habitus.
  - Chest x-ray films can be used to evaluate for cardiac, vascular, bone, and lung abnormalities and to assess device placement (i.e., endotracheal tube) and need for intervention.
  - Chest CT guidance can be used to drain fluid collections and obtain biopsies.
- Simple observation of the displays of an intubated patient who is being ventilated with a microprocessor-equipped ventilator provides information about the respiratory mechanics of the patient.
- Flexible bronchoscopy is used to evaluate the size, patency, and compression of the airway during respiration; to evaluate the anatomy/structure of the airway; and for removing or obtaining secretions from the lung.
- Rigid bronchoscopy is used for better evaluation of vocal cord paralysis, laryngeoesophageal clefts, and H-type tracheoesophageal fistulas. Removal of foreign bodies is performed more easily and safely with a rigid bronchoscope.

Introduction

The majority of children admitted to the pediatric intensive care unit (PICU) present with cardiorespiratory disease or an acute illness that may progress to involve the respiratory system, emphasizing the need for careful monitoring of respiratory parameters. Close respiratory examination and monitoring allow titration of therapies to minimize ventilator-induced injury, optimize patient–ventilator interaction, and aid in weaning from the ventilator.[1]

Physical Examination of the Respiratory System

Clinical assessment of respiratory function remains invaluable in the diagnosis and management of patients with respiratory failure despite all the technologic advances that have occurred in monitoring. Initial evaluation begins with assessment of the child's comfort and activity level. Coexisting nonpulmonary conditions, such as pain and anxiety, may make this assessment difficult. Observation of the child's body position, respiratory pattern, and body habitus provide important information as to his or her level of respiratory distress.

Often the child in respiratory distress assumes a body position of comfort. This may be splinting of the chest in a patient with pneumonia or assuming the "sniffing position" to maintain an open airway in a child with an upper airway obstruction. An infant is less independent and therefore is often held in position by the caregivers, irrespective of comfort.

The respiratory pattern provides information regarding the work of breathing in a distressed child. The respiratory rate varies with age, but an early sign of distress is tachypnea. Additional signs of increased work of breathing include grunting or irregular respirations, nasal flaring, use of accessory muscles of respiration (strap muscles of the neck), and retractions.

Inspection of the shape of the chest wall may reveal abnormalities that affect pulmonary function. Increased anteroposterior diameter can be seen in conditions associated with hyperinflation (asthma or cystic fibrosis). Scoliosis in severe cases can cause a reduction in lung volume. Neuromuscular disorders may be associated with an "A-shaped" chest and lung hypoplasia/dysplasia. Thoracic asymmetry may be associated with neuromuscular or skeletal deformities, pneumothorax, or paralyzed diaphragm. Fingers and toes should be examined for evidence of clubbing (painless enlargement of the connective tissues of the distal phalanges), which is nonspecific but may be indicative of chronic hypoxemia. Growth parameters and neurodevelopment should be obtained and compared to age-appropriate normal subjects to assist in evaluation of long standing or associated diseases.

Detection of cyanosis centrally (lips, tongue) or peripherally (nailbeds) may be difficult. Arterial oxygen tension must drop below 80 mmHg before cyanosis can be detected clinically. Cyanosis may be absent in severe anemia or missed in poor lighting. It also may be intermittent, seen only with exercise or change in position. Cyanosis that does not resolve with oxygen therapy may indicate right-to-left shunting of blood in the lungs or heart, or the formation of methemoglobin or sulfhemoglobin following ingestion of certain drugs.

Evaluation of breath sounds provides assessment of airflow through the tracheobronchial tree, presence of fluid in or obstruction of the airways, and conditions outside the lung and pleural space. The child's chest wall is thinner, which allows better access to breath sounds but impedes localization of the lesion as the breath sounds can be referred. Upper airway abnormalities may present with stridor or muffling of the voice. Bronchial breath sounds suggest consolidation, whereas wheezes result from narrowed airways. Crackles may be fine or coarse. They represent air bubbling through secretions and the reopening of closed airways. A friction rub may be heard when the inflamed surfaces of the pleura move against each other through the respiratory cycle. Breath sounds may be absent if there is a significant pleural effusion or complete lobar collapse resulting from a mucus plug or pneumothorax. Heart tones are often shifted away from the pneumothorax and toward the atelectasis because of complete airway obstruction. Assessment for pulsus paradoxus (exaggerated decrease in the pulse or systolic blood pressure with inspiration) should be made during the evaluation of severe airway obstruction or pulmonary embolus.

Although each assessment should include observation and a limited physical examination, it is recognized that interobserver repeatability of physical signs is poor and independent of the experience of the observer.[2] The assessments of clubbing, wheezes, friction rub, and crackles are the most reliable and reproducible.[2,3] The lack of accuracy of repeated physical examinations and the complexity of critically ill pediatric patients require adjunctive tests/assessments to monitor critically ill pediatric patients.

Radiography

Portable chest x-ray films are the most common films taken in the PICU. Technical quality of the chest radiograph affects the interpretation; therefore it is important to assess the film for adequacy of penetration, degree, and symmetry of lung inflation and degree of chest rotation. Chest x-ray films can be used to evaluate for cardiac, vascular, bone, and lung abnormalities, assessing device placement (i.e., endotracheal tube) and need for intervention.[4] Lateral decubitus films help identify and quantify pleural effusions, pneumothorax, and position of chest tubes/lines. Cross-table lateral films also may be used for these purposes but are harder to interpret. Chest computed tomography (CT) is used when details on the plain film are obscured by superimposition of structures or an opaque hemithorax. Chest CT guidance also can be used to drain fluid collections and obtain biopsies. High-resolution chest CT examines 1- to 1.5-mm slices at 10-mm intervals; therefore it can be used to illustrate lung parenchymal details better than conventional CT, which examines 7- to 10-mm slices at 10-mm intervals.[5] This detail can be helpful in distinguishing the pathologic process causing diffuse lung diseases that appear as diffuse lung shadowing on chest x-ray films. Chest ultrasound, ventilation/perfusion scanning, spiral CT, and magnetic resonance imaging may be useful adjutants depending on the disease process.

Evaluation of Gas Exchange

Episodic hypoxemia is common in critically ill adults.[6] Even very transient episodes of hypoxemia in adults are associated with increased mortality compared with adults without episodes of desaturation.[7] The frequency and impact of episodic hypoxemia in pediatrics has not been studied. Additionally, whether monitoring and early treatment of episodic hypoxemia will improve patient outcome remains unanswered, but continuous monitoring of oxygen saturation in the PICU has become the standard of care.

Noninvasive Respiratory Monitoring

Transcutaneous Oxygen and Carbon Dioxide Monitoring

Transcutaneous measurements reflect both gas exchange and skin perfusion. In this technique, a probe composed of a heater, an electrode, and a thermistor is applied to the patient's skin. The skin is warmed and softened to improve diffusion and permeability. This also causes capillaries to dilate, resulting in better approximation of arterial oxygen values. Several disadvantages limit the use of transcutaneous monitoring to the newborn population. Skin thickness increases with age, making transcutaneous measurements less predictable. Frequent electrode site changes are required to prevent local burns. Relatively frequent calibration and comparison with arterial blood gases are necessary. Because of these limitations and the ease of application of pulse oximetry and end-tidal carbon dioxide monitoring, transcutaneous monitoring has nearly been replaced.

Pulse Oximetry

Pulse oximetry is considered a significant technologic advance that has improved patient safety.[6,8,9] Its ease of application and accuracy have resulted in widespread use. Pulse oximetry is commonly used to detect hypoxemia and wean the oxygen concentration in patients on mechanical ventilation.

Pulse oximetry is based on the principles that (1) the pulsatile absorbance detected is arterial blood and (2) oxyhemoglobin and reduced hemoglobin have different absorption spectra.[6] Red (660-nm) and infrared (940-nm) wavelengths of light are used to determine the ratio of oxygenated to deoxygenated blood. Deoxygenated blood absorbs more red light, whereas oxygenated blood absorbs more infrared light. The two wavelengths are passed through an arterial bed, and the ratio of infrared and red light transmitted to the photodetector is determined. The ratio is calibrated against measurements of arterial oxygen saturations from human volunteers and their absorbance ratios.

Several factors may affect the accuracy of pulse oximetry. Pulse oximetry measures oxygen saturation (SaO_2). SaO_2 and PaO_2 are not linearly related; the oxyhemoglobin dissociation curve is sigmoid in shape (Figure 35–1). Large changes in PaO_2 at high levels of oxygen, the upper flat portion of the oxyhemoglobin dissociation curve, may occur with little change in saturation. Additionally, a reduction in oxygenation on the steep portion of the curve may not be appreciated as significant because only a small change in saturations will have occurred.[10] The accuracy of pulse oximetry falls with arterial oxygen saturations less than 70%.[11,12] At arterial oxygen saturations below 70%, pulse oximetry may be more appropriate for showing trends.[11]

Abnormal hemoglobins (carboxyhemoglobin, methemoglobin) that have similar absorbance spectra can lead to overestimation of the true SaO_2.[6] Patients with sickle cell anemia and acute vasoocclusive crisis have underestimation of SaO_2.[13] Intravenous dyes and certain

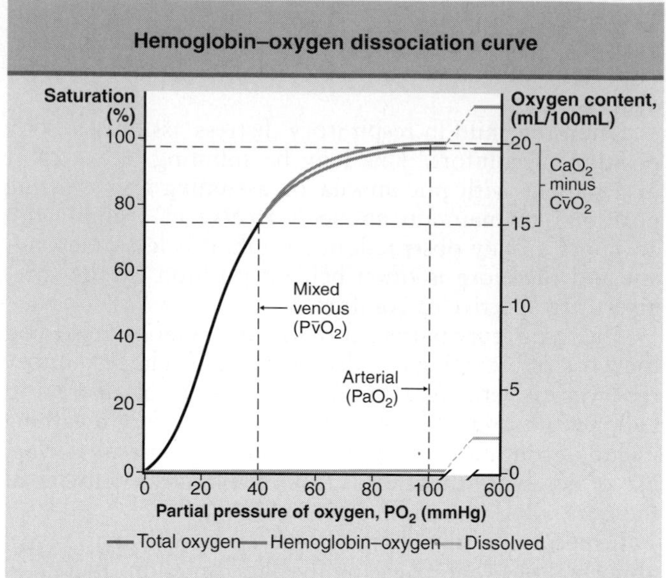

FIGURE 35–1 • Hemoglobin–oxygen (Hb-O_2) dissociation curve shows the percentage saturation of hemoglobin at each PO_2. When the hemoglobin concentration is known, the content of oxygen can be calculated. The total content includes the small additional content of oxygen in solution, which becomes significant at high levels of PO_2. The saturation scale on the **left** applies only to the Hb-O_2 line. The scale on the **right** shows content values for a normal hemoglobin level of 15 g/100 ml blood. (Modified from Hlastala MP: Blood gas transport. In Culver BH, editor: *The respiratory system.* Seattle, 1997, ASUW Publications. Redrawn in Albert RK, Spiro SG, Jett R, editors: *Clinical respiratory medicine,* ed 2. St. Louis, 2004, Mosby.)

colors of nail polish may falsely lower pulse oximetry readings.

Pulse oximetry sensors may be unable to distinguish true signal from background in low perfusions states that result in diminished pulsations (vasoconstriction, low cardiac output, hypothermia). This usually is displayed as an inadequate pulse message.[1] Motion artifact may cause inaccurate readings or false alarms.

The complications of pulse oximetry are rare. They include skin burns and pressure necrosis in newborns.[10] Limited understanding by health care providers of pulse oximetry may be an underrecognized problem.[14] In a survey of nurses and physicians, a significant percentage of respondents thought that the pulse oximeter measured PaO_2 and considered SpO_2 less than or equal to 88% acceptable.[14]

Capnography

End-tidal carbon dioxide monitoring is the noninvasive measurement of exhaled carbon dioxide at the plateau of the carbon dioxide waveform (Figure 35–2). End-tidal carbon dioxide concentration reflects $PaCO_2$, cardiac output, percent dead space, and airway time constants. In healthy subjects, the end-tidal carbon dioxide concentration is 1 to 5 mmHg less than the $PaCO_2$.[15] End-tidal carbon dioxide concentration represents the PCO_2 of all ventilated alveoli whether or not they are perfused. Therefore any condition that reduces pulmonary perfusion of ventilated alveoli increases the difference between

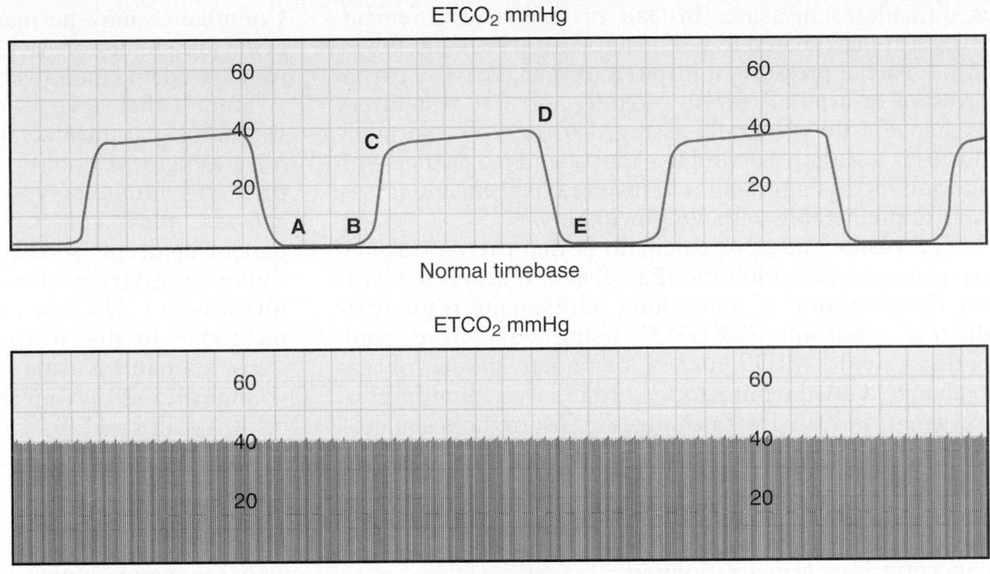

FIGURE 35–2 • Normal capnograph. *A-B* is dead space, *B-C* is start of expiration (mix of dead space and alveolar gas), *C-D* is the alveolar plateau with point *D* representing the end-tidal value, and *D-E* is the start of inhalation.

Pa_{CO_2} and end-tidal carbon dioxide. Comparison between end-tidal carbon dioxide concentration and Pa_{CO_2} helps to differentiate between change in alveolar ventilation, CO_2 production, or pulmonary perfusion as a cause of the change in end-tidal carbon dioxide concentration. Additionally, end-tidal carbon dioxide monitoring can be used to verify tracheal intubation, detect complete airway obstruction, and monitor ventilation during sedation.[16–19]

Sampling of exhaled carbon dioxide can be at the patient–ventilator interface (mainstream), diverted to a monitor (sidestream), or an intermediate connection.[11] The exhaled gas sample is exposed to various wavelengths of infrared light. The relative amount of light absorbed by the exhaled sample is compared with the amount of light absorbed by a sample that does not contain carbon dioxide. The difference between the two samples is the concentration of carbon dioxide. Carbon dioxide also can be measured semiquantitatively using a pH-sensitive indicator that changes from purple to yellow when exposed to carbon dioxide.[16]

Arterial Blood Gas Monitoring

Intermittent sampling of arterial blood can be obtained from a single arterial puncture or an indwelling arterial line. Although convenient and frequently used, they offer isolated data points of continuous physiologic changes. Because of limitations such as the spontaneous variability in patients over time, the fact that blood gas is often obtained after an event has occurred, and the significant amount of lag time in therapeutic decisions that may ensue, interest in the development and use of continuous arterial blood gas monitoring exists. The technology has progressed to the point where optical sensors are small enough to be used with a 20-gauge cannula, but considerable obstacles (mass-producing, affordable, high-technology probes that are reliable and accurate in diverse patient populations) need to be overcome before this is routine care.[20,21]

Evaluation of arterial blood gas provides information on the uptake of oxygen and disposal of carbon dioxide by the lung. In diseased lungs, additional information may be necessary to better understand and treat problems with gas exchange. Therefore indexes of oxygenation have been developed that use the data obtained from a blood gas to better define the efficiency of gas exchange and the causes of hypoxemia.

Venous blood that enters the arterial system without participating in gas exchange is termed *shunt*. Shunt flow may be intrapulmonary or extrapulmonary. Intrapulmonary shunt occurs when alveoli are being perfused but there is no inspired alveolar ventilation because the alveolus is collapsed or filled with fluid. Extrapulmonary shunting occurs when there is drainage of venous blood into the postcapillary pulmonary circulation through either anomalous (intracardiac right to left shunts) or normal (thebesian and bronchial veins) pathways. Approximately 3% of cardiac output is shunted in the normal individual. Most shunt flow is intrapulmonary in pulmonary disease. The magnitude of the shunt can be calculated using the following equation:

$$Q_s/Q_t = \frac{Cc_{O_2} - Ca_{O_2}}{Cc_{O_2} - Cv_{O_2}},$$

where Q_s = shunt, Q_t = total flow, Cc_{O_2} = pulmonary capillary oxygen content, Ca_{O_2} = arterial oxygen content, and Cv_{O_2} = mixed venous oxygen content. This requires measurement of a mixed venous sample collected from the right ventricle or the pulmonary outflow track (i.e., placement of a pulmonary artery catheter). This equation does not identify the site or cause of the shunt.

Calculation of the alveolar-arterial oxygen tension difference ($AaD_{O_2} = PA_{O_2} - Pa_{O_2}$) helps to differentiate hypoxemia caused by hypoventilation from diffusion abnormalities, ventilation/perfusion (V/Q) mismatch, or shunt. It has the advantage of not requiring mixed venous blood sampling, but it does require alveolar PA_{O_2}, which is difficult to measure. Instead of direct measurement, PAO_2 is approximated to be equal to $PIO_2 - PaCO_2/R$, where PIO_2 = partial pressure of inspired oxygen, $PaCO_2$ = partial pressure of arterial carbon dioxide, and R = respiratory exchange ratio (generally assumed to be 0.8). Normally $AaDO_2$ is less than 10 mmHg. $AaDO_2$ tends to change with age and increasing fraction of inspired oxygen, and it may vary unpredictably with V/Q inequality.[22,23]

The easiest index to calculate is the arterial inspired oxygen concentration ratio (PaO_2/FIO_2). It also is the basis for the definition of acute lung injury/acute respiratory distress syndrome (ARDS).[24] Using data from adult patients with ARDS and a computer model of gas exchange, Gowda and Klocke[23] found that all indexes of oxygenation varied with changes in inspired oxygen concentration, but the arterial inspired oxygen concentration ratio was the most stable of indexes studied. They noted that the majority of the variation in the arterial inspired oxygen concentration ratio occurred at inspired oxygen concentrations near to room air.[23]

Respiratory Mechanics

Institution of mechanical ventilation in a patient with acute respiratory failure may result in improvement and even normalization of blood gases and measures of ventilation without improving the underlying disease process. Assessment of respiratory mechanics can provide information on the status and progression of the disease process and information useful for minimizing ventilator-induced lung injury.

The development of microprocessor-equipped ventilators has simplified the measurement of respiratory mechanics. Simple observation of the displays of an intubated patient who is being ventilated with a microprocessor-equipped ventilator provides significant information about the respiratory mechanics of the patient. Inspection of the flow time trace provides evidence of the presence of auto-positive end expiratory pressure (autoPEEP) if the expiratory flow fails to stop (reach zero) prior to changing to inspiration. Inability of the patient to trigger the ventilator can be seen as "bumps" on expiration.

The simple maneuver of a rapid airway occlusion using the ventilator buttons can provide further information. The end-expiratory occlusion gives a direct measure of autoPEEP once a plateau in the airway pressure is reached.[25] The occlusion of the airway at end-inspiration for 5 seconds will measure the plateau pressure. The risk of barotrauma is thought to increase at plateau pressures greater than 35 cmH_2O. The plateau pressure also can be used to calculate the static compliance. *Static compliance* is the change in volume over the pressure change when flow has stopped in the airways and lung, measured as plateau pressure. Therefore the calculation of static compliance is $V_t/(P_{Plateau} - PEEP)$, where V_t = tidal volume, and PEEP = positive end-expiratory pressure. Dynamic compliance is the change in volume divided by the change in pressure when flow in the airway is zero but flow continues in the lung. It can be calculated at the bedside as $V_t/(PIP - PEEP)$, where PIP = peak inspiratory pressure. Dynamic and static compliance should be similar. Compliance may be markedly reduced in patients with acute lung injury or ARDS because of the presence of pulmonary edema and alveolar flooding.

Studies that have used pressure–volume curves to set ventilator parameters and compared survival outcome have generated interest in the clinical application of pressure–volume curves. Three methods can be used to generate these curves.[26] All methods require that the patient be deeply sedated and usually medically relaxed. This is necessary to eliminate the influence of the respiratory muscles. The first method used was the supersyringe method.[26] In this method, the lungs are inflated in a stepwise manner using a calibrated syringe of a known volume (1.5–2 L) from the resting volume to a maximum of 40 to 50 cmH_2O. The limitations of the method are that it takes a long time, the patient is disconnected repeatably from the ventilator, and the results may be influenced by oxygen consumption, changes in gas temperature, and humidity. Because of these limitations, its use is mainly limited to research.

The second method is the multiple occlusion technique.[26] The ventilator system is checked to ensure the absence of leaks. Multiple end-inspiratory occlusions are used to achieve different inflating volumes, each starting at the same lung volume. After several seconds of pause, the static pressure values are obtained, and the exhaled volume read off the ventilator after the occlusion is released. The volumes are plotted against the static pressures to make the pressure–volume curve. This is a fairly complex procedure that may not be well tolerated by the patient. In addition, the sequential inflations at different tidal breaths may modify the lung volume history and influence the shape of the curve.

The third method is the low-flow technique.[26] This method is based on the concept that the rate of airway pressure change is inversely related to the compliance of the respiratory system during a passive lung inflation with constant inspiratory flow (15 L/min). This method is rapid and reproducible and does not require that the patient be disconnected from the ventilator.

However generated, the pressure–volume curve is an S-shaped inspiratory curve of three segments (Figure 35–3). The lower inflection point is at the transition from the initial flat segment and the linear part of the curve. It is thought to reflect reopening of collapsed airways. The upper inflection point is at the transition of the linear part of the curve and the final portion of the curve. It is thought to reflect the start of overinflation. The portion of the curve between the upper and lower inflection points represents the target for ventilation in ARDS patients to reduce the potential for further lung injury.[27]

Endoscopy

Bronchoscopy and laryngoscopy are sometimes used in the PICU to visually examine the airway.

Direct endoscopy can be performed with a flexible or rigid bronchoscope.[28] Flexible bronchoscopy offers the advantages of requiring little sedation and can be done through the endotracheal tube. Flexible bronchoscopy is used to evaluate the size, patency, and compression of

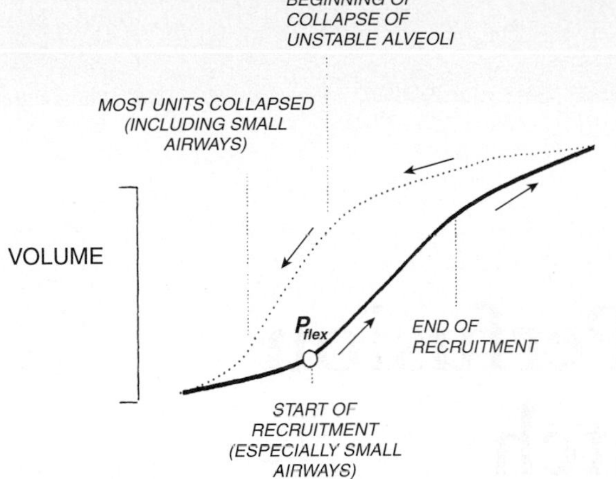

FIGURE 35-3 • The pressure-volume curve is an S-shaped inspiratory curve that can be divided into three sections. The lower inflection point (*P-flex*) is at the transition from the initial flat segment and the linear part of the curve. It is thought to reflect reopening of collapsed airways. The upper inflection point is at the transition of the linear part of the curve and the final portion of the curve. It is thought to reflect the end of recruitment and the start of overinflation. The portion of the curve between the upper and lower inflection points represents the target for ventilation in ARDS patients to reduce the potential for further lung injury. (From Albert RK, Spiro SG, Jett JR, editors: *Clinical respiratory medicine,* ed 2. St. Louis, 2004, Mosby.)

the airway during respiration. It also is useful for evaluating the anatomy/structure of the airway and for removing or obtaining secretions from the lung. Rigid bronchoscopy continues to have a role for several reasons. Visualization of the posterior aspects of the larynx and cervical trachea is difficult using a flexible bronchoscope. Therefore better evaluation of vocal cord paralysis, laryngeoesophageal clefts, and H-type tracheoesophageal fistulas are obtained with a rigid bronchoscope. Removal of foreign bodies is performed more easily and safely with a rigid bronchoscope.

Summary

A variety of methods for assessing pulmonary status and function have been reviewed. Use of the derived information may allow ventilator settings to be altered and better matched to patient demands and comfort. Better understanding and interpretation of respiratory monitoring may result in improved patient care.

REFERENCES

1. Jubran A: Advances in respiratory monitoring during mechanical ventilation. *Chest* 116:1416-1425, 1999.
2. Godfrey S, Edwards RHT, Campbell EJM, et al: Repeatability of physical signs of airways obstruction. *Thorax* 24:4-9, 1996.
3. Spiteri MA, Cook DG, Clarke SW: Reliability of eliciting physical signs and examination of the chest. Lancet i:873-875, 1988.
4. Quasney MW, Goodman DM, Billow M, et al: Routine chest radiographs in pediatric intensive care units. *Pediatrics* 107:241-248, 2001.
5. Ryu JH, Olson EJ, Midthun DE, Swensen SJ: Diagnostic approach to the patient with diffuse lung disease. *Mayo Clin Proc* 77:1221-1227, 2002.
6. Jubran A. Pulse oximetry. In Tobin MJ, editor: *Principles and practice of intensive care monitoring.* New York, 1998, McGraw-Hill.
7. Bowton DL, Scuderi PE, Haponik EF: The incidence and effect on outcome of hypoxemia in hospitalized medical patients. *Am J Med* 97:38-46, 1994.
8. Severinghaus JW, Astrup PB: History of blood gas analysis: VI. Oximetry. *J Clin Monit* 2:270-288, 1986.
9. Cote CJ, Notterman DA, Karl HW, et al: Adverse sedation events in pediatrics: a critical incident analysis of contributing factors. *Pediatrics* 105:805-814, 2000.
10. Poets CF, Southall DP: Noninvasive monitoring of oxygenation in infants and children: practical considerations and areas of concern. *Pediatrics* 93:737, 1994.
11. St. John RE, Thomson PD: Noninvasive respiratory monitoring. *Crit Care Nurs Clin North Am* 11:423-435, 1999.
12. Carter BG, Carlin JB, Tibballs J, et al: Accuracy of two pulse oximeters at low arterial hemoglobin-oxygen saturation. *Crit Care Med* 26:1128-1133, 1998.
13. Comber JT, Lopez BL: Evaluation of pulse oximetry in sickle anemia patients presenting to the emergency department in acute vasoocclusive crisis. *Am J Emerg Med* 14:16-18, 1996.
14. Stoneham MD, Saville GM, Wilson IH: Knowledge about pulse oximetry among medical and nursing staff. *Lancet* 344:1339-1342, 1994.
15. Jubran A, Tobin MJ: Monitoring during mechanical ventilation. *Clin Chest Med* 17:453-473, 1996.
16. Goldberg JS, Rawle PR, Zehnder JL, Sladen RN: Colorimetric end-tidal carbon dioxide monitoring for tracheal intubation. *Anesth Analg* 70:191-194, 1990.
17. Bhende MS, Allen WD: Evaluation of a Capno-Flo™ resuscitator during transport of critically ill children. *Pediatr Emerg Care* 18:414-416, 2002.
18. Poirier MP, Gonzalez Del-Rey JA, McAneney CM, DiGiulio GA: Utility of monitoring capnography, pulse oximetry, and vital signs in the detection of airway mishaps: a hyperoxemic animal model. *Am J Emerg Med* 16:350-352, 1998.
19. McQuillen KK, Steele DW: Capnography during sedation/analgesia in the pediatric emergency department. *Pediatr Emerg Care* 16: 401-404, 2000.
20. Shaprio BA: Clinical and economic performance criteria for intraarterial and extraarterial blood gas monitors, with comparison with in vitro testing. *Am J Clin Pathol* 104(suppl):S100-S106, 1995.
21. Weiss IK, Fink S, Harrison R, et al: Clinical use of continuous arterial blood gas monitoring in the pediatric intensive care unit. *Pediatrics* 103:440-445, 1999.
22. Gilbert R, Auchincloss JH, Kuppinger M, Thomas MV: Stability of the arterial/alveolar oxygen partial pressure ratio: effects of low ventilation/perfusion regions. *Crit Care Med* 7:267-271, 1979.
23. Gowda MS, Klocke RA: Variability of indices of hypoxemia in adult respiratory distress syndrome. *Crit Care Med* 25:41-45, 1997.
24. Bernard GR, Artigas A, Brigham KL, et al: The American-European consensus conference on ARDS: definitions, mechanism, relevant outcomes, and clinical trial coordination. *Am J Respir Crit Care Med* 149:818-824, 1994.
25. Rossi A, Polese G, Brandi G, Conti G: The intrinsic positive end expiratory pressure (PEEPi): physiology, implications, measurement, and treatment. *Intens Care Med* 21:522-536, 1995.
26. Maggiore SM, Brochard L: Pressure-volume curve in the critically ill. *Curr Opin Crit Care* 6:1-10, 2000.
27. Artigas A, Bernard GR, Carlet J, et al: The American-European Consensus Conference on ARDS, part 2. Ventilatory, pharmacologic, supportive therapy, study design strategies, and issues related to recovery and remodeling. *Am J Respir Crit Care Med* 157: 1332-1347, 1998.
28. Wood RE: The emerging role of flexible bronchoscopy in pediatrics. *Clin Chest Med* 22:311-317, 2001.

CHAPTER

36

Ventilation/Perfusion Mismatch

David J. Vaughan and Thomas V. Brogan

PEARLS

- Gravity plays an important role in determining the distribution of regional perfusion and ventilation, with both increasing down the lung.
- The heterogeneity of pulmonary blood flow and ventilation is greater than predicted by the gravitational model, following a fractal pattern.
- The hypoxemia found in patients with acute respiratory distress syndrome results from a significant proportion of cardiac output going to shunt.
- The hypoxemia among patients with asthma exacerbation results from areas of low ventilation/perfusion units, but shunt is very uncommon.
- Positive end-expiratory pressure decreases shunt by recruiting nonfunctional gas-exchanging units.
- Nitric oxide improves gas exchange by preferentially increasing blood flow to well-ventilated regions of the lung.

The primary function of the lung is to exchange oxygen and carbon dioxide between inspired air and blood. Efficient gas exchange requires the close matching of regional ventilation and perfusion (V_A/Q). Hypoxemia may be caused by intrapulmonary factors and/or extrapulmonary factors (Table 36–1). In children, mismatching of ventilation and blood flow within the lung causes most abnormalities of gas exchange. Lung units that are poorly ventilated in relation to blood flow (low V_A/Q) cause desaturation, whereas units with high V_A/Q ratios contribute to physiologic dead space but not to hypoxia (Figure 36–1). Traditional studies have supported the concept that V_A/Q matching is accomplished by gravitational gradients of both ventilation and perfusion. Newer data have shown that perfusion and ventilation are more heterogeneous than initially appreciated, and this heterogeneity serves to match ventilation and perfusion.

Distribution of Ventilation

Ventilation of the lung is heterogeneous, being influenced by multiple factors including gravity, posture, and even experimental technique. Gravity has been considered predominant because of the variation in pleural pressure from the apex to the base of the lung. The lung is a viscoelastic structure encased in the supporting chest wall, with gravity imposing a globular shape on the lung. Pleural pressure is more negative at the apex of the lung compared with the base, increasing approximately 0.25 cmH_2O per centimeter of vertical distance toward the lung base. Thus transpulmonary pressure is more marked at the apex. Large apical alveoli are located at the upper end of the normal pressure volume curve and distend less for a given pressure change, that is, they are less compliant. In the spontaneously breathing upright

TABLE 36–1

Intrapulmonary Factors	Extrapulmonary Factors
PRIMARY	PRIMARY
Ventilation/perfusion mismatch	Decreased minute ventilation
Shunt	Decreased cardiac output
Alveolar–end-capillary diffusion limitation	Decreased FIO_2
	SECONDARY
	Decreased P_{50}
	Decreased hemoglobin concentration
	Alkalosis

human, maximal gas distribution occurs at the base and progressively diminishes toward the lung apex.[1,2] This gradient also exists when inhalation occurs in the supine or lateral decubitus position, although to a lesser degree. Fast inspirations from functional residual capacity (at supranormal flow rates >1.5 L/s) may reverse this distribution with preferential ventilation of the upper parts of the lung.[3]

Heterogeneous ventilation may occur, independent of the aforementioned factors. The *time constant* (the product of resistance and compliance) is defined as the time required for inflation to 63% of final lung volume, inflation being indefinitely prolonged. Therefore a given lung unit with a slow time constant fills more slowly than one with a fast time constant, and it empties more slowly. Should the time constants of different lung units vary, as frequently happens in pulmonary illness, gas distribution is determined in part by the rate, duration, and frequency of inhalation.

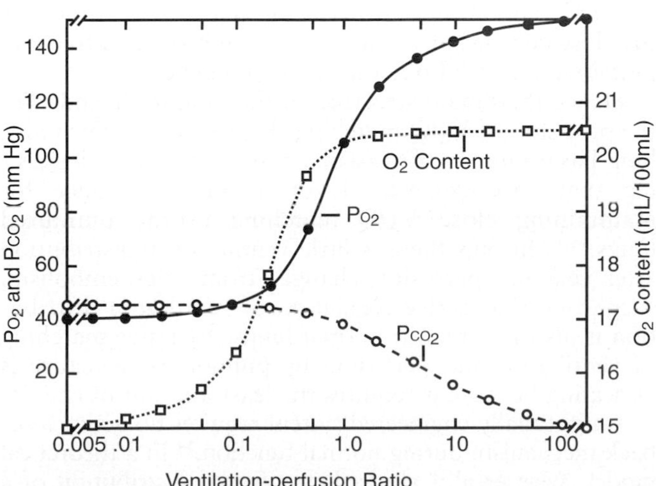

FIGURE 36–1 • Gas exchange in a single lung unit. Changes in P_{O_2}, P_{CO_2}, and end-capillary O_2 content in a lung unit as its ventilation/perfusion ratio is increased from shunt (V/Q = 0) to dead space (V/Q = ∞). Hemoglobin concentration is 14.8 g/dl.

Distribution of Perfusion

The predominant characteristic of the pulmonary circulation is that it is a low-pressure system. The mean pulmonary artery pressure (PPA) is approximately 15 mmHg, whereas the mean systemic arterial pressure is on the order of 100 mmHg. This implies that external pressures play a greater role in determining blood flow within the lung. According to the classic model of lung perfusion, gravity affects pulmonary blood flow (PBF) in a similar fashion but in the opposite direction to ventilation and to a much greater extent. In general, the dependent areas of lung receive more blood flow. The pulmonary artery pressure decreases by 1 cmH_2O per centimeter of vertical distance up the lung, so the driving pressure rapidly approaches zero with minimal blood flow to the apices. PPA may become negative. In the erect human, blood flow as measured by injected ^{131}xenon progressively increases from apex to base.[4]

The three-zone model of pulmonary blood flow has been widely used to explain the heterogeneity of perfusion within the lung (Figure 36–2).[4] Three variables compose the components of this model: pulmonary arterial pressure (PPA), alveolar pressure (PA), and pulmonary venous pressure (PV). The degree of blood flow within any area of the lung depends on the relative magnitudes of these pressures within that zone. Zone I (PA > PPA > PV) has negligible blood flow, as the higher alveolar pressure is believed to compress collapsible capillaries. This region is one of minimal gas exchange and "wasted" ventilation. Zone 1 conditions are rare except in cases of diminished pulmonary blood flow (e.g., hypotension, cardiac failure) or increased PA encountered during positive pressure ventilation. Zone II consists of the mid portions of the lungs in which PPA > PA > PV, where flow rate is

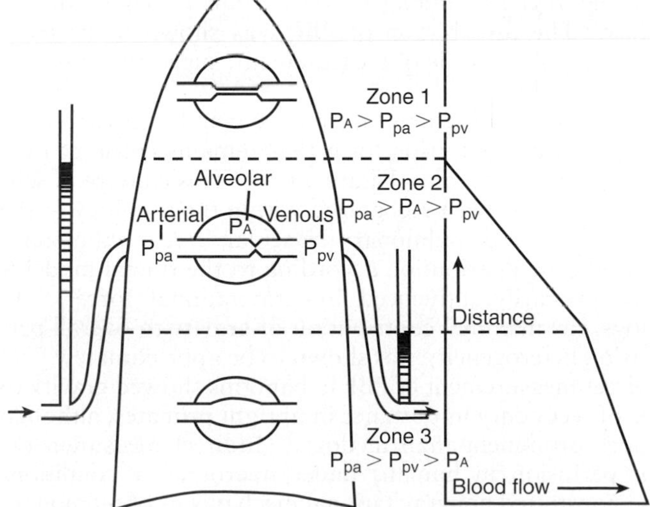

FIGURE 36–2 • Normal distribution of pulmonary blood flow: gravitational model. According to the model, the gravitational driving force for pulmonary blood flow increases down the lung. At the apex (zone 1), flow is absent as alveolar pressure (PA) exceeds pulmonary artery (PPA) and pulmonary venous (PV) pressures. In zone 2, flow is determined by the driving pressure (PPA – PA). Flow is constant and maximal in zone 3 because both PPA and PV exceed PA where the driving pressure is PPA – PV.

determined by the difference between pulmonary arterial and alveolar pressure. Venous pressure does not influence the flow rate. Blood flow progressively increases with descent through this zone, as PPA increases whereas PA remains relatively constant.

In zone II, the lower zones of the lung, PPA > PV > PA; therefore the arteriovenous pressure gradient (PPA – PV) determines flow rate. A zone 4 region in the most dependent areas of lung has also been described. In this region, transudated pulmonary interstitial fluid increases interstitial pressures, thereby reducing blood flow. This effect is exaggerated as lung volume diminishes from total lung capacity to residual volume.

Pulmonary blood flow in immature animals differs in several important ways from that in adult animals. Studies in piglets suggest that the pulmonary vascular bed is fully recruited,[5,6] with no contribution of Starling resistors in the pulmonary circulation during exposure to acute or chronic hypoxia. Furthermore, neonatal piglets show a relative hypoxemia and an increased dispersion of pulmonary blood flow (SDQ_p) among both high and low V_A/Q units compared with mature animals.

Fractal Model of Pulmonary Blood Flow and Ventilation

The gravitational model is a useful and accurate model of PBF. However, as studies used increasing power of resolution, PBF was shown to have greater heterogeneity than was described by the gravitational mode.[7–9] Blood flow in isogravitational planes was shown to be heterogeneous comparable with the heterogeneity of the entire lung, yet the gravitational model predicted uniform flow in such planes (Figure 36–3). This heterogeneity in PBF initially was considered random, but the regional flow distributions were shown to be correlated with neighboring regions tending to have similar magnitudes of flow.[9] The distribution of PBF was shown to be independent of the scale of measurement, suggesting a fractal nature of PBF.

A fractal structure or process can be described as having a characteristic form that remains constant over a magnitude of scales (Figure 36–4).[9] This concept of self-similarity has been recognized within the topology of the bronchial and pulmonary vascular trees. Pulmonary blood flow distribution according to the fractal model is not primarily influenced by gravitational forces.[10] In dogs, the maximal contribution of gravity to overall perfusion heterogeneity was shown to be approximately 7%. Direct measurement of PBF in baboons showed gravity to be of secondary importance in upright primates, although more prominent than in dogs.[11] Indirect measurements of perfusion in humans under microgravity conditions demonstrated nongravitational mechanisms of pulmonary perfusion in humans as well.[12] The asymmetry of flow at branches within the pulmonary arterial tree accounts for the heterogeneity of flow within isogravitational planes. Thus regions that share a parent or grandparent branch have more similar flows than branches that are separated by a greater distance. This fractal pattern of PBF extends down to the subacinar level of gas exchange.[13]

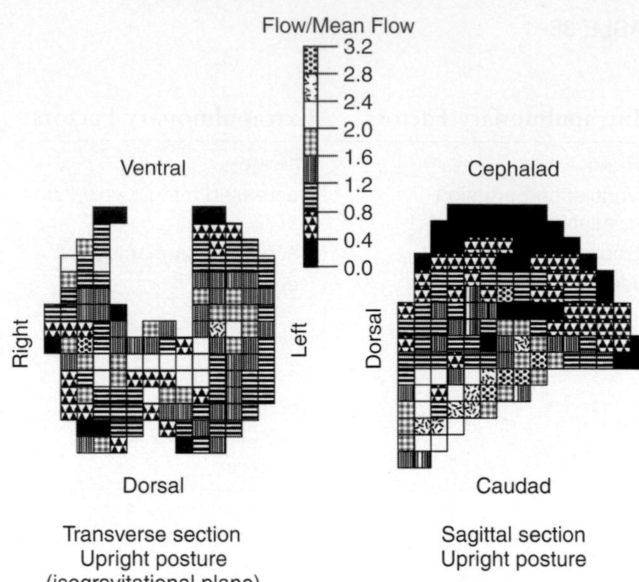

FIGURE 36–3 • Isogravitational heterogeneity of pulmonary blood flow. Reconstruction of transverse and sagittal plane from a single baboon animal during upright posture. Each *square* depicts location and relative blood flow to a piece of lung in a given plane. Heterogeneity of blood flow is present in isogravitational planes. Flow is not random; rather, neighboring pieces tend to have similar magnitudes of flow. Cephalad-caudad (gravitational) gradient is apparent in the sagittal section.

Fractal Model of Pulmonary Ventilation

The close correlation between regional ventilation and perfusion suggests that ventilation has spatial characteristics similar to regional perfusion. Using aerosolized fluorescent microspheres, regional ventilation was shown to be fractal[14] with similar heterogeneity to regional perfusion. The correlation in heterogeneities between ventilation and perfusion assures a narrow distribution of V_A/Q distributions in normal animals. Fractals possess large area/volume ratio and hence are well suited to the task of diffusion exchange. The high correlation between regional ventilation and perfusion may be explained by the close correlation of the developing bronchial tree and pulmonary arterial tree during organogenesis.[15]

Hence the innate structure of the lung itself underlies the precision of V_A/Q matching (Figure 36–5). Normally, lung basal pulmonary vascular tone is minimal, suggesting that vasoregulation is of minor importance for maintaining close V_A/Q matching in the uninjured lungs.[16,17] In pigs there is little ventilation redistribution after regional perfusion changes from microembolism, suggesting that active regulation of ventilation distribution is also minimal in normal lungs.[18] Passive matching of ventilation and perfusion by pulmonary structure is appealing because it requires the least amount of energy.

An optimally engineered system requires no active feedback mechanism during normal function.[14] In a theoretical model, West et al.[19] showed that fractal distribution of a substrate explains the $^1/_4$ allometric scaling law observed throughout nature. Their model was based, in part, on the assumption that the energy required to distribute a substrate throughout a region must be minimized for maximal

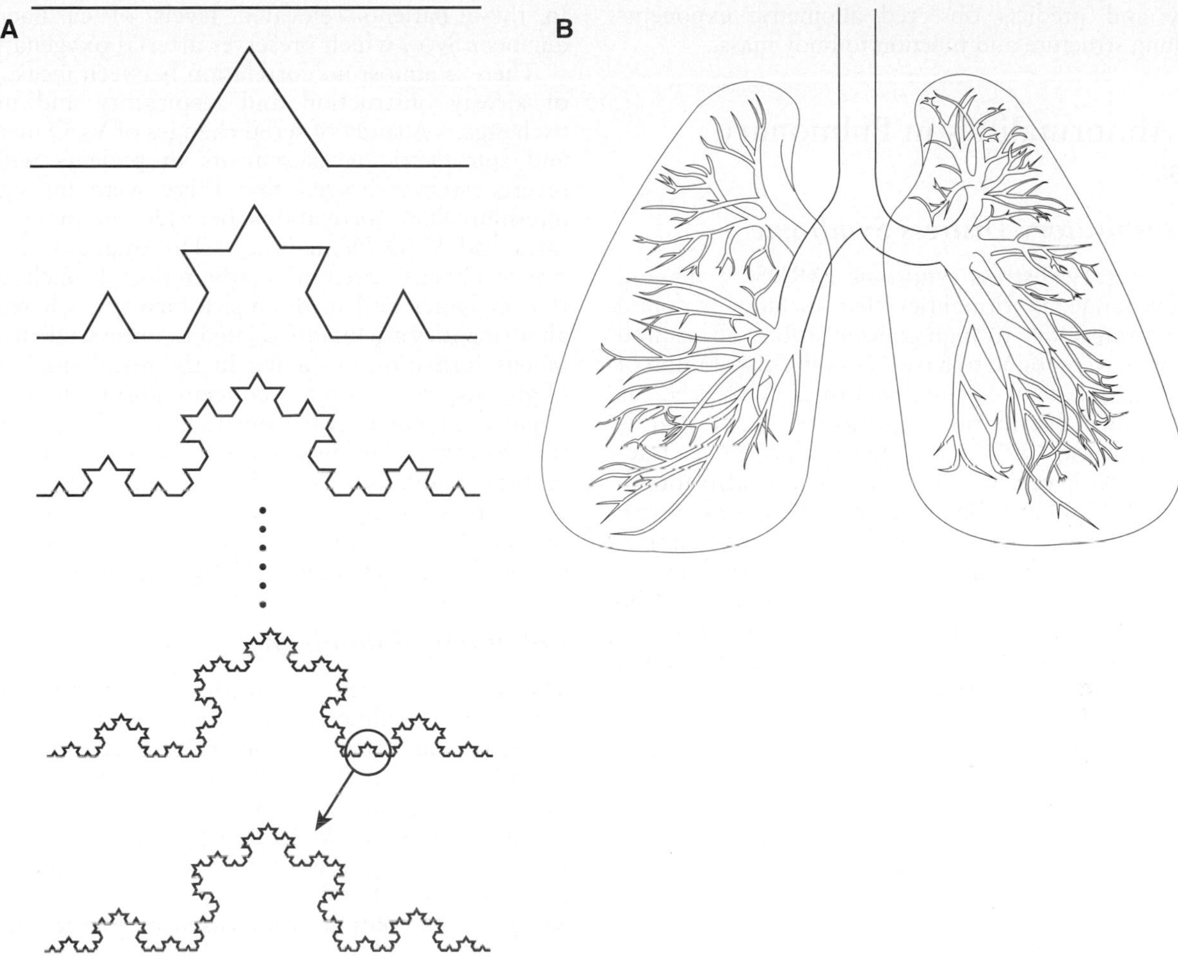

FIGURE 36–4 • Fractal structures. This curve is produced by a simple iterative transformation beginning with a straight line. At each step, the middle third of all lines is replaced with two segments, one-third length of the line, forming part of an equilateral triangle. An infinite number of iterations can be performed. Thus as increasing magnification reveals more detail, the overall appearance of the new segment remains similar to that of the previous segment. The pulmonary vascular (and bronchial) tree is a repetitive pattern of dichotomous branches that become progressively smaller and fill a predetermined area.

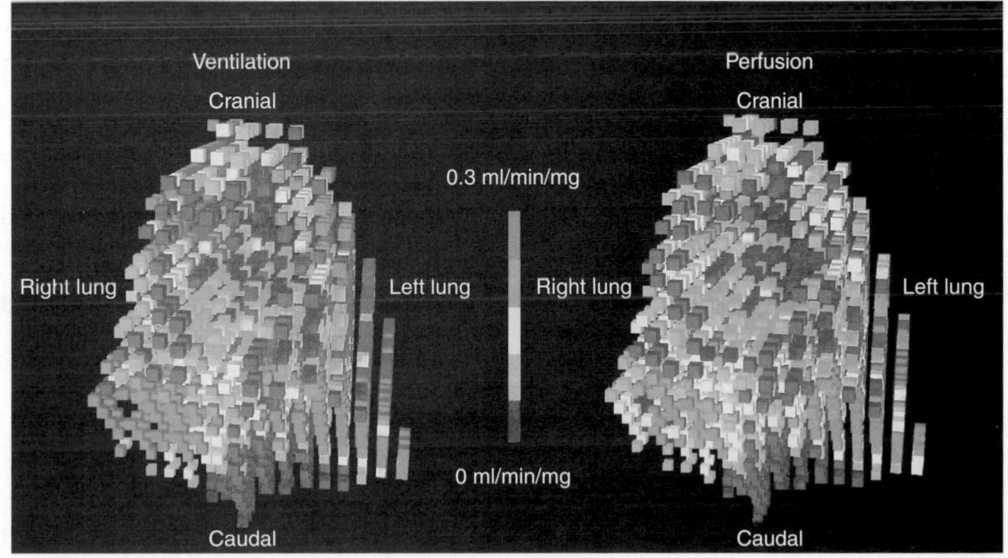

FIGURE 36–5 • Relative ventilation and perfusion maps. Regional ventilation and perfusion scaled to the measured minute ventilation and cardiac output in the pig. Both regional ventilation and perfusion show clustering in which adjacent units have similar flows. There is strong correlation in which areas of high ventilation receive high perfusion and areas of low ventilation receive low perfusion. (These pig lungs were examined in cubes of volume 1.5–2.0 cm^3.)

efficiency and predicts observed allometric exponents relating lung structure and function to body mass.

$\dot{V}_A/\dot{Q}$ Abnormalities in Pulmonary Disease

Acute Respiratory Distress Syndrome

Acute respiratory distress syndrome (ARDS) is marked by gas exchange abnormalities that include profound hypoxemia refractory to high concentrations of inspired O_2.[20] Patients were found to have a bimodal distribution of lung units. One had an essentially normal V_A/Q, whereas another smaller distribution represented shunt that is proportional to cardiac output.[20] In some patients, a fraction of units with very low V_A/Q ratios was also found. Areas of high V_A/Q may be observed and correlated with the level of alveolar pressure resulting from mechanical ventilation and the mechanical properties of the lung.

The large intrapulmonary shunt accounts for the hypoxemia of ARDS unresponsive to increases in inspired oxygen and is the result of alveolar flooding, atelectasis, and right-to-left shunt through a patent foramen ovale. The low V_A/Q units explain the increase in venous admixture with decreasing inspired fractional concentration of oxygen and may represent transient events with alveoli in the process of collapsing or reexpanding.[21] Diffusion impairment does not appear to contribute significantly to the gas exchange abnormalities in ARDS.

Pneumonia

Hypoxemia found in patients with pneumonia is multifactorial. Pure shunt was demonstrated in a canine model of pneumococcal lobar pneumonia in the first 48 hours of infection.[22] After 2 days, shunt resolved and perfusion was largely concentrated in alveoli with low V_A/Q ratios. The most common pattern of V_A/Q mismatching in patients with bacterial pneumonia severe enough to require mechanical ventilation was a combination of intrapulmonary shunt and increased perfusion to units with low V_A/Q ratios.[23] With 100% O_2 there was no increase in shunt. Similar findings were made in spontaneously breathing patients with less severe pneumonia.[24] Multiple inert gas elimination technique (MIGET) studies suggested no role for other factors such as intrapulmonary oxygen consumption, diffusion abnormalities, or postcapillary shunt resulting from increased bronchial blood flow.

Asthma

Ventilation/perfusion abnormalities have been found across the spectrum of asthmatic patients from those in clinical remission to those who are acutely ill. Asthmatic patients usually show a bimodal distribution of blood flow with normal units and large areas of low V_A/Q,[25] suggesting marked decreases in ventilation with preserved blood flow. There is little shunt even in severe asthmatics, indicating that collateral ventilation keeps lung units behind severely obstructed bronchioles open. In these patients, elevated levels of cardiac output augment $S\bar{v}O_2$, which preserves arterial oxygenation.

There is almost no correlation between measurements of airway obstruction and respiratory and inert gas exchange.[26] A study of serial changes of V_A/Q inequalities and spirometric measurements in patients with acute severe asthma showed that there were no significant interindividual correlations between maximum airflow rates and V_A/Q inequalities.[26] This suggests that spirometric changes predominantly reflect bronchoconstriction in larger and medium-size airways, whereas V_A/Q abnormalities are mainly related to events, edema, and/or mucus formation occurring in the distal small airways. High inspired oxygen concentrations may prevent hypoxic pulmonary vasoconstriction and place low V_A/Q regions at risk for absorption atelectasis, and high doses of bronchodilators may enhance the perfusion of low V_A/Q areas, exacerbating V_A/Q mismatch. However, the beneficial effects of bronchodilators on airway resistance outweigh the worsening in V_A/Q mismatch.

Pulmonary Embolism

The extent of ventilation/perfusion abnormalities in patients with pulmonary embolism is determined by the duration and extent of the mechanical obstruction of pulmonary blood flow.[27] In the acute phase (48 hours) of the disease, cardiac output is the predominant factor in the distribution of V_A/Q rather than redistribution of pulmonary blood flow to nonoccluded areas or increasing and redistributing ventilation to perfused areas.[28] When cardiac output is increased or preserved, there is increased perfusion of nonoccluded regions, producing low V_A/Q units. When cardiac output falls, blood flow through low V_A/Q compartments decreases and the V_A/Q ratios increase. The greater the obstruction, the larger the decline in cardiac output needed to prevent appearance of low V_A/Q units. The degree of V_A/Q mismatch and the level of hypoxemia show little correlation with the percent of vascular obstruction, and the reason is poorly understood.

Over the long term (>48 hours), intrapulmonary shunt probably as a result of atelectasis or alveolar filling appears to be an important determinant of hypoxemia, with V_A/Q inequality playing a relatively limited role.[28] Shunting across a patent foramen ovale also has been invoked. Vascular obstruction increases dead space. The correlation between mean pulmonary vascular obstruction and total dead space ventilation is strong. Yet the mean inert gas dead space has been found to be less than the percentage of obstruction observed by angiogram. In areas that have incomplete obstruction, there may be an increase in the V_A/Q ratio.

Primary Pulmonary Hypertension

V_A/Q inequalities tend to be moderate even in late stages of pulmonary hypertension.[29] Much of the cardiac output was distributed to lung units with almost normal V_A/Q ratios, whereas less than 10% perfused the underventilated or unventilated areas. When cardiac output is reduced, there often is hypoxemia as a result of low mixed venous Po_2. Oxygen, sodium nitroprusside, isoproterenol, or nifedipine worsened V_A/Q matching, but PaO_2 did not fall because of increased cardiac output. The resultant increase in Svo_2 raised the end-capillary Po_2.

Therapeutic Considerations

Positive End-Expiratory Pressure

Positive end-expiratory pressure (PEEP) decreases the proportion of shunt units by recruiting the nonfunctional gas-exchanging units, thereby improving functional residual capacity and arterial oxygenation. Additionally, by decreasing cardiac output (Q), PEEP produces a parallel fall in intrapulmonary shunt. However, even when Q is preserved, application of PEEP results in decreased shunt as a result of redistribution of blood flow from shunt units to normal units because of alveolar recruitment. With constant Q, PEEP decreases venous admixture and increases mixed venous Po_2.

PEEP also affects dead space.[21] Low levels of PEEP decrease dead space by reductions in shunt and midrange V_A/Q heterogeneity, but high levels of PEEP increase dead space. The increase in dead space with high PEEP results from overinflation of some lung units leading to compression of capillaries and increases in anatomic dead space.

Prone Positioning

The tight matching of perfusion and ventilation appears to improve during prone position.[30] MIGET analysis has shown that the improvement in arterial blood oxygenation often seen in the prone position in normal and injured lungs results from improved V_A/Q matching.[31] Using simultaneous aerosolized and injectable fluorescent microspheres, Mure et al.[32] showed that V_A/Q distribution becomes more uniform in the prone position because of increases in the homogeneity of V_A distribution and in the correlation between ventilation and perfusion. In some animals (dog, sheep) and in humans, there also appears to be a decrease in the heterogeneity of Q, as well as V, but this was not seen in pigs.

In ARDS and other lung injury models, nonaerated or poorly aerated positions of the lung are found mainly in the dependent areas. In contrast to ventilation, perfusion is largely gravity independent, especially in West zone 3 conditions. The majority of perfusion goes through dorsal lung regions whether in the prone or supine position. Consequently, perfusion is greatest to the dependent lung in the supine position and to the nondependent lung in the prone position. Positive pressure redistributes perfusion toward the dependent portion of the lungs by creating conditions of West zones 2 and 1. This redistribution may increase the vertical perfusion gradient in the supine position but may reduce it in the prone position. Additionally, the pleural pressure gradient is smaller in the prone position than in the supine position. These various physiologic factors contribute to the increase in the uniformity of perfusion in the prone position.

Effects of CO_2 and O_2

Changes in inspired O_2 can alter ventilation/perfusion relationships. Hypoxic pulmonary vasoconstriction reduces perfusion blood flow to poorly ventilated areas as alveolar Po_2 falls.[33,34] (A similar but less robust response is seen with decreased mixed venous Po_2.) The response to a local decrease in Po_2 can restore the local Po_2 only to half its previous level, and its efficiency is best when alveolar Po_2 is in the range of 70 to 90 mmHg.[34] Inspiration of 100% O_2 worsens V_A/Q mismatch substantially: the index of blood flow dispersion always increases significantly. In ARDS, units with low V_A/Q deteriorate to shunt secondary to absorption atelectasis.[35] The increase in shunt demonstrated with inhalation of 100% O_2 remained elevated 1 hour after returning to the original Fio_2. There may also be inhibition of hypoxic pulmonary vasoconstriction in shunt units secondary to increase in mixed venous Po_2. Interestingly, in neonatal piglets exposure to chronic hypoxia with resultant pulmonary hypertension did not significantly alter V_A/Q matching during room air or acute hypoxic gas breathing.[5,6]

Alterations in inspired or arterial CO_2 tensions affect V_A/Q ratios. Low concentrations of inspired CO_2 (3% to 5%) improve V_A/Q matching and perfusion heterogeneity in normal lungs.[36] In contrast, hypocapnia produces a deterioration in V_A/Q matching.[37] These changes in V_A/Q heterogeneity appear dependent on the increase in pH. Hypercapnia appears to improve oxygenation in injured lungs as well, but detailed analysis of V_A/Q relationships remains to be performed.[38]

In a study of low tidal volume ventilation with constant PEEP, allied with permissive hypercapnia, there was a deterioration of gas exchange with an increase in intrapulmonary shunt and cardiac output.[39] It is unclear what effects altering PEEP under similar circumstances would have on V_A/Q.

Nitric Oxide

NO improves gas exchange in acute lung diseases by preferentially increasing blood flow to well-ventilated regions of the lung. NO reaches the well-ventilated units, producing vasodilation and reducing shunt fraction.[40] Beneficial effects appear over a wide range of doses. NO does not appear to be beneficial in chronic lung diseases possibly because the structural damage precludes rapid vascular changes or because shunt is usually not found in such diseases.

REFERENCES

1. West JB: Regional differences in gas exchange in the lung of erect man. *J Appl Physiol* 17:893-898, 1962.
2. Hughes JMB, Grant BJB, Greene RE, et al: Inspiratory flow rate and ventilation distribution in normal subjects and in patients with simple bronchitis. *Clin Sci* 43:583-595, 1972.
3. Bake B, Wood L, Murphy B, et al: Effect of inspiratory flow rate on regional distribution of inspired gas. *J Appl Physiol* 37:8-17, 1974.
4. West JB, Dollery CT, Naimark A: Distributions of blood flow in isolated lung: relation to vascular and alveolar pressures. *J Appl Physiol* 19:713-724, 1964.

5. Gibson RL, Truog WE, Redding GJ: Hypoxic pulmonary vasoconstriction during and after infusion of group B Streptococcus in neonatal piglets. Vascular pressure-flow analysis. *Am Rev Respir Dis* 137:774-778, 1988.
6. Redding GJ, Gibson RL, Standaert TA, Truog WE: Regional pulmonary blood flow in piglets during group B streptococcal bacteremia. *Am Rev Respir Dis* 141:1209-1213, 1990.
7. Reed JH, Wood EH: Effect of body position on vertical distribution of pulmonary blood flow. *J Appl Physiol* 28:303-311, 1970.
8. Hakim TS, Dean GW, Lisbona R: Gravity independent inequality in pulmonary blood flow in humans. *J Appl Physiol* 63:1114-1121, 1987.
9. Glenny RW, Robertson HT: Fractal properties of pulmonary blood flow: characterization of spatial heterogeneity. *J Appl Physiol* 69:532-545, 1990.
10. Glenny RW, Lamm WJ, Albert RK, Robertson HT: Gravity is a minor determinant of pulmonary blood flow distribution. *J Appl Physiol* 71:620-629, 1991.
11. Glenny RW, Bernard S, Robertson HT, Hlastala MP: Gravity is an important but secondary determinant of regional pulmonary blood flow in upright primates. *J Appl Physiol* 86:623-632, 1999.
12. Prisk GK, Guy HJ, Elliot AR, West JB: Ventilatory inhomogeneity determined from multiple-breath washouts during sustained microgravity on Spacelab SLS-1. *J Appl Physiol* 70:2351-2367, 1994.
13. Glenny RW, Bernanrd S, Robertson HT: Pulmonary blood flow remains fractal down to the level of gas exchange. *J Appl Physiol* 89:742-748, 2000.
14. Altemeier WA, McKinney S, Glenny RW: Fractal nature of regional ventilation distribution. *J Appl Physiol* 88:1551-1557, 2000.
15. Weibel ER: Fractal geometry: a design principle for living organisms. *Am J Physiol Lung Cell Mol Physiol* 261:L361-L369, 1991.
16. Celermajer DS, Dollery C, Burch M, Deanfield JE: Role of the endothelium in the maintenance of low pulmonary vascular tone in normal children. *Circulation* 89:2041-2044, 1994.
17. Vaughan DJ, Brogan TV, Kerr ME, et al: Contributions of nitric oxide synthase isozymes to exhaled nitric oxide and hypoxic pulmonary vasoconstriction in rabbit lungs. *Am J Physiol Lung Cell Mol Physiol* 284:L834-L843, 2003.
18. Altemeier WA, Robertson HT, McKinney S, Glenny RW: Pulmonary embolization causes hypoxemia by redistributing regional blood flow without changing ventilation. *J Appl Physiol* 85:2337-2343, 1998.
19. West GB, Brown JH Enquist BJ: A general model for the origin of allometric scaling laws in biology. *Science* 276:122-126, 1997.
20. Dantzker DR, Brook CJ, Dehart P, et al: Ventilation-perfusion distribution in the adult respiratory distress syndrome. *Am Rev Respir Dis* 120:1039-1052, 1979.
21. Lamy M, Fallat RJ, Koeniger E, et al: Pathologic features and mechanisms of hypoxemia in adult respiratory distress syndrome. *Am Rev Respir Dis* 114:267-284, 1976.
22. Wagner PD, Laravuso RB, Goldzimmer E, et al: Distribution of ventilation-perfusion in dogs with normal and abnormal lungs. *J Appl Physiol* 38:1099-1109, 1975.
23. Gea J, Roca J, Torres A, et al: Mechanism of abnormal gas exchange in patients with pneumonia. *Anesthesiology* 75:782-789, 1991.
24. Lampron N, Lemaire F, Teisseire B, et al: Mechanical ventilation with 100% oxygen does not increase intrapulmonary shunt in patients with severe bacterial pneumonia. *Am Rev Respir Dis* 131:409-413, 1985.
25. Wagner PD, Dantzker DR, Iacovoni VE, et al: Ventilation-perfusion inequality in asymptomatic asthma. *Am Rev Respir Dis* 136:605-612, 1978.
26. Roca J, Ramis L, Rodriguez-Roisin R, et al: Serial relationships between ventilation-perfusion inequality and spirometry in acute severe asthma requiring hospitalization. *Am Rev Respir Dis* 137:1055, 1988.
27. Manier G, Castaing Y, Guenard H: Determinants of hypoxemia during the acute phase of pulmonary embolism in humans. *Am Rev Respir Dis* 132:332-338, 1985.
28. D'Alonzo GE, Bower HS, Dehart P, Dantzker DR: The mechanism of abnormal gas exchange in acute massive pulmonary embolism. *Am Rev Respir Dis* 128:170-172, 1983.
29. Dantzker DR, Bower JS: Pulmonary vascular tone improves V_A/Q matching in obliterative pulmonary hypertension *J Appl Physiol* 51:607-613, 1981.
30. Piehl MA, Brow RS: Use of extreme position changes in acute respiratory failure. *Crit Care Med* 4:13-14, 1976.
31. Beck KC, Vetterman J, Rehder K: Gas exchange in dogs in the prone and supine positions. *J Appl Physiol* 72:2292-2297, 1992.
32. Mure M, Domino KB, Lindahl SGE, et al: Regional ventilation-perfusion distribution is more uniform in the prone position. *J Appl Physiol* 88:1076-1083, 2000.
33. Duke HN: Site of action of anoxia on the pulmonary blood vessels of the cat. *J Physiol (Lond)* 125:393-382, 1954.
34. Grant BJB, Davies EE, Jones HA, Hughes JMB: Local regulation of pulmonary blood flow and ventilation/perfusion ratios in the coati mundi. *J Appl Physiol* 40:216-228, 1976.
35. Dantzker DR, Wagner PD, West JB: Instability of lung units with low $\dot{V}_A/\dot{Q}$ ratios during O_2 breathing. *J Appl Physiol* 38:886-895, 1975.
36. Swenson ER, Robertson HT, Hlastala MP: Effects of inspired carbon dioxide on ventilation-perfusion matching in normoxia, hypoxia, and hyperoxia. *Am J Respir Crit Care Med* 149:1563-1569, 1994.
37. Domino KB, Swenson ER, Hlastala MP: Hypocapnia-induced ventilation/perfusion mismatch: a direct CO_2 or pH-mediated effect? *Am J Respir Crit Care Med* 152(5 pt 1):1534-9, 1995.
38. Keenan RJ, Todd, TRJ, Wood W, Slutsky AS: Effects of hypercarbia on arterial and alveolar oxygen tensions in a model of gram negative pneumonia. *J Appl Physiol* 68:1820-1825, 1990.
39. Feihl F, Eckert P, Brimioulle S, et al: Permissive hypercapnia impairs pulmonary gas exchange in the acute respiratory distress syndrome. *Am J Respir Crit Care Med* 162:209-215, 2000.
40. Cooper CJ, Landzberg MJ, Anderson TJ, et al: Role of nitric oxide in local regulation of pulmonary vascular resistance in humans. *Circulation* 93:266-271, 1996.

CHAPTER

37

Mechanical Dysfunction of the Respiratory System

J. Julio Pérez Fontán

PEARLS

- As often occurs with systems that contain moving parts, most diseases of the respiratory system involve some sort of mechanical dysfunction that increases the pressure that the respiratory muscles must generate to change lung volume.
- The effort that the respiratory muscles must make to generate the increased demands is responsible for the majority of the acute signs and symptoms of the disease *(respiratory distress);* if the energy available to support this effort is insufficient to meet demands, gas exchange becomes disturbed and *respiratory failure* ensues.
- Volume changes during respiration are dictated primarily by the organism's need to take up oxygen and eliminate carbon dioxide; pressure chnages depend on the physical properties of the respiratory system's components, which are greatly affected by disease.
- Each type of mechanical derangement results in a distinctive pattern of breathing that tends to minimize energy expenditure. By inspecting the effort and frequency of the respiratory movements, the clinician can draw substantial inference on whether the derangement is primarily restrictive or obstructive.
- Restrictive disease increases inspiratory effort and lowers lung volume, sometimes to the point of rendering alveoli unstable. Newborns are particularly vulnerable to alveolar collapse because their highly compliant chest wall does not contribute to sustaining lung inflation.
- The diameter of an airway is determined by the transmural pressure and the mechanical characteristics of the airway wall. Transmural pressure is affected very differently by the phase of the breathing cycle, depending on whether an airway is intra- or extrathoracic. This is the reason why extrathoracic airway obstructions become excerbated during inspiration and intrathoracic obstructions become exacerbated during expiration.
- Considered in physical terms, even the healthy respiratory system is a very inefficient machine because a large proportion of the energy used to breathe is dissipated as heat without ever being converted to volume-pressure work in the lungs. Chest wall retractions and other disease-induced alterations in the configuration of the chest, malnutrition, and respiratory muscle fatigue add substantially to this inefficiency by increasing the amount of energy consumed per unit of alveolar ventilation.

Introduction

The normal function of the mammalian respiratory system requires that air and the gas byproducts of respiration move in and out of the gas-exchanging spaces of the lungs. This motion is achieved by a reciprocating pumplike mechanism that uses a specialized group of skeletal muscles (the respiratory muscles) to expand, and sometimes compress, the lungs. As often occurs with systems that contain moving parts, most diseases of the respiratory system in both children and adults involve some sort of mechanical dysfunction. The increased energy demands imposed by such dysfunction usually are responsible for the majority of the signs and symptoms of the disease and ultimately for the development of respiratory failure. Therefore any review of the pathophysiology of respiratory disease must first provide a basic understanding of respiratory mechanics in health and disease. This chapter provides such an understanding, focusing on the factors that determine both respiratory work and energy expenditure. Accordingly, the first portion of the chapter discusses the forces responsible for the volume-pressure behavior of the lungs and chest wall and how this behavior relates to the work of breathing in both normal and disease conditions. The second portion analyzes the elements that influence the translation of the work of breathing into energy expenditure, with special attention to those that define the efficiency of the respiratory system. Throughout the chapter, the unique characteristics of the developing respiratory system and the mechanical features that are relevant for the diagnosis and management of respiratory disease are highlighted.

Energy Expenditure in the Respiratory System

Like other thermodynamic systems, changes in the state of the respiratory system must be analyzed in terms of energy gains and losses. The first law of thermodynamics stipulates that when a certain amount of energy is added to a closed system by an external source (e.g., metabolism of fuels supplied by the circulation to the respiratory muscles), the resultant change in the system's internal energy (ΔU, the total change in all the kinds of energy possessed by the system's components) may be used to perform external work (W) or is transformed into heat (Q) in a manner that satisfies Equation 1:

$$\Delta U = W + Q \quad (1)$$

Consequently, only a portion of the energy that the respiratory muscles derive from metabolic substrates is transformed into respiratory work. This proportion varies depending on the system's efficiency (E), which is defined by Equation 2:

$$E = W/(W + Q) \quad (2)$$

The availability of energy to meet the demands imposed by the work of breathing is the ultimate determinant of whether the respiratory system can perform its function under physiologic conditions or in the presence of mechanical alterations caused by disease. Workload and efficiency define these demands and therefore are the relevant variables in the analysis of the mechanical function of the respiratory system.

Determinants of Respiratory Work

The external work done during a breath (dW) can be approximated by comparing the respiratory system with a cylindrical piston pump (Figure 37–1). If a constant force F causes the pump's piston to undergo a small linear displacement dx, the amount of work done by F can be computed as Equation 3:

$$dW = Fdx \quad (3)$$

In practical terms, however, it is much easier to measure the pressure inside the pump's cylinder (P) than to measure F. Because P = F/A (where A is the section area of the piston) and the volume displacement of the piston is dV = Adx, we can write Equation 4:

$$dW = PAdx = PdV \quad (4)$$

which, when integrated between volumes V_0 and V_1 to obtain work, yields Equation 5:

$$W = \int_{V_0}^{V_1} PdV \quad (5)$$

In simpler terms, the work done by the respiratory system and consequently the energy that must be supplied to the respiratory muscles to do this work are defined by the system's volume–pressure relationships.

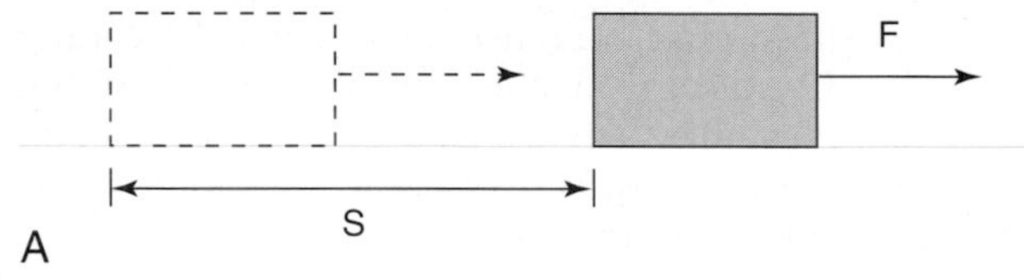

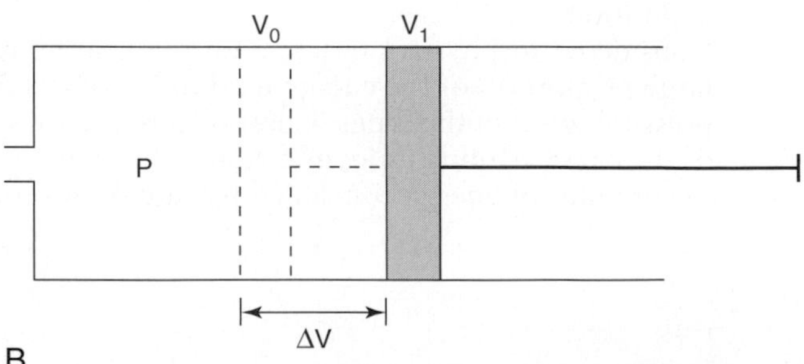

FIGURE 37–1 • **A,** The amount of work that a force must perform to move an object over a linear distance s is equivalent to the product F × s. **B,** Analogously, the work needed to produce a volume displacement ΔV in a piston pump is equivalent to the product of the pressure change inside the pump (the tridimensional analog of F) by ΔV (the tridimensional analog of s).

Volume–Pressure Relationships

Before analyzing the volume–pressure relationships of the various components of the respiratory system, it is helpful to clarify the terminology. Throughout this chapter, the term *thorax* is used in reference to all the moving components of the respiratory system, including the walls of the thoracic cavity (the rib cage), the abdomen, and the lungs themselves. Similarly, the term *chest wall* is used to indicate all the structures that form the enclosure of the lungs, including the thoracic wall, the diaphragm, the abdominal wall, and the abdominal organs. In addition, the volume–pressure relationships of the chest wall and, by extension, those of the thorax cannot be studied practically unless the respiratory muscles are relaxed. Otherwise it is impossible to separate the effects of the contractile force developed by the muscles from the mechanical changes that the muscle contraction imparts to the wall itself. Unless otherwise indicated, when we describe the volume–pressure relationships of the chest wall or thorax we are referring to the relationships measured in the course of a passive inflation or deflation.

The volume changes of the respiratory system can be easily measured with the help of devices such as spirometers or plethysmographs. For any breath, the thorax as a whole, the lungs, and the chest wall all undergo the same change in volume. If we use the subscripts TH, L, and W to represent the thorax, lung, and chest wall, we can write:

$$\Delta V_{TH} = \Delta V_L = \Delta V_W. \qquad (6)$$

The reason for this identity is the existence of a noncompressible and nondistensible boundary, the pleural space, which links the lungs to the chest wall and prevents both from changing volume independently of each other.

The pressures needed to inflate the thorax, the lungs, and the chest wall are, however, different from each other. Figure 37–2 shows graphically that, when the respiratory muscles are completely relaxed, the thorax, the lungs, and the chest wall are all held at their respective volumes by outward-acting pressure gradients across their walls. These pressure gradients or transmural pressures are defined by Equations 7, 8, and 9:

$$P_{TH} = P_A - P_B \qquad (7)$$

$$P_L = P_A - P_{pl} \qquad (8)$$

$$P_W = P_{pl} - P_B, \qquad (9)$$

where P_{TH} = thoracic transmural pressure, P_L = lung transmural pressure or transpulmonary pressure, P_W = chest wall transmural pressure, P_A = alveolar pressure, P_{pl} = representative pressure at the pleural surface, and P_B = atmospheric pressure (conventionally considered to be zero or reference). By adding Equations 8 and 9, it is easy to arrive at Equation 10:

$$P_{TH} = P_L + P_W, \qquad (10)$$

which reveals that the pressure necessary to hold the thorax at a given volume is equivalent to the sum of the pressures that would be necessary to hold the lungs and the chest wall independently at the same volume.

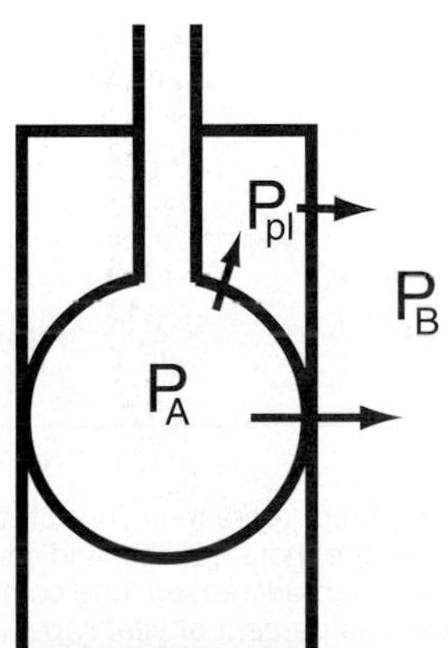

FIGURE 37–2 • Schematic representation of the thorax demonstrating the transmural pressures *(arrows)* that hold the thorax, lungs, and chest wall at a given volume. The transmural pressure of the thorax is the difference between alveolar (P_A) and atmospheric pressure (P_B). The transmural pressure of the lungs is the difference between P_A and pleural pressure (P_{pl}). The transmural pressure of the chest wall is the difference between P_{pl} and P_B.

Origin of the Mechanical Forces Acting on the Respiratory System

Volume changes within the respiratory system are dictated primarily by the organism's need to take up oxygen and eliminate carbon dioxide and therefore are determined by factors such as the physical activity or metabolic rate, which are independent of the condition of the lungs and chest wall. Pressure changes, on the other hand, depend on the physical properties of the respiratory system's constituents. For instance, elastic pressures result primarily from the tendency of cells and connective tissue elements, such as collagen and elastin fibers, to recover their original shape after being stretched during lung inflation. Airway resistive pressures overcome the adherence of the moving gas molecules to the airway walls (viscous pressures) and, to a lesser extent, compensate for the loss in gas kinetic energy at points where the movement and direction of the gas vary randomly (turbulence). Tissue-resistive pressures are applied primarily to produce molecular rearrangements in the tissue and at the gas–liquid alveolar interface as the lungs inflate and deflate. Finally, inertial pressures derive from the acceleration and deceleration of the gas and tissue contained in the thorax during breathing.

Disease induces alterations in all these physical phenomena. To relate these alterations to the disease's clinical manifestations, it is helpful to classify the physical phenomena (and the pressures that they originate) into nondissipative and dissipative, depending on whether the energy they consume or generate stays in or leaves the system. For instance, elasticity is nondissipative because the energy needed to overcome elastic forces during inspiration is accumulated in the tissues and then used to empty the lungs during expiration. Inertia also is nondissipative because the energy required to accelerate gas and tissue at the beginning of a breath is recovered as they decelerate later when the direction of thoracic movement is reversed. In contrast, resistance and viscoelasticity are dissipative: the energy consumed by the molecular interactions causing these phenomena is lost immediately as heat or used to generate durable changes in the molecular architecture of the lung tissue and lung–gas interface. As noted later, dissipative phenomena are responsible for the hysteresis (different behavior between inspiration and expiration) of the volume–pressure relationships of the respiratory system.

Nondissipative Pressure

Respiratory inertial pressures are negligible in the child during normal breathing; therefore we discuss only the elastic pressures.

Elastic Pressures: Static Volume–Pressure Relationships

Elastic pressures result from the tendency of the components of the lungs and chest wall to recover their original shape on deformation. Because this tendency increases proportionally to the magnitude of the deformation, elastic pressures are volume dependent. Thus they are most easily studied when the volume of the thorax is constant. Under these conditions, there is no flow of gas in the airways, and only the elastic pressures are operating in the respiratory system. Equations 7, 8, and 9 can be rewritten as (assuming $P_B = 0$):

$$P_{TH,el} = P_A \quad (11)$$

$$P_{L,el} = P_A - P_{pl} \quad (12)$$

$$P_{W,el} = P_{pl}, \quad (13)$$

where $P_{TH,el}$, $P_{L,el}$, and $P_{W,el}$ = elastic pressure or recoil generated by the thorax, lungs, and chest wall, respectively.

The volume–pressure relationships of the thorax, lungs, and chest wall are complex and cannot be described in a simple mathematical fashion. In the case of the lungs, for example, the relationship has a sigmoid shape, with pressure increasing rapidly relative to volume at low and high volumes and more slowly at middle volumes (Figure 37–3). Being a continuous function, however, each volume–pressure relationship has a defined slope at any given thoracic volume (dV/dP). This slope defines the *compliance* of the thorax, lungs, or chest wall for that particular volume, depending on whether dP is replaced by dP_{TH}, dP_L, or dP_W. Although a quick examination of Figure 37–3 reveals that both the lung and chest wall compliances defined in this manner vary markedly over the entire range of volumes, the ratio dV/dP is relatively constant at normal breathing volumes. Thus for these volumes, it is safe to write Equation 14:

$$\Delta P_{el} = \Delta V/C, \quad (14)$$

where ΔP_{el} = change in elastic recoil pressure of the lungs, chest wall, or thorax for a lung volume excursion ΔV, and C = compliance of the corresponding component. As lung volume decreases or increases beyond this linear range, dV/dP starts to decrease in a volume-dependent manner,[44] and the respiratory muscles must generate progressively larger pressures to produce the same volume change. Disease frequently causes the lungs to operate outside of their linear volume–pressure range, thereby increasing both the work of breathing and the energy needed to do it.

The elastic recoil of the thorax is equivalent to the total pressure that the respiratory muscles need to generate to produce a certain volume change. It can be calculated as the sum of the elastic recoils of the lungs and chest wall (see Equation 10). Recoil is a volume-dependent property that acts to change the lungs and chest wall volumes until they reach a certain *relaxation volume,* for which the recoil becomes zero (the intercept of the volume–pressure relationships with the ordinate in Figure 37–3). Just as they have different volume–pressure relationships, the lungs and the chest wall also have different relaxation volumes. In the adult, the relaxation volume of the lungs is lower than residual volume (the volume of gas contained in the lungs at the end of a forced expiration). The relaxation volume of the chest wall, by contrast, exceeds 50% of the vital capacity (the maximal volume of gas that can be inhaled from residual volume).

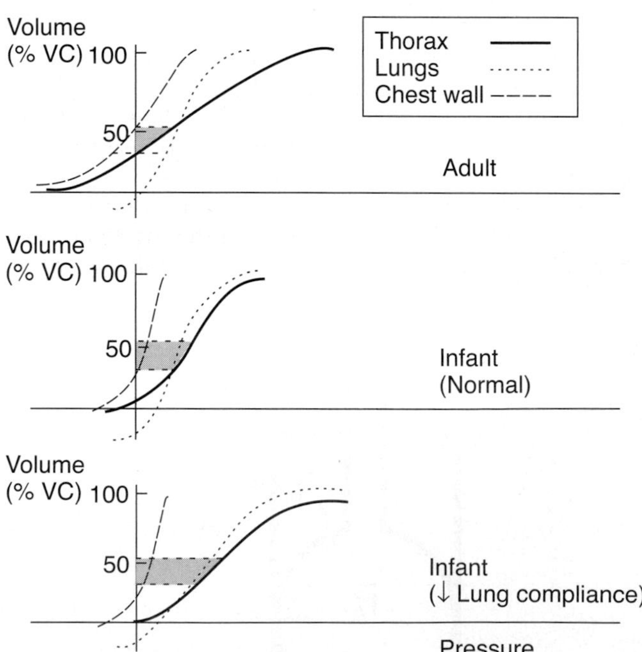

FIGURE 37–3 • Schematic representation of the static volume–pressure relationships of the thorax, lungs, and chest wall in the adult, normal infant, and infant with decreased lung compliance. Volume, on the **ordinates,** is shown as percent of vital capacity. Pressure, on the **abscissa,** represents the pressure across the thorax, lungs, and chest wall. The volume–pressure relationships of the lungs are similar in the adult and the normal infant. The volume-pressure relationship of the chest wall, however, is steeper in the infant, indicating a greater chest wall compliance. The *stippled area* between the volume–pressure curve of the thorax and the volume axis represents the elastic work done by the respiratory muscles for a breath starting at functional residual capacity (FRC).

Such discrepancy in the relaxation volumes of the lungs and chest wall has three important consequences. First, it forces the relaxation volume of the thorax as a whole to occupy a position intermediate between the relaxation volumes of the lungs and the chest wall (at approximately 35% of vital capacity). Under most circumstances, this volume coincides with the functional residual capacity (FRC), which is the volume contained in the lungs at the end of a tidal expiration. Second, as the thorax starts to rise above its relaxation volume during inspiration, the outward recoil of the chest wall contributes to the expansion of the lungs, thereby reducing the work that the respiratory muscles need to perform during normal breathing (Figure 37–3, *top*). Finally, at normal breathing volumes, the opposing actions of the lungs and chest wall recoils create a negative pressure at the boundaries of the lung tissue with the chest wall and the other intrathoracic structures. This negative pressure is an important contributor to the return of venous blood to the chest. The static volume–pressure relationships of the lungs and chest wall vary depending on their state of maturation and health (see Figure 37–3). In the infant, the chest wall generates remarkably little outward recoil within the normal range of breathing volumes.[1,16,40] Because the inward recoil of the lungs varies little with respect to lung size and age during development,[12,13,45] the relaxation volume of the infant's thorax is proportionally smaller than that of the adult (as shown in Figure 37–3 by the lower intercept of the volume–pressure relationship of the thorax and the ordinate). If, as occurs in the adult, the FRC coincided with this relaxation volume (15% of vital capacity compared with 35% in the adult), then the infant would be at a definite disadvantage in terms of alveolar stability and oxygenation. The newborns of most mammalian species, however, have developed physiologic strategies to maintain their FRC above the relaxation volume of the thorax. These strategies are generally directed at interrupting expiratory flow before expiration is complete and include shortening of the expiratory time,[35] contraction of adductor muscles of the glottis to retard exhalation,[11] and persistence of the tonic activity of the inspiratory muscles during expiration.[34] Being so dependent on the pattern of breathing, the FRC of the newborn and small infant is very vulnerable to changes in muscle coordination and tone. As an example, the decrease of tonic activity of the respiratory[34] and laryngeal muscles[17] associated with rapid eye movement (REM) sleep may cause a substantial reduction in thoracic lung volume at these ages.[19] Similarly, muscle weakness, anesthesia, deep sedation, and central nervous system depression in general tend to lower FRC below levels compatible with alveolar stability. Under such circumstances, alveoli close, and both the shunt fraction and the work of breathing increase.[22]

In addition to its effects on the FRC, the reduced outward recoil of the chest wall in the infant reduces the chest wall's contribution to lung expansion (Figure 37–3, *middle* and *bottom*). It also limits the amplitude of the pleural pressure variations as the lungs expand, an effect that helps to explain the surprising cardiovascular tolerance of many infants to the application of high levels of positive airway pressure.

Lungs–Chest Wall Interactions

As we have seen, the volume–pressure relationships of the lungs and chest wall are necessarily linked. Under normal conditions, lungs and chest wall cannot change volume independently and are simultaneously influenced by variations in the pressure at their boundary (P_{pl}). This lungs–chest wall interdependence is well illustrated by the effect of a pneumothorax on the volumes of the lungs and chest wall (Figure 37–4). When a certain volume of air enters the pleural space, the most immediate effect is an increase in the pleural pressure (ΔP). This increase causes the elastic recoils of the lungs and chest wall to change in a similar magnitude. The change, however, is in opposite directions: the recoil of the lungs ($P_A - P_{pl}$) decreases in a magnitude –ΔP, whereas the recoil of the chest wall ($P_{pl} - P_B$) increases in a magnitude ΔP. Because both lungs and chest wall must follow their respective volume–pressure relationships in response to the change in their transmural pressures, the volume of air originally introduced in the pleural cavity is divided into two components, one the volume by which the lungs collapse and the other the volume by which the chest wall expands. The absolute magnitude of these two components is dictated by the relationship between the volume–pressure relationships of the lungs and chest wall. If the compliance of the

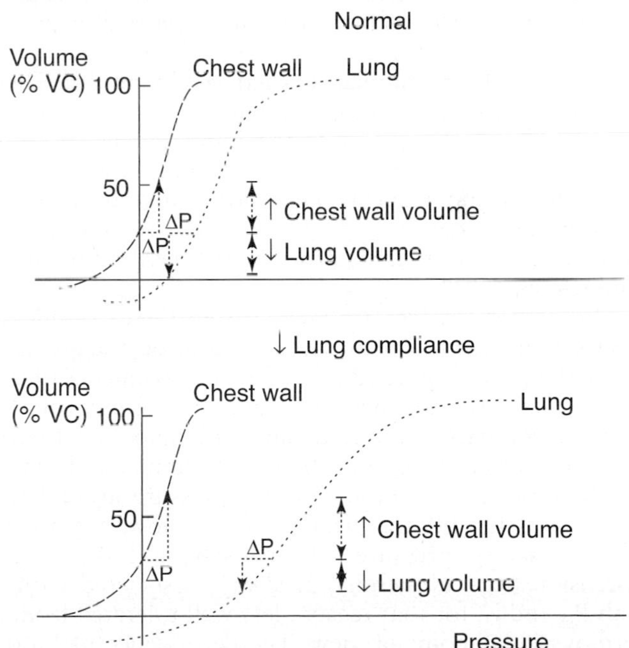

FIGURE 37–4 • Mechanical interdependence of the lungs and chest wall by comparing the effects of a pneumothorax on their respective volumes when lung compliance is normal **(top)** and reduced **(bottom).** Volumes, on the **ordinates,** are shown as a fraction of vital capacity *(VC).* Pressures, on the **abscissa,** represent the distending pressures of the lungs (alveolar – pleural pressure) and chest wall (pleural – atmospheric pressure). The introduction of a volume of gas into the pleural space raises pleural pressure by a magnitude ΔP, which depends on both the volume introduced and the volume–pressure characteristics of the chest wall. The increment in pleural pressure decreases both the distending pressure and the volume of the lungs and increases both the distending pressure and the volume of the chest wall.

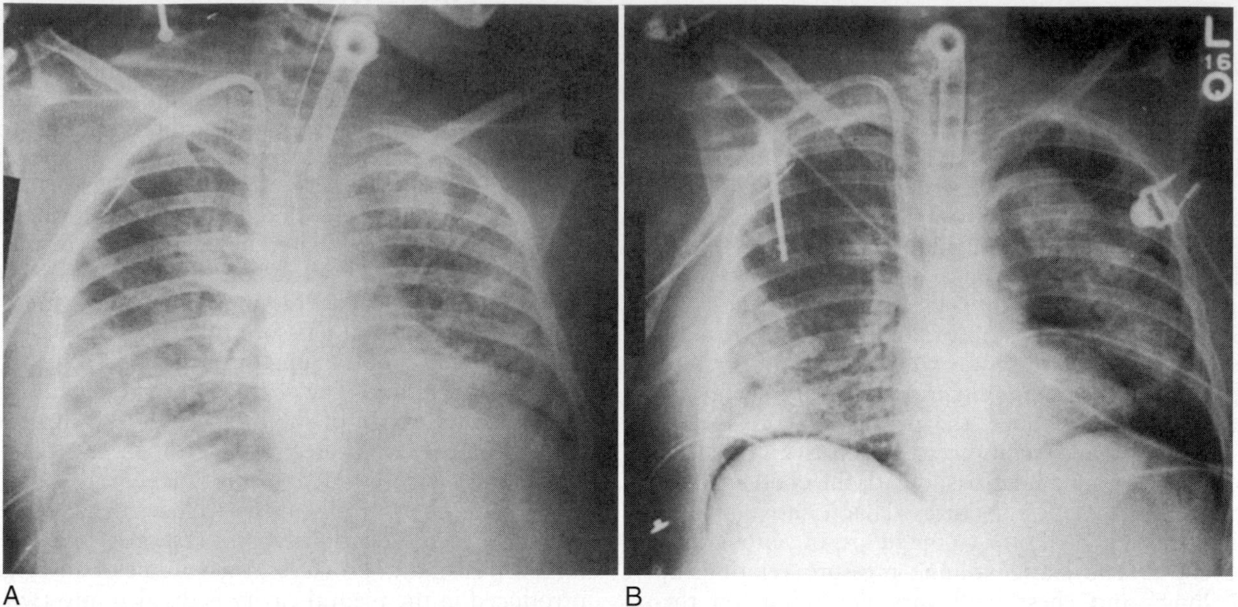

FIGURE 37–5 • Two chest radiographs illustrating the effect of a pneumothorax on the volumes of the lungs and chest wall in a 7-year-old child whose lung compliance was reduced by acute respiratory distress syndrome (ARDS). **A,** Diffuse densities are present. A chest tube has been placed in the right pleural space, but no pneumothorax is present. **B,** Obtained shortly after **A.** The patient had left tension and smaller right subpulmonic pneumothoraces. Consistent with the principles explained in Figure 37–3, note how, despite the increased recoil of the lungs and the elevated pleural pressure, the left lung experiences only a small decrease in volume. Also note how the left side of the rib cage appears to expand substantially to accommodate the volume of the pneumothorax.

chest wall exceeds the compliance of the lungs (as is usually the case in the infant), then the chest wall expands more than the lungs collapse. The difference is even greater when lung compliance is reduced by disease. Then (Figure 37–4, *bottom*) the chest wall absorbs the majority of the volume change while the lungs barely decrease their volume. This simple analysis explains why noncompliant lungs show surprisingly little collapse when a pneumothorax develops (Figure 37–5), a finding that is often mistakenly attributed to the "stiffness" of the lung parenchyma.

One important idea to emerge from these considerations is that, respiratory muscle activity aside, the pressure inside the pleural space (P_{pl}) is a direct consequence of the elastic recoil of the chest wall and the volume of the thoracic contents. As long as lung volume is not forced above its normal range and chest wall compliance is unaltered by disease, P_{pl} (and thus the pressure around the major vessels and the heart) remains low, regardless of the airway pressures. Conversely, excessive lung distension (e.g., in asthma) is always associated with a high P_{pl} and is, for that reason, less well tolerated from a cardiovascular point of view. The dependence of P_{pl} on chest wall compliance explains why premature infants and newborns have limited changes in P_{pl} during positive pressure ventilation, even if physiologic lung volumes are exceeded. A decreased chest wall compliance, on the other hand, always increases P_{pl} and, by causing a parallel increase in central venous pressure, reduces venous return to the heart. This is one reason why patients with abdominal distension typically have low cardiac output. Under these circumstances, relief of the distension (e.g., by paracentesis in patients with ascites) reduces pleural pressure and increases cardiac output.

Dissipative Forces

Dynamic Volume–Pressure Relationships

Until now, we have considered only the pressures generated when the thoracic volume is held constant. Analysis of the volume–pressure relationships of the thorax and its components becomes more complicated if the pressure changes generated by gas flow and by the movement of the lung and chest wall tissue as the lungs inflate and deflate also are considered. As discussed in the section discussing the Origin of Mechanical Forces, these pressure changes result from molecular interactions between the gas and the airway walls (friction), within the gas stream itself (turbulence), and among the components of the gas–liquid interface and the tissue (viscoelasticity[3,23]).

Regardless of their ultimate physical nature, all these molecular interactions have two characteristics in common. The first is that they always result in a net loss or dissipation of energy from the respiratory system. The lost energy can no longer be applied to perform work, and consequently dissipative pressure losses cause the volume–pressure relationships of the respiratory system to follow a different trajectory depending on the direction of the volume change. This property, known as *hysteresis,* is responsible for the development of loops when the volume–pressure relationships are plotted during breathing (Figure 37–6). In such graphic representation, the dissipative pressures can be easily identified as the horizontal distance between the volume–pressure point on the loop and the corresponding point on the elastic volume–pressure relationship. The work done against these pressures can be quantified as the total area enclosed by the loop.

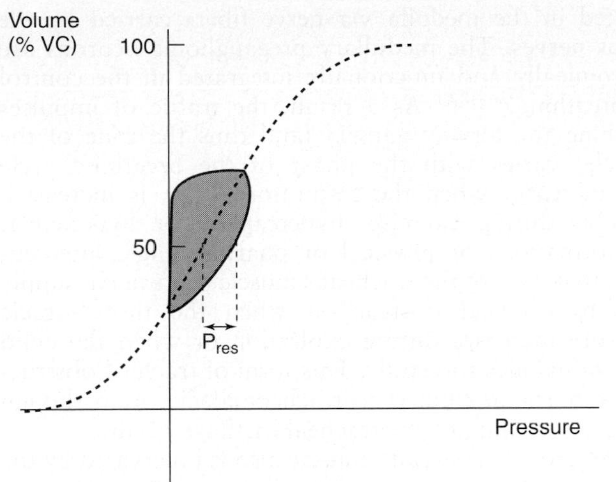

FIGURE 37–6 • Schematic representation of the volume–pressure relationship of the respiratory system during a single breath. Because energy is dissipated as the lungs change volume, the relationship follows a different trajectory during inspiration and expiration, forming a loop (hysteresis). The horizontal distance between any point in the loop and the line describing the elastic volume–pressure relationship of the respiratory system *(dashed line)* is the pressure needed to overcome the dissipative forces present at the point in the breath (P_{res}). The area enclosed by the loop *(shaded area)* is the amount of energy in overcoming these forces. The resistance of the respiratory system is calculated by dividing P_{res} by the airway flow.

The second characteristic common to all dissipative pressure losses is that they occur only when there is flow ($\dot{V}$) in or out of the lungs. The relationship between resistive pressure (P_{res}) and $\dot{V}$ in the respiratory system is also often assumed to be linear:

$$P_{res} = R\dot{V} \tag{15}$$

where R = flow resistance of the thorax, lungs, or chest wall. However, similar to elastic recoil, resistive pressure losses cannot be described with a single constant. In practice, R exhibits a complex dependence on flow rate, lung volume, and phase of the respiratory cycle. Understanding some of the reasons for this dependence is essential for recognizing airway obstruction.

Airway Dynamics

The airways behave like collapsible tubes rather than rigid pipes. At any time, the diameter of an airway is determined by both the transmural pressure (the pressure difference between the margin of the column of gas in the airway lumen and the outer surface of the airway) and the mechanical characteristics of the airway wall. Airway transmural pressure varies during breathing. Its variations result from the different effects of inspiration and expiration on the pressures inside and outside the airways. The pressure inside all airways undergoes qualitatively similar changes during each phase of the breathing cycle. During inspiration, for instance, there is a gradient of increasingly negative pressures from the mouth, where pressure is atmospheric (or the zero reference), to the alveolar spaces, where the pressure must be negative (or subatmospheric) for gas to flow in. The pressure inside the airways is always negative, independent of the airway's position in the airway branching tree. During expiration, alveolar pressure becomes positive and the gradient is inverted, with the pressures inside the airways being always positive but diminishing toward the mouth. In contrast, the pressure outside the airways is influenced in a different fashion by inspiration or expiration, depending on whether the airways are extrathoracic or intrathoracic. Extrathoracic airways are included in the tissues of the neck, where the pressure can be considered to be atmospheric (at least in nonobese individuals, in whom tissue gravitational forces are neutralized by the skeletal support of the neck). Most of the intrathoracic airways are embedded in the lung tissue, where multiple tethering elements transmit the stresses (or pressures) generated by the tissue recoil to the airway wall. Therefore the pressure outside the intrapulmonary airways approximates the pleural pressure[31] and, as we have seen, relates to lung volume in a manner that depends on the pressure–volume characteristics of the chest wall.

From the discussion in the previous paragraph, it follows that the effect of inspiration and expiration on airway caliber differs between the extrathoracic and intrathoracic airways. During inspiration, the extrathoracic airways (pharynx, larynx, and extrathoracic portion of the trachea) become narrower because the pressure inside their lumen decreases while the pressure immediately outside their walls is constant. The intrathoracic airways, however, become dilated because the pressure outside their walls (the pleural pressure) decreases more than the pressure inside their lumen. Conversely, during expiration, the extrathoracic airways dilate as their inside pressure becomes positive with respect to atmospheric pressure and the intrathoracic airways narrow as their inside pressure decreases with respect to pleural pressure.

It is important to understand that the narrowing of the intrathoracic airways during expiration is contingent on the existence of a pressure gradient from the alveoli to the mouth. As predicted by Equation 12, alveolar pressure (P_A) must always exceed pleural pressure (P_{pl}) by a magnitude equivalent to the elastic recoil of the lungs ($P_{L,el}$). As the gas progresses downstream during expiration, frictional pressure losses lower the pressure inside the airways. Eventually the cumulative pressure losses can be as large as $P_{L,el}$, and the pressure inside the airways becomes equal to P_{pl}. Beyond this *equal pressure point,*[32] airway transmural pressure is negative (i.e., the pressure outside exceeds the pressure inside the airway) and acts to collapse the airway. Depending on the airway's rigidity or compliance (see the following section) and diameter, airway collapse can lead to *expiratory flow limitation,* a situation in which gas flow can no longer increase, even if the subject makes a greater effort to raise alveolar pressure. In practice, flow limitation in the lungs is not only caused by the coupling of airway compliance and viscous pressure losses as described. Wave-speed flow limitation results from the fact that the velocity of gas flow through an airway cannot exceed the critical velocity with which disturbances or waves travel in the airway.[9,50] This critical velocity, which in an artery equals the velocity of the pulse wave, is directly proportional to the diameter of the airway and inversely proportional to the airway wall compliance.

Regardless of its mechanism, viscous or wave speed, flow limitation occurs at lower flows in the presence of airway obstruction and at low lung volumes, when airway diameter is minimal.

Airway Smooth Muscle and Compliance of the Airways

The effect of transmural pressure on the caliber of an airway depends on the mechanical characteristics of the airway itself or, more specifically, on its ability to undergo collapse or distension, a property that often is referred to as *airway wall compliance.* The structure of each segment of the airway tree has evolved to minimize luminal distortion in response to the varying stresses that act on the airway wall during breathing. The pharynx and larynx, for example, contain skeletal muscle, which stiffens their walls or dilates the pharyngeal lumen and the glottis during inspiration under the control of cranial nerves IX and X.[39] Loss of pharyngeal or laryngeal tone during sleep or after pharmacologic inhibition or injury of the controlling neurons is a common cause of upper airway obstruction during inspiration.

The smooth muscle of the trachea and bronchi has a similar function. For instance, the trachea is composed of a series of incomplete cartilaginous rings forming a relatively rigid arrangement that resists the collapsing effects of positive intrathoracic pressures during expiration. The rings leave a dorsal gap, where the wall of the trachea is soft. This weak point is bridged by the trachealis muscle, which, upon contracting, can approximate the edges of the cartilage rings and prevent the soft portion of the wall from bulging into the airway lumen (Figure 37–7). Like the smooth muscle in other airway segments, the trachealis muscle is innervated by local parasympathetic ganglia. The ganglia in turn receive inputs from parasympathetic preganglionic neurons located in the medulla via nerve fibers carried by the vagus nerves. The medullary preganglionic neurons are anatomically and functionally integrated in the control of breathing.[36–38,41] As a result, the traffic of impulses reaching the airway ganglia (and thus the tone of the muscle) varies with the phase of the breathing cycle and increases when the respiratory drive is increased, such as during exercise, hypercapnia, or hypoxemia. Malformations or physical or pharmacologic interventions that disrupt the trachealis muscle or its nerve supply lead to tracheal obstruction when the intrathoracic pressure increases during expiration or when the child cries or exhales forcefully. This form of tracheal obstruction often is attributed to tracheomalacia, even though no true softening of the tracheal cartilage occurs.

The bronchial smooth muscle also is innervated by the parasympathetic system. In cartilaginous bronchi, contraction of the smooth muscle fibers approximates the cartilage rings. Although this decreases the bronchial lumen, it also makes the airway stiffer and prevents it from collapsing when the transmural pressure decreases during expiration, coughing, or crying. In bronchioles, which in humans lack cartilage, contraction of the smooth muscle stiffens the airway walls as well. However, in these smaller airways, smooth muscle contraction may have a more important function of preventing excessive airway distension during inspiration.

Airway Obstruction

Airway obstruction causes an exaggeration of the normal breathing changes in airway caliber (Figure 37–8). Thus the

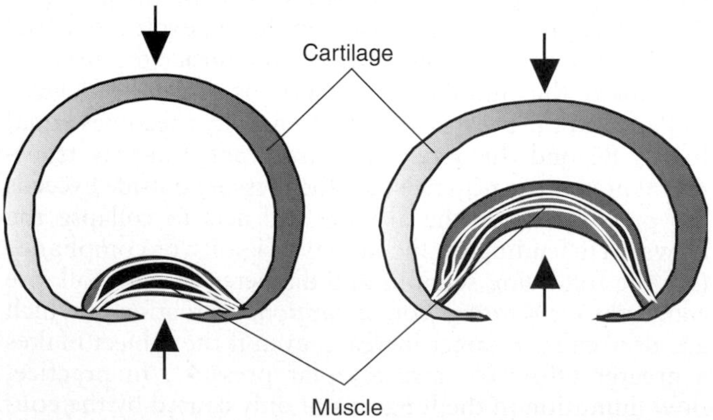

Cartilage
Muscle

FIGURE 37–7 • Schematic view of a coronal section of the trachea demonstrating the function of the trachealis muscle. **Left,** When the muscle contracts, the two ends of the horseshoe-shaped tracheal cartilages approximate, causing the trachea to become stiffer. **Right,** When the muscle loses tone or is disrupted in any other way, the increased pressure in the pleural space during expiration or forced exhalation causes the posterior tracheal membrane to bulge into the tracheal lumen. The resultant obstruction often is diagnosed as tracheomalacia.

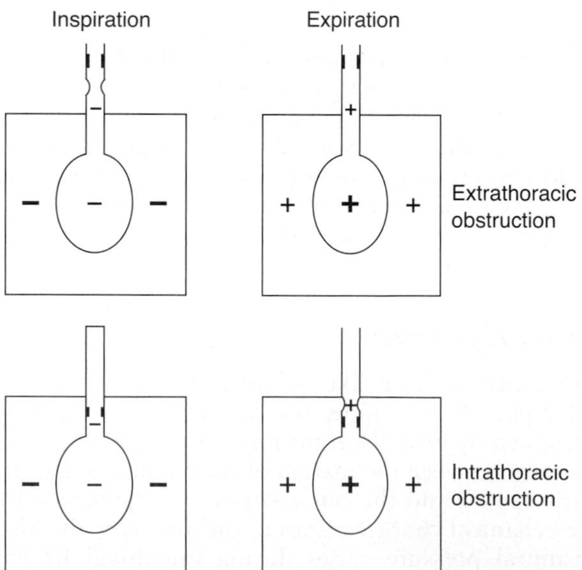

FIGURE 37–8 • Schematic representation of the effects of inspiration and expiration on the dimensions of the airways during extrathoracic and intrathoracic airway obstruction. Extrathoracic airway obstruction worsens during inspiration because the highly negative pressure inside the airway is unopposed by the atmospheric pressure outside the airway. Intrathoracic obstruction worsens during expiration because the positive pleural pressure outside the airways exceeds the pressure inside the airways downstream from the obstruction point. (Modified from Pérez Fontán JJ, Lister G. In Toulukian RJ, editor: *Pediatric trauma,* ed 2. St Louis, 1990, Mosby.)

clinical manifestations of the obstruction depend on its location (extrathoracic or intrathoracic) and the direction of flow (inspiratory or expiratory). When the obstruction is extrathoracic (e.g., croup, glossoptosis, tonsil or adenoid hypertrophy), the subject must create a more negative pressure inside the airway segment downstream from the obstruction to overcome the increased resistance during inspiration. Therefore this segment of the airway tends to collapse, worsening the obstruction and producing a characteristic turbulent noise (inspiratory stridor) as gas accelerates through the narrowest point and induces vibrations in the airway mucosa (in the process causing a Venturi effect that approximates the walls of the airway even further). The obstruction is relieved during expiration because the pressure inside the airway segment, now upstream from the obstruction, must become more positive with respect to atmospheric pressure to force gas flow through the obstruction.

When the obstruction is intrathoracic (e.g., extrinsic compression of the trachea and bronchi, tracheobronchomalacia, asthma), during inspiration, the pressure inside the airways downstream from the obstruction has to become more negative than that inside the airways upstream. However, no matter how negative, the pressure inside the airways still must be less negative than the pleural pressure (Equation 12), and therefore the transmural pressure remains positive. In contrast, during expiration the pressure inside the airway segment located between the obstruction and the thoracic outlet may become lower than pleural pressure at some point. This situation, coupled with the acceleration of flow at the obstructed segments, causes these airways to collapse and produce high-pitched vibrations (wheezing), expiratory delay, and dynamic hyperinflation.

Airway Dynamics During Positive Pressure Ventilation

The application of positive pressure in the airways changes the balance of pressures that determines airway caliber. When positive end-expiratory pressure (PEEP) is used, pressure inside the airways is positive (relative to the atmospheric pressure) during the entire respiratory cycle. As a result, any portion of the extrathoracic airway that is not bypassed by an endotracheal tube (or the entire extrathoracic airway when mask ventilation is used) is exposed to dilating stresses during both inspiration and expiration. The pressure inside the intrathoracic airways also increases with respect to pleural pressure, with the difference between these two pressures varying as a function of the increase in elastic lung recoil produced by the inflation. For this reason, PEEP has been proposed as a therapy to decrease airway resistance and gas trapping in patients with intrathoracic airway obstruction.[4,24,26] Although beneficial in some patients, in other patients PEEP increases lung volume, interferes with cardiovascular function, and ultimately decreases oxygen delivery to the tissues.[49] The individual variations in the response to PEEP of patients with airway obstruction may simply reflect differences in the mechanisms of dynamic hyperinflation. In patients who have gas trapping without expiratory flow limitation, proximal airway pressures (and thus also PEEP) are transmitted to the alveoli. As a result, their lung hyperinflation worsens.[24] In patients who have both gas trapping and expiratory flow limitation, in contrast, PEEP may not affect the pressures upstream of the flow-limiting point; therefore alveolar pressure and lung volume may not increase as much. The pressures inside the airways at the flow-limiting point and downstream increase, however, thereby improving the rate of lung emptying. The small diameter and high compliance of children's airways favor the development of flow limitation. Although PEEP is not recommended in every patient, its judicious use may be considered, under careful monitoring, to improve the mechanical function of the lungs of some selected infants and children with severe obstructive airway disease.

Compliance and Resistance as Factors in Regional Distribution of Gas Flow in the Lungs

From a mechanical perspective, the lungs constitute a parallel arrangement of acinary or multialveolar units, each supported by a conducting airway. The development of inequalities in the mechanical and gas-exchanging functions of these units is a fundamental factor in the manifestations of lung disease. To understand how mechanical inequality affects the distribution of ventilation in the lungs, it is essential to realize that the potential filling volume of any alveolar unit is determined by the unit's compliance. However, the actual filling volume during a breath depends on the rate at which the unit can fill relative to other units. This rate is a function of the unit's compliance and resistance and often is defined by their product, a constant with the dimension of time known as the time constant (represented by the Greek letter tau τ).

The mathematical formulations that describe the distribution of flow among units with different time constants can be complex. However, it is possible to make some basic predictions of how a certain flow pattern will influence the distribution of tidal volume among these units. Imagine a simplified lung composed of three units (Figure 37–9), one with a normal compliance and resistance (normal τ), another with a low compliance and a normal resistance (short τ), and the third with a normal compliance and a high resistance (long τ). As long as the inspiratory time is sufficiently long to allow equilibration of alveolar pressures within the lungs, a decelerating inspiratory flow pattern (pressure-controlled ventilation) will inflate all three units proportionally to their compliances, thus favoring the two units with normal compliance. If the inspiratory time is shortened, however, gas is still flowing at the end of inspiration. This situation results in pressure and inflation inequalities among the units, with a disproportionate portion of the tidal volume being directed to units with a short time constant (once again proportionally to their compliance) and away from the unit supplied by an obstructed airway. The effect of such a redistribution on gas exchange depends on the

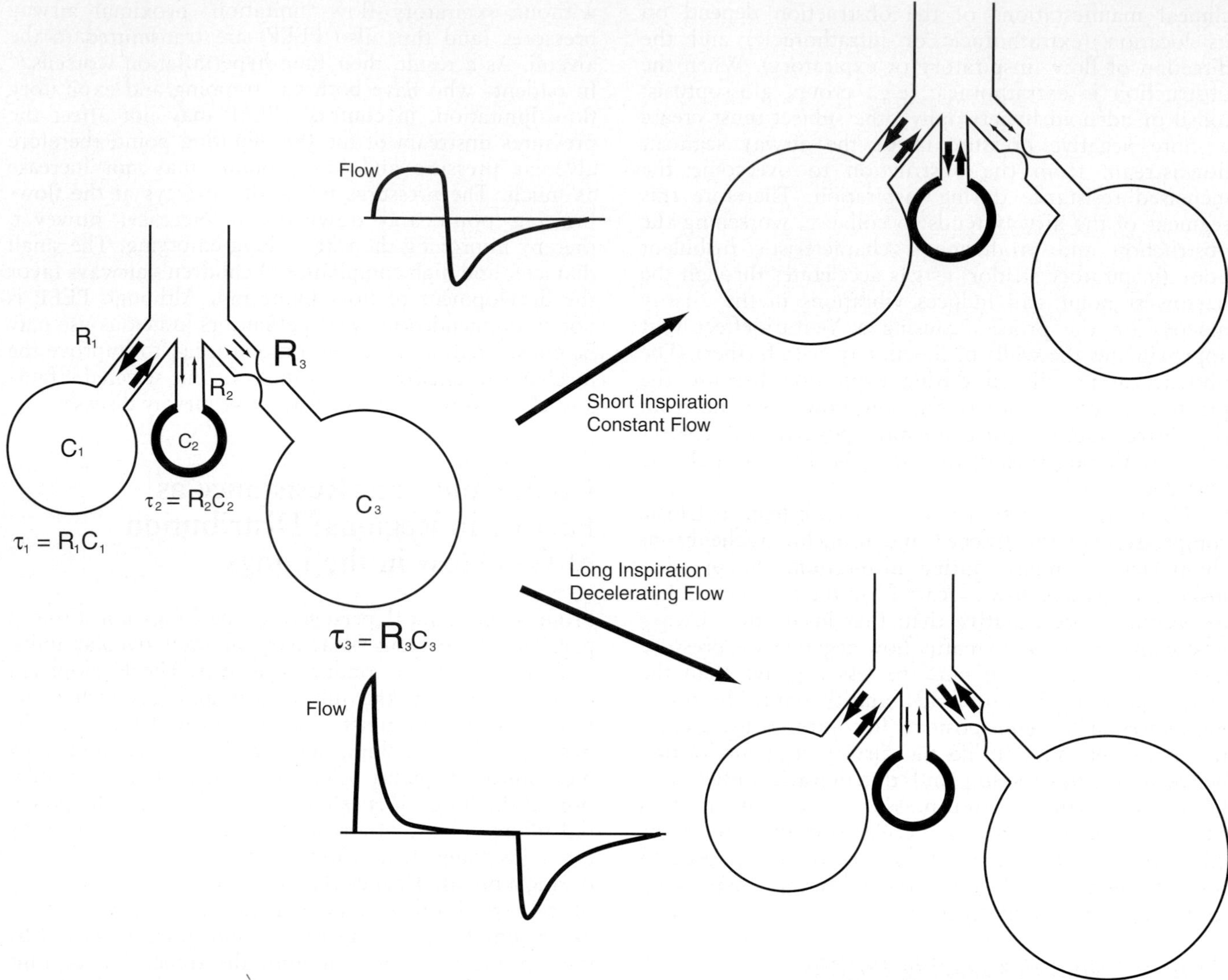

FIGURE 37–9 • Schematic representation of the lung showing the effects of ventilatory pattern on the distribution of inspiratory gas flow. The rate of inflation or deflation of an airway–alveolar unit can be characterized by a time constant (τ) equal to the product of its resistance *(R)* and compliance *(C)*. Three types of units are represented in the scheme: *1,* a normal unit with normal compliance and resistance (normal τ); *2,* a restrictive unit with decreased compliance and normal resistance (short τ); and *3,* an obstructed unit with normal compliance and increased resistance (long τ). Inflation with a decelerating pattern of flow *(lower arrow)* favors units with normal compliance *(1* and *3)*. Inflation with a short inspiratory time and a constant flow directs flow away from the unit with a long time constant *(3)*, causing the inflation of the other units *(1* and *2)* to be disproportionate with their compliance.

blood supply received by each type of unit and therefore is difficult to predict in diseased lungs.

Restrictive and Obstructive Respiratory Disease

As seen, inertial pressure losses are relatively insignificant at normal breathing frequencies in children, and viscoelastic pressure losses usually are lumped together with resistive pressure losses. Therefore the pressure that the respiratory muscles must generate to produce a certain volume excursion of the thorax (P_{TH}) can be simply considered the sum of elastic ($P_{TH,el}$) and resistive ($P_{TH,res}$) components:

$$P_{TH} = P_{TH,el} + P_{TH,res}. \quad (16)$$

Combining Equation 16 with Equations 14 and 15, we obtain a simplified form of the equation of motion of the respiratory system given in Equation 17:

$$P_{TH} = \Delta V_{TH}/C_{TH} + R_{TH} \times \dot{V}, \quad (17)$$

where ΔV_{TH}, C_{TH}, and R_{TH} = volume change, compliance, and resistance of the thorax, respectively.

Integration of Equation 16 with respect to dV_{TH} leads to Equation 18 for the total work done by the respiratory muscles (W_{TH}):

$$W_{TH} = W_{el} + W_{res}, \quad (18)$$

where W_{el} and W_{res} = works done to overcome elastic and resistive forces, respectively. When applying these formulations, it is important to realize that elastic and resistive forces do not always act in the same direction.

During inspiration, the respiratory muscles must generate the force to overcome both elasticity and resistance. Thus both W_{el} and W_{res} have the same sign and their effect on W_{TH} is additive. During expiration, however, the elastic recoil of the lungs normally provides the force needed to overcome resistance. W_{el} and W_{res} are of similar magnitude and opposite sign, and $W_{TH} = 0$. When there is intrathoracic airway obstruction, however, the absolute value of W_{res} often exceeds that of W_{el}. Under these circumstances, the expiratory value of W_{TH} is no longer negligible and the expiratory muscles must do the balance of the expiratory work.

The term *restrictive respiratory disease* encompasses all conditions in which W_{el} is primarily increased. Restrictive disease is caused by a decrease in thoracic compliance. Whether originating in the lungs or the chest wall, a decrease in thoracic compliance has two important mechanical consequences. First, the work of breathing increases, but only during inspiration; expiration continues to be passive and, in fact, takes place at a faster rate as elastic recoil increases. Second, the relaxation volume of the thorax and the FRC decrease (see Figure 37–3). This decrease in lung volume, which further reduces lung compliance, may be more pronounced in the infant, whose resting relaxation volume is already low. At low lung volumes, alveoli lack the support provided by the recoil of neighboring structures at higher volumes (a property known as *mechanical interdependence*) and become unstable. To prevent alveolar collapse, infants and small children with restrictive respiratory disease often close their glottis toward the end of expiration, causing each breath to end in a grunt. PEEP and continuous positive airway pressure are effective therapeutic modalities to achieve the same objective of preserving the end-expiratory inflation volume.[11,20,22,46] Deep lung inflations during positive pressure ventilation (often referred to loosely as *recruitment maneuvers*) may also maintain unstable alveoli open for a period of time.[30] This effect of volume history on alveolar volume decreases the work needed for spontaneous breaths following the inflation and explains some of the beneficial effects of intermittent mandatory ventilation in patients with restrictive lung disease.

Obstructive respiratory disease includes all conditions in which W_{res} is predominantly increased. The small caliber and high wall compliance of the developing airways[25] make the infant and child more susceptible to developing airway obstruction. Under normal breathing conditions the small caliber of the airways represents no mechanical disadvantage because gas flows are low (see Equation 15). When obstruction develops, however, airway resistance increases as an exponential function of the reduction in airway diameter. Because the same absolute decrease in caliber causes a much greater proportional reduction in airway diameter in a small than in a large airway, obstructive lesions tend to have more severe consequences in children than in adults. In addition, developing airways are more compliant than adult airways; therefore similar decreases in transmural pressure cause them to collapse more easily.

Determinants of Respiratory Efficiency

The respiratory system has a surprising ability to compensate for mechanical dysfunction. However, compensation does not come cheap. It raises the work of breathing in almost every instance, usually by combining increases in the force of contraction of the respiratory muscles with changes in ventilatory pattern. If the increase in work is sufficient to overcome the additional restrictive and obstructive loads applied on the respiratory system, minute alveolar ventilation and arterial PCO_2 are maintained within normal limits and respiratory failure is averted. In contrast, if the metabolic and contractile machinery of the respiratory muscles cannot meet the greater work demands, alveolar ventilation becomes insufficient to support gas exchange and respiratory failure ensues.

In the final analysis, the success or failure of the compensatory effort is a simple matter of balance between the energy resources available to the respiratory muscles and the energy demands imposed on these muscles. The energy resources are relatively well defined and limited by the blood supply of the muscles, their ability to metabolize substrates, and the internal efficiency of the muscle's metabolic apparatus.[42] The energy demands on the respiratory muscles are more variable, however, and depend on the workload these muscles must perform per unit of time (i.e., the power they must generate) and the overall efficiency with which the work is performed.

Power of Breathing and Breathing Frequency

Unlike work, which is a function of the volume–pressure characteristics of the thorax, respiratory power (work/time) is influenced by the pattern of breathing. It has been held for some time that, at any given time, each subject has an optimal breathing frequency at which minimum power is necessary to attain a certain minute alveolar ventilation.[8,27,33] Although this view has been challenged by those who believe that breathing frequency is adjusted to minimize average muscle force rather than power[7,28] (after all, there are no known energy or power receptors), it is a common clinical observation that different mechanical derangements result in distinctive patterns of breathing. These patterns generally agree with the principle of minimal power expenditure. For instance, patients with restrictive lung disease breathe rapidly and shallowly. In contrast, patients with airway obstruction breathe more slowly and prolong their inspiration or expiration, depending on whether the obstruction is extrathoracic or intrathoracic. By simply inspecting the effort and frequency of the breathing movements, the clinician can therefore assess not only the severity but also the specific nature of a patient's respiratory dysfunction. It is important to remember, however, that the low thoracic compliance of infants and small children mandates a relatively high breathing frequency at rest, even in the presence of airway obstruction. Nevertheless, severe tachypnea in a child with obstructive airway disease should always raise suspicions of an associated restrictive impairment. This distinction is best clarified by the following examples. A breathing frequency of 40 breaths/min can be considered low for a 3-month-old infant who has severe respiratory difficulty from bronchiolitis and is consistent with a predominantly obstructive dysfunction. On the contrary, a frequency of 100 breaths/min in the same infant would be indicative of a predominantly restrictive dysfunction, caused by either parenchymal involvement in the disease (e.g., pneumonitis or collapse) or severe distension of the lungs and chest wall caused by pulmonary hyperinflation.

Breathing Efficiency

In thermodynamic terms, *efficiency* is defined as the proportion of the free energy available within a system that is transformed into external work (Equation 2). This definition can be adapted for the respiratory system as given in Equation 19:

$$\text{Efficiency} = \text{Breathing power/Respiratory muscle energy consumption.} \quad (19)$$

In practice, the breathing power (work/time) almost always is calculated from the volume–pressure relationships of the lungs in spontaneously breathing subjects. The energy consumption of the respiratory muscles is estimated from their oxygen consumption, which in turn is computed as the difference between the total body oxygen consumptions measured during spontaneous and supported ventilation. Some obvious sources of energy consumption, which are not included in the breathing power, reduce the respiratory system's efficiency. For example, the work of breathing does not account for isometric activity of the respiratory and postural muscles, which is not proper work (no volume change) but consumes energy. Other forms of volume–pressure work usually are not taken into account when calculating respiratory efficiency, so they also become sources of inefficiency. For instance, the work performed to inflate the chest wall cannot be determined during spontaneous breathing when contraction of the muscles changes the wall's passive properties. Similarly, the work done to deform the rib cage is difficult to measure and often is ignored. Thus it is not surprising that the published efficiencies tend to be artifactually low.[6,33]

As defined by Equation 19 and by the considerations presented in the previous paragraph, the poor overall efficiency of the respiratory system implies that, during each breathing cycle, a substantial amount of energy derived from metabolic substrates is dissipated as heat and cannot be converted into volume–pressure work. Respiratory disease can increase this energy dissipation by various mechanisms leading to efficiency values as low as 1% to 3%.[6,15,48] Disease-induced alterations in chest wall configuration, for example, can limit the force generation by the muscles, thus interfering with the transformation of chemical energy into mechanical energy. Configurational changes also modify the spatial relationships of the muscles and can interfere with the transformation of mechanical energy into work. Finally, disease-related alterations in the contractile state of the muscles produced by fatigue or poor nutrition further decrease muscle force and the work of breathing without decreasing muscle energetic demands.

Alterations in Chest Wall Configuration

Diaphragmatic Configuration

The amount of force developed by a muscle depends on its resting length. An optimal resting length for which maximal force is developed can be defined for each muscle. In the case of the diaphragm, the optimal length is attained at thoracic volumes close to the normal FRC. At these volumes, the muscle has the shape of a dome-capped cylinder, a configuration that has several advantages.[10] First, diaphragmatic contraction shortens the cylinder in the axial direction,[5] producing a pistonlike motion that displaces more volume than if the diaphragmatic dome simply became flatter (assuming the same degree of fiber shortening). Second, the descent of the diaphragmatic dome increases the surface of contact between the rib cage and the lungs. Therefore the increase in lung surface produced by lung inflation can be accommodated without changing the shape of the lung or the chest wall. Finally, at normal breathing volumes, the sides of the diaphragmatic cylinder are apposed to the internal surface of the rib cage. This area of apposition establishes a mechanical link between intraabdominal pressure and lung volume.[29] As the diaphragm contracts during inspiration, intraabdominal pressure increases, pushing the lower portion of the rib cage forward and laterally. Thus diaphragmatic contraction has an additional contribution to lung inflation at low energy cost and may help to stabilize the lower rib cage against inspiratory distortion.

The configuration of the chest in the infant and small child minimizes these advantages. At these ages, the lower portion of the infant's rib cage has large anteroposterior and lateral diameters.[47] As a result, the insertions of the diaphragm are spread out, thereby reducing the axial shortening range of the muscle. Moreover, the lack of a substantial area of apposition of the diaphragm and rib cage abolishes the inspiratory and stabilizing effects of intraabdominal pressure on the rib cage.

Thoracic hyperexpansion and abdominal distension exaggerate these limitations by widening the diameters of the lower portion spreading out the diaphragmatic insertions. The length of the muscle fibers is diminished to a suboptimal length, and the force generated during inspiration is decreased. Abdominal distension has the additional disadvantage of raising intraabdominal pressure, which opposes diaphragmatic contraction and raises the work that the muscle has to do.

Rib Cage Distortion

Until now, we have assumed that the rib cage and abdomen have the same configuration during spontaneous breathing and passive inflation-deflation maneuvers. This assumption implies that all the various parts of the chest wall move with a single degree of freedom and that there are no volume shifts between parts. However, it has been known for quite some time that, under certain conditions, rib cage and abdomen can change volume independently of one another and even in opposite directions.[21] Under those conditions, the chest wall has multiple degrees of freedom and can undergo regional distortion.

Regional chest wall distortion results from the coupling of changes in pressure (pleural or intraabdominal) and the local compliances of the rib cage and abdominal wall. Rib cage distortion is more pronounced during inspiration, when pleural pressure decreases with respect to atmospheric pressure or the diaphragm pulls the rib cage by its costal insertions, forcing the thoracic wall inward in the expiratory direction. This inward movement of the rib cage causes visible retractions in areas where the chest wall has no bony support (intercostal, subcostal, or suprasternal spaces) or where the support has been abnormally weakened (e.g., costal fractures). Abdominal distortion, in contrast, usually involves alterations in the contractile state of the diaphragm or the abdominal wall muscles. When one hemidiaphragm becomes paralyzed, for example, the negative pleural pressure generated by other inspiratory muscles pulls the paralyzed muscle upward, into the rib cage, during inspiration. As a result, the abdominal wall of the affected side moves paradoxically in the inward direction, and the chest wall becomes distorted. As another example, contraction of the abdominal muscles stiffens the abdominal wall, raising intraabdominal pressure and shifting all volume changes to the rib cage during both inspiration and expiration.

The developing chest wall is particularly susceptible to distortion. As we have seen, the rib cage is very compliant in the newborn (see Figure 37–3).[16,40] Although this high compliance facilitates passage through the birth canal, it also promotes distortion of the rib cage during inspiration. In addition, the intercostal muscles, whose main contribution to breathing is to stabilize the rib cage by contracting simultaneously with the diaphragm, appear to have decreased tone at early ages, especially during REM sleep and in preterm infants.[19] Finally, the lack of a substantial area of apposition between the diaphragm and the rib cage removes the stabilizing effect of the intraabdominal pressure on the lower rib cage. Accordingly, infants tend to develop chest wall retractions in the presence of minimal mechanical lung dysfunction.

Chest wall distortion represents a pressure-induced change in volume, and therefore it constitutes a form of work. As noted earlier in this section, distortional work usually is not computed as part of the work of breathing because it has a measurable energy cost; it needs to be viewed as a source of respiratory inefficiency. Both the distortional work and its energy cost can be better understood if we analyze the volume–pressure relationships of the thorax in the particular case of rib cage retractions during inspiration. Regardless of whether such retractions are present, at any point in time, the volume change of the lungs (ΔV_L) must be equivalent to the sum of the volume changes of the rib cage (ΔV_{rc}) and abdomen (ΔV_{ab}).

$$\Delta V_L = \Delta V_{rc} + \Delta V_{ab}. \tag{20}$$

Consequently, if ΔV_L is to remain constant, decreases in ΔV_{rc} caused by rib cage retractions during inspiration must be accompanied by a proportional increase in ΔV_{ab}. If, as often occurs, ΔV_{rc} is negative, then ΔV_{ab} becomes greater than ΔV_L. Because the volume displacement of the diaphragm approximates ΔV_{ab}, chest wall retractions inevitably result in an increase in the diaphragmatic excursion. Considering that diaphragmatic work (W_{di}) is the integral of transdiaphragmatic pressure (intraabdominal pleural pressure or $P_{ga} - P_{pl}$, where P_{ga} = gastric pressure, which is often used to estimate intraabdominal pressure) with respect to the excursion volume of the diaphragm (V_{ab}), and the work done on the lungs (W_L) is the integral of transpulmonary pressure ($P_{\tilde{m}}\ P_{pl}$) with respect to tidal volume:

$$W_{di} = \int_{V_0}^{V_1} (P_{ga} - P_{pl})\, dV_{ab} \tag{21}$$

$$W_L = \int_{V_0}^{V_1} (P_A - P_{pl})\, dV_L \tag{22}$$

It is clear that W_{di} substantially exceeds W_L because P_{ga} is greater than P_m and dV_{ab} is greater than dV_L. It also is clear that W_{di} is greater when there are retractions than when there are no retractions because the latter increase dV_{ab}. The volume displacement of the diaphragm may be up to twice the tidal volume of the lungs in premature infants without apparent lung disease,[18] an increase that could be responsible for the poor weight gain and development of fatigue of infants recovering from the respiratory distress syndrome.

Alterations in Contractile State of the Respiratory Muscles

Respiratory efficiency is affected by the functional state of the respiratory muscles. Sustained increases in activity likely will eventually result in decreased contractile force and a lower minute alveolar ventilation, a condition often classified as *muscle fatigue.*[43] When muscle fatigue is present, the energy consumption of the muscle may be increased with respect to the actual work performed. Similar decreases in contractility without a decrease in energy consumption can be present in a variety of clinical situations. Some result from an imbalance between the energy demands of the muscle's contractile machinery and its substrate availability (e.g., shock).[2] Others are simply the expression of the inadequate coupling of the excitation–contraction processes inside the muscle cell or the chronic depletion of the muscle's energetic resources as a result of malnutrition.

Conclusion

Although the developing respiratory system has obvious mechanical disadvantages, the reader should not be left with the idea that infants and children are constantly on the brink of respiratory failure. Quite the contrary, they have a remarkable capability to tolerate respiratory disease. This capability is in great part based on a very proficient system of mechanical compensation. The information contained in this chapter is intended to provide an overview of the factors involved in both mechanical dysfunction and its compensation. Understanding these factors should permit a more rational approach to the therapy of respiratory disease in the critically ill child.

REFERENCES

1. Agostoni E, Mead J: Statics of the respiratory system. In Fenn WO, Rahn H, editors: Handbook of physiology I: respiration, vol 1. Washington, DC, 1964, American Physiologic Society.
2. Aubier M, Trippenbach T, Roussos C: Respiratory muscle fatigue during cardiogenic shock. J Appl Physiol 51:499, 1981.
3. Bachofen H, Duc G: Lung tissue resistance in healthy children. Pediatr Res 2:119, 1968.
4. Barach AL, Swenson P: Effect of breathing gases under positive pressure on lumens of small and medium-sized bronchi. Arch Intern Med 63:946, 1939.
5. Braun NMT, Arora NS, Rochester DF: Force-length relationship of the human diaphragm. J Appl Physiol 53:405, 1982.
6. Cherniack RM: The oxygen consumption and efficiency of the respiratory muscles in health and emphysema. J Clin Invest 38:494, 1959.
7. Clark JM, Sinclair RD, Lenox JB: Chemical and nonchemical components of ventilation during hypercapneic exercise in man. J Appl Physiol 48:1065, 1980.
8. Crossfill ML, Widdicombe JG: Physical characteristics of the chest and lungs and the work of breathing in different mammalian species. J Physiol (Lond) 158:1, 1961.
9. Dawson SV, Elliot EA: Wave-speed limitation on expiratory flow: a unifying concept. J Appl Physiol 43:498, 1977.
10. De Troyer A, Loring SH: Action of the respiratory muscles. In Macklem PT, Mead J, editors: *Handbook of physiology: the respiratory system.* Bethesda, 1986, American Physiologic Society.
11. Dueck R, Wagner PD, West JB: Effects of positive end-expiratory pressure on gas exchange in dogs with normal and edematous lungs. *Anesthesiology* 47:359, 1977.
12. Fagan DG: Post-mortem studies of the semistatic volume-pressure characteristics of infant's lungs. *Thorax* 31:534, 1976.
13. Fagan DG: Shape changes in static V-P loops for children's lungs related to growth. *Thorax* 32:198, 1977.
14. Fisher JT, Mortola JP, Smith JB, et al: Respiration in newborns: development of the control of breathing. *Am Rev Respir Dis* 125: 650, 1982.
15. Fritts HN Jr, Filler J, Fishman AP, et al: The efficiency of ventilation during voluntary hyperpnea: studies in normal subjects and in dyspneic patients with either chronic pulmonary emphysema or obesity. *J Clin Invest* 38:1339, 1959.
16. Gerhardt T, Bancalari E: Chest wall compliance in full term and premature infants. *Acta Paediatr Scand* 69:359, 1980.
17. Harding R, Johnson P, McClelland ME: The expiratory role of the larynx during development and the influence of behavioral state. In von Euler C, Lagercrantz H, editors: *Central nervous control mechanisms in breathing.* Oxford, 1979, Pergamon Press.
18. Heldt GP, McIlroy MB: Distortion of chest wall and work of diaphragm in preterm infants, *J Appl Physiol* 62:164, 1987.
19. Henderson-Smart DJ, Read DJC: Reduced lung volume during behavioral active sleep in the newborn. *J Appl Physiol* 46:1081, 1979.
20. Katz JA, Ozanne GM, Zinn SE, et al: Time course and mechanisms of lung-volume increase with PEEP in acute pulmonary failure. *Anesthesiology* 54:9, 1981.
21. Konno K, Mead J: Measurement of the separate volume changes of rib cage and abdomen during breathing. *J Appl Physiol* 22:407, 1967.
22. Kumar A, Falke KJ, Geffin B, et al: Continuous positive-pressure ventilation in acute respiratory failure. *N Engl J Med* 283:1430, 1970.
23. Ludwig MS, Dreshaj I, Solway J, et al: Partitioning of pulmonary resistance during constriction in the dog: effects of volume history. *J Appl Physiol* 62:807, 1987.
24. Marini JJ: Should PEEP be used in airflow obstruction? *Am Rev Respir Dis* 140:1, 1989.
25. Martin HB, Proctor DF: Pressure-volume measurements on dog bronchi. *J Appl Physiol* 13:337, 1958.
26. Martin JG, Shore S, Engel LA: Effect of continuous positive airway pressure on respiratory mechanics and pattern of breathing in induced asthma. *Am Rev Respir Dis* 126:812, 1982.
27. McIlroy MB, Marshall R, Christie RV: Work of breathing in normal subjects. *Clin Sci* 13:127, 1954.
28. Mead J: Control of respiratory frequency. *J Appl Physiol* 15:325, 1960.
29. Mead J: Functional significance of the area of apposition of diaphragm to rib cage. *Am Rev Respir Dis* 119:31, 1979.
30. Mead J, Collier C: Relation of volume history of lungs to respiratory mechanics in anesthetized dogs. *J Appl Physiol* 14:669, 1959.
31. Mead J, Takishima T, Leith D: Stress distribution in lungs: a model of pulmonary elasticity. *J Appl Physiol* 28:596, 1970.
32. Mead J, Turner JM, Macklem PT, et al: Significance of the relationship between lung recoil and maximum expiratory flow. *J Appl Physiol* 22:95, 1967.
33. Milic-Emili J, Petit JM: Mechanical efficiency of breathing. *J Appl Physiol* 15:359, 1960.
34. Muller N, Volgyesi G, Becker L, et al: Diaphragmatic muscle tone. *J Appl Physiol* 47:279, 1979.
35. Olinsky A, Bryan MH, Bryan AC: Influence of lung inflation on respiratory-control in neonates. *J Appl Physiol* 36:426, 1974.
36. Pérez Fontán JJ, Kinloch LP: Control of bronchomotor tone during perinatal development in sheep. *J Appl Physiol* 75:1486, 1993.
37. Pérez Fontán JJ, Kinloch LP, Donnelly DF: Integration of ventilatory and bronchomotor responses during chemoreceptor stimulation in developing sheep. *Respir Physiol* 111:1, 1998.
38. Pérez Fontán JJ, Diec CT, Velloff CR: Bilateral distribution of vagal motor and sensory nerve fibers in the rat's lungs and airways. *Am J Physiol* 279:713, 2000.
39. Pérez Fontán JJ: Mechanical function of the lungs and airways during hypoxia. In Lister G, Haddad GG, editors: *Tissue oxygen deprivation: from molecular to integrated function. Lung biology in health and disease series.* New York, 1996, Marcel Dekker.
40. Richard CC, Bachman L: Lung and chest wall compliance in apneic paralyzed infants. *J Clin Invest* 40:273, 1961.
41. Richardson CA, Herbert DA, Mitchell RA: Modulation of pulmonary stretch receptors and airway resistance by parasympathetic efferents. *J Appl Physiol* 57:1842, 1984.
42. Roussos C, Campbell EJM: Respiratory muscle energetics. In Macklem PT, Mead J, editors: *Handbook of physiology: the respiratory system.* Bethesda, 1986, American Physiologic Society.
43. Roussos C, Macklem PT: Inspiratory muscle fatigue. In Macklem PT, Mead J, editors: *Handbook of physiology: the respiratory system.* Bethesda, 1986, American Physiologic Society.
44. Salazar E, Knowles JH: An analysis of pressure volume characteristics of lungs. *J Appl Physiol* 19:97, 1964.
45. Stigol LC, Vawter GF, Mead J: Studies on elastic recoil of the lung in a pediatric population. *Am Rev Respir Dis* 105:552, 1972.
46. Suter PM, Fairley HB, Isenberg MD: Optimum end-expiratory airway pressure in patients with acute pulmonary failure. *N Engl J Med* 292:284, 1975.
47. Takahashi E, Atsumi H: Age differences in thoracic form as indicated by thoracic index. *Hum Biol* 27:65, 1955.
48. Thibeault DW, Clutario B, Auld PAM: The oxygen cost of breathing in the premature infant. *Pediatrics* 37:954, 1966.
49. Tuxen DV: Detrimental effects of positive end-expiratory pressure during controlled mechanical ventilation of patients with severe airflow obstruction. *Am Rev Respir Dis* 140:5, 1989.
50. Wilson TA, Rodarte JR, Bulter JP: Wave-speed and viscous flow limitation. In Macklem PT, Mead J, editors: *Handbook of physiology, respiration,* vol. 3, Bethesda, 1986, American Physiologic Society.

CHAPTER 38

Noninvasive Monitoring in Children

Daniel Rubens, Kenneth A. Schenkman, and Lynn D. Martin

PEARLS

- Many intensive care unit (ICU) patients are unusually sensitive to environmental temperature fluctuations. Temperature fluctuations in such patients may occur rapidly, and many have important effects on physiology and metabolism.
- Pulse oximeters measure only oxyhemoglobin and deoxyhemoglobin and ignore other forms of hemoglobin (methemoglobin, carboxyhemoglobin). Blood cooximeters, however, do account for these other species.
- The accuracy of the capnogram depends on the sampling site. If the tidal volume is small and the sample flow rate is large, the gas sample may be diluted by entrained fresh gas.
- The bispectral index monitor is a recently developed form of processed electroencephalogram that integrates various electroencephalographic descriptors into a single unitless number to assess the brain's response to hypnotic agents.

Monitoring, commonly the primary reason for admission to the intensive care unit (ICU), is designed to obtain frequent, repetitive, or continuous measurement of vital functions that are displayed at the bedside to allow prompt recognition of problems and early initiation of therapy. No single physiologic measurement or group of measures can completely convey the clinical condition of the patient. Clinical judgment often is subjective and hard to quantify. Monitoring provides objective criteria for the evaluation and treatment of physiologic deficiencies.

Noninvasive monitoring, in the form of vital signs (heart rate, respiratory rate, arterial pressure, and temperature), has been used routinely for all patients receiving care in the ICU since the birth of the specialty. Significant technologic improvements have been made with these critical monitoring systems over the past 4 decades. It has become increasingly apparent that accurate and continuous core temperature management adds much to the expected outcome in many settings. Two more recently introduced types of noninvasive monitoring, pulse oximetry and capnometry, have significantly impacted the practice of critical care medicine and become standards of care. Finally, new technology to noninvasively monitor physiologic function currently under development may significant decrease the need for more invasive monitoring and lessen the risk of therapies common in the ICU setting.

Vital Signs

Heart and respiratory rate, arterial pressure, and temperature are the simplest, most easily measured, and most commonly monitored and recorded physiologic variables in the ICU. Heart rate and respiratory rate are continuously recorded and displayed electronically. Changes in either of these variables reflect nonspecific alterations in cardiovascular and/or respiratory responses to physiologic function or pharmacologic intervention.

Electrocardiographic Monitoring

The electrocardiogram (ECG) evaluates the electrical events of cardiac contraction by sensing and recording voltage changes at the body surface. The body is assumed to be a homogeneous volume conductor with uniform geometry. The heart is represented by two charged electrodes: a dipole with one positive pole and one negative pole; this dipole is surrounded by a hypothetical equilateral triangle. This equivalent dipole measures the electrical activity of the heart (changes magnitude and orientation) throughout the cardiac cycle. The sides of the triangle, which represent the axes of the three standard limb leads, provide a triaxial frame of reference for spatial orientation of the cardiac electrical activity. When combined with the chest (V lead) recordings, the model provides frontal, sagittal, and horizontal components. This practice led to considerable information on the electrophysiology of the heart.

Blood Pressure Measurement

Like heart and respiratory rate, measurement of blood pressure is routine in the ICU. Accurate, continuous measurement of noninvasive blood pressure (NIBP) in infants and children can be challenging. Current methods of measuring NIBP are limited to auscultation, oscillometry, ultrasound, and the flush or return to flow.[1] Because of technical difficulties, routine, reliable measurements of NIBP in infants and children did not become possible until approximately 4 decades ago. Auscultatory determinations, even on an intermittent basis, can be difficult in infants. In the flush or return to flow technique, the distal extremity is compressed, facilitating blood drainage. An occluding cuff then is inflated proximally on the limb and gradually deflated. The systemic pressure is the pressure at which flow returns to the compressed distal extremity. Numerous subjective influences play a major role in accuracy. Other intermittent methods that can be used in the ICU include sensitive sound amplification systems. However, these devices are not commonly used. The most popular method used is based on the principle of oscillometry (e.g., Dinamap, Critikon, Tampa, FL), which automatically inflates and deflates the cuff and uses crystal microphones and piezoelectric crystals and the Doppler principle to measure and display systolic, mean, and diastolic pressures. During oscillometry, blood flow through an artery during cuff deflation causes the arterial wall to oscillate.[2] The rapid increase in oscillation amplitude represents systolic pressure whereas the sudden decrease in oscillation represents diastolic pressure. The period of maximum oscillation is used to estimate mean blood pressure. The needle bounce technique is another oscillometric method commonly practiced by flight nurses/physicians. An inflated distal or proximal extremity circumferential cuff is slowly deflated, and the first visible bounce corresponds to systolic pressure. Automatically obtained blood pressures by the oscillometric method compare favorably with those obtained via arterial cannulas in infants and children.[3–5] Oscillometric devices do not perform well if there is significant limb movement or in the presence of dysrhythmias.[1] Occlusive systems using frequent measuring intervals can be associated with problems after prolonged use.[1,6]

Doppler devices are extremely useful for determining blood pressure in small babies, particularly when shock is present. A small Doppler probe is placed over an extremity artery. Blood movement causes changes in exquisitely sensitive ultrasound reflectance. With a proximally applied cuff, which is slowly deflated, it is possible to read systolic pressure with the appearance of the first Doppler effect signal. Diastolic pressure is read when the strength and quality of the signal decrease. Correlation of these two pressures with arterial line numbers is good.[7] It is important to place the Doppler probe directly over an artery. Although the Doppler technique is easily utilized during surgery, its use in the ICU for continual monitoring is inconvenient. When an arterial line is not available and the automatic oscillometric device is not able to provide pressure readings, the Doppler technique can be used to obtain intermittent blood pressure in the ICU.

When measuring blood pressure in babies and children, it is important to select the appropriate-sized blood pressure cuff. Numerous cuff sizes are available. For the upper extremity, the cuff should occupy at least two thirds of the upper arm.[8] The cuff bladder circumferential dimension should be 20% greater than that of the extremity.[8] A cuff that is too small will result in falsely increased readings.[4,8] In contrast, an oversized cuff will artificially decrease blood pressure readings, but the magnitude of the error is small.[4]

Temperature Monitoring and Routine Temperature Management

Body temperature can dramatically alter physiology and metabolism. Monitoring of temperature is a routine part of the practice in the ICU. The accepted normal range of rectal temperature in children is from 36.1°C to 37.8°C.[9] This range is closely guarded by an intact thermoregulatory system that controls heat production and loss. However, many ICU patients can be considered poikilothermic, meaning they are unusually sensitive to environmental temperature fluctuations. A number of things may contribute to this tendency, including the presence of either endogenous or exogenous vasoactive influences, the administration of drugs that blunt the normal regulation of body temperature, and depression of the central nervous system, either endogenous or secondary to the administration of sedatives at moderate to high doses. This poikilothermic tendency also implies that temperature fluctuations in the patient may occur rapidly. For this reason, the continuous monitoring of true core temperature can be particularly useful in selected patients, including those patients with increased intracranial pressure or status epilepticus who are managed with high-dose pentobarbital and mechanical ventilation; patients with unstable hemodynamics after open heart surgery; patients with respiratory failure and extreme mechanical ventilation support; and, of course, patients being observed for development of malignant hyperthermia.

Temperature Monitoring Sites

Because core temperature is the principal thermoregulatory controller, monitoring core temperature is more useful than monitoring peripheral skin temperature.

Commonly used core temperature monitoring sites include the distal esophagus, tympanic membrane, pulmonary artery, and nasopharynx. These sites detect core temperature changes rapidly, in contrast to urinary bladder or rectal measurements, which are good reflections of core temperature during steady-state conditions.[10] Cutaneous temperature monitoring is the least reliable indicator of rapid core temperature changes, for example, as seen in malignant hyperthermia.[11] However, monitoring peripheral temperatures can be useful in defining core peripheral gradients in temperature and assist in tracking vasoconstriction and vasodilation. The ideal spot for continuous core temperature monitoring is a pulmonary artery catheter. An esophageal temperature probe positioned in the lower third of the esophagus and verified radiologically is a good alternative. In this position, the temperature sensor is immediately behind the left atrium and tracks true core temperature without significant time lag in the majority of situations. If a gastric tube with applied suction is present next to the temperature probe, it must be on the low intermittent setting or the temperature readings will be falsely lowered. Nasopharyngeal and tympanic membrane temperatures are good indicators of cerebral temperature but can be inaccurate secondary to temperature sensor positioning. Trauma to the nasopharynx or tympanic membrane may result in troublesome bleeding, especially where coagulation and platelet function are abnormal. Axillary and peripheral skin temperatures probably are the most convenient sites for monitoring, although they may be the most inaccurate secondary to skin perfusion. When continuous core temperature monitoring is desirable, the most reliable and convenient device is the lower esophageal temperature probe.

Pulse Oximetry

Pulse oximetry has become a standard monitoring modality for many aspects of medical care and is widely used throughout the modern hospital. In the ICU, pulse oximetry is routinely and continuously used to monitor most patients and has often been referred to as the fifth vital sign.[12] Of the advances in medical monitoring during the past several decades, pulse oximetry has undoubtedly had the largest positive impact on the clinical care of hospitalized patients. Despite the wide use of pulse oximetry throughout the hospital, many health care providers, including nurses and doctors, have a poor understanding of the underlying principles and limitations of pulse oximetry.[13,14]

Takuo Aoyagi, working for the Nihon Kohden Corporation in Japan, first proposed the theory for pulse oximetry in 1972. His idea was developed into a working oximeter, which subsequently was patented in Japan in 1974 and marketed as the world's first commercial pulse oximeter. In 1977 a fiberoptic-based pulse oximeter with improved accuracy was marketed by Minolta, and in 1982 Nellcor began marketing a pulse oximeter that ultimately became an industry standard.[15] Since then, numerous companies have produced and marketed pulse oximeters, and improvements in technology continue to improve the accuracy and reliability of these devices. Most recently, Masimo Corporation introduced pulse oximeters with technology that minimizes motion artifact.[16]

Principles of Pulse Oximetry

Pulse oximetry is based on the elegant observation that the attenuation of light passing through blood-perfused tissue changes with pulsation of blood, and that the alternating component of the light attenuation results from the composition of arterial blood. Figure 38–1 is a schematic diagram showing that the component of light attenuation as a result of pulsatility comes from arterial blood. This information can be analyzed to determine the hemoglobin saturation in the arterial blood. Absorption of light as a result of other tissue components and capillary and venous blood in the static portion of the signal is ignored in the analysis.

Light passing through a turbid media such as tissue is attenuated by absorption and scattering. If light scattering in tissue is assumed to be fairly constant, then measured changes in the attenuation of the transmitted light can be assumed to result from changes in absorption. Beer's Law describes the theoretical absorption of light as follows:

$$\text{Absorbance (OD)} = -\log_{10}(I/I_o) = \varepsilon bc, \qquad (1)$$

where I = light emerging from the sample, I_o = incident light illuminating the sample, ε = molar extinction coefficient of the specific absorbing species at a specific wavelength, b = path length (in centimeters) the light traverses, and c = molar concentration of the absorbing species. Thus changes in the concentration of an absorber, that is, oxyhemoglobin, results in changes in absorbance.

Hemoglobin has characteristic light-absorbing properties that change with oxygen binding. Figure 38–2 shows absorption spectra of oxyhemoglobin (oxyHb) and deoxyhemoglobin (deoxyHb) in the visible and near-infrared spectral region. At any given wavelength, there is a difference in absorption between oxyHb and deoxyHb except where the spectra cross, at wavelengths called *isosbestic wavelengths* where the absorption is the same for each state. At nonisosbestic wavelengths, the difference in absorption can be used to determine the fraction of oxyhemoglobin. Saturation of hemoglobin is defined as follows:

$$Hb_{sat} = [OxyHb]/([OxyHb] + [DeoxyHb]), \qquad (2)$$

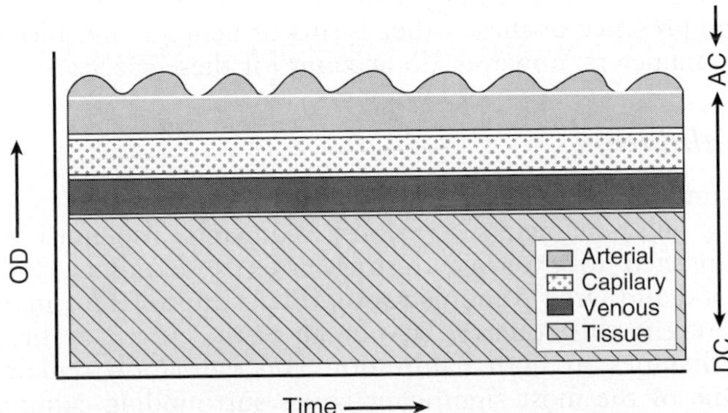

FIGURE 38–1 • Light passing through a pulsating tissue will be absorbed by multiple components of tissue and blood. The alternating component (AC) is composed only of arterial blood.

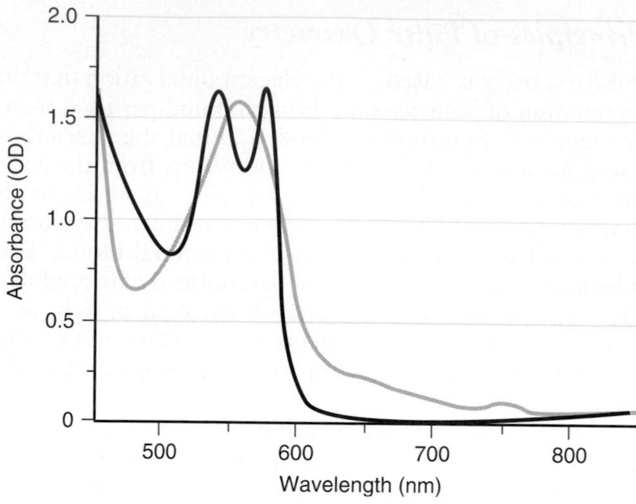

FIGURE 38–2 • Absorption spectra of hemoglobin in the visible and near infrared spectral region. The deoxy form of hemoglobin *(blue)* has a single peak in the visible and near-infrared region. Oxyhemoglobin *(red)* has two peaks in the visible region but no significant peak in the near-infrared region.

where Hb_{sat} = fractional saturation of hemoglobin, [oxyHb] = concentration of oxyhemoglobin, and [deoxyHb] = concentration of deoxyhemoglobin.

Pulse oximeters typically use two wavelengths of light to determine the saturation of hemoglobin, usually one around 660 nm in the visible light region and one around 940 nm in the near-infrared region.[17] The absorption around 940 nm is relatively low and fairly constant over the range of saturations; thus a change in absorbance at 660 nm can be referenced to the absorption at 940-nm wavelength and used to determine the saturation. Each pulse oximeter uses a complex algorithm to convert the change in absorbance at the two wavelengths to an absolute saturation value.

In the presence of other forms of hemoglobin, primarily carboxyhemoglobin or methemoglobin, the saturation of hemoglobin is correctly determined by the more complex relationship:

$$Hb_{sat} = [OxyHb]/([OxyHb] + [DeoxyHb] + [MetHb] + [CarboxyHb]), \quad (3)$$

where [metHb] = concentration of methemoglobin, and [carboxyHb] = concentration of carboxyhemoglobin. Pulse oximeters usually cannot accurately account for the presence of these other forms of hemoglobin. Blood cooximeters, however, do account for these species.

Validation

Numerous studies have been performed to validate existing pulse oximeters.[18–22] Pulse oximeters also must be subjected to extensive testing prior to obtaining U.S. Food and Drug Administration (FDA) approval for marketing in this country. Despite all of the current testing, difficulties in both calibration and validation remain. One of the most significant issues surrounding calibration is the development of an appropriate universal test that will accurately test the pulse oximeter for a wide range of potential clinical applications. Pulse oximeters must be accurate for a wide range of skin thickness and color and over a wide range of saturations. Pulse oximeter simulators and testing devices have been built to overcome some of these issues.[23–25] Clinical testing has been fairly extensive, and a number of studies have demonstrated the reliability of various pulse oximeters for specific clinical situations.[26–28] In general, pulse oximeters are most accurate at higher saturations, usually above 75%.[29–31]

Sources of Error

Although pulse oximetry is widely accepted as a valid clinical monitor and provides valuable minute-to-minute clinical data, pulse oximeters are subject to multiple potential sources of error. The most clinically significant source of error usually results from movement or "motion artifact," which, as most clinicians recognize, results in frequent and annoying false alarms. Other sources of error include dyshemoglobinopathies, interfering dyes or other pigments in the blood, ambient light, and poor tissue perfusion.

Minimizing motion artifact has been the subject of many of the recent advancements in technology used for the modern pulse oximeter. The Masimo Corporation has introduced signal extraction technology (Masimo SET) to decrease sensitivity of pulse oximeters to motion. This approach has improved the accuracy of pulse oximetry readings and has decreased the frequency of false alarms in clinical settings.[16,32–35]

The presence of interfering dyes or dyshemoglobinopathies is infrequently a clinical problem but can result in erroneous pulse oximetry readings. In methemoglobinemia, the iron in the heme groups in hemoglobin becomes oxidized from the ferrous (Fe^{2+}) state to the ferric (Fe^{3+}) state. The oxidized form of hemoglobin, called *methemoglobin,* cannot bind oxygen. Thus the presence of significant quantities of methemoglobin leads to tissue hypoxia because these molecules no longer participate in oxygen transport. However, light absorbance by methemoglobin more closely resembles oxyhemoglobin than deoxyhemoglobin at the measured wavelengths, erroneously leading the pulse oximeter to indicate a higher percent oxygen saturation than expected.[36,37] Similarly, the presence of carboxyhemoglobin may result in erroneous reading in pulse oximetry because carbon monoxide-bound hemoglobin also does not participate in oxygen transport.[38] Cooximeters account for the presence of both carboxyhemoglobin and methemoglobin, thus blood gas samples sent for cooximetry should correctly measure hemoglobin saturation in cases where measurable levels of either methemoglobin or carboxyhemoglobin are present or suspected. Fetal hemoglobin has a sufficiently similar absorbance spectrum to adult hemoglobin, such that the presence of fetal hemoglobin does not significantly affect the determined saturation.[39] The presence of bilirubin also does not appear to significantly affect pulse oximetry readings.[40]

Interfering light from the environment may adversely affect the accuracy of pulse oximeters,[35] although the extent of ambient light interference has been questioned for some of the pulse oximeters studied.[41] Shielding of the probe from ambient light is often used clinically to improve performance. Hypoperfusion also may limit the ability of pulse oximeters to adequately detect a pulsatile signal and can adversely affect reported saturation values.[18,35]

Probe Placement

Typically, pulse oximetry probes are placed on fingers or toes, where the light-emitting diodes are placed across the digit, opposite from the detector. For premature and small infants, the probe is often placed around the entire palm with good results. Because of scattering of light in tissue, pulse oximeter probes also can be used in a reflectance mode. In this manner, both light-emitting diodes and detectors are on the same surface and can be placed, for example, on the forehead.[42,43] Transesophageal probes have been designed and used for care of operative or critically ill patients with potentially poor peripheral perfusion.[44–46]

Cerebral Oximetry

The basic principles underlying pulse oximetry have been extended to determine hemoglobin saturation in the brain. Currently a small number of devices for determination of cerebral oxygenation are commercially available. Somanetics has an FDA-approved device available for pediatric use (INVOS 5100). Hamamatsu also makes a device, the NIRO 300, but it currently is not FDA approved.[47] These devices take advantage of the relative transparency of the skull and brain in the near-infrared spectral region. However, because these devices do not restrict analyses to a pulsatile component, the information provided comes from light absorption of hemoglobin in arterial, venous, and capillary blood and is contaminated to some extent by the presence of other light-absorbing molecules, primarily the cytochromes. Thus these devices provide a "relative" saturation value of cerebral oxygenation, which may have some correlation with clinical conditions,[48] but these devices currently do not report an absolute saturation value the way pulse oximeters do. Technical advances likely will improve the clinical utility of cerebral oximetry as the information provided becomes more reliable.

Muscle Oximetry

Optical spectroscopy has been used to assess muscle oxygenation with increasing success. Earlier approaches for determining muscle oxygenation have been limited by the similarity between optical absorbance spectra from hemoglobin and myoglobin. Many reports of tissue oxygenation as a combined hemoglobin plus myoglobin saturation have been reported.[49] Because hemoglobin and myoglobin have vastly different oxygen dissociation relationships,[50] a combined saturation may have little clinical significance. Successful distinction of myoglobin saturation from hemoglobin saturation has been reported, using a complex multiwavelength spectra analytic approach.[51,52] Because myoglobin is an intracellular oxygen-binding molecule in cardiac and skeletal muscle, myoglobin saturation can be used to determine intracellular oxygen tension. This approach has led to the determination of intracellular oxygen tension measurements in both cardiac and skeletal muscle in laboratory studies.[53–55] Technical advances using this approach likely will have a significant impact on clinical monitoring of critically ill and injured patients.

Capnometry and Capnography

Another monitoring technology routinely used in the critical care unit is the measurement of carbon dioxide. *Capnometry* is the measurement of the partial pressure (or concentration) of CO_2 in the patient's airway during the entire ventilatory cycle. A capnometer provides a numerical measurement of inspired and end-tidal P_{CO_2}. *Capnography* is the graphic display of the partial pressure or concentration of CO_2 as a waveform (capnogram), usually plotted as P_{CO_2} versus time. When the waveform display is calibrated, capnography includes capnometry.

Physiologic Basis

When ventilation and perfusion are well matched throughout the lung, Pa_{CO_2} and the partial pressure of end-tidal CO_2 (Pet_{CO_2}) are nearly equal, normally 40 mmHg. If a discrepancy between ventilation and perfusion exists, a difference between the Pa_{CO_2} and Pet_{CO_2}, also known as (a-et)ΔP_{CO_2}, occurs.

The capnogram displays the CO_2 concentration in the patient's airway over time (Figure 38–3). The essentials of a normal capnogram are (1) zero baseline during early exhalation, which reflects gas exhaled from the

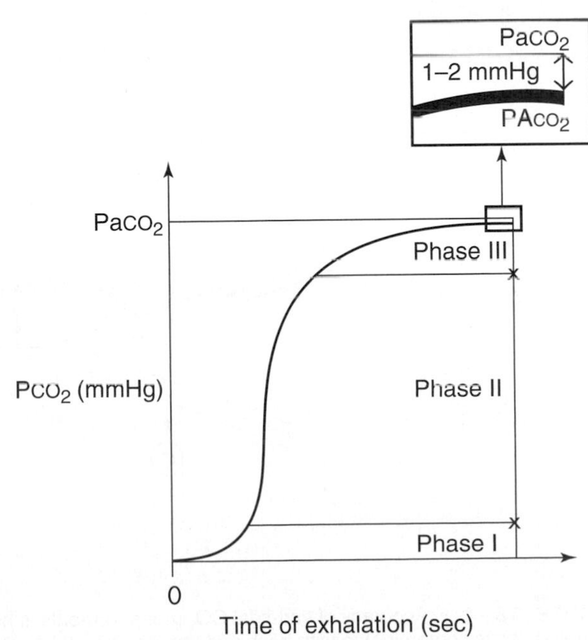

FIGURE 38–3 • Normal capnogram.

anatomic dead space; (2) sharp upstroke during midexhalation, which reflects the transition to alveolar gas; (3) relatively horizontal alveolar plateau (the final peak is also known as $PetCO_2$ because it reflects the end of expiration; prolonged exhalation caused by obstructive lung disease causes a steeper plateau); and (4) sharp downstroke and return to a zero baseline at the start of inhalation. A capnogram without these normal attributes suggests an anomaly in the patient's cardiopulmonary system, a malfunction in the airway, or a malfunction in the gas delivery system.[56]

Operating Principles of Capnometry

To measure the partial pressure of CO_2 in the airway, respiratory gas must be sampled. In the most common sampling method, gas is diverted from the airway and aspirated through a tube (sidestream) to the CO_2 monitor. Diverting capnometers allow true zero-PCO_2 reference measurements, which tend to produce dependable, drift-free performance and thus accurate CO_2 measurements. An alternative to the diverting instrument is the nondiverting or "mainstream" capnometer in which a special flow-through adapter and CO_2 monitor are placed on the patient's airway.

In the majority of stand-alone capnometers, CO_2 concentration is measured by infrared spectroscopy. By comparing absorption by the sample gas with absorption by the reference gas, the capnometer determines the amount of CO_2 in the sample gas, which it then displays as the CO_2 concentration. Raman scattering and mass spectrometry are alternative methods of PCO_2 measurement.

Clinical and Technical Issues

Both physiologic anomalies and technical factors can result in $PetCO_2$ values that do not approximate $PaCO_2$. For $PetCO_2$ to approximate $PaCO_2$, two assumptions must be met: (1) the lung units must empty fully with approximately equal time constants, and (2) ventilation and perfusion must be well matched in the lung units. Additionally, technical variables can produce $PetCO_2$ values that do not approximate $PaCO_2$. These include the design of the gas sampling system, the distance the gas must be transported, and the instrument's calibration methods.

Gas Sampling Issues

The gas sampling method used by a capnometer affects the accuracy of the capnogram and $PetCO_2$ measurements. Relevant factors include the location of the ventilatory circuit from which the gas is sampled, the distance over which the gas is transported before analysis, and the sample flow rate of the instrument. With a nondiverting or mainstream device, the CO_2 monitor is placed on the airway, so there is no need to divert gas from the airway. This sampling configuration typically is available only in infrared capnometers because only infrared CO_2 monitors can be designed small enough to fit on the airway. Another sampling configuration is seen in the proximal-diverting device. A lightweight, low-profile airway adapter is placed on the patient's airway, and gas is sampled from the airway and transported to the sensor, which is placed near the patient but not on the airway itself. A third sampling configuration is found in the distal-diverting device,

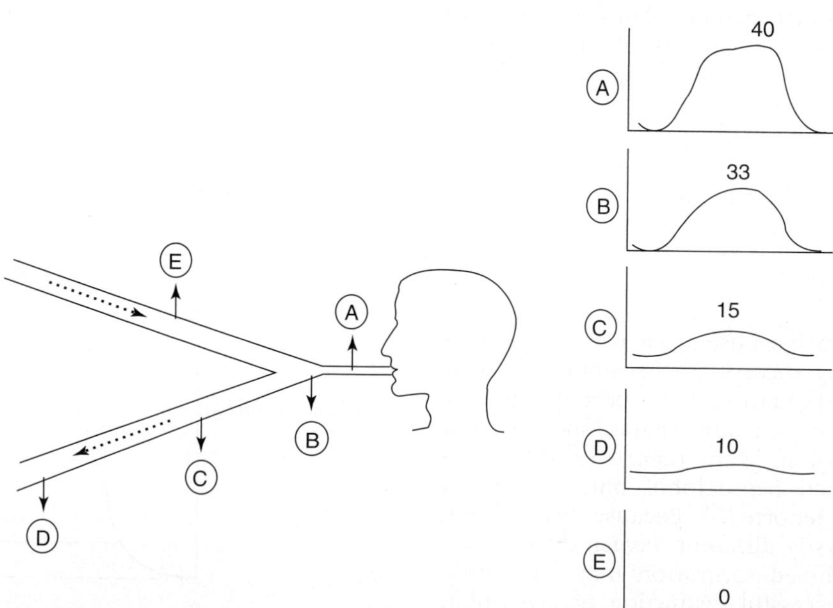

FIGURE 38–4 • Accuracy of end-tidal CO_2 measurements is highly dependent on obtaining good samples of expiratory gas from the patient. If sampled gas is contaminated with fresh gas from the breathing circuit, the measured values will not be accurate. The best samples are obtained from a site nearest to the source of CO_2, the patient (point *A*).

the classic "sidestream" capnometer. In a distal-diverting system, gas is sampled from the airway and transported to the CO_2 monitor, which is located in the display unit distal to the patient.

The accuracy of the capnogram, the $Petco_2$ measurements, and the displayed values depends on the sampling site (Figure 38–4). In continuous gas flow circuits, sampling in or at the endotracheal tube results in the most accurate values because there is little contamination with fresh gas from the breathing circuit (point A). The Y-connector of the breathing circuit is the next best sampling site (point B). However, if the fresh gas flow is large compared with the expiratory flow rate of the patient (as may be the case in neonates and small children), the capnogram and the $Petco_2$ values may be distorted as a result of dilution with the fresh gas flowing through the Y-connector. If gas is sampled "downstream" from the patient, the waveform and $Petco_2$ are increasingly diluted by fresh gas from the circuit (points C and D). If gas is sampled "upstream" from the patient in the fresh gas supply, none of the exhaled CO_2 is detected and the measured $Petco_2$ is zero (point E). Therefore the best sampling site is within the patient's endotracheal tube or at the tube connector, as far as possible from the Y-connector of the breathing circuit.[57]

In breathing circuits with intermittent flow (demand-valve ventilators) and in larger children with large exhaled tidal volumes, the capnogram and $Petco_2$ values usually are unaffected by minor changes in sampling location. If the tidal volume is small (e.g., as in infants and children) and the sample flow rate is large (i.e., >150 ml/min), the capnogram and $Petco_2$ measurements may be significantly diluted by the entrainment of fresh gas. Using a capnometer system with a low sample flow rate, typically less than 75 ml/min, restores the waveform and $Petco_2$ readings to more accurate values.

Dead-Space Ventilation

Dead space is the volume of gas in the airways and lung that participates in tidal breathing but does not participate in gas exchange. Obvious examples are the volume of the endotracheal tube and ventilator circuit (apparatus dead space) and the volume of the tracheal lumen and central airways (anatomic dead space). A less obvious but still an important source of error in critically ill patients is alveolar or physiologic dead space. This dead space is attributable to lung units in which ventilation greatly exceeds perfusion. Because perfusion to these lung units is inadequate, gas exchange in these overventilated, underperfused lung units is less efficient than normal.

Dead space (V_D/V_T) can be determined from a variant of the Bohr equation:

$$V_D/V_T = (Paco_2 - Petco_2)/Paco_2, \quad (4)$$

or

$$V_D/V_T = 1 - (Petco_2/Paco_2), \quad (5)$$

where $Petco_2$ is equal to use to calculate total (apparatus + anatomic + physiologic) dead-space fraction of tidal volume.

TABLE 38–1

Clinical Conditions Associated with Abnormalities in $ETco_2$

Increases in $ETco_2$
Sudden
Sudden increase in cardiac output
Release of a tourniquet
Injection of sodium bicarbonate
Gradual
Hypoventilation
Increased metabolism (carbon dioxide production)
Decreases in $ETco_2$
Sudden
Sudden hyperventilation
Sudden decrease in cardiac output
Massive pulmonary embolism
Air embolism
Ventilator disconnection
Ventilator circuit leakage
Obstruction of the endotracheal tube
Gradual
Hyperventilation
Decrease in metabolism (carbon dioxide production)
Decreased pulmonary perfusion
Absent $ETco_2$
Esophageal intubation
Accidental extubation

Modified from Tobin M: *JAMA* 264:244-251, 1990.

The peak value of CO_2 during exhalation is defined as end-tidal CO_2. In many clinical situations, dead-space ventilation is an appreciable fraction of tidal breathing, including severe respiratory dysfunction,[58] pulmonary hypoperfusion, pulmonary thromboembolism, and cardiac arrest (Table 38–1). In these conditions, the clinician using a capnometer may see a large arterial to end-tidal Pco_2 gradient (typically >10 mmHg). This gradient can be used as an indicator of severity of disease, and $Petco_2$ can be used to evaluate trends rather than a specific measure of alveolar Pco_2.

Differential Diagnosis of Abnormal Capnograms

The capnogram probably is the single most reliable and effective monitor for the presence of pulmonary ventilation. The integrity and function of both the patient's cardiopulmonary system and the breathing circuit are reflected by the capnogram, and malfunctions often can be detected by changes in the capnogram.[56,59]

Gradually Decreasing End-Tidal CO_2 Concentration

When the capnogram retains its normal morphology but there is a slow, progressive drop in $ETco_2$ (Figure 38–5), the possible causes include falling body temperature, slowly decreasing systemic or pulmonary perfusion, and hyperventilation. Sedation and neuromuscular blockade attenuate the normal body mechanisms for generating heat to preserve body temperature. As body temperature falls,

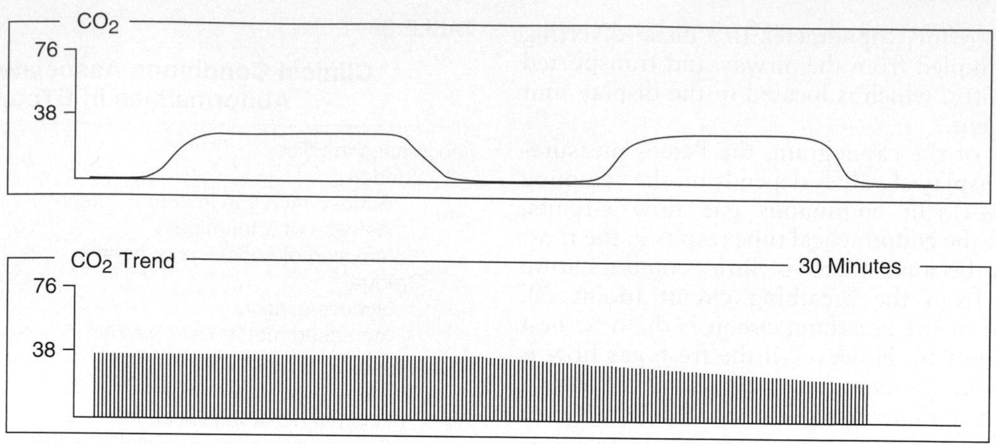

FIGURE 38–5 • Slow, progressive fall in end-tidal CO_2 occurs when CO_2 elimination exceeds CO_2 production or wasted ventilation increases slowly.

the patient's rate of metabolism and CO_2 production also fall. If ventilation is controlled and kept constant as body temperature decreases, alveolar CO_2 concentration and arterial P_{CO_2} decrease. This is reflected in the capnogram as a slow decrease in Pet_{CO_2} over many minutes. Another cause of decreasing Pet_{CO_2} is a fall in total body perfusion associated with blood loss or cardiovascular depression. As systemic and pulmonary perfusion crease, alveolar dead space increases with a resultant fall in Pet_{CO_2}.

Sustained Low End-Tidal CO_2 Concentrations without Plateaus

Occasionally, with no apparent malfunctions in the breathing circuit or in the patient's cardiopulmonary status, the capnogram shows sustained low Pet_{CO_2} values without a good alveolar plateau. In this situation, Pet_{CO_2} is not a good estimate of alveolar P_{CO_2}. The absence of a good alveolar plateau suggests that either full exhalation is not occurring before the beginning of the next breath or the patient's tidal volume is being diluted with fresh gas because of a small tidal volume, high aspirating sample rate, or high fresh gas dilution from the circuit. Several maneuvers are available to distinguish between these possibilities.

Incomplete emptying of the lungs may be suggested by adventitial sounds such as wheezing or large airway rhonchi with compromise of small airway patency caused by bronchospasm or secretions. If rhonchi are present, tracheal suctioning often corrects the partial obstruction and restores full exhalation. Bronchospasm may be treated with a variety of bronchodilators. An endotracheal tube that is kinked or partially obstructed by secretions may prevent full exhalation. Passing a suction catheter down the endotracheal tube usually confirms or eliminates this possibility. Gently squeezing the child's chest to assist with a forced exhalation often produces a waveform in which the CO_2 concentration continues to rise toward an alveolar plateau. If the plateau is present, the "squeeze end-tidal CO_2" value may be taken as a good estimate of alveolar CO_2 concentration.

When no signs of partial airway obstruction are present, another explanation for this type of capnographic waveform should be considered. In infants and other patients who have small tidal volumes, the aspirating sample rate may exceed the expiratory flow rate near the end of exhalation. When this occurs, the aspirating sample is diluted with fresh gas from the breathing circuit, resulting in a dropoff of the plateau and a fall in Pet_{CO_2} secondary to dilution. Reducing the flow rate of fresh gas or moving the sampling site closer to the endotracheal tube connector usually corrects the problem. In very small newborns, a sample rate of 100 to 250 ml/min may be too high to result in good plateaus despite instituting the preceding corrective measures. Then either a capnographic system having a very low sampling rate (50 ml/min) can be used or the capnogram can be used as a gross monitor of the integrity of the ventilatory circuit and trends in cardiopulmonary function rather than as an accurate estimate of alveolar ventilation.

Sustained Low End-Tidal CO_2 Concentration with Good Plateaus

In some circumstances, the capnogram demonstrates a low Pet_{CO_2} with a widened (a-et)ΔP_{CO_2} and preservation of a good alveolar plateau. This discrepancy may indicate that the capnograph is malfunctioning or miscalibrated. The clinician can evaluate this by sampling his or her own exhaled CO_2 and verifying that the Pet_{CO_2} concentration is between 5% and 6% (equivalent to approximately 38–46 mmHg). If the instrument is functioning properly and is well calibrated, a wide (a-et)ΔP_{CO_2} is an indication of excessive dead-space ventilation in the patient.

Exponential Decrease in End-Tidal CO_2

An exponential drop in Pet_{CO_2} that occurs within a short time (e.g., a dozen or so breaths) almost always signals a sudden and probably catastrophic event in the patient's cardiopulmonary system (Figure 38–6). The basis for this capnogram is a sudden and dramatic increase in

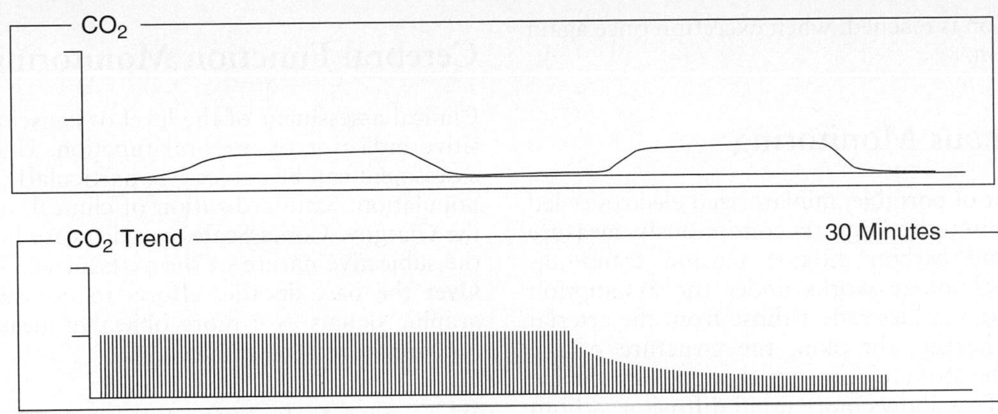

FIGURE 38–6 • Sudden, exponential decay in end-tidal CO_2 values almost always signals a potential catastrophe in the cardiopulmonary function of the child. The causative factor is a dramatic increase in wasted ventilation or dead space. Possible causative events include sudden hypotension such as that resulting from massive blood loss, circulatory arrest with continued pulmonary ventilation, and pulmonary embolism with thrombus or air.

alveolar dead-space ventilation. Possible causes include sudden hypovolemia, circulatory arrest with continued pulmonary ventilation, and pulmonary embolus with thrombus or air. Only after ruling out these catastrophic events and determining that the patient is hemodynamically stable should more mundane explanations for the exponential decay in $PetCO_2$ be considered. The most common noncatastrophic cause is an accidental increase in ventilation attributable to an incorrect ventilator adjustment, resulting in a gradual decrease in $PetCO_2$. However, it is important to note that even doubling the alveolar ventilation decreases the $PetCO_2$ to only half of the preadjustment value, not to the near-zero values that may accompany catastrophic cardiopulmonary events.

Gradual Increase in Both Baseline and End-Tidal CO_2

A gradual rise in both baseline and $ETCO_2$ value indicates previously exhaled CO_2 is being rebreathed from the circuit (Figure 38–7). In this situation, the inspiratory portion of the capnogram fails to reach the zero baseline, and there may actually be a premature rise in CO_2 concentration during the inspiratory phase of ventilation. $PetCO_2$ usually increases until a new equilibrium alveolar

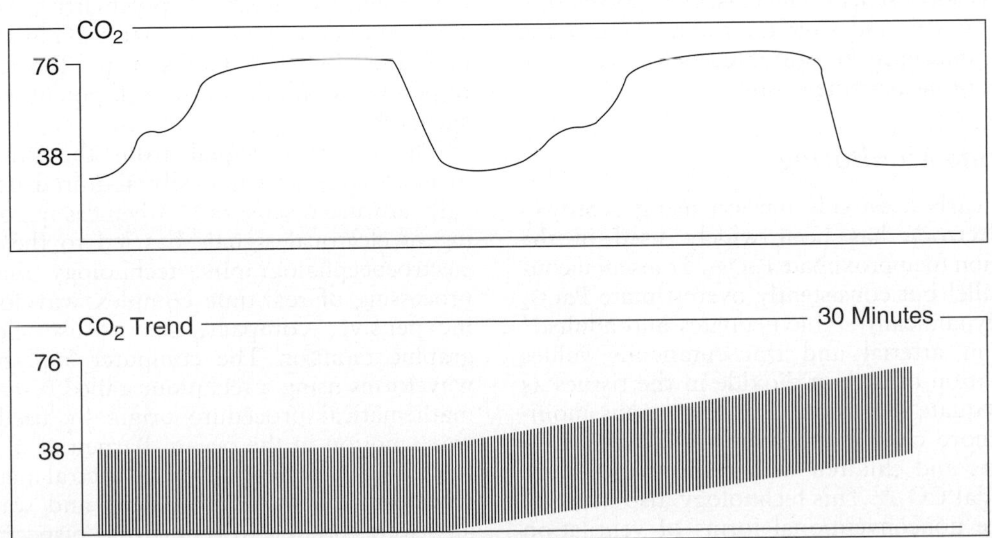

FIGURE 38–7 • Persistent elevation of the inspired CO_2 baseline and a rising end-tidal CO_2 value suggest that the child is rebreathing previously exhaled CO_2. In the intensive care unit, this pattern is often seen when the fresh gas supply to a breathing circuit becomes disconnected from the source.

CO_2 concentration is reached, when excretion once again equals production.

Transcutaneous Monitoring

The development of portable, miniaturized electrodes led to the use of this technology to continuously measure both oxygen and carbon dioxide tension transcutaneously. This technology works under the assumption that transcutaneous values reflect those from the arterial circulation. By heating the skin, the structure of the lipoproteins in the stratum corneum change from the gel to the sol state. This allows more rapid diffusion of both oxygen and carbon dioxide from the subcutaneous tissues to the surface of the electrode. However, the heating affects both tissue and blood by decreasing oxygen solubility, shifting the oxyhemoglobin dissociation curve to the right, and dilating local arterioles. Temperatures of 44°C to 45°C increase diffusion and prevent vasoconstriction in the local area of the skin.[60]

Oxygen Monitoring

Transcutaneous Clarke electrodes measure oxygen tension in a local segment of the heated skin. Because skin is the organ most responsive to adrenomedullary induced vasoconstriction, local oxygen tension may not be the same in all skin segments or other tissues. In essence, transcutaneous oxygen tension is only an indirect reflection of arterial oxygen tension; it is directly related to local tissue perfusion and oxygenation. Studies in both neonates and adults show that transcutaneous oxygen tension reflects PaO_2 in hemodynamically stable conditions but is appreciably lower than PaO_2 in patients with significant circulatory problems.

This technology has several limitations. Electrode placement must be changed every 4 to 6 hours to prevent thermal injury to the site of measurement or when readings become unstable. A thermal neutral environment to limit peripheral vasoconstriction increases the correlation between transcutaneous and arterial tensions. Finally, the electrode membranes must be calibrated before each use and each change of measurement site.

Carbon Dioxide Monitoring

Transcutaneous carbon dioxide tension using a Stowe-Severinghaus electrode has been widely used in the neonatal population to approximate $PaCO_2$. Transcutaneous CO_2 values parallel but consistently overestimate $PaCO_2$ values in hemodynamically stable neonates and adults.[61] The difference in arterial and transcutaneous values reflects accumulation of carbon dioxide in the tissues as a result of inadequate perfusion. Transcutaneous monitoring of CO_2 more closely approximates arterial CO_2 tension in infants and children with respiratory failure than does end-tidal CO_2.[62] This technology also is useful in settings where nonconventional forms of ventilation (high-frequency ventilation) preclude the use of end-tidal monitoring.

Cerebral Function Monitoring

Clinical assessment of the level of consciousness is a sensitive indicator of cerebral function. Unfortunately, the assessment can be subjective, particularly in the pediatric population. Standardization of clinical methods, such as the Glasgow Coma Scale, can decrease but not eliminate the subjective nature of the assessment of consciousness. Over the past decade, efforts to use electroencephalographic signals as a more objective measure of cerebral function have been pursued.

Bispectral Index Monitoring

The bispectral index (BIS) monitor is a recently developed form of processed electroencephalogram (EEG) that integrates various electroencephalographic descriptors, as an assessment of the brain response to hypnotic agents, into a single unitless number on a scale from 0 to 100. The technology processes and evaluates via fast Fourier transform analysis the common characteristic changes and waveform relationships that are seen on the EEG in response to the administration of sedative, hypnotic, and anesthetic agents. The development of this technology, which received FDA approval in 1996, was specifically directed toward the ability to measure or quantify these changes as they occurred in the target organ, the brain.

Historical Perspective and Development of the Electroencephalogram

Attempts to monitor the brain have a long history. Dr. Richard Caton, an English physician, described the first recognition of the EEG while mapping brain waves in animals.[63] The physiologic basis for the origin of the EEG potentials comes from the extracellular current flows associated with postsynaptic activity in the upper layers of the cerebral cortex.[64] A psychiatrist, Dr. Hans Berger, went on to describe the human EEG in a series of reports in 1929.[65] In 1937, Gibbs et al. reported that the EEG responded to administration of potent inhaled anesthetic agents.[66]

The electrical signal from the brain is measured in microvolts and is easily acquired using technologically advanced sensors.[67] Advances in computer processing of electrical signals has led to the development of electroencephalographic technology that allows rapid processing of real-time complex waveforms in a small, inexpensive, compact, easy-to-use electroencephalographic monitor. The computer analyzes the complex waveforms using a technique called *bispectral analysis,* a mathematical procedure originally used for describing wave motion in the ocean. Barnett et al.[68] described the first clinical applications of bispectral analysis of the EEG waveform during natural sleep and waking. Kearse et al.[69] were the first to report that bispectral analysis may predict anesthetic depth during narcotic induction of anesthesia.

Age-Related Maturation of the Electroencephalogram

Development of the normal EEG in infants and young children parallels brain maturation, with the most abrupt changes occurring between the early premature age and the first 3 months of life. Synapse formation continues after birth up to age 5, with the majority occurring (with gradual loss of neonatal patterns) in the first 3 months of life.[70] There are wide variations and developmental differences in the EEG of infants and children because of progressive development of the immature brain. Developmental maturation of the pediatric EEG, including changes in the power and frequency, progresses to that of the adult pattern in late adolescence. However, data on EEG changes produced by anesthetic drugs in the pediatric population are not available.[70,71] Bispectral index monitoring has yet to be validated for all pediatric patient age groups, particularly as age-related maturation differences in the EEG may affect the BIS algorithm.[72] Some evidence supports the validity of the algorithm in infants, but further studies in children younger than 1 year are needed.

Validation Studies

The BIS is a continuous form of complex processed EEG derived parameter, which has been validated in adults as a quantifiable, objective measure of the sedative, hypnotic drug effect on the central nervous system.[67,73] It has been shown to correlate with loss of consciousness, recall, and return to consciousness during general anesthesia. Glass et al.[74] established the strong correlation between the BIS value and level of sedation, as quantified by the Modified Observer's Assessment of Sedation Scale (MOAA/S). This same study also demonstrated the correlation between BIS values and measured plasma concentrations of propofol, alfentanil, midazolam, and isoflurane. They also tested for responsiveness and memory recall at targeted plasma concentrations and were able to determine the relationship between the BIS value and the probability of response to command and recall. These findings were confirmed in a subsequent study.[75]

Several studies have attempted to determine the clinical validity in infants and children; however, methods used to validate BIS performance in adults are difficult to replicate in children. The BIS range guidelines were developed based largely on responsiveness and recall data that were obtained from studies of adult volunteers who were maintained at various steady-state plasma concentrations of anesthetic, hypnotic agents. These studies cannot easily be conducted in children. The first report comparing the dose responses of sevoflurane to BIS values in infants and children scheduled for elective surgery showed that both pediatric and adult populations had awake BIS values between 90 and 100 that decreased precipitously after induction of anesthesia.[76] A second study found that the correlation between BIS and end-tidal sevoflurane concentration in children is very similar to that observed in adults.[77] No differences in BIS values between infants (0–2 years) and children (2–12 years) at similar clinical levels of anesthesia were seen. An end-tidal concentration-response difference between the two age groups is consistent with existing data regarding minimum alveolar concentration required to prevent movement with stimulus. The same age-related difference has been demonstrated for halothane minimum alveolar concentration.[78]

Utility Studies

The utility of the BIS as a clinical parameter to measure the depth of sedation or hypnosis has been well established through a multitude of adult clinical studies using inhalation anesthesia.[75,79] The titration of propofol to a specific BIS range during surgery resulted in a wide range of patient benefits compared with a standard practice (non-BIS–titrated) group. These benefits included a reduction in the amount of anesthetic agent used, faster emergence and shorter time to postanesthesia care unit (PACU) discharge eligibility, and higher levels of patient orientation on arrival in the PACU as assessed by blinded observers. Similar results were achieved in a variety of studies conducted using all of the commonly administered anesthetic, hypnotic agents.[80–82]

A growing number of observational and clinical utility studies in the pediatric population have demonstrated promising results with use of the current BIS algorithm in both infants and children. Experience to date suggests that BIS monitoring in children and infants provides similar benefits as those achieved in the adult population, with respect to improved sedative, hypnotic drug administration and recovery profiles.[83–85] However, not all agree. A subsequent study showed a weaker correlation between BIS and sevoflurane concentration in infants.[86] During scoliosis surgery, BIS was used as a predictor of voluntary patient movement to verbal command.[72] These investigators in a separate study recorded BIS values at various clinical endpoints during cardiac surgery with cardiopulmonary bypass in children and found results similar to those observed in adults.[87] A later study revealed large interpatient variability of BIS at different levels of anesthetic depth, which may limit the applicability of BIS to pediatric anesthesia.[88]

Summary of Bispectral Index Related Studies in Critical Care

After the clinical introduction of BIS into operating rooms, this technology naturally found its way into the ICU. Numerous studies in both adults and children have been published. Initial reports in both populations suggested good correlation between objective sedation scores and BIS.[89,90] One such study in children showed that the BIS and COMFORT scale measurements were highly correlated ($R^2 = 0.89$).[91] Others demonstrated a strong correlation between the Ramsay Sedation Score and BIS in nonparalyzed children for sedation monitoring.[92] They also noted the inadequacy of the Ramsay Sedation Score and bedside nursing assessment in the presence of chemical paralysis in their ability to recognize adequate or inadequate sedation states accurately. Others found the correlation between sedation scores and BIS was suboptimal and inconsistent in the heterogeneous ICU population.[93,94] Reliance on the BIS as the sole monitor of sedation may result in excessive sedation, primarily because of high levels of muscular activity.[95]

Although BIS monitoring is a well-established clinical parameter in the adult surgical population, its use and application in the critical care and pediatric arenas is still under investigation. Unfortunately, validation studies are very unlikely to ever be attempted in children. Several preliminary clinical studies of BIS monitoring in both the operating room and the ICU have demonstrated possible clinical utility and efficacy for improved sedation titration, decreased drug usage, strong sedation score correlation, and greater accuracy and reliability in sedation assessment for paralyzed children.

Conclusion

Noninvasive monitors, such as pulse oximetry and capnometry, have become standards of care in the critical care environment. Thus it becomes important to understand key clinical and technical issues that determine how these instruments can be used most effectively. These noninvasive technologies provide early warning of potential catastrophic events and facilitate early intervention. Concerns for complications related to invasive monitors will continue to drive the search for newer and better devices for noninvasive physiologic monitoring and will enlarge even more the "safety net" of vital monitoring.

REFERENCES

1. Sanford TJ, Jones BR, Ty Smith N: Noninvasive blood pressure measurement. *Anesth Clin North Am* 6:721, 1988.
2. Ramsey M III: Noninvasive blood pressure monitoring methods and validation. In Gravenstein JS, Newbauer RS, Ream AK, et al, editors: *Essential noninvasive monitoring in anesthesia.* Orlando, 1980, Grune & Stratton.
3. Friesen RJ, Lichtor JL: Indirect measurement of blood pressure in neonates and infants utilizing an automatic noninvasive oscillometric monitor. *Anesth Analg* 60:742, 1981.
4. Kimble KJ, Darnall RA, Yelderman M: An automated oscillometric technique for estimating arterial pressure in critically ill newborns. *Anesthesiology,* 54:423, 1981.
5. Park MK, Menard SM: Accuracy of blood pressure measurement by the Dinamap monitor in infants and children. *Pediatrics* 79:907, 1987.
6. Betts EK: Hazards of automatic noninvasive blood pressure monitoring. *Anesthesiology* 55:717, 1981.
7. Waltemath CL, Preuss DD: Determination of blood pressure in low-flow states by the Doppler technique. *Anesthesiology* 34:77, 1971.
8. Burch GE, Shewey L: Sphygmomanometric cuff size and blood pressure recordings. *JAMA* 225:1215, 1973.
9. Du Bois EF: *Fever and the regulation of body temperature.* Springfield, Ill, 1948, Charles C. Thomas.
10. Cork RC, Vaughan RW, Humphrey LS: Precision and accuracy of intraoperative temperature monitoring. *Anesth Analg* 62:211, 1983.
11. Iaizzo PA, Kehler CH, Zink RS, et al: Thermal response in acute porcine malignant hyperthermia. *Anesth Analg* 82:782, 1996.
12. Tremper KK: Pulse oximetry's final frontier. *Crit Care Med* 28: 1684-1685, 2000.
13 Stoneham MD, Saville GM, Wilson IH: Knowledge about pulse oximetry among medical and nursing staff. *Lancet* 344: 1339-1342, 1994.
14. Kruger PS, Longden PJ: A study of a hospital staff's knowledge of pulse oximetry. *Anaesth Intensive Care* 25:38-41, 1997.
15. Aoyagi T, Miyasaka K: Pulse oximetry: its invention, contribution to medicine, and future tasks. *Anesth Analg* 94:S1-S3, 2002.
16. Goldman JM, Petterson MT, Kopotic RJ, Barker SJ: Masimo signal extraction pulse oximetry. *J Clin Monit Comput* 16:475-483, 2000.
17. Alexander CM, Teller LE, Gross JB: Principles of pulse oximetry: theoretical and practical considerations. *Anesth Analg* 68: 368-376, 1989.
18. Morris RW, Nairn M, Torda TA: A comparison of fifteen pulse oximeters. part I: a clinical comparison; part II: a test of performance under conditions of poor perfusion. *Anaesth Intensive Care* 17:62-73, 1989.
19. Praud JP, Carofilis A, Bridey F, et al: Accuracy of two wavelength pulse oximetry in neonates and infants. *Pediatr Pulmonol* 6:180-182, 1989.
20. Severinghaus JW, Naifeh KH: Accuracy of response of six pulse oximeters to profound hypoxia. *Anesthesiology* 67:551-558, 1987.
21. Van de Louw A, Cracco C, Cerf C, et al: Accuracy of pulse oximetry in the intensive care unit. *Intensive Care Med* 27: 1606-1613, 2001.
22. van Oostrom, JH, Melker RJ: Comparative testing of pulse oximeter probes. *Anesth Analg* 98:1354-1358, 2004.
23. Hornberger C, Matz H, Konecny E, et al: Design and validation of a pulse oximeter calibrator. *Anesth Analg* 94:S8-S12, 2002.
24. Kastle SW, Konecny E: Determining the artifact sensitivity of recent pulse oximeters during laboratory benchmarking. *J Clin Monit Comput* 16:509-522, 2000.
25. Weininger S: Designing a pulse oximeter safety standard. *Anesth Analg* 94:S4-S7, 2002.
26. Iyer P, McDougall P, Loughnan P, et al: Accuracy of pulse oximetry in hypothermic neonates and infants undergoing cardiac surgery. *Crit Care Med* 24:507-511, 1996.
27. Nickerson BG, Sarkisian C, Tremper K: Bias and precision of pulse oximeters and arterial oximeters. *Chest* 93:515-517, 1988.
28. Walsh MC, Noble LM, Carlo WA, Martin RJ: Relationship of pulse oximetry to arterial oxygen tension in infants. *Crit Care Med* 15:1102-1105, 1987.
29. Bohnhorst B, Peter CS, Poets CF: Pulse oximeters' reliability in detecting hypoxemia and bradycardia: comparison between a conventional and two new generation oximeters. *Crit Care Med.* 28:1565-1568, 2000.
30. Carter BG, Carlin JB, Tibballs J, et al: Accuracy of two pulse oximeters at low arterial hemoglobin-oxygen saturation. *Crit Care Med* 26:1128-1133, 1998.
31. Fanconi S: Reliability of pulse oximetry in hypoxic infants. *J Pediatr* 112:424-427, 1988.
32. Barker SJ: "Motion-resistant" pulse oximetry: a comparison of new and old models. *Anesth Analg* 95:967-972, 2002.
33. Barker SJ, Shah NK: The effects of motion on the performance of pulse oximeters in volunteers (revised publication). *Anesthesiology* 86:101-108, 1997.
34. Malviya S, Reynolds PI, Voepel-Lewis T, et al: False alarms and sensitivity of conventional pulse oximetry versus the Masimo SET technology in the pediatric postanesthesia care unit. *Anesth Analg* 90:1336-1340, 2000.
35. Trivedi NS, Ghouri AF, Shah NK, et al: Effects of motion, ambient light, and hypoperfusion on pulse oximeter function. *J Clin Anesth* 9:179-183, 1997.
36. Reynolds KJ, Palayiwa E, Moyle JT, et al: The effect of dyshemoglobins on pulse oximetry: part I, theoretical approach and part II, experimental results using an in vitro test system. *J Clin Monit* 9:81-90, 1993.
37. Watcha MF, Connor MT, Hing AV: Pulse oximetry in methemoglobinemia. *Am J Dis Child* 143:845-847, 1989.
38. Hampson NB: Pulse oximetry in severe carbon monoxide poisoning. *Chest* 114:1036-1041, 1998.
39. Harris AP, Sendak MJ, Donham RT, et al: Absorption characteristics of human fetal hemoglobin at wavelengths used in pulse oximetry. *J Clin Monit* 4:175-177, 1988.
40. Ralston AC, Webb RK, Runciman WB: Potential errors in pulse oximetry. III: Effects of interferences, dyes, dyshaemoglobins and other pigments. *Anaesthesia* 46:291-295, 1991.
41. Fluck RR Jr, Schroeder C, Frani G, et al: Does ambient light affect the accuracy of pulse oximetry? *Respir Care* 48:677-680, 2003.

42. Cheng EY, Hopwood MB, Kay J: Forehead pulse oximetry compared with finger pulse oximetry and arterial blood gas measurement. *J Clin Monit* 4:223-226, 1988.
43. Dassel AC, Graaff R, Meijer A, et al: Reflectance pulse oximetry at the forehead of newborns: the influence of varying pressure on the probe. *J Clin Monit* 12:421-428, 1996.
44. Kyriacou PA, Powell S, Langford RM, Jones DP: Esophageal pulse oximetry utilizing reflectance photoplethysmography. *IEEE Trans Biomed Eng* 49:1360-1368, 2002.
45. Ramirez FC, Padda S, Medlin S, et al: Reflectance spectrophotometry in the gastrointestinal tract: limitations and new applications. *Am J Gastroenterol* 97:2780-2784, 2002.
46. Vicenzi MN, Gombotz H, Krenn H, et al: Transesophageal versus surface pulse oximetry in intensive care unit patients. *Crit Care Med* 28:2268-2270, 2000.
47. Andropoulos DB, Stayer SA, Diaz LK, Ramamoorthy C: Neurological monitoring for congenital heart surgery. *Anesth Analg* 99:1365-1375, 2004.
48. Haitsma IK, Maas AI: Advanced monitoring in the intensive care unit: brain tissue oxygen tension. *Curr Opin Crit Care* 8: 115-120, 2002.
49. Boushel R, Piantadosi CA: Near-infrared spectroscopy for monitoring muscle oxygenation. *Acta Physiol Scand* 168:615-622, 2000.
50. Schenkman KA, Marble DR, Burns DH, Feigl EO: Myoglobin oxygen dissociation by multiwavelength spectroscopy. *J Appl Physiol* 82:86-92, 1997.
51. Schenkman KA, Marble DR, Burns DH, Feigl EO: Optical spectroscopic method for in vivo measurement of cardiac myoglobin oxygen saturation. *Appl Spectrosc* 53:332-338, 1999.
52. Schenkman KA, Marble DR, Feigl EO, Burns DH: Near-infrared spectroscopic measurement of myoglobin oxygen saturation in the presence of hemoglobin using partial least-squares analysis. *Appl Spectrosc* 53:325-331, 1999.
53. Marcinek DJ, Ciesielski WA, Conley KE, Schenkman KA: Oxygen regulation and limitation to cellular respiration in mouse skeletal muscle in vivo. *Am J Physiol Heart Circ Physiol* 285:H1900-H1908, 2003.
54. Marcinek DJ, Schenkman KA, Ciesielski WA, Conley KE: Mitochondrial coupling in vivo in mouse skeletal muscle. *Am J Physiol Cell Physiol* 286:C457-C463, 2004.
55. Schenkman KA, Beard DA, Ciesielski WA, Feigl EO: Comparison of buffer and red blood cell perfusion of guinea pig heart oxygenation. *Am J Physiol Heart Circ Physiol* 285:H1819-H1825, 2003.
56. Swedlow DB: Capnometry and capnography: the anesthesia disaster warning system. *Semin Anesth* 5:194, 1986.
57. Gravenstein N, Lampotang S, Beneken J: Factors influencing capnography in the Bain circuit. *J Clin Monit* 1:6, 1985.
58. Yamanaka M, Sue D: Comparison of arterial-end-tidal Pco_2 difference and dead space/tidal volume ratio in respiratory failure. *Chest* 92:832, 1987.
59. St John RE: Exhaled gas analysis. Technical and clinical aspects of capnography and oxygen consumption. *Crit Care Nurs Clin North Am* 1:669, 1989.
60. Tremper KK, Waxman K, Shoemaker WC: Transcutaneous oxygen monitoring of critically ill adults with and without low flow shock. *Crit Care Med* 7:526-531, 1979.
61. Tremper KK, Shoemaker WC, Shippy CR, et al: Transcutaneous PCO_2 monitoring in adults patients in the ICU and operating room. *Crit Care Med* 9:752-755, 1981.
62. Tobias JD, Meyer DJ: Noninvasive monitoring of carbon dioxide during respiratory failure in toddlers and infants: end-tidal versus transcutaneous carbon dioxide. *Anesth Analg* 85:55-58, 1997.
63. Caton R: The electric currents of the brain. *BJM* 2:278, 1875.
64. Martin JH: The collective electrical behavior of cortical neurons: the electroencephalogram and the mechanisms of epilepsy. In Kandel ER, Schwartz JH, Jessell TM, editors: *Principles of neural science*, ed 3. New York, 1991, Elsevier.
65. Berger H: Uber das elektroekephalogramm des menchen. *Arch Pyschiat Nervenkr* 87:527-570, 1929.
66. Gibbs FA, Gibbs EL, Lennox WG: Effect on the electroencephalogram of certain drugs which influence nervous activity. *Arch Internal Med* 60;154-166, 1937.
67. Rampil IJ: A primer for EEG signal processing in anesthesia. *Anesthesiology* 89:980-1002, 1998.
68. Barnett TP, Johnson LC, Naitoh P, et al: Bispectrum analysis of electroencephalogram signals during waking and sleeping. *Science* 172:401-402, 1971.
69. Kearse LA, Manberg P, DeBros F, et al: Bispectral analysis of electroencephalogram during induction may predict hemodynamic responses to laryngoscopy and intubation. *Electroenecephalography Clin Neurophysiol* 90:194-200, 1994.
70. Witte H, Putsche P, Eiselt M, et al: Multimodal time-variant signal analysis of neonatal EEG burst patterns. *Medinfo* 9(pt 2): 1250-1254, 1998.
71. Eeg-Olofsson O: Longitudinal developmental course of electrical activity of brain. *Brain Dev* 2:33-44, 1980.
72. Brustowicz RM, Bacsik J, Sullivan L, et al: The bispectral index and explicit recall during the intraoperative wake-up test for scoliosis surgery. Anesth Analg 94:1474-1478, 2002.
73. Sigl J, Chamoun N: An introduction to bispectral analysis for the EEG. J Clin Monit 10:392-404, 1994.
74. Glass PSA, Bloom M, Kearse L, et al: Bispectral analysis measures sedation and memory effects of propofol, midazolam, isoflurane and alfentanil in healthy volunteers. Anesthesiology 86:836-847, 1997.
75. Vernon JM, Lang E, Sebel P, Manberg P: Prediction of movement using bispectral electroencephalographic analysis during propofol/alfentanil anesthesia. Anesth Analg 80:780-785, 1995.
76. Denman WT, Swanson EL, Rosow D, et al: Pediatric evaluation of the bispectral index (BIS) with end-tidal sevoflurane concentrations in infants and children. Anesth Analg 90:872-877, 2000.
77. Katoh T, Suzuki A, Ikeda K: Electroencephalographic derivatives as a tool for predicting the depth of sedation and anesthesia induced by sevoflurane. Anesthesiology 88:642-650, 1998.
78. Gregory GA, Eger EI II, Munson ES: The relationship between age and halothane requirement in man. Anesthesiology 30:488-491, 1969.
79. Sebel PS, Lang E, Rampil IJ, et al: A multicenter study of the bispectral electroencephalogram analysis for monitoring anesthetic effect. Anesth Analg 84:891-899, 1997.
80. Flaishon R, Windsor A, Sigl J, Sebel PS: Recovery of consciousness after thiopental or propofol. Anesthesiology 86: 613-619, 1997.
81. Gan TJ, Glass PS, Windsor A, et al: Bispectral index monitoring allows faster emergence and improved recovery from propofol, alfentanil, and nitrous oxide anesthesia. Anesthesiology 87: 808-815, 1997.
82. Song D, Joshi G, White PF: Titration of volatile anesthetics using bispectral index facilitates recovery after ambulatory anesthesia. Anesthesiology 87:842-848, 1997.
83. Bannister C, Brosius K, Meyer B: The effect of BIS monitoring on emergence, PACU discharge and anesthetic utilization in children receiving sevoflurane anesthesia. Anesth Analg 92:877-881, 2001.
84. Degoute, CS, Macabeo C, Dubreuil C, et al: EEG bispectral index and hypnotic component of anaesthesia induced by sevoflurane: comparison between children and adults. Br J Anaesth 86: 209-212, 2001.
85. Wallenborn L, Radow L, Wild DO: BIS monitoring in children: volatile induction and maintenance of anaesthesia versus total intravenous anaesthesia. Paediatr Anaesth 12:91-102, 2002.
86. Davidson AJ, McCann M, Prabhakar D, et al: The differences in the bispectral index between infants and children during emergence from anesthesia after circumcision surgery. Anesth Analg 93:326-330, 2001.
87. Laussen PC, Murphy JA, Zurakowski D, et al: Bispectral index monitoring in children during mild hypothermic cardiopulmonary bypass. Paediatr Anaesth 11:567-573, 2001.
88. Rodriguez RA, Hall LE, Duggan S, Splinter WM: The bispectral index does not correlate with clinical signs of inhalational anesthesia during sevoflurane induction and arousal in children. Can J Anaesth 51:411-416, 2004.
89. Courtman SP, Wardurgh A, Petros AJ: Comparison of the bispectral index monitor with the Comfort score in assessing level of sedation of critically ill children. Intensive Care Med 29: 2239-2246, 2003.
90. Berkenbosch JW, Fichter CR, Tobias JD: The correlation of the bispectral index monitor with clinical sedation scores during mechanical ventilation in the pediatric intensive care unit. Anesth Analg 94:506-511, 2002.

91. Crain N, Slonim A, Pollack M: Assessing sedation in the pediatric intensive care unit by using BIS and the COMFORT scale. Pediatr Crit Care Med 3:11-14, 2002.
92. Aneja R, Heard AM, Fletcher JE, Heard CM: Sedation monitoring of children by the bispectral index in the pediatric intensive care unit. Pediatr Crit Care Med 4:60-64, 2003.
93. Frenzel D, Greim CA, Sommer C, et al: Is the bispectral index appropriate for monitoring the sedation level of mechanically ventilated surgical ICU patients? Intensive Care Med 28:178-183, 2002.
94. Nasraway SA Jr, Wu EC, Kelleher RM, et al: How reliable is the bispectral index in critically ill patients? A prospective, comparative, single-blinded observer study. Crit Care Med 30:1483-1487, 2002.
95. Vivien B, Di Maria S, Ouattara A, et al: Overestimation of bispectral index in sedated intensive care unit patients revealed by administration of muscle relaxant. Anesthesiology 99:9-17, 2003.

CHAPTER 39

Specific Diseases of the Respiratory System: Upper Airway

David S. Jardine and Lynn D. Martin

PEARLS

- Diseases leading to compromise of the airway are the most frequent cause of cardiac arrest in pediatric patients. A small reduction in the caliber of the smaller child's airway may lead to a life-threatening reduction of airflow.
- Laryngomalacia is the most common congenital anomaly of the larynx. Infants tend to outgrow this problem during the first year of life; however, the condition may be of sufficient severity in some infants that activities such as feeding are compromised.
- The trachea may be compressed by the presence of an abnormal vascular structure. Children affected by this problem may have such diverse symptoms as stridor, wheezing, lobar atelectasis, or recurrent pulmonary infections.
- The practice of treating laryngotracheobronchitis with corticosteroids is standard of care, especially for hospitalized patients. A meta-analysis in which the efficacy of corticosteroids was evaluated suggests that corticosteroids may reduce the need for endotracheal intubation and hasten improvement in the first 24 hours of illness.
- Epiglottitis, a bacterial infection of the supraglottic tissues historically caused by *Haemophilus influenzae* type B, is now most frequently caused by group A β-hemolytic streptococcus.
- Patients with bacterial tracheitis usually do not respond to inhaled racemic epinephrine, have a higher fever, and appear very ill.

Diseases leading to compromise of the airway are the most frequent cause of cardiac arrest in pediatric patients. Prompt recognition of these illnesses can lead to timely intervention and improve the outcome of these patients. The small size of the infant's trachea makes airway obstruction more likely and particularly dangerous. The normal anteroposterior diameter of the infant's glottis is 4.5 mm. One millimeter of circumferential tracheal edema reduces the glottic lumen to 30% of its normal size. Poiseuille's law stipulates that laminar flow of gas through a tube is inversely proportional to the fourth power of the radius of the lumen:

$$R = \frac{8ln}{\pi r^4}$$

where R is the resistance to gas flow, l is the length of the tube, n is the viscosity of the gas, and r is the radius. Unfortunately, airflow through a narrowed trachea is usually turbulent, which worsens the situation because resistance to turbulent flow of gas past an obstruction is inversely proportional to the fifth power of the radius of the lumen.[1,2] Gas exchange will be dramatically reduced by minor degrees of impingement on an infant's trachea. This means that a child will not tolerate lesions that would not even produce symptoms in an adult.

Initial Management

Once the diagnosis of upper airway obstruction is made, efforts should be undertaken to minimize disturbing the patient unless the respiratory embarrassment is severe enough to be life threatening. Airway obstruction often worsens when infants and children are alarmed during a diagnostic evaluation. Humidified oxygen should be administered through a nasal cannula or facemask. These devices may frighten younger children who may more readily accept oxygen delivered through flexible tubing held by the parent. If the child will tolerate placement of a pulse oximeter probe, this provides a noninvasive way of evaluating oxygenation. If oxygen saturation through pulse oximeter measurement is within an acceptable range (≥95%), arterial blood gas determination may be unnecessary. An arterial blood gas is useful to identify the patient who may be hypercapnic, but this will usually be at the price of further upsetting the child.

After upper airway obstruction has been diagnosed, a combination of physical and radiographic findings may help localize the lesion. With identification of the anatomic site of the lesion, the diagnostic possibilities are greatly narrowed. During the diagnostic evaluation, the child may sit in the parent's lap if this reduces anxiety. This position usually does not interfere with the diagnostic evaluation, such as lateral neck and chest radiography. The dose of radiation to a nonpregnant parent is small and should be of little concern.

If it is thought to be safe, examination of the patient's head and neck may reveal the cause of the illness. Depending on the patient's condition, the degree of respiratory embarrassment may be quantified with a rating scale (Table 39–1). One of the primary benefits of using such a scale is that signs of respiratory obstruction are systematically sought and objectively documented. This information may be valuable in helping to define the course of the patient's illness and the response to treatment.

The initial evaluation should allow one to make important triage decisions about management and further evaluation of the patient with upper airway compromise. Depending on the severity of the illness, a decision must be made about which diagnostic tests will be undertaken. In the case of severe respiratory compromise, it may be necessary to plan for invasive procedures (endotracheal intubation or operative intervention) while the diagnostic evaluation is being performed. Finally, it should not be forgotten that pulmonary edema might follow relief of severe upper airway obstruction.[3] Postobstructive pulmonary edema may be severe enough to require vigorous therapy, including endotracheal intubation, mechanical ventilation, and positive end-expiratory pressure.

Congenital Malformations

A variety of congenital malformations can affect the pediatric airway. Many of these become evident in the delivery room. Some congenital malformations do not present until the child is older and somatic growth has made the airway impairment more evident.

Choanal Atresia

Choanal atresia is estimated to occur about once in every 5000 to 8000 live births.[4] Unilateral choanal atresia, the most common form,[4] may not be diagnosed at the time of delivery. Bilateral choanal atresia usually results in respiratory distress shortly after birth because infants are preferential nasal breathers until 2 to 5 months of age. Many infants breathe only through their nose and do not open their mouth when the nasal passages are occluded. Bilateral choanal atresia (Fig. 39–1) is diagnosed through examination of the naris with the mouth closed. If no airflow is present, a presumptive diagnosis of choanal atresia is established. Some authorities advocate passing a thin, flexible catheter through the naris. This will confirm the diagnosis of choanal atresia; however, if the symptoms are resulting from choanal stenosis, edema formation following even minor trauma of the nasal mucosa after catheter placement may lead to complete occlusion of the nasal airway and worsening of respiratory distress. Surgery is indicated for the correction of bilateral choanal

TABLE 39–1

Subjective Assessment of Clinical Severity of Laryngotracheobronchitis

	0	1	2	3
Stridor	None	Mild	Moderate at rest	Severe on inspiration and expiration or none with markedly decreased air entry
Retractions	None	Mild	Moderate	Severe, marked use of accessory muscles
Air entry	Normal	Mild decrease	Moderate decrease	Marked decrease
Color	Normal	Normal (0 score)	Normal (0 score)	Dusky or cyanotic
Level of consciousness	Normal	Restless when disturbed	Anxious, agitated; restless when undisturbed	Lethargic, depressed

From Davis HW, Gartner JC, Galvis AG et al: Acute upper airway obstruction: croup and epiglottis, *Pediatr Clin North Am* 28:859, 1981.

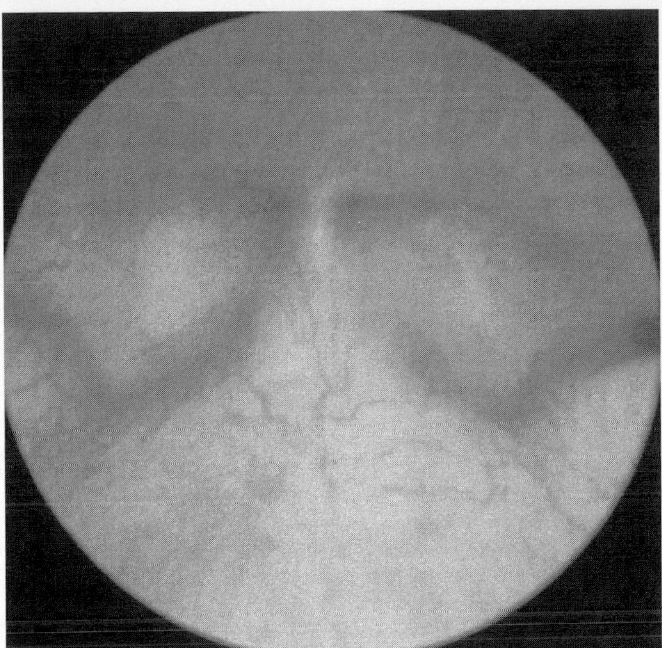

FIGURE 39–1 • Choanal atresia before repair. View of choanal atresia from posterior nasopharynx. There is complete absence of choanae. (Courtesy Andrew F. Inglis, Jr.)

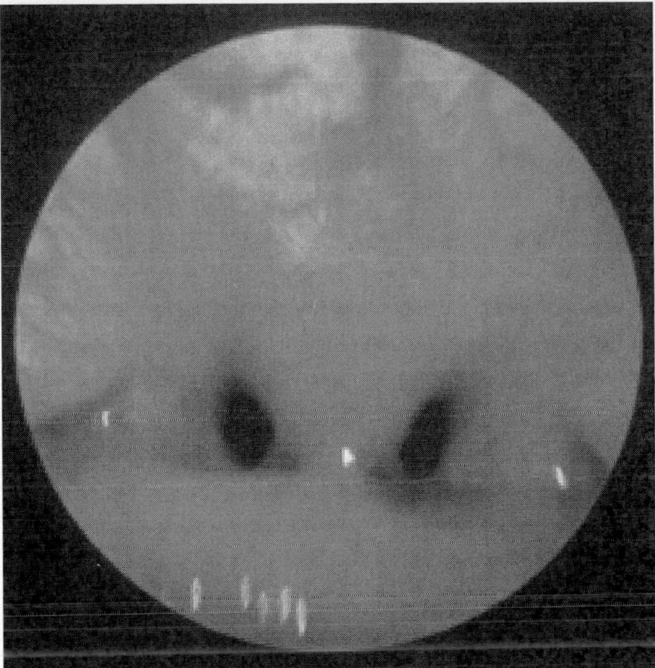

FIGURE 39–2 • Choanal atresia after repair. View from the posterior of nasopharynx showing patency of choanae after surgery. (Courtesy Andrew F. Inglis, Jr.)

atresia if the infant has symptoms[5] (Fig. 39–2). Topical application of mitomycin to inhibit fibroblast proliferation has been shown to be an effective adjunct to surgical repair of choanal atresia.[6]

Although choanal atresia is the most common cause of nasal airway obstruction, midline nasal masses such as meningoencephaloceles, gliomas, or dermoid tumors can also cause obstruction. Because these lesions may originate from within the cranial vault, computed tomography (CT) scanning or magnetic resonance imaging (MRI) should be performed before a biopsy or surgical correction of the abnormality is attempted.[7]

Laryngomalacia

Laryngomalacia is the most common congenital anomaly of the larynx. The infant has inspiratory stridor that is exacerbated by crying or distress. Although no gross anatomic abnormalities are present, the laryngeal cartilages lack their usual rigidity. When the larynx is observed during fiberoptic examination of the glottis, the arytenoid cartilages and supraglottic structures collapse inward (toward the glottis) during inspiration, leading to inspiratory stridor. These abnormalities can be graphically observed with fiberoptic laryngoscopy, which shows the dynamic component with obstruction during inspiration and full airflow during expiration. In some patients with laryngomalacia, gastroesophageal reflux may be the primary cause of the airway compromise, whereas in others it may be a significant cofactor exacerbating preexisting neurologic or anatomic abnormality.[8] The respiratory embarrassment associated with this problem is usually minor and self-limited, although hypoxia and hypercapnia have been documented.[9] Infants tend to outgrow this problem during the first year of life; however, the condition may be severe enough in some infants that activities such as feeding are compromised. In the most severe cases, surgical intervention with laser excision may be necessary.[10, 11] The goal is to relieve airway obstruction by excision of tissue that collapses into the glottis during inspiration.

Laryngeal Webs, Stenosis, and Tumors

Laryngeal webs usually occur at the level of the glottis. They are generally thin membranes of soft tissue that partially occlude the tracheal opening, producing symptoms of feeble cry and dyspnea shortly after birth (Fig. 39–3). Surgical lysis of these lesions corrects the problem. Laryngeal cysts and laryngocele are soft tissue masses that protrude into the glottic lumen (Fig. 39–4). The resulting respiratory compromise is usually recognized as inspiratory stridor. Treatment is surgical excision of the lesion.

Another lesion presenting as inspiratory stridor is congenital laryngotracheal (subglottic) stenosis. This is the third most frequent cause of stridor in infants. The infant with this problem may have symptoms when newborn but often comes to medical attention later when the tracheal edema produced by a minor respiratory infection causes severe inspiratory stridor. This may be initially diagnosed as croup (laryngotracheobronchitis) but is noted to recur with each subsequent upper respiratory infection. Although the diagnosis of laryngotracheal stenosis may be made radiographically, it is usually established with bronchoscopy. If endotracheal intubation is necessary, a smaller than normal endotracheal tube should be used to reduce trauma and ischemia of the subglottic tissues. Depending on the severity of the lesion, surgical

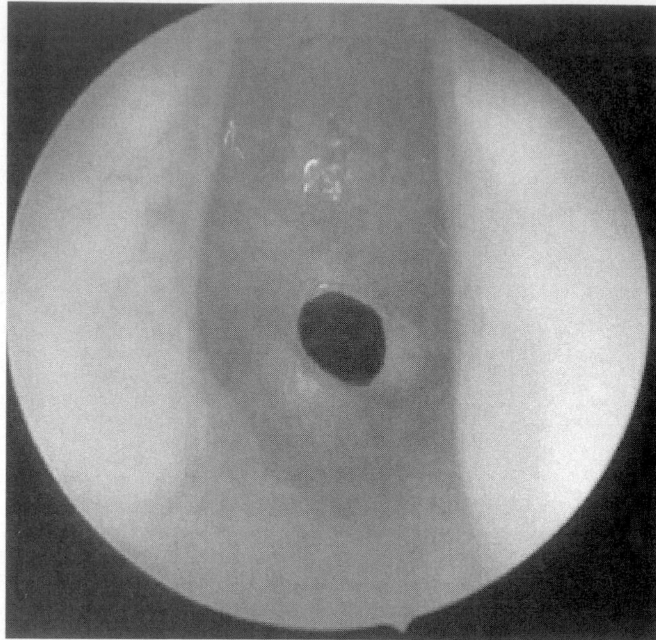

FIGURE 39–3 • A laryngeal web occludes most of the tracheal lumen in this patient. This web, which is a thin membrane of soft tissue at the level of the glottis, has many of the features that are typical of this class of lesions. (Courtesy Andrew F. Inglis, Jr.)

intervention may be necessary (see the discussion about acquired laryngotracheal [subglottic] stenosis for details of the surgical procedures).

Soft tissue masses may reduce the caliber of the tracheal lumen, either by extrinsic compression, as happens with a cystic hygroma, or by growth into the tracheal lumen from the tracheal wall, as happens with a hemangioma. Although these lesions may be present at birth, they often do not produce symptoms for the first few months until the growing lesion further impinges on the trachea.

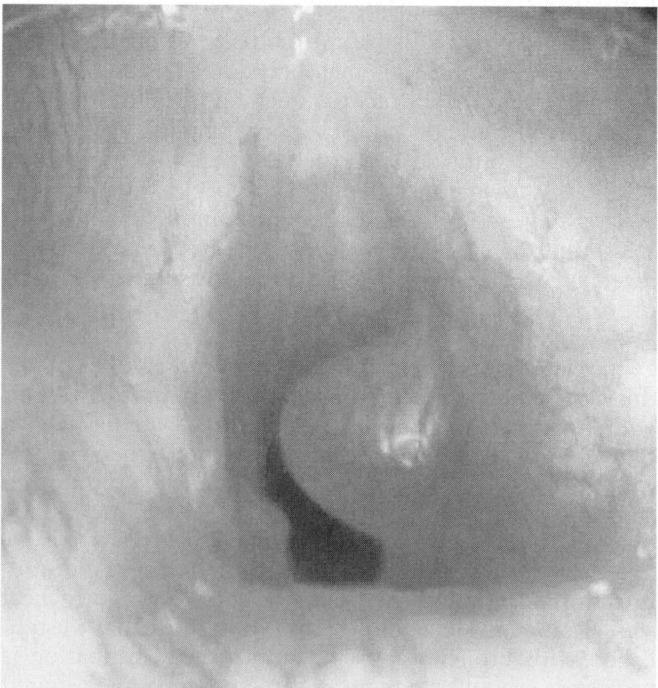

FIGURE 39–4 • A large laryngeal cyst protrudes from the lateral wall of the trachea, just below the level of the glottis. (Courtesy Andrew F. Inglis, Jr.)

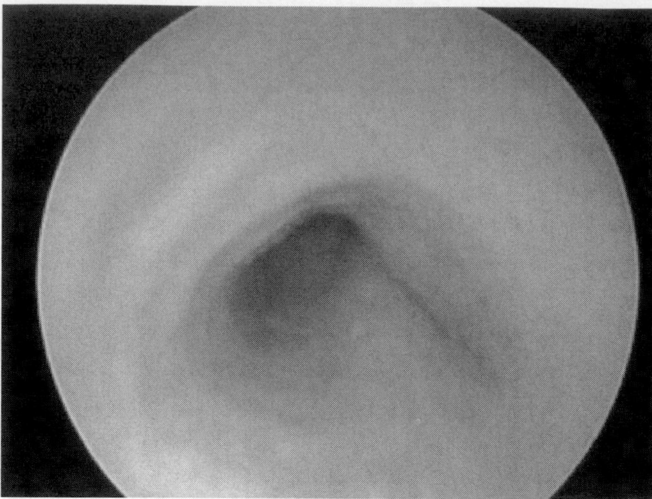

FIGURE 39–5 • The lateral portion of the tracheal lumen is severely compressed by the impingement of the vascular ring. (Courtesy Andrew F. Inglis, Jr.)

Vascular Impingement on the Trachea

The trachea may be compressed by the presence of an abnormal vascular structure. Children affected by this problem may have such diverse symptoms as stridor, wheezing, lobar atelectasis, or recurrent pulmonary infections. The innominate artery is the most common vessel causing tracheal compression.

Vascular rings and enlarged pulmonary arteries are also known to cause tracheal compression, as are a variety of other vascular abnormalities. These lesions may cause recurrent respiratory infections but often do not cause stridor or swallowing problems. Because of this it is difficult to recognize a vascular ring as the underlying cause of illness.[12] Careful inspection of the chest radiograph may reveal indentation of the trachea, but often this sign is absent. Barium swallow has been the historic method of diagnosing vascular impingement of the trachea (Fig. 39–5). CT scanning and MRI have rapidly become the diagnostic modality of choice (Figs. 39–6 and 39–7).[13] These noninvasive methods are effective at showing complex three-dimensional cardiovascular anatomy, especially the extracardiac morphology. Treatment involves surgical correction of the vascular anomaly in severe cases. Respiratory distress may persist postoperatively because prolonged compression of the trachea has made the affected segment softer and collapsible. In severe cases, the tracheomalacia may severely compromise the patient and may be improved by surgical intervention to prevent tracheal collapse.[14]

Bronchomalacia and Intrathoracic Tracheomalacia

During normal respiration, the upper airway is subject to cycles of positive and negative intraluminal pressure. The cartilaginous components of the upper airway are

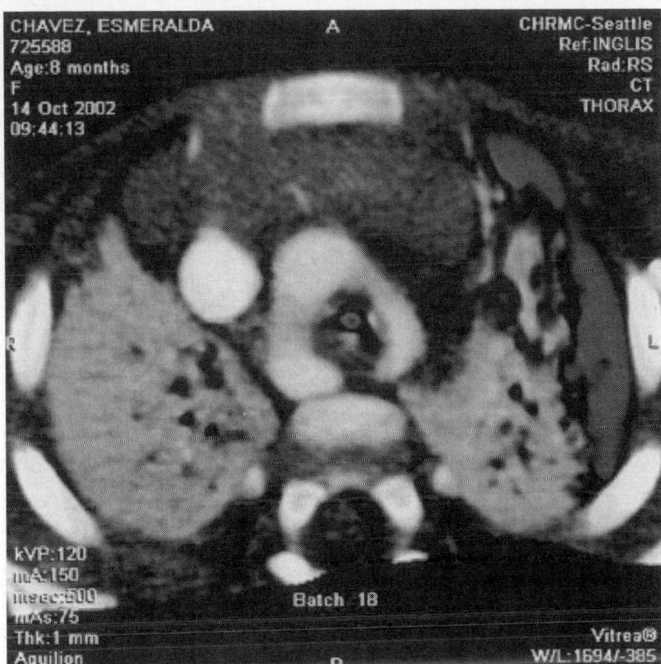

FIGURE 39–6 • Contrast computed tomography scan showing vascular ring encircling and compressing the trachea (*arrow* indicates vascular ring encircling trachea). (Courtesy Andrew F. Inglis, Jr.)

rigid ringlike structural elements that resist the tendency to collapse caused by the cycling of pressure within the airway lumen. When these structures lack their characteristic rigidity, the mechanics of breathing are altered. The symptoms produced by these changes depend on the location of the damaged cartilages. Characteristically,

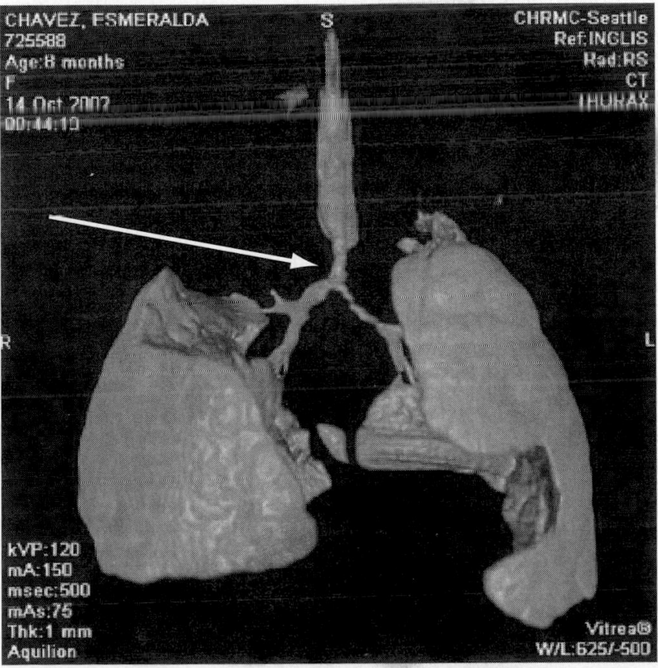

FIGURE 39–7 • High-resolution three-dimensional reconstruction of computed tomography scans clearly shows severe tracheal compression caused by vascular ring (*arrow* indicates tracheal narrowing caused by vascular ring).

intrathoracic cartilaginous lesions impede exhalation. Diagnosis of this problem may be made through observation of collapse of the upper airways during active exhalation, such as occurs while crying. Collapse can be observed with several diagnostic modalities including fluoroscopy, flexible or rigid bronchoscopy, and ultrafast CT scanning.[15]

Although these lesions may be congenital, many of the cases of tracheomalacia and bronchomalacia seen in the pediatric intensive care unit (PICU) are the result of an infectious or mechanical insult to the trachea. Recent investigations of infants with bronchopulmonary dysplasia and persistent respiratory problems revealed that some of these infants had bronchomalacia alone or in combination with tracheomalacia.[16,17] The obstructive symptoms produced by these lesions may be relieved by continuous positive airway pressure to maintain patency of the airway during exhalation.[18] The level of continuous positive airway pressure necessary to improve respiratory function may be assessed clinically (relief of obstructive symptoms), mechanically (measurement of flow-volume loops), or bronchoscopically (maintenance of airway patency throughout the respiratory cycle).[19] With sufficient time, many of these infants outgrow their respiratory difficulties. As an alternative to tracheostomy and positive airway pressure, some have advocated surgical intervention with pericardial flap aortopexy[20] or metallic airway stents.[21]

Infectious Processes

A variety of infectious processes may affect the pediatric airway. Poiseuille's law dictates that airway compromise from the swelling that accompanies an infectious process is greater in infants and young children than it is in adults. A small reduction in the caliber of the smaller child's airway may lead to a life-threatening reduction of airflow.

Laryngotracheobronchitis

Laryngotracheobronchitis (croup) is a common childhood infection. It is caused by a variety of infectious agents; parainfluenza virus A, adenovirus, and respiratory syncytial virus are the most common. This is a seasonal illness, happening mainly during the winter, and it most commonly affects children from age 6 months to 3 years. There is frequently a history of prodromal infection accompanied by an unusual cough (described as sounding like the bark of a seal). Swelling of the tracheal mucosa in the subglottic region causes airway compromise (Fig. 39–8). Medical attention is usually sought when the child develops inspiratory stridor and respiratory distress. Various scales have been devised to quantify the severity of the stridor to document the progression of the illness and the response to therapy (Table 39–1). Radiographically, the trachea is seen to have a gradual progressive narrowing of its lumen, reaching the narrowest point just below the vocal cords (the "steeple sign") (Fig. 39–9). The upper glottis as seen on a lateral neck radiograph is normal.

Exposing the child to cold or misty air often dramatically improves the symptoms. When the illness is refractory to these measures, racemic epinephrine has been shown to produce dramatic reduction of airway obstruction. This probably is accomplished by stimulation of the α-adrenergic receptors producing vasoconstriction and resulting in diminished tracheal edema. Rebound tracheal edema may occur several hours later as the effect of the racemic epinephrine dissipates. Because this problem is unpredictable, the child should be admitted to the hospital for observation after racemic epinephrine has been used.

The practice of treating laryngotracheobronchitis with corticosteroids is widespread, especially for hospitalized patients.[22] Oral, intramuscular, and nebulized corticosteroids have been shown to be beneficial in randomized, blinded trials.[23,24] Multiple meta-analyses in which the efficacy of corticosteroids were evaluated suggest that corticosteroids reduced the need for endotracheal intubation or inhaled epinephrine, hasten improvement in the first 24 hours of illness, shorten the duration of hospitalization, and reduce the frequency of readmission.[25-27]

Mixtures of helium and oxygen (heliox) have proven beneficial in settings with airway narrowing and turbulent air flow.[28] Because this gas mixture is less dense than air, turbulent flow past the airway obstruction is facilitated, resulting in lower airway resistance and improved gas exchange. The efficacy of this therapy depends on the quantity of helium present in the gas mixture. Gas mixtures containing less than 60% helium show little benefit compared with air. This limits the application of this therapy to patients who can tolerate a fractional concentration of oxygen in inspired gas (FiO_2) of 40% or less. To avoid the risk of hypoxemia, mixtures of 79% helium and 21% oxygen are commercially available. If supplemental oxygen is required, additional oxygen can be added to this mixture; care must be taken not to exceed an FiO_2 of 40%. Because the density of this gas mixture is different than air or oxygen, specially calibrated flow meters are necessary. No adjustment is necessary if an oxygen electrode is used to measure the FiO_2. This mixture must be delivered through a facemask. Delivery through a nasal cannula or an infant Oxyhood is ineffective.[29] In the latter case, a concentration gradient of helium and oxygen is rapidly established, with the greatest concentration of helium at the top of the hood. A recent randomized study has shown that heliox will result in similar improvements in severe croup as compared with racemic epinephrine.[30]

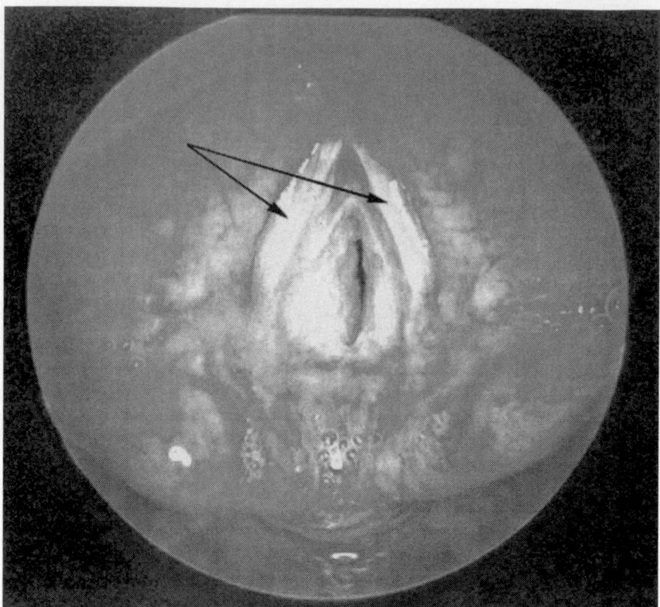

FIGURE 39–8 • Laryngotracheobronchitis. Below the level of the vocal cords the trachea appears swollen and the tracheal walls are covered with purulent material (vocal cords are indicated by *arrows*). (Courtesy Bruce Benjamin, MD.)

Endotracheal intubation is occasionally necessary when laryngotracheobronchitis proves refractory to

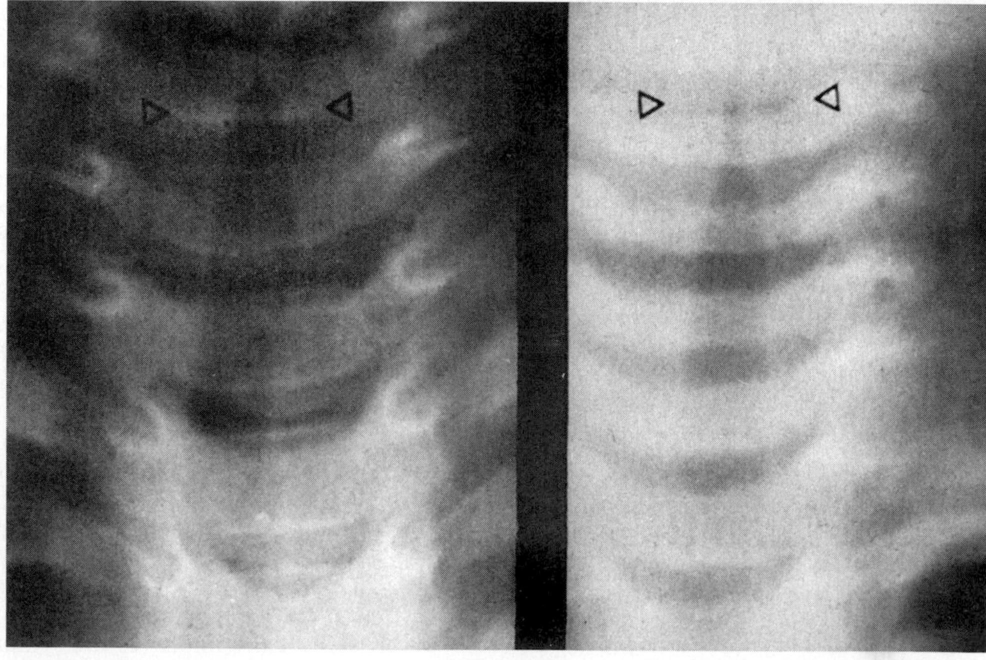

FIGURE 39–9 • Anteroposterior radiograph of the neck. *Left,* A normal tracheal air column (between the *arrows*). *Right,* Trachea narrowed by laryngotracheobronchitis.

TABLE 39–2

Characteristics of Laryngotracheobronchitis, Bacterial Tracheitis, and Epiglottitis

	Laryngotracheobronchitis	Bacterial tracheitis	Epiglottitis
Age	3 mo-3 yr	6 mo-12 yr	2 yr-7 yr
Onset	Gradual	Intermediate	<24 hr
Fever	Usually low	Usually high	High
Cough	Characteristic "barking"	Characteristic "barking"	None
Sore throat	None	Usually absent	Often severe
Drooling	No	No	Usually
Posture	Any position	Any position	Sitting forward, mouth open, drooling
Voice	Normal	Normal or hoarse	Muffled
Appearance	Nontoxic	Toxic	Toxic
Seasonal distribution	Usually winter, epidemic	Throughout the year	Throughout the year

medical intervention. The use of tracheostomy to treat life-threatening laryngotracheobronchitis is much less common now than formerly. Unless merited by special circumstances, such as severe subglottic stenosis in association with laryngotracheobronchitis, tracheostomy offers no advantages over endotracheal intubation. For placement of the endotracheal tube to be facilitated and for injury to the tracheal mucosa to be reduced, the endotracheal tube should be of a smaller size than would normally be used. If the tracheal edema is severe, even a small tube may fit tightly in the trachea.

Later, when an audible leak around the endotracheal tube is present, the trachea may be extubated with a high probability that reintubation will not be necessary.[31] If a leak does not become audible after 2 to 4 days, it is our practice to extubate the trachea because prolonged intubation may increase the risk for subglottic injury. Racemic epinephrine is commonly needed to treat stridor after extubation. If a patient should have especially severe or recurrent laryngotracheobronchitis, an anatomic lesion causing tracheal narrowing should be suspected.

Epiglottitis

Epiglottitis, a bacterial infection of the supraglottic tissues caused by *Haemophilus influenzae* type B and other organisms, is frequently confused with laryngotracheobronchitis because both present with inspiratory stridor and respiratory distress. Historically, epiglottitis was an infection seen primarily in younger children, but the widespread use of *H. influenzae* type B vaccine has greatly reduced the frequency of this infection and altered its presentation. After release of the vaccine, the overall incidence of epiglottitis has fallen from 10.9 per 10,000 hospital admissions to 1.8 per 10,000 admissions, and the average age of the patient with epiglottitis has risen from 35.5 months to 80.5 months.[32] During this same period, the frequency of identification of *H. influenzae* type B as the causative agent has fallen from 76% to 25%. Group A β-hemolytic streptococcus is now identified as the cause of epiglottitis in many patients and is clinically indistinguishable from epiglottitis caused by *H. influenzae* type B.[32] Although most cases of epiglottitis are caused by infectious pathogens, thermal injury from ingesting hot liquids can also cause epiglottitis.[33] Several points serve to distinguish epiglottitis from laryngotracheobronchitis (Table 39–2).

A radiograph of the anteroposterior and lateral neck will help to distinguish epiglottitis from laryngotracheobronchitis. In epiglottitis, the anteroposterior view of the trachea appears normal, but a lateral neck radiograph shows a markedly swollen and edematous epiglottis (Fig. 39–10). All diagnostic tests, such as radiography, must be accomplished with minimum stress to the patient.

Management of epiglottitis is a multidisciplinary undertaking, involving pediatric intensive care specialists, anesthesiologists, and otolaryngologists. When a child with presumed epiglottitis is admitted to the emergency department, this team should be notified in anticipation of taking the child to the operating room to secure his or her airway. As the team members are being notified, lateral radiographs of the neck may be obtained if tolerated by the patient. This may be done with the child sitting on the parent's lap to minimize the child's anxiety. The diagnostic evaluation of the patient should proceed expeditiously, while care is taken to disturb the patient as little as possible. Attempts to directly examine the oropharynx

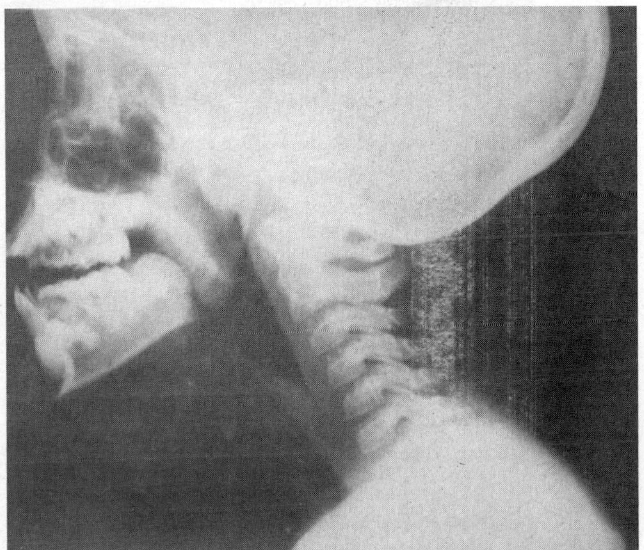

FIGURE 39–10 • Lateral radiograph of the neck of a patient with epiglottitis. Note the large, swollen epiglottis.

or to start an intravenous line should be discouraged. The apprehension caused by these events may lead to tracheal obstruction by the enlarged epiglottis. If the patient will tolerate it, humidified oxygen should be administered, preferably through a plastic hose held by the parent.

If the diagnosis of epiglottitis is strongly suspected or confirmed on the lateral neck x-ray film, the child should go to the operating room as quickly as possible. In the operating room, the patient is anesthetized with an inhaled anesthetic (sevoflurane or halothane) and oxygen while the patient is spontaneously breathing. Once the patient has been anesthetized, an intravenous catheter is inserted and a laryngoscopy is performed (Fig. 39–11). It may be exceedingly difficult to obtain a direct view of the glottis and trachea because of the large swollen epiglottis. Nevertheless, it is almost always possible to pass an endotracheal tube through the edematous tissues and into the trachea. Nasotracheal intubation is preferred to orotracheal intubation because the tube is more readily secured to the face, the patient cannot bite the tube, and salivation is decreased. An otolaryngologist should be in the operating room and ready to do an emergency tracheostomy if an airway cannot be secured by endotracheal intubation, although this is rarely necessary. As with laryngotracheobronchitis, endotracheal intubation is preferred to tracheostomy because it has been shown that complications are more common when a tracheostomy has been routinely used to treat epiglottitis. After the airway is secured, blood cultures and cultures of the epiglottis are obtained, and antibiotic therapy is initiated with a penicillinase-resistant antibiotic because of the high incidence of *H. influenzae* resistance to ampicillin.

In the PICU, patients usually require endotracheal intubation for 24 to 72 hours while the swollen epiglottis returns to normal size. The patient may be allowed to breathe spontaneously through the endotracheal tube or may undergo mechanical ventilation. Variable amounts of sedation are usually necessary. Extraepiglottic sites of *H. influenzae* infection are common. In one series, pneumonia occurred in 25% of patients with epiglottitis.

Peritonsillar Abscess

The initial presentation of peritonsillar abscess may resemble that of epiglottitis, but the age of the child with peritonsillar abscess is older—usually in the early second decade of life. The child may have a muffled voice and drooling. If the abscess is of sufficient size, the child may also experience respiratory distress. Unlike epiglottitis, children with peritonsillar abscess often experience trismus. If the abscess is fluctuant, surgical incision and drainage may be indicated. Although trismus may be of concern in evaluation of the patient for anesthesia, there is usually no anatomic restriction of jaw movement. Once the patient has been anesthetized, the mouth may be easily opened. Extubation is almost always possible after the abscess has been drained unless there is severe inflammation and swelling extending well beyond the tonsillar bed. Intraoral ultrasound examination has been

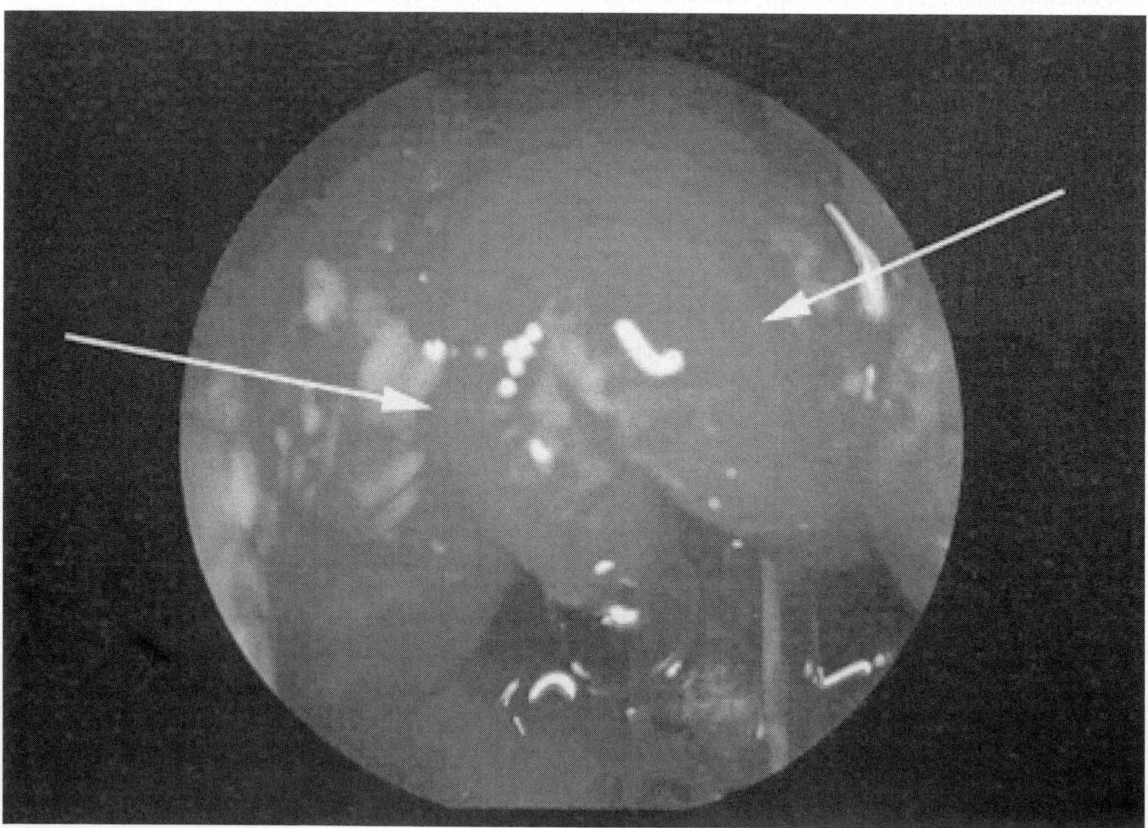

FIGURE 39–11 • Epiglottitis causing a severely swollen epiglottis (between the *arrows*). In the lower portion of the picture, the endotracheal tube can be seen. (Courtesy Andrew F. Inglis, Jr.)

suggested to be a useful test to differentiate abscess from cellulitis.[34]

Retropharyngeal Abscess

Almost 90% of children with retropharyngeal abscess are younger than 6 years.[35] Patients may have fever, dysphagia, drooling, muffled voice, and respiratory distress. The similarity to epiglottitis has occasionally led to misdiagnosis of this disease. In contrast to those with epiglottitis, most patients have a sore throat for several days before becoming ill with fever and increased pharyngeal discomfort. During examination of the oropharynx, the posterior pharyngeal wall may be observed to bulge, but most commonly, the findings are unremarkable. Palpation of the posterior pharyngeal wall should be avoided because it may cause rupture of the abscess with possible spillage of the contents into the tracheobronchial tree. An inspiratory radiograph of the lateral neck may show thickening of the prevertebral soft tissue, and occasionally an air fluid level may be present (Fig. 39–12). A chest radiograph should be obtained to evaluate possible mediastinal extension of the infection. If the chest radiograph or clinical findings are not convincing, CT is often performed, although these radiologic studies have limitations.[36]

A short trial of antibiotic therapy is often indicated before any decision is made to proceed with surgical drainage of the abscess.[37] Surgical treatment of this lesion is drainage of the abscess after the patient has been anesthetized and an endotracheal tube has been inserted to protect the patient from pulmonary aspiration of the purulent fluid. The organisms most often isolated are *Staphylococcus aureus, Micrococcus aureus,* group A β-hemolytic streptococci, and anaerobic organisms.[35]

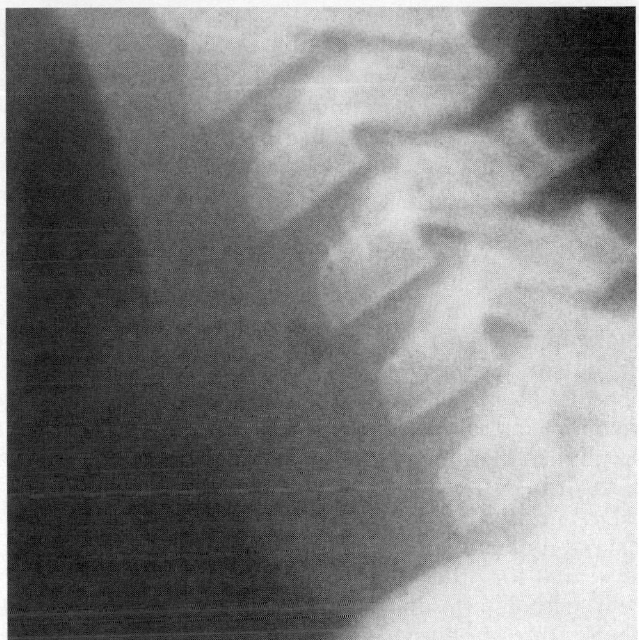

FIGURE 39–12 • Lateral radiograph of the neck of a patient with retropharyngeal abscess. Note the thickening of the prevertebral soft tissue and the radiolucent area caused by the presence of air in the tissue.

Bacterial Tracheitis

Since 1979, published reports of bacterial tracheitis have increased in frequency.[38] Although this illness resembles laryngotracheobronchitis, inspiratory stridor caused by tracheitis is not improved after administration of racemic epinephrine. Characteristically, the children have an upper respiratory tract illness lasting from several hours to several days and have a fever at the time of presentation.[38] In contrast to those with laryngotracheobronchitis, patients with bacterial tracheitis usually have a higher fever and may appear very ill (Table 39–2). Because of the clinical similarity of bacterial tracheitis to viral laryngotracheobronchitis, these patients are treated with racemic epinephrine but fail to respond. Bronchoscopy shows normal supraglottic structures, subglottic edema, and purulent secretions in the trachea.[39] Because of the severity of airway compromise, endotracheal intubation is often necessary. A more recent publication suggests that the condition is becoming less morbid with a less frequent need for airway instrumentation.[40]

Bacterial agents associated most commonly with this illness include *S. aureus, H. influenzae* type B, and pneumococcus.[41] Some authors think that bacterial superinfection with these agents follows a viral respiratory infection, often caused by parainfluenza.[38] The injury to the respiratory epithelium caused by the virus may predispose the patients to bacterial superinfection. The most common complication of bacterial tracheitis is pneumonia, which is observed in approximately 60% of patients with this illness. Antibiotics are an important aspect of therapy and should be directed by the results of bacterial cultures obtained during bronchoscopy or immediately after endotracheal intubation.

Laryngeal Papillomatosis

The laryngeal papilloma is the most common benign tumor of the larynx during childhood. Despite its nonmalignant structure, the propensity of this tumor to cause respiratory obstruction may result in injury to the patient or death. The onset of symptoms occurs between infancy and 4 years of age. New onset of infection is less frequent after age 5 years. The most common medical complaint in these children is voice change, which occurs in more than 90% of the patients. Airway obstruction is present in almost half of the patients, although it is mild in many of these individuals. The presence of inspiratory stridor may misdirect the diagnostician to think that the child has laryngotracheobronchitis. Diagnosis is typically made with laryngoscopy (Fig. 39–13).

Little is know about the immunological mechanisms involved in laryngeal papillomavirus infection, but cellular immunity is considered a more important mechanism than humoral immunity.[42] Better understanding of human papillomavirus infection is hampered by the lack of a good experimental model in which the entire viral life cycle can take place.

The treatment for this illness is surgical excision of the polyps. Induction of anesthesia in the child with severe airway obstruction may be hazardous because it may be difficult or impossible to ventilate the child's lungs after loss of consciousness. Although patients characteristically require multiple surgical resections of these lesions (an average of 11 resections over the course of the disease), the mortality with this illness is low. Carbon dioxide laser vaporization of the papillomata is widely used. During laser excision of lesions caused by a similar viral agent, anogenital condylomas, medical personnel have become infected with the virus, presumably from viable virus particles carried in the smoke plume.[43] Although this has caused concerns about the spread of infection after excision of laryngeal papillomatosis, test results of the smoke plume have been negative for viral DNA.[44] Despite this, careful scavenging of the plume is routine in most centers where this operation is performed.

Despite modern surgical treatments, recurrence of laryngeal papillomata is relatively common and has prompted the search for other treatment options. Adjunctive treatment with interferon-α has been shown to reduce the relapse rate in both children and adults.[45] Molecular analysis has recently shown that patients infected with human papillomavirus-11 were sensitive to interferon treatment as opposed to those with human papillomavirus-6.[46] This difference is likely due to the ability of human papillomavirus-6 to inhibit the induction of an interferon-responsive promoter element.

Vocal Cord Paralysis

Vocal cord paralysis in pediatric patients may be either present at birth or acquired later. The recurrent branch of the superior laryngeal nerve, which in turn originates from the tenth cranial nerve, innervates the vocal cords. Paralysis of the vocal cords produces a paramedian or median position of the vocal cords. Patients with vocal cord paralysis may be able to phonate because the thyroid muscle may serve as a tensor of the vocal cords and is not affected in most cases of vocal cord paralysis.

Most patients with vocal cord paralysis have inspiratory stridor, although asthma has been initially diagnosed in some patients because of perceived expiratory wheezing. Vocal cord paralysis is a well-recognized complication of thoracic surgery.[47] Congenital cord paralysis is a common anomaly of the larynx. Cord paralysis may be unilateral or bilateral. Left-sided cord paralysis is somewhat more common than right-sided cord paralysis because of the lengthy path followed by the left recurrent laryngeal nerve. A neurological disorder, such as brainstem compression by an Arnold-Chiari malformation, should be considered when acquired vocal cord paralysis is evaluated among pediatric patients. Brain tumors have rarely caused vocal cord paralysis.[48]

The treatment of vocal cord paralysis is primarily supportive. If a specific lesion may be addressed medically or surgically (such as decompression of the brainstem in Arnold-Chiari malformation), such therapy should be undertaken. Occasionally, respiratory embarrassment is of sufficient magnitude to merit surgical intervention with an external arytenoidopexy, an arytenoidectomy, or a tracheostomy. A recent meta-analysis suggests that an external arytenoidopexy and an external arytenoidectomy are equivalently effective and that the two combined are significantly more effective than carbon dioxide ablative procedures.[49] For cord paralysis resulting from birth trauma and other

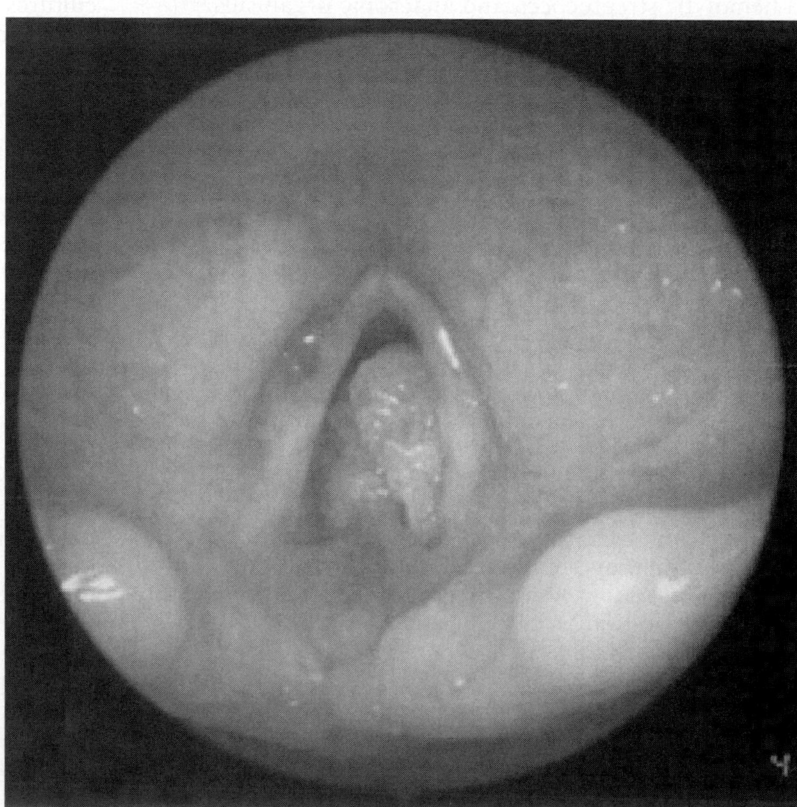

FIGURE 39–13 • Large, pedunculated papilloma is seen just below the vocal cords. These papillomas almost completely occluded the tracheal lumen and produced marked respiratory distress. (Courtesy Andrew F. Inglis, Jr.)

traumatic causes, the only course is to wait and hope that cord function returns as the affected nerve regenerates.

Intrathoracic Mass Lesions Causing Respiratory Obstruction

The intrathoracic trachea may be compressed by a variety of anterior mediastinal masses. Because the symptoms produced by a malignant mass impinging on the trachea can worsen dramatically over several days, the child with respiratory compromise resulting from a mediastinal mass deserves rapid evaluation and aggressive medical therapy.

Before caring for a child with this problem, the parents should be asked if the child refuses to lie in certain positions. The child's reluctance to recline in a given position may be caused by airway compromise from the mass. Forcing the child to lie down may result in airway compromise or even death.[50] Endotracheal intubation is indicated only if respiratory function becomes severely compromised. Unfortunately, this measure may be of little benefit because the lesion may compress the bronchi distal to the tip of the endotracheal tube.[51] In addition, it may be impossible to ventilate the child's lungs after muscle relaxants have been administered to facilitate placement of the endotracheal tube. Factors associated with the airway compromise are (1) anterior location of the mediastinal mass, (2) histological diagnosis of lymphoma, (3) symptoms and signs of superior vena cava syndrome, (4) radiological evidence of vessel compression or displacement, (5) pericardial effusion, and (6) pleural effusion.[52]

Trauma

Postextubation Stridor

After endotracheal intubation that lasts more than a few hours, postextubation stridor is a relatively common problem in pediatric patients and is most frequently caused by laryngeal edema. Estimates of the frequency of postextubation stridor in children vary widely. Most authors cite figures of less than 2% to 15%,[53,54] although the incidence may be as high as 37% in patients with trauma or burns.[55]

In addition to audible stridor, patients with this problem show decreased air movement; flaring of the alae nasi; and in more severe cases, decreased arterial oxygen saturation and mental status changes. The severity of these signs reliably indicates the severity of airway obstruction.[56]

Several risks are associated with the development of postextubation stridor. Endotracheal tube size plays an important role because too large an endotracheal tube may compress the tracheal mucosa, and this compression causes submucosal ischemia. When the endotracheal tube is removed, the injured tissue may swell and partially obstruct the larynx. Endotracheal tube movement within the trachea may also result in tissue injury and swelling. Whether stridor occurs depends on the extent of the swelling and the diameter of the child's airway. Small patients are more likely to have postextubation stridor because a larger proportion of their airway is obstructed with a given degree of swelling and because of the unfavorable characteristics of turbulent flow through small passages. Lack of an audible leak of air around the endotracheal tube is frequently used as a predictor of postextubation stridor in children. A recent study suggests that may be valid only in children ages 7 years and older.[57]

Uncuffed endotracheal tubes are often recommended for children younger than 8 years because of concern that the presence of an endotracheal tube cuff may contribute to the risk of postextubation stridor. The subglottic region is the narrowest portion of the airway in this age group and will often provide an adequate seal around the endotracheal tube. Although cuffed endotracheal tubes are not frequently used in children younger than 8 years, there may not be compelling reasons to avoid the use of such endotracheal tubes. Data regarding the harmful effects of cuffed endotracheal tubes were derived from tubes with high-pressure, low-volume cuffs, which are likely to cause submucosal tracheal ischemia. These endotracheal tubes have been replaced by low-pressure, high-volume cuffs that seal the trachea by providing a larger area of contact with the mucosa at a lower pressure, resulting in less submucosal ischemia. When such endotracheal tubes are used, the risk of postextubation stridor appears no greater than when uncuffed endotracheal tubes are used.[53] Because cuffed endotracheal tubes may provide a better seal than uncuffed endotracheal tubes, they can be useful in delivering higher pressures needed in patients with noncompliant lungs who require mechanical ventilation.

Postextubation stridor has a greater risk of developing in children with trisomy 21; as many as one third of these patients have stridor after extubation. There appear to be several causes for this problem, including hypotonia and facial abnormalities, such as a large tongue.

Although most cases of postextubation stridor are caused by laryngeal edema, when this problem persists, other causes should be sought. Anatomical airway anomalies, which may not be visible during endotracheal intubation (such as a tracheal hemangioma), may cause persistent postextubation stridor. Vocal cord paralysis is one of the more common causes of persistent postextubation stridor and may be caused by increased intracranial pressure,[58] brainstem compression, trauma to the brainstem after neurosurgery, or recurrent laryngeal nerve during thoracic surgery.[47]

The therapy of postextubation stridor is aimed at reducing airway edema. Racemic epinephrine and dexamethasone are the most widely used therapeutic agents. Racemic epinephrine, delivered by aerosol nebulizer, probably works by stimulation of α-adrenergic receptors; this stimulation causes vasoconstriction, which, in turn, reduces tracheal edema. Racemic epinephrine works rapidly, so improvement, when it occurs, should be observed within a few minutes of completion of therapy. Mixtures of helium and oxygen have also proven helpful in the treatment of postextubation stridor.[59]

The practice of using dexamethasone to treat postextubation stridor is widespread, although the efficacy of this therapy remains controversial. Although data from animal studies suggest that corticosteroid use at the time of extubation may reduce tracheal edema, inflammation, and capillary dilation, several human studies have failed to show reduction of postextubation stridor after corticosteroid use.[60-62] Nevertheless, many practitioners think that dexamethasone (or an equivalent dose of another steroid) will ameliorate postextubation stridor, especially if the medication is administered several hours before extubation.

In most cases, postextubation stridor is self-limited, but occasionally, endotracheal intubation may be necessary. If the degree of airway obstruction before reintubation was severe, postobstructive pulmonary edema may be observed and should be treated with positive end-expiratory pressure. When reintubation is contemplated, the size of the previous endotracheal tube should be determined, and a smaller endotracheal tube should be selected in the hope of preventing additional tracheal injury. Ideally, the trachea should remain intubated until a leak around the endotracheal tube is observed, indicating resolution of the laryngeal edema.

Acquired Laryngotracheal (Subglottic) Stenosis

Laryngotracheal (subglottic) stenosis may be congenital, but acquired subglottic stenosis is a well-described complication following endotracheal intubation (Fig. 39–14). This process is multifactorial. It appears to result from an interaction of several elements, including individual susceptibility, movement of the endotracheal tube, size of the endotracheal tube, and duration of intubation. Many think that choosing the smallest tube that allows adequate ventilation and pulmonary toilet reduces the risk of subglottic stenosis. Fortunately, the incidence of this complication in neonates appears to be decreasing.[63] It is also thought that nasotracheal intubation may reduce movement of the endotracheal tube within the trachea and diminish tracheal trauma. It has been reported that subglottic stenosis occurs infrequently after nasotracheal intubation with a proper-sized endotracheal tube. Gastroesophageal reflux is frequently present and perhaps plays a significant role in the development of laryngotracheal stenosis.[64]

Mild subglottic stenosis may be treated expectantly. Parents should be counseled to be aware that stridor may occur with respiratory infections. More severe forms of subglottic stenosis must be treated surgically. A complex array of surgical options is available.[65] When reconstruction is attempted, it should occur at a younger age (younger than 25 months) so that the child's speech and language development is not impaired.[66] Although this approach will avoid the need for tracheotomy and facilitate speech and language development, this recommendation may be at the price of laryngotracheal reconstruction failure and requirement for revision procedures. Postoperative management of these patients is frequently complicated by the need to maintain an artificial airway with minimal movement for many (5 to 14) days. This commonly requires the administration of sedatives, analgesics, and occasionally neuromuscular blocking agents. Fortunately, improvements in postoperative care have resulted in improved outcomes after laryngotracheal reconstruction.[67]

Foreign Body Aspiration

Airway obstruction may be produced by aspiration of a variety of foreign bodies, with nuts being one of the largest offenders in children.[68] Most of the patients aspirating foreign bodies are ages 1 to 3 years with more than 95% being younger than 10 years. Less than 30% of patients aspirating foreign bodies receive medical attention within the first 24 hours, with many patients experiencing a significant delay before seeking medical attention. A clear history of foreign body aspiration may be elicited from 40% to 80% of the patients.[69] Patients with an aspirated foreign body may initially be symptom free or may have a cough, wheezing, and evidence of respiratory embarrassment. Patients without symptoms who do not seek medical attention may have a persistent cough and ultimately pneumonia distal to the obstructed bronchus. Recurrent bouts of pneumonia may lead to bronchiectasis if the foreign body is not removed.

The airway may be blocked anywhere from the posterior pharynx to the bronchi. The symptoms produced by foreign body aspiration vary according to the site of the foreign body and the degree of obstruction it produces. Foreign bodies of the extrathoracic airway characteristically produce inspiratory stridor. Foreign bodies lodged in the intrathoracic trachea and bronchi tend to produce wheezing.

Radiographic evaluation should include inspiratory and expiratory radiographs because a single anteroposterior radiograph will be unremarkable in 18% of children with an aspirated foreign body (Fig. 39–15).[69] If the foreign body is producing ball valve bronchial obstruction, hyperinflation of the involved lung will be seen during the expiratory radiogram. Many foreign bodies are not radiopaque, so failure to see a foreign body on the chest radiograph cannot exclude this diagnosis. If a suspicion

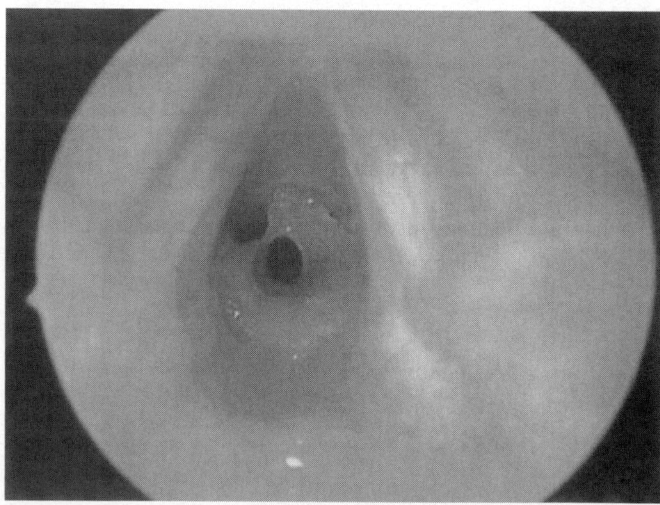

FIGURE 39–14 • A cicatricial ring is shown just below the glottis. This was caused by trauma from prolonged endotracheal intubation. (Courtesy Andrew F. Inglis, Jr.)

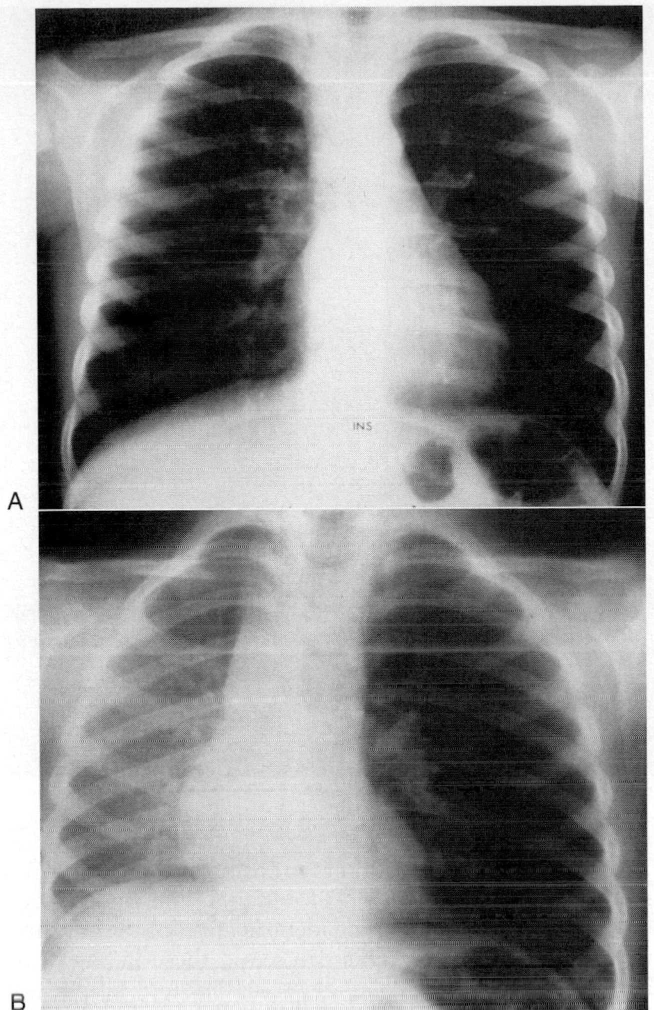

FIGURE 39–15 • **A,** Inspiratory chest radiograph with foreign body present in left mainstem bronchus. The left lung is slightly hyperinflated but could be considered normal. **B,** Expiratory chest radiograph with foreign body present in left mainstem bronchus. The left lung is clearly hyperinflated because of air trapping by the foreign body. (Courtesy Eric Effmann, MD.)

of an aspiration is high, a bronchoscopy is warranted (Fig. 39–16).

Foreign bodies are removed from the tracheobronchial tree with a bronchoscope.[70] Depending on the material, this may be a difficult procedure, although improvement in bronchoscopes in recent years has greatly facilitated this undertaking. Cardiopulmonary bypass has been successfully used to support a patient who had extensive foreign body aspiration. Occasionally, bronchoscopic extraction is unsuccessful, and a pulmonary lobectomy is required.

Traumatic Injury to the Airway

Traumatic injury to the upper airway may be divided into two broad categories: oral facial trauma and laryngeal/tracheal trauma. Patients with obvious oral facial trauma may be at risk for upper airway obstruction. Even if the patients have no sign of respiratory distress at the time of presentation, swelling of soft tissues and hemorrhaging to the airway may lead to airway compromise.

Patients who must undergo operative intervention to treat their traumatic injuries need careful evaluation of their airway, including radiographs and CT scan examination. Traumatic injuries may make intubations in the trachea difficult in these patients. For this reason, sedation is to be avoided and endotracheal intubation with the patient awake should be considered. This may be accomplished with direct laryngoscopy after local anesthesia has been applied to the patient's oropharynx. In more difficult cases, it may be necessary to use a fiberoptic bronchoscope to guide the endotracheal tube into the trachea.

Postoperatively, patients undergoing repair of facial trauma may have their jaw wired shut. These patients should undergo extubation only when fully awake after resolution of their airway and facial edema. Instruments to open the wires should always be kept at the patient's bedside. Emesis may present a grave hazard in these patients.

Injury to the larynx and trachea may occur after blunt trauma such as automobile accidents or after penetrating trauma. Blunt trauma to the neck may lead to fracture of the cartilaginous rings supporting the trachea or to disruption of the tracheal mucosa. In the latter case, attempted endotracheal intubation may worsen a partial tracheal transection and create an airway emergency.[71] Signs of laryngeal injury include dyspnea, altered phonation, pain on swallowing, hoarseness, swelling, and subcutaneous emphysema of the neck. The development of subcutaneous emphysema after blunt trauma to the neck suggests that a laryngeal fracture or tracheal tear has occurred. The quantity of air in the subcutaneous tissues does not correlate with the severity of the injury. Establishment of an adequate airway is an essential consideration. Acute trauma of the larynx is often treated with placement of a tracheostomy before surgical repair of the larynx.

Blunt thoracic trauma can cause tracheal or bronchial disruption. Most commonly, these are "blowout" injuries that result in tracheobronchial disruption. These injuries usually occur near the carina, and most involve mainstem bronchi.[72] Because children have flexible ribs, severe intrathoracic injuries can occur without rib fractures. The signs of tracheobronchial disruption include persistent air leak, failure to expand the lung with thoracostomy tube drainage, and massive atelectasis (from failure to conduct gas through an injured bronchus). Diagnosis of these injuries is usually made with bronchoscopy. Although small tracheobronchial disruptions may be managed conservatively, most of these lesions require surgical repair.[72]

Burn Injury to the Upper Airway

Thermal injury to the upper airway may complicate the management of a patient with burns. The presence of facial burns and singed nasal hairs, hoarseness, or inspiratory stridor should suggest the possibility of burn injury to the upper airway. Although respiratory compromise may not be present at the time of admission, it may develop later as swelling of the injured airway becomes more severe. Because of the efficient cooling capacity of the upper air

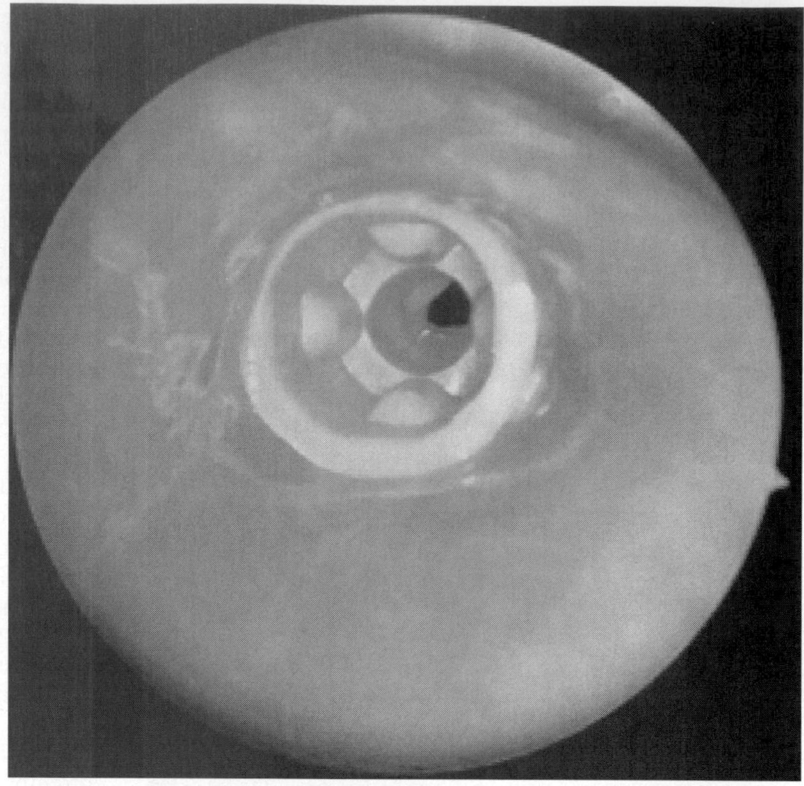

FIGURE 39–16 • Hollow plastic foreign body in patient's trachea. Because the lumen of the foreign body was aligned with the tracheal lumen, severe respiratory embarrassment did not occur. (Courtesy Andrew F. Inglis, Jr.)

passages, thermal injury to the airway below the vocal cords is uncommon, occurring in less than 5% of all hospitalized patients with burns.

Evidence of respiratory embarrassment in a patient with burns should be rapidly evaluated. Neck radiographs and fiberoptic examination of the larynx may show swelling of the soft tissues of the airway. If these findings are present, endotracheal intubation should be expeditiously performed to secure the airway before obstruction occurs. Because of the risk of infection, attempts are made to avoid tracheostomy placement in the patient with burns. Upper airway embarrassment is often accompanied by smoke inhalation injury to the lower airway, resulting in hypoxemia and hypercapnia. The products of combustion result in severe carbon monoxide intoxication or cyanide poisoning, both of which have nonspecific symptoms but require prompt medical therapy.[73]

Angioedema

Angioedema is a well-demarcated localized edema involving the deep layers of skin, including the subcutaneous tissue. Angioedema may occur in response to a variety of systemic disorders, including allergic reactions that are mediated with immunoglobulin E, anaphylactic and anaphylactoid reactions, and other illnesses. Angioedema may lead to swelling of the soft tissue of the face, particularly the eyes and lips. If this should involve the soft tissues of the upper respiratory tract, laryngeal obstruction may result. Administration of subcutaneous epinephrine may dramatically reduce swelling caused by this condition. Occasionally, respiratory embarrassment caused by this condition is so severe that endotracheal intubation is warranted. The evaluation of patients with this disorder should be directed at (1) the identification of the causative agents so that the patients can avoid these in the future and (2) the anatomical site of presentation to allow stratification of airway risk and planning of appropriate triage for airway intervention.[74]

Tracheostomy

Indications for the placement of a tracheostomy fall into three broad, frequently overlapping categories: airway obstruction, assisted ventilation, and pulmonary toilet. Pediatric anatomical anomalies that may necessitate tracheostomy are most often manifested in the neonatal period or in infancy, although some may not appear until childhood. The most common abnormalities include vocal cord paralysis (congenital and postbirth injury), subglottic stenosis, tracheal stenosis, cystic hygroma, tracheal hemangioma, and laryngeal cyst. The accurate diagnosis of these problems is frequently made during bronchoscopic examination of the larynx and trachea while the patient is anesthetized. If the obstruction is of sufficient magnitude, consideration should be given to doing a tracheostomy at the time of bronchoscopy.

Infants may require a tracheostomy because of the need for prolonged periods of assisted ventilation. The advent of neonatal intensive care has enabled small preterm infants to survive despite severe respiratory illness. Many of these patients will need lengthy periods of mechanical ventilation to treat infant respiratory distress syndrome and bronchopulmonary dysplasia. Prolonged intubation may lead to subglottic stenosis.[75] For a reduction in the frequency of this complication, a tracheostomy may be performed. The optimal timing of tracheostomy for children who need long-term intubation is controversial. In many neonatal ICUs, infants needing mechanical ventilatory support for more than 30 to 45 days will undergo a tracheostomy. Placement of a tracheostomy is not a trivial matter with several large studies showing a tracheostomy-related mortality rate of 0.5% to 0.7%.[76,77] One recent study provided evidence that long-term tracheostomy is associated with airway inflammation (number of cells, neutrophils), more frequent bacteria, and reduced concentration of surfactant protein-D.[78]

The decline of polio in the United States during the decade following 1950 dramatically decreased the number of tracheostomies performed to facilitate mechanical ventilation and pulmonary toilet. Nevertheless, several pediatric diseases predictably lead to prolonged neuromuscular failure. Infants with infant botulism may have prolonged neuromuscular weakness and may undergo a tracheostomy to simplify management of mechanical ventilation. Similarly, older children with Guillain-Barré syndrome and respiratory failure may need a tracheostomy if a lengthy course of mechanical ventilation is expected. The use of tracheostomy has been advocated to promote pulmonary toilet and improve ventilation during the treatment of flail chest.

The timing of the tracheostomy will depend on several issues, including the patient's underlying illness and the severity of the condition that makes tracheostomy necessary. If possible, emergency tracheostomy under unfavorable conditions should be avoided because the complications are more common in this setting. Percutaneous placement of a tracheostomy has been widely used in the adult population; however, experience in children remains limited. One small retrospective series suggests that placement in the ICU can be done safely with adherence to sound techniques and prudent patient selection.[79]

Postoperative Nursing Care

Care from attentive, trained nurses is essential for the well-being of the patient with a tracheostomy. Until a tract of granulation tissue has formed in the stoma between the cervical and tracheal epithelium, precautions should be taken to prevent the accidental displacement of the tracheostomy tube. Although stay sutures simplify replacement of the tracheostomy tube, this procedure may be difficult, especially in an emergency situation with a struggling patient. A hastily replaced tube may be incorrectly located in the pretracheal soft tissue resulting in asphyxiation. If positive-pressure ventilation is attempted with the tube in this position, subcutaneous and mediastinal emphysema may be followed by a life-threatening tension pneumothorax. Because of these risks, patients routinely stay in the ICU for 5 to 7 days postoperatively. Smaller children have arm restraints placed to prevent them from pulling at the tracheostomy tube. If necessary, sedation is given until the child grows accustomed to the tracheostomy and the tract matures with the formation of granulation tissue. If accidental displacement of the tracheostomy tube does occur, replacement may be facilitated with a gentle insertion of a 0 Miller laryngoscope blade into the stoma and the identification of the tracheal lumen before the tube is passed.

Besides avoiding accidental displacement of the tracheostomy, the nurse must constantly monitor the patient for obstruction of the tracheostomy tube. The tube may be obstructed by dried tracheal mucus. Sometimes the patient's chin may obstruct the tube. Humidified gas may be administered to prevent drying and inspissation of secretions.

Complications

Any operation on the airway involves risk. The complication rate after tracheostomy has been reported to be 10% to 30%, with a death rate of 3%. Early postoperative complications include air leak, hemorrhage, and aspiration. Air leak is seen more often in children than in adults and may be life threatening. The risk of complications declines as the patient ages. Some life-threatening complications, such as accidental decannulation or tracheostomy tube obstruction, may occur anytime after the placement of a tracheostomy. The safety and well-being of patients with a tracheostomy require constant vigilance to prevent these mishaps.

Swallowing dysfunction after tracheostomy may lead to aspiration of saliva and food. This may be due in part to anchoring of the trachea to the skin of the neck, preventing the cephalad movement of the trachea during swallowing. Children who have a tracheostomy often have difficulty learning to eat. The high frequency of pneumonia observed after tracheostomy may be in part due to the problem of recurrent aspiration. Aerophagia, another form of swallowing dysfunction, occurs with modest frequency in pediatric patients after tracheostomy.

Late complications include granulation tissue formation, tracheal stenosis, infection of the stoma, pneumonia, fused vocal cords, and distal tracheomalacia. Although infection of the stoma and distal tracheomalacia may be evident before decannulation, granulation formation and fused vocal cords may not be apparent until decannulation is attempted. An uncommon, but particularly dangerous late complication is erosion of the tracheostomy tube into the innominate artery.

Decannulation

Problems at the time of decannulation occur in up to 36% of children. These difficulties are most frequent in patients younger than 1 year. Structural abnormalities that result in decannulation problems include subglottic stenosis, tracheomalacia at the tracheostomy site, granuloma tissue obstructing the trachea, and fused vocal cords. If respiratory distress is encountered during decannulation, it should not be attributed to the patient's psychological dependence on the tracheostomy tube. Evaluation of the airway with bronchoscopy or a lateral neck radiograph is important. Psychological factors should not be considered until structural causes of respiratory embarrassment have been eliminated.

REFERENCES

1. Badgwell JM, McLeod ME, Friedberg J: Airway obstruction in infants and children, *Can J Anaesth* 34:90, 1987.
2. Freezer N, Butt W, Phelan P: Steroids in croup: do they increase the incidence of successful extubation? *Anaesth Intensive Care* 18:224, 1990.
3. Galvis AG, Stool SE, Bluestone CD: Pulmonary edema following relief of acute upper airway obstruction, *Ann Otolaryngol* 89: 124-128, 1980.
4. Nemechek AJ, Amedee RG: Choanal atresia, *J La State Med Soc* 146:337-340, 1994.
5. Friedman NR, Mitchell RB, Bailey CM, et al: Management and outcome of choanal atresia correction, *Int J Pediatr Otorhinolaryng* 52:45-51, 2000.
6. Prasad M, Ward RF, April MM, et al: Topical mitomycin as an adjunct to choanal atresia repair, *Arch Otolaryngol Head Neck Surg* 128:398-400, 2002.
7. Coates H: Nasal obstruction in the neonate and infant, *Clin Pediatr (Phila)* 31:25-29, 1992.
8. Matthews BL, Little JP, McGuirt WF Jr., Koufman JA: Reflux in infants with laryngomalacia: results of 24-hour double-probe pH monitoring. *Otolarygol Head Neck Surg* 120:860-864, 1999.
9. McCray BB, Crockett DM, Wagener JS, Thies DJ: Hypoxia and hypercapnia in infants with mild laryngomalacia, *Am J Dis Child* 142:896-899, 1988.
10. McClurg FL, Evans DA: Laser laryngoplasty for laryngomalacia, *Laryngoscope* 104(3 Pt 1):247-252, 1994.
11. Toynton SC, Saunders MW, Bailey CM: Aryepiglottoplasty for laryngomalacia: 100 consecutive cases, *J Laryngology Otology* 115:35-38, 2001.
12. van Aalderen WM, Hoekstra MO, Hess J, et al: Respiratory infections and vascular rings, *Acta Paediatr Scand* 79:477-480, 1990.
13. Haramati LB, Glickstein JS, Issenberg HJ, et al: MR imaging and CT of vascular anomalies and connections in patients with congenital heart disease: significance in surgical planning, *Radiographics* 22:337-347, 2002.
14. deLorimier AA, Harrison MR, Hardy K, et al: Tracheobronchial obstructions in infants and children. Experience with 45 cases, *Ann Surg* 212:227-289, 1990.
15. Brody AS, Kuhn JP, Seidel FG, Brodsky LS: Airway evaluation in children with use of ultrafast CT: pitfalls and recommendations, *Radiology* 178:181-184, 1991.
16. Greenholz S, Hall R, Lilly J, Shikes R: Surgical implications of bronchopulmonary dysplasia, *J Pediatr Surg* 22:1132-1136, 1987.
17. Miller R, Woo P, Kellman R, Slagle T: Tracheobronchial abnormalities in infants with bronchopulmonary dysplasia, *J Pediatr* 111:779-782, 1987.
18. Denneny JCI: Bronchomalacia in the neonate, *Ann Otol Rhinol Laryngol* 94(5 Pt 1):466-469, 1985.
19. Miller R, Pollack M, Murphy T, Fink R: Effectiveness of continuous positive airway pressure in the treatment of bronchomalacia in infants: a bronchoscopic documentation, *Crit Care Med* 14: 125-127, 1986.
20. Koyluoglu G, Gunay I, Ceran C, Berkan O: Pericardial flap aortopexy: an easy and safe technique in the treatment of tracheomalacia. *J Cardiovascular Surgery* 43:295-297, 2002.
21. Furman RH, Backer CL, Dunham ME, et al: The use of balloon-expandable metallic stents in the treatment of pediatric tracheomalacia and bronchomalacia, *Arch Otolaryngol Head Neck Surg* 125:203-207, 1999.
22. Geelhoed GC: Croup, *Pediatr Pulmonol* 23:370-374, 1997.
23. Johnson DW, Jacobson S, Edney PC, et al: A comparison of nebulized budesonide, intramuscular dexamethasone, and placebo for moderately severe croup, *N Engl J Med* 339: 498-503, 1998.
24. Klassen TP, Craig WR, Moher D, et al: Nebulized budesonide and oral dexamethasone for treatment of croup: a randomized controlled trial, *JAMA* 279:1629-1632, 1998.
25. Ausejo M, Saenz A, Pham B, et al: The effectiveness of glucocorticoids in treating croup: meta-analysis, *BMJ* 319:595-600, 1999.
26. Kairys SW, Olmstead EM, O'Connor GT: Steroid treatment of laryngotracheitis: a meta-analysis of the evidence from randomized trials, *Pediatrics* 83:683-693, 1989.
27. Russell K, Wiebe N, Saenz A, et al: Glucocorticoids for croup, *Cochrane Database of Systematic Reviews* (1):CD001955, 2004.
28. Duncan PG: Efficacy of helium-oxygen mixtures in the management of severe viral and post-intubation croup, *Canadian Anaesth Soc J* 26:206-212, 1979.
29. Stillwell PC, Quick JD, Munro PR, Mallory GB, Jr: Effectiveness of open-circuit and oxyhood delivery of helium-oxygen, *Chest* 95: 1222-1224, 1989.
30. Weber JE, Chudnofsky CR, Younger JG, et al: A randomized comparison of helium-oxygen mixture (Heliox) and racemic epinephrine for the treatment of moderate to severe croup, *Pediatrics* 107:E96, 2001.
31. Adderley RJ, Mullins GC: When to extubate the croup patient: the "leak" test, *Can J Anaesth* 34(3 Pt 1):304-306, 1987.
32. Gorelick MH, Baker MD: Epiglottitis in children, 1979 through 1992. Effects of *Haemophilus influenzae* type b immunization, *Arch Pediatr Adolesc Med* 148:47-50, 1994.
33. Harjacek M, Kornberg AE, Yates EW, Montgomery P: Thermal epiglottitis after swallowing hot tea, *Pediatr Emerg Care* 8:342-344, 1992.
34. Molteni RA: Epiglottis: incidence of extraepiglottis and pneumonia: report of 72 cases and review of the literature, *Pediatrics* 58:526-531, 1976.
35. Scott PMJ, Loftus WK, Kew J, et al: Diagnosis of peritonsillar infections: a prospective study of ultrasound, computerized tomography and clinical diagnosis, *J Laryngology Otology* 113:229-232, 1999.
36. Morrison JE, Pashley NRT: Retropharyngeal abscesses in children: a 10-year review, *Pediatr Emerg Care* 4:9-11, 1988.
37. Brechtelsbauer PB, Garetz SL, Gebarski SS, Bradford CR: Retropharyngeal abscess: pitfalls of plain films and computed tomography, *Am J Otolaryngol* 18: 258-262, 1997.
38. Lalakea ML, Messner AH: Retropharyngeal abscess management in children: current practices, *Otolaryngol Head Neck Surg* 121: 398-405, 1999.
39. Donnelly BW, McMillan JA, Weiner LB: Bacterial tracheitis: report of eight new cases and review, *Rev Infect Dis* 12:729-735, 1990.
40. Eckel HE, Widemann B, Damm M, Roth B: Airway endoscopy in the diagnosis and treatment of bacterial tracheitis in children, *Int J Pediatr Otorhinolaryngol* 27:147-157, 1993.
41. Bernstein T, Brilli R, Jacobs B: Is bacterial tracheitis changing? a 14-month experience in a pediatric intensive care unit, *Clin Infectious Dis* 27:458-462, 1998.
42. Dudin AA, Thalji A, Rambaud C-A: Bacterial tracheitis among children hospitalized for severe obstructive dyspnea, *Pediatr Infect Dis J* 9:293-295, 1990.
43. Aaltonen LM, Rihkanen H, Vaheri A: Human papillomavirus in larynx, *Laryngoscope* 112:700-707, 2002.
44. Hallmo P, Naess O: Laryngeal papillomatosis with human papillomavirus DNA contracted by a laser surgeon. *Eur Arch Otorhinolaryngol* 248:425-427, 1991.
45. Abramson AL, DiLorenzo TP, Steinberg BM: Is papillomavirus detectable in the plume of laser-treated laryngeal papilloma? *Arch Otolaryngol Head Neck Surg* 116:604-607, 1990.
46. Deunas L, Alcantud V, Alvarez F, et al: Use of interferon-a in laryngeal papillomatosis: eight years of the Cuban national programme, *J Laryngol Otol* 111:134-140, 1997.
47. Garcia-Millian R, Santos A, Perea SE, et al: Molecular analysis of resistance to interferon in patients with laryngeal papillomatosis, *Cytokines Cell Mol Ther* 5:79-85, 1999.
48. Zbar RIS, Chen AH, Behrendt DM, et al: Incidence of vocal fold paralysis in infants undergoing ligation of patent ductus arteriosus, *Ann Thorac Surg* 61:814-816, 1996.
49. Ross DA, Ward PH: Central vocal cord paralysis and paresis presenting as laryngeal stridor in children, *Laryngoscope* 100:10-13, 1990.
50. Brigger MT, Hartnick CJ: Surgery for pediatric vocal cord paralsis: a meta-analysis, *Otolaryngol Head Neck Surg* 126:349-355, 2002.
51. Yamashita M, Chin I, Horigome H, et al: Sudden fatal cardiac arrest in a child with an unrecognized anterior mediastinal mass, *Resuscitation* 19:175-177, 1990.
52. Montange F, Truffa B-J, Pichard E: Airway obstruction during anaesthesia in a child with a mediastinal mass, *Can J Anaesth* 37:271-272, 1990.
53. Lam JC, Chui CH, Jacobsen AS, et al: When is a mediastinal mass critical in a child? An analysis of 29 patients, *Pediatr Surg Int* 20:180-184, 2004.

54. Deakers TW, Reynolds G: Cuffed endotracheal tubes in pediatric intensive care, *J Pediatr* 125:57-62, 1994.
55. Rivera R, Tibballs J: Complications of endotracheal intubation and mechanical ventilation in infants and children, *Crit Care Med* 20:193-199, 1992.
56. Kemper KJ, Benson MS, Bishop MJ: Predictors of postextubation stridor in pediatric trauma patients, *Crit Care Med* 19:352-355, 1991.
57. Kemper KJ, Benson MS, Bishop MJ: Interobserver variability in assessing pediatric postextubation stridor, *Clin Pediatr (Phila)* 31:405-408, 1992.
58. Mhanna MJ, Zamel YB, Tichy CM, Super DM: The "air leak" test around the endotracheal tube, as a predictor of postextubation stridor, is age dependent in children, *Crit Care Med* 30:2639-2643, 2002.
59. Chaten FC, Lucking SE, Young ES, Mickell JJ: Stridor: intracranial pathology causing postextubation vocal cord paralysis, *Pediatrics* 87:39-43, 1991.
60. Darmon JY, Rauss A, Dreyfuss D et al: Evaluation of risk factors for laryngeal edema after tracheal extubation in adults and its prevention by dexamethasone. A placebo-controlled, double-blind, multicenter study [see comments], *Anesthesiology* 77:245-251, 1992.
61. Ferrara TB, Georgieff MK, Ebert J, Fisher JB: Routine use of dexamethasone for the prevention of postextubation respiratory distress, *J Perinatol* 9:287-290, 1989.
62. Tellez DW, Galvis AG, Storgion SA, et al: Dexamethasone in the prevention of postextubation stridor in children, *J Pediatr* 118:289-294, 1991.
63. Walner DL, Loewen MS, Kimura RE: Neonatal subglottic stenosis—incidence and trends, *Laryngoscope* 111:48-51, 2001.
64. Cotton RT, McMurray JS: Laryngotracheal stenosis. New perspectives, *Pediatr Pulmonol* 18:64-66, 1999.
65. Zalzal GH, Choi SS, Patel KM: Ideal timing of pediatric laryngotracheal reconstruction, *Arch Otolaryngol Head Neck Surg* 123:206-208, 1997.
66. Yellon RF, Parameswaran M, Brandom BW: Decreasing morbidity following larygotracheal reconstruction in children, *Int J Pediatr Otorhinolaryngol* 41:145-154, 1997.
67. Weissberg D, Schwartz I: Foreign bodies in the tracheobronchial tree, *Chest* 91:730-733, 1987.
68. Wolach B, Raz A, Weinberg J, et al: Aspirated foreign bodies in the respiratory tract of children: eleven years experience with 127 patients, *Int J Pediatr Otorhinolaryngol* 30:1-10, 1994.
69. Mantel K, Butenandt I: Tracheobronchial foreign body aspiration in childhood, *Eur J Pediatr* 145:211-216, 1986.
70. Kadish H, Schunk J, Woodward GA: Blunt pediatric laryngotracheal trauma: case reports and review of the literature, *Am J Emerg Med* 12:207-211, 1994.
71. Hancock BJ, Wiseman NE: Tracheobronchial injuries in children, *J Pediatr Surg* 26:1316-1319, 1991.
72. Ruddy RM: Smoke inhalation injury, *Pediatr Clin North Am* 41:317-336, 1994.
73. Ishoo E, Shah UK, Grillone GA, et al: Predicting airway risk in angioedema: staging system based on presentation, *Otolaryngol Head Neck Surg* 121:263-268, 1999.
74. Nau TW, Gates GA, Escobedo MB: Management of neonatal subglottic stenosis, *Otolaryngol Clin North Am* 19:153-162, 1986.
75. Carr MM, Poje CP, Kingston L et al: Complications in pediatric tracheostomies, *Laryngoscope* 111(11 Pt 1):1925-1928, 2001.
76. Wetmore RF, Marsh RR, Thompson ME, Tom LW: Pediatric tracheostomy: a changing procedure? *Ann Otology Rhinol Laryngol* 108(7 Pt 1):695-699, 1999.
77. Griese M, Felber J, Reiter K, et al: Airway inflammation in children with tracheostomy, *Pediatr Pulmonol* 37:356-361, 2004.
78. Klotz DA, Hengerer AS: Safety of pediatric bedside tracheostomy in the intensive care unit, *Arch Otolaryngol Head Neck Surg* 127:950-955, 2001.

CHAPTER 40

Asthma

Alexandre T. Rotta

PEARLS

- Acute exacerbations of asthma are responsible for a significant number of admissions to the pediatric intensive care unit. Complete understandings of asthma pathophysiology and of the clinical implications of severe airflow obstruction are paramount in the management of patients with acute asthma.
- Patients with severe acute asthma exacerbations should be aggressively managed in the emergency department with inhaled β agonists, ipratropium bromide, and corticosteroids. Those who fail to improve or further deteriorate should be admitted to the intensive care unit for a higher level of monitoring and escalation of therapy. Standard treatments include administration of fluids and oxygen, β agonists by intermittent or continuous nebulization, ipratropium bromide, parenteral corticosteroids, and intravenous infusion of a β_2 agonist. Other therapies available in the intensive care unit include intravenous infusions of magnesium sulfate, methylxanthines, and breathing helium-oxygen mixtures. Failure to respond to treatment can lead to further deterioration and the development of respiratory insufficiency, necessitating intubation and mechanical ventilatory support. These patients should be ventilated with a strategy that avoids high lung volumes that result from dynamic hyperinflation. Selected patients may benefit from inhalational anesthetics for bronchodilatation or from bronchoscopy to relieve airway obstruction or atelectasis resulting from mucous plugging.
- Aggressive medical treatment and a ventilation strategy that minimizes dynamic hyperinflation result in low morbidity and near-zero mortality in severe acute asthma.

Introduction/Definition

Asthma is a highly prevalent chronic disease that affects both children and adults and is the most common medical emergency in the pediatric population. Because of its significant impact on childhood health, asthma has been the focus of a number of government and private programs and initiatives, sharing the objective of improved surveillance.[1] Despite adequate treatment and access to medical care, patients with asthma are at risk for episodic acute deteriorations in pulmonary function commonly known as *reactive airway disease exacerbations* or *asthma attacks*. These attacks vary greatly in severity, ranging from mild episodes that are easily managed in the outpatient setting with intensification of bronchodilator therapy to severe episodes with intense airway obstruction that rapidly evolve to respiratory failure.

The term *status asthmaticus* has been used to denote a more severe form of asthma attack, but its definition varies widely among different authors. To some, status asthmaticus is an asthma attack that does not respond to initial treatments with bronchodilators,[2,3] whereas to others it indicates severe asthma that leads to respiratory failure and requires mechanical ventilatory support.[4] For the purposes of this text, status asthmaticus is defined as an asthma attack that fails to respond to initial doses of nebulized β_2-adrenergic and anticholinergic agents and a corticosteroid and that requires admission to the hospital for continuation of treatment. Patients who experience relentless progression of respiratory signs and symptoms, requiring admission to the intensive care unit (ICU), are defined as having near-fatal asthma.[5,6]

Epidemiology and Risk Factors

Asthma is the most common chronic illness in childhood, affecting approximately 4.8 million children and adolescents in the United States, or 6.9% of persons younger than 18 years.[7] Asthma is also the most common discharge diagnosis in children's hospitals, accounting for 10% to 30% of all admissions and more than 500,000 admissions each year in the United States alone.[8] The prevalence of asthma worldwide is highly variable, with greater than 20-fold differences in prevalence of symptoms encountered among centers located in various parts of the world.[9] The highest prevalence rates for asthma are found in the United Kingdom, Australia, New Zealand, and the Republic of Ireland; very low prevalence rates occur in eastern Europe, the Indian subcontinent, and China.[9] Race is a significant factor in determining prevalence and severity of asthma in children and young adults. African Americans are three to four times more likely than Caucasians to be hospitalized for asthma and have a higher death rate.[7]

Asthma prevalence and mortality have increased steadily for the past 25 years in the United States.[1] However, while the rate of asthma-related outpatient and emergency department visits continue to increase, asthma hospitalizations and death rates appear to be declining.[1] Whether or not this decline will be sustained during the current decade is yet to be seen.

The incidence of asthma-related respiratory failure requiring mechanical ventilation is difficult to determine because of variability in diagnostic criteria and reporting practices. Nonetheless, up to 36% of adult patients admitted to an inner-city medical ICU with near-fatal asthma require invasive mechanical ventilation.[10] This figure appears to be significantly lower for children, considering that only 22 (10.2%) of 237 patients treated for near-fatal asthma underwent mechanical ventilation in our own pediatric ICU over a 2-year period, and that 14 (8.6%) of 163 patients required intubation in another study.[11]

The majority of asthmatic patients who suffer respiratory failure or arrest do so during the first stages of therapy or prior to arrival in the emergency department.[11] Therefore early identification and close monitoring of patients at high risk for near-fatal asthma could be advantageous. High-risk patients often have a history of ICU admissions,[12] mechanical ventilation,[3,12] seizures or syncope during an attack,[13] $Pa{CO_2}$ greater than 45 torr,[3,12] attacks precipitated by food,[13] or a history of rapidly progressive and sudden respiratory deterioration.[2] These patients are likely to use more than two canisters of β-agonist metered-dose inhalers per month[14] and often are poorly compliant or receiving insufficient steroid therapy.[15,16] Denial or failure to perceive the severity of an attack are factors frequently associated with near-fatal asthma.[17,18] Although unquestionably some patients at risk for near-fatal asthma simply ignore early warning signs and do not seek adequate therapy, a subgroup of patients actually lacks normal perception of disease severity. Some patients with near-fatal asthma exhibit reduced chemosensitivity to hypoxia and blunted perception of dyspnea.[19] Other patients have a decreased perceptual sensitivity of inspiratory muscle loads and display abnormal respiratory-related evoked potentials.[20,21] Nonwhite residents of inner-city areas with limited access to health care contribute a substantial percentage of cases of near-fatal asthma and asthma-related deaths in the United States. In this country, black children are four to six times more like to die of asthma than their white counterparts.[1,7]

Although many of these high-risk factors are commonly present in patients with near-fatal asthma, they fail to prospectively identify a significant number of cases. In one study, 33% of patients who died of asthma were judged to have a history of trivial or mild asthma, whereas 32% had never been admitted to the hospital with asthma exacerbation.[2] Some of these patients may in fact have what likely represents a distinct clinical entity known as *sudden asphyxial asthma,* a condition marked by acute onset of severe airway obstruction and hypoxia that rapidly leads to cardiorespiratory arrest in patients known to have only mild asthma or no asthma history at all.[22,23]

Pathophysiology

Asthma is primarily an inflammatory disease and, as such, is marked by highly redundant pathways and complex interactions among inflammatory cells, mediators, and the airway epithelium[24] (Figure 40–1). Functionally, asthma is characterized by variable airflow obstruction and airway hyperresponsiveness associated with airway inflammation. Pathologically, it is marked by mast cell degranulation, accumulation of eosinophils and CD4 lymphocytes, hypersecretion of mucus, thickening of the subepithelial collagen layer, and smooth muscle hypertrophy and hyperplasia.[25,26]

Mast cells, eosinophils, macrophages, and T lymphocytes are central to the derangements that occur during an acute attack (see Figure 40–1). The usual cascade begins with the activation and degranulation of mast cells in response to allergens or topical insults. The mast cells in turn promote activation of T lymphocytes by presenting these cells to the allergenic particles. The inflammatory process is then amplified by T-lymphocyte release of cytokines and chemokines. There is increasing evidence that airway inflammation in asthma is the result of T-lymphocyte activation with the production of T_H2 cytokines, such as interleukin (IL)-4, IL-5, IL-8, and IL-13.[26,27] The presence of these T_H2 cytokines leads to further augmentation of the inflammatory process through overexuberant production of immunoglobulin E (IgE) by B cells, stimulation of airway epithelial cells, and eosinophil chemotaxis. IgE stimulates mast cells to release leukotrienes, whereas interleukins (particularly IL-5) promote maturation and migration of activated eosinophils into the airway.[28] This highly inflammatory milieu results in stimulation of airway epithelial cells and continued augmentation of the inflammatory process by further

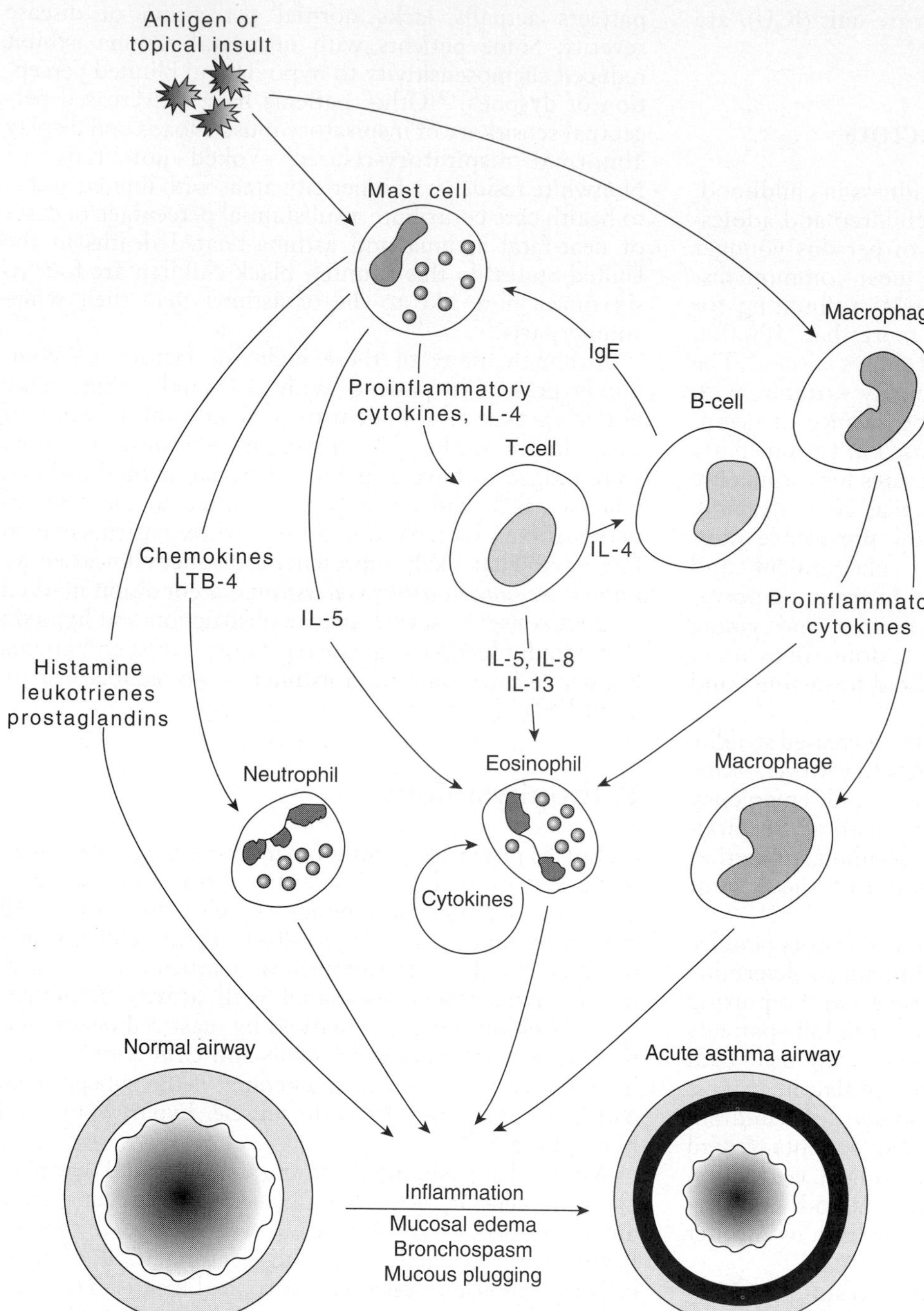

FIGURE 40–1 • Cellular and humoral mediators that lead to mucosal edema, bronchospasm, and mucous plugging in acute asthma. *IL,* Interleukin; *LTB-4,* leukotriene B-4.

release of leukotrienes, prostaglandins, nitric oxide, adhesion molecules, and platelet-activating factor. This process results in overproduction of mucus and epithelial cell destruction that lead to airway plugging and denudation of the airway surface. Epithelial denudation is known to expose nerve endings, resulting in hyperirritable airways[29] that become more susceptible to spasm and obstruction when challenged by subsequent exposure to allergens,[30] inhaled irritants such as cigarette smoke and pollution,[31,32] respiratory tract infections,[33] psychological stress,[34] and exercise,[35] among other insults.

Inflammation-mediated edema, mucus hypersecretion, airway plugging, and bronchospasm lead to the severe airway obstruction seen in patients with status asthmaticus and near-fatal asthma. The resulting obstruction and increased airway resistance create an impediment for inspiratory and expiratory gas flow, which leads to deranged pulmonary mechanics and increased lung volumes.

Airway plugging can result in ventilation/perfusion mismatching and increased oxygen requirements. Hypoxemia is common in patients with a severe asthma attack, but it is generally easily corrected with supplemental oxygen[36] and only weakly correlated with pulmonary function test abnormalities.[37] More frequently, airway plugging and obstruction lead to regional alveolar hyperinflation associated with reduced perfusion, resulting in a significantly increased pulmonary dead space. Most such patients exhibit an increased respiratory rate in attempt to achieve a higher minute volume and compensate for the ventilation abnormality. Unfortunately, in patients with more severe disease, airway obstruction also results in significant prolongation of expiratory time, which, coupled with initiation of inspiration prior to completion of the previous exhalation, leads to dynamic hyperinflation, gas trapping, and the development of abnormally high lung volumes[38] (Figure 40–2).

The higher lung volumes that result from incomplete alveolar emptying and dynamic hyperinflation serve as an adaptation mechanism to allow for higher expiratory flows than would have been possible at lower, more physiologic lung volumes. This is accomplished, however, at a high energy cost. Expiration becomes an active process, and the use of accessory muscles is required to overcome the high resistances to airflow both during inspiration and exhalation.[39] During a severe attack, inspiratory transpulmonary pressures in excess of 50 cmH_2O may be generated, compared with approximately 5 cmH_2O during normal breathing.[40] The increased muscle work is accompanied by an increase in blood flow to the diaphragm, but this often is insufficient to meet the much greater metabolic demands.[41] Failure to promptly relieve the airway obstruction and reduce the work of breathing eventually leads to respiratory muscle fatigue, inadequate ventilation, and respiratory failure.

States of advanced airway obstruction and dynamic hyperinflation typical of severe asthma attacks have a significant impact on the circulatory system. The highly negative intrapleural pressures generated by spontaneously breathing patients during inspiration favor transcapillary edema fluid movement into the airspaces.[39] They also cause a phasic increase in left ventricular afterload and a decrease in cardiac output[42] that is clinically manifested as pulsus paradoxus.[43] Right ventricular afterload may be increased during severe asthma as a result of pulmonary vasoconstriction related to hypoxia and acidosis. A state of increased pulmonary vascular resistance secondary to dynamic hyperinflation can also increase right ventricular afterload, further impacting cardiac output.[43–45]

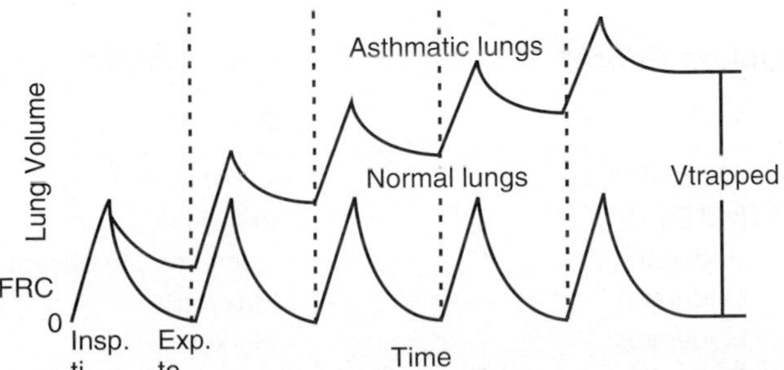

FIGURE 40–2 • Mechanics of dynamic pulmonary hyperinflation in the setting of severe airflow obstruction. The next inspiration begins before complete exhalation, leading to gas trapping and increased end-expiratory lung volume. (From reference 38.)

Clinical Assessment

History

The sick child with asthma usually presents with complaints of difficulty breathing and shortness of breath. The presence of these complaints in a child with known previous episodes of asthma exacerbations is highly suggestive of the diagnosis. A significant percentage of children have a history of a coexisting viral upper respiratory infection, whereas some describe exposure to known allergic triggers. Circumstances permitting, time should be taken to inquire about the presence of high-risk factors (Box 40–1) for near-fatal asthma and the adequacy of maintenance intercrisis therapy.

Physical Examination

Children with severe forms of acute asthma commonly present with tachypnea, diaphoresis, increased use of accessory muscles, and nasal flaring. Sick nonverbal children may appear anxious, agitated, or simply unable to be distracted from the task of breathing. Older children often assume a tripod sitting position and may voice a sensation of impending doom. Speech flow is truncated by the need to inspire. The presence of intercostal, subcostal, and suprasternal retractions; nasal flaring; inability to speak in sentences; and agitation are signs of impending respiratory failure. Evolution or persistence of these signs is followed by slower labored breathing, confusion or obtundation, and respiratory arrest.

Wheezing is a common clinical finding in patients with acute asthma exacerbations. It is the audible manifestation of the transmitted turbulence to airflow in the intrathoracic intrapulmonary airways. Wheezing may be predominantly expiratory as a result of the dynamic phasic compression of conducting airways, but it also can be biphasic. Wheezing in severe asthma usually

BOX 40–1

Risk Factors for Near-Fatal Asthma

Medical Factors
- Previous asthma attack with:
  - Admission to intensive care unit
  - Respiratory failure and mechanical ventilation
  - Seizures or syncope
  - $Paco_2$ >45 torr
  - High consumption (>2 canisters per month) of β-agonist metered-dose inhalers
  - Underuse of corticosteroid therapy

Psychosocial Factors
- Denial or failure to perceive severity of illness
- Associated depression or other psychiatric disorder
- Noncompliance
- Dysfunctional family unit
- Inner-city residents

Ethnic Factors
- Nonwhite children (black, Hispanic, other)

Modified from Werner HA: *Chest* 119:1913-1929, 2001.

is symmetrical. An asymmetrical distribution suggests regional mucous plugging, atelectasis, pneumothorax, or the presence of a foreign body. The degree of wheezing correlates poorly with disease severity,[46] as wheezes are heard only in the presence of airflow. As such, a patient with severe airway obstruction and very limited airflow may have a silent chest on arrival to the emergency department and develop loud wheezes after effective therapy is instituted. Likewise, a patient with loud wheezes that continues to worsen may develop a silent chest as a prelude to respiratory failure.

Objective assessment of disease severity is important in evaluating response to therapy. Wood et al.[47] developed a practical clinical asthma score composed of five variables with three different grades that allows for semiquantitative assessment of disease severity (Table 40–1). This clinical asthma score has been shown to correlate well with the need for prolonged bronchodilator therapy and hospitalization.[48] However, although clinical asthma scores seem to be useful for assessing the severity of an attack, they are not as effective in prospectively identifying patients who require prolonged hospitalization or who develop complications and subsequent disability.[49,50]

A less frequently used but more objective method of assessing disease severity and progression in patients with severe asthma is measurement of pulsus paradoxus. Originally described by Adolf Kussmaul[51] in a patient with constrictive pericarditis, pulsus paradoxus is also observed in conditions where pleural pressure swings are exaggerated, such as status asthmaticus and near-fatal asthma. The simplest definition of pulsus paradoxus is an exaggeration of the physiologic inspiratory decrease in systolic blood pressure[52] (Figure 40–3). It has been suggested that the term *pulsus paradoxus* is inappropriate to describe this phenomenon,[53] because an accentuated inspiratory decrease in systolic pressure in the same direction of the normally occurring change cannot be described as a paradox. However, the true paradox described by Kussmaul[51] was "the presence of a pulse slight and irregular, disappearing during inspiration and returning upon expiration despite the continued presence of the cardiac impulse during both respiratory phases."[52] Several mechanisms have been implicated as contributors to pulsus paradoxus in asthma, and it is likely that various mechanisms contribute differently depending on the adequacy of intravascular volume, the magnitude of pleural pressure swings, the degree of pulmonary hyperinflation, and the state of cardiac contractility. These include increased left ventricular afterload from highly negative intrapleural pressure[54]; decreased left ventricular preload as a result of inspiratory blood pooling in the pulmonary vasculature[55]; impaired left ventricular diastolic filling caused by a leftward shift of the interventricular septum resulting from increased venous return to the right heart[56]; constraint of cardiac filling because of longitudinal inspiratory deformation of the pericardium[43]; and increased right ventricular afterload with decreased filling of the left ventricle as a result of hyperinflation, acidosis, and hypoxia.[57] The pulsus paradoxus can be easily measured in the spontaneously breathing patient by transducing pressure signals from an indwelling arterial catheter or using a manual sphygmomanometer. In the latter, the cuff is inflated 20 mmHg above the systolic pressure and then deflated until the first Korotkoff sounds are heard (systolic blood pressure). Initially, Korotkoff sounds are heard only during expiration. The cuff is then carefully deflated until the point where the sounds are heard equally during both inspiration and expiration. The difference between the highest systolic pressure and the pressure at which all Korotkoff sounds are heard is the magnitude of the pulsus paradoxus. During normal breathing this difference is less than 5 mmHg, but it is generally greater than 10 mmHg during acute asthma exacerbations and greater than 20 mmHg in patients with more severe disease.[58] Changes in the magnitude of pulsus paradoxus during the course of therapy are good indicators of disease severity.[43,58]

Patients with status asthmaticus frequently have a palpable liver with normal liver span on physical examination. This sign is more pronounced in patients with significant hyperinflation and is explained by caudal displacement of the liver by the flattened diaphragm.

Radiography

Chest radiography is not routinely indicated in spontaneously breathing patients known to have asthma. However, this is a valuable diagnostic tool in patients suspected of having a pneumothorax or pneumomediastinum,

TABLE 40–1

Clinical Asthma Evaluation Score*

	0	1	2
Pa_{O_2} (torr) *or*	70–100 in 21% O_2	<70 in 21% O_2	<70 in 40% O_2
Cyanosis	None	In 21% O_2	In 40% O_2
Inspiratory breath sounds	Normal	Unequal	Decreased to absent
Accessory muscles used	None	Moderate	Maximal
Expiratory wheezing	None	Moderate	Marked
Cerebral function	Normal	Depressed or agitated	Coma

From Wood DW, Downes JJ, Lecks HI: *Am J Dis Child* 123:227-228, 1972.

*A score of 5 or more is thought to be indicative of impending respiratory failure. A score of 7 or more with Pa_{CO_2} >65 torr indicates existing respiratory failure.

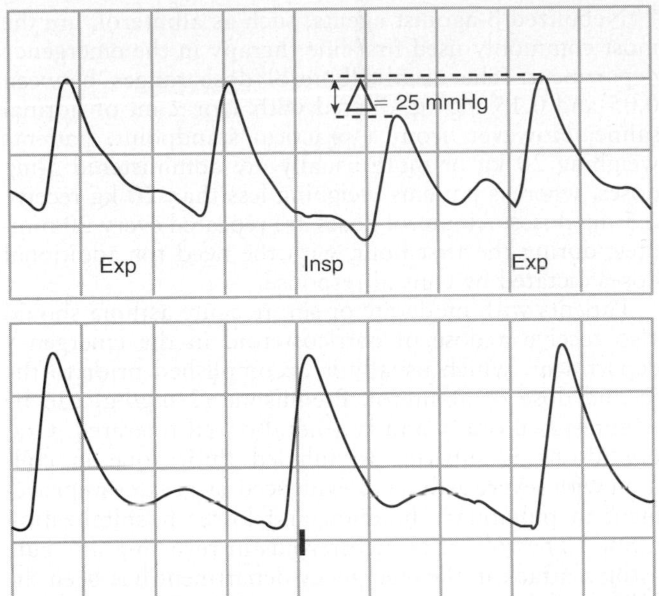

FIGURE 40–3 • Pressure recording from a radial artery catheter of a spontaneously breathing patient with airway obstruction. **Upper panel:** Abnormally high pulsus paradoxus of 23 mmHg is measured as the difference (Δ) in systolic blood pressure between expiration *(Exp)* and inspiration *(Insp)*. **Lower panel:** Normal slight physiologic variation of the systolic blood pressure as a function of the respiratory cycle 12 hours after onset of treatment.

pneumonias, or clinically important atelectasis and in children presenting with a first episode of wheezing in whom anatomic abnormalities (vascular rings, right-sided aortic arch) or foreign bodies are suspected. A chest radiograph should be obtained in patients who are sick enough to require monitoring and treatment in the ICU to exclude the possibility of unsuspected extrapulmonary air and airspace disease.

Laboratory Data

Arterial Blood Gas Analysis

Arterial blood gas measurements provide objective information on the adequacy of ventilation and oxygenation of the asthmatic patient. The typical blood gas abnormality encountered in the early phase of asthma is relative hypoxemia with hypocapnia (Pa_{CO_2} <35 torr) reflecting hyperventilation.[59] With worsening of airway obstruction, Pa_{CO_2} measurements return to the normal range of approximately 40 torr. However, this "normal" Pa_{CO_2} should not be viewed as reassuring when taken in the context of prolonged expiratory time, tachypnea, and accessory muscle use.[60] In fact, Pa_{CO_2} greater than 40 torr in a patient with status asthmaticus should be interpreted as a sign of evolving respiratory muscle fatigue and warrants close clinical observation. Sicker patients often exhibit a mixed respiratory and metabolic acidosis.[61] Lactic acidosis is frequently encountered in these patients and is thought to represent exaggerated lactate production by the respiratory muscles and tissue hypoxia.[62]

The decision of whether or not to intubate a child with asthma should not rest on the arterial blood gas measurements but on the overall clinical status. As such, routine arterial blood gas determinations are not a critical component of the evaluation of a spontaneously breathing child with status asthmaticus. In contrast, asthmatic children undergoing mechanical ventilation require frequent blood gas measurements to monitor disease progression and the adequacy of ventilatory support.

Electrolytes and Complete Blood Count

Routine chemistry and blood counts are generally not revealing in patients with status asthmaticus. Children who present with a more protracted asthma attack may have evidence of dehydration with elevated blood urea nitrogen as a result of decreased oral fluid intake and increased insensible water losses. Patients undergoing repeated treatments with nebulized or intravenous (IV) β agonists might show evidence of hypokalemia from intracellular potassium shifts. The blood cell count usually is normal, although some atopic patients exhibit elevated eosinophil counts. The presence of leukocytosis in some patients does not necessarily indicate infection and likely is related to adaptive stress or the administration of exogenous corticosteroids.

Muscle Enzymes

At least one third of patients with acute severe asthma exhibit an elevated plasma creatine kinase (CK) level.[63,64] Although such elevations seem to be more pronounced in patients with marked acidemia or those presenting with more severe respiratory insufficiency,[65] a convincing correlation between disease severity and CK elevation has not been established.[63] Myoglobin, a heme protein present in skeletal and cardiac muscle, is also found in patients with near-fatal asthma.[63] Some patients with near-fatal asthma develop elevations of CK-MB isoenzyme, suggesting a possible myocardial injury. This certainly is a plausible scenario, considering many patients are hypoxemic, acidotic, have high myocardial energy demand, and are receiving medications with cardiac side effects. However, plasma myoglobin and CK-MB elevations cannot be solely attributed to myocardial injury because the lungs and respiratory muscles are also known sources of these substances.[66] Cardiospecific troponin T is a very sensitive and specific marker of myocardial cell damage[67] and should be used preferentially to address the question of cardiomyocyte involvement in patients with severe asthma.

Electrocardiography

Patients with status asthmaticus or near-fatal asthma with significant airway obstruction and hyperinflation may exhibit a change in the mean frontal P-wave vector. A P-wave axis greater than 60 degrees has been associated with hyperinflation in both pediatric and adult patients with airway obstruction and is thought to represent positional atrial changes caused by inferior displacement of the diaphragm.[68,69]

Twelve-lead electrocardiography and continuous cardiac monitoring are valuable tools in the care of patients with near-fatal asthma in the ICU environment. These patients usually receive high doses of β-agonist drugs and may show evidence of hypokalemia (low-voltage T waves) or cardiac arrhythmias.[70,71] The already increased myocardial energy demand state resulting from airway obstruction is compounded by the chronotropic and vasodilatory effects inherent to β-agonist drugs and may lead to myocardial ischemia, particularly in adult patients with restricted coronary perfusion. Pediatric patients may also exhibit electrocardiographic (ECG) and enzymatic evidence of myocardial ischemia, particularly during treatment with IV isoproterenol.[72,73] However, despite the fact that a study reported a high percentage (66%) of patients exhibited nonspecific ST-segment changes or other criteria suggestive of ischemia, these changes were not well correlated with initiation of terbutaline therapy or elevations in cardiac troponin T.[74]

Spirometry

Measurement of peak expiratory flow rates can be used to estimate the degree of airway obstruction and response to therapy in patients presenting to the emergency department with an acute asthma attack. Use of this simple technique is less ubiquitous to the pediatric ICU environment because sick patients with severe respiratory distress simply may be unable to perform an adequate maneuver. Measurements also may not be reliable in younger patients who are incapable of coordinating a rapid forced expiratory effort.

Treatment

Initial Management in the Emergency Department

Pediatric patients with mild acute asthma exacerbations generally are managed in the emergency department with one or more doses of an inhaled β agonist, such as albuterol (salbutamol). Many of these patients also receive a dose of an oral corticosteroid, such as prednisone, and are sent home to complete a 3- to 5-day course of therapy. These patients with mild disease generally respond well to initial treatment and do not require the attention of a pediatric intensivist.

Patients with moderate or severe acute asthma attacks require aggressive management from the outset, including the prehospital setting. Because most patients with moderate or severe attacks have enough intrapulmonary shunt to result in clinically measurable hypoxemia, supplemental oxygen therapy should be initiated in patients with an oxygen saturation measured by pulse oximetry (Spo_2) lower than 95%. It should be obvious that use of supplemental oxygen will cause an increase in Spo_2 but will have no impact on ventilation. Therefore one must not incorrectly assume that ventilation is adequate in a patient with normal Spo_2 during supplemental oxygen therapy.

Nebulized β-agonist agents, such as albuterol, are the most commonly used first-line therapy in the emergency department. The usual albuterol dose ranges between 0.05 and 0.15 mg/kg, diluted with 1 or 2 ml of normal saline. However, from a practical standpoint, patients weighing 20 kg or more usually are administered 5-mg doses, whereas patients weighing less than 20 kg receive 2.5-mg doses. Albuterol doses are repeated every 20 minutes, during the first hour, with the need for additional doses dictated by clinical response.

Patients with moderate or severe acute asthma should also receive a dose of corticosteroid in the emergency department, which usually is accomplished prior to the second dose of albuterol. Prednisone (2 mg/kg) can be administered orally and is generally well tolerated. Oral prednisone is superior to inhaled fluticasone in children with severe asthma as evidenced by greater improvement in pulmonary function and lower hospitalization rates.[75] The role of corticosteroids in reversing an acute asthma attack in the emergency department has been the subject of debate, considering that these drugs require at least 4 to 6 hours for peak effects.[76,77] However, regardless of considerations about onset of action, acute suppression of inflammation is a cornerstone of acute asthma treatment and should be initiated as early as possible. Sicker patients with severe asthma exacerbations, those unable to tolerate oral medication because of respiratory distress or emesis, or those with a history of nausea during intensive β-agonist therapy should receive parenteral corticosteroids, such as methylprednisolone (2 mg/kg IV, followed by 0.5–1 mg/kg/dose IV every 6 hours).

Inhaled or nebulized anticholinergic agents, such as ipratropium bromide, are now considered an important adjunct in the treatment of moderate and severe asthma exacerbations in the emergency department. In patients treated with one dose of a corticosteroid, use of ipratropium bromide (500 μg/2.5 ml) in conjunction with the second and third albuterol (salbutamol) doses has been associated with greater clinical improvement[78] and reduced hospitalization rates in comparison with corticosteroid and albuterol (salbutamol) alone.[79]

Admission Criteria

The majority of patients with an acute asthma exacerbation respond to treatment in the emergency department and are discharged home. Among the patients whose symptoms persist despite initial treatment, most can be safely managed in the general pediatric inpatient ward. Indications for hospitalization from the emergency department are poorly defined but may include (1) inadequate response to three or four aerosol treatments; (2) relapse within 1 hour of receiving aerosols and steroids; (3) persistent Spo_2 less than 91% in room air; (4) need for oxygen therapy; (5) significant reduction in peak expiratory flow rate; (6) unreliable family or patient unable to comply with outpatient treatment; and (7) multiple visits for the same episode.[6,80] Patients who require higher levels or monitoring or more invasive and aggressive treatment or who deteriorate during hospitalization in the general pediatric ward should be admitted to the pediatric ICU.

Management in the Intensive Care Unit

General

Patients with near-fatal asthma who are admitted to the ICU represent a heterogeneous group and, as such, require different levels of monitoring, technology, and treatments. However, all patients who are sick enough to warrant admission to the ICU should be attached to a monitor capable of displaying continuous ECG tracing, respiratory rate, noninvasive blood pressures, and Sp_{O_2}. Sicker patients who require frequent blood draws or monitoring of pulsus paradoxus will benefit from an indwelling arterial catheter. Patients in respiratory failure requiring mechanical ventilation should have adequate central venous access and a Foley catheter in addition to the more basic instrumentation.

Oxygen

Sick patients with asthma are likely to exhibit hypoxemia as a result of intrapulmonary shunts caused by mucus plugging and atelectasis. Therefore humidified oxygen should be offered both as a carrier gas for nebulizations and continuously between treatments. Supplemental oxygen can be safely incorporated into the treatment algorithm because, unlike what is observed in some adult patients with chronic obstructive pulmonary disease and hypercarbia, no evidence suggests that supplemental oxygen suppresses the respiratory drive in children with near-fatal asthma.

Fluids

Patients with near-fatal asthma usually present in a state of decreased total body water, resulting from decreased oral fluid intake and increased insensible water losses. Therefore most patients require some degree of volume expansion. This need should be carefully balanced with the consideration that overhydration must be avoided because of the propensity for transcapillary fluid migration and alveolar flooding exhibited by some patients with large swings in intrathoracic pressures. The need for rapid fluid expansion often becomes obvious shortly after intubation of patients with low intravascular volumes receiving IV β agonists.

Beta Agonists

The β-agonist properties of the sympathomimetic agents cause bronchial smooth muscle relaxation and hence bronchodilatation. These agents can also increase diaphragmatic contractility, enhance mucociliary clearance, and inhibit bronchospastic mediators from mast cells.[81] Therefore β agonists are the mainstay of pharmacotherapy in near-fatal asthma. β_2-receptor selectivity is desirable to avoid side effects of nonselective α- and β_1-adrenergic receptor stimulation. However, despite β_2 selectivity, cardiovascular side effects remain a dose-limiting factor. The relative potency of various agents for the β_2 receptor is as follows: isoproterenol > fenoterol > albuterol > terbutaline > isoetharine > metaproterenol.[82] Of these agents, only albuterol and terbutaline are widely used in clinical practice, with some centers still using isoproterenol in selected occasions.

Once bound to the β-adrenergic receptor, β agonists activate adenyl cyclase resulting in increased intracellular cyclic adenosine monophosphate (cAMP) levels, which leads to bronchial and vascular smooth muscle relaxation. Dose-response curves demonstrate that large dose increases fail to enhance bronchodilation significantly; however, as the degree of bronchial constriction increases, the bronchodilation dose-response curve shifts to the right, indicating the need for a higher dose to achieve the desired response.[82]

In near-fatal asthma, parenteral and aerosol routes of administration are used exclusively. Traditional therapy for acute asthma previously included subcutaneous doses of epinephrine, but this practice is no longer widely used because of the development of newer, more selective β agonists with longer duration of action and fewer side effects.

The most frequent untoward side effects of β agonists are skeletal muscle tremor, nausea, and tachycardia. These side effects are common to both nonselective and selective β agonists administered by IV and inhalational routes. Other cardiovascular side effects include blood pressure instability (predominantly diastolic hypotension) and cardiac dysrhythmias.[83,84] Myocardial ischemia has been well documented as a complication of IV isoproterenol administration to children with near-fatal asthma.[72,85] However, continuous IV infusions of terbutaline appear to be safe and are not associated with significant cardiotoxicity.[74] Prolongations of the QTc interval and hypokalemia have been observed during IV infusions of β agonists.[81] Hypokalemia occurs in the setting of relatively stable total body potassium. It is the result of intracellular potassium shifting that results, at least in part, from an increased number of sodium-potassium pumps and not from augmented potassium elimination.[86] Therefore supraphysiologic potassium supplementation is rarely necessary.

Albuterol

Albuterol is the most β_2-specific aerosol agent available in the United States. It usually is administered every 20 minutes during the initial phase of treatment at a dose of 0.05 to 0.15 mg/kg. The optimal dose and frequency of albuterol (salbutamol) are controversial because less than 1% of the nebulized drug is deposited in the lung.[87] Moreover, spontaneous tidal volume, breathing pattern, and technique are unpredictable yet major determinants of drug delivery. After the initial series of three albuterol (salbutamol) treatments, patients who require nebulizations more frequently than every 1 hour should be started on continuous albuterol nebulization.

Continuous albuterol nebulization appears to be superior to repeated intermittent dosing[88,89] and has not been shown to cause significant cardiotoxicity.[82] A small prospective randomized study in children with near-fatal asthma and impending respiratory failure indicated that children treated with continuous albuterol had more rapid clinical improvement and shorter hospitalizations compared with children treated with intermittent albuterol doses.[89] Continuous albuterol was also associated with more efficient allocation of respiratory therapist time[89] and could offer the added advantage of more hours of uninterrupted sleep to patients who often are already exhausted.[90] The usual dose of continuous albuterol (salbutamol) ranges between 0.15 and 0.45 mg/kg/hour, with a maximum dose of 20 mg/hour. However, doses as high as 40 to 50 mg/hour have been advocated by some for severe status asthmaticus.[53]

The availability of treating patients with levalbuterol has generated some controversy. Albuterol is a 50:50 mixture of R-albuterol (levalbuterol), the active enantiomer that causes bronchodilation, and S-albuterol, which was thought to be inactive in humans. The Food and Drug Administration has approved levalbuterol, the pure R-isomer, as a preservative-free nebulizer solution.[91] The purported advantage of using levalbuterol over albuterol stems from the fact that S-albuterol has a longer elimination half-life than R-albuterol and may not be completely inert.[92,93] However, the notion that S-albuterol is not inert and capable of adverse effects is not universally accepted.[94–96] The randomized clinical studies in children with asthma failed to show definitive evidence that levalbuterol is superior to a regular racemic albuterol. Furthermore, R-albuterol is significantly more expensive than albuterol.[97] Considering the paucity of clinical evidence supporting the use of levalbuterol, routine use of this expensive drug in children with near-fatal asthma cannot be recommended at this time.

Intravenous albuterol is not available in the United States. However, the efficacy of albuterol infusions in patients with severe asthma has been well established in countries where the IV preparation is available.[98–100]

Terbutaline

Terbutaline is a relatively selective β_2-agonist with a mechanism of action similar to albuterol. It is the most commonly used parenteral β agonist in the United States and is available for nebulization, subcutaneous injection, and IV use. Because of its lower β_1-receptor affinity, subcutaneous administration of terbutaline has largely supplanted the use of epinephrine in severe acute asthma. The use of subcutaneous terbutaline is limited in the pediatric ICU environment, reserved for patients with acute worsening of the respiratory status who do not have vascular access and in whom access cannot be easily obtained. Subcutaneous terbutaline is more commonly used in the acute management of very sick patients in the emergency department and in the prehospital setting. The usual subcutaneous terbutaline dose is 0.01 mg/kg/dose (maximum 0.25 mg) subcutaneously every 20 minutes for three doses, as necessary.

Terbutaline is more commonly used in the ICU environment through the IV route. This therapy is indicated for patients with near-fatal asthma who fail to improve or show signs of deterioration during treatment with nebulized β_2 agonists, ipratropium bromide, and steroids. The usual IV terbutaline doses are 0.1 to 10 μg/kg/min, IV as a continuous infusion,[83] prepared in 0.9% normal saline or D_5W. In our clinical experience, however, most patients are started on 1 μg/kg/min and the dose is titrated to effect, with doses higher than 4 μg/kg/min rarely necessary. Patients receiving doses lower than 1 μg/kg/min can be given a loading dose of 10 μg/kg over 10 minutes to accelerate the onset of action.

Anticholinergics

Anticholinergics have become an important part of the treatment of children with severe acute asthma. The prototypical anticholinergic agent used in asthma is ipratropium bromide, a quaternary ammonium compound formed by the introduction of an isopropyl group to the N atom of atropine. Considering bronchial smooth muscle tone is influenced by the parasympathetic tone, ipratropium bromide can produce bronchodilation by inhibition of cholinergic-mediated bronchospasm.[101] An unexpected but important property of ipratropium bromide is the lack of negative effect on ciliary bronchial epithelium, unlike the marked inhibition of ciliary beating and mucociliary clearance produced by atropine.[101]

As stated on page 594, in the Initial Management in the Emergency Department section, 250-μg doses of nebulized ipratropium bromide can be used every 20 minutes during the first hour in the emergency department. The recommended dose for continuation therapy is 250 to 500 μg, given every 6 hours. After inhalation, peak responses usually develop over 30 to 90 minutes, and clinical effects may persist for more than 4 hours.[101] Systemic effects are minimal because less than 1% of an inhaled dose of ipratropium bromide is absorbed into the circulation. However, extrapulmonary effects, such as mydriasis and blurred vision, as a result of topical ocular absorption of the drug have been reported.[102,103]

Corticosteroids

Corticosteroids play a central role in the treatment of status asthmaticus and near-fatal asthma, considering that these are predominantly inflammatory conditions. Glucocorticosteroids modulate airway inflammation by a number of mechanisms, including direct interaction with cytosolic receptors and glucocorticosteroid response elements in gene promoters and indirect effects on binding of transcription factors, such as nuclear factor-kappa B (NF-κB), and on other cell signaling processes, such as posttranscriptional events.[104] Gene products suppressed by glucocorticosteroids include a wide range of cytokines (IL-1, IL-2, IL-3, IL-4, IL-5, IL-6, IL-7, IL-8, IL-11, IL-12, IL-13, tumor necrosis factor (TNF)-α, granulocyte-macrophage colony-stimulating factor [GM-CSF]), adhesion molecules (intracellular adhesion molecule [ICAM]-1, vascular cell adhesion molecule [VCAM]-1), and inducible enzymes including NO synthase (iNOS) and cyclooxygenase-2 (COX-2).[105] Transcription of other genes, such as lipocortin-1 and the β_2-adrenergic receptor, may be enhanced.[105] Glucocorticosteroids also decrease airway mucus production, reduce inflammatory cell infiltration and activation, and attenuate capillary permeability.[106–109]

In children with status asthmaticus or near-fatal asthma, glucocorticosteroids should be administered by the IV route. The oral route can be used in selected cases, but inhaled glucocorticosteroids play no role in the treatment of the sick hospitalized patient.[24] The most common agent used in the United States is methylprednisolone, because of its wide availability as an IV preparation and lack of mineralocorticoid effects. The usual dose of methylprednisolone is 0.5 to 1 mg/kg/dose, administered intravenously every 6 hours. Hydrocortisone, an agent with both glucocorticoid and mineralocorticoid activity, can be used as an alternative at doses of 2 to 4 mg/kg/dose, intravenously every 6 hours. Short courses of steroids usually are well tolerated without significant side effects.[108] However, hypertension, hyperglycemia, mood disorders, and serious viral infections, such as fatal varicella, have been reported in previously well asthmatic patients receiving glucocorticosteroids.[108,110,111] Duration of corticosteroid therapy is dictated by severity of illness and clinical response. Once initiated, treatment in patients with status asthmaticus or near-fatal asthma is generally continued for 5 to 7 days. Longer treatment courses necessitate gradual weaning of the drug to decrease the chances of symptomatic adrenal insufficiency or relapse.[112] Prophylaxis with an H_2 blocker should be considered because of the possibility of steroid-associated gastritis and gastric perforation.[113]

Magnesium Sulfate

Magnesium is a physiologic calcium antagonist that causes smooth muscle relaxation as a result of inhibition of calcium uptake. Magnesium has been known for more than 60 years to cause bronchorelaxation in patients with asthma,[114] but only more recently has it been incorporated as an adjunct in the treatment of patients with severe asthma. Numerous reports, case series, and randomized controlled trials have suggested clinical improvement when asthmatic patients with severe airway obstruction receive IV magnesium sulfate infusions in the emergency department or ICU.[115–120] Magnesium appears to be as effective as albuterol when delivered by nebulization[121] and has been successfully used as a liquid vehicle for albuterol nebulization.[122,123]

The indication for IV magnesium sulfate in children with status asthmaticus or near-fatal asthma is still controversial because of the paucity of randomized, controlled trials. Some studies suggest that magnesium sulfate infusions are associated with significant improvements in short-term pulmonary function,[124,125] whereas another study failed to show improvement in disease severity or a reduction in hospitalization rates.[126] The usual dose of magnesium sulfate in children with status asthmaticus or near-fatal asthma is 25 to 40 mg/kg/dose, intravenously, infused over 20 to 30 minutes.[124,125] Patients should be carefully monitored for adverse effects during the infusion, which include hypotension, nausea, and flushing. Serious toxicity involving cardiac arrhythmias, muscle weakness, areflexia, and respiratory depression has not been reported with the use of magnesium sulfate in acute asthma, as directed. Intravenous infusion of magnesium sulfate under controlled conditions appears to be safe, and a subset of patients with status asthmaticus and near-fatal asthma clearly responds to this mode of therapy.[115,120,124,125,127] However, systematic reviews of the published randomized controlled trials suggest there is insufficient evidence to support the routine use of magnesium sulfate in every case of severe acute asthma.[128,129]

Methylxanthines

Methylxanthines, as the name implies, are substances formed by the methylation of xanthine, such as caffeine, theobromine, and theophylline. The water solubility of methylxanthines is very low but can be greatly enhanced by formation of complexes with a variety of compounds. Most notably, the combination of theophylline and ethylenediamine yields aminophylline, a water-soluble salt. A large number of methylxanthine derivatives have been developed, but only theophylline and aminophylline are relevant to the treatment of patients with asthma.

The exact molecular mechanism of theophylline-mediated bronchodilation is unclear but is thought to involve, at least in part, its action as a phosphodiesterase 4 inhibitor, reducing the degradation of cAMP, which in turn mediates cellular responses that result in bronchial smooth muscle relaxation.[130] Other mechanisms of action have been proposed, including inhibition of inhibiting phosphoinositide 3-kinase activity,[131] adenosine receptor antagonism,[132] increasing histone deacetylase activity,[133] stimulation of endogenous catecholamine release,[134] prostaglandin antagonism,[135] and alterations in intracellular calcium mobilization.[136] Theophylline is also known to cause inhibition of afferent neuronal activity,[137] thereby leading to inhibition of bronchospasm mediated by reflex activation of cholinergic pathways. Theophylline has antiinflammatory and immunomodulatory actions[138,139] and is known to augment diaphragmatic contractility and increase respiratory drive.[140,141]

The bronchodilator effects of theophylline in isolated human bronchial preparations in vitro occur at concentrations greater than 70 μmol/L, which is capable of inducing a 50% reversal of bronchoconstriction.[142] Such high local concentrations presumably would be achieved with plasma levels greater than 10 to 20 μg/ml.[143] In clinical practice, however, this range poses a difficult problem because of the narrow window between therapeutic levels and toxicity, which often overlap. The half-life of theophylline ranges from 3 to 7 hours.[144,145] Therefore theophylline is generally administered as a continuous IV infusion to avoid significant fluctuations in serum concentrations. Aminophylline is equivalent to 80% theophylline and is also administered by continuous IV infusion. When a decision is made to initiate therapy with theophylline or aminophylline, a loading dose is given to achieve serum levels between 10 and 20 μg/ml. Assuming a normal average volume of distribution, a 1 mg/kg dose of theophylline (1.25 mg/kg of aminophylline) raises the serum concentration by 2 μg/ml. The loading dose should be administered over 20 minutes and should be followed immediately by the continuous infusion of the drug. Patients with normal hepatic and cardiac function can be started on empiric doses as follows: infants younger than 6 months: 0.5 mg/kg/hour; infants 6 months to 1 year: 0.85 to 1 mg/kg/hr; children 1 to 9 years: 1 mg/kg/hour; children older than 9 years: 0.75 mg/kg/hour. Patients with compromised hepatic and cardiovascular function should be started at a dose of 0.25 mg/kg/hour. Obese patients should have doses calculated by ideal body weight to prevent toxicity. Serum drug levels should be monitored 30 to 60 minutes after the loading dose and frequently during the continuous infusion, considering that steady-state concentrations are not achieved until approximately five half-lives, which corresponds to 24 to 36 hours of infusion.

A number of studies in adults and children with acute asthma indicate that therapy with theophylline or aminophylline is of no clinical benefit.[146–148] More recently, a randomized, double-blinded, placebo-controlled trial tested the efficacy of aminophylline in children with near-fatal asthma in the ICU environment.[11] This study found that aminophylline treatment resulted in significantly improved physiologic outcomes, such as oxygenation and pulmonary function testing, but did not decrease ICU length of stay and was associated with side effects such as nausea and vomiting.[11] Considering that the narrow therapeutic window (10–20 μg/ml) often overlaps the toxicity (>15 μg/ml), questionable evidence of clinical efficacy, and the fact that methylxanthines have been associated with serious side effects ranging from nausea, vomiting, and fever to dyskinesias, seizures, and death, enthusiasm for these agents has decreased significantly in the past decade. Although methylxanthines are still used as first-line agents in many parts of the world, they have been reserved for occasional selected patients who fail to respond to maximal therapy with β agonists, steroids, anticholinergics, and other adjuncts in North America.

Helium-Oxygen Mixtures

Helium is a biologically inert gas that is less dense than any other known gas except hydrogen and is about one seventh as dense as air. The medicinal application of helium and oxygen mixtures (heliox) in the treatment of asthma and extrathoracic airway obstruction has been known for approximately 7 decades.[149] Because of its low density, heliox has the potential to facilitate laminar gas flow and, therefore, decrease the work of breathing in situations associated with high airway resistance. Thus it provides a theoretical benefit to patients with obstructive lesions of the extrathoracic and intrathoracic airways. Several reports advocate the benefit of heliox in the management of children with extrathoracic airway obstruction.[150,151] The role of heliox in patients with asthma is less clear.

Research using heliox mixtures has demonstrated a greater percentage of lung particle retention and a greater delivery of albuterol from both metered-dose inhalers and nebulizers,[152,153] suggesting that one of the beneficial effects of heliox use in asthma is improved deposition of aerosolized drugs.[154] Heliox has been recommended by some as a useful adjunct in the adult patient with severe asthma, both during spontaneous breathing and during mechanical ventilation.[155–158] Anecdotal reports suggest that heliox is associated with improvement in pulmonary function in children with acute asthma.[159] However, a small randomized crossover trial of heliox in spontaneously breathing patients with severe asthma failed to show improvement in pulmonary function or dyspnea scores.[160] Additionally, a systematic review of seven prospective, controlled trials in children and adults failed to provide support for the use of heliox in patients with moderate or severe acute asthma.[161] The paucity of well-executed, randomized, controlled studies makes it impossible to assess the therapeutic effect of heliox in children with asthma at this time. In addition, should heliox be beneficial in some patients, the duration of administration and optimal helium-oxygen mixture remain undetermined. Until more sound information emerges, heliox remains an unproved therapy for pediatric asthma,[53] and its use should be restricted to individual attempts in selected patients with severe refractory near-fatal asthma who did not respond to more conventional treatments.[162] The need to use 80:20 or 70:30 helium-oxygen mixtures to take full advantage of the lower gas density properties may further thwart the use of heliox in sicker patients who exhibit significant hypoxemia.

Ketamine

Ketamine hydrochloride is a dissociative anesthetic agent available in solution for IV or intramuscular administration. The term *dissociative anesthetic* is derived from the strong feeling of dissociation from the environment that is experienced by the subject to whom it is administered. After IV administration, a sensation of dissociation is generally experienced within 15 seconds and unconsciousness becomes apparent after another 30 seconds. This is followed by intense analgesia that lasts approximately 40 to 60 minutes and amnesia that may persist for up to 2 hours. Some patients, particularly older children, may experience a postanesthesia emergence reaction with confusion, agitation, and hallucinations. Usual ketamine doses do not significantly affect hypoxic or hypercarbic respiratory drive.[163] Pharyngeal and laryngeal reflexes are maintained, and, although the cough reflex is somewhat depressed, airway obstruction does not normally occur. Aside from its anesthetic properties, ketamine exerts a number of other effects, including sialorrhea. It increases airway secretions, cardiac output, heart rate, blood pressure, metabolic rate, cerebral blood flow, and intracranial pressure.[164] Pulmonary vascular resistance is not altered, and hypoxic pulmonary vasoconstriction is preserved. Ketamine inhibits bronchospasm and lowers airway resistance, presumably through blockage of N-methyl-D-aspartate receptors in airway smooth muscle.[165] The bronchodilatory effect of ketamine makes it an attractive agent in patients with asthma who require sedation and anesthesia for intubation or mechanical ventilation.[166,167] Some controversy exists regarding the use of ketamine in nonintubated patients with near-fatal asthma, with the goal of avoiding the need for mechanical ventilation. Limited evidence suggests this may be a viable strategy in selected patients.[168,169] In our experience, the administration of ketamine to nonintubated children with severe refractory asthma frequently precedes the need to intubate and is rarely associated with significant and noticeable clinical improvement. For this reason, attempts at administering ketamine to nonintubated children with severe refractory asthma should always take place in the ICU under strictly monitored conditions and with personnel capable of rapidly establishing an airway for initiation of ventilatory support.

Ketamine usually is administered as an IV bolus of 2 mg/kg, followed by a continuous infusion of 1 to 2 mg/kg/hour. The resulting sialorrhea and increased airway secretions can be attenuated by administration of glycopyrrolate or atropine. The concurrent use of benzodiazepines may attenuate the agitation and hallucinations in patients who experience emergence reactions following ketamine anesthesia.

Mechanical Ventilation

Indications

Only a minority of patients with near-fatal asthma admitted to the pediatric ICU (approximately 8%) require endotracheal intubation. The indications for intubation are not precisely defined, and the decision to proceed with intubation is largely based on clinical judgment. Absolute indications are obvious and include cardiac or respiratory arrest, profound hypoxemia, and respiratory failure. The decision to intubate should not be based solely on blood gas results. However, the presence of a mixed respiratory and metabolic acidosis, persistent hypoxemia, and agitation or obtundation, despite adequate therapeutic efforts, indicate impending respiratory arrest and signal the urgent need to proceed with intubation and mechanical ventilation.

Older patients may benefit from attempts to attenuate respiratory muscle fatigue with a trial of noninvasive ventilation.[170] However, the use of bilevel positive airway pressure requires patient cooperation and a well-fitted and sealed mask, which may prove difficult, if not impossible, to achieve in the anxious and agitated child with impending respiratory failure.

Intubation

The intubation of patients with severe near-fatal asthma is complicated by the fact that these patients are, by definition, fatigued, acidotic, and often also hypoxemic or agitated. Once the decision to intubate is reached, the procedure should be promptly performed by someone skilled and experienced in rapid sequence intubation. Intubation should be preceded by the administration of an anesthetic, such as an opiate, propofol, or ketamine; a benzodiazepine; and a neuromuscular blocker. Ketamine is the preferred anesthetic because of its bronchodilatory properties. Our preference is to use ketamine with a benzodiazepine, such as midazolam or lorazepam, to ensure adequate sedation and reduce the risk of hallucinations during emergence from anesthesia. Propofol may cause bronchodilatation and could be used as an alternative to ketamine, although this drug currently is not approved in the United States for continued use for anesthesia in the pediatric ICU after induction. Among the opiates, fentanyl is a widely available choice; morphine should be avoided because it is associated with histamine release and could, at least in theory, contribute to the allergic and inflammatory process. A rapid-acting neuromuscular blocker such as succinylcholine should be used to induce chemical paralysis. Alternatively, a nondepolarizing neuromuscular blocker, such as vecuronium, rocuronium, or cisatracurium, can be used. The patient should be preoxygenated with 100% oxygen by face mask during spontaneous breathing. Assisted breathing with a bag-mask apparatus should be avoided, and cricoid pressure should be maintained throughout the procedure to reduce the risk of aspiration. Whenever possible, a nasogastric tube should be placed in advance to decompress the stomach.

A cuffed endotracheal tube should be introduced and its placement confirmed by a colorimetric method or capnography, auscultation, and chest radiograph. In young children (younger than 8 years), an uncuffed tube may be used instead, but it must be well fitted to tolerate the high airway pressures generated without allowing for a substantial leak. Special attention to the manual ventilation technique is needed in order to avoid fast rates that often are inadvertently applied immediately following intubation. Rapid respiratory rates applied to intubated children with severe airway obstruction lead to a state of high lung volume, significant dynamic hyperinflation, hypoxemia, and hemodynamic instability (hypotension). These patients require slow respiratory rates with very prolonged expiratory times in order to allow for adequate gas exchange and lung volumes. A helpful maneuver is to establish the timing of the next inspiration by using a stethoscope to auscultate for the disappearance of expiratory wheezes, thus marking the end of the previous exhalation. The occurrence of desaturation and hypotension following intubation should prompt an equipment check and confirmation of tube placement. A tension pneumothorax must be considered in patients with hypoxemia and hypotension who fail to rapidly improve after fluids and optimization of ventilation (or brief endotracheal tube disconnection), particularly when unequal breath sounds are present.

Ventilator Settings

The goal of mechanical ventilation in acute asthma should be to reverse hypoxemia (if present), relieve respiratory muscle fatigue, and maintain a level of alveolar ventilation compatible with an acceptable pH, while avoiding iatrogenic hyperinflation and levels of intrathoracic pressure that could adversely affect cardiac output.[6] Therefore the choice of mechanical ventilator settings must take into consideration the significant derangements of lung mechanics and function that are inherent to severe acute asthma. Attempts to achieve a normal Pa_{CO_2} would require fast respiratory rates, high minute volumes, and very high airway pressures, which are associated with the development of barotrauma (pneumothorax and pneumomediastinum) and very high mortality.[171–173] A paradigm shift in the ventilatory management of asthmatic patients occurred with the introduction of strategy of controlled hypoventilation reported by Darioli and Perret.[174] Their strategy resulted in no mortality in 34 episodes of mechanical ventilation in 26 patients and significantly lower complication rates in comparison with historical controls.[174] This approach used tidal volumes between 8 and 12 ml/kg and targeted peak airway pressures up to 50 cmH_2O. Tidal volumes were further reduced if the peak pressure limit could not be respected and higher $Pa{CO_2}$ measurements were tolerated. A similar approach using respiratory rates lower than 12 breaths per minute, tidal volumes between 8 and 12 ml/kg, peak inspiratory pressures of 40 to 45 cmH_2O, and permissive hypercapnia also resulted in very few complications and no mortality or long-term morbidity in 19 mechanically ventilated children with near-fatal asthma.[175]

From a simplified perspective, the modes of ventilatory support for patients with severe acute asthma can be divided between pressure and volume preset. No definitive evidence exists to suggest that one particular mode of ventilation is superior to the other. However, to safely ventilate the asthmatic patient, the characteristics of each mode must be understood. Pressure control modes use a decelerating gas flow and have the advantage of ensuring that a particular inspiratory pressure limit is respected. The main disadvantage of pressure control modes is that tidal volumes can vary greatly with changes in airway resistance and the state of hyperinflation. Volume control modes deliver a constant tidal volume, provided there is no significant air leak. An added advantage of volume control is that it allows for comparison of peak inspiratory pressure and plateau pressure measurements (peak-to-plateau pressure), which can serve as a longitudinal indicator of airway resistance and response to therapy. For these measurements, the plateau pressure is obtained by performing an inspiratory hold (a feature ubiquitous to most ventilators) and is then compared with peak inspiratory pressure (Figure 40–4). An increasing peak-to-plateau pressure indicates increasing airway resistance, whereas a decreasing peak-to-plateau pressure suggests response to therapy. A disadvantage of volume control ventilation is that patients can develop very high lung volumes if exhalation is incomplete, because tidal volumes remain constant breath to breath. The option of using pressure-regulated volume control, a mode available in some ventilators, offers some of the advantages of pressure control and of volume control, including optimal inspiratory gas flow, assured tidal volumes, and minimized airway pressures.

Use of positive end-expiratory pressure (PEEP) in intubated asthmatics has been the focus of controversy. Externally applied PEEP may benefit patients with expiratory flow limitation resulting from dynamic compression of small airways by moving the equal pressure point, stenting collapsed or severely narrowed airways, and enabling decompression of upstream alveoli.[176] The application of low levels of PEEP that are, by definition, lower than the level of auto PEEP may also relieve dyspnea by facilitating ventilator triggering and synchronization for intubated patients capable of drawing spontaneous breaths.[176,177] However, as elegantly demonstrated by Tuxen,[178] use of PEEP in chemically paralyzed patients with severe airflow obstruction was uniformly associated with higher lung volumes, increased airway and intrathoracic pressures, and circulatory compromise (Figure 40–5).

Our personal preference is to use the volume control synchronized mandatory ventilation (SIMV) mode, with tidal volumes of 8 to 12 ml/kg, to generate peak inspiratory pressures ≤45 cmH_2O and plateau pressures ≤30 cmH_2O (tidal volume may require further reduction to achieve these pressures in some patients). Respiratory rate is initially set between 6 and 12 breaths per minute, and inspiratory time is set between 1 and 1.5 seconds, allowing for expiratory times between 4 and 9 seconds. PEEP is set at zero for the patient under neuromuscular blockade. With intensification of therapy and clinical improvement, neuromuscular blockade is stopped and trigger

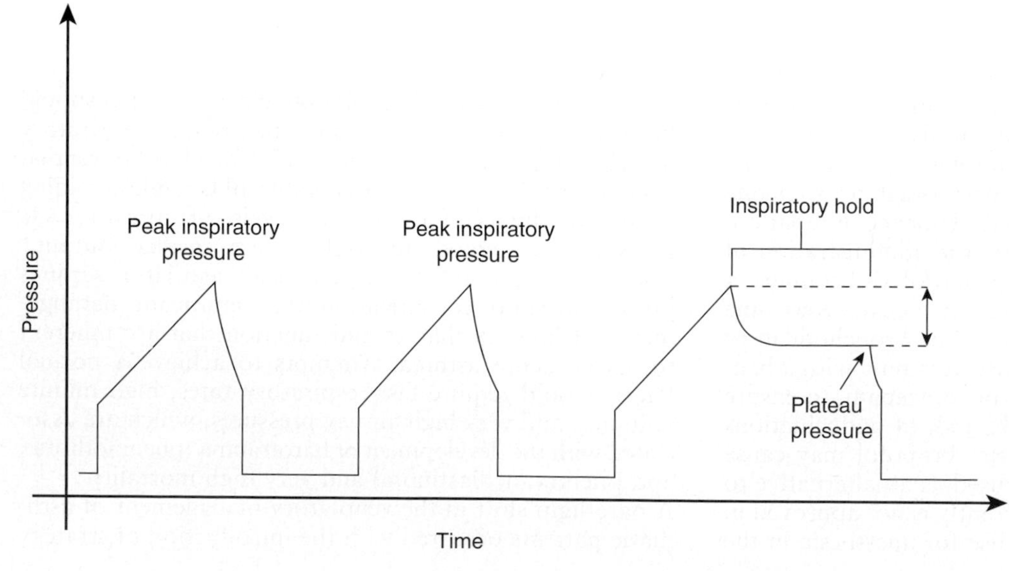

FIGURE 40–4 • Schematic representation of the airway pressure waveform over time during volume control ventilation. The peak-to-plateau pressure difference *(double-headed arrow)* is obtained after an inspiratory hold by comparing the peak pressure and the measured plateau pressure.

FIGURE 40–5 • Schematic representation of the measurement of V_{EI} both on and off positive end-expiratory pressure (PEEP) by a period of apnea during steady-state ventilation. *A,* V_{EI} measured with PEEP left on; *B,* V_{EI} measured with PEEP turned off. *FRC,* functional residual capacity; *FRC_{PEEP},* functional residual capacity resulting from PEEP; *V_{EI},* end-inspiratory lung volume above FRC; *V_T,* tidal volume; *$V_{trapped}$,* volume of trapped gas above FRC. (From reference 178.)

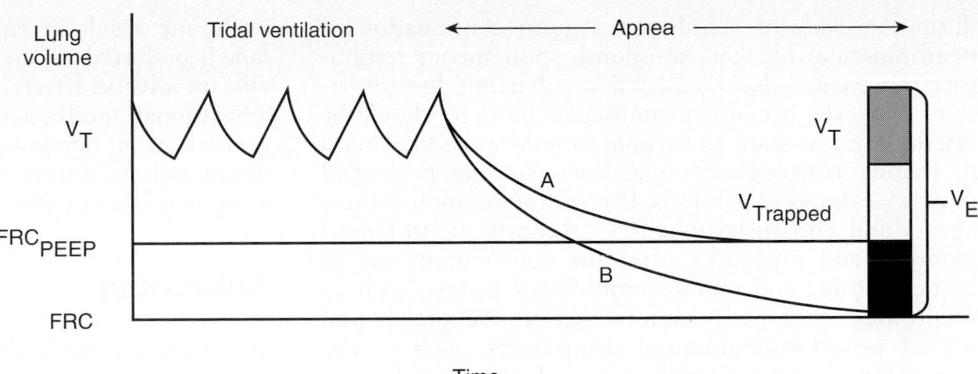

sensitivity for spontaneous breaths is optimized. A low level of PEEP (lower than the measured auto-PEEP and never in excess of 8 cmH_2O) is applied to facilitate synchronization between patient and machine, and spontaneous breaths are aided by the application of pressure support.

Use of high-level pressure support in the management of spontaneously breathing intubated asthmatics with the goal of reducing inspiratory work while allowing the patient to actively assist with exhalation is an intriguing strategy that warrants further study.[179]

Ventilatory Monitoring

Regardless of the chosen mode of ventilation, patients with near-fatal asthma undergoing mechanical ventilation require very close monitoring. Frequent auscultation can provide valuable information regarding symmetry of breath sounds (pneumothorax, mucus plugging) and optimal length of exhalation. Monitoring modules capable of analyzing and displaying permutations of important variables, such as pressure, volume, flow, and time, can provide important information that assists in the optimization of ventilatory settings (Figure 40–6). Monitoring peak-to-plateau pressure differences allows for inferences regarding airway resistance and response to treatment. The shape of the capnography curve may also provide insights regarding adequacy of lung emptying (Figure 40–7), while integrated volumetric capnography can track changes in alveolar dead space over time.

Analgesia, Sedation, and Muscle Relaxation

Patients with near-fatal asthma undergoing mechanical ventilation require adequate analgesia and sedation to avoid tachypnea, breath stacking, and ventilator dyssynchrony, particularly in the setting of hypercapnia. Ketamine is the anesthetic agent of choice because of its bronchodilatory properties. Its use with continuous infusions of midazolam or lorazepam can provide deep sedation while decreasing the chance of postanesthetic emergence reactions. When opiates are used, fentanyl is the preferred agent because morphine can cause histamine release and theoretically aggravate an acute attack.

Muscle relaxation with neuromuscular blockers should be maintained following initiation of mechanical ventilation until satisfactory gas exchange and clinical stability are achieved. Patients who exhibit hypercapnia

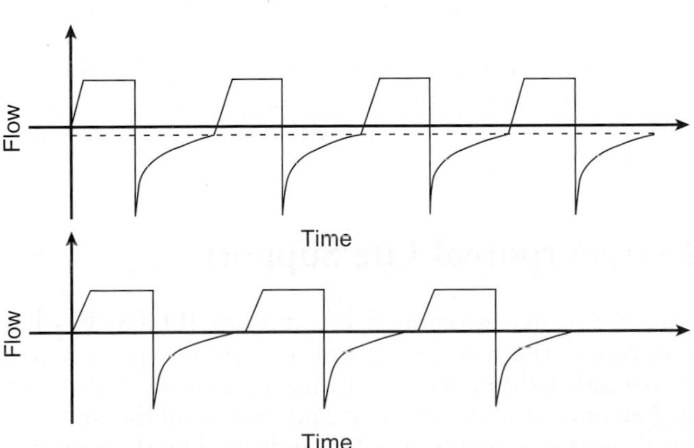

FIGURE 40–6 • Schematic representation of the airway flow tracing over time during volume control ventilation. **Upper panel:** Expiratory flow does not return to zero prior to the initiation of the following breath, resulting in auto-PEEP. **Lower panel:** Expiratory flow returns to baseline prior to initiation of the following breath after optimization of ventilator settings (lower respiratory rate and longer expiratory time).

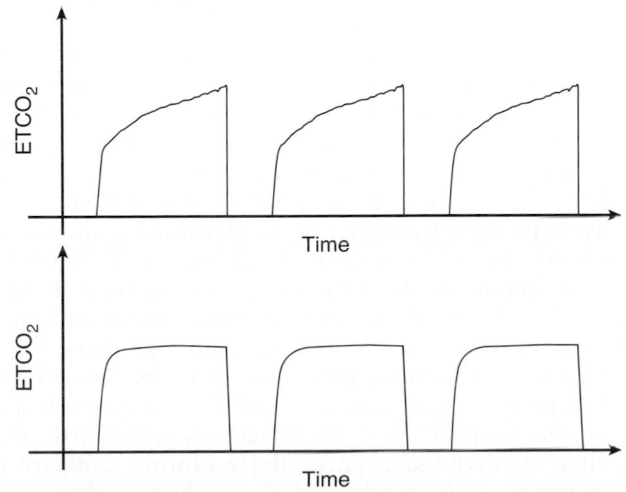

FIGURE 40–7 • Schematic representation of a capnogram in near-fatal asthma **(upper panel)** and under normal conditions **(lower panel).** Severe airflow obstruction in near-fatal asthma is manifested by sloping of the expiratory phase tracing and absence of a plateau, suggesting incomplete exhalation prior to the following inspiration.

during mechanical ventilation require continuation of neuromuscular blockers to abolish spontaneous respiratory movements that could worsen dynamic hyperinflation. However, use of neuromuscular blockers should be discontinued as soon as feasible to reduce the likelihood of serious neurologic complications, such as prolonged muscle weakness or paralysis, from the association of these agents and corticosteroids.[180–185] Reports of prolonged paralysis and myopathy after the concomitant use of corticosteroids and aminosteroid-based agents, such as vecuronium and pancuronium, led to the preferential use of benzylisoquinolinium compounds, such as cisatracurium, in patients with asthma. However, this combination may not be completely safe, as prolonged muscle weakness has been observed in a patient treated with cisatracurium and corticosteroids.[186]

Inhalational Anesthetics

Inhalational anesthetics have been used in the treatment of mechanically ventilated patients with refractory near-fatal asthma for their bronchodilatory effects.[187] The exact mechanism responsible for bronchodilatation during inhalational anesthesia is unknown but may involve direct inhibition of vagal tone.[188] Various agents have been used successfully in both adult and pediatric patients with refractory near-fatal asthma, including halothane,[189–191] isoflurane,[192–196] enflurane,[197] and sevoflurane.[198,199] Although halothane is often recommended as an agent of choice, little evidence in humans suggests it is more effective than other agents.[200,201] Sevoflurane compares favorably with halothane and appears to be less noxious to human airways than isoflurane or enflurane.[202,203]

Inhalational anesthetics can be delivered by means of an anesthesia machine that feeds into the low-pressure gas port of a conventional mechanical ventilator or via a dedicated anesthesia ventilator with its own vaporizer. Attention should be taken to ensure proper disposal of exhaled gases into a scavenger system to prevent release of the anesthetic agent into the ICU environment. A monitor capable of continuously analyzing inspiratory and expiratory drug concentrations is helpful in ascertaining the actual amount delivered and signaling interruptions in therapy, such as those caused by an empty vaporizer reservoir or inadvertent failure to resume therapy after a refill. Usual doses range from 0.5% to 2% and should be titrated for effect. Clinical response usually can be observed within 15 to 30 minutes of initiation of treatment.

Therapy for refractory near-fatal asthma with inhaled anesthetic should be performed only in a well-monitored ICU environment, under the direction of personnel experienced in the administration of these agents and their adverse effects. Patients treated with halothane often experience significant hypotension as a result of myocardial depression and require rapid fluid expansion and inotropic support.[204,205] Halothane is associated with cardiac arrhythmias, particularly during concurrent administration of epinephrine,[206,207] which explains why many physicians prefer a nonarrhythmogenic alternative such as isoflurane. Isoflurane does not have negative inotropic effects but may still cause hypotension because of vasodilatation.[162] Considering that halothane and isoflurane result in equivalent bronchodilation, isoflurane is preferred for use in children because of its less significant adverse effects. The use of subanesthetic doses of inhalational anesthetics in attempts to avoid mechanical ventilation in spontaneously breathing patients with severe asthma during maximal medical treatment is an intriguing strategy that warrants further study.[208]

Antibiotics

In children, acute asthma exacerbations are frequently triggered by a concurrent viral infection. As such, antibiotics are not indicated as part of the standard treatment strategy. A subset of school-age children may present to the hospital with shortness of breath, accessory muscle use, hypoxemia, and expiratory wheezing caused by *Mycoplasma pneumoniae* pneumonia that simulates an acute asthma exacerbation. These patients have bilateral interstitial disease on chest radiograph and should be treated with appropriate antibiotics such as a macrolide.

Patients with near-fatal asthma who require intubation and prolonged mechanical ventilation should be monitored for the development of nosocomial infections. The presence of fever and abundant thick white or purulent tracheal secretions should warrant a Gram stain and cultures to guide appropriate antibiotic coverage.

Bronchoscopy

Increased bronchial secretions and mucus plugging may contribute to continued deterioration observed in some patients with severe acute asthma who fail to respond to maximal therapy.[209,210] Mucous plugging and casts can cause atelectasis of large segments and worsen the heterogenicity of ventilation and dynamic hyperinflation. Thus a small percentage of mechanically ventilated patients with severe near-fatal asthma may require selective suction of mucus plugs, casts, or thick secretions by bronchoscopy.[211] The combination of bronchial lavage with mucolytic agents, such as N-acetylcysteine[212] or recombinant human deoxyribonuclease,[213,214] and aggressive selective suction through a bronchoscope may be beneficial in patients with clinically significant mucous plugging who fail to respond to maximal therapy and traditional tracheal suction.

Extracorporeal Life Support

The use of extracorporeal life support (ECLS) has been reported in the management of the very few patients with near-fatal asthma who continue to exhibit a profound degree of clinical instability despite maximal therapy.[215–218] Such cases are most unusual, as indicated by the very small number patients with acute asthma as the primary diagnosis in the Extracorporeal Life Support Organization registry (0.83%, i.e., 59 of 7110 pediatric and adult ECLS runs)[219] in contrast to the more than 470,000 annual admissions for asthma in the United States.[1] Interestingly, the survival for near-fatal asthma supported by ECLS is approximately 88%, which is remarkable considering that the vast majority of these patients were extraordinarily sick and had not responded to all forms of aggressive treatment.

Prognosis

The prognosis of patients with status asthmaticus or near-fatal asthma who receive proper medical therapy is excellent. Better understanding of the pathophysiology of airway obstruction and dynamic hyperinflation, coupled with improved mechanical ventilation strategies and aggressive pharmacologic treatment, has reduced the ICU mortality rate to nearly zero in these patients.[220–222] Asthma fatalities still occur in patients with sudden onset of severe airway obstruction who do not come to medical attention prior to developing respiratory failure or cardiorespiratory arrest.[6,223] The treatment plan for patients admitted to the hospital with status asthmaticus or near-fatal asthma should be carefully reviewed prior to discharge to ensure adequate outpatient therapy, education, and follow-up, in an attempt to reduce the likelihood of a preventable recurrence.

REFERENCES

1. Mannino DM, Homa DM, Akinbami LJ, et al: Surveillance for asthma—United States, 1980-1999. *MMWR Surveill Summ* 51: 1-13, 2002.
2. Robertson CF, Rubinfeld AR, Bowes G: Pediatric asthma deaths in Victoria: the mild are at risk. *Pediatr Pulmonol* 13:95-100, 1992.
3. Mountain RD, Sahn SA: Clinical features and outcome in patients with acute asthma presenting with hypercapnia. *Am Rev Respir Dis* 138:535-539, 1988.
4. Afzal M, Tharratt RS: Mechanical ventilation in severe asthma. *Clin Rev Allergy Immunol* 20:385-397, 2001.
5. Fitzgerald JM, Macklem PT: Proceedings on a workshop on near fatal asthma. *Can Respir J* 2:113-125, 1995.
6. Bohn D, Kissoon N: Acute asthma. *Pediatr Crit Care Med* 2:151-163, 1995.
7. CDC: Asthma mortality and hospitalization among children and young adults-United States, 1980-1993. *MMWR* 45:350-353, 1996.
8. American Academy of Allergy, Asthma, and Immunology: Pediatric asthma: predicting best practices. *AAAAI* 2-4, 1999.
9. Warner JO: Worldwide variations in the prevalence of atopic symptoms: what does it all mean? *Thorax* 54(suppl 2):S46-S51, 1999.
10. Afessa B, Morales I, Cury JD: Clinical course and outcome of patients admitted to an ICU for status asthmaticus. *Chest* 120: 1616-1621, 2001.
11. Yung M, South M: Randomised controlled trial of aminophylline for severe acute asthma. *Arch Dis Child* 79:405-410, 1998.
12. Turner MO, Noertjojo K, Vedal S, et al: Risk factors for near-fatal asthma. A case-control study in hospitalized patients with asthma. *Am J Respir Crit Care Med* 157:1804-1809, 1998.
13. Strunk RC, Mrazek DA, Fuhrmann GS, LaBrecque JF: Physiologic and psychological characteristics associated with deaths due to asthma in childhood. A case-controlled study. *JAMA* 254:1193-1198, 1985.
14. Spitzer WO, Suissa S, Ernst P, et al: The use of beta-agonists and the risk of death and near death from asthma. *N Engl J Med* 326:501-506, 1992.
15. Kolbe J, Vamos M, Fergusson W, Elkind G: Determinants of management errors in acute severe asthma. *Thorax* 53:14-20, 1998.
16. Ordonez GA, Phelan PD, Olinsky A, Robertson CF: Preventable factors in hospital admissions for asthma. *Arch Dis Child* 78: 143-147, 1998.
17. Birkhead G, Attaway NJ, Strunk RC, et al: Investigation of a cluster of deaths of adolescents from asthma: evidence implicating inadequate treatment and poor patient adherence with medications. *J Allergy Clin Immunol* 84:484-491, 1989.
18. Martin AJ, Campbell DA, Gluyas PA, et al: Characteristics of near-fatal asthma in childhood. *Pediatr Pulmonol* 20:1-8, 1995.
19. Kikuchi Y, Okabe S, Tamura G, et al: Chemosensitivity and perception of dyspnea in patients with a history of near-fatal asthma. *N Engl J Med* 330:1329-1334, 1994.
20. Kifle Y, Seng V, Davenport PW: Magnitude estimation of inspiratory resistive loads in children with life-threatening asthma. *Am J Respir Crit Care Med* 156:1530-1535, 1997.
21. Davenport PW, Cruz M, Stecenko AA, Kifle Y: Respiratory-related evoked potentials in children with life-threatening asthma. *Am J Respir Crit Care Med* 161:1830-1835, 2000.
22. Saetta M, Thiene G, Crescioli S, Fabbri LM: Fatal asthma in a young patient with severe bronchial hyperresponsiveness but stable peak flow records. *Eur Respir J* 2:1008-1012, 1989.
23. Sur S, Crotty TB, Kephart GM, et al: Sudden-onset fatal asthma. A distinct entity with few eosinophils and relatively more neutrophils in the airway submucosa? *Am Rev Respir Dis* 148:713-719, 1993.
24. Kercsmar CM: Current trends in management of pediatric asthma. *Respir Care* 48:194-205, 2003; discussion 205-208.
25. Wardlaw AJ, Brightling C, Green R, et al: Eosinophils in asthma and other allergic diseases. *Br Med Bull* 56:985-1003, 2000.
26. Kay AB: Pathology of mild, severe, and fatal asthma. *Am J Respir Crit Care Med* 154:S66-S69, 1996.
27. Brightling CE, Symon FA, Birring SS, et al: TH2 cytokine expression in bronchoalveolar lavage fluid T lymphocytes and bronchial submucosa is a feature of asthma and eosinophilic bronchitis. *J Allergy Clin Immunol* 110:899-905, 2002.
28. Panzer SE, Dodge AM, Kelly EA, Jarjour NN: Circadian variation of sputum inflammatory cells in mild asthma. *J Allergy Clin Immunol* 111:308-312, 2003.
29. Laitinen LA, Heino M, Laitinen A, et al: Damage of the airway epithelium and bronchial reactivity in patients with asthma. *Am Rev Respir Dis* 131:599-606, 1985.
30. Platts-Mills TA, Rakes G, Heymann PW: The relevance of allergen exposure to the development of asthma in childhood. *J Allergy Clin Immunol* 105:S503-S508, 2000.
31. Morkjaroenpong V, Rand CS, Butz AM, et al: Environmental tobacco smoke exposure and nocturnal symptoms among inner-city children with asthma. *J Allergy Clin Immunol* 110:147-153, 2002.
32. Hijazi Z: Environmental pollution and asthma. *Pediatr Pulmonol Suppl* 16:205-207, 1997.
33. Papadopoulos NG, Psarras S, Manoussakis E, Saxoni-Papageorgiou P: The role of respiratory viruses in the origin and exacerbations of asthma. *Curr Opin Allergy Clin Immunol* 3:39-44, 2003.
34. Schmaling KB, McKnight PE, Afari N: A prospective study of the relationship of mood and stress to pulmonary function among patients with asthma. *J Asthma* 39:501-510, 2002.
35. Melo RE, Sole D, Naspitz CK: Exercise-induced bronchoconstriction in children: montelukast attenuates the immediate-phase and late-phase responses. *J Allergy Clin Immunol* 111:301-307, 2003.
36. Rodriguez-Roisin R, Ballester E, Roca J, et al: Mechanisms of hypoxemia in patients with status asthmaticus requiring mechanical ventilation. *Am Rev Respir Dis* 139:732-739, 1989.
37. Roca J, Ramis L, Rodriguez-Roisin R, et al: Serial relationships between ventilation-perfusion inequality and spirometry in acute severe asthma requiring hospitalization. *Am Rev Respir Dis* 137: 1055-1061, 1988.
38. Levy BD, Kitch B, Fanta CH: Medical and ventilatory management of status asthmaticus. *Intensive Care Med* 24:105-117, 1998.
39. Stalcup SA, Mellins RB: Mechanical forces producing pulmonary edema in acute asthma. *N Engl J Med* 297:592-596, 1977.
40. Pride NB, Permutt S, Riley RL, Bromberger-Barnea B: Determinants of maximal expiratory flow from the lungs. *J Appl Physiol* 23: 646-662, 1967.
41. Martin JG, Shore SA, Engel LA: Mechanical load and inspiratory muscle action during induced asthma. *Am Rev Respir Dis* 128: 455-460, 1983.
42. Buda AJ, Pinsky MR, Ingels NB Jr, Daughters GT 2nd, Stinson EB, Alderman EL: Effect of intrathoracic pressure on left ventricular performance. *N Engl J Med* 301:453-459, 1979.

43. Jardin F, Farcot JC, Boisante L, et al: Mechanism of paradoxic pulse in bronchial asthma. *Circulation* 66:887-894, 1982.
44. Simmons DH, Linde LM, Miller JH, O'Reilly RJ: Relation between lung volume and pulmonary vascular resistance. *Circ Res* 9:465, 1961.
45. Williams MH, Zohman LR: Cardiopulmonary function in bronchial asthma: a comparison with chronic pulmonary emphysema. *Am Rev Respir Dis* 81:173, 1960.
46. McFadden ER Jr, Kiser R, DeGroot WJ: Acute bronchial asthma. Relations between clinical and physiologic manifestations. *N Engl J Med* 288:221-225, 1973.
47. Wood DW, Downes JJ, Lecks HI: A clinical scoring system for the diagnosis of respiratory failure. Preliminary report on childhood status asthmaticus. *Am J Dis Child* 123:227-228, 1972.
48. Keogh KA, Macarthur C, Parkin PC, et al: Predictors of hospitalization in children with acute asthma. *J Pediatr* 139:273-277, 2001.
49. van der Windt DA, Nagelkerke AF, Bouter LM, et al: Clinical scores for acute asthma in pre-school children. A review of the literature. *J Clin Epidemiol* 47:635-646, 1994.
50. Baker MD: Pitfalls in the use of clinical asthma scoring. *Am J Dis Child* 142:183-185, 1988.
51. Kussmaul A, Stern MT: Ueber schwielge mediastino-pericarditis und den paradoxen puls. *Berl Klin Wochenschr* 38, 1873.
52. Bilchick KC, Wise RA: Paradoxical physical findings described by Kussmaul: pulsus paradoxus and Kussmaul's sign. *Lancet* 359: 1940-1942, 2002.
53. Werner HA: Status asthmaticus in children: a review. *Chest* 119: 1913-1929, 2001.
54. Summer WR, Permutt S, Sagawa K, et al: Effects of spontaneous respiration on canine left ventricular function. *Circ Res* 45:719-728, 1979.
55. Hitzig WM: On mechanisms of inspiratory filling of the cervical veins and pulsus paradoxus in venous hypertension. *J Mt Sinai Hosp* 8:625, 1942.
56. Dohrnhorst AC, Howard P, Leathart GL: Pulsus paradoxus. *Lancet* 1:746-748, 1952.
57. Edmunds AT, Godfrey S: Cardiovascular response during severe acute asthma and its treatment in children. *Thorax* 36:534-540, 1981.
58. Knowles GK, Clark TJ: Pulsus paradoxus as a valuable sign indicating severity of asthma. *Lancet* 2:1356-1359, 1973.
59. McFadden ER Jr, Lyons HA: Arterial-blood gas tension in asthma. *N Engl J Med* 278:1027-1032, 1968.
60. Weiss EB, Faling LJ: Clinical significance of PaCO2 during status asthma: the cross-over point. *Ann Allergy* 26:545-551, 1968.
61. Mountain RD, Heffner JE, Brackett NC Jr, Sahn SA: Acid-base disturbances in acute asthma. *Chest* 98:651-655, 1990.
62. Appel D, Rubenstein R, Schrager K, Williams MH Jr: Lactic acidosis in severe asthma. *Am J Med* 75:580-584, 1983.
63. Lovis C, Mach F, Unger PF, et al: Elevation of creatine kinase in acute severe asthma is not of cardiac origin. *Intensive Care Med* 27:528-533, 2001.
64. Burki NK, Diamond L: Serum creatine phosphokinase activity in asthma. *Am Rev Respir Dis* 116:327-331, 1977.
65. Villard J, Magnenat J, Jolliet P, Chevrolet J: Acidose métabolique et augmentation de la créatine kinase dans l'asthme aigu sévère: rôle possible des muscles respiratoires. *Réan Urg* 2:259-266, 1993.
66. Tsung SH: Several conditions causing elevation of serum CK-MB and CK-BB. *Am J Clin Pathol* 75:711-715, 1981.
67. Gerhardt W, Katus H, Ravkilde J, et al: S-troponin T in suspected ischemic myocardial injury compared with mass and catalytic concentrations of S-creatine kinase isoenzyme MB. *Clin Chem* 37:1405-1411, 1991.
68. Krishnan SS, Stewart J, Amin N, et al: Electrocardiographic prediction of hyperinflation in children. *Am J Respir Crit Care Med* 156:2011-2014, 1997.
69. Silver HM, Calatayud JB, Ireland T: Estimation of lung function from the electrocardiogram in chronic obstructive pulmonary disease. *J Electrocardiol* 6:235-242, 1973.
70. Udezue E, D'Souza L, Mahajan M: Hypokalemia after normal doses of neubulized albuterol (salbutamol). *Am J Emerg Med* 13:168-171, 1995.
71. Keller KA, Bhisitkul DM: Supraventricular tachycardia: a complication of nebulized albuterol. *Pediatr Emerg Care* 11:98-99, 1995.
72. Maguire JF, O'Rourke PP, Colan SD, et al: Cardiotoxicity during treatment of severe childhood asthma. *Pediatrics* 88:1180-1186, 1991.
73. Matson JR, Loughlin GM, Strunk RC: Myocardial ischemia complicating the use of isoproterenol in asthmatic children. *J Pediatr* 92:776-778, 1978.
74. Chiang VW, Burns JP, Rifai N, et al: Cardiac toxicity of intravenous terbutaline for the treatment of severe asthma in children: a prospective assessment. *J Pediatr* 137:73-77, 2000.
75. Schuh S, Reisman J, Alshehri M, et al: A comparison of inhaled fluticasone and oral prednisone for children with severe acute asthma. *N Engl J Med* 343:689-694, 2000.
76. Rowe BH, Keller JL, Oxman AD: Effectiveness of steroid therapy in acute exacerbations of asthma: a meta-analysis. *Am J Emerg Med* 10:301-310, 1992.
77. Rowe BH, Spooner C, Ducharme FM, et al: Early emergency department treatment of acute asthma with systemic corticosteroids. *Cochrane Database Syst Rev* CD002178, 2000.
78. Qureshi F, Zaritsky A, Lakkis H: Efficacy of nebulized ipratropium in severely asthmatic children. *Ann Emerg Med* 29:205-211, 1997.
79. Qureshi F, Pestian J, Davis P, Zaritsky A: Effect of nebulized ipratropium on the hospitalization rates of children with asthma. *N Engl J Med* 339:1030-1035, 1998.
80. Geelhoed GC, Landau LI, Le Souef PN: Evaluation of SaO2 as a predictor of outcome in 280 children presenting with acute asthma. *Ann Emerg Med* 23:1236-1241, 1994.
81. Undem BJ, Lichtenstein LM: Drugs used in the treatment of asthma. In Hardman JG, Limbird LE, Gilman AG, editors. *Goodman & Gilaman's the pharmacological basis of therapeutics.* New York, 2001, McGraw-Hill.
82. Kelly HW: New beta 2-adrenergic agonist aerosols. *Clin Pharm* 4:393-403, 1985.
83. Stephanopoulos DE, Monge R, Schell KH, et al: Continuous intravenous terbutaline for pediatric status asthmaticus. *Crit Care Med* 26:1744-1748, 1998.
84. Katz RW, Kelly HW, Crowley MR, et al: Safety of continuous nebulized albuterol for bronchospasm in infants and children. *Pediatrics* 92:666-669, 1993.
85. Maguire JF, Geha RS, Umetsu DT: Myocardial specific creatine phosphokinase isoenzyme elevation in children with asthma treated with intravenous isoproterenol. *J Allergy Clin Immunol* 78:631-636, 1986.
86. Tveskov C, Djurhuus MS, Klitgaard NA, Egstrup K: Potassium and magnesium distribution, ECG changes, and ventricular ectopic beats during beta 2-adrenergic stimulation with terbutaline in healthy subjects. *Chest* 106:1654-1659, 1994.
87. Fok TF, Monkman S, Dolovich M, et al: Efficiency of aerosol medication delivery from a metered dose inhaler versus jet nebulizer in infants with bronchopulmonary dysplasia. *Pediatr Pulmonol* 21:301-309, 1996.
88. Montgomery VL, Eid NS. Low-dose beta-agonist continuous nebulization therapy for status asthmaticus in children. *J Asthma* 31:201-207, 1994.
89. Papo MC, Frank J, Thompson AE: A prospective, randomized study of continuous versus intermittent nebulized albuterol for severe status asthmaticus in children. *Crit Care Med* 21: 1479-1486, 1993.
90. Ackerman AD: Continuous nebulization of inhaled beta-agonists for status asthmaticus in children: a cost-effective therapeutic advance? *Crit Care Med* 21:1422-1424, 1993.
91. Levalbuterol for asthma. *Med Lett Drugs Ther* 41:51-53, 1999.
92. Johansson F, Rydberg I, Aberg G, Andersson RG: Effects of albuterol enantiomers on in vitro bronchial reactivity. *Clin Rev Allergy Immunol* 14:57-64, 1996.
93. Walle T, Eaton EA, Walle UK, Pesola GR: Stereoselective metabolism of RS-albuterol in humans. *Clin Rev Allergy Immunol* 14:101-113, 1996.
94. Asmus MJ, Hendeles L, Weinberger M, et al: Levalbuterol has not been established to have therapeutic advantage over racemic albuterol. *J Allergy Clin Immunol* 110:325, 2002; author reply 325-328.
95. Ramsay CM, Cowan J, Flannery E, et al: Bronchoprotective and bronchodilator effects of single doses of (S)-salbutamol, (R)-salbutamol and racemic salbutamol in patients with bronchial asthma. *Eur J Clin Pharmacol* 55:353-359, 1999.

96. Cockcroft DW, Swystun VA: Effect of single doses of S-salbutamol, R-salbutamol, racemic salbutamol, and placebo on the airway response to methacholine. *Thorax* 52:845-848, 1997.
97. Asmus MJ, Hendeles L: Levalbuterol nebulizer solution: is it worth five times the cost of albuterol? *Pharmacotherapy* 20: 123-129, 2000.
98. Browne GJ, Penna AS, Phung X, Soo M: Randomised trial of intravenous salbutamol in early management of acute severe asthma in children. *Lancet* 349:301-305, 1997.
99. Bohn D, Kalloghlian A, Jenkins J, et al: Intravenous salbutamol in the treatment of status asthmaticus in children. *Crit Care Med* 12:892-896, 1984.
100. Pirie J, Cox P, Johnson D, Schuh S: Changes in treatment and outcomes of children receiving care in the intensive care unit for severe acute asthma. *Pediatr Emerg Care* 14:104-108, 1998.
101. Gross NJ: Ipratropium bromide. *N Engl J Med* 319:486-494, 1988.
102. Woelfle J, Zielen S, Lentze MJ: Unilateral fixed dilated pupil in an infant after inhalation of nebulized ipratropium bromide. *J Pediatr* 136:423-424, 2000.
103. Kizer KM, Bess DT, Bedford NK: Blurred vision from ipratropium bromide inhalation. *Am J Health Syst Pharm* 56:914, 1999.
104. Peters-Golden M, Sampson AP: Cysteinyl leukotriene interactions with other mediators and with glucocorticosteroids during airway inflammation. *J Allergy Clin Immunol* 111:S37-S42, 2003; discussion S43-S48.
105. Barnes PJ, Adcock I: Anti-inflammatory actions of steroids: molecular mechanisms. *Trends Pharmacol Sci* 14:436-441, 1993.
106. Dworski R, Fitzgerald GA, Oates JA, Sheller JR: Effect of oral prednisone on airway inflammatory mediators in atopic asthma. *Am J Respir Crit Care Med* 149:953-959, 1994.
107. Peters-Golden M, Thebert P: Inhibition by methylprednisolone of zymosan induced leukotriene synthesis in alveolar macrophages. *Am Rev Respir Dis* 135:1020-1026, 1987.
108. Dunlap NE, Fulmer JD: Corticosteroid therapy in asthma. *Clin Chest Med* 5:669-683, 1984.
109. Fuller RW, Kelsey CR, Cole PJ, et al: Dexamethasone inhibits the production of thromboxane B2 and leukotriene B4 by human alveolar and peritoneal macrophages in culture. *Clin Sci (Lond)* 67:653-656, 1984.
110. Welch MJ: Inhaled steroids and severe viral infections. *J Asthma* 31:43-50, 1994.
111. Koh YI, Choi IS, Shin IS, et al: Steroid induced delirium in a patient with asthma: report of one case. *Korean J Intern Med* 17: 150-152, 2002.
112. Schimmer BP, Parker KL: Adrenocorticotropic hormone; adrenocortical steroids and their synthetic analogs; inhibitors of the synthesis and actions of adrenocortical hormones. In Hardman JG, Limbird LE, Gilman AG, editors. *Goodman & Gilaman's the pharmacological basis of therapeutics.* New York, 2001, McGraw-Hill.
113. Dayton MT, Kleckner SC, Brown DK: Peptic ulcer perforation associated with steroid use. *Arch Surg* 122:376-380, 1987.
114. Haurry VG: Blood serum magnesium in bronchial asthma and its treatment by administration of magnesium sulfate. *J Lab Clin Med* 26, 1940.
115. Rodrigo G, Rodrigo C, Burschtin O: Efficacy of magnesium sulfate in acute adult asthma: a meta-analysis of randomized trials. *Am J Emerg Med* 18:216-221, 2000.
116. Schiermeyer RP, Finkelstein JA: Rapid infusion of magnesium sulfate obviates need for intubation in status asthmaticus. *Am J Emerg Med* 12:164-166, 1994.
117. Dib JG, Engstrom FM, Sisca TS, Tiu RM: Intravenous magnesium sulfate treatment in a child with status asthmaticus. *Am J Health Syst Pharm* 56:997-1000, 1999.
118. Pabon H, Monem G, Kissoon N: Safety and efficacy of magnesium sulfate infusions in children with status asthmaticus. *Pediatr Emerg Care* 10:200-203, 1994.
119. Okayama H, Okayama M, Aikawa T, et al: Treatment of status asthmaticus with intravenous magnesium sulfate. *J Asthma* 28: 11-17, 1991.
120. Sydow M, Crozier TA, Zielmann S, et al: High-dose intravenous magnesium sulfate in the management of life-threatening status asthmaticus. *Intensive Care Med* 19:467-471, 1993.
121. Mangat HS, D'Souza GA, Jacob MS: Nebulized magnesium sulphate versus nebulized salbutamol in acute bronchial asthma: a clinical trial. *Eur Respir J* 12:341-344, 1998.
122. Nannini LJ Jr, Pendino JC, Corna RA, et al: Magnesium sulfate as a vehicle for nebulized salbutamol in acute asthma. *Am J Med* 108:193-197, 2000.
123. Hughes R, Goldkorn A, Masoli M, et al: Use of isotonic nebulised magnesium sulphate as an adjuvant to salbutamol in treatment of severe asthma in adults: randomised placebo-controlled trial. *Lancet* 361:2114-2117, 2003.
124. Ciarallo L, Sauer AH, Shannon MW: Intravenous magnesium therapy for moderate to severe pediatric asthma: results of a randomized, placebo-controlled trial. *J Pediatr* 129:809-814, 1996.
125. Ciarallo L, Brousseau D, Reinert S: Higher-dose intravenous magnesium therapy for children with moderate to severe acute asthma. *Arch Pediatr Adolesc Med* 154:979-983, 2000.
126. Scarfone RJ, Loiselle JM, Joffe MD, et al: A randomized trial of magnesium in the emergency department treatment of children with asthma. *Ann Emerg Med* 36:572-578, 2000.
127. Glover ML, Machado C, Totapally BR: Magnesium sulfate administered via continuous intravenous infusion in pediatric patients with refractory wheezing. *J Crit Care* 17:255-258, 2002.
128. Rowe BH, Bretzlaff JA, Bourdon C, et al: Magnesium sulfate for treating exacerbations of acute asthma in the emergency department. *Cochrane Database Syst Rev* CD001490, 2000.
129. Rowe BH, Bretzlaff JA, Bourdon C, et al: Intravenous magnesium sulfate treatment for acute asthma in the emergency department: a systematic review of the literature. *Ann Emerg Med* 36:181-190, 2000.
130. Nicholson CD, Shahid M: Inhibitors of cyclic nucleotide phosphodiesterase isoenzymes—their potential utility in the therapy of asthma. *Pulm Pharmacol* 7:1-17, 1994.
131. Foukas LC, Daniele N, Ktori C, et al: Direct effects of caffeine and theophylline on p110 delta and other phosphoinositide 3-kinases. Differential effects on lipid kinase and protein kinase activities. *J Biol Chem* 277:37124-37130, 2002.
132. Feoktistov I, Biaggioni I: Adenosine A2b receptors evoke interleukin-8 secretion in human mast cells. An enprofylline-sensitive mechanism with implications for asthma. *J Clin Invest* 96: 1979-1986, 1995.
133. Ito K, Lim S, Caramori G, et al: A molecular mechanism of action of theophylline: induction of histone deacetylase activity to decrease inflammatory gene expression. *Proc Natl Acad Sci U S A* 99:8921-8926, 2002.
134. Higbee MD, Kumar M, Galant SP: Stimulation of endogenous catecholamine release by theophylline: a proposed additional mechanism of action for theophylline effects. *J Allergy Clin Immunol* 70:377-382, 1982.
135. Horrobin DF, Manku MS, Franks DJ, Hamet P: Methyl xanthine phosphodiesterase inhibitors behave as prostaglandin antagonists in a perfused rat mesenteric artery preparation. *Prostaglandins* 13:33-40, 1977.
136. Kolbeck RC, Speir WA Jr, Carrier GO, Bransome ED Jr: Apparent irrelevance of cyclic nucleotides to the relaxation of tracheal smooth muscle induced by theophylline. *Lung* 156: 173-183, 1979.
137. Barlinski J, Lockhart A, Frossard N: Modulation by theophylline and enprofylline of the excitatory non-cholinergic transmission in guinea-pig bronchi. *Eur Respir J* 5:1201-1205, 1992.
138. Ward AJ, McKenniff M, Evans JM, et al: Theophylline: an immunomodulatory role in asthma? *Am Rev Respir Dis* 147: 518-523, 1993.
139. Kidney J, Dominguez M, Taylor PM, et al: Immunomodulation by theophylline in asthma. Demonstration by withdrawal of therapy. *Am J Respir Crit Care Med* 151:1907-1914, 1995.
140. Aubier M, De Troyer A, Sampson M, et al: Aminophylline improves diaphragmatic contractility. *N Engl J Med* 305:249-252, 1981.
141. Ashutosh K, Sedat M, Fragale-Jackson J: Effects of theophylline on respiratory drive in patients with chronic obstructive pulmonary disease. *J Clin Pharmacol* 37:1100-1107, 1997.
142. Rabe KF, Tenor H, Dent G, et al: Phosphodiesterase isozymes modulating inherent tone in human airways: identification and characterization. *Am J Physiol* 264:L458-L464, 1993.
143. Spina D: Theophylline and PDE4 inhibitors in asthma. *Curr Opin Pulm Med* 9:57-64, 2003.
144. Weinberger M, Hendeles L, Ahrens R: Clinical pharmacology of drugs used for asthma. *Pediatr Clin North Am* 28:47-75, 1981.
145. Weinberger M: The pharmacology and therapeutic use of theophylline. *J Allergy Clin Immunol* 73:525-540, 1984.

146. Strauss RE, Wertheim DL, Bonagura VR, Valacer DJ: Aminophylline therapy does not improve outcome and increases adverse effects in children hospitalized with acute asthmatic exacerbations. *Pediatrics* 93:205-210, 1994.
147. Rodrigo C, Rodrigo G: Treatment of acute asthma. Lack of therapeutic benefit and increase of the toxicity from aminophylline given in addition to high doses of salbutamol delivered by metered-dose inhaler with a spacer. *Chest* 106:1071-1076, 1994.
148. Goodman DC, Littenberg B, O'Connor GT, Brooks JG: Theophylline in acute childhood asthma: a meta-analysis of its efficacy. *Pediatr Pulmonol* 21:211-218, 1996.
149. Barach AL: The use of helium in the treatment of asthma and obstructive lesions in the larynx and trachea. *Ann Intern Med* 9:739-765, 1935.
150. Kemper KJ, Ritz RH, Benson MS, Bishop MS: Helium-oxygen mixture in the treatment of postextubation stridor in pediatric trauma patients. *Crit Care Med* 19:356-359, 1991.
151. Weber JE, Chudnofsky CR, Younger JG, et al: A randomized comparison of helium-oxygen mixture (Heliox) and racemic epinephrine for the treatment of moderate to severe croup. *Pediatrics* 107:E96, 2001.
152. Hess DR, Acosta FL, Ritz RH, et al: The effect of heliox on nebulizer function using a beta-agonist bronchodilator. *Chest* 115:184-189, 1999.
153. Goode ML, Fink JB, Dhand R, Tobin MJ: Improvement in aerosol delivery with helium-oxygen mixtures during mechanical ventilation. *Am J Respir Crit Care Med* 163:109-114, 2001.
154. Habib DM, Garner SS, Brandeburg S: Effect of helium-oxygen on delivery of albuterol in a pediatric, volume-cycled, ventilated lung model. *Pharmacotherapy* 19:143-149, 1999.
155. Gluck EH, Onorato DJ, Castriotta R: Helium-oxygen mixtures in intubated patients with status asthmaticus and respiratory acidosis. *Chest* 98:693-698, 1990.
156. Shiue ST, Gluck EH: The use of helium-oxygen mixtures in the support of patients with status asthmaticus and respiratory acidosis. *J Asthma* 26:177-180, 1989.
157. Kass JE, Castriotta RJ: Heliox therapy in acute severe asthma. *Chest* 107:757-760, 1995.
158. Manthous CA, Hall JB, Caputo MA, et al: Heliox improves pulsus paradoxus and peak expiratory flow in nonintubated patients with severe asthma. *Am J Respir Crit Care Med* 151:310-314, 1995.
159. Kudukis TM, Manthous CA, Schmidt GA, et al: Inhaled helium-oxygen revisited: effect of inhaled helium-oxygen during the treatment of status asthmaticus in children. *J Pediatr* 130:217-224, 1997.
160. Carter ER, Webb CR, Moffitt DR: Evaluation of heliox in children hospitalized with acute severe asthma. A randomized crossover trial. *Chest* 109:1256-1261, 1996.
161. Rodrigo GJ, Rodrigo C, Pollack CV, Rowe B: Use of helium-oxygen mixtures in the treatment of acute asthma: a systematic review. *Chest* 123:891-896, 2003.
162. Tobias JD, Garrett JS: Therapeutic options for severe, refractory status asthmaticus: inhalational anaesthetic agents, extracorporeal membrane oxygenation and helium/oxygen ventilation. *Paediatr Anaesth* 7:47-57, 1997.
163. Hirshman CA, McCullough RE, Cohen PJ, Weil JV: Hypoxic ventilatory drive in dogs during thiopental, ketamine, or pentobarbital anesthesia. *Anesthesiology* 43:628-634, 1975.
164. Evers AS, Crowder M: General anesthetics. In Hardman JG, Limbird LE, Gilman AG, editors. *Goodman & Gilaman's the pharmacological basis of therapeutics*. New York, 2001, McGraw-Hill.
165. Sato T, Hirota K, Matsuki A, et al: The role of the N-methyl-D-aspartic acid receptor in the relaxant effect of ketamine on tracheal smooth muscle. *Anesth Analg* 87:1383-1388, 1998.
166. L'Hommedieu CS, Arens JJ: The use of ketamine for the emergency intubation of patients with status asthmaticus. *Ann Emerg Med* 16:568-571, 1987.
167. Nehama J, Pass R, Bechtler-Karsch A, et al: Continuous ketamine infusion for the treatment of refractory asthma in a mechanically ventilated infant: case report and review of the pediatric literature. *Pediatr Emerg Care* 12:294-297, 1996.
168. Sarma VJ: Use of ketamine in acute severe asthma. *Acta Anaesthesiol Scand* 36:106-107, 1992.
169. Strube PJ, Hallam PL: Ketamine by continuous infusion in status asthmaticus. *Anaesthesia* 41:1017-1019, 1986.
170. Meduri GU, Cook TR, Turner RE, et al: Noninvasive positive pressure ventilation in status asthmaticus. *Chest* 110:767-774, 1996.
171. Scoggin CH, Sahn SA, Petty TL: Status asthmaticus. A nine-year experience. *JAMA* 238:1158-1162, 1977.
172. Westerman DE, Benatar SR, Potgieter PD, Ferguson AD: Identification of the high-risk asthmatic patient. Experience with 39 patients undergoing ventilation for status asthmaticus. *Am J Med* 66:565-572, 1979.
173. Picado C, Montserrat JM, Roca J, et al: Mechanical ventilation in severe exacerbation of asthma. Study of 26 cases with six deaths. *Eur J Respir Dis* 64:102-107, 1983.
174. Darioli R, Perret C: Mechanical controlled hypoventilation in status asthmaticus. *Am Rev Respir Dis* 129:385-387, 1984.
175. Cox RG, Barker GA, Bohn DJ: Efficacy, results, and complications of mechanical ventilation in children with status asthmaticus. *Pediatr Pulmonol* 11:120-126, 1991.
176. Marini JJ: Should PEEP be used in airflow obstruction? *Am Rev Respir Dis* 140:1-3, 1989.
177. Stewart TE, Slutsky AS: Occult, occult auto-PEEP in status asthmaticus. *Crit Care Med* 24:379-380, 1996.
178. Tuxen DV: Detrimental effects of positive end-expiratory pressure during controlled mechanical ventilation of patients with severe airflow obstruction. *Am Rev Respir Dis* 140:5-9, 1989.
179. Wetzel RC: Pressure-support ventilation in children with severe asthma. *Crit Care Med* 24:1603-1605, 1996.
180. Road J, Mackie G, Jiang TX, et al: Reversible paralysis with status asthmaticus, steroids, and pancuronium: clinical electrophysiological correlates. *Muscle Nerve* 20:1587-1590, 1997.
181. Lacomis D, Smith TW, Chad DA: Acute myopathy and neuropathy in status asthmaticus: case report and literature review. *Muscle Nerve* 16:84-90, 1993.
182. Douglass JA, Tuxen DV, Horne M, et al: Myopathy in severe asthma. *Am Rev Respir Dis* 146:517-519, 1992.
183. Barohn RJ, Jackson CE, Rogers SJ, et al: Prolonged paralysis due to nondepolarizing neuromuscular blocking agents and corticosteroids. *Muscle Nerve* 17:647-654, 1994.
184. Leatherman JW, Fluegel WL, David WS, et al: Muscle weakness in mechanically ventilated patients with severe asthma. *Am J Respir Crit Care Med* 153:1686-1690, 1996.
185. Tousignant CP, Bevan DR, Eisen AA, et al: Acute quadriparesis in an asthmatic treated with atracurium. *Can J Anaesth* 42: 224-227, 1995.
186. Davis NA, Rodgers JE, Gonzalez ER, Fowler AA III: Prolonged weakness after cisatracurium infusion: a case report. *Crit Care Med* 26:1290-1292, 1998.
187. Rooke GA, Choi JH, Bishop MJ: The effect of isoflurane, halothane, sevoflurane, and thiopental/nitrous oxide on respiratory system resistance after tracheal intubation. *Anesthesiology* 86:1294-1299, 1997.
188. Brown RH, Mitzner W, Zerhouni E, Hirshman CA: Direct in vivo visualization of bronchodilation induced by inhalational anesthesia using high-resolution computed tomography. *Anesthesiology* 78:295-300, 1993.
189. O'Rourke PP, Crone RK: Halothane in status asthmaticus. *Crit Care Med* 10:341-343, 1982.
190. Padkin AJ, Baigel G, Morgan GA: Halothane treatment of severe asthma to avoid mechanical ventilation. *Anaesthesia* 52: 994-997, 1997.
191. Rosseel P, Lauwers LF, Baute L: Halothane treatment in life-threatening asthma. *Intensive Care Med* 11:241-246, 1985.
192. Johnston RG, Noseworthy TW, Friesen EG, et al: Isoflurane therapy for status asthmaticus in children and adults. *Chest* 97: 698-701, 1990.
193. Bierman MI, Brown M, Muren O, et al: Prolonged isoflurane anesthesia in status asthmaticus. *Crit Care Med* 14:832-833, 1986.
194. Revell S, Greenhalgh D, Absalom SR, Soni N: Isoflurane in the treatment of asthma. *Anaesthesia* 43:477-479, 1988.
195. Otte RW, Fireman P: Isoflurane anesthesia for the treatment of refractory status asthmaticus. *Ann Allergy* 66:305-309, 1991.
196. Rice M, Hatherill M, Murdoch IA: Rapid response to isoflurane in refractory status asthmaticus. *Arch Dis Child* 78:395-396, 1998.
197. Parnass SM, Feld JM, Chamberlin WH, Segil LJ: Status asthmaticus treated with isoflurane and enflurane. *Anesth Analg* 66: 193-195, 1987.

198. Bando H, Yoneda K, Yamamoto A, Suzuki Y: [Two cases of status asthmaticus successfully treated with inhaled sevoflurane]. *Arerugi* 46:602-604, 1997.
199. Ohyama A, Arai K, Isa Y, et al: [Comparison of the effects of halothane, isoflurane and sevoflurane in the treatment of severe asthmatic attack: a case report]. *Masui* 45:362-366, 1996.
200. Lehane JR, Jordan C, Jones JG: Influence of halothane and enflurane on respiratory airflow resistance and specific conductance in anaesthetized man. *Br J Anaesth* 52:773-781, 1980.
201. Heneghan CP, Bergman NA, Jordan C, et al: Effect of isoflurane on bronchomotor tone in man. *Br J Anaesth* 58:24-28, 1986.
202. Doi M, Ikeda K: Airway irritation produced by volatile anaesthetics during brief inhalation: comparison of halothane, enflurane, isoflurane and sevoflurane. *Can J Anaesth* 40:122-126, 1993.
203. Tanaka S, Tsuchida H, Nakabayashi K, et al: The effects of sevoflurane, isoflurane, halothane, and enflurane on hemodynamic responses during an inhaled induction of anesthesia via a mask in humans. *Anesth Analg* 82:821-826, 1996.
204. Merin RG, Kumazawa T, Luka NL: Dose-dependent depression of cardiac function and metabolism by inhalation anesthetics in chronically instrumented dogs. *Recent Adv Stud Cardiac Struct Metab* 11:473-480, 1976.
205. Merin RG, Kumazawa T, Luka NL: Myocardial function and metabolism in the conscious dog and during halothane anesthesia. *Anesthesiology* 44:402-415, 1976.
206. Zink J, Sasyniuk BI, Dresel PE: Halothane-epinephrine-induced cardiac arrhythmias and the role of heart rate. *Anesthesiology* 43:548-555, 1975.
207. Atlee JL 3rd, Bosnjak ZJ: Mechanisms for cardiac dysrhythmias during anesthesia. *Anesthesiology* 72:347-374.
208. Baigel G: Volatile agents to avoid ventilating asthmatics. *Anaesth Intensive Care* 31:208-210, 2003.
209. Millman M, Goodman AH, Goldstein IM, et al: Treatment of a patient with chronic bronchial asthma with many bronchoscopies and lavages using acetylcysteine: a case report. *J Asthma* 22: 13-35, 1985.
210. Noizet O, Leclerc F, Leteurtre S, et al: Plastic bronchitis mimicking foreign body aspiration that needs a specific diagnostic procedure. *Intensive Care Med* 29:329-331, 2003.
211. Beach FX, Williams NE: Bronchial lavage in status asthmaticus. A long term review after treatment. *Anaesthesia* 25:378-381, 1970.
212. Henke CA, Hertz M, Gustafson P: Combined bronchoscopy and mucolytic therapy for patients with severe refractory status asthmaticus on mechanical ventilation: a case report and review of the literature. *Crit Care Med* 22:1880-1883, 1994.
213. Durward A, Forte V, Shemie SD: Resolution of mucus plugging and atelectasis after intratracheal rhDNase therapy in a mechanically ventilated child with refractory status asthmaticus. *Crit Care Med* 28:560-562, 2000.
214. Greally P: Human recombinant DNase for mucus plugging in status asthmaticus. *Lancet* 346:1423-1424, 1995.
215. Shapiro MB, Kleaveland AC, Bartlett RH: Extracorporeal life support for status asthmaticus. *Chest* 103:1651-1654, 1993.
216. King D, Smales C, Arnold AG, Jones OG: Extracorporeal membrane oxygenation as emergency treatment for life-threatening acute severe asthma. *Postgrad Med J* 62:855-857, 1986.
217. Tajimi K, Kasai T, Nakatani T, Kobayashi K: Extracorporeal lung assist for patient with hypercapnia due to status asthmaticus. *Intensive Care Med* 14:588-589, 1988.
218. Mabuchi N, Takasu H, Ito S, et al: Successful extracorporeal lung assist (ECLA) for a patient with severe asthma and cardiac arrest. *Clin Intensive Care* 2:292-294, 1991.
219. Extracorporeal Life Support Organization Registry, August 2003.
220. Braman SS, Kaemmerlen JT: Intensive care of status asthmaticus. A 10-year experience. *JAMA* 264:366-368, 1990.
221. Bellomo R, McLaughlin P, Tai E, Parkin G: Asthma requiring mechanical ventilation. A low morbidity approach. *Chest* 105:891-896, 1994.
222. Kearney SE, Graham DR, Atherton ST: Acute severe asthma treated by mechanical ventilation: a comparison of the changing characteristics over a 17 yr period. *Respir Med* 92:716-721, 1998.
223. Stein R, Canny GJ, Bohn DJ, et al: Severe acute asthma in a pediatric intensive care unit: six years' experience. *Pediatrics* 83: 1023-1028, 1989.

CHAPTER

41

Neonatal Respiratory Disease

James J. Cummings and William T. West

PEARLS

- Pulmonary or nonpulmonary disorders can lead to respiratory distress or failure.
- Respiratory distress presenting in the first hours of life is a common reason, second only to low birth weight, for admission to the intensive care nursery.
- The following factors are important in reducing complications and improving the outcome of neonates with respiratory distress: early recognition of respiratory distress, the ability to distinguish respiratory disorders from normal neonatal transition, and prompt intervention as indicated.
- Fetal lung fluid must be cleared from the airways to allow normal breathing after birth.
- As a group, pulmonary air leaks are more common during the neonatal period than at any other time of life. The two most common leaks are pneumothorax and pneumomediastinum.
- In most cases, what is called *pulmonary hemorrhage* is actually the most severe manifestation of pulmonary edema rather than vascular disruption. True pulmonary hemorrhage in a neonate is rare and is almost always terminal.
- Substantial abnormalities of the lung can exist antenatally with little or no clinical indication until delivery of the neonate because in utero, the organ of gas exchange is the placenta rather than a functioning lung.
- In addition to respiratory distress syndrome, many other clinical disorders may be associated with "functional" surfactant deficiency.
- Infants with "classic" bronchopulmonary dysplasia (BPD) typically require a high degree of ventilatory and oxygen support beyond age 1 week, are slow to wean, and have episodes of bronchospasm or desaturation. The goal of treatment is to promote growth while simultaneously supporting respiratory needs and minimizing further injury to the lungs.
- In the neonate, significant congenital heart disease typically presents in one of two ways: (1) cyanosis with minimal or no respiratory distress or (2) cardiorespiratory failure.

Overview

Effective gas exchange within the lung requires both adequate ventilation and perfusion. Determinants of ventilation include the ventilatory "pump" (e.g., central drive, muscle strength, and chest wall recoil),[1] compliance of the lung and chest wall, and resistance to airflow within the airways. Determinants of perfusion include the circulatory pump (right ventricular output) and pulmonary vascular resistance. A disorder in any one or a combination of these determinants can lead to respiratory insufficiency. Clearly then, a variety of disorders, either pulmonary or nonpulmonary, can lead to respiratory insufficiency.

Acute or Early-Onset Respiratory Disorders

Respiratory distress presenting in the first hours of life is a common reason, second only to low birth weight, for admission to the intensive care nursery. Even in the current era of surfactant replacement, high-frequency ventilation (HFV), extracorporeal membrane oxygenation (ECMO), and nitric oxide inhalation, morbidity and mortality due to acute respiratory disorders can be high. Early recognition of respiratory distress in the neonate, the ability to distinguish respiratory disorders from normal neonatal transition (see later), and prompt intervention when indicated are all important in reducing complications and improving the outcome of neonates with respiratory distress.

Delayed Clearance of Fetal Lung Liquid

Fetal lung fluid, actively produced and critical for normal fetal lung development,[2] must be readily cleared from the airways to allow normal breathing after birth. On the basis of results from animal studies, the relative volume of liquid within potential airspaces, which remains constant in utero, is approximately 20 to 30 ml/kg near term and is the result of a balance between net accumulation within the lung (production minus reabsorption) and efflux out the trachea into the amniotic cavity.[3] In the hours to days before delivery, net accumulation diminishes, and during labor, reabsorption predominates.[4] As a result, extravascular lung liquid (i.e., liquid within the airspaces and interstitium) decreases. Any excess fluid remaining within the airspaces at the time of delivery is further removed as air entry into the lung displaces liquid from the airways into the interstitium. Residual liquid within the interstitium is then taken up into the circulation over the next several hours. Excessive extravascular liquid will lead to impairment of gas exchange, interstitial liquid pressure can compress small airways leading to atelectasis and gas trapping, and excess liquid within airspaces will impair alveolar gas exchange.[5]

The processes that control clearance of excess extravascular fetal lung liquid during the perinatal period have been elucidated through experiments with fetal animals that were chronically instrumented.[3] Fetal lung liquid production and reabsorption are the result of active ion transport[6] and are presumably hormonally regulated. Although β-adrenergic agents such as terbutaline and epinephrine enhance Na^+ ion and thus liquid reabsorption,[7,8] β-adrenergic blockade does not inhibit the reabsorption of lung liquid during spontaneous labor and delivery in animal studies.[9,10] Other hormones of parturition, such as vasopressin, may be important as well.[11,12] The pulmonary circulation is also a key factor; not only does interstitial liquid drain directly into the circulation,[13,14] but the dramatic increases in pulmonary blood flow seen after birth may enhance reabsorption of liquid from fetal airspaces.[15] The onset of breathing not only increases the surface area for liquid reabsorption, but also is associated with the opening of pores through which liquid can readily enter the interstitium.[16] Drainage of interstitial liquid is generally complete by the end of neonatal transition (4 to 6 hours). Interstitial liquid appears to be directly absorbed during microcirculation, and this process is governed by Starling forces; the contribution of lymphatic drainage is negligible.[3]

Interference with this process of liquid removal from the airspaces and interstitium leads to impaired gas exchange and respiratory distress with a variable clinical presentation. Excess liquid within the airspaces reduces compliance and increases intrapulmonary shunting; this results in tachypnea and mild-to-moderate hypoxemia. The chest radiograph may show opaque areas similar to neonatal pneumonia or surfactant-deficient respiratory distress syndrome (RDS). This picture is often described as "prolonged neonatal transition" or "delayed extrauterine adaptation." Excess interstitial liquid reduces compliance and compresses small airways; this leads to the clinical signs of tachypnea and air-trapping. The chest radiograph may show streaky densities within the lung, fluid collection within interlobar fissures, or even small pleural effusions; the lungs will also appear hyperinflated because of gas trapping. This clinical picture is often labeled *retained fetal lung liquid* or *transient tachypnea of the newborn.*[5]

Taken together, these clinical entities resulting from delayed fetal lung liquid clearance represent the most common type of respiratory disorder in the neonate and occur in 5% to 10% of all neonates. Typically, affected infants are term or near term and have persistent tachypnea beyond the immediate perinatal period. Infants born precipitously, or by cesarean delivery, are at highest risk for this disorder. Of note, infants who have been stressed in utero or whose mothers have been receiving β-mimetics are less likely to have retained lung liquid. Preterm infants with this condition may be mistakenly assumed to have surfactant-deficient RDS; supportive treatment is similar, although surfactant therapy has not been studied in this condition. Because neonatal pneumonia can also present with tachypnea, an oxygen requirement, and a "wet" chest radiograph, infants with retained lung liquid who have symptoms are often treated with antibiotics. The clinical severity of this disorder can vary widely, and although most infants need only supplemental oxygen, others may require intubation and mechanical ventilation for 12 to 24 hours. Supplemental Oxygen requirement should last no more than 24 to 48 hours, but tachypnea may persist for several days.

Pulmonary Air Leak Syndromes

Pulmonary air leak syndrome encompasses a spectrum of disease including pneumothorax, pneumomediastinum, pneumopericardium, subcutaneous emphysema, pneumoperitoneum, and pulmonary interstitial emphysema (PIE). As a group, pulmonary air leaks are more common during the neonatal period than at any other time of life. The two most common types of air leaks—pneumothorax and pneumomediastinum—occur spontaneously in 1% to 2% of term neonates.[17] Preterm infants with surfactant-deficient respiratory distress had previously reported rates of air leaks in excess of 30%[18]; these rates fell rapidly with the advent of surfactant therapy in the 1980s but still remain around 5%.[19] Infants with meconium aspiration or hypoplastic lungs have much higher rates of air leaks. Although techniques such as HFV and extracorporeal membrane oxygenation have markedly reduced the incidence of air leaks associated with these disorders, the rates still remain high, at 25% to 30%.[20,21]

The pathophysiological cause of pulmonary air leaks has been hypothesized for many years as the uneven filling and redistribution of air in the lung; overdistension of more compliant air spaces leads to rupture. The alveoli most susceptible to this injury are those that border on arterioles and other structural elements of the lung; uniform protection by surrounding alveoli is lacking. After rupture of the alveolus or terminal airspace, air escapes into the lung interstitium and tracks along the vascular sheaths toward the hilum. For reasons that remain unclear, in the preterm infant the air may dissect within the interstitium (PIE).[22] More commonly, the air breaks through the pleural reflections at the hilum (pneumomediastinum) and from there gains access to various potential compartments: the pleural cavity (pneumothorax), the pericardial reflection (pneumopericardium), and the soft tissue planes of the neck (subcutaneous emphysema), or across the diaphragmatic apertures and into the peritoneal space (pneumoperitoneum).

In the past, pulmonary air leaks most commonly occurred as a result of excessive ventilatory pressures due to either aggressive mechanical ventilation (barotrauma) or air-trapping caused by partial airway obstruction with meconium or other debris (ball-valving). Now, air leaks are more commonly seen during the recovery phase of acute respiratory disease, when lung compliance dramatically improves and pressure-limited ventilation leads to excessive tidal volumes (volutrauma). This explains the clinical observations that air leaks tend to occur during the recovery phase of RDS[23] and that the incidence of air leaks actually increased during early trials of surfactant therapy.[24] Both observations underscore the need to closely monitor ventilatory volumes and wean pressure aggressively as compliance improves; these observations also suggest that volume-limited ventilation may be safer during the recovery phase of acute neonatal respiratory disease, although this theory has not been studied.

Pneumomediastinum is one of the most common air leaks and, considering the pathways by which air will track, is often the harbinger of further air leaks. Infants with isolated pneumomediastinum generally have few or no symptoms, other than low-density widening of the mediastinum, which is visible on chest x-ray film. Distention of the mediastinum has the potential to compress the great vessels and compromise circulation. This rarely occurs in clinical practice because air will usually track into the soft tissues of the neck or rupture into the pleural spaces before reaching the pressure needed for circulatory compromise.

Pneumothorax is a clinically common and more worrisome form of pulmonary air leak. The initial signs of pneumothorax reflect the decreased compliance of the lung due to compression. If compromise is minimal, the infant will maintain minute ventilation by simply increasing ventilatory rate (tachypnea); if that is insufficient, the infant will increase the use of accessory muscles (retractions) in an effort to improve tidal volume. If positive pressure within the pleural space builds to the point of vascular compromise (i.e., tension pneumothorax), cardiac return will decrease, and the heart rate will rise in an attempt to compensate for diminished stroke volume. Eventually, blood pressure may fall, and if oxygen delivery cannot be maintained, bradycardia and arrest will ensue.

Pneumopericardium is a rare but often life-threatening form of pulmonary air leak. The clinical signs closely resemble those of tension pneumothorax, but diminished heart sounds are invariably present. Clinical deterioration is often sudden and severe, and differentiation from pneumothorax is often difficult because usually no time is available to obtain a chest radiograph. Mortality may be as high 80%.

Pneumoperitoneum occurs when air dissects from the chest through a foramen of the diaphragm. This generally results in few if any symptoms or problems, other than possible confusion with a perforated viscus. Pneumoperitoneum is usually distinguished from bowel perforation by the clinical history of a prior pneumomediastinum or pneumothorax, especially with a lack of gastrointestinal symptoms. Although it usually requires no treatment, pneumoperitoneum can compromise ventilation. In that case, aspiration of air from the pneumoperitoneum is not only therapeutic but also diagnostic; oxygen tension in ventilatory gas is markedly higher than that in bowel gas.

PIE is a more severe manifestation of the same pathophysiological origin that leads to the rest of the air leak syndromes. In this case, the air accumulates in the interstitial space instead of tracking toward the hilum. This produces compression of the airways and vasculature, making ventilation more difficult. This forces the need for higher airway pressures to maintain open airways, which increases the air leak and therefore the PIE. Avoiding this escalation of therapy has become the primary principle in the treatment of PIE.

The approach to management of air leaks in infants is similar to that in older children. Pneumothorax, pneumopericardium, and occasionally pneumoperitoneum are acute, life-threatening emergencies because they can seriously impair cardiac output by decreasing venous return. A high degree of suspicion for air leaks in a patient who has a sudden cardiovascular deterioration for no apparent reason is critical for prompt diagnosis. Transillumination of the relatively translucent neonatal chest wall with an intensely focused light source is a quick and useful tool to diagnose a large pneumothorax. Immediate aspiration of the air, preferentially with a large-bore angiocatheter, without radiographic confirmation should be done if the infant is severely compromised. Clinical signs of compromise, not the radiographic interpretation of percent size or extent, should dictate treatment. An unstable or recurrent pneumothorax may require a thoracostomy tube. Cardiac tamponade due to a pneumopericardium may be suggested by distant heart tones and hypotensive shock with a normal-appearing electrocardiogram (ECG) tracing (so-called electromechanical dissociation). Pneumomediastinum is often asymptomatic and rarely benefits from drainage, even in the presence of symptoms. PIE occurs predominantly in preterm infants and often leads to a vicious cycle of increasing ventilator delivery pressures to open alveoli compressed by extrinsic air, which in turn leads to more extravasation of air and further collapse. Conventional treatment of PIE, including positioning, selective mainstem intubation, and steroids, has been unsatisfactory.[22,25] HFV, which occurs with the reduction of high inspiratory airway pressures and the maintenance of alveolar patency, appears to be the ventilatory mode of choice in managing infants with PIE[26] and refractory pneumothoraces.[27]

Pulmonary Hemorrhage

The term *pulmonary hemorrhage* is often misapplied in the neonatal intensive care setting. True pulmonary hemorrhage in a neonate is rare and is almost always terminal. In most cases, what is called *pulmonary hemorrhage* is actually the most severe manifestation of pulmonary edema rather than vascular disruption.[28] This distinction has been shown with the comparison of the hematocrit of blood with the amount of the hemorrhagic fluid suctioned from the airway.[29] The airway fluid will be generally 15 to 20 points lower than whole blood in the same patient at that time. Finding whole blood in the airway is rare and is usually due to trauma from suctioning.

Similar to older children and adults, factors that alter Starling forces within the pulmonary microcirculation will predispose the lung to hemorrhagic pulmonary edema. These include increased perfusion pressure (e.g., left ventricular failure), increased blood flow (e.g., from a left-to-right shunt across a patent ductus arteriosus [PDA]), increased microvascular permeability (e.g., associated with sepsis or oxygen toxicity), and decreased oncotic pressure (e.g., protein malnutrition, water overload). Most infants who have pulmonary hemorrhage will have more than one risk factor present. In the neonate, the factors most commonly associated with hemorrhagic pulmonary edema are those that increase pulmonary blood flow, such as a left-to-right shunt or treatment with surfactants.[28,30]

The diagnosis of hemorrhagic pulmonary edema is presumptively made when the appearance of bloody secretions within the endotracheal tube coincides with acute respiratory deterioration that requires increased oxygen and ventilatory support. The chest radiograph is the key to diagnosis; homogeneous, diffuse haziness or fluffy infiltrates are signs that best indicate hemorrhagic pulmonary edema. Focal opacities on radiograph require an alternative explanation such as pneumonia or upper airway trauma with subsequent aspiration of blood.

Although the diagnosis of hemorrhagic pulmonary edema is relatively straightforward, management can be challenging. The most important approach to managing hemorrhagic pulmonary edema is to establish high positive end-expiratory pressure (PEEP); this not only effectively reduces alveolar flooding but also improves oxygenation and left ventricular function. Although the airway must be kept clear, frequent suctioning not only may be traumatic but also can aggravate the condition by reducing PEEP. Some have advocated administration of epinephrine or iced saline via the endotracheal tube, but the efficacy of this method is questionable and epinephrine may worsen the condition by elevating pulmonary vascular pressures. Aggressive volume resuscitation should also be avoided for the same reason. Antibiotics should be considered if sepsis is clinically suspected, but the efficacy of prophylactic antibiotics to prevent bacterial contamination of the airways is unproven. If more common causes such as PDA or volume overload are not present, a coagulopathy should be considered and treated accordingly. Even with aggressive management, mortality from hemorrhagic pulmonary edema can exceed 25%.

Pneumonia

The lungs represent the most commonly affected organ in neonatal sepsis. Bacterial or viral infection of the neonate may begin in utero, either by transplacental passage or, more commonly, ascending infection from the maternal genital tract. A delay from the time of rupture of the amniotic membranes until delivery increases the risk of an ascending infection, although some organisms may invade through intact membranes. Cervical bacterial colonization with group B streptococci or primary herpesviral cervical infection during pregnancy increases the risk of transmitting those diseases; however, routine cervical cultures taken during pregnancy often do not reliably predict the actual flora at the time of delivery. Also, infants born vaginally are invariably colonized with organisms from the vaginal canal and typically swallow organisms during vaginal passage. Cesarean delivery is not necessarily protective because fetuses may swallow contaminated amniotic fluid or aspirate organisms in utero. Infection occurring during the perinatal period may not present clinically for several days; thus infections congenitally acquired are obscured from infections postnatally acquired (i.e., nosocomial).

Organisms that cause perinatal pneumonias, then, are typically those found in the genital tract of the mother and include streptococci (groups A, B, and D), gram-negative rods (e.g., *Escherichia coli* and *Klebsiella* species), *Listeria monocytogenes*, *Ureaplasma*, genital hemophilus, and herpesvirus. Less commonly, maternal viral infections due to adenovirus, enteroviruses, or varicella can be vertically transmitted to the fetus. If pneumonia occurs beyond the perinatal period, typical nosocomial pathogens such as *Staphylococcus* and *Pseudomonas* species, in addition to the pathogens previously listed, and atypical pathogens, such as tuberculosis, should be considered as possible causes. Although perinatal tuberculosis is rare compared with other causes of neonatal pneumonia, the increasing prevalence of this disease in women of child-bearing age increases the likelihood of new cases[31]; in congenitally acquired cases the mother may be symptom free.[32] Perinatal infection with other organisms, most typically *Chlamydia*, may not present for several weeks.

Congenital pneumonia can be difficult to diagnose because clinical symptoms and radiographic signs may be nonspecific. Although congenital infections are generally introduced through the respiratory tract, symptoms are rarely limited to those of pneumonia; the neonate is particularly prone to rapid dissemination of either bacterial or viral infections and typically has signs of sepsis or meningitis in addition to respiratory distress. The chest radiograph may initially appear normal, except for some slight streakiness or hyperinflation, or may be so opaque as to be confused with surfactant-deficient RDS.

Meconium aspiration with resultant severe chemical pneumonitis may be indistinguishable radiographically from bacterial pneumonia. Heart failure, or obstructed anomalous pulmonary venous drainage, can also present with a clinical and radiographic picture similar to pneumonia/sepsis.

Congenitally acquired pneumonia/sepsis can be a rapidly fatal disease, especially in the case of group B streptococcal or herpesviral infections for which mortality rates as high as 50% have been reported.[33,34] A high degree of suspicion is therefore important because prompt treatment may be lifesaving. Although antibiotics are routinely used in neonates with suspected pneumonia or sepsis, antiviral therapy should be considered if the infant has systemic signs such as shock or disseminated intravascular coagulation or is not responding to initial therapy.

Meconium Aspiration Syndrome

Passage of meconium in utero is generally considered a sign of fetal distress. The stress can be acute, as in the case of cord compression during labor, or chronic, as in the case of preeclampsia. Moderate distress occurring during labor results in passage of meconium during the final stages of delivery (terminal meconium), whereas more severe or chronic distress results in passage in utero, with resultant staining of the amniotic fluid and fetus. The incidence of meconium staining, as a more significant marker of fetal distress, occurs in 10% to 20% of all deliveries and is most common in postmature infants.[35] There also appears to be a maturational aspect to the ability to pass meconium because it is rarely observed in fetuses younger than 36 weeks' gestation.[35]

Not only is meconium-stained amniotic fluid a sign of antenatal distress, but it also can cause subsequent difficulties in the neonate. The contaminated amniotic fluid may be aspirated by the fetus, either in utero or during passage through the birth canal, and lead to subsequent respiratory distress. Meconium is a lipid and protein-rich substance that is highly irritating to mucous membranes of the distal airways, resulting in a chemical pneumonitis.[36] Dissolved meconium may travel down the respiratory tree and inactivate pulmonary surfactant; this inactivation leads to a functional surfactant deficiency.[37,38] More particulate meconium will remain trapped in small airways, and this leads to a ball-valve type of gas trapping. In most cases, the meconium is gradually removed from the respiratory tract through phagocytosis, and normal pulmonary function returns in 5 to 7 days. In more severe cases, meconium aspiration syndrome may lead to respiratory failure and even death despite aggressive intervention.

Infants with meconium aspiration are typically postmature, with elongated nails; peeling skin; and staining of the umbilical cord, skin, and nails. Respiratory distress develops soon after birth, although the infant may be initially depressed if meconium passage occurred in response to a recent asphyxial episode in utero. Gas trapping may lead to a barrel-shaped appearance to the chest, and signs of respiratory distress may be severe. Chest radiographs often show characteristic patchy densities, hyperinflation, and areas of collapse. Air leaks are especially common. Aspiration of blood during delivery results in a similar clinical and radiographic picture; however, blood aspiration usually has a much milder course.[39]

Treatment of meconium aspiration syndrome is supportive; infants are recognized as being at increased risk for having persistent pulmonary hypertension (see section on Persistent Pulmonary Hypertension of the Newborn). Supplemental oxygen support to maintain arterial oxygen saturation, endotracheal suctioning to clear remaining meconium, and ventilatory techniques to minimize gas trapping are commonly used. HFV may be helpful in preventing subsequent air leaks. Antibiotics are commonly used because distinguishing the clinical and radiographic picture from sepsis may be hard and because damage to the airways may predispose to subsequent bacterial infection. Surfactant therapy is currently being explored as an adjunctive therapy, after initial encouraging results in a recent pilot studies.[40,41] Despite the intense inflammatory nature of meconium aspiration, the utility of steroids remains unclear,[35] although results of a recent animal study suggest that antenatal treatment may be helpful.[42]

An important step in the treatment of meconium aspiration syndrome is prevention. When meconium staining of the amniotic fluid is observed, special care should be taken at delivery to suction out the infant's nose and mouth before the initiation of breathing. In addition, a physician or nurse skilled in neonatal intubation should be present at the delivery to perform endotracheal suctioning and give respiratory support if indicated. For years, controversy existed about which infants should receive aggressive suctioning or whether this type of intervention is truly preventive.[36] On the basis of results from a large, randomized clinical study,[43] suctioning should be limited to infants who are not vigorous at delivery.[44] Still, it can be argued that distressed fetuses may aspirate in utero, long before delivery, and that severe complications such as persistent pulmonary hypertension are more likely the result of the antecedent stress and are not due to meconium aspiration per se. Nevertheless, encouraging data from retrospective studies, with minimal iatrogenic morbidity due to airway manipulation, support the current attempts at prevention.[36]

Surfactant-Deficient Respiratory Distress Syndrome

For years, infants born preterm were recognized as being at increased risk for severe, occasionally lethal respiratory distress that presented within minutes to hours of age. In the past, the term commonly used to describe the acute neonatal lung disease was *hyaline membrane disease* (HMD), a pathological description of abnormal protein deposition in the alveolar linings of preterm infants who died after the onset of this disease. Today this disorder is commonly referred to as *respiratory distress syndrome* (RDS); this term emphasizes the clinical instead of the pathological presentation because hyaline membranes generally develop only in those now rare infants who eventually succumb to the disease. Recognizing that this disorder is primarily due to inadequate surfactant production, some authors prefer the term *surfactant-deficient respiratory distress syndrome* to differentiate the pathophysiological origins of this disorder from other types of neonatal respiratory distress such as transient tachypnea or retained fetal lung liquid.

Pulmonary surfactant disperses at the air-liquid interface on the inner surface of the alveolus, reduces surface tension at that interface, and prevents alveolar collapse at end-expiration. Surfactant is produced by type II alveolar epithelial cells and is a phospholipid and glycoprotein composite with phospholipid as the surface-active agent and glycoproteins aiding in surface adsorption, spreading, and metabolism of surfactant.[45] Maturation of the pulmonary surfactant system is generally not complete until the latter part of the third trimester of fetal life, but it can be induced by intrauterine stress, by maternal steroid therapy, and after preterm delivery. The incidence of surfactant deficiency at birth is inversely related to gestational age; approximately 50% of infants born between 30 and 36 weeks' gestation will be surfactant-deficient, and virtually all infants born before 28 weeks' gestation will be affected to some degree.[46]

Surfactant-deficient alveoli are more prone to collapse, and this leads to diffuse atelectasis, reduced ventilatory compliance, and intrapulmonary shunting. Infants with surfactant deficiency have stiff, noncompliant lungs and require significant distending pressure in order for the lungs to be ventilated. Neonates will have tachypnea, retractions, and expiratory grunting; these symptoms indicate RDS. Preterm infants with RDS have significant morbidity, although some complications may be primarily a result of prematurity per se. Short-term complications can be life-threatening and include pulmonary air leaks, pulmonary hemorrhage, and intracranial hemorrhage. Infants with RDS are at risk for later complications including necrotizing enterocolitis and chronic lung disease. Infants who require prolonged intubation and mechanical ventilation are also at risk for subglottic injury including subglottic stenosis and tracheomalacia. Before surfactant therapy, mortality from RDS exceeded 20%[47]; now infants rarely succumb to RDS unless severe complications develop.[48-50]

Assessment of fetal lung maturity, using phospholipid analysis of amniotic fluid and maternal steroid therapy, both introduced in the mid 1970s, have reduced the incidence of RDS in infants born before term. In the past decade, exogenous surfactants given to high-risk infants at or soon after birth (so-called prophylaxis therapy) have further contributed to this reduction. Treatment with surfactants in neonates with symptoms during the first few days of life (so-called rescue therapy) has significantly reduced the clinical severity of RDS and improved survival.[19] Currently, clinical research is directed at refining surfactant therapy for RDS; issues include prophylactic versus rescue dosing, dosing interval, timing and method of administration, and type of surfactant (see section on Surfactant Replacement). Unfortunately, although surfactant therapy has reduced some short-term complications such as pulmonary air leaks, the incidence of long-term morbidity remains unchanged; in part, this is due to increased survival of preterm infants with extremely low birth weight (<1000 g).[48,49]

Surfactant Protein B Deficiency

Pulmonary surfactant consists of surface-active phospholipid and a small amount (≈10% by weight) of protein.[45] Various surfactant-associated proteins (SPs) have been identified. SP-A and SP-D are large-molecular-weight, hydrophilic glycoproteins that do not appear to be important for lowering surface tension, but which may modulate surfactant metabolism or serve an immunological role. On the other hand, SP-B and SP-C are small, hydrophobic glycoproteins that promote spreading of surfactant across an air-liquid interface, which is an essential prerequisite for surfactant to function. A deficiency of either SP-B or SP-C markedly interferes with natural surfactant function in animal models.[45]

Congenital alveolar proteinosis is a rare disease entity with histopathological similarities to alveolar proteinosis in older children and adults.[51] The clinical course of congenital alveolar proteinosis, however, is markedly different, characterized by rapid progression to death within several hours to days. A clustering of cases within families has suggested a genetic basis for this disorder; the condition in older children and adults is thought to result from a nonspecific alveolar injury. Pulmonary lavage has been helpful in adults and some children with alveolar proteinosis, but it has not been studied in infants with congenital disease.[52] Extracorporeal support has not altered the long-term prognosis of infants with this condition.[53]

In the past 10 years, several cases of congenital alveolar proteinosis have been described in which SP-B and its messenger protein have been shown to be totally absent.[54,55] These same investigators have subsequently isolated a single gene mutation (121ins2) in several families who have had one or more affected children.[56] Adult humans heterozygous for this mutation have normal pulmonary function,[57] whereas homozygous cases are uniformly lethal within days of life. Affected infants respond only transiently to exogenous surfactants that contain SP-B[58]; to date, the only survivors are those who have undergone lung transplant. A novel splicing mutation has been reported, which results in less severe, nonlethal disease.[59]

Congenital Malformations of the Lung

In utero, the organ of gas exchange is the placenta. As such, fetal viability does not depend on a functioning lung. Not surprisingly, substantial abnormalities of the lung can exist antenatally with little or no clinical indication until delivery of the neonate when the lung must assume the placental function of gas exchange.

Pulmonary Hypoplasia

Both static and dynamic expansion of the fetal lung appears to be an important determinant of normal fetal lung development.[60] Static lung expansion occurs as a result of fetal lung liquid production. Epithelial cells within the lung actively secrete fluid into the lung lumen, distending the future airspaces. An intraluminal pressure gradient above amniotic fluid pressure is maintained by glottic regulation of fluid efflux from the trachea into the amniotic cavity, thus keeping the lungs expanded at a fluid volume that approximates postnatal functional residual capacity.[61] Failure to maintain this distention, either by inadequate production or excessive drainage of fetal lung liquid, leads to developmental hypoplasia. Dynamic lung expansion occurs during fetal breathing movements, which are rhythmic in nature and occur with increasing frequency during the latter part of gestation.[62] Absent or abnormal fetal breathing also appears to result in pulmonary hypoplasia.[60]

Pulmonary hypoplasia, unlike pulmonary agenesis or aplasia (see later), can occur anytime during gestation. Hypoplastic lungs are small in volume and DNA content relative to body size and have reduced numbers of alveoli, bronchioles, and arterioles per unit mass.[60] Although the pathophysiological origin is not well understood, pulmonary hypoplasia is thought to result from impairment of normal fetal lung expansion and generally occurs in conjunction with one of the following conditions: (1) space-occupying lesions within the hemithorax, such as a diaphragmatic hernia, or massive pleural effusions associated with fetal hydrops; (2) an inadequate thoracic cage, as in asphyxiating thoracic dystrophy or achondrogenesis; (3) a deficiency of amniotic fluid (oligohydramnios), due to either leakage (e.g., preterm rupture of fetal membranes) or to underproduction (e.g., renal dysplasia)[21]; (4) inadequate vascular supply to the developing lung, as may be seen with pulmonary artery atresia, hypoplastic right heart, or tetralogy of Fallot; (5) lack of the fetal breathing movements that normally occur throughout the latter part of gestation; and (6) chromosomal anomalies such as trisomy 13 or 18. Pulmonary hypoplasia may occur in the absence of any of these conditions, but such cases of primary isolated pulmonary hypoplasia are rare.[60]

Infants with pulmonary hypoplasia generally have signs of respiratory failure in the immediate newborn period. Reduced lung volumes impair ventilation and lead to hypercarbia, and decreased surface area for gas exchange (due to decreased alveoli) leads to hypoxemia. A decreased cross-sectional area of the vasculature makes these infants particularly susceptible to pulmonary hypertension, which further exacerbates the hypoxemia. The chest radiograph in infants with pulmonary hypoplasia should show low lung volumes but may otherwise be unremarkable. The severity of the respiratory distress depends on the degree of hypoplasia and the presence of associated problems such as fetal hydrops or cyanotic heart disease. The most common association is renal dysplasia or agenesis; in these cases infants have a history of moderate to severe oligohydramnios and have severe respiratory distress and compression deformities of the face and extremities (Potter's syndrome).[63]

Treatment of infants with pulmonary hypoplasia is supportive, and outcome depends on the severity of the hypoplasia and the presence of any associated lethal anomalies such as renal agenesis or achondrogenesis. The lungs of infants with severe pulmonary hypoplasia may be extremely difficult to ventilate, and pneumothoraces are common because of the need for high distending pressures. HFV may be an effective means of ventilating these infants' lungs through a combination of high ventilatory rates with extremely low tidal volumes.

Congenital Diaphragmatic Hernia

Failure of the pleuroperitoneal canal to close at 6 to 8 weeks' gestation results in a diaphragmatic defect that allows gastrointestinal structures to travel into the thoracic cavity as the intestines return from outside the fetus to the abdominal cavity.[64] The resulting mass effect in the chest exerts a negative influence on ipsilateral lung growth, characterized by a quantitative reduction in airways and their associated preacinar arteries. Congenital diaphragmatic hernia occurs in approximately 1 in 3000 births and is the most common cause of pulmonary hypoplasia in the neonate.[65] The defect occurs on the left side in 80% to 85% of cases; the reason is that closure of the right pleuroperitoneal membrane normally precedes the left during fetal development. Because herniation often occurs before the tenth week of gestation when normal gut rotation occurs, malrotation is common. Nongastrointestinal anomalies are found in approximately 25% of cases; the most common involve the cardiovascular system, where virtually any kind of defect has been reported.[64-66] Other associated anomalies include esophageal atresia, trisomies (13, 18 and 21), Turner's syndrome, neural tube defects, and renal anomalies.

Clinical presentation of congenital diaphragmatic hernia depends on the degree of pulmonary hypoplasia present (see section on Pulmonary Hypoplasia). In addition, the abdomen is often scaphoid because of a paucity of abdominal contents. As the infant cries and swallows air, the degree of lung compression may worsen, and an infant appearing healthy at delivery may undergo decompensation within minutes. The chest radiograph will show a cystic lesion in the lower lung field, often extending upward along the lateral chest wall. Initially, while the intestines remain fluid filled, the radiograph may be similar to that seen with pulmonary sequestrations or fluid-filled cysts (see later); as the infant swallows more air, the radiographic findings can be confused with congenital emphysema or even a pneumothorax. Small or right-sided defects in infants may not present for weeks or even months; indeed, occasional cases have been diagnosed incidentally during childhood when chest radiographs are obtained for other reasons. Today, with the widespread use of antenatal sonography, most cases are diagnosed before birth, and significant confusion is avoided in the delivery room.

Initial management focuses on stabilization, including immediate intubation and gastrointestinal decompression. Ventilation by bag and mask should be avoided because this will only introduce more gas into the gastrointestinal tract. As with pulmonary hypoplasia, the clinical course is usually complicated by persistent pulmonary hypertension, which accounted for mortality rates as high as 80%.[67] With the advent of ECMO this number has dropped somewhat but is still significant.[68] HFV appears to have particular merit for this condition and may have improved mortality independent of bypass technology.[66,69] Surfactant therapy may have a role in the management of these infants; in a lamb model of congenital diaphragmatic hernia, the contralateral nonhypoplastic lung is functionally immature.[70]

Surgical management of congenital diaphragmatic hernia remains somewhat controversial, with some advocating immediate repair[71] and others advocating immediate placement on ECMO and later repair[65]; increasingly, experts support an individualized approach to the timing of surgery.[66,72] In any case, early, aggressive cardiorespiratory stabilization is associated with improved outcome.[65,73] Attempts at intrauterine intervention, either to close the defect or to encourage lung growth through temporary blocking of the fetal lung liquid egress at the trachea, have been disappointing; fetal surgery is associated with an unacceptably high incidence of complications, including recurrence of the defect, preterm delivery, and miscarriage.[66,74] In infants with significant pulmonary hypoplasia who require ECMO, distending the lung with perfluorochemical can promote lung growth.[75]

Cystic Adenomatoid Malformation

Cystic adenomatoid malformation (CAM) is a relatively infrequent lesion, estimated at 1 in 30,000 pregnancies.[76] It results from abnormal mesenchymal proliferation and failure of maturation of bronchiolar structures early in gestation.[77,78] The resultant adenomatous overgrowth leads to the development of cysts and suppression of alveolar growth. The cysts are almost always multiple, and in more than 95% of cases the cystic malformations lie within a single lobe. There is no lobar predilection. Histologically, the lesions are notable for the preponderance of elastic tissue and for a lack of cartilage. The cysts communicate directly with the tracheobronchial tree and with each other.

CAMs have been divided into three types, which vary both in anatomical and clinical characteristics. Type 1 CAM, which accounts for about half the cases, occurs as a few, large (>2 cm) cysts, usually 1 to 4 in number, or a single large cyst surrounded by much smaller "satellite" cysts. Type 2 CAM, which accounts for about 40% to 45% of the cases, consists of multiple, small (<2 cm), evenly spaced cysts scattered throughout the affected area. Compared with type 1 CAM, type 2 cysts are associated with a much higher incidence (about 25%) of anomalies in other organs, particularly within the genitourinary tract (e.g., renal dysgenesis). Type 3 CAM, which accounts for less than 10% of cases, occurs as large collections of numerous tiny cysts; the affected area can be large, and this type often leads to early cardiovascular compromise, resulting in fetal hydrops or immediate postnatal complications.

Depending on the type, CAM presents during the neonatal period in 50% to 85% of infants, but presentation can be delayed for up to several years. Occasionally cases are discovered on chest radiographs taken for other reasons; many lesions are now detected prenatally during routine sonography. The most common presentation is respiratory distress that results from obstruction, although infection of the cyst leading to recurrent lobar pneumonias can occur as well. The elastic walls of the cyst allow easy expansion on inspiration, but the lack of cartilaginous support results in premature closure during exhalation, leading to a ball-valve type of respiratory compromise.

Chest radiograph findings are variable and depend somewhat on the type of CAM. In the neonate a solid, space-occupying mass will appear, becoming air-filled over the next several hours or days. In types 1 and 2 multiple air-filled cysts may become apparent. This appearance can be easily confused with diaphragmatic hernia; placement of a nasogastric (NG) tube to determine the location of the stomach and intestines and absence of a scaphoid abdomen will help rule this out. The multiple small cysts of type 3 CAM cannot be delineated on a chest radiograph; in this case CT of the chest can be helpful.

Treatment of infants with symptoms may require positive pressure ventilation; in some infants PEEP may facilitate emptying of the cysts. Definitive treatment is surgical removal of the affected lobe; infants without symptoms still carry a high risk of expansion or infection of the cyst if left untreated.[76]

Prognosis depends on the type and extent of the CAM. The large type 3 lesions are more likely to cause immediate distress and carry a higher mortality, especially if associated with pulmonary hypoplasia or fetal hydrops.[76] The prognosis in type 2 CAM depends on the presence and nature of associated anomalies. In addition, malignant transformation of CAM has been reported.[64,77] Most cases of CAM, however, carry a good prognosis.[76,79]

Bronchogenic Cysts

Bronchogenic cysts occur as a result of anomalous budding of the ventral or tracheal diverticulum of the foregut during the sixth week of gestation, with subsequent separation from the normally developing bronchi by the sixteenth week of gestation.[77,78] If separation occurs early (<12 weeks), the bronchogenic cyst tends to be located in the mediastinum (most common type); if separation occurs later, it is more likely to occur in the peripheral pulmonary parenchyma. The cyst walls are cartilaginous and receive either systemic or pulmonary blood supply depending on their location. Bronchogenic cysts are more common in males, are usually singular, are more commonly right-sided, and are generally less than 10 cm in diameter. They generally do not communicate with the airway and remain fluid filled; this differentiates them from pulmonary parenchymal cysts.

Bronchogenic cysts generally do not present in the neonatal period unless they are large, expand rapidly, or are located near major airways; in these cases infants may have moderate to severe respiratory distress. More commonly the young child will have recurring episodes of wheezing or infection; occasionally, asymptomatic bronchogenic cysts are visualized on chest radiographs taken for other reasons.

Chest radiographs can readily disclose most bronchogenic cysts.[80] The cyst typically appears as a round or oval water-density mass, commonly in the mediastinal or perihilar area; if the cyst has been infected, an air-fluid level may be present. Mediastinal bronchogenic cysts usually appear just beneath the carina and extend to the right. Pulmonary bronchogenic cysts are usually sharply circumscribed and appear toward the periphery; two thirds of these will be located in the lower lobes, with no right or left predilection. About 25% of bronchogenic cysts may be difficult to visualize with a chest radiograph; in these cases CT cannot only delineate the lesion but can also discern associated anomalies, such as a pulmonary sequestration (see later).[77,80]

Treatment may require ventilatory support for infants with symptoms; in all cases surgical resection is indicated. Prognosis for infants with bronchogenic cysts, whether mediastinal or pulmonary, is good.[81]

Pulmonary Parenchymal Cysts

Pulmonary parenchymal cysts are thought to represent a disorder of bronchial growth,[77,78] although they may also be acquired.[82] Like adenomatoid malformations and bronchogenic cysts, congenital cysts arise early in fetal life; pulmonary parenchymal cysts are thought to develop at a time when completion of the terminal bronchioles and development of the alveoli are occurring. Pulmonary cysts are typically thin walled, singular, multilocular, and located in the periphery. Unlike bronchogenic cysts, some communication usually exists between the pulmonary cyst and the tracheobronchial tree; approximately 75% will thus become air filled. Like adenomatoid malformations, pulmonary cysts contain mostly elastic tissue and little or no cartilage.

Although pulmonary cysts are generally small (1 to 2 cm in diameter), they can expand dramatically and thus are much more likely to be symptomatic than are bronchogenic cysts. As with adenomatoid malformations, the lack of cartilaginous support leads to air-trapping. Unlike adenomatoid malformations, pulmonary cysts are rarely associated with other anomalies. Rupture of a peripheral cyst can result in a pneumothorax. Rarely, multiple cysts can occur and involve both lungs in an extensive fashion; these cases are generally fatal within the perinatal period.

Chest radiographs typically reveal the thin-walled, round cysts with an air density. Often faint strands of lung tissue can be seen within the cysts. A large pulmonary cyst may be confused with congenital lobar emphysema; in this case CT should easily distinguish the cystic nature of the former.[80]

Reports of spontaneous resolution of pulmonary cysts have been infrequent. As with other cystic lesions of the lung, however, surgical resection of the affected lobe is usually indicated.[77,82]

Pulmonary Sequestrations

Like bronchogenic cysts, pulmonary sequestrations are thought to result from an abnormal budding of the foregut, which retains its embryonic systemic arterial connections.[77,78] Thus a sequestration is a mass of nonfunctioning, ectopic pulmonary tissue with its own blood supply. Pulmonary sequestrations are divided into two types, which are histologically similar. Extralobar sequestrations are surrounded by their own separate pleura, and intralobar sequestrations have no separate pleural covering.

Extralobar sequestrations account for about 25% of cases, are more common (90%) on the left side, are more common in males (80%), and are usually located in a subpulmonic location. Extralobar sequestrations have a high (50% to 60%) association with other anomalies, including direct esophageal communication, bronchial atresia, colonic duplication, pulmonary hypoplasia, and diaphragmatic hernia. Most cases of extralobar sequestration become evident in infancy; presentation ranges from fetal hydrops with massive pleural effusions and pulmonary hypoplasia to recurrent lower respiratory infections (particularly if there is a gastrointestinal communication).

Intralobar sequestrations are the more common type (75%); they are usually left sided (65% to 70%) and typically occur in the lower lobes. Association with other anomalies is less common. Most cases are asymptomatic and are found on chest radiographs obtained for other reasons. Symptomatic cases typically present in late childhood with recurrent infections.

Distinguishing between extralobar and intralobar sequestrations on chest radiographs may be difficult; both can appear as either solid or cystic structures, although extralobar lesions are more often solid and intralobar lesions are more often cystic.[80] Delineation of the vascular supply to the sequestration is important, not only to differentiate extralobar sequestrations from adenomatoid malformations, but to guide surgical management; in the past few years, magnetic resonance imaging has replaced arteriography for obtaining this information.[80] Some authors recommend a study of the gastrointestinal tract, particularly if communication with the sequestration is suspected.

As with other cystic lesions of the lung, surgical removal is indicated. Whereas extralobar sequestrations can be removed en bloc owing to their separate pleural covering, intralobar sequestrations require lobectomy.[64]

Congenital Lobar Emphysema

Congenital lobar emphysema is an unusual disorder characterized by overdistension of a pulmonary lobe caused by air-trapping. The term *emphysema* is misapplied because usually no emphysematous destruction of the alveoli occurs; thus many authors favor the term *congenital lobar overinflation*.[64,77,78] Although clinical and radiographic findings are typical of a ball-valve type of obstruction, evidence for this is found in less than 25% of cases; in most cases the cause for the air-trapping is unknown. Intrinsic bronchial obstruction may be due to a deficiency of cartilaginous support or an intraluminal mass such as a mucous plug. Extrinsic bronchial obstruction usually results from an underlying cardiovascular abnormality, such as a vascular sling or, rarely, a PDA. Intrathoracic masses, such as an enlarged lymph node or a bronchogenic cyst, can lead to extrinsic obstruction as well.

Congenital lobar emphysema is more common in males and typically occurs in the upper lobes or the right middle lobe; less than 1% of cases occur in the lower lobes.

Up to 20% of the cases have bilateral involvement. Associated cardiovascular anomalies are common; rib cage anomalies and aplasia/dysplasia of the kidneys have been reported in a small percentage of cases. In most infants with congenital lobar emphysema, the condition presents within the first month of life; about one third of infants have symptoms within hours of birth. Symptoms relate directly to the degree of overinflation. Typically, infants have mild to moderate tachypnea, asymmetric inflation of the chest, and cyanosis. Chest radiograph reveals the overinflated lobe with ipsilateral atelectasis and flattening of the hemidiaphragm; also, there may be a mediastinal shift away from the affected side. CT may be helpful in identifying the cause of obstruction, if one is present. Lobectomy is the definitive treatment, but controversy exists as a result of reports of spontaneous resolution in some cases.[64,77] If the infant is minimally distressed, careful observation may be indicated.

Pulmonary Agenesis and Aplasia

Pulmonary agenesis and aplasia, both rare and highly lethal disorders, have similar underlying causes, which differ from those of pulmonary hypoplasia.[78] Pulmonary agenesis and aplasia result from an arrest of development of the primitive lung during embryonic life. Obviously, the earlier in development that the arrest occurs, the more severe the defect. In pulmonary agenesis, the bronchial tree, pulmonary parenchyma, or pulmonary vasculature does not develop. In pulmonary aplasia there is a rudimentary bronchial pouch. The resulting lesion may involve one lobe or the entire lung; focal or bilateral defects are rare.

Clinical presentation is variable. If the defect is focal and isolated, the infant may be symptom free, but usually some mild respiratory distress is present. Chest radiograph reveals unilateral lung or lobar collapse with a shift of mediastinal structures, and this result leads to a suspicion of bronchial or bronchiolar obstruction. Misdiagnosis may subject the infant to the unnecessary risks of bronchoscopy when CT is readily diagnostic.[83]

Prognosis depends on the degree of pulmonary involvement, a history of recurrent pulmonary infections, and the presence of associated anomalies.[78] Bilateral defects are invariably lethal. If the defect is focal, the remaining normal lung tends to hypertrophy to compensate. Still, mortality rates exceed 50%, generally because of the presence of associated malformations, which are common. Right-sided defects have a poorer prognosis than left-sided lesions, partly because of a higher association with other anomalies and partly because of an increased risk for disseminating infection; it has also been suggested that right-sided lesions produce a greater mediastinal shift, distorting the trachea and great vessels.[84,85] Associated anomalies in the cardiovascular, gastrointestinal, genitourinary, central nervous, and musculoskeletal systems have all been described. Repeated lower respiratory infections result in progressive pulmonary debilitation and also increase the risk for death. If the defect is isolated to a single lobe, surgical resection will reduce symptoms and lessen the chance for infection.[78]

Special Treatment Considerations for Acute Respiratory Failure

Surfactant Replacement

As previously mentioned, a natural surfactant is a composite of phospholipids and glycoproteins. Natural surfactants are remarkably similar in composition across animal species. In fact, the natural surfactants in current clinical use are derived from either bovine or porcine lungs. Earlier concerns regarding sensitization to foreign animal proteins have not been substantiated in nearly two decades of clinical use. Human surfactant, purified and concentrated from pooled amniotic fluid, has also been studied clinically and is effective. The tremendous costs and limited available supplies, however, make human surfactant unsuitable for general use. An entirely synthetic surfactant consisting of dipalmitoyl phosphatidylcholine (DPPC) (the major phospholipid in natural surfactants), tyloxapol (a detergent, to aid spreading), and hexadecanol (an alcohol, to stabilize the suspension), was the first in clinical use in the United States. In head-to-head randomized comparison trials, however, natural surfactants result in more rapid and sustained clinical improvement.[86,87]

As previously noted, exogenous surfactant therapy has significantly decreased the incidence of RDS, decreased the severity and morbidity due to RDS, and improved the survival of low-birth-weight infants. Numerous surfactants are available for use in the United States; three natural surfactant preparations are used clinically for premature infants at risk for RDS, whereas a newer synthetic product is currently being evaluated in clinical trials. Although surfactant therapy is now established for the treatment of RDS, several clinical trials are still ongoing in which researchers are examining issues of timing and administration, and continuing to explore differences between the various preparations. Regarding the latter point, natural surfactants are compositionally different from each other; in particular, differences in SP-B content appear to translate into clinical differences such as onset and duration of activity and resistance to inhibition.[88]

In addition to RDS, many other clinical disorders can be associated with "functional" surfactant deficiency. There is increasing evidence that conditions such as meconium aspiration, persistent pulmonary hypertension, hemorrhagic pulmonary edema, congenital diaphragmatic hernia, pulmonary hypoplasia, acute respiratory distress syndrome (ARDS), pneumonia, bronchiolitis, and asthma are associated with surfactant dysfunction and inactivation and might theoretically benefit from exogenous surfactant therapy.[41,89-95] Animal and clinical studies of these potential applications are ongoing.

High-Frequency Ventilation

Over the past decade, a new generation of positive pressure ventilators has evolved for clinical use (see Chapter 44). Despite many fundamental differences among these ventilators, they have been collectively grouped under the rubric of high-frequency ventilation (HFV) because they all use supraphysiological (>60/min) ventilator rates. For an in-depth review, please refer to several articles listed at the end of this chapter.[27,96-99] Basically, four types of HFV are in clinical use: in one type, conventional ventilators are used, and in the other three, highly specialized pressure ventilators specifically designed for high-frequency use are used. The first type of HFV, high-frequency positive pressure ventilation (HFPPV), uses conventional pressure ventilators at nonconventional rates (60 to 150 breaths per minute). The second type uses a highly pressurized intermittent jet of gas that is delivered at rates of 120 to 600 Hz; this is called *high-frequency jet ventilation* (HFJV). High-frequency flow interruption (HFFI), the third type, uses higher frequency (600 to 1200 Hz) pulses of gas at somewhat lower pressures than HFJV. The last type of HFV uses rates similar to HFFI but uses an oscillating diaphragm or piston that provides active instillation and withdrawal of gas; this is called *high-frequency oscillatory ventilation* (HFOV).

Although the effects of ventilator settings have been well studied in HFV, the actual mechanics of gas exchange during HFV are less well understood. Similar to conventional ventilation, oxygenation is affected primarily by inspired oxygen concentration and mean airway pressure. Although ventilation is affected by volume and frequency, the effect of volume is much more pronounced than with conventional ventilation, and the effect of frequency is contrary to what would be expected because it inversely affects tidal volume.[27,99] In general practice, frequency is not a critical variable within the ranges afforded by the high-frequency ventilator and is not further adjusted during HFV use.

One advantage HFV has over conventional ventilation is the ability for high-end expiratory pressures to be used without the need for high-inspiratory pressures to maintain normal tidal volumes. Although this varies to some extent from one type of high frequency ventilator to another, it generally allows one to adjust mean airway pressure more or less independently of tidal volume. This is particularly desirable when there is a significant discrepancy between oxygenation and ventilation in an infant, such as the neonate with idiopathic persistent pulmonary hypertension whose lungs may be easy to ventilate but who is marginally oxygenated with 100% oxygen. Another advantage of HFV is the ability to use low, usually subphysiological tidal volumes. The use of low volumes prevents overdistension and rupture of more compliant alveoli, thereby reducing the risk of pneumothorax. Furthermore, in the face of ongoing air leak, HFV reduces air flow across existing air leaks, not only promoting their closure but also enabling more effective ventilation in situations such as severe PIE or a bronchopleural fistula.[27,96,97]

Complications that have been reported with HFV use include hypotension; pulmonary hypertension; tracheobronchitis; and, in preterm infants, intraventricular hemorrhage.[27,96-99] The use of excessive airway pressures may impede cardiac return and increase pulmonary vascular resistance, so hyperinflation must be avoided. Reports of necrotizing, sometimes lethal, tracheobronchitis, a complication recognized during the early years of HFV use, are now rare, presumably because of better attention to humidification and avoidance of excessive mean airway pressures. Some studies have suggested that HFOV increases the risk of intracranial hemorrhage in preterm infants, perhaps because of alterations in cerebral blood flow and drainage.[100-102] Researchers in several other clinical studies have found no such association,[69,103-108] and researchers in two studies in animals found no differences in the effects of HFV and conventional ventilation on the cerebral circulation.[109,110] In any case, a specific advantage of HFV over conventional pressure ventilation in preterm infants with RDS, other than managing air leaks, has yet to be demonstrated.[27,96,97]

Extracorporeal Membrane Oxygenation

Similar in many respects to cardiopulmonary bypass as practiced during open heart surgery, ECMO evolved from classic bypass technology with the advent of membrane oxygenators that could operate for days without significantly disrupting blood cells and plasma proteins. First applied in adults with pulmonary failure, then in premature neonates with RDS, initial experience with ECMO was disappointing.[111] ECMO did not reduce mortality in ARDS and was associated with a high risk of intracranial hemorrhage in preterm infants. Nevertheless, subsequent use in term infants with cardiorespiratory failure, particularly those with persistent pulmonary hypertension and congenital diaphragmatic hernia who failed conventional therapies, has led to its increasing application in this area, despite the absence of controlled clinical trials.[112] In addition, the use of ECMO in older children and adults has also received a resurgence of interest (see Chapter 47). The technical description, aspects of clinical management, and potential complications of ECMO are covered later in this book and are not detailed here.

Nitric Oxide Inhalation

In mammals, vascular smooth muscle relaxation is in large part induced by nitric oxide, which is released by adjacent endothelial cells in response to flow and shear stimuli and stimulates guanylate cyclase to produce cyclic guanosine monophosphate (cGMP), a potent vasodilator. Inhaled nitric oxide causes significant pulmonary vascular vasorelaxation without a significant systemic effect because it is rapidly scavenged by hemoglobin as it enters the pulmonary microvascular circulation. In addition, inhaled nitric oxide selectively vasodilates those lung units that are better ventilated, optimizing ventilation-perfusion matching. Inhaled nitric oxide is approved for use in term and near-term (>34 weeks' gestation) infants with persistent pulmonary hypertension (see later); although it does not alter long-term outcome in this condition, it significantly reduces the need for rescue treatment for ECMO (see Chapter 43).

While nitric oxide inhalation has received much interest in the management of term infants with persistent pulmonary hypertension, other applications continue to be evaluated. Animal studies suggest that nitric oxide may have a significant role in the successful perinatal transition to air-breathing.[113,114] Clinical studies suggest that inhaled nitric oxide may be beneficial in infants with surfactant-deficient respiratory distress syndrome, particularly those who do not respond to exogenous surfactant therapy.[115,116] The basis for these studies lies in the observation that pulmonary hypertension is not confined to term neonates, but has been reported in preterm infants with RDS as well.[117,118] In addition, recent work has shown that nitric oxide production modulates basal pulmonary vascular tone in preterm animals.[119]

Many questions regarding nitric oxide use remain to be answered before it can be approved for clinical use in preterm infants with RDS. Recognized clinical complications include methemoglobinemia (because of its high affinity for hemoglobin) and prolonged bleeding times;[120] the toxicity of nitric oxide metabolites includes the potential for injury to the pulmonary epithelium and surfactant system as well.[121] In time, the intense amount of ongoing basic research in nitric oxide biochemistry and clinical trials in both adults and children will begin to answer important questions about dosing, safety, and efficacy.[122,123]

Liquid Ventilation

Liquid ventilation with perfluorochemicals, a complete departure from traditional ventilation with gases, is one of the latest advances in ventilatory management for the neonate. Specific advantages of liquid instead of gas expansion of the lungs were first demonstrated in the 1920s, but application to the clinical setting was hampered by the poor solubility of most liquids for oxygen and carbon dioxide and technical difficulties in achieving liquid tidal volume exchange. The introduction of perfluorochemicals, which have high solubility for respiratory gases, and the development of specific liquid ventilators enabled researchers to study liquid ventilation in animals in the 1970s.[124] The demonstration that complete tidal liquid movement was not necessary to capitalize on the advantages of liquid ventilation[125] made liquid ventilation a clinical reality in the 1990s. *Partial liquid ventilation* is the term applied to conventional gas tidal volume ventilation superimposed on liquid-filled alveoli (i.e., alveoli filled to functional residual capacity).

Filling the alveoli with liquid removes the air-liquid interface normally present, markedly reducing surface tension and maintaining alveoli stability and eliminating the need for alveolar surfactant. Perfluorochemicals may also act as a mechanical PEEP, holding the alveoli open because of the higher density of the liquid. Therefore partial liquid ventilation offers the potential to manage infants with respiratory distress due to surfactant deficiency or dysfunction, in which exogenous surfactant replacement has failed or becomes impractical (e.g., heterogeneous lung disease such as ARDS). In animal models, perfluorochemicals also reduce neutrophil accumulation and inflammatory responses to lung injury[126-129] and inhibit hydrogen peroxide and free radical production by macrophages.[130] Studies in animals also show that partial liquid ventilation leads to marked improvements in respiratory mechanics compared with conventional ventilation strategies.[131-135] Limited clinical trials and individual case reports have also been encouraging.[136-144]

Chronic Pulmonary Disease

Chronic Lung Disease (Bronchopulmonary Dysplasia)

Sometimes neonates with acute lung disease do not fully recover and go on to have chronic respiratory insufficiency manifested by continued need for ventilatory support, oxygen support, or both. The first description of a chronic respiratory disease in neonates was in 1967 by Northway, who reported long-term radiographic and clinical outcomes of 32 low-birth-weight infants with acute respiratory disease.[142] The infants described by Northway progressed from the acute respiratory disease (typically, HMD) requiring mechanical ventilation to a chronic phase with persistent oxygen requirement and respiratory distress, often resulting in right ventricular failure and death. He coined the term *bronchopulmonary dysplasia* (BPD) to describe the pathological findings in these infants at autopsy. Over the years, this term has been loosely applied to include a wider variety of infants with chronic lung disease, most of whom survive[143,144]; as with HMD, application of a term that emphasizes the clinical instead of the pathological findings may be more apropos. Such a term is still wanting, and because *chronic lung disease* is nonspecific, many still use the term BPD to refer to these infants.[145]

Whatever term is used to describe these infants, the epidemiological and pathological origins of BPD have changed dramatically since Northway's first description 35 years ago.[146] Because of improvements in the management of severe RDS, pulmonary hypertension, and even pulmonary hypoplasia, barotrauma is much less common and the incidence of so-called classic BPD, as described by Northway, is rapidly diminishing. In its wake is a new population of infants with chronic lung disease: extremely-low-birth-weight (<1000 g) infants who without today's advancements in medicine and technology could not have survived in Northway's time. These infants typically have a relatively mild course of acute respiratory disease and usually wean to minimal ventilatory support, oxygen support, or both within the first 72 hours of life. The oxygen requirement, however, tends to persist for weeks, months, or even years, and these infants are at extreme risk for respiratory exacerbations. Although mortality is rare, those who die with this "new" type of BPD typically do not show severe lung injury with marked fibrosis and cellular proliferation, as seen in infants with classic BPD. Instead, one finds arrested lung development, with evidence of both impaired vascular and alveolar growth.[147,148]

The pathophysiological cause of chronic lung disease after relatively mild acute respiratory disease in these extremely low-birth-weight infants may, in part, relate to an increased sensitivity and abnormal responsiveness of the immature airways to injury.[146,148-161] It has been suggested that preterm birth during the late canalicular stage (24 to 27 weeks' gestation) leads to an arrest of normal lung development[149]; this is consistent with the observation that "normal" preterm infants (i.e., without clinical evidence of lung disease) have dysfunction of terminal respiratory units and higher elastic recoil than term infants at comparable postmenstrual ages.[152] This arrested development sets the stage for disordered repair when the immature lung is subjected to postnatal injury, perhaps by oxidants, infection, or ventilatory trauma.[153] Inflammation clearly plays a role in the development of BPD[154]; indeed, there is evidence that this may begin in utero.[149] Mediators of epithelial lung injury include a variety of cytokines, including interleukin-1β (IL-1β), IL-6, and IL-8[150]; in addition, impaired signaling of growth factors such as vascular endothelial growth factor (VEGF) has been implicated.[155,156] Given these considerations, it is likely that the pathogenesis of BPD, particularly in the extremely-low-birth-weight infant, is multifactorial in nature.

Generally, the incidence of BPD increases with decreasing gestational age; at less than 28 weeks' gestation the incidence is approximately 40% and approaches 90% for infants at less than 26 weeks' gestation.[143,144] Additional risk factors include maternal infection, neonatal sepsis, and PDA.[157] Although better monitoring, improved ventilation strategies, and new technologies have all had a positive impact on reducing the incidence and severity of BPD in the more mature neonate, increased survival of extremely low-birth-weight infants has increased the overall prevalence of this condition in neonatal intensive care graduates.

The clinical presentation of BPD depends on the severity and extent of the acute lung injury. In classic BPD, infants typically require a high degree of ventilatory and oxygen support beyond age 1 week. These infants are slow to wean, require supplemental oxygen for weeks to months, and have episodes of bronchospasm or desaturation. Infants with severe BPD can have varying degrees of right ventricular failure or, in less severe cases, simply display fluid intolerance. The chest radiograph will be abnormal, showing areas of increased density interspersed with areas of hyperinflation or even cystic development.

In the new type of BPD, onset is much more insidious. For the first 2 to 3 weeks of life, these extremely low-birth-weight infants appear stable on minimal ventilatory and oxygen support, but then their need for increased ventilatory and oxygen support slowly develops. These infants often have episodes of apnea, desaturation, or carbon dioxide retention. There may be increased secretions from the endotracheal tube as well. The chest radiograph may show areas of atelectasis, but more commonly it is clear in the early stages or simply shows a minimal, homogeneous increase in density in both lung fields. Depending on clinical signs, confounding conditions such as a PDA, pneumonia, or aspiration must be considered and ruled out.

Treatment of BPD is generally supportive. The goal of treatment is to promote lung growth while simultaneously supporting respiratory needs and minimizing further injury to the lungs. Supplemental oxygen should be used for infants with oxygen saturations below 93% in room air.[158] Bronchodilators may be helpful particularly during exacerbations because there is often a large airway component to BPD.[159] Fluid restriction or diuretics may be helpful in infants with evidence of cor pulmonale or fluid intolerance. At initial presentation infants often receive a few days of antibiotics until infection is ruled out. Infants with pulmonary insufficiency have increased energy needs,[160] making nutritional support particularly important, although it is often overlooked.[161]

An approach aimed at reducing the inflammation and ongoing fibrotic injury is the use of steroids; although earlier study results have shown that intravenous dexamethasone reduces the severity of BPD and improves respiratory outcome in older premature infants,[162,163] concerns have been raised regarding long-term safety, particularly from studies that included younger and more immature infants.[164-166] Because of these observations and a growing body of data that question the safety of high-dose steroids in extremely premature animals, the Academy of Pediatrics Committee on the Fetus and Newborn has recommended that steroid use for BPD be within the context of well-designed, randomized trials until issues of long-term efficacy and safety are more clear.[167] Unfortunately, given the rapid and sustained response that many infants with BPD have to steroids, there is significant controversy over this recommendation, particularly as it applies to the older or less premature infant with significant pulmonary disability.

What is clear is that infants who receive these long courses of steroids for BPD usually show chemical evidence of adrenal suppression, which may last for several months[162]; infants who receive steroids for more than several days should also receive supplementation at times of increased stress (e.g., surgery, infection). It is also apparent that inhaled steroids offer no particular advantage over intravenous dosing, except for ease of administration.[168] Potential new therapies to prevent or reduce the severity of BPD include synchronous mode ventilation, HFV, antioxidants, nitric oxide, antiproteases, vitamin A, and antenatal therapy with steroids and thyrotropin-releasing hormone; however, to date, study results have been inconclusive.[106-108,146,151,161,169-172]

The long-term outcome for infants with classic BPD has improved over the years, although these infants remain at risk for significant morbidity and mortality.[145,157] Infants typically require supplemental oxygen for the first several months of life, and some may require chronic diuretic and bronchodilator use. High-caloric formulas should be considered for those infants who cannot tolerate fluid loading. Rehospitalizations due to respiratory exacerbations, often brought on by infection, are common during the first 2 years of life.[173] Those with relatively uncomplicated courses will gradually improve and by school age often have normal lung function.[157]

The long-term outcome for extremely low-birth-weight infants with new BPD is less clear. Although these infants often require little or no respiratory support at the time of discharge from the neonatal intensive care unit (NICU), there are fewer data on long-term outcome because extremely low-birth-weight infants rarely survived to discharge before the advent of surfactant replacement therapy in the 1980s. If these infants indeed have an arrest of lung epithelial and vascular development due to preterm birth, long-term cardiorespiratory function remains unclear. Similar to infants with classic BPD, these infants are at increased risk for rehospitalization due to pulmonary infection and reactive airway disease,[174] but they may also be at increased risk for long-term pulmonary dysfunction.[175-177]

Mortality due to BMD has markedly improved over the past decade but remains high in infants with complicating conditions (such as cardiovascular disease) or in those with intercurrent respiratory infections, particularly with respiratory syncytial virus (RSV) or adenovirus. Passive immunization against RSV is now possible and is recommended for high-risk premature neonates [178]; however, it is costly and is not uniformly protective.[179,180] Minimizing exposure to environmental hazards whether infectious or irritant (e.g., from kerosene burners or cigarette smoke) cannot be overemphasized.[170]

Congenital Defects of the Lymphatics

Congenital defects of the lymphatics include congenital chylothorax and congenital pulmonary lymphangiectasia (or lymphangioma), which are rare, unrelated conditions. Congenital chylothorax is thought to be due to a failure of peripheral and central lymphatic channels to fuse, or perhaps a rupture of inadequately fused channels at birth.[181,182] Most affected infants have symptoms within hours of birth. Progressive respiratory compromise develops as fluid accumulates in the hemithorax. Drainage is both diagnostic and therapeutic; initially the lymphocyte-rich fluid is clear but becomes opaque when milk feedings are introduced. Nutritional support is critical because of the tremendous loss of protein in the chylous drainage. Most cases self-resolve in 2 to 3 weeks; occasionally, an attempt at surgical closure of the thoracic duct is indicated, although it is not always successful.

Pulmonary lymphangiectasia can be a primary condition or secondary dilation of pulmonary lymphatics due to obstructed pulmonary venous flow.[181,182] A primary lymphangiectasia can be isolated, which is termed *congenital pulmonary lymphangiectasia,* or can be part of a generalized condition, which includes intestinal lymphangiectasia and in which pulmonary involvement is less severe. Congenital pulmonary lymphangiectasia is thought to result from failure of connective tissue elements to normally regress during fetal lung development. In some cases, a hereditary pattern has been suggested. Affected infants usually have symptoms soon after birth; however, some may remain symptom free for several weeks. Infants are usually born at term and have tachypnea and cyanosis; infants born preterm may be mistaken as having surfactant-deficient RDS. Radiographs generally reveal streaky reticular densities as a result of engorged lymphatics; occasionally a finer, "ground-glass" appearance may be confused with surfactant deficiency. Pleural effusions have been reported but are unusual. The condition is progressive and untreatable; most infants die within days, but an occasional survivor beyond infancy has been reported.

Nonpulmonary Conditions that Result in Respiratory Disease

Many nonpulmonary disorders may present with respiratory distress in the neonate (Box 41–1). Conditions that affect the control or mechanics of breathing, the patency or integrity of the upper airway, perfusion to and from the lung, or acid-base balance can present with increased respiratory effort or signs of respiratory insufficiency (i.e., respiratory acidosis or hypoxemia). The clinical and radiographic picture may be consistent with an underlying pulmonary pathological condition, but nonpulmonary causes must be considered, particularly if an infant is gravely ill or not responding to conventional treatments. In many of these nonpulmonary conditions, a delay in diagnosis can lead to irreversible injury and, in some cases, to death despite maximal cardiorespiratory support. Box 41–1 lists many of these conditions; some specific conditions are described in more detail.

BOX 41–1

Nonpulmonary Conditions That Cause Respiratory Distress in the Newborn

DISORDERS OF RESPIRATORY CONTROL

Central hypoventilation disorder
Apnea

AIRWAY OBSTRUCTION/PATENCY

Choanal stenosis/atresia
Mandibular hypoplasia/micrognathia
Vocal cord injury
Subglottic hemangioma
Laryngeal web/stenosis
Laryngomalacia
Tracheobronchomalacia
Tracheoesophageal fistula
Vascular compression

INTERFERENCE WITH RESPIRATORY MECHANICS

Neuromuscular disorders
Phrenic nerve injury
Eventration of the diaphragm
Pleural effusion
Chest wall anomalies

PERFUSION ABNORMALITIES

Persistent pulmonary hypertension of the newborn
Hyperviscosity
Congenital heart disease

DISORDERS OF ACID-BASE BALANCE

Metabolic disorders (e.g., organic acidemias)
Intestinal bicarbonate wasting
Renal bicarbonate wasting
Sepsis
Iatrogenic metabolic acidosis/alkalosis

Apnea of Prematurity

Apnea is one of the most common respiratory problems encountered in the neonatal population. The incidence of apnea is inversely proportional to the gestational age at birth, and more than 75% of infants born before 27 weeks will have apnea at some point in their NICU stay. Apnea can be broadly classified as physiological (i.e., apnea of prematurity) or pathological (i.e., resulting from an underlying disorder such as sepsis).

There are three main types of apnea. The first is *central apnea,* which results from decreased central responsiveness to respiratory stimuli, such as hypoxia and hypercarbia. This responsiveness improves as the infant matures and approaches term. This type of apnea is characterized by cessation of respiratory effort, which usually occurs at the end of exhalation. The second type of apnea is called *obstructive apnea* because of an anatomical or physiological restriction of the airway. Common examples include tracheomalacia or Pierre Robin syndrome. The respiratory pattern of obstructive apnea demonstrates increasing respiratory effort with little to no air movement. *Mixed apnea* represents the third type of apnea. Initially the infant has what appears to be a central apnea, but when a respiratory effort is made, an obstructive pattern is revealed. The obstructive pattern is thought to result from gradual airway collapse during the initial central apneic portion of the episode. Most apneic episodes lasting longer than 20 seconds fall into this category.

Apnea of prematurity is a diagnosis of exclusion, and pathological causes such as hypoglycemia, hypoxemia, hypothermia or hyperthermia, infection, left-to-right shunt, and intracranial hemorrhage should be ruled out. Of particular concern is new-onset apnea in a previously symptom-free infant. Apnea also increases in response to less stressful stimuli, such as immunizations or an ophthalmoscopic examination. Apnea in a term or near-term infant is almost always pathological.

Isolated apnea may be treated with simple tactile stimulation in many cases. Infants who remain apneic after stimulation may require some blow-by oxygen or even positive pressure breaths for a short time. Repeated episodes may benefit from methylxanthine therapy. Caffeine is currently the agent of choice because of a long plasma half-life and low toxicity. Nasal continuous positive airway pressure (CPAP) may also be tried in an attempt to improve aeration of the lungs and help keep the airway open. Some infants, especially those who are still very premature, may require reintubation and ventilation until their respiratory control becomes more mature.

Choanal Atresia/Stenosis

Choanal obstruction due to failure of bony or membranous regression is the most common supralaryngeal congenital defect. It occurs in approximately 1 in 5000 live births. Choanal atresia is often associated with defects in other organs or with syndromes that include other craniofacial anomalies; choanal stenosis is almost always an isolated finding. Choanal atresia is usually unilateral, typically on the right side, and is twice as common in females. Associated findings include a high-arched palate, thickening of the vomer, and medial bowing of the lateral wall of the nose. Clinical presentation depends on the degree of obstruction; bilateral choanal atresia or severe bilateral stenosis will present in the newborn period, whereas unilateral cases or mild stenosis may not present for weeks, months, or years. Infants with symptoms are typically distressed during times of sleep or feeding, when nasal breathing is preferential. Clinical presentation in infants with unilateral obstruction or mild stenosis may occur only when the nares become obstructed, as with the passage of an NG tube or inflammation during an upper respiratory infection. With occlusion of the patent nares, an infant can suddenly decompensate, with signs of severe respiratory distress.

Infants in severe distress may require elective intubation if an oral airway is insufficient or cannot be easily maintained. Direct visualization of the obstruction is best performed by an otolaryngologist using a fiberoptic scope. A cranial CT scan can determine the presence and thickness of the bony plate within the nasal cavity, which is an important surgical consideration. Definitive treatment generally involves drilling through the bony plate and stenting the nasal passage with tubes for 6 weeks to allow proper healing. A high degree of suspicion is key to diagnosing and properly treating this disorder, and if true choanal atresia is present, associated anomalies must be ruled out.

Mandibular Hypoplasia

Mandibular hypoplasia compromises the airway by not allowing sufficient room for the tongue, particularly when the infant is in the supine position. This allows the normal-sized tongue to fall back into the posterior oropharynx and obstruct the airway. This condition is often apparent by observing the position of the chin relative to the rest of the face; the chin will be small (micrognathia) and displaced backward (retrognathia). The palate must be visualized in a patient with mandibular hypoplasia because these patients often have a posterior cleft palate (Pierre Robin syndrome). Management of the airway is usually accomplished with prone positioning, but occasionally CPAP is necessary to maintain hypopharyngeal patency. As the infant grows, relative airway obstruction decreases.

Laryngomalacia

Laryngomalacia is the most common cause of stridor in the neonate. It is thought to result from redundant soft tissue or delayed development of neuromuscular control. Similar to infants with mandibular hypoplasia, infants tend to have more symptoms in the supine position because this allows relatively unsupported anterior tissue to drop into hypopharynx, and this causes obstruction. Affected infants may be stridulous, however, only during periods of crying or distress. Treatment includes prone positioning, and resolution is common by age 1 to 2 years.

Vocal Cord Paralysis

Vocal cord paralysis can be unilateral or bilateral. Unilateral cord paralysis usually presents with a weak or sometimes hoarse cry. Obstructive symptoms, such as stridor or retractions, are less severe and less common. The infant may also cough or choke while feeding because of an inability to prevent aspiration while swallowing. The most common causes are stretch injury during delivery or recurrent laryngeal nerve injury during ductus ligation; thus left-sided paralysis or paresis is most common. Symptoms from unilateral cord paralysis usually improve over a few weeks or months with no intervention.

Bilateral cord paralysis represents a more serious problem and is usually the result of an intracranial pathological condition, such as Chiari malformation, intracranial hemorrhage, or hypoxic-ischemic encephalopathy. These infants may have near total airway obstruction and will have moderate to severe stridor. Most will require tracheostomy to maintain a patent and reliable airway.

Subglottic Hemangioma

Congenital hemangiomas just below the level of the vocal cords are another relatively common cause of stridor in the neonate. These lesions may produce an expiratory wheeze as well. Positional changes tend to have little effect on the severity of the symptoms. Superficial, capillary hemangiomas on the skin of the neck are often present, suggesting the diagnosis. For acute exacerbations, systemic steroids may be used to reduce tissue swelling and improve airway patency; however, symptomatic infants eventually require surgical removal of the lesions. The availability of laser surgery has markedly reduced the need for tracheostomy in children with subglottic hemangioma.

Tracheobronchomalacia

Tracheobronchomalacia is characterized by abnormally compliant airway cartilage, leading to intermittent collapse of the airways during normal respiration. Specific classification depends on the area(s) involved (e.g., tracheomalacia, tracheobronchomalacia, and bronchomalacia). Infants can be mildly or severely affected, depending on the extent of involvement and the ability of surrounding supporting tissues to maintain airway patency. Affected infants generally have symptoms in the newborn period, but presentation may be delayed for many days or weeks if the defect is mild. In these milder cases, infants may remain symptom free until an intercurrent infection leads to increased airway secretions and increased work of breathing. Symptoms include expiratory wheezing and respiratory distress including tachypnea and retractions, and the infant may receive a mistaken diagnosis of reactive airway disease; however, the use of bronchodilators may actually worsen the condition. A chest radiograph may show hyperinflation; definitive diagnosis is made by direct visualization, typically with flexible bronchoscopy. Treatment is supportive because airway compromise generally lessens as the infant grows; however, more severe cases may require stenting with CPAP or even surgical plication. Tracheostomy alone may not be helpful if the affected area extends beyond the proximal trachea. A high association with other congenital anomalies, including tracheoesophageal fistula (see later) must also be kept in mind; a history of recurrent coughing or choking requires further investigation.

Tracheoesophageal Fistula

Tracheoesophageal fistula (TEF) occurs in approximately 1 in 4500 live births, making it one of the most common congenital malformations. Usually isolated, it can be associated with other anomalies including complex syndromes like VATER (*v*ertebral defects, *a*nal atresia, *T*EF, *e*sophageal atresia, and *r*enal anomalies), VACTERL (VATER plus cardiac and upper limb defects), and CHARGE (*c*oloboma, *h*eart defect, choanal *a*tresia, mental *r*etardation, genital hypoplasia, *e*ar anomalies, and deafness). In the absence of a more generalized syndrome, TEF is also associated with isolated cardiac defects, which may present in up to 50% of cases. Whether as part of a syndrome or an isolated anomaly, TEF usually is associated with esophageal atresia; however, in 5% to 7% of cases there is no associated esophageal atresia (so-called H-type TEF).

TEF and an associated esophageal atresia and TEF as part of a more general disorder invariably present in the immediate newborn period; infants with isolated H-type fistula can remain clinically silent for many weeks or even months. Although relatively rare (approximately 1 in 100,000 live births), an H-type fistula must be suspected in any infant who coughs during feedings and has recurrent pneumonitis; in preterm infants it can present as apnea spells with no other signs. The diagnosis of an H-type fistula can be difficult but is best found by a cine esophagram; in cases where this study is inconclusive, bronchoscopy may be necessary. Successful repair and preservation of pulmonary function depends on early diagnosis.

Vascular Compression

Vascular compression of the trachea or mainstem bronchus can result from improper regression of the embryonic branchial arch arteries during fetal development. The most common anomaly is a vascular "ring" consisting of a double aortic arch, in which the vessel completely encircles the trachea and esophagus. Other variants include an ectopic aortic arch (passing behind the esophagus) or an aberrant origin of the right brachiocephalic artery.

Vascular rings will cause inspiratory stridor and expiratory wheezing, neither of which change appreciably with the infant's position. Intermittent worsening of symptoms is sometimes seen when feeding as boluses passing down the esophagus, further compressing the trachea. Feeding difficulty may also be present because of esophageal compression.

An abnormally shaped mediastinum on chest film often provides a clue to this diagnosis. Endoscopy may identify tracheal or esophageal compression. Echocardiogram may define the nature of the vascular anomaly; cardiac catheterization is sometimes necessary. Decisions regarding surgical correction of this defect depend on the relative compromise of the trachea and esophagus; however, the degree of compression may actually worsen as the infant grows.

Phrenic Nerve Paralysis

Stretch injury to the cervical nerve roots C3-C5 during delivery can lead to temporary paralysis of the hemidiaphragm; avulsion of the nerve roots will lead to a permanent injury. Most commonly on the right, this type of injury is associated with birth trauma; brachial plexus injury or Horner's syndrome is present in 70% to 80% of cases and clavicular fracture is common. Infants at highest risk are those with estimated birth weights of more than 4 kg, shoulder dystocia, or difficult breech presentations. There is diminished ventilation on the affected side, and the infant may be tachypneic or even cyanotic if severely compromised. The chest radiograph will show a varying degree of atelectasis with a raised hemidiaphragm on the affected side and the heart and mediastinum shifted toward the contralateral side. Fluoroscopy will show that the paralyzed diaphragm elevates during inspiration and descends on expiration (paradoxical movement). Treatment is supportive in most cases because function usually returns spontaneously in several weeks; in cases of avulsion or permanent dysfunction surgical plication may be necessary.

Eventration of the Diaphragm

The normal diaphragm consists of three layers: a muscular layer sandwiched between the pleural and peritoneal layers. Congenital dysplasia or absence of the muscular layer is a rare disorder that results in a nonfunctioning diaphragm that is highly stretchable. Partial defects are more common and most often on the right side; complete defects are more common on the left side and often associated with anomalies of other organs. Under normal abdominal pressure, viscera easily push the affected diaphragm upward into the hemithorax; in utero this may lead to pulmonary hypoplasia (although this is usually mild), whereas after birth this will cause respiratory compromise by affecting lung expansion. Radiographic and fluoroscopic findings are similar to those of a paralyzed diaphragm, but the clinical history of birth trauma or associated injuries is usually absent. With large defects the appearance of bowel apparently in the thoracic cavity on chest radiograph may be mistaken for a diaphragmatic hernia; however, close inspection will reveal the thin, overlying diaphragmatic pleura. Treatment is supportive; defects that remain symptomatic beyond the neonatal period may require plication.

Pleural Effusion

Collection of fluid within the pleural cavity, if excessive, can result in significant respiratory embarrassment. Pleural effusions in the neonate can result from inflammation, transudation, or frank leakage from disrupted vessels (either vascular or lymphatic). Small pleural effusions are normal during the first hours of life, as fetal lung liquid is cleared from the airspaces, but large effusions or persistence beyond the first day of life is abnormal. Large effusions can result in significant respiratory compromise; although initial management is similar regardless of the cause, successful long-term management depends on accurately identifying the source of the pleural effusion.

The most common cause of symptomatic pleural fluid accumulation in the infant is a chylothorax. Occurring at a rate of about 1 in 10,000 children, a chylothorax may result from a congenital malformation (see previous text) or, less commonly, from damage during a surgical procedure. It occurs more frequently on the right side instead of the left and is rarely bilateral. Although a chest radiograph can detect the effusion, definitive diagnosis is made by analysis of the fluid. Chyle is similar to other serous effusions except for the preponderance of lymphocytes. The presence of lipid confirms the diagnosis, but it may be absent if the infant has not been enterally fed in the past few days. Chylothorax usually regresses spontaneously, although serial thoracenteses or thoracostomy tube placement may be necessary for several days or weeks to manage respiratory symptoms; in those cases chyle production can be reduced with a restriction of the infant's diet to a formula that contains only medium chain triglycerides. Surgical intervention in cases of persistent chylothorax is not always successful.

Hydrothorax can be either exudative or transudative. Exudative pleural effusions typically are infectious in origin, whereas transudative effusions follow the same pathophysiological origin as pulmonary edema in the neonate (see previous text). Hemothorax occurs most commonly after intercostal vessel perforation during thoracostomy tube or subclavian venous catheter placement; in most cases the hemorrhage is self-resolved. More common than either hydrothorax or hemothorax, however, is the extravasation of parenteral nutritional fluid from a central venous catheter with its tip in the subclavian vein or the superior vena cava. This so-called "hyperalthorax" is thought to occur either by erosion of the catheter through the vessel wall or, more likely, by alterations in local vascular permeability induced by the hyperosmolar fluid. Indeed, most reported cases have occurred when dextrose concentrations in excess of 15% are infused, and the effusion fluid that is removed by thoracentesis typically is nonhemorrhagic. Regardless of cause, all three types of pleural effusion can result in dramatic respiratory compromise but respond readily to percutaneous drainage; a thoracostomy tube is rarely indicated.

Congenital Anomalies of the Chest Wall

Thoracic cage abnormalities represent a group of uncommon but often overlooked cause of respiratory distress in the neonate and can be classified as either structural or functional. Structural abnormalities may be limited to the sternum or involve the entire thoracic cage. Sternal deformities include pectus excavatum, a relatively common but usually benign condition, and complete separation of the sternum, which usually leads to ectopia cordis and is usually lethal. Generalized structural abnormalities invariably involve some degree of thoracic restriction and pulmonary hypoplasia; many of these are intrinsically lethal or are part of a more generalized, lethal disorder. Some conditions, however, such as achondroplasia and Ellis-van Creveld syndrome, are compatible with normal life. Functional anomalies result from dysfunction of the chest wall musculature. Like structural defects, they can be isolated to the thoracic cage, but more often they are part of a systemic disorder, such as congenital muscular dystrophy, glycogen storage disease, or myasthenia gravis.

Most infants with thoracic cage abnormalities are recognized in the immediate newborn period, although a relatively protuberant abdomen may distract the clinician from the primary problem. Infants with restricted thoracic cages (either structural or functional) will have tachypnea and retractions; the radiograph will show a narrow, elongated thoracic cage with high clavicles and low hemidiaphragms. Treatment is supportive; in the absence of severe pulmonary hypoplasia or an underlying lethal disorder, infants may do relatively well, although they often require mechanical ventilation for a limited duration.

Persistent Pulmonary Hypertension of the Neonate

In the fetus, the organ of gas exchange is the placenta, not the lung. Thus placental blood flow is high, whereas pulmonary blood flow is minimal. To achieve this, blood returning to the right side of the heart must be directed to the systemic (and thus, placental) circulation. This is accomplished by two principal right-to-left shunts in the fetus: the foramen ovale, which shunts blood from the right to left atrium, and the ductus arteriosus, which shunts blood from the pulmonary artery to the descending aorta. These shunts result in less than 10% of the combined fetal ventricular output going to the lungs.

At birth, dramatic changes must occur within the lung if the fetus is to make a successful transition from placental to pulmonary gas exchange. Not only must liquid be removed from potential airspaces (see section on Delayed Clearance of Fetal Lung Liquid), but also blood flow must be redirected. After inflation of the lungs with air and dramatic increases in oxygen tension within the lungs, there is a marked increase in cyclic nucleotides within the pulmonary vascular smooth muscle, leading to vasodilatation.[183,184] The resultant drop in pulmonary vascular resistance leads to a tenfold increase in pulmonary blood flow.[185] This causes left atrial pressure to exceed right atrial pressure, allowing the one-way flap across the foramen ovale to close. Flow across the ductus arteriosus reverses, and this, combined with the increase in oxygen tension in the blood, leads to gradual closure of the ductus over the first few hours of life.

In the syndrome of persistent pulmonary hypertension of the newborn (PPHN), this transition of the pulmonary circulation fails to occur normally (see Chapter 43). Pulmonary vascular resistance and pulmonary arterial pressure remain high and blood flow continues to bypass the lungs as in fetal life. (This is why the term *persistent fetal circulation* has been used, although it is not strictly correct because there is no longer any placental/umbilical circulation as in the fetus.) PPHN is associated with many neonatal disorders, including RDS, meconium aspiration, air leak syndromes, perinatal asphyxia, congenital sepsis, and structural lung disease such as pulmonary hypoplasia or alveolar-capillary dysplasia. PPHN can also be idiopathic. Infants with PPHN can be moderately or severely affected, depending on the degree of shunting. PPHN is often a self-limited disease, but this may take several days; meanwhile, severe hypoxemia can lead to significant morbidity. Mortality can be as high as 50% to 60%; it has improved significantly with the advent of new treatment modalities such as HFV and extracorporeal bypass, which allow the infant more time to spontaneously recover.[68,69,98,99,111,112,186-188]

Hyperviscosity Syndrome

Neonates with polycythemia (central hematocrit >65%) are at risk for abnormally high blood viscosity, which interferes with perfusion to vital tissues. Polycythemia can occur in several situations, including twin–twin transfusion, maternal–fetal transfusion, delayed cord-clamping, home delivery, maternal diabetes, small-for-gestational-age infants, postmature infants, and infants with Down syndrome or Beckwith-Wiedemann syndrome. Symptoms generally relate to the degree of hyperviscosity and can range from tachypnea to apnea, listlessness to irritability, and jitteriness to seizures. Hyperviscosity syndrome presents in the first few hours of infants' lives, and the presentation can mimic that in infants with congenital pneumonia, meconium aspiration, persistent pulmonary hypertension, or congenital heart disease. Affected infants are at risk for ongoing thrombotic injury unless the condition is reversed by partial blood volume exchange.

Congenital Heart Disease

In the neonate, significant congenital heart disease typically presents in one of two ways: (1) cyanosis with minimal or no respiratory distress or (2) cardiorespiratory failure. Cyanotic lesions, such as transposition of the great vessels or tetralogy of Fallot, usually present in an infant who is blue but comfortable. Characteristically, congenital cyanotic heart disease is suspected in such an infant, even if a murmur is absent, particularly if the infant remains desaturated or hypoxemic in 100% oxygen. Less common in the neonate are those conditions that lead to early failure, such as an atrioventricular canal defect or a large ventricular septal defect. These infants are generally not cyanotic but are pale with marked respiratory distress and often a loud murmur; chest radiographs may show the classic signs of cardiomegaly and pulmonary vascular congestion.

In some types of congenital heart disease there is an overlap in presentation, and infants will appear cyanotic and have signs of respiratory distress such as tachypnea and perhaps even retractions. This type of presentation, common with hypoplastic left heart syndrome and total obstructed anomalous pulmonary venous return, may initially be confused with sepsis, pneumonia, meconium aspiration, or even RDS. Total anomalous pulmonary venous return (TAPVR) deserves particular mention because it cannot be detected in utero; it is often missed postnatally, even on repeated echocardiograms. In fact, this condition is the most common, potentially correctable cardiac lesion for which neonates are mistakenly placed on ECMO. To diagnosis TAPVR, one must keep a high index of suspicion, particularly in a term or near-term infant who has a clinical and radiographic picture of surfactant-deficient respiratory distress or group B streptococcal sepsis. If TAPVR is suspected and echocardiograms are not confirmatory, these infants must have a cardiac catheterization to make the diagnosis.

REFERENCES

1. Watchko JF, Mayock DE, Standaert TA et al: The ventilatory pump: neonatal and developmental issues, Adv Pediatr 38:109-134, 1991.
2. Alcorn D, Adamson TM, Lambert TF et al: Morphological effects of chronic tracheal ligation and drainage in the fetal lamb lung, J Anat 123:649-60, 1977.
3. Bland RD: Formation of fetal lung liquid and its removal near birth. In Polin RA, Fox WW, editors: Fetal and neonatal physiology, vol 2, Philadelphia, 1998, WB Saunders.
4. Jain L: Alveolar fluid clearance in developing lungs and its role in neonatal transition, Clin Perinatol 26:585-599, 1999.
5. Avery ME, Gatewood OB, Brumley G: Transient tachypnea of the newborn, Am J Dis Child 111:380-385, 1966.
6. Olver RE, Strang LB: Ion fluxes across the pulmonary epithelium and the secretion of lung liquid in the foetal lamb, J Physiol 241: 327-357, 1974.
7. Walters DV, Olver RE: The role of catecholamines in lung liquid absorption at birth, Pediatr Res 12:239-242, 1978.
8. Olver RE, Ramsden CA, Strang LB et al: The role of amiloride-blockable sodium transport in adrenaline-induced lung liquid reabsorption in the fetal lamb, J Physiol 376:321-340, 1986.
9. McDonald JV, Gonzales LW, Ballard PL et al: Lung b-adrenoreceptor blockade affects perinatal surfactant release but not lung water, J Appl Physiol 60:1727-1733, 1986.
10. Chapman DL, Carlton DP, Nielson DW et al: Changes in lung liquid during spontaneous labor in fetal sheep, *J Appl Physiol* 76: 523-530, 1994.
11. Wallace MJ, Hooper SB, Harding R: Regulation of lung liquid secretion by arginine vasopressin in fetal sheep, *Am J Physiol* 258: R104-111, 1990.
12. Cummings JJ, Carlton DP, Poulain FR et al: Vasopressin effects on lung liquid volume in fetal sheep, *Pediatr Res* 38:30-35, 1995.
13. Raj JU, Bland RD: Lung liquid clearance in newborn lambs: effect of pulmonary microvascular pressure elevation, *Am Rev Respir Dis* 134:305-10, 1986.
14. Cummings JJ, Carlton DP, Poulain FR et al: Hypoproteinemia slows lung liquid clearance in young lambs, *J Appl Physiol* 74: 153-160, 1993.
15. Cummings JJ: Simultaneous increase in pulmonary blood flow and decrease in lung liquid production in late gestation fetal lambs, *Am Rev Respir Dis* 147:A417, 1993.
16. Egan EA, Dillon WP, Zorn S: Fetal lung liquid absorption and alveolar epithelial solute permeability in surfactant deficient, breathing lambs, *Pediatr Res* 18:566-570, 1984.
17. Miller MJ, Fanaroff AA, Martin RJ: The respiratory system: other pulmonary problems. In Fanaroff AA, Martin RJ, editors: *Neonatal-perinatal medicine, vol 2,* St Louis, 1992, Mosby.
18. Ogata ES, Gregory GA, Kitterman JA et al: Pneumothorax in respiratory distress syndrome: incidence and effect on vital signs, blood gases and pH, *Pediatrics* 58:177-182, 1976.
19. Mercier CE, Soll RF: Clinical trials of natural surfactant extract in respiratory distress syndrome, *Clin Perinatol* 20:711-735, 1993.
20. Wiswell TE: Advances in the treatment of the meconium aspiration syndrome, *Acta Paediatrica* 90:28-30, 2001.
21. Kilbride HW, Thibeault DW: Neonatal complications of preterm premature rupture of membranes. Pathophysiology and management, *Clin Perinatol* 28:761-785, 2001.
22. Plenat F, Vert P, Didier F et al: Pulmonary interstitial emphysema, *Clin Perinatol* 5:351-371, 1978.
23. Madansky DL, Lawson EE, Chernick V et al: Pneumothorax and other forms of pulmonary air leak in newborns, *Am Rev Resp Dis* 120:729-737, 1979.
24. Gormally SM, Clarke TA, Krishnan A et al: Surfactant therapy in respiratory distress syndrome: the effect of a learning curve in improving outcome, *Irish J Med Sci* 162:458-461, 1993.
25. Swingle HM, Eggert LD, Bucciarelli RL: New approach to management of unilateral tension pulmonary interstitial emphysema in premature infants, *Pediatrics* 74:354-357, 1984.
26. Keszler M, Donn SM, Bucciarelli RL et al: Multicenter controlled trial comparing high-frequency jet ventilation and conventional ventilation in newborn infants with pulmonary interstitial emphysema, *J Pediatr* 119:85-93, 1991.
27. Keszler M, Durand D: Neonatal high frequency ventilation: past, present, and future, *Clin Perinatol* 28:579-607, 2001.
28. van Houten J, Long W, Mullett M et al: Pulmonary hemorrhage in premature infants after treatment with synthetic surfactant: an autopsy evaluation, *J Pediatr* 120:S40-S44, 1992.
29. Cole VA, Normand ICS, Reynolds EOR, et al.: Pathogenesis of hemorrhagic pulmonary edema and massive pulmonary hemorrhage in the newborn, *Pediatr* 51:175-186, 1973.
30. Kluckow M, Evans N: Ductal shunting, high pulmonary blood flow, and pulmonary hemorrhage, *J Pediatr* 137:68-72, 2000.
31. Akinbami LJ, Selby DM, Slonim AD: Hepatosplenomegaly and pulmonary infiltrates in an infant, *J Pediatr* 139:124-129, 2001.
32. Correa AG: Unique aspects of tuberculosis in the pediatric population, *Clin Chest Med* 18:89-98, 1997.
33. Schuchat A, Oxtoby M, Cochi S et al: Population-based risk factors for neonatal group B streptococcal disease: results of a cohort study in metropolitan Atlanta, *J Infect Dis* 162:672-677, 1990.
34. Whitley R, Arvin A, Prober C et al: Predictors of morbidity and mortality in neonates with herpes simplex virus infections, *N Engl J Med* 324:450-454, 1991.
35. Greenough A: Meconium aspiration syndrome-prevention and treatment, *Early Hum Dev* 41:183-192, 1995.
36. Wiswell TE, Bent RC: Meconium staining and the meconium aspiration syndrome, *Pediatr Clin NA* 40:955-981, 1993.
37. Lam BC, Yeung CY, Fu KH et al: Surfactant tracheobronchial lavage for the management of a rabbit model of meconium aspiration syndrome, *Biol Neonate* 78:129-138, 2000.
38. Herting E, Rauprich P, Stichtenoth G et al: Resistance of different surfactant preparations to inactivation by meconium, *Pediatr Res* 50:44-49, 2001.
39. Gordon E, South M, McDougall PN et al: Blood aspiration syndrome as a cause of respiratory distress in the newborn infant, *J Pediatr* 142:200-202, 2003.
40. Auten RL, Notter RH, Kendig JW et al: Surfactant treatment of full-term newborns with respiratory failure, *Pediatrics* 87: 101-110, 1991.
41. Lam BC, Yeung CY: Surfactant for meconium aspiration syndrome: a pilot study, *Pediatrics* 103:1014-1018, 1999.
42. Holopainen R, Laine J, Halkola L et al: Dexamethasone treatment attenuates pulmonary injury in piglet meconium aspiration, *Pediatr Res* 49:162-168, 2001.
43. Wiswell TE, Gannon CM, Jacob J et al: Delivery room management of the apparently vigorous meconium-stained neonate: results of the multicenter, international collaborative trial, *Pediatrics* 105:1-7, 2000.
44. Niermeyer S, Kattwinkel J, Reempts PV et al: International Guidelines for Neonatal Resuscitation: an excerpt from the guidelines 2000 for cardiopulmonary resuscitation and emergency cardiovascular care: international consensus on science, *Pediatrics* 106:E29, 2000.
45. Holm BA, Waring AJ: Designer surfactants: the next generation in surfactant replacement, *Clin Perinatol* 20:813-829, 1993.
46. Jobe AH, Ikegami M: Surfactant metabolism, *Clin Perinatol* 20:683-696, 1993.
47. Krauss AN: Recent advances in hyaline membrane disease, *Pediatr Ann* 12:24-30, 1983.
48. Malloy MH, Freeman DH: Respiratory distress syndrome mortality in the United States, 1987 to 1995, *J Perinatol* 20:414-420, 2000.
49. Lemons JA, Bauer CR, Oh W et al: Very low birth weight outcomes of the National Institute of Child Health and Human Development Neonatal Research Network, January 1995 through December 1996, *Pediatrics* 107:e1-e8, 2001.
50. Clark RH, Auten RL, Peabody J: A comparison of the outcomes of neonates treated with two different natural surfactants, *J Pediatr* 139:828-831, 2001.
51. Coleman M, Dehner LP, Sibley RK et al: Pulmonary alveolar proteinosis: an uncommon cause of chronic neonatal respiratory distress, *Am Rev Respir Dis* 121:583-586, 1980.
52. Mahut B, deBlic J, LeBourgeois M et al: Partial and massive lung lavages in an infant with severe pulmonary alveolar proteinosis, *Pediatr Pulmonol* 13:50-53, 1992.
53. Moulton SL, Krous HF, Merritt TA et al: Congenital pulmonary alveolar proteinosis: failure of treatment with extracorporeal life support, *J Pediatr* 120:297-302, 1992.

54. deMello DE, Nogee LM, Heyman S, et al: Molecular and phenotypic variability in the congenital alveolar proteinosis syndrome associated with inherited surfactant protein B deficiency, *J Pediatr* 125:43-50, 1994.
55. Nogee LM, deMello DE, Dehner LP et al: Brief report: deficiency of pulmonary surfactant protein b in congenital alveolar proteinosis, *N Engl J Med* 328:406-410, 1993.
56. Nogee LM, Garnier G, Singer L et al: A mutation in the surfactant protein B gene responsible for fatal neonatal respiratory disease in multiple kindreds, *J Clin Invest* 93:1860-1863, 1994.
57. Yusen RD, Cohen AH, Hamvas A: Normal lung function in subjects heterozygous for surfactant protein-B deficiency, *Am J Respir Crit Care Med* 159:411-414, 1999.
58. Hamvas A, Cole FS, deMello DE et al.: Surfactant protein B deficiency: antenatal diagnosis and prospective treatment with surfactant replacement, *J Pediatr* 125:356-361, 1994.
59. Dunbar III AE, Wert SE, Ikegami M et al: Prolonged survival in hereditary surfactant protein B (SP-B) deficiency associated with a novel splicing mutation, *Pediatr Res* 48:275-282, 2000.
60. Sherer DM, Davis JM, Woods JR: Pulmonary hypoplasia: a review, *Obstet Gynecol Surv* 45:792-803, 1990.
61. Fewell JE, Hislop AA, Kitterman JA et al: Effect of tracheosotomy on lung development in fetal lambs, *J Appl Physiol* 55:1103-8, 1983.
62. Rigatto H: Maturation of breathing control in the fetus and newborn infant. In Beckerman RC, Brouillette RT, Hunt CE, editors: *Respiratory control disorders in infants and children*, Baltimore, 1992, Williams & Wilkins.
63. Thomas IT, Smith DW: Oligohydramnios, cause of the nonrenal features of Potter's syndrome, including pulmonary hypoplasia, *J Pediatr* 84:811-817, 1974.
64. Devine PC, Malone FD: Noncardiac thoracic anomalies, *Clin Perinatol* 27:865-900, 2000.
65. Lally KP: Congenital diaphragmatic hernia, *Curr Opin Pediatr* 14:486-490, 2002.
66. Bohn D: Congenital diaphragmatic hernia, *Am J Respir Crit Care Med* 166:911-915, 2002.
67. Cullen ML, Klein MD, Philippart AI: Congenital diaphragmatic hernia, *Surg Clin NA* 65:1115-1137, 1985.
68. Van Meurs KP, Robbins ST, Reed VL, et al: Congenital diaphragmatic hernia: long-term outcome in neonates treated with extracorporeal membrane oxygenation, *J Pediatr* 122:893-899, 1993.
69. Clark RH, Yoder BA, Sell MS: Prospective, randomized comparison of high-frequency oscillation and conventional ventilation in candidates for extracorporeal membrane oxygenation, *J Pediatr* 124:447-454, 1994.
70. Wilcox DT, Glick PL, Karamanoukian H, et al: Pathophysiology of congenital diaphragmatic hernia v. effect of exogenous surfactant therapy on gas exchange and lung mechanics in the lamb congenital diaphragmatic hernia model. *J Pediatr* 124:289-293, 1994.
71. Okuyama H: Inhaled nitric oxide with early surgery improves the outcome of antenatally diagnosed congenital diaphragmatic hernia. *J Pediatr Surg* 37:1188-1190, 2002.
72. Moyer V, Moya F, Tibboel R, et al: Late versus early surgical correction for congenital diaphragmatic hernia in newborn infants, *Cochrane Database Syst Rev* 3:CD001695 PMID 10908506, 2002.
73. Nakayama DK, Motoyama EK, Tagge EM: Effect of preoperative stabilization on respiratory system compliance and outcome in newborn infants with congenital diaphragmatic hernia, *J Pediatr* 118:793-799, 1991.
74. Harrison MR, Adzick NS, Longaker MT, et al: Successful repair in utero of a fetal diaphragmatic hernia after removal of herniated viscera from the left thorax, *N Engl J Med*, 322:1582-1589, 1990.
75. Walker GM, Kasem KF, O'Toole SJ, et al: Early perfluorodecalin lung distension in infants with congenital diaphragmatic hernia, *J Pediatr Surg* 38:17-20, 2003.
76. Laberge JM, Flageole H, Pukash D, et al: Outcome of the prenatally diagnosed congenital cystic adenomatoid lung malformation: a Canadian experience, *Fetal Diagn Ther* 16:178-186, 2001.
77. Hernanz-Schulman M: Cysts and cystlike lesions of the lung, *Radiol Clin N A* 31:631-649, 1993.
78. Kravitz RM: Congenital malformations of the lung, *Pediatr Clin NA* 41:453-472, 1994.
79. Duncombe GJ, Dickinson JE, Kikiros CS: Prenatal diagnosis and management of congenital cystic adenomatoid malformation of the lung, *Am J Obstet Gynecol* 187:950-954, 2002.
80. Williams HJ, Johnson KJ: Imaging of congenital cystic lung lesions, Paediatr Respir Rev 3:120-127, 2002.
81. Ryckman FC, Rosenkrantz JG: Thoracic surgical problems in infancy and childhood, Surg Clin N A 65:1423-1454, 1985.
82. Kugelman A, Weinger-Abend M, Miselevich I, et al: Acquired pulmonary cysts in the newborn infant, Pediatr Pulmonol 24:298-301, 1997.
83. Bentsianov BL, Goldstein NA, Giuste R, et al: Unilateral pulmonary agenesis presenting as an airway lesion, Arch Otolaryngol 126:1386-1389, 2000.
84. Bromley B, Benacerraf BR: Unilateral lung hypoplasia: report of three cases, J Ultrasound Med 16:599-601, 1997.
85. Shaw TR: Displacement of the heart caused by pulmonary agenesis, Heart 88:277, 2002.
86. Horbar JD, The National Institute of Child Health and Human Development Neonatal Research Network: a multicenter randomized trial comparing two surfactants for the treatment of neonatal respiratory distress syndrome, J Pediatr 123:757-766, 1993.
87. Hudak ML, Matteson EJ, Baus JA, et al: Infasurf v exosurf for the prophylaxis of RDS: a ten center randomized double-masked comparison trial, Pediatr Res 35:231A, 1994.
88. Cummings JJ: Surfactant therapy in neonates and beyond, RT Magazine 77-84, 1999.
89. Khammash H, Perlman M, Wojtulewicz J, et al: Surfactant therapy in full-term infants with severe respiratory failure, Pediatrics 92:135-139, 1993.
90. Lotze A, Mitchell BR, Bulas DI, et al: Multicenter study of surfactant (beractant) use in the treatment of term infants with severe respiratory failure, J Pediatr 132:40-47, 1998.
91. Willson DF, Zaritsky A, Bauman LA, et al: Instillation of calf lung surfactant extract (calfactant) is beneficial in pediatric acute hypoxemic respiratory failure, *Crit Care* 27:188-195, 1999.
92. Marraro GA, Luchetti M, Galassini EM, et al: Natural surfactant supplementation in ARDS in paediatric age, *Minerva Anestesiol* 65:92 97, 1999.
93. Golombek SG, Truog WE: Effects of surfactant treatment on gas exchange and clinical course in near-term newborns with RDS, *J Perinat Med* 28:436-442, 2000.
94. Tibby SM, Hatherill M, Wright SM, et al: Exogenous surfactant supplementation in infants with respiratory syncytial virus bronchiolitis, *Am J Respir Crit Care Med* 162:1251-1256, 2000.
95. Notter RH, Apostolakos M, Holm BA, et al: Surfactant therapy and its potential use with other agents in term neonates, children, and adults with acute lung injury, Persp Neonatol 1:4-20, 2000.
96. Cotten M, Clark RH: The science of neonatal high-frequency ventilation, *Respir Care Clin N Am* 7:611-631, 2001.
97. Keszler M, Durand DJ: Neonatal high-frequency ventilation: past, present, and future, *Clin Perinatol* 28:579-607, 2001.
98. Frantz ID III: High-frequency ventilation [abstract], *Crit Care Med* 21(Suppl 9):S370, 1993.
99. Clark RH: High-frequency ventilation, J Pediatr 124:661-670, 1994
100. Group HS: Randomized study of high-frequency oscillatory ventilation in infants with severe respiratory distress syndrome. J Pediatr 122:609-619, 1993
101. Wiswell TE, Graziani LJ, Kornhauser MS, et al: High-frequency jet ventilation in the early management of respiratory distress syndrome is associated with a greater risk for adverse outcomes, *Pediatrics* 98:1035-1043, 1996.
102. Moriette G, Paris-Llado J, Walti H, et al: Prospective randomized multicenter comparison of high-frequency oscillatory ventilation and conventional ventilation in preterm infants of less than 30 weeks with respiratory distress syndrome, *Pediatrics* 107: 363-372, 2001.
103. Ogawa Y, Miyasaka K, Kawano T, et al: A multicenter randomized trial of high frequency oscillatory ventilation as compared with conventional mechanical ventilation in preterm infants with respiratory failure, *Early Hum Dev* 32:1-10, 1993.
104. Gertsmann DR, Minton SD, Stoddard RA, et al: The Provo multicenter early high-frequency oscillatory ventilation trial: improved pulmonary and clinical outcome in respiratory distress syndrome, *Pediatrics* 98:1044-1057, 1996.
105. Keszler M, Modanlou HD, Brudno DS, et al: Multi-center controlled clinical trial of high-frequency jet ventilation in preterm infants with uncomplicated respiratory distress syndrome, *Pediatrics* 100:593-599, 1997.

106. Plavka R, Kopecky P, Sebron V, et al: A prospective randomized comparison of conventional mechanical ventilation and very early high frequency oscillatory ventilation in extremely premature newborns with respiratory distress syndrome, *Intensive Care Med* 25:68-75, 1999.
107. Courtney SE, Durand DJ, Asselin JM, et al: High-frequency oscillatory ventilation versus conventional mechanical ventilation for very-low-birth-weight infants, *N Engl J Med* 347:643-652, 2002.
108. Johnson AH, Peacock JL, Greenough A, et al: High-frequency oscillatory ventilation for the prevention of chronic lung disease of prematurity, *N Engl J Med* 347:633-642, 2002.
109. Todd MM, Toutant SM, Shapiro HM: The effects of high-frequency ventilation on intracranial pressure and brain surface movement in cats, *Anesthesiology* 54:496-504, 1981.
110. Walker AM, Brodecky VA, dePreu ND, et al: High frequency oscillatory ventilation compared with conventional mechanical ventilation in newborn lambs: effects of increasing airway pressures on intracranial pressures, *Pediatr Pulmonol* 12:11-16, 1992.
111. Klein MD, Whittlesey GC: Extracorporeal membrane oxygenation, *Pediatr Clin N A* 41:365-384, 1994.
112. Kanto WP: A decade of experience with neonatal extracorporeal membrane oxygenation, *J Pediatr* 124:335-347, 1994.
113. Cummings JJ: Nitric oxide decreases lung liquid production in fetal lambs. *J Appl Physiol* 83:1538-1544, 1997.
114. Abman SH, Kinsella JP, Parker TP, et al: Physiologic roles of nitric oxide in the perinatal pulmonary circulation. In Weir EK, Archer SL, Reeves JT, eds: Fetal and neonatal pulmonary circulations. New York, 1999, Futura.
115. Van Meurs KP, Rhine WD, Asselin JM, et al: Response of premature infants with severe respiratory failure to inhaled NO. *Pediatr Pulmonol* 24:319-323, 1997.
116. Kinsella JP, Walsh WF, Bose C, et al: Randomized controlled trial of inhaled nitric oxide in premature neonates with severe hypoxemic respiratory failure. *Lancet* 354:1061-1065, 1999.
117. Walther FJ, Benders MJ, Leighton JO: Persistent pulmonary hypertension in premature neonates with severe respiratory distress syndrome. *Pediatr* 90:899-904, 1992.
118. Watchko JF: Persistent pulmonary hypertension in a very low birthweight preterm infant. *Clin Pediatr* 24:592-595, 1985.
119. Kinsella JP, Ivy DD, Abman SH: Inhaled nitric oxide improves gas exchange and lowers pulmonary vascular resistance in severe experimental hyaline membrane disease. *Pediatr Res* 36:402-408, 1994.
120. Zapol WM, Rimar S, Gillis N, et al: Nitric oxide and the lung. *Am J Respir Crit Care Med* 149:1375-1380, 1994.
121. Abman SH, Kinsella JP: Nitric oxide in the pathophysiology and treatment of neonatal pulmonary hypertension. 4:1-11, 1994.
122. Kinsella JP: Inhaled nitric oxide: current and future uses in neonates. *Semin Perinatol* 24:387-395, 2000.
123. Abman SH, Kinsella JP: Is there a role for nitric oxide therapy in premature neonates? 2:4-16, 2001.
124. Greenspan JS, Wolfson MR, Shaffer TH: Liquid ventilation, *Sem Perinatol* 24:396-405, 2000.
125. Fuhrman BP, Paczan PR, DeFrancisis M: Perfluorocarbon associated gas exchange, *Crit Care Med* 19:712-723, 1991.
126. Rotta AT, Steinhorn DM: Partial liquid ventilation reduces pulmonary neutrophil accumulation in an experimental model of systemic endotoxemia and acute lung injury, *Crit Care Med* 26:1707-1715, 1998.
127. Colton DM, Till GO, Johnson KJ, et al: Neutrophil accumulation is reduced during partial liquid ventilation, *Crit Care Med* 26:1716-1724, 1998.
128. Merz U, Klosterhalfen B, Hausler M, et al: Partial liquid ventilation reduces release of leukotriene B4 and interleukin-6 in bronchoalveolar lavage surfactant-depleted newborn pigs, *Pediatr Res* 51:183-189, 2002.
129. Haeberle HA, Nesti N, Dieterich HJ, et al: Perflubron reduces lung inflammation in respiratory syncytial virus infection by inhibiting chemokine expression and nuclear factor-kappa B activation, *Am J Resp Crit Care Med* 165:1433-1438, 2002.
130. Steinhorn DM, Papo MC, Rotta AT, et al: Liquid ventilation attenuates pulmonary oxidative damage, *J Crit Care* 14:20-28, 1999.
131. Leach CL, Fuhrman BP: Perfluorocarbon associated gas exchange (PAGE) in surfactant deficiency. *ARRD* 145:A454, 1992.
132. Degraeuwe PL, Thunnissen FB, Jansen NJ, et al: Conventional gas ventilation, liquid-assisted high-frequency oscillatory ventilation, and tidal liquid ventilation in surfactant-treated preterm lambs, *Int J Artif Organs* 23:754-764, 2000.
133. Vazquez de Anda GF, Lachmann RA, Verbrugge SJ, et al: Partial liquid ventilation improves lung function in ventilation-induced lung injury, *Euro Resp J* 18:93-99, 2001.
134. Lewis DA, Colton D, Johnson K, et al: Prevention of ventilator-induced lung injury with partial liquid ventilation, *J Pediatr Surg* 36:1333-1336, 2001.
135. Jeng M, Kou YR, Sheu CC, et al: Effects of partial liquid ventilation with FC-77 on acute lung injury in newborn piglets, *Pediatr Pulmonol* 33:12-21, 2002.
136. Leach CL, Greenspan JS, Rubenstein SD, et al: Partial liquid ventilation with perflubron in premature infants with severe respiratory distress syndrome, *N Engl J Med* 335:761-767, 1996.
137. Hirschl RB, Conrad S, Kaiser R, et al: Partial liquid ventilation in adult patients with ARDS: a multicenter phase I-II trial, *Ann Surg* 228:692-700, 1998.
138. Fedora M, Nekvasil R, Seda M, et al: Partial liquid ventilation in the therapy of pediatric acute respiratory distress syndrome, *Bratisl Lek Listy* 100:481-485, 1999.
139. Sands TL, Miller KJ, Fischer J: Liquid ventilation: a case study, *Am J Crit Care* 9:397-402, 2000.
140. Dani C, Reali MF, Bertini G, et al: Liquid ventilation in an infant with persistent interstitial pulmonary emphysema, *J Perinatal Med* 29:158-162, 2001.
141. Hirschl RB, Croce M, Gore D, et al: Prospective, randomized, controlled pilot study of partial liquid ventilation in adult respiratory distress syndrome, *Am J Resp Crit Care Med* 165:787-787, 2002.
142. Northway WH, Rosan RC, Porter DY: Pulmonary disease following respiratory therapy of hyaline membrane disease: bronchopulmonary dysplasia, *N Engl J Med* 276:357-368, 1967.
143. Bancalari E, Gerhardt T: Bronchopulmonary dysplasia, *Pediatr Clin North Am* 33:1-23, 1986.
144. O'Brodovich HM, Mellins RB: Bronchopulmonary dysplasia: unresolved neonatal acute lung injury, *Am Rev Respir Dis* 132:694-709, 1985.
145. Jobe AH, Bancalari E: Bronchopulmonary dysplasia: a NICHD/NHLBI/ORD workshop summary, *Am J Respir Crit Care Med* 163:1723-1729, 2001.
146. Kennedy KA: Epidemiology of acute and chronic lung injury, *Semin Perinatol* 17:247-252, 1993,
147. Jobe AJ: The new BPD: an arrest of lung development, *Pediatr Res* 46:641-643, 1999.
148. Bland RD, Coalson JJ: *Chronic lung disease of infancy,* New York, 2000, Dekker.
149. Jobe AH, Ikegami M: Mechanisms initiating lung injury in the preterm, *Early Hum Dev* 53:81-94, 1998.
150. Speer CP: New insights into the pathogenesis of pulmonary inflammation in preterm infants, *Biol Neonate* 79:205-209, 2001.
151. Rozycki HJ: Oxygen, oxygen radicals, and inflammation in the development of chronic lung disease, Journal 12:1-8, 2002.
152. Hjalmarson O, Sandberg K: Abnormal lung function in healthy preterm infants, *Am J Respir Crit Care Med* 165:83-87, 2002.
153. Clark RH, Gerstmann DR, Jobe AH, et al: Lung injury in neonates: causes, strategies for prevention, and long-term consequences, *J Pediatr* 139:478-486, 2001.
154. Copland IB, Post M: Understanding the mechanisms of infant respiratory distress and chronic lung disease, *Am J Resp Cell Mol Biol* 26:261-265, 2002.
155. Bhatt AJ, Pryhuber GS, Huyck H, et al: Disrupted pulmonary vasculature and decreased vascular endothelial growth factor, Flt-1, and TIE-2 in human infants dying with bronchopulmonary dysplasia, *Am J Respir Crit Care Med* 164:1971-1980, 2001.
156. Lassus P, Turanlahti M, Heikkilä P, et al: Pulmonary vascular endothelial growth factor and Flt-1 in fetuses, in acute and chronic lung disease, and in persistent pulmonary hypertension of the newborn, *Am J Respir Crit Care Med* 164:1981-1987, 2001.
157. Vaucher YE: Bronchopulmonary dysplasia: an enduring challenge, *Pediatr Rev* 23:349-358, 2002.
158. Poets CF: When do infants need additional inspired oxygen? A review of the current literature, *Pediatr Pulmonol* 26:424-428, 1998.
159. Panitch HB, Shaffer TH: Developmental airway structure and function in health and chronic lung injury. In Coalson JJ, Bland RD, eds.: *Chronic lung disease of early infancy,* New York, 1999, Marcel Dekker, pp 535-568.

160. Denne SC: Energy expenditure in infants with pulmonary insufficiency: is there evidence for increased energy needs? *J Nutr* 131: 935S-937S, 2001.
161. Bancalari E, Sosenko I: Pathogenesis and prevention of neonatal chronic lung disease: recent developments, *Pediatr Pulmonol* 8: 109-116, 1990.
162. Cummings JJ, D'Eugenio DB, Gross SJ: A controlled trial of dexamethasone in preterm infants at high risk for bronchopulmonary dysplasia, *N Engl J Med* 320:1505-1510, 1989.
163. Harkavy KL, Scanlon JW, Chowdry PK, et al: Dexamethasone therapy for chronic lung disease in ventilator- and oxygen-dependent infants: a controlled trial, *J Pediatr* 115:979-983, 1989.
164. Garland JS, Alex CP, Pauly TH, et al: A three-day course of dexamethasone therapy to prevent chronic lung disease in ventilated neonates: a randomized trial, *Pediatrics* 104:91-99, 1999.
165. O'Shea TM, Kothadia JM, Klinepeter KL, et al: Randomized placebo-controlled trial of a 42-day tapering course of dexamethasone to reduce the duration of ventilator dependency in very low birth weight infants: outcome of study participants at 1-year adjusted age, *Pediatrics* 104:15-21, 1999.
166. Shinwell ES, Karplus M, Reich D, et al: Early postnatal dexamethasone treatment and increased incidence of cerebral palsy, *Arch Dis Child Fetal Neonatal Ed* 83:F177-F181, 2000.
167. Committee on Fetus and Newborn: postnatal corticosteroids to treat or prevent chronic lung disease in preterm infants, *Pediatrics* 109:330-338, 2002.
168. Suchomski SJ, Cummings JJ: A randomized trial of inhaled versus intravenous steroids in ventilator-dependent preterm infants. J Perinatol 22:196-203, 2002
169. Mazursky JE, Klein JM: Techniques to counter neonatal pulmonary disease, *Contemp OB GYN* ???: 11-27, 1994.
170. Rush MG, Hazinski TA: Current therapy of bronchopulmonary dysplasia, *Clin Perinatol* 19:563-590, 1992.
171. Truog WE, Jackson JC: Alternative modes of ventilation in the prevention and treatment of bronchopulmonary dysplasia, *Clin Perinatol* 19:621-647, 1992.
172. Jankov RP, Negus A, Tanswell AK: Antioxidants as therapy in the newborn: some words of caution, *Pediatr Res* 50:681-687, 2001.
173. Fulhman L, Bayley J, Borawski-Clark E, et al: Hospitalization as a measure of morbidity among very low birth weight infants with chronic lung disease, *J Pediatr* 128:447-452, 1994.
174. Evans M, Palta M, Sadek M, et al: Associations between family history of asthma, bronchopulmonary dysplasia, and childhood asthma in very low birth weight children, *Am J Epidemiol* 148: 460-466, 1998.
175. Gross SJ, Iannuzzi DM, Kveselis DA, et al: Effect of preterm birth on pulmonary function at school age: a prospective controlled study, *J Pediatr* 133:188-192, 1998.
176. Subhedar NV, Shaw NJ: Changes in pulmonary arterial pressure in preterm infants with chronic lung disease, *Arch Dis Child Fetal Neonatal Ed* 82:F243-F247, 2000.
177. Hofhuis W, Huysman MWA, van der Wiel EC, et al: Worsening of VmaxFRC in infants with chronic lung disease in the first year of life, *Am J Respir Crit Care Med* 166:1539-1543, 2002.
178. Committee on Infectious Diseases, and Committee on Fetus and Newborn: Revised indications for the use of palivizumab and respiratory syncytial virus immune globulin intravenous for the prevention of respiratory syncytial virus infections, *Pediatrics* 112:1447-1452, 2003.
179. Lee SL, Robinson JL: Questions about palivizumab (Synagis), *Pediatrics* 103:535, 1999 (comment).
180. Carter BS: Palivizumab (synagis): counting "costs" and values, *Pediatrics* 106:1168-1169, 2000.
181. Huber A, Schranz D, Blaha I, et al: Congenital pulmonary lym phangiectasia, *Pediatr Pulmonol* 10:310-313, 1991.
182. Scully RE, Mark EJ, McNeely WF, et al: Case records of the Massachusetts General Hospital case 13-1992, *N Engl J Med* 326:875-884, 1992.
183. Cornfield DN, Chatfield BA, McQueston JA, et al: Effects of birth-related stimuli on L-arginine-dependent pulmonary vasodilation in ovine fetus, *Am J Physiol* 262:H1474-H1481, 1992.
184. Morin III FC, Tiktinsky MH: Oxygenation increases fetal pulmonary blood flow via endothelium dependent vasodilation, *Pediatr Res* 31:1405A, 1992.
185. Heymann MA: Control of the pulmonary circulation in the perinatal period, *J Develop Physiol* 6:281-90, 1984.
186. Durand DJ, Asselin JM, Courtney SE, et al: Randomized study of high-frequency oscillatory ventilation in infants with severe respiratory distress syndrome, *J Pediatr* 122:609-619, 1993.
187. Subramanian KNS, Keszler M, Hoy G: ECMO for severe neonatal respiratory failure, *Technol* 21-37, 1987.
188. Perez-Benavides F, Boynton B, Desai NS: Persistent pulmonary hypertension (PPHN): comparison of conventional treatment vs. extracorporeal membrane oxygenation (ECMO) in neonates fulfilling Bartlett's criteria, *Clin Res* 38:A65A, 1990.

CHAPTER

42

Pneumonitis and Interstitial Disease

Daiva Parakininkas and Tom B. Rice

PEARLS

- Most pediatric pulmonary parenchymal disease is secondary to an infectious agent.
- Clinical evaluation for parenchymal lung disease in the pediatric patient should include a search for symptoms and signs associated with pulmonary disease, such as difficulty with feeding, exercise intolerance, chest pain, cough, tachypnea, dyspnea, cyanosis, orthopnea, clubbing of the nail beds, weight loss, and lethargy.
- Factors predisposing to bacterial pneumonia include increased number of siblings, parental smoking, preterm delivery, urban residence, poor socioeconomic status, airway foreign body, impaired immune response, congenital and anatomic lung defects, abnormalities of the tracheobronchial tree, cystic fibrosis, and congestive heart failure.
- Viral agents are the leading cause of lower respiratory tract infection in infants and children.
- Three major clinical syndromes are associated with lower respiratory tract viral illness: (1) bronchitis, (2) bronchiolitis, and (3) pneumonia.
- Fungal infections are important in the differential diagnosis of pulmonary infections, particularly in immune compromised children and in healthy children exposed to pathogens in a particular geographic or environmental setting.
- Three forms of disease patterns in pneumocystosis are (1) childhood/adult, (2) infantile, and (3) chronic fibrosing observed in some human immunodeficiency virus-infected patients.
- Chemical pneumonitis and/or pneumonia may be acquired by (1) aspiration, (2) inhalation, (3) ingestion, or (4) injection.
- Pulmonary hemorrhage is a potentially life-threatening event that can occur at any age. Clinical presentation varies from massive fatal hemoptysis to silent bleeding with respiratory distress and anemia.

Pneumonitis, or inflammation of the lung parenchyma, is perhaps the most common cause of life-threatening lower respiratory tract disease in pediatric patients. Although pneumonitis may result from noninfectious processes (Box 42–1), most pediatric pulmonary parenchymal disease is secondary to an infectious agent. Pneumonitis may involve the pleura, interstitium, and airways; *pneumonia* by definition must include alveolar consolidation. Whereas early parenchymal lung injury is associated with increased cellularity with minimal fibrosis, advanced disease is characterized by extensive fibrosis and destruction of gas exchange units. Physiologic changes may include the following: low lung volumes, diminished lung compliance, impaired gas exchange, and airflow limitation. This chapter addresses the principal potential causes of pediatric pulmonary parenchymal disease, including alveolar and interstitial disorders.

Pathogenesis

Regardless of the cause, pneumonitis often follows a common pathogenesis. The initial parenchymal injury can result from mechanisms that directly damage the

BOX 42–1

Etiology of Pediatric Interstitial Lung Disease

- Infectious
  - Bacteria
  - Virus
  - Mycoplasma
  - Chlamydia
  - Rickettsia
  - Protozoa
  - Fungus
- Noninfectious
  - Acute lung injury
    - Chemical agents
    - Physical agents
  - Radiation
  - Drugs
  - Congenital lymphangiectasia
  - Metabolic disorders
  - Bronchopulmonary dysplasia
  - Hypersensitivity pneumonitis
  - Cardiovascular causes
  - Collagen/vascular disorders
  - Mixed connective tissue disorders
  - Idiopathic pulmonary fibrosis
  - Pulmonary hemorrhage syndromes
  - Pulmonary hemosiderosis
  - Pulmonary veno-occlusive disease
  - Desquamative interstitial pneumonia
  - Lymphocytic infiltrative disorders
    - Lymphocytic interstitial pneumonitis
    - Familial erythrophagocytic lymphohistiocytosis
    - Angioimmunoblastic lymphadenopathy
  - Sarcoidosis
  - Inherited diseases
  - Malignancy
    - Leukemia
    - Hodgkin disease
    - Non-Hodgkin lymphoma
  - Histiocytosis X

endothelium or epithelial cells. Other agents may injure the lung indirectly by one or more of the following:

1. Generation of toxic radicals
2. Recruitment of inflammatory cells (e.g., neutrophils)
3. Activation of complement and/or release of chemotactic factors

If these processes go unchecked, alterations may occur in the lung parenchyma and connective tissues leading to end-stage fibrosis. This is characterized by severe destruction of gas exchange units and airways and the development of parenchymal cystic lesions.

Pathophysiology

Changes in lung volumes in pulmonary parenchymal disease depend primarily on the intensity of the alveolitis and stage of the disease process. Acute severe pneumonitis with an intense alveolitis is characterized by moderate-to-severe reduction in both vital capacity (VC) and total lung capacity (TLC). It also is associated with a reduction in pulmonary compliance. In the early stages, patients with chronic interstitial diseases involving the lung parenchyma often have normal VC and TLC. There is subsequent reduction in lung volumes and pulmonary compliance as the disease progresses and pulmonary fibrosis ensues.[44] Expiratory flow rates usually are preserved in pneumonitis involving the lung parenchyma, and major obstructive defects, although reported, are rare. The carbon monoxide diffusing capacity (DLCO), one of the earliest and most sensitive tests of parenchymal inflammation, is diminished in interstitial lung disease (ILD). A reduction in DLCO is not specific and may be found with other parenchymal disorders. In early parenchymal disease, resting arterial oxygen tension may be normal, but there is often mild alveolar hyperventilation with reduction in alveolar carbon dioxide tension and widening of the alveolar-arterial oxygen gradients ($PAO_2 - PaO_2$). With exercise, hypoxemia and an increased $PAO_2 - PaO_2$ become exaggerated because of ventilation/perfusion (V/Q) imbalance. V/Q mismatch is attributed to regional alterations of flow, altered parenchymal compliance, and increased obstruction to pulmonary airflow. Progressive alveolitis and subsequent derangement of gas exchange lead to deterioration of ventilatory efficiency and markedly increased work of breathing. Adequate oxygenation may become impossible even with the use of high-flow supplemental oxygen. Resting hypercapnia, pulmonary hypertension, and eventual right ventricular dysfunction with heart failure are common sequelae.[128,132,179]

Diagnosis

The diagnosis of parenchymal lung disease in the pediatric patient may be quite challenging because of extreme variability in the presentation of disease. Clinical evaluation of the child should include a search for symptoms and signs associated with pulmonary disease, such as difficulty with feeding, exercise intolerance, chest pain, cough, tachypnea, dyspnea, cyanosis, orthopnea, clubbing of the nail beds, weight loss, and lethargy. In the child with diffuse alveolar disease, auscultative findings may be normal unless significant consolidation or small airway involvement is present. Fine crackles that may be heard throughout the chest late in inspiration are a characteristic finding of small airway disease. These rales are produced by the opening of occluded small peripheral airways.

Laboratory Diagnosis

The chest radiograph is critical in the diagnosis and management of pulmonary parenchymal disease. In children with ILD the radiographic features classically present in adults may be absent. Computed tomographic scan,[59,64,138] gallium lung scanning, and bronchoalveolar lavage (BAL)[8,31,47] are useful techniques in the diagnosis and management of diseases involving the lung parenchyma. Pulmonary function testing is important and usually can be performed reliably in children older than 4 years.[28,44]

Bacterial Pneumonitis

Bacterial infections of the lower respiratory tract continue to account for a significant number of hospital admissions. The frequency of bacteria as etiologic agents of lower respiratory tract infection varies from 10% to 50%, depending upon the study population and the methods of evaluation used.[109,137] In a large study of pediatric patients with lower respiratory tract infection, an etiologic agent was identified in nearly 50% of the patients. Bacteria accounted for 10% to 15% of the causative agents identified.

Factors predisposing to bacterial pneumonia include increased number of siblings, parental smoking, preterm delivery, urban residence, and poor socioeconomic status. Hospitalization also increases risk because of the clustering of ill patients in confined areas, administration of immunosuppressive therapy, and various medical and surgical interventions that enhance colonization and infection. Additional factors that increase susceptibility to bacterial pneumonia include airway foreign body,[108] impaired immune response,[35,87,101,164,209] congenital and anatomical lung defects, abnormalities of the tracheobronchial tree, cystic fibrosis,[211] and congestive heart failure.

Definition

Bacterial pneumonia is an inflammatory process of the lungs that may involve interstitial tissue and pleura in its evolution but always progresses to alveolar consolidation.

Pathophysiology

Pneumonia occurs when pulmonary defense mechanisms are disrupted and bacteria invade the respiratory system by aspiration or hematogenous spread. In most instances pneumonia appears to be a consequence of aspiration of a high inoculum of pathogenic bacteria. Viruses are often responsible for enhancing the susceptibility of the respiratory tract to bacterial infection. Less frequently bacterial pneumonia may be the result of defects in host immunity because of young age, underlying immune dysfunction, or immunosuppressive therapy. Pneumonia also may occur when host defenses are mechanically disrupted because of tracheostomy or endotracheal intubation. The presence of respiratory pathogens in the terminal bronchioles and alveoli induces an outpouring of edema fluid and large numbers of leukocytes into the alveoli.[73,128] Macrophages subsequently remove cellular and bacterial debris. The infectious process may extend further within the lung segment, or it may disseminate through infected bronchial fluid to other areas of the lung. The pulmonary lymphatic system enables bacteria to reach the bloodstream or visceral pleura.

With consolidation of lung tissue, VC and lung compliance markedly decrease, and intrapulmonary right-to-left shunt and V/Q mismatch occur, resulting in hypoxia. Subsequently, pulmonary hypertension may occur because of significant oxygen desaturation and hypercapnia, often leading to cardiac overload.

Clinical Features

Signs and symptoms of bacterial pneumonia vary with the individual pathogen, age and immunologic condition of the patient, and severity of the illness. Clinical manifestations, especially in newborns and infants, may be absent. General or nonspecific complaints include fever, chills, headache, irritability, and restlessness. Individual patients may have gastrointestinal complaints including nausea, vomiting, diarrhea, abdominal distension, or pain. Specific pulmonary signs include nasal flaring, retractions, tachypnea, dyspnea, and occasionally apnea.

Tachypnea is the most sensitive index of disease severity. The sleeping respiratory rate is often a valuable guide to diagnosis. On auscultation, diminished breath sounds are frequently noted. Fine crackles that may be heard in children and older patients are commonly absent in infants. Because of the relatively small size of the child's thorax and the thin chest wall, broad transmission of the breath sounds occurs, and the classic findings of consolidation are often obscured. Pleural inflammation may be accompanied by chest pain at the site of inflammation. This pleuritic pain may cause "splinting" restricting chest wall movement during inspiration and reducing lung volume.

Extrapulmonary infections that may be present in some children include abscesses of the skin or soft tissue *(Staphylococcus aureus);* conjunctivitis, sinusitis, otitis media, and meningitis (*Streptococcus pneumoniae* or *Haemophilus influenzae*); and epiglottitis *(H. influenzae)*.

Radiographic Features

Bacterial pneumonia is typically characterized by defined areas of consolidation with either segmental or lobar involvement. Lobar consolidation is the most characteristic, but multilobed disease is not unusual. The findings of pleural effusion, pneumatocele, or abscess are also strongly indicative of a bacterial infection. Staphylococcal pneumonia is suggested by rapid clinical and radiographic progression of disease, particularly in a young infant. Evidence of an abscess or pneumatocele further suggests a diagnosis of staphylococcal or gram-negative pneumonia such as *Klebsiella*. Group A streptococcal pneumonia may initially present with a diffuse interstitial pattern prior to the development of consolidation. Except for *Pseudomonas,* which may have a diffuse nodular appearance in the lower lobes, pneumonias caused by gram-negative organisms have no specific radiographic pattern. Anaerobic pulmonary infection is also associated with lung abscesses or air fluid levels.

Diagnosis

Bacterial pneumonia is suggested by fever, leukocytosis (>15,000 white blood cells), and increased band forms on the peripheral blood smear. Examination of the sputum may be helpful in establishing the diagnosis of bacterial pneumonia; however, it often is difficult to obtain a satisfactory sputum sample in pediatric patients unless transtracheal aspiration or bronchoscopy is used. Transtracheal aspiration, although useful in adolescents and adults, is associated with significant complications in infants and young children. If a sputum sample is obtained (an adequate specimen must have >25 polymorphonuclear cells and <25 epithelial cells per high-power field), the Gram stain should be examined for a predominant bacterial pathogen, and cultures should be done with the appropriate antibiotic susceptibility studies. Counterimmune electrophoresis (CIE) performed on sputum specimens has proved helpful in establishing the diagnosis in both adults and children. Bacterial pneumonia is accompanied by bacteremia in a significant number of cases; hence blood cultures should be obtained prior to initiation of antibiotic therapy. Circulating antigens in *S. pneumoniae* and *H. influenzae* may be detected in the blood with CIE,[51] polymerase chain reaction,[102,124,125] or latex agglutination.[37,176]

If a significant pleural effusion is present, a diagnostic thoracentesis should be performed for the purposes of Gram stain and culture. Culturing pleural fluid has a relatively high yield in patients who have not received previous antibiotic therapy. If the Gram stain of pleural fluid is negative, CIE or latex agglutination should be performed because bacterial antigen may be detected in the fluid even after the initiation of antibiotics.

Bronchoalveolar lavage should be considered in the management of a severely ill child in order to make a prompt diagnosis.[31,47] This is essential for progressive disease that has responded poorly to initial therapy or for the child with underlying immunodeficiency for whom empirical antibiotic treatment may be hazardous. In such instances, if the BAL is nondiagnostic, then lung aspiration or biopsy should be considered.[158] Material may be obtained through closed-needle biopsy, percutaneous needle aspiration, or open lung biopsy. Positive results for such procedures in carefully selected cases identify an etiologic agent in 30% to 75% of cases, with open lung biopsy having the highest yield.[53,164]

Specific Pathogens

Group B Streptococci

Group B streptococci can cause infection in people of any age; however, these organisms are common pathogens in infants younger than 3 months.[159] Early-onset illness is often associated with maternal fever at the time of delivery, prolonged rupture of membranes, amnionitis, prematurity, and low birth weight.

Infected neonates usually manifest clinical symptoms within the first 6 to 12 hours of life. Symptoms include fever, respiratory distress, apnea, tachypnea, and hypoxemia. By 12 to 24 hours of age, signs of cardiovascular collapse are often apparent. Frequently, the syndrome of pulmonary hypertension of the newborn is present, and pulmonary or intracranial hemorrhage may become the terminal event.

Isolation of the organism establishes the diagnosis. Cultures from blood and cerebrospinal fluids must be obtained in all instances of suspected group B streptococcal pneumonia. Rapid diagnostic techniques have been helpful in providing early diagnoses. The radiographic findings in neonates with group B streptococcal pneumonia can be either a lobar (40%) or a diffuse reticulonodular pattern with bronchograms similar to findings of respiratory distress syndrome.

Aggressive cardiovascular and ventilatory support is usually required, particularly in the early stages of disease. Antibiotic therapy should include a combination of ampicillin or penicillin and an aminoglycoside.

Although in the past the mortality seen with group B streptococcal pneumonia could be as high as 50% to 60%, recent studies suggest improvement with prompt initiation of therapy and even better outcomes with maternal prophylaxis.[178] Some infants experience a second episode of infection 1 to 2 weeks after discontinuation of antibiotic therapy. Infants with group B streptococcal pneumonia and meningeal involvement (30%) may demonstrate significant neurologic deficits (20% to 50%).

Streptococcus Pneumoniae

Streptococcus pneumoniae is a gram-positive diplococcus with at least 84 sera types; however, 80% of the serious infections are caused by only 12 sera types. Streptococci are a major cause of pneumonia in the United States. Victims are usually infants younger than 2 years with a peak age between 3 and 5 months. Patients with asplenia, functional hyposplenia, or malignancy or those receiving immunosuppressive drugs are at special risk of developing invasive disease.[130]

The radiographic finding in infants often is a patchy bronchopneumonia. Lobar consolidation is not uncommon. Penicillin is the drug of choice in the treatment of streptococcal pneumonia. However, organisms relatively resistant to penicillin occur in 3% to 40% of culture-positive patients recorded in studies from different parts of the United States.[160] In such instances, pneumonias have been effectively treated with vancomycin or high-dose β-lactam cephalosporins such as cefuroxime, ceftriaxone, or cefotaxime. Disease resulting from penicillin-resistant pneumococci should be considered in patients who received therapy with β-lactam antibiotics.[114,189]

The heptavalent pneumococcal conjugate vaccine (PCV) is recommended for all children age 2 to 23 months. It also is recommended for certain children age 24 to 59 months. Pneumococcal polysaccharide vaccine is recommended in addition to PCV for certain high-risk groups.[94]

Haemophilus Influenzae

Haemophilus organisms are small, nonmotile, gram-negative rods that occur in both encapsulated and nonencapsulated forms. Approximately 90% to 95% of invasive disease is caused by the encapsulated sera type B. A pleural effusion or empyema is detected in nearly 40% of patients with *H. influenzae* pneumonia. There is an extremely high incidence of bacteremia in this disease.

Serious complications such as epiglottitis, meningitis, and pericarditis can be diagnosed in 15% to 20% of patients. Cellulitis, anemia, and septic arthritis occur infrequently.

In a hospitalized patient, administration of the combination of ampicillin and chloramphenicol or a single cephalosporin such as cefuroxime, cefotaxime, or ceftriaxone is effective therapy.[76,160] Mortality in appropriately treated patients is generally considered less than 5% and often is related to associated meningitis, epiglottitis, or pericarditis rather than the pneumonic process itself. Hib conjugate vaccine is an important measure in reducing the incidence of *Haemophilus*-related disease and should be administered to all children.[56,160,183]

Staphylococcal Pneumonia

Primary *Staphylococcus aureus* pneumonia has decreased in frequency over recent years but still accounts for approximately 25% of cases in young infants. The incidence of secondary or metastatic dissemination has increased since 1972. Patients with primary pneumonia present with fever and respiratory symptoms, whereas those with metastatic disease often present with fever, generalized toxicity, and musculoskeletal symptoms. There is often a preceding upper respiratory tract infection in patients presenting with primary staphylococcal pneumonia.[19,225] Pleural effusion or empyema develops in nearly 80% of the patients with primary staphylococcal pneumonia and is extremely common in patients with metastatic disease. It is not unusual for patients with staphylococcal pneumonia to remain bacteremic long after the initiation of appropriate antibiotic therapy.

Radiographic findings of *S. aureus* pneumonia differ according to the stage of disease. They vary from minimal changes to consolidation (most common) and are associated with pleural effusion (50%–60%) or pneumothorax (21%). Pneumatoceles usually appear during the convalescent stage and may persist for prolonged periods in asymptomatic patients. Antibiotic therapy should be administered intravenously and include a drug resistant to inactivation. Strong consideration should be given to providing antibiotic coverage for methicillin-resistant *S. aureus*, which can account for 1% to 30% of isolates, depending on the prevalence in the area.[97] The duration of therapy usually is lengthier in staphylococcal disease than for other bacterial pneumonias consisting of 21 days or more. Mortality of staphylococcal pneumonia varies from 23% to 33%. Increased mortality usually is associated with younger age, inappropriate initial antimicrobial therapy, or failure to drain an empyema appropriately.

Mycoplasma Pneumonia

Mycoplasma organisms are the smallest free-living microorganisms. They lack a cell wall and are pleomorphic. Mycoplasma is an uncommon cause of pneumonia in children younger than 5 years but is the leading cause of pneumonia in school-age children and young adults. Illness can range from a mild upper respiratory tract infection to tracheobronchitis to pneumonia. Symptoms include malaise, low-grade fevers, and headache. Ten percent of children develop a rash, usually maculopapular. Cough, if it develops, usually occurs within a few days and may continue 3 to 4 weeks. The cough is initially nonproductive but then may become productive and usually is associated with widespread rales on physical examination. Roentgenographic abnormalities vary but usually are bilateral and diffuse.[160]

Isolation of *Mycoplasma* by culture is complicated by the requirement for special enriched broth or agar media, which are not widely available, and is successful in only 40% to 90% of cases requiring 7 to 21 days. A fourfold increase in antibody titer between acute and convalescent sera is diagnostic but lengthy, providing only a retrospective diagnosis. Complement fixation and immunofluorescent and several enzyme immunoassay antibody tests have been developed but have been of limited diagnostic value.[160] Serum cold agglutinins with titers of 1:32 or greater are present in more than 50% of patients with pneumonia by the beginning of the second week of illness. A polymerase chain reaction (PCR) test has been developed but is not widely available. Where available, PCR has become an important means of diagnosing *M. pneumoniae* infections in clinical practice and allows for institution of therapy directed at the causative pathogen.[163] Treatment of upper respiratory tract infections or acute bronchitis is rarely indicated, but treatment with erythromycin or another macrolide such as azithromycin is indicated for pneumonia or otitis media.

Miscellaneous Etiologic Agents

Pneumonia resulting from group A streptococcus accounts for less than 1% of all bacterial pneumonias. This disease is found in older children (median age 5–6 years), and nearly all patients are bacteremic and toxic at the time of diagnosis. Associated findings may include anemia, hyponatremia, and respiratory distress often accompanied by pleural effusion or empyema. There is often a positive history of a preceding viral infection.

Gram-Negative Bacteria

Pneumonia caused by gram-negative enteric bacteria, especially *Pseudomonas*, almost always is found in patients with underlying pulmonary disease, compromised immune status, or those receiving prolonged respiratory therapy.[32,49] It is a frequent cause of nosocomial infection in critical care units. These organisms can produce a severe necrotizing pneumonia that is associated with an increase in morbidity.[92]

Legionella Pneumophila

Pneumonia secondary to *Legionella pneumophila* has been reported infrequently in the pediatric age group.[21,30,66,142] The onset of this disease is characterized by high unremitting fever, chills, and a nonproductive cough.[30] Extrapulmonary manifestations include gastrointestinal symptoms such as diarrhea, liver involvement, and confusion.

Chest radiographs typically consist of peripheral nodular infiltrates and pleural effusions. Cavitation occurs only in immunosuppressed individuals. Death in the normal host is unusual if prompt therapy with azithromycin or erythromycin is initiated.

Anaerobic Bacteria

Pneumonia secondary to anaerobic upper respiratory flora is uncommon in healthy children. When it does occur, it is frequently associated with risk factors such as underlying pulmonary disease, central nervous system disorder including seizures, postanesthetic state, and aspiration of a foreign body. Lung abscess and empyema are frequent complications in anaerobic bacterial pneumonias.

Complications

The mortality in uncomplicated bacterial pneumonia is less than 1%. Death is more common in children with complicated disease or an underlying disorder. The most frequent complications of bacterial pneumonia are pleural effusion and empyema (Table 42–1). Thoracentesis should always be performed if fluid is present in order to facilitate an etiologic diagnosis and to establish the character of the fluid. Tube thoracostomy is indicated if a large amount of fluid is present and is producing respiratory compromise or if purulent fluid is obtained by thoracentesis. Empyema may extend locally to involve pericardium, mediastinum, or chest wall. Evidence of empyema extension should be considered in the child unresponsive to antibiotic therapy.[158]

TABLE 42–1

Major Sequelae/Life-Threatening Complications Associated with Bacterial Infections

Complication/Sequelae	Organism
Necrotizing pneumonia	Anaerobic, GNB
Respiratory failure	GBS
Shock	GBS, SP, H. flu, GNB
Apnea	GBS
Pneumothorax	H. flu
Pneumatoceles	H. flu. Anaerobic, Staph, SP, GAS
Abscess (lung)	Staph, SP, anaerobic
Pleural effusion	H. flu, GAS, SP, Staph
Empyema	H. flu, Staph, SP
Epiglottitis	H. flu, GAS
Meningitis	H. flu, GBS, SP
Encephalopathy	Legionella
Pericarditis	H. flu
Bone/joint	H. flu, Staph
Kidneys	Staph

GAS, Group A streptococcus; *GBS*, group B streptococcus; *GNB*, gram-negative bacteria; *H. flu, Haemophilus influenzae*; *SP, Streptococcus pneumoniae*; *Staph, Staphylococcus aureus*.

When tube thoracostomy/surgical drainage is required, it should be discontinued as soon as drainage has substantially decreased. For patients with staphylococcal empyema, streptococcal pneumonia, or *H. influenzae* empyema, 3 to 7 days of drainage usually is sufficient. Patients with empyema require prolonged antimicrobial therapy and careful follow-up.

Pneumothorax and pneumatoceles can be seen with almost any bacterial pneumonia but are especially common with staphylococcal disease.[19] Such pneumatoceles require no special therapy and usually resolve. Lung abscess is an infrequent complication of *H. influenzae* and pneumococcal pneumonia and is most often encountered with staphylococcal disease or anaerobic bacteria.

Prognosis usually is excellent even in severe bacterial pneumonia complicated by empyema. Long-term follow-up of children with empyema has demonstrated remarkably few, if any, residual pulmonary function abnormalities and remarkable clearing of chest roentgenograms. In contrast to adults with empyema, children seldom require surgical procedures such as decortication. However, follow-up chest radiographs should be obtained on all patients with bacterial pneumonia in order to document complete resolution. Such radiographic follow-up studies probably are not indicated until at least 6 to 8 weeks following the initiation of antibiotic therapy.

Therapy

Therapy for bacterial pneumonia should include appropriate intravenous antibiotic treatment directed toward the specific pathogen if known (Table 42–2). Localized or compartmental complications such as empyema, lung abscess, pericarditis, or septic joints require appropriate surgical drainage and antibiotic therapy. Prevention via immunization or chemoprophylaxis has changed the incidence and epidemiology of pneumonitides significantly. Options for immunization, active or passive, and chemoprophylaxis for various etiologic agents are listed in Table 42–3.

Viral Pneumonitis

Infection is the most common cause of pulmonary interstitial disease in children, and viral agents are the leading cause of lower respiratory tract infection in infants and children. The viral agents listed in Table 42–4 account for the greatest percentage of pediatric pulmonary disease. Nearly 85% of all hospitalizations of children younger than 15 years occur during outbreaks of parainfluenza, respiratory syncytial, or influenza virus.

The diagnosis of a viral pneumonia in children is frequently based on the clinical presentation, epidemiologic setting, and exclusion of bacterial pathogens by negative cultures. A specific agent is identified in only approximately 50% of cases of presumed viral pneumonia. Pediatric viral respiratory tract infections occur most commonly during the winter, with distinct peaks during midwinter and early spring. Closed population groups provide for greater spread of respiratory viruses and increased recognition of viral pneumonias.

TABLE 42–2

Bacterial Pneumonia Therapy

Disease/Organism	Therapy
UNDETERMINED ORGANISMS	
Serious, life-threatening pneumonia, nonsuppressed host	Cefotaxime or ceftriaxone + azithromycin
	Bronchial lavage or needle aspiration of lung may be necessary to establish diagnosis
Suppressed neutropenic host	Imipenem/meropenem
	Or
	Piperacillin or ceftazidime + aminoglycoside ± clindamycin
	Vancomycin not included in initial therapy unless high suspicion, ampho not used unless still febrile after 3 days/high suspicion. Bronchial lavage, needle/open biopsy may be necessary to establish diagnosis
Lung abscess	Clindamycin
	Or
	Ticarcillin/clavulanate
	Or
	Piperacillin/tazobactam
SPECIFIC ORGANISMS	
Pneumonia with empyema	
Streptococcus pneumoniae, group A strep	
Penicillin susceptible	Cefotaxime or ceftriaxone + chest tube drainage
Penicillin resistant	Vancomycin ± rifampin + chest tube drainage
Staphylococcus	
Methicillin sensitive	Nafcillin or oxacillin + chest tube drainage
Methicillin resistant	Vancomycin + chest tube drainage
Pneumonia without empyema	
Haemophilus influenzae	Ampicillin or cefotaxime or ceftriaxone + chloramphenicol
Klebsiella pneumonia	Cefotaxime or ceftriaxone
Escherichia coli, Enterobacter	Aminoglycoside or cephalosporin
Legionella	Azithromycin or erythromycin ± rifampin
Pseudomonas	Aminoglycoside + anti-*Pseudomonas* penicillin
	Or
	Aminoglycoside + ceftazidime
Mycoplasma pneumoniae	Erythromycin *or* azithromycin *or* Clarithromycin

Pathophysiology

The mechanism of infection for most respiratory viruses appears to be a progressive spread from the larger airways to the alveoli. The respiratory epithelial cell is the major target of cytopathic effect. The normal ciliated columnar epithelium may become markedly dysplastic with loss of the overlying cilia.[15] Areas of ulceration then occur as segments of the mucosal surface desquamate into the bronchial lumen. Impaired mucociliary clearance occurs and altered stimulation of nerves mediating bronchial smooth muscle tone leads to increased airway resistance. Enhanced mucus formation along with mucosal debris may lead to obstruction of the bronchioles, luminal narrowing, distal air trapping, and hyperinflation of various lung segments. In advanced disease with complete small airway obstruction, atelectasis results, causing hypoxemia as a result of intrapulmonary shunting and V/Q imbalance.

In severe viral pneumonia, widespread parenchymal injury caused by a necrotizing alveolitis may occur. Alveolar round cell infiltrates occur often, with subsequent hyaline membrane formation and intraalveolar hemorrhage, which produces extensive parenchymal destruction and diminished lung compliance, decreased lung volumes, and intrapulmonary shunting.[9]

Diagnosis

Although the clinical presentations of illness by respiratory viruses overlap, presumptive diagnosis of the specific etiology is based on clinical presentation; setting; and, most importantly, epidemiologic information. In the past, virus isolation or seroconversion was necessary for definitive diagnosis. Today many respiratory viral infections can be diagnosed using new techniques.

Viral specimens should be obtained as early as possible during the period of greatest viral excretion. Nasopharyngeal washings or swabs of the throat are most widely used. Cultures may be negative in up to 40% of patients during acute viral respiratory tract disease; failure to isolate a virus is not definitive evidence against the diagnosis of viral pneumonia. Serologic tests including complement

TABLE 42–3

Preventive Measures

Organism	Immunization	Chemoprophylaxis
Cytomegalovirus	IVIG: Prophylaxis in seronegative transplant patients	Ganciclovir or valganciclovir
Haemophilus influenzae type b	Capsular polysaccharide vaccine *Or* Conjugate vaccine	Rifampin in the face of incomplete immunization and exposure
Influenza	Inactivated virus produced in chicken embryos	Oseltamivir (A or B) *Or* Amantadine/rimantadine (A)
Measles	Live virus vaccine *Or* IVIG for immunocompromised patients	None
Streptococcus pneumonia	Purified capsular polysaccharide antigens of 23 pneumococcal serotypes vaccine *Or* Multivalent protein conjugate vaccine	Penicillin VK for functional or anatomic asplenia until age 5 years
Pneumocystis carinii	None	Trimethoprim-sulfamethoxazole *Or* Pentamidine *or* dapsone
RSV	RSV-IVIG *Or* Palivizumab (monoclonal antibody)	None
Group B Strep	None	Intrapartum antibiotics

IVIG, intravenous immuneglobulin; *RSV*, respiratory syncytial virus.

fixation, hemagglutination inhibition, enzyme-linked solid-phase assays (enzyme-linked immunosorbent assays), and antibody assays have been used in the diagnosis of viral infection. Histologic evidence of infection in biopsy or postmortem specimens may be helpful, particularly when intranuclear inclusions are documented. Rapid diagnostic techniques focus on detection of the virus or its components in the sample. These new techniques include refinements in the use of immunofluorescence, enzyme immunoassay (EIA), time-resolved fluoroimmunoassay, latex agglutination assays, and use of nucleic acid hybridization methods, such as deoxyribonucleic acid (DNA) probes and polymerase chain reaction.[40,191,199] Three major clinical syndromes are associated with lower respiratory tract viral illness:

1. Bronchitis: Acute bronchitis is a febrile illness associated with a new productive cough. Symptoms of upper respiratory tract infection may be present. Acute bronchitis can adversely affect respiratory function, particularly in patients with chronic pulmonary impairment, leading to hospitalization of individuals with marginal lung function.
2. Bronchiolitis: Symptoms result from airflow obstruction caused by localized inflammation of the terminal respiratory bronchioles. The development of cough; tachypnea with intercostal retractions; fine, moist, inspiratory crackles; and expiratory wheezes are characteristic. Hypoxemia and cyanosis are often present.[93]
3. Pneumonia: Primary viral pneumonia is frequently a mild illness characterized by a mild cough and one or more segmental infiltrates on chest radiograph. Usually a self-limited process in some individuals, the pneumonic process may progress with extensive parenchymal injury, diffuse interstitial alveolar infiltrates, and severe hypoxemia. Bacterial superinfection is heralded by increased temperature, change in sputum, and signs of localized consolidation several days after initial onset of symptoms.

Radiographic Findings

Differentiation of bacteria from viral pneumonia cannot be made solely on the radiographic appearance. Children with presumed viral pneumonia, however, may have several radiographic findings, including the following:

1. Peribronchial thickening and perihilar linear densities
2. Partial lobar or patchy involvement in multiple areas of lung

TABLE 42–4

Viral Agents Associated with Pediatric Interstitial Lung Disease

Agent	Frequency
Respiratory syncytial virus	+++++
Parainfluenza virus	++++
Adenovirus	+++
Influenza virus	+++
Cytomegalovirus	+
Enterovirus	+
Rhinovirus	+
Measles	+

3. Shifting regional infiltrates
4. Areas of hyperinflation and atelectasis

Hilar adenopathy is usually absent. Diffuse bilateral infiltrates similar to those reported in adult respiratory distress syndrome (ARDS) have been found in severe influenza and adenovirus pneumonias. Pleural effusions can occur in both adenovirus and parainfluenza pneumonias. Pulmonary calcifications/nodules have been described in the convalescent phase of varicella and measles.

Specific Pathogens

We will review the most common viral pathogens that cause pneumonitis in children but have elected to exclude such viruses as Hantavirus that are beyond the scope of this chapter. Please refer to more up-to-date journal articles for specific pathogens of interest (see also Chapter 88).[105,125]

Respiratory Syncytial Virus

Respiratory syncytial virus (RSV) is the most common cause of bronchiolitis and pneumonia in the United States in children between the ages of 6 months and 3 years. The disease produced by RSV varies from upper respiratory tract infection to severe bronchiolitis and pneumonia with wheezing and respiratory failure.[93] Higher mortality and greater severity with prolonged symptoms occur in infants and children with underlying cardiopulmonary disease, especially those with pulmonary hypertension and those receiving chemotherapy or immunosuppressive therapy.[78,87,166] Signs of RSV pneumonia include wheezing, dyspnea, pulmonary infiltrates, and areas of atelectasis and hyperinflation on the chest radiograph. Respiratory syncytial virus infection may result in increased airway reactivity and airway resistance that persists for months. Significant respiratory tract shedding of virus continues for up to 21 days from the onset of illness. Nosocomial spread of RSV infection is common, and early diagnosis and appropriate isolation techniques are critical in hospitalized patients.

Methods for diagnosis of RSV include viral isolation in cell culture, immunofluorescence of exfoliated nasopharyngeal epithelial cells for detection of RSV antigens, and EIA for detection of RSV antigens in nasal secretions.[6,17]

Polymerase chain reaction technology is now available for diagnosis of RSV illness. All hospitalized patients with bronchiolitis and RSV pneumonia should be monitored for hypoxia, hypercarbia, and need for ventilatory assistance. Supportive care includes the use of humidified oxygen. Mechanical ventilation for respiratory failure usually is well tolerated. Extracorporeal membrane oxygenation has been used successfully in infants not responding to conventional ventilation. Some studies have documented clinical improvement in some infants using bronchodilators. Use of steroids, although theoretically inviting to reduce the inflammatory response, has not proved efficacious.[139] Ribavirin, an antiviral agent, has been used in the treatment of children with severe RSV pneumonitis, but its clinical effectiveness remains controversial.[1,26,43,71,86,144,169,182] Passive immunoprophylaxis has proved useful in high-risk populations in preventing RSV infection, as has palivizumab, a humanized mouse monoclonal antibody.[160] The incidence of bacterial superinfection in RSV disease is low; therefore prophylactic antibiotics are not recommended for RSV disease. It is not unusual for an infant with RSV to require hospitalization for 7 to 10 days following the onset of illness. Nearly 20% of infants with RSV have a prolonged course, with symptoms lasting for several weeks. Long-term complications of RSV infection and bronchiolitis include asthma and chronic obstructive pulmonary disease. Results of pulmonary function testing conducted in children 10 years following bronchiolitis revealed evidence of small airway disease and increased bronchial reactivity.[123,161,184,214]

Parainfluenza Virus

Parainfluenza virus (types 1 and 2) is more often associated with laryngotracheobronchitis and croup than with pneumonia (usually type 3). Parainfluenza is second only to RSV as an etiology of lower respiratory tract disease responsible for hospitalization of children.[110,212,213] The pneumonia associated with parainfluenza usually is mild; however, fatal cases with prolonged viral shedding have been reported in severe combined immunodeficiency disease.[39,215] Repeat infection occurs in nearly 50% of patients by age 30 months, although they result in progressively milder illness. Parainfluenza virus, such as RSV, has demonstrated ability to elicit an immunoglobulin (Ig)E-specific antibody response.[89] Rapid identification of parainfluenza virus by either fluorescent or enzyme-linked immunologic techniques is possible, but results are variable depending upon viral type and antisera used.

Adenovirus

Adenoviruses are responsible for approximately 3% of the pneumonias occurring in children. Clinical features are similar to other viral pneumonias except that the onset of illness is often gradual, occurring over several days. Of the 38 serotypes, types 3, 4, and 7 are the most common causes of lower respiratory tract disease in children. Adenovirus type 7 is most commonly associated with severe pneumonitis in infants and children and has significant mortality and morbidity.[57,186,223,225] Massive pleural effusion, rhabdomyolysis, and myoglobinuria have been reported with adenovirus type 21. Many infants with documented adenovirus respiratory tract infection develop chronic pulmonary disease manifested as persistent atelectasis, bronchiectasis, and recurrent pneumonitis with areas of hyperinflation and interstitial fibrosis. Bronchiectasis and restrictive lung disease have been documented in children following acute adenovirus infection. Fatal cases of adenovirus and pneumonia can occur even in previously healthy young individuals. Disseminated adenovirus occurs and usually is associated with infection by serotype 3, 7, or 21. It occurs most frequently in infants younger than 18 months and usually involves the heart, pericardium, liver, pancreas, kidneys, central nervous system, and skin.[150] Treatment for adenoviral infection is supportive.

Influenza

Influenza is a common cause of acute ILD in children, especially during epidemic years. There are three antigenically distinct influenza viruses—types A, B, and C—with periodic antigenic drifts and shifts that allow for repeated epidemics.[29,46,79,185,208] Pathologically, influenza virus infection is similar to RSV in that the virus destroys ciliated respiratory epithelial cells with subsequent edema and an acute inflammatory response.

Influenza infection is often associated with myalgia, encephalopathy, and cardiac involvement. Children with influenza typically have a more sudden onset of "toxic" signs than those with other viral diseases. Influenza has been associated with Reye syndrome and with significant bacterial suprainfections.[16]

Prevention of influenza disease is possible with either administration of influenza vaccine or recently developed oseltamivir (influenza A and B) or amantadine hydrochloride and its closely related analogue rimantadine (influenza A). One study showed efficacy of aerosolized ribavirin in the treatment of influenza B.[115,116] Clinical signs of uncomplicated influenza pneumonia include coryzal symptoms followed by dyspnea, fever, cyanosis, and wheezing. In patients who develop bacterial infection there often is a period of apparent improvement before a sudden worsening that is heralded by the production of purulent sputum, return of fever, and development of pulmonary consolidation.[180] Diagnosis of influenza pneumonia may be made by culture of the virus from respiratory secretions or by serologic techniques. Rapid diagnosis by using immunofluorescence of exfoliated nasopharyngeal cells may be helpful.

Measles

The prevalence of measles pneumonia is difficult to determine accurately because respiratory symptoms are nearly universal in this illness. In cases where radiographs have been obtained, a fine reticular infiltrate was present, as compared with the nodular infiltrates in children with atypical measles. Most children develop moist crackles, and approximately 20% have expiratory wheezes and hypoxia. Although the clinical syndrome usually resolves over 1 to 2 weeks, both radiographic and pulmonary function abnormalities may persist for months. Severe life-threatening tracheitis may occur during the course of measles or bacterial suprainfection.[81,147,154]

Human Immunodeficiency Virus

Human immunodeficiency virus (HIV) infection in children most commonly presents with recurrent bacterial infections. The major morbidity and mortality in pediatric acquired immune deficiency syndrome (AIDS) are associated with lung disease, ranging from opportunistic infections such as *Pneumocystis carinii* pneumonia to entities such as chronic interstitial pneumonitis.[172,200] Treatment for specific pulmonary pathogens are discussed throughout this chapter, but specific guidelines for HIV/AIDS treatment are lengthy, rapidly changing, and beyond the scope of this chapter. More specific and current information regarding HIV/AIDS are available at *www.aidsinfo.nih.gov/guidelines.* This website provides easy access to the latest information regarding HIV/AIDS clinical research, HIV treatment and prevention, and medical practice guidelines. This information can also be obtained by phone 1-800-HIV-0440 within the United States or 1-301-519-0459 outside the United States or by mail at AIDS Info, P.O. Box 6303, Rockville, MD 20849-6303.

Complications

The actual mechanisms by which viruses predispose the lung to secondary bacterial infection are not precisely understood. Viruses are capable of altering both cellular and noncellular defenses of the respiratory tract. Viral infection of the epithelial cells appears to predispose the upper respiratory tract mucosa to bacterial colonization by allowing bacterial pathogens to adhere to injured cells.[15] Viral infection may cause significant impairment of both intracellular killing and ingestion of bacteria by the pulmonary macrophage. Significant defects in polymorphonuclear leukocyte chemotaxis and phagolysosome fusion occur during acute viral infection. The greatest impairment of macrophage function occurs 1 week after onset of viral infection, which correlates with the peak incidence of bacterial suprainfection. Thus suprainfection during the course of viral lower respiratory tract disease appears to be the result of a combination of the cytopathic effects of the virus on the respiratory mucosa and various alterations in host immune response.

Significant life-threatening complications of viral lower respiratory tract disease are noted in Box 42–2. Respiratory failure with viral pneumonitis resembling ARDS is frequently seen in the pediatric critical care unit. It is often associated with influenza or adenovirus but can occur with varicella or cytomegalovirus (CMV).

A number of techniques are available for establishing viral diagnosis. In the critical care setting, the decision to undertake these diagnostic measures should be guided by how awareness of the specific viral illness will affect the clinical management. Potential benefits include (1) a guide to selection of appropriate antiviral therapy and avoidance of unnecessary treatments with antibiotics and (2) initiation of appropriate infection control measures and use of vaccine or drug prophylaxis.

Direct isolation of viruses is a sensitive method of diagnosis early in the course of disease when a large number of infectious particles are present in respiratory secretions. Nasopharyngeal washings are the preferred specimens for viral cultures because large quantities of secretions for culture are easily available. Unfortunately, viral isolation may require up to 2 weeks for positive culture results. The more commonly used methods for viral diagnosis involve detection of viral antigens present in the respiratory secretions. These antigen-detection techniques using radioimmune or enzyme-linked assays can detect all riboviruses and adenoviruses that commonly produce lower respiratory tract infections. Antibody detection has also been successfully used in the diagnosis of lower respiratory tract viral disease (CMV pneumonia).[188] A major advantage of tests capable of detecting viral

BOX 42-2

Major Sequelae/Life-Threatening Complications Associated with Viral Pneumonitis

Subacute sclerosing panencephalitis: Measles
Guillain-Barré syndrome: Influenza, varicella
Reye syndrome: Influenza, varicella-zoster virus (VZV)
Encephalitis: Adenovirus, measles, RSV, CMV
Seizures: Influenza
Bacterial superinfection: Influenza, VZV, Epstein-Barr (EBV), measles
Asthma: RSV, parainfluenza, rhinovirus
Apnea: RSV, influenza
Bronchiolitis obliterans: Influenza, adenovirus, measles
Chronic obstructive pulmonary disease: RSV
Fatal pneumonitis: Influenza, measles, adenovirus, RSV, parainfluenza, CMV
Tracheitis, life-threatening: Measles, parainfluenza
Appendicitis: Adenovirus, measles
Intussusception: Adenovirus, CMV
Hepatitis: Adenovirus, influenza measles, CMV
Nephritis: Adenovirus, influenza, measles
Myocarditis: Adenovirus, influenza, measles
Pericarditis: Adenovirus, influenza, measles
Arthritis: Adenovirus
Deafness: Adenovirus
Keratoconjunctivitis: Adenovirus
Myositis: Influenza
Stevens-Johnson syndrome: Measles
Coagulopathy: Measles
Thrombocytopenia: Measles, CMV

CMV = cytomegalovirus; RSV = respiratory syncytial virus.

components is that these studies can be performed rapidly with results made available to the critical care physician in hours, therefore allowing timely management.

Serologic testing is a slower but much less expensive method of viral diagnosis. Serologic testing or diagnosis depends upon demonstrating a rising IgG antibody titer between acute and convalescent sera. Although serologic data may provide a diagnosis, they are of little value in guiding therapeutic critical care interventions.

Prevention

Vaccination

Influenza vaccine is directed at the currently circulating antigenic types of influenza A and B strains. Because of antigenic drift, it is necessary to revaccinate on a yearly basis. The Centers for Disease Control recommends influenza vaccine administration for groups at special risk for complications of influenza such as children with chronic cardiac, pulmonary, or metabolic disorders and health care workers capable of nosocomial spread to high-risk patient groups. Palivizumab is a monoclonal antibody vaccine directed against RSV. Current recommendations are to administer this vaccine to high-risk infants during the RSV season.[160] Passive immunization is also available for some viruses that can be associated with pneumonitis (see Table 42–3 for further details).

Chemoprophylaxis

Amantadine, rimantadine, and oseltamivir are approved for prophylaxis of viral respiratory tract infection caused by influenza. Amantadine and rimantadine have been shown to be effective prophylaxis for influenza A; however, they are not active against influenza B. Oseltamivir, unlike amantadine and rimantadine, has activity against both influenza A and B. All three drugs are recommended for individuals at high risk for serious influenza infection who have not been vaccinated or who have received the vaccine within 2 weeks of the onset of an epidemic. They are also recommended for those who may not develop appropriate immune response following vaccination and for individuals who cannot receive the influenza vaccine because of allergic reactions.[201,219] Zanamivir also has activity against influenza A and B but is not yet approved for use as a prophylactic agent.[104]

Therapy

A number of antiviral agents inhibit the replication of respiratory viruses in vitro, and some of these drugs have been used clinically in both experimental and naturally occurring respiratory infections (Table 42–5). In varicella or zoster, acyclovir reduces the period of viral shedding and the time needed to heal skin lesions, and it can prevent dissemination of localized zoster in immunocompromised children. Thus the use of acyclovir in immunosuppressed patients can be justified by the low toxicity of the drug and the potential severity of the illness. Amantadine hydrochloride can be used to treat influenza A virus infections. Numerous studies have demonstrated that amantadine shortens the course of illness in uncomplicated influenza infections in otherwise healthy children if initiated within the first 48 hours of the disease. Amantadine is not effective against influenza B. Oseltamivir and zanamivir both are effective against influenza A and B and have been shown to reduce the severity and duration of illness.[91,202] Rimantadine has not been approved for therapeutic use in children.

Ganciclovir (DHPG) is an antiviral drug with significant activity against CMV.[84] It has been used successfully in immunocompromised patients with disseminated CMV and pneumonia.[181] Symptomatic infection of the lower airway with herpes viruses is rare. When it occurs it usually does so in an immunosuppressed child. Antiviral therapy for herpes viruses include acyclovir, foscarnet, and adenine arabinoside.[203] Ribavirin is a synthetic nucleoside analogue licensed for use in aerosol form for treatment of severe RSV infection. This therapy may shorten the course of the illness and improve oxygenation in high-risk patients. A few children with severe combined immune deficiency have been treated with ribavirin with resulting clinical improvement and decrease in viral shedding. Ribavirin aerosol may be effective in shortening the course of both influenza A and B in infections in college students, and it is possible that parainfluenza and measles virus can be treated with ribavirin.[194] Various case reports

TABLE 42–5

Antiviral Agents Used in Viral Pneumonia

Agent	Indication	Route	Side Effects
Acyclovir	HSV, varicella Prophylaxis/treatment	IV, PO	Phlebitis, seizures, leukopenia, renal dysfunction
Valacyclovir renal	HSV, varicella Prophylaxis/treatment	PO	Bone marrow suppression, renal failure
Ganciclovir	CMV in immunocompromised host Prophylaxis/treatment	IV, PO	Renal failure, bone marrow suppression, seizure
Valganciclovir	CMV prophylaxis	PO	Same as ganciclovir
Amantadine	Influenza A Prophylaxis/treatment	PO	Nausea, dizziness, ataxia, diarrhea
Rimantadine	Influenza A Prophylaxis	PO	Similar to amantadine
Zanamivir	Influenza A and B Treatment, prophylaxis under study	Diskhaler	Bronchospasm
Oseltamivir	Influenza A and B Prophylaxis/treatment	PO	Nausea, vomiting, vertigo
RSV-IVIG	RSV prophylaxis (high-risk population)	IV	Allergic, fluid overload, not approved for CCHD
Palivizumab	RSV prophylaxis	IM	Anaphylaxis
Ribavirin	RSV (?parainfluenza, influenza A and B, measles)	Small particle aerosol	Conjunctival edema
Foscarnet	CMV retinitis, HSV resistant to acyclovir	IV	Renal dysfunction, nausea, bone marrow suppression
Pleconaril (under investigation)	Enterovirus and rhinovirus Prophylaxis/treatment	PO	Under investigation

CCHD, cyanotic congenital heart disease; *CMV*, cytomegalovirus; *HSV*, herpes simplex virus; *RSV*, respiratory syncytial virus.

of treatment in seriously ill adults with complicated viral infections suggest that ribavirin may be effective treatment. Overall, the documented therapeutic benefit of antiviral agents has been inconclusive. Improvement is most apparent when the therapy was initiated early after the onset of infection. Future investigations are necessary to define the optimum dose/route of antiviral agents for each respiratory virus/pneumonia and to clarify the ability of antiviral therapy to modify serious lower respiratory tract infection in high-risk infants and children.

Fungal Pneumonitis

Fungal infections are becoming increasingly important in the differential diagnosis of pulmonary infections, particularly in immunocompromised hosts. The majority of pulmonary mycotic infections occur in two microbiologic and clinical groups (Box 42–3). In general, different patient groups are at risk for infection because of either opportunistic or pathogenic dimorphic pulmonary fungi. Primary pulmonary mycotic infections generally infect healthy children exposed to the pathogen in a particular geographic or environmental setting, whereas the opportunistic mycoses occur in immune compromised

BOX 42–3

Major Pulmonary Mycoses

PRIMARY (ENDEMIC; PATHOGENIC TO NORMAL CHILDREN)

Dimorphic Soil

- Histoplasmosis
- Blastomycosis
- Coccidioidomycosis
- Paracoccidioidomycosis
- Sporotrichosis

Nondimorphic Soil

- Cryptococcosis

OPPORTUNISTIC (UBIQUITOUS; ABNORMAL HOST)

- Aspergillosis
- Mucormycosis
- Candidiasis

children.[13,38,196] The increase in opportunistic fungal infections can be attributed to numerous factors, including the following:

1. Selection of fungal organisms as flora by the use of broad-spectrum antibiotics
2. Leukopenia secondary to cytotoxic agents
3. Suppression of humoral and cell-mediated immunity by cytotoxic and suppressive therapy
4. Increased use of immune suppressive drugs in patients with organ transplant or collagen vascular disease
5. Increasing number of patients with AIDS
6. Increased number of invasive surgical procedures in hospitalized children, which create portals of entry for fungi[209]

Primary Pulmonary Fungi

Fungi that cause primary pulmonary infection in otherwise healthy hosts are generally endemic mycoses found in a particular geographic distribution. The four major mycoses in this group are histoplasmosis, blastomycosis, coccidiomycosis, and paracoccidiomycosis.[35,168] Chemiluminescent DNA probes are available for identification of blastomycosis, coccidioidomycosis, and histoplasmosis. We review these primary pulmonary mycoses in the following section but exclude paracoccidiomycosis because this infection occurs primarily in South America, Central America, and Mexico. For information regarding paracoccidiomycosis infections please refer to up-to-date journal articles.[197]

Pathogenesis

The dimorphic fungi cause infection following inhalation of spores (conidia) into the pulmonary system. In the lower respiratory tract the conidia transform into the yeast phase, which is susceptible to phagocytosis by the pulmonary macrophages. These yeast forms may persist in the nonimmune host. As the yeast-laden macrophages are transported via the lymphatics to the peribronchial and mediastinal lymph nodes, hematogenous dissemination may occur. However, with the primary pulmonary infection in the immunocompetent host, extrapulmonary infection is rare.

Progressive primary pulmonary infection in the absence of host defenses (immune compromised, infant) may lead to seeding of extrapulmonary sites, dissemination, and death if left untreated. Cellular immunity is the primary host defense against these deep mycoses, many of which are subclinical and require no therapy. However, children with severe, life-threatening infections should be treated (Table 42–6).

TABLE 42–6

Antifungal Therapy

Drug	Indications	Route	Side Effects
Amphotericin B (AmB)	All life-threatening mycosis, empirical therapy in febrile granulocytopenic patients	IV	Fever, chills, nephrotoxicity, anemia, hypokalemia, thrombophlebitis
Ampho B lipid complex	Failure or intolerance to AmB, organ transplant with renal insufficiency	IV	Same as AmB with decreased nephrotoxicity and infusion-related adverse events
Ampho B cholesteryl sulfate			
Ampho B liposomal			
Flucytosine (5-FC)	With AmB for life-threatening infections with *Cryptococcus, Candida* (central nervous system, ophthalmitis, disseminated, renal) or invasive disease refractory to AmB	PO	Neutropenia with elevated serum levels (if levels are not available this agent should not be used)
Ketoconazole	Not indicated for acute treatment of severe invasive disease, alternative for mild blastomycosis, histoplasmosis, candida, or coccidioidomycosis	PO	Nausea, vomiting, hepatotoxicity, testosterone synthesis blockade
Miconazole	Deep infection: *Pseudallescheria* and *Scedosporium*	IV	Cardiac dysrhythmias, cardiovascular collapse with rapid infusion
Fluconazole	*Cryptococcus, Candida* (question in critically ill), coccidiomycosis	PO	Nausea, vomiting, dizziness
Itraconazole	Non–life-threatening, blastomycosis, sporotrichosis, histoplasmosis, paracoccidioidomycosis	PO	Pediatric dosage not yet established, nausea, hypokalemia, edema, hypertension, adrenal insufficiency, epigastric pain
Voriconazole	*Aspergillus* and *Cryptococcus,* resistant *Candida* species	IV	Visual changes, fever, nausea, vomiting, elevated liver enzymes
Caspofungin	Treatment for resistant *Aspergillus* and possible combination therapy for *Candida* and endemic mycoses	IV	Fever, phlebitis, nausea, headache, elevated liver enzymes

Histoplasmosis

Histoplasmosis is caused by *Histoplasma capsulatum,* which is endemic in the east-central United States, particularly the Mississippi and Ohio River valleys. Primary pulmonary histoplasmosis is asymptomatic in more than 50% of patients. Patients usually become ill 2 weeks following exposure, manifesting influenza-like illness with fever, chills, myalgia, headache, and a nonproductive cough. Occasionally children have a skin rash, arthritis, and erythema nodosum.

The chest radiograph may show patchy areas of pneumonitis and prominent hilar adenopathy. After exposure to an usually heavy inoculum, a more diffuse pulmonary involvement may occur with extensive nodular infiltrates. These children frequently have significant dyspnea and may progress to respiratory failure. The chest radiograph frequently returns to normal after a primary pulmonary infection; however, a number of residual abnormalities may be seen, including multiple nodules with a dense core of calcium (a target lesion), scattered calcifications within lymph nodes, and occasionally small "buckshot" calcifications scattered throughout both lung fields.[82]

Diagnosis

The skin test is of epidemiologic value but useless in individual case diagnosis because a positive test only indicates prior exposure to this disease. Direct smears of the sputum also are not helpful for diagnosis. Most cases are recognized by serology studies and include immunodiffusion (M and H bands) and complement fixation. Unfortunately, the immune diffusion test is relatively insensitive and a response may be delayed following a primary infection. The complement fixation test is more sensitive but less specific.[34] A titer of 1:32 or higher against the yeast antigen is diagnostic if the clinical picture suggests histoplasmosis. Children with rapidly progressive pneumonia not responding to antibacterial antibiotic therapy or those in impending respiratory failure need urgent diagnosis, and invasive procedures such as BAL, diagnostic lung aspiration, or open lung biopsy are necessary to obtain the required information.

Complications

Disseminated histoplasmosis refers to progressive extrapulmonary infection that occurs most frequently in children younger than 2 years and in patients with altered cellular immunity.[101,126] The clinical features of disseminated disease include fever, weight loss, hepatosplenomegaly, cough, diarrhea, gastrointestinal ulcers, and skin lesions. Anemia, leukopenia, and thrombocytopenia may occur secondary to bone marrow involvement in young children and may lead to rapid death. Chronic disseminated disease, uncommon and insidious, may present as a nonspecific afebrile illness without cough or radiographic abnormalities. Occasionally, disseminated histoplasmosis presents as a localized infection involving the central nervous system. Chorioretinitis and pleural effusion, along with isolated gastrointestinal findings involving terminal ileum, can occur.

Treatment

The usual primary pulmonary infection requires no treatment. Amphotericin B should be used for severe infection, especially if it is life threatening or associated with respiratory failure. On clinical improvement, itraconazole should be given to complete the course of therapy. Chronic cavitary histoplasmosis can be treated with intravenous amphotericin B or a long-term course of oral itraconazole or ketoconazole. Pericarditis therapy should include antiinflammatory agents such as indomethacin or aspirin. Failure of pericarditis to improve with nonsteroidal antiinflammatory medication should not prevent use of a brief course of steroids because steroid use does not appear to predispose to dissemination.[143,145,217]

Blastomycosis

Blastomycosis is endemic to the southeastern region of the United States but extends northward along the western shores of Lake Michigan across to northern Wisconsin and Minnesota and into Canada. An intimate exposure to an infected site is required for infection rather than the casual exposure often found with histoplasmosis and coccidioidomycosis.[112,113,175] Most pediatric cases of blastomycosis occur in older children and adolescents in rural areas.

The pathophysiology is similar to that of histoplasmosis. The clinical course of primary pulmonary blastomycosis is variable. The symptoms are similar to those of acute bacterial pneumonia and include high fever, cough with productive purulent sputum, occasional pleuritic chest pain, and myalgias. Such symptoms generally last 2 to 3 weeks.

The chest radiograph frequently demonstrates patchy areas of alveolar consolidation affecting one or both lower lobes. Pleural effusions and cavitation can occur but are unusual. A rather dense lobar infiltrate similar to pneumococcal pneumonia is uncommon but occurs more frequently in pulmonary blastomycosis than with other pulmonary fungi. Clearing of the chest x-ray film may take 3 to 4 months.

Blastomycosis is not always self-limited, and progressive pulmonary infection can occur with acute dissemination to distant sites. In such instances the child remains febrile and toxic with rather rapid progression. Diffuse pulmonary involvement with acute miliary spread can lead to rapid respiratory failure and radiographic findings of acute respiratory distress syndrome.

Children may have asymptomatic primary pulmonary blastomycosis that is diagnosed only with reactivation blastomycosis involving the skin, bones, or other distant organ sites. Reactivation blastomycosis appears to be most common in the first 1 or 2 years immediately after the initial pulmonary infection and probably occurs in less than 5% of all infected patients. A chronic form of pulmonary blastomycosis may occur in patients who have no significant history of acute pneumonia but present with respiratory symptoms that have persisted for weeks or months. These individuals have chronic cough, productive sputum, nocturnal fevers, night sweats, weight loss, and dyspnea. Chest radiographs in chronic blastomycosis may reveal a single large mass, often perihilar in location. A more common finding is a fibronodular infiltrate with small cavities and fibrosis radiating toward the hila. Such findings mimic tuberculosis.

Diagnosis

There is no reliable skin test for pulmonary blastomycosis. Sputum and material aspirated from BAL, lung aspiration, skin, or bone lesions may be examined directly after potassium hydroxide (KOH) digestion, and the pathognomonic yeast forms are identified. Such positive direct smears provide a rapid, accurate, inexpensive test. Serologic tests include immunodiffusion using purified antigen. The complement fixation test is less sensitive and less specific than the immunodiffusion test.[36] Most acute cases are diagnosed by direct sputum smears or from BAL. Needle aspiration under fluoroscopy usually is diagnostic in the severely ill child; lung biopsy (either from needle or open) and histopathology are necessary in some instances.

Complications

Patients whose illnesses are clinically similar to bacterial pneumonia frequently have a self-limited process. Life-threatening progressive respiratory failure similar to ARDS can occur. In such instances, diagnosis and therapy including mechanical ventilation must be initiated promptly. Dissemination occurs only in the most severe cases.[80,218] With dissemination, characteristic skin lesions (raised, crusted) may occur on the face and upper extremities. In disseminated disease, bone involvement often includes spine, ribs, and skull. The prostate, epididymis, or testes may be involved.

Treatment

Acute pulmonary blastomycosis does not require treatment in all cases. Treatment with intravenous amphotericin should be given if the patient is severely ill or progressive illness occurs. Oral itraconazole and ketoconazole have been used for treatment of chronic pulmonary blastomycosis (similar to tuberculosis) but should not be used for severe, life-threatening infections.[48,195]

Coccidioidomycosis

Coccidioidomycosis is a relatively common infection that occurs primarily in the southwestern United States. Sixty percent of patients with primary pulmonary infection have no or minimal symptoms. Pathogenesis is similar to that of histoplasmosis and other dimorphic fungi infections. Children 5 years or younger have a higher frequency of progressive disease than do older children and healthy adults. The clinical course of coccidioidomycosis is a flulike illness usually associated with fever, cough, and chest pain. There may be a transient maculopapular eruption similar to erythema nodosum in children. Radiographic abnormalities range from hilar adenopathy to patchy infiltrates with pleural effusion.

Diagnosis

Diagnostic studies include skin testing, which has some usefulness if the patient has compatible respiratory illness and a past negative skin test. Direct smears of KOH-digested sputum are helpful if characteristic spherules are found. Antibody detection through complement fixation may be a useful measure of severity of disease.[36] In cases of suspected coccidioidal meningitis, complement fixation tests on cerebrospinal fluid should be obtained because many patients have a negative spinal fluid culture with positive complement fixation studies. Use of chemiluminescent DNA probes may aid in rapid diagnosis.

Complications

Complications include chronic progressive coccidioidal pneumonia, which is similar to tuberculosis but is uncommon in pediatric patients. Disseminated coccidioidomycosis does occur and is often accompanied by persistent fever and rapid progression with development of meningitis, bony lesions, and skin and soft tissue disease. A fulminant primary miliary spread of disease with severe respiratory failure and diffuse lung involvement has been observed in patients with altered immune status. The disseminated disease frequently has an insidious onset, following the primary pulmonary infection by weeks. The meninges are the most worrisome site of extrapulmonary involvement because coccidioidal meningitis requires intrathecal amphotericin B therapy and cure is unlikely.[10,42,67,131,193,218]

Treatment

If the infection causes prolonged fever, progressive pulmonary disease, significant mediastinal adenopathy, or disseminated lesions, antifungal therapy with amphotericin B should be initiated. Ketoconazole has been used in skeletal, cutaneous, and other localized infection but not for meningitis. Coccidiomeningitis is the most difficult complication of this disease to treat; it requires intrathecal and systemic therapy with amphotericin B.

Opportunistic Pulmonary Mycoses

Pulmonary Aspergillosis

Invasive pulmonary aspergillosis occurs almost exclusively in immunocompromised patients.[35,118,152,167,190] Despite treatment, unless the underlying immune defect is ameliorated, invasive pulmonary aspergillosis is often fatal. Many cases are nosocomially acquired, usually in hospitals undergoing renovation or new construction.[175] Children with hematologic malignancies (myelogenous and lymphocytic leukemia) or organ transplantation are at the highest risk for development of invasive disease, presumably because of the abnormal immune cells and the cyclic neutropenia induced by repeated doses of chemotherapy. Cardiac and bone marrow transplants are at higher risk for aspergillosis infection than renal transplants.

Neutropenia is an important risk factor for development of aspergillosis because both the absolute neutrophil count and duration of neutropenia have been related to the incidence of infection. Steroids and immune suppressive drugs also appear to predispose to invasive aspergillosis.[85] Immune and myelosuppressed patients exposed to heavy aerosol concentrations of aspergillosis spores have an increased chance of developing invasive pneumonia. Efforts should be made to eliminate the risk of airborne conidospores in patient areas. If such elimination is not possible, then susceptible patients should be moved away from areas of excavation or construction.

Clinical signs of invasive aspergillosis are nonspecific. The usual presentation includes pulmonary infiltrates and fever that do not respond to empirical antibacterial therapy. Patients may exhibit dyspnea, a nonproductive cough, pleuritic chest pain, and pleural friction rubs. Symptoms usually are difficult to identify in small children, and auscultatory changes usually are found only with advanced disease. Hemoptysis is uncommon in children.

Diagnosis

Radiographs of the chest reveal virtually any infiltrative pattern, including patchy infiltrates, necrotizing pneumonitis, miliary nodules, and lung abscesses. Early findings may include a round, patchy pneumonia that progresses to a wedge-shaped density characteristic of pulmonary infarctions.[153] Definitive diagnosis of invasive pulmonary aspergillosis requires histopathologic identification of fungus in tissue specimens.[69] Positive sputum cultures do not prove the presence of invasive disease even in compromised hosts, although isolation should be taken seriously and multiple positive cultures should be considered strong evidence of fungal infection in immune compromised patients. Serologic antibody tests have no value in the diagnosis of invasive aspergillosis. In severely ill children, fiberoptic bronchoscopy with bronchial lavage is the initial diagnostic test of choice in patients with suspected pneumonitis. If the results of fiberoptic bronchoscopy are nondiagnostic, a lung biopsy (open or needle) may be required.

Complications

Untreated invasive pulmonary aspergillosis usually is fatal in immunocompromised patients. Fatality rates greater than 80% are reported; however, survival may improve if appropriate therapy is initiated early in the disease. Death usually results from progressive pneumonitis, pulmonary infarction, and massive hemoptysis. On rare occasion, endocarditis, osteomyelitis, meningitis, or infection of the eye or orbit occurs.

Treatment

Therapy with amphotericin B should be initiated early in the course of the disease. Surgical resection usually is not indicated in the treatment of critically ill patients with uncontrolled disease. However, it may be considered in patients who have only partial response to antifungal therapy or with relapsing disease in a well-defined lung segment or those identified with massive hemoptysis. In critically ill patients unresponsive to therapy or who develop aspergillosis while receiving amphotericin B, the addition of flucytosine or rifampin may be helpful.[95] Use of the lipid formulations of amphotericin is indicated in patients who are intolerant or refractory to conventional amphotericin for reasons such as renal toxicity or persistent infusion-related adverse events.[221] Itraconazole is an option for use after an initial course of amphotericin B.[41] Change from amphotericin to the oral itraconazole must take into account the patient's status. New antifungals such as voriconazole have shown in vitro activity against *Aspergillus* and are in phase II or III trials.[18,111]

Pulmonary Candidiasis

Of all the opportunistic pulmonary mycoses, candidiasis may be the most difficult to diagnosis and treat effectively because the *Candida* organism routinely colonizes the upper respiratory tract, resulting in positive cultures without significant disease. The prevalence of *Candida* pneumonitis has increased remarkably in the past 3 decades, secondary to the increased usage of broad-spectrum antibiotic therapy, immunosuppressive drugs, indwelling vascular lines, prosthetic devices, and organ transplantation.

Pathogenesis

Pulmonary candidiasis may occur by hematogenous seeding of the lung parenchyma from a distal infected site or through direct invasion of inhaled or aspirated organisms. *Candida* acquired through the hematogenous route demonstrates pulmonary lesions, which are diffuse, bilateral, and miliary. The endobronchial form of infection does not have a significant interstitial component such as that seen with a hematogenous form. The endobronchial form radiographically demonstrates pulmonary lesions that are small, asymmetrical, patchy, and frequently found in the lower lobes.

Diagnosis

There are no pathognomonic signs and symptoms of pulmonary candidiasis. The diagnosis should be considered in an immunocompromised febrile patient with a pulmonary lesion, particularly if broad-spectrum antibiotics were used without a response. Oral pharyngeal involvement (thrush) indicates the patient is harboring the organism in an invasive stage. Retinal lesions on ophthalmoscopic examination may help identify invasive *Candida*. A cutaneous lesion often seen in invasive *Candida* is a discrete erythematous papule with an erythematous halo. The radiographic findings of *Candida* pneumonia are nonspecific. Early in the course of infection, patients have normal chest radiographs. The isolation of *Candida* in culture from an otherwise sterile body fluid or tissue and the identification of the organism in a biopsy specimen are diagnostic of invasive *Candida*. Serologic studies are of no diagnostic value. Tests for antibody, antigen, and metabolite detection remain investigational at this time. Proof of *Candida* pneumonia requires tissue examination or evaluation of alveolar lavage or protected brush samples from bronchoscopy as direct evidence of tissue invasion. If these studies fail to identify the disease process, the diagnosis of pulmonary candidiasis may be established with lung biopsy.

Complications

As with other mycoses, pulmonary candidiasis may be complicated by systemic dissemination affecting other organs. Concomitant infection with other organisms, particularly bacteria, is not uncommon.

Treatment

Effective treatment includes correction of the patient's immunosuppression in addition to administration of amphotericin B. The concomitant and synergistic effect of flucytosine has been demonstrated with amphotericin B for most *Candida* species and is recommended for use in critically ill patients.

Pneumocystis Carinii Pneumonia

Pneumocystis carinii, which probably is a protozoan, produces a unique infection. In the early stages of the infection with cysts, trophozoites are found distributed within the alveoli, most commonly adjacent to the alveolar septum. Usually in this phase no clinical signs or symptoms are evident. With extension of infection, the number of organisms increases and bilateral diffuse distribution occurs throughout the lungs. Eventually desquamation of the alveolar septal cells occurs, with subsequent phagocytosis of the organisms by the alveolar macrophages. Minimal inflammation occurs in discrete areas of the alveolar septum at this stage of the disease, and a child may or may not be symptomatic. Ultimately the alveolar septum becomes thickened with inflammatory cells producing the clinical manifestations of childhood pneumocystosis.[50] In the infantile form there is extensive involvement of alveolar septa with plasma cell and lymphocyte infiltration. The normal septal thickness may be increased 5 to 20 times, which results in occupation of much of the alveolus by the distended septum.

Clinical Features

The three forms of disease patterns in pneumocystosis are the childhood/adult form, the infantile form, and a more chronic fibrosing form observed in some HIV-infected patients.[210] The typical child/adult type of pneumocystosis occurs in children beyond infancy suffering from congenital or acquired immunodeficiency disorders or from malignancies and in organ transplant recipients.[135,148,174] Clinical symptoms of pneumonitis include fever, cough, tachypnea, cyanosis, flaring of the nasal ala, and retractions. Chest auscultation usually reveals no adventitious sounds until the terminal stage of infection, at which time bilateral crackles may be present. The chest roentgenogram may initially be normal and changes only late in the course.[99]

In the infantile form of pneumocystosis, symptoms often begin insidiously, and presentations include poor feeding, failure to thrive, and diarrhea. Increasing tachypnea may be detected, with respiratory rates frequently in the range of 80 to 120 breaths per minute. A dry, nonproductive cough with increased retractions and flaring of the nasal alae becomes prominent. Diffuse crackles may be heard bilaterally on auscultation of the chest, and most infants remain afebrile. The clinical course in neonates and infants may be quite rapid, with progressive cyanosis and death secondary to respiratory failure within days. More commonly, however, the course extends over a period of several weeks, with a mortality rate varying from 20% to 50% without treatment.[25,174]

The chronic fibrosing type of *Pneumocystis* pneumonia identified in HIV patients is associated with the presence of long-standing symptoms, localized radiologic changes, and interstitial fibrosis.[210]

Diagnosis

A definitive diagnosis requires documentation of *P. carinii* in lung tissue. The standard surgical open lung biopsy provides histologic details; however, the necessity for general anesthesia presents additional risk, particularly in the critically ill child. Identification of the organism in sputum is sufficient for the diagnosis, but inducing and obtaining sputum in young children often are difficult; in such cases bronchoscopy should be considered.[98] Fiberoptic bronchoscopy with BAL, although not achieving yields as high as open lung biopsy, offers a useful and safe alternative to open biopsy.[31,47,53] Transthoracic percutaneous needle aspirate and thoracoscopy have been used successfully and can be obtained without the use of a general anesthetic.[3,146] However, pneumothorax can be expected in up to 30% of children. Once a specimen is obtained, it can be stained with one of the array of preparations by which the organism can be confidently identified. Molecular techniques have been developed for detection of the organism based on PCR techniques amplifying *P. carinii* DNA and have been shown to be sensitive and specific detection methods. PCR assays can be applied to BAL samples, sputum, and nasopharyngeal aspirates with success.[207] Serum lactate dehydrogenase usually is elevated in patients with *P. carinii* pneumonia and appears to be related to the degree of lung injury.[103]

The chest radiograph may often be normal early in the course of *P. carinii* pneumonia. However, as the disease progresses, the pattern demonstrates a diffuse bilateral alveolar disease process with hyperinflation and eventually development of air bronchograms. The bilateral densities are frequently more intense in the middle and lower lung fields. Only late in the course of disease do the upper lung fields become involved. Atypical lesions have been reported, including pneumonitis limited to lobar areas. Pneumatoceles and pleural effusions have been reported.[96]

Complications

Pneumocystis carinii usually remains localized to the lungs, even with extensive disease. A disseminated form has been documented, with recovery of the organism from extrapulmonary sites including bone marrow, liver, and spleen. Life-threatening complications that can arise in patients with *P. carinii* pneumonitis include pneumothorax and pneumomediastinum. Pneumothorax, both spontaneous and iatrogenic, occurs frequently in patients with *P. carinii* pneumonitis. Some evidence indicates that upper lobe predominance of pneumothorax may be more frequent in those previously treated with inhaled pentamidine. Pneumomediastinum, with associated respiratory failure, may be noted in those receiving assisted ventilation.

Treatment

Therapy for *P. carinii* should include specific anti-*Pneumocystis* chemotherapy, inhibition of the pulmonary inflammatory response, and enhancement of the immunologic status of the patient.[75,77,133,134,187,206] Several drugs have been used for treatment of pneumocystosis (Table 42–7).

Trimethoprim-sulfamethoxazole (TMP-SMX) may be administered either orally or intravenously and is the drug of choice for treatment of this disease.[131,132] The second most widely used drug for treatment of *P. carinii* pneumonitis is pentamidine isethionate.[119,187] Its effectiveness has been well documented over several years, but it does have an increased number of undesirable side effects and treatment failures compared with TMP-SMX.[148,206] Administration of a corticosteroid such as prednisone should occur at the initiation of specific anti-*Pneumocystis* therapy to improve survival and attenuate or prevent the initial decline in oxygenation. In addition to the specific therapies, efforts should be made to reverse the immune dysfunction that allowed occurrence of *P. carinii*, that is, reduce or discontinue immunosuppressive medications.

Chemical Pneumonitis

A large number of chemical and physical agents may produce intense inflammation of the lower respiratory tract in children. Chemical pneumonitis and/or pneumonia may be acquired in several different ways, such as aspiration, inhalation, ingestion, or injection.

Aspiration Pneumonia

Aspiration pneumonia is composed of a diverse group of disorders that have in common the soiling of the lower respiratory tract by foreign, nongaseous substances. For purposes of this chapter, neither the solid foreign body nor the infectious component of aspiration is discussed.

Gastroesophageal reflux (GER) has been defined as the retrograde passage of stomach contents into the esophagus. This condition may be asymptomatic, or it may be associated with significant regurgitation and vomiting, esophagitis, failure to thrive, and anemia.[204] Aspiration into the pulmonary tree can cause significant complications including apnea, pulmonary fibrosis, severe necrotizing pneumonias, recurrent bronchospasm, and death. Diminished lower esophageal sphincter pressure is often the result of physiologic immaturity; hence GER is more frequent in younger infants. This disorder also occurs in older children, especially those with central nervous and neuromuscular dysfunction. Other high-risk pediatric populations include patients with congenital abnormalities of the tracheal-bronchial tree and those with severe chronic pulmonary disease (Box 42–4).

Pathophysiology

The association of GER and lung disease has been well documented; however, the actual cause and effect of the relationship has not been firmly established. Massive aspiration of gastric fluid produces direct injury to the mucosal surface of the respiratory tract, resulting in diffuse alveolar damage, hemorrhage, and necrotizing bronchiolitis. This may be followed by a rapid interstitial reaction resulting in an acute inflammatory polymorphonuclear cell infiltration involving the interalveolar septa. Bronchiolitis obliterans and fibrosis can occur. In severe instances the initial onset of disease closely resembles that of ARDS with similar outcomes. Repeated aspiration of small amounts of gastric contents may lead to recurrent pneumonia, airway hyperreactivity,

TABLE 42–7

***Pneumocystis Carinii* Pneumonitis Therapy**

Drug	Route	Duration of Therapy (Days)	Comments
TMP-SMX	IV/PO	21	DOC
Pentamidine isethionate	IV	21	DOC
TMP + dapsone	PO	21	Alternative
Trimetrexate + folinic acid	IV	21	Alternative
Clindamycin + primaquine	PO	21	Alternative
Atovaquone	PO	21	Alternative
Prednisone	IV/PO	21	Adjunctive agent

DOC, drug of choice; *TMP-SMX,* trimethoprim-sulfamethoxazole.

BOX 42–4

Pulmonary Aspiration and Gastroesophageal Reflux: Associated Disorders

ASSOCIATED DISORDERS

- Bronchopulmonary dysplasia
- Asthma
- Cystic fibrosis
- Infantile apnea

CENTRAL NERVOUS SYSTEM

- Convulsive disorders
- Anoxic encephalopathy
- Neurologic impairment
- Myopathies

CONGENITAL MALFORMATIONS

- Tracheoesophageal fistula
- Hiatal hernia

GENERAL

- Failure to thrive
- Achalasia
- Cardiopulmonary resuscitation
- Emergency surgery

bronchitis, and bronchiectasis with eventual fibrosis and involvement of the pulmonary interstitium.

Clinical Findings

Clinical symptoms of GER vary with age.[202] In older children, heartburn, acid/bitter taste, retrosternal pain, or abdominal pain may be reported. Infants may be irritable and exhibit stridor, poor sleeping patterns, or intermittent apnea. Esophagitis can lead to microcytic anemia because of repeated episodes of gastrointestinal blood loss. Chronic respiratory symptoms may include coughing, wheezing with choking episodes occasionally resulting in apnea, or life-threatening events similar to those seen in sudden infant death syndrome. In the hospitalized pediatric patient, significant aspirations may occur during or after general anesthesia. Severe aspiration may be seen in patients receiving tube feedings secondary to displacement of the feeding catheter.

Findings on chest radiograph may vary from slight hyperinflation to a pattern of diffuse interstitial and alveolar densities. In mild cases a picture of bilateral diffuse infiltrates compatible with ARDS may be seen. Although a barium esophagogram can help to evaluate esophageal motility and detect esophagitis, it reflects only a single point in time. Therefore a negative study does not rule out the presence of GER. Radionuclide scans permit observation of esophageal function following administration of a radioactive tracer. Thus the frequency and severity of reflux and information on esophageal and gastric dysmotility may be obtained. If delayed aspiration occurs, the radionuclide may be observed in the lung fields on a delayed scan.[74] Esophageal motility and intraluminal pressures may be measured by esophageal manometry. Intraesophageal pH measurement is helpful in that it allows long-term monitoring of acid reflux by detecting frequency, duration, and intensity of reflux.[23,27] Esophagoscopy also is useful for assessing the extent of mucosal injury by allowing direct visualization and obtaining a mucosal biopsy. Use of BAL for assessment of lipid-laden macrophages has been useful in establishing or corroborating the diagnosis of aspiration in difficult patients.[23,27]

Treatment

Treatment of GER frequently includes placing the patient in an upright prone position and use of thickened feedings. Antacid preparations, omeprazole, cimetidine, ranitidine, and other inhibitors of H_2 gastroreceptors may be helpful to decrease acid production and neutralize its effects on the esophageal mucosa. Omeprazole has rarely been associated with electrolyte disturbances. It also has been reported to possibly result in atrophic gastritis with prolonged use, but its use continues to increase despite these possible side effects.[88,90,106,120,220] Metoclopramide is used prior to meals to help improve lower esophageal function and aid gastric emptying. With the suspension of cisapride from the marketplace as an effective prokinetic agent secondary to potentially fatal toxicity, interest in erythromycin as a prokinetic agent has resurfaced and many trials are evaluating its dose and efficacy are under way.[33] Bronchodilators are frequently used to treat bronchospasm associated with GER. Theophylline decreases the lower esophageal sphincter pressure; therefore aerosolized β_2 agonists are preferred. In instances where medical therapy was attempted and failed or in life-threatening situations, antireflux surgery is indicated. In such instances a fundoplication, partial plication, or percutaneous gastrojejunostomy is the appropriate treatment of choice.[53,205] The most favorable outcome and lowest morbidity in such instances are achieved when surgery is delayed until the patient is adequately nourished and optimal pulmonary status has been obtained.

Inhalation Injury

Acute inhalation injuries are a leading cause of fatalities in pediatric patients. Smoke inhalation accounts for the largest number of pediatric lives lost each year. A significant number of inhalation injuries as a result of irritant gases occur through industrial or household accidents.[151] Serious pulmonary inhalation injury may be manifested immediately or delayed in onset.[170,173,177] (Table 42–8).

Pathogenesis

Direct injury to the mucosal surface is the most common mode of pulmonary injury. Inhalation of noxious substances may cause extensive physical damage to the lungs and seriously impair subsequent gas exchange. The epithelial cells of air passages may become necrotic and desquamate, causing marked airway obstruction. Bronchospasm caused by irritation from the inhaled gases or particles may lead to further airway obstruction. Severe damage to

TABLE 42–8

Irritant Gases

Agent	Exposure/Environment
DIRECT MUCOSAL INJURY	
Acrolein	Plastic, rubber, textiles
Ammonia	Fertilizer, refrigerants, explosives
Chlorine	Bleaching, disinfectant
Formaldehyde	Disinfectant, paper, photography
Hydrogen chloride	Refining, dye making
Hydrogen fluoride	Etching, petroleum
Nitrogen dioxide	Welding, fertilizer, farming
Phosgene	Insecticide, dyes, chemicals
Sulfur dioxide	Bleaching, refrigeration
ASPHYXIATION INJURY	
Carbon dioxide	Mining, foundry
Carbon monoxide	Smoke, foundry, mining
Natural gas	Mining, petroleum

the basement membrane may occur and cause subsequent leakage of intravascular fluid and blood into the alveolar and interstitial spaces. Injury may occur at all levels of the respiratory tract, depending upon the physical and chemical properties of the irritant, the agent concentration, duration of exposure, and breathing pattern of the individual exposed.[2,65,170] The clinical course usually has three phases: (1) the acute phase, which occurs within minutes or hours of the insult, resulting in pulmonary edema, hypoxemia, and respiratory failure; (2) the delayed phase, which occurs within the first few days and may include continuing effects of the lung injury such as pulmonary edema, airway obstruction, and superinfection; and (3) the phase in which long-term sequelae may be noted because of the hypoxic or ischemic injury to other organ systems and recurrent pulmonary problems secondary to reactive airways disease or interstitial fibrosis.

Clinical Findings

Clinical manifestations are nonspecific for inhalation of various irritant gases and may differ, depending on the individual child. Injury of the airways may be manifested as upper airway obstruction resulting in laryngotracheitis, bronchitis, and upper airway edema. More peripheral airway obstruction may present with classic findings of asthma and airway edema with hypersecretion. In cases of massive exposure the presenting symptoms may be those associated with acute respiratory distress syndrome, manifested by profound ventilation/ perfusion mismatch, cyanosis, dyspnea, and respiratory failure. Severe nasopharyngeal and laryngeal edema with hypersecretion may present as stridor.[2,173] Chest radiograph findings are nonspecific, ranging from scattered areas of atelectasis and infiltrate to dense bilateral alveolar infiltrates.

Treatment

Prompt physical removal from the offending agent and maintenance of upper airway patency are imperative. Endotracheal intubation is a high-risk procedure, and meticulous attention must be directed toward maintaining proper pulmonary toilet and removal of upper airway secretions and debris from the artificial airway once it is secured.

Oxygenation should be closely monitored. High oxygen concentrations, mechanical ventilation, and use of positive end-expiratory pressure may be necessary in the event of acute respiratory failure because the diminished compliance and formation of pulmonary edema occur rapidly. Use of steroids may be justified in the treatment of patients who have been exposed to oxides of nitrogen; however, use after exposure to other irritant gases has not been validated.

Bronchoscopy may be indicated and useful in assessing the severity of airway injury and an aid to endotracheal intubation and treatment of major areas of atelectasis. However, use of BAL usually is not indicated except in instances where significant particulate or carbonaceous material is likely. Humidification of air and oxygen mixtures to thin secretions is necessary, and chest percussion/postural drainage may help to mechanically clear the airways.

Use of prophylactic antibiotics in inhalation injuries is not recommended. If pulmonary infection is suspected, prompt therapy with broad-spectrum antimicrobial agents should be started. Use of bronchodilators is advocated because of a high incidence of bronchospasm. No critical studies have evaluated this therapy in inhalation injury; however, the risk associated with its use is low, and administration to the child with obvious airflow obstruction is warranted. Use of aerosolized β_2 agonists is preferred. Special attention is required in the presence of smoke inhalation with regard to treatment of carbon monoxide poisoning. Hyperbaric oxygen, if available, or sustained administration of 100% oxygen is recommended in the initial treatment of patients with significant carbon monoxide intoxication. Development of upper or lower airway edema may necessitate intubation and mechanical ventilatory support.[70,121,170] Administration of artificial surfactant may be beneficial in patients who develop ARDS.[157] Use of prophylactic steroids and antibiotics for smoke inhalation victims is not recommended, especially if burn injuries are present because complications are more frequent.

Prognosis

The prognosis of children with acute pulmonary injury produced by inhalation of toxic gases is generally good. Restrictive and obstructive pulmonary function abnormalities have been observed following recovery. Residual defects such as bronchiolitis obliterans, bronchiectasis, and reactive airways disease have been observed following smoke inhalation.

Ingestion/Injection of Pharmacologic Agents

Several chemotherapeutic agents and other commonly used drugs have potentially serious pulmonary toxicity (Box 42–5). Pulmonary toxicity is thought to be a direct effect in most instances, but immunologic and

BOX 42–5

Pharmacologic Agents Associated with Pulmonary Toxicity

CYTOTOXIC AGENTS

Antibiotics

Bleomycin: IP/PF, H, PEFF
Mitomycin C: IP/PF, PE, PEFF

Alkylating Agents

Cyclophosphamide: IP/PF, PE, B
Chlorambucil: IP/PF
Melphalan: IP/PF

Antimetabolites

Methotrexate: IP/PF, PE, H, PEFF
Azathioprine: IP/PF
G-mercaptopurine: IP/PF
Cytosine arabinoside: IP/PF, PE
Nitrosoureas
Carmustine: PF

NONCYTOTOXIC AGENTS

Amiodarone: IP/PF
Carbamazepine: H, B
Gold salts: IP/PF, H
Nitrofurantoin: AH, PEFF, H, B, IP/PF
Diphenylhydantoin: H
Sulfasalazine: H, FA, BO, B
Penicillamine: DA, AH, H, BO

AH = Alveolar hemorrhage; B = bronchospasm; BO = bronchiolitis obliterans; DA = diffuse alveolitis; FA = fibrosing alveolitis; H = hypersensitivity lung reaction; IP = interstitial pneumonitis; PE = pulmonary edema; PEFF = pleural effusion; PF = pulmonary fibrosis.

hypersensitivity mechanisms also may be involved. Toxicity may occur during therapy or after discontinuation of the agent.[171] The development of blebs in the capillary endothelium is followed by an interstitial fibrinous edema and mononuclear cell response with eventual hyaline membrane formation. Some studies have shown a significant decrease in type 1 pneumocytes with evolution of type 2 pneumocytes, septal thickening, and a proliferation of fibrous tissue with a decrease in the number of alveolar septa. Pleural thickening may accompany the pneumonitis.

Diagnosis/Clinical Findings

Characteristic clinical features of drug-induced pulmonary disease include fever, malaise, dyspnea, and a nonproductive cough. Initial radiographic studies may be normal but usually demonstrate a diffuse alveolar and/or interstitial involvement. Pulmonary function studies may be of either an obstructive or restrictive pattern. Hypoxemia enhanced by exercise is an early and clinically important finding because interstitial pneumonitis and pulmonary fibrosis constitute a major portion of drug-induced pulmonary disease. Histologic examination of lung tissue is frequently indicated to confirm the clinical diagnosis and to rule out other potential causes of pneumonitis such as *Pneumocystis,* viral, or fungal infections that often occur in children treated with these agents.

Other complications such as hypersensitivity lung disease, noncardiogenic pulmonary edema, bronchiolitis obliterans, alveolar hemorrhage, and pleural effusion may occur in these patients. Persistent and fatal lung dysfunction may follow drug-induced pulmonary damage. Therapy should be directed at early recognition of the problem, discontinuation of the offending agent, and supportive therapy. The benefit of steroid use for treatment of lung injury caused by pharmacologic agents has not been well defined. In severe life-threatening disease, steroids are frequently used.

Idiopathic Interstitial Lung Disease

Interstitial lung disease of undetermined etiology is rare in adults but is even more uncommon in children. Histologic classification of this type of ILD can be somewhat confusing. Interstitial lung disease has been divided into several categories including usual interstitial pneumonitis (UIP), desquamative interstitial pneumonitis (DIP), and lymphoid interstitial pneumonitis (LIP). Usual interstitial pneumonitis, initially described by Hamman and Rich, is a relentlessly progressive form of ILD. The histopathologic lesion is heterogeneous, ranging from alveolitis associated with lymphocytic and plasma cell infiltration to an end-stage interstitial fibrosis and hyaline membrane formation. Typically, a variety of lesions are present throughout the lung, with mildly involved areas next to severely affected areas. DIP, as originally characterized by Liebow, is a form of ILD that is more responsive to corticosteroids than is UIP. The histologic picture in DIP is somewhat more monotonous than that seen in UIP. Macrophages are the primary inflammatory cells that fill the alveolus, although histiocytes, lymphocytes, eosinophils, and plasma cells are also present. Hyaline membrane formation is not seen in DIP, and the structural integrity of the alveolar unit usually is maintained. Fan and Langston[62] estimated the ratio of DIP to UIP in children was estimated to be 1:3, or approximately 10% of the incidence in adults. LIP, usually insidious in onset, appears secondary to infiltration of the interstitium by plasma cells, mature lymphocytes, and histiocytes. There is no evidence of epithelial or endothelial necrosis. Testing for specific polyclonal B lymphocytes can help separate LIP from other lymphocytic diseases. Detailed discussion of these disorders and their management is beyond the scope of this chapter but can be found in various review articles.[12,61,62,63,64,179] Patients who do not respond to medical therapy should be considered candidates for lung transplantation.

Pediatric Pulmonary Hemorrhage

Pulmonary hemorrhage (PH) is a potentially life-threatening event that can occur at any age. The clinical presentation varies from massive fatal hemoptysis to silent bleeding with respiratory distress and anemia. Rapid determination of the etiology of the PH and institution of specific therapy are often difficult. This section examines the less common causes of PH. Pulmonary hemorrhage resulting from trauma and infection will not be discussed.

Definition

Pulmonary hemorrhage is defined as extravasation of blood into airways and/or lung parenchyma. Massive PH in adults is defined as blood loss of 600 ml or more in 24 hours.[52,122,149] In infants, Esterly and Oppenheimer[58] characterized massive PH as the involvement of at least two pulmonary lobes by confluent foci of extravasated erythrocytes. Loss of 10% of a patient's circulating blood volume into the lungs regardless of age causes a significant alteration in cardiorespiratory function and should be considered massive. The diagnosis of PH following an episode of silent bleeding is established by pulmonary hemosiderosis, which is the abnormal accumulation of iron within lung parenchyma and alveolar macrophages.

Pathophysiology

Accumulation of blood in the airways following a significant episode of PH creates multiple problems. These include production of a diffusion barrier resulting in hypoxemia and reduction in the diameter of involved airways, which in turn increases airway resistance and may lead to airway obstruction.

Reduction in pulmonary compliance and impairment of ventilation may occur.[14,45] These changes in respiratory function increase both the ventilatory and myocardial work necessary to maintain a normal arterial oxygen tension. Interstitial fibrosis that develops following repeated episodes of PH results in reduced carbon monoxide diffusion and diminished static and dynamic lung compliance.

Etiology

Classification of the etiologies of PH provides a simple framework to proceed with diagnostic and therapeutic interventions (Box 42–6). Diffuse PH usually is associated with less total blood loss and can occur from either immune or nonimmune mechanisms. Diffuse, immune PH typically affects adolescents and, less commonly, school-age children. Focal PH is commonly responsible for massive PH and carries a mortality rate greater than 50%.[100,149] Focal PH typically affects preschool children but may occur in infancy.

Diffuse/Nonimmune Pulmonary Hemorrhage

Pulmonary hemorrhage in the neonate occurs in 0.7 to 4 per 1000 live births and is present in 6% to 26.3% of neonates at postmortem examination. Risk factors associated with PH in the neonate include asphyxia, infection/sepsis, central nervous system injury, weight less than 1500 g and/or small-for-gestational age, male sex, congenital heart disease, idiopathic respiratory distress syndrome, and coagulation disorders.[22,222] Intraalveolar hemorrhage

BOX 42–6

Causes of Pulmonary Hemorrhage

DIFFUSE

Nonimmune

- Neonatal
- Congenital heart disease
- Hematologic

Immune

- Lower respiratory and renal
  - Goodpasture syndrome
  - Idiopathic rapid progressive glomerulonephritis
- Upper and lower respiratory and renal
  - Wegener granulomatosis
- Multisystem organ involvement
  - Systemic lupus erythematosus
  - Polyarteritis nodosa
  - Behçet syndrome
  - Henoch-Schönlein syndrome
  - Rheumatoid arthritis

FOCAL

- Foreign body aspiration and chronic retention
- Sequestration
- Arteriovenous fistula
- Bronchogenic and gastroenteric cysts
- Thrombus or embolus
- Neoplasms: angiomas, adenomas

appears to occur more commonly in neonates of older gestational age. Pulmonary hemorrhage in neonates as a primary occurrence is uncommon.[22] Pathogenesis of PH in the neonate is considered to result from the development of persistent pulmonary hypertension with right-to-left intracardiac shunting of blood, secondary to hypoxia and acidosis. Left ventricular failure ensues, causing an increase in pulmonary capillary pressure and subsequently disruption of pulmonary capillary and alveolar membranes. Severe central nervous system injury may indirectly affect cardiac function, causing increased left ventricular end-diastolic pressure.[11]

Severe hemoptysis and life-threatening PH are very rare in the preadolescent child with congenital heart disease. However, a drastic increase in pulmonary capillary pressure in children with pulmonary atresia, unilateral pulmonary venous atresia, total anomalous pulmonary venous drainage, mitral stenosis, cor triatriatum, or hypoplastic left heart syndrome may result in massive PH.[11,198]

Although the lungs are an infrequent site for early manifestations of primary bleeding disorders,[52,58] a coagulopathy should be ruled out during the management of any patient with PH. In patients with leukemia, PH occurs most frequently when the platelet count is lower than 10,000/mm.

Diffuse/Immune Pulmonary Hemorrhage

The classic clinical triad of hemoptysis, microcytic hypochromic anemia, and diffuse alveolar-filling opacities on chest radiograph (Figure 42–1) is found in most episodes of PH in this category. Although the lung may be the only organ affected, more frequently multiple organs are involved. In patients with PH, establishing which extrapulmonary organs are involved by the disease helps to narrow the differential diagnosis of which of the immune-mediated disorders is most likely present.

Diffuse parenchymal bleeding without evidence of extrapulmonary involvement occurs in idiopathic pulmonary hemosiderosis, Heiner syndrome, and drug-induced PH. Idiopathic pulmonary hemosiderosis, a disease of childhood, is a diagnosis of exclusion. Clinically, episodes of PH recur, with 30% to 50% of patients eventually dying of exsanguination and/or respiratory failure.[24,83] Microscopic examination of the lungs is compatible with nonspecific injury rather than a specific cause such as vasculitis or immune deposits.[192] Heiner syndrome, which affects children between the ages of 6 months and 2 years, usually manifests other symptoms, such as chronic rhinitis, recurrent otitis media, and growth retardation.[11,123] Tests for precipitating antibodies to milk proteins are positive. Symptoms resolve when milk and milk products are eliminated from the diet.[11]

Although uncommon, exposure to or inhalation of D-penicillamine,[169] lymphangiography dye, trimellitic anhydride, cocaine, and exogenous surfactant[129,155,165] has been associated with development of PH. Acute PH of an undetermined etiology occurring in infants has been reported.[4,5]

Idiopathic rapidly progressive glomerulonephritis (GN) is usually a disease of older adults (mean age 55–60 years).[83] In children with PH and either proteinuria, hematuria, or red cell casts, Goodpasture syndrome is the most likely etiology. The presence of a linear immunofluorescent staining of Ig and C3 along glomerular capillary walls and antibasement membrane antibody (ABMA) in the serum confirms the diagnosis of Goodpasture syndrome. Renal biopsy is the preferred primary method of confirming the diagnosis because an ABMA assay is not readily available at most institutions. AMBA is a cytotoxic plasma

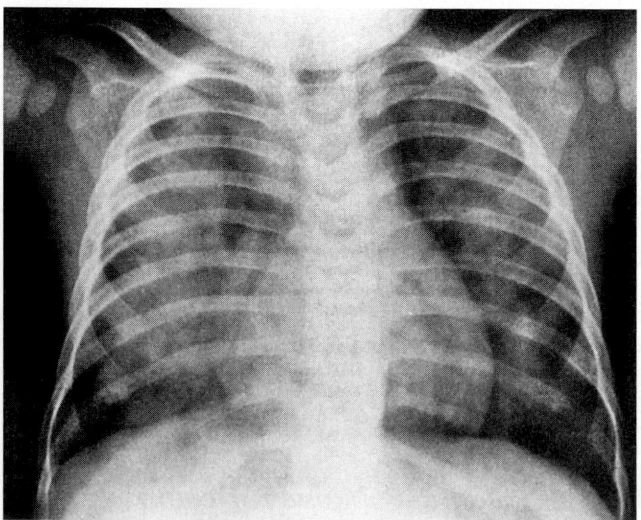

FIGURE 42–1 • Chest x-ray film of a patient with diffuse, immune pulmonary hemorrhage.

Ig that reacts immunologically with components of alveolar and glomerular basement membrane. Stress failure of pulmonary capillaries because of alteration of the alveolar and glomerular basement membrane may contribute to the likelihood of PH in these patients.[216] Fifty percent of patients with Goodpasture syndrome die of asphyxia secondary to massive PH. The presence of sinusitis and/or bilateral, multiple cavitary pulmonary nodules and evidence of GN in patients with PH help distinguish Wegener granulomatosis from the other vasculitides.[65] The immune-mediated causes of PH with multisystem organ involvement often have characteristic physical findings to suggest the diagnosis. Serositis, arthritis, facial erythema, fever, and glomerulonephritis are present prior to the development of PH in patients with systemic lupus erythematosus (SLE).[83,141] Ten percent of all cases of immune-mediated PH are associated with SLE.[83] The onset of PH in SLE is abrupt. Pulmonary histology may or may not reveal a small vessel vasculitis characterized by neutrophilic infiltration of vessel walls and necrosis of capillaries and alveolar septa. Renal histology shows a vasculitis represented by focal and segmental GN with absent or minimal immune deposits.[140] The majority of SLE patients with PH die.[192]

Pulmonary hemorrhage has been reported with most of the vasculitides, but the incidence is much lower than in the SLE population. Constitutional signs and symptoms, such as musculoskeletal involvement, blood dyscrasias, and dermatitis, are the predominant clinical features of polyarteritis nodosa, the second most likely vasculitis-associated disease to cause PH.[192] A segmental necrotizing (granular pattern) vasculitis is the characteristic lesion of polyarteritis nodosa, with PH a dominant feature.[127,136] Recurrent uveitis, mucocutaneous ulcerations, and genital ulcerations in a patient with PH suggests Behçet syndrome as the etiology. Other clinical features seen with Behçet syndrome include arthritis, gastrointestinal disease, cardiovascular involvement, and central nervous system disease.[54,55] A necrotizing vasculitis of small- to medium-size arteries and veins and thromboses of the terminal vascular beds or vena cava confirm the diagnosis.

Although PH is an extremely rare complication of Henoch-Schönlein purpura or syndrome (when abdominal pain and arthritis precede the purpura), it should be treated aggressively because it may be fatal. A few patients with rheumatoid arthritis have developed syndromes resembling idiopathic pulmonary hemosiderosis without evidence of vasculitis or renal disease.[192]

Focal Pulmonary Hemorrhage

Congenital malformations that may be responsible for PH during infancy include angiomas[11] and bronchogenic and gastroenteric cysts. Angiomas are located in the subglottic area and present with symptoms of airway obstruction by age 6 months in almost 90% of cases. Bronchogenic cysts arise from abnormal branching of the tracheobronchial tree, are lined with ciliated columnar epithelium, filled with mucoid fluid, and if in communication with the airway may demonstrate an air-fluid level. They are prone to infection and may bleed if contiguous vessels erode. Gastroenteric cysts, which are enteric duplication cysts lined with gastric mucosa, produce acid peptic secretions that may erode through adjacent vessels to cause bleeding.

Pulmonary sequestration, arteriovenous fistula, and bronchial adenomas are congenital malformations that may present in childhood or later life with PH. With its tendency to become recurrently infected, a sequestered lobe may suffer erosion into its systemic arterial supply, causing massive PH.[11] Pulmonary arteriovenous fistula with or without telangiectasia (isolated or familial) may produce massive PH during childhood, but this usually does not occur until adulthood.[68,162] Adenomas are highly vascular tumors that, with minor trauma or inflammation, can cause PH.

Acquired causes of focal PH include aspiration of an organic foreign body and development of a pulmonary arterial thrombus or embolus.[11,52] A patient presenting with PH and wheezing should lead the clinician to suspect a diagnosis of foreign body aspiration. Prolonged retention of an organic foreign body leads to hyperplasia of tortuous bronchial vessels, varicosities, and bronchiectasis, any of which may cause PH. Thrombi or emboli may develop in postoperative immobile children with central venous or pulmonary catheters, the adolescent female using oral contraceptives, or the patient with homozygous deficiency of antithrombin III, protein S, and protein C. Children with cystic fibrosis may develop focal PH secondary to bronchiectasis.

BOX 42–7

Treatment of Pulmonary Hemorrhage

GENERAL

- Admission to pediatric intensive care unit
- Positioning (intermittent Trendelenburg)
- Oxygen supplementation
- Mechanical ventilation (positive end-expiratory pressure)
- Hemodynamic monitoring
- Hemostasis replacement therapy
- Endobronchial tamponade (Fogarty catheter, cuffed endotracheal tube)

SPECIFIC

Immune

- Corticosteroids
- Other immunosuppressive agents (azathioprine, cyclophosphamide)
- Plasmapheresis (Goodpasture syndrome)
- Bilateral nephrectomy
- Deferoxamine, milk-free diet

Focal

- Surgical resection
- Selective embolization of bronchial vessels

Treatment

General

The primary objectives in treatment of PH are twofold: (1) to rapidly control the bleeding to prevent tissue hypoxia and/or ischemia secondary to air way obstruction and exsanguination and (2) to stabilize hemodynamics to prevent further damage to the kidneys or other extrapulmonary organs by the underlying disorder.[14,156] Initial management of the patient with severe PH should occur in the setting of a critical care unit because of the potential lethality of this event (Box 42–7). General care measures include use of Trendelenburg position as tolerated, oxygen supplementation, mechanical ventilation, and hemostasis therapy when indicated. The Trendelenburg position may assist clots to propagate superiorly and exit the airway. This position may not be well tolerated by patients with respiratory or cardiac embarrassment. Positive end-expiratory pressure during mechanical ventilation may become necessary to reverse hypoxemia and may provide a measure of tamponade to the site of hemorrhage.[149] Coagulation factors should be administered when indicated to lessen the severity of bleeding. Hemodynamic monitoring with a pulmonary arterial catheter may be beneficial in some instances because high pulmonary artery occlusion pressure may worsen PH of any etiology. Short-term control of bleeding may be obtained with insertion, under direct vision, of a balloon-tipped (Fogarty) catheter into the affected portion of the airway. Right upper lobe bleeding is best managed by intubating the left mainstem bronchus with a cuffed endotracheal tube and inflating the cuff of the tube. Utilization of a "double lumen" or Carlens-type endotracheal tube may also be helpful in isolating the bleeding segment. However, the diameter of these tubes precludes their use in smaller children, and proper positioning may prove difficult.[14,117] Rigid bronchoscopy not only is the best means of identifying the source and type of bleeding but also has therapeutic applications.[14,107] The rigid scope readily establishes an adequate airway and can be used for large-volume isotonic saline lavage and for suctioning large volumes of blood. Fiberoptic bronchoscopy should be reserved for diagnostic purposes, including definitive identification of the bronchopulmonary segments involved and BAL. Bronchoalveolar lavage provides useful information by permitting culture of the lavage for bacteria, fungi, mycobacteria, and viruses and quantitative assessment of the hemosiderin content of the alveolar lavage. Interpreting the presence or absence of hemosiderin-laden macrophages should be done cautiously because they may not appear for up to 48 hours following an acute episode of bleeding and usually disappear by 2 weeks.

Specific

Despite the different etiologies in the category of immune-mediated PH, the response to corticosteroid therapy is swift (within 24–48 hours) as assessed by transfusion requirements, hemoglobin concentration, hemoptysis, and absence of new infiltrates.[192] Although controlled clinical trials have not been performed to validate this temporal relationship suggestive of therapeutic benefit, the risk of administering a short course of high-dose corticosteroids in this setting is low. Hence, corticosteroids adrenocorticotropic hormone [ACTH] (10–25 units/day), methylprednisolone (2–4 mg/kg/day), or hydrocortisone (4 mg/kg/day) should be administered early in a patient with an acute, life-threatening episode of immune-mediated PH. Once remission is achieved, corticosteroids should be tapered until they are discontinued or until symptoms recur.

In cases of inadequate response to corticosteroids alone, other immunosuppressive agents (azathioprine, cyclophosphamide, chlorambucil) have been administered with some success in the immune-mediated PH syndromes.[11] Azathioprine (1.2–5 mg/kg/day) with prednisone (5–20 mg every 6 hours) is a typical treatment combination. Cyclophosphamide is the drug of choice for treatment of Wegener granulomatosis.[7,60,72,140]

Once a specific diagnosis is made for the various etiologies of immune-mediated PH, directed therapies are available, including immunosuppression and plasmapheresis. These therapies are beyond the scope of this chapter and are discussed in the literature.[60,72,140]

Administration of intravenous vasopressin to a patient with massive hemoptysis may temporarily control the bleeding. Surgical resection of a bleeding focus remains the procedure of choice if feasible. Surgical resection is the generally recommended treatment of uncorrectable, unilateral pulmonary vein atresia, bronchiectatic lung secondary to foreign body, recurrent infection, and vascular tumors.[14] Severe bleeding at the time of resection resulting in single lung ventilation increased mortality from 12% to 25% in one series. Pulmonary embolectomy should be considered for patients with an acute large embolus, especially if fibrinolysis is contraindicated.[14,20,224]

For focal PH secondary to increased bronchial circulation, selective embolization or occlusion of bronchial vessels with glass microspheres, small pledgets of absorbable gelatin sponge, or polyvinyl alcohol sponge may provide temporary hemostasis. Embolization should be considered in the unstable or poor surgical candidate with focal PH. Complications of embolization include inadvertent central nervous system or coronary artery occlusion and transverse myelitis with resulting paraplegia.

Summary

Pulmonary hemorrhage that does not occur in the familiar setting of trauma or infection can be classified according to extent of pulmonary involvement, that is, diffuse or focal. Pulmonary hemorrhage occurs most commonly during the neonatal period as a result of diffuse, nonimmune mechanisms. Pulmonary hemorrhage in the neonate is a preterminal complication of severe disorders of the cardiovascular and respiratory systems. The best initial approach to diagnosis and specific therapy in the older child is determining the extent of extrapulmonary organ involvement. Diseases that lead to focal hemorrhage are more likely to cause massive hemoptysis, typically affect younger children, and may be amenable to surgical resection. If the suspected cause of PH is a diffuse, immune-mediated process, a trial of corticosteroids should be administered early because of the rapid, dramatic response seen with some disorders. A systematic approach to diagnosis in PH will improve the odds of a favorable outcome for patients with this rare phenomenon.[14,117]

REFERENCES

1. American Academy of Pediatrics Committee on Infectious Disease: Reassessment of the indications for ribavirin therapy. *Pediatrics* 97:137, 1996.
2. Ainslie G: Inhalational injuries produced by smoke and nitrogen dioxide. *Respir Med* 87:169, 1993.
3. Angelillo Mackinlay T, Lyons G, et al: VATS debridement versus thoracotomy in the treatment of loculated post-pneumonia empyema. *Ann Thorac Surg* 61:1626, 1996.
4. Anonymous: Acute pulmonary hemorrhage among infants-Chicago, April 1992-November 1994. *MMWR* 44:67, 1995.
5. Anonymous: Acute pulmonary hemorrhage/hemosiderosis among infants-Cleveland, January 1993-November 1994. *MMWR* 43:881, 1995.
6. Baker KA, Ryan ME: RSV infection in infants and young children. What's new in diagnosis, treatment, and prevention? *Postgrad Med* 106:97-99, 103-14, 107-18, 1999.
7. Ball JA, Young KR Jr: Pulmonary manifestations of Goodpasture's syndrome. Antiglomerular basement membrane disease and related disorders. *Clin Chest Med* 19:777-791, ix, 1998.
8. Balough K, McCubbin M, et al: The relationship between infection and inflammation in the early stages of lung disease from cystic fibrosis. *Pediatr Pulmonol* 20:63, 1995.
9. Becroft, D: Bronchiolitis obliterans, and other sequelae of adenovirus type 21 infection in young children. *J Clin Pathol* 24:72, 1971.
10. Bennett J: Antifungal agents. In Mandell G, Douglas R, Bennett J, editors: *Principles and practice of infectious diseases.* New York, 1990, Churchill Livingstone.
11. Boat T: Pulmonary hemorrhage and hemoptysis. In Chernick V, Boat T, editors: *Kendig's disorders of the respiratory tract in children.* Philadelphia, 1998, WB Saunders.
12. Bokulic R, Hilman B: Interstitial lung disease in children. *Pediatr Clin North Am* 41:543, 1994.
13. Bueno J, Ramil C, et al: Current management strategies for the prevention and treatment of cytomegalovirus infection in pediatric transplant recipients. *Paediatr Drugs* 4:279-290, 2002.
14. Cahill B, Ingbar D: Massive hemoptysis. Assessment and management (review). *Clin Chest Med* 15:147, 1994.
15. Carson J, Collier A, et al: Acquired ciliary defects in nasal epithelium of children with acute viral upper respiratory tract infections. *N Engl J Med* 312:463, 1985.
16. Cate TR: Impact of influenza and other community-acquired viruses. *Semin Respir Infect* 13:17-23, 1998.
17. Chan KP: An update of rapid diagnosis of infectious diseases. II—Virus. *Singapore Med J* 35:407-410, 1994.
18. Chandrasekar PH, Cutright J, et al: Efficacy of voriconazole against invasive pulmonary aspergillosis in a guinea-pig model. *J Antimicrob Chemother* 45:673-676, 2000.
19. Chartrand S, McCracken G: Staphylococcal pneumonia in infants and children. *Pediatr Infect Dis J* 1:19, 1982.
20. Cipolli M, Perini S, et al: Bronchial artery embolization in the management of hemoptysis in cystic fibrosis. *Pediatr Pulmonol* 19:344, 1995.
21. Claesson BA, Trollfors B, et al: Etiology of community-acquired pneumonia in children based on antibody responses to bacterial and viral antigens. *Pediatr Infect Dis J* 8:856-862, 1989.
22. Coffin C, Schechtman K, et al: Neonatal and infantile pulmonary hemorrhage: an autopsy study with clinical correlation. *Pediatr Pathol* 13:583, 1993.
23. Colombo J, Hallberg T, et al: Time course of lipid-laden pulmonary macrophages with acute and recurrent milk aspiration in rabbits. *Pediatr Pulmonol* 12:95, 1992.
24. Colombo J, Stolz S: Treatment of life-threatening primary pulmonary hemosiderosis with cyclophosphamide. *Chest* 102:959, 1992.
25. Contini C, Villa M, et al: Detection of *Pneumocystis carinii* among children with chronic respiratory disorders in the absence of HIV infection and immunodeficiency. *J Med Microbiol* 47:329-333, 1998.

26. Cooper KE: The effectiveness of ribavirin in the treatment of RSV. *Pediatr Nurs* 27:95-98, 2001.
27. Corwin R, Irwin R: The lipid-laden alveolar macrophage as a marker of aspiration in parenchymal lung disease. *Am Rev Respir Dis* 132:576, 1985.
28. Cottin V, Tebib J, et al: Pulmonary function in patients receiving long-term low-dose methotrexate. *Chest* 109:933, 1996.
29. Couch RB, Kasel J, et al: Influenza: its control in persons and populations. *J Infect Dis* 153:431, 1986.
30. Couvreur J, Dournon E, et al: [Legionnaires' disease in children. Epidemiological survey with a new case report and review of the literature]. *Ann Pediatr* 33:379-384, 1986.
31. Croce M, Fabian T, et al: Using bronchoalveolar lavage to distinguish nosocomial pneumonia from systemic inflammatory response syndrome: a prospective analysis. *J Trauma* 39:1134, 1995.
32. Crouch Brewer S, Wunderink R, et al: Ventilator-associated pneumonia due to Pseudomonas aeruginosa. *Chest* 109:1019, 1996.
33. Curry JI, Lander TD, et al: Review article: erythromycin as a prokinetic agent in infants and children. *Aliment Pharmacol Ther* 15:595-603, 2001.
34. Davies S: Serodiagnosis of histoplasmosis. *Semin Respir Infect* 1:9, 1986.
35. Davies S, Sarosi G: Aspergillosis in the immunosuppressed patient. In Al-Doory Y, Wagner G, editors: *Aspergillosis.* Springfield, Ill, 1985, Charles C. Thomas.
36. Davies S, Sarosi G: Role of serodiagnostic tests and skin tests in diagnosis of fungal disease. *Clin Chest Med* 8:135, 1987.
37. Becker JA, Ascher DP, et al: False-negative urine latex particle agglutination testing in neonates with group B streptococcal bacteremia. A function of improper test implementation? *Clin Ped* 32:467-471, 1993.
38. De La Rosa GR, Champlin RE, et al: Risk factors for the development of invasive fungal infections in allogeneic blood and marrow transplant recipients. *Transplant Infect Dis* 4:3-9, 2002.
39. Delage G, Brochu P, et al: Giant-cell pneumonia caused by parainfluenza virus. *J Pediatr* 94:426, 1979.
40. Dennehy P: Rapid diagnosis of viral infections. In Hilman B, editor: *Pediatric respiratory disease.* Philadelphia, 1993, WB Saunders.
41. Denning DW: Invasive aspergillosis. *Clin Infect Dis* 26:781-803, 1998; quiz 804-805.
42. Deresinski SC: Coccidioidomycosis: efficacy of new agents and future prospects. *Curr Opin Infect Dis* 14:693-696, 2001.
43. DeVincenzo JP: Therapy of respiratory syncytial virus infection. *Pediatr Infect Dis J* 19:786-790, 2000.
44. Diaz R, Chiodo A, et al: Pulmonary function patterns in children with interstitial lung disease. *Am Rev Respir Dis* 139:A474, 1989.
45. Donald K, Edwards R, et al: Alveolar capillary basement membrane lesions in Goodpasture's syndrome and idiopathic pulmonary hemosiderosis. *Am J Med* 59:642, 1975.
46. Dowell SF, Kupronis BA, et al: Mortality from pneumonia in children in the United States, 1993 through 1996. *N Engl J Med* 342:1399-1407, 1993.
47. Drent M, van Nierop M, et al: A computer program using BALF-analysis results as a diagnostic tool in interstitial lung diseases. *Am J Respir Crit Care Medicine* 153:736, 1996.
48. Drutz D: Systemic fungal infections: diagnosis and treatment, part I. *Infect Dis Clin North Am* 2:779, 1988.
49. Dunn M, Wunderink R: Ventilator-associated pneumonia caused by Pseudomonas infection (review). *Clin Chest Med* 16:95, 1995.
50. Dutz W, Post C, et al: Cellular reaction to Pneumocystis carinii. *Z Kinderheilkd* 114:1-11, 1973.
51. Edward E, Coonrod J: Coagglutination and counterimmunoelectrophoresis for detection of pneumococcal antigens in the sputum of pneumonia patients. *J Clin Microbiol* 11:488, 1980.
52. Edwards J, Matthay K: Hematologic disorders affecting the lungs. *Clin Chest Med* 10:723, 1989.
53. Ellis M, Spence D, et al: Open lung biopsy provides a higher and more specific diagnostic yield compared to bronchoalveolar lavage in immunocompromised patients. Fungal Study Group. *Scand J Infect Dis* 27:157, 1995.
54. Erkan F: Pulmonary involvement in Behcet disease. *Curr Opin Pulm Med* 5:314-318, 1999.
55. Erkan F, Kiyan E, et al: Pulmonary complications of Behcet's disease. *Clin Chest Med* 23:493-503, 2002.
56. Eskola J: Use of conjugate vaccines to prevent meningitis caused by Haemophilus influenzae type b or Streptococcus pneumoniae. *J Hosp Infect* 30(suppl):313, 1995.
57. Esteban RE, Jimenez AM, et al: [Etiology of acute respiratory infections in 87 hospitalized children]. *Rev Clin Esp* 196:82-86, 1996.
58. Esterly SR, Oppenheimer EH: Massive pulmonary hemorrhage in the newborn. I. *J Pediatr* 69:3-11, 1966.
59. Evlogias N, Leonidas J, et al: Severe cystic pulmonary disease associated with chronic Pneumocystis carinii infection in a child with AIDS. *Pediatr Radiol* 24:606, 1994.
60. Falk RJ, Nachman PH, et al: ANCA glomerulonephritis and vasculitis: a Chapel Hill perspective. *Semin Nephrol* 20:233-243, 2000.
61. Fan L: Evaluation and therapy of chronic interstitial pneumonitis in children (review). *Curr Opin Pediatr* 6:248, 1994.
62. Fan LL, Langston C: Chronic interstitial lung disease in children. *Pediatr Pulmonol* 16:184, 1993.
63. Fan LL, Mullen A, et al: Clinical spectrum of chronic interstitial lung disease in children. *J Pediatr* 121:867, 1992.
64. Fann L: Evaluation and therapy of chronic interstitial pneumonitis in children (review). *Curr Opin Pediatr* 6:248, 1994.
65. Fauci AS, Haynes BF, et al: Wegener's granulomatosis: prospective clinical and therapeutic experience with 85 patients for 21 years. *Ann Intern Med* 98:76-85, 1983.
66. Feklisova LV, Vasil'eva VI, et al: [Legionella infections in children]. *Pediatriia* 3:28-32, 1990.
67. Feldman BS, Snyder LS: Primary pulmonary coccidioidomycosis. *Semin Respir Infect* 16:231-237, 2001.
68. Ference B, Shannon T, et al: Life-threatening pulmonary hemorrhage with pulmonary arteriovenous malformations and hereditary hemorrhagic telangiectasia. *Chest* 106:1387, 1994.
69. Fisher B, Armstrong D, et al: Invasive aspergillosis: progress in early diagnosis and treatment. *Am J Med* 71:571, 1981.
70. Fitzpatrick J, Cioffi WJ, et al: Predicting ventilation failure in children with inhalation injury. *J Pediatr Surg* 29:1122, 1994.
71. Fixler DE: Respiratory syncytial virus infection in children with congenital heart disease: a review. *Pediatr Cardiol* 17:163-168, 1996.
72. Fox HL, Swann D: Goodpasture syndrome: pathophysiology, diagnosis, and management. *Nephrol Nurs J* 28:305-310, 2001; quiz 311-2.
73. Fujita J, Yamadori I, et al: Distribution of human neutrophil elastase in diffuse alveolar damage and pneumonia in a case of neonatal sepsis. *Respir Med* 89:505, 1995.
74. Ghaed N, Stein M: Assessment of a technique for scintographic monitoring of pulmonary aspiration of gastric contents in asthmatics with gastroesophageal reflux. *Ann Allergy* 42:306, 1979.
75. Gigliotti F, Ballou L, et al: Purification and initial characterization of a Pneumocystis carinii surface antigen capable of inducing protective antibody. *Pediatr Res* 23:369A, 1988 (abstract).
76. Gilbert D, Moellering RJ, et al: *The Sanford guide to antimicrobial therapy.* Hyde Park, 2002, Sanford.
77. Glassroth J: Empiric diagnosis of Pneumocystis carinii pneumonia. *Am J Respir Crit Care* Med 152:1433, 1995.
78. Glezen W: Viral pneumonia as a cause and result of hospitalization. *J Infect Dis* 147:765, 1983.
79. Glezen W, Decker M, et al: Acute respiratory disease associated with influenza epidemics in Houston. *J Infect Dis* 115:1119, 1987.
80. Goldman M, Johnson PC, et al: Fungal pneumonias. The endemic mycoses. *Clin Chest Med* 20:507-519, 1999.
81. Gray MM, Hann IM, et al: Mortality and morbidity caused by measles in children with malignant disease attending four major treatment centres: a retrospective review. *Br Med J Clin Res Ed* 295:19-22, 1987.
82. Graybill OJ: Histoplasmosis and AIDS. *J Infect Dis* 158:623, 1988.
83. Gross T, Lynch J: Alveolar hemorrhage syndromes. *Pulm Crit Care Update* 5:1, 1990.
84. Treatment of serious cytomegalovirus infections with 9-(1,3-dihydroxy-2-propoxymethyl)guanine in patients with AIDS and other immunodeficiencies. Collaborative DHPG Treatment Study Group. *N Engl J Med* 314:801, 1986.
85. Gustafson T, Schaffer W, et al: Invasive aspergillosis in renal transplant recipients: correlation with corticosteroid therapy. *J Infect Dis* 148:230, 1983.

86. Hall C, McBride J, et al: Ribavirin treatment of respiratory syncytial viral infection in infants with underlying cardiopulmonary disease. *JAMA* 254:3047, 1985.
87. Hall C, Powell K, et al: Respiratory syncytial virus infection in children with compromised immune function. *N Engl J Med* 315:77, 1986.
88. Hallerback B, Unge P, et al: Omeprazole or ranitidine in long-term treatment of reflux esophagitis. The Scandinavian Clinics for United Research Group. *Gastroenterology* 107:1305, 1994.
89. Harmon A, Harmon M, et al: Evidence of interferon production in the hamster lung after primary or secondary exposure to parainfluenza virus type 3. *Am Rev Respir Dis* 125:706, 1982.
90. Hassall E: Wrap session: is the Nissen slipping? Can medical treatment replace surgery for severe gastroesophageal reflux disease in children? *Am J Gastroenterol* 90:1212, 1995.
91. Hayden F, Osterhaus A, et al: Efficacy and safety of the neuraminidase inhibitor Zanamivir in the treatment of influenza virus infections. GG167 Influenza Study Group. *N Engl J Med* 337:874-880, 1997.
92. Henderson A, Kelly W, et al: Fulminant primary *Pseudomonas aeruginosa* pneumonia and septicaemia in previously well adults (review). *Intensive Care Med* 18:430, 1992.
93. Henderson F, Clyde WJ, et al: The etiologic and epidemiologic spectrum of bronchiolitis in pediatric practice. *J Pediatr* 183:179, 1995.
94. Herrera GA, Smith P, et al: National, state, and urban area vaccination coverage levels among children aged 19-35 months—United States, 1998. *MMWR Surveill Summ* 49:1-26, 2000.
95. Holleron W, Wilbur J, et al: Empiric amphotericin B therapy in patients with acute leukemia. *Rev Infect Disease* 7:619, 1985.
96. Horowitz M, Schiff M, et al: *Pneumocystis carinii*: pleural effusion. *Am Rev Respir Dis* 148:232, 1993.
97. Hryniewicz W: Epidemiology of MRSA. *Infection* 27(suppl 2): S13-S16, 1999.
98. Huang L, Hecht F, et al: Suspected *Pneumocystis carinii* pneumonia with a negative induced sputum examination. *Am J Respir Crit Care Med* 151:1866, 1995.
99. Hughes W: *Pneumocystis carinii* pneumonitis. In Chernick V, editor: *Kendig's disorders of the respiratory tract in children.* Philadelphia, 1990, WB Saunders.
100. Ingbar D, White D: Acute respiratory failure. *Crit Care Clin* 4:11, 1988.
101. Johnson P, Sarosi G, et al: Progressive disseminated histoplasmosis in patients with the acquired immunodeficiency syndrome. *Semin Respir Infect* 1:1, 1986.
102. Jordens J, Leaves N, et al: Polymerase chain reaction-based strain characterization on noncapsulate *Haemophilus influenzae*. *J Clin Microbiol* 31:2981, 1993.
103. Kagawa F, Kirsch C, et al: Serum lactate dehydrogenase activity in patients with AIDS and *Pneumocystis carinii* pneumonia. *Chest* 94:1031, 1988.
104. Kaiser L, Henry D, et al: Short-term treatment with Zanamivir to prevent influenza: results of a placebo-controlled study. *Clin Infect Dis* 30:587-589, 2000.
105. Kaplan SL: Newer pediatric pathogens. *Adv Pediatr* 46:189-206, 1999.
106. Karjoo M, Kane R: Omeprazole treatment of children with peptic esophagitis refractory to ranitidine therapy. *Arch Pediatri Adolesc Med* 149:267, 1995.
107. Kato R, Sawafuji M, et al: Massive hemoptysis successfully treated by modified bronchoscopic balloon tamponade technique. *Chest* 109:842, 1996.
108. Kennedy G, Kanter R, et al: Can early bacterial complications of aspiration with respiratory failure be predicted? *Pediatr Emerg Care* 8:123, 1992.
109. Khampirad T, Glezen W: Clinical and radiologic assessment of acute lower respiratory tract disease in infants and children. *Semin Respir Infect* 2:130, 1987.
110. Kimmel K, Wyde P, et al: Evidence of a T-cell-mediated cytotoxic response to parainfluenza virus type 3 pneumonia in hamsters. *J Reticuloendothel Soc* 31:71, 1982.
111. Kirkpatrick WR, McAtee RK, et al: Efficacy of voriconazole in a guinea pig model of disseminated invasive aspergillosis. *Antimicrob Agents Chemother* 44:2865-868, 2000.
112. Klein B, Vergeront J, et al: Epidemiologic aspects of blastomycosis, the enigmatic systemic mycosis. *Semin Respir Infect* 1:29, 1986.
113. Klein B, Vergeront J, et al: Isolation of Blastomyces dermatitidis in soil associated with a large outbreak of blastomycosis in Wisconsin. *N Engl J Med* 314:529, 1986.
114. Klein M: Multicenter trial of cefpodoxime proxetil vs. amoxicillin-clavulanate in acute lower respiratory tract infections in childhood. International Study Group. *Pediatr Infect Dis J* 14(suppl 4):S19, 1995.
115. Knight V, Gilbert B: Ribavirin aerosol treatment of influenza. *Infect Dis Clin North Am* 1:441, 1987.
116. Knight V, McClung H, et al: Ribavirin small-particle aerosol treatment of influenza. *Lancet* 2:945, 2000.
117. Knott-Craig C, Oostuizen J, et al: Management and prognosis of massive hemoptysis. Recent experience with 120 patients. *J Thorac Cardiovasc Surg* 105:394, 1993.
118. Kontoyiannis DP, Bodey GP: Invasive aspergillosis in 2002: an update. *Eur J Clin Microbiol Infect Dis* 21:161-172, 2002.
119. Kovacs J, Masur H: Pneumocystis carinii pneumonia: therapy and prophylaxis. *J Infect Dis* 158:254, 1988.
120. Kuipers E, Lundell L, et al: Atrophic gastritis and *Helicobacter pylori* infection in patients with reflux esophagitis treated with omeprazole or fundoplication. *N Engl J Med* 334:1018, 1996.
121. Kulling P: Hospital treatment of victims exposed to combustion products. *Toxicology Lett Spec* 283:64-65, 1992.
122. Kumar S, et al: Pulmonary hemorrhage in a young infant. *Ann Allergy* 62:209, 1989.
123. Larouch V, Rivard G, et al: Asthma and airway hyper-responsiveness in adults who required hospital admission for bronchiolitis in early childhood. *Respir Med* 94:288-294, 2000.
124. Leaves N, Falla T, et al: 1995 The elucidation of novel capsular genotypes of *Haemophilus influenzae* type b with the polymerase chain reaction. *J Med Microbiol* 43:120, 1995.
125. Lee LM, Henderson DK: Emerging viral infections. *Curr Opin Infect Dis* 14:467-480, 2001.
126. Leggiadro R, Barrett F, et al: Disseminated histoplasmosis in infancy. *J Pediatr Infect Dis* 7:799, 1988.
127. Lhote F, Cohen P, et al: Microscopic polyangiitis: clinical aspects and treatment. *Ann Med Intern* 147:165-177, 1996.
128. Linden A, Desmecht D, et al: Pulmonary ventilation, mechanics, gas exchange and haemodynamics in calves following intratracheal inoculation of *Pasteurella haemolytica. Zentralblatt Veterinarmedizin-Reihe A* 42:531, 1995.
129. Long W, Corbet A, et al: Retrospective search for bleeding diathesis among premature newborn infants with pulmonary hemorrhage after synthetic surfactant treatment. The American Exosurf Neonatal Study Group I and the Canadian Exosurf Neonatal Study Group. *J Pediatr* 120(2 pt 2):S45, 1992.
130. Lossos I, Breuer R, et al: Bacterial pneumonia in recipients of bone marrow transplantation. A five-year prospective study. *Transplantation* 60:672, 1995.
131. Lu I, Dodds E, et al: New antifungal agents. *Semin Respir Infect* 17:140-50, 2002.
132. Marshall B, Hanson C, et al: Role of hypoxic pulmonary vasoconstriction in pulmonary gas exchange and blood flow distribution. 2. Pathophysiology. *Intensive Care Med* 20:379, 1994.
133. Martin M, Cox P, et al: A comparison of the effectiveness of three regimens in the prevention of Pneumocystis carinii pneumonia in HIV infected patients. *Arch Intern Med* 152:523, 1992.
134. Masur H, Cheigh J, et al: Prevention and treatment of Pneumocystis pneumonia. *N Engl J Med* 327:1853, 1992.
135. Mato SP, Van Dyke R: Pulmonary infections in children with HIV infection. *Semin Respir Infect* 17:33-46, 2002.
136. Matsumoto T, Homma S, et al: The lung in polyarteritis nodosa: a pathologic study of 10 cases. *Hum Pathol* 1993;24:717-724, 1993.
137. McCarthy P, Spiesel S, et al: Radiographic findings and etiologic diagnosis in ambulatory childhood pneumonias. *Clin Pediatr* 20:686, 1981.
138. McDonagh J, Greaves M, et al: High resolution computed tomography of the lungs in patients with rheumatoid arthritis and interstitial lung disease. *Br J Rheumatol* 33:118, 1994.
139. McIntosh K: Respiratory syncytial virus. In: Nelson W, Behrman R, et al., editors: *Nelson's textbook of pediatrics.* Philadelphia, 1996, WB Saunders.
140. Merkel F, Netzer KO, et al: Therapeutic options for critically ill patients suffering from progressive lupus nephritis or Goodpasture's syndrome. *Kidney Int Suppl* 64:S31-S38, 1998.

141. Miller R, Salcedo J, et al: Pulmonary hemorrhage in pediatric patients with systemic lupus erythematosus. *J Pediatr* 108:576, 1986.
142. Millunchick E, Floyd J, et al: Legionnaires disease in an immunologically normal child. *Am J Dis Child* 135:1065, 1981.
143. Mocherla S, Wheat LJ: Treatment of histoplasmosis. *Semin Respir Infect* 16:141-148, 2001.
144. Moler F, Steinhart C, et al: Effectiveness of ribavirin in otherwise well infants with RSV associated respiratory failure. *J Pediatr* 128:422, 1996.
145. Montgomerie J, Edwards J, et al: Mycoses study group: treatment of blastomycosis and histoplasmosis with ketoconazole. *Ann Intern Med* 103:861, 1985.
146. Nasim A, Akhtar R, et al: Video-thoracoscopic lung biopsy in diagnosis of interstitial lung disease. *J R Coll Surg Edinburgh* 40:22, 1995.
147. Navarro EE, Gonzaga NC, et al: Clinicopathologic studies of children who die of acute lower respiratory tract infections: mechanisms of death. *Rev Infect Dis* 12(suppl 8):S1065-S1073, 1990.
148. Neville K, Renbarger J, et al: Pneumonia in the immunocompromised pediatric cancer patient. *Semin Respir Infect* 17:21-32, 2002.
149. Noseworthy T, Anderson B: Massive hemoptysis. *Can Med J Assoc* 135:1097, 1986.
150. Odio C, McCracken GH Jr, et al: Disseminated adenovirus infection: a case report and review of the literature. *Pediatr Infect Dis* 3:46-49, 1984.
151. O'Kane G: Inhalation of ammonia vapor. *Anesthesia* 38:1208, 1983.
152. Oren I, Goldstein N: Invasive pulmonary aspergillosis. *Curr Opin Pulm Med* 8:195-200, 2002.
153. Orr O, Myerowitz R, et al: Patho-radiologic correlation of invasive pulmonary aspergillosis in the compromised host. *Cancer* 41:2028, 1978.
154. Pancham J. Complications of measles. *Nursing Times* 82:46-47, 1986.
155. Pandit P, Dunn M, et al: Surfactant therapy in neonates with respiratory deterioration due to pulmonary hemorrhage. *Pediatrics* 95:32, 1995.
156. Patel U, Pattison C, et al: Management of massive haemoptysis (review). *Br J Hosp Med* 52:74, 1994.
157. Perez-Benavides F, Riff E, et al: Adult respiratory distress syndrome and artificial surfactant replacement in the pediatric patient. *Pediatr Emerg Care* 11:153, 1995.
158. Peter G: The child with pneumonia: diagnostic and therapeutic considerations. *Pediatr Infect Dis J* 7:453, 1988.
159. Philip A: The changing face of neonatal infection: experience at a regional medical center. *Pediatr Infect Dis J* 13:1098, 1994.
160. Pickering L, Peter G, et al: *Red book*. Elk Grove Village, Ill, 2000, American Academy of Pediatrics.
161. Piedimonte G. The association between respiratory syncytial virus infection and reactive airway disease. Respir Med 96(suppl B):S25, 2002.
162. Pouwels H, Janevski B, et al: Systemic to pulmonary vascular malformation (review). *Eur Respir J* 5:1288, 1992.
163. Principi N, Esposito S: Mycoplasma pneumoniae and Chlamydia pneumoniae cause lower respiratory tract disease in paediatric patients. *Curr Opin Infect Dis* 15:295-300, 2002.
164. Prober C, Whyte H, et al: Open lung biopsy in immunocompromised children with pulmonary infiltrates. *Am J Dis Child* 138:60, 1984.
165. Raju T, Langenberg P: Pulmonary hemorrhage and exogenous surfactant therapy: a meta-analysis. *J Pediatr* 123:603, 1993.
166. Ray C, Holber C, et al: Acute lower respiratory illness during the first three years of life: potential roles for various etiologic agents. *Pediatr Infect Dis J* 12:10, 1993.
167. Reichenberger F, Habicht JM, et al: Diagnosis and treatment of invasive pulmonary aspergillosis in neutropenic patients. *Eur Respir J* 19:743-755, 2002.
168. Rippon J: *Medical mycology: the pathogenic fungi and the pathogenic actinomycetes*. Philadelphia, 1988, WB Saunders.
169. Rodriquez W, Parrott R: Ribavirin aerosol treatment of serious respiratory syncytial virus infections in infants. *Infect Dis Clin North Am* 1:425, 1987.
170. Rorison D, McPherson S: Acute toxic inhalations. *Emerg Med Clin North Am* 10:409, 1992.
171. Rosenow E, Myers J, et al: Drug-induced pulmonary disease: an update. *Chest* 102:239-250, 1992.
172. Rubinstein A, Morecki R, et al: Pulmonary disease in children with acquired immune deficiency syndrome and AIDS-related complex. *J Pediatr* 108:498-503, 1986.
173. Ruddy R: Smoke inhalation injury. *Pediatr Clin North Am* 41:317, 1994.
174. Russian DA, Levine SJ: *Pneumocystis carinii* pneumonia in patients without HIV infection. *Am J Med Sci* 321:56-65, 2001.
175. Sarubbi F, Kopf H, et al: Increased recovery of Aspergillosis flavus from respiratory specimens during hospital construction. *Am Rev Respir Dis* 125:33, 1982.
176. Saubolle M, Wright R: Comparative value of urine latex agglutination for detection of four bacterial antigens. Inter-science Conference on Antimicrobial Agents and Chemotherapy, New Orleans, Louisiana, 1986.
177. Scannell G, Waxman K, et al: Respiratory distress in traumatized and burned children. *J Pediatr Surg* 30:612, 1995.
178. Schrag SJ, Zywicki S, et al: Group B streptococcal disease in the era of intrapartum antibiotic prophylaxis. *N Engl J Med* 342:15-20, 2000.
179. Sharief N, Crawford O, et al: Fibrosing alveolitis and desquamative interstitial pneumonitis. *Pediatr Pulmonol* 17:359, 1994.
180. Sheibel S, Hayden F: Stay alert for the serious sequelae of influenza. *J Respir Dis* 6:21, 1985.
181. Shepp D, Danliker P, et al: Activity of 9-[2-hydroxy1 (hydroxymethyl) ethoxymethyl] guanine in the treatment of cytomegalovirus pneumonia. *Ann Intern Med* 103:368, 1985.
182. Shigeta S: Recent progress in antiviral chemotherapy for respiratory syncytial virus infections. *Exp Opin Investig Drugs* 9:221-235, 2000.
183. Shinefield H, Black S: Postlicensure surveillance for Haemophilus influenzae type b invasive disease after use of Haemophilus influenzae type b oligosaccharide CRM197 conjugate vaccine in a large defined United States population: a four-year eight-month follow-up. *Pediatr Infect Dis J* 14:978, 1995.
184. Sigurs N: Epidemiologic and clinical evidence of a respiratory syncytial virus-reactive airway disease link. *Am J Respir Crit Care Med* 163(3 pt 2):52-56, 2001.
185. Simonsen L, Clarke MJ, et al: The impact of influenza epidemics on mortality: introducing a severity index. *Am J Public Health* 87:1944-1950, 1997.
186. Simsir A, Greenebaum E, et al: Late fatal adenovirus pneumonitis in a lung transplant recipient. *Transplantation* 65:592-594, 1998.
187. Smego R Jr, Nagar S, et al: A meta-analysis of salvage therapy for Pneumocystis carinii pneumonia. *Arch Intern Med* 161: 1529-1533, 2001.
188. Smith I, Holley K, et al: Cytomegalovirus studies of autopsy tissue I. Virus isolation. *Ann Clin Pathol* 63:854, 1975.
189. Sniadack D, Schwartz B, et al: Potential interventions for the prevention of childhood pneumonia: geographic and temporal differences in serotype and serogroup distribution of sterile site pneumococcal isolates from children-implications for vaccine strategies. *Pediatr Infect Dis J* 14:503, 1995.
190. Soubani AO, Chandrasekar PH: The clinical spectrum of pulmonary aspergillosis. *Chest* 121:1988-1999, 1988.
191. Specter SC, Hodinka RL, et al: Clinical Virology Manual. Washington, D.C., 2000, American Society of Microbiology.
192. States LJ, Fields JM : Pulmonary hemorrhage in children. *Semin Roentgenol* 33:174-186, 1998.
193. Stevens DA, Shatsky SA: Intrathecal amphotericin in the management of coccidioidal meningitis. *Semin Respir Infect* 16:263-269, 2001.
194. Stogner SW, King JW, et al: Ribavirin and intravenous immune globulin therapy for measles pneumonia in HIV infection. *South Med J* 86:1415-1418, 1993.
195. Sugar AM: Overview: antifungal combination therapy. *Curr Opin Investig Drugs* 2:1364-1365, 2001.
196. Sullivan KM, Dykewicz CA, et al: Preventing opportunistic infections after hematopoietic stem cell transplantation: the Centers for Disease Control and Prevention, Infectious Diseases Society of America, and American Society for Blood and Marrow Transplantation Practice Guidelines and beyond. *Hematology* 392, 2001.

197. Sutton DA, Fothergill AW, et al: *Guide to clinically significant fungi*. Baltimore, 1998, Williams & Wilkins.
198. Swischuk L, Heureux P: Unilateral pulmonary vein atresia. *Am J Radiol* 135:667, 1980.
199. Takimoto S, Grandien M, et al: Comparison of enzme-linked immunosorbent assay, indirect immunofluorescence assay, and virus isolation for detection of respiratory viruses in nasopharyngeal secretions. *J Clin Microbiol* 29:470, 1987.
200. Thomson BJ, Dalgleish AG: Human retroviruses and pediatric disease. *Arch Dis Child* 62:631-634, 1987.
201. Tominack R, Hayden F: Rimantadine hydrochloride and amantadine hydrochloride use in influenza A virus infections. *Infect Dis Clin North Am* 1:459, 1987.
202. Treanor J, Hayden F, et al: Efficacy and safety o the oral neuraminidase inhibitor Oseltamivir in treating acute influenza: a randomized controlled trial. US Oral Neuraminidase Study Group. *JAMA* 283:1016-1024, 2000.
203. Van Dyke R: Antiviral therapy for pulmonary infections. In Hilman B, editor: *Pediatric respiratory disease*. Philadelphia, 1993, WB Saunders.
204. Vandenplas Y: Diagnosis and treatment of gastroesophageal reflux disease in infants and children. *Can J Gastroenterol* 14(suppl D): 26D-34D, 2000.
205. Vandenplas Y, Hegar B: Diagnosis and treatment of gastro-oesophageal reflux disease in infants and children. *J Gastroenterol Hepatol* 15:593-603, 2000.
206. Vasconcelles M, Bernardo M, et al: Aerosolized pentamidine as Pneumocystis prophylaxis after bone marrow transplantation is inferior to other regimens and is associated with decreased survival and an increased risk of other infections. *Biol Blood Marrow Transplant* 6:35-43, 2000.
207. Wakefield A: *Pneumocystis carinii*. *Br Med Bull* 61:175-188, 2002.
208. Wallach FR: Infectious disease. Update on treatment of pneumonia, influenza, and urinary tract infections. *Geriatrics* 56:43-47, 2001.
209. Walsh T, Pizzo P: Fungal infections in granulocytopenic patients current approaches to classification, diagnosis and treatment. In Holmgerg K, Meyer R, editors: *Diagnosis and therapy of systemic mycoses*. New York, 1989, Raven Press.
210. Wassermann K, Pothoff G, et al: Chronic *Pneumocystis carinii* pneumonia in AIDS. *Chest* 104:667, 1993.
211. Webb A: The treatment of pulmonary infection in cystic fibrosis (review). *Scand Infect Dis* 96(suppl):24, 1995.
212. Welliver R, Wong D, et al: Natural history of parainfluenza virus infection in childhood. *J Pediatr* 101:180, 1982.
213. Welliver R, Wong D, et al: Role of parainfluenza virus-specific IgE in pathogens of croup and wheezing. *J Pediatr* 101:889, 1982.
214. Welliver R, Wong D, et al: The development of respiratory syncytial virus-specific IgE and the release of histamine in nasopharyngeal secretions after infection. *N Engl J Med* 305: 841, 1981.
215. Wenzel R, McCormick D, et al: Parainfluenza pneumonia in adults. *JAMA* 221:294, 1972.
216. West J, Mathieu-Costello O: Stress failure of pulmonary capillaries in the intensive care setting (review). *Schweiz Med Wochenschr* 20:751, 1992.
217. Wheat J, Sarosi G, et al: Practice guidelines for the management of patients with histoplasmosis. Infectious Diseases Society of America. *Clin Infect Dis* 30:688-695, 2000.
218. Wheat LJ, Goldman M, et al: State-of-the-art review of pulmonary fungal infections. *Semin Respir Infect* 17:158-181, 2002.
219. Whitley R: Viral encephalitis. *N Engl J Med* 323:242-250, 1990.
220. Wilde M, McTavish D: Omeprazole. An update of its pharmacology and therapeutic use in acid-related disorders. *Drugs* 48:91, 1994.
221. Wong-Beringer A, Jacobs RA, et al: Lipid formulations of amphotericin B: clinical efficacy and toxicities. *Clin Infect Dis* 27:603-618, 1998.
222. Yeung C: Massive pulmonary hemorrhage in neonatal infection. *Can Med J Assoc* 114:135, 1976.
223. Zahradnik J: Adenovirus pneumonia. *Semin Respir Infect* 2:104, 1987.
224. Zhang J, Cui Z, et al: Bronchial arteriography and transcatheter embolization in the management of hemoptysis. *Cardiovasc Interv Radiol* 17:276, 1994.
225. Zhang ZJ, Wang ZL, et al: Acute respiratory infections in childhood in Beijing: an etiological study of pneumonia and bronchiolitis. *Chin Med J* 99:695-702, 1986.

CHAPTER

43

Diseases of Pulmonary Circulation

Vasanth H. Kumar and Frederick C. Morin III

PEARLS

- Multiple factors influence normal growth and development of the pulmonary vasculature in utero, which is critical for achieving successful transition to postnatal life.
- The onset of ventilation and lung inflation at birth with a resultant increase in oxygen tension decreases pulmonary vascular resistance (PVR), which is essential for establishing normal postnatal circulatory pattern.
- Elevated PVR resulting from either vasoconstriction or structural remodeling of the pulmonary vasculature characterizes persistent pulmonary hypertension of the newborn (PPHN).
- An increase in pulmonary vascular smooth muscle can occur in utero or after birth, resulting from peripheral extension of the smooth muscle into vessels that do not normally contain muscle layers, contributing to the pathology of PPHN.
- The gold standard in defining PPHN rests on the echocardiographic findings of right to left shunting of blood at the foramen ovale and/or ductus arteriosus, as well as estimates of pulmonary arterial pressures (PAP).
- In children, it is important to establish an accurate diagnosis with respect to etiology, because therapy may vary with etiology of pulmonary hypertension (PHT).
- Exertional dyspnea, chest pain, syncope, frequent fatigue, and dizziness are some of the typical symptoms of pulmonary hypertension in children.
- Overall exercise capacity, symptoms as assessed by WHO classification, and hemodynamic parameters of right ventricular function help in deciding the therapy for pulmonary hypertension in children.
- High frequency oscillatory ventilation, surfactant therapy, and nitric oxide have decreased considerably the need for extracorporeal membrane oxygenation (ECMO) in infants with PPHN.
- Even though prostacyclin is the mainstay of therapy of pulmonary hypertension in children, newer analogues of prostacyclin, phosphodiesterase (PDE) inhibitors, and endothelin receptor antagonists have widened the medical choices available in the management of these children.
- Aggressive medical therapy combined with early recognition of lung transplant candidates will improve quality of life and survival of children with pulmonary hypertension.

Etiology and Treatment of Pulmonary Hypertension

This chapter addresses the neonatal and pediatric aspects of pulmonary hypertension (PHT). First, unique aspects of fetal and postnatal development of pulmonary vasculature, transitional circulation, and developmental regulation of pulmonary vascular tone are discussed. This background helps in understanding the pathophysiology and treatment of pulmonary vascular disorders in newborns and children.

Developmental Pulmonary Vascular Anatomy

Embryology

The vascular network of the developing endodermal pair of lung buds is derived from the surrounding mesenchyme of the splanchnic mesoderm beginning at 4 weeks of gestation. These vessels accompany the developing airways, differentiate into arteries, and join the larger pulmonary arteries that originate from the sixth aortic arch. By week 9 of gestation, with each airway generation there is an accompanying artery, and by week 16 of gestation, the number of preacinar airways and accompanying arteries is complete. Thereafter, as the acini develop (terminal bronchiole, respiratory bronchiole, alveolar ducts, and alveoli), so do the accompanying arteries. Intraacinar arterial development accompanies alveolar growth, which begins in utero and continues through the first 3 years postnatally. The pulmonary vasculature increases dramatically in both number and surface area during the last few months of fetal life, and capillary growth appears to play a key role in the formation of new alveoli. The veins arise separately within the loose mesenchyme of the lung septa and subsequently connect to the developing left atrium.

Distinctions can be recognized between the proximal and distal pulmonary vasculature both in terms of their embryonic origins and the morphogenetic processes by which they develop. The sixth branchial arch is the embryonic origin of the proximal pulmonary vasculature, and it develops by the process of vasculogenesis. Vasculogenesis is the differentiation and segregation of angioblasts within the mesenchyme, which forms early vascular channels (arteries, veins, and lymphatics), depending on local influences from the epithelium and the mesenchyme. The lung mesenchyme is the embryonic origin of the distal vasculature, which develops by angiogenesis. Angiogenesis is the formation of new vessels from preexisting vascular channels by proliferation and migration of endothelial cells at the tips, which form multiple capillary sprouts. Abnormal maturation or maturational arrest in pulmonary arterial development is reflected in functional derangement that can appear in the newborn period. Persistent pulmonary hypertension of the newborn (PPHN) has been reported in association with pulmonary arterial maturational arrest at week 5 of gestation.[1] Normal growth and development of the pulmonary circulation in utero is critical for achieving successful transition to postnatal life.

Multiple factors influence development and growth of pulmonary vasculature in utero, including growth factors. Growth factors such as vascular endothelial growth factor[2] and fibroblast growth factor[3] appear to be responsible for orderly growth and branching morphogenesis of blood vessels. Growth and matrix production (especially elastin and collagen) in blood vessels are regulated by insulin-like growth factor-1[4] and transforming growth factor-β.[5] Quantity, timing, and location are critical determinants of the net effects of these agents. The balance of proteases and antiproteases also determines the regulation of growth factor interaction with cell surface molecules. Other factors that modulate structural vascular development include adhesion molecules, cytokines, extracellular matrix interactions, and later in gestation hemodynamic stimuli, nutrients, and hormonal influences. The mechanical stress that endothelial cells must withstand may be the predominant force responsible for development of large vessels after onset of circulation.[6]

Vascular Smooth Muscle

In the normal fetal and term lung, fully muscularized thick-walled preacinar arteries extend to the level of terminal bronchioles, whereas the intraacinar arteries (i.e., those accompanying respiratory bronchioles) are partially muscular (surrounded by a spiral of muscle) or nonmuscular. Arteries at alveolar ducts and alveolar walls are nonmuscular. Preacinar arteries in the fetus late in gestation and in the newborn have thicker coats of smooth muscle relative to the arterial diameter than do similar arteries in adults, although the fetus actually has less distal extension of smooth muscle in smaller arteries than do older children or adults. Figure 43–1 shows the diagrammatic representation of the extension of arterial smooth muscle within the acinus as a function of age.

Experimental studies suggest that the immediate postnatal period is characterized by rapid recruitment of small alveolar duct and alveolar wall vessels, which appear to be functionally and structurally closed in the prenatal period.[7] There is also progressive dilation of muscular arteries. Within a few days, the smallest muscular arteries (<250 μm) dilate and their walls thin to adult levels. By age 4 months, this process has included the largest pulmonary arteries at the hilum. As intraacinar arteries increase in external diameter, muscle extends peripherally. At first, nonmuscular arteries become partially muscular and later become fully muscularized. In infancy, vessels at the alveolar duct level are still largely nonmuscular, but in childhood they become partially muscularized and in the adult they are fully muscularized.[8] Alveolar wall arteries remain largely nonmuscular, even in the adult. Nonmuscularized arteries in utero contain precursors of smooth muscle cells (SMCs), called *pericytes* or *intermediate cells*, which undergo early differentiation into mature SMCs in response to different stimuli, such as chronic hypertension, increasing vascular tone, and reactivity. An increase in intrauterine vascular smooth muscle, resulting from peripheral extension of smooth muscle into vessels that do not normally contain muscle layers, may contribute to the pathophysiology of PPHN. Neonates who die of PHT may have a striking distal extension of smooth

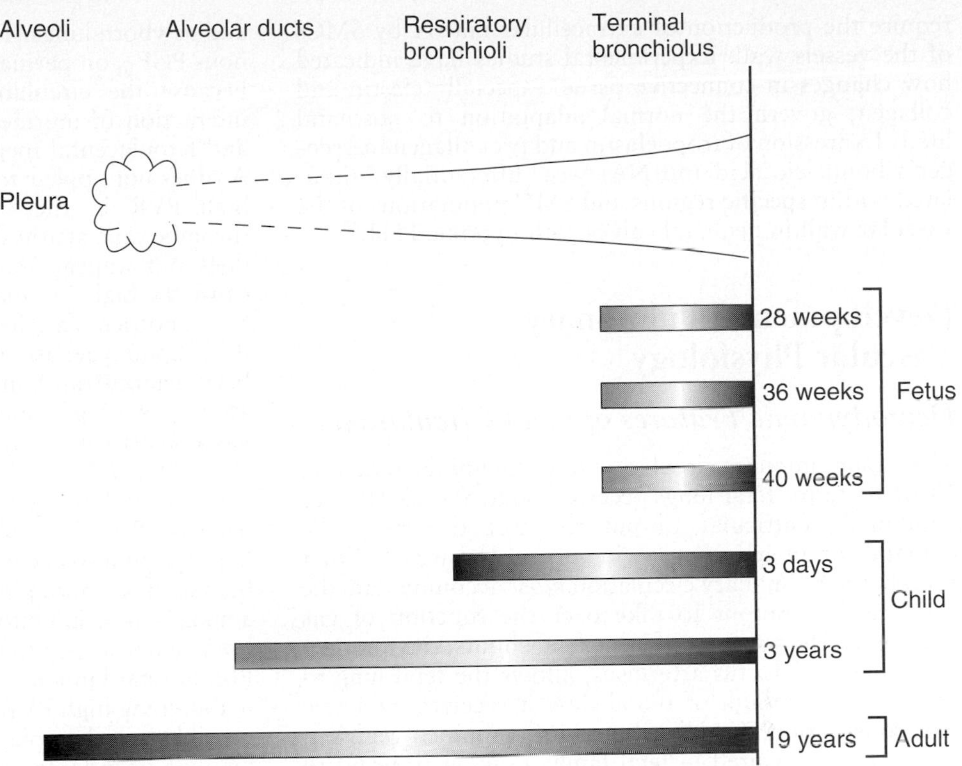

FIGURE 43–1 • "Extension" of muscular arteries within the acinus. In the fetus, muscular arteries are not found with the respiratory bronchiolus or beyond. During childhood, they extend further, until they reach distal alveoli in the adult. The acinus is the respiratory unit supplied by a terminal bronchiolus. (From Reid L: *Am Rev Respir Dis* 199: 531, 1979.)

muscle in the intraacinar region, thickening of the media and adventitia, and excessive accumulation of the matrix protein in the pulmonary vessels.[9] The increase in vascular smooth muscle and its peripheral extension can occur either prenatally or postnatally. In utero ductal ligation 1 to 2 weeks prior to delivery results in severe PHT at birth associated with distal extension of vascular smooth muscle in newborn lambs[10] (Figure 43–2). Hypoxia at birth prevents remodeling of the smooth muscle of the preacinar arteries. Increased muscularization of the pulmonary arteries has been described in infants dying of severe meconium aspiration syndrome (MAS) with PPHN.

Newborn SMCs underexpress many of the contractile proteins thought to be important in SMC contraction, compared with adult SMCs. Maturation of the vessel wall is accompanied by a transition of actin, a major contractile protein from a β-nonmuscle isoform to a smooth muscle specific α-type protein. Even though pulmonary artery protein content is unaltered by persistent PHT in fetal sheep, there is a decrease in expression of both smooth muscle myosin heavy-chain isoform and an increase in nonmuscle isoform myosin heavy-chain B.[11] The acquisition of contractile phenotype by SMCs in mature vessel walls is associated with an increased ability to contract and relax and decreased potential for cell replication. The fact that neonatal SMCs underexpress many of the contractile and cytoskeletal proteins found in fully mature SMCs may contribute to the rapid hyperplastic response observed in the neonatal vascular wall in response to stress. SMCs produce the bulk of the connective tissue, particularly elastin and collagen, which constitute a major part of large pulmonary arteries. Elastin provides for vascular distensibility, whereas collagen is necessary for vascular integrity. Vascular integrity and continued cell differentiation also

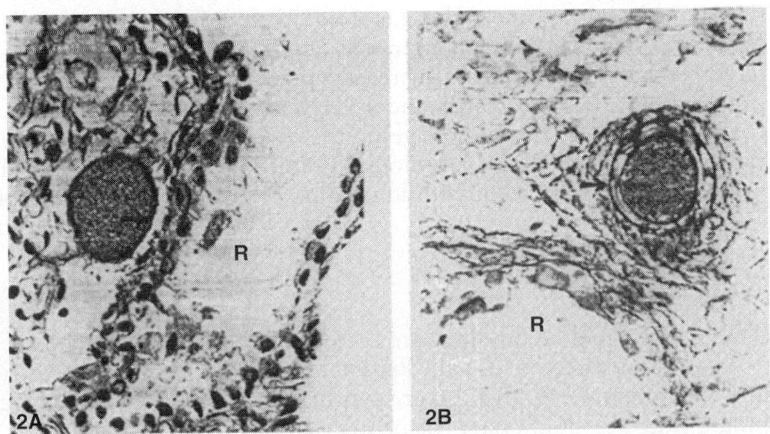

FIGURE 43–2 • Photomicrograph of branches of the pulmonary artery associated with respiratory bronchioles. The lumen of each artery is filled with densely staining barium-gelatin particles. **A,** Pulmonary artery (25 μm ED) with a single elastic lamina *(arrow)* and a nonmuscular arterial wall from a control lamb. **B,** Pulmonary artery (28.5 μm ED) with a double elastic lamina *(arrows),* muscularized arterial wall, and adventitial fibrosis from a lamb in which the ductus arteriosus was ligated for 15 days in utero. *R,* Respiratory bronchiole. Paraffin embedded section (4 μm) stained with Miller elastic stain. (From Wild LM, Nickerson PA, Morin FC III: *Pediatr Res* 25:251-257, 1989.)

require the production of extracellular matrix by SMCs of the vessels wall. Experimental studies have indicated how changes in connective tissue, especially elastin and collagen, govern the normal adaptation to postnatal life.[12] Expression of tropoelastin and procollagen messenger ribonucleic acid (mRNA) was differentially stimulated within specific regions and SMC populations of the vascular wall in neonatal calves with hypoxic PHT.[12]

Developmental Pulmonary Vascular Physiology

Hemodynamic Features of Fetal Circulation

The fetal pulmonary circulation fulfills a unique function. Close to term, fetal lungs receive about 5% to 10% of combined ventricular output to meet the metabolic demands of an actively growing organ, but with the first breath, the pulmonary circulation must accommodate the total cardiac output to take over the function of gas exchange. The presence of large fetal shunts, the foramen ovale and the ductus arteriosus, allows the fetal lung to regulate the amount of blood flow it receives by active vasoconstriction. The distribution of combined ventricular output, measured in fetal lambs ranging from 60 to 150 days gestational age, indicates that the lungs receive only about 3.5% of total output at 0.4 term, but the fraction increases to almost 8% at term.[13] This remarkable increase in fetal pulmonary perfusion presumably is related to growth of the fetal lung. The lung increases in weight by sixfold from midgestation to term,[14] and the number of pulmonary vessels increases more than tenfold.[15] Thus the tremendous increase in cross-sectional area of pulmonary vasculature permits pulmonary blood flow (PBF) to increase throughout gestation. However, PBF remains relatively constant when corrected for wet lung weight with advancing gestation.[16] A gradual increase in pulmonary arterial pressure (PAP), accompanied by a relatively constant flow per unit lung tissue, reveals increasing fetal pulmonary vascular resistance (PVR) with advancing gestation.[16] A major part of this increase comes from elevated pulmonary vascular tone associated with low Po_2 in the fetal lung.[16–18] Maintaining high PVR in utero is important because the function of gas exchange is performed not by the lungs but by the placenta. Thus in utero the PBF is apparently regulated at a level of perfusion that is necessary to meet the metabolic demands of the fetal lung. Ligation of ductus arteriosus of fetal lamb several days before delivery causes increased pulmonary artery pressure (PAP) before birth and PPHN after birth.[19–21] It also produces anatomic changes in the distal pulmonary vascular bed similar to pathologic alterations reported in human neonates dying with idiopathic PPHN.[10]

Regulation of Pulmonary Vascular Tone In Utero

Arachidonic acid metabolites are some of the most powerful vasoconstrictors known. Prostaglandin $F_{2\alpha}$ ($PGF_{2\alpha}$) and thromboxane A_2 (TXA_2) are synthesized by the fetal lung[22] and are pulmonary vasoconstrictors in the fetal and newborn lungs. The effects of exogenous and endogenous $PGF_{2\alpha}$ on perinatal circulation are difficult to assess because the circulatory response involves a complex interaction of uterine, umbilical, and ductal blood flow and fetoplacental metabolism of $PGF_{2\alpha}$.[23] Thromboxane A_2 does not appear to be responsible for maintenance of high PVR in the fetus.[24] Blocking prostaglandin or thromboxane synthesis does not decrease PVR.[25] Thus it does not appear that prostaglandins or thromboxane cause the high vascular tone of the fetal lung.

Leukotrienes are formed from arachidonic acid through the 5-lipooxygenase pathways. Lipoxygenase activity has been demonstrated in human fetal lung as early as 12 to 18 weeks of gestation.[26] LTC4 and LTD4 are potent vasoconstrictors of systemic and pulmonary circulations of newborn lambs.[27] Leukotriene inhibition using an experimental antagonist (FPL55712) has been shown to decrease PVR in fetal lambs by 45%.[28] It also reverses hypoxic pulmonary vasoconstriction in newborn lambs[29] but not in newborn piglets.[30] Infusion of piriprost (U60257), a lipoxygenase inhibitor, directly into pulmonary artery has been demonstrated to reduce PVR by 87% and to increase PBF in fetal lambs.[31] The specific role of leukotrienes in maintaining high PVR in immature fetuses is unclear. It is possible that they play a role in pathologic states such as hypoxia or inflammation.

One mechanism that does contribute to high PVR in fetal lamb as it approaches term is vasoconstriction in response to low oxygen tension.[18] Decreasing oxygen tension in fetuses at 103 to 104 days of gestation does not increase PVR, but it doubles resistance in fetuses at 132 to 138 days. Conversely, increasing oxygen tension does not change PVR before 100 days of gestation, but it decreases resistance markedly and increases blood flow to normal newborn levels at 135 days of gestation.[16]

Endothelins (ETs) are 21-residue peptides,[32] whose role in regulating vascular tone and vasomotor responses has been studied intensively in the past decade. Three distinct ET isoforms have been described: endothelin-1 (ET-1), endothelin-2 (ET-2), and endothelin-3 (ET-3), cleaved from ET precursors big ET-1, big ET-2, and big ET-3, respectively, by an ET-converting enzyme. Endothelin-1 synthesized by vascular endothelial cells is a potent vasoconstrictor,[33] and its effects on both animal and human studies vary with the tone of the pulmonary vessels, dose of ET-1, and the maturation of vessels.[34,35] Both ET-1 and ET-2 have been shown to dilate the fetal (normally high tone) pulmonary vasculature and constrict the bed when the tone is reduced by ventilation.[36] Thus it appears that the response of pulmonary vasculature to ETs is tone dependent. Currently two receptor subtypes, ET_a and ET_b, are thought to mediate responses to ETs. The ET_b receptor plays a role in vasodilation and ET_a receptor in vasoconstriction. Some investigators suggest a significant role for ET_{b1} receptor in vasodilation and, ET_{b2} receptor and ET_a receptor in vasoconstriction.[37,38] Vasoconstriction induced by ET-1 is mediated by prostaglandins[39] and calcium,[40] whereas the vasodilator properties are mediated by potassium[41] and endothelium-derived nitric oxide (NO).[37,42] ET-1 may play a role in the change that occurs in the pulmonary vasculature at birth.[43,44] Two studies have attempted to define the role of ET receptor subtypes in response to ET-1 in chronically instrumented fetal sheep.[45,46] Endothelin-1 may play a role in maintaining high vascular resistance of the fetal lung. However, ET_{b1} receptors mediate vasodilator responses to ET-1 in the fetus, and there is a suggestion that abundance of ET_{b1} receptors may be of physiologic importance in decreasing PVR at birth.[46] It is possible that prenatally endogenous ET-1 primarily stimulates ET_a receptors to cause vasoconstriction and that ET_{b1} receptors are less active in fetal life.[45]

Transitional Circulation

The first stage of transitional circulation is essentially a fetal pulmonary circulation that is characterized by high pressure and low flow because of both passive and active elevation of PVR. The passive resistance most likely is related to compression of pulmonary capillaries by fetal lung liquid, but there is also a high degree of active vasomotor tone resulting from hypoxic stimuli. This hypoxic increase in active pulmonary vascular tone is a dominant feature in the behavior of pulmonary vasculature at all stages of development but is more active in the fetus, perhaps because of a relatively much larger vascular muscle mass than in the adult. Thus PVR exceeds systemic vascular resistance (SVR), resulting in right atrial and ventricular pressures exceeding left atrial and ventricular pressures. High PVR results in right-to-left shunting of blood across the foramen ovale, and most of the blood ejected by the right ventricle flows across the ductus arteriosus into the descending aorta. Persistence of elevated PVR after birth without the benefit of placental oxygenation results in profound hypoxemia that characterizes PPHN.

The second stage of normal transition is accomplished when the fluid-filled fetal lungs are distended with air during the first breath. A rapid decrease in PVR occurs with mechanical distension of the pulmonary vascular bed. The entry of air into the alveoli improves oxygenation of the pulmonary vascular bed, further decreasing PVR. At birth PVR decreases dramatically. This leads to an eightfold increase in PBF. The increase in PBF raises left atrial pressures above right atrial pressures, closing the foramen ovale. SVR increases at birth, in part because of removal of the low resistance bed of the placenta. As PVR becomes less than systemic, flow across the ductus reverses. Within the first 5 minutes after birth, oxygen-induced vasodilation and lung expansion decrease PVR to approximately half of systemic resistance. Over the first few hours after birth, the ductus arteriosus closes, largely in response to the increase in oxygen tension. At this point the normal postnatal circulatory pattern is established.

The third stage of transitional circulation occurs for 12 to 24 hours after birth and accounts for the greatest reduction in PVR. In the final phase of neonatal pulmonary vascular transition, further decline in PVR is accompanied by rapid structural remodeling of the entire pulmonary bed from the main pulmonary arteries to the capillaries. During this remodeling, changes in SMC shape and geometric orientation cause luminal enlargement. Maturation of smooth muscle function, thinning of endothelial cells, and more gradual changes in elastic and connective tissue occur over the next few weeks.

Factors Responsible for Decrease in Pulmonary Vascular Resistance at Birth

The onset of ventilation and inflation of lungs at birth with a resultant increase in oxygen tension in the lungs leads to a decrease in PVR. Each of these stimuli has been shown to decrease vascular resistance and increase blood flow in the lungs of fetal lambs.[47] Increasing oxygen tension alone decreased PVR and increased blood flow to the fetal lungs quantitatively as expected at birth.[16] Inflation of lungs with gas may decrease resistance, at least in part by mechanical effects. Oxygen may dilate in part by direct effects on vascular smooth muscle.[48]

The drop in PVR soon after birth is accompanied with by production of prostacyclin (PGI_2) and NO. Arachidonic acid metabolites such as prostaglandins are potent pulmonary vasodilators in the fetus. PGI_2 synthesized by endothelial cells appears to relax smooth muscle by producing cyclic adenosine monophosphate (cAMP). PGI_2 and its metabolites are more potent vasodilators than PGE_2. Even though blockade of prostaglandin synthesis either by indomethacin[49] or meclofenamate[25] blunts the decrease in PVR, the magnitude of the role of PGI_2 at birth has been questioned. Pretreatment of fetal lamb with the cyclooxygenase inhibitor indomethacin decreased PGI_2 production and prevented the late fall in PVR,[49,50] but it does not disrupt the transition to gas exchange. The role of cyclooxygenase and PGI_2 in the transitional circulation may have clinical implications. Persistent pulmonary hypertension of the newborn has been observed in infants of mothers receiving aspirin or nonsteroidal antiinflammatory drugs that inhibit cyclooxygenase activity. In this situation, the inhibitor acts through prenatal constriction of the ductus arteriosus[51] or by decreasing PGI_2 synthesis at birth. The cAMP signal transduction pathway is shown in Figure 43–3.

Acetylcholine, bradykinin,[52] and histamine[53] are fetal pulmonary vasodilators, which in many species act by an endothelium-dependent mechanism. They stimulate the production of NO by vascular endothelium. NO activates soluble guanylate cyclase to produce the second messenger cyclic guanosine monophosphate (cGMP). cGMP induces relaxation of vascular smooth muscle through activation of a cGMP-dependent protein kinase that produces a lowering of intracellular calcium, in part through activation of potassium channel.[54] There is strong evidence that NO is an important mediator of the decrease in PVR at birth. NO is a potent dilator of the fetal pulmonary circulation.[55–57] The dilation of fetal pulmonary circulation caused by an increase in oxygen tension is mediated in large part by endogenous synthesis of NO.[58] Prolonged administration of L-NA in late gestation lambs to block endogenous NO synthesis does not affect basal PVR but markedly blunts the decrease in PVR observed at birth.[59]

The purines adenosine triphosphate (ATP) and adenosine are potent pulmonary vasodilators in the fetal lambs that may also be involved at birth.[60,61] Studies of the

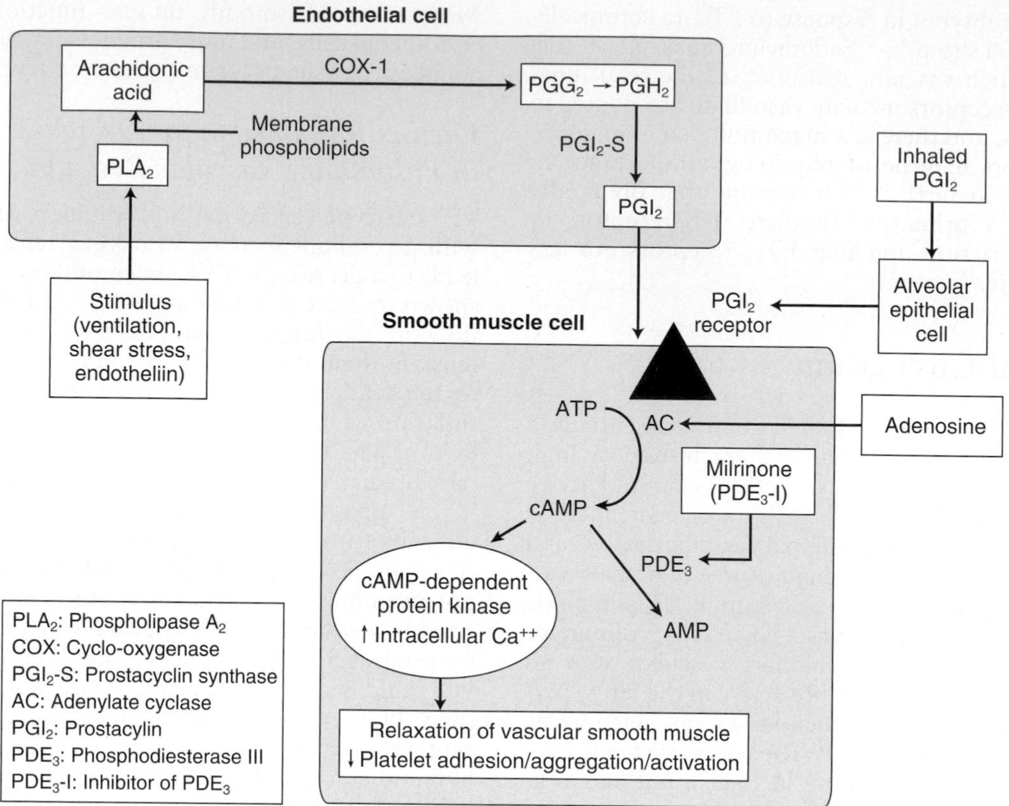

FIGURE 43–3 • Cyclic adenosine monophosphate signal transduction pathway of vasodilation. *AC,* Adenylate cyclase; *COX,* cyclooxygenase; *PDE_3,* phosphodiesterase III; *PDE_3-I,* PDE_3 inhibitor; *PGI_2,* prostacyclin; *PGI_2-S,* prostacyclin synthase; *PLA_2,* phospholipase A_2.

pulmonary effects of adenosine, ATP, and their antagonists indicate that adenosine and ATP play a significant role in the mediation of oxygen-induced pulmonary vasodilation in fetal lambs.[61] A small increase in blood adenosine levels in fetal lambs results in an increase in PBF to postnatal levels. ATP-induced relaxation is via the P_{2y} receptor, whereas adenosine stimulates the P_1-A_2 receptors on pulmonary arteries and veins, eliciting vasodilatation via endothelial synthesis of NO.[62] ATP can also induce the release of prostacyclin via the P_{2y} receptor, which may contribute to vasodilation in some vascular beds, although it does not appear to work through this mechanism in fetal lambs.[60] Adenosine infusion appeared to improve oxygenation in term infants with PPHN,[63] but its use requires confirmation in a larger trial.

Persistent Pulmonary Hypertension of the Newborn

Pathophysiology

Elevated PVR resulting from either vasoconstriction or structural remodeling of the pulmonary vasculature characterizes PPHN. This leads to PHT causing right-to-left shunting of blood across the foramen ovale and ductus arteriosus, resulting in hypoxemia. Numerous disease states with diverse etiologies can result in a similar final physiology. About 10% of cases with PPHN are idiopathic, with no associated pulmonary airspace pathology. However, PPHN is usually associated with other acute respiratory conditions, such as MAS, respiratory distress syndrome (RDS), pneumonia, or congenital diaphragmatic hernia (CDH). Hypoxemia in these conditions can be due to ventilation/perfusion (V/Q) mismatch and intrapulmonary, as well as extrapulmonary, right-to-left shunting of blood. In some newborns with hypoxic respiratory failure, a single mechanism predominates (e.g., extrapulmonary right to left shunting in idiopathic PPHN). However, more commonly, several of these mechanisms contribute to hypoxemia. In MAS, obstruction of the airways by meconium results in decreasing V/Q ratios and increasing intrapulmonary right-to-left shunt. Other segments of the lungs may be overventilated relative to perfusion, causing increased physiologic dead space. The same patient may also have severe PHT with extrapulmonary right-to-left shunting at the ductus arteriosus and foramen ovale. The PHT in MAS may result from the alveolar hypoxia, from inflammatory mediators, or from abnormal pulmonary vascular muscularization.

Pneumonia or meconium aspiration may release inflammatory mediators that induce vasoconstriction. Vasoconstrictors such as leukotrienes, platelet-activating factor, thromboxanes,[64] and ET-1[65] have been found to be elevated in infants with PPHN. Chronic intrauterine ET_A receptor blockade following ductal ligation, decreased PAP in utero, decreased right ventricular hypertrophy, and distal muscularization of small pulmonary arteries increased the fall in PVR at delivery in newborn lambs with PPHN.[66] Thus ET_A receptor stimulation might contribute to the pathogenesis and pathophysiology of perinatal PHT.[66] Derangements in the NO pathway of vasodilation can also result in the physiologic characteristics of PPHN. Hypoxia-induced PHT in rats is associated with loss of endothelium derived relating factor (EDRF) activity in pulmonary vessels, with rapid recovery upon return to a normoxic environment.[67] Pulmonary endothelial nitric oxide synthase (eNOS) gene and protein expression and enzyme activity are decreased in fetal lambs with PHT.[68] In addition, the response to stimulators of eNOS is lost in the ductal ligation PPHN lamb model.[69] Because NO both vasodilates and inhibits vascular smooth muscle growth, diminished eNOS expression may contribute to both abnormal vasoreactivity and excessive muscularization of pulmonary vessels in fetal PHT.[68] In newborn lambs with PHT, the vascular response to NO itself is also diminished,[70] whereas the response to cGMP is normal.[69,70] Thus the decreased responsiveness appears to result from decreased vascular smooth muscle sensitivity to NO at the level of soluble guanylate cyclase. The cGMP pathway of signal transduction is shown in Figure 43–4.

Pulmonary hypertension sometimes occurs because of an abnormal pulmonary vascular bed despite the absence of alveolar hypoxia and hypercapnia and of lung inflammation. These infants can be grouped according to the degree of muscularization and the number of pulmonary arteries.[71] In infants with hypoplastic lungs as in CDH and oligohydramnios sequence, PPHN may arise primarily as a consequence of decreased number of vessels causing decreased cross-sectional area of the pulmonary vascular bed, leading to flow restriction. Patients with alveolar capillary dysplasia may have a similar vascular hypoplasia. These cases may be complicated by increased muscularization of the vessels.

Pulmonary arterial muscularization with increased thickness of the muscular coat in preacinar arteries and extension of the muscle into intraacinar arteries is seen in infants dying of PPHN even in the first days of life compared with infants dying of nonrespiratory causes.[72] PPHN has been reported in infants of mothers who received indomethacin, aspirin, or other prostaglandin synthesis inhibitors resulting in closure of the ductus arteriosus. Prenatal closure of the ductus arteriosus causes immediate and sustained PHT.[19,20] Several studies found that lambs with prenatal closure of ductus arteriosus have increased muscularization of pulmonary vasculature and physiologic characteristics of PPHN.[10,19] Other stresses that tend to raise fetal arterial pressure are also associated with elevated PVR in newborn lambs.[73,74] One study found that chronic in utero hypoxemia enhanced muscularization and medial hypertrophy.[75] It is also possible that the abnormal muscularization occurs postnatally. Neonatal pulmonary vessels not only exhibit a greater vasoconstrictive response than adult pulmonary vessels but also possess a unique ability to undergo rapid changes in architecture, particularly the ability to hypertrophy muscle.[76] If the usual decline in vascular resistance at birth was disrupted by acute perinatal stress, such as asphyxia, sepsis, MAS, or acidosis leading to release of local vasoactive mediators such as leukotriene, thromboxane,[77] and ET, high PVR would be maintained. This could block the normal postnatal remodeling, and increased muscularization of the pulmonary vasculature might rapidly ensue.

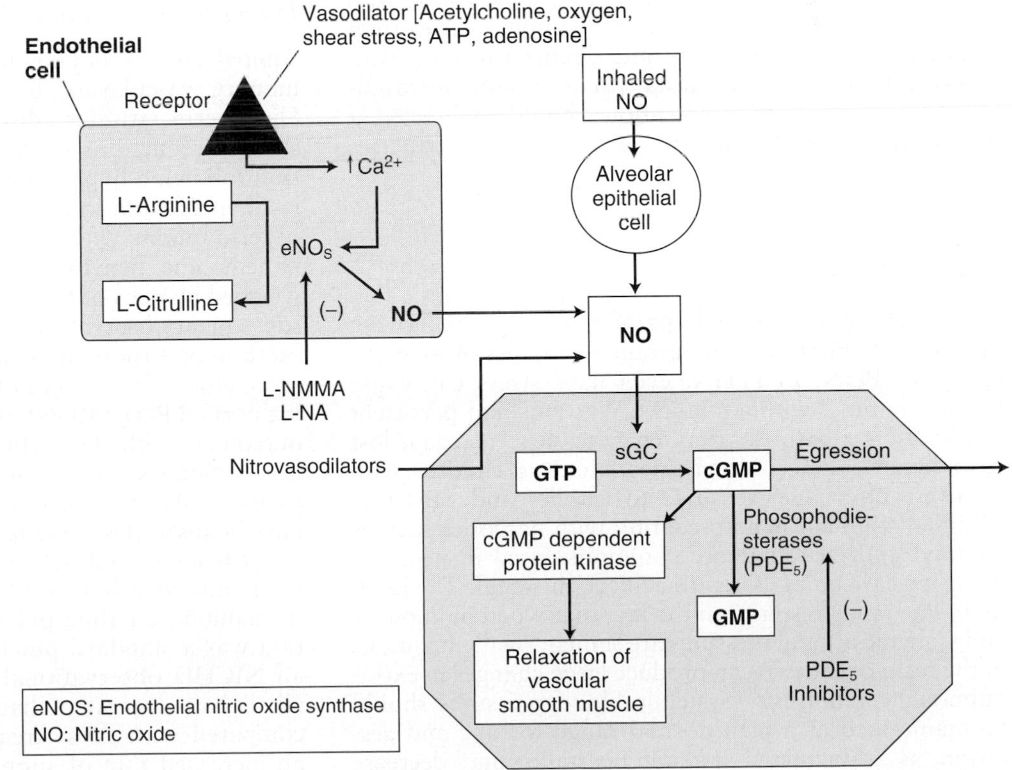

FIGURE 43–4 • Cyclic guanosine monophosphate signal transduction pathway of vasodilation.

Presentation

PPHN must be included in the differential diagnosis of hypoxic respiratory failure in term or near-term infants. Prenatal and perinatal history may provide clues to the etiology of PPHN. These include the presence of meconium, acidosis, and asphyxia at delivery, maternal risk factors for infection such as prolonged rupture of membranes, maternal fever, or positive group B Streptococcus status. Maternal use of over-the-counter medications that contain prostaglandin synthesis inhibitors such as aspirin may be important. Postmaturity also appears to be a risk factor. The neonate with PPHN is often extremely labile, with frequent desaturation episodes. Wide swings in arterial Po_2, without changes in ventilator settings, should suggest the possibility of PPHN. Lability can also occur in the face of significant parenchymal disease when V/Q mismatch is severe. Auscultation may reveal a single S_2, which can be loud, and systolic murmur of tricuspid regurgitation. Chest x-ray findings may vary depending on the etiology of PPHN. Hypoxemia out of proportion to the degree of parenchymal disease severity on chest radiography should suggest PPHN. Measurement of preductal and postductal arterial oxygenation can confirm PPHN. A difference in arterial $Po_2 \geq 20$ mmHg or oxygen saturation ≥ 10 should be considered significant. Minimal or no difference in oxygen tension does not exclude PPHN because shunting at the atrial level produces no ductal gradient and probably is the most common site of shunting. Thus in clinical practice, the gold standard in defining PPHN rests on the echocardiographic findings of right-to-left shunting of blood at the foramen ovale and/or the ductus arteriosus, as well as estimates of PAP. Elevated PVR alone does not cause hypoxemia. Doppler measurements of atrial and ductal level shunts provide essential information when managing a newborn with hypoxic respiratory failure. For example, left-to-right shunting at the foramen ovale and ductus arteriosus with marked hypoxemia suggests predominant intrapulmonary shunting, and interventions should be directed at optimizing lung inflation.

Treatment

General Measures

Understanding the dynamic pathophysiology underlying right-to-left shunting is important to successful management of PPHN. In PPHN, even mild stress can cause Po_2 to plummet within minutes. Vigorous and persistent resuscitative measures are often necessary to regain lost vasorelaxation. Accordingly, neonates and children with PHT are often very sensitive to activity and agitation. Minimal stimulation and sedation with narcotics such as fentanyl and morphine are commonly used in neonatal intensive care units (ICUs) to achieve this goal. The lability in Pao_2 may result from the fact that when pulmonary and systemic arterial pressures are similar, small alterations in the ratio of the two can produce large changes in extrapulmonary shunting.[78] Systemic blood pressures should be maintained at a high normal range for age and gestation, as an increased systemic resistance may decrease the degree of right-to-left shunting. Hypotension resulting from hypovolemia should be treated aggressively with volume replacement. If hypotension persists despite volume replacement, inotropic support with dopamine, dobutamine, and epinephrine may be required. All patients with PHT benefit from a core group of therapies that includes management of hypothermia, hypocalcemia, acidosis, hypoglycemia, and polycythemia. In case of PHT resulting from perinatal asphyxia, correcting alveolar hypoxia, hypercarbia, and metabolic acidosis with administration of 100% oxygen, conventional ventilation, and a buffer should restore normal pulmonary vasodilation. Surprisingly, there have been few prospective randomized trials of most of the therapeutic modalities advocated for treatment of PPHN. Older therapies such as hyperventilation and alkalosis were introduced into clinical practice based on animal studies or short-term studies that included very small numbers of patients and used physiologic response rather than patient outcome as the endpoint. Only newer therapies of inhaled nitric oxide (iNO) and extracorporeal membrane oxygenation (ECMO) have been rigorously evaluated in controlled clinical trials. In a National Institute of Child Health and Human Development (NICHD) observational study,[79] use of hyperventilation varied among the 12 NICHD centers from 33% to 92%, whereas alkali infusion ranged from 27% to 93%. Similar variation was seen in the use of inotropic agents (46%–100%) and intravenous vasodilators (13%–81%). High-frequency ventilation (HFV) use ranged from 0% to 73%, and ECMO use varied from 0% to 85%. Some of the variation is expected given the wide range of pathophysiology contributing to PPHN. A more likely explanation for the wide variation seen, however, is the overall lack of proven efficacy of many of these therapies.

Hyperventilation and Alkali Infusion

Animal studies documented the sensitivity of the pulmonary vasculature to both hypoxia and acidosis.[80] Short-term studies during cardiac catheterizations showed reductions in PAP and elevation of oxygen tension following hyperventilation.[78,81] Based on these studies, hyperventilation became the mainstay of ventilation of term infants with hypoxic respiratory failure. In some patients the benefits of hyperventilation may be outweighed by risks of barotrauma or volutrauma. However, subsequent observations have raised concern of impaired cerebral perfusion and neurosensory deafness at extremes of alkalosis.[82,83] Studies of infants with PPHN maintaining normal Pco_2 (40–60 mmHg) indicate similar or better outcomes with less chronic lung disease.[84,85] Many neonatologists have moved away from the practice of hyperventilation in neonates with PPHN. Animal studies have shown the beneficial effects of hyperventilation result from altered pH rather than from changes in Pco_2 or minute ventilation.[86,87] Until recently, alkali infusion to maintain alkaline pH to induce pulmonary vasodilation was a standard practice in many neonatal ICUs. In an NICHD observational study, the group treated with alkali had a greater chance of treatment with ECMO compared with those treated with hyperventilation and an increased rate of supplemental oxygen at 28 days.[79]

Alkali infusion increases CO_2 production, necessitating higher ventilator support. Lack of patient outcome data with both hyperventilation and alkali infusion and availability of better therapeutic options have led to less use of these management strategies.

Pulmonary Hypertension after the Newborn Period

After the newborn period, PHT is defined as a mean PAP of more than 25 mmHg at rest or more than 30 mmHg during exercise. Pulmonary arterial hypertension (PAH) may be initially caused by increased flow, as in some cases of congenital heart disease (CHD), or increased resistance in the pulmonary vascular bed, as in primary pulmonary hypertension (PPH). Primary pulmonary hypertension is an uncommon disease that predominantly affects young people in whom no cause for PHT can be identified. In secondary PHT, a coexisting disease or stimulus can been identified that presumably explains the PHT. Per World Health Organization (WHO) reclassification in 1998, the term *pulmonary arterial hypertension* refers to a disease spectrum with a similar clinical and pulmonary histopathology that includes PPH and PHT, which cannot be distinguished from PPH. This includes patients with PPH, both sporadic and familial, as well as PAH associated with collagen vascular disorders, congenital systemic-to-pulmonary shunts, human immunodeficiency virus (HIV), CHD, and appetite suppressants. Most of the initial abnormalities in PAH were identified by clinical observations. These observations then were linked to advances in our understanding of SMC physiology, endothelial and platelet dysfunction, vascular remodeling, and genetics to provide insights into the pathophysiology of PAH. It is important to establish an accurate diagnosis with respect to etiology of PHT because therapy may vary with etiology. For instance, thromboembolic disease often is amenable to surgery with excellent results from thromboendarterectomy. Similarly, secondary PAH may result from a left-sided heart lesion with pulmonary venous hypertension.

Pathophysiology

The mechanisms responsible for development of PAH are complex and incompletely understood. In individuals with PPH, hyperreactive lung vessels in which various stimuli initiate vasoconstriction may explain the subsequent development of characteristic vascular lesions.[88] Possibly the same mechanisms underlie the pathophysiology of Eisenmenger syndrome. The vascular endothelium is regarded as an important source of locally active mediators that contribute to control of vasomotor tone. Thromboxane/PGI_2 and NO/ET-1 system are two of the important balances that control pulmonary vasomotor tone. Endothelial injury/dysfunction may lead to vascular remodeling and progressively increasing vascular obstruction and obliteration. Risk factors that are associated with development of PPH include use of anorexic drugs, family history of PHT, infection with HIV, cirrhosis, and use of cocaine or intravenous drugs.[89]

Studies have demonstrated the interaction between NO (a vasodilator) and ET-1 (a potent vasoconstrictor) both produced by the vascular endothelium. It appears that they have opposing regulatory pathways.[90] Mechanism of action of the ET system is summarized in Figure 43–5. Of the two ET-1 receptors, ET_a receptors expressed mainly in the smooth muscle mediate vasoconstriction and cell proliferation, whereas ET_b receptors expressed mainly in the endothelial cells are important for clearance of ET-1, endothelial cell survival, release of NO and prostacyclin, and inhibition of endothelin-converting enzyme-1 (ECE-1).[91,92] In experimental studies of hypoxia-induced[93] and monocrotaline-induced PHT,[94] chronic ET receptor blockade lowered PAP and the incidence of vascular and pulmonary injury and improved NO-mediated pulmonary vasodilation. Studies in L-ω-nitroarginine methyl ester (L-NAME) hypertension suggest that ET-1 is linked to dysfunction of the L-arginine/NO pathway[95] because ET_a selective[96] but not combined ET blockade[97] improves endothelial function. Thus selective inhibition of ET_a receptors improves the endothelial L-arginine/NO pathway, which agrees with observations in humans.[98]

ET-1 expression in pulmonary tissue is increased in patients with primary and secondary PHT.[99] ET-1 increases at high altitudes in mountaineers and correlates with pulmonary pressures and oxygen tension.[100] ET increases even more in mountaineers prone to high-altitude pulmonary edema.[101] Increased local production[99] and elevated circulating levels of ET[102] have been demonstrated in patients with Eisenmenger syndrome,[103] PPH,[104] and PAH associated with CHD.[105] Increased expression of ET-1 in pulmonary arteries has been demonstrated in patients with PHT.[106] Lung specimens collected from patients with primary and secondary PHT have showed similar expression of nitric acid synthase-1 (NOS-1) in both normal and diseased lungs, whereas abundant expression of ECE-1 was present in diseased vessels. The precise role of elevated ET-1 in pulmonary hypertensive disorders needs to be understood.

Prostacyclin (PGI_2) is a powerful vasodilator[107] and inhibitor of platelet aggregation,[108] whereas TXA_2 is a vasoconstrictor and induces platelet aggregation[109] leading to microvascular thrombus formation and hence vascular injury. As TXA_2 and PGI_2 have opposing effects on platelet aggregation and pulmonary vascular smooth muscle, an imbalance in their biosynthesis could contribute to the progressive increase in PVR seen in older untreated patients with pulmonary hypertensive CHD.[110] Decreased urinary excretion of 2,3-dinor-6-keto-prostaglandin $F_{1\alpha}$, a metabolite of PGI_2, occurs in patients with PPH.[111] A decrease in expression of the enzyme PGI_2 synthase (PGI_2-S) in the lung may be an important manifestation of pulmonary endothelial dysfunction in severe PHT. Different-size pulmonary arteries express PGI_2-S differently, and loss of expression of PGI_2-S may be one of the phenotypic alterations present in the pulmonary endothelial cells in severe PAH.[112] Pulmonary PGI_2-S overexpression in transgenic mice protects against development of hypoxic PHT.[113] PGI_2-S may play a major role in modifying the pulmonary vascular response to injury. Intratracheal transfer of human PGI_2-S gene has been shown to augment pulmonary prostacyclin synthesis, ameliorate MCT-induced PHT,

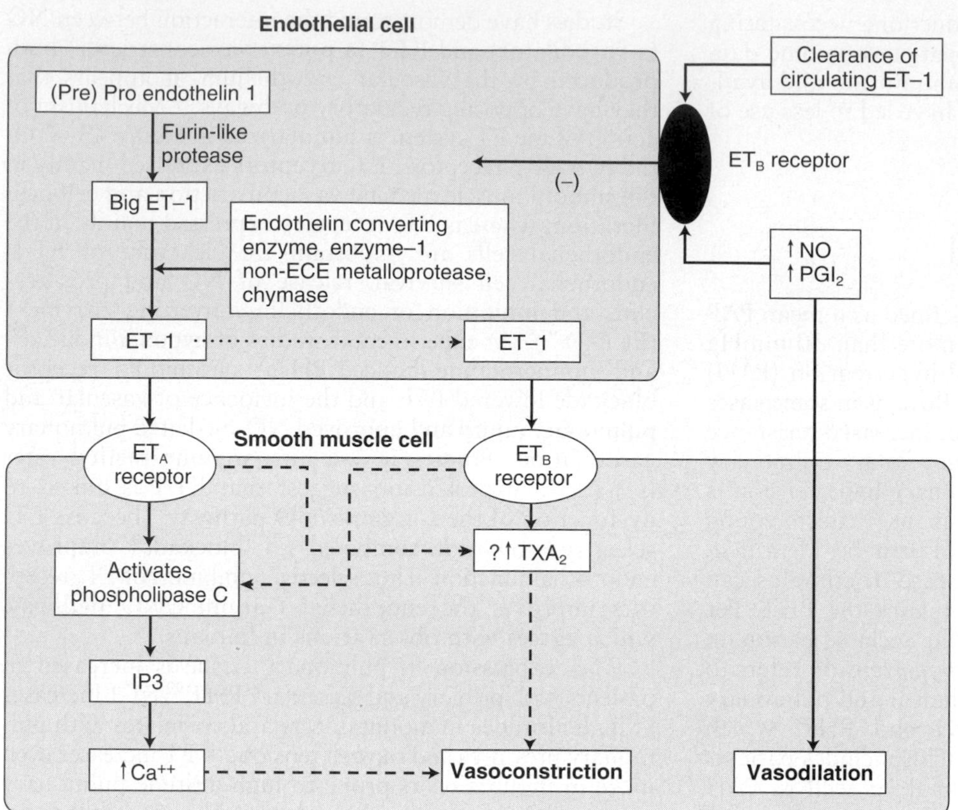

FIGURE 43–5 • Vascular effects of endothelin-1.

and improve survival in monocrotaline (MCT) rats.[114] These experiments have important pathogenetic and therapeutic implications in the management of severe PHT.

Potassium (K^+) channels play an important part in SMC electrophysiology, which has implications for the development of PAH (Figure 43–6). There are several types of K^+ channels, including voltage-gated (Kv), inward rectifier (K_{ir}), and calcium-sensitive (K_{ca}) channels. Inhibition of Kv channels results in accumulation of positively charged K^+ ions within the cell, hence depolarizing the cell and activating the voltage-gated, L-type calcium channel.[115] Calcium then enters the cell, activating the contractile apparatus, leading to vasoconstriction and possibly initiating cell proliferation. Acute hypoxia seems to initiate vasoconstriction in part by inhibiting the Kv channel in pulmonary artery SMCs.[115] There are nine families of Kv channels (Kv1–Kv9), each with many members (Kv1.1–Kv1.6). In humans with PPH but not those with secondary PH, Kv1.5 mRNA levels are reduced in pulmonary artery SMCs.[116] This down-regulation of Kv1.5 is associated with inhibition of the K^+ current, membrane depolarization, and elevation of cytosolic calcium. Thus decreased expression or function of K^+ channels in pulmonary artery SMCs in PPH patients could initiate

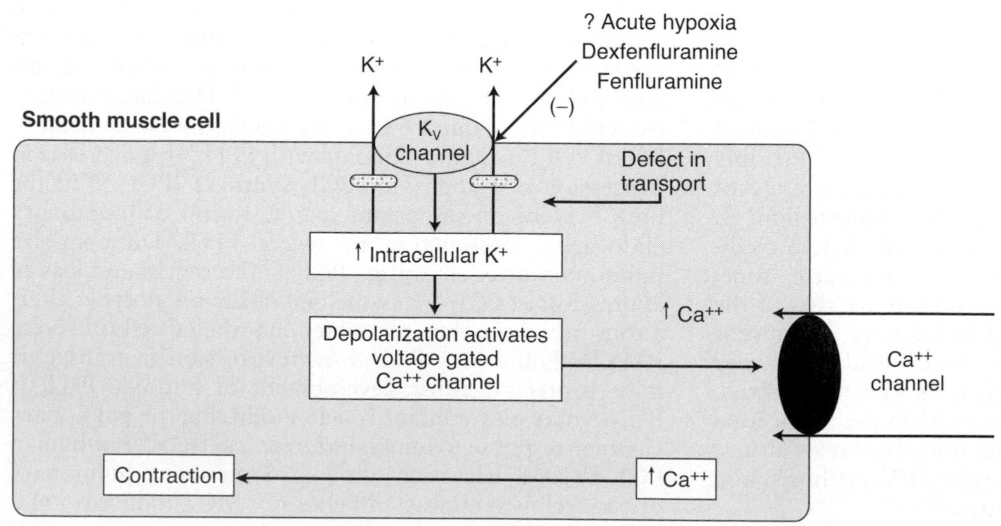

FIGURE 43–6 • Summary of the defect in voltage-gated potassium channel leading to smooth muscle contraction.

and/or maintain pulmonary vasoconstriction and play a role in the pathogenesis of PPH.[116] Use of anorexic agents such as aminorex, fenfluramine, and dexfenfluramine is associated with development of PPH,[89] and these agents are thought to act by blocking the Kv channel.[117] Kv2.1 is inhibited by dexfenfluramine, a weight loss drug that is associated with the development of PAH.[117] Anorexigen-induced Kv channel inhibition and membrane depolarization can contribute to pulmonary vasoconstriction.[118,119] In addition to its effects on Ca^{2+} entry via the L-type Ca^{2+} channel, dexfenfluramine promoted vasoconstriction by enhancing Ca^{2+} release from the sarcoplasmic reticulum.[120] Fenfluramine reduces Kv1.5 mRNA levels by 50% in pulmonary artery SMCs from normotensive patients,[121] suggesting that inhibited gene transcription and expression of Kv channels play important roles in anorexigen-induced PAH.

Matrix metalloproteinases (MMPs) and extracellular matrix are thought to be important in vascular remodeling and hence proliferation of SMCs. Endothelial abnormalities early in the course of PAH may permit extravasation of factors that stimulate SMC production of vascular serine elastase.[122,123] This results in liberation of matrix-bound SMC mitogens, such as basic fibroblast growth factor, and enhances matrix degradation by activating other MMPs. The MMPs stimulate the production of mitogenic cofactor, tenascin, leading to phosphorylation of growth factor receptors and SMC proliferation. When MMPs are inhibited, tenascin levels fall, leading to apoptosis.[122] Direct inhibition of MMP-2 and serine elastases leads to complete regression of experimental PHT in rats,[124] suggesting they regulate vascular tone. MMP-2 and MMP-9 can activate platelets,[125] and intravascular MMP-2 can enhance the formation of vasoconstrictors and inhibit the action of endogenous vasodilators.[126]

A number of other less well-studied factors are potentially involved in the pathogenesis of PHT. Abnormalities of thrombomodulin/protein C anticoagulant system with a decrease in soluble thrombomodulin and an increase in fibrinolytic inhibitor plasminogen activator 1 have been noted in patients with PPH.[127] Whether hypercoagulability occurs in response to PAH or can actually initiate PAH is unclear, but it likely contributes to disease progression. Serotonin (5-hydroxytryptamine [5-HT]) and serotonin transporter (5-HTT) have been shown to promote development of hypoxic PHT by stimulating pulmonary artery SMC growth.[128] 5-HTT activity may play a role in the pathogenesis of pulmonary artery SMC proliferation in PPH, and a 5-HTT polymorphism may confer susceptibility to PPH.[129] Familial PPH is a rare autosomal dominant disorder with reduced penetrance that has been mapped to chromosome 2q33. Reports of familial PPH associated with BMPR2 gene mutations suggest bone morphogenetic protein-signaling pathway to be defective at least in some patients with familial PPH.[130,131] Figure 43–7 shows a schematic representation of the main features in the pathogenesis of PHT. Figure 43–8 shows some typical changes that occur in PPH.

Pulmonary Vascular Anatomy

Heath-Edward introduced the first comprehensive classification of PAH based on histopathology of pulmonary vasculature,[132] in children with CHD or idiopathic PHT (Table 43–1). *Grade I* referred to changes seen in patients with CHD associated with PHT from birth. *Grades II* to *IV* were classified as a result of raised PAP. *Grades V* and *VI* often overlap and represent advanced disease. Rabinovitch introduced a morphometric classification

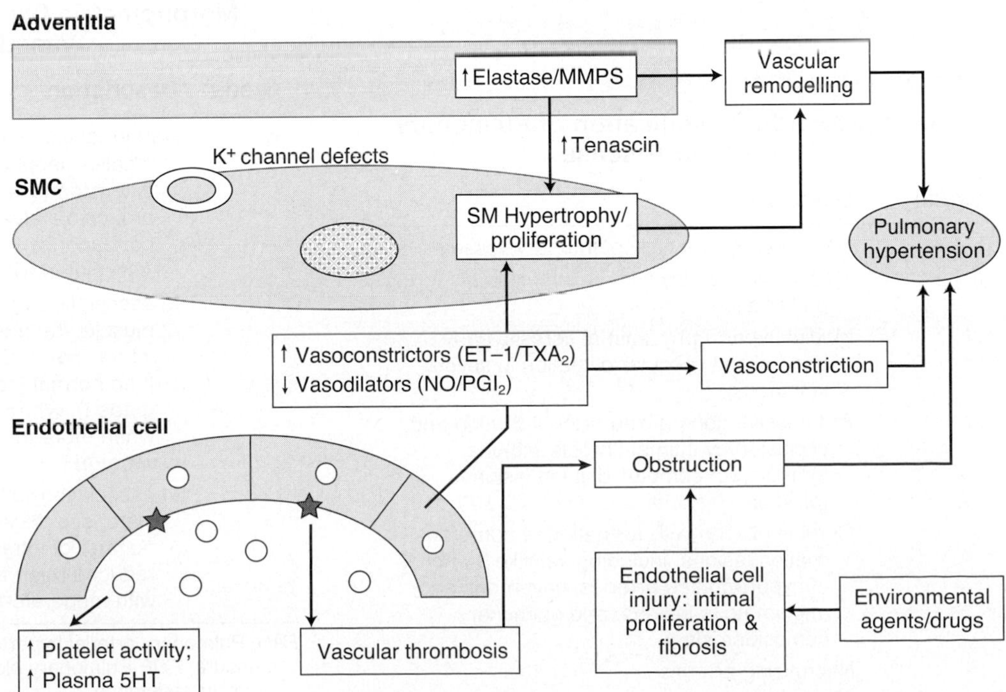

FIGURE 43–7 • Major pathways of pulmonary hypertension.

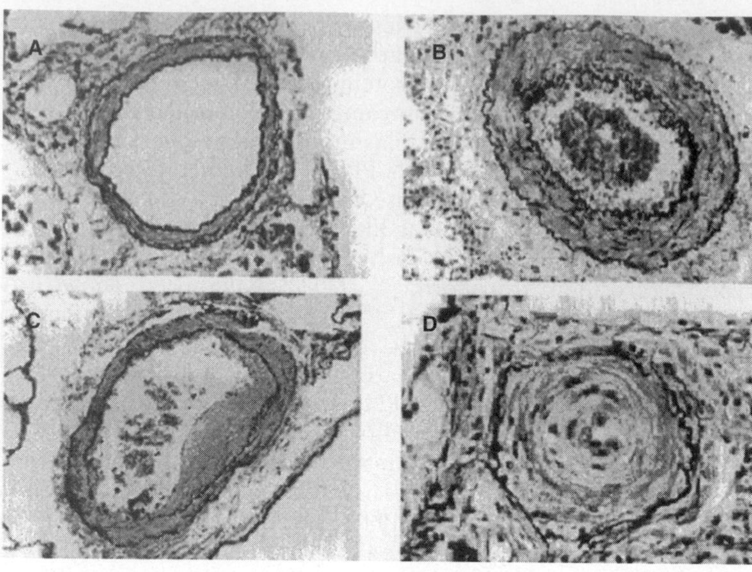

FIGURE 43–8 • A, Normal small pulmonary artery with typically thin muscular wall. **B–D** show some of the changes that can occur in primary pulmonary hypertension. **B,** Wall or small pulmonary artery thickens. **C,** Fibrous or scarred tissue appears on inner wall of small pulmonary artery. **D,** Bands of scarred tissue build up on inner wall of small pulmonary artery, substantially narrowing the blood vessel.

system in 1978, by studying lung biopsies of 50 patients with CHD (Table 43–2). The presence and severity of pathologic lesions correlated with increased PBF, elevated PAP, and elevated PVR. The most familiar patterns of pulmonary vascular lesions begin with medial hypertrophy followed by cellular proliferation and concentric laminar intimal fibrosis. Eventually dilatated lesions, fibrinoid necrosis, and plexiform lesions develop, and the disease is referred as *Eisenmenger syndrome*.[133] The progressive vascular lesions that occur in patients with PPH are identical to those that occur with CHD involving systemic to pulmonary shunts.[132] Based on these findings, similar therapeutic approaches have been used with children who have PPH and those with PAH associated with CHD.

In CHD, morphologic criteria[134] and pulmonary hemodynamics are both used to determine the stage beyond which surgical correction is no longer indicated because established disease will cause an unacceptably high operative risk or will continue to progress despite surgical repair.[135] Abnormalities in muscularization and growth of pulmonary arteries obtained at biopsy during surgical repair from patients with CHD correlated with preoperative hemodynamic data of increased PBF, pressure, and resistance.[134] Pulmonary vascular structural changes assessed by morphometry[134] (see Table 43–2) and Heath-Edward classification[132] (see Table 43–1) in lung tissue obtained by biopsy at the time of surgical repair correlated with the postoperative hemodynamic findings of PAP and PVR measured 1 day and 1 year after surgery.[136] On the first

TABLE 43–1

Heath-Edwards Classification of Pulmonary Vascular Disease

Grade	Description
I	Retention of fetal-type pulmonary vessels
II	Medial hypertrophy with cellular intimal proliferation
III	Medial hypertrophy, intimal fibrosis, early generalized vascular dilatation in severe instances
IV	Progressive generalized arterial dilation and occlusion by intimal fibrosis with the formation of complex dilation lesions (plexiform lesions)
V	Chronic dilation with formation of numerous dilation lesions, including veinlike branches of hypertrophied arteries, cavernous and angiomatous lesions, and pulmonary hemosiderosis
VI	Necrotizing arteritis

TABLE 43–2

Rabinovitch-Haworth-Castenada Morphometric Classification of Pulmonary Vascular Disease

Grade	Description
A	Abnormal extension of smooth muscle along smaller peripheral arteries with intraacinar extension (arteries accompanying respiratory bronchiole alveolar duct and alveolar wall) corresponds to Heath-Edwards grade 1. Associated with ↑ PBF without evidence of ↑ PAP.
B	In association with abnormal extension of the muscle, the medial muscular coat of the intraacinar and preacinar arteries is thicker than normal (corresponds to Heath-Edwards grade I). When mild, not associated with PAH; when more than twice normal, associated with PAH.
C	In association with abnormal extension and increased thickness of the muscular coat, the number of intraacinar and preacinar arteries is reduced (high alveolar-arterial ratio). Associated with moderate-to-severe elevation in PVR.

PAH, Pulmonary arterial hypertension; *PAP,* Pulmonary arterial pressure; *PBF,* Pulmonary blood flow; *PVR,* Pulmonary vascular resistance.

postoperative day, increases in mean PAP were uncommon in patients with morphometric grades A or B (mild) biopsy findings. Mean PAP was commonly elevated in those with grade B (severe) or C (mild or severe) (Heath-Edward grade I) and was more frequently elevated in those with grade II findings. Moderate-to-severe elevation of mean PAP was invariably present in patients with Heath-Edwards grade III regardless of morphometric grades. One year after repair, mean PAP and PVR were normal in all patients whose conditions were surgically corrected before age 9 months regardless of the severity of pulmonary vascular changes. PAP and PVR were increased in all patients whose conditions were repaired after age 2 years with grade C morphometric findings and to a severe degree if associated with Heath-Edward grade III. Thus although Heath-Edward grade usually can be used to identify patients at risk for PHT in the early postoperative period, both the morphometric and Heath-Edward grades, as well as age of the patient at the time of repair, can be used to determine whether PAP and PVR eventually return to normal or remain elevated.

Congenital Heart Disease

Pulmonary vascular disease remains a significant cause of morbidity and mortality in children with CHD. Congenital heart lesions resulting in increased PBF or pulmonary venous obstruction produce pulmonary artery smooth muscle hypertrophy and hyperplasia and pulmonary vasoconstriction.[137] Unless PHT is treated by either medical or surgical means, pulmonary vasoconstriction may persist, progress to vascular obliteration, and produce high morbidity. Pulmonary hypertensive crisis in the immediate postoperative period is a life-threatening complication in children with certain types of CHD, despite good surgical repair.[138] Even though early surgical repair has been advocated to prevent later pulmonary vascular obstructive disease, it does not abolish this occurrence of PHT in the immediate postoperative period.[139] Microemboli, platelet aggregation, complement activation, pulmonary leukosequestration, excess production of vasoactive mediators, atelectasis, and hypoxia during cardiopulmonary bypass all contribute to elevated PVR in the immediate postoperative period. The effects on the pulmonary vasculature may be insidious over several hours, presenting as low cardiac output and right heart failure or more acutely as pulmonary hypertensive crisis. In such situations, PAP increases to systemic or suprasystemic levels, systemic blood pressure falls, and arterial oxygen saturation drops. In one large center, half of the postoperative cardiac children who had pulmonary hypertensive crises died during their hospitalization.[140] In the newborn, parenchymal lung disorders including pulmonary edema, intrapulmonary shunting, and pneumonia may coexist with heart disease, resulting in hypoxic respiratory failure following cardiopulmonary bypass.

Pulmonary endothelial damage is an early histologic event in children with CHD and PHT.[141] Reduced pulmonary vasodilation to acetylcholine demonstrates physiologic impairment of endothelial function in these children.[142] Loss of local eNOS activity may be one of the contributing factors in postoperative pulmonary hypertensive crisis. It has been suggested that cardiopulmonary bypass may also contribute to endothelial dysfunction. Arteries with endothelial damage are particularly sensitive to exogenous NO, and response to iNO in the postoperative period suggests that the capacity for smooth muscle relaxation and pulmonary vasodilatation is intact in these children.[143] Even though NO-induced vasodilation varies among children with PHT and elevated PVR, a decline in selective response seems to parallel the progression of established vascular disease and thus may help in selecting patients for operation.[143a] An increased number of ET_a receptors in lung arteries and lung parenchyma has been noted in patients with increased PVR and low PBF.[144] Up-regulation of the ET-1 system may play a role in the pathogenesis of secondary PHT associated with CHD in children.[144]

Presentation

There is often no correlation between the time PPH is thought to have started, the age at which it is diagnosed, and the severity of symptoms. The disease seems to progress fairly rapidly, especially in children. Frequent fatigue, dyspnea, dizziness, and fainting spells are the typical early symptoms. Some other symptoms include edema of legs, cyanosis, palpitations, and chest pain. Examination findings compatible with PHT in children include jugular venous distension, tricuspid regurgitation murmur, loud second heart sound at the base of the heart, and diastolic murmur of pulmonary regurgitation (Graham Steell murmur). Exertional dyspnea, chest pain, and syncope result from the inability to increase cardiac output in the presence of increased oxygen demands. In infants and children with PAH, PAP is increased at rest and increases further after exercise. In a clinical setting, findings of Doppler echocardiography infer the diagnosis of PHT. The definitive diagnosis requires direct measurements of PAP by cardiac catheterization. Based on criteria from the National Institute of Health, a mean PAP greater than 25 mmHg at rest (>30 mmHg with exercise) is the standard for diagnosis of PH.[145] Initially the right ventricle hypertrophies to maintain cardiac output at rest, although the ability to increase cardiac output during exercise may be impaired. As pulmonary vascular disease progresses, right ventricular dysfunction ensues, resulting in right heart failure. Although the left heart is not directly affected by pulmonary vascular disease, progressive right heart dilatation can impair left ventricular filling.[146] Pulmonary function tests (PFT) and exercise testing are important not only for diagnosis but also for monitoring progression of the disease. Chest x-ray film, PFTs, and sleep study help rule out pulmonary causes of PHT. A V/Q scan can help distinguish PPH from PHT caused by thromboembolic disorder in the lung. Other tests that may help in the diagnosis include autoantibody testing for collagen vascular disorders, HIV testing, and PFTs in cases of portopulmonary hypertension. Factors that help in deciding the type of treatment include hemodynamic parameters of right ventricular function, extent of symptoms as assessed by WHO classification, and overall exercise capacity. Exercise capacity of more than 75% of predicted value might identify patients likely to respond well to vasodilator treatment.[147] Depending on the degree of physical limitation by symptoms, the functional level of patients is graded from I to IV, with higher grades representing severe disease and worse prognosis (Table 43–3). This is known as the WHO functional classification and is an adaptation of the New York Heart Association (NYHA) functional classification of congestive heart failure.

Low concentrations of antithrombin III, protein S, or protein C might be genetic in origin or result from consumption coagulopathy.[127,148] Screening siblings for familial forms of PHT once the diagnosis is confirmed in a given patient should be part of evaluation. Accurate measurement of PVR is a key component in evaluating the operability of CHD and assessing the severity of PPH. Even though invasive measurements of flow and PA pressures are the gold standard, noninvasive measurements are useful in frequent assessment during follow-ups and to facilitate monitoring individual patient responses. PAPs are estimated during echocardiography by continuous-wave Doppler measurement of the tricuspid regurgitant jet velocity. More recently velocity propagation within the main pulmonary artery, which can be quantified using color M-mode imaging, has been used to measure PVR.[149] The degree of right ventricular function determines the duration of survival of patients with PAH. The prognosis of untreated PAH is extremely poor, with the condition often complicated by right ventricular failure.

Treatment

General Measures

Treatment of PPH is usually treatment for life. The therapeutic regimen must be tailored to each child and adjusted according to the clinical and hemodynamic response. Optimizing the management of these children improves quality of life and survival. Conventional treatment of children with PPH consists of anticoagulant and oral vasodilator treatment, usually a calcium channel blocker and supplemental oxygen.[150] Anticoagulation with warfarin has been shown to be beneficial in these patients.[151] In a later study, anticoagulant therapy had a positive influence on long-term survival and a significant improvement in quality of life in patients with PPH, particularly in patients with a history of anorectic drug intake.[152]

Therapy in secondary PHT is directed at the cause of PAH. Closure of the heart defect resolves the PAH secondary to increased PBF. Management of pulmonary venous hypertension includes controlling left ventricular failure and relieving the cause of venous obstruction (commonly left heart obstructive lesions). Medical management includes administering oxygen, diuretics, and cardiac glycosides. Vasodilator therapy is the mainstay of management of pulmonary vascular obstruction. Even small reductions in right ventricular afterload following vasodilator therapy produces substantial improvement in right ventricular output in patients with PHT. The goal of vasodilator therapy in patients with PAH is to reduce PAP and increase cardiac output without symptomatic systemic hypotension. Therapeutic options in PHT depend on the etiology of the disease, severity of functional impairment, and response to vasodilators at right heart catheterization. The response to vasodilators is important in making a decision for surgical correction (lung or heart-lung transplantation). Severe intractable cases of left ventricular dysfunction may need heart transplantation.

TABLE 43–3

WHO Functional Classification of Pulmonary Hypertension

Class	Description
I	Patients with pulmonary hypertension but without resulting limitation of physical activity. Ordinary physical activity does not cause undue dyspnea or fatigue, chest pain, or near-syncope.
II	Patients with pulmonary hypertension resulting in slight limitation of physical activity. They are comfortable at rest. Ordinary physical activity causes undue dyspnea or fatigue, chest pain, or near-syncope.
III	Patients with pulmonary hypertension resulting in marked limitation of physical activity. They are comfortable at rest. Less than ordinary activity causes undue dyspnea or fatigue, chest pain, or near-syncope.
IV	Patients with pulmonary hypertension with inability to carry out any physical activity without symptoms. These patients manifest signs of right heart failure. Dyspnea and/or fatigue may be present even at rest. Discomfort is increased by any physical activity.

Specific Therapies

Most of the therapies discussed in the following sections have been attempted in patients of varying ages and diagnosis, so we organize the therapies primarily by treatment rather than by age or disease.

Lung Recruitment Strategies

Surfactant. If the cause of PPHN is RDS secondary to atelectasis and the attendant alveolar hypoxia, exogenous surfactant may be administered. Near-term and term infants delivered by elective repeat cesarean section may be one subset of patients who are at risk for deficiency or dysfunction of surfactant and progressive hypoxic respiratory failure.[153] Clinical reports suggest that surfactant therapy improves oxygenation in term infants with RDS, pneumonia, and MAS.[154,155] Both in patients and in fetal lamb model of CDH, surfactant deficiency may cause atelectasis and alveolar hypoxia, exacerbating PHT and hypoxemia.[156,157] Surfactant therapy has been shown to reduce PVR and increase PBF in the lamb model of CDH.[158] Hypoxic respiratory failure in patients with adult RDS or acute lung injury is associated with surfactant deficiency and dysfunction,[159–163] and administration of surfactant may be beneficial in these patients.[164,165] However, a study of continuous administration of aerosolized synthetic surfactant to patients with sepsis-induced adult respiratory distress syndrome (ARDS) showed no significant effect on 30-day survival, length of ICU stay, duration of mechanical ventilation, or physiologic function.[166]

High-Frequency Ventilation. Many clinicians use HFV to manage infants with PPHN. Considering the important role of parenchymal lung disease in specific disorders resulting in PPHN, adequate lung inflation and optimal ventilation are as essential as pharmacologic vasodilator therapy. In the case of inhaled vasodilators, optimal inflation and ventilation may be necessary for drug delivery. Infants with PPHN from a variety of causes have been successfully treated with HFV.[167] HFV decreases $Pa{CO_2}$ and, in case of oscillator, has increased oxygenation in infants with PPHN. High-frequency oscillatory ventilation (HFOV) may improve oxygenation through safer use of higher mean airway pressures to maintain lung volume and prevent atelectasis. Two studies have evaluated the effectiveness of HFV compared with conventional ventilation in rescuing infants with respiratory failure and PPHN from potential ECMO therapy.[168,169] Neither mode of ventilation was more effective in preventing ECMO in these infants. In clinical pilot studies using iNO, combination of HFOV and iNO resulted in the greatest improvement in oxygenation in some newborns who had severe PPHN complicated by diffuse parenchymal lung disease and underinflation.[170] A randomized controlled trial demonstrated that treatment with HFOV and iNO was often successful in patients who failed to respond to HFOV or iNO alone in severe PPHN, and the differences in responses were related to the specific disease associated with PPHN.[171] Studies of HFV in patients with ARDS revealed no important advantage over conventional forms of mechanical ventilation.[172,173]

Vasodilators

Calcium Channel Blockers. Calcium channel blockers are the drugs most frequently used for treatment of PHT outside of the neonatal period. The response to calcium channel blockers is better in children than in adults with PPH. Acute response to the vasodilator drug (usually NO, PGI_2, adenosine, or acetylcholine) during cardiac catheterization helps determine the desirability of using chronic oral calcium channel blockers. A positive response to a vasodilator is taken as a decrease in mean PAP of 20% or more with no fall in cardiac index. The response to acute vasodilator testing is higher in children compared with adults (41% vs. 12% in adults).[174] The acute response in children is also age dependent. Oral calcium channel blockers help reduce PAP in approximately 40% of children with PPH.[175] In the remaining 60%, acute vasodilator testing with agents such as iNO or IV prostacyclin failed to demonstrate responsiveness, and these children have not benefited from chronic oral calcium channel blocker therapy.[175] Chronic calcium channel blocker therapy improved survival and quality of life in children who acutely respond to vasodilator drug testing.[176] The 5-year survival rate of patients treated with chronic oral calcium channel blockade who respond acutely to vasodilator testing was 97% versus 35% for those who do not respond acutely.[175] Chronic use of calcium channel blockers in patients with fixed PVR and unfavorable hemodynamics may worsen right heart failure. Regular, noninvasive monitoring of PAP and cardiac function is an essential part of the management of these patients.

Intravenous Prostacyclin. The ultimate treatment of PPHN involves specific relaxation of the pulmonary vasculature. No intravenous vasodilator is completely specific for the pulmonary circulation. Thus intravenous vasodilators are often unsuccessful in the management of PPHN because of systemic hypotension. The commonly used intravenous vasodilators include tolazoline, sodium nitroprusside, and prostacyclin. Tolazoline has been used most extensively in both animal and human studies,[177] but systemic hypotension and gastric bleeding have limited its usefulness. Among many other intravenous vasodilators, prostacyclin (PGI_2) probably is the next most widely studied. Even though PGI_2 has been used extensively for treatment of adult PPH, some of the first reports of its use were in pediatric patients and newborns with PHT.[178,179] Intravenous PGI_2 decreased PAP and PVR in infants with PPHN.[178,180] However, systemic hypotension has limited its usefulness in the management of infants with PPHN.

Prostacyclin (sodium epoprostenol, also called Flolan) has been studied extensively over the past decade in patients with PPH[174,175,181,182] and secondary PHT.[183] Chronic administration of prostacyclin usually is well tolerated, with minimal decrease in systemic pressures and modest decrease in PAP. Higher doses can lead to high cardiac output states, suggesting it has important positive inotropic effects.[181] In patients who are nonresponders to short-term vasodilator testing and responders who do not improve on calcium channel blockers, continuous intravenous infusion of PGI_2 improves survival.[175] Long-term continuous IV prostacyclin has been shown to improve survival, quality of life, and exercise capacity and to significantly reduce PAP in children with PPH.[175,184] Ongoing studies suggest that in some children who previously were believed to have fixed pulmonary vascular disease with irreversible obstruction may be reversible with long-term IV prostacyclin, perhaps via remodeling of the pulmonary vascular bed.[175,185] Although in the late 1980s and early 1990s the aim of chronic prostacyclin therapy was to act as a bridge to lung or heart-lung transplantation,[186] now continuous prostacyclin is being used as an alternative therapy to transplantation in selected children.[174] Chronic PGI_2 infusion improves hemodynamics and quality of life in patients with PHT associated with CHD who do not respond to conventional therapy.[187] Continuous intravenous prostacyclin is the only one of the "specific" therapies currently approved for use in chronic PHT. However, this therapy has drawbacks. Tolerance develops in some patients, requiring dose escalation resulting in additional adverse events and increased drug costs. More importantly, complications associated with administration of PGI_2 include risk of serious infections, catheter thrombosis, and rebound PAH because of pump failure with subsequent interruptions in therapy. For these reasons, alternative prostacyclin analogues are under investigation, including iloprost, beraprost, and treprostinil. These agents exhibit the same action as PGI_2, producing potent pulmonary vasodilation and inhibiting platelet aggregation[188,189]; however, each agent is administered by a different route. Beraprost is stabilized for oral administration. Beraprost reduces PVR in patients with PPH[190–192] and may be effective in the treatment of secondary precapillary PHT.[193] Oral administration of beraprost sodium may improve exercise capacity and ventilatory efficiency in patients with both primary and chronic thromboembolic PHT.[194] Treprostinil is approved by the U.S. Food and

Drug Administration. It is an analogue of epoprostenol but has increased half-life, can be delivered by subcutaneous route, and is stable at room temperature. In a double-blind randomized trial, chronic subcutaneous infusion of treprostinil improved indices of dyspnea, signs and symptoms of PHT, and hemodynamics and had an acceptable safety profile in patients with PAH.[195]

Inhaled Prostacyclin and its Analogues. Inhaled PGI_2 is a more selective pulmonary vasodilator than the intravenous preparation. It has been studied only recently in infants with PPHN.[196,197] In both these small studies, inhaled PGI_2 reduced PAP with no systemic side effects in infants with PPHN.[196,197] Inhaled PGI_2 improved oxygenation in four infants with PPHN refractory to iNO.[197] Systematic study of this drug by inhalation has not been reported in newborn animals or infants with PPHN. Its ease of administration, lack of toxicity, and inexpensive delivery system compared with iNO makes it a potentially useful drug in the management of PPHN.

Inhaled PGI_2 has been used in acute management of PHT in infants and children with acute lung injury.[198] Aerosolization of prostacyclin or its stable analogue iloprost causes selective pulmonary vasodilatation, increases cardiac output, and improves venous and arterial oxygenation in patients with severe PHT.[199] Thus it may offer a new strategy for treatment of this disease. Long-term treatment with aerosolized iloprost has been shown to be safe and has sustained effects on exercise capacity and pulmonary hemodynamics in patients with PPH.[200] In a placebo-controlled trial, iloprost inhalation (2.5 μg or 5 μg per inhalation; median dose 30 μg/day) improved pulmonary hemodynamics and quality of life in patients with severe PHT.[201] Inhaled iloprost is a significant advance over intravenous PGI_2 in the management of PAH. Aerosolized iloprost might be an alternative to NO for early testing of vascular reactivity and for postoperative treatment of acute PHT in children with CHD.[202] Its short half-life and frequent inhalations indicate it is not an ideal candidate for chronic treatment of PPH in children.

Nitric Oxide. The FDA has approved iNO for use in neonates with PPHN.[203] The physiologic rationale for using iNO for treatment of PPHN[204,205] and in children with PHT[206,207] is based upon its ability to achieve potent and sustained pulmonary vasodilation without decreasing systemic vascular tone.[204,205] It has been widely used as an early test of vasodilator response in patients with chronic PAH and in the short-term treatment of patients with PAH resulting from a variety of conditions.[208] The acute responsiveness to iNO seems to predict the subset of patients who might be responsive to oral calcium channel blockers and thus is a relatively safe and easy test to perform during cardiac catheterization.[209] The experience with long-term use of NO in children with PAH is limited. However, iNO is expensive and requires a fairly sophisticated delivery and monitoring system. Nonetheless, iNO dilates the pulmonary circulation while avoiding unwanted and dangerous systemic vasodilation and is economical and extremely effective in the management of PHT in critically ill patients in ICUs.[210]

Three randomized trials on the use of iNO in newborns with PPHN and respiratory failure were published in 1997. In a randomized, controlled clinical trial of patients with PPHN reported by Roberts et al.,[211] oxygenation doubled in 58% of treated patients in response to 80 ppm iNO. In addition, twice the proportion of the treated group avoided ECMO compared with the control group. In the Neonatal Inhaled Nitric Oxide Study (NINOS), 235 infants greater than 34 weeks of gestation diagnosed with hypoxic respiratory failure were randomized to 20 ppm iNO or control. Infants whose partial pressure of arterial oxygen increased by 20 mmHg or less were studied for a response to 80 ppm iNO or control gas. The end point of this trial was death or ECMO. Although the mortality rate was no different in either treatment arm, there was a 40% reduction in need for ECMO among iNO-treated infants compared with controls.[212] In a study by Kinsella et al.,[171] 205 infants with PPHN were randomized to iNO and conventional ventilation or to HFOV alone. Those who failed either therapy received the combination of iNO and HFOV. Treatment with HFOV in combination with iNO was successful in some patients who did not respond to one treatment alone. The differences were partly related to the specific disease associated with PPHN.[171] As adequate lung inflation appears to be necessary for optimal response to iNO, lung recruitment strategies with HFOV would augment the response to iNO. Clark et al.[203] reported a 38% reduction in ECMO and no difference in mortality among 248 infants randomized to receive 20 ppm iNO for 24 hours followed by 5 ppm for no more than 96 hours. A meta-analysis of the results of seven randomized trials of iNO use in newborns with PPHN demonstrated that 58% of hypoxic near-term and term infants responded to iNO within 30 to 60 minutes.[213] Mortality was not reduced in any of the NO studies analyzed, but ECMO used as a rescue therapy in nonresponders was. Studies in newborn lambs have shown that prolonged administration of NO increased survival rates without increasing the incidence of acute lung injury in lambs with PPHN.[214]

NO by itself is toxic at higher concentrations. Potential side effects include methemoglobinemia, pulmonary edema, and platelet dysfunction. NO reacts with superoxide anion to form peroxynitrite, which causes lipid peroxidation and other oxidative injury to cell membranes. NO_2 is even more toxic. Careful monitoring of both NO and NO_2 levels during administration is mandatory. As the optimal dosing and timing of iNO administration remains unclear and the potential toxicities are dose related, lower doses might afford both safety and efficacy in the management of these infants. Two studies using 2 ppm iNO yielded contradictory results. In one study, 2 ppm iNO diminished the clinical response to 20 ppm.[215] In the other study, the initial exposure to a very low dose did not compromise the response to higher doses.[216] Some patients had elevated methemoglobin levels at 80 ppm but not at 40 or 20 ppm.[217] The results of randomized controlled trials support the use of iNO at starting does of 20 ppm in near-term and term infants. In responders the dose is generally decreased progressively over hours to days. The dose needed to raise arterial Po_2 is lower than the dose needed to maximally decrease PAP. In summary, iNO offers substantial benefit to a large proportion of near-term and term newborns with hypoxic respiratory failure who do not respond to ventilatory support, lung recruitment, and oxygen.

Outcome of infants treated with iNO collectively supports both the efficacy and safety of this mode of treatment.[218,219] Reports identify significant medical and neurodevelopmental sequelae of PPHN with or without iNO and point out the necessity for coordinated multidisciplinary follow-up for these infants. The overall rate of neurodevelopmental handicap in infants treated with NO was 46%, with 25% mildly affected and 21% severely affected at age 1 year in one study.[218] In another study, mild and severe neurodevelopmental handicaps were 14% and 12% at age 1 year and 9% and 12% at age 2 years.[219] Sensory neural hearing loss was present in 6% to 19% of infants with PPHN treated with iNO.[218,219] No difference was noted between control and treatment groups for these outcomes. Published reports on use of iNO in ECMO centers have not substantiated early concerns that iNO would adversely affect outcome by delaying ECMO utilization.[211,212] NO treatment may play an important role in stabilizing patients before ECMO is initiated, thus improving the chances of ECMO cannulation without further clinical deterioration. The committee on Fetus and Newborn, American Academy of Pediatrics, has suggested that iNO use be limited to tertiary care centers where ECMO is available.[220] In non-ECMO centers, a system should be in place to continue iNO during transport even if a response occurs, as not all physiologic responders avoid ECMO. For the same reason, the combination of HFOV and iNO should be used cautiously in non-ECMO centers.

Inhaled nitric oxide has been used to assess the vasodilator capacity of the pulmonary vascular bed in children with CHD and elevated PVR.[143,221] Low-dose iNO (2–20 ppm) has been effective in the management of postoperative PHT following corrective surgery in infants with CHD.[222] Nitric oxide at higher doses (20–80 ppm) produced selective pulmonary vasodilatation in children with CHD and PHT.[223] Hemodynamic benefit with NO has been shown in newborns with total anomalous pulmonary venous connection or congenital mitral stenosis and in postoperative patients with preexisting left-to-right shunts and other lesions.[224] It can be used to help discriminate anatomic obstruction to PBF from pulmonary vasoconstriction, and it may be used in the treatment or prevention of pulmonary hypertensive crisis after cardiopulmonary bypass in neonates.[224,225] ECMO support for severe cardiopulmonary failure after cardiac surgery in newborns and children has been advocated in many centers.[226] A trial of NO may diminish the need for ECMO in these patients.[227,228] In children with PHT and CHD, both NO and aerosolized iloprost were equally effective in selectively lowering PVR through an increase in cGMP or cAMP, respectively.[202]

Phosphodiesterase Inhibitors. Type 5 phosphodiesterase (PDE5) is primarily responsible for degradation of cGMP to inactive metabolite GMP. The gene encoding PDE5 is abundantly expressed in the lungs of perinatal rats and is available to participate in the mammalian pulmonary vascular transition to extrauterine life.[229] PDE5 appears to be particularly abundant in pulmonary vessels. One way of augmenting the concentration of cGMP in pulmonary vessels is by inhibiting the activity of PDE5. E4021, an ultraselective PDE5 inhibitor, selectively dilates the pulmonary circulation and increases oxygenation in newborn lambs with PPHN.[230] Sildenafil is a potent and selective inhibitor of cGMP-specific PDE5[231] and has been shown to cause selective pulmonary vasodilatation in an ovine model of acute PHT.[232]

Several agents that inhibit PDE5 augment the response to NO.[233–238] PDE5 inhibition by either intravenous[235,238,239] or inhaled[236] zaprinast augments and prolongs responses to NO in awake lambs with PPHN or PHT. It enhances the effect of NO in small arteries.[240] Dipyridamole, a nonselective PDE5 inhibitor, in combination with iNO augments the decrease in PVR index and blunts the severity of acute hypoxic pulmonary vasoconstriction in children with PHT.[241] When administered alone to children with PH, dipyridamole reduces PVR index (PVRI) primarily through an increase in cardiac index.[241] Dipyridamole may have clinical utility in some patients with severe PHT who demonstrate partial responsiveness to iNO. Systemic hypotension was a major side effect with intravenous dipyridamole in lambs with PPHN.[242] Dipyridamole enhanced the response to iNO, although transiently in two infants with CDH and PPHN.[243]

Although iNO causes sustained decreases in PVR, it may be complicated by adverse hemodynamic effects after abrupt withdrawal.[207] The occurrence of these events is highly variable and may be transient and resolve over time or may necessitate higher inspired oxygen for a period of time. Exogenous NO may produce a negative feedback with rapid reduction of pulmonary vascular smooth cGMP when iNO is abruptly withdrawn. Decreased endogenous NO synthesis,[244] increase in endogenous vasoconstrictor such as ET,[99] or increase in degradation of cGMP by PDE5 may contribute to this adverse effect.[233] Children with higher PAP who are treated with iNO for a longer duration may be at increased risk for adverse hemodynamic effects of NO withdrawal. PDE5 inhibitors, by sustaining the levels of cGMP, may facilitate weaning from NO. Dipyridamole acutely attenuated the adverse hemodynamic effects of rapid withdrawal of iNO in children with PHT after surgery for CHD[237] and facilitated weaning from NO in an infant with PPHN.[245] Rebound PHT caused by withdrawal of iNO was markedly attenuated by sildenafil in two patients.[246]

Endothelin Receptor Antagonists. Although it is not clear that increased ET-1 production is the etiology of PAH, its role as a mediator of PAH seems certain. Both nonselective (ET_A and ET_B receptor) and selective (ET_A receptor) antagonists are being evaluated in animal and clinical studies. Bosentan (Tracleer), an oral antagonist of both ET_A and ET_B receptors, is the most widely studied in clinical trials. In a placebo-controlled randomized trial, bosentan increased exercise capacity and improved hemodynamics in patients with PHT.[247] Patients given bosentan had a reduced Borg dyspnea index and an improved WHO functional class indicating exercise tolerance.[247] In another large double-blind, placebo-controlled multicenter study, bosentan given for 16 weeks was well tolerated, improved exercise tolerance, and increased time to clinical worsening.[248] Studies of the physiologic and long-term effects of bosentan in children appear to be warranted. Postoperative elevation of PVR in infants and children after corrective surgery for CHD was responsive to BQ123, an ET_A receptor antagonist.[249,250] Increased levels of ET-1 predict the response to therapy.[249] As with other drugs, intravenous administration is associated with systemic hypotension and must be used with caution.[250] Close monitoring and cautious use with bosentan are required because of potentially serious hepatotoxicity and teratogenicity.

Other Therapies

Inhibition of thromboxane with an orally active agent failed to improve exercise capacity or hemodynamics in a small group of patients with PPH. In addition, the incidence of severe leg pain precluded its use in this disorder.[251] ANP also causes pulmonary vasodilation in some children with PHT secondary to CHD.[221] Its nonselective effects may limit the utility of ANP as more selective vasodilators become available. Digoxin may be a potentially useful medication for patients who present with right ventricular failure either with isolated PHT or in combination with left ventricular systolic failure.[252] Digoxin modestly increased cardiac output in patients with PHT and right ventricular failure.[252] In patients with symptomatic cor pulmonale secondary to pulmonary vascular disease, atrial septostomy can improve symptoms and may serve as a palliative bridge to heart and/or lung transplantation.[253,254]

Combined Therapies

Combining two agents may be clinically useful. As noted earlier while discussing PDE inhibitors, agents that inhibit degradation of cGMP (PDE5 inhibitors) may act synergistically with iNO. Similarly, inhibiting PDE3, which is a principal metabolizer of cAMP, might be expected to augment the response to PGI_2. Inhaled milrinone, either alone or in combination with inhaled PGI_2, selectively dilated the pulmonary vasculature without systemic effects in cardiac surgical patients with PHT.[255] Intravenous milrinone augmented the response to iNO in an experimental model of PHT.[256] As the pathophysiologic mechanisms responsible for PHT are complex, combination therapy seems attractive enough to merit further evaluation in carefully designed clinical trials.[257]

Extracorporeal Membrane Oxygenation

If the heart and lungs cannot support the newborn, they can be bypassed with ECMO. Several randomized trials have indicated improved survival of infants supported with ECMO. In a large prospective trial conducted in the United Kingdom, 121 infants with severe respiratory failure were randomized to ECMO or conventional management.[258] Survival in the ECMO-treated patients was significantly greater than in the control group (68% vs. 41% in the control group). Neurologic outcome was similar among survivors of either treatment arm, indicating ECMO likely did not contribute to morbidity in this group of critically ill infants. ECMO has been shown to be both clinically[258] and economically[259] justifiable for mature newborn infants with severe respiratory failure. ECMO is not a specific treatment for any disease but rather a method of supportive treatment, in which the patient is kept alive while the lungs and their vasculature recover. As newer treatment modalities including HFOV, surfactant therapy, and NO have become available for treatment of hypoxemic respiratory failure, ECMO use in newborns has decreased considerably.[260,261] Because of serious inherent risks, such as systemic and intracranial hemorrhage, the procedure presently is reserved for newborn infants with reversible pulmonary disease in whom alternative therapies have failed. However, ECMO should be initiated before the infant is moribund. ECMO can be a useful posttransplant support device, particularly in patients undergoing lung transplants.[262]

Heart-Lung Transplantation

Prior to the availability of PGI_2 as long-term therapy, lung transplantation was the only option for survival for patients with severe PHT. Single-lung, double-lung, and heart-lung transplantation have all been advocated as the operation of choice in patients with PPH. Transplantation is offered after maximal therapeutic effort with vasodilators, and oxygen has been attempted and when the estimated 2-year survival is less than 50%.[263] Most centers now perform bilateral lung or heart-bilateral lung transplantation for patients with PPH. Intravenous PGI_2 has been used as a bridge to stabilize the patient until transplantation is accomplished. Of the 70 lung transplants performed in 1997, PHT accounted for 7% of infants and 18% of older children requiring transplantation.[264] Survival rates have improved considerably in the 1990s, suggesting both technical improvements and earlier referral for transplantation. Data from the International Society for Heart and Lung Transplantation (January 1998–December 2001) indicate an overall survival following lung transplant of 70% to 80% at 1 year and 50% at 3 years in children younger than 17 years. Survival in all patients with PPH following lung transplant was 72% at 1 year and 58% at 3 years. In a single-center study, survival following heart-lung transplant in patients with PPH was 72% at 1 year, 67% at 2 years, and 42% at 5 years.[265] As outcomes for infants listed for lung or heart-lung transplantation are similar to those of children, very young age should not be considered a contraindication to lung or heart-lung transplantation.[266] Earlier diagnosis and listing may decrease pretransplant mortality.[266] Even though the early outcome following lung transplantation has improved considerably, long-term complications including infections, bronchiolitis obliterans, and complications of immunosuppression remain significant problems.[267] Aggressive medical therapy combined with early recognition of lung transplant candidates will improve quality of life and overall survival of these children.

REFERENCES

1. Goldstein JD, et al: Unusual vascular anomalies causing persistent pulmonary hypertension in a newborn. *Am J Cardiol* 43:962-968, 1979.
2. Drake CJ, Little CD: Exogenous vascular endothelial growth factor induces malformed and hyperfused vessels during embryonic

neovascularization. *Proc Natl Acad Sci U S A* 92:7657-7661, 1995.
3. Klein S, et al: Basic fibroblast growth factor modulates integrin expression in microvascular endothelial cells. *Mol Biol Cell* 4: 973-982, 1993.
4. Wolfe BL, et al: Insulin-like growth factor-I regulates transcription of the elastin gene. *J Biol Chem* 268:12418-12426, 1993.
5. Liu JM, Davidson JM: The elastogenic effect of recombinant transforming growth factor-beta on porcine aortic smooth muscle cells. *Biochem Biophys Res Commun* 154:895-901, 1988.
6. Risau W: Embryonic angiogenesis factors. *Pharmacol Ther* 51: 371-376, 1991.
7. Hall SM, Haworth SG: Normal adaptation of pulmonary arterial intima to extrauterine life in the pig: ultrastructural studies. *J Pathol* 149:55-66, 1986.
8. Hislop A, Reid L: Pulmonary arterial development during childhood: branching pattern and structure. *Thorax* 28:129-135, 1973.
9. Belik J, et al: Pulmonary hypertension and vascular remodeling in fetal sheep. *Am J Physiol* 66(6 pt 2):H2303-H2309, 1994.
10. Wild LM, Nickerson PA, Morin FC III: Ligating the ductus arteriosus before birth remodels the pulmonary vasculature of the lamb. *Pediatr Res* 25:251-257, 1989.
11. Chapados R, Steinhorn R, Kamm K, et al: Increased pulmonary artery myosin heavy chain-B expression and decreased force generation occur in persistent pulmonary hypertension. *Pediatr Res* 37:389A, 1995.
12. Prosser IW, et al: Regional heterogeneity of elastin and collagen gene expression in intralobar arteries in response to hypoxic pulmonary hypertension as demonstrated by in situ hybridization. *Am J Pathol* 135:1073-1088, 1989.
13. Rudolph AM, Heymann MA: Circulatory changes during growth in the fetal lamb. *Circ Res* 26:289-299, 1970.
14. Cassin S, et al: The vascular resistance of the foetal and newly ventilated lung of the lamb. *J Physiol* 171:61-79, 1964.
15. Levin DL, et al: Morphological development of the pulmonary vascular bed in fetal lambs. *Circulation* 53:144-151, 1976.
16. Morin FC III, Egan EA: Pulmonary hemodynamics in fetal lambs during development at normal and increased oxygen tension. *J Appl Physiol* 73:213-218, 1992.
17. Dawes GS, Mott JC: The vascular tone of the fetal lung. *J Physiol* 164:465-477, 1962.
18. Heymann MA: Control of the pulmonary circulation in the perinatal period. *J Dev Physiol* 6:281-290, 1984.
19. Abman SH, Accurso FJ: Acute effects of partial compression of ductus arteriosus on fetal pulmonary circulation. *Am J Physiol* 257(2 pt 2):H626-H634, 1989.
20. Morin FC III: Ligating the ductus arteriosus before birth causes persistent pulmonary hypertension in the newborn lamb. *Pediatr Res* 25:245-250, 1989.
21. Morin FC III, Egan EA: The effect of closing the ductus arteriosus on the pulmonary circulation of the fetal sheep. *J Dev Physiol* 11:283-287, 1989.
22. Cassin S, et al: Leukotrienes and prostaglandins in fetal lung liquid. *J Appl Physiol* 68:2214-2222, 1990.
23. Leffler CW, Tyler TL, Cassin S: Responses of pulmonary and systemic circulations of perinatal goats to prostaglandin F2 alpha. *Can J Physiol Pharmacol* 57:167-173, 1979.
24. Clozel M, et al: Thromboxane is not responsible for the high pulmonary vascular resistance in fetal lambs. *Pediatr Res* 19: 1254-1257, 1985.
25. Velvis H, Moore P, Heymann MA: Prostaglandin inhibition prevents the fall in pulmonary vascular resistance as a result of rhythmic distension of the lungs in fetal lambs. *Pediatr Res* 30:62-68, 1991.
26. Saeed SA, Mitchell MD: Arachidonate lipoxygenase activity in human fetal lung. *Eur J Pharmacol* 78:389-391, 1982.
27. Schreiber MD, Heymann MA, Soifer SJ: The differential effects of leukotriene C4 and D4 on the pulmonary and systemic circulations in newborn lambs. *Pediatr Res* 21:176-182, 1987.
28. Soifer SJ, et al: Leukotriene end organ antagonists increase pulmonary blood flow in fetal lambs. *Am J Physiol* 249(3 pt 2): H570-H576, 1985.
29. Schreiber MD, Heymann MA, Soifer SJ: Leukotriene inhibition prevents and reverses hypoxic pulmonary vasoconstriction in newborn lambs. *Pediatr Res* 19:437-441, 1985.
30. Leffler CW, Mitchell JA, Green RS: Cardiovascular effects of leukotrienes in neonatal piglets. Role in hypoxic pulmonary vasoconstriction? *Circ Res* 55:780-787, 1984.
31. Heymann MA, et al: Leukotriene synthesis inhibition increases pulmonary blood flow in fetal lambs. *Chest* 93(3 suppl):117S, 1988.
32. Yanagisawa M, et al: A novel potent vasoconstrictor peptide produced by vascular endothelial cells. *Nature* 332:411-415, 1988.
33. Luscher TF: Endothelin: systemic arterial and pulmonary effects of a new peptide with potent biologic properties. *Am Rev Respir Dis* 146(5 pt 2):S56-S60, 1992.
34. Wong J, et al: Developmental effects of endothelin-1 on the pulmonary circulation in sheep. *Pediatr Res* 36:394-401, 1994.
35. Luscher TF: Endothelium-derived vasoactive factors and regulation of vascular tone in human blood vessels. *Lung* 168(suppl): 27-34, 1990.
36. Cassin S, et al: Tone-dependent responses to endothelin in the isolated perfused fetal sheep pulmonary circulation in situ. *J Appl Physiol* 70:1228-1234, 1991.
37. Wong J, et al: Endothelin-1 vasoactive responses in lambs with pulmonary hypertension and increased pulmonary blood flow. *Am J Physiol* 269(6 pt 2):H1965-H1972, 1995.
38. Elton TS, et al: Normobaric hypoxia stimulates endothelin-1 gene expression in the rat. *Am J Physiol* 263(6 pt 2):R1260-R1264, 1992.
39. de Nucci G, et al: Pressor effects of circulating endothelin are limited by its removal in the pulmonary circulation and by the release of prostacyclin and endothelium-derived relaxing factor. *Proc Natl Acad Sci U S A* 85:9797-9800, 1988.
40. Mann J, Farrukh IS, Michael JR: Mechanisms by which endothelin 1 induces pulmonary vasoconstriction in the rabbit. *J Appl Physiol* 71:410-416, 1991.
41. Pinheiro JM, Malik AB: K^+ATP-channel activation causes marked vasodilation in the hypertensive neonatal pig lung. *Am J Physiol* 263(5 pt 2):H1532-H1536, 1992.
42. Tod ML, Cassin S: Endothelin-1-induced pulmonary arterial dilation is reduced by N omega-nitro-L-arginine in fetal lambs. *J Appl Physiol* 72:1730-1734, 1992.
43. Ziegler JW, et al: The role of nitric oxide, endothelin, and prostaglandins in the transition of the pulmonary circulation. *Clin Perinatol* 22:387-403, 1995.
44. Radunovic N, et al: Fetal and maternal plasma endothelin levels during the second half of pregnancy. *Am J Obstet Gynecol* 172(1 pt 1):28-32, 1995.
45. Ivy DD, Kinsella JP, Abman SH: Physiologic characterization of endothelin A and B receptor activity in the ovine fetal pulmonary circulation. *J Clin Invest* 93:2141-2148, 1994.
46. Wong J, Fineman JR, Heymann MA: The role of endothelin and endothelin receptor subtypes in regulation of fetal pulmonary vascular tone. *Pediatr Res* 35:664-670, 1994.
47. Teitel DF, Iwamoto HS, Rudolph AM: Changes in the pulmonary circulation during birth-related events. *Pediatr Res* 27(4 pt 1): 372-378, 1990.
48. Cornfield DN, et al: Oxygen causes fetal pulmonary vasodilation through activation of a calcium-dependent potassium channel. *Proc Natl Acad Sci U S A* 93:8089-8094, 1996.
49. Leffler CW, Tyler TL, Cassin S: Effect of indomethacin on pulmonary vascular response to ventilation of fetal goats. *Am J Physiol* 234:H346-H351, 1978.
50. Tyler T, et al: The effects of indomethacin on the pulmonary vascular response to hypoxia in the premature and mature newborn goat. *Proc Soc Exp Biol Med* 150:695-698, 1975.
51. Turner GR, Levin DL: Prostaglandin synthesis inhibition in persistent pulmonary hypertension of the newborn. *Clin Perinatol* 11: 581-589, 1984.
52. Frantz E, et al: Bradykinin produces pulmonary vasodilation in fetal lambs: role of prostaglandin production. *J Appl Physiol* 67: 1512-1517, 1989.
53. Truog RD, Accurso FJ, Wilkening RB: Fetal pulmonary vasodilation by histamine: response to H1 and H2 stimulation. *Dev Pharmacol Ther* 14:180-186, 1990.
54. Archer SL, et al: Nitric oxide and cGMP cause vasorelaxation by activation of a charybdotoxin-sensitive K channel by cGMP-dependent protein kinase. *Proc Natl Acad Sci U S A* 91:7583-7587, 1994.
55. Abman SH, et al: Role of endothelium-derived relaxing factor during transition of pulmonary circulation at birth. *Am J Physiol* 259(6 pt 2):H1921-H1927, 1990.
56. Iwamoto J, Morin FC III: Nitric oxide inhibition varies with hemoglobin saturation. *J Appl Physiol* 75:2332-2336, 1993.

57. Tiktinsky MH, Cummings JJ, Morin FC III: Acetylcholine increases pulmonary blood flow in intact fetuses via endothelium-dependent vasodilation. *Am J Physiol* 262(2 pt 2):H406-H410, 1992.
58. Tiktinsky MH, Morin FC III: Increasing oxygen tension dilates fetal pulmonary circulation via endothelium-derived relaxing factor. *Am J Physiol* 265(1 pt 2):H376-H380, 1993.
59. Fineman JR, et al: Chronic nitric oxide inhibition in utero produces persistent pulmonary hypertension in newborn lambs. *J Clin Invest* 93:2675-2683, 1994.
60. Konduri GG, et al: Purine nucleotides contribute to pulmonary vasodilation caused by birth-related stimuli in the ovine fetus. *Am J Physiol* 272(5 pt 2):H2377-H2384, 1997.
61. Konduri GG, Gervasio CT, Theodorou AA: Role of adenosine triphosphate and adenosine in oxygen-induced pulmonary vasodilation in fetal lambs. *Pediatr Res* 33:533-539, 1993.
62. Steinhorn RH, et al: Endothelium-dependent relaxations to adenosine in juvenile rabbit pulmonary arteries and veins. *Am J Physiol* 266(5 pt 2):H2001-H2006, 1994.
63. Konduri GG, et al: Adenosine infusion improves oxygenation in term infants with respiratory failure. *Pediatrics* 97:295-300, 1996.
64. Dobyns EL, et al: Eicosanoids decrease with successful extracorporeal membrane oxygenation therapy in neonatal pulmonary hypertension. *Am J Respir Crit Care Med* 149(4 pt 1):873-880, 1994.
65. Langleben, D, et al: Endothelin-1 in acute lung injury and the adult respiratory distress syndrome. *Am Rev Respir Dis* 148(6 pt 1): 1646-1650, 1993.
66. Ivy DD, et al: Prolonged endothelin A receptor blockade attenuates chronic pulmonary hypertension in the ovine fetus. *J Clin Invest* 99:1179-1186, 1997.
67. Adnot S, et al: Loss of endothelium-dependent relaxant activity in the pulmonary circulation of rats exposed to chronic hypoxia. *J Clin Invest* 87:155-162, 1991.
68. Shaul PW, et al: Pulmonary endothelial NO synthase gene expression is decreased in fetal lambs with pulmonary hypertension. *Am J Physiol* 272(5 pt 1):L1005-L1012, 1997.
69. McQueston JA, et al: Chronic pulmonary hypertension in utero impairs endothelium-dependent vasodilation. *Am J Physiol* 268 (1 pt 2):H288-H294, 1995.
70. Steinhorn RH, Russell JA, Morin FC III: Disruption of cGMP production in pulmonary arteries isolated from fetal lambs with pulmonary hypertension. *Am J Physiol* 268(4 pt 2):H1483-H1489, 1995.
71. Geggel RL, Reid LM: The structural basis of PPHN. *Clin Perinatol* 11:525-549, 1984.
72. Murphy JD, et al: The structural basis of persistent pulmonary hypertension of the newborn infant. *J Pediatr* 98:962-967, 1981.
73. Drummond WH, Bissonnette JM: Persistent pulmonary hypertension in the neonate: development of an animal model. *Am J Obstet Gynecol* 131:761-763, 1978.
74. Soifer SJ, Kaslow D, Roman C, Heymann MA: Umbilical cord compression produces pulmonary hypertension in newborn lambs: a model to study the pathophysiology of persistent pulmonary hypertension in the newborn. *J Dev Physiol* 9:239-252, 1987.
75. Goldberg SJ, et al: The effects of maternal hypoxia and hyperoxia upon the neonatal pulmonary vasculature. *Pediatrics* 48:528-533, 1971.
76. Reid LM: Structure and function in pulmonary hypertension. New perceptions. *Chest* 89:279-288, 1986.
77. Hammerman C, et al: Prostanoids in neonates with persistent pulmonary hypertension. *J Pediatr* 110:470-472, 1987.
78. Drummond WH, et al: The independent effects of hyperventilation, tolazoline, and dopamine on infants with persistent pulmonary hypertension. *J Pediatr* 98:603-611, 1981.
79. Walsh-Sukys MC, et al: Persistent pulmonary hypertension of the newborn in the era before nitric oxide: practice variation and outcomes. *Pediatrics* 105(1 pt 1):14-20, 2000.
80. Rudolph AM, Yuan S: Response of the pulmonary vasculature to hypoxia and H^+ ion concentration changes. *J Clin Invest* 45: 399-411, 1966.
81. Peckham GJ, Fox WW: Physiologic factors affecting pulmonary artery pressure in infants with persistent pulmonary hypertension. *J Pediatr* 93:1005-1010, 1978.
82. Bifano EM, Pfannenstiel A: Duration of hyperventilation and outcome in infants with persistent pulmonary hypertension. *Pediatrics* 81:657-661, 1988.
83. Hendricks-Munoz KD, Walton JP: Hearing loss in infants with persistent fetal circulation. *Pediatrics* 81:650-656, 1988.
84. Dworetz AR, et al: Survival of infants with persistent pulmonary hypertension without extracorporeal membrane oxygenation. *Pediatrics* 84:1-6, 1989.
85. Wung JT, et al: Management of infants with severe respiratory failure and persistence of the fetal circulation, without hyperventilation. *Pediatrics* 76:488-494, 1985.
86. Lyrene RK, et al: Alkalosis attenuates hypoxic pulmonary vasoconstriction in neonatal lambs. *Pediatr Res* 19:1268-1271, 1985.
87. Morin FI: Hyperventilation, alkalosis, prostaglandins and the pulmonary circulation of the newborn. *Appl Physiol* 61:2088-2094, 1986.
88. Wagenvoort CA, Wagenvoort N: Primary pulmonary hypertension: a pathologic study of the lung vessels in 156 clinically diagnosed cases. *Circulation* 42:1163-1184, 1970.
89. Abenhaim L, et al: Appetite-suppressant drugs and the risk of primary pulmonary hypertension. International Primary Pulmonary Hypertension Study Group. *N Engl J Med* 335:609-616, 1996.
90. Miller VM, Burnett JC Jr: Modulation of NO and endothelin by chronic increases in blood flow in canine femoral arteries. *Am J Physiol* 263(1 pt 2):H103-H108, 1992.
91. Luscher TF, Barton M: Endothelins and endothelin receptor antagonists: therapeutic considerations for a novel class of cardiovascular drugs. *Circulation* 102:2434-2440, 2000.
92. Yanagisawa M: The endothelin system. A new target for therapeutic intervention. *Circulation* 89:1320-1322, 1994.
93. Chen SJ, et al: Endothelin-receptor antagonist bosentan prevents and reverses hypoxic pulmonary hypertension in rats. *J Appl Physiol* 79:2122-2131, 1995.
94. Prie S, Stewart DJ, Dupuis J: Endothelin A receptor blockade improves nitric oxide-mediated vasodilation in monocrotaline-induced pulmonary hypertension. *Circulation* 97:2169-2174, 1998.
95. Panza JA, et al: Effect of increased availability of endothelium-derived nitric oxide precursor on endothelium-dependent vascular relaxation in normal subjects and in patients with essential hypertension. *Circulation* 87:1475-1481, 1993.
96. d'uscio LV, et al: Blood pressure-independent effects of chronic selective ETa-receptor blockade in L-name-induced hypertension. *J Hypertens* 16(suppl 2):S90, 1998.
97. Moreau P, et al: Blood pressure and vascular effects of endothelin blockade in chronic nitric oxide-deficient hypertension. *Hypertension* 29:763-976, 1997.
98. Verhaar MC, et al: Endothelin-A receptor antagonist-mediated vasodilatation is attenuated by inhibition of nitric oxide synthesis and by endothelin-B receptor blockade. *Circulation* 97:752-756, 1998.
99. Giaid A, et al: Expression of endothelin-1 in the lungs of patients with pulmonary hypertension. *N Engl J Med* 328:1732-1739, 1993.
100. Goerre, S, et al: Endothelin-1 in pulmonary hypertension associated with high-altitude exposure. *Circulation* 91:359-364, 1995.
101. Sartori C, et al: Exaggerated endothelin release in high-altitude pulmonary edema. *Circulation* 99:2665-2668, 1999.
102. Stewart DJ, et al: Increased plasma endothelin-1 in pulmonary hypertension: marker or mediator of disease? *Ann Intern Med* 114:464-469, 1991.
103. Cacoub P, et al: Endothelin-1 in primary pulmonary hypertension and the Eisenmenger syndrome. *Am J Cardiol* 71:448-450, 1993.
104. Yoshibayashi M, et al: Plasma endothelin concentrations in patients with pulmonary hypertension associated with congenital heart defects. Evidence for increased production of endothelin in pulmonary circulation. *Circulation* 84:2280-2285, 1991.
105. Allen SW, et al: Circulating immunoreactive endothelin-1 in children with pulmonary hypertension. Association with acute hypoxic pulmonary vasoreactivity. *Am Rev Respir Dis* 148: 519-522, 1993.
106. Giaid A: Nitric oxide and endothelin-1 in pulmonary hypertension. *Chest* 114(3 suppl):208S-212S, 1998.
107. Gerber JG, et al: Moderation of hypoxic vasoconstriction by infused arachidonic acid: role of PGI2. *J Appl Physiol Respir Environ Exerc Physiol* 49:107-112, 1980.
108. Bunting S, et al: Arterial walls generate from prostaglandin endoperoxides a substance (prostaglandin X) which relaxes strips of mesenteric and coeliac arteries and inhibits platelet aggregation. *Prostaglandins* 12:897-913, 1976.

109. Hamberg M, Svensson J, Samuelsson B: Thromboxanes: a new group of biologically active compounds derived from prostaglandin endoperoxides. *Proc Natl Acad Sci U S A* 72: 2994-2998, 1975.
110. Adatia I, et al: Thromboxane A2 and prostacyclin biosynthesis in children and adolescents with pulmonary vascular disease. *Circulation* 88(5 pt 1):2117-2122, 1993.
111. Christman BW, et al: An imbalance between the excretion of thromboxane and prostacyclin metabolites in pulmonary hypertension. *N Engl J Med* 327:70-75, 1992.
112. Tuder RM, et al: Prostacyclin synthase expression is decreased in lungs from patients with severe pulmonary hypertension. *Am J Respir Crit Care Med* 159:1925-1932, 1999.
113. Geraci MW, et al: Pulmonary prostacyclin synthase overexpression in transgenic mice protects against development of hypoxic pulmonary hypertension. *J Clin Invest* 103:1509-1515, 1999.
114. Nagaya N, et al: Gene transfer of human prostacyclin synthase ameliorates monocrotaline-induced pulmonary hypertension in rats. *Circulation* 102:2005-2010, 2000.
115. Weir EK, Archer SL: The mechanism of acute hypoxic pulmonary vasoconstriction: the tale of two channels. *FASEB J* 9:183-189, 1995.
116. Yuan XJ, et al: Attenuated K^+ channel gene transcription in primary pulmonary hypertension. *Lancet* 351:726-727, 1998.
117. Patel AJ, Lazdunski M, Honore E: Kv2.1/Kv9.3, a novel ATP-dependent delayed-rectifier K^+ channel in oxygen-sensitive pulmonary artery myocytes. *EMBO J* 16:6615-6625, 1997.
118. Michelakis ED, et al: Dexfenfluramine elevates systemic blood pressure by inhibiting potassium currents in vascular smooth muscle cells. *J Pharmacol Exp Ther* 291:1143-1149, 1999.
119. Weir EK, et al: A role for potassium channels in smooth muscle cells and platelets in the etiology of primary pulmonary hypertension. *Chest* 114(3 suppl):200S-204S, 1998.
120. Reeve HL, et al: Dexfenfluramine increases pulmonary artery smooth muscle intracellular $Ca2^+$, independent of membrane potential. *Am J Physiol* 277(3 pt 1):L662-L666, 1999.
121. Wang J, et al: Action of fenfluramine on voltage-gated K^+ channels in human pulmonary-artery smooth-muscle cells. *Lancet* 352:290, 1998.
122. Cowan KN, Jones PL, Rabinovitch M: Elastase and matrix metalloproteinase inhibitors induce regression, and tenascin-C antisense prevents progression, of vascular disease. *J Clin Invest* 105:21-34, 2000.
123. Rabinovitch M: It all begins with EVE (endogenous vascular elastase). *Isr J Med Sci* 32:803-808, 1996; discussion 809-810.
124. Cowan KN, et al: Complete reversal of fatal pulmonary hypertension in rats by a serine elastase inhibitor. *Nat Med* 6:698-702, 2000.
125. Fernandez-Patron C, et al: Differential regulation of platelet aggregation by matrix metalloproteinases-9 and -2. *Thromb Haemost* 82:1730-1735, 1999.
126. Fernandez-Patron C, Radomski MW, Davidge ST: Vascular matrix metalloproteinase-2 cleaves big endothelin-1 yielding a novel vasoconstrictor. *Circ Res* 85:906-911, 1999.
127. Welsh CH, et al: Coagulation and fibrinolytic profiles in patients with severe pulmonary hypertension. *Chest* 110:710-717, 1996.
128. Eddahibi S, et al: Treatment with 5-HT potentiates development of pulmonary hypertension in chronically hypoxic rats. *Am J Physiol* 272(3 pt 2):H1173-H1181, 1997.
129. Eddahibi S, et al: Serotonin transporter overexpression is responsible for pulmonary artery smooth muscle hyperplasia in primary pulmonary hypertension. *J Clin Invest* 108:1141-1150, 2001.
130. Deng Z, et al: Familial primary pulmonary hypertension (gene PPH1) is caused by mutations in the bone morphogenetic protein receptor-II gene. *Am J Hum Genet* 67:737-744, 2000.
131. Lane KB, et al: Heterozygous germline mutations in BMPR2, encoding a TGF-beta receptor, cause familial primary pulmonary hypertension. The International PPH Consortium. *Nat Genet* 26:81-84, 2000.
132. Heath D, Edwards JE: The pathology of hypertensive pulmonary vascular disease: a description of six grades of structural changes in the pulmonary arteries with special reference to congenital cardiac septal defects. *Circulation* 18:533-547, 1958.
133. Wood P: The Eisenmenger syndrome or pulmonary hypertension with reversed central shunt. *Br Med J* 46:701-709, 1958.
134. Rabinovitch M, et al: Lung biopsy in congenital heart disease: a morphometric approach to pulmonary vascular disease. *Circulation* 58:1107-1122, 1978.
135. Blackstone EH, et al: Optimal age and results in repair of large ventricular septal defects. *J Thorac Cardiovasc Surg* 72:661-679, 1976.
136. Rabinovitch M, et al: Vascular structure in lung tissue obtained at biopsy correlated with pulmonary hemodynamic findings after repair of congenital heart defects. *Circulation* 69:655-667, 1984.
137. Haworth SG, Reid L: Structural study of pulmonary circulation and of heart in total anomalous pulmonary venous return in early infancy. *Br Heart J* 39:80-92, 1977.
138. Wheller J, et al: Diagnosis and management of postoperative pulmonary hypertensive crisis. *Circulation* 60:1640-1644, 1979.
139. Hanley FL, et al: Repair of truncus arteriosus in the neonate. *J Thorac Cardiovasc Surg* 105:1047-56, 101993.
140. Hopkins RA, et al: Pulmonary hypertensive crises following surgery for congenital heart defects in young children. *Eur J Cardiothorac Surg* 5:628-634, 1991.
141. Hall SM, Haworth SG: Onset and evolution of pulmonary vascular disease in young children: abnormal postnatal remodelling studied in lung biopsies. *J Pathol* 166:183-193, 1992.
142. Celermajer DS, Cullen S, Deanfield JE: Impairment of endothelium-dependent pulmonary artery relaxation in children with congenital heart disease and abnormal pulmonary hemodynamics. *Circulation* 87:440-446, 1993.
143. Wessel DL, et al: Use of inhaled nitric oxide and acetylcholine in the evaluation of pulmonary hypertension and endothelial function after cardiopulmonary bypass. *Circulation* 88(5 pt 1):2128-3821, 1993.
143a. Berner M, Beghetti M, Spahr-Schopfer I, Oberhansli I, Friedl B: Inhaled nitric oxide to test the vasodilator capacity of the pulmonary vascular bed in children with long-standing pulmonary hypertension and congenital heart disease. *Am J Cardiol* 77:532-535, 1996.
144. Lutz J, et al: Endothelin-1- and endothelin-receptors in lung biopsies of patients with pulmonary hypertension due to congenital heart disease. *Clin Chem Lab Med* 37:423-428, 1999.
145. Rich S, et al: Primary pulmonary hypertension. A national prospective study. *Ann Intern Med* 107:216-223, 1987.
146. Rubin LJ: Primary pulmonary hypertension. *Chest* 104:236-250, 1993.
147. Rhodes J, et al: Hemodynamic correlates of exercise function in patients with primary pulmonary hypertension. *J Am Coll Cardiol* 18:1738-1744, 1991.
148. D'Angelo A, et al: Brief report: autoimmune protein S deficiency in a boy with severe thromboembolic disease. *N Engl J Med* 328:1753-1757, 1993.
149. Shandas R, et al: Development of a noninvasive ultrasound color M-mode means of estimating pulmonary vascular resistance in pediatric pulmonary hypertension: mathematical analysis, in vitro validation, and preliminary clinical studies. *Circulation* 104:908-913, 2001.
150. Bowyer JJ, et al: Effect of long term oxygen treatment at home in children with pulmonary vascular disease. *Br Heart J* 55:385-390, 1986.
151. Fuster V, et al: Primary pulmonary hypertension: natural history and the importance of thrombosis. *Circulation* 70:580-587, 1984.
152. Frank H, et al: The effect of anticoagulant therapy in primary and anorectic drug-induced pulmonary hypertension. *Chest* 112: 714-721, 1997.
153. Keszler M, et al: Severe respiratory failure after elective repeat cesarean delivery: a potentially preventable condition leading to extracorporeal membrane oxygenation. *Pediatrics* 89(4 pt 1): 670-672, 1992.
154. Auten RL, et al: Surfactant treatment of full-term newborns with respiratory failure. *Pediatrics* 87:101-107, 1991.
155. Lotze A, et al: Multicenter study of surfactant (beractant) use in the treatment of term infants with severe respiratory failure. Survanta in Term Infants Study Group. *J Pediatr* 132:40-47, 1998.
156. Glick PL, et al: Pathophysiology of congenital diaphragmatic hernia. III: Exogenous surfactant therapy for the high-risk neonate with CDH. *J Pediatr* Surg 27:866-869, 1992.
157. Glick PL, et al: Pathophysiology of congenital diaphragmatic hernia II: the fetal lamb CDH model is surfactant deficient. *J Pediatr* Surg 27:382-387, 1992; discussion 387-388.
158. Wilcox DT, et al: Pathophysiology of congenital diaphragmatic hernia. V. Effect of exogenous surfactant therapy on gas exchange and lung mechanics in the lamb congenital diaphragmatic hernia model. *J Pediatr* 124:289-293, 1994.

159. Holm BA, Matalon S: Role of pulmonary surfactant in the development and treatment of adult respiratory distress syndrome. *Anesth Analg* 69:805-818, 1989.
160. Lewis JF, Jobe AH: Surfactant and the adult respiratory distress syndrome. [published erratum appears in *Am Rev Respir Dis* 147:following 1068, 1993]. *Am Rev Respir Dis* 147:218-233, 1993.
161. Petty TL, et al: Characteristics of pulmonary surfactant in adult respiratory distress syndrome associated with trauma and shock. *Am Rev Respir Dis* 115:531-536, 1977.
162. Petty TL, et al: Abnormalities in lung elastic properties and surfactant function in adult respiratory distress syndrome. *Chest* 75:571-574, 1979.
163. Gregory TJ, et al: Surfactant chemical composition and biophysical activity in acute respiratory distress syndrome. *J Clin Invest* 88:1976-1981, 1991.
164. Lachmann B: Animal models and clinical pilot studies of surfactant replacement in adult respiratory distress syndrome. *Eur Respir J Suppl* 3:98s-103s, 1989.
165. Richman PS, et al: The adult respiratory distress syndrome: first trials with surfactant replacement. *Eur Respir J Suppl* 3: 109s-111s, 1989.
166. Anzueto A, et al: Aerosolized surfactant in adults with sepsis-induced acute respiratory distress syndrome. Exosurf Acute Respiratory Distress Syndrome Sepsis Study Group. *N Engl J Med* 334:1417-1421, 1996.
167. Carlo WA, et al: High-frequency jet ventilation in neonatal pulmonary hypertension. *Am J Dis Child* 143:233-238, 1989.
168. Clark RH, Yoder BA, Sell MS: Prospective, randomized comparison of high-frequency oscillation and conventional ventilation in candidates for extracorporeal membrane oxygenation. *J Pediatr* 124:447-544, 1994.
169. Engle WA, et al: Controlled prospective randomized comparison of high-frequency jet ventilation and conventional ventilation in neonates with respiratory failure and persistent pulmonary hypertension. *J Perinatol* 17:3-9, 1997.
170. Kinsella JP, Abman SH: Clinical approaches to the use of high-frequency oscillatory ventilation in neonatal respiratory failure. *J Perinatol* 16(2 pt 2 suppl):S52-S55, 1996.
171. Kinsella JP, et al: Randomized, multicenter trial of inhaled nitric oxide and high-frequency oscillatory ventilation in severe, persistent pulmonary hypertension of the newborn. *J Pediatr* 131 (1 pt 1):55-62, 1997.
172. Holzapfel L, et al: Comparison of high-frequency jet ventilation to conventional ventilation in adults with respiratory distress syndrome. *Intensive Care Med* 13:100-105, 1987.
173. Schuster DP, Klain M, Snyder JV: Comparison of high frequency jet ventilation to conventional ventilation during severe acute respiratory failure in humans. *Crit Care Med* 10:625-630, 1982.
174. Barst RJ: Treatment of primary pulmonary hypertension with continuous intravenous prostacyclin. *Heart* 77:299-301, 1997.
175. Barst RJ, Maislin G, Fishman AP: Vasodilator therapy for primary pulmonary hypertension in children. *Circulation* 99: 1197-1208, 1999.
176. Rich S, Kaufmann E, Levy PS: The effect of high doses of calcium-channel blockers on survival in primary pulmonary hypertension. *N Engl J Med* 327:76-81, 1992.
177. Goetzman BW, et al: Neonatal hypoxia and pulmonary vasospasm: response to tolazoline. *J Pediatr* 89:617-621, 1976.
178. Lock JE, et al: Use of prostacyclin in persistent fetal circulation. *Lancet* 1:1343, 1979.
179. Watkins WD, et al: Prostacyclin and prostaglandin E1 for severe idiopathic pulmonary artery hypertension. *Lancet* 1:1083, 1980.
180. Eronen M, et al: Prostacyclin treatment for persistent pulmonary hypertension of the newborn. *Pediatr Cardiol* 18:3-7, 1997.
181. Rich S, McLaughlin VV: The effects of chronic prostacyclin therapy on cardiac output and symptoms in primary pulmonary hypertension. *J Am Coll Cardiol* 34:1184-1187, 1999.
182. Barst RJ, et al: A comparison of continuous intravenous epoprostenol (prostacyclin) with conventional therapy for primary pulmonary hypertension. The Primary Pulmonary Hypertension Study Group. *N Engl J Med* 334:296-302, 1996.
183. McLaughlin VV, et al: Compassionate use of continuous prostacyclin in the management of secondary pulmonary hypertension: a case series. *Ann Intern Med* 130:740-743, 1999.
184. Channick RN, et al: Pulsed delivery of inhaled nitric oxide to patients with primary pulmonary hypertension: an ambulatory delivery system and initial clinical tests. *Chest* 109:1545-1549, 1996.
185. McLaughlin VV, et al: Reduction in pulmonary vascular resistance with long-term epoprostenol (prostacyclin) therapy in primary pulmonary hypertension. *N Engl J Med* 338:273-277, 1998.
186. Barst RJ, et al: Survival in primary pulmonary hypertension with long-term continuous intravenous prostacyclin. *Ann Intern Med* 121:409-415, 1994.
187. Rosenzweig EB, Kerstein D, Barst RJ: Long-term prostacyclin for pulmonary hypertension with associated congenital heart defects. *Circulation* 99:1858-1865, 1999.
188. Murai T, et al: Effect of beraprost sodium on peripheral circulation insufficiency in rats and rabbits. *Arzneimittelforschung* 39:856-859, 1989.
189. Murata T, et al: General pharmacology of beraprost sodium. 2nd communication: effect on the autonomic, cardiovascular and gastrointestinal systems, and other effects. *Arzneimittelforschung* 39:867-876, 1989.
190. Ichida F, et al: Acute effect of oral prostacyclin and inhaled nitric oxide on pulmonary hypertension in children. *J Cardiol* 29: 217-224, 1997.
191. Nagaya N, et al: Effect of orally active prostacyclin analogue on survival of outpatients with primary pulmonary hypertension. *J Am Coll Cardiol* 34:1188-1192, 1999.
192. Okano Y, et al: Orally active prostacyclin analogue in primary pulmonary hypertension. [published erratum appears in *Lancet* 350:1406, 1997]. *Lancet* 349:1365, 1997.
193. Ono F, et al: Hemodynamic and hormonal effects of beraprost sodium, an orally active prostacyclin analogue, in patients with secondary precapillary pulmonary hypertension. *Circ J* 67:375-378, 2003.
194. Nagaya N, et al: Oral beraprost sodium improves exercise capacity and ventilatory efficiency in patients with primary or thromboembolic pulmonary hypertension. *Heart* 87:340-345, 2002.
195. Simonneau G, et al: Continuous subcutaneous infusion of treprostinil, a prostacyclin analogue, in patients with pulmonary arterial hypertension: a double-blind, randomized, placebo-controlled trial. *Am J Respir Crit Care Med* 165:800-804, 2002.
196. Bindl L, Fahnenstich H, Peukert U: Aerosolised prostacyclin for pulmonary hypertension in neonates. *Arch Dis Child Fetal Neonat Ed* 71:F214-F216, 1994.
197. Kelly LK, et al: Inhaled prostacyclin for term infants with persistent pulmonary hypertension refractory to inhaled nitric oxide. *J Pediatr* 141:830-832, 2002.
198. Walmrath D, et al: Direct comparison of inhaled nitric oxide and aerosolized prostacyclin in acute respiratory distress syndrome. *Am J Respir Crit Care Med* 153:991-996, 1996.
199. Olschewski H, et al: Aerosolized prostacyclin and iloprost in severe pulmonary hypertension. *Ann Intern Med* 124:820-824, 1996.
200. Hoeper MM, et al: Long-term treatment of primary pulmonary hypertension with aerosolized iloprost, a prostacyclin analogue. *N Engl J Med* 342:1866-1870, 2000.
201. Olschewski H, et al: Inhaled iloprost for severe pulmonary hypertension. *N Engl J Med* 347:322-329, 2002.
202. Rimensberger PC, et al: Inhaled nitric oxide versus aerosolized iloprost in secondary pulmonary hypertension in children with congenital heart disease: vasodilator capacity and cellular mechanisms. *Circulation* 103:544-548, 2001.
203. Clark RH, et al: Low-dose nitric oxide therapy for persistent pulmonary hypertension of the newborn. Clinical Inhaled Nitric Oxide Research Group. *N Engl J Med* 342:469-474, 2000.
204. Kinsella JP, et al: Low-dose inhalation nitric oxide in persistent pulmonary hypertension of the newborn. *Lancet* 340:819-820, 1992.
205. Roberts JD, et al: Inhaled nitric oxide in persistent pulmonary hypertension of the newborn. *Lancet* 340:818-819, 1992.
206. Pepke-Zaba J, et al: Inhaled nitric oxide as a cause of selective pulmonary vasodilatation in pulmonary hypertension. *Lancet* 338:1173-1174, 1991.
207. Kinsella JP, et al: Selective and sustained pulmonary vasodilation with inhalational nitric oxide therapy in a child with idiopathic pulmonary hypertension. *J Pediatr* 122(5 pt 1):803-806, 1993.

208. Snell GI, et al: Inhaled nitric oxide used as a bridge to heart-lung transplantation in a patient with end-stage pulmonary hypertension. *Am J Respir Crit Care Med* 151:1263-1266, 1995.
209. Ricciardi MJ, et al: Inhaled nitric oxide in primary pulmonary hypertension: a safe and effective agent for predicting response to nifedipine. *J Am Coll Cardiol* 32:1068-1073, 1998.
210. Petros AJ, Turner SC, Nunn AJ: Cost implications of using inhaled nitric oxide compared with epoprostenol for pulmonary hypertension. *J Pharm Technol* 11:163-166, 1995.
211. Roberts JD, Jr, et al: Inhaled nitric oxide and persistent pulmonary hypertension of the newborn. The Inhaled Nitric Oxide Study Group. *N Engl J Med* 336:605-610, 1997.
212. Anonymous: Inhaled nitric oxide in full-term and nearly full-term infants with hypoxic respiratory failure. The Neonatal Inhaled Nitric Oxide Study Group. [published erratum appears in *N Engl J Med* 337:434, 1997]. *N Engl J Med* 336:597-604, 1997.
213. Finer NN, Barrington KJ: Nitric oxide for respiratory failure in infants born at or near term. [update in *Cochrane Database Syst Rev* 2001:CD000399; PMID: 11405963]. *Cochrane Database Syst Rev* 2000:CD000399.
214. Zayek M, et al: Effect of nitric oxide on the survival rate and incidence of lung injury in newborn lambs with persistent pulmonary hypertension. *J Pediatr* 123:947-952, 1993.
215. Cornfield DN, et al: Randomized, controlled trial of low-dose inhaled nitric oxide in the treatment of term and near-term infants with respiratory failure and pulmonary hypertension. *Pediatrics* 104(5 pt 1):1089-1094, 1999.
216. Finer NN, et al: Randomized, prospective study of low-dose versus high-dose inhaled nitric oxide in the neonate with hypoxic respiratory failure. *Pediatrics* 108:949-955, 2001.
217. Davidson D, et al: Inhaled nitric oxide for the early treatment of persistent pulmonary hypertension of the term newborn: a randomized, double-masked, placebo-controlled, dose-response, multicenter study. The I-NO/PPHN Study Group. *Pediatrics* 101 (3 pt 1):325-334, 1998.
218. Lipkin PH, et al: Neurodevelopmental and medical outcomes of persistent pulmonary hypertension in term newborns treated with nitric oxide. *J Pediatr* 140:306-310, 2002.
219. Rosenberg AA, et al: Longitudinal follow-up of a cohort of newborn infants treated with inhaled nitric oxide for persistent pulmonary hypertension. *J Pediatr* 131(1 pt 1):70-75, 1997.
220. Anonymous: American Academy of Pediatrics. Committee on Fetus and Newborn. Use of inhaled nitric oxide. *Pediatrics* 106 (2 pt 1):344-345, 2000.
221. Ivy DD, et al: Atrial natriuretic peptide and nitric oxide in children with pulmonary hypertension after surgical repair of congenital heart disease. *Am J Cardiol* 77:102-105, 1996.
222. Miller OI, et al: Very low dose inhaled nitric oxide: a selective pulmonary vasodilator after operations for congenital heart disease. *J Thorac Cardiovasc Surg* 108:487-494, 1994.
223. Roberts JD Jr, et al: Inhaled nitric oxide in congenital heart disease. *Circulation* 87:447-453, 1993.
224. Atz AM, Wessel DL: Inhaled nitric oxide in the neonate with cardiac disease. *Semin Perinatol* 21:441-455, 1997.
225. Atz AM, et al: Inhaled nitric oxide in children with pulmonary hypertension and congenital mitral stenosis. *Am J Cardiol* 77: 316-319, 1996.
226. Kulik TJ, et al: Outcome-associated factors in pediatric patients treated with extracorporeal membrane oxygenator after cardiac surgery. *Circulation* 94(9 suppl):II63-II68, 1996.
227. Journois D, et al: Inhaled nitric oxide as a therapy for pulmonary hypertension after operations for congenital heart defects. *J Thorac Cardiovasc Surg* 107:1129-1135, 1994.
228. Goldman AP, et al: Nitric oxide might reduce the need for extracorporeal support in children with critical postoperative pulmonary hypertension. *Ann Thorac Surg* 62:750-755, 1996.
229. Sanchez LS, et al: Cyclic-GMP-binding, cyclic-GMP-specific phosphodiesterase (PDE5) gene expression is regulated during rat pulmonary development. *Pediatr Res* 43:163-168, 1998.
230. Dukarm RC, Morin RJFC III, Perry BJ, Steinhorn RH: The cGMP-specific phosphodiesterase inhibitor E4021 dilates the pulmonary circulation. *Am J Respir Crit Care Med* 160:858-865, 1999.
231. Boolell M, et al: Sildenafil, a novel effective oral therapy for male erectile dysfunction. *Br J Urol* 78:257-261, 1996.
232. Bigatello LM, et al: Sildenafil can increase the response to inhaled nitric oxide. *Anesthesiology* 92:1827-1829, 2000.
233. Cohen AH, et al: Inhibition of cyclic 3′-5′-guanosine monophosphate-specific phosphodiesterase selectively vasodilates the pulmonary circulation in chronically hypoxic rats. *J Clin Invest* 97:172-179, 1996.
234. Braner DA, et al: M&B 22948, a cGMP phosphodiesterase inhibitor, is a pulmonary vasodilator in lambs. *Am J Physiol* 264(1 pt 2):H252-H258, 1993.
235. Ichinose F, et al: Prolonged pulmonary vasodilator action of inhaled nitric oxide by Zaprinast in awake lambs. *J Appl Physiol* 78:1288-1295, 1995.
236. Ichinose F, et al: Selective pulmonary vasodilation induced by aerosolized zaprinast. *Anesthesiology* 88:410-416, 1998.
237. Ivy DD, et al: Dipyridamole attenuates rebound pulmonary hypertension after inhaled nitric oxide withdrawal in postoperative congenital heart disease. *J Thorac Cardiovasc Surg* 115:875-882, 1998.
238. Thusu KG, Morin FC III, Russell JA, Steinhorn RH: The cGMP phosphodiesterase inhibitor zaprinast enhances the effect of nitric oxide. *Am J Respir Crit Care Med* 152(5 pt 1):1605-1610, 1995.
239. Ziegler JW, et al: Dipyridamole, a cGMP phosphodiesterase inhibitor, causes pulmonary vasodilation in the ovine fetus. *Am J Physiol* 269(2 pt 2):H473-H479, 1995.
240. Steinhorn RH, Gordon JB, Tod ML: Site-specific effect of guanosine 3′,5′-cyclic monophosphate phosphodiesterase inhibition in isolated lamb lungs. *Crit Care Med* 28:490-495, 2000.
241. Ziegler JW, et al: Effects of dipyridamole and inhaled nitric oxide in pediatric patients with pulmonary hypertension. *Am J Respir Crit Care Med* 158(5 pt 1):1388-1395, 1998.
242. Dukarm RC, et al: Pulmonary and systemic effects of the phosphodiesterase inhibitor dipyridamole in newborn lambs with persistent pulmonary hypertension. *Pediatr Res* 44:831-837, 1998.
243. Thebaud B, et al: Dypiridamole, a cGMP phosphodiesterase inhibitor, transiently improves the response to inhaled nitric oxide in two newborns with congenital diaphragmatic hernia. *Intensive Care Med* 25:300-303, 1999.
244. Giaid A, Saleh D: Reduced expression of endothelial nitric oxide synthase in the lungs of patients with pulmonary hypertension. *N Engl J Med* 333:214-221, 1995.
245. al-Alaiyan S, al-Omran A, Dyer D: The use of phosphodiesterase inhibitor (dipyridamole) to wean from inhaled nitric oxide. *Intensive Care Med* 22:1093-1095, 1996.
246. Atz AM, Wessel DL: Sildenafil ameliorates effects of inhaled nitric oxide withdrawal. *Anesthesiology* 91:307-310, 1999.
247. Channick RN, et al: Effects of the dual endothelin-receptor antagonist bosentan in patients with pulmonary hypertension: a randomised placebo-controlled study. *Lancet* 358:1119-1123, 2001.
248. Rubin LJ, et al: Bosentan therapy for pulmonary arterial hypertension. [published erratum appears in *N Engl J Med* 346:1258, 2002]. *N Engl J Med* 346:896-903, 2002.
249. Schulze-Neick I, et al: The endothelin antagonist BQ123 reduces pulmonary vascular resistance after surgical intervention for congenital heart disease. *J Thorac Cardiovasc Surg* 124:435-441, 2002.
250. Prendergast B, et al: Early therapeutic experience with the endothelin antagonist BQ-123 in pulmonary hypertension after congenital heart surgery. *Heart* 82:505-508, 1999.
251. Langleben D, et al: Effects of the thromboxane synthetase inhibitor and receptor antagonist terbogrel in patients with primary pulmonary hypertension. *Am Heart J* 143:E4, 2002.
252. Rich S, et al: The short-term effects of digoxin in patients with right ventricular dysfunction from pulmonary hypertension. *Chest* 114:787-792, 1998.
253. Nihill MR, O'Laughlin MP, Mullins CE: Effects of atrial septostomy in patients with terminal cor pulmonale due to pulmonary vascular disease. *Cathet Cardiovasc Diagn* 24:166-172, 1991.
254. Kerstein D, et al: Blade balloon atrial septostomy in patients with severe primary pulmonary hypertension. *Circulation* 91:2028-2035, 1995.
255. Haraldsson SA, Kieler-Jensen N, Ricksten SE: The additive pulmonary vasodilatory effects of inhaled prostacyclin and inhaled

milrinone in postcardiac surgical patients with pulmonary hypertension. *Anesth Analg* 93:1439-1445, 2001.
256. Deb B, Bradford K, Pearl RG: Additive effects of inhaled nitric oxide and intravenous milrinone in experimental pulmonary hypertension. *Crit Care Med* 28:795-799, 2000.
257. Channick RN, Rubin LJ: Combination therapy for pulmonary hypertension: a glimpse into the future? *Crit Care Med* 28: 896-897, 2000.
258. Anonymous: UK collaborative randomised trial of neonatal extracorporeal membrane oxygenation. UK Collaborative ECMO Trail Group. *Lancet* 348:75-82, 1996.
259. Roberts TE: Economic evaluation and randomised controlled trial of extracorporeal membrane oxygenation: UK collaborative trial. The Extracorporeal Membrane Oxygenation Economics Working Group. *BMJ* 317:911-915, 1998; discussion 915-916.
260. Kennaugh JM, et al: Impact of new treatments for neonatal pulmonary hypertension on extracorporeal membrane oxygenation use and outcome. *J Perinatol* 17:366-369, 1997.
261. Hintz SR, et al: Decreased use of neonatal extracorporeal membrane oxygenation (ECMO): how new treatment modalities have affected ECMO utilization. *Pediatrics* 106:1339-1343, 2000.
262. Kirshbom PM, et al: Use of extracorporeal membrane oxygenation in pediatric thoracic organ transplantation. *J Thorac Cardiovasc Surg* 123:130-136, 2002.
263. Bridges ND: Lung transplantation in children. *Curr Opin Cardiol* 13:73-77, 1998.
264. Boucek MM, et al: The Registry of the International Society of Heart and Lung Transplantation: Second Official Pediatric Report—1998. *J Heart Lung Transplant* 17:1141-1160, 1998.
265. Whyte RI, et al: Heart-lung transplantation for primary pulmonary hypertension. *Ann Thorac Surg* 67:937-941, 1999; discussion 941-942.
266. Ro PS, Spray TL, Bridges ND: Outcome of infants listed for lung or heart/lung transplantation. *J Heart Lung Transplant* 18:1232-1237, 1999.
267. Gaynor JW, et al: Update on lung transplantation in children. *Curr Opin Pediatr* 10:256-261, 1998.

CHAPTER 44

Mechanical Ventilation and Respiratory Care

Shekhar T. Venkataraman

PEARLS

- Modern pediatric respiratory care requires a major institutional commitment in resource allocation for the state-of-the-art management of the patient undergoing mechanical ventilation.
- A team approach among the physician, the nurse, the respiratory therapist, and the family is required, in which the role and responsibilities of each of the team members is clearly defined and respected.
- Everyone is equally important for the care of the patient undergoing mechanical ventilation. Physician's medical expertise is of no value in the absence of appropriate nursing care and respiratory therapy.
- As new technologies are developed, every team member must become familiar with them so that they can be applied safely and effectively.
- Family involvement is crucial to provide emotional and psychological support to the child.

Applied Respiratory Physiology

Air gets in, air gets out; oxygen is taken up, carbon dioxide is eliminated; this is the essence of breathing, spontaneous or otherwise.

Lung Volumes and Capacities

Tidal volume is the volume of gas that is moved in and out of the lungs per breath. The normal tidal volume is 6 to 8 ml/kg, regardless of age. Total lung capacity (TLC) is the volume of gas present in the lung with maximal inflation. The normal range for TLC is 60 to 80 ml/kg. Vital capacity is the volume of gas that can be maximally expired from TLC. The normal vital capacity is about 30 to 40 ml/kg in infants and 45 to 55 ml/kg in adults. Functional residual capacity (FRC) is the volume of gas that is present in the lung at the end of expiration. FRC results from the balance between forces that favor alveolar collapse and maintain alveolar inflation. The normal FRC is about 30 ml/kg. Residual volume is the volume of gas present in the lung at the end of a maximal expiratory effort and cannot be expelled from the lung. Closing capacity (CC) refers to the volume of gas present in the lung at which small conducting airways begin to collapse. When FRC exceeds CC, the small airways and the alveoli remain open because the lung volume remains above CC. On the other hand, when CC exceeds FRC, the small airways and alveoli tend to collapse. In children older than 6 years, FRC exceeds CC. In infants and in children younger than 6 years, CC exceeds FRC. This explains the propensity for atelectasis in infants and young children.

Physiology of Inflation and Deflation

Thoracic structures impede lung inflation. Therefore a certain amount of force is required to overcome this impedance. One of the major determinants of impedance to lung inflation is elasticity of the lung and chest wall. Compliance, a measure of elasticity, is defined as the change in volume per unit change in transmural pressure. Lung compliance is defined as the change in lung volume for a unit change in transalveolar pressure (alveolar pressure minus the pleural pressure). Chest compliance is the change in thoracic cage volume produced by a unit change in transthoracic pressure (ambient pressure minus the pleural pressure). Specific lung compliance refers to lung compliance that is normalized to the lung volume or body weight and is similar in children and adults. Disease processes that result in an abnormal lung or chest wall compliance are given in Box 44–1. The second major determinant of impedance to lung inflation is airway resistance. Airway resistance is defined as the change in transpulmonary pressure (proximal airway pressure minus the alveolar pressure) required to produce a unit flow of gas through the airways of the lung. In the infant, the airway resistance is equally distributed between the upper and lower airways. With increasing age, most of the airway resistance resides in the upper airways. Two additional factors impede inflation. One is inertia of the respiratory gas, or inertance.[1] The other is the frictional resistance to deformation of the lungs, thoracic cage, and abdominal contents.[1] Frictional resistance is also known as the *nonelastic viscous resistance*. Therefore taking into consideration all the forces that impede lung inflation, the total pressure (Ptp) required to inflate the lung can be mathematically expressed as follows:

$$\text{Ptp} = \text{PCompliance} + \text{Presistance} + \text{PInertance} + \text{PFrictional resistance},$$

where PCompliance is the pressure required to overcome the compliance of the respiratory system, PResistance is the pressure required to overcome the resistance of the airways, PInertance is the pressure required to overcome inertance, and PFrictional resistance is the pressure required to overcome the frictional resistance to deformation of the lungs, thoracic cage, and abdominal contents. PCompliance = volume/compliance = volume × elastance, where elastance is the reciprocal of compliance.

$$\text{PResistance} + \text{PFrictional resistance} = \text{total resistance} \times \text{flow}$$

Normally, the PInertance and PFrictional resistance are negligible. In certain pathological conditions, such as pulmonary edema, interstitial lung disease, and pulmonary fibrosis, frictional resistance may be increased. Therefore with the effect of inertance neglected, a simplified equation of motion can be expressed as follows:

$$\text{Ptp} = (\text{volume/compliance}) + (\text{resistance} \times \text{flow}) \text{ or } (\text{elastance} \times \text{volume}) + (\text{resistance} \times \text{flow})$$

It takes a finite amount of time to inflate the lung with a given volume of gas. This factor is directly proportional to the compliance and the resistance. Time constant is the product of compliance and resistance, and it defines the time taken to cause a given change in lung volume with a constant distending pressure. The rate of inflation and deflation of the lung is normally exponential; one time constant is the time taken to cause a 63% change in volume, and three time constants is the time taken to cause a 95% change in volume.[1] For the most part expiration is passive because of the elastic recoil of the lung. Elastic recoil of the lung is attributable to alveolar surface tension and tissue elasticity. Surface tension is greatest at high lung volumes, and lowest at FRC. Elastic recoil of the lung provides most of the force required to expel the gas from the lungs. Again, the time taken to expel a certain tidal volume depends on the time constant of the respiratory system. Because inspiratory and expiratory resistances are different, inspiratory and expiratory time constants may be different.

BOX 44–1

Factors Associated with Decreased Total Respiratory Compliance

DECREASED LUNG COMPLIANCE

- Surfactant deficiency or alteration
  - Respiratory distress of the newborn
  - Adult respiratory distress syndrome
- Interstitial inflammation
  - Diffuse pneumonitis
  - Fibrosis
- Pulmonary edema
  - Alveolar edema
  - Interstitial edema
- Hyperinflation
  - Airway obstruction—both upper and lower
  - Excessive CPAP/PEEP or auto-PEEP
- Atelectasis

DECREASED CHEST COMPLIANCE

- Restrictive pleural disease
  - Pleural collection of air or fluid
  - Fibrosis
- Increased intercostal muscle tone
  - Upper motor neuron disease
  - Drugs
- Restrictive chest diseases
  - Deformations—kyphosis, scoliosis, or both
  - Ankylosis
  - Restrictive bandages

DIAPHRAGMATIC RESTRICTION

- Abdominal distension
- Abdominal binding
- Increased abdominal pressure—peritoneal dialysis, post-laparotomy, etc.

CPAP, continuous positive airway pressure; *PEEP*, positive end-expiratory pressure.

Work of Breathing

During normal tidal breathing, the work of breathing is performed entirely by the inspiratory muscles (Fig. 44–1), and almost all of the work is performed during inspiration. Nearly half of the work of breathing during inspiration is dissipated as heat to overcome frictional resistance to deformation.[1] The remaining inspiratory work is stored as potential energy that is used to perform the expiratory work. Increased airway resistance and decreased chest and lung compliances would require a greater Ptp to inflate the lung to the same lung volume. This imposes a greater workload on the respiratory muscles and increases the oxygen cost of breathing. When the oxygen supply-demand balance to the respiratory muscles is perturbed, respiratory failure may ensue because of muscle fatigue.

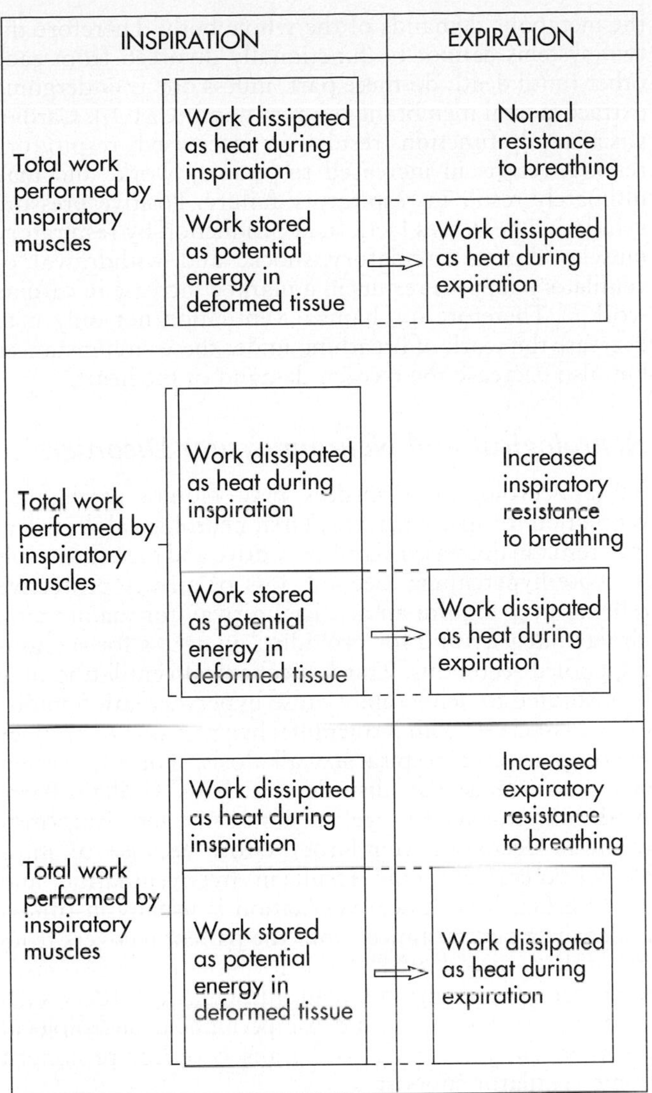

FIGURE 44–1 • Work of breathing of respiratory muscles. The area in each box represents the amount of work performed. The left side shows the total amount of work performed with normal resistance, and increased inspiratory and expiratory resistances to breathing. (Reproduced with permission from Nunn JF: *Applied respiratory physiology,* ed 3, London, 1987, Butterworths.)

Determinants of Gas Exchange

The determinants of systemic arterial oxygenation are inspired oxygen concentration and tension, lung volume, cardiac output, ventilation-perfusion (V/Q) matching, and the magnitude of venous admixture or intrapulmonary shunting. Lung volumes are increased during inspiration and fall during expiration. During expiration, the presence of alveolar surfactant prevents alveolar collapse. A critical opening pressure is required to maintain both the patency of the terminal airways and alveolar volume. When the airway pressure is below the critical opening pressure, the terminal airway closes and the alveoli collapse because of continued absorption of gases into the bloodstream. Surfactant deficiency, loss, or alteration promotes alveolar collapse and increases the critical opening pressure. In parenchymal lung disease, which is characterized by an increased critical closing pressure, alveoli collapse during expiration if the airway pressures cannot be maintained above the critical opening pressure. Alveolar collapse leads to inadequate oxygenation due to increased intrapulmonary shunting resulting from (V/Q) mismatch.

Inadequate ventilation results from a minute alveolar ventilation that is insufficient to meet the metabolic production of carbon dioxide. Partial pressure of arterial carbon dioxide ($Paco_2$) reflects the balance between metabolic production of carbon dioxide and its elimination. Failure of carbon dioxide elimination usually results from hypoventilation due to decreased central drive, lower airway obstruction, parenchymal disease, and muscle weakness (Box 44–2). Increased metabolic production of carbon dioxide usually results from hypermetabolic states and excessive caloric intake, especially high carbohydrate alimentation.

Indications for Mechanical Ventilation

Respiratory Failure

The primary indication for institution of assisted ventilation is respiratory failure. Apnea or respiratory arrest is an extreme form of respiratory failure and an absolute indication for mechanical ventilation. Respiratory failure is generally defined as the presence of (1) inadequate oxygenation, (2) inadequate ventilation, or (3) both. Inadequate oxygenation, objectively, is defined as partial pressure of arterial oxygen (Pao_2) less than 60 torr in room air. Oxygenation can also be expressed as the ratio of Pao_2 to Fio_2 (fractional concentration of oxygen in inspired gas). Inadequate oxygenation is defined as a Pao_2-Fio_2 ratio of less than 300. Other indexes include an alveolar-to-arterial oxygen gradient of more than 300 torr with an

BOX 44–2

Causes of Ventilatory Pump Failure

DECREASED RESPIRATORY MUSCLE CAPACITY

Decreased respiratory center output (CNS disorders)
Phrenic nerve injury
Decreased muscle strength or endurance
- Malnutrition
- Prolonged neuromuscular blockade
- Muscle fatigue
- Electrolyte abnormalities

INCREASED RESPIRATORY MUSCLE LOAD

Increased work of breathing
- Hyperinflation
- Lower airway obstruction
- Decreased respiratory system compliance

Increased ventilatory requirements
Increased carbon dioxide production (e.g., excessive carbohydrate intake)
- Increased dead space
- Hypercatabolic states (e.g., sepsis)

CNS, central nervous system.

FiO_2 of 1 and a calculated or measured intrapulmonary shunt fraction greater than 15%. Inadequate oxygenation due to intrapulmonary shunting can be overcome with the addition of increased inspired oxygen concentration, provided the magnitude of the shunt is less than 15% (Fig. 44–2). Intrapulmonary shunt can be decreased by with the reexpansion of collapsed alveoli or with the decrease of the fraction of pulmonary blood flow going to the collapsed alveolar segments. Inadequate ventilation is defined as $PaCO_2$ greater than 50 torr in the absence of chronic hypercapnia. Impending respiratory failure characterized by rapidly rising $PaCO_2$, progressive respiratory distress, $PaCO_2$ out of proportion to the respiratory effort, or fatigue of respiratory muscles is a relative indication for mechanical ventilation. Intubation and institution of mechanical ventilation under these circumstances are likely to be more controlled than when full-blown respiratory failure develops. Therefore in critically ill children, establishing mechanical ventilation before respiratory failure develops is preferable. Chronic respiratory failure is defined as requirement for mechanical ventilation for more than 28 days. Children with chronic lung disease often fail to grow despite adequate caloric intake. In these patients, mechanical ventilation may decrease the work of breathing enough to allow the child to grow.

Cardiovascular Dysfunction

Moderate to severe cardiovascular dysfunction is another major indication for mechanical ventilation. The cardiovascular and respiratory systems must act in concert to maintain adequate gas exchange and thereby meet the metabolic demands of the whole body. Therefore the two systems cannot be functionally divorced from each other (until death do these part, unless one is undergoing extracorporeal membrane oxygenation [ECMO]). Cardiovascular dysfunction results in decreased respiratory reserve, results in increased respiratory work, and may ultimately result in respiratory failure. Positive pressure ventilation decreases lactic acid production by respiratory muscles during circulatory shock, and withdrawal of ventilatory support results in a marked increase in cardiac work.[2,3] Therefore mechanical ventilation not only may decrease the work of breathing under these circumstances but also decrease the oxygen demand of the heart.

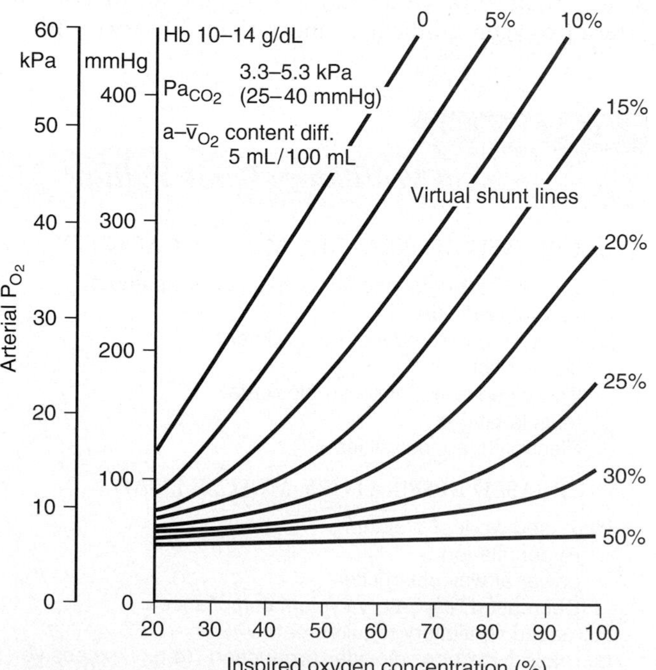

FIGURE 44–2 • Iso-shunt diagram. This shows the relationship among the magnitude of intrapulmonary shunt, the inspired oxygen concentration, and the arterial oxygen tension for a hypothetical patient. (Reproduced with permission from JF Nunn: *Applied respiratory physiology,* ed 3, London, 1987, Butterworths.)

Neurological and Neuromuscular Disorders

Acute neurological disorders may require mechanical ventilation for many reasons. First, neurological disorders may result in decreased ventilatory drive and therefore result in acute hypercapnia. Second, loss of airway protective reflexes may require an artificial airway for maintaining airway integrity and for providing an access for suctioning pooled secretions. Third, mechanical ventilation may be instituted to deliberately cause hyperventilation in disorders associated with intracranial hypertension to produce hypocapnia and respiratory alkalosis. Fourth, certain acute neuromuscular disorders such as Guillain-Barré syndrome, transverse myelitis, botulism, and drugs may result in decreased ventilatory effort because of muscle weakness and may result in hypoventilation and hypercarbia. Mechanical ventilation is usually instituted under these circumstances until the patient recovers from the primary disorder. Mechanical ventilation is also instituted for various chronic neuromuscular disorders such as muscular dystrophy and for permanent neurological disorders such as spinal cord transection for prolonged home ventilator support.

Design and Functional Characteristics of Mechanical Positive-Pressure Ventilators

A detailed review of the physical characteristics and functional design of ventilators is beyond the scope of this chapter, and the reader is referred to several excellent reviews on this subject.[4-8] Chatburn[7] first proposed a scheme to classify mechanical ventilators on the basis of the input power, control scheme, and the output variables (Box 44–3). Subsequent modifications to include newer modes of ventilation are described elsewhere.[8] The following is a brief summary that incorporates some of the elements of Chatburn's classification. A ventilator is a mechanical device that is used to move gas into the lungs by increasing Ptp. Positive pressure ventilators create Ptp by raising the mean airway pressure (Paw) above the intrapleural pressure (Ppl), whereas negative pressure ventilators create Ptp by decreasing Ppl below Paw. A ventilator can also be thought of as a machine that performs external work, i.e., movement of gas into the lungs. For this work to be performed, energy is applied to the ventilator, which is

BOX 44–3

Outline of Ventilator Classification System

I. Input
  A. Electric
    1. AC
    2. DC (battery)
  B. Pneumatic
II. Power Conversion and Transmission (drive mechanism)
  A. Compressor
    1. External
    2. Internal
  B. Motor and linkage
    1. Electric motor/rotating crank and piston rod
    2. Electric motor/rack and pinion
    3. Electric motor/direct
    4. Compressed gas/direct
  C. Output control valves
    1. Electromagnetic poppet valve
    2. Pneumatic poppet valve
    3. Electromagnetic proportional valve
    4. Pneumatic diaphragm
III. Control Scheme
  A. Control circuit
    1. Mechanical
    2. Pneumatic
    3. Fluidic
    4. Electric
    5. Electronic
  B. Control variables and waveforms
    1. Pressure
    2. Volume
    3. Flow
    4. Time
  C. Phase variables
    1. Trigger variable
    2. Limit variable
    3. Cycle variable
    4. Baseline variable
  D. Modes of ventilation and conditional variables
IV. Output
  A. Pressure
    1. Rectangular
    2. Exponential
    3. Sinusoidal
    4. Oscillating
  B. Volume
    1. Ramp
    2. Sinusoidal
  C. Flow
    1. Rectangular
    2. Ramp: a) ascending ramp, b) descending ramp
    3. Sinusoidal
  D. Effects of the patient circuit
V. Alarm Systems
  A. Input power alarms
    1. Loss of electric power
    2. Loss of pneumatic power
  B. Control circuit alarms
    1. General systems failure (ventilator-inoperative)
    2. Incompatible ventilator settings
    3. Inverse I:E ratio
  C. Output alarms
    1. Pressure
    2. Volume
    3. Flow
    4. Time
      a) high/low ventilatory frequency
      b) high/low inspiratory time
      c) high/low expiratory time (high expiratory time = apnea)
    5. Inspired Gas
      a) high/low inspired gas temperature
      b) high/low FIO_2

Reproduced from Chatburn RL: *Classification of mechanical ventilators, respiratory care equipment*, Philadelphia, 1995, JB Lippincott.
FIO_2, fractional concentration of oxygen in inspired gas; *I:E*, inspiratory-to-expiratory time ratio.

modified, transferred, and directed in a predetermined manner. All ventilators include an input power, a drive system, a control system, a cycling mechanism, and a system to provide positive end-expiratory pressure (PEEP).[4-8] The accessories include a heated humidifier and an oxygen blender. The input power provides the energy to operate the ventilator and is usually electric or pneumatic. The drive system provides the force required to generate a gas flow. For gas flow to be provided, a pressure gradient needs to be created between the ventilator and the lungs. This is most commonly accomplished with compressed gases at high pressures from wall outlets or cylinders or a small compressor designed to be used with individual ventilators. Alternatively, some ventilators have a built-in compressor such as a piston and cylinder (e.g., Emerson IMV), a diaphragm (e.g., Engtrom Erica), a system of bellows (Siemens Servo 900C), or a rotating vane (Bear 2). When a ventilator depends on an external source of compressed gases to power the ventilator, it acts mainly as a control system and will not function if the external source fails. On the other hand, a ventilator that has an internal compressor does not need an external source of gas to inflate the lung. The pressure generated within the ventilator can be thought of as the driving pressure that forces the gas into the lungs through the conducting system involving the ventilator circuit and the patient's airways. During mechanical ventilation, Ptp may be generated either by the ventilator or a spontaneous breath or a combination of both. Therefore the equation of motion can be reexpressed as:

$$\text{Ptp} = \text{Pmus} + \text{Pvent} = (\text{elastance} \times \text{volume}) + (\text{resistance} \times \text{flow}),$$

where Pmus is the pressure exerted by the respiratory muscles and Pvent is the pressure exerted by the ventilator. Compliance and resistance are assumed to remain constant during lung inflation and are called *parameters*. Pressure, volume, and flow in the respiratory system change with time and are therefore referred to as *variables*. Figure 44–3 shows the classification scheme that is based on the equation of motion.

A ventilator can also be viewed as a form of mechanical controller that "controls" either pressure (in a pressure generator) or flow (in a flow generator). A pressure generator is a ventilator that generates a fixed pattern of pressure within the ventilator and at the mouth regardless of the lung conditions, whereas the flow waveform is free to vary. This occurs when the generated pressure is low (generally between 20 and 50 cm H_2O), which results in a high initial flow rate that decays to zero as the alveolar pressure approaches the generated pressure. The generated pressure can be constant, nonconstant, increasing, or decreasing. The Hand-E-Vent (Ohio Medical Products), Bird Asthmatik (Bird Corporation), the Bennett PR-1, and the Bennett PR-2 ventilators are examples of pressure generators. A flow generator is a ventilator that generates a high driving pressure (3 to 50 psig corresponding to 200 to 3500 cm H_2O) and controls the inspiratory flow of gas into the patient by interposing a high series resistance system between the generated pressure and the patient. The flow generated may be constant, nonconstant, increasing, or decreasing.

The pattern of gas flow from the ventilator to the patient depends on the driving mechanism and the driving pressure in the ventilator. Three distinct flow patterns can be recognized: (1) a constant flow, (2) a decelerating flow, and (3) a sinusoidal or sine-wave flow (Figs. 44–4, 44–5, and 44–6). A constant inspiratory flow is generated when the driving pressure is very high (e.g., 50 psig) relative to the airway pressure. The drive mechanism is usually a high-pressure gas system (compressed air or oxygen at 10 to 50 psig). The driving force may exceed 1000 cm

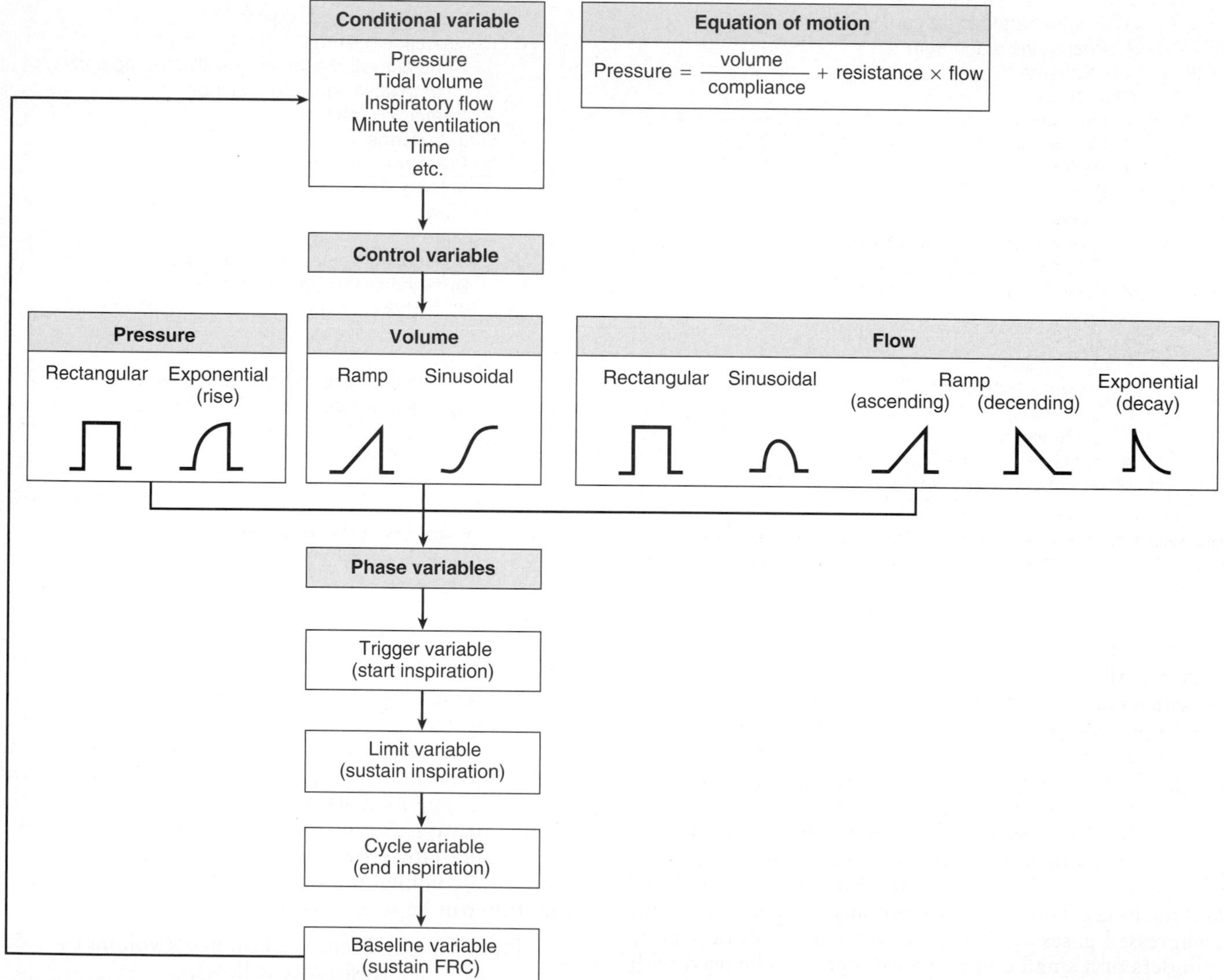

FIGURE 44–3 • Chatburn classification system based on a mathematical model known as the *equation of motion* for the respiratory system. This model indicates that during inspiration the ventilator is able to directly control one and only one variable at a time (e.g., pressure, volume, or flow). Some common waveforms provided by current ventilators are shown for each control variable. Pressure, volume, flow, and time are also used as phase variables that determine the parameters of each ventilatory cycle (e.g., trigger sensitivity, peak inspiratory flow rate or pressure, inspiratory time, and baseline pressure). (Reproduced with permission from Chatburn RL: *Classification of mechanical ventilators, respiratory care equipment,* Philadelphia, 1995, JB Lippincott.)

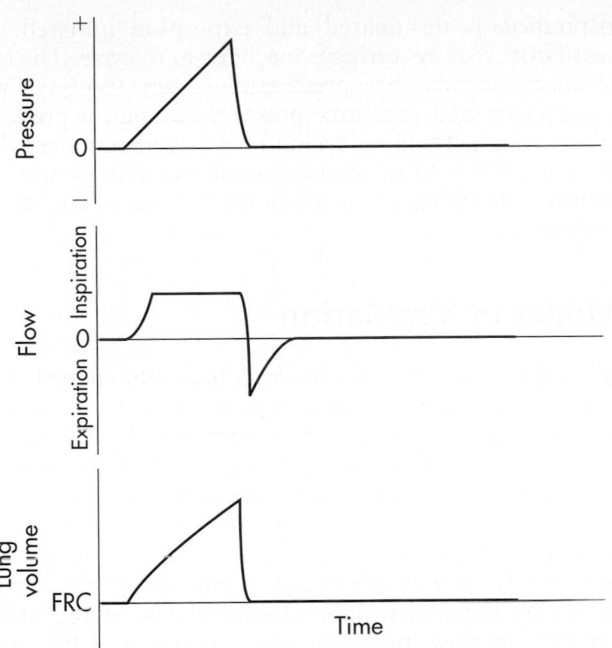

FIGURE 44–4 • Constant inspiratory flow. The flow quickly reaches a plateau and remains constant throughout the inspiratory phase. The airway pressure and lung volume increases relatively linearly. (Reproduced with permission from Kirby RR, Smith RA, Desautels DA: *Mechanical ventilation,* New York, 1985, Churchill Livingstone.)

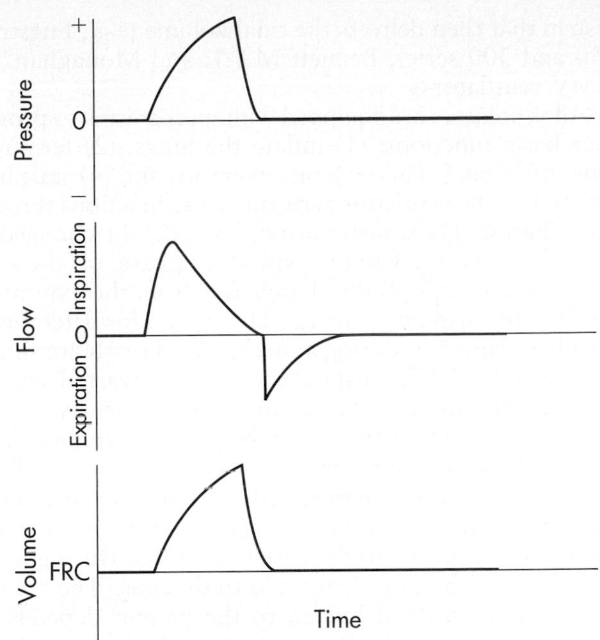

FIGURE 44–5 • Decelerating inspiratory flow. Inspiratory flow is maximal early in inspiration and gradually falls to zero at the end of inspiration. The airway pressure and lung volume rise exponentially. (Reproduced with permission from Kirby RR, Smith RA, Desautels DA: *Mechanical ventilation,* New York, 1985, Churchill Livingstone.)

H_2O and is severalfold higher than the typical proximal airway pressure that is required to inflate the lungs. An adjustable resistance controls the pressure and the flow to the proximal airway. The airway pressure and lung volume increase linearly until inspiration is terminated. Bird Mark 7 and Monaghan 225/SIMV are examples of high pressure drive systems with constant inspiratory flows. Constant flow can also be generated by a linear-driven piston, which moves at a constant rate of speed during inspiration (e.g., Bourns LS 104-150 Infant Ventilator). A decelerating inspiratory flow is created when the driving pressure is relatively low (<60 cm H_2O). In this case, a pressure-reducing valve controls the driving pressure to the desired level. As the airway pressure and lung volume increase during inspiration, the pressure gradient between the drive mechanism and the proximal airway decreases. Consequently, as inspiration continues, the inspiratory flow from the ventilator decreases and finally stops at the end of inspiration. The Bennett PR-1 and PR-2 are examples of low-pressure drive systems that produce decelerating inspiratory flows. A sine-wave or sinusoidal inspiratory flow is created when the drive mechanism is a rotary driven piston. As the rotary wheel turns, the piston is moved to and fro in the cylinder in an accelerating and then a decelerating fashion. The inspiratory flow produced also has a similar profile. Emerson 3-PV and 3-MV ventilators are examples of rotary piston devices. The notion that one specific flow pattern is more beneficial than the others is controversial. A detailed description of this topic is beyond the scope of this chapter, and the reader is referred to several excellent reviews.[4-8] Ventilators can also be classified as a single-circuit or a double-circuit device. A single-circuit device refers to a ventilator in which the gases go directly from the drive mechanism to the patient (e.g., Emerson-PV and 3-MV models, Bird Mark series, and the Siemens Elema 900 series ventilators). On the other hand, a double-circuit device refers to a system in which the drive mechanism is used to compress another

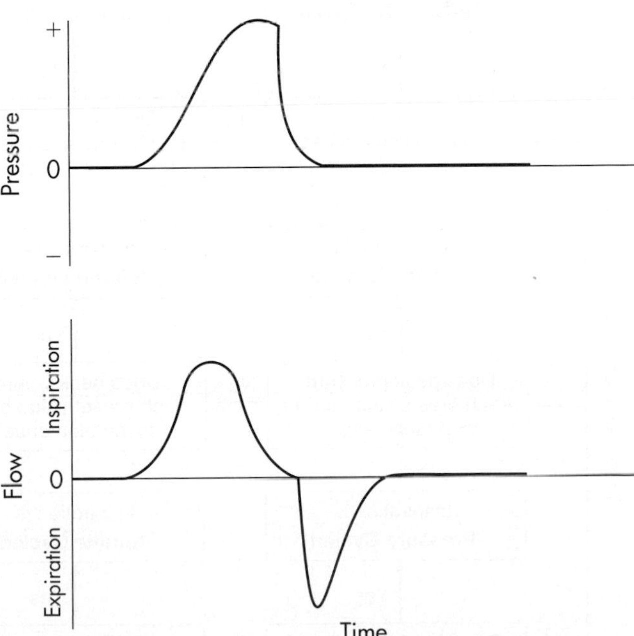

FIGURE 44–6 • Sinusoidal or "sine-wave" inspiratory flow. Inspiratory flow increases gradually and then falls gradually to zero. The airway pressure and lung volume increase in an S-shaped fashion. (Reproduced with permission from Kirby RR, Smith RA, Desautels DA: *Mechanical ventilation,* New York, 1985, Churchill Livingstone.)

system that then delivers the tidal volume (e.g., Engstrom 150 and 300 series, Bennett MA-1, and Monaghan225/ SIMV ventilators).

All ventilators are equipped with mechanisms to provide four basic functions: (1) inflate the lungs, (2) terminate lung inflation, (3) allow lungs to empty, and (4) start lung inflation.[6] The ventilator performs these functions through four phases: (1) the inspiratory phase, (2) the changeover from the inspiratory to the expiratory phase, (3) the expiratory phase, and (4) the changeover from the expiratory phase to the inspiratory phase. The criteria for determining the phase variables during a mechanical breath are shown in Figure 44–7. The inspiratory phase is started when a variable measured in the circuit or at the airway reaches a preset value. This variable can be pressure, volume, flow, or time. This is called the *trigger variable.* Pressure- or flow-triggering requires a patient effort. On the other hand, time-triggered breaths do not require a patient effort but can be synchronized to the patient's efforts. During inspiration, a tidal breath is delivered to the lung. The volume of the tidal breath delivered to the patient depends on several factors: (1) the Ptp generated, (2) the compliance and resistance of the ventilator circuit, (3) the impedance to inflation of the patient's lungs, (4) leaks in the circuit, (5) leaks around the endotracheal tube, and (6) limitation or regulation of inspiratory phase variables (pressure, flow, or volume). Limitation or regulation of the inspiratory pressure, volume, or flow does not terminate inspiration. Modern ventilators such as the Siemens Servo 300 can control more than one phase variable during inspiration. Termination of inspiration depends on the cycling mechanism. *Cycling* refers to the mechanism by which inspiration is terminated and expiration initiated. All ventilators require a trigger mechanism to cycle. The trigger for cycling may be a predetermined time (time-cycling), a predetermined pressure (pressure-cycling), a predetermined volume (volume-cycling), or a predetermined flow (flow-cycling). Most conventional ventilators used in infants and children today are time-cycled or volume-cycled ventilators.

Modes of Ventilation

When the termination of a breath is under the control of the mechanical ventilator, then it is referred to as a *mandatory breath.* A mandatory breath may be initiated by the ventilator with a preset frequency or minute ventilation, or it can be initiated by the patient. A mandatory breath is always cycled by a preset time, pressure, or volume and is not under the control of the patient. Whether the mandatory breath is initiated by the ventilator or by the patient, the characteristics of the breath (changes in flow, pressure, and volume) and the inspiratory time of the breath are the same. *Assist-control* refers to a mode of ventilation when a patient receives a combination of ventilator-initiated and patient-initiated mandatory breaths. The total number of mechanical breaths will be the sum of the preset frequency of ventilator breaths and the number of patient-triggered breaths. For example, if the preset frequency is 15 breaths per minutes and the patient triggers an additional 15 breaths per minute, the total number of mandatory breaths will be 30 breaths per minute. When the initiation and termination

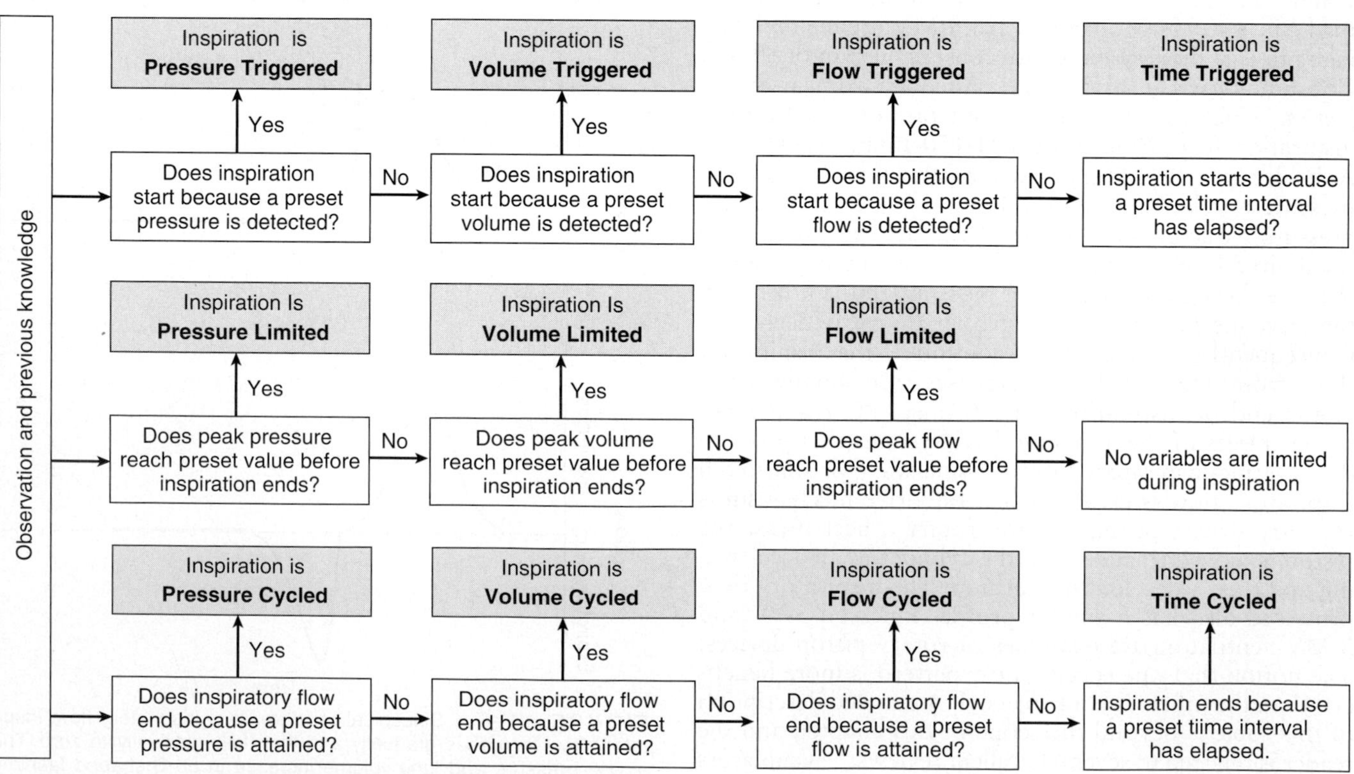

FIGURE 44–7 • Criteria for determining phase variables during a ventilator-assisted breath. (Reproduced from Chatburn RL: *Classification of mechanical ventilators, respiratory care equipment,* Philadelphia, 1995, JB Lippincott.)

of a breath is under the control of the patient's breathing efforts, it is referred to as *spontaneous breaths*. A spontaneous breath with an inspiratory pressure that is greater than the expiratory pressure is referred to as a *supported* or an *assisted mechanical breath*. For an assisted breath, the patient must initiate a breath, and then the ventilator is triggered to provide a positive pressure breath. The trigger can be either pressure or flow. When all minute ventilation is provided by the ventilator, it is referred to as *total ventilatory support*. When some of the minute ventilation is provided by spontaneous breathing and the rest by the ventilator, it is referred to as *partial ventilatory support*. Minute ventilation provided by ventilator-initiated mandatory breaths is referred to as *controlled mechanical ventilation*, and that provided by assisted mechanical breaths (patient-initiated) is referred to as *assisted mechanical ventilation* (AMV). When spontaneous breathing is responsible for the entire minute ventilation without any assistance from the ventilator, then it is referred to as *complete spontaneous breathing*. Total ventilatory support is provided when the patient does not take any spontaneous efforts because of a primary disease process (e.g., quadriplegia, muscle disease), pharmacological therapy (e.g., induced neuromuscular blockade), or suppression of spontaneous breathing efforts (e.g., hyperventilation). When all breaths are mandatory breaths, it is referred to as *continuous mandatory ventilation* (CMV). Total ventilatory support is provided entirely by CMV. On the other hand, partial ventilatory support can be provided by CMV, AMV, or a combination of both.

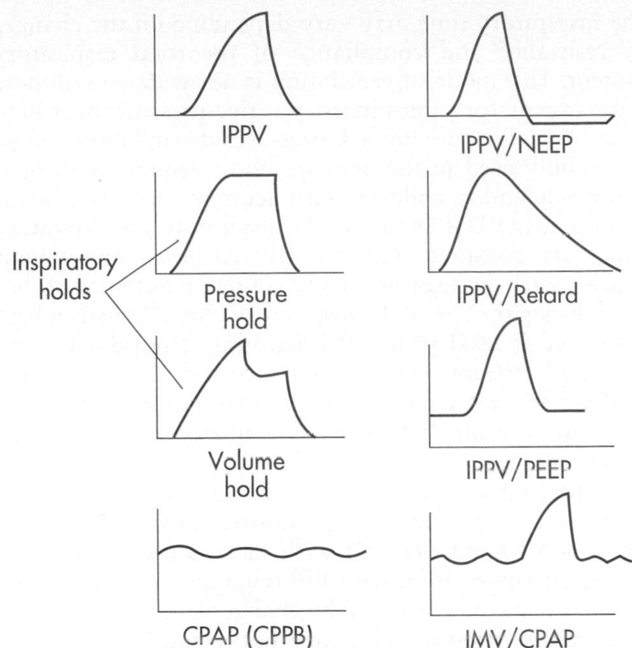

FIGURE 44–8 • Pressure-time curves of some of the mandatory modes of ventilation. (Reproduced with permission from Kirby RR, Smith RA, Desautels DA: *Mechanical ventilation,* New York, 1985, Churchill Livingstone.)

Mandatory Mechanical Ventilation

The two most common forms of controlled mechanical ventilation are pressure-regulated and volume-regulated ventilation. Figure 44–8 shows pressure-time curves for some of the mandatory modes of ventilation.

Volume-Regulated Mandatory Breaths

Volume-regulated ventilation can be delivered either by volume-cycled breath, where inspiration is terminated after a preset volume is delivered and inspiratory time is allowed to vary, or by volume-regulated time-cycled breaths, where the cycling mechanism is preset time and the tidal volume delivered is regulated by adjusting the inspiratory flow rate. In volume-regulated ventilation, the tidal volume is delivered throughout inspiration. The peak inspiratory pressure (PIP) is variable and depends on the flow rate, the total resistance, and the total compliance of the ventilator circuit and the patient's lungs. Changes in resistance or compliance will be reflected by an increase in PIP, and the ventilator can be set to alarm at a pressure limit that is generally set 5 to 10 cm above the PIP.

Most modern ventilators deliver the preset tidal volumes reliably, but the tidal volumes delivered to the patient on a breath-to-breath basis may not always be constant. The tidal volume delivered by the ventilator is distributed between the ventilator circuit, the airways, and the patient's lungs. The compliances and resistances of the ventilator circuit, the endotracheal or tracheostomy tube, and the patient independently and together affect the distribution of tidal volume delivered by the ventilator. A decrease in the compliance or an increase in the resistance of the ventilator circuit will affect the actual tidal volume delivered to the patient. The ventilator circuit includes an internal volume and the external tubing. The actual tidal volume or the effective tidal volume (VTeff) delivered to the patient can be approximated by the following formula: VTeff = VTdel – Cvent (PIP – PEEP), where VTdel is tidal volume delivered by the ventilator and Cvent is the compliance of the ventilator circuit. VTdel is equal to the inspired tidal volume, when there is no leak in the total respiratory system. When there is a leak in the system, however, such as with the use of uncuffed endotracheal tubes, then VTdel is less than the inspired tidal volume. A gain in resistance or compliance of the ventilator circuit, the endotracheal tube, or the patient's airways or lungs will increase the time constant to inflation. If the inspiratory time is less than five times the time constant of the whole respiratory system, which includes the ventilator circuit and the patient's airways, then the VTdel will be less than the preset tidal volume. During inspiration, after the tidal volume is delivered, an inspiratory hold will maintain inspiratory pressure and prolong the duration of inspiration (see Fig. 45–8). During exhalation, expiratory flow curves depend on the type of expiratory resistance or PEEP valve in the system.

Pressure-Regulated Mandatory Breaths

Pressure-regulated ventilation can be either pressure-cycled or pressure-limited time-cycled ventilation. In pressure-cycled ventilators, inspiration is terminated when a preset pressure limit is reached. In this mode of ventilation, the inspiratory time may vary depending on the changes in resistance and compliance of the total respiratory system. This mode of ventilation is not widely used these days except for intermittent positive-pressure breathing treatments. Pressure-limited, time-cycled ventilation is most commonly used in the neonate with respiratory distress syndrome and in children with acute respiratory distress syndrome (ARDS). In this mode, inspiratory and expiratory times are constant, and the PIP reaches a preset limit quickly early in inspiration and is then maintained at that level during the rest of the inspiratory phase. Usually a high flow rate is used (4 to 10 L/kg/min). The tidal volume delivered depends on the compliance and resistance of the ventilator circuit and the patient's lungs. Pressure-controlled ventilation results in higher mean airway pressure for the same amount of minute ventilation. Figure 44–9 shows the time course of changes in airway pressure, inspiratory flow, and lung volume with normal lungs, lungs with decreased compliance and with increased resistance. As shown in Figure 44-9, with PIP remaining the same, lung volume delivered is affected by changes in lung compliance and airways resistance. Factors that would increase mean airway pressure during pressure-controlled ventilation are shown in Figure 44–10.

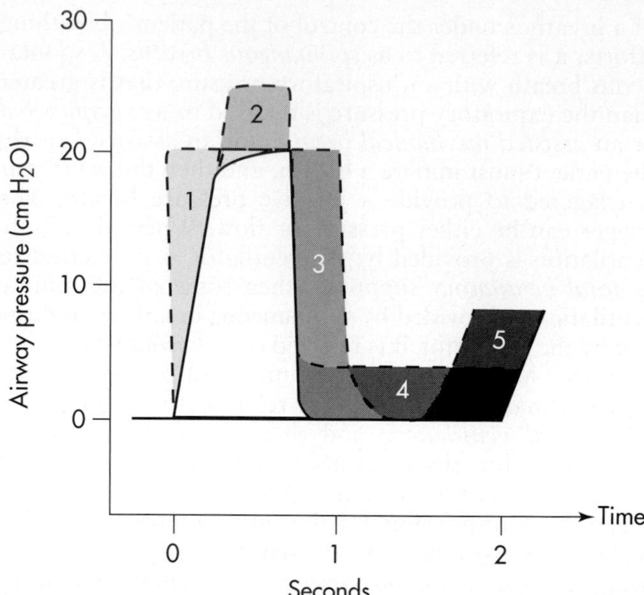

FIGURE 44–10 • Factors that increase mean airway pressure during pressure controlled ventilation: (1) increased inspiratory flow rate, (2) increased preset pressure limit, (3) increased inspiratory time, (4) increased PEEP, and (5) increased ventilator rate. Note that with each maneuver, the area under the curve increases. Area under the curve represents mean airway pressure. (Reproduced with permission from Goldsmith JP, Karotkin EH, editors: *Assisted ventilation of the neonate,* Philadelphia, 1988, WB Saunders.)

Continuous Flow versus Demand Flow

Some ventilators that can provide pressure-regulated ventilation have both inspiratory and expiratory valves. Once PIP is reached, both inspiratory and expiratory valves close and the lung is held in inflation until the end of inspiration. For use in infants, ventilators have been modified to provide continuous flow throughout the respiratory cycle. A continuous flow device refers to a ventilator in which the flow of respiratory gas occurs throughout the respiratory cycle. Most infant ventilators are continuous flow devices (e.g., Infant Star, Baby Bird). In most continuous flow infant ventilators, inspiratory valves are lacking, and the cycling is controlled by the exhalation valve. Closure of the exhalation valve begins inspiration, and the flow of gas going through the circuit is diverted to the patient. If the inspiratory flow rate is low (1 to 3 L/kg) and if the PIP is not limited, the tidal volume delivered by the patient can be calculated from the inspiratory flow rate and the inspiratory time. This would result in a time-cycled, volume-regulated breath. For pressure-control ventilation, the flow rates used are usually higher (4 to 10 L/kg). Once the preset PIP is reached, the excess flow is vented through a pressure relief valve, and the lungs are maintained in inflation throughout the rest of inspiration. During exhalation there is continuous flow of gas, allowing the patient to breathe from the circuit rather than open a demand valve. A demand flow ventilator refers to a ventilator that allows inspiratory flow of gas to the patient between ventilator breaths through a demand valve that is opened by the patient's inspiratory efforts. Work of breathing is higher with a demand flow ventilator compared with a continuous flow device because of the effort required to open the demand valve.

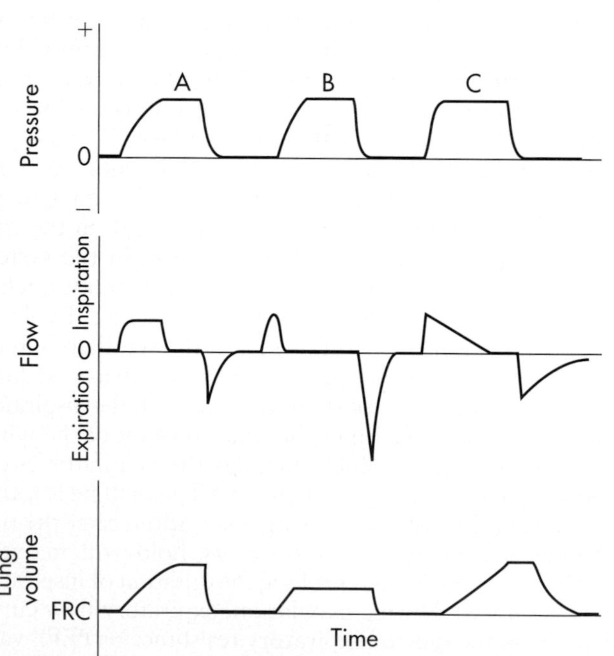

FIGURE 44–9 • Pressure-control ventilation. Inspiratory flow pattern is constant. Airway pressure and lung volume rise relatively linearly. The airway pressure reaches a preset pressure limit and does not change throughout inspiration. Lung volume follows the time course of the pressure curve with a slight lag. **A,** Normal lung. **B,** Lung with decreased compliance. **C,** Lung with increased resistance. With decreased compliance the tidal volume delivered is decreased. With increased resistance, it takes longer to deliver the tidal volume. (Reproduced with permission from Kirby RR, Smith RA, Desautels DA: *Mechanical ventilation,* New York, 1985, Churchill Livingstone.)

Intermittent Mandatory Ventilation

Intermittent mandatory ventilation (IMV) refers to a pattern of controlled ventilation in which spontaneous breathing is permitted. Between mandatory machine breaths, the patient can breathe spontaneously and the required gas flow is delivered through either a continuous flow or a demand system. The concept of IMV where spontaneous breathing occurred with a preset mechanical ventilator rate was first developed by Kirby et al[9] in 1971 with the use of a continuous flow circuit in the management of respiratory distress syndrome of the neonate. IMV was first described by Downs et al[10] in 1973 to describe a mode of ventilation that allowed the patient to breathe spontaneously with a preset ventilator rate. The spontaneous breaths are not assisted by a ventilator breath. Therefore the tidal volumes generated by the spontaneous breaths depend on the patient's effort alone and not on the ventilator support. The total ventilatory support time and duration of weaning were significantly reduced in infants using IMV compared with CMV.[11,12] Two systems are currently available to deliver IMV: one uses continuous flow, and the other uses a demand valve. Ventilators such as the InfantStar incorporate a continuous flow circuit that can be adjusted to the inspiratory flow demand of the patient. The ideal flow rate would result in minimal pressure swings associated with spontaneous inspiration and expiration. Most modern ventilators incorporate a demand valve that needs to be opened to satisfy the inspiratory flow requirements of the patient. This increases the inspiratory work of breathing. This can be minimized by the application of a small amount of pressure support. When IMV is synchronized to the patient's inspiratory efforts, it is referred to as *synchronized IMV* (SIMV) (Fig. 44-11). The ventilator accomplishes this by creating a timing window just before the next mandatory breath is scheduled to be delivered. If the patient takes a spontaneous breath in this timing window and the ventilator senses this breath on the basis of the trigger sensitivity, then the mandatory breath is synchronized with the patient's effort. Each time a synchronized breath is delivered, the machine recomputes the time required to deliver the next mandatory breath. In SIMV, the total number of mandatory breaths will only be equal to the preset frequency of mandatory breaths. SIMV breaths can be both volume regulated or pressure limited.

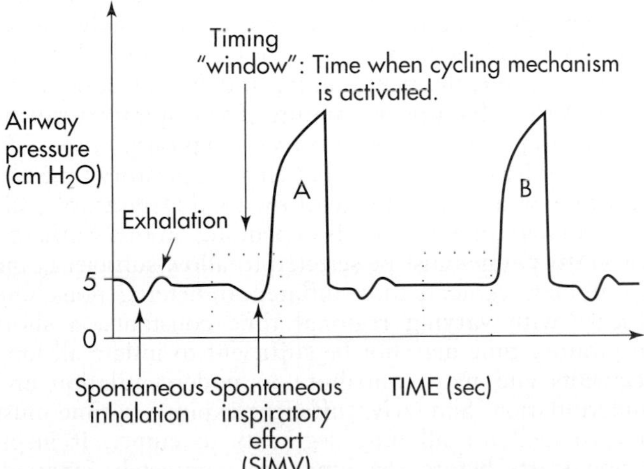

FIGURE 44–11 • Synchronized intermittent mandatory ventilation (SIMV). At set intervals, the ventilator's timing circuit becomes activated and a timing "window" appears (*shaded area*). If the patient initiates a breath in the timing window, then the ventilator will deliver a mandatory breath. If no spontaneous effort occurs, then the ventilator will deliver a mandatory breath a fixed time after the timing window. (Reproduced with permission from Kirby RR, Smith RA, Desautels DA: *Mechanical ventilation,* New York, 1985, Churchill Livingstone.)

CPAP/PEEP

CPAP (continuous positive airway pressure) refers to the maintenance of positive airway pressure throughout the respiratory cycle with no positive pressure breaths being delivered to the patient. Positive end-expiratory pressure (PEEP) refers to the maintenance of positive airway pressure above atmospheric pressure at the airway opening at end expiration.[13] CPAP/PEEP can be applied by a variety of devices. These include (1) an underwater column, (2) a water-weighted diaphragm, (3) a venturi valve, (4) a spring-loaded valve, (5) a pressurized exhalation valve, (6) a magnetic valve, and (7) a fixed or adjustable orifice. Devices that retard expiratory flows (e.g., venturi valve, fixed or adjustable orifice) tend to produce higher mean airway pressure than those that do not retard expiratory flow rates.

CPAP may be provided by several means:

1. Endotracheal CPAP[5,14]: This is the most reliable method of applying CPAP. The advantages of endotracheal CPAP are precise control of airway pressure and FiO_2; access to the airway for tracheobronchial toilet; maintenance of enteral feeding through a nasogastric tube; and, if necessary, immediate institution of mechanical ventilation. The disadvantages are those associated with those of endotracheal intubation and the long-term presence of an artificial airway.
2. Nasal CPAP: Specially designed nasal prongs,[15] a single cannula or a shortened uncuffed endotracheal tube inserted into the nasopharynx, and nasal masks[16] provide a means of applying CPAP. Because of the location in the nasopharynx, there will be a loss of pressure in the hypopharynx so that the actual CPAP delivered to the trachea may vary. This technique is easy to apply and can be instituted by less-skilled personnel. This technique is most useful in infants who are obligatory nose breathers. Mouth breathing reduces the efficiency of this technique considerably. Nasal prongs are more prone to obstruction with thick secretions and require proper humidification and frequent suctioning. Nasal prongs have also been reported to increase the work of breathing.[17]
3. Face mask CPAP: A tight-fitting mask is placed on the face covering the nose and the mouth. CPAP is provided with the application of positive airway pressure to the mask. This technique is only useful in patients who are alert and cooperative, without a tendency for nausea and vomiting. A tight-fitting mask may produce pressure lesions on the face if applied too tight. Gastric distention with vomiting and aspiration are potential problems.

The primary effect of CPAP/PEEP is an increase in FRC due to the increased Ptp. In lung diseases characterized by increased closing volume and decreased FRC, alveoli are unstable and tend to collapse. Recruitment of collapsed alveoli requires a Ptp greater than that required to sustain inflation once the alveoli are open. An increase in FRC above the closing volume restores this balance, prevents alveolar collapse, and maintains alveolar stability (Fig. 44–12). This reduces the magnitude of V/Q mismatching because of improved distribution of alveolar ventilation.[18,19] Airway closure and alveolar collapse can be prevented if the level of CPAP/PEEP is above the critical opening pressure. In lung disease with nonuniform or heterogeneous parenchymal involvement, CPAP/PEEP may hyperinflate normal lung segments, and this hyperinflation results in redistribution of blood toward the diseased segments, increasing intrapulmonary shunt on one hand and increasing alveolar dead space on the other (Fig. 44–13).

Selection of Parameters for Mandatory Breaths

The first parameter is the tidal volume. A practical approach to determining an adequate tidal volume is to evaluate the desired degree of chest expansion during manual ventilation and to reproduce that when the patient is connected to the ventilator. A desirable VTeff for most patients is 8 to 10 ml/kg. Patients with normal lung compliance may require a preset tidal volume of 12 to 15 ml/kg to produce a VTeff of 8 to 10 ml/kg. Patients with lung disease may require a preset tidal volume of 14 to 15 ml/kg to produce an effective tidal volume of 8 to 10 ml/kg because more volume will be lost in the ventilator circuit because of higher inflating pressures. A VTeff larger than 18 ml/kg is not generally recommended. The end-inspiratory alveolar

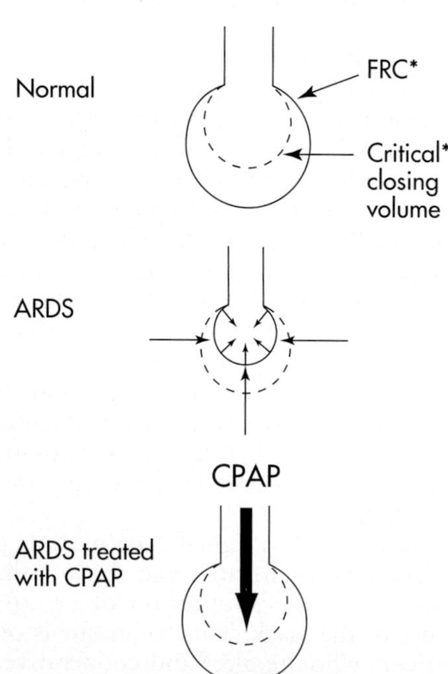

FIGURE 44–12 • Effect of CPAP on FRC. In normal lungs **(A),** FRC is greater than critical closing volume. In ARDS **(B),** FRC is less than critical closing volume. CPAP restores FRC to be greater than critical closing volume and prevents alveolar collapse. *ARDS,* Acute respiratory distress syndrome; *CPAP,* continuous positive airway pressure; *FRC,* functional residual capacity. (Reproduced with permission from Kirby RR, Smith RA, Desautels DA: *Mechanical ventilation,* New York, 1985, Churchill Livingstone.)

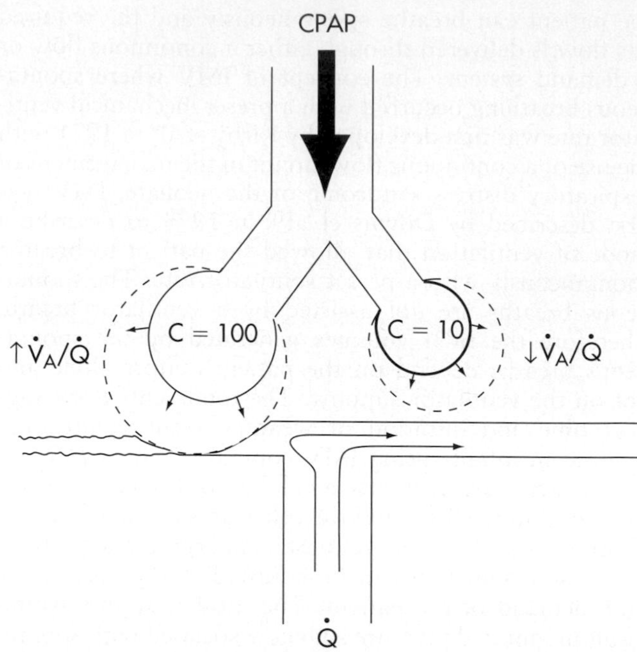

FIGURE 44–13 • Effect of CPAP on nonhomogenous lung disease. CPAP increases FRC in the lung segment with decreased ventilation-perfusion ratio (VA/Q) and decreases shunt reaction. CPAP overdistends lung segments with high VA/Q and redistributes blood toward the segments with low VA/Q increasing the amount of shunt. The net effect depends on the balance between the two. *CPAP,* continuous positive airway pressure; *FRC,* functional residual capacity; *VA/Q,* alveolar ventilation and perfusion. (Reproduced with permission from Kirby RR, Smith RA, Desautels DA: *Mechanical ventilation,* New York, 1985, Churchill Livingstone.)

pressure should not exceed 40 cm of H_2O. During mechanical ventilation, end-inspiratory alveolar pressure can be estimated through the measurement of the end-inspiratory airway pressure with an end-inspiratory hold maneuver.

Ventilator rate is the next parameter to be selected. The rate selected depends on the age of the patient and the ventilatory requirements of the patient and may subsequently be adjusted according to the $Pa{CO_2}$. The initial ventilator rate for a newborn infant usually ranges from 25 to 30 breaths per minute; for a 1 year old, between 20 and 25 breaths per minute; and for an adolescent, from 15 to 20 breaths per minute. The inspiratory time is selected to provide an inspiratory-to-expiratory time (I:E) ratio of at least 1:2 in most patients. Inspiratory time can be set either as a percentage of the total respiratory cycle or as a fixed time in seconds depending on the ventilator. Inspiratory time must be selected to allow sufficient time for all lung segments to be inflated. In heterogenous lung disease with varying regional time constants, a short inspiratory time may not be sufficient to inflate all lung segments and may contribute to underventilation and underinflation. Similarly, sufficient expiratory time must be provided for all lung segments to empty. If inspiration starts before the lung has completely emptied, this will result in air-trapping and inadvertent positive end-expiratory pressure. The I:E ratio can be adjusted according to the pathophysiological cause of the lung disease. In infants with bronchiolitis and in children with asthma, the expiratory time may have to be lengthened to avoid air-trapping.

PEEP is the next parameter to be selected. The level of PEEP will depend on the clinical circumstance. During volume-controlled ventilation, the application of PEEP results in higher PIP, mean airway pressure, and mean lung volumes. The goals of PEEP are (1) increasing FRC above closing volume to prevent alveolar collapse, (2) maintaining stability of alveolar segments, (3) improving oxygenation, and (4) reducing work of breathing. The optimum PEEP is the level at which there is an acceptable balance between the desired goals and undesired adverse effects. The desired goals are (1) reduction in inspired oxygen concentration to "nontoxic" levels (usually < 50%); (2) maintenance of PaO_2 or SaO_2 (arterial oxygen saturation) of more than 60 mmHg or more than 90%, respectively; (3) improvement of lung compliance; and (4) maximal oxygen delivery.[20-22] Arbitrary limits cannot be placed on the level of PEEP or mean airway pressure that will be required to maintain adequate gas exchange. When the level of PEEP is high, peak inspiratory pressure may be limited to prevent it from reaching dangerous levels that contribute to air leaks and barotrauma. The level of PEEP selected for patients with lower airway obstruction is controversial. There are two schools of thought: "low PEEP" and "high PEEP." Low PEEP advocates usually apply a PEEP of 3 to 5 cm H_2O because of the concern for pulmonary barotrauma from air-trapping and alveolar hyperinflation. In lower airway disease, air-trapping often results in an end-expiratory alveolar pressure that is higher than the proximal airway pressure because of incomplete emptying of the alveoli. This results in "auto-PEEP" or "inadvertent PEEP." End-expiratory lung volume and therefore the level of alveolar inflation will not be affected by the level of proximal set PEEP as long as it is less than the amount of auto-PEEP. In adults with severe asthma, high levels of PEEP, which is closer to the level of auto-PEEP, have been shown to decrease the magnitude of air-trapping and work of breathing without significant complications.[23-25] In children with tracheomalacia or bronchomalacia, PEEP decreases the airway resistance by distending the airways and preventing dynamic compression during expiration.

FiO_2 is the next parameter to be selected. FiO_2 is adjusted to maintain an adequate PaO_2. High concentration of oxygen can produce lung injury and should be avoided. The exact threshold of inspired oxygen that increases the risk of lung injury is not clear. An FiO_2 less than 0.5 is generally considered safe. In patients with parenchymal lung disease with significant intrapulmonary shunting, the major determinant of oxygenation is lung volume, which is a function of the mean airway pressure. With a shunt fraction of more than 20%, oxygenation may not be substantially improved by higher concentrations of oxygen.

Assisted Mechanical Ventilation

As defined previously, all assisted ventilation requires the patient to trigger the ventilator to provide a breath. With assisted ventilation, every breath that reaches a trigger threshold will result in a mechanical breath that is predetermined. There are two forms of assisted ventilation: with one, the ventilator controls the termination of the breath by triggering mandatory breaths (assist-control mode), and with the other the triggering and termination of the breath is under the control of the patient. For complete assisted ventilation with the assist-control mode, the ventilator preset frequency ("ventilator rate") is set to zero. Following is a description of the most common mode of assisted ventilation that is used today.

Pressure-Support Ventilation

Pressure-support ventilation (PSV) is a form of assisted ventilation in which the ventilator assists the patient's own spontaneous effort with a mechanical breath with a preset pressure limit. Figure 44–14 shows the important components of a pressure support breath. As with any form of support that is designed to respond to the patient's effort, the inspiratory pressure assist of PSV requires a signal to trigger the demand valve to initiate flow.[26] The patient's spontaneous breath creates a negative pressure (pressure-triggering) or a change in flow through the circuit (flow-triggering), which triggers the ventilator to deliver a breath. With initiation, the machine delivers high inspiratory flow to achieve a peak airway pressure level that is selected by the operator.[27-29] The pressure-limit stays constant as long as the patient's

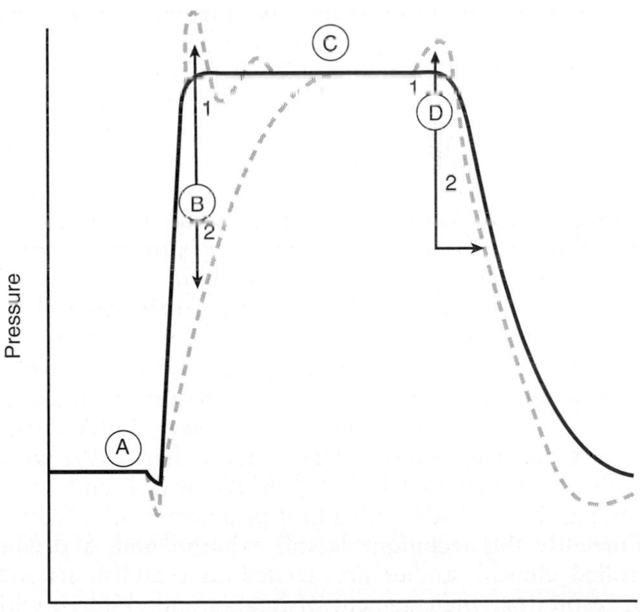

FIGURE 44–14 • Components of a pressure-support breath. *Point A* is the patient's effort indicated by a negative deflection. When the ventilator senses this trigger (change in pressure or flow), it will deliver flow to reach the desired pressure-support level (*Point B*) as rapidly as possible. Ventilator-delivered flow is then servo-adjusted to patient demand to maintain this pressure plateau (*Point C*). Inspiration is terminated when a minimal flow criterion is reached (*Point D*) and airway pressure returns to baseline. (Reproduced from MacIntyre NR: Pressure support ventilation. Mechanical ventilation and assisted Respiration. In Grenvik A, Downs J, Rasanen J, Smith R, editors: *Contemporary, management in critical care,* New York, 1991, Churchill Livingstone.)

inspiratory effort is maintained with a variable gas flow rate from the ventilator.[28,29] As inspiration continues, the inspiratory flow rate decreases. A threshold reduction in the flow rate is a signal for the termination of the inspiratory assist, with the opening of an expiratory valve, after which passive exhalation occurs.[27-29] The termination signal can be a predetermined percentage of the peak inspiratory flow (10% or 25%) or a fixed flow (usually 5 L/min).[30-32] Many ventilators also incorporate backup flow termination criteria, such as the duration of inspiration greater than 5 seconds or an increase in the airway pressure above the set pressure support level (e.g., when a patient attempts to cough). In summary, PSV is patient triggered, pressure limited, and flow cycled. PSV is entirely dependent on the patient's effort; if the patient becomes apneic, the ventilator will not provide any mechanical breath.

Other Modes of Ventilation

Airway Pressure Release Ventilation

Airway pressure release ventilation (APRV) is a method of mechanical ventilation introduced by Downs and Stock.[33] The circuit includes a CPAP device and a mechanism to release airway pressure periodically to some desired low pressure. Simplistically, this can be thought of as pressure-limited, time-cycled ventilation, in which the preset pressure limit is equal to the level of CPAP required and the PEEP is usually ambient pressure or a selected lower airway pressure, with reversal of inspiratory-expiratory ratio. Spontaneous breathing occurs at both levels of airway pressure. In the original description, the device incorporated a CPAP circuit that allowed for sufficient continuous flow of gas to maintain spontaneous ventilation. Minute ventilation occurs with both spontaneous breaths and the periodic inflation and deflation that occur with the two levels of airway pressure. Gas exchange can occur throughout the respiratory cycle. Several studies with acute respiratory failure have shown that APRV results in improvement in gas exchange with much lower airway pressures.[34-37] Lower airway pressures are the consistent major advantage of ARPV. Because airway pressures are lower, APRV results in less adverse cardiovascular effects than IMV, when both are added to CPAP.[34,36] APRV was found to be comparable to IMV with PEEP in critically ill infants.[37] Currently this technique is still experimental, and controlled clinical studies are needed to establish its role in respiratory management of infants and children with lung disease.

Mandatory Minute Volume Ventilation

Mandatory minute volume ventilation (MMV) was first introduced by Hewlett et al[38] in 1977. In this mode, the patient is guaranteed a preset delivered minute ventilation. If the spontaneous minute ventilation exceeds the preset value, then the ventilator reduces the rate to zero and does not deliver a mechanical breath. If there is no spontaneous minute ventilation, then the ventilator will deliver sufficient breaths to match the preset minute ventilation. If the spontaneous minute ventilation is insufficient to match the preset value, then the ventilator will provide the remainder of the minute ventilation. Different mechanisms are used by manufacturers to achieve this goal. In the Ohmeda CPU1 ventilator, the preset minute ventilation is compared with the patient's total minute ventilation (spontaneous and mechanical) every 24 cycles and then adjusted. In the Engstrom Erica ventilator, it is done on a breath-by-breath basis. Currently there is not much experience with MMV in pediatric patients. The indications of MMV are in patients after abdominal surgery, especially with complications; patients who are recovering from respiratory muscle paralysis (e.g., Guillain-Barré syndrome, myositis, myasthenia gravis); and patients who have widely fluctuating respiratory drive (encephalopathy).

Dual Control Modes

Dual control modes are newer modes that allow the ventilator to control pressure or volume on the basis of a feedback loop. They cannot control both at the same time, but rather one or the other. There are currently two techniques for performing dual control. In both of these techniques, there is an attempt made to ensure a certain target tidal volume. These can be classified as dual-control within a breath or dual control breath-to-breath. Dual-control within a breath uses a measured input to switch from pressure control to volume control in the middle of the breath so that the targeted volume is delivered within the same breath. In the dual control breath-to-breath, if the delivered tidal volume is not equal to targeted tidal volume, the ventilator will adjust the pressure level of subsequent pressure-limited breaths to achieve the targeted tidal volume (either pressure control mandatory breath or a pressure support breath). The example of a dual-control within a breath is volume-assured pressure support (VAPS). Examples of the dual control breath-to-breath modes are volume support (Servo 300), variable pressure support (Venturi), and pressure-regulated volume control (Servo 300). In dual-control breath-to-breath mode, the ventilator operates either in pressure-support or pressure-control mode. Some of these modes are described.

Dual Control within a Breath

These modes allow the ventilator to deliver a pressure-controlled breath or switch from a pressure-controlled breath to a volume-controlled breath within the breath. This is shown in Figure 44–15. This mode is referred to as VAPS (Bird 8400ST and Tbird, Bird Corp., Palm Springs, CA) and pressure augmentation (PA) (Bear 1000). Both of these techniques can operate during mandatory breaths (pressure-limited time-cycled) or pressure-supported breaths. During VAPS and PA, the clinician must set the respiratory frequency, peak flow, PEEP, inspired oxygen concentration, trigger sensitivity, and minimum desired tidal volume. During VAPS or PA, the ventilator's inspiratory flow waveform is constant (square). Additionally, the pressure support setting must be set. During pressure

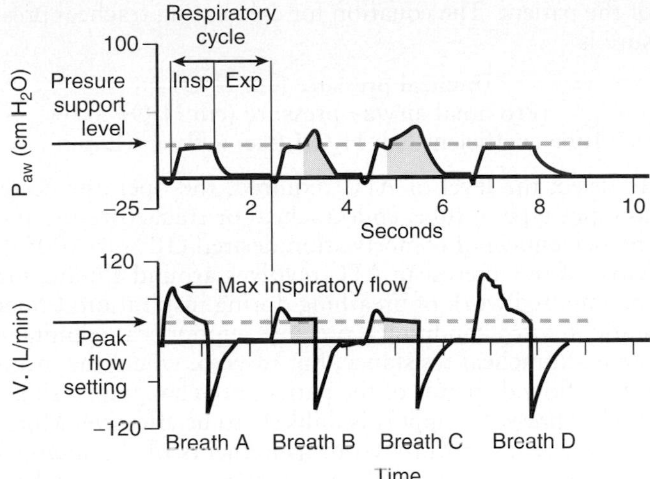

FIGURE 44–15 • Pressure and flow waveforms illustrating volume-assured pressure support (VAPS). (Reproduced with permission from Branson RD, MacIntyre NR: Dual-control modes of mechanical ventilation, *Respir Care* 41:294-305, 1996.)

support, VAPS and PA can be considered a safety net that always supplies a minimum tidal volume. A VAPS or PA breath may be initiated by the patient or time triggered. Once the breath is triggered, the ventilator attempts to reach the pressure support setting as quickly as possible. This portion of the breath is the pressure control portion and is associated with a rapid variable flow, which may reduce the work of breathing. As this pressure level is reached, the ventilator's microprocessor determines the volume that has been delivered from the machine (note: this is not exhaled tidal volume), compares this measurement with the desired tidal volume, and determines whether the minimum desired tidal volume will be reached. If the ventilator determines that the ultimate delivered tidal volume will be equivalent to the set tidal volume, the breath is delivered as a pressure support breath. If the ventilator determines that the ultimate delivered tidal volume will be less than the set tidal volume, then the breath changes from a pressure-limited to a volume-limited breath. At that point inspiratory flow remains constant, and the ventilator increases the inspiratory time until the desired volume has been delivered. Inspiratory pressure will increase above the set pressure support setting. Setting the high pressure alarm remains important during VAPS. If pressure increases abruptly, the high-pressure alarm setting is reached, and the breath is pressure cycled (Fig. 44–15). VAPS breath can allow the patient a tidal volume larger than the set volume.

Mandatory Dual Control Breath-to-Breath Modes

Dual-control breath-to-breath mode with mandatory pressure-limited time-cycled breaths is referred to as pressure-regulated volume control (PRVC) (with Siemens 300), adaptive pressure ventilation (APV) (with Hamilton Galileo), autoflow (Evita 4), or variable pressure control (Venturi), depending on the manufacturer. In this form of pressure-limited, time-cycled ventilation, delivered tidal volume is used as a feedback control for continuously adjusting the pressure limit. All breaths in these modes are time or patient triggered, pressure limited, and time cycled. One difference between devices is that the Siemens 300 only allows PRVC in the CMV mode. The newer Servo-i ventilator and the other ventilators allow dual control breath to breath with CMV or SIMV. During SIMV, the mandatory breaths are the dual control breaths. PRVC is selected on the mode selector switch, and the desired tidal volume is set. A "test breath" is delivered, and total system compliance is calculated. The next three breaths are delivered at a pressure limit that is 75% of that necessary to achieve the desired tidal volume on the basis of the compliance calculation. The ensuing breaths increase or decrease the pressure limit at less than 3 cm H_2O per breath in an attempt to deliver the desired tidal volume. The pressure limit fluctuates between 0 cm H_2O above the PEEP level and 5 cm H_2O below the upper-pressure alarm setting. The ventilator sounds an alarm if the tidal volume and maximum pressure limit settings are incompatible. With changes in lung compliance and resistance, the delivered tidal volume may not be equivalent to the set tidal volume. If the delivered tidal volume is less than the set tidal volume, the pressure-limit is increased to achieve the set tidal volume until the pressure limit is equal to a level 5 cm H_2O below the upper pressure limit alarm. The upper pressure-limit alarm must be adjusted with this in mind. It should be set to the maximum allowable pressure plus 5 cm of H_2O. When the delivered tidal volume is larger than the set tidal volume, then the ventilator will lower the pressure limit to achieve the set tidal volume. There is no lower limit for the reduction in the pressure-limit level. This mode of ventilation appears to be most beneficial when there are rapid changes in lung compliance (such as after surfactant administration[38-41]). Clinically controlled trials are required to evaluate the benefits of PRVC ventilation in acute lung disease, in ventilation of healthy lungs (i.e., in patients undergoing neurosurgical procedures), and during weaning from the ventilator.

Assisted Dual-Control Breath-to-Breath Mode

Dual control breath to breath in the pressure support mode is simply closed loop pressure support ventilation, with tidal volume as the input variable. It is referred to as volume support (Siemens 300) and variable pressure support (Venturi). All breaths are patient triggered, pressure limited, and flow cycled. Volume support is selected with the mode selector switch, and the desired tidal volume is set. The ventilator initiates volume support by delivering a "test breath" with a peak pressure of 5 cm H_2O when a patient effort is sensed. The delivered tidal volume is measured, and total system compliance is calculated. The subsequent three breaths are delivered at a peak inspiratory pressure of 75% of the pressure calculated to deliver the minimum tidal volume. Each subsequent breath uses the previous calculation of system compliance to manipulate peak pressure to achieve the desired tidal volume. From breath to breath, the maximum pressure change is less than 3 cm H_2O and can range from 0 cm H_2O above PEEP to 5 cm H_2O below the high-pressure alarm setting.

The primary cycling mechanism is flow cycling of the pressure-supported breath. Similar to the PRVC mode previously described, the pressure-support level is adjusted to maintain the set tidal volume with changes in compliance and resistance. In addition to the volume-support settings, a mandatory ventilator frequency must be set. This frequency is set according to the age of the patient; the frequency for ages younger than 6 months is 16 to 20 breaths per minute; for 6 months to 2 years, 14 to 18 breaths per minutes; for 2 to 5 years, 12 to 16 breaths per minute; and for older than 5 years, 10 to 16 breaths per minute. A secondary cycling mechanism is activated if inspiratory time exceeds 80% of the set total cycle time. There is also a relationship between the set ventilator frequency and tidal volume. The minute ventilation calculated by the set tidal volume and the backup ventilator rate gives the minimum minute ventilation that needs to be achieved. If the patient is breathing at a frequency faster than the set ventilator rate, then the only adjustment that is made by the ventilator is to manipulate the pressure-support level to achieve the desired tidal volume. The total minute ventilation in this instance will be larger than the minimum level that needs to be achieved. When the patient's breathing rate is less than the set frequency, then the total minute ventilation will decrease to a level below the set minimum level. Then, the tidal volume target is automatically increased by raising the pressure-support level up to a maximum of 150% of the initial set value. If the tidal volume has to be increased beyond the 150% of the initial set value or the minute ventilation cannot be maintained at the set minimum level, then the ventilator will alarm and switch to the PRVC mode to ensure that at least the set minimum minute ventilation is delivered.

AutoMode

AutoMode combines mandatory and assisted dual control breath-to-breath modes. The patient's effort or lack of breathing effort determines whether the breaths are flow cycled or time cycled. AutoMode is available on the Siemens 300A ventilator. Simplistically, AutoMode can be thought of as the combination of volume support and PRVC in a single mode. When the patient is breathing spontaneously, then the patient is in volume-support mode. If the patient becomes apneic or is paralyzed, the ventilator provides PRVC. The apneic threshold setting is 12 seconds for adults, 8 seconds for children, and 5 seconds for neonates. The change from PRVC to volume support or from volume support to PRVC is accomplished at equivalent peak pressures.

Automatic Tube Compensation

Automatic tube compensation (ATC) is a technique of overcoming the imposed work of breathing caused by artificial airways available in the Evita 4 ventilator. It accomplishes this by using the known resistive characteristics of the artificial airways. ATC is essentially pressure support in which the ventilator adjusts the pressure support to compensate for the imposed work of breathing by the artificial airways and the flow demand of the patient. The equation for calculating tracheal pressure is

$$\text{Tracheal pressure (cm } H_2O) = \\ \text{(Proximal airway pressure (cm } H_2O) - \\ \text{Tube coefficient (cm } H_2O\text{/L/sec)} \times \text{flow}^2 \text{ (L/min)}.$$

To select the level of ATC required, the operator needs to input type of tube, endotracheal or tracheostomy, and the percentage of compensation desired (10% to 100%). Most of the interest in ATC revolves around eliminating the imposed work of breathing during inspiration. Under static in vitro conditions, pressure support can eliminate the endotracheal resistance, but in vivo, where the inspiratory flow demands of the patient are changing, a single level of pressure support is unlikely to be effective. Moreover, there are no in vivo measurements of the minimal pressure support needed to overcome the endotracheal tube resistance. During periods of tachypnea, the level of pressure support no longer eliminates work imposed by the endotracheal tube. Additionally, the resistance of the endotracheal tube creates a condition early in the breath in which ventilator flow is high, tracheal pressure remains low, and undercompensation for imposed work occurs.[42] Late in the breath, when pressure begins to equilibrate during the pressure plateau, pressure support tends to overcompensate, prolong inspiration, and exacerbate overinflation.[42] During expiration, however, there is also a flow-dependent pressure decrease across the tube. ATC also compensates for this flow-resistive component and may reduce expiratory resistance and unintentional hyperinflation. During expiration, the calculated tracheal pressure is greater than airway pressure.

Proportional Assist Ventilation

Proportional assist ventilation (PAV) is a mode of mechanical ventilation that is based on the equation of motion. The design of PAV allows the ventilator to change the pressure output (pressure control) to always perform work proportionally to patient effort. PAV is simply PSV in which the level of pressure support is adjusted as a multiple of the sum of the volume and flow signals. The ventilator tries to maintain a constant percentage of work performed by the patient per breath irrespective of the volume of the breath or the inspiratory flow of the breath. Currently, there are major issues of interface and accurate breath-to-breath measurement of elastance and resistance and the need to take into account the confounding effects of endotracheal tube resistance, level of auto-PEEP, and the problem of nonlinearity of elastance and resistance.

Approach to Mechanical Ventilation Based on Underlying Pathophysiology

Primary Respiratory Muscle Failure ("Respiratory Pump Failure")

The primary difficulty in these disorders is inadequate ventilation due to weakness of the respiratory muscles (pump failure). Tidal volumes and ventilatory rates are set to provide normal minute ventilation to maintain normocarbia.

Complete control of ventilation may result in disuse muscle atrophy and complicate weaning from mechanical ventilation. Therefore spontaneous breathing should be encouraged as much as possible. Assisted ventilation is a useful mode of ventilation in these disorders because the trigger sensitivity can be adjusted to encourage spontaneous breathing on the one hand and prevent muscle fatigue on the other. FiO_2 is usually kept to a minimum (<0.3) because these disorders are not associated with inadequate oxygenation. In chronic hypoventilation, hypercarbia is often acceptable, provided the arterial pH is within the normal range. PEEP is usually set at a relatively low level (3-5 cm H_2O).

Disorders with Airway Obstruction

Provision of an artificial airway relieves respiratory distress due to upper airway obstruction (e.g., epiglottitis, croup). Respiratory failure due to lower airway obstruction poses a special problem during mechanical ventilation. Depression of cardiac output and hypotension may occur during intubation because of the institution of positive airway pressure to already hyperinflated lungs. This causes further impedance to venous return and increased pulmonary vascular resistance. Volume-controlled ventilation is the preferred mode of ventilation. Inspiratory-expiratory ratio should be at least 1:2. The expiratory time required depends on the severity of the lower airway obstruction. If the expiratory time is inadequate to empty the lung, "auto-PEEP" or "inadvertent PEEP" will result. Inadvertant PEEP results in air-trapping and hyperinflation with its attendant complications. The use of low levels of PEEP compared with high levels has been described previously.

Parenchymal Lung Disease

ARDS, idiopathic respiratory distress syndrome (IRDS), and interstitial pneumonias are examples of parenchymal lung disorders that are characterized by a reduction in FRC, an increase in closing volume above FRC, and diffuse subsegmental atelectasis. These diseases are characterized primarily by inadequate oxygenation due to V/Q mismatching and intrapulmonary shunting. Therapy should be directed toward maintaining lung volumes above closing volume throughout the respiratory cycle, increasing FRC above closing volume, and reducing V/Q mismatching and intrapulmonary shunting. The most effective method of achieving these goals is with an increase of mean lung volume, which is usually obtained with an increase of the mean airway pressure. During spontaneous breathing without any ventilatory assistance, CPAP is the most reliable method to increase lung volume. CPAP is effective in improving oxygenation in IRDS[14] and ARDS.[43,44] During positive-pressure breathing, the level of PEEP required to maintain adequate oxygenation primarily depends on the severity of the underlying lung disease. The degree of intrapulmonary shunting, ventilation-perfusion mismatching, alveolar edema, alveolar collapse, and decreased compliance is directly proportional to the severity of lung disease. As the severity of lung disease increases, the airway pressures required to maintain adequate gas exchange also increase. Therefore arbitrary limits cannot be placed on the level of PEEP or mean airway pressure that will be necessary to maintain adequate gas exchange. Tidal volumes should be limited to 6 to 8 ml/kg. Studies in adults, including the ARDSNetwork study, have demonstrated that using high tidal volumes of 12 ml/kg is detrimental to patient outcome.[45,46] When high levels of PEEP are used, PIP may reach levels that contribute to pulmonary air leak and barotrauma. Attempts to decrease PIP with the reduction of tidal volume will result in decreased mean airway pressure, mean lung volume, and decreased minute ventilation. With a high airway pressure maintained throughout inspiration, pressure-control ventilation may provide higher mean airway pressure and maintain a higher mean lung volume compared with volume-control ventilation. A general rule of thumb is to consider switching to pressure-limited time-cycled ventilation when PEEP requirement is more than 10 cm H_2O. For hyperinflation to be avoided, the end-inspiratory pause pressure should not exceed 35 cm H_2O. Hypercapnia may be permitted under these circumstances provided arterial pH is adequate (permissive hypercapnia).

It has been recommended that the optimal PEEP should be set above the critical closing or critical opening pressure of the airways. This can be deduced by the lower inflection point generated with static pressure-volume loops (Fig. 44–16). As the lung is inflated from zero end-expiratory pressure, in many lungs there is an abrupt change in compliance as denoted by the "lower inflection point." It is generally thought that this is the critical opening pressure of the airways above which the alveoli and airways remain open. As the lung is further inflated in increments, the pressure-volume slope increases and then abruptly changes direction as noted in Figure 45–16

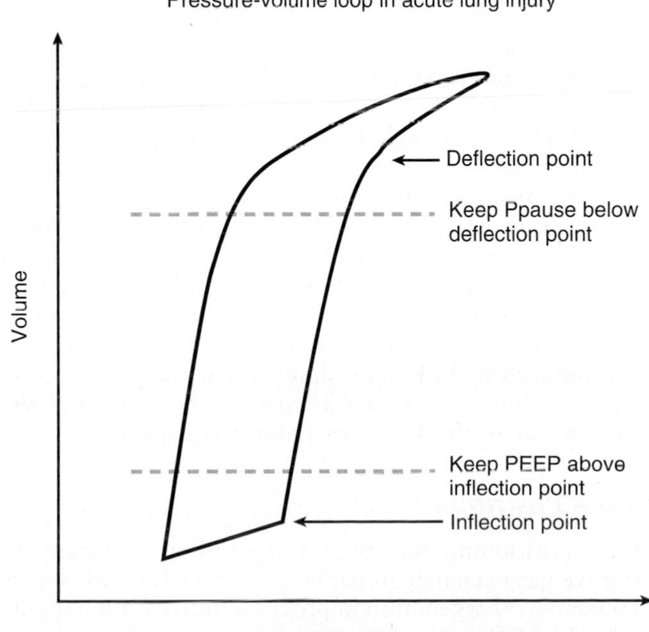

FIGURE 44–16 • Optimal PEEP and peak alveolar pressure setting in ALI/ARDS on the basis of static pressure-volume loop. The goal is to keep the PEEP level above the lower inflection point and to keep the end-inspiratory pause pressure below the upper inflection point.

as the "upper inflection point." It is generally thought that the upper inflection point reflects overdistension of the alveoli. The general recommendation is to keep the PEEP level above the lower inflection point and to keep the end-inspiratory pause pressure below the upper inflection point. Currently, bedside use of static pressure-volume loops to set PEEP is not a standard practice in infants and children. Therefore the level of PEEP should be set by titrating the level of PEEP and selecting the level by the maximal level of improvement in oxygenation compliance seen without affecting systemic hemodynamics. The repeated collapse and reopening of the lung units at low lung volume have been shown to contribute to ventilation-induced lung injury. A strategy combining recruitment maneuvers, low-tidal volume, and higher PEEP has been shown to decrease the incidence of barotrauma or volutrauma.[47-51]

Alveolar Recruitment and Derecruitment

Alveolar recruitment with maintenance of lung volume by preventing derecruitment during mechanical ventilation is a goal in ventilating the lungs of patients with acute lung injury (ALI) and ARDS. The benefits of optimal lung recruitment and prevention of derecruitment are (1) a reduction in the intrapulmonary shunt fraction and venous admixture resulting in an improvement in arterial oxygenation; (2) improvement in lung compliance; and (3) prevention of repeated alveolar collapse and reopening, which may ameliorate or prevent ventilator-induced lung injury. The primary determinants of alveolar recruitment and derecruitment are transpulmonary pressure and PEEP, respectively. Mean airway pressure has been shown to be an excellent marker of mean alveolar pressure.[52] Increasing mean airway pressure will improve oxygenation if there is alveolar recruitment. Currently several techniques of alveolar recruitment have been described in the literature. These include manual inflation to high airway pressures, the increase of PEEP in a stepwise manner, application of a sign maneuver, the use of pressure-limited time-cycled ventilation with a high peak inspiratory pressure, and the combination of titrated levels of PEEP with increased inflation pressures. Ventilatory sighs are effective in recruiting alveoli in ARDS.[53] They are effective, however, only from an optimal level of PEEP that does not result in derecruitment. At optimal PEEP, a sigh maneuver increases end-expiratory lung volume and improves oxygenation.[54] Gattinoni et al[55,56] showed and quantified alveolar recruitment induced by PEEP and showed that the primary role of tidal volume inflation was to open the lung and the primary role of PEEP was to avoid derecruitment.

Prone Positioning

Prone positioning has been proposed as a means to improve gas exchange in patients with ARDS with severe hypoxemia. Oxygenation improves in most adult patients with ALI/ARDS when they are placed prone.[57-61] A large, multicenter trial of proning for almost 7 hours a day did not show improvement in mortality rates in patients with ALI/ARDS; however, a post hoc analysis suggested improvement in those patients with the most severe hypoxemia.[60] A recent multicenter trial of proning for almost 20 hours a day also suggested improvement in this patient subgroup[62] that did not reach statistical significance. Bruno et al[63] reported the short-term effects of 1 to 2 hours of prone positioning in children with respiratory failure. They found that only 28% of the patients had a significant improvement in oxygenation.[63] On the other hand, Curley, Thompson, and Arnold,[64] in a preliminary single-center study in children with ALI/ARDS, showed that oxygenation improved with prone positioning in 84% of patients without any critical incident. Relvas, Silver, and Sagy[71] also reported a retrospective study on the effects of prone positioning in children with ARDS and showed that the improvement in oxygenation was much more sustained if the duration of prone positioning was between 18 and 24 hours than when the duration of prone positioning was between 6 and 10 hours. Although some patients benefit by an improvement in oxygenation, there are currently no data on its efficacy in improving patient outcome. Although the magnitude of the response varies widely from marginal to dramatic, there is no adequate model predicting where a particular patient with ARDS will fall in the spectrum. Furthermore, patients' response times vary from immediate to several hours. As a result, little is known about the optimal time period to maintain the prone position. Some patients respond to a return to a supine position after a trial of prone positioning by reverting to their original oxygenation, others have a reduction in oxygenation that is better than the original supine value, and some patients show an improvement. A multicenter trial in children has been currently completed, and the results are expected. Prone positioning may have potentially life-threatening complications, including accidental dislodgement of the endotracheal tube and central venous catheters. Marcano, Silver, and Sagy[66] reported that prone positioning resulted in cephalad movement of the endotracheal tube within the trachea in children with ARDS ranging from 10% to 57% of their thoracic tracheal length. Their study also suggested that if the tip of the endotracheal tube is not deeper than one third of the thoracic tracheal length before prone positioning, it might slide into the cervical trachea as a result of prone positioning.[66]

Unilateral Lung Disease or Severely Differential Lung Disease

Unilateral or asymmetrical lung disease in infants and children poses special problems during mechanical ventilation. Some of these patients may have severe intrapulmonary shunts leading to hypoxemia requiring mechanical ventilation. Because of regional differences in compliance and resistance, the time constants for inflation and deflation may vary widely between lung segments. During conventional ventilation, tidal volume delivered tends to preferentially inflate the more compliant lung and underventilate the stiffer, more affected lung. This may result in overinflation of the relatively "normal" lung and cause redistribution of pulmonary blood flow away from the hyperinflated lung, thus exaggerating the ventilation-perfusion mismatching. Such overinflation may contribute to further barotrauma. In such circumstances, with unilateral or asymmetrical lung disease, simultaneous independent lung ventilation (SILV) may allow each lung to be ventilated according to its needs without affecting the opposite lung. Currently, ILV can be generally indicated in the treatment of unilateral lung disease, such as unilateral atelectasis or consolidation, emphysema, pneumonia, pneumothorax, and bronchopulmonary fistula. In postoperative care, ILV can be used for lung reexpansion after thoracic surgery, for correction of V/Q mismatch in the lung remaining dependent during surgery, and for the treatment of pulmonary complications arising during anesthesia and surgery (e.g., pneumothorax or aspiration syndrome).[67-73] A new possible indication for ILV can be the selective administration of drugs to one lung, such as antibiotics or surfactant. SILV requires a bilumen tube with one tube being the longer "bronchial" tube and the other shorter "tracheal" tube. Usually, the bronchial tube is advanced into the right main stem bronchus so that both lungs can be ventilated separately. In adults, SILV has been shown to be useful in the treatment of unilateral lung disease.[67-70] In infants and children, SILV has been limited because of the lack of a suitable bilumen tube. Marraro[71] reviewed their experience with SILV in infants and children younger than 1 year with a bilumen tube developed in their department, but it is currently available through Portex Ltd. (Mythe, Kent, UK). The indications included bronchopneumonia with unilateral prevalence, unilateral pneumonia, lobar atelectasis, and diaphragmatic hernia. Nine of 41 patients treated with SILV had rapid improvement in lung disease, whereas the other 32 recovered more slowly. No major complications were attributed to SILV. In newborns and infants, it is possible to provide ILV with a double-lumen endotracheal tube manufactured by Portex as special equipment. In children older than 6 to 8 years, selective bronchial intubation is possible using a cuffed double-lumen tube similar to that used in adults (26- to 28-Fr Bronchocath Mallinckrodt, Bronchoport Rusch). The Marraro Paediatric Endobronchial Bilumen Tube, produced by SIMS-Portex, may be used in neonates and children age 2 to 3 years.[72] It is uncuffed to maximize the internal diameter of the tube and has no carinal hook; this minimizes tracheal trauma.[71-73] ILV requires two ventilators that permit the application of different modes of ventilation and different PEEP levels for each lung. Synchronization of the beginning of the inspiratory phase and the inspiratory time can avoid mediastinal shifts that impede venous return and reduce cardiac output.[71-73]

Heart Failure

The goals in respiratory management in congestive heart failure are prevention and relief of alveolar collapse from alveolar and interstitial edema due to pulmonary vascular congestion, as well as decreased oxygen demand on the heart with a reduction in the work of breathing. CPAP/PEEP will provide relief of atelectasis. Hyperinflation should be avoided because it may increase pulmonary vascular resistance and increase right ventricular afterload. The oxygen cost of breathing can be reduced with a decrease in the work of breathing. This can be provided by a judicious combination of controlled ventilation and sedation. By unloading the respiratory muscles, AMV can also reduce the work of breathing. In extreme cases, muscle relaxation by neuromuscular blockers may provide additional reduction in oxygen cost of breathing. As a general principle, the greater the inotropic support a heart needs, the greater should be the respiratory support provided. Tidal volumes should be generally maintained on the lower range (8 to 12 ml/kg). In adults with congestive heart failure, positive intrathoracic pressure has been shown to improve cardiac output.[74,75] This effect has been attributed to decreased left ventricular afterload provided by positive airway pressure.

Postoperative Management after Repair of Congenital Heart Disease

After open heart surgery, many infants and children require mechanical ventilation during the postoperative period. The duration of requirement of mechanical ventilation depends on several factors such as age of the patient, complexity of the cardiac lesion, complexity of the operative procedure, duration of bypass, duration of circulatory arrest, and postoperative cardiopulmonary status. Prolonged intubation and mechanical ventilation are more likely in children younger than 1 year of age, with more complex heart lesions, prolonged bypass and prolonged circulatory arrest times, and postoperative respiratory failure and hemodynamic instability. In the immediate postoperative period, patients should be supported with controlled mechanical ventilation until hemodynamic functions improve. Adequate PEEP should be applied to prevent and relieve atelectasis. Initially, the ventilator rate should be appropriate for the age. As the hemodynamic function improves, the rate can be weaned, as dictated by the clinical status. The choice of ventilatory parameters depends on the goals for each patient. In patients with pulmonary hypertension or pulmonary vascular disease, hyperventilation to provide respiratory alkalosis will decrease pulmonary vascular resistance and right ventricular afterload. In patients with marginal cardiac output, high airway pressures are to be avoided. In patients who have undergone a Fontan procedure, early extubation is desirable, and if that is not possible, then spontaneous ventilation should be encouraged. Because these patients are totally dependent on venous return for their cardiac output, airway pressures must be kept at a minimum. High intrathoracic pressure may not only impede venous return, but also decrease pulmonary blood flow from increased pulmonary vascular resistance.

Diseases with Abdominal Distention

The presence of abdominal distention poses a special problem. Positive intraabdominal pressure tends to elevate the diaphragm, decrease Ptp in the lung bases, and decrease alveolar lung volumes in the lung bases. For normal lung volumes to be maintained, a greater Ptp has to be generated. This increases the airway pressures during positive pressure ventilation and increases work of breathing during spontaneous breathing. During positive pressure ventilation, a higher Ptp may cause hyperinflation of the apical regions while restoring normal volumes in the bases. Therapy should be directed primarily toward reducing the intraabdominal pressure.

Neurological and Neuromuscular Diseases

Hyperventilation with respiratory alkalosis is an effective method of reducing intracranial pressure. High intrathoracic pressure may impede venous return from the brain by increasing central venous pressures. Therefore high levels of PEEP are to be avoided. The goals of respiratory support in patients with acute neuromuscular diseases that are self-limiting are (1) provision of respiratory assistance to maintain adequate minute ventilation and (2) avoidance of disuse muscle atrophy from mechanical ventilation. Spontaneous breathing must be encouraged as much as possible. Neuromuscular blockade must be avoided.

Patient-Ventilator Asynchrony

When the patient is capable of spontaneous breathing or allowed to breathe spontaneously, monitoring and titrating mechanical ventilation to either minimize or eliminate patient-ventilator asynchrony are important. One of the primary goals of mechanical ventilation is to reduce the patient's work of breathing. This can be achieved only if the patient's respiratory muscles and the ventilator act in a coordinated manner. The patient should not be attempting to inspire when the ventilator is in the expiratory phase and should not be attempting to exhale when the ventilator is attempting to deliver a breath. When the ventilator phase (inspiration or expiration) is not synchronized completely with the phase of the spontaneous breath, it is referred to as *asynchrony.* When the ventilator phase is only partially not synchronized with the spontaneous breath, it is referred to as *dyssynchrony.* The interplay between the respiratory pump and the ventilator can occur either within one breath or on a breath-to-breath basis.

Use of Neuromuscular Blockade

Neuromuscular blockers are often used as adjunctive therapy to mechanical ventilation. Although spontaneous breathing is to be encouraged as much as possible, respiratory muscle paralysis becomes necessary at times as an aid to mechanical ventilation. The indications for the use of neuromuscular blocking agents during mechanical ventilation are (1) asynchrony between the patient and the ventilator; (2) use in controlled ventilation; (3) a decrease in oxygen demand of skeletal muscles, especially in patients with hemodynamic instability; and (4) prevention of coughing, especially in patients with intracranial hypertension. Ideally, ventilator breaths should be synchronized with spontaneous breaths. Asynchrony between mechanical ventilation and spontaneous breathing is common, especially in small infants. The most common form of asynchrony is active exhalation during a ventilator-delivered inspiratory breath. This has several detrimental effects. These are increased expiratory work of breathing, decreased overall minute ventilation with hypercarbia, patient discomfort, and increased risk for air leak.[76,77] Patients exhibiting asynchrony during mechanical ventilation have shown improved oxygenation and ventilation after neuromuscular blockade.[78,79] Neuromuscular blockade is also used in patients when ventilation is to be controlled so that the appropriate minute ventilation is delivered. Paralysis of respiratory muscles may also be required in patients after congenital heart surgery to reduce the oxygen demand on the heart. Prolonged neuromuscular blockade is to be avoided because it tends to promote muscle atrophy. This, in turn, will prolong weaning from mechanical ventilation.

Special Techniques of Respiratory Support

Altering Inspired Oxygen and Carbon Dioxide Concentration

A low alveolar oxygen tension increases pulmonary vascular resistance (hypoxic pulmonary vasoconstriction), and a high alveolar oxygen tension decreases pulmonary vascular resistance.[80] With certain types of congenital heart disease such as hypoplastic left heart syndrome, it is critical to control pulmonary blood flow and prevent pulmonary overflooding. One approach is to decrease the FiO_2 to less than 0.21 with a blending of room air with nitrogen. The exact FiO_2 delivered must be monitored to avoid administering excessively low inspired oxygen. The other approach, especially in patients undergoing mechanical ventilation, both preoperatively and postoperatively, is to increase the inspired carbon dioxide concentration ($FiCO_2$).[81] Increased $FiCO_2$ also increases pulmonary vascular resistance. During mechanical ventilation, increased $FiCO_2$ allows one to hyperventilate and prevent atelectasis without producing hypocarbia. One of the difficulties with a boost in $FiCO_2$ is increased spontaneous ventilatory drive due to an increased $PaCO_2$. This increases the work of breathing and with marginal cardiac reserve may impose undue strain on the heart. Therefore in spontaneously breathing patients, neuromuscular blockade and total ventilatory support may be necessary with increased $FiCO_2$ to avoid an increased workload on the heart.

Helium-Oxygen Mixture

Helium-oxygen mixture has much lower density compared with oxygen-nitrogen mixture and offers a reduced resistance to breathing. This property has been used in the successful treatment of upper airway obstruction after extubation in children.[82] I have used helium-oxygen mixture in upper airway obstruction due to laryngotracheobronchitis and postextubation subglottic edema in infants and children. Helium is usually administered in at least 30% to 40% oxygen through a tight-fitting face mask. Use of an Oxygood is not indicated because helium tends to separate and layer at the top of the Oxyhood with the patient breathing very little helium. Recently, helium-oxygen mixture has been shown to improve gas exchange in neonates with respiratory distress syndrome.[83] Oxygenation should be monitored during administration of helium-oxygen mixture to avoid hypoxia, especially in neonates.[84] In adults, helium-oxygen mixture has also been used in the management of severe lower airway obstruction in asthma. Because ventilator transducers are calibrated with an air-oxygen mixture, the true volumes delivered tend to be different from preset values. Therefore when helium-oxygen mixture is administered through the ventilator, direct volume measurements are necessary to ensure that the appropriate VTeff is being delivered.

Inhaled Nitric Oxide

Inhaled nitric oxide produces selective pulmonary vasodilation. Indications for inhaled nitric oxide include diaphragmatic hernia, pulmonary hypertension after repair of congenital heart disease, primary pulmonary hypertension, and isolated right heart failure. In babies with severe hypoxemia and pulmonary hypertension, inhaled nitric oxide rapidly increases arterial oxygen tension without causing systemic hypotension.[85-88] Randomized controlled studies showed that nitric oxide inhalation safely improves arterial oxygen levels and decreases the need for extracorporeal membrane oxygenation (ECMO) therapy.[85-88] Oxygenation improves in approximately 50% of infants receiving nitric oxide. In addition, Kinsella and Abman[89] showed that high-frequency ventilation seems to augment the response to inhaled nitric oxide probably by better recruitment of alveoli. In children with ALI/ARDS, Ream et al[90] showed an improvement in oxygenation in more than two thirds of the patients. Researchers of a randomized controlled trial of inhaled nitric oxide in children with acute hypoxemic respiratory failure have also reported an improvement in oxygenation.[91] Results from several adult studies, however, showed that several participants failed to show any improvement.[92-95] In these multicenter studies in children and adults, there were no differences in ventilator-free days and no effect on mortality between treatment groups. Because only some patients seem to respond to inhaled nitric oxide, the staff at Children's Hospital of Pittsburgh has devised a protocol for the judicious use of inhaled nitric oxide: a 2-hour trial of inhaled nitric oxide with 20 to 40 ppm is administered to infants and children with ALI/ARDS with hypoxemic respiratory failure. A good response is defined as improvement in PaO_2/FiO_2 ratio of greater than 100%. A partial response is defined as an improvement in PaO_2/FiO_2 ratio between 50% and 100%. If the response is less than 50%, the patient is considered a nonresponder. Inhaled nitric oxide is then continued in only those patients who show a partial or good response. Nitric oxide binds to hemoglobin to produce methemoglobin. Therefore methemoglobin levels should be monitored during administration of nitric oxide. In addition, nitric oxide combines with oxygen to form nitrogen dioxide. Nitrogen dioxide is known to cause lung injury. Therefore the concentration of nitrogen dioxide should be monitored in the inspired gas to keep it below 1 to 2 ppm.

Noninvasive Mechanical Ventilation

Conventional mechanical ventilation provided through endotracheal intubation or a tracheostomy is a life-saving technique in the management of patients with respiratory failure. Endotracheal intubation and tracheostomy are associated with complications including injury to the airway and nosocomial infections. In addition, mechanical ventilation of children with endotracheal intubation often requires use of sedatives with its attendant side effects and complications. Noninvasive ventilation refers to a technique of respiratory support that is provided without an artificial airway in the trachea. Noninvasive ventilation can be provided with either positive or negative pressure ventilators.[96-100] The advantages of noninvasive mechanical ventilation are (1) avoidance of an artificial airway, (2) greater acceptance by patient and families, (3) decreased use of sedation, and (4) positive effects on appearance and speech. Not all patients are candidates for noninvasive mechanical ventilation. The indications for noninvasive mechanical ventilation are (1) static or slowly progressive neuromuscular disease, (2) central hypoventilation syndromes (congenital and acquired), (3) static or slowly progressive restrictive chest diseases (kyphoscoliosis), (4) chronic respiratory failure from parenchymal lung disease, and (5) chronic obstructive lung disease. In adults, it has been shown that the probability of continuing noninvasive mechanical ventilation was very high in patients with scoliosis, previous poliomyelitis, and neuromuscular disorders.[97]

Noninvasive Positive-Pressure Ventilation

Noninvasive positive-pressure ventilation (NPPV) can be provided through a tight-fitting face mask, through a nasal mask, or through a mouthpiece. Mechanical ventilation can be provided through ventilators used with endotracheal ventilation or specially designed ventilators for noninvasive use. Patient-triggered positive pressure breath can be either volume preset or pressure preset. The Bi-Level Positive Airway Pressure (Bi-PAP) ventilator (Respironics, Inc., Murrysville, PA) is a more recent innovation. The Bi-PAP ventilator is a low-pressure, electrically driven unit with electronic pressure control. It is pneumatically powered and electrically controlled, using a moderate gas pressure (20-44 cm H_2O) source that electrically regulates the pressure down to low gas pressure. It is primarily intended to augment or assist patient's own spontaneous efforts. It senses the patient's effort by monitoring airflow and supplies pressurized air during inspiration (inspiratory positive airway pressure [IPAP]) or exhalation (expiratory positive airway pressure [EPAP]) or both (Bi-PAP). Air flow is sensed in the patient circuit with a flow transducer. The flow data are analyzed to derive a signal proportional to the instantaneous flow rate in the circuit. This signal is composed of flow into the patient's lungs and flow due to leaks in the patient circuit. These data are continually processed, and adjustments are automatically made to trigger thresholds. There are four modes: (1) the spontaneous mode, in which the unit cycles between IPAP and EPAP in response to patient triggering and the rate and depth of breathing is controlled by the patient; (2) the spontaneous/timed mode, in which the unit cycles between IPAP and EPAP levels in response to patient triggering and if the patient fails to initiate an inspiration, the unit will deliver positive pressure breaths at a preset frequency; (3) timed mode, in which the unit provides positive pressure breaths with EPAP at a preset frequency and the patient may breathe spontaneously; and (4) CPAP mode. Modifications to this original design include the provision of a backup rate. A detailed description of the various ventilators that are currently in use for long-term noninvasive ventilation is beyond the scope of this chapter.

Indications and Clinical Studies in Children

Not all patients are candidates for noninvasive mechanical ventilation. The indications and contraindications for use of NPPV are shown in Box 44–4. In adults, it has been shown that the probability of continuing noninvasive mechanical ventilation was high in patients with scoliosis, previous poliomyelitis, and neuromuscular disorders.[97] NPPV has been used extensively in adults with obstructive sleep apnea, chronic obstructive lung disease, chronic respiratory insufficiency due to skeletal or neuromuscular disorders, and central hypoventilation.[98-100] In adults, the addition of NPPV to standard care in the setting of acute hypoxemic respiratory failure reduced the rate of endotracheal intubation, ICU length of stay, and ICU mortality.[101]

Bi-PAP has been used successfully in children with respiratory insufficiency.[102-106] Padman, Lawless, and Von Nessen[102] observed significant improvement in hospital days, respiratory rate, heart rate, serum bicarbonate, arterial carbon dioxide, dyspnea, activity tolerance, and quality of sleep. In 1995 Fortenberry et al[104] reported on a retrospective study on the efficacy and complications of Bi-PAP in 28 children with acute hypoxemic respiratory insufficiency. Bi-PAP significantly decreased respiratory rate and improved both oxygenation and ventilation. The use of Bi-PAP decreased hospitalization rate and increased patient comfort.[104] Only 3 of 28 patients required intubation or reintubation.[104] Padman et al[105] conducted a prospective study in 34 patients with impending failure, all of whom required airway or oxygenation/ventilation support and required admission to the pediatric ICU. A decrease in respiratory rate, heart rate, and dyspnea score, and an improvement in oxygenation were noted in more than 90% of patients studied. The frequency of intubation in these patients was only 8%.[105] Birnkrant, Pope, and Eiben[107] reported their experience with Bi-PAP in six patients with spinal muscular atrophy and three patients with other causes of respiratory failure. This uncontrolled study showed that in these patients noninvasive pressure ventilation facilitated extubation. These studies show that noninvasive ventilation is useful in providing respiratory support in patients who would be considered candidates for endotracheal intubation and positive pressure mechanical ventilation. These studies, though uncontrolled, also suggest that endotracheal intubation can be avoided in these patients. Some have advocated that noninvasive ventilation be provided to prevent respiratory failure in patients with progressive neuromuscular disease. A recent randomized study showed, however, that preventive nasal positive pressure ventilation did not improve respiratory handicap and reduced survival in patients with Duchenne's muscular dystrophy with a forced vital capacity between 20% and 50% predicted.[108] On the other hand, Vianello et al[109] reported improved survival for patients with advanced Duchenne's muscular dystrophy with chronic respiratory failure who were treated with nasal intermittent positive pressure ventilation compared with an unventilated group. Therefore selection of patients is crucial because not all patients can benefit from NPPV.

BOX 44–4

Indications and Contraindication for Noninvasive Positive Pressure Ventilation

INDICATIONS

- Abnormalities of central ventilatory control
  - Congenital
  - Acquired
- Rib-cage abnormality
  - Congenital abnormalities
  - Ankylosing spondylitis
- Neuromuscular disease affecting respiratory muscles
  - Anterior horn cell disease
  - Guillain-Barré syndrome
  - Phrenic nerve disease or injury
  - Myasthenia gravis
  - Muscle diseases
- Abnormalities of the spine
  - Kyphoscoliosis
- Primary lung disease
  - Acute pulmonary edema
  - Acute lung injury
  - Infection
  - Obstructive pulmonary disease
  - Cystic fibrosis
- Other diseases
  - Primary pulmonary hypertension

CONTRAINDICATIONS

- Absolute
  - Hemodynamic instability
  - Patients at risk for aspiration
  - Inability to clear secretions
- Relative
  - Inability to properly fit the mask
  - Uncooperative patient
  - Morbid obesity

Negative Pressure Ventilation

Design and Modes of Negative Pressure Ventilators

All negative pressure ventilators have a chamber in which subatmospheric pressure is generated and a pump that generates this pressure. The chamber may cover only the chest and the upper abdomen (cuirass) or all the extracranial portions of the body (tank respirator, isolette, or a body suit). The tank respirator has both the chamber and the pump in one unit. In all other cases the two units are separate. The cuirass can be prefabricated or custom designed to fit the contours of the chest. Custom-designed cuirasses are especially useful in patients with skeletal or spinal deformities. All body suits fit over a hard shell similar to the cuirass placed over the chest and the upper abdomen. Most negative pressure pumps in use today are pressure cycled. Some volume-cycled pumps have been used, but their use has been limited because the pump cannot compensate for the variable amounts of air leak. Additionally, some ventilators provide an inspiratory assist mode. Currently there are four modes of negative pressure application: (1) cyclical negative pressure, (2) negative/positive pressure, (3) continuous negative extrathoracic pressure (CNEP), and (4) negative pressure/CNEP. Cyclical negative pressure ventilation refers to a mode in which the ventilator generates the preset subatmospheric pressure during inspiration while expiration is passive. Negative/positive pressure ventilation refers to a mode that is a combination of negative pressure during inspiration with positive pressure during expiration. CNEP refers to a mode in which a constant subatmospheric pressure is provided throughout the respiratory cycle and the patient breathes spontaneously. Negative pressure/CNEP refers to a mode in which negative pressure inspiratory cycles are superimposed on CNEP.

Clinical Applications

Box 44–5 shows the indications, advantages, disadvantages, contraindications, and clinical side effects of negative pressure ventilation. In the 1960s and 1970s, several controlled and uncontrolled studies showed that negative pressure ventilation was effective in the management of neonatal respiratory syndrome.[110-112] The utility of this technique, though, was limited because of problems such as upper airway obstruction, difficulties in achieving access to patients, difficulties in achieving an adequate seal, sores from the neck seal, and inability to maintain an adequate neutral thermal environment. Negative pressure ventilation has been reintroduced in the treatment of neonatal respiratory distress syndrome. A recent randomized control study showed that application of CNEP was associated with fewer intubations and decreased the total duration of oxygen therapy.[113] CNEP was, however, associated with a slightly higher (not statistically significant) mortality, cranial sound abnormalities, and pneumothoraces. Further studies are warranted to assess the utility and safety of negative pressure ventilation in neonatal respiratory distress syndrome.

Respiratory Dysfunction and Failure

During the polio epidemics in the 1930s and 1940s, negative pressure tank ventilators reduced mortality in patients with spinal polio.[114-116] There has been a resurgent interest in negative pressure ventilation in patients with neuromuscular diseases and skeletal deformities. In adults with kyphoscoliosis and neuromuscular disorders with chronic hypoventilation, intermittent use of negative pressure ventilation, mostly nocturnal, decreased or reversed day-time symptoms of hypoventilation and gas exchange abnormalities.[117,118] These studies show that negative pressure ventilation is useful in acute or chronic respiratory failure associated with skeletal or neuromuscular disorders.

BOX 44–5

Indications, Advantages, Disadvantages, and Contraindications of Negative Pressure Ventilation

INDICATIONS

- Parenchymal lung disease
  - Respiratory distress of the neonate
  - Interstitial pneumonias
  - Acute respiratory distress syndrome
  - Acute pulmonary edema
- Respiratory pump failure
  - Poliomyelitis
  - Neuromuscular diseases
  - Skeletal deformities
  - Persistent flail chest deformity
- Cardiovascular disorders
  - After Fontan-type operations
  - Repair of total cavopulmonary connection
  - Tetralogy of Fallot
  - Phrenic nerve palsy after pediatric cardiac surgery

ADVANTAGES

- Avoidance of intubation or tracheostomy
- Preservation of physiological functions such as speech, cough, swallowing, and feeding
- Allows fiberoptic bronchoscopy to be performed without disconnection from the ventilator
- Promote venous return by creating negative intrathoracic pressure

DISADVANTAGES

- Ventilators are noisy
- Access to patient is difficult
- Tank ventilators produce abdominal pooling of blood resulting in hypotension (tank shock)
- Regulation of inspiratory-expiratory ratio is difficult (more recent ventilators such as the Hayek negative pressure ventilator allow for regulation of inspiratory-expiratory ratio and application of negative end-expiratory pressure)
- Ventilators are difficult to sterilize
- Lack of protection of the upper airway, especially in unconscious patients or those with bulbar dysfunction
- Upper airway obstruction—can be minimized with an oral airway
- Difficulty in achieving an adequate seal
- Discomfort

CONTRAINDICATIONS

- Gastrointestinal bleeding
- Rib fracture
- Recent abdominal surgery
- Uncooperative patients
- Sleep apnea syndrome
- Neurological disorders with bulbar syndrome

CLINICAL SIDE EFFECTS

- Tiredness
- Musculoskeletal pain or tightness
- Esophagitis
- Rib fractures and pneumothorax
- Impaired sleep quality
- Poor compliance

Isolated case reports in adults have been published about the use of CNEP in adult respiratory distress syndrome and in persistent flail chest deformity.[119-122] CNEP has been used to assist ventilation in children with diffuse alveolar disease and progressive respiratory failure.[123-125]

Cardiovascular Disorders

In 1993 Raine et al[126] published a pilot study of 10 children with respiratory failure and found that CNEP introduced exclusively or in conjunction with intermittent positive pressure ventilation did not produce large changes in cardiac output. In patients undergoing Fontan-type operations, pulmonary blood flow and cardiac output increases with spontaneous inspiration, and positive pressure ventilation decreases antegrade pulmonary blood flow and any increase in pulmonary valvular incompetence in patients with restrictive function of the right side of the heart after repair of tetralogy of Fallot.[127] In children after repair of total cavopulmonary connection and tetralogy of Fallot and after Fontan-type procedures, negative pressure ventilation provided with a Hayek external high-frequency oscillator (Breasy Medical Equipment, London, UK) improved cardiac output by 42% to 46% almost entirely by an increase in stroke volume with improvement in mixed venous oxygen saturation.[128] Additionally, the systemic and pulmonary vascular resistances decreased significantly. A similar finding was observed in children after transcatheter occlusion of an asymptomatic patent ductus arteriosus and after open heart surgery.[129] In 1992 Raine et al[130] reported findings of an uncontrolled study that showed that negative pressure ventilation with either CNEP or intermittent negative pressure ventilation is a viable alternative to positive pressure ventilation in patients with phrenic nerve palsy after pediatric cardiac surgery by reducing the need for diaphragmatic plication and facilitating weaning from positive pressure ventilation. These findings show that negative pressure ventilation is a useful technique in selected patients after cardiac surgery when positive pressure ventilation is not desirable or results in unwanted hemodynamic effects.

High-Frequency Ventilation

Definitions

High-frequency ventilation (HFV) refers to diverse modes of ventilation characterized in general by supraphysiological ventilatory frequencies (>60 cycles/min) and low tidal volumes (less than or equal to physiological dead space during conventional ventilation). Four distinct methods of HFV are recognized: high-frequency positive pressure ventilation (HFPPV), high-frequency jet ventilation (HFJV), high-frequency oscillatory ventilation (HFOV), and high-frequency chest wall oscillation (HFCWO).

1. *HFPPV:* HFPPV was first described by Oberg and Sjostrand in 1969[131] and refers to ventilation at a frequency of 60 to 100 cycles per minute with a tidal volume of 3 to 4 ml/kg using a ventilator with a small internal dead space, low internal compliance, and minimal compression of gases within the ventilator. HFPPV was initially instituted by insufflation through a catheter positioned within the endotracheal tube, with expiration occurring through an expiratory valve connected to the outer orifice. Since 1973, a pneumatic valve, based on the Coanda or wall effect, was developed in which the gas mixture was intermittently delivered through a sidearm branching off the main channel of the pneumatic valve connector (Fig. 44–17). This main channel remains open for insertion of a bronchoscope or a laryngoscope.
2. *HFJV:* HFJV, which was first described by Sanders in 1967[132] to assist bronchoscopy, refers to delivery of inspiratory gases through a jet injector at a high velocity into the trachea at a rate of 100 to 400 cycles per minute (Fig. 44–18). Tidal volumes delivered are usually 3 to 5 ml/kg.
3. *HFOV:* HFOV was first described by Lunkenheimer in 1972[133] and refers to ventilation at frequencies of 900 to 3600 cycles per minute, with an alternating positive and negative pressure in the airway. This oscillatory flow may be produced by a piston pump or a diaphragm with tidal volumes of 1 to 3 ml/kg (Fig. 44–19).
4. *HFCWO:* HFCWO was first described by Zidulka et al in 1983[134] and refers to a method of ventilation in which a rigid harness surrounds the chest and is oscillated at a frequency of 180 to 600 cycles per minute; minute ventilation is controlled with adjustment of the inflation pressure and frequency. A variant of HFCWO is high-frequency body surface oscillation (HFBSO), in which the body is encased in an air-tight tank.

Only HFPPV, HFJV, and HFOV have been extensively used clinically.

Mechanism of Gas Flow in High-Frequency Ventilation in the Normal Lung

The exact mechanism of gas transport in HFV is currently not clear. It is possible that each mode of ventilation may have differing mechanisms of gas flow from the proximal airway to the alveoli. If gas flow to the lungs is increased more than 200 times the minute volume of oxygen demand, the lung parenchyma can be made to oscillate.[135,136] At ventilatory frequencies less than 7 Hz, regional alveolar ventilation depends on segmental compliance and airway resistance. At a ventilatory frequency greater than 7 Hz, a frequency-dependent excitation of the lung parenchyma and airway conduits occurs,[137] and at frequencies greater than 10 Hz, ventilation becomes independent of regional compliance. When the gas in the airways is oscillated at high frequency, the airways begin to undergo spatial oscillation inside the chest. These oscillations are composed of periodic changes in length and width, movements of curved or angular bronchi, and wave motions in the bronchi. When the frequency of oscillation approaches the natural resonant frequency of the lung structures, the oscillations of the airways and the lung parenchyma are amplified. These result in shaking and squeezing of the neighboring parenchyma, resulting in intraparenchymal and interparenchymal gas mixing.[138]

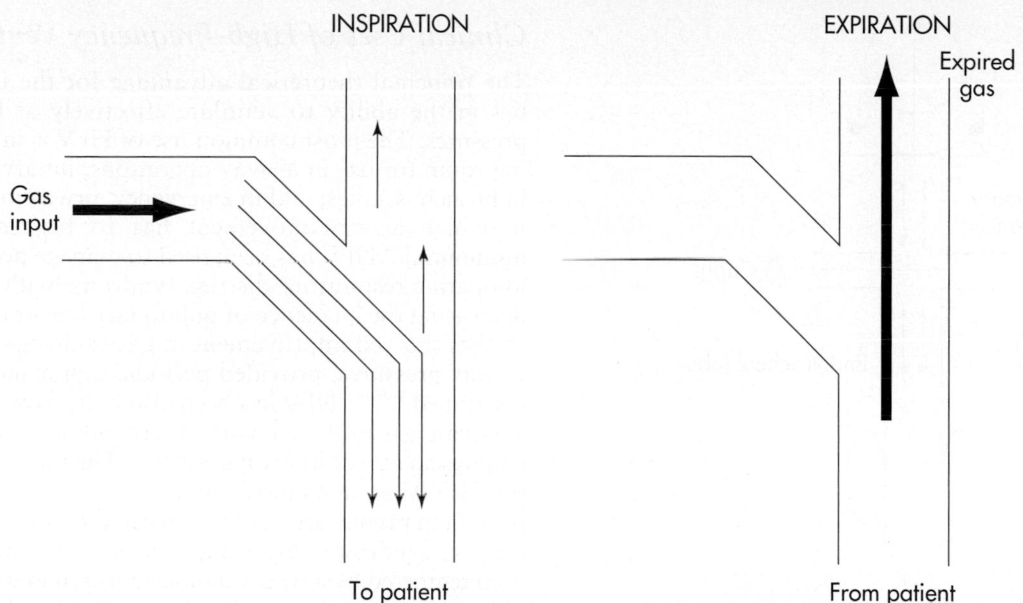

FIGURE 44–17 • High-frequency positive pressure ventilator. The inspiratory limb is angled so that the inspiratory gas can be directed to the patient. During inspiration, some gas escapes through the expiratory limb, preventing entrainment. During expiration, the gas flows out into the expiratory limb. (Reproduced with permission from Shoemaker WC, Ayres S, Grenvik A, Holbrook PR, Thompson WL, editors: *The textbook of critical care,* Philadelphia,1989, WB Saunders.)

Other mechanisms involved in gas transport during HFV include accelerated axial dispersion, increased collateral flow through pores of Kohn, intersegmental gas mixing or pendelluft phenomenon, Taylor dispersion, asymmetrical gas flow profiles, and gas mixing within the airway due to the nonlinear pressure-diameter relationship of the bronchi.

Parameters to Be Selected

High-Frequency Jet Ventilation

The main controls in HFJV are the driving pressure inspiratory time, and rate. The driving pressure is usually initiated a low PSI and gradually increased to reach the desired mean airway pressure. Inspiratory time is usually kept to a minimum at 20%. A higher inspiratory time may be used but may result in air-trapping. The rate can be adjusted up to 600 breaths per minute depending on the jet ventilator used. PEEP is applied through a separate bias flow circuit with continuous flow. FiO_2 delivered to the patient is adjusted through regulation of the inspired oxygen concentration of the bias flow circuit. In certain circumstances, conventional ventilation can be combined with HFJV. Here, conventional ventilation provides "sigh breaths" of approximately 10 to 12 ml/kg to prevent atelectasis and maintain lung volumes during HFJV. The size of each breath increases with a higher driving pressure, increased inspiratory time, and a decreased frequency. Because there is entrainment of gas with HFJV, it is difficult to predict the effect of ventilator parameters on minute ventilation. Ventilation is most effective when the jet catheter is close to the carina. The main concerns with HFJV are airway injury and air-trapping. Airway injury can be minimized with placement of the tip of the catheter sufficiently proximal in the endotracheal tube and without close placement close to the carina. Air-trapping can be avoided with the minimal inspiratory time and the lowest driving pressure.[139]

High-Frequency Oscillatory Ventilation

The main controls in HFOV are mean airway pressure, oscillatory pressure amplitude, bias flow, frequency, and inspiratory time. With piston-driven oscillators, piston-centering is an additional control mechanism. Mean airway pressure determines the mean lung volume of the lung. Oscillatory amplitude is the total change in pressure

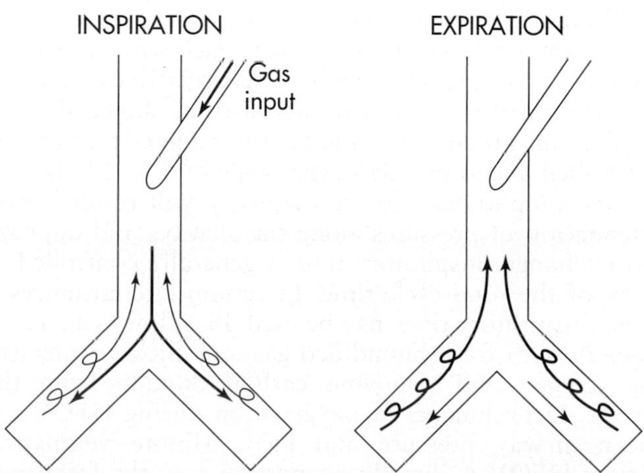

FIGURE 44–18 • High-frequency jet ventilator. Gas is introduced into the trachea at a high pressure through a small catheter. Arrows represent coaxial and turbulent flow patterns. (Reproduced with permission from Shoemaker WC, Ayres S, Grenvik A, Holbrrok PR, Thompson WL, editors: *The textbook of critical care,* Philadelphia, 1989, WB Saunders.)

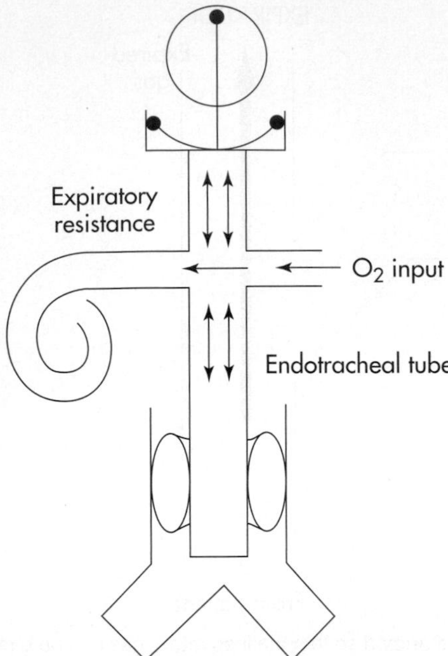

FIGURE 44–19 • High-frequency oscillation system. Uses a reciprocating pump (*top*) to oscillate a column of gas that is a mixture of inspired and expired gases. Excess gas is vented through the overflow side port (left). (Reproduced with permission from Shoemaker WC, Ayres S, Grenvik A, Holbrook PR, Thompson WL, editors: *The textbook of critical care,* Philadelphia, 1989, WB Saunders.)

around the mean airway pressure produced by forward and backward displacement of the piston. The pressures developed in the patients' airways are considerably dampened because of the impedance of the endotracheal tube. Similarly, the pressure profile is further dampened in the distal airways because of the impedance of the proximal airways. If the oscillatory frequency approaches the natural resonant frequency of the lung and airways, then there may be amplification of the pressure waves. The oscillatory amplitude determines the volume displacement with each stroke of the piston. If the volume of gas displaced is less than the dead space of the airways and lungs, then there is little chest displacement. If sufficient chest displacement is seen with each stroke, then the volume of gas displaced tends to be larger than the physiological dead space and results in some direct alveolar ventilation. Frequency is the next parameter that can be controlled and is usually in the range of 5 to 10 Hz. For a given amplitude, a lower frequency will result in less attenuation of pressures along the airways and improve gas exchange. Inspiratory time is generally controlled at 33% of the total cycle time. In certain circumstances a lower inspiratory time may be used. Bias flow is a continuous flow of fresh humidified gas and allows replenishing oxygen and removing carbon dioxide from the circuit. Determinants of oxygenation during HFOV are mean airway pressure and FiO_2. Minute ventilation during HFOV is directly proportional to the frequency and the square of the tidal volume. The primary determinant of ventilation is oscillatory amplitude. Decreasing the frequency to reduce attenuation and increasing the inspiratory time are less effective strategies to improve carbon dioxide elimination.

Clinical Uses of High-Frequency Ventilation

The principal theoretical advantage for the use of HFV lies in the ability to ventilate effectively at low airway pressures. The most common use of HFV is in the operating room for use in airway operations; in laryngoscopies; in bronchoscopies; and in emergency airway management, in which airway movement has to be reduced to a minimum.[139] HFV has been used to manage neonates with idiopathic respiratory distress syndrome with the goal of decreasing the incidence of pulmonary barotrauma. Initial studies showed improvement in gas exchange with lower airway pressures, provided periodic sigh maneuvers were performed.[140-143] HFV has been also been shown to support adequate gas exchange with severe pulmonary interstitial emphysema (PIE) in neonates.[144,145] The initial enthusiasm for HFOV as a method for reducing pulmonary barotrauma in premature neonates with idiopathic respiratory distress syndrome requiring mechanical ventilation has been tempered by a recent multicenter trial in which HFOV did not prove to be superior to conventional mechanical ventilation.[146] One area of relatively proven benefit of HFV is in the management of bronchopleural fistulae. HFJV has proven useful in the management of bronchopleural fistula, with consistent improvement in arterial blood gas, when conventional ventilation had previously failed.[147]

Recent studies have suggested a role for HFV in children after cardiac surgery and with ARDS.[148-153] HFJV has been shown to improve cardiac function after a Fontan procedure.[148] HFJV and HFOV have been shown to improve oxygenation and ventilation compared with conventional ventilation in children with respiratory failure.[150-153] There are many reported strategies with the use of HFV: (1) "high lung volume strategy," which requires HFV to be provided at a mean airway pressure that is at least 3 to 5 cm higher than with conventional ventilation; (2) combined HFV and conventional ventilation (usually used with HFJV), in which conventional tidal breaths are interposed during HFV usually at a rate of 5 to 8 breaths per minute; or (3) application of HFV at the same mean airway pressure as conventional ventilation. The high lung volume strategy seems to be the most promising one at least for HFOV.

Respiratory Care During Mechanical Ventilation

Pulmonary Hygiene

The fundamental goals of pulmonary hygiene are clearance of secretions and prevention and relief of atelectasis. The most effective method of clearing secretions is a combination of changing body position and vigorous coughing by the patient.[154] When the patient is unable to cough effectively, it is common practice to resort to chest physiotherapy and active suctioning of the trachea. Suctioning the trachea usually requires disconnecting the patient from the ventilator, passage of a suction catheter into the endotracheal tube, and application of suction to the catheter while the catheter is withdrawn from the endotracheal tube. In patients with marginal oxygenation, suctioning may result in hypoxia; arrhythmias; hemodynamic instability; and, in rare instances, cardiac arrest.[155-157] This can be prevented by prior hyperoxygenation. Suctioning may also result in cardiac arrhythmias. Chest physiotherapy refers to a variety of respiratory maneuvers performed to aid in the clearance of airway secretions and promoting lung expansion. These are (1) postural drainage, (2) chest percussion and chest vibration, and (3) deep breathing exercises. The efficacy of chest physiotherapy in patients who have undergone intubation is unclear. In adults, some studies have shown a benefit when all the components of the chest physiotherapy regimen are performed.[158] In children with cystic fibrosis, no additional benefit was provided by chest physiotherapy maneuvers when compared with spontaneous coughing.[159] Recently, several devices have been proposed as an adjunct to the standard chest physiotherapy. They include an intrapulmonary percussive ventilator (IPV); a mechanical insufflator-exsufflator (CoughAssist); the FLUTTER mucous clearance device and Acapella devices; intermittent positive pressure breathing (IPPB); mechanical percussors; and the ABI Vest, formerly known as the ThAIRapy Vest.

The IPV is used in mechanized chest physical therapy; the IPV device delivers high-flow jets of air to the airways by a pneumatic flow interrupter at a rate of 100 to 300 cycles per minute through a mouthpiece. The patient controls variables such as inspiratory time, peak pressure, and delivery rates. Initial studies showed that in children with cystic fibrosis, IPV was as effective as standard aerosol and chest physiotherapy.[160,161]

IPV was recently reported to improve atelectasis in children, compared with conventional chest physiotherapy.[162] A more recent study suggests that IPV may be more beneficial in secretion clearance in children with cystic fibrosis.[163] The mechanical insufflator-exsufflator (CoughAssist) is a portable electric device that uses a blower and a valve to alternately apply a positive and then a negative pressure to a patient's airway to assist the patient in clearing retained bronchopulmonary secretions. This device attempts to simulate a cough. Air is delivered to and from the patient through a breathing circuit incorporating a flexible tube; a bacterial filter; and a facemask, a mouthpiece, or an adapter to a tracheostomy or endotracheal tube. Miske et al[164] reported that in children with neuromuscular disease and impaired cough, the use of a mechanical insufflator-exsufflator was safe, well tolerated, and effective in preventing pulmonary complications. The FLUTTER mucous clearance device and Acapella device are small handheld devices that provide positive expiratory pressure (PEP.) Exhaling through the device creates oscillations, or "flutter," in pressures in the airway resulting in loosening of mucus. Other PEP devices are used with a small volume nebulizer and function in conjunction with medication delivery. A recent Cochrane review concluded that there was no clear evidence that PEP was a more or less effective intervention overall than other forms of physiotherapy, and there was limited evidence that PEP was preferred by participants compared with other techniques.[165] IPPB devices use pressure to passively fill the lungs when a breath is initiated. An incorporated manometer and mechanical valves serve to terminate the flow of inspired air when a predetermined pressure is reached on inhalation. IPPB breathing circuits are designed to nebulize inhaled medication. Most IPPB devices are powered by compressed air and are not suitable for home use. Mechanical percussors are typically electrical devices used in lieu of a caretaker's hands for chest percussion or vibration. Conventional chest physiotherapy is both labor intensive and time consuming. A high-frequency chest wall vibrating/oscillating device is currently available (The ABI Vest). Arens et al[166] showed that in hospitalized patients with cystic fibrosis, high-frequency chest compression with the vest conventional chest physiotherapy was equally safe and effective when used during acute pulmonary exacerbations.

Humidification Systems

During spontaneous breathing, inspired air is warmed and almost completely humidified as it passes through the upper airways.[167] The use of an endotracheal or a tracheostomy tube bypasses the natural warming and humidifying functions of the upper airway. The mucosal surface below the artificial airway must then provide both humidification and heat to the inspired air. This may adversely affect mucociliary clearance.[168,169] If the inspired gases are not warmed to the body temperature, insensible water loss in the lung is increased. All gases used in respiratory therapy are dry with no moisture. Therefore these gases must have moisture added to them during delivery to the patients. When a gas is warmed, its relative humidity decreases.

Humidifiers can be classified into those that provide only humidity and those that provide both heat and humidity. There are several types of nonheated simple humidifiers. The simplest in design is the pass-over or blow-by humidifier. The second type is the bubble humidifier, probably the most common device used in respiratory therapy. In this device, the gas is directed below the surface of the water and allowed to bubble to the surface. A jet-humidifier produces an aerosol; humidity is provided by evaporation of the aerosol particles. An underwater jet humidifier uses a combination of jet and bubble humidification principles. In the clinical setting, the amount of humidity provided by the simple humidifiers is about the same. Although the more efficient humidifiers increase humidification, they also tend to cool the inspired air. Therefore the absolute humidity delivered tends to be similar among the simple humidifiers. Relative humidity of 100% at room temperature is less than 40% relative humidity at body temperature. When inspired gases are humidified with one of these devices, the balance of the moisture is provided by the airway mucosa. Therefore when the upper airway is bypassed by the presence of an artificial airway, then the inspired gases must be additionally heated to provide 100% humidity at body temperature. The factors that determine the efficiency of humidifying devices depend on (1) time of contact with the gas and water, (2) temperature of both the gas and water, and (3) the surface area of contact of the gas–water interface. The efficiency of humidification increases as the time of contact increases and as the surface area of contact increases. Increasing the temperature of the inspired gas before delivery decreases the humidity that needs to be provided by the airway mucosa and adds to patient comfort. Heated humidifiers use the same principle as the simple humidifiers and have in addition a heating element. The relative humidity with these systems can be as high as 100%. The heating system can be servo-controlled to adjust the heat according to the relative humidity.

Aerosol Therapy

Aerosolized drug administration is often used in the treatment of infants and children with respiratory diseases including reversible lower airway obstruction, pneumonias due to *Pneumocystis carinii* and respiratory syncytial virus, and hyaline membrane disease. Common drugs used as aerosol agents include beta-2 agonists, atropine, ipratropium bromide, cromolyn sodium, antiviral agents, corticosteroids, antibiotics, surfactant, pentamidine, and mucolytics. A drug aerosol increases the therapeutic index of the drug by delivering it directly to the site of action with minimal side effects. The factors that affect deposition of aerosol particles are gravity, viscosity of the gas, kinetic activity of the particles, particle inertia, physical nature of the particle, temperature and humidity of the aerosol, and the ventilatory pattern. Compared with that in adults, deposition of aerosolized particles in infants and children is poor because of factors such as a small airway caliber, greater airway resistance, high respiratory rate with a short inspiratory time, increased chest wall compliance, ineffective coordination effort, and inconsistent breathholding maneuvers. Despite poor aerosol deposition, a clinical response to inhaled medications can often be seen. The dose and the delivery method should be individualized to each patient to ensure a good clinical response.

Nebulizers are devices that generate aerosols. Particle size has to be at least 1 to 5 μm for deposition in the distal airways. Currently, four types of delivery systems are available for clinical use that generate medication aerosols. These are the jet nebulizers (small volume and large volume nebulizer), ultrasonic nebulizers, metered-dose inhalers, and dry-powder inhalers. A jet nebulizer uses the Bernoulli principle to create an aerosol. The size of the particle depends on the jet flow rate and the size of the capillary tube. Baffles placed in the path of the aerosols tend to remove larger particles, allowing delivery of smaller particles to the patient. A pneumatic nebulizer is a device that creates the aerosol using the same principle as the jet nebulizer, but the aerosol particles are carried to the patient by a main gas flow. A pneumatic nebulizer may be a mainstream nebulizer in which the aerosol is generated in the path of the main gas flow or a sidestream nebulizer in which the aerosol is generated in a separate chamber and carried passively into the path of the main gas flow. The ultrasonic nebulizer uses a piezoelectric crystal that produces a highly concentrated output of aerosol particles and has been used primarily for cough and sputum production or bronchoprovocational challenges. Ultrasonic nebulizers have not been routinely used for drug delivery in infants and children. With the replacement of the saline solution with medication, however, the highly concentrated output from the ultrasonic nebulizer may perform better than a small-volume nebulizer in accomplishing greater deposition of medications in children. The metered-dose inhaler uses a pressurized canister that dispenses a single bolus of aerosolized medication. Such inhalers are convenient, cost-effective, and versatile, and generally have an effective deposition rate of 10% to 15%. The canister is activated into the spacer and the medication remains suspended in the chamber until the patient inhales. A dry-powder inhaler delivers a large bolus of medication during a single inspiration maneuver and produces therapeutic effects similar to a metered-dose inhaler and an aerosol nebulizer. The dry-powder medication, released from a capsule and deposited into a small canister, is delivered to the lungs during inspiration. The inspired flow rate causes a turbulent state within the canister, and the powder is directed toward the respiratory tract.

Aerosolized medications are often delivered through mechanical ventilators for the treatment of bronchospasm. Aerosol delivery is inefficient when delivered through a ventilator. The endotracheal tube is the most significant barrier to effective delivery. The smaller the inner diameter of the tube, the less efficient is aerosol delivery. The nebulizer is most effective when it is synchronized to fill the inspiratory limb of the circuit with aerosolized particles during the exhalation phase of ventilation, thereby improving the delivery of medication during the subsequent inspiration. The inspiratory portion of the circuit serves as a spacer chamber, similar to the spacer used for metered dose inhalers. Some current ventilators offer a synchronized nebulization capability, in which a portion of the preset inspiratory gas is diverted to power the nebulizer. The effects of added volume delivered to the inspiratory limb should be taken into account and minimized with the addition of a pressure relief valve to the circuit. Metered-dose inhalers can be equally effective as nebulizers during mechanical ventilation.

Weaning from Mechanical Ventilation

Weaning from mechanical ventilation is defined as liberation from mechanical ventilation while spontaneous breathing is allowed to assume the responsibility for effective gas exchange. Weaning can be considered a success when a patient can maintain effective gas exchange, with complete spontaneous breathing and without any mechanical assistance. Weaning can be considered a failure when spontaneous efforts are incapable of sustaining effective gas exchange without mechanical ventilator support. *Extubation* is defined as the removal of an endotracheal tube. The timing of extubation should coincide with an assessment that the patient is capable of maintaining effective gas exchange without any mechanical ventilator support. Avoiding both premature extubation and unnecessary prolongation of mechanical ventilation is important.

When the indications that were met for provision of mechanical ventilation are no longer present, then the patient can be weaned from mechanical ventilation.

Weaning should start (1) when the underlying disease process is improving; (2) when gas exchange is adequate; (3) when no conditions exist that impose an undue burden on the respiratory muscles, such as cardiac insufficiency, severe hyperinflation, severe malnutrition, and multiple organ system failure; and (4) when the patient is capable of sustaining spontaneous ventilation as ventilator support is decreased without expending an excessive amount of energy. It is the patient who dictates the initiation of the weaning process and the pace of the weaning process. Patients cannot be arbitrarily forced to wean. Improvement of the underlying disease process can be assessed with measurement of indices of gas exchange, pulmonary mechanics, ventilation perfusion relationships, and x-ray findings. The patient's ability to take over the responsibility from the ventilator depends on several factors: (1) respiratory muscle strength, (2) stability of the cardiovascular system, (3) work of breathing, (4) general nutritional status of the patient, and (5) the presence or absence of an underlying hypercatabolic state (e.g., sepsis). Weaning cannot be accomplished unless all of these factors are optimal. The pathophysiological determinants of weaning outcome include the following: (1) adequacy of pulmonary gas exchange; (2) respiratory drive; (3) respiratory muscle performance and capacity; (4) respiratory muscle load; (5) amount of dead-space ventilation; and (6) work of breathing and ventilatory requirements. Box 44–6 shows the specific parameters to be met before initiating weaning.

There are currently two approaches to weaning. One is the "traditional" method of slowly reducing the ventilator support, including inspired oxygen concentration, to a minimal acceptable level and then assessing the patient's readiness to extubate. The other is the "modern" concept of assessing the patient's readiness to extubate as soon as the patient meets criteria to initiate weaning.

BOX 44–6

Criteria To Be Met Before Initiating Weaning

1. Alert mental status
2. Good cough and gag reflexes
3. Core temperature below 38.5° C
4. Spontaneous respiratory effort
5. pH 7.32 to 7.47
6. Partial pressure of arterial oxygen (Pa_{O_2}) higher than 60 mmHg or pulse oximetry reading less than 95%
7. Fractional inspired oxygen (Fi_{O_2}) of 0.50 or less
8. Positive end-expiratory pressure (PEEP) less than or equal to 7 cm H_2O
9. Partial pressure of carbon dioxide (Pa_{CO_2}) less than 50 mmHg
10. No further need for vasoactive agents
11. No clinical need for increased ventilator support in the past 24 hours
12. No planned operative procedures requiring heavy sedation in the next 12 hours

Traditional Method of Weaning

In the traditional method, the exact sequence of the weaning process will be dictated by the clinical circumstance. At each step of weaning, the patient must demonstrate an ability to sustain effectiveness of breathing. Minute ventilation is reduced primarily with a decrease in the ventilator rate. Mean airway pressure is then reduced to a minimum with a decrease in CPAP/PEEP. Most children are currently weaned with SIMV or IMV alone, with SIMV and added pressure support, or with pressure support alone. Despite earlier indications that weaning with IMV was useful,[10,169,170] current studies do not advocate weaning with IMV in adults.[171,172] In infants, provision of a continuous flow device has been shown to decrease work of breathing and aid in weaning.[10] PSV has been advocated as a weaning mode because it can result in better synchrony between the patient and the ventilator than IMV, volume-assisted ventilation, or pressure control ventilation.[173-176] Pressure support will allow ventilatory muscle loads to be returned gradually during the weaning process.[173-176] Because each breath is assisted, it alters the pressure-volume relationship of the respiratory muscles in such a way as to improve its efficiency.[173-176] The parameters that can be manipulated to titrate the muscle loading are the magnitude of the trigger threshold and the preset pressure limit. PEEP is provided to maintain FRC and prevent alveolar collapse. The amount of pressure support to be provided depends on the clinical circumstance. PSVmax, or the maximum pressure support needed to reduce the respiratory work to zero, requires a pressure limit that delivers a VTeff of about 10 to 12 ml/kg. PSVmax is not necessary at the start of weaning. The level of pressure support that should be selected should allow for spontaneous respiration without undue exertion and still result in normal minute ventilation. No strict criteria can be established; they have to be applied and titrated on an individual basis. Weaning of PSV is accomplished with a decremental reduction of the pressure limit. Similar to that previously mentioned in the weaning guidelines, with each wean, the effect of weaning on muscle loading has to be evaluated clinically. An increase in respiratory rate is an early indication of increasing muscle load. Retractions and use of accessory muscles would indicate a more severe muscle load. If respiratory rate increases during the weaning process, the level of pressure support should be increased until there is reduction in the respiratory rate. A relative contraindication to the use of PSV is a high baseline spontaneous respiratory rate. There is a finite lag time involved from the initiation of a breath to the sensing of this effort and from the sensing to the delivery of a mechanical breath. In infants breathing at a relatively fast rate (>50 breaths per minute), this lag time may be too long, and this may result in asynchrony between the patient and the ventilator.

Modern Method of Weaning

The premise underlying the modern method is that not all patients require a prolonged weaning process. If patients meet the criteria for weaning as outlined in Box 44–7,

BOX 44–7

Criteria for Terminating a Spontaneous Breathing Trial

1. Inability to maintain gas exchange
   Pulse oximeter saturations less than 95% with 40% inspired oxygen
   Needing more than 50% inspired oxygen to maintain oxygen saturations greater than 95%
2. Inability to maintain effective ventilation
   Measured exhaled tidal volume less than 5 ml/kg ideal body weight*
   An increase in $Paco_2$ greater than 50 mmHg or an increase of more than 10 mmHg
   Respiratory acidosis with pH less than 7.3
3. Increased work of breathing
   Respiratory rate outside of the acceptable range for their age

for age <6 months	20-60/min
6 months-2 years	15-45/min
2-5 years	15-40/min
>5 years	10-35/min

   Use of accessory respiratory muscles
      Intercostals/suprasternal/supraclavicular retractions
      A paradoxical breathing pattern
4. Other signs of distress
   Diaphoresis
   Anxiety
   Heart rate higher than the 90th percentile for a given age
   Change in mental status (agitation or somnolence)
   Systolic blood pressure lower than the 3rd percentile for a given age

If a patient has any of these signs at any time during the breathing trial, the trial should be terminated and mechanical ventilation should be reinstituted.
*Ideal body weight was estimated as the 50th percentile for age and sex from National Center for Health Statistics growth charts and was the weight used for adjustment of all respiratory parameters during the test and within the protocol groups of the study.
$Paco_2$, partial pressure of carbon dioxide.

they can be subjected to a spontaneous breathing trial (SBT) to test their readiness to extubate. If the SBT is successful, then the patient is ready to be extubated. If the patient fails an SBT, ventilation is continued until the patient is able to successfully tolerate an SBT. The criteria for terminating a SBT are shown in Box 45–7. Esteban et al[171] showed that 76.2% of patients successfully underwent a 2-hour trial of spontaneous breathing, and 89.4% of them immediately underwent extubation. In a recently completed randomized, controlled trial of weaning modes in children, 42% of the patients initially tested with a minimal pressure-support trial passed the test and underwent extubation.[177] These studies validate the modern method of weaning patients from mechanical ventilation.

Spontaneous Breathing Trial

Currently, there are three methods of SBTs. These are (1) T-piece trials, (2) CPAP trials, and (3) minimal pressure-support trials.[171,172,177-180] In T-piece trials, the patient is removed from the ventilator but does not undergo extubation. Humidified supplemental oxygen is provided to the airway without any positive pressure support through a T-piece (Fig. 44–20). In this system, a corrugated tubing from the nebulizer/humidifier attaches to one end of the T-piece, and an extension of corrugated tubing attaches to the other end of the T-piece. The flow rate should be adjusted to produce a constant mist coming from the extension piece on the T-tube both during inspiration and expiration so that the patient's minute ventilation is matched by the device. Roughly, this corresponds to about three times the minute ventilation of the patient.

The SBT can also be conducted without removing the patient from the ventilator with a low level (e.g., 5 cm H_2O) of CPAP or with a low level of PSV. Randolph et al[175] described a minimal pressure support technique in which the level of pressure support was adjusted for the endotracheal tube size (3 to 3.5 mm = pressure support of 10 cm H_2O; 4 to 4.5 mm = pressure support of 8 cm H_2O; >5 mm = pressure support of 6 cm H_2O). On the other hand, in a study comparing minimal pressure support with T-piece trials, Farias et al[179] used a pressure support of 10 cm H_2O for all patients. The duration of the trial can range from 30 minutes to 2 hours.

The proponents of a "minimal pressure support" approach to the SBT speculate that this overcomes the resistance to breathing through the artificial airway. Ishaaya, Nathan, and Belman[181] showed that minimal pressure support based on in vitro studies overestimated the amount of support required to overcome the resistance of the endotracheal tube and ventilator circuitry. There are no measurements in vivo validating this concept in children. In one study of adults, the authors reported a similar resistance to breathing through the upper airway after extubation as that with the endotracheal tube in place.[182] Resistance through the artificial airway is affected by many factors, including the inspiratory flow of the patient, the inner diameter of the tube, the use of either an endotracheal or a tracheostomy tube, and the presence of secretions in the tube. In children, Farias et al[179] recently compared two methods of SBT, one with pressure support of 10 cm H_2O and the other with a T-piece circuit. The extubation failure was not different between the two groups.[179]

Physicians are reluctant to subject infants and young children to a trial of complete spontaneous breathing with either CPAP or a T-piece circuit because of concern about the work of breathing imposed by the endotracheal tube and the breathing circuit. It is still common for infants and children to undergo extubation from a "low" level of ventilator support. Studies in children, however, have shown that when the fraction of minute ventilation provided by the ventilator is more than 30, the risk of extubation failure is increased.[183,184] This suggests that there is an overestimation of the ability of children to breathe spontaneously when they undergo extubation from a low level of ventilator support. The studies by Farias et al[178-180] have shown that SBTs with a T-piece circuit are well tolerated by children. Therefore it is crucial that the ability to breathe effectively be determined with complete spontaneous breathing without ventilator support. An important dictum to remember is that "the test for extubation readiness is not extubation."[185]

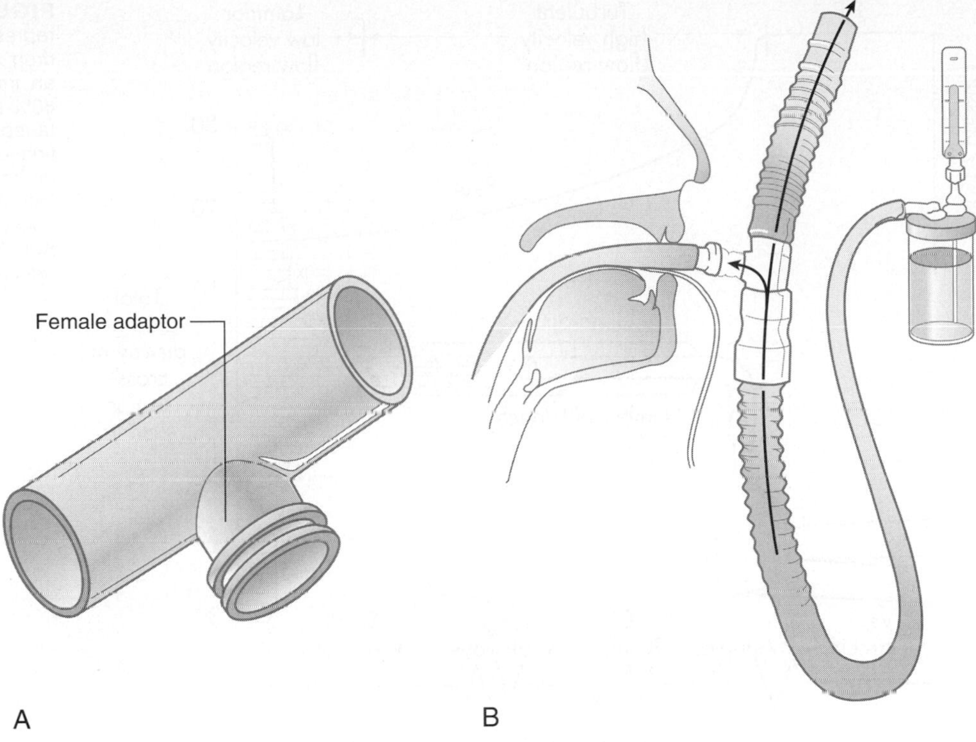

FIGURE 44–20 • T-piece circuit. (Reproduced with permission from Kofke WA: Postoperative respiratory care techniques. Part III. Weaning from mechanical ventilation and oxygen therapy, *Curr Rev RACN* 13:161, 1992.)

Extubation

When SBT is successful, the patient can undergo extubation and be liberated from mechanical ventilation. The patient must be awake, be alert, and have airway protective reflexes. The patient must be breathing effectively, without undue exertion. Adequate gas exchange with a relatively low FiO_2 must be established. A stable cardiovascular system must be established. Metabolic, nutritional, and electrolyte balance must be ensured. Airway pressures must be reduced to a minimum. At the time of extubation, it is possible to estimate the risk of reintubation with simple bedside measures of respiratory function.[183,184] A low risk is defined as an extubation failure rate of less than 10%, and a high risk of failure is defined as an extubation failure rate of at least 25%.[183,184] Table 44–1 lists the threshold values for the respiratory parameters with identified low- and high-risk values.[183,184] Additional parameters that may be useful in determining eligibility for extubation are an intrapulmonary shunt fraction less than 15% (requires pulmonary artery catheterization), a physiological dead space less than 40%, a vital capacity of at least 15 mL/kg, and a maximum negative inspiratory force of at least 30 cm H_2O.

Weaning Problems

Farias et al[178] distinguish between two types of failure: trial failure and extubation failure. *Trial failure* is defined as a failure to sustain effective gas exchange and breathing during a trial of spontaneous breathing while the patient is still intubated. *Extubation failure* is defined as the requirement for reintubation within 48 hours after extubation. Some patients take longer than others to wean. Factors that prolong the weaning process are (1) slow resolution of the underlying disease process, (2) ventilatory pump failure, and (3) psychological factors. In many instances, weaning is delayed because of the slow resolution of the underlying disease process. Ventilatory pump failure can be due to increased respiratory work load, decreased respiratory muscle capacity, or a combination of both. Decreased ventilatory drive may result from respiratory center dysfunction caused by sedative agents; neurological disease, particularly if it affects the brainstem; sleep deprivation; and metabolic alkalosis. Phrenic nerve injury usually results as a complication of birth trauma or operative procedures involving the heart

TABLE 44–1

Threshold Values for Low- and High-Risk of Reintubation for Bedside Parameters of Respiratory Function

Respiratory Parameter	<10%	<25%
Spontaneous tidal volume (ml/kg)	>6.5	<3.5
FiO_2	<0.3	>0.4
Mean airway pressure (cm H_2O)	<5	>8.5
Peak inspiratory pressure (cm H_2O)	<25	>30
Dynamic compliance (ml/kg/cm H_2O)	>0.9	<0.4
Fraction of the total minute ventilation provided by the ventilator (%)	<20	>30
Mean inspiratory flow (ml/kg/sec)	>14	<8

Respiratory parameters were measured just before extubation. Risk of reintubation is percent of patients who underwent reintubation within 48 hours of extubation.

FiO_2, fractional concentration of oxygen in inspired gas.

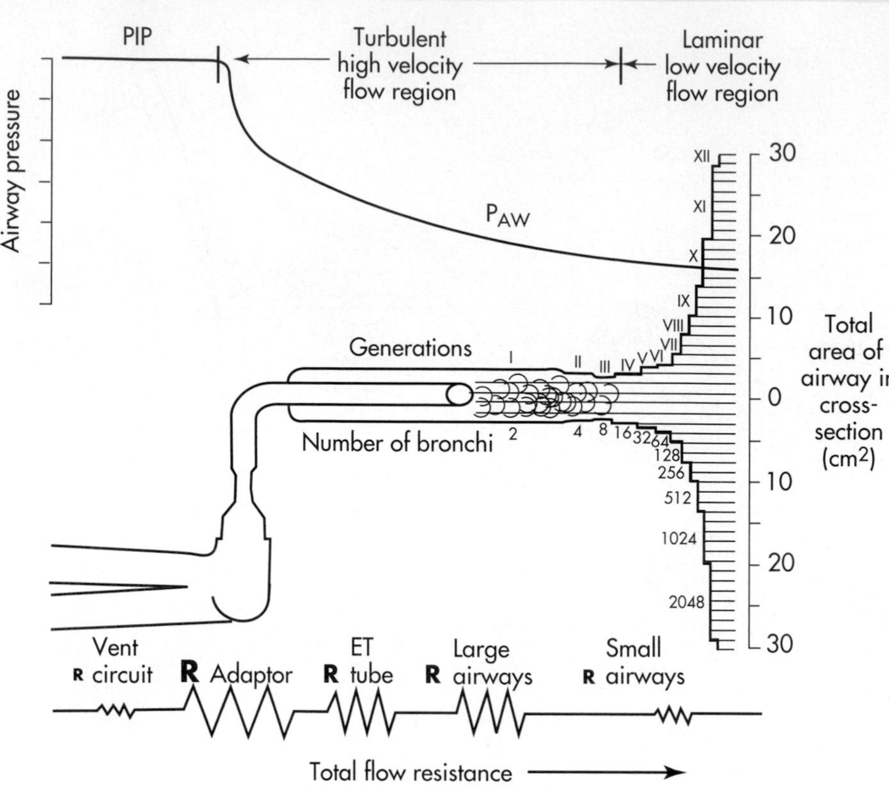

FIGURE 44–21 • Schematic and graphic representation of resistances and pressure drop across the entire respiratory system in an intubated patient. Approximately 60% to 80% of the total airway resistance in a spontaneously breathing patient resides within the first few generations of bronchi. Addition of an endotracheal tube and the ventilator circuit increases the resistance to breathing. (Reproduced with permission from Goldsmith JP, Karotkin EH, editors: *Assisted ventilation of the neonate,* Philadelphia, 1988, WB Saunders.)

and other thoracic structures.[186-189] This may result in either paresis or paralysis of one or both hemidiaphragms. When muscle weakness is present, weaning should generally be slow, allowing sufficient time for regaining muscle strength and endurance. Muscle training through an incremental increase in muscle work can be achieved by a gradual increase in the trigger threshold for assisted ventilation. Ventilatory requirements can be reduced with a decrease in carbon dioxide production with a reduction in excess caloric intake. Muscle loading may occur during IMV because of patient asynchrony. Asynchrony between the patient's breathing and the mechanical breaths may occur during both phases of the respiratory cycle. When the patient exhales while the ventilator delivers a mechanical breath, the airway pressures will be higher and the mechanical breath is wasted. This increases the work of breathing during exhalation. Prolonged asynchrony may result in muscle fatigue and may contribute to prolonged weaning. Considering nonrespiratory factors that may affect extubation failure is important. In a study by Khamiees et al,[190] although all patients passed an SBT, poor cough strength and endotracheal secretions were synergistic in predicting extubation failure.

Tracheostomy and Weaning

Most airway resistance resides in the upper airways. The presence of an endotracheal tube markedly increases the airway resistance (Fig. 44–21) and contributes to the work of breathing. Tracheostomy may aid in the weaning by several mechanisms. First, it reduces airway resistance by bypassing the upper airway. This reduces the work of breathing. Second, it increases patient comfort and allows better interaction between the patient and the caretakers, especially the parents. Third, it increases nursing comfort. Tracheostomy is not without risk. The procedure and complications of tracheostomy are described in detail elsewhere. Immediate complications are those related to bleeding, those related to pulmonary air leak, and those associated with anesthesia. Long-term complications include infections of the trachea and the lung, granuloma formation with subglottic stenosis from scarring, erosion of the trachea, and bleeding from erosion into a major thoracic vessel (e.g., innominate artery).

REFERENCES

1. Nunn JF: *Applied respiratory physiology,* ed 3, London, 1987, Butterworths & Co.
2. Aubier M, Viires N, Syllie G, et al: Respiratory muscle contribution to lactic acidosis in low cardiac output, *Am Rev Respir Dis* 126: 648, 1982.
3. Shepard FM, Arango LA, Simmons JG, et al: Hemodynamic effects of mechanical ventilation in normal and distressed lambs: a comparison of negative pressure and positive pressure respirators, *Biol Neonate* 19:83, 1971.
4. Kirby RR, Smith RA, Desautels DA: *Mechanical ventilation,* New York, 1985, Churchill Livingstone..
5. McPherson SP: *Respiratory therapy equipment,* St Louis, 1985, CV Mosby.
6. Dupuis YG: *Ventilators: theory and clinical application,* ed 2, St Louis, 1992, Mosby–Year Book.
7. Chatburn RL: A new system for understanding mechanical ventilators, *Respir Care* 36:1123-1155, 1991.
8. Chatburn RL, Primiano FP Jr: A new system for understanding modes of mechanical ventilation, *Respir Care* 46:604-621, 2001.
9. Kirby RR, Robison EJ, Schulz J, et al: A new pediatric volume ventilator, *Anesth Analg* 50:533-537, 1971.
10. Downs JB, Klein EF Jr, Desautels D, et al: Intermittent mandatory ventilation: a new approach to weaning patients from mechanical ventilators, *Chest* 64:331-335, 1973.
11. Kirby RR: Intermittent mandatory ventilation in the neonate, *Crit Care Med* 5:18-22, 1977.

12. Fricker HS, Palla C, Mettler M: Intermittent mandatory ventilation in the treatment of the idiopathic respiratory distress syndrome of newborns, *Schweiz Med Wochenschr* 110:251-255, 1980.
13. Pulmonary terms and symbols. A report of the ACCP-STS Joint Committee on Pulmonary Nomenclature, *Chest* 67: 583-593, 1975.
14. Gregory GA, Kitterman JA, Phibbs RH, et al: Treatment of idiopathic respiratory-distress syndrome with continuous positive airway pressure, *N Engl J Med* 284:1333-1340, 1971.
15. Kattwinkel J, Fleming D, Cha CC, et al: A device for administration of continuous positive airway pressure by nasal route, *Pediatrics* 52:131-134, 1973.
16. Sullivan CE, Issa FG, Berthon-Jones M, et al: Reversal of obstructive sleep apnoea by continuous positive airway pressure applied through the nares, *Lancet* 1:862-865, 1981.
17. Goldman SL, Brady JP, Dumpit FM: Increased work of breathing associated with nasal prongs, *Pediatrics* 64:160, 1979.
18. Dantzker DR, Brook CJ, Dehart P, et al: Ventilation-perfusion distributions in the adult respiratory distress syndrome, *Am Rev Respir Dis* 120:1039-1052, 1979.
19. Pontoppidan H, Geffin B, Lowenstein E: Acute respiratory failure in the adult, *N Engl J Med* 287:690, 743, 799, 1972.
20. Suter PM, Fairley HB, Isenberg MD: Optimal end-expiratory airway pressure in patients with acute pulmonary failure, *N Engl J Med* 292:284, 1975.
21. Civetta JM, Barnes TA, Smith LO: "Optimal PEEP" and intermittent mandatory ventilation in the treatment of respiratory failure, *Respir Care* 20:551, 1975.
22. White MK, Galli SA, Chatburn RL, et al: Optimal positive end-expiratory pressure therapy in infants and children with acute respiratory failure, *Pediatr Res* 24:217, 1988.
23. Beasley JM, Jones SE: Continuous positive airway pressure in bronchiolitis, *Br Med J* 283:1506, 1981.
24. Martin JG, Shore S, Engel LA: Effect of continuous positive airway pressure on respiratory mechanics and pattern of breathing in induced asthma, *Am Rev Respir Dis* 126:812, 1982.
25. Qvist J, Anderson JB, Pemberton M, et al: High level PEEP in severe asthma, *N Engl J Med* 307:1347, 1982.
26. MacIntyre NR: Respiratory function during pressure support ventilation, *Chest* 89:677-683, 1986.
27. MacIntyre NR, Nishimura M, Usada Y, et al: The Nagoya conference on system design and patient-ventilator interactions during pressure support ventilation, *Chest* 97:1463-1466, 1990.
28. MacIntyre NR, Ho LI: Effects of initial flow rate and breath termination criteria on pressure ventilation, *Chest* 99:134-138, 1991.
29. Marini JJ, Smith TC, Lomb VJ: External work output and force generation during synchronized intermittent mechanical ventilation, *Am J Respir Crit Care Med* 138:1169-1170, 1988.
30. Ho LI, MacIntyre NR: Pressure supported breaths: ventilatory effects of breath initiation and breath termination design characteristics, *Crit Care Med* 17:26, 1989.
31. Braschi A, Sala Gallini G, et al: Relationship between sensitivity of the expiratory trigger and breathing pattern during pressure support ventilation, *Am J Respir Crit Care Med* 130:361, 1989.
32. Banner MJ, Blanch P, Desautels DA: Mechanical ventilators. In Kirby RR, Banner MJ, Downs JB, editors: *Clinical applications of ventilatory support*, New York, 1990, Churchill Livingstone.
33. Downs JB, Stock MC: Airway pressure release ventilation: a new concept in ventilatory support, *Crit Care Med* 15:459, 1987.
34. Rasanen J, Downs JB, Stock MC: Cardiovascular effects of conventional positive pressure ventilatio and airway pressure release ventilation, *Chest* 92:390, 1987.
35. Rasanen J, et al: Airway pressure release ventilation: a multicenter trial, *Anesthesiology* 71:A1078, 1989.
36. Rasanen J, Downs JB, Stock MC: Cardiovascular effects of of conventional positive pressure ventilation and airway pressure release ventilation, *Chest* 93:911, 1988.
37. Stock MC, Downs JB, Frolicher DA: Airway pressure release ventilation, *Crit Care Med* 15:462, 1987.
38. Hewlett AM, Platt AS, Terry VG: Mandatory minute volume. A new concept in weaning from mechanical ventilation, *Anaesthesia*. 32:163-169, 1977.
39. Marraro G, Casiraghi G, Galbiati AM: A study of pressure regulated volume control ventilation in natural surfactant treated infants with RDS, Ped Res 4(suppl):223A, 1321, 1995.
40. Hazelzet JA, Petru R, Ouden CD, et al: New modes of mechanical ventilation for severe respiratory failure, *Crit Care Med* 21(suppl 9l):S366–S367, 1993.
41. Kocis KC, Dekeon MK, Rosen HK, et al: Pressure-regulated volume control vs volume control ventilation in infants after surgery for congenital heart disease, *Pediatr Cardiol* 22:233-237, 2001,
42. MacIntyre N, Branson RD: *Mechanical ventilation*, Philadelphia, 2001, WB Saunders.
43. Tyler DC: Positive end-expiratory pressure. A review, *Crit Care Med* 11:300, 1983.
44. Weisman IM, Rinaldo JE, Roger RM: Positive end-expiratory pressure in adult respiratory failure, *N Engl J Med* 307:1381, 1982.
45. Amato MB, Barbas CS, Medeiros DM, et al: Effect of a protective-ventilation strategy on mortality in the acute respiratory distress syndrome, *N Engl J Med* 338:347-354, 1998.
46. Acute Respiratory Distress Syndrome Network: Ventilation with lower tidal volumes as compared to traditional tidal volumes for acute lung injury and the acute respiratory distress syndrome, *N Engl J Med* 342:1301-1308, 2000.
47. Dreyfuss D, Saumon G: Barotrauma is volutrauma, but which volume is the one responsible? *Intensive Care Med* 18:139-141, 1992.
48. Dreyfuss D, Saumon G: Role of tidal volume, FRC and end-inspiratory volume in the development of pulmonary edema following mechanical ventilation, *Am Rev Respir Dis* 148:1194-1203, 1993.
49. Lachmann B: Open the lung and keep the lung open, *Intensive Care Med* 18:319-321, 1992.
50. Slutsky AS: Lung injury caused by mechanical ventilation, *Chest* 116(suppl): 9S-15S, 1999.
51. Clark RH, Slutsky AS, Gerstmann DR: Lung protective strategy of ventilation in the neonate: what are they? *Pediatrics* 105:112-114, 2000.
52. Fuhrman BP, Smith-Wright DL, Venkataraman S, et al: Proximal mean airway pressure: a good estimator of mean alveolar pressure during continuous positive-pressure breathing, *Crit Care Med* 17:666-670, 1989.
53. Pelosi P, Cadringher P, Bottino P, et al: Sigh in acute respiratory distress syndrome, *Am J Respir Crit Care Med* 159:872-880, 1999.
54. Rimensberger PC, Cox PN, Frndova H, et al: The open lung during small tidal volume ventilation: concepts of recruitment and "optimal" positive end-expiratory pressure, *Crit Care Med* 27:1946-1952, 1999.
55. Gattinoni L, Mascheroni D, Torresin A, et al: Morphological response to PEEP in acute respiratory failure: a computerized tomography study, *Intensive Care Med* 12:137-143, 1986.
56. Gattinoni L, Pesenti A, Avalli L, et al: Pressure-volume curve of total respiratory system in acute respiratory failure: computed tomographic scan study, *Am Rev Respir Dis* 136:730-736, 1987.
57. Stocker R, Stein S, Ecknauer E, et al: Prone positioning and low-volume pressure-limited ventilation improve survival in patients with severe ARDS, *Chest* 111:1008-1017, 1997.
58. Lamm WJ, Albert RK: Mechanism by which prone position improves oxygenation in acute lung injury, *Am J Respir Crit Care Med* 150:184-193, 1994.
59. Jolliet P, Chevrolet JC: Effects of the prone position on gas exchange and hemodynamics in severe acute respiratory distress syndrome, *Crit Care Med* 26:1977-1985, 1998.
60. Gattinoni L, Pesenti A, Taccone P, et al: Effect of prone positioning on the survival of patients with acute respiratory failure, *N Engl J Med* 345:568-573, 2001.
61. Chatte G, Sab JM, Dubois JM, et al: Prone position in mechanically ventilated patients with severe acute respiratory failure, *Am J Respir Crit Care Med* 155:473-478, 1997.
62. Mancebo J, Fernandez R, Gordo F, et al: Prone vs supine position in ARDS patients: results of a randomized multicenter trial, *Am J Respir Crit Care Med* 167:A180, 2003.
63. Bruno F, Piva JP, Garcia PC, et al: Short-term effects of prone positioning on the oxygenation of pediatric patients submitted to mechanical ventilation, *J Pediatr (Rio J)* 77:361-368, 2001.
64. Curley MAQ, Thompson JE, Arnold JH: The effects of early and repeated prone positioning in pediatric patients with acute lung injury, *Chest* 118:156-163, 2000.
65. Relvas MS, Silver PC, Sagy M: Prone positioning of pediatric patients with ARDS results in improvement in oxygenation if maintained > 12 h daily, *Chest* 124:269-274, 2003.

66. Marcano BV, Silver P, Sagy M: Cephalad movement of endotracheal tubes caused by prone positioning pediatric patients with acute respiratory distress syndrome, *Pediatr Crit Care Med* 4:186-189, 2003.
67. Powner DJ, Eross B, Grenvik A: Differential lung ventilation with PEEP in the treatment of unilateral pneumonia, *Crit Care Med* 5:170, 1977.
68. Carlon GC, Ray C, Klein R, et al: Criteria for selective positive end-expiratory pressure and independent synchronized ventilation of each lung, *Chest* 74:501, 1978.
69. Rivara D, Burgain JL, Rieuf P, et al: Differential ventilation in unilateral lung disease: effects on respiratory mechanics and gas exchange, *Intensive Care Med* 5:189, 1979.
70. Baehrendtz S, Santesson J, Bindselv L, et al: Differential ventilation in acute bilateral lung disease. Influence on gas exchange and central haemodynamic, *Acta Anaesthesiol Scand* 27: 270, 1983.
71. Marraro G: Simultaneous independent lung ventilation in pediatric patients, *Crit Care Clinics* 8: 131, 1992.
72. Marraro G: Synchronized independent lung ventilation in pediatric age. *ACP Appl Cardiopulm Pathophys* 2:283-288, 1987.
73. Marraro G: Selective endobronchial intubation in paediatrics: the Marraro paediatric bilumen tube, *Paediatr Anaesth* 4:255-258, 1994.
74. Buda AJ, Pinsky MR, Ingels NB Jr, et al: Effect of intrathoracic pressure on left ventricular performance, *N Engl J Med* 301:453, 1979.
75. Pinsky MR, Summer WR: Cardiac augmentation by phasic high intrathoracic pressure support, *Chest* 84:370, 1983.
76. Greenough A, Morley C, Davis J: Interaction of spontaneous respiration with artificial respiration in preterm babies, *J Pediatr* 103:769, 1983.
77. Stark AR Bascom R, Frantz ID III: Muscle relaxation in mechanically ventilated infants, *J Pediatr* 94:439, 1979.
78. Crone RK, Favorito J: The effects of pancuronium bromide on infants with hyaline membrane disease, *J Pediatr* 97:991, 1980.
79. Runkle B, Bancalari E: Acute cardiopulmonary effects of pancuronium bromide in mechanically ventilated newborn infants, *J Pediatr* 104:615, 1984.
80. Fishman AP: Vasomotor regulation of the pulmonary circulation, *Ann Rev Physiol* 42:211, 1980.
81. Jobes DR, Nicolson SC, Steven JM, et al: Carbon dioxide prevents pulmonary overcirculation in hypoplastic left heart syndrome, *Ann Thorac Surg* 54:150, 1992.
82. Kemper KJ, Ritz RH, Benson MS, et al: Helium-oxygen mixture in the treatment of post-extubation stridor in pediatric trauma patients, *Crit Care Med* 19:356, 1991.
83. Elleau C, Galperine RI, Guenard H, et al: Helium-oxygen mixture in respiratory distress syndrome: a double-blind study, *J Pediatr* 122:132, 1993.
84. Brett WW, Koren G, England S, et al: Hypoxia associated with helium oxygen therapy in neonates, *J Pediatr* 106:474, 1985.
85. Inhaled nitric oxide and hypoxic respiratory failure in infants with congenital diaphragmatic hernia. The Neonatal Inhaled Nitric Oxide Study Group (NINOS), *Pediatrics* 99:838-845, 1997.
86. Roberts JD Jr. Fineman JR, Morin FC III, et al: Inhaled nitric oxide and persistent pulmonary hypertension of the newborn. The Inhaled Nitric Oxide Study Group, *N Engl J Med* 336:605-610, 1997.
87. Cornfield DN, Maynard RC, deRegnier RA, et al: Randomized, controlled trial of low-dose inhaled nitric oxide in the treatment of term and near-term infants with respiratory failure and pulmonary hypertension, *Pediatrics* 104(5 pt 1):1089-1094, 1999.
88. Clark RH, Kueser TJ, Walker MW, et al: Low-dose nitric oxide therapy for persistent pulmonary hypertension of the newborn. Clinical Inhaled Nitric Oxide Research Group, *N Engl J Med* 342:469-474 2000.
89. Kinsella JP, Abman SH: High-frequency oscillatory ventilation augments the response to inhaled nitric oxide in persistent pulmonary hypertension of the newborn: Nitric Oxide Study Group, *Chest* 114(suppl 1):100S, 1998.
90. Ream RS, Hauver JF, Lynch RE, et al: Low-dose inhaled nitric oxide improves the oxygenation and ventilation of infants and children with acute, hypoxemic respiratory failure, *Crit Care Med* 27:989-96, 1999; comment in *Crit Care Med* 27:871-872, 1999.
91. Dobyns EL, Cornfield DN, Anas NG, et al: Multicenter randomized controlled trial of the effects of inhaled nitric oxide therapy on gas exchange in children with acute hypoxemic respiratory failure, *J Pediatr* 134:406-412, 1999.
92. Dellinger RP, Zimmerman JL, Taylor RW, et al: Effects of inhaled nitric oxide in patients with acute respiratory distress syndrome: results of a randomized phase II trial. Inhaled Nitric Oxide in ARDS Study Group, *Crit Care Med* 26:15-23, 1998.
93. Michael JR, Barton G, Saffle SR, et al: Inhaled nitric oxide versus conventional therapy: effect on oxygenation in ARDS, *Am J Respir Crit Care Med* 157:1372–1380, 1998.
94. Troncy E, Collet J-P, Shapiro S, et al: Inhaled nitric oxide in acute respiratory distress syndrome: a pilot randomized controlled study, *Am J Respir Crit Care Med* 157:14831488, 1998.
95. Lundin S, Mang H, Smithies M, et al: Inhalation of nitric oxide in acute lung injury: results of a European multicentre study, *Intensive Care Med* 25: 911–919, 1999.
96. Bach JR. A comparison of long-term ventilatory support alternatives from the perspective of the patient and caregiver, *Chest* 104:1702-1706, 1993.
97. Simonds AK, Elliot MW: Outcome of the domiciliary nasal intermittent positive pressure ventilation in restrictive and obstructive disorders, *Thorax* 50:604-609, 1995.
98. Brochard L, Mancebo J, Wysocki M, et al: Noninvasive ventilation for acute exacerbations of chronic obstructive pulmonary disease, *N Engl J Med* 333:817-822, 1995.
99. Hill NS: Noninvasive ventilation. Does it work, for whom, and how? *Am Rev Respir Dis* 147:1050-1055, 1993.
100. Bach JR: Mechanical exsufflation, noninvasive ventilation, and new strategies for pulmonary rehabilitation and sleep disordered breathing, *Bull N Y Acad Med* 68:321-340, 1992.
101. Keenan SP, Sinuff T, Cook DJ, et al: Does noninvasive positive pressure ventilation improve outcome in acute hypoxemic respiratory failure? A systematic review, *Crit Care Med* 32:2516-2523, 2004.
102. Padman R, Lawless S, Von Nessen S: Use of BiPAP by nasal mask in the treatment of respiratory insufficiency in pediatric patients: preliminary investigation, *Pediatr Pulmonol* 17:119-123, 1994.
103. Akimbola OA, Servant GM, Custer JR, et al: Noninvasive bi-level positive pressure ventilation: management of two pediatric patients, *Respir Care* 38:1092-1098, 1993.
104. Fortenberry JD, Del Toro J, Jefferson LS, et al: Management of pediatric acute hypoxemic respiratory insufficiency with bilevel positive pressure (BiPAP) nasal mask ventilation, *Chest* 108: 1059-1064, 1995.
105. Padman R, Hyde C, Foster P, et al: The pediatric use of bilevel positive airway pressure therapy for obstructive sleep apnea syndrome: a retrospective review with analysis of respiratory parameters, *Clin Pediatr* 41:163-169, 2002.
106. Padman R, Lawless ST, Kettrick RG: Noninvasive ventilation via bilevel positive airway pressure support in pediatric practice, *Crit Care Med* 28:169-173, 1998.
107. Birnkrant DJ, Pope JF, Eiben RM: Pediatric noninvasive nasal ventilation. *J Child Neurol* 12:231-236, 1997.
108. Raphael JC, Chevret S, Chastang C, et al: Randomised trial of preventive nasal ventilation in Duchenne muscular dystrophy. French Multicentre Cooperative Group on Home Mechanical Ventilation Assistance in Duchenne de Boulogne Muscular Dystrophy, *Lancet* 343:1600-1604, 1994.
109. Vianello A, Bevilacqua M, Salvador V, et al: Long-term nasal intermittent positive pressure ventilation in advanced Duchenne's muscular dystrophy, *Chest* 105:445-448, 1994.
110. Bancalari E, Gerhardt T, Monkus E: Simple device for producing continuous negative pressure in infants with IRDS, *Pediatrics* 52:128-131, 1973.
111. Outerbridge EW, Roloff DW, Stern L: Continuous negative pressure in the management of severe respiratory distress syndrome, *J Pediatr* 81:384-391, 1972.
112. Alexander G, Gerhardt T, Bancalari E: Hyaline membrane disease. Comparison of continuous negative pressure and nasal positive airway pressure in its treatment, *Am J Dis Child* 133:1156-1159, 1979.
113. Samuels MP, Raine J, Wright T, et al: Continuous negative extrathoracic pressure in neonatal respiratory failure, *Pediatrics* 98:1154-1160, 1996.
114. Brahdy MB, Lenarsky M: Respiratory failure in acute epidemic poliomyeltis, *J Pediatr* 8:420-433, 1936.
115. Crone NL: The treatment of acute poliomyelitis with the respirator, *N Engl J Med* 210:621-623, 1934.

116. Wilson JL: Acute anterior poliomyelitis, *N Engl J Med* 206: 887-893, 1932
117. Splaingard ML, Frates RC Jr, Jefferson LS, et al: Home negative pressure ventilation: report of 20 years of experience in patients with neuromuscular disease, *Arch Phys Med Rehabil* 66:239-242, 1985.
118. Goldstein RS, Stradling JR: An artifact induced by negative pressure ventilation, *Chest* 101:563-565, 1992.
119. Sanyal SK, Bernal R, Hughes WT, et al: Continuous negative chest-wall pressure. Successful use for severe respiratory distress in an adult, *JAMA* 236:1727-1728, 1976.
120. Sawicka EH, Spencer GT, Branthwaite MA: Management of respiratory failure complicating pregnancy in severe kyphoscoliosis: a new use for an old technique? *Br J Dis Chest* 80:191-196, 1986.
121. Morris AH, Elliott CG: Adult respiratory distress syndrome: successful support with continuous negative extrathoracic pressure, *Crit Care Med* 13:989-990, 1985.
122. Hartke RH Jr, Block AJ: External stabilization of flail chest using continuous negative extrathoracic pressure, *Chest* 102:1283-1285, 1992.
123. Sanyal SK, MacGaw D, Hughes WT: Continuous negative chest-wall pressure as therapy for severe respiratory distress in an older child: preliminary observations, *J Pediatr* 85:230-232, 1974.
124. Sanyal SK, Mitchell C, Hughes WT, et al: Continuous negative chest-wall pressure as therapy for severe respiratory distress in older children, *Chest* 68:143-148, 1975.
125. Sanyal SK, Avery TL, Thapar MK, et al: Continuous negative chest-wall pressure therapy for assisting ventilation in older children with progressive respiratory insufficiency, *Acta Paediatr Scand* 66:451-456, 1977
126. Raine J, Redington AN, Benatar A, et al: Continuous negative extrathoracic pressure and cardiac output—a pilot study, *Eur J Pediatr* 152:595-598, 1993.
127. Shapiro SH, Ernst P, Gray-Donald K, et al: Effect of negative pressure ventilation in severe chronic obstructive pulmonary disease, *Lancet* 340:1425-1429, 1992; comment in *Lancet* 340:1440-1441, 1992.
128. Shekerdemian LS, Bush A, Shore DF, et al: Cardiopulmonary interactions after Fontan operations: augmentation of cardiac output using negative pressure ventilation, *Circulation* 96:3934-3942, 1997
129. Shekerdemian LS, Bush A, Lincoln C, et al. Cardiopulmonary interactions in healthy children and children after simple cardiac surgery: the effects of positive and negative pressure ventilation, *Heart* 78:587-593, 1997.
130. Raine J, Samuels MP, Mok Q, et al: Negative extrathoracic pressure ventilation for phrenic nerve palsy after paediatric cardiac surgery, *Br Heart J* 67:308-311, 1992.
131. Öberg PA, Sjostrand U: Studies of blood pressure regulation. Common carotid artery clamping in studies of the carotid-sinus baroreceptro control of the systemic blood pressure, *Acta Physiol Scand* 75:276, 1969.
132. Sanders RD: Two ventilating attachments for bronchoscopes, *Del Med* 39:170, 1967.
133. Lunkenheimer P, Rafflenbeul W, Keller H, et al: Application of transtracheal pressure oscillations as modification of "diffusion respiration," *Br J Anaesth* 44:627, 1972.
134. Zidulka A, Gross D, Minami H, et al: Ventilation by high-frequency chest wall compression in dogs with normal lungs, *Am Rev Respir* Dis 127:709, 1983.
135. Allen JL, Frantz ID III, Fredberg JJ: Heterogeneity of mean alveolar pressure during high-frequency oscillations, *J Appl Physiol* 62:223, 1987.
136. Fredberg JJ, Keefe DH, Glass GM, et al: Alveolar pressure nonhomogeneity during small-amplitude high-frequency oscillation, *J Appl Physiol* 57:788, 1984.
137. Lunkenheimer PP, Frieling G, Mersch FJ, et al: High frequency oscillation: paradigm of inhomogeneous alveolar ventilation, *Acta Anaesthesiol Scand (Suppl)* 90:13, 1989.
138. Gavriely N, Solway J, Drazen JM, et al: Radiographic visualization of airway wall movement during oscillatory flow in dogs, *J Appl Physiol* 58:645, 1985.
139. Klain M: Clinical applications of high frequency jet ventilation in high frequency ventilation in intensive care and during surgery. In Carlon GC, Howland WS, editors: *Lung biology in health and disease,* New York, 1985, Marcel Dekker.
140. Bohn D: High frequency oscillation, *Br J Anaesth* 63(7 suppl 1): 16S-23S. ???.
141. Bryan AC: Use of high frequency ventilation in HMD, *Acta Anaesth Scand* 90:124, 1989.
142. Frantz ID, Werthammer J, Stark AR: High frequency ventilation in premature infants with lung disease: adequate gas exchange at low tracheal pressure, *Pediatrics* 71:483, 1983.
143. Marchak BE, Thompson WK, Duffty P, et al: Treatment of RDS by high frequency oscillatory ventilation: a prelimiany report, *J Pediatr* 99:287, 1981.
144. Harris TR: High frequency jet ventilation treatment of neonates with life-threatening restrictive lung disease, *Pediatr Res* 17:316A, 1983.
145. Ng NPK, Easa D: Management of interstitial emphysema by high frequency low positive pressure hand ventilation in the neonate, *J Pediatr* 95:117, 1979.
146. HiFi Study Group: High frequency oscillatory ventilation compared with conventional mechanical ventilation in the treatment of respiratory failure in preterm infants: assessment of pulmonary function at 9 months of corrected age, *J Pediatr* 116: 933, 1990.
147. Turnbull AD, Carlon G, Howland WS, et al: High frequency ventilation in major airway or pulmonary disruption, *Ann Thorac Surg* 32:468, 1980.
148. Meliones JN, Bove EL, Dekeon MK, et al: High-frequency jet ventilation improves cardiac function after the Fontan procedure, *Circulation* 84(suppl 5):III364-III368, 1991.
149. Kocis KC, Meliones JN, Dekeon MK, et al: High-frequency jet ventilation for respiratory failure after congenital heart surgery, *Circulation* 86(suppl):II127-II32, 1992.
150. Berner ME, Rouge JC, Suter PM: Combined high-frequency ventilation in children with severe adult respiratory distress syndrome, *Intensive Care Med* 17:209-214, 1991.
151. Rosenberg RB, Broner CW, Peters KJ, et al: High-frequency ventilation for acute pediatric respiratory failure, *Chest* 104: 1216-1221, 1993.
152. Arnold JH, Truog RD, Thompson JE, et al: High frequency oscillatory ventilation in pediatric respiratory failure, *Crit Care Med* 21:272-278, 1993.
153. Arnold JH, Hanson JH, Toro-Figuero LO, et al: Prospective, randomized comparison of high-frequency oscillatory ventilation and conventional mechanical ventilation in pediatric respiratory failure, *Crit Care Med* 22:1530-1539, 1994.
154. Deboeck C: Cough versus chest physiotherapy, *Am Rev Respir Dis* 129:182, 1984.
155. Kerem E, Yatsiv I, Goitein KJ: Effect of endotracheal tube suctioning on arterial blood gases in children, *Intensive Care Medicine* 16:95, 1990.
156. Cordero L Jr, Hon EH. Neonatal bradycardia following nasopharyngeal stimulation, *J Pediatr* 78:441, 1979.
157. Nickolson MS: Cardiac arrest during therapeutic tracheal suction, *Anesth Analg* 39:568, 1960.
158. Mackenzie CF, Shin B: Evaluation of respiratory physical therapy, *N Engl J Med* 301:665, 1979.
159. Rossman CM, Waldes R, Sampson D, et al: Effect of chest physiotherapy on the removal of mucus in patients with cystic fibrosis, *Am Rev Respir Dis* 126:131, 1982.
160. Natale JE, Pfeifle J, Homnick DN: Comparison of intrapulmonary percussive ventilation and chest physiotherapy. A pilot study in patients with cystic fibrosis, *Chest* 105:1789-1793, 1994.
161. Homnick DN, White F, de Castro C: Comparison of effects of an intrapulmonary percussive ventilator to standard aerosol and chest physiotherapy in treatment of cystic fibrosis, *Pediatr Pulmonol* 20:50-55, 1995.
162. Deakins K, Chatburn RL: A comparison of intrapulmonary percussive ventilation and conventional chest physiotherapy for the treatment of atelectasis in the pediatric patient, *Respir Care* 47:1162-1167, 2002.
163. Newhouse PA, White F, Marks JH, et al: The intrapulmonary percussive ventilator and flutter device compared to standard chest physiotherapy in patients with cystic fibrosis, *Clin Pediatr (Phila)* 37:427-432, 1998.
164. Miske LJ, Hickey EM, Kolb SM, et al: Use of the mechanical in-exsufflator in pediatric patients with neuromuscular disease and impaired cough, *Chest* 125:1406-1412, 2004.

165. Elkins MR, Jones A, Schans C: Positive expiratory pressure physiotherapy for airway clearance in people with cystic fibrosis, *Cochrane Database Syst Rev* (1):CD003147, 2004.
166. Arens R, Gozal D, Omlin KJ, et al: Comparison of high-frequency chest compression and conventional chest physiotherapy in hospitalized patients with cystic fibrosis, *Am J Respir Crit Care Med* 150:1154-1157, 1994.
167. Ingelstedt S: Studies on the conditioning of the air in the respiratory tract, *Acta Otolaryngol* 56(131 suppl):1-80, 1956.
168. Egan DF: *Aerosol and humidity therapy in fundamentals of respiratory therapy,* ed 3, St. Louis, 1977, CV Mosby.
169. Klein EF Jr: Weaning from mechanical breathing with intermittent mandatory ventilation, *Arch Surg* 110:345, 1975.
170. Downs JB, Douglas ME, Sanfelippo PM, et al: Ventilatory pattern, intrapleural pressure, and cardiac output, *Anesth Analg* 56:88, 1977.
171. Esteban A, Frutos F, Tobin MJ, et al: A comparison of four methods of weaning patients from mechanical ventilation, *N Engl J Med* 332:345-350, 1995.
172. Brochard L, Rauss A, Benito S, et al: Comparison of three methods of gradual withdrawal from ventilatory support during weaning from mechanical ventilation, *Am J Respir Crit Care Med* 150: 896-903, 1994.
173. MacIntyre NR: Pressure-support ventilation. In Grenvik A, Downs JB, Rasanen J, Smith R, editors: *Contemporary management in critical care,* New York, 1991, Churchill Livingstone.
174. MacIntyre NR, Leathermann NE: Mechanical loads on the ventilatory muscles: a theoretical analysis, *Am Rev Respir Dis* 139: 968, 1989.
175. MacIntyre NR, Leatherman NE: Ventilatory muscle loads and the frequency-tidal volume pattern during respiratory pressure assisted (pressure supported) ventilation, *Am Rev Respir Dis* 141: 327, 1990.
176. MacIntyre NR: Respiratory function during pressure support ventilation, *Chest* 89:677, 1986.
177. Randolph AG, Wypij D, Venkataraman ST, et al; Pediatric Acute Lung Injury and Sepsis Investigators (PALISI) Network: Effect of mechanical ventilator weaning protocols on respiratory outcomes in infants and children: a randomized controlled trial, *JAMA* 288:2561-2568, 2002.
178. Farias JA, Alia I, Esteban A, et al: Weaning from mechanical ventilation in pediatric intensive care patients, *Intensive Care Med* 24: 1070-1075, 1998.
179. Farias JA, Retta A, Alia I, et al: A comparison of two methods to perform a breathing trial before extubation in pediatric intensive care patients, *Intensive Care Med* 27:1649-1654, 2001.
180. Farias JA, Alia I, Retta A, et al: An evaluation of extubation failure predictors in mechanically ventilated infants and children, *Intensive Care Med* 28:752-757, 2002.
181. Ishaaya AM, Nathan SD, Belman MJ: Work of breathing after extubation, *Chest* 107:204-209, 1995.
182. Straus C, Louis B, Isabey D, et al: Contribution of the endotracheal tube and the upper airway to breathing workload, *Am J Respir Crit Care Med* 157, 23-30, 1998.
183. Khan N, Brown A, Venkataraman ST: Predictors of extubation success and failure in mechanically ventilated infants and children, *Crit Care Med* 24: 1568-1579, 1996.
184. Venkataraman ST, Khan N, Brown A: Validation of predictors of extubation in mechanically ventilated infants and children, *Crit Care Med* 28:2991-2996, 2000.
185. Venkataraman ST: Weaning and extubation in infants and children: religion, art, or science, *Pediatr Crit Care Med* 3:203-205, 2002.
186. Greene W, L'Heureux P, Hunt CE: Paralysis of the diaphragm, *Am J Dis Child* 129:1402, 1975.
187. Zhao HX, D'Agostino RS, Pitlick PT, et al: Phrenic nerve injury complicating closed cardiovascular procedures for congenital heart disease, *Ann Thorac Surg* 39:445, 1985.
188. Lynn AM, Jenkins JG, Edmonds JF, et al: Diaphragmatic paralysis after pediatric cardiac surgery: a retrospective analysis of 34 cases, *Crit Care Med* 11:280, 1983.
189. Mickell JJ, Oh KS, Siewers RD, et al: Clinical implications of postoperative unilateral phrenic nerve paralysis, *J Thoracic Cardiovasc Surg* 76:297, 1978.
190. Khamiees M, Raju P, DeGirolamo A, et al: Predictors of extubation outcome in patients who have successfully completed a spontaneous breathing trial, *Chest* 120:1262-1270, 2001. Ovid Full Text Bibliographic Links Library.

CHAPTER

45

Ventilator-Induced Lung Injury

Jean-Damien Ricard, Didier Dreyfuss, Alexandre T. Rotta, and Georges Saumon

PEARLS

- Although essential to the support of patients with respiratory failure, mechanical ventilation can be associated with the development of pulmonary tissue injury, termed *ventilator-induced lung injury* (VILI).
- The concept of VILI has been elegantly tested in the research laboratory in both normal and diseased lungs, where the individual contribution of various factors, such as tidal volume, positive end-expiratory pressure, and overall state of lung distension can be determined. Lung volume at the end of inspiration (i.e., the overall degree of lung distension) probably is the main determinant of VILI severity.
- Experimental and clinical data support the idea that reasoned tidal volume reduction designed to prevent volutrauma can be advantageous in the management of these patients.

Mechanical ventilation is essential for the basic life support of patients with respiratory failure. However, several potential drawbacks and complications have been identified.[1] Experimental studies have shown that some patterns of ventilation may produce subtle tissue damages that resemble the early stages of acute respiratory distress syndrome (ARDS), so-called *ventilator-induced lung injury* (VILI).[2] This issue has received significant attention in the clinical field.[3–7] This chapter describes pathophysiologic events that lead to VILI and places these observations into a clinical perspective of ventilatory management of patients with ARDS.

Evidence for Ventilator-Induced Lung Injury

Ventilation of Intact Lungs

High Lung Volume Ventilator-Induced Lung Injury

Webb and Tierney[8] found that rats subjected to ventilation with a peak airway pressure of 45 cmH_2O rapidly developed pulmonary edema, whereas those ventilated for a longer time with a peak airway pressure 14 cmH_2O did not. Edema severity and rate of development increased in direct proportion with peak airway pressure magnitude. It was later confirmed that such a ventilation strategy produces endothelial and epithelial cell damage and lung capillary permeability alterations that result in a nonhydrostatic pulmonary edema.[9] The respective role of increased airway pressure and increased lung volume was clarified by showing that mechanical ventilation with large or low tidal volume (V_T) but with identical (45 cmH_2O) peak airway pressures did not result in the same lung alterations.[10] Pulmonary edema was evident in rats subjected to high V_T but not in rats in which lung distension was limited by thoracoabdominal strapping[10] (Figure 45–1). Furthermore, animals ventilated with high V_T but with negative airway pressure by means of an iron lung still developed pulmonary edema, thus demonstrating that excessive airway pressure is not the causal factor of this type of injury.[10] Because VILI depended predominantly on end-inspiratory volume, it was termed *volutrauma*.[11,12] The pressure corresponding to end-inspiratory volume is the "plateau" end-inspiratory occlusion airway pressure, and its clinical

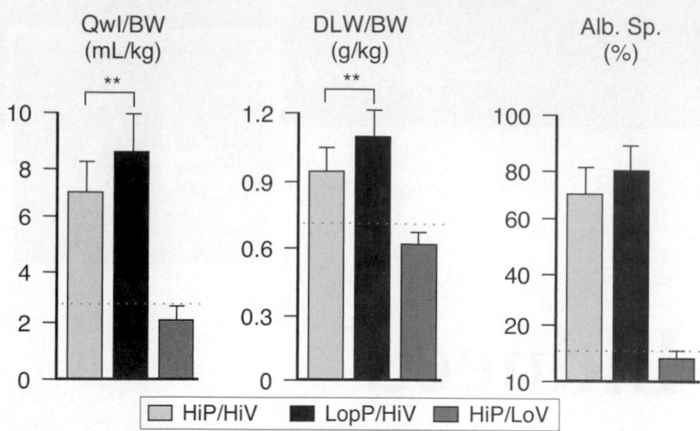

FIGURE 45–1 • Comparisons of the effects of high-pressure–high-volume ventilation *(HiP-HiV)* with those of negative inspiratory airway pressure high tidal volume ventilation (iron lung ventilation, *LoP-HiV)* and of high-pressure–low-volume ventilation (thoraco-abdominal strapping, *HiP-LoV)*. *Dotted lines* represent the upper 95% confidence limit for control values. See Figure 45–3 for details on edema indices. Permeability edema occurred in both groups receiving high V_T ventilation. Animals ventilated with a high peak pressure and a normal V_T had no edema. (From Dreyfuss D, Soler P, Basset G, Saumon G: *Am Rev Respir Dis* 137:1159-1164, 1988.)

importance was emphasized in a Consensus Conference on mechanical ventilation.[13]

Several investigators reached the same conclusions in other species using different protocols. Hernandez et al.[14] compared lung capillary filtration coefficients (a measure of capillary permeability to water) of rabbits ventilated with different peak airway pressures with those of animals ventilated with the same airway pressures but with restriction of thoracoabdominal excursions by plaster casts placed around the chest and the abdomen. The capillary filtration coefficient was normal in animals ventilated at a peak pressure of 15 cmH_2O, increased by 31% for a peak pressure of 30 cmH_2O and by 430% for a peak pressure of 45 cmH_2O in animals without restriction, whereas no increase was found in those with plaster casts.[14] Carlton et al.[15] confirmed this observation in lambs. Besides lung distension, the rate at which volume varies (which determines peak but not plateau inspiratory pressure) may also affect microvascular permeability. Peevy et al.[16] determined the capillary filtration coefficient of isolated perfused rabbit lungs ventilated with various V_T and inspiratory flow rates. They observed that a high flow rate increased the filtration coefficient (approximately six times baseline value) despite the application of a small V_T. This increase was similar to that found with ventilation with a markedly higher V_T and the same peak airway pressure because of lower inspiratory flow rate.[16]

Taken together, these experimental studies demonstrated that large tidal volumes more than high intrathoracic pressures promote ventilator-induced lung edema in intact animals.

Low Lung Volume Ventilator-Induced Lung Injury

Unlike volutrauma, ventilation at low lung volumes does not seem to injure healthy lungs. Intact animals tolerate mechanical ventilation with physiologic V_T and low levels of positive end-expiratory pressure (PEEP) for prolonged periods of time without any apparent damage. Taskar et al.[17] showed that the repetitive collapse and reopening of terminal units during 1 hour of mechanical ventilation does not result in appreciable lung damage, although it does alter gas exchange and reduce compliance, as generally does spontaneous ventilation under deep anesthesia.

Ventilation of Damaged Lungs

High-Volume Lung Injury

Several investigators evaluated the effect of overdistension on damaged lungs. These studies consistently demonstrate the increased susceptibility of diseased lungs to the detrimental effects of some patterns of mechanical ventilation.

Early studies were performed on isolated lungs. Bowton and Kong[18] showed that isolated perfused rabbit lungs injured by oleic acid gained significantly more weight when ventilated with V_T of 18 ml/kg, in comparison with ventilation with V_T of 6 ml/kg. Hernandez et al.[19] used the rabbit model to compare the effects of oleic acid alone, mechanical ventilation alone, and their combination on lung capillary filtration coefficient and wet-to-dry weight ratio. Measurements were made on isolated lungs sampled subsequently to in vivo stress. Injury markers were not significantly affected by low doses of oleic acid or mechanical ventilation with a peak inspiratory pressure of 25 cmH_2O for 15 minutes. However, the filtration coefficient increased significantly when oleic acid injury was followed by mechanical ventilation. Wet-to-dry weight ratio was also significantly higher than in lungs subjected to oleic acid injury or ventilation alone. The same investigators also showed that surfactant inactivation by dioctyl succinate exacerbates the increase in filtration coefficient produced by ventilating isolated blood-perfused rabbit lungs with peak pressures of 30 to 45 cmH_2O.[20] Light microscopic examination of the lungs of animals subjected to ventilation or surfactant inactivation alone showed only minor abnormalities (minimal hemorrhage and vascular congestion), in contrast to the severe damage (edema and flooding, hyaline membranes, and extensive alveolar hemorrhage) observed when the insults were combined. These results suggested that high volume/pressure ventilation favors VILI in abnormal isolated lungs and that it might occur at lower airway pressure. Whether this could also occur in lungs in situ was investigated by comparing the effects of different patterns of mechanical ventilation in rats with α-naphthylthiourea (ANTU)-injured lungs.[21] ANTU infusion alone caused moderate permeability pulmonary edema. Mechanical ventilation alone resulted in a permeability edema, the severity of which was related to V_T magnitude. Thus it was possible to calculate the theoretical amount of edema that would result from ventilating ANTU-diseased lungs with a given V_T by summing up the separate effect of mechanical ventilation and ANTU. However, lungs of animals injured by ANTU had more edema than predicted when they were ventilated with a high V_T (45 ml/kg), indicating the two insults acted in synergy. Even slight lung alterations, such as those produced by spontaneous ventilation during prolonged anesthesia (which inactivates surfactant and promotes focal atelectasis[22,23]), were sufficient to exacerbate the harmful effects of high-volume ventilation[21] (Figure 45–2). The extent to which lung mechanical properties are altered prior to ventilation is a key factor in this synergy. The amount of pulmonary edema produced by high-volume mechanical ventilation in animals given ANTU, or that had undergone prolonged anesthesia, was inversely proportional to respiratory system compliance measured at the very beginning of high-volume mechanical ventilation.[21] Thus the more severe the lung abnormalities were before ventilation, the more severe was the subsequent VILI. The reason for this synergy requires clarification. The presence of lung regions with alveolar edema in animals given this harmful high V_T ventilation was their most evident difference from animals ventilated with lower, less harmful V_T.[21] Because alveolar flooding reduced the number of alveoli available for ventilation, these open alveoli were more prone to overinflation, were more vulnerable to injury, and were at risk for flooding. This in turn would further reduce aerated lung volume and result in a positive injury feedback. The same reasoning applies to prolonged anesthesia, during which aerated lung volume probably was gradually reduced by atelectasis.[21] Both flooding and atelectasis decrease compliance, leaving fewer alveoli open, the "baby lung" effect. It is not surprising that the lower the compliance was before ventilation, the more severe were lung alterations induced by high-volume ventilation.[21] Thus uneven distribution of ventilation during acute lung injury[24] favors regional overinflation and injury. To further substantiate this finding, rats were ventilated with V_T up to 33 ml/kg after alveolar flooding was produced by instilling saline into the trachea. Flooding with saline did not significantly affect microvascular permeability when V_T was low. In agreement with the expectation, capillary permeability alterations were more important in flooded than in normal animals subjected to a high V_T. There were also correlations between both end-inspiratory (plateau) airway pressure and the pressure at which the "lower inflection point" was found on the volume–pressure curve and capillary permeability changes in flooded animals ventilated with a high V_T.[25] Thus changes in capillary permeability caused by lung overinflation are more severe in barely recruitable (and less compliant) lungs.

Low Lung Volume Injury

There likely is an increase in trapped gas volume during pulmonary edema and acute lung injury because of airway closure from surfactant dysfunction.[26] Under such conditions, the slope of the inspiratory limb of the respiratory system volume–pressure curve often displays a sharp increase at low lung volume. This change is thought to reflect the sudden and massive opening of units previously excluded from the ventilation and has been termed the *lower inflection point* (Figure 45–3). The importance of this phenomenon is more often appreciated in terms of arterial oxygenation, as setting PEEP above the pressure of this inflection point usually results in a decrease in shunt and increase in PaO_2.[27–30]

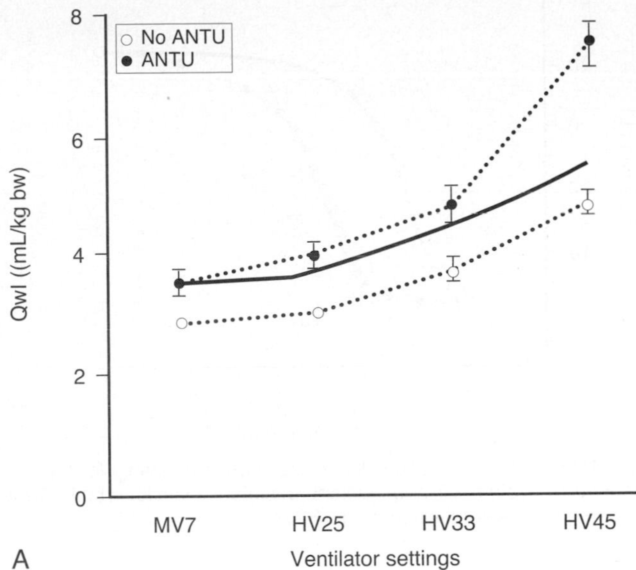

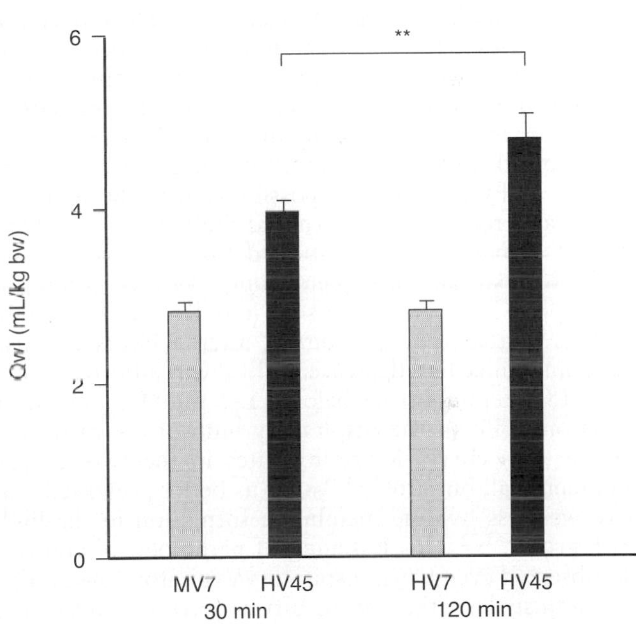

FIGURE 45–2 • Interaction between previous lung alterations and mechanical ventilation on pulmonary edema. **A,** Effect of previous toxic lung injury. Extravascular lung water *(Qwl)* after mechanical ventilation in normal rats *(open circles)* and in rats with mild lung injury produced by α-naphthylthiourea *(ANTU) (closed circles)*. V_T varied from 7 to 45 ml/kg BW. *Solid line* represents the Qwl value expected for the aggravating effect of ANTU on ventilation edema assuming additivity. ANTU did not potentiate the effect of ventilation with V_T up to 33 ml/kg BW. In contrast, ventilation at 45 ml/kg BW V_T resulted in an increase in edema that greatly exceeded additivity, indicating synergy between the two insults. **B,** Effect of lung functional alteration by prolonged anesthesia. Intact rats were anesthetized and breathed spontaneously for 30 or 120 minutes prior to mechanical ventilation with 7 ml/kg BW *(open bars)* or 45 ml/kg BW *(shaded bars)* V_T in intact rats. Qwl of animals ventilated with a high V_T was significantly higher than in those ventilated with a normal V_T. Qwl was not affected by the duration of anesthesia in animals ventilated with a normal V_T. In contrast, 120 minutes of anesthesia before high V_T ventilation resulted in a larger increase in Qwl than did 30 minutes of anesthesia. $^{**}p < 0.01$. (From Dreyfuss D, Soler P, Saumon GL: *Am J Respir Crit Care Med* 151:1568-1575, 1995.)

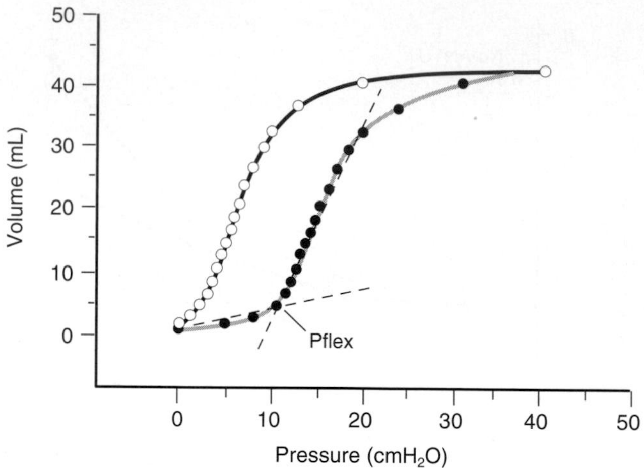

FIGURE 45–3 • Static volume–pressure relationship for the total respiratory system of a surfactant depleted juvenile rabbit. *Arrow* indicates the lower inflexion point *(Pflex)*.

Attention has focused only recently on the possibility that pulmonary lesions may be aggravated if this inflection point lies within the V_T. Experimental evidence for this was initially provided by studies comparing conventional mechanical ventilation with high-frequency oscillatory ventilation in premature or surfactant-depleted lungs. Studies performed on such lungs ventilated with various levels of PEEP support the possibility that the repeated closure and reopening of terminal units also cause lung injury.[31–33] Sykes et al[31,32] studied this issue ventilating rabbits with surfactant-depleted lungs. V_T was set but not stated; peak inspiratory pressure initially was 15 mmHg but was increased to 25 mmHg after 5 hours because lung compliance had decreased. PEEP was adjusted either above (8–12 mmHg) or below (1–2 mmHg) the lower inflection point of the inspiratory limb of the pressure–volume (PV) curve. Mortality rates in the two groups were identical, but arterial PaO_2 was better preserved and there was less hyaline membrane formation in the high PEEP group.[31,32] This lessening of pathologic alterations was observed even when inspiratory/expiratory time ratios were adjusted so that mean airway pressures were the same in the low and high PEEP groups.[32] Muscedere et al[33] reported similar results in isolated, unperfused, saline lavaged rabbit lungs ventilated with a low V_T (5–6 ml/kg) and with PEEP set below or above the inflection point. However, Sykes et al[34] found no such injury in vivo in rabbits whose lungs had been injured with hydrochloric acid. It is often thought that the lower inflection point on the PV curve reflects the recruitment of collapsed zones (that are found predominantly in dependent areas of lung[35,36]) and that this recruitment persists during further lung expansion. Martynowicz et al[37] challenged the reality of the repetitive collapse–reexpansion phenomenon during tidal ventilation and reevaluated the significance of the lower inflection point on the PV curve.

They studied the regional expansion of oleic acid-injured lungs using the parenchymal marker technique in dogs. They found that the gravitational distribution of volume at functional residual capacity was not affected and not associated with a decrease in parenchymal volume of the dependent regions. In addition, they found that the between-region asynchrony of tidal expansion was not influenced by oleic acid injury. Their findings therefore did not support the hypothesis that the exaggerated gravitational gradient present in injured lungs produces atelectasis by compression of the dependent lung, cyclic recruitment and collapse, and ultimately shear stress injury.[37]

They propose that displacement of air–liquid interfaces along the tracheobronchial tree causes the lower inflection point on the PV curve and conclude that this knee on the curve reflects the mechanics of partially fluid-filled alveoli with constant surface tension and not the abrupt opening of airways or atelectatic parenchyma.[38] Therefore whether injury caused by the repetitive reopening of collapsed terminal units and the protective effect of PEEP is restricted to the peculiar situation of surfactant depletion by broncho-alveolar lavage remains unsettled.

In the clinical field, the negative results of the ALVEOLI (*A*ssessment of *L*ow Tidal *V*olume and *E*levated End-Expiratory Pressure to Obviate *L*ung *I*njury) trial (*http://www.ardsnet.org/alveoli.php*) cast some doubt on the clinical existence of repetitive opening and closing lung injury.[39]

Roles of Tidal Volume, Positive-end-expiratory Pressure, and Overall Lung Distension

The influence of PEEP on acute lung injury, and more specifically on ventilator-induced pulmonary edema, must be studied in the context of the level of V_T. Indeed, PEEP increases functional residual capacity (FRC) and prevents lung derecruitment, but it also increases end-inspiratory volume when V_T is kept constant, thus possibly favoring overinflation. PEEP application may depress hemodynamics and affect lung fluid balance. Therefore close analysis of the numerous studies performed to clarify the relationships between PEEP, oxygenation, and extravascular lung water accumulation during hydrostatic or permeability edema must take into account the experimental approach used, that is, intact animals or isolated lungs (for which lung water content differ) and whether or not V_T is reduced at high PEEP (which affects end-inspiratory lung volume).

Effects of Positive End-Expiratory Pressure When Tidal Volume Is Kept Constant

Application of PEEP may result in lung overinflation if it causes a significant change in FRC, by raising end-inspiratory volume. Overinflation affects preferentially the more distensible areas that receive the bulk of ventilation, which may explain the lack of reduction or even the worsening of edema reported following PEEP application in most experiments.[40] PEEP does not affect the severity of hydrostatic[41] or permeability[41,42] edema in intact animals, although it improves oxygenation[41] because of recruitment of flooded alveoli (Figure 45–4). In isolated ventilated-perfused lungs, PEEP aggravates edema fluid

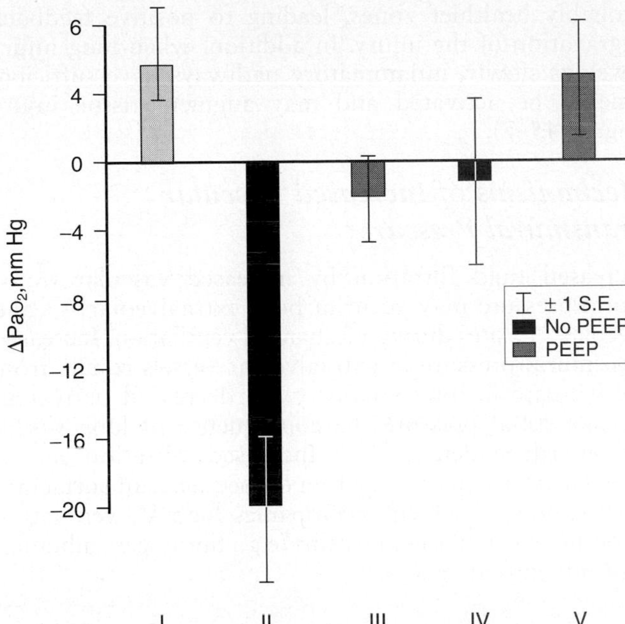

FIGURE 45–4 • Change in arterial oxygen tension (ΔPaO_2, mmHg) during 1-hour period between the initial and final measurements for groups I (control), II, and III (severe hydrostatic pulmonary edema, without and with positive end-expiratory pressure [PEEP], respectively), and IV and V (moderate pulmonary edema, without and with PEEP, respectively). The difference between ΔPaO_2 for groups II and III is significant ($p < 0.01$). (From Hopewell PC, Murray JF: *J Appl Physiol* 40:568-574, 1976.)

accumulation[43] (Figure 45–5). Thus when V_T is held constant, increasing FRC with PEEP affects edema formation differently in isolated lungs versus intact animals. In intact animals, the lack of effect of PEEP suggests a balance between PEEP-induced increase in end-inspiratory lung volume (which decreases interstitial pressure and increases filtration pressure in extra-alveolar vessels) and reduced lung perfusion because of elevated intrathoracic pressure (which decreases filtration pressure). In contrast, constant perfusion rate of isolated-perfused lung preparations favors edema formation.[43]

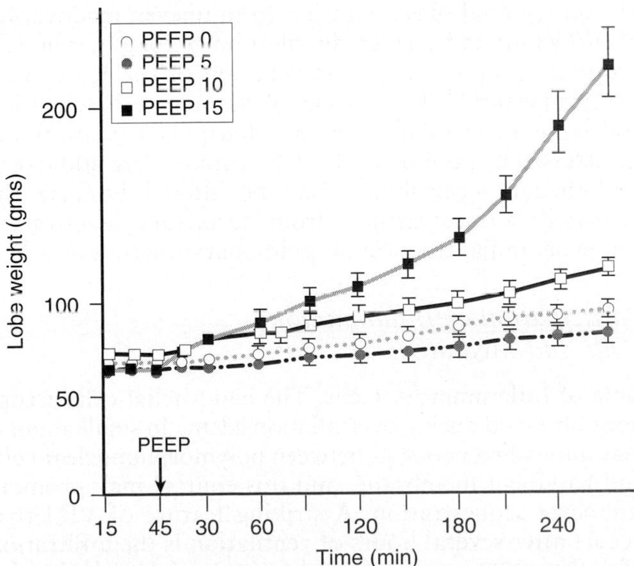

FIGURE 45–5 • Effect of three levels of positive end-expiratory pressure (PEEP) on water accumulation in hydrochloric acid-injured ventilated-perfused dog pulmonary lobes. The highest PEEP resulted in a further increase in pulmonary edema. (From Toung T, Saharia P, Permutt S, et al: *Surgery* 82:279-283, 1977.)

Effects of Positive End-Expiratory Pressure When Tidal Volume Is Reduced

When PEEP is applied but edema is less severe, end-inspiratory lung volume is kept constant by decreasing V_T[2] (Figure 45–6). Webb and Tierney[8] showed that edema was less pronounced during ventilation with a peak airway pressure of 45 cmH_2O when 10 cmH_2O PEEP was applied. The authors attributed this beneficial effect of PEEP to preservation of surfactant activity. It was later shown that although PEEP decreased the amount of edema, it did not prevent the changes in capillary permeability.[10] However, animals ventilated with PEEP had no alveolar damage in contrast to those ventilated without PEEP. The only cellular alterations found in animals ventilated with PEEP were of capillary endothelial blebs.[10] The observed preservation of the epithelial layer has received no satisfactory explanation. It may be that PEEP prevented fluid movement in terminal units, thereby decreasing shear stress at this level. Similar observations have been made by other investigators in intact animals[44,45] and in perfused canine lobes.[46]

The hemodynamic alterations induced by PEEP probably play an important role in lessening edema severity.

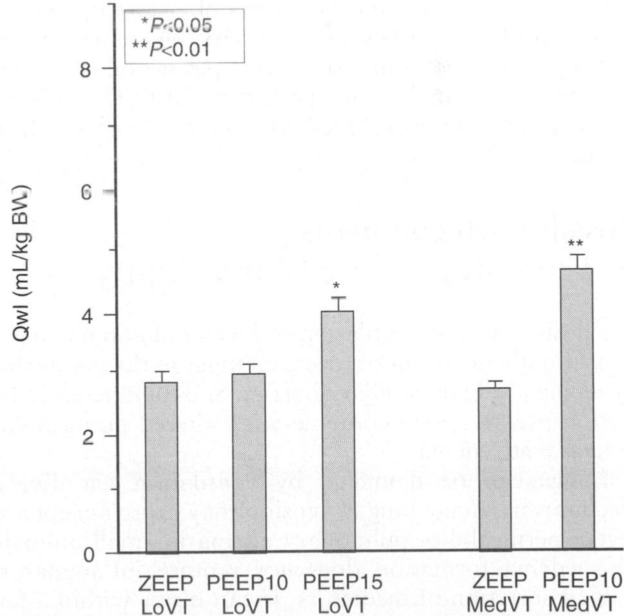

FIGURE 45–6 • Effect of increasing positive end-expiratory pressure (PEEP) from 0 to 15 cmH_2O during ventilation with two different V_T values (7 ml/kg BW: Lo V_T and 14 ml/kg BW: Med V_T). Pulmonary edema (as evaluated by increases in extravascular lung water) occurred when PEEP was increased. PEEP required to produce edema varied with V_T: 15 cmH_2O PEEP during ventilation with low V_T and 10 cmH_2O PEEP during ventilation with moderately increased V_T. $^*p < 0.05$; $^{**}p < 0.01$ vs. ZEEP and the same V_T. (From Dreyfuss D, Saumon G: *Am Rev Respir Dis* 148:1194-1203, 1993.)

Application of PEEP produces an increase in mean intrathoracic pressure, which adversely affects cardiac output[47,48] (see Chapter 24). Edema was more severe when the hemodynamic alterations induced by PEEP were corrected with dopamine infusion in rats subjected to high peak airway pressure ventilation with 10 cmH_2O PEEP.[49] The amount of extravascular lung water was correlated with systemic blood pressure, suggesting that restoration of cardiac output increased filtration pressure and was responsible for edema aggravation. The reduction of edema and severity of cellular damage by PEEP during ventilation-induced pulmonary edema may be linked to reduced tissue stress (decreased volume–pressure excursion), movement of foam in distal airways, preservation of surfactant activity, and decrease in capillary filtration.

Importance of Overall Lung Distension

Lung volume at the end of inspiration (i.e., overall degree of lung distension) probably is the main determinant of VILI severity. Rats ventilated with low V_T and 15 cmH_2O PEEP developed pulmonary edema, whereas rats ventilated with the same V_T but 10 cmH_2O PEEP did not[49] (see Figure 45–6). Similarly, doubling this V_T in the presence of 10 cmH_2O PEEP produced pulmonary edema, whereas it did not in animals ventilated without PEEP. Thus the safety of a given V_T depends on how much the FRC is simultaneously increased.

In conclusion, permeability edema and ventilation-induced lung injury occur when some as yet undetermined threshold of lung overinflation is reached. This can occur when V_T is excessive for the PEEP applied. In contrast, when PEEP is added or increased while end-inspiratory pressure is held constant, it slows the development of edema and diminishes the severity of tissue injury, although changes in microvascular permeability are not prevented.[10,49] Finally, the application of PEEP increases end-inspiratory (plateau) pressure, so there is risk of edema occurrence.[49]

Possible Mechanisms of Ventilator-Induced Lung Injury

It is now clear that ventilation-induced pulmonary edema is essentially the result of severe changes in the permeability of the alveolar–capillary barrier. Small increases in filtration pressure may combine with altered permeability to aggravate edema.

Lungs can be damaged by ventilation via diverse mechanisms. Acute lung distension may cause abrupt and severe permeability pulmonary edema in small animals. This edema formation does not require inflammatory cells or secretion of mediators. It can occur within a few minutes. Edema develops more slowly in larger animals for the same plateau pressure, rendering its interruption more complex. A low lung volume injury may progressively aggravate the problem. Further, ventilation without PEEP may reduce aerated lung volume and gradually worsen mechanical nonuniformity. This lung inhomogeneity in turn promotes overinflation of the more compliant and probably healthier zones, leading to positive feedback aggravation of the injury. In addition, when lung injury develops slowly, inflammatory pathways have sufficient time to be activated and may augment tissue injury (Figure 45–7).

Mechanisms of Increased Vascular Transmural Pressure

Increased fluid filtration by increased vascular transmural pressure may occur at both extraalveolar[50,51] and alveolar[52–54] sites during mechanical ventilation. Increased transmural pressure in extraalveolar vessels results from the increase in lung volume, with decreased perivascular interstitial pressure the consequence of lung vascular interdependence.[47,55,56] Increased filtration across alveolar microvessels may be a consequence of surfactant inactivation,[8,54] which accompanies high V_T ventilation or occurs when plasma proteins (e.g., fibrinogen, albumin) transude into airspaces.

Mechanisms of Altered Permeability

Although capillary permeability changes are obvious and severe during VILI, their underlying mechanisms are not fully understood and probably are multifactorial. Not only the severity but also the mechanisms of lung injury may vary with the extent and duration of lung overdistension.

Effects of Surfactant Inactivation

In addition to its effects on fluid filtration, surfactant inactivation and elevated alveolar surface tension may increase alveolar epithelial permeability to small solutes. Surfactant inactivation by detergent aerosolization increases diethylenetriamine-pentaacetic acid (DTPA) clearance in rabbits[57] and dogs.[58] This effect was ascribed to pulmonary inhomogeneity and regional overexpansion from uneven inactivation of surfactant and uneven distribution of lung mechanical properties, rather than to elimination of surfactant barrier properties.[58] The effects of surfactant inactivation and large V_T ventilation on alveolocapillary permeability (as assessed by pulmonary DTPA clearance) are additive.[59] Endothelial permeability may be altered because the increased surface tension from surfactant inactivation augments radial traction on pulmonary microvessels.[54]

Participation of Inflammatory Cells and Mediators

Role of Inflammatory Cells. The endothelial cell disruptions observed during overinflation edema in small animals may allow direct contact between polymorphonuclear cells and basement membrane, and this contact may promote leukocyte sequestration. A striking feature of VILI that occurs after several hours of ventilation is the infiltration of inflammatory cells into the interstitial and alveolar spaces. In one of the earliest studies on this subject, Woo and Hedley-White[60] observed that overinflation produced edema in open-chest dogs, and that leukocytes accumulated

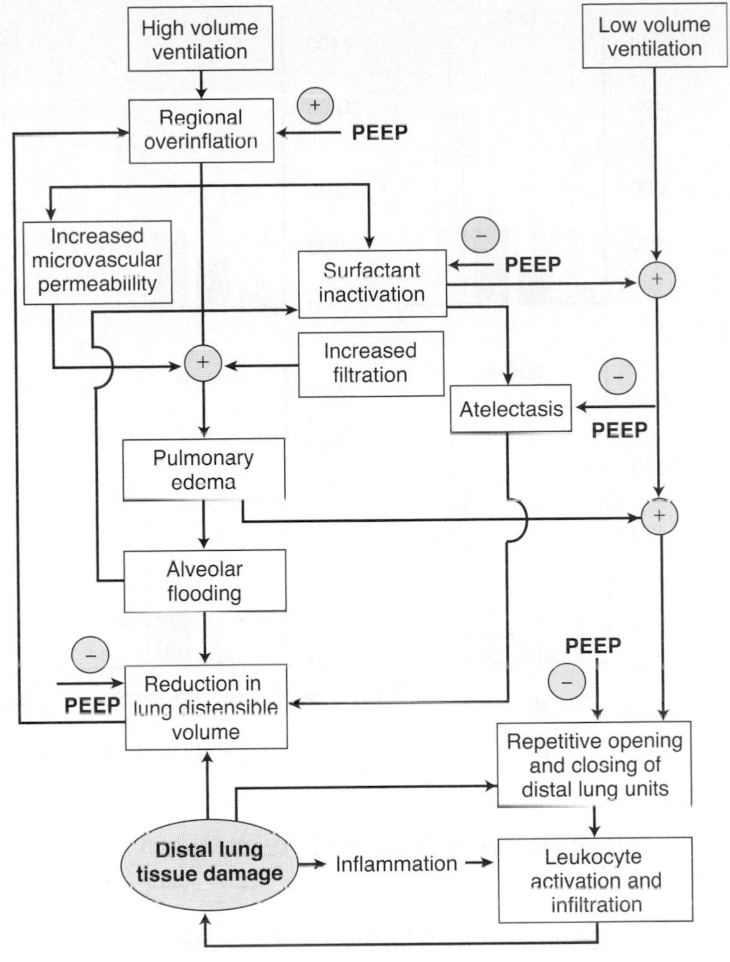

FIGURE 45–7 • Flow diagram summarizing the contributors to mechanical ventilation-induced lung injury. Positive end-expiratory pressure generally opposes injury or edema formation *(minus sign)* except when it contributes to overinflation *(plus sign)*. (From Dreyfuss D, Saumon G: *Am J Respir Crit Care Med* 157:294-323, 1998.)

in the vasculature and macrophages in the alveoli. Further studies confirmed these results[61] and showed that high transpulmonary pressure increased the transit time of leukocytes in the lungs of rabbits.[62] Conversely, when animals are depleted of neutrophils, high-volume pulmonary edema is less severe than in nondepleted animals.[63] Protracted ventilation in small mammals also recruits leukocytes in lungs that may contribute to VILI.[64]

Role of Inflammatory Mediators. The role of inflammatory cytokines and chemokines in the course of VILI has been the subject of studies and is a matter of debate.[65,66] Tremblay et al[67] examined the effects of different ventilatory strategies on the level of several inflammatory mediators in bronchoalveolar lavage fluid of isolated rat lungs ventilated with different end-expiratory pressures and V_T. High V_T ventilation (40 ml/kg) with zero end-expiratory pressure resulted in considerable increases in tumor necrosis factor (TNF)-α, interleukin (IL)-1β, IL-6, and macrophage inflammatory protein (MIP)-2 (Figure 45–8). Unfortunately, results from this study have not been replicated by another group using the same ex vivo lung model[68] (Figure 45–9). It is worth noting that stretching in vitro human alveolar macrophages[69] or A549 epithelial cells[70] led to no TNF-α release but to release of IL-8. In vivo studies of intact animals show that high-volume mechanical ventilation that produces very severe pulmonary edema does not induce release of TNF-α.[68,71] Studies on TNF-α mRNA also yield conflicting results, as Takata et al[72] showed large increases in TNF-α mRNA in the intraalveolar cells of surfactant-depleted rabbits after 1 hour of conventional mechanical ventilation with peak inspiratory and end-expiratory pressures of 28 and 5 cmH_2O, respectively (resulting in a mean airway pressure of 13 cmH_2O), whereas Imanaka et al[73] showed no increase in lung tissue TNF-α mRNA of rats ventilated by high pressure (45 cmH_2O peak inspiratory pressure). The only mediator that is constantly found in the different experimental studies is MIP-2 (or IL-8, depending on the experimental model). The presence of this neutrophil chemoattractant mediator in lungs subjected to high-volume ventilation is in agreement with the well-documented recruitment of neutrophils that occurs after long-term ventilation.[61,74–76] In vivo inhibition of MIP-2–ligand interactions led to a marked reduction in neutrophil sequestration and lung injury in mice subjected to high-volume ventilation for 6 hours.[64]

In addition to increasing the amount of cytokines in the lung, it has been suspected that overinflation during mechanical ventilation promotes the release of cytokines[77,78] or bacteria[79,80] into the blood, thus giving a causative role for mechanical ventilation in multiorgan dysfunction.[81,82] However, this hypothesis remains to be proven.[83]

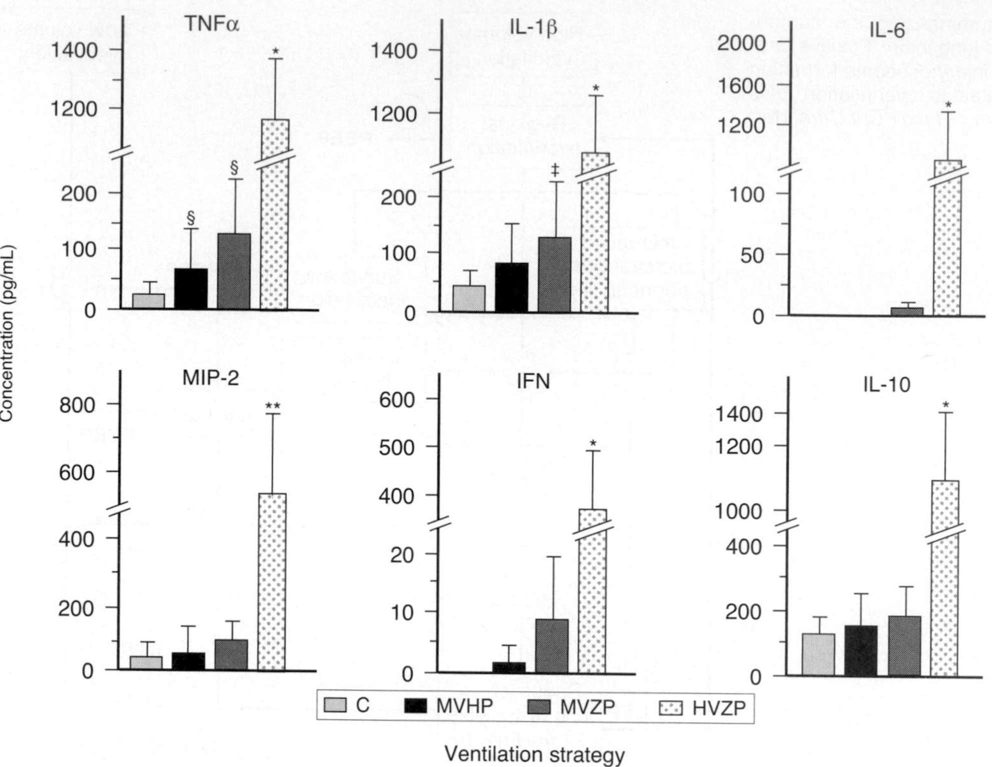

FIGURE 45–8 • Effect of different ventilatory strategies on cytokine concentrations in lung lavage of isolated unperfused rat lungs. Four ventilator settings were used: controls (*C*, normal V_T), moderate V_T + high positive end-expiratory pressure (PEEP) *(MVHP)*, moderate V_T + zero PEEP *(MVZP)*, and high V_T + zero PEEP *(HVZP)* resulting in the same end-inspiratory distension as MVHP. Major increases in cytokine concentrations were observed with HVZP. (From Tremblay L, Valenza F, Ribeiro SP, et al: *J Clin Invest* 99: 944-952, 1997.)

New Insights into Ventilator-Induced Lung Injury

Cellular Response to Mechanical Strain

The cellular response to mechanical strain has been the focus of growing interest and has been comprehensively reviewed.[84] Parker et al.[85] studied the different signal transduction pathways that might be involved in the microvascular permeability increases observed during experimental VILI. They found that gadolinium (which blocks stretch-activated nonselective cation channels) abolished the increases in vascular permeability induced by high airway pressure.[86] The authors concluded that stretch-activated cation channels might initiate the increase in permeability induced by mechanical ventilation through increases in intracellular Ca^{2+} concentration. To further explore the involvement of this pathway, the same team showed that Ca^{2+}/calmodulin–myosin light-chain kinase inhibitors significantly attenuate the vascular permeability increase induced by high-pressure mechanical ventilation in an isolated perfused rat model.[87] High-volume ventilation of isolated rat lungs leads to release of nitrogen-reactive species.[88] Nitric oxide participates in the control of endothelial permeability, and nitric oxide overproduction results in increases in endothelial permeability and blebs at the ultrastructural level very similar to those observed after periods of high-volume ventilation.[89] Taken together, these results suggest that the increase in microvascular permeability may not simply be a passive physical phenomenon (a "stress failure"[90,91]) but, at least in part, the result of a biochemical process.

Maintenance of plasma membrane integrity is essential in the face of mechanical stress. Vlahakis et al.[92] reported a previously unknown response of alveolar epithelial cells to deformation. Membrane lipids were labeled to study deformation-induced lipid trafficking and observed in a direct manner under laser confocal microscopy to examine cellular response to deforming forces. A 25% stretch deformation resulted in lipid transport to the plasma membrane that ensured cell integrity by increasing its surface area. This lipid trafficking occurred in all cells, in contrast with plasma breaks, which were seen in only a small percentage of cells. The authors concluded that deformation-induced lipid trafficking serves in part to repair plasma breaks, and that this could be viewed as a cytoprotective mechanism against plasma membrane stress failure seen during VILI.[10,91] Other investigators have focused on the relative importance of deformation frequency, duration, and amplitude in stress-induced cell injury.[93] Exposing rat primary alveolar epithelial cells to cyclic deformation (25%, 37%, and 60% increase in membrane surface area [ΔSA]) led to significantly greater cell death in comparison with static deformation. To investigate the relative importance of peak deformation magnitude and cyclic deformation amplitude on deformation-induced injury, cells were subjected to cyclic deformation amplitudes of 12% and 25% ΔSA superimposed on a static deformation of 25% ΔSA, thus resulting in a peak deformation magnitude of 37% and 50% ΔSA, respectively. Interestingly, the authors found that limiting the deformation amplitude resulted in significant reductions in cell death at identical peak deformations (Figure 45–10). From these results, an analogy can be drawn with experiments that showed a decrease in lung injury when V_T was reduced with a constant PEEP level, thus reducing end-inspiratory lung volume.[49]

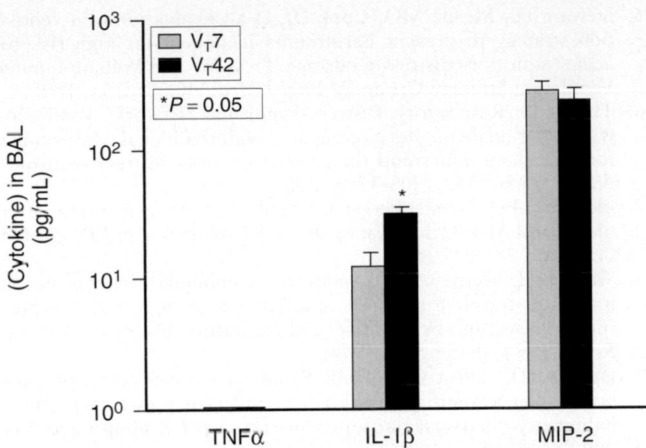

FIGURE 45–9 • Effect of different ventilatory strategies on cytokine concentrations in lung lavage. Tumor necrosis factor (TNF)-α, interleukin (IL)-1β, and macrophage inflammatory protein (MIP)-2 concentrations in broncho-alveolar lavage fluid (BALF) of rats ventilated for 2 hours with 7 ml/kg V_T and 3 cmH_2O positive end-expiratory pressure (PEEP) (V_T7) and 42 ml/kg V_T and PEEP (V_T42). TNF-α was undetectable whatever the ventilation strategy. IL-1β and MIP-2 were found in small amounts. IL-1β was slightly higher (*$p = 0.05$) in BALF of rats ventilated with the larger V_T. (Note that 100 signifies a value below the detection threshold). (From Ricard J-D, Dreyfuss D, Saumon G: *Am J Respir Crit Care Med* 163:1176-1180, 2001.)

Influence of Capnia on Ventilator-Induced Lung Injury

Deleterious effects of hypocapnia have been extensively reviewed.[94] In addition to detrimental effects on ischemia/reperfusion lung injury of hypocapnia[95] and of buffering hypercapnic acidosis,[96] experimental studies suggest that hypercapnic acidosis may protect from acute increase in capillary permeability resulting from overinflation[88] and/ or inflammation during VILI.[97]

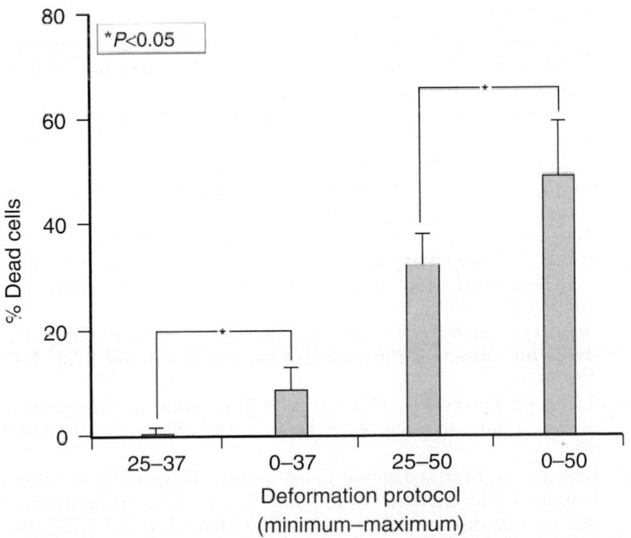

FIGURE 45–10 • Relative importance of deformation magnitude and amplitude. Deformations were applied for 60 minutes at 15 cpm. Data are given as mean ± SD. Reducing the amplitude to 12% ΔSA or 25% ΔSA significantly reduced cell death when maximum deformation was held at 37% ΔSA or 50% ΔSA, respectively. *$p < 0.05$. (From Tschumperlin DJ, Oswari J, Margulies SS: *Am J Respir Crit Care Med* 162:357-362, 2000.)

Strategies To Reduce Ventilator-Induced Lung Injury: Use of the Pressure–volume Curve

The ARDS network trial[6] has undisputedly shown that reducing V_T from 12 to 6 ml/kg resulted in a 22% reduction of mortality (Figure 45–11). By protocol, the same reduction of V_T was applied to all patients allocated to the low V_T group. However, it has been repeatedly shown that the pressure and volume considered safe for some ARDS patients may cause lung overdistension in other patients.[35,36,98,99] Conversely, arbitrary settings may result in an unnecessary reduction in V_T, which a meta-analysis has suggested might be harmful.[7] It has been suggested that information from the inspiratory pressure–volume curve of the respiratory system could be used to tailor ventilator settings. For instance, the presence of an opening pressure (lower inflection point) could be used to adjust the PEEP.[27-29] In addition to improving oxygenation, PEEP reduces the severity of VILI[10] and may lessen the damage produced by the repeated opening and closing of lung units in surfactant-depleted lungs.[31,33,100] However, PEEP may favor overinflation if V_T is not reduced.[2,101] It has been proposed that V_T be adjusted to keep end-inspiratory pressure below the upper inflection point (UIP) of the pressure volume curve.[3,98,99] The UIP, often seen in patients with ARDS, has been ascribed to overinflation[98,99] or to the end of recruitment[102,103] during lung expansion. However, whether or not ventilator settings that would result in pressure–volume excursions above the UIP are deleterious remains unsettled and has never been assessed experimentally. The impact of pulmonary edema and the resulting decrease in ventilatable lung volume on the inspiratory limb of the respiratory system volume–pressure curve has not yet been evaluated. A better understanding of its significance is required before the

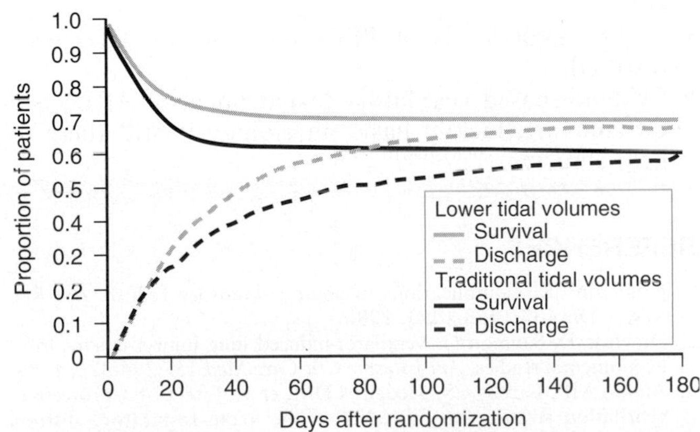

FIGURE 45–11 • Probability of survival and of being discharged home and breathing without assistance during the first 180 days after randomization in patients with acute lung injury and acute respiratory distress syndrome. (From The Acute Respiratory Distress Syndrome Network: *N Engl J Med* 342:1301-1308, 2000.)

UIP can be used to set V_T in patients. An experimental study was designed to examine several hypotheses.[104] The first was that reduction in ventilatable lung volume not only decreases compliance[36,105] but also affects the position of the UIP. The second was that the development of edema alters the volume–pressure curve by causing distal airway obstruction. The third was that individual characteristics of the volume–pressure curve reflect the susceptibility of the lungs to the deleterious effects of high-volume ventilation. The first two hypotheses were tested by obstructing the distal airways of rats by instilling a viscous liquid and comparing the shape of their volume–pressure curves to those of intact rats. The authors found that changes in the shape of the volume–pressure curve (relationship between compliance, volume at which the upper inflection point was seen, and end-inspiratory pressure) were similar whether they resulted from viscous fluid instillation or pulmonary edema. To test the third hypothesis, volume–pressure curves obtained prior to mechanical ventilation with a high V_T were examined with respect to the amount of pulmonary edema resulting from this overinflation in lungs injured by ANTU. The authors found that the higher the compliance and the volume of the UIP before ventilation, the less severe the resulting edema after overinflation. Taken together, these results suggest that the position of the UIP is a marker of ventilatable lung volume and is both influenced by, and predictive of, the development of edema during mechanical ventilation.

Conclusion and Clinical Applications

The experimental concept of VILI has been shown to be relevant to outcome in ARDS.[6] However, a uniform reduction in V_T for every ARDS patient may not be appropriate.[7] For the time being and until further evidence, the following conclusions can be put forth:

- Drastic V_T reduction may not be justified for *every* ARDS patient.
- Reasoned V_T reduction, designed to prevent volutrauma, should be guided by the lung's mechanical properties as measured on the respiratory system volume–pressure curve.
- Use of high levels of PEEP has not, to date, been justified.
- Evidence-based ventilatory management of ARDS is a difficult art; luckily basic physiology is still there to help clinicians.[39,65,106,107]

REFERENCES

1. Pingleton SK: Complications of acute respiratory failure. *Am Rev Respir Dis* 137:1463-1493, 1988.
2. Dreyfuss D, Saumon G: Ventilator-induced lung injury: lessons from experimental studies. *Am J Respir Crit Care Med* 157:294-323, 1998.
3. Amato MB, Barbas CS, Medeiros DM, et al: Effect of a protective-ventilation strategy on mortality in the acute respiratory distress syndrome. *N Engl J Med* 338:347-354, 1998.
4. Brochard L, Roudot-Thoraval F, Roupie E, et al: Tidal volume reduction for prevention of ventilator-induced lung injury in acute respiratory distress syndrome. The Multicenter Trial Group on Tidal Volume reduction in ARDS. *Am J Respir Crit Care Med* 158:1831-1838, 1998.
5. Stewart TE, Meade MO, Cook DJ, et al: Evaluation of a ventilation strategy to prevent barotrauma in patients at high risk for acute respiratory distress syndrome. Pressure- and Volume-Limited Ventilation Strategy Group. *N Engl J Med* 338:355-361, 1998.
6. The Acute Respiratory Distress Syndrome Network: Ventilation with lower tidal volumes as compared with traditional tidal volumes for acute lung injury and the acute respiratory distress syndrome. *N Engl J Med* 342:1301-1308, 2000.
7. Eichacker PQ, Gerstenberger EP, Banks SM, et al: A metaanalysis of ALI and ARDS trials testing low tidal volumes. *Am J Respir Crit Care Med* 28:28, 2002.
8. Webb HH, Tierney DF: Experimental pulmonary edema due to intermittentpositive pressure ventilation with high inflation pressures. Protection by positive end-expiratory pressure. *Am Rev Respir Dis* 110:556-565, 1974.
9. Dreyfuss D, Basset G, Soler P, Saumon G: Intermittent positive-pressure hyperventilation with high inflation pressures produces pulmonary microvascular injury in rats. *Am Rev Respir Dis* 132: 880-884, 1985.
10. Dreyfuss D, Soler P, Basset G, Saumon G: High inflation pressure pulmonary edema. Respective effects of high airway pressure, high tidal volume, and positive end-expiratory pressure. *Am Rev Respir Dis* 137:1159-1164, 1988.
11. Dreyfuss D, Saumon G: Barotrauma is volutrauma, but which volume is the one responsible? *Intensive Care Med* 18:139-141, 1992 (editorial).
12. Dreyfuss D, Soler P, Saumon G: Spontaneous resolution of pulmonary edema caused by short periods of cyclic overinflation. *J Appl Physiol* 72:2081-2089, 1992.
13. Slutsky AS: Consensus conference on mechanical ventilation: January 28–30, 1993 at Northbrook, Illinois, USA. *Intensive Care Med* 20:64-79, 1994.
14. Hernandez LA, Peevy KJ, Moise AA, Parker JC: Chest wall restriction limits high airway pressure-induced lung injury in young rabbits. *J Appl Physiol* 66:2364-2368, 1989.
15. Carlton DP, Cummings JJ, Scheerer RG, et al: Lung overexpansion increases pulmonary microvascular protein permeability in young lambs. *J Appl Physiol* 69:577-583, 1990.
16. Peevy KJ, Hernandez LA, Moise AA, Parker JC: Barotrauma and microvascular injury in lungs of nonadult rabbits: effect of ventilation pattern. *Crit Care Med* 18:634-637, 1990.
17. Taskar V, John J, Evander E, et al: Healthy lungs tolerate repetitive collapse and reopening during short periods of mechanical ventilation. *Acta Anaesthesiol Scand* 39:370-376, 1995.
18. Bowton DL, Kong DL: High tidal volume ventilation produces increased lung water in oleic acid-injured rabbit lungs. *Crit Care Med* 17:908-911, 1989.
19. Hernandez LA, Coker PJ, May S, et al: Mechanical ventilation increases microvascular permeability in oleic acid-injured lungs. *J Appl Physiol* 69:2057-2061, 1990.
20. Coker PJ, Hernandez LA, Peevy KJ, et al: Increased sensitivity to mechanical ventilation after surfactant inactivation in young rabbit lungs. *Crit Care Med* 20:635-640, 1992.
21. Dreyfuss D, Soler P, Saumon GL: Mechanical ventilation-induced pulmonary edema. Interaction with previous lung alterations. *Am J Respir Crit Care Med* 151:1568-1575, 1995.
22. Huang YC, Weinmann GG, Mitzner W: Effect of tidal volume and frequency on the temporal fall in compliance. *J Appl Physiol* 65: 2040-2047, 1988.
23. Ward HE, Nicholas TE: Effect of artificial ventilation and anaesthesia on surfactant turnover in rats. *Respir Physiol* 87:115-129, 1992.
24. Tsang JY, Emery MJ, Hlastala MP: Ventilation inhomogeneity in oleic acid-induced pulmonary edema. *J Appl Physiol* 82:1040-1045, 1997.
25. Dreyfuss D, Martin-Lefevre L, Saumon G: Hyperinflation-induced lung injury during alveolar flooding in rats: effect of perfluorocarbon instillation. *Am J Respir Crit Care Med* 159:1752-1757, 1999.
26. Hughes JMB, Rosenzweig DY: Factors affecting trapped gas volume in perfused dog lungs. *J Appl Physiol* 29:332-339, 1970.
27. Falke KJ, Pontoppidan H, Kumar A, et al: Ventilation with end-expiratory pressure in acute lung disease. *J Clin Invest* 51:2315-2323, 1972.
28. Suter PM, Fairley B, Isenberg MD: Optimum end-expiratory airway pressure in patients with acute pulmonary failure. *N Engl J Med* 292:284-289, 1975.

29. Matamis D, Lemaire F, Harf A, et al: Total respiratory pressure-volume curves in the adult respiratory distress syndrome. *Chest* 86:58-66, 1984.
30. Benito S, Lemaire F: Pulmonary pressure-volume relationship in acute respiratory distress syndrome in adults: role of positive end-expiratory pressure. *J Crit Care* 5:27-34, 1990.
31. Argiras EP, Blakeley CR, Dunnill MS, et al: High peep decreases hyaline membrane formation in surfactant deficient lungs. *Br J Anaesth* 59:1278-1285, 1987.
32. Sandhar BK, Niblett DJ, Argiras EP, et al: Effects of positive end-expiratory pressure on hyaline membrane formation in a rabbit model of the neonatal respiratory distress syndrome. *Intensive Care Med* 14:538-546, 1988.
33. Muscedere JG, Mullen JB, Gan K, Slutsky AS: Tidal ventilation at low airway pressures can augment lung injury. *Am J Respir Crit Care Med* 149:1327-1334, 1994.
34. Sohma A, Brampton WJ, Dunnill MS, Sykes MK: Effect of ventilation with positive end-expiratory pressure on the development of lung damage in experimental acid aspiration pneumonia in the rabbit. *Intensive Care Med* 18:112-117, 1992.
35. Gattinoni L, Pelosi P, Crotti S, Valenza F: Effects of positive end-expiratory pressure on regional distribution of tidal volume and recruitment in adult respiratory distress syndrome. *Am J Respir Crit Care Med* 151:1807-1814, 1995.
36. Gattinoni L, Pesenti A, Avalli L, et al: Pressure-volume curve of total respiratory system in acute respiratory failure. Computed tomographic scan study. *Am Rev Respir Dis* 136:730-736, 1987.
37. Martynowicz MA, Minor TA, Walters BJ, Hubmayr RD: Regional expansion of oleic acid-injured lungs. *Am J Respir Crit Care Med* 160:250-258, 1999.
38. Wilson TA, Anafi RC, Hubmayr RD: Mechanics of edematous lungs. *J Appl Physiol* 90:2088-2093, 2001.
39. Hubmayr RD: Perspective on lung injury and recruitment: a skeptical look at the opening and collapse story. *Am J Respir Crit Care Med* 165:1647-1653, 2002.
40. Rizk NW, Murray JF: PEEP and pulmonary edema. *Am J Med* 72:381-383, 1982.
41. Hopewell PC, Murray JF: Effects of continuous positive-pressure ventilation in experimental pulmonary edema. *J Appl Physiol* 40: 568-574, 1976.
42. Luce JM, Huang TW, Robertson HT, et al: The effects of prophylactic expiratory positive airway pressure on the resolution of oleic acid-induced lung injury in dogs. *Ann Surg* 197:327-336, 1983.
43. Toung T, Saharia P, Permutt S, et al: Aspiration pneumonia: beneficial and harmful effects of positive end-expiratory pressure. *Surgery* 82:279-283, 1977.
44. Corbridge TC, Wood LDH, Crawford GP, et al: Adverse effects of large tidal volume and low PEEP in canine acid aspiration. *Am Rev Respir Dis* 142:311-315, 1990.
45. Colmenero Ruiz M, Fernández Mondéjar E, Fernández Sacristán MA, Rivera Fernández R, Vazquez Mata G: PEEP and low tidal volume ventilation reduce lung water in porcine pulmonary edema. *Am J Respir Crit Care Med* 155:964-970, 1997.
46. Bshouty Z, Ali J, Younes M: Effect of tidal volume and PEEP on rate of edema formation in in situ perfused canine lobes. *J Appl Physiol* 64:1900-1907, 1988.
47. Permutt S: Mechanical influences on water accumulation in the lungs. In Fishman AP, Renkin EM, editors: *Pulmonary edema*. Bethesda, 1979, American Physiological Society.
48. Luce JM: The cardiovascular effects of mechanical ventilation and positive end-expiratory pressure. *JAMA* 252:807-811, 1984.
49. Dreyfuss D, Saumon G: Role of tidal volume, FRC, and end-inspiratory volume in the development of pulmonary edema following mechanical ventilation. *Am Rev Respir Dis* 148:1194-1203, 1993.
50. Iliff LD: Extra-alveolar vessels and edema development in excised dog lungs. *Circ Res* 28:524-532, 1971.
51. Albert RK, Lakshminarayan S, Kirk W, Butler J: Lung inflation can cause pulmonary edema in zone I of in situ dog lungs. *J Appl Physiol* 49:815-819, 1980.
52. Pattle RE: Properties, function and origin of the alveolar lining layer. *Nature (Lond)* 175:1125-1126, 1955.
53. Clements JA: Pulmonary edema and permeability of alveolar membranes. *Arch Environ Health* 2:280-283, 1961.
54. Albert RK, Lakshminarayan S, Hildebrandt J, Kirk W, Butler J: Increased surface tension favors pulmonary edema formation in anesthetized dogs' lungs. *J Clin Invest* 63:1015-1018, 1979.
55. Howell JBL, Permutt S, Proctor DF, Riley RL: Effect of inflation of the lung on different parts of pulmonary vascular bed. *J Appl Physiol* 16:71-76, 1961.
56. Benjamin JJ, Murtagh PS, Proctor DF, et al: Pulmonary vascular interdependence in excised dog lobes. *J Appl Physiol* 37:887-894, 1974.
57. Jefferies AL, Kawano T, Mori S, Burger R: Effect of increased surface tension and assisted ventilation on 99mTc-DTPA clearance. *J Appl Physiol* 64:562-568, 1988.
58. Nieman G, Ritter-Hrncirik C, Grossman Z, et al: High alveolar surface tension increases clearance of technetium 99m diethylene-triamine-pentaacetic acid. *J Thorac Cardiovasc Surg* 100:129-133, 1990.
59. John J, Taskar V, Evander E, et al: Additive nature of distension and surfactant perturbation on alveolocapillary permeability. *Eur Respir J* 10:192-199, 1997.
60. Woo SW, Hedley-White J: Macrophage accumulation and pulmonary edema due to thoracotomy and lung overinflation. *J Appl Physiol* 33:14-21, 1972.
61. Tsuno K, Miura K, Takeya M, et al: Histopathologic pulmonary changes from mechanical ventilation at high peak airway pressures. *Am Rev Respir Dis* 143:1115-1120, 1991.
62. Markos J, Doerschuk CM, English D, et al: Effect of positive end-expiratory pressure on leukocyte transit in rabbit lungs. *J Appl Physiol* 74:2627-2633, 1993.
63. Kawano T, Mori S, Cybulsky M, et al: Effect of granulocyte depletion in a ventilated surfactant-depleted lung. *J Appl Physiol* 62: 27-33, 1987.
64. Belperio JA, Keane MP, Burdick MD, et al: Critical role for CXCR2 and CXCR2 ligands during the pathogenesis of ventilator-induced lung injury. *J Clin Invest* 110:1703-1716, 2002.
65. Ricard J-D, Dreyfuss D: Cytokines during ventilator-induced lung injury: a word of caution. *Anesth Analg* 93:251-252, 2001.
66. Dreyfuss D, Ricard J-D, Saumon G: On the physiologic and clinical relevance of lung borne cytokines during ventilator-induced lung injury. *Am J Respir Crit Care Med* 167:1467-1471, 2003.
67. Tremblay L, Valenza F, Ribeiro SP, et al: Injurious ventilatory strategies increase cytokines and c-fos m-RNA expression in an isolated rat lung model. *J Clin Invest* 99:944-952, 1997.
68. Ricard J-D, Dreyfuss D, Saumon G: Production of inflammatory cytokines during ventilator-induced lung injury: a reappraisal. *Am J Respir Crit Care Med* 163:1176-1180, 2001.
69. Pugin J, Dunn I, Jolliet P, et al: Activation of human macrophages by mechanical ventilation in vitro. *Am J Physiol* 275:L1040-L1050, 1998.
70. Vlahakis NE, Schroeder MA, Limper AH, Hubmayr RD: Stretch induces cytokine release by alveolar epithelial cells in vitro. *Am J Physiol* 277:L167-L173, 1999.
71. Verbrugge SJC, Uhlig S, Neggers SJCM, et al: Different ventilation strategies affect lung function but do not increase tumor necrosis factor-α and prostacyclin production in lavaged rat lungs in vivo. *Anesthesiology* 91:1834-1843, 1999.
72. Takata M, Abe J, Tanaka H, et al: Intraalveolar expression of tumor necrosis factor-alpha gene during conventional and high-frequency ventilation. *Am J Respir Crit Care Med* 156:272-279, 1997.
73. Imanaka H, Shimaoka M, Matsuura N, et al: Ventilator-induced lung injury is associated with neutrophil infiltration, macrophage activation, and TGF-ss1 mRNA upregulation in rat lungs. *Anesth Analg* 92:428 436, 2001.
74. Matsuoka T, Kawano T, Miyasaka K: Role of high-frequency ventilation in surfactant-depleted lung injury as measured by granulocytes. *J Appl Physiol* 76:539-544, 1994.
75. Sugiura M, McCulloch PR, Wren S, et al: Ventilator pattern influences neutrophil influx and activation in atelectasis-prone rabbit lung. *J Appl Physiol* 77:1355-1365, 1994.
76. Imai Y, Kawano T, Miyasaka K, et al: Inflammatory chemical mediators during conventional ventilation and during high frequency oscillatory ventilation. *Am J Respir Crit Care Med* 150:1550-1554, 1994.
77. von Bethmann AN, Brasch F, Nusing R, et al: Hyperventilation induces release of cytokines from perfused mouse lung. *Am J Respir Crit Care Med* 157:263-272, 1998.
78. Chiumello D, Pristine G, Slutsky AS: Mechanical ventilation affects local and systemic cytokines in an animal model of acute respiratory syndrome. *Am J Respir Crit Care Med* 160:109-116, 1999.

79. Nahum A, Hoyt J, Schmitz L, et al: Effect of mechanical ventilation strategy on dissemination of intratracheally instilled Escherichia coli in dogs. *Crit Care Med* 25:1733-1743, 1997.
80. Verbrugge SJ, Sorm V, van't Veen A, et al: Lung overinflation without positive end-expiratory pressure promotes bacteremia after experimental Klebsiella pneumoniae inoculation. *Intensive Care Med* 24:172-177, 1998.
81. Slutsky AS, Tremblay LN: Multiple system organ failure. Is mechanical ventilation a contributing factor? *Am J Respir Crit Care Med* 157:1721-1725, 1998.
82. Dreyfuss D, Saumon G: From ventilator-induced lung injury to multiple organ dysfunction? *Intensive Care Med* 24:102-104, 1998 (editorial).
83. Pugin J: Is the ventilator responsible for lung and systemic inflammation? *Intensive Care Med* 28:817-819, 2002.
84. Dos Santos CC, Slutsky AS: Mechanisms of ventilator-induced lung injury: a perspective. *J Appl Physiol* 89:1645-1655, 2000.
85. Parker JC, Townsley MI, Rippe B, et al: Increased microvascular permeability in dog lungs due to high peak airway pressures. *J Appl Physiol* 57:1809-1816, 1984.
86. Parker JC, Ivey CL, Tucker A: Gadolinium prevents high airway pressure-induced permeability increases in isolated rat lungs. *J Appl Physiol* 84:1113-1118, 1998.
87. Parker JC: Inhibitors of myosin light chain kinase and phosphodiesterase reduce ventilator-induced lung injury. *J Appl Physiol* 89:2241-2248, 2000.
88. Broccard AF, Hotchkiss JR, Vannay C, et al: Protective effects of hypercapnic acidosis on ventilator-induced lung injury. *Am J Respir Crit Care Med* 164:802-806, 2001.
89. Schubert W, Frank PG, Woodman SE, et al: Microvascular hyperpermeability in caveolin-$1^{-/-}$ knock-out mice. Treatment with a specific nitric-oxide synthase inhibitor, L-name, restores normal microvascular permeability in Cav-1 null mice. *J Biol Chem* 277: 40091-40098, 2002.
90. West JB, Tsukimoto K, Mathieu Costello M, Prediletto R: Stress failure in pulmonary capillaries. *J Appl Physiol* 70:1731-1742, 1991.
91. Fu Z, Costello ML, Tsukimoto K, et al: High lung volume increases stress failure in pulmonary capillaries. *J Appl Physiol* 73:123-133, 1992.
92. Vlahakis NE, Schroeder MA, Pagano RE, Hubmayr RD: Deformation-induced lipid trafficking in alveolar epithelial cells. *Am J Physiol* 280:L938-L946, 2001.
93. Tschumperlin DJ, Oswari J, Margulies SS: Deformation-induced injury of alveolar epithelial cells: effects of frequency, duration and amplitude. *Am J Respir Crit Care Med* 162:357-362, 2000.
94. Laffey JG, Kavanagh BP: Hypocapnia. *N Engl J Med* 347:43-53, 2002.
95. Laffey JG, Engelberts D, Kavanagh BP: Injurious effects of hypocapnic alkalosis in the isolated lung. *Am J Respir Crit Care* 162:399-405, 2000.
96. Laffey JG, Engelberts D, Kavanagh BP: Buffering hypercapnic acidosis worsens acute lung injury. *Am J Respir Crit Care Med* 161:141-146, 2000.
97. Sinclair SE, Kregenow DA, Lamm WJ, et al: Hypercapnic acidosis is protective in an in vivo model of ventilator-induced lung injury. *Am J Respir Crit Care Med* 166:403-408, 2002.
98. Roupie E, Dambrosio M, Servillo G, et al: Titration of tidal volume and induced hypercapnia in acute respiratory distress syndrome. *Am J Respir Crit Care Med* 152:121-128, 1995.
99. Dambrosio M, Roupie E, Mollet JJ, et al: Effects of positive end-expiratory pressure and different tidal volumes on alveolar recruitment and hyperinflation. *Anesthesiology* 87:495-503, 1997.
100. Rotta AT, Gunnarsson B, Fuhrman BP, et al: Comparison of lung protective ventilation strategies in a rabbit model of acute lung injury. *Crit Care Med* 29:2176-2184, 2001.
101. Ranieri VM, Mascia L, Fiore T, et al: Cardiorespiratory effects of positive end-expiratory pressure during progressive tidal volume reduction (permissive hypercapnia) in patients with acute respiratory distress syndrome. *Anesthesiology* 83:710-720, 1995.
102. Hickling KG: The pressure-volume curve is greatly modified by recruitment. A mathematical model of ARDS lungs. *Am J Respir Crit Care Med* 158:194-202, 1998.
103. Jonson B, Richard JC, Straus C, et al: Pressure-volume curves and compliance in acute lung injury: evidence of recruitment above the lower inflection point. *Am J Respir Crit Care Med* 159:1172-1178, 1999.
104. Martin-Lefèvre L, Ricard J-D, Roupie E, et al: Significance of the changes in the respiratory system pressure-volume curve during acute lung injury in rats. *Am J Respir Crit Care Med* 164:627-632, 2001.
105. Gibson GJ, Pride NB: Pulmonary mechanics in fibrosing alveolitis: the effects of lung shrinkage. *Am Rev Respir Dis* 116: 637-647, 1977.
106. Mead J, Takishima T, Leith D: Stress distribution in lungs: a model of pulmonary elasticity. *J Appl Physiol* 28:596-608, 1970.
107. Dreyfuss D, Saumon G: Evidence-based medicine or fuzzy logic: what is best for ARDS management? *Intensive Care Med* 28: 230-234, 2002.

CHAPTER

46

Acute Respiratory Distress Syndrome in Children

Jean-Christophe Mercier, Stéphane Dauger, Philippe Durand, and Etienne Javouey

PEARLS

- The incidence of acute lung injury and acute respiratory distress syndrome is low in children.
- Insults leading to acute lung injury and acute respiratory distress syndrome are similar to those observed in adults such as direct lung injury including pneumonia, gastric content aspiration, lung contusion, hydrocarbon ingestion, lung contusion, and smoke inhalation or indirect injury including near-drowning, multiple emergent transfusions, and sepsis.
- Endothelial and epithelial injury is critical to diffuse alveolar damage and pulmonary edema.
- Acute lung injury resolution can be hastened by strategies that activate apical epithelial sodium channel-type channels and basal Na^+/K^+-ATPase channels, including β-adrenergic agents and nitric oxide.
- As ventilator-induced lung injury is now recognized to play a major role in the outcome, ventilator strategies aim to limit both tidal volume less than 8 to 10 ml/kg and pause inspiratory pressure less than 25 to 30 cmH_2O with permissive hypercarbia and to use sufficient levels of positive end-expiratory pressure to achieve optimal lung recruitment (7–9 ribs on chest x-ray film).
- Whereas no adjunct therapies including high-frequency oscillatory ventilation, prone positioning, and inhaled nitric oxide therapy have demonstrated significant benefits, they are currently used in clinical practice to limit both barotraumata and oxygen toxicity. Likewise, surfactant replacement trials have failed to demonstrate long-term benefits, and despite no conclusive trials extracorporeal life support is still used in some centers as last resort.
- Noninvasive ventilation can be valuable in the management of respiratory failure in immunocompromised children, given the high mortality observed when tracheal intubation and mechanical ventilation are required.
- Although no conclusive data have emerged from appropriately designed trials, some evidence suggests that steroids used at the late fibrosing stage of the acute respiratory distress syndrome are of benefit.

Definitions

The acute respiratory distress syndrome is a common and devastating clinical syndrome of acute lung injury that affects both medical and surgical patients. In 1967, Ashbaugh et al[1] described 12 adults with acute-onset tachypnea and cyanosis refractory to oxygen therapy, diffuse infiltrates on chest x-ray film, and decreased lung compliance. Initially called the *"adult" respiratory distress syndrome,* this entity now is called the *"acute" respiratory distress syndrome* (ARDS) because it does occur in children[2–5] and in newborns.[6]

Because the initial definition lacks specific diagnostic criteria, controversy existed over the incidence and natural history of the syndrome. Some investigators attempted to exclude cardiogenic causes of pulmonary edema by requiring a "normal" pulmonary capillary wedge pressure and specified that values range from 12 mmHg or less[7] to less than 18 mmHg.[8] In 1988, an expanded definition was proposed that quantified the respiratory impairment through a four-point lung-injury scoring system that was based on the degree of infiltration evident on the chest x-ray film, the ratio of the partial pressure of arterial oxygen to the fraction of inspired oxygen (Pao_2/Fio_2), the level of positive end-expiratory pressure (PEEP), and the decrease in static lung compliance.[9] Mild-to-moderate acute lung injury was defined by a lung injury score less than 2.5 and severe lung injury (ARDS) by a score greater than 2.5. Although the lung injury scoring system has been widely used to quantify the severity of lung injury in clinical trials, it cannot be used to predict the outcome during the first 24 to 72 hours after onset of ARDS. In contrast, when used 4 to 7 days after onset of the syndrome, scores greater than 2.5 may be predictive of a complicated course and the need for prolonged mechanical ventilation.

Furthermore, the direct (e.g., aspiration, fat embolism, drug ingestion, toxic gas inhalation, infectious pneumonia) or indirect (e.g., sepsis, acute pancreatitis, multiple blood transfusions, disseminated intravascular coagulation) cause of the acute lung injury was thought to influence the outcome as well as the presence or absence of nonpulmonary organ dysfunction. However, the former concept was later challenged.[10]

In 1994, the American-European Consensus Conference Committee proposed a new definition (Table 46–1).[11] The consensus definition had two advantages. First, it recognized that the severity of clinical lung injury varies. Patients with less severe hypoxemia (defined as $Pao_2/Fio_2 \geq 200$ and ≤ 300) were considered to have "acute lung injury," and those with more severe hypoxemia (defined as $Pao_2/Fio_2 < 200$) were considered to have "acute respiratory distress syndrome." Earlier recognition of patients with acute lung injury was supposed to facilitate earlier enrollment of patients in clinical trials. Second, the definition was simple to apply in the clinical setting because measurement of static compliance was abandoned. However, the new definition did not take into account other important factors that influence the outcome, such as optimization of ventilation including PEEP level,[12,13] a significant improvement in blood gas exchange within the first 24 hours,[14] the underlying cause, and whether other organ systems were affected.[15] Nevertheless, the widespread acceptance of both the 1988 lung injury scoring system and the 1994 consensus definition has improved the standardization of clinical research and trials.

Pathogenesis

Endothelial and Epithelial Injury

The alveolar–capillary barrier is formed of two separate cellular linear barriers, the *vascular endothelium* and the *alveolar epithelium*.[16] The acute phase of acute lung injury and the adult respiratory distress syndrome are characterized by the influx of protein-rich edema fluid into the airspaces as a consequence of increased permeability of the alveolar–capillary barrier.[17] The importance of endothelial injury and increased vascular permeability to the formation of pulmonary edema that characterize the early phase of ARDS are well established.

The critical role of epithelial injury to both the development of and recovery from ARDS is now recognized.[18] Loss of epithelial integrity has numerous consequences. First, the diffuse alveolar damage contributes to alveolar flooding. Second, epithelial injury disrupts normal epithelial fluid transport and impedes removal of edema fluid from the alveolar space. Alveolar fluid clearance has been found to be impaired in the majority of patients with acute lung injury and ARDS.[19] Third, alveolar type II cell injury impedes surfactant production and turnover, contributing to the characteristic surfactant abnormalities.[20] Finally, the inflammatory cascade is activated with release of numerous mediators. Activated macrophages secrete proinflammatory cytokines, including tumor necrosis factor-α, interleukin (IL)-1, IL-6, and IL-8, which act locally to stimulate chemotaxis and activate neutrophils.[21] Neutrophils adhere to the injured capillary endothelium and marginate through the interstitium into the airspace. Neutrophils can, in turn, release oxidants, proteases, leukotrienes, and many other proinflammatory molecules (Figure 46–1).

Role of Cytokines

A complex network of cytokines and other proinflammatory compounds are thought to initiate and amplify the inflammatory response in acute lung injury and ARDS. Regulation of cytokine production may be influenced by extrapulmonary factors, including microbial products, lipopolysaccharide endotoxins, and macrophage inhibitory factor, which has been found in high concentrations in the bronchoalveolar lavage fluid of patients with this syndrome.[22] Not only is the production of proinflammatory cytokines important but also the balance between the proinflammatory and antiinflammatory mediators.[23] Several endogenous inhibitors of proinflammatory

TABLE 46–1

American–European Consensus Conference Definitions of Acute Lung Injury (ALI) and Acute Respiratory Distress Syndrome (ARDS)

Criteria	Timing	Pao_2/Fio_2	Chest X-Ray Film	Pulmonary Wedge Pressure
ALI	Acute onset	≤300	Bilateral infiltrates	≤18 mmHg or absence of clinical evidence of left atrial hypertension
ARDS	Acute onset	≤200	Bilateral infiltrates	≤18 mmHg or absence of clinical evidence of left atrial hypertension

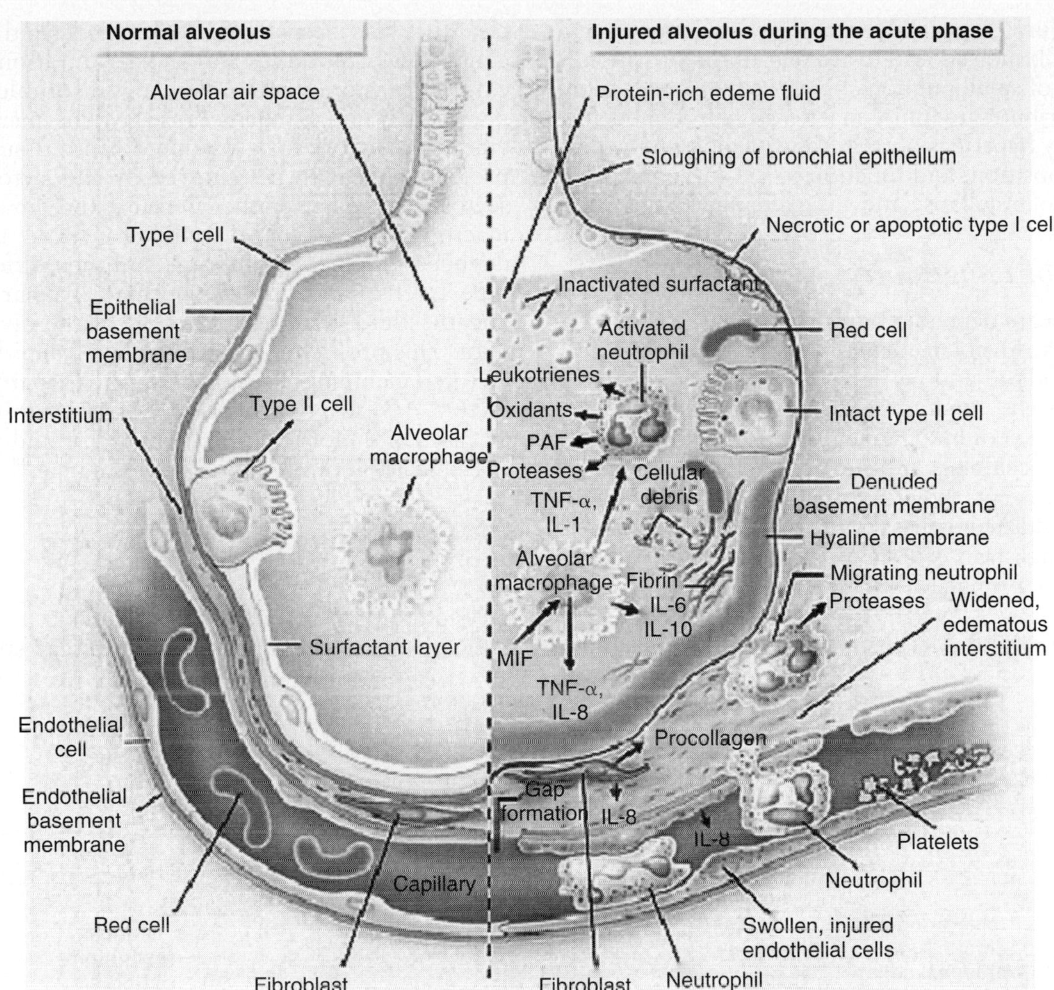

FIGURE 46–1 • Normal alveolus **(left)** and injured alveolus in the acute phase of acute lung injury and acute respiratory distress syndrome. In the acute phase of the syndrome **(right)**, there is sloughing of both the bronchial and alveolar epithelial cells, with formation of protein rich hyaline membranes on the denuded basement membrane. Neutrophils are shown adhering to the injured capillary endothelium and marginating through the interstitium into the airspace, which is filled with protein-rich edema fluid. In the airspace, an alveolar macrophage is secreting cytokines interleukin (IL)-1, IL-6, IL-8, and IL-10, and tumor necrosis factor (TNF)-α, which act locally to stimulate chemotaxis and activate neutrophils. Macrophages also secrete other cytokines, including interleukin-1, IL-6, and IL-10. Interleukin-1 can also stimulate the production of extracellular matrix by fibroblasts. Neutrophils can release oxidants, proteases, leukotrienes, and other proinflammatory molecules, such as platelet-activating factor (PAF). A number of antiinflammatory mediators are present in the alveolar milieu, including IL-1–receptor antagonist, soluble TNF receptor, autoantibodies against IL-8, and cytokines such as IL-10 and IL-11 (not shown). The influx of protein-rich edema fluid into the alveolus has led to the inactivation of surfactant. *MIF,* Macrophage inhibitory factor. (From Ware LB, Matthay MA: *N Engl J Med* 342:1334-1349, 2000.)

cytokines have been described, including soluble tumor necrosis factor receptor, IL-1 receptor antagonist, and antiinflammatory cytokines such as IL-10 and IL-11. However, the critical role of cytokines in acute lung injury and ventilator-induced lung injury has been challenged.[24]

Role of Ventilator-Induced Lung Injury

Although high fractions of inspired oxygen have long been considered potentially toxic to the lung, accumulating experimental evidence indicates that high volumes and pressures can injure the lung, causing increased permeability edema in the uninjured lung[25] and enhanced edema in the injured lung.[26] Initial theories focused on capillary stress failure as a result of alveolar distension.[27] More recently, alveolar distension associated with the repeated collapse and reopening of alveoli was shown to initiate a cascade of proinflammatory cytokines.[28] As most patients with acute lung injury who die do so from multisystem organ failure, it has been postulated that ventilator-induced lung injury plays a key role in determining the negative clinical outcome of patients exposed to mechanical ventilation.[29] The term *cellular biotrauma* has been coined to describe the process by which mechanical stress produced by mechanical ventilation leads to up-regulation of an inflammatory response.[30] Thus cells are required to sense mechanical forces and activate opposite intracellular signaling pathways able to release (1) growth factors and surfactant when forces are "physiologic" (e.g., fetal or postnatal lung breathing), and (2) proinflammatory cytokines when forces are "pathologic" (e.g., barotrauma or volutrauma resulting from either excessive inspiratory positive pressures or tidal volumes).[31] Multiple other pathways can perpetuate or inhibit lung injury. Abnormalities of the coagulation system and impaired fibrinolysis lead to alveolar fibrin formation,[32] and occlusion of small pulmonary vessels by platelet-fibrin thrombi contributes to pulmonary vascular remodeling and pulmonary hypertension.[33,34] Abnormalities in the production, composition, and function of the surfactant contribute to alveolar collapse and gas exchange anomalies.[35]

Resolution of Lung Injury

Prognosis appears dependent on resolution of the pathologic processes. Alveolar edema is resolved by the active transport of sodium and perhaps chloride from the distal airspaces into the lung interstitium (Figure 46–2).[36,37] Apical epithelial sodium channel-type channels and basal Na^+/K^+-ATPase channels appeared to be highly regulated by β-adrenergic agents, whereas amiloride-sensitive sodium transport is modulated by basal nitric oxide.[38] Water follows passively through transcellular water channels, the aquaporins, located primarily on type I cells.[39] Lung fluid clearance is impaired in the majority of patients with acute lung injury and ARDS, but maximal alveolar fluid clearance has been found to be associated with significantly lower mortality and shorter duration of mechanical ventilation.[40] Removal of insoluble protein is particularly important because hyaline membranes provide a framework for growth of fibrous tissue.[41] Insoluble proteins appear to be removed by endocytosis and transcytosis, alveolar epithelial cells, and phagocytosis by macrophages.[42] Type II cells proliferate to cover the denuded basement membrane and then differentiate into type I cells, restoring the normal alveolar architecture and the fluid transport function of the alveolar epithelium. This proliferation is controlled by epithelial growth factors, including keratinocyte and hepatocyte growth factors.[43] New blood vessels are formed mostly as a result of vascular endothelium growth factor and contribute to normalization of the blood gas exchange.[44]

Fibrosing Lung Injury

After the initial phase of acute lung injury and ARDS, progression to fibrotic lung injury usually occurs 5 to 10 days after onset of the disorder. The alveolar space becomes

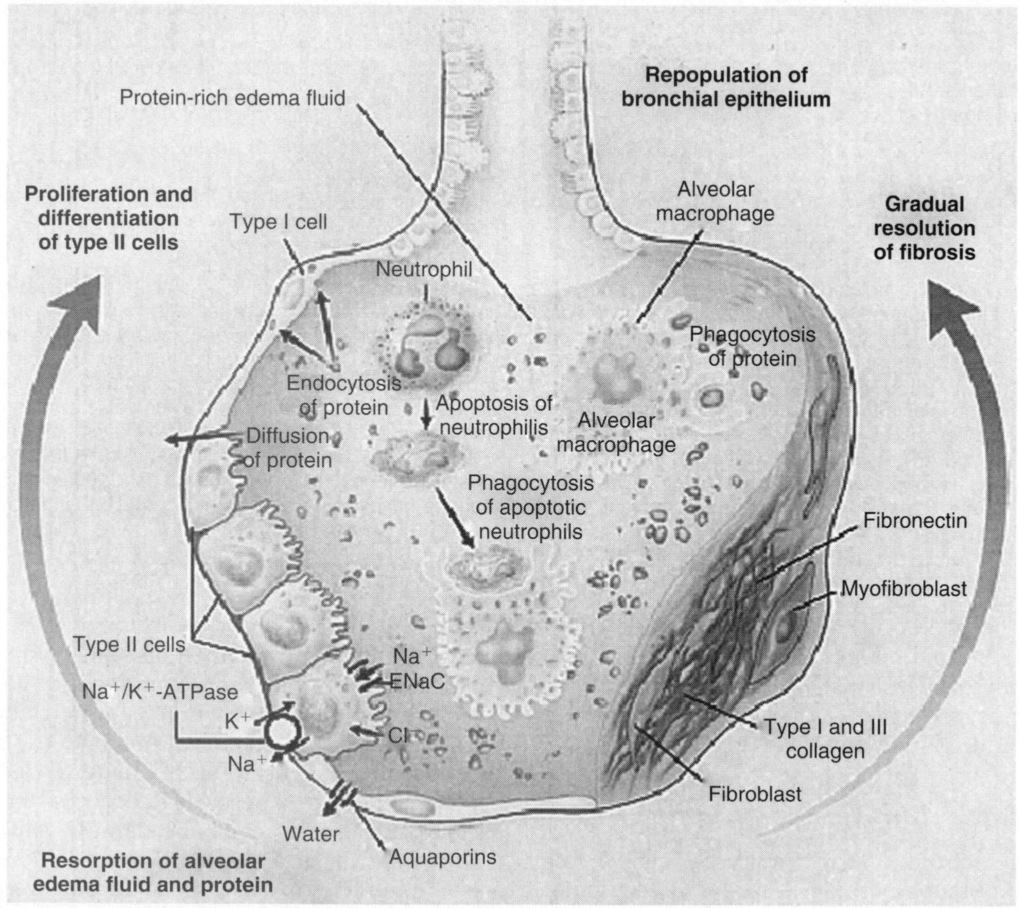

FIGURE 46–2 • Mechanisms important in the resolution of acute lung injury and acute respiratory distress syndrome. On the **left** side of the alveolus, the alveolar epithelium is being repopulated by the proliferation and differentiation of alveolar type II cells. Resorption of alveolar edema fluid is shown at the base of the alveolus, with sodium and chloride being transported through the apical membrane of type II cells. Sodium is taken up by the epithelial sodium channel (ENaC) and through the basolateral membrane of type II cells by the sodium pump (Na^+/K^+-ATPase). The relevant pathways for chloride transport are unclear. Water is shown moving through water channels, the aquaporins, located primarily on type I cells. Some water may cross by a paracellular route. Soluble protein probably is cleared primarily by paracellular diffusion and secondarily by endocytosis by alveolar epithelial cells. Macrophages remove insoluble protein and apoptotic neutrophils by phagocytosis. On the **right** side of the alveolus, the gradual remodeling and resolution of intraalveolar and interstitial granulation tissue and fibrosis are shown. (From Ware LB, Matthay MA: *N Engl J Med* 342:1334-1349, 2000.)

filled with fibroblasts and procollagen III peptide, of which the early appearance in the alveolar space has been associated with an increased risk of death.[45] The finding of marked fibrosing alveolitis on lung biopsy (or autopsy) correlates with an increased risk of death.[46] The mechanisms underlying resolution of the inflammatory-cell infiltrates and fibrosis are unclear. Apoptosis is thought to play a major role in clearance of neutrophils from the injured lung, as high concentrations of the markers of apoptosis have been shown in the bronchoalveolar lavage fluid taken from patients with ARDS.[47,48] Antiinflammatory cytokines and proteases likely play a major role.

Clinical Features

Incidence and Etiology

The incidence of acute lung injury and ARDS ranges from 1% to 5% of pediatric intensive care admissions.[49–54] However, ARDS now appears to be a relatively rare disease in children, perhaps because of stricter definitions or changing diagnostic criteria over the years. Within a 6-month period in nine large pediatric intensive care units across North America, 1096 (17.1%) of 6403 admissions required mechanical ventilator support for a minimum of 24 hours. Of these patients, 701 (64%) met criteria other than primary respiratory failure to require mechanical support, including 13.5% upper airway obstruction, 11.5% cyanotic congenital heart disease, 9.7% life support restriction, and 5.5% chronically ventilated. In the 395 children who were eligible for respiratory failure studies, 62.4% had an acute primary diagnosis of pulmonary disease, 14.2% neurologic disease, and 8.9% cardiac disease. Chronic underlying conditions were present in 43.2% of patients. The most common acute diagnosis was bronchiolitis in infants (43.6%) and pneumonia in children 1 year and older (24.5%). ARDS was identified in only 9 (5.7%) and 14 (9.7%) of the children with primary lung disease younger than 1 year and older than 1 year, respectively. Thus ARDS actually occurred in 23 children of 6403 admissions, which is a true incidence of 0.36%.[55]

Insults causing acute lung injury or ARDS may either directly or indirectly injure the lung. Causes of direct lung injury include pneumonia, gastric content aspiration, lung contusion, hydrocarbon ingestion, and smoke inhalation. Near-drowning, multiple emergent transfusions, and sepsis lead to acute lung injury as part of multiorgan failure. Sepsis is the more common and lethal predisposing condition associated with ARDS, whether it is related to community infection, such as severe meningococcal shock; nosocomial infection, such as ventilator-associated pneumonia[56]; or serious underlying conditions, such as immunocompromised states.[57]

Clinical Course

The clinical course of acute lung injury and ARDS parallels the histopathologic abnormalities. Clinical changes that occur first are tachypnea, dyspnea, agitation, and hypoxemia. These findings usually develop rapidly during a period of hours but can evolve over 1 to 5 days.[58] As the lung becomes edematous and consolidated, tachypnea and hypoxemia are caused by progressive restrictive lung disease and respiratory muscle fatigue. Chest x-ray film shows diffuse bilateral alveolar opacities, sometimes accompanied by small pleural effusion (Figure 46–3). However, computed tomographic scans reveal juxtaposition of abnormal dense lung regions and more functional lucent regions. Dense lung regions often develop in the dependent regions of the lung, reflecting collapse of the edematous lung with secondary atelectasis, whereas aerated regions usually prevail in nondependent areas.[59] Lung function measurements show reduced functional residual capacity. Total lung compliance is reduced, but compliance of the small regions of functional lung is normal. Hypoxemia results from intrapulmonary shunting and the regions with low ventilation/perfusion relationships. These regions can be recruited in response to PEEP, thereby improving oxygenation.[60]

During the fibroproliferative phase, lung compliance is reduced by progressive lung fibrosis, and the effects of PEEP on oxygenation are less impressive. Lung parenchyma becomes better aerated despite accentuated interstitial markings indicative of fibrosis. At this stage, carbon dioxide retention is not uncommon. Requirements for mechanical ventilation may be prolonged for weeks, and clinical recovery usually requires a few months in children.[61] Although pediatric survivors of acute hypoxemic respiratory failure perceive no limitation in lifestyle, significant abnormalities in lung function including bronchoreactivity have been found.[62] Likewise, adult survivors of ARDS have persistent functional disability 1 year after discharge from the intensive care unit. Most patients have extrapulmonary conditions, with muscle wasting and weakness being most prominent.[63]

Oxygenation and Ventilator Strategy

Most patients with acute lung injury and ARDS require supplemental oxygen and mechanical ventilation. However, these interventions can themselves produce lung injury and worsen ARDS.

Cellular toxicity of the oxygen has been well established in both animals and humans. However, high levels of oxygen appear to be surprisingly well tolerated in patients with acute respiratory failure, even for several days.[64] The reasons for this phenomenon are unclear. Antioxidant defense mechanisms have been found to be more efficient in primates than in rats.[65] Furthermore, prior lung exposure to endotoxin or cytokines (i.e., tolerance phenomenon) has been shown to protect animals exposed to 100% oxygen for several days compared with naive animals who died rapidly.[66]

Ventilator-induced lung injury has been the subject of intensive experimental and human research (see Chapter 45). Traditionally, mechanical ventilation was delivered in an effort to normalize arterial blood gases. Tidal volumes of 10 to 15 ml/kg of body weight were used to normalize $Pa{CO_2}$ values. After numerous experimental studies clearly demonstrated that excessive tidal volume traumatized lung structures, particularly when functioning lung volume is reduced to an aerated "baby lung" surrounded by extensive consolidation area, an international conference addressed factors likely responsible for ventilator-induced lung injury.[67] Several clinical trials evaluated lower ventilator settings as a means to minimize

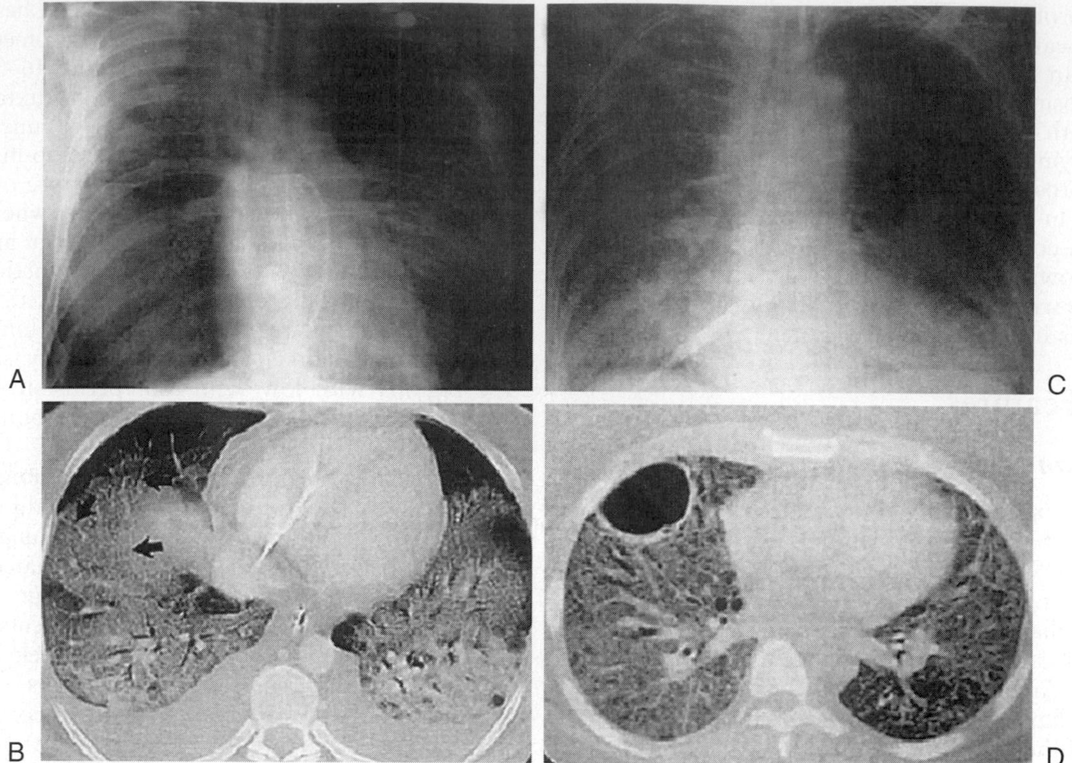

FIGURE 46–3 • Radiographic and computed tomographic findings in the acute exudative phase **(A, C)** and the fibrosing alveolitis phase **(B, D)** of acute lung injury and acute respiratory distress syndrome. *Arrow* indicates thickened interlobular septa, consistent with pulmonary edema. (From Goodman LR: *Radiol Clin North Am* 34:33-46, 1996.)

ventilator-induced lung injury and pulmonary fibrosis, even at the expense of normal blood gas exchange, with little success other than one preliminary study.[68–71] In the culmination of this research, the ARDS Network trial ultimately reported convincing improved clinical outcomes with a lung protection ventilator strategy, compared with standard treatment for ARDS in 861 adults.[72] The study group received 4 to 6 ml/kg of predicted body weight tidal volume and positive plateau pressure less than 30 cmH_2O, compared with 11 to 12 ml/kg tidal volume and positive plateau pressure less than 50 cmH_2O in the control group. PEEP was adjusted to minimize Fio_2 but maintain oxygen saturation between 88% and 95%. $Paco_2$ values were allowed to rise, but pH was maintained higher than 7.15. Adult patients receiving a lung protection strategy had significantly reduced mortality (31% vs. 40%), fewer hospital days with extrapulmonary organ failure, and increased ventilator-free days (55% vs. 66%) over the first 28 hospital days compared with the control group. However, the marked improvement in significant outcomes was later criticized when it appeared that the control group purposely may have received higher than normal tidal volume.[73] Indeed, the lack of difference in significant outcomes observed in all previous trials but one may have been related to the relatively limited tidal volume of approximately 10 ml/kg used in the control group. A fierce debate ensued and was summarized in two successive commentaries.[74,75]

Positive end-expiratory pressure maximizes alveolar recruitment, improves oxygenation insufficiency, and minimizes the need for oxygen supplementation, thereby minimizing iatrogenic oxygen toxicity. Early use of PEEP does not prevent the development or progression of ARDS.[76] In animal models of acute lung injury, tidal volumes delivered without PEEP increase the shear stress between interfacing normal and injured regions, creating neutrophilic inflammation and cytokine release similar to ARDS.[77] However, PEEP can also overdistend the normal lung and compromise hemodynamic function[78] (Figure 46–4). Intensivists have therefore searched for the "best" PEEP that maximizes lung compliance and oxygenation efficiency yet minimizes overdistension and reduced cardiac output.[79] For years, the issue of how to set up optimal PEEP remained controversial, until a new trial of the ARDS Network demonstrated that in patients with acute lung injury and ARDS who receive a tidal volume of 6 ml/kg of predicted body weight and an end-inspiratory plateau-pressure limit of 30 cmH_2O, clinical outcomes were similar whether lower (8.3 ± 3.2 cmH_2O) or higher (13.2 ± 3.5 cmH_2O) PEEP were used throughout days 1 to 4.[80] Practical guidelines for ventilator settings in acute lung injury or ARDS are given in Table 46–2.

Prone positioning is another method for recruiting atelectatic-dependent zones of the lung. Several mechanisms have been proposed to account for this effect, including an increase in end-expiratory lung volume, better ventilation/perfusion matching, and regional changes in ventilation associated with alterations in chest-wall mechanics.[81] Prone positioning was shown to improve overall oxygenation in most patients, including children with acute respiratory failure.[82,83] However, although prone positioning improved oxygenation, it did not improve survival in a multicenter,

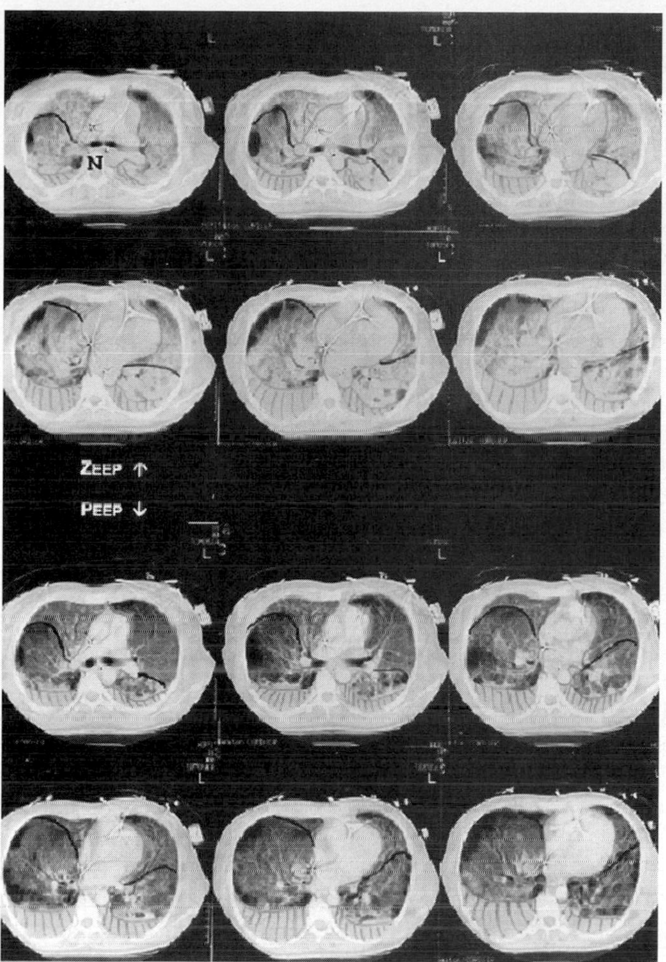

FIGURE 46–4 • Divergent effects of positive end-expiratory pressure (PEEP, **lower panels**) compared with zero end-expiratory pressure (ZEEP, **upper panels**) on regional lung recruitment assessed by computed tomography. **A,** Acute diffuse form of acute respiratory distress syndrome (ARDS) **(left side panels). B,** "Lobar" form **(right side panels).** PEEP induced marked lung recruitment of the edematous zones but marked overdistension of aerated zones in pneumonia. *Black line* indicates the scissura and *hatched area* the pleural effusion. (From Puybasset L, Gusman P, Muller JC, et al. *Am J Respir Crit Care Med* 158:1644-1655, 1998.)

randomized trial that enrolled 304 adult patients with acute lung injury or ARDS.[84]

Permissive Hypercapnia

Permissive hypercapnia is a well-accepted consequence of lung protection strategies of ventilator support. Goals of management are to allow gradual increase in $Paco_2$, that is, no more than 5 mmHg increase per hour, and to avoid acute severe acidosis.[85] $Paco_2$ values of 65 to 85 mmHg are well tolerated in most patients, although additional sedation may be necessary to reduce air hunger and dyspnea. Permissive hypercapnia is contraindicated in children with suspected increased intracranial pressure and those with sickle cell disease.

High-frequency oscillatory ventilation (HFOV) reflects the extreme form of reduced tidal volume delivery, providing 1 to 2 ml/kg inspiratory volumes at frequencies of 5 to 15 Hz. Amplitudes of oscillation are set to minimize hypercapnia (HFOV is often very efficient in normalizing hypercapnia), whereas mean airway pressure is set to maximize lung inflation and oxygen efficiency. In a prospective, randomized, crossover study involving 70 children with either diffuse alveolar disease and/or air leak syndrome, children receiving HFOV alone had better survival (94% vs. 60%), fewer days with supplemental oxygen, and chronic lung disease less often (11% vs. 30%) compared with the control group.[86] Fifty-eight percent of children who did not respond to conventional ventilation crossed over to HFOV and survived, whereas 18% of those who crossed over to conventional ventilation because of persistent respiratory failure survived. Parallel to the emerging consensus that ventilator-induced lung injury was preventable, use of HFOV has increased significantly in patients with severe pediatric respiratory failure. A multicenter randomized trial compared HFOV with conventional ventilation in 148 adults with ARDS. Although an early but not sustained improvement in Pao_2/Fio_2 was observed in the HFOV group, no other significant differences were seen in oxygenation failure, ventilation failure, barotrauma, and survival at day 30.[87]

Adjunct Therapies

Adjunct therapies aim at improving lung function and minimizing the risks of ventilator support.

Surfactant replacement therapy aims to reinflate collapsed areas of the lung, improve compliance, and reduce intrapulmonary shunting, thereby leading to reductions in morbidity and mortality. Surfactant not only is decreased in quantity but also is functionally abnormal in patients with ARDS.[88] Based on the similarities with neonatal respiratory distress syndrome, several anecdotal case reports and then results of phase II trials were encouraging. However, a multicenter randomized trial of 725 adult patients with sepsis-induced ARDS who received continuous aerosolization of a synthetic surfactant (Exosurf, Glaxo Wellcome) for up to 5 days showed no significant effect on 30-day survival, length of stay in the intensive care unit, duration of mechanical ventilation, or physiologic function.[89] The lack of effect was attributed perhaps to low-level alveolar deposition and absence of surfactant protein. Therefore natural surfactant was tested in a limited number of children with severe ARDS and led to sustained improvement in oxygenation in the subgroup of children without pneumonia and Pao_2/Fio_2 greater than 65.[90] In two international combined randomized double-blind trials involving 448 adult patients with ARDS of various causes, up to four intratracheal doses of a recombinant protein C based-surfactant given within a period of 24 hours failed to improve survival.[91] However, patients who received surfactant had greater improvement in gas exchange during the 24-hour treatment period than patients who received standard therapy alone, suggesting the potential benefit of a longer treatment course.

Fluid management and hemodynamic support[92] are critical in the management of acute lung injury and ARDS, both of which are associated with sepsis.[93] Assessment of vascular volume status is not easy,[94] and its management is particularly difficult when large amounts of fluid must

TABLE 46–2

Recommendations for Ventilator Settings in the Acute Respiratory Distress Syndrome

For Conventional Mechanical Ventilation		
Mode		Volume or pressure controlled Airway pressure release ventilation preferred when preservation of spontaneous ventilation is desired
Tidal volume	6–10 ml/kg	Permissive hypercapnia (increase <5 mmHg per hour) $Paco_2$ 65–85 mmHg well tolerated unless increased intracranial pressure Arterial pH >7.15
End-inspiratory plateau-pressure	<30 cmH_2O	Above this limit, increased risks of barotrauma and air leaks
PEEP	10–15 cmH_2O	Lower PEEP levels, if heterogeneous lung injury Higher PEEP levels, if diffuse lung injury Consider early prone positioning (6–12 hours)
Respiratory rate	20–60 breaths/min	Adjusted to age; higher than normal may limit hypercapnia
Inspiratory/expiratory ratio	1:2 to 1:1	Check for inadvertent PEEP
Fio_2	<60%–80%	Depends upon how the diseased lung may be recruited Pao_2 40–60 mmHg, Spo_2 85%–95%
For High-Frequency Oscillatory Ventilation		
Amplitude pressure	30–50 cmH_2O	To achieve visible chest vibrations
Mean airway pressure	15–30 cmH_2O	To achieve adequate chest recruitment (7–9 ribs)
Respiratory rate	3–10 Hz	Decrease to increase tidal volume (usually not measured)
Inspiratory/expiratory ratio	1:3 to 1:1	1:1 more appropriate in diffuse lung injury
Fio_2	<60%–80%	Depends upon whether the lung may be recruited

FiO_2, fraction of inspired oxygen; *PEEP,* positive end-expiratory pressure.

be administered to treat septic shock at the same time that capillary leak promotes accumulation of extravascular lung water. An ongoing large-scale randomized trial by the ARDS Network is under way to compare the effects of restricted versus more liberal fluids. Fluid-refractory shock clearly affects the outcome of ARDS, as the need for vasopressors was found to be associated with increased mortality in adult patients with ARDS.[95,96] Both pulmonary hypertension associated with ARDS and excessive airway pressures may significantly increase right ventricular afterload.[97] Despite inherent shortcomings, transthoracic or transesophageal echocardiography is probably the most useful technique for assessing cardiac function in patients mechanically ventilated for ARDS.[98] Right ventricular dysfunction may be improved by cautiously decreasing PEEP or limiting inadvertent PEEP by reducing the respiratory rate and adjusting the inspiratory/expiratory ratio. Persistent cor pulmonale should prompt considering use of specific pulmonary vasodilators such as inhaled nitric oxide (iNO) and/or systemic vasopressors such as norepinephrine because right ventricular function critically depends on right coronary perfusion pressure.[99]

Inhaled nitric oxide at 1 to 20 ppm relaxes pulmonary vascular smooth muscle. Inhaled nitric oxide clinically reduces elevated pulmonary artery pressures and improves arterial oxygenation by increasing blood flow to the lung regions that remained functional, thereby improving matching of perfusion to ventilation.[100,101] Effective doses in adults with ARDS varied from a few parts per million to efficiently reduce pulmonary hypertension to a few parts per billion (ppb) to significantly improve oxygenation.[102] Responsiveness to such low doses of NO suggests that tracheal intubation inadvertently creates an NO deficiency state by preventing autoinhalation of NO from the upper respiratory airways.[103] However, efficient doses appeared to be higher (5–20 ppm) in children and neonates.[104] Although iNO may also benefit alveolar neutrophil function and cytokine release,[105] several clinical trials enrolling adults with ARDS of various causes were unable to demonstrate any significant improvement in survival.[106–110] Likewise, in children with severe hypoxemic respiratory failure, although iNO at 20 ppm acutely improved oxygenation and lowered mean pulmonary artery pressure,[111] there was no clear effect on survival.[112] As 35% of children who initially did not respond to iNO did so after lung volumes were increased by HFOV, combined use of HFOV and iNO may provide more predictable improvement in children with ARDS.[113]

Extracorporeal life support (ECLS) provides both gas exchange and circulatory support for patients with life-threatening acute lung injury and ARDS and allows the lung to rest from mechanical ventilation. ECLS can be provided by venoarterial or venovenous bypass techniques, using artificial membranes or hollow fibers to provide oxygen and remove carbon dioxide and intravascular fluid. In a retrospective case-cohort study of 331 children with respiratory failure, 53 children who received ECLS were compared with 53 diagnosis- and risk-matched children who did not receive ECLS. The ECLS patients had a 26% mortality rate, whereas those who were treated in standard fashion had a mortality rate of 49%.[114] In 84 adults with ARDS, ECLS was used in an algorithm of care when patients worsened despite a ventilator protective strategy, prone positioning, and iNO therapy.[115] Eighty-five percent of patients who did not require ECLS had 83% survival. Of the 13 patients who had ECLS,

62% survived. Overall survival was 80%, suggesting that combination of treatments can improve ARDS-related survival.

Ventilator-acquired pneumonia is the most common late complication of acute lung injury and ARDS. Prolonged intubation, frequent suctioning, and suboptimal nutritional status all contribute to ventilator-associated pneumonia.[116] This infection is frequently polymicrobial and commonly includes *Streptococcus pneumoniae, Staphylococcus* species, and *Pseudomonas aeruginosa* or other multiresistant gram-negative rods that are frequently encountered in intensive care units that do not have a restrictive antibiotic policy. Diagnosis of ventilator-acquired pneumonia is difficult and often based on fever, purulent aspect of the sputum, new infiltrates, and blood gas exchange worsening. Identification of the responsible germs usually requires use of protected brush or bronchoalveolar lavage under fibroscopic guidance,[117] but these procedures are not easy in small children. Eight and 15 days of appropriate antibiotic therapy have been found equally effective treatment of ventilator-associated pneumonia.[118] Mortality from nosocomial pneumonia in these patients reportedly is as high as 80%.

Corticosteroids are used extensively in acute respiratory failure,[119] including the most serious forms of acute lung injury or ARDS.[120] In a first study, Meduri et al.[121] treated nine adult patients with ARDS of 7 days' duration with 2 mg/kg methylprednisolone qid, then stepwise decreased doses. Eight patients improved after 5 days of treatment, and six survived.[121] In a second study, the authors treated 25 new patients similar to the 8 previous patients.[122] Steroids 2 mg/kg qid were initiated on day 15 of mechanical ventilation, with slow weaning over 6 weeks. After 1 week, blood gas exchange improved, with 76% survival. Interestingly, survival was 86% in the 21 responders compared with 25% in the four nonresponders. In a small randomized trial of adult patients with severe ARDS who failed to improve after day 7 of mechanical ventilation, improvement in lung injury and multiple organ dysfunction scores and reduced mortality were observed after prolonged methyl-prednisolone treatment.[123] However, the efficacy and safety of corticosteroid therapy at the fibrosing stage of ARDS are not yet proved, and a large randomized trial by the ARDS Network (Late Steroid Rescue Study [LaSRS] with a planned enrollment of 180 patients) is under way to demonstrate whether this treatment has beneficial effects.

Noninvasive Ventilation

The *pulmonary complications of solid organ and hematopoietic stem cell transplantation* have been reviewed.[124] Paramount among these are pulmonary complications, which arise as a consequence of the immunosuppressed status of the recipient and from such factors as the initial surgical insult of organ transplantation, the chemotherapy and radiation conditioning regimens that precede hematopoietic stem cell transplantation, and alloimmune mechanisms mediating host-versus-graft and graft-versus-host responses. Worsening of the respiratory status by a bacterial or viral process is often indistinguishable from acute lung injury or ARDS. Thus sepsis workup should encompass blood cultures, tracheal fluid aspirates at intubation, bronchoalveolar lavage, and viral tests by immunofluorescence or polymerase chain reaction of the blood, urine, stools, tracheal aspirates, or bronchoalveolar fluid. Pneumocystis pneumonia is frequently seen in this context, and it is important to rapidly isolate the organism usually by bronchoalveolar lavage because the association of prolonged trimethoprim-sulfamethoxazole and short-term steroids are regularly efficacious.[125] Otherwise, the prognosis of immunocompromised patients with acute lung injury or ARDS severe enough to require tracheal intubation and mechanical ventilation is poor in all the series.

Avoiding intubation and mechanical ventilation is a major goal in the management of respiratory failure in immunocompromised patients. A prospective, randomized trial of intermittent noninvasive ventilation compared with standard treatment with supplemental oxygen and no ventilatory support was conducted in 52 immunocompromised adult patients with pulmonary infiltrates, fever, and an early stage of hypoxemic respiratory failure.[126] Periods of noninvasive ventilation set in the pressure support mode delivering 7 to 10 ml/kg tidal volume at a respiratory rate fewer than 25 breaths per minute and PEEP stepwise increased by 2 cmH_2O up to 10 cmH_2O through a face mask lasted at least 45 minutes and alternated every 3 hours with periods of spontaneous breathing. Each group of 26 adult patients included 15 patients with hematologic cancer and neutropenia. Fewer patients in the noninvasive ventilation group than in the standard treatment group required tracheal intubation (12 vs. 20, $p = 0.03$), died in the intensive care unit (10 vs. 18, $p = 0.03$), or died in the hospital (13 vs. 21, $p = 0.02$).

In *immunocompetent patients*, despite initially rather negative results,[127] there has been renewal of interest in noninvasive ventilation in the early stages of acute lung injury and ARDS. In a small randomized trial, 20 (62%) of 32 patients in the noninvasive ventilation group and 15 (47%) of 32 in the conventional ventilation group had improved Pao_2/Fio_2 within the first hour of ventilation.[128] Ten patients in the noninvasive ventilation group subsequently required tracheal intubation. Twenty-three patients in the noninvasive ventilation group (72%) and 17 in the conventional ventilation group (53%) survived their stay in the intensive care unit (odd ratio 0.4, 95% confidence interval 0.1–1.4, $p = 0.19$), and 22 and 16, respectively, were discharged from the hospital. In a larger trial, 105 patients with severe acute hypoxemic respiratory failure were allocated to noninvasive ventilation (n = 51) or high-concentration oxygen therapy (n = 54).[129] Compared with oxygen therapy, noninvasive ventilation decreased the need for intubation (25% vs. 39%, $p = 0.028$) and increased the cumulative 90-day survival ($p = 0.025$). Multivariate analysis showed that noninvasive ventilation was independently associated with decreased risks of intubation, reduced risks of septic shock, and improved 90-day survival. Likewise, the same beneficial effect of noninvasive ventilation was confirmed in another trial not yet fully reported.[130] However, in a later preliminary study of 93 children with diverse causes of acute respiratory failure treated either initially or during weaning, use of noninvasive positive pressure ventilation appeared to reduce the rate of endotracheal intubation, except in the nine children with ARDS.[131] Moreover, several adult intensivists, experts in that field, have cautioned that noninvasive positive pressure ventilation might actually delay the timing of endotracheal intubation, which may become more hazardous in a hypoxic patient.

The *success of noninvasive ventilation* critically depends upon several factors, including the choice of face mask,[132] replacement of the filter humidifier by a heated humidifier,[133] removal of any device that adds extra dead space, and use of a ventilator having a sensitive inspiratory trigger and built-in algorithm for correcting leaks.[134] The most frequently used ventilatory mode is pressure support ventilation in combination with the necessary level of PEEP to recruit the lung, but the "airway pressure release ventilation" mode is increasingly used.

Conclusion

Substantial progress has been made in our understanding of acute lung injury and ARDS. Significant actions have been made to reduce the aggressiveness of mechanical ventilation: reduction of tidal volume to a safer margin of 6 to 10 ml/kg, maintenance of end-inspiratory plateau pressure less than 30 cmH_2O, acceptance of permissive hypercapnia, and use of a reasonable level of PEEP that allows decrease of Fio_2 to safe margins. If respiratory failure worsens despite these actions, prone positioning and HFOV to optimize lung recruitment, iNO therapy to reduce pulmonary hypertension and prevent cor pulmonale, and ECLS may all be helpful to buy time while the underlying pathology recovers. Mortality remains high, particularly when there is associated sepsis and evolving multiple organ dysfunction. Further research is needed to better understand the genetic polymorphisms that favor the occurrence of acute lung injury and ARDS and the mechanisms of alveolar fluid clearance and lung healing that may hasten recovery from acute lung injury.

REFERENCES

1. Ashbaugh DG, Bigelow DB, Petty TL, Levine BE: Acute respiratory distress in adults. *Lancet* 2:319-323, 1967.
2. Lyrene RK, Truog WE: Adult respiratory distress syndrome in a pediatric intensive care unit: predisposing conditions, clinical course, and outcome. *Pediatrics* 67:790-795, 1981.
3. Pfenninger J, Gerber A, Tschappeler H, Zimmermann A: Adult respiratory distress syndrome in children. *J Pediatr* 101:352-357, 1982.
4. Nussbaum E: Adult-type respiratory distress syndrome in children. Experience with seven cases. *Clin Pediatr* 22:401-406, 1983.
5. Effman EL, Merten DF, Kirks DR, et al: Adult respiratory distress syndrome in children. *Radiology* 157:69-74, 1985.
6. Faix RG, Viscardi RM, DiPietro MA, Nicks JJ: Adult respiratory distress syndrome in full-term newborns. *Pediatrics* 83:971-976, 1989.
7. Fowler AA, Hamman RF, Good JT, et al: Adult respiratory distress syndrome: risk with common predispositions. *Ann Intern Med* 98: 593-597, 1983.
8. Simmons RS, Berdine GG, Seidenfeld JJ, et al: Fluid balance and the adult respiratory distress syndrome. *Am Rev Respir Dis* 135:924-929, 1987.
9. Murray JF, Matthay MA, Luce JM, Flick MR: An expanded definition of the adult respiratory distress syndrome. *Am Rev Respir Dis* 138:720-723, 1988.
10. Gattinoni L, Pelosi P, Pedoto A, et al: Acute respiratory distress syndrome caused by pulmonary and extrapulmonary disease: different syndromes? *Am J Respir Crit Care Med* 158:3-11, 1998.
11. Bernard GR, Artigas A, Brigham KL, et al., and the Consensus Committee: The American-European consensus conference on ARDS: Definitions, mechanisms, relevant outcomes, and clinical trial coordination. *Am J Respir Crit Care Med* 149:818-824, 1994; *Intensive Care Med* 20:225-232, 1994.
12. Villar J, Perez-Mendes L, Kacmarck R: Current definitions of acute lung injury and the acute respiratory distress syndrome do not reflect their true severity and outcome. *Intensive Care Med* 25:930-935, 1999.
13. Estenssoro E, Dubin A, Laffaire E, et al: Impact of positive end-expiratory pressure on the definition of acute respiratory distress syndrome. *Intensive Care Med* 29:1936-1942, 2003.
14. Guinard N, Beloucif S, Gatecel C, et al: Interest of a therapeutic optimization strategy in severe ARDS. *Chest* 111:1000-1007, 1997.
15. Brun-Buisson C, Minelli C, Bertolini G, et al: Epidemiology and outcome of acute lung injury in European intensive care units. *Intensive Care Med* 30:51-61, 2004.
16. West JB: Thoughts on the pulmonary blood-gas barrier. *Am J Physiol* 285:L501-L513, 2003.
17. Pugin J, Verghese G, Widmer M-C, Matthay MA: The alveolar space is the site of intense inflammatory and profibrotic reactions in the early phase of acute respiratory distress syndrome. *Crit Care Med* 27:304-312, 1999.
18. Wiener-Kronish JP, Albertine KH, Matthay MA: Differential responses of the endothelial and epithelial barriers of the lung in sheep to Escherichia coli endotoxin. *J Clin Invest* 27:304-312, 1999.
19. Ware LB, Matthay MA: Alveolar fluid clearance has been found to be impaired in the majority of patients with acute lung injury and the acute respiratory distress syndrome. *Am J Respir Crit Care Med* 163:1376-1383, 2001.
20. Greene KE, Wright JR, Steinberg KP, et al: Serial changes in surfactant-associated proteins in lung and serum before and after onset of ARDS. *Am J Respir Crit Care Med* 160:1843-1850, 1999.
21. Pittet JF, Mackersie RC, Martin TR, Matthay MA: Biological markers of acute lung injury: prognostic and pathogenetic significance. *Am J Respir Crit Care Med* 155:1187-1205, 1997.
22. Donnelly SC, Haslett C, Reid PT, et al: Regulatory role for macrophage migration inhibitory factor in acute respiratory distress syndrome. *Nat Med* 3:320-323, 1997.
23. Martin TR: Cytokines and the acute respiratory distress syndrome (ARDS): a question of balance. *Nat Med* 3:272-273, 1997.
24. Dreyfuss D, Ricard JD, Saumon G: On the physiologic and clinical relevance of lung-borne cytokines during ventilator-induced lung injury. *Am J Respir Crit Care Med* 167:1467-1471, 2003.
25. Dreyfuss D, Soler P, Basset G, Saumon G: High inflation pressure pulmonary edema: respective effects of high airway pressure, high tidal volume, and positive end-expiratory pressure. *Am Rev Respir Dis* 137:1159-1164, 1988.
26. Dreyfuss D, Soler P, Saumon G: Mechanical ventilation-induced pulmonary edema: interactions with previous lung alterations. *Am J Respir Crit Care Med* 151:1568-1575, 1995.
27. Fu Z, Costello ML, Tsukimoto K, et al: High lung volume increases stress failure in pulmonary capillaries. *J Appl Physiol* 73:123-133, 1992.
28. Tremblay L, Valenza F, Ribeiro SP, et al: Injurious ventilatory strategies increase cytokines and c-fos m-RNA expression in an isolated rat lung model. *J Clin Invest* 99:944-952, 1997.
29. Slutsky AS, Tremblay LN: Multiple system organ failure: is mechanical ventilation a contributing factor? *Am J Respir Crit Care Med* 157:1721-1725, 1998.
30. Dos Santos CC, Slutsky AS: Mechanisms of ventilator-induced lung injury: a perspective. *J Appl Physiol* 89:1645-1655, 2000.
31. Liu M, Tanswell AK, Post M: Mechanical force-induced signal transduction in lung cells. *Am J Physiol* 277:L667-L683, 1999.
32. Gunther A, Mosavi P, Heineman S, et al: Alveolar fibrin formation caused by procoagulant and depressed fibrinolytic capacities in severe pneumonia: comparison with the acute respiratory distress syndrome. *Am J Respir Crit Care Med* 161:454-462, 2000.
33. Zapol W, Jones R: Vascular components of ARDS. Clinical pulmonary hemodynamics and morphology. *Am Rev Respir Dis* 136: 471-474, 1987.

34. Leeman M, Naeije R: La circulation pulmonaire dans le syndrome de détresse respiratoire aiguë. *Reanimation* 13:131-135, 2004.
35. Lewis JF, Jobe AH: Surfactant and the adult respiratory distress syndrome. *Am Rev Respir Dis* 147:218-233, 1993.
36. Snajdder JI, Factor P, Ingbar D: Lung edema clearance: role of Na^+-K^+-ATPase. *J Appl Physiol* 93:1860-1866, 2002.
37. Matthay MA, Folkesson HG, Clerici C: Lung epithelial fluid transport and the resolution of pulmonary edema. *Physiol Rev* 82:569-600, 2002.
38. Hardiman KM, McNicholas-Bevensee CM, Fortenberry J, et al: Regulation of amiloride-sensitive Na^+ transport by basal nitric oxide. *Am J Respir Cell Mol Biol* 30:720-728, 2004.
39. Bhattacharya J: The alveolar water gate. *Am J Physiol* 286: L257-L258, 2004.
40. Ware BL, Matthay MA: Lung fluid clearance is impaired in the majority of patients with acute lung injury and the adult respiratory distress syndrome. *Am J Respir Crit Care Med* 163: 1376-1383, 2001.
41. Bitterman PB: Pathogenesis of fibrosis in acute lung injury. *Am J Med* 92:39S-43S, 1992.
42. Folkesson HG, Matthay MA, Westrom BR, et al: Alveolar epithelial clearance of protein. *J Appl Physiol* 80:1431-1435, 1996.
43. Ware LB, Matthay MA: Keratinocyte and hepatocyte growth factors in the lung: role in lung development, inflammation and repair. *Am J Physiol* 282:L924-L940, 2002.
44. Thickett DR, Armstrong L, Millar AB: A role for vascular endothelial growth factor in acute and resolving lung injury. *Am J Respir Crit Care Med* 166:1332-1337, 2002.
45. Chestnutt AN, Matthay MA, Tibayan FA, Clark JG: Early detection of type III procollagen peptide in acute lung injury: pathogenetic and prognostic significance. *Am J Respir Crit Care Med* 156:840-845, 1997.
46. Martin C, Papazian L, Payan MJ, et al: Pulmonary fibrosis correlates with outcome in adult respiratory distress syndrome: a study in mechanically ventilated patients. *Chest* 107:196-200, 1995.
47. Ware LB, Geiser T, Nuckton T, Matthay MA: Elevated levels of markers of apoptosis in the biological fluids of patients with early acute lung injury. *Am J Respir Crit Care Med* 161:A380, 2000 (abstract).
48. Martin TR, Nakamura M, Matute-Bello G: The role of apoptosis in acute lung injury. *Crit Care Med* 31(suppl 4):S184-S188, 2003.
49. Lyrene RK, Truog WE: Adult respiratory distress syndrome in a pediatric intensive care unit: predisposing conditions, clinical course and outcome. *Pediatrics* 67:790-795, 1981.
50. Pfenninger J, Gerber A, Tschappeler H, Zimmermann A: Adult respiratory distress syndrome in children. *J Pediatr* 101:352-357, 1982.
51. Timmons OD, Dean JM, Vernon DD: Mortality rates and prognostic variables in children with adult respiratory distress syndrome. *J Pediatr* 119:896-899, 1991.
52. Davis SL, Fuhrman DP, Costarino AT: Adult respiratory distress syndrome in children: associated disease, clinical course, and predictors of death. *J Pediatr* 123:35-45, 1993.
53. Costil J, Cloup M, Leclerc F, et al: Acute respiratory distress syndrome (ARDS) in children: Multicenter collaborative study of the French group of pediatric intensive care. *Pediatr Pulmonol* 11(suppl):106-107, 1995.
54. Peters MJ, Tasker RC, Kiff KM, et al: Acute hypoxemic respiratory failure in children: case mix and the utility of respiratory severity indices. *Intensive Care Med* 24:699-705, 1998.
55. Randolph AG, Meert KL, O'Neil ME, et al., for the Pediatric Acute Lung Injury And Sepsis Investigators Network: The feasibility of conducting clinical trials in infants and children with acute respiratory failure. *Am J Respir Crit Care Med* 167:1334-1340, 2003.
56. Fagon JY, Chastre J: Ventilator-associated pneumonia. *Am J Respir Crit Care Med* 165:867-903, 2002.
57. DeBruin W, Notterman DA, Magid M, et al: Acute hypoxemic respiratory failure in infants and children: clinical and pathologic characteristics. *Crit Care Med* 20:1223-1234, 1992.
58. Hudson LD, Milberg JA, Anardi D, Maunder RJ: Clinical risks for the development of the acute respiratory distress syndrome. *Am J Respir Crit Care Med* 151:293-301, 1995.
59. Gattinoni L, Cairon P, Pleosi P, Goodman L: What has computed tomography taught us about the acute respiratory distress syndrome? *Am J Respir Crit Care Med* 164:1701-1711, 2001.
60. Gattinoni L, Pelosi P, Crotti S, Valenza F: Effects of positive end-expiratory pressure on regional distribution of tidal volume and recruitment in adult respiratory distress syndrome. *Am J Respir Crit Care Med* 151:1807-1814, 1995.
61. Golder NDB, Lane R, Tasker RC: Timing of recovery of lung function after severe hypoxemic respiratory failure in children. *Intensive Care Med* 24:530-533, 1998.
62. Weiss I, Ushay M, DeBruin W, et al: Respiratory and cardiac function in children after acute hypoxemic respiratory failure. *Crit Care Med* 24:148-154, 1996.
63. Herridge MS, Cheung AM, Tansey CM, et al., for the Canadian Critical Care Trials Group: One-year outcomes in survivors of the acute respiratory distress syndrome. *N Engl J Med* 348:683-693, 2003.
64. Capellier G, Beuret P, Clement G, et al: Oxygen tolerance in patients with acute respiratory failure. *Intensive Care Med* 24: 422-428, 1998.
65. Clerch LB, Massaro D, Berkovitch A: Molecular mechanisms of antioxidant enzyme expression in lung during exposure to and recovery from hyperoxia. *Am J Physiol* 274:L313-L319, 1998.
66. Berg JT, Allison RC, Prasad VR, Taylor AE: Endotoxin protection of rats from pulmonary oxygen toxicity: possible cytokine involvement. *J Appl Physiol* 68:549-553, 1990.
67. American Thoracic Society, the European Society of Intensive Care Medicine, the Société de Réanimation de Langue Française: International consensus conference in intensive care medicine: ventilator-associated lung injury in ARDS. *Am J Respir Crit Care Med* 160:2118-2124, 1999.
68. Brochard L, Roudot-Thoraval F, Roupie E, et al: Tidal volume reduction for prevention of ventilator-induced lung injury in acute respiratory distress syndrome. Multicenter trial group on tidal volume reduction in ARDS. *Am J Respir Crit Care Med* 158: 1831-1838, 1998.
69. Amato MB, Barbas CS, Medeiros DM, et al: Effect of a protective-ventilation strategy on mortality in the acute respiratory distress syndrome. *N Engl J Med* 338:347-354, 1998.
70. Stewart TE, Meade MO, Cook DJ, et al., and the Pressure- and Volume-Limited Ventilation Strategy Group: Evaluation of a ventilation strategy to prevent barotrauma in patients with high risk for acute respiratory distress syndrome. *N Engl J Med* 338:355-361, 1998.
71. Brower RG, Shanholtz CB, Fessler HE, et al: Prospective, randomized, controlled clinical trial comparing traditional versus reduced tidal volume ventilation in acute respiratory distress syndrome patients. *Crit Care Med* 27:1492-1498, 1999.
72. Acute Respiratory Distress Syndrome Network: Ventilation with lower tidal volumes for acute lung injury and the acute respiratory distress syndrome. *N Engl J Med* 342:1301-1308, 2000.
73. Eichacker PQ, Gerstenberger EP, Banks SM, et al: Meta-analysis of acute lung injury and acute respiratory distress syndrome trials testing low tidal volumes. *Am J Respir Crit Care Med* 166:1510-1514, 2002 (see correspondence 167:612-613, 933-936, 2003).
74. Steinbrook R: How best to ventilate? Trial design and patient safety in studies of the acute respiratory distress syndrome. *N Engl J Med* 348:1393-1401, 2003.
75. Steinbrook R: Trial design and patient safety? The debate continues. *N Engl J Med* 349:629-630, 2003.
76. Pepe PE, Hudson LD, Carrico CJ: Early application of positive-end expiratory pressure in patients at risk for the adult respiratory distress syndrome. *N Engl J Med* 311:281-286, 1984.
77. Chiumello D, Pristine G, Slutsky AS: Mechanical ventilation affects local and systemic cytokines in an animal model of acute respiratory distress syndrome. *Am J Respir Crit Care Med* 160:109-116, 1999.
78. Rouby JJ, Puybasset L, Nieszkowska A, Lu Q: Acute respiratory distress syndrome: lessons from computed tomography of the whole lung. *Crit Care Med* 31(4 suppl):S285-S295, 2003.
79. Suter PM, Fairley B, Isemberg MD: Optimum end-expiratory airway pressure in patients with acute pulmonary failure. *N Engl J Med* 292:284-289, 1975.
80. ARDS Clinical Trials Network: Higher versus lower positive end-expiratory pressures in patients with the acute respiratory distress syndrome. *N Engl J Med* 351:327-336, 2004.
81. Pelosi P, Tubiolo D, Mascheroni D, et al: Effects of the prone position on respiratory mechanics and gas exchange during acute lung injury. *Am J Respir Crit Care Med* 157:387-393, 1998.

82. Curley MA, Thompson JE, Arnold JH: The effects of early and repeated prone positioning in pediatric patients with acute lung injury. *Chest* 118:156-163, 2000.
83. Kornecki A, Frndova H, Coates AL, Shemie SD: Randomized trial of prolonged prone positioning in children with acute respiratory failure. *Chest* 119:211-218, 2001.
84. Gattinoni L, Tognoni G, Pesenti A, et al., for the Prone-Supine Study Group: Effect of prone positioning on the survival of patients with acute respiratory failure. *N Engl J Med* 345: 568-573, 2001.
85. Feihl F, Perret C: Permissive hypercapnia. How permissive should we be? *Am J Respir Crit Care Med* 150:1722-1737, 1994.
86. Arnold JH, Hanson JH, Togo-Figuero LO, et al: Prospective, randomized comparison of high-frequency oscillatory ventilation and conventional mechanical ventilation in pediatric respiratory failure. *Crit Care Med* 22:1530-1539, 1994.
87. Derdak S, Mehta S, Stewart TE, et al., and the Multicenter Oscillatory Ventilation for Acute Respiratory Distress Syndrome Trial (MOAT) Study Investigators. High-frequency oscillatory ventilation for acute respiratory distress syndrome in adults: a randomized, controlled trial. *Am J Respir Crit Care Med* 166: 801-808, 2002.
88. Hallman M, Spragg R, Harell JH, et al: Evidence of lung surfactant abnormality in respiratory failure. Study of bronchoalveolar lavage phospholipids, surface activity, and plasma myoinositol. *J Clin Invest* 70:673-683, 1982.
89. Anzueto A, Baughman RP, Guntupalli KK, et al., for the Exosurf Acute Respiratory Distress Syndrome Sepsis Study Group: Aerosolized surfactant in adults with sepsis-induced acute respiratory distress syndrome. *N Engl J Med* 334:1417-1421, 1996.
90. Möller JC, Schaible T, Roll C, et al., and the surfactant ARDS Study Group: Treatment with bovine surfactant in severe acute respiratory distress syndrome in children: a randomized multicenter study. *Intensive Care Med* 29:437-446, 2003.
91. Spragg RG, Lewis JF, Walmrath HD, et al: Effect of recombinant protein C-based surfactant on the acute respiratory distress syndrome. *N Engl J Med* 351:884-892, 2004.
92. Carcillo JA, Fields AI, American College of Critical Care Medicine Task Force Committee Members: Clinical practice parameters for hemodynamic support of pediatric and neonatal patients in septic shock. *Crit Care Med* 30:1365-1378, 2002.
93. Brun-Buisson C, Minelli C, Bertolini G, et al: Epidemiology and outcome of acute lung injury in European intensive care units. Results from the ALIVE study. *Intensive Care Med* 30:51-61, 2004.
94. Michard F, Boussat S, Chemla D, et al: Relation between respiratory changes in arterial pulse pressure and fluid responsiveness in septic patients with acute circulatory failure *Am J Respir Crit Care Med* 162:134-138, 2000.
95. Vieillard-Baron A, Girou E, Valente E, et al: Predictors of mortality in acute respiratory distress syndrome. Focus on the role of right heart catheterization. *Am J Respir Crit Care Med* 161:1597-1601, 2000.
96. Page B, Vieillard-Baron A, Beauchet A, et al: Low stretch ventilation strategy in acute respiratory distress syndrome: eight years of clinical experience in a single center. *Crit Care Med* 31:765-769, 2003.
97. Schmitt JM, Vieillard-Baron A, Augarde R, et al: Positive end-expiratory pressure titration in acute respiratory distress syndrome patients: impact on right ventricular outflow impedance evaluated by pulmonary artery Doppler flow velocity measurements. *Crit Care Med* 29:1407-1412, 2001.
98. Vieillard-Baron A, Prin S, Chergui K, et al: Echo-Doppler demonstration of *cor pulmonale* at the bedside in the medical intensive care unit. *Am J Respir Crit Care Med* 166:1310-1319, 2002.
99. Vieillard-Baron A, Prin S, Chergui K, et al: Hemodynamic instability in sepsis. Bedside assessment by Doppler echocardiography. *Am J Respir Crit Care Med* 168:1270-1276, 2003.
100. Rossaint R, Falke KJ, Lopez F, et al: Inhaled nitric oxide for the adult respiratory distress syndrome. *N Engl J Med* 328:399-405, 1993.
101. Pison U, Lopez FA, Heidelmeyer CF, et al: Inhaled nitric oxide reverses hypoxic pulmonary vasoconstriction without impairing gas exchange. *J Appl Physiol* 74:1287-1292, 1993.
102. Gerlach H, Rossaint R, Pappert D, Falke KJ: Time-course and dose-response of nitric oxide inhalation for systemic oxygenation and pulmonary hypertension in patients with adult respiratory distress syndrome. *Eur J Clin Invest* 23:499-502, 1993.
103. Gerlach H, Rossaint R, Pappert D, et al: Autoinhalation of nitric oxide after endogenous synthesis in nasopharynx. *Lancet* 343:518-519, 1994.
104. Demirakça S, Dötsch J, Knothe C, et al: Inhaled nitric oxide in neonatal and pediatric acute respiratory distress syndrome: dose-response, prolonged inhalation, and weaning. *Crit Care Med* 24: 1913-1919, 1996.
105. Chollet-Martin S, Gatecel C, Kermarrec N, et al: Alveolar neutrophil functions and cytokine levels in patients with the adult respiratory distress syndrome during nitric oxide inhalation. *Am J Respir Crit Care Med* 153:985-990, 1996.
106. Dellinger RP, Zimmerman JL, Taylor RW, et al., and the Inhaled Nitric Oxide in ARDS Study Group: Effects of inhaled nitric oxide in patients with acute respiratory distress syndrome: results of a randomized phase II trial. *Crit Care Med* 26:15-23, 1998.
107. Troncy E, Collet JP, Shapiro S, et al: Inhaled nitric oxide in acute respiratory distress syndrome. A pilot randomized controlled study. *Am J Respir Crit Care Med* 157:1483-1488, 1998.
108. Michael JR, Barton RG, Saffle JR, et al: Inhaled nitric oxide versus conventional therapy. *Am J Respir Crit Care Med* 157: 1372-1380, 1998.
109. Lundin S, Mang H, Smithies M, et al: Inhalation of nitric oxide in acute lung injury: results of a European multicentre study. The European Study Group of Inhaled Nitric Oxide. Inhalation of nitric oxide in acute lung injury: results of a European multicentre study. *Intensive Care Med* 25:911-919, 1999.
110. Taylor RW, Zimmerman JL, Dellinger RP, et al., for the Inhaled Nitric Oxide in ARDS Study Group: Low-dose inhaled nitric oxide in patients with acute lung injury: a randomized controlled trial. *JAMA* 291:1603-1609, 2004.
111. Abman SH, Griebel JL, Parker DK, et al: Acute effects of inhaled nitric oxide in children with severe hypoxemic respiratory failure. *J Pediatr* 124:881-888, 1994.
112. Dobyns EL, Cornfield DN, Anas NG, et al: Multicenter randomized controlled trial of the effects of inhaled nitric oxide therapy on gas exchange in children with acute hypoxemic respiratory failure. *J Pediatr* 134:406-412, 1999.
113. Dobyns EL, Anas NG, Fortenberry JD, et al: Interactive effects of high-frequency oscillatory ventilation and inhaled nitric oxide in acute hypoxemic respiratory failure in pediatrics. *Crit Care Med* 30:2425-2429, 2002.
114. Green TP, Timmons OD, Fackler JC, et al, for the Pediatric Critical Care Study Group: The impact of extracorporeal membrane oxygenation on survival in pediatric patients with acute respiratory failure. *Crit Care Med* 24:323-329, 1996.
115. Ullrich R, Lorber C, Roder G: Controlled airway pressure therapy, nitric oxide inhalation, prone positioning, and extracorporeal membrane oxygenation (ECMO) as components of an integrated approach to ARDS. *Anesthesiology* 91:1577-1585, 1999.
116. Combes A, Figliolini C, Trouillet JL, et al: Incidence and outcome of polymicrobial ventilator-associated pneumonia. *Chest* 121: 1618-1623, 2002.
117. Torres A, Ewig S: Diagnosing ventilator-associated pneumonia. *N Engl J Med* 350:433-435, 2004.
118. Chastre J, Wolff M, Fagon JY, et al., for the PneumA Trial Group. Comparison of 8 vs 15 days of antibiotic therapy for ventilator-associated pneumonia in adults. A randomized trial. *JAMA* 290: 2588-2598, 2003.
119. Jantz MA, Sahn SA: Corticosteroids in acute respiratory failure. *Am J Respir Crit Care Med* 160:1079-1100, 1999.
120. Bernard GR: Corticosteroids, the "terminator" of all untreatable serious pulmonary illness. *Am J Respir Crit Care Med* 168: 1409-1410, 2003.
121. Meduri GU, Belenchia JM, Estes RJ, et al: Fibroproliferative phase of ARDS, clinical findings and effects of corticosteroids. *Chest* 100:943-952, 1991.
122. Meduri GU, Headley S, Tolley E, et al: Plasma and BAL cytokine response to corticosteroid rescue treatment in late ARDS. *Chest* 108:1315-1325, 1995.
123. Meduri UG, Headley AS, Golden E, et al: Effect of prolonged methylprednisolone therapy in unresolving acute respiratory distress syndrome. *JAMA* 280:159-165, 1998.

124. Kotloff RM, Ahya VN, Crawford SW: Pulmonary complications of solid organ and hematopoietic stem cell transplantation. *Am J Respir Crit Care Med* 170:22-48, 2004.
125. Thomas CF Jr, Limper AH: Pneumocystis pneumonia. *N Engl J Med* 350:2487-2498, 2004.
126. Hilbert G, Gruson D, Vargas F, et al: Noninvasive ventilation in immunosuppressed patients with infiltrates, fever, and acute respiratory failure. *N Engl J Med* 344:481-487, 2001.
127. Wysocki M, Tric L, Wolff MA, et al: Noninvasive ventilatory support ventilation in patients with acute respiratory failure. *Chest* 107:761-768, 1995.
128. Antonelli M, Conti G, Rocco M, et al: A comparison of noninvasive positive-pressure ventilation and conventional mechanical ventilation in patients with acute respiratory failure. *N Engl J Med* 339:429-435, 1998.
129. Ferrer M, Esquinas A, Leon M, et al: Noninvasive ventilation in severe hypoxemic respiratory failure. A randomized clinical trial. *Am J Respir Crit Care Med* 168:1438-1444, 2003.
130. Guisset O, Gruson D, Vargas F, et al: Noninvasive ventilation in acute respiratory distress syndrome patients. *Intensive Care Med* 29:S124, 2003 (abstract).
131. Essouri S, Chevret L, Durand P, et al: Noninvasive positive pressure ventilation in one pediatric intensive care unit: a promising approach of respiratory support. *Pediatr Crit Care Med* 6:245, 2005 (abstract).
132. Gregoretti C, Confalonieri M, Navalesi P, et al: Evaluation of patient skin breakdown and comfort with a new face mask for noninvasive ventilation: a multi-center study. *Intensive Care Med* 28:278-284, 2002.
133. Lellouche F, Maggiore SM, Deye N, et al: Effect of the humidification device on the work of breathing during noninvasive ventilation. *Intensive Care Med* 28:1582-1589, 2002.
134. Richard JC, Carlucci A, Breton L, et al: Bench testing of pressure support ventilation with three different generations of ventilators. *Intensive Care Med* 28:1049-1057, 2002.

CHAPTER

47

Extracorporeal Life Support

Heidi J. Dalton

PEARLS

- Venoarterial access for extracorporeal membrane oxygenation has been the most common cannulation technique because it provides both respiratory and cardiac support.
- Venovenous cannulation for ECMO is currently preferred for patients with adequate cardiac function.
- In venoarterial ECMO, desaturated venous blood is drained from the body and reinfused into a large artery after being oxygenated in the ECMO circuit.
- Venovenous ECMO differs from venoarterial in that blood is both withdrawn and returned into the venous circulation of the patient.
- The use of ECMO in neonatal respiratory failure has fallen as new methods of support such as inhaled nitric oxide, surfactant, and high-frequency oscillation have been developed.
- As experience with ECMO support in older patients has grown, expansion to clinical situations such as cancer, sepsis, burns, and trauma has occurred.
- The largest area of growth of extracorporeal support is in patients with cardiogenic shock or following repair of congenital heart defects.
- One quickly expanding area of extracorporeal support is as a means of resuscitation in cardiac arrest. Initial reports of survival are encouraging.
- Improvements in extracorporeal pumps, cannula, circuitry, and oxygenators are making ECMO safer and easier to use.
- A randomized, controlled trial of ECMO in adults with respiratory failure will be complete soon and will offer new information as to the potential benefit of ECMO in older patients.

Aided by the discovery of heparin in 1916[1] and advances in the technology of membrane oxygenators, extracorporeal life support (ECLS) has changed dramatically since John Gibbon first supported a cat whose pulmonary artery was occluded with a clamp using a machine of his own design in the early 1950s.[2] Although early experiences with the use of cardiopulmonary bypass during operations on the heart were mixed, as experience and technology continued to advance, the field of cardiopulmonary bypass expanded at a rapid rate.[3–5] Today, the dreams of men such as Gibbon have been realized, as extracorporeal support for the heart and lungs is used daily throughout the world. Nowhere is the impact of cardiopulmonary bypass seen more clearly than in pediatrics, where increasingly intricate intracardiac repairs of once lethal congenital heart defects are performed with the aid of cardiopulmonary bypass every day.

As experience with bypass techniques in the operating suite grew, investigation began of its use in supporting cardiopulmonary failure in patients outside the operating room.[6,7] Infants with severe respiratory disease or pulmonary hypertension were one of the groups in which use of a temporary cardiopulmonary bypass system seemed appropriate. This technique of modified cardiopulmonary bypass came to be known as *extracorporeal membrane oxygenation* and abbreviated as ECMO.[8] Although premature infants had an unacceptably high incidence of intracranial hemorrhage as a result of the systemic heparinization required, infants older than 35 weeks of gestation with respiratory failure were successfully supported with ECMO.[9,10] An abandoned infant with severe hypoxemia named *Esperanza* (Hope) by her caregivers was among the first placed on ECMO by Bartlett in 1976. Today, Esperanza is a grown woman with children of her own. Efforts to organize and collate data on patients treated with ECMO resulted in the formation of the Extracorporeal Life Support Organization (ELSO). In 2004 ELSO celebrated its 15th anniversary. This largely volunteer network of physicians, surgeons, nurses, respiratory therapists, and others with an interest in ECLS has more than 100 centers as members and contains data on more than 29,000 patients treated with ECLS throughout the world.[11]

As more patients have been treated and techniques refined, the procedures and management of ECMO patients have evolved to allow it to be offered to patient groups previously excluded from consideration.[12–14] Despite multiple attempts to define specific selection criteria for ECMO candidates, no well-defined and universally applied criteria exist. The decision as to when a patient should be placed on ECMO remains a decision often made empirically at the bedside based on the clinician's experience. Similarly, although there is little complete standardization of ECMO circuit design, cannulation techniques, and patient management, the general principles remain fairly constant and differences between centers are minor. The following represents general practice, my experience, and a review of the literature. For more detailed information on ECLS, the reader is directed to the excellent text regarding this subject published by ELSO.

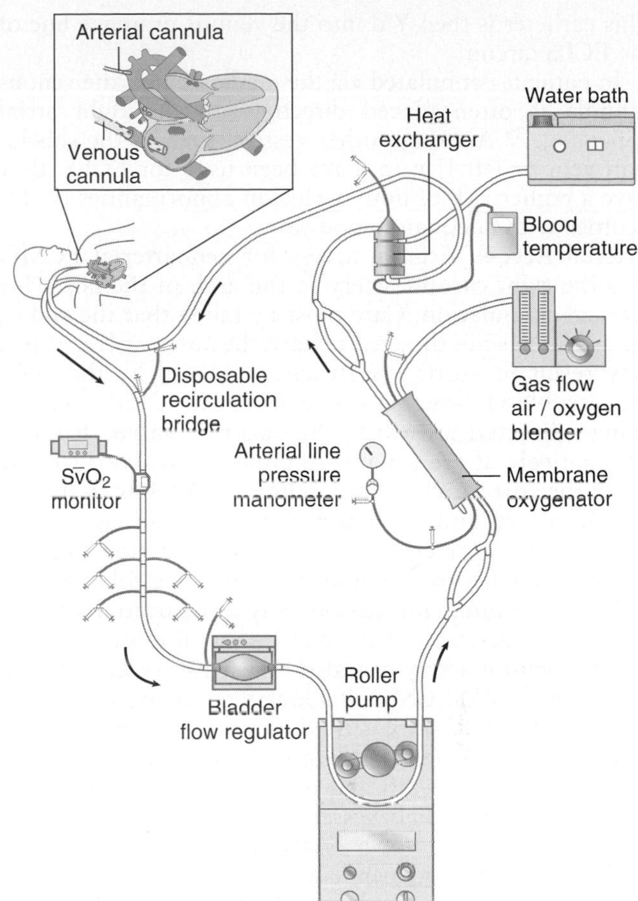

FIGURE 47–1 • Venoarterial extracorporeal life support via cervical cannulation. (M. Dowhy, with permission) (Courtesy Children's Hospital Pittsburgh, or Fuhrman & Zimmerman, *Critical Care*, ed 2, St. Louis, 1998, Mosby.)

Materials and Methods

Cannulation Techniques

Several modes of ECMO, or extracorporeal life support as it is also known, have been developed that differ according to cannulation site and minor physiologic principles. However, the basic circuit is similar for all modes. Patients are cannulated by either the venoarterial or venovenous mode. Venoarterial access is the most common mode of ECMO support and is discussed first.

Venoarterial Extracorporeal Membrane Oxygenation

Venous Access. In venoarterial ECMO, desaturated systemic venous blood is drained from the body and reinfused into a large artery after it has been oxygenated in the ECMO circuit (Figure 47–1). As the right atrium contains the largest amount of venous blood in the body, it is the usual site accessed for ECMO cannulation. The internal jugular (IJ) vein is a large vessel with a fairly short, straight course to the right atrium and thus is preferred during cervical cannulation. To augment cerebral venous drainage in patients cannulated via the right IJ, some centers also place a smaller cannula retrograde in the vessel to the level of the jugular venous bulb at the base of the skull. This catheter can facilitate cerebral venous drainage and provide a means of monitoring jugular venous oxygen saturation. Some clinicians believe that monitoring jugular venous saturation provides information on adequacy of oxygen delivery to the brain and that it is valuable during ECMO, although this is relatively controversial. This cannula is then connected by a Y-shaped connector into the venous drainage line.[15,16]

In older children and adults, the femoral vessels can be used for cannulation.[17] Venous access is obtained from the saphenous or femoral vein into the inferior vena cava (IVC) or the cannula can be advanced further up the IVC to the right atrial–IVC junction. Although femoral vein cannulation diverts less venous return to the pump than a catheter positioned in the right atrium, the amount of blood drained is often adequate to meet the patient's needs. The age and size of patients who are candidates for femoral cannulation are generally confined to adolescents and adults. Some surgeons suggest that if the child is old enough to walk and run, the femoral vessels are of adequate size to consider femoral cannulation. The author has successfully used femoral vessels in a 13-kg, 6-year-old child without difficulty. For patients with femoral venous access who exhibit venous stasis or obstruction of the extremity distal to the cannula, a similar catheter to that used for jugular venous drainage can be placed down the leg via the saphenous or femoral vein to augment decompression of the leg and augment venous return.

This catheter is then Y'd into the venous drainage line of the ECLS circuit.

In patients cannulated via the mediastinum, the venous cannula is often placed directly into the right atrial appendage.[18] Although other vessels, such as the subclavian vein or left IJ vein, have been used for ECLS, they have a higher risk of limb perfusion abnormalities or difficulties with adequate blood flow.

Arterial Access. Arterial access for venoarterial ECMO uses the right carotid artery to the arch of the aorta for cervical cannulation. Care must be taken that the end of the cannula is not directed toward the aortic valve, as this may result in aortic insufficiency induced by the high-velocity blood flow returning from the ECMO circuit being directed toward the aortic valve leaflets. Alternatively, if the arterial cannula is advanced too far down the aortic arch, it can occlude blood flow to the left carotid artery and the brain. Concern over use of the carotid artery for cervical ECMO cannulation and the potential for neurologic abnormalities or stroke later in life is a predominant reason why venoarterial ECMO may be less desirable than venovenous support.

The femoral artery can also be used for access during venoarterial (VA) ECMO. If a long femoral artery cannula that reaches the thorax is used, good oxygenation to the upper body is assured but resistance to flow will be elevated.[19] If a short femoral artery cannula is used, it normally sits in the iliac vessels. The amount of arterial return reaching the upper body, heart, and brain in this mode of ECMO is dependent on antegrade flow out of the native left heart and the retrograde flow from the ECMO arterial return. In patients with severe cardiac dysfunction, arterial return from the ECMO circuit flows further up the aorta and may predominate. In patients with good cardiac function, the majority of upper body arterial flow may be from native left heart ejection. Arterial flow from low-lying ECMO cannulas with good native heart function may thus preferentially flow to the lower body. This arterial flow will mix with venous return from the lower body before the oxygenated blood flows through the cardiopulmonary circuit and out the aorta. In patients with impaired gas exchange, the amount of venous mixing prior to reaching the ascending aorta reduces the amount of oxygen that is delivered to the upper body (heart and brain). Thus the PaO_2 and arterial oxygen saturations in the upper body may be lower than that obtained with cervical VA ECMO. Concern over limited oxygen delivery to the brain has resulted in slow acceptance of VA ECMO with a low-lying femoral arterial cannula. Successful use of ECMO has been achieved, however, with this mode. Monitoring of obtained oxygenation with a pulse oximeter on the ear or nose of the patient is a good safety precaution to assess the amount of oxygenated flow getting to the head during this mode of ECMO. Echocardiography can often determine the extent of retrograde aortic flow versus native heart ejection. Femoral arterial cannulation can also be associated with impaired flow to the distal limb and resultant ischemia. A small "feeder" cannula can be directed distally down the leg artery and then Y'd into the arterial cannula to improve perfusion. Additionally, placement of a 14-gauge catheter into the posterior tibial artery, which is then Y'd into the arterial side of the ECMO circuit, can also provide distal limb perfusion.

In mediastinal cannulation, the arterial return cannula usually is placed into the aortic arch under direct vision.[20] During mediastinal cannulation, patients with severe left ventricular dysfunction who cannot open the aortic valve to eject blood often have a left atrial venting catheter placed to allow decompression of the left heart. This prevents pulmonary venous hypertension, which can lead to severe pulmonary edema or hemorrhage. This catheter can be Y'd into the venous drainage of the ECLS circuit to provide adequate left heart decompression. Patients with intact sternums who require left atrial decompression often are taken to the cardiac catheterization suite for a blade atrial septostomy that then allows the left heart to decompress into the right atrium and the blood to be drained into the venous ECMO cannula.[21]

Other arterial access sites, such as the subclavian, have been used but have experienced difficulty with limb perfusion. One report described successful use of the axillary artery by means of a Gore-Tex graft placed into the side of the vessel for venoarterial support in adult lung transplant patients supported by ECMO.[22]

Venovenous Extracorporeal Membrane Oxygenation

Venovenous ECMO differs from venoarterial ECMO in that blood is both withdrawn and reinfused into the patient's venous circulation (Figure 47–2). Cannulation can be introduced via either the cervical or femoral vessels.[23]

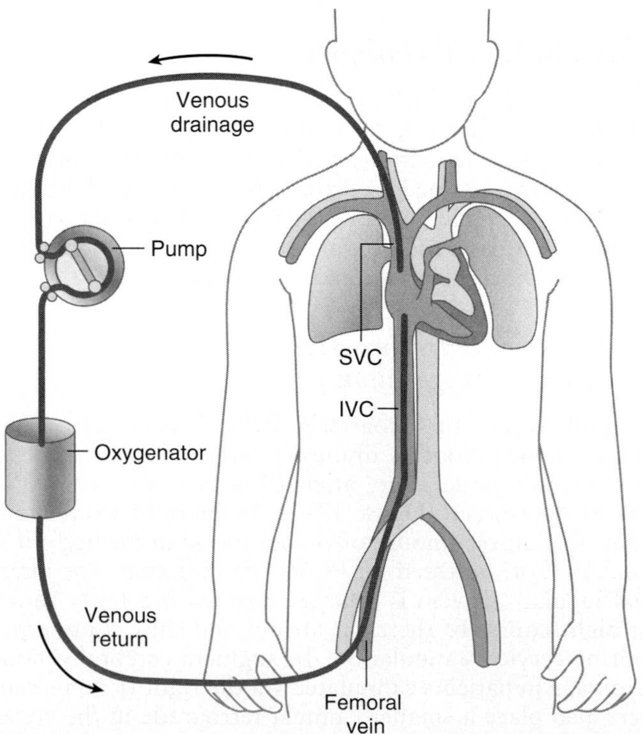

FIGURE 47–2 • Venovenous extracorporeal life support. Note superior vena cava *(SVC)* to right atrium as venous outflow tract and femoral vein to inferior vena cava *(IVC)* as inflow tract. Outflow and inflow drainage and reinfusion directions can be reversed.

A double-lumen, single cannula exists in sizes up to 18F, which can support a child up to about 12 kg.[24] This cannula is placed into the right IJ vein and requires only one surgical site. The drainage and infusion lumens in this cannula are separated by a distance of a few centimeters. In patients too large for double-lumen cannulas, two access sites are required. The right IJ and the femoral vein provide access sites in the majority of patients. Patients with venovenous cannulation may have venous blood drained from the right atrium via the IJ vein or from the IVC via the femoral vein. Although more venous drainage usually can be obtained from a cervical cannula (which usually is shorter and larger than can be placed into the femoral vein), the femoral site may prove adequate. Older children and adults also may have bilateral saphenous or femoral cannulations performed, with one cannula placed into the high IVC and the other ending in the low IVC or iliac vessels[25] (Figure 47–3). Current research is under way to develop larger double-lumen, single cannulas that can be used for IJ or femoral cannulation in large patients and adults. If these techniques are perfected, the application of extracorporeal support likely will become more attractive in older patients.

Several features unique to venovenous cannulation are important to understand. First, because blood is both withdrawn and reinfused into the venous circulation, adequate native cardiac function must exist to provide the "pumping" of oxygenated ECMO return to the patient's systemic circulation. One factor that may influence cardiac function during venovenous ECMO is that well-oxygenated blood returning from the ECMO circuit will enter the right heart. This highly oxygenated blood may reduce pulmonary artery pressure by reducing pulmonary vascular resistance, which in turn may improve right heart function.[26] Likewise, highly saturated blood ejected from the left ventricle to the coronary arteries may improve myocardial blood flow and improve cardiac performance. For these reasons, some clinicians will first try venovenous ECMO in patients with cardiac dysfunction and transition to venoarterial ECMO if support is inadequate. Other clinicians prefer to use venoarterial ECMO preferentially if cardiac dysfunction exists.

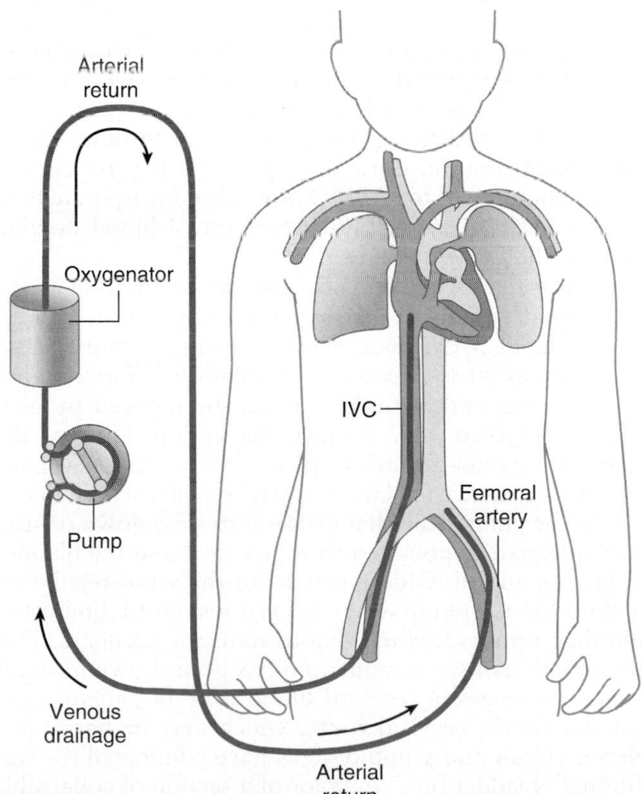

FIGURE 47–3 • Modified venoarterial extracorporeal membrane oxygenation circuit. Bilateral femoral venous and arterial cannulation for extracorporeal life support.

Another feature of venovenous ECMO is that because blood is withdrawn and reinfused into the venous side of the circulation, some of the return coming from the ECMO circuit will be drained by the venous drainage cannula before it goes through the patient's heart into the systemic circulation. This phenomenon is known as *recirculation,* and it can be a major limiting factor in providing adequate patient support with venovenous ECMO.[27] With double-lumen cannulas placed via the right IJ to the right atrium, careful orientation of the inflow lumen toward the tricuspid valve may limit recirculation. With two-site venous cannulation, recirculation can be limited to some degree by ensuring that some distance separates the end tips of the drainage and infusion cannulas in the body. Recirculation also can be reduced by draining from the femoral vein cannula and reinfusing into the right IJ vein cannula. The extent of recirculation can be estimated by following the venous saturation in the ECLS circuit—high levels of recirculation will elevate the displayed venous saturation on the drainage line because some of the highly saturated return from the ECLS circuit is immediately drawn out by the drainage cannula. Whether venovenous cannulation will provide adequate capture of the patient's cardiac output for ECMO support is dependent on how large the cannulas are, where they lie in the vessel, and how much overall ECMO support the patient requires.[28]

Percutaneous Cannulation

Although the historical approach to vessel access has been via an open procedure with placement of cannulas under direct vision, kits for percutaneous placement now exist in many sizes. These kits use a modified Seldinger technique with obturators increasing in size to dilate the vessel. Once the appropriate size is reached, the cannula is passed into the vessel over the largest obturator.[29]

Percutaneous cannulation carries with it the inherent risks of potentially tearing a large vessel during cannulation. Although percutaneous cannulation in some centers is performed by nonsurgical personnel, surgical backup to perform an immediate cutdown for control of bleeding from a disrupted vessel may be necessary. Despite the obvious fear of vessel disruption, few reports of patients receiving percutaneous access have actually noted this as a complication. In one early series of 21 patients cannulated percutaneously, only 18% required any pursestring suturing around the cannulation site for bleeding, and none suffered vessel disruption.[30] Percutaneous cannulation avoids the need for an open surgical site, thus decreasing surgical site bleeding and risk of infection.

Decannulation

Decannulation involves removal of surgically placed cannulas and repair of the operative site, with or without vessel repair. Vessels used in traditional open venotomy or arteriotomy ECMO can often be repaired at decannulation, although this approach is not used universally. Whether avoiding ligation or repairing cannulated vessels results in long-term improvement in blood flow or reduced risk of stroke from thrombosis or infarct is unknown.[31–35] The longest follow-up study of repaired carotid vessels found restenosis or occlusion in 24%. Patients with reconstructed vessels had less neuroradiologic abnormalities or cerebral palsy than unrepaired historical controls, although these data represent a small, single-center report and is not a randomized study.[36]

Percutaneously placed cannulas are merely withdrawn at decannulation while gentle pressure is applied to the site until hemostasis is obtained. Vessels accessed percutaneously are not usually ligated either at initiation or decannulation from ECMO.

Heparin is discontinued at decannulation, and normalization of coagulation usually occurs within a few hours. Protamine can be used for reversal of heparin-induced coagulation effects if desired, although the risk-to-benefit ratio of this approach must be considered. Patients may develop deep venous thrombosis after ECLS has been discontinued, especially if femoral cannulation is used. This may be an additional reason why heparinization should not be reversed.

Venous Reservoir and Venous Saturation Monitor

Following cannulation, venous ECMO blood flows by gravity through the attached tubing to a reservoir called the *bladder.* The bladder historically is a 30- to 50-ml oblong device that sits at the lowest point of the ECMO circuit and allows blood to collect and be drawn from it to the pump head. It also acts as an air trap and normally has access ports to allow aspiration of any air collected in the bladder chamber. The output of the ECMO circuit is determined primarily by the amount of venous blood that can be withdrawn from the patient to enter the circuit. The venous drainage to the bladder is gravity dependent, generated by the pressure difference between the column of blood in the venous cannula and the reservoir. Thus the siphon effect of venous return is augmented by elevating the patient higher above the venous reservoir.[37] Because the venous cannula can drain only as much blood as is available at the cannulation site, adequate systemic venous return must be maintained. In addition to systemic hypovolemia, any process that limits right atrial filling, such as pneumothorax or pneumopericardium, will impede drainage to the ECMO circuit.[38] Changes in venous and arterial tone may alter right atrial and venous filling pressures and affect the amount of venous drainage that can be obtained. The bladder can be used as a servo-regulating device that helps to match forward flow to venous return.

Most centers use some type of venous saturation monitoring device along the venous drainage line. Following venous saturation over time gives information regarding the adequacy of oxygen delivery. Especially in patients receiving ECLS for cardiac support and who have minimal lung injury, care must be taken in interpreting the observed venous saturation. The presence of left atrial drains or left-to-right intracardiac shunts may increase the observed venous saturation in the ECLS drainage line but may not reflect overall venous saturation in the body. Measuring venous saturation as an index of oxygen delivery and consumption balance from another site not involved with the ECLS circuit is recommended in this circumstance.

Pumps

The majority of ECMO centers use a roller head pump during extracorporeal support. This device contains steel roller heads enclosed in a box (the *pump housing*). The heads rotate and push against the ECMO circuit tubing, which is threaded through the box. The piece of tubing in contact with the roller heads is called the *raceway* and is generally composed of a special material called *super-Tygon,* which is less likely to rupture under the wear and tear induced by the roller heads. Blood contained in the tubing is advanced forward by the motion of the roller heads. The amount of blood advanced from the raceway is dependent on the number of revolutions of the roller heads, the tubing size, and the occlusion between the heads and the tubing. Too little contact between the roller heads and the tubing (loose occlusion) decreases the amount of blood advanced, whereas excessive pressure of the roller heads against the tubing (tight occlusion) obstructs blood from moving forward and causes excessive wear on the tubing, which may result in rupture. The correct occlusion is set by measuring the displacement of fluid during roller head rotation during setup of the ECMO circuit. Newer pumps used for ECMO now often incorporate flow probes that display the actual amount of blood flowing through the ECMO circuit.

Loss of venous return with continuous rotation of the roller heads results in generation of high negative pressure in the ECMO tubing that can lead to hemolysis and cavitation as air is drawn out of solution.[39] The collapse of the tubing and cannula that can be induced by high negative pressure can damage the endothelium of the vessel or the right atrium. To protect the patient as venous return is lost and the bladder starts to collapse, a signal is sent to the pump head that causes it to slow down or stop until adequate venous return is achieved and the bladder is once again full. Older versions of the servo-regulation system stop the pump whenever venous return diminishes and then restarts it when venous return is adequate. This on/off action of servo-regulation has been shown to result in acute changes in cerebral blood flow in patients cannulated via the cervical route, which may be harmful.[40] Newer circuit and pump designs have eliminated the traditional “bladder box” in favor of a section of collapsible tubing that performs a similar servo-regulating function. Elimination of the bladder reduces the potential for clot formation. It also removes a potential site for air trapping, however, which was easily accomplished with the older cylindrical bladder design. In the new systems, as venous return to the ECMO circuit diminishes, the collapsible tubing signals the roller heads to slow down and then speed up again once adequate venous return is obtained. This may decrease the on/off action of the roller head pump and potentially limit the acute changes in blood flow noted with the older style of servo-regulation. Newer pumps may be able to provide pulsatile flow, which may be useful in maintaining normal perfusion patterns to the body. The nonpulsatile nature of venoarterial ECMO flow has been suggested as a factor in renal dysfunction that has been noted in patients treated with venoarterial ECMO. The pulsatile flow of the newer pumps has yet to be effectively linked to native heart ejection, although this is a goal in the future. Roller pumps generate high pressure in the circuit distal to the raceway/roller heads. Thus acute interruption to forward flow, as may occur with kinking of the arterial cannula or elevated resistance to blood flow on the high pressure side of the circuit, can result in immediate and potentially lethal circuit rupture. Monitoring of the high-pressure side of the ECMO circuit is almost universal, with critical high limits for arterial line pressure determined based on tubing size and pump flow. Pressures below 300 to 350 mmHg are desired. Newer pump systems provide safety mechanisms to stop the ECMO pump if line pressure limits are exceeded. Some centers use filters in the ECMO circuit prior to blood return to the patient that can help detect air bubbles or trap debris. Although this seems practical, in reality these devices may be so sensitive that they result in many episodes of stopping ECMO to check alarms or maintain the filters. This may harm the patient and is one reason why air detectors or filters are not used universally.

Centrifugal pumps are also used for ECMO support, although much less commonly than roller head pumps. Centrifugal pump heads are shaped like a cone and contain a spinning rotor that is controlled by magnets within and without the cone.[41,42] Blood enters the cone at the apex and is propelled tangentially to the base of the pump head, where it is expelled. The longer blood sits in the centrifugal head and the faster the head spins, the more hemolysis will be created. It also is postulated that development of blood clots in the membrane oxygenator over time increases outflow resistance, which may increase hemolysis within the rotor head. Hemolysis has limited the use of centrifugal pumps. Use of low- resistance, hollow-fiber oxygenators may help this particular problem.

Because blood flow to and from the centrifugal head is identically affected by gravity, centrifugal circuits can be placed at any level relative to the patient. This makes transporting the patient on ECMO easier than with roller head devices. The active suction effect of centrifugal heads can create levels of negative pressures as high as −200 to −700 within the venous inlet tubing. The amount of negative pressure generated by centrifugal pumps can result in hemolysis or endothelial damage to cannulated vessels. Thus noting when adequate venous return is diminishing and understanding the function of centrifugal pumps are keys to safe and appropriate use of this form of support.[43,44] Blood flow from centrifugal devices is nonpulsatile, which raises concerns about secondary organ dysfunction. One potential advantage of centrifugal pumping devices is that air and debris are trapped within the vortex of the pump head and may be less likely to embolize to the patient than with roller head circuits. This is countered by some reports that centrifugal pumps generate more microbubbles than roller head devices, although this has not been confirmed.[45] Centrifugal circuits contain a flow probe that displays how much blood is being returned to the patient. They do not require servo-regulation devices to change the speed of the rotating heads as inflow directly alters outflow. Another advantage of centrifugal pumps is that in case of occlusion of the circuit past the centrifugal head, no high backpressure is exerted that will result in rupture of the circuit. Obstruction to forward flow, however, will result in increased hemolysis from the blood trapped in the centrifugal head. The components of ECMO circuits used with centrifugal pumps can be completely heparin coated, which may limit bleeding or need for exogenous heparin. Although centrifugal pumps are easy to set up and operate, lack of familiarity with them compared with roller head pumps is another reason why they are less common in ECMO practice. Centrifugal pumps that are safer and more efficient are currently entering the marketplace; this may increase the use of these devices for extracorporeal support.

Advances in ECLS likely will be drawn from continuing work with artificial heart or ventricular support devices. One intriguing report from Japan noted successful use of a self-regulating ECMO device that contained two sac-type blood pumps that are placed in parallel and use compressed air to eject blood. This pump is completely self-regulated and provides pulsatile ECMO return. Three neonatal patients with respiratory failure were supported successfully with this device in Japan.[46]

Whether by semiocclusive contact between pump roller heads and ECMO tubing or by advancement through a centrifugal head, blood moves past the pumping device to the membrane oxygenator, where gas exchange occurs. Oxygenated blood then flows through a heat exchanger, where it is rewarmed or cooled depending on the clinical situation, and then returns to the patient.

Membrane Oxygenator

Currently, the predominant membrane oxygenator consists of a silicone membrane envelope (with a plastic spacer screen inside) wound in a spiral fashion around a polycarbonate spool. Gas flows through the interior of the envelope, and blood flows between the turns in the membrane envelope. Blood flow to the membrane lung is controlled by the pump setting.

Gas exchange in the membrane oxygenator is determined by the permeability of the membrane to oxygen and carbon dioxide (their diffusion coefficients), the available membrane surface area, the pressure gradient for oxygen or carbon dioxide between the gas compartment and the blood, and the amount of time gas and blood interface across the membrane.[47] Viscosity, temperature, and pH of the blood can also influence the amount of oxygen binding to the blood as it passes through the oxygenator. Each membrane has a predetermined maximum blood flow above which the thickness of the blood film limits oxygenation. Blood or gas flow in excess of the manufacturer's specifications may generate high pressure within the membrane oxygenator, which may cause it to rupture. If the blood side of the envelope ruptures, blood escapes into the gas side of the envelope and drips out through the gas exit port at the bottom of the oxygenator (this is colloquially called a *nosebleed*). Small breaks in the integrity of the blood–gas barrier with little bleeding can be tolerated because the small tear usually clots off. More vigorous bleeding often requires an emergent oxygenator change. Rupture of the gas side of the envelope from excessive gas pressure can result in transfer of air to the blood phase of the membrane. This is a true emergency that requires immediate stopping of ECMO and replacement of the oxygenator. Although an uncommon complication, massive air embolus and death to the patient can occur in this scenario.

Countercurrent gas and blood flows in the oxygenator provide optimal gas exchange by maintaining the pressure gradient for oxygen transfer from gas to blood along the entire length of the membrane surface. The gravitational gas flow through the membrane also helps remove the condensation that forms when warm blood flows by cooler gas in the membrane. Water droplets are expelled from the membrane surface via the gas exhaust port. Membrane failure can be characterized by a decrease in the capacity to remove carbon dioxide or to oxygenate blood. Membrane failure may result from clot formation on the membrane, which decreases the available surface area for gas exchange; excess condensation in the membrane lung ("pulmonary edema"); or technical defects in the membrane itself. A difference greater than 100 torr between the estimated PaO_2 in membrane gas and that in blood leaving the oxygenator blood may indicate early membrane failure. Membrane failure can also be predicted when the pressure drop between blood entering the membrane and leaving it increases and becomes greater than 100 torr. This may indicate clotting in the membrane oxygenator with restriction to blood flow. Initially, increasing the PO_2 in the membrane gas may augment diffusion of oxygen across the available surface area into the blood and maintain adequate oxygenation. Increasing the flow rate of gas across the membrane may also help remove condensation and improve gas diffusion. When these methods fail or the pressure difference between entry and exit of blood in the oxygenator continues to rise, the oxygenator may need to be replaced. Although the exact timing for membrane oxygenator failure varies, they are not generally rated for use beyond 7 days. Replacement of the oxygenator is usually a quick and uncomplicated process.

Hollow-fiber oxygenators are becoming more available for ECMO use. These devices are microporous and have long thin fibers. Blood flows either between the inside or the outside of the fibers. These devices have a lower resistance to blood flow and a lower priming volume than the traditional silicone membrane lung, which makes them faster and easier to prime.[48] Early versions of these oxygenators were plagued by plasma leakage difficulties that resulted in very short lifespans for the oxygenator and limited their use. Newer versions hold promise as in vivo studies have shown excellent gas exchange, little hemolysis, and durability of days to weeks without failure from plasma leakage. European versions of hollow-fiber oxygenators now last for weeks at a time. Currently, however, only 5% of centers surveyed use hollow-fiber oxygenators for routine ECMO use.[49] The major use for these devices is to treat patients who are acutely deteriorating or arresting. Hollow-fiber oxygenators are faster to prime and are well suited to this situation.

Other Points

One concern with ECMO circuitry is the potential for leeching of high levels of di(2-ethylhexyl)phthalate (DEHP) from the polyvinyl tubing over time, thus increasing the patient's exposure to this chemical. One neonatal ECMO circuit evaluation noted that high levels of DEHP were found on routine roller head use over time.[50] High levels of DEHP have been shown to cause sterility and endocrine abnormalities in rats. A follow-up report of 22 neonatal ECMO patients who are now 14 to 16 years old found no abnormalities in observed genital development; sex hormone levels; or thyroid, renal, or hepatic function.[51]

Work with heparin bonded tubing has resulted in several commercially available products. Although none has proved to effectively reduce the need for systemic heparin administration on a long-term basis, short periods (<24 hours) of support without heparin have been achieved without clotting of the circuit or observable thrombosis in the patient. Complete heparin-bonded ECMO circuits that include a hollow-fiber oxygenator are now available and are used especially in rapid-deployment ECMO situations to lessen or prevent the need for anticoagulation.

Patient Populations Treated with Extracorporeal Life Support

The demographics of patients who have received ECMO support over time are given in Table 47–1.

Neonatal Cardiopulmonary Failure

Most patients treated with ECMO were neonates with severe respiratory failure with overall survival of 77%. Common diagnoses include meconium aspiration syndrome, respiratory distress syndrome, sepsis, and persistent pulmonary hypertension of the newborn (PPHN). With the exception of the last group, most of these infants suffer from a combination of pulmonary parenchymal and vascular dysfunction that leads to impaired gas exchange.[52] The diagnosis, outcome, and mode of ECMO applied in neonatal patients are given in Table 47–2.

Because vasodilation in the pulmonary circuit depends on alveolar oxygen tension (PaO_2) and pH, any process that results in hypoxia or acidosis can cause persistently high pulmonary vascular resistance, failure of the foramen ovale and ductus arteriosus to close, right-to-left shunting, and profound cyanosis. Obstruction to pulmonary venous drainage or abnormalities in the pulmonary vascular circuit also can result in pulmonary hypertension. Whatever the cause, the resulting systemic arterial desaturation may

TABLE 47–1

Total Numbers of Extracorporeal Life Support Patients

Group	Total Cases	Survive to Discharge or Transfer	
NEONATAL			
Respiratory	19,061	14,681	77%
Cardiac	2,215	841	38%
ECPR	151	65	43%
PEDIATRIC			
Respiratory	2,762	1,536	56%
Cardiac	2,936	1,256	43%
ECPR	282	111	39%
ADULT			
Respiratory	972	515	53%
Cardiac	474	156	33%
ECPR	132	50	38%
Total	28,985	19,211	66%

Data modified from ELSO International Summary, July 2004.
ECPR, Extracorporeal cardiopulmonary resuscitation.

depress myocardial performance, worsen acidosis, and perpetuate the dysfunctional circulation. The impact of parenchymal lung disease and PPHN varies among infants, but the circulatory contribution to hypoxia of PPHN is commonly very important.

When medical therapies fail to relieve hypoxia and pulmonary hypertension in an infant, ECMO may be an effective means of support. ECMO provides adequate gas exchange and circulatory support without further exposure to high oxygen concentrations or high airway pressures, thus fostering healing of damaged lungs. The circulatory changes that result from initiation of ECMO also lower pulmonary vascular resistance. Draining right atrial blood reduces right atrial pressure and promotes closure of the foramen ovale. In addition, the reduced blood flow to the pulmonary vascular bed decreases pulmonary flow, reduces pulmonary artery pressure, and relieves right-to-left shunting through the patent ductus arteriosus. Well-oxygenated blood flowing left-to-right through the patent ductus arteriosus promotes its closure. By relieving hypoxia, hypercapnia, and acidosis, ECMO promotes relaxation of pulmonary vascular tone. Normal regression in the amount and extent of smooth muscle found in the pulmonary arteriolar vessels begins.[53] These changes allow the transition to a mature circulation. The infant remains on ECMO until the parenchymal lung disease heals sufficiently to allow adequate gas exchange. Pulmonary function tests indicate, however, that infants are commonly weaned from ECMO with only moderate improvement in mechanical lung function.[54] These observations support the impression that circulatory abnormalities contribute importantly to neonatal "respiratory" failure and may partially explain the dramatic difference in outcome between neonates and older patients treated with ECMO.

Infants with congenital diaphragmatic hernia comprise a special subgroup of patients treated with ECMO for severe pulmonary hypertension and respiratory failure.[55,56] Severe pulmonary hypertension or lung hypoplasia leads to approximately 50% mortality even with ECMO support.[57] Morphologic examination, better understanding of the pathophysiology of this lesion, and stabilization with ECMO as needed preoperatively has improved

TABLE 47–2

Neonatal Extracorporeal Life Support for Respiratory Failure

Primary Diagnosis	Total Cases	Number Surviving	Percent Surviving
NEONATAL CASES BY DIAGNOSIS			
Congenital diaphragmatic hernia	4,491	2,367	53
Meconium aspiration syndrome	6,560	6,160	94
Persistent pulmonary hypertension of the newborn/persistent fetal circulation	2,914	2,287	78
Infant respiratory distress syndrome	1,380	1,161	84
Sepsis	2,384	1,794	75
Other	1,567	1,003	64
Mode	**Total Cases**	**Number Surviving**	**Percent Surviving**
NEONATAL MODE OF EXTRACORPOREAL LIFE SUPPORT			
VA	13,301	9,882	74
VV	276	220	80
VVDL	3,537	3,053	86
VA(+V)	1,159	868	75
VV → VA	544	360	66
VVDL+V	410	346	84

Data modified from ELSO International Summary, July 2004.
VA, Venoarterial; *VV,* venovenous; *VVDL,* venovenous double lumen.

survival in some centers in this challenging group of patients.[58–61]

As alternative support methods such as high-frequency ventilation, surfactant, and inhaled nitric oxide have been developed and their use accepted in the neonatal population, the need for ECMO support has declined.[62] Neonatal ECMO cases now number approximately 800 per year, down from the peak of 1500 cases per year in the early 1990s. Survival has also decreased in the neonatal population over the past few years. This is speculated to be related to delays in institution of ECMO while other, less-invasive therapies were attempted. Infants who do not respond to all other therapies and require ECMO thus may be sicker than in years past when ECMO was the only "rescue" therapy available. Although this explanation seems logical, in an evaluation of the ELSO registry data, there was no difference in outcome between infants who received treatment with inhaled nitric oxide, high-frequency ventilation, or both prior to ECMO and those who did not.[63] Similarly, there was no statistical difference in measures of respiratory severity such as $AaDo_2$ or oxygenation index in the past few years. An alternative explanation is that use of ECMO has expanded from "simple" neonates with respiratory failure to now include a variety of neonates with comorbidities that may influence survival.

Pediatric and Adult Patients

Approximately 200 nonneonatal pediatric patients receive ECMO each year for severe respiratory failure, with an overall survival rate of 53% (Table 47–3).[64] Most patients suffer from severe hypoxia, hypercapnia, or intractable air leaks. Pulmonary dysfunction resulting from bacterial or viral pneumonia, aspiration syndromes, intrapulmonary hemorrhage, acute respiratory distress syndrome, and other poorly defined disorders have been successfully treated with ECMO. The uncertainties accompanying the use of ECMO in neonates, who compose a homogeneous group relative to other age groups, are compounded in older children. The enormously heterogeneous older pediatric population spans nearly two decades of physiologic development, and cardiorespiratory failure develops from a multitude of different disorders. Furthermore, many patients have varying degrees of multiple organ failure along with respiratory disease at the time ECMO is instituted. Resolution of both lung disease and secondary organ dysfunction must occur to achieve survival. These factors result in lower survival rates in older patients treated with ECMO than rates achieved in the neonatal patient population.[65]

Despite attempts to define predictive models for ECMO candidacy and institution, none has proved universally applicable. The clinician still most often relies on clinical judgment at the bedside to determine when conventional medical therapy has failed. Perhaps the largest change in nonneonatal ECMO in the past few years is the variety of patients to whom it has been applied. Patients with recent trauma, tracheal injury requiring reconstruction, burns, smoke inhalation, severe sepsis, immunocompromised patients, and toxic ingestions with cardiopulmonary collapse are some of the types of patients who may have been excluded from ECMO support a few years ago but have now received successful ECMO therapy.[66–69] The multiple exclusion criteria used in the early days of ECMO have now been fairly well eliminated, and each potential patient is considered on a case-by-case basis. Even patients with known bleeding disorders, such as hemophilia, have received ECMO support.[70]

Perhaps one group in which ECMO is still cautiously avoided or rarely applied is patients with malignancy and bone marrow transplant. The continued high mortality in these patients when respiratory failure develops, however,

TABLE 47–3

Extracorporeal Life Support for Pediatric Respiratory Failure

Primary Diagnosis	Total Cases	Number Surviving	Percent Surviving
PEDIATRIC CASES BY DIAGNOSIS			
Bacterial pneumonia	290	157	54
Viral pneumonia	728	457	63
Aspiration pneumonia	168	110	65
ARDS	348	188	54
Acute respiratory failure, non-ARDS	605	286	47
Other	671	359	54
Mode	**Total Cases**	**Number Surviving**	**Percent Surviving**
PEDIATRIC MODE OF EXTRACORPOREAL LIFE SUPPORT			
VA	1663	851	51
VV	510	328	64
VVDL	283	200	71
VA(+V)	89	42	47
VV → VA	163	74	45
VVDL+V	44	32	73

ARDS, Acute respiratory distress syndrome; *VA*, venoarterial; *VV*, venovenous; *VVDL*, venovenous double lumen.
Data modified from ELSO International Summary, July 2004.

has caused several clinicians to advocate for application of ECMO at an early stage of disease to determine if outcome can be improved. A review of ECMO use in 30 cancer patients from 58 centers noted an overall survival in 37%. Of seven patients with bone marrow transplant who received ECMO, 2 (29%) patients survived.[71]

The potential impact of ECMO on patients suffering from or at risk for developing multiple system failure is intriguing. Rather than being a treatment restricted to patients with only respiratory failure, ECMO can provide circulatory support as well. It can readily be combined with hemofiltration to augment renal function, provide stable hemodynamics to allow use of plasmapheresis or plasma exchange, allow use of hepatic support devices, or be coupled with a variety of these adjunct therapies. As a consequence, ECMO may benefit patients with established multisystem dysfunction. Implementation of ECMO during multiple organ systems failure now occurs under a variety of conditions, with resolution of organ dysfunction and good outcome obtained in some patients.[72] Furthermore, because it avoids the circulatory derangements that often result from extreme forms of mechanical ventilation and provides systemic perfusion without the need for high dose levels of inotropic agents, ECMO may prevent damage to other systems.

Adult patients have received ECMO support, although only a minority of patients (Table 47–4). Several attempts at randomized trials of ECMO use in adults did not show benefit of ECMO and to many clinicians the lack of benefit argued against consideration of ECMO use in adults.[73] However, all of these studies had design and procedure flaws that may have affected results. Although not randomized trials, multiple reports of successful use of ECMO in adults exist.[74,75] In one report of ECMO use in 255 adults with severe respiratory failure, 68% were weaned off ECMO support and 53% survived to discharge. Multivariate analysis noted that age, gender, pH less than 7.10, number of pre-ECMO ventilator days, and pre-ECMO PaO_2/FIO_2 were associated with outcome.[76] Other reports of successful use of ECMO in adult burn patients, trauma, myocardial infarct with arrest, and a variety of other disease processes exist in the literature. The large size of adult patients makes them ideal for venovenous ECMO support, which may be important in older patients. The need to use the carotid artery for ECMO support in older patients has been another reason why clinicians have avoided ECMO in this age group. Advances in ECMO technology and a newly funded grant by the National Institutes of Health to develop large double-lumen single cannulas that can be used in adult-size patients may make ECMO a more attractive and accepted modality in this population. The lack of adult ECMO centers and poor awareness of the technique and potential benefits among adult clinicians are major obstacles to acceptance of ECMO use in adults. Currently, many pediatric ECMO centers (including my own) are opening their ECMO programs to adults and trying to teach adult caregivers about the potential benefits of ECMO in selected patients. Alternative support techniques, such as the implantable artificial lung, are close to clinical application and may provide rescue modalities for adult respiratory failure.[77–79]

Extracorporeal Membrane Oxygenation for Myocardial Dysfunction

Perhaps the largest expansion in application of ECMO has been in patients with cardiogenic shock or following repair of congenital heart defects.[80–82] The International ELSO Registry lists more than 6000 patients who received ECMO for cardiac failure, predominantly following surgical repair of congenital heart defects (Table 47–5).[83] Outcome of neonatal and pediatric patients notes that 56% are successfully weaned from ECMO and 40% are discharged alive from the hospital. Adult cardiac patients have slightly decreased survival, with 47% weaned off ECMO and 36% discharged from the hospital.

Although center-specific factors separating patients with myocardial dysfunction who will die from those who will recover adequate function without such invasive support have been put forth in the literature, none has been universally accepted.[84–87] Patients with evidence of low cardiac output and shock (including low urine output, poor perfusion, hypotension, elevated cardiac filling pressures, and low mixed venous oxygen saturation) despite maximal respiratory and pharmacologic support are candidates for ECMO rescue. The absence of clear criteria for using ECMO and the reluctance to initiate such invasive support often delay use until cardiac arrest has occurred.

TABLE 47–4

Extracorporeal Life Support for Adult Respiratory Failure

Primary Diagnosis	Total Cases	Number Surviving	Percent Surviving
ADULT CASES BY DIAGNOSIS			
Bacterial pneumonia	186	97	52
Viral pneumonia	87	54	62
Aspiration pneumonia	32	18	56
ARDS, postoperative/trauma	132	68	52
ARDS, not postoperative/trauma	196	100	51
Acute respiratory failure, non-ARDS	55	35	64
Other	317	154	49

ARDS, Acute respiratory distress syndrome.
Data modified from ELSO International Summary, July 2004.

TABLE 47–5

Extracorporeal Life Support for Cardiac Failure: Cardiac Runs by Diagnosis

Age Group	Total Runs	Survived	Percent Survived
0–30 Days			
Congenital defect	2006	719	36
Cardiac arrest	24	5	21
Cardiogenic shock	22	11	50
Cardiomyopathy	72	48	67
Myocarditis	27	11	41
Other	168	74	44
31 Days to < 1 Year			
Congenital defect	1318	548	42
Cardiac arrest	25	6	24
Cardiogenic shock	11	4	36
Cardiomyopathy	61	28	46
Myocarditis	33	18	55
Other	155	65	42
1 Year to < 16 Years			
Congenital defect	740	297	40
Cardiac arrest	49	19	39
Cardiogenic shock	34	11	32
Cardiomyopathy	200	108	54
Myocarditis	96	60	63
Other	260	113	43
16 Years and Older			
Congenital defect	42	12	29
Cardiac arrest	43	9	21
Cardiogenic shock	74	34	46
Cardiomyopathy	73	25	34
Myocarditis	14	9	64
Other	297	92	31

Data modified from ELSO International Summary, July 2004.

As a result, a significant number of patients treated with ECMO have recovered from myocardial function only to die of hypoxic/ischemic encephalopathy suffered before ECMO was started.

One trend in cardiac patients is to consider ECMO earlier in the course of dysfunction. Availability of ECMO is now a mandatory portion of many cardiac surgical programs. As newer and smaller cardiac assist devices are developed for pediatric patients, the need for ECMO support in this population may wane but, at this time, ECMO provides the most readily available support technique for cardiac failure over a wide range of patient ages and sizes.[88,89]

Most patients requiring ECMO for circulatory support have undergone VA ECMO because of its capacity to bypass the heart. Although many patients are cannulated through the carotid and jugular vessels, transthoracic cannulation is performed frequently in postoperative patients. Use of the femoral vessels also is feasible. Patients with very severe left ventricular dysfunction may require an additional cannula to decompress the left ventricle. After evidence of myocardial recovery on ECMO, patients are tested on progressively lower flows, with assessment of myocardial function by echocardiography and observation of systemic blood pressure, perfusion, blood gas tensions, and mixed venous oxygen saturation. When a patient exhibits good ventricular function and adequate systemic circulation at low flow, ECMO is discontinued and the patient returned to conventional therapy.

Most patients recover myocardial function within 72 hours of ECMO support. In most reports, patients whose myocardial function has not improved substantially within 24 to 72 hours of rest on ECMO are not likely to recover cardiac function sufficient to support life.[90,91] Transplantation may be an option in these patients if their underlying cardiac anatomy and general clinical condition make them appropriate candidates.[92] Cardiac patients with good respiratory function may not routinely require ventilator support. Such patients may require only low levels of ventilator support or even be extubated during ECMO. This may alleviate the need for heavy sedation to maintain endotracheal tube position.

Myocarditis and cardiomyopathy are two categories of nonsurgical cardiac failure that have increasingly received ECLS support. Although it may be difficult acutely to differentiate cardiomyopathy from viral myocarditis, both diseases may benefit from mechanical support with ECMO or ventricular assist devices (VADs) that create a stable hemodynamic milieu where the heart can "rest" and recover. Data from the ELSO registry reveals approximately 52% survival in cardiomyopathy/myocarditis patients who receive ECLS support. In a review of 15 children with viral myocarditis supported with ECMO (n = 12) or VADs (n = 3), overall survival was 80%.[93] Nine of the 15 patients recovered cardiac function and were able to be weaned successfully from mechanical support. Follow-up after 0.9 to 5.3 years found normal ventricular function in these children. Cardiac transplantation was required in the six other patients, with overall survival of 83%. The need for transplantation was noted to be higher in the early study period, perhaps reflecting the common belief that patients without recovery of myocardial function within 24 to 72 hours of ECLS were unlikely to be able to be weaned off mechanical support. Although this notion holds true for postoperative cardiac failure patients in the majority of circumstances, it now is recognized that nonsurgical patients should be treated differently. Adequate ventricular recovery may occur after a prolonged period of mechanical support and obviate the need for transplantation. The median duration of mechanical support in the 15 myocarditis patients reported was 140 hours, with a range of 48 to 400 hours. Persistent elevation of central venous pressure and multiple organ dysfunction despite ECLS support for 24 hours were markers of poor prognosis or need for transplantation.

To obtain more specific information regarding cardiac ECMO, an addendum to the ELSO registry form was developed several years ago. Now in use for about 3 years, this addition allows for more specific determination of cardiac ECMO prognostic factors, diagnoses, complications, and outcomes.

Extracorporeal Membrane Oxygenation for Resuscitation

One extreme form of cardiac support is among the fastest expanding use of ECMO at the current time. This type of support is termed *extracorporeal cardiopulmonary resuscitation* (ECPR), or ECMO during cardiac arrest. Designed as a resuscitative tool for patients in cardiac arrest, ECPR use has been reported in more than 400 neonates, children, and adults, with an overall survival to discharge rate of 36%. To facilitate expedient access to ECMO support for ECPR, in situations of acute deterioration or whenever there is insufficient time or personnel for routine ECMO, many centers maintain a "rapid deployment" ECMO circuit setup that either is preprimed with a crystalloid solution or can be primed within a very short period. Other centers use a portable, centrifugal bypass perfusion system that is also easily set up within 10 to 20 minutes. Both methods often use a hollow-fiber membrane oxygenator, which is less difficult and faster to prime for use than a traditional silicone-coated membrane lung used in routine ECMO. Although ECPR is still new enough that definitive information on patient selection, management, and outcome is not available, the initial reports seem to be encouraging, especially in cardiac patients with acute, witnessed arrests who can be placed on ECMO support in a very short time frame.[94,95]

Patient Selection Criteria

Various mortality prediction criteria have been put forth as indicators of when ECMO rescue is best applied, although many of these criteria have been derived from small series of historical data for respiratory failure patients or extrapolated from neonatal respiratory failure data.[95–99] Attempts to provide universally accepted criteria for institution of ECMO have proved difficult.

The predominant listed criteria for placing a pediatric patient on ECMO remains "failure to respond." Although there is no strict definition of what "failure to respond" entails, the basic premise may be interpreted as the clinician who is caring for the patient determining that current support is insufficient and death is imminent without ECMO rescue. More than 50% of pediatric ECMO patients reported to the ELSO registry have "failure to respond" as the major criteria for initiation of ECMO.

The majority of patients who are placed on ECMO have not responded to less invasive methods of respiratory support. Such methods of support often include conventional mechanical ventilation in pressure-control or pressure-regulated volume control modes, high positive end-expiratory pressure (PEEP), high-frequency ventilation (HFV), surfactant, or inhaled nitric oxide. An evaluation of the ELSO registry noted that in pediatric patients who received ECMO, use of both inhaled nitric oxide and HFOV prior to ECMO was associated with poorer outcome than in patients who received neither or only one of these modalities prior to ECMO.[100] Examples of selection criteria for ECLS may include the following:

1. Requirement for F_{IO_2} > 60% to maintain arterial oxygen saturation > 85% – 90% despite high PEEP
2. Mean airway pressures > 20 cmH_2O on conventional mechanical ventilation
3. Mean airway pressures > 25–35 cmH_2O on high-frequency ventilation
4. Evidence of ongoing barotrauma in the form of air leak or pulmonary interstitial edema
5. Oxygenation index (OI) > 40, where OI = (100 × [Mean airway pressure × F_{IO_2}])/Pa_{O_2}
6. Mechanical ventilation < 7–14 days
7. Lack of an underlying irreversible illness
8. Lack of known significant neurologic damage
9. Lack of an ongoing bleeding diathesis
10. Inability to ventilate

There has been concern that respiratory severity indices reported in the past are not applicable to today's respiratory failure patients, although there are few reports comparing past severity indices to outcome in the current era. One report examined the current utility of respiratory severity indices used in the past for potential ECMO eligibility in 118 children with acute hypoxemic respiratory failure.[100] Indices examined included AaD_{O_2}, OI, Pa_{O_2}/F_{IO_2}, ventilation index, and mean airway pressure (Paw), as well as individual ventilator settings and arterial blood gas values. When risk of mortality based on respiratory severity indices was compared with actual mortality observed in these 118 children, survival was much better than would have been predicted based on historical data.[101] As an example, OI > 40 has been associated with > 80% risk of death in the past. Although only 15 patients reached OI > 40 in this study, the positive predictive risk of mortality in these patients was 40%, significantly lower than predicted by past reports. AaD_{O_2} > 450 for 24 hours, Paw > 23, or AaD_{O_2} > 420 had positive predictive value for mortality of 32% to 40%. Using logistic regression, no respiratory parameter (AaD_{O_2}, OI, Paw, ventilator settings, or blood gas values) was independently correlated with death. All deaths were associated with multiorgan system failure, coincident pathology, or perceived treatment futility leading to limitation or withdrawal of care. The overall mortality of these 118 children was 22%, with no previously healthy child dying of respiratory failure. Nonconventional therapies applied included high-frequency ventilation in 25 (21%) of 119 (survival 64%), surfactant administration in 15 (31%) of 119 (survival 73%), inhaled nitric oxide in 38 (32%) of 119 (survival 69%), and ECMO in 4 (3%) of 119 (survival 75%) patients.

Gas Exchange and Oxygen Delivery

Oxygenation

The difference between the partial pressure of oxygen (P_{O_2}) in the gas supplied to the oxygenator and that in the patient's systemic venous blood provides the "driving pressure" across the membrane lung. As an example, 30% oxygen blended into the gas entering the oxygenator results in an estimated Pa_{O_2} of approximately 228 torr at sea level. P_{O_2} of venous blood entering the oxygenator depends on the difference between oxygen delivery and consumption in the patient but usually is approximately

40 torr. The driving pressure for oxygen diffusion into the blood thus would be approximately 188 torr (228 torr − 40 torr = 188 torr), which usually is adequate to achieve 100% saturation of hemoglobin. Higher oxygen concentrations in the gas phase may be necessary to compensate for loss of membrane surface area over time to maintain hemoglobin saturation. Once oxyhemoglobin saturation exceeds 95%, however, higher oxygen concentration in the sweep gas results in a higher PO_2 in postoxygenator blood but a negligible increment in overall oxygen content. For this reason, oxygen concentration in sweep gas usually is adjusted to maintain an oxygen saturation of approximately 95% in postoxygenator blood.

Carbon Dioxide Exchange

The pressure gradient for carbon dioxide between blood and gas is less than that for oxygen. The partial pressure of carbon dioxide in the body usually is low (the venous partial pressure of carbon dioxide, $PvCO_2$, is 45–55 torr), so the pressure difference between the blood and gas phase in the oxygenator is much less than with oxygen. Despite the small pressure difference, the membrane's high diffusion coefficient for carbon dioxide (at least six times that for oxygen) allows excellent carbon dioxide removal, even at low flow rates. To eliminate more carbon dioxide, the gas flow in the membrane must be increased, much as alveolar ventilation must increase to eliminate carbon dioxide from the body under physiologic conditions. Carbon dioxide removal is also limited by the surface area across which gas exchange can occur. Thus increased carbon dioxide clearance may be obtained by using larger oxygenators or using more than one oxygenator in parallel in the circuit. Conversely, to prevent excessive CO_2 removal and hypocapnia in small infants and neonates, carbon dioxide may be blended into the gas mixture to further reduce the partial pressure difference between blood and gas and maintain normocarbia.

Oxygen Delivery

During venoarterial ECMO, both increasing oxygen delivery and increasing the patient's PaO_2 and arterial saturation can be accomplished by increasing the ECMO flow rate. This diverts more of the systemic venous return into the ECMO circuit for oxygenation while proportionally decreasing the amount of venous blood that enters the diseased pulmonary circuit. The result of increasing ECMO flow is an increase in oxygen delivery provided by the circuit and an elevation in measured systemic arterial saturation and PaO_2. Another means to change the ratio of native blood flow to that from the ECMO circuit is to decrease the overall blood volume in the patient. During cardiopulmonary bypass, filling pressures and overall blood volume can be adjusted by removal of blood volume into the bypass circuit. Circulating volume is also frequently decreased by modified ultrafiltration. During ECMO, these same principles can be followed: excessively high filling pressures can be lowered by simple removal of blood volume from the circuit and diuretics, and renal replacement strategies can be used to control fluid balance. Care must be taken, however, to avoid decreasing circulating volume excessively, as this in turn may cause tissue hypoperfusion or an increase in oxygen extraction.

Systemic oxygen delivery is defined as the product of cardiac output and arterial oxygen content.[102] By altering the amount of cardiac output diverted from the patient to the ECMO circuit, venoarterial ECMO can be "complete" or "partial." In the patient on "complete" VA ECMO, the cardiopulmonary circuit is almost totally bypassed and oxygen delivery is determined by the product of pump flow and the oxygen content of blood leaving the oxygenator. Most centers use partial venoarterial ECMO because adequate systemic oxygenation can be achieved by diverting less than 100% of cardiac output to the ECMO circuit. Studies have suggested that complete bypass of the pulmonary circuit may lead to pulmonary alkalosis or ischemia and cause direct damage of the pulmonary capillary bed.[103] Microsphere studies have shown that the majority of coronary artery perfusion comes from native left heart ejection during ECMO, which is another reason to avoid total bypass.[104] Monitoring of adequate oxygen delivery is aided by following venous saturation.[105] Most ECMO circuits contain a sensor along the venous return line that measures and displays venous saturation. Other centers use an in-dwelling blood gas monitor for the same purpose. Low venous saturation and other markers such as elevated lactate, poor perfusion, decreased urine output, and mental status changes may indicate need for improved oxygen delivery. If ECMO flow cannot be increased to provide adequate support, an additional drainage cannula to improve ECMO flow may be necessary.

In patients cannulated via the venovenous route, reduced systemic oxygenation resulting from less bypass obtained in this mode and the effect of recirculation is observed compared with patients with venoarterial ECMO. Persistent signs of inadequate oxygen delivery or continued hemodynamic instability with venovenous ECMO may require conversion to venoarterial ECMO. Patients with venovenous ECMO support or who have a left atrial communication to the ECMO circuit may have artificially high measured venous saturations because of mixing of well-oxygenated blood with systemic venous return. Following venous saturations from another site in the body may be helpful in monitoring adequacy of support in this circumstance.

One novel means to improve oxygenation to the head and upper body in patients cannulated through bilateral femoral veins is to add another venous cannula via the right IJ to the right atrium. Connecting this cannula into the inflow return side of the ECMO circuit will increase the amount of oxygenated bypass directly returning to the right heart. This may improve overall oxygen delivery to the patient while still avoiding the need for arterial vessel cannulation.

Loose occlusion of the roller heads against the raceway tubing can lead to less blood being propelled forward through the ECMO circuit and reduce systemic oxygen delivery. Although this is an uncommon problem, failure to recognize the condition can be harmful to the patient. Persistent vasodilation, which occurs with sepsis, may require the administration of low levels of vasoconstricting agents to maintain adequate central venous pressures and adequate pump return without massive fluid administration.

Patient Management

Screening

Infants who are candidates for ECMO undergo routine cranial ultrasonography to identify existing intracranial hemorrhage.[106,107] The presence of hemorrhage greater than that confined to the germinal matrix (grade I) is a contraindication to ECMO because heparinization may cause additional bleeding. Older patients may have evaluation of intracranial bleeding by ultrasound if an open fontanelle is present. Computed tomography (CT) can be useful if the patient is stable enough to undergo such an examination. Frequently, however, older patients are not stable enough to undergo CT scan, and clinical neurologic evaluation may be hampered by sedation or neuromuscular blockade prior to ECMO. The decision to place a patient on ECMO is made on best assessment of neurologic function. Echocardiography usually is performed prior to ECMO to determine if hypoxia is the result of structural defects in the heart that may be better served by surgical repair than by ECMO support. Echocardiography is also used to detect the presence and direction of central shunts and to assess myocardial function.[108,109]

Cannulation and Initiation of Extracorporeal Life Support

Guidelines for selecting cannula size and circuit components based on patient weight are given in Table 47–6A for cardiac patients and Table 47–6B for respiratory failure patients.

Cannulation usually is performed at the bedside, with the patient receiving a combination of local anesthetics and intravenous analgesics, sedatives, and neuromuscular blocking drugs. An initial bolus of heparin (usually 50–200 U/kg) and continued heparin infusion ensures systemic anticoagulation for the duration of ECMO. Activated clotting time, measured at the bedside, provides a gauge for adjusting the heparin dose to avoid either catastrophic clotting in the circuit or bleeding complications.[110] The ECMO flow initially is begun at 50 ml/kg/min and increased in 50 to 100-ml increments. In infants, a rate of 100 to 200 ml/kg/min usually provides adequate perfusion and oxygenation, although patients in a state of high cardiac output, such as sepsis, may require more. Use of high-flow ECMO is recommended for patients with single-ventricle physiology and a systemic-to-pulmonary artery shunt to provide adequate circulation for both systemic and pulmonary organs.[111] Pediatric patients usually require about 90 ml/kg/min of ECMO flow to maintain adequate oxygen delivery, and adult patients require rates of 70 ml/kg/min. Estimates of flow needs can be predicted using cardiac index data based on body surface area. One caution in estimating ECMO flow in this manner is that patients with sepsis or multiple organ dysfunction may require flows that are much higher than predicted. These factors must be taken into account when selecting cannula size, as cannula size larger than predicted by body surface area may be required. Patients with sepsis or critical illness may require flows that are higher than predicted from body surface area algorithms. In venoarterial ECMO, the arterial waveform provides a rough estimate of the degree of bypass provided by the ECMO circuit. Because ECMO flow is nonpulsatile, increasing flow and decreasing left ventricular output result in flattening of the arterial wave contour. Severe myocardial dysfunction also may cause a flattened wave contour. This effect must be kept in mind when waveform contour is used to monitor the extent of bypass.

Priming

Priming the ECMO circuit prior to initiation is accomplished with a crystalloid solution that is then replaced with blood. Because required blood usually has been citrated

TABLE 47–6A

Sample Components for Cardiac ECLS Based on Patient Weight

	Weight (kg)					
	2.5–6	**6–12**	**12–25**	**25–40**	**40–70**	**70+**
Tubing pack (inch)	1/4	1/4	3/8	3/8	1/2	1/2
Raceway (inch)	1/4–3/8	3/8	3/8–1/2	1/2	1/2	1/2
Oxygenator	0800	1500	I-2500	I-3500	I-4500	I-4500 × 2
Venous cannula (F)	10–15	14–19	17–19	19–21	19–23	19–29
Chest venous cannula (F)	16	20	22	24–28	28–32	32–36
Arterial cannula (F)	8–12	12–15	14–17	17–21	17–21	19–23
Blood prime (U PRBC)*	1	1–2	2–3	3–4	4	4–5

Modified from University of Michigan, Ann Arbor, Michigan, and Children's National Medical Center, Washington, DC.
These are guidelines only; individual variables must be considered!
Estimates are for roller head pump with silicone membrane oxygenator.
All cannula references are for Biomedicus.
*Consider adding albumin 25% 200 ml after crystalloid priming. Also may add fresh-frozen plasma 50 ml/U packed red blood cells (PRBC).
ECLS, extracorporeal life support.

TABLE 47–6B

Sample Components for Respiratory Failure Extracorporeal Life Support Based on Patient Weight for Respiratory Failure Patients

	Weight (kg)					
	2.5–6	6–12	12–25	25–40	40–70	70+
Tubing pack (inch)	1/4	1/4	3/8	3/8	1/2	1/2
Raceway (inch)	1/4	1/4–3/8	3/8	1/2	1/2	1/2
Oxygenator(s)	0800	1500	I-2500	I-3500	I-4500	I-4500 × 2
Venous cannula (F)	10–15†	14–18†	15–19	19–21	19–23	19–29
Arterial cannula (F)	8–12	12–15	14–17	17–21	17–21	19–23
Blood prime (U/PRBC)*	1	1–2	2–3	3–4	4	4–5

Modified from University of Michigan, Ann Arbor, Michigan, and Children's National Medical Center, Washington, DC.
These are guidelines only; individual variables must be considered!
Estimates are for roller head pump with silicone membrane oxygenator.
All cannula references are for Biomedicus; shortest cannula available in specified sizes except DLC.
*Consider adding albumin 25% 200 ml after crystalloid priming. Also may add fresh-frozen plasma 50 ml/U packed red blood cells (PRBCs).
†V-V DLC available 12F, 15F, 18F by Origen, 14F by Kendall.

and stored, it may be acidotic, calcium depleted, and have a high potassium level. Addition of calcium (usually as calcium chloride), bicarbonate or THAM (tromethamine), and heparin is performed during the priming procedure. Electrolytes should be measured in the priming blood before bypass is begun, as disturbances of cardiac rhythm or frank cardiac arrest can occur upon initiation of ECMO.[112] Hyperkalemia exists almost universally in the ECMO-primed circuit despite buffering by calcium and bicarbonate. The potassium level rarely causes systemic effects once the ECMO prime is diluted with the patient's intrinsic blood volume. As an example, if a neonatal patient with a blood volume similar to that of the ECMO circuit has a potassium level of 3 and the ECMO prime has a potassium level of 7, the circulating potassium level may be approximately 5 on ECMO initiation. This likely will not cause systemic or cardiac effects. Larger patients with blood volumes proportionally much less than that of the ECMO circuit will have less risk of hyperkalemia or hypocalcemia. Use of the freshest blood available may lessen the degree of hyperkalemia in the primed circuit. Rarely, hyperkalemia may be of such concern that blood must be washed prior to ECMO use or the primed ECMO circuit cannot be used until the potassium level is reduced. In this circumstance, replacement of blood in the circuit with fresh-frozen plasma or albumin is done to lower the circulating potassium concentration in the prime.

Patient Management During Extracorporeal Life Support

Hypovolemia causes low central venous pressures and results in decreased venous return to the circuit. This can be easily corrected with fluid administration. Increased oxygen delivery also can be accomplished by increasing the pump flow rate, which increases blood diverted into the ECMO circuit for oxygenation. Anemia can be corrected with transfusion of blood products. Maintenance of hematocrit of 30% to 40% usually is sufficient to sustain adequate oxygen content.[113,114] Treatment of sepsis requires identification of the responsible organisms and initiation of antibiotic therapy.

Intermittent administration of packed red blood cells to maintain adequate blood volume and hematocrit will be required.[115–117] Fresh-frozen plasma may be given intermittently to provide adequate clotting factors and help prevent excessive bleeding.[118] Platelet sequestration in the ECMO circuit is a constant problem. Historically, platelet counts of 80,000 to 100,000/mm^3 have been maintained routinely on ECMO to deter bleeding, but now multiple examples exist of patients placed on ECMO with thrombocytopenia of 30,000/mm^3 or lower in whom massive bleeding was not a problem. Although patients often require frequent platelet transfusions, the capacity of transfusions to increase platelet counts to high levels may be limited in patients such as those with cancer. In such patients, lower platelet counts may be allowed and a careful watch for bleeding maintained. Another problem identified with ECMO, especially for prolonged runs, is heparin-induced thrombocytopenia (HIT). HIT should be suspected in any patient receiving heparin who develops a drop in platelet count that is unresponsive to platelet transfusion or continues to fall without an identified reason. Although HIT usually develops 5 to 15 days after initial exposure to heparin, it can occur immediately in patients with previous exposure to heparin, such as cardiac surgical patients. HIT associated with immune response to heparin can result in severe thrombocytopenia and thrombotic complications. The only "cure" is removing heparin exposure from the patient. During ECMO, this necessitates use of other anticoagulation methods. Currently, lepirudin and argatroban are the two alternatives that have been discussed with regard to ECMO, although neither is widely used in the pediatric population in general.[119–121] Lepirudin is a derivative of the leech anticoagulant hirudin. Two reports of its use during ECMO noted no bleeding or clotting complications. It is rapid, has a relatively short half-life of 1.3 hours, and is dosed on weight. One pediatric report used 0.1 mg/kg bolus dosing followed by an infusion of 0.12 mg/kg/hour and monitoring to maintain the activated partial thromboplastin time at twice the control level. It is relatively contraindicated in renal failure. Argatroban is also a direct thrombin inhibitor approved for use in HIT. It is metabolized predominantly by the liver but excreted normally even in severe renal failure. One report of two infants with CDH and HIT treated with argatroban at a dose of 0.5 to 10 μg/kg/min to maintain activated clotting times (ACTs) around 200 seconds had no associated bleeding or thrombotic complications. Another report of thrombin production in ECMO circuits comparing heparin-prepared circuits with argatroban-primed circuits found that the circuits with argatroban had less thrombin generation.[122] Thrombocytopenia resulting from platelet antibodies has been described.

Adequate nutrition is essential for healing and is provided as total parenteral nutrition (TPN), enteral feeding, or a combination of both. The old concern of lipids potentially causing either platelet malfunction (bleeding) or increased lung damage from metabolism of arachidonic acid seems to have died away. Lipids have anecdotally been associated with shortened lifespans and with development of cracks in stopcocks used to connect the lipid infusion line to the ECMO circuit.[123] Use of lipids may be associated with shortened lifespans of hollow-fiber oxygenators. Enteral feeding has been shown to be safe and effective during ECMO and may limit the need for TPN with its associated complications.[124,125] It currently is popular to maintain strict fluid balance in critically ill patients, and ECMO is no exception. The use of diuretics to promote urine excretion, concentration of fluids to balance intake and output, and hemofiltration in patients with renal insufficiency are other important aspects of patient care.[126,127] Use of continuous renal replacement therapies has become commonplace during ECMO to maintain fluid balance, support failing kidneys, and potentially clear "bad humours" from the blood. One abstract noted that continuous renal replacement therapy (continuous venovenous hemofiltration [CVVH]) was used in 27 (32%) of 84 pediatric ECMO patients, usually for fluid overload. Overall survival was 75% for respiratory failure patients. Of these 84 patients, 27 were matched for age, diagnosis, and PRISM III score with ECMO patients who did not receive CVVH. Improved fluid balance over time, less diuretic use, and faster time to reach caloric intake goals were noted in patients receiving renal replacement. There was no difference in survival (67% CVVH, 82% non-CVVH, $p = 0.352$), duration of ventilation post-ECMO, or need for potassium supplementation between groups.[128] Data from the ELSO registry shows that approximately 30% of pediatric and adult ECMO patients receive renal replacement by either hemofiltration or dialysis, although elevations of creatinine greater than 1.5 were reported in only 15% of pediatric patients. Other adjunct extracorporeal therapies such as plasmapheresis or liver support systems have been used successfully during ECMO.[129]

The optimal ventilatory management for patients on ECMO is not known, and each center may have its own preference for how to treat the lungs during ECMO. Minimizing further barotrauma or oxygen toxicity and providing an environment that promotes lung healing are basic goals. For neonatal patients on venoarterial ECMO, most centers use ventilator settings with low peak inspiratory pressure ([PIP] 25–30 cmH_2O), PEEP (5 cmH_2O), intermittent mandatory ventilation (IMV) rate (6–12 breaths/min), and fraction of inspired oxygen (FIO_2 0.21). Lung volume decreases dramatically with such settings in most ECMO patients, resulting in generalized opacification on the chest radiograph. Maintaining lung expansion and functional residual capacity with higher levels of PEEP (10–15 cmH_2O) have noted shorter ECMO durations in one neonatal study, and this approach is used frequently at many centers.[130] Given the evidence supporting the role of atelectasis in ongoing cytokine production, maintaining some lung distension with PEEP even during ECMO seems prudent. In older patients, use of PEEP with reduced peak airway pressures, low ventilator rates, and low concentrations of inspired oxygen are the predominant method of support. Commonly, PEEP levels in the range of 5 to 15 cmH_2O, PIP less than 30 cmH_2O, and breath rates of 10 to 12 with inspired oxygen concentrations between 30% and 40% are reported in the pediatric and adult ECMO literature.

Patients with barotrauma and persistent air leaks even at low distending airway pressures on ECMO may benefit from a period of total apnea to allow the lungs to rest.[131] Allowing airway pressure to equilibrate with atmospheric pressure has been used successfully to promote healing of ruptured parenchyma within 48 to 72 hours. Reinflation is accomplished by lavage to remove accumulated secretions, hand ventilation to begin recruiting collapsed alveoli, and then resumption of mechanical ventilation to complete alveolar reexpansion. Use of high-frequency ventilation to improve lung recruitment, bronchoscopy to remove inspissated secretions, and prone positioning to improve lung mechanics have all been used successfully in ECMO patients.

At high flow rates in venoarterial ECMO, minimal blood enters the pulmonary circuit. Manipulating ventilator settings, especially in diseased lungs with impaired gas exchange, has little effect on blood gas tensions. Oxygenation and carbon dioxide elimination depend on the function of the ECMO circuit. With venovenous cannulation, less overall bypass is obtained and the systemic oxygenation provided by ECLS is less than with venoarterial access. Thus arterial oxygen saturations are lower with venovenous support. Although the majority of patients do well with saturations in the 80s, monitoring of adequate oxygen delivery by following lactate, venous saturation, urine output, metabolic acid-base balance, and mental status is recommended.

Increasing oxygenation over time may herald recovery of native pulmonary function. As the lungs heal, compliance and tidal volume increase.[132] The radiograph of the lung fields gradually improves from atelectatic opacification to increasing lung aeration. Increasing concentration and absolute volume of expired carbon dioxide also heralds improved alveolar–capillary gas exchange. These changes, along with evidence of decreasing pulmonary artery pressure (indicating resolution of right-to-left intracardiac shunting), may signal that the patient is ready to be weaned from ECMO.[133]

Maintaining patient comfort during ECMO can be a challenge, especially in prolonged ECMO runs. Sedation and analgesia are provided by routine medications, such as morphine, fentanyl, midazolam, and lorazepam. If lorazepam infusions are used, intermittent osmolality and osmol gap should be calculated to prevent propylene glycol toxicity.[134] Medications may be absorbed by the membrane oxygenator, and patients can become tolerant to the drugs over time.[135] The extraordinary amount of medications some patients require has led some centers to use anesthesia gas into the membrane oxygenator, although a protocol for appropriate scavenging of these gases must be developed for use. European centers are facile in maintaining patients in a "normal" awake status such that they can play games, read books, and even eat during their ECMO course. Nursing and family support play a major role in the success of providing ECMO with little sedation.

Weaning from Extracorporeal Membrane Oxygenation

A patient can be weaned from ECMO in several ways. The most common mode involves reducing the ECMO flow rate in increments every 1 to 2 hours provided arterial and mixed venous oxygen saturations remain adequate. Once ECMO flow is reduced to provide only about two thirds of cardiac output, ventilator support is increased (PIP 20–30 cmH_2O, IMV 20–30, PEEP 5 cmH_2O, FIO_2 30%–40%). Weaning continues to an ECMO flow of 50 to 100 ml/min in infants or an estimated 10% of cardiac output. If the patient remains physiologically stable with acceptable blood gas tensions at this low flow, the ECMO cannulas are clamped and the infant is observed off ECMO support for a short time. If respiration and circulation remain stable during the trial, the cannulas are removed and the patient is returned to conventional therapy. Quicker weaning methods involve decreasing ECMO flow in larger increments over shorter periods of time, similar to the procedure performed during cardiopulmonary bypass in the operating room.[136]

Complications

Complications that occur during ECMO can be mechanical or patient related. The most common adverse events reported to the ELSO Registry are listed in Table 47–7 for respiratory failure patients and Table 47–8 for cardiac patients.

Bleeding

Bleeding from systemic heparinization required with ECMO is the major complication associated with ECMO.[137] Bleeding occurs predominately from cannulation or surgical sites, but intracranial hemorrhage is the most dreaded site for bleeding occurrence. Intracranial bleeding occurs in approximately 11% of patients overall, with the highest rate in the neonatal patient and the lowest rate in the adult population. Bleeding occurring outside the head that cannot be controlled with medical means requires surgical investigation. Although there are obvious risks of surgical intervention in a bleeding patient who is systemically anticoagulated, many operative repairs have been accomplished during ECMO support.[138] Initial attempts to control bleeding focus on decreasing the rate of heparin infusion and lowering ACT levels. Limitation of heparin may put the circuit at risk for increased clotting, especially at lower flow levels. This must be balanced against the bleeding risk. Medications to help prevent clot breakdown in the patient are also used. Aminocaproic acid (Amicar) has historically been the predominant medication used during ECMO.[139] An antifibrinolytic amino acid, Amicar displaces plasminogen from fibrin and inhibits clot breakdown. Although a survey found a wide range of doses used, I have commonly followed a dosage scheme of 100 mg/kg as a load followed by an infusion of 25 to 50 mg/kg/hour. Although used in ECMO centers for many years, a randomized controlled trial of Amicar versus placebo in neonates found no difference between groups with regard to need for transfusion or need for

TABLE 47–7

Mechanical and Patient-Related Complications for Respiratory Population

Complication	Neonatal Respiratory	Pediatric Respiratory	Adult Respiratory
MECHANICAL			
Oxygenator failure	5.7 (55)	13.8 (44)	18.2 (43)
Tubing rupture	0.7 (74)	3.8 (47)	4.0 (30)
Pump malfunction	1.8 (68)	3.1 (47)	4.1 (37)
Cannula problems	11.1 (70)	14.2 (48)	10.7 (42)
PATIENT-RELATED			
Gastrointestinal hemorrhage	1.7 (46)	4.0 (25)	4.3 (26)
Cannula site bleeding	6.1 (68)	9.2 (60)	11.5 (47)
Surgical site bleeding	6.1 (46)	16.0 (47)	22.4 (35)
Hemolysis	12.2 (68)	8.8 (42)	5.3 (28)
Brain death	1.0 (0)	6.0 (0)	3.8 (0)
Seizures: clinically determined	10.9 (62)	7.3 (35)	2.0 (45)

Data modified from ELSO International Summary, July 2004.
Table entries are in percent reported (percent survival).

TABLE 47–8

Mechanical and Patient-Related Complications for the Cardiac Population

Complication	0–30 days	31 Days to <1 Year	1 Year to <16 Years	16 Years and Older
MECHANICAL				
Oxygenator failure	7.2 (23)	7.2 (28)	9.1 (37)	16.4 (27)
Tubing rupture	0.7 (31)	1.1 (24)	2.0 (30)	0.9 (20)
Pump malfunction	1.3 (32)	1.9 (26)	2.2 (42)	1.8 (36)
Cannula problems	6.7 (33)	5.9 (35)	6.4 (31)	6.8 (32)
PATIENT-RELATED				
Gastrointestinal hemorrhage	0.9 (5)	1.8 (14)	2.8 (23)	2.4 (15)
Cannula site bleeding	6.8 (27)	6.7 (23)	10.7 (44)	12.9 (30)
Surgical site bleeding	31.0 (29)	33.9 (36)	31.3 (42)	31.9 (27)
Hemolysis	10.8 (24)	9.9 (33)	8.5 (35)	8.1 (34)
Brain death	1.3 (0)	5.1 (0)	9.5 (0)	7.9 (0)
Seizures: clinically determined	9.7 (29)	11.0 (24)	6.8 (21)	4.8 (12)

Modified from the ELSO International Summary, July 2004.

circuit changes because of thrombosis. More recently, aprotinin has become the favored agent in many centers.[140] A serine protease inhibitor, aprotinin is antifibrinolytic, inhibits protein C and factors Va and VIIIa in the extrinsic coagulation pathway, and inhibits the intrinsic pathway. It also preserves platelet function, reduces vascular permeability, and has been suggested to decrease the inflammatory response to cardiopulmonary bypass. It has not been compared in a randomized fashion to Amicar or placebo during ECMO, but many centers now use it as their first agent in bleeding patients. Aprotinin is administered as a loading dose of 10,000 U/kg and continued at an infusion rate of 10,000 U/kg/hour. Circuit thromboses may be noted with use of Amicar or aprotinin. Several reports of intractable bleeding in patients on ECMO have commented on the benefits of factor VIIa, although the data with this medication are too sparse to recommend it without further investigation.[141] Discontinuation of heparin to help control intractable bleeding can be beneficial and has been used for variable periods up to 36 hours or more without significant clotting in the ECMO circuit.[142] Larger patients with faster ECMO flow rates are more likely to tolerate discontinuation of heparin without significant clotting. It is wise, however, to have a backup circuit readily available if clotting does occur and the ECMO system requires an emergent replacement.

Infection

Infection is another potential complication of ECMO.[143] Colonization of indwelling catheters, selective adherence of bacteria to polyurethane surfaces, sequestration of bacteria from the body's normal antibody and phagocytic defense mechanisms, and the patient's prior debilitated state are all factors that may increase the risk of infection.[144,145] Successful therapy may be difficult without eliminating invasive equipment, most significantly the ECMO cannulas. Viral infection from blood transfusions may occur. The risk may be limited by minimizing the exposure to blood products from multiple donors by administering multialiquoted, sequentially dispensed units of packed red cells. Although sepsis, either preexisting or developing on ECMO, was once seen as a reason to exclude patients from ECMO support, several reports have demonstrated that sepsis can be cleared and septic patients successfully treated with ECMO. In fact, the most recent guidelines for hemodynamic support of pediatric patients with septic shock note that ECMO should be considered in patients with refractory catecholamine-resistant shock.[146] Although there is still some debate over whether patients in high cardiac output shock will receive any benefit from augmenting cardiac output further with ECMO, such patients have been treated successfully with ECMO support.

Long-Term Outcome

Patients undergoing ECMO are at risk for neurologic damage from hypoxia, acidosis, hypotension, induced alkalosis prior to ECMO, and hemorrhage or ischemia related to systemic heparinization and alterations in cerebral blood flow following ligation of the carotid artery and IJ vein.[147–152] Nevertheless, two thirds of neonatal survivors appear to have normal neurodevelopmental outcome. The remaining third suffer from mild-to-severe deficits in motor or cognitive function. Sensorineural hearing loss has been noted in 23% of patients, an incidence comparable to that in infants with persistent pulmonary hypertension treated conventionally. The long term effects of carotid artery and jugular vein ligation are unknown.

Severe chronic respiratory disease in patients treated with ECMO is uncommon.[153] Most reports relate an incidence of bronchopulmonary dysplasia (defined as the need for oxygen beyond the first month of life) from 4% to 27%. Most cases occurred in patients who had required extreme ventilator settings for more than 7 days before ECMO rescue. A follow-up report of neonates treated with ECMO and evaluated 10 to 15 years post-ECMO found that although the ECMO patients had some diminished lung function by pulmonary function testing, they had similar aerobic capacity and were able to reach anaerobic exercise goals similar to those of age-matched healthy controls.[154]

Of 2700 pediatric respiratory ECMO patients listed in the registry through January 2004, 6% of patients had intracranial infarct or hemorrhage found on CT examination. Brain death occurred in 6% of the patients, and 7% of patients had reported seizures. Long-term neurologic outcome data are missing in the pediatric population. Few centers maintain regular follow-up clinics, and patients are often referred for ECMO from distant sites, which makes follow-up difficult. In one report of 15 pediatric and four adult patients, 58% survived to discharge. Patients were evaluated using the Pediatric Cerebral Performance Category (PCPC, which measures cognitive impairment) and the Pediatric Overall Performance Category (POPC, which measures functional morbidity). Overall, 64% of survivors had normal PCPC scores, 27% had mild disabilities, and 9% had moderate cognitive disability. Functional morbidity was normal in 27%, whereas 45% had mild disability, 18% had moderate disability, and 9% had severe disability.[155] In another small series of 26 patients followed 1 to 3 years after ECMO, 38% of preschool-age children were described as normal and 31% had observed abnormalities. Four patients (31%) who had prior neurologic dysfunction remained at baseline following ECMO. Among children who were of school age, 77% were described as normal by parental report.[156] More specific neurologic follow-up in the pediatric age groups is needed.

Neurologic complications in cardiac patients who receive ECMO parallel those of respiratory failure patients. Six percent of patients developed brain death, 2% had intracranial infarct, and 4% had intracranial hemorrhage. Because many cardiac patients are in a state of prolonged low cardiac output or sudden cardiac arrest prior to ECMO, the ability to assess neurologic function once ECMO is instituted is vitally important. Paralysis and sedation should be minimized until a neurologic examination can occur. This information is especially important in patients who are being listed for transplantation to avoid transplanting a viable organ into an inappropriate recipient.

One report of 64 cardiac ECMO patients found that 28 (44%) had neurologic complications.[157] Seizures occurred in 18 patients (28%), 3 patients (5%) had embolus or thrombus, 9 patients (14%) had an intraventricular hemorrhage higher than grade 2, and 13 patients (20%) had anoxic encephalopathy. In 68% of patients with neurologic complications, hemodynamic compromise had occurred prior to ECMO. Five patients had evidence of neurologic complication prior to ECMO, 30% of patients with neurologic complications had received cardiopulmonary resuscitation prior to ECMO, and 14% had several hours of low cardiac output prior to ECMO. Sixty-nine percent of patients who were electively removed from ECMO had neurologic and/or multisystem organ failure.

The long-term follow-up of children with cardiac disease who required mechanical circulatory support during a decade of experience at Children's Hospital, Boston has been analyzed.[158] Thirty-seven children (26 ECMO and 11 VAD survivors) were followed for an average of more than 4 years. Only a single patient in either group died, for an overall long-term survival of 95%. Eighty percent of the patients in both groups were described as exhibiting good-to-excellent general health. Both low weight at the time support was originally instituted and long duration of hypothermic circulatory arrest in operative patients were associated with poor neurologic outcome. The majority of patients with these characteristics were supported with ECMO. Neurologic impairment of moderate-to-severe degree was noted in more than 60% of the ECMO patients and 20% of VAD survivors. Adverse neurologic outcomes were not associated with presupport cardiac arrest, carotid cannulation, or carotid reconstruction. Other series have noted neurologic complications in 205 to 30% of cardiac ECMO patients. Survivors are generally described as "normal" neurologically, although the extent of examination or radiologic assessment of the brain is typically unknown.

Longer-term evaluation of patients surviving ECLS and comparison to patients with similar disease severity and diagnosis are imperative to adequately interpret neurologic outcome.[159]

The Future

Use of ECMO in neonatal patients with respiratory failure has been accepted medical practice for many years. The current extension of ECLS systems to older pediatric and adult patients in a variety of clinical settings highlights the changes that have occurred in the ECLS environment. Progress in renal replacement, liver support and plasmapheresis, and the development of new cardiac support devices applicable to pediatrics may expand the use of ECMO or related techniques overall. Additionally, the development of small portable systems for cardiopulmonary resuscitation may herald a new age of extracorporeal support. Technical advances in ECLS equipment continue to make such support safer and more efficient. Venovenous ECMO techniques have been refined and used successfully in patients from neonatal to adult age groups. Single-cannula, double-lumen catheters for venovenous ECMO may obviate the risks of arterial cannulation and offer the benefit of requiring only one surgical site for venous access. Heparin-bonded circuits may decrease the need for systemic anticoagulation and the risk of hemorrhagic complications.

Until the day when medical science makes obsolete the need for ECLS, research into ways to make it safer and more efficient should continue.

REFERENCES

1. McLean J: The thromboplastic action of cephalin. *Am J Physiol* 41:250, 1916.
2. Hill JD, Gibbon JH Jr: Development of the first successful heart lung machine. *Ann Thorac Surg* 34:337, 1982.
3. Clowes GH, Hopkins AL, Neville WE: An artificial lung dependent upon diffusion of oxygen and carbon dioxide through plastic membranes. *J Thorac Surg* 32:630, 1956.

4. Page US, Bigelow JC, Carter CR, Swank RL: Emboli (debris) produced by bubble oxygenators. Removal by filtration. *Ann Thorac Surg* 18:164, 1974.
5. Kolobow T, Bowman RL: Construction and evaluation of an alveolar membrane artificial lung. *Trans Am Soc Artif Intern Organs* 9:243, 1963.
6. Gille JP: Respiratory support by extracorporeal circulation with a membrane artificial lung. *Bull Physiopathol Respir* 10:373, 1974.
7. Sinard JM, Bartlett RH: Extracorporeal membrane oxygenation (ECMO): prolonged bedside cardiopulmonary bypass. *Perfusion* 5:239-249, 1990.
8. Bartlett RH, Gazzaniga AB, Jeffries MR, et al: Extracorporeal membrane oxygenation (ECMO) cardiopulmonary support in infancy. *Trans Am Soc Artif Intern Organs* 22:80, 1976.
9. Short BL, Pearson GD: Neonatal extracorporeal membrane oxygenation: a review. *J Intensive Care Med* 1:48, 1986.
10. Heiss KF, Bartlett RH: Extracorporeal membrane oxygenation: an experimental protocol becomes a clinical service. *Adv Pediatr* 36:117, 1989.
11. International ECMO Registry Report of the Extracorporeal Life Support Organization (ELSO), Ann Arbor, Michigan, January 2004.
12. Kolobow T: An update on adult extracorporeal membrane oxygenation-extracorporeal CO_2 removal. *ASAIO Trans* 34:1004, 1988.
13. Stork E: Extracorporeal membrane oxygenation in the newborn and beyond. *Clin Perinatol* 15:815, 1988.
14. Stolar CJ, Dillon PW: Extracorporeal membrane oxygenation for neonatal respiratory failure. *Surg Annu* 19:111-122, 1987.
15. Skarsgard ED, Salt DR, Lee SK, Extracorporeal Life Support Organization: Venovenous extracorporeal membrane oxygenation in neonatal respiratory failure: does routine, cephalad jugular drainage improve outcome? *J Pediatr Surg* 39:672-676, 2004.
16. Pettignano R, Labuz M, Gauthier TW, et al: The use of cephalad cannulae to monitor jugular venous oxygen content during extracorporeal membrane oxygenation. *Crit Care* 1:95-99, 1997.
17. Snider MT, Campbell DB, Kofke WA, et al: Venovenous perfusion of adults and children with severe acute respiratory distress syndrome. The Pennsylvania State University experience from 1982-1987. *ASAIO Trans* 34:1014, 1988.
18. Pennington DG, Merjavy JP, Codd JE, et al: Extracorporeal membrane oxygenation for patients with cardiogenic shock. *Circulation* 70:130, 1984.
19. Van Meurs KP, Mikesell GT, Seale WR, et al: Maximum blood flow rates for arterial cannulae used in neonatal ECMO. *ASAIO Trans* 36:M679, 1990.
20. Rogers AJ, Trento A, Siewers RD, et al: Extracorporeal membrane oxygenation for postcardiotomy cardiogenic shock in children. *Ann Thorac Surg* 47:903-906, 1989.
21. Seib PM, Faulkner SC, Erickson CC, et al: Blade and balloon atrial septostomy for left heart decompression in patients with severe ventricular dysfunction on extracorporeal membrane oxygenation. *Catheter Cardiovasc Interv* 46:179-186, 1999.
22. Moazami N, Moon MR, Lawton JS, et al: Axillary artery cannulation for extracorporeal membrane oxygenator support in adults: an approach to minimize complications. *J Thorac Cardiovasc Surg* 126:2097-2098, 2003.
23. Andrews AF, Klein MD, Toomasian JM, et al: Venovenous extracorporeal membrane oxygenation in neonates with respiratory failure. *J Pediatr Surg* 18:339-346, 1983.
24. Rais-Bahrami K, Walton DM, Sell JE, et al: Improved oxygenation with reduced recirculation during venovenous ECMO: comparison of two catheters. *Perfusion* 17:415-419, 2002.
25. Dalton HJ: Extracorporeal membrane oxygenation in the new millennium: forging ahead or fading out? *New Horizons* 1999.
26. Roberts N, Westrope C, Pooboni SK, et al: Venovenous extracorporeal membrane oxygenation for respiratory failure in inotrope dependent neonates. *ASAIO J* 49:568-571, 2003.
27. Habashi NM, Borg UR, Reynolds HN: Low blood flow extracorporeal carbon dioxide removal (ECCO2R): a review of the concept and a case report. *Intensive Care Med* 21:594-597, 1995.
28. Rich PB, Awad SS, Crotti S, et al: A prospective comparison of atrio-femoral and femoro-atrial flow in adult venovenous extracorporeal life support. *J Thorac Cardiovasc Surg* 116:628-632, 1998.
29. Chen YS, Ko WJ, Lin FY: Insertion of percutaneous ECMO cannula. *Am J Emerg Med* 18:184-185, 2000.
30. Foley DS, Swaniker F, Pranikoff T, et al: Percutaneous cannulation for pediatric venovenous extracorporeal life support. *J Pediatr Surg* 35:943-947, 2000.
31. Campbell LR, Bunyapen C, Kanto WP, et al: Right common carotid artery ligation in extracorporeal membrane oxygenation. *J Pediatr* 113:110, 1988.
32. Schumacher RE, Barks JD, Johnston MV, et al: Right-sided brain lesions in infants following extracorporeal membrane oxygenation. *Pediatrics* 82:155, 1988.
33. Adolph V, Bonis S, Falterman K, Arensman R: Carotid artery repair after pediatric extracorporeal membrane oxygenation. *J Pediatr Surg* 25:867, 1990.
34. Karl TR, Iyer KS, Sano S, Mee RB: Infant ECMO cannulation technique allowing preservation of carotid and jugular vessels. *Ann Thorac Surg* 50:488, 1990.
35. Crombleholme TM, Adzick NS, deLorimier AA, et al: Carotid artery reconstruction following extracorporeal membrane oxygenation. *Am J Dis Child* 144:872, 1990.
36. Desai SA, Stanley C, Gringlas M, et al: Five-year follow-up of neonates with reconstructed right common carotid arteries after extracorporeal membrane oxygenation. *J Pediatr* 134:428-433, 1999.
37. Engel M, Dalton HJ: Extracorporeal life support in children. *J Pediatr Respir Care* 5:115-125, 2003.
38. Zwischenberger JB, Bowers RM, Pickens GJ: Tension pneumothorax during extracorporeal membrane oxygenation. *Ann Thorac Surg* 47:868, 1989.
39. Steinhorn RH, Isham-Schopf B, Green TP: Hemolysis during long-term extracorporeal membrane oxygenation. *J Pediatr* 115:625, 1989.
40. Van Heijst A, Liem D, Van Der Staak F, et al: Hemodynamic changes during opening of the bridge in venoarterial extracorporeal membrane oxygenation. *Pediatr Crit Care Med* 2:265-270, 2001.
41. Yamagishi T, Kunimoto F, Isa Y, et al: Clinical results of extracorporeal membrane oxygenation (ECMO) support for acute respiratory failure: a comparison of a centrifugal pump ECMO with a roller pump ECMO. *Surg Today* 34:209-213, 2004.
42. Allison PL, Kurusz M, Graves DF, Zwischenberger JB: Devices and monitoring during neonatal ECMO: survey results. *Perfusion* 5:193-201, 1990.
43. Palatianos GM, Dewanjee MK, Kapadvanjwala M, et al: Cardiopulmonary bypass with a surface-heparinized extracorporeal perfusion system. *ASAIO Trans* 36:M476, 1990.
44. Matsuwaka R, Matsuda H, Kaneko M, et al: Experimental evaluation of a heparin coated ECMO system simplified with a centrifugal pump. *ASAIO Trans* 36:M473, 1990.
45. Tamari Y, Lee TP, Baker T, et al: Bubble counts: centrifugal vs. roller pump with and without a venous bladder. 13th Annual ELSO Conference 2002, Scottsdale Arizona.
46. Seo T, Ando H, Ito T, et al: Development of disposable self-regulating blood pumps and automatically-controlled portable extracorporeal membrane oxygenation systems for neonatal extracorporeal membrane oxygenation. *Artif Organs* 27:192-198, 2003.
47. SciMed Membrane Oxygenators Instruction Manual, SciMed Life Systems, Minneapolis, Minnesota.
48. Kawahito S, Motomura T, Glueck J, Nose Y: Development of a new hollow fiber silicone membrane oxygenator for ECMO: the recent progress. *Ann Thorac Cardiovasc Surg* 8:268-274, 2002.
49. Lawson DS, Walczak R, Lawson AF, et al: North American neonatal extracorporeal membrane oxygenation (ECMO) devices: 2002 survey results. *J Extracorpor Technol* 36:16-21, 2004.
50. Karle VA, Short BL, Martin GR, et al: Extracorporeal membrane oxygenation exposes infants to the plasticizer, di(2-ethylhexyl) phthalate. *Crit Care Med* 25:696-703, 1997.
51. Rais-Bahrami K, Nunez S, Revenis ME, et al: Follow-up study of adolescents exposed to di(2-ethylhexyl) phthalate (DEHP) as neonates on extracorporeal membrane oxygenation (ECMO) support. *Environ Health Perspect* 112:1339-1340, 2004.
52. Dalton HJ, Heulitt MJ: Extracorporeal membrane oxygenation. *Respir Care* 43:966-977, 1998.
53. Murphy JD, Rabinovitch M, Goldstein JD, et al: The structural basis of persistent pulmonary hypertension of the newborn infant. *J Pediatr* 98:962, 1981.
54. Koumbourlis AC, Motoyama EK, Thompson AE: Lung changes during and after ECMO for meconium aspiration syndrome. *Crit Care Med* 18:S245, 1990.

55. Van Meurs KP, Newman KD, Anderson KD, Short BL: Effect of extracorporeal membrane oxygenation on survival of infants with congenital diaphragmatic hernia. *J Pediatr* 117:954, 1990.
56. Levin DL: Congenital diaphragmatic hernia: a persistent problem. *J Pediatr* 111:390, 1987.
57. ECMO Registry of the Extracorporeal Life Support Organization, Ann Arbor, Michigan, January 2004.
58. Geggel RL, Murphy JD, Langleben D, et al: Congenital diaphragmatic hernia: arterial structural changes and persistent pulmonary hypertension after surgical repair. *J Pediatr* 107:457, 1985.
59. Connors RH, Tracy T Jr, Bailey PV, et al: Congenital diaphragmatic hernia repair on ECMO. *J Pediatr Surg* 25:1043, 1990.
60. Tibboel D, Bos AP, Pattenier JW, et al: Pre-operative stabilisation with delayed repair in congenital diaphragmatic hernia. *Z Kenderchir* 44:139-143, 1989.
61. Doyle NM, Lally KP: The CDH Study Group and advances in the clinical care of the patient with congenital diaphragmatic hernia. *Semin Perinatol* 28:174-184, 2004.
62. Tulenko DR: An update on ECMO. *Neonatal Netw* 23:11-18, 2004.
63. Dalton HJ, Rycus P: Unpublished data. Extracorporeal Life Support Organization, 2002.
64. ECMO Registry of the Extracorporeal Life Support Organization, Ann Arbor, Michigan, January 2004.
65. O'Rourke PP, Crone RK: Pediatric applications of extracorporeal membrane oxygenation. *J Pediatr* 116:393, 1990.
66. Fortenberry JD, Meier AH, Pettignano R, et al: Extracorporeal life support for posttraumatic acute respiratory distress syndrome at a children's medical center. *J Pediatr Surg* 38:1221-1226, 2003.
67. Szocik J. Rudich S, Csete M: ECMO resuscitation after massive pulmonary embolism during liver transplantation. *Anesthesiology* 97:763-764, 2002.
68. Sheridan RL, Schnitzer JJ: Management of the high risk pediatric burn patient. *J Pediatr Surg* 36:1308-1312, 2001.
69. Linden V, Karlen J, Olsson M, et al: Successful extracorporeal membrane oxygenation in four children with malignant disease and severe *Pneumocystis carinii* pneumonia. *Med Pediatr Oncol* 32:25-31, 1999.
70. Thiagarajan RR, Roth SJ, Margossian S, et al: Extracorporeal membrane oxygenation as a bridge to cardiac transplantation in a patient with cardiomyopathy and hemophilia A. *Intensive Care Med* 29:985-988, 2003.
71. Gow KW, Heard ML, Heiss KF, et al: Extracorporeal membrane oxygenation (ECMO) in children with malignancy. 20th Annual CNMC Symposium on ECMO and Advanced Respiratory Therapies, Keystone, Colorado, A23; 2004.
72. MacLaren G, Pellegrino V, Butt W, et al: Successful use of ECMO in adults with life-threatening infections. *Anaesth Intensive Care* 32:707-710, 2004.
73. Zapol WM, Snider MT, Hill JD, et al: Extracorporeal membrane oxygenation in severe acute respiratory failure. A randomized prospective study. *JAMA* 242:2193-2196, 1979.
74. Gattinoni L, Kolobow T, Tomlinson T, et al: Low frequency positive pressure ventilation with extracorporeal carbon dioxide removal (LFPPV-ECCO$_2$R): an experimental study. *Anesth Analg* 57:470, 1978.
75. Kolla S, Awad SS, Rich PB, et al: Extracorporeal life support for 100 adult patients with severe respiratory failure. *Ann Surg* 226: 544-564, 1997.
76. Hemmila MR, Rowe SA, Boules TN, et al: Extracorporeal life support for severe acute respiratory distress syndrome in adults. *Ann Surg* 240:595-605, 2004.
77. Kolobow T: An update on adult extracorporeal membrane oxygenation: extracorporeal CO$_2$ removal. *Trans Am Soc Artif Intern Organs* 34:1004, 1988.
78. Alpard SK, Zwischenberger JB, Tao W, et al: Reduced ventilator pressure and improved P/F ratio during percutaneous arteriovenous carbon dioxide removal for severe respiratory failure. *Ann Surg* 230:215-224, 1999.
79. Kolobow T: The artificial lung: the past. A personal retrospective. *ASAIO J* 50:xliii-xlviii, 2004.
80. Dalton HJ, Siewers RD, Fuhrmana BP, et al: Extracorporeal membrane oxygenation for cardiac rescue in children with severe myocardial dysfunction. *Crit Care Med* 21:1020-1028, 1993.
81. Rogers AJ, Trento A, Siewers RD, et al: Extracorporeal membrane oxygenation for postcardiotomy cardiogenic shock in children. *Ann Thorac Surg* 47:903, 1989.
82. Weinhaus L, Canter C, Noetzel M, et al: Extracorporeal membrane oxygenation for circulatory support after repair of congenital heart defects. *Ann Thorac Surg* 48:206, 1989.
83. International Registry of the Extracorporeal Life Support Organization, January 2004.
84. Galantowica M, Stolar C: Extracorporeal membrane oxygenation for peri-operative support in pediatric heart transplantation. Extracorporeal Life Support Organization Charter Meeting, Ann Arbor, Michigan, 48A, 1989.
85. Klein MD, Whittlesey GC, Shaheen KW, et al: Predictors of mortality in children following repair of congential heart defects. ELSO Charter Organization Meeting, Ann Arbor, Michigan, 49A, 1989.
86. Undar A, McKenzie ED, McGarry MC, et al: Outcomes of congenital heart surgery patients after extracorporeal life support at Texas Children's Hospital. *Artif Organs* 28:963-966, 2004.
87. Kolovos NS, Bratton SL, Moler FW, et al: Outcome of pediatric patients treated with extracorporeal life support after cardiac surgery. *Ann Thorac Surg* 76:1435-1441, 2003.
88. Chaturvedi RR, Macrae D, Brown KL, et al: Cardiac ECMO for biventricular hearts after paediatric open heart surgery. *Heart* 90:545-551, 2004.
89. Duncan B, Hraska V, Jonas R: Mechanical circulatory support in children with cardiac disease. *J Thorac Cardiovasc Surg* 117:529-542, 1999.
90. Kanter KR, Pennington DG, Wever TG, et al: Extracorporeal membrane oxygenation for postoperative cardiac failure in children. *J Thorac Cardiovasc Surg* 93:27-35, 1987.
91. Klein MD, Shaheen KW, Whittlesey GC, et al: Extracorporeal membrane oxygenation for the circulatory support of children after repair of congenital heart disease. *J Thorac Cardiovasc Surg* 100:498-505, 1990.
92. del Nido P, Armitage J, Fricker J: Extracorporeal membrane oxygenation support as a bridge to pediatric heart transplantation. *Circulation* 90:II67-II69, 1994.
93. Duncan BW, Bohn DJ, Atz AM, et al: Mechanical circulatory support for the treatment of children with acute fulminant myocarditis. *J Thorac Cardiovasc Surg* 122:440-448, 2001.
94. del Nido PJ, Dalton HJ, Thompson AE, Siewers RD: Extracorporeal membrane oxygenator rescue in children during cardiac arrest after cardiac surgery. *Circulation* 86(5 suppl):II300-II-304, 1992.
95. Morris MC, Wernovsky G, Nadkarni VM: Survival outcomes after extracorporeal cardiopulmonary resuscitation instituted during active chest compressions following refractory in-hospital pediatric cardiac arrest. *Pediatr Crit Care Med* 5:440-446, 2004.
96. Marsh TD, Wilkerson SA, Cook LN: Extracorporeal membrane oxygenation selection criteria: partial pressure of arterial oxygen versus alveolar-arterial oxygen gradient. *Pediatrics* 82:162, 1988.
97. Beck R, Anderson KD, Pearson GD, et al: Criteria for extracorporeal membrane oxygenation in a population of infants with persistent pulmonary hypertension of the newborn. *J Pediatr Surg* 21:297, 1986.
98. Ortiz RM, Cilley RE, Bartlett RH: Extracorporeal membrane oxygenation in pediatric respiratory failure. *Pediatr Clin North Am* 34:39, 1987.
99. Nading JH: Historical controls for extracorporeal membrane oxygenation in neonates. *Crit Care Med* 17:423, 1989.
100. Dalton HJ, Rycus P: Unpublished data, Extracorporeal Life Support Registry, Ann Arbor, Michigan, 2004.
101. Peters MJ, Tasker RC, Kiff KM, et al: Acute hypoxemic respiratory failure in children: case mix and the utility of respiratory severity indices. *Intensive Care Med* 24:699-705, 1998.
102. Gilbert EM, Haupt MT, Mandanas RY, et al: The effect of fluid loading, blood transfusion and catecholamine infusion on oxygen delivery and consumption in patients with sepsis. *Am Rev Respir Dis* 134:873, 1986.
103. Kolobow T, Spragg RG, Pierce JE: Massive pulmonary infarction during total cardiopulmonary bypass in unanesthetized spontaneously breathing lambs. *Int J Artif Organs* 4:76, 1981.
104. Secker-Walker JS, Edmonds JF, Spratt EH, Conn AW: The source of coronary perfusion during partial bypass for extracorporeal membrane oxygenation (ECMO). *Ann Thorac Surg* 21:138-143, 1976.

105. Mims BC: Physiologic monitoring of SO_2 monitoring. *Crit Care Nurs Clin North Am* 1:619, 1989.
106. Babcock DS, Han BK, Weiss RG, Ryckman FC: Brain abnormalities in infants on extracorporeal membrane oxygenation: sonographic and CT findings. *AJR Am J Roentgenol* 153:571, 1989.
107. Taylor GA, Fitz CR, Kapur S, Short BL: Cerebrovascular accidents in neonates treated with extracorporeal membrane oxygenation: sonographic-pathologic correlation. *AJR Am J Roentgenol* 153:355, 1989.
108. Kimball TR, Weiss RG, Meyer RA, et al: Color flow mapping to document normal pulmonary venous return in neonates with persistent pulmonary hypertension being considered for extracorporeal membrane oxygenation. *J Pediatr* 114:433, 1989.
109. Martin GR, Short BL: Doppler echocardiographic evaluation of cardiac performance in infants on prolonged extracorporeal membrane oxygenation. *Am J Cardiol* 62:929, 1988.
110. Green TP, Isham-Schopf B, Steinhorn RH, et al: Whole blood activated clotting time in infants during extracorporeal membrane oxygenation. *Crit Care Med* 18:494, 1990.
111. Jaggers JJ, Forbes JM, Shah AS, et al: Extracorporeal membrane oxygenation for infant postcardiotomy support: significance of shunt management. *Ann Thorac Surg* 69:1476-1483, 2000 May.
112. Meliones JN, Moler FW, Custer JR, et al: Normalization of priming solution ionized calcium concentration improves hemodynamic stability of neonates receiving venovenous ECMO. *ASAIO J* 41:884-888, 1995.
113. Mink RB, Pollack MM: Effect of blood transfusion on oxygen consumption in pediatric septic shock. *Crit Care Med* 18:1087, 1990.
114. Gilbert EM, Haupt MT, Mandanas RY, et al: The effect of fluid loading, blood transfusion and catecholamine infusion on oxygen delivery and consumption in patients with sepsis. *Am Rev Respir Dis* 134:873, 1986.
115. Bjerke HS, Kelly RE Jr, Foglia RP, et al: Decreasing transfusion exposure risk during extracorporeal membrane oxygenation (ECMO). *Transfus Med* 2:43-49, 1992.
116. Zavadil DP, Stammers AH, Willett LD, et al: Hematological abnormalities in neonatal patients treated with extracorporeal membrane oxygenation. *J Extra Corpor Technol* 30:83-90, 1998.
117. McCoy-Pardington D, Judd WJ, Knafl P, et al: Blood use during extracorporeal membrane oxygenation. *Transfusion* 30:307-309, 1990.
118. Plotz F: Extracorporeal membrane oxygenation and clotting revisited. *J Pediatr* 130:847-848, 1997.
119. Dager WE, Gosselin RC, Yoshikawa R, Owings JT: Lepirudin in heparin-induced thrombocytopenia and extracorporeal membranous oxygenation. *Ann Pharmacother* 38:598-601, 2004.
120. Deitcher SR, Topoulos AP, Bartholomew JR, Kichuk-Chrisant MR: Lepirudin anticoagulation for heparin-induced thrombocytopenia. *J Pediatr* 140:264-266, 2002.
121. Mejak B, Giacomuzzi C, Heller E, et al: Argatroban usage for anticoagulation for ECMO on a post-cardiac patient with heparin-induced thrombocytopenia. *J Extra Corpor Technol* 36:178-181, 2004.
122. Young G, Yonekawa KE, Nakagawa P, Nugent DJ: Argatroban as an alternative to heparin in extracorporeal membrane oxygenation circuits. *Perfusion* 19:283-288, 2004.
123. Buck ML, Ksenich RA, Wooldridge P: Effect of infusing fat emulsion into extracorporeal membrane oxygenation circuits. *Pharmacotherapy* 17:1292-1295, 1997.
124. Scott LK, Boudreaux K, Thaljeh F, et al: Early enteral feedings in adults receiving venovenous extracorporeal membrane oxygenation. *J Parenter Enteral Nutr* 28:295-300, 2004.
125. Piena M, Albers MJ, Van Haard PM, et al: Introduction of enteral feeding in neonates on extracorporeal membrane oxygenation after evaluation of intestinal permeability changes. *J Pediatr Surg* 33:30-34, 1998.
126. Lochan S, Adeniyi-Jones S, Assadi F: Coadministration of theophylline enhances diuretic response to furosemide in infants during extracorporeal membrane oxygenation: a randomized controlled pilot study. *J Pediatr* 133:86-89, 1998.
127. Foland JA, Fortenberry JD, Warshaw BL, et al: Fluid overload before continuous hemofiltration and survival in critically ill children: a retrospective analysis. *Crit Care Med* 32:1771-1776, 2004.
128. Hoover NG, Fortenberry JD, Heard M, et al: Continuous venovenous hemofiltration use in pediatric respiratory failure patients on ECMO: a case-control study. 20th Annual CNMC Symposium on ECMO and Advanced Respiratory Therapies, Keystone, Colorado, A24, 2004.
129. Daimon S, Umeda T, Michishita I, et al: Goodpasture's-like syndrome and effect of extracorporeal membrane oxygenator support. *Intern Med* 33:569-573, 1994.
130. Keszler M, Subramanian KN, Smith YA: Pulmonary management during extracorporeal membrane oxygenation. *Crit Care Med* 17:495-500, 1989.
131. Frattalone J, Fuhrman BP, Thompson AE: Treatment of air leak during extracorporeal membrane oxygenation: total apneic lung rest. *Clin Res* 35:912A, 1987.
132. Kugelman A, Saiki K, Platzker AC, Garg M: Measurement of lung volumes and pulmonary mechanics during weaning of newborn infants with intractable respiratory failure from extracorporeal membrane oxygenation. *Pediatr Pulmonol* 20:145-151, 1995.
133. Tanke R, Daniels O, Van Heyst A, et al: The influence of ductal left-to-right shunting during extracorporeal membrane oxygenation. *J Pediatr Surg* 37:1165-1168, 2002.
134. Yaucher NE, Fish JT, Smith HW, Wells JA: Propylene glycol-associated renal toxicity from lorazepam infusion. *Pharmacotherapy* 23:1094-1099, 2003.
135. Arnold JH, Truog RD, Orav DJ: Tolerance and dependence in neonates sadated with fentanyl during extracorporeal membrane oxygenation. *Anesthesiology* 73:1136-1140, 1990.
136. Cronin J: Cycling: an alternative method for weaning ECMO. CNMC National ECMO Symposium, Breckenridge, Colorado, 69, 1990.
137. Sell LL, Cullen ML, Whittlesey GC, et al: Hemorrhagic complications during extracorporeal membrane oxygenation: prevention and treatment. *J Pediatr Surg* 21:1087, 1986.
138. Fortenberry JD, Meier AH, Pettignano R, et al: Extracorporeal life support for posttraumatic acute respiratory distress syndrome at a children's medical center. *J Pediatr Surg* 38:1221-1226, 2003.
139. Downard CD, Betit P, Chang RW, et al: Impact of AMICAR on hemorrhagic complications of ECMO: a ten-year review. *Pediatr Surg* 38:1212-1216, 2003.
140. Jamieson WR, Dryden PJ, O'Connor JP, et al: Beneficial effect of both tranexamic acid and aprotinin on blood loss reduction in reoperative valve replacement surgery. *Circulation* 96(9 suppl): II-96-II-100, 1997.
141. Verrijckt A, Proulx F, Morneau S, Vobecky S: Activated recombinant factor VII for refractory bleeding during extracorporeal membrane oxygenation. *J Thorac Cardiovasc Surg* 127:1812-1813, 2004.
142. Shanley CJ, Hultquist KA, Rosenberg DM, et al: Prolonged extracorporeal membrane circulation without heparin. Evaluation of the Medtronic Minimax oxygenator. *ASAIO J* 38:M311-M316, 1992.
143. Schutze GE, Heulitt MJ: Infections during extracorporeal life support. *J Pediatr Surg* 30:809-812, 1995.
144. Brody J: Altered lymphocyte subsets during cardiopulmonary bypass. *Am J Clin Pathol* 87:66628, 1987.
145. Zach TL: Leukopenia associated with extracorporeal membrane oxygenation in newborn infants. *J Pediatr* 116:440-444, 1990.
146. Carcillo JA, Fields AI, American College of Critical Care Medicine Task Force Committee Members: Clinical practice parameters for hemodynamic support of pediatric and neonatal patients in septic shock. *Crit Care Med* 30:1365-1378, 2002.
147. Adolph V, Ekelund C, Smith C, et al: Developmental outcome of neonates treated with extracorporeal membrane oxygenation. *J Pediatr Surg* 25:38, 1990.
148. Matamoros A, Anderson JC, McConnell J, et al: Neurosonographic findings in infants treated by extracorporeal membrane oxygenation (ECMO). *J Child Neurol* 4(suppl):S52, 1989.
149. Krummel TM, Greenfield LJ, Kirkpatrick BV, et al: The early evaluation of survivors after extracorporeal membrane oxygenation for neonatal pulmonary failure. *J Pediatr Surg* 19:585, 1984.
150. Towne BH, Lott IT, Hicks DA, et al: Long-term follow-up of infants and children treated with extracorporeal membrane oxygenation (ECMO): a preliminary report. *J Pediatr Surg* 20:410, 1985.

151. Lott IT, McPherson D, Towne B, et al: Long-term neurophysiologic outcome after neonatal extracorporeal membrane oxygenation. *J Pediatr* 116:343, 1990.
152. Hofkosh D, Clouse H, Smith-Jones J, et al: Ten years of ECMO: neurodevelopmental outcome among survivors. *Pediatr Res* 27: 246A, 1990.
153. Koumbourlis AC, Motoyama EK, Mutich RL: Lung mechanics during and after extracorporeal membrane oxygenation for meconium aspiration syndrome. *Crit Care Med* 20:751-756, 1992.
154. Boykin AR, Quivers ES, Wagenhoffer KL, et al: Cardiopulmonary outcome of neonatal extracorporeal membrane oxygenation at ages 10-15 years. *Crit Care Med* 31:2380-2384, 2003.
155. Heulitt MJ, Moss MM, Walker WM: Morbidity and mortality in pediatric patients with respiratory failure. *Extracorporeal Life Support Meeting* 41, 1993.
156. Fajardo EM: Outcome and follow-up of children following extracorporeal life support. In Zwischenberger JB, Barlett RH, editors: ECMO: Extracorporeal cardiopulmonary support in critical care. Ann Arbor, 1975, Extracorporeal Life Support Organization.
157. Kulik T, Moler F, Palmisano J: Outcome-associated factors in pediatric patients treated with extracorporeal membrane oxygenator after cardiac surgery. *Circulation* 94:II63-II68, 1996.
158. Ibrahim AE, Duncan BW, Blume ED, Jonas RA: Long-term follow-up of pediatric cardiac patients requiring mechanical circulatory support. *Ann Thorac Surg* 69:186-192, 2000.
159. Lanksa MJ, Lanksa DJ, Horwitz SJ, Aram DM: Presentation, clinical course, and outcome of childhood stroke. *Pediatr Neurol* 7:333-341, 1991.

CHAPTER 48

Development, Structure, and Function of the Brain and Neuromuscular Systems

Michael V. Johnston

PEARLS

- Virtually all the neurons of the brain are "born" before birth, and most of the neurons in the forebrain are born in the first half of gestation.
- The blood-brain barrier is well developed at birth in full-term infants but is more permeable in preterm infants. Immaturity of the blood-brain barrier is one factor that contributes to the relatively high incidence of intracranial hemorrhage in preterm infants.
- A variety of diseases may attack one component of the peripheral nerve selectively.
- The immature brain has greater plasticity or ability to recover following brain injuries than the adult brain.
- In contrast to structural and biochemical events, which mature from spinal cord upward toward the cortex, the infant's behavioral repertoire develops from the head downward.
- Although a large number of disorders may disrupt the developing nervous system, a smaller number present as specific syndromes in critically ill children, based on their tendency to involve specific parts of the nervous system.
  - Seizures, language disorders, and altered levels of consciousness are primary signs of disorders of the cerebral cortex.
  - Choreoathetosis (writhing, dancelike movements of the tongue and extremities) may be produced by a variety of toxic, infectious, and immunologic abnormalities, such as rheumatic fever.
  - Dystonia (rigid, fixed postures of the neck, back, and extremities) reflects a basal ganglia disorder and is frequently seen following ingestion of drugs, such as phenytoin and major tranquilizers.
  - Disruption in the physiology of cerebrospinal fluid is relatively common in the intensive care unit and can present as increased intracranial pressure.
  - The cerebellum is subject to a variety of acute disorders that usually produce a stereotyped cluster of signs, including limb ataxia, intention tremor, hypotonia, decreased reflexes, and nystagmus.
  - A variety of cranial nerve disorders may be seen in the critical care unit. These may involve the eye muscles, jaw and face, tongue, gag reflex, swallowing, hoarseness, airway, and shoulder.
  - Disorders of the spinal cord usually produce a combination of motor abnormalities in the lower extremities associated with a discrete sensory level and abnormalities of bowel and bladder function.
  - Muscle disorders usually present with severe muscle weakness but with relatively preserved deep tendon reflexes.

The nervous system, more than virtually any other organ system in the body, undergoes striking changes in cellular development during childhood. Although some of the changes in the central nervous system that occur during maturation, such as the length of axons connecting the brain with the spinal cord, are simply related to growth, many others involve fundamental changes in organization. For example, evidence indicates that during the postnatal period more connections between neurons are formed than are needed in adulthood.[6] The infant at age 2 to 3 years has approximately twice as many interneuronal connections within the cerebral cortex as the adult, and these synaptic connections are pruned selectively during maturation. This observation implies that the brain undergoes reorganization during development and that its response to stress or injury is dependent on age.

The fundamental elements of the central nervous system include neurons, blood vessels, and the supporting structures or glia.[9,13] These cellular elements are replicated and differentiate according to a fairly rigid, genetically determined program. The relationship between the major developmental features of these elements is shown in Figure 48–1.

Cellular Development

Neurons

Virtually all the neurons of the brain are "born" before birth, and most of the neurons in the forebrain are born in the first half of gestation. Neurons originate in areas of germinal epithelium adjacent to the midline ventricular system of the brain and then migrate outward into the positions they will occupy later in life. The neuron cell body contains most of its protein synthetic machinery, which includes the nucleus and the ribosomes attached to the endoplasmic reticulum. The ribosomes in neurons stain darkly with cresyl violet histologic stain and are referred to as *Nissl substance.* Proteins synthesized in the cell body are transported down into the axon and the nerve terminal. There is an active flow of proteins within the axon both anterograde into the nerve terminal and retrograde into the cell body.

Neurons communicate with each other using neurotransmitter chemicals released from nerve terminals (Table 48–1). Neurotransmitters usually are packaged within vesicles in the axon terminal and are released in response to depolarization of the nerve terminal by an action potential propagated along the axon (Figure 48–2). The neurotransmitter's "message" is decoded on adjacent neurons by specific neurotransmitter receptors located on dendrites or cell bodies.[3,8] Interaction of a neurotransmitter with a receptor alters the function of neurons by two basic mechanisms: opening specific ion channels and activation of second messenger systems (see Chapter 103). For example, release of acetylcholine and interaction with nicotinic receptors at the neuromuscular junction causes a prominent inward sodium current through activated ion channels. Another example is the neurotransmitter system, which uses the excitatory amino acid glutamate. L-Glutamate activates a receptor that causes entry of sodium and calcium into the neuron and allows passage of potassium out of the neuron. The same neurotransmitters that activate ion channels can also activate distinct membrane receptors that are coupled to the production of second messenger chemicals such as inositol phosphates (phosphoinositide turnover) and cyclic adenosine monophosphate. These second messenger substances in turn trigger intracellular events within the neuron.

Evidence indicates that neurotransmitter circuitry may be complex. Many neurons release two distinct neurotransmitter substances that modulate each other's effect. Developmental patterns of specific neurotransmitter circuits contribute to this complexity. Although some neurotransmitter pathways are less active in the immature brain than in adults, others appear to be even more active in the infant than in the adult. For example, excitatory amino acid pathways are especially active in the neonatal period. This activity can be demonstrated by measuring the activity of glutamate-stimulated second messenger systems and activity of ion channels.[7,14]

The biochemical pattern of neuronal development can be examined by assessing the biochemical markers for specific neurotransmitter systems.[7] These studies in animal brains and to a limited extent in human postmortem brains also reveal a stepwise pattern of development. For example, in the cerebral cortex, neurotransmitter systems that originate in the brainstem, including the noradrenergic and serotonin neurons, develop relatively early in the fetal and neonatal period. Their development in the early postnatal period is considerably more advanced than the development of neurons that reside entirely within the cerebral hemispheres, such as the inhibitory γ-aminobutyric acidergic (GABAergic) neurons. Among the last central neuronal systems to differentiate are those that use the neurotransmitter acetylcholine. These biochemical changes in neurotransmitter synthetic enzymes and other biochemical markers for specific neurons are correlated with anatomic changes in axonodendritic development. This evidence indicates that age has an important influence on the organization and function of the developing brain.

Developmental changes in the morphology and biochemical characteristics of neurotransmitters, especially the major excitatory transmitter glutamate and the prominent inhibitory γ-aminobutyric acid (GABA), have important influences on the immature brain's response to medications, stress, and injury. These two neurotransmitters are closely interrelated because GABA is formed by enzymatic decarboxylation of glutamate. The process is dependent on the vitamin cofactor pyridoxal phosphate. Deficiency of pyridoxine or an abnormal requirement for the vitamin, pyridoxine dependency, causes excessive accumulation of glutamate and seizures. After release from synaptic terminals, glutamate and GABA are rapidly taken up again by sodium and energy-dependent transporters on perisynaptic glia. Glucose uptake in the brain has been shown to be tightly linked to cycling of glutamate and GABA at synapses.[12] Excessive stimulation of excitatory amino acid receptors (Figure 48–3) can cause "excitotoxic" injury from insults, such as hypoxia-ischemia, which cause excessive levels of glutamate in the brain's extracellular fluid.

Patterns of selective damage to certain regions of the brain, such as the cerebral cortex, basal ganglia, and

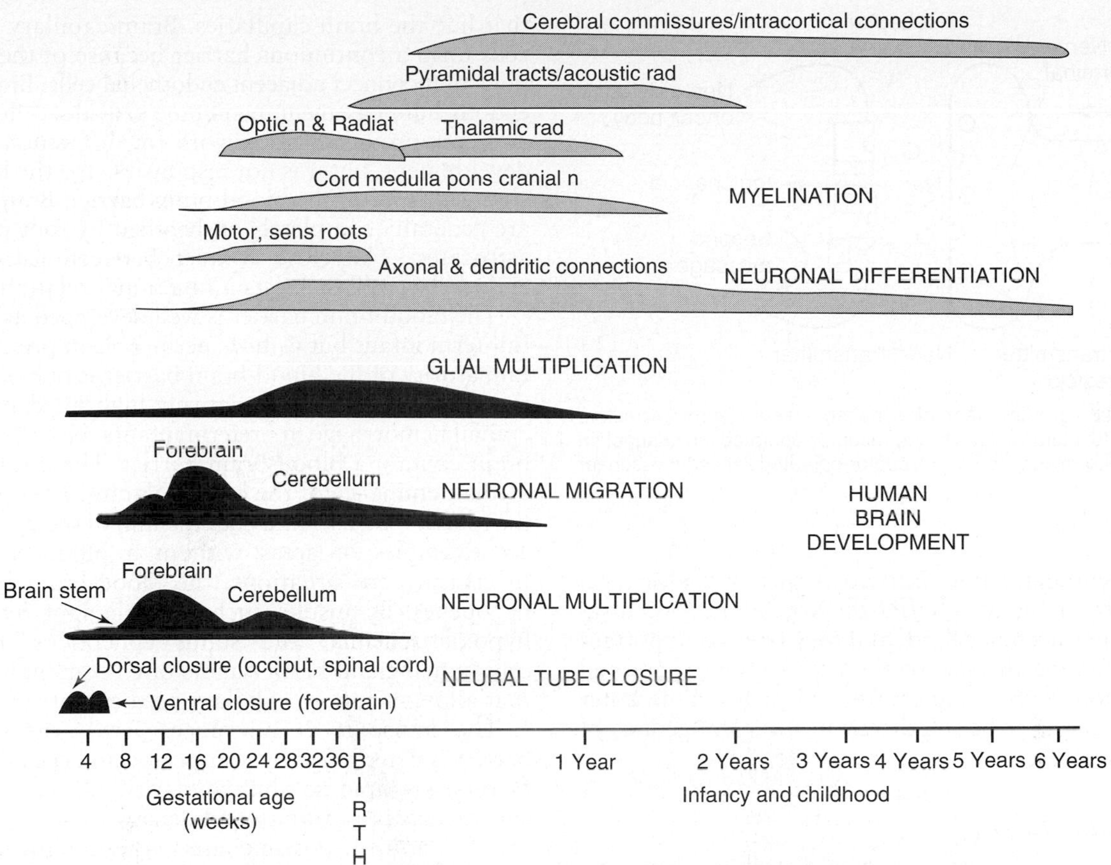

FIGURE 48–1 • Time course of major events in human brain development. The configuration of the curves indicates approximate times of peak activity in development of individual elements. (Redrawn from Gregory GA, editor: *Pediatric anesthesia.* New York, 1989, Churchill Livingstone.)

hippocampus, can be related to changes in the distribution and type of glutamate receptors during development.[14]

Glia

Glial cells are the major support structures within the brain that also serve important homeostatic functions.[1,13] Glia cells are separated into macroglia and microglia. *Macroglia* are the major supporting cells and include astrocytes, oligodendrocytes, and ependymal cells. *Microglia* are phagocytic cells that are activated after injury or infection. The astrocytes, oligodendrocytes, and ependymal cells each have specialized functions. Ependymal cells line the ventricular system of the brain. Oligodendrocytes form the myelin that ensheathes axons. Astrocytes extend foot processes, which have a close relationship with blood vessels and neurons. During embryonic development, certain glia serve as guides for the migration of immature neurons

TABLE 48–1

Neurotransmitters Used in the Nervous System Grouped by Selected Neuronal Pathways

Neurotransmitter	Pathway	Function
Acetylcholine	Neuromuscular junction	Nicotinic receptor: muscle contraction
	Preganglionic autonomic synapses	Nicotinic receptor: stimulate sympathetic and parasympathetic fibers
	Postganglionic parasympathetic fibers	Muscarinic: smooth muscle contraction
	Basal forebrain to cortex; brainstem	Muscarinic: memory and learning; regulation of breathing
Norepinephrine	Pons to cerebral cortex; spinal cord	Alerting cerebral cortex
Serotonin	Midbrain to cerebral cortex	Regulation of sleep and attention
Dopamine	Midbrain to basal ganglia and cerebral cortex	Regulate movement and attention
γ-Aminobutyric acid (GABA)	Interneurons in cerebral cortex	Inhibitory
Glutamate	Many pathways; intracortical, corticospinal, corticostriatal	Excitatory

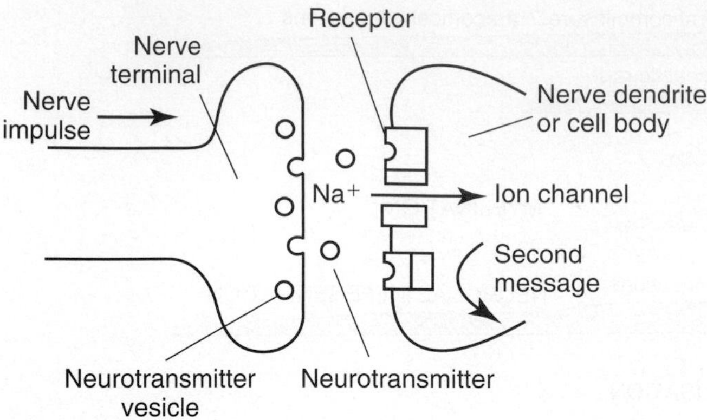

FIGURE 48–2 • Diagram of synapse where neurotransmitters are released to interact with either a receptor-operated ion channel (in this case a sodium channel) or a receptor-operated second messenger system.

from the neuroepithelium into areas such as the cerebral cortex. Certain glia also buffer the potassium concentration of the extracellular fluid, and they have an important role in regulating the size of the extracellular space and concentration of neurotransmitters. Changes in the water content of glia may be important in the pathogenesis of cerebral edema.

Blood-Brain Barrier

The capillary endothelial blood-brain barrier limits the movement of polar solutes, including drugs and proteins, between the blood and the brain.[1] The barrier between the bloodstream and the brain is formed by endothelial cells that line the brain capillaries. Brain capillary endothelial cells form a continuous barrier because of the tight junctions that connect adjacent endothelial cells. Brain capillary endothelium basement membrane provides cellular support and may provide a framework for differentiation during development, but it is not responsible for the biochemical characteristics of the blood-brain barrier. Brain capillaries are generally completely ensheathed by foot processes of astrocytes. The close contact between astrocytes and endothelial cells suggests a functional relationship.

The blood-brain barrier is well developed at birth in the full-term infant but is more permeable in preterm infants. Immaturity of the blood-brain barrier is one of the factors that contributes to the relatively high incidence of intracranial hemorrhage in preterm infants. Not all areas of the brain contain a blood-brain barrier. The pituitary gland, median eminence of the hypothalamus, area postrema of the fourth ventricle, and endothelium of the choroid plexus are examples of areas without a blood-brain barrier. In critical care situations, the blood-brain barrier may be opened by insults such as malignant hypertension, hypoxia-ischemia, and status epilepticus. Endothelial cells in malignant brain tumors often contain fenestrations that allow enhanced capillary permeability.

The transport of substances across the blood-brain barrier is determined by nonspecific and specific transport factors: (1) lipid solubility/polarity, (2) size of capillary surface area, (3) affinity and density of specific transport carriers, and (4) possible enzymatic modification within endothelial cells. A major nonspecific factor that determines the ability of substances to cross the blood-brain barrier is lipid solubility. Oxygen, carbon dioxide, and lipid-soluble drugs such as nicotine, ethanol, inhalation and barbiturate

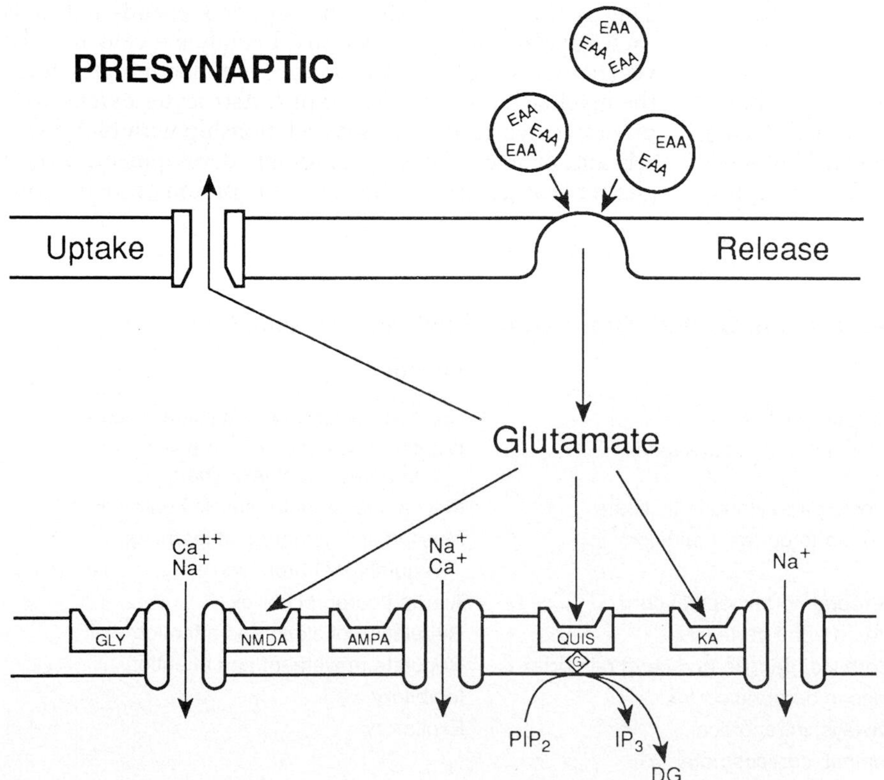

FIGURE 48–3 • Diagram of the glutamate synapses that transmit most of the excitatory neuronal activity in the brain. Glutamate is the principal excitatory amino acid *(EAA)* neurotransmitter released from presynaptic nerve terminals. Glutamate is usually taken up rapidly (uptake site) so that it does not overstimulate postsynaptic neurons. Glutamate's flexible dicarboxylic acid structure can fit comfortably into one of numerous excitatory amino acid subtypes. The α-amino-3-hydroxy-5-methyl-4-isoxazolepropionate *(AMPA)* and kainate *(KA)* receptors open sodium channels and mediate much of the "fast" excitation in the brain. Some types of AMPA receptors conduct some calcium, but more calcium is fluxed through N-methyl-D-aspartate *(NMDA)*-type channels. The NMDA channels require both depolarization of the neuronal membrane and receptor occupancy by glutamate to open. Glycine is also required as a cotransmitter to open the NMDA channel. The distribution of different receptor subtypes varies in different regions of the brain. Seizures and neuronal injury can occur through excessive stimulation of glutamate receptors (excitotoxicity), especially of the NMDA receptor. *QUIS,* Quisqualate.

anesthetics, and diazepam all cross the blood-brain barrier readily because of their high lipid solubility. In contrast, many antibiotics including penicillin do not cross well. Water readily crosses the blood-brain barrier, but sugars such as mannitol cross approximately 100 times less readily. This difference provides a method for dehydrating brain tissue in order to control cerebral edema (see Chapter 52).

Several molecules with low lipid solubility pass readily across the blood-brain barrier because of specific transport mechanisms. Although glucose and mannitol have similar biochemical characteristics, the brain extraction of glucose is 30 times greater than that of mannitol. Glucose is carried across the blood-brain barrier and into neurons by a group of genetically distinct facilitated biochemical transporters.[4] Another example of a carrier mechanism is the one for large neutral amino acids. A common carrier mechanism transports the amino acids phenylalanine, tyrosine, L-dopa, leucine, isoleucine, valine, and methionine. An excess of one of these amino acids restricts the transport of the others because of competition for the carrier.

The blood-brain barrier also has specific transport mechanisms for controlling the transport of sodium and potassium across the capillary endothelium. One of the transport mechanisms uses the enzyme sodium/potassium adenosine triphosphatase (ATPase). This system is a large consumer of energy. Appropriately, brain capillary endothelial cells contain a relatively large number of mitochondria. The high energy requirement of brain capillaries makes them vulnerable to metabolic disturbances that lead to disruptions in ion homeostasis and cerebral edema.

Peripheral Nerve

Peripheral nerves are formed from mixtures of sensory, motor, and autonomic fibers. Motor and autonomic fibers form the ventral root; sensory fibers form the posterior dorsal root attached to the spinal cord (Figure 48–4). These two roots join in the peripheral nerve a short distance outside the spinal cord. The sensory and autonomic axons emanate from cell bodies within sensory or autonomic ganglia outside the central nervous system, but motor axons extend from cell bodies with the spinal cord or brainstem. The myelin sheath around axons is provided by Schwann cells that gradually, during development, wrap thin concentric layers of plasmalemma and cytoplasm around the axon. The myelin is divided into segments by the nodes of Ranvier, which are the gaps between individual Schwann cells (Figure 48–5). Saltatory conduction of electricity from one node of Ranvier to another enhances the efficiency of conduction of nerve impulses. Axons of different diameters are grouped together within the connective tissue that makes up the peripheral nerve. Among the largest axons are those that conduct position and vibratory sensation. Fibers that conduct pain sensation tend to be smaller and unmyelinated.

A variety of diseases may attack one component of the peripheral nerve selectively. Disorders of the cell body lead to secondary degeneration of the axon. This process occurs in motor neuron diseases such as Werdnig-Hoffmann disease. Disruption of the peripheral nerve and axon leads to a secondary reaction in the cell body. Regeneration of peripheral nerve occurs readily if the myelinated tunnel is preserved.

Neuromuscular Junction

The neuromuscular junction is the point of attachment of the motor axon to the muscle. The junction contains the axonal nerve terminal from which acetylcholine is released and a number of junctional folds in the muscle membrane on which nicotinic cholinergic receptors are located. The motor endplate is formed early in fetal life, approximately around week 10 of gestation. The location of nicotinic receptors and junctional regions is

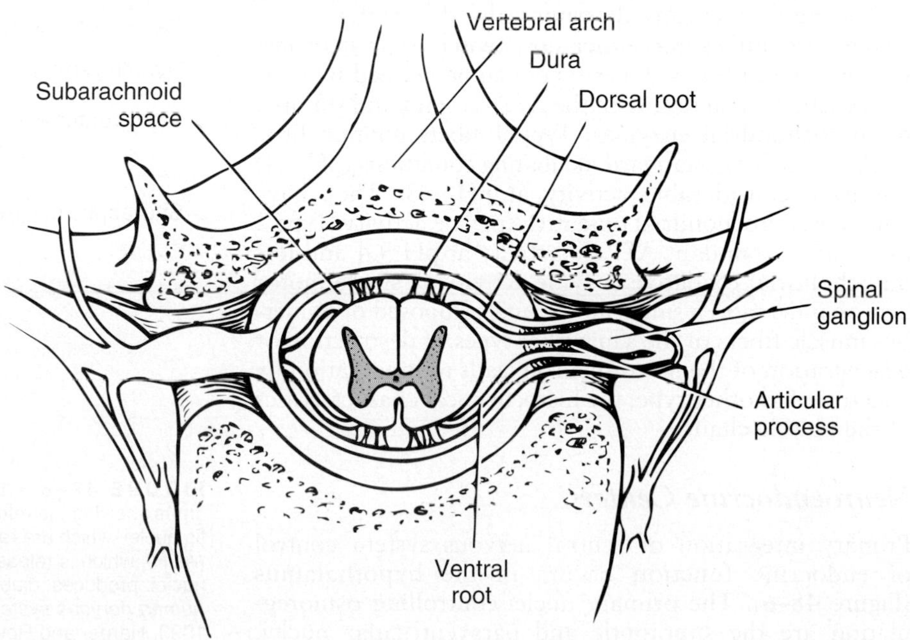

FIGURE 48–4 • Diagram of a spinal column segment showing vertebral body and spinal cord with nerve roots and peripheral nerve. (Redrawn from Barr ML: *The human nervous system: an anatomical viewpoint,* ed 2. Philadelphia, 1993, Harper and Row.)

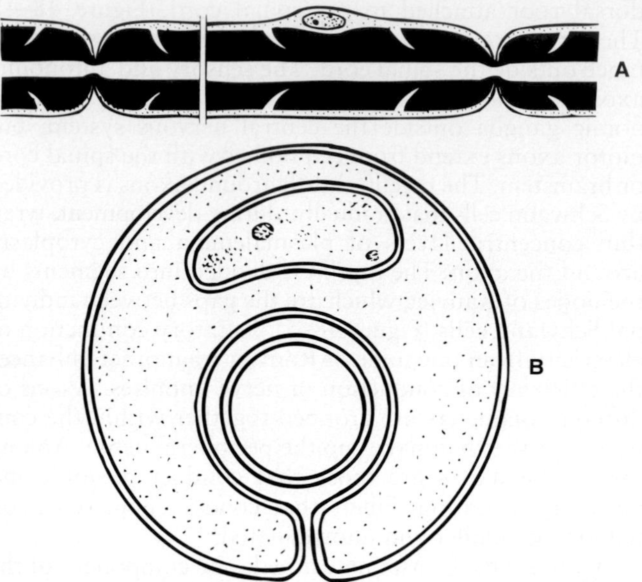

FIGURE 48–5 • Schematic drawing of nerve with myelin sheath as seen in longitudinal **(A)** and cross-section **(B)**. (Redrawn from Barr ML: *The human nervous system: an anatomical viewpoint,* ed 2. Philadelphia, 1993, Harper and Row.)

dependent on a trophic influence of innervation by immature motor axons.

Muscles

Muscles are derived from myoblasts that differentiate from mesoderm at approximately 5 weeks of gestation and fuse to form myotubes at approximately 7 weeks of gestation.[1] The first neuromuscular contacts are formed at approximately 10 weeks of gestation. Motor nerves that are present at 8 weeks of development stimulate muscle proliferation and fiber-type differentiation. Muscle fibers gradually increase in length and diameter during childhood.

The motor neurons determine the differentiation of primary myotubes into either slow twitch (type 1) or fast twitch (type 2) fibers. Fiber types can be defined by their histochemical reaction with the ATPase stain and staining for mitochondrial enzymes. Type 1 fibers contain little ATPase activity at standard incubating conditions (pH 9.4) but have considerable activity at pH 4.3. They have abundant mitochondrial oxidative enzyme activity. Type 2 fibers have abundant ATPase activity at pH 9.4 and less mitochondrial oxidative enzyme activity. A single motor neuron innervates a single motor unit composed of numerous muscle fibers of the same fiber types. If destruction or degeneration of the motor neuron leads to innervation by an axon of another type, the histochemical characteristics of the muscle change.

Neuroendocrine Centers

Primary integration of central nervous system control of endocrine function occurs in the hypothalamus (Figure 48–6). The primary nuclei controlling osmoregulation are the supraoptic and paraventricular nuclei. Cell bodies in this region project axons into the neurohypophysis, where vasopressin is released. Corticotropin-releasing factor, thyrotropin-releasing hormone, and growth hormone-releasing factor are the most important hormones released from the hypothalamus into the pituitary portal circulation to control secretion of the pituitary hormones, adrenocorticotrophin (ACTH), thyroid-stimulation hormone, and growth hormone. Other important hypothalamic nuclei control temperature, feeding, and sleep. Neuroendocrine control mechanisms become established quite early in fetal development and are essential for homeostatic regulation.

Autonomic Nervous System

The autonomic nervous system includes sympathetic and parasympathetic divisions.[5] Preganglionic sympathetic axons are projected from cell bodies of neurons in the lateral portion of thoracic segments and the first two lumbar segments of the spinal cord and enter the paravertebral sympathetic chain. The sympathetic trunk consists of longitudinally arranged ganglia along the spinal column. Extensions of these axons or postganglionic sympathetic fibers innervate the viscera.

The sympathetic innervation of the iris is especially important because it is commonly disrupted, producing pupillary constriction and ptosis (Horner syndrome). The iris is innervated by sympathetic fibers exiting at the T1-T2 level that pass through the superior cervical ganglion and extend up along the carotid artery to the orbit.

The parasympathetic system originates from levels of the spinal cord above and below the sympathetic system. Preganglionic parasympathetic fibers exit from the brainstem with cranial nerves III, VII, IX, and X and from S2-S4.

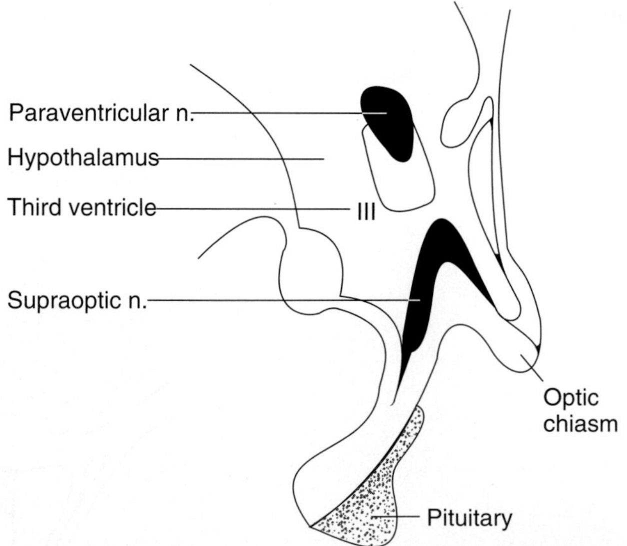

FIGURE 48–6 • Diagram of sagittal section through the hypothalamus showing the relative position of the paraventricular and supraoptic nuclei, which are responsible for production of antidiuretic hormone *(ADH),* which is released into the posterior pituitary. Damage to these nuclei produces diabetes insipidus. (Redrawn from Barr ML: *The human nervous system: an anatomical viewpoint,* ed 2. Philadelphia, 1993, Harper and Row.)

Parasympathetic fibers from the vagus nerve innervate widespread areas in the heart, lungs, and visceral organs.

Neuroblasts for the sympathetic and parasympathetic ganglia originate in the neural crest. Neural crest cells migrate from their position above the neural tube ventrolaterally to reach their final positions. The local environment in which neural crest cells find themselves determines the final commitment to a sympathetic or parasympathetic neurotransmitter phenotype.

Acetylcholine and norepinephrine are the primary neurotransmitters in the autonomic nervous system. Acetylcholine is released from preganglionic fibers in both sympathetic and parasympathetic ganglia to act at nicotinic acetylcholine receptors. Postganglionic parasympathetic nerve fibers release acetylcholine, which stimulates muscarinic receptors. Postganglionic sympathetic fibers release norepinephrine except in sweat glands, where acetylcholine is released. Four classes of adrenergic receptors (α_1, α_2, β_1, and β_2) have been identified (see Chapters 23 and 111).

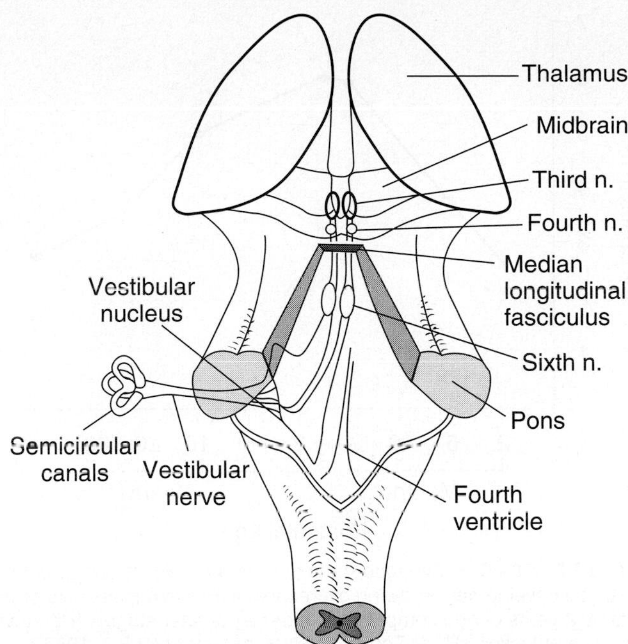

FIGURE 48–7 • Diagram of brainstem from the top with cerebellum and forebrain cut away showing vestibular nuclei, median longitudinal fasciculus *(MLF),* and input from vestibular nerve. This circuit is responsible for coordination of eye movement produced by head movement or caloric stimulation of the semicircular canals. Stimulation of the vestibular nuclei sends impulses along the MLF that activate the ipsilateral sixth nerve (lateral rectus) and contralateral third nerve (medial rectus) to move the eyes to one side. (Redrawn from Martinez Martinez PFA: *Neuroanatomy.* Philadelphia, 1982, WB Saunders.)

Anatomic Development

Neural Tube, Crest, and Spinal Cord

The general pattern of brain development follows a caudal to rostral pattern so that morphologic development of the spinal cord occurs before development of the cerebral cortex[10] (see Figure 48–1). By the end of week 4 of gestation, the edges of the neural plate destined to form the spinal cord have folded and fused into a tube.

Establishment of the basic form of the divided cerebral ventricular system takes place several weeks later. Birth defects that cause spina bifida occur within the first month of gestation, whereas anomalies of the cerebral ventricles occur at about the same time or a few weeks later.

Sequential Development of Brain Regions

The major developmental events in the central nervous system take place in overlapping waves that progress up the neuraxis from the spinal cord through the medulla, pons, midbrain, diencephalon, and cerebral hemispheres. Two events that contribute to the major increase in the brain's mass in the postnatal period are myelination and elaboration of neuronal axons and dendrites and their connections (see Figure 48–1). The process of axon myelination is particularly prominent because it gives the developing brain its characteristic division into white matter and gray matter. Among the first areas of the brain to myelinate are the motor and sensory roots, followed by the spinal cord, medulla, pons, and cranial nerves. One of the earlier tracts to myelinate within the brainstem is the median longitudinal fasciculus, which connects the third and sixth cranial nerve nuclei with the vestibular system (Figure 48–7). Myelination of the optic and thalamic tracts is followed by myelination of the pyramidal tracts, which is generally advanced by age 18 months. The intracortical and commissural tracts in the cerebral hemispheres are among the last to myelinate.

Myelination of axons is an important anatomic and physiologic milestone because it enhances the speed and efficiency of impulse flow. However, equally important is the elaboration of the connections between axons and dendrites in the brain. During this process, more interneuronal synaptic connections are created in the immediate postnatal period than are needed for later life.[6] The pattern of synaptic overproduction of synapses in the visual cortex in the human is shown in Figure 48–8. This pattern of formation of interneuronal connection appears to play an important role in development of brain function and probably also is related to the response of the brain to injury. The immature brain has greater plasticity or ability to recover following brain injuries than the adult brain, and this capacity is related in part to the redundancy in connections created by this developmental pattern.[8]

Brain Metabolism and Cerebral Blood Flow

Autoregulation is the descriptive term applied to the mechanisms that link brain blood flow with brain metabolism. The concept of pressure autoregulation states that cerebral blood flow is maintained relatively constant over wide ranges of arterial blood pressure.[2] Both local and global injuries can disrupt pressure autoregulation, which can result in blood flow changing passively with changes in arterial pressure.

Chemical autoregulation is the principle that relates changes in arterial P_{CO_2} and arterial P_{O_2} to changes in cerebral blood flow. A change in cerebral blood flow of 2 ml/100 g/min occurs for each 1 torr change in arterial P_{CO_2}. These changes appear to result from alterations in

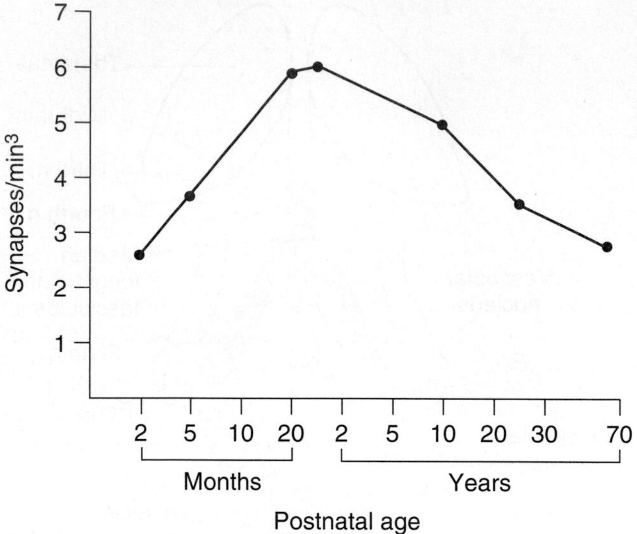

FIGURE 48–8 • Synapse density in human visual cortex during postnatal development showing overexpression of synapses at approximately 2 years of age compared with earlier or later stages. (Redrawn from Huttenlocker PR, deCourten CH: *Hum Neurobiol* 6:1, 1987.)

TABLE 48–2

Major Developmental Milestones

Age	Development
1 month	Visual contact with objects, faces
2 months	Social smile
3 months	Head control
4 months	Reach for objects
5 months	Roll both ways
6 months	Sitting
7 months	Crawling, babbling
8 months	Support weight on legs
9–14 months	Stand, cruise, walk; "ma-ma," "da-da," pincer grasp
2 years	50 words
3 years	Tricycle; 250 words

cerebral interstitial pH,[18] which in turn causes local vessels to constrict or dilate. Arterial PO_2 has no effect on cerebral blood until it falls below 50 torr, after which cerebral blood flow increases dramatically in proportion to the degree of hypoxia (see Chapter 52).

Cerebral blood flow also increases or decreases, depending on the metabolic requirements present at any given time. A variety of potential mediators of metabolic regulation have been espoused, including hydrogen ion,[11] potassium ion,[17] adenosine,[19] prostaglandins,[15] and nitric oxide (see Chapter 17). Viscosity of the blood can affect its flow.[2] In the presence of hyperviscosity, brain blood flow can be markedly altered. Clinical manifestations of this condition can be seen with polycythemia of infancy or with polycythemia secondary to chronic cyanotic heart disease.

The intimate and intricate relationship between metabolism and blood flow is well maintained in the absence of injury. When brain tissue is injured from any of a variety of causes, autoregulatory mechanisms linking blood flow and metabolism are altered. Depending on the nature of the injury and its severity, autoregulatory mechanisms may recover. Loss of these mechanisms is an indication of severe injury, and their failure to resume function is an ominous prognostic sign (see Chapter 17).

Clinical Correlates of Postnatal Neuromuscular Development

Developmental Milestones

Infants develop gross motor, fine motor, social, and language skills according to a relatively standard developmental program that is summarized in Table 48–2.[10] In contrast to structural and biochemical events, which mature from spinal cord upward toward the cortex, the infant's behavioral repertoire develops from the head downward. Full-term newborn infants are able to follow a large red object held in front of their eyes, and by age 6 weeks infants usually are able to track through a 90-degree arc. By age 6 to 8 weeks, most infants develop a social smile. Laughing in response to playful activity usually is apparent by 3 to 4 months. At the same time, the infant usually has acquired good head control, and head lag is no longer present. The infant's ability to reach for and hold onto objects usually is delayed until about 4 months. One month later, at 5 months, the infant is generally able to roll over from back to front and from front to back.

Most infants are able to sit briefly by 6 months, and by 9 months most infants are able to sit well without support. Many infants crawl by age 7 months, although this can be quite variable. Control of the legs and support of weight develop about the same time as sitting, and most infants are able to stand by 8 months and to walk between 9 and 14 months.

Although gross motor milestones are important indicators of development, abnormalities in them may indicate an isolated motor problem rather than difficulty with overall psychomotor development. For example, delay in walking with preservation of other milestones may indicate an isolated upper motor neuron lesion, as is found in cerebral palsy, or a neuromuscular disorder, such as muscular dystrophy. Delays in social milestones, such as smiling, laughing, and cooing, and delays in speech development are more sensitive indicators of defects in cognitive function. Speech development proceeds from cooing to babbling in the first few months of life. Most normally developing infants are able to say "ma-ma" and "da-da" by age 11 months, and by age 1 year they are able to respond to a simple sentence. Two-year-olds usually have a vocabulary of about 50 words and are able to put together a two-word sentence; 3-year-olds have a vocabulary of more than 200 words. Development of fine motor skills also is related to psychomotor ability. Development of a pincer grasp between the thumb and index finger is an important fine motor skill, and delays in this ability may be indicative of serious psychomotor delays.

Changes in Reflexes

Several changes in neurologic signs occur during infancy and early childhood. The Moro response, in which arms and legs are suddenly brought symmetrically to the midline in response to a startle or to a backward movement of the head, usually disappears within several weeks of delivery and usually is abnormal beyond age 6 weeks. The parachute response, in which an infant throws the hands outward when held with the head down, usually develops at 9 to 11 months. Deep tendon reflexes in infants usually are fairly brisk, and some clonus often can be elicited in the first 6 months of life. Babinski responses usually are elicited until between ages 12 and 18 months. At this time the asymmetry in Babinski responses is a more important indicator of abnormality than its presence alone.

Anatomic Localization: Physiology and Function

Although a large number of disorders may disrupt the developing nervous system, a smaller number present as specific syndromes in critically ill children, based on their tendency to involve specific parts of the nervous system. The structures commonly involved in brain disorders in children are shown as a diagram in Figure 48–9 and in magnetic resonance images of the brain in Figures 48–10, 48–11, and 48–12. This section briefly focuses on disorders that are relatively common in the intensive care unit and correlates them with their localization within the nervous system.

Cerebral Cortex

Seizures, language disorders, and altered levels of consciousness are primary signs of disorders of the cerebral cortex. Seizures (see Chapter 55) probably do not originate from any deeper structure of the brain. Aphasia, either inability to produce language (motor aphasia or Broca aphasia) or receptive aphasia (Wernicke aphasia), indicates a primary disorder of specific areas of cerebral cortex in the dominant (usually left) cerebral hemisphere. Aphasia must sometimes be distinguished from dysarthria, in which speech is produced but is distorted or garbled. Occasionally, hesitancy to speak can be produced by mesial frontal lobe lesions. Coma is produced by bilateral lesions of the cerebral cortex or damage to the brainstem reticular activation system[16] (see Chapter 54).

Basal Ganglia

Disorders of the basal ganglia include choreoathetosis and dystonia. Choreoathetosis (writhing, dancelike movements of the tongue and extremities) may be produced by a variety of toxic, infectious, and immunologic abnormalities such as rheumatic fever. Dystonia (rigid, fixed postures of the neck, back, and extremities) reflects a basal ganglia disorder and is frequently seen following ingestion of drugs, such as phenytoin and major tranquilizers. It also may follow hypoxic-ischemic encephalopathy or other brain insults.

Cerebral Spinal Fluid Pathways and Hydrocephalus

Disruption in the physiology of cerebrospinal fluid (CSF) is relatively common in the intensive care unit and presents

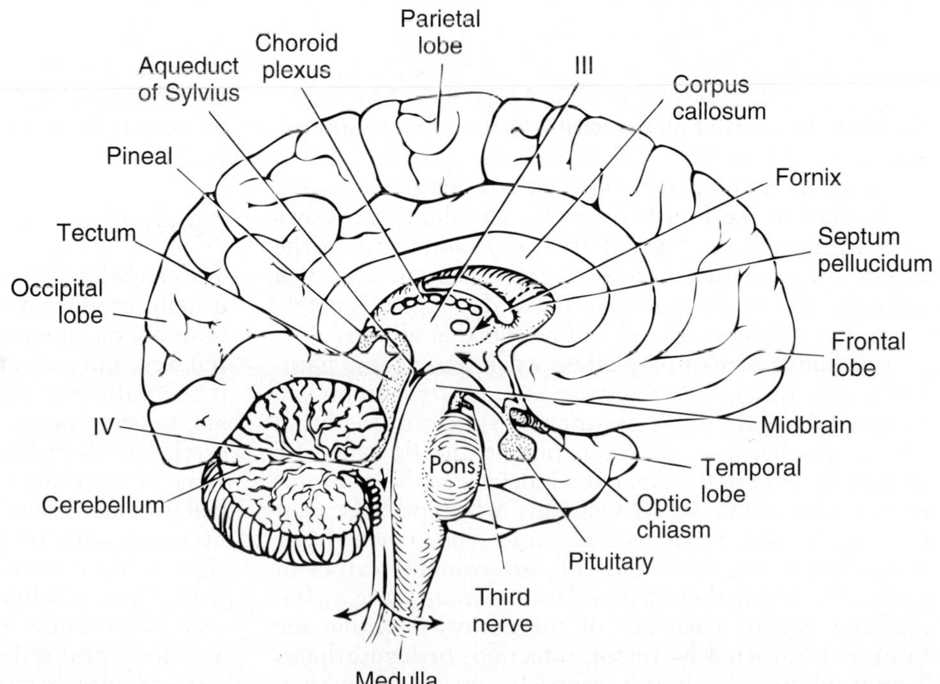

FIGURE 48–9 • Midsagittal view of the brain showing important structures and flow of cerebrospinal fluid (CSF) *(arrows)*. CSF produced by the choroid plexus flows from each lateral ventricle through the foramina of Monro into the third ventricle (III), then caudally through the aqueduct of Sylvius into the fourth ventricle (IV). CSF leaves the fourth ventricle for the foramina of Luschka and Magendie and then circulates upward around the base of the brain and up over the convexities.

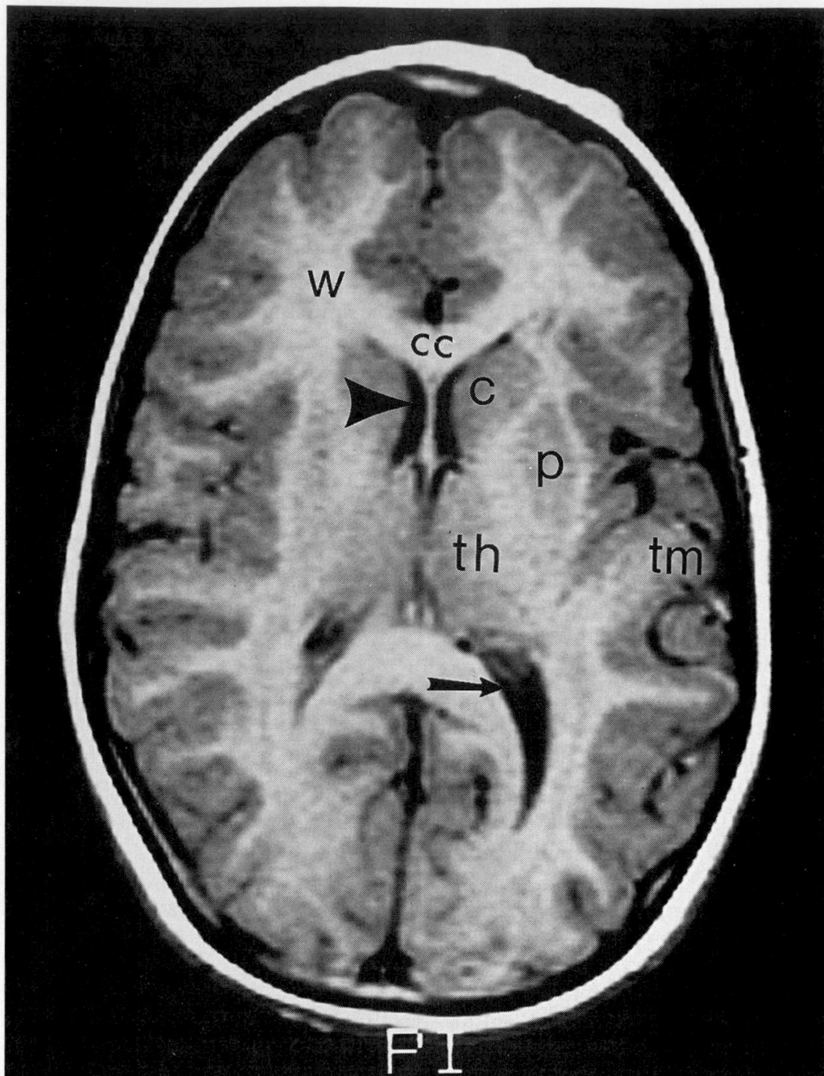

FIGURE 48–10 • Normal magnetic resonance image of the brain of a 7-year-old child showing a horizontal section with nose at top. The cerebrospinal fluid is *black* in this T1-weighted image. The *black triangle* points to the frontal horn of the left lateral ventricle, separated from the frontal horn on the other side by the septum pellucidum. The *arrow* posteriorly points to the occipital horn of the right lateral ventricle. White matter consisting of myelinated nerve fibers is *white,* whereas gray matter including neurons is *gray.* *c,* Caudate nucleus; *cc,* corpus callosum; *p,* putamen; th, thalamus; tm, temporal lobe; *w,* white matter.

as hydrocephalus (see Chapter 53). Most of the CSF is produced in the choroid plexus within the cerebral ventricles. It travels through the brain's ventricular system as shown in Figure 48–9 and passes outward through the foramina in the roof of the fourth ventricle. The fluid then flows upward around the base of the brain and up over the cerebral convexities, where a great deal is absorbed through the arachnoid villi. Each day approximately 500 ml of CSF is produced and resorbed at all ages.

Two kinds of hydrocephalus occur when these pathways are disrupted. *Communicating hydrocephalus* usually dilates the entire ventricular system of the brain and occurs because of a reduction in the flow of CSF around the base of the brain or a blockage in the reabsorption over the convexities. Meningitis, which produces scar tissue in the basilar cisterns, and intracerebral hemorrhage, which blocks the arachnoid villi, are common causes of communicating hydrocephalus. *Noncommunicating hydrocephalus* occurs when one of the pathways within the brain is obstructed by tumor, infection, or hemorrhage. Tumor within the fourth ventricle, as occurs with a medulloblastoma, may produce dilation of the third and lateral ventricles. Congenital obstruction of the aqueduct of Sylvius between the third and fourth ventricles is a fairly common cause of congenital hydrocephalus.

Cerebellum

The cerebellum is subject to a variety of acute disorders that usually produce a stereotyped cluster of signs, including limb ataxia, intention tremor, hypotonia and decreased reflexes, and nystagmus. Ataxic gait usually is prominent if the patient is able to walk. Both the nystagmus and ataxia occur on the same side as the lesion. Occasionally cerebellar disorders may be so severe and abrupt that some of these signs are missing. For example, acute cerebellar hemorrhage may produce acute loss of consciousness and signs of brainstem dysfunction.[16] In this case, signs of dysfunction of cranial nerves closely associated with the cerebellum and brainstem are usually found, such as weakness in the abducens or facial nerve and an absent corneal reflex (fifth cranial nerve).

Cerebellar hemorrhage is a life-threatening disorder that usually demands prompt neurosurgical attention.

Cerebellar abscess is uncommon in the United States but occurs frequently with disseminated tuberculosis. Drug intoxication with anticonvulsants or sedatives frequently produces acute disturbances of the cerebellum that cause ataxia. Postinfectious disorders such as acute cerebellar ataxia may cause acute cerebellar signs, and brain tumors including medulloblastoma and cerebellar astrocytoma produce acute cerebellar disease that may lead to admission to the critical care unit (see Chapter 53).

Brainstem and Cranial Nerves

A variety of cranial nerve disorders may be seen in the critical care unit. Anosmia as a result of disruption of the first cranial nerve from head injury is fairly common, although seldom tested for. Trauma to the optic nerve frequently causes loss of vision and may be associated with swelling of the optic nerve head resembling papilledema. Optic neuritis produces a similar picture. However, true papilledema from increased intracranial pressure does not usually cause visual impairment, although the blind spot may enlarge.

Cranial Nerves III, IV, and VI

Abnormalities in the eye muscles controlled by the third, fourth, and sixth cranial nerve are often valuable signs in the intensive care unit. A list of these nerves, the muscles they control, and oculomotor abnormalities produced by lesions in the nerves is given in Table 48–3. Focal injury to the third, fourth, and sixth cranial nerves is common with infectious diseases such as meningitis. Herniation of the uncus of the temporal lobe between the tentorium and brainstem frequently causes third nerve injury, usually in association with coma. A more subtle lesion of the third nerve is produced by aneurysmal dilation of the posterior communicating artery, which dilates the pupil by compressing the parasympathetic fibers on the outside of the nerve. Sixth nerve palsy is a common nonspecific finding in increased intracranial pressure of any cause.

Two maneuvers used to test these cranial nerves, the doll's eye or oculocephalic maneuver and caloric testing, deserve special attention[16] (see Chapter 50).

Cranial Nerves V, VII, and VIII

The fifth cranial nerve from the pons controls motor function of the jaw and serves facial and corneal sensation. The corneal reflex is commonly tested to establish brainstem function. The seventh and eighth (facial and vestibuloacoustic) cranial nerves also emanate from the pons. Although the eighth nerve is commonly disrupted in disorders such as meningitis, it is not frequently of localizing value in the intensive care unit. When function of the seventh nerve is disrupted in upper motor neuron lesions of the opposite hemisphere to produce facial palsy, the forehead is usually spared. Complete peripheral paresis of the seventh nerve results in complete weakness of the entire side of the face. Bilateral seventh nerve weakness is commonly found in Guillain-Barré syndrome.

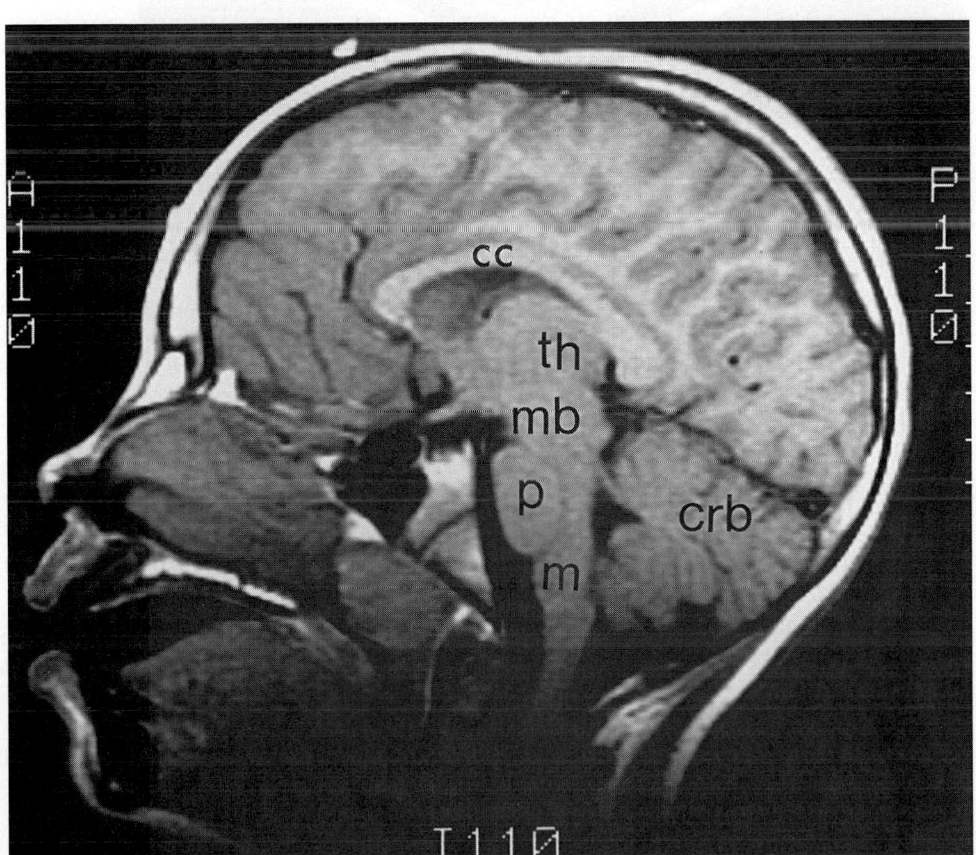

FIGURE 48–11 • Midsagittal magnetic resonance image of the same brain shown in Figure 48–10 showing the posterior fossa structures, the brainstem, and cerebellum. *cc,* Corpus callosum; *crb,* cerebellum; *m,* medulla oblongata; *mb,* midbrain; *p,* pons; *th,* thalamus.

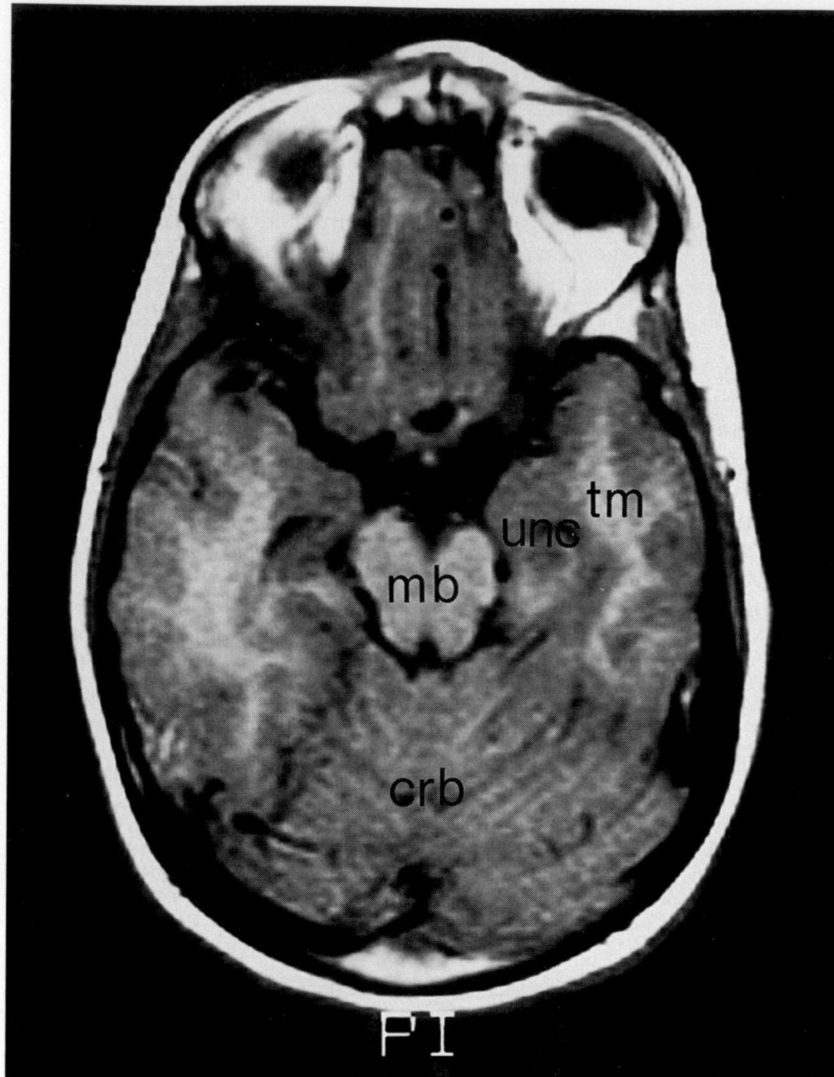

FIGURE 48–12 • Lower horizontal cut of magnetic resonance image of brain shown in Figures 48–10 and 48–11. The image shows the location of the uncus *(unc)* of the medial temporal lobe *(tm)* almost touching the midbrain *(mb)*. The location of the cerebellum *(crb)* is shown behind the brainstem. Swelling of the brain from cerebral edema can cause herniation of the uncus downward between the tentorium and the brainstem, leading to compression of the third cranial nerve with pupillary dilation. The third nerve emerges ventrally from the midbrain at approximately this level, accounting for the frequency of third nerve palsy in uncal herniation.

Cranial Nerves IX, X, XI, and XII

The ninth and tenth cranial nerves occasionally are affected by disorders of the posterior fossa but more frequently are paralyzed in neuropathic disorders such as Guillain-Barré syndrome or by local inflammation and trauma. This causes loss of gag, swallowing, hoarseness, and inability to protect the airway. The eleventh cranial nerve can be affected by infectious processes such as mononucleosis but is quite unusual. This causes loss of shoulder shrug. Similarly, focal neuropathic abnormalities of the twelfth nerve may produce deviation of the tongue to the same side. It is unusual for the twelfth nerve to be affected in isolation. Asymmetrical abnormalities of the cranial nerves may be produced by intrinsic neoplasms such as brainstem gliomas.

Spinal Cord

Disorders to the spinal cord are often difficult to diagnose and may be mistaken for other problems. However, rapid treatment is important for preserving function. Disorders of the spinal cord usually produce a combination of motor abnormalities in the lower extremities associated with a discrete sensory level and abnormalities of bowel and bladder function. Any patient with a segmental motor disorder such as paraplegia or paralysis of all four extremities should be suspected of having a spinal cord lesion.

TABLE 48–3

Abnormalities in Eye Movements Produced by Cranial Nerve Lesions

Cranial Nerve	Muscle	Lesion
III	Levator for eyelids	Eye out
	Superior, inferior rectus	Eye down
	Ciliary	Dilated pupil
IV	Superior oblique	Vertical diplopia; eye cannot be turned down and inward
VI	Lateral rectus	Eye in

Once the lesion is suspected, the search for sensory level and abnormalities of sphincter function can be started.

Several spinal cord syndromes following compression, trauma, or ischemia have been delineated. Anterior spinal artery ischemia produced by meningitis or trauma causes damage in the anterior half of the spinal cord. This region disrupts motor areas of the cord but spares more dorsal sensory pathways. Brown-Séquard syndrome is produced by lateral hemisection of the cord. In this syndrome, position sense is impaired below the lesion on the side of damage, but pain and temperature are disturbed on the opposite side. Occasionally the central core of the cervical spinal cord is preferentially damaged by contusive trauma, resulting in more weakness in the arms than the legs. This may be seen in flexion extension injuries of the cervical cord, as occurs in diving accidents.

Peripheral Nerves

The primary abnormalities of peripheral nerves that present in the intensive care unit are acute or subacute neuropathies or polyradiculoneuropathies.[1] Guillain-Barré syndrome (see Chapter 56) is a particularly important disorder that disrupts nerve roots near the spinal cord. A variety of other infectious, inflammatory, and toxic disorders produce peripheral neuropathies. The major clinical signs of peripheral neuropathy are focal abnormalities in sensation or motor function and diminished deep tendon reflexes.

Neuromuscular Junction

Neuromuscular junction abnormalities (see Chapter 56) should be suspected in any patient with progressive waxing and waning weakness or fatigability.[1] Neuromuscular junction abnormalities usually do not affect the reflexes unless the patient is quite weak, and a high clinical suspicion is necessary, combined with electrodiagnostic testing.

Muscle Disorders

Muscle disorders usually present with severe muscle weakness but with relatively preserved deep tendon reflexes. A number of patients with neuromuscular disorders come to the intensive care unit because of respiratory failure after a chronic course (see Chapter 56). Other disorders may present with acute muscular paralysis because of an underlying myopathy. Occasionally patients present with metabolic myopathies with or without myoglobinuria. One example of a metabolic myopathy is mitochondrial disorders associated with defects in the respiratory chain enzymes[1] (see Chapter 69). Myopathies usually present with preserved reflexes, although the muscle weakness may be so profound that reflexes cannot be elicited. Another condition that may produce acute muscle weakness is polymyositis, which may follow a viral infection such as influenza B.

REFERENCES

1. Asbury AK, McKhann GM, McDonald WI: *Diseases of the nervous system.* Philadelphia, 1986, Ardmore Medical Books.
2. Bruce DA: Cerebrovascular dynamics. In James HE, Anas NG, Perkin RM, editors: *Brain insults in infants and children.* Orlando, 1985, Grune & Stratton.
3. Cooper JR, Bloom FE, Roth RH: *The biochemical basis of neuropharmacology.* New York, 1986, Oxford University Press.
4. Gilman AG, Goodman LS, Gilman A: *The pharmacological basis of therapeutics,* New York, 1980, Macmillan Publishing Co.
5. Dwyer DS, Vannucci SJ, Simpson IA: Expression, regulation, and functional role of glucose transporters (GLUTs) in brain. *Int Rev Neurobiol* 51:159, 2002.
6. Huttenlocker PR, deCourten CH: The development of synapses in striate cortex of man. *Hum Neurobiol* 6:1, 1987.
7. Johnston MV: Biochemistry of neurotransmitters in cortical development. In Peters A, Jones EA, editors: *Cerebral cortex, vol. 7.* New York, 1988, Plenum Press.
8. Johnston MV, Nishimura A, Harum K, Pekar J, Blue ME: Sculpting the developing brain. *Adv Pediatrics* 48:1, 2001.
9. Kandel ER, Schwartz JH, editors: *Principles of neural science.* New York, 1985, Elsevier.
10. Kandt R, Johnston MV, Goldstein G: The central nervous system: basic comments. In Gregory EA, editor: *Pediatric anesthesia.* New York, 1989, Churchill Livingstone.
11. Krause GS, White BC, Aust SD, et al: Brain cell death following ischemia and reperfusion: a proposed biochemical sequence. *Crit Care Med* 16:714, 1988.
12. Magistretti PJ, Pellerin L, Rothman DL, Shulman RG: Energy on demand. *Science* 283:496, 1999.
13. Martinez Martinez PFA: *Neuroanatomy.* Philadelphia, 1982, WB Saunders.
14. McDonald JW, Johnston MV: Physiological and pathophysiological roles of excitatory amino acids during central nervous system development. *Brain Res Rev* 15:41, 1990.
15. Paul KS, Whalley ET, Forster C, et al: Prostacyclin and cerebral vessel relaxation. *J Neurosurg* 57:334, 1982.
16. Plum F, Posner JB: *The diagnosis of stupor and coma,* ed 3. Philadelphia, 1982, FA Davis.
17. Raichle ME: The pathophysiology of brain ischemia. *Ann Neurol* 13:2, 1983.
18. Siesjo BK: Cerebral circulation and metabolism. *J Neurosurg* 60:883, 1984.
19. Winn HR, Rubio R, Berne RM: The role of adenosine in the regulation of cerebral blood flow. *J Cereb Blood Flow Metab* 1:239, 1981.

CHAPTER

49

Neuroimaging

Dennis W. W. Shaw and Ed Weinberger

PEARLS

- Neonatal imaging
  - Ultrasound remains the primary modality for germinal matrix hemorrhage; routine screening has been recommended for all infants born before 30 weeks' gestation
  - Magnetic resonance (MR) is more sensitive than ultrasound to noncystic periventricular radiolucency, but impact on care has not been established
  - Acute computed tomography (CT) and conventional MR detection of hypoxic-ischemic injury (HII) in the term child depends on edema.
  - Diffusion-weighted-MR will be sensitive to acute ischemia in the neonate, even before swelling has developed
- Imaging: Ultrasound (US)
  Advantages
  - Portable
  - No ionizing radiation

  Disadvantages
  - User dependent
  - Except for transcranial Doppler (TCD) US, open fontanelle is needed

  Major applications
  - Germinal matrix hemorrhage
  - Ventricular size
  - General evaluation of cerebral parenchyma
- Imaging: CT
  Advantages
  - Fast, usually does not require sedation for head scans
  - More sensitive than US to many cerebral parenchymal diseases
  - Adequate assessment of cerebral neurosurgical emergencies

  Disadvantages
  - Less sensitive than MR with some exceptions (calcium including cortical bone; acute blood)
  - Uses ionizing radiation
  - Requires transport to scanner
- Imaging: MRI
  Advantages
  - Best parenchymal evaluation for most cerebral disorders
  - Multiplanar imaging
  - No ionizing radiation
  - Best assessment of spinal cord and para-axial tissues, whereas CT offers better assessment of bony integrity

  Disadvantages
  - Requires transport to scanner
  - Extended scan times often necessitate sedation in younger children and uncooperative patients

Safety requirements
- Patient, equipment, and attendant personnel must be screened before entering MR room
- Potentially fatal disruption of electrical devices (e.g., cardiac pacers)
- Metallic projectiles (e.g., ferromagnetic oxygen tanks)
- A website on MR safety is available (www.mrisafety.com)

- Imaging: Catheter Angiography

Advantages
- Best detail of cerebral vasculature
- Gives dynamic flow information (e.g., early draining vein confirming an arteriovenous malformation [AVM])

Disadvantages
- Ionizing radiation
- Invasive

Major applications
- Evaluation of AVM, aneurysm, and some vasculitis cases

Imaging Modality Overview

Multiple imaging modalities are available to investigate the neurologic status of the child in the intensive care unit (ICU). The selection of the most appropriate examination depends on weighing factors of modality sensitivity to the suspected disease, the degree of suspicion for a particular disease, the practicalities of the examination's complexity, and the child's condition. In this chapter the imaging modalities available are reviewed and followed by the disease processes most likely to be subject to neuroimaging evaluation.

Ultrasound

Standard cranial ultrasound (US) has been a mainstay in the neonatal ICU. US generates gray scale digital images from components of a US beam reflected off tissue interfaces, with no ionizing radiation, and bedside imaging can be performed with it. Cranial US has, however, a restricted window through which to visualize the brain, primarily through an open fontanelle, and is therefore limited for the most part to the first few months of life. US is sensitive to some intracranial pathologic conditions, including the detection of germinal matrix hemorrhage, evaluation of ventricular size, and severe white matter lesions in premature infants including cystic periventricular leukomalacia (PVL). It is less sensitive for conditions such as mild to moderate parenchymal ischemic changes, subarachnoid, punctate parenchymal hemorrhage, and subtle cerebral malformations. Extraaxial collections, especially lateral, can also be difficult to appreciate on US performed through a midline fontanelle.

Color Doppler US with the standard US machine uses the shift in frequency associated with reflection of the sound beam off an interface in motion (Doppler shift) to detect movement in the image field and assigns a color to those pixels with movement to distinguish them from those pixels without movement. The color (most often red and blue) assigned is different depending on whether the movement is away or toward the transducer, but the color assigned is arbitrary and arteries and veins are not necessarily red and blue, respectively. Color Doppler US allows for some investigation of the cerebral circulation, primarily through the open fontanelle. Transcranial Doppler (TCD) US uses the same Doppler shift to produce waveforms giving flow velocities and direction. TCD US has the advantage of being able to be performed through the thinner portions of the skull, primarily the temporal squamosa, in older children and adults. (Fig. 49–1; see color on insert). TCD US has been used in the evaluation of cerebral perfusion in patients with sickle cell disease. TCD US is generally sensitive to stenoses less than 50% in the central cerebral circulation, with the highest sensitivity and specificity being in the middle cerebral artery (MCA).[1]

Computed Tomography

Computed tomography (CT) scanning has increased sensitivity over US for many intracranial diseases, including most neurosurgical emergencies, and is not obviated by closing fontanelles. Imaging on modern scanners with multiarray detectors can be performed rapidly. CT, however, requires transporting the patient from the ICU and uses ionizing radiation (x-rays) to produce digital computer reconstructed images based on differences in tissue density. The choice of radiation parameters, slice thickness, postprocessing, and image viewing (window and level) must be tailored to the particular clinical question to optimize the imaging. Bone and other calcification have the highest density, and with the lowest density are, in decreasing order (nonadipose) soft tissue (such as brain), water (i.e., cerebrospinal fluid [CSF]), fat, and air. The difference in density between bone and brain is great, whereas the difference between brain and fat is less. The density difference between gray and white matter is much smaller but is sufficient to be appreciated with the appropriate window and leveling. As edema develops in nonfatty tissue, there is a decrease in density. Acute blood is of higher density than brain, and CT is sensitive in the detection of acute (generally less than

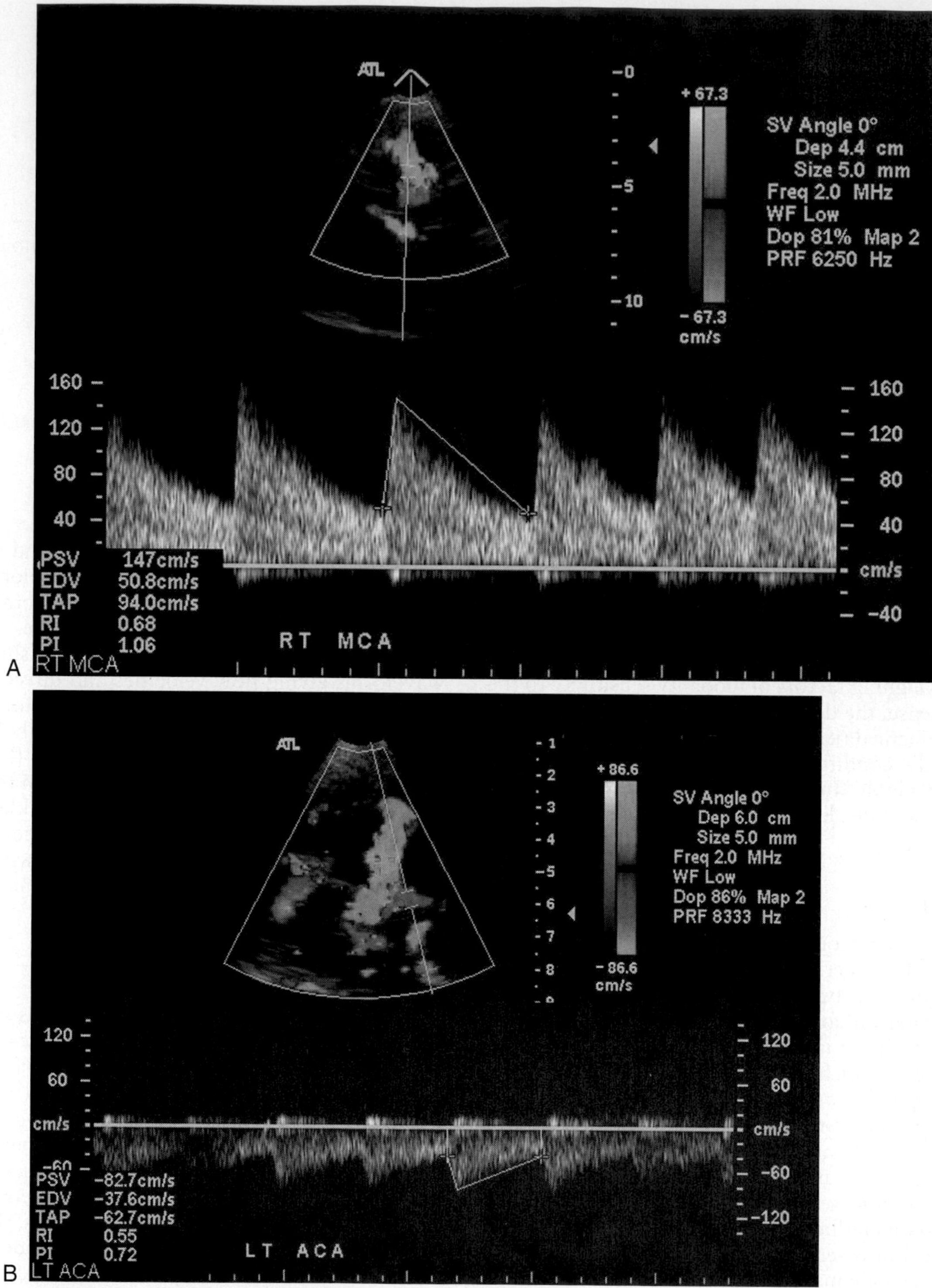

FIGURE 49–1 • Transcranial Doppler ultrasound images. Color and pulse Doppler waveforms from middle **(A)**, anterior **(B)** and posterior.

1 week old) parenchymal and subarachnoid hemorrhage (SAH) and in the evaluation of ventricular size and extra-axial collections.

Iodinated intravenous (IV) contrast can be used with CT to detect any integrity of the blood-brain barrier (BBB) differences in tissue perfusion. With the injection of IV contrast, transiently the vessels will become higher in density, with a variable rate of contrast leak into the tissues, depending on the local physiologic function. The rate of equilibration of contrast concentration between vessels and parenchyma is much slower in the brain because of the BBB. Contrast then is especially useful in the brain where changes in the normal BBB can reveal underlying disease. This increased density is also used to image arteries and venous structures with CT angiography (CTA). With the appropriate software, postprocessing of

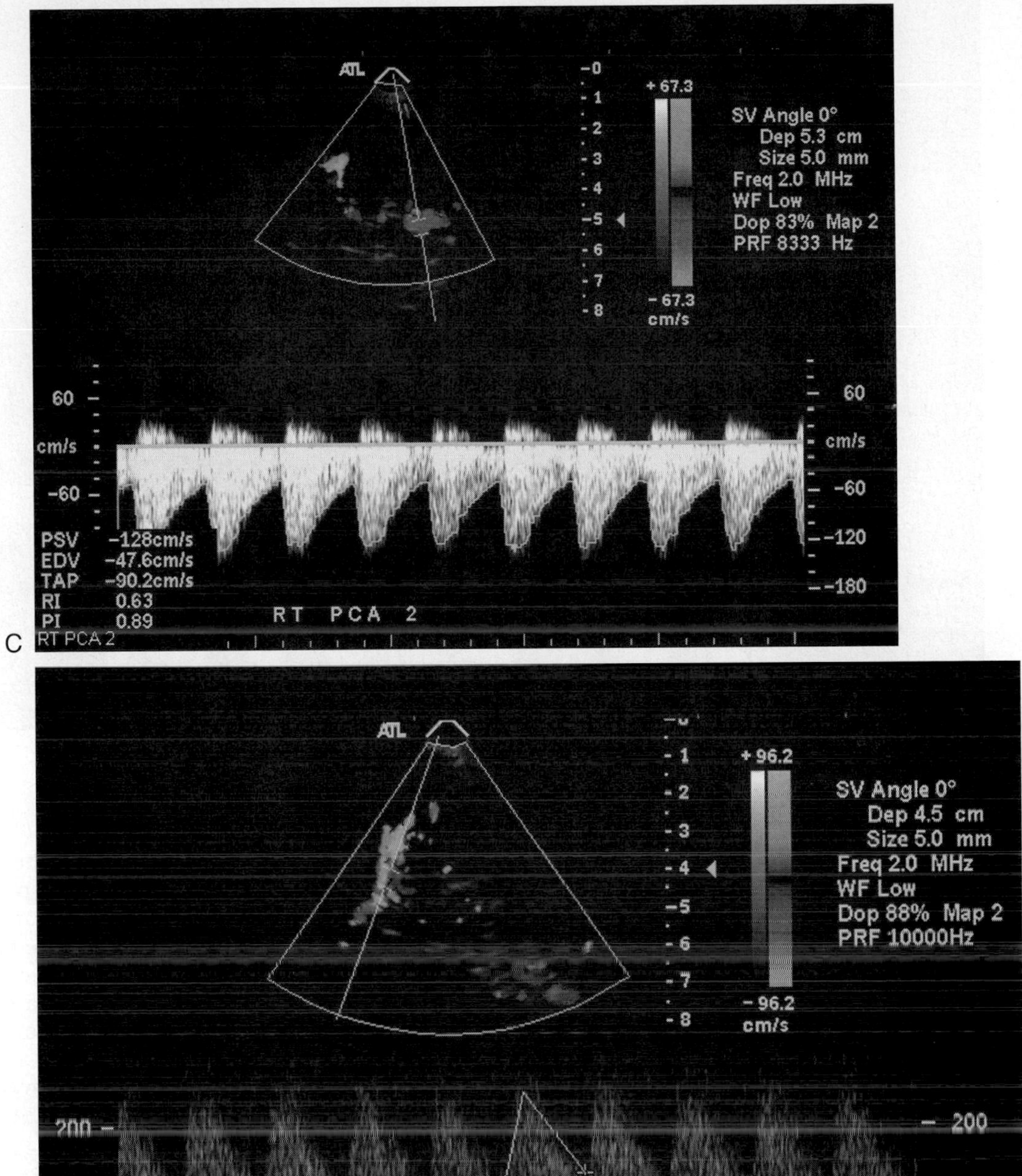

FIGURE 49–1 • Cont'd—**(C)** Cerebral arteries are shown. Abnormal middle cerebral (**D**) and terminal carotid.

the data can produce three-dimensional (3D) images of the vessels.

Xenon CT (XeCT) is a perfusion technique available in some centers. XeCT requires the apparatus to deliver xenon gas and additional software for the CT scanner.[2] Though capable of quantitative flow measurements, XeCT has largely been supplanted by relative flow measures from magnetic resonance (MR) perfusion techniques.

Magnetic Resonance Imaging

Magnetic resonance imaging (MRI) uses a high-field magnet in combination with radiofrequency pulses to produce images based on the nuclear resonance of hydrogen protons in tissue, primarily in water and fat. MRI provides the most sensitive measure of most (but not all) CNS diseases, and imaging can be obtained in any plane, unlike with CT.

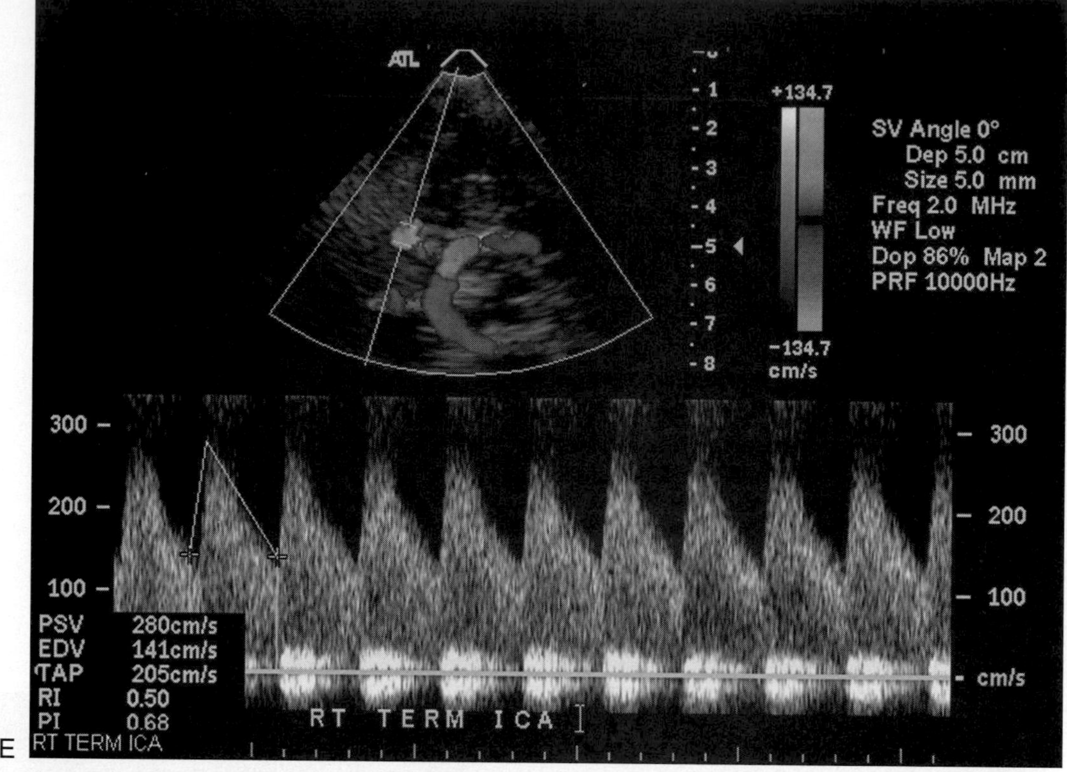

FIGURE 49–1 • Cont'd—(**E**) Waveforms in another patient with sickle cell disease. See color insert.

Imaging, however, requires patient transport to the scanner, as well as increased complexity and potential safety concerns primarily related to the high field magnets (typically 1.5 T) and long imaging sequences (1 to 10 minutes) provide the greatest tissue characterization, with several sequences in a complete study. MRI is particularly useful in evaluation of the posterior fossa and spinal cord, where beam hardening due to bone results in considerable artifact on CT.

MRI-compatible monitoring and life support systems must be used. Patients need to be screened for any internal hardware/implants that would preclude scanning, such as MRI-incompatible aneurysm clips. Electronic devices such as pacemakers are disrupted by the changing magnetic field occurring with imaging, and thus patients with such devices should not generally undergo MRI (www.upms.edu/mrsafety). Injuries and deaths due to failures to recognize these dangers have been reported. Most MRI sequences require imaging times in the range of minutes and are susceptible to motion degradation. For patients who cannot cooperate, deep sedation or anesthesia is often required.

MRI exploits nuclear characteristics of the hydrogen protons principally in tissue water referred to as T_1 (longitudinal relaxation) and T_2 (spin-spin relaxation). An imaging sequence includes both T_1 and T_2 components to create an image; however, the particular sequence can be formulated to be predominately one or the other (i.e., T_1 weighted or T_2 weighted [often referred to as simply T_1 or T_2 images]). Because most pathobiologic conditions result in some disturbance of water, these imaging parameters turn out to be sensitive to many diseases. Water, such as in the ventricles or globes, is dark on T_1-weighted images. Such water is bright on T_2-weighted images. One point to be aware of is that for the most part the signal intensity of any tissue being imaged on MRI is relative (unlike the absolute density measure in CT). Therefore the detection of disease depends on visualizing differences in intensity of one tissue relative to another.

FLAIR (fluid-attenuated inversion recovery) is a variation of T_2-weighted imaging in which the CSF is specifically rendered dark to enhance visibility of hyperintense disease in parenchyma adjacent to the CSF spaces. Fat is hyperintense on T_1-weighted sequences and also fairly bright on fast T_2-weighted sequences, which most scanners now use. In some situations it is advantageous to suppress the brightness of fat, which can be specifically done with some cost of increased time. Gradient MR images are often used for detection of hemorrhage, though these sequences generally also have more artifacts. The appearance of acute blood on CT is fairly straightforward; it appears hyperdense initially and becomes isodense in about a week. The appearance of blood on MRI is much more complex, and although it is generally detectable much longer on MRI, it can be difficult to appreciate hyperacute blood. Overall, the detection of calcium and hyperacute blood can be difficult with MRI, and CT is often better in this regard. IV contrast is also used in MRI, with similar application as seen in CT. In this case the contrast is a gadolinium chelate that shortens the T_1 relaxation time of nearby water. The result is that the water near gadolinium is hyperintense on T_1-weighted images. This effect can be used to detect differences in perfusion, especially

BBB disruption, which can be seen in many disorders including ischemia, inflammation/infection, and status epilepticus. Malignant and some benign brain tumors also show enhanced capillary permeability with enhancement following contrast. MR with gadolinium is about an order of magnitude more sensitive than CT with iodinated contrast in detecting BBB disruption. Some areas of the brain that lack BBB include the choroid plexus, the pituitary gland, and the median eminence; therefore these areas enhance normally.

Advanced Magnetic Resonance Techniques

Expanding techniques in MRI such as diffusion, perfusion, and spectroscopy are providing new information that is being used increasingly in the management of critically ill patients. Diffusion weighted MR (DWI) imaging is a technique sensitive to the molecular level motion of water.[3] Different cerebral diseases produce different types of edema (e.g., cytotoxic, vasogenic, interstitial). Evaluation of the molecular (Brownian) motion of water turns out to be a sensitive measure of some pathologic states, the most significant application currently being cytotoxic edema associated with the detection of ischemia.[4] Cytotoxic edema causes restriction of water diffusion with decrease in the apparent diffusion coefficient (ADC), which typically is viewed on the DWI image as increased signal intensity. In contrast to cytotoxic edema, vasogenic and interstitial edema increase water diffusion and therefore increase the ADC.

Detecting this molecular level motion requires strong, fast gradients, which have become more standard on newer MRI scanners, to allow sufficiently rapid scanning to effectively "freeze" the gross tissue motion, which normally swamps this molecular level motion. Care must be taken in interpreting the DWI image because it necessarily will have some T_2 weighting, and "T_2 shine through" can result in a focus of increased signal on the DWI image that does not represent restricted diffusion. Review of the calculated ADC map images should show a corresponding darkening in a focus of cytotoxic edema to confirm restricted diffusion. Also, the hyperintensity on DWI image may "pseudonormalize" for a period of several days after the ictus because of the development of associated vasogenic edema. Restricted diffusion due to infarct will generally resolve over the course of 1 to 3 weeks, and this allows for distinguishing a new infarct from older lesions. Restricted diffusion is not limited to ischemia and can be seen in other cerebral diseases.

Perfusion MR is increasingly being used in the evaluation of cerebral perfusion. The most widely available techniques use rapid scanning associated with a bolus of IV gadolinium contrast to measure first pass changes in signal intensity. These techniques give a relative measure of perfusion but not quantitative flow.

Conventional MRI is based on the signal intensities derived from the hydrogen bonded to oxygen in water and, to a lesser extent, from the hydrogen bonded to carbon in fat. With the appropriate software, MR can be used as a probe for hydrogen bonded to other molecules (termed *MR spectroscopy* [MRS]). The sensitivity is sufficient to detect molecules in the millimolar range, although at a much lower resolution than that used to detect water for imaging. The nonwater molecules are most commonly reported as ratios of signal peaks that correspond to one of several molecules. In the brain the most common peaks detected are N-acetyl aspartate (NAA); creatinine (Cr); choline (Cho); and, in some physiologic states, lactate. The MRS signal is either obtained from a single voxel (usually of several milliliters volume) or multiple voxels (which can be as small as 1 to 2 ml volume). Multivoxel MRS can be used to make low-resolution images termed *chemical shift imaging* (CSI) for some of the more prevalent peaks. The utility of MRS is still in evolution. Detection of lactate to evaluate newborn ischemia and some metabolic diseases are two of the more promising applications.

Magnetic Resonance Angiography

Fluid motion within tissue can be used by MR to image flow in vessels and CSF. This can be accomplished with and without contrast, although the contrast techniques are generally more sensitive for vascular flow. The MR angiogram can be tailored for artery (MRA) or vein (MRV) visualization, primarily based on flow direction, and is usually most effective if the area of interest can be narrowed (e.g., the circle of Willis), although newer techniques have greatly increased the area that can be covered in one scan (Fig. 49–2). The maximum resolution of MRA of slightly less than 1 mm is generally less than CTA where maximum resolution can be less than 0.25 mm.[5] In addition to the source images (all the thin slices obtained during the scan), various reconstructed images can be visualized, including 3D reformatted images from maximum intensity pixel (MIP) data (Fig. 49–3) and surface renderings, viewed from multiple projections. Many clinical cerebral arterial questions are now answered with MRA, and MRV of the cerebral venous system has largely replaced diagnostic catheter venograms.

Catheter Angiograms

Although significant inroads have been made in cerebral vascular evaluation with both CTA and MRA, when indicated, catheter angiography remains the gold standard for most vessel imaging. Angiography is basically a rapid series of radiographs (x-rays) obtained during injection of iodinated contrast directly into the arteries or veins being imaged. Most angiography equipment used now is digital. Digital subtraction angiography (DSA) images produced show the contrast opacified vessels with the background structures subtracted. Catheter angiography requires transport to and patient support in the angiography suite. Vessel access for arterial studies is usually through the femoral artery and has generally small but "nonzero" risk of vessel injury and embolization. In the very young, injury to the femoral artery is of greater concern, and although any acute risk to the limb is extremely uncommon, there has been documentation of relative diminished leg growth in some cases. Risks of neurologic complication are small but present, with the reported incidence of persistent defects typically ranging

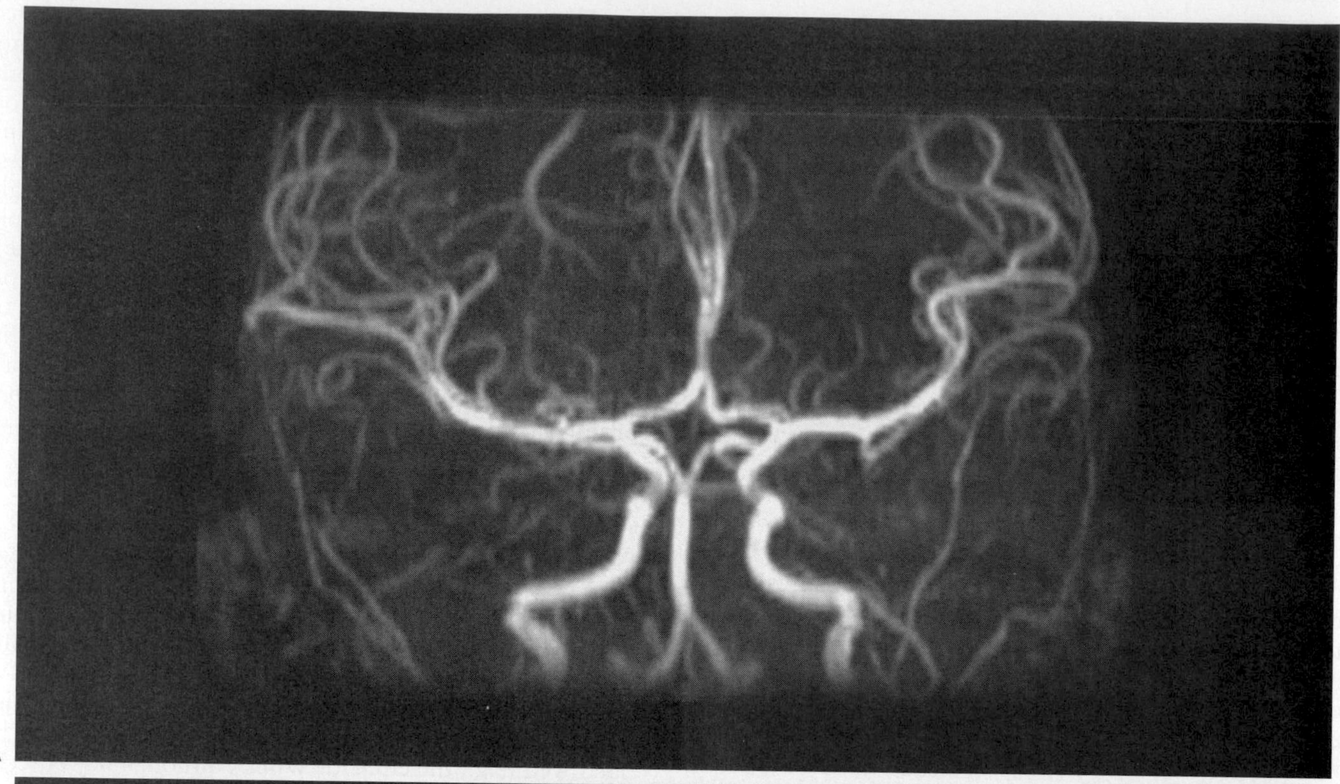

A

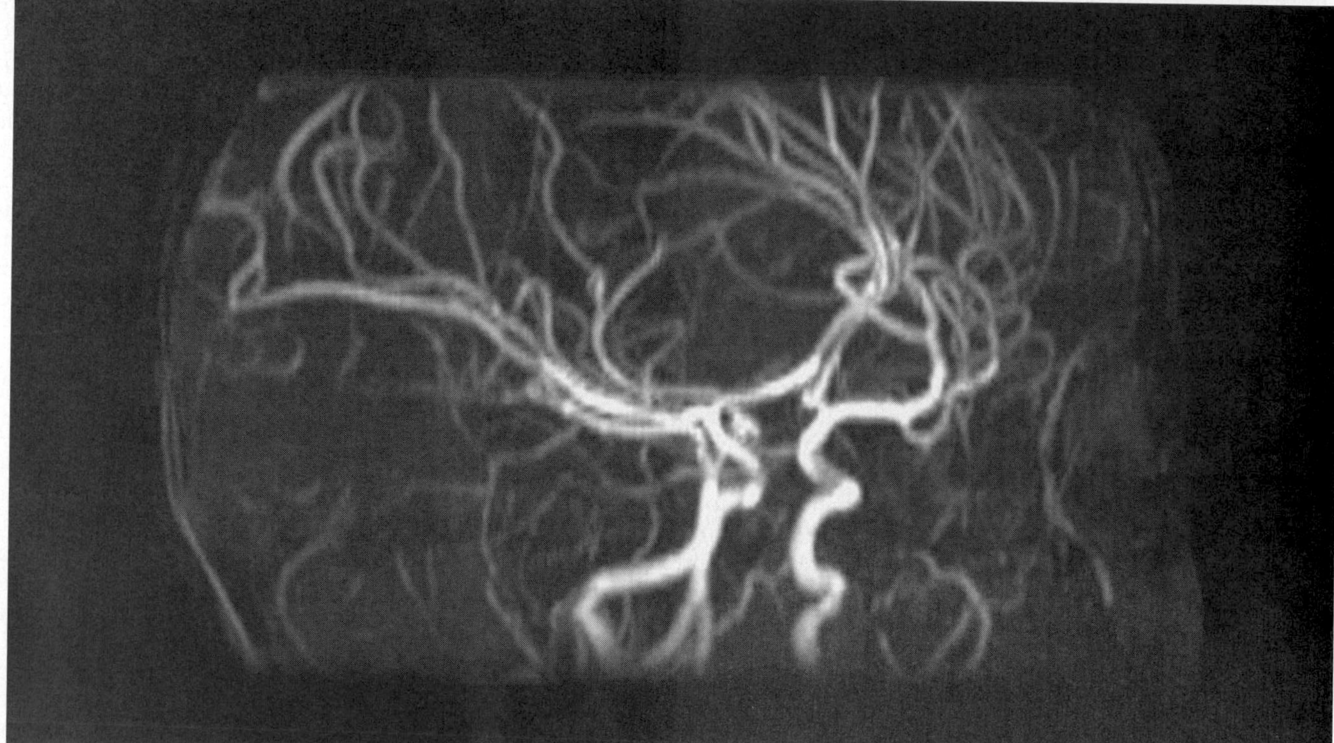

B

FIGURE 49–2 • Normal scans from magnetic resonance arteriography (MRA) and MR venography. Frontal **(A)** and lateral **(B)** maximum intensity pixel images from an MRA show normal appearance of anterior and posterior cerebral circulations.

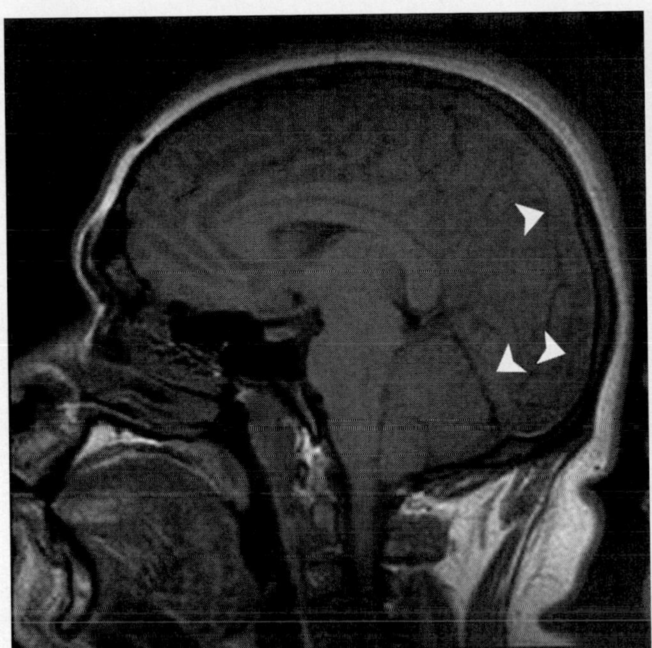

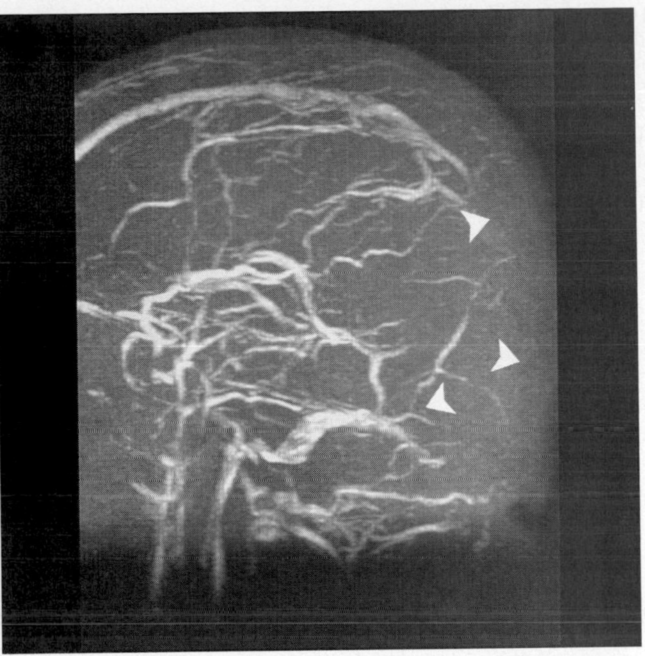

FIGURE 49–3 • Superior sagittal sinus (SSS) thrombosis on magnetic resonance venography (MRV). SSS and straight sinus thrombosis: sagittal T_1 MR image **(A)** shows intermediate signal intensity in sagittal and straight sinuses (*arrowheads*). No flow is seen on MRV **(B)** in these vessels (*arrowheads*). Compare with normal example in Figure 50–2.

from about 0.5% to 0.07%.[6,7] Therapeutic endovascular procedures carry higher risks but generally are used in lieu of riskier surgical procedures; at times they are the only avenue of treatment.

Myelography

Myelography involves radiographs (x-rays), CT, or both of the spine after opacification of the CSF by intrathecal injection of iodinated contrast, which is most commonly injected at the lumbar level. The myelogram has largely been replaced by MRI, which can show both extrathecal encroachment and intrathecal masses, as well as give signal characteristics of the spinal cord itself and any mass. Exceptions include either the inability to obtain an MR because of local field disruption most commonly from ferromagnetic spinal rods or MR incompatibility due to safety issues (e.g., pacemaker). CT remains better in evaluation of the bony spine column, particularly in trauma, although MRI is used in trauma to evaluate the soft tissues in the spinal column and the cord.

Nuclear Medicine

Most nuclear medicine studies involve injection of a small amount of radioactively labeled substance (radiotracer). Either the physiologic uptake and metabolism of the radiotracer are followed, or, as in the following studies, the movement of the radiotracer is followed with a gamma camera.

Ventriculoperitoneal (and ventriculoatrial) shunt function evaluation can include a nuclear medicine shunt study. One can assess the flow in the shunt by injecting a small amount of radiotracer in the shunt reservoir and following the movement of the activity with a gamma camera. Cerebral arterial perfusion is also assessed at times with an IV injection of a radiotracer, while the cerebrum undergoes imagine with the gamma camera. This technique has been most commonly used in the ICU in cases of suspected brain death, where acute cerebral swelling will exclude cerebral perfusion.

Preterm/Neonate Imaging

In the premature infant, US remains the primary modality for detection and follow-up of germinal matrix hemorrhage in the neonate to detect intraventricular extension and evaluate for hydrocephalus. (Fig. 49–4) Also, assessment can be made for white matter injury including PVL, although MRI will be more sensitive for noncystic PVL. MRI performed at about the third week of life has been reported as predictive of outcome at term.[8] Routine screening cranial US has been recommended for all infants of younger than 30 weeks' gestation, between days 7 and 14, and optimally should be repeated at 36 to 40 weeks after gestation.[9] Moderate to large parenchymal and extraaxial bleeds can also be detected on US. As mentioned earlier, smaller extraaxial collections, especially laterally, can be missed with US, as can small parenchymal hemorrhages.

As noted in Chapters 49 and 59, an understanding of hypoxic-ischemic encephalopathy in children is complicated by the developmental status of the child. The pattern of injury seen is determined by the characteristics of the insult and the maturational state of the brain. Metabolic demands and regions of selective vulnerability evolve during development. Grayscale US, widely used for intracranial imaging in the neonate, is relatively insensitive to

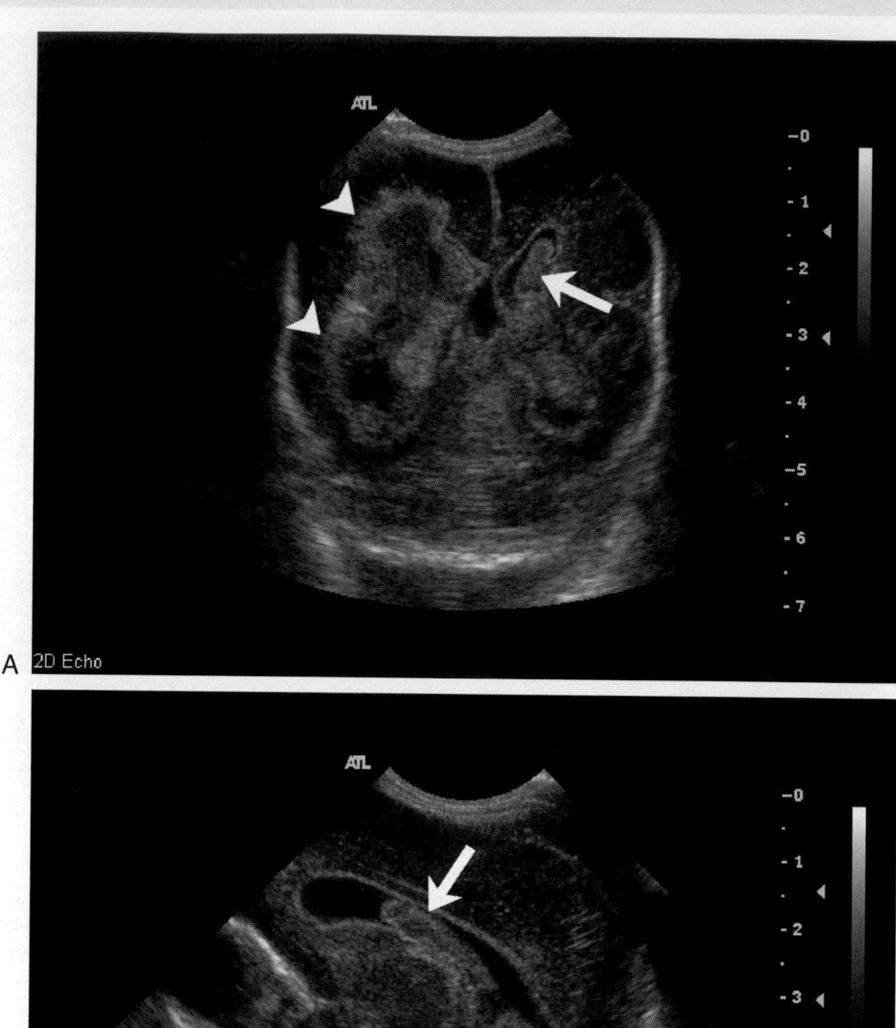

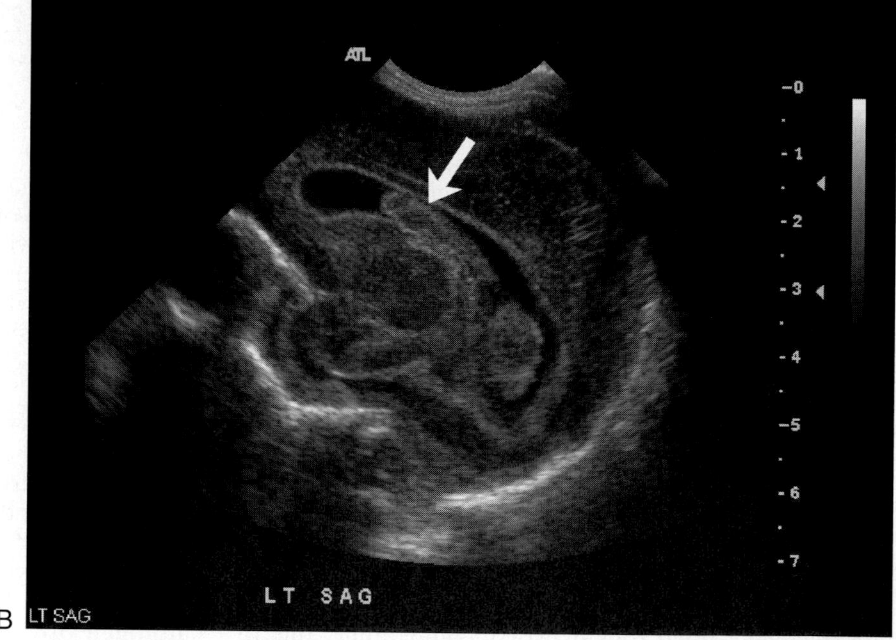

FIGURE 49–4 • Germinal matrix hemorrhage in a premature infant. Coronal **(A)** and left sagittal **(B)** ultrasound images through the anterior fontanelle demonstrate dilated lateral ventricles with intraventricular extension of clot on the left (*arrows*) and parenchymal extension on the right (*arrowheads*) consistent with a grade 3 bleed on the left and grade 4 on the right.

acute changes associated with hypoxic-ischemic injury (HII).[10] As edema develops, usually after several hours, increased echogenicity of brain parenchyma can be seen, but this is relative and often difficult to appreciate. Blood associated with a hemorrhagic infarct will also appear as increased echogenicity. As mass effect develops as a result of edema, ventricular and sulcal effacement can be seen. Later, vascular/perivascular mineralization can result in linear thalamic and basal ganglia echogenicities.[11] US Doppler evaluation of newborn ischemia has shown some utility. Brain perfusion can be investigated with determination of the resistive index (RI). The RI in the healthy neonate (0.75 +/– 0.10) is higher than that seen in the older infant before (0.65 +/– 0.5) and after (0.55 +/– 0.5) fontanelle closure.[10] A decrease in the RI to less than 0.60 24 hours after neonatal asphyxia, which is thought to result from a decrease in a vascular tone–associated loss of autoregulation, has been associated with a poorer outcome at 8 months to 1 year.[12] One half of the patients in this study with low resistance indexes had normal grayscale images. There is a differential to a low RI, however, including cardiac disease, extracorporeal membrane oxygenation (ECMO), ongoing hypoxia, hypercapnia, and technical mismeasurement issues. Increased fontanelle pressure can increase the RI measure by 20%; thus there is considerable user dependence to this application. If hyperemia persists, and as HII evolves, there is increasing cytotoxic edema that leads to increased intracranial pressure (ICP) and increased RI measurements. A high RI in the first day of life with neonatal insults suggests an in utero injury.

CT detection of acute ischemic injury also depends on edema that results from the injury. This is seen as decreased attenuation and loss of gray-white differentiation, usually several hours after an ictal episode.[13] Small or early infarcts can be missed with CT, and detection of ischemia in the neonate is made more difficult by the generally lower attenuation of the relatively watery unmyelinated newborn brain. As brain swelling develops in the first few days, there can be loss of CSF spaces seen as ventricular compression, sulcal effacement, and loss of perimesencephalic cisterns. Acute thrombotic stroke associated with arterial thrombosis can at times be appreciated acutely as a hyperdense artery, most commonly the MCA on noncontrast CT. Acute hemorrhage, such as with a hemorrhagic infarct, will be hyperdense initially on CT, evolving to isodense over the first week.

Standard MR sequences that exploit T_1 and T_2 relaxation times also depend on the development of edema to appreciate acute ischemic injury, which results in hyperintensity on T_2 weight images and hypointensity on T_1 weight images. Typically, this change takes at least several hours to develop. Although MR is generally more sensitive than CT in adults, evaluation of the neonate is again somewhat made more difficult by the lack of myelination, and as a result ischemia can be more conspicuous on CT than T_1- or T_2-weighted images (Fig. 49–5). FLAIR and

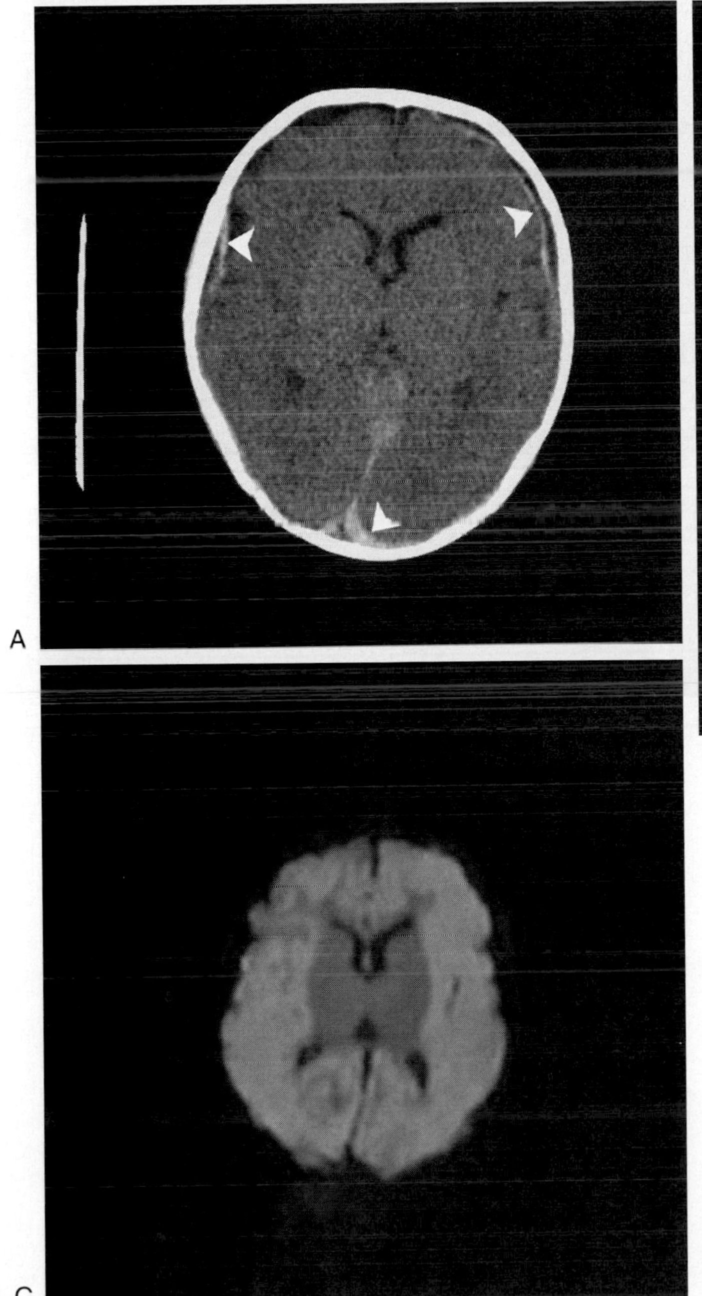

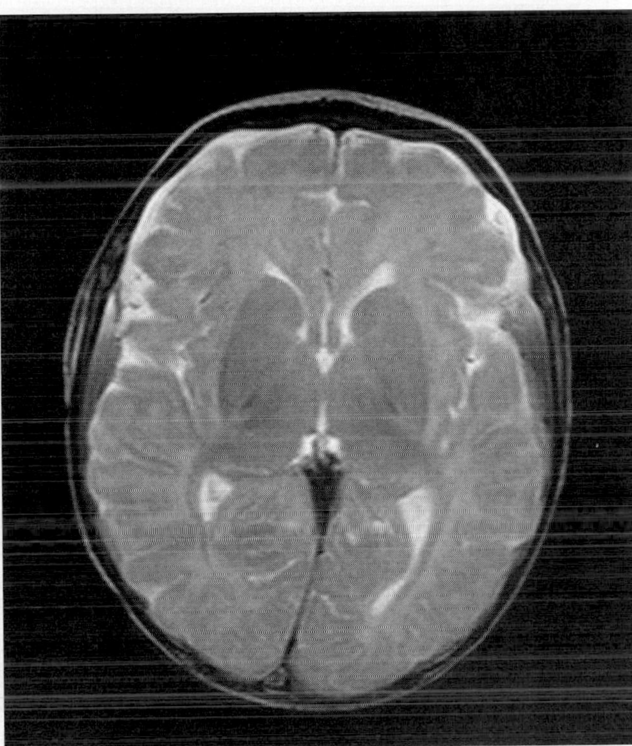

FIGURE 49–5 • Nonaccidental trauma with diffuse cerebral ischemia. Axial computed tomography (CT) without contrast **(A)**, axial T_2 magnetic resonance (MR) **(B)**, and diffusion-weighted MR image DWI **(C)**. CT **(A)** shows a thin layer of acute subdural blood (*arrowheads*) and diffuse loss of gray-white demarcation in the cerebral hemispheres. Although the T_2 **(B)** image is remarkably normal with appropriate lack of myelination in this 3-month-old child, the relative brightness of the cerebral hemispheres compared with the central gray on DWI **(C)** images is consistent with a diffuse ischemic insult.

short tau inversion recovery (STIR) imaging techniques have proved to be more sensitive than T_1 and T_2 to ischemic changes in adults.[14] More recently, DWI sequences, as previously discussed, have been shown to be acutely sensitive to the cytotoxic edema associated with ischemia.[4] This cytotoxic edema results in diminished diffusion of water in the affected area. Diffusion-weighted imaging (DWI) in experimental models can detect ischemia in minutes after onset as a region of restricted diffusion.[15] These sequences have become widely implemented in adults where acute differentiation of ischemic stroke from other neurologic disorders affords implementation of developing stroke therapies. The restricted diffusion associated with ischemia evolves over a 1- to 3-week period, at which time the diffusion image normalizes. If there is sufficient tissue destruction, the diffusion will ultimately be increased because of the greater free water following necrosis. This change in diffusion is also then useful to distinguish a new stroke, which will show decreased diffusion from an older lesion, which will have increased diffusion; both lesions may be of similar signal intensity on standard T_1 and T_2 imaging (Fig. 49–6).

There are some unresolved questions about transferring the adult experience with diffusion-weighted scanning to infants. Although researchers have found that diffusion changes may not precede T_2 changes in some neonatal animal models, in contrast to adults, this has not been the case in at least some infants who underwent imaging.[16]

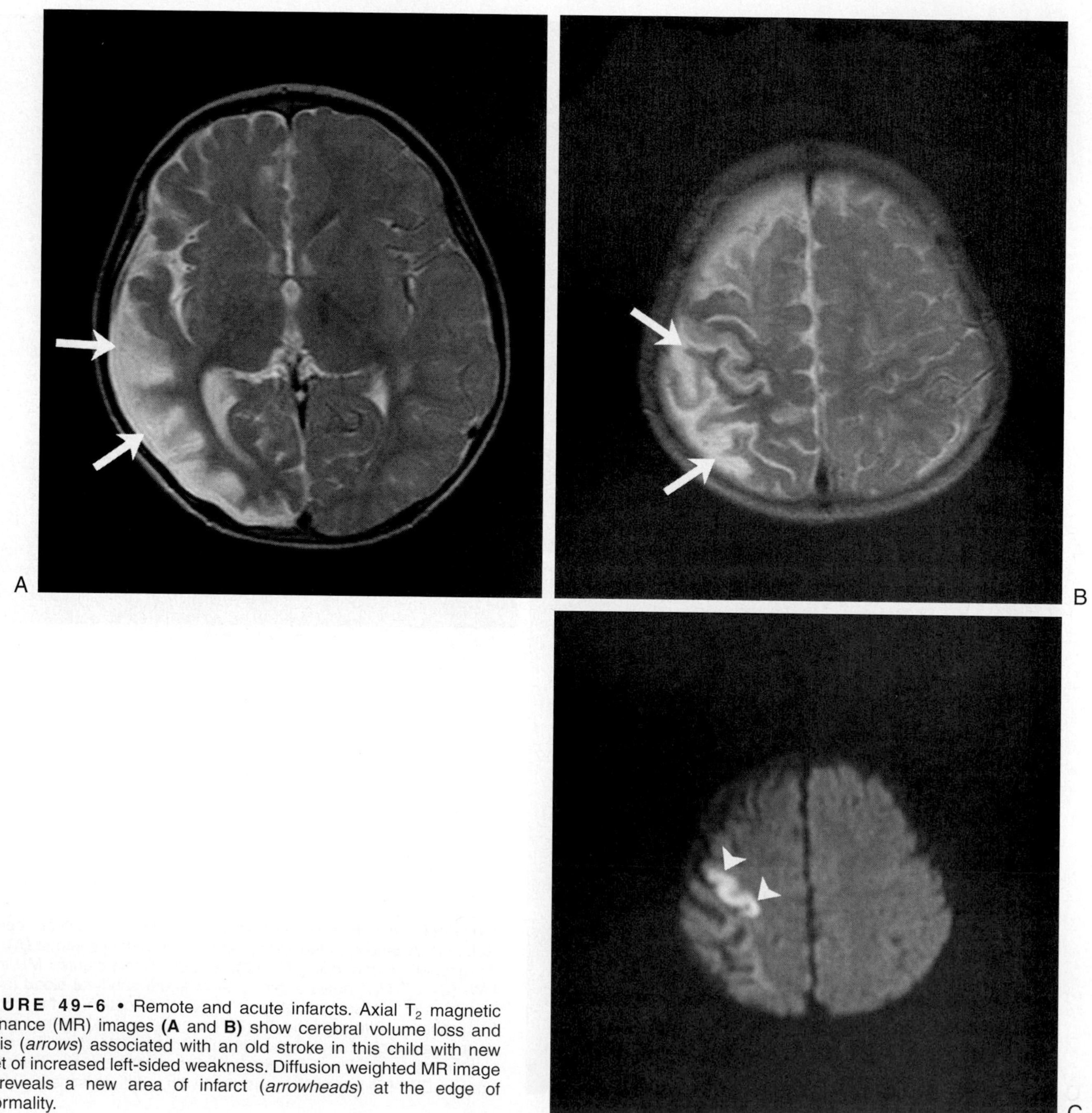

FIGURE 49–6 • Remote and acute infarcts. Axial T_2 magnetic resonance (MR) images **(A and B)** show cerebral volume loss and gliosis (*arrows*) associated with an old stroke in this child with new onset of increased left-sided weakness. Diffusion weighted MR image **(C)** reveals a new area of infarct (*arrowheads*) at the edge of abnormality.

The initial diffusion abnormality may increase over the first day, and the extent of diffusion abnormality can encompass both the core infarct and penumbra and thus potentially overestimate the ultimate infarct. Although most DWI experience has been with adults, DWI appears to be more sensitive than T_2 and FLAIR imaging and correlates well with at least short-term clinical outcome in neonates and infants.[17] The identification of lactate on MRS is also evolving as a potentially useful predictor of perinatal asphyxia severity, although there is considerable complexity in applying this technology.[14]

As mentioned previously, the pattern of HII varies with the cause of the insult and the developmental state of the brain. Early in utero insults result in tissue resorption, with the ability to mount a gliotic response not being seen until the third trimester. During early brain development insults can result in congenital malformations. HII in the early to mid-second trimester may result in polymicrogyria. In the 24- to 26-week gestation range, HII can preferentially injure the deep gray matter nuclei in the setting of total asphyxia. Perivascular leukomalacia (PVL) is the pattern of injury seen with prolonged partial hypoxia at 24 to 34 weeks. Typically with PVL on neonatal grayscale US there may be increased echogenicity in the periventricular white matter, an appearance that is indistinguishable at this stage from edema or from parenchymal hemorrhage, which can also be seen. As PVL progresses, there is cavitation of the involved white matter, and the collapse of these spaces results ultimately in the thinning of the white matter, particularly posteriorly. MRI is more sensitive to white matter injury than US is in the premature neonate, but it is not yet clear whether this increased sensitivity is of significant prognostic values. Ischemic insults to the term child demonstrate different patterns of injury, determined by the specifics of the insult and the vulnerability of various areas. Profound hypoxia in the term infant results in injury to the lateral thalamus and posterior putamen as well as areas that are most actively myelinating, particularly the perirolandic white matter and the associated corticospinal tracts and the white matter tracts associated with the occipital cortex. In contrast, a watershed pattern of injury, discussed later, develops with prolonged partial ischemia. Current recommendations for the encephalopathic term infant have included early CT to assess for intracranial hemorrhage, with consideration for MRI later in the first postnatal week to assess for extent of injury.[9]

Stroke in the Older Infant/Child

Although the imaging picture may not be specific, the diagnosis of acute stroke can be made, usually in combination with the clinical history.[18] The imaging pattern can be of help in determining a cause. A watershed distribution is consistent with a low flow/hypotensive cause (Fig. 49–7). Specifically, there are ischemic changes seen in the boundary regions between the major cerebral distributions (i.e., between anterior and middle cerebral and between middle and posterior cerebral arterial distributions). Lesions in multiple brachiocephalic vessel distributions suggest a central thrombotic source, although other causes such as a

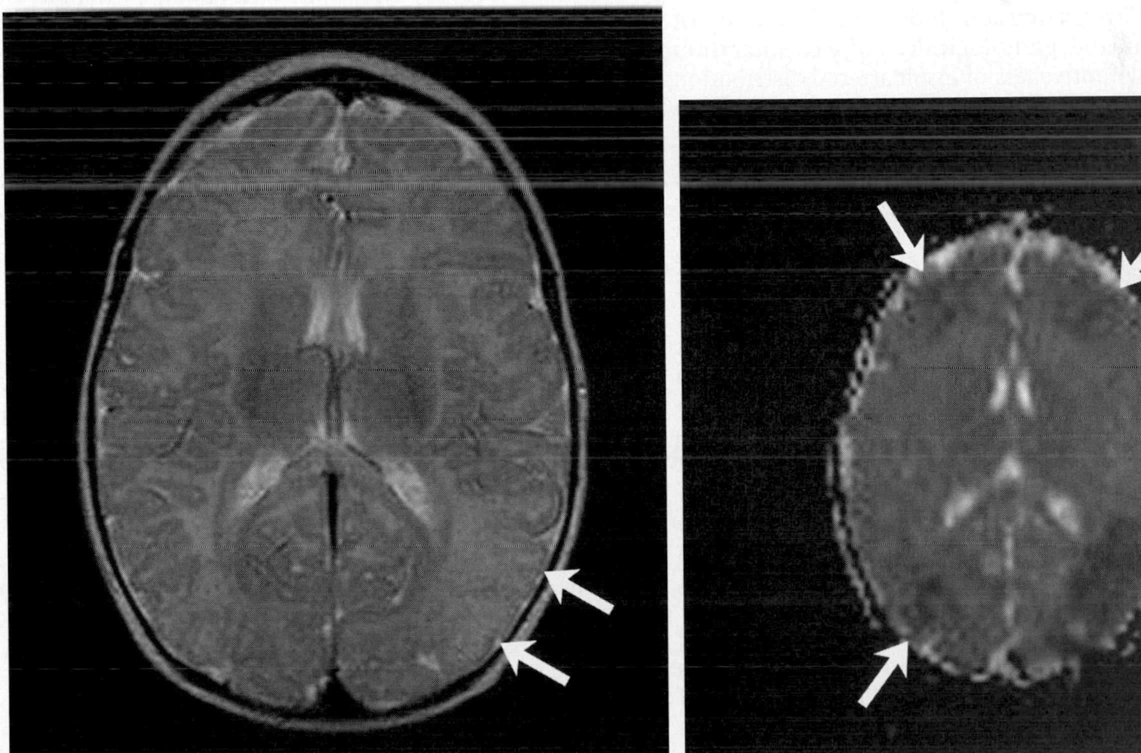

FIGURE 49–7 • Watershed infarct. Axial T_2 **(A)** shows some loss of the gray-white interface on the left posteriorly (*arrows*). Diffusion weight magnetic resonance **(B)** shows bilateral restricted diffusion consistent with ischemic injury in a watershed distribution (*arrows*).

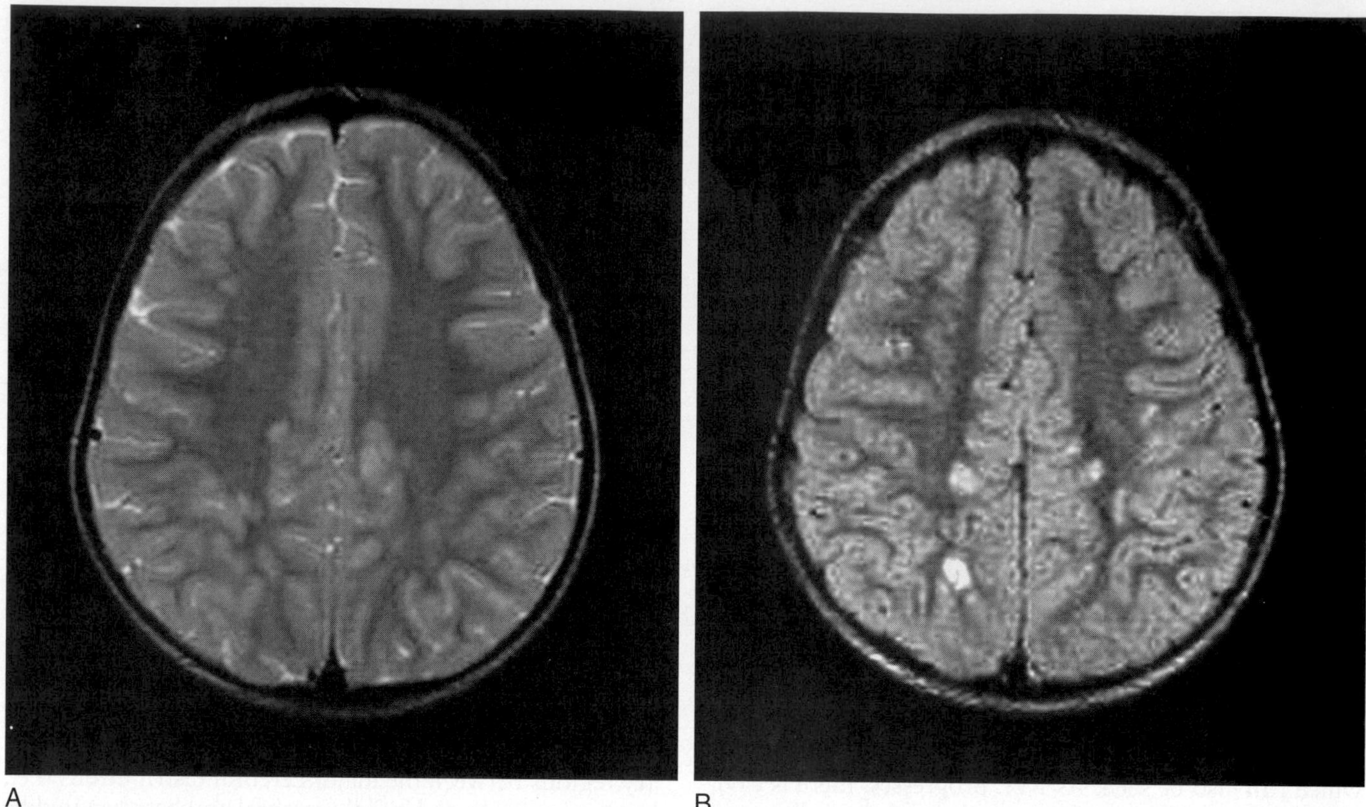

FIGURE 49–8 • Acute disseminated encephalomyelitis (ADEM). T_2 **(A)** and FLAIR **(B)** images show multiple foci of hyperintensity. In addition to ADEM, vasculitis and multiple emboli could have this imaging appearance.

vasculitis or demyelinating disease can also have this multiple vessel involvement (Fig. 49–8). Usually, an embolus will be seen at the gray-white junction and most commonly in the MCA distribution. Individual variability of boundary regions and pathologically induced alteration in flow limit the definitiveness of insult arterial distribution categorization.[19]

As discussed previously, DWI is useful in earlier imaging detection of cerebral infarcts (Fig. 49–9) and in distinguishing recent infarcts in a background of abnormality, such as prior infarcts (Fig. 49–6). The area of restricted diffusion on DWI is generally thought to represent irreversible injury, although there may be some cases where the lesions are at least potentially reversible. In the setting of acute stroke, perfusion MRI may have a contributory roll in demonstrating the total region of brain at risk and predicting the ultimate infarct extent.[20] The area of perfusion abnormality beyond that of diffusion abnormality most likely represents the penumbra, which is at risk but potentially salvageable. Etiologic workup of stroke in children includes a broad differential. Although catheter angiogram remains the gold standard and is necessary in some situations, the use of MRA and CTA for ruling out a vascular lesion has increased.

Arterial dissections can be diagnosed with MRI and MRA or with CTA. The visualization of methemoglobin in the false lumen with fat-saturated, T_1-weighted MRI detects most dissection cases, although subtle lesions can still require catheter angiogram for diagnosis. On CTA, the false lumen is detected by the absent or diminished enhancement compared with the true lumen. Suspicion for dissection is raised in the setting of multiple apparent embolic strokes in a single brachiocephalic distribution, with a history of appropriate trauma, although more rarely spontaneous dissections are seen. As mentioned earlier, emboli in multiple circulations raise questions of a more central cause, such as a heart valve vegetation.

Posterior Reversible Encephalopathy Syndrome

Loss of autoregulation in the older infant and child as seen in hypertensive encephalopathy, cytotoxic and immunosuppressive drug neurotoxicity, and thrombotic thrombocytopenia purpura typically involves a posterior and parasagittal distribution of T_2 hyperintensity, although it can involve the frontal lobes and brainstem.[21-23] Lesions are often relatively symmetrical with confluent lesions centered in the subcortical white matter that may demonstrate patchy enhancement (Fig. 49–10).[22] Because the underlying disease causes vasogenic edema, these lesions will not be bright on DWI. Ischemia can, however, be triggered by a severe increase in blood pressure, resulting in cytotoxic edema and therefore bright lesions on DWI. These lesions usually result in infarctions with a severity that often correlates with the prognosis.

Venous Infarct

The presence of blood in an area of cerebral infarct raises suspicion for a venous stroke, although an arterially

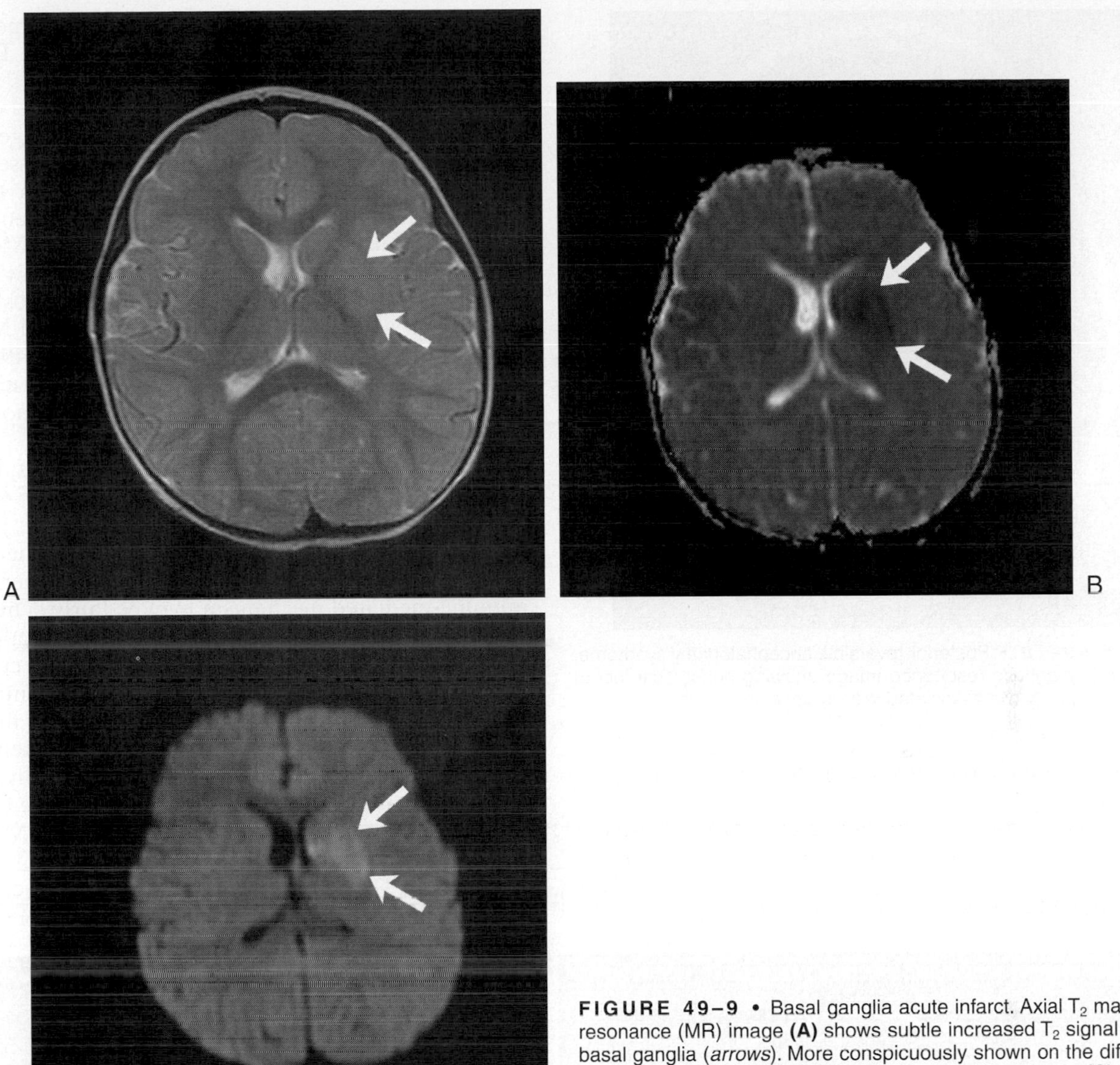

FIGURE 49–9 • Basal ganglia acute infarct. Axial T_2 magnetic resonance (MR) image **(A)** shows subtle increased T_2 signal in left basal ganglia (*arrows*). More conspicuously shown on the diffusion weighted MR **(B)** and apparent diffusion coefficient map **(C)** is restricted diffusion (*arrows*) associated with an early infarct involving the left caudate and lentiform nuclei infarct.

induced stroke can have associated hemorrhage. A nonarterial pattern infarct also raises suspicion of a venous stroke. In the setting of suspected venous stroke, evaluation of the cerebral venous system should be undertaken. US has limited utility in this setting, although evaluation of superior sagittal sinus (SSS) flow can be undertaken in the infant with an open fontanelle. CT evidence of venous clot can be detected as hyperdense venous sinuses acutely on noncontrast scans and as the "empty delta sign" (lower density in area of clot surrounded by enhancing blood) in the SSS on contrast-enhanced scans. This assessment can be problematic in the neonate in whom the venous sinuses appear normally dense on CT because of the normal low-density unmyelinated brain and typically higher hematocrit. The venous phase of a catheter angiogram has been classically used to most definitively look for venous sinus thrombosis. Catheter evaluation of the venous sinuses, however, has been effectively replaced with MRV techniques. Subacute clot in a venous sinus can also be evident on standard T_1- and T_2-weighted MRI, although acute clot can be more difficult to appreciate. MRV uses flow sensitive sequences that can effectively delineate the major venous sinuses (Fig. 49–3).

Vasculopathy/Vasculitis

Acquired vasculopathies can result from known infectious or noninfectious causes, or from unknown pathophysiologic origin, such as in primary cerebral vasculitis, which tends to involve medium and small vessels or Moyamoya syndrome, which shows greatest involvement of the central vessels. Vasculopathy involving large- and medium-size vessels can be seen on MRA, although more subtle irregularities and small vessel involvement still require catheter

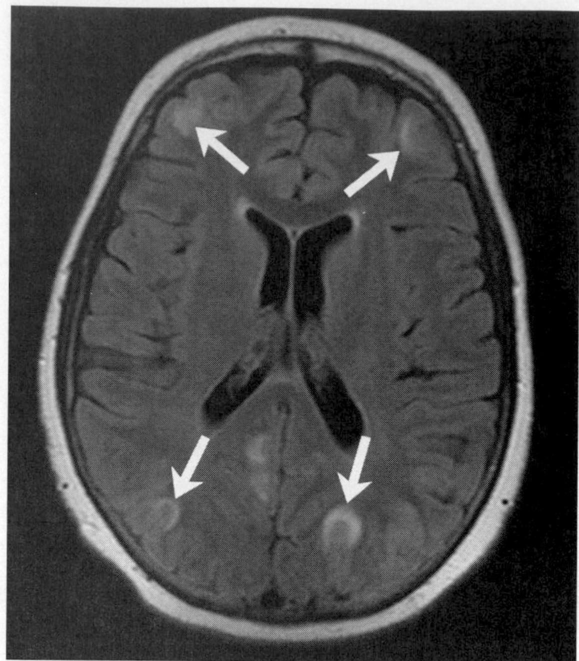

FIGURE 49–10 • Posterior reversible encephalopathy syndrome. Axial FLAIR magnetic resonance image showing subcortical foci of hyperintensity (*arrows*) associated with cyclosporin toxicity.

angiogram, which remains the gold standard imaging modality.

In a classic case of acute hemiplegia of childhood, a basal ganglia infarct that results from narrowing of the M1 segment and occlusion of lenticulostriate vessels is seen; cortical injury is less common. Narrowing typically of the terminal carotid and proximal M1 segment of the affected side can often be delineated on MRA. There also will be a lack of well-developed collaterals as is typical with Moyamoya syndrome, in which the vessel occlusion has been more slowly progressive over a longer period. Moyamoya syndrome denotes the pattern of vessel involvement, which can be of human association or course as following radiation, or of unknown cause when the term *Moyamoya disease* is used. More commonly Moyamoya syndrome will be bilateral, and MRI will show evidence of chronic ischemic insult. The enlarged lenticulostriate collaterals will generally be appreciable on a good MRA and as flow voids through the basal ganglia on (Fig. 49–11) MR images. These apparent flow voids need to be distinguished from enlarged perivascular spaces, which are not uncommon in this region.

Vasculitic changes can accompany infections, including meningitis, either through direct invasion of vessels or by an immune mechanism response to the particular pathogen. Parenchymal injury, if present, is mediated by ischemic changes. The pattern of involvement in the immune-mediated mechanism may be fairly symmetrical, as can be seen in acute disseminated encephalomyelitis (ADEM) or some metabolic diseases. Noninfectious vasculitides, including those associated with systemic disease (e.g., systemic lupus erythematosus [SLE] and in particular primary angiitis of the central nervous system [CNS]) can be more problematic in diagnosis. Typically, catheter angiogram and occasionally brain biopsy have been used to evaluate for questions of CNS vasculitis. Most cases of symptomatic vasculitis will show abnormality on standard MRI (T_2, FLAIR) sequences so that a completely normal MRI makes the likelihood of CNS vasculitis low.

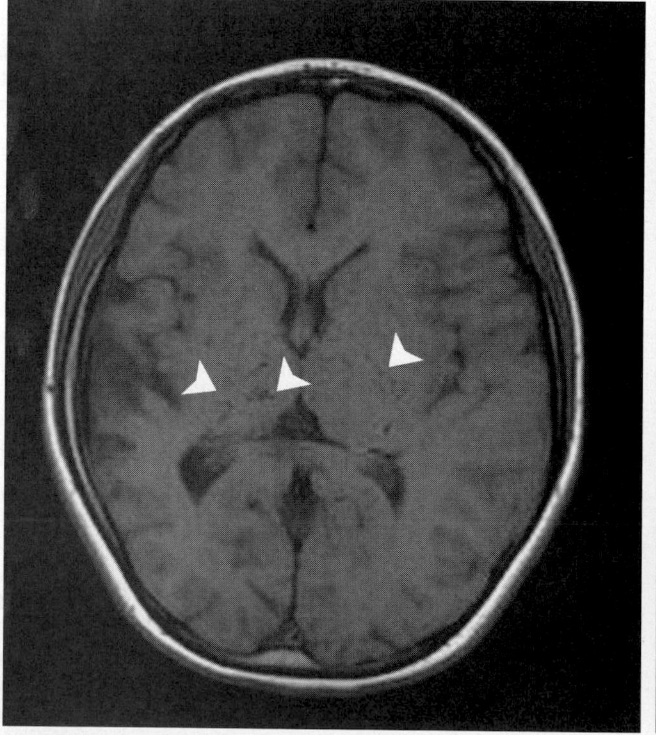

A

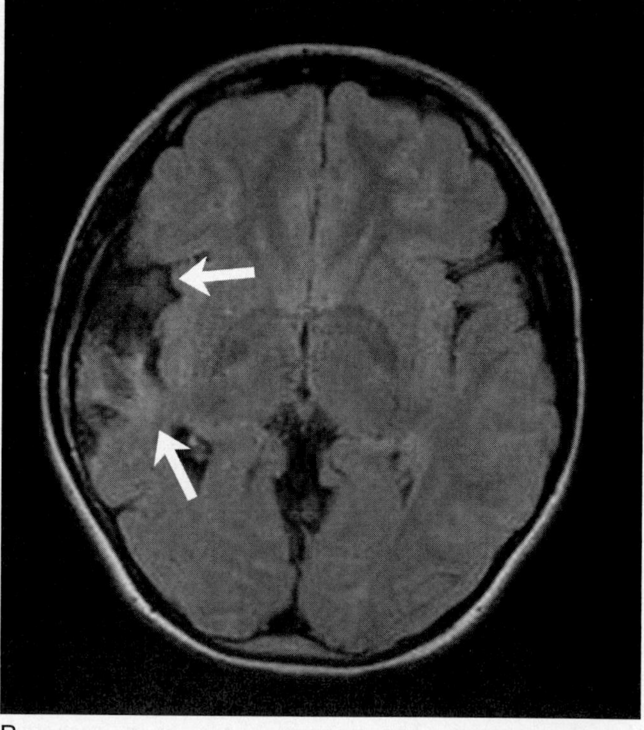

B

FIGURE 49–11 • Moyamoya syndrome in a 10-year-old girl. Axial T_1 **(A)** magnetic resonance (MR) image shows flow voids (*arrowheads*) associated with enlarged lenticulostriate colaterals. Axial FLAIR **(B)** also shows encephalomalacia from an old right middle cerebral artery stroke (*arrows*).

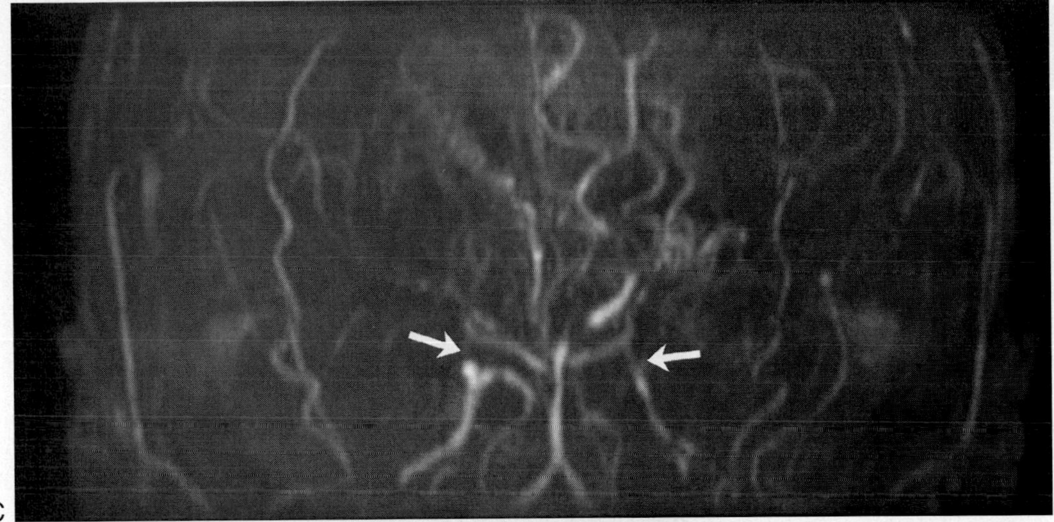

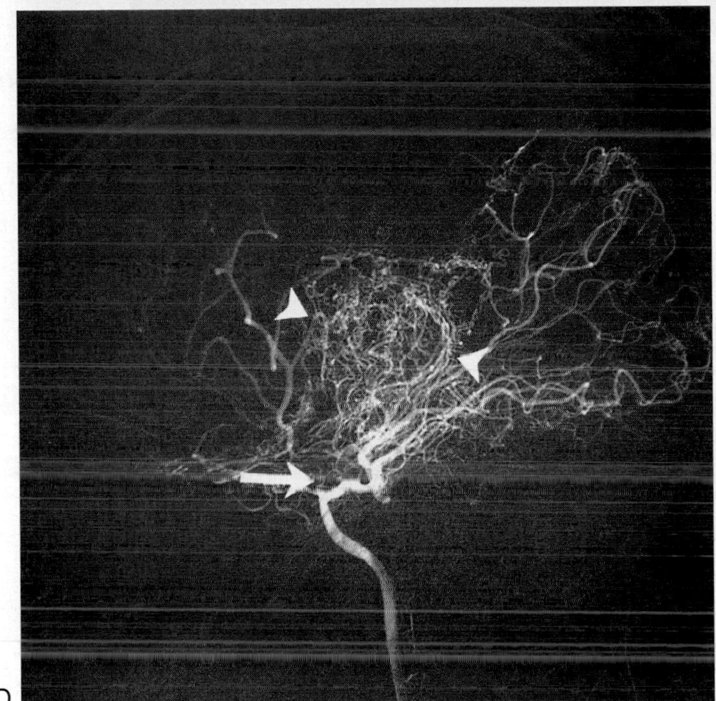

FIGURE 49–11 • Cont'd—Coronal **(C)** Maximum intensity pixel images from an MR arteriography (MRA) show no flow distal internal carotid arteries (ICAs) and abnormal posterior cerebral artery distributions as well (compare with normal MRA in **Fig. 50–2.**) Lateral view from a right ICA injection of a catheter angiogram **(D)** shows occlusion of the ICA below the siphon (*arrow*) and extensive thalamostriate collateral vessels (*arrowheads*).

Occasionally, however, there can be a vasculitic process in the presence of a normal MRI.[23] Furthermore, there are cases of CNS vasculitis in which the MRI is abnormal with a normal catheter angiogram.[25] Because medium and small vessels, which an MRA is less sensitive to, are often involved in the setting of CNS vasculitis, a catheter angiogram may be indicated in the setting of strong concern for vasculitis with a normal MRA and occasionally even normal MRI.

Vascular Malformations

Most AVMs and many aneurysms can be detected with a combination of MRI and MRA or CTA, although small lesions can be missed (Fig. 49–12). Catheter angiogram remains the gold standard for AVM diagnosis, confirming the flow dynamics and aneurysm, and will generally be required before surgical intervention. In the appropriate clinical setting such as a spontaneous SAH with an unknown etiology, abnormal images from MRI, MRA, or CTA, however, should not exclude a catheter angiogram. Arterial aneurysms are much less common in children than in adults; many of those seen are likely congenital or due to infection, in contrast to the typical acquired berry aneurysm seen in adults. As in adults, all but the smallest aneurysms can be seen on MRA or CTA, with CTA sensitivity for berry aneurysms in adult series reported in the range of 80% to 97%.[5] These studies, though, need to be of optimum resolution, generally targeted to the high-risk

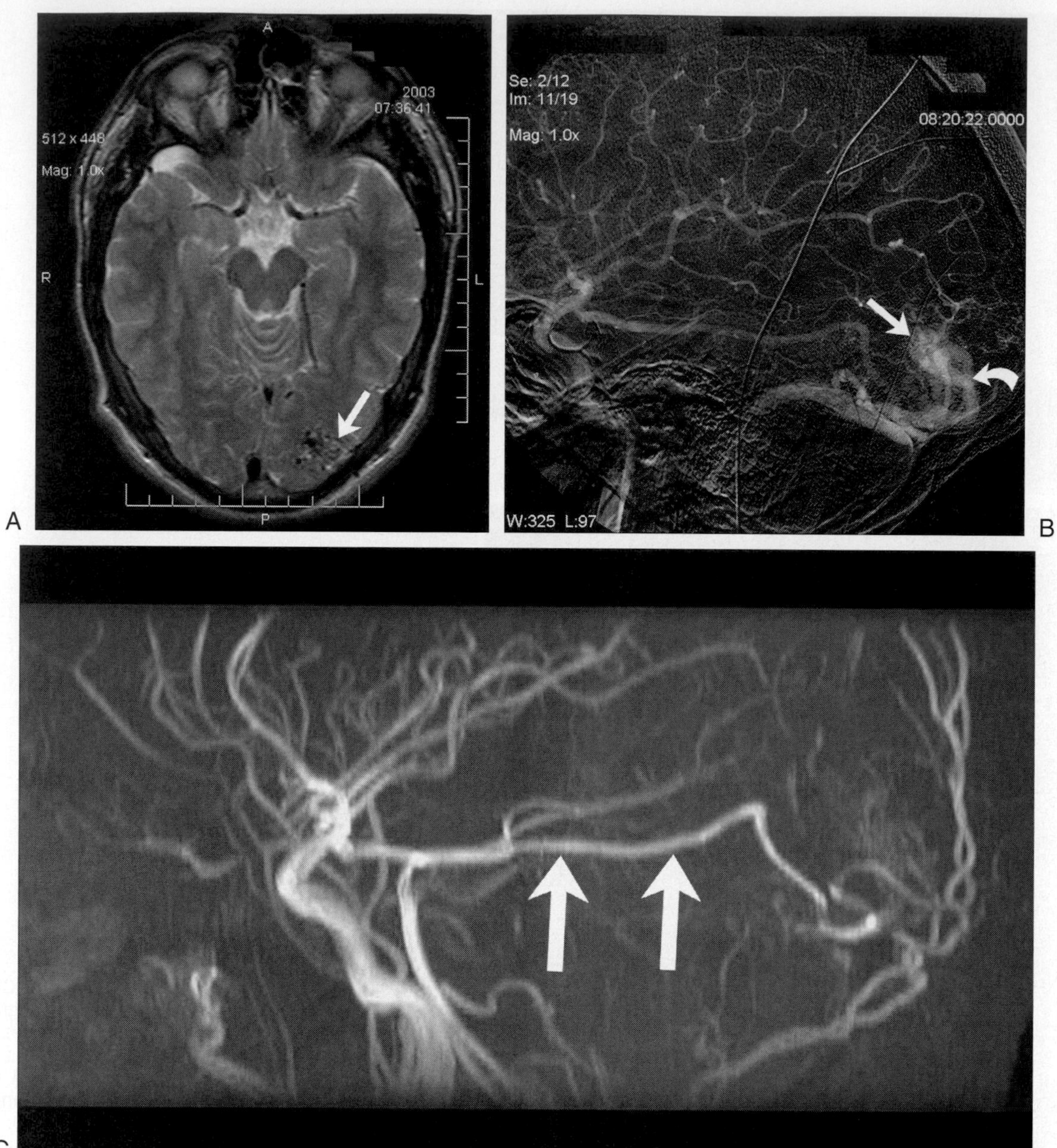

FIGURE 49–12 • A 14-year-old child with a left occipital arteriovenous malformation (AVM). Axial T_2 magnetic resonance (MR) image **(A)** shows a tangle of flow voids in the left occipital lobe (*arrow*). Lateral maximum intensity pixel image from an MR angiogram **(B)** shows an enlarged posterior cerebral artery branch (*arrows*), which feeds the area of abnormal vessels. Lateral view from catheter angiogram **(C)** confirms the presence of an AVM (*arrow*) and early draining veins (*curved arrow*).

locations for aneurysms in adults, which may not include less common aneurysm locations, which are seen with greater frequency in children. Angiographically occult lesions including capillary telangiectasia, cavernous malfunction, and developmental venous anomalies are seen on MR but are not usually of consequence, except the occasional large cavernous malformation.

A vein of Galen aneurysmal malformation (VGAM) is a misnomer because it is not the vein of Galen but a persistent embryonic vein that is dilated in association with a large fistula.[26] Those VGAMs presenting in the newborn period will manifest with cardiac symptoms resulting from the large shunt. Although the malformation can be seen with US, a CT scan is useful as a quick evaluation to visualize the malformation and determine the status of the cerebral cortex, which can have already been severely affected by birth. A noncontrast CT is sufficient because the density of blood (usually with an increased hematocrit) provides good contrast against the relatively less dense newborn brain (Fig. 49–13). In the presence of a VGAM,

MRI with MR angiography will give an overall vascular road map for planning endovascular intervention because the limited amount of contrast that can be used in a neonate requires any intervention to be directed.

Central Nervous System Infection

Imaging findings and the role of imaging in cerebral infection will depend on the organism and location of the infection (see also Chapter 58). The appearance will depend on the cell type infected and the host immune response. Infection can involve the subarachnoid spaces and meninges, the parameningeal spaces, or the brain parenchyma itself either primarily or secondarily. With bacterial meningitis the appearance on CT and MRI may range from normal to diffuse swelling with loss of gray-white differentiation and obliteration of ventricular and cisternal CSF spaces. Coxsackie virus, echovirus, and mumps infect the meninges more than the neurons, whereas poliovirus infects the neurons, particularly the motor neurons. Herpes simplex virus (HSV) type I has a predilection for the limbic system, most commonly affects the temporal lobes, and is the most common sporadic viral encephalitis.[27] HSV type II encephalitis is most commonly acquired at birth and does not display the predilection to the temporal lobes. Although MR is more sensitive than CT, a normal MR image still does not entirely exclude a viral encephalitis. In the clinical setting of suspected meningeal infection, CT may be indicated

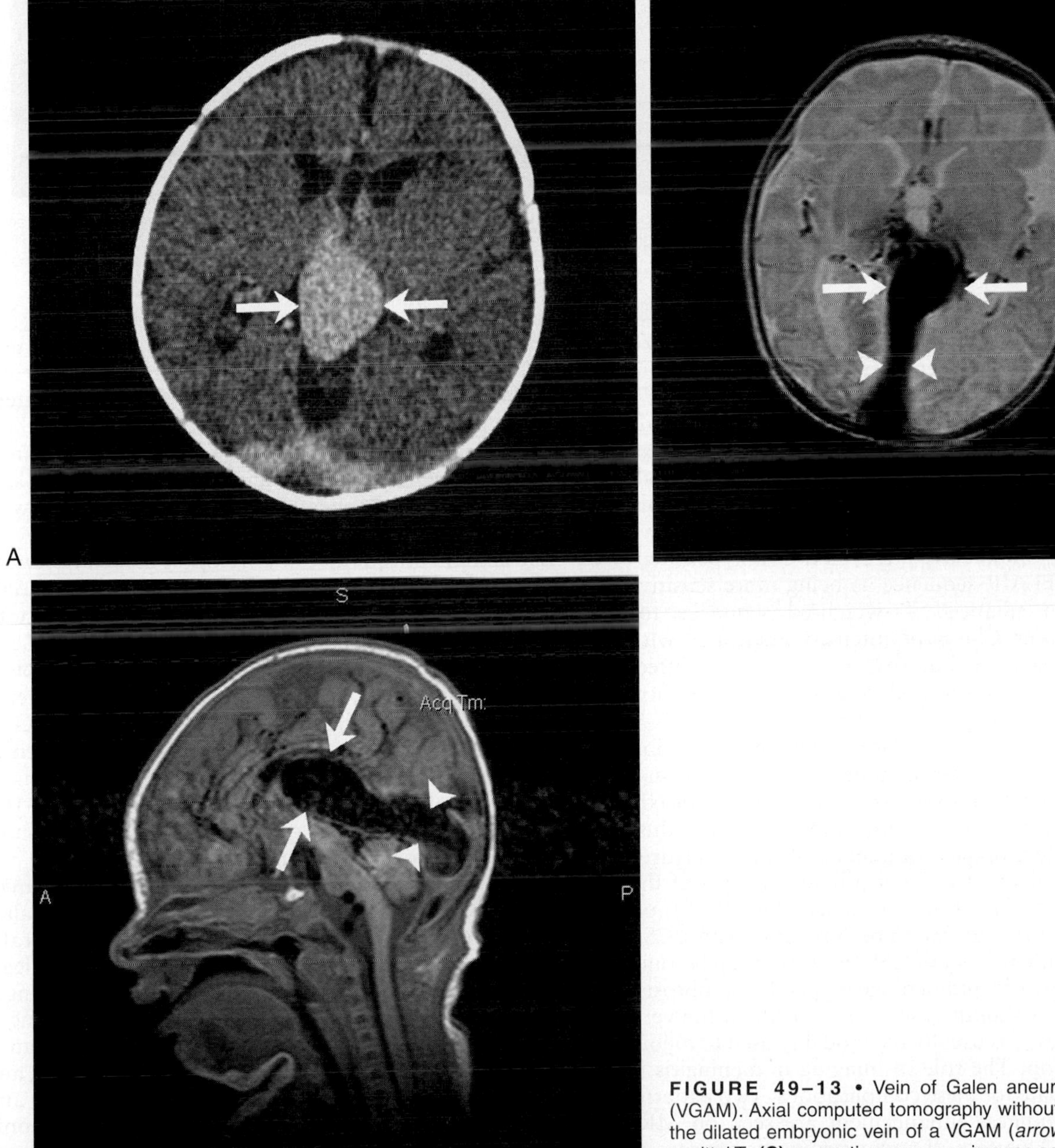

FIGURE 49–13 • Vein of Galen aneurysmal malformation (VGAM). Axial computed tomography without contrast **(A)** shows the dilated embryonic vein of a VGAM (*arrows*). Axial T_2 **(B)** and sagittal T_1 **(C)** magnetic resonance images again show the dilated embryonic vein (*arrows*) and the draining vein (*arrowheads*).

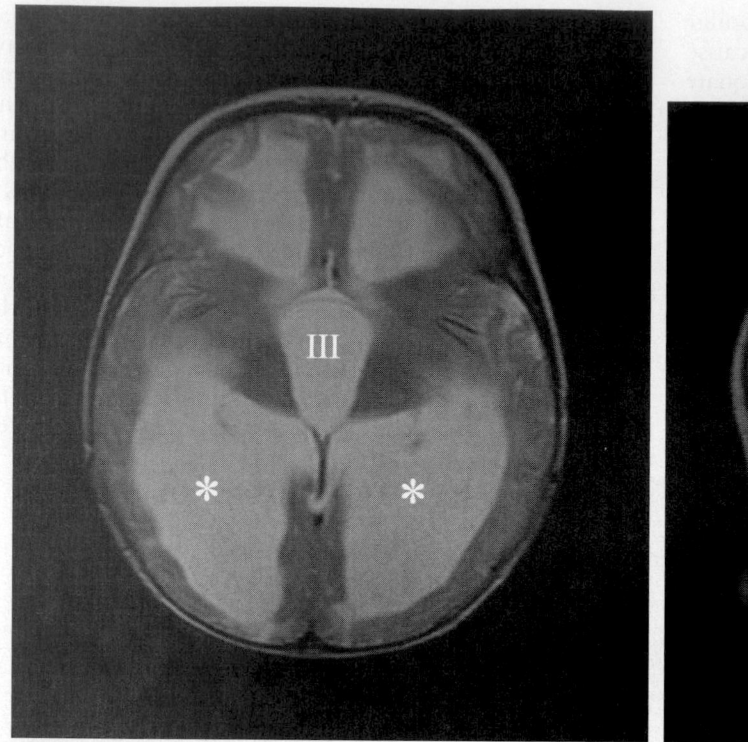

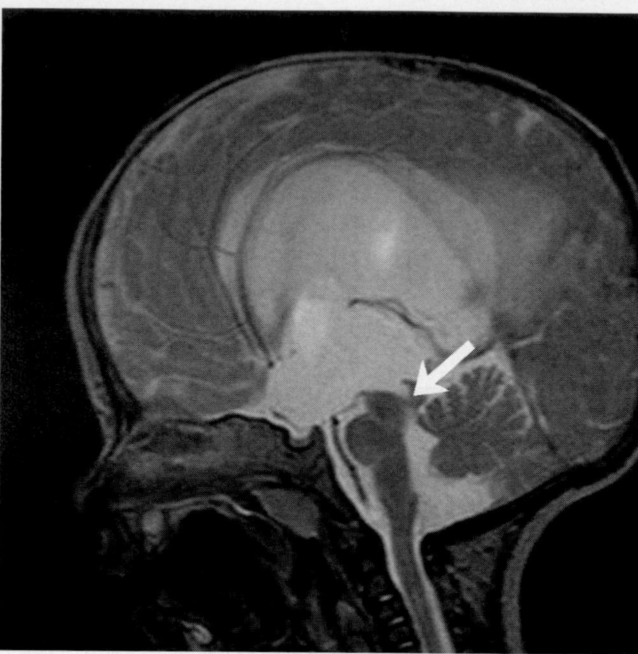

FIGURE 49–14 • Obstructive hydrocephalus following meningitis. Axial **(A)** and midline sagittal **(B)** T_2 magnetic resonance images show dilated lateral (*asterisks*) and third (III) ventricles that result from aqueductal level obstruction (*arrow*).

before lumbar puncture (LP) to exclude hydrocephalus or swelling, which would potentially preclude LP without neurosurgical consultation.

Imaging alone should not be used, however, to exclude meningeal infection. Particularly early in the setting of meningitis, contrast-enhanced CT is often normal. Although MRI with gadolinium is more sensitive, only 55% to 70% of those with proven meningitis have abnormal scans.[28] Some have advocated CSF hyperintensity on the MR FLAIR sequence as being more sensitive than gadolinium-enhanced T_1-weighted sequence for meningitis; however, CSF hyperintensity associated with supplemental oxygen and anesthesia, as well as noninfectious meningeal irritation and leptomeningeal tumor, render this finding less specific.[29,30]

Complications associated with meningeal infection include compromise of the BBB leading to vasogenic edema; arterial spasm that can cause ischemia with cytotoxic edema and eventual infarction; and hydrocephalus, potentially with development of interstitial edema. Hydrocephalus can be obstructive, typically at the level of the aqueduct or outlet of the fourth ventricle (Fig. 49–14) or, more commonly, communicating because of impaired CSF resorption. This impairment of CSF resorption can become permanent because of leptomeningeal-ependymal fibrosis, and it may require shunting. US can be used in the very young; otherwise, CT is usually the modality used to follow ventricular dilation. The role of imaging in meningitis is primarily to evaluate for these complications. Two patterns of abnormal meningeal enhancement are seen on MRI with meningitis. A pattern of pachymeningitis appears as diffuse linear thickening of the normal dural lining. This appearance, however, is not specific, as the same pattern can be seen in other settings including after surgery and occasionally following shunt revision. The other pattern is a leptomeningeal pattern of enhancement, where there is enhancement seen along the pia-arachnoid membranes, following the sulcal grooves. This pattern is also not specific, with a similar appearance being seen at times with leptomeningeal spread of tumor.

Extraaxial collections can develop in association with meningitis including subdural effusions and less commonly subdural abscesses. Effusions are crescentic collections that typically are isodense to CSF on CT and isointense to CSF on most MR sequences, although because the protein level may be increased, the collections may be hyperintense on FLAIR (Fig. 49–15). Subdural abscesses can be crescentic or lentiform when larger and typically slightly denser than CSF on CT. A rim of enhancement of variable thickness is generally better detected on MRI (Fig. 49–16). Subdural abscess can also occur as a direct extension of paranasal sinus or mastoid infection.

Infection of the brain parenchyma can take the form of a focal abscess(es) or a more diffuse encephalitis. Encephalitis in isolation or associated with meningitis will generally produce nonspecific cerebral parenchymal changes, at least on T_2 and FLAIR, and separation of ischemic changes associated with meningitis and encephalitis by imaging is problematic. A focal abscess will generally demonstrate a central focus of low density on CT and low T_1, high T_2, and FLAIR signal on MRI, with a ring of enhancement and variable surrounding edema (Fig. 49–17). More commonly in adults, there can be uncertainty with a ring-enhancing lesion between a possible brain abscess and a necrotic

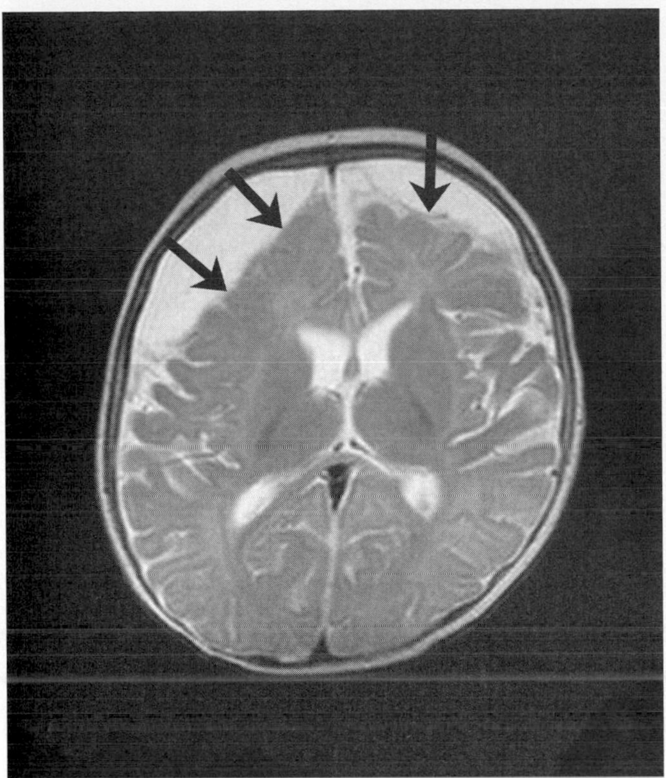

FIGURE 49–15 • Chronic subdural effusions following meningitis. Axial T_2 shows mass effect with sulcal compression associated with bifrontal subdural collections (*arrows*).

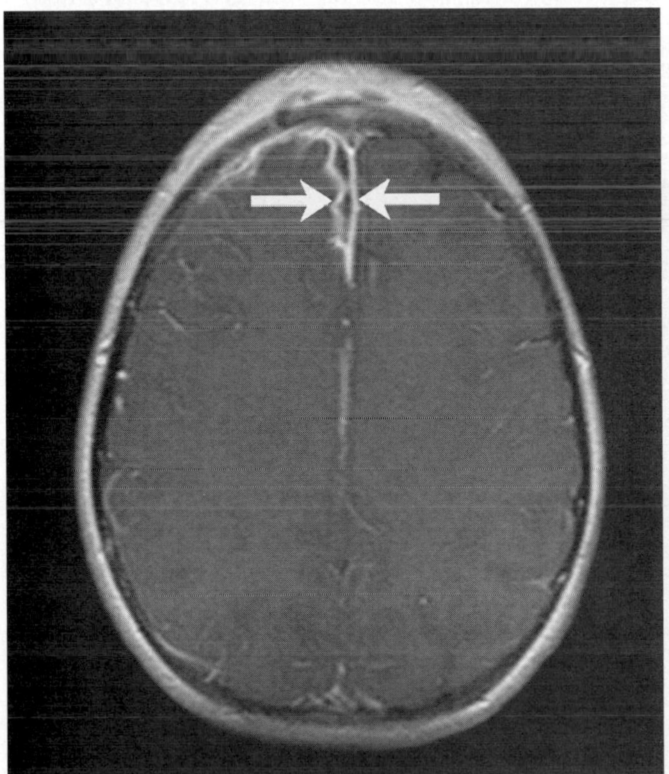

FIGURE 49–16 • Subdural abscess. Axial T_1 magnetic resonance image with gadolinium shows enhancement rim of a small right frontal paramedian subdural abscess (*arrows*).

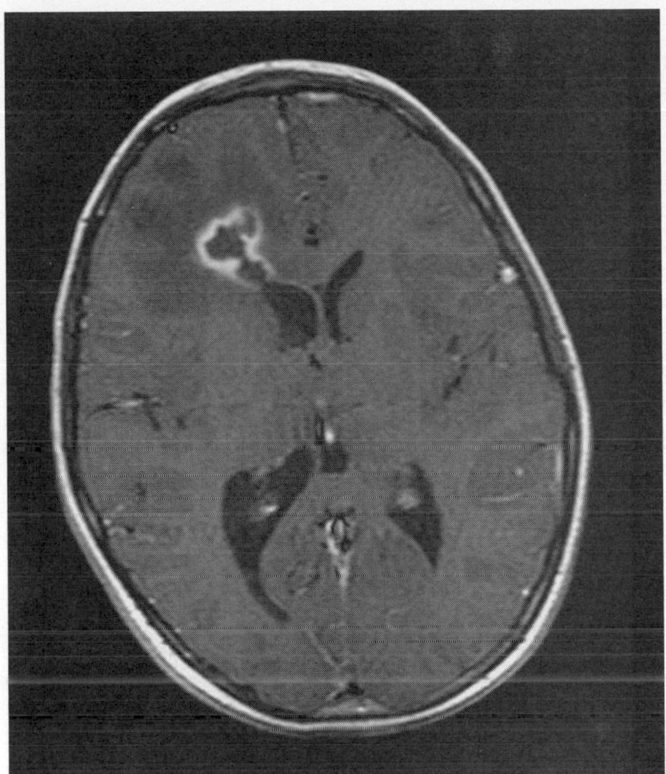

FIGURE 49–17 • Frontal brain abscess. Axial T_1 magnetic resonance image with gadolinium shows a right frontal lobe ring enhancing lesion with considerable surrounding edema with swelling.

tumor. The brain abscess will generally have a thinner rim of enhancement and on DWI the abscess will show restricted diffusion, while the necrotic tumor core will show increased diffusion. Exclusion of a meningeal or parameningeal abscess in the head can largely be accomplished with contrast-enhanced CT in which one is looking for a fluid collection with a surrounding enhancing rim, although occasionally a small collection can be missed on CT but detected on MRI. Evaluation for meningeal or parameningeal abscess in the spine should be approached with MRI.

Demyelinating Disease

Multiple sclerosis (MS) is much less common in children than in adults, whereas acute disseminated encephalomyelitis (ADEM) primarily occurs in children. ADEM can at times manifest with symmetrical involvement (Fig. 49–18) in which the imaging picture of ADEM overlaps with some metabolic diseases or the lesions can be scattered with a picture similar to vasculitis or emboli. (Fig. 50–9) The appearance of MS and ADEM can be similar. If lesions of multiple ages are present, this would be consistent with MS rather than with ADEM (Fig. 49–19). Demyelinating lesions are seen most commonly in white matter, but they do appear in gray matter as well. Acute demyelinating lesions can enhance. Acute lesions can also show restricted diffusion, which means that the appearance on DWI can mimic that of an acute ischemic lesion. Often, however,

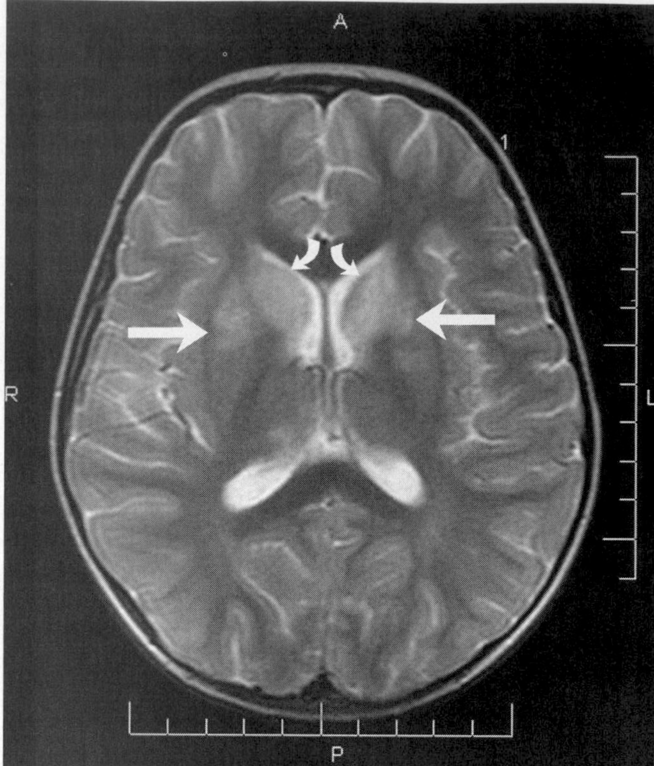

FIGURE 49–18 • Acute disseminated encephalomyelitis (ADEM). Axial T_2 magnetic resonance image shows symmetrical increased signal in caudate (*curved arrows*) and anterior lentiform nuclei (*arrows*) associated with ADEM.

the pattern of involvement is useful in distinguishing demyelinating disease (Fig. 49–20) from ischemic disease. The spinal cord can be involved with MS or ADEM although relatively rarely in isolation; thus imaging the brain to look for additional involvement can be useful in some cases to distinguish between a cord demyelinating process and infarct, which can have similar imaging pictures when the clinical scenario is not clear.

Trauma

CT remains the primary imaging modality in acute cerebral trauma and has the advantage of relative ease of scanning compared with MRI, including allowing non-MR compatible monitoring and life support equipment to be maintained while imaging. CT is sufficient for evaluation of most cerebral neurosurgical pathologic conditions, including the assessment of swelling and acute hemorrhage, both parenchymal and extraaxial. CT is generally more sensitive than MRI in detecting acute SAH and in the evaluation of bony injury (Fig. 49–21). CT is generally sufficient to detect cerebral swelling associated with herniation syndromes and therefore the potential need for neurosurgical intervention (Fig. 49–22). MRI is more sensitive for the detection of parenchymal injury and for more subtle extraaxial collections including more chronic epidural and subdural hematomas, which are common in nonaccidental trauma (NAT). MRI is indicated when there is doubt as to the presence of a subdural collection in the setting of suspected trauma. Also, in the setting of NAT, MRI can detect evidence of old parenchymal trauma/hemorrhage not seen on CT and give evidence of old

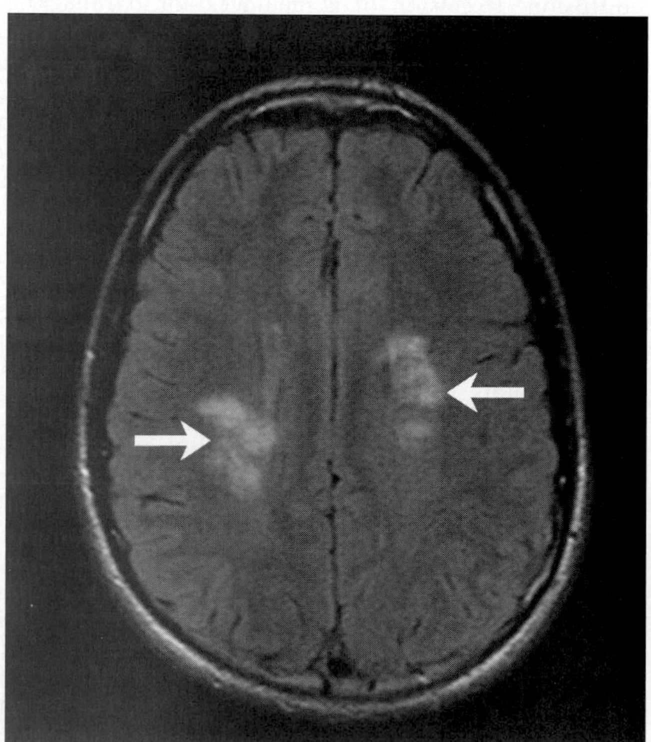

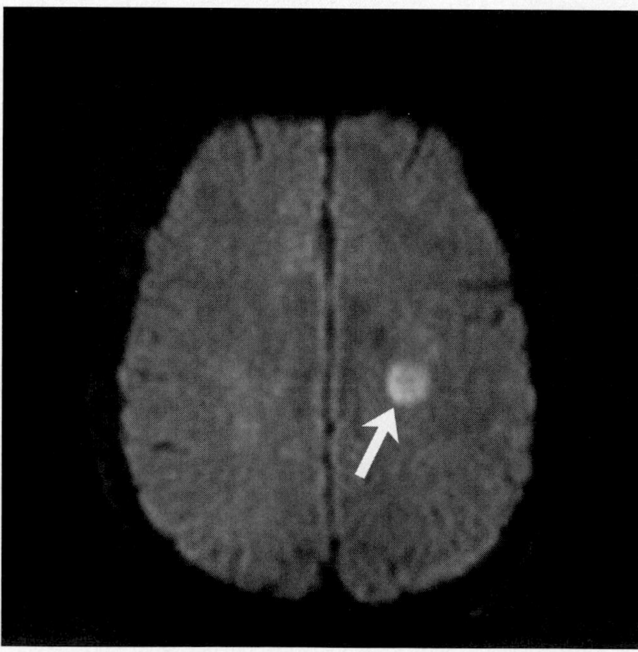

FIGURE 49–19 • Multiple sclerosis in a 16-year-old child. FLAIR magnetic resonance (MR) image **(A)** shows bilateral white matter lesions. Diffusion weighted MR **(B)** shows enhancement and diffusion restriction of acute lesion on the left (*arrow*).

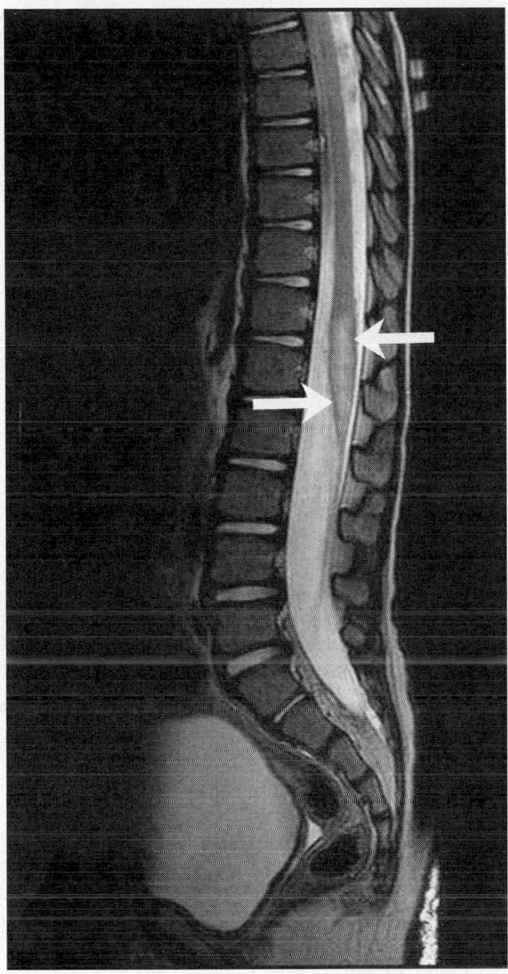

FIGURE 49–20 • Transverse myelitis. Sagittal T_2 magnetic resonance image of the distal cord shows central T_2 hyperintensity within the distal spinal cord (*arrows*) in this case of acute disseminated encephalomyelitis. Acutely, a spinal cord infarct could have this imaging appearance.

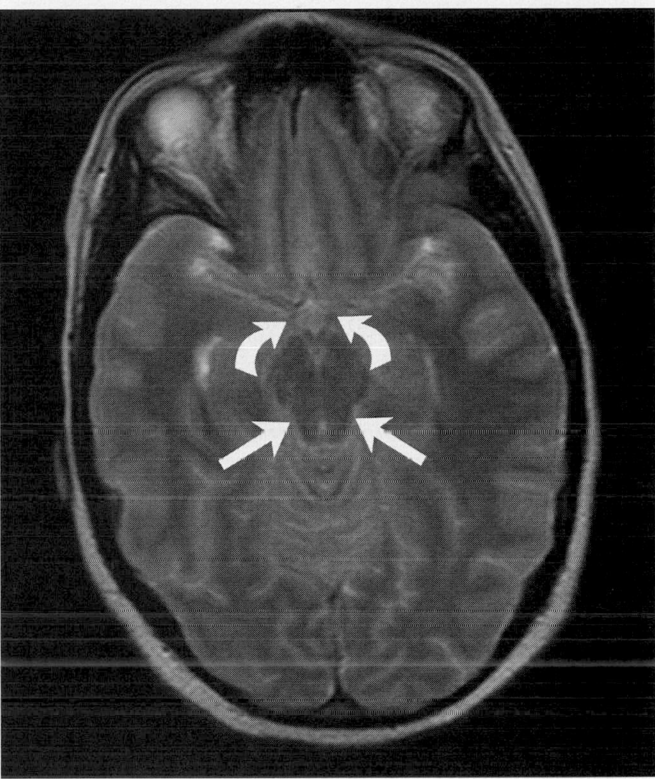

FIGURE 49–22 • Diffuse brain swelling with herniation. T_2 magnetic resonance image shows diffuse cerebral swelling with loss of ambient (*arrows*) and suprasellar cistern (*curved arrows*) cerebrospinal fluid spaces.

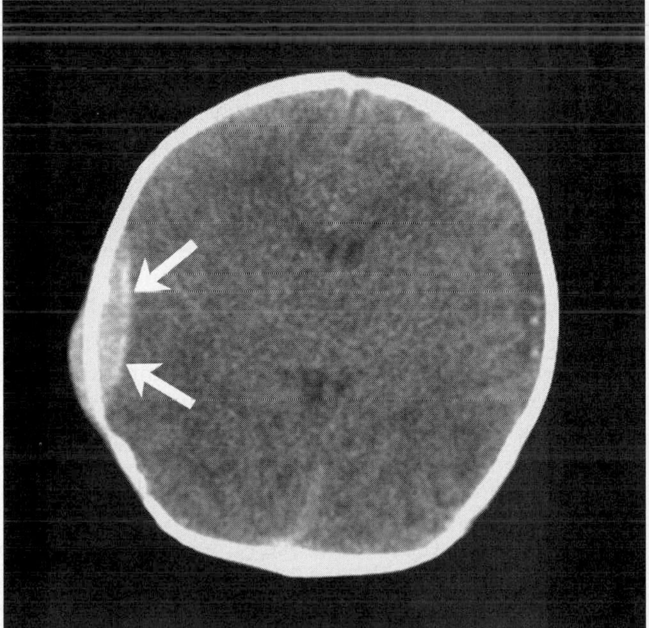

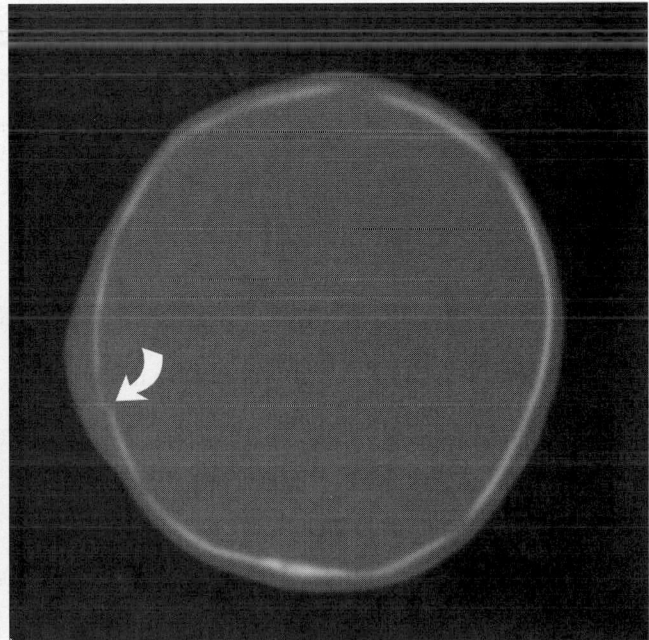

FIGURE 49–21 • Epidural hematoma with skull fracture. Computed tomography scan in brain **(A)** and bone **(B)** windows showing typical lentiform configuration of right-sided epidural hematoma (*arrows*). Bone window reveals an associated fracture (*curved arrow*).

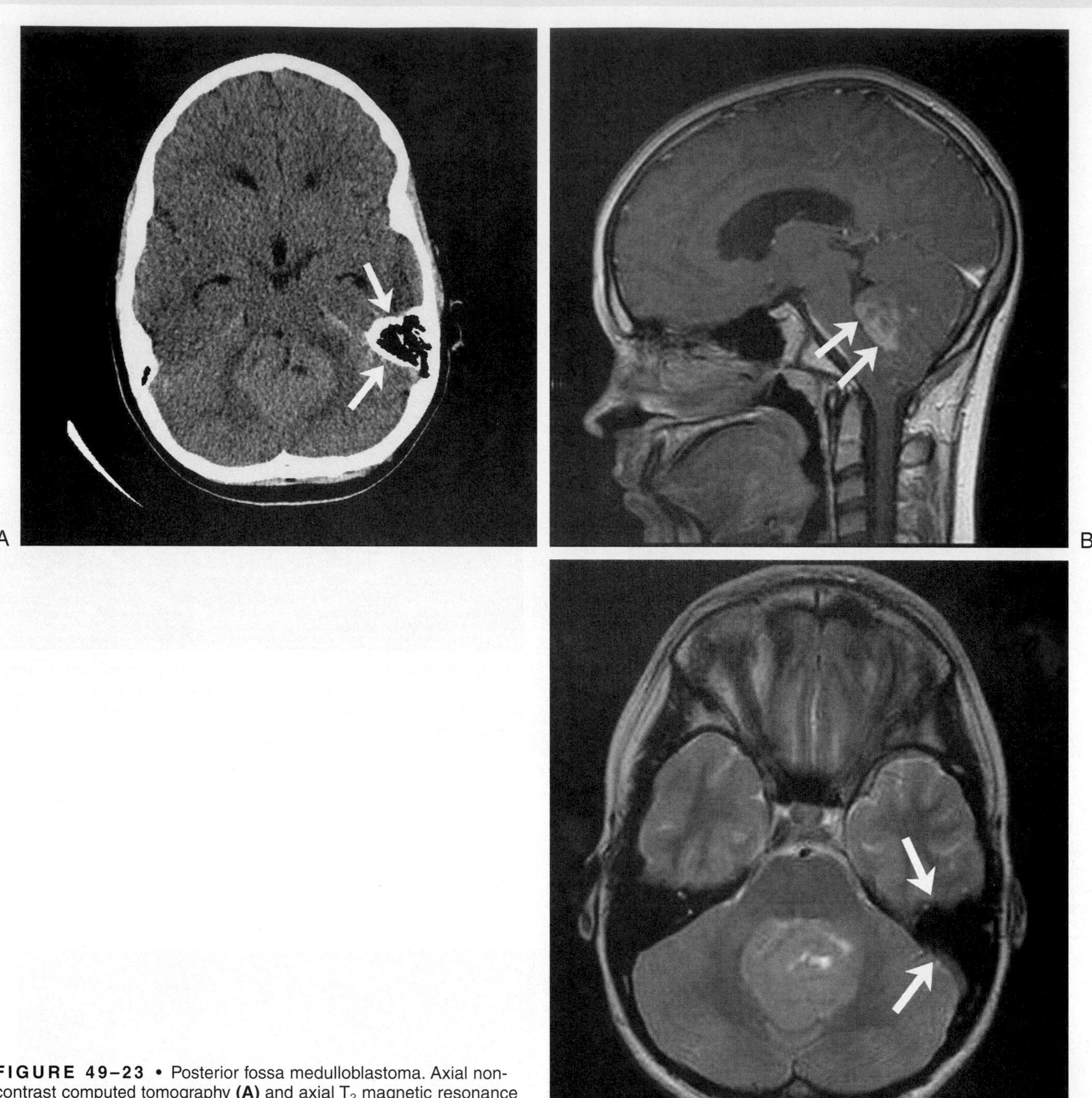

FIGURE 49–23 • Posterior fossa medulloblastoma. Axial noncontrast computed tomography **(A)** and axial T_2 magnetic resonance (MR) **(B)** show midline posterior fossa mass (*arrows*). Sagittal T_1 MR with gadolinium **(C)** shows enhancement in some of the tumor (*arrows*).

parenchymal hemorrhages (Fig. 49–5). In particular, gradient sequences can reveal evidence of old parenchymal hemorrhages. Bony injury of the spine is also better evaluated with CT, although cord compression and injury is better assessed with MRI.

Hydrocephalus

Hydrocephalus can be congenital or caused by hemorrhage, tumor, and meningitis. In the neonatal period, US is used as a screening tool in the evaluation of ventricular enlargement, in particular, that associated with germinal matrix hemorrhage. Beyond this period, most monitoring of ventricular size and shunts is accomplished with CT. In the initial evaluation of hydrocephalus, MRI can be helpful in determining the level and possible cause of CSF obstruction (Fig. 49–14). Acute hydrocephalus can be associated with evidence of transependymal CSF flow along the walls of the ventricular system, which is better appreciated on MRI. The absence of this appearance, however, does not reliably predict the absence of increased ventricular CSF pressure. Physiologic evaluation of shunt patency is also investigated with nuclear medicine shunt studies.

Tumor

Although cerebral tumors are best imaged with MRI (Fig. 49–23), the acute evaluation of a cerebral mass can be rapidly accomplished in the acute setting with CT, which will show the degree of mass effect and any impending herniation. Posterior fossa lesions, which are more common in children than in adults and predominate over supratentorial tumors in the 4- to 11-year-old range[31] and acute spinal cord symptoms possibly associated with a tumor, however, are best evaluated with MRI because of beam hardening at the skull base and spinal canal on CT.

Seizures

The CT imaging yield for a single self-limited seizure with no focal neurologic deficit is low, although most children currently will ultimately undergo scanning with CT or MRI. With focal neurologic deficit or prolonged seizure, the imaging yield increases. As discussed in Chapter 56, after seizures are controlled, MRI is indicated in the absence of a clinically apparent cause for the seizures. Abnormalities, however, particularly on MRI, may be secondary rather than reflecting the underlying cause of seizures. Prolonged seizures can be associated with transient enhancement due to BBB disruption and cytotoxic edema with hyperintensity on DWI that may be confused with stroke.

Conclusion

The ultimate selection of imaging will depend on clinical question(s), age and condition of the patient, and the locally available imaging technology. Consultation with radiologic colleagues is encouraged because the more the clinical situation is conveyed, the better tailored the imaging will be. This is particularly the case with the ever-increasing complexity of imaging modalities.

REFERENCES

1. Grant EG, El-Saden SM, Melany ML: Transcranial doppler. In McGahan JP, Goldberg BB, editors: *Diagnostic ultrasound: a logical approach*, Philadelphia, 1998, Lippincott Williams & Wilkins, pp 1037-1046.
2. Jungreis CA, Yonas H, Firlik AD, et al: Advanced CT imaging (functional CT), *Neuroimaging Clin N Am* 9:455-464, 1999.
3. Romero JM, Schaefer PW, Grant PE, et al: Diffusion MR imaging of acute ischemic stroke, *Neuroimaging Clin N Am* 12:35-53, 2002.
4. Gonzalez RG, Schaefer PW, Buonanno FS, et al: Diffusion-weighted MR imaging: diagnostic accuracy in patients imaged within 6 hours of stroke symptom onset, *Radiology* 210:155-162, 1999.
5. Tomandl BF, Kostner NC, Schempershofe M, et al: CT angiography ofintracranial aneurysms: a focus on postprocedures, *Radiographics* 24:637-655, 2004.
6. Heiserman JE, Dean BL, Hodak JA, et al: Neurologic complications of cerebral angiography, *AJNR Am J Neuroradiol* 15:1401-1407, discussion 1408-1411, 1994.
7. Cloft HJ, Joseph GJ, Dion JE: Risk of cerebral angiography in patients with subarachnoid hemorrhage, cerebral aneurysm, and arteriovenous malformation: a meta-analysis, *Stroke* 30:317-320, 1999.
8. DeBillon T, Nguyen S, Muet A, et al: Limitations of ultrasonography for diagnosing white matter damage in preterm infants, *Arch Dis Child Fetal Neonatal Ed* 88:F275-279, 2003.
9. Ment MR, Bada HS, Barnes P, et al: Practice parameter: neuroimaging of the neonate, *Neurology* 58:1726-1738, 2002.
10. Allison JW, Seibert JJ: Transcranial doppler in the newborn with asphyxia, *Neuroimaging Clin N Am* 9:11-16, 1999.
11. Hughes P, Weinberger E, Shaw DWW: Linear areas of echogenicity in the thalami and basal ganglia of neonates: an expanded association. Work in progress, *Radiology* 179:103-105, 1991.
12. Stark JE, Seibert JJ: Cerebral artery Doppler ultrasonography for prediction of outcome after perinatal asphyxia, *J Ultrasound Med* 13:595-600, 1994.
13. Gaskill-Shipley MF: Routine CT evaluation of acute stroke, *Neuroimaging Clin N Am* 9:411-422, 1999.
14. Barkovich AJ, Baranski K, Vigneron D, et al: Proton MR spectroscopy for the evaluation of brain injury in asphyxiated, term neonates, *AJNR Am J Neuroradiol* 20:1399-1405, 1999.
15. Schaefer PW, Grant PE, Gonzalez RG: Diffusion-weighted MR imaging of the brain, *Radiology* 217:331-345, 2000.
16. Tuor UI, Kozlowski P, Del Bigio MR, et al: Diffusion- and T2-weighted increases in magnetic resonance images of immature brain during hypoxia-ischemia: transient reversal posthypoxia, *Exp Neurol* 150:321-328, 1998.
17. Johnson AJ, Lee BC, Lin W: Echoplanar diffusion-weighted imaging in neonates and infants with suspected hypoxic-ischemic injury: correlation with patient outcome, *AJR Am J Roentgenol* 172:219-226, 1999.
18. Provenzale JM, Jahan R, Naidich TP, Fox AJ: Assessment of the patient with hyperacute stroke: imaging and therapy, Radiology 229:347-359, 2003.
19. van der Zwan A, Hillen B: Review of the variability of the territories of the major cerebral arteries, *Stroke* 22:1078-1084, 1991.
20. Grandin CB, Duprez TP, Smith AM, et al: Which MR-derived perfusion parameters are the best predictors of infarct growth in hyperacute stroke? Comparative study between relative and quantitative measurements, *Radiology* 223:361-370, 2002.
21. Lamy C, Oppenheim C, Meder JF, et al: Neuroimaging in posterior reversible encephalopathy syndrome, *J Neuroimaging* 14:89-96, 2004.
22. Port JD, Beauchamp NJ Jr: Reversible intracerebral pathologic entities mediated by vascular autoregulatory dysfunction, *Radiographics* 18:353-367, 1998.
23. Cooney MJ, Bradley WG, Symko SC, et al: Hypertensive encyphalopathy: complication in children treated for myeloproliferative disorders—report of three cases, *Radiology* 214:711-716, 2000.
24. Wasserman BA, Stone JH, Hellmann DB, et al: Reliability of normal findings on MR imaging for excluding the diagnosis of vasculitis of the central nervous system, *AJR Am J Roentgenol* 177:455-459, 2001.
25. Harris KG, Tran DD, Sickels WJ, et al: Diagnosing intracranial vasculitis: the roles of MR and angiography, *AJNR Am J Neuroradiol* 15:317-320, 1994.
26. Vein of Galen aneurysmal malformation: modern concept of vein of Galen aneurysmal malformation. In Lasjaunias P, editor: *Vascular diseases in neonates, infants and children: interventional neuroradiology management*, Berlin, 1997, Springer.
27. Shaw DW, Cohen WA: Viral infection of the CNS in children: imaging features, *AJR Am J Roentgenol* 160:125-133, 1993.
28. Kanamalla US, Ibarra RA, Jinkins JR: Imaging of cranial meningitis and ventriculitis, *Neuroimaging Clin N Am* 10:309-331, 2000.
29. Smith RR: Neuroradiology of intracranial infection, *Pediatr Neurosurg* 13:92-104, 1992.
30. Frigon C, Jardine DS, Weinberger E, et al: Fraction of inspired oxygen in relation to cerebrospinal fluid hyperintensity on FLAIR MR imaging of the brain in children and young adults undergoing anesthesia, *AJR Am J Roentgenol* 179:791, 2002.
31. Luh GY, Bird CR: Imaging of brain tumor in the pediatric population, *Neuroimaging Clin N Am* 9:691-716, 1999.

CHAPTER

50

Pediatric Neurologic Assessment and Monitoring

Gülay Pinar Alper and Ira Bergman

PEARLS

- The most important component of neurologic assessment of the patient in the pediatric intensive care unit (PICU) is serial evaluation of the level of consciousness.
- Any child with acute encephalopathy of unknown cause should undergo brain imaging. A magnetic resonance imaging (MRI) scan should be performed in a comatose patient if computed tomography (CT) is not diagnostic. An electroencephalogram (EEG) is another crucial tool of neuromonitoring that can provide immediate diagnosis and direct appropriate treatment in an unresponsive patient with no apparent underlying cause.

Every patient in the pediatric intensive care unit (PICU) requires a neurologic assessment. Systemic illnesses that transiently interrupt energy supply to the brain can permanently damage the brain. The goal of critical care management is to rapidly identify, prevent, and treat these brain insults. Neurologic dysfunction must be discriminated from sedation, residual anesthesia, neuromuscular blockade, and psychologic adjustment to the intensive care unit (ICU) environment. The most important component of neurologic assessment of the patient in the PICU is serial evaluation of the level of consciousness. In a child with altered consciousness, one must first determine when the child was last awake, alert, and functioning normally and then obtain a detailed chronology of the child's consciousness to the present moment. Parents, emergency medical technicians, and transport personnel may need to be interviewed. Often, this historical information is sufficient to make a neurologic diagnosis. Toxins, infections, metabolic diseases, and hypoxia tend to cause generalized cerebral dysfunction with relative sparing of the brainstem. Tumors, trauma, and focal ischemia tend to cause localized lesions that can affect either the cerebral hemispheres or the brain stem.

Observation

First, the child is observed. The child who is upset and fighting the nursing staff and equipment and whose eyes are open and looking about the room has a normal or, at worst, a mildly depressed mental state. A child lying with eyes closed in a comfortable sleeping posture may be asleep or have mild depression of consciousness. Yawning and spontaneous shifting of body positions indicate a minimal degree of unresponsiveness. Vocalization may persist in stupor and is the first response to be lost as coma appears. Restless movements of extremities, grasping, resistance to passive movement, grimacing, complex avoidance movements, or protective movements indicate that coma is not usually profound and that corticospinal and corticobulbar tracts are more or less intact. The child who lies still with eyes closed or, more ominously, with eyes a quarter open in a flaccid or stiff, invariant, unnatural posture has severe depression of consciousness and is at risk of permanent central nervous system (CNS) damage or death.

Seizures may be obvious or subtle and may be overlooked if the child is not watched carefully (see Chapter 55). Hallmarks of seizures are clonic movements of extremities, face, eyelids, or eyes and sudden interruptions of consciousness that occur repetitively in a stereotyped manner. During a seizure, the eyes are usually open, may appear to be staring straight ahead or fixed to one side, and may exhibit fine or coarse nystagmus. A focal motor seizure indicates that the corresponding corticospinal pathway is intact. If there is massive destruction of one cerebral hemisphere, focal seizures are rarely seen on the paralyzed side.

Asymmetries of spontaneous movement and posture are the best clues to hemiparesis in the unconscious patient. One leg that lies quietly in a flexed, abducted, and externally rotated posture probably indicates a hemiparesis on that side. A flattened corner of the mouth that does not elevate during spontaneous facial movements also indicates an ipsilateral hemiparesis. This side of the face may, however, produce a symmetrical grimace to noxious stimulation; this reaction stresses the importance of observation of spontaneous movements.

Tremors, myoclonus, and asterixis suggest metabolic disorders or drug or toxin effects. Choreoathetosis and dystonia imply basal ganglia dysfunction just as they do in an alert patient.

Visual and tactile hallucinations are most often due to toxins, drugs, or metabolic derangements. Olfactory and gustatory hallucinations suggest structural CNS disease. Auditory hallucinations are frequent in psychiatric illness.

Important recognizable respiratory patterns include Cheyne-Stokes respirations, central neurogenic hyperventilation, and gasping respirations (Biot's respiration). In Cheyne-Stokes respirations a period of hyperventilation with a crescendo-decrescendo pattern alternates with a shorter period of apnea. Cerebral, thalamic, or hypothalamic modulation of respirations has been lost, but brainstem control is intact. This pattern can also be observed in patients with congestive heart failure or primary respiratory disease. Midbrain disease yields central neurogenic hyperventilation, which consists of sustained, rapid deep breathing. Pulmonary disease, sepsis, metabolic acidosis (Kussmaul's respiration), and hepatic failure can produce a similar appearance. Central neurogenic hyperventilation produces respiratory alkalosis. Gasping respirations are irregularly irregular. They indicate dysfunction of the lower brainstem or medulla and will usually be followed by terminal apnea. Artificial ventilation must be instituted if life support is intended. Slow breathing can be observed in opiate or barbiturate intoxication and hypothyroidism. Determinants of respiration control are further discussed in Chapter 35.

Level of Consciousness and Mental Status

The child with depression of consciousness is assessed with a stepwise approach to judge the degree of depression. The child's name is called in a normal conversational tone to see if he or she is alert and will respond appropriately. If there is no response, one attempts to arouse the child using progressively intense stimuli. Responses consist of full arousal, partial arousal, localization and removal of the stimulus with one or both hands; withdrawal of the head and grimace; stereotyped flexion or extension of the arms with extension of the legs and arching of the back, other nonpurposeful stereotyped movements; and no response. Often a description of the patient's response to specific stimuli allows for the best assessment over time of a change in responsiveness. The pattern of change over time may suggest specific diseases or disease processes.

The degree of alertness or depression of consciousness can be quantitated with the Glasgow Coma Scale (Table 50–1). This scale has a special value as a measure by which to compare patients (or groups) to other cohorts of known prognosis. It has limited applicability to preverbal children.

General Neurologic Examination

A complete neurologic examination is outlined in Box 50–1.

Alteration of vital signs is important in the assessment of neurologic emergencies. Fever with coma suggests sepsis, pneumonia, bacterial meningitis or viral encephalitis. Hypothermia is observed in patients with barbiturate intoxication, hypothyroidism, cold exposure, and peripheral circulatory failure. Bradycardia may indicate intoxication from medications such as tricyclic antidepressants or anticonvulsants or intracranial pressure (ICP) if combined with hypertension and periodic breathing. Hypertension is important for hypertensive encephalopathy and again, in patients with Cushing

TABLE 50–1

The Glasgow Coma Scale

Activity	Best Response	Score
Eye opening	Spontaneous	4
	To command	3
	To pain	2
	None	1
Verbal	Oriented	5
	Confused	4
	Inappropriate words	3
	Incomprehensible sounds	2
	None	1
Motor response	Obeys commands	6
	Localizes pain	5
	Withdraws to pain	4
	Abnormal flexion to pain	3
	Abnormal extension	2
	None	1
	Total	3-15

BOX 50–1

Neurologic Examination

STATE OF CONSCIOUSNESS AND ALERTNESS

Oriented vs. confused
Spontaneous and stimulated interactions with environment
Eye opening, best motor and best verbal responses
Attention span

DEVELOPMENTAL EVALUATION

Language
Gross motor
Fine motor
Social

MENTAL STATUS EXAMINATION

Language: speech, comprehension, naming, repeating, writing, reading
Drawing
Math
Praxis
Memory
Fund of knowledge
Reasoning: similarities, proverbs
Judgment and humor
Mood
Hallucinations, delusions, obsessions

CRANIAL NERVES

I: Smell
II: Visual acuity, visual fields, fundi: discs, vessels, macula, background
III, IV, VI: Extraocular movement; pupillary reaction to light: direct and consensual, nystagmus, ptosis, strabismus
V: Masseters, pterygoids, facial sensation, corneals
VII: Orbicularis oris, oculi, frontalis; taste, anterior two thirds of tongue; stapedius, loss leads to hyperacusis
VIII: Hearing, vestibular responses
IX: Elevation of palate; gag reflex
X: Swallowing, movement of vocal cords
XI: Sternocleidomastoid, trapezius function
XII: Tongue movement, fasciculations

MOTOR

Strength: atrophy, fasciculations, weakness
Tone: passive, active, posture
Abnormal movements: tremor, chorea, athetosis, tics, myoclonus, seizures
Coordination: finger to nose, rapid alternating movements, heel to shin, ocular dysmetria, rebound
Gait: spontaneous, heel, toe, tandem, Romberg
Reflexes
Tendon jerks: knee, ankle, biceps, triceps, brachioradialis, pectorals, finger flexors
Superficial: abdominal, cremasteric, anal, Babinski's
Infants: suck, root, step, place, Moro, grasp
Frontal release: snout, grasp, root, suck, glabellar reflex

SENSORY

Touch, pin, temperature
Vibration, joint position sense, deep pressure
Double simultaneous stimulation, graphesthesia
Stereognosis, two-point discrimination, touch localization

triad. Hypotension is seen with septicemia, internal hemorrhage, barbiturate intoxication, Addison disease, or massive brain trauma.

Cutaneous Findings

Examination of the skin, skull, and neck is an essential adjunct to the neurologic examination. Cyanosis indicates inadequate oxygenation. Cherry-red coloration may be seen in carbon monoxide poisoning. Marked pallor suggests hemorrhage or hemolysis. Café au lait spots suggest neurofibromatosis and hypopigmented macules; facial angiomyofibromas and shagreen patches indicate tuberous sclerosis. Diffuse hyperpigmentation suggests Addison's disease. Petechiae and purpura are seen in meningococcemia, idiopathic thrombocytopenic purpura (ITP), thrombotic thrombocytopenic purpura (TTP), diffuse intravascular coagulation (DIC), and fat embolism. Bruises on the head or around the ears and eyes suggest head trauma. Bruises on the skin and thumb; and digital indentation marks on the chest and back; small circular (cigarette) burn wounds; belt marks; inflamed and scarred buttocks; and multiple retinal and subhyaloid hemorrhages indicate child abuse (Fig. 50–1) (see Chapter 106).

Meningeal Signs

In all but the deepest stage of coma, meningeal irritation (bacterial meningitis, subarachnoid hemorrhage [SAH]) will cause resistance to passive flexion of the neck. It may not develop for 12 to 24 hours after the onset of SAH. Cerebellar tonsillar herniation may also limit neck flexion. In infants, a bulging fontantelle is an important finding of meningeal irritation or increased ICP.

Motor Neuron Function

Lack of movement or decreased strength may be caused by disease of either the corticospinal tract or its neurons (the "upper motor neuron" [UMN]) or the peripheral neuromuscular apparatus, including the anterior horn cells (the "lower motor neuron" [LMN]) with their motor roots and peripheral nerves, the neuromuscular junctions, and the muscles. Destruction of the spinal cord leaves intact simple stereotyped reflex movements coordinated by local spinal reflexes below the level of the lesion. Destruction of the LMN leads to total absence of movement because it is the final common pathway producing muscle activity.

The corticospinal tract begins in the motor and premotor cortex anterior to the central sulcus, with some contribution from neurons in the postcentral gyrus. It descends through the central white matter of the cerebral hemispheres, the corona radiata, the cerebral peduncle, the basis pontis, and the pyramids of the medulla. It then decussates in the lower medulla and travels in the lateral funiculus of the spinal cord until it terminates on the anterior horn cells or interneurons closely associated with the anterior horn cells. Fibers controlling movement of the face decussate in the midbrain and pons before terminating on the appropriate motor nuclei in the brainstem. Muscles subserving movement of the jaw, pharynx, larynx, upper half of the face, neck, thorax, and abdomen

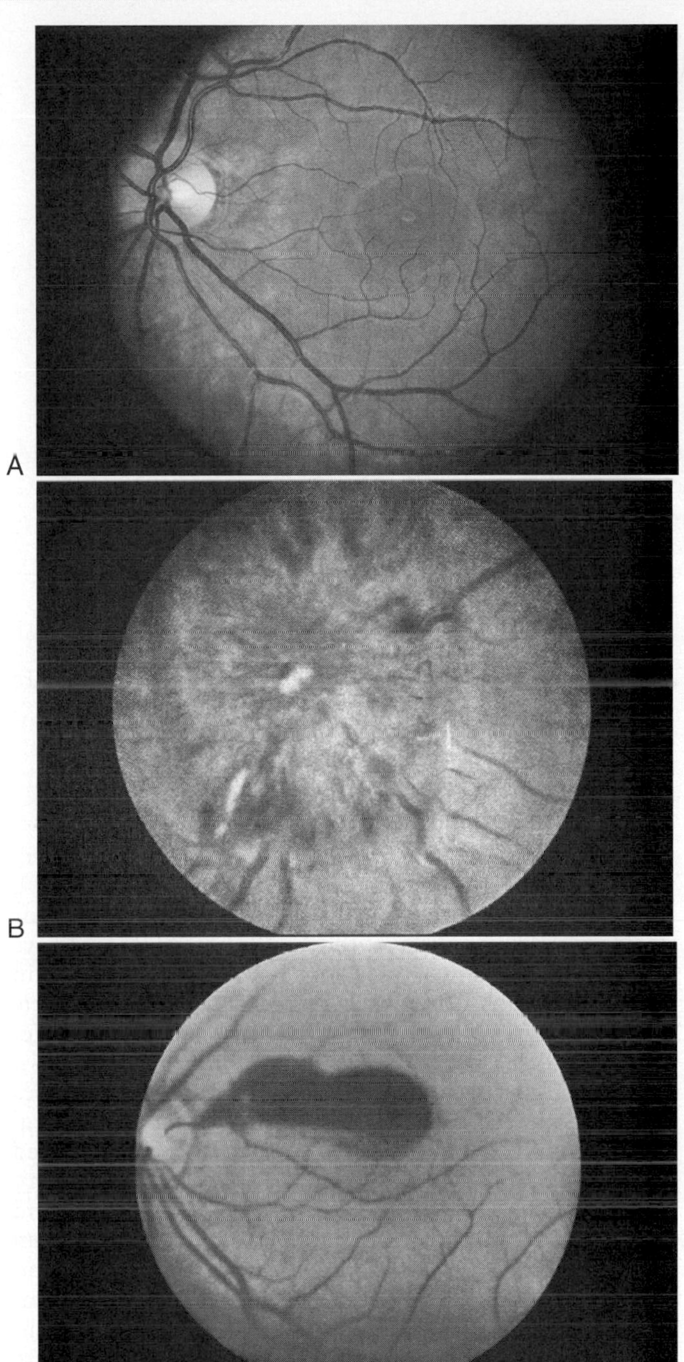

FIGURE 50–1 • **A,** Fundus photograph shows a normal fundus. **B,** Fundus photograph shows severe papilledema with loss of disc margins, tortuosity of vessels around the disc margins, and flame-shaped hemorrhages in and around the disc. **C,** Fundus photograph shows subhyaloid hemorrhage behind the vitreous.

are innervated from both cerebral hemispheres. Consequently, unilateral cerebral lesions lead only to weakness of the contralateral limbs and lower face. Lesions producing UMN weakness can be anatomically localized by their association with other deficits (Table 50–2).

Chronic UMN lesions usually produce hypertonic, hyperreflexive postured limbs; acute UMN lesions, however, yield flaccid limbs. Babinski's sign is usually strongly positive in acute disease and clearly indicates corticospinal tract (UMN) disease. In addition, hemiplegic weakness is likely to be caused by UMN disease.

Diseases of the LMN usually cause symmetrical hypotonic, hyporeflexive weakness and are discussed extensively in Chapter 56. The "topography" of weakness—namely, which muscles are most severely involved—can point toward specific diseases. In general, proximal weakness suggests myopathy, whereas distal weakness suggests neuropathy. Weakness of single muscles or muscle groups, except for ocular muscles, is almost always neuropathic.

Certain characteristics of postures and tone can define the level or locus of neurologic disability. Acute spinal cord disease may produce a flaccid, areflexive paralysis that simulates neuromuscular disease. A child who presents with an acute or subacute flaccid paraparesis is most likely to have either an acute cord syndrome, such as transverse myelitis or cord tumor, or the Guillain-Barré syndrome. The hallmarks of spinal cord disease are a sensory level, a motor level, disturbance of bowel and bladder function, and local spinal pain or tenderness.

Flaccid tone is noted with any acute lesion, in any location in the nervous system. Spastic tone, which is increased but more so in some phases of movement of the limbs than in others, is characteristic of chronic lesions of the corticospinal system. Rigid tone, in which the limb severely resists movement in any position ("lead pipe rigidity"), is noted with diseases of the basal ganglia. Decorticate posturing consists of adduction and stiff extension of the legs, flexion and supination of the arms, and fisting of the hands. It occurs when the midbrain and red nucleus control body posture without inhibition by diencephalon, basal ganglia, and cerebral cortex. Decerebrate posturing consists of stiff extension of legs, arms, trunk, and head with hyperpronation of lower arms and plantar flexion of the feet. It indicates pontine and vestibular nucleus control of posture without inhibition from more rostral structures. These postures may be exhibited unilaterally or bilaterally, indicating equal or unequal dysfunction of the two sides of the brain. Sometimes stereotyped rigid postures are shown that do not easily fall into the category of decerebrate or decorticate positions. These postures also indicate lack of cerebral and diencephalic control of upper brainstem motor reflexes. Lesions below the level of vestibular nuclei lead to flaccidity and abolition of all postures and movements. The coma is then usually profound and often progresses to brain death.

Reflexes

Reflexes to be tested include the tendon jerks, superficial abdominal, Babinski's sign, and frontal release. Deep tendon reflexes are depressed after an acute lesion. Asymmetrical stretch reflexes may indicate either an acute cerebral injury contralateral to the side with the depressed reflexes or an old injury contralateral to the side with the brisk reflexes. The presence of Babinski's reflex (i.e., dorsiflexion of the great toe in response to stimulation of the lateral plantar aspect of the foot) indicates acute or chronic injury to the corticospinal tract. Absence of superficial abdominal reflexes has the same meaning but is reliable only when the response is clearly

TABLE 50–2

Localization of Upper Motor Neuron Lesions

Signs	Localization
Aphasia Cortical sensory loss (graphesthesia, stereognosis, two-point discrimination) Gaze preference Unilaterally diminished opticokinetic nystagmus Visual field deficit	Cerebrum
Equal paralysis of face, arm, and leg Motor loss without sensory symptoms Motor loss with dense hemi-sensory deficit	Internal capsule
Hemiplegia with contralateral third nerve palsy (Weber's)	Midbrain
Hemiplegia with contralateral sixth or seventh nerve palsy (Millard-Gubler)	Pons
Spastic weakness, difficulty swallowing and phonating, incoordination	Medulla
Weakness of one leg with contralateral loss of pain and temperature sensibility (Brown-Séquard's)	Spinal cord
Paraplegia, sensory level, bowel and bladder dysfunction	Spinal cord

asymmetric. Frontal release signs include uncontrollable grasping, sucking, pursing of lips (snout), or exaggerated eye blinking (glabellar reflex) to local cutaneous stimulation. Presence of frontal release signs indicates that inhibitory fibers from contralateral portions of the frontal lobe are not functioning.

Cerebellar Function Testing

Gait is often difficult to test in the ICU because of patient illness and debilitation and attached equipment and catheters. Assessment of even two or three steps of spontaneous walking and then toe-and-heel walking, however, can be so rewarding that major efforts should be made to have the patient try to walk. Sitting balance should certainly be assessed in every awake patient. Finger-to-nose and heel-to-shin movements, rapid alternating movements of each hand and each foot, speech, and ocular movements provide further clues to cerebellar functioning. Ocular dysmetria consists of overshoots of the target or a series of ratchetlike undershooting movements to reach the target when the eyes are rapidly brought from fixation on one object to another.

Sensory Examination

Full sensory testing requires an alert, cooperative patient. An ominous finding is sensory loss in both legs. A spinal cord lesion must be strongly considered. The only sensory responses that can be tested in patients with depressed consciousness are gross responses to pain and the corneal reflex. Painful stimulation of a limb that produces a grimace indicates that the sensory message has reached the brainstem or higher centers. If painful stimulation produces withdrawal only of the limb stimulated, a spinal response is being observed. The sensory examination should be conducted with appropriate gentleness even in the comatose patient. Nasal stimulation with a cotton swab, cutaneous pricking with the cut end of a sterile wooden applicator, and gentle nail bed pressure are adequately painful stimulations. Pinching and sternal rubbing are not necessary.

Cranial Nerve Examination

The Pupillary Reactions

The pupillary reaction to light is a sturdy reflex that is abolished only by structural damage to the midbrain or third cranial nerve. Loss of the pupillary reflexes is always an ominous finding. Preservation of pupillary reflexes in the presence of deep coma suggests a metabolic-toxic cause. A unilaterally dilated pupil that does not constrict directly or consensually indicates oculomotor nerve palsy, whereas a pupil that does not constrict directly but does consensually indicates an optic nerve lesion. Unilateral oculomotor palsy in a comatose patient is often caused by an ipsilateral cerebral mass that produces uncal herniation. Horner's syndrome causes unilateral miosis and ptosis and is caused by unilateral lesions of the brainstem or hypothalamus or by dissection of the internal carotid artery. Hippus or fluctuating pupil size suggests metabolic encephalopathies. Small pupils are caused by pontine lesion and opiate and barbiturates; large pupils are caused by atropine and tricyclics.

Eye Movements

Eye movements are observed and then elicited with doll's head maneuver (DHM) (oculocephalic response) and cold caloric stimulation (oculovestibular response). In light coma of metabolic origin, the eyes rove conjugately from side to side in a random fashion. As coma deepens, these movements disappear and the eyes remain motionless in slightly exotropic positions. DHM involves turning the head from side to side to elicit horizontal eye movements and up and down to elicit vertical eye movements. Cold caloric stimulation of horizontal eye movements consists of placing the patient's head 30 degrees up from the horizontal position and then irrigating first one ear canal and then later the other with ice water. This produces intense dizziness, nausea, and vomiting in the awake patient and thus should be performed only in an unconscious patient. Regardless of the stimulus, eye movements fall into one of three patterns: (1) inhibited, (2) uninhibited, and (3) incomplete or absent. Awake persons can always move their eyes whenever and wherever they wish, either by making a quick jumping (i.e., saccadic) eye movement or by slowly following (i.e., pursuing) a target. Observation of the awake patient will reveal saccadic eye movements. DHM will produce inconsistent responses, depending on how patients direct their eyes. Nevertheless, at some time, saccadic eye movements will be observed, indicating that the cerebral cortex is functioning at least reasonably well. Cold caloric stimulation will produce nystagmus with the rapid phase contralateral to the ear that has been stimulated. This rapid phase is the equivalent of saccadic eye movements and also indicates good functioning of the cerebral cortex. The ears are irrigated separately several minutes apart. In comatose patients the fast "corrective" phase of nystagmus is lost and the eyes are tonically deflected to the side irrigated with cold water or away from the side irrigated with warm water. These vestibulo-ocular responses are lost or disrupted in brainstem lesions.

Uninhibited eye movements are seen in patients with intact brainstems but poorly functioning cerebrums. The normal oculomotor brainstem reflexes are not controlled or inhibited by the aware brain. There may be no spontaneous eye movements, or the eyes may spontaneously move slowly side to side. With DHM, the eyes move opposite to the direction of head movement at exactly the same pace, as if they were floating ball bearings within the orbits. To cold caloric stimulation, the eyes deviate fully and conjugately toward the ear that has been stimulated. Nystagmus is not observed.

Incomplete eye movements are observed when the brainstem, peripheral oculomotor nerves, neuromuscular junctions, or eye muscles are not functioning properly. With complete loss of oculomotor function, the eyes will remain in the center of the orbit, as if they are painted on, regardless of any stimulation. With partial loss, the paralyzed portions will be nonfunctioning, regardless of stimulation. For example, with a left third cranial nerve palsy, the left eye will not move medially at any time. In this example, if the patient is comatose and eye movements are otherwise uninhibited, DHM to the left or cold caloric stimulation of the right ear will result in a dysconjugate gaze, with the right eye moving fully laterally but the left eye stopping in the midline position.

Abnormal position of the eyes or pupils and failure of specific extraocular movements can localize the site of neurologic dysfunction (Table 50–3). Unilateral frontal lesions prevent voluntary eye movements to the contralateral side. Reflex eye movements induced by DHM or cold caloric stimulation, however, are intact. Pontine lesions may destroy the LMN center for conjugate horizontal gaze to the ipsilateral side. Neither voluntary nor reflex eye movements to that side are possible. Ocular bobbing consists of slow downward rolling of the eyes, followed by a quick jerk upward. In association with failure of voluntary and reflex horizontal eye movements, it indicates extensive pontine injury. Retraction nystagmus consists of sudden inward displacements of the globe caused by simultaneous contraction of all extraocular muscles. This or convergence nystagmus, with both eyes simultaneously deviating medially, indicates intrinsic or compressive lesions of the midbrain. Skew gaze, in which

TABLE 50–3

Eye Position, Extraocular Movements, Pupils, and Neurologic Lesions

EYE POSITION OR ABNORMAL MOVEMENT	SITE OF NEUROLOGIC LESION
To one side (gaze preference)	Frontal lobe ipsilateral to eye position or pons contralateral to eye position
Down and in	Thalamus or upper midbrain
Ocular bobbing	Pons
Retraction or convergence nystagmus	Midbrain
Oculomotor nerve palsy	Midbrain or herniation syndrome
Abducens nerve palsy	Unreliable localization
Internuclear ophthalmoplegia	Midbrain or pons
Dysconjugate or skew gaze	Brainstem
Absent vertical and retained horizontal movement	Midbrain
Absent horizontal and retained vertical movements	Pons
Absence of all extraocular movements, retained pupillary light reflex	Metabolic-toxic insult
PUPILS	
Small, reactive	Metabolic-toxic insult or thalamus, hypothalamus
Pinpoint, reactive	Pons
Midposition, fixed	Midbrain
Large, fixed	Oculomotor nerve or tectum of midbrain or mydriatic ophthalmic drops
Horner's syndrome	Lateral medulla or sympathetic pathways

one eye rests superior to the other, denotes dysfunction of some portion of the brainstem.

Abnormal eye movements may indicate an ongoing seizure activity. Eyes turn or jerk toward the convulsing site in focal seizures. Brisk, small amplitude, mainly vertical but occasionally horizontal eye movements are detectable by passive lid elevation in electrographic status epilepticus (without motor manifestations).

Fundoscopic Examination

Examination of the fundi may reveal hemorrhages or papilledema. Hemorrhages indicate either acute subarachnoid or subdural hemorrhage, cranial trauma from a direct blow or shaking injury, or malignant hypertension. Papilledema indicates raised ICP from any cause. Usually papilledema develops hours after the onset of the elevated ICP. Acute severe increases, however, as with SAH from a ruptured saccular aneurysm, can result in almost instantaneous papilledema (Fig. 50–1). Sometimes papilledema never develops, despite prolonged severe elevations of ICP.

Corneal Reflex

An abnormal corneal reflex may indicate either fifth nerve afferent disease (ipsilateral stimulation results in neither a direct nor consensual eye blink) or seventh nerve efferent disease (ipsilateral stimulation results in a brisk consensual but no direct response).

Unilateral weakness of eye closure, forehead movement, and mouth movement indicates peripheral seventh cranial nerve palsy, whereas failure to move only the mouth with preservation of upper face movements indicates a central corticospinal tract lesion rostral to the pons. Facial weakness may be noted during grimacing while responses to painful stimuli are evaluated.

Voluntary pharyngeal and laryngeal control is tested by asking the patient to speak and say "ah." In the absence of voluntary movement, a hypoactive gag indicates medullary or vagal dysfunction and a hyperactive gag indicates interruption of corticospinal inhibition to the medulla.

In a comatose patient or one whose consciousness is rapidly sinking, one must quickly determine whether the patient is experiencing raised ICP. Papilledema or third cranial nerve palsy are strong evidence of elevated ICP. More commonly, depressed consciousness accompanied by a characteristic progression of motor, oculomotor, pupillary, and respiratory signs, as detailed in Chapter 52, warns of incipient transtentorial herniation. Cranial computed tomography (CT) may reveal characteristic findings of cerebral edema, including hypodensity of cortical gray matter and subcortical white matter and obliteration of the cisterns surrounding the midbrain (Fig. 50–2).

Sedation and Paralysis

Neurologic examination of the pharmacologically paralyzed patient consists of examining the pupillary reflexes and fundi. As always, loss or slowing of the pupillary light reflex is an ominous finding. In addition to seeking

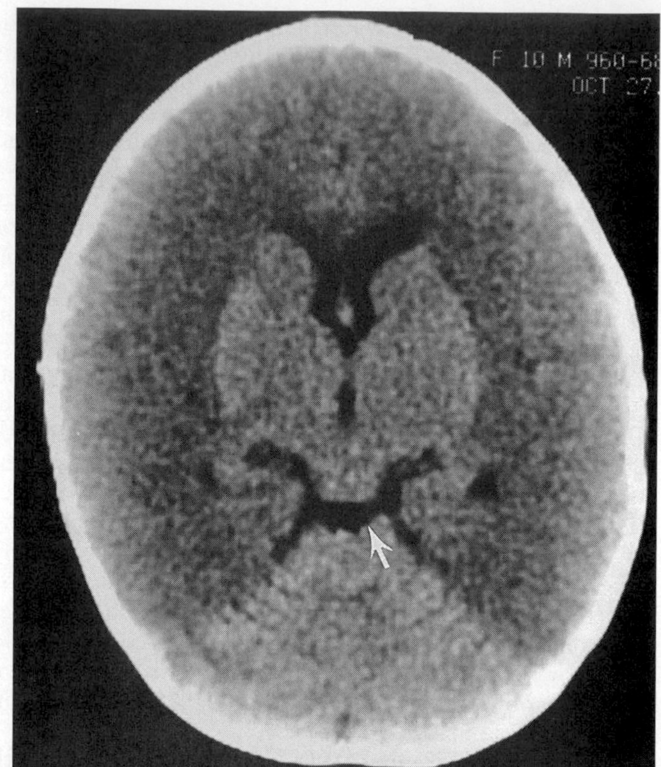

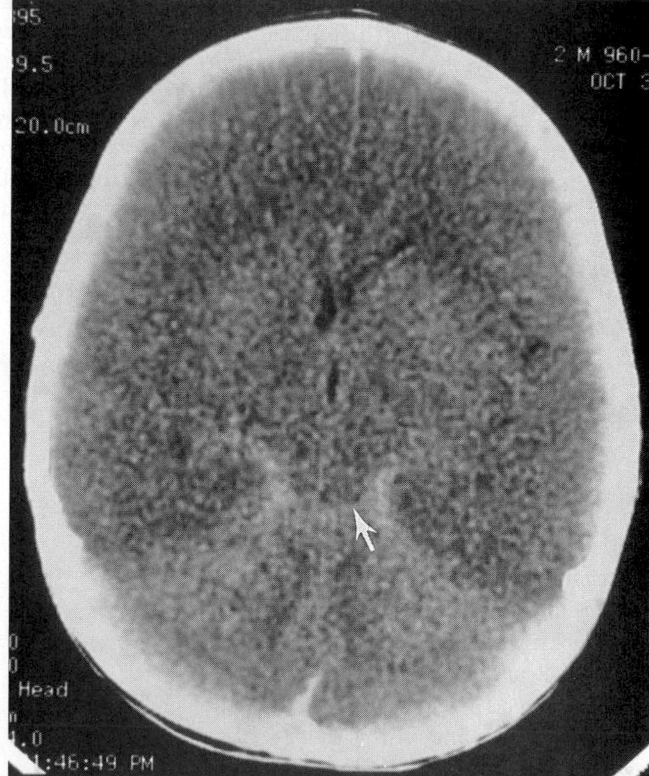

FIGURE 50–2 • A, Cranial computed tomography (CT) without contrast demonstrating hypodensity of the cortical gray matter and subcortical white matter in a patient with hepatic encephalopathy. The density of the basal ganglia and cerebellum are normal, and there is a normal contour of the ventricles and ambient cistern (*arrow*). **B,** Cranial CT shows severe cerebral edema in a patient with hepatic encephalopathy. There is severe hypodensity of the cortical gray matter and subcortical white matter, as well as hypodensity of the basal ganglia. There is severe compression of the frontal horns of the lateral ventricles and of the ambient cistern (*arrow*).

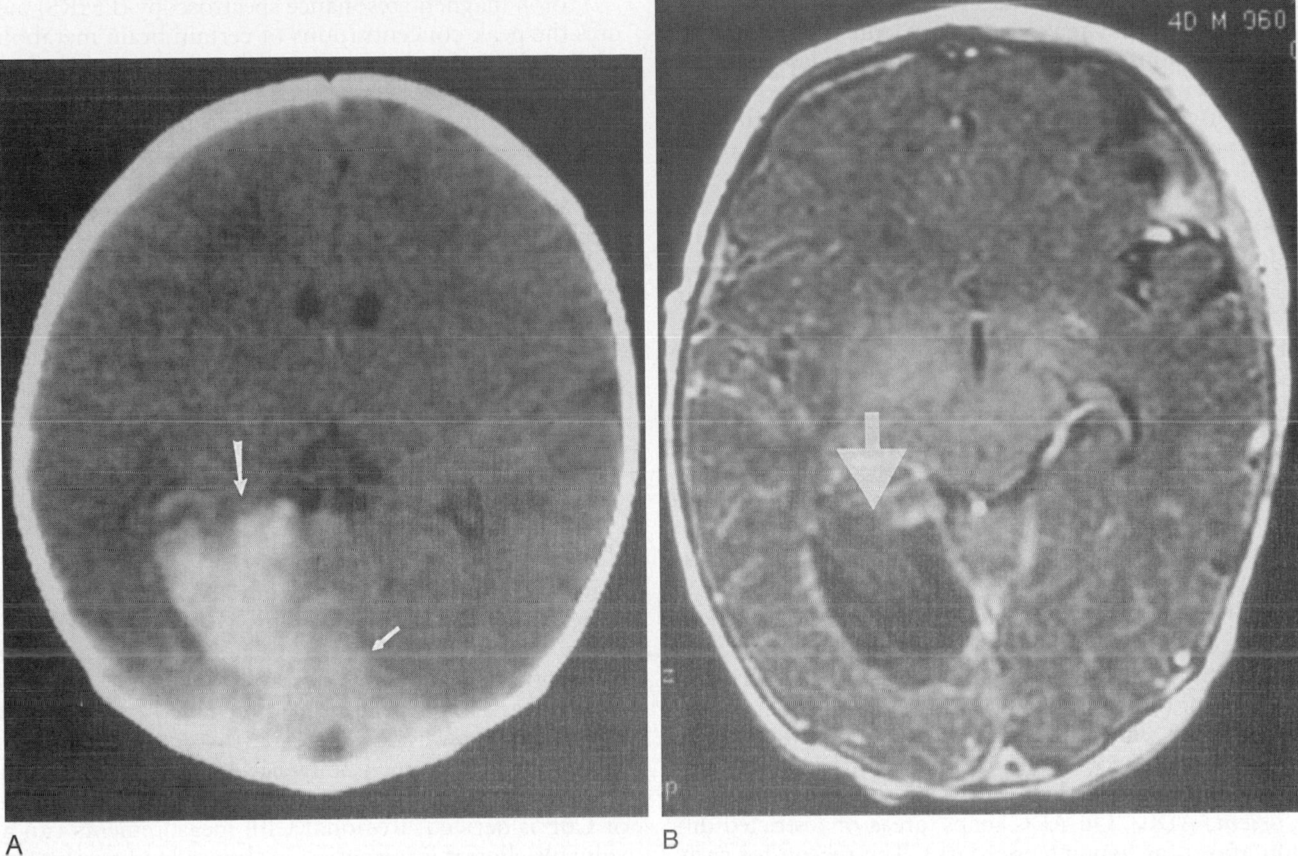

FIGURE 50–3 • **A,** Cranial computed tomography shows an acute right occipital intraparenchymal hemorrhage (*large arrow*) in a 2-day-old infant. Blood was also layered over the tentorium (*small arrow*). **B,** Cranial magnetic resonance imaging utilizing T_1 techniques in the same infant at age 3 days shows the acute intraparenchymal hemorrhage as a large low signal region (*arrow*). Intravenous contrast was administered, and no areas of abnormal vascularity are noted. The cause of the hemorrhage was not known.

a cause, an electroencephalogram (EEG) should be used to see if any electrocerebral activity remains. A contribution of neuromuscular blocking agents to patient flaccidity may be confirmed by transcutaneous nerve stimulation (see Chapter 115).

The neurologic state of the sedated patient is also very difficult to evaluate when sedation accumulates following days of consecutive use or when hepatic and renal failure slow metabolism of the sedating drugs. Sometimes examination is possible only after sedation has been stopped for several days.

Laboratory Adjuncts

Cranial Imaging

Any child with an acute encephalopathy of unknown cause should receive either a CT scan or magnetic resonance imaging (MRI). At this time, CT has the advantage of ready availability, rapid sequence times (< 10 seconds), and ease of interpretation. Diagnostic CT should be performed first without contrast and then with contrast. Contraindications to contrast are renal failure, incipient renal failure, or a history of allergy to contrast media. White (dense) lesions on the noncontrast study are either hemorrhage or calcification. In most patients in the ICU, these white areas represent hemorrhage (Fig. 50–3, *A*). Contrast enhancement indicates either local breakdown of the blood-brain barrier or excess vascularity and is associated with neoplasms, infections, inflammatory lesions, and subacute stroke.

Recently, MRI has supplemented or supplanted CT and other imaging modalities such as angiography, radioisotope brain scanning, and xenon blood flow. MRI measures radiofrequency signals rather than x-ray density, and lesions are either high- or low-signal intensity. After stimulation with a specific radiofrequency pulse, the tissue will return to its preexcited state by processes known as T_1 or T_2 relaxation. Imaging can concentrate on T_1 relaxation (cerebrospinal fluid [CSF] appears dark) or T_2 relaxation (CSF appears white). Acute hemorrhage (7 to 72 hours) appears isointense or hypointense on T_1 and hypointense on T_2 studies (Fig. 50–3, *B*). Early subacute hemorrhage (4 to 7 days) appears hyperintense on T_1 and still hypointense on T_2 studies. Late subacute (over 7 days) hemorrhage is hyperintense on both T_1 and T_2 images until hemosiderin formation, which appears as hypointense ring (over 6 weeks or a few months). Gradient echo (GRE) sequence is dark even in hyperacute stage (4 to 6 hours) and remains dark in all the stages of hemorrhage. Most other common lesions appear white on T_2-weighted studies. Small infarcts, infections, inflammatory areas, and demyelinating plaques are seen much more readily on MRI than on CT. In addition, MRI provides clear sagittal images that make it the procedure of choice for suspected lesions of the spinal cord or cervicomedullary junction. Fluid-attenuated inversion recovery (FLAIR) imaging uses T_2 weighted (T_2W), but CSF appears dark to make a sharper contrast between most lesions, which are white, and the cerebral ventricles, which now appear black. Special techniques have been developed for specific purposes. GRE and echo planar susceptibility-weighted imaging (EPI-SWI) detect the paramagnetic effects of blood-breakdown products (deoxyhemoglobin, ferritin, and hemosiderin), which appear dark on T_2W images. GRE MRI and EPI-SWI sequences allow visualization of petechial hemorrhages (microbleeds) that cannot be detected with head CT.[1,2] Magnetization transfer contrast (MTC) is useful in the assessment of myelination and demyelination. MTC imaging relies on detecting differences in relaxation properties of free and bound water; water protons bound to macromolecules such as those composing myelin. Diffusion-weighted images (DWIs) detect acute cytotoxic edema and can identify acute ischemic strokes as bright lesions within minutes of their occurrence.[3,5] It is useful in the detection of hypoxic-ischemic injury (Fig. 50–4). Hyperintense (bright) lesions on DWIs indicate a restriction in the diffusional movement of water and thus an increased water content of the region. The degree of water proton mobility can be quantified by a parameter known as the *apparent diffusion coefficient* (ADC). On ADC maps, areas of restricted diffusion appear as hypointense (dark). The reason for early decline in ADC is thought to be cytotoxic edema as a result of cellular energy failure causing a loss of ion homeostasis and subsequent shift of water to intracellular compartment. ADC findings persist 7 to 10 days after a completed stroke (gliotic tissue shows reverse signals). Irreversible ischemia is probably present if ADC values fall to 50% or less of surrounding brain tissue.[3] Newer techniques to visualize and evaluate the prognosis of stroke such as diffusion tensor imaging and blood oxygenation level-dependent functional MRI (BOLD-fMRI) are being developed.

The techniques of magnetic resonance angiography (MRA) and magnetic resonance venography (MRV) are excellent procedures to detect vascular occlusions in large- and medium-size vessels in the head and neck and cerebral aneurysms larger than 5 mm. Carotid artery dissection can be visualized by axial fat-saturated T_1W imaging in the neck, which will detect the presence of methemoglobin in the false lumen within the vessel wall. CT angiography (CTA) is an alternative to MRA and is also noninvasive. The procedure requires intravenous injection of iodine contrast and imaging with a spiral CT scanner. The enhanced blood vessels are extracted from a three-dimensional (3D) data set and can be displayed as two-dimensional (2D) images, which resemble conventional angiograms, or as 3D structures. Both CTA and MRA are accurate and easy to perform, but MRA is preferable because a contrast agent is not required and the procedure does not use ionizing radiation. Detection of small vessel vasculitis and small cerebral aneurysms requires the more invasive conventional angiography with selective catheterization of single cerebral arteries followed by iodinated contrast injection.

Proton magnetic resonance spectroscopy (PMRS) measures the peak concentrations of certain brain metabolites such as N-acetylaspartate, creatine, lactate, and choline in defined areas (voxels) of the brain. Changes may be nonspecific because of cerebral damage from demyelination and neuronal loss or specific such as elevation of lactate in mitochondrial encephalopathies, elevation of glutamine and glutamate in hyperammonemia, and elevation of glycine in hyperglycinemia.

Ultrasonography can be used to visualize the cerebral ventricles and brains of infants with open anterior fontanels. Although the resolution of the images is not as good as those seen with CT or MRI, the technique can be performed easily and noninvasively at the patient's bedside with a portable scanner.[6] Small hemorrhages or cysts and medium-sized infarcts or masses are readily identified.

Xenon Cerebral Blood Flow

Two methods use the heavy atom xenon to create images representing cerebral blood flow (CBF). One uses intravenous injection of the radionuclide ^{133}Xe and the other inhalation of a high-density stable nonradioactive xenon. In both techniques, the brain is scanned before, during, and after xenon administration; the arterial xenon concentration is measured noninvasively from end-tidal xenon concentration; and a computer-calculated measurement of CBF is derived. Regional CBF measurements can add valuable clinical information in the study of patients with stroke, global hypoxic ischemic injury, trauma, raised ICP, and suspected brain death. The utility of hyperventilation to treat raised ICP from trauma or hepatic encephalopathy can be tested by CBF reactivity to lowering of arterial partial pressure of carbon dioxide (pCO_2). Absence of CBF defined by calculated flow values less than 5 ml/100 g/min is a strong indicator of brain death. Measurement of CBF with xenon techniques, however, is not widely available and is likely to be replaced by MRI perfusion imaging. Similarly, the use of radioactively labeled compounds for brain scanning and assessment of CBF is being replaced by MRI.

Cerebrospinal Fluid

Analysis of CSF is essential when CNS infection is suspected (see Chapter 57). An interpretation of results is presented in Box 50–2. Differentiating a hemorrhagic CSF caused by a traumatic lumbar puncture (LP) from a true SAH may be difficult. In most cases of traumatic LP, the fluid clears significantly over time. If the fluid is spun immediately, the supernatant may be clear after a traumatic LP and xanthochromic with a SAH. Usually the person performing the LP has a good sense of whether the tap was traumatic or atraumatic.

LP should be avoided in patients with clinical evidence of raised ICP. Warning signs are papilledema or depression of consciousness with focal neurologic deficits. The danger in performing an LP in the face of raised ICP lies in the tear made in the lumbar dura by the spinal needle; CSF continues to leak from this tear for hours after the LP. Intradural pressure is thereby lowered below

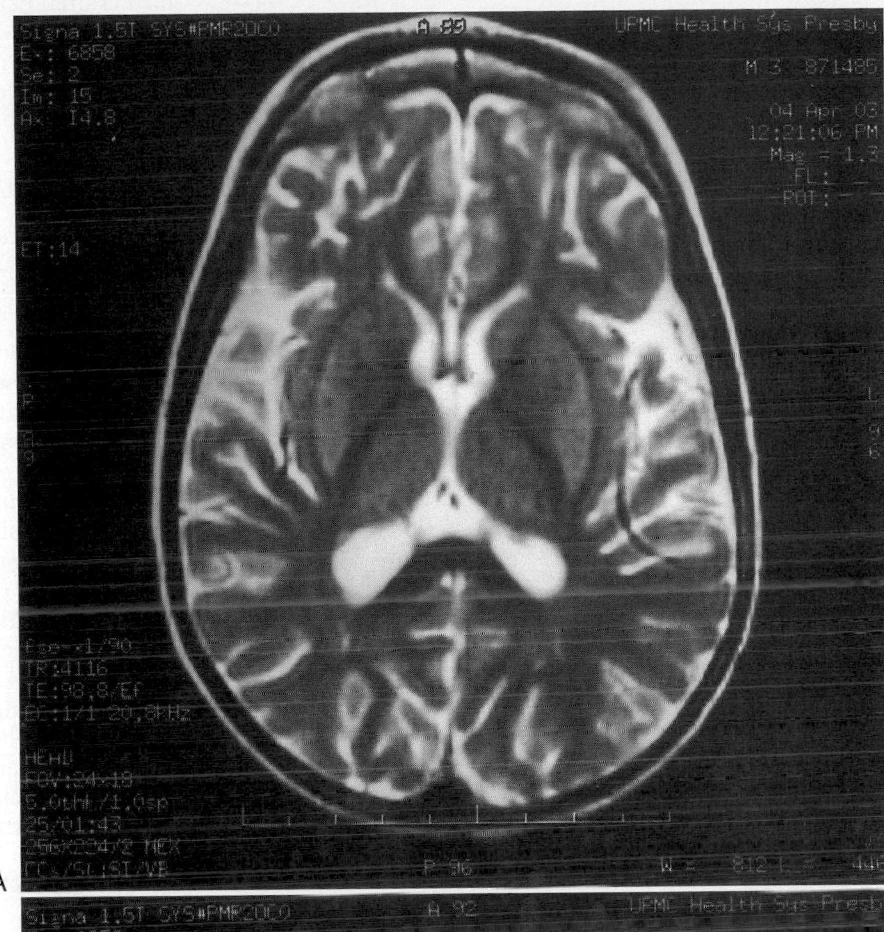

A

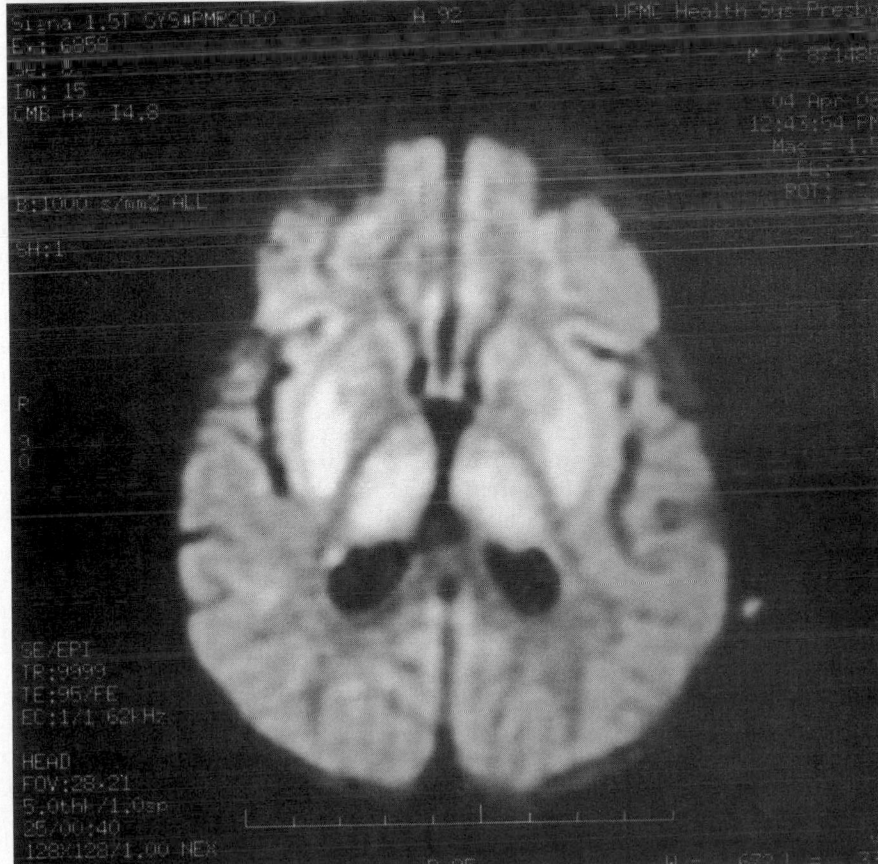

B

FIGURE 50–4 • **A,** An axial T_2-weighted image shows slightly increased signal on bilateral putamen after a hypoxic-ischemic event in a 3-year-old child. **B,** Diffusion-weighted image of the same patient obtained at the same time shows significant bright signals of bilateral putamen and thalami, indicating hypoxic-ischemic injury.

BOX 50-2

Rapid CSF Interpretation

	NORMAL CSF > 1 MONTH OLD	NORMAL CSF < 1 WK OLD
WBC count	< 5/μL	< 10 to 40
Protein	< 40 mg/dl	< 65-150
Glucose	> 2/3 blood glucose or > 40 mg/dl	> 2/3 blood glucose or > 40 mg/dl

↑ POLYMORPHONUCLEAR WBCs, ↓ GLUCOSE

Bacterial infection
Parasitic infection

↑ LYMPHOCYTES, ↑ GLUCOSE

Mycobacterial infection
Fungal infection
Carcinomatous meningitis
Sarcoidosis

↑ LYMPHOCYTES, NORMAL GLUCOSE

Viral infection
Parainfectious or postinfectious disease (e.g., ADEM)
Parameningeal infection
Lead intoxication

↑ CSF PROTEIN

Infection
Venous thrombosis
Hypertension
Spinal block (Froin's syndrome)
Guillain-Barré syndrome

MILD CSF PLEOCYTOSIS

Tumor
Infarction
Multiple sclerosis
Oligoclonal bands
↑ IgG index
↑ Myelin basic protein
Subacute bacterial endocarditis
CNS vasculitis

ADEM, acute disseminated encephalomyelitis; *CNS,* central nervous system, *CSF,* cerebrospinal fluid; *IgG,* immunoglobulin G; *WBC,* white blood cell.

the tentorium at a time when it is severely elevated above it. The CSF in the two compartments is not in free communication because cerebral contents have already begun to affect and block the tentorial notch. The increased differential results in further compression and herniation of thalamus and midbrain through the tentorial notch and eventually infarction of these vital structures. If raised ICP is suspected, CT may indicate critical compression by showing effacement of the cisterns around the midbrain, but a normal CT scan does not rule out elevated ICP.

Most patients with meningitis can safely receive an LP despite elevations of the ICP. The elevations are usually moderate, and the pressure is evenly distributed around the entire CNS. Symptoms include headache, vomiting, full fontanelle, and perhaps sixth cranial nerve palsy. If there are signs of incipient herniation, however, such as third cranial nerve palsy, poor pupillary reaction to light, or decerebrate or decorticate posturing, then LP must be deferred, even in these patients. Appropriate antibiotics are administered. Diagnosis emerges from blood cultures and testing of bacterial antigens in urine and blood.

Electroencephalogram

The EEG records the electrical activity of the surface of the brain from 20 scalp electrodes placed widely over the skull. Most of the recorded electrical activity has a frequency of 1 to 30 c/s and an amplitude of 5 to 200 μV. Two major types of abnormalities are seen: epileptiform activity and slowing. These abnormalities may be focal or diffuse. Epileptiform activity indicates a predisposition to produce seizures that either may be latent or expressed as a clinical seizure. Slowing and decreased amplitude of the electrical activity indicate brain dysfunction. The dysfunction may be reversible or irreversible and may have diverse causes such as stroke, mass lesions, metabolic or toxic effect, or postictal change.

The greatest utility of the EEG in the PICU lies in the assessment of seizure states or possible seizure states (see Chapter 55). Active seizure states almost always have concomitant ongoing epileptiform activity on the EEG. In patients pharmacologically paralyzed or deeply sedated with barbiturates, the EEG is the only test capable of determining the presence of seizures. Under these circumstances the administration of anticonvulsant medications can be guided by the persistence or disappearance of ictal activity on the EEG. Nonconvulsive status epilepticus (NCSE), which is found in 8% of neurologic patients with coma,[7] is another important indication of emergency EEG monitoring. NCSE can present with no overt signs of seizure activity and without motor manifestations; unless EEG is performed, the diagnosis of NCSE will be missed. Bedside EEG monitoring should be continued until electrographic status is abated.

Epileptiform activity is found interictally in 50% or more of patients with epilepsy and in 1% or less of the general population. Therefore an EEG with epileptiform activity found in a patient suspected of having seizures is a strong indicator that the patient does indeed have a seizure disorder.

Periodic complexes are sharp waves arising from the background at regular intervals. When they occur in one hemisphere, they are called *periodic lateralizing epileptiform discharges* (PLEDs) and most often are associated with a fresh infarct of that hemisphere. When localized to the temporal regions, periodic complexes suggest herpes encephalitis. The slow virus diseases, Creutzfeldt-Jakob disease, and subacute sclerosing panencephalitis (SSPE) are suggested by generalized periodic slow wave complexes with or without (not always time locked) associated myoclonic jerks. Frontal triphasic sharp waves are seen in patients with hepatic, uremic, and other metabolic encephalopathies. The presence of large amounts of fast activity (>13 Hz) usually indicates excessive sedative-hypnotic or barbiturate drug use.

Generalized bursts of sharp and slow waves followed by generalized amplitude suppression in a recurring pattern are called *burst suppression.* It is often seen following major hypoxic ischemic injuries to the brain.

Other rhythms that do not vary during an hour-long recording and do not change with auditory, visual, or tactile stimulation such as generalized alpha activity or spindle activity also indicate a global cerebral insult or sedative drug overdose. The EEG is used to monitor depth of coma when continuous high-dose barbiturate administration is used to treat critically raised ICP or status epilepticus. The barbiturate dose is increased until a burst-suppression pattern is obtained.

Absence of any cerebral electrical activity above 2 μV, in the absence of drug intoxication, usually indicates brain death. The ICU is a difficult environment in which to obtain an EEG free of electrical artifacts. When a clear, interpretable EEG is necessary to make the diagnosis of brain death, it is sometimes necessary to pharmacologically paralyze the patient, prevent anyone from walking in the vicinity of the bed, and briefly disconnect the ventilator and other life support systems from the patient. A normal waking EEG pattern found in a patient seemingly comatose indicates pharmacologic paralysis or conversion.

Evoked Potentials: Brainstem Auditory and Somatosensory

Click stimuli to the ear generate a series of five waveforms within 10 ms in the brainstem auditory structures: eighth cranial nerve, cochlear nucleus and superior olivary complex (low pons), lateral lemniscus (high pons), and inferior colliculus (midbrain). Electrical stimulation of large nerves in the upper limb generates a series of waveforms within 30 seconds in the large fiber somatosensory pathway: brachial plexus, upper cervical cord, dorsal column nuclei, thalamic nuclei, and contralateral primary sensory cortex. Similar waveforms are generated by stimulation of nerves in the lower limbs. These sensory-evoked potentials are of low amplitude and are separated and highlighted from the much higher voltage ongoing EEG activity by signal averaging. Stimuli are given repetitively, and a computer averages the new data acquired after each stimulus, with the average result from previous stimuli stored in its memory. The evoked potentials (EPs), which are time locked to the stimulus, summate, whereas the ongoing random activity averages to zero. The clinical utility of these evoked responses stems from the close relationship between the EP waveforms and the structural and functional integrity of specific anatomic structures. These EPs are consistently reproducible and are not influenced by the patient's state of arousal or medication. They can be utilized diagnostically to assess dysfunction of the auditory brainstem or somatosensory peripheral nerve, spinal cord, thalamic, and cerebral pathways. They can be repeated sequentially to monitor changes over time in the integrity of these pathways. They have not been widely used as cerebral monitoring devices in the ICU because the small amplitude of the EPs is more easily obscured by artifact than the larger EEG potentials; specialized personnel are required to maintain the systems, and only a limited portion of brain function is being surveyed.

BOX 50–3

Guidelines for the Determination of Brain Death in Children

A. HISTORY

Determination of the cause of coma to eliminate remediable and reversible conditions

B. PHYSICAL EXAMINATION

1. Coma and apnea must coexist
2. Absence of brainstem function
   i. Midposition or fully dilated pupils that do not respond to light
   ii. Absence of spontaneous eye movements, those induced by oculocephalic (doll's eye) and oculovestibular (caloric) testing
   iii. Absence of movement of bulbar musculature including facial and oropharyngeal muscles. Absence of corneal, gag, cough, sucking and rooting reflexes
   iv. Absence of respiratory effort with standardized testing for apnea
3. Patient must not be hypothermic or hypotensive. Toxic and/or metabolic encephalopathies must be ruled out including excessive sedation or neuromuscular paralysis
4. Flaccid tone and absence of spontaneous or induced movements, excluding spinal cord events such as reflex withdrawal or spinal myoclonus should exist
5. The examination should remain consistent with brain death throughout the observation and testing period

C. OBSERVATION PERIODS ACCORDING TO AGE

1. 7 days to 2 months: Two examinations and EEGs separated by at least 48 hours
2. 2 months to 1 year: Two examinations and two EEGs separated by at least 24 hours. A repeat examination and EEG are not necessary if a concomitant cerebral radionuclide angiographic study demonstrates no visualization of cerebral arteries
3. Older than 1 year: Two examinations 12 hours apart when an irreversible cause exists. At least a 24-hour observation period is required if it is difficult to assess the extent and reversibility of brain damage (such as hypoxic-ischemic encephalopathy). EEG and radionuclide angiography are optional.

Brain Death

A frequent issue in pediatric critical care is determination of brain death. The essential considerations in the diagnosis of brain death are (1) absence of cerebral functions (no reception and no response) (2) absence of brainstem functions including spontaneous respiration (by apnea testing) and (3) irreversibility of the state. Persistence of spinal reflexes does not exclude the diagnosis of brain death. Published guidelines in the report of the *Task Force for the Determination of Brain Death in Children*[8] are summarized in Box 50–3. Neonates and infants must be observed for prolonged intervals for failure to improve before a determination of brain death can be confidently made.

A properly performed EEG that shows electrocerebral silence is highly reliable in predicting brain death if CNS depressant drugs, toxic ingestion, metabolic disorders, or hypothermia are excluded. It remains one of the more well-validated confirmatory tests. In contrast, brainstem auditory evoked responses (BAERs) have not yet been shown to aid in the determination of brain death. Cerebral angiography, which documents no intracerebral filling at the level of entry of the carotid or vertebral artery to the skull, indicates brain death. Transcranial Doppler ultrasonography has a sensitivity of 91% to 99% and specificity of 100% in the determination of brain death. Nuclear imaging with technetium may reveal an absence of intracerebral uptake, and the correlation with conventional angiography in the diagnosis of brain death is good. The use of these methods, however, may include technical pitfalls.

REFERENCES

1. Greenberg S, Finklestein SP, Schaefer PW: Petechial hemorrhages accompanying lobar hemorrhage: detection by gradient-echo MRI, *Neurology* 46:1751-1754, 1996.
2. Kidwell C, Saver J, Villablanca JP, et al: Magnetic resonance imaging detection of microbleeds before thrombolysis: an emerging application, *Stroke* 33:95-98, 2002.
3. Hunter VJ: Magnetic resonance imaging in pediatric stroke. *Top Magn Reson Imaging* 13:23-38, 2002.
4. Jager HR: Diagnosis of stroke with advanced CT and MR imaging, *Br Med Bull* 56:318-333, 2000.
5. Guadagno JV, Calautti C, Baron J-C: Progress in imaging stroke: emerging clinical applications, *Br Med Bull* 65:145-157, 2003.
6. Bejar R, Coen R: Normal cranial ultrasonography in neonates. In James HE, Anas NG, Perkin RM, editors: *Brain insults in infants and children,* Orlando, 1985, Grune & Stratton.
7. Towne AR, Waterhouse EJ, Boggs JG, et al: Prevalence of nonconvulsive status epilepticus in comatose patients, *Neurology* 54: 340-345, 2000.
8. Report of Special Task Force. Guidelines for the determination of brain death in children. American Academy of Pediatrics Task Force on Brain Death in Children, *Pediatrics* 80:298-300, 1987.

SUGGESTED READINGS

American Electroencephalogram Society Guidelines for EEG 1-7 (revised 1985), *J Clin Neurophysiol* 3:131, 1986.

Barkovich AS: Techniques and methods in pediatric neuroimaging. In: Barkovich AS, editor: *Pediatric neuroimaging,* ed 3. Philadelphia, 2000, Lippincott Williams & Wilkins.

Chiappa KH, Hoch DB: Electrophysiologic monitoring. In Ropper AH, editor: *Neurological and neurosurgical intensive care,* ed 3, New York, 1993, Raven Press.

Holmes GL: *Diagnosis and management of seizures in children,* Philadelphia, 1987, WB Saunders.

Jordan KG: Continuous EEG monitoring in the neuroscience intensive care unit and emergency department, *J Clin Neurophysiol,* 16: 14-39, 1999.

Jordan KG: Nonconvulsive status epilepticus in brain injury, *J Clin Neurophysiol,* 16:332-340, 1999.

Meyer PG, Ducrocq S, Carli P. Pediatric neurologic emergencies, *Curr Opin Crit Care* 7:81-87, 2001.

Orrison WW: Computed tomography and magnetic resonance imaging. In Orrison WW, editor: *Introduction to neuroimaging,* Boston, 1989, Little Brown.

Osborn A: Intracranial hemorrhage. In Osborn A, editor: *Diagnostic neuroradiology,* St. Louis, 1994, Mosby-Year Book.

Pistoia F, Johnson DW, Darby JM, et al: The role of xenon CT measurements of cerebral blood flow in the clinical determination of brain death, *AJNR Am J Neuroradiol,* 12:97, 1991.

Plum F, Posner JB: *The diagnosis of stupor and coma,* Philadelphia, 1980, FA Davis.

Schneider S, Ashwal S: Determination of brain death in infants and children. In Swaiman KF, Ashwal S editors: *Pediatric neurology: principles and practice, vol 2,* ed 3, St Louis, 1999, Mosby.

Tasken RC: Neurological critical care, *Curr Opin Pediatr,*12:222-226, 2000.

Victor M, Ropper AH: Coma and related disorders of consciousness. In Victor M, Ropper AH, editors: *Adams and Victor's principles of neurology,* ed 7, New York, 2001, McGraw-Hill.

Wijdicks EFM: Current concepts: the diagnosis of brain death. *N Engl J Med* 344:1215-1221, 2001.

Wood JH: *Cerebral blood flow: physiologic and clinical aspects,* New York, 1987, McGraw-Hill.

CHAPTER

51

Congenital Malformations of the Brain and Spinal Cord

Stephanie Greene and Richard G. Ellenbogen

PEARLS

- Hydrocephalus is a common accompaniment to many central nervous system (CNS) malformations.
- Midline cutaneous abnormalities of the lumbosacral region seen above the gluteal cleft should prompt an evaluation for a spinal dysraphism.
- Once a patient has an intradural spinal dysraphism repair, he or she is at risk for spinal cord retethering for life.

Nearly 2000 congenital malformations of the central nervous system (CNS) have been identified. Almost 1% of all live births and an estimated 2% of all conceived pregnancies have CNS anomalies. Forty percent of infant deaths and 75% of fetal deaths are attributed to CNS malformations. Genetic defects, prenatal infection or irradiation, maternal medication use (e.g., antiepileptic drugs and thalidomide), and maternal disease (e.g., diabetes) have all been implicated as etiologic factors in these malformations.

An understanding of the embryologic development of the CNS is essential to an understanding of its congenital malformations (see also Chapter 48). The brain and spinal cord are formed through a complex series of embryologic stages to include dorsal induction, ventral induction, neuronal proliferation, migration, organization, and myelination. Various malformations appear at different stages of development, and knowledge of normal embryologic growth often provides insight into the development of the malformation.

The major class of congenital nervous system defects involves a failure of closure of the neural tube and can affect the spinal cord or the brain. Neural tube defects are one of the most commonly occurring of all congenital malformations and are seen in 1 to 5 per 1000 live births in the United States and, more frequently, in some other parts of the world. For a healthy couple with a child with a neural tube defect, the risk for subsequent offspring rises to 3% to 4%. The severity of the neural tube defect can vary from mild, as with spina bifida occulta, to severe, such as anencephaly. The primary embryologic abnormality is a failure of the neural folds to fuse in the midline to form the neural tube, with a secondary maldevelopment of the mesoderm, which normally forms the bony and muscular structures overlying the nervous tissue. The highest incidence of neural tube defects occurs in the British Isles, especially in people of Celtic origin, and the lowest incidence occurs in Japan. The highest rate of occurrence in the United States is found in Boston, particularly in people of Irish descent; thus the predisposition appears to be at least partially genetic in cause. The incidence has declined markedly over the past few decades, most likely because of the combined forces of the administration of prenatal folic acid and an increase in elective termination after the introduction of prenatal screening. Folic acid supplementation is estimated to have reduced the incidence of neural tube defects by up to 70%. Attempts to identify genetic susceptibility to these malformations have been focused on folic acid metabolism, although few polymorphisms have been identified within these candidate genes as significant risk factors. Several single nucleotide polymorphisms have been identified that appear to increase the risk of neural tube defects but only when present in conjunction with environmental and nutritional risk factors.[1] This chapter addresses the major brain malformations, followed by the major spinal cord malformations.

Embryology

Dorsal induction takes place during the first month of gestation and encompasses the formation of the neural tube from the neural plate. The neural folds first fuse to form the neural tube (thereby separating cutaneous from neural ectoderm) at the future craniocervical junction, and the fusion proceeds both rostrally and caudally from this point. The rostral neuropore closes on day 24, and the caudal neuropore closes on day 26 to terminate primary neurulation. Malformations that develop at this stage include anencephaly and myelomeningocele. Secondary neurulation begins immediately thereafter and includes the formation of the conus medullaris and filum terminale from the caudal cell mass by retrogressive differentiation. Disorders of secondary neurulation include the closed spinal dysraphisms.

The development of the prosencephalon is termed *ventral induction.* The cleavage of the prosencephalon into three primary vesicles (prosencephalon, mesencephalon, and rhombencephalon) occurs in the third week of gestation, and further subdivision into five secondary vesicles (telencephalon, diencephalon, mesencephalon or midbrain, metencephalon or cerebellum and pons, and myelencephalon or medulla and spinal cord) occurs at 5 weeks gestation. Holoprosencephaly and septo-optic dysplasia develop during ventral induction.

The proliferative stage occurs during the third month of gestation, when the telencephalon begins to differentiate into the cerebral cortex. The division of the future ventricular system into paired telencephalic vesicles separated by the foramina of Monro occurs in the sixth week. At 7 weeks, the cerebral hemispheres begin to enlarge, and the fibers of the internal capsule are first visible. Microcephaly and macrocephaly are potential consequences of aberrant proliferation.

Neurons migrate during the fourth and fifth months, forming the major pattern of sulci and gyri. The interhemispheric fissure is visible by 2 months gestation, and the Sylvian fissure is visible by 3.5 months. The central sulcus appears by 5 months gestation. Three cortical layers form. The subventricular zone, the innermost layer, is the layer of actively proliferating cells. The intermediate layer, the intermediate zone of His, consists of primitive white matter. The outer layer, the primordial plexiform layer, consists of bipolar neurons that eventually form layer I of the cortex. Newly formed neurons migrate outward so that the deeper layers of neurons are formed before the superficial layers, with the exception of layer I. Migration is complete by 20 weeks. Schizencephaly, agenesis of the corpus callosum, lissencephaly, pachygyria, microgyria, and heterotopias are products of disordered migration.

Organization of neurons begins at 6 months and continues until after birth. The differentiation of the six-layered cortex is completed during this stage. The glia proliferates, and synaptic contacts continue to form. Deranged neuronal organization is implicated in polymicrogyria, hypothalamic hamartoma, and Down's syndrome.

Myelination begins at 5 months gestation and is largely complete by the end of the second year of life. Some areas of the brain are not fully myelinated until the end of the third decade. Disorders of myelination are beyond the scope of this chapter but include aminoaciduria and leukodystrophies.

Congenital Malformation of the Brain

Anencephaly

The most severe, and most common, neural tube defect is anencephaly, comprising approximately 60% of neural tube defects. The embryologic defect is threefold: failure of closure of the rostral neuropore; failure of the development of the overlying mesoderm (dura and skull); and the exposure of neurons to amniotic fluid, resulting in the destruction of the developing forebrain. Anencephaly is 37 times more common in females than males, and the recurrence rate in families has been found to be 1% to 3% in the United States. The fetus has a small head and dysmorphic facies, with a flattened forehead, exophthalmos, and large ears, with relatively normal lower facial features (Fig. 51–1). A primitive vascular connective tissue known as the *area cerebrovasculosa* covers the defect. The brainstem and basal ganglia can usually be recognized on computed tomography (CT). Anencephaly can continue inferiorly to involve the length of the spinal column, a condition known as craniorachischisis; more commonly it is seen in conjunction with a lumbosacral myelomeningocele. These patients rarely survive more than a few days; most die in utero.

Hydranencephaly

Although it is often classified with anencephaly, hydranencephaly is actually the result of a destructive process, such as vasculitis, a hypercoagulable state, or a viral infection occurring after the third month of gestation. The point of commonality is bilateral infarction of the anterior circulation, supported by the fact that no filling of the carotids is seen on angiography. Hydranencephaly is defined as an absence of the telencephalon in the presence of normal structures supplied by the vertebrobasilar system, to include the basal ganglia, occipital lobes, cerebellum, and brainstem. The falx and interhemispheric fissure can often be recognized on ultrasound and CT (Fig. 51–2). This is an isolated defect and occurs sporadically in about 1 per 5000 pregnancies. A normal ultrasound in the first half of pregnancy is not incompatible with the development of hydranencephaly before birth. The condition must be

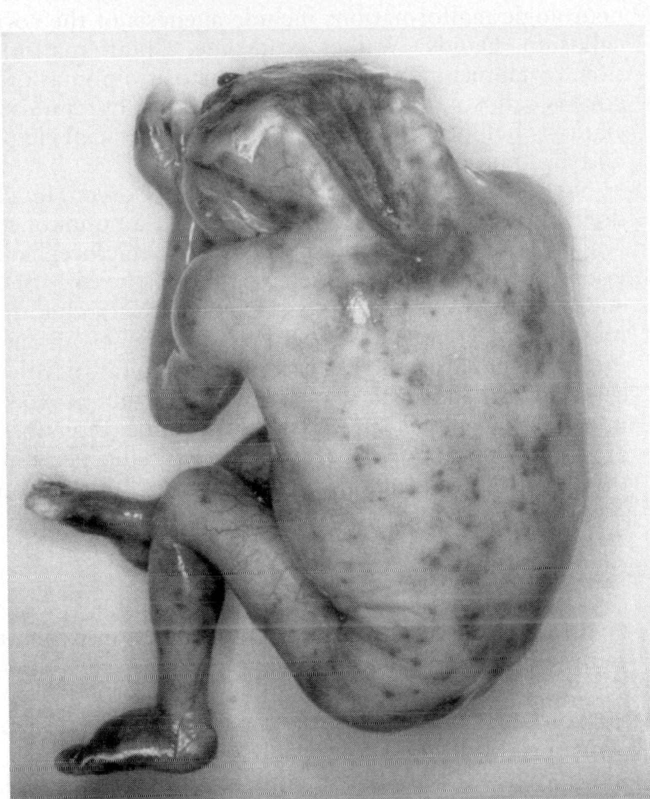
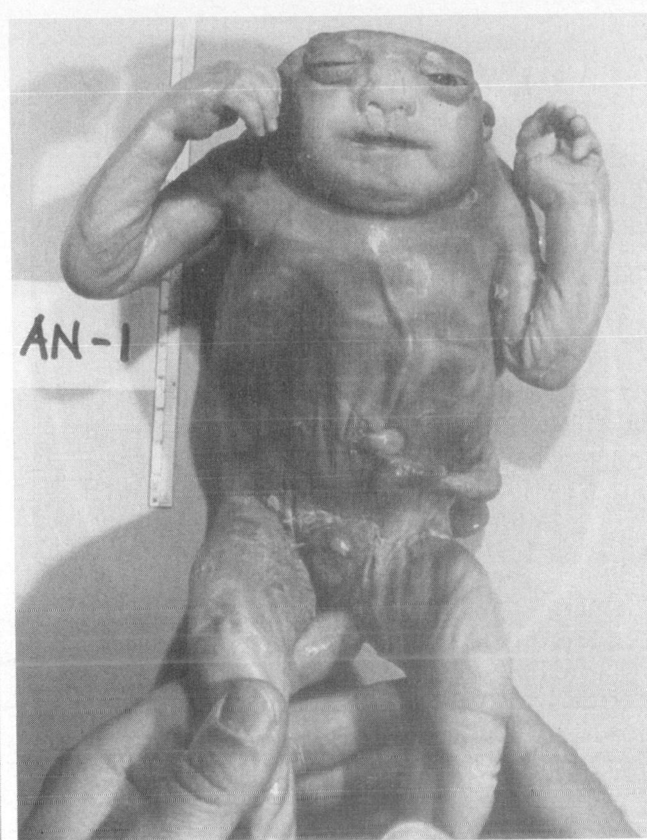

FIGURE 51–1 • Stillborn patient with anencephaly (photo courtesy of Ron Lemire, MD). Used with permission from eMedicine.com, Inc., 2004.

differentiated from severe hydrocephalus with magnetic resonance imaging (MRI); a thin cortical mantle is seen in patients with severe hydrocephalus. Shunting is often recommended to be used as a palliative procedure and to ease the care of the child. Infants with hydranencephaly usually die within 2 years and often within several months, but patients living as long as 10 years have been reported. They do not progress neurologically after birth.

Encephaloceles

Encephaloceles are another group of congential malformations conventionally grouped with the neural tube defects. This is unlikely to be strictly correct because they nearly always contain brain tissue that differentiates after neurulation is completed.[2] A delay in neurocutaneous disjunction past the time of closure of the anterior neuropore has been postulated.[3] The incidence of encephalocele is 10% more than that of myelomeningocele in live births worldwide[4,5] and is estimated at 1 per 10,000 live births. The rate of fetal loss is at least 70%, so the actual incidence is much higher.[6] There is no increased incidence in siblings or offspring of affected individuals, which suggests a significant environmental role in causation.[7] Implicated etiologic factors include maternal folate deficiency, fever, and ingestion of a variety of toxins.[8] Encephalocele has been associated with various spinal dysraphisms, particularly myelomeningocele and diastematomyelia.

Encephaloceles are skin-covered cystic lesions with bony and dural defects. Most are within a centimeter or two of the midline. The contents of the cyst are usually dysplastic tissue and cerebrospinal fluid (CSF); only 30% of those occurring in the United States contain cerebral cortex.[4] The contents of the sac, the presence of hydrocephalus, and the relationship of the venous sinuses to the sac must be elucidated by MRI before surgical repair is planned. The goals of surgery are repair of the dural and skull defects and cosmetic repair. The dysplastic tissue within the encephalocele is nearly always truncated at its base because it is thought to be nonfunctional and the volume is considered too large for safe return to the intracranial compartment. If the tissue within the sac is thought to be functional based on the MRI scan or inspection at the time of surgery, then every attempt is made to preserve it and to include shunting at the time of surgery to reduce the intracranial contents, or staged repair.[7]

The anatomic site of the encephalocele varies with the geographic location of the patient, and each subtype of encephalocele has unique characteristics. For example, 80% of encephaloceles in the United States are occipital. Occipital encephaloceles (Fig. 51–3) are more commonly seen in Western European countries, Japan, and Australia. The occipital encephalocele can be supratorcular or subtorcular; anomalies of the posterior fossa are common even in the supratorcular variant.[8] Sixty percent of occipital encephaloceles eventually require shunting for hydrocephalus. These encephaloceles are more common in girls. Ninety percent of the encephaloceles seen in Southeast Asia are frontoethmoidal (sincipital). Sincipital encephaloceles

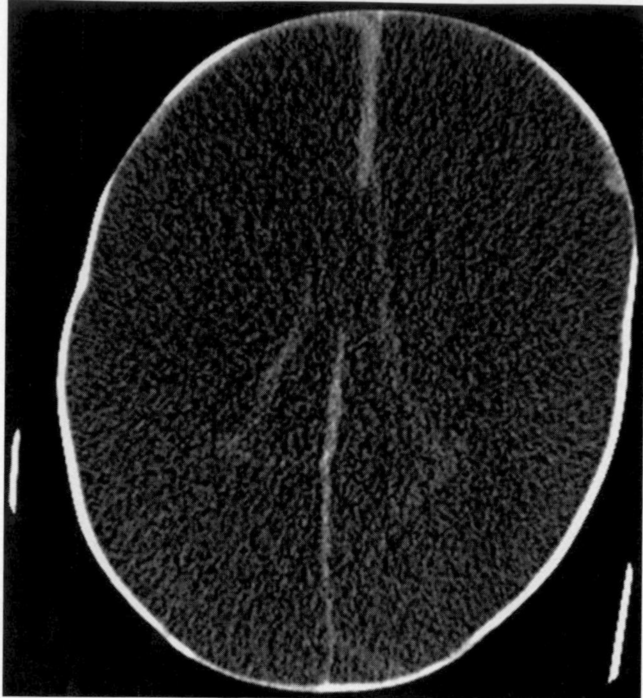

FIGURE 51–2 • Computed tomography of the head showing hydranencephaly. Note the preservation of the falx and interhemispheric fissure.

are also common in aboriginal Australians, in parts of India, and in southern Russia. These lesions are more often seen in males. Only 10% of sincipital encephaloceles require shunting for hydrocephalus. Basal encephaloceles are rare. The term *nasal glioma* actually refers to a basal encephalocele with an atretic stalk. These encephaloceles carry a 70% risk of significant endocrine abnormality. The associated location-specific features of the encephalocele play a great role in the outcome of the child with an encephalocele.[4,6,7]

Encephaloceles are occasionally associated with syndromes such as Meckel-Gruber (polydactyly, polycystic kidneys, holoprosencephaly, microophthalmia, retinal dysplasia, cardiac anomalies), Walker-Warburg,

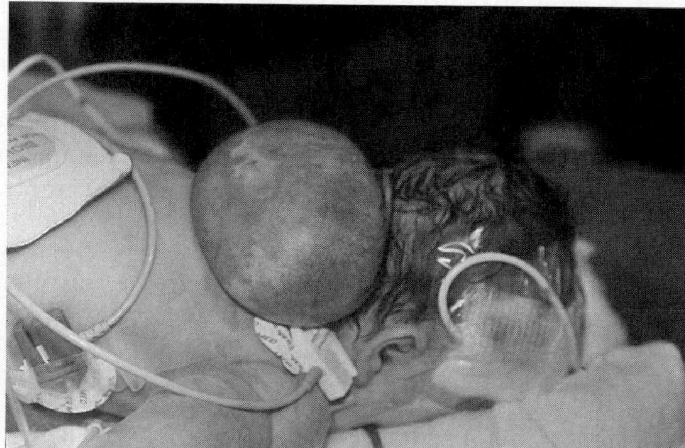

FIGURE 51–3 • Occipital encephalocele. Used with permission from eMedicine.com, Inc., 2004.

Goldenhar's, or amniotic band. Commonly associated neurologic malformations include agenesis of the corpus callosum, Dandy- Walker syndrome, Chiari malformation, myelomeningocele, craniosynostosis, lipomas of the corpus callosum, and holoprosencephaly. Systemic associations include renal agenesis, syndactyly, facial clefting, and arm and rib anomalies.[7,9,10]

Significant developmental disability is seen in children whose encephaloceles contain a large amount of cerebral cortex, particularly those who are also microcephalic.[11] Poor outcome has also been related to the size of the encephalocele and the presence of other CNS abnormalities. Hydrocephalus is only a negative prognostic factor if it is present at birth. Children with occipital encephaloceles have an 83% chance of significant mental or physical impairment, whereas those with sincipital encephaloceles are far more likely to be of normal intelligence unless they have associated CNS abnormalities or syndromic disorders.[7,10-13]

Hydrocephalus

Hydrocephalus is produced by an obstruction within the ventricular system, with the rare possible exception of choroid plexus papilloma as an example of overproduction of CSF. The obstruction can occur at the foramen of Monro, the aqueduct of Sylvius, or the foramina of Magendie or Luschka. Communicating hydrocephalus, or occlusion of the arachnoid villi that absorb CSF into the venous sinuses, is a condition suggested by diffuse enlargement of all ventricles and the subarachnoid spaces. It must be differentiated from benign extraaxial collections of infancy (these patients' head circumferences do not cross percentile lines on growth charts, and their families' head circumference measurements are also larger than average) and shaken baby syndrome (if a sudden increase in head circumference is found after a normal measurement at birth, an MRI should be obtained to evaluate these collections for blood).

The main causes of hydrocephalus are due to hemorrhage in a premature infant (beyond the scope of this chapter), myelomeningocele or tumor, and aqueductal stenosis. Those patients with aqueductal stenosis or a tumor obstructing the aqueduct who are older than 1 year of age are appropriate candidates for endoscopic third ventriculostomy. All others require a CSF diversion procedure, most commonly a ventriculoperitoneal (VP) shunt. In neonates weighing less than 2 kilograms, a ventriculo- subgaleal shunt or a McComb tapping reservoir may be placed until the risk of necrotizing enterocolitis decreases and a VP shunt can be placed. Shunt placement and revision are the most common group of procedures in pediatric neurosurgery.

Arachnoid Cysts

Arachnoid cysts are collections of CSF that develop within the arachnoid membrane itself because of a splitting or duplication; *intraarachnoid cyst* is actually a better term. True arachnoid cysts are congenital; secondary arachnoid cysts can develop after head injury or infection. The incidence by autopsy series is 5 per 1000. They certainly can expand with time, and this expansion may explain their delayed presentation in some circumstances. Spontaneous regression (and reappearance) of arachnoid cysts has been documented.[14] One-way valve effects have been postulated to explain their growth; alternatively, the cells lining the cyst may secrete fluid.[15,16] They occur more often in males (two thirds of patients) and on the left side of the brain.[17] The most common locations are the Sylvian fissure and posterior fossa, but they can occur in any location adjacent to a subarachnoid cistern. It is likely that most incidentally discovered lesions will remain asymptomatic.

Symptoms are most commonly related to hydrocephalus or raised intracranial pressure. Alternatively, arachnoid cysts may present as mass lesions. Suprasellar arachnoid cysts have been associated with the bobble-head doll syndrome and endocrine disorders. Arachnoid cysts are often discovered during the workup of symptoms that may or may not be related, such as headache, seizure, macrocrania, attention deficit disorder, minor head trauma, or learning disability, and so their surgical treatment must be undertaken with caution.

Traumatic hemorrhage into the cyst has been well-documented in large middle fossa arachnoid cysts. Although rare, bitemporal arachnoid cysts may be associated with glutaric aciduria type 1, and surgery can be dangerous in such patients.[18] Any patient with bitemporal arachnoid cysts should be screened for this disease. The evaluation of an arachnoid cyst mandates an MRI scan with gadolinium to assess for the possibility of a low-grade tumor (Fig. 51–4). Some cysts enhance with contrast administration, so the diagnosis of a neoplasm must rely on other factors such as peritumoral edema and intramural nodules.

Cysts causing mass effect or hydrocephalus should be operated on. Some advocate surgical treatment of asymptomatic lesions for prevention of traumatic hemorrhage. Surgical treatment most often involves fenestration of a cyst into an adjacent cistern or placement of a cystoperitoneal shunt; some favor direct microsurgical removal of the cyst wall, which can be difficult given the diaphanous nature of the arachnoid membrane and the well-reported ability of the cyst wall to reconstitute itself. Middle fossa arachnoid cysts have the highest likelihood of resolution postoperatively, and suprasellar cysts have the highest chance of recurrence.[19]

Dandy-Walker Syndrome

The classic Dandy-Walker malformation is defined as aplasia of the cerebellar vermis with a posterior fossa cyst that directly communicates with the fourth ventricle. The disorder of embryogenesis is thought to be either atresia of the foramina of Magendie and Luschka or a failure of regression of the inferior medullary velum. Variants are far more common than the classic malformation and involve hypoplasia, rather than complete aplasia, of the vermis. The group of classic malformations and the variants thereof comprise the Dandy-Walker syndrome. Ninety percent of these patients have hydrocephalus (Fig. 51–5). The posterior fossa is usually large, with an elevated torcular (confluence of sinuses). The differential diagnosis includes mega cisterna magna (normal vermis and fourth ventricle) and posterior fossa arachnoid cyst (compressed

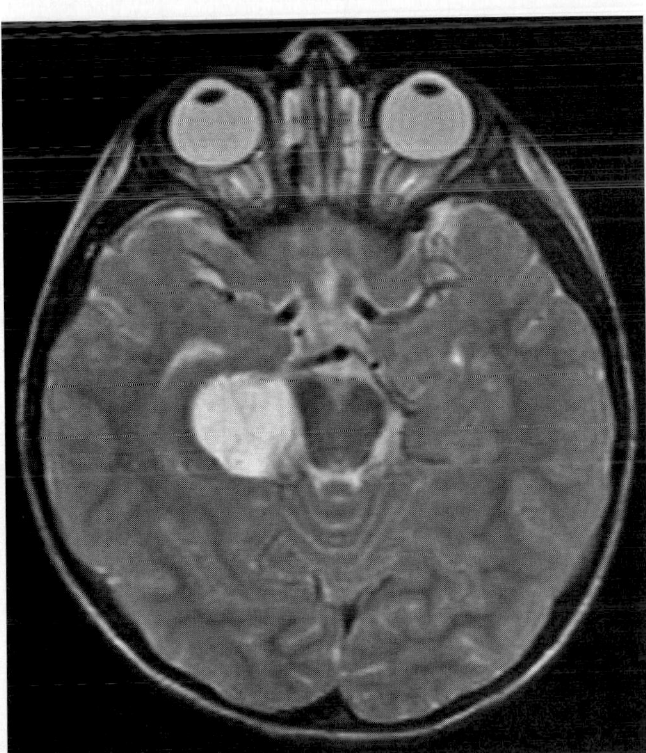

FIGURE 51–4 • T_2-weighted magnetic resonance image showing an arachnoid cyst of the choroidal fissure.

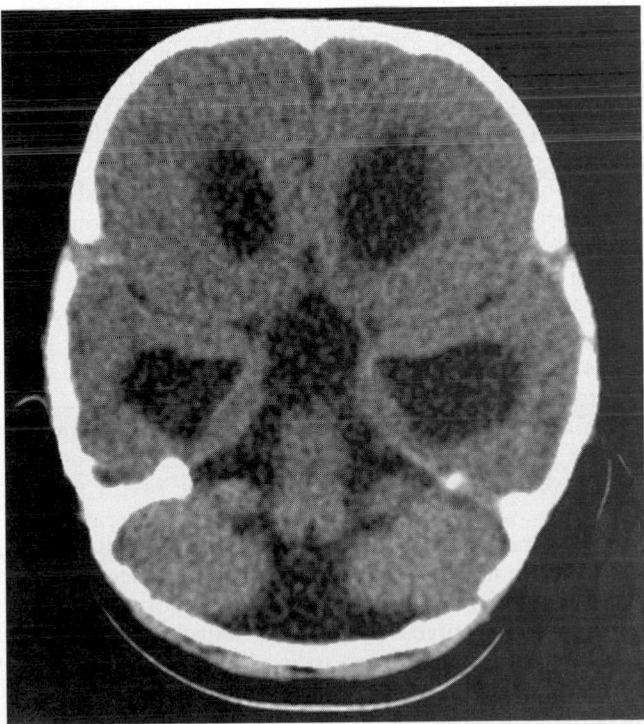

FIGURE 51–5 • Computed tomography of the head showing a Dandy-Walker variant and marked hydrocephalus.

fourth ventricle; the vermis may be difficult to identify). In the absence of hydrocephalus, these patients may be followed up clinically. If treatment is necessary, the posterior fossa cyst usually requires shunting in addition to the ventricles.

The prognosis of these patients is highly variable. Only 30% to 50% of children with Dandy-Walker syndrome have a normal intelligence quotient (IQ). The outcome does not depend on the size of the cyst, but it appears to depend more on the management of hydrocephalus and the presence of other associated anomalies. CNS anomalies include callosal agenesis, occipital encephalocele, heterotopias, and microcephaly. Associated systemic anomalies include cleft palate, microopthalmia, cardiac septal anomalies, and coarctation of the aorta. Critical to the determination of a patient's prognosis are a cranial MRI scan to search for other CNS anomalies and a thorough evaluation for systemic malformations.

Chiari Malformation

The Chiari malformations are a heterogeneous group of disorders classified together for historical reasons. This group of four congenital anomalies of the cerebellum and brainstem were initially described by Dr. Hans Chiari, a German pathologist, in the early 1890s. It has become apparent that each of these malformations has a distinct pathophysiologic origin and clinical presentation. All, however, result from a disproportion of the posterior fossa bony structure to the intradural contents.

Chiari malformation type I consists of cerebellar tonsillar herniation below the foramen magnum, into the upper cervical spinal canal. It is accompanied by syringomyelia in 50% to 75% of pediatric patients with symptoms; this usually resolves after successful surgical treatment of the Chiari I malformation. The age of presentation has become younger as the use of MRI has become more prevalent, but it can be anywhere from age 2 years to young adulthood. The classic headache is occipital and exacerbated by Valsalva's maneuvers. Neck pain, sensory changes in the upper extremities, and clumsiness are other common presenting complaints. Vertical nystagmus, scoliosis, and overt myelopathy may be seen on examination. These malformations are often asymptomatic, and these patients often have symptoms that are difficult to categorize. Although the presence of a radiographic Chiari I malformation is necessary for the diagnosis, the clinical symptoms determine whether an operation is required.

Chiari II is sometimes called the Arnold-Chiari malformation, in acknowledgment of an autopsy description by Dr. Arnold in 1894, although most of the original descriptive work was done by Dr. Chiari. This malformation is characterized by herniation of the cerebellar vermis and brainstem below the foramen magnum, accompanied by kinking of the cervicomedullary junction and in 20% of cases, syringomyelia (Fig. 51–6). Surgical treatment of the Chiari II malformation is less likely to result in resolution of the syrinx. This form occurs nearly exclusively in patients with myelomeningocele. Virtually all (99%) patients with myelomeningocele have a radiographic Chiari II malformation, but only those who have symptoms require treatment. Ninety percent of these patients have hydrocephalus. Today, the Chiari II malformation is one of the leading causes of death in pediatric patients with myelomeningocele, and it is responsible for death in 15% to 20% of these patients. Symptoms develop in one third of patients by age 5 years; one third of those patients die, most commonly, of respiratory failure. Symptomatic Chiari II malformation may present acutely with central or obstructive apnea, aspiration, stridor, nystagmus, and profound quadriparesis. Deterioration can progress to death in these circumstances, regardless of the type or acuity of treatment. Such a course is most common in children younger than 2 years and is not related to increased intracranial pressure.[20,21] Disorganized brainstem nuclei are often found in these patients during autopsy.[22] The Chiari malformation can also present subtly, with hoarseness, dysphagia, pneumonia, increasing nystagmus, or sensory changes in the upper extremities. The most common cause of new brainstem findings in a patient with a myelomeningocele is a shunt malfunction, and so shunt exploration is routinely undertaken before Chiari decompression.

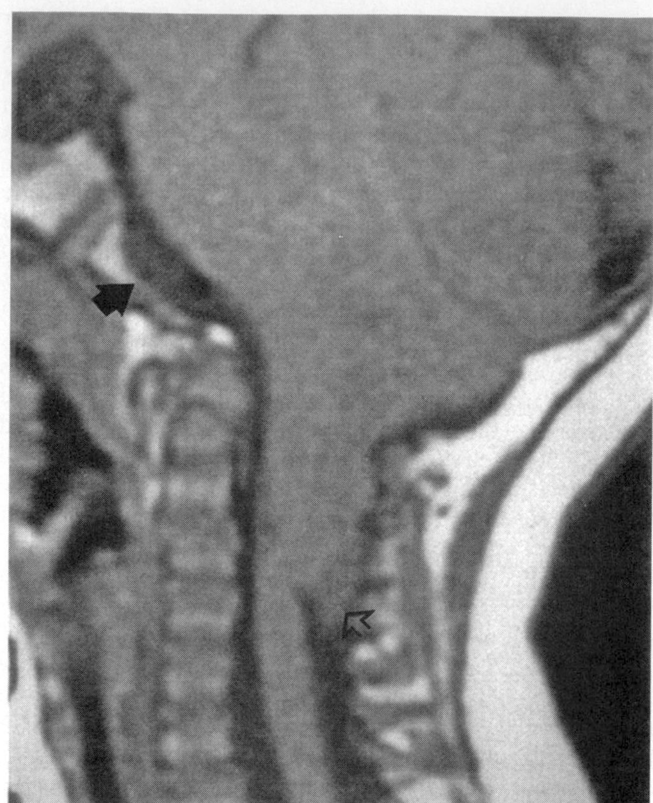

FIGURE 51–6 • Chiari type II malformation. Note the descent of the cerebellar tonsils to the level of C4 (*open arrow*). Used with permission from eMedicine.com, Inc., 2004.

Type III malformation is a posterior fossa encephalocele, with evagination of the cerebellum, lower brainstem, and fourth ventricle. Type IV is actually a cerebellar hypoplasia and is no longer considered part of the group of Chiari malformations.

Congenital Malformations of the Spinal Cord

Spina Bifida

Spina bifida is a failure of closure of the caudal neural tube. When the bony defect is covered by normal skin and no neural tissue is extruded through the bony defect, it is termed *spina bifida occulta.* If the bony defect contains a protruding sac of tissue, the term *spina bifida cystica* is used. This group is conventionally subdivided into closed and open defects. Open defects (spina bifida aperta) are covered by a thin reddish membrane called the *area medullovasculosa,* the margin of which blends into the more normal surrounding skin. If the sac contains meninges and CSF, but no neural elements, the term *meningocele* is applied. This is associated with normal findings of a neurologic examination, and the lesion is usually skin covered (although the skin may be dysplastic). These patients do not have an association with hydrocephalus or Chiari II malformation. If nervous tissue is contained in the sac, it is termed a *myelomeningocele;* these patients usually have both hydrocephalus and Chiari II malformations, although they are often symptom free at birth. Myelomeningocele comprises 95% of open spina bifida, and meningocele, 5%.[23]

Closed spinal dysraphisms are associated with cutaneous abnormalities in up to 50% of cases.[24] The skin lesion, such as a hairy patch (hypertrichosis), dermal sinus tract, dimple, or hemangioma, may be the only sign of an abnormality. The presence of these cutaneous stigmata above the gluteal fold should alert the clinician to investigate the possibility of an underlying spinal lesion. Dimples below the gluteal fold do not signify neurologic abnormalities. These patients may complain of weakness of one or both legs, atrophy of the musculature in the legs, loss of sensation, hyperreflexia, back pain, or gait abnormalities. Neurogenic bladder is the most common urologic problem these children have. Orthopedic anomalies include asymmetry in the length of the extremities, foot deformities, or neurogenic scoliosis. Imperforate anus is associated with intradural lesions in at least 10% of patients. Concerning lesions should be evaluated with ultrasound in the neonate or MRI in the older child. These studies may identify a tethered cord, diastematomyelia (split cord malformation), diplomyelia (duplication of the spinal cord), dermal sinus tract, or thickened filum terminale. X-ray film may reveal defects in the spinal laminae, hemivertebrae, scoliosis, widened interpedicular distance, or butterfly vertebrae. The surgical repair of these lesions is best undertaken prophylactically to preserve neurologic function.

The tethered spinal cord syndrome is a clinical syndrome made up of back or leg pain, sensory changes or motor weakness, increasing scoliosis, increasing incontinence or increasingly abnormal urodynamic studies in a patient with a low-lying conus medullaris and an intradural lesion in the (usually) lumbosacral spine. That lesion can be a repaired myelomeningocele, lipomyelomeningocele, thickened filum terminale, diastematomyelia, or dermoid cyst (Fig. 51–7).

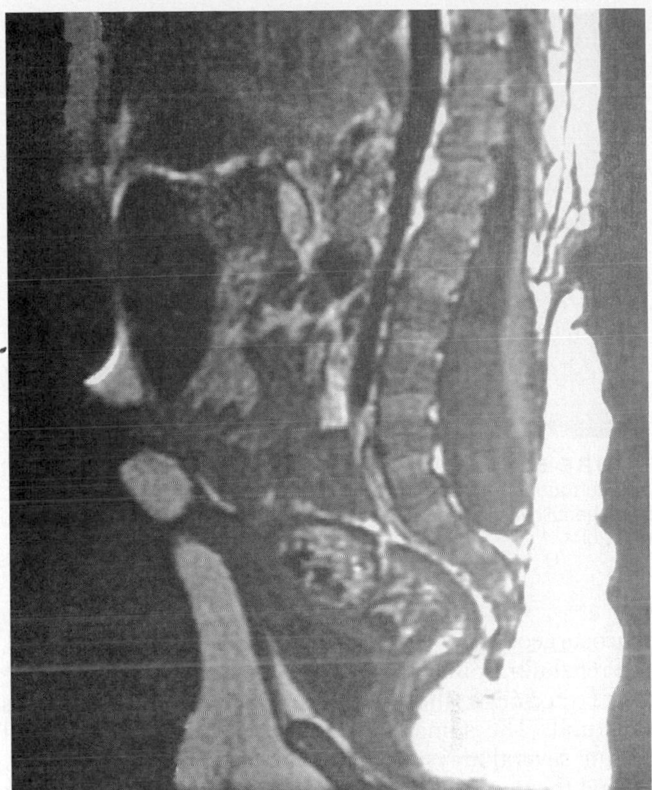

FIGURE 51–7 • Tethered spinal cord after myelomeningocele repair. The spinal cord is tethered at L5. Used with permission from eMedicine.com, Inc., 2004.

The symptoms often present after a period of rapid physical growth or intense exercise, leading to a hypothesis of a water-hammer effect of repeated trauma to the spinal cord leading to ischemia. Untethering can improve these symptoms, with incontinence being the most refractory to surgical treatment. The results of an operation are most impressive in children younger than 18 months and are better in patients with a shorter duration of symptoms before the operation.

Myelomeningocele

Myelomeningocele is a condition in which the neural placode protrudes through the bony and muscular defect to be visible at its junction with the cutaneous ectoderm (Fig. 51–8). The neural tube does not form at this point, and the spinal cord ends in this lesion. It is seen most commonly in the lumbar or lumbosacral region. Cardiac, intestinal, renal, urogenital, and orthopedic anomalies are common in these patients. Associated neurologic deficits include agenesis of the corpus callosum, heterotopias, and polymicrogyria. A prenatal diagnosis of myelomeningocele mandates a cesarean delivery because research has shown that children born via vaginal delivery were more than twice as likely to be born with severe paralysis, presumably as a result of birth trauma.[44] In the perinatal period, a patient with myelomeningocele should be evaluated by a team of physicians to include a neonatologist, pediatric geneticist, pediatric urologist, pediatric

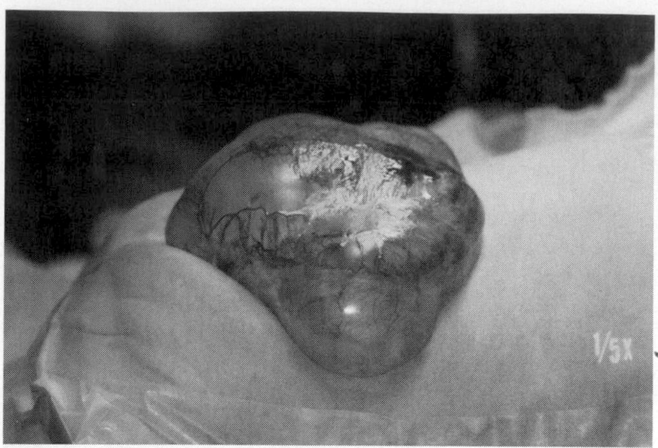

FIGURE 51–8 • Myelomeningocele. Note the sac of cerebrospinal fluid surrounding the neural placode on the dorsal surface and the area medullovasculosa. Used with permission from eMedicine.com, Inc., 2004.

neurosurgeon, and pediatric orthopedist. Cardiac, cranial, and renal ultrasounds should be performed, and the appropriate specialists should be consulted should anomalies be found. The spinal defect should ideally be repaired within several days, reapproximating the neural tube, closing the dura (which sometimes requires a patch graft), and closing the skin without tension (which sometimes requires a complicated skin closure, or more uncommonly, a kyphectomy).

Hydrocephalus and Chiari II malformations are common neurologic associations with myelomeningocele. Hydrocephalus is seen in 80% to 95% of patients with myelomeningocele; it is most common in thoracic myelomeningocele patients and least common in patients with sacral myelomeningoceles. It is significant in 20% at birth, and the placement of a VP shunt at the time of myelomeningocele closure is common. Syringomyelia is present in 40% to 80% of patients[26] and can cause rapid development of scoliosis. The formation of a syrinx can result from either a tethered spinal cord or a Chiari II malformation.

McLone and Naidich[27] proposed a unifying theory underlying the constellation of associated anomalies. The dorsal defect in the spinal cord, spinal canal, and skin allows the CSF to leak out into the amniotic fluid, creating a collapse of the primitive ventricular system. The failure of the ventricles to increase in size leads to a decrease in the size of the posterior fossa and subsequent herniation of the cerebellum upward and downward (Chiari II malformation). The arachnoid granulations, which normally absorb CSF back into the venous system, may not develop in these patients because of the dearth of circulating CSF, causing a condition called *communicating hydrocephalus*. (The usual causes of hydrocephalus in the patient with a myelomeningocele are obstruction of the fourth ventricle at its outlet and communicating hydrocephalus.)

Long-term function depends on a number of factors. Seventy-five percent of patients have normal intelligence. Cognitive ability in these patients is influenced most strongly by CNS infection. Children with shunts have an average IQ of 97, whereas those without shunts have an average IQ of 102. The average IQ drops by 24 points if a CNS infection occurs.[28] Eighty-five percent to 90% of these children require clean intermittent catheterization (CIC) for social continence, and anticholinergic drugs are often used. Bowel continence is achieved with a combination of medications, diet control, and enemas. As many as 50% of these children are sensitive to latex. Seventy-five percent can ambulate, sometimes with the assistance of bracing. Children with sacral lesions can usually walk, and those with thoracic lesions usually cannot. The degree of ambulation for patients with lumbar lesions varies significantly and often declines with age. The most common late deterioration results from a tethered spinal cord; 20% of these patients require a detethering operation later in life. The need for detethering can be suggested by the development of a syrinx, a decrease in lower extremity function, increasing scoliosis, gait difficulty, back pain, or a change in continence or urodynamic studies.

Spinal Lipomas

Spinal lipomas are the most common type of occult spinal dysraphism. The incidence of spinal lipoma is approximately one fifth that of neural tube defects[12] and is present in 1:4000 births. This category includes lipomyelomeningocele (84%), lipoma of the filum terminale (12%), and intradural lipoma (4%).[26] A spinal lipoma is defined as an intraspinal mass of adipose tissue that is contiguous with the adjacent spinal cord, usually at lumbosacral levels. These lesions are abnormalities of primary neurulation caused by focal premature disjunction of the neurocutaneous ectoderm.

Lipomyelomeningoceles are lipomas that attach to the spinal cord and protrude into the subcutaneous tissue through a bony defect. The mass may involve nerve roots or only the conus medullaris and filum terminale. The embryologic defect likely occurs between gestational days 28 and 48 and is thought to be a premature disjunction of the neural and cutaneous ectoderm, leaving the neural folds vulnerable to paraxial mesenchymal entry.[12] The presentation is of a skin-covered mass above the buttocks, often in infancy (Fig. 51–9). Seventy percent of these patients are female. They produce symptoms by tethering the spinal cord to the subcutaneous tissue and are ideally treated prophylactically. The goal of surgery is to detether the cord; some lipoma may be left behind to avoid injury to the spinal nerves. A patulous graft is placed over the dural opening to encourage formation of a large pool of CSF around the cord and nerve roots to limit the likelihood of retethering. The retethering rate is as high as 20% in some series.[4] Three percent to 6% of lipomyelomeningoceles are associated with Chiari I malformation.[29] Approximately 10% of these patients have scoliosis. Improvement in symptoms is seen in 26% of patients who were operated on, whereas another 51% remain stable. Significantly, 23% have a decline in symptoms.[30]

A lipoma of the filum terminale is caused by incomplete involution of the distal spinal cord during retrogressive differentiation. It is rarely associated with a cutaneous abnormality. The lipoma is completely intradural

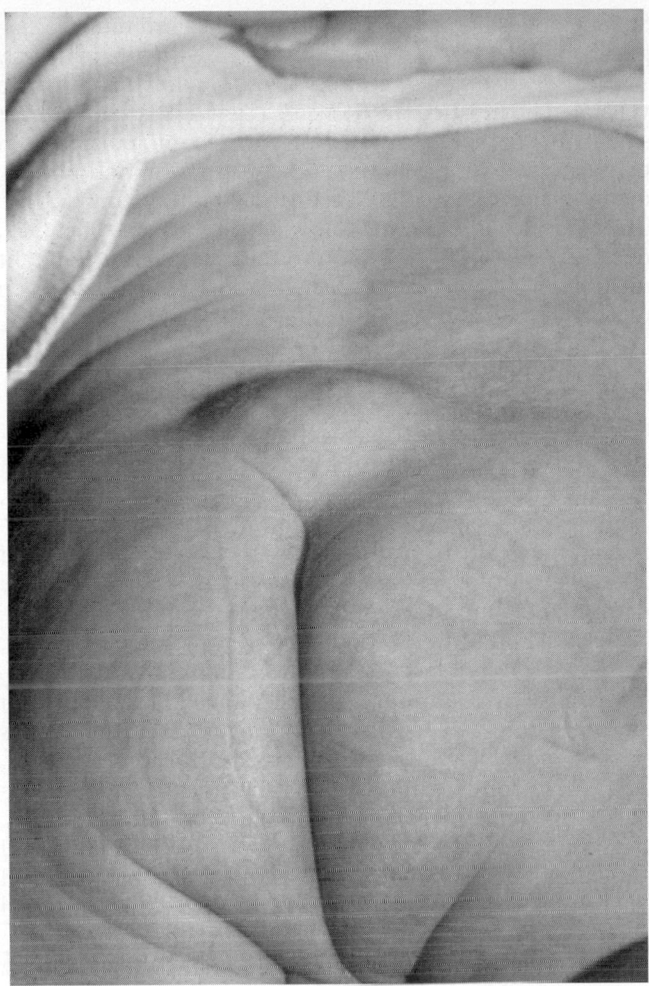

FIGURE 51–9 • Lipomyelomeningocele. The lesion on the left is pedunculated, the one on the right has a more typical appearance of a lipomyelomeningocele. Used with permission from eMedicine.com, Inc., 2004.

and causes spinal cord tethering. Ultrasound reveals a filum terminale more than 2 mm in diameter at the level of L5-S1 and decreased mobility of the spinal cord within the canal. It usually is associated with a low-lying conus medullaris, although it need not be. It is treated prophylactically to prevent deterioration in strength, sensation, or continence. It is seen in up to 88% of cases of imperforate anus. Urologic deficits are most likely to improve if an operation is performed before age 18 months.[28] Symptoms improve in more than one half of patients who are operated on.[30]

Intradural lipomas are fully contained within an intact dural sac. They are usually lumbosacral in origin and produce symptoms of tethered cord syndrome. They may rarely be intramedullary.

Dermal sinus tracts are tracts lined with epithelium leading from the skin to the intradural space. They are presumed to result from a focal failure of separation of the cutaneous from the neuroectoderm. This failure may lead to the development of a dermal sinus tract or into a mass composed of ectodermal elements (epidermoid cyst) or ectodermal and mesodermal elements (dermoid) without cutaneous extension. Dermoid cysts are more commonly seen in the midline, whereas epidermoids are more commonly seen at the cerebellopontine angle. Dermal sinus tracts are usually lumbosacral in location, but any location up to the occipital or even nasal region is possible. As the spinal cord ascends within the canal during development, the area of persistent adhesion elongates to form a tract. The most common presentation is of a midline dimple above the gluteal cleft with associated cutaneous anomalies. The tract extends superiorly. A well-described presentation is of recurrent bouts of meningitis. The tract must be excised completely; dermoid and epidermoid cysts must ideally be excised without spillage of their contents into the intradural space, which can cause chemical meningitis.

Neurenteric Cysts

Neurenteric cysts are thought to be remnants of the embryonic neurenteric canal and are a form of failure of midline notochordal fusion in which primitive streak cells remain trapped within a split notochord. They are cysts lined with mucin-secreting cuboidal or columnar epithelium found within the spinal canal, most commonly at the cervicothoracic junction and at the conus medullaris. They may be entirely within the spinal canal or communicate with the chest or abdomen. The intraspinal component may be intradural or intramedullary. The more complicated lesions often present as masses in the chest or abdomen, which are subsequently found to extend into the spinal canal; an alternative presentation is recurrent bouts of meningitis. Patients with entirely intraspinal cysts usually have myelopathy. Defects in the vertebral bodies are common, and diastematomyelia may be seen on MRI. The cyst must be surgically excised, and any communication with the thoracic or abdominal cavities must be abolished.

Diastematomyelia

Diastematomyelia is a condition in which a portion of the spinal cord is split into two hemicords for a variable length, with the two cords commonly reuniting at the distal limit of the abnormality (Fig. 51–10). If there is no distal reunion, the term diplomyelia is used instead. The hemicords may be separated by pia; dura; or a fibrous, cartilaginous, or bony spur. This is the most common form of failure of midline notochordal integration, with two separate notochords inducing the formation of two hemicords; the presence of an intervening spur depends on the pathway of differentiation of the intervening primitive streak cells. This condition rarely occurs in the absence of other anomalies of the vertebral system. At the minimum, a bifid spinous process is nearly always seen at the level of the split. Diastematomyelia occurs in 20% to 40% of patients with myelomeningocele. The abnormality is usually discovered during the evaluation of an associated spinal abnormality or of a cutaneous lesion. Rarely, it is diagnosed when a previously healthy patient has an unexplained neurologic deterioration. Seventy percent of the reported patients have been female. Because neurologic deterioration is a risk of surgical repair, treatment

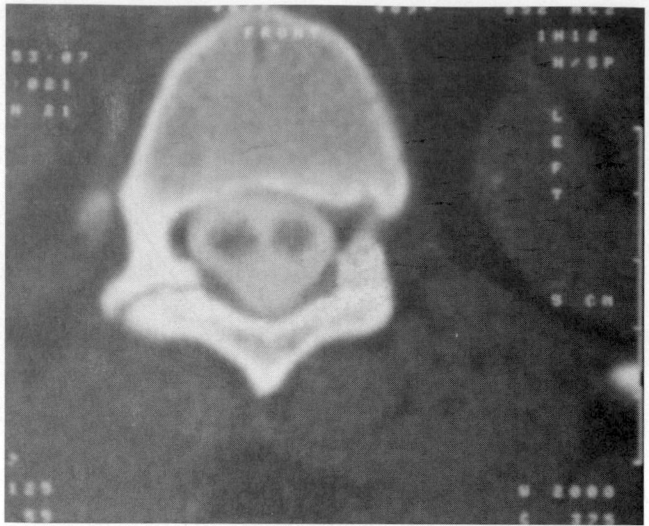

FIGURE 51–10 • Computed tomography myelogram showing the two hemicords of diastematomyelia.

consists of complete removal of the septum in patients with symptoms, or in those scheduled to undergo a scoliosis operation. The dura must be opened to ensure that the spinal cord is not tethered. Spurs have been reported to recur. Diastematomyelia is a congenital malformation rarely seen in isolation; vertebral anomalies are extremely common, and anomalies of other organ systems are not unusual.

Myelocystocele

Myelocystocele, a rare condition in which the spinal cord terminates in a dilation of the central canal, is often associated with bladder or cloacal exstrophy, anal atresia, scoliosis, and sacral agenesis. The embryologic defect is hypothesized to be a midline failure of retrogressive differentiation of the caudal cell mass. The dorsal aspect of the cord is attached to the cutaneous ectoderm, which produces a large skin-covered sac (Fig. 51–11). Subcutaneous lipomas are common. The cord must be surgically untethered, and the dura closed with a patch graft.

Nearly all of these lesions are dorsal, but 0.5% are ventral. The most common ventral variant is the anterior sacral meningocele, usually discovered in females as a pelvic mass. Symptoms include constipation and urinary incontinence. Surgical obliteration of the ostium of the meningocele via a laminectomy is the treatment of choice, to avoid the risks of erosion into the rectum with resultant meningitis and rupture during labor, which has been reported to be fatal.[21]

Caudal Agenesis

Caudal agenesis syndrome encompasses a range of anomalies from coccygeal spine dysgenesis to sirenomelia (absence of the lumbosacral spine and fused lower extremities). The embryologic abnormality is one of segmental maldevelopment of the notochord, with secondary failure of development of the associated mesoderm. It is associated with imperforate anus, genitourinary anomalies (hydronephrosis, duplication of mullerian ducts), renal dysplasia, pulmonary hypoplasia, and lower extremity dysplasia. Mothers with gestational diabetes have a 1% chance of giving birth to an infant with this syndrome. It is seen as a component of syndromes such as OEIS (omphalocele, cloacal exstrophy, imperforate anus, and spinal deformities), VACTERL (vertebral anomaly, imperforate anus, cardiac anomalies, tracheoesophageal fistula, renal anomalies and limb deformities), and the Currarino triad (sacral agenesis, anorectal malformation, and presacral mass [teratoma and/or meningocele]).[24, 31]

Malformations of the brain and spinal cord are among the most common congenital malformations. Nearly all of the malformations discussed in this chapter are related to a specific defect in embryogenesis. Hydrocephalus is commonly associated with many cranial malformations. The tethered cord syndrome is a common presentation for spinal anomalies. An understanding of these CNS malformations is essential for the critical care physician, pediatrician, and surgical specialist who care for these patients.

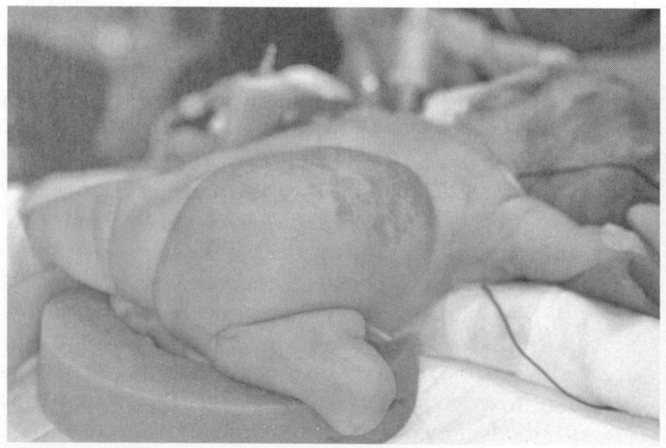

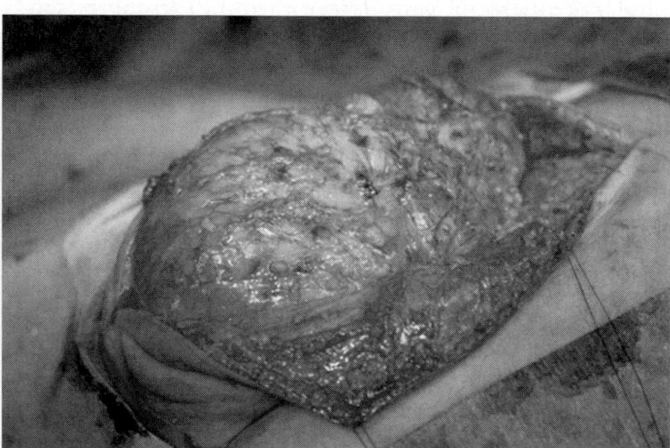

FIGURE 51–11 • Terminal myelocystocele. Note the extremity anomaly. **B**, Figure shows the lipoma commonly seen within the cyst (photo courtesy of Anthony Avellino, MD).

REFERENCES

1. Steinbok P, Cochrane DD: Cervical meningoceles and myelocystoceles: a unifying hypothesis, *Pediatr Neurosurg* 23: 317-322, 1995.
2. Gluckman TJ, George TM, McLone DG: Post-neurulation rapid brain growth represents a critical time for encephalocele formation: a chick model, *Pediatr Neurosurg* 25:130-136, 1996.
3. Hoving EW, Blaser S, Kelly E, et al: Anatomical and embryological considerations in the repair of a large vertex encephalocele, *J Neurosurg* 90:537-541, 1999.
4. Ellenbogen RG: Neural tube defects in the neonatal period, *eMedicine* 2003.
5. Ingraham FD, Swan H: Spina bifida and cranium bifidum. I. A survey of five hundred and forty-six cases, *N Engl J Med* 228:559-563, 1943.
6. Sever LE, Sanders M, Monsen R: An epidemiologic study of neural tube defects in Los Angeles County I. Prevalence at birth based on multiple sources of case ascertainment, *Teratology* 25:315-321, 1982.
7. Peter JC, Fieggen G: Congenital malformations of the brain—a neurosurgical perspective at the close of the twentieth century, *Childs Nerv Syst* 15:635-645, 1999.
8. Chapman TH, Swearingen B, Caviness VS: Subtorcular occipital encephaloceles. Anatomical considerations relevant to operative treatment, *J Neurosurg* 71:375-381, 1989.
9. Cohen MM Jr, Lemire RJ: Syndromes with cephaloceles, *Teratology* 25:161-172, 1982.
10. Martinez-Lage JF, Pusa M, Sola J, et al: The child with an encephalocele: etiology, neuroimaging and outcome, *Childs Nerv Syst* 12: 540-550, 1996.
11. Jiminez D, Barone CM: Encephaloceles, meningoceles, and dermal sinuses. In Albright AL, Pollack IF, Adelson PD, editors: *Principles and practice of pediatric neurosurgery,* New York 1999, Thieme Medical Publishers.
12. McLone DG. Congenital malformations of the central nervous system, *Clin Neurosurg* 47: 346-377, 2000.
13. Simpson BA, David DJ, White J: Cephaloceles: treatment, outcome and antenatal diagnosis, *Neurosurgery* 15:14-21, 1984.
14. MacDonald PJ, Rutka JT: Middle cranial fossa arachnoid cysts that come and go. A report of two cases and a review of the literature, *Pediatr Neurosurg* 26:48-52, 1997.
15. Go KG, Houthoff HG, Blaauw EH, et al: Arachnoid cysts of the sylvian fissure. Evidence of fluid secretion, *J Neurosurg* 60:803-813, 1984.
16. Gosalakkal JA: Intracranial arachnoid cysts in children: a review of pathogenesis, clinical features, and management, *Pediatr Neurol* 26:93-98, 2002.
17. Wester K: Gender distribution and sidedness of middle fossa arachnoid cysts: a review of cases diagnosed with computed imaging, *Neurosurgery* 31:940-944, 1992.
18. Lutcherath V, Waaler PE, Jellum E, et al: Children with bitemporal arachnoid cysts may have glutaric aciduria type 1 (GAT1); operation without knowing that may be harmful, *Acta Neurochir (Wien)* 142:1025-1030, 2000.
19. Richard KE, Dahl K, Sanker P: Long-term follow-up of children and juveniles with arachnoid cysts, *Childs Nerv Syst* 5:184-187, 1989.
20. Caldarelli M, Ceddia A, Di Rocco C, et al: Chiari type II malformation: a rare neurologic emergency, *J Pediatr Neurosci* 3:191-205, 1987.
21. Villarejo F, Scavone C, Blazques MG, et al: Anterior sacral meningocele: review of the literature, *Surg Neurol* 19:57-71, 1983.
22. Venes JL: Surgical considerations in the initial repair of meningomyelocele and the introduction of a technical midificaiton, *Neurosurgery* 17:111-113, 1985.
23. Swift DM, Carmel PW: Congenital intradural pathology, *Neurosurg Clin N Am* 1:551-566, 1990.
24. Rossi A, Cama A, Piatelli G, et al: Spinal dysraphism: MR imaging rationale, *J Neuroradiol* 31: 3-24, 2004.
25. Shurtleff DB, Lemire RJ: Epidemiology, etiologic factors, and prenatal diagnosis of open dysraphism, *Neurosurg Clin N Am* 6: 183-193, 1995.
26. Unsinn KM, Geley T, Freund MC, et al: US of the spinal cord in newborns: spectrum of normal findings, variants, congenital anomalies, and acquired diseases, *Radiographics* 20:923-938, 2000.
27. McLone DG, Naidich TP: Developmental morphology of the subarachnoid space, brain vasculature, and contiguous structures, and the cause of the Chiari II malformation, *Am J Neuroradiol* 13:463-482, 1992.
28. McLone DG: Continuing concepts in the management of spina bifida, *Pediatr Neurosurg* 18: 254-256, 1992.
29. Byrne RW, Hayes EA, George TM, et al: Operative resection of 100 spinal lipomas in infants less than 1 year of age, *Pediatr Neurosurg* 23:182-187, 1995.
30. La Marca F, Grant JA, Tomita T, et al: Spinal lipomas in children: outcome of 270 procedures, *Pediatr Neurosurg* 26:8, 1997.
31. Tortori-Donati P, Rossi A, Biancheri R, et al: Magnetic resonance imaging of spinal dysraphism, *Top Magn Reson Imaging* 12: 375-409, 2001.

CHAPTER 52

Intracranial Hypertension and Brain Monitoring

Robert C. Tasker and Marek Czosnyka

PEARLS

- As intracranial hypertension progresses, changes may occur in the vital signs, with an elevation of blood pressure, a decrease or an increase in pulse, and irregularity in the respiratory rhythm. These signs, sometimes associated with episodes of decerebrate rigidity, indicate the occurrence of transtentorial herniation or "coning" and imply the possibility of impending death if the process cannot be reversed.
- The continuous measurement of intracranial pressure (ICP) is an essential modality in most brain monitoring systems. After a decade of enthusiastic attempts to introduce newer modalities for brain monitoring (e.g., tissue oxygenation, microdialysis, cortical blood flow, transcranial Doppler (TCD) ultrasonography, and jugular bulb oxygen saturation), the measurement of ICP has become increasingly noticeable as a robust and only moderately invasive modality, and it can be realistically conducted in most critical care units.

In most organs in the human body the environmental pressure for blood perfusion is either low or coupled to atmospheric pressure. The environmental pressure for the brain differs in this respect because the brain is surrounded and protected by a stiff skull. Thus a rise in environmental pressure—intracranial pressure (ICP)—may impede blood flow and cause ischemia. In pediatric critical care, ICP may be of acute significance in a number of instances (e.g., traumatic brain injury, bacterial meningitis, and the Fontan circulation). In this chapter we consider how information from ICP monitoring helps our understanding and treatment of brain disorders.

Clinical Background

In critical illness, the early recognition and treatment of intracranial hypertension is important because it is a major cause of mortality and morbidity. An attempt should therefore be made to collate the clinical evidence for and against its presence. The early symptoms and signs of this complication, however, which are invariably subtle and nonspecific (Table 52–1), make this form of assessment somewhat limited. As discussed later, as intracranial hypertension progresses, changes may occur in the vital signs, with an elevation of blood pressure, a decrease or an increase in pulse, and irregularity in the respiratory rhythm. These signs, sometimes associated with episodes of decerebrate rigidity, indicate the occurrence of transtentorial herniation or "coning" and imply the possibility of impending death if the process cannot be reversed. Unfortunately recognition at this stage is often too late.

Brain tissue shifts may produce various "syndromes." First, transtentorial or cerebellar herniation may result in midbrain or medullary compression. Many of the clinical signs observed in association with herniation result from direct compression of structures by the impacted tissue

TABLE 52–1

Early, Subtle Symptoms and Signs of Raised Intracranial Pressure

	Infant	Child
General state	Poor feeding	Anorexia and nausea
	Vomiting	Vomiting
	Irritability to coma	Lethargy to coma
	Seizures	Seizures
Head/eyes	Full fontanelle	False localizing signs
	Scalp vein distention	
	False localizing signs	
Other	Altered vital signs	Altered vital signs
	Hypertension	Hypertension
	Pulmonary edema	Pulmonary edema

or are due to angulation of nerves or arteries against normal structures in the area. These herniations can cause increasing coma, with distortion of the brainstem leading to midbrain and pontine hemorrhages. Cerebellar herniation is likely to occur when the increase in ICP is maximal in the posterior fossa. Such herniation occurs more commonly downward, squeezing one or more of the cerebellar tonsils through the foramen magnum; compressing the medulla; and leading to neck stiffness, head tilt, lower cranial nerve palsies, respiratory irregularities, or sudden cardiorespiratory arrest. Cerebellar herniation may occur, though uncommonly, upward through the tentorial notch, causing midbrain compression and leading to paralysis of upward gaze, dilated and fixed pupils, and respiratory abnormalities.

When intracranial hypertension is more marked in the supratentorial compartment, for instance, with acute intracerebral hematoma, the temporal lobe on the affected side may be displaced into the tentorial notch and result in unilateral transtentorial herniation. The herniation may be more marked anteriorly (uncal) or posteriorly (hippocampal) and is usually accompanied by displacement of the ipsilateral cingulate gyrus under the falx (cingulate herniation). Clinical manifestations of this may include ipsilateral third nerve palsy, contralateral hemiparesis, respiratory irregularities, deepening coma with decerebrate posturing, and ultimately cardiorespiratory arrest.

Finally, when there is bilateral or general increase in ICP in the supratentorial compartment, as in diffuse cerebral edema, central transtentorial herniation may occur. This leads to impairment of upward gaze, pupillary constriction, hypertonus, and decerebrate posturing. Temperature irregularities and diabetes insipidus may develop, as might cardiorespiratory arrest eventually. A summary of the clinical features of "central syndrome" is given in Table 52–2.

TABLE 52–2

Clinical Features of Central Syndrome or Rostrocaudal Deterioration

Stage	Level of Consciousness	Respiration	Pupil Size and Reactivity	Oculocephalic and Oculovestibular Responses	Posture and Tone
Diencephalic (early to late) ↓	Agitation Drowsiness Stupor	Deep sighs or yawns Occasional pauses Cheyne-Stokes or periodic breathing	Small (1-3 mm) with brisk reaction to light	Conjugate at rest and respond quickly	Normal or slightly increased Generalized muscular hypertonus
Midbrain to upper pontine ↓	Coma	Central hyperventilation	Midposition (3-5 mm) with sluggish reaction to light	Dysconjugate	Decorticate posturing and increased tone
Lower pontine to upper medullary ↓	Deep coma		Midposition and fixed	Absent	Flaccid: (a) Retained bilateral extensor plantars (b) Occasional flexor responses in the lower limbs
Medullary (terminal)	Deep coma	Irregular breathing interrupted by deep sighs, gasps, and then terminal apnea	May be unequal	Absent	Flaccid

Modified from Plum F, Posner JB: *Diagnosis of stupor and coma,* Philadelphia, 1966, FA Davis.

Physiology of the Intracranial Vault

A physiologic process underlies the clinical picture of intracranial hypertension, and in this section of the chapter our intention is to familiarize the pediatric intensivist with new approaches to understanding the hydrodynamic function of the intracranial vault. In other words, what happens before brain tissue shifts occur? Most of the developments in this field have occurred in the setting of adult neurosurgery and critical care. In common with any aspect of physiology the tasks have been straightforward: Can it be measured? Can it be modeled? How do the models help in the understanding of the underlying homeostasis and the mechanism of derangement and perturbation? We highlight these topics and hope that the reader will see the obvious application to pediatric critical care; that is, our use of this form of cerebral monitoring and potential approaches to ICP assessment. In many specific conditions, however, knowledge is still lacking as to which parts of the adult-generated theory may be fully applicable to children.

Intracranial Pressure

The brain is an expansile structure that expands and contracts with each beat of the heart. Because there are no valves within the venous drainage from the brain, any changes in intrathoracic pressure are transmitted to ICP. Such phenomena can be seen and palpated simply through the examination of a baby's fontanelle and quantified with cerebrospinal fluid (CSF) pressure recording. Once the cranial sutures have fused, any change in cerebral blood volume (CBV) on the arterial-to-arteriolar side of the cerebral circulation must be compensated by either reduction in cerebral venous volume or by phasic movement of CSF out of the intracranial vault through the foramen magnum. Such expansion of the cerebral mantle with compression of the lateral ventricles during systole and movement of CSF through the aqueduct of Sylvius and to and fro through the foramen magnum was first visualized with pneumoencephalography. These changes can now be seen more easily with dynamic magnetic resonance imaging (MRI). Inevitably there is a lag phase between the systolic increase in CBV and the effect of the compensatory mechanisms so that CSF pressure increases to reflect, in part, the systolic waveform. The CSF pressure waveform is not an exact replica of the arterial waveform because it has been "filtered" by the combined effects of arterial wall compliance of the cerebral arteries, cerebrovascular resistance, and intracranial compliance (Fig. 52–1).[1]

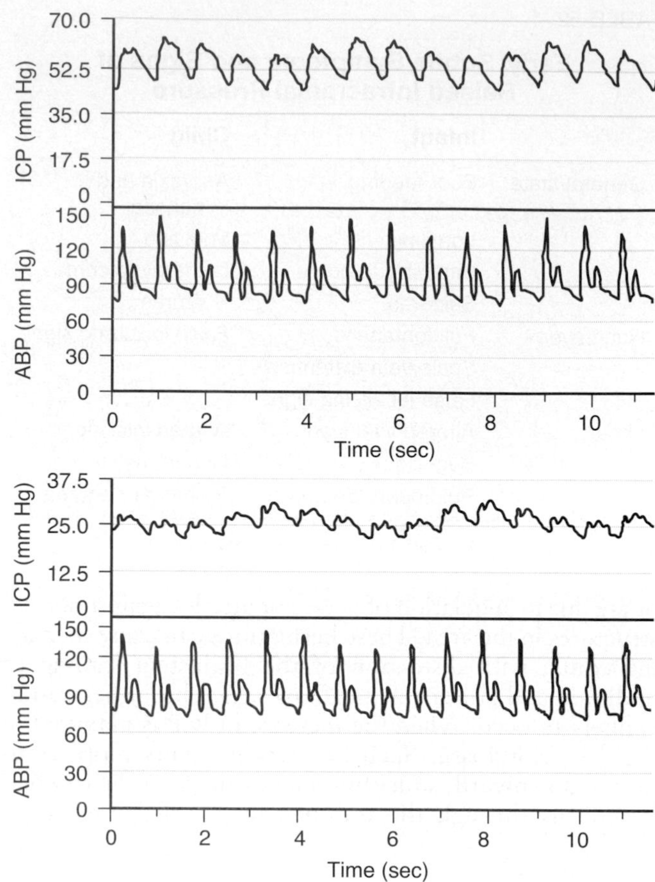

FIGURE 52–1 • Examples of waveforms of intracranial pressure (ICP) and arterial blood pressure (ABP) recorded at a high level of ICP (*upper plots*) and a lower level of ICP (*lower plots*). Note that the pattern of ABP waveform is relatively invariant, but ICP changes its shape considerably.[1]

Hydrodynamic Model of Intracranial Pressure

ICP is a function of the circulation of cerebral blood and CSF in which ICP is related to a vascular component ($ICP_{vascular}$) and a CSF component (ICP_{CSF}). There is considerable interest in modeling these relationships as an aid to understanding some of the complex phenomena seen in critically ill patients. The vascular component is difficult to express quantitatively.[2,3] It is probably derived from the pulsation of CBV that is detected and averaged by nonlinear mechanisms of regulation of CBV. More generally, multiple variables such as the arterial blood pressure (ABP), autoregulation, and cerebral venous outflow all contribute to the vascular component. In regard to the other component, circulation of CSF, 80% of CSF is the product of active secretion by the choroid plexus, and movement of interstitial fluid into the ventricles and subarachnoid space contribute the remainder. Drainage is largely passive via arachnoid villi and granulations into the superior sagittal sinus and spinal root sleeve venous drainage. Some drainage, which is currently unquantifiable, occurs through the olfactory bulb and mucosa into the deep cervical lymphatics. The equation by Davson, Hollingsworth, and Segal[4] shows the immediate relationships controlling CSF pressure, in which ICP_{CSF} = (resistance to CSF outflow) × (CSF formation) + (pressure in sagittal sinus). With these two components—vascular and CSF—taken together, Figure 52–2[5] shows the hydrodynamic model of cerebral blood flow (CBF) and CSF circulation, and the equivalent electrical circuit. This model can be used to interrogate CSF dynamics clinically (see later).

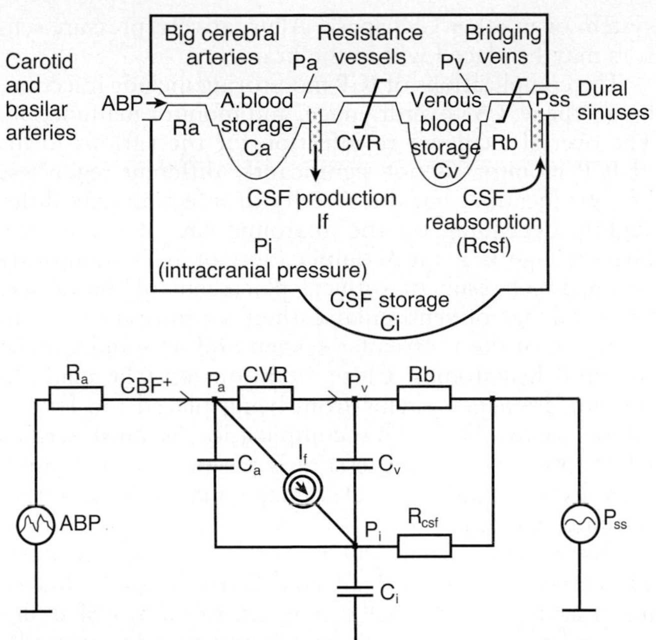

FIGURE 52–2 • Hydrodynamic model of cerebral blood and cerebrospinal fluid circulation (*upper plot*) and its electrical equivalent (*lower plot*).[5]

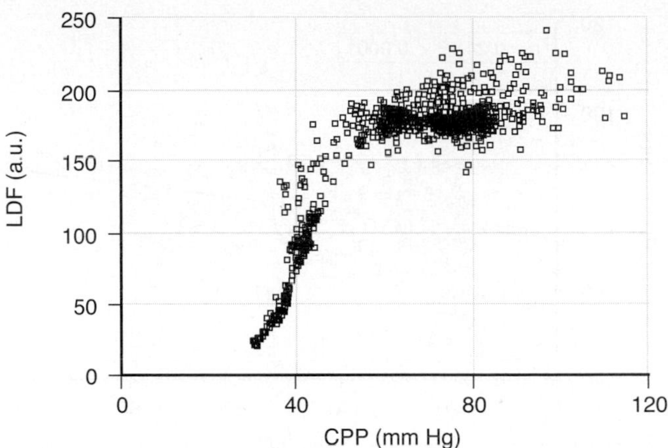

FIGURE 52–3 • Pressure autoregulation where cerebral blood flow (CBF) stays constant. CBF is measured with laser Doppler flowmetry (LDF) (y-axis). During changes in cerebral perfusion pressure (CPP) (x-axis) CBF remains constant until a critical threshold is reached, below which CBF falls passively with decreasing CPP.

Cerebral Vasodilatation and Cerebrospinal Fluid Pressure

Three major factors regulate CBF: cerebral perfusion pressure (CPP), partial pressure of arterial carbon dioxide ($PaCO_2$), and partial pressure of arterial oxygen (PaO_2). Hypercapnia causes cerebral vasodilatation, increases CBF, and increases ICP. Hypoxia also causes cerebral vasodilatation and a rise in ICP. Cerebral perfusion pressure is taken as the difference between mean ABP and ICP and represents the pressure gradient acting across the cerebrovascular bed; therefore it is an important factor in regulation of CBF.[6] Under normal circumstances, over a wide range of CPP, CBF is autoregulated (i.e., it remains constant when CPP varies). Thus in regard to the effect of this phenomenon on ICP, active cerebral arteriolar constriction occurs and ICP consequently falls to maintain CBF when ABP is increased (i.e., hypertension). At the other extreme, systemic hypotension (within the autoregulatory range) provokes cerebral vasodilatation and an increase in ICP. When autoregulation is defective, ICP increases and decreases with ABP (Figs. 52–3 and 52–4).[7]

In practice, measurement of ICP can be used to estimate the CPP when it is the most significant 'downstream' pressure acting on vascular perfusion. However, in some instances, venous pressure may be of more significance, such as critical Fontan circulation.

Cerebral Perfusion Pressure and Autoregulation

In adults, the lower limit for CPP is taken as a threshold of 60 to 70 mmHg. In children, however, it is evident from measurement of normal ABP that the lower limit for CPP must be lower than this adult level for much of childhood (Fig. 52–5).[7] A new concept that has arisen in the adult critical care literature is worth considering in this context. The idea is that there is an autoregulatory reserve that is considered as the difference between current mean CPP and the lower limit of autoregulation.[8,9] This reserve may become exhausted. Alternatively, it may change over time, and it has been argued that the border between adequate and nonadequate CPP should be assessed individually and frequently.

How is this done? Autoregulation of CBF may be assessed by artificial manipulation of ABP with medication but only at infrequent intervals and with the risk that the drugs used may have a direct cerebrovascular effect. Alternatively, transient hyperemia after transient carotid compression has been used as an all-or-none index of whether autoregulation is intact. A more sophisticated approach is to examine the effect of natural variation in ABP; however, this technique requires precise signal processing. For example, to date, the most robust clinical method is to monitor the slow fluctuations in ABP, which last from

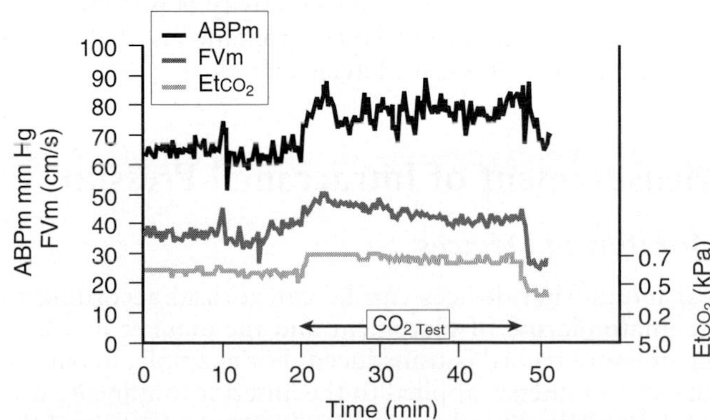

FIGURE 52–4 • Cerebral vessels dilate when arterial content of carbon dioxide (here measured with end-tidal carbon dioxide [$EtCO_2$]) increases. A rise in cerebral blood flow (here assessed with transcranial Doppler velocity [FVm]) also increases.[6] *ABPm,* mean blood pressure.

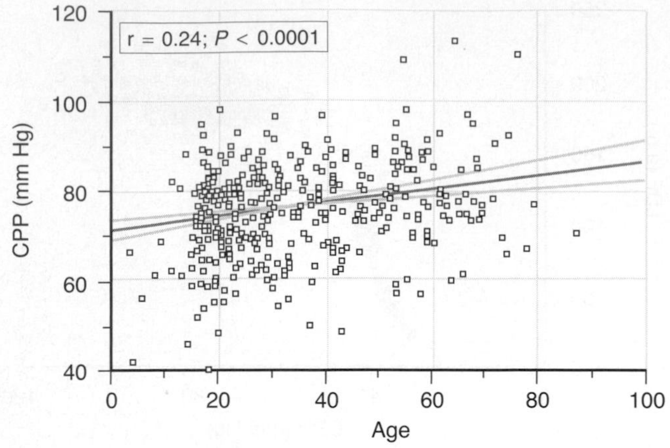

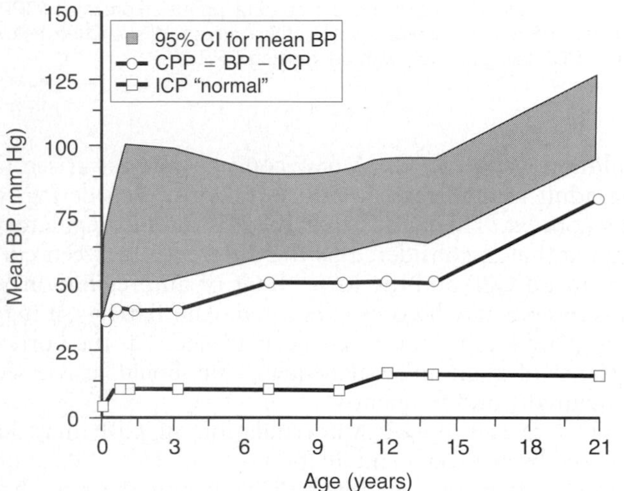

FIGURE 52–5 • The top panel shows the empirical relationship between cerebral perfusion pressure (CPP) and age in nearly 400 adults after head injury. The bottom panel shows estimated lower limit of CPP by age in the pediatric range on the basis of normal blood pressure (BP) and intracranial pressure (ICP) data.[7]

30 seconds to a few minutes, that are almost always present in patients who undergo ventilation[10]; the rate of change observed is usually sufficient to provoke a noticeable vasomotor response. Figure 52–6 shows that continuous monitoring of cerebrovascular reactivity is possible with this method even during large spontaneous ICP waves (B and plateau waves; see later).[11,12]

Measurement of Intracranial Pressure

Monitoring Devices

ICP monitoring devices can be categorized according to the anatomic site of placement and the manner in which the pressure record is transduced. For example, in babies, surface tonometry, applied to the anterior fontanelle, was an early method used for noninvasive transduction of the ICP waveform. This method, however, is limited because the force of applanation influences the pressure record. More standard approaches for the measurement of ICP rely on manometry of catheters placed in the ventricular system or in other CSF space. Alternatively, pressure sensors may be placed within the brain.

The complications of ICP monitoring include infection, hemorrhage, CSF overdrainage, and monitor malfunction. The overall incidence of infection for the various forms of ICP monitors is not significantly different regardless of their location, but the severity of infection may differ slightly depending on the anatomic site of the device. Hemorrhage is a rare complication of ICP monitoring and a direct result of surgical placement of the device. Overdrainage of ventricular catheters can result in rapid emptying of the ventricular system and accumulation of subdural hematomas. Close attention must be made to prevent drainage systems from being placed too low or falling to the floor. This complication is most serious when intraventricular pressure is monitored in children with hydrocephalus. Overdrainage may also result in pneumocephalus.

Overall, an intraventricular drain connected to an external pressure transducer is still considered the gold standard for measuring ICP.[13,14] ICP can be controlled by CSF drainage, and the transducer can be adjusted to zero externally. After 5 days of monitoring, however, the risk of infection starts to increase, with an overall risk estimated to be about 5%.[15] Insertion of the ventricular catheter may be difficult or impossible in cases of advanced brain swelling. As an alternative, modern catheter-tipped ventricular, subdural, or intraparenchymal microtransducers (most popular types: Camino ICP Bolt, Camino Laboratories, San Diego, Calif., and Codman MicroSensor, Johnson and Johnson Professional Inc, Raynham, Mass.) have been used. These are said to reduce infection rate and risk of hemorrhage[15] and have excellent metrologic property.[16] One disadvantage of microtransducer systems, however, is that they cannot,

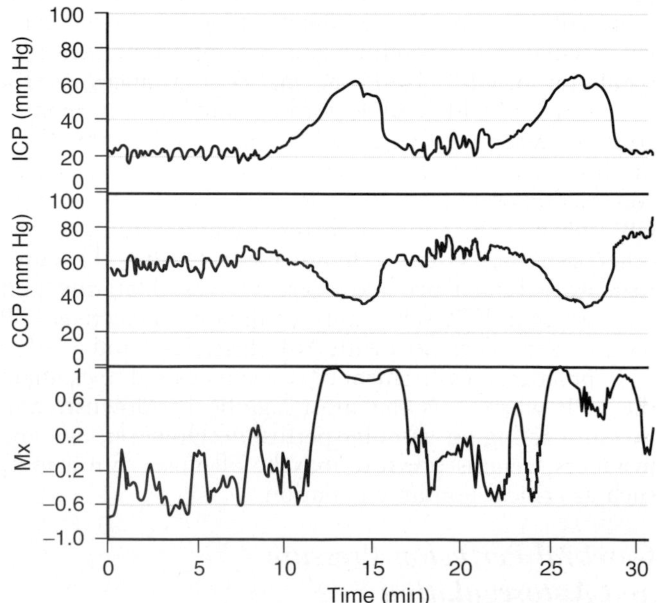

FIGURE 52–6 • Continuous monitoring of cerebral autoregulation during plateau waves of raised intracranial pressure (ICP). Positive values of the autoregulation index (Mx)[11] indicate faulty autoregulation. Autoregulation fails during the waves, when cerebral vasodilation occurs.[12] *CPP,* cerebral perfusion pressure.

in general, be readjusted to zero after insertion, and considerable zero drift can sometimes occur in long-term monitoring.[17]

Regarding other forms of monitoring, contemporary epidural sensors are much more reliable now than they were 10 years ago. Nevertheless the question as to whether epidural pressure can express ICP with confidence and under all circumstances is still unanswered. Lumbar CSF pressure is seldom measured in neurointensive care. This form of assessment of craniospinal dynamics is more often used in the assessment of hydrocephalus and benign intracranial hypertension. It is unreliable if the instantaneous value of the fluid column pressure is recorded; at least 30 minutes averaging in resting conditions (with a period of overnight monitoring as the gold standard) is the desired requirement. Finally, attempts to monitor ICP noninvasively are still in a phase of technical evaluation,[18] and the most promising methods are based on transcranial ultrasonography.[19-21]

Noninvasive Inference of Intracranial Pressure

It would be helpful to measure ICP or CPP without invasive transducers. To this end, transcranial Doppler (TCD) examination,[22] tympanic membrane displacement,[23] and ultrasound "time of flight"[20] techniques have been suggested. The description of TCD sonography by Aaslid, Markwalde, and Nornes[24] permitted bedside monitoring of one index of CBF, noninvasively, repeatedly, and even continuously. The problem has been that it is a "big tube technique," which measures flow velocity in branches of the circle of Willis, most commonly the middle cerebral artery (MCA). Compliant branches of the MCA can be compared with two physiologic pressure transducers. The pattern of blood flow within these tubes is certainly modulated by transmural pressure, that is, CPP and the distal vascular resistance (also modulated by CPP). What is the calibration factor and how should we compensate for unknown nonlinear distortion?

There is reasonable correlation between the pulsatility index of MCA velocity and CPP after head injury, but absolute measurements of CPP cannot be extrapolated.[25] Others have suggested that "critical closing pressure" derived from flow velocity and arterial pressure waveform approximated the value of ICP.[26] The accuracy of this method, however, has never been satisfactory.[27] Aaslid et al[28] suggested that an index of CPP could be derived from the ratio of the amplitudes of the first harmonics of the ABP and the MCA velocity (detected with TCD sonography) multiplied by mean flow velocity. Recently, a method for the noninvasive assessment of CPP has been reported, derived from mean ABP multiplied by the ratio of diastolic to mean flow velocity.[29,30] This estimator can predict real CPP—in the adult range (60 to 100 mmHg)—with an error of less than 10 mmHg for more than 80% of measurements. This is of potential benefit for the continuous monitoring of changes in real CPP over time in situations where direct measurement of CPP is not readily available. Finally, a more complex method aimed at the noninvasive assessment of ICP has been introduced and tested by Schmidt et al.[31] The method is based on the presumed linear transformation between ABP and ICP waveforms. All of these techniques still require validation in pediatric series.

Pressure Compartments

In a fluid-filled container, pressure is the same wherever one chooses to measure it within that space. Generally, uniformly distributed ICP can be seen only when CSF is circulating freely among all of its natural pools, equilibrating pressure everywhere. When little or no CSF volume is left (because of brain swelling), the assumption of one uniform value of ICP is questionable. (This is the reason that brain tissue shift and herniation occurs: they move down tissue pressure gradients.) It is worth remembering that with the commonly used catheter-tipped, intraparenchymal probes, the measurement of pressure is at a particular point, an area of cortex within a hemisphere, and the ICP may merely reflect pressure in that compartment rather than be representative of pressure within the ventricular system (i.e., real CSF pressure).[32]

Analysis of Intracranial Pressure

Normal Values in Intracranial Pressure Monitoring

Establishing a universal "normal value" for ICP is difficult because it depends on age, body posture, and clinical condition. In the horizontal position, a normal ICP value in healthy adults was reported to be within the range of 7 to 15 mmHg.[33] In the upright position ICP is a negative value, with a mean of around −10 mmHg but not exceeding −15 mmHg.[34] In infants and children, normal values for ICP, usually taken at the time of a "negative" diagnostic lumbar puncture, are lower than the adult values and are probably between 5 and 10 mmHg.

The definition of a raised ICP value depends on the specific disease. In hydrocephalus, a pressure above 15 mmHg can be regarded as elevated. After head injury, any pressure above 20 mmHg is considered abnormal, and aggressive treatment is usually started with values above 25 mmHg.[35] Also, in most cases, ICP varies with time. Decent averaging for at least 30 minutes is needed to calculate "mean ICP." The patient should be in a horizontal position during the measurement, and movement should be avoided.

Normal Trends in ICP and Waveform Analysis

Overnight monitoring, during natural sleep, provides a "grand average" with a good description of the dynamics of ICP. When monitored continuously in acute states (e.g., head injury, poor-grade subarachnoid hemorrhage, and intracerebral hematoma), changes in the time-averaged mean ICP may be classified into relatively few patterns (Fig. 52–7).[36] The first pattern, *low and stable ICP* (below 20 mmHg) is seen after uncomplicated head injury (Fig. 52–7, *A*). Such a pattern is also commonly seen in the initial period after brain trauma before brain swelling evolves. The second pattern, *high and stable ICP*

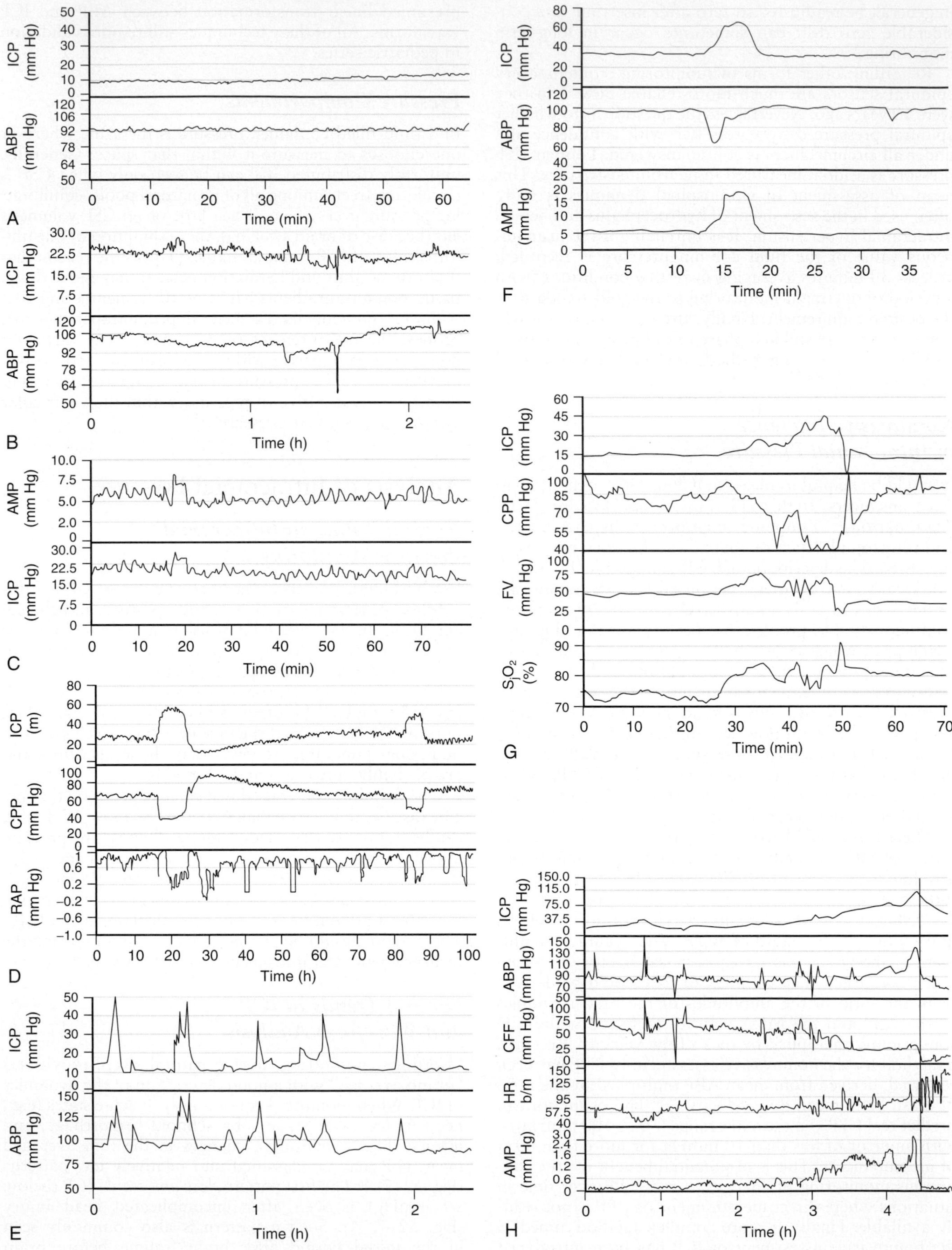
ICP (mm Hg)
50
40
30
20
10
0
ABP (mm Hg)
120
106
92
78
64
50
0
10
20
30
40
50
60
Time (min)
A
ICP (mm Hg)
30.0
22.5
15.0
7.5
0
ABP (mm Hg)
120
106
92
78
64
50
0
1
2
Time (h)
B
AMP (mm Hg)
10.0
7.5
5.0
2.0
0
ICP (mm Hg)
30.0
22.5
15.0
7.5
0
0
10
20
30
40
50
60
70
Time (min)
C
ICP (m)
80
60
40
20
0
CPP (mm Hg)
100
80
60
40
20
0
RAP (mm Hg)
1
0.6
0.2
−0.2
−0.6
−1.0
0
10
20
30
40
50
60
70
80
90
100
Time (h)
D
ICP (mm Hg)
50
40
30
20
10
0
ABP (mm Hg)
150
125
100
75
50
0
1
2
Time (h)
E
ICP (mm Hg)
80
60
40
20
0
ABP (mm Hg)
120
100
80
60
40
AMP (mm Hg)
25
20
15
10
5
0
0
5
10
15
20
25
30
35
Time (min)
F
ICP (mm Hg)
60
45
30
15
0
CPP (mm Hg)
100
85
70
55
40
FV (mm Hg)
100
75
50
25
0
S_jO_2 (%)
90
80
70
0
10
20
30
40
50
60
70
Time (min)
G
ICP (mm Hg)
150.0
115.0
75.0
37.5
0
ABP (mm Hg)
150
130
110
90
70
50
CFF (mm Hg)
100
75
50
25
0
HR b/m
150
125
95
57.5
40
AMP (mm Hg)
3.0
2.4
1.6
1.2
0.6
0
0
1
2
3
4
Time (h)
H

FIGURE 52–7 • Examples of intracranial pressure (ICP) recording in various clinical scenarios after head trauma[36]; note the different scales. **A,** Low and stable ICP: mean arterial blood pressure (ABP) is plotted in the bottom panel. **B,** Stable and elevated ICP: such a picture can be seen most of the time in patients with head injuries. **C,** B waves of ICP: these are seen both in mean ICP and spectrally resolved pulse amplitude of ICP (AMP). They are usually seen also in plot of time-averaged ABP but not always. **D,** Plateau waves of ICP: cerebrospinal compensatory reserve is usually low when waves are recorded (the correlation coefficient between AMP and mean ABP, RAP, is close to +1). At the top of the waves, during maximal vasodilatation, integration between pulse amplitude and mean ICP fails, as is indicated by fall in RAP. After the plateau wave, ICP usually falls below the baseline level and cerebrospinal compensatory reserve becomes better. **E,** High, spiky waves of ICP caused by sudden increases in ABP. **F,** Increase in ICP caused by temporary decrease in ABP. **G,** Increase in ICP of hyperemic nature: both blood flow velocity and jugular bulb oxygen saturation (S_jO_2) increase in parallel with ICP. **H,** Refractory intracranial hypertension: ICP increases within a few hours to 100 mmHg. The vertical line denotes the likely moment when the vasomotor centers in brainstem became ischemic. At this point the heart rate (HR) increased and cerebral perfusion pressure (CPP) decreased abruptly. Note that pulse amplitude of ICP (AMP) disappeared around 10 minutes before this terminal event.

(above 20 mmHg), is the most common picture to follow head injury (Fig. 52–7, *B*). The third pattern is *vasogenic wave,* that is, B waves (Fig. 52–7, *C*) and plateau waves (Fig. 52–7, *D*). The fourth pattern is *ICP waves* related to changes in ABP and hyperemic events (Fig. 52–7, *E* to *G*). The final pattern, *refractory intracranial hypertension* (Fig. 52–7, *H*), usually leads to death unless surgical decompression is undertaken.

In addition to these patterns, more information can be gained from analyzing the ICP waveform. The ICP waveform consists of three components, which overlap in the time domain but can be separated in the frequency domain (Fig. 52–8).[36,37] The pulse waveform has several harmonic components; of these the fundamental component has a frequency equal to the heart rate. The amplitude of this component (AMP) is useful for the evaluation of various indices. The respiratory waveform is related to the frequency of the respiratory cycle (8 to 20 cycles per minute). "Slow waves" are usually not as precisely defined as in Lundberg's original work[38]; that is, all components that have a spectral representation within the frequency limits of 0.05 to 0.0055 Hz (20 s to 3 min period) are considered

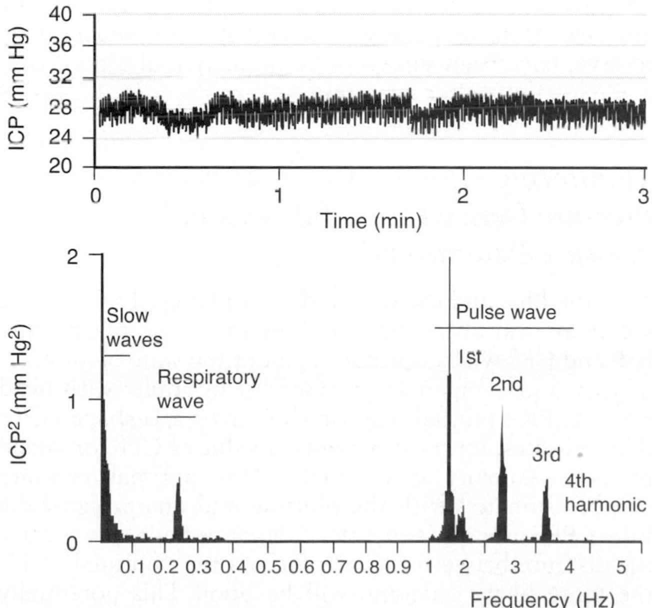

FIGURE 52–8 • Example of intracranial pressure (ICP) recording showing pulse, respiratory and "slow waves" overlapped in the time-domain (*upper panel*) and separated in the frequency domain (*lower panel*).[37]

slow waves. The magnitude of these waves can be calculated as the square root of the power of the signal, of the passband, or of the equivalent frequency range at the output of the digital filter.

Assessment of Pressure-Volume Compensatory Reserve

Theoretically, the compensatory reserve in intracranial hydrodynamics can be studied through the relation between ICP and changes in volume of the intracerebral space, known as the *pressure-volume curve.*[39,40] For example, the RAP index, an index of reserve based on the correlation coefficient (R) between AMP amplitude (A) and mean pressure (P), can be derived. This can be done in real-time with bedside computing to calculate the linear correlation between consecutive, time-averaged data points of AMP and ICP (usually 40 such samples) acquired over a reasonably long period to average over respiratory and pulse waves (usually 6- to 10-seconds epochs). The RAP index indicates the degree of correlation between AMP and mean ICP over short periods (~4 min). An RAP index close to 0 indicates lack of synchronization between changes in AMP and mean ICP. This denotes good pressure-volume compensatory reserve at low ICP (i.e., a change in volume produces little or no change in pressure) (Fig. 52–9).[41] When the RAP index rises to +1, AMP varies directly with ICP and indicates that the "working point" of the intracranial space shifts to the right toward the steep part of the pressure-volume curve. Here compensatory reserve is low; therefore any further rise in volume may produce a rapid increase in ICP. After head injury and subsequent brain swelling, the RAP index is usually close to +1. With any further increase in ICP, AMP decreases and RAP values fall below zero. This occurs when cerebral autoregulatory capacity is exhausted; the pressure-volume curve bends to the right, the capacity of cerebral arterioles to dilate in response to a fall in CPP is exhausted, and the arterioles tend to collapse passively. This indicates terminal cerebrovascular derangement with a decrease in pulse pressure transmission from the arterial bed to the intracranial compartment.

Cerebrovascular Pressure Reactivity

Another ICP-derived index is the pressure-reactivity index (PRx), which incorporates the idea of assessing cerebrovascular reaction by observing the response of ICP to slow spontaneous changes in ABP (see earlier text).[42]

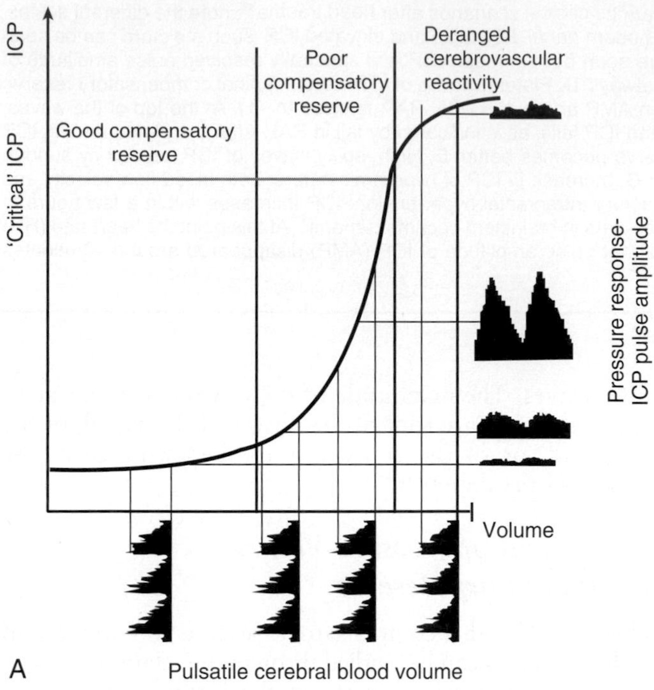

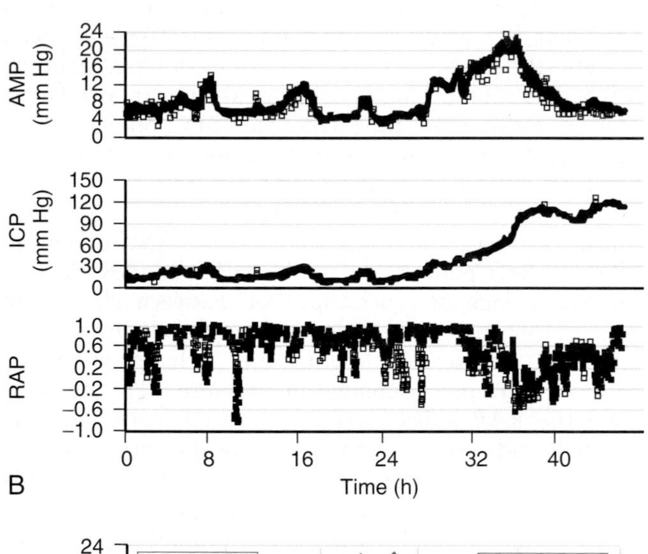

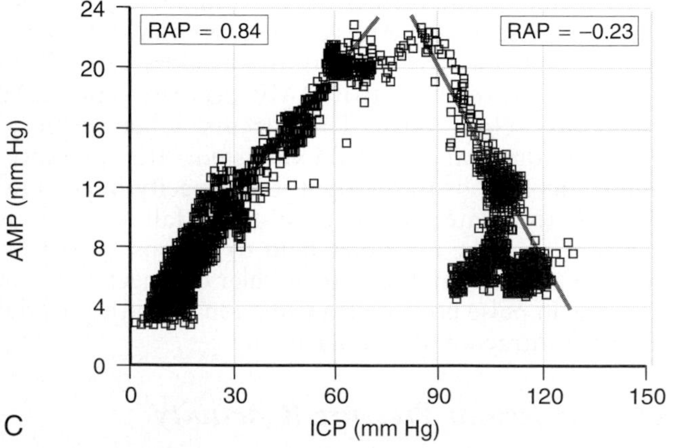

FIGURE 52–9 • A, In a simple model, pulse amplitude of intracranial pressure (ICP) (AMP, expressed along the y-axis on the right side of the panel) results from pulsatile changes in cerebral blood volume (expressed along the x-axis) transformed by the pressure-volume curve. This curve has three zones: a flat zone, expressing good compensatory reserve; an exponential zone, depicting poor compensatory reserve; and a flat zone again, seen at very high ICP (above the "critical" ICP) depicting derangement of normal cerebrovascular responses. The pulse amplitude of ICP is low and does not depend on mean ICP in the first zone. The pulse amplitude increases linearly with mean ICP in the zone of poor compensatory reserve. In the third zone, the pulse amplitude starts to decrease with rising ICP. **B,** Example of the relationship between AMP and mean ICP recorded during a 46-hour period, during which terminal intracranial hypertension developed. Pulse amplitude increased first proportionally to the change in ICP but started to decrease when ICP increased above 80 mmHg. **C,** The regression plot between AMP and ICP indicates a biphasic relationship of positive and negative slopes. The correlation coefficient between AMP and ICP (RAP) was positive before 32 hours, but negative after that, and this indicated terminal cerebrovascular deterioration.[41]

For example, when the cerebrovascular bed is normally reactive, any change in ABP produces an inverse change in CBV and thus ICP. When cerebrovascular reactivity is disturbed, changes in ABP are transmitted passively to ICP. Again, with the use of computational methods similar to those used for the calculation of the RAP index, PRx is determined with the calculation of the correlation coefficient between 40 consecutive, time-averaged data points of ICP and ABP. A positive PRx signifies a positive gradient of the regression line between the slow components of ABP and ICP, which is suggested as being associated with passive behavior of a nonreactive vascular bed (Fig. 52–10, *A*).[10] A negative value of PRx reflects a normally reactive vascular bed, as ABP waves provoke inversely correlated waves in ICP (Fig. 52–10, *B*). In practice, this index correlates well with TCD ultrasonography indices of autoregulation.[10] Also, abnormal values of both PRx and RAP, which are indicative respectively of poor autoregulation or deranged cerebrospinal compensatory reserve, have been shown to be predictive of a poor outcome in adults after head injury.[8]

Monitoring Optimal Cerebral Perfusion Pressure Derived from Intracranial Pressure Parameters

Both the PRx and the RAP index can be used to evaluate secondary variables that combine the value of absolute ICP and CPP with information about the state of autoregulatory and compensatory reserves. In adults with head trauma, PRx plotted against CPP gives a U-shape curve that indicates, for most patients, a value of CPP for which pressure-reactivity is optimal.[8] This optimal pressure can be estimated with the plotting and analyzing of the PRx-CPP curve in sequential 6-hour periods; the greater the distance between the current and the "optimal" CPP, the more likely outcome will be poor. This potentially useful method attempts to refine the current approach to CPP-oriented therapy: both too low (ischemia) and too high (hyperemia and secondary increase in ICP) CPP are detrimental. It has been suggested that CPP in adults

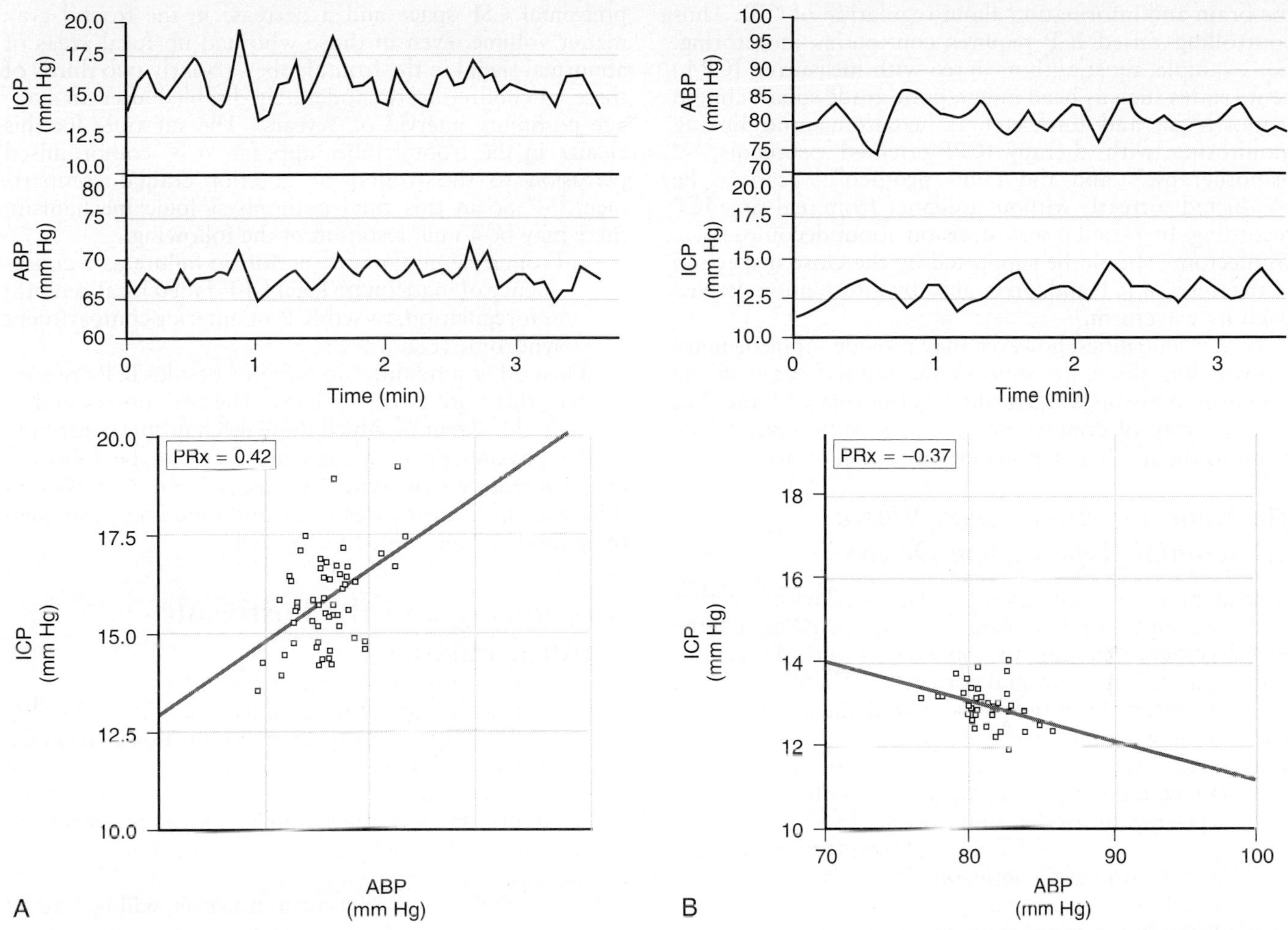

FIGURE 52–10 • Relationship between slow waves of arterial pressure (ABP) and intracranial pressure (ICP). **A,** Slow waves in ICP and ABP produce a positive correlation (*lower left panel*), giving a positive value of the pressure-reactivity index (PRx), which indicates loss of cerebrovascular reserve. **B,** Coherent waves both in ABP and ICP produced a negative correlation coefficient, when plotted on the regression graph (lower right), giving values of PRx clearly negative.

should be optimized to maintain CPP in the globally most favorable state.[8]

Quantifying the Cumulative ICP-CPP Insult to the Brain

In adults with severe head injury, there are a number of ways in which the cumulative insult to the brain can be quantified. For example, an average ICP above 25 mmHg during the whole period of monitoring doubles the risk of death.[8] Averaged values of the RAP index and the PRx are also strong predictors of fatal outcome. Both these indices suggest that good vascular reactivity is an important element of brain homeostasis, which enables the brain to protect itself against an uncontrollable rise in intracerebral volume. Also, a low value of slow waves of ICP is also indicative of a fatal outcome after head injury. Because each of these parameters—ICP, PRx, and the power of ICP slow waves—is an independent predictor of outcome, these three variables, although mutually correlated, should be considered jointly in any analysis.

In regard to mean CPP, it is now one of the variables that is actively targeted with treatment; therefore it has lost its predictive power for outcome. This fact does not mean that short-term decreases in CPP ("CPP insults") have become any more benign, but they are probably better managed now and do not frequently produce ischemia (see also Chapter 107).

The Clinical Utility of Intracranial Pressure Monitoring and Other Monitoring Modalities

The continuous measurement of ICP is an essential modality in most brain monitoring systems. After a decade of enthusiastic attempts to introduce newer modalities for brain monitoring (e.g., tissue oxygenation, microdialysis, cortical blood flow, TCD ultrasonography, and jugular bulb oxygen saturation), it is becoming increasingly obvious that ICP is robust, only moderately invasive, and can be realistically conducted in most critical care units. In previous sections of this chapter we have discussed that ICP measurement is a complex modality that contains information about compensatory mechanisms intrinsic to the brain and information about regulation of CBF. Thus controlling raised ICP requires continuous monitoring. For example, most authors agree with measuring ICP in acute states such as head injury, poor-grade subarachnoid hemorrhage, and intracerebral hematoma and linking monitoring with therapy. CPP-oriented protocols,[43,44] osmotherapy,[45] and the Lund protocol[9,46] cannot be conducted correctly without guidance from real-time ICP recording. In a similar way, decision about decompressive craniectomy should be supported by the close inspection of the trend of ICP and, preferably, by information derived from its waveform.[47]

Newer modalities, however, may provide supplementary information about the state of the injured brain in the comatose patient. We now discuss the role of these, but first, by way of context, some consideration should be given to the mechanisms underlying brain injury.

Mechanism of Brain Injury Where Intracranial Hypertension Occurs

In head injury, MRI commonly reveals focal lesions within the frontal and temporal lobes, the temporal poles, and the limbic system, including its connections with the orbitofrontal surface of the frontal cortex.[48,49] There are several injurious mechanisms whereby pathologic change may occur in these regions. In the temporal lobes or its connections, there may be manifestations of the following:

1. Direct high-speed impact injury with or without acceleration-deceleration forces. In this instance, the medial temporal lobe is vulnerable to mechanical deformation and contusion.[50]
2. Metabolic perturbation resulting from vascular or systemic factors such as hypoxia, ischemia, hypoglycemia, and seizures. In these head injury–related insults, there is a predilection for vulnerability within a structure in the temporal limbic system, the hippocampus.[51]
3. Diffuse axonal injury as a consequence of rotational forces at the time of injury affecting axonal integrity; thereafter there is secondary or postacute deafferentation or deefferentation of structures such as the hippocampus.[52,53]
4. Raised ICP with brain swelling resulting in pressure necrosis of the main cortical input to the hippocampus, to the parahippocampal gyrus, and against the free edge of the tentorium cerebelli.[54]

Each of these four mechanisms may result in injuries that, in the long-term, induce deficits in neuropsychologic function. However, only the fourth mechanism (pressure necrosis of the parahippocampal gyrus) depends on the development and presence of brain swelling.[54]

A fifth injurious mechanism, which is important in regard to morbidity, is best shown by the disease to the frontal lobes. Recent research in children suggests that emerging or developing executive functions may be particularly vulnerable when the frontal lobes are injured in childhood.[55,56] In the context of head injury, such an insult is not excluded by the absence of focal brain lesions detected with MRI. For example, Berryhill et al[57] used MRI-volumetric analysis to study pediatric survivors of severe head injury. Measurements in the frontal lobes disclosed an increase in the prefrontal CSF space and a decrease in the frontal gray matter volume, even in those who had no focal areas of abnormal signal in the frontal lobes. (Nearly two thirds of these 14 children were moderately disabled after an average postinjury interval of 3 years.) The substrate for this change in the frontal lobes appears to be compromised perfusion to the frontal or anterior cranial compartment.[58,59] So in this final pathophysiologic mechanism, there may be a manifestation of the following:

5. Frontal hemodynamic perfusion failure as a consequence of inadequate local CBF, failed local cerebral autoregulation, raised ICP, or anterior compartment syndrome (Fig. 52–11).

When other modalities to monitor besides ICP are considered, there are two problems. The first one is understanding the extent to which these mechanisms contribute to the physiologic derangements that can be followed in the intensive care unit. The second one is making a difference in patient assessment and outcomes, provided these mechanisms can be influenced.

Monitoring and the Postinsult Natural History

In a patient with a severe head injury, the value and utility of monitoring may serve a spectrum of functions. Given the five potential mechanisms outlined in the previous section (i.e., direct mechanical effect, metabolic perturbation, axonal injury, brain swelling, and hemodynamic perfusion failure), specific foci, whether for assessment or treatment, can be identified for monitoring. The potential for treatment, rather than for assessment, however, will be limited by the time course over which the pathophysiologic monitoring is enacted. For example, the following need to be considered: What processes occur at the time of injury, what are the subsequent epiphenomena of these events, and what are the secondary factors that are amenable to treatment and altered outcome?

Mechanisms 1 and 3 occur at the time of injury, and mechanism 2 starts during the interval between accident and arrival in the intensive care unit, although this may, in part, be avoidable with attention to emergency care and

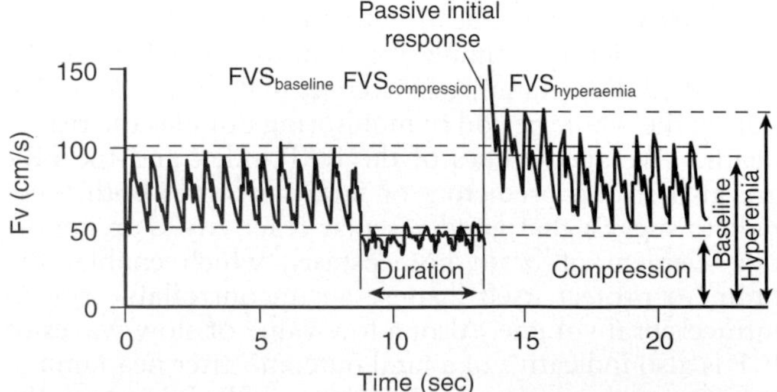

FIGURE 52–11 • Transient hyperemic response used test to assess autoregulation: middle cerebral artery (MCA) blood flow velocity (Fv) is measured with transcranial Doppler ultrasonography before, during, and after a 6-second compression of the carotid artery. Hyperemia after release of compression signifies properly functioning vascular reactivity.

life support.[60] Mechanisms 4 and 5 are processes in which treatment that is directed by intensive care monitoring presumably has the potential for altered outcome (i.e., focal brain tissue shifts and hemodynamic perfusion failure). One important issue, therefore, is the natural history of brain swelling and local compartment syndrome after severe head injury.

In traumatic head injury intracranial hypertension occurs when there is brain swelling or a hematoma occupying significant space. In those with severe traumatic injury and abnormalities shown with computed tomography (CT) on admission, there is a greater than 50% chance of raised ICP.[61,62] Furthermore, in adults, this complication may occur in those whose CT scans appear normal, particularly if two of the following three features are present: age older than 40 years, unilateral or bilateral motor posturing, or systolic ABP below 90 mmHg. In those who do not require neurosurgery, the natural history of this complication can be as short as 3 days, but not infrequently it lasts for 7 to 10 days.[63] Thus in regard to brain tissue shifts and frontal compartment perfusion failure, the potential of a postinsult "therapeutic window" exists, and this also implies a goal for monitoring-directed therapy.

Newer Modalities: Supplementary Monitoring to Intracranial Pressure

In the broadest sense, many of the recently reported modalities that are available for the process of monitoring can be grouped into the following categories: acute stress response and acute phase reaction, neurochemical protein markers of injury, substrate delivery and utilization, and clinical neurophysiology. Each of these is considered in relation to the literature on head injury because this is the most common reason for instituting ICP monitoring.

Acute Stress Response and Acute Phase Reaction

These data are concerned with assessing some systemic effect of or response to head injury. The magnitude of this reaction may reflect the severity of that injury, or possibly the reaction itself may be part of the pathologic mechanism. For example, experimentally, subsets of neurons from the hippocampus and frontal region have an exaggerated vulnerability to the combination of cell metabolic stress and endogenous steroids.[64,65]

In adults, the acute phase of illness after head injury is characterized by changes in plasma cortisol, which displays a gradient that is proportional to the degree of neurologic dysfunction. This is a phenomenon best observed 1 day after injury. For example, Woolf et al[66] reported that plasma cortisol concentration on admission was increased in all of their patients, irrespective of injury severity. The cortisol gradient, although flattened, was still present on day 4 and disappeared 3 days later, by which time mean cortisol concentration approached, but had not reached, normal values. In a more recent study, Koiv et al[67] studied both the adrenergic and glucocorticoid components of the stress response in 55 head-injured adults. Their observations suggested that head injury caused activation of both of these components, depending on the severity of trauma. An inverse correlation was found between the venous levels of epinephrine, norepinephrine, and the Glasgow Coma Scale (GCS) score, with a similar but weaker relationship in adrenocorticotrophic hormone (ACTH), cortisol, and GCS. In general, these changes in hormonal levels were present during the 1-week research period. In patients whose CT scans revealed serious alterations in the mesencephalic-diencephalic area, however, plasma catecholamines and ACTH levels were relatively low, but, at the same time, their cortisol levels obtained maximal values. A similar acute stress response has been reported in children with head injury,[68] suggesting that, as in adults, this is a coordinated systemic insult.

More recently, Kalabalikis et al[69] have looked at serum markers of the acute phase response in 45 children with head injury. They reported that there were changes in both interleukin-6 (IL-6) and C-reactive protein (CRP): peak serum IL-6 occurred 4 hours after injury and decreased over time, and CRP, although normal 4 hours after injury, reached a peak level at 48 hours after injury. There was no relationship between these profiles and outcome, but there was a relationship with the severity of injury. Those patients with more severe GCS had higher peaks in these serum markers. Taken together with the data on acute stress (see earlier text), clearly, acute head injury is accompanied by a neuroendocrine and systemic inflammatory response, the intensity of which is consistent with the severity of injury.

Neurochemical Protein Markers of Injury

There has been growing interest in markers that are concerned with broadly assessing tissue integrity and cell-specific injury. The clinical measurement of two proteins may serve this purpose.[70] Neuron-specific enolase (NSE), an enzyme involved in glycolysis localized in neurons and axonal processes, potentially escapes into the blood and CSF at the time of neural injury. (This enzyme is also found in erythrocytes.) S-100B protein, a calcium-binding protein localized to astroglia, may also be released from cells at the time of cerebral damage.

A number of clinical monitoring studies of these proteins have been undertaken in patients with head injury. For example, in patients with mild traumatic brain injury, de Kruijk et al[71] found that in blood samples taken shortly after trauma, the median and range of NSE levels were similar in patients ($n = 104$) and controls ($n = 92$). They found, however, that S-100B levels were significantly higher, particularly in those patients with trauma who were also vomiting. Ingebrigtsen et al[72] selected a similar group of 50 patients (i.e., GCS score of 13 to 15 and CT scan showing no abnormalities). They found that serum S-100B protein levels were highest immediately after the trauma and then declined each hour thereafter so that the level was undetectable 6 hours after injury. Four of the 5 patients with an MRI-detectable brain contusion had detectable levels of S-100B.

In patients with more severe injuries (GCS score = 8), Raabe et al[73] found that the level of S-100B in venous blood was higher in nonsurvivors, and on logistic regression, the S-100B level was an independent predictor of outcome along with age, GCS score, ICP, and CT scan findings. These authors also reported that persistent elevation of S-100B for 3 to 5 days occurred even in patients with favorable outcome and no signs of secondary insults.[37,73] Finally, in this class of patient, venous NSE appears to perform poorly as a diagnostic marker of severity.[74] Its level rises acutely in patients with both favorable and unfavorable outcome. With a cut-off level of more than 100 μg/L, the likelihood ratio for positively identifying unfavorable outcome is approximately 2 (i.e., specificity 0.96 and sensitivity 0.09), which is of indeterminate diagnostic impact.

In children, Berger et al[75] have followed the levels of S-100B and NSE in CSF samples from patients with inflicted and noninflicted trauma. Of note, these authors found that in both mechanisms of trauma there was a single peak in S-100B at approximately 27 hours after injury, but there was a difference in the profile for NSE. After an initial or transient peak in NSE (around 11 hours after injury) in both forms of insult, inflicted trauma had the additional feature of a sustained and delayed peak at around 63 hours after injury.

There is still a dilemma after these various facts about neurochemical protein markers of injury have been collated. Does the very nature of sustaining a head injury initiate a normal, yet insignificant transient release (albeit marked in CSF) of NSE and S-100B into the circulation, or are patterns of injury with varying mechanisms such as cerebral contusion in the case of S-100B and unappreciated hypoxia-ischemia or diffuse neuroaxonal injury in the case of NSE unable to be identified?

Substrate Delivery and Utilization

These measurements are about assessing, restoring, controlling, or supporting viability of the brain, a region of cerebral tissue, or specific cell types. For example, as already stated in a previous section of this chapter, there is evidence that, in a patient with head injury, the frontal lobes are susceptible to hemodynamic perfusion failure.[55–59] For the most effective therapy for the injured brain, continuously monitoring substrate delivery is desirable because interruption of substrate delivery is a major factor of vulnerability to ischemic damage. Like cerebrovascular stroke, the frontal perfusion defect in head injury is most evident in the white matter.[59] On further study with proton magnetic resonance spectroscopy (^{1}H-MRS), even in normal-appearing tissue, there is evidence of resulting cell-specific damage and reaction. Garnett et al[76,77] reported ^{1}H-MRS in 26 head-injured adults who were examined about 12 days after injury. In a posterior part of a normal-appearing frontal lobe containing predominantly white matter, they found a reduced ratio of N-acetylaspartate to creatine, which indicated neuroaxonal cell damage, and an increased ratio of choline to creatine and a ratio of myoinositol to creatine that reflected glial reaction and proliferation. Ashwal et al[78] have also observed similar ^{1}H-MRS abnormalities in children with head injuries.

Regional CBF and metabolism can be assessed more directly in the critically ill patient with a head injury with positron emission tomography (PET) scanning.[79] "Triple oxygen" scanning permits the quantification of CBV, regional CBF, regional cerebral metabolic rate of oxygen ($CMRO_2$), and regional oxygen extraction fraction (OEF). The three radiolabeled tracers include carbon monoxide labeled with oxygen-15 (^{15}O), water labeled with ^{15}O, and $^{15}O_2$ gas. One potential hope of such an assessment is that it would enable the evaluation of regional flow-metabolism coupling, which may be absent or deranged in injured or compromised brain tissue.[80,81] Unfortunately, the validity of this approach is in question because the current mathematical models for the measurement incorporating the kinetics of the oxygen tracers are limited by inherent interrelationships. For example, there is mathematical coupling in the derivation of CBV, CBF, OEF, and $CMRO_2$. The derivation of CBF incorporates CBV data. The derivation of OEF incorporates CBF data. Finally, $CMRO_2$ is derived from the multiplication of OEF, CBF, and the rate of oxygen delivered to the tissue. Despite this theoretical failing, the technology has enabled some validation of another technique used in the assessment of hemodynamic perfusion failure, brain tissue oxygenation with microsensors (see later).

Jugular bulb oxygen saturation (S_jO_2) is currently the most popular technique used to measure cerebral oxygenation. There are, however, several shortcomings with this form of monitoring, not the least of which is that this is a global measure insensitive to small, though important, regional changes. The relatively recent development of implantable tissue oxygen and pH microsensors (and the approval of NeuroTrend [Codman, Raynham, Mass.] by the Food and Drug Administration) has meant that more direct regional assessments are now being made. The questions, though, are what is normal tissue oxygen tension and what does it mean? Recent reports in adults indicate that the threshold for abnormality is around 10 mmHg, [82–84] although the validity and appropriateness of using such an exact measure has been questioned by Gupta et al.[79] These investigators used PET scanning in 19 adults with head injuries to validate the reading of brain tissue oxygen pressure (P_tO_2) from a NeuroTrend sensor inserted into the frontal region. End-capillary oxygen tension (P_vO_2) was calculated from OEF (see earlier text) in a 20-mm region of interest around the sensor and compared with P_tO_2. No correlation was found between the absolute values of P_tO_2 and P_vO_2. In contrast, a significant correlation was obtained between the change in P_tO_2 and the change in P_vO_2 produced by a decrease in arterial carbon dioxide by approximately 1 kPa (7.5 mmHg). These authors, therefore, could only conclude that such monitoring be used to assess, in real time, the changes attributable to a particular intervention.

The final level of perfusion information in this category, tissue biochemical metabolic markers, can be provided by cerebral microdialysis. Currently, this approach is used predominantly for research purposes,[85] although it has been applied to monitoring during aneurysm neurosurgery to define the limits of vascular clipping.[86] This technology enables bedside measurement (usually hourly in the case of head injury) of levels of cerebral dialysate glucose, lactate, pyruvate, glutamate, and glycerol. Typically, glucose level and lactate-pyruvate ratio are used as indices of inadequate substrate delivery, altered metabolism, and ischemia. The potential importance of such measurements is illustrated by an observation reported by Bergsneider et al in 1997.[87] In 28 adults with severe head injuries, within the first week of injury, [^{18}F]-fluorodeoxyglucose-PET assessment of local cerebral metabolic rate of glucose revealed that 56% of the patients had presumptive evidence of tissue hyperglycolysis; that is, glucose utilization that measures two standard deviations above expected levels both regionally and globally in pericontusional tissue. In regard to dialysate increases in glutamate and glycerol, these are used as indices of cumulative tissue responses to secondary ischemic events such as intracranial hypertension, systemic hypotension, seizures, and contusions.[88–90] Before definite clinical utility, however, issues such as the specificity of these changes need to be resolved. For example, it is difficult to assess the significance of a small or moderate change in lactate, or lactate-pyruvate ratio, in the absence of knowing tissue pH and redox state. Also, if measurements are to be made hourly—dialysate flow rate of 0.3 µl/min is the most common—then what does a change represent: a concurrent acute event, a prolonged ongoing event, or an acute event that has now resolved but with abnormal tissue biochemistry (see also Chapter 107)?

Transcranial Doppler Ultrasonography and Assessment of Autoregulation

There are a number of uses for TCD ultrasonography in the assessment of cerebrovascular health. In the field of adult neurocritical care there has been much progress in applying this technology to head injury practice. The following discussion highlights the key issues. TCD ultrasonography provides noninvasive measurement of blood flow velocity in basal cerebral arteries.[24] Most data have been derived from the MCA. This vessel is readily accessible to the ultrasonographer; it is the most convenient for probe fixation and long-term monitoring, and it delivers the largest percentage of supratentorial blood. Although the blood flow velocity cannot express a baseline volume of flow, dynamic changes of CBF are usually reflected in the TCD readings.[24,91] The response of blood flow velocity to a critical decrease in CPP is sensitive and usually immediate (Fig. 52–11). It is this high dynamic resolution and close correlation with other hemodynamic modalities that has encouraged the development of the technique in clinical practice.

Increased baseline flow velocity (>100 cm/s) may indicate cerebral vasospasm or hyperemia.[92,93] Uncoupling between CBF and flow velocity in vasospasm has been documented both experimentally and clinically.[94] For example, if the ratio of flow velocity in the insonated artery to the velocity in the ipsilateral internal carotid artery is greater than 3, vasospasm is likely. A ratio lower than 2 indicates hyperemia as the cause for accelerated blood flow.[91] After severe head injury, cerebral autoregulation is frequently disturbed, although the extent of this disturbance may fluctuate with time.[8,10]

1. *Static test of autoregulation:* Methods for the static assessment of autoregulation rely on measurement of MCA blood flow velocity during changes in mean ABP induced by a vasopressor infusion. The static rate of autoregulation (SoR) can be calculated as the percentage increase in vascular resistance divided by the percentage rise in ABP. A SoR of 100% indicates fully intact autoregulation, whereas an SoR of 0% indicates fully depleted autoregulation.
2. *TCD reactivity to changes in carbon dioxide concentration:* Testing for carbon dioxide cerebrovascular reactivity has been shown to have an important application in the assessment of severe head injuries and other cerebrovascular conditions. Many authors have shown that cerebral vessels are reactive to changes in carbon dioxide when cerebral autoregulation had been impaired.[95] Carbon dioxide reactivity correlates significantly with outcome after head injury.[96] In patients with exhausted cerebral compensatory reserve, however, hypercapnia may provoke substantial changes in ICP. Therefore this method cannot be used without consideration of patient safety, particularly if baseline ICP is already elevated.
3. *Dynamic test of autoregulation:* Aaslid et al[97] have described a method in which a step decrease in ABP is achieved by the deflation of compressed leg cuffs while TCD flow velocity in the MCA is simultaneously monitored. An index called the *dynamic rate of autoregulation* (RoR) describes how quickly cerebral vessels react to the sudden fall in blood pressure.[97] The RoR is thought to express the autoregulatory reserve and, in adult volunteers, has been shown to correlate with blood carbon dioxide concentration in volunteers.[98]
4. *Transient hyperemic response test:* Short-term compression of the common carotid artery produces a marked decrease in MCA blood flow velocity in the ipsilateral hemisphere. During compression, the distal cerebrovascular bed dilates if autoregulation is intact. On release of the compression, transient hyperemia, which lasts for a few seconds, occurs until the distal cerebrovascular bed constricts to its former diameter. This sequence of events, which underlies the transient hyperemic response test, indicates a positive autoregulatory response (Fig. 52–11). In head injury, preliminary results show a positive correlation between the presence of a hyperemic response and outcome.[99]
5. *Continuous analysis of TCD ultrasonography with respiratory waves:* An interesting method of deriving the autoregulatory status from natural fluctuations in MCA blood flow velocity involves the assessment of phase shift between the superimposed respiratory and ABP waves during deep breathing.[100] A 0-degree phase shift indicates absent autoregulation, whereas a phase shift of 90 degrees indicates intact autoregulation. Such an approach may allow for the continuous assessment of autoregulation without performing potentially hazardous test maneuvers on arterial pressure.
6. *Continuous analysis of TCD flow velocity waveform:* In patients with severe head injuries, CPP monitoring can be correlated with mean blood flow velocity continuously. For example, consecutive CPP samples (averaged over 5-second periods) can be assessed with average flow velocity (collected over

5-minute epochs). The correlation coefficient (named *mean index* [Mx]) may be positive or negative, and the regression line describing the relationship between the systolic-, mean-, and diastolic-flow velocity and the CPP may be used for assessment. A positive correlation coefficient signifies positive association of flow velocity with CPP; a negative correlation coefficient signifies a negative association. In head injury, group analysis has shown that clinical outcome depends on the averaged autoregulation indices.[11] Furthermore, time analysis has shown that failure of autoregulation is a strong, independent predictor of fatal outcome after head injury.[101]

Clinical Neurophysiology

In comparison with the other categories already discussed, these data are unique in that they can provide some assessment of what the brain produces—activity. This may take the form of its global integrity (e.g., general brain activity) or of some specific electrophysiologic function (e.g., dysrhythmic or seizure activity and sensory pathway performance).

In comatose states, the electroencephalogram (EEG) can provide useful information about the severity and distribution of altered function of the cerebral cortex. Multiple factors, however, may affect the level of such activity, and in the context of pediatric head injury, the signals reflect the summed effects of brain temperature, cerebral perfusion, metabolic state, anesthesia, and drug action on the normal background activity expected for age or stage of brain development. Therefore while the technique itself is sensitive, the changes observed are generally not that specific, particularly when one considers the range of variables that will lead to altered EEG activity. Serial EEGs, however, can provide important, albeit intermittent, assessment of changes in cerebral function.[102] Alternatively, automated, signal-processed, continuous EEG can be used for uninterrupted surveillance of brain function. Various methods of displaying modified EEG data in an understandable and interpretable form have been developed and reported on,[103,104] although the value of these methods in the identification of those with likely poor prognosis has been questioned in recent studies. For example, in adults with severe head injury (n = 103, GCS score = 8), Moulton, Brown, and Konasiewicz[105] reported that signal-processed EEG data could not be relied on to base critical management decisions. In contrast, Thielen et al[106] found that in a group of 32 adults with head injuries (GCS score ≤8), a cut-off of EEG-silence ratio, which was derived from a mathematically processed EEG, at 20% was of high diagnostic impact in the identification of the Glasgow Outcome Scale (GOS) category at 6 months (GOS 4-5 compared with GOS 1-3). (The sensitivity was 0.91, the specificity was 0.91, and the likelihood ratio was < 0.1.) Finally, Murdoch-Eaton, Darowski, and Livingston[107] have reported a similar experience with continuous monitoring in 108 children with a variety of brain insults, although the presence of seizure activity featured highly in the prognostication.

In addition to the identification of background EEG activity (which, as discussed, has limited specificity) in the patient with head injury, identifying seizure activity may be more pertinent because its presence will result in a change in therapy. In this regard, Vespa et al[108] undertook continuous EEG monitoring in 94 adults with moderate-to-severe brain injuries. Convulsive and nonconvulsive seizures occurred in 22% of the patients, with 6 individuals displaying electrical status epilepticus. In more than half of the patients the seizures were diagnosed solely on the EEG monitoring. Of particular concern was the finding that these seizures occurred despite the unit's use of prophylactic anticonvulsant therapy. In another EEG study of comatose patients (n = 236), including children, Towne et al[109] also found that nonconvulsive status epilepticus was underrecognized, occurring in 8% of their comatose patients without signs of seizure activity. Finally, in children with head injury, Chiaretti et al [110] reviewed their clinical experience in 125 patients, 12% of whom had seizures within 24 hours of trauma. Taken together with the adult EEG studies, there certainly appears to be some merit in characterizing the role of seizure monitoring in children with head injuries, particularly because anticonvulsant prophylaxis seems to be failing to confer protection, and we can easily provide a remedy.

Somatosensory evoked potentials (SEPs) are widely used to assess neurophysiologic function in patients with severe head injury.[105] The strong predictive value of these potentials in comatose patients has been demonstrated in a number of pediatric series. The bilateral absence of the cortical components of the SEP is usually regarded as an ominous sign, invariably indicating a poor outcome. For example, Carter et al[111] recently reported on a series of 105 children with severe brain injury, in whom they had long-term (5 years) functional and health status outcomes. For bilaterally absent SEP responses the positive likelihood ratio of identifying unfavorable functional outcome was approximately 15 (specificity 0.96, sensitivity 0.57, and high diagnostic impact). The results for health status were of equally high diagnostic impact. The question that arises, though, is: Are these data sufficient for influencing practice, or should such assessment merely be used for stratifying patient prognosis at an early stage?

In 1997 Pohlmann-Eden et al[112] reviewed 18 studies in which the predictive value of SEPs in 758 comatose patients was analyzed. They identified 300 reports of patients with bilateral loss of cortical SEP responses, and of these patients, 286 died or remained in a vegetative state. Two of the remaining 16 surviving patients had a good outcome with functional independence; both were children.[113,114] In 1999, Schwarz et al[115] reported on four adults who survived despite bilateral loss of the cortical SEP; three of these patients had excellent outcome. Most recently, Wohlrab et al[116] reviewed 53 children with bilateral absent cortical SEP, 13 of whom had sustained severe head injury. Thirty of 53 children (57%) died within the first 4 weeks, and another 8 children within 4 years of the event (i.e., a total of 72%). Of the 15 surviving children (6 of whom had severe head injury), 2 children remained in a persistent vegetative state, 9 children had severe deficits (2 of these were head injuries), and 4 children had mild or moderate deficits (all of these were head injuries). Interestingly, 30 of the 53 children underwent repeated examinations, and in 8 of these, unilateral or bilateral cortical responses reappeared. Taken together, the poor prognostic implications of bilateral loss of SEPs are indisputable. Nevertheless the occurrence of recovery from, in the main, transiently absent cortical responses indicates that this finding alone does not imply irreversible dysfunction of the somatosensory pathway in the severely head-injured child. Absent SEPs should be interpreted carefully, particularly in conjunction with hypothermia, deep sedation, intoxication, or decompressive craniectomy.[117]

REFERENCES

1. Pickard JD, Czosnyka M, Steiner LA: Raised intracranial pressure, In Hughes RAC, editor: *I: neurological emergencies*, London, 2003, BMJ Publishing Group.
2. Marmarou A, Maset AL, Ward JD, et al: Contribution of CSF and vascular factors to elevation of ICP in severely head-injured patients, *J Neurosurg* 66:883-890, 1987.
3. Czosnyka M, Richards HK, Czosnyka Z, et al: Vascular components of cerebrospinal fluid compensation, *J Neurosurg* 90:752-759, 1999.
4. Davson H, Hollingsworth G, Segal MB: The mechanism of drainage of the cerebrospinal fluid, *Brain* 93:665-678, 1970.
5. Czosnyka M, Piechnik S, Richards HK, et al: Contribution of mathematical modelling to the bedside tests of cerebrovascular autoregulation, *J Neurol Neurosurg Psychiatry* 63:721-731, 1997.
6. Miller JD, Stanek A, Langfitt TW: Concepts of cerebral perfusion pressure and vascular compression during intracranial hypertension, *Prog Brain Res* 35:411-432, 1972.
7. Tasker RC: Neurocritical care and traumatic brain injury, *Indian J Pediatr* 68:257-266, 2001.
8. Steiner LA, Czosnyka M, Piechnik SK, et al: Continuous monitoring of cerebrovascular pressure reactivity allows determination of optimal cerebral perfusion pressure in patients with traumatic brain injury, *Crit Care Med* 30:733-738, 2002.
9. Asgeirsson B, Grande PO, Nordstrom CH: A new therapy of post-trauma brain oedema based on haemodynamic principles for brain volume regulation, *Intensive Care Med* 20:260-267, 1994.
10. Czosnyka M, Smielewski P, Kirkpatrick P, et al: Continuous assessment of the cerebral vasomotor reactivity in head injury, *Neurosurgery* 41:11-19, 1997.
11. Czosnyka M, Smielewski P, Kirkpatrick P, Menon DK, Pickard JD: Monitoring of cerebral autoregulation in head-injured patients, Stroke 1996, 27:829-834.
12. Czosnyka M, Smielewski P, Piechnik S, et al: Hemodynamic characterization of intracranial pressure plateau waves in head-injured patients, *J Neurosurg* 91:11-19, 1999.
13. Guillaume J, Janny P: Manometrie intracranienne continué interest de la methode et premiers resultants, Rev Neurol (Paris) 84:131-142, 1951.
14. Lundberg N: Continuous recording and control of ventricular fluid pressure in neurosurgical practice, *Acta Psychiatr Neurol Scand* 36(suppl 149):1-193, 1960.
15. Ghajar J: Intracranial pressure monitoring techniques, *New Horizions* 3:395-399, 1995.
16. Czosnyka M, Czosnyka Z, Pickard JD: Laboratory testing of three intracranial pressure microtransducers, *Neurosurgery* 38:219-224, 1996 (technical report).
17. Piper I, Barnes A, Smith D, et al: The Camino intracranial pressure sensor: is it optimal technology? An internal audit with a review of current intracranial pressure monitoring technologies, *Neurosurgery* 49:1158-1164, 2001.
18. Reid A, Marchbanks RJ, Martin R, et al: Mean intracranial pressure monitoring by an audiological technique-a pilot study, *J Neurol Neurosurg Psychiatry* 52:610-612, 1989.
19. Schoser BG, Riemenschneider N, Hansen HC: The impact of raised intracranial pressure on cerebral venous hemodynamics: a prospective venous transcranial Doppler ultrasonography study, *J Neurosurg* 91:744-749, 1999.
20. Petkus V, Ragauskas A, Jurkonis R: Investigation of intracranial media ultrasonic monitoring model, *Ultrasonics* 40:829-833, 2002.
21. Schmidt B, Klingelhofer J, Schwarze JJ, et al: Noninvasive prediction of intracranial pressure curves using transcranial Doppler ultrasonography and blood pressure curves, *Stroke* 28:2465-2472, 1997.
22. Schoser BG, Riemenschneider N, Hansen HC: The impact of raised intracranial pressure on cerebral venous hemodynamics: a prospective venous transcranial Doppler ultrasonography study, *J Neurosurg* 91:744-749, 1999.
23. Reid A, Marchbanks RJ, Martin R, et al: Mean intracranial pressure monitoring by an audiological technique-a pilot study, *J Neurol Neurosurg Psychiatry* 52:610-612, 1989.
24. Aaslid R, Markwalder TM, Nornes H: Noninvasive transcranial Doppler ultrasound recording of flow velocity in basal cerebral arteries, *J Neurosurg* 57:769-774, 1982.
25. Chan KH, Miller JD, Dearden NM, et al: The effect of changes in cerebral perfusion pressure upon middle cerebral artery blood flow velocity and jugular bulb venous oxygen saturation after severe brain injury, *J Neurosurg* 77:55-61, 1992.
26. Dewey RC, Pieper HP, Hunt WE: Experimental cerebral hemodynamics. Vasomotor tone, critical closing pressure, and vascular bed resistance, *Neurosurgery* 41:597-606, 1974.
27. Czosnyka M, Smielewski P, Piechnik S, et al: Critical closing pressure in cerebrovascular circulation, *J Neurol Neurosurg Psychiatry* 66:606-611, 1999.
28. Aaslid R, Lundar T, Lindegaard K-F, et al: Estimation of cerebral perfusion pressure from arterial blood pressure and transcranial Doppler recordings. In: Miller JD, Teasdale GM, Rowan JO, Galbraith SL, Mendelow AD, editors: *Intracranial pressure VI*, Berlin, 1986, Springer-Verlag.
29. Czosnyka M, Matta BF, Smielewski P, et al: Cerebral perfusion pressure in head-injured patients: a noninvasive assessment using transcranial Doppler ultrasonography, *J Neurosurg* 88:802-808, 1998.
30. Schmidt EA, Czosnyka M, Matta BF, et al: Non-invasive cerebral perfusion pressure (nCPP): evaluation of the monitoring methodology in head injured patients, *Acta Neurochir Suppl* 76:451-452, 2000.
31. Schmidt B, Klingelhofer J, Schwarze JJ, et al: Noninvasive prediction of intracranial pressure curves using transcranial Doppler ultrasonography and blood pressure curves, *Stroke* 28:2465-2472, 1997.
32. Wolfla CE, Luerssen TG, Bowman RM, et al: Brain tissue pressure gradients created by expanding frontal epidural mass lesion, *J Neurosurg* 84:642-647, 1996.
33. Albeck MJ, Borgesen SE, Gjerris F, et al: Intracranial pressure and cerebrospinal fluid outflow conductance in healthy subjects, *J Neurosurg* 74:597-600, 1991.
34. Chapman PH, Cosman ER, Arnold MA: The relationship between ventricular fluid pressure and body position in normal subjects and subjects with shunts: a telemetric study, *Neurosurgery* 26:181-189, 1990.
35. Carney NA, Chesnut R, Kochanek PM: Guidelines for the acute medical management of severe traumatic brain injury in infants, children, and adolescents, *Pediatr Crit Care Med* 4:S25-S27, 2003.
36. Czosnyka M, Pickard JD: Monitoring and interpretation of intracranial pressure, *J Neurol Neurosurg Psychiatry* 75:813-821, 2004.
37. Raabe A, Menon DK, Gupta S, et al: Jugular venous and arterial concentrations of serum S-100B protein in patients with severe head injury: a pilot study, *J Neurol Neurosurg Psychiatry* 65:930-932, 1998.
38. Lundberg N: Continuous recording and control of ventricular fluid pressure in neurosurgical practice, Acta Psychiatr Neurol Scand 36(suppl 149):1-193, 1960.
39. Lofgren J, von Essen C, Zwetnow NN: The pressure-volume curve of the cerebrospinal fluid space in dogs, *Acta Neurol Scand* 49: 557-574, 1973.
40. Avezaat CJ, van Eijndhoven JH, Wyper DJ: Cerebrospinal fluid pulse pressure and intracranial volume-pressure relationships, *J Neurol Neurosurg Psychiatry* 42:687-700, 1979.
41. Balestreri M, Czosnyka M, Steiner LA, et al: Intracranial hypertension: what additional information can be derived from ICP waveform after head injury? *Acta Neurochir*,
42. Muizelaar JP, Ward JD, Marmarou A, et al: Cerebral blood flow and metabolism in severely head-injured children, *Autoregulation. Neurosurg* 71:72-76, 1989.
43. Rosner MJ, Rosner SD, Johnson AH: Cerebral perfusion pressure: management protocol and clinical results, *J Neurosurg* 83:949-962, 1995.

44. Patel HC, Menon DK, Tebbs S, et al: Specialist neurocritical care and outcome from head injury, *Intensive Care Med* 28:547-553, 2002.
45. Bullock R. Mannitol and other diuretics in severe neurotrauma, *New Horizons* 3:448-452, 1995.
46. Grande PO: The "Lund concept" for treatment of severe brain trauma: a physiological approach. In *Yearbook of intensive care and emergency medicine,* Vincent J-L, ed. Springer-Verlag, 806-820, 2004.
47. Whitfield PC, Patel H, Hutchinson PJ, et al: Bifrontal decompressive craniectomy in the management of posttraumatic intracranial hypertension, *Br J Neurosurg* 15:500-507, 2001.
48. Levin HS, Amparo E, Eisenberg HM, et al: Magnetic resonance imaging and computerized tomography in relation to the neurobehavioural sequelae of mild and moderate head injuries, *J Neurosurg* 66:706-713, 1987.
49. Wallesch CW, Curio N, Kutz S, et al: Outcome after mild-to-moderate blunt head injury: effects of focal lesions and diffuse axonal injury, *Brain Injury* 15:401-412, 2001.
50. Sweeney JE: Non impact brain injury: grounds for clinical study of the neuropsychological effects of acceleration forces, *Clinical Neuropsychologist* 6:443-457, 1992.
51. Kotapka MJ, Graham DI, Adams JH, et al: Hippocampal pathology in fatal human head injury without high intracranial pressure, *J Neurotrauma* 11:317-324, 1994.
52. Gale SD, Johnson SC, Bigler ED, et al: Nonspecific white matter degeneration following traumatic brain injury, *J International Neuropsychol Soc* 1:17-28, 1995.
53. Tate DF, Bigler ED: Fornix and hippocampal atrophy in traumatic brain injury, *Learn Mem* 7:442-446, 2000.
54. Adams JH, Graham DI: The relationship between ventricular fluid pressure and the neuropathology of raised intracranial pressure, *Neuropathol Appl Neurobiol* 2:323-332, 1976.
55. Stuss D: Biological and psychological development of executive functions, *Brain Cogn* 20:8-23, 1992.
56. Garth J, Anderson V, Wrennall J: Executive function following moderate to severe frontal lobe injury: impact of injury and age at injury, *Pediatr Rehabil* 1:99-108, 1997.
57. Berryhill P, Lilly MA, Levin HS, et al: Frontal lobe changes after severe diffuse closed head injury in children: a volumetric study of magnetic resonance imaging, *Neurosurgery* 3 7:392-399, 1995.
58. Abu-Judeh HH, Parker R, Singh M, et al: SPET brain perfusion imaging in mild traumatic brain injury without loss of consciousness and normal computed tomography, *Nucl Med Commun* 20:505-510, 1999.
59. Vinjamuri S, O'Driscoll K: Significance of white matter abnormalities in patients with closed head injury, *Nucl Med Commun* 21: 645-649, 2000.
60. Sharples PM, Storey A, Aynsley-Green A, et al: Avoidable factors contributing to death of children with head injury, *BMJ* 300:87-91, 1990.
61. Narayan RK, Kishore PRS, Becker DP, et al: Intracranial pressure: to monitor or not to monitor? A review of our experience with severe head injury, *J Neurosurg* 56:650-659, 1982.
62. Ghajar J: Traumatic brain injury, *Lancet* 356:923-929, 2000.
63. Natale JE, Joseph JG, Helfaer MA, et al: Early hyperthermia after traumatic brain injury in children: risk factors, influence on length of stay, and effect on short-term neurologic status, *Crit Care Med* 28:2608-2615, 2000.
64. Ajilore OA, Sapolsky RM: Application of silicon microphysiometer to tissue slices: detection of metabolic correlates of selective vulnerability, *Brain Res* 752:99-106, 1997.
65. Lathe R: Hormones and the hippocampus, *J Endocrinol* 169:205-231, 2001.
66. Woolf PD, Cox C, Kelly M, et al: The adrenocortical response to brain injury: correlation with the severity of neurologic dysfunction, effects of intoxication and patient outcome, *Alcoholism* 14:917-921, 1990.
67. Koiv L, Merisalu E, Zilmer K, et al: Changes of sympatho-adrenal and hypothalamo-pituitary-adrenocortical system in patients with head injury, *Acta Neurol Scand* 96:52-58, 1997.
68. Fanconi S, Kloti J, Meuli M, et al: Dexamethasone therapy and endogenous cortisol production in severe pediatric head injury, *Intensive Care Med* 14:163-166, 1988.
69. Kalabalikis P, Papazoglou K, Gouriotis D, et al: Correlation between serum IL-6 and CRP levels and severity of head injury in children, *Intensive Care Med* 25:288-292, 1999.
70. Kochanek PM, Clark RS, Ruppel RA, et al: Biochemical, cellular, and molecular mechanisms in the evolution of secondary damage after severe traumatic brain injury in infants and children: lessons learned from the bedside, *Pediatr Crit Care Med* 1:4-19, 2000.
71. de Kruijk JR, Leffers P, Menheere PP, et al: S-100B and neuron-specific enolase in serum of mild traumatic brain injury patients. A comparison with healthy controls, *Acta Neurol Scand* 103: 175-179, 2001.
72. Ingebrigtsen T, Waterloo K, Jacobsen EA, et al: Traumatic brain damage in minor head injury: relation of serum S-100 protein measurements to magnetic resonance imaging and neurobehavioural outcome, *Neurosurger* 45:468-475, 1999.
73. Raabe A, Grolms C, Sorge O, et al: Serum S-100B protein in severe head injury, *Neurosurger* 45:477-483, 1999.
74. Raabe A, Grolms C, Seifert V: Serum markers of brain damage and outcome prediction in patients after severe head injury, *Br J Neurosurg* 13:56-59, 1999.
75. Berger RP, Pierce MC, Wisniewski SR, et al: Neuron-specific enolase and S100B in cerebrospinal fluid after severe traumatic brain injury in infants and children, *Pediatrics* 109:E31, 2002.
76. Garnett MR, Blamire AM, Rajagopalan B, et al: Evidence for cellular damage in normal-appearing white matter correlates with injury severity in patients following traumatic brain injury. A magnetic resonance spectroscopy study, *Brain* 123:1403-1409, 2000.
77. Garnett MR, Blamire AM, Corkill RG, et al: Early proton magnetic resonance spectroscopy in normal-appearing brain correlates with outcome in patients following traumatic brain injury, *Brain* 123:2046-2054, 2000.
78. Ashwal S, Holshouser BA, Shu SK, et al: Predictive value of proton magnetic resonance spectroscopy in pediatric closed head injury, *Pediatric Neurol* 23:114-125, 2000.
79. Gupta AK, Hutchinson PJ, Fryer T, et al: Measurement of brain tissue oxygenation performed using positron emission tomography scanning to validate a novel monitoring method, *J Neurosurg* 96:263-68, 2002.
80. Obrist WD, Langfitt TW, Jaggi JL, et al: Cerebral blood flow and metabolism in comatose patients with acute head injury. Relationship to intracranial hypertension, *J Neurosurg* 61:241-253, 1984.
81. Menzel M, Doppenberg EMR, Zauner A, et al: Increased inspired oxygen concentration as a factor in improved tissue oxygenation and tissue lactate levels after severe human head injury, *J Neurosurg* 91:1-10, 1999.
82. Meixensberger J, Kunze E, Barcsay E, et al: Clinical cerebral microdialysis: brain metabolism and brain tissue oxygenation after acute brain injury, *Neurol Res* 23:801-806, 2001.
83. Imberti R, Bellinzona G, Langer M: Cerebral tissue PO2 and SjvO2 changes during moderate hyperventilation in patients with severe traumatic brain injury, *J Neurosurg* 96:97-102, 2002.
84. Gupta AK, Al-Rawi PG, Hutchinson PJ, et al: Effect of hypothermia on brain tissue oxygenation in patients with severe head injury, *Br J Anaesth* 88:188-192, 2002.
85. Hillered L, Persson L: Theory and practice of microdialysis—prospect for future clinical use, *Acta Neurochir Suppl (Wien)* 75:3-6, 1999.
86. Hutchinson PJ, Al-Rawi PG, O'Connell MT, et al: Monitoring of brain metabolism during aneurysm surgery using microdialysis and brain multiparameter sensors, *Neurol Res* 21:352-358, 1999.
87. Bergsneider M, Hovda DA, Shalmon E, et al: Cerebral hyperglycolysis following severe traumatic brain injury in humans: a positron emission tomography study, *J Neurosurg* 86:241-251, 1997.
88. Persson L, Hillered L: Chemical monitoring of neurosurgical intensive care patients using intracerebral microdialysis, *Neurosurg* 76:72-80, 1992.
89. Mendelowitsch A, Sekhar LN, Wright DC, et al: An increase in extracellular glutamate is a sensitive method of detecting ischaemic neuronal damage during cranial base and cerebrovascular surgery. An in vivo microdialysis study, *Acta Neurochir Suppl (Wien)* 140:349-355, 1998.
90. Hutchinson PJ, Al-Rawi PG, O'Connell MT, et al: On-line monitoring of substrate delivery and brain metabolism in head injury, *Acta Neurochir Suppl (Wien)* 76:431-435, 2001.
91. Lindegaard KF, Grolimund P, Aalid R, et al: Evaluation of cerebral AVM's using transcranial Doppler ultrasound, *J Neurosurg* 65:335-344, 1986.

92. Compton JS, Teddy PJ. Cerebral arterial vasospasm following severe head injury: a transcranial Doppler study, *Br J Neurosurg* 1:435-439, 1987.
93. Aaslid R, Huber P, Nornes H: Evaluation of cerebrovascular spasm with transcranial Doppler ultrasound, *J Neurosurg* 60:37-41, 1984.
94. Nelson RJ, Perry S, Hames TK, et al: Transcranial Doppler ultrasound studies of cerebral autoregulation and subarachnoid hemorrhage in the rabbit, *J Neurosurg* 73:601-610, 1990.
95. Envoldsen EM, Jensen FT: Autoregulation and CO2 responses of cerebral blood flow in patients with acute severe head injury, *J Neurosurg* 48:689-703, 1978.
96. Steiger HJ, Aaslid R, Stooss R, et al: Transcranial Doppler monitoing in head injury: relationships between type of injury, flow velocities, vasoreactivity and outcome, *Neurosurgery* 34:79-85, 1994.
97. Aaslid R, Lindegaard KF, Sorteberg W, et al: Cerebral autoregulation dynamics in humans, *Stroke* 20:45-52, 1989.
98. Smielewski P, Czosnyka P, Kirkpatrick P, et al: Assessment of cerebral autoregulation using carotid artery compression, *Stroke* 27: 2197-2203, 1996.
99. Smielewski P, Czosnyka M, Kirkpatrick P, et al: Evaluation of transient hyperaemic response test in head injured patients, *J Neurosurg* 86:773-778, 1997.
100. Diehl RR, Linden D, Lucke D, et al: Phase relationship between cerebral blood flow velocity and blood pressure. A clinical test of autoregulation, *Stroke* 26:1801-1804, 1995.
101. Czosnyka M, Smielewski P, Piechnik S, et al: Cerebral autoregulation following head injury, *J Neurosurg* 95:756-763, 2001.
102. Tasker RC, Boyd S, Harden A, et al: Monitoring in non-traumatic coma. Part II: electroencephalography, *Arch Dis Child* 63:895-899, 1988.
103. Talwar D, Torres F: Continuous electrophysiologic monitoring of cerebral function in the pediatric intensive care unit, *Pediatr Neurol* 4:137-147, 1988
104. Tasker RC, Boyd S, Harden A, et al: The cerebral function analysing monitor in paediatric medical intensive care: application and limitations, *Intensive Care Med* 16:60-68, 1990.
105. Moulton RJ, Brown JI, Konasiewicz SJ: Monitoring severe head injury: a comparison of EEG and somatosensory evoked potentials, *Can J Neurol Sci* 25:S7-S11, 1998.
106. Thielen HJ, Ragaller M, Tscho U, et al: Electroencephalogram silence ratio for early outcome prognosis in severe head trauma, *Crit Care Med* 28:3522-3529, 2000.
107. Murdoch-Eaton D, Darowski M, Livingston J: Cerebral function monitoring in paediatric intensive care: useful features for predicting outcome, *Dev Med Child Neurol* 43:91-96, 2001.
108. Vespa PM, Nuwer MR, Nenov V, et al: Increased incidence and impact of nonconvulsive and convulsive seizures after traumatic brain injury as detected by continuous electroencephalographic monitoring, *J Neurosurg* 91:750-760, 1999.
109. Towne AR, Waterhouse EJ, Boggs JG, et al: Prevalence of nonconvulsive status epilepticus in comatose patients, *Neurology* 25: 340-345, 2000.
110. Chiaretti A, De Benedictis R, Polidori G, et al: Early posttraumatic seizures in children with head injury, *Childs Nerve Syst* 16:862-866, 2000.
111. Carter BG, Taylor A, Butt W: Severe brain injury in children: long-term outcome and its prediction using somatosensory evoked potentials (SEPs), *Intensive Card Med* 25:722-728, 1999.
112. Pohlmann-Eden B, Dingethal K, Bender HJ, et al: How reliable is the predictive value of SEP (somatosensory evoked potentials) patterns in severe brain damage with special regard to bilateral loss of cortical responses? *Intensive Care Med* 23:301-308, 1997.
113. De Meirleir LJ, Taylor MJ: Prognostic utility of SEPs in comatose children, *Pediatr Neurol* 3:78-82, 1987.
114. Taylor MJ, Farrell EJ: Comparison of the prognostic utility of VEPs and SEPs in comatose children, *Pediatr Neurol* 5:145-150, 1989.
115. Schwarz S, Schwab S, Aschoff A, Hacke W: Favorable recovery from bilateral loss of somatosensory evoked potentials, *Crit Care Med* 27:182-187, 1999.
116. Wohlrab G, Boltshanser E, Schmitt B: Neurological outcome in comatose children with bilateral loss of cortical somatosensory evoked potentials, *Neuropediatrics* 32:271-274, 2001.
117. Beca J, Cox PN, Taylor MJ, et al: Somatosensory evoked potentials for prediction of outcome in acute severe brain injury, *J Pediatr* 126:44-49, 1995.

CHAPTER 53

Postoperative Neurosurgical Intensive Care

Hector E. James

PEARLS

- In infancy, untreated hydrocephalus will usually present with progressive macrocrania and a full fontanelle; it will subsequently cause loss of appetite, irritability, and further clinical deterioration.
- In childhood, hydrocephalus may present with progressive headaches, loss of appetite, vomiting, and irritability.
- Furosemide reduces ICP through two mechanisms: (1) it interferes with cerebrospinal fluid production for up to approximately 6 hours after its administration, and (2) it also extracts brain water and reduces brain bulk.
- In reconstruction of the calvarial vault in infancy, the primary postoperative concerns are blood loss and hypovolemia.
- Children and adolescents with a Chiari type I or type II malformation may have occipital cervical headaches that are recurrent and progressive, and intermittent or continuous with extension of the neck and head. Children and adolescents may have progressive difficulty with airway control in the form of aspiration, may have "recurrent pneumonia and bronchitis," may have difficulty with swallowing and gagging with liquids, and may be able to swallow solid foods better than liquids. Snoring and stertorous breathing when sleeping are not uncommon.
- Tumors of the central nervous system are the most common type of tumors in childhood. The incidence of primary tumors is approximately 2.13 to 2.45 cases per 100,000 in a population younger than 15 years. Approximately 70% of the tumors in children occur in the posterior fossa, whereas in adults, most tumors occur in the supratentorial compartment.
- The best way to control diabetes insipidus is with crystalline antidiuretic hormone (vasopressin) administered in an intravenous drip. This short-acting agent ceases to act if the drip is discontinued, within 15 to 20 minutes. It permits an adequate calibration and monitoring of urine output during the first hours/days of the onset of diabetes insipidus.

Hydrocephalus and Arachnoid Cysts

The term *hydrocephalus* refers to an enlargement of the ventricular system due to an imbalance between the production and reabsorption of cerebrospinal fluid (CSF). This condition can be due to an obstruction within the ventricular system (obstructive hydrocephalus) or to an impairment of circulation in the subarachnoid spaces and reabsorption in the arachnoid granulations (communicating hydrocephalus). Hydrocephalus, as previously defined, must be differentiated from an enlargement of the ventricular system due to volume loss of brain parenchyma (hydrocephalus ex vacuo), which may occur after a stroke and brain disruption. Congenital hydrocephalus may present with macrocrania at birth or progressive cranial enlargement, postnatally. The potential causes of hydrocephalus (e.g., tumors, subarachnoid hemorrhage that results from trauma or ruptured vascular malformation, infection, and inflammation [meningitis]) are multiple. These causes may present at any age.[1]

Cranial arachnoid cysts are collections of CSF that may be causing mass effect and displacement of structures due to progressive expansion. Arachnoid cysts may be congenital and slowly expand over the development of the child or may follow traumatic head injuries due to disruption of the arachnoid.[2] Arachnoid cysts may be present in any part of the intracranial compartment. If they are close to CSF pathways, such as in the posterior fossa, they may interfere with the circulation of spinal fluid within the aqueduct of Sylvius or the fourth ventricle. As a consequence, not only might they create mass effect because of their presence, but there may be a gradual elevation of intracranial pressure (ICP) due to obstruction of the CSF circulation.

Clinical Presentation

The clinical presentation of hydrocephalus will vary according to whether it occurs in an infant or in a child and whether the child has a CSF shunt in place.[1] In infancy, untreated hydrocephalus will usually present with progressive macrocrania and a full fontanelle, and it will subsequently cause loss of appetite, irritability, and further clinical deterioration. In childhood, the hydrocephalus may present with progressive headaches, loss of appetite, vomiting, and irritability. Macrocrania may or may not be present, depending on the rapidity of the development of the hydrocephalus. In children with posterior fossa tumors, the hydrocephalus may be more insidious and progressive, and at some point, the patient may have acute clinical deterioration due to severe impairment of CSF circulation. Hydrocephalus may present in infants and in adolescents in a progressive and insidious fashion with mild symptoms that are often ignored. Usually, these patients do have macrocrania and a head circumference over the 98th percentile on the head circumference chart. They may have intermittent headaches, progressive loss of learning skills, loss of appetite, and diminished activity.

In patients who have been treated for hydrocephalus, there may be acute clinical deterioration that is characterized by rapid loss of appetite, headache, nausea, and vomiting. Impairment of consciousness may occur acutely. In chronic shunt malfunction, progressive macrocrania may be present; patients may also have intermittent headaches and may be unable to perform regular day-to-day activities. Early morning vomiting may be part of the presentation.[1]

Cranial arachnoid cysts may present in infancy with progressive macrocrania and distortion of part of the cranium, if the mass effect is significant. In children and adolescents, arachnoid cysts may present with progressive signs of increased ICP with or without macrocrania. Acute rupture of an arachnoid cyst following trauma with acute herniation can occur in large cysts because the rupture into the subdural space can create a sudden mass effect and displacement of structures.[2,3]

The diagnosis of the previous conditions is usually promptly and effectively achieved by neuro imaging with cranial computed tomography (CT) or cranial magnetic resonance imaging (MRI).

Treatment

There are two primary forms of treatment of progressive enlargement of the ventricular system and progressive hydrocephalus: with a shunt and without a shunt. With shunt placement (ventriculoperitoneal, lumboperitoneal, ventriculovascular, ventriculopleural, or ventriculogallbladder shunt systems) the CSF fluid is taken to another site of reabsorption such as the peritoneal cavity, where the CSF will reenter the circulation through absorption in the peritoneal wall.[1] Many commercial forms of CSF shunt systems are available. The familiarity of the individual shunt systems and the method used to evaluate them depend on the treating neurosurgeon. Because so many commercial variations of reservoirs and valves are available, other physicians or allied health providers have difficulty determining, either through inspection or palpation, what is actually in place in each patient. Swelling around the shunt site due to CSF leakage may be a form of presentation for a shunt malfunction. In the presence of a fever, it may also indicate an infection of the CSF shunt system.[1]

Programmable shunts are currently being used. The child with a programmable shunt can undergo imaging with cranial CT. If, however, cranial MRI is to be used, the treating neurosurgeon must be made aware of this because the shunt will need to be reprogrammed after MRI. This is due to the possibility that the valve mechanism may be activated and the pressure in the system may be changed.

Hydrocephalus may be treated without shunt systems; instead, a neuroendoscopic third ventriculostomy is performed.[4] In this procedure, the floor of the third ventricle is perforated under direct vision with the endoscope, and the CSF pathways are opened up to the subarachnoid spaces of the skull base. The reason for this is that the CSF, which did not have access to the subarachnoid space (such as in narrowing of the aqueduct of Sylvius), will now go to the site of reabsorption, in the arachnoid granulations. The patients are followed up both through clinical visits and through imaging to determine if the CSF has indeed been reabsorbed. Consequently, no hardware is visible in these patients, and attempts to check the shunt systems through imaging are of no value.

Symptomatic cranial arachnoid cysts may be treated with shunt systems, as with hydrocephalus, or a neuroendoscopic opening into the subarachnoid pathways or ventricular system can be created. The method depends on the cysts' location. Also, their walls can be excised with open craniotomy.[5]

Pediatric Intensive Care Unit Monitoring and Care

Primary Management Issues

Patients who have been admitted to the pediatric intensive care unit (PICU) with acute clinical deterioration from shunt malfunction or progressive hydrocephalus need to have their respiratory patterns and ventilation closely monitored. Impairment of ventilation due to progressive intracranial hypertension will generate a vicious cycle of a further increase of arterial carbon dioxide, a further increase of cerebrovascular dilatation, and a further rise of ICP. Seizures may further interfere with adequate ventilation, worsen the clinical status, and lead to acute decompensation. Obtunded patients need to undergo intubation, undergo adequate ventilation, and have access to prompt decompression of the CSF pathways. At times, shunt puncture in those patients who have shunts in place may alleviate the ICP. This will only occur, however, if the obstruction is distal to the puncture site, such as in the peritoneal catheter in ventriculoperitoneal shunts. Prompt neurosurgical evaluation and treatment are mandatory.

The correct diagnosis is usually made through examination of the patient's history and confirmed with neuroimaging, such as with cranial CT scan. The neurosurgeon will explore the shunt in these situations and determine which portion is malfunctioning and which is correct. Isolated seizures in an otherwise healthy child with a shunt do not indicate a shunt malfunction. Seizures should be effectively treated and the airway maintained to prevent cerebral hypoxia (see also Chapter 55).

Children who have undergone a shunt revision or a CSF pathway procedure such as a third ventriculostomy need to be monitored closely at first because the shunt system may acutely obstruct owing to hemorrhage at the time of the operation. The neurologic monitoring should be accompanied by close observation of respiration and vital signs. If the patient is not recovering from the neurosurgical intervention the way that is expected, repeat neuroimaging should be promptly performed. Hemorrhage at the time of the operation may complicate the recovery because of hematoma formation and mass effect. A seizure may occur after a shunt revision and should be appropriately and effectively treated; again, the priority should be maintaining adequate ventilation.

Secondary Management Issues

Short-term recovery from a shunt revision may not be possible not only because of the combination of intracranial hypertension at the time of shunt revision, but also because of the prolonged effect of intracranial hypertension, reduction of cerebral perfusion, and cerebral ischemia, before the shunt revision. An encephalopathy may follow, and the patient may have a poor return of consciousness and neurologic function. Repeat neuroimaging needs to be done at this point to confirm that the CSF shunt is functioning correctly. Adequate ventilation and support need to be maintained in these situations at all times. The blood pressure needs to be supported to maintain cerebral perfusion pressure. These encephalopathies may be complicated by postoperative seizures.

In the face of acute neurologic deterioration in the PICU, an airway needs to be established if it is not already present. Prompt neurosurgical consultation should take place. A single dose of furosemide at 1 mg/kg is adjuvant treatment in these situations. Furosemide reduces ICP through two mechanisms: (1) it interferes with CSF production for up to approximately 6 hours after its administration, and (2) it also extracts brain water and reduces brain bulk.[6,7] Furosemide is preferred over mannitol. Acetazolamide should not be an agent of choice in acute deterioration from shunt malfunction. Acetazolamide, if given intravenously, can raise the arterial carbon dioxide tension and will therefore increase cerebral blood flow, with a consequent increase in cerebral blood volume. Consequently, ICP will be elevated further.[8]

If an encephalopathy is suspected or if seizures are suspected, an electroencephalogram (EEG) or continuous EEG monitoring may be useful. Continuous "electrical" seizures may be detected only with an EEG.

Craniosynostosis and Craniofacial Disorders

Craniosynostosis is the premature closure of the sutures of the calvarial vault.[9] *Craniofacial dysostosis* is the premature closure of the sutures of the cranium and of the skull base and facial sutures.[10] Both of these conditions present in various forms, depending on the sutures involved and the underlying disease. Craniosynostosis may be an intrauterine positional deformity due to constraint.[11] Craniofacial disorders are usually familial, but sporadic mutations exist. Craniofacial disorders also present in various forms and, consequently, in various syndromal patterns (see also Chapter 51).[9,10,12]

Craniosynostosis most commonly involves the sagittal (interparietal) suture. Consequently, the cranium is elongated in the anterior-posterior axis, and the disorder is readily recognizable. Other forms of craniosynostosis involve the coronal suture and the sutures of the frontal skull base, which create a frontal flattening (frontal plagiocephaly). Premature closure of the lambda suture (occipital parietal) can cause flattening and asymmetry of the posterior aspect of the cranium (occipital plagiocephaly). These disorders need to be differentiated from postnatal benign positional deformities. These may occur when infants are allowed to lie for prolonged periods of time on the back of their heads.

Craniofacial disorders may present with or without other anomalies. The association of craniofacial disorder with syndactyly may be readily seen in Apert's syndrome. More common are the disorders in which the digits are shaped abnormally, such as short and stubby, without syndactyly, as seen in syndromes such as Saethre-Chotzen, Crouzon, and Pfeiffer's.

Clinical Presentation

The particular association of the disorders of the cranium and face with or without digit abnormalities allows for a prompt diagnosis of these disorders. They may be confirmed with radiologic examination, such as plain x-ray films of the cranium and face, and with CT.

Treatment

The primary reason for treatment is to allow for adequate growth of the brain because this organ is growing early in life. Seventy-five percent of total brain growth is achieved by age 18 to 19 months (see also Chapter 48). Release of the sutures and reconstruction of the calvarium are indicated to permit for this. The second reason for surgical correction is for the cosmetic correction of the underlying disorder.

In craniosynostosis, the correction takes place primarily in the calvarial vault with a variety of surgical procedures, depending on the underlying disease process. Open operations and endoscopic operations are performed according to the underlying disease and the surgeon's choice.

Craniofacial disorders require a more complex approach that is usually staged according to the severity of the disease process and the underlying disorder. Reconstruction of the calvarium is usually performed in infancy to permit for brain growth, whereas the reconstruction of the craniofacial anomaly usually takes place at a later age to permit correction of the midface and periorbital regions, as well as any further remodeling that is needed for the calvarium.

Pediatric Intensive Care Unit Monitoring and Care: Craniosynostosis Postoperative Care

Primary Management Issues

In reconstruction of the calvarial vault in infancy, the primary postoperative concerns are those of blood loss and hypovolemia. The infants have had (or not) significant blood loss that has usually been replaced during surgery. The osteotomy sites and dural surfaces, however, may continue to ooze under the scalp in the first 12 to 18 hours after surgery. Accordingly, observation of the vital signs and frequent monitoring of the hematocrit are important. In addition, because of the stress of surgery in these infants, systemic acidosis may be present. Monitoring of the blood gases and bicarbonate may detect underlying metabolic acidosis that should be readily corrected. Further blood loss and hypovolemia necessitate blood product replacement. On admission to the PICU from the postanesthesia care unit, the pediatric intensivist needs to document that there is blood available in case of the need for further transfusions.

In most situations, by the following day, the intravascular volume has stabilized, and there is no further hemorrhage. Some surgeons place drains to the subgaleal space to allow for drainage of blood and serum products to minimize postoperative cranial deformity. This accentuates the blood loss, and the hematocrit needs to be followed frequently.

Secondary Management Issues

Facial and calvarial swelling is common because of the migration of serum and blood products from the area of the operation and, at times, from impediment of lymphatic drainage. Swelling usually starts the day after the operation, is maximized on the second or third day, and then resolves spontaneously. Palpebral swelling is not uncommon if the operation involved the frontal and temporal regions. Because it will spontaneously resolve, the swelling requires no specific treatment other than reassurance to the family that this is the natural postoperative course. Infants are usually irritable immediately after the operation, primarily because they are hungry. Formula or breast milk needs to readily follow if an oral electrolyte solution (Pedialyte) or water is being readily tolerated.

In most of the situations, surgical pain is not a persistent problem. After the child is well fed, there is less need for analgesics. The use of analgesics that lead to sedation and depression of consciousness should be minimized.

Pediatric Intensive Care Unit Monitoring and Care: Craniofacial Dysostosis Postoperative Care

Primary Management Issues

Craniofacial dysostosis corrective surgery is usually a lengthier intervention and is followed by significant blood loss. The intensivist needs to document that there will be blood available for postoperative management for the first 12 to 18 hours on admission to the PICU. Hypovolemia may be present, and the patient's vital signs and blood pressure need to be monitored closely. These patients should have an arterial line in place, unless it was a limited surgical intervention. A bladder catheter needs to be in place to document urinary output.

If the operation involved the patient's midface, the airway needs to be closely monitored because upper airway irritation or hemorrhage may be present. If the patient is intubated, intubation should probably be maintained until the following morning to ascertain that hemostasis has normalized. Frequent blood gas and hematocrit monitoring is imperative during the first 8 to 12 hours of the operation and subsequently is less needed. If scalp drains are in place, the hematocrit needs to be closely monitored. These may exaggerate blood loss.

Because of the facial operation, postoperative pain is more common with craniofacial dysostosis surgery than with craniosynostosis surgery. Morphine sulfate needs to be administered as needed, but respiration and adequate ventilation need to be ascertained.

Secondary Management Issues

Facial swelling and swelling around the calvarium may be present and may worsen by the second or third day. This swelling, in most situations, starts to improve by the fourth or fifth postoperative day. Palpebral swelling may be severe, and it also tends to improve promptly.

The osteotomy sites often involve sinuses such as the ethmoidal and frontal. Infection may occur. The patient is usually receiving broad-spectrum antibiotics. If the dura was interrupted during the operation, close monitoring for CSF leakage is important. Meningitis may present itself acutely with a febrile course that persists and then worsens. In these situations, a lumbar puncture is mandatory to obtain CSF cultures. Appropriate antibiotic treatment needs to be instituted and adjusted according to the results of the Gram stain and cultures.

Brain swelling may occur in these patients. Because the calvarium is usually not completely closed, however, altered intracranial compliance may not be a major issue. If this is a significant concern, the surgeon may opt to place an ICP monitoring device at the end of the operative procedure. This is then removed when the ICP stabilizes in the postoperative course.

ICP monitoring may be of significant use in the patients whose lungs are mechanically ventilated and who are paralyzed. Additional information is readily given by the ICP monitor when ventilation is inadequate and there is elevation of the arterial carbon dioxide. Ventilation may be adjusted to correct ICP (see also Chapter 52).

By the second or third day, the clinical course of these patients usually stabilizes and airway and blood loss are of less concern. The patient may be transferred out of the PICU.

Chiari Malformation

The congenital malformations of the posterior fossa that are globally encompassed under the title *Chiari malformation* are discussed in this section. These are disorders in which the posterior fossa structures are restricted in their space and, as a consequence, are herniating through the foramen magnum caudally and through the incisura rostrally (see also Chapter 51). Chiari[13] described pathologic specimens that are known as the following malformations: type I, type II, type III, and type IV.

In type I, there is a descent of the cerebellar tonsils into and below the foramen magnum. In type II, the cerebellar tonsils, descent is accompanied by the cerebellar vermis and the lower portion of the fourth ventricle. There is upward herniation of the superior portion of the cerebellar vermis into the incisura. In type III, the associated malformations of type II are accompanied by an occipital/cervical encephalocele. Type IV, as described by Chiari, was a pathologic specimen in which there was hypoplasia of the cerebellum. This malformation is probably unrelated to the previously described disorders.

At approximately the same time as Chiari, Arnold[14] described the disorder that is now known at Chiari type II in patients with spina bifida (myelomeningocele). Consequently, common usage of the term *Arnold-Chiari malformation* is a description of the type II Chiari malformation in patients with spina bifida.

Syringomyelia, a disorder of CSF circulation within the spinal cord, is frequently associated with the Chiari malformation. Syringomyelia is a cavitation of the central portion of the spinal cord that may involve all the spinal cord or segments of the same.[15] The term *hydromyelia* is used interchangeably with syringomyelia in most clinical situations.[15] Some use the term *hydromyelia* to refer to dilatation of the normal central canal inside the spinal cord; syringomyelia is a disruption of the ependymal lining of the central canal and a progressive enlargement and cavitation of spinal cord.

The actual cause of this disease process is subject to speculation. The Chiari malformation is seen with neuroimaging in all patients with myelomeningocele. Less than 10% to 15% of patients, however, reveal the signs and symptoms of the Chiari malformation.

Clinical Presentation

The clinical presentation varies according to the severity of the disease, the age of the patient at presentation, and the presence or absence of associated anomalies. Children and adolescents with a Chiari type I or type II malformation may have occipital cervical headaches that are recurrent and progressive and intermittent or continuous with arching of the neck. They may have progressive difficulty with airway control in the form of aspiration, may have "recurrent pneumonia and bronchitis," may have difficulty with swallowing and gagging with liquids, and may be able to swallow solid foods better than liquids. Snoring and stertorous breathing are not uncommon during sleep. The disease progresses gradually and steadfastly. The examination reveals an impaired gag reflex and abnormal amounts of saliva in the mouth and posterior airway as the patient is unable to protect the airway because of the abnormal gag and swallowing reflex. Dysesthesias and unusual sensation in the upper extremities and trunk may be present. In other patients, it may present associated with long tract signs and ataxia of gait. Clumsiness and wasting of musculature of the upper extremities accompanied by weakness may be noted.

In infants and children, progressive Chiari type I or type II malformation may present with recurrent occipital cervical headaches, and in younger children it may present with irritability and neck extension. The neck extension and irritability are thought to be due to pressure on the dura mater of the foramen magnum.[16]

Treatment

The treatment for decompensating Chiari malformation is occipital/cervical decompression to relieve the pressure on the posterior fossa structures and the cervical medullary junction. This is done through removal of bone in the posterior arch of C-1 or C-2 or others if the tonsillar herniation is below the C-2 level. The technique used by most has been opening and patching the dura to expand the posterior fossa and the cervical spine. In children, treatment may be performed with bone decompression of the occipital bone and the posterior elements of the cervical spine without durotomy.[17] The reason is that the elasticity of the dura is still retained, and it may "stretch" after the bone elements are removed.[17] Some of the children have decompensated enough to have required a tracheostomy for airway control, before the intervention. In some situations, the tracheostomy may be removed at a later date.

Children with spina bifida and Chiari malformation who are decompensating clinically with signs and symptoms of a deteriorating posterior fossa pressure may have an acute or chronic malfunction of the ventriculoperitoneal shunt. The ventricular enlargement and the intracranial hypertension create further pressure on the posterior fossa structures and further herniation, which creates the symptoms of Chiari malformation. These children need an immediate revision of the ventriculoperitoneal shunt—not a posterior fossa operation.

Pediatric Intensive Care Unit: Monitoring and Care

Primary Management Issues

Both the primary management in the patient with decompensating Chiari malformation and the postoperative management in the form of decompression or shunt revision involve maintaining a patent airway and adequate ventilation. If the patient has undergone extubation before returning to the PICU after the operation, copious secretions may be present because of the previous aspiration of saliva into the airway. Underlying pneumonia and atelectasis may be present. Intensive pulmonary toilet is important in these situations with frequent endotracheal suction. If the patient's airway is inadequate, reintubation is mandatory. In some situations, the swallowing reflex and protection of the airway may take a long time to improve after the operation, and a tracheostomy may be mandatory.

For immediate postoperative management, an arterial line for continuous monitoring of blood gases is imperative. This will facilitate adequate monitoring of ventilation.

Patients who have undergone a posterior fossa exploration need to be monitored closely, even if they are doing clinically well, in the first 10 to 12 hours after the operation because postoperative hematoma formation may occur in the surgical area, with acute compression of the cervical medullary junction. Level of consciousness does not always signal that the posterior fossa is decompressed. Patients may be alert but have progressive brainstem compression and suddenly have a rapid dysfunction of the respiratory center. These patients need to be monitored carefully in the PICU by experienced physician, nursing, and allied health personnel who can reestablish the airway if sudden decompensation occurs.

Patients who have undergone a revision of the CSF shunt system for a decompensating Chiari malformation require similar close monitoring. Sudden obstruction of the shunt in the immediate postoperative period will exacerbate the respiratory difficulty and embarrassment of the airway.

Secondary Management Issues

As the patient steadily recovers in the PICU from the decompression or shunt revision, the patient should be transferred into an intermediate care unit facility for airway monitoring, pulmonary toilet, and acute rehabilitation. The patient should undergo physical and occupational therapy as soon as possible to try to return to the preoperative clinical status. Pulmonary medicine may need to be prescribed when the patient moves from PICU care to intermediate care until any pulmonary difficulties have improved. Ongoing assessment of swallowing capabilities, reinstitution of feedings, and general support are necessary in these patients.

An immediate improvement of the patient who has had significant swallowing and airway difficulties following a decompression will not occur in most situations. Any acute neurologic deterioration in the postoperative management of the patient mandates an immediate study with neuroimaging to ascertain that acute hydrocephalus has not occurred or recurred. Delay in revision of the shunt system or decompression of the CSF pathways may seriously affect outcome. Close communication between the pediatric neurosurgery staff and the pediatric critical care staff is imperative in these patients.

Because Chiari malformation is not a well-known disease and the consequences of it are usually difficult to assess for inexperienced health care personnel, ongoing education and communications among the pediatric neurosurgery staff, PICU faculty and staff, and allied health personnel should be part of the quality improvement process of any PICU. In addition, latex precautions are needed in all children with spina bifida and associated conditions because of the potential complications from allergic reactions to latex products.[18]

Brain Tumors and Arteriovenous Malformations

Tumors of the central nervous system are the second most common type of tumors in childhood. The incidence of primary tumors is approximately 2.13 to 2.45 cases per 100,000 in a population younger than 15 years.[19] Approximately 70% of the tumors in children occur in the posterior fossa, whereas in adults, most tumors occur in the supratentorial compartment.[19] Astrocytomas are the most common tumors in childhood; overall, they comprise approximately 50% of the tumors, followed closely by the primitive neuroectodermal tumor (medulloblastoma) and then by ependymomas.[20] In the pediatric population, the astrocytomas, compared with those that occur in the adult population, prefer the midline, so they are most commonly located in the cerebellar vermis region when in the posterior fossa and in and around the third ventricle when they are in the supratentorial compartment. The most common locations for the medulloblastoma and the ependymoma are in the posterior fossa, in and around the fourth ventricle.

Supratentorial tumors are more common than infratentorial tumors in children younger than 2 years.[21] In children with ages between 2 and 15 years, the posterior fossa is the most common location for tumors.

Approximately 6% of tumors in childhood will present with acute hemorrhage. Hemorrhage in a tumor may cause acute neurologic deterioration due to the underlying altered compliance from the tumor mass itself and then the acute aggregate of elevation of ICP from the hemorrhage.

Arteriovenous malformations (AVMs) most commonly present with hemorrhage in adults with ages between age 30 and 35 years.[22] In the second decade of childhood, however, there is also a peak incidence of AVM ruptures.[23] Once an AVM is diagnosed, the risk of hemorrhage is 2% to 4% per year of life by some reports.[24] The mortality from rupture of an AVM is estimated between 20%

and 30%; one third of the survivors will have a persistent neurologic impairment.[24] Approximately 90% of the AVMs are in the supratentorial compartment.[24]

Clinical Presentation

Brain tumors: Because most brain tumors are in the posterior fossa, most patients show progressive signs and symptoms of increased ICP due to obstructive hydrocephalus. Patients may have intermittent emesis, which usually, but not always, occurs in the morning, accompanied by headache, loss of appetite, and hypoactivity. In infants, the characteristic presenting sign is increasing head circumference. If the presentation is due to acute hemorrhage, sudden neurologic deterioration will be present. In the supratentorial compartment, presentation is usually with progressive macrocrania in infants and seizures with or without hemiparesis. Tumors in the third ventricle region, such as astrocytoma or craniopharyngioma, may present with progressive visual impairment; the most noticeable sign is a child bumping into objects. Older children will have headaches and hypoactivity. Suprasellar tumors may present with polydipsia and polyuria (diabetes insipidus).

Arteriovenous malformation: AMVs may present with recurrent seizures, especially if they are in the cerebral hemispheres; mass effect due to the large size of the malformation presenting then, with progressive macrocrania in infants; and cardiac failure. The latter is due to cardiac overload when there is a significant arteriovenous shunt. Those who have hemorrhage will also have acute neurologic deterioration, with or without seizures and hemiparesis.

The diagnosis is made with cranial neuroimaging with CT or MRI scans. Vascular lesions such as AVMs are subsequently studied with magnetic resonance angiography (MRA) or cerebral angiography, to better delineate the pathologic anatomy (see also Chapter 49). Embolization techniques are often used to treat the vascular malformations with or without subsequent surgery. Vascular tumors may also be embolized to reduce the blood flow through them and maximize the therapy. The surgical interventions for brain tumors and AVMs may be lengthy. The patient usually enters the PICU with some degree of systemic acidosis and may have had significant blood loss.

Pediatric Intensive Care Unit Monitoring and Care

Primary Management Issues

Close monitoring of the neurologic status and ventilation in those patients who undergo extubation is mandatory. Sudden neurologic deterioration after the operation may occur because of seizures, hemorrhage, and collection of hematoma and mass effect in the surgical area. Acute hydrocephalus may occur, especially in those patients who have had CSF shunts in place before the intervention. The shunt may suddenly become obstructed with blood and debris from the operation.

Ascertaining that airway and ventilation is adequate is mandatory, especially in the first 12 hours after the operation. Hypoventilation will lead to hypercarbia, and this in turn will lead to an acute rise in ICP. In some situations, the surgeon may place at the end of the surgical procedure an ICP monitor to assist in postoperative management.

Patients who have undergone posterior fossa operations are at higher risk of sudden embarrassment of the airway because of pressure effect on the brainstem. Consequently, the neurologic surgeon may opt to maintain endotracheal intubation overnight to better control the airway in the case of any postoperative complications. Maintenance of an arterial line for frequent sampling of blood gases and electrolytes is important.

Elevation of the head of the bed at approximately 10 degrees will improve venous return from the cerebral circulation to the right atrium and will then assist in reducing ICP. The patient's blood pressure must be properly supported to maintain adequate cerebral perfusion. Sudden hypotension will facilitate ischemia and cytotoxic edema in the areas that have already been affected by the surgical intervention, and the peritumoral or mass effect. If acute neurologic deterioration or lack of improvement of level of consciousness and neurologic function is noted, the patient should promptly undergo a CT scan. This scan is used to determine whether there is postoperative clot formation, mass effect, or acute hydrocephalus.

If ICP is being monitored, any persistent elevations of ICP over 15 mmHg should be of concern. Cerebral perfusion pressure should be maintained in children and in young adults over 60 mmHg. Frequent repositioning and turning side to side and back (side to side in bed can be in the oblique position rather than full side to side) will help with pulmonary toilet and reduce the risk of atelectasis.

Seizures may present with subtle abnormal motor movements such as twitching of the thumb and part of the face and subsequently spread to involve the arm, shoulder, and rest of the body. Close monitoring for abnormal motor movements is imperative in the first 10 to 12 hours after the operation, especially in patients who have undergone a supratentorial surgical procedure. Prompt control of the seizures is mandatory. This means ensuring that ventilation is adequate at all times. If there is significant impairment of level of consciousness, the patient should undergo reintubation at the same time the patient receives the necessary anticonvulsant therapy. The most rapid way to control seizures in children for the most part is with the use of a short-acting anticonvulsant. The airway, however, needs to be properly maintained. Phenobarbital load at 5 mg/kg followed shortly thereafter by another load at 5 mg/kg administered intravenously slowly will control seizures for the most part in infants. No anticonvulsant agents should be given too rapidly so as not to reduce blood pressure. Cerebral perfusion pressure needs to be maintained and not interfered with in the acute postoperative period. Ultra–short-acting anticonvulsants may be promptly and effectively used, as long as the patient has an endotracheal tube in place. A dose of diazepam at 0.25 mg/kg slowly administered intravenously so as not to interfere with blood pressure is an effective way of controlling acute tonic-clonic seizures in the patient who has an endotracheal tube in place. In patients who are maintaining good oxygenation and good ventilation and have a focal tonic-clonic seizure, an alternative is the administration of fosphenytoin load at 5 to 10 mg/kg by slow intravenous infusion. This medication is less likely to interfere with the level of consciousness (see also Chapter 55).

Patients in the postoperative craniotomy phase should not be fed immediately. They may be given small amounts of clear liquids if they are alert. There is the potential for acute neurologic deterioration or seizures in the first 6 to 10 hours after the operation.

Secondary Management Issues

The syndrome of inappropriate antidiuretic hormone secretion (SIADH) may occur at 24 to 48 hours after the operation.[25] This may account for neurologic deterioration at 1 or 2 days postoperatively, with or without seizure presentation. The sudden shift of the water into the nervous system due to the drop in serum osmolality will magnify any perisurgical/peritumor edema. The already altered compliance from the underlying disease process may be magnified by the sudden shift in water, into the neurons and glia. The syndrome needs to be promptly recognized and treated. Close monitoring of serum electrolytes and osmolality is mandatory in patients undergoing postoperative craniotomy. Initial treatment is prompt reduction of intravenous fluid administration. Patients undergoing postoperative craniotomy should be maintained with intravenous fluid solutions of dextrose (5%) and normal saline. If the serum osmolality and serum sodium level drops with administration of these solutions, intravenous fluids should be reduced to one-third maintenance or less. In the face of further reduction of serum osmolality and serum sodium level, 3% hypertonic saline may be administered (5 to 10 ml/kg).

The clinical picture may be complicated by the salt wasting syndrome, also known as cerebral salt wasting.[26] In these situations, 3% hypertonic saline is the treatment of choice. Serum sodium should be maintained between 140 and 150 mEq/L, and serum osmolality should be maintained over 290 mOsm/L. Seizures should be promptly and effectively treated with anticonvulsants in the presence of a reduced serum osmolality. If the serum osmolality and serum sodium level are not corrected, however, the anticonvulsant treatment will be ineffective. Slow liberalization of fluids and reduction of the hypertonic saline will allow for correction of the abnormal state, usually in 2 to 3 days.

If not already present, diabetes insipidus may occur after removal of suprasellar tumors. This may not happen immediately after the operation; it may have a delayed onset of 12 to 24 hours after the surgical intervention. Some of the antidiuretic hormone may be stored in the posterior pituitary gland, and the diabetes insipidus may not start until after the stored antidiuretic hormone is released. Because of the surgical intervention, interruption of the antidiuretic hormone flow from its site of production in the nucleus paraventricularis of the hypothalamus is not uncommon after surgical procedures in the suprasellar region. This may be transient, but often it is permanent. Prompt recognition of the onset of diabetes insipidus is important to manage the patient's postoperative state. Sudden urine output in large amounts is accompanied by a reduction of the urine specific gravity below 1.005. This should lead to a prompt realization that diabetes insipidus is taking place. Serum osmolality will rapidly rise above 300 mOsm/L. The patient may become acutely dehydrated, the reduction of blood pressure will reduce cerebral perfusion pressure, and it may lead to cerebral ischemia.

Diabetes insipidus, once initiated, may not be permanent; and administration of the long-acting diuretic hormone may be accompanied by a release of further antidiuretic hormone from the posterior pituitary gland; and a sudden retention of water may lead to sodium shift and reduction of serum osmolality. This pendular swing may complicate postoperative cerebral edema and lead to further seizures. Consequently, the best way to control diabetes insipidus is with crystalline antidiuretic hormone (vasopressin) administered in an intravenous drip. This short-acting agent will cease to act if the drip is discontinued, within 15 to 20 minutes. It will permit an adequate calibration and monitoring of urine output during the first hours/days of the onset of diabetes insipidus. The vasopressin drip should be prepared with 20 units, diluted, and started with 0.1 to 0.3 ml per dose. The drip should be titrated to maintain a normal urine output. If the urine output suddenly decreases, the drip should be titrated down or halted. When the urine output starts once more, specific gravity will better determine if there is antidiuretic hormone present and circulating. The vasopressin drip should be restarted when the urine output starts to increase again and specific gravities are below 1.005. After 24 to 48 hours, the intravenous drip may be replaced by the nasal antidiuretic hormone spray or the antidiuretic hormone tablets, according to the determined needs of each patient. Some patients may have a partial antidiuretic hormone deficit and not a total deficit. Pediatric endocrinology consultation will assist in the management under these circumstances.

Some patients who underwent posterior fossa surgery will have difficulty with swallowing and speech. Initial consultation for speech therapy and occupational therapy should be placed while the patient is in the PICU for baseline assessment and follow-up. In those patients in whom the airway remains unstable, a tracheostomy may be necessary to initiate rehabilitation measures until the neurologic status is improved and stabilized.

Physical therapy consultation needs to occur in the PICU for patients who manifest motor weakness, paralysis, or severe spasticity. Acute rehabilitation measures initiated in the PICU not only facilitate patient care, but also allow for a progressive evaluation of the response to therapy and necessary adjustments, for subacute and long-term care. For the first few days after a craniotomy, the patient should be closely monitored by PICU staff and transitioned accordingly from the PICU to an intermediate or "step-down care" unit. Complications such as seizures, aspiration, and infection may occur at any time in the postoperative period.

REFERENCES

1. James HE: Hydrocephalus in infants and children: a clinical review, *Am Fam Physician* 45:733-742, 1992.
2. Harsh GR IV, Edwards MSB, Wilson CB: Intracranial arachnoid cysts in children, *J Neurosurg* 64:835-842, 1986.

3. Page AC, Mohan D, Paxton RM: Arachnoid cysts of the middle fossa predispose to subdural hematoma formation: fact or fiction? *Acta Neurochir Suppl* 42:210-215, 1988.
4. Feng H, Huang G, Lia X, et al: Endoscopic third ventriculostomy in the management of obstructive hydrocephalus: an outcome analysis, *J Neurosurg* 100:626-633, 2004.
5. Ciricillo SF, Cogen PH, Harsh GR, et al: Intracranial arachnoid cysts in children: a comparison of the effects of fenestration and shunting, *J Neurosurg* 74:230-235, 1991.
6. Pollay M: Formation of spinal fluid: relations or studies of isolated choroid plexus to the standing gradient hypothesis, *J Neurosurg* 42:665-673, 1975.
7. Reed DJ: The effects of furosemide on cerebrospinal fluid flow in rabbits, *Arch Int Pharmacodys Ther* 178:324-330, 1969.
8. Knopp LM, Atkinson JR, Ward AA Jr: Effect of Diamox on cerebrospinal fluid pressure of cat and monkey, *Neurology* 7:119-123, 1957.
9. Shillito JD, Matson DD: Craniosynostosis: a review of 519 surgical patients, *Pediatrics* 41:829-853, 1968.
10. Tessier P: Relationship of craniostenosis to craniofacial dysostosis and to faciostenosis, *Plastic Reconst Surg* 48:224-237, 1971.
11. Higginbottom MC, Jones KL, James HE: Intrauterine constraint and craniosynostosis, *Neurosurgery* 6:39-44, 1980.
12. Cohen MM: Genetic prospectives and craniosynostosis and syndromes with craniosynostosis, *J Neurosurg* 47:886-898, 1977.
13. Chiari H: Ube Veranderungen des Kleinhirns, des Pons und der Medulla Oblongata in Folge von Congenitaler Hydrocephalie des Grosshirns, *Denksehr Akad Wiss, Wien* 63:71-116, 1896.
14. Arnold J: Myelocyste Transposition von Gewebskeimen und Sympodie, *Beitr Path Anat* 16:1-28, 1894.
15. Isu T, Iwasaka Y, Akino M, et al: Hydrosyringomyelia associated with Chiari I malformation in children and adolescents, *Neurosurgery* 26:591-597, 1990.
16. Greenlee DW, Donovan KA, Hasan DM, et al: Chiari I malformation in the very young child: the spectrum of presentations and experience in 31 children under 2 years of age, *Pediatrics* 110:1212-1219, 2002.
17. James HE, Brant A: Treatment of the Chiari malformation with bone decompression without durotomy in children and young adults, *Childs Nerv Syst* 18:202-206, 2002.
18. Nieto A, Estornell F, Mazon A, et al: Allergy to latex in spina bifida: a multivariate study of associated factors in 100 consecutive patients, *J Allergy Clin Immunol* 98:501-507, 1996.
19. Boring CC, Squires TS, Tong T: Cancer statistics, *Cancer J Clin* 42: 19-38, 1992.
20. Kornbluth PL, Walker MD, Cassady JR. *Neurological oncology*, Philadelphia, 1987, Lippincott.
21. Buetow PC, Smirniotopoulos JG, Done S: Congenital brain tumors: a review of 45 cases, *AJAR* 11:793-799, 1990.
22. Foster DMC, Steiner L, Hakanson S: Arteriovenous malformation of the brain: a long-term clinical study, *J Neurosurg* 37:562-570, 1972.
23. Gerosa MA, Cappellotto P, Licata C, et al: Cerebral arteriovenous malformation in children (56 cases). *Childs Brain* 8:356-371, 1981.
24. Perret G, Nishioka H: Arteriovenous malformations: an analysis of 545 cases of cranio-cerebral malformations and fistulae reported to the Cooperative Study, *J Neurosurg* 25:467-490, 1966.
25. Barrter FC, Schwartz WB: The syndrome of inappropriate secretion of antidiuretic hormone, *Am J Med* 42:790-806, 1967.
26. Kappy MS, Gannong CA: Cerebral salt wasting in children: the role of atrial natriuretic hormone, *Adv Pediatr* 43:271-308, 1996.

CHAPTER 54

Coma and Depressed Sensorium

Anthony L. Pearson-Shaver and Renuka Mehta

PEARLS

- A Glasgow Coma Scale (GCS) of less than 15 in children should be taken seriously.
- The ABCs (airway, breathing, and circulation) should be the priority during management of a child with coma.
- Spinal tap should be deferred until a raised intracranial pressure (ICP) has been ruled out.
- Blood glucose level should be checked urgently during the initial presentation of coma.
- When in doubt, it is better to protect the airway and control cerebral blood flow electively.
- Unequal pupillary size is a sign of uncal herniation.
- The goal of therapy should be the prevention of secondary brain injury.

Coma, a state of unresponsiveness and unconsciousness, presents as a result of many disorders ranging from structural central nervous system (CNS) disorders to diffuse systemic abnormalities. As a medical emergency, coma presents a challenge to providers because optimal care requires timely intervention; however, information is frequently limited during the initial evaluation. Knowledge of CNS anatomy and structures responsible for consciousness provide helpful clues as one attempts to interpret physical findings and optimize patient care. A careful general physical examination with a focused neurologic examination can suggest the diagnosis, aid in the location of lesions, guide therapeutic intervention, and determine prognosis. Further adjunctive radiologic and laboratory evaluation will then confirm physical findings. Therefore we discuss CNS anatomy, the pathophysiology of coma, historical and physical findings that aid in localization of lesions, the emergent management and evaluation of patients with altered level of consciousness LOC, and the prognosis of patients with coma.

Pathophysiology

Coma may be simplistically described as a lack of consciousness. Plum and Posner[1] describe coma as a "state of unarousable psychological responsiveness." *Consciousness* is a set of neural processes that allow an individual to perceive, comprehend, and act on the internal and external environment.[1,2] Two neurophysiologic functions, *arousal* and *awareness*, have discrete neuroanatomic locations and are integrated in the conscious person.[3] *Arousal* describes the degree to which an individual appears to be able to interact within the environment.

Awareness reflects the depth and content of the arousal state. When one is aware, one is alert (or aroused) and cognizant of self and surroundings. Sleeping and waking are common examples of different states of arousal. Although coma and sleep both abolish conscious interaction with the environment, they differ physiologically. Sleep is an active physiologic process with several distinct stages. During sleep, mechanisms for arousal remain intact. Coma, however, occurs because of impairment of physiologic components responsible for arousal. The comatose patient is not able to consciously interact.

Anatomy of Arousal and the Ascending Reticular Activating System

Arousal occurs by nonspecific physiologic mechanisms that can be selectively impaired by toxins, anesthetics, or physical destruction of the brainstem. Neuroanatomically, the ascending reticular activating system (ARAS) and related structures responsible for arousal are primarily located in the brainstem within the paramedian tegmental gray matter immediately ventral to the pons. Three ARAS principle pathways have been identified. Communication among the ARAS, the cortex, and the limbic system occurs via pathways connecting the thalamic reticular nucleus, the cortex, the hypothalamus, the basal forebrain, and the brainstem median raphe (locus caeruleus).[4] The ARAS receives collaterals from and is stimulated by every major somatic and sensory pathway directly or indirectly; thus it is best regarded as a physiologic rather than an anatomic entity. This explains why patients with large discrete lesions (brain tumors) may be entirely alert, whereas those with anatomically undetectable but biochemically widespread lesions (e.g., hepatic encephalopathy) may be comatose.

Depression of the level of arousal occurs by direct brainstem-diencephalic injury involving the ARAS or lesions causing bilateral cerebral dysfunction. Conscious behavior depends on the interplay between the cerebral cortex and ARAS—neural components required for arousal and awareness.[1] Because the brain maintains a rich network of connections among the cortex, the ARAS, and the brainstem, patients with large discrete lesions might be alert on presentation, though localized neurologic deficits are noted on physical examination. On the other hand, patients with only minimal exposure to CNS depressants may have a depressed sensorium.

Level of Arousal

Precise use of definitions and descriptions of the levels of consciousness (LOC) improves communication among health care providers and makes interpreting changes in a patient's condition easier.[1,5,6,7] Box 54–1 lists definitions for LOC. *Lethargy,* a term in common use among the lay population, does not appear to have the expected precision that health care workers might expect. *Stedman's Medical Dictionary* (1995, Williams & Wilkins) defines lethargy as "A state of deep and prolonged unconsciousness, resembling profound slumber, from which one can be aroused but into which one immediately relapses." *Dorland's Medical Dictionary* (2001, WB Saunders) defines lethargy as "A lowered level of consciousness, with drowsiness, listlessness and apathy." *Stedman's* definition is most consistent with Posner and Plum's definition of "obtundation," whereas the *Dorland's* definition appears most similar to "clouding of consciousness." Given the differences in definition offered by these two respected medical references, it is clear that the use of the term *lethargy* is ambiguous at best. It is best for health care workers to avoid the use of the term when describing patients with a reduced LOC. Numerous scoring systems have been developed to assess acute neurologic conditions. By far the most useful is the Glasgow Coma Scale (GCS). Developed as part of a series of outcome scales to evaluate the prognosis of adults who have sustained head injury, the use of the GCS has been expanded to evaluate all patients who have sustained neurologic injury. Its use as a general means of neurologic assessment is detailed in Chapter 50 and in Chapter 99. A GCS of 8 or less has been used as an alternative definition of coma. A number of other scales have been used to assess the severity of illness and coma (e.g., Liege coma scale, Apache II scale, Reye's syndrome). The GCS has gained wider acceptance because of its ease and familiarity.[8] A modified GCS has been devised that is more applicable to infants and is described in detail in Chapter 99.

BOX 54–1

Levels of Consciousness Defined

1. **Clouding of consciousness**—impaired capacity to think clearly and to remember current stimuli.
2. **Delirium**—disturbed consciousness with motor restlessness, disorientation, and hallucination.
3. **Obtundation**—reduced alertness; person appears to sleep but responds to verbal or tactile stimuli.
4. **Stupor**—markedly reduced alertness; person only responds to noxious stimuli.
5. **Coma**—no response to even noxious stimuli and person will not utter understandable words.

Identification of Cause

Coma may present as part of the progression of a known neurologic illness or the unpredictable consequence or complication of a known systemic disease, or it may result from an unexpected event or illness.[5] An accurate history of the events and circumstances before the onset of the symptoms and information concerning medical history and medication use may be invaluable in determining the cause of coma. This information could quickly lead to the most appropriate diagnostic testing and treatment. As in most pediatric diseases, the differential diagnosis of coma is age related, as listed in Box 54–2. Common causes of coma seen in the pediatric population are listed in Box 54–3.

The initial assessment of the comatose patient should start with an evaluation of airway patency, the adequacy of ventilation, and the status of the patient's perfusion. As in any resuscitation, problems should be addressed as they are discovered. A complete set of vital signs including core temperature and oxygen saturation is an important adjunct to the assessment of the coma patient. General assessment of the neurologic status is in order. Pupillary response, respiratory pattern, stimuli required to elicit a response, and the general character of the response should be noted. Many practitioners assign an initial GCS at this time.

Observing the respiratory pattern before endotracheal intubation in patients who require airway management is important. The rate, depth, and regularity of respiration depend on a complex interplay of chemical and neural control systems that operate automatically and respond to changes in arterial gas tensions and arterial pH. In the comatose patient, abnormality may occur in rate and in the pattern. A low respiratory rate is associated with the use of CNS depressants (e.g., alcohol, barbiturates, benzodiazepines, and narcotics) and leads to hypoventilation. Hypopnea can also be associated with elevated intracranial

BOX 54–2

Differential Diagnosis of Altered Mental Status at Various Ages

INFANT

Infection
Inborn error of metabolism
Metabolic
Abuse
Trauma

CHILD

Ingestion
Infection
Intussusception
Seizure
Abuse
Trauma

ADOLESCENT

Ingestion
Intentional
Trauma
Drug/alcohol overdose

pressure (ICP). Though tachypnea is commonly seen in pediatric patients as a physiologic response to hypoxia, metabolic acidosis, or fever, central hyperventilation can be a sign of brainstem herniation. Observance of the respiratory pattern can assist in localizing a lesion. The respiratory pattern is determined by observation but should be interpreted in the light of arterial blood gas results. Anatomic correlations between areas of injury and the resultant respiratory patterns can be found in Table 54–1.

Unless evaluation proves otherwise, shock that occurs coincidentally with coma is due to a hemodynamic disturbance; hypotension accompanying coma is seen in systemic diseases rather than isolated CNS injury (e.g., shock, sepsis, certain drug ingestions, myocardial injury or failure, and adrenal insufficiency). Hypertension is suggestive of an intracranial structural lesion or raised ICP. The patient with systemic hypertension and coma should be evaluated for the possibility of primary hypertensive encephalopathy.

Signs of trauma should be sought after initial assessment of the comatose patient. Cervical immobilization should be maintained until trauma has been excluded or cervical spine has been cleared through radiographic and physical examinations. The patient should be completely exposed to allow a visual appraisal of swelling, lacerations, bruises, and other obvious signs of trauma. Blood or clear fluid noted in the nose or ears suggests a basilar skull fracture. Injuries with characteristic patterns (e.g., cigarette burns, glove and stocking burns), characteristic shapes, and characteristic locations (e.g., finger marks on buttocks, bruises over ear lobes) suggest child abuse.

After the ABCs (airway, breathing, and circulation) have been addressed, it is appropriate to evaluate the patient's LOC.[6] Because a diminished LOC requires either reticular

BOX 54–3

Causes of Impaired Consciousness and Coma

METABOLIC/TOXIC

Hypoxia-ischemia

Shock
Cardiac or pulmonary failure
Near drowning
Carbon monoxide poisoning
Strangulation

Metabolic Disorders

Hypoglycemia
Acidosis
Hyperammonemias
Uremia

Fluid and Electrolyte Imbalance

Endocrine Disorders

Thyroid dysfunction, adrenal insufficiency, hypoparathyroidism

Hypertensive Encephalopathy

Vitamin Deficiency (thiamin, pyridoxine, niacin)

Mitochondrial Disorders

Exogenous Toxins and Poisons

Poisoning in Munchausen by Proxy Syndrome

Infection

Bacterial
Viral
Rickettsial

PAROXYSMAL DISORDERS

STRUCTURAL/INTRINSIC

Trauma

Concussion
Cerebral contusion
Epidural hematoma
Subdural hematoma/effusion
Intracerebral hematoma
Diffuse axonal injury

Neoplasms

Vascular Disease

Cerebral infraction
  Thrombosis
  Embolism
Cerebral hemorrhage
  Arteriovenous malformation
  Aneurysm
Vasculitis
Trauma to carotid or vertebral A in the neck

Focal Infection

Cerebritis
Abscess

Hydrocephalus

TABLE 54–1

Respiratory Patterns in Patients with Altered Mental Status

Respiratory Pattern	Description	Location of Injury
Posthyperventilation apnea	10 sec of apnea after 5 deep breaths	Bilateral hemispheric dysfunction
Cheyne-Stokes respiration	Rhythmic waxing and waning if respiratory amplitude	Bilateral hemispheric dysfunction
Central reflex hyperpnea	Continuous deep breathing	Bilateral hemispheric dysfunction; injury to lower midbrain or upper pons
Apneustic respiration	Prolonged "inspiratory cramp"	Pons
Ataxic respiration	Infrequent irregular breaths	Lower pons, upper medulla
Ondine's curse	Failure of involuntary respiration with retained voluntary respiration	Medulla
Apnea	No respiratory effort	Medulla to C4, peripheral nerves, neuromuscular junction

system or bilateral hemispheric dysfunction, testing the structures immediately adjacent to reticular system provides clues to the cause of coma and directs subsequent investigations.[2] Physical examination findings and their expected anatomic correlates are presented in Table 54–2. A thorough examination should precede any radiographic or laboratory studies, which should be used as adjunctive aids to diagnosis.

The neurologic examination of a comatose patient differs from that of an awake, communicative subject. Although attention is given to posture, movement, and respiration, it must be systematic to document a baseline, define the lesion, and begin to determine prognosis. The presence or absence of focal lateralizing neurologic signs sharply shortens the differential diagnosis. If a single anatomic lesion can explain all the signs, then the differential shrinks to the structural CNS causes. If there is neuroanatomic inconsistency, then toxic and metabolic causes, as described in Box 54–4, are likely. Focal dysfunction may be misinterpreted as altered LOC (i.e., a patient with receptive aphasia who is misdiagnosed as confused or psychotic).[9]

History and presenting symptoms should be evaluated in the context of neurologic findings. Taken together, history and presenting symptoms help determine the cause of diminished LOC. The level of neurologic injury is often best defined by the motor examination (Table 54–2), associated eye findings (Table 54–2), and respiratory pattern (see Fig. 54–2). Figure 54–1 shows the neuroanatomy of corticospinal tracts. The figure primarily presents the upper and lower motor neuron lesions; however, note that cranial nerve (CN) nuclei are frequently associated with important features of the corticospinal tracts. Because these anatomic relationships exist, associated CN and motor findings provide clues to the location of lesions. Injuries above lower medulla result in ipsilateral motor findings.

Eye Examination

Specific eye findings can help to localize the level of lesions and prognosis. Pupillary changes are informative during the examination of a comatose patient because the anatomic areas responsible for consciousness are adjacent to those that control pupillary response. Distinguishing between pupillary dilatation caused by disease or injury and that caused by medication is important. When structural lesions are present, primary pupillary changes are due to the location of the lesion. The pupillary examination may be modified by secondary injuries such as increased ICP (see Fig. 54–2). Pupillary pathways are relatively resistant to metabolic insults; therefore the presence or absence of a light reflex is helpful in distinguishing between structural injuries and metabolic disease. Pupillary reactivity is preserved in metabolic disease.

An assessment of the fundi is important to note the presence of papilledema and retinal hemorrhages. Papilledema is a late sign of increased ICP, and its absence does not rule out raised ICP. Signs of papilledema include blurring of the margins of the optic disc and a decrease in venous pulsations. *Blurring first occurs at the medial margins of the optic disc and progresses laterally.* Retinal hemorrhages are most commonly associated with child abuse, though they may be seen following cardiopulmonary resuscitation. Hemorrhages in the retina appear as perivascular collections of blood that may coalesce to include large areas of the retina. Retinal hemorrhages appear to be associated only with significant head injury that disrupts retinal blood vessels among the internal limiting membrane, the ganglion cell layer, and vessels in the nerve fiber layer of the retina.

The oculocephalic responses (doll's eye reflex and the caloric responses) are two specific maneuvers used when the comatose child is evaluated; they are described in Chapter 50. Positive or normal oculocephalic responses indicate that the brainstem is intact. Conjugate deviation of the eyes is noted toward the side of cerebral lesions and away from the side of brainstem lesions. The corneal reflex is a good test of mid and low pontine function. The mechanism is described in Chapter 50.

Supratentorial Lesions Leading to Coma

The supratentorial compartment mainly contains the cortex, thalamus, and other structures above the midbrain (Fig. 54–2 and Fig. 54–3). Asymmetrical findings on physical examination are indicative of cortical lesions. Given a "focal" or asymmetrical examination, hemiparesis suggests a lesion in a contralateral upper motor neuron pathway. Hypotonia, a diminished LOC, and equally reactive pupils

TABLE 54–2

Clinical Findings Correlated with the Level of CNS Injury

Dysfunction	Response to Noxious Stimuli	Pupils	Eye Position and Movements	Breathing	Motor Findings for Structural Lesions
Both cortices	Withdrawal	Small, reactive	Extraocular movements can be elicited; ipsilateral deviation in frontal lobe lesion	Posthyperventilation apnea or Cheyne-Stokes respiration	
Thalamus	Decorticated posturing	Equal and small, unless the optic tract is also damaged	Eyes deviated down and in toward the side of the lesion	Same as above	Contralateral hemiparesis
Midbrain	Decorticated or decerebrate posturing	Midposition, fixed to light, spontaneous fluctuation	Nystagmus may be present Absent vertical but retained horizontal Loss of ability to adduct; both eyes may be deviated laterally and down in CN III damage	Usually same as above; potential for central reflex hyperpnea	Hemiplegia with contralateral 3rd CN palsy
Pons	Decerebrate posturing	Bilateral pinpoint pupils, reactive to light (especially with midline pontine hemorrhage); Horner's syndrome with lateral lesions	Ocular bobbing Absent conjugate horizontal movements with retained vertical movements and accommodation; often eyes are deviated medially, CN VII damage	May exhibit central reflex hyperpnea, cluster (Biot's) breathing, or apneustic breathing	Hemiplegia with contraleteral 6th and/or 7th CN palsy
Medulla	Weak leg flexion (or none)	Nonreactive, normal size Small Horner's syndrome with lateral lesions	Usually no effect on spontaneous eye movements; may interfere with reflex responses, nystagmus	Rarely, ataxic respiration, apnea if respiratory centers involved	Flaccid weakness with difficulty swallowing, phonating, and incoordination
Spinal cord	None	Normal reaction, abnormal response if brain-stem affected	Normal response	Normal	Flaccid weakness, loss of bowel and bladder control

CN, cranial nerve; *CNS,* central nervous system.

are likely to be localized to a cortical lesion on the contralateral side. Acute unilateral cortical lesions often dampen alertness but do not lead to stupor or coma. Expansion of cortical lesions resulting in raised ICP may reduce blood flow to other areas of the brain and cause the LOC to diminish.

Cortical lesions associated with contralateral thalamic lesions present with contralateral hemiparesis, decorticate (flexor) posturing, a "down and in" (inferiorly and medially) gaze deviation, and small reactive pupils. Decorticate posturing (tonic flexion of upper extremities and tonic extension, adduction, and internal rotation of lower extremities) reflects a lesion above the midbrain.

Sudden changes in the LOC of an otherwise healthy child should make one consider vascular lesions such as cerebrovascular accidents, arteriovenous malformations, bleeding CNS tumors, or ruptured berry aneurysms. Acute sinusitis may result in intracerebral or subdural empyemas because of direct extension of the infection or from hematogenous spread of the organism. A history of fever associated with a diminished LOC may suggest meningoencephalitis associated with any number of organisms. The diminished LOC associated with infection may be a consequence of hemodynamic disturbances caused by the systemic inflammatory response, vascular compromise caused by the mass of an expanding intracranial fluid collection, or poor perfusion that results from vasculitis caused by the infection.

Evaluation of the cardiovascular system of patients with changes in the LOC is important. Murmurs, gallops, and dysrhythmias are suggestive of cardiac lesions that may lead to strokes or intracranial abscesses. Heart lesions associated with right to left shunts, endocarditis, and dysrhythmias may cause emboli that compromise blood flow to the brain. Intravenous therapy has been implicated in the embolism of air bubbles and particles in these patients.

When traumatic injury occurs, coma may occur at the moment of impact or it may be preceded by a lucid interval suggesting an expanding epidural hematoma. For a complete discussion of traumatic brain injuries, see Chapter 99.

BOX 54–4

Characteristics of Coma Caused by Structural and Metabolic Lesions

STRUCTURAL LESIONS

Supratentorial Lesions

Initial focal signs
Retro-caudal progression
Neurologic examination is asymmetrical

Infratentorial Lesions

Brainstem symptoms are often seen initially
Sudden onset of coma
Cranial nerve abnormalities
Alteration of the respiratory pattern

TOXIC, METABOLIC, INFECTIOUS LESIONS

Confusion/stupor often precede signs
Symmetrical examination
Pupillary reactions preserved
Respiratory pattern is often altered (e.g., Cheyne-Stokes breathing)

Several systemic illnesses may result in changes in a patient's LOC. As previously mentioned, metabolic illnesses present with generalized findings. Focal neurologic findings associated with systemic illness and a decreased LOC are common because of vascular consequences of the primary disease. Alterations in the LOC in patients with underlying systemic lupus erythematosus, sickle cell anemia, nephrotic syndrome, homocystinuria, leukemia, and coagulation disorders such as protein C and S deficiency suggest cerebral infarction resulting from vascular obstruction. Patients with generalized petechia and purpura due to thrombocytopenic purpura may have intracranial bleeding. Hypoxic insults and injuries to vertebral or carotid arteries cause cerebral infarction as a consequence of vascular disruption. A period of lucidity is often noted in patients after an acute vascular incident. Stupor and coma develop as brain swelling increases ICP and blood supply to the midbrain and brainstem are compromised.

Venous obstruction caused by thrombosis in the venous sinuses of the brain causes blood flow to diminish by creating a pressure gradient that the intraarteriolar pressure cannot overcome. Venous sinus thrombosis can be seen after severe dehydration and hypercoagulable states, particularly in young infants with histories of vomiting and diarrhea. Orbital cellulitis has been associated with cavernous venous thrombosis.

Although uncommon, diminished LOC may occur because of bleeding, convulsions, or rapidly rising ICP as a result of brain tumor. A history of headache may suggest elevated ICP resulting from hydrocephalus or neoplasm but may be seen in migraine syndrome with impaired consciousness. The presence of neurocutaneous lesions (such as the depigmented areas seen in tuberous sclerosis) suggests that seizures or intracranial masses are the cause of diminished LOC.

BOX 54–5

Diagnostic Evaluation in Patient with Coma

TESTS TO FACILITATE SUPPORTIVE THERAPY

Arterial blood gas
Urea, electrolytes and creatinine, Ca, Mg
Blood glucose
Osmolality of plasma and urine
Urine for ketones, sugar, and pH
Complete blood count
Coagulation screen
Blood culture, urine culture, tracheal culture
Blood levels of anticonvulsants
Virology
Chest radiograph
Electrocardiogram
Electroencephalogram
Cerebral imaging CAT scan, MRI scan
Brainstem auditory-, visual-, and somatosensory-evoked potentials

TESTS TO IDENTIFY A SPECIFIC DIAGNOSIS

CSF examination
Toxicology screen
Blood ammonia
Blood pyruvate and lactate
Amino acid profile
Organic acid analysis
Porphyrins
Liver function tests
Carnitine
Serum lead level
Serum cortisol
Skeletal survey
Cerebral imaging

Ca, calcium*; CAT,* computed axial tomography; *CSF,* cerebrospinal fluid; *Mg,* magnesium; *MRI,* magnetic resonance imaging.

Subtentorial Lesions Leading to Coma

The subtentorial compartment is the area beneath the tentorium that contains most of the brainstem, the cerebellum, the exit sites for most of the CNs, and passages for cerebrospinal fluid (CSF) movement (Fig. 54–2 and Fig. 54–3). Injury and insult can alter function of these components by either destruction or compression. Brainstem lesions are capable of creating immediate loss of consciousness due to the proximity of the ARAS. The relationship of CNs to the brainstem is described in Figure 54–3.

Lesions in the brainstem may be due to demyelinating diseases, cerebrovascular diseases, neoplasm, or head trauma. Uncal herniation can occur after head trauma as a result of rapidly expanding subdural or epidural hematomas. Fever, vomiting, and LOC are noted in patients with brainstem and cerebellar infarction. Cerebrovascular lesions disrupt blood supply causing brainstem dysfunction. Headache, vomiting, and gait unsteadiness before the LOC develops suggest the presence of a tumor.

The brainstem contains a number of structures that are compactly arranged. Because of this arrangement, a single

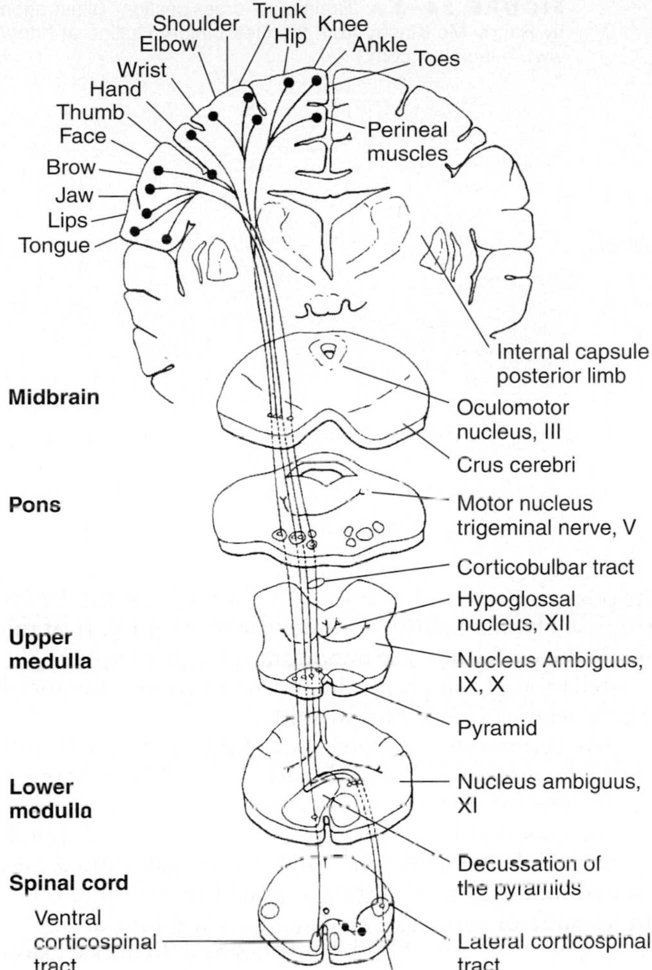

FIGURE 54–1 • The pyramidal system. (From Gilman S, Newman S: *Manter and Gantz's clinical neuroanatomy and neurophysiology,* ed 9, Philadelphia,1996, FA Davis.)

lesion can result in several abnormalities. As mentioned earlier, because of the proximity of nerve tracts and CN nuclei, the resultant association of symptoms can assist in localization of lesions. Because the CN nuclei innervate ipsilateral structures and the long tracts innervate contralateral structures, unilateral brainstem lesions frequently result in ipsilateral CN dysfunction and contralateral hemiplegia and hemisensory loss. Considering the CNs involved can further identify the level of injury, midbrain lesions commonly affect CN III. Lesions in the pons affect CNs V, VI, or both. Medullary lesions tend to affect CN XII.

Midbrain lesions frequently present with hemiplegia contralateral to the lesion and an ipsilateral midposition, nonreactive pupil due to third CN palsy. Third CN palsy generally causes both eyes to deviate laterally or inferiorly and laterally. When gaze is deviated down and out, the patient is said to have the "setting sun sign." Decerebrate or extensor posturing is elicited in response to noxious stimuli in patients with midbrain lesions. This complex yet abnormal response consists of tonic extension of the upper extremities and extension, adduction, and internal rotation of lower extremities.

Contralateral hemiplegia and medial deviation of the ipsilateral eye (CN VI) are hallmarks of medial lesions in the caudal portion of the pons. The ipsilateral pupil remains small and reactive to light. Midline pontine hemorrhages, however, may cause bilateral pinpoint pupils. Extension of caudal midline pontine lesions can cause a peripheral facial paralysis. If a patient has a lesion in a more rostral portion of the pons, ipsilateral CN V lesions might be noted with loss of the ipsilateral corneal reflex. A lesion in this area might also affect some uncrossed fibers from the corticobulbar and corticotectal tracts. In addition to contralateral hemiplegia, these patients will display paralysis of the superficial facial muscles on the side contralateral to the lesion.

Although hypertonia is a feature of preexisting corticospinal tract injury, it can be seen in acute injury to the midbrain or the pons. When the more rostral corticospinal tract is disrupted, the vestibulospinal motor system continues to exert tonic influence on the spinal cord. Consequently, these patients exhibit decerebrate posturing to noxious stimuli. Acute lesions often cause extensor posturing regardless of anatomic location. Decorticated and decerebrate posturing may occur in combination. These facts render posturing less reliable for localization of CNS lesions. Though not always reliable for localization, posturing suggests that cortical control centers are not functioning.

Patients with hemiplegia, swallowing difficulties, problems with phonation, nonreactive normal-sized pupils, and normal extraocular eye movements are likely to have an injury to the medulla. CNs VIII to XII exit the brainstem in the area of the medulla. Consequently, medullary lesions are associated with dysfunctional bulbar muscles, such as speech and swallowing. If respiratory centers are affected, patients may have apnea. If the medullary injury is to the dorsal portion of the medulla, patients may have hypotonia and ataxia on the side of the lesion.

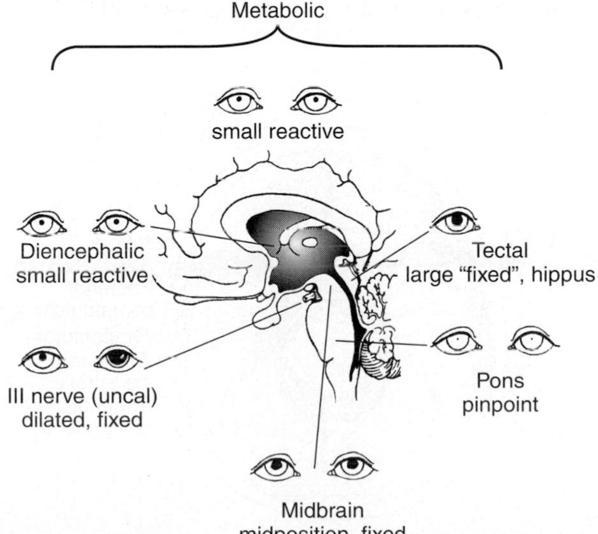

FIGURE 54–2 • Pupils in the comatose patient. (From Plum F, Posner JB: *The diagnosis of stupor and coma,* ed 3, Philadelphia, 1982, FA Davis.)

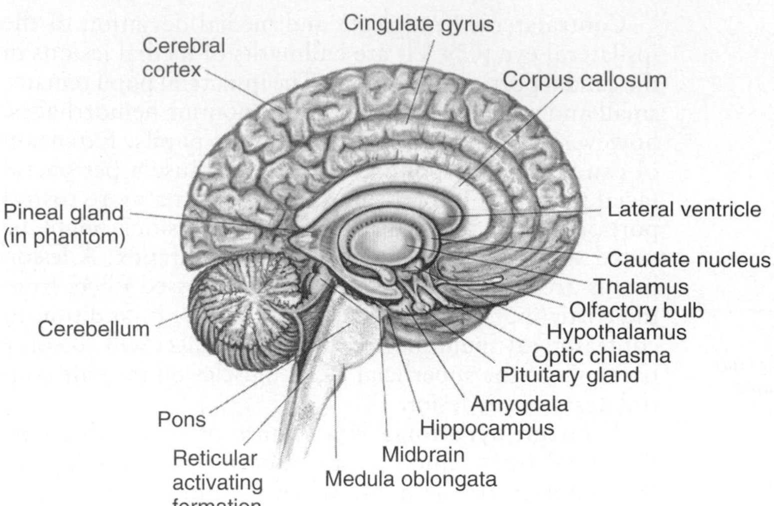

FIGURE 54–3 • "Brain map–cross section." (Illustration by Randy Mc Kinsey from the Head Injury Hotline at http://www.headinjury.com.)

Cerebellar lesions usually produce coma by brainstem compression. Cerebellar signs in confused patients should raise suspicions of intoxication or nutritional deficiency (e.g., vitamin B_{12}).

Herniation Syndromes

Expanding mass lesions develop at the expense of one of the CNS compartments (brain, blood, or CSF). Herniation occurs when the brain is subjected to pressure gradients that cause portions of it to flow from one intracranial compartment to another. Although the brain has substantial elasticity, the arteries and veins responsible for its blood supply are relatively fixed in space, creating a risk that brain shifts will cause moving portions to lose their blood supply. The supratentorial compartment is connected to the subtentorial compartment via the tentorium cerebelli, which passes through tentorial notch (Fig. 54–4). Located in the tentorial notch are the midbrain; the third CN; and several arteries including choroidal arteries, the posterior cerebral arteries, and the superior cerebellar arteries. The cerebellum occupies the posterior part of the notch. Proximity of these important structures explains the constellation of symptoms that occur when supratentorial lesions lead to transtentorial shifts.

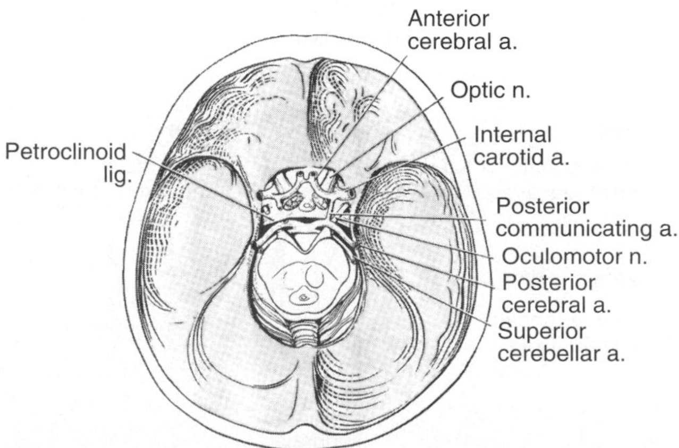

FIGURE 54–4 • The floor of anterior and middle fossa, showing the tentorial notch and relationship of the third CN nerve with other intracranial structures. (From Plum F, Posner JB: *The diagnosis of stupor and coma*, ed 3, Philadelphia, 1982, FA Davis.)

Two herniation syndromes are principally important: *central herniation* and *uncal herniation*. Central herniation occurs when diffuse brain swelling or a centrally located mass causes the diencephalon to move caudally through the tentorial notch. Figure 54–5 shows the remote and catastrophic effects of certain supratentorial lesions leading to shift of intracranial structure via tentorial notch. Dysfunction of the ARAS and cerebral hypoperfusion cause the alteration of consciousness. Patients become initially less alert and later progress to stupor and coma. Diencephalic dysfunction initially produces small reactive pupils because sympathetic output from the hypothalamus is lost. At this stage, decorticate (flexor) posturing may be spontaneous or elicited by noxious stimuli, and Cheyne-Stokes respiration is noted. Recognizing this constellation of symptoms is important because herniation at this stage is reversible without severe consequences.

As rostral-caudal progression of central herniation continues into the midbrain and pons, the likelihood of reversibility markedly decreases. As the midbrain begins to fail, pupils enlarge to midposition, and decerebrate (extensor) posturing is noted. Attempts to elicit horizontal eye movements with either cerebro-ocular reflex or cerebro-vestibular reflex fail, and the respiratory rhythm becomes irregular. The patient becomes overtly comatose. Further progression affects the medullary respiratory centers. Virtually all brainstem reflexes are absent, and death becomes imminent. The initial cardiovascular response to diminished brainstem perfusion is hypertension, which leads to reflex bradycardia. Classic Cushing's reflex responses are seen after herniation syndromes develop.

Uncal herniation occurs when a lateral expanding cerebral mass pushes the uncus and hippocampal gyrus over the lateral edges of the tentorium. As the diencephalon begins to shift away from the mass, consciousness begins to diminish and ipsilateral third CN palsy develops.

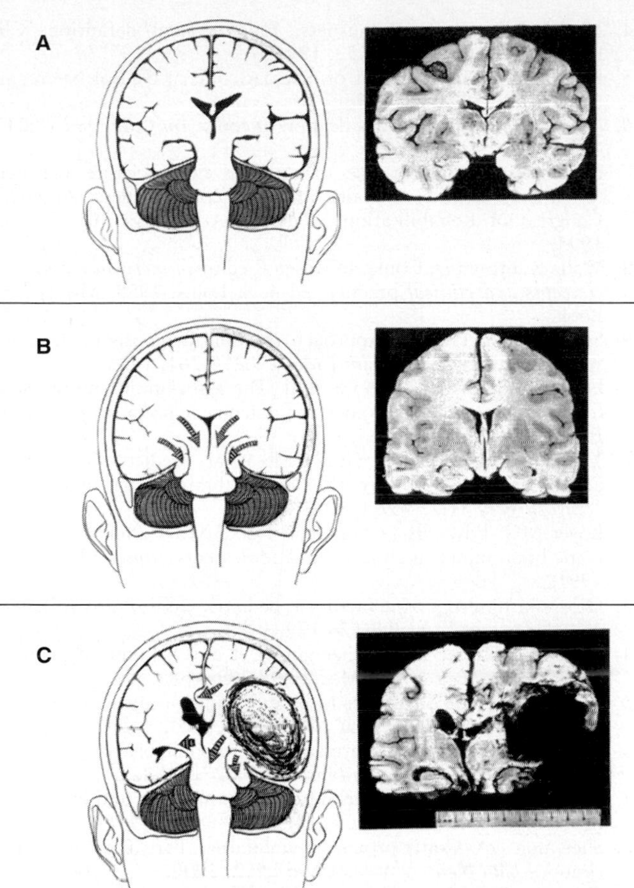

FIGURE 54–5 • **A,** Intracranial shifts from supratentorial lesions. The relationships of various supratentorial and infratentorial compartments seen in the coronal section. **B,** Central transtentorial herniation. **C,** Uncal and transtentorial herniation. (From Plum F, Posner JB: *The diagnosis of stupor and coma*, ed 3, Philadelphia, 1982, FA Davis.)

When the CN III is compressed against the tentorial notch, the papillary fibers, located most peripherally in the nerve, are primarily damaged, resulting in large pupils. A unilateral dilated pupil, often without severe impairment of consciousness, and contralateral hemiparesis are the hallmark findings of uncal herniation. Other findings, such as impaired ocular motility, may take some time to develop. Once present, symptoms may proceed rapidly. Some patients have bilateral pupillary dilatation presumably because of distortion of CN III anatomy and midbrain ischemia. At this point, uncal herniation begins to affect midbrain and upper pons, producing fixed pupils and extensor posturing. Further progression is indistinguishable from central herniation.

Cerebellar tonsillar herniation is seen in patients with posterior fossa masses, which cause compression of the brainstem, CN dysfunction, and obstructive hydrocephalus. As the pressure gradient across the foramen magnum increases, cerebellar tonsils may be pushed through the foramen. Medullary compression affects respiratory centers in the medulla with resultant apnea. Patients with cerebellar tonsillar herniation may complain of neck pain before losing consciousness. Upward transtentorial herniation syndrome occurs as well. This is usually seen in patients undergoing ventriculostomy for relief of hydrocephalus. Contents of the posterior fossa herniate into the diencephalic region.

Outcome

The major causes of pediatric coma involve anoxic-ischemic encephalopathy and trauma. In a study by Levi et al,[10] the prognostic indicators for traumatic coma are associated with the injury, the admission GCS score, the presence of a mass with persistent increased ICP, and the presence of diffuse axonal injury. In their study, Michaud et al[11] found that the most significant predictor of disability was the GCS score at 72 hours and the level of oxygenation in the emergency department. In children, improvement can continue over a very protracted time, even several years, long beyond the time that most adult patients will have reached the plateau of their recovery.[12] Orlowski[13] developed a scoring system for evaluating prognosis in submersion based on five unfavorable prognostic factors: age younger than 3 years, estimated submersion more than 5 minutes, no attempts at resuscitation for 10 minutes, coma on admission to the emergency department, and severe acidosis with arterial blood gas pH = 7.10. A score of less than or equal to 2 was associated with 90% chance of recovery, but a score greater than or equal to 3 points was associated with only a 5% chance of recovery.

Cardiopulmonary arrests are far less common in children, and outcome statistics are generally pessimistic. In hospital settings, cardiopulmonary arrests occur mainly in face of severe pulmonary and cardiac diseases. Respiratory arrests without cardiac arrests were associated with a 25% mortality; by contrast cardiopulmonary arrest are associated with an 83% to 87% mortality.[14] Factors associated with 100% mortality are duration of asystole more than 15 minutes and administration of more than one dose of epinephrine.[15] The best predictor of survival beyond 24 hours was a patient's prearrest CNS status (76% of patients are alert before resuscitation compared with 30% who are comatose before resuscitation). In a retrospective study of cardiopulmonary resuscitation, 64% of attempts were initially successful, 48% were associated with more than 24 hours of survival, and only 31% were followed up since discharge from the intensive care unit (ICU).[16] The prognosis for outpatient arrests is gloomier yet. O'Rourke[17] reported the results of 34 children who were apneic and pulseless in the emergency department. None of these patients survived to be discharged home; 27 patients died, 5 remained in a persistent vegetative state (PVS), and 2 were severely disabled and were admitted to long-term care facilities.

Ethical Consideration

Coma prognostication is done to help parents and families understand the extent of injury and to help the health care team make management decisions.[18] If within the acute period there is a high probability of death without regaining consciousness, withdrawal of support might be reasonable. By contrast, a decision to withdraw support based on a high probability of survival with severe motor or mental disability is ultimately a judgment about "quality of life." A decision to withdraw support in this case implies that life with severe disability is worse than no life at all. Shewmon, Holmes, and Byrne[19] suggest that it is not possible to precisely judge the outcome of vegetative patients. Given this assertion, life and death judgments based on quality of life issues may not have a place in pediatrics. Age-specific differences in the ability of children to cope with and adapt to injury suggest that care must be taken when making decisions to withdraw therapy after acute injury. It has been noted that younger children adapt better to physical and mental disability, and these adaptations are better incorporated into family life. Expressions such as "mild, moderate, or severe disability" can subjectively describe levels of neurologic dysfunction. Categories such as "favorable or unfavorable" convey value judgments. Thus it is important to use appropriate terminology for coma prognosis. Parents of children with disabilities tend to strongly disagree with subjective and judgmental terminology even if at the time of the brain insult they felt utterly incapable of learning to cope with such an outcome. Thus with respect to ethical implications, as well as the neurobiology of coma prognosis, the adage holds true: children are not miniature adults.

REFERENCES

1. Plum F, Posner J: *The diagnosis of stupor and coma,* ed 3, Philadelphia, 1980, FA Davis.
2. Bleck TP: Level of consciousness and attention. In Goetz C.G., editor: *Textbook of clinical neurology,* ed 1, Philadelphia, 1999 WB Saunders.
3. Howsepian AA: The 1994 Multi-Society Task Force consensus statement on the Persistent Vegetative State: a critical analysis, *Issues Law Med* 12:3-29, 1996.
4. Niedermeyer E: Consciousness: function and definition, Clin Electroencephalogr 25:86-93, 1994.
5. Bates D: The management of medical coma, J Neurol Neurosurg Psychiatr 56:589-598, 1993.
6. Bozza Marrubini M: Classification of coma, *Int Care Med* 10:217, 1984.
7. Recommendations for use of uniform nomenclature pertinent to patients with severe alterations in consciousness. American Congress of Rehabilitation Medicine, *Arch Phys Med* 76:205, 1995.
8. Wolfe R, Brown D: Coma. In Rosen P, editor: *Emergency medicine: concepts and clinical* practice, ed 4, St Louis. 1998, Mosby-Year Book.
9. Samuels MA. Practical approach to coma diagnosis in the unresponsive patient, *Cleve Clin J Med* 59:257-261, 1992.
10. Levi L, Guilburd JN, Linn S et al. The association between skull fracture, intracranial pathology and outcome in pediatric head injury, *Br J Neurosurg* 5:617-625, 1991.
11. Michaud LJ, Rivara FP, Grady MS et al. Predictors of survival and severity of disability after severe brain injury in children, *Neurosurgery* 31:254-264, 1992.
12. Boyer MG, Edwards P: Outcome 1 to 3 years after severe traumatic brain injury in children and adolescents, *Injury* 22:315-320, 1991.
13. Orlowski JP: Prognostic factors in pediatric cases of drowning and near-drowning, *JACEP* 8:176-179, 1979.
14. Lewis JK, Minter MG, Eshelman SJ et al. Outcome of pediatric resuscitation, *Ann Emerg Med* 2:297-299, 1983.
15. Gillis J, Dikerson D, Rieder M et al: Results of inpatient pediatric resuscitation, *Crit Care Med* 14:469-471, 1986.
16. Von Seggern K, Egar M, Fuhrman BP: Cardiopulmonary resuscitation in pediatric ICU, *Crit Care Med* 14:275-277, 1986.
17. O'Rourke PP: Outcome of children who are apneic and pulseless in the emergency room, *Crit Care Med* 14:466-468, 1986.
18. Shewmon DA: Coma prognosis in children. Part II: clinical application, *J Clin Neurophysiol* 17:467-472, 2000.
19. Shewmon DA, Holmes GL, Byrne PA: Consciousness in congenitally decorticate children: developmental vegetative state as self-fulfilling prophecy, *Dev Med Child Neurol* 41:364-374, 1999.

CHAPTER 55

Status Epilepticus

Elizabeth J. Donner, Cecil D. Hahn, and Sam D. Shemie

PEARLS

- Convulsive and nonconvulsive seizures cause neuronal injury on a hypoxic-ischemic basis related to intense neuronal metabolic demand and cardiorespiratory compromise.
- Later to treat, harder to cease. Early diagnosis and aggressive intervention for any seizure activity, convulsive or nonconvulsive, are more important than the time-related definitions that differentiate status epilepticus (SE) from refractory SE.
- Practitioners in the intensive care unit (ICU) should distinguish SE from its underlying cause and view it as one of the clinical expressions of severe brain disease that threatens life through impairment of airway control and respiratory function. Once the intubation and mechanical ventilation are established, outcome is primarily related to the underlying brain disease and the ability to control seizures.
- ICU practitioners should resist the temptation to rely on judging seizure control in SE on the basis of clinical motor activity alone; clinical examination can be unreliable or confounded by subtle findings, and subclinical SE may commonly occur. Electroencephalography (EEG) provides real-time information regarding brain activity and is invaluable in the evaluation of patients with SE to allow for direct correlation of patient behavior, neural activity, and titration of anticonvulsants.
- The pharmacologic treatment of sustained and refractory SE should be titrated to EEG endpoints. The limitations of high-dose therapies (e.g. barbiturate or benzodiazepine) are generally related to cardiovascular toxicity rather than to any predefined upper limit of dosing.

Definition

Status epilepticus (SE) is a life-threatening medical emergency. In children, SE often necessitates urgent treatment and monitoring in the pediatric intensive care unit (ICU) and requires that the pediatric intensivist be comfortable with the diagnosis and management of this common condition.

The International League Against Epilepsy defines SE as a seizure that persists for a sufficient length of time or is repeated enough to produce a fixed and enduring epileptic condition.[1] From the practical perspective of the treating physician, this definition has been difficult to apply. A more commonly used clinical definition includes duration of seizure activity, specifying SE as seizures lasting 30 minutes or longer, which is based on the theory that neuronal damage may begin after 30 minutes of continuous seizures. No clinical data support the 30-minute rule, however, and more recent definitions of SE include a shorter duration of seizure activity. An operational definition has been proposed, in which generalized convulsive SE in adults and children older than 5 years is "greater than or equal to 5 minutes of continuous seizures or two or more discrete seizures between which there is incomplete recovery of consciousness."[2] This has been supported by clinical studies showing that most secondarily generalized convulsive seizures in adults last less than 5 minutes[3]; these results suggest that seizures lasting more than 5 minutes should be regarded as more significant. Similar data in children have shown that new-onset seizures cluster by duration; most seizures (76%) last less than 5 minutes and 24% last longer, with a mean duration of 31 minutes.[4] The shorter duration definition of SE remains controversial, however, because although it is less common for seizures to persist beyond 5 minutes, it has also been shown that seizures lasting 10 to 29 minutes that stop spontaneously are associated with a significantly lower mortality than seizures lasting beyond 30 minutes.[15] Thus before the definition of SE includes a seizure duration of less than 30 minutes, further study and discussion are required.

Regardless of the definition of SE, there is a consensus in the medical community that continuous or prolonged seizures require urgent intervention. Children with prolonged seizures should receive prompt and aggressive treatment with the aim of stopping seizures as soon as possible.

Classification of Status Epilepticus

SE should be classified with the same terminology used for seizure classification. The most recent International League Against Epilepsy Proposed Diagnostic Scheme for People with Epileptic Seizures and with Epilepsy[6] identifies two major categories that may be applied to both self-limited and continuous seizures.

Generalized seizures refer to seizures originating from both cerebral hemispheres. Consciousness is usually impaired. This includes seizures with motor movements and absence seizures during which there may be no convulsive signs. Electroencephalography (EEG), however, indicates seizure onset in both cerebral hemispheres. *Focal seizures*, (previously referred to as *partial seizures*) are those in which the first clinical and EEG changes indicate seizure onset in one area of the cerebral cortex. Generalized seizures that begin as focal seizures are termed *secondarily generalized seizures*. *Complex focal seizures* are associated with an impairment of consciousness. *Simple focal seizures* have no impairment of consciousness. When simple focal seizures are prolonged and have a focal motor component, the term *epilepsia partialis continua* is used.[7] These same terms are also used to describe continuous seizures and SE. Although the distinction between generalized and focal seizures is helpful to predict the cause and outcomes of SE, the differentiation may require EEG and has limited utility in the acute clinical situation.

A more clinically useful classification scheme involves categorizing SE by the presence of motor movements. (Box 55–1). *Generalized convulsive SE* (GCSE) consists of continuous clonic or tonic motor activity with bilateral epileptiform discharges on the EEG. As GCSE progresses, the motor movements are reduced and may be characterized only by subtle twitching of the limbs, face, or trunk. This is termed *subtle GCSE*.

Nonconvulsive SE (NCSE) consists of continuous electrographic seizures with no motor movements. This may occur after prolonged GCSE. NCSE also refers to SE consisting of absence seizures or focal onset seizures that do not produce motor movements.

In children, an additional category, *febrile SE,* may be considered. SE occurring in association with fever represents one form of complex febrile convulsions.

Finally, SE may also be classified with respect to cause. *Symptomatic* implies a known cause for SE and can be further divided into *acute symptomatic* and *remote symptomatic* on the basis of cause. Examples of acute symptomatic causes include toxic and infectious causes. Remote symptomatic SE is most often associated with a long-standing history of epilepsy or remote central nervous system (CNS) insult. The term *idiopathic* SE is used when there is no known or suspected cause for the seizures.

Nonepileptic seizures, also known as nonepileptic events or psychogenic or pseudoseizures, may also present as SE. Patients with and without a prior history of epileptic seizures may have nonepileptic SE. In this situation, EEG may be necessary for diagnosis to confirm the absence of abnormal electrical discharges in the brain.

BOX 55–1

Modified Classification of Status Epilepticus

GENERALIZED STATUS EPILEPTICUS

Convulsive
Nonconvulsive (i.e., absence or following prolonged convulsive)

FOCAL STATUS EPILEPTICUS

Simple: without altered consciousness
Complex: with altered consciousness

From Riviello JJ: *Status epilepticus.* American Academy of Neurology, Child Neurology Course, Denver, 2002.

Epidemiology of Status Epilepticus

Incidence

Two population-based studies have examined the incidence of SE in the United States. The incidence of SE in Richmond, Va.,[8] was determined to be 41 per 100,000 population, and in Rochester, Minn.,[9] the incidence was 18 per 100,000 population. The difference may reflect a different racial composition in the communities studied; in the Richmond study, the incidence of SE was higher in the nonwhite population.

The incidence of SE peaks during young and old age. In infants younger than 1 year, the incidence of SE may be as high as 150/100 000.[8] Furthermore, the incidence is more than twofold higher in children younger than 5 years than in those older than 5 years. SE was found to be the admission diagnosis of 1.6% of children admitted to a pediatric ICU.[10]

Cause

One of the largest series of SE in children was published in 1970. This review of 239 cases of SE in children identified 47% of cases to be symptomatic (26% acute symptomatic, 21% remote symptomatic) and the remaining 53% of cases to be idiopathic, including febrile SE.[11] The cause of SE is age dependent; infection plays a larger role in the cause of SE in children. In a 1996 Richmond, Va., study, the three major causes of SE in children were infection with fever, remote symptomatic cause, and low anticonvulsant drug levels (Table 55–1).[8] The three major causes in adults were low antiepileptic drug (AED) levels, remote symptomatic cause, and stroke.[8] The cause also differs among younger and older children. Febrile and acute symptomatic SE are more common in children younger than 2 years, whereas idiopathic and remote symptomatic causes are most common in older children.[10,12]

In children with first seizures, 12% have SE,[13] and in a study of 613 children with newly diagnosed epilepsy, 9.1% had provoked or unprovoked SE before the diagnosis of epilepsy.[14] Children who had SE before a diagnosis of epilepsy were most likely to have remote symptomatic epilepsy.

Outcome

Mortality

Practitioners in the ICU should distinguish SE from its underlying cause and view it as one of the clinical expressions of severe brain disease that threatens life through impairment of airway control and respiratory function. Once the intubation and mechanical ventilation are established, outcome is primarily related to the underlying brain disease and the ability to control seizures. Age and cause are strong predictors of outcome in SE, reflecting the fact that morbidity and mortality are more related to the underlying disorder than to the seizures. Mortality as high as 23% has been reported in SE in adults[15]; however, in a study of 193 children with SE, only 7 children (3.6%) died within 3 months of the SE. The etiology of SE was the strongest predictor of mortality. All deaths that occurred were associated with an acute CNS insult or progressive encephalopathy, and no children with unprovoked or febrile SE died.[16] Similar findings were documented in a study of 40 cases of pediatric SE, in which mortality was 10% and the cause of SE in all children who died was acutely life threatening.[17] Refractory SE carries higher risks of significant morbidity and mortality (see section on Refractory SE later).

TABLE 55–1

Causes of SE in Children from the Richmond, Va., SE Database[8]

Cause	% of SE
Non-CNS infection	52
Remote symptomatic	38
Low AED level	21
Cerebrovascular disease	10
Metabolic	7
Hypoxia	5
Idiopathic	5
CNS infection	2
Drug overdose	2

AED, antiepileptic drug; *CNS*, central nervous system; *SE*, status epilepticus.

Subsequent Development of Epilepsy

Epilepsy, defined as recurrent unprovoked seizures, is a potential long-term complication of SE. The risk of epilepsy development after SE in children ranges from 26% to 36%.[17,18] Like mortality, the development of epilepsy after SE is strongly related to the cause of SE. In children with acute symptomatic SE, the risk for development of subsequent unprovoked seizures was found to be 41%, 3 times higher than that for children with self-limited acute symptomatic seizures. This risk was highest in children with anoxic encephalopathy, followed by structural then metabolic causes.[19]

In contrast, children with a first unprovoked seizure presenting as SE were not more likely than children with self-limited first unprovoked seizures to have recurrent seizures.[13] Furthermore, the increased risk of developing epilepsy after febrile SE is generally reported to be small to none.[16–18,20]

Pathophysiology

The exact mechanism that permits a seizure to become sustained is not known. Theoretically, either a failure of routine neuronal inhibition or an excess of excitation is required. Much of the research in this area has focused on the failure of neuronal inhibition. γ-Aminobutyric acid (GABA) is the major inhibitory neurotransmitter in the CNS, and observations from animal studies suggest that a deficit in GABA inhibition or altered GABA receptor function[21] may permit excessive excitation and the prolongation of seizures. Clinically this may be shown by the poor response of prolonged seizures to the GABA agonists, benzodiazepines.[22] A role in seizure termination for the endogenous inhibitory neuropeptides has also been proposed, possibly implicating these molecules in the failure of neuronal inhibition in SE.

Neuronal injury in SE appears related to traditional hypoxic-ischemic mechanisms. Early in SE, there is an increase in neuronal metabolic demand with a compensatory increase in cerebral blood flow (CBF) and brain oxygenation. Later in SE, the homeostatic mechanisms appear unable to keep up with the high cerebral metabolic demand and autoregulation of CBF fails, so that increased mean arterial pressure is required to maintain adequate brain perfusion. As blood pressure falls, there is subsequent reduction in brain parenchymal oxygenation. In the face of increased neuronal metabolic demand, uncontrolled muscular contractions, hyperthermia, and impaired airway control, both impaired oxygenation and ventilation contribute to the mismatch between metabolic supply and demand. Pathologic neuronal injury has been shown, however, to occur even when these other factors are controlled and before CBF is reduced, presumably because of a relation to unmet neuronal metabolic demand in isolation.

Further evidence suggests that it is the excessive excitation that results in the neuronal injury associated with SE. Glutamate is the major excitatory neurotransmitter in the CNS, and glutamate agonists are used to induce seizures in experimental animal models of SE. Studies have implicated both the N-methyl-D-aspartate (NMDA) and α-amino-3-hydroxy-5-methyl-4-isoxazole-propionic acid (AMPA) glutamate receptors in the pathophysiology of SE.[23] The NMDA receptor may have a dual function in the pathophysiology of SE. Magnesium (Mg) blocks the NMDA channel when it is in its normal state. With depolarization, Mg no longer blocks the channel, and calcium, which is allowed to flow into the cell, produces further depolarization. Thus the NMDA receptor is activated when the cell is depolarized and responds by further depolarizing the cell, sustaining the excitation. This process has also been implicated in SE-induced neuronal injury, as the accumulation of intracellular calcium activates pathologic processes resulting in both necrotic and apoptotic cell death.[24,25]

Diagnosis

The clinical presentation of SE is variable, depending on seizure type and the baseline developmental and medical status of the child. Diagnosis depends on the identification of continuous or repetitive seizures, which is usually straightforward in the presence of convulsive seizures. After prolonged convulsive seizures, however, the motor manifestations often diminish, and differentiating between continuous nonconvulsive seizures and the postictal state is difficult. Furthermore, patients with NCSE, including absence SE, may be difficult to identify by history and physical examination alone. These patients can have intermittent altered awareness and continuous lethargy or unresponsiveness with or without subtle myoclonic jerks of the face or limbs. In such cases, EEG monitoring may be critical. EEG monitoring can also be used to identify nonepileptic or psychogenic SE. Although uncommon, prolonged delays in the EEG-based diagnosis of nonepileptic SE can lead to unnecessary medical intervention.[26]

EEG measures extracellular electrical activity generated by cortical neurons. Data are collected with a standard array of scalp electrodes and translated for visual display onto a paper or digital record. Because EEG provides real-time information regarding brain activity, it is invaluable in the evaluation of patients with SE. EEG allows for direct correlation between patient behavior and neural activity. A trained neurologist or neurophysiologist should perform EEG interpretation. Movement and muscle artifact can resemble seizure activity leading to misinterpretation of the EEG. Cerebral function monitors (CFMs), single-channel amplitude electroencephalograms, are commercially available; they provide a more gross assessment of brain activity than standard EEG. These devices have been used to identify background brain activity and generalized seizures in neonates and adults.[27,28] CFMs can be applied and interpreted by trained ICU staff and thereby can provide improved accessibility over EEG. Because of the complex nature of EEG in children, however, many pediatric ICUs perform EEG monitoring for SE under the supervision of a neurologist or neurophysiologist.

Abnormal waveforms on EEG can be divided into two categories: epileptiform abnormalities and nonepileptiform abnormalities. *Epileptiform abnormalities* are abnormal discharges associated with an increased risk of seizures, including sharp waves, spikes, polyspikes, and spike and slow wave discharges. When present between seizures, these waveforms are identified as interictal abnormalities. Seizures, or ictal abnormalities, may have various appearances on EEG, but usually include widespread epileptiform discharges (Fig. 55–1, A). In generalized SE, these abnormal discharges are seen in both hemispheres. In focal SE, the epileptiform discharges are usually confined to one brain region.

Nonepileptiform abnormalities are not necessarily associated with a risk of seizure but suggest some CNS dysfunction. Slow waves are a nonspecific finding, which suggests a structural or functional abnormality, and are often seen after a seizure or SE. The location of slow waves after a seizure may aid in the differentiation between generalized and focal seizures. Generalized slow waves are associated with a diffuse encephalopathy.

Two further EEG patterns are of particular relevance to the treatment of prolonged seizures. *Burst-suppression* is characterized by brief bursts of mixed spikes, sharp waves and slow waves followed by longer periods of relative EEG flattening (Fig. 56–1, *B*). An *isoelectric* EEG pattern refers to a low voltage record, with no discernable cortical activity (Fig. 56–1, *C*). Both burst-suppression and isoelectric EEG patterns can be seen in coma and may carry a poor prognosis in certain clinical situations. In the treatment of SE, however, these patterns are often used to monitor the response to treatment and are a desired endpoint of adequate seizure control (see section on refractory SE later).

Refractory Status Epilepticus

Refractory status epilepticus (RSE) is characterized by seizures that persist beyond 60 minutes and fail to respond to first- and second-line therapy. In adults, SE may be refractory in 9% to 31% of patients and carries an increased rate of morbidity and mortality.[16,29] In children, the incidence of RSE has not been well documented; however, in a large series of children with SE, 26% of the children had seizures lasting more than 60 minutes.[16] Pediatric mortality from RSE has been reported to be 16% to 32%.[30,31] As with all SE, outcome appears to be related to cause, with deaths occurring predominantly in acute symptomatic cases.[30,31]

Prolonged therapy for sustained RSE may be required. Although it is virtually always possible to control seizures with high-dose seizure-suppressive medications, complete seizure remission is not always possible when these high-dose medications are withdrawn.

There is a particularly severely affected group of patients who have seizures that persist for more than 24 hours; this has been termed *sustained refractory status epilepticus*. The outcome of acute symptomatic RSE in seven children who received long-term high-dose seizure suppressive medication was reported to be uniformly poor, with all children having medically intractable epilepsy and developmental deterioration.[32] We have reviewed seven cases of acute symptomatic sustained RSE. In these cases, sustained RSE is most often associated with viral encephalitis or a postinfectious process.

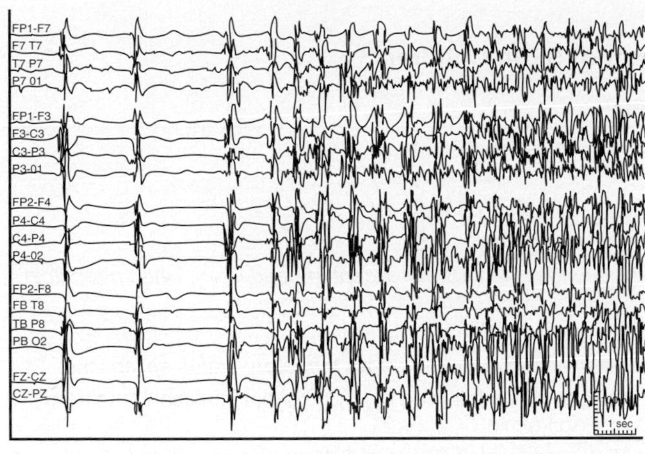

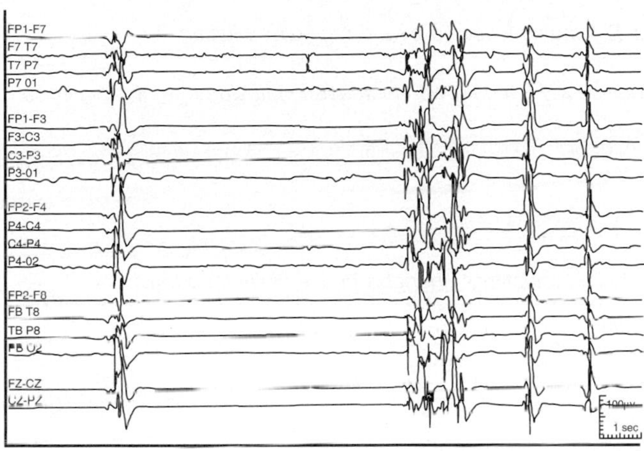

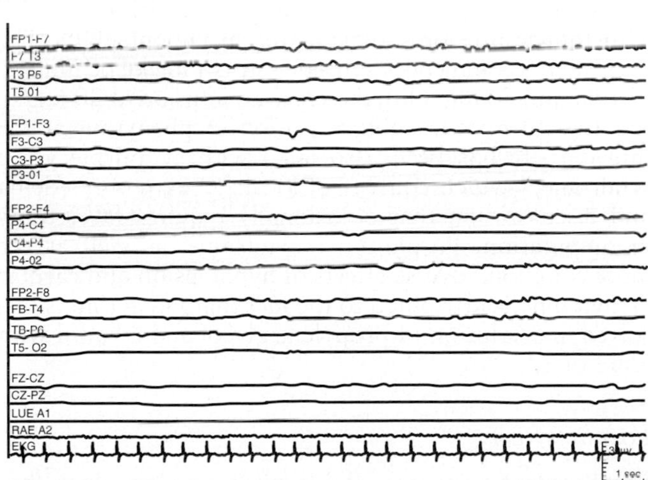

FIGURE 55–1 • Electroencephalography in status epilepticus (SE). **A,** A generalized seizure evolving. **B,** Burst-suppression pattern in a patient treated with high-dose suppressive medication for SE. **C,** Isoelectric pattern in a patient treated with high-dose suppressive medication for SE.

This experience shows that SE persisting longer than 24 hours identifies a prolonged course with our patients requiring high-dose seizure suppressive medication for up to 108 days. Outcome was consistently poor, with 57% mortality and severe disability in the surviving children.

Treatment of Status Epilepticus

The principal goal of therapy in SE is to abort the seizure before irreversible neuronal injury occurs. In experimental models of SE, irreversible neuronal injury begins after 20 minutes to 1 hour of continuous seizure activity, despite the maintenance of adequate brain oxygenation and perfusion. Furthermore, there is evidence that SE becomes more difficult to control as its duration increases.[22,33] Therefore prompt and aggressive pharmacologic management is paramount. For prompt and effective management, the formulation of an institutional protocol for SE management is invaluable. The protocol for the treatment of SE at The Hospital for Sick Children in Toronto, Canada,[34] is shown in Table 55–2.

General Supportive Measures

The initial approach to therapy should always focus on securing the airway and maintaining adequate ventilation and circulation. Patients should be positioned on their sides with the head below the torso to minimize the risk of aspiration. An oral or nasopharyngeal airway should be inserted. If oxygenation is inadequate, early intubation may be required, in which case only short-acting neuromuscular blocking agents and sedatives should be used to avoid compromising the neurologic assessment. Vital signs should be checked at frequent intervals, including the patient's heart rate, blood pressure, and temperature. A cardiac monitor and transcutaneous oxygen saturation monitor should be applied. A rapid test of blood glucose should be performed, and hypoglycemia should be treated with intravenous dextrose. In parallel with the efforts to abort the seizure, investigations into the cause should be undertaken as soon as the patient's medical condition permits (see later).

Initial Management

Most AEDs used to treat SE have the potential to compromise airway control and respiratory drive and therefore should be used with necessary precautions. Table 55–3 provides details of the drugs used in the treatment of SE.

Benzodiazepines

Benzodiazepines are considered the first-line agents for the initial therapy of prolonged seizures and SE. Benzodiazepines enhance inhibitory neurotransmission by binding to a specific benzodiazepine site on the $GABA_A$ receptor. Lorazepam and diazepam have been shown to be equally effective at aborting seizures.[35] Seizure recurrence is higher with diazepam because of rapid protein binding,[36] however, and this leads to an abrupt fall in the unbound (and pharmacologically active) serum diazepam concentration. For these reasons, lorazepam has become the drug of choice in many centers for the initial management of SE.[22] Intravenous administration of benzodiazepines is the preferred route because of its rapid onset of action, but alternatives include buccal administration of the sublingual preparation and rectal administration of the

TABLE 55–2

Protocol for the Drug Treatment of SE in Children[34]

Time from Seizure Onset	Drug	Dosage
5 min	Lorazepam	0.1 mg/kg, max 4 mg, PR/IV
For children under 18 months, consider pyridoxine 100 mg/IV		
10 min	Lorazepam	0.1 mg/kg, max 4 mg, PR/IV
15 min	Phenytoin	20 mg/kg, max 1g, IV
The order of phenytoin and phenobarbital can be interchanged in infants younger than 18 mo except in head injury when phenytoin should be used first line.		
35 min	Phenobarbital	20 mg/kg, max 1 g, IV
If seizures persist for more than 10 min after administration of phenobarbital, continue treatment as refractory status epilepticus:		
45 min	Midazolam	0.15 mg/kg IV bolus followed by 2 µg/kg/min infusion then titrate to max 24 µg/kg/min
Titrate midazolam to seizure control by increasing by 2 µg/kg/min every 5 min and with boluses of 0.15 mg/kg as needed.		
If no seizures in 48 hr, taper midazolam by 1 µg/kg/min every 15 min.		
Persistent seizures in the face of midazolam	*Thiopentone*	*Bolus 2-4 mg/kg followed by 2-4 mg/kg/hr infusion*
Based on EEG suppression of epileptiform discharges; use additional boluses of 2 mg/kg with increase in infusion rate of 1 mg/kg/hr every 30 min to 6 mg/kg/hr as needed.		
Discontinue midazolam and phenobarbital once thiopentone infusion started.		
Maintain phenytoin at therapeutic level.		
Consider vasopressor support.		
Monitor thiopentone levels.		
If no seizures for 48 hr, taper thiopentone over 12 hr in 25% decrements and reinstitute phenobarbitone while tapering.		

EEG, electroencephalography; *IV,* intravenous; *PR,* rectal; SE, status epilepticus.

liquid form. Diazepam may be rectally administered in a commercially available gel preparation. Buccal midazolam may be an equally effective and more socially acceptable alternative to rectal diazepam.[37]

Barbiturates

Phenobarbital and other barbiturates enhance inhibitory neurotransmission by binding to a specific barbiturate site on the $GABA_A$ receptor. Phenobarbital and phenytoin are generally considered second-line agents for the treatment of SE and are usually administered when benzodiazepines do not promptly abort the seizure. Advantages of phenobarbital include a relatively rapid infusion time and efficacy against a wide spectrum of seizure types, including generalized tonic-clonic, absence, myoclonic, and focal seizures. The predominant drawbacks of phenobarbital are sedation, respiratory depression, and hypotension. Phenobarbital is the primary AED used in neonatal seizures, although phenytoin appears to be equally effective.[38]

Phenytoin

Phenytoin blocks the fast repetitive firing of neurons through the use-dependent inhibition of voltage-gated sodium channels. Advantages of phenytoin include minimal sedation and respiratory depression at therapeutic levels. The main disadvantage of phenytoin is that it must be infused relatively slowly to minimize the risk of cardiac arrhythmia, infusion site pain, and thrombophlebitis. The maximum recommended infusion rate is 1 mg/kg per minute (maximum, 50 mg/min); therefore an infusion of 20 mg/kg requires 20 minutes. Extravasation of phenytoin at the infusion site has been associated with a "purple glove syndrome," which consists of localized extremity edema and discoloration that occasionally requires fasciotomy or amputation. Purple glove syndrome, as well as the more common adverse effects of hypotension and cardiac arrhythmia, is attributed to the fact that phenytoin is dissolved in a solution of propylene glycol and ethanol with a pH of 12.

Fosphenytoin

Fosphenytoin, a water-soluble phenytoin pro-drug, has several advantages over phenytoin and has been widely adopted in the United States. Fosphenytoin may be administered intramuscularly or intravenously. The maximal recommended infusion rate is 150 mg phenytoin equivalents per minute, and the pro-drug has a 7-minute half-life of conversion to phenytoin.[39] Although it remains to be proven that the greater speed of administration of fosphenytoin results in improved seizure control over phenytoin, fosphenytoin is often preferred because it is better tolerated at the infusion site, carries a lower risk for cardiac arrhythmia and hypotension, and has not been associated with the purple glove syndrome.[40] The higher

TABLE 55–3

Drugs Used in the Treatment of Status Epilepticus

Drug	Initial dose	Maximum single dose	IV administration	Onset of action	Half-life	Principal adverse effects in short-term use
Lorazepam	0.05-0.1 mg/kg IV	4 mg IV	0.5 mg/min	1-3 min	Neonates: 40 hr Children: 10 hr	Sedation, hypotension, bradycardia, respiratory depression, paradoxical hyperactivity
Diazepam	0.05-0.3 mg/kg IV	<5 yr: 5 mg ≥5 yr: 10 mg	0.1 mg/kg/min	1-3 min	Neonates: 50-95 hr Infants: 40-50 hr Children: 15-20 hr	Sedation, hypotension, bradycardia, respiratory depression, paradoxical hyperactivity, thrombophlebitis
Phenobarbital	15-20 mg/kg IV	1 g	1 mg/kg/min to max. 60 mg/min	5 min	Neonates: 45-200 hr Infants: 20-133 hr Children: 37-73 hr	Hypotension, sedation, respiratory depression, paradoxical hyperactivity, immunosuppression
Pentobarbital IV	5-12 mg/kg	100 mg	1 mg/kg/hr and titrate	1 min	25 hr	Sedation, bradycardia, hypotension, cardiac arrhythmia, respiratory depression, laryngospasm
Phenytoin	15-20 mg/kg IV	1 g	1 mg/kg/min, to max. 50 mg/min		7-42 hr (first-order kinetics do not apply)	Dysarthria, ataxia, sedation, hypotension, cardiac arrhythmia, thrombophlebitis, purple glove syndrome
Fosphenytoin	15-20 mgPE/kg IV	1g PE	3 mgPE/kg/min to max. 150 mgPE/min		12-29 hr (first-order kinetics do not apply)	Dysarthria, ataxia, sedation, hypotension, bradycardia, tachycardia
Valproic acid	15-20 mg/kg IV	25 mg/kg	5 mg/kg/min		Children >2 mo: 7-13 hr Children 2-14 yr: 3.5-20 hr	Hypotension, cardiac arrhythmia, hepatitis, pancreatitis
Paraldehyde	200-400 mg/kg PR	10 g PR	n/a		4-10 hr	Rectal irritation, lung toxicity
Midazolam	0.15 mg/kg IV	0.15 mg/kg	1 mg/kg/min, titrate to max. 24 mg/kg/min	1-5 min	Neonates: 4-12 hr Children: 3-4 hr	Sedation, hypotension, bradycardia, respiratory depression, apnea, laryngospasm, paradoxical hyperactivity
Propofol	2-5 mg/kg IV		1-15 mg/kg/hr		1.5-12 hr	Sedation, hypotension, bradycardia, respiratory depression, bronchospasm, hallucinations, pain when injected, metabolic acidosis; sudden cardiac deaths have been reported in children
Ketamine	0.5-2 mg/kg IV		0.5 mg/kg/min	30 sec	2.5 hr	Hypertension, increased intracranial pressure, hallucinations, vomiting, laryngospasm
Thiopental	2-4 mg/kg IV		Titrate up to 6 mg/kg/hr	30-60 sec	14-34 hr	Sedation, hypotension, respiratory depression, accumulation due to lipid solubility, extravasation causes skin necrosis due to pH of 10.6
Isoflurane	0.5-1% v/v		n/a			Respiratory depression, hypotension, arrhythmias, malignant hyperthermia, laryngospasm, coughing (due to pungent odor)
Lidocaine	2-3 mg/kg IV	200-300 mg	3-10 mg/kg/hr, up to 50 mg/min		1.5-2 hr in adults	Sedation

IV, intravenous; PE, phenytoin equivalents, PR, rectal.

cost of fosphenytoin and the lack of definitive evidence for superior efficacy, however, may limit its widespread use, despite the suggestion by phamacoeconomic analysis that fosphenytoin is cost-effective.[41]

Paraldehyde

Paraldehyde is an alternative to phenytoin and phenobarbital for the treatment of early SE and may also be used for RSE. The primary advantages of paraldehyde are its wide spectrum of efficacy for different seizure types and relatively modest respiratory depressant effect. Disadvantages of paraldehyde include limited availability (particularly of the intravenous formulation), its irritant effect on the rectal mucosa, and its unpleasant pungent odor. Paraldehyde is usually administered rectally, diluted in an equal volume of mineral or cooking oil at a dose of 200 to 400 mg/kg. Intravenous administration is possible but difficult because paraldehyde may dissolve plastic intravenous tubing and decompose into acetaldehyde and acetic acid when exposed to air and light. Plastic syringes may be used safely, however, for rectal administration, if this is performed promptly. Pulmonary toxicity, which is likely due to the partial excretion of paraldehyde through the lungs, has been reported; therefore the drug should be used with caution in patients with significant pulmonary disease.[39]

Treatment of Refractory Status Epilepticus

SE that persists beyond 1 hour despite AED therapy is considered refractory. Conventional AEDs have low efficacy in RSE, and although conventional AEDs should be continued during this treatment phase, higher-dose or higher-potency agents are required. Therapeutic options include high-dose benzodiazepines, barbiturates, propofol, valproic acid, ketamine, lidocaine, and inhalational anesthetic agents. Currently the evidence is insufficient to conclude which of these high-dose seizure suppressive medications has superior efficacy in the treatment of RSE.[30] High-dose midazolam is the preferred initial approach at the Toronto Hospital for Sick Children because of accumulated historic experience of profound cardiovascular depression with high-dose barbiturates.

Goals of Therapy

In the treatment of RSE, as in SE, the goal is termination of all clinical and electrographic seizure activity, and thus continuous EEG monitoring is required. ICU practitioners should resist the temptation to assess seizure control on the basis of clinical signs alone because the clinical examination can be unreliable or confounded by the subtle findings of NCSE. In the case of RSE, however, the exact target of therapy as titrated to the EEG remains controversial. In addition to seizure suppression, it is generally recommended to escalate therapy to achieve a burst-suppression pattern on EEG. The rationale for achieving burst-suppression is that profound suppression of brain activity may have a protective effect and "break the cycle" of seizures, thus reducing the chance of seizure recurrence on tapering of medications.[43] Debate remains about what is the recommended length of the periods of suppression and how long the burst suppression pattern should be maintained. Furthermore, because there is concern that seizures may persist even interspersed with a burst-suppression pattern, some experts recommend an isoelectric EEG pattern.[33] As a general approach, once seizure control or burst-suppression has been accomplished, a suggested practice is to maintain burst-suppression for at least 12 hours before a medication taper is attempted. If seizures recur on medication taper, then therapy is reinstated to achieve burst-suppression for at least another 48 hours.

High-Dose Barbiturates

Barbiturates including pentobarbital, thiopental, and phenobarbital are widely used medications for RSE that may also have neuroprotective effects.[44] Pentobarbital is the best-studied drug, and the most data are available on its use. Pentobarbital is administered as an intravenous loading dose of 5 to 12 mg/kg, followed by a continuous infusion of 1 mg/kg per hour, increasing as needed to a maximum rate of 10 mg/kg per hour. Breakthrough seizures may be treated with additional boluses of 3 to 5 mg/kg.[39] High-dose phenobarbital is an alternative to pentobarbital. Phenobarbital may be given in incremental boluses of 10 mg/kg, without reference to a predetermined maximum level or dose, until seizures are suppressed. There appears to be no maximum dose beyond which further doses are ineffective, and serum levels of up to 344 μg/ml (1490 μmol/L) have been reported.[45] The main drawback of all of the barbiturates in high doses is the high risk of cardiovascular depression and hypotension. This frequently requires inotropic and vasopressor therapy and in rare instances, cardiopulmonary resuscitation. In addition, the need for mechanical ventilation and the time to regain consciousness are also greater with barbiturates than with benzodiazepines.[30] Among the barbiturates, phenobarbital probably carries the lowest risk of hypotension and respiratory depression.[45] Finally, there is evidence that high-dose, prolonged barbiturate therapy is immunosuppressive, and thus particular vigilance for nosocomial infections is indicated.[46,47]

High-Dose Benzodiazepines

Midazolam is a short-acting benzodiazepine with an efficacy equal to pentobarbital in controlling RSE.[48] It is administered as a loading dose of 0.2 mg/kg, followed by a continuous infusion beginning at 1 μg/kg per minute. The infusion rate may be increased as tolerated to a maximum of 24 μg/kg per minute, although even higher infusion rates have been reported. The advantages of midazolam include a rapid onset of action, a short half-life, and a lower incidence of cardiovascular depression and need for vasopressors than with pentobarbital.[30,49]

The major disadvantage of midazolam is the need for escalating doses due to tachyphylaxis. High-dose infusions of diazepam and lorazepam represent other alternatives.[50,51]

Propofol

The $GABA_A$ agonist propofol is an anesthetic agent with potent anticonvulsant properties that is widely used for the treatment of RSE. Propofol may be given as a loading dose of 2 to 5 mg/kg, followed by an infusion of 1 to 15 mg/kg per hour titrated to achieve electrographic seizure control or burst-suppression.[52] The advantage of propofol is its short half-life; however, rapid taper of propofol can precipitate seizures.[53] The main side effects of propofol are respiratory depression and hypotension due to myocardial depression. Early concerns about a possible proconvulsant effect of propofol have been largely allayed.[54,55] High-dose propofol infusions should be limited to short duration in children, generally not beyond 6 to 12 hours, because of reported, but rare, toxicity characterized by refractory lactic acidemia, lipemia, and bradyarrhythmias.[56,57]

Valproic Acid

Intravenous valproic acid may have a useful role in RSE, but there is relatively little evidence to support its use.[58] In one case series, the authors reported on the efficacy of intravenous valproic acid for generalized convulsive and nonconvulsive in children. They recommended a loading dose of 20 mg/kg, given at a concentration of 75 mg/L, followed by an infusion at 1 to 4 mg/kg per hour, depending on the patient's state of hepatic induction (1 mg/kg per hour for noninduced, 2 mg/kg hour in the presence of polyanticonvulsant therapy, and 4 mg/kg per hour for high-dose pentobarbital).[59] In a subsequent retrospective review of 40 children (18 with SE), the researchers reported on the safety and efficacy of valproic acid when administered at loading doses of 25 mg/kg (in valproate-naive patients) and infused at rates of 2 to 3 mg/kg per minute.[60] No significant changes were noted in heart rate or rhythm, blood pressure, or liver enzymes. One patient complained of a transient tremor after the infusion.

Inhalational Anesthetics

The efficacy of inhalational anesthetics for SE refractory to high-dose benzodiazepines and barbiturates is described in several reports.[61,62] Inhalational anesthetics have the advantage of being easily titratable; however, prolonged use (particularly of halothane) may cause organotoxicity. Hemodynamic compromise is seen with all of these agents, particularly halothane, and all patients who have been reported required vasopressors. In adults, isoelectric EEGs have required isoflurane concentrations of 1.5% to 2 %.[63] The use of inhalational anesthetics in the ICU setting is complicated by the need for a proper gas scavenging system and supervision by anesthesia-trained staff.

Ketamine and Lidocaine

Ketamine is a unique NMDA antagonist that has been reported to have anticonvulsant and neuroprotective properties. There is a case report of its efficacy for SE refractory to high-dose benzodiazepines and barbiturates.[64] Lidocaine, given as an intravenous bolus or continuous infusion, is another treatment option, although not widely used.[65]

Pyridoxine

Pyridoxine (vitamin B_6) is a cofactor for both glutamic acid decarboxylase and GABA transaminase, the enzymes required for the synthesis and metabolism of GABA in the brain. Pyridoxine dependency and pyridoxine deficiency are rare disorders (prevalence ~1/300,000 in the United Kingdom) that usually present in the neonatal or infantile period but may present as late as age 2.5 years.[66] Patients with these disorders have intractable seizures that are refractory to conventional anticonvulsant medications but respond promptly to pyridoxine. Therefore a trial of pyridoxine should be considered in any child who is seen before age 3 years with recurrent seizures or SE, particularly if refractory to conventional anticonvulsants.[66] Isoniazid poisoning is another clinical scnario in which pyridoxine may be the only effective anticonvulsant therapy.[67]

Surgical Treatment

When SE is refractory to multiple medical treatments, including high-dose barbiturates and benzodiazepines, surgical intervention has been considered. Focal cortical resections may be indicated if a focal structural abnormality can be identified on neuroimaging, particularly if there is concordance with the location of ictal and interictal EEG discharges. Corpus callosotomy has also been attempted for SE that is generalized or cannot be localized. The evidence for either of these approaches is limited to case reports.[68,69] Implantation of a vagal nerve stimulator may be another therapeutic option, although it is rarely considered in the acute situation.[70]

Investigations

Investigation of the cause of SE should proceed in parallel with treatment because the optimal treatment, including prevention of recurrent SE, requires an understanding of the cause of the seizure. Box 55–2 outlines the spectrum of investigations that should be considered in patients with SE and their rationale.

Acknowledgments

We would like to thank Ms. Angela Trope for her contribution to Table 56–3 and acknowledge the Hospital for Sick Children Foundation and the Duncan L. Gordon Fellowship for their support of Dr. Hahn.

BOX 55–2

Investigation of the Patient with Status Epilepticus

To be performed in all patients with status epilepticus:

- Serum glucose, electrolytes, calcium, magnesium
- Blood gas, serum osmolality
- Toxicology screen (serum and urine)
- Antiepileptic drug levels
- Complete blood count (RBC, differential WBC, platelet count)
- Liver enzymes, serum ammonium
- Blood culture
- Lumbar puncture, including
  - Opening pressure
  - Cell count, Gram stain, smear for acid fast bacilli
  - Viral and bacterial cultures
  - PCR for herpesvirus
- EEG, preferably continuous monitoring with video
  - To monitor for subtle or subclinical seizures
  - To guide antiepileptic drug therapy
  - To localize the epileptogenic brain region (focal slowing or epileptiform activity)

To be considered in patients with status epilepticus:

- Structural neuroimaging (CT, MRI)
  - To diagnose acute infarction, hemorrhage, vascular malformation, encephalitis, abscess, neurocysticercosis, neoplasm
  - In nonlesional cases, may localize the epileptogenic zone by evidence of focal edema in the affected cortical region
  - To assess the degree of cerebral edema and diagnose impending uncal or transtentorial herniation
  - MR angiography may identify CNS vasculitis, especially in medium or large vessel disease
- Functional neuroimaging (PET, SPECT)
  In nonlesional cases, may identify the epileptogenic zone
- Cerebral angiography
  To identify small vessel CNS vasculitis, which may not be visible on MR angiography
- Rheumatological workup for vasculitides
- ESR, C-reactive protein, rheumatoid factor, serum complement levels, antineurotrophil cytoplasmic antibodies
- Brain biopsy
  - To diagnose cerebral vasculitis (granulomatous compared with nongranulomatous)
  - To identify malformations of cortical development

CNS, central nervous system; *CT,* computed tomography; *EEG,* electroencephalography; *ESR,* erythrocyte sedimentation rate; *MRI,* magnetic resonance imaging; *PCR,* polymerase chain reaction; *PET,* positron emission tomography; *RBC,* red blood cell; *SPECT,* single photon emission computed tomography; *WBC,* white blood cell.

REFERENCES

1. International League Against Epilepsy: Proposal for revised classification of epilepsies and epileptic syndromes, *Epilepsia* 30:389, 1989.
2. Lowenstein DH, Bleck T, Macdonald RL: It's time to revise the definition of status epilepticus, *Epilepsia* 40:120, 1999.
3. Theodore W, Porter R, Albert P: The secondarily generalized tonic-clonic seizure: a videotape analysis, *Neurology* 44:1403, 1994.
4. Shinnar S, Berg AT, Moshe SL, et al: How long do new-onset seizures in children last? *Ann Neurol* 49:659, 2001.
5. DeLorenzo RJ, Garnett LK, Towne AR, et al: Comparison of status epilepticus with prolonged seizure episodes lasting from 10 to 29 minutes, *Epilepsia* 40:164, 1999.
6. Engel J: A proposed diagnostic scheme for people with epileptic seizures and with epilepsy: Report of the ILAE task force on classification and terminology, *Epilepsia* 42:796, 2001.
7. International League Against Epilepsy: Proposal for revised clinical and electrographic classification of epileptic seizures, *Epilepsia* 22: 489, 1981.
8. DeLorenzo RJ, Hauser WA, Towne AR, et al: A prospective, population-based epidemiologic study of status epilepticus in Richmond, Virginia, *Neurology* 46:1029, 1996.
9. Hesdorffer DC, Logroscino G, Cascino G, et al: Incidence of status epilepticus in Rochester, Minnesota, 1965-1984, *Neurology* 50: 735, 1998.
10. Lacroix J, Deal C, Gautheier M, et al: Admissions to a pediatric intensive care unit for status epilepticus: a 10-year experience, *Crit Care Med* 22:827, 1994.
11 Aicardi J, Chevrie JJ: Convulsive status epilepticus in infants and children. A study of 239 cases, *Epilepsia* 11:179, 1970.
12. Shinnar S, Pellock JM, Moshe SL, et al: In whom does status epilepticus occur: age-related differences in children, *Epilepsia* 38:907, 1997.
13. Shinnar S, Berg AT, Moshe SL, et al: The risk of seizure recurrence after a first unprovoked afebrile seizure in childhood: an extended follow-up, *Pediatrics* 98:216, 1996.
14. Berg AT, Shinnar S, Levy SR, et al: Status epilepticus in children with newly diagnosed epilepsy, *Ann Neurol* 45:618, 1999.
15. Towne AR, Pellock JM, Ko D, et al: Determinants of mortality in status epilepticus, *Epilepsia* 35:27, 1994.
16. Maytal J, Shinnar S, Moshe SL, et al: Low morbidity and mortality in status epilepticus in children, *Pediatrics* 83:323, 1989.
17. Barnard C, Wirrell E: Does status epilepticus in children cause developmental deterioration and exacerbation of epilepsy? *J Child Neurol* 14:787, 1999.
18. Eriksson KJ, Koivikko MJ: Status epilepticus in children: aetiology, treatment, and outcome, *Develop Med Child Neurol* 39:652, 1997.
19. Hesdorffer DC, Logroscino G, Cascino G, et al: Risk of unprovoked seizure after acute symptomatic seizure: effect of status epilepticus, *Ann Neurol* 44:908, 1998.
20. van Esch A, Ramlal IR, van Steensel-Moll HA, et al: Outcome after febrile status epilepticus, *Develop Med Child Neurol* 38:19, 1996.
21. Kapur J MacDonald R: Rapid seizure-induced reduction of benzodiazepine and Zn^{2+} sensitivity of hippocampal dentate granule cell GABA A receptors, *J Neurosci* 17:7532, 1997.
22. Treiman DM, Meyers PD, Walon NY, et al: A comparison of four treatments for generalized convulsive status epilepticus, *N Engl J Med* 339:792, 1998.
23. Kapur J: Status epilepticus in epileptogenesis, *Curr Opin Neurol* 12:191, 1999.
24. Fountain NB: Status epilepticus: risk factors and complications, *Epilepsia* 41:S23, 2000
25. Fountain NB, Lothman EW: Pathophysiology of status epilepticus. *J Clin Neurophysiol* 12:326, 1995.
26. Tuxhorn IEB, Fischbach HS: Pseudostatus epilepticus in childhood, *Pediatr Neurol* 27:407, 2002.
27. Altafullah I, Asaikar S, Torres F: Status epilepticus: clinical experience with two special devices for continuous cerebral monitoring, *Acta Neurol Scand* 84:374, 1991.
28. Toet MC, van der Meij W, de Vries LS, et al: Comparison between simultaneously recorded amplitude integrated electroencephalogram (cerebral function monitor) and standard electroencephalogram in neonates, *Pediatrics* 109:772, 2002.
29. Bleck TP: Advances in the management of refractory status epilepticus, *Crit Care Med* 21:955, 1993.
30. Gilbert DL, Gartside PS, Glauser TA: Efficacy and mortality in treatment of refractory generalized convulsive status epilepticus in children: a meta-analysis, *J Child Neurol* 14:602, 1999.
31. Sahin M, Menache CC, Holmes GL, et al: Outcome of severe refractory status epilepticus in children, *Epilepsia* 42:1461, 2001.
32. Sahin M, Menache CC, Holmes GL, et al.: Prolonged treatment for acute symptomatic refractory status epilepticus: outcome in children, *Neurology* 61:398, 2003.
33. Bleck TP: Refractory status epilepticus in 2001, *Arch Neurol* 59:188, 2002.
34. Nolan M, Elliott I, Trope K, et al: Guidelines for management of status epilepticus in infants (age > 1 month), children and adolescents, Unpublished manuscript, 2004.

35. Qureshi A, Wassmer E, Davies P et al: Comparative audit of intravenous lorazepam and diazepam in the emergency treatment of convulsive status epilepticus in children, *Seizure* 11:141, 2002.
36. Cock HR, Schapira AH: A comparison of lorazepam and diazepam as initial therapy in convulsive status epilepticus, *QJM* 95:225, 2002.
37. Scott RC, Besag FM, Neville BG: Buccal midazolam and rectal diazepam for treatment of prolonged seizures in childhood and adolescence: a randomised trial, *Lancet* 353:623, 1999.
38. Painter MJ, Scher MS, Stein AD et al: Phenobarbital compared with phenytoin for the treatment of neonatal seizures, *N Engl J Med* 341:485, 1999.
39. Bleck TP: Management approaches to prolonged seizures and status epilepticus, *Epilepsia* 40:S59, 1999.
40. Wheless JW: Pediatric use of intravenous and intramuscular phenytoin: lessons learned, *J Child Neurol* 13:S11, 1998.
41. Graves N: Pharmacoeconomic considerations in treatment options for acute seizures, *J Child Neurol* 13:S27, 1998.
42. Levy RH: *Antiepileptic drugs*, ed 5, Philadelphia, 2002, Lippincott Williams & Wilkins.
43. Krishnamurthy KB, Drislane FW: Depth of EEG suppression and outcome in barbiturate anesthetic treatment for refractory status epilepticus, *Epilepsia* 40:759, 1999.
44. Mikati MA, Holmes GL, Chronopoulos A et al: Phenobarbital modifies seizure-related brain injury in the developing brain, *Ann Neurol* 36:425, 1994.
45. Crawford TO, Mitchell WG, Fishman LS et al: Very-high-dose phenobarbital for refractory status epilepticus in children, *Neurology* 38:1035, 1988.
46. Devlin EG, Clarke RS, Mirakhur RK et al: Effect of four I.V. Induction agents on t-lymphocyte proliferations to PHA in vitro, *Br J Anaesth* 73:315, 1994.
47. Neuwelt EA, Kikuchi K, Hill SA et al: Barbiturate inhibition of lymphocyte function. Differing effects of various barbiturates used to induce coma, *J Neurosurg* 56:254, 1982.
48. Holmes GL and Riviello JJ: Midazolam and pentobarbital for refractory status epilepticus, *Pediatr Neurol* 20:259, 1999.
49. Igartua J, Silver P, Maytal J et al: Midazolam coma for refractory status epilepticus in children, *Crit Care Med* 27:1982, 1999.
50. Labar DR, Ali A, Root J: High-dose intravenous lorazepam for the treatment of refractory status epilepticus, *Neurology* 44:1400, 1994.
51. Singhi S, Banerjee S, Singhi P: Refractory status epilepticus in children: role of continuous diazepam infusion, *J Child Neurol* 13:23, 1998.
52. Stecker MM, Kramer TH, Raps EC et al: Treatment of refractory status epilepticus with propofol: clinical and pharmacokinetic findings, *Epilepsia* 39:18, 1998.
53. Finley GA, MacManus B, Sampson SE et al: Delayed seizures following sedation with propofol, *Can J Anaesth* 40:863, 1993.
54. Bevan JC: Propofol-related convulsions, *Can J Anaesth* 40:805, 1993.
55. Cheng MA, Tempelhoff R, Silbergeld DL et al: Large-dose propofol alone in adult epileptic patients: electrocorticographic results, *Anesth Analg* 83:169, 1996.
56. Bray RJ: Propofol infusion syndrome in children, *Paediatr Anaesth* 8:491, 1998.
57. Cray SH, Robinson BH, Cox PN: Lactic acidemia and bradyarrhythmia in a child sedated with propofol, *Crit Care Med* 26:2087, 1998.
58. Yamamoto LG, Yim GK: The role of intravenous valproic acid in status epilepticus, *Pediatr Emerg Care* 16:296, 2000.
59. Hovinga CA, Chicella MF, Rose DF et al: Use of intravenous valproate in three pediatric patients with nonconvulsive or convulsive status epilepticus, *Ann Pharmacother* 33:579, 1999.
60. Yu KT, Mills S, Thompson N et al: Safety and efficacy of intravenous valproate in pediatric status epilepticus and acute repetitive seizures, *Epilepsia* 44:724, 2003.
61. Kofke WA, Young RS, Davis P et al: Isoflurane for refractory status epilepticus: a clinical series, *Anesthesiology* 71:653, 1989.
62. Sharpe MD, Young GB, Mirsattari S et al: Prolonged desflurane administration for refractory status epilepticus, *Anesthesiology* 97:261, 2002.
63. Ropper AH, Kofke WA, Bromfield EB et al: Comparison of isoflurane, halothane, and nitrous oxide in status epilepticus, *Ann Neurol* 19:98, 1986.
64. Sheth RD, Gidal BE: Refractory status epilepticus: response to ketamine, *Neurology* 51:1765, 1998.
65. Pascual J, Ciudad J, Berciano J: Role of lidocaine in managing status epilepticus, *J Neurol Neurosurg Psychiatry* 55:49, 1992.
66. Baxter P: Epidemiology of pyridoxine dependent and pyridoxine responsive seizures in the UK, *Arch Dis Child* 81:431, 1999.
67. Nelson L, Rella J, Hoffman R: Status epilepticus, *N Engl J Med* 339:409, 1998.
68. Gorman DG, Shields WD, Shewmon DA et al: Neurosurgical treatment of refractory status epilepticus, *Epilepsia* 33:546, 1992.
69. Ma X, Liporace J, O'Connor MJ et al: Neurosurgical treatment of medically intractable status epilepticus, *Epilepsy Res* 46:33, 2001.
70. Winston KR, Levisohn P, Miller BR et al: Vagal nerve stimulation for status epilepticus, *Pediatr Neurosurg* 34:190, 2001.

CHAPTER

56

Acute Neuromuscular Diseases and Disorders

Maria B. Weimer and Ann Henderson Tilton

PEARLS

- Some causes of acute flaccid paralysis in childhood
  - Guillain-Barré syndrome (GBS)
  - Botulism
  - Tick paralysis
  - Periodic paralyses
  - Organophosphate poisoning
- Risk factors for respiratory failure in GBS
  - Elevated cerebrospinal fluid (CSF) protein in first week of disease
  - Short time interval between prodrome and onset of GBS symptoms
  - Cranial nerve involvement
- Myasthenia gravis symptoms
  - Ptosis
  - Diplopia
  - Pupillary sparing
  - Weakness that waxes and wanes
- Asbury criteria for GBS
  - Required criteria
    - Progressive motor weakness of more than one limb
    - Areflexia
  - Supportive criteria
    - Symmetry of symptoms
    - Mild sensory changes
    - Cranial nerve involvement
    - Autonomic symptoms
    - Recovery begins 2 to 4 weeks after symptom progression discontinues
- Differential diagnosis in hypokalemic periodic paralysis
  - Bartter's syndrome
  - Corticosteroids
  - Diuretics
  - Hyperaldosteronism
  - Laxatives
  - Licorice
  - Renal tubular acidosis

- Amphotericin B
- p-Aminosalicylic acid
- Alcoholism
- Villous adenoma
- Acute management of hypokalemic periodic paralysis
  - Oral potassium is preferred unless there is an inability to swallow or there are cardiac symptoms
  - Avoid intravenous fluids with dextrose or physiological saline
  - Vigilant cardiac monitoring
  - Serial potassium levels
  - Serial muscle strength examinations
- Botulism symptoms
  - Clinical symptoms
    - Weak cry
    - Poor suck and swallow
    - Decreased tone
    - Decreased reflexes
    - Weakness in descending pattern
    - Constipation
  - Autonomic symptoms
    - Tachycardia
    - Fluctuating blood pressure
    - Urinary retention
    - Decreased tears and saliva
    - Flushed skin or pallor

Neuromuscular diseases, which encompass the entire motor unit, may have similar presentations initially and must be deciphered in a methodical manner. The motor unit consists of the anterior horn cell, which is located in the spinal cord and terminates in a motor nerve, the myelin associated with the nerve, the neuromuscular junction, and the muscle that the nerve innervates. Any disruption of function in this pathway may produce weakness of some variety. Neuropathies and myopathies have similar clinical findings such as weakness and decreased or absent reflexes. These disease processes may be distinguished, however, by sensory abnormalities and the distribution of the weakness. Neuromuscular junction defects may have reflexes present, as in myasthenia gravis, or absent reflexes, as seen in tick paralysis. The presentation of these diseases, family history, inciting factors including recent illnesses or travel, and the clinical course help the clinician narrow the etiological possibilities.

This chapter is devoted to acute neuromuscular diseases that present to a pediatric intensive care unit. A variety of neuromuscular illnesses exist; therefore this chapter begins with the most common disorders presenting to the pediatric intensive care unit. Weakness due to spinal cord or other central nervous system abnormalities are discussed in a separate chapter.

Guillain-Barré Syndrome

The most common of the acute neuromuscular diseases to present to the intensive care unit is Guillain-Barré syndrome (GBS). When given the history of an ascending paralysis, a clinician can easily place GBS in the differential diagnosis; however, this history may be difficult to obtain, particularly if the patient is a small child or an infant. GBS is the most common cause of acute flaccid paralysis in children. The incidence is estimated to be 0.38 to 1.1 per 100,000 in a population younger than 15 years.[1,2] A prodromal respiratory or gastrointestinal illness is commonly found in the history. The prodromal illnesses may include *Campylobacter jejuni* and cytomegalovirus (CMV). In one study, 70% of patients reported an illness before the onset of symptoms with 26% having documented CMV.[3]

The neurological symptoms typically present with progressive paralysis that is relatively symmetrical and may evolve to all extremities. Other symptoms include varying degrees of hyporeflexia or areflexia, or even respiratory embarrassment. Other presentations may include acute ataxia, pain, or cranial neuropathies.[4,5] In one study, risk factors for patients requiring ventilation included cranial nerve involvement, elevated cerebrospinal fluid (CSF) protein during the first week of illness, and a short period between antecedent illness and onset of symptoms.[6]

Autonomic symptoms, which may be overlooked, are also present in some cases. Autonomic instability, particularly cardiac arrhythmias, increase the morbidity of this disease. Cardiac monitoring of the R-R interval with reduction of beat-to-beat variability may possibly identify patients at risk for fatal arrhythmia.[7] Cardiac arrhythmias induced by tracheal tube manipulation have been reported.[8]

Asbury and Cornblath[9] have established criteria for the diagnosis of GBS. Per their criteria, the features that are required for the diagnosis include progressive motor weakness of more than one limb and areflexia. Symptoms that are strongly supportive of GBS include the relative symmetry of symptoms, mild sensory symptoms, cranial nerve involvement, autonomic symptoms, and recovery that usually begins 2 to 4 weeks after symptom progression discontinues. Sphincter disturbances rarely occur early in the course of GBS and are usually transient.[10]

Diagnostic studies include examination of the CSF and nerve conduction studies. The CSF reveals elevated protein amid a relative paucity of white blood cells (WBCs), usually less than 10 cells per milliliter with the protein increasing after the first week of symptoms.[9] Electrodiagnostic testing reveals motor conduction velocities in the demyelinating range, conduction block, temporal dispersion, and prolonged F waves. Bradshaw and Jones[4] reported that conduction block and temporal dispersion occurred in 74% of the patients.

If the symptoms are severe, treatment options for GBS include plasmapheresis and intravenous immunoglobulin (IVIg). The decision of which therapy to apply is controversial because there has not been a large randomized study performed in children. Plasmapheresis may be technically difficult in young or very small children; therefore immunoglobulin may be used with more ease. Results from one adult study in which the two methods were compared showed that 53% of the patients treated with immunoglobulin improved by one or more grades on the functional scale at 4 weeks compared with 34% of the patients treated with plasmapheresis.[11] Favorable improvement in pediatric patients treated with immunoglobulin has been reported in several small series.[12-15] The standard immunoglobulin dosing is 2 g/kg divided in two to five doses given over 2 to 5 successive days. The initial treatment course is usually divided over 4 to 5 days. If additional courses of IVIg are necessary, a 2-day protocol is often well tolerated.

Several GBS variants exist. The best known are the Miller-Fisher variant and acute inflammatory axonal polyneuropathy, the axonal form of GBS. The neurological triad found in the Miller Fisher syndrome includes ataxia, areflexia, and ophthalmoparesis. Miller Fisher syndrome has been linked to immunoglobulin G (IgG) antibodies against ganglioside GQ1b.[16] In some *C. jejuni* strains, molecular mimicry exists between the surface epitopes and ganglioside GQ1b.[17] The GQ1b ganglioside is thought to cross-react in the brainstem area of the ophthalmic cranial nerves.[18] The axonal form of GBS has been associated with a more prolonged recovery than the classic form of GBS, due to axonal involvement.

Myasthenia Gravis

Myasthenia gravis (MG) has many forms that may present in the pediatric population. The juvenile form of MG is the most common and is clinically identical to the autoimmune adult form of MG. Overall, however, juvenile MG is rare and comprises 10% of all cases of MG in Western populations. Antibodies directed toward the acetylcholine receptor (AchR) at the postsynaptic neuromuscular junction cause this form of the disease. These antibodies result in blockade of the AchR, increase the degradation of the AchR, and also result in complement damage to the AchR.[19] Fenichel[20] reported that 75% of cases occur after age 10 years; however, this age of onset has been debated in recent years.[21,22] AchR antibodies are found less frequently in juvenile MG compared with adult autoimmune MG and are more easily shown in the postpubertal patient population.[23] Anticholinesterase antibody levels should be drawn, however, in all patients with suspected MG.

The most common heralding symptoms of weakness in MG include ptosis (with pupillary sparing) and diplopia (from restricted eye movements). These symptoms wax and wane, and the weakness may generalize to the extremities. The two clinical forms of juvenile MG are ocular and generalized. In ocular MG, symptoms include ptosis and diplopia, but the weakness does not progress to other areas of the body. Generalized MG may begin with ocular symptoms and progress to generalized weakness, usually within 1 year of onset; however, generalized weakness may be the initial presentation. The exact prevalence of generalized compared with ocular forms of juvenile MG is disputed. As in adults with MG, pediatric patients have the fewest symptoms in the morning or after rest, with increasing fatigability with exercise being a hallmark of this disease. The most troublesome symptoms seen in generalized MG are those involving bulbar and respiratory muscles, which may result in difficulty chewing or swallowing and exercise intolerance.

When a patient is suspected to have MG, the best diagnostic bedside test is the edrophonium (Tensilon) challenge. Edrophonium is an intravenous short-acting anticholinesterase preparation. The dosing in infants is 0.15 mg/kg and 0.2 mg/kg in older children. Only 10% of the entire dose is given initially so that the clinician can observe for muscarinic side effects. Atropine (0.015 to 0.04 mg/kg) should be available for these possible side effects, which include bradycardia and respiratory distress secondary to bronchial secretions and bronchospasm. After the trial dose is tolerated, the entire dose is then given. The patient should be observed during the trial for changes in ptosis or fatigability. The onset of action is approximately 30 to 90 seconds after intravenous push and remains for approximately 5 minutes. Many clinicians also perform a blinded placebo trial of normal saline.

The neurodiagnostic study used in patients with suspected MG is repetitive nerve stimulation. This study is best performed on proximal muscles, although distal muscles are often studied. The confirmatory finding on repetitive nerve stimulation is a 10% decrement in amplitude of the compound muscle action potential.

Treatment of MG begins with anticholinesterase medications. The symptoms of MG usually respond to pyridostigmine bromide (Mestinon), the most common oral form of anticholinesterase medication. The dosage of pyridostigmine bromide is 7 mg/kg per day divided 4 to 6 times daily as needed for symptoms. Immunosuppressant agents, including prednisone, azathioprine, and cylclophosphamide, are rapidly added to the regimen for pyridostigmine nonresponders. Prednisone is usually initiated at 1 to 2 mg/kg per day. Clinicians must be careful with the use of prednisone because it may exacerbate weakness on initiation.

Many studies have suggested that thymectomy is best early in the course of MG.[23-25] Because of the spontaneous remission rate reported by Rodriquez et al[26] as 22.4 per 1000 person-years, however, many clinicians are reluctant to proceed with early thymectomy, particularly with young children.

Myasthenic crisis is an exacerbation of myasthenic symptoms requiring ventilatory assistance. In adult MG, myasthenic crisis has been reported to occur in 15% to 20% of patients, with 74% having their first crisis within 2 years of disease presentation.[27,28] Researchers of one pediatric study of 30 patients with juvenile MG reported that one third of these patients had at least one episode of crisis.[29] Crisis duration in adults has been reported to have a median duration of 13 days by Thomas et al.[28] Initial therapy during crisis includes ventilation, which provides rest for the weakened patient. Anticholinesterase medications should be discontinued because they increase secretions, which could lead to mucous plugging. Myasthenic crisis is most commonly heralded by infection in 38% of patients; however, 30% of patients have no obvious trigger for their crisis other than respiratory or bulbar weakness.[28] A thorough investigation for the cause of crisis should be undertaken. The mortality rate has fallen with improvements in health care; however, Thomas et al[28] recently reported a 10% mortality rate in patients with myasthenic crisis.

Plasmapheresis and IVIg (2 g/kg over 2 to 5 days) also play a role in the treatment of myasthenic crisis and acute exacerbations of myasthenic symptoms. In adult crisis, plasmapheresis has been shown to be more efficacious than IVIg; however, plasmapheresis has more deleterious side effects, including cardiovascular and infectious complications.[30] In the first randomized adult trial between plasmapheresis and IVIg, there was no significant difference between the two treatments; however, this study also included myasthenic exacerbations, as well as crisis.[31] Only small numbers of juvenile MG exacerbations or crisis treated with IVIg have been reported.[32,33] These reports have been favorable for IVIg in acute exacerbations of MG.[32,33] Therefore IVIg should be considered for treatment in myasthenic crisis or exacerbation, in patients in whom plasmapheresis is not feasible.

Cholinergic crisis must also be a consideration in a patient with an MG exacerbation. Cholinergic crisis occurs with an overdose of anticholinesterase drugs in patients with MG. The overdose causes depolarization of skeletal muscles and muscarinic side effects, including increased secretions, diarrhea, lacrimation, sweating, and bradycardia. These symptoms will improve on withdrawal of the anticholinesterase medications. Some authors think that cholinergic crisis is rarely the cause for worsening myasthenic symptoms.[27,34]

The clinician must always be cautious when initiating new medications in the patient with MG. Many drugs interfere with the neuromuscular junction; the best known are the aminoglycoside medications. Although not well recognized, steroids can also exacerbate weakness in a patient with MG. For this reason, one must be cautious when beginning prednisone in the patient with refractory MG, observing closely for any initial increased weakness. Other antibiotics that have been implicated in the worsening of myasthenic symptoms include ampicillin, ciprofloxacin, clindamycin, erythromycin, sulfonamide, tetracycline, and the peptide antibiotics (polymyxin A and B, and colistin). Cardiovascular medications including the antiarrhythmics (quinidine, procainamide, and lidocaine) and beta-blockers (propanolol, timolol, and others) have also been reported to worsen symptoms. Thyroid replacement medications and phenytoin may also cause problems. The neuromuscular junction blockers, including vecuronium, pancuronium, and succinylcholine, should be used with caution because the effects of these medications are prolonged in patients with MG.[34,35]

Additional immune diseases have been associated in approximately 16% of patients with juvenile MG.[26] The autoimmune diseases may include asthma, rheumatoid arthritis, juvenile diabetes mellitus, hyperthyroidism, and chronic inflammatory demyelinating polyneuropathy.[21,26,36] Seizures have also occurred in 4% to 12% of patients with juvenile MG, although the exact cause is not known.[21,26]

Congenital and Transient Neonatal Myasthenia Gravis

The other forms of MG are congenital MG and neonatal transient MG. Neonatal transient MG is unique in neonates who are born to mothers with autoimmune MG. Neonates can manifest symptoms of neonatal transient MG even if the mothers were symptom free during pregnancy and delivery. Neonatal transient MG occurs in approximately 12% of infants born to mothers with MG.[37] If a mother with MG gives birth to an infant with neonatal MG, her subsequent neonates are also at increased risk of having this transient disorder. Neonatal MG usually resolves in the first few weeks after birth, when the maternally derived antibody level diminishes in the neonate. Results from several studies have shown that even symptom-free infants born to mothers with MG have elevated titers of AchR antibodies[38]; however, the reason some infants appear to be more susceptible than others for having transient neonatal MG is not known. Therefore no correlation exists between transferred maternal antibodies and development of neonatal transient MG in the neonate.[39] The antibody concentration of the symptom-free neonate appears to rapidly decrease when compared with the antibody concentration of a neonate with symptoms.[39] The symptoms of neonatal transient MG usually include hypotonia, feeding problems (particularly fatigue), weak cry, and respiratory difficulty. The treatment of these symptoms is supportive, with anticholinesterase medications used for severe symptoms.

Congenital MG usually presents in childhood, with symptoms similar to those of juvenile MG. Many defects are responsible for causing symptoms in congenital MG, including congenital abnormalities resulting in presynaptic, synaptic, or postsynaptic defects of the neuromuscular junction.[40] Congenital MG is always negative for Ach antibody, and a family history of congenital MG may or may not be present. The inheritance of congenital MG may be autosomal recessive or dominant, or sporadic.[40] Treatment of congenital MG is different from the treatment of juvenile MG because immunosuppression obviously does not play a role. Symptoms of congenital MG may or may not respond to anticholinesterase medications.

Tick Paralysis

The clinician must always entertain tick paralysis in the differential diagnosis of acute flaccid paralysis in children. On presentation, patients with tick paralysis may be mistakenly diagnosed with GBS. The treatment of the two diseases is distinct; therefore a high index of suspicion for tick paralysis should be maintained.

Affected patients are usually between the ages of 1 and 5 years. Dworkin et al[41] reported that in a review of 33 patients with tick paralysis, 82% were younger than 10 years and 76% were female. The longer hairstyles have been speculated to be the cause of this female preponderance. A thorough search of the patient should ensue because more than one tick may be attached. The ticks most commonly implicated in North America are *Dermacentor andersoni* (wood tick) and *Dermacentor variabilis* (dog tick)[42]; however, other types of ticks have also been documented. In Australia, the most common tick variety to cause paralysis is *Ixodes holocyclus*.[42] The cause of the weakness is a neurotoxin, which is secreted in the saliva of the gravid female tick. The neurotoxin is produced during the engorgement phase of feeding after mating. The neurotoxin inhibits the release of Ach at the presynaptic terminal.[42]

The symptoms in North American hosts begin with vague complaints of fatigue, irritability, and pain. Vague symptoms may not begin until approximately 5 days after tick attachment, but they progress rapidly.[43] Symptoms may also include cerebellar signs such as ataxia.[43] If the tick remains attached, a symmetrical ascending flaccid paralysis with areflexia develops. Subsequently, cranial nerve symptoms of bulbar and facial weakness and respiratory involvement occur. No systemic features are seen in tick paralysis. Patients are afebrile with normal vital signs, erythrocyte sedimentation rate (ESR), CSF, and mental status. The removal of the tick results in the rapid reversal of symptoms, usually within 24 hours.

On discovery, the tick needs to be promptly removed. Removal of the tick is performed with blunt curved forceps or tweezers. The tick should be grasped at the point of attachment, as close to the skin as possible. The tick should be pulled upward with steady pressure. Twisting or jerking motions may cause parts of the tick to break off, particularly the mouthparts. The tick should not be handled with bare hands. Needham[44] evaluated various methods of tick removal including fingernail polish, petroleum jelly, 70% isopropyl alcohol, and a hot kitchen match. None of these passive techniques induced tick detachment.

Tick paralysis is more severe in Australia than in North America. The presenting symptoms are similar to those in the North American cases; however, ocular involvement with noncreative pupils has been described.[45] The flaccid paralysis may take days to evolve, unlike in North American hosts. The major difference in Australian tick paralysis occurs after the tick is removed. The Australian patients must be carefully observed because maximal weakness may not occur until 48 hours after tick removal.[45] Another distinguishing feature of Australian tick paralysis is the possible use of an antitoxin for treatment. The antitoxin, a canine hyperimmune serum, is used cautiously in humans because of potential reactions, including serum sickness.[45] The efficacy of the antitoxin remains uncertain because no controlled studies have been performed.[45]

Periodic Paralyses

Several forms of periodic paralyses exist including hypokalemic, hyperkalemic, and normokalemic periodic paralysis. Most forms of the periodic paralyses have a family history of the disease. The weakness, eventually resulting in paralysis, is associated with potassium response or potassium serum levels.

Hypokalemic Periodic Paralysis

Hypokalemic periodic paralysis (HypoPP) is the most common form of the periodic paralyses. The presentation of HypoPP usually occurs within the second decade of life. The number of attacks, which may be frequent, usually decreases as patients get older. The occurrence of HypoPP is 1 in 100,000 people. The inheritance pattern of HypoPP is autosomal dominant with males more frequently affected, but one third of cases are sporadic.[46] The most common mutation in familial HypoPP is the dihydropyridine receptor in the voltage sensitive Ca^{++} channel, located on chromosome 1q.[47]

The onset of symptoms in HypoPP usually occurs after the consumption of a high-carbohydrate meal or after vigorous exercise followed by rest. Other provoking factors include cold temperature, emotional stress, menses, and pregnancy.[48] In one study of a large affected family, Chinese food was specifically cited as a specific provocative factor.[48] Weakness usually begins during sleep with the patient noticing weakness on awakening. The weakness may progress to flaccid paralysis of all limbs with areflexia and normal sensation. The weakness usually begins proximally in the legs then progresses distally before involvement in the upper extremities. Cranial nerve function remains normal with swallowing and respiratory function rarely affected. The patient remains alert with a normal mental status during the attack, and sensation remains intact. The weakness usually lasts a few hours but may last several days. On noticing the initial symptoms of mild muscle cramping or "heaviness", however, some patients are able to abort an attack with light exercise.[49] Sudden death from cardiac arrhythmias or respiratory failure has been reported.[50,51] During paralytic attacks, patients have minimal urine output with decreased potassium excretion and absent defecation.[48,52] In HypoPP, myotonia confined to the eyelids has been described.[53] Before this report, myotonia was described as occurring only with hyperkalemic periodic paralysis.

The diagnosis of HypoPP can be confirmed with the identification of hypokalemia during an attack. Laboratory testing during HypoPP reveals a markedly diminished potassium level. Although serum potassium levels are decreased, the total body amount of potassium remains normal. The decreased potassium level is due to a shift of the potassium into the muscle cells, resulting in inexcitable muscle cells.[54] During an attack, potassium levels usually fall below 3, but levels below 2 are found.[55] Secondary causes of hypokalemia such as Bartter's syndrome, corticosteroids, diuretics, hyperaldosteronism, laxatives, licorice, renal tubular acidosis, amphotericin B, p-aminosalicylic acid, alcoholism, and villous adenoma must be ruled out[56].

The paralytic attack may be reversed with normalization of the potassium level. The clinician must be careful when correcting the potassium level, remembering that the total body amount of potassium remains normal. Correction with oral potassium (0.2 to 0.4 mmol/kg every 15 to 30 minutes) should be considered. Patients with cardiac symptoms or an inability to swallow, however, require parental potassium.[46] While the potassium level is corrected, vigilant cardiac monitoring, serial potassium levels, and muscle strength examinations should be used. Intravenous fluids with dextrose or physiological saline should be avoided because they may prolong an attack or even induce cardiac arrhythmias.[56,57] Griggs, Resnick, and Engel[56] reported that 5% mannitol solution should be considered as a diluent for intravenous potassium replacement.

Links et al[48] studied a large kindred with HypoPP and showed that all family members older than 50 years had permanent muscle weakness. Muscle biopsy specimens from patients with HypoPP reveal vacuoles in the muscle fibers.[51] Vacuolar changes in the muscle have also been shown in family members of HypoPP who have not had any paralytic attacks.[48] Links et al[48]concluded from a large kindred study that all patients eventually exhibit permanent muscle weakness but only 60% may have paralytic attacks.

Once a patient is known to have HypoPP, prophylactic medications should be initiated. Acetazolamide has been shown to prevent future attacks in patients with and without a family history of the disease when they take daily doses of 250 to 750 mg.[58] Some patients, however, have been reported to have an exacerbation of attacks when taking acetazolamide.[59] Another report revealed acetazolamide prophylaxis improved strength between attacks in 80% of patients who displayed persistent weakness between paralytic attacks.[58] Daily oral potassium chloride does shorten the duration of the attacks but does not appear to prevent attacks.[58] Other medications used for prophylaxis of attacks include triamterene and spironolactone in patients not responsive to acetazolamide.[58,59] Other considerations for the prevention of attacks include avoidance of high-sodium, high-carbohydrate meals; prolonged rest; and arduous exercise.

Thyrotoxic periodic paralysis is another entity of weakness with concomitant hypokalemia. As the name implies, a thyrotoxic state is the impetus of this disease. It is mostly found in adult Asian males, although it has been reported in the Asian American pediatric population.[60] The purpose of treatment of this disease is to alleviate the hyperthyroid state.

Hyperkalemic Periodic Paralysis

The term *hyperkalemic periodic paralysis* (HyperPP) may be misleading because high, normal, and low levels of potassium have been reported in these attacks.[61] The name HyperPP actually correlates to the response these patients have to potassium. HyperPP is also referred to as *potassium-sensitive PP,* which may be more appropriate and less confusing. HyperPP is autosomal dominant with the gene located on chromosome 17q, affecting the alpha subunit of the sodium channel.[62,63] Sporadic cases have also been reported.[64] HyperPP usually presents in the first decade of life.

Rest after exercise is the most common provoking feature. Other provoking factors include cold temperatures and meal skipping. The pattern of weakness is similar to HypoPP: the legs are usually affected before the arms, with symmetrical weakness. A normal sensory examination is found in patients during an attack. Weakness during the attacks varies from mild to flaccid quadriplegia with areflexia, but respiratory weakness rarely occurs. The usual length of attacks is shorter than that of HypoPP attacks, usually resolving in a few hours, but they may last days. Myotonia and Chvostek's sign are often found in these patients.

Light exercise can prevent an attack. An attack may be provoked by potassium intake and relieved by glucose intake. Most attacks do not require treatment. In the rare severe attack, however, intravenous glucose can be used.[65] Cardiac monitoring is important if medical intervention is needed because cardiac arrhythmias may occur.[66]

Prophylactic therapy should be considered in these patients because permanent muscle weakness does develop over time.[67] Muscle biopsy specimens reveal vacuoles in the muscle cells.[61] Acetazolamide and thiazides have been used for prophylaxis of this disease.[68]

Normokalemic Periodic Paralysis

Normokalemic periodic paralysis (NormPP) is a disputed phenomenon. Patients with NormPP have normal potassium levels during an attack and have been shown to be potassium sensitive.[69] Provoking factors include cold temperatures, alcohol intake, and stress.[69] The kindred described by Poskanzer and Kerr[69] also displayed autosomal dominant inheritance. Therefore it has been argued that this is actually HyperPP, which is also known to display normal values of potassium during an attack. Recently, Chinnery et al[70] studied a descendant of the original family with NormPP as reported by Poskanzer and Kerr. Molecular testing in this patient revealed the same point mutation that is commonly found in HyperPP. Treatment of this disease is similar to the treatment of HyperPP.

Botulism

Infantile botulism is a syndrome predominately found in infants ages 6 days to 12 months.[71] Infantile botulism is different from foodborne botulism, in which the preformed toxin is actually ingested. In infantile botulism, *Clostridium botulinum* enters the body as a spore through ingestion, germination occurs, and the organism begins to produce the neurotoxin that is the cause of the symptoms.[72] In mouse models, the relationship of the gut and the spores are important, with the pH of the gut and the transient lack of competitive intestinal flora being essential in allowing the spores to germinate.[71] Infants appear to be susceptible, as are adults who have abnormal intestinal flora from abdominal surgery, gut abnormalities, or antibiotic use.[73-76]

When discussing the risk factors for botulism, the clinician must consider various sources of the spores. Most cases of infantile botulism occur in California, Pennsylvania, and Utah. In one report, more than 75% of the patients with botulism had *C. botulinum* in their home environment.[77] Other sources include soil disruption from cultivation or construction and parental occupations that involve soil exposure.[78] The consumption of honey and corn syrup is a risk factor; therefore infants younger than 12 months should not be fed these products. Breast-feeding remains controversial in its role in botulism.[79] In one study of 44 patients with botulism, 100% of the patients were breast-fed.[7, 8] Nevertheless, breast milk has been cited as a protective influence against botulism.[80] Arnon et al[80] reported that of the 10 patients who died of sudden infant death syndrome (SIDS) that was linked to *C. botulinum* infection, 8 were fed formula exclusively, and the remaining 2 patients had not received breast milk 10 weeks before their death. Arnon et al[80] concluded that breast-fed infants are not completely protected from botulism but appear to have diminished severity of the disease at onset.

The botulinum toxin irreversibly binds at the presynaptic segment of the neuromuscular junction, inhibiting Ach release and causing neuromuscular weakness. The autonomic system is also affected because the toxin binds the Ach mediated preganglionic parasympathetic and sympathetic synapses, as well as the postganglionic parasympathetic synapse.[81]

The most common symptoms include weak cry, poor suck and feeding, decreased tone with decreased reflexes, weakness in a descending pattern, and constipation.[81] Autonomic symptoms, which are the initial symptoms in botulism, include constipation, tachycardia, fluctuating blood pressure, urinary retention, decreased tears and saliva, and flushed skin or pallor.[71,82] L'Hommedieu and Polin[82] proposed an algorithm of symptoms beginning with tachycardia and constipation progressing to loss of head control, difficulty feeding, and weak cry. A depressed gag reflex is followed by peripheral muscle weakness and finally, diaphragmatic weakness. Because of the combination of autonomic and neuromuscular symptoms, the infant with botulism may be mistaken to be septic or dehydrated. Enlarged, sluggishly reactive pupils may also be present but are less common than the other autonomic symptoms.[83]

The most concerning consequence of botulism is respiratory embarrassment. Schreiner, Field, and Ruddy[81] reported only 24% of the patients reviewed did not require ventilation or an artificial airway. Patients have also become apneic during certain procedures, including lumbar puncture and intravenous catheter placement.[81] Hypoxic ischemic encephalopathy resulting from respiratory arrest has also been described.[83] Other complications that have been described include syndrome of inappropriate secretion of antidiuretic hormone (SIADH), urinary tract infections, pneumonia, and autonomic instability.[81] Aminoglycosides exacerbate the neuromuscular blockade and should be avoided in botulism[84] L'Hommedieu et al[84] reported that in five patients with botulism who received aminoglycosides, clinical deterioration was apparent in all.

The diagnosis of botulism is clinical but confirmed by isolation of the organism or toxin in stool. Electromyography (EMG) in patients with botulism reveals decreased compound motor action potential (CMAP) amplitude and facilitation of the CMAP amplitude with high-frequency repetitive motor nerve stimulation.[85]

The management of patients with botulism is supportive until axonal sprouting reestablishes the neuromuscular junction. The median length of hospital stay was 27 to 37 days; patients were connected to a ventilator for a median of 13 to 16 days.[77,83,86] In respiratory compromise, mechanical ventilation should be instituted until the patient regains protective reflexes and respiratory strength. If the patients are unable to tolerate oral feeds, nasogastric or nasojejunal feeding should be initiated. The resolution of symptoms occurs in the reverse pattern of presentation, with return of head control appearing to be a reliable measure of improving muscle function.[82]

Diphtheria

Although at the turn of the century diphtheria was the leading killer of children, the United States currently reports fewer than 10 cases of diphtheria annually. There have been epidemics in developing countries. The former Soviet Union had a dramatic resurgence of diphtheria with approximately 48,000 cases reported in 1994.[87]

Although there are several forms of diphtheria, the most common in children is the upper respiratory tract infection. The initial mild infection of the pharyngeal area is followed by tonsillar membrane formation. The pseudomembrane may cover the airways and pharynx to the main bronchi down into the smaller bronchi. The exudate consists of necrotic epithelium and fibrin, as well as numerous colonies of the bacterium. It can lead to aspiration and ultimately closing of the airway. Extensive soft tissue edema and lymph node enlargement occur.[88]

A toxic myocardiopathy is estimated to occur in 10% to 25% of patients and is responsible for 50% to 60% of the deaths.[89] This often arises in the second to third week of illness when the affected individual is improving. Abnormalities of the myocardium, the conductive system, and the pericardium occur. The conductive disturbances are in response to the toxin.[90] Cardiac ectopy is 100% sensitive and specific to predict fatal outcome in children with severe diphtheria.[89]

When there is severe disease, neuropathy is seen in approximately three fourths of the patients.[88] In a classic case of diphtheria, local paralysis of the soft palate occurs 2 to 3 weeks after the beginning of the oropharyngeal infection. Weaknesses of the pharyngeal, facial, and ocular nerves follow. The symmetrical polyneuropathy has a varied onset from 10 days to 3 months following the oropharyngeal infection. The axonal and demyelinating neuropathies are based on the circulating toxins and range from motor weakness to sensory abnormalities in a stocking glove distribution.[88,89]

The distal ascending weakness and spinal fluid findings are described as being "indistinguishable" from GBS.[89] Additionally, there can be dysfunction of the autonomic function with associated hypertension and cardiac failure, although this is rare. Typically, there is complete recovery.

Diagnostically, cultures should be obtained from the nose, throat, and the infected mucocutaneous area. Giving the antitoxin is critical even when there is only a presumptive diagnosis. If the antitoxin is administered on the first day, the mortality is 1% compared with a mortality of 20% if administration is delayed until the fourth day.[89] Immunoglobulin preparations have also been hypothesized as helpful. The only antimicrobials that have had prospective studies proving efficacy are penicillin and erythromycin.[89]

Airway complications should be anticipated, as should the probability of congestive heart failure and, ultimately, malnutrition. Studies have revealed no difference in the occurrence of carditis, neuritis, or death in those receiving steroids. Additionally, digitalis is associated with increased occurrence of arrhythmias. Overall prognosis depends on multiple variables including the delay in the administration of the antitoxin along with the immunization status and age of the individual. The fatality rate of 10% for respiratory tract diphtheria has not changed in 50 years.[89]

Acute Intermittent Porphyria

The most common of the four types of porphyria is acute intermittent porphyria (AIP). The clinical symptoms in acute attacks span multiple medical subspecialties and may be precipitated by numerous medications, hormonal variations, calorie restrictions, and alcohol. It most commonly occurs in females with the age of onset between 15 and 40 years and rarely occurs before puberty.[91]

An acute neuropathy is seen in approximately 40% of acute AIP attacks.[92-94] The neuropathy typically follows the onset of the attack by 1 to 4 weeks but may do so as late as 11 weeks. Although paresthesias and distal sensory changes may be a prodromal finding, the motor signs are much more prominent. Typically, the patient has proximally symmetrical upper extremity weakness, but it may advance to involve the lower extremities. Generalized weakness is documented in approximately 42% of patients,[92] In AIP's most dramatic setting, the patient can have a rapid progression of weakness, which leads to a flaccid involvement of all four extremities and respiratory compromise. When cranial nerves are involved, VII and X are the most frequently affected. Vascular compromise has been documented in individuals with vision loss, which may be monocular or total. Although this vision loss is usually transient, it can be permanent.[92]

AIP is often difficult to diagnose. The patient's chief complaints are typically nonspecific abdominal and back pain. This colicky pain often leads to the consideration of surgical intervention. Very helpful in the differential is that AIP is not associated with temperature elevation, leukocytosis, or rebound tenderness.[92] Neurological and psychiatric symptoms often accompany the onset of attack.

Another important issue is significant hyponatremia and associated seizures, which may be further precipitated by the use of intravenous fluids containing dextrose and water. Cardiovascular complications include hypertension and tachycardia. In its most extreme case, there may be significant hypertension with associated hypertensive encephalopathy and ischemic changes. Intravenous infusion of magnesium sulfate may be helpful.[91] Another major concern is nutrition with avoidance of the catabolic state. In the event that nutrition is required intravenously, high glucose solutions with dextrose are recommended. Enteral feeding is preferred, with carbohydrates providing 50% to 60% of the energy needs.[91]

Diagnostically in AIP, urine and stool can be tested for alpha aminolevulinic acid (ALA). Also there is a marked elevation of urinary porphobilinogen (PBG). In the blood, PBG deaminase is helpful in that its level is abnormal even between the acute attacks.[91]

AIP should be a consideration in the differential diagnosis of progressive weakness. It is most often confused with GBS. The ascending qualities, which are classic in GBS, are rare in acute porphyria. Additionally, acute porphyria does not have elevation of the CSF protein or abnormalities of the cellular contents. The associated abdominal discomfort and tachycardia that are seen in porphyria would not be anticipated in GBS. Differential considerations should include lead intoxication and hereditary tyrosinemia as well.[92]

Elder and Hift[91] provided a recent review of AIP therapy. The two recommended approaches are carbohydrate loading and administration of heme. If the patient has severe symptoms such as seizures, hyponatremia, and the beginnings of neuropathy, then aggressive therapy is begun as early in the crisis as possible. In mild attacks it may be possible to wait 24 hours to determine if the attack will spontaneously reverse. Carbohydrate loading is delivered as a 20% glucose solution provided via a central venous catheter. Studies that support the use of heme are primarily noncontrolled and have difficulty reaching statistical significance, but the overall consensus is that it does provide significant efficacy. Daily measurements of urinary ALA or PBG may be a helpful monitor.

Spinal Muscular Atrophy

Spinal muscular atrophy (SMA), a disease of the anterior horn cell, is most commonly inherited in an autosomal recessive manner. SMA has three subtypes that present in childhood, and an autosomal dominant and X-linked inheritance has been reported. The combined incidence of all forms of SMA has been estimated as 1 case in 6000 to 25,700 live births.[95,96] SMA is the second most common fatal disease with an autosomal recessive pattern of inheritance after cystic fibrosis.[95] The most severe form, formerly known as Werdnig-Hoffmann disease and now more commonly referred to as SMA type I, usually presents shortly after birth. SMA type I presents before age 6 months and is defined by the patient never being able to achieve independent sitting. SMA type II, which usually presents between ages 6 and 18 months, is characterized by the patient sitting but never standing or walking.

In SMA type III, these patients do stand independently and walk. The gene for SMA has been localized to chromosome 5q11.2-13.3.[97]

In SMA type I, the examination reveals a floppy baby with proximal weakness greater than distal. The lower extremities are more affected than the upper extremities, and the only spontaneous movement in these infants may be in the hands and feet. When supine, the infant will assume a frog-legged position. Polyminimyoclonus, a fine tremor most easily visualized in the hands, may also be present in these patients. Areflexia, tongue fasciculations, facial weakness, and normal sensation are also found in these patients.[98,99] Retrospectively, some mothers will admit to decreased fetal movement during the pregnancy with the affected infant. Death usually occurs before age 2 years as a result of respiratory problems.[95] In patients with clinical symptoms within the first day of life, their life expectancy was between 2 and 6 months with a mean age at death slightly before 4 months.[100]

Patients with SMA type II usually have delayed motor milestones, after having normal motor development in infancy. Polyminimyoclonus is also present in these patients. Life expectancy is variable, with many patients not surviving past adolescence.[95] Life expectancy can be enhanced, however, with fastidious respiratory care.[101] Not surprising was the correlation that patients with an earlier onset of the disease had an earlier death.[102]

In SMA type III, weakness is again more proximal than distal with the lower extremities being more severely affected. The gait exhibited in these patients has a waddling quality, and lumbar lordosis is also prominent. Once the patient loses ambulation, the inability to raise hands above the head occurs.[103] If disease onset is after age 2 years, ambulation may continue to a median age of 44 years.[103] Ambulation continues to a median age of 12 years if the onset of symptoms occurs before age 2 years.[103] Life expectancy for patients with SMA type III may be the same as in the normal population because muscle weakness appears to stabilize in these patients.

Electrodiagnostic studies on these patients reveal normal motor conduction velocities. Over time, the amplitude of the compound muscle action potential may be decreased. Results from sensory nerve conduction studies are normal. EMG reveals both evidence of acute denervation with spontaneous activity and chronic denervative changes with polyphasic motor units. Muscle biopsy specimens reveal angulated fibers suggestive of denervation. The creatine phosphokinase (CPK) level may or may not be increased. Genetic testing may also be performed to confirm the diagnosis.

The respiratory complications are the most concerning aspect of this disease, which includes aspiration, pneumonia, and respiratory failure. Respiratory failure may even be the presenting symptom in SMA type I.[104] Respiratory muscle weakness results in restrictive lung disease with a weak cough and hypoventilation.[99] Hypercapnia is also a consequence of restrictive lung disease, so supplemental oxygen may have devastating consequences including apnea and death.[99] If supplemental oxygen is needed, conventional ventilation and noninvasive ventilation should be instituted.

Other complications may also occur over time. Scoliosis also complicates pulmonary function over time because of chest wall alterations. Other orthopedic issues such as contractures, particularly in the lower extremities, are also common. In addition, feeding difficulties play a prominent role, particularly in the developing infant with SMA type I. If nutrition is a concern, a feeding evaluation should be performed to rule out aspiration. Supplemental feeding through nasogastric tube or gastrostomy may be necessary.

Poliomyelitis

The paralytic form of polio represents only 1% to 2% of the actual infections. Aseptic meningitis represents less than 10% and is often thought to be a nonspecific illness. The remaining 90% to 95% of those affected have no apparent infection. The patients who will have paralytic disorder show very high fevers and significant muscle pain with the lack of reflexes. The paralysis rapidly progresses to complete loss of motor use asymmetrically in one or more extremities over a few hours. The distribution of weakness is classically proximal and in the lower extremities. Cranial nerve abnormalities have been reported in 5% to 35% of the patients. The loss of function peaks at 5 days. The disorder can be associated with bowel and bladder problems over the initial 3 days. Sensory abnormalities are rare. Physical examination reveals meningeal findings with changes in the reflexes both superficially and deep. One of the classic signs described in the early reports is the "head drop." As the examiner lifts the patient's shoulders and raises the trunk, the head often falls backward in a limp fashion. It is thought that this is not due to paralysis of the neck muscles because it can occur in the nonparalytic form. The clinical course may include significant respiratory muscle weakness. Involvement of the bulbar muscles, brainstem, and the respiratory center and cranial nerve involvement pose difficulties in breathing and paralysis of the pharynx and vocal cords. The respiratory compromise leads to most deaths in the paralytic form.[105] Typically, 50% of patients with any paralysis exhibit some degree of residual deficits, although most do improve. A 10% mortality is now reported in the patients with the paralytic from. Before ventilation, 60% of the individuals died.[105]

Throat and stool culture may reveal the poliovirus, which is shed early in the course of the throat and later from the stool. It is difficult to isolate from the spinal fluid in affected patients. Usually, the results of routine laboratory tests are unremarkable. The CSF findings are characteristic of aseptic meningitis. A white cell count between 20 and 300 cells is expected with predominantly lymphocytes and a normal glucose level. There may be normal or slightly elevated protein. In the first few hours after the onset of symptoms, polymorphonuclear leukocytes may predominate, but within 12 hours the predominance of lymphocytes is seen.[105]

There are numerous clinical manifestations of this disorder. In the viral myocarditis, the heart is extremely sensitive, and thus very small doses of digoxin must be initiated. Hypertension is well recognized and can be extensive enough to cause an encephalopathy. In the child with poliomyelitis, analgesics, including opiates, may be required for pain relief. Hot packs have been noted to be effective when applied every 2 to 4 hours. Constipation and bladder paralysis are major issues early in the course and should be monitored closely. Because of the risk of aspiration and airway compromise, a high level of vigilance must be maintained. If the patient demonstrates respiratory compromise, then a tracheostomy is indicated with accompanying mechanical ventilation.[105]

The use of antiviral agents is debated. Additionally, some authors argue that steroids are not indicated in enteroviral infections.[105]

Children with mild weakness generally have full recovery. If paralysis is present, the recovery is ongoing for 2 years with 80% realized by 6 months.[105] There are adults who have had new symptoms later in life after paralytic poliomyelitis. This involves weakness and muscle atrophy that is related to continued normal attrition of anterior horn cells.[106]

Polio-like Syndromes

Polio-like syndromes have been reported, and antiviral intervention has been advocated.[107] Interferon-α therapy within 24 hours of admission has been recommended on the basis of information from small case studies. The authors thought that it altered the course and that improvement was evident within 1 to 2 days. Also, MRI and proton magnetic resolution spectroscopy have been recommended to monitor the functional activity of the neurons. It is difficult to determine without further study whether the natural course would have been almost complete recovery or if it was in the fact the interferon α intervention that is responsible.[108] Overall prognosis in the nonpolio enteroviral infections is very good.[105]

Organophosphate and Carbamate Poisoning

The clinician must always maintain a high index of suspicion and consider poisonings in the differential diagnosis in patients with altered mental status, respiratory symptoms, or weakness (see also Chapters 98 and 99). Zweiner and Ginsburg[109] reported in their study of 37 children with organophosphate or carbamate poisonings that 43% of these patients were evaluated by their primary care doctor, and pesticide toxicity was not suspected. Therefore clinicians should always ask about exposure to toxic substances when taking a history. These patients, however, commonly do not have a known history of exposure. Exposure to these substances may occur as inhalation, ingestion, and dermal contact. In one study of 37 infants and children with organophosphate and carbamate poisonings, 76% of these patients ingested these substances (which were improperly stored), 16% had transcutaneous exposure (through contact with treated carpets, linens and lawns), and 8% were poisoned by an unknown etiology.[109] Cholinesterase, which is present in the neuromuscular junction, is irreversibly inhibited by organophosphates and reversibly inhibited by carbamate compounds. Therefore a constellation of muscarinic, nicotinic, and central nervous system symptoms may occur.

Muscarinic symptoms that occur include miosis, excessive salivation, sweating, lacrimation, diarrhea, urination, and bradycardia. In severe poisonings, flaccid paralysis with areflexia is common. In moderate poisonings, muscle fasciculations may be present. Central nervous system symptoms include coma and seizures; however, seizures are less common in carbamate toxicity.[110] Pulmonary symptoms including bronchoconstriction, increased pulmonary secretions, and wheezing have been reported.[111] In one study of 52 children with organophosphate or carbamate poisoning, 100% of these patients exhibited hypotonia, stupor, or coma.[112] With further analysis of the 16 patients with organophosphate poisoning, the other common symptoms included miosis (56%), salivation (37%), pulmonary edema (37%), diarrhea (30%), and bradycardia (25%).[112] Overall, carbamate poisonings are usually less severe and shorter in duration, although the symptoms are essentially the same as those found in organophosphate poisonings.[113]

In both forms of poisonings, atropine is used as an antidote for the muscarinic symptoms. Treatment with atropine, however, does not reverse the nicotinic symptoms, which include muscle weakness or respiratory failure. Atropine should be administered as quickly as possible and in adequate doses. In children older than 12 years, the dosing is 1 to 2 mg intravenously every 10 to 30 minutes.[111] In children younger than 12 years, the initial dose is 0.05 mg/kg with maintenance doses of 0.02 to 0.05 mg/kg over 10 to 30 minutes.[111] In organophosphate and carbamate poisonings, the atropine dose is 5 to 10 times greater than conventional atropine dosing.[111] Atropine should be continued until the muscarinic symptoms begin to abate. The signs of atropinization include mydriasis, tachycardia, and xerostomia, and they help provide parameters for adequate dosing.[114] Atropine should be continued for at least 24 hours after severe exposures and then tapered if symptoms are improving.[111]

If organophosphate and carbamate compounds are ingested, gastric lavage and activated charcoal should be initiated. If contaminated, the patient's skin and hair should be rinsed and cleansed thoroughly with soap, and the clothes should be changed to reduce further exposure.[110]

Pralidoxime chloride, the only cholinesterase reactivator in the United States, is an antidote for only the nicotinic symptoms of organophosphate poisonings; therefore atropine must be used concomitantly. Pralidoxime chloride does not help in carbamate exposures. The dosing for patients older than 12 years is 0.5 to 1 g of pralidoxime.[111] In patients younger than 12 years, the dose is 25 to 50 mg/kg.[111] Pralidoxime should be given intravenously over 15 to 30 minutes. If needed, the dose may be repeated every 10 to 12 hours, beginning 1 to 2 hours after the initial dose.[111]

After the antidotes are given, the mainstay of treatment is supportive. If necessary, ventilation should be provided until the patient regains respiratory strength. Suctioning of secretions in both the oropharynx and in the respiratory tree is essential. Seizures should be treated with diazepam or lorazepam. Cardiac monitoring should be implemented because complex ventricular arrhythmias may occur.[115] Death usually occurs as a result of respiratory arrest and pulmonary complications, including excessive secretions, edema, and bronchoconstriction.[111]

Diagnosis is based on clinical findings and response to antidote medications. Serum and red blood cell cholinesterase levels should be obtained to assist in the diagnosis of organophosphate poisoning. Treatment should be initiated immediately and not delayed while waiting for cholinesterase level results. Cholinesterase levels do not assist in the diagnosis carbamate exposure because the reversal of the enzyme occurs too rapidly to be quantified.

Rhabdomyolysis

Rhabdomyolysis refers to a process in which myoglobin is liberated from injured or damaged skeletal muscle into the urine and blood, resulting in myoglobinuria and myoglobinemia. Evidence of chronic rhabdomyolysis, the most common form in children, may be discovered incidentally during routine blood laboratory workups that include CPK levels.[116] Acute episodes of rhabdomyolysis also may result from a myriad of causes. The history of the patient is extremely important in the determination of the exact cause. Acute episodes of rhabdomyolysis may be fatal because of electrolyte abnormalities, cardiac arrhythmias, and renal damage, which occur during this process.

Watemberg et al[117] reviewed an extensive list of potential causes that included environmental factors (extreme cold or heat); viral and bacterial infections; and metabolic abnormalities including hypokalemia, hypernatremia, nonketotic hyperosmolar coma, and diabetic ketoacidosis. Other causes include excessive muscle activity as seen in convulsive seizures, extreme exertion, drugs, toxins, and venoms. Physical trauma, malignant hyperthermia, and metabolic myopathies are other potential causes of acute rhabdomyolysis.

The muscle symptoms found in rhabdomyolysis include severe weakness, hypoactive reflexes, tenderness, edema, cramps, and localized pain.[118] Muscle symptoms make the diagnosis more obvious; however, if the patient has decreased level of consciousness from metabolic abnormalities, trauma, drugs or seizures, these muscle symptoms may not be apparent.

The abnormal laboratory results found include myoglobinuria and profound elevation of serum CPK. Muscle cell destruction results in releasing potassium and phosphorous into the blood, with consequential hyperkalemia, hyperphosphatemia, and eventually hypocalcemia.[118,119] Elevations of adolase, uric acid, lactic dehydrogenase (LDH), and transaminase (SGOT [serum glutamate oxaloacetate transaminase] and SGPT [serum glutamate pyruvate transaminase]) levels also occur.[118,119]

Complications from rhabdomyolysis may affect the heart, kidneys, and ventilation. The severe myoglobinuria in rhabdomyolysis may result in acute tubular necrosis, which can be fatal. Alkalinization of the urine, hydration, and osmotic diuresis have been used to prevent renal damage.[119] Hypocalcemia, which results from the elevated potassium and phosphorous levels, may lead to cardiac arrhythmias. In Robotham and Haddow's review,[118] several types of cardiac disturbances were reported, including ventricular arrhythmias, intraventricular conduction delays, abnormal axis deviation, sinus bradycardias and tachycardias, ischemic changes, nonspecifc ST segment and T wave changes, and T wave changes associated with hyperkalemia. Compartment syndrome may also occur because of severe muscle edema and may require fasciotomy to prevent neurovascular compression.[119] If the diaphragm and intercostal muscles are affected, mechanical ventilation may be required. Bulbar weakness necessitating mechanical ventilation in rhabdomyolysis is rare.[119] Overall, it is unusual for muscle weakness to be permanent, with full muscle strength usually returning in 1 to 6 weeks.[119]

Several diseases that may result in recurrent rhabdomyolysis are briefly discussed here. McArdle's disease, a metabolic myopathy that also goes by the names type V glycogenosis and myophosphorylase deficiency, is predominantly autosomal recessive. Patients with this disease exhibit exercise intolerance, muscle stiffness, and myalgia.[120] Vigorous activity, including squatting, sprinting, and carrying heavy objects, may precipitate an episode of muscle rigidity with cramping and myoglobinuria resulting in rhabdomyolysis. Recognition of these symptoms will help make the diagnosis, prevent morbidity, and avoid recurrent rhabdomyolysis. Tarui's disease, also known as glycogenosis type VII and phosphofructokinase deficiency, is also autosomal recessive. The clinical picture is similar to that found in McArdle's disease resulting in rhabdomyolysis.[120]

Carnitine palmitoyltransferase (CPT) deficiency is an autosomal recessive disease. CPT catalyzes carnitine and fatty acid for transfer into the mitochondria. Rhabdomyolysis may be precipitated by prolonged exercise and fasting.[120] Prevention of rhabdomyolysis is the best treatment and consists of frequent meals of low-fat, carbohydrate-rich foods with avoidance of both fasting and prolonged exercise.[120]

Malignant Hyperthermia

Malignant hyperthermia (MH) is a disease that is associated with certain anesthetic agents, including inhalation anesthesia such as halothane and depolarizing muscle relaxant agents such as succinylcholine (see also Chapter 117). MH occurs in approximately 1 in 12,000 children with anesthesia.[121] MH has a variable clinical presentation as described by Kaus and Rockoff.[122] In classic MH, the symptoms include tachypnea, tachycardia, blood pressure abnormalities, cyanosis, mottling, and diaphoresis. Hypoxia, hypercapnia, metabolic acidosis, and muscle rigidity resulting in severe rhabdomyolysis also occur. The severe hyperthermia, which denotes the disease, may exceed more than 42° C. A second presentation of MH occurs after the administration of succinylcholine and results in an abrupt onset of generalized muscle rigidity, cardiac arrest, and rhabdomyolysis. An additional presentation is masseter muscle spasm, which occurs after the administration of halothane and succinylcholine, and results in severe contracture of the jaw that lasts 5 to 20 minutes.[122]

The treatment of MH, once it is identified, is immediate discontinuation of the offending drugs. Hyperventilation with 100% oxygen and administration of dantrolene sodium should be started immediately. Dantrolene sodium doses of 2.5 mg/kg should be given intravenously. If all of the symptoms have not resolved within 45 minutes of the initial dantrolene dose, an additional 7.5 mg/kg should be given intravenously.[121] Continued doses of 2.5 mg/kg every 6 hours should be given until the patient is stable. Cooling of the patient should also occur if dantrolene sodium does not relieve the hyperthermia. Monitoring for 24 hours after the initial episode should continue for fear of reoccurrence. Complications may include cardiac arrhythmias, renal failure, hepatic failure, disseminated intravascular coagulation, and neurological damage.[122] Prevention of future episodes is imperative. Patients should avoid succinylcholine and the halogenated inhaled anesthetic agents. The genetics of MH is not fully understood. First- and second-degree family members of patients who have or are suspected of having MH should be considered at risk for MH until a muscle biopsy is performed.[121] Some muscle diseases have been associated with MH including Duchenne's muscular dystrophy, Becker's muscular dystrophy, central core disease, myotonia congenita, King-Denborough syndrome, Schwartz-Jampel syndrome, and other muscular dystrophies.[122]

Neuroleptic Malignant Syndrome

Neuroleptic malignant syndrome (NMS) occurs in 0.5% to 1.4% of patients exposed to antipsychotic medications.[123,124] NMS has a constellation of signs and symptoms including hyperthermia, muscle rigidity, autonomic instability, tachycardia, tachypnea, diaphoresis, hypertension, and altered mental status.[125] Rhabdomyolysis may also be a component of this syndrome, which includes elevated CPK levels and myoglobinuria; therefore MH may be in the differential diagnosis. Another abnormal laboratory finding seen with NMS is leukocytosis.

Treatment of NMS includes immediate discontinuation of the antipsychotic medication. In a recent review article, Ty and Rothner[126] discuss the symptoms and treatment regimen in NMS, which includes levodopa and carbidopa, bromocriptine, dantrolene, and benzodiazepine derivatives. Levodopa and carbidopa manage the hyperthermia and may need to be continued for several days. Depending on body temperature and autonomic and extrapyramidal symptoms, bromocriptine at doses of 5 to 7.5 μg three times a day should be instituted. Dantrolene sodium reduces the muscular rigidity with the initial dose of 0.8 to 2.5 mg/kg intravenously every 6 hours. Finally, the benzodiazepine derivatives are useful to control the agitation in patients. Addonizio, Susman, and Roth[127] reviewed 115 patients, both pediatric and adult, with NMS. The mortality of these 115 patients was 11%. The medical complications in these 115 patients included cardiac arrest, seizures, sepsis, pulmonary embolism, and pulmonary edema, with pneumonia and renal failure being the most common at 15% and 8%, respectively. Fifty percent of the 115 patients received a neuroleptic for 7 days or less before the onset of symptoms; however, almost 3% of the patients had the onset of NMS after 360 days while taking this medication.

Inflammatory Myopathies

Dermatomyositis and Polymyositis

Dermatomyositis and polymyositis are inflammatory myopathies with symmetrical proximal muscle weakness that progress over weeks to months (see also Chapter 91). Denardo et al[128] reported the incidence of dermatomyositis and polymyositis was 0.4 per 100,000 children in the region studied and comprised 5% of all rheumatologic diseases referred to the centers that were reviewed. Five major criteria exist for the diagnosis of polymyositis/dermatomyositis as described by Bohan and Peter.[129] Of the five criteria, one clinical criterion is symmetrical proximal weakness that may include respiratory muscles. Another clinical criterion is dermatological, which includes the heliotrope rash and Gottron's sign. In addition, a scaly erythematous rash of the face, neck, upper torso, knees, elbows, and median malleoli is also present. The two laboratory criteria include elevation of skeletal muscle enzymes, including CPK and adolase, and a muscle biopsy specimen with evidence of necrosis of type I and II fibers, phagocyotosis, and inflammatory exudates. The electro diagnostic criterion includes EMG findings of spontaneous activity, myopathic motor units, and bizarre high-frequency repetitive discharges. Definitive diagnosis must include three or four criteria and the rash for dermatomyositis, and four criteria without the rash for polymyositis.

Systemic symptoms such as fatigue, lethargy, irritability, arthralgias, myalgias, weight loss, gastrointestinal discomfort, and low-grade fever may herald the onset of weakness.[130] Complications of dermatomyositis and polymyositis include respiratory problems such as chronic interstitial pulmonary fibrosis and pneumothorax; gastrointestinal involvement with decreased esophageal motility, gastric ulceration, and bleeding; and cardiac problems such as arrhythmias, abnormal electrocardiograms, and pericarditis.[130,131] The initial treatment of polymyositis and dermatomyositis is corticosteroids. The mortality of juvenile dermatomyositis is 3% in the United States.[132]

Benign Acute Childhood Myositis

Benign acute childhood myositis (BACM) is a self-limited process that usually affects boys more often than girls.[133] The presentation of muscular symptoms occurs after a prodrome of viral upper respiratory illness. An acute onset of severe muscle pain usually involving the calf muscles, difficulty walking, and increased CPK levels usually follows the prodrome. Mackay et al[133] describe the prodromal symptoms of fever, cough, headache, rhinorrhea, sore throat, and vomiting as being the most common symptoms. In the 41 episodes of BACM that Mackay et al[133] reported, 42% of those tested were confirmed to be caused by a virus, with 50% of those cases confirmed as being caused by influenza B. The mean CPK level was 14 times normal, but resolution of symptoms occurred within 1 week. BACM resolves rapidly. Bed rest may be necessary until the pain resolves; otherwise, no treatment is needed. This disease process rarely progresses into a severe life-threatening form.

REFERENCES

1. Rantala H, Uhari M, Niemela M: Occurrence, clinical manifestations, and prognosis of Guillain-Barre syndrome, *Arch Dis Child* 66:706-709, 1991.
2. Hart D, Rojas L, Rosario J, et al: Childhood Guillain-Barre syndrome in Paraguay, 1990 to 1991, *Ann Neuro* 36:859-863, 1994.
3. Ammache Z, Afifi A, Brown C, et al: Childhood Guillain-Barre syndrome: clinical and electrophysiologic features predictive of outcome, *J Child Neurol* 6:477-483, 2001.
4. Bradshaw D, Jones H: Guillain-Barre syndrome in children: clinical course, electrodiagnosis, and prognosis, *Muscle Nerve* 15:500-506, 1992.
5. Hood Guillain-Barre sydnrome: clinical presentation, diagnosis, and therapy, *J Child Neurol* 11:4-12, 1996.
6. Rantala H, Uhari M, Cherry J, et al: Risk factors of respiratory failure in children with Guillain-Barre syndrome, *Pediatric Neurol* 13: 289-292, 1995.
7. Oakley C: The heart in the Guillain-Barre syndrome, *BMJ* 288:94, 1984.
8. Emmons P, Blume W, DuShane J: Cardiac monitoring and demand pacemaker in Guillain-Barre syndrome, *Arch Neurol* 32:59-61, 1975.
9. Asbury A, Cornblath D: Assessment of current diagnostic criteria for Guillain-Barre syndrome, *Ann Neuro* 27(suppl):S21-S24, 1990.
10. Jones H: Guillain-Barre syndrome in children; *Curr Opin Pediatr* 7:663-668, 1995.
11. Van der Meche F, Schmitz P, Group tDG-BS: A randomized trial comparing intravenous immune globulin and plasma exchange in Guillain-Barre syndrome, *N Engl J Med* 326:1123-1129, 1992.
12. Al-Quadah A: Immunoglobulins in the treatment of Guillain-Barre syndrome in early childhood, *J Child Neurol* 9:178-180, 1994.
13. Shahar E, Roifman C, Shorer Z, et al: High-dose intravenous serum gamma globulins are effective in severe pediatric Guillain-Barre syndrome: a prospective follow-up study of 23 cases, *Ann Neurol* 36:503, 1994.
14. Vajsar J, Sloane A, Wood E, et al: Plasmapheresis vs intravenous immunoglobulin in childhood Guillain-Barre syndrome, *Arch Pediatr Adolesc Med* 148:1210-1212, 1994.
15. Korinthenberg R, Monting J: Natural history and treatment effects in Guillain-Barre syndrome: a multicentre study, *Arch Dis Child* 74:281-287, 1996.
16. Chiba A, Kusunoki S, Shimizu T, et al: Serum IgG antibody to ganglioside GQ1b is a possible marker of Miller Fisher syndrome, *Ann Neurol* 31:677-679, 1992.
17. Jacobs B, Endtz H, van der Meche F, et al: Serum anti-GQ1b IgG antibodies recognize surface epitopes on *Camplyobacter jejuni* from patients with Miller Fisher syndrome, *Ann Neurol* 37:260-264, 1995.
18. Chiba A, Kusunoki S, Obata H, et al: Serum anti-GQ1b IgG antibody is associated with ophthalmoplegia in Miller Fisher syndrome and Guillain-Barre syndrome: clinical and immunohistochemical studies, *Neurology* 43:1911-1917, 1993.
19. Drachman D: Myasthenia gravis, *N Engl J Med* 330:1797-1810, 1994.
20. Fenichel G: Myasthenia gravis, *Pediatr Ann* 18:432-438, 1989.
21. Snead O, Benton J, Dwyer D, et al: Juvenile myasthenia gravis, *Neurology* 30:732-739, 1980.
22. Afifi A, Bell W: Tests for juvenile myasthenia gravis: comparative diagnostic yield and prediction of outcome, *J Child Neurol* 8: 403-411, 1993.
23. Andrews P, Massey J, Howard J, et al: Race, sex, and puberty influence onset, severity, and outcome in juvenile myasthenia gravis, *Neurology* 44:1208-1214, 1994.
24. Youssef S. Thymectomy for myasthenia gravis in children, *J Pediatr Surg* 18:537-541, 1983.
25. Adams C, Theodorescu D, Murphy E, et al: Thymectomy in juvenile myasthenia gravis, *J Child Neurol* 5:215-218, 1990.
26. Rodriguez M, Gomez M, Howard F, et al: Myasthenia gravis in children: long-term follow-up, *Ann Neurol* 13:504-510, 1983.
27. Fink M. Treatment of the critical ill patient with myasthenia gravis. In Ropper A, editor, *Neurological and neurosurgical intensive care*, New York, 1993, Raven Press.
28. Thomas C, Mayer S, Gungor Y, et al: Myasthenic crisis: clinical features, mortality, complications, and risk factors for prolonged intubation, *Neurology* 48:1253-1260, 1997.
29. Anlar B, Ozdirim E, Renda Y, et al: Myasthenia gravis in childhood, *Acta Paedriatr* 85:838-842, 1995.
30. Qureshi A, Choudhry M, Akbar M, et al: Plasma exchange versus intravenous immunoglobulin treatment in myasthenic crisis, *Neurology* 52:629-632, 1999.
31. Gajdos P, Chevret S, Clair B, et al: Clinical trial of plasma exchange and high-dose intravenous immunoglobulin in myasthenia gravis, *Ann Neurol* 41:789-796, 1997.
32. Herrmann D, Carney P, Wald J: Juvenile myasthenia gravis: treatment with immune globulin and thymectomy, *Pediatr Neurol* 18:63-66, 1998.
33. Selcen D, Dabrowski E, Michon A, et al: High-dose intravenous immunoglobulin therapy in juvenile myasthenia gravis, *Pediatr Neurol* 22:40-43, 2000.
34. Mayer S: Intensive care of the myasthenic patient, *Neurology* 48(suppl 5):S70-S75, 1997.
35. Adams S, Mathews J, Grammer L: Drugs that may exacerbate myasthenia gravis, *Ann Emerg Med* 13:532-538, 1984.
36. Kimura K, Nezu A, Kimura S, et al: A case of myasthenia gravis in childhood associated with chronic inflammatory demyelinating polyradiculoneuropathy, *Neuropediatrics* 29:108-112, 1998.
37. Namba T, Brown S, Grob D: Neonatal myasthenia gravis: report of two cases and review of the literature, *Pediatrics* 45:488-504, 1970.
38. Ohta M, Matsubara F, Hayashi K, et al: Acetylcholine receptor antibodies in infants of mothers with myasthenia gravis, *Neurology* 31:1019-1022, 1981.
39. Lefvert A, Osterman P: Newborn infants to myasthenic mothers: a clinical study and an investigation of acetylcholine receptor antibodies in 17 children, *Neurology* 33:133-138, 1983.
40. Engel A, Ohno K, Milone M: Congenital myasthenic syndromes caused by mutations in acetylcholine receptor genes. *Neurology* 48(suppl 5):S28-S35, 1997.
41. Dworkin M, Shoemaker P, Anderson D: Tick paralysis: 33 human cases in Washington State, 1946-1996, *Clin Infect Dis* 29:1435-1439, 1999.
42. Greenstein P: Tick paralysis, *Med Clin North Am* 86:441-446, 2002.
43. Gorman R, Snead O: Tick paralysis in three children, *Clin Pediatr* 17:249-251, 1978.
44. Needham G: Evaluation of five popular methods for tick removal, *Pediatrics* 75:997-1002, 1985.
45. Grattan-Smith P, Morris J, Johnston H, et al: Clinical and neurophysiological features of tick paralysis, *Brain* 120:1975-1987, 1997.
46. Ahlawat S, Sachdev A: Hypokalaemic paralysis, *Postgrad Med J* 75: 193-197, 1997.
47. Ptacek L, Tawil R, Griggs R, et al: Dihydropyridine receptor mutations cause hypokalemic periodic paralysis, *Cell* 77:863-868, 1994.
48. Links T, Smit A, Molenaar W, et al: Familial hypokalemic periodic paralysis clinical, diagnostic and therapeutic aspects, *J Neurol Sci* 122:33-43, 1994.
49. Schiller T, Auerbach P: Hypokalemic periodic paralysis: two case reports, *Pediatr Emerg Care* 4:183-186, 1988.
50. Smith W: Periodic paralysis: report of two fatal cases, *J Nerv Men Dis* 90:210-215, 1937.
51. Talbott J: Periodic paralysis: a clinical syndrome, *Medicine* 20:85-143, 1941.
52. Pudenz R, McIntosh J, McEachern D: Role of potassium in familial periodic paralysis, *JAMA,* 111:2253-2258, 1938.
53. Resnick J, Engel W: Myotonic lid lag in hypokalaemic periodic paralysis, *J Neurol Neurosurg Psychiatry* 30:47-51, 1967.
54. Zierler K, Andres R: Movement of potassium into skeletal muscle during spontaneous attack in family periodic paralysis, *J Clin Invest* 36:730-737, 1957.
55. Charness M: Clinical conferences at The Johns Hopkins Hospital. Hypokalemic periodic paralysis, *Johns Hopkins Med J* 143:148-153, 1978.
56. Griggs R, Resnick J, Engel W: Intravenous treatment of hypokalemic periodic paralysis, *Arch Neurol* 40:539-540, 1983.
57. Kunin A, Surawicz B, Sims E: Decrease in serum potassium concentrations and appearance of cardiac arrhythmias during infusion of potassium with glucose in potassium-depleted patients, *N Engl J Med* 266:228-233, 1962.

58. Griggs R, Engel W, Resnick J: Acetazolamide treatment of hypokalemic periodic paralysis: prevention of attacks and improvement of persistent weakness, *Ann Internal Med* 73:39-48, 1970.
59. Torres C, Griggs R, Moxley R, et al: Hypokalemic periodic paralysis exacerbated by acetazolamide, *Neurology* 31: 1423-1428, 1981.
60. Miller J, Quillian W, Cleveland W: Nonfamilial hypokalemic periodic paralysis and thyrotoxicosis in a 16-year-old male, *Pediatrics* 100:412-414, 1997.
61. Gamstorp I: Adynamia episodica hereditaria, *Acta Paedriatr* 45(suppl 108):1-126, 1956.
62. George AL Jr, Ledbetter DH, Kallen RG, et al: Assignment of a human skeletal muscle sodium channel alpha-subunit gene (SCN4A) to 17q23.1-25.3, *Genomics* 9:555-556, 1991.
63. Fontaine B, Khurana T, Hoffman E, et al: Hyperkalemic periodic paralysis and the adult muscle sodium channel alpha-subunit gene, *Science* 250:1000-1002, 1990.
64. Dyken M, Timmons G: Hyperkalemic periodic paralysis with hypocalcemic episode, *Arch Neurol* 9:508-517, 1963.
65. Herman RH, McDowell MK: Hyperkalemic paralysis (adynamia episodica hereditaria). Report of four cases and clinical studies, *Am J Med* 35:749-767, 1963.
66. Lisak R, Lebeau J, Tucker S, et al: Hyperkalemic periodic paralysis and cardiac arrhythmia, *Neurology* 22:810-815, 1972.
67. McArdle B: Adynamia episodica hereditaria and its treatment, *Brain* 85:121-148, 1962.
68. Layzer R, Lovelace R, Rowland L: Hyperkalemic periodic paralysis, *Arch Neurol* 16:455-472, 1967.
69. Poskanzer D, Kerr D: A third type of periodic paralysis, with normokalemia and favourable response to sodium chloride, *Am J Med* 31:328-342, 1961.
70. Chinnery P, Walls T, Hanna M, et al: Normokalemic periodic paralysis revisited: does it exist? *Ann Neurol* 52:251-252. 2002.
71. Long S: Infant botulism, *Pediatr Infect Disease J* 20:707-709, 2001.
72. Midura T, Arnon S: Infant botulism: identification of Clostridium botulinum and its toxins in feces, *Lancet* 2:934-935, 1976.
73. Shapiro R, Hatheway C, Swerdlow D: Botulism in the United States: a clinical and epidemiologic review, *Ann Intern Med* 129:221-228, 1998.
74. Chia J, Clark J, Ryan C, et al: Botulism in an adult associated with food borne intestinal infection with Clostridium botulinum, *N Engl J Med* 315:239-241, 1986.
75. Griffin P, Hatheway C, Rosenbaum R, et al. Endogenous antibody production to botulinum toxin in an adult with intestinal colonization botulism and underlying Crohn's disease, *J Infect Dis* 175:633-637, 1997.
76. McCroskey L, Hatheway C: Laboratory findings in four cases of adult botulism suggest colonization of the intestinal tract, *J Clin Microbiol* 26:1052-1054, 1988.
77. Long S, Gajewski J, Brown L, et al: Clinical, laboratory, and environmental features of infant botulism in Southeastern Pennsylvania, *Pediatrics* 75:935-941, 1985.
78. Long S: Epidemiologic study of infant botulism in Pennsylvania: Report of the Infant Botulism Study group, *Pediatrics* 75:928-934, 1985.
79. Spika J, Shaffer N, Hargrett-Bean N, et al: Risk factors for infant botulism in the United States, *Am J Dis Child* 143:828-832, 1989.
80. Arnon S, Damus K, Thompson B, et al: Protective role of human milk against sudden death from infant botulism, *J Pediatr* 100: 568-573, 1982.
81. Schreiner M, Field E, Ruddy R: Infant botulism: a review of 12 years' experience at the Children's Hospital of Philadelphia, *Pediatrics* 87:159-165, 1991.
82. L'Hommedieu C, Polin R: Progression of clinical signs in severe infant botulism. Therapeutic implications, *Clinical Pediatr (Phila)* 20:90-95, 1981.
83. Thompson J, Glasgow L, Warpinski J, et al: Infant botulism: clinical spectrum and epidemiology, *Pediatrics* 66:936-942, 1980.
84. L'Hommedieu C, Stough R, Brown L, et al: Potentiation of neuromuscular weakness in infant botulism by aminoglycosides, *J Pediatr* 95:1065-1070, 1979.
85. Cornblath D, Sladky J, Sumner A: Clinical electrophysiology of infantile botulism, *Muscle Nerve* 6:448-452, 1983.
86. Wilson R, Morris J, Snyder J, et al: Clinical characteristics of infant botulism in the United States: a study of the non-California cases, *Pediatr Infect Dis* 1:148-150, 1982.
87. Perles Z, Nir A, Cohen E, et al: Atrioventricular block in a toxic child: do not forget diphtheria. *Pediatr Cardiol* 21:282-283, 2001.
88. Hadfield TL, McEvoy P, Polotsky Y, et al: The pathology of diphtheria, *J Infect Dis* 181(suppl 1):S10-22, 2000.
89. Overturf GD. *Corynebacterium diphtheria*. In Long SS, Pickering LK, Prober CG, editors: *Principles and practice of pediatric infectious diseases,* New York, 2003, Churchhill Livingstone.
90. Rosenberg RN, Prusiner SB, Dimauro S, Barchi RL: *The molecular and genetic basis of neurological disease*, ed 2, Boston, 1997, Butterworth-Heinemann.
91. Elder GH, Hift RJ: Treatment of acute porphyria, *Hos Med* 62:422-425. 2001.
92. Bissell DM. The Porphyrias:1255-1269.
93. Cavanagh JB, Ridley AR: The nature of the neuropathy complicating acute intermittent porphyria, *Lancet* 2:1023-1024, 1967.
94. Ridley A: The neuropathy of acute intermittent porphyria, *Q J Med* 8:307-309, 1969.
95. Talbot K: Spinal muscular atrophy, *J Inherit Metab Dis* 22:545-554, 1999.
96. Pearn JH: The gene frequency of acute Werdnig-Hoffmann disease (SMA type 1). A total population survey in North-East England, *J Med Genet* 10:260-265, 1973.
97. Brzustowicz L, Lehner T, Castilla L, et al: Genetic mapping of chronic childhood-onset spinal muscular atrophy to chromosome 5q11.2-13.3, *Nature* 344:540-541, 1990.
98. Iannaccone S, Browne R, Samaha F, et al: Prospective study of spinal muscular atrophy before age 6 years, *Pediatr Neurol* 9:187-193, 1993.
99. Iannaccone S, Burghes A: Spinal muscular atrophies, *Adv Neurol* 88:83-98, 2002.
100. Thomas N, Dubowitz V: The natural history of type I (severe) spinal muscular atrophy, *Neuromuscul Disord* 4:497-502, 1994.
101. Gozal D: Pulmonary manifestations of neuromuscular disease with special reference to Duchenne muscular dystrophy and spinal muscular atrophy, *Pediatr Pulmon* 29:141-150, 2000.
102. Zerres K, Rudnik-Schoneborn S, Forrest E, et al: A collaborative study on the natural history of childhood and juvenile onset proximal spinal muscular atrophy (type II and III SMA): 569 patients, *J Neurol Sci* 146:67-72, 1997.
103. Russman B, Buncher C, White M, et al: Function changes in spinal muscular atrophy II and III, *Neurology* 47:973-976, 1996.
104. McWilliam R, Gardner-Medwin D, Doyle D, et al: Diaphragmatic paralysis due to spinal muscular atrophy, *Arch Dis Child* 60: 145-149, 1985.
105. Feigin RD, Cherry JD: *Textbook of pediatric infectious diseases, vol* 2, ed 4, Philadelphia, 1998, WB Saunders.
106. Thorsteinsson G: Management of postpolio syndrome, *Mayo Clin Proc* 72:627-638, 1997.
107. Yoshimura K, Kurashige T: A case of poliomyelitis-like syndrome, *Brain Dev* 20:540-542, 1997.
108. Arya S: Antiviral therapeutic intervention in poliomyelitis-like syndrome, *Brain Dev* 21:567, 1999.
109. Zwiener R, Ginsberg C: Organophosphate and carbate poisoning in infants and children, *Pediatrics* 81:121-126, 1988.
110. Morgan D: *Recognition and management of pesticide poisinings,* Washington, D.C., 1976, U.S. Environmental Protection Agency Office of Pesticide Program.
111. Mortensen M: Management of acute childhood poisonings caused by selected insecticides and herbicides, *Pediatr Clin North Am* 33:421-445, 1986.
112. Lifshitz M, Shahak E, Sofer S: Carbamate and organophosphate poisoning in young children, *Pediatr Emerg Care* 15:102-103, 1999
113. Lifshitz M, Rotenberg M, Sofer S, et al: Carbamate poisoning and oxime treatment in children: a clinical and laboratory study, *Pediatrics* 93:652-655, 1994.
114. Goswamy R, Chaudhuri A, Mahashur A: Study of respiratory failure in organophosphate and carbamate poisoning, *Heart Lung* 23:466-472, 1994.
115. Tafuri J, Roberts J. Organophosphate poisoning, *Ann Emerg Med* 16:193-202, 1987.
116. Brumback R, Feeback D, Leech R: Rhabdomyolysis in childhood. A primer on normal muscle function and selected metabolic myopathies characterized by disordered energy production, *Pediatr Clin North Am* 39:821-858, 1992.
117. Watemberg N, Leshner R, Armstrong B, et al: Acute pediatric rhabdomyolysis, *J Child Neurol* 15:222-227, 2000.

118. Robotham J, Haddow J: Rhabdomyolysis and myoglobinuria in childhoood, *Pediatr Clin North Am* 23:279-301, 1976.
119. Chamberlain M. Rhabdomyolysis in children: a 3-year retrospective study, *Pediatr Neurol* 7:226-228, 1991.
120. Griggs R, Mendell J, Miller J: *Evaluation and treatment of myopathies,* Philadelphia, 1995, FA Davis.
121. Sessler D: Malignant hyperthermia, *J Pediatr* 109:9-14, 1986.
122. Kaus S, Rockoff M: Malignant hyperthermia, *Pediatr Clin North Am* 41:221-237, 1994.
123. Pope H, Keck P, McElroy S: Frequency and presentation of neuroleptic malignant syndrome in a large psychiatric hospital, *Am J Psychiatry* 143:1227-1232. 1986.
124. Knight M, Roberts R: Phenothiazine and butyrophenone intoxication in children, *Pediatr Clin North Am* 33:299-309, 1986.
125. Silva R, Munoz D, Alpert M et al: Neuroleptic malignant syndrome in children and adolescents, *J Am Acad Child Adolesc Psychiatry* 38:187-194, 1999.
126. Ty E, Rothner A: Neuroleptic malignant syndrome in children and adolescents, *J Child Neurol* 16:157-163, 2001.
127. Addonizio G, Susman V, Roth S: Neuroleptic malignant syndrome: review and analysis of 115 cases, *Biol Psychiatry* 22:1004-1020, 1987.
128. Denardo B, Tucker L, Miller L et al: Demography of a regional pediatric rheumatology patient population, *J Rheumatol* 21:1553-1561, 1994.
129. Bohan A, Peter J: Polymyositis and dermatomyositis, *N Engl J Med* 292:344-347, 1975.
130. Spiro A: Childhood dermatomyositis and polymyositis, *Pediatri Rev* 6:163-172, 1984.
131. Pachman L: Inflammatory myopathy in children, *Rheum Dis Clin North Am* 20:919-942, 1995.
132. Pachman L: Juvenile dermatomyositis. Pathophysiology and disease expression, *Pediatr Clin North Am* 42:1071-1098, 1995.
133. Mackay M, Kornberg A, Shield L et al: Benign acute childhood myositis: laboratory and clinical features, *Neurology* 53:2127-2131, 1999.

CHAPTER

57

Acute Pediatric Central Nervous System Infections

William G. Harmon, Frank Maffei, and Jeffrey S. Rubenstein

PEARLS

- With the successful implementation of vaccination against *Haemophilus influenzae,* the most commonly seen pathogenic meningeal bacteria are *Streptococcus pneumoniae* and *Neisseria meningitidis.*
- Successful treatment of bacterial meningitis involves eradication of the pathogenic organism and treatment of the both the systemic and the pathological derangements specific to the central nervous system.
- In bacterial meningitis, seizures in the first 48 hours of illness do not have prognostic significance.
- In herpes encephalitis, the patient's level of consciousness at the time of antimicrobial treatment offers the best prediction of outcome.

Acute Pediatric Central Nervous System Infections

Acute infections of the central nervous system (CNS) are relatively common in childhood and are often associated with significant mortality and morbidity. Bacterial meningitis, viral meningoencephalitis, viral encephalitis, and viral meningitis account for most childhood CNS infections. In the last decade, the etiological landscape of acute CNS infections has changed dramatically because of the development and widespread use of effective conjugate vaccines and the emergence of new CNS pathogens. Regardless of the causative agent, however, optimal care to children with acute CNS infection continues to provide the intensivist with a formidable and clinically significant challenge: management must successfully integrate treatments aimed at correcting or preventing a diverse group of systemic and intracranial pathophysiological abnormalities.

Bacterial Meningitis

Epidemiology

Bacterial meningitis (BM) is the most common life-threatening acute infectious disease of the CNS in children. It occurs mainly in infants and toddlers, although children and adults of all ages can be affected. Group B streptococci, gram-negative bacilli, and *Listeria monocytogenes* cause most cases of neonatal meningitis; *Streptococcus pneumoniae, Neisseria meningitidis,* and *Haemophilus influenzae* are the predominant pathogens in children older than 1 month. The following discussion focuses on nonneonatal meningitis.

Before the widespread use of the *H. influenzae* vaccine, the overall attack rate for BM was 3/100,000 with the highest rates occurring in infants younger than 1 year of age.[1] Recent decline in the incidence of BM to 1.25/100,000 is due to the successful introduction of *H. influenzae* type B vaccine. Incidence of *H. influenzae* type B meningitis has decreased from 3/100,000 in 1986 to current estimates of less than 0.2/100,000,[2,3] with an unchanging mortality (3% to 6%). Despite initial concerns that meningitis due to *S. pneumoniae* and *N. meningitidis* would rise in the post–*H. influenzae*-vaccine era, attack rates for both pathogens has remained stable (1.1/100,000 and 0.6/100,000, respectively).[2-4] Mortality from *S. pneumoniae* has declined from traditional estimates of 20% to 6% to 12%.[4-6] *N. meningitidis* meningitis without overt hemodynamic signs of septicemia has a mortality of approximately 3%. It is likely that the current use of a pneumococcal conjugate vaccine and the development of a more effective meningococcal vaccine will cause further declines in the occurrence of BM. Historically, *H. influenzae* was more frequently seen in the spring and fall; cases of meningitis as a result of *N. meningitidis* and *S. pneumoniae* occur mainly during the winter.

Uncommon pathogens causing nonneonatal BM include *Staphylococcus pyogenes*, aerobic gram-negative bacilli (i.e., *Pseudomonas aeruginosa*, *Salmonella* spp, *Klebsiella* spp, *Escherichia coli*, *Serratia marcescens*), *Propionibacterium acnes*, *Staphylococcus aureus*, and *Staphylococcus epidermidis*. CNS infection due to these organisms often occurs in the setting of impaired immunity, contiguous foci of infection, or disruption of anatomical barriers (e.g., traumatic brain injury, postneurosurgical complications). Meningitis caused by *Mycobacterium tuberculosis* is a devastating disease that occurs rarely and is the result of lymphohematogenous dissemination of the primary infection.

Pathophysiology

BM is almost always a systemic disease, with bacteria gaining entry to the CNS through the bloodstream. Pathogenic bacteria, however, can gain direct access to the CNS in two much less common ways: (1) through a rupture of an intracranial abscess and (2) across the dura mater, as a result of trauma, instrumentation, or extension from an extradural focus (e.g., otitis, sinusitis). Likely pathogens for nonhematogenously spread BM include streptococcal species, anaerobic species, and gram-negative bacilli.

Nasal colonization with potentially invasive bacteria initiates the most common pathogenesis of bacterial meningitis. Often, the bacterium is recently acquired. The presence of fimbriae or pili (*H. influenzae* and *N. meningitidis*) and the secretion of immunoglobulin A proteases (*S. pneumoniae, H. influenzae,* and *N. meningitidis*) increase the ability of bacteria to adhere to mucosal surfaces. Bacteria gain entry into the intravascular space by breaking down tight junctions between mucosal epithelial cells, or, alternatively, they are transported across the mucosal barrier by bacteria-directed endocytosis, as seen with *N. meningitidis*.[7] Although the exact sequence of events that encourages mucosal invasion in the setting of colonization is not completely understood, there is evidence that antecedent viral or mycoplasmal infection may predispose patients to this transformation. Once bacteria gain entry into the vascular space, bacterial survival is enhanced by the presence of a capsule. Encapsulation, present in *S. pneumoniae, H. influenzae N. meningitidis, E. coli,* and *Streptococcus agalcataie,* confers resistance to both neutrophil phagocytosis and the bactericidal action of the classic complement system.[8]

Bacterial penetration of the blood-brain barrier is also poorly understood, but it appears to be dependent on a sufficient bacterial inoculum (>1000 colony-forming units per milliliters of blood) aided by multiple inflammatory mediators liberated by invading pathogens and the host's own immune cells.[9] As a result, endothelial injury occurs and the integrity of the blood-brain barrier is lost. After entry into the CNS, bacteria replicate rapidly because host CNS defenses are inadequate to control bacterial invasion. Antibody-mediated opsonification is particularly ineffective in the CNS.[7,8,10] The inflammatory cascade that ensues is mediated by a variety of effector molecules. Reaction to bacterial invasion is heightened at the time of treatment with bactericidal antibiotics when cell wall components, teichoic acid and peptidoglycan, or lipopolysaccharide are released from *S. pneumoniae* or gram-negative bacteria, respectively.[11] Bacteria and bacterial byproducts in the cerebrospinal fluid (CSF) activate complement that promotes chemotaxis of leukocytes (neutrophils and macrophages) into the CSF, further exacerbating the endothelial cell damage.[12] Other chemokines, such as interleukin-8 (IL-8), macrophage inflammatory protein 2 (MIP–2), and monocyte chemotactic protein 1 (MCP-1), have been found to be potent neutrophil chemoattractants during meningitis.[13] During bacterial killing, neutrophils can cause further injury by releasing reactive oxygen species (ROS) such as superoxide, hydrogen peroxide, or hypochlorous acid. Peroxynitrite is formed when nitric oxide reacts with superoxide. ROS and peroxynitrite cause damage to neural cells by oxidation of cell membranes and intracellular proteins and nucleic acid.[10] Defensins, released from the primary granules of neutrophils, act as endogenous antibiotics with the ability to lyse bacteria; however, when present in high concentrations, these may also be cytotoxic to the host's cells.[14] Macrophages in the CNS release IL-1, tumor necrosis factor (TNF), and prostaglandin E_2 (PGE_2) in response to meningeal infection. IL-1 and TNF are present in the CSF of children with meningitis.[15] These cytokines, among others, directly kill neural cells, promote leukocyte chemotaxis, destroy the integrity of the blood-brain barrier (by acting pathologically on capillary endothelial cells), and induce the synthesis and release of arachidonic acid metabolites and proteolytic enzymes. PGE_2 is present in the CSF of experimental animals with meningitis and causes local vasodilation and increased capillary permeability.[16] Matrix metalloproteinases, a family of proteases produced by a variety of immune cells, also likely play a central role in disruption of the blood-brain barrier and ongoing neuronal injury in bacterial meningitis.[13,17]

Increased intracranial pressure (ICP) is a near universal finding in children with BM and is most severe in the first days after diagnosis and treatment, when the pathophysiological mechanisms causing it are exaggerated.[18] Early in the disease course, intracranial blood and parenchymal volumes are larger. Increased intracranial blood volume results from a loss of the ability to autoregulate cerebral blood flow (CBF), which often leads to discrete areas of relative hyperemia and hypoperfusion.[19] Cerebral edema occurs both as a direct result of the cytotoxic effects of bacteria, bacterial byproducts, cytokines, and lipid mediators (cytotoxic cerebral edema) and as a result of the increased capillary permeability that these materials cause (vasogenic cerebral edema). The increased transcapillary pressures that result from a loss of autoregulation exacerbate the vasogenic cerebral edema. Thrombosis of cerebral veins and dural sinuses can obstruct venous return (interstitial cerebral edema). Later in the course of the disease, obstruction of CSF outflow at the arachnoid villi[20] can lead to communicating hydrocephalus and subdural effusions or, rarely, empyemas.

Autopsy examinations of children who have died of BM confirm these observations.[21] An intense inflammatory infiltrate is seen in the subarachnoid space in all cases. Cerebral edema that causes transtentorial herniation is commonly seen. Vasculitis affecting the cerebral blood vessels is often noted[22,23]and can worsen an already irregular pattern of CBF or cause infarction if severe. Vasculitic changes have also been noted in the arterial supply of the brainstem in some series.[24]

Clinical Manifestations

Clinical Presentation

Infants and children with BM have acute onset of a febrile illness that can be accompanied by altered consciousness, headache with or without a stiff neck, photophobia, nausea and vomiting, anorexia, or seizures. Often the child has had an antecedent upper respiratory tract infection. A petechial or purpuric rash is commonly seen with meningitis caused by *N. meningitidis* and less frequently with *H. influenzae* disease. Other organs (e.g., pericardium, lung, joints) may be seeded at the time of dissemination of bacteria to the CNS; occasional patients may have concurrent symptoms. On examination, infants typically have fever, a bulging anterior fontanelle, an altered level of consciousness (usually lethargy or irritability), and hyperactive or hypoactive deep tendon reflexes. Older children also can have altered deep tendon reflexes and similar changes in consciousness but more reliably exhibit signs of meningeal irritation. Resistance to neck flexion indicates meningitis; meningoencephalitis; subarachnoid hemorrhage; space-occupying lesion in the posterior fossa; or, rarely, non-CNS disease, such as deep neck infections and pneumonia.[25] Meningeal irritation is also manifested by Brudzinski's and Kernig's signs. Brudzinski's sign is elicited by rapidly flexing the neck; immediate flexion of the legs at the hips and knees results. Bending the hips to right angles and then attempting to extend the legs at the knees elicit Kernig's sign; severe meningitis makes full extension impossible. Less commonly, an infant or child can have frank coma, pupillary changes, cranial nerve dysfunction, or an altered respiratory pattern (e.g., Cheyne-Stokes respirations, sustained hyperventilation, or hypoventilation). Although some of these findings can be seen after a seizure or as the result of metabolic disturbances associated with the systemic process, they are also suggestive of dangerous elevations of intracranial volume and pressure. Focal neurological deficits are present in 20% of children with BM. Papilledema can be present in all ages; its absence must not be taken as proof that the ICP is normal because of the acuity of the meningitic process. Any child with BM may show signs of circulatory failure (e.g., poor peripheral pulses and perfusion, oliguria, hypotension).

Lumbar Puncture and Laboratory Evaluation

The definitive diagnosis of BM is made with a culture of pathogenic organisms obtained from the CSF by lumbar puncture from any patient in whom the diagnosis of BM is a serious consideration unless a specific contraindication to the procedure exists.[26] Lumbar puncture should be performed with full cardiorespiratory monitoring with a small gauge spinal needle; only the minimum amount of CSF necessary for diagnostic testing should be withdrawn for culture and studies. If a focal CNS mass lesion is suspected or if the patient displays clinical signs of dangerous elevations in the ICP, the lumbar puncture may be delayed (this is described later). Nevertheless, antibiotic treatment, with or without corticosteroids, should not be postponed. Measures to lower ICP may be warranted (see also Chapter 52). Computed tomography (CT) of the head (assuming relative patient stability) may provide additional diagnostic information.

CSF obtained from a patient with suspected bacterial meningitis must be cultured. Although a positive culture is the sine qua non for diagnosis, up to 2 days may be required for the bacteria to grow adequately to be identified. Therefore for more immediate diagnostic information to be provided, the glucose and protein contents and white blood cell (WBC) counts of the spinal fluid should be quantified, and the fluid should be studied with Gram stain and examined for evidence of pathogenic bacteria. The CSF of an infant or child with untreated BM typically exhibits pleocytosis (>6 WBCs per microliter for a nonneonate) with absolute predominance of polymorphonuclear neutrophils (PMNs). PMNs are not normally found in the CSF of infants and children; more than one PMN per microliter should be considered abnormal. Because most children with viral meningitis will have a predominance of PMNs in the CSF at presentation, PMN predominance alone does not distinguish BM from viral meningitis.[27] CSF protein is elevated in children with BM (>40 mg/dl), and the CSF glucose/serum glucose ratio is depressed below normal (<66%). The CSF abnormalities seen in BM are usually not subtle; most children have a protein concentration greater than 100 mg/dl, a glucose concentration less than 20 mg/dl, and marked pleocytosis. In some settings, rapid diagnostic tests that use latex agglutination or countercurrent immunoelectrophoresis can also be useful in helping to confirm a diagnosis of BM by establishing the presence of bacterial antigen in the CSF. The CSF of children with meningitis caused by *M. tuberculosis* typically has markedly elevated protein and decreased glucose contents and a marked pleocytosis with a mononuclear predominance.

Administration of antibiotics to a patient with meningitis before diagnostic lumbar puncture has the potential to alter some of the CSF findings but, in general, will not completely obscure the correct diagnosis. Prediagnostic treatment with a course of oral antibiotics has been shown to sterilize the CSF of many patients with meningitis caused by *S. pneumoniae* and *N. meningitidis* but not to affect significantly the recovery of *H. influenzae*.[28] CSF sterilization after administration of intravenous antibiotics occurs rapidly (within 4 hours in cases of *S. pneumoniae* BM and within 2 hours in cases of *N. meningitidis* BM).[29] Despite pretreatment with appropriate intravenous antibiotics, the biochemical and cellular diagnostic measures are basically unaffected, although there may be a trend toward a decrease in the ratio of CSF PMNs to mononuclear cells, with an increasing length of oral pretreatment. Adjunctive diagnostic tests can be valuable in this setting.

Reasons for deferring lumbar puncture have been the subject of much controversy.[30-33] The suggested contraindications center on three themes: the presence of intracranial hypertension, cardiorespiratory instability, or a coagulopathy. A diagnostic lumbar puncture may acutely decrease spinal CSF pressure and therefore predispose to a shift of brain substance through the foramen magnum. It also has the potential to contribute to the pathogenesis of a herniation syndrome in a patient by worsening intracranial hypertension because the procedure requires that the patient be placed in a flexed posture. This positioning can both obstruct cerebral venous return (increasing cerebral blood volume and ICP) and interfere with ventilation (again increasing cerebral blood volume and ICP). The flexed posture can also adversely affect patients with cardiorespiratory instability by interfering with ventilation and by increasing systemic vascular resistance. Presence of a coagulopathy may predispose a patient to the development of a spinal epidural hematoma.

Currently it seems reasonable to defer lumbar puncture in a *small* number of selected patients with suspected BM. Specifically, patients with cardiorespiratory instability should have specimens for blood cultures obtained and be treated presumptively with antibiotics. Lumbar puncture can be attempted after hemodynamic stability is achieved. Patients with clear evidence of significantly increased ICP should be presumptively treated with antibiotics after a blood culture is obtained. Patients with a severe coagulopathy should have samples obtained for a blood culture and be given antibiotics empirically. Lumbar puncture should be undertaken when hemostatic function is restored.

Radiographic imaging studies are useful in some patients with BM. Head CT can help to assess the volume status of the intracranial compartment. The CT scan at the time of presentation may show cerebral edema (e.g., loss of the clarity of gray-white matter differentiation) or obliteration of ventricles and cisterns, or it can be totally normal.[34,35] Magnetic resonance imaging (MRI) techniques may become useful to assess brain water content, although they are currently much more cumbersome. Not surprisingly, one pilot study was unable to show clinical utility when scans were performed between 2 and 5 days after diagnosis.[36] Results of laboratory studies other than the lumbar puncture may be abnormal, and they are indicative of the systemic nature of the disease process. Blood culture results are positive for the offending organism in more than 85% of patients. The complete blood cell count may show any combination of anemia, thrombocytopenia, leukocytosis or leukopenia, or may be normal. Biochemical evidence of shock, sepsis, stress, and the syndrome of inappropriate secretion of antidiuretic hormone (SIADH) may be found in children with a large systemic component to their disease.

Clinical Course/Complications

Clinical manifestations of BM in children are easily related to the pathophysiological process of the infection. Most of the manifestations can be attributed either to the shock state, which can be associated with the bacteremic phase of the disease, or to the intracranial events that stem from bacterial invasion of the meninges. Although artificial at times, this classification provides a clearer understanding of the meningitic process and a framework for designing a cohesive management plan.

Systemic Manifestations

Signs of shock may be seen in up to one fifth of children with BM (see also Chapter 96) and are often manifest as end-organ failure rather than as overt circulatory collapse. Impaired circulatory function should be a concern in a child with meningitis who has any combination of an abnormal peripheral circulation, altered mental status, and oliguria. Shock in these patients is usually the result of sepsis and may involve alterations in preload, cardiac function, and afterload. Hemodynamic problems can be compounded by volume depletion because these children have often had symptoms of fever, anorexia, and vomiting during the time immediately before diagnosis. Disseminated intravascular coagulation can result either from shock or directly from the infectious process. Inadequately treated shock can lead to disastrous results by decreasing cerebral perfusion pressure (and CBF) or by leading to the development of the syndrome of multiple-organ system failure. (See also Chapter 97 and Chapter 96 for a complete discussion of the treatment of septic shock and multiple organ dysfunction syndrome.)

Pericardial and joint effusions occur both early and late in the course of the disease. Early in the course of meningitis, cultures of pericardial or joint fluid from affected patients are often positive for the meningeal pathogen. The effusions that occur a week or later into the course are usually sterile and may take up to a month to resolve.[26]

Manifestations in the Central Nervous System

All children with BM show some degree of evidence of CNS disease. Abnormal patterns of CBF and substrate utilization, elevated ICP, and the irritative effects of the infectious process and inflammatory response combine to cause a variable combination of altered consciousness, seizures, isolated cranial nerve palsies, and SIADH.

CBF patterns are abnormal in adult patients with meningitis[19] and in animal models of BM.[16,37] In children, CBF velocity has been found to be increased and global CBF decreased in the acute phase of BM.[38,39] The degree of CBF alteration may have prognostic significance because survivors without neurological sequelae have been found to have maintained CBF early in their course.[40] Children with meningitis have impaired autoregulation with marked regional variability in carbon dioxide responsiveness[38] and are more sensitive to the cerebral vasodilatory effects of hypercapnia. These changes can increase cerebral blood volume and increase the likelihood of intracranial hypertension, which raises the potential for local ischemia. These effects are further accentuated by systemic hypertension because the intravascular pressures are directly transmitted to the cerebral compartment. Autoregulation may be restored by mild hyperventilation (partial pressure of carbon dioxide [P_{CO_2}] of 32 to 36) in some patients.[19]

Evidence that ICP is elevated in patients with BM is incontrovertible; it is found on physical examination and by direct measurement. Physical findings in BM-associated ICP elevation can include any combination of a bulging anterior fontanelle, altered mental status, hyperreflexia with positive Babinski's sign, and pupillary and cranial nerve dysfunction.[41]

Direct assessment of ICP has used the measurement of opening pressure at the time of lumbar puncture (average ICP = 30.7 cm H_2O),[42] extradural measurement techniques validated by correlation with opening pressures (peak ICP = 20 to 32 cm H_2O),[43] and subdural and intraventricular techniques (average ICP = 41 cm H_2O).[44] This last study, in which all patients were deeply comatose, showed that the ICPs of children who died were significantly higher than those who survived (70 versus 19 cm H_2O). Most of the affected patients who recovered had normal ICPs by the fourth or fifth day of treatment.

Increased ICP clearly has the potential to harm the patient by causing further cerebral ischemia and can, if it is measured, provide a warning sign of impending cerebral herniation. Occurrence of cerebral herniation in a child with meningitis has grave prognostic implications. In one study of 307 pediatric patients with meningitis, children who showed clinical signs of herniation were more likely to die (17% versus 2.5%) and more likely to be left with serious neurological residua (27% versus 5.8%).[45] *The presence of an open anterior fontanelle does not protect infants from cerebral herniation.*

Seizures occur in up to one third of patients with meningitis and can be either generalized or focal. Seizures that occur within the first few days are usually generalized and can be attributed mainly to cortical irritation by the infectious process and products liberated by immune response; they have no prognostic implications. Seizures that occur later in the course of the disease are more likely to be focal and usually originate in cortical areas in which local ischemia or infarction has caused neuronal damage; these seizures may coexist with an abnormal neurological recovery.[26]

SIADH has been reported to occur in up to one half of children with meningitis and is likely caused by inflamatory or ischemic changes around the neurohypophysis that lead to release of antidiuretic hormone (ADH).[18] Patients with SIADH exhibit oliguria, hyponatremia, and an inappropriately high urine sodium concentration (see also Chapter 59). The hypo-osmolality that results can contribute to the development of cerebral edema. Differentiating SIADH from a patient's normal response to a decreased intravascular volume may represent a difficult diagnostic dilemma with real physiologic repercussions.

The clinical course of a patient whose condition is uncomplicated and who is adequately treated for BM is one of steady, gradual recovery of neurological function. Any worsening of neurological function should prompt an immediate investigation for its cause. CT is usually the diagnostic tool of choice because most CNS complications (e.g., secondary brain abscess, infarction, cerebral edema, vasculitis, subdural effusion, and abscess) have anatomical correlates. CT scanning is not useful as a screening or prognostic tool without the presence of neurological signs.[34,35] Cranial ultrasound can be useful in infants with an open fontanelle.[46] MRI may also be of use, but its utility can be limited by technical issues (e.g., length of time needed, need for mechanical ventilation, need for sedation in some patients).

Fever can be long lasting; the average duration of fever in *Haemophilus* disease is near 5 days.[47] Persistent fever, which lasts longer than 10 days, or recurrent fever, which occurs after a 24-hour afebrile period, requires investigation. Nosocomial infections (usually thrombophlebitis at an intravenous access site) and drug fever are the most common treatment-related causes. Although inadequate or incomplete antibacterial therapy, pneumonia, arthritis, pericarditis, and brain abscess are all clinical entities that should be considered, the most common cause of persistent fever directly related to the meningeal process is a subdural effusion.[26] These subdural collections are usually sterile but should be aspirated if the child shows signs of increased ICP or focal neurological signs or if there is clinical evidence suggesting that it is an empyema. Subdural effusions are most commonly seen in patients with *H. influenzae* disease.

Treatment Options

The overall aim of treatment for a patient with BM is survival with an intact CNS. For this goal to be met, multiple pathophysiological considerations must be weighed, and a cohesive plan organized. The infant or child with BM should be cared for in an intensive care setting whenever the resources available in the pediatric intensive care unit (PICU) will improve care. Although the need for ventilatory assistance, hemodynamic support, or ICP monitoring generally ensures a patient's admission to the PICU, it is often appropriate to admit a severely lethargic child with meningitis to the PICU for close observation of neurological status. The primary therapeutic options for an infant or child with meningitis can be grouped into three categories: optimization of the patient's overall physiological status, antibiotic therapies, and CNS-specific therapies.

Optimization of Physiological Status

As with any other life-threatening pediatric disease, the preservation of physiological status is centered on the maintenance of the patient's airway, breathing, and circulation (the ABCs). Because the pathophysiological process can be potentiated by hypercarbia (an increase in cerebral blood volume), by hypotension (a decrease in cerebral perfusion pressure), and by hypertension (an increase in cerebral blood volume and a worsening cerebral edema), the ABCs demand meticulous and ongoing attention in such patients to avoid secondary injury. The airway must be secured and ventilation assisted as needed if there is any suggestion of either failure to protect the airway or hypoventilation. Shock should be aggressively treated, first with restoration of intravascular volume and next with administration of inotropic or vasoactive support as indicated. (See Chapter 27 for a complete discussion of the therapy of shock.) The proper limits for treating hypertension are not clear, especially because systemic hypertension may be an appropriate response to raised ICP.

Careful attention must also be given to fluid and electrolyte balance. The overriding goal of fluid management must be the provision of an ongoing adequate intravascular volume, although this must be tempered by respect for the potential for SIADH and its complications to develop. Fluid restriction to two thirds of the calculated maintenance rate has been advocated for patients with meningitis whose course is uncomplicated to guard against the development of SIADH.[1] The course of most patients in the PICU is *not* uncomplicated and therefore demands a more individualized management scheme. It is prudent to administer dextrose-containing isotonic crystalloid at a rate appropriate to hydration status and to monitor serum (and urine) electrolytes frequently to assess for the onset of SIADH. SIADH should be treated with fluid restriction but never to the point of compromising the patient's intravascular volume status. Intravascular monitoring of central venous or pulmonary artery pressures may be useful in guiding fluid strategies. Hypoglycemia can occur, especially early in the disease process, and should be vigorously treated.

Antibiotic Therapy

Prompt administration of appropriate antibiotics is the basis of curative therapy for patients with BM. Because the causative organism and its sensitivities are not initially known, empirical therapy against all likely pathogens must be instituted. In recent years, the emergence of penicillin-resistant strains of *S. pneumoniae* has required modification of empiric antibiotic therapy in BM. The mechanism of resistance is due to alterations in pneumococcal binding proteins and is not based on β-lactamase production. Pneumococcal resistance varies geographically, with some areas reporting 30% of isolates found to be intermediately (minimum inhibitory concentration [MIC] range 0.1 to 1 µg /ml) or highly (MIC >2 µg/ml) resistant to penicillin.[48,49] Young age, day care attendance, frequent or prolonged antibiotic use, and immunosuppression can predispose children to pneumococcal resistance. Because of the changing susceptibility patterns, the combination of vancomycin (60 mg/kg per day divided every 6 hours) and a cephalosporin (cefotaxime 300 mg/kg per day divided every 8 hours or ceftriaxone 100 mg/kg/day divided every 12 or 24 hours) is appropriate initial therapy until bacterial identification and susceptibility have been established. Rifampin (20 mg/kg per day divided every 12 hours) can be used in place of the cephalosporin if a β-lactam allergy exists.[49] Once the organism is isolated, antibiotic therapy can be adjusted and made more specific. Duration of therapy should be tailored to the individual patient on the basis of clinical and microbiological data. In general, BM caused by *N. meningitidis* is treated for 7 days, whereas *S. pneumoniae* and *H. influenzae* require 10 to 14 days of systemic antibiotics. BM caused by gram-negative bacilli other than *H. influenzae* requires prolonged systemic antibiotics up to 21 days.[50]

CNS-Specific Therapies

Therapies aimed at the CNS with the goal of minimizing sequelae have their basis in control of ICP, seizures, and inflammation.

Therapy for Increased Intracranial Pressure. Anecdotal evidence that supports aggressive treatment of elevated ICP is readily available. Osmotherapy to reduce cerebral edema was shown to be of therapeutic value in selected cases.[51] Perhaps the most convincing evidence of the efficacy of ICP-related therapies is that mild hypocapnia may restore lost cerebral autoregulation in adults with meningitis.[19] No controlled trial of invasive techniques of monitoring and controlling ICP has been undertaken in patients with meningitis. (See Chapter 52 for a detailed description of the management of increased ICP.) Because of its invasive nature, current practice has been to limit the use of intracranial monitoring to patients with coma or signs of impending herniation syndrome.

Anticonvulsant Therapy. Seizures raise cerebral metabolic demand and ICP by increasing systemic blood pressure. At the very least, seizure activity should be promptly and aggressively treated after provisions are made for an adequate airway. Prophylaxis against seizures with an agent that does not decrease respiratory drive (e.g., phenytoin) may be indicated in severe cases of meningitis or in a patient with a history of seizure activity.

Antiinflammatory Therapy. The major effort at controlling the CNS inflammatory response has involved systemic administration of corticosteroids, specifically dexamethasone. Routine use of dexamethasone early in the course of BM remains controversial. Early reports have shown a benefit of adjunctive dexamethasone therapy in children with BM caused by *H. influenzae* type B.[52-55] Data regarding dexamethasone use in BM due to *S. pneumoniae* have been conflicting. A large prospective study showed a significant reduction in unfavorable outcomes and death in adult patients with penicillin-sensitive pneumococcal BM treated with dexamethasone.[56] A meta-analysis of dexamethasone use in BM from 1988 to 1996 showed a significant reduction in severe hearing loss when dexamethasone was given early in the course of pneumococcal meningitis.[57] Subsequent studies of children with pneumococcal meningitis, however, which included penicillin-resistant strains, revealed no beneficial effect of dexamethasone use.[5,58] With the recent introduction of the conjugate pneumococcal vaccine, further prospective trials in which the efficacy of dexamethasone in pneumococcal BM is investigated are unlikely to occur. Dexamethasone has not been shown to improve outcome in children with meningococcal BM. Current recommendations from the Committee on Infectious Diseases, American Academy of Pediatrics, are for dexamethasone treatment for infants and children with *H. influenzae* type B BM and individual consideration of dexamethasone for pneumococcal BM in children older than 6 weeks at a dose of 0.6 mg/kg per day in four divided intravenous infusions during the first 4 days of antibiotic treatment.[59] If used, the first dose of dexamethasone should be administered immediately before or at the time of the first dose of antibiotics.

Prognosis

Approximately 5% of children with BM die.[26] This mortality rate, which has been stable for the past decades, can be attributed to the occurrence of catastrophic intracranial events and to the sepsis syndrome and complications arising from it.

About one fourth of children have sequelae as a result of an episode of BM,[26] with BM due to *S. pneumoniae* carrying the greatest risk for significant morbidity.[60,61] This morbidity almost invariably takes the form of persistent neurological deficits. Moderate to severe sensorineural hearing loss is seen in up to 10% of survivors and is the most common serious sequelae. Behavioral abnormalities and developmental delay also are commonly seen in individual patients.[60] In patients with the most severe cases, damage to the cerebral cortex can be severe enough to cause a persistent vegetative state, cortical blindness, and any degree of loss of motor function. Onset of a new seizure disorder can either coexist with any of these sequelae or be an independent adverse outcome.

Prevention

The relatively high mortality and morbidity associated with BM demand that primary efforts are made to immunize at-risk populations and to prevent the spread of the disease with the use of prophylactic antibiotics, when appropriate. Current efforts at prevention involve immunization against *H. influenzae* and *S. pneumoniae* and prophylaxis of contacts of patients with *H. influenzae* or *N. meningitidis*.

All direct contacts of patients with *N. meningitidis* should receive prophylaxis orally with rifampin (10 mg/kg per dose [600 mg maximum] twice a day for 2 days) or receive intramuscular ceftriaxone (125 mg if age 12 years or younger; 250 mg if older than 12 years). A single 500-mg oral dose of ciprofloxacin can be used for prophylaxis of adult contacts. All household contacts of a child with *H. influenzae* meningitis should receive prophylaxis with rifampin (20 mg/kg [600 mg maximum] every day for 4 days) if there is another child younger than 4 years in the house. Prophylaxis for day care exposures should be individualized.[59]

Viral Meningoencephalitis

Epidemiology

With the success of immunization strategies designed to prevent bacterial meningitis, proportionately more infants and children with CNS infection appear in the PICU with viral meningoencephalitis. A survey of hospital discharge records showed that there were approximately 19,000 hospital admissions of adults and children per year for encephalitis in the United States over a 10-year period (1988 to 1997).[62] Despite many diagnostic advances over this period, no etiological agent was identified in a majority (59.5%) of these cases. Children younger than 1 year were at the greatest risk for the development of encephalitis and were more likely than adults to have a causative agent identified.

Encephalitis in the pediatric age group usually represents a rare complication of an otherwise common childhood viral infection. Herpes simplex virus (HSV) and varicella are most frequently associated with pediatric viral encephalitis, followed by arboviral (arthropod-borne virus) and other less common agents. HSV often causes moderate to severe CNS disease. Adenovirus, Epstein-Barr virus, cytomegalovirus (CMV), rubeola, rubella, and the nonpolio enteroviruses have all been associated with meningoencephalitis (Table 57–1). Respiratory syncytial virus (RSV) infection, ubiquitous in the PICU environment, has also been described as a cause of meningoencephalitis that results in encephalopathy and seizures.[63] Poliovirus can cause meningoencephalitis but is rarely seen because of aggressive immunization programs. Increasing data support *Mycoplasma pneumoniae* as a relatively common agent responsible for childhood encephalitis.[64] In the adult U.S. population, toxoplasmic encephalitis related to human immunodeficiency virus (HIV) is identified nearly as often as viral disease.

Worldwide and in the United States, arboviruses remain a common cause of identifiable infection. In the United States, eastern equine, western equine, St. Louis, and La Crosse encephalitis remain the predominant agents associated with seasonal mosquito-spread encephalitis in which an etiological agent is identified.[65] Epidemiological variables continually change, bringing new agents to the forefront. The West Nile virus subsequent to 1999 is one such example. Vaccination is available for prevention of several of the arboviral encephalitides (e.g., Japanese encephalitis); vaccine administration may be appropriate for those living in or traveling to endemic regions.

Pathophysiology

The pathophysiological processes of the viral encephalitides have not been clearly established. Arbovirus infections follow seasonal vector patterns and are usually seen during summer outbreaks. Other viral encephalitides do not have a seasonal occurrence. Each arbovirus has a predilection for a particular geographical area and age range of patient. For example, West Nile virus rarely affects children, with only two documented pediatric infections during the 1999 to 2000 outbreak.[66] In contrast, La Crosse virus typically causes encephalitis in the pediatric age group that can mimic the clinical and radiographic findings found with HSV disease.[67]

After introduction into the body, the virus is spread either by hematogenous or neuronal routes. The typical pattern begins with localized skin infection, followed by a transient primary viremia infecting the reticuloendothelial system. After replication in lymphatic tissues, a secondary viremia occurs leading to infection of other organs, including the CNS. With severe disease, striking inflammation of the cortical endothelium ensues, with perivascular lymphocytic infiltration and cerebral edema easily identifiable on light microscopy. Virus can often be isolated from the perivascular space by culture or identified with fluorescent antibody techniques.

HSV is thought to primarily invade the CNS from the nasopharynx through the olfactory system or, secondarily, to invade from the trigeminal ganglion, where it often is found in a dormant state.[68] Once HSV obtains access to the CNS and infection is established, the pathological processes (severe cerebral edema, eosinophilic intranuclear inclusions, and a lymphocytic meningeal infiltrate) favor the temporal and frontal cortical lobes.

TABLE 57–1

Causative Agents and Differential Diagnosis of Encephalitis/Aseptic Meningitis Syndromes

Viral Infections	Nonviral Infections	Inflammatory/Miscellaneous Etiologies
VIRUSES ASSOCIATED WITH CLINICAL ENCEPHALITIS	*Mycoplasma pneumoniae*	Toxic shock syndrome
Herpes simplex virus	Lyme disease	ADEM
Varicella	Rocky Mountain spotted fever	SLE
Arboviruses	Toxoplasmosis	SSPE
Eastern equine encephalitis	Leptospirosis	Reye's syndrome
Western equine encephalitis	Fungal	Rasmussen's encephalitis
St. Louis encephalitis	Tuberculosis	Other vasculitides
California encephalitis	Amoebic *(Naegleria fowleri)*	Tumors
Encephalitis		Subdural hematomas
West Nile virus		
La Cross Encephalitis		
Powassan		
Nipah		
Hendra		
Other regional agents		
Enterovirus 71		
Mumps		
CMV		
EBV		
Adenovirus		
RSV		
Influenza A, B		
Rabies		
HIV		
VIRUSES COMMONLY ASSOCIATED WITH ASEPTIC MENINGITIS		
Nonpolio enteroviral infections		
ECHO virus		
Coxsackie (enteroviruses are causative in 80%-90% of cases)		
Any of the above viruses (e.g., arboviruses, HSV) may be associated with milder forms of aseptic meningitis		

ADEM, acute demyelinating encephalomyelitis; *CMV,* cytomegalovirus; *EBV,* Epstein-Barr virus; *ECHO,* enteric cytopathic human orphan; *HIV,* human immunodeficiency virus; *HSV,* herpes simplex virus; *RSV,* respiratory syncytial virus; *SLE,* systemic lupus erythematosus; *SSPE,* subacute sclerosing panencephalitis;

With all of the viral encephalitides, T-cell mediated inflammation may lead to progressive gliosis in affected neuronal tissue. Apoptic neurons and glia have been detected in acute HSV and CMV encephalitis.[69] This suggests that viral-induced neuronal apoptosis, not just inflammatory tissue destruction, contributes to encephalitic acute brain injury; molecular biological advancements may allow future antiapoptosis-directed therapy (see also Chapter 93).

Many of the changes that occur with bacterial CNS infection (e.g., loss of cerebral vascular autoregulation, cerebral edema, localized ischemia, and increased ICP) occur in viral meningoencephalitis as well.[70] Brain single-photon emission computed tomography (SPECT) scanning has identified regional hyperperfusion in some patients with acute viral encephalitis; conversely, local ischemia indicative of a small vessel vasculitis has been shown in others.[71]

Clinical Manifestations

Clinical Presentation

Infants and children with viral meningoencephalitis have abrupt onset of any combination of fever, encephalopathy or other changes in cortical function, ataxia, seizures, headache, photophobia, nausea, and vomiting. Meningeal signs may be present, but they depend on the age of the patient and the degree of meningeal, compared with cerebral, involvement. Disease in infants and children with herpes encephalitis presents in a similar fashion, except that focal neurological signs and either focal or generalized seizures are more commonly seen.

Changes in cortical function serve to clinically differentiate viral meningoencephalitis from viral meningitis. Because the laboratory abnormalities seen in viral encephalitis can be nonspecific, it is important to consider other clinical entities that can present in a similar fashion.

Drug ingestions, trauma (e.g., child abuse), hepatic or renal failure, electrolyte abnormalities, lead toxicity, and Reye's syndrome can all cause an encephalopathy that may be hard to distinguish from viral or other infectious encephalopathies. Rheumatological disorders, stroke, vasculitides and postinfectious encephalomyelitis should also enter into the differential diagnosis when acute mental status changes are observed. Postinfectious encephalomyelitis typically follows a nonspecific viral illness. Demyelination is the prominent pathological or MRI finding with clinical symptoms reflecting the specific areas of brain involvement.

Laboratory Manifestations

A definitive diagnosis of viral meningoencephalitis can be made by identification of a pathogenic virus from CSF or brain tissue. CSF biochemical abnormalities (mildly decreased glucose and mildly elevated protein levels) and a mild pleocytosis (either polymorphonuclear or mononuclear) can be seen; conversely, the CSF can be totally normal.

Before the development of molecular techniques, laboratory detection of viral CNS infections relied on viral culture, comparison of acute and convalescent antibody titers, or brain biopsies. These standard laboratory tests often lack sensitivity or do not provide timely enough results to serve as a basis for acute therapeutic guidance. Molecular techniques such as the polymerase chain reaction (PCR) are now routinely used to identify a number of pathogenic viruses including HSV-1, HSV-2, varicella, CMV, and enteroviruses.[72] PCR of CSF is a highly sensitive (approximately 92%) and specific tool that has virtually replaced brain biopsy as the gold standard for HSV detection.[73] False-negative results can be seen, however, when CSF is obtained early in the course of the encephalitis. Serum antibody titers remain a useful method to diagnose less common arboviral infections; consultation with infectious disease and government health services can guide serological testing in a specific locale. Often these results are of greater epidemiological interest because they may not be available in real time.

Radiographic evaluation is indicated for many patients with altered mental status. Neuroimaging studies may provide a variety of diagnostic clues, aid acute therapeutic decision making, and provide prognostic information. A noncontrasted head CT scan often can be obtained quickly and can provide information regarding acute or chronic hemorrhage, fluid accumulations, cerebral edema, or mass effects. CT scans are often normal during the early presentation of the viral encephalitides. MRI scanning provides more detailed anatomical and functional data, often showing abnormalities at the time of clinical presentation. MRI can be useful in the evaluation of presumed encephalitis; however, this mode of imaging may be less available, requires longer scan times, and may necessitate the use of sedation to obtain adequate images in encephalopathic, agitated pediatric patients. Safe sedation practices focusing on airway management and maintenance of adequate hemodynamics must be ensured in the MRI suite (see also Chapter 116).

MRI often shows subtle edema and gyral swelling early in the course of encephalitis. Radiologic consultation may be particularly helpful to guide the application of ever-advancing imaging technology. MR spectroscopy, diffusion-weighted imaging, and SPECT scanning have been applied to evaluate acute encephalitis. Diffusion-weighted imaging may be particularly sensitive in defining the presence and extent of early encephalitic changes in infants and young children.[75] Parenchymal hemorrhage may develop, especially in association with HSV disease. Follow-up imaging is often normal in patients and shows complete clinical recovery. Conversely, encephalomalacia, brain atrophy, and ventricular enlargement may be present in those recovering from more severe disease with clinically apparent neurological residua.

Herpetic encephalitis represents a special diagnostic challenge because of the decreased morbidity and mortality associated with the early initiation of antiviral therapy. Physicians caring for a patient with an acute encephalopathy must have a high index of suspicion for HSV disease. Classically, HSV encephalitis is described as febrile illness associated with altered consciousness or seizures and focal temporal lobe involvement. Patients with herpetic encephalitis often show evidence of CNS hemorrhage with up to 1000 red blood cells per cubic microliter of CSF.[76] Electroencephalographic (EEG) tracings may indicate a characteristic pattern of sharp waves superimposed on a slow background in the temporal areas.[77] Most HSV-infected individuals show abnormal MRI findings in the inferomedial regions of one or both temporal lobes; these findings correlate closely with a positive HSV PCR.[78] Infants with severe HSV encephalitis may show generalized brain edema that can mimic the radiographic findings seen with diffuse hypoxic injury.

Clinical Course

The clinical courses of the different encephalitides vary. St. Louis encephalitis is typically a mild (or even asymptomatic) disease in infants and children. La Crosse encephalitis occurs in children and may be severe. Seizures are common, and approximately one fourth of patients subsequently have a permanent seizure disorder. Eastern equine encephalitis is less commonly seen but in general has an abrupt onset and catastrophic course. Seizures, coma, and signs of elevated ICP occur within 1 to 2 days of the onset of disease. Affected children usually either die or have severe neurological residua. Western equine encephalitis affects all ages, but the disease is more severe in younger infants. Seizures are common in these infants, about half of whom have significant neurological residua (90% of older children have a complete recovery). The acute portion of these arboviral diseases generally resolves within 1 to 2 weeks. Herpes encephalitis is a devastating disease if untreated or if the initiation of treatment is delayed. Seizures or coma and other signs of increased ICP occur as the disease progresses.

Treatment

Therapy for infants and children with encephalitis is largely supportive and similar to that required by patients with meningitis. Care must be taken to ensure that the patient has an adequate airway and adequate respiratory and circulatory function. Meticulous attention should be paid to electrolyte balance because SIADH, diabetes insipidus, and cerebral salt wasting have all been described in association with encephalitis. Finally, therapies specific to the CNS should be undertaken as needed. These therapies must include adequate control of seizures for all patients and may extend to ICP monitoring and the use of therapies designed to decrease ICP in selected patients. Decompressive craniectomy has been successfully used in the setting of severe encephalitis-induced intracranial hypertension.[79] Seizure control can be difficult in some instances. Continuous EEG monitoring can be useful for titration of barbiturate coma to burst suppression; prolonged mechanical respiratory support may be required.

Antiviral therapy with acyclovir has improved the outcome of patients with herpetic encephalitis from a previous horrendous 70% mortality and almost 100% serious neurological morbidity.[75,80] Acyclovir is more efficacious than vidarabine and is now considered the drug of choice. In a population of adults, infants, and children who were treated with acyclovir, 38% had returned to normal function, and 9% had moderate disability, which did not prevent them from returning to work, 6 months after diagnosis. Therapy was much more successful in patients who had a Glasgow Coma Scale score greater than 10 and in patients who were younger than 30 years.

Acyclovir is a relatively nontoxic drug with demonstrated efficacy for herpetic encephalitis. These factors mandate a low threshold for acyclovir treatment in a patient demonstrating clinical and radiographic findings consistent with HSV infection. HSV PCR has a high sensitivity and has replaced brain biopsy as the gold standard for diagnosis. Negative HSV PCR results have been reported, however, when obtained early (before day 3 to 4) in the course of illness. Therefore the clinician should interpret a negative result cautiously if other clinical data are suggestive of HSV infection, and a repeat CSF specimen should be analyzed before acyclovir treatment is stopped. With newer diagnostic techniques brain biopsy is reserved for those patients with undiagnosed, progressive disease unresponsive to empiric therapy.

A variety of other antiviral and antiinflammatory agents should be considered in specific settings. Acyclovir is also effective against varicella and should be administered to children with CNS disease induced by varicella-zoster virus.[81] Corticosteroids may be beneficial when there is evidence of an ongoing CNS inflammation or vasculitis. Ribavirin shows in vitro activity against several arboviruses (e.g., Nipah, West Nile) and has been used for treatment of Nipah outbreaks in Southeast Asia; recommendations for more widespread ribavirin use await further investigation.[82] Immunomodulatory therapies also hold promise as treatment for infectious encephalitis. Recombinant interferon-α has been applied to a few patients with Japanese encephalitis and is currently under investigation in placebo-controlled trials.[83] Influenza encephalitis has been increasingly reported, especially in Japanese children. A variety of antiinfluenza drugs, including oseltamivir and rimantadine, are potentially useful in this setting, pending further investigation. Pleconaril is a recently developed antiviral agent designed to bind to enteroviral capsid proteins and inhibit viral replication. Pleconaril shows a wide spectrum of antiviral activity and has shown a positive effect in early placebo-controlled trials against pediatric enteroviral meningitis.[84] Treatment with pleconaril may prove beneficial against more severe disease forms of enteroviral infections. Its use has been reported for enteroviral encephalitis, for poliomyelitis, for neonatal viral sepsis, and in children with inherited or acquired immunodeficiency.[85] Pleconaril has not been approved for widespread use in the United States.

Prognosis

The prognosis of patients with meningoencephalitis varies with the responsible pathogen and degree of neurological injury. As described previously, acyclovir treatment improves the prognosis of most patients with herpetic encephalitis, although the effect is not nearly as pronounced for patients who were comatose before the initiation of antiviral therapy.[80] Serial neuroimaging studies can often provide prognostic data to aid counseling individual patients and their families.

Viral Meningitis

Viruses are the causative agent for the overwhelming majority of cases of "aseptic meningitis," although other infectious processes, including Lyme disease, toxic shock syndrome, *Mycoplasma* infection, leptospirosis, toxoplasmosis, and Rocky Mountain spotted fever, may cause nonbacterial meningitis. Differentiation between meningitis and meningoencephalitis can be made pathologically or, less accurately, it can be made on the basis of the presence of encephalopathy. This clinical classification is somewhat artificial; there will always be some overlap between the two entities. Enteroviruses are the most common viral cause of pediatric meningitis, with enteric cytopathic human orphan (ECHO) virus and coxsackievirus the underlying agent in most cases.[86] This predominance explains the peak incidence of viral meningitis in the late summer and early fall. Less common viral causes of meningitis include mumps and agents that are more likely to cause meningoencephalitis, such as herpes simplex, arboviruses, CMV, Epstein-Barr virus, varicella, and adenovirus.

Viral meningitis is spread by person-to-person contact; the mouth and nose serve as the usual portal of entry. As with meningoencephalitis, many of the steps intermediate to invasion of the CNS are not completely established, but most infections are presumed to be bloodborne.

Clinical Manifestations

Clinical Presentation

Patients with viral meningitis have symptoms similar to those of patients with bacterial meningitis. Typically they have an acute onset of fever, lethargy or irritability, anorexia, and vomiting. Older children may report headache, stiff neck, or photophobia.

During examination, infants are often found to be lethargic or irritable and either hyperreflexic or hyporeflexic. They will have a bulging anterior fontanelle but may not have meningismus or meningeal signs. In addition to the mild mental status changes and changes in tendon reflexes that are often seen, children often have meningismus and meningeal signs.

The viruses that cause meningitis also have other clinical effects. Skin rashes (varicella, enteroviruses), diarrhea (enteroviruses), and upper respiratory tract infections (enteroviruses) commonly coexist with meningitis. Severe systemic disease (enteroviruses, adenovirus) and pericarditis or myocarditis (enteroviruses) rarely occur in patients with meningitis but can be life threatening.

Laboratory Manifestations

The major laboratory abnormalities seen in uncomplicated viral meningitis are found in the CSF. The CSF typically shows mild biochemical abnormalities (normal or slightly low glucose [30% to 50% of serum] and slightly elevated protein levels [50 to 100 mg/ml]) and a mild pleocytosis (10 to 1000 WBCs per cubic microliter). Lymphocytes tend to predominate in the CSF, but early in the course there may be a neutrophil predominance. This may make the differentiation between bacterial and viral meningitis difficult early in the disease. The possibility of withholding antibiotics for 6 to 8 hours and repeating the lumbar puncture has been advocated for some children and is a therapeutically sound option for the child who does not appear to be in a toxic state. Children who require admission to the PICU for meningitis are generally sicker and should be empirically treated with antibiotics until a bacterial process is ruled out.

Clinical Course

The clinical course of infants and children with viral meningitis is one of improvement. The disease process is generally self-limited and resolves over 7 to 14 days, although younger infants (younger than 6 months) may have a more difficult course and more CNS symptoms. These patients may have respiratory or circulatory compromise and are more likely to have seizures or a greatly decreased level of consciousness.

Treatment Options

Management of an infant or child with viral meningitis is largely supportive. As always, special care must be taken to maintain the ABCs. Beyond this, symptomatic therapy that may include control of seizures, antipyretics, and monitored rehydration should be undertaken as needed. As previously discussed, treatment with the antiviral agent pleconaril has been shown to decrease the severity and duration of meningitis symptoms. In the United States, however, pleconaril is not commercially available.

Prognosis

Smaller infants (younger than 3 months) who have an episode of viral meningitis are at risk for subtle neurological residua, such as learning and language disabilities.[87,88] The major cause of morbidity and mortality in older children is not related to CNS disease but rather to systemic effects of viremia (e.g., pneumonitis, carditis, hepatitis).

REFERENCES

1. Schlech WF III, Ward JI, Band JD, et al: Bacterial meningitis in the United States, 1978 through 1981. The National Bacterial Meningitis Surveillance Study, *JAMA* 253:1749, 1985.
2. Schuchat A, Robinson K, Wenger JD, et al: Bacterial meningitis in the United States in 1995. Active Surveillance Team, *N Engl J Med* 337:970, 1997.
3. Neuman HB, Wald ER: Bacterial meningitis at the Children's Hospital of Pittsburgh: 1988-1998. *Clin Ped* 40:595, 2001.
4. Dawson KG, Emerson JC, Burns JL: Fifteen years experience with bacterial meningitis, *Pediatr Infect Dis J* 18:816, 1999.
5. Arditi M, Mason EO Jr, Bradley JS, et al: Three-year multicenter surveillance of pneumococcal meningitis in children: clinical characteristics, and outcome related to penicillin susceptibility and dexamethasone use, *Pediatrics* 102:1087, 1998.
6. Stanek RJ, Mufson MA: A twenty-year epidemiological study of pneumococcal meningitis, *Clin Infect Dis* 28:1265, 1999.
7. Quagliarello V, Scheld WM: Bacterial meningitis: Pathogenesis, pathophysiology, and progress. *N Engl J Med* 327:864, 1992.
8. Tunkel AR, Scheld WM: Pathogenesis and pathophysiology of bacterial meningitis. *Clin Microbial Rev* 6:118, 1993.
9. Quagliarello VJ, Long WJ, Scheld WM: Morphological alterations of the blood-brain barrier with experimental meningitis in the rat, *J Clin Invest* 77:1084, 1986.
10. Nau R, Bruck W: Neuronal injury in bacterial meningitis: mechanisms and implications for therapy, *Trends Neurosci* 25:38, 2002.
11. Tauber MG, Shibl AM, Hackbarth CJ, et al: Antibiotic therapy, endotoxin concentration in cerebrospinal fluid, and brain edema in experimental *Escherichia coli* meningitis in rabbits. *J Infect Dis* 156:456, 1987.
12. Ernst JD: Complement: role of chemotaxis, *Pediatr Infect Dis J* 6(Suppl):1154, 1987.
13. Scheld WM, et al. Pathophysiology of bacterial meningitis: Mechanisms of neuronal injury, *J Infect Dis* 186(suppl):225, 2002.
14. Maffei FA, Heine RP, Whalen MJ, et al: Levels of antimicrobial molecules defensin and lactoferrin are elevated in the cerebrospinal fluid of children with meningitis. *Pediatrics* 103:987, 1999.
15. Mustafa MM, Ramilo O, Saez-Llorens X, et al: Cerebrospinal fluid prostaglandins, interleukin 1 beta, and tumor necrosis factor in bacterial meningitis. Clinical and laboratory correlations in placebo-treated and dexamethasone-treated patients, *Am J Dis Child* 144:883, 1990.
16. Tureen JH, et al. Effect of indomethacin on brain water content, cerebrospinal fluid white cell response and prostaglandin E_2 levels in cerebrospinal fluid in experimental pneumococcal meningitis, *Pediatr Infect Dis J* 6(suppl):1151, 1987.
17. Leppert D, Lindberg RL, Kappos L, et al: Matrix metalloproteinases: multifunctional effectors of inflammation in multiple sclerosis and bacterial meningitis. *Brain Res Rev* 36:249, 2001.
18. Kaplan SL, Feigin RD: The syndrome of inappropriate secretion of antidiuretic hormone in children with bacterial meningitis, *J Pediatr* 92:758, 1978.
19. Paulson OB, Brodersen P, Hansen EL, et al: Regional cerebral blood flow, cerebral metabolic rate of oxygen, and cerebrospinal fluid acid-base variables in patients with acute meningitis and with acute encephalitis. *Acta Med Scand* 196:191, 1974.
20. Scheld WM, Dacey RG, Winn HR, et al: Cerebrospinal fluid outflow resistance in rabbits with experimental meningitis. Alterations with penicillin and methylprednisolone, *J Clin Invest* 66:243, 1980.
21. Rorke LB, Pitts FW: Purulent meningitis—the pathologic basis of clinical manifestations, *Clin Pediatr* 2:64, 1963.
22. Gado M, Axley J, Appleton DB, et al: Angiography in the acute and post-treatment phases of *Haemophilus influenzae* meningitis, *Radiology* 110:439, 1974.
23. Thomas VH, Hopkins IJ: Arteriographic demonstration of vascular lesions in the study of neurologic deficit in advanced *Haemophilus influenzae* meningitis, *Dev Med Child Neurol* 14:783, 1972.

24. James AE Jr, Hodges FJ III, Jordan CE, et al: Angiography and cisternography in acute meningitis due to *Hemophilus influenzae, Radiology* 103:601, 1972.
25. Oostenbrink R, Moons KG, Theunissen CC, et al: Signs of meningeal irritation in the emergency department: how often bacterial meningitis? *Pediatr Emerg Care* 17:161, 2001.
26. Klein JO, Feigin RD, McCracken GH: Report of the task force on diagnosis and management of meningitis, *Pediatrics* 78(suppl):959, 1986.
27. Negrini B, Kelleher KJ, Wald ER: Cerebrospinal fluid findings in aseptic versus bacterial meningitis, *Pediatrics* 105:316, 2000.
28. Blazer S, Berant M, Alon U: Bacterial meningitis: effect of antibiotic treatment on cerebrospinal fluid, *Am J Clin Pathol* 80:386, 1983.
29. Kanegage JT, Soliemanzadeh P, Bradley JS: Lumbar puncture in pediatric bacterial meningitis: defining the time interval for recovery of cerebrospinal fluid pathogens after parenteral antibiotic pretreatment, *Pediatrics* 108:1169, 2001.
30. Addy DP: When not to do a lumbar puncture, *Arch Dis Child* 62: 873, 1987.
31. Heldrich FJ, Walker SH, Crosby RMN: Risk of diagnostic lumbar puncture in acute bacterial meningitis, *Pediatr Emerg Care* 2:180, 1986.
32. Rennick G, Shann F, deCampo J: Cerebral herniation during bacterial meningitis in children, *BMJ* 306:953, 1993.
33. Riordan FAI, Cant AJ: When to do a lumbar puncture, *Arch Dis Child* 87:235, 2002.
34. Cabral DA, Flodmark O, Farrell K, et al: Prospective study of computed tomography in acute bacterial meningitis, *J Pediatr* 111:201, 1987.
35. Kline MW, Kaplan SL: Computed tomography in bacterial meningitis of childhood, *Pediatr Infect Dis J* 7:855, 1988.
36. Lebel MH, Hoyt MJ, Waagner DC, et al: Magnetic resonance imaging and dexamethasone therapy for bacterial meningitis, *Am J Dis Child* 143:301, 1989.
37. Smith AL et al: Cerebral blood flow in experimental *Haemophilus influenzae B* meningitis, *Pediatr Infect Dis J* 6(suppl):1159, 1987.
38. Ashwal S, Stringer W, Tomasi L, et al: Cerebral blood flow and carbon dioxide reactivity in children with bacterial meningitis, *J Pediatr* 17:523, 1990.
39. Fassbender K, Ries S, Schminke U, et al: Inflammatory cytokines in CSF in bacterial meningitis: association with altered blood flow velocities in basal cerebral arteries, *J Neurol Neurosurg Psychiatry* 61:57, 1996.
40. Okten A, Ahmetoglu A, Dilber E, et al: Cranial Doppler ultrasonography as a predictor of neurologic sequelae in infants with bacterial meningitis, *Invest Radiol* 37:86, 2002.
41. Plum F, Posner JB: *The diagnosis of stupor and coma,* Philadelphia, 1980, FA Davis.
42. Dodge PR, Swartz MN: Bacterial meningitis—a review of selected aspects: II. Special neurologic problems, postmeningitic complications and clinicopathologic correlations, *N Engl J Med* 272:954, 1965.
43. McMenamin JB, Volpe JJ: Bacterial meningitis in infancy: effects on intracranial pressure and cerebral blood flow velocity, *Neurology* 34:500, 1984.
44. Rebaud P, Berthier JC, Hartemann E, et al: Intracranial pressure in childhood central nervous system infections, *Intensive Care Med* 14:522-525, 1988.
45. Horwitz SJ, Boxerbaum B, O'Bell J: Cerebral herniation in bacterial meningitis in childhood, *Ann Neurol* 7:524, 1980.
46. Gravois K: Sonographic evaluation of acute bacterial meningitis, *J La State Med Soc* 140:31, 1988.
47. Lin TY, Nelson JD, McCracken GH: Fever during treatment for bacterial meningitis, *Pediatr Infect Dis J* 3:319, 1984.
48. Tunkel AR, Scheld W: ??? In Mandell ???, editor: *Principles and practice of infectious disease,* ed 5, ???, 2000, Churchill Livingstone.
49. Therapy for children with invasive pneumococcal infections. American Academy of Pediatrics Committee on Infectious Disease, *Pediatrics* 99:289, 1997.
50. Quagliarello VJ, Scheld WM: Treatment of bacterial meningitis, *N Engl J Med* 336:708, 1997.
51. Williams CPS, Swanson AG, Chapman JT: Brain swelling with acute purulent meningitis—report of treatment with hypertonic intravenous urea, *Pediatrics* 34:220, 1964.
52. Lebel MH, Freij BJ, Syrogiannopoulos GA, et al: Dexamethasone therapy for bacterial meningitis. Results of two double-blind, placebo-controlled trials, *N Engl J Med* 319:964, 1988.
53. Odio CM, Faingezicht I, Paris M, et al: The beneficial effects of early dexamethasone administration in infants and children with bacterial meningitis, *N Engl J Med* 324:1525-1531 1991.
54. Schaad UB, Lips U, Gnehm HE, et al: Dexamethasone therapy for bacterial meningitis in children. Swiss Meningitis Study Group, *Lancet* 342:457, 1993.
55. Wald ER, Kaplan SL, Mason EO Jr, et al: Dexamethasone therapy for children with bacterial meningitis. Meningitis Study Group, *Pediatrics* 95:21, 1995.
56. de Gans J, van de Beek D; European Dexamethasone in Adulthood Bacterial Meningitis Study Investigators: Dexamethasone in adults with bacterial meningitis, *N Engl J Med* 347:1549, 2002.
57. McIntyre PB, Berkey CS, King SM, et al: Dexamethasone as adjunctive therapy in bacterial meningitis. A meta-analysis of randomized clinical trials since 1988, *JAMA* 278:925, 1997.
58. Molyneux EM, Walsh AL, Forsyth H, et al: Dexamethasone treatment in childhood bacterial meningitis in Malawi: a randomised controlled trial, *Lancet* 360:211, 2002.
59. Committee on Infectious Disease, American Academy of Pediatrics: *Report of the Committee on Infectious Disease,* Elk Creek Village, Ill, 2000, American Academy of Pediatrics.
60. Grimwood K, Anderson VA, Bond L, et al: Adverse outcomes of bacterial meningitis in school-age survivors, *Pediatrics* 95:646, 1995.
61. Kornelisse RF, Westerbeek CM, Spoor AB, et al: Pneumococcal meningitis in children: prognostic indicators and outcome, *Clin Infect Dis* 21:1390, 1995.
62. Khetsuriani N, Holman RC, Anderson LJ: Burden of encephalitis-associated hospitalization in the United States, 1988-1997, *Clin Infect Dis* 35:175-182, 2002.
63. Ng YT, Cox C, Atkins J, Butler IJ: Encephalopathy associated with respiratory syncytial virus bronchiolitis, *J Child Neurol* 16:105-108, 2001
64. CDC Division of Vector-Borne Infectious Diseases. *Information on arboviral encephalitides.* Available at http://www.cdc.gov./ncidod/dvbid/arbor/arbdet.htm. Accessed ???.
65. Bitnun A, Ford-Jones EL, Petric M, et al: Acute childhood encephalitis and *Mycoplasma pneumoniae, Clin Infect Dis* 32:1674-1684, 2001.
66. West Nile virus activity—United States, September 26-October 2, 2002, and investigations of West Nile virus infections in recipients of blood transfusion and organ transplantation, *MMWR Morb Mortal Wkly Rep,* 51: 884, 895, 2002.
67. McJunkin JE, DE Los Reyes EC, et al: La Crosse encephalitis in children, *N Engl J Med* 344; 801-807, 2001.
68. Corey L, Spear PG: Infections with herpes simplex virus (part 2), *N Engl J Med* 314:749, 1986.
69. DeBiasi RL, Kleinschmidt-DeMasters BK, Richardson-Burns S, et al: Central nervous system apoptosis in human herpes simplex virus and cytomegalovirus encephalitis, *J Infect Dis* 186:1547-1557, 2002.
70. Barnett GH, Ropper AH, Romeo J: Intracranial pressure and outcome in adult encephalitis, *J Neurosurg* 68:585, 1988.
71. Wakamoto H, Ohta M, Nakano N, et al: SPECT in focal enterovirus encephalitis: evidence for local cerebral vasculitis, *Ped Neurol* 23: 429-431, 2000.
72. Read SJ, Kurtz JB: Laboratory diagnosis of common viral infections of the central nervous system by using a single multiplex PCR screening assay, *J Clin Microbiol* 37: 1352-1355, 1999.
73. Atkins JT: HSV PCR for CNS infections: pearls and pitfalls, *Pediatr Infect Dis J* 18:823-824, 1999.
74. Weil AA, Glaser CA, Amad Z, et al: Patients with suspected herpes simplex encephalitis: rethinking an initial negative polymerase chain reaction result, *Clin Infect Dis* 34:1154-1157, 2002.
75. Teizeira J, Zimmerman RA, Haselgrove JC, et al: Diffusion imaging in pediatric central nervous system infections, *Neuroradiology* 43:1031-1039, 2001.
76. Olson LC, Buescher EL, Artenstein MS, et al: Herpesvirus infections of the human central nervous system, *N Engl J Med* 277:1271, 1967.
77. Illis LS, Taylor FM: The electroencephalogram in herpes simplex encephalitis, *Lancet* 1:650, 1970.
78. Domingues RB, Fink MC, Tsanaclis AM, et al: Diagnosis of herpes simplex encephalitis by magnetic resonance imaging and polymerase chain reaction assay of cerebrospinal fluid. *J Neurol Sci* 157:148-153, 1998.

79. Taferner E, Pfausler B, Kofler A, et al: Craniectomy in severe, life-threatening encephalitis: a report on outcome and long-term prognosis of four cases, *Intensive Care Med* 27:1426-1428, 2001.
80. Whitley RJ, Alford CA, Hirsch MS, et al: Vidarabine versus acyclovir therapy in herpes simplex encephalitis, *N Engl J Med* 314:144, 1986.
81. Gilden DH, Kleinschmidt-DeMasters BK, LaGuardia, et al: Neurologic complications of the reactivation of varicella-zoster virus, *N Engl J Med* 342:635-645, 2000.
82. Chong HT, Kamarulzaman A, Tan CT et al: Treatment of acute Nipah encephalitis with ribavirin, *Ann Neurol* 49:810-813, 2001.
83. Solomon T, Minh Dung N, Kneen R, et al: Japanese Encephalitis. *J Neurol Neurosurg Psychiatry* 68: 405-15, 2000.
84. Sawyer MH, Laez-Llorenz X, Aviles CL, et al: Oral pleconaril reduces the duration of and severity of enteroviral meningitis in children [abstract], Proceedings of the Academic Pediatric Society Annual Meeting, Elk Grove Village, Ill, 1999, Academic Pediatric Society.
85. Rotbart HA, Webster AD: Treatment of potentially life-threatening enterovirus infections with pleconaril, *Clin Infect Dis* 32:228-235, 2001.
86. Enterovirus surveillance—United States, 2000-2001, *MMWR Morb Mortal Wkl Rep* 51; 1047-1049, 2002.
87. Baker RC, Kummer AW, Schultz JR, et al: Neurodevelopmental outcome of infants with viral meningitis in the first three months of life, *Clin Pediatr (Phila)* 35:295-301, 1996.
88. Wilfert CM, Thompson RJ Jr, Sunder TR, et al: Longitudinal assessment of children with enteroviral meningitis during the first three months of life, *Pediatrics* 67:811, 1981.

CHAPTER

58

Hypoxic-Ischemic Encephalopathy: Pathobiology and Therapy of the Postresuscitation Syndrome in Children

Robert S. B. Clark, Yichen Lai, Robert W. Hickey, Peter J. Safar, and Patrick M. Kochanek

PEARLS

- Cardiac arrest in adult patients differs from cardiac arrest in pediatric patients in at least two important aspects:
  - Cardiac arrest in pediatric patients is predominantly due to asphyxial arrest, in contrast to adult patients, in whom it is predominantly due to ventricular dysrhythmias.
  - Developmental differences exist between pediatric and adult patients including ongoing synaptogenesis, lower cerebral blood flow (CBF) in neonates, and higher CBF in toddlers and children compared with adults, neurotransmitter receptor maturation, and higher energy expenditure in pediatric patients.
- Currently, optimal intensive care management can be summed up by targeting *normo*: *normo*tension, *normo*capnea, *normo*xemia, and *normo*glycemia. One apparent exception at this time is *normo*thermia.
- Two independent randomized clinical trials in adults with cardiac arrest showed a beneficial effect of mild-moderate whole body hypothermia,[1,2] prompting the International Liaison Committee on Resuscitation to recommend 12 to 24 hours of moderate hypothermia (32 to 34° C) for selected adults with cardiac arrest.[3]
- Currently, there is no cure for hypoxic-ischemic encephalopathy. It is likely that targeted therapies, spanning field interventions, intensive care, and rehabilitation, will be required to successfully prevent and treat hypoxic- ischemic encephalopathy in infants and children after cardiac arrest.

Since the previous edition of this chapter, significant advances in our understanding of mechanisms involved in hypoxic-ischemic encephalopathy have occurred. Clinical advances have not progressed, however, at nearly the same trajectory. Exceptions to this are the encouraging results from two clinical trials in adults after cardiac arrest in which postarrest hypothermia was found to improve neurological recovery.[1,2] These results have spurred renewed interest in the development of optimal strategies for the application of therapeutic hypothermia in infants and children after cardiopulmonary arrest. Direct translation from adult to pediatric cardiac arrest trials may be restricted because of notable differences between the two patient populations, however. These differences are discussed later. Although modest "breakthroughs" in adult patients and increasing depth and breadth of the understanding of mechanisms of hypoxic-ischemic encephalopathy provide hope, challenges remain because by and large, the likelihood of intact neurological survival in children with cardiopulmonary arrest remains small. A proven effective treatment protocol that reliably improves neurological recovery from hypoxic-ischemic encephalopathy after cardiopulmonary arrest in infants and children remains elusive. Despite numerous advances in critical care medicine, the optimal supportive care to maintain neuronal function and optimize recovery after cardiorespiratory arrest also remains controversial.

This uncertainty arises from the pathobiological complexity of cerebral injury and from the limitations in the clinical ability to monitor key metabolic and physiological parameters in the brain. Clinical stumbling blocks in the history of "brain resuscitation" have also slowed progress in the understanding of hypoxic-ischemic encephalopathy after cardiopulmonary arrest. Until recently, this entity was largely ignored as a specific disease process. First, brain resuscitation was dealt with as a single therapeutic paradigm regardless of the cause.[4] This resulted in the misguided application of results from studies of head trauma, stroke, Reye's syndrome, and cerebral protection to patients with cardiopulmonary arrest. Second, within cardiopulmonary arrest, causes and patient-relevant biological factors such as genetic influences and comorbidities are lumped together. Factors influencing neurological damage and recovery are clearly different depending on the cause (e.g., asphyxia, arrhythmia, hemorrhage, trauma, sepsis), age of the patient, interval between arrest and return of spontaneous circulation (ROSC), and effectiveness of cardiopulmonary resuscitation (CPR). Finally, the frustration encountered in dealing with the poor neurological outcomes that often occur in this syndrome has fostered the application or withholding of inadequately tested treatments. Adequate understanding of the pathobiology of hypoxic-ischemic encephalopathy after cardiopulmonary arrest in children can be derived only partially from the medical literature.

In this chapter, the pathobiology of hypoxic-ischemic encephalopathy is reviewed with emphasis on cellular mechanisms, pathophysiology, and histopathology. Differences between the most prevalent causes of cardiopulmonary arrest in children (asphyxia compared with cardiac arrhythmia) are examined, and an appraisal of traditional and novel therapies is presented, including reexamination of the potential for therapeutic hypothermia in infants and children after cardiopulmonary arrest. Any discussion of hypoxemic-ischemic encephalopathy in children is complicated not only by the specific mode of arrest in children but also by the unique nature of these young patients. The child's brain is still developing, adding another layer of variability in terms of age-specific pathological and reparative mechanisms, potential for therapies to afford benefit, evaluation of therapeutic effectiveness, and neurological outcome. Thus the effect of the host's immaturity on the pathobiology of postarrest encephalopathy also is examined.

Etiology

Asphyxia is the cause of most arrests and the primary cause of hypoxic-ischemic encephalopathy in children.[6,7] Asphyxial arrest most commonly results from submersion accidents, airway obstruction, aspiration, severe acute asthma, inhalation injury, or apnea syndromes. In asphyxial arrest, asystole or pulseless electrical activity is preceded and precipitated by a period of anoxic or hypoxemic perfusion.[7] In contrast, ventricular fibrillation (VF) is the most common cause of cardiopulmonary arrest in adults. In experimental animal models, VF-induced or potassium chloride (KCl)–induced cardiac arrest is used. In VF-induced cardiac arrest, respiration ceases shortly *after* loss of perfusion pressure. VF can also occur in children, but this occurs in fewer than 10% of pediatric patients with cardiopulmonary arrest. VF and asphyxial arrests differ in pathophysiology despite having been traditionally grouped as "cardiopulmonary arrests." Another related insult of interest to pediatricians is the perinatal hypoxic-ischemic insult. Models of graded hypoxia with or without ischemia in immature animals have been developed that resemble asphyxial arrest.[8,9] Recently, contemporary models of pediatric asphyxial arrest in rodents and piglets have been developed, which may lead to more etiology-specific evaluation of the postresuscitation syndrome in terms of mechanisms and relevant therapies.[10,11]

Cellular and Molecular Pathobiology

Mechanisms of Hypoxic-Ischemic Brain Injury

Cerebral neurons in culture can tolerate hours of extreme hypoxia. Although it takes about 160 minutes of exposure to an anoxic gas mixture for oxygen tension in the culture medium to reach 1 mmHg, cortical neurons tolerate 1 to 3 additional hours with little histological change.[12] If 1 mmol/L sodium cyanide is used to simulate immediate anoxia, hippocampal neurons become swollen and vacuolated within 20 to 60 minutes and begin to disintegrate in 4 hours. Similarly, even 1 hour of complete global brain ischemia in monkeys is followed by electrophysiological recovery of many neurons and significant recovery of some aspects of brain metabolism, such as protein synthesis.[13] Although the time limit for consistently normal outcome after normothermic primary cardiac arrest is unknown, it is certainly closer to 5 to 10 minutes than 1 to 3 hours. Restoration of integrated brain function, that is, "neurological recovery," differs markedly from physiological or metabolic brain recovery. In contrast to the relative cellular homogeneity in other organs, the functional specificity and interactions of neurons and glia in brain make patchy areas of cell death potentially devastating. This is evident in the neuropathology of dogs in persistent coma 1 week after a 10- to 15-minute cardiopulmonary arrest.

Scattered neuronal death is evident, but most neurons appear normal.[14]

Energy Failure

The brain depends on large amounts of substrate (glucose and lactate) because of its tremendous metabolic demands and paltry energy stores. Interruption of cerebral blood flow (CBF) results in loss of consciousness and electroencephalographic silence within seconds. Within 5 to 7 minutes, energy failure occurs, accompanied by disturbances of ion homeostasis in neurons and glial cells. Influx of sodium and water and efflux of potassium occur because the cells cannot maintain their energy-dependent electrochemical gradients. When the extracellular potassium concentration reaches 10 to 15 mmol/L, voltage-gated channels open and extracellular calcium influx occurs.[15]

If flow remains inadequate and energy failure persists, calcium-mediated events such as phospholipase and protease activation can lead to irreversible injury and neuronal cell death. Cerebral acidosis occurs, and intracellular pH decreases from 7 to 6.4.[15] If blood flow is restored, however, recovery of basal cellular metabolism (adenosine triphosphate [ATP] levels, protein synthesis, oxygen consumption) and pH occurs. This has been shown in brain tissue samples and intact brain measurements after global ischemic insults that result in persistent vegetative coma.[13]

After anoxia or ischemia, the recovery of aerobic metabolism is essential for recovery but is not in and of itself sufficient. The imbalance between aerobic and anaerobic metabolism and overdependence of neurons on lactate as a substrate[16] must be restored. Despite global metabolic recovery, certain neurons progress to cell death. After restitution of blood flow and oxidative metabolism after energy failure in the brain, cellular and molecular dysfunction progresses and can occur through at least two cellular processes, necrosis and programmed cell death (apoptosis).[17] Depending on the degree and duration of energy failure, cells may die by means of necrosis (complete energy failure), programmed cell death, or a spectrum of these processes.[18,19] These processes, coupled with the need to restore highly integrated function, explain the unfortunate clinical scenario of the persistent vegetative state despite restoration of normal function in other organ systems. The relationship of these two forms of cell death to selective vulnerability of neurons in brain is beginning to emerge.

Selective Vulnerability

Certain neurons, such as those in the CA_1 region of the hippocampus; cerebral cortex layers III and V; portions of the amygdaloid nucleus; the cerebellar Purkinje cells; and in infants, periventricular white matter regions and some brainstem nuclei, have long been known to be especially vulnerable to hypoxemic-ischemic insults.[20,21] Five minutes of complete global brain ischemia produces cell death in these regions that begins to appear between 48 and 72 hours after the insult, without apparent histological damage in other brain areas.

Transient calcium accumulation occurs in all cells during ischemia, but secondary irreversible accumulation occurs in the selectively vulnerable zones many hours later.[22] Electrophysiological studies show that delayed neuronal death is preceded by neuronal hyperactivity. It is hypothesized that ischemic and early postischemic calcium accumulation leads to a complex sequence of derangements in cellular metabolism such as protease activation and oxygen-derived free radical formation.[23] These conditions, in concert with excessive release of excitatory neurotransmitters (glutamate, aspartate) in these areas, lead to excitotoxicity and cell death. These findings are supported by work in neuronal culture showing that calcium influx accompanies cell death in the presence of anoxia or supraphysiological levels of excitatory amino acids such as glutamate[12,24] and that CA_1 cells are the most sensitive to glutamate-mediated injury.[25]

Of particular interest is that these intrinsically vulnerable cells do not have a unique vascular distribution.[26] They represent neither vascular watersheds nor hypoperfused zones. Death of these neurons after a threshold ischemic insult occurs in a delayed fashion after reperfusion and thus may be preventable, at least in part, by treatment.

Necrosis Compared with Programmed Cell Death (Apoptosis)

It is now known that cell death can occur by two distinct pathways, necrosis and programmed cell death (apoptosis).[27] Necrosis, which is characterized by denaturing and coagulation of cellular proteins, is the basic pattern of pathological cell death that results from progressive reduction in the cellular content of ATP (see Chapter 92).[27] Necrosis involves progressive derangements in energy and substrate metabolism that are followed by a series of morphological alterations, including swelling of cells and organelles; subsurface cellular blebbing; amorphous deposits in mitochondria; condensation of nuclear chromatin; and finally, breaks in plasma and organellar membranes.[27] It was traditionally assumed that all ischemic cell death occurred through this process and that selective vulnerability represented a specific predilection for the development of necrosis in certain neurons after transient ischemic insults. Researchers have shown, however, that cell death after hypoxic-ischemic insults can occur by a second pathway, programmed cell death, also known as *apoptosis*.[28] Development of programmed cell death usually requires new protein synthesis and the activation of endonucleases. Two distinct types of characteristic cleavage of DNA have been described. The most well-described involves cleavage by caspase activated deoxyribonuclease at linkage regions between nucleosomes to form fragments of double-stranded DNA.[29] This produces a pattern of DNA cleavage observed on Southern blot analysis termed *DNA laddering*. Recently, a unique pathway of programmed cell death resulting in large-scale DNA fragmentation induced by the apoptosis-inducing factor, a mitochondrial flavoprotein, has been reported after oxidative stress, traumatic brain injury, and neonatal hypoxia-ischemia.[30-32] The stimuli triggering programmed cell death are complex and multifactorial, involving extracellular surface receptors, cell signaling pathways, protease cascades, and mitochondrial and other organelle dysfunction. Selective vulnerable cell death in brain regions such as the CA_1 region of the hippocampus after transient global brain ischemia appears to occur by an apoptotic mechanism.[32] DNA extracted from the hippocampus of gerbils at 4 days after a threshold global ischemic insult shows a characteristic laddering pattern consistent with apoptotic cell death. Thus after a threshold ischemic insult, selective vulnerable neuronal death in the highly vulnerably CA_1 region of the hippocampus occurs by programmed cell death.

Li et al[34] reported that programmed cell death in the postischemic brain is not limited to scattered neuronal death in what have been traditionally deemed to be "selectively vulnerable regions," but is seen even in penumbral regions around evolving cerebral infarcts (Fig. 58–1). It is likely that the severity of the ischemic insult and other local factors determine whether an injured neuron recovers, undergoes programmed cell death, or dies a necrotic death. Importantly, several molecular and pharmacological interventions that interrupt programmed cell death have been reported to improve outcome after cerebral ischemia, including "pediatric" models.[34] The proportion of neuronal cell death that occurs by means of apoptosis compared with necrosis after cerebral ischemia remains controversial, however.[36,37] Moreover, it remains possible that treatments inhibiting apoptosis may simply convert cell death to necrosis.[38] Although speculative, it is possible that after cardiopulmonary arrest and resuscitation, a continuum exists in neurons from recovery to necrosis[19] that depends on the duration of the insult, the local milieu, and the given brain region. Nevertheless, in any given brain region, whether neuronal death is produced by necrosis, apoptosis, or both, a highly complex series of events appears to be involved during the arrest and after restoration of spontaneous circulation. A theoretical scheme of the mechanisms involved is given in Figure 58–2. Although studies showing improved functional recovery with treatments inhibiting programmed cell death after cerebral ischemia suggest that some salvaged neurons regain their integrative properties, it is also possible that some of the delayed apoptosis represents appropriate pruning of neurons that have lost their targets.

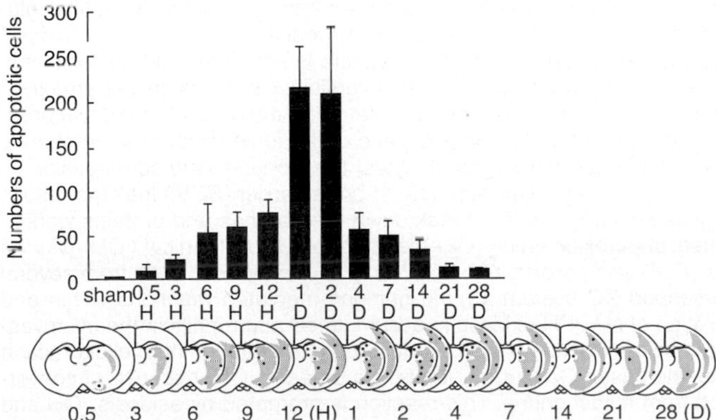

FIGURE 58–1 • Apoptotic cells in coronal brain sections in rats subjected to 2 hours of middle cerebral artery occlusion and between 0.5 and 28 days of reperfusion. *Top:* Progressive increase in the numbers of apoptotic cells occurs with increasing reperfusion time to peak at 24 hours. Apoptotic cells are still detectable even after 1 week of reperfusion, however. *Bottom:* Distribution of apoptosis (*dots*) and necrotic neurons (*hatched areas*). Apoptotic cells are localized predominately to inner boundary zone of infarction. (From Li et al[33].)

Reperfusion Injury

Reoxygenation and reperfusion are essential to recovery of any organ after ischemia. Experimental evidence suggests, however, that certain aspects of reperfusion result in tissue injury.[39,40] Reperfusion injury is a complex series of interactions between parenchyma and microcirculatory elements, resulting in detrimental effects that negate some fraction of the benefits of reperfusion. The magnitude of reperfusion injury varies with the organ in question and with the duration and type of hypoxic-ischemic insult.[41]

In many organs and in the brain after focal insults, progressive microcirculatory failure is thought to be an important aspect of reperfusion injury.[42] As suggested by the nonspecific vascular distribution of selectively vulnerable neurons, however, the brain may display a second unique setting for the evolution of reperfusion injury, the evolution of selectively vulnerable cell death. Four key mechanisms hypothesized to be important to reperfusion injury in the brain include (1) excitotoxicity and calcium accumulation, (2) protease activation, (3) oxygen radical formation, and (4) membrane phospholipid hydrolysis and mediator formation.

Excitotoxicity and Calcium Accumulation

Glutamate and aspartate are the major excitatory amino acid neurotransmitters in the mammalian central nervous system, but both also have neurotoxic properties. Pioneering studies by Rothman et al[43] showed in vitro that hypoxia-induced neuronal death is mediated by synaptic activity. Inhibition of synaptic glutamate release or blockade of glutamate receptors prevented the hypoxic neuronal injury. Glutamate is the major neurotransmitter in the selectively vulnerable zones and accumulates extracellularly in these regions after hypoxic or ischemic insults.[22] The mechanisms by which glutamate may harm neurons during ischemia and reperfusion are becoming more clearly defined.

Glutamate is released at the presynaptic terminal in response to neuronal stimulation and acts by binding to postsynaptic dendritic receptors. Two main classes of excitatory neurotransmitter receptors have been identified. One class consists of the ligand-gated ion channels ("ionotropic" receptors) and includes NMDA (N-methyl-D-aspartate), AMPA (α-amino-3-hydroxy-5-methyl-4-isoxazole propionic acid) or quisqualate, and kainate receptor subtypes. Toxicity caused by NMDA receptor activation is usually rapid, whereas AMPA or kainate receptor-mediated cell death is somewhat slower to develop.[44] The other class of excitatory neurotransmitter receptors includes the "metabotropic" receptors. These receptors are coupled with G proteins and modulate intracellular second messengers such as calcium, cyclic nucleotides, and inositol triphosphate.[45] When activated, the ionotropic glutamate receptors open sodium channels and may also have an important role in initiation and propagation of membrane depolarization and spreading depression.[46] With ionotropic receptor activation, rapid excitatory amino acid-mediated calcium accumulation occurs. In the face of ischemia this

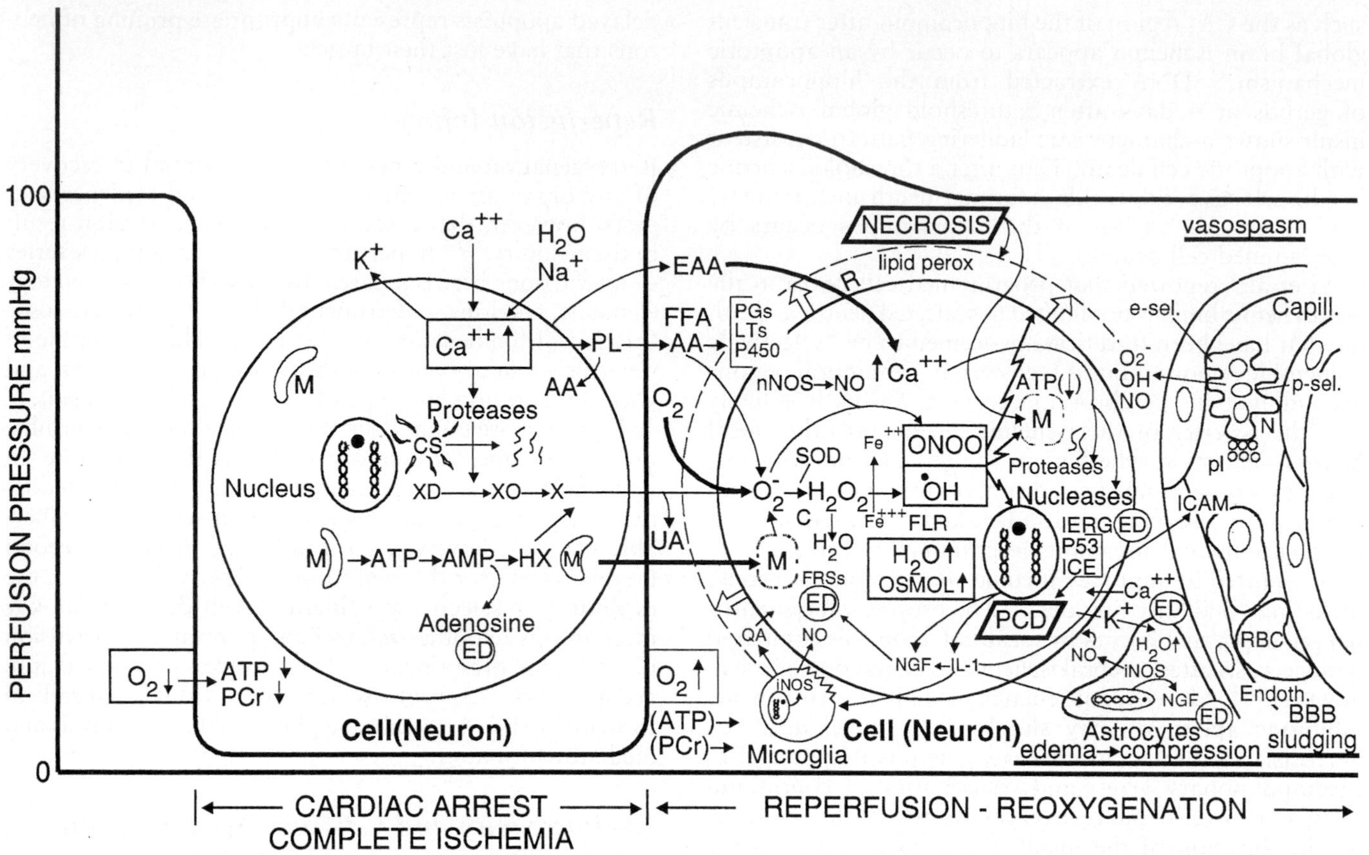

FIGURE 58–2 • Death of cells after temporary ischemia. Diagram of complex, partially hypothesized biochemical cascades in neurons during and after cardiac arrest.[45] Normally intracellular ($[Ca^{2+}]i$) to extracellular ($[Ca^{2+}]e$) calcium gradient is 1:10,000. Calcium regulators include calcium/magnesium ATPase, the endoplasmic reticulum (ER), mitochondria, and arachidonic acid (*AA*). With stimulation, different cell types respond with an increase in $[Ca^{2+}]i$ because of release of bound Ca^{2+} in the ER and influx of $[Ca^{2+}]e$, or both. During complete ischemic anoxia (cardiac arrest) (*left*), the level of energy (phosphocreatinine [*PCr*] and adenosine triphosphate [*ATP*]) decreases to near zero in all tissues at different rates, depending on stores of oxygen and substrate; it is fastest in the brain (~5 minutes) and slower in the heart and other vital organs. This energy loss causes membrane pump failure, which causes a shift of sodium (Na^+) ions, water (H_2O), and calcium ions (Ca^{2+}) from the extracellular into the intracellular space (cytosolic edema), and potassium (K^+) leakage from the intracellular into the extracellular space. Increase in $[Ca^{2+}]i$ activates phospholipase A_2, which breaks down membrane phospholipids (*PL*) into free fatty acids (*FFAs*), particularly arachidonic acid (*AA*). Increase in $[Ca^{2+}]i$ also activates proteolytic enzymes, such as calpain, which may disrupt the cytoskeleton (*CS*) and possibly the nucleus. In mitochondria (*M*) hydrolysis of ATP to adenosine monophosphate (*AMP*) leads to an accumulation of hypoxanthine (*HX*). Increased $[Ca^{2+}]i$ may enhance conversion of xanthine dehydrogenase (*XD*) to xanthine oxidase (*XO*), priming the neuron for the production of the oxygen free radical superoxide anion (O_2^-), although this pathway is of questionable importance in neurons (*X*, xanthine; *UA*, uric acid). Excitatory amino acid (*EAA*) neurotransmitters, particularly glutamate and aspartate, increase in extracellular fluid. Increased [EAA]e activates N-methyl-D-aspartate (NMDA) and non-NMDA receptors (*R*), thereby increasing calcium and sodium influx and mobilizing stores of $[Ca^{2+}]i$. Increased extracellular potassium activates EAA receptors by membrane depolarization. Glycolysis during hypoxia results in anaerobic metabolism and lactic acidosis, until all glucose is used (in the brain, during anoxia after ~20 minutes). This lactic acidosis, plus inability to wash out CO_2, results in mixed tissue acidosis that adversely influences neuronal viability. The net effect of acidosis on the cascades during and after ischemia is not clear. Mild acidosis may actually attenuate NMDA-mediated $[Ca^{2+}]i$ accumulation. Without reoxygenation, cells progress via first reversible, later irreversible structural damage, to necrosis at specific rates for different cell types. During reperfusion and reoxygenation (*right*), lactate and molecular breakdown products can create osmotic edema and rupture of organelles and mitochondria. Recovery of [ATP] and [PCr] and of the ionic membrane pump may be hampered by hypoperfusion as a result of vasospasm, cell sludging, adhesion of neutrophils (granulocytes) (*N*), and capillary compression by swollen astrocytes, which also help to protect neurons by absorbing extracellular potassium. Capillary (blood-brain barrier [*BBB*]) leakage results in interstitial (vasogenic) edema. Increased concentrations of at least four oxyradical species that break down membranes and proteins worsen the microcirculation and possibly also damage the nucleus that may be formed: superoxide anion (O_2.–) leading to hydroxyl radical (·OH) (via the iron-catalyzed $Fe^{+++} \rightarrow Fe^{++}$, Haber-Weiss/Fenton reaction); free lipid radicals (*FLR*) and peroxynitrite (*ONOO*–). O_2.⁻ may be formed from several sources: (1) directly from eicosanoid metabolism; (2) by the previously described XO system; (3) via quinone-mediated reactions within and outside the electron transport chain (from mitochondria [*M*]); and (4) by activation of NADPH-oxidase in accumulated neutrophils in the microvasculature or after diapedesis into tissue. Increased O_2.⁻ leads to increased hydrogen peroxide (H_2O_2) production as a result of intracellular action of superoxide dismutase (*SOD*). $[H_2O_2]$ is controlled by intracellular catalase. Increased O_2.⁻ further leads to increased ·OH, because of conversion of H_2O_2 to ·OH via the Haber-Weiss/Fenton reaction, with iron liberated from mitochondria. This reaction is promoted by acidosis. ·OH and ONOO– damage cellular lipids, proteins, and nucleic acids. Also, AA is metabolized by the cyclooxygenase pathways to prostaglandins (*PGs*) including thromboxane A_2, or by the lipoxygenase pathway to produce leukotrienes (*LTs*); and by the cytochrome P-450 pathway. These products can act as neurotransmitters and signal transducers in neuronal and glial cells and can activate thrombotic and inflammatory pathways in the microcirculation. Inflammatory reactions after ischemia have been shown to occur in extracerebral organs, focal brain ischemia, or brain trauma; to date, they have not been demonstrated after temporary complete global brain ischemia. Neuronal injury can signal interleukin-1 and other cytokines to be produced and trigger endogenous activation of microglia, with additional injury (*QA*, quinolinic acid). In addition, tissue or endothelial injury—particularly associated with necrosis—can signal the endothelium to produce adhesion molecules (intercellular [*ICAM*], e-selectin [e-sel], p-selectin [p-sel]), cytokines, chemokines, and other mediators, triggering local involvement of systemic inflammatory cells in an interaction

FIGURE 58–2 • Cont'd—between blood and damaged tissue. Reoxygenation restores [ATP] through oxidative phosphorylation, which may result in massive uptake of $[Ca^{2+}]i$ into mitochondria, which are swollen from increased osmolality. Thus mitochondria loaded with bound $[Ca^{2+}]$ may self-destruct by rupturing and releasing additional free radicals. Increased $[Ca^{2+}]i$ by itself and by triggering free radical reactions may result in lipid peroxidation, leaky membranes, and cell death. Neuronal damage can be caused, in part, by increased [EAA]*e* (excitotoxicity). During reperfusion, $[Ca^{2+}]i$ and increased [EAAs]*c* normalize. Their contribution to ultimate death of neurons is more likely through the cascades they have triggered during ischemia. During ischemia and subsequent reperfusion, loading of cells and calcium maldistribution in cells are thought to be the key trigger common to the development of cell death. This calcium loading signals a wide variety of pathological processes. Proteases, lipases, and nucleases are activated, which may contribute to activation of genes or gene products (i.e., interleukin-converting enzyme, [*ICE*] or *P53*) critical to the development of programmed cell death (*PCD*, i.e., apoptosis), or inactivation of genes or gene products normally inhibiting this process. Activation of neuronal nitric oxide synthase (*nNOS*) by calcium can lead to production of NO·, which can combine with superoxide to generate peroxynitrite (*OONO*⁻). $OONO^-$ and ·OH can lead to both DNA injury and PCD, or protein and membrane peroxidation and necrosis, respectively. Nerve growth factor (*NGF*), nuclear immediate early response genes (*IERG*) such as heat shock protein, free radical scavengers (*FRSs*), adenosine, and other endogenous defenses (*ED*) may modulate the damage. (Designed in 1995 by P. Safar, MD, and P. Kochanek, MD, with input from N. Bircher, MD, and J. Severinghaus, MD.)

calcium accumulation is exacerbated by cellular energy failure, which disables the Na^+/K^+-ATPase membrane pump and results in further calcium accumulation.[22] Reestablishment of the energy supply can reverse these changes. Delayed glutamate-related neuronal injury is most likely the result of activation of ionotropic receptors and subsequent calcium influx. Calcium influx causes death of neurons in culture under anoxic conditions or in the presence of glutamate.[22] The intracellular accumulation of calcium (1) activates proteases, lipases, and endonucleases resulting in the breakdown of membrane phospholipids; (2) activates neuronal nitric oxide synthase, resulting in nitric oxide production and, in the presence of superoxide, peroxynitrite formation; (3) damages mitochondria; (4) disrupts nucleic acid sequences; and (5) ultimately mediates cell death, either necrosis or apoptosis (Fig. 58–2). The disturbance of the finely regulated intracellular calcium homeostasis is now recognized as a possible final common pathway of neuronal death.[18,22,45,47] NMDA receptor activation has also been shown to stimulate superoxide anion production, which may contribute to cellular injury.[48] The NMDA and AMPA-receptor subtypes have been suggested to play key roles in ischemic brain injury. The potential implications of these mechanisms in regard to therapeutic manipulation of glutamate receptors, as well as calcium and sodium channels, are discussed later.

Protease Activation

One of the candidates for a critical role in neuronal injury as a result of increases in intracellular calcium concentration is protease activation. Protease activation may play a central role in mediating both necrosis and programmed cell death. With regard to necrosis, numerous calcium-dependent enzymes can become activated during ischemia and produce important structural injury to neurons. One class of calcium-dependent proteases, calpains, is cytosolic cysteine proteases that degrade numerous cytoskeletal protein components of neurotubules and neurofilaments, as well as activate protein kinase C and phospholipases. Inhibition of calpain activation has produced marked reduction in ischemic brain injury, particularly in cerebral infarcts after focal ischemia.[49] With regard to apoptosis, the caspase family may also play a pivotal role in the initiation of programmed cell death after cerebral ischemia and may have a more prominent role in the developing mammalian brain compared with the mature brain.[50]

Oxygen Radical Formation

Toxic oxygen radical species produced during postischemic reperfusion have been implicated as important contributors to "reperfusion injury" and delayed cell death.[40] The primary species of interest include superoxide anion, hydrogen peroxide, hydroxyl radical, and the reactive nitrogen species peroxynitrite.

The potential sources of oxygen radicals are many. Superoxide anion is produced by the electron transport chain during normal mitochondrial respiration. Mitochondrial dysfunction, as may occur under conditions of ischemia, produces increased generation of free radicals that may extend beyond the capacity of endogenous antioxidants leading to oxidative stress.[30] Metabolism of arachidonic acid (AA) compared with the cyclooxygenase pathway to form prostaglandins also produces superoxide anion as an enzymatic byproduct, and this also occurs to a lesser extent in the lipoxygenase and cytochrome P-450 pathways.[40,51] Accumulated neutrophils also can contribute superoxide anion via neutrophil reduced nicotinamide adenine dinucleotide phosphate (NADPH)–oxidase. Another potential oxygen radical source is xanthine oxidase (XO)–xanthine dehydrogenase (XD). Energy depletion is associated with conversion of ATP to adenosine diphosphate (ADP) and eventually to hypoxanthine. This ischemia- or anoxia-induced energy deprivation also causes conversion of XD to XO via calcium-activated proteases. In the presence of hypoxanthine and oxygen, which become available during reperfusion, XO produces superoxide anion. These XO-mediated reactions may occur in cerebral vascular endothelial cells, which are rich in XO.[40] The importance of XO in contribution to the generation of free radicals in human beings, however, has been challenged.[52,53] Auto-oxidation of circulating catecholamines or of neurotransmitter catecholamines may represent another potential source of oxygen radicals.

Another possible contributor to free radical generation is "delocalized" iron. Iron is normally transported in the blood tightly bound to transferrin and stored inside the cell bound to ferritin. In ischemic conditions with accompanying acidosis, however, iron may be displaced from its normal binding sites and can catalyze reactions that promote oxygen radical formation.[54] Most commonly implicated is the Haber-Weiss/Fenton reaction, whereby the potent hydroxyl radical is produced from superoxide anion and hydrogen peroxide in the presence of free iron.

Finally, nitric oxide is another free radical that contributes to both nitrosative and oxidative stress. Nitric oxide increases during ischemia through increased NMDA receptor stimulation, mediated by release of excitatory amino acids and subsequent calcium-mediated activation of neuronal nitric oxide synthase.[54] Nitric oxide, in the presence of superoxide, produces peroxynitrite.[55] Free radicals have also been associated directly with an increased release of excitatory amino acids and vice versa.[47,56] Not only do they participate in each other's release and formation, but they may act synergistically in causing tissue damage.

The brain may be particularly vulnerable to free radical injury for several reasons. One is the high concentration of polyunsaturated fatty acids, especially AA. As noted previously, free fatty acids (FFAs) are released throughout ischemia. On exposure to oxygen radical species, these FFAs are vulnerable to autocatalytic lipid peroxidation.[58] Cerebrospinal fluid (CSF) has low concentrations of iron-binding proteins; therefore iron released from injured neurons or glia is likely to contribute to these peroxidation reactions. Byproducts of these reactions, for example, malondialdehyde and conjugated dienes, have been used as markers of the extent of lipid peroxidation after brain injury (e.g., the thiobarbiturate assay). Lipid peroxides accumulate in the selectively vulnerable zones during reperfusion after transient forebrain ischemia.[54,59] The peroxides do not accumulate during the ischemic period itself or in areas that are not reperfused and thus are implicated in reperfusion injury.[60]

Investigators have also detected oxidative damage to brain proteins after reperfusion.[60] Others, however, have argued that the oxidized proteins detected in the previous study were oxidized during sampling and not as a result of ischemia.[58] Other investigators were also unable to detect oxidized nuclear material or mitochondrial DNA during cerebral ischemia.[61] These results were expected because of the compact structure of DNA and the presence of histones, which provide increased resistance to oxidative damage. There are two problems with these findings, however: (1) damage caused by oxidative stress can occur in the absence of lipid peroxidation[62] and (2) work in which apoptosis is investigated suggests that oxidation of regulatory proteins of transcription and translation of DNA may be an important intermediate step in propagation of neuronal cell death.[63,64] Application of newly refined techniques to quantify oxidative stress should help clarify this issue[65] and may assist in the evaluation of therapies to prevent oxidative stress-mediated brain damage produced during ischemia and reperfusion.

Membrane Phospholipid Hydrolysis and Mediator Formation

FFAs are released from neuronal membranes during ischemia, and the amount of FFAs released is proportional to the duration of ischemia. FFA release continues to change in proportion to duration of ischemia after the completion of energy failure.[66] FFAs are released by two distinct but related processes. First, phosphatidyl inositol is hydrolyzed by phospholipase C with the production of diacylglycerol (DAG) and inositol phosphates.[67,68] Phospholipase C–mediated hydrolysis begins during the initial moments of the ischemic insult and is related to neurotransmitter receptor stimulation. DAG is then hydrolyzed by lipases to FFA, predominantly AA and stearic acid. Second, other brain glycerophospholipids are hydrolyzed by phospholipase A_2, which is activated by increases in intracellular calcium concentration. FFA release and metabolism is not a generalized process in the neuronal membrane, but is concentrated in the synaptic regions and is thus related to excitotoxicity.[69]

The FFAs released then have potential detrimental effects during the postischemic period by three mechanisms. First, AA metabolism via the cyclooxygenase pathway contributes to oxygen radical production during reperfusion.[57] Second, FFAs and DAG directly increase membrane fluidity, inhibit adenosine triphosphatases (ATPases), increase neurotransmitter release, and uncouple oxidative phosphorylation. Third, enzymatic oxidation of AA during reperfusion by cyclooxygenase, lipoxygenase, or cytochrome P-450 produces a large number of bioactive lipids, including prostaglandins, thromboxanes, leukotrienes, and hydroxy fatty acids, many of which have detrimental effects (Fig. 58–2).

Endogenous Defenses

In response to the complex sequence of pathobiological events that evolve after brain injury, several "endogenous neuroprotectants" are produced, induced, or activated after ischemia, and their postulated or proven functions improve cell (specifically neuronal) survival in in vivo and in vitro models.

The heat shock proteins (Hsps) are one family of candidate neuroprotectants that are highly conserved among biological species and are induced in cells after a variety of stimuli. Thermal stress is the classic example; however, any insult that damages protein structure, including ischemic[70] and traumatic brain injury,[71] can produce an Hsp response. Simon et al[70] showed that after global ischemia the 72 kDa heat shock protein (Hsp 72) is temporally expressed in a pattern that mirrors the pattern of selective vulnerability in the model, seen first in the CA_1 region of the hippocampus, followed by CA_3, cortex, and thalamus, and finally in the dentate granule cells. Hsp72 is also induced in both gray and white matter of piglets after mild and severe hypoxia.[72] The Hsps have generated major interest as potential neuroprotectants because their prior induction by a sublethal stress can afford protection from subsequent injury. Transient whole-body hyperthermia reduces subsequent ischemic brain injury in both adult[73] and neonatal rats.[74] Furthermore, exogenous Hsp72 reduces glutamate toxicity in neuronal cell cultures.[75] Importantly, overexpression of Hsp72 reduces ischemic damage and programmed cell death after experimental stroke and global ischemia in vivo.[76-78]

Another potential mechanism for endogenous neuroprotection is the upregulation of genes that inhibit programmed cell death. The mammalian gene bcl-2, a proto-oncogene, can block apoptotic cell death[63] and perhaps necrotic cell death as well.[79] The bcl-2 gene is expressed in neurons surviving both focal and global ischemia[80,81] and is reduced in degenerating neurons after cardiopulmonary arrest in rats.[82] Viral transfection of bcl-2 reduces infarction after focal ischemia,[83] and upregulation of bcl-2 through ceramide administered 30 minutes after hypoxia-ischemia reduced the number of cells with DNA damage in immature rat brain.[84] Forced overexpression of the bcl-2 family member bcl-x-long also reduces tissue damage after focal cerebral ischemia in adult rats.[85] After traumatic brain injury in infants and children, CSF levels of bcl-2 are increased in patients who survive compared with those who die.[86]

Adenosine is an endogenous biochemical mediator that may serve a protective role after cerebral ischemia, particularly early after injury. Adenosine is increased in brain tissue after experimental ischemia[87] and in response to hypoxia,[88] hypotension,[89] and hypoglycemia.[90] The release of adenosine after ischemia could afford neuroprotection by a combination of several mechanisms. When bound to A2-receptors, adenosine is a potent cerebrovasodilator and inhibits platelet activation and neutrophil function.[91] Bound to A1-receptors, adenosine reduces neuronal metabolism and excitatory amino acid release and stabilizes postsynaptic membranes.[91] Thus the beneficial effects of adenosine after cerebral ischemia include improved regional blood flow, reduced local oxygen demand, attenuation of both excitotoxicity and calcium accumulation, and anti-inflammatory and rheological effects. Finally, adenosine agonists have been shown to improve survival of selectively vulnerable neurons after ischemia in many studies (reviewed in Rudolphi et al[92]).

Clinical Pathophysiology

Cerebral Blood Flow and Metabolism after Resuscitation

The pioneering studies in which global CBF and cerebral metabolic rate for oxygen ($CMRO_2$) were measured in animal models of global ischemia or cardiac arrest focused on the early postresuscitation period. In their classic study, Snyder et al[93] showed that after 15 minutes of global brain ischemia in dogs, CBF transiently increased to levels well above baseline (Fig. 58–3). Then, after 15 to 30 minutes, CBF progressively decreased to a level below normal for the remainder of the monitoring period (90 minutes). This pattern of "early" transient postischemic hyperemia and subsequent "delayed postischemic hypoperfusion" has been observed almost universally in global cerebral ischemia models, including both VF and asphyxial arrest.[94,95] The level of hyperemia and subsequent hypoperfusion vary in relation to the duration of the insult.[96] Although these phases of increased and decreased CBF characterize the net global effect, regional CBF is often inhomogeneous, particularly during postischemic hypoperfusion, when areas of decreased and increased perfusion may coexist.[97] Metabolism, as assessed with $CMRO_2$, is reduced during the early postischemic period and then progressively recovers to a level that varies, depending on the model used and on the duration of ischemia.[96,98] In some models,

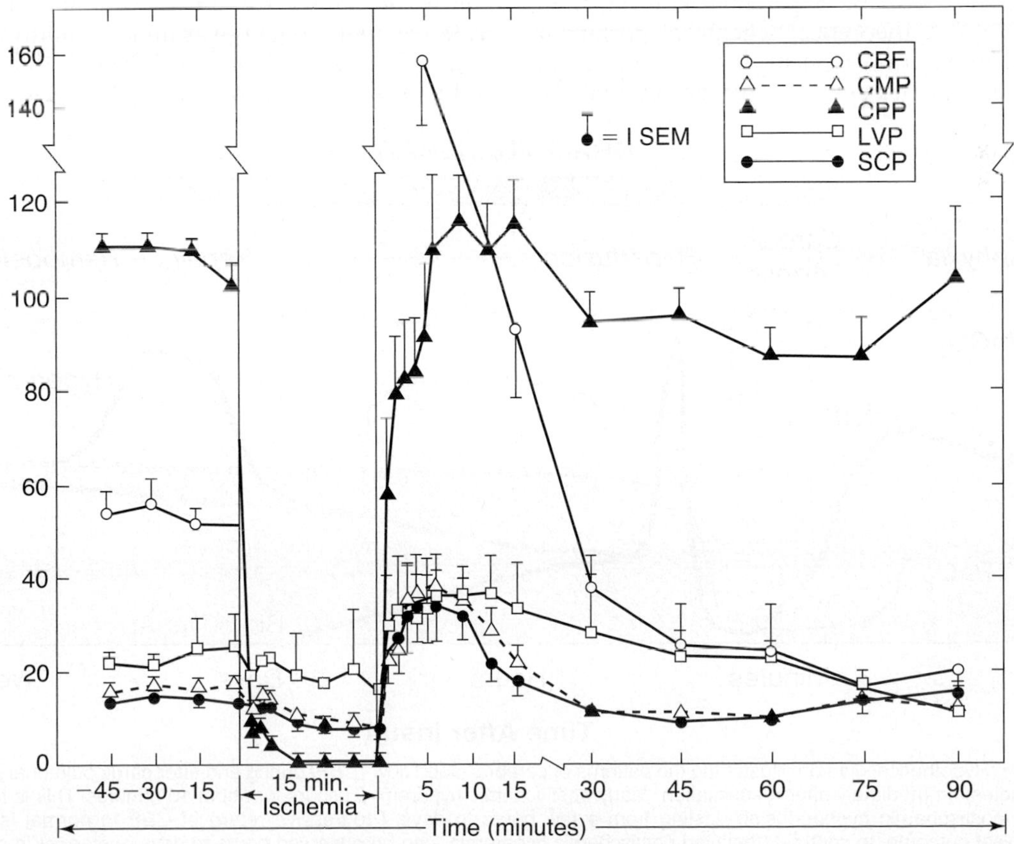

FIGURE 58–3 • Cerebral blood flow *(CBF)*, cisterna magna pressure *(CMP)*, cerebral perfusion pressure *(CPP)*, lateral ventricular pressure *(LVP)*, and supracortical pressure *(SCP)* measured before, during, and for 90 minutes after a 15-minute circulatory arrest in dogs. CBF data demonstrate that early postresuscitation hyperemia occurs, followed by hypoperfusion.

including VF arrest in dogs, significant recovery of $CMRO_2$ may occur during the first few hours, despite persistent postischemic hypoperfusion; this recovery creates the potential for a secondary ischemic insult during reperfusion. Whether this increase in $CMRO_2$ represents appropriate synaptic activity, seizures, or basal metabolism is not certain. In other models, global CBF and $CMRO_2$ are matched during the first few hours after ischemia.

Drugs such as nimodipine can increase CBF during the early postischemic hypoperfusion phase after global cerebral ischemia. $CMRO_2$ recovery is generally not increased by treatment.[99] Although nimodipine has been shown to be beneficial in patients after subarachnoid hemorrhage,[100] but not ischemic stroke,[101] the testing of strategies targeting early postarrest hypoperfusion deserves further study. Safar et al[102] have reported that a multifaceted treatment strategy to increase CBF ("flow promotion") and reduce CMR or $CMRO_2$ early after VF in dogs improved outcome. This was accomplished by use of cardiopulmonary bypass (CPB), mild hypothermia, hemodilution, and transient hypertension.

Immediately after cardiac arrest accompanied by restoration of systemic hemodynamic stability, transient global brain hyperemia occurs and is followed by a period of patchy hypoperfusion. The magnitude and duration of these alterations in flow appear to be related to the duration of the insult. In patients with good outcomes, global CBF recovers over the subsequent 24 to 72 hours, and carbon dioxide (CO_2) reactivity remains intact. Patients who do not regain consciousness or progress to brain death have absolute or relative CBF hyperemia with impaired CO_2 reactivity.[103,104] A theoretical scheme of postarrest global CBF and its relation to neurological outcome is presented in Figure 58–3. It must be recognized that the measurements of metabolism in the studies have traditionally been $CMRO_2$. Bergsneider et al[105] used positron emission tomography (PET) in patients after traumatic brain injury, however, and reported the occurrence of delayed hyperglycolysis in some comatose patients, suggesting a shift to anaerobic metabolism in injured brain in some patients.

Most studies in experimental animal models of asphyxial arrest suggest a similar pattern of CBF and $CMRO_2$ to that observed after VF cardiac arrest and global ischemia in the early postresuscitation period.[96,103] There are some exceptions, however.[106] Results from clinical studies of asphyxial arrest are scarce and somewhat conflicting with regard to the prognostic implications of high or low values of postarrest CBF on the basis of a single measurement; however, loss of CO_2 reactivity appears to be associated with poor outcome in all studies. In studies of children between 24 and 48 hours after near drowning, Ashwal et al[107] observed low CBF in the seven nonsurvivors and no relationship between CBF and partial pressure of arterial CO_2 ($PaCO_2$) in these patients. These results again suggested loss of CBF reactivity to changes in $PaCO_2$. In this study, hyperemia was not routinely observed in either survivors in a persistent vegetative state or in children who died, but only a single CBF measurement was made in these patients. Beyda[108] obtained serial measurements of postarrest xenon Xe 133 in a series of children who had asphyxial arrest from submersion accidents. Children with good neurological outcomes had slightly decreased CBF values at 12 hours that increased to normal during the subsequent 24 to 60 hours. In these children, CBF reactivity to CO_2 was intact. Children with eventual vegetative outcome or brain death exhibited hyperemia with loss or attenuation of CO_2 reactivity (Fig. 58–4).

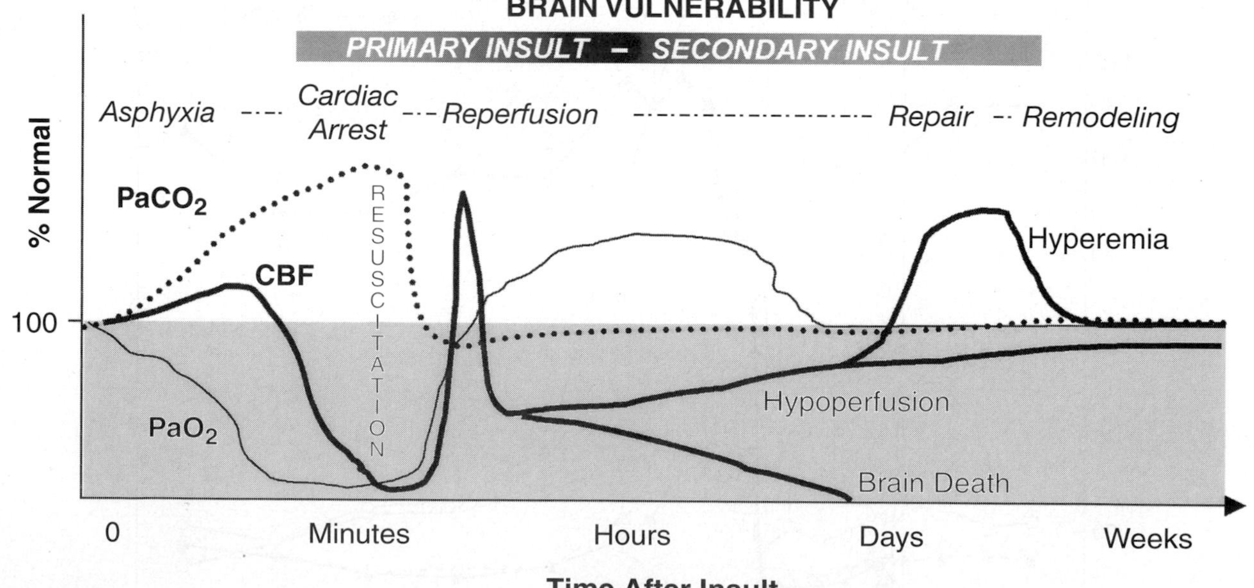

FIGURE 58–4 • Hypothetical diagram illustrating the patterns of cerebral blood flow *(CBF)* during and after cardiopulmonary arrest in humans (based on adult studies). Immediately after resuscitation, "early postischemic hyperemia" occurs for about 15 minutes. This is followed by patchy multifocal "delayed postischemic hypoperfusion" lasting from a few hours to days. Progressive return of CBF to normal is seen in patients with intact neurological outcome. In contrast, "delayed postischemic hyperemia" can be observed hours to days postarrest in patients with more severe insults.[101,105] This delayed hyperemia appears to be associated with disabled or vegetative outcome (in which CBF gradually decreases to near normal or below normal) or brain death (in which CBF decreases to no flow). It is unclear, however, if all patients with vegetative outcome or eventual brain death have delayed hyperemia.

This hyperemia progressed to low or normal flow over the following 12 to 72 hours in children with vegetative outcome and progressed to low and then no flow with the development of brain death. Although routine monitoring of CBF or CMR has not been applied extensively to the postarrest setting in children, the use of stable xenon-enhanced computed tomography (CT) and magnetic resonance spectroscopy could lead to the routine assessment of CBF and CMR and an improved understanding of pathophysiology.[109]

Histopathology of Hypoxic-Ischemic Encephalopathy

Ischemic neuronal change, as first described by Sommer in 1880 and later by Spielmeyer, involves a progression from extensive cellular microvacuolation to a cell that resembles a naked shrunken nucleus (Fig. 58–5).[13] As described by Brierley et al[26] "this type of neuronal damage is neither ubiquitous nor randomly distributed but is found in regions which exhibit selective vulnerability to hypoxic stress." As discussed previously, death of selectively vulnerable neurons (e.g., hippocampal CA_1) cannot be explained by vascular distribution. Remarkably, these clinical descriptions of cell shrinkage were consistent with programmed cell death rather than with necrosis. The connection between selective vulnerability and apoptosis, however, was made 100 years later.[33] Neuronal death after cardiopulmonary arrest is seen not only in the selectively vulnerable neurons but also as a subtle histopathological finding in the arterial boundary zones. These neurons (not otherwise selectively vulnerable) are in the most poorly perfused areas during or after resuscitation.[25] Neuronal death in the arterial boundary zones was elegantly described by Nemoto et al[110] in a monkey model of 16 minutes of complete global brain ischemia followed by 7 days of intensive care. Maximal damage appeared to be in the classically described selectively vulnerable zones, but neuronal death was also observed in the most distal distribution of the posterior cerebral artery and in the watershed zones of the anterior and middle cerebral arteries (Fig. 58–6). With sufficient injury in the arterial boundary zone, more severe findings such as microinfarction or laminar necrosis can be seen.[14,110]

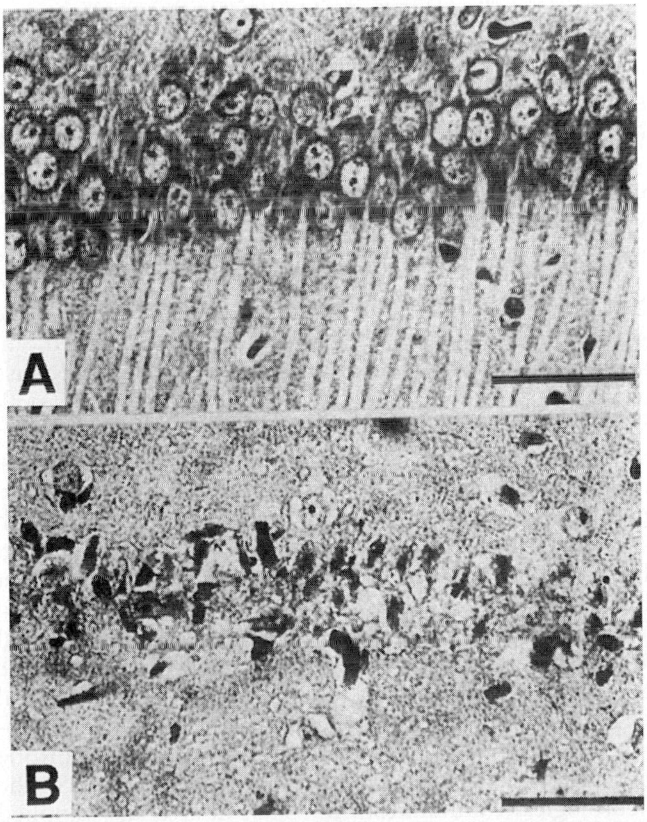

FIGURE 58–5 • Light micrograph of dorsal hippocampus in gerbils 7 days after 5 minutes sham ischemia **(A)** or global ischemia by carotid occlusion **(B)**. Ischemic neuronal change is seen with CA_1 neurons appearing as dark, shrunken nuclei without cytoplasm **(B)** by contrast with the normal-appearing nonischemic neurons **(A)**. Investigations by Nitatori et al[32] indicate that neuronal death in selective areas, after threshold ischemia insults, occurs via programmed cell death. (From Kuroiwa T, Bonnekoh P, Hossman KA: *Stroke* 21:1489, 1990.)

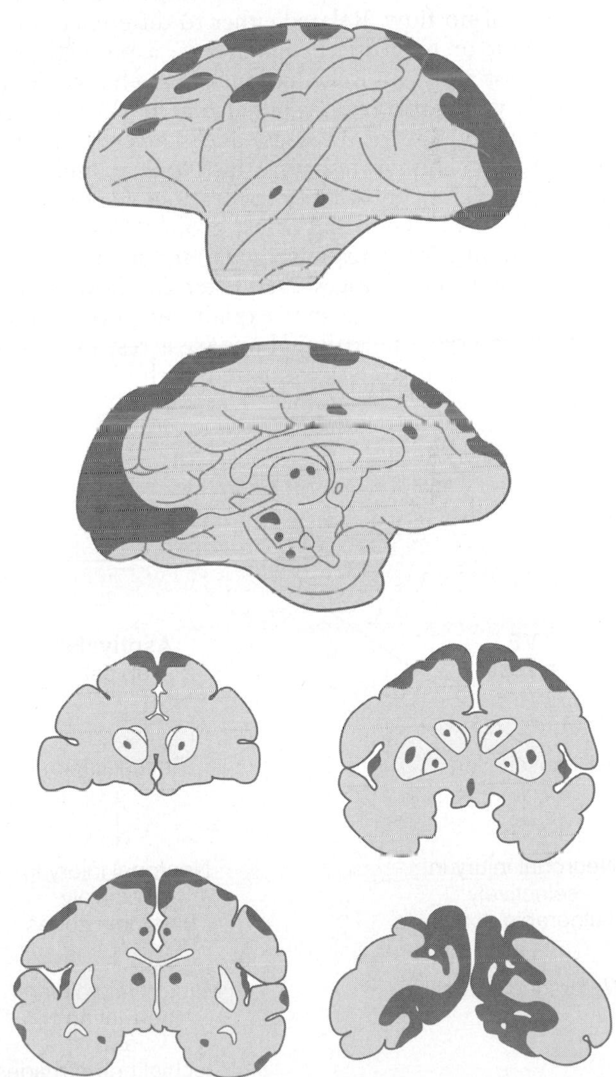

FIGURE 58–6 • Topographical distribution of cortical lesions 7 days after 16 minutes of global brain ischemia in rhesus monkeys. Neuronal death in areas with intrinsic selective vulnerability was most apparent in the distal distribution of the posterior cerebral artery. Damage in the watershed distributions of the anterior and middle cerebral arteries was less consistent.

As previously discussed, even in stroke, neuronal death in an ischemic penumbra can occur either by necrosis or apoptosis. Thus it appears that there may be a continuum between apoptosis and necrosis that may depend on a large number of factors, such as duration of the insult and brain region in question.[19] Whereas programmed cell death in a given area often affects only a small percentage of neurons, infarction affects all neurons and glia. Obviously, if the arrest time is long or if the postischemic conditions are sufficiently poor, infarction of the entire brain can occur.

Vaagenes et al[14] studied neuropathology after primary VF arrest of 10 minutes in dogs. Despite vegetative outcome at 96 hours, only scattered ischemic neuronal changes in the selectively vulnerable neurons and to a much lesser extent in the vascular watersheds were observed. Microinfarct formation was seen in only 5 of 18 dogs, suggesting that patchy ischemic neuronal change is sufficient for vegetative outcome. The Vaagenes group then compared this 10-minute VF arrest with an asphyxial episode (airway occlusion) that resulted in cardiac arrest with 7 minutes of no flow. Related either to differences in the initial insult or to postischemic events, asphyxial arrest resulted not only in ischemic neuronal change in the selectively vulnerable regions but also in marked microinfarct formation (30 of 32 dogs) and scattered petechial hemorrhages. This more severe histological injury was seen despite significantly *easier* restoration of spontaneous circulation in the asphyxial arrest group (Fig. 58–7). In addition, unlike VF arrest, asphyxial arrest caused some ischemic neuronal changes even after no flow of only 2 minutes. These findings may explain the poor outcome generally observed in cardiopulmonary arrest in children (usually asphyxial arrest) compared with that in adult series (VF arrest). After asphyxial cardiac arrest that results in long-term survival in both adult and pediatric-aged animals,[10,11,111] the pattern of neuronal death produced is similar to that reported in human studies[112] including that of the young victim of asphyxial cardiac arrest, Karen Ann Quinlan,[113] in whom a predilection for basal ganglial injury resulted in a persistent vegetative state.

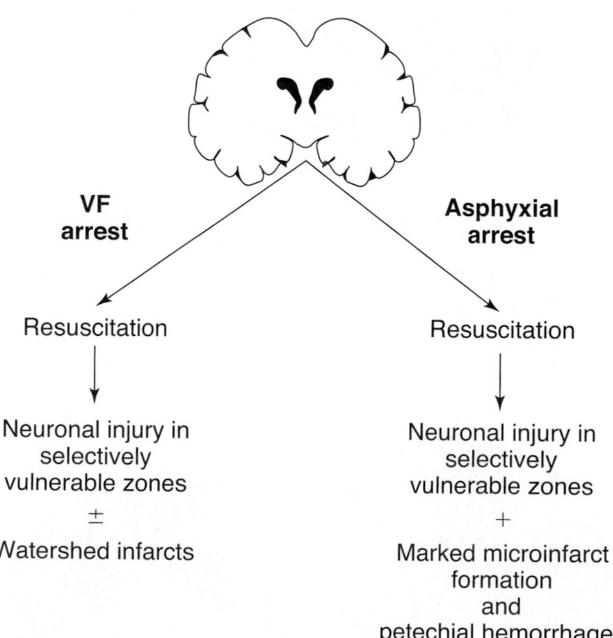

FIGURE 58–7 • Schematic diagram based on the work of Vaagenes et al[55] comparing the histological outcome of VF cardiac (adult) and asphyxial (pediatric) arrest. (From Kochanek PM: Novel pharmacologic approaches to brain resuscitation after cardiopulmonary arrest in the pediatric patient. In: *Critical Care Clinics*, Philadelphia, 1988, WB Saunders.)

*Clinical Outcome after Pediatric Cardiopulmonary Arrest**

Compared with results in adult series, survival and neurological outcome after cardiopulmonary arrest in infants and children are remarkably poor.[5,114,115] Most published data about the examination of out-of-hospital cardiopulmonary arrest in adults reveal about 11% to 12% "good" neurological outcome at 6 months after arrest, with *good* outcome generally defined as the ability to function independently.[116] A recent review in which the results from 44 studies totaling 3094 pediatric patients after cardiopulmonary arrest were summarized, showed favorable outcome (generally defined as nonvegetative) in only about 6% of patients.[6] In addition, after asphyxial arrest in children, clinical outcomes somewhere between vegetative and good, such as moderate disability or severe disability, are uncommon.[107,117] Survival after out-of-hospital arrest is 9% and after in-patient arrest is 24%, with an overall survival of 13%.[6] Furthermore, neurological outcome in pediatric patients surviving cardiac arrest is often overestimated with traditional outcome measures such as the Glasgow Outcome Score.[118] This high mortality and poor outcome after cardiorespiratory arrest in children generally represents out-of-hospital or unwitnessed full arrests. Recovery is much better in children who had witnessed arrests, cold water submersion, or isolated respiratory arrest, after which intact survival rates as high as 44% to 75% have been reported.[5,115,119,120] Nevertheless, these clinical data seem to bear out the severe neuropathological conditions observed in asphyxia-induced arrest in animal models because asphyxial arrest is the most common mode of arrest in all of the clinical pediatric series.[5,6,115,118-120]

Such factors as initial pH, number of epinephrine doses, and arrest duration have been examined in an attempt to predict outcome from cardiopulmonary arrest. Although sometimes predictive, this information can be misleading. For example, the time delay before analysis of the first blood sample can vary, as can estimates of arrest duration. With asphyxial arrest, even controlled experimental animal studies show that the time from asphyxia until cardiac arrest varies considerably. Currently, the most powerful individual predictor of neurological outcome after cardiorespiratory arrest is the neurological examination or one of several scoring systems based on selected aspects of the neurological examination. In 1985, Levy et al[121] applied multivariate analysis to variables from the neurological examination in a series of 210 comatose adults who were studied for at least 6 hours after a hypoxic-ischemic insult. None of the 15 patients who were in a vegetative state

*See also Chapters 112 and 113.

at 1 month regained independent function. In this retrospective study the combination of scores is from 2 weeks. The oculocephalic response and the 3-day motor response were able to identify all patients who gained independent function. This was true even for the 2 of 57 patients who remained in eyes-closed coma for 3 days and then ultimately regained independent function. Edgren et al[122] applied the Glasgow Coma Score (GCS) to assess outcome in 262 comatose adults who underwent cardiac arrest. A GCS less than 6 at 3 days after arrest predicted poor outcome (at 6 months) with no false-negative results. In a similar study of 216 adults who underwent out-of-hospital cardiac arrest, Mullie et al[122] found that a best GCS of less than 4 as early as 2 days after arrest predicted death or vegetative outcome in all but one patient. The condition of the one exception changed from a vegetative state to severe disability.

Although a few patients survive relatively intact despite poor prognosis, they likely represent cases of asphyxia without cardiac arrest, coma of an origin other than asphyxial arrest, unrecognized hypothermia, or an associated overdose of a cerebral protective drug. In two recent prospective trials, researchers examined the predictors of outcome after cardiopulmonary arrest in pediatric patients. In a series of 27 pediatric patients with hypoxic-ischemic encephalopathy, Robertson et al[118] found that a GCS of 3 and nonreactive pupils were predictive of adverse outcome. Sirbaugh et al,[124] whose result was consistent with asphyxia as the predominant cause of cardiac arrest in infants and children, found that the only factor that was positively associated with ROSC was endotracheal intubation. This would not support abandonment of the practice of ventilating the lungs of infants and children who were found pulseless and apneic but rather suggests that ventilation is crucial in this patient population.[125,126]

The electroencephalogram (EEG) also can provide prognostic information after cardiopulmonary arrest. Scollo-Lavizzari and Bassetti[127] retrospectively examined the relation between first postarrest EEG and clinical outcome in 408 cases. A five-grade classification was used to categorize EEGs. Although permanent severe neurological damage was observed in some patients with grade I EEG, none of the 208 patients with grade IV or V EEGs had a good neurological recovery.

Adjunctive prognostic information also can be derived from brain-derived protein levels in serum or cerebrospinal fluid (CSF). High serum levels of neuron-specific enolase (NSE) in comatose patients at 24 and 48 hours after cardiopulmonary arrest predict poor neurological outcome.[128] Martens et al[125] found that serum concentrations of the astrocyte-derived protein S-100B were superior to serum NSE (as well as CSF S-100B and NSE) in predicting which adult patients would regain consciousness after cardiac arrest.[129] In a recent study, researchers used a multimodal approach, combining serum concentrations of NSE, the astrocyte-derived protein S-100B, and somatosensory-evoked potentials (SEPs), prospectively in 27 adult patients after cardiac arrest and were able to predict all patients who did not regain consciousness.[130]

Researchers have used evoked potential monitoring in an attempt to provide early prognostic information about outcome after CPR. Madl et al[131] tested median nerve SEPs in 66 adults after successful resuscitation from cardiac arrest. They reported that the presence or absence and the latency of the cortical N70 peak reliably differentiated between bad and favorable outcome with 100% predictive ability. Testing was performed within 48 hours of resuscitation, which is a clinically relevant time frame. Auditory evoked response testing has been used in children with cardiac arrest after a submersion accident.[114] Normal evoked responses were observed in all children who recovered neurologically intact. Children who recovered with significant handicaps showed a reduction in wave V amplitude over time and prolonged wave I-V interpeak latencies.

Response of the Immature Brain to Cardiopulmonary Arrest

Clinical and laboratory studies suggest that the neurological outcome of newborn animals after a hypoxic-ischemic insult is favorable compared with that of adults, although this may be related to the ability of newborn animals to tolerate asphyxia systemically. This is most evident when neonatal and adult experimental models are compared. In newborn monkeys even 12 minutes of asphyxia did not result in cardiac arrest,[132] and in beagle puppies, 15 minutes of asphyxia produced hypotension but not cardiac arrest.[133] Asphyxial arrest in mature animal models generally occurs within 6 to 8 minutes.[14,94] Kirsch et al[134] showed that newborn piglets had better recovery of SEPs and less postarrest hypoperfusion than young adult pigs in the 2 hours after global cerebral ischemia. Thus not only does the cardiovascular response during asphyxia appear to be more robust in immature animals, but also the intrinsic sensitivity of the brain to a hypoxic-ischemic insult may be less. Studies suggest a selective vulnerability of the neonatal brainstem sensory nuclei to asphyxia.[132,135] This "selective vulnerability" may more correctly represent a relative lack of vulnerability of neonatal cerebral cortex to asphyxia because anoxic perfusion was tolerated for more than 12 minutes in immature monkeys, most of which showed no ischemic neuronal change.[132] Some mechanisms of secondary damage, however, such as excitotoxicity, appear to be more injurious in the immature.[136,137] Further complexity is added to processes such as excitoxicity when the immature brain is involved because some degree of excitatory stimulation is essential for neuronal survival and normal development.[138] Finally, greater plasticity in the immature brain may also allow for improved long-term recovery of function, although this may be more important in focal insults.[139,140]

The poor clinical outcome of infants and children who undergo cardiopulmonary arrest is probably related to specific mechanisms operating in the special setting of the asphyxial arrest. As the asphyxial arrest is developing, cardiac standstill is preceded by a variable period of severe hypoxia with increased CBF. During this period, severely hypoxic perfusion, a form of incomplete ischemia is produced, which can markedly increase cerebral lactate production.[141] The initial phase of asphyxia can also be accompanied by extreme stress during struggling, which could increase $CMRO_2$ and may be accompanied by systemic hyperglycemia.[107] The combination of hypoxic perfusion or incomplete hypoxia-ischemia and hyperglycemia can increase cerebral lactate concentration to 30 to 35 μmol/g and decrease tissue pH to levels as low as 6.05.[142-144] These lactate levels are much higher than those observed during even 30 minutes of complete ischemia (11 to 14 μmol/g) and are above the threshold of 20 to 25 μmol/g, at which lactic acid can produce local coagulation necrosis.[145] As suggested by the histopathological outcome studies previously discussed,[14] cardiac arrest or reperfusion may be particularly devastating to the brain in this milieu. Also, because of the relative resistance of the immature myocardium to asphyxia, it is easier to restore cardiovascular function in younger patients after longer durations of cardiac arrest than would be possible in adults. Total insult time (hypoxia plus anoxia plus cardiac arrest) is often very long. In adults with asystole or a pulseless bradycardia rather than VF, outcome is also poor.[146] Thus although pediatric intensivists have the apparent luxury of dealing with a somewhat resistant brain with more plasticity for functional recovery, this advantage is often trivial compared with the devastating pathobiology of the asphyxial arrest.[10,147]

Treatment of Cardiopulmonary Arrest

Field Interventions

Pediatric cardiac arrests are usually not as sudden in onset as in those in adults, and thus a window of opportunity exists during which interventions could potentially prevent cardiac arrest and subsequent poor outcome. As discussed, children sustaining isolated respiratory arrest have a mortality rate as low as 25%, whereas patients with cardiac arrests as a result of hypoxia have a high mortality.[6] Thus the sooner the recognition and interventions, the better are the chances for a good outcome. Prehospital emergency medical services (EMS) are capable of providing the earliest medical interventions and hold the greatest promise for improving outcome from prehospital pediatric cardiopulmonary arrest. EMS have developed sophisticated methods for dispatch and transport, but there are logistical limits to the rapidity with which they can provide basic interventions. Nationwide the average response time is well over 8 minutes, greater than the time required for an infant to progress from apnea to cardiac arrest. As a result, more advanced, traditionally hospital-based, and investigational interventions must also be administered in the prehospital setting in attempts to optimize outcome.

High-dose epinephrine therapy has been shown in many animal models to improve resuscitation rates.[148] A more recent study in a piglet model of asphyxial cardiac arrest, however, showed no improvement in survival or neurological outcome when high-dose epinephrine was used for resuscitation compared with standard dose.[149] Vasopressin may also be of value after cardiac arrest in pediatric patients because vasopressin alone and in combination with epinephrine increases CBF during resuscitation from VF compared with epinephrine alone.[150] The effects of high-dose epinephrine or vasopressin on long-term survival and neurological outcome in pediatric patients have not been established though. A small study in children with historical controls showed a beneficial effect on resuscitation and outcome in patients receiving high-dose epinephrine.[146] In contrast, a large multicenter trial with concomitant controls in adults was unable to show a beneficial effect of high-dose epinephrine.[152] Further, a recent meta-analysis of adult studies favored high-dose epinephrine in terms of ROSC, but favored a trend toward standard-dose epinephrine in terms of survival to hospital discharge.[153] The efficacy of pharmacological therapy during cardiopulmonary resuscitation (CPR) is probably limited by the minimal perfusion provided by standard CPR (see Chapter 113). Development and implementation of improved perfusion techniques for those undergoing cardiac arrest in the prehospital environment would provide an increased "therapeutic window" and thus a better chance of benefiting from advanced therapeutic techniques.

Controlled experimental or prospective clinical studies of intracranial pressure (ICP) monitoring or treatment after asphyxial arrest have not been performed. It could be predicted that ICP elevation would be more common after asphyxial arrest than after isolated global brain ischemia or VF arrest, given the severe histopathological conditions seen after asphyxial arrest and the long insult times from which the myocardium can recover in children. Sustained elevation of ICP (>20 mmHg) has been shown uniformly to predict poor outcome in four series of pediatric submersion accidents.[154-157] Unfortunately, as in VF arrest, the threshold for poor outcome from asphyxial arrest appears to be below the threshold for the occurrence of intracranial hypertension because some patients experience poor outcome despite normal ICP.[152] Although anecdotal cases of asphyxial arrest in patients with intact neurological outcome despite elevated ICP are occasionally discussed, in the series cited previously the ability to control ICP elevation did not result in meaningful survival.[155,157] Routine ICP monitoring and ICP-directed treatment are not currently recommended after asphyxial arrest,[117,155,157] Studies with ICP-directed therapy in the era of contemporary neurointensive care, however, have yet to be performed.

The blanket use of hyperventilation for cerebral resuscitation after cardiac arrest is currently out of favor. Only one laboratory study of cardiopulmonary arrest has shown a beneficial effect of hyperventilation. Vanicky et al[158] reported that 8 hours of hyperventilation reduced neuronal damage after cardiac arrest in dogs. Tissue was examined at 3 hours after arrest, however, and no long-term outcome was studied. The blind application of hyperventilation early after severe traumatic brain injury in adults worsened outcome.[159] The failure of ICP-directed therapy to improve outcome after cardiopulmonary arrest and the commonly observed period of hypoperfusion in the first hours to days after arrest seriously question the application of an intervention with the potential to further reduce CBF.[160,161] Although irreversible ischemic brain damage has never been shown with hyperventilation,[162] these data suggest that it is probably not wise to hyperventilate patients' lungs routinely after arrest, particularly during the period of postischemic hypoperfusion.[93,108,110] With the availability of stable-xenon CT CBF measurement, the effect of hyperventilation during the period of delayed postarrest hyperemia should be tested. Clinical studies suggest that postischemic hyperemia is accompanied by loss or severe attenuation of CBF response to alterations in $Paco_2$ resulting from severe ischemic insult.[104,108] Some postresuscitation patients with delayed hyperemia but intact CBF response to $Paco_2$ have been observed (Fig. 58–8).

The traditional approach to cerebral resuscitation has also recommended the use of hyperosmotic agents in the postarrest period,[102] although similar to hyperventilation, the blanket use of hyperosmotic agents after cardiac arrest is currently not in favor. Again, studies in the setting of cardiopulmonary arrest are lacking. In dogs subjected to 6 minutes of global ischemia, mannitol (2 g/kg) further reduced CBF during the postischemic hypoperfusion phase.[164] This unwanted effect of mannitol likely represents a result of dehydration because with more conventional doses, decreased blood viscosity after mannitol administration lowers cerebral blood volume but maintains CBF.[164] A few anecdotal reports in support of the use of albumin as an osmotic agent after cardiac arrest exist,[165,166] supported by several more recent experimental studies in models of global ischemia.[20] Administration of hypertonic saline improves myocardial blood flow and survival compared with standard resuscitation after VF in pigs.[168] These studies suggest that clinical trials on the effect of hypertonic solutions on outcome after cardiopulmonary arrest are warranted.

In clinical practice, patients are encountered who have been successfully resuscitated from an arrest of unknown etiology, have a clinical history suggestive of trauma, or demonstrate focal pupillary findings. In this setting it is appropriate to hyperventilate the lungs or administer mannitol until CT and clinical examination confirm the absence of trauma or a mass lesion.

Supportive Care in the Intensive Care Unit

In addition to maintenance of normal ventilation, arterial oxygenation, and blood pressure, several other aspects of supportive care are important to discuss because suboptimal treatment might adversely affect outcome.

Transient hyperglycemia commonly occurs after resuscitation from cardiac arrest. The optimal therapy or need for controlling blood glucose after resuscitation has not been established and is currently under investigation. Current recommendations are for the use of glucose-containing solutions during newborn resuscitations[109] because of evidence that hypoglycemia has synergistic deleterious effects, coupled with perinatal asphyxia.[169] Glucose-containing solutions are generally avoided in the resuscitation of the older child, given the association between hyperglycemia and poorer outcome after near drowning and traumatic brain injury in pediatric patients.[107,170] Although a cause and effect relationship between hyperglycemia and outcome in humans has not been established, in one of the recent clinical trials in which beneficial effects of hypothermia in adults after cardiac arrest are shown, hyperglycemia was associated with hypothermic treatment.[2] The optimal resuscitation fluid has not been established, particularly in pediatric patients beyond the neonatal period and before adolescence, but is likely to be age and perhaps mechanism dependent.

Although the optimal cerebral perfusion pattern for neuronal recovery remains to be defined,[102] blood pressure fluctuations, both high and low, adversely affect outcome. In their classic study of the neurological disease of systemic circulatory arrest in immature monkeys, Miller and Myers[132] found that systolic blood pressures at or below 50 mmHg during the reperfusion period had devastating effects on survival and neurological disease. This occurred even when the ischemic time was less than the 12-minute minimum that caused brain injury in their model. In contrast, Bleyaert et al[171] showed that intermittent episodes of hypertension (mean arterial pressure [MAP] 150 to 190 mmHg) induced with norepinephrine during the first 24 hours after 16 minutes of global brain ischemia in monkeys worsened neurological outcome. A beneficial

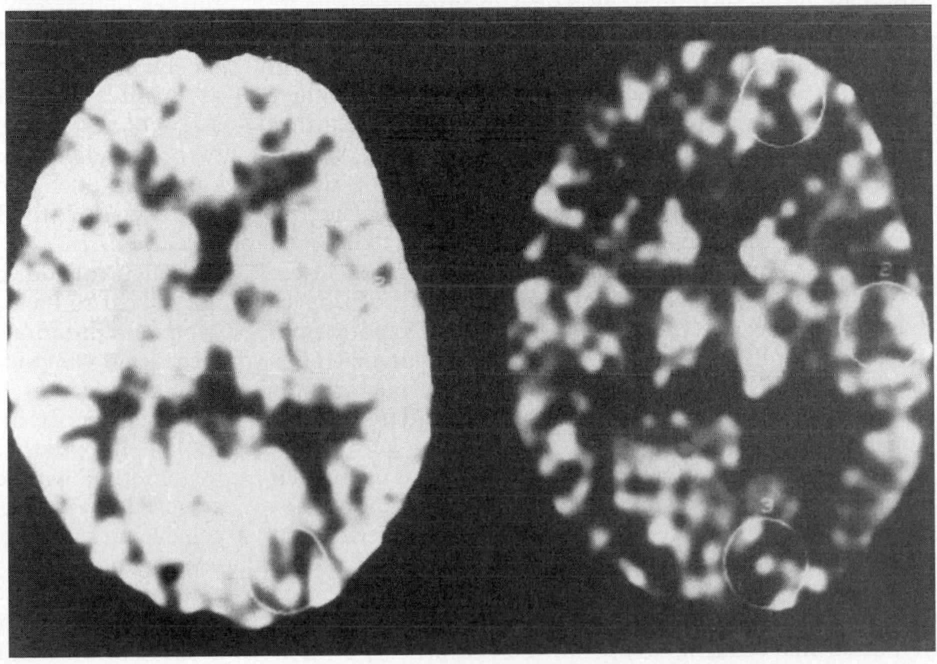

FIGURE 58–8 • Stable-xenon CT cerebral blood flow study in a comatose 6-year-old 3 days after cold-water submersion accident with asphyxial cardiorespiratory arrest. Delayed CBF hyperemia is represented as high-density white areas through the CT brain section shown on the left ($Paco_2$ ~40 mmHg). Flows (calculated from this scan) are in excess of 100 ml/100 g/min throughout the brain. Normal values are ~60 to 70 ml/100 g/min. Despite diffuse hyperemia, CBF reactivity to changes in $Paco_2$ remains intact. CBF values ranged from 50 to 60 ml/100 g/min *(right)* in areas sampled when $Paco_2$ was reduced to 29 mmHg with hyperventilation. Six months after the arrest, the child was moderately disabled but not in a vegetative state.

effect of transient hypertension during the immediate postresuscitation period has been suggested[5]: it has been hypothesized as improving flow in areas with microvascular sludging. Safar et al[102] suggested that transient hypertension was beneficial after cardiac arrest in dogs. It was applied as part of a multifaceted treatment protocol, however, and its specific benefit remains controversial.

Current and Novel Therapies

Postresuscitative Hypothermia

The effectiveness of hypothermia as a cerebral protective intervention (i.e., before arrest) is unquestioned. The beneficial effects of hypothermia applied immediately before and during cardiopulmonary arrest are also clearly shown by the clinical experience with cold-water submersion (near-drowning) accident victims.[117] By contrast, complications from the use of moderate hypothermia (30 to 34° C) after arrest and the apparent lack of a beneficial effect led to the abandonment of its routine application in the 1980s.[172]

Recently, however, two independent randomized clinical trials in adults who underwent cardiac arrest that show a beneficial effect of mild-moderate whole-body hypothermia have reignited an interest in the use of hypothermia as a neuroprotective strategy.[1,2] These studies prompted the International Liaison Committee on Resuscitation to recommend 12 to 24 hours of moderate (32 to 34° C) hypothermia for selected adults who underwent cardiac arrest.[3]

Although hypothermia after cardiac arrest has only recently been recommended, therapeutic hypothermia has been used to treat acute brain injury for more than a century.[173] Classically, the beneficial effect of hypothermia was thought to be primarily related to a reduction in oxidative metabolism. Rosomoff and Holaday[174] showed that with each decrement of 1° C, brain oxidative metabolism slows by 6.7%, a finding also seen in immature rats.[175] Moderate hypothermia (31° C) during neonatal hypoxia-ischemia maintains brain glucose and ATP concentration and reduces lactate production compared with normothermia (37° C) or mild hypothermia (34° C).[175] Taken together with the well-documented effects of hypothermia on neurological outcome, at least a partial contribution of the effect of hypothermia on cellular energetics in affording neuroprotection after cardiac arrest is supported. Given that mild hypothermia, which does not significantly lower oxygen consumption, provides some degree of neuroprotection, however, it seems more likely that hypothermia affects multiple mechanisms that influence outcome after cardiac arrest. These mechanisms include, but are not limited to, excitotoxicity, calcium fluxes, oxidative stress, and inflammation.

Although the composition of mechanisms by which hypothermia confers neuroprotection after cardiopulmonary arrest is still under debate, numerous experimental studies support further preclinical and clinical studies designed to optimize its application in humans. For instance, in both kinds of studies, researchers applied mild hypothermia, reducing temperature by as little as 2° C,[176] and delayed spontaneous hypothermia[177] neuronal death seen after cerebral ischemia in rats was reduced. Leonov et al[178] reported improved neurological recovery in dogs subjected to ice-water immersion of the cranium beginning 3 minutes after the onset of 12.5 minutes VF arrest, using CPB to maintain core temperature at 34° C for 1 hour. In this same canine VF arrest model, mild (34° C) or moderate (30° C) hypothermia was found to be protective, whereas deep (15° C) hypothermia worsened cerebral and cardiac outcome.[179] Relevant to pediatric cardiopulmonary arrest, postreatment with prolonged (24-hour) hypothermia improved neurological outcome in a piglet model of asphyxial cardiac arrest.[11]

Raising the question as to the need for further clinical trials in pediatric cardiopulmonary arrest in the era of contemporary intensive care are the two multicenter, randomized trials that show beneficial effects of hypothermia after cardiac arrest in adult patients.[1,2] In the European study by the Hypothermia after Cardiac Arrest Study Group, 137 of 275 patients were assigned to the hypothermic group. Mild hypothermia (32 to 34° C) was instituted with a median interval to target temperature of 105 minutes after ROSC. Patients were maintained at target temperature for 24 hours. Passive rewarming to a temperature above 36° C occurred over a median of 8 hours. Mortality at 6 months after arrest was 41% in the hypothermic group compared with 55% in the control group. The hypothermic group also had more patients with better neurological outcome assessed by the cerebral performance category (55% compared with 39% in the control group). In the Australian study by Bernard et al,[2] cooling was initiated in 77 patients in the field after ROSC. Mild hypothermia (33° C) was maintained for 12 hours, followed by active rewarming over 6 hours. Improved survival to discharge was observed in patients in the hypothermic group compared with patients in the normothermic group (49% compared with 26%).

Many questions and a few caveats remain. For instance, the timing, duration, and degree of hypothermia warrant further optimization, as well as which patients stand to benefit from treatment. With extrapolation from experimental studies, hypothermia should be initiated as soon as possible after resuscitation. Even when delayed for a few hours, though, mild hypothermia has been shown to be beneficial in animal models of cardiac arrest.[177] Current guidelines recommend that 12 to 24 hours of moderate (32 to 34° C) hypothermia for adults after cardiac arrest be instituted as quickly as possible.[3] Although this duration and degree of hypothermia does not appear to have any untoward effects, more profound depth and duration of hypothermia (28 to 32° C) increase the risk for complications such as arrhythmias, coagulopathy, and infection.[180]

Other important issues include the method and rate of cooling. In both the European and Australian studies, mild hypothermia was achieved by surface cooling, which was achieved over a period of hours. Other modalities that achieve target temperatures more rapidly deserve further investigation, such as peritoneal lavage, veno-venous or arteriovenous CPB, or novel internal cooling devices.[181,182] Recently Bernard et al[183] reported that administering a bolus of 30 ml/kg of ice-cold (4° C) lactated Ringer's solution intravenously safely and effectively decreased core temperature from 35.5 to 33.8° C in 22 adult patients after cardiac arrest. In a group of healthy volunteers, mild hypothermia (34.9 to 35.5° C) was attained after 40 ml/kg of ice-cold (4° C) normal saline was infused through an antecubital vein.[184] This method of core cooling might be the fastest, most practical way of inducing hypothermia in the field immediately after ROSC. Rapid rewarming and hyperthermia[185,186] should be avoided, and on the basis of available data, active rewarming of patients after cardiac arrest with mild-moderate spontaneous hypothermia (33 to 35° C) should be discouraged.

Finally, treatment of neonates with selective head cooling and mild systemic hypothermia after perinatal asphyxia appears safe,[187] and a multicenter randomized clinical trial of hypothermia for the treatment of perinatal asphyxia has recently been completed. If the results of this trial in which neonates with asphyxial cardiac arrest were examined are positive, coupled with the favorable results seen in adults with primarily VF arrest, any clinicians may be swayed to study or treat pediatric patients with asphyxial arrest and to implement a hypothermic treatment protocol for all patients with cardiac arrest and documented ventricular tachyarrhythmia (VT) or VF.

Inhibition of Postischemic Excitotoxicity

The observation in certain animal models that hypermetabolism accompanies postischemic hypoperfusion formed the basis for early clinical cerebroprotective strategies in the postarrest setting. Therapies directed at attenuating active cerebral metabolism ($CMRO_2$ resulting from synaptic transmission) were applied in the hope of reducing this secondary insult of hypoperfusion plus hypermetabolism. The cerebral protective effects of interventions that decrease cerebral metabolic rate *before* the onset of ischemia, such as barbiturates and hypothermia, are well established and clinically important.[188,189] The selective inhibitory effect of barbiturates on active $CMRO_2$ was particularly attractive. Therapeutic reductions in brain metabolism when applied *after* the insult, however, as in the "HYPER" therapy of the 1970 and 1980s, did not improve outcome.[172,190] This may have been the result of the relative lack of postarrest hypermetabolism in human beings.[103] In addition, adverse hemodynamic consequences of barbiturates and the ill effects of sustained hypothermia on immune function and blood flow may have counteracted any beneficial effects.

Death of selectively vulnerable neurons is mediated by local release of excitatory neurotransmitters with hypermetabolism and calcium accumulation. This has led to attempts to attenuate postischemic excitotoxicity more selectively through the administration of specific receptor antagonists. The failure of barbiturates to block NMDA-mediated excitotoxicity in vitro emphasized the need to test more specific agents. Many animal models of focal and global brain ischemia have been used to test the efficacy of both competitive and noncompetitive NMDA receptor antagonists. Most studies have shown beneficial effects on histological severity of ischemic damage, especially in the hippocampus, and several have shown benefits in survival.[191] After asphyxial arrest in piglets, alterations in NMDA receptor potentiation within the striatum may participate in striatal neuron degeneration.[192] An important consideration is the finding that beneficial effects of NMDA antagonists in the earlier rodent models of ischemia may have been related to mild systemic hypothermia induced by a central effect of these agents.[193] Blockade of non-NMDA receptors (e.g., AMPA and kainate receptors) with selective receptor-antagonists has shown the most consistent prevention of delayed neuronal cell loss in the hippocampal CA_1 region in models of global cerebral ischemia. In their report, however, Brambrink et al[194] suggest that treatment with the AMPA antagonist NBQX (chemical name, 2,3-dihydroxy-6-nitro-7-sulfamoyl- benzo(f)quinoxaline) in piglets worsened outcome after asphyxia. The exact role of excitatory neurotransmitter receptor and sodium channel blockade in both the selectively vulnerable zones and other areas of the brain remains to be more clearly defined,[195] particularly in established models of cardiac arrest. A final caveat is that clinical trials with antiexcitotoxic strategies to treat adult patients after stroke have been terminated for both futility and the possibility of adverse effects.[196]

Voltage-Operated Calcium Channel Antagonists

Calcium accumulation in neurons and release of stored intracellular calcium are pivotal events leading to irreversible cellular damage during the reperfusion phase after an ischemic insult. Calcium accumulation occurs through receptor-operated channels such as the NMDA receptor-activated channels, voltage-operated calcium channels, nonspecific membrane channels, and release of intracellular calcium through the inositol second-messenger pathway. Conflicting results have been obtained regarding the ability of the voltage-operated calcium channel antagonists (lidoflazine, nimodipine, nicardipine) to attenuate calcium accumulation in neurons after ischemia.[197] The contribution of the voltage-gated channels to postischemic calcium accumulation is apparently less than that of the agonist-operated channels in selectively vulnerable zones.

After encouraging animal investigations, Abramson et al[197]conducted a multicenter study of the effect of lidoflazine treatment in a blinded, randomized protocol in 505 adult patients after cardiopulmonary arrest. Lidoflazine did not significantly improve neurological outcome, which was normal in about 12% of patients.[152] Nimodipine increased CBF in humans at 3 hours after cardiac arrest in a blinded, randomized study.[198] A subsequent multicenter, placebo-controlled, randomized, double-blind trial of nimodipine after out-of-hospital cardiac arrest in adults, however, failed to demonstrate a beneficial effect on cognitive function in the survivors.[199] Adults who had a stroke also did not benefit from nimodipine.[101] Although clinical studies of nimodipine in asphyxial arrest have not been done, Ment et al[133] observed hypotension and decreased CBF with nimodipine in a perinatal asphyxia model.

A limitation of these studies is that they target only one of several redundant pathways contributing to cell death.

Thus some investigators argue for trials targeting multiple mechanisms or final common pathways.

Inhibitors of Oxygen Free Radical Mediated Injury

As previously noted, free radicals can damage membrane lipids, cellular proteins/enzymes, and DNA (see Chapter 99). The importance of damage to each brain component and subsequent contribution to triggering or mediating the final pathway of neuronal death remains to be defined. Studies in which superoxide dismutase (SOD) was used to reduce injury from ischemia have met with mixed results.[200,201] Manipulation of glutathione metabolism has also shown some promise.[202,203]

Antioxidant enzymes and water-soluble free radical scavengers do not easily penetrate the blood-brain barrier.[204] As a result, multiple strategies have been devised to modify these agents to improve availability and efficacy in the brain. Conjugation of polyethylene glycol (PEG) to both SOD and catalase improves drug half-life and reduces cerebral damage caused by ischemia.[205] Liposome-encapsulated SOD has also been shown to be beneficial.[206] An analog of glutathione, YM737, has been developed to allow for better penetration into cells. YM737 reduces brain damage caused by cerebral ischemia.[207] Ascorbic acid has been combined with α-tocopherol to form the compound EPC-K1. EPC-K1 has both protective and resuscitative effects on the brains of gerbils sustaining cerebral ischemia and reperfusion.[188]

Lipid-soluble agents rapidly cross the blood-brain barrier, a beneficial property for cerebral resuscitation. Administration of α-tocopherol after cerebral ischemia reduces ischemic neuronal damage in gerbils.[208] Lipid-soluble compounds termed "Lazaroids" have been developed to reduce iron-dependent lipid peroxidation after cerebral ischemia. The 21-aminosteroid Trilizad (U74006) has been most extensively investigated and is efficacious in reducing brain damage when given before both focal and global cerebral ischemia.[209] A promising new agent, U78517, is more potent than U74006 and may be more efficacious in ameliorating brain damage, especially after cerebral ischemia.[210]

Hydroxyl starch–conjugated deferoxamine that penetrates the blood-brain barrier and chelates transitional metals can reduce free radical production and brain injury.[211] PBN (chemical name, α-phenyl-N-tert-butyl-nitrone), a spin trap commonly used for quantitating free radical production, may have therapeutic use during ischemia and reperfusion.[212] A recent report, however, showed that PBN paradoxically increases DNA fragmentation in neurons after traumatic brain injury.[213] The antioxidant Tempol provides benefit above and beyond deep hypothermia in a dog model of hemorrhagic shock–induced cardiac arrest that produces cerebral ischemia.[214]

The amount of oxygen administered during resuscitation also appears to influence the severity of the free radical damage,[215,216] and oxidative stress was found to be increased in asphyxiated infants resuscitated with 100% oxygen compared with a group resuscitated with room air,[217] although hyperbaric oxygen has been shown to reduce histological damage after transient forebrain ischemia in rodents.[218] Two recent clinical studies have shown that resuscitation outcomes are similar between neonates resuscitated with 100% oxygen compared with room air[219,220]; however, in one of these studies the incidence of cerebral palsy was nonsignificantly higher in the group treated with room air compared with that in the 100% oxygen group (12% compared with 9%, respectively), as well as the incidence of neurological abnormalities reported (15% compared with 10%, respectively).[220] Therefore the optimal FiO_2 for resuscitating victims of cardiac arrest needs to be further examined.

Multifaceted antioxidant therapeutic strategies have also been used in experimental asphyxial arrest. Cerchiari et al[94] produced an asphyxial arrest in mature dogs with a 5- to 8-minute period of airway obstruction followed by 7 minutes of cardiac standstill. Dogs treated with deferoxamine and SOD showed improved recovery of somatosensory evoked response, but functional neurological outcome was not evaluated. Rosenberg et al[221] showed improved CBF and $CMRO_2$ at 2 hours after prolonged hypoxia (without arrest) in newborn lambs pretreated with PEG-SOD and PEG-catalase. Thiringer et al[222] produced asphyxia in fetal lambs by umbilical cord clamping and studied two insults: severe asphyxia (until asystole) or moderate asphyxia (10 minutes). Treatment with the radical-scavenging compounds methionine and mannitol and the calcium antagonist lidoflazine increased survival and improved postischemic CBF. Long-term follow-up studies with antioxidant therapies in asphyxial arrest models and clinical studies are lacking.

Interventions targeting pathways indirectly related to free radical generation may be beneficial for reducing oxidative stress in the brain. Hypothermia reduces lipid peroxidation and maintains endogenous antioxidant activity during reperfusion from global brain ischemia[223] and is a promising therapy for improving neurological outcome after cardiac arrest.[178] Acidosis during ischemia increases free radial production[224] and may inactivate endogenous antioxidants[225]; however, the role of buffer therapy is controversial.

Phospholipid-Derived Mediator Manipulation and Antiinflammatory Therapies

Although many avenues exist for manipulation of phospholipid-derived mediator formation after global cerebral ischemia or cardiorespiratory arrest, most studies have focused on the AA cascade. Prostaglandins potentiate the effects of excitatory amino acids, and inhibition of this effect may explain the protection afforded by these agents. Similarly, inhibition of superoxide anion synthesis during the metabolism of AA also may be an important mechanism for this effect. Alternatively, cyclooxygenase metabolites of AA are important regulators of normal CBF, especially in the immature brain,[226] and cyclooxygenase inhibitors increase CBF after global ischemia.[227] Pretreatment with cyclooxygenase inhibitors (indomethacin, piroxicam, diclofenac, or flubiprofen) before 5 minutes of global brain ischemia in gerbils attenuated selectively vulnerable cell death.[228] In contrast, inhibition of the lipoxygenase pathway did not prevent selectively vulnerable cell death.[228] Cyclooxygenase inhibitors (indomethacin or diclofenac), however, are not protective when given before 10 minutes of global ischemia;[230] indomethacin administration *after* ischemia does not increase CBF;[231] and the effect of resuscitation with cyclooxygenase inhibitors on CBF after cardiorespiratory arrest has not been studied. A limit to the clinical effectiveness of cyclooxygenase inhibitors may be that a burst of cyclooxygenase product formation occurs within seconds of reperfusion.[232] Nevertheless, Kuhn et al[233] showed improved 24-hour neurological outcome in dogs treated with ibuprofen after a 6-minute VF arrest. The 46% mortality rate in vehicle-treated dogs after 6 minutes of VF was excessively high, however, and affected outcome scoring. Jastremski et al[234] retrospectively assessed the impact of steroid use in the 262 patients who did not receive thiopental in the Brain Resuscitation Clinical Trial I. Four groups (no, low-, medium-, or high-dose steroid) were compared. No effect on mortality or neurological outcome was seen.

Identification of and agents targeting specific cyclooxygenase isoforms has led to a resurgence of investigation in this area. The inducible form of cyclooxygenase is formed after tissue injury (cyclooxygenase II [COX-2]).[235] Thus COX-2 may be a more appropriate therapeutic target, if prostanoids or AA metabolites play an important role in ischemic brain injury. Currently, their use as a neuroresuscitative therapy after cardiopulmonary arrest is unsupported.[230,236] Recent data suggesting that COX-2 is upregulated after asphyxia in neonates[237] support further testing of more specific agents as they are developed.

Futuristic Approaches

Neuronal Regeneration

Several trophic factors are synthesized by neurons and other parenchymal cells and are critical to cellular maintenance and regeneration. Nerve growth factor,[238] brain-derived neurotrophic factor,[239] and neurotrophin-3[240] have all been shown to be neuroprotective in models of neonatal hypoxia ischemia. Many others, including vascular endothelial growth factor, have been found to be upregulated after cerebral ischemia.[241] Recently, D'Cruz et al[242] found that hypothermia increases brain-derived neurotrophic factor after asphyxial cardiac arrest in adult rats, and this increase implies enhancement of trophic factors as one possible mechanism behind the protective effects of hypothermia seen in this model. Several of these trophic factors are now commercially available. Augmentation of neuronal regeneration either through trophic factor replacement or augmentation by other means after cardiopulmonary arrest is an unexplored area for future research.

Pharmacogenetic Strategies

The advancement of sophisticated molecular techniques has led to the identification of many constitutive and inducible genes that regulate cell death or survival after injury. Currently known "death-effector" genes include apoptosis-inducing factor, *p53, bax, Fas,* and genes that encode the caspase family of cysteine proteases. "Death-suppressor" genes include inhibitor-of-apoptosis proteins, *bcl-2, bcl-xL,* and genes that encode the heat shock and other stress proteins. Many of these genes have been shown to play a role in regulating neuronal survival after cerebral ischemia. Antisense oligodeoxynucleotides, viral transfection or other means of gene or protein transfection, and transgenic models (knockouts) have been used to selectively alter expression of a specific gene in vivo. Although current limitations involving toxicity of these techniques prevent clinical application at this time, further research may generate clinically relevant therapies targeting host responses at the gene level that prevent secondary injury and promote cell survival.

Extracorporeal Support

As previously suggested, CPB initiated immediately after VF arrest in dogs (with cannulae already in place) improves outcome when compared with standard resuscitation guided by advanced cardiac life support (ACLS).[243] CPB produced 64% survival after even 20 minutes of VF arrest, although all dogs were neurologically impaired. This supports the concept that cerebral and coronary perfusion failure during CPR extends insult time, although studies with vascular cannulation during resuscitation have not been reported. These studies would be important in light of the difficulty in obtaining this type of vascular access during arrest in children. Nevertheless, extracorporeal support allows control of postarrest blood flow and temperature, and the cardiovascular support provided might allow use of otherwise contraindicated therapies. Recently, Chen et al[244] reported a 32% survival rate in adult patients rescued with extracorporeal membrane oxygenation (ECMO) after prolonged cardiac arrest. A strikingly favorable 5.6% incidence of severe neurological deficit was reported in survivors within this study.

A multimodality approach, combining hypothermia with extracorporeal modalities in pediatric patients after cardiopulmonary arrest, particularly refractory or prolonged arrest, appears to be the next logical step. This is not a new concept. In 1984, Dr. Safar et al recommended research into "suspended animation for delayed resuscitation" for situations in which conventional resuscitation attempts were not successful. Recently, they reported survival without brain damage after clinical death of 1 to 2 hours in dogs using suspended animation.[245] In their canine exsanguinations–cardiac arrest model, deep hypothermia (10° to 20° C) was induced by infusion of ice-cold saline via the abdominal aorta. Postarrest resuscitation and hemodynamic support was provided by CPB. Mild hypothermia was subsequently maintained at 34° C. Using this protocol, they reported good neurological outcome on the basis of overall performance category score, neurological deficit score, and brain histological damage score. The histological differences between the groups were striking, with little evidence of neuronal damage in dogs treated with the suspended animation strategy (Fig. 58–9). The use of CPB allows ROSC after a prolonged down time and control of postarrest blood flow and temperature, providing that the cardiovascular support that

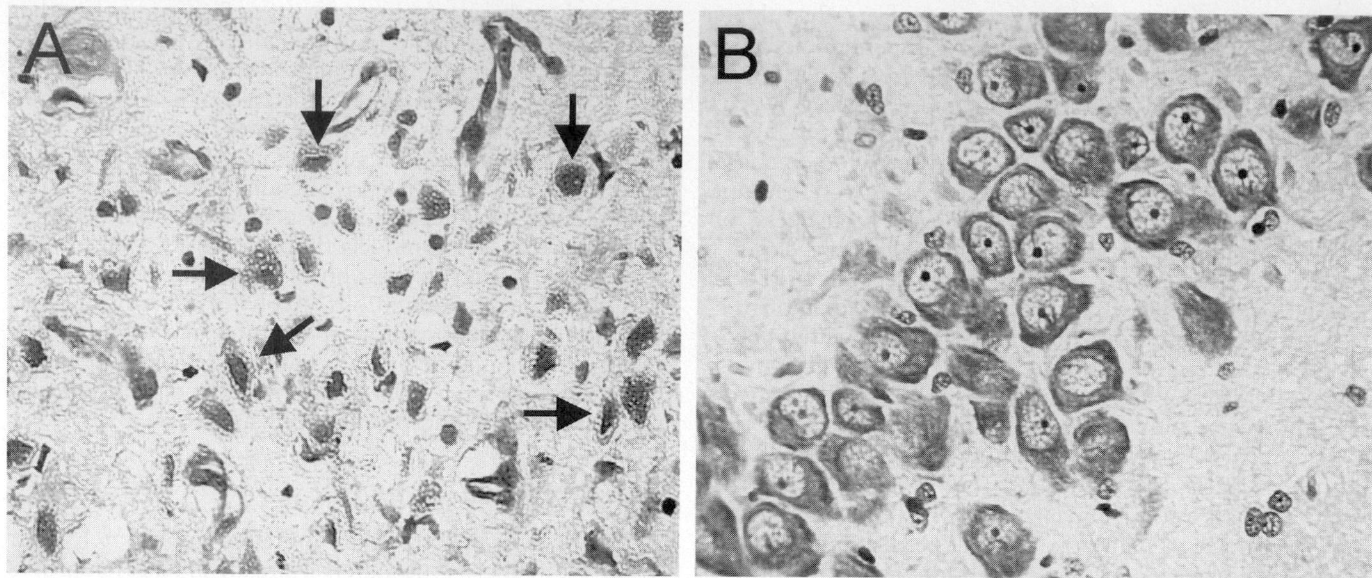

FIGURE 58–9 • With a "suspended animation" paradigm envisioned by Dr. Peter Safar, neuropathological damage typically produced by 60 min of no flow is dramatically reduced. The hippocampal region of dogs without treatment **(A)** compared with hypothermic intraaortic flush **(B)** is shown. Note extensive neuronal damage with evidence of DNA fragmentation (*arrows*) in Panel **A**.

many patients might require, particularly under conditions of more profound hypothermia, is available. Nagao et al[246] reported a 92% ROSC in 50 adult patients in whom standard CPR failed and who were rescued with CPB, followed by mild hypothermia (34° C) for a minimum of 2 days. These investigators also reported "good outcome" in 12 of the 23 long-term survivors. In the study by Chen et al,[244] hypothermia was not used with ECMO. Much of the mortality was attributed to multiple-organ failure (MOF) in this study. After a prolonged cardiopulmonary arrest, MOF is a common finding, sometimes ignored because the focus is generally on neurological status. Treatment of MOF will likely become necessary in the postresuscitation phase, particularly as effective cerebroprotective strategies are developed.

For patients at risk for the development of hypoxic-ischemic encephalopathy with MOF and coagulopathy, plasma exchange might be beneficial. Plasma exchange has been shown to reverse sepsis-induced MOF and effectively correct coagulopathy by removing cytokines and inflammatory mediators and restoring clotting homeostasis.[247] Granted, further clinical studies are needed; however, combining CPB, mild hypothermia, and plasma exchange would provide maximum therapeutic support after cardiopulmonary arrest, and all of these therapies are clinically used in pediatric patients. This concept of "therapeutic hibernation and plasma exchange" (HIBERPLEX) was introduced for recalcitrant shock in the pediatric population.[248] This approach could potentially provide neuroprotection, hemodynamic support, and reversal of MOF, thus targeting the major management challenges after prolonged cardiopulmonary arrest.

Summary

The social and economic impact of children left with persistent neurological injury after cardiorespiratory arrest is unacceptable. With the exception of near drowning, preventive approaches to this problem are unlikely to reduce significantly the occurrence of these multifactorial and largely unanticipated events. Improvements in prognostication after cardiopulmonary arrest are on the horizon with a more concerted application of existing methods and new techniques. The successful application of novel brain-oriented therapeutic approaches is somewhat more speculative but is likely to require intervention beginning in the prehospital setting or emergency department. Improved pathophysiologically guided stratification of patients after arrest is essential to determine which patients have resuscitative insults and, with optimal supportive care and prevention of secondary neuronal deterioration, potential for a good rather than vegetative outcome. Unfortunately, this group is unlikely to include most patients with asphyxial arrest and in any single institution represents a small number of cases per year. Biochemically guided, multifaceted pharmacological and mechanical approaches will almost certainly be required, with their application based on the temporal sequence of pathological events.

Acknowledgment

This chapter is dedicated to Peter J. Safar, the "Father of Modern-Day CPR," who passed away August 3, 2003. *Rest in Peace*.

REFERENCES

1. Hypothermia after Cardiac Arrest Study Group: Mild therapeutic hypothermia to improve the neurologic outcome after cardiac arrest, N Engl J Med 346:549-556, 2002.
2. Bernard SA, Gray TW, Buist MD, et al: Treatment of comatose survivors of out-of-hospital cardiac arrest with induced hypothermia, N Engl J Med 346:557-563, 2002.

application based on the temporal sequence of pathological events.

Acknowledgment

This chapter is dedicated to Peter J. Safar, the "Father of Modern-Day CPR," who passed away August 3, 2003. *Rest in Peace.*

REFERENCES

1. Hypothermia after Cardiac Arrest Study Group: Mild therapeutic hypothermia to improve the neurologic outcome after cardiac arrest, *N Engl J Med* 346:549-556, 2002.
2. Bernard SA, Gray TW, Buist MD, et al: Treatment of comatose survivors of out-of-hospital cardiac arrest with induced hypothermia, *N Engl J Med* 346:557-563, 2002.
3. Nolan JP, Morley PT, Vanden Hoek TL, et al: Therapeutic hypothermia after cardiac arrest: an advisory statement by the advanced life support task force of the International Liaison Committee on Resuscitation, *Circulation* 108:118-21, 2003.
4. Safar P: Cerebral resuscitation after cardiac arrest: a review, *Circulation* 74:111-138, 1986.
5. O'Rourke PP: Outcome of children who are apneic and pulseless in the emergency room, *Crit Care Med* 14:466-468, 1986.
6. Young KD, Seidel JS: Pediatric cardiopulmonary resuscitation: a collective review, *Ann Emerg Med* 33:195-205, 1999.
7. Reis AG, Nadkarni V, Perondi MB, et al: A prospective investigation into the epidemiology of in-hospital pediatric cardiopulmonary resuscitation using the international Utstein reporting style, *Pediatrics* 109:200-209, 2002.
8. Odden JP, Stiris T, Hansen TW, et al: Cerebral blood flow during experimental hypoxaemia and ischaemia in the newborn piglet, *Acta Paediatr Scand Suppl* 360:13-19, 1989.
9. Odden JP, Farstad T, Roll EB, et al: Cerebral blood flow autoregulation after moderate hypoxemia in the newborn piglet, *Biol Neonate* 65:367-377, 1994.
10. Fink EL, Alexander H, Marco CD, et al: Experimental model of pediatric asphyxial cardiopulmonary arrest in rats, *Pediatr Crit Care Med* 5:139-144, 2004.
11. Agnew DM, Koehler RC, Guerguerian AM, et al: Hypothermia for 24 hours after asphyxic cardiac arrest in piglets provides striatal neuroprotection that is sustained 10 days after rewarming, *Pediatr Res* 54:253-262, 2003.
12. Goldberg MP, Monyer H, Choi DW: Hypoxic neuronal injury in vitro depends on extracellular glutamine, *Neurosci Lett* 94:52-57, 1988.
13. Bodsch W, Barbier A, Oehmichen M, et al: Recovery of monkey brain after prolonged ischemia. II. Protein synthesis and morphological alterations, *J Cereb Blood Flow Metab* 6:22-33, 1986.
14. Vaagenes P, Safar P, Moossy J, et al: Asphyxiation versus ventricular fibrillation cardiac arrest in dogs. Differences in cerebral resuscitation effects–a preliminary study, *Resuscitation* 35:41-52, 1997.
15. Siesjo BK, Wieloch T: Cerebral metabolism in ischaemia: neurochemical basis for therapy, *BJA: Brit J Anaesth* 57:47-62, 1985.
16. Pellerin L, Magistretti PJ: Glutamate uptake into astrocytes stimulates aerobic glycolysis: A mechanism coupling neuronal activity to glucose utilization., *Proc Natl Acad Sci USA* 91:10625-10629, 1994.
17. Liou AK, Clark RS, Henshall DC, et al: To die or not to die for neurons in ischemia, traumatic brain injury and epilepsy: a review on the stress-activated signaling pathways and apoptotic pathways, *Prog Neurobiol* 69:103-142, 2003.
18. Choi DW: Ischemia-induced neuronal apoptosis, *Curr Opin Neurobiol* 6:667-672, 1996.
19. Portera-Cailliau C, Price DL, Martin LJ: Excitotoxic neuronal death in the immature brain is an apoptosis-necrosis morphological continuum., *J Comp Neurol* 378:70-87, 1997.
20. Bralet J, Schreiber L, Bouvier C: Effect of acidosis and anoxia on iron delocalization from brain homogenates, *Biochem Pharmacol* 43:979-983, 1992.
21. du Plessis AJ, Volpe JJ: Perinatal brain injury in the preterm and term newborn, *Curr Opin Neurol* 15:151-157, 2002.
22. Siesjo BK, Bengtsson F: Calcium fluxes, calcium antagonists, and calcium-related pathology in brain ischemia, hypoglycemia, and spreading depression: a unifying hypothesis, *J Cereb Blood Flow Metab* 9:127-140, 1989.
23. Katz LM, Callaway CW, Kagan VE, et al: Electron spin resonance measure of brain antioxidant activity during ischemia/reperfusion, *Neuroreport* 9:1587-1593, 1998.
24. Choi DW, Maulucci-Gedde M, Kriegstein AR: Glutamate neurotoxicity in cortical cell culture, *J Neurosci* 7:357-368, 1987.
25. Newell DW, Malouf AT, Franck JE: Glutamate-mediated selective vulnerability to ischemia is present in organotypic cultures of hippocampus, *Neurosci Lett* 116:325-330, 1990.
26. Brierley JB, Meldrum BS, Brown AW: The threshold and neuropathology of cerebral "anoxic-ischemic" cell change, *Arch Neurol* 29:367-374, 1973.
27. Buja LM, Eigenbrodt ML, Eigenbrodt EH: Apoptosis and necrosis. Basic types and mechanisms of cell death, *Arch Pathol Lab Med* 117:1208-1214, 1993.
28. Kerr JF, Wyllie AH, Currie AR: Apoptosis: a basic biological phenomenon with wide-ranging implications in tissue kinetics, *Br J Cancer* 26:239-257, 1972.
29. Cao G, Pei W, Lan J, et al: Caspase-activated DNase/DFF40 mediates apoptotic DNA fragmentation in transient cerebral ischemia and in neuronal cultures, *J. Neurosci,* 21:4678-4690, 2001.
30. Du L, Zhang X, Han YY, et al: Intra-mitochondrial poly-ADP-ribosylation contributes to NAD+ depletion and cell death induced by oxidative stress, *J Biol Chem*, 278:18426-18433, 2003.
31. Zhu C, Qiu L, Wang X, et al: Involvement of apoptosis-inducing factor in neuronal cell death after hypoxia-ischemia in the neonatal rat brain, *J Neurochem* 86:306-317, 2003.
32. Zhang X, Chen J, Graham SH, et al: Intranuclear localization of apoptosis-inducing factor (AIF) and large scale DNA fragmentation after traumatic brain injury in rats and in neuronal cultures exposed to peroxynitrite, *J Neurochem* 82:181-191, 2002.
33. Nitatori T, Sato N, Waguri S, et al: Delayed neuronal death in the CA1 pyramidal cell layer of the gerbil hippocampus following transient ischemia is apoptosis, *J Neurosci* 15:1001-1011, 1995.
34. Li Y, Chopp M, Jiang N, et al: Temporal profile of in situ DNA fragmentation after transient middle cerebral artery occlusion in the rat, *J Cereb Blood Flow Metab* 15:389-397, 1995.
35. Cheng Y, Deshmukh M, D'Costa A, et al: Caspase inhibitor affords neuroprotection with delayed administration in a rat model of neonatal hypoxic-ischemic brain injury, *J Clin Invest* 101:1992-1999, 1998.
36. MacManus JP, Buchan AM: Apoptosis after experimental stroke: fact or fashion? *J Neurotrauma* 17:899-914, 2000.
37. Deshpande J, Bergstedt K, Linden T, et al: Ultrastructural changes in the hippocampal CA1 region following transient cerebral ischemia: evidence against programmed cell death, *Exp Brain Res* 88:91-105, 1992.
38. Lemaire C, Andreau K, Souvannavong V, et al: Inhibition of caspase activity induces a switch from apoptosis to necrosis., *FEBS Lett* 425:266-270, 1998.
39. Kloner RA, Przyklenk K, Whittaker P: Deleterious effects of oxygen radicals in ischemia/reperfusion. Resolved and unresolved issues, *Circulation* 80:1115-1127, 1989.
40. Siesjo BK, Agardh CD, Bengtsson F: Free radicals and brain damage, *Cerebrovasc Brain Metab Rev* 1:165-211, 1989.
41. Opie LH: Reperfusion injury and its pharmacologic modification, *Circulation* 80:1049-1062, 1989.
42. Hallenbeck JM: Prevention of postischemic impairment of microvascular perfusion, *Neurology* 27:3-10, 1977.
43. Rothman S: Synaptic release of excitatory amino acid neurotransmitter mediates anoxic neuronal death, *J Neurosci* 4:1884-1891, 1984.
44. Dugan LL, Choi DW: Excitotoxicity, free radicals, and cell membrane changes, *Ann Neurol* 35 Suppl:S17-21, 1994.
45. Lipton SA, Rosenberg PA: Excitatory amino acids as a final common pathway for neurologic disorders, *N Engl J Med* 330:613-622, 1994.
46. Stys PK, Waxman SG, Ransom BR: Ionic mechanisms of anoxic injury in mammalian CNS white matter: role of Na+ channels and Na(+)-Ca2+ exchanger, *J Neurosci* 12:430-439, 1992.

47. Bellamy R, Safar P, Tisherman SA, et al: Suspended animation for delayed resuscitation, *Crit Care Med* 24:S24-47, 1996.
48. Lafon-Cazal M, Pietri S, Culcasi M, et al: NMDA-dependent superoxide production and neurotoxicity, *Nature* 364:535-537, 1993.
49. Bartus RT, Baker KL, Heiser AD, et al: Postischemic administration of AK275, a calpain inhibitor, provides substantial protection against focal ischemic brain damage, *J Cereb Blood Flow Metab* 14:537-544, 1994.
50. Gill R, Soriano M, Blomgren K, et al: Role of caspase-3 activation in cerebral ischemia-induced neurodegeneration in adult and neonatal brain, *J Cereb Blood Flow Metab* 22:420-430, 2002.
51. Kontos HA: Oxygen radicals from arachidonate metabolism in abnormal vascular responses, *Am Rev Respir Dis* 136:474-477, 1987.
52. Betz AL, Randall J, Martz D: Xanthine oxidase is not a major source of free radicals in focal cerebral ischemia, *Am J Physiol* 260:H563-568, 1991.
53. Lindsay S, Liu TH, Xu JA, et al: Role of xanthine dehydrogenase and oxidase in focal cerebral ischemic injury to rat, *Am J Physiol* 261:H2051-2057, 1991.
54. Komara JS, Nayini NR, Bialick HA, et al: Brain iron delocalization and lipid peroxidation following cardiac arrest, *Ann Emerg Med* 15:384-389, 1986.
55. Garthwaite J, Garthwaite G, Palmer RM, et al: NMDA receptor activation induces nitric oxide synthesis from arginine in rat brain slices, *Eur J Pharmacol* 172:413-416, 1989.
56. Beckman JS, Beckman TW, Chen J, et al: Apparent hydroxyl radical production by peroxynitrite: implications for endothelial injury from nitric oxide and superoxide, *Proc Natl Acad Sci U S A* 87:1620-1624, 1990.
57. Gilman SC, Bonner MJ, Pellmar TC: Free radicals enhance basal release of D-[3H]aspartate from cerebral cortical synaptosomes, *J Neurochem* 62:1757-1763, 1994.
58. Krause GS, DeGracia DJ, Skjaerlund JM, et al: Assessment of free radical-induced damage in brain proteins after ischemia and reperfusion, *Resuscitation* 23:59-69, 1992.
59. Bromont C, Marie C, Bralet J: Increased lipid peroxidation in vulnerable brain regions after transient forebrain ischemia in rats, *Stroke* 20:918-924, 1989.
60. Oliver CN, Starke-Reed PE, Stadtman ER, et al: Oxidative damage to brain proteins, loss of glutamine synthetase activity, and production of free radicals during ischemia/reperfusion-induced injury to gerbil brain, *Proc Natl Acad Sci U S A* 87:5144-5147, 1990.
61. White BC, Tribhuwan RC, Vander Laan DJ, et al: Brain mitochondrial DNA is not damaged by prolonged cardiac arrest or reperfusion, *J Neurochem* 58:1716-1722, 1992.
62. Cochrane CG: Mechanisms of oxidant injury of cells, *Mol Aspects Med* 12:137-147, 1991.
63. Hockenbery DM, Oltvai ZN, Yin XM, et al: Bcl-2 functions in an antioxidant pathway to prevent apoptosis, *Cell* 75:241-251, 1993.
64. Nagayama T, Lan J, Henshall DC, et al: Induction of oxidative DNA damage in the peri-infarct region after permanent focal cerebral ischemia, *J Neurochem* 75:1716-1728, 2000.
65. Bayir H, Kagan VE, Tyurina YY, et al: Assessment of antioxidant reserves and oxidative stress in cerebrospinal fluid after severe traumatic brain injury in infants and children, *Pediatr Res* 51:571-578, 2002.
66. Shiu GK, Nemmer JP, Nemoto EM: Reassessment of brain free fatty acid liberation during global ischemia and its attenuation by barbiturate anesthesia, *J Neurochem* 40:880-884, 1983.
67. Ikeda M, Yoshida S, Busto R, et al: Polyphosphoinositides as a probable source of brain free fatty acids accumulated at the onset of ischemia, *J Neurochem* 47:123-132, 1986.
68. Abe K, Kogure K, Yamamoto H, et al: Mechanism of arachidonic acid liberation during ischemia in gerbil cerebral cortex, *J Neurochem* 48:503-509, 1987.
69. Bazan NG, *Involvement of acachidonic acid and platelet-activating factor in the response of the nervous system to ischemia and convulsions*, in *Lipid mediators in ischemic brain damage and experimental epilepsy*, N.G. Bazan, Editor. 1990, Karger: Basel. p. kon.
70. Simon RP, Cho H, Gwinn R, et al: The temporal profile of 72-kDa heat-shock protein expression following global ischemia, *J Neurosci* 11:881-889, 1991.
71. Seidberg N, Clark RS, Zhang X, et al: Alterations in inducible 72 kilodalton heat shock protein and the chaperone cofactor BAG-1 in human brain after head injury, *J Neurochem* in press, 2002.
72. Murphy SJ, Song D, Welsh FA, et al: Regional expression of heat shock protein 72 mRNA following mild and severe hypoxia in neonatal piglet brain, *Adv Exper Med Biol* 471:155-163, 1999.
73. Chopp M, Chen H, Ho KL, et al: Transient hyperthermia protects against subsequent forebrain ischemic cell damage in the rat, *Neurology* 39:1396-1398, 1989.
74. Ota A, Ikeda T, Xia XY, et al: Hypoxic-ischemic tolerance induced by hyperthermic pretreatment in newborn rats, *J Soc Gynecol Invest* 7:102-105, 2000.
75. Lowenstein DH, Chan PH, Miles MF: The stress protein response in cultured neurons: characterization and evidence for a protective role in excitotoxicity, *Neuron* 7:1053-1060, 1991.
76. Hoehn B, Ringer TM, Xu L, et al: Overexpression of HSP72 after induction of experimental stroke protects neurons from ischemic damage, *J Cereb Blood Flow Metab* 21:1303-1309, 2001.
77. Tsuchiya D, Hong S, Matsumori Y, et al: Overexpression of rat heat shock protein 70 is associated with reduction of early mitochondrial cytochrome C release and subsequent DNA fragmentation after permanent focal ischemia, *J Cereb Blood Flow Metab* 23:718-727, 2003.
78. Kelly S, Zhang ZJ, Zhao H, et al: Gene transfer of HSP72 protects cornu ammonis 1 region of the hippocampus neurons from global ischemia: influence of Bcl-2, *Annals of Neurology* 52:160-167, 2002.
79. Kane DJ, Ord T, Anton R, et al: Expression of bcl-2 inhibits necrotic neural cell death, *J Neurosci Res* 40:269-275, 1995.
80. Chen J, Graham SH, Chan PH, et al: bcl-2 is expressed in neurons that survive focal ischemia in the rat, *Neuroreport* 6:394-398, 1995.
81. Shimazaki K, Ishida A, Kawai N: Increase in bcl-2 oncoprotein and the tolerance to ischemia-induced neuronal death in the gerbil hippocampus, *Neurosci Res* 20:95-99, 1994.
82. Krajewski S, Mai JK, Krajewska M, et al: Upregulation of bax protein levels in neurons following cerebral ischemia, *J Neurosci* 15:6364-6376, 1995.
83. Linnik MD, Zahos P, Geschwind MD, et al: Expression of bcl-2 from a defective herpes simplex virus-1 vector limits neuronal death in focal cerebral ischemia, *Stroke* 26:1670-4; discussion 1675, 1995.
84. Chen Y, Ginis I, Hallenbeck JM: The protective effect of ceramide in immature rat brain hypoxia-ischemia involves up-regulation of bcl-2 and reduction of TUNEL-positive cells, *J Cereb Blood Flow Metab* 21:34-40, 2001.
85. Cao G, Pei W, Ge H, et al: In Vivo Delivery of a Bcl-xL Fusion Protein Containing the TAT Protein Transduction Domain Protects against Ischemic Brain Injury and Neuronal Apoptosis, *J Neurosci* 22:5423-5431, 2002.
86. Clark RS, Kochanek PM, Chen M, et al: Increases in Bcl-2 and cleavage of Caspase-1 and Caspase-3 in human brain after head injury, *FASEB J* 13:813-821, 1999.
87. Phillis JW, Smith-Barbour M, O'Regan MH, et al: Amino acid and purine release in rat brain following temporary middle cerebral artery occlusion, *Neurochem Res* 19:1125-1130, 1994.
88. Morii S, Ngai AC, Ko KR, et al: Role of adenosine in regulation of cerebral blood flow: effects of theophylline during normoxia and hypoxia, *Am J Physiol* 253:H165-H175, 1987.
89. Laudignon N, Beharry K, Farri E, et al: The role of adenosine in the vascular adaptation of neonatal cerebral blood flow during hypotension, *J Cereb Blood Flow Metab* 11:424-431, 1991.
90. Ruth VJ, Park TS, Gonzales ER, et al: Adenosine and cerebrovascular hyperemia during insulin-induced hypoglycemia in newborn piglet., *Am J Physiol* 265:H1762-H1768, 1993.
91. Miller LP, Hsu C: Therapeutic potential for adenosine receptor activation in ischemic brain injury, *J Neurotrauma* 9 Suppl 2:S563-S5677, 1992.
92. Rudolphi KA, Schubert P, Parkinson FE, et al: Neuroprotective role of adenosine in cerebral ischaemia, *Trends Pharmacol Sci* 13:439-445, 1992.
93. Snyder JV, Nemoto EM, Carroll RG, et al: Global ischemia in dogs: intracranial pressures, brain blood flow and metabolism, *Stroke* 6:21-27, 1975.
94. Cerchiari EL, Hoel TM, Safar P, et al: Protective effects of combined superoxide dismutase and deferoxamine on recovery of cerebral blood flow and function after cardiac arrest in dogs, *Stroke* 18:869-878, 1987.
95. Rosenberg AA: Cerebral blood flow and O2 metabolism after asphyxia in neonatal lambs, *Pediatr Res* 20:778-782, 1986.

96. Michenfelder JD, Milde JH: Postischemic canine cerebral blood flow appears to be determined by cerebral metabolic needs, *J Cereb Blood Flow Metab* 10:71-76, 1990.
97. Wolfson SK, Jr., Safar P, Reich H, et al: Dynamic heterogeneity of cerebral hypoperfusion after prolonged cardiac arrest in dogs measured by the stable xenon/CT technique: a preliminary study, *Resuscitation* 23:1-20, 1992.
98. Sterz F, Leonov Y, Safar P, et al: Multifocal cerebral blood flow by Xe-CT and global cerebral metabolism after prolonged cardiac arrest in dogs. Reperfusion with open-chest CPR or cardiopulmonary bypass, *Resuscitation* 24:27-47, 1992.
99. Steen PA, Gisvold SE, Milde JH, et al: Nimodipine improves outcome when given after complete cerebral ischemia in primates, *Anesthesiology* 62:406-414, 1985.
100. Karinen P, Koivukangas P, Ohinmaa A, et al: Cost-effectiveness analysis of nimodipine treatment after aneurysmal subarachnoid hemorrhage and surgery, *Neurosurgery* 45:780-4; discussion 784-785, 1999.
101. Horn J, de Haan RJ, Vermeulen M, et al: Very Early Nimodipine Use in Stroke (VENUS): a randomized, double-blind, placebo-controlled trial, *Stroke* 32:461-465, 2001.
102. Safar P, Xiao F, Radovsky A, et al: Improved cerebral resuscitation from cardiac arrest in dogs with mild hypothermia plus blood flow promotion, *Stroke* 27:105-113, 1996.
103. Beckstead JE, Tweed WA, Lee J, et al: Cerebral blood flow and metabolism in man following cardiac arrest, *Stroke* 9:569-573, 1978.
104. Cohan SL, Mun SK, Petite J, et al: Cerebral blood flow in humans following resuscitation from cardiac arrest, *Stroke* 20:761-765, 1989.
105. Bergsneider M, Hovda DA, Shalmon E, et al: Cerebral hyperglycolysis following severe traumatic brain injury in humans: a positron emission tomography study, *J Neurosurg* 86:241-251, 1997.
106. Mujsce DJ, Christensen MA, Vannucci RC: Cerebral blood flow and edema in perinatal hypoxic-ischemic brain damage, *Pediatr Res* 27:450-453, 1990.
107. Ashwal S, Schneider S, Tomasi L, et al: Prognostic implications of hyperglycemia and reduced cerebral blood flow in childhood near-drowning, *Neurology* 40:820-823, 1990.
108. Beyda DH, *The prognostic value of measuring regional cerebral blood flow in the neuro-compromised paediatric patient*, in *Current problems in neurology: impact of functional imaging*, J. Wade, Editor. 1987, J Libbey. London.
109. Jacobs MM, Phibbs RH: Prevention, recognition, and treatment of perinatal asphyxia, *Clin Perinatol* 16:785-807, 1989.
110. Nemoto EM, Bleyaert AL, Stezoski SW, et al: Global brain ischemia: a reproducible monkey model, *Stroke* 8:558-564, 1977.
111. Katz L, Ebmeyer U, Safar P, et al: Outcome model of asphyxial cardiac arrest in rats, *J Cereb Blood Flow Metab* 15:1032-1039, 1995.
112. Ng T, Graham DI, Adams JH, et al: Changes in the hippocampus and the cerebellum resulting from hypoxic insults: frequency and distribution, *Acta Neuropathol (Berl)* 78:438-443, 1989.
113. Kinney HC, Korein J, Panigrahy A, et al: Neuropathological findings in the brain of Karen Ann Quinlan. The role of the thalamus in the persistent vegetative state, *N Engl J Med* 330:1469-1475, 1994.
114. Fisher B, Peterson B, Hicks G: Use of brainstem auditory-evoked response testing to assess neurologic outcome following near drowning in children, *Crit Care Med* 20:578-585, 1992.
115. Zaritsky A: Cardiopulmonary resuscitation in children, *Clin Chest Med* 8:561-571, 1987.
116. Earnest MP, Yarnell PR, Merrill SL, et al: Long-term survival and neurologic status after resuscitation from out-of-hospital cardiac arrest, *Neurology* 30:1298-1302, 1980.
117. Biggart MJ, Bohn DJ: Effect of hypothermia and cardiac arrest on outcome of near-drowning accidents in children, *J Pediatr* 117:179-183, 1990.
118. Robertson CM, Joffe AR, Moore AJ, et al: Neurodevelopmental outcome of young pediatric intensive care unit survivors of serious brain injury, *Pediatr Crit Care Med* 3:345-350, 2002.
119. Lewis JK, Minter MG, Eshelman SJ, et al: Outcome of pediatric resuscitation, *Ann Emerg Med* 12:297-299, 1983.
120. Torphy DE, Minter MG, Thompson BM: Cardiorespiratory arrest and resuscitation of children, *Am J Dis Child* 138:1099-1102, 1984.
121. Levy DE, Caronna JJ, Singer BH, et al: Predicting outcome from hypoxic-ischemic coma, *JAMA* 253:1420-1426, 1985.
122. Edgren E, Hedstrand U, Nordin M, et al: Prediction of outcome after cardiac arrest, *Crit Care Med* 15:820-825, 1987.
123. Mullie A, Verstringe P, Buylaert W, et al: Predictive value of Glasgow coma score for awakening after out-of-hospital cardiac arrest. Cerebral Resuscitation Study Group of the Belgian Society for Intensive Care, *Lancet* 1:137-140, 1988.
124. Sirbaugh PE, Pepe PE, Shook JE, et al: A prospective, population-based study of the demographics, epidemiology, management, and outcome of out-of-hospital pediatric cardiopulmonary arrest.[comment][erratum appears in Ann Emerg Med 1999 Mar;33(3):358], *Ann Emerg Med* 33:174-184, 1999.
125. Safar P, Bircher N, Pretto E, Jr., et al: Reappraisal of mouth-to-mouth ventilation, *Ann Emerg Med* 31:653-654, 1998.
126. Becker LB, Berg RA, Pepe PE, et al: A reappraisal of mouth-to-mouth ventilation during bystander-initiated cardiopulmonary resuscitation: a statement for Healthcare Professionals from the Ventilation Working Group of the Basic Life Support and Pediatric Life Support Subcommittees, American Heart Association, *Ann Emerg Med* 30:654-666, 1997.
127. Scollo-Lavizzari G, Bassetti C: Prognostic value of EEG in post-anoxic coma after cardiac arrest, *Eur Neurol* 26:161-170, 1987.
128. Meynaar IA, Straaten HM, van der Wetering J, et al: Serum neuron-specific enolase predicts outcome in post-anoxic coma: a prospective cohort study, *Inten Care Med* 29:189-195, 2003.
129. Martens P, Raabe A, Johnsson P: Serum S-100 and neuron-specific enolase for prediction of regaining consciousness after global cerebral ischemia, *Stroke* 29:2363-2366, 1998.
130. Zingler VC, Krumm B, Bertsch T, et al: Early prediction of neurological outcome after cardiopulmonary resuscitation: a multimodal approach combining neurobiochemical and electrophysiological investigations may provide high prognostic certainty in patients after cardiac arrest, *Eur Neurol* 49:79-84, 2003.
131. Madl C, Grimm G, Kramer L, et al: Early prediction of individual outcome after cardiopulmonary resuscitation, *Lancet* 341:855-858, 1993.
132. Miller JR, Myers RE: Neuropathology of systemic circulatory arrest in adult monkeys, *Neurology* 22:888-904, 1972.
133. Ment LR, Stewart WB, Duncan CC, et al: Beagle pup model of perinatal asphyxia: nimodipine studies, *Stroke* 18:599-605, 1987.
134. Kirsch JR, Helfaer MA, Blizzard K, et al: Age-related cerebrovascular response to global ischemia in pigs, *Am J Physiol* 259:H1551-H1558, 1990.
135. Roland EH, Hill A, Norman MG, et al: Selective brainstem injury in an asphyxiated newborn, *Ann Neurol* 23:89-92, 1988.
136. van Lookeren Campagne M, Verheul JB, Nicolay K, et al: Early evolution and recovery from excitotoxic injury in the neonatal rat brain: a study combining magnetic resonance imaging, electrical impedance, and histology, *J Cereb Blood Flow Metab* 14:1011-1023, 1994.
137. Johnston MV: Developmental aspects of NMDA receptor agonists and antagonists in the central nervous system, *Psychopharmacol Bull* 30:567-575, 1994.
138. Ikonomidou C, Bosch F, Miksa M, et al: Blockade of NMDA receptors and apoptotic neurodegeneration in the developing brain, *Science* 283:70-74, 1999.
139. Finger S, Almli CR: Brain damage and neuroplasticity: mechanisms of recovery or development? *Brain Res* 357:177-186, 1985.
140. Hicks SP, D'Amato CJ: Motor-sensory and visual behavior after hemispherectomy in newborn and mature rats, *Exp Neurol* 29:416-438, 1970.
141. Hoffman WE, Braucher E, Pelligrino DA, et al: Brain lactate and neurologic outcome following incomplete ischemia in fasted, nonfasted, and glucose-loaded rats, *Anesthesiology* 72:1045-1050, 1990.
142. Kalimo H, Rehncrona S, Soderfeldt B, et al: Brain lactic acidosis and ischemic cell damage: 2. Histopathology, *J Cereb Blood Flow Metab* 1:313-327, 1981.
143. Rehncrona S, Rosen I, Siesjo BK: Brain lactic acidosis and ischemic cell damage: 1. Biochemistry and neurophysiology, *J Cereb Blood Flow Metab* 1:297-311, 1981.
144. Simon R, Shiraishi K: N-methyl-D-aspartate antagonist reduces stroke size and regional glucose metabolism, *Ann Neurol* 27:606-611, 1990.

145. Kraig RP, Petito CK, Plum F, et al: Hydrogen ions kill brain at concentrations reached in ischemia, *J Cereb Blood Flow Metab* 7:379-386, 1987.
146. Myerburg RJ, Estes D, Zaman L, et al: Outcome of resuscitation from bradyarrhythmic or asystolic prehospital cardiac arrest, *J Am Coll Cardiol* 4:1118-1122, 1984.
147. Martin LJ, Brambrink A, Koehler RC, et al: Primary sensory and forebrain motor systems in the newborn brain are preferentially damaged by hypoxia-ischemia, *J Comp Neurol* 377:262-285, 1997.
148. Brown CG, Werman HA: Adrenergic agonists during cardiopulmonary resuscitation, *Resuscitation* 19:1-16, 1990.
149. Berg RA, Otto CW, Kern KB, et al: A randomized, blinded trial of high-dose epinephrine versus standard-dose epinephrine in a swine model of pediatric asphyxial cardiac arrest, *Crit Care Med* 24:1695-1700, 1996.
150. Voelckel WG, Lurie KG, McKnite S, et al: Effects of epinephrine and vasopressin in a piglet model of prolonged ventricular fibrillation and cardiopulmonary resuscitation, *Crit Care Med* 30:957-962, 2002.
151. Goetting MG, Paradis NA: High-dose epinephrine improves outcome from pediatric cardiac arrest, *Ann Emerg Med* 20:22-26, 1991.
152. Sutton-Tyrrell K, Snyder JV, Kelsey S, et al: Risk monitoring of randomized trials in emergency medicine: experience of the Brain Resuscitation Clinical Trial II, *Am J Emerg Med* 9:112-117, 1991.
153. Vandycke C, Martens P: High dose versus standard dose epinephrine in cardiac arrest - a meta-analysis, *Resuscitation* 45:161-166, 2000.
154. Dean JM, McComb JG: Intracranial pressure monitoring in severe pediatric near-drowning, *Neurosurgery* 9:627-630, 1981.
155. Nussbaum E, Galant SP: Intracranial pressure monitoring as a guide to prognosis in the nearly drowned, severely comatose child, *J Pediatr* 102:215-218, 1983.
156. Frewen TC, Sumabat WO, Han VK, et al: Cerebral resuscitation therapy in pediatric near-drowning, *J Pediatr* 106:615-617, 1985.
157. Sarnaik AP, Preston G, Lieh-Lai M, et al: Intracranial pressure and cerebral perfusion pressure in near-drowning, *Crit Care Med* 13:224-227, 1985.
158. Vanicky I, Marsala M, Murar J, et al: Prolonged postischemic hyperventilation reduces acute neuronal damage after 15 min of cardiac arrest in the dog, *Neurosci Lett* 135:167-170, 1992.
159. Muizelaar JP, Marmarou A, Ward JD, et al: Adverse effects of prolonged hyperventilation in patients with severe head injury: a randomized clinical trial, *J Neurosurg* 75:731-739, 1991.
160. Miller CL, Lampard DG, Alexander K, et al: Local cerebral blood flow following transient cerebral ischemia. I. Onset of impaired reperfusion within the first hour following global ischemia, *Stroke* 11:534-541, 1980.
161. Todd MM, Tommasino C, Shapiro HM: Cerebrovascular effects of prolonged hypocarbia and hypercarbia after experimental global ischemia in cats, *Crit Care Med* 13:720-723, 1985.
162. Cold GE: Does acute hyperventilation provoke cerebral oligaemia in comatose patients after acute head injury? *Acta Neurochir (Wien)* 96:100-106, 1989.
163. Arai T, Tsukahara I, Nitta K, et al: Effects of mannitol on cerebral circulation after transient complete cerebral ischemia in dogs, *Crit Care Med* 14:634-637, 1986.
164. Muizelaar JP, Ward JD, Marmarou A, et al: Cerebral blood flow and metabolism in severely head-injured children. Part 2: Autoregulation, *J Neurosurg* 71:72-76, 1989.
165. Moolten SE: Albumin therapy for brain swelling in cardiac arrest: a proposal, *Mt Sinai J Med* 46:277-287, 1979.
166. Cole F: Use of human serum albumini n cerebral edema following cardiac arrest, report of a case, *JAMA* 147:1563-1564, 1951.
167. Belayev L, Saul I, Huh PW, et al: Neuroprotective effect of high-dose albumin therapy against global ischemic brain injury in rats, *Brain Res* 845:107-111, 1999.
168. Breil M, Krep H, Sinn D, et al: Hypertonic saline improves myocardial blood flow during CPR, but is not enhanced further by the addition of hydroxy ethyl starch, *Resuscitation* 56:307-317, 2003.
169. Lubchenco LO, Bard H: Incidence of hypoglycemia in newborn infants classified by birth weight and gestational age, *Pediatrics* 47:831-838, 1971.
170. Chiaretti A, Piastra M, Pulitano S, et al: Prognostic factors and outcome of children with severe head injury: an 8-year experience, *Childs Nerv Syst* 18:129-136, 2002.
171. Bleyaert AL, Sands PA, Safar P, et al: Augmentation of postischemic brain damage by severe intermittent hypertension, *Crit Care Med* 8:41-47, 1980.
172. Bohn DJ, Biggar WD, Smith CR, et al: Influence of hypothermia, barbiturate therapy, and intracranial pressure monitoring on morbidity and mortality after near-drowning, *Crit Care Med* 14:529-534, 1986.
173. Phelps C, *Principles of Treatment*, in *Traumatic Injuries of the Brain and Its Membranes*, M. Critchley, et al., Editors. 1897, D. Appleton and Company: New York. p. 223.
174. Rosomoff HL, Holaday DA: Cerebral blood flow and cerebral oxygen consumption during hypothermia, *Am J Physiol* 179:85-88, 1954.
175. Yager JY, Asselin J: Effect of mild hypothermia on cerebral energy metabolism during the evolution of hypoxic-ischemic brain damage in the immature rat, *Stroke* 27:919-926, 1996.
176. Busto R, Dietrich WD, Globus MY, et al: Small differences in intraischemic brain temperature critically determine the extent of ischemic neuronal injury, *J Cereb Blood Flow Metab* 7:729-738, 1987.
177. Hickey RW, Ferimer H, Alexander HL, et al: Delayed, spontaneous hypothermia reduces neuronal damage after asphyxial cardiac arrest in rats, *Crit Care Med* 28:3511-3516, 2000.
178. Leonov Y, Sterz F, Safar P, et al: Mild cerebral hypothermia during and after cardiac arrest improves neurologic outcome in dogs, *J Cereb Blood Flow Metab* 10:57-70, 1990.
179. Weinrauch V, Safar P, Tisherman S, et al: Beneficial effect of mild hypothermia and detrimental effect of deep hypothermia after cardiac arrest in dogs, *Stroke* 23:1454-1462, 1992.
180. Tisherman SA, Rodriguez A, Safar P: Therapeutic hypothermia in traumatology, *Surg Clin N Am* 79:1269-1289, 1999.
181. Xiao F, Safar P, Alexander H: Peritoneal cooling for mild cerebral hypothermia after cardiac arrest in dogs., *Resuscitation* 30:51-59, 1995.
182. Behringer W, Safar P, Wu X, et al: Veno-venous extracorporeal blood shunt cooling to induce mild hypothermia in dog experiments and review of cooling methods, *Resuscitation* 54:89-98, 2002.
183. Bernard S, Buist M, Monteiro O, et al: Induced hypothermia using large volume, ice-cold intravenous fluid in comatose survivors of out-of-hospital cardiac arrest: a preliminary report, *Resuscitation* 56:9-13, 2003.
184. Frank SM, Raja SN, Bulcao C, et al: Age-related thermoregulatory differences during core cooling in humans, *Am J Physiol - Reg Integ Comp Physiol* 279:R349-354, 2000.
185. Hickey RW, Kochanek PM, Ferimer H, et al: Hypothermia and hyperthermia in children after resuscitation from cardiac arrest, *Pediatrics* 106:118-122, 2000.
186. Minamisawa H, Smith ML, Siesjo BK: The effect of mild hyperthermia and hypothermia on brain damage following 5, 10, and 15 minutes of forebrain ischemia, *Ann Neurol* 28:26-33, 1990.
187. Battin MR, Penrice J, Gunn TR, et al: Treatment of term infants with head cooling and mild systemic hypothermia (35.0 degrees C and 34.5 degrees C) after perinatal asphyxia, *Pediatrics* 111:244-251, 2003.
188. Kuroiwa T, Bonnekoh P, Hossmann KA: Therapeutic window of CA1 neuronal damage defined by an ultrashort-acting barbiturate after brain ischemia in gerbils, *Stroke* 21:1489-493, 1990.
189. Steen PA, Michenfelder JD: Mechanisms of barbiturate protection, *Anesthesiology* 53:183-185, 1980.
190. Detre K, Abramson N, Safar P, et al: Collaborative randomized clinical study of cardiopulmonary-cerebral resuscitation, *Crit Care Med* 9:395-396, 1981.
191. Albers GW, Goldberg MP, Choi DW: N-methyl-D-aspartate antagonists: ready for clinical trial in brain ischemia? *Ann Neurol* 25:398-403, 1989.
192. Guerguerian AM, Brambrink AM, Traystman RJ, et al: Altered expression and phosphorylation of N-methyl-D-aspartate receptors in piglet striatum after hypoxia-ischemia, *Brain Res Mol Brain Res* 104:66-80, 2002.
193. Buchan A, Li H, Pulsinelli WA: The N-methyl-D-aspartate antagonist, MK-801, fails to protect against neuronal damage caused by transient, severe forebrain ischemia in adult rats, *J Neurosci* 11:1049-1056, 1991.

194. Brambrink AM, Martin LJ, Hanley DF, et al: Effects of the AMPA receptor antagonist NBQX on outcome of newborn pigs after asphyxic cardiac arrest, *J Cereb Blood Flow Metab* 19:927-938, 1999.
195. Lysko PG, Webb CL, Yue TL, et al: Neuroprotective effects of tetrodotoxin as a Na+ channel modulator and glutamate release inhibitor in cultured rat cerebellar neurons and in gerbil global brain ischemia, *Stroke* 25:2476-2482, 1994.
196. Davis SM, Lees KR, Albers GW, et al: Selfotel in acute ischemic stroke: possible neurotoxic effects of an NMDA antagonist, *Stroke* 31:347-354, 2000.
197. Grotta JC, Picone CM, Earls R, et al: Calcium-calmodulin binding in ischemic rat neurons after calcium channel blocker therapy, *Stroke* 21:948-952, 1990.
198. Forsman M, Aarseth HP, Nordby HK, et al: Effects of nimodipine on cerebral blood flow and cerebrospinal fluid pressure after cardiac arrest: correlation with neurologic outcome, *Anesth Analg* 68:436-443, 1989.
199. Roine RO, Kajaste S, Kaste M: Neuropsychological sequelae of cardiac arrest, *JAMA* 269:237-242, 1993.
200. Helfaer MA, Kirsch JR, Haun SE, et al: Polyethylene glycol-conjugated superoxide dismutase fails to blunt postischemic reactive hyperemia, *Am J Physiol* 261:H548-553, 1991.
201. Lim KH, Connolly M, Rose D, et al: Prevention of reperfusion injury of the ischemic spinal cord: use of recombinant superoxide dismutase, *Ann Thorac Surg* 42:282-286, 1986.
202. Hayashi M, Slater TF: Inhibitory effects of ebselen on lipid peroxidation in rat liver microsomes, *Free Radic Res Commun* 2:179-185, 1986.
203. Kramer K, Voss HP, Grimbergen JA, et al: Glutathione mobilization during cerebral ischemia and reperfusion in the rat, *Gen Pharmacol* 23:105-108, 1992.
204. Ikeda Y, Anderson JH, Long DM: Oxygen free radicals in the genesis of traumatic and peritumoral brain edema, *Neurosurgery* 24:679-685, 1989.
205. Liu TH, Beckman JS, Freeman BA, et al: Polyethylene glycol-conjugated superoxide dismutase and catalase reduce ischemic brain injury, *Am J Physiol* 256:H589-593, 1989.
206. Chan PH: Antioxidant-dependent amelioration of brain injury: role of CuZn-superoxide dismutase, *J Neurotrauma* 9 Suppl 2:S417-423, 1992.
207. Kuribayashi Y, Naritomi H, Sasaki M, et al: Effects of L-ascorbic acid 2-[3,4-dihydro-2,5,7,8-tetramethyl-2-(4,8,12-trimethyltridecyl)-2H-1- benzopyran-6yl-hydrogen phosphate] potassium salt on cerebral energy state and consciousness recovery following transient forebrain ischemia in gerbils, *Arzneimittelforschung* 44:995-998, 1994.
208. Hara H, Kato H, Kogure K: Protective effect of alpha-tocopherol on ischemic neuronal damage in the gerbil hippocampus, *Brain Res* 510:335-338, 1990.
209. Perkins WJ, Milde LN, Milde JH, et al: Pretreatment with U74006F improves neurologic outcome following complete cerebral ischemia in dogs, *Stroke* 22:902-909, 1991.
210. Hall ED, Pazara KE, Braughler JM, et al: Nonsteroidal lazaroid U78517F in models of focal and global ischemia, *Stroke* 21:III83-87, 1990.
211. Rosenthal RE, Chanderbhan R, Marshall G, et al: Prevention of post-ischemic brain lipid conjugated diene production and neurological injury by hydroxyethyl starch-conjugated deferoxamine, *Free Radic Biol Med* 12:29-33, 1992.
212. Kotake Y: Pharmacologic properties of phenyl N-tert-butylnitrone, *Antiox Redox Signal* 1:481-499, 1999.
213. Lewen A, Skoglosa Y, Clausen F, et al: Paradoxical increase in neuronal DNA fragmentation after neuroprotective free radical scavenger treatment in experimental traumatic brain injury, *J Cereb Blood Flow Metab* 21:344-350, 2001.
214. Behringer W, Safar P, Kentner R, et al: Antioxidant Tempol enhances hypothermic cerebral preservation during prolonged cardiac arrest in dogs, *J Cereb Blood Flow Metab* 22:105-117, 2002.
215. Agardh CD, Zhang H, Smith ML, et al: Free radical production and ischemic brain damage: influence of postischemic oxygen tension, *Int J Dev Neurosci* 9:127-138, 1991.
216. Zwemer CF, Whitesall SE, D'Alecy LG: Cardiopulmonary-cerebral resuscitation with 100% oxygen exacerbates neurological dysfunction following nine minutes of normothermic cardiac arrest in dogs, *Resuscitation* 27:159-170, 1994.
217. Vento M, Asensi M, Sastre J, et al: Oxidative stress in asphyxiated term infants resuscitated with 100% oxygen, *J Pediatr* 142:240-246, 2003.
218. Rosenthal RE, Silbergleit R, Hof PR, et al: Hyperbaric oxygen reduces neuronal death and improves neurological outcome after canine cardiac arrest, *Stroke* 34:1311-1316, 2003.
219. Ramji S, Rasaily R, Mishra PK, et al: Resuscitation of asphyxiated newborns with room air or 100% oxygen at birth: a multicentric clinical trial, *Ind Pediatr* 40:510-517, 2003.
220. Saugstad OD, Ramji S, Irani SF, et al: Resuscitation of newborn infants with 21% or 100% oxygen: Follow-up at 18 to 24 months, *Pediatrics* 112:296-300, 2003.
221. Rosenberg AA, Murdaugh E, White CW: The role of oxygen free radicals in postasphyxia cerebral hypoperfusion in newborn lambs, *Pediatr Res* 26:215-219, 1989.
222. Thiringer K, Hrbek A, Karlsson K, et al: Postasphyxial cerebral survival in newborn sheep after treatment with oxygen free radical scavengers and a calcium antagonist, *Pediatr Res* 22:62-66, 1987.
223. Lei B, Tan X, Cai H, et al: Effect of moderate hypothermia on lipid peroxidation in canine brain tissue after cardiac arrest and resuscitation, *Stroke* 25:147-152, 1994.
224. Siesjo BK, Bendek G, Koide T, et al: Influence of acidosis on lipid peroxidation in brain tissues in vitro, *J Cereb Blood Flow Metab* 5:253-258, 1985.
225. Link EM: The mechanism of pH-dependent hydrogen peroxide cytotoxicity in vitro, *Arch Biochem Biophys* 265:362-372, 1988.
226. Chemtob S, Beharry K, Rex J, et al: Prostanoids determine the range of cerebral blood flow autoregulation of newborn piglets, *Stroke* 21:777-784, 1990.
227. Furlow TW, Jr., Hallenbeck JM: Indomethacin prevents impaired perfusion of the dogs's brain after global ischemia, *Stroke* 9:591-594, 1987.
228. Sasaki T, Nakagomi T, Kirino T, et al: Indomethacin ameliorates ischemic neuronal damage in the gerbil hippocampal CA1 sector, *Stroke* 19:1399-1403, 1988.
229. Nakagomi T, Sasaki T, Kirino T, et al: Effect of cyclooxygenase and lipoxygenase inhibitors on delayed neuronal death in the gerbil hippocampus, *Stroke* 20:925-929, 1989.
230. Koide T, Wieloch TW, Siesjo BK: Chronic dexamethasone pretreatment aggravates ischemic neuronal necrosis, *J Cereb Blood Flow Metab* 6:395-404, 1986.
231. Hallenbeck JM, Leitch DR, Dutka AJ, et al: Prostaglandin I2, indomethacin, and heparin promote postischemic neuronal recovery in dogs, *Ann Neurol* 12:145-156, 1982.
232. Minamisawa H, Terashi A, Katayama Y, et al: Brain eicosanoid levels in spontaneously hypertensive rats after ischemia with reperfusion: leukotriene C4 as a possible cause of cerebral edema, *Stroke* 19:372-377, 1988.
233. Kuhn JE, Steimle CN, Zelenock GB, et al: Ibuprofen improves survival and neurologic outcome after resuscitation from cardiac arrest, *Resuscitation* 14:199-212, 1986.
234. Jastremski M, Sutton-Tyrrell K, Vaagenes P, et al: Glucocorticoid treatment does not improve neurological recovery following cardiac arrest. Brain Resuscitation Clinical Trial I Study Group, *JAMA* 262:3427-3430, 1989.
235. Szczepanski A, Moatter T, Carley WW, et al: Induction of cyclooxygenase II in human synovial microvessel endothelial cells by interleukin-1. Inhibition by glucocorticoids, *Arthritis Rheum* 37:495-503, 1994.
236. Sapolsky RM: A mechanism for glucocorticoid toxicity in the hippocampus: increased neuronal vulnerability to metabolic insults, *J Neurosci* 5:1228-1232, 1985.
237. Toti P, C DEF, Schurfeld K, et al: Cyclooxygenase-2 immunoreactivity in the ischemic neonatal human brain. An autopsy study, *J Submicroscopic Cytol Pathol* 33:245-249, 2001.
238. Holtzman DM, Sheldon RA, Jaffe W, et al: Nerve growth factor protects the neonatal brain against hypoxic-ischemic injury, *Ann Neurol* 39:114-122, 1996.
239. Han BH, Holtzman DM: BDNF protects the neonatal brain from hypoxic-ischemic injury in vivo via the ERK pathway, *J Neurosci* 20:5775-5781, 2000.
240. Galvin KA, Oorschot DE: Continuous low-dose treatment with brain-derived neurotrophic factor or neurotrophin-3 protects striatal medium spiny neurons from mild neonatal hypoxia/ischemia: a stereological study, *Neuroscience* 118:1023-1032, 2003.

241. Pichiule P, Chavez JC, Xu K, et al: Vascular endothelial growth factor upregulation in transient global ischemia induced by cardiac arrest and resuscitation in rat brain, *Brain Res Mol Brain Res* 74:83-90, 1999.
242. D'Cruz BJ, Fertig KC, Filiano AJ, et al: Hypothermic reperfusion after cardiac arrest augments brain-derived neurotrophic factor activation, *J Cereb Blood Flow Metab* 22:843-851, 2002.
243. Safar P, Abramson NS, Angelos M, et al: Emergency cardiopulmonary bypass for resuscitation from prolonged cardiac arrest, *Am J Emerg Med* 8:55-67, 1990.
244. Chen YS, Chao A, Yu HY, et al: Analysis and results of prolonged resuscitation in cardiac arrest patients rescued by extracorporeal membrane oxygenation, *J Am Coll Cardiol* 41:197-203, 2003.
245. Behringer W, Safar P, Wu X, et al: Survival without brain damage after clinical death of 60-120 mins in dogs using suspended animation by profound hypothermia, *Crit Care Med* 31:1523-1531, 2003.
246. Nagao K, Hayashi N, Kanmatsuse K, et al: Cardiopulmonary cerebral resuscitation using emergency cardiopulmonary bypass, coronary reperfusion therapy and mild hypothermia in patients with cardiac arrest outside the hospital, *J Am Coll Cardiol* 36:776-783, 2000.
247. Stegmayr BG: Apheresis as therapy for patients with severe sepsis and multiorgan dysfunction syndrome, *Therapeutic Apheresis* 5:123-127, 2001.
248. Carcillo JA. *Management of recalitrant pediatric septic shock*. in *4th World Congress on Pediatric Intensive Care*. 2003. Boston, MA.

CHAPTER 59

Renal Structure and Function

Maury N. Pinsk and Victoria F. Norwood

PEARLS

- The efferent blood supply from a single glomerulus will contribute to the capillary vascular supply of tubules from different nephrons. This arrangement of the vascular supply explains the patchy distribution of tubular damage after ischemic injury.
- Combinations of angiotensin-converting enzyme inhibitors and nonsteroidal antiinflammatory drugs result in inhibition of afferent arteriolar vasodilation and inhibition of efferent arteriolar vasoconstriction. In low flow states, these agents can cause precipitous loss of glomerular filtration pressure and kidney function.
- Renal biopsy findings of effacement and fusion of the foot processes indicate podocyte injury, which is clinically apparent by proteinuria.
- The use of thiazide diuretics promotes calcium reabsorption because it limits the uptake of sodium from the luminal membrane. As intracellular sodium concentrations become lower, calcium reabsorption is favored by the basolateral sodium-calcium counterexchanger, which exports calcium while importing sodium across the membrane.

Renal Development

The human kidneys begin development in the third week of gestation, at which time they are primitive organs called *pronephroi*. These early kidneys are functional but regress as development progresses. As gestation continues in the fourth week, the secondary kidney elements, the mesonephroi, form from parallel strips of mesoderm along the paravertebral axis. The mesonephroi begin functioning between the sixth and tenth week of gestation before involution in a caudal-cranial direction beginning at 10 weeks' gestation. The definitive kidney, or metanephros, begins development at the fifth week of gestation and begins functioning between the tenth and fourteenth week. This kidney develops in the pelvis as the branching ureteric bud and undifferentiated metanephric mesenchyme interact in a complex series of reciprocal inductions.[1] These interactions lead to the formation of glomeruli, whereas vessels and tubules form from mesenchymal precursors, and distal tubules and collecting ducts derive from ureteric bud epithelium. This process occurs in a centrifugal fashion so that deeper corticomedullary nephrons form earliest in organogenesis, whereas the more peripheral cortical nephrons form later. As the metanephros develops, the maturing kidney ascends into the retroperitoneal space to its final location with the upper poles at the T12 vertebra. During the ascent, the systemic blood supply is derived from more cranial aspects of the aorta and from the lumbar renal arteries at the final position of the kidney. The ureters elongate and canalize during the ascent to maintain drainage to the bladder. By the time human nephrogenesis is complete at 34 weeks of gestation, repeated cycles of mesenchymal induction, ureteric branching, and morphogenesis result in approximately 1 million nephrons per kidney.

Renal Anatomy

Normal human kidneys reside in the retroperitoneal space at the level of T12 vertebra. The liver is superior to the right kidney and thus displaces it lower than the kidney on the left side. The spleen and stomach overlie the superior aspect of the left kidney. Kidneys, however, can be found in a variety of other locations as a result of alterations of the normal developmental program (reviewed by Abramson et al[7]). For example, failure of the kidney to ascend normally results in a pelvic kidney that has abnormal vascular supplies from the aorta and iliac vessels. Mesenchymal regions of the two kidneys coming in contact during early development likely cause fused kidneys, most commonly the horseshoe kidney. Partial or complete renal duplications comprise a variety of abnormalities that may arise from aberrant branching of the ureteric bud into the developing mesenchyme. Unilateral agenesis likely results from failure of ureteric bud development or abnormal mesenchymal induction, leading to regression of the metanephric mesenchyme and failed renal development.

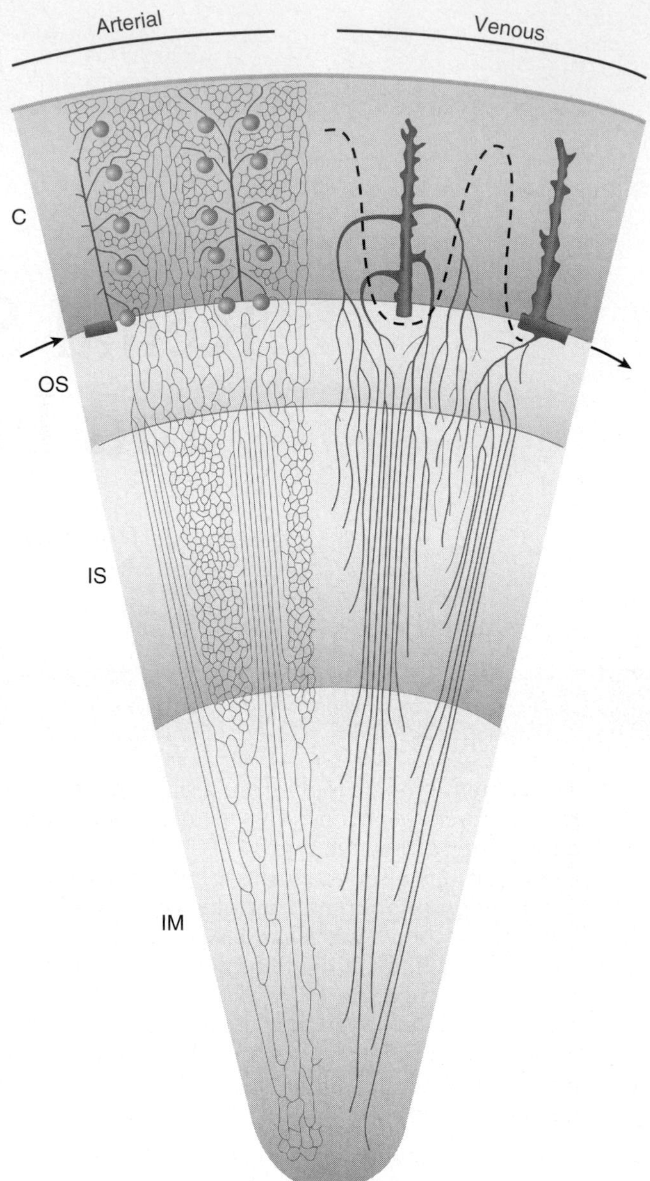

FIGURE 59–1 • The microvasculature of the mammalian kidney. Arterial supply (*left side*): The arcuate artery (*arrow*) travels parallel to the surface of the kidney, branching into interlobular arteries that travel toward the kidney surface, and further branches into afferent arterioles supplying each glomerulus. The efferent arterioles travel to the medulla forming the vasa rectae. Venous drainage (*right side*): Interlobular veins receive blood from the vasa rectae of the medulla and superficial cortex. Interlobular veins drain into arcuate veins and ultimately rejoin the systemic circulation via the renal vein. *C,* cortex, *OS,* outer stripe, *IS,* inner stripe, *IM,* inner medulla. (Modified from Kriz W, Lever AF. Renal countercurrent mechanisms: structure and function, *Am Heart J* 78:101-118, 1969; Rollhäuser H, Kriz W, Heinke W: Das Gefässsystem der Rattenniere, *Z Zellforsch* 64:381-403, 1964.)

The Renal Vasculature

Vascular Development

Markers of early vascular development are expressed in undifferentiated metanephric mesenchyme. This suggests that the blood supply to the nephron develops at least partially from precursors inherent to the maturing kidney.[3,4] Migration of committed endothelial cells into the developing glomerulus occurs in response to secreted factors such as platelet-derived growth factor β (PDGF-β) and vascular endothelial growth factor, as well as selective expression of the corresponding receptors.[4,5,8] Control of the corresponding branching of extraglomerular vessels is an area of active study and may involve branching from existing vessels, de novo vessel formation, or both processes. These actions appear to be regulated in part by the renin-angiotensin system.[6,7] Evidence to support this hypothesis stems from gene deletion studies of the renin-angiotensin cascade and experiments with pharmacological blockade of angiotensin II actions, in which the renal vasculature is rarified, blunted, and abnormally thickened.[6]

Vascular Anatomy

The arterial supply of the kidney branches from the main renal artery and enters the kidney in a series of rays called *interlobar arteries*. The interlobar vessels branch at the corticomedullary junction to run parallel to the surface of the kidney as arcuate arteries (Fig. 59–1, *left panel*). Arcuate arteries penetrate the cortex as interlobular arteries, which ascend into the cortex in a radial pattern. It is from the interlobular arteries that afferent arterioles of the glomeruli arise. After filtration across the glomerular tuft, blood exits the glomerulus by efferent arterioles, which travel to the surface of the cortex and eventually feed the peritubular capillary vascular beds, the vasa rectae. The efferent arteriole of a single nephron can supply blood to multiple vasa rectae. The postglomerular vasculature of the cortex is supplied by efferent arterioles from midcortical and superficial cortical nephrons, whereas the blood supply to the medulla is entirely derived from juxtamedullary efferent arterioles. The vasa rectae of the medulla branch as they descend toward the papilla of the kidney and form the complex meshwork of the medullary capillary vascular beds. Only a few vessels of the vasa rectae eventually reach the papillary tip.

Venous drainage of the vasa rectae is divided into two types: the vessels of the deep medulla ascend to join the arcuate veins at the corticomedullary junction, and those of the superficial medulla ascend into the cortex to join the cortical capillary network and ultimately the interlobular and arcuate veins (Fig. 59–1, *right side*). The arcuate veins join with the interlobar veins via the interlobular veins and finally drain into the main renal vein to join the main circulation.

Vascular Function

The kidneys are extraordinarily vascular organs; they receive 15% to 18% of cardiac output in the neonate and up to 20% of cardiac output in the adult.[9] Blood flow to the kidney is tightly regulated to ensure continued renal function over a range of blood pressures. Sympathetic α_1-receptors, myogenic contraction, and vasoactive mediators control vascular resistance and provide autoregulation of renal blood flow. Maintenance of glomerular filtration rate at the level of the glomerulus occurs by vasoconstriction of efferent arterioles in response to pressors such as angiotensin II, whereas afferent arterioles relax in response to vasodilators such as prostacyclin. In infants, the effect of vasoactive mediators on renal blood flow is blunted compared with adults. For example, circulating angiotensin II is elevated in the neonate, but the vasoconstrictor response to angiotensin II is reduced compared with adults.[10] Therefore infants have a decreased capacity to regulate renal blood flow, which explains their increased susceptibility to renal ischemia in hypotensive states.

The Nephron Unit

The nephron unit consists of a glomerular tuft, proximal tubule, loop of Henle, distal tubule, and collecting duct (Fig. 59–2). The proximal tubule is an extension of the urinary space of the glomerulus and courses into the loop of Henle. Two types of nephrons are characterized on the basis of the location of the glomerulus and the path of the loop of Henle: the juxtamedullary nephrons and the cortical nephrons. Most nephrons are cortical in location, have short loops of Henle that extend into the superficial medulla, and have a relatively low capacity to reabsorb solute and water. Juxtamedullary nephrons are fewer in number but have longer loops of Henle that extend deep into the medulla. Consequently, these nephrons absorb larger amounts of salt and water, generate steep osmotic gradients, and produce highly concentrated urine. Regardless of the location of the nephron, the loop of Henle returns to the cortex to become a distal tubule. The distal tubule then continues on to form the collecting duct, the final common pathway for several nephrons draining into the renal papilla.

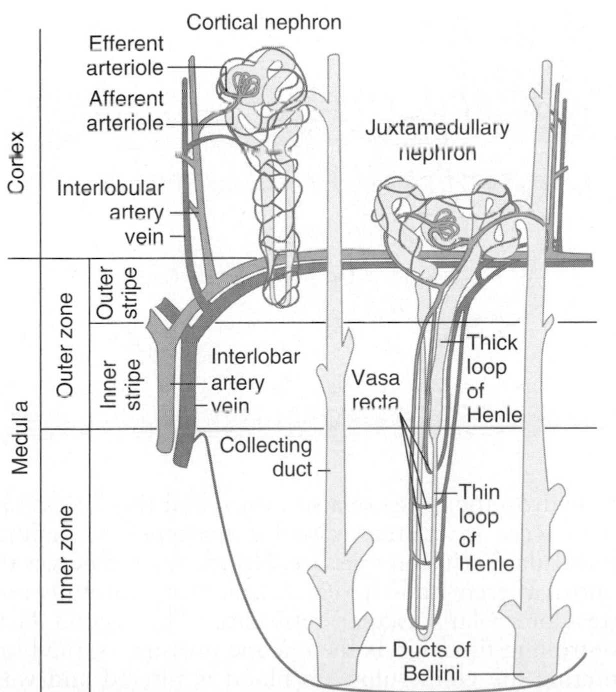

FIGURE 59–2 • The nephron structure. (From Guyton A: Formation of urine by the kidney: I. Renal blood flow, glomerular filtration, and their control. In Wonsiewicz M, editor: *Textbook of medical physiology,* ed 8, Philadelphia, 1991, WB Saunders.)

Nephron Development

Nephron development occurs through a complex, interactive series of processes that remains to be completely understood.[1] Nephron development begins with the outpouching of the ureteric epithelium, the ureteric bud. This precursor to the collecting duct encroaches on undifferentiated mesenchyme in the caudal retroperitoneal space and induces the development of an epithelial cell condensate, the precursor to the future glomerulus and tubule (Fig. 59–3). Simultaneously, factors within the metanephric mesenchyme induce the ureteric bud to continue branching. The epithelial condensate forms a vesicle, which convolutes progressively into a comma-shaped body and then an S-shaped body, signifying the development of the urinary space and early tubule segments. The terminal portion of the tubule is contributed by the ureteric bud derivatives and forms the collecting duct. The mechanisms by which the ureteric bud epithelial derivatives link to the corresponding mesenchymal derivatives in the distal nephron remain unknown. The glomerular capillary loops appear to form through the angiogenic processes of committed endothelial cells, and supporting mesangial cells develop from committed metanephric mesenchyme with myoblastic characteristics.[8] Nephrogenesis in the human is complete by the thirty-fourth week of gestation, but functional maturation continues into the second year of life.[1]

Glomerular Anatomy

The glomerular tuft consists of endothelial cells, specialized epithelial cells (podocytes), and supporting mesangial cells. Epithelial cells form the urinary compartment into which ultrafiltrate passes (Bowman's space). Endothelial cells and podocytes sit on opposite sides of the glomerular basement membrane, the entirety of which forms the filtration apparatus. The epithelial side is characterized by fingerlike extensions of the podocyte cell membrane that interdigitate to form a mesh on the glomerular basement membrane. Glomerular endothelial cells on the blood side of the filtration barrier are highly fenestrated, thereby enhancing solute and fluid transfer. Mesangial cells form the supporting network of the glomerular structure, provide some phagocytic function, and participate in control of glomerular filtration.

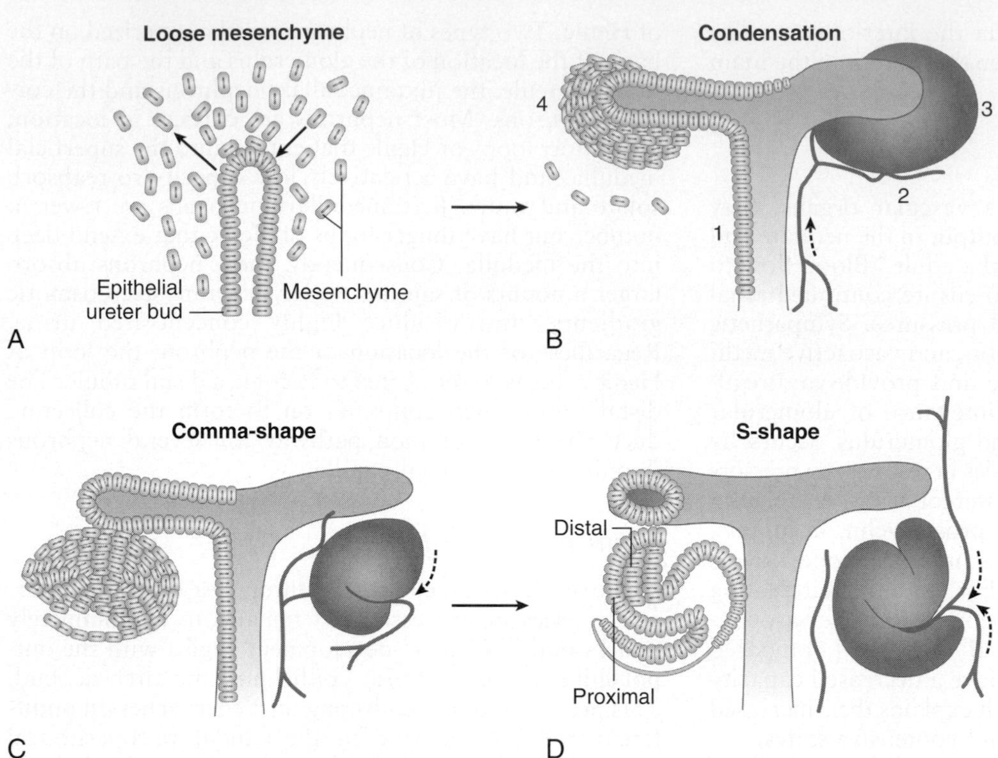

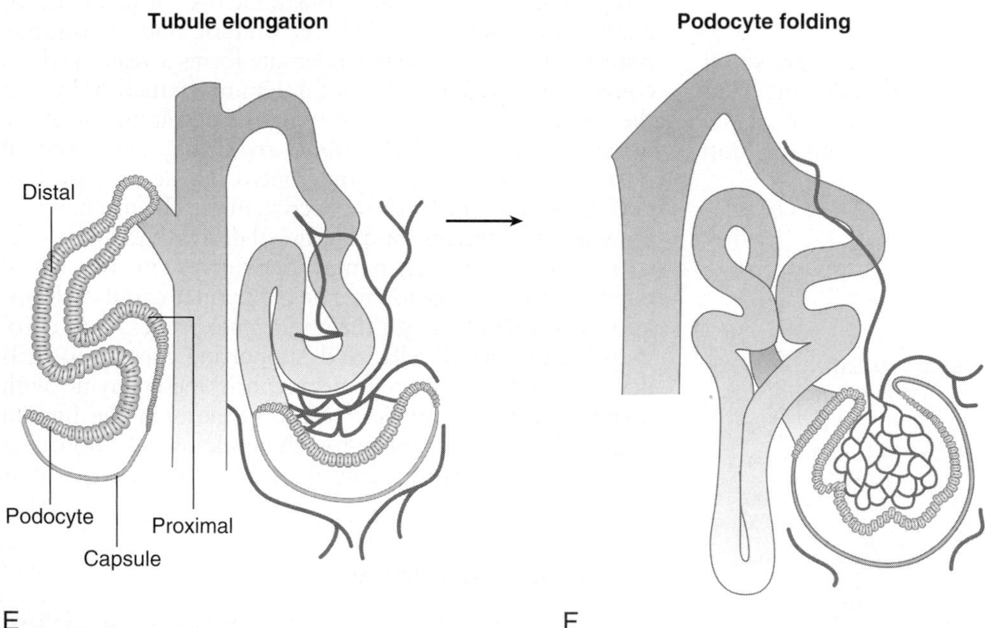

FIGURE 59–3 • Branching morphogenesis of the developing kidney. **A** and **B,** The ureteric epithelium interacts with the metanephric mesenchyme inducing condensation of the mesenchyme (*1* = ureteric epithelium, *2* = vasculature, *3* = undifferentiated mesenchyme, *4* = condensed mesenchyme [precursor to epithelium]). **C** and **D,** Infolding of the glomerular epithelium forms a comma-shaped body, followed by development of an S-shaped body. **E** and **F,** Infolding of the glomerular epithelium and vascular structures and elongation of the tubular elements form the completed nephron. The mature glomerular capillary network is likely initiated during **C** and **D.** (From Gomez RA, Norwood VF: Recent advances in renal development, *Curr Opin Pediatr* 11:136, 1999.)

Glomerular Function

Filtration is the primary function of the glomerulus. For filtration to occur, there must be a gradient across the glomerular basement membrane favoring the movement of filtrate to a low-pressure area. There are generally four factors that determine the quantity of filtrate obtained across the glomerular basement membrane (Fig. 59–4). First, hydrostatic pressure in the glomerular capillary drives filtration of fluid across the glomerular basement membrane. If the blood flow drops to the glomerulus, the hydrostatic pressure also drops, and this necessitates an increase in efferent vascular resistance to maintain glomerular perfusion pressure. Hormones and nerves that control afferent and efferent vascular tone carefully regulate glomerular vascular resistance. The second factor controlling filtration is the oncotic pressure of the blood entering the glomerulus. As blood is filtered and water leaves the vascular compartment to enter the urinary space, the oncotic pressure in the blood compartment rises, retarding the further passage of fluid across the glomerular

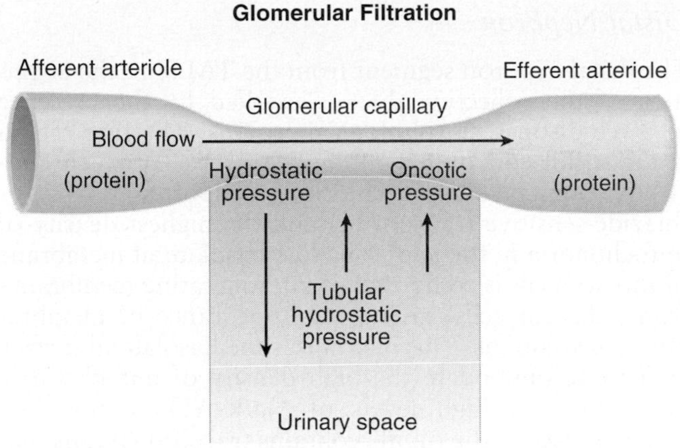

FIGURE 59–4 • Forces affecting ultrafiltrate formation in the isolated nephron. (From Brem A: An overview of renal structure and function. In Fuhrman BP, Zimmerman JJ, editors: *Pediatric critical care,* ed 2, Philadelphia, 1998, Mosby.)

basement membrane. In situations of low oncotic pressure, such as nephrotic syndrome, the initial rate of ultrafiltrate formation is increased because of low oncotic pressure. Low oncotic pressure, however, also causes a concomitant redistribution of intravascular volume into peripheral tissue spaces, resulting in decreased vascular hydrostatic pressure, thus causing ultrafiltrate production to drop. Lower hydrostatic pressure therefore balances the low oncotic pressure. The third factor determining the efficiency of ultrafiltrate formation is tubular hydrostatic pressure, or the resistance within the urinary space. This is an important factor limiting ultrafiltrate generation in the setting of urinary obstruction because tubular hydrostatic pressure can rise above the hydrostatic pressure of the blood compartment and arrest ultrafiltrate generation. The last important factor in the determination of ultrafiltrate formation relates to the intrinsic properties of the glomerular basement membrane. Both the area of available membrane surface and the efficiency of the membrane to filter affect the generation of ultrafiltrate. Physiologically, the "size" of the glomerular basement membrane can be determined at the whole kidney level or at the glomerular level. At the whole kidney level, the number of nephrons receiving adequate blood supply determines glomerular basement membrane area available for filtration. For example, shunting of blood from the cortex into the medulla, as seen in hepatorenal syndrome, effectively decreases the available glomerular basement membrane area by reducing the number of actively filtering nephrons. At the glomerular level, glomerular basement membrane area can be altered by mesangial cell function. In hypovolemic states, mesangial cell contraction is thought to decrease glomerular basement membrane area in response to hormonal mediators, resulting in decreased filtration and preservation of intravascular volume.[11] The efficiency of basement membrane filtration can also be affected by disease states including immune complex deposition or complement activation that disrupt the integrity of the membrane. Finally, selectivity of the filtration barrier is determined by the ability of the basement membrane to permit some materials to pass into the urine while restricting others to stay in the blood compartment. Selectivity appears to be the result of both size discrimination of the glomerular basement membrane and receptor-mediated uptake or degradation of solute by the podocyte. One such receptor, megalin, controls uptake of filtered albumin into the podocyte and subsequent trafficking of the protein back to the blood space or into degradation pathways. Disruption of the normal podocyte physiology alters this trafficking pathway and likely contributes to proteinuria during podocyte injury.[12]

Tubular Anatomy

Proximal Tubule

The proximal tubule consists of polarized epithelia with a distinctive apical brush border not seen in other parts of the tubule (Fig. 59–5). The brush border functions to increase the surface area of the luminal side of the cell so that maximal contact of the cell with the ultrafiltrate is made. Increased surface area facilitates reabsorption of solute and water, which occurs through an abundant variety of sodium-coupled transport proteins. Also on the brush border membrane are ion channels and ion exchange proteins that maintain electrochemical gradients across the apical membrane. On the basolateral aspect of the proximal tubular cells are located Na-K-ATPase proteins and a high density of mitochondria. It is through the Na/K-ATPase that favorable sodium gradients and electrochemical gradients are generated to facilitate transcellular and paracellular transport of solutes. The lateral membranes of the proximal tubule cells are characterized by the presence of cell–cell adhesion molecules called *tight junctions*. Tight junctions maintain the polarity of the proximal tubule cells by separating transport proteins on the apical side from the gradient-generating basolateral membrane proteins.

Loop of Henle

The cortical and juxtamedullary nephrons are defined by their position within the cortex but also by the length of the loop of Henle. The juxtamedullary nephrons have loops of Henle that extend deep into the hyperosmolar medulla, whereas most nephrons are cortical and have loops that reach only the mildly hyperosmolar outer medulla. The properties of the epithelial cells change throughout

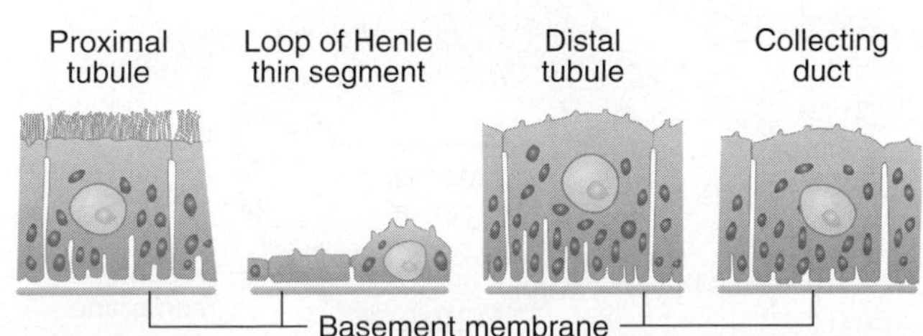

FIGURE 59–5 • Tubular epithelia from different tubular segments. (From Guyton A: Formation of urine by the kidney: II. Processing of the filtrate in the tubules. In Wonsiewicz M, editor: *Textbook of medical physiology,* ed 8, Philadelphia, 1991, WB Saunders.)

the length of the loop of Henle. The proximal portions have cells with prominent microvilli and permeable cell junctions that permit passage of fluid through and between cells (reviewed by Kriz and Kaissling[13]). The cells themselves are permeable to water and urea because of the presence of aquaporin-1 water channels and urea transporters. The distal sections of the loop of Henle consist of flat epithelia lacking microvilli and are devoid of aquaporin-1 channels and urea transporters. Thus the thin ascending limb of the loop of Henle is impermeable to water and urea but transports other solutes, largely in a paracellular fashion. An abrupt transition occurs at the beginning of the thick ascending limb of the loop of Henle (TALH). The TALH is impermeable to water but transports solute in an active, adenosine triphosphate (ATP)–dependent manner. These cells do not have prominent microvilli but do have dense tight junctions. These tight junctions allow solute, but not water, to move among cells into the basolateral space. TALH cells are characterized by the dense localization of mitochondria and Na/K-ATPase at the basolateral membrane that generate gradients for solute transport across the luminal surface. Compared with the proximal tubule, the TALH basolateral surface is larger than the luminal surface, accommodates a larger number of Na/K-ATPase pumps, and is more metabolically active than the proximal tubular epithelium (reviewed by Kriz and Kaissling[13]). At the distal end of the TALH, the tubule courses back toward its originating glomerulus. Here a small plaque of tall, narrow cells, the macula densa, contacts the vascular pole and extraglomerular mesangial cells (Fig. 59–6). The primary function of the macula densa cells (mentioned later) appears to be the detection of tubular chloride content and the regulation of glomerular filtration.

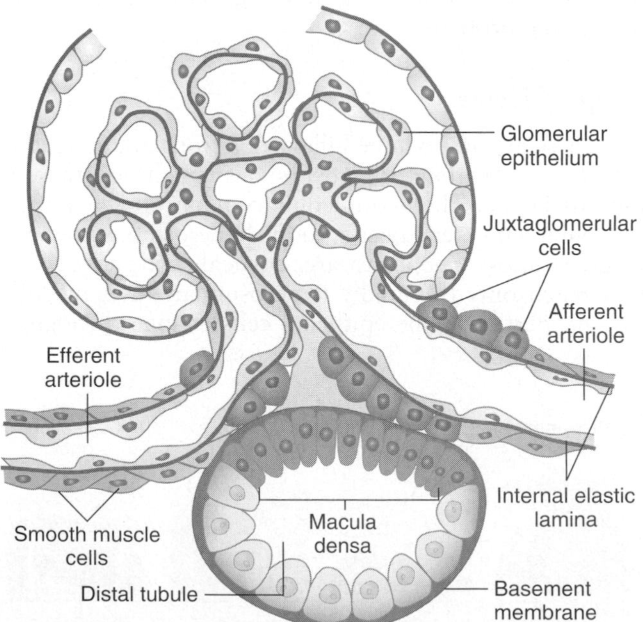

FIGURE 59–6 • Structure of the juxtaglomerular apparatus. (From Guyton A: Formation of urine by the kidney: I. Renal blood flow, glomerular filtration, and their control. In Wonsiewicz M, editor: *Textbook of medical physiology,* ed 8, Philadelphia, 1991, WB Saunders.)

Distal Nephron

The distal nephron segment from the TALH to the beginning of the collecting duct is marked by the presence of three distinct morphological regions. The first region is the distal convoluted tubule, the cells of which contain the luminal sodium chloride transporter (NCC2, or thiazide-sensitive transporter) and the highest density of mitochondria in the nephron. The basolateral membrane of this segment is composed of interdigitating membranes from adjacent cells, giving the appearance of membranous convolutions. This maximizes the basolateral surface area to accommodate the high density of mitochondria and allow for high levels of Na/K-ATPase function. Moving distally, the tubule contains transitional cells that have a smaller basolateral surface area and fewer mitochondria at the basolateral membrane. Transitional cells express both the NCC2 channel and the luminal epithelial sodium channel (ENaC), with the quantities of ENaC increasing and NCC2 decreasing with distal progression along the segment.[13] The next segment is the connecting tubule, where cells show even fewer mitochondria and smaller basolateral membranes. These cells are distinguished by a more flattened appearance, an expression of ENaC, and a luminal potassium channel (ROMK), but not NCC2. The basolateral membrane is expanded to some degree by infoldings of the basal membrane, but there is no interdigitation from neighboring cells. Because Ca/Mg-ATPase, a parathyroid hormone receptor, and a Na/Ca exchanger may also be found in the basolateral membrane, they may have a role in calcium homeostasis.[14-16] The last segment in the distal nephron is the collecting duct. The primary cells of this segment, the principal cells, are characterized by apical vacuoles, some of which store aquaporin-2 channels. They also contain mineralocorticoid receptors and apical sodium channels that function in sodium and potassium balance. The basolateral membrane is infolded but to a lesser degree than other cells in the region. These infolds diminish in cells of the medullary collecting duct compared with those in the cortical collecting duct. In the medullary portions of the collecting duct, urea transporters again appear.

Intercalated cells, α and β, exist as single cells interspersed throughout the distal nephron. These cells have prominent microfolds in the apical membrane, have high densities of mitochondria, and express several important membrane proteins such as the luminal H+-ATPase and H+/K+-ATPase, as well as cytoplasmic carbonic anhydrase, serving an integral role in acid-base balance. The essential difference between α- and β-intercalated cells is that cell polarity is opposite in the two cell types. In α-intercalated cells, the apical membrane contains an H+-ATPase, whereas the basolateral membrane contains bicarbonate and chloride exchangers, providing a mechanism for proton secretion.[17] The β-intercalated cell has proton-ATPase on the basolateral surface and a chloride channel (ClC3) on the apical surface, allowing bicarbonate secretion and proton reabsorption.[18] Generally, the α-subtype is located in the distal tubule and connecting tubule, whereas the ß-subtype predominates in the collecting duct.

Tubular Function

While the function of the glomerulus is filtration, the function of the tubule is to modify the ultrafiltrate to maintain metabolic balance. This is accomplished through the following outlined mechanisms but includes the reabsorption of water and solutes and excretion of waste products generated from daily metabolism.

Proximal Tubule

Solute and water are transported in the proximal tubule via both paracellular and transcellular routes (Fig. 59–7). Paracellular transport is a high-flux means of moving water and solute between cells along chemical or electrical gradients generated by the basolateral Na/K-ATPase. The mechanism for high flux movement of sodium out of the lumen is explained by a net luminal positive charge generated by the basolateral Na/K-ATPase and net anion reabsorption. The bulk of the sodium therefore follows an electrochemical gradient through paracellular pathways into the blood space. The same principle applies to other cations, such as calcium, which are passively reabsorbed down electrochemical gradients in the proximal tubule. Neutrally charged solutes, such as glucose, move between cells following concentration gradients, the transport becoming less effective more distally as the gradient dissipates. Water movement generally follows sodium movement and is facilitated by the high oncotic pressure of the peritubular capillary network. This favorable osmotic gradient allows for reabsorption of approximately 70% of the filtered water in the adult proximal tubule.

Transcellular movement of solute is a high-resistance method of sodium-coupled transport that results from electrochemical and concentration gradients established by the basolateral Na/K-ATPase (Fig. 59–7). The Na/K-ATPase pumps three sodium molecules into the basolateral extracellular milieu against a concentration gradient and imports two potassium molecules into the cell against a concentration gradient. The process, which is ATP dependent, establishes a low intracellular sodium concentration and permits luminal sodium entry along a concentration gradient coupled with solutes such as phosphate, glucose, amino acids, and organic acids. In a similar fashion, protons are exported from the luminal membrane by an Na-H+ exchanger that exploits the intracellular movement of sodium to facilitate the export of protons. Bicarbonate is indirectly absorbed through the activity of luminal carbonic anhydrase and the Na-H+ exchanger. The high oncotic pressure of the blood in the arterioles and early vasa recta drives transcellular water reabsorption in the proximal tubular cells via constitutively expressed aquaporin-1 channels that permit water to flow from lumen to vasculature.[19] Some proximal solute reabsorption is modifiable by hormone activity. Parathyroid hormone binding to the proximal tubule receptors activates several second messenger systems that ultimately result in decreased sodium-phosphate transporter activity and phosphate excretion.[20] The proximal tubule is also a site of hormone production with 1α-hydroxylase activity converting 25-hydroxyvitamin D to the active 1,25-dihydroxy form.

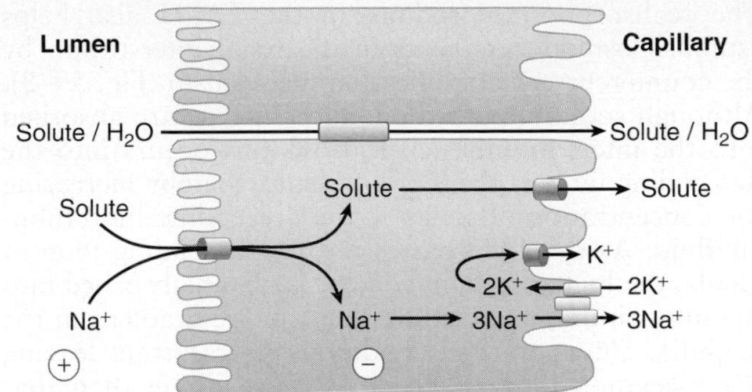

FIGURE 59–7 • Proximal tubule transport of solute and water. Apical solute reabsorption (glucose, amino acids, phosphate, and organic acids) is sodium coupled and follows an electrochemical gradient generated by basolateral Na+/K+-ATPase activity.

This conversion permits vitamin D to act in calcium and phosphate metabolism.[21]

Maturational development of the proximal tubule imparts functional differences in neonatal proximal tubules compared with those in adult kidneys. The relatively low outer cortical nephron blood flow in infancy results in a generalized decrease in proximal tubule resorptive capacity because fewer nephrons participate in active solute and water reabsorption. In the neonate, the proximal tubule is also shorter than that of adults, and the results are a smaller tubular resorptive surface area and an additional decrease in epithelial transport.[22] Sodium transport proteins and Na/K-ATPase are expressed in lower density during early life, also decreasing sodium and water resorptive capacity.[23] In addition, hormone receptors are expressed in fewer numbers or may have higher thresholds for activation in the neonate. For example, sodium-phosphate transporters of the premature neonate exhibit a relatively low sensitivity to parathyroid hormone, resulting in lower urinary excretion of phosphate and higher serum phosphate levels than those seen in adults.[24]

Loop of Henle

The loop of Henle plays an important role in establishing the osmotic gradients facilitating water reabsorption in the kidney. In the descending limb of the loop of Henle, the tubular epithelium is impermeable to solute but not water. Therefore as ultrafiltrate passes down the descending loop of Henle, ultrafiltrate becomes increasingly hyperosmolar as water leaves the luminal space. Water permeability decreases, however, in the ascending loop, and solute transporters become more prevalent, allowing the filtrate to become hypo-osmolar by the time it reaches the outer cortex. The thick ascending loop of Henle is responsible for roughly 25% of the total sodium reclamation in the kidney, primarily by the NKCC2 channel, which allows one sodium, one potassium, and two chloride ions to move from the tubular lumen into the cell.[25] Potassium subsequently leaks back into the lumen via the ROMK potassium channel, causing the lumen to become positively charged. This electrochemical gradient permits paracellular reabsorption of cations such as calcium and magnesium as they are propelled out of the tubular lumen.

The reabsorption of sodium in the TALH also helps establish osmotic gradients in the renal interstitium by the countercurrent amplification mechanism (Fig. 59–8). Although sodium, potassium, and chloride are absorbed into the interstitium, back leak of ions occurs into the descending limb of the loop of Henle, thereby increasing the concentration of solute in the descending limb tubular fluid. As this fluid passes into the ascending loop of Henle, the higher sodium content is also reabsorbed into the interstitium, augmenting the osmotic gradient in the medulla. Under normal conditions, ultrafiltrate leaving the ascending loop of Henle is more dilute than that entering the descending loop because of the proficient solute reabsorption in the late ascending limb. Loop diuretics such as bumetanide or furosemide block the NKCC2 channel function and impair the ability both to establish osmotic gradients and to reabsorb solute. The result is the production of large volumes of isotonic urine. In the immature kidney, the loop of Henle is relatively short and impedes the ability to set up steep osmotic gradients. Therefore neonatal urinary concentrating ability is relatively weak compared with that of the mature adult kidney. In addition, because renal blood flow is shunted away from the outer cortex in the neonate, the result is less sodium transport in the interstitium and the prevention of the establishment of high osmotic gradients.[26]

The thick ascending loop of Henle returns to its glomerulus of origin where the tubular epithelium is attached to the triangle between the efferent and afferent arteriole. The tubular epithelium in contact with the glomerulus contains about 15 to 20 cells in the form of a plaque,

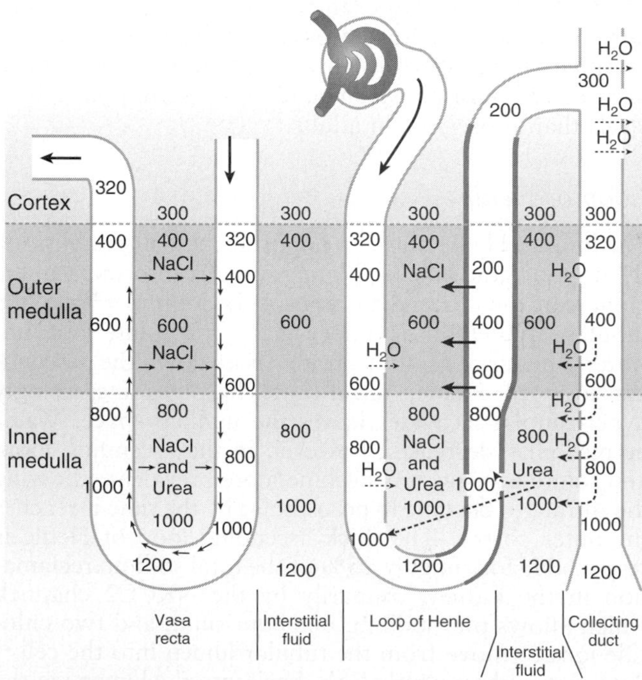

FIGURE 59–8 • The countercurrent amplification mechanism permitting urinary concentration. (From Guyton A: Renal and associated mechanisms for controlling extracellular fluid osmolality and sodium. In Wonsiewicz M, editor: *Textbook of medical physiology,* ed 8, Philadelphia, 1991, WB Saunders.)

called the *macula densa* (see Fig. 59–6). The macula densa actively reabsorbs sodium, potassium, and chloride through the NKCC2 channel and, in doing so, acts as a sensor of tubular chloride concentration.[27] This sensing mechanism is integral to the functioning of the juxtaglomerular apparatus, which consists of the macula densa, the afferent arteriole containing renin-producing granular cells, the efferent arteriole, and the extraglomerular mesangium. In response to low tubular chloride, such as in hypovolemia, the macula densa secretes chemical mediators (prostaglandins, nitric oxide, adenosine, and ATP) that trigger renin release from the granular cells in the afferent arteriole.[28,29] Similar effects can be induced by sympathetic nervous system stimulation and arteriolar baroreceptor activation.[28] Renin activity ultimately leads to the production of the potent vasoconstrictor angiotensin II, vascular smooth muscle contraction in the efferent arteriole, increased efferent arteriolar vascular resistance, and a rise in glomerular perfusion pressure.[28] The macula densa also signals the mesangial cells and neighboring smooth muscle cells to contract, and this contraction results in increased vascular tone and decreased effective filtration area of the glomerular basement membrane.[27]

Distal Tubule

The distal convoluted tubule is also a site of active sodium reabsorption and functions to help fine-tune the urinary filtrate. When tubular fluid enters the distal convoluted tubule, it is relatively dilute because of active solute reabsorption in the distal loop of Henle. Thus reabsorption of sodium and chloride in this segment occurs against a concentration gradient. Sodium and chloride are actively reabsorbed through the luminal thiazide-sensitive cotransporter following electrochemical gradients generated by the basolateral Na/K-ATPase.[30] Approximately 10% of filtered calcium is also reabsorbed from the luminal space in the distal convoluted tubule through parathyroid hormone activation of ATP-dependent calcium channels. Once inside the cell, calcium is sequestered by calbindin-D28k, a protein that facilitates the transport of calcium to the basolateral membrane. Calcium exits the cell through either a basolateral Na-Ca counterexchanger or Ca-ATPase.[31]

Collecting Duct

The collecting duct also functions to fine-tune the final composition of the renal ultrafiltrate adjusting sodium, potassium, and water content and acid-base balance. Approximately 5% of the filtered sodium is reabsorbed at this location and occurs through active transport. Sodium enters the cell through apical sodium channels (ENaC) and generates a luminal electronegative gradient (reviewed by Kriz and Kaissling[13]). Consequently, the excretion of cations such as potassium (principal cell) or protons (α-intercalated cell) is favored (Fig. 59–9). Because relatively little potassium is in the tubular fluid when it reaches this segment, potassium excretion down a concentration gradient is facilitated. As potassium is excreted, urine flow keeps the concentration in the tubular fluid low, and the favorable gradient is maintained. In states

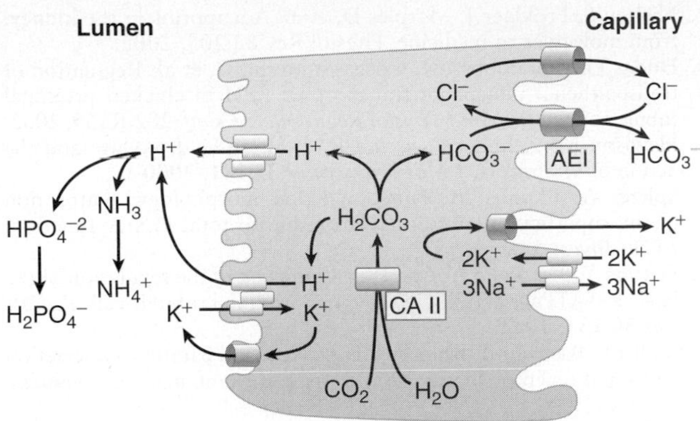

FIGURE 59–9 • Acid-base balance in the α-intercalated cell. Titratable acids in the urinary space capture actively secreted protons. This process is coupled with basolateral bicarbonate reabsorption through the anion exchange protein 1 (AE1) after intracellular carbonic anhydrase activity (CAII). Electrochemical gradients facilitating this process are generated both locally and by neighboring principal cells.

of low urine flow the tubular potassium concentration rises, the gradient is reduced, and potassium excretion decreases. Potassium excretion and sodium reabsorption are also enhanced by the presence of aldosterone. Binding of aldosterone to its receptor and subsequent translocation to the cell nucleus induces transcription of the luminal sodium channel and basolateral Na/K-ATPase.[2] More ENaCs on the luminal membrane tend to increase cell permeability to sodium, and this increase allows the tubular fluid to become more negatively charged after the influx of sodium. This process is facilitated by the increased activity and number of Na/K-ATPase pumps at the basolateral membrane, which creates larger electrical gradients. The net result is an increased capacity to excrete potassium or, in the hypokalemic state, an increased capacity to excrete protons.

The electrical gradient in the collecting duct also favors proton secretion into the tubular lumen, but the chemical gradient does not; the pH in the lumen can be as low as 5, whereas that of the intracellular space is 7.3. Excretion of protons occurs through an apical H+-ATPase in the α-intercalated cells and is also increased by aldosterone action in principal cells, as previously described. Protons secreted into the lumen are bound by ammonia to form NH_4^+ or by other titratable acids such as phosphate or sulfate. This sequestration lowers the concentration of free protons in the ultrafiltrate, prevents diffusion of protons back into the intracellular space, and ultimately promotes acid secretion.

The collecting duct is also responsible for establishing the final concentration of the urine by controlling water reabsorption. At the beginning of the medullary collecting duct, the ultrafiltrate remains relatively dilute and the cells are relatively impermeable to water and solute (see Fig. 59–8). In the setting of hypovolemia or hyperosmolarity, however, arginine vasopressin binds to V2 vasopressin receptors on the basolateral membrane of the medullary collecting duct cell. V2 receptor signaling results in aquaporin-2 channel migration from intracellular vesicles to the apical surface, and this increases tubular permeability to water. Because of the high interstitial osmolality, water is reabsorbed through the aquaporin channels along an osmotic gradient into the blood space; thus the urine is concentrated.[32]

Although largely established by active sodium reabsorption in the TALH, the medullary osmotic gradient is also maintained by the presence of urea gradients generated in the collecting tubule (see Fig. 59–8). As tubular fluid moves down the collecting duct, the water entering the interstitium allows the urine to become more concentrated and the urea concentration to rise. The interstitium, however, becomes less hyperosmolar with the influx of water. As the distal tubular permeability to urea increases distally, urea moves from an area of high concentration (the lumen) into an area of lower urea concentration (the interstitium).[33] The interstitium becomes more hypertonic with the influx of urea, and the concentrating mechanism of the interstitium is partially restored.

The Interstitium

The tubular interstitium is a poorly understood region of the kidney, both from developmental and functional standpoints. Although it is clear that the interstitium is important in maintaining osmotic and chemical gradients, other functions are only beginning to be completely elucidated. Erythropoietin, a hormone important in the production of normal red blood cell numbers, is produced by renal interstitial cells in response to low blood flow, low viscosity, or low oxygen-carrying capacity.[34] The interstitium is also a target of disease, with the result often being interstitial fibrosis. The mechanism of developing interstitial fibrosis in response to injury is thought to be cytokine mediated, particularly by transforming growth factor β (TGF-β). A number of chronic inflammatory processes may induce chronic renal insufficiency through development of interstitial fibrosis, a phenomenon that remains an area of active study.

Summary

Structural development of the human kidney implies that renal physiological processes change with maturation. Perfusion, tubular function, and hormonal responses are unique in young patients and affect the renal response in health and disease. Understanding the functions of the pediatric kidney at various stages of development is important in predicting therapeutic responsiveness in the critically ill child and in monitoring recovery from illness.

REFERENCES

1. Gomez RA, Norwood VF: Recent advances in renal development, *Curr Opin Pediatr* 11:135, 1999.
2. Eaton DC, Malik B, Saxena NC, et al: Mechanisms of aldosterone's action on epithelial Na + transport, *J Membr Biol* 184:313, 2001.
3. Robert B, St. John P, Abrahamson D: Direct visualization of renal vascular morphogenesis in *Flk-1* heterozygous mutant mice, *Am J Physiol* 275:F164, 1998.
4. Woolf A, Loughna S: Origin of the glomerular capillaries: is the verdict in? *Exp Nephrol* 6:17, 1998.
5. Leven P, Pekny M, Gebre-Medhin S, et al: Mice deficient for PDGF B show renal, cardiovascular, and hematological abnormalities, *Genes Dev* 8:1875, 1994.

6. Gomez RA: Role of angiotensin in renal vascular development, *Kidney Int Suppl* 67:s12, 1998.
7. Abrahamson DR, Robert B, Hyink D, et al: Origins and formation of microvasculature in the developing kidney, *Kidney Int* 67:s7, 1998.
8. Soriano P: Abnormal kidney development and hematological disorders in PDGF beta-receptor mutant mice, *Genes Dev* 8:1888, 1994.
9. Guyton A: Formation of urine by the kidney: I. Renal blood flow, glomerular filtration, and their control. In Wonsiewicz M, editor, *Textbook of medical physiology,* ed 8, Philadelphia, 1991, WB Saunders.
10. Robillard J, Gomez R, VanOrden D, et al: Comparison of the adrenal and renal responses to angiotensin II in fetal lambs and adult sheep, *Circ Res* 50:140, 1982.
11. Elger M, Sakai T, Kriz W: Role of mesangial cell contraction in adaptation of the glomerular tuft to changes in extracellular volume, *Pflugers Arch* 415:598, 1990.
12. Russo LM, Bakris GL, Comper WD: Renal handling of albumin: a critical review of basic concepts and perspective, *Am J Kidney Dis* 39:899, 2002.
13. Kriz W, Kaissling N: Structural organization of the mammalian kidney. In Seldin D, Giebisch G, editors, *The kidney: physiology and pathophysiology,* ed 3, Philadelphia, 2000, Lippincott Williams & Wilkins.
14. Riccardi D, Lee WS, Lee K, et al: Localization of the extracellular Ca+2-sensing receptor and PPTH/PTHrP receptor in rat kidney, *Am J Physiol* 271:F951, 1996.
15. Borke J, Caride A, Verma A et al: Plasma membrane calcium pump and 28-KDa calcium binding protein in rat kidney distal tubules, *Am J Physiol* 257:F842, 1989.
16. Reilly R, Shugrue C, Lattanzi D, et al: Immunolocalization of the Na+/Ca+2 exchanger in rabbit kidney, *Am J Physiol* 265:F327, 1993.
17. Madsen K, Kim J, Tisher C: Intracellular band 3 immunostaining in type A intercalated cells of rabbit kidney, *Am J Physiol* 262: F1015, 1992.
18. Al-Awqati Q: Plasticity in epithelial polarity of renal intercalated cell: targeting of the H(+)-ATPase and band 3, *Am J Physiol* 270: C1571, 1996.
19. Nielsen S, Froklaer J, Marples D, et al: Aquaporins in the kidney: from molecules to medicine, Physiol Rev 82:205, 2002.
20. Dudas PL, Villalobos AR, Gocek-Stutterlin G, et al: Regulation of transepithelial phosphate transport by PTH in chicken proximal tubule epithelium, *Am J Physiol Regul Integr Comp* 282:R139, 2002.
21. Hewison M, Zehnder D, Bland R, et al: 1a-Hydroxylase and the action of vitamin D, *J Mol Endocrinol* 25:141, 2000.
22. Spitzer A, Brandis M: Functional and morphologic maturation of the superficial nephrons: relationship to total kidney function, *J Clin Invest* 53:279, 1974.
23. Fukuda Y, Bertorello A, Aperia A: Ontogeny of the regulation of the Na+, K+-ATPase activity in the renal proximal tubular cell, *Pediatr Res* 30:131, 1991.
24. Mallet E, Basuyau JP, Brunelle P, et al: Neonatal parathyroid secretion and renal receptor maturation in premature infants, *Biol Neonate* 33:304, 1978.
25. Hebert S, Andreoli T: Control of NaCl transport in the thick ascending limb, *Am J Physiol* 246:F745, 1984.
26. Ichikawa I, Maddox D, Brenner BM: Maturational development of glomerular ultrafiltration in the rat, *Am J Physiol* 236:F465, 1979.
27. Matsunaga H, Yamashita N, Okuda T, et al: Mesangial cell ion transport and tubuloglomerular feedback, *Curr Opin Nephrol Hypertens* 3:518, 1994.
28. Bachmann S, Theilig F: Juxtaglomerular apparatus, nitric oxide, and macula densa signaling, *Adv Nephrol Necker Hosp* 30:95, 2000.
29. Nishiyama A, Navar LG: ATP mediates tubuloglomerular feedback, *Am J Physiol Regul Integr Comp Physiol* 283:R273, 2002.
30. Mount D, Delpire E, Gamba G: The electroneutral cation-chloride cotransporters, *J Exp Biol* 201(Pt 14):2091, 1998.
31. Bronner F: Renal calcium transport: mechanisms and regulation—an overview, *Am J Physiol* 257:F707, 1989.
32. Ward DT, Hammond TG, Harris HW: Modulation of vasopressin-elicited water transport by trafficking of aquaporin2-containing vesicles, *Annu Rev Physiol* 61:683, 1999.
33. Wade JB, Lee AJ, Liu J, et al: UT-A2: a 55-kDa urea transporter in thin descending limb whose abundance is regulated by vasopressin, *Am J Physiol Renal Physiol* 278:F52, 2000.
34. Wiesener MS, Eckardt KU: Erythropoietin, tumors and the von Hippel-Lindau gene: towards identification of mechanisms and dysfunction of oxygen sensing, *Nephrol Dial Transplant* 17:356, 2002.

CHAPTER

60

Electrolyte Management in Pediatric Critical Illness

Ellen G. Wood and Robert E. Lynch

Electrolyte management is one of the older areas of pediatric interventional medicine. There continue to be developments important to the management of childhood critical illness, and of course there continue to be questions and mysteries awaiting further elucidation.

This chapter takes a current look at relevant disturbances in sodium, potassium, magnesium, and phosphate during critical illness. Several developing areas deserve attention. The clinical entity of cerebral salt wasting syndrome is widely accepted and is clearly demonstrated in children,[1,2] but its mechanism is not yet understood. Central pontine myelinolysis may have a reversible phase,[3] and the process of myelinolysis is not restricted to the pons nor to patients with hyponatremia.[4] Some new drugs have been identified as causes of SIADH (syndrome of inappropriate secretion of antidiuretic hormone), and natural antidiuretic hormone (ADH) receptors can now be blocked experimentally. Genetic manipulation of aquaporin II channels involved in ADH function has further elucidated the mechanisms involved. The treatment of hyperkalemia with β_2 agonists has been examined further in both adults and children and has become an established form of therapy. The measurement of ionized magnesium is becoming more widespread, and its pertinence in critical illness is being explored.

Sodium

Sodium (Na) and its ions, chloride and bicarbonate, are the primary osmotic solutes that determine extracellular fluid (ECF) volume. They comprise more than 90% of the total solute in the ECF space. ECF sodium concentration is about 145 mEq/L, whereas intracellular fluid (ICF) sodium is only about 10 mEq/L. These concentrations are maintained by active transport mechanisms. Disturbances that significantly alter the ECF sodium concentration may have dramatic secondary effects on intracellular volume.

The regulation of sodium balance is determined by the relationship between sodium intake, renal sodium excretion, and extrarenal sodium losses. Pathological sodium retention may occur in disorders such as congestive heart failure (CHF), cirrhosis, and nephrosis without causing a significant alteration of ECF sodium concentration. A variety of other disorders may result in the development of either hyponatremia or hypernatremia and are addressed in the following sections.[44]

Hyponatremia

Pathophysiology and Etiology

Hyponatremia may occur in the presence of decreased, increased, or normal amounts of total body sodium.

Decreased Total Body Sodium. Total body sodium deficit with hyponatremia is generally associated with a total body water deficit that is less pronounced than the sodium loss. Intravascular volume depletion reduces the glomerular filtration rate (GFR). With a reduced GFR, fractional proximal tubular sodium reabsorption is increased and sodium delivery to the diluting distal nephron is decreased. In addition, ADH is released by nonosmotic and osmotic stimuli. Once the nonosmotic threshold is reached by a 5% to 10% reduction in volume, nonosmotic stimuli predominate.[5] Thus in the presence of hypovolemia, water is retained despite the development of hyponatremia and hypoosmolality.

Sodium deficit may occur through extrarenal or renal losses. In children extrarenal losses most often occur from vomiting and diarrhea. In critically ill patients, large extrarenal losses may result from fluid sequestration occurring with septicemia, peritonitis, pancreatitis, ileus, rhabdomyolysis, and burns. Transcutaneous losses also contribute in the patient with burns and in infants with cystic fibrosis. If renal function is preserved, these situations are associated with renal sodium conservation (urinary sodium <20 mEq/L or fractional excretion of sodium [FENa] <1%).

Renal losses include diuretic use, osmotic diuresis, various salt-losing renal diseases, and adrenal insufficiency.[6] Excessive diuretic use, especially with thiazides, may result in hyponatremia with hypovolemia and generally is associated with hypokalemic metabolic alkalosis.[6,7] Concentrated urine is produced by the equilibration of fluid in the collecting tubules with the hyperosmotic medullary interstitium, which in turn is generated by sodium chloride (NaCl) reabsorption without water in the ascending limb of the loop of Henle. Loop diuretics, therefore, alter concentrating ability by inhibiting NaCl reabsorption in the medullary ascending limb. Thiazides act in the cortex in the distal tubule and do not impair the ability of ADH to increase water reabsorption in the collecting tubules and collecting duct.[7] The resulting NaCl loss with water retention contributes to thiazide-associated hyponatremia.

Osmotic sodium and water losses occur in a child with uncontrolled hyperglycemia with glucosuria, with mannitol use, and less commonly after urea diuresis following relief of urinary tract obstruction. Sodium wasting is greater in the presence of massive ketonuria because the ketoacids are anions obligating cation losses. Hyperglycemia in mannitol, in addition to inducing urinary sodium and water losses, produces osmotic water movement from the ICF to the ECF; thus serum sodium concentration is further lowered. Sodium levels drop by about 1.5 mEq/L for every 100 mg/dl rise in the blood glucose level.[8]

Significant salt wasting may occur with several intrinsic renal diseases and may result in hyponatremia when associated with decreased access to water and sodium (Box 60–1). In the absence of these causes, adrenal insufficiency must be considered. Generally it is associated with hyperkalemia and decreased urinary potassium excretion. In each of the renal wasting states, urinary sodium excretion is generally greater than 20 mEq/L (FENa more than 1%).[6]

Cerebral salt wasting was reported in 1950, was attributed to SIADH in the 1690s and 1970s, and has been rediscovered over the last 20 years. Despite lingering skepticism, its clinical identity is accepted (Table 60–1). Patients typically have neurological injury with hemorrhage, infection, or mass and often undergo surgical procedures. The development of hyponatremia may be attributed to SIADH, but it is distinct in that large urine volumes contain very high sodium concentrations that lead to rapid depletion of both sodium and ACF volume. Secondary findings of hypovolemia develop and require volume restitution while attention is also given to careful repair of the hyponatremic-hypoosmotic condition.[1]

Atrial natruretic peptide has been elevated in many cases, but the release of brain natruretic peptide or other natruretic factors may be an important part of a multifactorial syndrome. Of particular interest is the sometimes noted aldosterone suppression and patient response to fludrocortisone therapy.[9] Occasional patients will have large urine outputs. Once serum sodium has been returned to low normal values, a cautious trial of fludrocortisone or even DDAVP (1-deamino-8-D-arginine vasopressin) may be appropriate in such difficult situations.

BOX 60–1

Causes of Hyponatremia

DECREASED TOTAL BODY SODIUM

Extrarenal

Vomiting/diarrhea
Fluid sequestration
  Septicemia, peritonitis, pancreatitis, ileus, burns, rhabdomyolysis
Cutaneous losses
  Burns, cystic fibrosis
Ventriculostomy drainage

Renal

Cerebral salt wasting
Diuretics
  Nonosmotic
    Thiazides > loop agents
Osmotic
Mannitol, glucose, urea
Tubulointerstitial diseases
Medullary cystic disease, obstructive uropathy, tubulointerstitial nephritis, chronic pyelonephritis, renal tubular acidosis, Kearns-Sayre syndrome
Adrenal insufficiency
Congenital adrenal hyperplasia, Addison's disease

INCREASED TOTAL BODY SODIUM

Congestive heart failure
Cirrhosis
Nephrotic syndrome
Advanced renal failure

NORMAL TOTAL BODY SODIUM

Syndrome of inappropriate ADH secretion
Glucocorticoid deficiency
Hypothyroidism
Infantile water intoxication
Abusive water intoxication

ADH, Antidiuretic hormone.

TABLE 60–1

Cerebral Salt Wasting Syndrome

Trigger	Subarachnoid hemorrhage or other acute intracranial injury or illness
Onset	Usually a few days after the injury
Signs	Falling serum Na^+, high urine output, high urine Na^+
Course	Without treatment, it proceeds to intravascular volume depletion, hypoperfusion, and hypotension
Treatment	Replace salt and water loss; restoring serum Na^+ may require 3% NaCl, furosemide, rarely fludrocortisone
Resolution	Days to weeks
Differential Dx	SIADH, adrenal insufficiency, osmotic diruesis

Dx, Diagnosis; *NaCl,* sodium chloride; *SIADH,* syndrome of inappropriate secretion of antidiuretic hormone.

Increased Total Body Sodium. Hyponatremia occurs when the increase in total body water exceeds the sodium retention. Four clinical situations are commonly seen: CHF, cirrhosis, nephrotic syndrome (NS), and advanced renal failure. In each of the first three clinical situations, controversy exists regarding the role of renal and extrarenal mechanisms in pathogenesis. In all four conditions, hyponatremia tends to be mild, asymptomatic, and non-progressive. These patients come to the intensive care units (ICUs) primarily for care of the other aspects of their chronic conditions.

Congestive Heart Failure. In a low CO animal model, renal sodium excretion is decreased primarily from the associated decrease in "effective" blood volume.[10] Similar changes occur in models of high cardiac output CHF. Stimulation of aortic and carotid vasoreceptors and right and left heart volume receptors may result in sodium retention through increased sympathetic activity and stimulation of the renin angiotensin aldosterone systems, producing increased renal vascular resistance, decreased GFR, and resultant decreased urinary sodium excretion. In addition, decreased aldosterone degradation and altered levels of other vasoactive and nonvasoactive substances result in the primary increased tubular sodium reabsorption. Impaired water excretion occurs from both nonosmotic ADH release and decreased distal renal tubular delivery of fluid.[11]

Cirrhosis. Early in cirrhosis increased intrahepatic pressure may initiate renal sodium retention before ascites formation. Later, peripheral vasodilation mediated with nitric oxide, multiple arteriovenous fistulae, and a decrease in the effective blood volume occur. These "decompensated" patients have higher levels of renin, aldosterone, vasopressin, and norepinephrine than "compensated" patients with cirrhosis.[6,12,13]

Nephrotic Syndrome. Hyponatremia is seen less frequently in patients with NS than in those with CHF or liver disease.[14] Humoral factors involved in patients with decreased central volume appear to be similar to decompensated patients with cirrhosis.[130] In addition, the release of atrial natriuretic factor (ANF) following albumin infusion appears to be a major trigger for diuresis and natriuresis.[14] The cause of hyponatremia in patients reported to have normal central volume status is unclear.

Renal Failure. As a diseased kidney loses nephrons, the remaining nephrons exhibit a dramatically elevated fractional sodium excretion in efforts to maintain sodium balance. Edema develops when larger quantities of sodium are ingested than can be excreted. The ability to excrete water is also impaired, primarily because of a dramatic decrease in the GFR. Hyponatremia occurs when water intake exceeds insensible losses plus the maximum volume that can be excreted.[5,6]

Normal Total Body Sodium. Hyponatremia with no evidence of hypovolemia or edema in the pediatric population is almost exclusively associated with SIADH, which results from many causes. Renal concentrating and diluting ability ultimately depends on the presence or absence of ADH to modulate water permeability in the collecting duct. Osmoreceptors for ADH reside in the anterior hypothalamus, responding to changes of as little as 1% in plasma osmolality. The nonosmotic stimuli that induce release are generally associated with changes in autonomic neural tone such as those that occur with physical pain, emotional stress, hypoxia, cardiac failure, adrenal insufficiency, and volume depletion. When stimuli for ADH release are competitive, the nonosmotic pathway appears to predominate. Vasopressin synthesized in the hypothalamus is transported in neurosecretory granules to the axonal bulbs in the median eminence and posterior pituitary gland and is released by exocytosis. After release, binding to V2 receptors occurs at the basolateral membrane of the collecting duct, increasing cyclic adenosine 3′, 5′-monophosphate (cAMP) formation, facilitating phosphorylation of aquaporin 2. Incorporation of aquaporin 2 containing vesicles into the apical (luminal) membrane increases cell permeability to reabsorptive water movement.[15]

Several categories of clinical diseases have been associated with SIADH, including central nervous system (CNS) and pulmonary disorders, malignancies, and side effects of numerous drugs.[136] Less commonly, ingestion of dilute formula and water intoxication,[16] postoperative states,[17] and endocrine disorders such as glucocorticoid deficiency and hypothyroidism have been associated with SIADH (Box 60–2).[16] SIADH should be considered when hyponatremia occurs in the absence of hypovolemia, edema, and other previously discussed causes (endocrine dysfunction, renal failure, drugs). Urine osmolality is inappropriately high compared with plasma osmolality. A urine osmolality of 200 to 250 mOsm does not rule out the diagnosis because a fall of 4 to 5 mEq/L below normal in serum sodium should maximally inhibit ADH secretion with a resultant urine osmolality of less than 100 mOsm. Urinary sodium is generally more than 20 mEq/L; however, it can be much less than 20 mEq/L in patients who are given a low sodium intake or in whom some degree of volume depletion occurs concurrently.[15]

Signs and Symptoms

The severity of signs and symptoms depends on the rapidity of development. Acute decreases in sodium are associated with lethargy, apathy, and disorientation often accompanied by nausea, vomiting, and muscle cramps. No predictable correlation exists between the degree of hyponatremia and its resulting symptoms. In general, however, most patients exhibit seizures and coma with acute falls in sodium to less than 120 mEq/L. Other signs include decreased deep tendon reflexes, pathological reflexes, pseudobulbar palsy, and Cheyne-Stokes respiratory pattern. Signs and symptoms are related to cellular swelling and resultant cerebral edema, which may be severe enough to result in herniation.[18] In animal studies, increases in brain water were more severe with acute than with chronic hyponatremia.[18] Patients who have hyponatremia over several days to weeks may be symptom free or may have nonspecific symptoms of nausea, vomiting, and lethargy.

Treatment

The correction of severe hyponatremia became a controversial issue.[18-24] It is generally agreed that severe

BOX 60–2

Conditions Associated with SIADH

CENTRAL NERVOUS SYSTEM

Meningitis
Encephalitis
Head trauma
Brain tumors
Brain abscess
Guillain-Barré syndrome
Hypoxia (neonatal)
Hydrocephalus
Rocky Mountain spotted fever
Vincristine
Salicylates
Cerebral thrombosis or hemorrhage
Subarachnoid or subdural hemorrhage
Acute psychosis
Peripheral neuropathy
Multiple sclerosis
Hypopituitarism

PULMONARY

Pneumonia
Positive-pressure
Asthma
Pneumothorax

TUMORS

Lymphoma, thymoma
Ewing's sarcoma, mesothelioma
Carcinoma (bronchogenic, duodenum pancreas, ureter, bladder, prostate)

DRUGS

ADH analogs
Chlorpropamide
Vincristine
Cyclophosphamide
Carbamazepine
Barbiturates
Colchicine
Haloperidol
Fluphenazine
Tricyclics, SSRIs
Clofibrate
Salicylates
Indomethacin, NSAID
Interferon
Ecstasy (MDMA)

MISCELLANEOUS

Infants (0-6 mo) receiving diluted feeding
Marathon runner
Postoperative, postprocedural patients

NSAID, Nonsteroidal antiinflammatory drug; *SIADH,* syndrome of inappropriate secretion of antidiuretic hormone; *SSRI,* selective serotonin reuptake inhibitor.

hyponatremia is associated with significant morbidity and mortality. Its treatment, however, has been associated with development of central pontine myelinolysis, the "osmotic demyelination syndrome."[19,21-24] Most studies have involved adult patients rather than infants or children. A decrease in the serum sodium concentration would be expected to cause a shift of water from the ECF to the ICF compartment, resulting in generalized cellular edema. When this swelling occurs in the brain, which is limited by the presence of meninges and the cranium, neurological symptoms are expected. In numerous studies authors have reported cerebral edema and herniation of the brainstem at postmortem examination with acute hyponatremia. This sequela has, however, not been reported in patients with hyponatremia over a more prolonged period. The results of several animal studies are the same: Brain cells prevent massive swelling when gradual hyponatremia is produced by the extrusion of electrolytes and other osmolites. Total brain amino acid content, particularly taurine, is strikingly decreased in hyponatremic rats with prolonged deficits. Brain water content is also lower in these animals. These data suggest that brain edema develops when the plasma-to-brain osmotic gradient reaches a critical level before these adaptive processes have been fully developed, suggesting a rationale of differentiating therapy between those patients who have acute hyponatremia and those in whom it has developed over a more prolonged period. Rapid correction of serum sodium concentration under acute circumstances should prevent the plasma-to-brain osmotic gradient from becoming critical and resulting in life-threatening cerebral edema. When adaptation of brain cells has already occurred, however, a rapid rise in serum sodium concentration may induce a shift of water from the ICF to the ECF compartment, resulting in brain dehydration and subsequent brain injury, that is, the osmotic demyelination syndrome.

Deep brain regions seem particularly sensitive to the dehydrating effects of rapid increases in serum osmolality. Originally noted in the pons, both pontine and extrapontine myelinolysis has been reported in children. Extrapontine sites have included the cerebellum, thalamus, lateral geniculate body, and hippocampus.[4,25]

Osmotic demyelination can occur without hyponatremia as a starting point. Thus large bolus doses of hypertonic saline may put the patient at risk regardless of starting sodium concentration. Rapid correction of hypernatremia is a possible cause of myelinolysis, which suggests pressure effects may be capable of causing damage to myelinated structures.

Symptoms of osmotic demyelination may include obtundation, quadriplegia, pseudobulbar palsy, seizures, and coma.[26] Individual cases have been reported in which these symptoms were appreciated, the patient's osmolarity was intentionally relowered significantly and corrected more slowly, and good neurological outcome was the result.[3,27,28]

Approaches to patients with hyponatremia should vary depending on whether this hyponatremia has developed acutely, has developed over 24 to 48 hours, or has developed over a longer period (i.e., chronic hyponatremia).[142,143] In planning treatment it is also critical to determine the presence or absence of CNS symptoms suggestive of cerebral edema. Development of CNS cellular swelling would seem more likely with acute hyponatremia or with severe chronic hyponatremia. In these patients, an initial small but rapid correction of serum sodium, about 5 mEq/L, should stabilize or begin to reverse cerebral swelling and avoid impending herniation. Subsequently, further correction of the hyponatremia should occur more slowly.[26]

A dose of 3% saline at 5 to 6 ml/kg would be expected to initially raise the serum sodium approximately 5 mEq/L. The subsequent correction rate for patients with acute hyponatremia with CNS symptoms or for any patient with chronic hyponatremia should raise the serum sodium no more than 0.5 mEq/L an hour. For patients with acute hyponatremia but no CNS symptoms, rates of 0.7 to 1 mEq/L an hour have been reported without patient morbidity or mortality. In many patients, a regimen of hypertonic 3% saline at 1 to 2 ml/kg an hour plus periodic administration of a loop diuretic results in an appropriate correction for those patients for whom "rapid" correction is safe. CNS symptoms that develop during correction suggest osmotic demyelination and have occurred most frequently in patients or experimental animals that are euvolemic rather than hypovolemic.[20-24] At least three patients have been reported who had symptoms of osmotic demyelination and whose course was subsequently reversed; their serum sodium was decreased to its nadir followed by a slower rate of correction resulting in recovery without neurologic sequelae.

ADH V2 receptor antagonists are undergoing trials for treatment of hyponatremia, particularly in fluid-retaining states. These promising agents increase urine volume and reduce urine osmolality. Further study of safety and efficacy will clarify their clinical utility.[140]

Several authors have reported that infants with acute hyponatremia may be at lower risk for neurological sequelae because of flexible suture lines permitting brain volume expansion.[20,23] Newborn puppies tolerate a more significant degree of swelling.[20] Sterns et al[23] have also noted no evidence of brain death or neurological sequelae in 37 patients with infantile water intoxication. Anecdotal evidence of those caring for critically ill children, however, suggests that this entity certainly does occur in infants.

In the patient in whom less severe hyponatremia (serum sodium 120-130 mEq/L) occurs, slow correction through water restriction, occasionally with the use of oral sodium supplements, is all that is required for normalization to occur. In the patient with hypovolemia, volume status clearly must be corrected in addition to the hyponatremia. As previously discussed, these patients seem to be at less risk for consequences of rapid correction of hyponatremia and for acute cerebral edema.

Hypernatremia

As is the case with hyponatremia, hypernatremia can develop with low, normal, or high total body sodium. History and weights are particularly important in evaluating the hydration state of patients with hypernatremia because a shift in the ICF to the ECF tends to obscure the physical findings of dehydration. Accurate assessment of total body sodium and water aids considerably in planning management, although the most important management principle is the frequent monitoring of the patient's progress with treatment adjustments as needed.

Low Total Body Sodium

Patients with low total body sodium have a loss of water in relative excess of sodium losses. Because the ECF space is hyperosmolar, water movement from the ICF occurs with resulting ICF dehydration. Therefore the ECF space is somewhat preserved until extreme degrees of hypovolemia have occurred. Losses of sodium and water may be extrarenal or renal (Box 60–3). In the pediatric patient, extrarenal causes are commonly seen from vomiting and diarrhea. Excessive sweating with inadequate replacement may also occur. Acute hypernatremic dehydration after treatment of an infant with large doses of activated charcoal in 70% sorbitol for theophylline toxicity has been described.[29] Sorbitol that remains in the gut acts as an osmotic agent; its drawing of free water into the lumen causes diarrhea. In these cases, urine osmolality is high, whereas urine sodium is low (<20 mEq/L) from renal conservation. Renal causes of hypernatremia include osmotic diuresis from mannitol, hyperglycemia, or increased urea excretion. In these cases, urine is either hypotonic or isotonic, whereas urine sodium is more than 20 mEq/L. One cause of hypernatremia in the neonate has been insufficient maternal lactation. Infants are

BOX 60–3

Causes of Hypernatremia

LOW TOTAL BODY SODIUM

Extrarenal Losses

Vomiting/diarrhea
Sweating
70% sorbitol

Renal Losses

Osmotic diuresis
  Mannitol, glucose, urea

Inadequate Intake

Insufficient lactation

NORMAL TOTAL BODY SODIUM

Extrarenal Losses

Respiratory insensible losses
Dermal insensible losses
  Fever
  Burns
  Radiant warmers
  Phototherapy

Renal

Diabetes insipidus
  Central
  Nephrogenic
  Hypodipsia (reset osmostat)

INCREASED TOTAL BODY SODIUM

Administration/ingestion of sodium
Improperly diluted formula
Near-drowning (seawater)

particularly susceptible to "hypernatremic dehydration" because their surface area/weight ratio is high and their relative renal immaturity results in greater water losses for excretion of a solute load compared with older children and adults.[30]

Normal Total Body Sodium

Loss of water occurs without excessive sodium losses in some conditions. Extrarenal causes include increased respiratory losses as may occur with tachypnea, hyperventilation, or mechanical ventilation with inadequate humidification and increased skin losses associated with fever, burns, extreme prematurity, or use of phototherapy or radiant warmers in the neonate without adequate water replacement. Renal losses result from acquired or congenital diabetes insipidus (DI), either central or nephrogenic. Acquired forms of DI are more commonly seen by the intensivist. Major insults resulting in central DI include head trauma, tumors, infections, hypoxic injury, neurosurgical procedures, and nontraumatic brain death. Often, in experimental animals and in humans, three stages occur: (1) an initial polyuric phase (hours to several days); (2) a period of antidiuresis probably due to ADH release from injured axons (hours to days); and (3) a second period of DI that may or may not resolve, depending on the location and extent of the injury.[30,31,145] Sudden onset of polyuria is characteristic, as is polydipsia (in the conscious patient). In the critically ill patient, lack of access to increased water may result in life-threatening hypernatremia. Patients with the rare congenital nephrogenic DI may have repeated bouts of hypernatremic dehydration, resulting from x-linked alteration of the vasopressin receptor V2 or the autosomal recessive changes in the aquaporin II water channel physiologically regulated by ADH.[32,33] Acquired forms are much more common, and fortunately manifestations are less severe. Causes are shown in Box 60–4.

Essential hypernatremia is a rare condition characterized by persistent hypernatremia unexplained by water loss, along with hypodipsia, partial DI, and a normal renal response to ADH. In most cases cerebral lesions around the hypothalamus have been associated with essential hypernatremia. These patients have been proposed to have "reset" osmoreceptors, with urinary concentration and dilution occurring at inappropriately high levels of plasma osmolality.[34]

BOX 60–4

Causes of Diabetes Insipidus

CENTRAL

Congenital

- Inherited
- Idiopathic

Acquired

- Head trauma
- Orbital trauma
- Tumors, suprasellar and intrasellar
- Infections
  - Encephalitis
  - Meningitis
  - Guillain-Barré syndrome
  - Hypoxia (infant)
- Post neurosurgical procedures
- Miscellaneous
  - Vascular
  - Cerebral aneurysms, thrombosis, hemorrhage
  - Histiocytosis
  - Granulomas
  - Nontraumatic brain death

NEPHROGENIC

Congenital

- VR_2 mutation, X linked
- AQP-2 mutation

Acquired

- Chronic renal failure
- Renal tubulointerstitial diseases
- Hypercalcemia
- K^+ depletion
- Drugs
  - Alcohol, lithium, diuretics, amphotericin B, methoxyflurane, demeclocycline
- Sickle cell disease
- Dietary abnormalities
  - Primary polydipsia, decreased sodium chloride intake, severe protein restriction or depletion

Increased Total Body Sodium

Hypernatremia with increased total body sodium is most often an iatrogenic problem. In the critical care unit, administration of hypertonic solutions of sodium bicarbonate during resuscitation efforts or as therapy of intractable metabolic acidosis is often responsible. Particularly at risk is the patient after cardiac arrest, when renal failure from hypoxic injury may ensue as well. Other causes include excessive hypertonic NaCl administration for treatment of hyponatremia, salt water near drowning, ingestion by infants of improperly diluted formula, inadvertent intravascular infusion of hypertonic saline in therapeutic abortion, and dialysis against a high sodium concentration. Normonatremic patients with massive edema who undergo a forced diuresis frequently become mildly hypernatremic as the induced urine may be hypotonic and water loss exceeds sodium loss.

Hypernatremia is purposely induced in patients with head trauma as a form of osmotherapy for control of intracranial hypertension. This approach is somewhat controversial but also somewhat promising. When the ECF osmolality of these patients is manipulated, the risks involved with rapid changes in either direction must be kept in mind.

Signs and Symptoms

Clinical manifestations of hypernatremia relate predominantly to the CNS. Marked irritability, a high-pitched cry, a decrease in sensorium varying from lethargy to coma, normal or increased muscle tone, and frank seizure activity occur in about two thirds of children with development of hypernatremia over 48 hours or more. Hyperglycemia and hypocalcemia may also occur.[35,36] In infants with acute hypernatremia, vomiting, fever, respiratory distress, spasticity, tonic-clonic seizure activity, and coma are common.[37,38] Death from respiratory failure occurred in experimental animals when serum osmolality reached about 430 mOsm/kg.[39] Mortality in children has ranged from 10% to about 45% with chronic and acute hypernatremia, respectively. Morbidity in survivors has also been high.[41]

Anatomical changes seen with the hyperosmolar state include loss of volume of brain cells with resultant tearing of cerebral vessels, capillary and venous congestion, subcortical or subarachnoid bleeding, and venous sinus thrombosis.[30,38] During the first 4 hours of experimental acute hypernatremia, brain water significantly decreases while the concentration of solutes (electrolytes and glucose) increases. A small portion of increased osmolality is not accounted for by the increase in electrolytes and glucose, termed *idiogenic osmoles*. By 48 hours, however, brain water has returned to normal with idiogenic osmoles (amino acids, polyhydric alcohols, and urea and trimethylamines) accounting for about 60% of the increased osmoles.[35,39]

The central demyelination syndrome has been seen in patients with hypernatremia. It remains unclear as to whether it results from a rapid rise in serum osmolality or from some other aspect of the clinical course.

Treatment

Whenever possible, therapy of hypernatremia should address correction of the underlying disease process as a primary goal. Treatment of infants and children with hypernatremic dehydration is by far the most controversial. In this situation, therapy with fluid providing free water in excess of electrolytes has generally been used after correction of shock or circulatory collapse.[6,30,38,40,41] Few data are available regarding the ideal rate of correction. Numerous fatal cases of cerebral edema have occurred with correction over a 24-hour period, however, leading to recommendations for correction over no less than a 48-hour period.[6,38,40-42] Sodium content of replacement intravenous fluids has ranged from one fifth to normal saline in 2.5% to 5% dextrose, with agreement that plasma osmolality should not be decreased more rapidly than 2 mOsm/hr.[38] Patients with serum sodium levels greater than 165 for more than 48 hours deserve particular care, and a correction rate of no more than 1 mOsm/hr may be appropriate. Thus corrections from extreme hypernatremia may take several days. This slower rate of correction appears to allow time for dissipation of idiogenic osmoles without development of cerebral edema. Estimated deficits, ongoing maintenance requirements, and additional excessive losses must be accounted for in calculations of amount of fluid replacement. Though not frequently required, calculation of tonicity balance may give an accurate analysis of the disturbance.

In a patient in whom DI is suspected and urgent care is not required, a water deprivation test is still the most accurate means of determining the type of abnormality present. In the ICU setting, however, this is often not a feasible approach. Central DI is a likely cause of hypernatremia, particularly in patients who have head trauma or have undergone a recent intracranial operation. In those patients, a trial of vasopressin is in order. Either aqueous vasopressin (shorter half-life) given subcutaneously or intravenously or DDAVP may be used. Aqueous pitressin may be given in a continuous infusion beginning at a rate of 0.5 mU/kg/hr with gradual sequential increase to 10 mU/kg/hr. An increase in urine osmolality to values exceeding that in serum suggests the diagnosis of central DI. Careful adjustments must be made in fluid administration to avoid iatrogenic hyponatremia. DDAVP is generally begun in a dosage ranging from 0.05 to 0.1 ml by spray once or twice daily.

In patients with increased total body sodium (and often hypervolemia), the goal is its removal. In patients with intact renal function, this may be accomplished with diuretics and a decrease in sodium administration. If renal failure is present, dialysis may be required.

Potassium

Presentation of deficient or excessive potassium (K) stores with resultant hypokalemia or hyperkalemia is common to the intensivist. Extracellular potassium with a general range of 3.5 to 5.5 mEq/L makes up only 2% of total body potassium, with concentrations in the intracellular compartments of 150 to 160 mEq/L.[43] Total body stores are estimated to be about 50 mEq/kg body weight.[44] The distribution of potassium between intracellular and extracellular compartments is maintained by numerous hormonal and nonhormonal factors.

The transcellular distribution of potassium establishes the resting membrane potential of cells. Factors involved in total body distribution include acid-base status, insulin, catecholamines, magnesium, and possibly aldosterone.[43,45,141] Acidemia raises the serum potassium, and alkalemia lowers its concentration. The type of acid-base disturbance (metabolic or respiratory), the duration of the disturbance, and the nature of the anion accompanying the hydrogen ion in metabolic acidosis, however, are important in determining what effect a particular acid-base disorder may have on potassium concentration.[46-48] The greatest effect occurs with mineral acids, where cellular permeability to accompanying anions is low so that hydrogen ions enter cells alone. In this case, potassium must move out of the cells to maintain electrical neutrality. In metabolic acidosis caused by organic acids such as lactate and β-hydroxybutyrate, however, hydrogen ions presumably enter cells with their accompanying anions so that cation exchange with potassium is not required.[46,47]

Hyperkalemia associated with diabetic ketoacidosis (DKA) may reflect the effects of hyperosmolality and decreased circulating insulin, rather than the acidemia itself.[43,45] Epinephrine initially causes serum potassium to rise, reflecting release from the liver, and then fall, as potassium moves into the cell.[49] This effect appears to be mediated by β receptors because it is abolished by β-adrenergic blocking drugs.[50] In rats with experimentally induced insulin deficiency, both epinephrine and the peripheral sympathetic nervous system have been shown to regulate cell potassium uptake.[51] Change in intracellular magnesium (mg^{++}) may affect the sodium-potassium adenosine triphosphatase (ATPase) pump and alter the transcellular distribution. An additional mechanism, mineralocorticoid-mediated potassium redistribution, has been demonstrated in glucocorticoid-replaced animals that have undergone adrenalectomies.[52] All of these mechanisms, however, are generally representative of fine-tuning in potassium homeostasis. Ultimately, potassium balance is regulated through excretion by the kidney and to a lesser extent the gastrointestinal (GI) tract.

Most of the filtered potassium is absorbed before the distal nephron in normal kidneys.[43] The potassium excreted in the urine then is mainly due to secretion in the distal convoluted tubule and cortical collecting duct. As with sodium, the kidney's capacity to vary potassium excretion is profound, ranging from a low of approximately 5 mEq/L to amounts exceeding 100 mEq/L of urine. Factors influencing renal potassium excretion include mineralocorticoid and glucocorticoid hormones, acid-base balance, anion effects, tubular fluid flow rate, sodium intake, potassium intake, ICF and plasma potassium concentrations, and diuretics.[43,45,52-54] Aldosterone is a major kaliuretic hormone. Metabolic acidosis decreases and metabolic alkalosis increases intracellular potassium activity in cells of the distal tubule, causing enhanced potassium secretion during alkalosis and reabsorption during acidosis.[53] Fluid delivery to the distal tubule probably enhances potassium secretion by two mechanisms: (1) the faster fluid moves past the secretory site, and a greater amount of potassium can be secreted. (2) Because tubular fluid potassium concentration decreases as flow rate increases, a favorable gradient for potassium movement is maintained at high flow rates.[45]

Hypokalemia

Causes of Hypokalemia

Hypokalemia without Potassium Deficit. The detection of a low serum potassium level may reflect a true deficit in total body stores or an apparent deficit from the shift of this ion from the ECF to the ICF pool. A shift to the ICF pool may occur in alkalemia,[43,45] exogenous administration and likely endogenous release of β-adrenergic agonists,[45,55,56] familial hypokalemic periodic paralysis,[57] barium poisoning,[58,148] and excess insulin.[59] In the case of alkalemia, potassium moves into the cell in exchange for H^+ in attempts to maintain extracellular pH. The pediatric patient with alkalemia may have a true potassium deficit in addition due to decreased potassium intake or increased losses. Numerous studies have confirmed an acute decrease in serum potassium after administration of β_2 agonists, including epinephrine and albuterol, presumably from cellular influx of potassium into skeletal muscle cells. Diuretic use in this situation appears to have additive effects.[60] Endogenous levels of epinephrine equal to or greater than levels obtained by exogenous administration have been reported in adults with acute myocardial infarction and recently in children after near drowning.[61]

Periodic paralysis is a rare autosomal dominant disorder presenting with intermittent episodes of profound muscle weakness associated with a sudden fall in serum potassium concentration precipitated by high-carbohydrate/low-potassium diet, exercise, infection, stress, or alcohol ingestion.[57] Barium poisoning has been reported to produce hypokalemia, paralysis, vomiting, and diarrhea.[58] Insulin produces potassium shifts into the liver in association with glycogen formation and into muscle cells.[59]

Hypokalemia with Potassium Deficit. A deficit in total body potassium may occur from decreased intake, from renal losses, or from GI losses. Poor intake coupled with increased GI or renal losses is common. Any history of geophagia in the toddler should be sought because ingested clay binds potassium in the GI tract.[62]

Renal Losses. Major categories that may be seen in the ICU setting include hyperaldosteronism, diuretic use, osmotic diuresis, use of various other drugs, renal tubular acidosis, magnesium deficiency, and recovery from acute renal failure (ARF).

Primary aldosteronism, congenital adrenal hyperplasia, adrenal adenoma, and familial idiopathic hyperaldosteronism are rare in children and even rarer in the pediatric ICU setting. Secondary hyperaldosteronism is common, however, either from volume depletion or from CHF, cirrhosis, or NS.[43,45] Patients with the latter conditions, however, rarely have severe hypokalemia unless they are additionally treated with diuretics. The infant with Bartter's syndrome may initially come to the ICU because of multiple metabolic derangements including hypokalemia, metabolic alkalosis, and often hypomagnesemia and hyperuricemia. Other findings include weakness, polyuria, and failure to thrive, with elevated renin and aldosterone levels in the absence of hypertension.[63] Other conditions associated with elevated renin secretion, secondary hyperaldosteronism, and hypokalemia include renal artery stenosis, malignant hypertension, renin-producing tumor, or Wilms' tumor. Osmotic diuresis from glucosuria is the primary cause of renal potassium wasting in DKA. Additional mechanisms include secondary hyperaldosteronism and increased distal tubular fluid delivery. The severity of hypokalemia is often masked by the shift of potassium from ICF to ECF space related to insulin deficiency, metabolic acidosis, and hypertonicity.[43,45]

If a brisk diuresis is induced by loop, thiazide, or osmotic diuretics, kaliuresis may result, and this may lead to acute hypokalemia. Use of combinations of these diuretics, in particular loop diuretics and metolazone, may accentuate potassium losses. Each agent leads to increased distal delivery of tubular fluid. Other drugs that induce excessive renal losses include amphotericin B (kaliuresis with reduced renal function and tubular injury); aminoglycosides, particularly gentamicin; and high-dose penicillin and carbenicillin, which produce an osmotic load in addition to acting as nonreabsorbable anions.[64]

Renal tubular acidosis, both proximal and distal types, is more likely to be seen in the pediatric wards than in the ICU setting. Also, hypomagnesemia causes renal potassium wasting that continues until correction of magnesium occurs.[65] Lysozymuria associated with acute leukemia has also resulted in massive renal potassium losses.[66]

Gastrointestinal Losses. Upper GI losses from vomiting or from nasogastric (NG) suction are frequently associated with hypokalemia, although they are rarely responsible for the total depletion seen. The gastric concentration of potassium ranges from 5 to 10 mEq/L.[43,45] Concomitant volume depletion and metabolic alkalosis associated with NaCl and hydrogen ion losses often result in secondary aldosteronism, however, and an increased filtered load of bicarbonate with resultant renal potassium losses. Diarrhea, regardless of cause, may result in large potassium losses, the amount lost being related to the volume of fluid lost. Other GI causes are listed in Box 60–5.

Signs and Symptoms

For the intensivist, cardiovascular and neuromuscular effects of potassium deficiency are of particular concern, although metabolic, hormonal, and renal effects may also occur.

Electrocardiographic (ECG) changes include T wave flattening or inversion, ST depression, and the appearance of a U wave. Finally, atrial and ventricular arrhythmias and conduction disturbances may occur. Resting membrane potential is increased, as are both the duration of the action potential and the refractory period. The decreasing of conductivity predisposes a patient to arrhythmias. Finally, threshold potential and automaticity are increased, and this increase makes automatic arrhythmias possible.[67-69]

Hypokalemia diminishes skeletal muscular excitability. This can present as a dynamic ileus or a skeletal muscle weakness initially worse in the lower extremities, and it can eventually affect the trunk and upper extremities, becoming severe enough to result in quadriplegia and respiratory failure.[70-73] Rhabdomyolysis has also been reported from decreased muscle blood flow, decreased glycogen stores, and altered Na/K-ATPase and membrane potential.[74] Autonomic insufficiency may also occur, generally manifested as orthostatic hypotension.

In patients with severe liver disease, hypokalemia may precipitate or exacerbate encephalopathy. Glucose intolerance in the presence of primary hyperaldosteronism and in certain patients receiving thiazide diuretics has been corrected with potassium repletion. Renal effects of hypokalemia include polyuria and polydipsia, renal structural changes with cellular vacuolization in the proximal tubule, and occasional interstitial fibrosis.

BOX 60–5

Causes of Hypokalemia

HYPOKALEMIA WITHOUT POTASSIUM DEFICIT

- Alkalosis
- β-Agonist, exogenous or endogenous
- Familial periodic paralysis
- Thyrotoxic periodic paralysis
- Barium poisoning
- Excessive insulin

HYPOKALEMIA WITH POTASSIUM DEFICIT

- Decrease intake
- Renal losses
  - Hyperaldosteronism
    - Primary or secondary
    - Barter's syndrome
    - Liddle's syndrome
    - Laxative and/or diuretic abuse
    - Licorice ingestion
  - Osmotic agents
  - Drugs
    - Caffeine
    - Diuretics
    - Amphotericin B
    - Aminoglycosides
    - High-dose penicillin, carbenicillin
  - Miscellaneous
    - Hypomagnesemia
    - Renal tubular acidosis
    - Toluene toxicity
- Extrarenal loses
  - Gastrointestinal
    - Vomiting, nasogastric suction
    - Diarrhea
    - Laxative abuse
    - Ureteral sigmoidostomy
    - Obstructed or long ileal loop

Treatment

Because of the wide spectrum of abnormalities resulting from marked potassium depletion, judicious correction is generally in order.[75] In the patient without life-threatening complications, the oral route is generally preferred for treatment, if possible, because this route is rarely associated with "overshoot" hyperkalemia if normal renal function exists. If, however, depletion is associated with digoxin use or with life-threatening complications, including cardiac arrhythmias, rhabdomyolysis, extreme weakness with quadriplegia, or respiratory distress, then urgent IV therapy is generally needed. Recommendations for IV dosage in the pediatric patient have ranged from infusions of 0.25 mEq/kg/hr to those as high as 1 mEq/kg/hr in the face of severe hypokalemia associated with DKA, arrhythmias, or quadriparesis and respiratory insufficiency. Continuous ECG monitoring is essential, as well as frequent physical examination and determination of serum potassium levels to avoid hyperkalemic complications. Preoperative repletion of diuretic-treated patients with cardiac disease may be beneficial.[76,77]

The potential for catastrophic drug error in replacing potassium is real. In most pediatric ICUs, patients with cardiovascular disease are given NG or IV supplements at serum levels of 3 to 4 mEq/L. Steps to decrease the chance of error include satellite pharmacy dosing, NG replacement when possible, use of a single solution concentration for all doses, and small aliquot solution containers. Continuing education regarding this risk for the pediatric ICU staff is essential. Patients who receive albuterol continuously are frequently mildly hypokalemic, but they rarely warrant potassium chloride replacement.

Hyperkalemia

Causes

Hyperkalemia may result from artifactual elevation; from redistribution of potassium from ICF to ECF space; or from increased intake, decreased losses, or both (Box 60–6).

BOX 60–6

Causes of Hyperkalemia

ARTIFACTUAL

Ischemic potassium loss from tourniquet use
In vivo red cell injury
In vitro hemolysis-profound leukocytosis, thrombocytosis

REDISTRIBUTION

Change in pH
Hypertonicity
Drugs
- Digoxin toxicity, β-blockers (β_2-inhibitory activity), succinylcholine, arginine, or lysine hydrochloride, chemotherapeutic agents, sodium fluoride, epsilon-amino caproic acid

TRUE POTASSIUM EXCESS

Increased Load

Exogenous
- IV infusion, PO supplements, potassium-containing salt substitutes, potassium penicillin, blood transfusion

Endogenous
- Tissue necrosis
  - Burns, trauma, rhabdomyolysis, intravascular coagulation
- Gastrointestinal bleeding
- Tumor cell lysis
- Reabsorption of hematoma

Decreased Excretion

Acute renal failure
Chronic renal failure
Mineralocorticoid deficiency
Addison's disease
Adrenal biosynthetic defects
- 21-Hydroxylase deficiency
- Desmolase deficiency
- 3-β-OH-Dehydrogenase deficiency

Aldosterone deficiency
Diabetes mellitus
Renal tubulointerstitial disease
Drugs
- Indomethacin, converting enzyme inhibitors, heparin, cyclosporine, tacrolimus, trimethoprim, pentamidine, amphotericin B

Renal tubular secretory deficit
- Pseudohypoaldosteronism

Sickle cell disease
Systemic lupus erythematosus
Renal allograft
Urinary tract obstruction
Very-low-birth-weight infants

Inhibition of Tubular Secretion

Drugs
- Spironolactone, triamterene, amiloride

Artifactual. Tight, prolonged tourniquet use produces spurious potassium elevation due to potassium release from ischemic muscle. Even more common is hemolysis of red cells with potassium release associated with capillary sticks. Here, serum is usually pink from the presence of free hemoglobin. Less commonly, in vitro release of potassium occurs from white blood cells (WBCs) (>100,000/mm^3) or platelets (>1,000,000/mm^3) and may result in increased serum, but not plasma, levels.[43,45]

Redistribution. In general, when extracellular pH falls, potassium exits from cells; the result is an increase in serum potassium. As mentioned earlier, metabolic acidosis from mineral acids has a more pronounced effect than that of organic acids. Plasma potassium does not change in parallel with the pH change; rather, it gradually rises even as extracellular pH returns to normal after acute acid loading. Respiratory acidosis does not usually cause marked changes in potassium concentration.[46,47,62]

Hypertonicity per se produces a shift of potassium from ICF to ECF. The best demonstration of this comes from studies of anephric animals in which potassium increased by 0.1 to 0.6 mEq/L for each increment of 10 mOsm/kg H_2O in tonicity. Hypertonicity causes cellular dehydration and therefore an increase in ICF potassium that favors increased passive diffusion out of cells.[43,45] Hypertonic mannitol is frequently used in the patient in the ICU who has acute oliguria or increased intracranial pressure. Particularly in the former situation, if potassium is already elevated, caution would seem advisable. In the patient with hyperglycemia, this mechanism is likely only one of several resulting in elevated serum levels.

Several commonly used drugs result in net movement of potassium from ICF to ECF. Cardiac glycosides inhibit the net uptake of K by cells by inhibiting Na/K-ATPas, with hyperkalemia commonly occurring in digitalis poisoning.[78] Other drugs include beta-blockers with β_2 activity[151] and the muscle relaxant succinylcholine.[78] This drug induces a prolonged dose-related increase in the ionic permeability of muscle, with subsequent efflux of potassium from muscle cells. Normal serum potassium concentration rises about 0.5 mEq/L. In patients with burns, muscle trauma, spinal injuries, certain neuromuscular diseases, near drowning, and closed head trauma, life-threatening hyperkalemia has been reported. Finally, familial hyperkalemic periodic paralysis appears to be related to potassium redistribution, although the cause of this rare disorder is unclear.[43,45]

Increased Load. Hyperkalemia due to an increased potassium load is unusual as long as renal function is normal. Transient elevations may be seen with inappropriate IV infusion, delivery of large volumes of cold stored blood, oral potassium supplements, salt substitutes containing potassium,[79] or large doses of potassium penicillin. Large endogenous loads of potassium are more likely in the patient who is in the ICU. The release of cellular potassium associated with tissue necrosis from burns, trauma, rhabdomyolysis, massive intravascular coagulopathy, massive hemolysis, or GI bleeding may lead to hyperkalemia.[43,45] Fatal hyperkalemia may occur during tumor lysis syndrome at initiation of tumor therapy or reabsorption of hematomas in the neonate. In many such patients, renal insufficiency, acidosis, or ECF contraction contributes to the development of life-threatening hyperkalemia.

Decreased Excretion. Hyperkalemia in ARF results from a profound reduction in the GFR, decreased distal water and solute delivery limiting Na/K exchange, and an insufficient time for renal and extrarenal adaptive mechanisms to develop. These are often associated with increased catabolism and metabolic acidosis. Nondiabetic chronic renal failure is rarely associated with hyperkalemia until the GFR falls below 5% to 10% of normal. Progressive, gradual impairment induces excretion of more potassium per remaining nephron. Other adaptations include increased stool loss and more rapid redistribution of potassium into cells.[43] Decreased mineralocorticoid activity regardless of origin causes hyperkalemia. Addison's disease, although rare in the pediatric ICU, may present in crisis with life-threatening hyperkalemia, as may adrenogenital syndromes. The syndrome of hyporeninemic hypoaldosteronism is commonly seen in adults; the classic example is the patient with diabetes mellitus and mild to moderate renal insufficiency.[78] Aldosterone production may be suppressed by heparin, angiotensin-converting enzyme inhibitors, prostaglandin inhibitors, tacrolimus, or cyclosporin.[79]

Renal tubular secretory defects occur in patients with pseudohypoaldosteronism presenting in children with failure to thrive, metabolic acidosis, hyperkalemia, and elevated aldosterone levels, as well as in rare patients with sickle cell disease, systemic lupus erythematosus, urinary tract obstruction, and renal allografts. Infants weighing less than 1000 g may have life threatening hyperkalemia in the absence of renal failure and increased sodium excretion in association with decreased potassium excretion.[80] Tubular immaturity with unresponsiveness to aldosterone has been postulated. Finally, potassium-sparing diuretics, trimethoprim, and pentamidine may produce hyperkalemia, particularly when used in combination with other drugs that decrease potassium excretion or in patients with renal insufficiency.[78]

Manifestations of Hyperkalemia

Cardiac abnormalities associated with hyperkalemia are the most likely abnormalities to produce life-threatening results. ECG signs include tall, peaked T waves in the precordial leads, followed by a decrease in amplitude of the R wave, bradycardia, widened QRS complexes, prolonged PR intervals, and decreased amplitude and disappearance of the P wave. Finally, the classic sine wave of hyperkalemia from the blending of the QRS complex with the P wave may appear. Realizing that ventricular arrhythmias or cardiac arrest may occur at any point in this progression and that progression may occur over a matter of minutes is extremely important.[81,82]

Treatment

Treatment of hyperkalemia depends on the level of plasma potassium and the state of neuromuscular irritability.[81] If the potassium is less than 6.5 mEq/L without ECG changes, discontinuation of exogenous potassium and drugs that decrease its excretion with close follow-up of potassium levels may be all that is necessary. In the patient with renal compromise, extra potassium may be eliminated with use of the potassium-binding agent sodium polystyrene sulfonate (Kayexalate) (oral, NG, or rectal doses of 1 to 2 g/kg in a sorbitol or dextrose solution). When administered rectally, sorbitol may not be necessary, and it should certainly not be given rectally in concentration greater than 20%. Highly concentrated sorbitol may cause severe proctitis and colonic injury.[83] Having the pharmacy stock a premixed 10% to 20% suspension of sodium polystyrene sulfonate and sorbitol allows either oral or rectal administration on short notice. If the potassium concentration is more than 6.5 mEq/L with associated ECG changes, additional measures are indicated. In the absence of digitalis toxicity, hyperkalemia with ECG changes should be treated with a secure and rapid IV infusion of calcium chloride or calcium gluconate. Hand injection with ECG monitoring is reasonable beginning with the administration of 10 mg/kg of calcium chloride (or gluconate equivalent) over 1 to 5 minutes. Infusion may be stopped if the electrocardiogram has normalized or if deterioration of the electrocardiogram seems to be precipitated by the potassium, suggesting a clinical scenario more complex than simple hyperkalemia. If the electrocardiogram improves but is not normalized by this calcium dose, additional calcium chloride may be given at a lower rate. It should be anticipated that ECG changes will recur in 15 to 30 minutes unless additional measures are taken immediately to treat the hyperkalemia. The effective calcium dose may be repeated as necessary to preserve cardiac function while additional treatments are in progress. Additional, rapidly effective treatments include nebulized albuterol (rapid neb or continuous neb of 0.1 to 0.3 mg/kg) or salbutamol (IV dose of 4 to 5 μg/kg over 20 minutes and repeated after 2 hours).[84,85,137]

Insulin and glucose are also rapidly helpful in redistributing potassium to the ICF. Glucose (1 g/kg) and insulin (0.2 U/g of glucose) may be given over 15 to 30 minutes and then infused continuously with a similar amount per hour. Blood glucose monitoring is essential because the relative glucose and insulin amounts may need adjustment.

Sodium bicarbonate (1 to 2 mEq/kg given intravenously) has been a part of the classic treatment of hyperkalemia. Its benefit, however, is more difficult to predict and slower in onset than that of the measures mentioned earlier.[86]

Sodium polystyrene sulfonate removes potassium and may be administered while dialysis arrangements are made. Sodium polystyrene sulfonate administered rectally must be retained for 15 to 30 minutes to be effective. If the oral route is available, it is generally more efficient.

In the patient with severely compromised renal function, these measures generally allow stabilization of potassium long enough to institute dialysis. Although hemodialysis is much more efficient for potassium removal than peritoneal dialysis, the latter may be more quickly instituted in many centers, particularly in the small infant in whom vascular access to support reasonable blood flow may be difficult to accomplish. In the absence of renal failure, loop diuretics or thiazide diuretics or both are useful for the increase of renal excretion.

If mineralocorticoid activity is deficient, the administration of fludrocortisone may be indicated. In patients with severe hyperglycemia and moderate hyperkalemia, early steps to improve glucose control should decrease ECF potassium shifts from hyperosmolality and decrease insulin.

Magnesium

Magnesium (Mg) deficiency, which leads to overt clinical symptoms and signs, is an increasingly recognized problem in the ICU setting.[138] Less than 1% of magnesium is in the ECF space, with the remainder distributed in the ICF space. More than 50% of ICF magnesium is located in bone; 20% in skeletal muscle; and the remainder, 30%, in other soft tissues. ECF forms include free ion (Mg^{2+}) (55% to 65%), magnesium complexed with anions (phosphate, oxalate, and citrate) (20% to 30%), and protein bound (5% to 20%).[87] Magnesium plays a key role in numerous metabolic processes, including cellular energy production, storage, and utilization involving adenosine triphosphate (ATP); the metabolism of protein, fat, and nucleic acids; and the maintenance of normal cell membrane function. It is also involved in neuromuscular transmission, cardiac excitability, and cardiovascular tone.[87,88]

Magnesium balance is maintained through intestinal absorption and renal excretion; 25% to 65% of ingested Mg is absorbed in the ileum. Absorption varies inversely with intake and is also affected by paracellular water reabsorption. Increased bowel water that is due to any cause results in decreased magnesium reabsorption. Regulation of renal excretion occurs by glomerular filtration and reabsorption. The bulk (50% to 60%) of filtered magnesium is reabsorbed in the ascending limb of the loop of Henle,[89] which results from active NaCl reabsorption. The threshold value for magnesium excretion varies between 1.5 and 2 mg/dl in different species. Thus if serum magnesium levels fall even slightly, renal excretion dramatically decreases under normal circumstances. Primary factors that increase renal magnesium excretion include ECF volume expansion; hypermagnesemia; hypercalcemia; metabolic acidosis; phosphate depletion; and various drugs including loop and osmotic diuretics, cisplatin, aminoglycosides, cyclosporin, and digoxin. Decreased excretion occurs with ECF volume depletion; with hypomagnesemia; with hypocalcemia, with hypothyroidism and metabolic alkalosis, to a lesser extent; and in response to parathyroid hormone (PTH). PTH effects, however, may be offset by the opposite effects of hypercalcemia.[87]

Hypomagnesemia

Clinically significant magnesium depletion may be present despite normal serum magnesium levels. Serum total magnesium correlates fairly well with bone concentration but may be normal in the presence of low tissue or muscle levels. Free, ionized magnesium is physiologically the most important form, but determination of total magnesium is still generally used. Critically ill children, however, are reported to frequently have low ionized magnesium despite normal total magnesium levels.[90] Ionized hypomagnesemia may be associated with more complicated postoperative conditions that occur after surgical correction of congenital heart disease.[91] A deeper investigation of the use of ionized magnesium measurements seems warranted.[92]

Magnesium depletion results in hypocalcemia, the association being reported in one study in 22% of hospitalized patients with hypocalcemia.[65] The mechanisms include the suppression of PTH secretion and bone resistance to PTH.[93] Hypokalemia has also been reported to occur in as many as 46% of adult patients with hypomagnesemia.[65,94] Magnesium deficiency impairs the Na/K pump allowing potassium loss from the ICF, which is in turn excreted in the urine.[67,94] Several studies have shown an inability to correct potassium until magnesium stores have been repleted.[94,95] Intracellular phosphate depletion in skeletal muscles has been described, again usually associated with phosphaturia.[96] Hypomagnesemia has been reported to occur in 60% to 65% of adult patients in an ICU.[97] Hypomagnesemia within 5 days of a cardiac operation in more than 80% of pediatric patients has been reported.[98]

Cause

Intensivists deal with hypomagnesemia most often in patients receiving loop diuretics or transplant immunosuppressives. Other causes must be considered.

Magnesium deficiency may be caused by decreased intake or increased losses. Although slight falls in serum magnesium levels may occur after 1 week of a deficient diet, a more sustained period of deprivation is generally necessary (30 to 80 days in human volunteers) for significant hypomagnesemia to occur.[99] In children, magnesium deficiency has been particularly common in protein-energy malnutrition and in anorexia nervosa. Intestinal malabsorption is a major cause of magnesium deficiency. Isolated familial primary hypomagnesemia occurs from selective malabsorption of magnesium.[100] Patients generally have symptoms in infancy, often with tetany and convulsions as a result of severe hypomagnesemia with consequent hypocalcemia and respond well to supplemental magnesium. Other causes associated with magnesium malabsorption include regional enteritis, ulcerative colitis, massive small bowel resection, generalized malabsorption syndromes, pancreatic insufficiency, and cystic fibrosis. In some of these cases, the formation of insoluble soaps due to the complexing of magnesium with unabsorbed fat is the postulated mechanism for hypomagnesemia.

Intrinsic renal tubular disorders associated with hypomagnesemia are rare in the ICU setting (Box 60–7). Drugs that induce renal magnesium wasting are more common causes and include aminoglycosides,[101] cisplatin,[102] amphotericin B, diuretics, cyclosporin A,[103] and tacrolimus.[104] Furosemide produces greater losses of magnesium than of sodium and calcium. Hypomagnesemia requiring supplementation is common in transplant recipients who receive cyclosporine or tacrolimus. Fractional excretion of magnesium and total excretion

BOX 60–7

Causes of Hypomagnesemia

DECREASED INTAKE

Low Mg++ TPN, IVF

INCREASED LOSSES

Gastrointestinal

Malabsorption
- Familial primary hypomagnesemia
- Small bowel disease
- Regional arteritis, ulcerative colitis, massive bowel resection
- Pancreatic insufficiency, pancreatitis
- Cystic fibrosis

Renal

Congenital renal magnesium wasting
Diffuse tubular disorders
Hypophosphatemia
Postrenal transplantation
Drugs: aminoglycosides, cisplatin, amphotericin B, diuretics, cyclosporine, tacrolimus, pentamidine, foscarnet, GM-CSG
Hypercalciuria
Diabetic ketoacidosis
Barter's syndrome
Hyperaldosteronism
Inappropriate ADH secretion

Miscellaneous

Epinephrine, β agonists
Thyrotoxicosis
Citrated blood transfusion (massive)
Burns
Alcoholism

ADH, antidiuretic hormone; *GM-CSF,* granulocyte-macrophage colony-stimulating factor; *IVF,* intravascular fluid; *TPN,* total parenteral nutrition.

are elevated. Patients with DKA may also have marked renal magnesium wasting during the acidotic period, as well as in early treatment. An increased urine calcium level, from whatever cause, is often associated with magnesium wasting from competitive inhibition of renal tubular reabsorption of magnesium in the ascending limb.

Signs and Symptoms

In addition to biochemical derangements associated with hypomagnesemia, a wide spectrum of other clinical disorders have been attributed to its depletion, including cardiac arrhythmias, increased sensitivity to digoxin, coronary spasm, hypertension, and neuromuscular derangements.

Arrhythmias include ventricular premature beats, ventricular tachycardia, torsade de pointes, and ventricular fibrillation.[105,106] Supraventricular arrhythmias are less common. Improvement in resistant ventricular arrhythmias following magnesium infusion has been reported,[105,106] although other metabolic derangements often coexist in such patients. Digoxin enhances magnesium secretion, and magnesium deficiency enhances myocardial cell uptake of digoxin. Both inhibit Na/K-ATPase with resultant ICF potassium depletion.

Depletion is thought to contribute to the development or worsening of hypertension by increasing vascular smooth muscle tone and reactivity. Increased cellular influx of calcium and decreased reuptake by sarcoplasmic reticula occur; the result is increased cytosolic calcium for activation of actin-myosin contractile proteins. Similar effects in coronary and cerebral vessels have also been observed.

Personality changes, including apathetic behavior and depression, have also been associated.[99] Neuromuscular changes may include tremors, fasciculations, spontaneous carpopedal spasm, muscle cramps, paresthesias, seizures, and coma.[99]

Treatment

Patients undergoing or at immediate risk of hypomagnesemic malignant ventricular arrhythmias or seizures can be given magnesium sulfate intravenously with careful monitoring. An IV infusion of 25 to 50 mg/kg per dose diluted to 10 mg/ml can be administered over 15 to 60 minutes. The rate of infusion should not exceed 150 mg/min. Doses may be repeated as needed depending on patient response. Complications of parenteral magnesium therapy include neuromuscular and respiratory depression, malignant arrhythmias, flushing, and hypotension.[98] Hypotension and malignant arrhythmias have been reported more frequently in young children who require close monitoring if IV replacement is used. Other routes of therapy include intramuscular magnesium sulfate, injections of which are painful, and oral therapy with magnesium oxide or citrate. In situations known to be associated with the development of hypomagnesemia, it seems particularly important to attempt to avoid deficiency by adequate magnesium intake before development of life-threatening symptoms.

Hypermagnesemia

Hypermagnesemia is seen much less commonly than hypomagnesemia. Magnesium infusions in status asthmaticus have become common, however, and may be associated with hypermagnesemia. The frequency and clinical importance of elevated blood levels of magnesium in these patients needs further investigation.

Cause

Hypermagnesemia occurs in patients with renal failure and is generally associated with iatrogenic administration of magnesium as antacids, cathartics, or enemas or through total parenteral nutrition (TPN) containing magnesium. In the absence of renal failure, the administration of large quantities of magnesium cathartics in the management of overdoses[107,108] and antacid use with increased peritoneal absorption of magnesium in the presence of a perforated viscus[109] are causes. Magnesium levels as high as 10 to 12 mEq/L have been reported.

Megadose vitamin-mineral supplementation, including magnesium oxide, has been fatal.[147]

Signs and Symptoms

Acute elevations of magnesium depress the CNS and the peripheral neuromuscular junction. Pseudocoma with fixed, dilated pupils has been reported.[149] Deep tendon reflexes are depressed at levels greater than 4 mEq/L with total disappearance along with flaccid quadriplegia at levels greater than 8 to 10 mEq/L. Hypotension, hypoventilation, and cardiac arrhythmias may also occur.[107-109] Moderate potassium elevations have been associated with prolonged magnesium infusions in occasional patients.

Treatment

Calcium acts as a direct antagonist to magnesium. Therefore in life-threatening situations associated with severe magnesium intoxication, intravenous calcium should be used as the initial therapy. Adults have been treated with 5 to 10 mEq of calcium in either the chloride or gluconate forms over 5 to 10 minutes, with doses repeated if necessary. An initial dose of calcium chloride at 10 mg/kg or an equivalent amount of calcium gluconate has been suggested for infants and children. Magnesium-containing medications obviously should be discontinued. If renal function is normal, IV furosemide may be administered to increase magnesium excretion with fluid replaced with half-normal saline. In patients with renal failure or severe toxicity, dialysis may be necessary for removal.[110]

Phosphorus

Virtually all of plasma phosphorus (P) is in the inorganic form, with a small organic component composed entirely of phospholipids bound to protein. Serum levels vary with age; approximate normal values (specific to the analytical instrument) are 4.8 to 8.2 mg/dl for neonates, 3.8 to 6.5 mg/dl for children aged 1 week to 3 years, 3.7 to 5.5 mg/dl for children aged 3 years to 12 years, and 2.9 to 5 mg/dl for adolescents aged 12 to 19 years.[111] Differences are thought to be related to more rapid rates of skeletal growth in the pediatric population. Most total body phosphorus resides in bone. More than 50% to 65% of ingested phosphorus is absorbed, primarily in the jejunum. Its absorption may be decreased by a high calcium intake or by ingestion of antacids, which bind phosphorus in the bowel. Urinary excretion depends primarily on oral intake. About 80% of the inorganic phosphorus is filtered, with reabsorption occurring predominantly in the proximal tubule by an active mechanism coupled to sodium transfer. Renal phosphorus reabsorption is decreased by PTH and by calcitonin with resultant phosphaturia. Glucose competitively inhibits phosphorus reabsorption. Glucocorticoids produce phosphaturia by a decrease in sodium-dependent transport in the proximal tubule and vitamin D, which may increase or decrease reabsorption, depending on conditions.[112, 113]

Phosphorus plays an important role in cellular structure and function, bone mineralization, and urinary acid excretion. The development of severe phosphorus depletion affects the availability of intracellular ATP for every production; depletes the erythrocyte of 2,3-diphosphoglycerate (2,3-DPG), with resultant tissue hypoxia; and impairs urinary acid excretion.[112, 114] The major acute effect of hyperphosphatemia is hypocalcemia; the long-term consequence is soft tissue calcification.

Hypophosphatemia

Hypophosphatemia as measured by serum or plasma levels may or may not indicate true phosphorus deficiency. Severely depressed levels of serum-measurable phosphorus may occur in the absence of true deficiency after transcellular shifts from the ECF to the ICF, whereas a moderate phosphorus deficiency may be indicated only by slightly decreased serum levels.[112,114] Moderate hypophosphatemia has been defined as levels between 1.5 and 2.5 mg/dl and severe hypophosphatemia as levels less than 1.5 mg/dl on serum determination. In general, only with severe deficiency of phosphorus do multiple symptoms occur, as well as overt cell dysfunction or necrosis. Risk is greatest when superimposed additional cellular injury exists.

Cause of Severe Hypophosphatemia

Although numerous abnormalities may result in moderate decreases in phosphorus levels, severe hypophosphatemia has been associated with only a handful of clinical syndromes. These include significant respiratory alkalosis, use of TPN, the nutritional refeeding syndrome, thermal burns, DKA, pharmacological binding of phosphorus in the gut, and alcohol withdrawal.[112,114] The increase in the ICF pH associated with acute respiratory alkalosis stimulates the enzymes of glycolysis, with subsequent depletion of ICF phosphorus. This is replaced by an influx from the ECF space. Although carbon dioxide diffuses across membranes much more readily than bicarbonate does, metabolic alkalosis rarely produces a fall in phosphorus levels, whereas levels as low as 0.3 mg/dl have been reported with respiratory alkalosis.[115] An absolute deficiency from malnutrition and transcellular shifts from the ECF to the ICF with an anabolic response to increasing caloric intake are the causes associated with TPN use.[112,114,116] In the pediatric population, the preterm infant is particularly susceptible. Nearly 80% of calcium-phosphorus assimilation in the fetus occurs in the last trimester of pregnancy. The preterm infant is therefore born deficient in total body phosphorus. When reasonable nutrition has been absent for even short periods or when phosphorus has not been provided in TPN, severe hypophosphatemia has occurred, associated in several cases with the development of hypercalcemia.[116] A similar situation may occur with the refeeding of patients who have significant protein calorie malnutrition.[76] As previously noted, an absolute phosphorus deficiency and transcellular shifts from the ECF to the ICF in the face of an anabolic response are responsible.

Significant hypophosphatemia occurred in five of nine infants and children with protein calorie malnutrition, which happened during the first 48 to 72 hours of refeeding.[117] Significant hypophosphatemia in burn patients during their recovery phase has been associated with the presence of respiratory alkalosis, diuresis of initially retained sodium and water, and acceleration of glycolysis.[112,114] As previously described, ECF phosphorus shifts to the ICF compartment when intracellular-free phosphorus has been used in phosphorylation of organic compounds such as occurs during glycolysis; oxidative phosphorylation; glycogenolysis; and synthesis of glycogen, protein, and phosphocreatine. Acidosis decomposes organic compounds within the cell with subsequent movement of inorganic phosphorus from ICF to ECF and excretion in the urine. Osmotic diuresis augments these losses. Decreased intake also commonly occurs. During treatment of DKA, renal phosphorus clearance generally increases with fluid administration. In addition, insulin therapy results in stimulation of glycolysis and anabolism with a shift of phosphorus back to the ICF.[114] Controversy currently exists regarding the need for phosphorus replacement in all patients hospitalized with DKA. It is generally now thought that if the acidosis has been present for only a few days, then rarely is there a severe phosphorus deficiency. Although levels may fall, they generally return to normal without extra phosphorus therapy. In the patient whose symptoms have been present for a number of days to weeks, however, severe deficiency may exist at the time of admission. These patients may have life-threatening complications of hypophosphatemia if not treated. In general, this subset of patients has low phosphorus levels on admission, whereas phosphorus levels are normal or increased at admission in less severely affected patients. Antacid therapy, used commonly in the ICU, may also result in profound hypophosphatemia, particularly when coupled with inadequate intake.[114,118] Aluminum hydroxide, magnesium hydroxide, and aluminum carbonate have been incriminated.

Signs and Symptoms of Severe Hypophosphatemia

Multiple organ systems may be affected by severe hypophosphatemia, including CNS, cardiac, musculoskeletal, hematological, renal, and hepatic abnormalities. Perhaps the greatest interest to the intensivist is the association of hypophosphatemia with respiratory muscle dysfunction.[112,114,118-121] Muscular weakness in humans[118] and diaphragmatic weakness in dogs[122] have been reported with experimental phosphorus depletion. Decreased diaphragmatic contractility in patients with hypophosphatemia with acute respiratory failure significantly improved as measured by transdiaphragmatic pressures during phrenic stimulation with treatment of hypophosphatemia.[119] The frequency of respiratory muscle weakness in patients with hypophosphatemia but without respiratory failure has also been examined; abnormal maximum inspiratory and expiratory pressures were found in 16 of 23 patients with hypophosphatemia compared with 0 of 11 controls with normophosphatemia.[120] Pressures normalized with phosphorus repletion. These data provide increasing evidence in adults that respiratory muscle function in phosphorus-depleted patients may be improved with normalization of phosphate stores.

Neurological symptoms initially include irritability and apprehension followed by weakness, peripheral neuropathy with numbness and paresthesias,[72,118] dysarthria, confusion, obtundation, seizures, and coma.[112,114,123] Reports in the literature include Guillain-Barré–like syndrome; diffuse slowing on electroencephalogram; and congestive cardiomyopathy,[124] which significantly improved with correction of phosphorus depletion. Experimentally, decreased CO, decreased ventricular ejection velocity, and increased left ventricular end diastolic pressure, which reversed with repletion, have been reported in dogs.[125] Again in dogs, phosphorus depletion produced by partial starvation and then refeeding of excessive calories resulted in profound phosphate depletion, markedly elevated creatine phosphokinase (CPK), and frank rhabdomyolysis.[126] In humans, rhabdomyolysis has been predominantly seen in alcoholic patients, in whom subtle myopathy was likely present, and rarely in patients with DKA or after TPN therapy.[112] Decreased levels of 2,3-DPG in red blood cells (RBCs) may depress P-50 (oxygen half-saturation pressure) values so that the release of molecular oxygen to peripheral tissues is decreased, with resultant tissue hypoxia.[127,128] Structural defects of RBCs have included rigidity and, rarely, hemolysis and have generally occurred when additional metabolic requirements such as metabolic acidosis or infection were placed on the RBC.[129] Decreased levels of ATP in neutrophils may result in decreased chemotaxis, phagocytosis, and bacterial killing.[130] The mechanisms underlying the development of metabolic acidosis include decreased phosphorus excretion, which thereby limits titratable acid excretion and decreased ammonia levels. Metabolic acidosis from phosphorus deficiency has been reported in children with malnutrition from diarrhea.

Treatment

As with other minerals and electrolytes, when oral therapy is potentially possible, it is the preferable route for administration. In patients with severe hypophosphatemia, IV therapy is often indicated. Little data exist in the pediatric literature as to dosage. Therefore most data are extrapolated from adult literature.[131,132] General recommendations in children with severe phosphorus depletion are to use 0.15 to 0.33 mmol/kg per dose (5-10 mg/kg per dose), given as a continuous infusion over at least 6 hours. Subsequent doses are generally calculated on the basis of response to this initial dosage. Either potassium or sodium phosphate may be administered with the attendant potential complications of hypernatremia or hyperkalemia. Other potential complications of therapy include hyperphosphatemia, metastatic deposition of calcium phosphate, hypocalcemia, potential nephrocalcinosis with renal failure, and hypotension.[131] Both sodium and potassium phosphate contain 3 mmol of phosphate per milliliter and 4 to 4.5 mEq of sodium or potassium, respectively. For oral administration, a combination product of sodium with potassium phosphate (Neutra-Phos) has been commonly used in the pediatric patient. One capsule supplies 8 mmol of phosphorus along with 7.1 mEq of sodium and potassium. Capsules can be reconstituted in water as well.

Hyperphosphatemia

Cause

Acute and chronic renal failure with decreased phosphorus excretion are the most common causes of hyperphosphatemia, with elevation in serum phosphorus occurring when the GFR is less than 30 ml/min. Extreme hyperphosphatemia associated with several deaths has been reported from the use of sodium phosphate enemas in infants and young children.[133] Abnormalities of intestinal anatomy or motility predisposing to retention of enemas occurred in 55% of patients, renal insufficiency occurred in 15%, and no predisposing problems were present in 30%. Lethal outcome was reported in pigs that received 20 ml/kg of these agents, which was equivalent to four pediatric-sized enemas in a 2-year-old child.[134] The administration of IV boluses of sodium or potassium phosphate rather than slow infusion may result in symptomatic hyperphosphatemia.[135]

Tumor lysis syndrome is an additional cause of hyperphosphatemia. It results from drug-induced lysis of tumor cells,[139,146] and is always a concern in a child with a lymphoid malignancy and substantial cellular mass. Initial chemotherapy or radiation of B-cell lymphoma is particularly likely to produce cell lysis and hyperphosphatemia along with hyperuricemia, ARF, hyperkalemia, metabolic acidosis, and hypocalcemia. Aggressive hydration and careful initiation of chemotherapy will usually result in a manageable degree of electrolyte abnormality. Urinary alkalinization to increase urate solubility is usually recommended but is being reexamined. Rasburicase is replacing allopurinol in the control of urate levels. Hemodialysis is an essential resource to have available if managing such a patient (Table 60–2).

TABLE 60–2

Tumor Lysis Syndrome

At risk	Lymphoid malignancies
High risk	Large tumor mass, B-cell lymphoma
	Renal compromise
Initiating event	Cytolytic chemotherapy
	Radiation therapy
Prophylaxis	Hydration, urinary alkalinization, allopurinol
	Gradual chemotherapy initiation, rasburicase
Serious disturbances	Hyperkalemia, hypocalcemia, acidosis, renal failure, hyperuricemia, hyperphosphatemia
Management	Obsessive electrolyte monitoring Hemodialysis available stat CVVHD helpful, may not be adequate

CVVHD, continuous veno-venous hemodialysis; *stat,* immediately.

Signs and Symptoms

The major clinical consequence of severe hyperphosphatemia is its associated hypocalcemia, as well as soft tissue deposition of calcium phosphate salts. Seizures, coma, and cardiac arrest have been reported, generally in the presence of both hypocalcemia and hyperphosphatemia. In one case report, however, seizures, malignant ventricular arrhythmias, and cardiac arrest with acute hyperphosphatemia alone were described.[135]

Treatment

In patients with life-threatening complications, fluid administration to increase renal phosphorus losses and intravenous calcium has been described.[133] Dialysis may be required as well in the patient with renal failure. Sodium phosphate enemas should be avoided in the infant and young child.

REFERENCES

1. Harrigan MR: Cerebral salt wasting syndrome, *Crit Care Clin* 17:125, 2001.
2. Bussmann C, Bast T, Rating D: Hyponatraemia in children with acute CNS disease: SIADH or cerebral salt wasting? *Child's Nerv Syst* 17:58, 2001.
3. Soupart A, Ngassa M, Decaux G: Therapeutic relowering of the serum sodium in a patient after excessive correction of hyponatremia, *Clin Nephrol* 51:383, 1999.
4. Menger H, Jorg J: Outcome of central pontine and extrapontine myelinolysis (n = 44), *J Neurol* 246:700, 1999.
5. Schrier RW, Berl T, Anderson RJ: Osmotic and nonosmotic control of vasopressin release, *Am J Physiol* 236:F321, 1979.
6. Kumar S, Berl T: Sodium, *Lancet* 352:220, 1998.
7. Szatalowicz VL, Miller PD, Lacher JW, et al: Comparative effect of diuretics on renal H_2O excretion in hyponatremic oedematous disorders, *Clin Sci* 62:235, 1982.
8. Katz MA: Hyperglycemia induced hyponatremia: calculation of expected serum sodium depression, *N Engl J Med* 289:843, 1973.
9. Sakarcan A, Bocchini J: The role of fludrocortisone in a child with cerebral salt wasting, *Pediatr Nephrol* 12:769, 1998.
10. Schrier RW, Humphreys MH: Factors involved in the antinatriuretic effects of acute constriction of the thoracic and abdominal inferior vena cava, *Circ Res* 29:479, 1971.
11. Szatalowicz VL, Arnold PA, Chaimovitz C, et al: Radioimmunoassay of plasma arginine vasopressin in hyponatremic patients with congestive heart failure, *N Engl J Med* 305:263, 1981.
12. Bichet DG, Groves RM, Schrier RW: Mechanisms of improvement of water and Na excretion by enhancement of central hemodynamics in decompensated cirrhotic patients, *Kidney Int* 24:788, 1983.
13. Epstein M: Atrial natriuretic factor in patients with liver disease, *Am J Nephrol* 9:89, 1989.
14. Tulassay T, Rascher W, Lang RE, et al: Atrial natriuretic peptide and other vasoactive hormones in nephrotic syndrome, *Kidney Int* 31:1391, 1987.
15. Smith DM, McKenna K, Thompson CJ: Hyponatremia, *Clin Endocrinol* 52:667, 2000.
16. David R, Ellis D, Gartner JC: Water intoxication in normal infants: role of antidiuretic hormone in pathogenesis, *Pediatrics* 68:349, 1981.
17. Chung HM, Kluge R, Schrier R, et al: Post operative hyponatremia. A prospective study, *Arch Intern Med* 146:333, 1986.
18. Arieff AI: Hyponatremia, convulsions, respiratory arrest, and permanent brain damage after elective surgery in healthy women, *N Engl J Med* 314:1529, 1986.
19. Cluitmans FHM, Meinders AE: Management of severe hyponatremia: rapid or slow correction? *Am J Med* 88:161, 1990.
20. Nattie EE, Edward WH: Brain and CSF water in newborn puppies during acute hypo- and hypernatremia, *J Appl Physiol* 51:1086, 1981.

21. Norenberg MD, Leslie KO, Robertson AS: Associations between rise in serum sodium and central pontine myelinolysis, *Ann Neurol* 11:128, 1982.
22. Sterns RH: Severe symptomatic hyponatremia: treatment and outcome. A study of 64 cases, *Ann Intern Med* 107:656, 1987.
23. Sterns RH, Thomas DJ, Herndon RM: Brain dehydration and neurologic deterioration after rapid correction of hyponatremia, *Kidney Int* 35:69, 1989.
24. Thurston JH, Hauhart RE: Brain amino acids decrease in chronic hyponatremia and rapid correction causes brain dehydration: possible clinical significance, *Life Sci* 40:2539, 1987.
25. Brown WD, Caruso JM: Extrapontine myelinolysis with involvement of the hippocampus in three children with severe hypernatremia, *J Child Neurol* 14:428.
26. Soupart A, Decaux G: Therapeutic recommendations for management of severe hyponatremia: current concepts on pathogenesis and prevention of neurologic complications, *Clin Nephrol* 46: 149, 1996.
27. Oya S, Tsutsumi K, Ueki K, et al: Reinduction of hyponatremia to treat central pontine myelinolysis, *Neurology* 57:1931, 2001.
28. Soupart A, Penninckx R, Stenuit A, et al: Reinduction of hyponatremia improves survival in rats with myelinolysis-related neurologic syndrome, *J Neuropathol Exp Neurol* 55:594, 1996.
29. Farley TA: Severe hypernatremic dehydration after use of an activated charcoal-sorbitol suspension, *J Pediatr* 109:719, 1986.
30. Finberg L: Hypernatremia (hypertonic) dehydration in infants, *N Engl J Med* 289:196, 1973.
31. Randall RV, Clark EC, Dodge HWJ, et al: Polyuria after operation for tumors in the region of the hypophysis and hypothalamus, *J Clin Endocrinol Metab* 20:1614, 1966.
32. Adrogue HJ, Madias NE: Hypernatremia, *N Engl J Med* 342: 1493, 2000.
33. Birnbaumer M: The V2 vasopressin receptor mutations and fluid homeostasis, *Cardiovasc Res* 51:409, 2001.
34. Dunn FL, Brennan TJ, Nelson AE, et al: The role of blood osmolality and volume in regulating vasopressin secretion in the rat, *J Clin Invest* 52:3212, 1973.
35. Lohr J, McReynolds J, Grimaldi T, et al: Effect of acute and chronic hypernatremia on myoinositol and sorbitol concentration in rat brain and kidney, *Life Sci* 43:271, 1988.
36. Stevenson RE, Bowyer FP: Hyperglycemia with hyperosmolar dehydration in nondiabetic infants, *J Pediatr* 77:818, 1970.
37. Finberg L: Pathogenesis of lesions in the nervous system in hypernatremic states. I. Clinical observations on infants, *Pediatrics* 23:40, 1959.
38. Lohr J, Springate J, Feld L: Seizures during correction of hypernatremic dehydration in an infant, *Am J Kidney Dis* 14:232, 1989.
39. Lockwood A: Acute and chronic hyperosmolality: effects on cerebral amino acids and energy metabolism, *Arch Neurol* 32:6263, 1975.
40. Macaulay D, Watson M: Hypernatremia as a cause of brain damage, *Arch Dis Child* 42:485, 1967.
41. Banister A, Siddiqi S, Hatcher GW: Treatment of hypernatremic dehydration in infancy, *Arch Dis Child* 50:179, 1975.
42. Belton K, Thomas SHL: Drug-induced syndrome of inappropriate antidiuretic hormone secretion, *Postgrad Med J* 76 :319, 2000.
43. Gabow PA, Peterson LN: Disorders of potassium metabolism. In Schrier RW, editor: *Renal and electrolyte disorders,* Boston, 1986, Little, Brown, and Co.
44. Patrick J: Assessment of body potassium stores, *Kidney Int* 11: 476, 1977.
45. Sterns RH, Cox M, Feig PU, et al: Internal potassium balance and the control of the plasma potassium concentration, *Medicine* 60:339, 1981.
46. Adrogue HJ, Madias NE: Changes in plasma potassium concentration during acute acid-base disturbances, *Am J Med* 71:456, 1981.
47. Oster JR, Perez GO, Castro A, et al: Plasma potassium response to acute metabolic acidosis induced by mineral and non-mineral acids, *Mineral Electrolyte Metab* 4:28, 1980.
48. Oster JR, Perez GO, Vaamonde CA: Relationship between blood pH and potassium and phosphorus during acute metabolic acidosis, *Am J Physiol* 235:F345, 1978.
49. DeFronzo RA, Bia M, Birkhead G: Epinephrine and potassium homeostasis, *Kidney Int* 20:83, 1981.
50. Todd EP, Vick RL: Kalenotropic effect of epinephrine: analysis with adrenergic agonists and antagonists, *Am J Physiol* 220:1964, 1971.
51. Bia MJ, Tyler KA, DeFronzo FT: Regulation of extrarenal potassium homeostasis by adrenal hormones in rats, *Am J Physiol* 242:F641, 1982.
52. Young DB, Paulsen WP: Interrelated effects of aldosterone and plasma potassium on potassium excretion, *Am J Physiol* 244: F28, 1983.
53. Stanton BA, Giebisch G: Effects of pH on potassium transport by renal tubular cells, *Am J Physiol* 242:F544, 1982.
54. Wright FS: Flow dependent transport processes: filtration, absorption, secretion, *Am J Physiol* 243:F1, 1982.
55. Brown MJ: Hypokalemia from beta-2-receptor stimulation by circulating epinephrine, *Am J Cardiol* 56:3D, 1985.
56. Struthers AD, Reid JL, Whitesmith R, et al: The effect of cardioselective and nonselective beta-adrenoreceptor blockade on hypokalemic and cardiovascular responses to adrenomedullary hormone in man, *Clin Sci* 65:143, 1983.
57. Buruma OJ, Bots GT, Went LN: Familial hypokalemic periodic paralysis. 50-year follow-up of a large family.*Arch Neurol* 42:28, 1985.
58. Glauser J: Cardiac arrhythmias, respiratory failure, and profound hypokalemia in a trauma patient, *Clevel Clin J Med* 68:401, 2001.
59. Minaker KL, Meneilly GS, Flier JS, et al: Insulin-mediated hypokalemia and paralysis in familial hypokalemic periodic paralysis, *Am J Med* 84:1001, 1988.
60. Lipworth BJ, McDevitt DG, Struthers AD: Prior treatment with diuretic augments the hypokalemic and electrocardiographic effects of inhaled albuterol, *Am J Med* 86:653, 1989.
61. Frank BS: Hypokalemia following fresh-water submersion injuries, *Pediatric Emerg Care* 3:158, 1987.
62. Severance HW Jr, Holt T, Patron NA, et al: Profound muscle weakness and hypokalemia due to clay ingestion, *South Med J* 81:272, 1988.
63. Bartter FC, Pronove P, Gill JR Jr, et al: Hyperplasia of the juxtaglomerular complex with hyperaldosteronism and hypokalemic alkalosis, *Am J Med* 33:88, 1962.
64. Stapleton FB, Nelson B, Vats TS, et al: Hypokalemia associated with antibiotic treatment, *Am J Dis Child* 130:1104, 1976.
65. Whang R, Tjien OO, Aikawa JK, et al: Predictors of clinical hypomagnesemia: hypokalemia, hypophosphatemia, hyponatremia and hypocalcemia, *Arch Intern Med* 144:1794, 1984.
66. O'Regan S, Kaplan BS, Chesney RW, et al: Hypokalemia in children with leukemia in relapse, *Am J Dis Child* 130:937, 1976.
67. Helfant RH: Hypokalemia and arrhythmias, *Am J Med* 80:13, 1986.
68. Kaplan NM: Our appropriate concern about hypokalemia, *Am J Med* 77:1, 1984.
69. Rosales AM, Walsh EP, Wessel DL, et al: Postoperative ectopic atrial tachycardia in children with congenital heart disease, *Am J Cardiol* 88:1169, 2001.
70. Alvarez J, Low RB: Acute respiratory arrest due to hypokalemia, *Ann Emerg Med* 17:288, 1988.
71. Comi G, Testa D, Cornelio F, et al: Potassium depletion myopathy: a clinical and morphological study of 6 cases, *Muscle Nerve* 8:17, 1985.
72. Kolski GB, Cunningham AS, Niemee PW, et al: Hypokalemia and respiratory arrest in an infant with status asthmaticus, *J Pediatr* 112:304, 1988.
73. Manary MJ, Keating JP, Hirschberg GE: Quadriparesis due to potassium depletion, *Crit Care Med* 14:750, 1986.
74. Knochel JP: Rhabdomyolysis and effects of potassium deficiency on muscle structure and function, *Cardiovasc Med* 3:247, 1978.
75. Pinski SL: Potassium replacement after cardiac surgery: it is not time to change practice, yet, *Crit Care Med* 27:2581, 1999.
76. Cohen HW, Madhavan S, Alderman MH: High and low serum potassium associated with cardiovascular events in diuretic-treated patients, *J Hypertens* 19:1315, 2001.
77. Wahr JA, Parks R, Boisvert D, et al: Preoperative serum potassium levels and perioperative outcomes in cardiac surgery patients, *JAMA* 281:2203, 1999.
78. Perazella MA: Drug-induced hyperkalemia: old culprits and new offenders, *Am J Med* 109:307, 2000.
79. Hoyt RE: Hyperkalemia due to salt substitutes, *JAMA* 256: 1726, 1986.
80. Gruskay J, Costarino AT, Polin RA, et al: Nonoliguric hyperkalemia in the premature infant weighing less than 1000 grams, *J Pediatr* 113:381, 1988.

81. Greenberg A: Hyperkalemia: treatment options, *Semin Nephrol* 18:46, 1998.
82. Mattu A, Brady WJ, Robinson DA: Electrocardiographic manifestations of hyperkalemia, *Am J Emerg Med* 18:721, 2000.
83. Rogers FB, Li SC: Acute colonic necrosis associated with sodium polystyrene sulfonate [Kayexalate] enemas in a critically ill patient: case report and review of the literature, *J Trauma* 51: 395, 2001.
84. Kemper MJ, Harps E, Hellwege HH: Effective treatment of acute hyperkalemia in childhood by short-term infusion of salbutamol, *Eur J Pediatr* 155:495, 1996.
85. McClure RJ, Prasad VK, Brocklebank JT: Treatment of hyperkalemia using intravenous and nebulised salbutamol, *Arch Dis Child* 70:126, 1994.
86. Allon M, Shanklin N: Effect of bicarbonate administration on plasma potassium in dialysis patients: Interactions with insulin and albuterol, *Am J Kidney Dis* 28:508, 1996.
87. Dacey MJ: Hypomagnesemic disorders, *Crit Care Clin* 17: 155, 2001.
88. Agus MSD, Agus ZS: Cardiovascular actions of magnesium, *Crit Care Clin,* 17:175, 2001.
89. Shareghi GR, Agus ZS: Magnesium transport in the cortical thick ascending limb of Henle's loop of the rabbit, *J Clin Invest* 65:759, 1982.
90. Fiser RT, Torres A, Butch AW: Ionized magnesium concentrations in critically ill children, *Crit Care Med* 26:2048, 1998.
91. Munoz R, Laussen PC, Palacio G: Whole blood ionized magnesium: age-related differences in normal values and clinical implications of ionized hypomagnesemia in patients undergoing surgery for congenital cardiac disease, *J Thorac Cardiovasc Surg* 119:891, 2000.
92. Huijgen HJ, Soesan M, Sanders R: Magnesium levels in critically ill patients, *Am J Clin Pathol* 114:688, 2000.
93. Anast CS, Winnacker JL, Forte LR, et al: Impaired release of parathyroid hormone in magnesium deficiency, *J Clin Endocrinol Metab* 42:707, 1976.
94. Whang R: Magnesium deficiency: pathogenesis, prevalence, and clinical implications, *Am J Med* 82(suppl 3A):24, 1987.
95. Whang R, Flink EB, Dyckner T, et al: Magnesium depletion as cause of refractory potassium repletion, *Arch Intern Med* 145:1686, 1985.
96. Cronin RE, Ferguson ER, Shannon WA Jr, et al: Skeletal muscle injury after magnesium depletion in the dog, *Am J Physiol* 243:113, 1982.
97. Ryzen E, Wagers PW, Singer FR, et al: Magnesium deficiency in a medical ICU population, *Crit Care Med* 13:19, 1985.
98. Weise KL, Thompson S, Besunder JB, et al: Hypomagnesemia after cardiac surgery in children: patterns and complications of treatment. Paper presented at the third Pediatric Critical Care Colloquium, October 26-28, 1989, Santa Monica, CA (abstract 28).
99. Shils ME: Experimental human magnesium depletion, *Medicine* (Baltimore) 48:61, 1969.
100. Stromme JH, Steen-Johnsen J, Harnaas K, et al: Familial hypomagnesemia—a follow up examination of three patients after 9-12 years of treatment, *Pediatr Res* 15:1134, 1981.
101. Zaloga GP, Chernow B, Pock A, et al: Hypomagnesemia is a common complication of aminoglycoside therapy, *Surg Gynecol Obstet* 158:561, 1984.
102. Bellin SL, Selim M: Cisplatin-induced hypomagnesemia with seizures: a case report and review of the literature, *Gynecol Oncol* 30:104, 1988.
103. Barton CH, Vaziri ND, Martin DC, et al: Hypomagnesemia and renal magnesium wasting in renal transplant recipients receiving cyclosporine, *Am J Med* 83:693, 1987.
104. Yanik G, Levine JE, Ratanatharathorn V: Tacrolimus (FK506) and methotrexate as prophylaxis for acute graft-versus-host disease in pediatric allogeneic stem cell transplantation, *Bone Marrow Transplantation* 26:161, 2000.
105. Boriss MN, Papa L: Magnesium: A discussion of its role in the treatment of ventricular dysrhythmia, *Crit Care Med* 16: 292, 1988.
106. Ramee SR, White CJ, Svinarich JT, et al: Torsades de pointes and magnesium deficiency, *Am Heart J* 109:164, 1985.
107. Fassler CA, Rodriguez M, Badesch DB et al: Magnesium toxicity as a cause of hypotension and hypoventilation. Occurrence in patients with normal renal function, *Arch Intern Med* 145:1604, 1985.
108. Jones J, Heiselman D, Dougherty J, et al: Cathartic-induced magnesium toxicity during overdose management, *Ann Emerg Med* 15:1214, 1986.
109. Zwanger ML: Hypermagnesemia and perforated viscus, *Ann Emerg Med* 15:1219, 1986
110. Harker HE, Majcher TA: Hypermagnesemia in a pediatric patient, *Anesth Analg* 91:1160, 2000.
111. Lockitch G, Halstead AS, Albersheim S, et al: Age- and sex-specific pediatric reference intervals for biochemistry analytes as measured with Ektachem-700 analyzer *Clin Chem* 34: 1623, 1988.
112. Berkelhammer C, Bear RA: A clinical approach to common electrolyte problems. 3. Hypophosphatemia, *Can Med Assoc J* 130:17, 1984.
113. Loffing J, Lotscher M, Kaissling B, et al: Renal Na/H exchanger NHE-3 and Na-PO4 cotransporter NaPi-2 protein expression in glucocorticoid excess and deficient states, *J Am Soc Nephrol* 9:1560, 1998.
114. Knochel JP: The clinical status of hypophosphatemia. An update, *N Engl J Med* 313:447, 1985.
115. Okel BB, Hurst JW: Prolonged hyperventilation in man. Associated electrolyte changes and subjective symptoms, *Arch Intern Med* 108:757, 1961.
116. Miller RR, Menke JA, Mentser MI: Hypercalcemia associated with phosphate depletion in the neonate, *J Pediatr* 105:814, 1984.
117. Mezoff AG, Gremse DA, Farrell MK: Hypophosphatemia in the nutritional recovery syndrome, *Am J Dis Child* 143:1111, 1989.
118. Lotz M, Zisman E, Bartter FC: Evidence for a phosphorous depletion syndrome in man, *N Engl J Med* 278:409, 1968.
119. Aubier M, Murciano D, Lecocguic Y, et al: Effect of hypophosphatemia in diaphragmatic contractility in patients with acute respiratory failure, *N Engl J Med* 313:420, 1985.
120. Gravelyn TR, Brophy N, Siegert C, et al: Hypophosphatemia-associated respiratory muscle weakness in a general inpatient population, *Am J Med* 84:870, 1988.
121. Newman JH, Neff TA, Ziporin P: Acute respiratory failure associated with hypophosphatemia, *N Engl J Med* 296:1101, 1977.
122. Planas RF, McBreyer RH, Koen PA: Effects of hypophosphatemia on pulmonary muscle performance, *Adv Exp Med Biol* 151: 283, 1982.
123. Yagnik P, Singh N, Burus R: Peripheral neuropathy with hypophosphatemia in a patient receiving intravenous hyperalimentation, *South Med J* 78:1381, 1985.
124. O'Connor LR, Wheeler WS, Bethune JE: Effect of hypophosphatemia on myocardial performance in man, *N Engl J Med* 297:901, 1977.
125. Fuller TJ, Nichols WW, Brenner BJ, et al: Reversible depression in myocardial performance in dogs with experimental phosphorus deficiency, *J Clin Invest* 62:1194, 1978.
126. Knochel JP, Barcenas C, Cotton JR, et al: Hypophosphatemia and rhabdomyolysis, *J Clin Invest* 62:1240, 1978.
127. Klock JC, Williams H, Mantzer WC: Hemolytic anemic and somatic cell dysfunction in severe hypophosphatemia, *Arch Intern Med* 134:360, 1974.
128. Lichtman MA, Miller DR, Cohen J, et al: Reduced red cell glycolysis, 2,3-diphosphoglycerate and adenosine triphosphate concentration, and increased hemoglobin—oxygen affinity caused by hypophosphatemia, *Ann Intern Med* 74:562, 1971.
129. Jacob HS, Amsden T: Acute hemolytic anemia with rigid red cells in hypophosphatemia, *N Engl J Med* 285:1446, 1971.
130. Craddock PR, Yawata Y, Van Santen L, et al: Acquired phagocytic dysfunction. A complication of the hypophosphatemia of parenteral hyperalimentation, *N Engl J Med* 290:1403, 1974.
131. Andres DL: Phosphorus administration in patients with profound hypophosphatemia, *Kidney Int* 25:551, 1984.
132. Kingston M and Al-Sibai MB: Treatment of severe hypophosphatemia, *Crit Care Med* 13:16, 1985.
133. Wason S, Tiller T, Cunha C: Severe hyperphosphatemia, hypocalcemia, acidosis, and shock in a 5 month old child following the administration of an adult Fleet enema, *Ann Emerg Med* 18: 696, 1989.
134. Martin RR, Lisehora GR, Braxton M, et al: Fatal poisoning from sodium phosphate enema. Case report and experiment study, *JAMA* 257:2190, 1987.
135. Nemer WF, Teba L, Schiebel F, et al: Cardiac arrest after acute hyperphosphatemia, *South Med J* 81:1068, 1988.

136. Abbot R: Hyponatremia due to antidepressant medications, *Ann Emerg Med* 12:708, 1983.
137. Allon M, Dunlay R, Copkney C: Nebulized albuterol for acute hyperkalemia in patients on hemodialysis, *Ann Intern Med* 110:426, 1989.
138. Chernow B, Bamberger S, Stoiko M: Hypomagnesemia in patients in postoperative intensive care, *Chest* 95:391, 1989.
139. Cohen LF, Balow JE, Magrath IT, et al: Acute tumor lysis syndrome, *Am J Med* 68:486, 1980.
140. Decaux G: Long term treatment of inappropriate secretion of antidiuretic hormone by the vasopressin antagonist conivaptan, urea, or furosemide, *Am J Med* 110:582, 2001.
141. DeFronzo RA, Sherwin RS, Dillingham M, et al: Influence of basal insulin and glucagon secretion in potassium and sodium metabolism, *J Clin Invest* 61:472, 1978.
142. DeFronzo RA, Thier SO: Pathophysiologic approach to hyponatremia, *Arch Intern Med* 140:897, 1980.
143. Gross P: Correction of hyponatremia, *Semin Nephrol* 21(3):269, 2001.
144. Gruskin AB, Baluarte HJ, Prebis JW, et al: Serum sodium abnormality in children, *Ped Clin North Am* 29(4):907, 1982.
145. Hollinshead WH: The interphase of diabetes insipidus, *Mayo Clin Proc* 39:92, 1964.
146. Jeha S: Tumor lysis syndrome, *Semin Hematal* 38(4)Suppl 10: 14, 2001.
147. McGuire JK, Kulkarni MS, Baden HP: Fatal hypermagnesemia in a child treated with megavitamin/megamineral therapy, *Pediatrics* 105(2), e18, 2000.
148. Phelan DM, Hagley SR, Guerrin MD: Is hypokalemia the cause of paralysis in barium poisoning? *Br Med J* 289:882, 1984.
149. Rizzo MA, Fisher M, Lock JP: Hypermagnesemic pseudocoma, Arch Intern Med 153:1130, 1993.
150. Tulassay T, Rascher W, Scharer K: Intra- and extrarenal factors of oedema formation in the nephrotic syndrome, *Pediatr Nephrol* 3:92, 1989.
151. Yang WC, Huang TP, Ho LT, et al: Beta-adrenergic mediated extrarenal potassium disposal in patients with end stage renal disease: effect of propranolol, *Mineral Electrolyte Metab* 12:186, 1986.

CHAPTER

61

Acid-Base Disorders

Hector Carrillo-Lopez, Adrian Chavez, Alberto Jarillo, and Victor Olivar

Physics, chemistry, and physiology of the acid-base balance are among the first subjects that are taught at medical school. They remain topics, however, about which physicians seem to display only a superficial knowledge. About 20 years ago, 70% of medical doctors at a university hospital answered, when inquired, that they needed no help in correctly interpreting arterial blood gases. They succeeded in only 40% of the cases presented to them, though.[1] It is likely that this situation still plagues hospitals worldwide.

The knowledge required for the proper interpretation of the patient's blood gas analysis or clinical picture remains one of the best examples of the close correlation between basic and clinical sciences. Currently, this statement contains more truth than ever because many exciting concepts in the field of acid-base physiology are evolving and are now being applied rather slowly but at an increasing pace in the clinical arena. Because intensivists spend much of their time managing problems related to fluids, electrolytes, and acid-base balance, a thorough but practical understanding of the physiology and pathophysiology of acid-base disorders is a central aspect of the expertise of the critical care practitioner.

This chapter represents an effort to summarize the useful aspects of the traditional approach to the understanding and management of the acid-base balance, along with a glimpse of the new physiological insight that allows a refreshing and deeper comprehension of the body's acid-base equilibrium. A brief review of the causes of acid-base disturbances in the pediatric critical care setting is included, and lactic acidosis is highlighted. Finally, a discussion of available therapies and their controversies closes the chapter.

Understanding Acid-Base Physiology: From Henderson-Hasselbalch to Stewart and Beyond

Most of the concepts of the acid-base physiology were developed in the early twentieth century[2-4] and are based mainly in the accepted definition of *acid*.[5,6] As early as 1887, Arrhenius had defined *acid* as a substance that, when dissolved in water, produces an increased concentration of hydrogen ions.[4,7] By 1900, Naunyn and others proposed that the acid-base status was, at least partially, determined by the concentration of some electrolytes, mainly sodium and chloride, which had been formerly described by Faraday as "base-forming cation" and "acid-forming anion," respectively.[4] These concepts were the main influence on the work of most of the more distinguished acid-base physiologists of those times, including Henderson in 1908, Hasselbalch in 1916, and Van Slyke in 1921. Van Slyke adopted and spread Naunyn's concepts and developed a method for determining gas concentration (total carbon dioxide [CO_2]) in blood.[4,6,8,9]

In the 1920s, Brönsted and Lowry stated that an "acid" is every molecule that contains hydrogen atoms and that is able to release them in a soluble manner; that is, an acid is a "proton-donor substance."[5, 6, 10] Thus an acid (HA) may dissociate and donate a proton (H^+) to the solution, forming the conjugate base (or anion) A^- in a reversible manner:

$$K' [HA] \Leftrightarrow [H^+] + [A^-] \qquad \text{Eq. 1}$$

where K' is the equilibrium or dissociation constant, particular to every different substance and influenced by the characteristics of the particular solution in which the reaction is taken place. Therefore a *base* is a molecule with the ability for accepting or "trapping" free hydrogen ions ("proton acceptor substance").[6] Examples include bicarbonate, hemoglobin, several proteins, and phosphates.

Whatever definition of acid is used, its validity depends on the given situation in which one is trying to understand or is explaining some event. In biological solutions such as plasma, the given situation is a water-based solution with tightly controlled solute concentrations. It is remarkable that, in this scenario, all the former acid definitions are valid[4] because water can supply both hydrogen and hydroxyl ions:

$$H_2O \Leftrightarrow H^+ + OH^- \qquad \text{Eq. 2}$$

According to the acid definition, the acidity of a solution is a measure of the chemical activity of hydrogen ions. In body fluids, this is proportional to the concentration of hydrogen ions [H^+].[11] Normal concentration of hydrogen ions in the extracellular fluid is extremely low, in the nanoequivalent (nEq) or nanomole (nmol) range (i.e., the order of magnitude of the [H^+] is in the millionth of a milliequivalent range [nanoequivalent = 10^{-9} equivalent = 10^{-6} milliequivalent]). The usual arterial blood [H^+] is about 40 nEq/L (or nmol/L) (i.e., 0.000040 mEq/L, with a normal range of 35 to 45 nEq/L [0.000035 to 0.000045 mEq/L or mmol/L]). In other words, serum [H^+] is about 3 millions times less than the serum sodium concentration.[12] Because hydrogen ion concentration in body fluids and tissues has a strong influence on the function of almost all enzymatic systems of the organism,[13,14] a tight regulation of its concentration is mandatory for the body.

Because these figures and units can be confusing or cumbersome for the clinician, the [H^+] value is usually expressed as pH units, which are obtained from the negative $\log_{10}$ of the hydrogen ion concentration in nanoequivalents per liter. This concept was developed by Sörenson and adapted by Karl Hasselbalch to clinical medicine in 1909.[12] The relationship between pH and [H^+][15] is shown in Table 61–1. A normal pH of 7.4 corresponds to a blood hydrogen ion concentration of 40 nEq/L. Because pH is the negative log of [H^+], it is important to remember that, as the hydrogen ion concentration increases, the pH value decreases and vice versa. Please note that the relationship is nonlinear, but it is almost linear over the narrow normal range of 7.35 to 7.45 (corresponding to 45 to 35 nEq/L of [H^+]).

An acid is "strong" when it dissociates its hydrogen ion easily because the corresponding base has a low affinity for it (high K′–dissociation constant value). "Weak" acids only partially dissociate because their corresponding base has high affinity for hydrogen ions (low K′value). When the latter is the case, both the acid and base forms of the parental molecule are present in the resulting solution in equimolar proportions. As a consequence, this solution has the ability to resist changes in acidity (or pH) after the addition of a strong acid or base. This solution, constituted by an acid-base pair, is known as a *buffer*, a term coined by Sörenson. The dissociation constant K′, as in the case of pH, can be expressed as $-\log_{10}K'$ and is termed *pK′*, which is a measure of the tendency of the acid-base pair to ionize. Strong acids have a low pK′ (high K′) and weak acids have high pK′ (low K′). A weak acid-base pair is more effective as a buffer in living systems when the pK′ is close to physiological pH.[11]

Physiological buffering systems may be classified into two general categories: the bicarbonate/carbonic acid (HCO_3^- / H_2CO_3) buffering system, which acts in both the extracellular space and inside the erythrocytes, and the nonbicarbonate buffers, which include hemoglobin and oxyhemoglobin, organic phosphates, inorganic phosphates, and plasma proteins. Extracellular buffers (HCO_3^-, plasma proteins) represent the body's first and immediate line of defense against any alteration of pH of the body fluids.[12] After extracellular buffering occurs, a second intracellular phase takes place, as long as intracellular buffers (intracellular proteins, dibasic phosphates, hemoglobin-oxyhemoglobin and carbonate in bones) reach buffering capacity over the next several hours.[16,17] The buffering systems cannot truly eliminate hydrogen ions from the body, but they tamper sudden changes in [H^+] (or pH) and "buy time" until a new balance can be achieved. Altogether, extracellular and intracellular buffers provide a volume of distribution close to that of the total body water to any exogenous acid load (or deficit). This represents a formidable capacity for resisting changes in pH.

Acid production in the body occurs in two major ways. The first one involves CO_2 production during oxidative metabolism of carbohydrates, fat, and amino acids, which is then hydrated by the cytoplasmic enzyme carbonic anhydrase to produce carbonic acid (H_2CO_3), a weak acid that dissociates in hydrogen ion and bicarbonate.

$$H^+ + HCO_3^- \Leftrightarrow H_2CO_3 \Leftrightarrow CO_2 + H_2O \qquad \text{Eq. 3}$$

The second pathway involves nonvolatile metabolic acids that are produced by the normal daily catabolic load (oxidation of sulfur containing amino acids, hydrolysis of pyrophosphate and orthophosphate esters) or during situations with incomplete catabolism of fat and carbohydrates, such as lactic acidosis or diabetic ketoacidosis. The free hydrogen ions are neutralized by extracellular and intracellular buffers, but because these acids are not in equilibrium in the normal plasma, they must be metabolized, mainly in the liver, and then excreted by the kidneys.[16]

The major acid-base buffering system in the blood is the bicarbonate/carbonic acid system, which has the tremendous advantage of its interconversion with CO_2, the volatile form of H_2CO_3. Any increase in [H^+] (or drop in pH) will shift the former reaction (Eq. 3) to the right. This fact allows that the pulmonary system can modify, with an increase in alveolar ventilation, the elimination rate of CO_2. This respiratory response is another line of defense and begins within minutes, but may not reach a steady state for 12 to 24 hours. This way of getting a fast and actual decrease of the acid component is a unique characteristic of the bicarbonate/carbonic acid buffering system. For the

TABLE 61–1

Relationship between [H^+] and pH

[H+] in nEq / L	pH	[H+] in nEq / L	pH
10	8.00	65	7.19
15	7.85	70	7.15
20	**7.70**	75	7.12
25	7.60	80	7.10
30	7.52	85	7.07
35	7.45	90	7.05
40	**7.40**	95	7.02
45	7.35	**100**	**7.00**
50	7.30	126	6.90
55	7.26	158	6.80
60	7.22		

other buffers, the addition or removal of hydrogen ions has the corresponding opposite effects on the buffer components, limiting the maximum buffering capacity. On the contrary, the capacity of the bicarbonate-CO_2 system is greatly increased because the lungs can eliminate a vast amount of CO_2 per day. Similarly, the kidneys can eliminate or regenerate bicarbonate, as needed, although their response is slower than that of the lungs.

The quantitative importance of the bicarbonate/carbonic acid buffering system was clearly noticed by Henderson when he developed his famous equation, modified by Hasselbalch shortly after. The Henderson-Hasselbalch equation[2,4] expresses the relationship of the bicarbonate/carbonic acid buffering system to pH[12,17]:

$$pH = pKa + \log ([HCO_3^-]/[H_2CO_3]) \qquad \text{Eq. 4}$$

The pH is equal to a constant (pKa, the $^-\log_{10}$ of Ka, the first dissociation constant for H_2CO_3, which has a value of 6.1 for human plasma in physiological conditions) plus log of the ratio of HCO_3^- (proton acceptor) to H_2CO_3 (proton donor). The modified Henderson-Hasselbalch equation takes into consideration that H_2CO_3 is in equilibrium with dissolved CO_2 and is rewritten as:

$$pH = pKa + \log ([HCO_3^-]/0.03 \times P_{CO_2} \qquad \text{Eq. 5}$$

where 0.03 stands for the solubility coefficient for carbon dioxide in blood at 37° C.

What the Henderson-Hasselbalch equation tells is how pH is affected by the change in the ratio of the concentration of nondissociated acid HA (in this case carbonic acid or P_{CO_2}) to the concentration of the conjugated base or anion A^- (in this case HCO_3^-). When pH is altered as the result of changes in the volatile component (increases or decreases of P_{CO_2}), clinically speaking, the change is referred to as *respiratory*. When pH is modified by changes in nonvolatile acids (e.g., lactic acid, ketoacids), it is referred to as *metabolic* in origin. The term *acidosis* is used to describe the process that tends to produce an increase in $[H^+]$, whether there is a change in pH. Alkalosis is the opposite; that is, the process that tends to produce a decrease in $[H^+]$, with or without changes in pH. Acidemia and alkalemia are the corresponding terms for those situations in which blood pH actually changes. Thus this equation allows disorders to be classified according to the primary type of acid being increased or decreased. For example, if a patient's pH is low (acidemia), then the patient will have either an increased P_{CO_2} or a P_{CO_2} within normal values. In the first case the condition is classified as *respiratory acidosis*. In the second situation, P_{CO_2} is not increased and thus there cannot be a respiratory acidosis. Therefore some nonvolatile acid must be the cause of the acidemia, which is then referred to as *metabolic acidosis*. If these examples are reversed, then alkalemia conditions can also be classified as resulting from either respiratory or metabolic alkaloses.

The Henderson-Hasselbalch equation is useful but has intrinsic limitations.[4,18] The first one is that it does not quantify the severity of the metabolic derangement as it does for the respiratory component. In a respiratory acidosis, the increase in the P_{CO_2} quantifies the derangement even when there are mixed disorders. The metabolic component can only be approximated, however, by the change in HCO_3^-. Although the relationship between P_{CO_2} and HCO_3^- provides a useful clinical guide for uncovering a metabolic origin of a given derangement, this is dampened because P_{CO_2}, H_2CO_3, and HCO_3^- are all interlinked (Eq. 3), so the bicarbonate will also increase if P_{CO_2} increases.[4,18] The second important characteristic of the Henderson-Hasselbalch equation is that it does not give information about any acids other than carbonic acid.[4,14,18-20]

Therefore since the first half of the twentieth century, several groups searched for methods to better identify acid-base changes independent of CO_2. In 1948 Singer and Hastings[21] developed the concept of "buffer base," defined as the sum of weak acid (buffer) anions in plasma including albumin, hemoglobin, and bicarbonate; they also defined *fixed acids* as nonbuffer anions, with chloride being one. This approach was essentially correct, but it was rather complex in a time before handheld calculators, computers, and personal digital assistants (PDAs).[4,20] The panorama did not change much until the mid 1950s, when a gradual shift of thinking appears to have followed a desire for clinical chemistry to adapt to the "newest" Brönsted-Lowry definition of acid as a "proton donor."[5,6,10,22,23] Using the Brönsted-Lowry definition, many physiologists dismissed defining chloride as an acid and sodium as a base,[6,22,23] arguing that there was an insufficient link between these and other electrolytes and the subsequent changes in hydrogen ions. Thus by accepting only Brönsted-Lowry acids while looking for factors controlling the nonrespiratory component of acid-base balance, many physiologists focused on the plasma bicarbonate concentration and the Henderson-Hasselbalch equation.[4] This was the beginning of the still dominant concept that plasma bicarbonate is not only an indicator of acid-base status, but also a main determinant of it.

Immersed in this bicarbonate-centered approach, investigators yielded basically three solutions for analyzing the "metabolic side" of the equation: the base excess method, the six bicarbonate "rules of thumb," and the use of anion gap (AG).[4,14,18,24-27]

As a further refinement and simplification of the former "buffer base," Siggaard-Andersen, from Copenhagen, developed the "base excess" method in the late 1950s.[3,28-32] *Base excess* (BE) is defined as the amount of strong acid (or strong base), in moles per liter (mol/L), that must be added to a whole blood sample to return the pH of the sample to 7.40, while the P_{CO_2} is maintained at 40 mmHg.[7,30,32,33] Therefore if the blood sample is normal (i.e., its pH is 7.4 and its P_{CO_2} is about 40 mmHg), the BE will be 0 mmol/L. Positive values mean literally an excess of metabolic bases; negative values mean an excess of metabolic acids.[32] For use of the BE in the clinical setting, a nomogram was developed, which was later mathematically transcribed to allow BE calculation by blood gas analyzers.[8] Several flaws soon appeared, however.[34-37] For clinical accuracy, other assumptions had to be incorporated (correction factors,[35] adjusted formulas,[4,35] nomogram modifications),[32] and remarkably an empiric estimate of hemoglobin concentration throughout the entire extracellular fluid space (whole blood plus interstitial fluid) had to be established. The chosen concentration was 50 g/L (5 g/dl).[32,35] This was known as *standard base excess* (SBE), a parameter reported nowadays by modern gas analyzers and used in the standard approach to acid-base balance (Table 61–2). Although SBE has good correlation with bicarbonate levels and quantifies the change in metabolic acid-base status in vivo, its accuracy depends on the 5 g/dl of hemoglobin assumption, and still it does not give information about the origin or mechanisms of the metabolic acid-base derangement because SBE is not a substance that can be regulated, absorbed, or excreted by the body.[18,19,38] In a "great trans-Atlantic debate,"[34,36,37] strong criticism from Schwartz and Relman from Boston yielded the six bicarbonate "rules of thumb"[18] (Table 61–3). The Henderson-Hasselbalch equation easily disclosed derangements into "respiratory" and "metabolic," the so-called simple derangements.[17] Because the body always seeks to tightly control $[H^+]$, however, several physiological responses become active over time, and then the relationship between $P{CO_2}$ and HCO^-_3 is modified so pH changes can be minimized. This minimization gives origin to more complex or "mixed" conditions.[17] Despite this, through careful examination of the changes that occur in $P{CO_2}$ and HCO^-_3 in relation to each other, it was possible to find patterns and to derive rules (the six rules of thumb) for uncovering mixed disorders and to differentiate acute from chronic respiratory unbalances. These rules describe the physiological compensation to acid-base changes to optimize acid-base homeostasis. With the expected physiological compensation allowed for, residual changes in CO_2 or bicarbonate are then seen as the mechanisms for changes in acid-base status (Tables 61–3 and 61–4).

The AG was introduced by Emmett and Narins,[39] Oh and Carroll,[40] and Oh et al[41] in 1977 as a complementary diagnostic tool for either SBE or bicarbonate rules of thumb approaches of metabolic disturbances. It is based on the principle of electroneutrality. Accordingly, serum positive-charged cations (sodium + potassium + calcium + magnesium) must equal anions (chloride + bicarbonate + proteins + sulfate + phosphate + organic acid anions). The AG has traditionally been simplified and is commonly defined as ([Na+] + [K+]) – ([Cl–] + [HCO3]) or even more; sometimes [K+] is suppressed and its effect neglected.[26] Typically, normal values are 16 mEq/L (if [K+] is included) or 12 mEq/L (without [K+]), with variations (plus/minus) of 2 to 4 mEq/L. These values may be influenced by the way the values of some of the parameters are measured, so it is always better to consult each institution's own expected "normal AG."[24,42] The AG is not useful for "quantification" of the metabolic derangement but can assist the clinician in the categorization of metabolic acidoses. Thus through the AG it is possible to differentiate hyperchloremic acidosis (normal AG) from "gap acidoses" (increased AG).[13,26,27] The last category includes all conditions of metabolic acidosis caused by increased concentrations of nonvolatile anions other than chloride, usually unmeasured (or unmeasurable), such as lactate, ketoacids, sulfates, phosphate and other anions in renal failure setting, salicylate, some β-lactam antibiotics, and acetate from parenteral nutrition (Table 61–5). Undoubtedly, the AG is a powerful tool in the hands of experienced clinicians.[27] For example, if the AG is clearly elevated, in the critical care setting the cause almost always will be one of these five: lactic acidosis, ketoacidosis, inborn error of metabolism, renal failure, or

TABLE 61–2

Standard Acid-Base Approach: Standard Acid-Base Parameters

pH	$-\log_{10}[H^+]$. Measured directly by electrode. Normal = 7.35 – 7.45.
$P{CO_2}$	Partial pressure of gaseous CO_2. Measured directly by electrode. Usually expressed in mmHg. Normal value: 35 to 45 mmHg (sea level, arterial blood).
$[HCO_3^-]$	A calculated parameter, derived from pH and $P{CO_2}$ values with a nomogram or the Henderson-Hasselbalch equation, or it is the difference between serum total CO_2 (CO_{2TOT}) and the dissolved CO_2 that equals $P{CO_2} \times 0.03$. Normal value: 22-28 mEq/L.
Base excess (BE or BE/D)	Also known as "base excess/deficit." Defined as the amount of strong base (negative base excess, or "base deficit") or strong acid (positive base excess) in mmol/L that would be needed to restore a pH of 7.4 ($[HCO_3^-]$ = 24 mmol/L) to a liter of whole blood equilibrated at $P{CO_2}$ = 40 mmHg. It is calculated strong by a nomogram or equation based on an experimental series of in vitro titrations of strong acid and base in whole blood samples at various $P{CO_2}$ levels. It excludes the effect of acute changes in $P{CO_2}$, so it loses accuracy if $P{CO_2}$ is abnormal.
Standard base excess (SBE)	A modification of base excess to allow equilibration across the entire extracellular fluid space (whole blood + interstitial fluid) and thus preserve accuracy at variable $P{CO_2}$ values. The new equation assumes an "average" concentration of hemoglobin through that space of 5 g/dl. Despite being a somewhat arbitrary figure, it indeed works in vivo.
CO_{2TOT} or $[CO_2]$	A serum chemistry measured value. Its components include HCO_3^-, dissolved gaseous CO_2, carbonic acid (H_2CO_3), carbamino CO_2, and carbonate. About 95% exists as HCO_3^-, and 4% to 5% as dissolved gaseous CO_2. Remaining species are negligible.
Anion gap (AG)	A calculated value that indicates the presence of "unmeasured" anions. AG = ([Na+] + [K+]) – ([Cl–] + $[HCO_3^-]$). Normal ≤ 16 mEq/L (see text).

Modified from Venticinque SG: Metabolic acidosis surrounding resuscitation. *7th Critical Care Refresher Course Cutting Edge Therapeutics.* San Antonio, 2003, Society of Critical Care Medicine.

TABLE 61–3

Standard Acid-Base Approach: Observational Standard Acid-Base Patterns

Primary Disorder	Expected Changes $[HCO_3^-]$ (mEq/L or mmol/L)	Expected Changes P_{CO_2} (mmHg)	Expected Changes SBE (mmol/L)
Metabolic acidosis	<22	$= (1.5 \times HCO_3^-) + (8 \pm 2)$ $= 40 + SBE$	<–5
Metabolic alkalosis	>26	$= (0.7 \times HCO_3^-) + (21 \pm 2)$ $= 40 + (0.6 \times SBE)$	>+5
Acute respiratory acidosis	$= [(P_{CO_2} - 40)/10] + 24$	> 45 or $\Delta pH = 0.008 \times (P_{CO_2} - 40)$	= 0
Chronic respiratory acidosis	$= [(P_{CO_2} - 40) / 3] + 24$	> 45 or $\Delta pH = 0.003 \times (PCO_2 - 40)$	$= 0.4 \times (PCO_2 - 40)$
Acute respiratory alkalosis	$= [(40 - P_{CO_2})/5] + 24$	<35 or $\Delta pH = 0.008 \times (40 - P_{CO_2})$	= 0
Chronic respiratory alkalosis	$= [(40 - P_{CO_2})/10] + 24$	< 35 or $\Delta pH = 0.017 \times (40 - P_{CO_2})$	$= 0.4 \times (P_{CO_2} - 40)$

Modified from Marino PL: *The ICU Book*, ed 2, Baltimore, 1998, Williams & Wilkins; Ichikawa I, Narins RG, Harris HW Jr: Regulation of acid-base homeostasis. In Ichikawa I, editor: *Pediatric Textbook of Fluids and Electrolytes,* Baltimore, 1990, Williams & Wilkins; Schlichtig R, Grogono AW, Severinghaus JW: Human PaCO2 and standard base excess compensation for acid-base imbalance. *Crit Care Med* 26: 1173-1179, 1998; and Kellum JA: Determinants of blood pH in health and disease. *Crit Care* 4:8-14, 2004.

poisoning/presence of some medication.[13] False-negative values are not rare, however.[13,18,25-27,43-48]

Proponents of the Brönsted-Lowry–based and bicarbonate-centered approaches could not prove that the previous approach was wrong.[4] It is remarkable that no one examined the role of water as a virtually inexhaustible source of hydrogen ion, as Peter Stewart later did.[4,14,18,49-51] Although pure water dissociates only slightly into H^+ and OH^- in plasma, the presence of electrolytes, CO_2, and other weak acids produces powerful electrochemical forces influencing water dissociation.[18] What was overlooked is that all weak acids in a given aqueous solution such as plasma can be inserted into a Henderson-Hasselbalch type of equation to calculate pH, just as Lawrence Henderson himself showed in 1908.[2] The reason is easy to understand: for a single solution containing several weak acids (as human plasma), all the weak acids are equilibrated with a single pool of hydrogen ions.

TABLE 61–4

Standard Acid-Base Approach: Additional Clues

1. A metabolic acid-base derangement exists if:
   a. pH is abnormal
   b. pH and P_{CO_2} have changed in the same direction (both increased or both decreased)
   c. Respiratory compensation is intact if Pa_{CO_2} resembles last two digits of pH
2. A respiratory acid-base derangement is overlapped if *any* of the following occurs:
   a. P_{CO_2} is reported within normal limits
   b. P_{CO_2} reported is higher than expected P_{CO_2} (respiratory acidosis overlapped)
   c. P_{CO_2} reported is lower than expected P_{CO_2} (respiratory alkalosis overlapped)
3. A respiratory acid-base derangement exists if:
   a. Pa_{CO_2} is abnormal
   b. P_{CO_2} and pH have changed in opposite directions (i.e., raised P_{CO_2} and decreased pH or vice versa)
4. If the change of pH is … (see formulas in Table 61–3)
   a. 0.008 × change in P_{CO_2}, there is no compensation; then the derangement is acute
   b. >0.003 but <0.008 × change in P_{CO_2}, there is a partial compensation
   c. 0.003 × change in P_{CO_2}, there is full compensation; then the derangement is chronic
   d. >0.008 × change in P_{CO_2}, there is a metabolic derangement overlapped
5. There is a mixed derangement (acidosis and alkalosis) if any of the following occurs:
   a. Pa_{CO_2} is abnormal and pH has not changed as expected or is within normal values
   b. pH is abnormal and Pa_{CO_2} has not changed as expected or is within normal values

Modified from Marino PL: *The ICU Book,* ed 2, Baltimore, 1998, Williams & Wilkins.

TABLE 61–5

Traditional Causes of Metabolic Acidosis

Anion Gap	
Increased	**Normal**
ENDOGEN SOURCE OF ACIDS	RENAL LOSS OF BICARBONATE
Lactic acidosis	Renal tubular acidosis
Glycogen storage disorders	Hypoaldosteronism
Uremia (chronic renal insufficiency)	Renal insufficiency
Ketoacidosis	Recovery phase of diabetic ketoacidosis
Diabetes	Urinary tract obstruction
Starvation	GASTROINTESTINAL LOSS OF BICARBONATE
ALCOHOLISM	Infective diarrhea and dehydration
EXOGENOUS ACIDS	Short bowel syndrome
Toxic ingestion/abuse	Small bowel, pancreatic or biliary drainage
Salicylates	Sulfamylon, cholestyramine
Ethanol	DRUGS
METHANOL	Potassium-sparing diuretics
Nonlegal drugs	Carbonic anhydrase inhibitors
Paraldehyde	Amphotericin B
	ACID INFUSION
	HCl, NH_4Cl, arginine HCl
	Intravenous hyperalimentation

Modified from Meliones JN, Wilson BG, Cheifetz IM et al: Respiratory monitoring. In Rogers MC, editor: *Textbook of Pediatric Critical Care,* ed 3, Baltimore, 1996, Williams & Wilkins.

This is called the *isohydric principle.*[4] Consider two buffer systems: bicarbonate/carbonic acid and phosphate/phosphoric acid:

$$H_2CO_3 \Leftrightarrow HCO_3^- + H^+ \; HPO_4^{2-} \Leftrightarrow H_2PO_4^- \qquad \text{Eq. 6}$$

Expressing the same concept in the Henderson-Hasselbalch way:

$$pKa_1 ++ \log([HCO_3^-]/[H_2CO_3]) = \mathbf{pH} = pKa_2 + \log([HPO^{2-}_4/[H_2PO_4^-]) \qquad \text{Eq. 7}$$

Thus according to the isohydric principle, the ratio of *any pair* of conjugate base or anion and its nondissociated acid will be able to *describe* the [H+] or pH.[4,52] This means that although the ratio of PCO_2 to bicarbonate can describe how the pH and acid-base status is, the system bicarbonate/carbonic acid is not necessarily the primary or underlying mechanism for explaining changes in pH (i.e., correlation and causation are not the same).[4,14,18]

Therefore it should be apparent that for aqueous solutions, water is the primary source of hydrogen ion, and thus the determinants of $[H^+]$ are the determinants of water dissociation. In the late 1970s and early 1980s, Peter Stewart proposed that Arrhenius' more general definition of an acid, along with Naunyn's ideas from 1900, is more useful to acid-base physiology than the Brönsted-Lowry definition.[49-51,53] Applying several basic principles of physical chemistry, particularly electroneutrality; conservation of mass; and dissociation equilibrium of partially dissociated substances (electrolytes and others),[25,49,53,54] Stewart developed a model of acid-base balance in which there are only three independent controlling variables of H^+ concentration: (1) the partial pressure of carbon dioxide (PCO_2); (2) the strong ion difference (SID), that is, the difference between the sums of all "strong" (fully dissociated, chemically non reacting) cations (Na^+, K^+, Ca^{2+}, Mg^{2+}) and all the strong anions (Cl^-, lactate$^-$, and others); and (3) concentration of nonvolatile weak acids, that is, for each of them, the sum of its dissociated and undissociated forms ($A_{TOT} = A^- + HA$).[25,50,51,54] The two most important plasmatic *strong* ions—completely dissociated ions—are sodium and chloride.[50,51,55,56] The most important weak acid—partially dissociated acid—is albumin, with a minor effect from phosphate.[54,56] "Independent variables" mean that PCO_2, SID, and A_{TOT} are causally related to the hydrogen ion, rather than being merely correlated. Therefore hydrogen ion and bicarbonate concentrations are totally dependent on these three factors, in association with the temperature-dependent dissociation constants of the weak acids and water, which are accepted as constants within physiological limits and thus are ignored.[4,53] What about bicarbonate and SBE? According to Stewart, the major use for bicarbonate rules of thumb and SBE is to determine the extent of the clinical acid-base disorder, rather than the mechanism.[4,51] Normal acid-base status occurs when the independent variables have normal values. Abnormality of one or more of the independent variables underlies all acid-base disturbances. Adjustment of the independent variables is the essence of all therapeutic interventions because none of the dependent variables (e.g., pH, BE, $[HCO_3^-]$) can be changed primarily or individually; the dependent variables change all of them simultaneously if, and only if, one or more of the independent variables changes.[25]

According to Stewart's approach, CO_2 holds its main roll as an independent determinant of pH, just as in the bicarbonate-EB-centered approaches (i.e., there are no changes in the understanding of the respiratory acid-base derangements). In normal conditions, alveolar ventilation is adjusted to maintain arterial PCO_2 between 35 and 45 mmHg. Therefore a respiratory acid-base disorder exists when alveolar ventilation decreases or increases out of proportion to CO_2 production. For example, in the critical care setting a patient has an acute elevation of PCO_2. The rise of the PCO_2, according to the Henderson-Hasselbalch equation (Eq. 5), will increase both H^+ and HCO_3^- concentrations. Therefore the change in HCO_3^- concentration is mediated by chemical equilibrium (Eq. 3) and not by any systemic adaptive response.[18] The total CO_2 concentration, and thus the HCO_3^- concentration, is determined by the PCO_2, which is in turn determined by the balance between alveolar ventilation and CO_2 production at tissue level. Therefore HCO_3^- cannot be regulated independently of PCO_2. Plasma bicarbonate concentration will always increase if PCO_2 increases, but this is not an alkalosis. Therefore the increased bicarbonate concentration is not "buffering" the rise of $[H^+]$, and there will be no change in the SBE. As CO_2 easily diffuses through membranes, there is always tissue acidosis.

If P_{CO_2} remains high, the body will attempt to compensate by altering another independent determinant of pH; the kidneys are the main organs involved in this compensation.[18]

Since Stewart's original papers, several refinements have been performed to the "physical chemical" approach to acid-base derangements.[4,14,18,19,25,26,57-59] In plasma, strong cations (mainly Na^+) outnumber strong anions (mainly Cl^-). Therefore SID is the difference between the sum of all strong cations and the sum of all strong anions.

$$SID = (Na^+ + K^+ Ca^{2+} + Mg^{2+}) - (Cl^- + lactate^-) \quad \text{Eq. 8}$$

This calculation of SID has been termed by some groups as the *apparent SID* (SIDa)[18,19,54,60] (see later) (see Table 61–7). In healthy humans this is normally between 38 and 42 mmol/L[4,18,19,25,54] but is usually substantially reduced in critical care illness, even when there is no evidence (by the traditional approach) of a metabolic acid-base derangement.[58] This lower SID in critical care patients is not surprising given the fact that the positive charge of the SID is balanced by the negative charges of A^- and total CO_2. Because P_{CO_2} is usually modified by the body for other reasons (e.g., hyperventilation in a patient that tends to be hypoxemic) and because hypoalbuminemia is the rule rather than the exception in these kinds of settings, A^- tends to be reduced, and this decrease leads to a reduction in SID to keep the normal pH. Thus a typical critical care patient might have an SID of 30 mEq/L rather than the "usual" 38 to 42 mEq/L. If this patient then has metabolic acidosis, the SID will decrease further. Also, the lower the baseline of the SID, the greater the susceptibility to a subsequent acid load.[13]

The principle of electroneutrality dictates that in aqueous solutions, the sum of all positive charges (cations) must equal the sum of all negative charges (anions). Both H^+ and OH^- behave as a weak cation and anion, respectively. Because practically all the cations in plasma are strong ions, except for H^+, only H^+ concentration can vary in response to changes in anions. On the other hand, there are several anions that are weak ions, and thus there are several "options" of anion molecules that can change their charges if cations change.[14,54] Thus the SID has a powerful electrochemical effect on water dissociation and on $[H^+]$. As the SID increases (strong cations in excess over strong anions) plasma becomes positively charged; then H^+, a weak cation, decreases (and pH increases) to maintain electrical neutrality; and alkalosis is produced. On the other hand, if the SID decreases (strong anions in relative excess over strong cations), plasma becomes negatively charged, more water is dissociated to have more H^+ for keeping electroneutrality, and acidosis is produced.[52] According to the principle of electroneutrality, blood plasma cannot be charged, so there should be remaining negative charges balancing the SID, coming from total CO_2 (HCO_3^-) and from two substances that act as nonvolatile weak acids. The concentrations in plasma should be large enough so that changes in them can produce significant acid disturbances: the weak acids (A^-) albumin and inorganic phosphate. Thus the SID can be derived as the sum of $[HCO_3^-]$ plus the negative electric charges contributed by albumin ($[Alb^-]$) and by inorganic phosphate ($[Pi^-]$).[21,25,60] For bedside purposes, the formula for SID can be simplified as follows[25,60]:

$$SID = [HCO_3^-] + 0.28 \times [Alb^-]\ (g/L) + 1.8 \times [Pi^-]\ (mmol/L) \quad \text{Eq. 9}$$

This calculation of SID is known by some authors as *effective SID* (SIDe) (see later)[54,61]. Factors 0.28 and 1.8 are the negative electric charges displayed by 1 g of albumin and 1 mmol of [Pi], respectively (0.6 if [Pi] is in milligrams per deciliter), in plasma at pH = 7.4.[60] The variation of these factors with the actual critical care patient's pH or with ion binding can be neglected.[25] Of course, the free OH^- that arouses from dissociated water has a theoretical role in SID. At physiological pH, however, OH^- contribution is so small that it can be ignored, as it is in the nanomole range.[18]

This approach has important physiological implications. For example, how is the SID regulated by the body? For the SID to be modified, an actual change in the relative concentrations of strong cations or anions must be made, with the kidneys as the primary organs in charge of such a change. The kidneys can excrete only small amounts of strong ion into the urine each minute though; therefore several minutes to hours are required for achieving a significant change of the SID. The control of the kidney is important and precise because every chloride ion filtered and not reabsorbed increases the SID. Acid handling of the kidney has traditionally focused on H^+ excretion and the role of NH_3 and NH_4^+.[11,62,63] Because water provides an essentially infinite source of H^+, however, its excretion per se is irrelevant. In fact, the H^+ net excretion by the kidney as water molecules is larger than the excretion as NH_4^+. Therefore the purpose of renal NH_4^+ production is to allow the excretion of Cl^- without the excretion of Na^+ or K^+. Thus NH_4^+ is important to systemic acid-base balance, not for its role as an H^+ carrier or for its direct action in the plasma (normal $[NH_4^+]$ is <0.01 mmol/L), but because it allows a "safe" excretion of Cl^-. the bicarbonate-EB [18,64]

Landing in the Clinical Arena

Undoubtedly, insight into acid-base balance and its disorders can go deeper, but is it useful for the busy clinician in the daily work at critical care units? Table 61–6 shows a proposal of an "independent-variables-based" classification of primary acid-base disturbances.[25,52] In this point of view, metabolic acid-base disorders can be caused by two types of abnormalities: abnormal SID and abnormal concentration of nonvolatile weak acids. The SID value can change in two general ways: First, this situation can be detected by abnormal $[Na^+]$ through excess or deficit of water in plasma, by which the strong cations and the strong anions are equally diluted or concentrated. These situations have been referred to as *dilutional acidosis* and *concentrational alkalosis*. These terms should not be confused with the older concepts of *contraction alkalosis* and dilution acidosis,[65] terms formerly used in reference to supposed acid-base consequences

TABLE 61–6

Classification of Primary Acid-Base Disturbances: Independent Variables–Oriented Approach

	Acidosis	Alkalosis
I. Respiratory	↑ Pa_{CO_2}	↓ Pa_{CO_2}
II. Nonrespiratory (metabolic)		
II-1. Abnormal SID		
a. Water excess/deficit	↓ SID, ↓ [Na^+]	↑ SID, ↑ [Na^+]
b. Imbalance of strong ions		
i. Chloride excess/deficit*	↓ SID, ↑ [Cl^-]	↑ SID, ↓ [Cl^-]
ii. Unidentified anion excess†	↓ SID, ↑ [XA^-]	—
II-2. Nonvolatile weak acids		
a. Serum albumin	↑ [Alb]‡	↓ [Alb]
b. Inorganic phosphate	↑ [Pi]	↓ [Pi]§

Modified from reference 25.

*Hyperchloremic acidosis and hypochloremic alkalosis.

†Includes several organic acids, endogenous and exogenous (e.g.,lactate, ketoacids, salicylate) in metabolic acidosis; also sulfate and other anions in chronic renal failure and unknown anions in conditions such as sepsis. Unlike anion gap, Pi is not included.

‡Component of acidosis in severe extracellular volume loss, such as in cholera.

§This source of alkalosis is clinically insignificant; the normal value of [Pi] (~ 1 mmol/L) cannot decrease enough to have an appreciable acid-base effect.

[A^-], concentration of unidentified strong anions; *[Alb]*, serum albumin concentration; *[Pi]*, inorganic phosphate concentration; *SID*, strong ion difference (Σ[strong cations] – Σ[strong anions]).

of decreased or increased extracellular fluid volume, respectively. Changes in volume do not change, by themselves, however, any of the variables that determine acid-base balance. The second way is by changing the total concentration of the strong anions only. This is true because concentrations of strong cations other than Na^+ are tightly regulated in extracellular fluids within narrow limits, for purposes unrelated to acid-base balance or osmolarity (e.g., K^+ and Ca^{2+} participation in electrical excitability of cellular membranes and neuromuscular plates).[25] This is the case of the acute expansion of extracellular volume with normal saline solution (sodium chloride [NaCl] 0.9%), which may result in hyperchloremic acidosis.[66-68] The understanding of this condition has improved through the physical chemical comprehension of the acid-base equilibrium: saline causes acidosis not through "dilution" of bicarbonate,[65] but rather by its Cl^- content, which decreases the SID and produces an increase in water dissociation and in [H^+]. This occurs despite equal amounts of Na^+ and Cl^- in saline solution because in plasma, sodium and chloride concentrations are different. Therefore when large amounts of NaCl in solution are infused, they will have a proportionally greater effect on total body chloride than on total body sodium.[18,55,64,66-68,70] In the sepsis setting, there appear to be unexplained sources of Cl^-. Kellum[13,18] and coworkers have hypothesized that this sourceless chloride comes from intracellular and interstitial compartments as a result of the partial loss of Donnan equilibrium due to albumin leaving the intravascular space owing to endothelial damage.[13,18] Of course, in addition to Cl^-, several other strong ions may be present in critically ill patients. Lactate is, no doubt, the most important one,[71-73] but ketones, medications, poisons (β-lactam antibiotics, salicylates, illegal drugs, methanol) and sulfates in the chronic renal failure setting can also be present.[20,72] According to Fencl et al,[25] all these anions, the so-called unmeasured or unidentified anions or XA^- have pK′ values at least three orders of magnitude lower than plasma pH; therefore they are always 99.9% or more dissociated and must be included in the SID definition because they do not behave as weak anions. According to Fencl et al[25] unlike the AG, XA^- does not include inorganic phosphate. The SID derived from Σ (strong cations) – Σ (strong anions) (Eq, 8) has been termed the SIDa because this calculation is precise but only in the healthy individual[19,26,54] (Table 61–7). The SID estimated from the value of the remaining negative charge (Eq. 9) has been termed the SIDe because it should include all the *remaining* anions needed for keeping electroneutrality of plasma. According to Kellum and coworkers, neither SIDa nor SIDe is a precise estimate of the "true SID," although they are nearly identical in healthy individuals. Kellum and coworkers coined the term and concept of *strong ion gap* (SIG)[38,74-77] (Table 61–7). These investigators advocate SIG use in situations in which SIDa and SIDe are not equal. Blood samples from certain patients often encountered in the critical care setting may contain unmeasured strong ions (e.g., ketones, sulfates, organic acids from inborn errors of metabolism), making the SIDa an inaccurate estimate of the "true" SID or SIDe. Similarly, these same kind of patients may have abnormal weak ions (such as proteins) that could make the SIDe inaccurate as well. According to Kellum et al,[77] when SIDa and SIDe are not equal, SIG could be useful.[54,73] It is calculated as follows:

$$SIG = SIDa - SIDe \qquad \text{Eq. 10}$$

By convention, SIG is *positive* when unmeasured anions exceed unmeasured cations and *negative* when unmeasured cations exceed unmeasured anions. In ideal theoretical conditions, it would be possible for the sum of strong cations and weak anions to cancel each other out, with an SIG equal to zero, but plenty of unmeasured ions would still present. For practical purposes, however, most SIGs are positive (anions > cations).[19] Unexplained anions, and in some case cations, have been found in the circulation of patients with various diseases and in animal models.[78-80] SIG concept is similar to the unidentified strong acids (XA^-) described by Fencl et al.[25] Nevertheless, SIG will change if unmeasured *weak* anions or acids (A_x^-) are present as well, so actual SIG in such a case would be $A_x^- + XA^-$.[18,19,25] Both SID (calculated as SIDe) and SIG have been evaluated as prognostic markers in

TABLE 61–7

Common Concepts in the Physical-Chemical Approach to Acid-Base Balance

Variable	Comment
Total CO_2(CO_{2TOT})	CO_{2TOT} includes not only HCO_3^- but also dissolved CO_2, carbonic acid (H_2CO_3), and CO^{2-}_3. Because the difference between CO_{2TOT} and HCO_3^- is about 1 mEq/L at physiological pH, for clinical purposes they are taken almost as equivalents.
Strong cations (Na^+, K^+ Ca^{2+}, Mg^{2+})	All cations that dissociate in aqueous solution
Strong anions (Cl^-, lactate$^-$)	All anions that dissociate in aqueous solution
Strong ion difference (SID)	It is the difference between the sum of all strong cations and the sum of all strong anions. Theoretically, it equals the following: SID = (Na^+ + K^+ Ca^{2+} + Mg^{2+}) – (Cl^- + lactate$^-$) In healthy individuals, plasma SID is 38 to 42 mmol/L. According to the principle of electroneutrality, blood plasma cannot be charged, so there should be remaining negative charges balancing the SID, coming from total CO_2 (HCO_3^-) and from the weak acids albumin and inorganic phosphate. Thus SID can also be derived from the sum of [HCO_3^-] plus the negative electric charges contributed by albumin ([Alb^-]) and by inorganic phosphate ([Pi^-]): SID = [HCO_3^-] + 0.28 × [Alb^-] (g/L) + 1.8 × [Pi^-] (mmol/L)
Apparent strong ion difference (SIDa)	The theoretical definition of SID: SID = (Na^+ + K^+ Ca^{2+} + Mg^{2+}) – (Cl^- + lactate$^-$) with the understanding that some "unmeasured ions" might also be present.
Effective strong ion difference (SIDe)	The determination of SID from the value of the remaining negative charge: SID = [HCO_3^-] + 0.28 × [Alb^-] (g/L) + 1.8 × [Pi^-] (mmol/L) It is equivalent to the "buffer base" concept described in the 1950s
Strong ion gap (SIG)	A term coined by Kellum and co-workers, its use is advocated in situations in which SIDa and SIDe are not equal. It is calculated as: SIG = SIDa – SIDe. By convention, SIG is *positive* when unmeasured anions exceed unmeasured cations and *negative* when unmeasured cations exceed unmeasured anions SIG is similar to Fencl's concept of unidentified strong anions (XA^-), but SIG will also change if unmeasured weak acids (A_x^-) are present, so actual SIG in such a case would be A_x^- + XA^-
Nonvolatile weak acids (A_{TOT}); A^- is sometimes used as equivalent concept (see comment)	Nonvolatile acids with pKa almost equal to the physiological pH of 7.4 and therefore almost not dissociated in plasma. The concentration of each one of these acids, is the sum of its dissociated and undissociated forms: A_{TOT} = AH + A^-). The two nonvolatile weak acids with great enough concentrations in plasma for having influence on acid-base status are albumin and inorganic phosphate; A^- value can be approximated by: 2 (albumin in g/dL) + 0.5 (phosphate in mg/dL). In a healthy individual, A^- concentration is near the value of the "normal" anion gap; if one is a purist, A^- is not an independent variable because it may change with alterations in SID and PCO_2; rather, A_{TOT} is the true independent variable
Unmeasured (or unidentified) anions (XA^-; other used abbreviation is UMA)	Includes organic acids, such as lactate (if not measured), and ketoacids, as the main "self-acids" that are often abnormally high in the critical care setting; sulfates and other acids may be high in the chronic renal failure setting; in inborn errors of metabolism, less common organic acids may appear; salicylate, formate, and other drug or toxic-derived acids can be responsible for acidosis in some patients; all these XA^- are strong acids
Tissue acids (TAs)	It equals the unmeasured (or unidentified) anions (XA^-) plus lactate (if this was actually measured); a value of TA >5 mEq/L has been used for defining significant tissue acidosis; increased XA^- has been defined as >3 mEq/L

both children and adults, with good predictive capability of both indexes, in most publications.[24,25,47,57,81-85] This evaluation is not universally accepted because some groups have found no further benefit of the "new" approach.[83,86,87] The common parameters and terms used in the physical-chemical approach of the acid-base balance are depicted in Table 61–7.

Finally, as already explained, there are normally only two substances that act as nonvolatile weak acids with large enough concentrations for influencing [H^+]: albumin and inorganic phosphate. It is possible to see that changes in these three independently variable quantities, [Alb], [Pi], and SID, can have additive or offsetting effects on the metabolic acid-base balance (Table 61–6). Such offsetting effects may result in normal values of the dependent variables pH, [HCO_3^-] and SBE, whereas some independent variables are abnormal. If that would be the case, such a condition could not be considered a normal acid-base status, despite the absence of acidemia or alkalemia. Although the loss of weak acid (A^-) from the plasma space is an alkalinizing process, there is no evidence that the body regulates A^- directly to maintain acid-base balance, nor is there evidence that clinicians should treat hypoalbuminemia as an acid-base derangement.[18] There is now enough evidence (and agreement), however, that hypoalbuminemia does influence the efficacy of traditional diagnostic tools as AG and SBE, and therefore it is now wise to make the proper corrections, particularly in the critical care setting,[13,14,18-20,25,26,43,47,57,59] where hypoalbuminemia is nearly ubiquitous, particularly in pediatric patients.[25,26,43,54,88] Figge et al showed that in most patients, the AG could be corrected as follows:

$$AG_{CORRECTED} = AG_{OBSERVED} + 2.5\ [\text{normal albumin g/dL}] - [\text{observed albumin g/dL}], \quad \text{Eq. 10}$$

or

$$AG_{CORRECTED} = AG_{OBSERVED} + 0.25\ [\text{normal albumin g/L}] - [\text{observed albumin g/L}]$$

considering normal albumin as 3.2 to 4.5 g/dl.

According to Kellum,[13,14] however, if serum phosphate is abnormal, the correction will not be so accurate. Therefore it is also recommended to include phosphate concentration in the correction formula if phosphate is "significantly" abnormal:

$$AG_{EXPECTED} - 2\ (\text{albumin g/dl}) + 0.5\ (\text{phosphate mg/dl}) \quad \text{Eq. 11}$$

or

$$AG_{EXPECTED} - 0.2\ (\text{albumin g/L}) + 1.5\ (\text{phosphate mmol/L})$$

Recently, a simplified and combined Fencl-Stewart approach to correct the hypoalbuminemia effect on the SBE was developed and tested in children in a pediatric intensive care unit (ICU) with apparent success.[57] Further simplifications, without losing accuracy, have been achieved by Dr. Story's group.[59] So far, their recommendations, designed to facilitate the clinical application of the Stewart approach, need the determination of four variables: (1) the SBE (mmol/L = mEq/L) obtained from a blood gas analyzer and BE effects of (2) NaCl, (3) albumin, and (4) unmeasured ions to resolve three equations:

$$\text{NaCl effect (mEq/L)} = [Na^+] - [Cl^-] - 38 \quad \text{Eq. 12A}$$

$$\text{Albumin effect (mEq/L)} = 0.25 \times [42 - \text{albumin (g/L)}] \quad \text{Eq. 12B}$$

$$\text{Unmeasured ion effect (mEq/L)} = \text{SBE} - \text{NaCl effect} - \text{albumin effect} \quad \text{Eq. 12C}$$

These four variables, along with the P_{CO_2}, allow a simple examination of the BE effects of the most important of Stewart's independent factors: CO_2, SID (NaCl), and total weak acid concentration (i.e., ≅ albumin). The unmeasured ion effect may be due to strong ions, such as sulphate or acetate,[57] or weak acids, such as phosphate, ketoacids, or polygelatin, used for priming circuits in cardiopulmonary bypass in some hospitals, as recently demonstrated.[19,80,82,86,89-91] Special situations, such as proteolysis associated with sepsis, may release organic and inorganic acids, some of which are poorly defined. Some of these acids are present in ill patients, and then their presence as unmeasured anions may serve as a marker of organ dysfunction.

Although these concepts are just being applied to patients, including children,[26,43,47,61,87,92,93] and at first glance seem complicated and akin to rocket science,[75,94] there is no doubt that this approach is here to stay,[95] so clinicians should cope with it and master it. After all, clinician-scientists are always looking for causation, not just correlation. In addition, other more practical and less philosophical reasons exist. In the critical care setting, clinicians cannot always use the traditional assessments to determine the causes of metabolic acidosis (Table 61–5) for several reasons on the basis of what has been discussed so far in the text.[20,96]

- The AG is an insensitive indicator of unmeasured anions, particularly in the critical care patient
- Mechanism and contribution of resuscitation fluids relative to the patient's acidosis have not been given enough attention
- The diverse mechanisms of lactic acidosis, which are often applicable in critical care patients, are not mentioned
- The concept that uncharacterized anions may be contributing to metabolic acidosis in this setting is not signaled

Although several of these issues can be addressed within the traditional acid-base physiology, the physical chemical approach facilitates understanding the many *why*'s. One radical difference is in how the following issues are analyzed and answered by the two approaches. The "traditional," "time-honored," "common sense" knowledge includes the following:

- Metabolic alkalosis seen with severe emesis or nasogastric tube losses is due to a loss of H^+
- Metabolic acidosis seen in persistent postpyloric fluid losses is due to a loss of bicarbonate
- An acidosis caused by large volume fluid administration is caused by dilution of bicarbonate
- Sodium bicarbonate ($NaHCO_3$) therapy corrects metabolic acidosis by contributing HCO_3^- to the body.

The physical chemical approach has thrown these long-held explanations to the garbage can, at least for now. Now we are aware that pH has no relationship with any total body loss or gain of H^+ and HCO_3, that our already known independent variables act through changing the dissociation of water, and that the resultant concentrations of H^+ and HCO_3^-, and the pH are merely effects rather than the cause of the acid-base derangements.

In the critical care unit, acid-base disorders are often considered more important for what they tell the clinician about the patient than for any harm that is directly provoked by the acid-base imbalance. Hatherill et al[87,97] recently reinforced this concept because they showed that mortality, more than the magnitude of metabolic acidosis (estimated by the BE), was more closely related to the nature of acid-base disorders. They found that hyperlactatemia, and not elevation on unmeasured anions (SIG) or BE, is predictive of a poor outcome. Despite this reliable data from children with shock, it is generally accepted that acid-base derangement may cause damage, severe damage indeed, in certain circumstances.[13,98-100]

The obvious examples are the extreme conditions of pH (<7 or >7.7). It is also important, however, to consider how fast the acid-base derangement is evolving, along with the specific expected consequences of the alteration in specific patients. For example, in a patient who depends on vasopressors, hypotension due to alkalosis,[101] either respiratory and iatrogenic in origin for overzealous hand-bagging of the patient, or metabolic as a consequence of intestinal fluid losses caused by a mechanically obstructed jejunum, can be catastrophic. Another typical example is the spontaneously breathing patient with metabolic acidosis, who tries to compensate by increasing minute ventilation; if the patient gets tired, there is the possibility that hypoxemia develops along with a respiratory component of the acidosis. In such cases, the underlying disorder must be treated, but one must also provide immediate treatment for the acid-base derangement itself. In summary, the main expected physiological effects of acidemia and alkalemia are as follows:

Acidemia initially causes sympathetic and adrenal stimulation, an effect that is counterbalanced, as the drop in pH becomes more and more severe, by a depressed responsiveness of adrenergic receptors to circulating catecholamines.[98,102-105] In isolated animal heart preparations and in isolated human ventricle muscle, there is no doubt that acidosis reduces contractile function.[106,107] The net influence of acidosis in the whole animal and in real patients, however, is more complicated to discern, and depending on the experimental or clinical model, it has been found that acidosis caused myocardial contractility to remain constant, decrease marginally, or transiently rise and then fall[108] (i.e., the whole-body response to acidosis is much less clearly detrimental in real patients). In many studies of patients undergoing permissive hypercapnia, a pH less than 7.2 was well tolerated,[109-111] as it is in youngsters with diabetic ketoacidosis,[112] children and adults with supercarbia,[113,114] and those with grand mal seizures.[115,116] Thus it is now clear that the effect of acidosis may differ according to type, magnitude, and time of onset.[87] Three types of extracellular acidosis—inorganic, respiratory, and lactic—may have disparate effects on left ventricular function in a model of isolated rabbit hearts.[117] Lactic acidosis caused a significant increase in the time to peak left ventricular pressure while retarding ventricular relaxation. This reinforced the concept that lactate ions have an independent and deleterious effect on myocardial function.[117] These findings make sense when they are extrapolated (with some reserve) to clinical grounds. Despite the frequent coincidence of clinical shock and metabolic acidosis, the striking discordance between the clinical course and outcome of patients with lactic acidosis compared with those who have ketoacidosis or ventilatory failure, suggests that the low pH itself is important but not crucial for the presentation of the hemodynamic collapse of these patients.[103,108] Therefore the net effect on ventricular performance, heart rhythm, and vascular tone depends on the relative effects of many, sometimes competing, influences. In general terms, severe acidemia (pH <7.10 according to the most, pH <7.20 according to others)[98,103] is associated with decreased cardiac performance that provokes a drop in cardiac output, along with decreased vascular reactivity that manifests itself as arterial vasodilatation and venous constriction.[98,118] An important effect in the critical care setting is the marked increase in cerebral blood flow due to acute respiratory acidemia.[113,118,119] When P_{CO_2} is abruptly increased in excess of 70 mmHg, loss of consciousness and seizures can be seen, probably due to the abrupt lowering of intracellular pH.[98] In patients connected to a mechanical ventilator with acute respiratory distress syndrome (ARDS) and treated with the "permissive hypercapnia" approach (i.e., intentional hypoventilation), the gradual rise of the P_{CO_2} is, generally speaking, well tolerated.[109,110] Intentional hypoventilation has been documented as having no significant effect on cardiac output, oxygen delivery, or vascular resistances, both pulmonary and systemic, and the current practice does not generally include an attempt to alkalinize the blood to compensate for respiratory acidosis.[108] Of course, patients with increased intracranial pressure are not candidates to this approach.[119] Other potential effects of acidemia include endogenous catecholamine, aldosterone, and parathyroid hormone stimulation; insulin resistance; increased free radical formation; increased protein degradation; gut barrier dysfunction; further respiratory depression; decreased sensorium; hyperkalemia; hypercalcemia; and hyperuricemia.[13,98] In regard to the effect of extracellular acidemia on inflammatory response and immune infection, recent research has indicated that different acids produce different effects, despite similar extracellular pH.[100]

When associated with severe alkalemia (pH > 7.60), both metabolic and respiratory alkalosis lower blood pressure and cardiac output. The potential deleterious effects of this drop in systemic and regional blood flow may be aggravated by the increased hemoglobin oxygen affinity (shift to the left of the oxyhemoglobin dissociation curve), particularly in the acute alkalosis. In the chronic alkalemia this effect is counterbalanced by an increase in the 2,3-diphosphoglyceric acid concentration in red cells.[99] Cerebral circulation responds dramatically to alkalemia with marked vasoconstriction. Cerebral blood flow may drop in response to an acute hyperventilation, at about 50% of the basal flow, at P_{CO_2} of 20 mmHg. This effect has been used as an emergency management of an impending raise of intracranial pressure but has the risk of producing an excessive drop of blood flow in the most affected areas of the brain, with the increased possibility of ischemia and subsequent cerebral infarct.[119] Because both metabolic and respiratory alkalemia may provoke abrupt transcellular membrane shifts of several electrolytes, mainly potassium and calcium, the net effect is an increase in neuromuscular irritability and excitability. The occurrence of seizures and severe cardiac arrhythmias has been reported, mainly if pH is around 7.7.[62,101]

Metabolic Acidosis

Lactic Acidosis

The classic approach to metabolic acidosis is to classify the disorders as those with either a normal AG or an elevated AG (Table 61–5). A revised list of the causes of metabolic acidosis that recognizes new paradigms, perhaps more suitable for the critical care patient, is presented in Tables 61–8 and 61–9. The popular classification of hyperlactatemia as type A (associated with decreased tissue oxygen delivery) or type B (adequate tissue oxygen delivery) is maintained, however, because of its simplicity, which is not necessarily a reflection of the disease.[120]

TABLE 61–8

Causes of Metabolic Acidosis in Critically Ill Patients

A. Accumulation of unmeasured anions (estimated by $AG_{CORRECTED}$)
  1. Type A hyperlactatemia (↓↓ tissue O_2 delivery)
    a. Hypodynamic shock or inadequate resuscitation
    b. Ischemic tissue (e.g., bowel or extremity)
    c. Severe anemia
    d. Severe hypoxemia
    e. Carbon monoxide poisoning
  2. Type B hyperlactatemia (abnormal pyruvate metabolism or aerobic metabolism)
    a. Hypermetabolism
      i. Increased aerobic glycolysis
      ii. Increased protein catabolism
      iii. Hematological malignancies
    b. Thiamine deficiency
    c. Toxins and drugs
    d. Congenital
    e. Decreased lactate clearance
  3. Ingested toxins and drugs or their metabolic byproducts
    a. Methanol, formic acid, ketoacids, lactate
    b. Ethylene glycol, glycolic acid, oxalic acid
    c. Ethanol
    d. Salicylate, salicylic acid, acetic acid
    e. Paraldehyde
  4. Renal failure: accumulation of phosphates, sulphates, and organic ions
  5. Unidentified anions in sepsis
  6. Ketoacids (diabetic, alcoholic, starvation)
    a. Acetoacetate
    b. β-hydroxybutyrate
B. Excessive chloride administration
  1. Normal saline or hypertonic saline resuscitation
  2. HCl administration
C. Renal causes
  1. Renal tubular acidosis
  2. Hypoaldosteronism
D. Parenteral hyperalimentation
E. Postpyloric gastrointestinal fluid losses
F. Drugs
  1. Acetazolamide
  2. Amphotericin B
  3. K+-sparing diuretics

TABLE 61–9

Causes of Lactic Acidosis

A. Type A: inadequate tissue oxygen delivery
  1. Hypodynamic shock or inadequate resuscitation
  2. Ischemic tissue (mesentery or extremity)
  3. Severe hypoxemia
  4. Severe anemia
  5. Carbon monoxide poisoning
B. Type B: adequate tissue oxygen delivery (abnormal pyruvate metabolism or aerobic metabolism)
  1. Alterations in cellular metabolism
    a. Hypermetabolism
      i. ↑ Aerobic glycolysis
      ii. ↑ Protein catabolism
      iii. Sepsis and hematological malignancies
    b. Post–cardiopulmonary bypass
    c. Burn injury
    d. Hematological malignancy
    e. End-organ failure (liver, lungs)
    f. Diabetes mellitus
    g. Thiamine deficiency
    h. Mitochondrial myopathies
    i. Severe alkalosis/hyperventilation
  2. Increased oxygen consumption
    a. Strenuous exercise
    b. Grand mal seizure, status epilepticus
    c. Malignant hyperthermia
    d. Neurological malignant syndrome
    e. Severe asthma
    f. Pheochromocytoma
  3. Ingested toxins and drugs or their metabolic byproducts:
    a. Epinephrine
    b. Propofol
    c. Terbutaline
    d. Salicylate
    e. Acetaminophen
    f. Cocaine
    g. Ethanol
    h. Methanol
    i. Cyanide (nitroprusside)
    j. Zidovudine (AZT)
    k. Biguanides (metformin)
    l. Ethylene-glycol, glycolic acid, oxalic acid
    m. Others
  4. Congenital
    a. Glucose-6-phosphate deficiency
    b. Fructuose-1,6-diphosphate deficiency
    c. Pyruvate carboxylase deficiency
    d. Pyruvate dehydrogenase deficiency
    e. Oxidative phosphorylation defects
  5. Decreased lactate clearance
    a. Fulminant hepatic failure
  6. d-Lactate
    a. Short gut syndrome
    b. Antibiotic induced

Significant overlap exists among many of the causes and are grouped under specific categories.

Among all metabolic acidoses, lactic acidosis in the ICU unit signals trouble, regardless of patient age.[13,73,87,97,121-123] Hyperlactatemia is defined as a lactate level between 2 and 5 mmol/L, whereas lactic acidosis is said to be present when lactate level exceeds 5 mmol/L and the arterial pH is less than 7.35. These definitions are arbitrary, though.[20,124] Blood lactate concentration, both in terms of the magnitude of the lactate elevation and in terms of the duration of its persistence, has been shown to correlate with mortality in patients, both pediatric and adults, and can occur as a result of septic shock, as a result of hemorrhagic shock, after a pediatric cardiac operation, in neonates receiving ventilation, and during necrotizing enterocolitis.[13,20,87,97,123-125] Therefore lactate measurement has become commonplace in "point of care" blood gas analyzers used at bedside in modern ICUs, both as a therapeutic guide and as a prognostic marker,[87,97,126,127] particularly during the early phases of resuscitation of clinically recognizable or uncompensated shock when tissue hypoperfusion is the rule.

Lactate represents the end product of anaerobic metabolism (i.e., it is a product of pyruvate reduction via the enzyme lactate dehydrogenase and the reduced nicotinamide hypoxanthine dinucleotide/nicotinamide hypoxanthine dinucleotide [NADH/NAD] cofactor system [see also Chapter 67]). It derives primarily from skeletal muscle, gut, brain, and circulating erythrocytes, with a production of about 1 mmol/kg/h. The healthy liver uptakes most lactate and recycles it through three primary options: conversion back to glucose (Cori cycle); oxidation back to pyruvate, which subsequently can be oxidized to CO_2 via the Krebs cycle; or transamination into alanine.[12,124,128,129]

Causes of hyperlactatemia and lactic acidosis are numerous in the critical care setting: cardiac arrest, shock, hypoxia, ARDS, certain inborn errors of metabolism (see also Chapter 69), status epilepticus, hematological malignancies with high "tumoral" burden, toxin exposure, and regional ischemia (e.g., extensive necrosis of tissue as in patients with trauma).[13,120,129,130-133] Other causes or associations, such as epinephrine infusion and liver failure, must not be overlooked[72] (Tables 61–8 and 61–9). Type A lactic acidosis (i.e., associated with or caused by inadequate tissue oxygen delivery) seems to be the most frequent cause encountered in critical care patients.[120,130,131] A decrease in oxygen availability at tissue and cellular levels results in an impairment in oxidative phosphorylation, which results in an increase of the intracellular levels of NADH, which facilitates the cofactor in the conversion of pyruvate to lactate.[131,134] This mechanism is clear and easily understandable by the busy clinician seeking prompt explanations for what he or she is facing in the critical care unit. Using blood lactate concentration as evidence of tissue hypoxia, however, is, at best, an oversimplification.[135] For example, in septic shock, intravascular volume depletion, oxygenation impairment, myocardial depression, and mitochondrial dysfunction all contribute to lactic acidosis in this setting.[13,80,90,134-136] Moreover, correlation of lactate levels in terms of rate of increase, magnitude of the increase, and persistence is a well-known prognostic marker in both children and adults[13,89,97,123] and is clinically used for gauging the response to treatment.[126] Lactic acidosis is thought to correlate with the oxygen debt, with the magnitude of hypoperfusion, and with the severity of shock.[87,123] This view, however, has been increasingly challenged by several observations.[13,72,76,131,134-139] First, even "resuscitated" patients who have sepsis, with acceptable or frankly elevated global, or tissue oxygen delivery, can experience persistent elevations in serum lactate.[135] Second, it has been shown that in sepsis, even in uncompensated shock, resting muscle does not produce lactate; on the contrary, there is now evidence that it actually may behave as a lactate consumer during endotoxemia.[13,72] Of course, during hypoperfusion several tissues are a clear source of lactic acid. For example, underperfused intestine can release lactate but not if mesenteric perfusion is maintained.[13,137] In the severe sepsis/septic shock setting, after the initial resuscitation with fluid and vasoactive/inotropic drugs, systemic oxygen transport is typically preserved or increased rather than decreased.[72] Therefore some alternative explanations for hyperlactatemia have emerged.[13,72,134] In the sepsis setting, endotoxin (and perhaps several cytokines) inhibits pyruvate dehydrogenase, the enzyme that catalyzes pyruvate to acetyl coenzyme A as a substrate for the Krebs cycle. Increased aerobic metabolism, however, may be more relevant than metabolic defects or anaerobic metabolism.[13,72,134] Therefore the pathogenesis of hyperlactatemia in patients with sepsis is complex and may involve changes in intermediary metabolism and accelerated glycolytic flux, the modulation of which, in terms of its rate and efficiency, seems to be governed by the redox state of cytoplasm and mitochondria through accumulation.[140,141] In addition, lactate levels may fluctuate in response to exogenous catecholamines, particularly epinephrine,[13,72,132,140,142] which clearly increases lactate levels through stimulation of glycogenolysis and glycolytic flux with a resultant increase in pyruvate production. This effect does not occur with norepinephrine or dobutamine infusions and is not related to decreased tissue perfusion, although there is a catabolic effect with epinephrine.[72,134] Several studies suggest that the lung may be a major source of lactate produced in severe sepsis/septic shock[125,130,134,138] and that decreased lactate clearance by the liver is also an important component of sepsis-associated hyperlactatemia and lactic acidosis.[143-145] Thus instead of being caused by cellular oxygen debt, the persistent lactate elevations often seen in patients with sepsis (and in patients after trauma resuscitation or after a cardiac operation) may be a consequence of the severe physiological, inflammatory, and metabolic stresses that these patients usually have.[72,76,143,146] This is the so-called stress hyperlactatemia that probably reflects the degree of physiological insult perpetrated by the severe sepsis or injury.[72,131,132,134,143,146] From this viewpoint, it is not surprising that lactate levels correlate so well with outcome and survival.[87,97,135] Given the complex and incompletely understood metabolism of lactate in sepsis, however, the belief that lactate levels can be accurately used as a stand-alone marker of outcome and mortality is probably naive.[54,121,135,136] Although the source and pathophysiological interpretation of lactic acidosis are matters of discussion, no question exists about the ability of lactate accumulation to produce acidemia. Given its pKa of 3.9, which indicates that 3162 molecules are dissociated for every one that is not within clinically encountered pH, lactic acid behaves as a strong ion within clinically encountered pH. Therefore the accumulation of lactate (a strong anion) without the addition of an important strong cation such as sodium will be expected to lower the SID, increase [H^+], and decrease the pH. Lactic acidosis would also be expected to be associated with increased adenosine triphosphate (ATP) hydrolysis, another source of hydrogen ions. Because the body can produce and clear lactate rapidly, it functions as one of the most dynamic components of the SID (Eq. 8).

Type B lactic acidoses are probably operative in many clinical circumstances where the so-called type A lactic acidoses have traditionally been invocated. Particularly in the patient with sepsis, lactic acidosis may be associated with a variety of coexisting mechanisms.[72,134,135] In addition, there likely exists significant overlap between many of these mechanisms; thus categorization of these mechanisms is a real challenge. Accordingly, classification of lactic acidosis into type A and type B represents a practical ("clinically useful") categorization that does not entirely reflect the actual disease. A potentially useful method for distinguishing anaerobically produced lactate from other sources is to measure the whole blood pyruvate concentration. The normal lactate to pyruvate ratio is 10:1. Because pyruvate is reduced to lactate during anaerobic metabolism, the ratio of lactate to pyruvate increases. Therefore if this ratio is higher than 25:1, it is considered evidence of anaerobic metabolism.[140] Unfortunately, pyruvate is unstable in solution, and an accurate measurement in the clinical setting is therefore difficult to obtain. Thus the clinical usefulness of this approach is reduced.[13]

Despite that, lactic acidosis is a common finding in sepsis and is considered one of the main causes of metabolic acidosis in this setting; the magnitude of the accumulation of lactate does not always account for the whole of the acid-balance derangement observed.[72] Therefore the increase in the AG seen in severe sepsis is often substantially greater than the lactate concentration. This finding has led to the active search of the so-called unexplained anions.[18,78,80,87,90] Several mechanisms have been advocated for the fact that as much as 15% to 50% of the increased AG is not due to the increased lactate: Donnan equilibrium alterations due to sepsis-mediated endothelial damage and a switch from a hepatic anion-uptake state to an anion-release state during endotoxemia have been the main explanations advanced.[18,78,79,90,131,134] Accumulation of molecules such as succinate, citrate, and formate has also been implicated.[18,134]

In addition to epinephrine, numerous drugs and toxins encountered in critical care medicine may cause or contribute to increased lactate, with or without acidemia. Likewise, drugs associated with the release of endogenous catecholamines, such as cocaine, can stimulate lactate production.[147] A similar mechanism is advocated in patients with pheochromocytoma.[148,149] Sodium nitroprusside remains a key vasodilator drug. Because it is metabolized to cyanide, this toxin may accumulate if excessive drug is administered or impaired cyanide clearance occurs, as in the setting of renal failure setting. In such cases, mitochondrial respiratory chain activity may be inhibited and lactate production increased.[150]

There are some other conditions in which lactic acidosis or hyperlactatemia may occur. As noted previously, in acute lung injury (ALI) and ARDS, lactate levels may be high even in the absence of shock or sepsis.[130,138] In ALI/ARDS the lung is an important source of lactate.[130,134] This was first evidenced by higher lactate levels in arterial blood than in the mixed blood obtained from patients with ALI/ARDS,[130,134,151,152] a phenomenon not seen in patients with other serious lung diseases.[153] Nevertheless it has been shown that the lung is a source of lactate production in patients receiving mechanical ventilation after cardiopulmonary bypass.[154] Potential mechanisms of lactate production by the injured lung may include not only the onset of anaerobic metabolism in hypoxic zones, but also direct cytokine effects on pulmonary cells and a stress-induced enhancement of glycolysis and lactate synthesis by both the parenchymal and nonparenchymal cells (e.g., endothelial cells and inflammatory cells infiltrating lung tissue such as macrophages and neutrophils).[134,138,150-152,154] A similar mechanism is operative in wound tissue, the intestine, and the liver in patients with trauma.[145]

Hyperlactatemia, lactic acidosis, or both occur in about 80% of cases of acute liver failure.[155] It is feasible that this can be explained not only by a decreased hepatic clearance of systemically produced lactic acid, but also by an increased hepatic production of lactate.[131,145,156,157] In animal models a hypermetabolism associated with lactate accumulation has been observed in organs rich in mononuclear phagocytes, especially the liver and spleen. Meszaros et al[158] observed the largest increase in glucose metabolism (and therefore in lactate increase) in Kupffer's cells (6.7-fold increase) followed by infiltrated neutrophils (5.4-fold), and endothelial cells (2.7-fold). In 10 adult patients, Murphy et al[157] showed that, before liver transplant, both the liver and intestine were net producers of lactate. After transplantation, the grafted liver became a net consumer of lactate as evidenced by a negative lactate gradient between hepatic and portal venous blood. The intestinal bed, however, continued to produce lactate after transplantation, but arterial blood levels dropped back to normal values.[157] Thus before transplant, hyperlactatemia and lactic acidosis were due to both defective clearance of lactate by the sick liver and to an increased lactate production resulting from hepatic inflammation in addition to lactate released from the intestine, the lung, and other organs participating in this multisystem problem.[157, 159] Cessation of hepatic lactate release after transplantation was the result not only of improved lactate clearance, but also of the removal of a large body of activated, lactate-producing inflammatory cells.[156]

In status asthmaticus, 1% of patients admitted to a pediatric ICU had lactic acidosis.[160] This incidence is lower than that reported in adults with acute severe asthma,[161,162] which is around 25% to 30%. Pathogenesis of lactic acidosis in this setting seems to be multifactorial and includes contributions from lactate production by overwhelmed respiratory muscles, tissue hypoxia, a hyperadrenergic state, and the metabolic effect of pharmacological

β_2 agonists.[160,161,163] Muscle participation does not seem to be so important, however, because lactic acidosis has been described even in patients with asthma who were receiving muscle relaxants.[163] In head trauma, it is possible to find lactic acidosis in arterial blood samples, both as an effect of polytrauma and hemorrhagic shock and as a manifestation of severe traumatic brain injury. Arterial to jugular venous blood lactate difference has been shown to correlate with the severity of the brain trauma, and it has been argued that it is useful as a prognostic marker, both in children and in adults.[164] At the regional level, elevated lactate concentration is usually the rule in edema associated with brain trauma.[165]

Salicylate intoxication is a special situation in which lactic acidosis may play an important role (see also Chapter 99). Although salicylate toxicity occurs less frequently now than in the past because of the increased use of alternative antipyretics in young children, it must still be considered in therapeutic situations (e.g., rheumatic diseases), as well as in cases of overdose. Salicylates directly or indirectly affect most organ systems in the body by uncoupling oxidative phosphorylation, inhibiting Krebs cycle enzymes, and inhibiting amino acid synthesis.[166] These derangements can result in variable acid-base patterns: respiratory alkalosis, mixed respiratory alkalosis plus metabolic acidosis, or (less commonly) simple metabolic acidosis.[98] Respiratory alkalosis is caused by direct stimulation of the respiratory center by salicylates, leading to hyperventilation and a compensatory alkaluria, with both potassium and bicarbonate excreted in the urine.[166] This first phase may last for several hours after ingestion in adolescents but may be overlooked in young infants. During the next 12 to 24 hours (or less in younger patients), hypokalemia develops and urinary excretion of hydrogen ion starts. This "paradoxical aciduria" occurs despite continued respiratory alkalosis and aggravates the clinical manifestations because a higher percentage of salicylate in acidic urine remains in the unionized form, which is reabsorbed from the glomerular filtrate. Soon after the hypokalemia onset, dehydration and progressive metabolic acidosis develop. The metabolic acidosis is mainly due to lactic acid, but ketoacids and other metabolic acids also participate. As metabolic acidosis ensues, more acidic urine is produced, and the plasma salicylate level may be even higher than in early phases because of the inability to excrete the drug in urine.[98] Chronic salicylate poisoning has been described, in which the patient usually has metabolic acidosis and a "pseudosepsis" syndrome similar to some inborn errors of metabolism.[167]

A curious form of lactic acidosis is the so-called D-lactic acidosis. The lactic acid produced by mammals is a levoisomer; some bowel bacteria produce a dextroisomer.[168] D-lactate derived from bacterial fermentation in the bowel lumina may reach systemic circulation and lead to metabolic acidemia, especially if liver function (and thus lactate clearance) is suboptimal. D-lactic acidosis must be considered in patients with a history of intestinal disease who have neurological findings such as confusion and ataxia, and high AG metabolic acidosis, with normal L-lactate levels. Symptoms worsen after high-carbohydrate meals or tube hyperalimentation. In patients with short bowel syndrome, there is not only an overgrowth of bacteria but also accumulation of carbohydrates in the colon.[169] Therefore the development of the syndrome requires some of the following: (1) carbohydrate malabsorption with increased delivery of these compounds to the colon; (2) colonic bacteria flora producing D-lactic acid; (3) ingestion of large amounts of carbohydrate; (4) diminished colon motility, allowing time for bacterial fermentation; and (5) impaired D-lactate metabolism.[169] Treatment focuses on decreasing gut bacteria overgrowth antibiotics and the avoidance of high-carbohydrate or lactose feeding.[170]

Other Forms of Metabolic Acidosis Associated with an Increased Anion Gap

Ketoacidosis is another common cause of increased AG acidosis. Ketones are formed by beta oxidation of fatty acids, a process that increases substantially in insulin-deficient states. In the pediatric intensive care setting, this is most often seen in patients with diabetes mellitus with overproduction and underutilization of acetone and β-hydroxybutyric and acetoacetic acids (ketone bodies), which accumulate in plasma. This problem is exacerbated because of the glucosuria-mediated diuresis and intravascular volume contraction. Ketoacidosis is also seen in various inborn errors of amino acid and organic acid metabolism, and a mixed ketoacidosis and lactic acidosis are seen with glycogen storage disease type I (glucose-6-phosphate deficiency) (see also Chapter 69).

The pediatric critical care physician should be aware of a condition often called *late metabolic acidosis of prematurity.*[171] Although its incidence is greater in the premature infant when compared with that in the term infant (20% compared with 5%), the capacity of less well-developed renal tubules to excrete H^+ and to concentrate is a fairly common situation during the first month of life. This level of renal tubular development is adequate for the breast-fed infant, but if the protein intake or solute load is excessive, the capacity may be exceeded. This appears particularly true during periods of stress.

When chronic renal insufficiency develops, hyperchloremic metabolic acidosis may initially occur because of impaired ammonia generation. When the glomerular filtration rate falls below 20 ml/min, the kidneys are incapable of excreting fixed acids; the resulting accumulation of sulfates among other acids may increase the AG. These acidoses are usually mild, producing an excess AG of approximately 10 mEq/L. A mixed metabolic acidosis (high + normal AG mechanisms) is not uncommon in this setting.[63,172] If the patient has sepsis or another condition associated with hypermetabolism, however, the rate of acid generation increases and the acidosis may become rather severe. The SID decreases, and because of the lack of renal compensation, some intervention must be taken. Patients who do not yet require dialysis and those who are between their dialytic processes are often given $NaHCO_3$ (provided there is no hypernatremia or sodium potassium citrate). In the case that bicarbonate is contraindicated, a dialytic process is in order (see later).

Hyperchloremic Acidoses: The Normal Anion Gap Metabolic Acidoses

These alterations occur either as a result of an increase in chloride concentration relative to strong cations (especially sodium) or because of the loss of cations with retention of chloride (Table 61–6). When the pH drops, the normal response by the kidney is to increase chloride excretion. Failure to do so identifies the kidney as the problem,[13,173] as in renal tubular acidosis (RTA). Extrarenal causes of hyperchloremic acidosis include exogenous chloride loads and loss of cations from the lower gastrointestinal tract without proportional losses of chloride, as in secretory diarrhea, but also in conditions in which loss of small bowel, biliary, or pancreatic secretions are present (such as drainage from ostomies, tubes, or fistulas).[12,63,129]

The defect in all types of RTAs is an inability to excrete chloride in proportion to sodium, although the reason depends on the specific type of RTA.[174,175] Treatment largely depends on whether there are losses of sodium that can be replaced with $NaHCO_3$ or whether the kidney will require mineralocorticoid replacement. Distal RTA (type 1) presents with a urine pH of 6 or greater with mild to severe episodes of acidosis. Proximal RTA (type 2) also is seen in patients with urine pH of 6 or greater, usually only with mild episodes of acidosis. Type 4 (hyperkalemic) RTA is most frequently associated with pseudohypoaldosteronism but may also be seen with primary aldosterone deficiency as in the 21-hydroxylase deficiency in congenital adrenal hyperplasia.[176,177] A more detailed discussion of RTA is beyond the scope of this chapter. It is worth mentioning, however, that both urinary AG and urinary strong ion difference (uSID = $[uNa^+ + uK^+] - [uCl^-]$) are useful in the diagnosis of hyperchloremic metabolic acidosis.[13,178]

In the critical care unit there are often mandatory therapeutic interventions that can cause (or at least be associated) with hyperchloremic metabolic acidosis. The more common of such interventions are parenteral nutrition, isotonic saline (0.9% NaCl) infusion or boluses, and certain drugs that behave as anion exchangers during their elimination by the kidneys. Parenteral formulas contain weak anions, such as acetate, in addition to chloride. If an insufficient amount of weak anions is provided, plasma $[Cl^-]$ increases, SID decreases, and acidosis results.[13,179] As already mentioned, a similar condition can arise if isotonic saline is generously used for hemodynamic resuscitation (Table 61–6).[25,66-68,179]

Also of importance to the intensivist is iatrogenic RTA caused by the nephrotoxicity of amphotericin B and to a lesser extent aminoglycosides. Kidney alterations due to amphotericin B include decreased glomerular filtration rate, distal tubulopathy with urinary loss of potassium and magnesium, RTA, loss of urine concentration ability, and sometimes Fanconi's syndrome.[180,181] Nephrotoxicity is dose dependent and duration dependent.[182] The mechanisms involved in nephrotoxicity include the deoxycholate vehicle for amphotericin B, reduction in renal blood flow and glomerular filtration rate, increased salt concentration at the macula densa, interaction of amphotericin B with ergosterol in the cell membrane, and apoptosis in proximal tubular cells and medullary interstitial cells.[180,181] The following risk factors for such toxicity have been proposed for pediatric population: dose of 35 mg or larger, male sex, chronic renal disease, and use of amikacin or cyclosporine. Patients with more than two risk factors showed an incidence of moderate-to-severe nephrotoxicity of 29%.[183] Accordingly, such patients should be considered as potential candidates for alternative antifungal therapy. Salt loading is the only measure proven by a controlled prospective study to ameliorate amphotericin B nephrotoxicity in humans, including extremely low-birth-weight infants.[184,185] Trimethoprim-sulfamethoxazole is another antimicrobial that has been related to RTA.[186]

Another rare cause of normal AG metabolic acidosis that may be seen in the ICU is acetazolamide, a carbonic anhydrase inhibitor used occasionally to decrease cerebral spinal fluid production in conditions of hydrocephalus and more frequently to stimulate renal bicarbonate wasting. This drug decreases hydrolysis of H_2CO_3 to CO_2 and H_2O, resulting in a decrease of renal HCO_3^- reabsorption. It has recently been described that in humans and in an animal model, acetazolamide can produce severe lactic acidosis with an increased lactate-to-pyruvate ratio, ketosis with a low β-hydroxybutyrate-to-acetoacetate ratio, and a urinary organic acid profile typical of pyruvate carboxylase deficiency.[187] This "acquired enzymatic injury" stems from the inhibition of mitochondrial carbonic anhydrase type V, which provides bicarbonate to pyruvate carboxylase and can produce Krebs cycle damage. Some of these patients improved dramatically after packed red blood transfusion; the improvement was likely related to the citrate anticoagulant.[187]

Treating Metabolic Acidosis

How is metabolic acidosis treated? Should metabolic acidosis be treated? This topic remains controversial, except in the more basic approach: *treat the underlying cause*. Certain acidoses have specific therapies, such as insulin and fluids for the patient with diabetic ketoacidosis, $NaHCO_3$ for patients with the classic distal RTA, and fomepizole for methanol intoxication.[103] These cases are beyond the scope of this chapter. The following discussion focuses on lactic acidosis.

The clinician has been taught to fear acidemia. The rationale for such a fear is essentially the hypothetical deleterious effect of low pH on cellular function and hemodynamics. Because proteins underlie the function and structure of the cells and because they all contain areas of both positive and negative charge, it is a fact that they are sensitive to the H^+ concentration of their environment. Therefore a decrease in arterial pH might be expected to have important detrimental effects on a host of bodily functions.[103,108] It is simplistic, though, to assume that the arterial blood pH reflects the intracellular pH, which seems likely to be more relevant. Further clouding the value of arterial blood pH may be different acid-base states in different cells of a single organ or within different organs of a single patient.[44,108,188] Mitochondrial pH may even be more crucial than cytoplasmic pH because this is the site of energy production.[189] Once the diversity of microcirculations and tissue metabolism throughout the body is taken into account, the meaning of a single arterial blood pH is rather limited.[103,108] Although arterial blood gas information is needed for the assessment of pulmonary gas exchange, a significant widening of the arteriovenous differences in pH and P_{CO_2} has been observed in patients with severe circulatory failure, such as shock and cardiac arrest.[188] Thus in the presence of severe hypoperfusion, the hypercapnia and acidemia at the level of the tissues are better detected in central venous blood than in arterial blood samples because they directly reflect the average acid-base status of the venous blood returning from the tissues, and not merely the pulmonary function.[152,188] Therefore both arterial and central venous blood samples are needed to assess acid-base status in patients with severe hemodynamic compromise. In treating a critically ill child, sometimes one has to rely on capillary samples for blood gas analyses. There is significant correlation in pH, P_{CO_2}, partial pressure of oxygen (P_{O_2}), SBE, and HCO_3^- among arterial, central venous, and capillary blood gases, but a poor correlation in P_{O_2} in the presence of hypotension. Thus capillary and venous blood gas measurements may be useful alternatives to arterial samples when an arterial line is not in place, for acid-base balance monitoring, but they are not useful for monitoring P_{O_2}.[190]

Sodium Bicarbonate

$NaHCO_3$ administration had long been the standard therapy for metabolic acidosis including lactic acidosis,[98,191-193] although its safety and efficacy came under scrutiny only in the 1980s and still continues.[194,195] Accumulated data have challenged the traditional arguments for bicarbonate use and provided evidence against its safety and efficacy.[103,118,195]

It seems self-evident that adding bicarbonate to acidic blood will raise the pH; however, the reality is more complex. In agreement with Equation 8, the administration of $NaHCO_3$ increases the SID (which tends to raise the pH) because sodium is a strong cation and bicarbonate is a weak anion, but in agreement with Equation 3, it is an anion that rapidly converts to carbonic acid and then to CO_2 (which tends to lower the pH).[13,196,197] Therefore $NaHCO_3$ may increase arterial pH if, and only if, alveolar ventilation is not limited. Otherwise, the risk of "paradoxal acidemia" after bicarbonate administration is not negligible.[98,103,108,194,197,198] The final effect of $NaHCO_3$ on intracellular pH depends on changes in P_{CO_2} in the medium bathing the cells, which are influenced by the extracellular nonbicarbonate buffering capacity.[197] These cells are usually depressed in the critically ill patient in whom $NaHCO_3$ is administered. In addition, bicarbonate administration may promote metabolic reactions that may themselves alter not only P_{CO_2}, but also the total concentration of weak acids and the SID. In fact, it has been documented that bicarbonate can increase the production of lactic acid in both animals and humans.[108,191] Mechanisms to explain this remain speculative but include a shift in the oxyhemoglobin-saturation relationship[108]; enhanced anaerobic glycolysis probably mediated by the pH-sensitive enzyme phosphofructokinase; and changes in hepatic blood flow or lactate uptake.[72,108] Altogether however, animal and human studies and time-honored clinical experience have shown that arterial pH can be raised and even normalized with $NaHCO_3$,[108,118] yet multiple compartments separated by membranes of differing permeabilities exist. Thus even when $NaHCO_3$ added to the central veins reliably elevates the arterial pH, its effect can be "erratic" at tissue and cellular levels. For example, in the cerebrospinal fluid and intracellular spaces the pH may drop further, without concordance with an already alkalemic arterial blood sample.[188,195] This could happen because CO_2 raised by the bicarbonate infusion may readily diffuse across cell membranes and the blood-brain barrier, whereas bicarbonate cannot. Therefore despite its ability to increase blood pH when given intravenously, bicarbonate fails to augment the intracellular pH reliably.[197,198] In most animal models and in most organs studied so far, including the brain in healthy human volunteers, intracellular pH decreases with bicarbonate administration.[108]

Results of human studies in which researchers examined the impact of bicarbonate administration during cardiopulmonary resuscitation in which lactic acidosis or respiratory acidosis is expected have uniformly shown no benefit in terms of survival and hemodynamic recovery. Several studies have shown a deleterious effect in this setting, and many others (including one study with class III evidence) have shown no discernable effects.[118,189,195] This is why the American Heart Association no longer recommends routine administration of bicarbonate during cardiopulmonary resuscitation.[195] Its use is considered only after effective ventilation, chest compressions, and epinephrine are established in the prolonged arrest scenario[99] and for cases in which bicarbonate is a "specific" therapeutic intervention (e.g., hyperkalemia, hypermagnesemia, tricyclic antidepressant poisoning, and sodium channel blocker poisoning).[199]

The rationale for bicarbonate use is to mitigate the adverse hemodynamic consequences of acidemia. In two randomized, controlled trials of $NaHCO_3$ therapy in critical adult patients with lactic acidosis, there was no benefit from bicarbonate compared with NaCl in improving global hemodynamics or the cardiovascular response to infused catecholamines.[118,196] This finding is rather easy to apply to children, although not that easy in infants and neonates for whom there is insufficient evidence from randomized, controlled trials to determine whether infusion of base or fluid bolus reduces morbidity and mortality of metabolic acidosis.[200] Both adult studies indicated that bicarbonate is no more effective than saline in improving heart rate, central venous pressure, pulmonary artery pressure, mixed venous hemoglobin saturation, systemic oxygen delivery, oxygen consumption, arterial blood pressure, pulmonary artery occlusion pressure, and cardiac output.[103,118,196] These findings suggest that the commonly observed hemodynamic response to bicarbonate administration in patients treated with inotropic/vasoactive drug infusions may simply be due to preload augmentation rather than enhanced catecholamine responsiveness.[108] When the most severely acidemic subset of patients (those with pH in the range of 6.9 to 7.2) was analyzed separately, the findings persisted.[196] This result does not support the common practice of withholding bicarbonate from patients with mild acidemia but of allowing its administration in those patients with "severe" acidemia.[98,192,193] On the contrary, if the negative effects of bicarbonate infusion are real, it could be expected that this sicker subset of patients would have more profound paradoxical intracellular acidosis.[108,198,201,202] In addition, $NaHCO_3$ is not free of negative side effects. The main effects relate to fluid and sodium load that can cause hypervolemia, hyperosmolarity, and hypernatremia.[194] $NaHCO_3$ given as a rapid intravenous (IV) bolus can cause a transient decrease in arterial blood pressure and a transient rise in intracranial pressure, probably related to its hypertonicity.[98,108] This effect is ameliorated when bicarbonate is administered as a slow IV infusion. Regardless of the infusion rate, IV administration of bicarbonate can cause sudden shifts of several cations through cell membrane–mediated mechanisms. This is advantageous in treating hyperkalemia,[199] but it also can be dangerous because bicarbonate lowers ionized calcium.[196] "Overshoot" alkalosis, in which an abrupt and poorly tolerated transition from severe acidemia to alkalemia develops, can result from overly aggressive bicarbonate "correction."[98]

Therefore the decision whether to use bicarbonate can become a difficult one because it is a choice between a long-standing but unproven therapy with potential deleterious effects and reliance on limited studies.[118] Because of the lack of data supporting bicarbonate use in human beings and of the evidence of deleterious effects, the use of bicarbonate is not recommended in lactic acidosis regardless of the pH.[103,108,194] Nevertheless many clinicians still use $NaHCO_3$. Certainly, it will always be prudent to adjust the clinical decision to the specific characteristics of each patient, keeping pros and cons in mind. Thus the decision to give "bicarbonate correction" must be based on the best clinical judgment mixed with a knowledge of the available evidence. This science and art approach to the individual patient can be summarized in the clinician's answer to the following questions, modified from Forsythe and Schmidt[108]:

1. Is the level of low pH a clear and present hazard or danger to this patient?
2. Is there a reasonable expectation that increasing the blood pH with $NaHCO_3$ will have some beneficial effect?
3. Is there a particular and specific risk to this patient from the known potential negative effects of $NaHCO_3$?
4. Is the mechanism of the acidosis suitable for being treatment with $NaHCO_3$, or can the acidosis be exacerbated?

There are no recipes for answering these questions.[103,108]

Salicylate intoxication represents a special setting. Because the risk of death and the severity of neurological manifestations depend on the concentration of salicylates in the central nervous system, therapy is directed at limiting further drug absorption by administering activated charcoal in the emergency department and promoting the exit of the drug from the cerebral tissue by increasing the alkalinity of the blood, which also will raise urine pH and therefore inhibit salicylate reabsorption. Thus this represents a special case of lactic acidosis in which $NaHCO_3$ is clearly indicated for two reasons: (1) to establish a high urinary flow rate along with other fluids and (2) to promote salicylate excretion. The target-pH of the urine is 7 to 7.5. Hemodialysis is reserved for severe cases, especially those involving renal dysfunction.

If the science and art decision is to administer $NaHCO_3$, some time-honored clinical clues are valuable. $NaHCO_3$ dose is best estimated with either the SBE or the bicarbonate level derived from P_{CO_2} measured by the blood gas analyzer:

$$\text{Total body base deficit} = \text{SBE} \times \text{body weight (Kg)} \times 0.3 \quad \text{Eq 13A}$$

$$HCO_3^- \text{ deficit (mEq)} = 0.3 \times \text{body weight (Kg)} \times [HCO_3^- \text{ expected} - HCO_3^- \text{ observed}] \quad \text{Eq 13B}$$

The distribution volume of bicarbonate is 0.3, or 30% of the lean body weight. The theoretical distribution volume of $NaHCO_3$ equals the extracellular fluid volume, which grossly represents 60% of the body weight (70% in young infants), and therefore it can be argued that the correct arithmetic factor should be 0.6 (or 0.7) rather than 0.3. Time-honored experience has shown, however, that as the starting point, bicarbonate or SBE correction with 0.3 ("half correction") will suffice in most cases and will avoid unnecessary risks from excessive load of solutes and fluid as well as the overshoot alkalemia.[98] It should be taken into account that the usual $NaHCO_3$ preparation available worldwide has a concentration of 0.88 mEq/ml, with pH = 8 and 1461 mOsm/kg. Therefore bicarbonate is ideally administered through a central venous line or diluted with distillated water.

Alternative Alkalinizing Agents

Concern about the CO_2-producing effect of bicarbonate led to the development of Carbicarb, which consists of equimolar concentrations of $NaHCO_3$ and sodium carbonate.[98,203] Carbicarb raises the SID and thus increases the pH far more than bicarbonate, with much less rise in P_{CO_2}, so Carbicarb limits but does not eliminate the generation of CO_2.[98] The risks of hypervolemia and hypertonicity are similar to those of bicarbonate. Animal studies have shown stabilization of serum lactate levels and improved acid-balance profile both in blood and at the intracellular level.[204] Carbicarb administration also resulted in a significant increase in cardiac index when compared with normal saline and $NaHCO_3$, although neither Carbicarb nor $NaHCO_3$ prevented the progressive reduction in myocardial cell pH in an animal model of ventricular fibrillation.[205] Although Carbicarb more consistently increases intracellular pH, studies of its effects on hemodynamics have yielded conflicting results.[98,103,108] Although Carbicarb is not currently available for clinical use, there is no doubt that it deserves further research.[170]

THAM (tris[hydroxymethyl]aminomethane), also known as tromethamine and tris buffer, is an amino alcohol that behaves as a weak base (pKa 7.8). It exists in neutral form at physiological pH. It crosses lipid membranes and penetrates cells easily. Therefore it has the potential to raise both intracellular and central nervous system pH. In addition, THAM's buffering action occurs without producing CO_2, and thus is not dependent on pulmonary function. Protonated THAM is excreted by the kidneys. Despite THAM's being commercially available for several decades, there are few studies establishing THAM's clinical efficacy. In animal models, THAM incompletely buffered metabolic acidosis but significantly improved contractility and relaxation in an isolated rabbit heart model.[103] Nevertheless, THAM has not been documented to be clinically more efficacious than bicarbonate. In humans, from neonates to adults, there are several anecdotal reports but no clinical trials of THAM's efficacy in metabolic (lactic) acidosis.[98,108] This paucity of information and the report of several serious side effects, including hypekalemia, hypoglycemia, local extravasation injury, and hepatic necrosis in neonates, have limited its widespread use. Recently, THAM has been proposed for respiratory acidosis associated with permissive hypercapnia in patients with ARDS (see later).

Of particular relevance for lactic acidosis is dichloroacetate (DCA), a simple compound that reduces plasma lactic acid concentration. DCA is not a buffer but a stimulator of pyruvate dehydrogenase, the enzyme that catalyzes the oxidation of pyruvate to acetyl–coenzyme A (CoA), facilitating its entry to the Krebs cycle and thus decreasing lactate production and promoting the clearance of accumulated lactate.[103,206] In addition, DCA promotes myocardial glucose utilization and contractility.[207] Initial data from both children and adults were promising,[208] but a large controlled clinical trial in adults with severe lactic acidosis showed that DCA treatment resulted in statistically significant but clinically unimportant changes in arterial-blood lactate concentrations and pH. It also failed in altering hemodynamics or survival.[209] Renewed interest in DCA has arisen from its potential applications for attenuating lactic acidosis in certain congenital errors of metabolism, particularly defects in mitochondrial energy metabolism,[210-212] and lactic acidosis due to severe malaria in children.[213]

Dialytic procedures may be indicated in some cases of metabolic acidosis that are refractory to bicarbonate or in cases in which there are serious limitations in the amount of fluid or sodium load that can be administered to the patient, a common situation in the pediatric critical care unit (see also Chapter 65). Uncompensated metabolic acidosis (pH <7.1) remains one of the acknowledged criteria for the initiation of renal replacement therapy in the pediatric ICU.[214] Peritoneal dialysis is often not the best choice, particularly in lactic acidosis associated with hypoperfusion. In this setting the hypoperfused peritoneal membranes may not be efficient for supporting enough peritoneal flux, and the increase in intraabdominal pressure may contribute to a further drop of cardiac output. If peritoneal dialysis is chosen, bicarbonate-buffered peritoneal dialysis solution provides some advantages over the conventional lactate-buffered peritoneal dialysis solution both in terms of pH control and in mesothelial cell preservation.[214] Most critically ill patients lack the hemodynamic stability to tolerate intermittent hemodialysis. Hemofiltration and hemodiafiltration are better options. In patients with metabolic acidosis, hemofiltration techniques replace plasma water, which is low in bicarbonate concentration, with a solution that contains an above-normal bicarbonate (or lactate or acetate) concentration. Such anions are then transformed into CO_2, which is removed by ventilation. This exchange contributes to the correction of acidosis. If such oxidizable anions are not fully extracted and metabolized by the liver and, therefore remain in plasma, their ability to correct acidosis is lost. They accumulate in blood and fail to increase the SID adequately; this results in acidosis.[215] Such an effect (i.e., iatrogenic hyperlactatemia with acidification of plasma) is typically seen in patients with liver failure.[215] In such patients it is mandatory to use bicarbonate-based replacement fluids. In addition, the effect of lactate-based replacement fluid on blood lactate concentration can be misleading in patients who have sepsis with lactic acidosis. Additionally, it appears that lactate clearance through the hemofilter is small compared with endogenous clearance. Therefore despite the fact that hemofiltration has been advocated for the treatment of lactic acidosis, kinetic studies of lactate removal do not suggest that such removal can counteract lactate production in any meaningful way.[139] A detailed discussion of renal replacement therapies is provided in Chapter 65.

Metabolic Alkalosis

Metabolic alkalosis is reported to occur in about 50% of all acid-base disorders as described in one classic report.[216] This high incidence can be ascribed to the almost ubiquitous use of chloruretic diuretics and to the common occurrence of vomiting and nasogastric suction. It is difficult to attribute a figure of mortality or morbidity directly to metabolic alkalosis, although 80% mortality has been previously reported when the pH was less than 7.65. This does not necessarily indicate a cause-effect relationship.[217]

In the classic approach to acid-base derangements, metabolic alkalosis is generated by net gain of base (primarily bicarbonate) or loss of nonvolatile acid from the extracellular fluid, usually hydrochloric acid (HCl) by vomiting or enhanced renal acid excretion promoted by diuretics or aldosterone excess, and is often accompanied by hypochloremia and hypokalemia.[101,170] Bicarbonate or base loading, whether exogenous or endogenous (as in bone dissolution in severe osteolysis), is rarely the single cause of metabolic alkalosis. Such transient states may occur during and immediately after an IV infusion of $NaHCO_3$ or an equivalent base (e.g., citrate anticoagulant in transfused packed red blood cells).[218] This situation may also occur after the successful treatment of ketoacidosis or lactic acidosis because these organic anions are metabolized to bicarbonate and after the successful correction of hypercapnia in respiratory acidosis, before the kidney can excrete the bicarbonate previously retained for compensation. Because it is unusual for alkali to be added to the body, metabolic alkalosis generally involves a "generative" stage, in which the loss of acid usually causes alkalosis,[101,170,219] and a "maintenance" stage, in which the kidneys fail to compensate by excreting HCO_3^- because of volume contraction, low glomerular filtration rate, or depletion of chloride or potassium or some external influence such as diuretics or endogenous aldosterone.[170,218,220,221] Accordingly, the "traditional" therapeutic approach was based on the idea of inducing urinary bicarbonate wasting.[101] On the basis of the research by Galla and others,[62,220,222] however, this approach has been questioned for almost two decades for several reasons. First, the pathophysiology of metabolic alkalosis is far from being homogeneous and indeed may vary over time. Second, metabolic alkalosis may be accompanied by a total deficit of bicarbonate, and thus bicarbonaturia may not be the correct approach to deal with metabolic alkalosis.[62] Third, the mechanism that maintains an elevated bicarbonate concentration may change during the natural history of metabolic alkalosis despite unchanging alkalemia.[62,218,220] Thus the importance of performing the analysis of metabolic alkalosis through a quantitative interpretation of events with attention to the electroneutrality in three compartments, extracellular fluids, intracellular fluids, and urine, has been claimed.[62] Stewart's physical chemical analysis addresses these issues. In this approach, metabolic alkalosis occurs as a result of an increase in the SID or a decrease in the circulating anions (Table 61–6). These changes can occur because of a loss of anions (e.g., Cl^- from the stomach, albumin from the plasma), which represents the most common mechanism, or because of retention of cations by the kidney.[13] Metabolic alkalosis has been classified by the primary organ system involved, the response to therapy, or the underlying disease.[12,101,218] For the critical care environment it may be more convenient to classify it according to the response to therapy. Thus it seems practical to follow the physical chemical approach and use the serum chloride concentration (the most commonly anion involved) as the key variable for such a classification.[13,18] Sometimes the loss of Cl^- is temporary and can be treated effectively by replacing it; this type of metabolic alkalosis is known as *chloride-responsive*. This represents the most frequently encountered metabolic alkalosis in the pediatric critical care unit, and it is also the most severe. In other cases, hormonal mechanisms produce ongoing losses of Cl^-. In this situation, the Cl^- deficit can be offset only temporarily, at best, by Cl^- administration. Therefore this form of metabolic alkalosis is said to be *chloride-resistant*.[13,18,218] Urine chloride concentration can be helpful for distinguishing these disorders.

Chloride-responsive disorders are the result of Cl^- losses from gastric drainage or persisting vomiting, as in pyloric stenosis and other causes of upper gastrointestinal obstruction. They also may occur as a consequence of the administration of loop diuretics.[99] Both persisting vomiting and excessive diuretics generate some degree of dehydration, with volume contraction and secondary stimulation of aldosterone release, which in turn leads to increased tubular Na^+ reabsorption (an alkalinizing process, because it increases the SID) and to increased urinary loss of K^+.

Chloride-resistant disorders are so called because of ongoing urinary chloride losses that will provoke a drop in plasma chloride and thus induce metabolic alkalosis, despite the apparent success of an IV infusion of chloride transiently raising plasma levels. The hallmark of this group of disorders is an increased urine Cl^- concentration, usually more than 20 mEq/L.[13,182,218,223] Commonly, excessive chloride losses are the result of increased mineralocorticoid activity, and therefore treatment requires a search for the underlying disorder and, if possible, a specific therapeutic intervention. Among the most important causes of chloride-resistant disorders are the group of diseases with mineralocorticoid excess, which includes primary and secondary aldosteronism, congenital adrenal hyperplasia (17α-hydroxylase deficiency), renin-secreting tumors, and Cushing's syndrome; the group of impaired chloride-associated sodium transport including Bartter's and Gitelman's syndromes; the group of drug-induced hypokalemic alkalosis including diuretics, high-dose glucocorticoids, fludrocortisone, aminoglycosides, and licorice; and the miscellaneous group, which includes Liddle's syndrome, 11β-hydroxysteroid dehydrogenase deficiency, and salt-losing nephropathy, among others.[13,218,223-225] For further details about these specific disorders, the reader is referred to other sources.[177,182,218,226] The cause of normotensive hypokalemic metabolic alkalosis sometimes is not apparent from the patient's history. In this setting, it is always useful to consider that in most cases, metabolic alkalosis of extrarenal origin is usually associated with a low urinary chloride excretion. Thus random urine chloride/creatinine ratio is usually low in this group of patients but is within or above normal reference values in metabolic alkalosis of renal origin.[223]

Other special causes of metabolic alkalosis include the extrarenal chloride-resistant forms with normal or decreased urine chloride, such as cystic fibrosis[227] and congenital chloride diarrhea, which is a recessively inherited disorder of chloride transport in the distal ileum and colon.[228] In both disorders a huge extrarenal chloride loss occurs (through sweat or diarrhea), and urine chloride may be low, normal, or high, depending on the patient's renal function and clinical situation.

Finally, metabolic alkalosis may occur as the SID increases as a consequence of the gain of cations rather than anion depletion. The most common clinical situation in the critical care setting is the IV administration of strong cations without strong anions, such as for massive blood transfusion. In this case, sodium is administered predominantly with citrate (a weak anion) instead of chloride. A similar mechanism of metabolic alkalosis occurs when the parenteral nutrition contains excess sodium acetate (another weak anion) and insufficient chloride to balance the sodium load.[13] Excessive infusion of some gelatins used as plasma volume expanders and sodium lactate (as in Ringer's solution) can also cause metabolic alkalosis. The milk-alkali syndrome is now a rare cause of this derangement.

Treating Metabolic Alkalosis

Regardless of the type of metabolic alkalosis, the first step for its proper management is to moderate or stop the process that generated the problem, even if only temporarily.[99] For example, if continuation of gastric drainage is required, the loss of gastric fluid can be reduced though the administration of H_2 receptor blockers or inhibitors of the gastric H^+/K^+-ATPase. If it is not possible to withdraw diuretics, it may be possible to use potassium-sparing compounds (e.g., spironolactone, amiloride), which decrease distal acidification and curtail potassium excretion. The administration of bicarbonate or its precursors such as lactate, citrate, and acetate (all of them are weak anions) should be discontinued; these compounds are commonly present in IV and dialytic solutions, transfused blood and blood derivatives, and parenteral nutrition, respectively. If drugs with mineralocorticoid activity are being administered, their indication and dose should be reassessed.

According to the physical chemical approach, it is not necessary to focus on ameliorating the existing hyperbicarbonatemia or increasing urinary bicarbonate wasting.[99] The treatment is simply to replace Cl^-. Saline plus KCl infusion are usually the best choice because of the typical coexisting volume depletion and hypokalemia.[13,101] As previously stated, the administration of normal saline is effective despite the release of equal amounts of Na^+ and Cl^- because this results in larger relative increases in Cl^- concentration compared with Na^+ concentration (see earlier). Treatment of severe chloride-responsive metabolic alkalosis can be a real challenge without the presence of either volume depletion or hypokalemia and in patients with cardiac or renal dysfunction.[99] For example, potassium chloride can induce hyperkalemia in patients with renal failure. In these patients, decreasing or adjusting the diuretic regimen, adding acetazolamide, and cautiously administering NaCl and potassium chloride may suffice.[99] If the pace of correction of the alkalemia needs to be accelerated, Hcl can be infused intravenously as a 0.1 to 0.2 N solution (i.e., one containing 100 to 200 mmol of hydrogen per liter). This intervention, which is rarely needed, is safe and effective for the symptomatic rapid relief of severe metabolic alkalosis. Because of its sclerosing properties and its hyperosmotic concentration, Hcl must be infused through a central venous line at an infusion rate of no more than 0.2 mmol/kg/h or up to 20 to 50 mmol/h,[99] with arterial pH monitored every hour. Although an alternative infusion through a peripheral IV line was described decades ago, this route is not advisable in the pediatric population.[229] The calculation of the amount of Hcl solution to be infused is based on a distribution volume equivalent to 30% of the body weight. Thus HCl dosage can be calculated with either the SBE or the bicarbonate difference in a manner similar to the bicarbonate administration formula (Eqs. 13A and 13B):

$$\text{Total body BE} = \text{SBE} \times \text{body weight (kg)} \times 0.3 \qquad \text{Eq 14A}$$

$$HCO_3^- \text{ “excess” (mEq)} = 0.3 \times \text{body weight (kg)} \times [HCO_3^- \text{ observed} - HCO_3^- \text{ desired}] \qquad \text{Eq 14B}$$

In both formulas, the result is millimoles of HCl to be administered. If this intervention is contraindicated, not effective, or not available, and the alkalemia is severe with no hope of quick control, hemodialysis or hemodiafiltration can rapidly correct severe alkalemia and volume overload. If unstable hemodynamics coexist, the same goals can be achieved by continuous arteriovenous or venovenous hemodiafiltration (see also Chapter 65).

Respiratory Acid-Base Derangements

Although the underlying pathological process may vary, the respiratory acid-base derangements always have the same mechanism: alveolar ventilation is increased or decreased out of proportion to CO_2 production (Table 61–6). CO_2 arises either from the cellular metabolism or by the titration of HCO_3^- by metabolic acids. Normal CO_2 production by the body (and its excretion by the lungs) is impressive (about 220 ml/min or about 317 L/day in a 70-kg adult equivalent to 15,000 mmol of carbonic acid per day) compared with the 500 mmol/day of all nonrespiratory acids that are handled by the kidneys and gut.[13] Pulmonary ventilation is adjusted by the respiratory center in the brainstem in response to changes in $Pa{CO_2}$, pH, and $Pa{O_2}$, although respiratory drive can be influenced by other neural (anxiety, wakefulness) and nonneural factors (e.g., exercise, muscle strength) and also can be altered in some pathological situations (cystic fibrosis, asthma, and congenital central hypoventilation syndrome).[230-232] The precise and real-time match of alveolar minute ventilation to CO_2 production allows stable $Pa{CO_2}$ levels of 35 to 45 mmHg at sea level. Accuracy of the central control allows the body to adjust $Pa{CO_2}$ in compensation for alterations in arterial pH produced by metabolic acidosis or alkalosis in predictable ways (Tables 61–3 and 61–4). When this normal respiratory system is disrupted or overwhelmed, $Pa{CO_2}$ deviates from normal and the respiratory acid-base disturbances are initiated. Respiratory acidosis is produced by CO_2 retention leading to hypercapnia (elevation of $Pa{CO_2}$). Respiratory alkalosis is produced by hyperventilation, leading to a drop in $PaCO_2$ (i.e., hypocapnia). As soon as $Pa{CO_2}$ increases or decreases, plasma and intracellular buffers change dissociation to maintain a stable pH, the effect of which is fully manifested within 15 to 30 minutes. If the alteration in $Pa{CO_2}$ is sustained for more than 6 to 12 hours, renal mechanisms induce far larger changes in bicarbonate concentration, reaching maximal impact within 3 to 5 days. These renal effects lead to a new steady state for the pH. The two responses to the primary alterations in $Pa{CO_2}$, plasma plus tissue buffers and the renal response, permit description of the respiratory acid-base derangements into acute and chronic phases.[233] Thus *acute* respiratory acidosis or alkalosis involves the immediate plasma and intracellular buffer response to hypercapnia or hypocapnia, whereas *chronic* respiratory acidosis or alkalosis involves the renal response.

Respiratory Acidosis

Respiratory acidosis occurs whenever the CO_2 elimination by the lungs is lower than the CO_2 production by the tissues, resulting in a “positive balance” of CO_2, which in turn increases $Pa{CO_2}$ to a new equilibrium determined by the altered relationship between CO_2 production and alveolar ventilation. Because increases in CO_2 production alone are not sufficient to overcome the normal ability of the lungs to increase alveolar ventilation,[233] what is central to all forms of respiratory acidosis is a failure of alveolar ventilation and CO_2 excretion to increase in response to a rising $Paco_2$. Nevertheless an increase in CO_2 production in the face of fixed ventilation, which may occur in the critical care setting in patients receiving mechanical hypoventilation with a high load of carbohydrates in their parenteral nutrition, can result in respiratory acidosis.[233] This may also happen if a patient with hypoventilated lungs becomes febrile (acute hypermetabolism).

Immediately, the increase in $Paco_2$ increases both the hydrogen ion and bicarbonate concentrations in blood (Eqs. 3, 4, and 5). This is in agreement with the physical chemical explanation of acid-base interactions and is in opposition with the long-held concept that the change in bicarbonate concentration is mediated simply by the dissociation of H_2CO_3 into H^+ and HCO_3^-, not by an active physiological adaptation response.[4,13,18,25] Therefore the increase in $[HCO_3^-]$ occurs as a consequence of physical chemical principles and does not "buffer" the increase in $[H^+]$. The only immediate buffering activity in hypercapnia comes from the nonbicarbonate plasma and intracellular buffers.[197] Because of the increase in bicarbonate (a weak anion), no change in the SID is produced, and thus no change occurs in the SBE.[18,25] Because CO_2 is produced within the cells and because CO_2 can freely diffuse across the lipophilic cellular membranes, intracellular acidosis always occurs with respiratory acidosis.[197,198] If the $Paco_2$ remains increased, active compensatory mechanisms are activated, and the SID increases to restore $[H^+]$ toward normal. Primarily, respiratory acidemia compensation is accomplished by removal of Cl^- from the plasma space. Because movement of Cl^- into the tissues or red blood cells results in a drop of intracellular pH, Cl^- must be removed from the body to achieve a lasting effect on the SID. As stated before in this chapter, the kidneys are the most important organ for this task. Because every chloride ion that is filtered and not reabsorbed increases the SID (and the pH), Cl^- removal by the kidney must be highly accurate. The role of ammonium in this process is preeminent, not as a hydrogen ion carrier or a potential buffer, but for the excretion of Cl^- without loss of Na^+ or K.[18,64,74] Thus when renal function is intact, Cl^- is eliminated in the urine, and after a few days, the SID increases to the level necessary to return blood pH near 7.35. This amount of time is required by the physiological constraints of the system, but that is not entirely a disadvantage because this rate of response is useful to avoid being oversensitive to transient changes in alveolar ventilation. In any case, the compensation results in an increased pH for any degree of hypercarbia. Thus according to the Henderson-Hasselbalch equation (Eqs. 4 and 5), the increased pH will result in an increased HCO_3^- concentration for a given Pco_2. Therefore the so-called adaptive increase in $[HCO_3^-]$ to hypercapnia actually results from the increase in pH, and *it is not* the cause for the increase in the pH, which actually occurred from the increase in the SID as a consequence of the removal of chloride. Although the change in HCO_3^- concentration is *a convenient and reliable marker* for the metabolic compensation (Tables 61–3 and 61–4), *it is not the mechanism*. This understanding is more than semantic because only changes in the independent variables of acid base balance (Pco_2, SID and A_{TOT}) can affect the plasma hydrogen ion concentration and $[HCO_3^-]$ is not an independent variable.[13,18,108]

Acute respiratory acidosis develops as a consequence of the impaired function of one or more of the three participants in the ventilatory function: central nervous system; neural (peripheral), muscular, and skeletal structures; and lungs (airway and alveoli). Central nervous system depression can occur as a consequence of severe head trauma causing brain edema, from metabolic diseases, from some infectious diseases, from intentional sedation, or from the pharmacological effect of other legal and illegal drugs. Neuromuscular function impairment, damage to efferent nerves or to the muscles of respiration, is seen in some electrolyte disturbances (hypophosphatemia, hypokalemia), in some diseases (e.g., myasthenia gravis, Guillain-Barré syndrome, Werdnig-Hoffmann disease, Duchenne's muscular dystrophy), and in ventilatory restriction (as in patients with rib fractures and flail chest, and in patients with increased intraabdominal hypertension from ascites, from closure of congenital abdominal wall defects). Airway and parenchymal lung disease are the most common causes of acute CO_2 retention, as in respiratory obstructive disease, either acute or chronic (croup, asthma, bronchiolitis, bronchopulmonary dysplasia) and alveolar injury, such as that occurring in pneumonia or pulmonary edema (cardiogenic or not cardiogenic). According to the alveolar gas equation (Eq. 15), this last group of conditions also produces primary hypoxemia, not only hypercapnia:

$$P_AO_2 = PIO_2 - Paco_2/R \qquad \text{Eq. 15}$$

where P_AO_2 is the alveolar oxygen partial pressure; PIO_2 is the inspired oxygen tension (about 150 mmHg in ambient air); and R is the respiratory coefficient, usually assumed to be 0.8. The alveolar gas equation predicts that the rise in the $Paco_2$ will cause obligatory hypoxemia in patients breathing room air, as $Paco_2$ increases, P_AO_2 decreases in a predictable fashion. Thus this equation predicts that if the patient is in ambient air, acute hypercapnia of approximately 80 to 90 mmHg will impose a life-threatening decrease in the Pao_2.[98] Under these circumstances, it is hypoxemia, not hypercapnia or acidemia, that poses the principal threat to life. The already mentioned conditions that cause the failure of the lungs to eliminate CO_2 can also be grouped into two types of ventilatory disorders.[233] The first or "pure" hypoventilation occurs as a result of brainstem or neuromuscular dysfunction (the so-called respiratory pump) or because of extrapulmonary restrictive lung compromise, such as rib cage malformations and limited diaphragmatic movement due to increased intraabdominal pressure. In this setting, the lung simply fails to move enough air in and out to exchange CO_2 and oxygen. As a result, Pao_2 falls in proportion to the rise in $Paco_2$. In the second and more common situation in the critical care setting, alveolar hypoventilation is the result of the imbalance between perfused and hypoventilated segments of a damaged lung (i.e., ventilation-perfusion inequality). In this setting, a fall in Pao_2 often precedes hypercapnia, and when hypercapnia finally develops, the reduction in Pa_{O_2} is proportionally greater than the rise in Pa_{CO_2}.[98] With both types of ventilatory defects, however, hypoxemia is a concurrent finding when hypercapnia is present.[13,233]

Chronic respiratory acidosis is most often associated with chronic lung disease (e.g., bronchopulmonary dysplasia) or chest diseases with abnormal chest wall mechanics (chest congenital deformities, kyphoscoliosis), but it can also be caused by chronic upper airway obstruction (e.g., obstructive sleep apnea syndrome and craniofacial disorders),[234,235] chronic neuromuscular diseases (e.g., Duchenne's muscular dystrophy), or chronic central nervous system problems (congenital central hypoventilation syndrome).[231,232] Respiratory decompensation in patients with these conditions usually results from recently acquired infection, use of narcotics, or uncontrolled oxygen therapy.[236] These additional factors superimpose an acute element of CO_2 retention and acidemia on the already elevated chronic CO_2 baseline disorder. Progressive narcosis and coma (i.e., hypercapnic encephalopathy) can ensue. On the basis of the preeminent renal participation in the ultimate compensation of hypercapnia, one should expect that patients with renal disease (with difficulties excreting chloride) will have a defective adaptation to chronic hypercapnia.

Treating Respiratory Acidosis

As stated before, the main threat to life in respiratory acidosis comes from associated hypoxemia, not from the level of hypercapnia or acidemia. Consequently, oxygen administration represents a critical element in the management of respiratory acidosis. Although hypoxemia is not expected in children with previously healthy lungs,[237] caution must be taken when uncontrolled concentrations of oxygen are administered to some patients with hypercarbia, particularly in those with chronic lung disease, in whom exaggerated oxygen supplementation could depress respiratory drive and provoke further increase in Pa_{CO_2}.[236,238,239] This occurs because chronic hypercapnia is thought to downregulate CO_2 chemoreceptor sensitivity, which means that these patients are more dependent on hypoxic drive to maintain adequate spontaneous ventilation.[240] Thus hypoventilation (and hypercapnia), may worsen if unrestricted (and excessive) oxygen is administered. This phenomenon has been described mainly in adults with chronic obstructive pulmonary disease and acute asthma,[236,239] but it may also occur in children with chronic lung disease.[238] It should be emphasized, however, that the correction of hypoxia overrides strategies to avert oxygen-related hypercapnia, which normally tends to be of small clinical significance in children.[241] Thus immediate actions should focus on securing a patent airway and restoring adequate oxygenation by delivering an oxygen-enriched gas mixture. Oxygen administration alone, however, is almost never enough as a single therapeutic measure. Thus the hypoventilation must be treated directly. Whenever feasible, treatment must be directed to the underlying cause. Sometimes it is possible to solve the primary cause of hypoventilation rather quickly (e.g., relief of obstruction from croup with racemic epinephrine, reversal of narcotics with naloxone, resolution of bronchial spasm with some β_2 agonist). In such cases, it may be possible to avoid positive pressure ventilation. It is more common, though, to need some form of respiratory support. Generally speaking, mechanical ventilation is indicated when the patient is at risk of instability, the patient is already unstable, or the central nervous system function shows a trend toward deterioration. When respiratory muscle fatigue is impending, further deterioration must be avoided utilizing positive pressure ventilation. The classic "rule of the 50s" (i.e., 50 mmHg of Pa_{O_2} and Pa_{CO_2} as a guide for endotracheal intubation) should not be interpreted literally. It is not the absolute value of Pa_{CO_2} (or Pa_{O_2}) that is important but rather the clinical condition and perceived trajectory of the patient.

In chronic hypercapnia, management of the respiratory decompensation depends on the cause, severity, and rate of progression of the hypercapnia.[98] Immediate treatment of pulmonary infection with proper antibiotics, bronchodilator therapy, and removal of secretions can offer considerable benefit. The ventilatory drive can be optimized by minimizing the use of tranquilizers and sedatives, by gradually reducing supplemental oxygen (aiming for a Pa_{O_2} of about 60 mmHg), and by correcting a superimposed metabolic alkalosis.[98] The "aggressive" approach that favors the early implementation of positive pressure ventilation is often appropriate for patients with acute respiratory acidosis.[242] For those patients with chronic diseases that limit pulmonary reserve, however, a more conservative approach is often advisable and possible because of the great difficulty often encountered in weaning such patients from ventilators. If the patient is obtunded or unable to cough and if hypercapnia and acidemia are worsening, mechanical ventilation should be instituted. Noninvasive mechanical ventilation (NIV) with a nasal or facial mask is being used with increasing frequency in children both with moderately severe acute respiratory failure and with hypercapnic respiratory failure resulting from acute exacerbations of chronic lung disease.[243-245] Despite the fact that most experience with this technique comes from the adult population[246-248] and despite the limited pediatric experience,[242,243,249] its application in children is growing both in acute situations within the critical care unit and in cases of chronic hypercapnic and hypoxemic respiratory failure of various causes, which are encountered in intermediate care wards and in children's home environments.[243,249-252] Today, NIV is used even in small children younger than 1 year.[245,253] Although NIV is contraindicated in the presence of hemodynamic instability, this method has several claimed advantages, including its noninvasiveness, easy-to-use equipment, fewer complications from the reduced use of endotracheal tubes (infections possibly included), delayed need for tracheostomy in neuromuscular ventilatory failure, and easier weaning from mechanical ventilation.[243,250] Also, surprisingly, it is not routinely rejected by children.[250,252] The main disadvantages include gastric distention, facial skin redness (or even necrosis), and transient hypoxemia.[242,243]

When Pa_{CO_2} is increased and minute ventilation is normal or increased, the respiratory muscles are failing to generate sufficient alveolar ventilation to eliminate the CO_2 being produced. The means of correcting this disease include augmenting alveolar ventilation by increasing tidal volume or respiratory rate and reducing CO_2 production by decreasing the work of breathing.[246] Respiratory muscle failure can occur when the work of breathing is normal (e.g., numerous acute or chronic neuromuscular problems) or increased (e.g., patients with asthma or the obesity hypoventilation syndrome) and presumably because of inadequate delivery of oxygen to the respiratory muscles (e.g., patients with cardiogenic pulmonary edema). When Pa_{CO_2} is increased and minute ventilation is low, the level of consciousness is generally impaired. Such patients usually require intubation for airway protection in addition to ventilatory assistance, unless the hypercapnia can be reversed within minutes with NIV.[243,246] Hypoxemia is treated with F_{IO_2} augmentation (the lower the $\dot{V}A/\dot{Q}$, the less the effect) and through the recruitment of airspaces with an increase of the transpulmonary pressure applied at end-exhalation (continuous positive airway pressure [CPAP]).[242] The usual ventilatory strategy for hypercapnia is to increase minute ventilation, which should gradually return the Pa_{CO_2} toward baseline values, while the excretion of excess bicarbonate by the kidneys is accomplished (on the assumption that chloride is provided). By contrast, an overly rapid reduction in the Pa_{CO_2} risks the development of posthypercapnic alkalosis, with potentially serious consequences. Should posthypercapnic alkalosis develop, it can be ameliorated with chloride in the form of sodium or potassium salt with the aim of decreasing the SID or through the administration of acetazolamide, the bicarbonate-wasting diuretic that will provoke enhanced renal chloride reabsorption.[18,98] Finally, it is always convenient to reduce CO_2 production. This can be achieved through reduction of the carbohydrate load in parenteral and sometimes in enteral nutrition, through aggressive control of hyperthermia, and through adequate sedation or analgesia in anxious or combative patients.

What alternatives are there for those patients with intractable hypercapnia? One possible option not yet routinely available is intratracheal pulmonary ventilation, a method in which an intratracheal catheter with a reversed continuous flow of gas at its tip (away from the lungs) facilitates flushing CO_2 from the proximal dead space. Marked reductions in Pa_{CO_2}, ranging from 37% to 71%, and improvement in baseline pH were achieved with this intervention in five moribund neonatal and pediatric patients with uncontrollable hypercapnia who were receiving ventilation.[254] Another possible approach is the extracorporeal removal of CO_2. A promising phase I clinical study of total extracorporeal arteriovenous CO_2 removal was recently concluded in eight adult patients either with acute hypercapnic respiratory failure or with hypoxemic respiratory failure managed with permissive hypercapnia.[255]

Permissive Hypercapnia

The ultimate treatment for respiratory acidosis is to increase minute ventilation, a measure that often requires mechanical ventilation support. This ventilation support may have consequences for the patient's respiratory, cardiovascular, neurological, and metabolic conditions that must not be overlooked. In the last decade, a deep concern has emerged regarding the pulmonary effects of positive pressure ventilation. The ARDS Network study[256] showed that in patients with ALI and ARDS, mechanical ventilation with a lower tidal volume than that traditionally used resulted in decreased mortality and decreased the number of ventilator-free days. Thus the former standard practice of prescribing tidal volumes of 10 to 15 ml/kg (two to three times the physiological volume) or programming high-peak pressures as needed to achieve normocarbia (i.e., Pa_{CO_2} 35-45 mmHg) is gradually being abandoned.[257-259] Because in many patients with respiratory acidosis lung dysfunction already exists, it is usually not possible to achieve normocapnia values without producing alveolar distension (the so-called volutrauma) or auto positive end-expiratory pressure (auto-PEEP).[98] Accordingly, in the critically ill patient with some sort of lung disease, normalizing the Pa_{CO_2} comes at the cost of volutrauma or barotrauma (i.e., the alveolar distension and collapse cycle that is now known to be associated with tissue injury, increased microvascular permeability, and lung rupture).[260] Thus the current practice for both adults and children favors the use of lower tidal volumes (5 to 8 ml/kg or less), with plateau or peak pressures no higher than 20 cm H_2O above the baseline (PEEP). With this approach, there is increasing evidence that the lungs may have better outcomes,[256,259] but an increase in the Pa_{CO_2} might ensue. This "controlled hypoventilation" is known as *permissive hypercapnia*.[257,258] There is now a growing experience with this approach, mainly from adult patients with ARDS[109,110], or status asthmaticus,[111] but the appearance of pediatric reports is also increasing.[113,251,257,259,261,262] In most of these reports, in both children and adults, hypercapnia and acidemia are tolerated to avoid alveolar overdistention, which has resulted in lower morbidity and respiratory deaths than those with the conventional mechanical ventilation approach.[259,261,263] For example, permissive hypercapnia in burned children was associated with similar rates of barotrauma and pneumonia as in historic controls, but reduced the incidence of respiratory deaths.[259] Similar data have been generated in neonates. A Danish study of mechanical ventilation for extremely premature and extremely low-birth-weight infants reported that infants treated with early nasal CPAP and permissive hypercapnia had comparable survival rates and sensorineural outcome, in comparison with infants treated with the traditional mechanical ventilation approach; however, the incidence of chronic lung disease was lower than that reported with conventional treatment.[262] Carlo et al[261] also observed a reduction in the incidence of bronchopulmonary dysplasia with this approach. In sedated adults with ARDS who received ventilation, rapid intentional hypoventilation (pH falling from 7.40 to 7.26 in 30 to 60 minutes) lowered systemic vascular resistance and increased cardiac output.[110] Mean systemic arterial pressure and pulmonary vascular resistance did not change. In children, several groups have shown that hypoventilation improves arterial oxygenation after bidirectional superior cavopulmonary anastomosis.[263,264]

In these patients, moderate hypercapnia with respiratory acidosis was also shown to reduce oxygen consumption and arterial lactate levels.[264]

How low can the pH drop? How high can the Pa_{CO_2} rise? Actually, in many studies of adult patients undergoing permissive hypercapnia, a pH well below 7.20 has been tolerated.[109] The feared consequences of acidemia, projected from the experience with patients having lactic acidosis (and, usually, concomitant sepsis), failed to materialize. With data now available from many adults who consented to hypoventilation, the systemic hemodynamic effects are small, even as the pH falls to 7.15; the typical adult patient experiences no change or small increases in cardiac output and blood pressure. Patients whose pH falls below 7 are fewer in number, so firm conclusions cannot be drawn, but they similarly tolerate their acidemia. What is the limit of hypercapnia for pediatric patients? Mazzeo et al[265] described a case of prolonged severe hypercapnia with acidemia occurring during an episode of near-fatal asthma in an 8-year-old boy, followed by complete recovery. Ten hours after admission, this boy reached a Pa_{CO_2} of 293 mmHg, with a pH of 6.77 and a Pa_{O_2} of 65 mmHg. Despite this supercarbia[113] lasting more than 14 hours, associated with severe neck, subcutaneous, and mediastinal emphysema, no hemodynamic instability was seen. This case illustrates the cardiovascular and neurological tolerance to prolonged supercarbia in a child with previously healthy cardiovascular and neurological systems.[113,265] This might not be the case for the typical critically ill child scenario with multiple system involvement, though.[263] For example, Tasker and Peters[266] reported on a child with combined meningococcal sepsis and meningitis, cerebral edema, and ARDS, in whom significant acidemia was not well tolerated. Nevertheless, cautious induction of pH down to 7.32 and of a Pa_{CO_2} less than 45 mmHg was tolerated acutely without significant brain hyperemia. The authors used jugular venous oxygen saturation monitoring for titration of the effect of the Pa_{CO_2} level on the brain.[265] With the development of metabolic compensation and normal pH, higher levels of Pa_{CO_2} could be eventually tolerated by the edematous brain. The message is clear: it is mandatory to individually assess every case. Balancing Pa_{CO_2} and pH in the face of multiple organ involvement, some of them with contradictory needs, represents a daily challenge for the pediatric intensivist. The final decision must be taken on solid clinical grounds and with appropriate available monitoring.[263] High levels of Pa_{CO_2} may cause increased respiratory drive and discomfort in the neurologically intact patient, necessitating heavy sedation and sometimes neuromuscular blockade. There are several potential contraindications to the use of permissive hypercapnia: brain edema, intracranial hypertension, seizures, and pulmonary hypertension.[98] Although there has been some discussion on the topic,[98] the current practice of permissive hypercapnia does not generally include an attempt to alkalinize the blood to compensate for respiratory acidosis.[13] In this setting, THAM could be more useful than bicarbonate because the Pa_{CO_2} will not rise with THAM. Weber et al[267] studied the effect of THAM on systemic hemodynamics in 12 adults with ARDS in whom permissive hypercapnia was induced with a target Pa_{CO_2} of 80 mmHg. In the control group (no attempt for correcting pH), hypercapnia had several deleterious effects: reduced systemic vascular resistance, mean arterial pressure and myocardial contractility, and increased cardiac output and pulmonary artery pressure. Patients who received THAM experienced significantly less myocardial depression when compared with control patients, and the effects of hypercapnia on mean arterial pressure and mean pulmonary artery pressure were ameliorated. The administration of THAM to 10 patients with acidosis and ALI caused significant improvements in arterial pH and base deficit, as well as a decrease in Pa_{CO_2} that could not be attributed to the mechanical ventilation.[268] When the ventilator is used to correct respiratory acidosis, the end-inspiratory plateau and auto-PEEP pressures should be monitored routinely to detect any adverse effects of hyperventilation.

What is the place of permissive hypercapnia in children nowadays? Several specific concerns regarding the safety of hypercapnia still remain, particularly in the pediatric population. Currently, protective ventilatory strategies that involve hypercapnia are clinically acceptable, provided the clinician is primarily targeting reduced tidal alveolar stretch.[251,263] There are insufficient clinical data to suggest that hypercapnia per se should be independently induced, nor do outcome data exist to support the practice of buffering hypercapnic acidosis.[251] Rapidly advancing basic scientific investigations should better delineate the advantages, disadvantages, and optimal use of hypercapnia in children in the near future.

Respiratory Alkalosis

If alveolar ventilation rises out of proportion to CO_2 production, then arterial P_{CO_2} falls. Indeed, for any given rate of CO_2 production, an increase in alveolar ventilation always reduces Pa_{CO_2}.[233] In the ICU environment, hyperventilation occurs in a number of pathological conditions, including salicylate intoxication, early sepsis, hypoxic respiratory disorders, hepatic failure, fever, certain central nervous system alterations, and pain or anxiety. The sole presence of respiratory alkalosis is a bad prognosis sign because mortality increases in direct proportion to the severity of the hypocapnia.[99] The detrimental effects of hypocapnia have been described in many settings (e.g. in premature infants in whom it has been associated with poor neurological outcome[269]; in children after severe traumatic brain injury, in whom a relationship between hypocarbia and cerebral ischemia and infarcts have been described[270]; and in children after a cardiopulmonary bypass procedure).[263]

As in acute respiratory acidosis, acute respiratory alkalosis elicits a secondary change in plasma bicarbonate that has two components.[233] A small to moderate acute decrease in the bicarbonate concentration occurs; this is dictated by the Henderson-Hasselbalch equation (Eqs. 4 and 5) and is also due to some tissue buffering.[94,233] If hypocapnia persists, the SID will begin to decrease as a result of renal chloride reabsorption, which is associated with a larger decrease of bicarbonate and a rise in urine pH.[13,99,233,271] By 48 to 72 hours of evolution, the SID assumes a new, lower, steady state. This occurs because renal adaptation to hypocapnia "backtitrates" the nonbicarbonate buffers, an action that decreases SID and tends to return pH toward normal values, usually with an increased chloride serum concentration.[233]

Usually, blood pH does not exceed 7.55 in most cases of respiratory alkalosis, and severe manifestations of alkalemia are unusual. Therefore management is directed to the underlying cause. Marked alkalemia can occur in certain circumstances, however, such as with inappropriately set ventilators, central nervous system disorders, and some psychiatric diseases, and is uncommon in children.[99] Typically, these mild acid-base changes are clinically more important for what they can alert the clinician to, in terms of the underlying disease, than for any threat they may pose to the patient. Accordingly, specific measures directed to compensate the pH are not usually required. The anxiety-hyperventilation syndrome, more commonly seen in adolescents in the emergency department than in the critical care unit, can be an exception. In such cases, an active therapeutic approach with assistance from the hospital's psychological team is required. In rare cases, sedation may be necessary.

Pseudorespiratory Alkalosis

Arterial hypocapnia does not necessarily imply respiratory alkalosis or the secondary and compensatory response to metabolic acidosis.[99] The presence of arterial hypocapnia in patients with profound circulatory shock has been termed *pseudorespiratory alkalosis*[272] or, simply, *venoarterial carbon dioxide gradient*.[188,272-274] This condition can be seen when alveolar ventilation is relatively preserved but profound cardiovascular depression exists. In such conditions, the severely reduced pulmonary blood flow limits the CO_2 delivered to the lungs for excretion. On the other hand, the increased ratio of ventilation to perfusion and the increased pulmonary transit time result in the removal of a larger-than-normal amount of CO_2 per unit of blood traversing the pulmonary circulation.[274] Thus despite decreased CO_2 delivery to the lungs, a situation that provokes a significant elevation of the mixed venous blood CO_2, arterial normocapnia or frank hypocapnia may be noted. Overall CO_2 excretion is markedly decreased, however, and the CO_2 balance of the body is positive, a phenomenon that is the hallmark of respiratory acidosis. Marked tissue acidosis is reflected in mixed venous blood acidemia, usually involving both metabolic and respiratory components.[13,99,233,274] The metabolic component derives from tissue hypoperfusion and hyperlactatemia. This is accompanied by an arterial pH that ranges from mildly acidic to the frankly alkaline. This venous-arterial P_{CO_2} gradient increases as cardiac index decreases.[99,188,272,273] In animal models, both venous-arterial P_{CO_2} gradient and venous-arterial pH difference increase as oxygen delivery declines. In septic shock, an elevated venous-arterial P_{CO_2} gradient is seen in those patients with low cardiac output and in those with pulmonary disease who cannot eliminate CO_2.[273] In patients with cardiogenic shock, the venous-arterial P_{CO_2} gradient decreases as hemodynamic variables improve with dobutamine, a phenomenon also seen in pediatric septic shock with myocardial depression. In this setting, arterial oxygen saturation may appear to be adequate despite tissue hypoxemia because of the shift to the left of the oxygen-hemoglobin dissociation curve caused by hypocapnia. This condition is rapidly fatal unless cardiac output is rapidly corrected.

Mixed Acid-Base Derangements

Coexisting metabolic acidosis and respiratory acidosis can be seen in several clinical conditions (e.g., during cardiopulmonary arrest, in chronic lung disease complicated with pneumonia and septic shock, in renal and pulmonary insufficiency, and as a consequence of certain toxic agents that may provoke both neural depression [and hypoventilation] and cardiocirculatory collapse [and metabolic acidosis]).[99] Treatment must be targeted, as usual, to the underlying causes. In addition, both components of the acid-based derangement must be addressed. The first step will always be ABCs: to secure the airway, to provide oxygenation and controlled hyperventilation, and to infuse fluids or vasoactive-inotropic agents according to the clinical conditions of the given patient. Administration of an alkalinizing agent should be considered only after hyperventilation has begun and on the basis of results of the arterial blood gas analysis.

Alkalemia of both metabolic and respiratory origin may occur in several complex settings, such as in patients with chronic liver disease in whom hyperventilation ensues as the initial manifestation of pneumonia. This hypocapnia appears in a patient in whom metabolic alkalosis is common because of vomiting or gastric drainage, hypokalemia, diuretics, or alkali administration.[99] Mixed alkalosis may also occur in patients with chronic renal insufficiency in whom primary hypocapnia develops. In this setting, inappropriately high plasma bicarbonate levels occur as a consequence of the nonexistent renal adaptive response. This situation is seen despite the patient's dialysis program because the dialytic procedures are an alkalinizing influence and are much less effective in compensating alkalemia than acidemia.[214,215] This effect can be minimized by switching the patient from peritoneal dialysis to hemodiafiltration or hemodialysis.

Some Other Important Considerations

A couple of decades ago, the so-called point of care (POC) testing technology became increasingly available in the ICUs as gas analyzers evolved quickly from rather simple devices to more complex machines with multiparametric capabilities. Thus electrolyte (Na, K, Ca, Cl, and Mg) and even lactate[276] analysis are available at bedside, in addition to the pH, P_{CO_2}, and P_{O_2}. The busy critical care practitioner confidently uses this POC technology for AG and SID calculations, assuming that the technology used has limited or no impact. The problem of method-related errors, arising from different measurement technologies, however, was clearly shown in patients by Morimatsu et al.[127] These researchers showed significant differences between AG and SID calculations derived from

POC analyzers and the same calculations derived from the central hospital laboratory automated blood biochemistry analyzers.[83,127] Mean values for sodium and chloride (but not for potassium) differed significantly; in some cases they led to a diverging assessment of the acid-base or electrolyte status. In this prospective study, 46% of the patients whose AG value was out of the reference range with one technology showed a value within the normal range with the other. Moreover, because all parameters used for diagnosis of nonrespiratory acid-base disturbances are calculated quantities, their utility greatly depends on the accuracy and precision of each of the measured primary values used in the particular calculation. Thus the tolerable values of inaccuracy may also have a strong influence on AG and SID calculations. For example, the mean ± SD (SD%) for the electrolyte concentrations in plasma include sodium, 142 ± 2.8 (2.0%); potassium, 4.5 ± 0.2 (3.7%); chloride, 103 ± 4.1 (4%) (mEq/L); and lactate, 1.5 ± 0.1 (6%) mmol/L (CL). With these figures, the normal value of the SID ([Na + K] − [Cl^- − $lactate^-$]) is calculated as 42 ± 5.0 mmol/L, with the high SD secondary to error propagation. This could be an explanation of some conflicting results in regard to the ability of the SID, SIG, and AG to predict survival.[81-83,86,91,276] In comparison, the normal SBE is 0 ± 2.2 mmol/L, calculated at pH 7.40 ± 0.02, P_{CO_2} 40 ± 1.6 mm Hg (4%), standard hemoglobin, and full oxygen saturation. The SBE has less potential for cumulative errors, but one must not overlook the "artificial" concept of the SBE.[7,30,35,85,276] Because of this potential imprecision,[277] it is probably wise to rely on the SBE and bicarbonate rules of thumb as the primary approach for metabolic acidosis and to use the SID, lactate, and corrected-for-albumin-AG as secondary parameters for a detailed differential diagnosis (see Table 61–6).[278]

Conclusion

What then is the role of the physical chemical approach to acid-base management in the contemporary pediatric ICU? Some researchers have examined if the Stewart approach, later modified by Figge, Fencl, and Watson, offers some clinical advantage over traditional approaches.[25] Although the physical chemical approach is still developing, some generalizations can be made. From a theoretical standpoint, this "new" way offers a more precise estimate of the acid-base physiology. The later modifications to the Stewart's approach by Figge, Fencl, and Watson[25,26,279] allow detection of metabolic acidosis not apparent by the application of the traditional AG. Differences between the Stewart and traditional approaches for determining unmeasured anions are narrowed significantly if the traditional AG is corrected for albumin concentration and measurement of lactate is taken into consideration.[81] The SID approach, however, is possibly more expensive than the traditional approach, and the calculation of the variables for the SID are more cumbersome than those of the traditional approach.[81,83] Thus it is possible that the busy clinician may (and will) resist to change for practical reasons. The clinician may also consider that the physical chemical approach is not sufficiently better than a critical assessment of the BE, the AG, or pH/PCO_2 nomograms. Interpretation of acid-base derangements will always be a mix of art, knowledge, and clinical competence, so it is up to the physician to put all the available information together in the context of the individual patient and the natural course of his or her disease. If the new approach proves in time to be adequate for diagnostic, therapeutic, and prognostic purposes, then the cumbersome calculations could be automated by hospital laboratory programs to increase availability and usage by clinicians. There are already some useful tools and resources on the World Wide Web (noted after references). Meanwhile, both the SBE and bicarbonate rules of thumb can be clinically useful, but the pediatric intensivist must not confound these practical tools with pathophysiological accuracy.

REFERENCES

1. Broughton JO Jr, Kennedy TC: Interpretation of arterial blood gases by computer, *Chest* 65:148, 1984.
2. Henderson LJ: The theory of neutrality regulation in the animal organism, *Am J Physiol* 21:427, 1908.
3. Severinghaus JW, Astrup P, Murray JF: Blood gas analysis and critical care medicine, *Am J Respir Crit Care Med* 157:S114, 1998.
4. Story DA: Bench-to-bedside review: a brief history of clinical acid-base. *Crit Care* 8:253, 2004.
5. Brönsted JN: The acid basic functions of molecules and its dependency on the electric charge types, *J Phys Chem* 30:777, 1926.
6. Relman A: What are 'acids' and 'bases'? *Am J Med* 17:435, 1954.
7. Mizock BA: Utility of standard base excess in acid-base analysis, *Crit Care Med* 26:1146, 1998.
8. Siggaard-Andersen O: The van Slyke equation, *Scand J Clin Lab Invest Suppl* 37:15, 1977.
9. Van Slyke DD, Neill JM: The determination of gases in blood and other solutions by vacuum extraction and manometric measurement. *J Biol Chem* 61:523, 1924.
10. Lowry TM: The electronic theory of valency. 1. The origin of acidity. *Trans Farad Soc* 20:13, 1924.
11. Ichikawa I, Narins RG, Harris Jr W: Regulation of acid-base homeostasis. In Ichikawa I, editor: *Pediatric textbook of fluids and electrolytes,* Baltimore, 1990, Williams & Wilkins.
12. Narins RG, Krishna GG, Ikemiyashiro JYD, et al: The metabolic acidoses. In Narins RG, editor: *Maxwell & Kleeman's clinical disorders of fluid and electrolyte metabolism,* ed 5, New York, 1994, McGraw-Hill.
13. Kellum JA: Acid-base disorders. In Fink MP, Abraham E, Vincent JL et al, editors: *Textbook of critical care,* ed 5, Philadelphia, 2005, Elsevier Saunders.
14. Kellum JA: Acid-base physiology in the post-Copernican era, *Curr Opin Crit Care Med* 5:429, 1999.
15. Astrup P, Bie P, Engell HC: Salt and water in culture and medicine. Copenhagen: Radiometer, 1993:51.
16. Brewer ED: Disorders of acid-base balancem *Pediatr Clin North Am* 37:429, 1990.
17. Narins RG, Emmett M: Simple and mixed acid-base disorders: a practical approach, *Medicine* 59:161, 1980.
18. Kellum JA: Determinants of blood pH in health and disease, *Crit Care* 4:6, 2000.
19. Kellum JA: Making strong ion difference the "Euro" for bedside acid-base analysis. In Vincent JL, editor: *Yearbook of intensive care & emergency medicine,* Berlin, 2005, Springer-Verlag.
20. Venticinque SG: Metabolic acidosis surrounding resuscitation. *Critical care refresher course 'cutting edge therapeutics,'* Des Plaines, 2003, Society of Critical Care Medicine.
21. Singer RB, Hastings AB: An improved clinical method for the estimation of disturbances of the acid-base balance of human blood, *Medicine* (Baltimore) 27:223, 1948.
22. Christensen H: Anions versus cations, *Am J Med* 27:163, 1957.
23. Frazer S, Stewart C: Acidosis and alkalosis: a modern view, *J Clin Pathol* 12:195, 1959.

24. Durward A, Tibby S, Skellett S, et al: The strong ion gap predicts mortality in children following cardiopulmonary bypass surgery, *Pediatr Crit Care Med* 6:281, 2005.
25. Fencl V, Jabor A, Kazda A, et al: Diagnosis of metabolic acid-base disturbances in critically ill patients, *Am J Respir Crit Care Med* 162:2246, 2000.
26. Figge J, Jabor A, Kazda A, et al: Anion gap and hypoalbuminemia, *Crit Care Med* 26:1807, 1998.
27. Reilly RF, Anderson RJ: Interpreting the anion gap, *Crit Care Med* 26: 1771, 1998.
28. Astrup P, Jorgensen K, Siggard-Andersen O: Acid-base metabolism: new approach, *Lancet* 1:1035, 1960.
29. Grogono AW, Byles PH, Hawke W: An *in vivo* representation of acid-base balance, *Lancet* 1:499, 1976.
30. Kofstad J: Base excess: a historical review—has the calculation of base excess been more standardized the last 20 years? *Clin Chim Acta* 2001; 307: 193.
31. Severinghaus JW: Acid-base balance nomogram—a Boston-Copenhagen détente, *Anesthesiology* 45:539, 1976.
32. Siggaard-Andersen O: The pH-log pCO_2 blood acid-base nomogram revised, *Scand J Clin Lab Invest* 14:598, 1962.
33. Siggaard-Andersen O, Foch-Andersen N: Base excess or buffer base (strong ion difference) as measure of a non-respiratory acid-base disturbance, *Acta Anaesthesiol Scand* 39(suppl 106):123, 1995.
34. Bunker JP: The great trans-Atlantic acid-base debate, *Anesthesiology* 26:591, 1965.
35. Schlichtig R, Grogono AW, Severinghaus JW: Human $PaCO_2$ and standard base excess compensation for acid-base imbalance, *Crit Care Med* 26:1173, 1998.
36. Schwartz, WB, Relman AS: A critique of the parameters used in the evaluation of the acid-base disorders, *N Engl J Med* 268: 1383, 1963.
37. Severinghaus JW: Siggaard-Andersen and the "Great Trans Atlantic Acid Base Debate," *Scand J Clin Lab Invest Suppl* 214: 99, 1993.
38. Kellum JA: Metabolic acidosis in the critically ill: lessons from physical chemistry, *Kidney Int* 53(suppl 66):S81, 1998.
39. Emmett M, Narins RG: Clinical use of anion gap, *Medicine* (Baltimore) 56:38, 1997.
40. Oh MS, Carroll HJ: The anion gap, *N Engl J Med* 297:814, 1977.
41. Oh MS, Carroll HJ, Goldstein DA, et al: Hyperchloremic acidosis during the recovery phase of diabetic ketoacidosis, *Ann Intern Med* 89:925, 1978.
42. Winter SD, Pearson JR, Gabow PA, et al: The fall of the serum anion gap, *Arch Intern Med* 150:311, 1990.
43. Durward A, Mayer A, Skellet S, et al: Hypoalbuminemia in critically ill children: incidence, prognosis, and influence on the anion gap, *Arch Dis Child* 88:419, 2003.
44. Elisaf MS, Tsatsoulis AA, Katopodis KP, et al: Acid-base and electrolyte disturbances in patients with diabetic ketoacidosis, *Diabetes Res Clin Pract* 34:23, 1996.
45. Gabow PA: Disorders associated with an altered anion gap, *Kidney Int* 27:472, 1985.
46. Gabow PA, Kaehny WD, Fennessey PV, et al: Diagnostic importance of an increased serum anion gap, *N Engl J Med* 303: 854, 1980.
47. Hatherill M, Waggie Z, Purves L, et al: Correction of the anion gap for albumin in order to detect occult tissue anions in shock, *Arch Dis Child* 87:526, 2002.
48. Levraut J, Bounatirou T, Ichai C, et al: Reliability of anion gap as an indicator of blood lactate in critically ill patients, *Intensive Care Med* 23:417, 1997.
49. Reeves RB: Commentary on review article by Dr. Peter Stewart, *Can J Physiol Pharmacol* 61:1442, 1983.
50. Stewart PA: *How to understand acid-base. A quantitative acid-base primer for biology and medicine.* New York, 1981, Elsevier, pp 1–286. An Internet version review through *http://www.acidbase.org.*
51. Stewart PA: Modern quantitative acid-base chemistry, *Can J Physiol Pharmacol* 61:1444, 1983.
52. Fencl V, Leith DE: Stewart's quantitative acid-base chemistry: applications in biology and medicine, *Respir Physiol* 91:1, 1993.
53. Stewart PA: Independent and dependent variables of acid-base control, *Respir Physiol* 33:9, 1978.
54. Rhodes A, Cusack RJ: Arterial blood gas analysis and lactate, *Curr Opin Crit Care Med* 6:227, 2000.
55. Durward A, Skellett S, Mayer A, et al: The value of the chloride:sodium ratio in differentiating the aetiology of metabolic acidosis, *Intensive Care Med* 27:828, 2001.
56. Gilfix BM, Bique M, Magder S: A physical chemical approach to the analysis of acid-base balance in the clinical setting, *J Crit Care* 8:187, 1993.
57. Balasubramanyan N, Havens PL, Hoffman GM: Unmeasured anions identified by the Fencl-Stewart method predict mortality better than base excess, anion gap, and lactate in patients in the pediatric intensive care unit, *Crit Care Med* 27:1577, 1999.
58. Rocktaeschel J, Morimatsu H, Uchino S, et al: Acid-base status of critically ill patients with acute renal failure: analysis based on Stewart-Figge methodology, *Crit Care* 7:R60, 2003.
59. Story DA, Morimatsu H, Bellomo R: Strong ions, weak acids and base excess: a simplified Fencl-Stewart approach to clinical acid-base disorders, *Br J Anaesth* 92:54, 2004.
60. Figge J, Mydosh T, Fencl V: Serum proteins and acid-base equillibria: a follow-up, *J Clin Lab Med* 120:713, 1992.
61. Gunnerson KJ, Kellum JA: Acid-base and electrolyte analysis in critically ill patients: are we ready for the new millennium? *Curr Opin Crit Care* 9:468, 2003.
62. Kamel SK, Cheema-Dhadli S, Halperin ML: Metabolic aspects of metabolic acidosis and metabolic alkalosis. In: Narins RG, editors: *Maxwell & Kleeman's clinical disorders of fluid and electrolyte metabolism,* ed 5, New York, 1994, McGraw-Hill.
63. Moe OW, Rector FC Jr, Alpern RJ: Renal regulation of acid-base metabolism. In Narins RG, editor: *Maxwell & Kleeman's clinical disorders of fluid and electrolyte metabolism,* ed 5, New York, 1994, McGraw-Hill.
64. Leblanc M, Kellum JA: Biochemical and biophysical principles of hydrogen ion regulation. In Ronco C, Bellomo R, editors: *Critical care nephrology,* Dordrecht, 1998, Kluwer Academic Publishers.
65. Garella S, Chang BS, Kahn SI: Dilution acidosis and contraction alkalosis: review of a concept, *Kidney Int* 8:279, 1975.
66. Kellum JA, Bellomo R, Kramer DJ, et al: Etiology of metabolic acidosis during saline resuscitation in endotoxemia, *Shock* 9:364, 1998.
67. Prough DS, Terry White R: Acidosis associated with peri-operative saline administration. Dilution or delusion? *Anesthesiology* 93:1167, 2000.
68. Waters JH, Gottlieb A, Schoenwald P, et al: Normal saline versus lactated Ringer's solution for intra-operative fluid management in patients undergoing abdominal aortic aneurysm repair: an outcome study, *Anesth Analg* 93:817, 2001.
69. Story DA: Intravenous fluid administration and controversies in acid-base, *Crit Care Resusc* 1:151, 1999.
70. Story DA, Bellomo R: The acid-base physiology of crystalloid solutions, *Curr Opin Crit Care* 5:436, 1999.
71. Aduen JF, Burritt MF, Murray MJ: Blood lactate accumulation: hemodynamics and acid base status, *J Intens Care* 17:180, 2002.
72. Bellomo R, Ronco C: The pathogenesis of lactic acidosis in sepsis, *Curr Opin Crit Care* 5:452, 1999.
73. Kaplan LJ, Frangos S: Clinical review: Acid-base abnormalities in the intensive care unit, *Crit Care* 2005; 9:198.
74. Karim Z, Attmane-Elakeb A, Bichara M: Renal handling of $NH4^+$ in relation to the control of acid-base balance by the kidney, *J Nephrol* 2002;15 Suppl 5:S128.
75. Kellum JA: Closing the gap on unmeasured anions, *Crit Care* 7:219, 2003.
76. Kellum JA: Lactate and pHi: our continued search for markers of tissue distress, *Crit Care Med* 26:1783, 1998.
77. Kellum JA, Kramer DJ, Pinsky MR: Strong ion gap: a methodology for exploring unexplained anions, *J Crit Care* 10:51, 1995.
78. Kellum JA, Bellomo R, Kramer DJ, et al: Hepatic anion flux during acute endotoxemia, *J Appl Physiol* 78:2212, 1995.
79. Kirschbaum B: Increased anion gap after liver transplantation, *Am J Med Sci* 313:107, 1997.
80. Mecher C, Rackow EC, Astiz M, et al: Unaccounted for anion in metabolic acidosis during severe sepsis in humans, *Crit Care Med* 19:705, 1991.
81. Carreira F, Anderson RJ: Assessing metabolic acidosis in the intensive care unit: does the method make a difference? *Crit Care Med* 32:1227, 2004.
82. Kaplan LJ, Kellum JA: Initial pH, base deficit, anion gap, strong ion difference, and strong ion gap predict outcome from major vascular injury, *Crit Care Med* 2004; 32: 1120.

83. Moviat M, van Haren F, van der Hoeven H: Conventional or physicochemical approach in intensive care unit patients with metabolic acidosis, *Crit Care* 7:R41, 2003.
84. Murray DM, Olhsson V, Fraser JI: Defining acidosis in postoperative cardiac patients using Stewart's method of strong ion difference, *Pediatr Crit Care Med* 5:240, 2004.
85. Schlichtig R: [Base excess] vs [strong ion difference]. Which is more helpful? *Adv Exp Med Biol* 411:91, 1997.
86. Cusack RJ, Rhodes A, Lochhead P, et al: The strong ion gap does not have prognostic value in critically ill patients in a mixed medical/surgical adult ICU, *Intensive Care Med* 28:864, 2002.
87. Hatherill M, Waggie Z, Purves L, et al: Mortality and the nature of metabolic acidosis in children with shock, *Intensive Care Med* 29:286, 2003.
88. Salem MM, Mujais SK: Gaps in the anion gap, *Arch Intern Med* 152:1625, 1992.
89. Hayhoe M, Bellomo R, Liu G, et al: The aetiology and pathogenesis of cardiopulmonary bypass-associated metabolic acidosis using polygeline pump prime, *Intensive Care Med* 25:680, 1999.
90. Rackow EC, Mecher C, Astiz ME, et al: Unmeasured anion during severe sepsis with metabolic acidosis, *Circ Shock* 30:107, 1990.
91. Rocktaeschel J, Morimatsu H, Uchino S, et al: Unmeasured anions in critically ill patients: can they predict mortality? *Crit Care Med* 31:2131, 2003.
92. Kaplan LJ: It's all in the charge... *Crit Care Med* 33:680, 2005.
93. Kellum JA: Unknown anions and gaps in medical knowledge, *Pediatr Crit Care Med* 6:373, 2005.
94. Zaritsky A: Unmeasured anions: déjà vu all over again? *Crit Care Med* 27:1672, 1999.
95. Bellomo R, Ronco C: New paradigms in acid-base physiology, *Curr Opin Crit Care* 5:427, 1999.
96. Iberti TJ, Leibowitz AB, Papadakos PJ: Low sensitivity of the anion gap as a screen to detect hyperlactemia in critically ill patients, *Crit Care Med* 18:275, 1990.
97. Hatherill M, McIntyre AG, Wattie M, et al: Early hyperlectataemia in critically ill children, *Intensive Care Med* 26:314, 2000.
98. Adrogué HJ, Madias NE: Management of life-threatening acid-base disorders: first of two parts, *N Engl J Med* 338: 26, 1998.
99 Adrogué HJ, Madias NE: Management of life-threatening acid-base disorders: second of two parts, *N Engl J Med* 338: 107, 1998.
100. Kellum JA, Song M, Li J: Science review: extracellular acidosis and the immune response: clinical and physiologic implications, *Crit Care* 8:331, 2004.
101. Sabatini S, Kurtzman NA: Metabolic alkalosis. In Narins RG, editor: *Maxwell & Kleeman's clinical disorders of fluid and electrolyte metabolism,* ed 5, New York, 1994, McGraw-Hill.
102. Davies AO: Rapid desensitization and uncoupling of human beta-adrenergic receptors in an in vitro model of lactic acidosis, *J Clin Endocrinol Metab* 59:398, 1984.
103. Gehlbach BK, Schmidt GA: Bench-to-bedside review: treating acid-base abnormalities in the intensive care unit—the role of buffers, *Crit Care* 8:259, 2004.
104. Marsh JD, Margolis TI, Kim D: Mechanism of diminished contractile response to catecholamines during acidosis, *Am J Physiol* 254:H20, 1988.
105. Nakanishi T, Okuda H, Kamata K, et al: Influence of acidosis on inotropic effect of catecholamines in newborn rabbit hearts, *Am J Physiol* 253: H1441, 1987.
106. Komukai K, Brette F, Orchard CH: Electrophysiological response of rat atrial myocytes to acidosis, *Am J Physiol Heart Circ Physiol* 283:H715, 2002.
107. Thatte HS, Rhee JH, Zagarins SE, et al: Acidosis-induced apoptosis in human and porcine heart, *Ann Thorac Surg* 77:1376, 2004.
108. Forsythe SM, Schmidt GA: Sodium bicarbonate for the treatment of lactic acidosis, *Chest* 117:260, 2000.
109. Feihl F, Perret C: Permissive hypercapnia: how permissive should we be? *Am J Respirt Crit Care Med* 150:1722, 1994.
110. Thorens JB, Jolliet P, Ritz M, et al: Effects of rapid permissive hypercapnia on hemodynamics, gas exchange, and oxygen transport and consumption during mechanical ventilation for the acute respiratory distress syndrome, *Intensive Care Med* 22:182, 1996.
111. Tuxen DV, Williams TJ, Scheinkestel CD, et al: Use of a measurement of pulmonary hyperinflation to control the level of mechanical ventilation in patients with acute severe asthma, *Am Rev Respir Dis* 146:1136, 1992.
112. Gamba G, Oseguera J, Castrejon M, et al: Bicarbonate therapy in severe diabetic ketoacidosis. A double blind, randomized, placebo controlled trial, *Rev Invest Clin* 43:234, 1991.
113. Goldstein B, Shannon DC, Todres ID: Supercarbia in children. Clinical course and outcome, *Crit Care Med* 18:166, 1990.
114. Potkin RT, Swenson ER: Resuscitation from severe acute hypercapnia: determinants of tolerance and survival, *Chest* 102: 1742, 1992.
115. Glaser GH: Medical complications of status epilepticus, *Adv Neurol* 34:395, 1983.
116. Lipka K, Bulow HH: Lactic acidosis following convulsions, *Acta Anaesthesiol Scand* 47:616, 2003.
117. Berger DS, Fellner SK, Robinson KA, et al: Disparate effects of three types of extracellular acidosis on left ventricular function, *Am J Physiol* 276:H582, 1999.
118. Mathieu D, Neviere R, Billard V, et al: Effects of bicarbonate therapy on hemodynamics and tissue oxygenation in patients with lactic acidosis: a prospective, controlled, clinical study, *Crit Care Med* 19:1352, 1991.
119. Adelson PD, Bratton SL, Carney NA, et al: Guidelines for the acute medical management of severe traumatic brain injury in infants, children, and adolescents. Chapter 12. Use of hyperventilation in the acute management of severe traumatic brain injury, *Pediatr Crit Care Med* 4: S45, 2003.
120. Mizock BA, Falk JL: Lactic acidosis in critical illness, *Crit Care Med* 20:80, 1992.
121. Deshpande SA, Platt MP: Association between blood lactate and acid-base status and mortality in ventilated babies, *Arch Dis Child* 76:15, 1997.
122. Gauthier PM, Szerlip HM: Metabolic acidosis in the intensive care unit, *Crit Care Clin* 18:289, 2002.
123. Hatherill M, Sajjanhar T, Tibby SM, et al: Serum lactate as a predictor of mortality after paediatric cardiac surgery, *Arch Dis Child* 77:235, 1997.
124. Geheb MA, Kruse JA, Haupt MT, et al: Fluid and electrolyte abnormalities in critically ill patients: fluid resuscitation, lactate metabolism, and calcium metabolism. In Narins RG, editor: *Maxwell & Kleeman's clinical disorders of fluid and electrolyte metabolism,* ed 5, New York, 1994, McGraw-Hill.
125. Shruti A, Anil S, Dhiren G, et al: Role of lactate in critically ill children, *Ind J Crit Care Med* 8:173, 2004.
126. Chernow B, Aduen J, Bernstein WK: Lactate: the ultimate blood test in critical care? In Parker MM, Shapiro MJ, Porembka DT, editors, *Critical care state of the art,* Fullerton, CA, 1995, Society of Critical Care Medicine.
127. Morimatsu H, Rocktächel J, Bellomo R, et al: Comparison of point-of-care versus central laboratory measurement of electrolyte concentrations on calculations of the anion gap and the strong ion difference, *Anesthesiology* 98:1077, 2003.
128. Kleinman JG, Lemann Jr J: Acid production. In Narins RG, editor: *Maxwell & Kleeman's clinical disorders of fluid and electrolyte metabolism,* ed 5, New York, 1994, McGraw-Hill.
129. Narins RG: Acid-base disorders: definitions and introductory concepts. In Narins RG, editor: *Maxwell & Kleeman's clinical disorders of fluid and electrolyte metabolism,* ed 5, New York, 1994, McGraw-Hill.
130. Mizock BA: Lung injury and lactate production: a hypoxic stimulus? *Crit Care Med* 27:2585, 1999.
131. Mizock BA: Metabolic derangements in sepsis and septic shock, *Crit Care Clin* 16:319, 2000.
132. Mizock BA: Significance of hyperlactemia without acidosis during hypermetabolic stress, *Crit Care Med* 25:1780, 1997.
133. Riley LJ Jr, Ilson BE, Narins RG: Acute metabolic acid-base disorders, *Crit Care Clin* 5:699, 1987.
134. Iscra F, Gullo A, Biolo G: Bench-to-bedside review: lactate and the lung, *Crit Care* 4:327, 2002.
135. Gutierrez G, Wulf ME: Lactic acidosis in sepsis: a commentary, *Intensive Care Med* 22:6, 1996.
136. James JH, Luchette FA, McCarter FD, et al: Lactate as an unreliable indicator of tissue hypoxia in injury or sepsis, *Lancet* 354: 505-508, 1999.
137. Bellomo R, Kellum JA, Pinsky MR: Transvisceral lactate fluxes during early endotoxemia, *Chest* 110:198, 1996.

138. Kellum JA, Kramer DJ, Lee K, et al: Release of lactate by the lung in acute lung injury, *Chest* 111:1301, 1997.
139. Luft FC: Lactic acidosis update for critical care clinicians, *J Am Soc Nephrol* 12(suppl 17):S15, 2001.
140. Levy B, Sadoune LO, Gelot AM, et al: Evolution of lactate/pyruvate and arterial ketone body ratios in the early course of catecholamine-treated septic shock, *Crit Care Med* 28:114, 2000.
141. Mizock BA: Redox pairs, tissue hypoxia, organ dysfunction, and mortality, *Crit Care Med* 28:270, 2000.
142. Totaro RJ, Raper RF: Epinephrine-induced lactic acidosis following cardiopulmonary bypass, *Crit Care Med* 25:1693, 1997.
143. Levraut J, Ciebiera JP, Chave S, et al: Mild hyperlactatemia in stable septic patients is due to impaired lactate clearance rather than overproduction, *Am J Respir Crit Care Med* 157:1021, 1998.
144. Madger S: Pathophysiology of metabolic acid-base disturbances in patients with critical illness. In Ronco C, Bellomo R, editors: *Critical care nephrology,* Dordrecht, 1998, Kluwer Academic Publishers.
145. Mizock BA: The hepatosplanchnic area and hyperlactatemia: a tale of two lactates, *Crit Care Med* 29:447, 2001.
146. Raper RF, Cameron G, Walker D, et al: Type B lactic acidosis following cardiopulmonary bypass, *Crit Care Med* 25:46, 1997.
147. Conlee RK, Kelly KP, Ojuka EO, et al: Cocaine and exercise: alpha-1 receptor blockade does not alter muscle glycogenolysis or blood lactacidosis, *J Appl Physiol* 88:77, 2000.
148. Bornemann M, Hill SC, Kidd GS II: Lactic acidosis in pheochromocytoma, *Ann Intern Med* 105:880, 1986.
149. Bravo EL, Gifford RW Jr: Pheochromocytoma, *Endocrinol Metab Clin North Am* 22:329, 1993.
150. Meyer S, Baghai A, Sailer NL, et al: Lactic acidosis caused by sodium nitroprusside in a newborn with congenital heart disease, *Eur J Pediatr* 164:253, 2005.
151. Routsi C, Bardouniotou H, Delivoria Ioannidou V, et al: Pulmonary lactate release in patients with acute lung injury is not attributable to lung tissue hypoxia, *Crit Care Med* 27:2469, 1999.
152. Weil MH, Michael S, Rackow EC: Comparison of blood lactate concentration in central vein, pulmonary artery and arterial blood, *Crit Care Med* 15:489, 1987.
153. DeBacker D, Creteur J, Zhang H, et al: Lactate production by the lungs in acute lung injury, *Am J Respir Crit Care Med* 156:1099, 1997.
154. Bendjelid K, Treggiari MM, Romand JA: Transpulmonary lactate gradient after hypothermic cardiopulmonary bypass, *Intensive Care Med* 30:817, 2004.
155. Bihari D, Gimson AES, Lindridge J, et al: Lactic acidosis in fulminant hepatic failure, *J Hepatol* 1:405, 1985.
156. Chang DM: Hyperlactatemia in acute liver failure: decreased clearance versus increased production, *Crit Care Med* 29: 2225, 2001.
157. Murphy ND, Kodakat SK, Wendon JA, et al: Liver and intestinal lactate metabolism in patients with acute hepatic failure undergoing liver transplantation, *Crit Care Med* 29:2111, 2001.
158. Meszaros K, Bojta J, Bautista AP, et al: Glucose utilization by Kupffer cells, endothelial cells, and granulocytes in endotoxemic rat liver, *Am J Physiol* 260:G7, 1991.
159. Walsh TS, McLellan S, Mackenzie SJ, et al: Hyperlactatemia and pulmonary lactate production in patients with fulminant hepatic failure, *Chest* 116:471, 1999.
160. Yousef E, McGeady SJ: Lactic acidosis and status asthmaticus: how common in pediatrics? *Ann Allergy Asthma Immunol* 89:585, 2002.
161. Mountain RD, Heffner JE, Brackett Jr NC, et al: Acid-base disturbances in acute asthma, *Chest* 98:651, 1990.
162. Rodrigo GJ, Rodrigo C: Elevated plasma lactate level associated with high dose inhaled albuterol therapy in acute severe asthma, *Emerg Med J* 22:404, 2005.
163. Manthous CA: Lactic acidosis in status asthmaticus, *Chest* 119:1599, 2001.
164. Perez A, Minces PG, Schnitzler EJ, et al: Jugular venous oxygen saturation or arteriovenous difference of lactate content and outcome in children with severe traumatic brain injury, *Pediatr Crit Care Med* 4:33, 2003.
165. Utenberg AW, Stover J, Kress B, et al: Edema and brain trauma, *Neuroscience* 129:1021, 2004.
166. Krause DS, Wolf BA, Shaw LM: Acute aspirin overdose: mechanisms of toxicity, *Ther Drug Monit* 14:1441, 1991.
167. Leatherman JW, Schmitz PG: Fever, hyperdynamic shock, and multiple-system organ failure. A pseudo-sepsis syndrome associated with chronic salicylate intoxication, *Chest* 100:1391, 1991.
168. Anonymous: The colon, the rumen, and D-lactic acidosis, *Lancet* 336:599, 1990.
169. Uribarri J, Oh MS, Carroll HJ: D-lactic acidosis. A review of clinical presentation, biochemical features, and pathophysiologic mechanisms, *Medicine* (Baltimore) 77:73, 1998.
170. DuBose TD Jr: Metabolic acidosis and alkalosis. In Fink MP, Abraham E, Vincent JL et al, editors: *Textbook of critical care,* ed 5, Philadelphia, 2005, Elsevier Saunders.
171. Kalhoff H, Diekmann L, Hettrich B, et al: Modified cow's milk formula with reduced renal acid load preventing incipient late metabolic acidosis in premature infants, *J Pediatr Gastroenterol Nutr* 25:46, 1997.
172. Emmett M, Narins RG: Mixed-acid-base disorders. In Narins RG, editor: *Maxwell & Kleeman's clinical disorders of fluid and electrolyte metabolism,* ed 5, New York, 1994, McGraw-Hill.
173. Miller L, Waters JH: Mechanism of hyperchloremic nonanion gap acidosis, *Anesthesiology* 87:1009, 1997.
174. Battle D, Flores G: Underlying defects in distal renal tubular acidosis: new understandings, *Am J Kidney Dis* 27:869, 1996.
175. Igarashi T, Sekine T, Watanabe H: Molecular basis of proximal renal tubular acidosis, *J Nephrol* 15(suppl 5):S135, 2002.
176. Bergstein JM: Renal tubular acidosis. In Behrman RE, Kliegman RM, Jenson HB, editors: *Nelson textbook of pediatrics,* ed 16, Philadelphia, 2000, WB Saunders.
177. Root AW, Shulman DI: Clinical adrenal disorders. In Pescovitz OH, Eugster EA, editors: *Pediatric endocrinology: mechanisms, manifestations, and management.* Philadelphia, 2004, Lippincott Williams & Wilkins.
178. Battle DC, Hizon M, Cohen E, et al: The use of the urinary anion gap in the diagnosis of hyperchloremic metabolic acidosis, *N Engl J Med* 318:594, 1988.
179. Story DA, Liskaser F, Bellomo R: Saline infusion, acidosis, and the Stewart approach, *Anesthesiology* 92:624, 2000.
180. Fanos V, Cataldi L: Amphotericin B-induced nephrotoxicity: a review, *Chemother* 12:463, 2000.
181. Goldman RD, Koren G: Amphotericin B toxicity in children, *J Pediatr Hematol Oncol* 26:421, 2004.
182. Hanna JD, Scheinman JI, Chan JC: The kidney in acid-base balance, *Pediatr Clin North Am* 42:1365, 1995.
183. Harbarth S, Pestotnik SL, Lloyd JF, et al: The epidemiology of nephrotoxicity associated with conventional amphotericin B therapy, *Am J Med* 111:528, 2001.
184. Holler B, Omar SA, Farid MD, et al: Effects of fluid and electrolyte management on amphotericin B-induced nephrotoxicity among extremely low birth weight infants, *Pediatrics* 113: e608, 2004.
185. Sawaya BP, Briggs JP, Schnermann J: Amphotericin B toxicity: the adverse consequences of altered membrane properties, *J Am Soc Nephrol* 6:154, 1995.
186. Hemstreet BA: Antimicrobal-associated renal tubular acidosis, *Ann Pharmacother* 38:1031, 2004.
187. Filippi L, Bagnoli F, Margollici M, et al: Pathogenic mechanism, prophylaxis, and therapy of symptomatic acidosis induced by acetazolamide, *J Investig Med* 50:125, 2002.
188. Adrogué HJ, Rashad MN, Gorin AB, et al: Assessing acid-base status in circulatory failure. Differences between arterial and central venous blood, *N Engl J Med* 320:1312, 1989.
189. Bonventre JV, Cheung JY: Effects of metabolic acidosis on viability of cells exposed to anoxia, *Am J Physiol* 1985; 249: C149.
190. Yildizdas D, Yapicioglu H, Yilmaz HL, et al: Correlation of simultaneously obtained capillary, venous, and arterial blood gases op patients in a paediatric intensive care unit, *Arch Dis Child* 89:176, 2004.
191. Biebuyck JF: Sodium bicarbonate in the treatment of subtypes of acute lactic acidosis: physiologic considerations, *Anesthesiology* 72:1064, 1990.
192. Hindman BJ: Sodium bicarbonate in the treatment of subtypes of acute lactic acidosis: physiologic considerations, *Anesthesiology* 72:1064, 1990.
193. Narins RG, Cohen JJ: Bicarbonate therapy for organic acidosis: the case for its continued use, *Ann Intern Med* 106:615, 1987.

194. Ammari AN, Schulze KF: Uses and abuses of sodium bicarbonate in the neonatal intensive care unit, *Curr Opin Pediatr* 14:151, 2002.
195. Levy MM: An evidence-based evaluation of the use of sodium bicarbonate during cardiopulmonary resuscitation, *Crit Care Clin* 14:457, 1998.
196. Cooper DJ, Walley KR, Wiggs BR, et al: Bicarbonate does not improve hemodynamics in critically ill patients who have lactic acidosis. A prospective, controlled clinical study, *Ann Intern Med* 112:492, 1990.
197. Levraut J, Giunti C, Ciebiera J-P, et al: Initial effect of sodium bicarbonate on intracellular pH depends on the extracellular non-bicarbonate buffering capacity, *Crit Care Med* 29:1033, 2001.
198. Cuhaci B, Lee J, Ahmed Z: Sodium bicarbonate and intracellular acidosis: myth or reality? *Crit Care Med* 29:1088, 2001.
199. Hazinski MF, Zaristsky A, Nadkarni VM, et al, editors: PALS Provider Manual. Chapter 5: Fluid therapy and medications for shock and cardiac arrest. Dallas: American Heart Association. 2002: 27.
200. Lawn C, Weir F, McGuire W: Base administration or fluid bolus for preventing morbidity and mortality in preterm infants with metabolic acidosis, *Cochrane Database Syst Rev* 18:CD003215, 2005.
201. Ritter JM, Doktor HS, Benjamin N: Paradoxical effect of bicarbonate on cytoplasmic pH, *Lancet* 335:1243, 1990.
202. Waters JH, Gottlieb A, Sprung J: Bicarbonate administration is potentially harmful in patients with moderate acidosis, *Anesth Analg* 95:256, 2002.
203. Sun JH, Filley GF, Hord K, et al: Carbicarb: an effective substitute for HCO_3^- for the treatment of acidosis, *Surgery* 102:835, 1987.
204. Kucera RR, Shapiro JI, Whalen MA, et al: Brain effects of HCO_3^- and Carbicarb in lactic acidosis, *Crit Care Med* 17: 1320, 1989.
205. Kette F, Weil MH, von Planta M, et al: Buffer agents do not reverse intramyocardial acidosis during cardiac resuscitation, *Circulation* 81:1660, 1990.
206. Shangraw RE, Jahoor F: Mechanism of dichloroacetate-induced hypolactatemia in humans with or without cirrhosis, *Metabolism* 53:1087, 2004.
207. Stacpoole PW: The pharmacology of dichloroacetate, *Metabolism* 38:1124, 1989.
208. Stacpoole W, Lorenz AC, Thomas RG, et al: Dichloroacetate in the treatment of lactic acidosis, *Ann Intern Med* 108:58, 1988.
209. Stacpoole PW, Wright EC, Baumgartner TG, et al: A controlled clinical trial of dichloroacetate for treatment of lactic acidosis in adults. The Dichloroacetate-Lactic Acidosis Study Group. *N Engl J Med* 327:1564, 1992.
210. Duncan GE, Perkins LA, Theriaque DW, et al: Dichloroacetate therapy attenuates the blood lactate response to submaximal exercise in patients with defects in mithocondrial energy metabolism, *J Clin Endocrinol Metab* 89:1733, 2004.
211. Stacpoole PW, Barnes CL, Hurbanis MD, et al: Treatment of congenital lactic acidosis with dichloroacetate, *Arch Dis Child* 77:535, 1997.
212. Stacpoole PW, Nagaraja NV, Hutson AD: Efficacy of dichloroacetate as a lactate-lowering drug, *J Clin Pharmacol* 43:683, 2003.
213. Agbenyega T, Planche T, Bedu-Addo G, et al: Population kinetics, efficacy, and safety of dichloroacetate for lactic acidosis due to severe malaria in children, *J Clin Pharmacol* 43:386, 2003.
214. Bellomo R, D'Intini V, Ronco C: Renal replacement therapy in the ICU. In Fink MP, Abraham E, Vincent JL et al, editors: *Textbook of critical care,* ed 5, Philadelphia, 2005, Elsevier Saunders.
215. Tan HK, Bellomo R: The effect of continuous hemofiltration on acid-base physiology, *Curr Opin Crit Care* 5:443, 1999.
216. Hodgkin JE, Soeprono FF, Chan DM: Incidence of metabolic alkalemia in hospitalized patients, *Crit Care Med* 8:725, 1980.
217. Anderson LE, Henrich WL: Alkalemia-associated morbidity and mortality in medical and surgical patients, *South Med J* 80: 729, 1987.
218. Galla JH: Metabolic alkalosis, *J Am Soc Nephrol* 11:369, 2000.
219. Jacobson HR, Seldin DW: On the generation, maintenance, and correction of metabolic alkalosis, *Am J Physiol* 244:F425, 1983.
220. Galla JH, Bonduris DN, Luke RG: Effects of chloride and extracellular fluid volume on bicarbonate reabsorption along the nephron in metabolic alkalosis in the rat: reassessment of the classical hypothesis of the pathogenesis of metabolic alkalosis, *J Clin Invest* 80:41, 1987.
221. Sabatini S, Kurtzman NA: The maintenance of metabolic alkalosis: factors which decrease bicarbonate excretion, *Kidney Int* 25: 357, 1984.
222. Norris SH, Kurtzman NA: Does chloride play an independent role in the pathogenesis of metabolic alkalosis? *Semin Nephrol* 8:101, 1988.
223. Mersin SS, Ramelli GP, Laux-End R, et al: Urinary chloride excretion distinguishes between renal and extrarenal metabolic alkalosis, *Eur J Pediatr* 154:979, 1995.
224. Devendra D, Rowe PA: Unexplained hypokalemia and metabolic alkalosis, *Postgrad Med J* 77:e4, 2001.
225. Rodriguez-Soriano J, Vallo A: Salt-losing nephropathy associated with inappropriate secretion of atrial natriuretic peptide? A new clinical syndrome, *Pediatr Nephrol* 11:565, 1997.
226. Schurman SJ, Shoemaker LR: Bartter and Gitelman syndromes, *Adv Pediatr* 47:223, 2000.
227. Fustik S, Pop-Jordanova, Slaveska N, et al: Metabolic alkalosis with hypoelectrolytemia in infants with cystic fibrosis, *Pediatr Int* 44:289, 2002.
228. Badawi MH, Zaki M, Ismail EA, et al: Congenital chloride diarrhea in Kuwait: a clinical reappraisal, *J Trop Pediatr* 44: 296-299, 1998.
229. Knutson OH: New method for administration of hydrochloric acid in metabolic alkalosis, *Lancet* 1:953, 1983.
230. Bureau MA, Lupien L, Begin R: Neural drive and ventilatory strategy of breathing in normal children, and in patients with cystic fibrosis and asthma, *Pediatrics* 68:187, 1981.
231. Chen ML, Keens TG: Congenital central hypoventilation syndrome: not just another rare disorder, *Paediatr Respir Rev* 5:182, 2004.
232. Macey PM, Woo MA, Macey KE, et al: Hypoxia reveals posterior thalamic, cerebellar, midbrain, and limbic deficits in congenital central hypoventilation syndrome, *J Appl Physiol* 98:958, 2005.
233. Gennari FJ: Respiratory acidosis and alkalosis. In Narins RG, editor: *Maxwell & Kleeman's clinical disorders of fluid and electrolyte metabolism,* ed 5, New York, 1994, McGraw-Hill.
234. Blum RH, McGowan FX Jr: Chronic upper airway obstruction and cardiac dysfunction: anatomy, pathophysiology, and anaesthetic implications, *Pediatr Anaesth* 14:75, 2004.
235. Francois G, Culée C: Le syndrome d'apnées obstructives liées au sommeil chez le nourrisson et l'enfant. [Obstructive sleep apnea syndrome in infants and children], *Arch Pediatr* 2000; 7:1088-1102.
236. Chien JW, Ciufo R, Novak R, et al: Uncontrolled oxygen administration and respiratory failure in acute asthma, *Chest* 117:728, 2000.
237. Schiff M: Control of breathing in asthma, *Clin Chest Med* 1:85, 1980.
238. Rodrigo GJ, Rodrigo C, Werner HA: Status asthmaticus in children: evidence-based recommendations, *Chest* 121: 667, 2002.
239. Rodrigo GJ, Rodríguez-Verde M, Peregalli V, et al: Effects of short-term 28% and 100% oxygen on $PaCO_2$ and peak expiratory flow rate in acute asthma, *Chest* 124:1312, 2003.
240. Wallis C: Non-invasive home ventilation, *Paediatr Respir Rev* 1:165, 2000.
241. Ting JY: Hypercapnia and oxygen therapy in older asthmatic patients, *Eur J Emerg Med* 11:355, 2004.
242. Priestley MA, Helfaer MA: Approaches in the management of acute respiratory failure in children, *Curr Opin Pediatr* 16: 293-298, 2004.
243. Akingbola OA, Hopkins RL: Pediatric noninvasive ventilation, *Pediatr Crit Care Med* 2:164-169, 2001.
244. Madden BP, Kariyawasam H, Siddiqi AJ, et al: Noninvasive ventilation in cystic fibrosis patients with acute or chronic respiratory failure, *Eur Respir J* 19:310, 2002.
245. Padman R, Lawless ST, Kettrick RG: Noninvasive ventilation via bilevel positive airway pressure support in pediatric practice, *Crit Care Med* 26:169-173, 1998.
246. International Consensus Conferences in Intensive Care Medicine: Noninvasive positive pressure ventilation in acute respiratory failure, *Am J Respir Crit Care Med* 163:283, 2001.
247. Keenan SP, Brake D: An evidence-based approach to noninvasive ventilation in acute respiratory failure, *Crit Care Clin* 14: 359, 1998.

248. Lightowler JV, Wedzicha JA, Elliott MW, et al: Non-invasive positive pressure ventilation to treat respiratory failure resulting from exacerbations of chronic obstructive pulmonary disease: Cochrane systematic review and meta-analysis, *BMJ* 326:185, 2003.
249. Carvalho WB, Fonseca MCM: Noninvasive ventilation in pediatrics: we still do not have a consistent base, *Pediatr Crit Care Med* 5:408, 2004.
250. Bach JR, Niranjan V, Weaver B: Spinal muscular atrophy type 1. A noninvasive respiratory management approach, *Chest* 117: 1100, 2000.
251. Laffey JG, O'Croinin D, McLoughlin P, et al: Permissive hypercapnia—role in protective lung ventilatory strategies, *Intensive Care Med* 30:347, 2004.
252. Thill PJ, McGuire JK, Baden HP, et al: Noninvasive positive-pressure ventilation in children with lower airway obstruction, *Pediatr Crit Care Med* 5:337, 2004.
253. Vermeulen F, de Halleux Q, Ruiz N, et al: Ventilation non invasive en réanimation pédiatrique: un debut d'expérience [Starting experience with non-invasive ventilation in paediatric intensive care unit], *Ann Fr Anesth Reanim* 22:716, 2003.
254. Makhoul IR, Bar-Joseph G, Blazer S, et al: Intratracheal pulmonary ventilation in premature infants and children with intractable hypercapnia, *ASAIO J* 44:82, 1998.
255. Conrad SA, Zwischenberger JB, Grier LR, et al: Total extracorporeal arteriovenous carbon dioxide removal in acute respiratory failure: a phase I clinical study, *Intensive Care Med* 27:1340, 2001.
256. The Acute Respiratory Distress Syndrome Network: Ventilation with lower tidal volumes as compared with traditional tidal volumes for acute lung injury and the acute respiratory distress syndrome, *N Engl J Med* 342:1301, 2000.
257. Marraro GA: Innovative practices of ventilatory support with pediatric patients, *Pediatr Crit Care Med* 4:8, 2003.
258. Redding GJ: Current concepts in adult respiratory distress syndrome in children, *Curr Opin Pediatr* 13:261, 2001.
259. Sheridan RL, Kacmarek RM, McEttrick MM, et al: Permissive hypercapnia as a ventilatory strategy in burned children: effect on barotrauma, pneumonia, and mortality, *J Trauma* 39:854, 1995.
260. Ware LB, Matthay MA: Medical progress: the acute respiratory distress syndrome, *N Engl J Med* 342:1334, 2000.
261. Carlo WA, Stark AR, Wright LL, et al: Minimal ventilation to prevent bronchopulmonary dysplasia in extremely low birth weight infants, *J Pediatr* 141:370, 2002.
262. Kamper J, Feilberg JN, Jorgensen N, et al; Danish ETFOL Study Group. The Danish National Study in infants with extremely low gestational age and birthweight (the ETFOL study): respiratory morbidity and outcome, *Acta Paediatr* 2004; 93:225.
263. Frey B: Hypercapnic acidosis is mostly good for critically ill children: Also after cardiopulmonary bypass? *Crit Care Med* 33:1154, 2005.
264. Li J, Hoskote A, Hickey C, et al: Effect of carbon dioxide on systemic oxygenation, oxygen consumption, and blood lactate levels after bidirectional superior cavopulmonary anastomosis, *Crit Care Med* 33:984, 2005.
265. Mazzeo AT, Spada A, Pratico C, et al: Hypercapnia: what is the limit in paediatric patients? A case of near-fatal asthma successfully treated by multipharmacological approach, *Paediatr Anaesth* 14:596, 2004.
266. Tasker RC, Peters MJ: Combined lung injury, meningitis, and cerebral edema: how permissive can hypercapnia be? *Intensive Care Med* 24:616, 1998.
267. Weber T, Tschemich H, Sitzwohl C, et al: Thrometamine buffer modifies the depressant effect of permissive hypercapnia on myocardial contractility in patients with acute respiratory distress syndrome, *Am J Respir Crit Care Med* 162:1361, 2000.
268. Kallet RH, Jasmer RM, Luce JM, et al: The treatment of acidosis in acute lung injury with tris-hydroxymetheyl aminomethane (THAM), *Am J Respir Crit Care Med* 161:1149, 2000.
269. Greisen G, Vannucci RC: Is periventricular leucomalacia a result of hypoxic-ischemic injury? Hypocapnia and the preterm brain, *Biol Neonate* 79:194, 2001.
270. Skippen P, Seear M, Poskitt K, et al: Effect of hyperventilation on regional cerebral blood flow in head-injured children, *Crit Care Med* 25:1402, 1997.
271. Krapf R, Beeler I, Hertner D, et al: Chronic respiratory alkalosis: the effect of sustained hyperventilation on renal regulation of acid-base equilibrium, *N Engl J Med* 324:1394, 1991
272. Adrogué HJ, Rashad MN, Gorin AB, et al: Arteriovenous acid-base disparity in circulatory failure: studies on mechanism, *Am J Physiol* 257:F1087, 1989.
273. Bakker J, Vincent JL, Gris P, et al: Veno-arterial carbon dioxide gradient in human septic shock, *Chest* 101:509, 1992.
274. Weil MH, Rackow EC, Trevino R, et al: Difference in acid-base state between venous and arterial blood during cardiopulmonary resuscitation, *N Engl J Med* 315:153, 1986.
275. Slomovitz BM, Lavery RF, Tortella B, et al: Validation of a hand-held lactate device in determination of blood lactate in critically injured patients, *Crit Care Med* 26:1523, 1998.
276. Zander R, Lang W: Base excess and strong ion difference: clinical limitations related to inaccuracy, *Anesthesiology* 100:459, 2004.
277. Story DA, Poustie S, Bellomo R: Comparison of three methods to estimate plasma bicarbonate in critically ill patients: Henderson-Hasselbalch, Enzymatic, and Strong-Ion-Gap, *Anaesth Intensive Care* 29:585, 2001.
278. Brill SA, Stewart TA, Brundage SI, et al: Base deficit does not predict mortality when secondary to hyperchloremic acidosis, *Shock* 17:459, 2002.
279. Watson PD. Modeling the effects of proteins on pH in plasma, *J Appl Physiol* 86:1421, 1999.

SOME USEFUL RESOURCES ON THE WORLD WIDE WEB

(a) Using Stewart for clinical gain! The Worldwide Intensivist. *http://www.anaesthesist.com/icu/elec/ionz/useful1.htm* A place for practical acid-base understanding, using Stewart's approach. Useful links. It is a good place for beginners.

(b) The physicochemical approach to acid-base (Putting things together). *http://www.anaesthesist.com/icu/elec/ionz/.htm* Also a good place. In spite of rather passionate argumentation, it is mandatory for approaching the physical-chemical approach!!

(c) A basic approach to body pH. The Worldwide Intensivist. *http://www.anaesthesist.com/icu/elec/ionz/Stewart.htm* A place with good academic level and easy-to-read reviews, with emphatic defense of the physicochemical approach. Includes some useful tools for calculating SID and several interesting links.

(d) All about physical-chemical approach including original work by Stewart.
http://www.acidbase.org A place for acid-base fans (i.e., physical chemical approach fans). Good contents (including tutorials, cases and access to original articles) and links. A full Internet edition adapted from the 1981 publication of Peter A. Stewart's classic *How to Understand Acid-Base* is available free!!

(e) Acid Base Physiology. *http://www.anaesthesiamcq.com/AcidBaseBook/ABindex.php* An unforgivable. Includes traditional and quantitative approaches.

(f) Acid-Base Tutorial. *http://www.acid-base.com* A complete review of traditional and physical-chemical approaches. Good contests, several interactive simulators.

(g) The acid base pHorum. *http://www.ccm.upmc.edu/education/resources/pHorum/htlm* Provided by the University of Pittsburgh's Department of Critical Care Medicine and run by John Kellum. That tells everything. Wonderful, truly scientific place with reviews, examples, tools (SIG calculator), links, and more. It is devoted to Stewart's (and Kellum's) approach. Contributions by Fencl, Figge, and other authors can be accessed through an excellent set of references.

(h) The Figge-Fencl quantitative physicochemical model of human acid-base physiology. *http://www.figgefencl.org* Excellent reviews and tutorials.

CHAPTER

62

Tests of Renal Function

Wayne R. Waz

PEARLS

- Current methods for accurately determining renal function at the bedside need to be improved.
- The use of plasma creatinine in empirical equations for estimation of glomerular filtration rate (GFR), combined with Doppler ultrasound imaging, provides practical bedside assessment of renal status in patients in the intensive care unit (ICU).
- Early detection of impending renal insufficiency may lead to earlier hemodynamic and pharmacological interventions and improve outcomes.
- The use of cystatin C as a plasma marker and the use of combined clinical and laboratory scoring systems may help achieve the goal of early detection.

Glomerular Function

Acute renal failure (ARF) associated with multiple organ dysfunction syndrome is a major cause of death in critically ill patients. Earlier detection of impending renal failure may improve outcomes: it allows earlier intervention with dialysis or continuous renal replacement therapies along with application of newer pharmacological interventions designed to prevent, delay, or repair renal damage. Essential to assessment of renal status is the accurate and reproducible measurement of glomerular filtration rate (GFR). Gold standard measurement of GFR with inulin clearance is time consuming, technically impractical, and expensive; thus any attempts to assess GFR necessarily involve estimates. Each of the GFR measurement estimates discussed later has technical or clinical limitations, some of which may be more relevant in the ICU setting than in other settings, such as monitoring of chronic renal insufficiency, answering research questions, or aiding in decisions about initiation of end-stage renal disease therapies. Unfortunately, most currently available methods of estimation favor long-term measurement of renal function, detecting relatively large changes over weeks or months, and their shortcomings become particularly obvious in the critical care setting. The ideal GFR measurement in the ICU should include the following characteristics:

1. Able to measure early changes in GFR
2. Able to measure small changes over relatively short periods (hours and days as opposed to weeks or months), with rapid result turnaround time
3. Able to aid in medication dosing, particularly medications for which blood levels are not readily available
4. Not influenced by patient volume status
5. Not influenced by patient nutritional status
6. Reliable for pediatric patients
7. Minimally invasive
8. Inexpensive

Although no currently available method addresses all of these needs, it is useful to consider each one's strengths and weaknesses (Table 62–1). Currently available measurement techniques include clearance techniques, estimate of clearance with plasma markers, enhanced estimate of clearance with plasma markers with empirical equations, and imaging techniques. Regardless of the technique used, the goal is to estimate GFR, with normal pediatric values on the basis of age (Table 62–2).

TABLE 62-1

Comparison of Glomerular Filtration Rate Determination Methods

Method	Detect early and small changes	Assist medication dosing	Independent of volume status	Independent of nutritional status	Reliable in pediatrics	Minimally invasive	Inexpensive
C_{inulin}	+	+++	+++	+++	+++	+	+
$C_{creatinine}$	+	++	+	+	++	++	+++
$C_{iohexol}$	+	++	+	+++	+++	++	+
$C_{isotope}$	+	++	+	+++	+++	++	+
C_{drug}	+	++	+	+++	?	++	++
$P_{creatinine}$	+	++	+	+	++	+++	+++
$P_{cystatin\ C}$	+++	++	+++	+++	+++	+++	?
Schwartz*	+	++	+	+	+++	+++	+++
Leger†	+	++	+	+	+++	+++	+++
Cockroft-Gault‡	+	++	+	+	++	+++	+++
MDRD§	+	++	+	+	+	+++	+++

Data modified from *Schwartz GJ, Brion L, Spitzer A: The use of plasma creatinine concentration for estimating glomerular filtration rate in infants, children, and adolescents, *Pediatr Clin North Am* 34:571, 1987; †Leger F, Bouissou F, Coulais Y et al: Estimation of glomerular filtration rate in children, *Pediatr Nephrol* 17:903-907, 2002; ‡Cockroft DW, Gault MH: Prediction of creatinine clearance from serum creatinine, *Nephron* 16:31-41, 1976; §Gault MH, Longerich LL, Harnett JD et al: Predicting glomerular function from adjusted serum creatinine, *Nephron* 62:249-256, 1992 and Levey AS, Bosch JP, Lewis JB et al: A more accurate method to estimate glomerular filtration rate from serum creatinine: a new prediction equation, *Ann Intern Med* 130: 461-470, 1999
MDRD, Modification of Diet in Renal Disease Study.

Clearance Techniques: Inulin, Creatinine, Isotope, Iohexol, and Drugs

Glomerular filtration is traditionally measured as plasma clearance of a substance that is freely filtered at the glomerulus and is neither secreted nor absorbed by the renal tubules. The ideal substance, which either is intrinsic to the patient or is introduced intravenously, also maintains plasma levels that are independent of the patient's volume and nutritional status. Clearance of any substance (x) is measured with the equation:

$$C_x = U_x V / P_x$$

where C_x = clearance of x, U_x = urine concentration of x, V = urine flow rate (milliliter per minute), and P_x = plasma concentration of x. (Note that urine and plasma concentrations of x must be in the same units.) Clearances in humans are traditionally measured in ml/minute, representing the volume of plasma cleared of the substance of interest per minute, and normalized to a body surface area of 1.73 m^2.

Although inulin clearance remains the gold standard for definitive measurement of GFR, the technique is impractical; it requires continuous infusion of inulin to maintain a constant plasma level, accurately timed blood and urine levels, urinary catheterization, water diuresis, and laborious laboratory measurement techniques. It is not currently used in clinical practice.

Creatinine clearance, traditionally measured over 24 hours (although some investigators have studied times as short as 30 minutes for critically ill patients) is widely available and easily measured. The major obstacle is the inability to accurately collect a timed urine specimen. Creatinine clearance is measured with the following equation:

$$(U_{creatinine} \times U_{volume}) / (P_{creatine} \times \text{time}) \times 1.73\ m^2 / \text{Patient's BSA}$$

Where:
$U_{creatine}$ and $P_{creatine}$ are in mg/dl
U_{volume} is in ml
Time is in minutes

TABLE 62–2

Normal Values of Glomerular Filtration Rate[43]

Age		GFR-mean (ml/min/1.73m²)	GFR-range (ml/min/1.73m²)
Neonates <34 wk gestational age	2-8 days	11	11-15
	4-28 days	20	15-28
	30-90 days	50	40-65
Neonates >34 wk gestational age	2-8 days	39	17-60
	4-28 days	47	26-68
	30-90 days	58	30-86
1-6 mo		70	39-114
6-12 mo		103	49-157
12-19 mo		127	62-191
2 yr-adult		127	89-165

GFR, glomerular filtration rate.

Urine collection should start with an empty bladder, be timed to the nearest minute, and include urine voided at the end of the collection period. For patients with rapidly changing plasma creatinine values, measure at the beginning and end of collection period and average the values. Urine collection times shorter than 24 hours, ranging from 30 minutes to 3 hours,[1] have proved reliable and reproducible and may justify the added effort in select patients for whom accurate estimation of true GFR, rather than monitoring of individual patient changes over time, is important. Creatinine clearance following treatment with cimetidine, a substance that blocks tubular secretion of creatinine and thus improves accuracy of GFR determination, correlates well with inulin clearance with urine collection times as short as 2 hours.[2]

Isotope clearance studies, including chromium-labeled ethylenediamine tetraacetic acid (^{51}Cr-EDTA), ^{99m}Tc-diethylenetriaminepentaacetic acid (DTPA), ^{99m}Tc-mercaptoacetyltriglycine (MAG3), ^{125}I-iothalamate, and iodothalamate are accurate, and clearance values may be obtained either with plasma clearance studies or with gamma-camera imaging disappearance curves.[3] All of these substances, like inulin, meet the ideal criteria for accurate estimation of GFR. Furthermore, isotope clearance methods do not require urine collection and can be calculated with relatively few blood samples. Edema and third-space fluid loss, common in the ICU setting, however, impairs the accuracy of isotope methods because tracers have an increased volume of distribution. Despite advantages, more widespread clinical use is hampered by radiation exposure (for both patients and for staff handling specimens), the need for multiple blood samples, and cost. Detailed guidelines for the use of isotope clearance studies in children have been published.[4]

Plasma clearance of the contrast medium iohexol can also be used to estimate GFR. Like inulin and the radionuclide substances, iohexol is an ideal molecule for measurement of GFR, and laboratory measurement methods do not require the use of radiation. Like measurement with the isotope methods, however, accurate measurement of GFR requires multiple blood samples, particularly for patients with a GFR less than 40 ml/min,[5] and currently, iohexol measurement is not widely available for most ICUs.

Clearance of drugs with elimination primarily through glomerular filtration may be used to estimate GFR. Aminoglycoside plasma clearance estimates GFR with less error than the Cockroft-Gault equation[6] and can provide additional information for patients receiving those drugs. No pediatric data are available.

In general, clearance studies provide the most accurate measurement of GFR[7] but are not sufficiently superior to plasma markers, particularly when used with empirical equations, to justify the added effort and expense. In a study directly comparing 30-minute creatinine clearance, 24-hour creatinine clearance, and estimation using the Cockroft-Gault equation to inulin clearance in adult medical ICU patients, Robert et al[8] found that the Cockroft-Gault equation (using clinical adjustments: see Table 62–3) resulted in more accurate prediction of GFR than either 30-minute or 24-hour creatinine clearances. This study, however, included only hemodynamically stable patients at one point in time, and others have argued that creatinine clearances measured over short periods (30 to 120 minutes) may be more sensitive to early changes in GFR as renal function begins to deteriorate.[9] Whether the value of this information justifies the added effort and expense is still being studied.

Estimate of Clearance with Plasma Markers

The most commonly used and widely available estimate of GFR in clinical use is measurement of plasma creatinine. Although laboratory measurement of creatinine is fast, inexpensive, and readily available, problems with creatinine measurement exist. The main assumption that must be made when creatinine is used as a marker of GFR is that creatinine varies only as a result of changes in GFR. This assumption is not true, particularly for patients in the ICU. Serum creatinine represents equilibrium among production, glomerular filtration, and excretion. Both low and high intrinsic creatinine production influences plasma creatinine measurements. A low plasma creatinine clearance overestimates GFR for patients with poor nutritional status or prolonged immobilization, and a high creatinine clearance underestimates GFR in patients in catabolic states with rapid changes in muscle mass. For patients with unstable (and rapidly changing) renal function, creatinine measurements at one point in time may not correlate with a patient's current (real-time) renal function. Particularly important to note for patients early in their ICU course is that creatinine may remain at normal levels until the GFR falls below 50 ml/min/1.73 m^2. Creatinine is not only filtered at the glomerulus but is also secreted by renal tubules. Thus a lower serum value is created, and this value results in an overestimate of true GFR for patients with impaired renal function. Drugs that block tubular secretion of creatinine (e.g., trimethoprim, cimetidine, pyrimethamine, salicylates) will increase the serum creatinine value. In laboratories where the Jaffe reaction for creatinine determination is used, plasma chromogens (e. g., glucose, protein, keto acids, ascorbic acid, barbiturates, cephalosporin antibiotics) falsely increase values, particularly in patients with a low GFR. In laboratories where creatinine is measured with enzymatic methods, these drug interactions do not occur but may be influenced by flucytosine and by plasma glucose concentrations greater than 1000 mg/dl.[10] Creatinine has sites of extrarenal elimination, particularly metabolism by intestinal flora, resulting in overestimates of GFR. Despite these limitations, measurement of serum creatinine remains the most widely used method of estimating GFR in the clinical setting.

Cystatin C is gaining interest as a serum marker of GFR. Cystatin C is a cysteine protease inhibitor with a low molecular weight (13.359 kDa) and 120 amino acid residues. In humans, it is found in all nucleated cells and is produced at a constant rate.[11] It is filtered by the glomerulus, with some tubular reabsorption and catabolism, and serum levels are highly correlated with GFR.[12] Serum cystatin C levels are sensitive to changes in GFR and to tubular damage. Urine concentration is low and measurement of urine concentration is difficult because of degradation, so urinary excretion and clearance values are unlikely to be clinically available. Nevertheless, because cystatin C provides GFR estimates that are independent of

TABLE 62–3

Empirical Equations for Estimating Renal Function

Schwartz*	GFR (ml/min/1.73 m^2)	$\frac{k \times \text{length (cm)}}{S_{Cr}\text{ (mg/dl)}}$
Leger	GFR (ml/min)	$\frac{[56.7 \times \text{body weight (kg)} + 0.142 \times \text{length (cm)}]}{P_{Cr}\ (\mu M)}$
Cockroft-Gault†	C_{Cr} (ml/min)	$\frac{(140\text{-age}) \times \text{weight (kg)} (\times 0.85 \text{ if female})}{72 \times S_{Cr}\text{ (mg/dl)}}$
MDRD	GFR (ml/min/1.73 m^2)	$170 \times S_{Cr}^{-0.999} \times BUN^{-0.170} \times Alb^{+0.318} \times age^{-0.176} \times (0.762 \text{ if female}) \times (1.180 \text{ if black})$

*k = a proportionality constant that is age dependent (k = 0.33 for low birth weight during first year of life, k = 0.45 for term AGA during first year of life, k = 0.55 for children older than 1 year and for adolescent girls, and k = 0.7 for adolescent boys).
† Use the lower of ideal or total body weight and the higher of actual serum creatinine or corrected creatinine to 1 mg/d (85 μmol/L). Modified from Cockroft DW, Gault MH: Prediction of creatinine clearance from serum creatinine, *Nephron* 16:31-41, 1976.
AGA, appropriate for gestational age; *Alb,* albumin; *BUN,* blood urea nitrogen; *C_{Cr},* creatinine clearance; *GFR,* glomerular filtration rate; *MDRD,* Modification of Diet in Renal Disease Study; *P_{Cr},* plasma creatinine; *S_{Cr},* serum creatinine.

sex, nutritional status, muscle mass, inflammatory states, fever, malignancy, and age, it may prove to be superior to creatinine in the ICU setting. A particular value in the ICU setting is the ability of cystatin C to measure smaller changes in GFR than can be detected by creatinine.[13]

Cystatin C levels may prove to be particularly valuable in infants. Fischbach et al[14] noted that infants younger than 18 months had higher mean values than older children. These values suggested the need for age-specific data for children younger than 18 months. Although creatinine values typically reach a nadir around 4 months of age and increase to adult values by ages 15 to 17, cystatin C levels are relatively high at birth (and higher in preterm than term neonates), fall over the first year of life, and then remain constant into and through adulthood. These levels more accurately reflect developmental changes in GFR seen in infancy and childhood.[15] Reference levels are currently being developed that confirm the finding of higher levels in premature and term neonates.[16-18] Uncertainty remains regarding the precise age at which adult reference levels may be used (probably somewhere between 1 and 3 years).

In some patients, cystatin C has proved to be superior to creatinine as a marker of small, early changes in GFR, such as in children with malignancy after induction chemotherapy,[19] patients with spinal cord injury,[20] elderly patients (ages 69 to 92 years),[21] patients with early diabetic nephropathy,[22,23] patients undergoing renal transplants,[24] and patients with spina bifida,[25] but it may not be reliable in patients with thyroid disease[26] or with ketoacidosis,[27] As more widespread and universally acceptable reference ranges are developed and laboratory techniques are standardized, clinical use of cystatin C should increase.

Enhanced Estimate of Clearance with Plasma Markers with Empirical Equations

The use of empirical equations improves the accuracy of creatinine-based GFR estimates; they provide closer approximations of true GFR than measurement of plasma creatinine alone (Table 62-3). Because most equations are based on some combination of height, ideal body weight, BSA, age, and sex, parameters that are unlikely to change during a typical ICU stay, they do not offer an improved ability to monitor for small and early changes in GFR. The most commonly used equation in pediatrics is the Schwartz formula.[28] More recently, Leger et al[29] used a population pharmacokinetic approach to improve the correlation of a plasma creatinine-based estimate when compared with a reference standard of ^{51}Cr-EDTA clearance, and showed the following:

$$\text{Estimated GFR} = [56.7 \times \text{body weight (kg)} + 0.142 \times \text{length (cm)}]/\text{plasma creatinine } (P_{Cr})\ (\mu\text{mol})$$

This equation produced estimates of GFR that were less biased and more precise than those obtained from the Schwartz formula. It also improves reliability over the Schwartz formula at those ages when a patient is in transition from one "k" value to another. In the Leger study, however, GFR data were obtained from patients with chronic renal disease, and Schwartz studied children with normal renal function. Further prospective study of the Leger formula is needed before its more widespread acceptance.

For adult patients, the most commonly used equations are the Cockroft-Gault equation,[30,31] which estimates creatinine clearance in milliliters per minute, and the more recently established equations from the Modification of Diet in Renal Disease Study (MDRD),[32,33] which estimate glomerular filtration rate in milliliters per minute per 1.73 m^2. Like the pediatric equations, all are limited by the use of serum creatinine as the primary marker of renal function. Modification of the Cockroft-Gault equation to account for the unique situation in patients in the ICU led to improved accuracy of the equation.[8] Robert et al recommend using the lower of ideal or total body weight and the higher of actual serum creatinine or corrected creatinine to 1 mg/dl (85 μmol/L). In a direct comparison of the Schwartz formula, Cockroft-Gault equation, and MDRD equations with inulin clearance in 198 children (two kidneys, one kidney, transplant kidney) and 116 adults (single kidney, transplant kidney), Pierrat et al[34] concluded that for all patients older than 12 years, the Cockroft-Gault equation provided the best estimate of GFR corrected for a BSA of 1.73 m^2, with 95% of the results between +40 ml/min/1.73 m^2 for children older than 12 years and +30 ml/min/1.73 m^2 for adults. No equation emerged as superior for children 12 years or younger, and a direct comparison between the Schwartz and Leger estimates is needed.

Because of the wide availability of computerized laboratory and patient information systems, many hospital laboratories are now reporting GFR or creatinine clearance in addition to serum creatinine values. It is important to check with the laboratory to see which equation is being used.

Because all empirical equations use serum creatinine as a marker of renal function, all are subject to the previously mentioned limitations of plasma creatinine as a marker of GFR. If plasma cystatin C measurement replaces creatinine measurement, new empirical formulas with cystatin C are likely to more accurately approximate true GFR, particularly in a typical patient in the ICU with rapidly changing hemodynamic, volume, and nutritional status. Comparison of the following cystatin C–based formula:

$$\log(\text{GFR}) = 1.962 + [1.123 \times \log(1/\text{cystatin C})]$$

with the Schwartz formula in 536 pediatric patients showed the cystatin C–based formula to be a better predictor of GFR,[35] although these results have not yet been duplicated.

Imaging Techniques: Doppler Ultrasound, Radionuclide Scans, and Functional Magnetic Resonance Imaging

Information from GFR estimates may be enhanced with imaging studies. Because of the inability of current techniques to detect early and small changes in renal function, functional imaging studies may emerge as a valuable tool. Currently available Doppler ultrasound can provide information about renal anatomy, vascular supply, cortical blood flow, and urine outflow obstruction. It is performed noninvasively at the patient's bedside with no radiation exposure, and it should be considered in any patient at risk for (or experiencing) renal insufficiency. With the development of contrast media for ultrasound and improved hardware and software, renal status may be able to be assessed with increasing resolution. As the ability to detect early changes in renal function improves, an earlier role for ultrasound may emerge. Studies should be performed to indicate whether baseline ultrasound studies at the time of ICU admission might be of value in patients whose history and reason for admission suggest a risk for progressive renal impairment.

Although able to provide detailed anatomical and functional information, radionuclide scanning requires that patients be transported to a site where gamma-camera scanning is available. Many patients who would benefit from such information are too unstable for transport. Radionuclide scans can be divided into two types: those that provide better functional information (dynamic imaging) and those that provide better anatomical definition (static imaging). Although the availability of the different isotopes varies by location, most functional studies are performed with technetium 99m-labeled DTPA or MAG3. Although both provide good dynamic and split renal function data, MAG3 provides better images in patients with decreased GFR. An advantage of DTPA, however, is that it is not significantly handled by the renal tubules; thus plasma clearances can be used to measure GFR. If better anatomical definition is needed, particularly diagnoses of cortical scarring or pyelonephritis, technetium 99m-labeled dimercaptosuccinic acid (DMSA) or glucoheptonate are preferred but do not provide functional data. In general, radionuclide scanning is useful for specific diagnosis of primary renal problems such as obstruction, renovascular hypertension, renal transplant imaging, and cortical scarring but provides little benefit over ultrasound in assessing patients in the ICU with ARF.[36]

Although not currently available for clinical use, emerging technologies in MRI angiography and three-dimensional imaging may provide rapid, accurate, and noninvasive assessment of GFR, regional renal blood flow, and renal parenchymal oxygenation status. These allow more complete evaluation of changes in renal status.[37,38]

The Present State and the Future of Glomerular Filtration Rate Measurement in Critical Care

The lack of progress in measuring GFR reflects the absence of improved outcomes for patients in the ICU with ARF over the past 30 years. Currently, measurement of creatinine, augmented with the use of empirical equations, comes closest to meeting all the criteria outlined at the beginning of the chapter (see Table 62–1). When more accurate measurement of GFR is needed, isotope or iohexol clearance techniques should be considered, although cost will be a barrier in many settings. Accuracy can be improved with the comparison of these methods with drug clearance studies for some pharmaceuticals, but currently pediatric data are lacking. Although cystatin C is superior to creatinine for most anticipated ICU uses, laboratory testing is not generally available for clinicians. Ultrasound with Doppler imaging remains an important component of renal status assessment. Although other imaging modalities may provide more detailed functional information, their practical utility is limited by the need to transport patients to an imaging site outside the ICU.

Current techniques for measuring changes in GFR do not meet the criteria outlined at the beginning of this chapter for predicting severity, duration, and need for (and timing of) interventions in patients in the ICU patients who have ARF. To improve the ability to predict and react to changes in renal function, Mehta and Chertow[39] (Table 62-4) have proposed a clinical and laboratory classification system similar to other organ-specific scoring systems. Their proposed classification scheme grades four categories:

1. Preexisting susceptibility to renal disease
2. The nature and timing of renal insult
3. The response of biomarkers of GFR, tubular damage, and physiological measures (urine output)
4. The end-organ consequences to nonrenal organs

If this or a similar classification scheme receives wide acceptance among clinicians and investigators, better

TABLE 62–4

Proposed Classification of Acute Renal Dysfunction[39]

Domain		Stage 1	Stage 2	Stage 3	Stage 4
Susceptibility		None	Known preexisting kidney disease (CKD stage 2)* baseline GFR 60 to 89 ml/min/1.73 m^2	Preexisting kidney disease (CKD stages 3 and above); baseline GFR <60 ml/min/ 1.73 m^2	Preexisting kidney disease (CKD stage 2 or 3 or above) GFR <89 ml/min/ 1.73 m^2 + presence of one risk factor†
Insult					
	Nature	Known	Known	Unknown	Unknown
	Timing	Within 24 hr	24-48 hr	>48 hr	Unknown
Response‡					
	Biomarker: creatinine, GFR	Creat increase 0.5 to 1 mg/dl, GFR decrease 25 to 49%	Creat increase 1 to 2 mg/dl, GFR decrease by 50 to 74%	Creat increase >2.0 mg/dl, GFR decrease >75%	Creat increase >3.0 mg/dl, GFR <10 ml/min/ 1.73 m^2
	Physiological: urine output	0.5 ml/kg/hr for 3 hr	<0.5 ml/kg/hr for 12 to 23 hr	0.3 ml/kg/hr for 24 hr or anuria for 12 hr	Anuria
End-organ consequences: nonrenal organs failing§		None	Single organ	Two organs	>2 organs

*K/DOQI Clinical Practice Guidelines for Chronic Kidney Disease (CKD).[44]
†Risk factors include diabetes mellitus with microalbuminuria, dehydration, multiple myeloma, congestive heart failure, and decompensated cirrhosis.
‡Based on consensus RIFLE criteria proposed by ADQI.[45]
§Respiratory, cerebrovascular, neurological, hematological, liver, on the basis of organ system failure criteria.
Creat, creatinine; *GFR,* glomerular filtration rate

data, better timing of interventions, and ultimately better outcomes for critically ill patients with ARF may be forthcoming. At the time of this writing, a specific classification system is not currently in widespread use. Nevertheless, evaluating patients with a combination of history, laboratory, and clinical measurements has intuitive value and may lead to earlier nephrology consultation and initiation of renal replacement therapies for selected patients, as well as improved timing regarding the use of emerging therapies targeted at ameliorating ARF. Of the four listed categories, the development of biomarkers other than creatinine, particularly cystatin C, is likely to significantly improve the ability to manage patients with impending renal failure. Further improvement in GFR estimation will include the use of improved empirical equations with newer biomarkers. The ability to detect early hemodynamic and toxic injury, thus the ability to predict ARF failure before any changes in biomarkers occur, will improve with the use of functional imaging studies.

Detection of Tubular Injury

Although GFR determination remains the most widespread index of renal function, assessment of renal tubular status contributes to the differential diagnosis of ARF and assists in clinical management. A common dilemma in the ICU is the distinction between prerenal azotemia and intrinsic renal acute tubular necrosis (ATN). This distinction is particularly relevant when hemodynamic and fluid management is planned. Tests for renal tubule damage include direct markers of tubular damage and functional tests; that is, those that distinguish whether the kidney is responding appropriately to nonrenal disturbances. Currently no direct markers of tubular damage are in widespread clinical use, but candidates currently under investigation include beta$_2$-microglobulin, retinol-binding protein, Clara cell protein, and beta-N-acetyl glucosaminidase.[40] In the absence of direct urine or blood tests for tubule damage, a combination of functional studies and clinical measurements is routinely used. Laboratory and clinical assessment is outlined in Table 62-5. Functional measurement is limited by the use of medications that alter tubule function, particularly diuretics that increase urinary sodium excretion (and thus the fractional excretion of sodium [FENa]) even in the face of decreased renal perfusion. A goal of ongoing research is to provide urine or plasma markers that improve the ability to localize primary sites of renal damage following different types of renal insult.

Another clinical setting in which tests of tubular function are needed occurs in patients with persistent normal anion gap metabolic acidosis (hyperchloremia). As with the distinction between prerenal azotemia and ATN,

TABLE 62–5

Dehydration/Reduced Renal Perfusion vs. Acute Tubular Necrosis

	Dehydration/ ↓↓perfusion		*Acute tubular necrosis*	
	Child	**Neonate**	**Child**	**Neonate**
U_{Na}(mEq/L)	<10	≤20	>50	>50
FENa (%)[1]	≤1	≤2.5	>2	>3
U_{osm}	≥500	≥350	≤300	≤300
U/P_{osm}	≥1.5	≥1.2	0.8-1.2	0.8-1.2
BUN/creat	>20	>10	Both ↑	Both ↑
Fluid push	Urine ⇑	Urine ⇑	No Δ	No Δ

*FENa = fractional excretion of sodium: $[(U_{Na} \times P_{creat}) / (P_{Na} \times U_{creat})] \times 100\%$.

BUN, blood urea nitrogen; *creat,* creatinine; U_{Na}, urinary sodium; U_{osm}, urinary osmolality; U/P_{osm}, urine and plasma osmolality.

an analogous distinction can be made between patients whose kidneys are responding appropriately to nonrenal acid production and those whose kidneys are contributing to the problem (renal tubular acidosis [RTA]). A complete discussion of RTA is beyond the scope of this section and has been reviewed in detail.[41,42] Methods for assessment of proximal and distal renal tubular acidification mechanisms are summarized in Table 62-6.

Routine urinalysis and microscopic examination of the urine should not be forgotten because they can provide clues to the different causes of renal damage (Table 62-7). For improved quantification of urinary protein excretion, without the need for timed urine collections, a spot urine protein/creatinine ratio correlates well with 24-hour urine protein excretion in children and adults. A normal protein/creatinine ratio is less than 0.20, with values from 0.21 to 2 considered to be moderate proteinuria and values greater than 2 considered to be in the nephrotic range. Magnesium, usually defined as urinary albumin excretion rates from 20 to 200 μg/min on a timed urine specimen (amounts below the detection limit of standard test strips), is commonly used to detect incipient renal disease in patients with diabetes mellitus and is being studied in patients with hypertension. Whether detection of microalbuminuria in the ICU setting may serve as an early indicator of tubular or glomerular damage needs to be studied.

Other Potentially Useful Renal Function Tests

Various clinical and laboratory findings may require the use of other renal function measurements. Although a discussion of the physiology behind these measurements is beyond the scope of this chapter, several commonly used equations are presented here for reference. For the following equations, Na^+, HCO_3^-, and Cl^- are measured in milliequivalents per liter; blood urea nitrogen (BUN) and glucose are measured in milligrams per deciliter; and all weights are in kilograms.

Anion gap (serum) = $[Na^+] - ([Cl^-] + [TCO_2])$

Corrected serum sodium in hyperglycemia = $[Na^+] + ([\text{glucose}] - 100) \times 1.6/100$

Calculated serum osmolality = $2 \times [Na^+] + [\text{glucose}]/18 + [\text{BUN}]/2.8$

Electrolyte deficit = (desired value − patient value) × weight × distribution factor

Distribution factor = 0.4-0.5 for HCO_3^-, 0.6-0.7 for Na^+, and 0.2-0.3 for Cl^-

Free water deficit = (Patient $[Na^+]$ − desired $[Na^+]$) / desired $[Na^+] \times 0.6 \times$ weight

TABLE 62–6

Evaluation of Renal Tubular Acidification Mechanisms

Proximal tubular function: Fractional Excretion of Bicarbonate $\frac{(U_{bicarbonate} \times P_{creatinine})}{(P_{bicarbonate} \times U_{creatinine})} \times 100\%$ Should be <15% in patients with corrected acidosis. Need plasma creatinine, plasma bicarbonate (from VBG or CBG), urine creatinine, urine bicarbonate (from urine collected anaerobically and sent to blood gas lab)	Distal tubular function: Urine anion gap: (Na + K) – CL If Na + K is lower than Cl, it suggests presence of another cation, presumably NH_4^+, and normal distal tubular acidification. If Na + K is greater than Cl, it suggests NH_4^+ and absence of possibility of distal RTA Urine-to-blood PCO_2 gradient = $UPCO_2 - B\ PCO_2$ In a patient with corrected acidosis, a difference of 20 or more suggests adequate distal tubular acidification. For this, urine PCO_2 is needed (collected anaerobically and sent to blood gas lab) and blood PCO_2 (from VBG or CBG)

Order the following to perform calculations: VBG or CBG; plasma creatinine; urine Na, K, Cl, and creatinine; and urine "gas." To obtain urine gas, either use catheterized specimen immediately collected in blood gas syringe and capped and processed as soon as possible, or for clean catch specimen, have patient void into container with mineral oil and collect urine into blood gas syringe from beneath mineral oil. The evaporation of carbon dioxide from specimen will alter results and make them uninterpretable.

CBG, capillary blood gases; *Cl,* chloride; *K,* potassium; *Na,* sodium; PCO_2, partial pressure of carbon dioxide; *RTA,* renal tubular acidosis; *VBG,* venous blood gases.

TABLE 62–7

Urinalysis Findings in Acute Renal Failure[46]

Prerenal azotemia	Acute Tubular Necrosis	Cortical Necrosis	Interstitial Nephritis	Glomerulonephritis	Obstruction
Increased specific gravity, normal urinalysis	Granular casts, epithelial cells, epithelial casts, pigmenturia	Gross or microscopic hematuria, proteinuria	Pyuria, WBC casts, eosinophiluria	Gross or microscopic hematuria, RBC casts, proteinuria	Normal urinalysis

RBC, red blood cell; *WBC* white blood cell.

REFERENCES

1. Herget-Rosenthal S, Kribben A, Pietruck F, et al: Two by two hour creatinine clearance-reproducible and valid, *Clin Nephrol* 51: 348-354, 1999.
2. Hellerstein S, Berenbom M, Alon US, et al: Creatinine clearance following cimetidine for estimation of glomerular filtration rate, *Pediatr Nephrol* 12:49-54, 1998.
3. Peters AM, Gordon I: Quantitative assessment of the urinary tract with radionuclides. In Barrat TM, Avner ED, Harmon WE, editors: *Pediatric nephrology,* ed 4, Baltimore, 1999, Williams and Wilkins.
4. Piepsz A, Colarinha P, Gordon I, et al: Paediatric Committee of the European Association of Nuclear Medicine: Guidelines for glomerular filtration rate determination in children, *Eur J Nucl Med* 28:BP31-BP36, 2001.
5. Gaspari F, Perico N, Remuzzi G: Measurement of glomerular filtration rate, *Kidney Int Suppl* 63: S151-S154, 1997.
6. Zarowitz BJ, Robert S, Peterson EL: Prediction of glomerular filtration rate using Aminoglycoside clearance in critically ill medical patients, *Ann Pharmacother* 26:1205-1210, 1992.
7. Hjorth L, Wiebe T, Karpman D: Correct evaluation of renal glomerular filtration rate requires clearance assays, *Pediatr Nephrol* 17:847-851, 2002.
8. Robert S, Zarowitz BJ, Peterson EL, et al: Predictability of creatinine clearance estimates in critically ill patients, *Crit Care Med* 21:1487-1495, 1993.
9. Sladen RN: Accurate estimation of glomerular filtration in the intensive care unit: another Holy Grail? *Crit Care Med* 21: 1424-1427, 1993.
10. Andreev E, Koopman M, Arisz L: A rise in plasma creatinine is not a sign of renal failure: which drugs can be responsible? *J Intern Med* 246:247-252, 1999.
11. Reed CH: Diagnostic applications of cystatin C, *Br J Biomed Sci* 57:323-329, 2000.
12. Randers E, Erlandsen EJ: Serum cystatin C as an endogenous marker of the renal function—a review, *Clin Chem Lab Med* 37(4): 389-395, 1999.
13. Dworkin LD: Serum cystatin C as a marker of glomerular filtration rate, *Curr Opin Nephrol Hypertens* 10:551-553, 2001.
14. Fischbach M, Graff V, Terzic J, et al: Impact of age on reference values for serum concentration of cystatin C in children, *Pediatr Nephrol* 17:104-106, 2002.
15. Finney H, Newman DJ, Thakkar H, et al: Reference ranges for plasma cystatin C and creatinine measurements in premature infants, neonates, and older children, *Arch Dis Child* 82:71-75, 2000.
16. Harmoinen A, Ylinen E, Ala-Houhala M, et al: Reference intervals for cystatin C in pre- and full-term infants in children, *Pediatr Nephrol* 15:105-108, 2000.
17. Montini G, Cosmo L, Amici G, et al: Plasma cystatin C values and inulin clearances in premature neonates, *Pediatr Nephrol* 16: 463-464, 2001.
18. Bokenkamp A, Dietrich C, Schumann G: Pediatric reference values for cystatin C revisited, *Pediatr Nephrol* 13:367-368, 1999.
19. Al-Tonbary YA, Hammad AM, Zaghloul HM, et al: Pretreatment cystatin C in children with malignancy: can it predict chemotherapy-induced glomerular filtration rate reduction during the induction phase? *J Pediatr Hematol Oncol* 26:336-341, 2004.
20. Jenkins MA, Brown DJ, Ierino FL, et al: Cystatin C for estimation of glomerular filtration rate in patients with spinal cord injury, *Ann Clin Biochem* 40(Pt 4):364-368, 2003.
21. O'Riordan SE, Webb MC, Stowe HJ, et al: Cystatin C improves the detection of mild renal dysfunction in older patients, *Ann Clin Biochem* 40(Pt 6):648-655, 2003.
22. Shimizu A, Horikoshi S, Rinnno H, et al: Serum cystatin C may predict the early prognostic stages of patients with type 2 diabetic nephropathy, *J Clin Lab Anal* 17:164-167, 2003.
23. Buysschaert M, Joudi I, Wallemacq P, et al: Comparative performance of serum cystatin-c versus serum creatinine in diabetic subjects, *Diabetes Metab* 29(4 Pt 1):377-383, 2003.
24. Poge U, Stoschus B, Stoffel-Wagner B, et al: Cystatin C as an endogenous marker of glomerular filtration rate in renal transplant patients, *Kidney Blood Press Res* 26:55-60, 2003.
25. Pham-Huy A, Leonard M, Lepage N, et al: Measuring glomerular filtration rate with cystatin C and beta-trace protein in children with spina bifida, *J Urol* 169:2312-2315, 2003.
26. Fricker M, Wiesli P, Brandle M, et al: Impact of thyroid dysfunction on serum cystatin C, *Kidney Int* 63:1944-1947, 2003.
27. Holmquist P, Torffvit O, Sjoblad S: Metabolic status in diabetes mellitus affects markers for glomerular filtration rate, *Pediatr Nephrol* 18:536-540, 2003.
28. Schwartz GJ, Brion L, Spitzer A: The use of plasma creatinine concentration for estimating glomerular filtration rate in infants, children, and adolescents, *Pediatr Clin North Am* 34:571, 1987.
29. Leger F, Bouissou F, Coulais Y, et al: Estimation of glomerular filtration rate in children, *Pediatr Nephrol* 17:903-907, 2002.
30. Cockroft DW, Gault MH: Prediction of creatinine clearance from serum creatinine, *Nephron* 16:31-41, 1976.
31. Gault MH, Longerich LL, Harnett JD, et al: Predicting glomerular function from adjusted serum creatinine, *Nephron* 62: 249-256, 1992.
32. Levey AS, Bosch JP, Lewis JB, et al: A more accurate method to estimate glomerular filtration rate from serum creatinine: a new prediction equation. Modification of Diet in Renal Disease Study Group, *Ann Intern Med* 130: 461-470, 1999.
33. Vervoort G, Willems HL, Wetzels JF: Assessment of glomerular filtration rate in healthy subjects and normoalbuminuric diabetic patients: validity of a new (MDRD) prediction equation, *Nephrol Dial Transplant* 17:1909-1913, 2002.
34. Pierrat A, Gravier E, Saunders C, et al: Predicting GFR in children and adults: a comparison of the Cockcroft-Gault, Schwartz, and modification of diet in renal disease formulas, *Kidney Int* 64: 1425-1436, 2003.
35. Filler G, Lepage N: Should the Schwartz formula for estimation of GFR be replaced by cystatin C formula? *Pediatr Nephrol* 18: 981-985, 2003.
36. Woolfson RG, Neild GH: Renal nuclear medicine: can it survive the millennium? *Nephrol Dial Transplant* 13:12-14, 1998.
37. Knesplova L, Krestin GP: Magnetic resonance in the assessment of renal function, *Eur Radiol* 8:201-211, 1998.
38. Dagher PC, Herget-Rosenthal S, Ruehm SG, et al: Newly developed techniques to study and diagnose acute renal failure, *J Am Soc Nephrol* 14: 2188-2198, 2003.
39. Mehta RL, Chertow GM: Acute renal failure definitions and classification: time for change? *J Am Soc Nephrol* 14: 2178-2187, 2003.

40. Delanghe J: Use of specific urinary proteins as diagnostic markers for renal disease, *Acta Clin Belg* 52:148-153, 1997.
41. Rodriguez-Soriano J: New insights into the pathogenesis of renal tubular acidosis—from functional to molecular studies, *Pediatr Nephrol* 14:1121-1136, 2000.
42. Rodriguez-Soriano J, Vallo A: Renal tubular acidosis, *Pediatr Nephrol* 4:268-275, 1990.
43. Suzuki MM: Nephrology. In Siberry GK, Iannone R, editors: *The Harriet Lane handbook,* ed 15, Baltimore, 2000, Mosby.
44. National Kidney Foundation: K/DOQI clinical practice guidelines for chronic kidney disease: evaluation, classification, and stratification, *Am J Kidney Dis* 39(2 suppl 1): S1-S266, 2002.
45. Kellum J, Levin N, Bouman C, et al: Developing a consensus classification system for acute renal failure, *Curr Opin Crit Care* 8: 509-514, 2002.
46. Andreoli S: Management of acute renal failure. In Barrat TM, Avner ED, Harmon WE, editors: *Pediatric nephrology,* ed 4, Baltimore, 1999, Williams and Wilkins.

CHAPTER

63

Renal Pharmacology

Douglas L. Blowey

PEARLS

- For situations when the goal is the maintenance of a serum concentration close to the steady state level throughout the dosing interval, a decrease in the size of the dose while the normal dosing interval is maintained will decrease the variation between the serum drug concentration peak and trough.
- With the exception of spironolactone, diuretics must reach the renal tubular fluid to produce a pharmacological effect.
- Loop diuretics decrease sodium reabsorption by inhibiting the electroneutral Na/K/2Cl cotransporter located on the apical cell membrane in the ascending limb of Henle.
- Spironolactone prevents the binding of aldosterone to a cytosolic receptor resulting in decreased activity of Na/K-ATPase and a decrease in the number of apical sodium channels.
- The continuous infusion of a loop diuretic is more efficient than intermittent high doses and avoids the high and low serum concentrations associated with toxicity and resistance.

The kidney plays a central role in many physiological processes that directly have an impact on drug action and disposition, and the kidney is also an important target for drug therapy in the critically ill child. The key functions of the kidney are the elimination of endogenous and exogenous substances from the body, including drug and drug metabolites, and the maintenance of body fluid composition and volume. The glomerular and tubular mechanisms that carry out these functions are directly and indirectly influenced by the function of other organs. For example, congestive heart failure decreases the adequacy of arterial blood flow and is detected by sensors located throughout the circulatory system. The sensed reduction in effective arterial blood volume triggers a complex neurohormonal response that decreases kidney blood flow, increases sodium and water retention in the kidney, and further aggravates the edema associated with congestive heart failure. Conversely, the accumulation of drugs, drug metabolites, metabolic waste products, and alterations in body fluid composition and volume associated with kidney failure may have deleterious effects on the function of other vital organs and physiological systems.

Kidney Function and Drug Disposition

Abnormal kidney function can affect the amount of drug present at the site of action and the magnitude of the drug response. A clear understanding of the effects of abnormal kidney function on drug disposition and action is important because abnormal kidney function is common in the critically ill child and alterations in drug disposition or action may result in suboptimal therapeutic efficacy or serious adverse events.

The pharmacological effect of a therapeutic agent is determined by the amount and time that the active drug component (e.g., parent drug or drug metabolite) is present at the site of action and the responsiveness of the target organ to the drug. Only the free, unbound form of a drug can exert a pharmacological effect through interaction with receptors. The disposition of a drug after administration is determined by the formulation and route of administration, the rate and extent of absorption from the site of administration, the extent of distribution in the body fluids and tissues, the rate and extent of metabolism, and the rate and route of elimination. Drug disposition and response are further influenced by the genetic, physiological, and pathological constitution of the ill child.[1, 2] Pharmacokinetics is the mathematical expression of drug disposition, and pharmacodynamics describes the magnitude of response to a drug. The determination of pharmacokinetic parameters is an invaluable tool for designing individualized drug-dosing regimens in children with kidney failure or critical illnesses that may alter drug disposition (see also Chapter 113).

Although decreased kidney elimination of drugs and drug metabolites is the most obvious consequence of altered kidney function, kidney failure or the associated coexisting conditions may affect drug absorption, distribution, and metabolism (Table 63-1).[3,4] The mechanisms that govern drug removal by the kidneys are glomerular filtration, tubular secretion, and tubular reabsorption. These processes are altered in children with kidney disease, as well as other organ dysfunction. Each of the kidney's one million nephrons consists of a tuft of capillaries (glomerulus) enveloped by an epithelial-lined capsule (Bowman's space) that drains into a contiguous tubular system. As blood flows through the glomerular capillaries, fluid and small solutes, including drugs and drug metabolites not bound to plasma proteins, pass through the glomeruli into Bowman's space. The volume of water and accompanying solute that is filtered through the glomeruli per unit time is the glomerular filtration rate (GFR) and is the most important measure of kidney function (see also Chapter 64). The GFR is estimated with the measurement of the rate that the kidney removes a substance from the blood (e.g., renal clearance). The measured substance may be an endogenous compound (e.g., creatinine [Cr]), an exogenous compound that is specifically administered to measure the GFR (e.g., inulin, isotope), or a compound primarily eliminated by glomerular filtration that is administered as part of clinical care (e.g., gentamicin).[5] The clearance of Cr corrected for body surface area (BSA) is the most common method used to estimate the GFR. Creatinine clearance (C_{Cr}), expressed in milliliters per minute per 1.73 m^2, is calculated with the measurement of the amount of Cr in an accurately timed urine collection and a midcollection plasma Cr.

$$CCr = \frac{\{\text{Urine Cr [mg/dl]} \times \text{[urine volume (ml)/time (min)]}\} \times 1.73\ m^2}{\text{Plasma Cr (mg/dl) BSA } (m^2)}$$

C_{Cr} is low at birth and rapidly increases during the first 2 weeks of life followed by a steady rise until adult values are reached by 8 to 12 months.[6,7].

Although not as accurate as a timed urine collection, C_{Cr} can be quickly estimated with the measurement of the child's serum Cr and length with the following equation[8]:

$$C_{Cr} = \frac{\text{Length (cm) K}}{\text{Plasma Cr (mg/dl)}}$$

where K represents the Cr production rate and varies with age (0.45, term neonate; 0.55, child; and 0.7, adolescent boy). It is important to understand that the normal relationships among serum Cr, length, and GFR are altered in disturbances of Cr biosynthesis (e.g., muscular disease and malnutrition) or in clinical settings where the serum Cr is rapidly changing (e.g., acute renal failure, recovery from renal failure, and dialysis). In these situations, a timed urine collection is required for an accurate estimate of the GRF.

The total amount of drug eliminated from the body by the kidneys is a composition of the amount of drug filtered across the glomeruli, the amount actively secreted into the filtrate by the renal tubules, and the renal tubular reabsorption. For drugs and drug metabolites that are primarily eliminated by glomerular filtration, the rate of elimination mirrors kidney function (C_{Cr}). As such, when kidney function declines, the reduced drug elimination results in drug accumulation in the body. For example, gentamicin is an aminoglycoside that is eliminated primarily by glomerular filtration with an elimination half-life of around 2 hours in children and adults with normal kidney function and 4 to 12 hours in infants because of the well-characterized developmental immaturity of kidney function.[6,7] A 75% reduction of the GFR (e.g., C_{Cr} = 30 ml/min/1.73 m^2) in a 5-year-old child receiving intravenous (IV) gentamicin will prolong the elimination half-life to 8 hours. Unless adjustments are made in the dosing regimen to account for the decreased kidney elimination, gentamicin will accumulate to toxic serum concentrations (Fig. 63-1). Because albumin and other large molecules do not pass through the glomeruli, large drugs and drugs bound to plasma proteins normally do not pass through the glomeruli and are not effectively removed by glomerular filtration but may be efficiently eliminated by the kidney through renal tubular secretion (e.g., furosemide).

TABLE 63–1

Potential Alterations of Drug Distribution in Kidney Failure

PK Parameter	Effect	Proposed Mechanism
Absorption	↓	Edema of GI tract, uremic N/V, delayed gastric emptying
		Drug interaction–phosphate binders, histamine blockers
		Altered GI pH
Distribution	↑	Increased unbound drug fraction
		Hypoalbuminemia (nephrosis, malnutrition)
		Uremic changes in albumin structure
Metabolism	↓ ↑	Inhibition of CYP 450 metabolism (liver, intestine, kidney)
		Drug interaction
		Direct inhibition by "uremic" milieu
		Induced CYP 450 metabolism
Excretion	↓	Decreased GFR
		Decreased tubular secretion
		Increased tubular reabsorption

CYP 450, cytochromes P450; *GFR*, glomerular filtration rate; *GI*, gastrointestinal; *N/V*, nausea and vomiting; *PK*, pharmacokinetic.

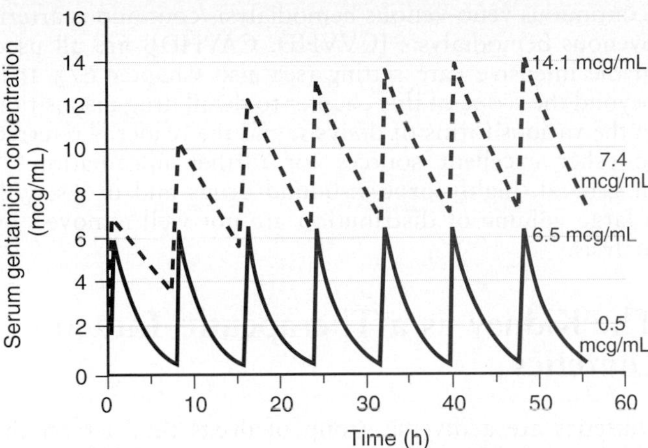

FIGURE 63–1 • Gentamicin concentration-time profile in a 5-year-old child receiving 2.5 mg/kg intravenously every 8 hours. The solid line represents the concentration-time profile in a child with normal kidney function (e.g., 120 ml/min/1.73 m²), and the dashed line represents the concentration-time profile in a child with a creatinine clearance of 30 ml/min/1.73 m².

The active renal tubular secretion of drugs and drug metabolites by relatively nonspecific anionic and cationic transport systems in the proximal tubule can contribute substantially to the amount of drug eliminated by the kidney. The renal tubular secretion of a drug may be inhibited by other drugs or endogenous substrates that use the same nonspecific transport systems. For example, probenecid blocks the tubular secretion of many drugs by the organic anion transporter and is of clinical utility as an adjuvant to antibiotic therapy and the prevention of drug-induced nephrotoxicity.[9-11] The coadministration of probenecid and penicillin-type antibiotics results in higher and more prolonged serum penicillin levels because of the inhibition of penicillin secretion by the renal tubule. The increased penicillin exposure may enhance the therapeutic efficacy of penicillin.[12,13] Nephrotoxicity is the major dose-limiting adverse effect of the antiviral agent cidofovir and is in part mediated by the proximal tubular transport of cidofovir by the organic anion system. Coadministration of probenecid restricts the proximal renal tubular uptake of cidofivir and decreases the incidence of nephrotoxicity.[10] Reabsorption is the passive diffusion of nonionized (noncharged) drug from the filtrate into the renal tubular cell. Basic urine (e.g., urine pH >7.5) favors the ionized form of acidic drugs and limits reabsorption, whereas reabsorption of basic drugs is enhanced in basic urine because the nonionized form of the drug is favored. Urinary alkalinization is used to enhance the elimination of salicylates and possibly barbiturates in overdose situations (see also Chapters 101 and 102).[14]

Drug Dosing in Kidney Disease

Drugs and drug metabolites that are predominately eliminated by the kidney will accumulate to higher serum drug concentrations in patients with decreased kidney function if adjustments are not made to the drug-dosing regimen. A systematic approach to individualized drug therapy in children with kidney failure will ensure maximal therapeutic efficacy and minimize toxicity (Box 63-1). The first step in designing a rational individualized dosing regimen is an estimation of the child's kidney function with measurement of the C_{Cr} as described in the previous section. The next step is to evaluate the effect of kidney failure on the drug disposition characteristics for all of the drugs prescribed to the child. Reference books such as the *Pediatric Dosage Handbook*,[15] *Physicians Desk Reference,* and *Micromedex* are excellent beginning sources for information about drug disposition in kidney failure. Unfortunately, there is little pharmacokinetic information about drug disposition in children with kidney failure. Estimates from adult patients with kidney failure are cautiously used; the potential changes in drug disposition that occur with development are kept in mind.[16] The most important information for designing an optimal dosing regimen is the amount of drug that is eliminated by the kidneys in individuals with normal kidney function. If one assumes that drug protein binding, distribution, and metabolism are not greatly altered in kidney failure, an assumption that is likely true for most drugs, then a dosage adjustment factor (Q) can be estimated:

$$Q - 1\ [\%\ \text{excreted unchanged} \times 1 - \frac{\text{Child's } C_{Cr}\ (\text{ml/min/1.73 m}^2)}{\text{Normal } C_{Cr}\ (120\ \text{ml/min/1.73 m}^2)}]$$

Once the need for a dosage adjustment has been established and the adjustment factor (Q) calculated, the best method of adjustment, whether it be a change in the size of the dose or the length of the dosing interval, is selected on the basis of the known relationships between the peak and trough drug concentrations and clinical response or toxicity. Figure 63–2 shows the concentration-time profiles for two different IV gentamicin dosing regimens in a child with a measured C_{Cr} of 30 ml/min/1.73 m². About 95% of gentamicin is excreted unchanged in the urine, and the dosage adjustment factor is calculated as:

$$[Q = 1\ [0.95 \times (1 - \frac{30\ \text{ml/min/1.73 m}^2}{120\ \text{ml/min/1.73 m}^2})] = 0.30$$

When the dosing interval is increased and the size of the drug dose remains unchanged (Fig. 63–2, solid line),

BOX 63–1

Guidelines for Drug Dosing in Kidney Failure

1. Estimate the glomerular filtration rate
2. Determine the percentage of drug eliminated by the kidney
3. Calculate the dosage adjustment factor (Q)
4. Adjust the dose size or dosing interval
5. Monitor response
6. Monitor therapeutic drug (when available)

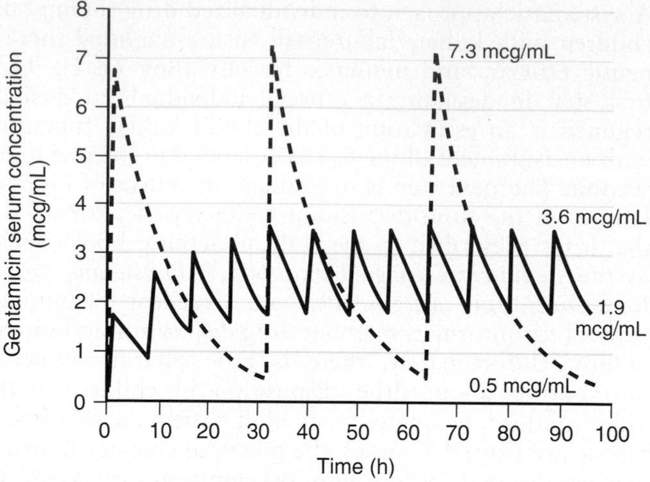

FIGURE 63–2 • Gentamicin concentration-time profile in a child with a creatinine clearance of 30 ml/min/1.73 m^2 receiving gentamicin intravenously. The dashed line represents the concentration-time profile when the dosing interval is adjusted to 32 hours (normal dosing interval [8 hour] ÷ dosing adjustment factor [0.3]), and the size of the dose remains unchanged (2.5 mg/kg). The solid line represents the concentration-time profile if the dose is adjusted to 0.625 mg/kg (normal dose [2.5 mg/kg] × dosing adjustment factor [0.3), and the dosing interval remains unchanged (8 hours).

the steady state peak and trough drug concentration are similar to those seen in children with normal renal function; however, there is a prolonged period when the serum gentamicin concentration is above and below the average steady state concentration. This dosing regimen may be inappropriate for drugs that should be maintained at a relatively stable serum concentration, such as cephalosporins or antihypertensive medications. For situations when the goal is the maintenance of a serum concentration close to the steady state level throughout the dosing interval, a decrease in the size of the dose while the normal dosing interval is maintained will decrease the variation between the serum drug concentration peak and trough (Fig. 63–2, *solid line*). The dosing adjustments are estimates based on many assumptions, and the final step in individual therapy is close monitoring of clinical efficacy and toxicity. When available, the measurement of serum drug concentrations and determination of pharmacokinetic parameters is invaluable for individual drug therapy, especially in agents with a narrow therapeutic index.

Dialysis

Some form of dialysis is used in about 3% of children admitted to the intensive care unit. Drug elimination in children receiving dialysis is a composite of nonrenal drug elimination, residual kidney elimination, and the added elimination provided by dialysis. The efficiency of a given dialysis modality to eliminate drug depends on the physiochemical characteristics of the drug and the form and characteristics of the dialysis procedure. Hemodialysis, peritoneal dialysis, hemofiltration (continuous veno-venous hemodialysis/continuous arteriovenous hemodialysis [CVVH/CAVH]) and hemodiafiltration (continuous veno-venous hemodialysis/continuous arteriovenous hemodialysis [CVVHD, CAVHD]) are all used in the intensive care setting (see also Chapter 67). It is beyond the scope of this chapter to detail drug disposition in the various forms of dialysis, and the reader is referred to other excellent sources for further information.[4,17] In general, highly protein-bound drugs and drugs with a large volume of distribution are not well removed by dialysis.

The Kidney as a Therapeutic Target: Diuretics

Diuretics are a diverse group of drugs that act on the kidney to increase salt and water excretion. In the intensive care setting, diuretics are commonly prescribed for mobilization of excess body fluid, treatment of cerebral edema, and hypertension. Less common indications include congestive heart failure, disorders of calcium metabolism, glaucoma, and drug overdoses. Diuretics are grouped into five classes according to the primary site of action: osmotic diuretics and carbonic anhydrase inhibitors act in the proximal tubule; loop diuretics act in the thick ascending limb of Henle; thiazide and thiazide-like diuretics act in the distal tubule; and potassium-sparing diuretics act in the collecting ducts.

Renal tubular cells transport solute and water from the apical cell membrane (tubular fluid) to the basolateral cell membrane (blood side). The reabsorption of sodium is central to the kidney's ability to reabsorb water and other solutes (e.g., glucose, amino acids, bicarbonate). Apical cell sodium entry is mediated by channels that permit sodium to enter by diffusion or facilitated by specific transport proteins located on the apical cell membrane. In all renal tubular cells, the Na/K-ATPase located on the basolateral membrane maintains the low intracellular sodium concentration that favors sodium movement from the tubular fluid into the renal tubular cell. Diuretics inhibit sodium reabsorption by blocking sodium channels or sodium transport proteins located on the apical cell membrane at discrete sites along the nephron. Because sodium reabsorption occurs in a sequential manner along the nephron, the combination of diuretics with different sites of action (e.g., loop diuretic plus a thiazide diuretic) has a synergistic effect on sodium reabsorption. The additional osmotic force associated with the increased urinary sodium causes a rise in urine volume. The diuresis is associated with a decrease in vascular volume that stimulates movement of sodium and water from the interstitial space into the vascular space, as well as stimulation of counterregulatory pathways (e.g., renin-angiotensin-aldosterone system) that serve to maintain an adequate extracellular fluid volume.

With the exception of spironolactone, diuretics must reach the renal tubular fluid to produce a pharmacological effect. Because diuretics are extensively bound to plasma proteins, their entry into the tubular fluid depends on proximal tubular secretion. The organic anion transporters actively secrete carbonic anhydrase inhibitors, loop diuretics, and thiazide diuretics, whereas the organic cation transporters actively secrete amiloride and triamterene.

Mannitol is freely filtered at the glomerulus, and spironolactone has a complex mechanism of action that does not require entry into the tubular fluid for pharmacological effect.

The response to diuretics is determined by the amount and time course of drug reaching the site of action and the sensitivity of the active site to the diuretic. The concentration-response curve (Fig. 63-3) depicts the relationship between the urinary excretion rate of loop and thiazide diuretics and diuretic response. The S-shaped curve shows that for each diuretic there is a minimal concentration that must be reached at the site of action before any response is noted (therapeutic threshold) and that there is a maximal response (ceiling) above which no further response will occur even if more drug reaches the site of action. The amount and time course of drug reaching the site of action, and thus effect, are influenced by the route and frequency of administration, as well as drug and disease states that modify the amount of diuretic reaching the tubular fluid or the tubular response to the diuretic. An example is the twofold to threefold increase in loop diuretic dosage required for response in patients with decreased kidney function. In kidney failure, the entry of loop diuretics into the tubular fluid is limited by decreased drug delivery to the organic anion transporters due to decreased renal blood flow and competitive inhibition of diuretic transport by "uremic toxins." Adequate tubular fluid diuretic concentration and response can be achieved with the administration of high doses of diuretic[18] but at the risk of increasing ototoxicity, particularly with concurrent aminoglycoside administration.[19,20]

Loop diuretics, such as furosemide, bumetanide, and torsemide, are the most potent diuretics because a large percentage of sodium is reabsorbed in the ascending limb of Henle. Loop diuretics decrease sodium reabsorption by inhibiting the electroneutral Na/K/2Cl cotransporter located on the apical cell membrane in the ascending limb of Henle. Loop diuretics increase sodium delivery to the distal tubular segments and diminish water reabsorption by increasing the tubular fluid osmotic force and disrupting the generation of a hypertonic medullary interstitium.

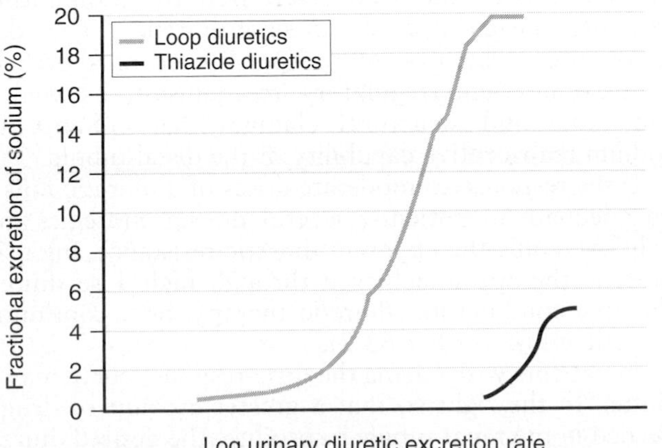

FIGURE 63–3 • Concentration-response curve depicting the relationship between the urinary diuretic excretion rate and the excretion of sodium in the urine.

The potential for profound fluid and electrolyte loss with loop diuretics mandates close monitoring of body fluid volume and serum electrolytes during therapy.

The increased delivery of sodium to the distal nephron segments has three significant physiological consequences. First, because sodium reabsorption in the thick ascending limb results in a lumen-positive transepithelial voltage that drives passive magnesium and calcium reabsorption, inhibition of sodium reabsorption by loop diuretics diminishes the transepithelial voltage and causes an increase in the urinary excretion of calcium and magnesium. Long-term use of loop diuretics is associated with hypomagnesaemia, hypercalciuria, and calcium-based kidney stones.[21-23] On the other hand, the enhanced urinary excretion of magnesium and calcium observed with loop diuretics is clinically beneficial in the treatment of hypercalcemia and hypermagnesemia.[24,25] The second physiological consequence of increased sodium delivery to the distal nephron segments is enhanced potassium secretion. Sodium reabsorption by the principal cell in the collecting duct favors potassium secretion into the tubular fluid and promotes hypokalemia.[26,27] Finally, the increased sodium delivery to the distal nephron is associated with acute and chronic adaptive processes that enhance distal sodium reabsorption and diminish diuretic efficacy.[28]

The loop diuretics display similar efficacy but differ slightly in pharmacokinetic characteristics. Bumetanide and torsemide are almost completely absorbed after oral administration, whereas the absorption of furosemide is extremely variable with an average bioavailability of 50%.[29,30] Therefore when IV furosemide is switched to oral furosemide, the dose is increased to account for the decreased absorption. The onset of diuretic effect is within minutes of IV administration of a loop diuretic and 30 to 60 minutes after oral administration. The duration of diuretic effect is short (2 to 6 hours),[26,31,32] and this often results in the need for multiple doses or a continuous infusion to achieve the desired effect.

Thiazide and thiazide-like diuretics such as chlorothiazide, hydrochlorothiazide, metolazone, and chlorthalidone decrease sodium reabsorption by inhibiting the Na/Cl cotransporter located on the apical membrane in the distal tubule. The thiazide diuretics are less effective than the loop diuretics (Fig. 63–3) because less sodium reabsorption occurs in the distal tubule as compared with the ascending limb of Henle. Thiazide diuretics have a synergistic effect on fluid and electrolyte excretion when combined with loop diuretics.[33-35] The different thiazide diuretics have similar efficacy, and the main difference resides in potency and duration of action. Metolazone and chlorthalidone display a longer duration of effect than chlorothiazide and hydrochlorothiazide; however, the biological effect of thiazides is prolonged compared with their elimination rates and are usually dosed once or twice a day. Thiazides are relatively ineffective in renal failure because of the decreased delivery of drug into the tubular fluid and the limited distal tubule sodium reabsorption. In contrast to the calciuric effect of loop diuretics, thiazide diuretics enhance calcium reabsorption and may have a beneficial effect in children with nephrocalcinosis/nephrolithiasis and hypercalciuria. Thiazides have a greater propensity than other diuretics to cause hypokalemia.

The potassium-sparing diuretics triamterene and amiloride decrease sodium reabsorption by blocking the apical membrane sodium channel in the principal cells of the cortical collecting duct. Sodium reabsorption in the cortical collecting duct results in a transepithelial voltage that favors the secretion of potassium and hydrogen ions. Although potassium-sparring diuretics can enhance diuresis, particularly in patients receiving loop or thiazide diuretics, the main clinical benefit of these agents is a reduction in the potassium excretion induced by loop and thiazide diuretics. Spironolactone prevents the binding of aldosterone to a cytosolic receptor resulting in decreased activity of Na/K-ATPase and a decrease in the number of apical sodium channels. Spironolactone is effective in primary and secondary hyperaldosteronism (e.g., liver disease). Potassium-sparing diuretics are not recommended in patients with renal failure because of the propensity for hyperkalemia.

Osmotic diuretics are nonelectrolytes that are freely filtered at the glomerulus and poorly reabsorbed or, in the case of glucose, present in amounts that exceed the tubular reabsorptive capacity. Mannitol is the prototypical osmotic diuretic, and its therapeutic effectiveness is directly related to the mannitol dose being large enough to raise the plasma and tubular fluid osmolality. The extraction of water from the intracellular compartments to the extracellular fluid volume that is associated with mannitol administration is clinically useful in cerebral edema, glaucoma, and the prevention of dialysis dysequilibrium syndrome. The mannitol-induced expansion of the extracellular fluid volume may be sufficient to perpetuate congestive heart failure, pulmonary edema, and significant hyponatremia in patients with renal failure in whom the half-life of mannitol is prolonged and the ability to excrete free water is limited.[36]

Carbonic anhydrase catalyzes the dehydration of carbonic acid to water and carbon dioxide, as well as the reverse hydration reaction. Acetazolamide is the prototypical carbonic anhydrase inhibitor and is more clinically useful for its extrarenal effects than its diuretic effects. Acetazolamide is used to treat glaucoma, acute mountain sickness, and occasionally epilepsy. The effectiveness of the carbonic anhydrase inhibitor (CAI) is limited by the metabolic acidosis that develops because of the bicarbonate loss in the urine.

Diuretic Resistance

An inadequate diuretic response results from disease- or drug-related alterations in diuretic pharmacokinetics or phamacodynamics, high dietary salt intake,[37] or adaptive processes[28] (Table 63-2). During diuretic-induced extracellular volume depletion, short-term and long-term adaptive processes serve to protect the intravascular volume; however, when these adaptive processes interfere with the diuretic responsiveness before the desired reduction in the extracellular fluid volume is achieved, they contribute to diuretic resistance.

Short-term adaptation results from enhanced postdiuretic sodium retention. The brisk diuresis associated with diuretics activates counterregulatory pathways that serve to enhance sodium reabsorption and maintain extracellular fluid volume. Counterregulatory mechanisms involved in the short-term adaptation to diuretics include a decrease in atrial natriuretic peptide, increased renal sympathetic activity, increased antidiuretic hormone, a stimulated rennin-angiotensin-aldosterone system, and a reduced GFR. The balance favors sodium and water excretion when the diuretic concentration in the renal tubular fluid is sufficient to inhibit sodium reabsorption. When the concentration of diuretic in the tubular fluid is below the threshold needed to elicit sodium excretion, the balance favors sodium and water reabsorption. In patients receiving a generous salt intake, which may be either dietary or associated with obligate fluids or medications, the postdiuretic sodium reabsorption may compensate entirely for the diuretic-induced sodium losses with an end-result of no change in the extracellular fluid volume. Long-term adaptation occurs after several days of diuretic use and is characterized by a diminished response to each successive dose of diuretic.[37] The adaptation occurs because of the persistence of short-term adaptation counterregulatory mechanisms, as well as functional and structural changes that enhance the sodium reabsorptive capability of the distal tubule.[38,39]

If the response to moderate doses of a diuretic fails to be adequate in patients, several dosing strategies may help overcome the apparent diuretic resistance. Intensive diuretic therapy is achieved through high-dose diuretic therapy, combination diuretic therapy, or a continuous diuretic infusion (Box 63-2).

In patients with edema the dose-response curve may be shifted to the right so that a greater amount of drug is needed in the renal tubule to produce the desired diuretic response. In patients who have renal failure or patients who receive drugs that inhibit the secretion of diuretic from the blood into the renal tubule, the dose response

TABLE 63–2

Causes of Diuretic Resistance

Noncompliance
Medication, salt restriction
Poor absorption of medication
Poorly absorbed formulation (e.g., furosemide oral)
Disease-induced changes in absorption
Impaired excretion of diuretic
Renal failure, renal transplant
Drug interactions: NSAIDs, probenecid
Protein binding in renal tubule
NS
Hemodynamic
Shock, hypoxemia
Drugs: NSAIDs, antihypertensive drugs
Change in dose response
CHF, NS, cirrhosis
Adaptive responses

CHF, Congestive heart failure; *NS,* nephrotic syndrome; *NSAID,* nonsteroidal antiinflammatory drug.

BOX 63–2

Intensive Diuretic Therapy

1. High-dose diuretic therapy
2. Combination of diuretic therapy
3. Continuous infusion diuretic therapy

curve is normal, but the problem lies in the inability to get a sufficient concentration of diuretic into the renal tubule. In both situations, an intermittent high-dose diuretic regimen may overcome the impaired rate of tubular secretion and increase the urinary diuretic concentration in an amount sufficient to elicit a response. High-dose therapy is associated with an increased risk of fluid and electrolyte abnormalities and a risk of toxicity related to high blood concentrations. Loop diuretic ototoxicity is more common with rapid infusion of high doses, especially when furosemide is combined with other ototoxic drugs.[35]

Because sodium reabsorption in the kidney is sequential and many of the adaptive processes increase sodium reabsorption distal to the site of diuretic action, combination therapy with diuretics that inhibit the distal tubule with loop inhibitors is effective. Part of the effectiveness of combination diuretic therapy resides in the longer duration of effect for thiazides that prevents the post diuretic sodium reabsorption noted with the shorter-acting loop diuretics. Fluid and electrolyte abnormalities are more common with combination drug therapy (Box 63-3).

The final strategy to overcome diuretic resistance is a continuous infusion of a loop diuretic. The continuous infusion of a loop diuretic is more efficient than intermittent high doses and avoids the high and low serum concentrations associated with toxicity and resistance.[40-43] Continuous infusions result in steady diuretic effect and may avoid the rapid hemodynamic changes and stimulation of counterregulatory process associated with rapid changes in extracellular fluid volume. A loading dose of diuretic is recommended at initiation and with each upward dosing adjustment to ensure a prompt response. The diuretic response may be further augmented by the addition of a distally acting diuretic.

BOX 63–3

Common Adverse Effects Associated with Diuretics

1. Volume depletion
2. Electrolyte abnormalities
   Hyponatremia
   Hypokalemia (loop and thiazide diuretics)
   Hyperkalemia (potassium-sparing diuretics)
   Hypomagnesemia (loop diuretics)
3. Hypercalciuria (loop diuretics)
4. Ototoxicity (loop diuretics, especially furosemide)

Prevention/Reversal of Acute Renal Failure

Acute renal failure in the pediatric intensive care unit is generally associated with diminished renal perfusion caused by hypovolemia, hypotension, or decreased cardiac output. Acute renal failure is also associated with nephrotoxins such as radiocontrast agents, antibiotics (e.g., vancomycin), and chemotherapeutic agents (e.g., cisplatin). With the exception of simple saline hydration, little evidence suggests that in humans, mannitol, furosemide, or dopamine prevents the development of acute renal failure in high-risk patients or changes the outcome in patients with established acute renal failure.[44-47] Nevertheless, the use of high-dose furosemide alone or in combination with low-dose dopamine might increase urine output and ease patient care by improving fluid management and permitting for increased nutrition.

REFERENCES

1. Leeder JS, Kearns GL: Pharmacogenetics in pediatrics, *Pediatr Clin North Am* 44:55-77, 1997.
2. MacLoed S: Drug disposition and action in disease. In: Radde I, MacLoed S, editors, *Pediatric pharmacology and therapeutics*, Chicago, 1993, Mosby.
3. Blowey D, Kearns G, Lalkin A: Special considerations in the prescribing of medications for the pediatric CAPD/CCPD patient In: Fine R, Alexander S, Warady B, editors, *CAPD/CCPD in children*, Boston, 1998, Kluwer Academic Publishers.
4. Olyaei A, de Mattos A, Bennett W: Prescribing drugs in renal disease. In: Brenner B, editor, *The kidney*, Philadelphia, 2000, WB Saunders.
5. Koren G, James A, Perlman M: A simple method for the estimation of glomerular filtration rate by gentamicin pharmacokinetics during routine drug monitoring in the newborn, *Clin Pharmacol Ther* 38:680-685, 1985.
6. Arant BS Jr: Developmental patterns of renal functional maturation in the human neonate, *J Pediatr* 92:705-712, 1978.
7. van den Anker JN, Schoemaker R, Hop W, et al: Ceftazidime pharmacokinetics in preterm infants: effects of renal function and gestational age, *Clin Pharmacol Ther* 58:650-659, 1995.
8. Schwartz G, Brion L, Spitzer A: The use of plasma creatinine concentration for estimating glomerular filtration rate in infants, children, and adolescents, *Pediatr Clin North Am* 34:571-590, 1987.
9. Jacobs C, Kaubisch S, Halsey J, et al: The use of probenecid as a chemoprotector against cisplatin nephrotoxicity, *Cancer* 67:1518-1524, 1991.
10. Lacy S, Hitchcock M, Lee W, et al: Effect of oral probenecid coadministration on the chronic toxicity and pharmacokinetics of intravenous cidofovir in cynomolgus monkeys, *Toxicol Sci* 44: 97-106, 1988.
11. Lalezari J, Holland G, Kramer F, et al: Randomized, controlled study of the safety and efficacy of intravenous cidofovir for the treatment of relapsing cytomegalovirus retinitis in patients with AIDS, *J Acquir Immune Defic Syndr Hum Retrovirol* 17:339-344, 1998.
12. Holmes K, Karney W, Harnisch J, et al: Single-dose aqueous procaine penicillin G therapy for gonorrhea: use of probenecid and cause of treatment failure, J Infect Dis 127(4):455-460, 1973.
13. Odugbemi T: An open evaluation study of sulbactam/ampicillin with or without probenecid in the treatment of gonococcal infections in Lagos, *Drugs* 35(suppl 7):89-91, 1988.
14. Prescott L, Balali-Mood M, Critchley J, et al: Diuresis or urinary alkalinisation for salicylate poisoning, *Br Med J (Clin Red Ed)* 285:1383-1386, 1982.
15. Taketomo CK, Hodding JH, Kraus DM: *Pediatric dosage handbook*, ed 6, Hudson, Ohio, 1999, Lexi-Comp.
16. Kearns G: Pediatric pharmacokinetics. In: Ritschel W, Kearns G, editors, *Handbook of basic pharmacokinetics*, Washington, DC, 1999, American Pharmaceutical Association.

17. Reetze-Bonorden P, Bohler J, Keller E: Drug dosage in patients during continuous renal replacement therapy, *Clin Pharmacokinet* 24:362-379, 1993.
18. Voelker J, Cartwright-Brown D, Anderson S, et al: Comparison of loop diuretics in patients with chronic renal insufficiency, *Kidney Int* 32:572-578, 1987.
19. Brummett R, Bendrick T, Himes D: Comparative ototoxicity of bumetanide and furosemide when used in combination with kanamycin, *J Clin Pharmacol* 21(11-12 Pt 2):628-636, 1981.
20. Gallagher K, Jones J: Furosemide-induced ototoxicity, *Ann Intern Med* 91:744-745, 1979.
21. Downing G, Egelhoff J, Daily D, et al: Furosemide-related renal calcifications in the premature infant. A longitudinal ultrasonographic study, *Pediatr Radiol* 21:563-565, 1991.
22. Ryan M, Devane J, Ryan M, et al: Effects of diuretics on the renal handling of magnesium, *Drugs* 28(suppl 1):167-181, 1984.
23. Sutton R: Diuretics and calcium metabolism, *Am J Kidney Dis* 5: 4-9, 1985.
24. Bilezikian J: Clinical review 51: management of hypercalcemia, *J Clin Endocrinol Metab* 77:1445-1449, 1993.
25. Suki W, Yium J, Von Minden M, et al: Acute treatment of hypercalcemia with furosemide, *N Engl J Med* 283:836-840, 1970.
26. Engle M, Lewy J, Lewy P, et al: The use of furosemide in the treatment of edema in infants and children, *Pediatrics* 62:811-818, 1978.
27. Flamenbaum W, Friedman R: Pharmacology, therapeutic efficacy, and adverse effects of bumetanide, a new "loop" diuretic, *Pharmacotherapy* 2:213-222, 1982,
28. Ellison D: Adaptation to diuretic drugs. In: Seldin D, Giebisch G, editors, *Diuretic agents: clinical physiology and pharmacology,* Boston, 1997, Academic Press.
29. Grahnen A, Hammarlund M, Lundqvist T: Implications of intraindividual variability in bioavailability studies of furosemide, *Eur J Clin Pharmacol* 27:595-602, 1984.
30. Peterson R, Simmons M, Rumack B, et al: Pharmacology of furosemide in the premature newborn infant, *J Pediatr* 97:139-143, 1980.
31. Marshall J, Wells T, Letzig L, et al: Pharmacokinetics and pharmacodynamics of bumetanide in critically ill pediatric patients, *J Clin Pharmacol* 38:994-1002, 1998.
32. Repetto H, Lewy J, Braudo J, et al: The renal functional response to furosemide in children with acute glomerulonephritis, *J Pediatr* 80:660-666, 1972.
33. Arnold W: Efficacy of metolazone and furosemide in children with furosemide-resistant edema, *Pediatrics* 74:872-875, 1984.
34. Segar J, Robillard J, Johnson K, et al: Addition of metolazone to overcome tolerance to furosemide in infants with bronchopulmonary dysplasia, *J Pediatr* 120:966-973, 1992.
35. Sica D, Gehr T: Diuretic combinations in refractory oedema states: pharmacokinetic-pharmacodynamic relationships, *Clin Pharmacokinet* 30:229-249, 1996.
36. Borges H, Hocks J, Kjellstrand C: Mannitol intoxication in patients with renal failure, *Arch Intern Med* 142:63-66, 1982.
37. Wilcox C, Mitch W, Kelly R, et al: Response of the kidney to furosemide. I. Effects of salt intake and renal compensation, *J Lab Clin Med* 102:450-458, 1983.
38. Kobayashi S, Clemmons D, Nogami H, et al: Tubular hypertrophy due to work load induced by furosemide is associated with increases of IGF-1 and IGFBP-1, *Kidney Int* 47:818-828, 1995.
39. Loon N, Wilcox C, Unwin R: Mechanisms of impaired natiuretic response to furosemide during prolonged therapy, *Kidney Int* 36:682-689, 1989.
40. Klinge J, Scharf J, Hofbeck M, et al: Intermittent administration of furosemide versus continuous infusion in the postoperative management of children following open heart surgery, *Intensive Care Med* 23:693-697, 1997.
41. Rudy DW, Voelker JR, Greene PK, et al: Loop diuretics for chronic renal insufficiency: a continuous infusion is more efficacious than bolus therapy, *Ann Intern Med* 115:360-366, 1991.
42. Singh N, Kissoon N, Al Mofada S, et al: Comparison of continuous versus intermittent furosemide administration in postoperative cardiac patients, *Crit Care Med* 20:17-21, 1992.
43. van der Vorst M, Ruys-Dudok van Heel I, Kist-van Holthe J, et al: Continuous intravenous furosemide in haemodynamically unstable children after cardiac surgery, *Intensive Care Med* 27: 711-715, 2001.
44. Brown C, Ogg C, Cameron J: High dose furosemide in acute renal failure: a controlled trial, *Clin Nephrol* 15:90-96. 1981.
45. Gubern J, Sancho J, Simo J, et al: A randomized trial on the effect of mannitol on postoperative renal function in patients with obstructive jaundice, *Surgery* 103:39-44, 1988.
46. Minuth A, Terrell J Jr, Suki W: Acute renal failure: a study of the course and prognosis of 104 patients and of the role of furosemide, *Am J Med Sci* 271:317-324, 1976.
47. Solomon R, Werner C, Mann D, et al: Effects of saline, mannitol, and furosemide to prevent acute decreases in renal function induced by radiocontrast agents, *N Engl J Med* 331: 1416-1420, 1994.

CHAPTER

64

Glomerulotubular Dysfunction and Acute Renal Failure

Deborah P. Jones, Russell W. Chesney, and Aaron L. Friedman

PEARLS

- Acute renal failure (ARF) in the critically ill child is often associated with cardiovascular instability, which if prolonged, exhausts the normal renal compensatory responses to maintain renal blood flow (RBF) and glomerular filtration.
- Because tubular blood flow, and thus oxygen delivery to this vital epithelium, depends on postglomerular blood flow, prolonged vasoconstriction of glomerular arterioles results in tubular necrosis.
- Nephrotoxic drugs, sepsis, and overzealous use of diuretics are common comorbid conditions that further contribute to renal injury.
- Attention to cardiovascular status and the avoidance of unnecessary nephrotoxic agents such as aminoglycosides, nonsteroidal antiinflammatory drugs (NSAIDs), and contrast agents may avoid further renal injury in the child with established renal failure.
- In the case of pigment nephropathy, which is another common cause of ARF in the critically ill patient, aggressive volume administration with a forced diuresis and alkalinization of the urine may help prevent renal tubular cell injury. If needed, continuous renal replacement therapies may aid in pigment removal.

Pathophysiology of Acute Renal Failure

Physiology of Glomerular Filtration

Glomerular filtration rate (GFR) is the product of the filtration rate of the individual nephrons and the number of functioning nephrons.[1] The filtration rate of a single nephron, that is, single nephron glomerular filtration rate (SNGFR), is determined by the properties of the glomerular capillary wall and the Starling forces of the glomerular capillaries (Fig. 64–1).

$$\text{SNGFR} = \text{Kf} \times (\Delta P - \Delta\pi) = \text{Kf} \times P_{UF}$$

The Kf is a capillary wall property known as the *ultrafiltration coefficient* and is the product of the surface area available for filtration and the hydraulic conductivity of the membrane (see Fig. 64–1). The Starling forces (or pressures) that affect filtration are the hydraulic pressure in the glomerular capillary (P_{gc}), the hydraulic pressure in Bowman's space (P_{bs}), the oncotic pressure of the glomerular capillary (π_{gc}), and the oncotic pressure in Bowman's space (π_{bs}), which is usually zero because the ultrafiltrate is essentially protein free.[2] P_{gc} favors filtration; P_{bs} and π_{gc} are opposing forces to filtration. The mean ultrafiltration pressure (P_{uf}) is the difference between the net change in hydraulic pressure and the net change in the oncotic pressure. Thus SNGFR may be modified by any process that changes glomerular capillary pressures, glomerular membrane

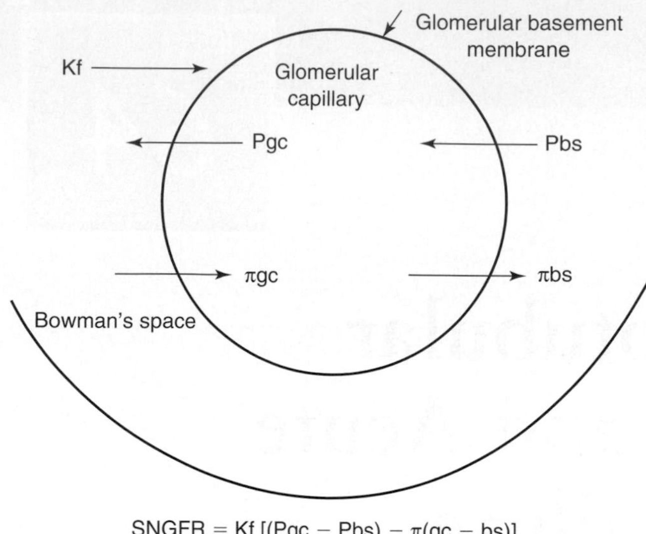

FIGURE 64–1 • Schematic representation of forces that determine single-nephron glomerular filtration rate *(SNGFR).* See text for definitions.

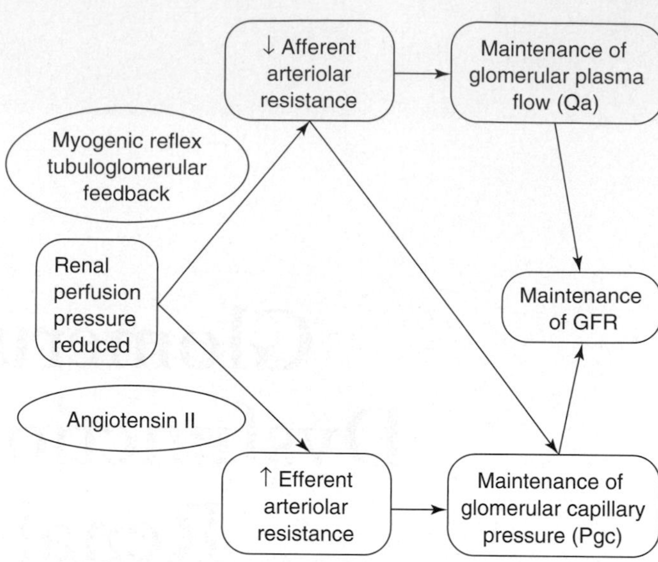

FIGURE 64–2 • Mechanisms of autoregulation. (With permission from Badr KF, Ichikawa I: Prerenal failure: a deleterious shift from renal compensation to decompensation, *N Engl J Med* 319:623, 1988.)

characteristics, or the surface area available for filtration.

Mechanisms of Renal Adaptation

The kidneys are responsible for water and electrolyte homeostasis through filtration of plasma at the glomerular membrane and reabsorption of water and electrolytes from the renal tubular epithelium. *Acute renal failure* (ARF) is defined as loss of renal capacity for filtration and tubular reabsorption, a state that becomes clinically apparent when there is a reduction in urine flow and retention of nitrogenous wastes, electrolytes, and fluid. The loss of filtration and tubular reabsorption is the end result of a continuum of renal adaptive changes that function to preserve renal perfusion and glomerular filtration. Eventually, the kidney can no longer compensate, and renal failure ensues.

In simple terms, glomerular filtration depends on adequate blood flow. The kidneys receive approximately 20% to 30% of total cardiac output. The fraction of cardiac output perfusing the kidneys is related to the ratio of renal vascular resistance (RVR) and systemic vascular resistance.[3,4] Renal blood flow (RBF) is determined by systemic blood pressure (SBP) and RVR, a relationship expressed by the formula RBF = SBP/RVR.[3,4] The kidney has adaptive mechanisms, referred to as *autoregulation,* that maintain constant renal perfusion pressure by alterations in RVR in the face of changes in systemic vascular resistance or intravascular volume. When SBP is within the normal physiological or autoregulatory range, the kidney can maintain constant blood flow and GFR by dilation of the preglomerular or afferent arteriole.

A reduction in renal perfusion pressure is accompanied by afferent arteriolar dilation, which reduces RVR and increases RBF (Fig. 64–2). At least two mechanisms are responsible for this smooth muscle relaxation of the afferent arteriole: the myogenic reflex and the tubuloglomerular feedback system. A reduction in transmural pressure is sensed by the arteriolar wall, which stimulates relaxation of vascular smooth muscle, termed the *myogenic reflex.*[3] The tubuloglomerular feedback system is operational following a reduction of plasma flow. When water and solute delivery to the macula densa are reduced, the juxtaglomerular apparatus responds by relaxing the smooth muscle of the adjacent afferent arteriole. Thus a reduction in cardiac output or effective intravascular volume is accompanied by vasodilation at the preglomerular arteriole, which, in turn, reduces RVR, thereby restoring RBF.

During states of reduced cardiac output or intravascular volume depletion, the systemic vasoconstrictors, angiotensin II and vasopressin, are released to help preserve vascular tone. The kidney counteracts the renal vasoconstrictor activity of angiotensin II and increased sympathetic tone through the intrarenal production of vasodilatory prostaglandins such as prostaglandin I_2.[5] These locally produced autacoids may attenuate renal vasoconstrictive forces and thereby preserve renal perfusion. Another prostaglandin, thromboxane A_2, is a potent vasoconstrictor.[5] In addition, prostaglandins may also modify the renal vasoconstrictive action of vasopressin, which is secreted by the pituitary gland in response to a decreased effective plasma volume.[2] Studies in animal models of congestive heart failure have provided evidence that enhanced prostaglandin synthesis is required for preservation of renal perfusion and GFR. Patients with congestive heart failure receiving prostaglandin synthetase inhibitors such as nonsteroidal antiinflammatory drugs (NSAIDs) have potentiation of renal ischemia because of an increase in renal vasoconstriction not antagonized by intrarenal prostaglandin synthesis.[6] Endothelial cells may also control the local vascular tone by the release of endothelium-derived relaxation factors (EDRFs), which are vasodilatory, and the potent vasoconstrictor endothelin.[7]

Constriction of the postglomerular capillary sphincter, the efferent arteriole, in the face of reduced RBF serves to increase the filtration fraction and preserve GFR, although this occurs at the expense of renal plasma flow, which may be further reduced. The increase in RVR may also contribute to the maintenance of cardiac output and SBP.

Vasoconstriction at the efferent arteriole is mediated by angiotensin II and, to a lesser extent, by the action of the adrenergic system by epinephrine.[8,9] Elevation in postglomerular arteriolar resistance may be blocked by the angiotensin-converting enzyme inhibitors. Whenever converting enzyme inhibitors are administered to the patient who requires efferent arteriolar constriction to maintain GFR, renal decompensation often results.[10]

Reductions in effective intravascular volume and cardiac output are accompanied by increased activity of the sympathetic nervous system and the renin-angiotensin-aldosterone system and increased circulating levels of vasopressin.[11-13] These neural and hormonal systems signal the kidneys to increase the reabsorption of sodium and water to help restore the deficient intravascular volume, increase cardiac output, and consequently improve RBF. In summary, even with a reduction in effective intravascular volume, whether through volume depletion or in states such as sepsis or cardiac failure, the kidney maintains glomerular filtration by afferent arteriolar vasodilation and efferent arteriolar constriction. The kidney's homeostatic mechanisms, however, are not without limitation. The autoregulatory ability of the afferent arteriole is maximal once the mean SBP falls below 80 mmHg. The renal autoregulatory range appears to be age dependent because younger animals can autoregulate over lower pressure ranges.[14] The range of perfusion pressure over which the kidney can autoregulate may be limited in certain conditions so that vasodilation is maximal with a minor reduction in mean arterial blood pressure. Examples include extracellular fluid depletion, renal ischemia, or renal vascular disease (e.g., hypertension, diabetes, atherosclerosis).

As the stimulus for release of vasoconstrictors continues, afferent arteriolar constriction rather than vasodilation may predominate, and the result is a decrease in filtration rate and renal plasma flow. Constriction of the afferent arteriole may be stimulated by increased sympathetic nervous system activity and increased levels of endogenous or exogenous circulating catecholamines such as dopamine or norepinephrine.[11] Thus the administration of these inotropic agents may actually compromise the kidney's adaptive mechanisms. Excessive vasoconstriction eventually results in diminished filtration rate and oxygen delivery to the kidney.[4]

Pharmacological agents may alter renal perfusion by changing SBP through an action on systemic vasculature or by direct effects on renal vasculature (Box 64–1).[4] Vasodilators such as hydralazine lower SBP without changing renal perfusion pressure because the decrease in SBP is accompanied by decreased RVR. Conversely, epinephrine increases SBP but decreases RBF by its vasoconstrictor effect on intrarenal blood vessels.

BOX 64–1

Vasoactive Substances in the Renal Vasculature

1. ↑ Renal Vascular Resistance/↓ Renal Blood Flow
   - Epinephrine
   - Norepinephrine
   - Angiotensin II
   - Arachidonic acid
   - Thromboxane A_2
2. ↓ Renal Vascular Resistance/↑ Renal Blood Flow
   - Prostaglandin E_1
   - Prostaglandin E_2
   - Dopamine
   - Furosemide
   - Angiotensin-converting enzyme inhibitors
   - Bradykinin
   - Isoproterenol
   - Acetylcholine

Data from Hostetter TH, Brenner BM: Renal circulatory and nephron function in experimental acute renal failure. In Brenner BM, Lazarus JM, editors: *Acute renal failure,* ed 2, New York, 1988, Churchill Livingstone.

Pathogenesis of Reduced Glomerular Filtration Rate in Acute Renal Failure

The mechanisms responsible for GFR reduction in acute renal injury have been studied extensively with experimental models of ARF designed to mimic states encountered clinically. In most cases, more than one mechanism is operational in mediating hypofiltration. Whereas one factor may have greater importance in the initiation of injury and decreased filtration, other factors are involved in the sustained reduction in GFR during the maintenance phase of ARF. Four major mechanisms result in reduced GFR during ARF[15]: reduced blood flow, decreased Kf, tubular obstruction, and backleakage of tubular fluid (Figs. 64–3 and 64–4). Each factor is discussed regarding its role in both the initiation and maintenance phases of ARF.

A reduction in RBF can be demonstrated during the initiation phase of many forms of ARF and seems to play a predominant role in ischemic injury and rhabdomyolysis.[15, 16] This relatively straightforward mechanism for hypofiltration was initially thought to adequately explain the reduction in GFR; however, studies have shown that restoration of RBF, even during the initiation phase, rarely restores GFR to normal.[17] Proposed theories for the reduction of RBF include (1) a proportional increase in the afferent and efferent arteriolar resistances in response to activation of the renin-angiotensin system, (2) vascular endothelial cell swelling and damage with release of vasoactive peptides such as endothelin, and (3) hyperemic congestion of the medullary peritubular capillaries.

Kf may be reduced in both nephrotoxic and ischemic forms of renal failure. Endothelial or mesangial cell swelling reduces the surface area available for filtration. Altered permeability induced by humoral factors such as angiotensin II

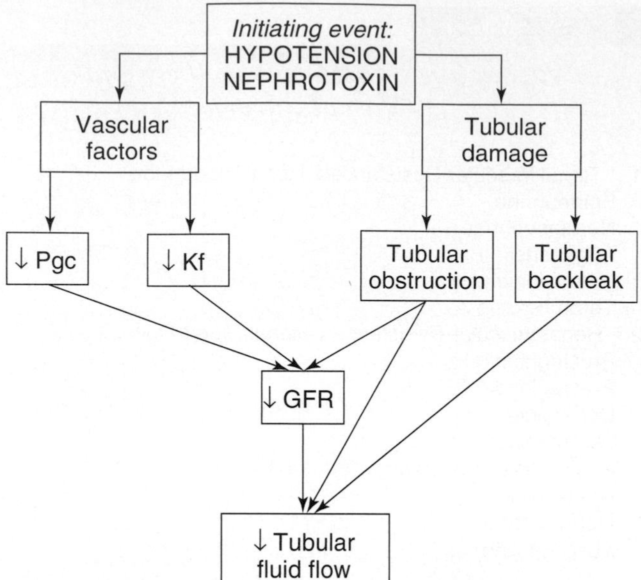

FIGURE 64–3 • Pathophysiological mechanisms for filtration failure during the initiation and maintenance phases of acute renal failure.

and vasopressin may also decrease Kf.[18] Circulating levels of both hormones are increased during ARF.

Renal tubular cells are the primary site of injury in both ischemia and nephrotoxin-induced renal injury.[19] Tubular cell injury may be sublethal or lethal and result in cell necrosis. Once this injury occurs, cells detach from the supporting basement membrane and obstruct the tubule lumen. In addition, even with sublethal injury, tight junctions may be disrupted, and the intact layer may be lost. The loss of epithelial integrity allows backleakage of ultrafiltrate, which contains creatinine and urea, through paracellular pathways into the renal interstitium, creating further diminution of excretory function and reduced urine formation. Necrosis of a selected region of the renal tubule is accompanied by tubular obstruction and eventual filtration failure by that entire unit or nephron.

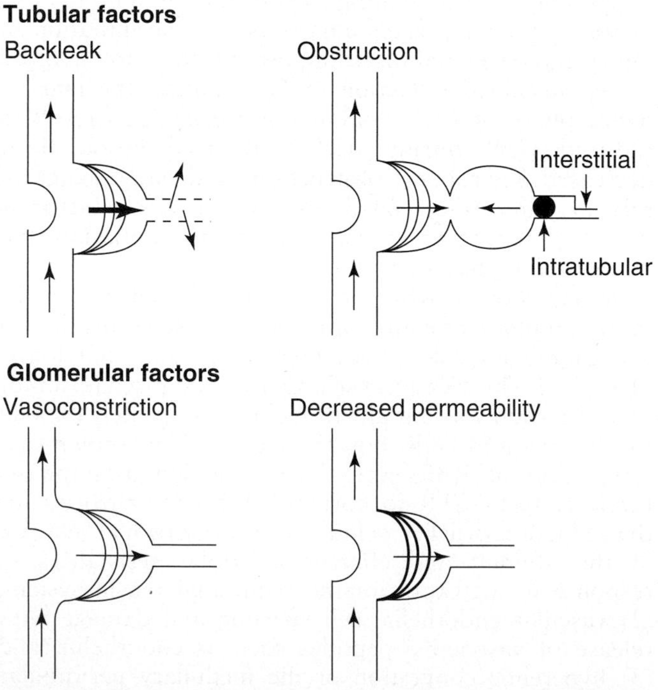

Intratubular obstruction occurs in most forms of acute renal injury either as a contributing factor in the initiation phase or during the maintenance phase.[15] Tubular obstruction with cellular debris and precipitated protein is a prominent finding in both the initiation and maintenance phases of ischemic injury. In the case of nephrotoxic injury, the degree of injury may determine the extent of tubular obstruction. In an experimental model of gentamicin nephrotoxicity, the drug dose was positively correlated with the contribution of tubular obstruction to reduced GFR.[20]

Tubular obstruction and loss of epithelial integrity caused by tubular cell injury result in the backleakage of tubular fluid and solutes. Excretion of solute and fluid is decreased, and this decrease possibly signals a further reduction in the GFR by stimulation of the tubuloglomerular feedback mechanism.[15] Backleakage of fluid involves tubular factors and is not a result of hypofiltration, although it does impair the excretory function of the kidney. Consequently, a falsely low estimation of actual GFR may occur because tubular fluid containing urea and creatinine leaks back into the vascular space and interstitium. Prevention of the tubular obstruction may alter the course of renal failure, even in those states in which the primary mechanism of injury is not obstruction.

To aid in the comprehension of ARF, we have divided the process into three phases[21]: (1) an initiation phase in which the primary mechanism of injury is operational, (2) a maintenance phase during which renal function remains poor and other factors may contribute to sustained injury, and (3) a recovery phase during which there is regeneration of cells and restoration of function. Although the primary initiating event may be hypoperfusion with ischemia, often it involves multiple contributing factors, which mediate additional cellular damage, usually through alterations in energy supply. From a clinical perspective, it may be most helpful to consider acute renal dysfunction syndromes according to the cause of the inciting event; however, it is equally vital to understand the other contributing mechanisms that ultimately affect outcome.

Recently, endothelial injury and vascular dysfunction have been postulated to occur during the initiation and particularly during the maintenance phases of ARF. Although most studies have focused on the tubular cell as the primary site of injury leading to dysfunction, recent studies have provided insight into the potential role for endothelial injury in continued reduced RBF and altered vascular function.[22] Sutton, Fisher, and Molitoris[22] propose that an additional phase be added to the current

Tubular factors
Backleak
Obstruction
Interstitial
Intratubular
Glomerular factors
Vasoconstriction
Decreased permeability

FIGURE 64–4 • Schematic representation of proposed mechanisms for filtration and excretory failure in acute renal failure. (Modified with permission from Thurau K, Mason J, Gstraunthaler G: Experimental acute renal failure. In Seldin DW, Giebisch G, editors: *The kidney: physiology and pathophysiology,* New York, 1985, Raven Press.)

model for ARF: after the initiation phase, an extension phase occurs that is due to microvascular injury related to ischemic damage to endothelial cells, infiltration of leukocytes, and activation of the coagulation system. This process is thought to predominate in the cortico-medullary and outer medullary microvessels and may occur in the face of early tubular cell regeneration so that limiting the extension process provides a potential mechanism for aiding recovery.

Mechanisms of Renal Cell Injury

The renal tubular cell expends energy in the form of adenosine triphosphate (ATP) to maintain a high intracellular concentration of potassium and a low intracellular concentration of sodium. This concentration gradient depends on the continuous activity of the Na^+/K^+-ATPase and is the driving force for the reabsorption of sodium. Active reabsorption of sodium is the primary driving force for water reabsorption and the coupled transport of amino acids, carbohydrates, organic acids, and other compounds. Thus all transport functions, as well as many other vital cell functions, depend on normal activity of the Na^+-K^+ pump, which, in turn, depends on an adequate supply of energy. In addition, membrane fluidity or integrity is important to transport functions in tubular cells. Processes that result in alterations in the membrane or in the supply of energy are common final pathways for renal tubular cell death (Fig. 64–5).

A decrease in the cellular ATP content occurs in many forms of renal injury,[23] possibly as the result of primary alterations in the cell's ability to perform oxidative phosphorylation or the end result of other perturbations (see Chapter 68). Heterogeneity exists in the susceptibility of nephron segments to oxygen deprivation with more

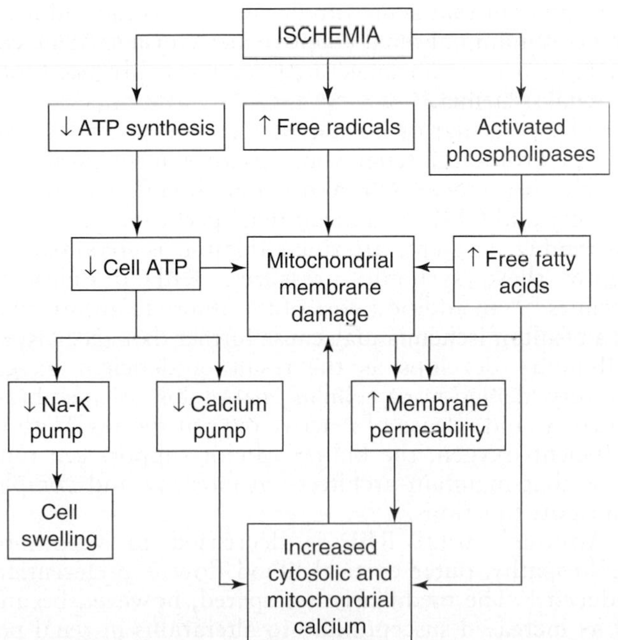

FIGURE 64–5 • Mechanism of cellular injury. (With permission from Epstein FH, Brown RS: Acute renal failure: a collection of paradoxes, *Hosp Pract (Off Ed)* 23:142, 1988.)

distal segments being relatively resistant. This is related to the greater glycolytic capacity of the distal tubule compared with the proximal tubule, which relies on oxygen-consuming pathways for ATP generation. Therefore the net result of renal injury is usually a depletion of energy in the form of ATP, with the inability of the cell to perform vital functions, including transport and maintenance of cell integrity.

Cellular injury may be modified by the requirements made on its energy stores.[23] If more transport is required of the cell, more energy is consumed, and less energy is left for cell maintenance. Evidence exists to support this theory. If transport requirements are reduced by the administration of diuretics or by the stimulation of the glomerulotubular feedback mechanism, then further injury may be attenuated. The feedback mechanism, whereby there is reduction of GFR in the face of reduced reabsorption by the proximal tubule, is a protective signal that conserves cell energy by reducing metabolic demands made on the cell.

Heat shock proteins (Hsps) are a family of proteins that appear to protect cells from injury as a result of hyperthermia, ischemia, or toxins (see Chapter 93). The Hsp induction by sublethal thermal stress has been found to attenuate subsequent injury in the kidney.[24-26] Renal transplants from animals that underwent short-term hyperthermia had better initial function and subsequent survival.[25] Furthermore, in cultured inner medullary collecting duct cells, induction of Hsp1 by preconditioning hyperthermia attenuated the alterations in mitochondrial function and glycolysis, which were observed after cells were exposed to high temperatures. Investigations into potential mechanisms to use this natural cell defense mechanism are under way.

The ability of renal tubular epithelial cells to undergo regeneration determines in large part the degree of renal recovery. Therefore much work has recently been done to study ways that cells regenerate and mechanisms that might enhance recovery. Early in ischemic injury there is induction of early response genes such as *c-fos* and *Egr-1*.[27,28] By 2 days after ischemia, the proliferating cell nuclear antigen is detected, followed by expression of other dedifferentiated cell markers, which seem to be a sign of early recovery.[28] Other cells appear to undergo apoptosis or cell death (see Chapter 93). Postischemic regeneration seems to be a recapitulation of early renal tubular cell development. Growth factors such as insulin-like growth factor-I (IGF-I) and epidermal growth factor 1 (EGF-1) have been associated with enhanced recovery as well. Renal levels of hepatocyte growth factor (HGF) increase after two models of renal failure, postnephrectomy and CCl4 injection, and this increase supports a role for HGF in renal repair.[29] Exogenous EGF has been shown to enhance renal tubular cell regeneration and to lessen the severity and duration of hypoxia and toxin-induced renal failure. EGF receptor levels increase within hours of postischemic injury in the rat. Elevation of soluble EGF occurs along with morphological evidence of tubular injury within 12 hours of ischemia, which is followed by cell proliferation and a decrease in soluble EGF by 24 to 48 hours after ischemia.

Alterations in Cell Membranes

Membrane phospholipids have a structural function and affect membrane permeability, as well as the activity of membrane transport systems.[30] These compounds are regulated in part by the activity of phospholipases, which release free fatty acids from phospholipids. Several mechanisms related to acute cell injury may alter phospholipase activity and thereby change membrane phospholipids and membrane integrity: altered intracellular calcium homeostasis, depletion of ATP, and lipid peroxidation.[22] Increased phospholipase activity has been associated with an abnormal increase in permeability of the inner mitochondrial membrane, which ultimately results in disruption of mitochondria and loss of the ability to produce adequate energy.

Cellular Calcium Homeostasis

Increased intracellular calcium is commonly found in cell injury (see Chapter 93). It is not, however, a consistent finding in all models of renal injury.[31] Techniques to study changes in the subcellular distribution of calcium have allowed time-related changes to be assessed. In the rat proximal tubule, steady-state hypoxia is accompanied by a prompt increase in cytosolic free calcium, which precedes the appearance of membrane damage. The increase in calcium is reversed with reoxygenation.[32] Increased cellular calcium may activate phospholipases, as previously mentioned; alter the cytoskeleton and cause injury by allowing cell swelling; or affect membrane permeability at the plasma membrane, the mitochondrial membrane, or the endoplasmic reticulum. Alterations in mitochondrial function that occur as a result of calcium loading of this organelle have been extensively studied. Excess mitochondrial calcium is associated with changes in the permeability of the inner mitochondrial membrane with loss of the electrochemical gradient and the capacity for oxidative phosphorylation. In addition, changes in enzyme activity and mitochondrial levels of nucleotides may exist (see Chapters 93 and 97).

Production of Free Radicals

Renal cell damage induced by inflammation or oxygen deprivation may be mediated, in part, by oxygen free radicals that are generated by several cell processes (see Chapter 97). The net result is increased intracellular calcium and ultimately changes in membrane-related functions.[22]

Tubular Cell Energy Metabolism

After exposure to a variety of nephrotoxins or ischemia, renal cortical ATP levels are reduced even before changes in membrane integrity and cell death occur.[22,33,34,35] In ischemic injury, alterations in renal perfusion may result in decreased oxygen delivery to tubular epithelium. Direct mitochondrial damage has been postulated to be the primary event in many forms of nephrotoxic injury.[22] Other nephrotoxins interfere with energy production by the inhibition of enzymes along the citric acid cycle. In this way, toxins impair energy production. ATP levels decrease immediately after ischemia, with concomitant increases in ATP hydrolysis products. Reflow is associated with a gradual increase in cell ATP levels.

Classification of Acute Glomerulotubular Dysfunction

Hemodynamically Mediated Acute Renal Failure

Renal hypoperfusion with ischemia is a common form of acute renal damage, especially in the setting of the intensive care unit (ICU). This form of renal injury is often accompanied by oliguria and results from alterations in renal perfusion after a period of hypoxia, hypotension, cardiac dysfunction, or any condition that promotes hemodynamic instability, decreased effective plasma volume, or both states. This condition is commonly referred to as *acute tubular necrosis* because it is characterized by necrosis of tubule cells; however, this is a nonspecific term that may also define nephrotoxic injury. A preferred term is *vasomotor nephropathy* or *hemodynamically mediated renal failure*.[36] The same physiological alterations that initiate renal injury in this form of nephropathy may potentiate renal failure in conditions whose primary inciting event may not have been vascular. This is discussed in more detail later in this chapter.

Vasomotor nephropathy commonly follows a period of renal compensatory changes that may be termed preprerenal failure and prerenal failure,[3] which are discussed in the preceding section on physiology. When the kidney has fully used normal compensatory mechanisms, renal oxygen delivery is critically impaired, and this impairment results in cell damage or tubular cell necrosis. Thus it is apparent that acute tubular necrosis is the end result of a continuum of renal adaptive mechanisms. Acute cortical necrosis is an exaggerated and more advanced form of renal ischemia.[37]

When vascular or hemodynamic abnormalities persist or are profound, renal compensatory mechanisms are unable to preserve RBF and maintain sufficient oxygen delivery and GFR. At a mean renal perfusion pressure of 80 mmHg, afferent, arteriolar dilation is maximal and below these systemic pressures, RBF dramatically declines.[3,36] In addition, loss of the ability to autoregulate as a result of ischemia may cause further damage.[23] Renal cell injury develops as the result of deficient oxygen delivery, depletion of cellular energy, loss of membrane integrity, and release of reactive oxygen species. Without sufficient oxygen, the kidney cannot support cell functions that maintain architectural integrity and complex transport functions.

Although total RBF is decreased in vasomotor nephropathy, outer cortical blood flow is preferentially reduced.[37] The medulla is not spared, however, because of its increased susceptibility to alterations in renal perfusion.[23,38] Oxygen delivery to this segment of the kidney is precarious. Medullary partial pressure of oxygen (PO_2) is approximately 10 mmHg in the rat and dog.

This oxygen level approaches the critical minimum level required to support oxidative phosphorylation and ATP synthesis for cell function. In general, however, the proximal tubule sustains the greatest injury. The renal arteriogram of human subjects with vasomotor nephropathy reveals marked narrowing of the arcuate arteries and absence of peripheral vasculature, providing further evidence for the marked vascular resistance enhancement.[36]

The primary event in vasomotor nephropathy is injury of the renal tubule. The initiation of this injury, however, is microvascular in origin. Maximal renal compensation with marked efferent and afferent arteriolar vasoconstriction reduces glomerular plasma flow with resulting hypofiltration and compromises postglomerular blood supply to the renal tubule. Tubular cell necrosis with sloughing of tubular cells into the lumen results in obstruction of flow and backleakage of filtrate through the injured epithelium. Alterations in tubular cell function in cells receiving sublethal or lethal injury increase fluid and salt delivery distally, and this increase signals the glomerulotubular feedback system to cause vasoconstriction of the afferent arteriole and limit the fraction of plasma filtered at the glomerulus.[3,36] Although the initial reduction in GFR is the result of decreased RBF and tubular factors such as obstruction and backleakage, continued hypofiltration during the maintenance phase is related primarily to continued vasoconstriction and renal hypoperfusion.[15,36] Recovery from postischemic ARF is biphasic. Initially, an increase in GFR occurs with relief of tubular obstruction and subsequently improved filtration in association with renal vasodilation.

Oliguria in the presence of renal hypoperfusion has been referred to as acute renal success by investigators who propose that the response of an intelligent organ to a perceived reduction in blood flow is to reduce fluid and electrolyte losses by vasoconstriction to reduce the fraction of plasma filtered and by maximal reabsorption of fluid and salt to restore the circulation (Fig. 64–6).[39] In addition, increased distal delivery of water and solutes because of tubular cell necrosis reflects failure of the renal tubule to absorb what is filtered. The appropriate response of an intact nephron is to reduce filtration by release of angiotensin II into the interstitium. Angiotensin II mediates arteriolar vasoconstriction, which decreases glomerular plasma flow, and retraction of the glomerular tuft, which reduces Kf, the net effect being decreased glomerular filtration.[19,38]

The classic form of hemodynamically mediated ARF was oliguric, by definition; however, nonoliguric acute vasomotor nephropathy is increasingly recognized.[38,40] This form of less severe disease has been referred to as attenuated *acute tubular necrosis* and has allowed the recognition of three stages of ARF that actually represent a continuum of worsening disease: First, abbreviated renal insufficiency occurs after a single event of renal hypoperfusion, such as aortic cross-clamping, in the face of adequate volume repletion and SBP. This syndrome is characterized by an acute drop in the GFR with gradual return to normal within a few days. The inability to concentrate the urine or to conserve sodium provides evidence of tubular injury. The second phase or form is referred to as *overt renal failure*. An example of this

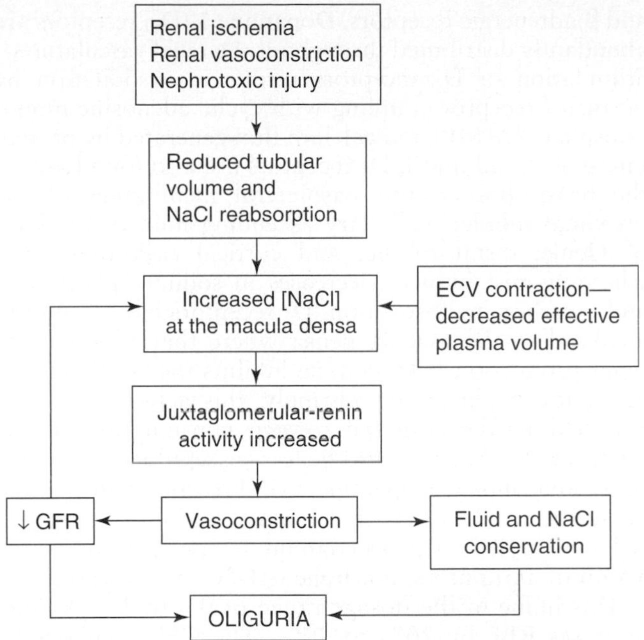

FIGURE 64–6 • Revised tubuloglomerular feedback and its role in potentiating oliguria and reduced glomerular filtration rate.

situation is aortic cross-clamping followed by continued renal hypoperfusion because of poor cardiac function. A more prolonged period of hypofiltration lasts for several days to weeks with a gradual return of the GFR. If recovery of renal perfusion is impaired by repeated episodes of hypotension, sepsis, or hypoxia, the third pattern may be observed in which a protracted course may be observed and chances for recovery may be doubtful.[40] One situation in which the last example could exist is aggressive hemodialysis (ultrafiltration) with hypovolemia and, consequently, renal hypoperfusion in the recovering phase of renal failure. Clinical experience has supported this theory (see Chapter 65). Patients with multiple renal insults have a more protracted course and increased morbidity.[41]

Attenuation of Acute Renal Failure

Prevention or attenuation of ARF has been the subject of numerous studies because most agree that protection of the kidney from damage or enhancing recovery after damage would be preferable to currently available supportive therapies. Protective agents have been studied extensively with animal models of acute renal injury. Some of these agents have ultimately been used in clinical situations with variable success. In general, methods to reduce renal injury have been aimed at manipulation of RVR or alteration of the metabolic processes of the renal tubular cell.[42]

Dopamine

Dopamine, infused in low intravenous doses, increases RBF, increases GFR, and increases sodium excretion. The renal actions of dopamine are exerted by two major classes of dopamine receptors at high doses: α-adrenergic and β-adrenergic receptors. Dopamine 1 (D_1) receptors are abundantly distributed throughout the renal vasculature.[43] Stimulation of D_1 receptors results in vasodilation by means of receptor coupling with cyclic adenosine monophosphate (cAMP) and calcium flux generated by protein kinase A. In addition, D_1 receptors are also found within the brush border and basolateral membranes of the proximal tubule; medullary ascending limb of the loop of Henle; distal tubule; and cortical collecting ducts where agonist induces decreases in sodium, phosphate, and bicarbonate absorption. D_1 receptors have also been localized to the macula densa where they may modify renin production.[43] Dopamine inhibits the Na/K-ATPase along the nephron. Interestingly, this action would be expected to decrease the oxygen consumption of the renal tubule; thus it would be less susceptible to ischemic or hypoxic injury. Dopamine 2 (D_2) receptors are present along the renal tubule. In the inner medulla, a subclass, D_2k is coupled to prostaglandin E_2 and attenuates the action of antidiuretic hormone (ADH) in this segment.

Dopamine in the dosage range of 0.5 to 2 μg/kg/min increases RBF by 20% to 40%. The GFR increases by 5% to 20%, an effect related to enhanced glomerular ultrafiltration by a preferential vasodilation at the afferent arteriole.[43] This is thought to be related to a dopamine-induced increase in local angiotensin production, which attenuates the dopamine-induced vasodilation at the efferent but not the afferent arteriole. The increase in medullary blood flow observed with dopamine results in a decrease in the urea concentration within the medullary interstitium and contributes to the limited concentrating ability of the dopamine-stimulated renal tubule.

The observed increase in urinary flow is thought to be related primarily to the tubular actions rather than the vascular actions of dopamine. At higher doses, dopamine stimulation of receptors results in decreased sodium and fluid excretion, as well as renal vasoconstriction. Dopamine clearance is decreased in the presence of renal or liver dysfunction.[43] Dopamine increases the creatinine clearance and urine volume in patients with ischemic ARF, especially when there is coexisting cardiac dysfunction. Dopamine should be used cautiously in neonates because the renal vascular response to dopamine is age dependent,[44] although administration of dopamine (0.5 to 2 μg/kg/min) to premature neonates with respiratory distress syndrome and renal insufficiency was reported to result in improved creatinine clearance without major side effects.[45]

Diuretics

Loop diuretics and mannitol have been used in the oliguric phase of prerenal and renal failure as a means of increasing urine flow; however, these agents rarely improve the GFR or the morbidity associated with ARF.[46] Mannitol may attenuate renal failure if it is given before the insult or immediately afterward.[47,48] Loop diuretics, such as furosemide, if given along with a potentially nephrotoxic agent, may increase the renal excretion of the agent and reduce associated nephrotoxicity. Mannitol has been shown to ameliorate nephrotoxicity related to gentamicin, amphotericin B, cisplatin, and myoglobin. A specific beneficial effect is doubtful, however, because acute saline loading alone provides similar protection. When tubular obstruction plays a major role, mannitol may increase tubular flow enough to wash obstructing debris downstream. It seems reasonable to use mannitol and potentially furosemide in the initial phases of oliguria when ARF may not be established; these agents provide little benefit and may increase toxicity in sustained oliguria as a result of tubular necrosis.

Calcium Entry Blockers

These agents may prevent renal insufficiency through their vasodilatory action on renal vasculature, as well as inhibition of calcium entry. The calcium channel blockers verapamil, nitrendipine, diltiazem, and nisoldipine have been administered to various animal models of ischemic injury with some success in the prevention or attenuation of renal failure. Minimal protection is observed, however, if they are administered after ischemia.[42,49,50,51] Calcium entry blockers had a beneficial effect in endotoxin-mediated ARF.[52] This effect was postulated to be a result of an antagonism of platelet-activating factor.[53] The perfusion of cadaveric renal grafts before transplantation with diltiazem was associated with improved graft survival compared with control subjects.[54] Preoperative administration of calcium channel blockers to adults undergoing cardiac surgical procedures did not provide any obvious protection from the development of ARF.[55]

Prostaglandins

Vasoconstrictive forces in the renal vasculature may result from the action of vasoconstrictor prostaglandins and are counteracted by the vasodilatory substances.[42,56] Infusion or stimulation of the vasodilatory prostaglandins or inhibition of the vasoconstrictor prostaglandins seems to be a reasonable approach. Prostacyclin provided protection during ischemia in a rat model.[56] Administration of the thromboxane synthetase inhibitor OKY-046 partially ameliorated hypofiltration in a rat model of ischemic renal failure.[57] In addition, the administration of the free radical scavengers dimethylthiourea and superoxide dismutase attenuated renal insufficiency and reduced thromboxane levels.

Renin-Angiotensin Antagonists

Administration of saralasin, an angiotensin II receptor antagonist, either before or after ischemia was not beneficial in the rat model.[58] Blockade of angiotensin production by the conversion of enzyme inhibition with enalapril or captopril was not successful in preventing ARF.[59] Although captopril did prevent a fall in RBF, in one study the GFR actually dropped.[42]

Adenosine and Adenosine Triphosphate

Renal ischemia results in the depletion of cellular adenine nucleotides and increased levels of adenosine, an agent implicated as a mediator of local vasoconstriction.[60] Adenosine may also have protective tubular effects during ischemia because it inhibits solute reabsorption in the medullary thick ascending limb of the loop of Henle.[23] Theophylline, which is a competitive inhibitor of adenosine receptors, partially prevents the hypofiltration following ischemia in the rat.[42]

Infusion of ATP–magnesium chloride (ATP-$MgCl_2$) after renal ischemia promotes more rapid cellular recovery and attenuates renal injury.[60] Exogenous ATP, adenosine diphosphate (ADP), adenosine monophosphate (AMP), and adenosine preserve renal tubular cell metabolism during anoxia by protecting the membrane from disruption and providing precursors for rapid synthesis of ATP during reperfusion.[33,35]

Atrial Natriuretic Factor

Atrial natriuretic factor (ANF) has direct effects on glomerular hemodynamics and GFR.[61] ANF dilates arcuate, interlobular, and proximal afferent arterioles, and it relaxes mesangial cells.[62] In a rat model of rhabdomyolysis, administration of ANF improved GFR and enhanced sodium and water excretion.[1] In addition, ANF improved GFR and maintained cell energy levels during ischemic injury.[63] ANF preserves glomerular filtration and cellular ATP levels in experimental models of ARF by its effect on glomerular hemodynamics.

Free Radical Scavengers

Reactive oxygen species have been proposed as a cause of cellular injury in many forms of ARF.[42,64] The conversion of xanthine to hypoxanthine during reoxygenation produces free radicals. Antioxidants and xanthine oxidase inhibition (allopurinol) have proved to attenuate renal injury in many models of ARF.

Thyroxine

Thyroxine reduces renal injury in a number of experimental models when given before the injury, immediately after, or 24 hours after ischemia.[51] The mechanism by which thyroxine preserves both glomerular and tubular function is not completely understood; however, the rate of recovery of cellular ATP levels was much more rapid in animals given thyroxine after ischemic ARF. Isolated mitochondria from rats subjected to 45 minutes of ischemia exhibited decreased mitochondrial ADP transport. Administration of thyroxine was associated with significantly enhanced ADP transport.[65] The investigators speculated that part of the ATP depletion associated with ischemic injury might be the result of decreased mitochondrial uptake of the ATP precursor, ADP. The administration of thyroxine at 5 to 6 ng/kg/day for 5 to 10 days in eight children with ARF resulted in the recovery of renal function in all but one child, who died of the original disease.[66] A subsequent report of six children treated in a similar manner revealed similar findings.[67]

Glycine

The amino acids glycine and alanine have recently been shown to have cytoprotective effects against injury in anoxia-hypoxia and chemotherapy-induced renal failure.[64] The mechanism of cytoprotection is not understood but does not appear to involve preservation of intracellular ATP levels. Studies performed in cultured proximal tubular cells indicate that glycine and alanine may stimulate the expression of Hsp genes and increase Hsp proteins, which protect cells from injury. The cytoprotective effect was not observed with other amino acids and was independent of cellular ATP levels in this model of renal injury.[68] Incubation of isolated renal tubules with glycine during hypoxia was associated with increased levels of glutathione, as well as increased cell ATP, although these did not appear to account fully for the protective effect of glycine.[64] In addition, administration of glycine prevented renal injury in rats treated with nephrotoxic doses of cisplatin.[69]

Treatment of Acute Renal Failure

Rapid and severe deterioration of renal function can have a profound effect on body fluid homeostasis and on blood pressure. The nature of these alterations often requires intensive care management regardless of the precise underlying diagnosis. A wide variety of renal diseases may result in ARF. The most urgent aspects of ARF are (1) hyperkalemia, (2) severe hypertension, (3) severe plasma and extracellular volume expansion leading to heart failure and pulmonary edema, (4) unremitting metabolic acidosis, (5) hypocalcemia/hyperphosphatemia, and (6) uremia. Each item in the list is frequently used as an indication for dialysis, but in fact it could be viewed as an indication for intensive care and consideration of dialysis.[70]

*Hyperkalemia**

The major reason for the development of hyperkalemia (serum potassium concentration more than 6 mEq/L) is the release (or infusion, or both) of potassium into the extracellular space at a rate greater than the kidney's ability to excrete potassium. The fact that ARF and oliguria have developed does not mean that hyperkalemia will develop. By the same token, hyperkalemia may develop rapidly in situations of extensive tissue destruction even without oliguria and "full-blown" ARF. Thus in the clinical situation of a crush injury or the tumor lysis syndrome, hyperkalemia should be anticipated and careful anticipatory monitoring begun.

Severe Hypertension

Hypertension is frequently associated with renal disease. The two main mechanisms by which renal disease leads to hypertension, especially accelerated hypertension, are (1) plasma volume expansion caused by the failure to excrete sodium chloride and water and (2) hyperreninemia associated with decreased renal perfusion. For a more complete discussion of hypertension and its treatment, see Chapter 66.

*See Chapter 60.

Plasma and Extracellular Volume Expansion

Plasma and extracellular volume expansion are associated with renal failure. With an abrupt decline in GFR, even "normal" amounts of sodium and water intake expand the extracellular and plasma volumes. Depending on the cardiac status of the patient, the serum albumin level, and the degree of capillary permeability, this extracellular and plasma volume expansion may be manifest as peripheral edema, hypertension, or congestive heart failure and pulmonary edema. In situations of hypertension or congestive heart failure, the treatment involves two principles. The first is to reduce to as low a level as possible the amount of sodium the patient receives. This requires attention to diet, intravenous or hyperalimentation solutions, and drugs. The second principle is to remove extracellular fluid. If the patient's renal function permits (glomerular filtration of approximately 15 ml/min or higher), then diuretics, especially loop diuretics such as furosemide, bumetanide, or ethacrynic acid, will help to stimulate a diuresis that should improve the blood pressure or the congestive heart failure. In children with more severe renal disease, diuretic therapy does not result in diuresis, and dialysis will be necessary.

Severe Metabolic Acidosis

Severe metabolic acidosis is encountered when renal function abruptly ceases. The kidney is responsible for the excretion of hydrogen ion and the regeneration of bicarbonate. When renal function rapidly deteriorates, then the extracellular concentration of hydrogen ion increases, and this increase leads to acidosis and low serum bicarbonate concentrations. This problem is exacerbated by conditions that increase the production of hydrogen ion and its release into the extracellular fluid. Conditions such as sepsis, severe trauma, burns, extensive abdominal disease or surgery, and hemolysis are all examples in which hypoxia, high H^+ ion production and/or release into the extracellular space, and a decline in RBF and the GFR are combined. The result is severe metabolic acidosis (see Chapter 61).

Hypocalcemia/Hyperphosphatemia

Defects in mineral metabolism are evident in patients with ARF. These patients appear to have secondary hyperparathyroidism accompanied by skeletal resistance to parathyroid hormone (PTH). The major factors contributing to increased PTH secretion are hypocalcemia and reduced values of calcitriol (1,25-dihydroxycholecalciferol) (Fig. 64–7; see Chapter 70). Hypocalcemia arises from hyperphosphatemia as a result of dietary load, cellular breakdown, and reduced renal phosphate excretion; reduced synthesis of calcitriol; down-regulation of skeletal cell receptors for PTH; and acidosis.[71] Diminished circulating values of calcitriol and hypocalcemia augment PTH synthesis and secretion, with the result that both hypocalcemia and hyperphosphatemia are found, similar to changes in chronic renal failure.

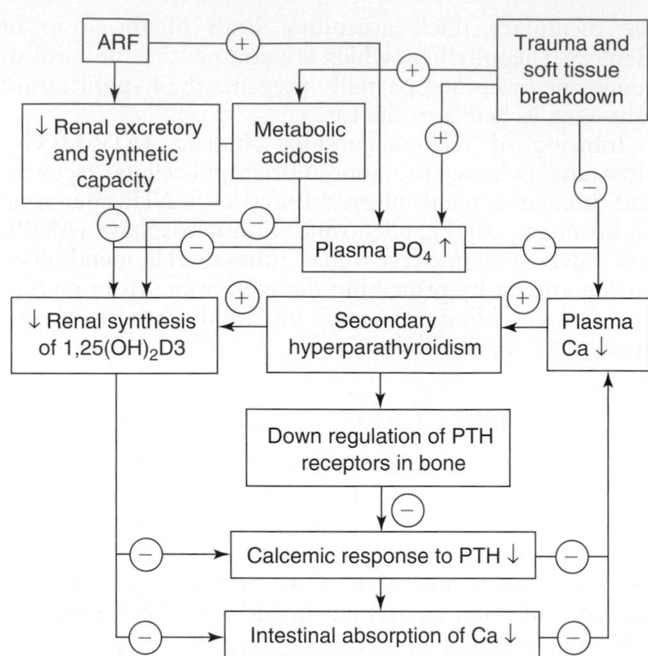

FIGURE 64–7 • Mechanisms that contribute to altered mineral metabolism in acute renal failure.

Of interest, these changes in divalent minerals can be found within hours of the onset of ARF; therefore an impaired movement of divalent ions across muscle and other tissue membranes, particularly after injury that causes muscle damage and ARF, is suggested. These ionic changes are accentuated as ARF progresses and the kidney is less able to excrete phosphorus, potassium, and protons. An implication of these changes in serum calcium and phosphorus is a potential aggravation of hyperkalemic cardiotoxicity. Finally, the persistent hyperparathyroidism and increased synthesis of calcitriol are responsible, in part, for the hypercalcemia that may occur during the recovery phase of ARF.

Uremia

ARF involves all organ systems to some degree. The symptoms of uremia are frequently vague and difficult to quantitate. They include central nervous system (CNS) manifestations such as lethargy, confusion, seizures, and obtundation and also gastrointestinal manifestations such as anorexia, nausea, and vomiting. These symptoms plus metabolic derangements often lead to the initiation of dialysis.

An important consideration in ARF is the role of the kidney in the metabolism, elimination, and detoxification of endogenous and exogenous materials. Any drugs given must be reviewed because the dosing interval or the dose of drug may need to be altered in renal failure (see Chapters 63 and 110). Endogenous substances generally are more slowly metabolized or excreted. For example, the hormone gastrin is metabolized by the proximal tubule after being filtered by the glomerulus. The resultant persistent high circulating levels of gastrin may explain the higher incidence of gastritis and ulcer disease seen in patients with renal failure.

Specific Renal Diseases That May Lead to Acute Renal Failure

Hemolytic Uremic Syndrome

Hemolytic uremic syndrome (HUS) is characterized by thrombotic microangiopathy with platelet aggregation and fibrin deposition in small vessels in the kidney, gut, CNS, and elsewhere. The hemolytic anemia is related predominantly to shearing of red blood cells as they pass through involved vessels. In the typical form of the disease a triggering infectious agent has been reported frequently. Most recently *Escherichia coli* (0157:H7) has been implicated in a large number of cases of typical (epidemic) forms of HUS.[26,72] In many institutions the most common cause of ARF is the hemolytic-uremic syndrome.[73,74] The syndrome is defined by the presence of anemia (hemolysis), thrombocytopenia, and impaired renal function.

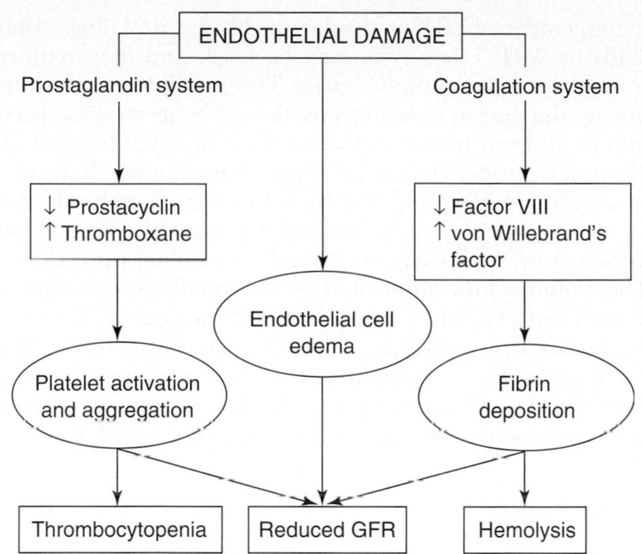

FIGURE 64–8 • Pathophysiology of microangiopathic disease.

Clinical Signs

Typical HUS usually presents in "epidemics" and is characterized by a prodrome of bloody diarrhea. Children with HUS are older than 1 year and younger than 10 years (typically, 18 months to 3 years). The important presenting features of bloody diarrhea, fever, lethargy, decreased urine output, and paleness should lead to a suspicion of HUS. Laboratory evaluation will verify the diagnosis.

Thrombotic vascular diseases such as HUS and thrombotic thrombocytopenic purpura are characterized by microangiopathic anemia, thrombocytopenia, and azotemia. The predominant finding is glomerular capillary obstruction with endothelial cell swelling and fibrin thrombi. Small vessels of the gut, CNS, and elsewhere may be involved. The development of HUS has been associated with bacterial and viral infections, oral contraceptives, cyclosporin A, and complement abnormalities.[58,75,76] The final common pathway, regardless of the initiating agent, is endothelial cell injury. As noted, development of HUS is commonly associated with infection with a verotoxin-producing strain of *E. coli* (0157:H7), as well as a strain of *Shigella* that produces a similar toxin.[77] Other bacteria may elaborate neuraminidase whose action exposes the Thomsen-Friedenreich antigen on glomeruli, red blood cells, and platelets, and this promotes agglutination of erythrocytes and aggregation of platelets within the glomerulus.[75,76] Endotoxin alone appears to play a direct role in endothelial cell injury. Animal models in which two injections of endotoxin (generalized Shwartzman reaction) are used show marked intracapillary fibrin deposition, which can be prevented by anticoagulants.

Once the endothelium is injured and the subendothelial region is exposed, a sequence of events is set into motion that serves to amplify the initial endothelial damage (Figure 64–8).[78] Platelets adhere to the subendothelial space, and a release reaction follows that activates additional platelets and initiates fibrin deposition. Both endothelial cell and platelet factors are involved in the propagation of intraglomerular fibrin deposition and coagulation. Direct injury of the endothelial cell may initiate coagulation by release of tissue factor or exposure of the basement membrane. Evidence suggests that the endothelial cells in patients with HUS have reduced ability to produce prostacyclin (PGI_2), a potent vasodilator and inhibitor of platelet aggregation. Some patients with HUS lack a plasma factor that stimulates PGI_2 production. In addition, there is decreased glomerular fibrinolytic activity because of a circulating inhibitor of plasminogen activator. Interestingly, this fibrinolysis inhibitor is removed from the circulation by dialysis.[76] Platelet count and survival time are decreased in patients with HUS, and occasionally there is evidence of platelet activation.

HUS is a heterogeneous group of disorders that have a common result. As a means of differentiating the pathogenesis and clinical outcome, the following classification scheme has been proposed[75]:

1. The classic form presents in infants or small children after a prodrome of bloody diarrhea that may involve the verotoxin-producing strain of *E. coli*.
2. The postinfectious form is associated with an identified infectious agent such as *Shigella* or *Salmonella* or with endotoxemia.
3. Hereditary forms have been recognized that have both autosomal dominant and recessive modes of inheritance. These patients probably lack a plasma factor necessary for PGI_2 production or have a prostacyclin inhibitor.
4. An immunologically mediated form is characterized by low plasma C3 and activation of the alternative complement pathway. This form may also be familial.
5. A so-called secondary form is related to known predisposing conditions such as lupus, scleroderma, chemotherapy, malignant hypertension, and renal irradiation.
6. A form related to pregnancy or use of oral contraceptives is characterized by arterial microangiopathy.

Immediate life-threatening aspects of HUS are numerous.[74] ARF is a major problem, and the basic management of HUS is similar to that for any illness that leads to ARF. Hemolysis may be brisk and may require transfusions on a daily basis. The aim of transfusions during the period of hemolysis should be to prevent heart failure and not to return the hematocrit value to normal. Thrombocytopenia may be severe but only rarely results in significant bleeding, and therefore platelets should not be given unless clearly needed to stop bleeding or in anticipation of invasive (especially vascular) procedures. The volume infused should be as small as possible; it should not exceed 15 ml/kg per body weight. Some have suggested that platelets play an important role in the pathophysiology of this disorder. It is further suggested that infusing platelets may actually prolong or worsen the intravascular deposition characteristic of HUS.

Complications

Other organ system involvement may lead to serious complications. CNS involvement may reflect the metabolic effects of uremia and can be manifested by lethargy, somnolence, stupor, coma, or seizures. Seizures, paresis, and even CNS hemorrhages can result from vascular damage and CNS vessel occlusion. Gastrointestinal involvement has also been well documented.[79] Liver enzyme elevations, abdominal pain, intestinal obstruction, and bowel perforation have all been reported. These possibilities must be considered and evaluated when appropriate. In some instances, the diagnosis of HUS has been made after abdominal exploration.

Therapy

In recent years therapy has been conservative, aimed at preventing deterioration and carefully managing such complications as ARF, anemia, and CNS and abdominal symptoms. Furthermore, any therapy would have to show a dramatic benefit to improve on a complete recovery rate of more than 90%.

Comprehensive supportive care has clearly resulted in a dramatic decline in the mortality from HUS (40% in the 1950s to 5% to 10% in the 1980s).[74] Nevertheless, therapy specifically aimed at HUS has been attempted because vascular platelet plugging and fibrin deposition in arterioles is part of the pathophysiology.

Heparin, fibrinolytics, and antiplatelet drugs (aspirin, dipyridamole) have all been attempted. In general, reports demonstrate lack of benefit and, in the cases of heparin and fibrinolytics, increased harm from increased bleeding.[74] Fresh frozen plasma infusion was suggested because of the finding that serum from some patients with HUS cannot generate normal amounts of prostaglandin or does not demonstrate normal antithrombotic and antiplatelet function.[80] All these defects could account for the thrombotic microangiopathy of HUS. Fresh frozen plasma might provide the missing factors that could ultimately reduce microangiopathy. Unfortunately, studies in patients did not demonstrate a beneficial effect.[81] Plasmapheresis has not been tested as carefully as fresh frozen plasma infusion in patients with typical HUS. Currently, plasmapheresis must be viewed as untested and not recommended.[82]

Vitamin E therapy has been proposed after findings of abnormal lipid peroxidation and low vitamin E activity in patients with HUS. Anecdotal studies suggested some benefit, but controlled, albeit small, studies have not shown benefit.[83,84]

Most recently, intravenous immunoglobulin G (IgG) infusions have received attention on the basis of studies in adults that showed IgG can inhibit platelet aggregation.[85] This presumably would diminish thrombotic microangiopathy and reduce the period of time of thrombocytopenia. Controlled studies have not been completed. The preliminary data suggest a shorter period of thrombocytopenia but, as yet, little information on reductions in other morbidities of HUS.[86]

Prognosis

The prognosis for the "typical" form of HUS is good. Most series report 3% to 5% mortality rates and an additional 3% to 5% with chronic changes such as chronic renal disease, persistent hematuria/proteinuria, and chronic hypertension. Thus more than 90% of children with the typical form of HUS recover completely.

Acute Glomerulonephritis

Nearly every form of glomerulonephritis has been reported to present as ARF (Box 64–2). In some instances the renal insufficiency may be the result of an immunological process leading to acute inflammation (e.g., acute poststreptococcal glomerulonephritis). In others, intravascular volume depletion may play a prominent role in ARF (e.g., minimal change nephrotic syndrome).

In general, glomerulonephritis is initiated by immunological events within the glomerulus followed by mechanisms that result in damage to the glomerulus.[77,87] Glomerular disease results from the deposition of immune complexes composed of (1) antibodies to nonrenal antigens that localize within the glomeruli and form in situ immune complexes; (2) circulating soluble immune complexes that are trapped within the mesangium or subendothelial space; or (3) antibody to antigens within the glomerulus, either as normal glomerular antigens or as neoantigens induced by inflammation or infection. Antibody deposits promote injury

BOX 64–2

Acute Nephritis and Acute Renal Failure

- Acute poststreptococcal glomerulonephritis
- Membranoproliferative glomerulonephritis
- Rapidly progressive glomerulonephritis
- Minimal change nephrotic syndrome
- Henoch-Schönlein purpura
- Immunoglobulin A nephropathy
- Hemolytic uremic syndrome
- Systemic lupus erythematosus
- Vasculitis
- Nephritis associated with bacterial infection

by activation of inflammatory cells or by their direct interaction with glomerular cells. The result is mesangial cell proliferation, capillary wall and basement membrane injury, and extracapillary proliferation of epithelial cells, a process known as *crescent formation.*

Immune complexes mediate glomerular injury in two ways (Fig. 64–9): through direct membrane damage by the membranolytic membrane attack complex (C5b-9) or by stimulation of glomerular localized inflammatory cells.[77] The degree of inflammatory cell participation may depend on the site of immune complex deposition within the glomerulus. Subendothelial deposits appear to elicit the most intense inflammatory response. Neutrophils are recruited in response to C5a, platelet-activating factor, leukotriene B4, and other products released from damaged cells. Neutrophils adhere to the glomerular endothelium or denuded subendothelial space, become activated, and release additional toxic mediators such as reactive oxygen species and proteinases. Monocytes and macrophages are also effector cells in many forms of glomerular immune injury. Macrophages produce prostaglandins, tumor necrosis factor, growth factors, complement components, and coagulants. The macrophage is particularly important in the pathogenesis of crescentic glomerulonephritis, which is a common form of glomerulonephritis presenting in ARF. In crescentic glomerulonephritis, macrophages enter Bowman's space through breaks in the glomerular basement membrane, release procoagulants that induce fibrin deposition, and also release growth factors that stimulate the proliferation of parietal epithelial cells. The cluster of epithelioid cells, called a *crescent,* eventually crowds and chokes off the glomerulus; thus glomerular function is compromised. In addition to damage promoted by circulating cells, glomerular mesangial cells may proliferate in response to immune complexes, C5b-9, endotoxin, and growth factors and thus reduce the surface area available for filtration. Mesangial cells produce prostaglandins, tissue necrosis factor, oxidants, proteases, and extracellular matrix, which intensify the inflammatory response.

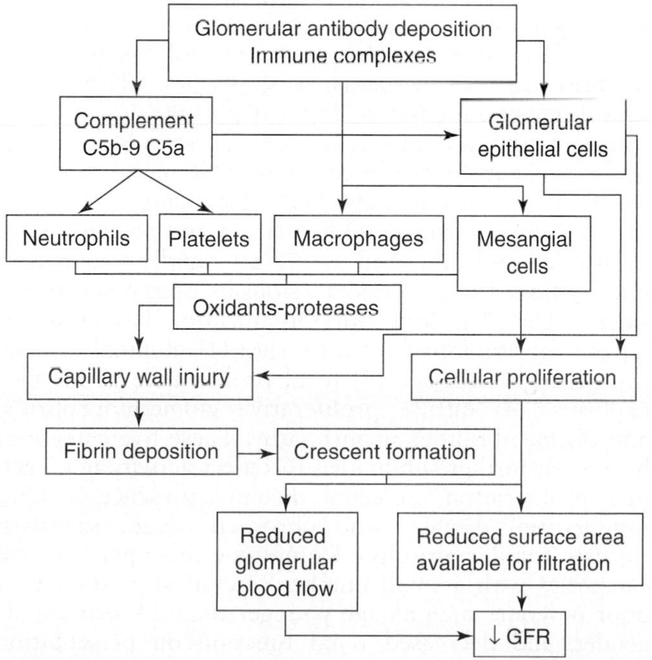

FIGURE 64–9 • Pathogenesis of immune-mediated glomerulonephritis and physiological sequelae. (Modified with permission from Couser WG: Mediation of immune glomerular injury, *J Am Soc Nephrol* 1:13, 1990.)

The physiological abnormalities observed in acute glomerulonephritis are the consequence of glomerular cell proliferation, fibrin deposition, and crescent formation.[88] Hypofiltration occurs as a result of decreased glomerular blood flow, as well as a decrease in the Kf. Arteriolar vasoconstriction, capillary obstruction by thrombi, and endothelial cell edema compromise glomerular blood flow. Both afferent and efferent arteriolar vasoconstriction is observed in experimental forms of acute glomerulonephritis. Neither the renin-angiotensin system nor the prostaglandin system is thought to contribute to this vasoconstriction. Evidence suggests vasoconstrictive substances may be released as a consequence of complement activation. In addition, the adrenergic nervous system may mediate vasoconstriction. Reduction in RBF is a less important factor than intrinsic changes in the glomerulus because the reduction in the GFR is disproportionate to the reduction in renal plasma flow.

A reduction in the Kf has been observed in many experimental forms of glomerulonephritis.[89] Initially the hydraulic permeability is reduced in response to the elaboration of compounds such as angiotensin II, prostaglandins, vasopressin, histamine, and bradykinin. These compounds may also stimulate the contraction of mesangial cells and consequently reduce the surface area for filtration. Proliferation of mesangial and epithelial cells further reduces the surface area available for filtration. Infiltration of the glomerulus by circulating inflammatory cells further impairs glomerular blood flow.

Salt and water retention commonly observed with acute glomerulonephritis is the result of a decreased GFR, not increased tubular reabsorption, as once proposed. The renin-angiotensin system is thought not to play a role in the positive salt and water balance. In general, the presentation of glomerulonephritis as ARF implies a virulent form of disease known as *rapidly progressive* or *crescentic glomerulonephritis.* Although *rapidly progressive* refers to a clinical characteristic and *crescentic* to a pathological feature, the two are commonly coincidental in the presentation of ARF. A classification of rapidly progressive glomerulonephritis is presented in Box 64–3. Four prototypical conditions serve as examples of acute renal disease that may result in the need for intensive care.

Acute Poststreptococcal Glomerulonephritis

This condition is well known to pediatricians. An association between glomerulonephritis and scarlet fever was known in the eighteenth century. In the early twentieth century, however, a clear connection between streptococcal infections and glomerulonephritis was established.[10] The disease is most frequent between the ages of 2 and 12 years. It is seen as a sporadic event or in epidemics. It appears that only certain strains of streptococci lead

BOX 64-3

Classification of Rapidly Progressive, Crescentic Glomerulonephritis

Antiglomerular basement membrane antibody mediated
With pulmonary hemorrhage (Goodpasture's syndrome)
Without pulmonary hemorrhage
Immune complex mediated
Postinfectious
Systemic lupus erythematosus
Henoch-Schönlein purpura
Immunoglobulin A nephropathy
Membranoproliferative glomerulonephritis
Pauciimmune
Polyarteritis nodosa
Wegener's granulomatosis
Idiopathic

Data from Jennette JC, Falk RJ: Diagnosis and management of glomerulonephritis and vasculitis presenting as acute renal failure, *Med Clin North Am* 74:893, 1990.

to glomerulonephritis, thus the term *nephritogenic streptococcus*.[90]

The mechanism(s) by which nephritogenic streptococci cause glomerular injury is similar to that seen with "shunt nephritis." It is generally accepted that immune complexes with the participation of complement and other inflammatory mediators cause glomerular inflammation. The precise nature of the bacterial antigen and its site of formation (circulation compared with in situ in the glomerulus) remain areas of study.[91]

Clinical Signs. The usual sites of infection are the upper respiratory tract, skin, or both. A long-standing observation is that the latent period is 7 to 14 days if the infection is in the upper respiratory tract and 21 to 40 days if the infection is on the skin. Subclinical cases may be common; they are estimated to be 2 to 19 times as frequent as clinical cases.[90]

Symptomatic cases usually present with an acute nephritic syndrome: edema, hypertension, hematuria, and oliguria. Other important clinical features include proteinuria, red cell casts, and abnormal urinary red cell morphological findings, all markers of glomerular injury. Pulmonary edema may also be present, especially if significant salt and water retention are present and if hypertension is severe. Nonspecific findings include malaise, anorexia, abdominal pain, nausea, and vomiting. (This presentation is seen with other forms of acute glomerulonephritis.) Patients may have ARF.

Laboratory Findings. Laboratory findings at the time of presentation or early in the course include high serum IgG levels and low serum complement levels, especially C3 and CH50. In general, the alternate pathway of complement is the mechanism of complement activation, although on occasion C2 and C4 may be depressed as well. Complement levels return to normal in 4 to 6 weeks. Therefore if complement levels remain depressed for 6 to 8 weeks after the onset of acute glomerulonephritis, another diagnosis should be strongly entertained (systemic lupus erythematosus or membranoproliferative glomerulonephritis). Antistreptolysin O (ASO) titer is often elevated at the onset of the nephritic picture. The ASO titer response after skin infections is poor; however, antihyaluronidase and antideoxyribonuclease B (anti-DNAase B) detect a recent streptococcal infection in nearly all cases.

Treatment. Treatment is based on the patient's symptoms and is directed at preventing or reducing salt and water retention and hypertension. All patients should have salt and water restriction unless dehydration is obvious (an unusual situation). Approximately 50% to 60% of patients require treatment for hypertension. Diuretics, angiotensin-converting enzyme inhibitors, and potent vasodilators should be considered. Five percent of patients may require dialysis for congestive heart failure, hypervolemia, or encephalopathy.[90]

Prognosis. The long-term prognosis in acute poststreptococcal glomerulonephritis is a matter of debate. The mortality rate is approximately 0.5%, and death usually results from severe hypertension and encephalopathy or heart failure. Studies by Baldwin et al[92,93] suggested that the long-term prognosis generally thought to be excellent was in fact not necessarily so. They suggested 50% of patients had evidence of renal disease in long-term studies. Other authors, however, have suggested more limited chronic renal disease.[94,95] Studies with follow-up of 10 to 15 years suggest that chronic renal failure develops in approximately 1% of patients. A second consensus conclusion is that the prognosis is better in children than in adults.[90] Longer-term follow-up is needed.

Systemic Lupus Erythematosus

Systemic lupus erythematosus (SLE) is a protean illness affecting many organ systems. In some instances intensive care is needed for such aspects of SLE as nephritis, cerebritis, carditis, serositis, or sepsis (see Chapter 91). This discussion focuses on lupus nephritis.

Even within a relatively narrow aspect of SLE such as nephritis, great heterogeneity exists. Glomerulonephritis develops in approximately 75% of patients with SLE.[96] This may range from mild hematuria and proteinuria to nephrotic syndrome and rarely to rapidly progressive renal failure. The patterns of lesions in lupus nephritis are varied. The World Health Organization has classified lupus nephritis into five categories: (1) minimal disease, (2) mesangial disease, (3) focal proliferative glomerulonephritis, (4) diffuse proliferative glomerulonephritis, and (5) membranous nephropathy. These five categories have been further subdivided to reflect activity (e.g., cellular proliferation, crescents, thrombi, presence of tubulointerstitial disease) and chronicity (e.g., sclerosis, fibrosis, tubular atrophy). Combining these pathological categories with a small number of clinical predictors of poor outcome such as age younger than 24 years, male gender, and decreased renal function on presentation has permitted a more careful assessment of therapeutic interventions.[97]

Clinical Signs. The broad variation in clinical manifestations may reflect individual expression of similar immunopathological mechanisms or different immunopathological mechanisms presenting as a similar constellation of clinical manifestations. It is clear that SLE represents the overproduction of antibodies against multiple "self"-antigens. Patients with lupus have high titers of antinuclear antibodies and in particular anti–double-stranded DNA antibodies, which are often seen in SLE nephritis. The factors that lead to the abundant production and activation of relevant B cells are unclear. Certainly hormonal influence must be important because most patients with SLE are women. Environmental factors may be important in cases of SLE induced by drugs or viruses and the known association of SLE with ultraviolet light exposure. Other important factors are suggested by the higher than normal T helper/T suppressor cell ratio. Many of those act in concert to result in abundant antibody production and the deposition of complexes in target organs such as the kidney.[52]

Clinically, patients with SLE nephritis who require intensive care probably have rapidly progressive glomerulonephritis or ARF.[97] Their presentation includes many of the following features: hypertension; active urinary sediment with proteinuria, hematuria, and casts; oliguria or rarely anuria; intravascular volume expansion; and declining renal function with rising serum creatinine, hyperkalemia, and metabolic acidosis. Unlike the glomerulonephritis described previously, treatment should include management of renal dysfunction as previously outlined and management aimed at the SLE itself. Renal biopsy may be useful.[98] When in doubt, a biopsy specimen may help distinguish acute tubular necrosis from glomerulonephritis. A biopsy specimen will ascertain the degree of interstitial involvement, which may suggest drug toxicity. Biopsy can be useful in determining long-term treatment and prognosis.

Treatment. In the intensive care setting, treatment directed at rapidly progressive or diffuse proliferative SLE nephritis consists of high dose bolus corticosteroid (usually methylprednisolone) at a dosage of 10 to 20 mg/kg intravenously (IV) given 3 to 5 times in a daily or every-other-day regimen.[99] This therapy is associated with hypertension. Other treatments have included plasmapheresis; antiplatelet drugs such as dipyridamole; and immunosuppressives including azathioprine, cyclophosphamide, or other alkylating agents, and methotrexate. Recent data from the National Institutes of Health and others have suggested significant benefit of monthly cyclophosphamide in maintaining renal function.[100,101]

Prognosis. The long-term prognosis for children with SLE nephritis is unclear. Regardless, patients and families must expect persistent evidence of renal injury such as hematuria, proteinuria, hypertension, and even reduced renal function such as a diminished GFR. Further, patients may have relapsing episodes of nephrotic syndrome or acute glomerulonephritis.

Other Glomerulonephritides

Two other forms of glomerulonephritis may result in the need for intensive care therapy. These are antiglomerular basement membrane (anti-GBM) antibody disease (Goodpasture's syndrome) and Wegener's granulomatosis. Although rare in children, both conditions can result in ARF. Therapy should be directed at the general condition of ARF as discussed previously in addition to specific therapy.

In the case of anti-GBM antibody disease, patients may have both renal disease and pulmonary disease, often pulmonary hemorrhage. Treatment includes corticosteroids, plasmapheresis, and immunosuppressives, mainly alkylating agents. Despite therapy, end-stage renal disease develops in some patients. Recurrences of anti-GBM antibody disease in renal allografts have also been reported.102 Vasculitic syndromes associated with renal disease include Wegener's granulomatosis and so-called antineutrophil cytoplasm antibody (ANCA) associated diseases. ANCA is an autoantibody that is found in one of two patterns in many forms of vasculitis and serves as a potentially useful diagnostic tool. Wegener's granulomatosis is characterized by granulomatous vasculitis that attacks the lungs, the respiratory tract including sinuses and trachea, and the kidneys. This condition may be difficult to diagnose, and biopsy may be the only means of determining the diagnosis if the plasma ANCA is negative. Five children with ANCA-associated glomerulonephritis and renal failure have been described.[103] Nonspecific systemic illness commonly preceded the presentation of ARF. In two of the five, renal function recovered; the other three required long-term dialysis. Cyclophosphamide has been shown to be beneficial in the treatment of the renal disease of Wegener's granulomatosis, and plasmapheresis is also of potential benefit in crescentic forms, although it is not widely used because of frequent complications.[104]

Nephrotic Syndrome and Acute Renal Failure

ARF is an uncommon complication of primary nephrotic syndrome in children but may occur as a result of intravascular volume depletion, bilateral renal venous thrombosis, or drug-induced renal toxicity.

The clinical scenario is one in which the child has a low serum albumin level and edema (increased extracellular volume). These patients have stable and often normal plasma volumes despite low oncotic pressure. Should an acute illness (e.g., gastroenteritis) occur, however, intravascular volume depletion and ARF may develop rapidly. Patients with nephrotic syndrome who have fluid losses or are unable to take in fluids should be admitted to the hospital, and intravenous administration of albumin plus maintenance and replacement fluids should be considered. The use of intravenous albumin helps to maintain the intravascular volume and reduces the edema that might develop during fluid therapy.[87,105] In some children with nephrosis and ARF, no cause for reduced GFR can be found. In a recent report of four children with idiopathic ARF associated with primary nephrotic syndrome, three had evidence of peritonitis at presentation, two had minimal change nephrotic syndrome, and two had focal segmental glomerulosclerosis.[106] All four children required dialysis for treatment of marked anasarca. Renal biopsies performed during ARF in three of the four children showed tubular ischemic injury. Removal of fluid with diuretics or dialysis/hemofiltration was associated with recovery of function. Together these observations support renal ischemia as a potential mechanism for renal failure.[106,107] One mechanism proposed that severe edema of the kidney results in compression of renal tubules and vessels, producing a drastically reduced GFR. In most cases, renal failure is reversible.

Tubulointerstitial Disease

Acute Tubulointerstitial Nephritis

Acute tubulointerstitial nephritis (ATIN) is a clinical syndrome characterized by inflammation of the renal interstitium accompanied by interstitial edema and renal tubular injury. ATIN may be caused by numerous drugs, infectious agents, and systemic illnesses.[108-110] A partial list of causes can be found in Box 64–4.

In most cases, ATIN is immunological in origin. Most of understanding of the pathogenesis has been obtained from animal models. Three phases have been described for ATIN.[110, 111] The initial phase involves recognition of a nephritogenic antigen located in the interstitium. The antigen may be a normal component of the interstitium, a modified constituent, drug induced, or infection induced. Loss of host tolerance is thought to be required for the initial phase to occur. The immune regulatory phase is characterized by the activation of T-helper lymphocytes, which induce differentiation of T and B cells that directly injure the interstitium. The inability of the host to counteract this response with T-suppressor cells permits T- and B-cell activation to go unabated. In the effector phase, both humoral and cell-mediated components contribute to tissue injury. Antibodies to tissue antigens promote injury by activation of the complement cascade, chemotaxis, and cell-mediated cytotoxicity. IgE is also produced, which may recruit eosinophils or mast cells. Mononuclear cell infiltration produces tissue injury by release of proteases and lymphokines. Eosinophils also damage surrounding tissue by release of proteases, leukotrienes, and toxic oxygen species.

BOX 64–4

Primary Causes of Acute Tubulointerstitial Nephritis

Drugs
Infections
Septicemia
Leptospirosis
Candidiasis
Malignant infiltration
Lymphoma
Leukemia
Systemic diseases
Systemic lupus erythematosus
Sarcoidosis

From Grunfeld J, Kleinknecht D, Droz D: Acute interstitial nephritis. In Schrier RW, Gottshalk CW, editors: *Diseases of the kidney,* ed 4, Boston, 1988, Little, Brown.

Several theories have been proposed to explain the reduced GFR[110]: (1) the "clogged drain," (2) the capillary bed, and (3) vascular tone hypotheses. The clogged drain theory proposes that tubular obstruction caused by luminal debris and interstitial edema results in increased pressure in Bowman's space and decreased pressure favoring filtration. Interstitial inflammation results in injury to the blood supply of the tubules (capillary bed hypothesis). Because these vessels are postglomerular, the increased resistance and reduced surface area associated with vessel injury result in an increase in efferent arteriolar pressure and a reduction in the pressure gradient across the glomerulus with a resultant drop in the GFR.[108] Decreased sodium reabsorption by injured proximal tubular epithelial cells reduces the medullary interstitial osmolality, which impairs the ability to concentrate the urine. Thus an increased volume of filtrate is delivered distally, stimulating the juxtaglomerular apparatus to increase angiotensin II production (vascular tone hypothesis). The net result is vasoconstriction and a diminished GFR.[108]

Pathologically, diffuse or patchy infiltration of the renal interstitium by lymphocytes, plasma cells, eosinophils, and edema of the interstitial space is observed. Eosinophils are usually indicative of an acute phase, whereas epithelioid granulomas with giant cells and fibroblasts or fibrosis indicate chronic disease. Tubules may have mild structural alterations or marked necrosis with loss of brush border.[110] Drug-induced interstitial nephritis is the most common form of ATIN in adults and children. Eight of 13 pediatric patients described in one series[112] and 38 of 57 in another series of children[113] with interstitial nephritis had drug-related causes of ATIN. Numerous drugs have been associated with ATIN. The fl-lactamines are the most frequently associated with ATIN with methicillin being the prototype, although ampicillin is the most common offending drug in pediatric series. NSAIDs are increasingly recognized as a cause of acute renal dysfunction.

Clinically apparent disease usually develops days to weeks after exposure to the inciting drug or agent but may be immediate.[114] Drug-induced tubulointerstitial disease is localized predominantly to the cortex, whereas infectious or infiltrative disorders more commonly localize to the medulla. The functional abnormality often indicates the primary site of tubular injury (Box 64–5).[115, 116] Damage involving mainly the proximal tubule results in the wasting of bicarbonate, phosphate, glucose, amino acids, and uric acid. Distal tubular involvement may be manifest as hyperkalemic renal tubular acidosis as a result of impaired secretion of both K^+ and H^+. A nephrogenic diabetes insipidus can result with medullary involvement.

Although ATIN is primarily a disease of the renal interstitium and tubule with lack of glomerular structural alterations, the GRF may also be reduced. Of 13 children described by Ellis et al[112] and Andreoli,[117] 12 had a creatinine clearance of less than 50 ml/min/1.73 m. ARF resulting from ATIN may be oliguric. Other clinical signs of ATIN are fever and rash. ATIN usually resolves with removal of the offending agent, although occasionally chronic renal insufficiency may result.[109, 112]

BOX 64–5

Patterns of Tubular Dysfunction

Cortex
- Proximal
  - ↓Reabsorption of
    - Glucose = glycosuria
    - Bicarbonate = acidosis
    - Uric acid = uricosuria
    - Amino acids = aminoaciduria
- Distal
  - ↓ Secretion of H^+, K^+ = acidosis/hyperkalemia
  - ↓ Reabsorption of Na^+ = increased fractional excretion of sodium

Medulla
- Impaired ability to concentrate = polyuria
- ↓ Reabsorption of Na^+ = increased fractional excretion of sodium

Data from Eknoyan G: Acute renal failure associated with tubulointerstitial nephropathies. In Brenner BM, Lazarus JM, editors: *Acute renal failure,* ed 2, New York, 1988, Churchill Livingstone.

Toxic Metabolic-Mediated Nephropathy

Toxic nephropathy, or drug-induced renal dysfunction, is initially a disorder of the renal tubule; however, significant tubular damage eventually results in alterations in glomerular function. Factors that contribute to the high susceptibility of the kidney to nephrotoxic injury include its constant exposure to potentially harmful compounds, the large surface area available for exposure and uptake of potentially harmful compounds, the concentration of tubular fluid drug that may result in passive concentration of a toxin within the renal tubule, dependence on a high metabolic rate to maintain tubular function, and possession of transport systems that may actually concentrate drugs or toxins within the tubular cell.[118] Certain nephrotoxins may preferentially damage certain nephron segments, depending on the area of maximal exposure, the location of specific uptake systems, and the nephronal location of specific intracellular sites that are susceptible to the toxin.[118]

*Urate Nephropathy and Tumor Lysis Syndrome**

Elevated urinary uric acid is usually the result of an elevated filtered load of uric acid, although forms of abnormal tubular handling of urate may also be associated with hyperuricosuria in the absence of hyperuricemia. Uric acid is poorly soluble and may precipitate within the renal tubule, resulting in obstruction of the tubular lumen. The most common clinical setting for urate nephropathy is in the tumor lysis syndrome, which results from the increased production and release of purines from tumor cells with precipitation in the urinary space.[119] Occasionally, ARF with extreme hyperuricemia may be the initial symptom in lymphoproliferative malignancies.[119] Hyperuricemia may also occur with sickle cell anemia, rhabdomyolysis, radiocontrast, cardiopulmonary bypass, and genetic causes. The primary feature of urate nephropathy is deposition of urate crystals within the distal tubules and collecting ducts. There may be secondary changes in the medullary interstitium. The urinary concentration of uric acid and the urine pH determine the solubility and thus the likelihood of urate precipitation.[119] This syndrome is usually reversible or preventable with forced diuresis and alkalinization of the urine plus administration of diuretics such as mannitol or furosemide.

Tumor lysis syndrome occurs at the initiation of antineoplastic therapy for large, rapidly growing tumors that are sensitive to therapy.[105,120] Occasionally, it is the result of tumor necrosis before the onset of therapy.[119] The intracellular products of malignant cells are released as a result of cytolysis and result in hyperuricemia, hyperphosphatemia, and hyperkalemia. Hyperxanthinemia may develop, especially in patients treated with allopurinol. This condition should be anticipated, especially with acute leukemia and high white blood cell counts ($>10^6/\mu l$), large lymphomas, and Burkitt's lymphoma. Severity of the condition depends on the tumor burden, the rapidity of cell necrosis, and renal function. Prior renal insufficiency greatly increases the chances of development of ARF with tumor lysis.

The basic pathophysiological events are (1) high concentrations of uric acid, phosphate, potassium, and xanthine in the blood, leading to (2) high filtered loads and high urinary concentrations of each, leading to (3) crystallization, (4) tubular obstruction, (5) decreased urine output, (6) renal insufficiency or failure, and (7) hyperphosphatemia and can result in hypocalcemia as well (see Chapter 74).

Treatment

Treatment is outlined in Box 64–6. An important and potentially protective first step in therapy is anticipation. Patients who are likely to have the rapid killing of large numbers of tumor cells should have phosphorus and potassium removed from intravenous solutions and markedly reduced in their diets. Allopurinol should be started, preferably before antineoplastic agents

BOX 64–6

Treatment of Tumor Lysis Syndrome and Crush Injury

- Anticipation
- Decrease intravenous and oral potassium and phosphorus administration
- Increase oral or intravenous fluid administration; replace urine losses to maintain vigorous diuresis
- Diuretics, especially loop diuretics to increase urine output
- Intravenous mannitol
- Maintain urine pH 6.5 to 7; may require bicarbonate administration
- Dialysis

*See Chapter 74.

are administered. Although xanthines may also crystallize in urine, xanthines are more soluble in urine than uric acid.[119] When allopurinol reduces uric acid production, the chances for renal tubular obstruction are reduced. The administration of high fluid volumes, both IV and orally, leads to high urine volumes, another cornerstone of treatment to prevent or diminish the effect of tumor lysis. High urine volumes decrease the concentration of potential obstructing compounds such as calcium phosphate, uric acid, or xanthines. Techniques for creating a forced diuresis include high-volume intravenous infusion with or without the use of a loop diuretic (e.g., furosemide) or mannitol infusion. If a diuretic or intravenous mannitol is used, urine volume should be replaced to guarantee continued high urine volumes. Another frequently suggested therapy is urinary alkalinization. The rationale is that uric acid is more soluble in an alkaline pH. Urine pH need only be raised to 6.5 to 7 but not above 7. Urine pH above 7 facilitates the crystallization of other products (e.g., calcium phosphate). It must be recognized that a patient with a falling urine output and rising serum creatinine level, despite the measure noted previously, may require dialysis.

Pigment Nephropathy

Rhabdomyolysis and hemolysis are associated with renal injury in the form of acute tubular necrosis and the appearance of free hemoglobin or myoglobin in the plasma and urine.[121,122] ARF associated with rhabdomyolysis or hemolysis is commonly referred to as *pigment-induced nephropathy* because of the myoglobinuria or hemoglobinuria associated with these clinical disorders. Renal injury resulting from rhabdomyolysis or hemolysis, however, involves initiating factors in addition to pigmenturia. Much of the knowledge of ARF is the result of observations made during World War II, when rhabdomyolysis that resulted from "crush syndrome" was commonly encountered as a cause of ARF.[121,123] Animal models of myoglobinuric and hemoglobinuric ARF have provided additional insight into the pathogenesis of this form of acute renal injury.

Because rhabdomyolysis is accompanied by the release of many muscle constituents in addition to myoglobin, it may be difficult to differentiate whether the renal injury that occurs after rhabdomyolysis is entirely related to the pigmenturia or to other factors released during muscle necrosis.[122] The primary mechanisms that cause renal tubular toxicity related to exposure to heme protein are renal vasoconstriction, intraluminal cast formation, and direct heme protein-induced cytotoxicity.[122] Please refer to reference 122 for an in-depth discussion of the biochemical events involved in the cellular injury in rhabdomyolysis.

Rhabdomyolysis may occur in association with traumatic muscle injury, as well as nontraumatic causes such as drug intoxication,[124] hyperpyrexia,[125] vascular occlusion, carbon monoxide poisoning, diabetic ketoacidosis, primary muscle diseases, or prolonged seizures.[121,126,127] Traumatic muscle injury, referred to as *crush syndrome,* is characterized by hypotension in addition to rhabdomyolysis. Water and electrolytes are lost into damaged muscle, and this leads to diminished intravascular volume. As discussed later in this section, renal hypoperfusion and aciduria potentiate myoglobinuria-induced tubular injury. Arterial thrombi within the extremity may produce tissue damage as a result of ischemia with myoedema and release of myoglobin when the circulation is restored.[128] Nontraumatic rhabdomyolysis has been reported in patients with metabolic or inflammatory muscle disorders such as McArdle's syndrome, Tarui's disease, carnitine palmitoyl transferase deficiency, dermatomyositis, and polymyositis.[121,127] Diabetic ketoacidosis, burns, and poisoning with copper sulfate, zinc phosphate, or mercuric chloride may also result in myoglobinuria.[121]

Prolonged coma has been associated with rhabdomyolysis. The pressure from a patient's own weight with or without the addition of hypnotic drugs may result in myonecrosis. Drugs such as heroin, methadone, methamphetamine, chlorpromazine, carbon monoxide, ethanol, methanol, quinine, and barbiturates have been associated with the development of myoglobinuria.[21,129,130] The cause of myoglobinuria after the use of hypnotic drugs may be related to the coma induced rather than a direct action of the drug itself. Cocaine has been associated with myoglobinuria and renal failure.[124] Heat stress, hyperpyrexia, and exercise may also induce myoglobinuria and ARF (see Chapter 101).[15,131,132]

Rhabdomyolysis complicates infections such as influenza, coxsackievirus, herpesviruses, gram-negative sepsis, shigellosis, and Rocky Mountain spotted fever.[76,121,133] Myoglobinuria may be a major contributing factor in the development of ARF after asphyxia in neonates.[134,135]

Hemolysis with associated hemoglobinuria is unlikely to result in ARF unless accompanied by conditions resulting in renal hypoperfusion (acidosis, sepsis, dehydration, and hemorrhage).[121] Any condition associated with the lysis of red blood cells may produce hemoglobinuria. Pigment-induced ARF presents in a manner similar to other forms of acute tubular toxicity or vasomotor nephropathy. The severity of the electrolyte disturbance may be out of proportion to the reduction in GFR because of the release of other muscle constituents such as uric acid, phosphorus, and potassium. Hypocalcemia is commonly associated with rhabdomyolysis and is the result of several phenomena, including hyperphosphatemia, skeletal resistance to PTH, and possibly impaired 1,25-dihydroxyvitamin D synthesis.[136] Hypercalcemia may complicate the recovery phase because calcium is mobilized after its deposition in damaged muscle.

The pathogenesis of pigment-induced nephropathy is not entirely understood. When released into the circulation, hemoglobin binds to haptoglobin (up to 100 mg/dl plasma) and myoglobin binds to α_2-globulin (up to 23 mg/dl).[121] The appearance of pigment in the urine depends on the amount of the substance released into the plasma, the concentration of the binding protein available, the GFR, urine flow, and the extent of renal tubular reabsorption of the pigment.[121]

Pigment-induced nephropathy may induce renal injury by several potential mechanisms: intratubular obstruction from precipitation of proteins and heme pigments, alterations in renal hemodynamics, and direct tubular toxicity. The formation of intratubular casts is a hallmark feature of pigment nephropathy and is also a predominant pathological finding. Although some animal studies have failed to demonstrate direct renal toxicity of isolated myoglobin, evidence suggests that the intravenous injection of myoglobin is associated with a reduction in GFR and a concomitant increase in RVR as a result of both afferent and efferent vasoconstriction.[137] Aciduria may be a prerequisite for the development of renal injury with myoglobinuria, possibly because when the urine pH is 5.6 or lower, ferrihemate is formed from either hemoglobin or myoglobin. This compound has been shown to be directly injurious to the renal tubule.[138] Newer theories have proposed that renal injury may be mediated by iron in the ferric state, which promotes lipid peroxidation and the release of hydroxyl radical. Deferoxamine, an iron chelator, reduces renal injury in animal models of hemoglobin- and myoglobin-induced renal injury.[122]

Therapy for crush injury or rhabdomyolysis includes the administration of large fluid volumes and forced diuresis with potent diuretics, mannitol, or both. Mannitol infusions may have a second, theoretical advantage in that mannitol appears to be a free radical scavenger and therefore may reduce free radical–mediated injury. Maintaining urine pH between 6.5 and 7 is also helpful. As with tumor lysis, diligent attention to urine output and measures of renal function (e.g., serum creatinine) should alert the practitioner to the need for dialysis. CVVH (continuous venovenous hemofiltration) removes myoglobin, and this modality offers an excellent alternative to conventional dialysis in the treatment of ARF that results from pigment nephropathy.[139]

Aminoglycoside Nephrotoxicity

Aminoglycoside antibiotics are a commonly used class of drugs associated with nephrotoxicity.[94] Certain risk factors predispose to aminoglycoside toxicity, many of which are seen in the pediatric ICU population. These include the following:

1. Drug dose and duration of drug administration
2. Age—the neonatal and the geriatric populations are more prone to toxicity
3. Presence of renal insufficiency
4. Concomitant nephrotoxic drug administration, in particular, such drugs as amphotericin B, certain cephalosporins, and cyclosporine
5. Extracellular volume depletion
6. Potassium depletion

Aminoglycosides are excreted primarily by glomerular filtration; however, reabsorption by the renal tubular cell occurs after charge interaction of these strongly cationic drugs with the brush border of the proximal tubule, followed by transport into the cell by pinocytosis directed to lysosomes.[35,140] Although less significant, gentamicin may be reabsorbed from the basolateral surface of the tubular cell. Accumulation of the drug within the lysosome results in phospholipid hydrolysis and the formation of electron-dense myeloid bodies.[141] The combined processes of basolateral uptake and brush border accumulation contribute to the high concentration of drug in the renal tubular cell.[142]

The major pathological finding in aminoglycoside nephrotoxicity is tubular cell necrosis, which involves the most proximal segments of the nephron, the convoluted tubule, and pars recta (S1 and S2).[22,29] The earliest finding is an increase in the number of lysosomes, followed by alterations in the brush border architecture and mitochondrial swelling.[143] This process may be patchy or diffuse. Even during continued aminoglycoside administration, tubular cell regeneration can be found.

Aminoglycoside nephrotoxicity may initially exhibit subtle tubular or glomerular dysfunction and occasionally progresses to oliguric ARF. The earliest clinically detectable abnormality is enzymuria, which results from loss of brush border membrane segments bearing the enzymes. Tubular damage produces a Fanconi-like syndrome with proximal tubular wasting of glucose, phosphate, amino acids, and bicarbonate, as well as numerous ions including magnesium.[84,120] Urine volume may actually be increased with mild-to-moderate tubular toxicity because of a vasopressin-resistant concentrating defect. Renal dysfunction may be initially detected after a rise in the serum creatinine concentration or serum drug levels; however, severe sustained renal dysfunction has been described.[144]

The GFR may decrease after gentamicin administration in the absence of tubular necrosis as a result of angiotensin II–mediated afferent arteriolar vasoconstriction. The potentiating of the vasoconstriction and hypofiltration by the prostaglandin synthetase inhibitors provides indirect evidence for a palliative role of locally produced vasodilatory prostaglandins in this form of nephrotoxic injury.[145] In addition to the microvascular and tubular changes, Kf is decreased because of a decrease in the number and density of glomerular capillary wall fenestrae.[146, 147]

The relative toxicity of the aminoglycosides is neomycin > gentamicin> tobramycin > amikacin.[29] Several factors may contribute to or predispose to aminoglycoside nephrotoxicity. Drug dosage and duration of therapy, particularly repeated and prolonged courses, determine the severity of the tubular toxicity. Concomitant administration of other nephrotoxic drugs, concomitant administration of cationic amino acids, volume depletion, potassium depletion, endotoxemia, hypokalemia, and hyperphosphatemia further potentiate renal injury.[29,140,148] Nephrotoxicity may be attenuated by increased dietary calcium intake, alkalinization, solute diuresis, calcium channel blockers, or captopril.[140]

Prevention of aminoglycoside toxicity involves the prudent use of aminoglycosides. As indicated by these predisposing factors, patients in the pediatric ICU are at great risk because many of the factors are likely to be present during concurrent aminoglycoside administration. Therefore aminoglycosides should be used only when truly indicated. Careful dosing schedules reduce toxicity. Avoiding full dosing during periods of volume contraction is important. Finally, recognizing the interaction of certain drugs with each other allows for anticipation of renal toxicity. For example, furosemide enhances renal aminoglycoside toxicity by favoring volume contraction.

Amphotericin B

Amphotericin B is an antifungal agent that exerts its effect by interaction with membrane sterols. This chemical interaction is the basis for its antifungal action and its renal toxicity.[29] Amphotericin B has two major pathophysiological effects on the kidney: renal tubular cell injury, mainly of the distal renal tubule, and an acute afferent arteriolar vasoconstriction.[141]

Unlike virtually all of the other tubular toxins, the primary tubular site of amphotericin B–induced injury is the distal tubule.[29] The interaction of this drug with membrane cholesterol leads to the formation of aqueous pores, which greatly increase the permeability of the normally tight epithelium of the distal tubule. This increase results first in a backleakage of H^+, Na^+, and Cl^- and then in a vasopressin-resistant polyuria.[29,117] Increased permeability to Cl^- may stimulate increased tubuloglomerular feedback and reduce the GFR, ultimately resulting in renal ischemia and azotemia. In a canine model, amphotericin administration was accompanied by a decrease in urine flow and the GFR within 1 hour, accompanied by increased RVR as a result of afferent arteriolar constriction.[149] Aminophylline's blocking of the gentamicin-induced vasoconstriction suggested a role for adenosine as a potential mediator.[150]

Amphotericin B nephrotoxicity may become clinically evident as a reduction in the GFR or as distal tubular dysfunction with metabolic acidosis (related to the distal type of renal tubular acidification defect), salt wasting, polyuria, or hypokalemia.[29, 140] Nephrotoxicity is predictable and usually reversible, although irreversible azotemia has been observed with large doses. Severity of tubular toxicity and hypofiltration is proportional to the cumulative dose. In adults, a cumulative dose exceeding 5 g was associated with significant renal dysfunction, whereas patients who received less than a 600-mg cumulative dose rarely had renal toxicity.[151] Newborn infants are equally susceptible to amphotericin nephrotoxicity.[152] Concomitant use of diuretics and abnormal pretreatment renal function increases the risk for development of amphotericin toxicity.[29, 151]

Sodium loading appears to have a beneficial effect on amphotericin B–induced nephrotoxicity[29]; that is, it maintains intravascular volume and reduces renal vasoconstriction. Mannitol has been shown to ameliorate nephrotoxicity in animal studies, but the benefit of this agent in humans has not been clearly demonstrated.[153,154]

Calcineurin Inhibitors

Cyclosporine and tacrolimus are used extensively in transplant recipients and for other renal diseases. The mechanisms for renal toxicity are (1) a proximal tubulopathy that may manifest as proteinuria, bicarbonate or electrolyte wasting, and enzymuria and (2) a toxic effect on endothelial cells that results in a reduction of the GFR and hypertension. Toxicity appears to be dose related.[88,155]

Radiocontrast Agents

Radiographic contrast agents are triiodinated benzoic acid derivatives, usually the sodium or methylglucamine salts, of detrizoate or iothalamate. Contrast agents are freely filtered at the glomerulus, with the kidney as the primary organ responsible for their excretion. Some concentration of the drug may occur within the renal tubular cell, but most of a bolus of contrast material is rapidly excreted into the urine.[156]

The incidence of nephrotoxicity after use of radiocontrast agents is approximately 2% in the general population of patients, [156] but certain groups may be at increased risk of ARF after radiocontrast administration. Risk factors include preexisting renal insufficiency, diabetes mellitus, multiple myeloma, dehydration, proteinuria, and hyperuricemia.[29] Preexisting renal dysfunction is associated with a much greater occurrence of ARF. Of those individuals who have renal insufficiency after radiocontrast administration, 50% to 75% of the adults studied have evidence of preexisting renal dysfunction, which was defined as a serum creatinine concentration of 2 to 3 mg/dl.[156] Dehydration insufficient to induce renal injury alone may be an additional risk factor.

Nephrotoxicity may be mild with minimal clinical symptoms. Most cases are manifested as nonoliguric acute renal dysfunction, although renal injury may be more severe with typical oliguric renal failure. The peak rise in the serum creatinine level usually occurs at 3 to 5 days after contrast administration with return to baseline by 10 to 14 days. If nephrotoxicity is severe, pronounced oliguria may be evident within 24 hours of the injection. Pathological changes are localized to the proximal tubular cell in the form of pronounced vacuolization, termed *osmotic nephrosis.*[144] This is one form of acute tubular toxicity that is characterized by a low fractional excretion of sodium.[29]

Measures to reduce nephrotoxicity from radiocontrast agents include the administration of saline and oral acetylcysteine prior to contrast agents. A randomized trial compared 0.45% saline alone with 0.45% saline, mannitol and furosemide.[157] The group that received saline plus diuretics experienced a significantly higher serum creatinine at 48 hours after contrast. In a trial in which patients were randomized to 0.45% or 0.9% saline, researchers found that the isotonic saline was superior in prevention of contrast nephropathy.[158] Although results from some trials have shown acetylcysteine to be beneficial as a protective agent,[159] other results have not.[160] Patients with chronic renal failure who underwent coronary interventions were randomized to hemofiltration or isotonic saline administration.[161] Only 5% of the group receiving hemofiltration experienced a significant increase in creatinine compared with 50% in the saline group.

*Hepatorenal Syndrome**

Hepatorenal syndrome (HRS) represents a distinct category of renal failure because of its unique pattern

*See Chapter 81.

of systemic and renal hemodynamic alterations. HRS is initiated by stresses such as gastrointestinal hemorrhage, sepsis, paracentesis, or a surgical procedure in the patient with preexisting hepatic disease. Reduction in the GFR occurs as the result of intense renal vasoconstriction, which severely impairs RBF. Intensity of renal vasoconstriction appears to correlate to the degree of liver dysfunction.[162] Systemic vascular resistance is low, and intravascular volume is increased in this setting. Volume expansion is unsuccessful in restoration of renal perfusion.

Two major hypotheses exist for the functional reduction of RBF.[162] One theory proposes that renal vasoconstriction is the appropriate physiological response to shunting of blood away from the kidney to other vital organs. Hypofiltration, however, does not appear to be related to the effective plasma volume in this setting. A second theory proposes that renal vasoconstriction is the result of an abnormal neural response or alteration in the synthesis or degradation of a hormone. Abnormalities in the plasma concentration, metabolism, or tissue responsiveness of several vasoactive substances have been reported (Box 64–7).[19,102] In addition, abnormalities in the neural control of renal vascular tone have been advanced as a mechanism for the reduction of RBF.

Intrahepatic receptors respond to the increase in hepatic sinusoidal pressure with enhanced afferent hepatic nerve activity, which increases renal sympathetic nerve activity.[163] Increased renal release of norepinephrine and epinephrine has been observed in patients with cirrhosis and correlates with the intrahepatic sinusoidal pressures.[164] Thus the hypofiltration of HRS is the expression of a reversible, functional disturbance in vascular tone. This theory is supported by clinical examples. Renal function improves in patients with HRS after liver transplantation. Kidneys from donors with HRS function normally when transplanted into recipients with normal liver function.[165] Unfortunately, once oliguria is present, therapy for HRS has been largely unsuccessful. Differentiating the syndrome from potentially reversible causes of ARF in this clinical setting is most important.

BOX 64–7

Vasoactive Substances in the Hepatorenal Syndrome

INCREASED

- Renin (C)
- Angiotensin II (C)
- Norepinephrine (C)
- Vasopressin (C)
- Prostaglandin E_2 (D)
- Prostaglandin I_2 (D)
- Substance P (C)
- Vasoactive intestinal peptide (C)
- Endotoxin (C)
- False neurotransmitters (octopamine) (D)

DECREASED

- Prekallikrein (D)
- Bradykinin (D)

C, Vasoconstrictor effect; *D*, vasodilatory effect.
Modified from Epstein M: Acute renal failure in liver disease. In Molitoris BA, Finn WF, editors: Acute renal failure, Philadelphia, 2001, WB Saunders.

*Acute Renal Failure after Bone Marrow Transplantation**

Renal dysfunction is commonly observed in patients after bone marrow transplantation. Numerous potential causes include nephrotoxic drugs such as cyclosporine, amphotericin B, aminoglycosides, as well as sepsis. Approximately half of patients who undergo bone marrow transplantation experience a reduction in GFR, and 25% may require dialysis.[166] Risk factors for development of ARF are use of amphotericin B and sepsis, as well as fluid retention and hepatic failure.[166] Because renal biopsy commonly fails to show structural abnormality or glomerular disease, the assumption is that renal failure is related to vascular causes, particularly an HRS, in some cases. Prognosis is poor, with an 84% mortality rate among the group of patients with renal failure requiring dialysis, 37% of those with significant elevation of the serum creatinine level, compared with 17% in patients without significant renal insufficiency.[166]

Urinary Tract Obstruction

Obstruction of urine flow may result in ARF, although unilateral obstruction rarely causes ARF unless there is a single kidney or disease in the other kidney. Both unilateral and bilateral ureteral obstruction is accompanied by an initial increase in RBF caused by afferent arteriolar vasodilation.[167] Relaxation of the preglomerular capillary sphincter is mediated by the local release of vasodilatory prostaglandins.[168,169] Administration of indomethacin, a cyclooxygenase inhibitor, results in a marked reduction in the GFR after a decrease in glomerular plasma flow and an increase in both afferent and efferent arteriolar resistances.[170] This indicates an important role of vasodilatory prostaglandins in the maintenance of the GFR. If the obstruction persists, RBF progressively decreases as afferent arteriolar resistance increases because of the overriding action of angiotensin II and thromboxane.[170] This vasoconstriction may actually protect the kidney from damage during the period of obstruction. Intratubular pressure rises after ureteral obstruction; this pressure is translated to the glomerulus as increased pressure in Bowman's space. The contribution of this increased force opposing filtration to the decrease in the GFR is probably inconsequential because the intratubular pressure rise is transient.[167] In addition, the elevation in Bowman's space pressure is negated by an increase in the glomerular capillary pressure, which increases the GFR. RBF is redistributed from the outer to the inner cortex and results in relative ischemia of the renal medulla.[167]

*See Chapter 76.

BOX 64–8

Causes of Urinary Tract Obstruction

Tumors
Cystic diseases
Calculi
Ureteropelvic junction obstruction
Posterior urethral valves
Megaureter
Prune belly syndrome
Retroperitoneal fibrosis
Ureterocele
Neurogenic bladder
Duplicated ureters

Data from Badr KF, Brenner BM: Renal circulatory and nephron function in experimental obstruction of the urinary tract. In Brenner BM, Lazarus JM, editors: *Acute renal failure,* ed 2, New York, 1988, Churchill Livingstone.

Various clinical causes of urinary tract obstruction are listed in Box 64–8.[168] The most important factors determining recovery of renal and tubular function are the degree and severity of the obstruction. Treatment consists of decompression of the urinary collecting system by removal of the obstruction or by urinary diversion. Relief of obstruction is accompanied by a marked diuresis resulting from increased RBF and abnormal tubular function. The increase in urine volume is related to a concentrating defect caused by loss of the medullary gradient and unresponsiveness of the renal tubule to vasopressin.[171] Hydrogen ion and potassium secretion may also be impaired, and the result is a distal type of renal tubular acidosis with hyperkalemia.[172]

This chapter has reviewed the major factors that contribute to the development of ARF, both in its oliguric and nonoliguric forms. Also indicated are the clinical settings in which ARF may occur. In addition, treatment modalities have been discussed. Clearly, the challenge in ARF is the development of novel therapeutic strategies that will more directly intervene in the disease process and that can have an impact on the cellular and metabolic mechanisms that contribute to renal cell injury. Certain current investigations were discussed because they may lead to clinical trials during the next 10 years. Included among these agents are calcium channel blockers, adenine nucleotides, thyroid hormone, and oxyradical scavengers because they may modulate the full expression of renal cell injury. Only with understanding of the pathophysiological mechanisms in ARF can these potential therapeutics be applied in a clinical setting to the care of pediatric patients.

REFERENCES

1. Heidbreder E, Schafferhans K, Schramm D, et al: Toxic renal failure in the rat: beneficial effects of atrial natriuretic factor, *Klin Wochenschr* 64(suppl 6):78, 1986.
2. Yared A, Kon V, Ichikawa I: Mechanism of preservation of glomerular perfusion and filtration during acute extracellular fluid volume depletion: importance of intrarenal vasopressin-prostaglandin interaction for protecting kidneys from constrictor action of vasopressin, *J Clin Invest* 75:1477, 1985.
3. Badr KF, Ichikawa I: Prerenal failure: a deleterious shift from renal compensation to decompensation, *N Engl J Med* 319:623, 1988.
4. Yared A, Ichikawa I: Regulation of renal blood flow and glomerular filtration rate. In Ichikawa I, editor: *Pediatric textbook of fluids and electrolytes,* Baltimore, 1990, Williams & Wilkins.
5. Schlondorff D, Ardaillou R: Prostaglandins and other arachidonic acid metabolites in the kidney, *Kidney Int* 29:108, 1986.
6. Halliday HL, Hirata T, Brady JP: Indomethacin therapy for large patent ductus arteriosus in the very low birth weight infant: results and complications, *Pediatrics* 64:154, 1979.
7. Kon V, Yoshioka T, Fogo A, et al: Glomerular actions of endothelin in vivo, *J Clin Invest* 83:1762, 1989.
8. Ichikawa I, Pfeffer JM, Pfeffer MA, et al: Role of angiotensin II in the altered renal function of congestive heart failure, *Circ Res* 55:669, 1984.
9. Kon V, Yared A, Ichikawa I: Role of renal sympathetic nerves in mediating hypoperfusion of renal cortical microcirculation in experimental congestive heart failure and acute extracellular volume depletion, *J Clin Invest* 76:1913, 1985.
10. Mujais SK, Fouad FM, Textor SC, et al: Transient renal dysfunction during initial inhibition of converting enzyme in congestive heart failure, *Br Heart J* 52:63, 1984.
11. Edwards RM: Segmental effects of norepinephrine and angiotension II on isolated renal microvessels, *Am J Physiol* 244:F526, 1983.
12. Hall JE, Guyton AC, Jackson TE, et al: Control of glomerular filtration rate by the renin-angiotensin system, *Am J Physiol* 233: F366, 1977.
13. Ichikawa I, Brenner BM: Importance of efferent arteriolar vascular tone in regulation of proximal tubule fluid reabsorption and glomerulotubular balance in the rat, *J Clin Invest* 65:1192, 1980.
14. Chevalier RL, Kaiser DL: Autoregulation of renal blood flow in the rat: effects of growth and uninephrectomy, *Am J Physiol* 244: F483, 1984.
15. Hostetter TH, Brenner BM: Renal circulatory and nephron function in experimental acute renal failure. In Brenner BM, Lazarus JM, editors: *Acute renal failure,* ed 2, New York, 1988, Churchill Livingstone.
16. Thurau K, Mason J, Gstraunthaler G: Experimental acute renal failure. In Seldin DW, Giebisch G, editors: *The kidney: physiology and pathophysiology,* New York, 1985, Raven Press.
17. Patak RV, Fadem SZ, Lifschitz MD, et al: Study of factors which modify the development of norepinephrine-induced acute renal failure in the dog, *Kidney Int* 15:227, 1979.
18. Brenner BM, Dworkin LD, Ichikawa I: Glomerular ultrafiltration. In Brenner BM, Rector FC Jr, editors: *The kidney,* ed 3, Philadelphia, 1986, WB Saunders.
19. Brezis M, Rosen S, Epstein FH: *Acute renal failure.* In Brenner BM, Rector FC Jr, editors: *The kidney,* ed 3, Philadelphia, 1986, WB Saunders.
20. Neill MA, Tarr PI, Clausen CR, et al: *Escherichia coli* 0157:H7 or the predominant pathogen associated with the hemolytic uremic syndrome: a prospective study in the Pacific Northwest, *Pediatrics* 80:37, 1987.
21. Gaudio KM, Siegel NJ: Pathogenesis and treatment of acute renal failure, *Pediatr Clin North Am* 34:771, 1987.
22. Sutton TA, Fisher CJ, Molitoris BA: Microvascular endothelial injury and dysfunction during ischemic acute renal failure, *Kidney Int* 62:1539, 2002.
23. Epstein FH, Brown RS: Acute renal failure: a collection of paradoxes, *Hosp Pract (Off Ed)* 23:157, 1988.
24. Borkan SC, Emami A, Schwartz JH: Heat stress protein-associated cytoprotection of inner medullary collecting duct cells from rat kidney, *Am J Physiol* 265:F333, 1993.
25. Ezell C: Hot stuff: medical applications of the heat shock response, *J NIH Res* 8:43, 1995.
26. Nissim I, Hardy M, Pleasure J, et al: A mechanism of glycine and alanine cytoprotective action: stimulation of stress-induced HSP70 mRNA, *Kidney Int* 42:775, 1992.
27. Schaudies RP, Nonclercq D, Nelson L, et al: Endogenous EGF as a potential renotrophic factor in ischemia-induced acute renal failure, *Am J Physiol* 265:F425, 1993.
28. Witzgall R, Brown D, Schwarz C, et al: Localization of proliferating cell nuclear antigen, vimentin, c-Fos, and clusterin in the postischemic kidney. Evidence for a heterogenous genetic response among nephron segments, and a large pool of mitotically active and dedifferentiated cells, *J Clin Invest* 93:2175, 1994.

29. Coggins CH, Fang LS-T: Acute renal failure associated with antibiotics, anesthetic agents and radio-contrast agents. In Brenner BM, Lazarus JM, editors: *Acute renal failure,* ed 2, New York, 1988, Churchill Livingstone.
30. Green D, Fry M, Blondin G: Phospholipids as the molecular instruments of ion and solute transport in biological membranes, *Proc Natl Acad Sci U S A* 77:257, 1980.
31. Schrier RW, Arnold PE, Van Putten VJ, et al: Cellular calcium in ischemic acute renal failure: role of calcium entry blockers, *Kidney Int* 32:313, 1987
32. Kribben A, Wieder ED, Wetzels JF, et al: Evidence for role of cytosolic free calcium in hypoxia-induced proximal tubule injury, *J Clin Invest* 93:1922, 1994.
33. Mandel LJ, Takano T, Soltoff SP, et al: Mechanisms whereby exogenous adenine nucleotides improve rabbit renal proximal function during and after anoxia, *J Clin Invest* 81:1255, 1988.
34. Siegel NJ, Glazier WB, Chaudry IH, et al: Enhanced recovery from acute renal failure by post-ischemic infusion of adenine nucleotides and magnesium chloride in rats, *Kidney Int* 17: 338, 1980.
35. Weinberg JM, Davis JA, Lawton A, et al: Modulation of cell nucleotides levels of isolated kidney tubules, *Am J Physiol* 254:F311, 1988.
36. Oken DE: Hemodynamic basis for human acute renal failure (vasomotor nephropathy), *Am J Med* 76:702, 1984.
37. Hollenberg NK, Epstein M, Rosen SM, et al: Acute oliguric renal failure in man: evidence for preferential renal cortical ischemia, *Medicine (Baltimore)* 47:455, 1968.
38. Brezis M, Rosen S, Silva P, et al: Renal ischemia: a new perspective, *Kidney Int* 26:375, 1984.
39. Thurau K, Boylan JW: Acute renal success: the unexpected logic of oliguria in acute renal failure, *Am J Med* 61:308, 1976.
40. Myers BD, Moran SM: Hemodynamically mediated acute renal failure, *N Engl J Med* 314:97, 1986.
41. Rasmussen HH, Bels LS: Acute renal failure: multivariate analysis of causes and risk factors, *Am J Med* 73:211, 1982.
42. Burke TJ, Schrier RW: Acute renal failure. In Gonick HC, editor: *Current nephrology,* Chicago, 1990, Year Book.
43. Seri I: Cardiovascular, renal, and endocrine actions of dopamine in neonates and children, *J Pediatr* 126:333, 1995.
44. Pelayo JC, Fildes RD, Jose PA: Age-dependent renal effects of intrarenal dopamine infusion, *Am J Physiol* 247:R212, 1984.
45. Tulassay T, Seri I, Machay T, et al: Effects of dopamine on renal functions in premature neonates with respiratory distress, *Int J Pediatr Nephrol* 4:19, 1983.
46. Burke TJ, Arnold PE, Schrier RW: Prevention of ischemic acute renal failure with impermeant solutes, *Am J Physiol* 244: F646, 1983.
47. Graziani G, Cantaluppi A, Casati S, et al: Dopamine and furosemide in oliguric acute renal failure, *Nephron* 37:39, 1984.
48. Rigden SP, Dillon MJ, Kind PR, et al: The beneficial effect of mannitol on postoperative renal function in children undergoing cardiopulmonary bypass surgery,*Clin Nephrol* 21:148, 1984.
49. Hock CE, Su JY, Lefer AM: Salutory effects of nitrendipine, a new calcium entry blocker, in hemorrhagic shock, *Eur J Pharmacol* 97:37, 1984.
50. Malis CD, Cheung JY, Leaf A, et al: Effects of verapamil in models of ischemic acute renal failure in the rat, *Am J Physiol* 245: F735, 1983.
51. Siegel NJ: Ask the expert, *Pediatr Nephrol* 4:358, 1990.
52. Balow JE: Lupus as a renal disease, *Hosp Pract (Off Ed)* 22:129, 1988.
53. Wang J, Dunn MJ: Platelet activating factor mediates endotoxin-induced acute renal insufficiency in rats, *Am J Physiol* 253: F1283, 1987.
54. Wagner K, Albrecht S, Neumayer HH: Prevention of delayed graft function in cadaveric kidney transplantation by a calcium antagonist: preliminary results of two prospective randomized trials, *Transplant Proc* 18:510, 1986.
55. Hull RW, Hasbargen JA: No clinical evidence for protective effects of calcium channel blockers against acute renal failure, *N Engl J Med* 313:1477, 1985 (letter).
56. Finn WF, Hak LJ, Grossman SH: Protective effect of prostacyclin on post ischemic acute renal failure in the rat, *Kidney Int* 32: 479, 1987.
57. Kaufman RP Jr, Anner H, Kobzik L, et al: A high plasma prostaglandin to thromboxane ratio protects against renal ischemia, *Surg Gynecol Obstet* 165:404, 1987.
58. Schuldt HH, Oesterwitz IT: Experimental studies on the modifiability of ischemic acute renal failure by saralasin, *Z Urol Nephrol* 78:619, 1985 (German).
59. Koelz AM, Bertschin S, Hermle M, et al: The angiotensin converting enzyme inhibitor enalapril in acute ischemic renal failure in rats, *Experimentia* 44:172, 1988.
60. Gaudio KM, Stromski M, Thulin G, et al: Postischemic hemodynamics and recovery of renal adenosine triphosphate, *Am J Physiol* 251:F603, 1986.
61. Zeidel ML: Renal actions of atrial natriuretic peptide. In Brenner BM, Stein JH, editors: *Contemporary issues in nephrology,* New York, 1989, Churchill Livingstone.
62. Fried TA, McCoy RN, Osgood RW, et al: Effect of atriopeptin II on determinants of glomerular filtration rate in the in vitro perfused dog glomerulus, *Am J Physiol* 250:F119, 1986.
63. Shaw SS, Weidmann P, Hodler J, et al: Atrial natriuretic peptide protects against acute ischemic renal failure in the rat, *J Clin Invest* 80:1232, 1987.
64. Weinberg JM, Davis JA, Abarzua M, et al: Cytoprotective effects of glycine and glutathione against hypoxic injury to renal tubules, *J Clin Invest* 80:1446, 1987.
65. Boydstun I, Najjar S, Kashgarian M, et al: Postischemic thyroxin stimulates renal mitochondrial adenine nucleotide translocator activity, *Am J Physiol* 268:E651, 1995.
66. Straub E: Effects of l -thyroxin in acute renal failure, *Res Exp Med (Berl)* 168:81, 1976.
67. Straub E: Influences of thyroid hormones on kidney function. In Hesch RD, editor: *The low T3 syndrome,* London, 1981, Academic Press.
68. Nissenson AR, Baraff LJ, Fine RN, et al: Poststreptococcal acute glomerulonephritis: fact and controversy, *Ann Intern Med* 91:76, 1979.
69. Epstein FH, Silva P, Spokes K, et al: Prevention with glycine of acute renal failure caused by cis-platinum, *Kidney Int* 37:480, 1990.
70. Feld LG, Springate JE, Fildes RD: Acute renal failure: II, management of suspected and established disease, *J Pediatr* 109:567, 1986.
71. Better OS, Winaver J: Acute renal failure. In Arieff A, DeFronzo R, editors. *Fluid, electrolyte, and acid-base disorders,* New York, 1995, Churchill Livingstone.
72. Karmali MA, Petric M, Lim C, et al: The association between idiopathic hemolytic uremic syndrome and infection by verotoxin-producing *Escherichia coli, J Infect Dis* 151: 775, 1985.
73. Neugarten J, Aynedjian HS, Bank N: Role of tubular obstruction in acute renal failure due to gentamicin, *Kidney Int* 24:330, 1983.
74. Siegler RL: Management of hemolytic-uremic syndrome, *J Pediatr* 112:1014, 1988.
75. Drummond KN: Hemolytic uremic syndrome–then and now, *N Engl J Med* 312:116, 1985.
76. Remuzzi G, Missaui R, Marchesi D: Treatment of hemolytic uremic syndrome with plasma, *Clin Nephrol* 12:279, 1979.
77. Couser WG: Mediation of immune glomerular injury, *J Am Soc Nephrol* 1:13, 1990.
78. Bergstein JM: Glomerular fibrin deposition and removal, *Pediatr Nephrol* 4:78, 1990.
79. Whitington PF, Friedman AL, Chesney RW: Gastrointestinal disease in hemolytic uremic syndrome, *Gastroenterology* 76: 728, 1979.
80. Remuzzi G, Bertani T: Thrombotic thrombocytopenic purpura, hemolytic uremic syndrome and acute cortical necrosis. In Schrier RW, Gottshalk CW, editors: *Diseases of the kidney,* ed 4, Boston, 1988, Little, Brown.
81. Loirat C, Sonsino E, Hunglais N, et al: Treatment of hemolytic uremic syndrome with fresh frozen plasma: a prospective trial from the French Society of Pediatric Nephrology, *Pediatr Nephrol* 1:C52, 1987.
82. Hakim RM, Schulmen G, Churchill WH, et al: Successful management of thrombocytopenia, microangiopathic anaemia and acute renal failure by plasmapheresis, *Am J Kidney Dis* 5:170, 1985.
83. Powell HR, McCredie DA, Taylor CM, et al: Vitamin E treatment of haemolytic uraemic syndrome, *Arch Dis Child* 59:401, 1984.

84. Powell HR, Milner LS: A randomly selected trial of vitamin E in the haemolytic uremic syndrome (HUS). Paper presented at the Tenth International Congress of Nephrology, London, 1987.
85. Lian ECY, Mui PTK, Siddiqui FA: Inhibition of platelet aggregating activity in thrombotic thrombocytopenic purpura plasma by normal adult immunoglobulin G, *J Clin Invest* 73:548, 1984.
86. Sheth KJ, Gill JC, Leichter H: High dose immunoglobulin (Ig) infusions in hemolytic uremic syndrome (HUS), *Kidney Int* 31: 217, 1987.
87. Jennette JC, Falk RJ: Diagnosis and management of glomerulonephritis and vasculitis presenting as acute renal failure, *Med Clin North Am* 74:893, 1990.
88. Myers BD, Ross J, Newton L, et al: Cyclosporine associated chronic nephropathy, *N Engl J Med* 311:699, 1984.
89. Blantz RC, Wilson CB: Acute effects of antiglomerular basement membrane antibody on the process of glomerular filtration in the rat, *J Clin Invest* 58:899, 1976.
90. Rodriguez-Iturbe B: Epidemic poststreptococcal glomerulonephritis, *Kidney Int* 25:129, 1984.
91. Nelson EG: Pathogenesis and therapy of interstitial nephritis, *Kidney Int* 35:1257, 1989.
92. Baldwin DS: Poststreptococcal glomerulonephritis: a progressive disease? *Am J Med* 27:49, 1976.
93. Baldwin DS, Gluck MC, Schacht RG, et al: The long term course of poststreptococcal glomerulonephritis, *Ann Intern Med* 80: 342, 1974.
94. Potter EV, Lipschultz SA, Abidh S, et al: Twelve to seventeen year following of patients with poststreptococcal acute glomerulonephritis in Trinidad, *N Engl J Med* 307:725, 1982.
95. Vogl W, Renke M, Mayer-Eichberger D, et al: Long-term prognosis for endocapillary glomerulonephritis of poststreptococcal type in children and adults, *Nephron* 44:58, 1986.
96. Balow JE, Austin HA: Renal disease in systemic lupus erythematosus, *Rheum Dis Clin North Am* 14:117, 1988.
97. Balow JE, Austin HA, Tsokos G, et al: Lupus nephritis, *Ann Intern Med* 106:79, 1987.
98. McCluskey RT: The value of renal biopsy in lupus nephritis, *Arthritis Rheum* 25:867, 1982.
99. Donadio JV Jr, Holley KE, Ferguson RH, et al: Treatment of diffuse proliferative lupus nephritis with prednisone and combined prednisone and cyclophosphamide, *N Engl J Med* 299:1151, 1978.
100. Austin HA, Klippel JH, Balow JE, et al: Therapy of lupus nephritis: a controlled trial of prednisone and cytotoxic drugs, *N Engl J Med* 314:614, 1986.
101. McClone WJ, Golbus J, Zeides W, et al: Clinical and immunological effects of monthly administration of intravenous cyclophosphamide in severe lupus erythematosus, *N Engl J Med* 318:1423, 1988.
102. Johnson JP, Moore J Jr, Austin HA, et al: Therapy of antiglomerular basement antibody disease: analysis of prognostic significance of clinical pathologic and treatment factors, *Medicine (Baltimore)* 64:219, 1985.
103. Ellis EN, Wood EG, Berry P: Spectrum of disease associated with anti-neutrophil cytoplasmic autoantibodies in pediatric patients, *J Pediatr* 126:40, 1995.
104. Hall SL, Miller LC, Duggan E, et al: Wegener granulomatosis in pediatric patients, *J Pediatr* 106:739, 1985.
105. Stapleton FB, Strother DR, Roy S III, et al: Acute renal failure at onset of therapy for advanced stage Burkett lymphoma and B cell acute lymphoblastic lymphoma, *Pediatrics* 82:863, 1988.
106. Sakarcan A, Timmons C, Seikaly MG: Reversible idiopathic acute renal failure in children with primary nephrotic syndrome, *J Pediatr* 125:723, 1994.
107. Springate JE, Coyne JF, Karp MP, et al: Acute renal failure in minimal charge nephrotic syndrome, *Pediatrics* 80:946, 1987.
108. Eknoyan G: Acute renal failure associated with tubulointerstitial nephropathies. In Brenner BM, Lazarus JM, editors: *Acute renal failure,* ed 2, New York, 1988, Churchill Livingstone.
109. Grunfeld J, Kleinknecht D, Droz D: Acute interstitial nephritis. In Schrier RW, Gottshalk CW, editors: *Diseases of the kidney,* ed 4, Boston, 1988, Little, Brown.
110. Neild G: The haemolytic uraemic syndrome: a review, *Q J Med* 241:367, 1987.
111. Revert L, Montoliu J: Acute interstitial nephritis, *Semin Nephrol* 8:82, 1988.
112. Ellis D, Fried WA, Yunis EJ, et al: Acute interstitial nephritis in children: a report of 13 cases and review of the literature, *Pediatrics* 67:862, 1981.
113. Hawkins EP, Beray P, Silva F: Tubulointerstitial nephritis in children: clinical, morphologic, immunohistochemical and lectin studies. Southwest Pediatric Nephrology Study Group, *Am J Kidney Dis* 14:466, 1987.
114. Koskomies O, Holmberg C: Interstitial nephritis of acute onset, *Arch Dis Child* 60:752, 1985.
115. Cogan MC, Arieff AI: Sodium wasting, acidosis and hyperkalemia induced by methicillin interstitial nephritis: evidence for selective distal tubular dysfunction, *Am J Med* 64:500, 1978.
116. Cogan MG: Tubulointerstitial nephropathies: a pathophysiologic approach, *West J Med* 132:134, 1980.
117. Andreoli T: On the anatomy of amphotericin B-cholesterol pores in lipid bilayer membranes, *Kidney Int* 4:337, 1973.
118. Weinberg JM: The cellular basis of nephrotoxicity. In Schrier RW, Gottshalk CW, editors: *Diseases of the kidney,* ed, 4, Boston, 1988, Little, Brown.
119. Jones DP, Mahmoud H, Chesney RW: Tumor lysis syndrome: pathogenesis and management, *Pediatr Nephrol* 9:206, 1995.
120. Cohen LF, Balow JE, Margath II: Acute tumor lysis syndrome, *Am J Med* 68:486, 1980.
121. Dubrow A, Flamenbaum W: Acute renal failure associated with myoglobinuria and hemoglobinuria. In Brenner BM, Lazarus JM, editors: *Acute renal failure,* ed 2, New York, 1988, Churchill Livingstone.
122. Zager RA: Rhabdomyolysis and myoglobinuric renal failure, *Kidney Int* 49:314, 1996.
123. Mitchell RM, Freeman J: Crush syndrome: the management of hypovolemia and renal complications, *Aust N Z J Surg* 39: 155, 1969.
124. Pogue VA, Nurse HM: Cocaine-associated acute myoglobinuric renal failure, *Am J Med* 86:183, 1989.
125. Schrier RW, Henderson HS, Tisher CC, et al: Nephropathy associated with heat stress and exercise, *Ann Intern Med* 67: 356, 1967.
126. Grossman RA, Hamilton RW, Morse BM, et al: Nontraumatic rhabdomyolysis and acute renal failure, *N Engl J Med* 291: 807, 1974.
127. Robotham JL, Haddow JE: Rhabdomyolysis and myoglobinuria in childhood, *Pediatr Clin North Am* 23:279, 1976.
128. Haimovich H: Arterial embolism, myoglobinuria and renal tubular necrosis, *Arch Surg* 100:639, 1970.
129. Cadnapaphornchai P, Taber S, McDonald FD: Acute drug-associated rhabdomyolysis: an examination of its diverse renal manifestations and complications, *Am J Med Sci* 280:66, 1980.
130. Loughridge LW, Leader LP, Broron DAL: Acute renal failure due to muscle necrosis in carbon monoxide poisoning, *Lancet* 2:349, 1958.
131. Jackson RC: Exercise-induced renal failure and muscle damage, *Proc R Soc Med* 63:4, 1970.
132. Vertel RM, Knochel JP: Acute renal failure due to heat injury: an analysis of ten cases associated with a high incidence of myoglobinuria, *Am J Med* 43:435, 1967.
133. Morgensen JL: Myoglobinuria and renal failure associated with influenza, *Ann Intern Med* 80:302, 1974.
134. Haftel AJ, Eichner J, Haling J, et al: Myoglobinuric renal failure in a newborn infant, *J Pediatr* 93:1015, 1978.
135. Kojima T, Kobayashi T, Matsuzaki S, et al: Effects of perinatal asphyxia and myoglobinuria on development of acute, neonatal renal failure, *Arch Dis Child* 60:908, 1985.
136. Llach PP, Felsenfeld AJ, Haussler MR: The pathophysiology of altered calcium metabolism in rhabdomyolysis-induced acute renal failure: interactions of parathyroid hormone, 25-hydroxycholecalciferol, and 1,25-dihydroxycholecalciferol, *N Engl J Med* 305:117, 1981.
137. Ayer G, Grandchamp A, Wyler T, et al: Intrarenal hemodynamics in glycerol-induced myohemoglobinuric acute renal failure in the rat, *Circ Res* 29:128, 1971.
138. Braun SR, Weiss FR, Keller AI, et al: Evaluation of the renal toxicity of heme proteins and their derivatives: a role in the genesis of acute tubular necrosis, *J Exp Med* 131:443, 1970.

139. Nicolau D, Feng YS, Wu AH, et al: Myoglobin clearance during continuous veno-venous hemofiltration with or without dialysis, *Int J Artif Organs* 21:205, 1998.
140. Mendosa SA: Nephrotoxic drugs, *Pediatr Nephrol* 2:466, 1988.
141. Porter GA, Bennett WM: Nephrotoxic acute renal failure due to common drugs, *Am J Physiol* 274:F1, 1981.
142. Senekjian HO, Knight TF, Weinman EJ: Micropuncture study of the handling of gentamicin by the rat kidney, *Kidney Int* 19:416, 1981.
143. DeBroe ME, Paulus GJ, Verpooten GA, et al: Early effects of gentamicin, tobramycin, and amikacin on the human kidney, *Kidney Int* 25:643, 1984.
144. Cronin RE: Aminoglycoside nephrotoxicity: pathogenesis and prevention, *Clin Nephrol* 11:251, 1979.
145. Higa EM, Schor N, Boim MA, et al: Role of the prostaglandin and kallikrein-kinin systems in aminoglycoside-induced acute renal failure, *Braz J Med Biol Res* 18:355, 1985.
146. Avasthi PS, Evan AP, Huser JW, et al: Effect of gentamicin on glomerular ultrastructure, *J Lab Clin Med* 98:444, 1981.
147. Baylis C, Rennke HR, Brenner BM: Mechanisms of the defect in glomerular ultrafiltration associated with gentamicin administration, *Kidney Int* 12:384, 1977.
148. Zager RA: Gentamicin nephrotoxicity in the setting of acute renal hypoperfusion hypotension potentials, *Am J Physiol* 254:F574, 1988.
149. Cheng J, Witty RT, Robinson RR, et al: Amphotericin B nephrotoxicity: increased renal resistance and tubule permeability, *Kidney Int* 22:626, 1982.
150. Gerkens J, Heidemann HT, Jackson EK, et al: Effect of aminophylline on amphotericin B nephrotoxicity in the dog, *J Pharmacol Exp Ther* 224:609, 1983.
151. Fisher MA, Talbot GH, Maislin G, et al: Risk factors for amphotericin B-associated nephrotoxicity, *Am J Med* 87:547, 1989.
152. Baley J, Kleegman R, Fanaroff A: Disseminated fungal infections in very low birth weight infants: therapeutic toxicity, *Pediatrics* 73:153, 1984.
153. Bullock WE, Luke RG, Nuttall CE, et al: Can mannitol reduce amphotericin B nephrotoxicity? Double-blind study and description of a new vascular lesion in kidneys, *Antimicrob Agents Chemother* 10:555, 1976.
154. Hellebusch AA, Salama F, Eadie E: The use of mannitol to reduce the nephrotoxicity of amphotericin B, *Surg Gynecol Obstet* 134:241, 1972.
155. Bennett WM, Pullian JP: Cyclosporine nephrotoxicity, *Ann Intern Med* 99:851, 1983.
156. Cronin RE: Radiocontrast media-induced acute renal failure. In Brenner BM, Lazarus JM, editors: *Acute renal failure,* ed 2, New York, 1988, Churchill Livingstone.
157. Solomon R, Werner C, Mann D, et al: Effects of saline, mannitol, and furosemide on acute decreases in renal function induced by radiocontrast agents, *N Engl J Med* 331: 1416, 1994.
158. Mueller C, Buerkle G, Buettner H, et al: Prevention of radiocontrast media associated nephropathy. Randomized comparison of 2 hydration regimens in 1620 patients undergoing coronary angioplasty, *Arch Intern Med* 162:329, 2002.
159. Tepel M, van der Giet M, Schwarzfeld C, et al: Prevention of radiocontrast agent induced reductions in renal function by acetylcysteine, *N Engl J Med* 343:180, 2000.
160. Briguori C, Manganelli F, Scarpato P, et al: Acetylcysteine and contrast agent-associated nephrotoxicity, *J Am Coll Cardiol* 40:298, 2002.
161. Marenzi G, Marana I, Lauri G, et al: The prevention of radiocontrast-agent induced nephropathy by hemofiltration, *N Engl J Med* 49:1333, 2003.
162. Epstein M: Acute renal failure in liver disease. In Molitoris BA, Finn WF, editors: *Acute renal failure,* Philadelphia, 2001, WB Saunders.
163. Dworkin LD, Ichikawa I, Brenner BM: Hormonal modulation of glomerular function, *Am J Physiol* 244:F95, 1983.
164. Kostreva DR, Castaner A, Kanipine JP: Reflex effects of hepatic baroreceptor on renal and cardiac sympathetic nerve reactivity, *Am J Physiol* 238:R390, 1980.
165. Koppel J, Coburn JW, Mims MM, et al: Transplantation of cadaveric kidneys from patients with hepatorenal syndrome: evidence for the functional nature of renal failure in advanced liver disease, *N Engl J Med* 280:1367, 1969.
166. Zager RA, O'Quigley J, Zager BK, et al: Acute renal failure following bone marrow transplantation: a retrospective study of 272 patients *Am J Kidney Dis* 13:210, 1989.
167. Badr KF, Brenner BM: Renal circulatory and nephron function in experimental obstruction of the urinary tract. In Brenner BM, Lazarus JM, editors: *Acute renal failure,* New York, 1988, Churchill Livingstone.
168. Morrison AR, Benabe EJ: Prostaglandins and vascular tone in experimental obstructive nephropathy, *Kidney Int* 19: 786, 1981.
169. Whinnery MA, Shaw JO, Beck N: Thromboxane B2 and prostaglandin E2 in the rat kidney with unilateral ureteral obstruction, *Am J Physiol* 242:F220, 1984.
170. Klotman PE, Smith SR, Volpp BD, et al: Thromboxane synthetase inhibition improves function of hydronephrotic rat kidneys, *Am J Physiol* 254:F282, 1986.
171. Campbell HT, Bello-Reuss E, Klahr S: Hydraulic water permeability and transepithelial voltage in the isolated perfused rabbit cortical collecting tubule following acute unilateral ureteral obstruction, *J Clin Invest* 75:219, 1985.
172. Thirakomen K, Kozlov N, Arruda JA, et al: Renal hydrogen ion secretion after release of unilateral ureteral obstruction, *Am J Physiol* 231:1233, 1976.

CHAPTER

65

Pediatric Renal Replacement Therapy in the Intensive Care Unit

Jordan M. Symons and Stuart L. Goldstein

PEARLS

- Earlier initiation of renal replacement therapy may improve outcome.
- Peritoneal dialysis remains an excellent form of acute pediatric renal replacement therapy.
- Hemodialysis is the modality of choice for rapid correction of fluid or metabolic imbalance.
- Continuous renal replacement therapy (CRRT) can establish and maintain fluid and metabolic control even in unstable patients.
- Patients receiving renal replacement therapy require careful monitoring of fluid and electrolyte balance and nutritional needs.
- Coordination between the critical care and nephrology staff is essential for the successful care of patients requiring renal replacement therapy.

Renal replacement therapy has a growing role in the pediatric intensive care unit (ICU).[1] Volume overload and metabolic imbalance can complicate the course of critically ill patients, especially those with multiorgan dysfunction.[2] Some patients with overall normal renal function may have metabolic imbalance or intoxication that overwhelms baseline renal capacity. Improving techniques coupled with the realization that early supportive therapy may improve outcomes have combined to expand the use of renal replacement for critically ill pediatric patients.

Renal Failure and Other Indications for Renal Support

Acute Renal Failure

Acute renal failure (ARF) can be defined as an acute decrease in the glomerular filtration rate (GFR). Oligoanuria is a frequent but not essential component of ARF. Common causes of ARF in the critically ill patient include hypoperfusion of the kidneys (leading to so-called prerenal azotemia), hypotension or shock causing renal ischemic injury or acute tubular necrosis (ATN), nonspecific renal involvement as part of a sepsis syndrome or multiorgan dysfunction, and renal injury from nephrotoxins such as antibiotics and radiocontrast media (see also Chapter 63 and Chapter 67).

Patients with even mild ARF can have volume overload, electrolyte imbalance, and metabolic derangement. Such complications can be particularly detrimental to the care of the critically ill patient. All modalities of renal replacement therapy can correct these abnormalities.

Acute Intoxication and Metabolic Disorders

Hemodialysis can rapidly remove many ingested toxins and is often the therapy of choice for severe intoxication. Hemodialysis and hemofiltration techniques can also remove endogenously generated toxins, as seen with inborn errors of metabolism (see also Chapters 109 and Chapter 110).

Renal Support

Diminished renal function is a common component of multiorgan dysfunction syndrome. Studies in adults strongly suggest increased morbidity in critically ill patients with renal failure.[3,4] Early intervention with renal replacement therapy has been shown to improve the outcome of critically ill adults[5]; a recent study supports this concept for pediatric patients receiving continuous renal replacement therapy (CRRT).[6] The concept of early "renal support" for patients in the ICU to limit metabolic derangement and prevent volume overload[7] has gained wider acceptance in both the adult and pediatric critical care arenas.

Conservative Management

Conservative management of ARF includes optimization of clinical status with the maintenance of fluid balance, renal perfusion, cardiac output, and adequate blood pressure. Nephrotoxin exposure should be limited. Judicious use of diuretics can greatly augment the patient's ability to maintain fluid balance. Fluids may need to be restricted to prevent fluid overload. The patient will require careful dietary management to provide sufficient nutrition in a smaller daily fluid volume and to avoid excess delivery of substances normally cleared through the kidney (e.g., potassium, phosphorus). Conservative management avoids the potential risks associated with renal replacement modalities; many pediatric patients with milder renal dysfunction can be managed successfully without dialysis or filtration. As noted previously, however, there is support for the use of renal replacement early in the ICU course. Data show improved outcomes for pediatric patients receiving CRRT who had less fluid overload at initiation of therapy,[6] suggesting a survival advantage for patients who begin CRRT earlier rather than later. Adults who received more vigorous ultrafiltration regimens while undergoing CRRT were more likely to survive than matched counterparts who underwent less aggressive CRRT.[5] Although the best time to initiate renal replacement for the patient in the ICU remains unclear, there is a growing consensus to avoid unnecessary delay.

Basic Physiology of Dialysis and Ultrafiltration

The physical principles of molecular movement across a semipermeable membrane underlie peritoneal dialysis, hemodialysis, and hemofiltration modalities. The following brief review summarizes the basic mechanisms of particle and water removal for all forms of renal replacement therapy.

Diffusion describes the movement of dissolved particles across a semipermeable membrane from an area of high concentration to an area of low concentration (Fig. 65–1).

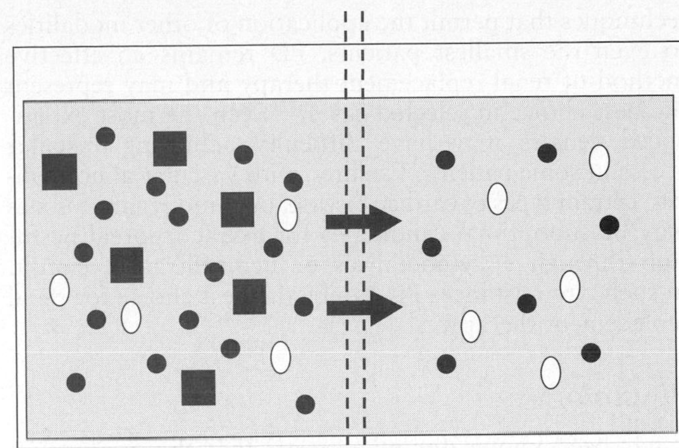

FIGURE 65–1 • Diffusion. Particles move across the semipermeable membrane from an area of higher concentration to an area of lower concentration. Smaller particles diffuse more freely, whereas larger particles are relatively restricted.

This physical principle operates in all renal replacement modalities in which dialysate is used. Diffusion favors the movement of smaller particles and is most rapid when the concentration gradient across the semipermeable membrane is greatest; diffusion stops when the concentrations achieve equilibrium.

Convection occurs when dissolved particles pass across a semipermeable membrane due to the effects of a pressure gradient (Fig. 65–2). Particles that are smaller than the pores of the membrane can pass freely, whereas larger particles are restricted. Because particles and water are moving together, the removed solution is isotonic to the original.

Ultrafiltration describes the movement of water across the semipermeable membrane due to pressure. Convection occurs with ultrafiltration.

Peritoneal Dialysis

Peritoneal dialysis (PD) has been a standard form for renal replacement therapy for many years.[8-11] Despite improving

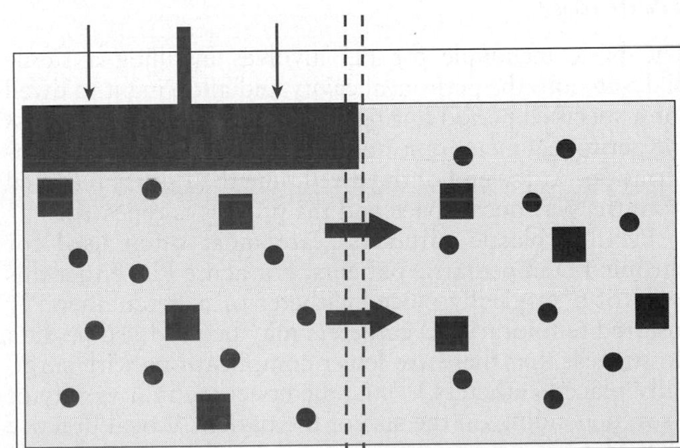

FIGURE 65–2 • Convection. Particles move across the semipermeable membrane, carried by ultrafiltered water, because of the effect of pressure. All particles up to the cutoff size of the membrane move relatively equally. The concentration of the effluent is equal to that of the original solution.

techniques that permit the application of other modalities to even the smallest patients, PD remains an effective method of renal replacement therapy and may represent the best choice in selected cases.[12] Even the most experienced centers may have difficulty achieving vascular access in some patients. Children with vascular abnormalities, certain types of cardiac disease, or hemodynamic issues may be suboptimal candidates for extracorporeal perfusion through a hemodialysis or hemofiltration circuit. In such circumstances PD can be the best choice for renal replacement therapy.

Physiology

It has been known for many years that the peritoneum can be used as a dialyzing membrane.[13] Instillation of a dialysate into the peritoneal space permits diffusion of particles out of the blood and into the dialysate across the peritoneum, which acts as a semipermeable membrane. Through the use of a hypertonic solution, water also passes across the membrane, generating an ultrafiltrate. Water movement will also tend to drag particles across the peritoneum by convection. After the dwell is complete, the spent dialysate is drained from the abdomen, and fresh dialysate may be introduced.

Indications

PD can remove excess fluid and provide volume control in the patient with oligoanuria. As compared with fluid removal with intermittent hemodialysis, fluid removal with PD is much slower. Manipulation of dialysate osmolality and dwell time can adjust the quantity of volume removed. The slow, steady ultrafiltration achieved with PD may be preferable to the rapid fluid removal seen in intermittent hemodialysis, particularly in the unstable, critically ill patient.

Similar to volume control, PD provides slow and relatively continuous metabolic control. It is an effective method for correction of uremia. Manipulation of the PD prescription can improve clearances.

Technique

The basic technique for PD involves instilling a sterile dialysate into the peritoneal cavity and allowing it to dwell for a specified period during which particles diffuse across the peritoneal membrane and water moves across by ultrafiltration. At the end of the dwell time the fluid is removed from the peritoneal space and the process is repeated.

Flexible plastic catheters[14] are most often used for chronic PD in pediatric patients. For acute PD, either this form of a surgically placed catheter or a percutaneously inserted temporary PD catheters may be used; some data do suggest that there are fewer complications with surgically placed catheters.[15-17] Catheters come in a variety of sizes, depending on the size of the patient. Local practice often determines who will insert the catheters when they are needed; the procedure requires expertise to ensure proper function of the catheter.

Peritoneal dialysate comes in standardized, sterile bags with premixed formulations; pharmacy preparation is unnecessary. Because most patients with renal failure have metabolic acidosis, the dialysate contains base, usually in the form of lactate. Thus the PD system will remove unwanted particles and can also act as a source of electrolytes. Lactate absorption can lead to complications, especially in critically ill infants; in such settings dialysate with bicarbonate may need to be used.[18] This may require extemporaneous preparation by the local pharmacy.

Ultrafiltration in PD is accomplished by osmotic pressure, usually through the presence of dextrose in the dialysate. Dialysates come with standardized concentrations of dextrose; the choices vary somewhat between the United States and Europe. Dialysate with higher concentrations of dextrose will cause greater ultrafiltration for each exchange of fluid.

Dialysate should be warmed to body temperature before instillation. This is particularly important in small patients who can have hypotension associated with cold dialysate infusion.[19]

Initial exchanges with a new PD catheter should use relatively lower volumes of dialysate (10 to 20 ml/kg; <500 ml/m^2) to limit the chance of leak from the operative site. Volumes may increase gradually over the next few days or weeks to 1100 ml/m^2.[19]

Longer periods between exchanges provide more time for equilibration of dialyzable particles and for ultrafiltration. Although shorter dwell times may not maximize mass transport for a given dwell periods, they may permit more dialysis and ultrafiltration in a 24-hour period by allowing more exchanges per day. Initial dwell periods of 30 to 60 minutes can be adjusted later on the basis of clinical status.

Peritoneal dialysate can be instilled by hand or with the use of a cycler, a device that will automatically fill and empty the patient's abdomen with dialysate on a preprogrammed schedule. The cycler also contains a warmer for the dialysate and monitoring systems to record effluent volumes. Several brands of cycler are currently available. Programming limitations may prevent the use of a cycler for some patients who require very small fill volumes or very short dwell times.

The importance of sterile technique when performing PD cannot be overemphasized. Appropriate technique limits the risk of infectious complications, which could be fatal in a critically ill patient.

Disadvantages and Complications

The PD technique requires placement of a peritoneal catheter and a sufficiently maintained intraabdominal status to permit infusion of dialysate with successful diffusion and ultrafiltration. Patients who have undergone an abdominal operation or have had abdominal complications may be poor candidates for PD.

Invasion of the peritoneal space puts the patient at risk for peritonitis, a potentially serious complication. Careful attention to sterile technique is an essential part of successful PD therapy. Peritonitis must always be considered in a PD patient with a fever or cloudy effluent. Dialysate should be analyzed for cell count, Gram stain, and bacterial culture if infection is suspected. Empirical or specific antibiotic therapy can be placed in the dialysate to treat peritonitis via the intraperitoneal route.[20]

Dialysate can fail to fill or drain through the PD catheter because of a number of potential problems, including kinking, fibrin plugs, omental obstruction, or catheter malposition. Percutaneously inserted temporary dialysis catheters are more prone to malfunction than are surgically placed catheters.[16] Abdominal x-ray images can confirm appropriate positioning of the catheter and allow kinks to be checked. Some success has been reported with thrombolytic agents to treat fibrin plugging.[21] Revision or replacement of the catheter may need to be considered if simple maneuvers do not correct the malfunction.

Perforation of abdominal or pelvic structures can occur, either at the time of initial catheter placement or later.[16] Although this is a relatively uncommon event, significant morbidity can result.

PD is a suboptimal choice for those patients who require rapid correction of metabolic abnormalities, immediate removal of circulating toxins, or rapid ultrafiltration for acute complications of fluid overload. Hemodialysis would be the preferred modality.

Fluid leak is seen most often with dwell volumes that are too large, especially in the period immediately after catheter placement.[22] Lower fill volumes should be used. Fluid leak into the thorax can compromise respiration. External fluid leak around the catheter increases the risk of infection.

Intensive Care Unit Issues

Patients undergoing PD can lose protein into the dialysate. Nutritional support must provide sufficient protein to compensate for this loss. High dextrose concentrations in the dialysate can cause hyperglycemia; insulin may be necessary. Indwelling dialysate causes increased intraabdominal pressure that can complicate care of the critically ill patient. Diaphragmatic excursion may be limited, and venous return can be reduced. Stomach compression can lead to gastroesophageal reflux. Although patients undergoing long-term PD who receive fewer daily exchanges usually require maximal fill volumes to achieve adequate dialysis, patients undergoing short-term PD may do better using submaximal fill volumes with more frequent exchanges provided around the clock.

Intermittent Hemodialysis

Intermittent hemodialysis (IHD) has been the traditional form of renal replacement therapy in the ICU. The technique is well established for pediatric patients.[23-25] IHD offers the advantages of high efficiency for rapid metabolic correction and fluid removal. Its very advantages, however, may limit IHD's usefulness in the critically ill patient. IHD for infants and small children can be technically difficult and demanding. IHD may be the therapy of choice for some critically ill pediatric patients; successful treatment in this setting requires experienced personnel.

Physiology

The dialyzer used in IHD is an artifical semipermeable membrane. The most common design used today is the hollow-fiber dialyzer. It consists of a plastic cartridge traversed by several thousand thin hollow fibers, each with microscopic fenestrations that permit the passage of water and other small molecules. Dialyzers vary in their surface area, permeability, priming volume, and membrane composition; numerous dialyzers are available commercially. Choosing different dialyzer characteristics permits adjustment of the dialysis prescription to the clinical situation.

Successful hemodialysis requires sufficiently high blood flow to allow adequate dialysis and ultrafiltration with a minimal risk of clotting. Dialysis efficiency falls off dramatically with lower blood pump speeds; this may require extended time on dialysis to compensate. Consequently, high-quality vascular access is essential for successful hemodialysis.

While blood flows through the hollow fibers of the dialyzer, dialysate flows through the cartridge in the space surrounding the hollow fibers. Particles move by diffusion from the blood across the semipermeable membrane into the dialysate. Use of high-flow dialysate with maximal blood flow through the dialyzer permits intermittent hemodialysis to remove particles more efficiently than any other renal replacement therapy.

Increasing blood flow, dialysate flow, or dialyzer size will increase the rate of diffusion. Because diffusion favors the movement of small particles over large particles, large molecules or small molecules bound to larger molecules (such as albumin) will not dialyze well. In addition, intracellular particles will move into the vascular compartment on the basis of individual cell membrane transport characteristics; this may limit the rate at which dialysis can remove particles that do not reside within the vascular compartment.

Ultrafiltration on hemodialysis occurs because of hydrostatic pressure across the membrane, which forces water out of the blood. Dissolved particles will travel with the water, leaving by convection. Using IHD, dialysis staff can control the rate of ultrafiltration with precision and can achieve high rates of ultrafiltration.

Analogous to the process of diffusion, ultrafiltration during IHD removes fluid only from the vascular compartment. Extravascular or “third space” fluid must move into the vascular compartment for removal by ultrafiltration. When the rate of movement from the extravascular space is slower than the rate of ultrafiltration, intravascular depletion can occur even though total body water remains elevated (Fig. 65–3). This “two-compartment” model represents a potential limitation of rapid ultrafiltration during IHD, especially in the critically ill patient.

Indications

Thanks to its high efficiency, hemodialysis is the best modality for rapid particle removal. IHD is indicated for the treatment of toxic ingestions, many serious drug

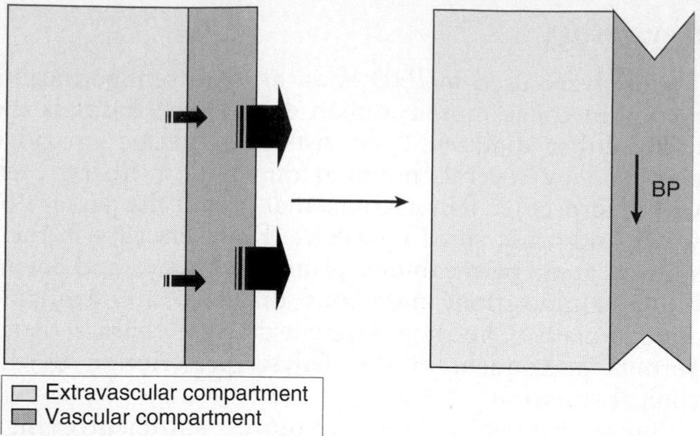

FIGURE 65–3 • Two-compartment model of ultrafiltration. The rate of water removal from the vascular compartment by ultrafiltration (*large arrows*) exceeds the rate of refilling from the extravascular compartment (*smaller arrows*), and this process leads to relative vascular volume depletion and hypotension.

overdoses, and metabolic derangements that lead to the overproduction of endogenous toxins such as ammonia (see also Chapters 72,109, and 110).[26-30]

The IHD system can perform ultrafiltration more rapidly than any other renal replacement modality. Consequently it is often the best choice for the treatment of critical volume overload.

Profound metabolic imbalance, such as seen with critical hyperkalemia, can be corrected most quickly with IHD. Patients with oncological problems such as tumor lysis syndrome may require IHD to correct rapidly the multiple metabolic abnormalities and to aid clearance of uric acid, which can cause renal failure (see also Chapter 78).[31, 32]

Technique

Vascular access is the first step for successful hemodialysis. Double-lumen catheters for hemodialysis come in a variety of sizes; occasionally, two single-lumen catheters at separate sites are needed for small infants. Catheters can be placed in jugular, femoral, or subclavian positions (see also Chapter 15). The jugular vein is preferred for access that will be required for more than a few sessions. Surgical support may be needed for patients where percutaneous placement is difficult.

Most patients receiving IHD will require heparin for anticoagulation. Some may be able to undergo successful dialysis with little or no heparin because of coagulopathy related to their systemic disease. Staff members often monitor clotting times during the IHD session to determine the need for heparin.

Blood pump rate is chosen based on the patient's clinical status and the quality of the vascular access. Smaller patients with smaller catheters must often run with blood pump speeds less than 100 ml/min; infants may run as low as 25 to 50 ml/min. Larger patients can tolerate faster blood pump speeds. Higher blood flow rates permit greater mass transfer of particles out of the patient in a given period.

The chosen dialyzer should provide sufficient clearance to achieve the goals of the dialysis session. Smaller patients receive dialysis with smaller dialyzers to limit extracorporeal blood volume and reduce the risk of dialyzer clotting with slower blood flow rates.

Small patients or those with unstable blood pressure may require priming of the IHD circuit with saline, albumin, or reconstituted whole blood. The development of dialysis machines with volumetric ultrafiltration control allows for accurate and safe IHD in neonates and infants, for whom small inaccuracies in ultrafiltration volumes could potentially lead to severe fluid imbalances. Dialysate concentrations of electrolytes can be adjusted to some extent on the basis of the clinical situation. The length of the IHD session will vary depending on the clinical situation and goals of the therapy. Mathematical models permit estimation of dialytic clearance and can be used to structure session length. The rate at which the patient can tolerate ultrafiltration is often the limiting factor in IHD for critically ill patients. Sessions may need to be extended to achieve ultrafiltration goals without significant hypotension.

Disadvantages and Complications

The principal disadvantage of IHD is the requirement for vascular access. Acceptable access can be difficult to achieve in critically ill children. Complications related to the access can include infection, bleeding, and thrombosis.

IHD's benefit of high efficiency with rapid fluid and particle removal can also lead to difficulties in the ICU setting. Critically ill patients may not tolerate the rapid ultrafiltration and metabolic shifts of IHD.

Smaller patients or those with unstable blood pressure may require priming of the extracorporeal circuit to limit hemodynamic stress at dialysis initiation. For infants in whom the extracorporeal volume is relatively much larger, priming may need to be done with a blood/albumin mix, and this exposes the patient to blood products.

Most IHD sessions require systemic anticoagulation with heparin, which can be difficult to manage in a critically ill child. Heparin exposure can complicate bleeding and cause heparin-induced thrombocytopenia. With careful monitoring of clotting times and circuit performance during the session, it is possible to perform IHD without heparin. The risk of clot formation in the IHD circuit rises, however, when heparin is not used.

Intensive Care Unit Issues

Patients receiving IHD as ongoing renal replacement therapy in the ICU require special attention to fluid and electrolyte balance. One should limit potassium and phosphorus delivery and may need to limit total daily fluids because ultrafiltration only occurs intermittently. Medication doses and schedule may require adjustment because of poor excretion with renal failure and subsequent rapid removal on dialysis (see also Chapter 119).

Continuous Renal Replacement Therapy

CRRT is a generic term applied to several techniques of extracorporeal renal support.[33] Similar to IHD in the use of a blood pump and hemofilter, the various subcategories of CRRT differ in their reliance on diffusion, convection, or a combination of the two for molecular clearance.

CRRT is becoming more popular as a method of renal support for pediatric patients.[34,35] Technological improvements in catheters, blood pumps, and ultrafiltration control mechanisms permit the application of CRRT to even the smallest infants.[36]

Physiology

The CRRT hemofilter is similar to that used for IHD. CRRT membranes traditionally have been more porous to permit greater removal of water. Numerous hemofilters are available commercially; most membranes are made from either polysulfone or polyacrylonitrile.

Both convection and diffusion can be used to remove particles during CRRT. Dialysate allows diffusion, which favors the movement of smaller molecules. High rates of ultrafiltration will remove both small and larger particles by convection, up to the limits of the membrane. With high ultrafiltration rates to achieve better convective clearance, the patient may need to receive replacement of volume and electrolytes to compensate for that lost in ultrafiltrate.

Because of slower flow rates, the clearance achieved with CRRT is significantly lower than that of IHD. Continuous therapies, however, make up for this lower efficiency through the extended time of the treatment. Compared with a 3 or 4-hour IHD session, CRRT running 24 hours a day can achieve equivalent daily clearance with less metabolic variation.

CRRT nomenclature continues to evolve. Recent consensus[37] has defined the names of various subcategories of CRRT on the basis of vascular access and primary method of particle clearance (convection, diffusion, or both). Because most CRRT in pediatric patients is a pump-assisted veno-venous method, the most commonly used terms are continuous veno-venous hemofiltration (CVVH), which uses high convective clearance requiring replacement fluids; continuous veno-venous hemodialysis (CVVHD), which uses dialysate for diffusion but minimal additional convection; and continuous veno-venous hemodiafiltration (CVVHDF), which uses both dialysate and replacement fluids for combined diffusion and high-grade convection.

Indications

As a result of the slow, continuous removal of fluid, CRRT is particularly well suited to the treatment of volume overload in critically ill patients. Whereas IHD will attempt to reach an ultrafiltration goal within a relatively short therapeutic session, CRRT allows continuous ultrafiltration that can help maintain cardiovascular stability.

CRRT is useful to maintain metabolic balance through ongoing removal of unwanted particles. Although it is less efficient than IHD, CRRT's continuous nature can avoid daily fluctuations inherent in the use of an intermittent modality. In addition, CRRT can be used as a secondary method to maintain metabolic balance after rapid correction with IHD.[38]

For those patients with diminished renal function and decreased urinary output, CRRT can permit administration of the daily load of fluids required to deliver medication and nutrition. This modality can maintain the patient in more stable balance compared with IHD, in which the patient has progressive volume overload in between IHD sessions and then must achieve the ultrafiltration goal in a brief treatment period.

Technique

As for IHD, successful CRRT requires adequate vascular access (see also Chapter 15). Given the relatively large extracorporeal volume, smaller patients may require priming of the CRRT circuit with blood/albumin mix.[39] Larger, more stable patients can successfully initiate CRRT with saline prime.

Earlier methods with arterio-venous access have largely been abandoned in favor of veno-venous CRRT. Older systems with adapted blood and fluid pumps linked together extemporaneously have been replaced by dedicated CRRT machinery. Several CRRT systems are available, and newer machines will be brought to market soon. This latest generation of CRRT machines permits much greater accuracy for blood pump speed, fluid delivery, and ultrafiltration control.

Anticoagulation

Adequate anticoagulation is essential for successful CRRT.[40] Currently, most patients treated with CRRT receive systemic heparin, regional citrate, or no added anticoagulation.

Systemic heparinization has been the traditional form of anticoagulation used in CRRT. This is a proven method that functions well. Disadvantages include systemic anticoagulation with risk of bleeding, risk of heparin-induced thrombocytopenia, and the need for frequent monitoring and adjustment of the heparin dose.

Regional citrate anticoagulation is becoming increasingly popular for CRRT in both adult and pediatric patients. Citrate, introduced into the CRRT circuit, chelates calcium, which is a required cofactor in both the intrinsic and extrinsic arms of the clotting cascade. Calcium is infused back into the patient through a separate central access to prevent systemic hypocalcemia. Citrate is metabolized to bicarbonate, acting as a source of base. Several protocols have been developed for regional citrate anticoagulation in CRRT.[41-43] The systems are stable and require less monitoring than heparin-based anticoagulation. Disadvantages include the potential for acid/base imbalance, the risk of hypercalcemia or hypocalcemia, citrate overload due to poor metabolism or diminished clearance, and the need for additional central access for high rates of calcium delivery.

Many critically ill patients have disorders of coagulation as a part of their multiple organ system injury and can undergo CRRT without exogenous anticoagulation. Increased clotting of the CRRT circuit in such patients may be a sign of improving clinical status.

Patient and vascular access size can limit blood pump rate. The current generation of CRRT machines can run at lower blood pump speeds with greater accuracy than earlier systems.

Many brands of hemofilter are available for CRRT. Larger surface areas will permit more rapid ultrafiltration and clearance by convection. Of particular interest in the pediatric patient are reports of profound hypotensive events related to the use of a type of polyacrylonitrile hemofilter known as the AN-69 membrane.[44,45] This reaction, occurring rapidly when the patient's blood comes in contact with the hemofilter, is thought to be related to the release of bradykinin in response to the low pH of blood used to prime the CRRT circuit. Smaller patients and those with metabolic acidosis seem to be at greatest risk. Maneuvers to adjust pH within the circuit and limit this reaction have been described.[45]

Dialysate and Infused Fluids

Nearly all of the current CRRT machines use premade, fully mixed dialysate rather than generating dialysate online from concentrates (during IHD the dialysate is generated online). The physician is therefore faced with the choice of using commercially available dialysate or requesting extemporaneously prepared dialysate from local pharmacy services. There are a limited number of approved dialysates available commercially for CRRT. Because of the volume of production and commercial quality control, their use may limit the potential for error with extemporaneous solution.[43] They may also be more cost-effective when compared with local pharmacy expense.

Even fewer commercially prepared options exist for replacement fluids in CRRT, and programs will often choose to have the local pharmacy prepare fluids for infusion. Selections vary from normal saline to complex electrolyte solutions designed to approximate physiological levels. More complex solutions may require preparing components in separate bags that mix at the time of infusion to limit the chance of precipitation. Simpler systems may not meet all the needs of electrolyte balance, but more complicated schemes may have a greater risk for error.

Replacement fluids are infused to the CRRT system either before the hemofilter ("prefilter" or "predilution") or after ("postfilter" or "postdilution"). Prefilter delivery will reduce convective clearance at a given ultrafiltration rate because the blood entering the hemofilter will be diluted by the replacement fluid. This reduction, however, can be easily overcome with an increase of the ultrafiltration rate. Furthermore, prefilter replacement permits significantly higher ultrafiltration rates because it limits hemoconcentration within the hemofilter and thus lessens the chances of filter clotting. Some CRRT machines will permit either prefilter or postfilter delivery of replacement fluids, whereas others have a fixed location for replacement fluids.

Clearance

CRRT blood pump, dialysate, and replacement fluid rates tend to be lower overall than those used in IHD. Consequently, clearance rates are lower but total daily clearance increases because the therapy is continuous. In most prescriptions, the limiting factor in CRRT clearance is the dialysate or replacement fluid flow rate[46]; greater rates of clearance can often be achieved with an increase in the rate of dialysate or replacement fluid. Data suggest that increased convective clearance achieved with higher rates of ultrafiltration and replacement fluids can improve survival.[5] Slower blood pump speeds can also potentially limit clearances.

Slow, steady ultrafiltration to gradually achieve fluid balance and then maintain it is the hallmark of CRRT. Slow ultrafiltration can permit movement of extravascular fluid into the vascular space at a rate roughly equal to the ultrafiltration rate, and this allows greater mobilization of fluid while the risk of acute intravascular volume depletion and hypotension is limited. Ultrafiltration rates must be chosen on the basis of clinical status of the patient and fluid balance goals; frequent reevaluation is often necessary.

Disadvantages and Complications

Like IHD, CRRT requires the placement of vascular access, which can be difficult in infants and small children. Continuous extracorporeal perfusion and anticoagulation carry risks of bleeding and infection. Some patients experience blood pressure instability despite the slow method of ultrafiltration. Continuous exposure to heparin can lead to heparin-induced thrombocytopenia. Patients receiving citrate anticoagulation are at risk for acid/base disturbance or hypocalcemia. Citrate overload can cause low patient ionized calcium with normal or high total calcium levels, the so-called calcium gap or citrate lock.[43,47,48] This occurs when excess citrate binds free calcium in the patient. Under these circumstances, citrate delivery should be reduced.

Intensive Care Unit Issues

Continuous clearance on CRRT, particularly with convective modalities, can cause profound electrolyte deficiencies. Careful attention must be paid to appropriate replacement of electrolytes lost through CRRT. Similarly, nitrogen losses on CRRT can be high.[49] Patients require increased nutritional support during CRRT therapy. Medication dosages often require adjustment because of losses through the CRRT system. Coordination between the ICU staff and nephrology staff is essential to establish appropriate goals for fluid removal and metabolic control.

Summary

Pediatric patients who need renal replacement therapy represent a special challenge. Multiple modalities are available and the best choice may be dictated by the clinical situation and local expertise. Careful attention to fluid and electrolyte balance and appropriate nutritional support and close interaction between critical care and nephrology personnel will yield the best outcomes.

REFERENCES

1. Mentser M, Bunchman T: Nephrology in the pediatric intensive care unit, *Semin Nephrol,* 18:330-340, 1998.
2. Lowrie LH: Renal replacement therapies in pediatric multiorgan dysfunction syndrome, *Pediatr Nephrol,* 14:6-12, 2000.
3. Levy EM, Viscoli CM, Horwitz RI: The effect of acute renal failure on mortality. A cohort analysis, *JAMA,* 275:1489-1494, 1996.
4. Chertow GM, Levy EM, Hammermeister KE, et al: Independent association between acute renal failure and mortality following cardiac surgery, *Am J Med,* 104:343-348, 1998.
5. Ronco C, Bellomo R, Homel P, et al: Effects of different doses in continuous veno-venous haemofiltration on outcomes of acute renal failure: a prospective randomised trial, *Lancet,* 356: 26-30, 2000.
6. Goldstein SL, Currier H, Graf C, et al: Outcome in children receiving continuous venovenous hemofiltration, *Pediatrics,* 107:1309-1312, 2001.
7. Mehta RL: Indications for dialysis in the ICU: renal replacement vs. renal support, *Blood Purif,* 19:227-232, 2001.
8. Rhoads JE: Peritoneal lavage in the treatment of renal insufficiency, *Am J Med Sci,* 196:642-644, 1938.
9. Frank HA, Seligman AM, Fine J: Treatment of uremia after acute renal failure by peritoneal irrigation, *JAMA,* 130:703-706, 1946.
10. Bloxsum A, Powell N: The treatment of acute temporary dysfunction of the kidneys by peritoneal irrigation, *Pediatrics,* 1:52-57, 1948.
11. Feldman W, Baliah T, Drummond KN: Intermittent peritoneal dialysis in the management of chronic renal failure in children, *Am J Dis Child,* 116:30-36, 1968.
12. Flynn JT, Kershaw DB, Smoyer WE, et al: Peritoneal dialysis for management of pediatric acute renal failure, *Perit Dial Int,* 21: 390-394, 2001.
13. Putnam T: The living peritoneum as a dialyzing membrane, *Am J Physiol,* 63:548-565, 1922-1923.
14. Tenckhoff H, Schechter H: A bacteriologically safe peritoneal access device, *Trans Am Soc Artif Intern Organs,* 14:181-187, 1968.
15. Wong SN, Geary DF: Comparison of temporary and permanent catheters for acute peritoneal dialysis, *Arch Dis Child,* 63: 827-831, 1988.
16. Huber R, Fuchshuber A, Huber P: Acute peritoneal dialysis in preterm newborns and small infants: surgical management, *J Pediatr Surg,* 29:400-402, 1994
17. Chadha V, Warady BA, Blowey DL, et al: Tenckhoff catheters prove superior to cook catheters in pediatric acute peritoneal dialysis, *Am J Kidney Dis,* 35:1111-1116, 2000.
18. Nash MA, Russo JC: Neonatal lactic acidosis and renal failure: the role of peritoneal dialysis, *J Pediatr,* 91:101-105, 1977.
19. Warady B, Fivush B, Alexander S: Peritoneal dialysis. In Barratt T, Avner E, Harmon W, editors, *Pediatric nephrology,* ed 4, Baltimore, 1999, Lippincott Williams & Wilkins.
20. Warady BA, Schaefer F, Holloway M, et al: Consensus guidelines for the treatment of peritonitis in pediatric patients receiving peritoneal dialysis, *Perit Dial Int,* 20:610-624, 2000.
21. Shea M, Hmiel SP, Beck AM: Use of tissue plasminogen activator for thrombolysis in occluded peritoneal dialysis catheters in children, *Adv Perit Dial,* 17:249-252, 2001.
22. Leblanc M, Ouimet D, Pichette V: Dialysate leaks in peritoneal dialysis, *Semin Dial,* 14:50-54, 2001.
23. Donckerwolcke RA, Bunchman TE: Hemodialysis in infants and small children, *Pediatr Nephrol,* 8:103-106, 1994.
24. Sadowski RH, Harmon WE, Jabs K: Acute hemodialysis of infants weighing less than five kilograms, *Kidney Int,* 45:903-906, 1994.
25. Fischbach M, Terzic J, Menouer S, et al: Hemodialysis in children: principles and practice, *Semin Nephrol,* 21:470-479, 2001.
26. Elshihabi I, Brzowski A, Kaye C et al.: Efficiency of hemodialysis therapy for a urea cycle defect in a neonate, *Clin Nephrol,* 43: 208-209, 1995.
27. Bunchman TE, Valentini RP, Gardner J, et al: Treatment of vancomycin overdose using high-efficiency dialysis membranes, *Pediatr Nephrol,* 13:773-774, 1999.
28. Brophy PD, Tenenbein M, Gardner J, et al: Childhood diethylene glycol poisoning treated with alcohol dehydrogenase inhibitor fomepizole and hemodialysis, *Am J Kidney Dis,* 35:958-962, 2000.
29. Brown MJ, Shannon MW, Woolf A, et al: Childhood methanol ingestion treated with fomepizole and hemodialysis, *Pediatrics,* 108:E77, 2001.
30. Gitomer JJ, Khan AM, Ferris ME: Treatment of severe theophylline toxicity with hemodialysis in a preterm neonate, *Pediatr Nephrol,* 16:784-786, 2001.
31. Sakarcan A, Quigley R: Hyperphosphatemia in tumor lysis syndrome: the role of hemodialysis and continuous veno-venous hemofiltration, *Pediatr Nephrol,* 8:351-353, 1994.
32. Jaing TH, Hsueh C, Tain YL, et al: Tumor lysis syndrome in an infant with Langerhans cell histiocytosis successfully treated using continuous arteriovenous hemofiltration, *J Pediatr Hematol Oncol,* 23:142-144, 2001.
33. Bellomo R, Ronco C: Continuous renal replacement therapy in the intensive care unit, *Intensive Care Med,* 25:781-789, 1999.
34. Belsha CW, Kohaut EC, Warady BA: Dialytic management of childhood acute renal failure: a survey of North American pediatric nephrologists, *Pediatr Nephrol,* 9:361-363, 1995.
35. Warady BA, Bunchman T: Dialysis therapy for children with acute renal failure: survey results, *Pediatr Nephrol,* 15:11-13, 2000.
36. Symons JM, Brophy PD, Gregory MJ, et al: Continuous renal replacement therapy in children up to 10kg, *Am J Kidney Disease,* 41:984-989, 2003.
37. Ronco C, Bellomo R: Continuous renal replacement therapy: evolution in technology and current nomenclature, *Kidney Int Suppl,* 66:S160-S164, 1998.
38. McBryde KD, Brophy PD, Gregory MJ, et al: Renal replacement therapy in metabolic disturbances. Abstract presented at the ASN/ISN World Congress of Nephrology, San Francisco, October 2001.
39. Parekh RS, Bunchman TE: Dialysis support in the pediatric intensive care unit, *Adv Ren Replace Ther,* 3:326-336, 1996.
40. Abramson S, Niles JL: Anticoagulation in continuous renal replacement therapy, *Curr Opin Nephrol Hypertens,* 8:701-707, 1999.
41. Mehta RL, McDonald BR, Aguilar MM, et al: Regional citrate anticoagulation for continuous arteriovenous hemodialysis in critically ill patients, *Kidney Int,* 38:976-981, 1990.
42. Palsson R, Niles JL: Regional citrate anticoagulation in continuous venovenous hemofiltration in critically ill patients with a high risk of bleeding, *Kidney Int,* 55:1991-1997, 1999.
43. Bunchman TE, Maxvold NJ, Barnett J, et al: Pediatric hemofiltration: Normocarb dialysate solution with citrate anticoagulation, *Pediatr Nephrol,* 17:150-154, 2002.
44. Smoyer WE, Gardner AV, Mottes TA, et al: Early experience with the safety and effectiveness of the Cobe PRISMA for pediatric CRRT, *Blood Purif,* 18:80, 2000.
45. Brophy PD, Mottes TA, Kudelka TL, et al: AN-69 membrane reactions are pH-dependent and preventable, *Am J Kidney Dis,* 38:173-178, 2001.
46. Clark WR, Ronco C: CRRT efficiency and efficacy in relation to solute size, *Kidney Int Suppl,* 72:S3-S7, 1999.
47. Meier-Kriesche HU, Finkel KW, Gitomer JJ, et al: Unexpected severe hypocalcemia during continuous venovenous hemodialysis with regional citrate anticoagulation, *Am J Kidney Dis,* 33:e8, 1999.
48. Meier-Kriesche HU, Gitomer J, Finkel K, et al: Increased total to ionized calcium ratio during continuous venovenous hemodialysis with regional citrate anticoagulation, *Crit Care Med,* 29:748-752, 2001.
49. Maxvold NJ, Smoyer WE, Custer JR, et al: Amino acid loss and nitrogen balance in critically ill children with acute renal failure: a prospective comparison between classic hemofiltration and hemofiltration with dialysis, *Crit Care Med,* 28:1161-1165, 2000.

CHAPTER 66

Hypertension in the Pediatric Intensive Care Unit

Arno Zaritsky and Dale Whitby

PEARLS

- Hypertensive emergencies require immediate intervention to reduce the blood pressure to prevent progression of end-organ damage, whereas hypertensive urgencies are treated using an approach designed to control blood pressure over several hours.
- Elevated blood pressure may result from stimuli that increase cardiac output, systemic vascular resistance, or both. If systemic vascular resistance falls in concert with an increase in the cardiac output, blood pressure does not change.
- Although hypervolemia is a common cause of hypertensive urgencies or emergencies, pressure diuresis may render some patients relatively hypovolemic, producing hemoconcentration and further marked activation of the renin-angiotensin-aldosterone system. Further volume depletion may actually worsen hypertension by stimulating a further increase in systemic vascular resistance with the potential for organ ischemia.
- In clinical practice, mean arterial pressure of patients with critical hypertension should be lowered acutely by no more than 25%. Although the autoregulatory range may be restored toward normal after several hours, an acute decrease in pressure may result in a sudden fall in cerebral blood flow leading to cerebral ischemia.
- The goals of therapy should be based on duration of symptoms, baseline blood pressure, rapidity of onset and severity of hypertension, and concomitant clinical findings.
- Hypertension when present in children in the pediatric intensive care (PICU) is most often related to pain, agitation, positive fluid balance, drug effect, or occasionally unrecognized seizure. For patients with hypertension admitted to the PICU, renal causes are most frequent and may be clinically silent, such as renovascular hypertension.

This chapter addresses the diagnosis, pathophysiology, and management of hypertension as it applies to practice in the pediatric intensive care unit (PICU). Readers are referred to several comprehensive reviews for consideration of the causes and treatment of hypertension outside the critical care unit.[1–3]

Definitions of Terms

Updated age-appropriate norms for blood pressure[1] and guidelines for the diagnosis and treatment of urgent and emergent hypertension have been published.[1,4,5] The values associated with severe hypertension are given in

Table 66–1, but emergent hypertension is a clinical diagnosis that is not associated with specific systolic or diastolic values. Note that the upper range of normal blood pressure is based on the child's gender and height percentile in the updated blood pressure tables.[1]

In general, hypertensive crises are designated as hypertensive urgencies or hypertensive emergencies.[4–6] *Hypertensive urgencies* are characterized by markedly increased blood pressure but no evidence of end-organ damage. *Hypertensive emergencies* are defined as elevations of blood pressure resulting in hypertension-related end-organ damage. Organs most affected include the central nervous system (hypertensive encephalopathy, retinal vasculopathy-induced visual changes, cerebral infarction and hemorrhage); the cardiovascular system (congestive heart failure, myocardial ischemia, aortic dissection); and the kidneys, with an active urine sediment (proteinuria, pyuria, and hematuria) with or without acute renal insufficiency. Hypertensive emergencies require immediate intervention to reduce the blood pressure to prevent progression of end-organ damage, whereas hypertensive urgencies are treated using an approach designed to control blood pressure over several hours.

Accelerated hypertension and *malignant hypertension* were used frequently in the past to describe hypertension, where *accelerated hypertension* is characterized by retinopathy (exudates, hemorrhages, arteriolar narrowing, and spasm).[7] The previous four-stage Keith classification[8] was updated to three stages (Table 66–2) based on data showing that the previous categorization did not correlate with the severity of vasculopathy as assessed by fluorescein angiography.[7] *Malignant hypertension* is an antiquated term that refers to accelerated hypertension with the additional finding of papilledema. The term *malignant hypertension* adds little value to the clinician and is essentially the same as a hypertensive emergency; therefore some authors suggest the term *malignant hypertension* no longer be used.

TABLE 66–1

Hypertension by Age

	Boys		Girls	
Age (years)	Systolic BP (mmHg)	Diastolic BP (mmHg) Boys	Systolic BP (mmHg)	Diastolic BP (mmHg)
1	103	56	104	58
2	106	61	105	63
3	109	65	107	67
4	111	69	108	70
5	112	72	110	72
7	115	76	113	75
9	118	79	117	77
11	121	80	121	79
13	126	81	124	81
15	131	83	127	83
17	136	86	129	84

Based on the 50th percentile for height[1], where hypertension is defined as the 95th percentile for blood pressure.

TABLE 66–2

Classification of Hypertensive Retinopathy

Grade of Retinopathy	Retinal Signs	Systemic Associations*
None	No detectable signs	
Mild	Generalized arteriolar narrowing, focal arteriolar narrowing, arteriovenous nicking, opacity of arteriolar wall, or a combination of these signs	Modest association with risk of clinical stroke, subclinical stroke, coronary heart disease, and death
Moderate	Hemorrhage (blot, dot or flame shaped), micro-aneurysm, cotton-wool spot, hard exudates, or a combination of these signs	Strong association with risk of clinical stroke, subclinical stroke, cognitive decline, and death from cardiovascular causes
Malignant	Signs of moderate retinopathy plus swelling of the optic disk	Strong association with death

From Wong TY, Mitchell P: *N Engl J Med* 351:2310-2317, 2004.
*Systemic associations are referenced to identified risks in adults. Data in children are not available.

Measurement of Blood Pressure

The first step in identifying urgent hypertension is accurate determination of the blood pressure. The main techniques used to determine blood pressure in the intensive care unit (ICU) are the auscultatory method, Doppler method, oscillometric method, and invasive hemodynamic monitoring.

The *auscultatory method* is uncommonly used in many ICUs. It uses a blood pressure cuff to obstruct the artery. On deflation, turbulent flow develops and becomes laminar as deflation proceeds. These changes in flow and turbulence are appreciated as Korotkoff sounds when a stethoscope is placed over the vessel.[1,9] Phase I, the reappearance of sound with deflation, represents systole, and diastole is interpreted as phase IV (muffling) or phase V (disappearance) as the pressure in the bladder falls. The latter now is recommended as the diastolic blood pressure rather than phase IV.[1] Because this method depends on flow, it can be affected by arterial wall compliance. Meticulous technique is required to provide reproducible measures, and use of the bell of the stethoscope is recommended because it allows auscultation of softer sounds.[9–11] It is recommended that the cuff cover approximately 75% of the upper arm[1,2]; however, data suggest that the labels on blood pressure cuffs are often misleading and do not lead to selection of the correct size cuff.[12] If the cuff is too small, determinations will factitiously suggest elevated blood pressure.

Doppler devices use the apparent change in frequency of a reflected ultrasound pulse to infer the velocity of the target. The Doppler shift corresponds to the turbulent flow, appreciated as Korotkoff sounds, which diminishes when near-laminar flow predominates.[13] Reliability may be compromised if position is not maintained.[11] As with the auscultatory method, selection of appropriate cuff size for the extremity is crucial.

The *oscillometric method* is quite similar to manual sphygmomanometry in that it uses cuff inflation to occlude a vessel and then proceeds with stepped deflation. Small vibrations in the wall of the artery during the turbulent flow of systole are detected as oscillations in cuff pressure. The mean blood pressure is determined directly by the device, and proprietary algorithms are used to calculate the systolic and diastolic blood pressure, which can lead to discrepancies between oscillometric pressure measurements and those made by auscultation or invasive monitoring.[1] The mean blood pressure obtained by oscillometric devices correlates well with invasively measured blood pressure.[1]

Invasive catheters are fluid-filled tubes connected to a pressure transducer, a device consisting of a thin flexible diaphragm connected to a strain gauge and capable of converting the pressure transmitted to an electrical signal (see Chapter 38). The most common source of inaccuracy in this technique is the influence of electrical damping on reported blood pressure. An overdamped signal underestimates both systolic and diastolic blood pressures, but mean arterial pressure may be accurate. An underdamped system overestimates systolic blood pressure, especially with a hyperdynamic circulation, but does not change mean arterial blood pressure.[14] This often is recognized as a narrow peaked pressure wave and wide pulse pressure. Invasive blood pressure measured in the lower extremity is higher than in the upper extremities secondary to the physics of blood pressure wave transmission,[15] and systolic blood pressure increases the further the catheter is from the heart.[15]

Each technique has both strengths and weaknesses; the choice of technique must be determined within the context of the clinical situation, weighing the risks and benefits of invasive versus noninvasive methods. Doppler and oscillometric devices are more reliable in reporting systole than diastole. The mean blood pressure from an invasive arterial catheter is least altered by electrical damping artifact. When values are in doubt, confirmation of blood pressure by more than one technique is indicated before embarking on therapeutic interventions. In addition, four extremity blood pressures should be obtained to rule out a coarctation or other causes of aortic obstruction leading to isolated upper extremity hypertension.

Pathophysiology

Because of the prevalence of hypertension in adults and the resultant substantial morbidity and mortality, intensive investigation has expanded our understanding of the regulation of blood pressure, the causes of hypertension, and its consequences on various organ systems. The following discussion focuses on three aspects of pathophysiology especially relevant to hypertension in the critical care unit: (1) the kidney and its role in regulation of blood pressure, (2) the control of arterial vascular resistance, and (3) the regulation of cerebral vascular resistance.

Renal Regulation of Blood Pressure

The regulation of sodium and water balance is a central mechanism of blood pressure control. Abnormalities in this system are involved in many forms of hypertension[1,16] (see Chapter 62).

Hemodynamics of the Kidney

Regulation of sodium, the principal extracellular solute, controls extracellular fluid volume. As extracellular fluid volume increases, blood pressure increases, particularly if systemic vascular resistance simultaneously increases in response to angiotensin; sympathetic nervous system activation; and increased vasopressin release, which often accompanies renal dysfunction. In the normal kidney an increase in blood pressure increases renal excretion of sodium and water, which are respectively termed *pressure natriuresis* and *pressure diuresis*. With prolonged hypertension, extracellular fluid may be depleted, leading to a somewhat paradoxical state of hypertension and hypovolemia.

In addition to the hydrostatic effects of increased blood pressure on the glomerulus, a number of vasoactive substances may alter the glomerular filtration rate and renal blood flow by modulating resistances of the afferent and efferent arterioles, which affects the hydrostatic driving pressure at the glomerulus.

Renin

Renin converts angiotensinogen to angiotensin I, which is converted to angiotensin II leading to renin's action. Renin is synthesized in the juxtaglomerular apparatus in response to hemodynamic, hormonal, and biochemical signals. Renin synthesis and release is stimulated by sodium depletion, decreased perfusion pressure, sympathetic nerve stimulation, and β-adrenergic agonists. Conversely, sodium excess, increased perfusion pressure, with resultant stretching of afferent arterioles, central sympathetic nervous system depressants, and β-adrenergic antagonists inhibit renin release.

Angiotensin-Converting Enzyme

Angiotensin-converting enzyme (ACE) is a widely distributed enzyme whose principal effect is the conversion of angiotensin I to the potent vasoconstrictor angiotensin II.[17] ACE also inactivates the vasodilator bradykinin, providing a two-pronged mechanism to increase blood pressure.

Angiotensin II and Aldosterone

Angiotensin II production and plasma concentration vary in reciprocal fashion to sodium intake in normal individuals. Thus increased sodium intake leads to a fall in angiotensin II concentration, and decreased sodium intake is followed by an increase in angiotensin II concentration. Angiotensin II is a potent vasoconstrictor and indirectly increases vascular tone by stimulating norepinephrine release from sympathetic nerves.[18] In addition, through angiotensin receptors, angiotensin II stimulates the production and release of aldosterone, renal reabsorption of sodium, cardiac cellular growth, proliferation of vascular smooth muscle, central activation of the sympathetic nervous system, stimulation of vasopressin release, and inhibition of renin release from the kidney.[19] The increased aldosterone production and release in turn increases tissue sensitivity to angiotensin. Aldosterone is synthesized from cholesterol in the adrenal cortex and promotes renal sodium reabsorption, principally in the cortical collecting tubule, and renal secretion of potassium in exchange for reabsorption of filtered sodium. A pathologic excess of renin, aldosterone, or both substances can culminate in a vicious cycle of impaired renal perfusion and resultant further increase in renin and thus angiotensin II production.

Focal impairment of renal blood flow with release of renin and subsequent increase in circulating angiotensin II underlie many types of childhood hypertension.[20] Thromboembolic phenomena from umbilical or central vascular catheters may impair renal perfusion,[20,21] and coarctation of the aorta is associated with high peripheral renin activity.[22] In children, hyperreninemia usually is associated with identifiable renal lesions,[21,22] but hypertension also can occur with normal or low renin activities.[21]

As a corollary of Ohm's Law (Q = P/R), mean blood pressure is determined by cardiac output and systemic vascular resistance, as seen in Equation 1:

$$\text{Blood pressure} = \text{Cardiac output} \times \text{Systemic vascular resistance} \quad (1).$$

Thus elevated blood pressure may result from stimuli that increase cardiac output, systemic vascular resistance, or both. If systemic vascular resistance falls in concert with an increase in the cardiac output, blood pressure does not change. A common cause of increased cardiac output is activation of the sympathetic nervous system, often in concert with an increase in intravascular volume. At the same time, sympathetic nervous system activation further increases systemic vascular resistance, exacerbating the rise in blood pressure. Equation 1 also illustrates why the therapeutic approach to hypertension depends on reducing systemic vascular resistance and often suppressing or reducing sympathetic nervous system activation. Without the latter being suppressed, the drop in systemic vascular resistance mediated by a vasodilator may be compensated by an increase in sympathetic activation with a resultant increase in cardiac output and no net reduction in blood pressure.

An acute increase in intravascular volume is a frequent cause of acute decompensation of blood pressure control in a patient with chronic hypertension, particularly in the setting of stimuli that increase sympathetic nervous system and/or renin-angiotensin-aldosterone system activation. Although hypervolemia is a common cause of hypertensive urgencies or emergencies, pressure diuresis may render some patients relatively hypovolemic, producing hemoconcentration and further marked activation of the renin-angiotensin-aldosterone system.[23] Further volume depletion may actually worsen hypertension by stimulating a further increase in systemic vascular resistance with the potential for organ ischemia. Thus diuretics and fluid restriction are not standard therapy for patients who present in hypertensive crisis; they are reserved for those patients with clinically apparent fluid overload.[5,6,23]

Two other mediators, arginine vasopressin and natriuretic peptides (atrial and B-type), participate in regulation of volume status and vascular reactivity, but their role in the pathogenesis of hypertension is not well defined, and no therapeutic interventions specifically target these mediators for treatment of hypertension. Arginine vasopressin, released by the posterior pituitary as a result of increased plasma osmolarity, stimulates renal water reabsorption. Volume expansion produces stretching of the atria releasing atrial natriuretic peptide and the ventricle releasing B-type natriuretic peptide. Both natriuretic peptides suppress renin secretion by increasing cyclic guanosine 3′,5′-monophosphate (cGMP) in the juxtaglomerular cells, increase sodium excretion by blocking renal tubular sodium reabsorption, and increase renal blood flow.[24,25] Natriuretic peptides also dilate vessels preconstricted by other vasoactive agents, such as norepinephrine, angiotensin II, and arginine vasopressin, and appear to have complex effects on stimulating changes in vascular smooth muscle.[24,25]

Multiple interrelated mediators arising in the kidney or related to renal regulation of salt and water balance contribute to maintenance of blood pressure. Nonrenal regulation of arterial resistance is also an integral part of blood pressure homeostasis.

Nonrenal Effectors of Arterial Vascular Resistance

Nitric oxide, now recognized as a ubiquitous biologic effector,[26–28] is a labile, short-lived gas produced from arginine through nitric oxide synthases. These synthases are distinguished by cellular distribution and by the requirement for calcium as a cofactor. The constitutive isoform of nitric oxide synthase is believed most responsible for basal vasomotor tone, although inducible nitric oxide synthase may have a role. Nitric oxide is released continuously from arteries and arterioles but not veins. In addition, other mediators function through the nitric oxide system. For instance, bradykinin stimulates the release of nitric oxide to produce vasodilation. Nitric oxide diffuses from the endothelium to the vascular smooth muscle cell, where it produces its vasodilatory effect in part by increasing the intracellular concentration of cGMP through stimulation of soluble guanylyl cyclase. Nitric oxide that diffuses from the local endothelial environment is rapidly bound by hemoglobin, forming nitrosohemoglobin and then methemoglobin. This affinity for the heme moiety explains the formation of cGMP, as soluble guanylyl cyclase has a heme moiety, as does nitric oxide synthase, allowing for negative feedback of nitric oxide production. Thus hypertension need not be attributed only to a direct vasoconstrictor effect but also may be related to loss of basal nitric oxide vasodilation. Therapeutic agents, such as sodium nitroprusside and nitroglycerin, produce their systemic vasodilator action by stimulating nitric oxide production (see management).

Endothelin-1 (ET-1) is a pleiotropic 21-amino-acid peptide hormone with potent biologic activity produced primarily by the endothelium. Synthesis of ET-1 is stimulated by the major signals of cardiovascular stress, such as vasoactive agents (e.g., angiotensin II, norepinephrine, vasopressin, and bradykinin), cytokines (e.g., tumor necrosis factor-α and transforming growth factor-β), and other factors, including thrombin and mechanical stress. Endothelin is a potent vasoconstrictor, is proinflammatory, promotes fibrosis, and has mitogenic potential, important factors in the regulation of vascular tone, arterial remodeling, and vascular injury.[29,30] These effects are mediated via two receptor types, ETA and ETB. Inhibition of these receptors may provide new therapeutic interventions for treatment of hypertension.[29]

Autoregulation of Cerebral Blood Flow

Cerebral autoregulation is the process by which cerebral blood flow is maintained at a stable level over a wide range in blood pressure.[31] If blood pressure rises to levels beyond the autoregulatory range, particularly if the rise in blood pressure is rapid, cerebral blood flow and hydrostatic capillary pressure may rise suddenly, leading to cerebral edema and neuronal injury (see Chapter 52). Fortunately, hypertensive encephalopathy appears to be relatively uncommon in children.[32,33]

When blood pressure decreases, cerebral vessels dilate to maintain cerebral blood flow until they become maximally dilated. Further reduction in blood pressure decreases cerebral blood flow. Similarly, cerebral vessels constrict in the context of rising blood pressure until maximum vasoconstriction is attained. Note that Equation 1 can be rearranged to Cardiac output = Blood flow = Mean blood pressure ÷ Systemic vascular resistance; thus blood flow is constant as long as the rise in perfusion pressure is matched by a proportional rise in systemic vascular resistance. At high blood pressures that exceed the autoregulatory range, cerebral vessels dilate, with a resultant increase in cerebral blood flow.[31] The high flow and perfusion pressure injure the microcirculation, leading to endothelial injury with breakdown of the blood-brain barrier, plasma exudation, and cerebral edema. Pathologic findings following severe hypertensive encephalopathy include cerebral microinfarctions, petechial hemorrhages, fibrinoid necrosis of cerebral arterioles, and cerebral edema.

Cerebral blood flow is generally reported to be 50 ml/min/100 g of brain across a mean arterial pressure range of approximately 50 to 70 mmHg at the low end to 120 or perhaps even 170 mmHg.[23,31] With chronic hypertension this curve shifts to the right, in that autoregulation may fail below a mean arterial pressure of 110 mmHg.[23,31] The lower limit of autoregulation usually is 25% below the prevailing mean arterial blood pressure.[23,31] Similarly, the upper limit of autoregulation is considered to be 30% to 40% above the basal mean arterial pressure.[34] Thus in clinical practice, mean arterial pressure in patients with critical hypertension should be lowered acutely by no more than 25%.[4–6,23] The other reason to lower pressure slowly is that the autoregulation range shifts to the right when pressure is chronically elevated. Although the autoregulatory range may be restored toward normal after several hours, an acute decrease in pressure may result in a sudden fall in cerebral blood flow, leading to cerebral ischemia.

Numerous mechanisms may influence cerebral vascular tone.[31,34] The myogenic hypothesis holds that the smooth muscle of the cerebral arteries and arterioles changes tone reflexly, as evidenced by the near-immediate response to changes in blood pressure. Proponents of the metabolic hypothesis point to the proportionality between cerebral blood flow and cortical metabolic activity. The neurogenic hypothesis implicates the sympathetic nervous system as the primary arbiter of cerebral vascular tone. This last hypothesis is supported by the exaggerated diminution in cerebral blood flow when hemorrhage occurs with an intact sympathetic nervous system compared with hemorrhage after sympathectomy and by the presence of adrenergic receptors on cerebral vessels.[31,34]

There are other modulators of cerebral blood flow. Intracranial pressure markedly affects blood flow; initially increased intracranial pressure is matched by increased blood pressure, maintaining cerebral blood flow. An increase in hematocrit, perhaps by increasing blood viscosity, lowers blood pressure. Cerebral blood flow is inversely related to arterial oxygen saturation and directly related to arterial carbon dioxide content.[23,31,34] The importance of blood viscosity, oxygen saturation, and carbon dioxide content on cerebral blood flow may increase in patients in whom cerebral autoregulation is altered by hypertension.

At least two theories have been articulated for the failure of autoregulation at extremes of blood pressure.[6,23,31,34,35] Exaggerated vasoconstriction may lead to cerebral ischemia at very high systemic blood pressures.[36] Alternatively, hypertensive encephalopathy may represent a sudden breakthrough in blood flow.[6,23,34,35] The breakthrough theory is supported by data demonstrating pressure-forced vasodilation at blood pressures greater than the upper limit of autoregulation and by magnetic resonance imaging diffusion-weighted imaging consistent with vasogenic rather than cytotoxic edema.[33–35] The latter would be expected if intensive vasoconstriction caused ischemic brain injury. As described by the breakthrough theory, severe hypertension can produce increased cerebral blood flow when blood pressure exceeds the upper limit of autoregulation. Blood-brain barrier disruption with edema and extravasation of plasma proteins may accompany regional or global increased cerebral blood flow.[23,34,37] This cerebral edema may produce secondary ischemia. The clinical findings of headache, nausea, vomiting, and neurologic deterioration reflect these intracranial events.

Evaluation

Primary (also called *essential)* hypertension is unusual in the PICU, although the frequency is increasing with the current epidemic of obesity.[1] In children, hypertension is more often secondary to other conditions. Although identification of the cause of hypertension is important to determining eventual therapy, initial therapy for a hypertensive emergency or urgency typically focuses on symptomatic treatment of the elevated blood pressure. A thorough history, targeted physical examination, and a few diagnostic tests identify patients with severe hypertension requiring emergent therapy. The initial examination should focus on signs of injury of the cardiovascular, neurologic, renal, and ocular systems.

In the critical care unit, inadequately treated pain and agitation probably are the most common causes of elevated blood pressure values, particularly systolic hypertension. Without a high degree of suspicion, this circumstance may be difficult to detect, particularly if neuromuscular blockade is also administered. Concurrent tachycardia is a useful clue to this condition, as is tearing of the eye with noxious interventions. Inadequate sedation and analgesia in concert with pharmacologic paralysis is an underrecognized problem in clinical practice.

The combination of hypertension and tachycardia may occur in occult seizures. Diagnosis of this entity is difficult if the patient is receiving a muscle relaxant. An electroencephalogram may be the only way to make the diagnosis.

Hypertension secondary to drug effect is common, especially when high-dose corticosteroids are administered for conditions such as organ transplant rejection or immunologic disorders. Other drugs associated with increased blood pressure include ethanol, nicotine, caffeine, theophylline, nonsteroidal antiinflammatory drugs, decongestants, atropine, and antihistamines.[38] Sympathomimetics may be implicated, including dopamine and dobutamine, as well as other stimulants such as ephedrine, terbutaline, phenylephrine, agents used for treatment of ADHD, and illicit agents such as cocaine and methamphetamine.[38] Over-the-counter drugs may include ephedrine, caffeine, pseudoephedrine, or combinations of these agents. Many of the over-the-counter weight loss products and energy-enhancing products contain medications that can increase blood pressure. Early in the evaluation of hypertension in the ICU, the complete medication list for the patient should be scrutinized for any agents that may produce elevated blood pressure (see Chapter 99).

The patient's fluid balance for the past several days should be reviewed. Apparently innocuous discrepancies between input and output when noted for a single day may cumulatively produce significant fluid overload after several days. As noted previously, fluid retention alone usually does not cause hypertension in the absence of other renal, cardiovascular, or central nervous system problems that raise systemic vascular resistance, cardiac output, or both.

Figure 66–1 shows an algorithm for evaluating and directing the treatment of hypertension. The signs and symptoms resulting from hypertension often reflect the rapidity of onset, underlying cause, and concurrent organ dysfunction. General symptoms include generalized weakness, malaise, and fatigue. Cardiac symptoms are uncommon but may include acute heart failure with pulmonary edema secondary to acute left ventricular failure. Rarely pediatric patients present solely with abdominal symptoms, such as abdominal pain or vomiting.[39] Neurologic symptoms often are the presenting complaint in hypertensive emergencies. Symptoms include headache, dizziness, confusion, nausea, vomiting, and visual complaints such as blurred vision or cortical blindness.[4–6,23,40] With more severe involvement, there may be focal ischemic symptoms and focal or generalized seizures.

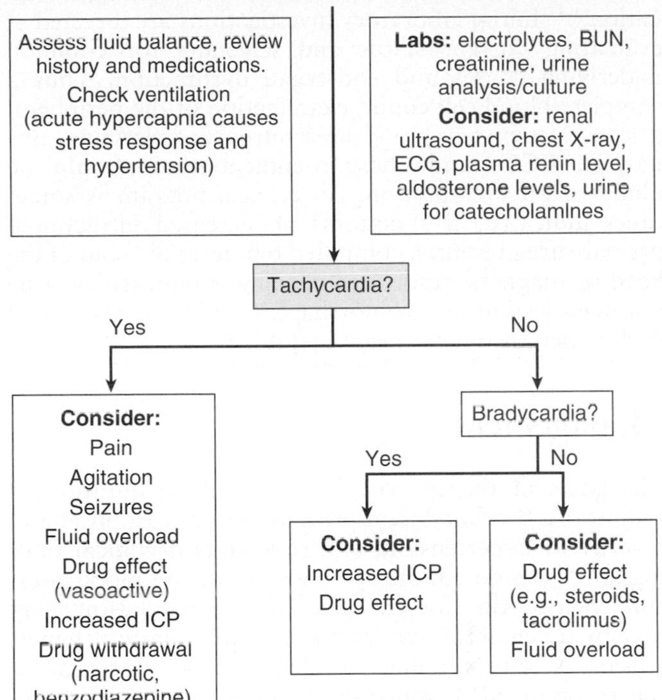

FIGURE 66–1 • Evaluation of hypertension in the pediatric intensive care unit. *BUN*, Blood urea nitrogen; *ECG*, electrocardiogram; *ICP*, intracranial pressure.

Evidence can be obtained from physical examination and laboratory studies of other organ involvement, including chest x-ray film showing signs of congestive heart failure (e.g., pulmonary edema, cardiomegaly), proteinuria, hematuria, renal casts, azotemia, and microangiopathic anemia or anemia consistent with chronic disease. Microangiopathic hemolytic anemia is secondary to diffuse endothelial cell injury with disseminated activation of the coagulation system. Hypokalemic metabolic alkalosis may develop secondary to volume depletion and secondary hyperaldosteronism.

Any aspect of the history or physical examination may reveal the cause of hypertension in a previously normotensive individual. Relevant historic information includes family history for cardiovascular and renal disease and tumors with familial predisposition, such as pheochromocytoma.[1] The medical history should include a review of the perinatal course (including use of umbilical catheters in the neonatal period), growth failure or weight loss, complete description of initial symptoms, history of altered sympathetic tone (pallor, flushing, sweating, palpitations), dysuria, nocturia, and use of licit and illicit drugs.[1] The physical examination should include blood pressure measurements in all extremities; evaluation for cutaneous lesions; a search for evidence of endocrine dysfunction; eye ground examination; complete cardiovascular examination including quality of distal pulses, cardiac examination, and search for bruits; abdominal examination for masses; and neurologic evaluation.[1,41] Initial laboratory investigations are directed at evaluating current status and screening for common underlying causes and end-organ dysfunction. Thus a complete blood cell count, examination of the peripheral smear, electrolytes, blood urea nitrogen, creatinine, urinalysis, ECG, and chest roentgenogram should be obtained on presentation. An echocardiogram is sometimes indicated. If symptoms of increased intracranial pressure are present, a computed tomographic scan of the head or magnetic resonance imaging is indicated to rule out mass lesions and hemorrhage. Conditions associated with hypertension are listed in Table 66–3.

TABLE 66–3

Causes of Hypertension in Children
RENAL
Glomerulonephritis, acute or chronic
Hemolytic-uremic syndrome
Henoch-Schönlein purpura
Acute renal failure
Obstructive uropathy
Congenital defects (polycystic kidneys, multicystic kidneys)
Renovascular disease
Perirenal masses
Renal tumors (Wilms disease)
Collagen vascular disease
Trauma
CARDIOVASCULAR AND HEMATOLOGIC
Polycythemia
Anemia
Coarctation of the aorta
Hypoplasia of abdominal aorta
Patent ductus arteriosus (systolic hypertension only)
ENDOCRINE AND METABOLIC
Pheochromocytoma
Congenital adrenal hyperplasia
Hyperthyroidism
17-Hydroxylase deficiency syndrome
Hyperaldosteronism
Neuroblastoma
Cushing disease
Hyperparathyroidism
Acute intermittent porphyria
Hypercalcemia
NEUROLOGIC
Space-occupying central nervous system lesion
Increased intracranial pressure
Dysautonomia (Riley-Day syndrome)
Guillain-Barré syndrome
Catecholamine excess from spinal cord disease
DRUG INGESTION AND ABUSE
Sympathomimetics (amphetamines, ephedrine, phenylephrine eyedrops, lysergic acid diethylamide [LSD], cocaine)
Glucocorticoids and mineralocorticoids
Heavy metals
Birth control pills
Rebound after withdrawal of antihypertensive agents (especially clonidine and beta-blockers)
Nonsteroidal antiinflammatory agents
Ergot alkaloids
Ingestion of tyramine in conjunction with a monoamine oxidase inhibitor
Cyclosporine and tacrolimus
MISCELLANEOUS
Burns
Stevens-Johnson syndrome
Preeclampsia, eclampsia
Orthopedic injuries and procedures
Essential hypertension

Management

The goals of therapy should be based on duration of symptoms, baseline blood pressure, rapidity of onset and severity of hypertension, and concomitant clinical findings.[5,23,41] As noted, abrupt lowering of the blood pressure below the lower limit of autoregulation may precipitate cerebral hypoperfusion, particularly if hypertension is long-standing. For hypertensive emergencies, the recommended approach is use of agents that can be titrated readily to achieve the desired endpoint of decreasing the mean arterial pressure by not more than 20% to 25% or decreasing the diastolic pressure to 100 to 110 mmHg, whichever is higher, over 2 to 3 hours.[5,6,23,41] Because some patients presenting with hypertensive emergencies are volume depleted, as has been discussed, initial therapy generally uses antihypertensive agents as opposed to diuretics and fluid restriction. To properly titrate intravenous agents and avoid toxicity in patients with a hypertensive emergency, blood pressure should be monitored invasively because cuff pressures may not be reliable as previously noted. In some patients with signs of volume overload, particularly in the child with renal failure, acute hemodialysis with fluid removal often is helpful in restoring baseline blood pressure. After the hypertensive emergency has been addressed, institution of chronic therapy with appropriate agents should begin based on the etiology of the child's hypertension.

Specific Agents

Table 66–4 lists the characteristics of specific antihypertensive agents. Table 66–5 lists agents based on the etiology of hypertension. The indications, pharmacology, adverse effects, and dosage are reviewed for the agents commonly used to treat hypertensive emergencies and urgencies in children.

Vasodilators

Sodium nitroprusside was the drug of choice for hypertensive emergencies for many years because it has a rapid onset and short (<5 minute) duration of action. Unfortunately, it also has a slowly excreted metabolite (thiocyanate) that accumulates in renal failure, and its

TABLE 66–4

Antihypertensive Agents

Drug	Mechanism	Dose	Route	Comments
Captopril	ACE inhibitor	Infants: 0.1–0.5 mg/kg/dose Child: 0.3–0.5 mg/kg/dose	Oral every 6–12 hours	Contraindicated if obstruction to renal blood flow Monitor potassium (hyperkalemia risk) Cough and angioedema
Clonidine	Central α_2-adrenergic agonist	3–10 μg/kg/dose up to 25 μg/kg/day	Oral every 6–8 hours	Caution if altered mentation Frequently causes sedation
Diazoxide	Direct vasodilator	1–3 mg/kg (maximum 150 mg)	IV infusion; may repeat in 5–15 min	Hypotension and reflex tachycardia Hyperglycemia (inhibits insulin release)
Enalapril/ enalaprilat	ACE inhibitor	Enalapril: 0.1–0.5 mg/kg/day Enalaprilat: 5–10 μg/kg/dose	Oral: Every 12 hours IV: repeat q6–8h as needed	Same as captopril, except cough and angioedema are rare
Esmolol	Selective β_1-adrenergic blocker	500 μg/kg bolus followed by infusion of 50–250 μg/kg/min	IV bolus and infusion	Avoid in patients with asthma, chronic obstructive pulmonary disease, bradycardia, and heart failure May cause profound bradycardia
Fenoldopam	Dopamine receptor agonist	0.2–0.8 μg/kg/min	IV infusion	Increases renal perfusion and urine output
Hydralazine	Direct vasodilator	0.2–0.6 mg/kg/dose (maximum initial dose 20 mg)	IV, IM	Give every 4 hours by IV bolus Associated with lupus-like reaction in slow acetylators Reflex tachycardia and fluid retention common
Labetalol	Combined β- and α-adrenergic receptor blocker (7:1 relative potency for β- over α-antagonism)	0.2–1 mg/kg bolus (up to 40-mg initial dose); repeat 0.15 mg/kg q5–15 min Infusion of 0.25–3 mg/kg/hour	IV bolus or infusion	Contraindicated in asthma and overt heart failure May cause infusion-limiting bradycardia
Nicardipine	Inhibition of L-type calcium channels	0.5–5 μg/kg/min; increase by 0.5 μg/kg/min every 10–15 min as needed	IV infusion	May cause reflex tachycardia. Should be infused centrally (high rate of phlebitis peripherally)
Nifedipine	Inhibition of L-type calcium channels	0.25 mg/kg (maximum dose 10 mg)	Oral or feeding tube (not sublingual)	May cause significant fall in blood pressure
Nitroprusside	Stimulation of NO in both arterial and venous circulation	0.5–8 μg/kg/min	Intravenous infusion	Reflex tachycardia occurs frequently Monitor cyanide levels (or lactate) Consider coadministration of sodium thiosulfate
Nitroglycerin	Relatively selective NO stimulation in veins	0.5–5 μg/kg/min	Intravenous infusion	No active metabolite but relatively weak arterial dilator
Phentolamine	Nonselective α-adrenergic receptor blocker	0.05–0.1 mg/kg IV bolus 5–15 mg in adults	IV bolus	Used for pheochromocytoma
Trimethaphan camsylate	Blocks acetylcholine in both sympathetic and cholinergic ganglia reducing sympathetic activity; also a peripheral vasodilator	50–150 μg/kg/min	IV infusion	Reflex tachycardia May cause weakness and apnea with high doses

Agents are listed alphabetically and compiled from several sources.[1,41,53,60,91]
ACE = angiotensin-converting enzyme; *IM* = intramuscular; *IV* = intravenous.

TABLE 66–5

Drug Selection Based on Etiology of Hypertensive Emergency/Urgency

Type of Emergency	Drugs of Choice	Alternate Second Line	Relative Contraindications
Hypertensive encephalopathy	Nicardipine Nitroprusside	Labetalol	Trimethaphan, clonidine
Intracranial hemorrhage	Labetalol Nicardipine	Nitroprusside	Vasodilators with reflex sympathetic stimulation (e.g., hydralazine, diazoxide, short-acting nifedipine)
Left ventricular failure and pulmonary edema	Nitroprusside ± loop diuretics ± ACE inhibitor	Nitroglycerin, fenoldopam	Labetalol, β-adrenergic blockers, verapamil
Adrenergic crisis	Nitroprusside ± beta-blockers, phentolamine Clonidine (if centrally mediated hypertension such as narcotic withdrawal)	Labetalol	Monotherapy with beta-blockers Contraindicated with cocaine-induced hypertension
Dissecting aortic aneurysm	Beta-blockers ± nitroprusside, trimethaphan	Labetalol, verapamil	Vasodilators with reflex sympathetic stimulation
Eclampsia	Hydralazine, labetalol Nicardipine	Nifedipine	ACE inhibitor, nitroprusside
HYPERTENSIVE URGENCIES			
Acute renal failure	Labetalol, minoxidil ± beta-blocker	ACE inhibitor, diuretics, or hemofiltration (if volume overloaded)	Nitroprusside (to limit risk of thiocyanate toxicity)
Perioperative hypertension (if not a result of pain, agitation)	Nitroglycerin, nitroprusside ± beta-blocker Enalaprilat or nicardipine for coarctation of aorta	Labetalol, nicardipine, fenoldopam	

*Modified from several sources.[40,92]
ACE = angiotensin-converting enzyme.

desired pharmacologic action often is antagonized to some extent by reflex stimulation of the sympathetic nervous system and renin-angiotensin-aldosterone system. Sodium nitroprusside stimulates nitric oxide production in vascular smooth muscle, resulting in a balanced reduction of venous and arteriolar vascular tone. Cardiac output is generally maintained, provided intravascular volume is adequate. By relaxing both arteriolar and venous smooth muscle, renal blood flow and glomerular filtration rate are maintained while renin release increases.[42] Often heart rate and cardiac contractility increase secondary to increased sympathetic stimulation. Nitroprusside may be used for treatment of hypertensive encephalopathy, but there is concern that it may increase intracranial pressure secondary to cerebral vasodilation. In addition, safer agents, such as nicardipine or labetalol, are more commonly used to treat hypertensive encephalopathy.[6,23]

In addition to reflex tachycardia, fluid retention may occur secondary to peripheral venodilation, and oxygenation may worsen, especially in patients with parenchymal lung disease secondary to loss of hypoxic pulmonary vasoconstriction. Nitroprusside is contraindicated in eclampsia because of the risk of fetal cyanide toxicity.

Nitroprusside nonenzymatically reacts with hemoglobin to form cyanide and methemoglobin. The half-life of cyanide is 20 to 60 minutes.[43,44] It usually is converted to thiocyanate by the enzyme rhodanese (E.C. 2.8.1.1) (thiosulfate:cyanide sulfur transferase). Thiocyanate is renally excreted, with a half-life of 3 days in healthy patients and 9 days in patients with renal failure.[43,44] Thus thiocyanate toxicity is a concern in children with renal impairment. In patients with normal renal function, thiocyanate toxicity is associated with longer-term use; thiocyanate levels may require monitoring if doses exceeding 70 mg/kg have been given (corresponding to a dose of 5 μg/kg/min for almost 10 days) or if there is concurrent renal insufficiency. Thiocyanate toxicity is characterized by tinnitus, blurred vision, confusion, psychotic behavior, nausea, abdominal pain, hyperreflexia, and seizures.[43] Thiocyanate also inhibits iodine uptake by the thyroid and may produce hypothyroidism.

Because the liver is the major source of rhodanese, patients with liver failure may develop signs and symptoms of cyanide intoxication upon nitroprusside administration. Early signs of cyanide toxicity include metabolic acidosis, hyperpnea, giddiness, confusion, palpitations, and headache, followed by vomiting, bradycardia, hypotension, coma, convulsions, and apnea.[44,45] Because the rate-limiting step of cyanide detoxification to thiocyanate usually is the need for a sulfur donor, coadministration of sodium thiosulfate as a sulfur donor increases the rate of reaction of rhodanese, removing cyanide from circulation so that it no longer binds to cytochrome *c*. A solution of 0.1%

sodium nitroprusside and 1% sodium thiosulfate, or a 1:10 ratio by weight, in light-protected tubing is given according to the usual dosing guidelines for sodium nitroprusside.[43–45] Alternatively, hydroxocobalamin (vitamin B_{12a}) can be used to trap the cyanide ion by forming cyanocobalamin.[46] Of note, intravenous methylene blue is contraindicated in treating methemoglobinemia attributable to cyanide toxicity because the conversion of methemoglobin to hemoglobin may liberate large amounts of cyanide.[46] Because of its potential toxicity, sodium nitroprusside is not appropriate for chronic therapy. It may be used for short-term blood pressure control, but its use is clearly falling out of favor.

Diazoxide is a direct selective arterial vasodilator. Pure arterial vasodilation often is associated with marked reflexive increases in heart rate, cardiac output, rate of pressure change (dp/dt, a marker of increased contractility), and shear stress in the aorta. Thus diazoxide is contraindicated in left ventricular failure and aortic dissection.[47] Severe hyperglycemia and fluid retention have been described following administration.[48] Rapid bolus administration of a large dose previously was recommended to overcome protein binding of the drug, but this may produce precipitous hypotension and tissue ischemia.[41,49] Although a continuous infusion has been used,[40] it is difficult to titrate drug effect and overshoot may occur; therefore this agent is no longer recommended for hypertensive emergencies or urgencies.[50]

Hydralazine causes direct arteriolar smooth muscle relaxation through mechanisms that increase the intracellular concentration of cGMP, although this is not consistently observed.[51] It is less potent than diazoxide and has a more variable effect.[40] Like diazoxide, hydralazine may cause reflex tachycardia, increased cardiac output and stroke work, and increased dp/dt. Thus it may worsen left ventricular failure and is contraindicated in the presence of aortic aneurysm or dissection. Following an intramuscular or intravenous dose, there is an initial latent period of 5 to 15 minutes, followed by a progressive (often precipitous) fall in blood pressure that lasts for up to 12 hours. Although the circulating half-life of the drug is approximately 3 hours, the half-time of its effect on blood pressure is variable and ranges from 3 to 100 hours. Hydralazine binds to the walls of muscular arteries, which may explain the drug's prolonged pharmacologic effect. Although it was used commonly in the past,[41] hydralazine should not be used in the management of hypertensive emergencies because of its prolonged and unpredictable antihypertensive effects and the inability to effectively titrate its hypotensive effect. Hydralazine is metabolized by acetylation in the liver, and there is genetic variability in the efficiency of this process.[52]

Ganglionic Blockers

Trimethaphan camsylate blocks both cholinergic and adrenergic ganglia, decreasing sympathetic nervous system effects on the peripheral vascular bed. Unlike other vasodilators, this action inhibits reflex activation of heart rate and contractility and may be useful in settings where β-adrenergic blockers are contraindicated, such as patients with asthma, severe chronic lung disease, bradycardia, and heart failure. Because trimethaphan decreases blood pressure without increasing cerebral blood flow, it may be useful when increased intracranial pressure is problematic. With an onset in 1 to 2 minutes and duration of approximately 10 minutes, this agent must be given by continuous infusion. Tachyphylaxis may develop within 48 hours.[40] Use of trimethaphan can lead to ileus and bladder atony, and trimethaphan is contraindicated in eclampsia because of an increased risk of meconium ileus.[47]

Drugs Affecting the Adrenergic Nervous System

β-Adrenergic antagonists differ in terms of cardioselectivity, lipid solubility, potency, half-life, and metabolism.[53] Beta-blockers without intrinsic sympathomimetic activity or concurrent α-blocking characteristics cause increased systemic vascular resistance by inhibition of β_2-adrenergic receptors, decreased cardiac output mediated by β_1-adrenergic blockade, and reduced renal blood flow and glomerular filtration rate[1,41,53]; thus they are not indicated as first-line therapy for most hypertensive emergencies. An exception is hypertension related to coarctation of the aorta, where control has been achieved with beta-blockade, often combined with a vasodilator.[54] Use of nonselective β-adrenergic antagonists, such as propranolol, is not recommended because β_2-adrenergic receptors mediate bronchial dilation, vascular smooth muscle relaxation, and suppression of renin secretion.

Esmolol is a selective β_1-receptor blocker with a short half-life in children (1.5–5 minutes)[55,56] and therefore is most easily titratable. Following intravenous administration by bolus and constant infusion, the onset of action is within 60 seconds, with rapid clearance by esterases located in red blood cell membranes. The half-life is approximately 5 minutes, but the duration of effect is 10 to 30 minutes. Esmolol has been used alone and in combination with vasodilator agents to treat postoperative hypertension in children.[41,54]

Labetalol blocks both β-adrenergic and α-adrenergic receptors, although its β-adrenergic blockade effect is approximately seven times more potent.[57–59] This results in a reduction of systemic vascular resistance and relative inhibition of the reflex tachycardia and contractility seen with nonselective vasodilators.[58] The onset of action occurs within 2 to 5 minutes following an intravenous bolus dose, with peak effect at 5 to 15 minutes.[40,57,59] Labetalol can be given by bolus or infusion and can be used in many types of hypertensive emergency. The duration of action is approximately 2 to 4 hours in most patients; therefore repeat doses are often required. As long as small bolus doses are given, acute changes in blood pressure likely will not occur. An oral form exists for long-term therapy after the hypertensive emergency is addressed. Labetalol is effective in treating hypertension attributable to pheochromocytoma and may be used safely during pregnancy.[40,59,60] Like other β-adrenergic blockers, labetalol may induce significant hyperkalemia in patients with renal failure and existing high potassium concentrations.[61]

Phentolamine and phenoxybenzamine are direct α_2-adrenergic receptor antagonists. These agents are best used for disorders characterized by excessive catecholamine activity, such as pheochromocytoma.[40,62] Intravenous phentolamine has an onset of action of 1 to 2 minutes and duration of 3 to 10 minutes following bolus administration and thus is given by infusion. Because it has no β-adrenergic blocker activity, reflex tachycardia and increased contractility may occur. Phenoxybenzamine is an oral agent for more long-term blood pressure control and is often used preoperatively in patients with pheochromocytoma.[62]

Clonidine binds to central α_2 and imidazole receptors, resulting in suppression of sympathetic outflow.[53,63] Clonidine is available as a patch, oral formulation, or injection for epidural use; dexmedetomidine is an intravenous α_2-adrenergic agonist used for short-term sedation, but there is little experience with its use for hypertensive emergencies.[64] Like clonidine, dexmedetomidine may stimulate peripheral α_2-adrenergic receptors resulting initially in increased vascular tone followed by a fall in blood pressure and heart rate.[64] Diuresis and natriuresis result from the central effect of α_2-adrenergic agonists.[63] Oral clonidine has an onset of action of 30 to 60 minutes and a duration of action of 8 to 24 hours and therefore is not indicated for acute blood pressure reduction. It has been used for treatment of hypertensive urgencies.[6,40]

Fenoldopam is a selective dopamine agonist that acts at the D-1 receptor.[65,66] D-1 stimulation increases intracellular cAMP through G protein-coupled activation of adenylate cyclase. The latter leads to a decrease in intracellular calcium concentration and thus relaxation of vascular smooth muscle tone. D-1 receptors are most prominently located in the splanchnic and renal vascular beds, with a reduced density in the coronary and cerebral circulations. Thus agonist stimulation of these receptors reduces vascular resistance and increases splanchnic and renal blood flow.[66] D-1 receptors are also located on renal tubular cells, which when activated inhibit sodium reabsorption. The net renal effect of fenoldopam is significant enhancement of renal perfusion and sodium excretion.

Fenoldopam was approved by the U.S. Food and Drug Administration in 1997 for short-term (<48 hour) treatment of hypertensive emergencies. Additional labeling approving its use in children was issued in mid-2004. Because of receptor down-regulation, the effect of fenoldopam is reduced when the infusion is extended beyond 48 hours. The drug has a short half-life of 5 to 10 minutes and thus can be titrated to effect with infusion adjustments every 15 to 20 minutes as needed.

In clinical trials, fenoldopam was equivalent to nitroprusside in lowering systolic and diastolic blood pressures in patients with severe hypertension.[67–69] However, fenoldopam selectively increases renal blood flow compared with nitroprusside.[69] In patients with hypertension and renal dysfunction, fenoldopam, but not nitroprusside, improved renal blood flow and creatinine clearance.[70] Fenoldopam also has been used in the management of postoperative hypertension. Although it is equally effective to nitroprusside, the treatment cost with fenoldopam is much higher.[67]

There are limited data on use of fenoldopam in children, including a small case series,[71] and on its use for inducing controlled hypotension in the operating room.[72] The drug company's information suggests onset is more rapid in children with a half-life as short as 3 minutes. Doses greater than 0.8 μg/kg/min did not produce greater reductions in blood pressure and were more likely to result in reflex tachycardia.

Angiotensin-Converting Enzyme Inhibitors

ACE inhibitors competitively inhibit ACE, the endogenous enzyme that converts angiotensin I to the potent vasoconstrictor angiotensin II. Captopril has been widely studied in children,[53,73] and its potency and duration of action vary by age. Enalapril is a prodrug converted to the active form enalaprilat, primarily in the liver; thus peak serum concentrations are delayed until 3 to 4 hours after administration.[74] Enalapril appears to be a useful agent for blood pressure control in children.[75] The main concern about ACE inhibitors is their effects on worsening renal blood flow when there is obstruction to renal artery blood flow, so they are generally contraindicated in this setting.[23,41,50] Captopril has a more rapid onset of action because it is the active form of the drug and does not require hepatic metabolism, as does enalapril. Despite this more rapid onset, captopril is generally used for long-term hypertension control rather than treatment of hypertensive emergencies because of its prolonged and sometimes unpredictable pharmacologic effects and duration of action. Other ACE inhibitors, such as lisinopril and quinapril, are used for hypertension in children, but they have not been studied in hypertensive urgencies or emergencies.

Enalaprilat is the only ACE inhibitor available in an intravenous preparation. Several case series report that it is useful for controlling hypertensive urgencies and emergencies, particularly after repair of aortic coarctation.[76] ACE inhibitors should not be used in hypovolemic patients because these agents may cause a rapid fall in blood pressure and precipitate acute ischemic renal injury. In addition, a potentially deadly side effect of all ACE inhibitors is the development of hyperkalemia through their action of inhibiting aldosterone production.

Calcium Channel Blockers

Type I calcium channel blockers have a tertiary amine group and are used primarily as antidysrhythmic agents (e.g., verapamil and diltiazem), whereas type II drugs possess a dihydropyridine nucleus and are potent vasodilators.[77] Calcium channel blockers also promote natriuresis.[52] Nifedipine was widely used for hypertensive emergencies because of its rapid onset and short duration of action.[41] Although sublingual use is common, there is no advantage to giving the drug by this route because only a small amount of drug is absorbed sublingually, whereas oral (or nasogastric) administration, especially in the absence of food, results in rapid absorption and onset of action.[52,53] In adults, nifedipine is no longer administered for hypertensive emergencies secondary to concern that it increases the risk of myocardial and cerebral ischemic injury secondary to the rapid fall in blood pressure.[78] Despite the widespread assumption of safety in children, nifedipine frequently results in a significant uncontrolled fall in blood pressure in hypertensive children. In a case series of 117 children, 35% of the doses resulted in a fall in mean arterial pressure greater than the desired upper range decline of 25%.[78] Similarly, in a review of 1746 doses of nifedipine in 166 pediatric patients, systolic blood pressure decreased by a mean of 17% and a maximum of 63%. Diastolic blood pressure decreased by a mean of 28% and a maximum of 89%. Adverse events included a change in neurologic status in six cases and hypotension in two cases.[79] As long as the dose was no more than 0.25 mg/kg, a significant fall in blood pressure was not observed.[80]

Nicardipine is a newer parenteral dihydropyridine calcium channel blocker that has been effective in the management of hypertensive emergencies and urgencies in children and adults,[40,81,82] including neonates and premature infants.[83,84] It has a rapid onset of action, on the order of 10 of 15 minutes, and short half-life of about 40 minutes. Its clearance is directly related to hepatic blood flow.[85] In a double-blind trial of acute hypertension, nicardipine was equally efficacious compared with nitroprusside in adults.[82] Nicardipine has added advantages over nitroprusside because nicardipine reduces the risk of brain ischemia[86] and does not pose the risk of cyanide or thiocyanate toxicity. Nicardipine is effective for hypertensive crises secondary to renal failure[87] and was effective in the treatment of hypertension in children after repair of aortic coarctation.[88] It is safe and effective in patients with aortic dissection.[89]

Nicardipine is generally safe but must be administered by a central venous line because there is a relatively high rate of thrombosis with peripheral administration. In addition, the drug cannot be highly concentrated, sometimes resulting in a significant fluid load in a hypertensive patient who is already fluid overloaded. Like other dihydropyridines, nicardipine has few direct myocardial effects, and cardiac output typically increases with administration. Like a host of other drugs, nicardipine interferes with cyclosporine metabolism, resulting in increased cyclosporine concentration.[90]

Summary

Hypertension when present in children in the PICU is most often related to pain, agitation, positive fluid balance, drug effect, or occasionally unrecognized seizure. For patients with hypertension admitted to the PICU, renal causes are most frequent and may be clinically silent, such as renovascular hypertension. Hypertension as a primary diagnosis is less common, although its prevalence is increasing in concert with the rise in type II diabetes in obese adolescents. An organized approach to clinical and laboratory examination often yields the cause and distinguishes between hypertensive urgency and hypertensive emergency. Treatment of a hypertensive emergency is directed at controlled reduction of blood pressure not to exceed 25% of the baseline mean arterial pressure. The rate of blood pressure reduction is within minutes to hours in patients with a hypertensive emergency versus hours to 1 day in children with a hypertensive urgency.

REFERENCES

1. National High Blood Pressure Education Program Working Group on High Blood Pressure in Children and Adolescents: The fourth report on the diagnosis, evaluation, and treatment of high blood pressure in children and adolescents. *Pediatrics* 114: 555-576, 2004.
2. National High Blood Pressure Education Program Working Group on Hypertension Control in Children and Adolescents: Update on the 1987 Task Force Report on High Blood Pressure in Children and Adolescents: a working group report from the National High Blood Pressure Education Program. *Pediatrics* 98:649-658, 1996.
3. Chobanian AV, Bakris GL, Black HR, et al: The Seventh Report of the Joint National Committee on Prevention, Detection, Evaluation, and Treatment of High Blood Pressure: the JNC 7 report. *JAMA* 289:2560-2572, 2003.
4. Cherney D, Straus S: Management of patients with hypertensive urgencies and emergencies. *J Gen Intern Med* 17:937-945,2002.
5. Elliott WJ: Hypertensive emergencies. *Crit Care Clin* 17: 435-451, 2001.
6. Vaughan CJ, Delanty N: Hypertensive emergencies. *Lancet* 356:411-417, 2000.
7. Wong TY, Mitchell P: Hypertensive retinopathy. *N Engl J Med* 351:2310-2317, 2004.
8. Scheie HG: Evaluation of ophthalmoscopic changes of hypertension and arteriolar sclerosis. *AMA Arch Ophthalmol* 49: 117-138, 1953.
9. O'Sullivan J, Allen J, Murray A: The forgotten Korotkoff phases: how often are phases II and III present, and how do they relate to the other Korotkoff phases? *Am J Hypertens* 15:264-268, 2002.
10. Prineas RJ, Jacobs D: Quality of Korotkoff sounds: bell vs diaphragm, cubital fossa vs brachial artery. *Prev Med* 12: 715-719, 1983.
11. Reeves RA: The rational clinical examination. Does this patient have hypertension? How to measure blood pressure. *JAMA* 273:1211-1218, 1983.
12. Arafat M, Mattoo TK: Measurement of blood pressure in children: recommendations and perceptions on cuff selection. *Pediatrics* 104:e30, 1999.
13. Carr JJ, Brown JM: *Introduction to biomedical equipment technology*, ed 2. Englewood Cliffs, NJ, 1993, Regents/Prentice Hall.
14. Perloff WH: Invasive measurements in the PICU. In Fuhrman BP, Zimmerman JJ, editors: *Pediatric critical care*. St. Louis, 1992, Mosby.
15. Nelson LD, Snyder JV: Technical problems in data acquisition. In Snyder JV, Pinsky MR, editors: *Oxygen transport in the critically ill*. Chicago, 1987, Year Book Medical Publishers.
16. Blumenfeld JD: Renal and cardiac complications of hypertension. *Clin Symp* 46:3-32, 1994.
17. Wong J, Patel RA, Kowey PR: The clinical use of angiotensin-converting enzyme inhibitors. *Prog Cardiovasc Dis* 47:116-130, 2004.
18. Weir MR, Dzau VJ: The renin-angiotensin-aldosterone system: a specific target for hypertension management. *Am J Hypertens* 12:205S-213S, 1999.
19. Contreras F, de la Parte MA, Cabrera J, et al: Role of angiotensin II AT1 receptor blockers in the treatment of arterial hypertension. *Am J Ther* 10:401-408, 2003.
20. Dillon MJ: Renovascular hypertension. *J Hum Hypertens* 8: 367-369, 1994.
21. Dillon MJ: The diagnosis of renovascular disease. *Pediatr Nephrol* 11:366-372, 1997.
22. Guillery EN, Robillard JE: The renin-angiotensin system and blood pressure regulation during infancy and childhood. *Pediatr Clin North Am* 40:61-79, 1993.
23. Blumenfeld JD, Laragh JH: Management of hypertensive crises: the scientific basis for treatment decisions. *Am J Hypertens* 14: 1154-1167, 2001.
24. Baxter G: The natriuretic peptides. *Bas Res Cardiol* 99:71-75, 2004.
25. Ahluwalia A, MacAllister R, Hobbs A: Vascular actions of natriuretic peptides. *Bas Res Cardiol* 99:83-89, 2004.
26. Li H, Forstermann U: Nitric oxide in the pathogenesis of vascular disease. *J Pathol* 190:244-254, 2000.
27. Zhou MS, Schulman IH, Raij L: Nitric oxide, angiotensin II, and hypertension. *Semin Nephrol* 24:366-378, 2004.

28. Moncada S, Higgs A: The L-arginine-nitric oxide pathway. *N Engl J Med* 329:2002-2012, 1993.
29. Touyz RM, Schiffrin EL: Role of endothelin in human hypertension. *Can J Physiol Pharmacol* 81:533-541, 2003.
30. Lariviere R, Lebel M: Endothelin-1 in chronic renal failure and hypertension. *Can J Physiol Pharmacol* 81:6076-21,2003.
31. Paulson OB, Strandgaard S, Edvinsson L: Cerebral autoregulation. *Cerebrovasc Brain Metab Rev* 2:161-192, 1990.
32. Wright RR, Mathews KD: Hypertensive encephalopathy in childhood. *J Child Neurol* 11:193-196, 1996.
33. Jones BV, Egelhoff JC, Patterson RJ: Hypertensive encephalopathy in children. *AJNR Am J Neuroradiol* 18:101-106, 1997.
34. Phillips SJ, Whisnant JP: Hypertension and the brain. The National High Blood Pressure Education Program. *Arch Intern Med* 152:938-945, 1992.
35. Schwartz R, Mulkern R, Gudbjartsson H, Jolesz F: Diffusion-weighted MR imaging in hypertensive encephalopathy: clues to pathogenesis. *AJNR Am J Neuroradiol* 19:859-862, 1998.
36. Sundgren P, Edvardsson B, Holtas S: Serial investigation of perfusion disturbances and vasogenic oedema in hypertensive encephalopathy by diffusion and perfusion weighted imaging. *Neuroradiology* 44:299-304, 2002.
37. Sokrab TE, Johansson BB, Kalimo H, Olsson Y: A transient hypertensive opening of the blood-brain barrier can lead to brain damage. Extravasation of serum proteins and cellular changes in rats subjected to aortic compression. *Acta Neuropathol (Berl)* 75:557-565, 1988.
38. Ziegler MG: Antihypertensive therapy. In Chernow B, editor: *The pharmacologic approach to the critically ill patient,* ed 2. Baltimore, 1988, Williams & Wilkins.
39. Van Why SK, Boydstun, II, Gaudio KM, Siegel NJ: Abdominal symptoms as presentation of hypertensive crisis. *Am J Dis Child* 147:638-641, 1993.
40. Varon J, Marik PE: The diagnosis and management of hypertensive crises. *Chest* 118:214-227, 2000.
41. Fivush B, Neu A, Furth S: Acute hypertensive crises in children: emergencies and urgencies. *Curr Opin Pediatr* 9:233-236, 1997.
42. Tinker JH, Michenfelder JD: Sodium nitroprusside: pharmacology, toxicology and therapeutics. *Anesthesiology* 45:340-353, 1976.
43. Schulz V: Clinical pharmacokinetics of nitroprusside, cyanide, thiosulphate and thiocyanate. *Clin Pharmacokinet* 9:239-251, 1984.
44. Hall VA, Guest JM: Sodium nitroprusside-induced cyanide intoxication and prevention with sodium thiosulfate prophylaxis. *Am J Crit Care* 1:19-25, 1992.
45. Rindone JP, Sloane EP: Cyanide toxicity from sodium nitroprusside: risks and management [published erratum appears in *Ann Pharmacother* 1992;26:1160. *Ann Pharmacother* 26:515-519, 1992.
46. Zerbe NF, Wagner BK: Use of vitamin B12 in the treatment and prevention of nitroprusside-induced cyanide toxicity. *Crit Care Med* 21:465-467, 1993.
47. Calhoun DA, Oparil S: Treatment of hypertensive crisis. *N Engl J Med* 323:1177-1183, 1990.
48. Koch-Weser J: Diazoxide. *N Engl J Med* 294:1271-273, 1976.
49. Neuman J, Weiss B, Rabello Y, et al: Diazoxide for the acute control of severe hypertension complicating pregnancy: a pilot study. *Obstet Gynecol* 53:50S-55S, 1979.
50. Grossman E, Ironi AN, Messerli FH: Comparative tolerability profile of hypertensive crisis treatments. *Drug Saf* 19:99-122, 1998.
51. Vidrio H, Fernandez G, Medina M, et al: Effects of hydrazine derivatives on vascular smooth muscle contractility, blood pressure and cGMP production in rats: comparison with hydralazine. *Vascul Pharmacol* 40:13-21, 2003.
52. Kirsten R, Nelson K, Kirsten D, Heintz B: Clinical pharmacokinetics of vasodilators. Part I. *Clin Pharmacokinet* 34:457-482, 1998.
53. Sinaiko AR: Pharmacologic management of childhood hypertension. *Pediatr Clin North Am* 40:195-212, 1993.
54. Wiest DB, Garner SS, Uber WE, Sade RM: Esmolol for the management of pediatric hypertension after cardiac operations. *J Thorac Cardiovasc Surg* 115:890-897, 1998.
55. Wiest DB, Trippel DL, Gillette PC, Garner SS: Pharmacokinetics of esmolol in children. *Clin Pharmacol Ther* 49:618-623, 1991.
56. Cuneo BF, Zales VR, Blahunka PC, Benson DW Jr: Pharmacodynamics and pharmacokinetics of esmolol, a short-acting beta-blocking agent, in children. *Pediatr Cardiol* 15:296-301, 1994.
57. Lund-Johansen P: Pharmacology of combined alpha-beta-blockade. II. Haemodynamic effects of labetalol. *Drugs* 28(suppl 2):35-50, 1984.
58. Lund-Johansen P: Hemodynamic effects of beta-blocking compounds possessing vasodilating activity: a review of labetalol, prizidilol, and dilevalol. *J Cardiovasc Pharmacol* 11(suppl 2): S12-S17, 1988.
59. Kirsten R, Nelson K, Kirsten D, Heintz B: Clinical pharmacokinetics of vasodilators. Part II. *Clin Pharmacokinet* 35:9-36, 1998.
60. Temple ME, Nahata MC: Treatment of pediatric hypertension. *Pharmacotherapy* 20:140-150, 2000.
61. McCauley J, Murray J, Jordan M, et al: Labetalol-induced hyperkalemia in renal transplant recipients. *Am J Nephrol* 22:347-351, 2002.
62. Stenstrom G, Haljamae H, Tisell LE: Influence of pre-operative treatment with phenoxybenzamine on the incidence of adverse cardiovascular reactions during anaesthesia and surgery for phaeochromocytoma. *Acta Anaesthesiol Scand* 29:797-803, 1985.
63. Gales MA: Oral antihypertensives for hypertensive urgencies. *Ann Pharmacother* 28:352-358, 1994.
64. Coursin DB, Maccioli GA: Dexmedetomidine. *Curr Opin Crit Care* 7:221-226, 2001.
65. Hegde SS, Ricci A, Amenta F, Lokhandwala MF: Evidence from functional and autoradiographic studies for the presence of tubular dopamine-1 receptors and their involvement in the renal effects of fenoldopam. *J Pharmacol Exp Ther* 251: 1237-1245, 1989.
66. Murphy MB, Murray C, Shorten GD: Fenoldopam—a selective peripheral dopamine-receptor agonist for the treatment of severe hypertension. *N Engl J Med* 345:1548-1557, 2001.
67. Devlin JW, Seta ML, Kanji S, Somerville AL: Fenoldopam versus nitroprusside for the treatment of hypertensive emergency. *Ann Pharmacother* 38:755-759, 2004.
68. Panacek EA, Bednarczyk EM, Dunbar LM, et al: Randomized, prospective trial of fenoldopam vs sodium nitroprusside in the treatment of acute severe hypertension. Fenoldopam Study Group. *Acad Emerg Med* 2:959-965, 1995.
69. Pilmer BL, Green JA, Panacek EA, Elliot WJ, Murphy MB, Rutherford W, Nara AR: Fenoldopam mesylate versus sodium nitroprusside in the acute management of severe systemic hypertension. *J Clin Pharmacol* 33:549-553, 1993.
70. Shusterman NH, Elliott WJ, White WB: Fenoldopam, but not nitroprusside, improves renal function in severely hypertensive patients with impaired renal function. *Am J Med* 95:161-168, 1993.
71. Strauser LM, Pruitt RD, Tobias JD: Initial experience with fenoldopam in children. *Am J Ther* 6:283-288, 1999.
72. Tobias JD: Controlled hypotension in children: a critical review of available agents. *Paediatr Drugs* 4:439-453, 2002.
73. Sinaiko A, Kashtan C, Mirkin B: Antihypertensive drug therapy with captopril in children and adolescents. *Clin Exp Hypertens* 8:829-839, 1986.
74. Wells T, Rippley R, Hogg R, et al: The pharmacokinetics of enalapril in children and infants with hypertension. *J Clin Pharmacol* 41:1064-1074, 2001.
75. Wells T, Frame V, Soffer B, et al: A double-blind, placebo-controlled, dose-response study of the effectiveness and safety of enalapril for children with hypertension. *J Clin Pharmacol* 42:870-880, 2002.
76. Rouine-Rapp K, Mello DM, Hanley FL, et al: Effect of enalaprilat on postoperative hypertension after surgical repair of coarctation of the aorta. *Pediatr Crit Care Med* 4:327-332, 2003.
77. Flynn JT, Pasko DA: Calcium channel blockers: pharmacology and place in therapy of pediatric hypertension. *Pediatr Nephrol* 15:302-316, 2000.
78. Grossman E, Messerli FH, Grodzicki T, Kowey P: Should a moratorium be placed on sublingual nifedipine capsules given for hypertensive emergencies and pseudoemergencies? *JAMA* 276:1328-1331, 1996.
79. Egger DW, Deming DD, Hamada N, et al: Evaluation of the safety of short-acting nifedipine in children with hypertension. *Pediatr Nephrol* 17:35-40, 2002.
80. Blaszak RT, Savage JA, Ellis EN: The use of short-acting nifedipine in pediatric patients with hypertension. *J Pediatr* 139:34-37, 2001.
81. Flynn JT, Mottes TA, Brophy PD, et al: Intravenous nicardipine for treatment of severe hypertension in children. *J Pediatr* 139:38-43, 2001.

82. Halpern NA, Goldberg M, Neely C, et al: Postoperative hypertension: a multicenter, prospective, randomized comparison between intravenous nicardipine and sodium nitroprusside. *Crit Care Med* 20:1637-1643, 1992.
83. Gouyon JB, Geneste B, Semama DS, et al: Intravenous nicardipine in hypertensive preterm infants. *Arch Dis Child Fetal Neonatal Ed* 76:F126-F127, 1997.
84. Milou C, Debuche-Benouachkou V, Semama DS, Germain JF, Gouyon JB: Intravenous nicardipine as a first-line antihypertensive drug in neonates. *Intensive Care Med* 26:956-958, 2000.
85. Graham DJ, Dow RJ, Hall DJ, et al: The metabolism and pharmacokinetics of nicardipine hydrochloride in man. *Br J Clin Pharmacol* 20(suppl 1):23S-28S, 1985.
86. Kittaka M, Giannotta SL, Zelman V, et al: Attenuation of brain injury and reduction of neuron-specific enolase by nicardipine in systemic circulation following focal ischemia and reperfusion in a rat model. *J Neurosurg* 87:731-737, 1997.
87. Tenney F, Sakarcan A: Nicardipine is a safe and effective agent in pediatric hypertensive emergencies. *Am J Kidney Dis* 35: E20, 2000.
88. Nakagawa TA, Sartori SC, Morris A, Schneider DS: Intravenous nicardipine for treatment of postcoarctectomy hypertension in children. *Pediatr Cardiol* 25:26-30, 2004.
89. Kim KH, Moon IS, Park JS, et al: Nicardipine hydrochloride injectable phase IV open-label clinical trial: study on the antihypertensive effect and safety of nicardipine for acute aortic dissection. *J Int Med Res* 30:337-345, 2002.
90. Campana C, Regazzi MB, Buggia I, Molinaro M: Clinically significant drug interactions with cyclosporin. An update. *Clin Pharmacokinet* 30:141-179, 1996.
91. Sinaiko AR: Hypertension in children. *N Engl J Med* 335: 1968-1973, 1996.
92. Kitiyakara C, Guzman NJ: Malignant hypertension and hypertensive emergencies. *J Am Soc Nephrol* 9:133-142, 1998.

CHAPTER

67

Cellular Bioenergetic Pathways and Processes

Gregory A. Hollman and Waldemar E. Storm

PEARLS

- The three primary components regulating cellular respiration are the ATP/ADP ratio, the NADH/NAD ratio (redox state), and oxygen availability.
- Critical illness is accompanied by a number of bioenergetic disturbances, which include insufficient NADH availability (PARP-1 activation), disturbances in electron transport (cytochrome aa_3 dysfunction), and dissipation of the inner mitochondrial membrane electrochemical gradient.
- Hypoglycemia and hypoxemia represent extremes in insufficient substrate delivery to the respiratory chain and trigger similar disturbances in mitochondrial dysfunction.
- Disturbances in cellular bioenergetic processes (energy metabolism) are primary mechanisms leading to organ dysfunction in critical illness.

Organisms, composed of material which is characterized by the utmost inconstancy and unsteadiness, have somehow learned the methods of maintaining constancy and keeping steady in the presence of conditions, which might reasonably be expected to prove profoundly disturbing.

Walter B. Cannon, 1932[13]

Homeostasis is the ability of an organism to maintain a dynamic steady state despite perturbations in its external or internal environment. It is secured by the pathways governing cellular energy metabolism. Through a network of multienzyme reactions, the chemical energy of nutrient molecules is transformed into useful energy utilized by the cell to maintain internal order and perform work-related functions. The processes and components that link energy-yielding to energy-requiring processes are highly regulated and tightly coupled and consist of the metabolic substrates that fuel cellular respiration (nutrient molecules and oxygen) and the elements that compose the respiratory chain: oxidation-reduction (redox) reactions, electrochemical gradients, and adenosine triphosphate (ATP) synthesis.

This chapter focuses on the key bioenergetic processes and pathways utilized by the organism to extract, transform, and deliver useful energy. The major metabolic pathways involved in the oxidation of metabolic fuels and the components of the respiratory chain—redox reactions, electrochemical gradients and ATP synthesis—are discussed. The metabolic signals regulating cellular respiration and cellular bioenergetic disturbances relevant to critical care practice are addressed.

Basic Bioenergetic Processes

Cellular metabolism consists of a series of coordinated enzymatic steps involved in the extraction, transformation, and utilization of chemical energy. Chemical reactions are characterized by two types: those that produce energy *(exergonic)* and those that consume energy *(endergonic)*. *Exergonic processes* release energy and in living organisms are exemplified by a complex, highly ordered state progressing "naturally" to a less complex, disordered state. Catabolic processes are a specific type of exergonic reaction that results in release of free energy during the degradation of complex nutrient molecules to simpler and less organized endproducts. Conversely, *endergonic reactions* require energy input in order to transition from a disordered state to a more highly structured level. Biosynthetic processes are examples of endergonic reactions in which basic elemental molecules are organized into larger complex macromolecules. Within living organisms, exergonic and endergonic reactions are tightly coupled in time and space and driven by the energy needs of the system (Fig. 67–1).

Free Energy and Work

Living organisms use energy to maintain self-order and a dynamic state of responsiveness to internal and external perturbations. As such, the living organism functions far from an equilibrium position, a state upheld through the extraction and use of high-energy, complex fuels from the environment. The ability of the organism to use the potential energy in complex fuels for maintaining homeostasis is essential to their viability. The amount of chemical energy from nutrient molecules available for work is termed *useful* or *free energy* and designated by the letter G. The quantity of free energy accessible to the organism during nutrient metabolism is termed the *free energy change* and designated by ΔG, where −ΔG indicates an exergonic process. The magnitude of ΔG is determined by how far reactants and products are displaced from their equilibrium position. In biologic systems, chemical reactions have a standard free energy change (ΔG°) traditionally expressed in kilocalories per mole under standard conditions of temperature and pressure:

$$-\Delta G\text{: exergonic. } \Delta G^\circ -2.3\ RT \log K_{eq} \qquad K_{eq} = \frac{[C]\,[D]}{[A]\,[B]}$$
$$+\Delta G\text{: endergonic}$$

where K_{eq} = equilibrium constant when concentrations of reactants [A] and [B] and products [C] and [D] are at equilibrium, R = the gas constant, and T = absolute temperature. Concentrations of reactants displaced far from equilibrium release large amounts of energy as the chemical reaction progresses toward an equilibrium state. Large free energy changes enhance the amount of work *(W)* that can be performed by the organism ($-\Delta G = W_{max}$). Much of the free energy generated and used by the organism occurs during the combustion of carbohydrates, fats, and proteins during cellular metabolism. The living organism conserves and transforms the energy of metabolic fuels into work primarily via three bioenergetic processes: redox reactions, membrane electrochemical gradients, and phosphate group transfer.

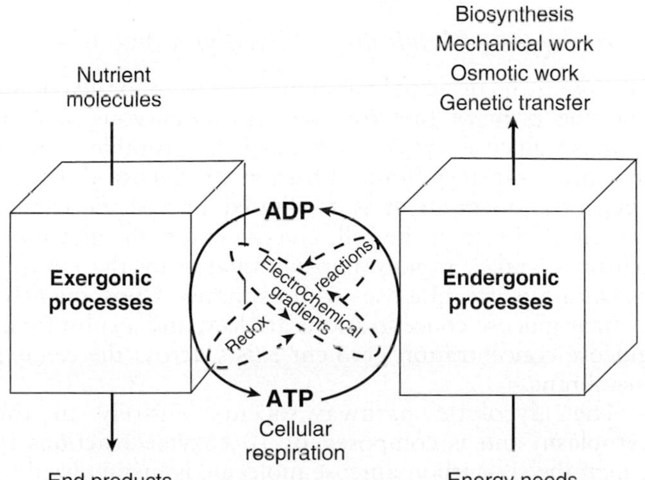

FIGURE 67–1 • Overview of cellular metabolism. The potential energy of complex nutrient fuels is extracted and coupled with ATP to drive energy-requiring biologic processes. The bulk of this energy is generated and transformed during cellular respiration. During cellular respiration, three bioenergetic processes are linked to ultimately couple exergonic processes to endergonic processes: oxidative-reduction (redox) reactions, electrochemical gradients, and ATP synthesis.

Biologic Free Energy Transformations

Oxidation-Reduction Reactions

Redox reactions are chemical reactions in which electrons are transferred from one chemical species to another. Redox reactions are ubiquitous in biologic systems and are responsible, directly or indirectly, for all work performed by the organism.[35] Electron flow from one molecule to another occurs by one of four different mechanisms: direct electron transfer, hydrogen transfer, hydride ion transfer (hydrogen atom with two electrons, H:), and direct reaction with oxygen. Free energy (−ΔG) is released during electron flow through redox reactions and is transformed and utilized to conduct useful biologic work, including creation of electrochemical gradients, facilitation of muscle contractions, and synthesis of macromolecules. The mitochondrial electron transport chain is fueled by hydride ions (H:) originating from the high-energy electron intermediates reduced nicotinamide dinucleotide (NADH) and flavine adenine dinucleotide ($FADH_2$) and is an example of a series of redox reactions whose free energy release is linked to the formation of an electrochemical gradient and the eventual synthesis of ATP.

Membrane Electrochemical Gradients

Biologic membranes separate one compartment from another and function as permeability barriers to molecules, selectively allowing passage of some while restricting others. As a result, depending on a compound's characteristics, differences in concentration, osmotic pressure, or electrical charge are established across cellular membranes. In the case of ions, transmembrane differences in both concentration and electrical charge are created and result in the generation of an electrochemical gradient across the cellular membrane. The transmembrane electrochemical potential difference is a source of energy, the magnitude of which is customarily expressed in millivolts and analogous to an electrical current generated by a battery. During cellular respiration, ion flow down the electrochemical gradient (proton motive force) is coupled to a number of work functions, including mechanical rotation of ATP synthase and the synthesis of ATP in the respiratory chain.

Phosphate Group Transfer (Adenosine Triphosphate Turnover)

Energy released during the oxidation of nutrient compounds ultimately is conserved in the form of ATP. ATP is a high-energy phosphate compound consisting of a nitrogen-containing organic base (adenine), a sugar (ribose), and three phosphate groups. Under standard conditions, hydrolysis of ATP's terminal phosphate group yields approximately 7.3 kcal/mol[35]:

$$\text{ATP} \bullet H_2O\ (\rightarrow)\ \text{ADP} \bullet \text{Pi}\ (\Delta G° \approx -7.3\ \text{kcal/mol})$$

The basic work-related cellular processes requiring ATP input include (1) biosynthesis of macromolecules, (2) coupling of actin-myosin filaments (mechanical work), (3) transmembrane transport of solutes (osmotic work), and (4) transfer of genetic information[35] (see Fig. 67–1).

Two unique characteristics of ATP form the basis of its ability to function as the primary energy exchanger within the body. First, ATP, like many phosphorylated compounds, is metabolically active and, when coupled to chemical reactions, allows these pathways to proceed with a release of free energy.[35] ATP has an intermediate $\Delta G°$, placing it in an ideal position to function as a carrier of phosphate groups between super-high-energy phosphate compounds and low-energy phosphate compounds. The process in which ATP shuttles phosphate groups between molecules is referred to as *substrate level phosphorylation* and is the primary mechanism for energy transfer during glycolysis.

The second unique aspect of ATP metabolism is that [ATP]/[ADP] ratios are maintained approximately 10^8-fold higher than their equilibrium position. Thus the actual ΔG of ATP in biologic systems is ≈ −15 kcal/mol, twofold greater than its standard free energy change of ≈ 7.3 kcal/mol. Consequently, coupling of ATP to an endergonic reaction pulls the reaction to completion as the high [ATP]/[ADP] ratio "flows downward" toward equilibrium. In addition, the [ATP]/[ADP] ratio serves as an indicator of the cell's energy state and is continuously monitored and maintained in biologic systems. The significance of the [ATP]/[ADP] ratio as an important marker of the cellular energy state is examined more fully in the section on regulation of cellular metabolism.

Central Catabolic Pathways

Complete oxidation of nutrient fuels is accompanied by a large release of free energy, the vast majority of which occurs in the mitochondria. Although the initial catabolic steps vary among the different fuels (e.g., carbohydrates vs. fats), all nutrient molecules eventually converge to a common mitochondrial pathway (Fig. 67-2). In general, nutrient fuels are metabolized through the following common stages[35]:

I. Generation of the two-carbon acetyl-coenzyme A (acetyl-CoA) molecule following glycolysis, β-oxidation of fatty acids, and amino acid catabolism
II. Generation of energy-rich electron carriers in the form of NADH and FADH2 in the Krebs cycle
III. Synthesis of ATP in the respiratory chain

Initial oxidation and breakdown of carbohydrates, fats, and proteins result in the generation of the two-carbon acetyl-CoA molecule in the mitochondria. Acetyl-CoA is the common endproduct of nutrient metabolism prior to entry into the Krebs cycle. Acetyl-CoA is metabolized in the Krebs cycle, generating high-energy electron intermediates, primarily in the form of NADH and $FADH_2$. Electron pairs originating from NADH and $FADH_2$ are delivered to a series of redox reactions in the inner mitochondrial membrane, the electron transport chain. Free energy is released as electrons "flow down" the electron transport chain and is utilized to establish an electrochemical proton gradient across the inner mitochondrial membrane and synthesize ATP during cellular respiration.

Stage I: Formation of Acetyl-Coenzyme A

Most of the major catabolic pathways of carbohydrate, lipid, and protein metabolism coalesce to the formation of acetyl-CoA in the mitochondria (see Figure 67–2). Metabolism of each of these metabolic fuels during this first stage is described here. Because of the critical role of glucose in energy metabolism in virtually all tissues, glucose metabolism is highlighted.

Carbohydrate Metabolism: Glycolysis (Fig. 67-3)

Glucose is the principal metabolic substrate for glycolysis and the primary fuel for the central nervous system. Cellular glucose uptake is a passive, saturable process in which transmembrane diffusion of glucose down its concentration gradient is facilitated by specific carrier proteins.[63] Once in the cell, glucose enters the glycolytic pathway and is rapidly phosphorylated by the enzyme hexokinase to glucose 6-phosphate. Consequently, cellular glucose concentrations are low, and a substantial glucose concentration gradient exists across the cellular membrane.[28]

The glycolytic pathway occurs entirely in the cytoplasm and is composed of 10 enzyme reactions in which the six-carbon glucose molecule is metabolized to two three-carbon pyruvate molecules. All nine glycolytic intermediates are ionized and phosphorylated compounds. These physicochemical properties inhibit transmembrane diffusion out of the cell and provide a source of phosphate for ATP synthesis. Overall, the full sequence of glycolysis is irreversible and exergonic in which the free energy in the glucose molecule is extracted and utilized to synthesize a net two molecules of ATP.

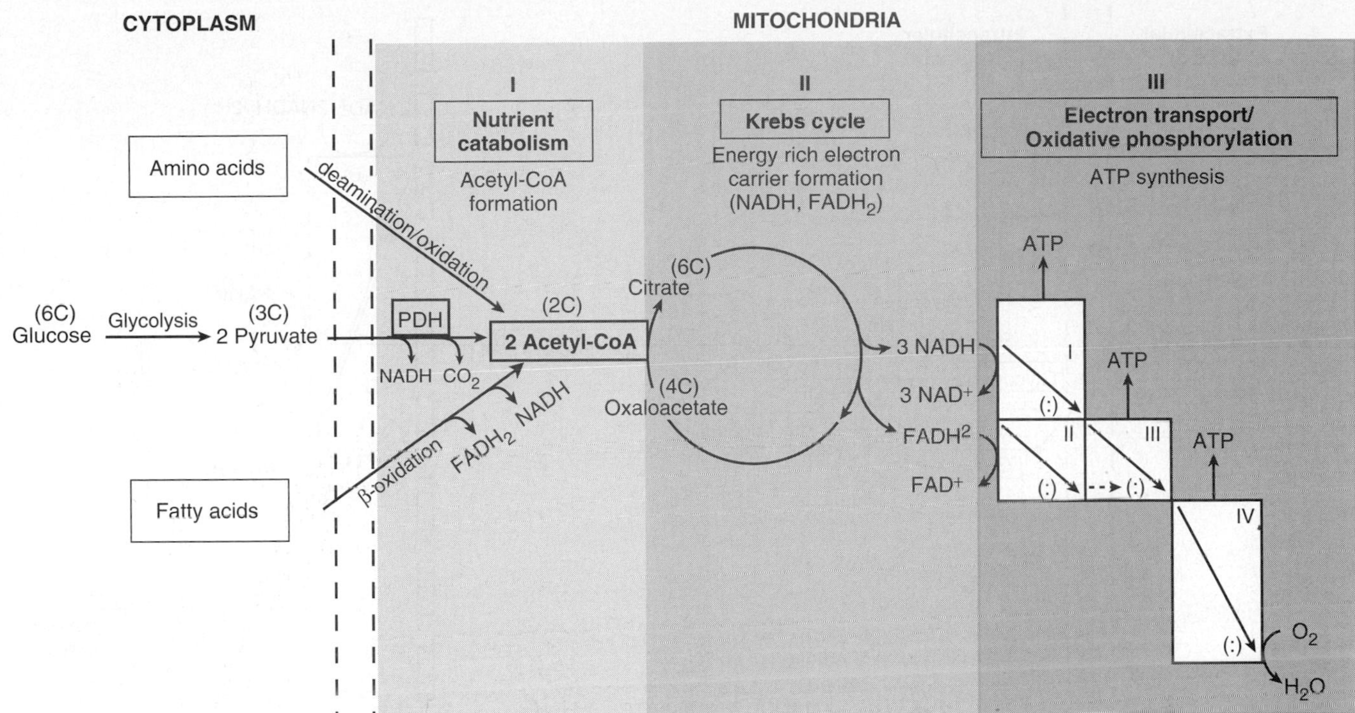

FIGURE 67–2 • Catabolism of nutrient molecules. Nutrient fuel catabolism undergoes three distinct steps. Step I results in the formation of the two-carbon acetyl-CoA molecule. Step II, the Krebs cycle, generates high-energy electron intermediates in the form of NADH and $FADH_2$ that eventually deliver electron pairs to the respiratory chain. Step III consists of the electron transport chain and oxidative phosphorylation. Free energy released during electron transport is linked to the formation of an electrochemical gradient (proton motive force) across the inner mitochondrial membrane. Ion flow down the electrochemical gradient drives the synthesis of ATP. I, II, III, and IV compose the four complexes of the electron transport chain. Three sites along the respiratory chain are associated with ATP synthesis.

Glycolysis is composed of both an endergonic (preparatory) stage and an exergonic stage (Fig. 67–3). The first five reactions of glycolysis compose the endergonic stage, in which two ATP molecules are used to break down the six-carbon glucose molecule to two three-carbon glyceraldehyde 3-phosphate molecules. The first and third reactions of glycolysis consume one molecule of ATP each and are considered the "priming" steps of glycolysis. When coupled with ATP, these reactions proceed with a large loss of free energy and are irreversible under normal cellular conditions. The energy-requiring stage of glycolysis is completed upon generation of two glyceraldehyde 3-phosphate molecules.

The final five steps of glycolysis are associated with the release of energy that eventually is coupled to the synthesis of four molecules of ATP. Glycolytic reactions 6 and 9 generate the super-high-energy phosphate molecules 1,3-biphosphoglycerate and phosphoenolpyruvate. Both compounds donate phosphate groups to generate ATP, a process referred to as substrate level phosphorylation, in reactions 7 and 10. The sixth reaction is also involved in the synthesis of the high-energy electron carrier NADH. NADH eventually transfers its electrons to the mitochondrial respiratory chain by way of the malate-aspartate shuttle system. The final reaction of glycolysis results in the production of two pyruvate molecules. This irreversible and highly regulated reaction is catalyzed by the enzyme pyruvate kinase. The fate of pyruvate now depends on the presence or absence of oxygen, the latter leading to lactate formation.

In summary, glycolysis is characterized by three distinct metabolic processes:

1. Breakdown of the six-carbon glucose molecule to two three-carbon pyruvate molecules
2. Synthesis of a net two ATP molecules from super-high-energy phosphate compounds (substrate level phosphorylation)
3. Generation of four electrons (two electron pairs) as two hydride ions (H:) transported via NADH to the mitochondrial respiratory chain

Regulation of Glycolysis. The rate of cellular glucose uptake and metabolism through glycolysis is regulated by the cell's energy needs and nutrient requirements.[20,50] As such, cellular concentrations of ATP and its metabolites and certain nutrient substrates target specific regulatory enzyme steps and determine the pace of glucose flux through the glycolytic chain. Overall, high levels of ATP and certain metabolic intermediates inhibit specific glycolytic enzymes and decrease glucose flow through glycolysis. These key regulatory enzyme reactions compose the rate-limiting "gates" of glycolysis and tend to accumulate reactants far in excess of products. Thus these enzymatic control points displace reactant and product concentrations far from equilibrium and are exergonic and irreversible in vivo. Although all nine glycolytic reactions are crucial to the metabolism of glucose, four enzyme steps, identified by an asterisk in Figure 67-3, in particular determine the rate of glucose flux through glycolysis. All of these reactions are associated with large $-\Delta G$, some stoichiometrically coupled with ATP.

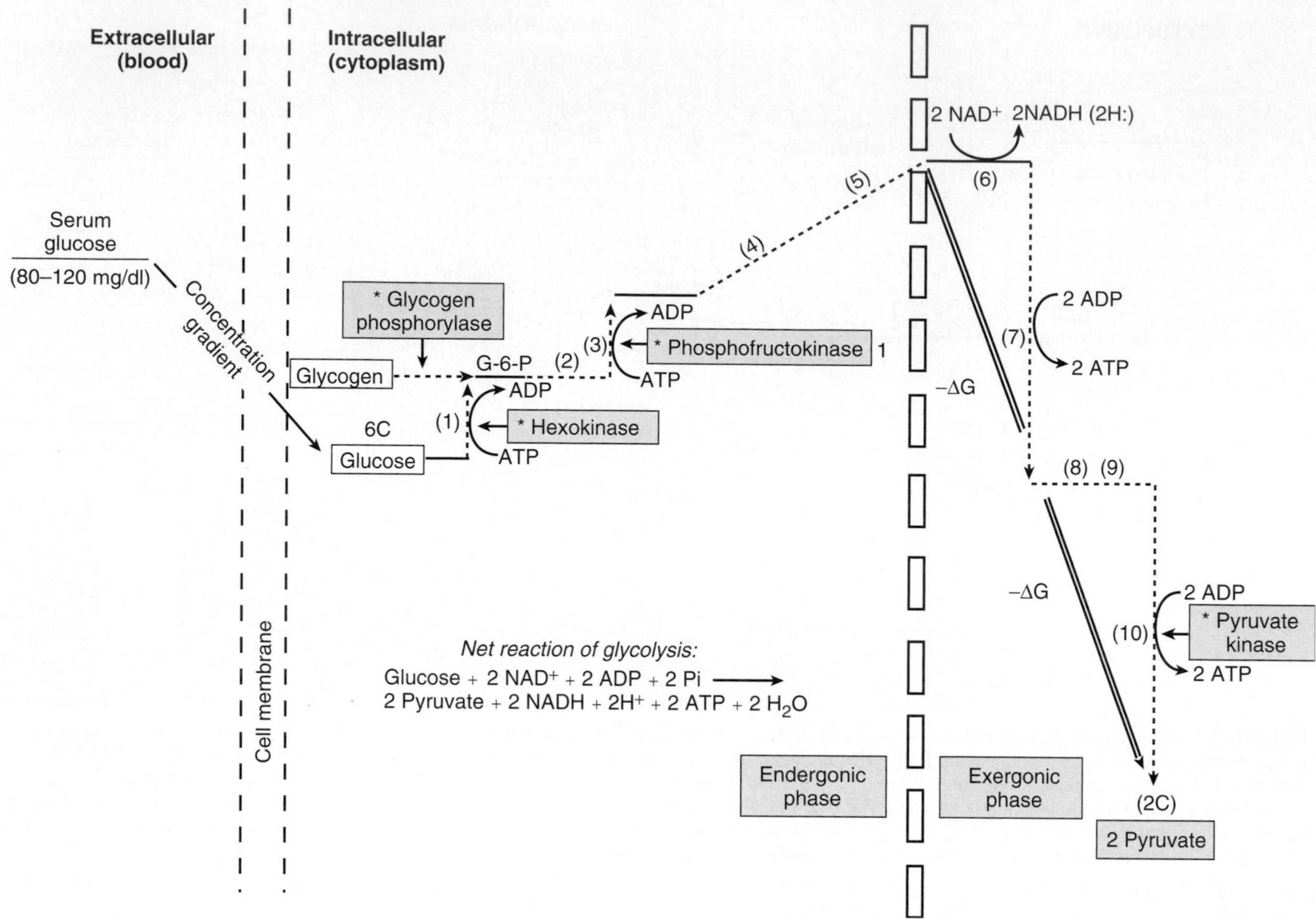

FIGURE 67–3 • Glycolysis consists of an endergonic (preparatory phase) and an exergonic phase. Cellular glucose entry proceeds down a significant concentration gradient from blood to cytoplasm. Glucose is rapidly phosphorylated in the cell to glucose 6-phosphate (G-6-P) by hexokinase. Both hexokinase and phosphofructokinase-1 are coupled to ATP hydrolysis and are irreversible in vivo. The final five reactions of glycolysis compose the exergonic phase in which a total of four molecules of ATP are generated. Pyruvate kinase catalyzes the final reaction in glycolysis and is linked to the formation of two molecules of ATP. Glycogen phosphorylase mobilizes glucose residues from glycogen. Numbers 1 through 10 designate each of the 10 enzyme steps in glycolysis. The four key regulatory steps are glycogen phosphorylase, hexokinase, phosphofructokinase-1, and pyruvate kinase.

1. Hexokinase (step 1) catalyzes the entry of glucose into glycolysis and is the principal determinant of cellular glucose entry and the glycolytic rate. Following entry into the cell, glucose is rapidly phosphorylated by hexokinase to glucose 6-phosphate (G-6-P). Hexokinase is fully saturated at normal serum glucose concentrations and typically functions at a maximal rate. As a consequence, cellular glucose concentrations are very low.[28] Hexokinase is allosterically inhibited by elevated concentrations of its product glucose 6-phosphate.[35] In contrast to other cells such as muscle, the liver contains an isoenzyme of hexokinase called *glucokinase.* Glucokinase also catalyzes the reaction glucose to glucose 6-phosphate but is not inhibited by elevated glucose 6-phosphate levels. In the presence of "excess" glucose, the liver can channel cellular glucose away from glycolysis to the formation of glycogen. Consequently, the liver directs glucose to one of two pathways: glycolysis or glycogen synthesis.
2. Glycogen phosphorylase provides a point of entry for glucose into the glycolytic pathway (muscle) or serum (liver). Although a number of carbohydrate pathways feed into the glycolytic sequence, mobilization of stored glycogen (a glucose polymer) in muscle and liver by glycogen phosphorylase provides the most readily available and rapid source of glucose to the glycolytic chain and in some organs (liver) the serum. Glycogen is sequentially cleaved by glycogen phosphorylase to glucose 1-phosphate when additional carbohydrate substrate is required for energy needs. Glucose-1-phosphate subsequently enters the glycolytic pathway as glucose 6-phosphate following its metabolism by phosphoglucomutase. Glycogen phosphorylase is a highly regulated enzyme that exists in both an active phosphorylated form (phosphorylase a) and a less active dephosphorylated form (phosphorylase b). Glycogen breakdown is determined by the ratio of active to inactive forms, and under resting conditions most of the enzyme is in the inactive b form. The fate of glucose residues from glycogen depends on which organ is examined, muscle versus liver.

During stress, circulating epinephrine facilitates glycogen breakdown in muscle through a cyclic adenosine monophosphate (AMP)-mediated phosphorylation of phosphorylase b to the active phosphorylase a. Alternatively, sufficient supplies of ATP and glucose-6-phosphate inhibit glycogen breakdown. Regulation of glycogen phosphorylase by AMP from increased ATP breakdown during muscle contraction allosterically alters phosphorylase b to a more active form. Conversion of phosphorylase b to a more active form facilitates the mobilization of glucose residues from glycogen to glycolysis.

In contrast, glycogen breakdown in the liver typically is in response to low serum glucose levels. Unlike skeletal muscle, the liver contains the enzyme glucose 6-phosphatase, which catalyzes the removal of phosphate from glucose 6-phosphate to form free glucose that can directly enter the serum. In response to low blood sugar, glucagon is released and, in a mechanism similar to epinephrine-mediated glycogen breakdown in muscle, converts phosphorylase b to phosphorylase a, increasing glycogen breakdown and formation of free glucose. In liver, glycogen phosphorylase is under allosteric regulation by glucose. Elevated serum glucose facilitates the conversion of the active to the inactive form by directly binding to the regulatory site of glycogen phosphorylase. In this manner, glycogen breakdown in the liver is inhibited in the presence of elevated serum glucose concentrations.

3. Phosphofructokinase-1(step 3) is the enzymatic step that commits glucose to the glycolytic pathway. Prior to this step, glucose may be channeled to other secondary pathways, namely, the pentose phosphate and uridine diphosphate glucuronate pathways. Phosphofructokinase-1 metabolizes fructose 6-phosphate to fructose 1,6-biphosphate and is under complex allosteric regulation, controlled primarily by the cellular energy state.[5] ATP, a substrate in this reaction, and citrate allosterically inhibit this step, thereby reducing the glycolytic rate. On the other hand, increased levels of AMP and adenosine diphosphate (ADP), indicators of high ATP turnover and energy deficit, enhance this enzyme step and facilitate glucose flux through glycolysis.
4. Pyruvate kinase (step 10) catalyzes the final reaction in glycolysis. In this step, phosphoenolpyruvate is metabolized to pyruvate and ATP is synthesized. Because pyruvate is a common substrate to a number of metabolic pathways, this enzyme reaction affects many aspects of cellular metabolism.[40] Like other key glycolytic reactions, pyruvate kinase is allosterically regulated by barometers of the cellular energy state. ATP inhibits this enzyme step by reducing the affinity of the enzyme to its substrate. Similarly elevated acetyl-CoA levels as a result of sufficient nutrient fuel availability slows down this reaction.

Pyruvate dehydrogenase (PDH) is the enzyme step linking glycolysis (cytoplasm) to cellular respiration (mitochondria) (see Fig. 67-2). Under aerobic conditions, pyruvate enters the mitochondria still retaining more than 90% of the total free energy within the original glucose molecule.[35] Pyruvate is metabolized to acetyl-CoA, CO_2, and NADH by the enzyme pyruvate dehydrogenase,[51] the "gateway" into the mitochondria. PDH is a multienzyme complex consisting of three different catalytic enzymes and five coenzymes. Overall the reaction consists of five enzymatic steps in which hydrogen atoms and acetyl groups are transferred from one enzyme to the next by way of sulfhydryl groups located on the coenzyme lipoic acid. The conversion of pyruvate to acetyl-CoA is under complex regulatory control and is irreversible under cellular conditions. PDH activity is controlled by the energy state of the cell through feedback regulation. Inactivation of PDH is mediated through phosphorylation of the enzyme complex by PDH kinase. Inhibition of PDH activity occurs with elevated ratios of NADH/NAD^+, ATP/ADP, and acetyl-CoA/CoA. Change in the acetyl-CoA/CoA (redox) ratio has been implicated as the main regulator of PDH activity in skeletal muscle mitochondria.[59,60] Conversely, dephosphorylation of PDH by PDH phosphatase activates this enzyme complex.

Lipid Metabolism

Fatty acids are primarily oxidized by β-oxidation in the mitochondria, in which two-carbon units are removed sequentially from the carboxyl terminal. Free fatty acids (FFAs) must first enter the cell prior to oxidation. Entry of long-chain fatty acids into mitochondria is dependent on a membrane transport system for which carnitine is the carrier molecule. Medium-chain fatty acids and ketone bodies, on the other hand, enter the mitochondrion without carnitine. Within the mitochondrion, β-oxidation proceeds through a series of steps that result in cleavage of fatty acids at the β-carbon to produce acetyl-CoA and a saturated acyl-CoA two carbons shorter than the original. The acyl-CoA formed in the reaction reenters the oxidative pathway to undergo further degradation. Each set of oxidation reactions results in the production of one acetyl-CoA, one reduced flavoprotein ($FADH_2$), and one NADH. Acetyl-CoA subsequently enters the Krebs cycle and is metabolized to CO_2 and H_2O, while $FADH_2$ and NADH transport electron pairs to the electron transport chain.

Lipid metabolism is closely regulated so that lipid uptake or output for oxidation can be achieved as rapidly as required. Lipid from adipose tissue cycles continuously between triglycerides and FFAs.[39] The tendency for net triglyceride synthesis versus FFA release is regulated by plasma concentrations of specific hormones and substrates. When glucose and insulin concentrations are high (e.g., after a meal), lipoprotein lipase is stimulated, releasing FFAs from chylomicrons and lipoproteins. FFAs subsequently enter the adipocyte, resulting in the synthesis and storage of triglycerides. In contrast, in starvation, catecholamines and glucagon stimulate a hormone-sensitive lipase, resulting in a net breakdown of fat. FFAs are consequently released from intracellular triglyceride stores into the circulation and are either used directly by peripheral tissues as fuel for the Krebs cycle or transported to the liver to be converted to the ketone bodies acetoacetate, β-hydroxybutyrate, and acetone. Under circumstances of low substrate availability, oxaloacetate is channeled through gluconeogenesis to maintain serum glucose concentrations instead of being recycled in its reaction with acetyl-CoA into the Krebs cycle. As a consequence, acetyl-CoA accumulates in the liver and is used in the formation of ketone bodies. Ketone body formation occurs when two acetyl-CoA molecules undergo condensation to form acetoacetate. Acetoacetate is reduced to β-hydroxybutyrate in a reaction that oxidizes NADH to NAD^+. In this manner, despite the diversion of FFAs away from the Krebs cycle, the liver is able to continue oxidation of FFAs in the form of ketones. During prolonged starvation, up to 80% of fatty acids are converted in the liver to ketone bodies and provide more than half of the central nervous system's energy needs.[10] Ketone body formation is promoted by increased glucagon and decreased insulin. Ketone bodies acetoacetate and β-hydroxybutyrate are substrates for oxidative phosphorylation in most tissues, including heart, kidney, brain, and skeletal muscle, by reconversion to acetyl-CoA and subsequent entry into the Krebs cycle.

Protein Metabolism

Although typically protected as a fuel source, amino acids also can be oxidized in times of energy need. Ten of the 20 amino acids enter the Krebs cycle by way of acetyl-CoA in one manner or another, whereas others enter through various Krebs cycle intermediates, usually α-ketoglutarate and succinyl-CoA.

Body protein stores are in a dynamic state of turnover, continuously being synthesized and catabolized.[35] There is a high metabolic cost (between 10% and 40% of the resting metabolic expenditure) for this constant flux of amino acids. However seemingly wasteful this process appears, it actually is adaptive in affording the organism the flexibility to change protein structure and function in response to metabolic need.[35] The protein turnover rate is subject to significant hormonal and substrate influences.

Normally amino acid oxidation is far less than glycolysis or fatty acid oxidation. Consequently the contribution of protein to total energy expenditure is small. In starvation, however, decreased insulin levels permit increased amino acid release from skeletal muscle, chiefly as alanine, which feeds gluconeogenesis. In early starvation, this process is adaptive in providing precursors for glucose synthesis required by glucose-dependent organs.[11] However, after 4 to 6 weeks of starvation glucose oxidation is markedly reduced and amino acid catabolism diminishes as the central nervous system adjusts to utilizing ketone bodies for energy.[10,11] Such central nervous system energy substrate conversion is inhibited in stress starvation associated with systemic inflammatory response syndrome (interleukin [IL]-6, IL-2) (see Chapter 68).

Although amino acid oxidation is increased in stress states, it is rare for amino acid oxidation to account for more than 20% of total energy expenditure.[19] Critically ill, septic adult patients may lose up to 20 g of urinary nitrogen per day (125 g of protein), which at 4 kcal/g protein amounts to a loss of 500 kcal/day. Quantities in smaller infants and children are correspondingly less. Despite the relatively small contribution of amino acids to energy expenditure, the net metabolic cost of increased protein turnover, reflecting inefficient gluconeogenic cycling of carbon skeletons, incomplete oxidation of pyruvate, and urea synthesis, is high in terms of energy use and nitrogen loss.[2] Energy to fuel these and other metabolically expensive processes derives predominantly from β-oxidation of fatty acids.[46,49]

Step II: Generation of Energy-Rich Electron Carriers: The Krebs Cycle (Fig. 67-4)

The Krebs cycle is a vortex for carbohydrate, lipid, and protein metabolism. Acetyl-CoA is the primary entry port for metabolic fuels to the Krebs cycle, but α-ketoglutarate, fumarate, and oxaloacetate are other sites of entry, particularly for amino acids. The Krebs cycle is a series of redox reactions in which acetyl-CoA is metabolized to CO_2, and energy-rich electron carriers NADH and $FADH_2$. Electrons from NADH and $FADH_2$ fuel the electron transport/oxidative phosphorylation chain.[35] NADH provides the major source of electrons transported to the electron transport chain and is generated from NADH-linked dehydrogenase reactions in the Krebs cycle, as well as glycolysis, fatty acid oxidation, and amino acid catabolism. Thus along with its role as a portal of entry for nutrient molecules undergoing oxidative metabolism, the other primary function of the Krebs cycle is to extract and channel high-energy electrons to the final stage of cellular respiration.

The Krebs cycle is a "circular" pathway consisting of a series of nine redox reactions in which oxaloacetate serves as both the substrate and product. The first step catalyzes the formation of the six-carbon citrate molecule from the two-carbon acetyl-CoA and four-carbon oxaloacetate. This reaction is catalyzed by the enzyme citrate synthetase and is the rate-limiting step of the Krebs cycle.[35] Reactions 4, 5, and 9 are dehydrogenase reactions that generate a total of three molecules of NADH. An additional high-energy electron-carrying molecule is synthesized in the form of $FADH_2$ in step 7 of the cycle. With each "revolution," two carbon molecules (ostensibly acetate in acetyl-CoA) are cleaved from the six-carbon citrate skeleton, forming two molecules of CO_2 and regenerating the four-carbon oxaloacetate molecule. Guanosine triphosphate is synthesized in the sixth step of the Krebs cycle and is subsequently converted to ATP by the action of nucleoside diphosphokinase.

In summary, two molecules of acetyl-CoA (derived per molecule of glucose) enter the Krebs cycle and are oxidized in two "revolutions" to generate a total of six molecules of NADH, two molecules of $FADH_2$, and two molecules of ATP. The fuel substrate that entered the cycle as acetyl-CoA is completely oxidized to CO_2 and water.

Stage III: Synthesis of Adenosine Triphosphate: Electron Transport/ Oxidative Phosphorylation

The electron transport/oxidative phosphorylation chain is fueled by pairs of electrons originating from the molecules of NADH and $FADH_2$. Each pair of electrons proceeds from a higher-energy state to a lower-energy state down a series of electron-shuttling reactions, the respiratory chain. Molecular oxygen, the final electron acceptor, completes the electron transport chain by irreversibly accepting electrons from cytochrome aa_3 and forming water. The free energy released as electrons flow down the respiratory chain generates a proton gradient across the inner mitochondrial membrane. This electrochemical gradient (proton motive force) provides the free energy necessary for ATP synthesis.

The electron transport chain, located in the inner mitochondrial membrane, is a series of electron-carrying proteins arranged in order of an increasing tendency to accept electrons. Chemically it is a sequence of redox reactions located between the initial electron donor (NADH or $FADH_2$) and the final electron acceptor oxygen. The tendency for electrons to transfer from one protein to another reflects the difference in energy states between the electron donor and electron acceptor. Electron flow down the respiratory chain is associated with a large release of free energy ($-\Delta G \approx 53$ kcal/mol).[18] Four complexes of electron-carrying molecules (I, II, III, and IV) constitute the electron transport chain and are arranged in a specific sequence (Fig. 67–2). Complex IV is composed of cytochrome aa_3 and reacts directly with molecular oxygen in the third and final site of ATP synthesis. In this final electron transfer, molecular oxygen is converted to water. Three sites along the respiratory chain release sufficient energy to synthesize ATP (energy-conserving sites). Thus for each pair of electrons entering the respiratory chain, three ATP molecules are produced.

In 1961 Mitchell[42] proposed a mechanism by which the free energy released during electron transport is coupled to the synthesis of ATP. This mechanism, termed *chemiosmotic coupling,* recognized the membrane as an essential feature in linking these two processes. Since that time, the chemiosmotic hypothesis has been used to explain the transfer of energy during electron transport and oxidative phosphorylation. The three features essential to this mechanism are (1) a membrane-bound redox chain (electron transport chain), (2) a semipermeable "coupling" membrane (inner mitochondrial membrane), and (3) an ATP-synthesizing enzyme (ATP synthase)[43] (Fig. 67–5).

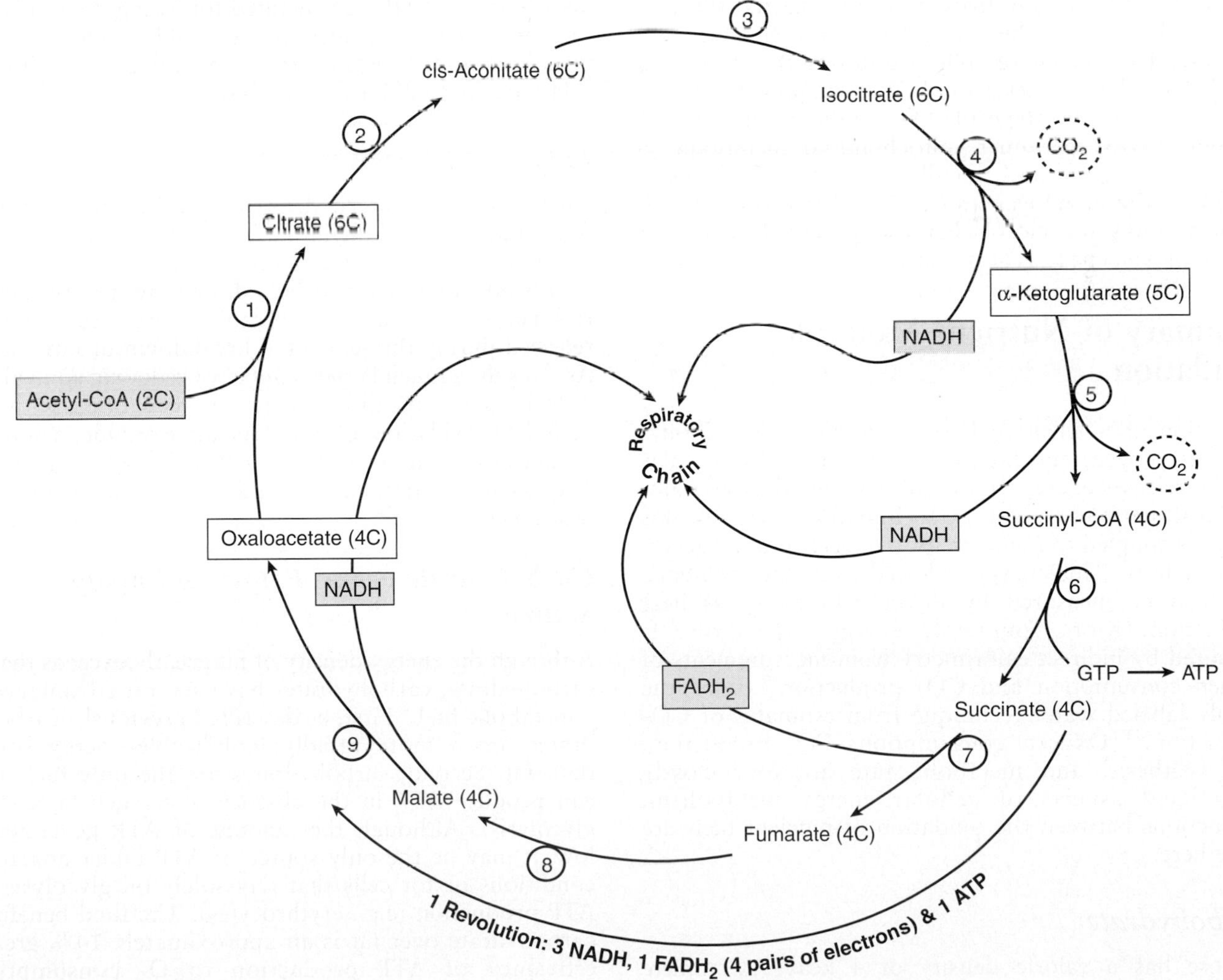

FIGURE 67–4 • The Krebs cycle is a series of redox reactions that generate the energy-rich electron intermediates NADH and $FADH_2$ as fuel for the respiratory chain. The Krebs cycle also functions as a common channel for all nutrient molecules entering cellular respiration.

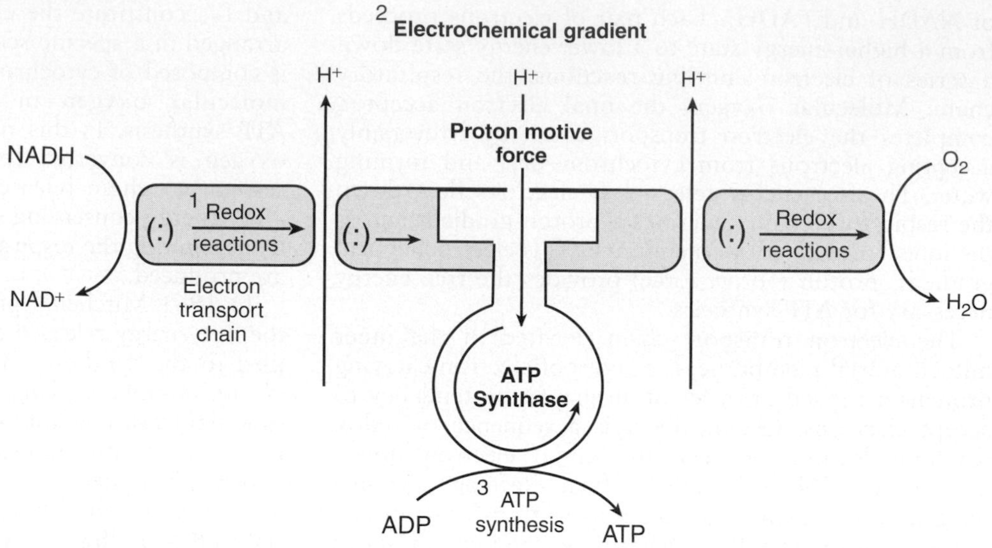

FIGURE 67–5 • Chemiosmotic coupling mechanism during cellular respiration. Components of cellular respiration include a "coupling" inner mitochondrial membrane and three bioenergetic mechanisms that transforms the potential energy of nutrient fuels into ATP synthesis: (1) redox reactions in the electron transport chain, (2) an electrochemical gradient, and (3) ATP synthesis by ATP synthase.

The free energy generated as electrons flow down the respiratory chain is used to translocate protons (H^+) from the matrix of the mitochondria to the outside of the inner mitochondrial membrane,[15] establishing an electrochemical gradient. Protons flow down the membrane electrochemical gradient and back into the matrix through specific channels in the ATP-synthesizing enzyme ATP synthase. The free energy released during this process is coupled to the synthesis of ATP from phosphate and ADP.[35] During this stage of ATP synthesis, the flow of protons across the inner mitochondrial membrane is directly utilized to mechanically rotate specific subunits of ATP synthase. In this manner, the rotary torque of ATP synthase links the electrochemical potential energy of proton movement to ATP synthesis.[22,48]

Summary of Nutrient Molecule Oxidation

Oxidation of nutrient fuel stores, particularly carbohydrates (glycogen) and fats, in the presence of molecular oxygen releases energy, commonly expressed as kilocalories (kcal) per mole of substrate. In biologic systems, this energy is coupled to the formation of ATP and the generation of heat. This energy, referred to as the *metabolic rate,* can be measured by direct calorimetry as heat production. More commonly energy expenditure is measured by indirect calorimetry from measurements of oxygen consumption and CO_2 production[38] or by the doubly labeled water technique from estimates of CO_2 production.[53] Oxygen consumption, CO_2 production, ATP synthesis, and metabolic rate are four closely interrelated aspects of cellular energy metabolism. Distinctions between the oxidation of nutrient fuels are made here.

Carbohydrate

Glucose has a caloric density of 4 kcal/g. Complete oxidation of glucose during aerobic metabolism yields 686 kcal and the formation of 38 moles of ATP[35]: $C_6H_{12}O_6 + 6O_2 + 38\ ADP \rightarrow 6CO_2 + 6H_2O + 38ATP$ ($-\Delta G$ = 686 kcal/mole). Twenty-four of the 38 ATP molecules are synthesized on complete oxidation of the two acetyl-CoA molecules entering the Krebs cycle. An additional 12 ATP are generated following the oxidation of four NADH molecules (two from PDH and two from glycolysis) in the respiratory chain. A net two additional ATPs are formed during glycolysis.

Fats

Fat has a higher caloric density (7 kcal/g) than carbohydrate and, when taking into account the amount of water required for glycogen deposition, fat has an eightfold energy advantage over carbohydrate in terms of kilocalories per mass. Thus considerably more free energy is released during the sequential breakdown of fatty acids. As a result, a much larger number of reducing equivalents NADH (close to three times) are generated with the complete oxidation of fats. As an example, complete oxidation of the 16-carbon fatty acid palmitate yields 2380 kcal, consumes 23 O_2, and generates a net 129 ATP molecules.

Carbohydrate versus Fat as an Energy Source

Although the energy density of fat greatly exceeds that of carbohydrate, carbohydrates have several advantages as a metabolic fuel.[6] First, as described previously, carbohydrates are a more rapidly mobilizable energy source than fat. Second, carbohydrates are the only fuels that can produce ATP in the absence of oxygen (anaerobic glycolysis). Although the amount of ATP generated is low, it may be the only source of ATP under anaerobic conditions or for cells that rely solely on glycolysis for ATP production (e.g., erythrocytes). The final benefit of carbohydrate over fat is an approximately 14% greater efficiency of ATP production to O_2 consumption. As noted earlier, complete oxidation of glucose consumes

6 moles of O_2 while producing 38 moles of ATP, an ATP production to O_2 consumption ratio of 3.1:1. In contrast, oxidation of palmitic acid generates 129 ATP and consumes 23 O_2, an ATP:O_2 ratio of 2.8:1.[6] Although the greater oxidative efficiency of carbohydrate metabolism over fat metabolism may seem small, this may be particularly advantageous under circumstances of low oxygen availability.

Regulation of Cellular Metabolism

(Fig. 67-6)

Cellular energy metabolism is closely regulated by the energy needs of the organism. Beginning as pools of potential energy, nutrient molecules are channeled through specific pathways and converge to the formation of acetyl-CoA. Acetyl-CoA in a reaction with oxaloacetate forms the six-carbon molecule citrate, from which high-energy electron intermediates (NADH) are generated in the Krebs cycle. Electron pairs flow down a series of cascading redox reactions, releasing sufficient energy to form an electrochemical gradient across the inner mitochondrial membrane. Electrical and chemical energy drive the mechanical rotation of the enzyme ATP synthase from which ATP is synthesized. ATP exits the mitochondria and provides chemical energy to perform work.

Mitochondrial oxidative phosphorylation is the primary energy-producing pathway under aerobic conditions, generating more than 95% of the total ATP requirements of the cell. The three constituents involved in the net overall reaction of cellular respiration include (1) ATP and its hydrolytic byproducts; (2) NADH, the endproduct of nutrient fuel breakdown; and (3) cellular oxygen, the final electron acceptor in cellular respiration (Fig. 67–6).[7,14,29] The net reaction of cellular respiration is given by the following reaction: NADH + H^+ + 3ADP + 3 Pi + 1/2O_2 NAD^+ + 3ATP + H_2O. Although the precise mechanisms that control cellular respiration are not fully understood, there is general agreement that these three components are the major regulatory parameters that control the cell's energy needs.[7,25,29]

ATp/ADP Ratio: The Cellular Energy State

The ratio of ATP to its hydrolytic byproducts ADP and Pi is an indicator of the cell's energy state and is the most important determinant of the cellular respiratory rate.[14] Synthesis of ATP in mitochondria is matched closely to the utilization of ATP by endergonic reactions.[1] ATP must be transported from mitochondria to the cytoplasm to be made available for cellular work. On the other hand, ADP must also be returned to the mitochondria from the cytoplasm for resynthesis of ATP. Adenine nucleotide translocase, located in the mitochondrial membrane, performs both functions. The transport process catalyzed by adenine nucleotide translocase is driven by the inner mitochondrial membrane proton gradient and accelerates with increases in cellular respiration. Thus adenine nucleotide translocase is an important enzymatic reaction controlling the overall rate of cellular respiration.[33]

Under normal conditions, the cell maintains an almost fully phosphorylated system, such that the ratio of ATP/ADP is approximately 100:1. Increased ATP utilization decreases the ATP/ADP ratio, increases ADP and Pi levels, and provides metabolic feedback to increase the rate of oxidative phosphorylation.[7,29]

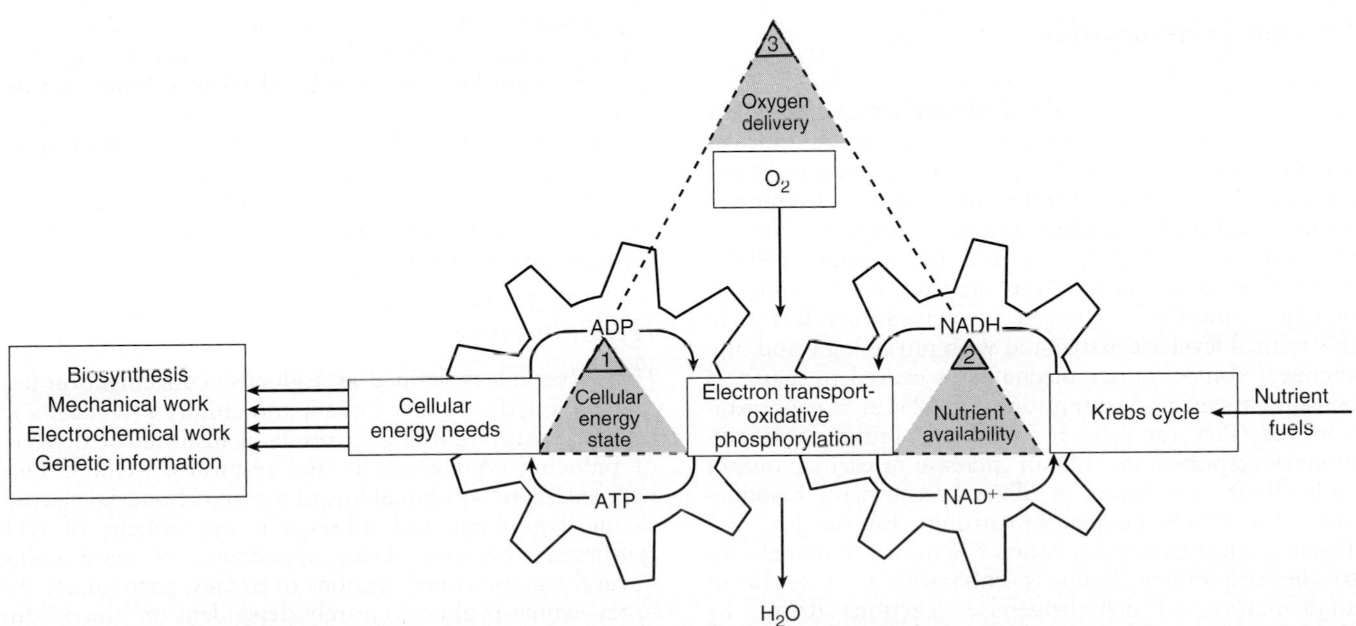

FIGURE 67–6 • Regulation of cellular metabolism. The three key components regulating cellular respiration are (1) the *cellular energy state* defined as the ATP/ADP and Pi ratio, (2) the availability of nutrient molecules *(redox state)* defined as the NADH/NAD ratio, and (3) oxygen availability. Flux of substrate through cellular respiration is influenced by the *supply* of nutrient molecules and the *demands* of work-related functions.

This feedback results in an increased flux of NADH and oxygen to the electron transport chain, supplying the necessary substrates required for increased oxidative phosphorylation.[14]

NADH:NAD$^+$: The Redox State (Nutrient Availability)

Oxidation of nutrient molecules (i.e., carbohydrates, fatty acids, and amino acids) generates NADH, the primary reducing agent for the respiratory chain.[1] The ratio of reduced NADH to its oxidized byproduct NAD is a marker of nutrient fuel availability and the redox state of the cell. Increases in substrate input (e.g., fatty acids) raise mitochondrial NADH concentrations and stimulate oxidative phosphorylation.[7,29] Similarly, increases in cellular energy demand (e.g., increased ATP utilization) are accompanied by an increase in delivery of NADH to the respiratory chain.[50] Reductions in NADH/NAD$^+$ and/or acetyl-CoA/CoA ratios, indicators of insufficient substrate and a reduced redox state, also stimulate NAD-linked dehydrogenase reactions in the Krebs cycle and in the β-oxidation of fatty acids.[7] Thus feedback control of dehydrogenase reactions in fatty acid oxidation and the Krebs cycle plays an important role in controlling the rate of oxidative phosphorylation.[7,45]

The overall rate of the Krebs cycle is primarily determined by the first step in which oxaloacetate and acetyl-CoA are catalyzed to form citrate by the enzyme citrate synthetase. Activity of this enzyme is enhanced by increased concentrations of the reactants oxaloacetate and acetyl-CoA and is inhibited by elevated levels of the product citrate and elevated ratios of NADH/NAD$^+$ and ATP/ADP. Other Krebs cycle dehydrogenase reactions that produce NADH and $FADH_2$ are subject to feedback inhibition by increased NADH/NAD$^+$ ratios as well.

Oxygen Concentration

Tissue oxygen delivery is an elaborate and highly regulated system. Oxygen proceeds down a partial pressure gradient, ultimately reaching its lowest level of approximately 3.8 to 22.5 mmHg in the mitochondria. At this point, 80% to 90% of total body oxygen consumption occurs. Although variable among tissues, the critical intramitochondrial PO_2 required to maintain cellular respiration at a constant rate appears to be approximately 1 mmHg.[14] Oxygen concentrations less than this critical level are associated with physiologic and biochemical compensatory mechanisms geared to maintain constant oxygen consumption and ATP at a concentration necessary for cellular viability.[14] Initial cardiopulmonary responses include an increase in cardiac output and minute ventilation, capillary recruitment, vasodilation, and altered hemoglobin affinity for oxygen.[9,31,54] Tissue oxygen extraction ratios rise and NADH delivery to the respiratory chain is enhanced as a result of augmentation of dehydrogenase reactions driven by changes in the NADH/NAD$^+$ redox state. These physiologic and biochemical responses maintain sufficient ATP concentrations.[14,65]

Extreme Substrate (Energy) Insufficiency: Oxygen Lack and Hypoglycemia

Oxygen Lack

Accompanying severe reductions in oxygen concentration, the cell makes a transition from zero-order to first-order oxygen kinetics and oxygen consumption becomes contingent on oxygen delivery (oxygen dependence).[14,56,65] Insufficient tissue oxygen concentrations result in enhanced synthesis of ATP by anaerobic glycolysis. Anaerobic glycolysis results in the conversion of one molecule of glucose to two molecules of lactate. In the final reaction of anaerobic glycolysis, pyruvate is reduced to lactate by lactate dehydrogenase, a step that reoxidizes NADH to NAD$^+$. Lactic acidosis that accompanies anaerobic glycolysis originates from the release of one hydrogen atom during hydrolysis of ATP.[44] The metabolism of one mole of glucose via anaerobic glycolysis generates 47 kcal and two molecules of ATP. Although anaerobic glycolysis is considerably less energy efficient, in the short term it can provide the cell with an alternative mode to reoxidize NADH to NAD$^+$ in the absence of oxygen and supplies a continued, albeit meager, source of ATP for cellular metabolic needs.

Early on, oxygen lack results in reduction of cytochrome aa_3[27] and decreases in oxidative phosphorylation and ATP synthesis. Reduction in the ATP/ADP and NADH/NAD$^+$ ratios increases cellular glucose uptake and induction of specific glycolytic enzymes that enhance the flow of substrate through glycolysis. This process is accompanied by an increase in lactate production.[32] Further decline in oxygen delivery results in overall decreases in ATP turnover and eventual hydrolysis of ATP by ATP synthase.[55] ATP and ADP are further hydrolyzed to their purine nucleotide products xanthine and hypoxanthine[26] as a means of extracting all available energy to meet metabolic demands. As oxygen concentrations continue to fall, mitochondrial membrane permeability increases (mitochondrial permeability transition [MPT]), diminishing the proton electrochemical gradient across the inner mitochondrial membrane.[36] Ultimately this process uncouples oxidative phosphorylation and severely impairs ATP synthesis, leading to loss of cell function and integrity.

Hypoglycemia

Hypoglycemia is defined as a glucose concentration less than 50 mg/dl in older infants and children. It results in cellular energy failure as a result of insufficient delivery of reducing equivalents to the respiratory chain. Like hypoxia, there is eventual loss of the mitochondrial electrochemical gradient and subsequent impairment of ATP synthesis.[21] Because of the importance of maintaining normal glucose concentrations to tissues, particularly the brain, which is almost entirely dependent on glucose for energy metabolism, it is not surprising that the organism has constructed an elaborate hormonal response to decreasing glucose levels that occurs long before hypoglycemia occurs.[4] Insulin levels decrease significantly at glucose levels of 80 to 85 mg/dl. Later, as glucose concentrations fall to 65 to 75 mg/dl, glucagon and epinephrine secretion is enhanced to increase glucose production through glycogenolysis.

Because of the importance of glucose for brain energy metabolism, a number of animal studies have examined the metabolic effects of hypoglycemia on the central nervous system. Characteristically, evidence of changes in brain energy metabolism occur at glucose levels of 40 to 45 mg/dl. At glucose concentrations less than 45 mg/dl, hexokinase is less than fully saturated and cellular glucose entry diminishes.[47] Using ^{31}P-nuclear magnetic resonance spectroscopy in a newborn piglet model, glucose levels less than 40 mg/dl decreased phosphorylation potentials measured as the phosphocreatine/inorganic phosphate ratio.[30] Further decline in glucose levels to 20 mg/dl resulted in energy failure as phosphocreatine/inorganic phosphate ratios dropped to <1. Electroencephalogram isoelectricity also occurs in severe hypoglycemia and is accompanied by an increase in NADH oxidation as a result of insufficient delivery of electron intermediates to the respiratory chain.[47] Prolonged hypoglycemia delays return of high-energy phosphate molecules and normal oxygen consumption despite normalization of glucose levels.

Bioenergetic Disturbances in Critical Illness

Disturbances in cellular bioenergetic pathways have been applied to better understand the metabolic aberrations in critical illness. A number of studies have demonstrated morphologic damage in mitochondria and functional derangements in hypoxic/ischemic and sepsis models.[16,23,37] *Cytopathic hypoxia* is the term used to describe the cellular energy disturbances leading to impairment of mitochondrial function and ATP synthesis.[23] Disruption in cellular energy metabolism may be secondary to any number of abnormalities consequential to the transduction and flow of energy during cellular respiration, such as reduced delivery of NADH or oxygen (see earlier discussion) to the respiratory chain, impairment of electron flow during electron transport, disruption of the inner mitochondrial electrochemical gradient, or direct impairment of ATP synthesis. Each of these mechanisms alone or in combination has been implicated in the bioenergetic dysfunction seen in critical illness, particularly sepsis (Fig. 67–7).

1. *Diminished NADH Availability:* Diminished NADH delivery to the respiratory chain may be the consequence of several different mechanisms: changes in nutrient fuel metabolism (see Chapter 68), interruptions of specific enzymatic steps in substrate metabolism (e.g., PDH), or impairments of NADH synthesis and /or consumption. Several animal studies have demonstrated impaired PDH activity in septic shock.[41,60,61] Elevated ratios of phosphorylated PDH (inactive form) to unphosphorylated (active form) because of increased PDH kinase activity have been implicated as one of the mechanisms causing reduced PDH function.[62] Consequently, delivery of glycolytic intermediates to the mitochondria is impaired and NADH synthesis is reduced.

Reactive oxygen species can result in disturbances of cellular respiration. The potent oxygen radical peroxynitrate, produced from the reaction of nitric oxide and superoxide, causes single-strand DNA breakage and results in activation of the enzyme

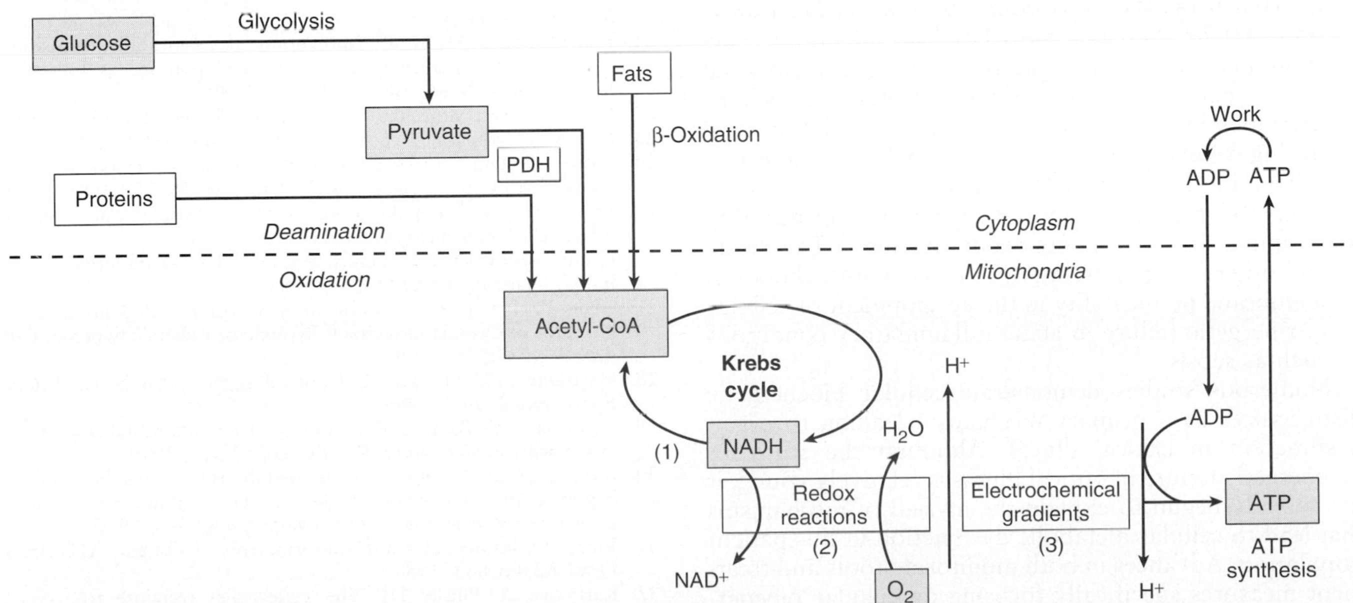

FIGURE 67–7 • Bioenergetic disturbances in critical illness. Bioenergetic disturbances affecting cellular respiration in critical illness include (1) insufficient delivery of NADH to the respiratory chain, (2) disruption of redox reactions in the electron transport chain, and (3) disruption of the electrochemical gradient across the mitochondrial membrane, all of which result in impaired ATP production. *PDH,* Pyruvate dehydrogenase.

poly(ADP-ribose)polymerase-1 (PARP-1). PARP-1 activation has been implicated in a number of pathophysiologic states, including anoxic/ischemic injury, hypoglycemia, and septic shock.[3,52,57,58,64] PARP-1 repairs DNA through a process that cleaves NAD^+ to ADP-ribose and nicotinamide, thereby consuming NAD^+ during the reparative process. Although this process repairs DNA, it ultimately may impair ATP production by depleting the cell of high-energy reducing equivalents (NADH) for the respiratory chain.

2. *Dysfunction of the Electron Transport Chain:* Dysfunction of individual redox reactions within the electron transport chain has been connected to disturbances in cellular metabolism, particularly in animal models of sepsis and anoxic/ischemic injury. Of these, cytochrome aa_3, the final step in the electron transport chain, has been examined most extensively. Several studies have demonstrated a discordance between the cytochrome aa_3 redox state and tissue oxygen levels. Using near infrared spectroscopy in animal models of sepsis, measurements of cytochrome aa_3 were found to be less oxidized, indicative of decreased cytochrome aa_3 function and impaired delivery of electrons to molecular oxygen.[12,24] Although the mechanism of cytochrome aa_3 dysfunction remains speculative, several reports have demonstrated that nitric oxide impairs cellular respiration by reversibly inhibiting cytochrome oxidase in competition with oxygen.[8] In addition, the formation of peroxynitrite from the reaction of nitric oxide with superoxide has been demonstrated to inhibit and/or injure complexes I, II, and IV and ATP synthase within the respiratory chain.[8]
3. *Disruption of the Mitochondrial Electrochemical Gradient:* Studies implicate disruption of the electrochemical gradient across the inner mitochondrial membrane as a mechanism of energy failure in models of oxidative stress and sepsis.[17,34,66] This disturbance, referred to as the *mitochondrial permeability transition (MPT),* increases mitochondrial membrane permeability and literally short-circuits the membrane electrochemical gradient across the inner mitochondrial membrane. As a consequence, formation of ATP during cellular respiration is disrupted. Cyclosporin, a potent inhibitor of MPT, has been demonstrated to attenuate the mitochondrial membrane permeability in animal models of acute endotoxemia.[17] This study and others suggest an important role in mitochondrial membrane permeability in the development of cellular bioenergetic failure in acute inflammatory conditions such as sepsis.

Numerous studies demonstrate cellular bioenergetic disturbances as a primary mechanism leading to organ dysfunction in critical illness. Although the study of bioenergetic failure in critical illness is relatively young, it has already begun to explain the myriad of mechanisms that lead to cellular metabolic dysfunction in this patient population. Advances in both monitoring tools and treatment measures specifically focusing on cellular bioenergetic disturbances undoubtedly will shed further light on the basic mechanisms of critical illness and organ failure.

REFERENCES

1. Balaban RS: Regulation of oxidative phosphorylation in the mammalian cell. *Am J Physiol* 258:C377, 1990.
2. Beisel WR, Wannemacher RW: Gluconeogenesis, ureagenesis, and ketogenesis during sepsis. *J Parenter Enterol Nutr* 4:277, 1980.
3. Boulos M, et al: Impaired mitochondrial function induced by serum from septic shock patients is attenuated by inhibition of nitric oxide synthase and poly (ADP-ribose) synthase. *Crit Care Med* 31:353, 2003.
4. Bolli GB, Fanelli CG: Hypoglycemic disorders. *Endocrinol Metab Clin* 28:1, 1999.
5. Brindle KM, et al: Studies of metabolic control using NMR and molecular genetics. *J Mol Recogn* 10:187, 1997.
6. Brosnan JT: Comments on metabolic needs for glucose and the role of gluconeogenesis. *Eur J Clin Nutr* 53:S107, 1999.
7. Brown GC: Control of respiration and ATP synthesis in mammalian mitochondria and cells. *Biochem J* 284:1, 1992.
8. Brown GC: Nitric oxide and mitochondrial respiration. *Biochim Biophys Acta* 1411:351, 1999.
9. Bryan-Brown CW: Blood flow to organs: parameters for function and survival in critical illness. *Crit Care Med* 16:170, 1988.
10. Bursztein S, Elwyn DH, Askanazi J, Kinney JM: *Energy metabolism, indirect calorimetry, and nutrition.* Baltimore, Maryland, 1989, Williams & Wilkins.
11. Cahill GF: Starvation in man. *N Engl J Med* 282:668, 1970.
12. Cairns CB, et al: Evidence for early supply independent mitochondrial dysfunction in patients developing multiple organ failure after trauma. *J Trauma* 42:532, 1997.
13. Cannon WB: *The wisdom of the body.* New York, 1932, WW Norton.
14. Connett RJ, et al: Defining hypoxia: a systems view of VO2, glycolysis, energetics and intracellular PO2. *J Appl Physiol* 68:833, 1990.
15. Cross RL: The mechanism and regulation of ATP synthesis by F1-ATPases. *Am Rev Biochem* 50:681, 1981.
16. Crouser ED, et al: Endotoxin-induced mitochondrial damage correlates with impaired respiratory activity. *Crit Care Med* 30:276, 2002.
17. Crouser ED, et al: Cyclosporin A ameliorates mitochondrial ultrastructural injury in the ileum during acute endotoxemia. *Crit Care Med* 30:2722, 2002.
18. Dickerson RE: Cytochrome c and the evolution of energy metabolism. *Sci Am* 242:137, 1980.
19. Duke JH, et al: Contribution of protein to caloric expenditure following injury. *Surgery* 68:168, 1970.
20. Eto K, et al: Role of NADH shuttle system in glucose-induced activation of mitochondrial metabolism and insulin secretion. *Science* 283:981, 1999.
21. Ferrand-Drake M, et al: Mitochondrial permeability transition induced DNA-fragmentation in the rat hippocampus following hypoglycemia. *Neuroscience* 90:1325, 1999.
22. Fillingame RH: Molecular rotary motors. *Science* 286:1687, 1999.
23. Fink MP: Cytopathic hypoxia. *Crit Care Clin* 17:219, 2001.
24. Forget AP, et al: *Escherichia coli* endotoxin reduces cytochrome aa_3 redox status in pig skeletal muscle. *Crit Care Med* 28:3491, 2000.
25. From AHL, et al: Regulation of oxidative phosphorylation in the intact cell. *Biochemistry* 29:3731, 1990.
26. Grum CM: Evidence of adenosine triphosphate degradation in critically ill patients. *Chest* 88:763, 1985.
27. Guery BPH, et al: Redox status of cytochrome a,a3: A noninvasive indicator of dysoxia in regional hypoxic or ischemic hypoxia. *Crit Care Med* 27:576, 1999.
28. Haymond MW, Sunehag A: Controlling the sugar bowl. *Pediatr Endocrinol* 28:663, 1999.
29. Heineman FW, Balaban RS: Control of mitochondrial respiration in the heart in vivo. *Annu Rev Physiol* 52:523, 1990.
30. Imai T, et al: Cerebral energy metabolism in insulin induced hypoglycemia in newborn piglets: *in vivo* ^{31}P-nuclear magnetic resonance spectroscopy. *Acta Paediatr Jpn* 38:343, 1996.
31. Jones DP: Intracellular diffusion gradients of O2 and ATP. *Am J Physiol* 250:C663, 1986.
32. Karimova A, Pinsky DJ: The endothelial response to oxygen deprivation: biology and clinical implications. *Intensive Care Med* 27:19, 2001.
33. Klingenberg M: The ADP-ATP translocation in mitochondria, a membrane potential controlled transport. *J Membr Biol* 56:97, 1980.

34. Kowaltowski AJ, et al: Mitochondrial permeability transition and oxidative stress. *FEBS Lett* 495:12, 2001.
35. Lehninger AL, Nelson DL, Cox MM: *Principles of biochemistry,* ed 2. New York, 1993, Worth Publishers.
36. Lemasters JJ, et al: The mitochondrial permeability transition in toxic, hypoxic and reperfusion injury. *Mol Cell Biochem* 174:159, 1997.
37. L'Her E, Sebert P: A global approach to energy metabolism in an experimental model of sepsis. *Am J Respir Crit Care Med* 164:1444, 2001.
38. Makk LJ, et al: Clinical application of the metabolic cart to the delivery of total parenteral nutrition. *Crit Care Med* 18:1320, 1990.
39. Masoro EJ: Fat metabolism in normal and abnormal states. *Am J Clin Nutr* 30:1311, 1977.
40. Mattevi A, et al: The allosteric regulation of pyruvate kinase. *FEBS Lett* 389:15, 1996.
41. Mela-Riker L, Tavakoli H: Mitochondrial function in shock. *Am J Emerg Med* 2:2, 1983.
42. Mitchell P: Coupling of phosphorylation to electron and hydrogen transfer by a chemiosmotic type of mechanism. *Nature* 191: 144, 1961.
43. Mitchell P: Keilin's respiratory chain concept and its chemiosmotic consequences. *Science* 206:1148, 1979.
44. Mizock BA: Controversies in lactic acidosis. Implications in critically ill patients. *JAMA* 258:497, 1987.
45. Moreno-Sanchez R, Hogue BA, Hansford RC: Influence of NAD linked dehydrogenase activity on flux through oxidative phosphorylation. *Biochem J* 268:421, 1990.
46. Nanni GJ, et al: Increased lipid fuel dependence in the critically ill septic patient. *J Trauma* 24:14, 1984.
47. Nehlig A: Cerebral energy metabolism, glucose transport and blood flow: changes with maturation and adaptation to hypoglycaemia. *Diabetes Metab* 23:18, 1997.
48. Noji H, Yoshida M: The rotary machine in the cell, ATP synthase. *J Biol Chem* 276:1665, 2001.
49. Nordenstrom J, et al: Free fatty acid mobilization and oxidation during total parenteral nutrition in trauma and infection. *Ann Surg* 198:725, 1983.
50. Oliver S: Demand management in cells. *Nature* 418:33, 2002.
51. Patel MS, Roche TE: Molecular biology and biochemistry of pyruvate dehydrogenase complexes. *FASEB J* 4:3224, 1990.
52. Pulido EJ, et al: Inhibition of PARS attenuates endotoxin-induced dysfunction of pulmonary vasorelaxation. *Am J Physiol* 277: L769, 1999.
53. Schoeller DA: Recent advances from application of doubly labeled water to measurement of human energy expenditure. *J Nutr* 129:1765, 1999.
54. Schumacker PT: Hypoxia, anoxia, and O_2 sensing: the search continues. *Am J Physiol Lung Cell Mol Physiol* 283:L918, 2002.
55. St. Pierre J, Brand MD, Boutilier RG: Mitochondria as ATP consumers: cellular treason in anoxia. *Proc Natl Acad Sci U S A* 97:8670, 2000.
56. Sugano T, Oshino N, Chance B: Mitochondrial functions under hypoxic conditions: the steady states of cytochrome c reduction and of energy metabolism. *Biochim Biophys Acta* 347:340, 1974.
57. Suh SW, et al: Hypoglycemic neuronal death and cognitive impairment are prevented by poly (ADP-ribose) polymerase inhibitors administered after hypoglycemia. *J Neurosci* 23: 10681, 2003.
58. Szabo C, et al: Endothelial dysfunction in a rat model of endotoxic shock: importance of the activation of poly (ADP-ribose) synthetase by peroxynitrite. *J Clin Invest* 100:723, 1997.
59. Vary TC, et al: Regulation of glucose metabolism by altered pyruvate dehydrogenase activity. I: potential site of insulin resistance. *J Parenter Enterol Nutr* 10:351, 1986.
60. Vary TC, et al: Effect of sepsis on activity of pyruvate dehydrogenase complex in skeletal muscle and liver. *Am J Physiol* 250:E634, 1986.
61. Vary TC, Martin LF: Potentiation of decreased pyruvate dehydrogenase activity by inflammatory stimuli in sepsis. *Circ Shock* 39:299, 1993.
62. Vary TC, Hazen S: Sepsis alters pyruvate dehydrogenase kinase activity in skeletal muscle. *Mol Cell Biochem* 198:113, 1999.
63. Vidal-Puig A, O'Rahilly S: Controlling the glucose factory. *Nature* 413:125, 2001.
64. Virag L, Szabo C: The therapeutic potential of poly (ADP-Ribose) polymerase inhibitors. *Pharmacol Rev* 54:375, 2002.
65. Wilson DF, et al: The oxygen dependence of cellular energy metabolism. *Arch Biochem Biophys* 195:485, 1979.
66. Zoratti M, Szabo I: The mitochondrial permeability transition. *Biochem Biophys Acta* 1241:139, 1995.

CHAPTER

68

Nutrition in the Critically Ill Child

Nilesh Mehta and Leticia Castillo

PEARLS

- Accurate assessment of nutritional status and provision of individually tailored optimal nutrition to the critically ill child are important but elusive goals of pediatric critical care. Malnutrition and obesity are prevalent in the critical care population and have a significant influence on the outcome of critical illness. Furthermore, the hypermetabolic stress response places demands on the critically ill child that must be met with evidence-based nutrient supplementation.
- Early enteral nutrition has been shown to decrease infectious episodes and decrease length of hospital stay in critically ill patients.
- Although widespread in its application, parenteral nutrition is associated with mechanical, infectious, and metabolic complications and hence should be used only in carefully selected patients.
- No conclusive data on the beneficial effects of immune-enhancing diets have been established. Proponents of immunonutrition argue that the inability to achieve goal volume of enteral feeds in most of the studies may be responsible for the lack of favorable effect on outcomes.
- Prolonged fluid resuscitation is a major factor hindering the achievement of estimated energy requirements despite maximizing the energy content of feeds. Other contributing factors are interruption of feeds for procedures, enteral feed intolerance, and cooling.
- If the necessary conditions are met, the doubly labeled water technique is currently the best method for estimating energy expenditure because expired gas analysis is not required and serial measurements of stable isotopes in urine samples provide an objective assessment of energy expenditure over a period of 4 to 21 days. However, the doubly labeled water technique for determining energy expenditure is difficult to use in critically ill children because it requires fluid balance in the steady state.
- The metabolic response to critical illness results in glucose and lipid intolerance and increased protein breakdown. This condition results in weight reduction and rapid loss of lean body mass. Supply of adequate nutritional intake under these circumstances is challenging, yet recovery of critically ill patients depends on their ability to utilize energy substrates and synthesize new proteins.
- Malnutrition in critically ill patients also results from a hypermetabolic state, which is a consequence of the stress response. In contrast to starvation, during the inflammatory response, supply of glucose does not reduce protein breakdown and nitrogen loss.
- During starvation, nitrogen loss can be suppressed by administration of glucose, which reduces gluconeogenesis and conserves nitrogen in proportion to the amount of glucose supplied. Therefore starvation protein catabolism is a reversible process if energy intake is provided. This characteristic differentiates starvation from a hypermetabolic state.
- Malnutrition is associated with increased physiologic instability and need for increased quantity of care in the ICU.

Critically ill pediatric patients frequently present with altered nutritional states. Malnutrition is prevalent among critically ill patients with a prolonged and/or protracted clinical course. Alternatively, severely overweight critically ill children with adult-type pathology are being admitted to the pediatric intensive care unit (PICU). Supply of optimal nutrition for the critically ill child is an important but elusive goal of pediatric critical care. Malnutrition in the PICU results from starvation because of poor nutritional support, but also as part of the hypermetabolic state often experienced by critically ill patients.[19] Nutritional intake in critically ill children must account for the complex demands placed by the hypermetabolic stress response.

Malnutrition in the Pediatric Critically Ill Patient

The prevalence of malnutrition in children admitted to the ICU has remained largely unchanged over the last two decades. An estimated 24% of children admitted to the PICU show signs of acute and/or chronic malnutrition on admission.[38] In addition, 84% of the PICU patients present with conditions that affect growth. Pollack and colleagues[70] reported 19% and 18% prevalence of acute and chronic malnutrition, respectively, in a cohort of children admitted to the intensive care unit (ICU) in 1982. Nutritional status affects physiologic responses and influences outcome. Malnutrition is associated with increased physiologic instability and the need for increased quantity of care in the ICU.[69]

Starvation

The initial adaptive response to fasting involves increased glycolysis, which is directed at maintaining glucose for the brain and other glucose-dependent tissues, including erythrocytes, bone marrow, and the renal medulla. Once glycogen is exhausted, free fatty acids (FFAs) are mobilized from fat stores, with production of ketones. Protein breakdown is increased to facilitate the release of amino acids, especially alanine and glutamine, from muscle and enhance gluconeogenesis so that glucose is provided for the brain and glucose-dependent tissues. Fatty acid oxidation provides energy for gluconeogenesis and other organ systems. Insulin acts as the major regulator of peripheral lipolysis and proteolysis, whereas the main effect of glucagon is focused on hepatic glycogenolysis and gluconeogenesis, stimulating glycogen hydrolysis and hepatic uptake of alanine. Alanine release from muscle proteolysis represents the major substrate for hepatic gluconeogenesis. Additional gluconeogenic substrates include glutamine, lactate, and glycerol. Lactate, the endproduct of glycolysis, may lead to glucose synthesis by way of the Cori cycle using energy derived from oxidation of FFAs. In addition, the glycerol derived from the hydrolysis of triglycerides is readily converted to glucose.

Survival during prolonged starvation requires a reduction in proteolysis and, therefore, a reduction in glucose utilization. This occurs with the progressive decline in the rate of gluconeogenesis, decreased metabolic rate, and increased ketone utilization by the central nervous system. The brain begins to metabolize more ketones and keto acids as starvation progresses and glucose availability decreases. As starvation proceeds and fat is mobilized for energy, progressively fewer fatty acids are fully oxidized, and metabolism is directed toward ketone body formation. In addition, the ketone bodies block complete oxidation of glucose by inhibiting the activity of pyruvate dehydrogenase, and this block likely plays a further regulatory role in the switch in energy substrate from glucose to fatty acids and ketones that occurs late during starvation.[59] Elevated ketone levels apparently inhibit amino acid catabolism, resulting in reduced output of alanine, thereby reducing hepatic gluconeogenesis from muscle-derived amino acids. Thus the requirement for glucose is reduced and protein conservation is enhanced. However, ongoing demand for some glucose continues. During prolonged starvation, the kidney becomes a significant source of glucose by means of gluconeogenesis using glutamine as a substrate. Alanine, the prime substrate for liver gluconeogenesis, and glutamine, the prime substrate for renal gluconeogenesis, both are derived from muscle protein catabolism. Increased ketone bodies provide a major energy substrate to replace glucose, especially for the brain. If starvation is not reversed, protein catabolism persists and involves all protein compartments, including heart, lungs, and intestine, resulting in significant organ dysfunction and increasing morbidity and mortality. During starvation, nitrogen loss can be suppressed by administration of glucose, which reduces gluconeogenesis and conserves nitrogen in proportion to the amount of glucose supplied.[64] Therefore starvation protein catabolism is a reversible process if energy intake is provided. This characteristic differentiates starvation from a hypermetabolic state.

Hypermetabolic State

Malnutrition in critically ill patients also results from a hypermetabolic state, which is a consequence of the stress response. In contrast to starvation, during the inflammatory response, supply of glucose does not reduce protein breakdown and nitrogen loss.[80]

Etiology of the stress response is multifactorial. Neuroendocrine profile, release of cytokines, and other molecular mechanisms influence the metabolic response to stress.

Neuroendocrine Mechanisms that Affect Metabolic Processes During the Stress Response

The stress response has been well characterized in other sections of this book (see Chapters 70, 84, and 95). Hence this chapter focuses on metabolic aspects of the stress response and its consequences. The stress response affects the nutritional and metabolic condition of the critically ill pediatric patient through a series of neuroendocrine responses involving increased autonomic sympathetic nervous system activity with release of catecholamines and increased pituitary release of a host of hormones, among these, adrenocorticotrophic hormone (ACTH) and growth hormone (GH) have well-established functions in the stress response. Release of these hormones influences the mobilization and use of nutrients as substrates. Release of catecholamines inhibits insulin secretion and peripheral insulin action and stimulates glucagon and ACTH production. Pituitary stimuli release ACTH with subsequent increases in corticosteroid production by the adrenals, which inhibit insulin activity. Cortisol acts directly on adipose tissue to mediate lipolysis and release of FFAs. Cortisol also influences the hyperglycemic state by (1) facilitation of amino acid mobilization from skeletal muscle, (2) stimulation of glucagon production, and (3) augmentation of catecholamine-induced hepatic glycolysis.[45] The stress response also induces release of aldosterone, with resultant retention of sodium and water, whereas stimulation of the posterior pituitary produces vasopressin, with resultant water retention and antidiuresis. The hypothalamus regulates neurologic (autonomic nervous system) and endocrine mechanisms (pituitary gland). Autonomic activity with regard to water intake, food intake, temperature control, and stress response is integrated at the level of the hypothalamus.[46] In addition, visceral sensory pathways and chemoreceptors play important roles in mediating the stress response.

Release of epinephrine results in increased glucose and FFA levels and suppression of insulin, which normally would increase in response to the elevated glucose level. Norepinephrine release results in a more moderate rise in glucose and FFA levels without a similar reduction of the insulin response. The mechanism of the catecholamine effect on insulin secretion has been related to the presence of both alpha- and beta-receptors on the pancreatic islet cells.[40]

Epinephrine and norepinephrine induce peripheral insulin resistance, which is an additional mechanism mediating hyperglycemia observed with severe stress. Catecholamines also induce release of glucagon. The elevated glucagon level acts on skeletal muscle to mobilize amino acids for hepatic gluconeogenesis. Therefore the combination of elevated glucagon levels and suppressed insulin levels may be of major importance in the regulation of hepatic gluconeogenesis and hyperglycemia in the critically ill patient.[87]

Although GH plays an important role in inducing an anabolic response during the stress response, the metabolic interactions between anabolic and catabolic networks are not well established.[51] Whereas administration of recombinant human growth hormone was shown to increase the mortality of critical ill adult patients,[83] strict glycemic control has resulted in increased survival (see Chapter 70).[48,88]

Cellular Mechanisms that Affect Metabolic Processes During the Stress Response

Another important mechanism of the stress response involves production of pro-inflammatory cytokines, which play multiple functions (see Chapters 84, 95, 96, and 97). The metabolic response to stress involves an altered balance among catabolic and anabolic systems. Proinflammatory cytokines induce many of the metabolic responses observed during stress. Tumor necrosis factor (TNF), interleukin (IL)-1, and IL-6 are among those mediators that exert major influence on regulation of energy substrate and protein metabolism, stimulation of lipolysis, and synthesis of acute-phase reactants by the liver. TNF-α, IL-1, and IL-6 all contribute to regulation of hepatocyte secretory protein synthesis, including fibrinogen, α_1-antiprotease inhibitor, and haptoglobin. TNF, IL-1, and IL-6 can also stimulate hepatic fatty acid synthesis.[33] Proinflammatory cytokines act through their membrane-bound receptors, which activate intracellular signaling pathways. Activation of nuclear factor-kappa B (NF-κB) leads to transcriptional activation of TNF-α and IL-1β in a positive feedback loop that leads to the secretion of these cytokines in various tissues (see Chapters 84 and 96). In skeletal muscle, IL-1β increases expression of the ubiquitin conjugating enzymes (E3 ligases) atrogin-1 and muscle ring finger protein-1 (MURF-1), which leads to increased ubiquitination and muscle breakdown. In addition, TNF-α increases reactive oxygen species (ROS) generation and enhances ubiquitination, which further augments muscle breakdown.[72] TNF-α inhibits insulin receptor–substrate interaction and mediates insulin resistance. Release of insulin-like growth factor (IGF-1) inhibits the IL-1β–mediated expression of E3 ligases and therefore reduces ubiquitination and muscle breakdown. However, the balance between anabolic and catabolic stimuli is altered during the stress response, with predominance of catabolic signals. Other cytokines, such as leptin and ghrelin, are released by adipose tissue and regulate energy metabolism; they also may be altered during the inflammatory response.[60] Leptin is a member of the IL-6 superfamily of proteins. It modifies gene expression and the synthetic pathway of appetite-stimulating (orexigenic) and appetite-suppressing (anorexigenic) molecules in the hypothalamus and, therefore, controls adipocyte energy stores. Ghrelin is the endogenous ligand of the GH-releasing peptide receptor and has anabolic effects. Both cytokines and the nervous system have the capacity to cause the neuroendocrine changes affecting the metabolic stress response.

Metabolic Consequences of the Stress Response

The metabolic response to stress involves alteration in protein and energy metabolism (summarized in Table 68–1 and Figure 68–1). Carbohydrate metabolism in the critically ill patient presents with insulin resistance and increased glycolysis, gluconeogenesis, and hyperglycemia. Extensive literature reports on the toxic effects of glucose exist.[47] Van den Berghe and coworkers[88] demonstrated increased mortality in critically ill, hyperglycemic, postoperative surgical patients. With regard to lipid metabolism, inhibition of lipoprotein lipase is mediated by cytokines,[61] hypertriglyceridemia, and increased lipolysis resulting in lipid intolerance. Protein metabolism is altered. Protein catabolism is increased with reprioritization of protein synthesis. This condition results in increased synthesis of acute-phase reactant proteins such as C-reactive protein, α_1-acid glycoprotein, haptoglobin, α_1-antitrypsin, α_2-macroglobulin, ceruloplasmin, and fibrinogen. Synthesis of these proteins in the liver or white blood cells

TABLE 68–1

Metabolic Characteristics of the Critically Ill Patient

Protein Metabolism	Glucose Metabolism	Lipid Metabolism
Increased protein turnover	Increased gluconeogenesis	Inhibition of lipoprotein lipase
Reprioritization of protein synthesis	Insulin resistance	Hypertriglyceridemia
Increased proteolysis	Hyperglycemia	Lipolysis
Lack of proteolysis response to administration of protein or energy	IGF-1 decreases; IGFBP-1 increases	

is mediated, at least in part, by IL-1.[24] The acute-phase protein response is nonspecific, and increased acute-phase protein concentrations are measurable shortly after the onset of stress response. Plasma concentrations of other proteins, including transferrin and albumin, decrease with injury or sepsis. This decline is not simply a result of decreased synthesis. In fact, in septic children the rates of both synthesis and degradation of protein increases.[13] The fall in albumin level results, in part, from an increase in transcapillary leakage. This is the result of increased vascular permeability promoted in part by TNF-1α and IL-1. Marked hypoalbuminemia in severe injury and sepsis is also related to large and frequently sustained increases in extracellular and extravascular water.

Increased release of glucogenic amino acids contributes to increased gluconeogenesis. Furthermore, protein breakdown is not suppressed by administration of adequate caloric intake. However, administration of protein increases protein synthesis without decreasing protein breakdown, but overall protein balance becomes less negative. With resolution of a hypermetabolic stress response, an anabolic phase typically follows, with increased release of GH and IGF-1. Supply of adequate nutrition is essential for this recovery phase.

In summary, the metabolic response to critical illness results in glucose and lipid intolerance and increased protein breakdown. This condition results in weight reduction and rapid loss of lean body mass. Supply of adequate nutritional intake under these circumstances is challenging, and yet recovery of critically ill patients depends on their ability to utilize energy substrates and synthesize new proteins.

Metabolic, endocrine, and immune responses are responsible for the increased resting energy requirements of critically ill children. Respiratory compromise involving loss of respiratory muscle mass; cardiac dysfunction and arrhythmias involving loss of myocardial muscle tissue; and intestinal dysfunction involving loss of the gut barrier contribute to the morbidity and mortality of critical illness. Protein breakdown may continue for an extended period of time, in an attempt to provide amino acids for gluconeogenesis and for production of glucose as the preferred energy substrate for the brain, erythrocytes,

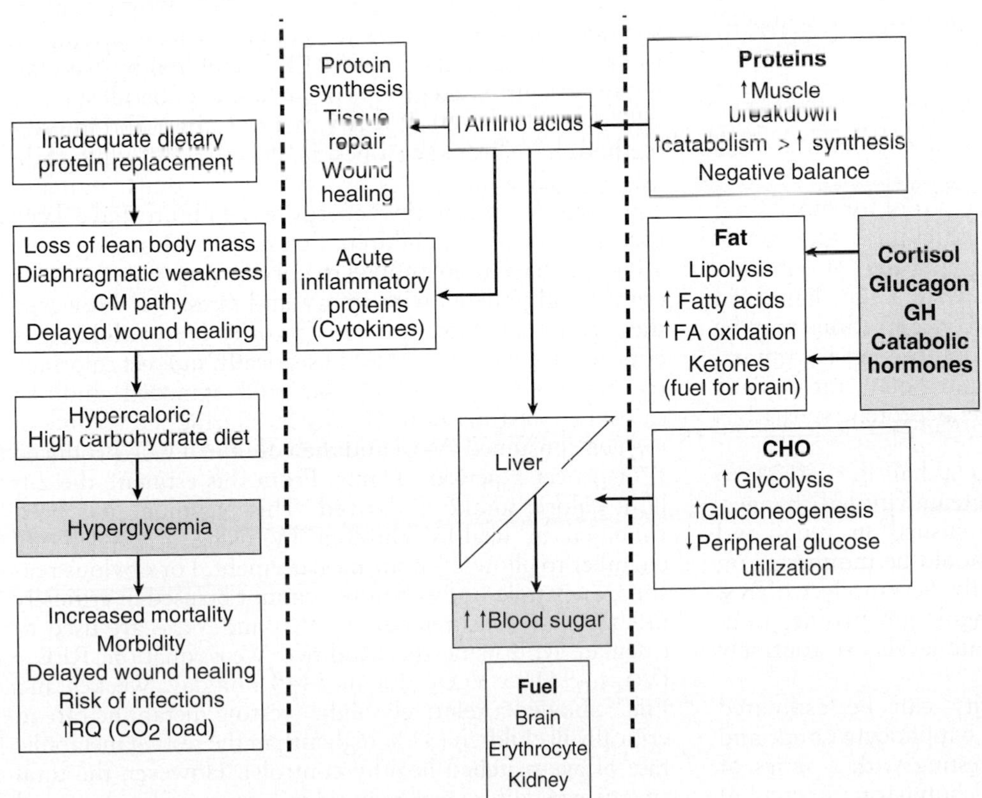

FIGURE 68–1 • Metabolic stress response. *CHO,* carbohydrate; *CM pathy,* cardiomyopathy; *FA,* fatty acid; *GH,* growth hormone; *RQ,* respiratory quotient.

and renal medulla. Tissue repair following trauma and surgical stress also relies on a continuous pool of amino acids derived from protein turnover. Increased fat oxidation reflects the premiere role of fatty acids as an energy source during critical illness. The beneficial effects of the acute metabolic response to illness/injury must be considered in relation to the harmful consequences of a persistently severe catabolic response. Critically ill children are particularly vulnerable to the harmful effects of a protracted catabolic state. Children have decreased glycogen stores and higher resting energy expenditure (REE) compared with adults. Nutritional therapy should aim to support the metabolic changes occurring during the acute catabolic stage and replenish the necessary substrates upon return to anabolism.

Assessment of Nutritional Status

Assessment of the nutritional status in the critically ill child is vital but challenging, and clinicians use a combination of anthropometric and laboratory data to diagnose undernourishment. Carefully elicited past history with details of weight gain, dietary history, recent illness, and medications allows identification of risk factors for preoperative malnutrition. Weight on admission to the hospital is important and may be the only measure of the actual dry weight before capillary leak syndrome results in edema and weight gain. Weight changes during the ICU admission should be interpreted in the context of fluid therapy, diuresis, and other causes of volume alterations. Physical examination should be directed toward specific signs of nutritional and metabolic deficiencies. Hair, skin, eyes, mouth, and extremities may reveal stigmata of protein-energy malnutrition or vitamin and mineral deficiencies.

Laboratory Tests

Serum albumin is frequently used as a tool for nutritional assessment in the ICU. Levels less than 2.2 g/dl reflect malnutrition. However, the long half-life of albumin (14–20 days) makes it less responsive to acute changes in nutritional status. Serum albumin concentrations may be affected by albumin infusion, dehydration, sepsis, trauma, and liver disease, independent of nutritional status. Thus its reliability as a marker of visceral protein status has been questioned.

Prealbumin (transthyretin) has a half-life of 24 to 48 hours and may reflect more acute nutritional changes. Prealbumin concentration is diminished in renal and liver disease. Chemistry profiles should be monitored on admission and repeated periodically. Serum electrolytes, blood urea nitrogen, glucose, coagulation profile, iron, magnesium, calcium, and phosphate levels are routinely monitored.

Adequacy of cellular immunity can be estimated through the measurement of total lymphocyte count and by delayed-type hypersensitivity testing with a series of common antigens (e.g., *Candida,* trichophyton, tuberculin)

Visceral proteins are rapid turnover proteins produced in the liver. Circulating levels of visceral protein are low in the setting of malnutrition, inflammatory states, and impaired hepatic synthetic function. Cytokines released during stress response modify liver synthetic activity, promoting the release of acute-phase reactant proteins. Acute-phase reactant proteins are elevated during stress and may be used to longitudinally monitor the inflammatory response.

Assessing Energy Expenditure in Critically Ill Patients

Recommendations for pediatric nutritional requirements have traditionally focused on the supply of nutrients for growth. Current recommendations for nutritional requirements of the critically ill child are derived from limited data, based on studies in healthy children and based on limited methodologic approaches.[62] Although the Food Agricultural Organization and the World Health Organization (WHO) have recommended that energy requirements and dietary recommendations be based on measurements of energy expenditure, such measurements are difficult to accomplish in the critically ill patient.

The components of total energy expenditure include (1) REE 70%, (2) diet-induced thermogenesis 10%, and (3) energy expended during physical activity 20%. The sum of these components determines the energy requirement for an individual. Previous recommendations for energy requirements were based on estimates of basal metabolic rate or REE derived by either indirect calorimetry or standard equations.[79,90] REE estimates have a large individual variability, and their estimation using the WHO predictive equations is unreliable, particularly in underweight subjects.[20,39,62] Newer equations have attempted to improve the prediction of REE in children by accounting for weight-based groups or including pubertal staging, with variable success.[35,62] A variety of direct and indirect methods have been developed as objective and valid methods for measuring energy expenditure in adults. Standard equations for estimating energy expenditure have been used in critically ill children. Stress factors ranging from 1.0 to 2.7 have been applied to correct these equations for critically ill patients with injury and stress.[22,85] However, these equations have not satisfactorily been validated in critically ill children.[16,18,68,85] Historically, indirect calorimetry has been regarded as the gold standard. Indirect calorimetry estimates the EE by measuring the volume of oxygen consumed (V_{O_2}) and the volume of CO_2 produced (V_{CO_2}) over a period of time. From this estimate the 24-hour caloric intake is derived. This technique has been validated in healthy children by using a whole-body chamber to allow 24-hour measurement. For obvious reasons, the whole-body chamber cannot be used in critically ill children. Measurements of V_{O_2} and V_{CO_2} are used to calculate REE using the Modified Weir equation: $REE = [V_{O_2}\ (3.941) + V_{CO_2}\ (1.11)]\ 1440$ min/day. Weekes and Elia[89] showed a relatively higher resting metabolic rate in critically ill children (37% higher than the resting metabolic rate of age-matched healthy controls). However, the total energy expenditure was reduced in a group of head-injured children receiving enteral nutrition.[89] Energy expenditure was noted to decrease over time and returned to normal after the second week of injury. It is difficult to determine the caloric needs of critically ill patients because many reported studies have been conducted on heterogeneous populations under various conditions. In critically ill mechanically ventilated children, use of sedation and muscle paralysis decreases the component of energy requirement related to physical activity,[30] and caloric needs in the critically ill child may be lower than previously considered. Indirect calorimetry may be unreliable or inaccurate in the critically ill child, in the setting of air leaks around the endotracheal tube, ventilator circuit, or through a chest tube. High inspired oxygen fraction ($FiO_2 > 0.6$) also affects indirect calorimetry. Therefore the use of indirect calorimetry in the critically ill patient is limited to a group of patients with lesser acuity of disease.

Another method of energy expenditure determination is based on the use of doubly labeled water. Stable isotope technique has been available for many years and was first applied for energy expenditure measurement in humans by Schoeller and van Santen[78] in 1982. Isotope studies using doubly labeled water have since been validated and following intense and skeptical scrutiny have now been established as a "gold" standard for total energy expenditure estimation with widespread application.[43,74–77] In this method, stable isotopes of water (^2H_2O and $H_2{}^{18}O$) are administered orally. They mix with the body water and the ^{18}O is lost from the body as both water and CO_2, while the ^2H is lost from the body only as water. The difference in the rates of loss of the isotopes ^{18}O and ^2H from the body reflects the rate of CO_2 production, which can be used to calculate the total energy expenditure. This method has advantages in children because of its noninvasive nature. However, isotope decay is measured over two half-lives of the isotope, and hence the technique only gives an average estimate of total energy expenditure over a period of a few days. Analytical errors in the mass spectrometric estimation of isotope enrichment, isotope fractionation during CO_2 formation or vaporization of water, and the calculation of total body water or respiratory quotient are factors that might introduce errors in the estimation of total energy expenditure with this technique. If the necessary conditions are met, the doubly labeled water technique is currently the best method for estimating energy expenditure because expired gas analysis is not required, and serial measurements of stable isotopes in urine samples provide an objective assessment of energy expenditure over a period of 4 to 21 days. However, the doubly labeled water technique for determination of energy expenditure is difficult to use in critically ill children because it requires fluid balance in the steady state. This is a major problem in the critically ill child with active capillary "leak" syndrome. Hence decreased urinary output, capillary leak syndrome, use of diuretics, or fluid overload exclude the use of this technique. The isotope costs and availability may be concerns, and the doubly labeled water technique cannot measure brief periods of peak energy expenditure. Estimated caloric needs for critically ill children are based on predictive equations for age, weight, and height and are corrected for a stress factor. Although not ideal, this is currently the best estimate of energy needs in critically ill children requiring ventilatory support with higher oxygen concentrations and/or air leaks.

Nutritional Requirements in Critically Ill Children

Estimating nutritional requirements in critically ill children are a challenging endeavor. Fluid balance is an important factor in the early phase of critical illness, and it limits nutritional intake. Intolerance to lipid and glucose administration and increased protein breakdown add to the challenge of providing adequate nutritional support. Yet recovery from critical illness requires adequate protein synthesis and metabolic support.

An initial prescription of a low-volume, concentrated formula with electrolyte content individually tailored to normalize any existing electrolyte imbalance is commonly used. Sodium, potassium, phosphate, magnesium, and calcium must be addressed in these calculations and should be frequently monitored in the critically ill child. Hypomagnesemia is associated with cardiac rhythm disturbances. Hypophosphatemia may lead to hemolytic anemia, weakness, and respiratory muscle dysfunction, prolonging efforts to wean mechanical ventilatory support. Renal failure may cause a rapid rise of electrolytes, such as potassium and phosphate, and must be accounted for when prescribing electrolyte requirements. Initial nutritional support may contain glucose in adequate quantities to supply caloric requirement. However, "adequate" caloric requirement is based on the needs of healthy children and corrected for stress factor. Hence, the adequacy of nutritional support is not based on direct data obtained in critically ill pediatric patients. Data have shown that excessive administration of caloric intake is deleterious. Normoglycemic control should be achieved and may require use of insulin, given the presence of insulin resistance. The role of tight glycemic control in adult ICU patients and its application in pediatrics are reviewed later in this chapter.

Ideally, calculation of initial nutrient requirements and its prescription requires careful assessment of (1) initial nutritional status and (2) extent of injury or insult during current ICU admission. Specific nutrient requirements (specific amino acids or fatty acids) or micronutrient requirements have not been determined in critically ill patients, adults, or children. Hence, evidence-based nutritional support for critically ill children is limited.

Protein and Energy Requirements (Macronutrients)

Energy Requirements

The role of caloric supply during the acute phase of critical illness has been examined, and investigators have proposed hypocaloric diets during this period.[58,66] Administration of high-calorie (glucose-load) diets in this early phase may exacerbate hyperglycemia, increase carbon dioxide generation with increased load on the respiratory system, promote hyperlipidemia resulting from increased lipogenesis, and result in a hyperosmolar state. Hypocaloric diets may have a protein-sparing effect and have demonstrable benefits in critically ill obese patients. Basal or resting energy expenditure may be calculated using existing standard equations such as the Harris-Benedict equation.[25] The addition of stress factor to account for hypercatabolism in the critically ill patient has been challenged because it may result in overfeeding.[62] It is uncertain if administration of lower caloric intakes are appropriate for the critically ill pediatric patient. However, overfeeding critically ill children is associated with net lipogenesis, hepatic steatosis, liver dysfunction, and increased CO_2 production and difficulty in ventilator weaning.[55] Obtaining accurate measurements by indirect calorimetry in ventilated patients is feasible, as long as FiO_2 does not exceed 0.6 and air leaks are not present. The optimal substrate required for maintenance of energy needs is mixed fuel (glucose and fat). The proportion of each varies according to the clinical situation. However, 55% to 65% of nonprotein calories are commonly provided as carbohydrates and 35% to 45% as fat. In the absence of adequate lipid supplementation in the diet, critically ill children, who have depleted lipid stores at baseline, are likely to suffer essential fatty acid deficiency.[67] Lipid administration is generally restricted to 30% to 40% of the total calories, and after an initial prescription of 1 g/kg/day it may be gradually increased to 2 to 4 g/kg/day, depending on the tolerance level. Triglyceride levels should be regularly monitored for lipid tolerance. Concentrated lipid formulas (Intralipid 20%) should be used, given the limitation on fluid volume for administration of nutritional support. Uncertainties about the ideal caloric regimen must be addressed by future studies. Table 68–2 lists the macronutrient requirements for healthy children.

TABLE 68–2

Recommended Energy and Protein Allowances

	Age (years)	Energy (kcal/kg/day)	Protein (g/kg/day)
Infants	0–0.5	115	2.2
	0.5–1.0	105	2.0
Children	1–3	100	1.8
	4–6	85	1.5
	7–10	86	1.2
Males	11–14	60	1.0
	15–18	42	0.8
Females	11–14	48	1.0
	15–18	38	0.8

From the Food and Nutrition Board, National Academy of Science, National Research Council, ed 9. Washington, DC, 1980.

Hyperglycemia in Critical Illness: Role of Glycemic Control

Hyperglycemia is present during the posttraumatic state and in critical illness.[19] The etiology of hyperglycemia during the stress response is multifactorial. The neuroendocrine response to stress is partly responsible. In addition, insulin resistance during critical illness is well established.

Data suggest a strong correlation between hyperglycemia and mortality.[47,50] The Leuven study demonstrated improved outcomes in a cohort consisting predominantly of postcardiac surgery patients in an adult ICU by implementing strict glycemic control using insulin infusion.[88] Insulin infusion was titrated in the treatment group to achieve arterial blood glucose levels below 110 mg/dl. Average blood glucose levels of 150 to 160 mg/dl were achieved in the control group in which patients received insulin infusion for blood glucose levels greater than 200 mg/dl. Mortality was reduced by 43% in the treatment group with tight glycemic control (Fig. 68–2). Significant improvements in overall hospital mortality, new-onset renal dysfunction, bacteremia, red cell transfusion requirement, and critical illness neuropathy also were demonstrated. Krinsley[48] successfully implemented a nursing-led insulin protocol, designed to maintain blood glucose levels below 140 mg/dl, in a heterogeneous cohort of adult ICU patients. The treatment group in this study had a 29.3% decrease in mortality compared with historical controls (matched for disease type and severity) without increase in the frequency of hypoglycemia or resources used. Although these two studies firmly established the correlation between glycemic control and intensive care mortality in adults, questions regarding the true mechanism(s) responsible for this beneficial effect and the ideal blood glucose level remain unanswered. The short-term actions of insulin, an anabolic hormone, are induction of protein synthesis, energy production through glucose uptake and oxidation, and energy storage through glycogen synthesis and lipogenesis. Some of these actions are mediated through the PI3K signaling pathway.[14] Compensatory hyperinsulinemia as a result of insulin resistance is mediated mainly through the (MAPK) pathway.[56] The long-term actions of insulin are mainly focused on differentiation and growth, also involving synthesis of transcription factors and translation, prenylation, potentiation of growth factors and anti-apoptosis, and differentiation of adipocytes and vascular smooth muscle cells.

Alternatively, an absolute or relative insulin deficiency results in catabolism with proteolysis and lipolysis. There will be a lack of adequate energy production, switching from glucose oxidation to lipid oxidation and utilization of ketones, which is a short-term compensation that becomes detrimental over a longer period. In addition, hyperglycemia has multiple detrimental effects, including poor healing, acquired immunodeficiency including a poor antiinflammatory response, dehydration, and electrolyte disturbances. The exact molecular mechanisms whereby insulin resistance occurs are not well elucidated, but alterations in the insulin signaling pathways have been suspected, mainly at the PI3K signaling pathway, which mediates the acute actions of insulin. Interestingly, the

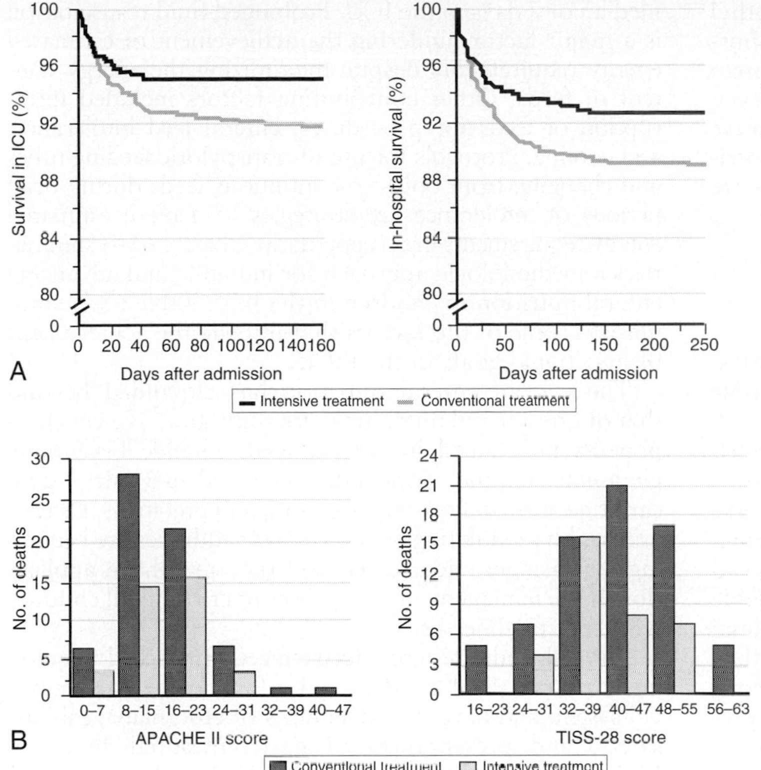

FIGURE 68–2 • A, Kaplan-Meier curves showing cumulative survival of patients who received intensive insulin treatment or conventional treatment in the intensive care unit (ICU) in the Leuven trial.[1] (From van den Berghe G, Wouters P, Weekers F, et al: *N Engl J Med* 345:1359, 2001.) **B,** Number of deaths in the intensive care unit according to the Acute Physiology and Chronic Health Evaluation (APACHE II) score **(top)** and the Simplified Therapeutic Intervention Scoring System (TISS-28) score **(bottom)** in the first 24 hours.[1] Higher APACHE II scores indicate more severe illness, and higher TISS-28 scores indicate a higher number of therapeutic interventions. (From van den Berghe G, Wouters P, Weekers F, et al: *N Engl J Med* 345:1359, 2001.)

MAPK signaling pathway, which mediates the long-term actions of insulin, remains unchanged during insulin resistance.[56] In addition, insufficient translocation of GLUT-4 transporters to the plasma membrane limits glucose uptake by adipocytes and myocytes. This insufficient uptake increases blood glucose, causing a compensatory increase in insulin by pancreatic B cells. Insulin resistance results in compensatory hyperinsulinemia and activation of prenyltransferases with increased activities of prenylated Ras and Rho signaling pathways and resultant potentiation of mitogenicity at different cellular targets, such as vascular smooth muscle and endothelial cells and inability to counteract growth factors.

Aggressive insulin therapy enhances the acute actions of endogenous insulin and results in improved protein synthesis, stimulation of energy production, and counteraction of the detrimental effect of hyperglycemia. However, the ultimate goal of therapy in the setting of insulin resistance is to improve insulin sensitivity rather than to increase the insulin dose with the goal of overcoming insulin resistance.

No data exist for similar benefits in the pediatric age group. The incidence of hyperglycemia in the pediatric intensive care population is high and is associated with increased mortality and length of stay.[23,81] A multicenter trial evaluating the beneficial role of an aggressive glycemic control in this population is being conducted. However, in the absence of definitive data, caution concerning the desired glucose level for pediatric patients is necessary.

Protein Requirements

Protein turnover is increased several-fold in critically ill children. Children have reduced macronutrient reserves with less than half the protein content of adults.[71] Furthermore, in response to acute stress, redistribution of amino acids from skeletal muscle to the liver (for gluconeogenesis), wound (for tissue repair), and other tissues for inflammatory response occurs. Increased net protein degradation has been demonstrated in the postoperative period and with extracorporeal membrane oxygenator support.[44] Supply of adequate proteins and energy intake improve protein balance by increasing protein synthesis, although protein breakdown is not affected. The amount of protein required to maintain a positive nitrogen balance may vary according to the severity of illness. Furthermore, the ideal amount and proportion of amino acids required during critical illness are not known. This is relevant because amino acids and other nutrients not only serve a nutritional role but also are actively involved in physiologic and pathophysiologic processes and may act as pharmacologic agents.[65] Nitrogen balance varied in critically ill patients receiving different amounts of branched-chain amino acids in parenteral formula.[27] Sulfur amino acid metabolism in septic children is impaired, and the rates of cysteine oxidation are decreased and plasma cysteine fluxes are increased, suggesting increased protein breakdown to supply cysteine and spared cysteine catabolism by decreased rates of oxidation.[53] Further studies to determine the individual requirement of specific amino acids under catabolic conditions are necessary, particularly in view of the important functions of amino acids, not only in protein synthesis but as signaling molecules[26,92] and precursors for important substrates such as glutathione[82] and methyl group donors.[52] Alternatively, excessive protein administration could be deleterious. Neonates with higher protein intakes have been shown to develop azotemia, pyrexia, and possible long-term detrimental effects on cognitive development.[28,29] Hence further studies on specific nutritional and functional requirements of amino acids are needed.

Micronutrient Requirements

Micronutrients play significant physiologic roles. Beneficial effects of micronutrients such as fat-soluble vitamins (A, D, E, and K), water-soluble vitamin (C), zinc, selenium, and folic acid have been described in selected groups of patients in well-defined settings. Presumed safety of micronutrients and probably exaggerated efficacy and generalized applicability to heterogeneous populations are factors that may be responsible for the widespread prescription of these compounds.[11] Commercially available antioxidant nutrients need to be scrutinized for optimal dosage and side effects in the clinical setting where they are most likely to be beneficial. Hospitalized patients, especially those with critical illness, currently receive these additives in accordance with Food and Nutrition Board recommendations for daily allowances.

Enteral Nutrition in Critically Ill Children

Early enteral nutrition has been shown to decrease infectious episodes and decrease length of hospital stay in critically ill patients.[93] Pediatric studies have shown successful implementation of early enteral nutrition.[9,10,15] Intolerance to enteral feeds may be a limiting factor, and supplementation with parenteral nutrition (PN) in this group of patients allows earlier optimal nutritional intake. In a subgroup of critically ill patients, total PN may be required for a period before initiation of enteral feeds. However, many studies have shown inability to achieve nutritional goals. In a study examining the endocrine and metabolic response of children with meningococcal sepsis, goal nutrition was achieved in only 25% of cases.[21,73] Taylor and colleagues reviewed nutritional delivery in a group of 95 children in a PICU over a 12-month period and made similar observations. Nutrition was delivered by enteral (54.0%) and parenteral routes (9.5%). Why doesn't this add up to 100%? Children received a median of 58.8% (range 0% to 277%) of their estimated energy requirements in this review. Enteral feeding was interrupted on 264 occasions to allow clinical procedures. Consistently underachieved enteral nutrition goals are thought to be responsible for the absence of beneficial effect in multiple studies and a meta-analysis of the efficacy of immunonutrition in preventing infection.[3]

Rogers and colleagues[73] reviewed nutritional intake in 42 patients admitted to a tertiary-level PICU over 458 ICU days. When actual energy intake was compared with estimated energy requirement, only 50% of patients had received full estimated energy requirements after a median of 7 days in the ICU. Prolonged fluid resuscitation is a major factor hindering the achievement of estimated energy requirements despite maximizing the energy content of feeds. Other contributing factors included interruption of feeds for procedures, enteral feed intolerance, and cooling. Protocols for use of transpyloric feeding tubes and changing from bolus to continuous feeds during brief periods of intolerance are strategies to achieve estimated energy requirements in this population. Figure 68–3 summarizes a methodologic approach for initiating and advancing enteral nutrition in children in the ICU. Table 68–3 summarizes some of the factors that impede the achievement of nutritional goals in the PICU.

The role of enteral nutrition has expanded beyond that of growth and nutritional rehabilitation. Newer components introduced in enteral feeds include L-arginine, glutamine, taurine, nucleotides, ω-3 and ω-6 fatty acids, carnitine, growth factors, probiotics, and prebiotics. Disease and health modulating effects of these additives are becoming increasingly understood, and they may have application in the management of a subset of critically ill children with specific illnesses.

Enterally administered feeds meet nutritional requirements in critically ill children with a functional gastrointestinal system and have the advantages of cost, manageability, safety, and preservation of gastrointestinal function. Early introduction of enteral feeds in critically ill patients helps to achieve positive protein and energy balance and restores nitrogen balance during the acute hypermetabolic state of illness. Enteral nutrition elicits release of growth factors and hormones that maintain gut integrity and function.[8] Despite its perceived benefits, current practice in ICUs indicates a significant proportion of eligible patients are deprived of enteral feeds.[36] An aggressive protocol for early intragastric feeding was applied to 71 critically ill children, using full-strength enteral formula started within 12 hours of enrollment and advanced to target volumes of energy intake.[10] In this study, increases in caloric intake were well tolerated by the children and reached predicted basal metabolic rate by day 1 and predicted REE by day 4. Children who were successfully fed had a lower mortality than those who did not respond to the early poststress intragastric feeding. The majority of children who did not respond to the early enteral feeding strategy were sicker and exhibited nonreversible septic shock and significantly lower ejection fractions on echocardiography.

Enteral feedings are indicated early in the course of critical illness if peristalsis has been established. Postpyloric feedings are recommended because of gastric distension and hypomotility. Feeds can be administered into the stomach or jejunum with the aid of feeding tubes inserted nasally or orally. Intragastric or intrajejunal feeding tube tip placement should be confirmed by radiography. Softer tubes constructed from silicone or polyurethane may be inserted using stylets at the bedside. Insertion of jejunal feeding tubes may require fluoroscopic or endoscopic guidance.

Postpyloric tubes provide the opportunity to feed a subset of children for whom intragastric feeding has not succeeded or is deemed unsafe. Postpyloric feeding is increasingly adopted to feed children with reflux or delayed gastric emptying who are at risk for aspiration. Placement is not always successful, and a variety of novel

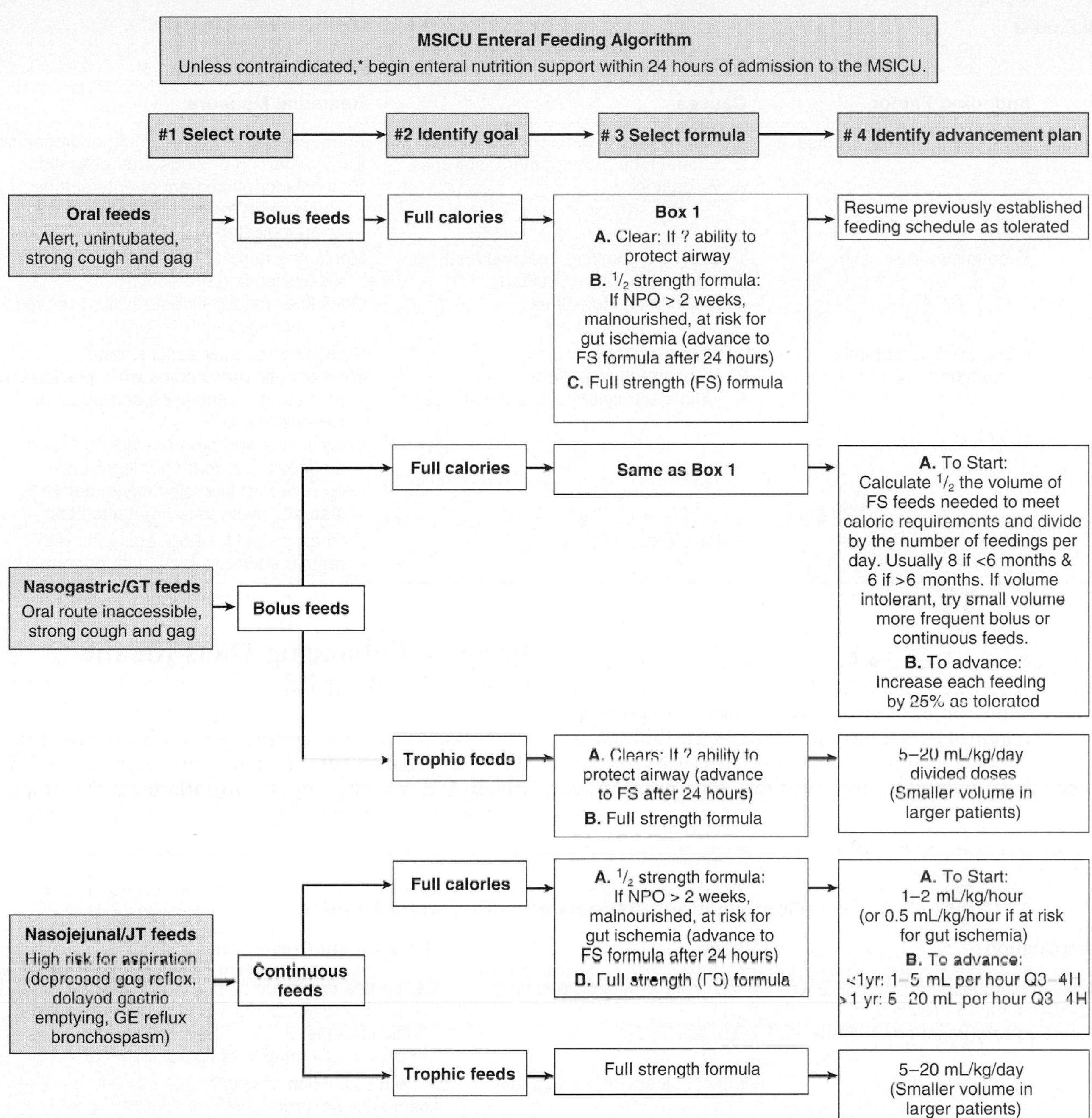

FIGURE 68–3 • Enteral feeding algorithm. Medical Surgical Intensive Care Unit (MSICU), Boston Children's Hospital.

techniques have been used to facilitate postpyloric placement. These methods rely on gravity and gut peristalsis to advance the tube tip past the pylorus. Because difficulty in tube placement can be anticipated in some patients, endoscopy or fluoroscopy guidance should be used, which avoids the rare occurrence of adverse events (such as perforation) and pancreatitis seen during blind enteral tube placement.

Surgical placement of gastrostomy or jejunostomy tubes allows long-term enteral feeding and administration of drugs in selected patients during intensive care and after discharge from the ICU. The advent of percutaneously placed gastric and jejunal tubes has minimized cost, time, and morbidity. Stoma site infection, obstruction, and tube dislodgment are common complications and must be identified and managed early. Tube tip malposition is frequently encountered with any of these devices either at placement or during the course of its use. Bedside screening methods for ascertainment of correct tip position range from auscultation during air insufflation

TABLE 68–3

Factors Impeding the Achievement of Nutritional Goals in the PICU

	Impeding Factor	Causes	Remedial Measure
1	Interrupted enteral nutrition	1. Procedures: diagnostic/therapeutic 2. Enteral tube placement/transpyloric vs. gastric	Adequate planning and timing of procedure Early restarting of feeds after cessation Protocols for placement of enteral tubes and support for transpyloric placement when indicated
2	Feed intolerance	1. Diarrhea, vomiting, residual feed 2. Acute abdomen: infectious/ postinflammatory/ileus	Monitoring narcotic use/early minimal enteral feeding protocols Guidelines for significant residual volume and management of feeds
3	Interrupted parenteral nutrition	1. Central venous access 2. Bloodstream infections 3. Fluid/electrolyte/glucose imbalance	Dedicated vascular access team Strict aseptic precautions while placing and accessing central lines dedicated for parenteral use Surveillance and prompt evidence-based diagnosis and management of BSI Daily review of fluid/electrolyte/metabolic status to allow parenteral alteration
4	Late initiation of feeds	1. Failure to prescribe	Protocol-based feeding regimens, with regular audit to assess unit performance

to ultrasound-guided tip localization. However, feeds should be held when malposition of tip is suspected; when in doubt, radiographic confirmation of correct tip position should be obtained before recommencing feeds. Table 68–4 summarizes some complications associated with enteral feeding and highlights intervention and prevention measures.

Immune-Enhancing Diets for the Critically Ill Child

In 1996, Bone and colleagues[6] outlined the role of the compensatory antiinflammatory response (CARS), which follows the initial proinflammatory response by the body challenged with an insult or infection

TABLE 68–4

Complications Associated with Enteral Feeding

Complication	Causes	Management/Prevention
Pulmonary intubation (sedated, muscle relaxed, or neurologically impaired children)	Incorrect placement/dislodgment	Appropriate technique Use radiographic/ultrasound/surgical assistance in difficult cases Immediate confirmation of tip position
Tip malposition in the gut	Incorrect placement/dislodgment	Correct estimation of length Adequately secured tube Screening tip position when in doubt
Accidental tube removal	Inadequately secured tube Noncompliant patient	Tube secured Exit marking on tube recorded at placement and checked Restraining for brief periods
Local inflammation, skin breakdown or infection	Poor stoma care Leaking stoma Tight-fitting tube	Prompt identification of any discoloration or skin breakdown at stoma at tube entry site Surveillance for skin integrity
Bowel obstruction/volvulus	Mechanical tube-related problem	Immediate surgical consult Discontinue tube feeds
Perforation	Repeated (blind) unsuccessful tube placement attempts Ulcer disease/friable gastric mucosa Stiff tubes/improper stylet use	Appropriate tube type and placement technique Abandon procedure when not successful after two good attempts Refer for surgical, endoscopic, ultrasound-guided technique Prompt recognition of perforation (monitor vital signs, abdominal examination, radiography) and surgical consultation

(see Chapters 95, 96, and 97). The antiinflammatory response was believed to be the second phase of a biphasic, highly coordinated inflammatory response and was aimed at keeping the proinflammatory response under control. It is clear that immunomodulation plays a significant role in the nature of response to infectious insult and impacts outcome in children with sepsis admitted to the ICU. Therapies aimed at modulating or stimulating the immune response have yet to be validated.

Immune-enhancing diets (IEDs) have been available for many years, and their role in the care of critically ill patients remains controversial. Table 68–5 lists immunonutrients and their key functions. An increasing number of studies examining the effect of IEDs in various clinical populations and related meta-analyses continue to provide conflicting conclusions. Methodologic flaws in conducting initial studies and the heterogeneous nature of the IED formulations used do not allow for dispelling current doubts regarding the safety and efficacy of these diets. The commercially available diets contain a mixture of compounds in varying doses, and the role of individual compounds is impossible to interpret. There are no pediatric studies evaluating the role of nutrition-based immunonutrition in critically ill children.

In a meta-analysis of randomized clinical trials examining the efficacy of enteral immunonutrients in adult patients, Heyland and colleagues[37] selected 22 human studies, which included 2419 subjects. There was no difference in mortality between the two groups, although patients who received enteral immunonutrition had a decreased incidence of nosocomial infections and decreased length of hospital stay compared with patients who received standard enteral formula. The authors analyzed a subgroup of 13 trials involving critically ill patients. Duration of hospital stay was decreased in the experimental arm in this subgroup (treatment effect −0.47 days; 95% confidence interval [CI] −0.93 to −0.01 days). When this subgroup of investigations was further subdivided into trials using experimental formulas with high arginine versus those using lower arginine content, mortality was noted to be higher in the studies using relatively lower arginine content formulas (RR 2.13; 95%CI, 1.08–4.21). A statistically nonsignificant trend toward decreased infectious complications in the high arginine group was reported. The high arginine group was associated with a shorter duration of hospitalization. This overview did not address the issue of the cost of intervention. Although an overall effect on mortality was not seen with immunonutrition intervention, some studies in the overview showed contrasting results. The study by Bower et al.[7] (n = 296) comparing IMPACT with Osmolite HN formula in critically ill adults demonstrated increased mortality (15.7%) in the immunonutrition (IMPACT) group versus control group (8.4%). A subgroup analysis of patients designated as septic at baseline showed that mortality in the experimental arm (IMPACT) was almost three times higher (11/45 [25%]) than that in the control arm (4/45 [8.9%]).

A multicenter trial comparing enteral immunonutrition with PN conducted an interim subgroup analysis based on some reports suggestive of increased mortality

TABLE 68–5

Commonly Used Immunonutrients and Their Key Functions

Nutrient	Comments	Key Functions or Effects
Arginine	Endogenous synthesis is decreased in trauma and sepsis	Precursor of polyamines and nucleic acids Precursor of amino acids involved in connective tissue synthesis Precursor of nitric oxide Secretagogue for growth hormone, prolactin, and insulin Increases number of T cells and enhances T-cell function Improves wound healing
Glutamine	Most prevalent free amino acid in the human body Synthesized mainly in skeletal muscle Catabolic conditions are associated with marked decline in skeletal muscle and plasma concentrations	Precursor of purines,pyrimidines, nucleotides, and amino sugars Precursor of glutathione Major metabolic fuel for enterocytres, colonocytes, and immune cells Most important substrate for renal ammoniagenesis Protects structural and functional integrity of intestinal mucosa Maintains or augments cellular immune functions, especially those associated with cell-mediated immunity
Branched chain amino acids		Precursor of glutamine
n-3 Fatty acids	Readily incorporated into cell membranes, often at the expense of the n-6 arachidonic acid Subject to ready peroxidation because of high degree of unsaturation (therefore important to maintain appropriate antioxidant status)	Antagonize production of inflammatory eicosanoids from the n-6 arachidonic acid Precursor of alternative family of eicosanoids, often with only weak biologic effects Antiinflammatory Can prevent immunosuppression in some situations
Nucleotides	De novo synthesis is impaired in catabolic states	Precursors of ribonucleic acid and deoxyribonucleic acid Protects structural and functional integrity of intestinal mucosa Maintains or augments cellular immune functions, especially those associated with cell-mediated immunity

in critically ill patients receiving immunonutrition.[5] Interestingly, the study was discontinued after the interim analysis. Analysis of 39 patients with sepsis or septic shock included in this interim analysis indicated mortality in the immunonutrition enteral arm (8/18 [44.4%]) was three times higher than that in the PN arm (3/21 [14.3%]).

Decreased length of hospital stay and decreased nosocomial infections in the treatment group were beneficial secondary outcomes reported by each of the three reviews/meta-analyses of studies examining the use of IEDs. In summary, no conclusive data on the beneficial effects of IEDs have been established. Proponents of immunonutrition argue that the inability to achieve goal volume of enteral feeds in most of the studies may be responsible for the lack of favorable effect on outcomes. ICU patients are heterogeneous, and timing of intervention may be important in this subgroup of patients. Severity of illness in some patients may not be amenable to manipulation by immunonutrients, and careful selection of patients is essential to demonstrate benefit in subgroups.

Future research should investigate the role of individual nutrients in select groups of patients. Dose response effect then identifies the essential components of immunonutrition at the correct doses. Future studies are required to prove if a critical volume must be reached in order to demonstrate a beneficial effect of these immunonutrients. Until then, generalized use of immunonutrition in broad ICU populations and children is not advisable. The immune-enhancing effect of individual components of these formulations has not been tested. Arginine, n-3 polyunsaturated fatty acids, glutamine, and nucleic acid concentrations distinguish the commercially available IEDs.

Arginine is a conditionally essential amino acid. It becomes essential in the setting of sepsis.[62] Subgroup analyses have shown that adult studies using immunonutrition solutions containing higher arginine concentrations (>12 g/L) are more likely to show a beneficial effect compared with studies with low arginine content (6 g/L) in IEDs.[37]

Glutamine is an abundant amino acid that may become conditionally essential during critical illness when demand outstrips availability. It may have significant immune-enhancing effects in addition to its role in tissue repair and integrity. Glutamine has also been added to enteral feeds as an immunomodulating agent. A Spanish study of 11 ICUs and 84 adult patients with active inflammation (predominantly septic) compared glutamine-enriched enteral feed with a control matched for nonprotein calories/nitrogen ratio. Although ICU mortality and length of stay remained unchanged, the incidence of nosocomial pneumonia decreased from 33% to 14%. Griffith reported improved survival at 6 months and decreased costs per survivor in the treatment arm of a study comparing glutamine-enriched PN to isonitrogenous and isocaloric control nutrition in 84 critically ill adults. Following enteral administration, there is a 50% splanchnic extraction of this amino acid, which attenuates its blood levels attained by this route. A large meta-analysis by Novak and colleagues[63] confirmed a larger benefit from parenteral administration compared with enteral glutamine intake. Overall, the studies investigating glutamine in IED have shown no major side effects, and this relatively inexpensive additive may be a promising immune nutrient in critically ill patients with anticipated mortality benefits in treatment groups.

Parenteral Nutrition

PN or hyperalimentation bypasses the gut, allowing intravenous administration of macronutrients and micronutrients to meet the nutritional requirements of the body, either partly (as a supplement to enteral feeds) or entirely (total PN). PN is indicated in children who are unable to tolerate enteral feeds for prolonged periods. In the setting of intact intestinal function, PN is not indicated if enteral feeds alone can maintain nutrition. Although widespread in its application, PN is associated with mechanical, infectious, and metabolic complications and hence should be used only in carefully selected patients. In minimally stressed children who cannot tolerate enteral feeds, peripheral PN may be the best option.

Fluid and electrolyte status guides the initial PN prescription. Fluid restrictions limit the amount of calories delivered despite use of a concentrated formula. PN should not be used for replacing ongoing losses.

PN should be prescribed daily and after reviewing levels of electrolytes and blood sugar in order to allow adjustments in the macronutrient and micronutrient composition. The patient's hydration, size, age, and underlying disease dictate the amount of the fluid to be administered.

Carbohydrates

Carbohydrates are the major nonprotein source of energy. D-Glucose is provided in the monohydrate form for intravenous administration and yields 3.4 kcal/g. The concentration of the dextrose solution should not exceed 10% for peripheral administration. In the setting of central venous access, a range of concentrations (5% to 40%) can be prepared. Higher glucose concentration makes the solutions hyperosmolar and may cause phlebitis or thrombosis and decrease the lifespan of the vessel when PN is administered peripherally through a vein. Blood glucose estimations must be followed carefully given the increased incidence of hyperglycemia, especially in young infants. Carbohydrate is started at 5 to 8 mg/kg/min. Gradually increasing the carbohydrate load allows appropriate endogenous insulin response and prevents fluctuations in blood sugar. Abrupt cessation of PN may result in hypoglycemia and should be anticipated and avoided.[49] Fat is supplied as intralipid, which provides the other source of calories in PN and reduces carbon dioxide production and water retention that is seen when carbohydrate is the sole source of calories.[2,54]

Amino Acids

One gram of protein yields 4 kcal. Initial recommended dosage range from 0.5 to 3 g/kg/day is based on age, disease state, and individual requirements. Usual concentrations available are between 1% and 4%, although patients with hepatic disease, renal insufficiency, and children with metabolic diseases (e.g., maple syrup urine disease) should receive appropriately modified concentrations. TrophAmine contains a higher percentage of branched-chain amino acids and a small amount of glycyl-cysteine. This solution is mainly used in the neonatal population. It is recommended and used in patients with hepatic encephalopathy and in children on long-term PN (e.g., short bowel), although data supporting this application are scarce.

There is an increasing interest in the use of glutamine in PN. Glutamine along with cysteine as glycyl-cysteine are precursors for glutathione, which is a major antioxidant. Glutamine is also a precursor for nucleotide synthesis, and although it is a nonessential amino acid, it can become conditionally essential, especially in catabolic states such as sepsis and trauma. Glutamine has a short shelf life. However, its applicability has been widespread. It has been introduced in PN solutions for its presumed benefits, such as restoration of protein and nitrogen balance, attenuation of gastrointestinal mucosal atrophy, reduction of bacterial translocation, and bacteremia after chemotherapy. The National Institute of Child Health and Development (NICHD) neonatal research network did not find significant differences in outcomes when a multicenter study randomized 1430 extremely-low-birth-weight neonates to PN containing 20% glutamine or an isonitrogenous control. However, pediatric burn patients have been shown to have deficient peripheral glutamine production. In a double-blinded randomized control trial, glutamine-enhanced PN reduced gram-negative bacteremia in severely burned patients.[31]

Lipids

Lipids are an integral part of PN and provide energy through fatty acid oxidation. Lipids are usually started at 0.5 to 1 g/kg and advanced to a maximum intake of 3 g/kg or a maximum 60% of total kilocalories. Lipid calories allow for lower concentration of carbohydrate (lower osmolarity of PN). Lipid emulsions are available as 10% (1.1 kcal/ml) or 20% (2 kcal/ml). Intralipid prevents or treats essential fatty acid deficiency. The total lipid usually is delivered over an 18- to 24-hour period through separate tubing using a Y connector near the infusion site. Delivery of amino acid, glucose, and lipid (three-in-one) is no longer recommended for neonatal patients because of the risk of calcium phosphate precipitation being obscured by lipid in the preparation.

Lipids are a crucial source of nutrition in parenteral formulas. Traditionally considered a calorie-dense nutrient and a source of essential fatty acids, lipids in intravenous feeding regimens have added advantages, such as providing a more balanced energy expenditure and facilitating better respiratory function parameters. Fatty acid derivatives are major biologic modulators.[12] The linoleic acid load, as a consequence of predominantly soy-based lipid in current formulations, results in increased arachidonic acid production and decreased production of eicosapentaenoic acid (EPA) and docosahexanoic acid (DHA).[42] Increased arachidonic acid levels may increase the proinflammatory cytokine production and activity. EPA levels may influence the production of antiinflammatory cytokines,[12] and DHA has been shown to lower blood pressure, improve endothelial function, and elevate levels of high-density and low-density lipoproteins.[91] Thus DHA and EPA, found in fish and fish oils, are essential fatty acids for humans. In an attempt to decrease the linoleic acid intake, soy-based oil has been partly replaced by medium-chain triglycerides, olive oil, or fish oil in intravenous emulsions. The metabolic roles of n-3 polyunsaturated fatty acids are emerging. Parenteral fish oils may have immune modulatory function and have been applied for their beneficial effect in the perioperative period following major abdominal surgery.[34,86] Further research examining the efficacy and safety of different triglycerides, derived from medium-chain triglycerides, olive oil, and fish oils, will allow their application in specific disease conditions. Furthermore, in this era of *nutrigenomics,* the effect of fatty acids on genes and proteins is being increasingly elucidated and will influence clinical practice. In the future, designer lipid formulations and molecules may be applied in parenteral or enteral nutrition regimens for their beneficial effects in specific disease conditions.

Electrolytes/Minerals and Trace Elements

All solutions typically are prepared with minimum acetate (i.e., all salts are added as chloride) unless prescribed otherwise. It is possible to prescribe an all-acetate solution with no chloride. Calcium and phosphorus precipitate when their concentrations exceed an allowable limit, related to the solubility index of $(Ca)_3(PO_4)_2$ and the pH of the solution. Selenium may not be routinely added to PN. A serum selenium level is obtained if a patient requires PN for more than 30 days without enteral intake. Multivitamins and trace elements are routinely added to the PN, and recommended intakes are elucidated elsewhere.[32] Heparin usage in PN is practiced in many centers and has been shown to decrease catheter-related sepsis.[4] Heparin in concentrations of 0.5 to 1 U/ml is thought to prevent thrombosis and possibly phlebitis in peripheral lines, although there are no controlled trials showing significant benefit of heparin usage in PN.

Biochemical Monitoring

A PN profile is recommended at initiation of therapy and weekly thereafter. The profile includes serum levels of sodium, potassium, chloride, glucose, carbon dioxide, blood urine nitrogen, creatinine, albumin, magnesium, phosphate, total and direct bilirubin, and transaminases. For children requiring PN for more than 30 days, selenium, iron, zinc, copper and carnitine levels should be checked. Daily vital statistics and routine anthropometry must be monitored to ensure adequate growth and development. Critical care units benefit from the expertise of a dedicated nutritionist, who should be consulted on a regular basis to guide optimal nutritional intake of patients.

Central venous access is required for delivery of hyperosmolar PN solutions into a large-bore vein with high-volume blood flow, to prevent thrombosis and phlebitis (see Chapter 15). The incidences of infective and life-threatening complications related to indwelling central lines have necessitated extreme caution with central PN use.[1,17,94] Central lines should be placed by experienced operators and line tip position confirmed by radiography before the lines are used for PN delivery. It is recommended that central line tips be positioned outside the cardiac chambers at all times. Central lines are recommended for delivery of infusates with osmolarity greater than 900 mOsm/L (10% dextrose, 2% amino acids with standard additives).

Nutritional Support of Obese Critically Ill Children

Overweight/obesity continues to increase in children and adolescents, and annual obesity-related hospital costs in 6- to 17-year-olds have reached $127 million per year. Overweight children and adolescents are increasingly being diagnosed with impaired glucose tolerance and type II diabetes, and they show early signs of the insulin resistance syndrome and cardiovascular risk. Obesity is a common medical condition affecting a significant number of critically ill children. Obesity can range from simply being overweight without associated major medical risk to morbid obesity with severe associated morbidity. Obesity is diagnosed in children based on body mass index (BMI). Even though the BMI z-score is optimal for assessing adiposity, it is not necessarily the best scale for measuring change in adiposity, as the within-child variability over time depends on the child's level of adiposity. Obesity is classified as follows: *overweight* BMI 25–30 kg/m^2, *obesity* BMI 30–40 kg/m^2, and *morbid obesity* BMI ≥40 kg/m^2. Centralization of body fat is associated with metabolic syndrome. Metabolic syndrome is observed in obese children and is characterized by visceral obesity, insulin resistance, and dyslipidemia. There is a high risk for type II diabetes and cardiovascular complications in patients with metabolic syndrome.[84] Grossly overweight patients are prone to sleep apnea syndrome, restrictive lung disease, venous thrombosis, musculoskeletal degenerative disorders, hepatic steatosis, and metabolic disorders associated with bariatric surgery.

The metabolic response to stress in obese critically ill patients is complex, given that it occurs in a population with preexisting major metabolic and endocrine alterations. In critically ill obese patients, the pattern of substrate oxidation is mainly protein and glucose, with decreased fat oxidation.[41] Extent of protein breakdown is greater than in nonobese critically ill adults. No data on metabolic abnormalities of obese children are available.

In the adult critically ill population, hypocaloric nutrition estimated for ideal weight has been recommended.[58] The limited adult literature suggest that protein requirements are higher in critically ill adult obese patients. It is recommended that fat be administrated sparingly, mainly to prevent essential fatty acid deficiency.[57] No data on the best nutritional support of critically ill obese children are available.

Drug–Nutrient Interactions in the Critically Ill Patient

Dietary components have a significant interaction with the pharmacokinetic and pharmacodynamic properties of various drugs used in the ICU (see Chapter 112). Considerations of wide ranges in body surface area and developmental changes influence drug distribution, metabolism, and dosing in the pediatric population. The nutritional status and intake in the critically ill child can impact absorption, distribution, metabolism, transport, and excretion of drugs. It is important for the pediatric intensivist to be mindful of these complex and not entirely predictable interactions. A dedicated pharmacist in the critical care unit is desirable to review the myriad of potential drug–nutrient interactions and has already become an indispensable part of a multidisciplinary critical care team. Table 68–6 summarizes mechanisms of drug–nutrient interactions.

Conclusion

Accurate assessment of nutritional status and provision of individually tailored optimal nutrition to the critically ill child are important but elusive goals of pediatric critical care. Malnutrition and obesity are prevalent in the critical care population and have significant influence on the outcome of critical illness. Furthermore, the hypermetabolic stress response places demands on the critically ill child that must be met with evidence-based nutrient supplementation.

TABLE 68–6

Mechanisms of Drug–Nutrient Interactions

Effect of Malnutrition and Nutritional Interventions on Drug Therapy	Effects of Drugs on Nutritional Status
Altered absorption of drug from gastrointestinal tract	Decreased appetite
Altered plasma protein levels and drug-binding capacity	Altered gastrointestinal mucosa, pH, and enzymatic function
Changes in GFR and clearance of drug	Decreased absorption and gastrointestinal motility
Tissue–receptor alterations	Induction of drug metabolism enzymes
Up-regulation of enzymes metabolizing drugs	Micronutrient deficiencies (folate deficiency)
Altered drug distribution (obesity with increased adipose tissue affects lipophilic drug distribution)	Altered plasma protein binding, receptor block, or competing with excretion
	Drug-induced fluid and electrolyte alterations

Interest in immune-modulating effects of nutrients, micronutrient supplementation, and the role of newer sources of lipid formulations has advanced the fields of enteral and parenteral nutrition.

The role of strict glycemic control in reducing mortality in critical care units has suggested a new standard of care in adult ICUs. Biochemical monitoring will allow safe implementation of the various macronutrients and micronutrients in the diet. Pediatric intensivists should be mindful of the various drug–nutrient interactions in the critical care population. In the future, patients will benefit from individually tailored nutritional regimens suited to the type and stage of their illness.

REFERENCES

1. Agarwal KC, Khan MA, Falla A, et al: Cardiac perforation from central venous catheters: survival after cardiac tamponade in an infant, *Pediatrics* 73:333, 1984.
2. Askanazi J, Nordenstrom J, Rosenbaum SH, et al: Nutrition for the patient with respiratory failure: glucose vs. fat, *Anesthesiology* 54: 373, 1981.
3. Atkinson S, Sieffert E, Bihari D: A prospective, randomized, double-blind, controlled clinical trial of enteral immunonutrition in the critically ill. Guy's Hospital Intensive Care Group, *Crit Care Med* 26:1164, 1998.
4. Bailey MJ: Reduction of catheter-associated sepsis in parenteral nutrition using low-dose intravenous heparin, *BMJ* 1:1671, 1979.
5. Bertolini G, Iapichino G, Radrizzani D, et al: Early enteral immunonutrition in patients with severe sepsis: results of an interim analysis of a randomized multicentre clinical trial, *Intensive Care Med* 29:834, 2003.
6. Bone RC, Grodzin CJ, Balk RA: Sepsis: a new hypothesis for pathogenesis of the disease process, *Chest* 112:235, 1997.
7. Bower RH, Cerra FB, Bershadsky B, et al: Early enteral administration of a formula (Impact) supplemented with arginine, nucleotides, and fish oil in intensive care unit patients: results of a multicenter, prospective, randomized, clinical trial, *Crit Care Med* 23:436, 1995.
8. Briassoulis G, Tsorva A, Zavras N, et al: Influence of an aggressive early enteral nutrition protocol on nitrogen balance in critically ill children, *J Nutr Biochem* 13:560, 2002.
9. Briassoulis G, Zavras N, Hatzis T: Malnutrition, nutritional indices, and early enteral feeding in critically ill children, *Nutrition* 17:548, 2001.
10. Briassoulis GC, Zavras NJ, Hatzis MT: Effectiveness and safety of a protocol for promotion of early intragastric feeding in critically ill children, *Pediatr Crit Care Med* 2:113, 2001.
11. Bristow A, Qureshi S, Rona RJ, et al: The use of nutritional supplements by 4-12 year olds in England and Scotland, *Eur J Clin Nutr* 51:366, 1997.
12. Calder PC, Deckelbaum RJ: Fat as a physiological regulator: the news gets better, *Curr Opin Clin Nutr Metab Care* 6:127, 2003.
13. Castillo L, Yu YM, Marchini JS, et al: Phenylalanine and tyrosine kinetics in critically ill children with sepsis, *Pediatr Res* 35:580, 1994.
14. Ceolotto G, Bevilacqua M, Papparella I, et al: Insulin generates free radicals by an NAD(P)H, phosphatidylinositol 3′-kinase-dependent mechanism in human skin fibroblasts ex vivo, *Diabetes* 53: 1344, 2004.
15. Chellis MJ, Sanders SV, Webster H, et al: Early enteral feeding in the pediatric intensive care unit, *JPEN J Parenter Enteral Nutr* 20:71, 1996.
16. Chwals WJ, Bistrian BR: Predicted energy expenditure in critically ill children: problems associated with increased variability, *Crit Care Med* 28:2655, 2000.
17. Collier PE, Ryan JJ, Diamond DL: Cardiac tamponade from central venous catheters. Report of a case and review of the English literature, *Angiology* 35:595, 1984.
18. Coss-Bu JA, Klish WJ, Walding D, et al: Energy metabolism, nitrogen balance, and substrate utilization in critically ill children, *Am J Clin Nutr* 74:664, 2001.
19. Cuthbertson D: Intensive-care-metabolic response to injury, *Br J Surg* 57:718, 1970.
20. Daly JM, Heymsfield SB, Head CA, et al: Human energy requirements: overestimation by widely used prediction equation, *Am J Clin Nutr* 42:1170, 1985.
21. de Groof F, Joosten KF, Janssen JA, et al: Acute stress response in children with meningococcal sepsis: important differences in the growth hormone/insulin-like growth factor I axis between nonsurvivors and survivors, *J Clin Endocrinol Metab* 87:3118, 2002.
22. Elwyn DH, Kinney JM, Askanazi J: Energy expenditure in surgical patients, *Surg Clin North Am* 61:545, 1981.
23. Faustino EV, Apkon M: Persistent hyperglycemia in critically ill children, *J Pediatr* 146:30, 2005.
24. Fleck A, Colley CM, Myers MA: Liver export proteins and trauma, *Br Med Bull* 41:265, 1985.
25. Frankenfield DC, Muth ER, Rowe WA: The Harris-Benedict studies of human basal metabolism: history and limitations, *J Am Diet Assoc* 98:439, 1998.
26. Gaczynska M, Osmulski PA, Gao Y, et al: Proline- and arginine-rich peptides constitute a novel class of allosteric inhibitors of proteasome activity, *Biochemistry* 42:8663, 2003.
27. Garcia-de-Lorenzo A, Ortiz-Leyba C, Planas M, et al: Parenteral administration of different amounts of branch-chain amino acids in septic patients: clinical and metabolic aspects, *Crit Care Med* 25:418, 1997.
28. Goldman HI, Freudenthal R, Holland B, et al: Clinical effects of two different levels of protein intake on low-birth-weight infants, *J Pediatr* 74:881, 1969.
29. Goldman HI, Liebman OB, Freudenthal R, et al: Effects of early dietary protein intake on low-birth-weight infants: evaluation at 3 years of age, *J Pediatr* 78:126, 1971.
30. Goran MI, Kaskoun M, Johnson R: Determinants of resting energy expenditure in young children, *J Pediatr* 125:362, 1994.
31. Gore DC, Jahoor F: Deficiency in peripheral glutamine production in pediatric patients with burns, *J Burn Care Rehabil* 21:171, 2000; discussion 172.
32. Greene HL, Hambidge KM, Schanler R, et al: Guidelines for the use of vitamins, trace elements, calcium, magnesium, and phosphorus in infants and children receiving total parenteral nutrition: report of the Subcommittee on Pediatric Parenteral Nutrient Requirements from the Committee on Clinical Practice Issues of the American Society for Clinical Nutrition, *Am J Clin Nutr* 48:1324, 1988.
33. Hardin TC: Cytokine mediators of malnutrition: clinical implications, *Nutr Clin Pract* 8:55, 1993.
34. Heller AR, Rossel T, Gottschlich B, et al: Omega-3 fatty acids improve liver and pancreas function in postoperative cancer patients, *Int J Cancer* 111:611, 2004.
35. Henry CJ, Dyer S, Ghusain-Choueiri A: New equations to estimate basal metabolic rate in children aged 10-15 years, *Eur J Clin Nutr* 53:134, 1999.
36. Heyland DK, Cook DJ, Guyatt GH: Enteral nutrition in the critically ill patient: a critical review of the evidence, *Intensive Care Med* 19:435, 1993.
37. Heyland DK, Novak F, Drover JW, et al: Should immunonutrition become routine in critically ill patients? A systematic review of the evidence, *JAMA* 286:944, 2001.
38. Hulst J, Joosten K, Zimmermann L, et al: Malnutrition in critically ill children: from admission to 6 months after discharge, *Clin Nutr* 23:223, 2004.
39. Hunter DC, Jaksic T, Lewis D, et al: Resting energy expenditure in the critically ill: estimations versus measurement, *Br J Surg* 75:875, 1988.
40. Iversen J: Adrenergic receptors and the secretion of glucagon and insulin from the isolated, perfused canine pancreas, *J Clin Invest* 52:2102, 1973.
41. Jeevanandam M, Young DH, Schiller WR: Obesity and the metabolic response to severe multiple trauma in man, *J Clin Invest* 87:262, 1991.
42. Jensen CL, Chen H, Fraley JK, et al: Biochemical effects of dietary linoleic/alpha-linolenic acid ratio in term infants, *Lipids* 31:107, 1996.
43. Jones PJ, Winthrop AL, Schoeller DA, et al: Validation of doubly labeled water for assessing energy expenditure in infants, *Pediatr Res* 21:242, 1987.
44. Keshen TH, Miller RG, Jahoor F, et al: Stable isotopic quantitation of protein metabolism and energy expenditure in neonates on- and post-extracorporeal life support, *J Pediatr Surg* 32:958, 1997.

45. Kinney JM, Elwyn DH: Protein metabolism and injury, *Annu Rev Nutr* 3:433, 1983.
46. Koizumi K MC: The autonomic nervous system and its role in controlling visceral activities. In VB M, editor: *Medical physiology.* St Louis, 1974, Mosby.
47. Krinsley JS: Association between hyperglycemia and increased hospital mortality in a heterogeneous population of critically ill patients, *Mayo Clin Proc* 78:1471, 2003.
48. Krinsley JS: Effect of an intensive glucose management protocol on the mortality of critically ill adult patients, *Mayo Clin Proc* 79: 992, 2004.
49. Krzywda EA, Andris DA, Whipple JK, et al: Glucose response to abrupt initiation and discontinuation of total parenteral nutrition, *JPEN J Parenter Enteral Nutr* 17:64, 1993.
50. Laird AM, Miller PR, Kilgo PD, et al: Relationship of early hyperglycemia to mortality in trauma patients, *J Trauma* 56:1058, 2004.
51. Lang CH, Frost RA: Role of growth hormone, insulin-like growth factor-I, and insulin-like growth factor binding proteins in the catabolic response to injury and infection, *Curr Opin Clin Nutr Metab Care* 5:271, 2002.
52. Leiper J, Vallance P: Biological significance of endogenous methylarginines that inhibit nitric oxide synthases, *Cardiovasc Res* 43: 542, 1999.
53. Lyons J, Rauh-Pfeiffer A, Ming-Yu Y, et al: Cysteine metabolism and whole blood glutathione synthesis in septic pediatric patients, *Crit Care Med* 29:870, 2001.
54. Macfie J, Smith RC, Hill GL: Glucose or fat as a nonprotein energy source? A controlled clinical trial in gastroenterological patients requiring intravenous nutrition, *Gastroenterology* 80:103, 1981.
55. MacIntyre NR, Cook DJ, Ely EW, Jr, et al: Evidence-based guidelines for weaning and discontinuing ventilatory support: a collective task force facilitated by the American College of Chest Physicians; the American Association for Respiratory Care; and the American College of Critical Care Medicine, *Chest* 120:375S, 2001.
56. Martinez-deMena R, Obregon MJ: Insulin increases the adrenergic stimulation of 5′ deiodinase activity and mRNA expression in rat brown adipocytes; role of MAPK and PI3K, *J Mol Endocrinol* 34:139, 2005.
57. McCarthy MC, Cottam GL, Turner WW, Jr: Essential fatty acid deficiency in critically ill surgical patients, *Am J Surg* 142:747, 1981.
58. McCowen KC, Friel C, Sternberg J, et al: Hypocaloric total parenteral nutrition: effectiveness in prevention of hyperglycemia and infectious complications—a randomized clinical trial, *Crit Care Med* 28:3606, 2000.
59. McGarry JD, Foster DW: Regulation of ketogenesis and clinical aspects of the ketotic state, *Metabolism* 21:471, 1972.
60. Meier U, Gressner AM: Endocrine regulation of energy metabolism: review of pathobiochemical and clinical chemical aspects of leptin, ghrelin, adiponectin, and resistin, *Clin Chem* 50:1511, 2004.
61. Muhammad TS, Hughes TR, Cryer A, et al: Regulation of macrophage lipoprotein lipase by cytokines, *Biochem Soc Trans* 26:S253, 1998.
62. Muller MJ, Bosy-Westphal A, Klaus S, et al: World Health Organization equations have shortcomings for predicting resting energy expenditure in persons from a modern, affluent population: generation of a new reference standard from a retrospective analysis of a German database of resting energy expenditure, *Am J Clin Nutr* 80:1379, 2004.
63. Novak F, Heyland DK, Avenell A, et al: Glutamine supplementation in serious illness: a systematic review of the evidence, *Crit Care Med* 30:2022, 2002.
64. O'Connell RC, Morgan AP, Aoki TT, et al: Nitrogen conservation in starvation: graded responses to intravenous glucose, *J Clin Endocrinol Metab* 39:555, 1974.
65. Palmer RH: Lipid-lowering drugs and low-fat diets, *Curr Concepts Nutr* 12:101, 1983.
66. Patino JF, de Pimiento SE, Vergara A, et al: Hypocaloric support in the critically ill, *World J Surg* 23:553, 1999.
67. Paulsrud JR, Pensler L, Whitten CF, et al: Essential fatty acid deficiency in infants induced by fat-free intravenous feeding, *Am J Clin Nutr* 25:897, 1972.
68. Phillips R, Ott L, Young B, et al: Nutritional support and measured energy expenditure of the child and adolescent with head injury, *J Neurosurg* 67:846, 1987.
69. Pollack MM, Ruttimann UE, Wiley JS: Nutritional depletions in critically ill children: associations with physiologic instability and increased quantity of care, *JPEN J Parenter Enteral Nutr* 9:309, 1985.
70. Pollack MM, Wiley JS, Kanter R, et al: Malnutrition in critically ill infants and children, *JPEN J Parenter Enteral Nutr* 6:20, 1982.
71. Reichman B, Chessex P, Verellen G, et al: Dietary composition and macronutrient storage in preterm infants, *Pediatrics* 72:322, 1983.
72. Reid MB, Li YP: Tumor necrosis factor-alpha and muscle wasting: a cellular perspective, *Respir Res* 2:269, 2001.
73. Rogers EJ, Gilbertson HR, Heine RG, et al: Barriers to adequate nutrition in critically ill children, *Nutrition* 19:865, 2003.
74. Schoeller DA: Recent advances from application of doubly labeled water to measurement of human energy expenditure, *J Nutr* 129:1765, 1999.
75. Schoeller DA, Hnilicka JM: Reliability of the doubly labeled water method for the measurement of total daily energy expenditure in free-living subjects, *J Nutr* 126:348S, 1996.
76. Schoeller DA, Kushner RF, Jones PJ: Validation of doubly labeled water for measuring energy expenditure during parenteral nutrition, *Am J Clin Nutr* 44:291, 1986.
77. Schoeller DA, Ravussin E, Schutz Y, et al: Energy expenditure by doubly labeled water: validation in humans and proposed calculation, *Am J Physiol* 250:R823, 1986.
78. Schoeller DA, van Santen E: Measurement of energy expenditure in humans by doubly labeled water method, *J Appl Physiol* 53: 955, 1982.
79. Schofield WN: Predicting basal metabolic rate, new standards and review of previous work, *Hum Nutr Clin Nutr* 39(suppl 1): 5, 1985.
80. SF L: Host metabolic response to injury. In Gallin JI FA, editors: *Advances in host defense mechanisms,* vol 6. New York, 1986, Raven Press.
81. Srinivasan V, Spinella PC, Drott HR, et al: Association of timing, duration, and intensity of hyperglycemia with intensive care unit mortality in critically ill children, *Pediatr Crit Care Med* 5: 329, 2004.
82. Stipanuk MH: Metabolism of sulfur-containing amino acids, *Annu Rev Nutr* 6:179, 1986.
83. Takala J, Ruokonen E, Webster NR, et al: Increased mortality associated with growth hormone treatment in critically ill adults, *N Engl J Med* 341:785, 1999.
84. Tenenbaum A, Fisman EZ, Motro M: Metabolic syndrome and type 2 diabetes mellitus: focus on peroxisome proliferator activated receptors (PPAR), *Cardiovasc Diabetol* 2:4, 2003.
85. Tilden SJ, Watkins S, Tong TK, et al: Measured energy expenditure in pediatric intensive care patients, *Am J Dis Child* 143: 490, 1989.
86. Tsekos E, Reuter C, Stehle P, et al: Perioperative administration of parenteral fish oil supplements in a routine clinical setting improves patient outcome after major abdominal surgery, *Clin Nutr* 23:325, 2004.
87. Van den Berghe G: Insulin therapy for the critically ill patient, *Clin Cornerstone* 5:56, 2003.
88. van den Berghe G, Wouters P, Weekers F, et al: Intensive insulin therapy in the critically ill patients, *N Engl J Med* 345:1359, 2001.
89. Weekes E, Elia M: Observations on the patterns of 24-hour energy expenditure changes in body composition and gastric emptying in head-injured patients receiving nasogastric tube feeding, *JPEN J Parenter Enteral Nutr* 20:31, 1996.
90. White MS, Shepherd RW, McEniery JA: Energy expenditure measurements in ventilated critically ill children: within- and between-day variability, *JPEN J Parenter Enteral Nutr* 23:300, 1999.
91. Woodman RJ, Mori TA, Burke V, et al: Effects of purified eicosapentaenoic and docosahexaenoic acids on glycemic control, blood pressure, and serum lipids in type 2 diabetic patients with treated hypertension, *Am J Clin Nutr* 76:1007, 2002.
92. Xu G, Kwon G, Cruz WS, et al: Metabolic regulation by leucine of translation initiation through the mTOR-signaling pathway by pancreatic beta-cells, *Diabetes* 50:353, 2001.
93. Zaloga GP: Early enteral nutritional support improves outcome: hypothesis or fact? *Crit Care Med* 27:259, 1999.
94. Ziegler M, Jakobowski D, Hoelzer D, et al: Route of pediatric parenteral nutrition: proposed criteria revision, *J Pediatr Surg* 15:472, 1980.

CHAPTER

69

Inborn Errors of Metabolism

Laurie Smith and Cary O. Harding

PEARLS

- Unexpected and unexplained clinical deterioration in a previously healthy infant or child is an important clue to the presence of an inborn error of metabolism.
- Loss of previously attained developmental milestones during childhood is an important clue to the presence of a neurodegenerative disorder such as lysosomal storage disease.
- Blood glucose less than 40 mg/dl is distinctly unusual after the first 24 hours of life, particularly in infants who have started feeding, and should be thoroughly investigated.
- Laboratory evaluation for inborn error of metabolism should be undertaken in any child with a suggestive clinical history regardless of the results of newborn screening. A normal newborn screen, although perhaps reassuring, does not rule out the possibility of an IEM.

Metabolism can be defined as the sum of all biochemical processes that convert food to protoplasm and subsequently convert protoplasm to small molecules and energy. An *inborn error of metabolism* (IEM) is an inherited deficiency of any critical step in metabolism. Although genetic deficiency of catalytic enzymes in intermediate metabolic pathways is the classic paradigm for IEM, the pathophysiology of metabolic disorders may involve abnormalities of any number of cellular processes, including transmembrane transport, cell signaling, cell differentiation and development, energy production, and others. Many IEMs are individually rare, although a few, including phenylketonuria (PKU) and medium-chain acyl-coenzyme A (acyl-CoA) dehydrogenase deficiency (MCADD), a defect in fatty acid oxidation, exhibit a population incidence approaching 1:10,000 live births.[9,14] Specific IEMs may be more common in certain ethnic groups with a history of relative reproductive isolation. Collectively, the population incidence of all IEMs may approach 1:1500 live births, depending upon how broadly IEM is defined. Many IEMs are associated with catastrophic illness necessitating advanced life support. Although IEM may present very rarely within the professional lifetime of the average medical practitioner, critically ill children with IEM will not be uncommon visitors to the pediatric intensive care unit, especially in a tertiary care center.

The key to successful treatment of IEM is the initial suspicion and timely diagnosis of the disorder.[6] Certain features of the clinical history, physical signs and symptoms, and results of routine laboratory studies often suggest the possibility of IEM. Second-tier screening metabolic studies provide further evidence for the presence of a disorder. The results of routine neonatal screening studies may suggest a specific disorder prior to development of any diagnostic suspicion on the part of the clinician or even prior to the onset of symptoms in the neonate. In the case of a critically ill child with a suspected metabolic disease or with an abnormal neonatal screening test result for a specific metabolic disorder, immediate consultation with a biochemical geneticist, even if only by telephone, is paramount. The genetic consultant helps direct the diagnostic laboratory evaluation and recommends nonspecific emergency treatment, if any is warranted, prior to the availability of the definitive diagnostic studies. Communication among the intensivist, genetic consultant, and biochemical genetic diagnostic laboratory is critical to achieving the timely and correct diagnosis of IEM. A satisfactory clinical outcome for the affected child is completely dependent upon the collaborative efforts of this tripartite team approach.

Several published reviews on the diagnosis and treatment of IEM provide an exhaustive list of known disorders.[27,36] Rather than recapitulate an encyclopedia of possible diseases, this chapter presents a diagnostic rationale based upon specific clinical symptom complexes that are likely to occur in the critically ill child. Algorithms for the differential diagnosis of specific clinical scenarios are given in support of this rationale. Symptoms often begin during early infancy in the biochemically most severe IEM; naturally, these IEMs with neonatal onset are the focus of our discussion in this chapter. However, "milder" or late-onset variants of virtually every IEM have been described with onset of symptoms occurring at all ages, even during adulthood. Some IEMs uniformly present after the neonatal period; age of symptom onset (late infancy, childhood, or adulthood) often is an important clue to the specific diagnosis. The clinical presentation, diagnostic workup, and treatment of neonatal onset disorders provide a paradigm for the evaluation and management of possible IEM in a child of any age.

Pathophysiology of Inborn Errors of Metabolism

Under the classic paradigm, an IEM is associated with deficiency of a specific protein, often a catalytic enzyme, involved in a critical metabolic pathway (Fig. 69–1). This deficiency leads to a block in the pathway and the accumulation of the enzyme substrate. In this model, three distinct pathogenic mechanisms are possible proximate causes of the symptoms associated with an IEM. The specific pathogenic mechanism involved in any given IEM dictates the appropriate treatment strategy. First, accumulation of the substrate may lead to toxic effects at very high levels; successful therapy requires effective elimination of the substrate or a method to block its toxic effects. An appropriate example for this mechanism is PKU, in which elevated phenylalanine levels adversely affect neuronal development, and the reduction of tissue phenylalanine content through dietary phenylalanine restriction largely prevents the major clinical features of PKU.[26] Second, deficiency of the reaction product, should it be a critically important metabolite, may lead to disease. Supplementation with the essential metabolite, if possible, may cure the disease. Biotin is a required cofactor for four distinct carboxylase enzymes. Deficiency of free biotin develops in the face of genetic biotinidase deficiency and leads to symptoms of multiple carboxylase deficiency. Supplementation with oral biotin completely prevents the clinical manifestations of biotinidase deficiency.[4] The final pathogenic mechanism involves the conversion of the enzyme substrate, through normally quiescent alternative pathways, to toxic secondary metabolites. Elimination or decreased production of these secondary metabolites may improve disease symptoms. For example, tyrosinemia type I (fumarylacetoacetate hydrolase [FAH] deficiency) is associated with recurrent attacks of abdominal pain and paresthesias reminiscent of acute intermittent porphyria. The accumulating substrate, fumarylacetoacetic acid, is converted through secondary pathways to succinylacetone, and succinylacetone in turn inhibits the heme synthetic pathway and causes porphyria-like symptoms. Pharmacologic inhibition of the tyrosine catabolic pathway proximal to the block at FAH decreases the production of fumarylacetoacetic acid and succinylacetone and alleviates the pathology associated with these toxic compounds.[31]

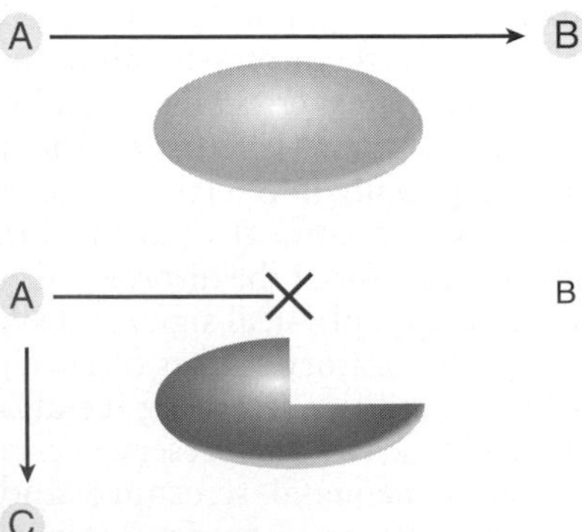

FIGURE 69–1 • Inborn error of metabolism paradigm. Normally, in a given step of intermediate metabolism with intact enzymatic activity, the substrate *A* is efficiently converted to the product *B*. In an inborn error of metabolism, deficiency of enzyme activity may lead to excessive accumulation of the substrate; critical deficiency of the product; or production of an alternative, potentially toxic metabolite *C* through normally quiescent pathways.

Inheritance of Inborn Errors of Metabolism

IEMs are heritable disorders. The majority of diseases are inherited in an autosomal recessive pattern, yielding a 25% recurrence risk in future offspring. The gene defects associated with several IEMs are located on the X chromosome. These IEMs, such as ornithine transcarbamoylase deficiency and glycerol kinase deficiency, are inherited in an X-linked pattern. These IEMs are most severe in males, but carrier females may be symptomatic, although usually with less severe or late-onset disease as a result of skewed X chromosome inactivation. Mutations for several mitochondrial disorders are found on mitochondrial deoxyribonucleic acid (mtDNA). Because mtDNA is exclusively passed from mothers to their offspring, these IEMs exhibit a maternal inheritance pattern but often with variable penetrance and expressivity. Prenatal diagnosis is possible for many IEMs. In addition to allowing for appropriate medical therapy, the timely diagnosis of an IEM in a sick infant or child is important for genetic counseling purposes.[15]

Signs and Symptoms of Inborn Errors of Metabolism

Clinical signs and symptoms frequently associated with IEM are listed in Table 69–1. The symptom repertoire of the critically ill infant is limited, and the clinical presentation of metabolic disorders often is nonspecific. It is for this reason that the diagnosis of an IEM may be easily missed. To maintain maximum diagnostic sensitivity for IEM, the clinician must maintain a high level of suspicion and be willing to initiate screening metabolic laboratory studies with little provocation. As was true for appendectomies in the era prior to the advent of ultrasound-based diagnosis of appendicitis, a certain number of nondiagnostic metabolic laboratory workups in sick children must be performed to ensure ascertainment of individuals with inherited metabolic disorders. In particular, IEM should be a strong diagnostic consideration in any neonate who has become catastrophically ill following a period of normalcy. This presentation may be clinically indistinguishable from bacterial or viral sepsis, and the nonspecific supportive therapy provided to potentially septic infants (fluid and glucose administration) may alleviate the symptoms and mask the presence of an IEM. Diagnostic metabolic laboratory studies are most likely to provide definitive information if performed on clinical samples obtained at initial presentation and before any therapy is initiated. Failure to obtain the necessary specimens at this time may miss an important diagnostic window of opportunity. Many children with IEM have been saved initially by intensive but nonspecific treatment but then suffered clinical relapse or even death in the absence of the correct diagnosis. Certainly, the possibility of an IEM should be considered in any child for whom the clinical picture suggests sepsis but the laboratory evaluation for sepsis is negative. Unfortunately, bacterial sepsis is often a complicating factor in critically ill children with IEM. For example, *Escherichia coli* infection (including pyelonephritis, bacteremia, or meningitis) is frequently detected at presentation in infants with galactosemia. The astute clinician remains ever vigilant for the signs and symptoms that may suggest an inherited metabolic disorder.

Recurrent episodes of vomiting and dehydration in response to fasting or intercurrent illness are an important clue to IEM in older infants and children. Feeding difficulties and failure to thrive are common chronic complications. Children with unexplained hypotonia, developmental delay, or movement disorder should be evaluated for possible IEM. Inherited neurodegenerative disorders, such as the lysosomal storage diseases, stereotypically cause developmental regression, specifically loss of previously attained developmental milestones. Several IEMs are associated with major physical anomalies (Table 69–2). When present, these anomalies are exceedingly valuable in suggesting a specific diagnosis and directing the diagnostic evaluation. More commonly, the child with IEM is morphologically normal, and the presenting symptoms are nonspecific. The clinician must then rely upon screening laboratory tests to evaluate the potential for IEM.

TABLE 69–1

Signs and Symptoms of Inborn Errors of Metabolism

Acute illness after period of normal behavior and feeding (hours to weeks)
Recurrent decompensation with fasting, intercurrent illness, or specific food ingestion
Unusual body odor
Persistent or recurrent vomiting
Failure to thrive
Apnea or tachypnea
Jaundice
Hepatomegaly or liver dysfunction
Lethargy or coma
Sepsis
Unexplained hemorrhage or strokes
Developmental delay with unknown etiology
Developmental regression
Seizures, especially if seizures are intractable
Hypotonia
Chronic movement disorder (ataxia, dystonia, choreoathetosis)
Family history of unexplained death or recurrent illness in siblings
Parental consanguinity

Laboratory Evaluation of Suspected Inborn Errors of Metabolism

Abnormal results of routine laboratory studies may provide clues to the presence and type of IEM (Table 69–3). In our experience, highly informative but sometimes subtle laboratory abnormalities are often overlooked, especially in a busy intensive care unit or hospital ward. For instance, a clinically relevant newborn screening result may have been sent to the primary care provider or birth hospital but not efficiently communicated to the intensive care unit, in a different hospital, to which the now critically ill infant has been admitted. It is imperative to verify the infant's screening results with the primary care provider or newborn screening laboratory (Box 69–1). Calculation of the anion gap, another example of a routine and highly informative result, is key to the differential diagnosis of metabolic acidosis. The absence of urine ketones in hypoglycemic children older than 2 weeks strongly suggests impaired ketogenesis as a consequence of either hyperinsulinism or fatty acid oxidation disorder. On the other hand, fatty acid oxidation and ketogenesis are incompletely developed in neonates. The presence of ketones in urine of infants younger than 2 weeks is very unusual even during fasting or hypoglycemia and suggests the presence of an unusual ketoacid, such as those excreted in maple syrup disease or the organic acidemias. Ketoacids, organic acids, and sugars such as galactose or fructose increase urine specific gravity. Urine specific gravity >1.020 in any neonate or in well-hydrated older children suggests the unexpected presence of an osmotically active substance. Routine urinalysis at many hospitals

TABLE 69–2

Physical Anomalies Associated with Inborn Errors of Metabolism

Dysmorphic facial features	Peroxisomal disorders Glutaric aciduria type II Smith-Lemli-Opitz syndrome Menkes syndrome Lysosomal storage disorders
Structural brain anomalies	Glutaric aciduria type II (cortical cysts) Pyruvate dehydrogenase deficiency (cortical cysts, agenesis of the corpus callosum) Glycosylation disorders (cerebellar agenesis)
Macrocephaly	Glutaric aciduria type I (with subdural effusions) Canavan disease Alexander disease
Cataracts	Galactosemia Peroxisomal disorders Mitochondrial disorders Lowe syndrome
Pigmentary retinopathy including cherry red spots	Peroxisomal disorders Lysosomal storage disorders Long chain 3-hydroxyacyl-CoA dehydrogenase deficiency
Lens dislocation	Homocystinuria Sulfite oxidase deficiency Molybdenum cofactor deficiency
Renal cysts	Glutaric aciduria type II Peroxisomal disorders Mitochondrial disorders
Ambiguous genitalia	Congenital adrenal hyperplasia Smith-Lemli-Opitz syndrome
Skeletal abnormalities	Menkes disease Homocystinuria Peroxisomal disorders Lysosomal storage diseases
Hair or skin abnormalities	Menkes disease Holocarboxylase synthetase deficiency Biotinidase deficiency Argininosuccinic aciduria Phenylketonuria

may not include use of the Clinitest to detect reducing substances. Urine Chemstrips utilize a colorimetric glucose oxidase-based method to specifically detect glucose. This test does not react with any other sugar (galactose or fructose). However, some bedside glucose monitoring systems do react with galactose or fructose; inappropriately elevated capillary blood "glucose" accompanied by a normal venous glucose as measured by chemistry analyzer suggests the presence of a sugar other than glucose in the blood. A comatose infant with a blood urea nitrogen (BUN) level below the limits of detection may have an inherited defect in the urea cycle. Blood ammonia measurement is crucial to confirming that suspicion. Failure to check the blood ammonia level has caused missed diagnoses, failure to appropriately treat hyperammonemia, and further morbidity and mortality in comatose infants with urea cycle disorders or organic acidemias. Finally, bacterial sepsis and meningitis are more common causes of severe lethargy and coma in infants than is IEM, but bacterial infection may also be a complicating feature in severely ill infants with IEM. Infants with galactosemia, for example, are particularly prone to pyelonephritis, bacteremia, sepsis, or meningitis, often with *E. coli*. Antibiotic therapy without diagnosis and specific treatment of the underlying disorder may be useful in the short term but does not mitigate long-term IEM-specific effects.

Suspicion of an IEM based upon clinical and routine laboratory findings should initiate specialized biochemical testing (Table 69–4). In the case of severely ill infants or when the clinical suspicion of IEM is very high, consultation with a biochemical geneticist, even if only by phone, is strongly advised to help direct the laboratory investigation and initial therapy. When the clinical presentation is nonspecific, that is, catastrophic illness in a previously well child without signs of any particular IEM, the "shotgun" diagnostic evaluation should minimally include plasma amino acid analysis, urine organic acid analysis by gas chromatography-mass spectrometry, and a so-called *urine metabolic screen*. The battery of qualitative assays included in a urine metabolic screen differs among laboratories, and the ordering clinician should be aware of which tests and disorders are included in the repertoire of the diagnostic laboratory chosen. Furthermore, although diagnostic laboratories in the United States must meet CLIA requirements and often are accredited by the College of American Pathologists (CAP), the testing methodologies used, the quality of diagnostic testing for IEM, and more problematically the availability of laboratory-associated consultants with experience in the diagnosis and treatment of IEM vary widely among laboratories. Although the ability of clinicians to direct clinical specimens toward specific diagnostic laboratories may be inhibited by contractual arrangements between the hospital and large referral laboratories, the critically ill patient is best served by diagnostic evaluation carried out in a timely manner by an experienced biochemical genetics laboratory, with laboratory staff available by phone for expert consultation on interpretation of test results.

The specific clinical presentation or specific screening laboratory findings may direct the intensivist or biochemical geneticist to order other more specialized metabolic tests (see Table 69–4). These analyses may provide diagnostic confirmation for specific disorders and supportive evidence alone for others. For several IEMs, confirmation of diagnosis may require enzyme activity analysis in tissue (red blood cells, lymphocytes, cultured skin fibroblasts, liver, or skeletal muscle depending upon the specific disorder in question) or molecular DNA testing for a specific gene defect. In general, these tertiary tests, which are often difficult, labor intensive, and expensive, should be ordered following consultation with a biochemical geneticist. In some instances, confirmatory diagnostic

TABLE 69–3

Initial Laboratory Evaluation of Suspected Inborn Errors of Metabolism

Laboratory Test	Abnormality	Disorder
Check newborn screen!		Multiple disorders (differs in each state)
Complete blood count (CBC)	Neutropenia	Organic acidemias Glycogenosis type Ib
	Macrocytic anemia	Cobalamin defects
	Pancytopenia	Congenital lactic acidoses
Electrolytes	Metabolic acidosis	Glycogenoses Organic acidemias FAO disorders MSUD Congenital lactic acidoses
Blood gas	Metabolic acidosis	Same as above
	Metabolic alkalosis	Urea cycle disorders
Glucose	Hypoglycemia	Glycogenoses FAO disorders Gluconeogenic defects Liver disease (galactosemia, fructosemia, other)
Blood urea nitrogen (BUN)	Low or undetectable BUN (with hyperammonemia)	Urea cycle disorders
Transaminases (ALT, AST)	Liver dysfunction	Galactosemia Fructosemia Tyrosinemia α_1-Antitrypsin deficiency FAO disorders Organic acidemias Congenital lactic acidosis Congenital disorders of glycosylation
Total and direct bilirubin	Hyperbilirubinemia	Galactosemia Fructosemia Tyrosinemia α_1-Antitrypsin deficiency Congenital lactic acidoses
Uric acid	Elevated serum uric acid	Glycogenoses Purine disorders
Ammonia	Hyperammonemia	Urea cycle disorders FAO disorders Organic acidemias
Lactate	Lactic acidemia	Congenital lactic acidosis Glycogenoses Fructosemia Gluconeogenic defects
Urinalysis		
Odor	Unusual odor	Phenylketonuria MSUD Organic acidemias
Color		
pH		
Specific gravity	Inappropriately high specific gravity as a result of metabolites	Organic acidemias Galactosemia Fructosemia
Ketones	Ketosis	MSUD Organic acidemias
Reducing substances (Clinitest)	Reducing substances	Galactosemia Fructosemia
Cerebrospinal fluid	Meningitis	May be comorbid feature, along with sepsis, in any severely ill child with inborn error of metabolism *Escherichia coli* sepsis/meningitis particularly frequent in galactosemia

FAO, Fatty acid oxidation; MSUD, maple syrup urine disease.

BOX 69–1

Screening Metabolic Laboratory Studies for Children with Suspected Inborn Errors of Metabolism

- Plasma amino acid analysis
  Minimum 2 ml blood in a heparin tube
- Urine organic acid analysis
- Urine metabolic screen
  Minimum 10 ml urine

biochemical or molecular tests are available only through specialized research laboratories.

Postmortem Evaluation of a Child with Suspected Inborn Errors of Metabolism

Some IEMs, particularly those exacerbated by fasting, may present as sudden infant death. For many IEMs, acute metabolic compensation may be rapid and lethal despite intensive medical intervention. The time after clinical presentation but prior to death may be insufficient to execute an adequate metabolic evaluation. Disease diagnosis is still possible postmortem and is important for fully understanding the cause of death and determining recurrence risk in the family. A protocol for postmortem evaluation of an infant or child with suspected IEM is given in Table 69–5. Many of the biochemical genetic analyses recommended for acutely ill children are still valid on postmortem specimens. Valuable information may be learned from amino acid, carnitine, and acylcarnitine analyses in blood and from metabolic screening and organic acid analysis in urine (Box 69–2). However, collection of blood and urine may not be possible postmortem, especially if the autopsy is performed many hours after death. In these instances, metabolic testing may be obtained on alternative specimens such as vitreous humor or bile. In the event that screening biochemical studies suggest a specific diagnosis, disease confirmation by enzyme analysis in tissue is highly desirable. Many enzymes can be assayed in cultured fibroblasts; viable fibroblasts may be cultured from skin or Achilles tendon samples obtained as late as 24 hours after death. Biopsies of other organs may be necessary for analysis of certain other enzymes. Muscle, liver, and kidney specimens may be obtained postmortem for enzymatic analysis, but most enzymatic activities in solid organs deteriorate rapidly following death. Collection of specimens as soon as possible after death is critical for valid enzyme analyses.

TABLE 69–4

Biochemical Genetic Laboratory Studies

Specimen	Test	Disorder
Blood	Plasma quantitative amino acid analysis	Aminoacidopathies
	Plasma carnitine	Organic acidemias FAO disorders
	Plasma acylcarnitine profile	Organic acidemias FAO disorders
	Serum transferrin electrophoresis	Congenital disorders of glycosylation
Urine	Metabolic screen	
	Ketones	
	Reducing substances	Galactosemia, fructosemia
	Ferric chloride	Phenylketonuria (PKU)
	Dinitrophenylhydrazine	PKU, Maple syrup disease
	2,4-nitrosonaphthol	Tyrosinemia
	Cyanide-nitroprusside	Sulfur-containing amino acids
	Qualitative mucopolysaccharides	Mucopolysaccharidoses
	Qualitative amino acid Chromatography	Multiple disorders
	Organic acid analysis	Organic acidemias FAO disorders
	Acylglycine profile	Organic acidemias FAO disorders
	Quantitative mucopolysaccharide measurement and electrophoresis	Mucopolysaccharidoses
	Qualitative sulfites (Sulfitest) or quantitative sulfocysteine	Sulfite oxidase deficiency Molybdenum cofactor deficiency
	Quantitative purines, pyrimidines	Disorders of purine or pyrimidine metabolism

FAO, Fatty acid oxidation.

TABLE 69–5

Postmortem Biochemical Genetic Evaluation

To be performed on any deceased infant <1 year for which the cause of death is not apparent or any child with suspected IEM. Analyses are most reliable if obtained within 6 hours after death.

1. Contact newborn screening laboratory for results of neonatal screening.
2. Obtain a 3-mm punch biopsy of skin or Achilles tendon for fibroblast culture.
   A. Prepare skin with chlorhexidine (Hibiclens) or alcohol. Do not use Betadine because it may inhibit fibroblast growth.
   B. Use sterile technique.
   C. Store biopsy specimen in sterile RPMI culture media (if available) at room temperature. May be stored in sterile nonbacteriostatic saline for up to 24 hours prior to culture if culture media is not readily available.
   D. Send to cytogenetics or biochemical genetics laboratory for culture, possible enzyme analyses, and frozen storage.
3. Collect blood via cardiac puncture (≈5 ml per tube).
   A. One red top tube at room temperature. Collect and store serum at –70° C.
      I. Comprehensive metabolic panel (potassium, lipids, uric acid may not be accurate postmortem)
      II. If hypoglycemic, insulin, growth hormone, and cortisol levels
   B. One green top (sodium heparin) at room temperature. Collect and store plasma at –70° C.
      I. Plasma amino acid analysis
      II. Plasma carnitine levels
      III. Plasma acylcarnitine profile
   C. One green top (sodium heparin) at room temperature for cytogenetic (karyotype) analysis.
   D. If storage disorder suspected, one green top (sodium heparin) at 4° C (wet ice) for leukocyte isolation and diagnostic enzyme analyses.
   E. One lavender top (EDTA) tube at room temperature for CBC.
   F. One yellow top (ACD) tube for DNA isolation and possible mutation analysis.
   G. If infant <1 year, spot whole blood onto newborn screening filter paper card for repeat screen.
   H. Blood lactate and ammonia may not be accurate postmortem.
4. Collect urine (10–20 ml) by suprapubic tap or by swabbing the bladder interior with cotton swab.
   A. Urinalysis
   B. Urine reducing substances
   C. Urine metabolic screen
   D. Urine organic acid analysis
   E. If storage disorder suspected, quantitative urine mucopolysaccharide and oligosaccharide analysis
5. If urine is unobtainable, organic acid analysis may be performed on vitreous humor collected by needle aspiration from an eye. Freeze vitreous humor at –70° C.
6. If blood is unobtainable, collect bile (2–3 ml) via puncture of the gallbladder for acylcarnitine profile. Store at –20° C.
7. Collect several biopsies (2 g each) from skeletal muscle, cardiac muscle, kidney, and liver.
   A. For routine histology, biopsies should be submitted fresh to the pathology laboratory.
   B. For enzyme analyses, biopsies should be wrapped in aluminum foil, placed in a labeled small specimen container, and immediately frozen in liquid nitrogen. Store at –70° C.

Modified from Steiner 2001.

Emergency Treatment of Children with Suspected Inborn Errors of Metabolism

Laboratory investigation of suspected IEM may require several days to complete, given that the biochemical genetics laboratory may be physically remote from the treating hospital and many of the tests involve complex specimen preparation and analysis. A general approach to emergency treatment of children with suspected IEM while awaiting diagnostic studies is given in Table 69–6. For many IEMs associated with acute catastrophic illness, elimination of the offending metabolite is the key to therapy. Immediate cessation of oral feedings, to stop protein or fat intake, will begin to limit toxin production in disorders of amino acid or fatty acid metabolism. Adequate energy intake as carbohydrate must be supplied, usually parenterally, until a specific diagnosis and definitive treatment plan are available. Dextrose infusion at a high rate suppresses catabolism and reduces the consumption of endogenous protein or fatty acid stores. In extremely recalcitrant cases, insulin infusion drives anabolism and further decreases toxin production. Acute metabolic decompensation in some IEMs (e.g., maple syrup disease) is associated with mild peripheral insulin resistance. Insulin administration (often as little as 0.01–0.05 U/kg/hour given by continuous intravenous [IV] infusion or subcutaneous bolus injection) overcomes this

BOX 69–2

Postmortem Metabolic Evaluation

- Blood
  Electrolytes, glucose
  Amino acid analysis
  Organic acid analysis
  Acylcarnitine profile
- Bile
  Acylcarnitine profile
- Vitreous humor
  Organic acid analysis
  Acylcarnitine profile
- Urine
  Organic acid analysis
  Qualitative metabolic screen
- Liver and skeletal muscle:
  Samples frozen at –80°C for possible enzyme analysis
- Skin biopsy or Achilles tendon
  Fibroblast culture for enzyme or DNA studies

resistance and has an immediate impact upon metabolic control. Some clinicians also use anabolic agents such as growth hormone or testosterone to acutely suppress protein and fat catabolism. In certain types of congenital lactic acidosis, particularly defects of pyruvate metabolism, carbohydrate infusion worsens lactic acidosis. Replacement of some carbohydrate with fat as an intralipid infusion may partly reduce blood lactate levels, but infants with this degree of sensitivity to glucose infusion often are difficult to treat and suffer high mortality. Severe hyperammonemia that does not respond to dietary protein restriction and dextrose infusion must be treated by hemodialysis. Ammonia clearance with exchange transfusion or peritoneal dialysis is insufficient to adequately decrease blood ammonia levels. If the results of specialized biochemical genetic diagnostic tests are expected within 2 to 3 days, then parenteral dextrose infusion alone should be adequate to maintain nutrition until a more definitive treatment plan is available. Beyond 3 days, developing essential amino acid and fatty acid deficiencies may induce catabolism of endogenous protein and fat. To prevent this occurrence, enteral or parenteral nutrition with minimal amounts of protein (0.5 g/kg body weight/day) and lipid (20% of total energy intake) should be considered. Empiric administration of cofactors such as the B vitamins is not harmful and may improve metabolite clearance, particularly in disorders caused by deficiency of enzymes that require specific cofactors. Carnitine is required for transport of long-chain fatty acids across the mitochondrial membrane and serves a secondary role in the disposal of excess and potentially toxic acyl-CoA species. Secondary carnitine deficiency is commonly associated with acute metabolic decompensation in organic acidemias and fatty acid oxidation defects. L-Carnitine administration prevents secondary carnitine deficiency and may improve clearance of toxic metabolites; it is lifesaving in specific inherited dilated cardiomyopathies.

TABLE 69–6

Emergency Treatment of Suspected Inborn Error of Metabolism

Goal	Action
Suppress toxic metabolite production	Discontinue oral feedings
Correct fluid imbalance and electrolyte abnormalities	Appropriate intravenous fluid management
Correct hypoglycemia	Intravenous dextrose-containing fluid infusion
Correct metabolic acidosis	Intravenous hydration alone if pH >7.2 Add IV bicarbonate if pH <7.2: Sodium bicarbonate (1 mEq/ml solution), 1 mEq/kg IV push at <1 mEq/min. May be repeated 3× until pH >7.2. Maximum dose 7mEq/kg/24 hours
Correct hyperammonemia	Suppress protein catabolism (see below) Hemodialysis
Treat infection	Appropriate infectious disease laboratory evaluation and antibiotic therapy
Suppress protein and lipid catabolism	Infuse D_{10}1/2NS at 1.5–2× maintenance: Add insulin if hyperglycemic If severe, unrelenting acidosis, consider growth hormone or testosterone therapy to promote anabolism
Empiric cofactor administration	L-Carnitine 25–50 mg/kg/every 6 hours IV if organic acidemia or FAO disorder suspected or cardiomyopathy present B vitamin complex 100 mg each day Vitamin B_{12} 1 mg IM 1× if macrocytic anemia
Maintain nutritional status (if without enteral feeds > 2 days and without diagnosis of a specific inborn error metabolism)	Enteral feeds or parenteral hyperalimentation to include: Protein 0.5 g/kg/day only Lipid, 20% of total energy intake Carbohydrate to provide at least the minimum necessary total energy intake

Classification of Inborn Errors of Metabolism by Clinical Presentation

As mentioned previously, the clinical presentation of IEM in neonates provides a paradigm for the suspicion and evaluation of potential IEM at all ages. The classification outlined here is adapted and expanded to include late-onset disorders from a neonatal IEM classification system first described by Jean-Marie Saudubray and colleagues.[32,34]

IEM can be classified into one of three groups by pathogenic mechanism. In *group 1* IEMs, the production or catabolism of complex molecules is disturbed. The lysosomal storage and peroxisomal disorders are included in this group. The symptoms of these disorders include permanent and progressive somatic and neurologic abnormalities that develop in utero, are often clinically apparent at birth, and are unaffected by food intake. This group is often distinguished by the presence of somatic abnormalities such as dysmorphic features or hepatosplenomegaly. Typical clinical features, potential neonatal and late-onset diagnoses, and confirmatory diagnostic tests are listed in Table 69–7.

In *group 2* IEMs, the symptoms are caused by defects in the production or utilization of energy. This group includes the congenital lactic acidoses, glycogenoses, gluconeogenic defects, and fatty acid oxidation disorders. *In group 3* IEMs, clinical symptoms are caused by progressive intoxication in a previously well infant because of accumulation of toxic metabolites proximal to a metabolic block. Often, neonatal onset IEM in groups 2 and 3 can be distinguished by the time of clinical onset relative to birth. The symptoms of a block in energy production or utilization (group 2) may present within hours after birth, whereas symptoms of intoxication (group 3) develop over the first week of life with increasing food intake and accumulation of toxic metabolites. However, variants of many of these disorders may not become clinically apparent for several months or even years after birth.

Group 2 Inborn Errors of Metabolism

Systemic or tissue-specific impaired energy production from food substrates is the unifying feature of disorders classified in group 2. Generalized profound neurologic dysfunction, including severe central hypotonia, coma, and seizures, sometimes with peripheral spasticity or abnormal movements, typifies the clinical presentation. Children with these disorders present with similar clinical phenotypes but are easily separated into four subgroups (A–D) based upon associated results of routine laboratory studies (Table 69–8). Severe refractory generalized motor seizures, often beginning within the first hours after birth, sometimes even prenatally, are the hallmark of subgroup A. Routine laboratory studies (glucose, blood pH, electrolytes, ammonia) are generally normal unless the infant is near *extremis* and secondary metabolic abnormalities are present. Several inherited disorders are associated with this phenotype; diagnostic differentiation depends upon clinical evaluation by an experienced pediatric neurologist or geneticist and the judicious use of specialized diagnostic laboratory tests. All infants with refractory seizures should undergo a pyridoxine challenge (100 mg pyridoxine given intravenously during electroencephalographic [EEG] monitoring).[7] In true pyridoxine dependency, the EEG pattern (characterized by generalized spike and burst-suppression patterns) normalizes within minutes after pyridoxine infusion.

The amino acid glycine is an abundant neurotransmitter within the central nervous system (CNS). Inherited deficiency of the glycine cleavage system, which removes glycine from its receptor in the neuronal synapse, causes severe unrelenting generalized seizures and profound

TABLE 69–7

Features of Group 1 Inborn Errors of Metabolism

Clinical Features	Associated Laboratory Findings	Possible Diagnoses	Specialized Diagnostic Tests
Hepatosplenomegaly Coarse facies Macroglossia Fetal hydrops Macular cherry red spots Bone changes (dysostosis multiplex) Abnormal muscle tone (hypotonia/hypertonia) ± Chronic diarrhea ± Failure to thrive	Liver dysfunction (elevated transaminases, cholestatic jaundice) No acidosis Normal ammonia Normal glucose	Neonatal onset G_{M1} gangliosidosis I cell disease Sialidosis Galactosialidosis Niemann-Pick type A Mucopolysaccharidosis VII (Sly syndrome) Congenital disorders of glycosylation Later onset Tay-Sachs disease Krabbe disease Other Mucopolysaccharidoses Niemann-Pick B or C	Urine mucopolysaccharides Urine oligosaccharides Serum transferrin electrophoresis Enzyme analysis in lymphocytes or fibroblasts
Hepatomegaly Dysmorphic facies Severe hypotonia Large anterior fontanelle Seizures Bone changes (epiphyseal calcific stippling)	Liver dysfunction (elevated transaminases, cholestatic jaundice) No acidosis Normal ammonia Normal glucose Adrenal insufficiency	Peroxisomal disorders Zellweger syndrome Neonatal Adrenoleukodystrophy Others	Plasma very-long-chain fatty acid analysis Functional and genetic analysis of fibroblasts

TABLE 69–8

Features of Group 2 Inborn Errors of Metabolism

Clinical Features	Associated Laboratory Findings	Possible Diagnoses	Specialized Diagnostic Tests
SUBGROUP A			
Profound neurologic dysfunction Severe hypotonia Seizures	No acidosis Normal ammonia Normal glucose	Nonketotic hyperglycinemia Sulfite oxidase or molybdenum cofactor deficiency Pyridoxine-responsive seizures Peroxisomal disorders Respiratory chain disorders Congenital disorders of glycosylation (CDG) Cholesterol synthesis defects Neurotransmitter synthesis defects	Plasma and CSF amino acid analysis Urine sulfocysteine Urine oxypurines Pyridoxine challenge Plasma very-long-chain fatty acid analysis (peroxisomal) Blood and CSF lactate Plasma acylcarnitine profile Urine organic acid analysis Serum transferrin electrophoresis (CDG) Plasma sterols (cholesterol) Neurotransmitters (blood, urine, CSF)
SUBGROUP B			
Neurologic dysfunction Hypotonia Seizures With severe acidosis ± Liver dysfunction ± Dilated cardiomyopathy	Severe acidosis Lactic acidosis ± Ketosis ± Hypoglycemia ± Anemia	Congenital lactic acidoses Pyruvate dehydrogenase Pyruvate carboxylase Krebs cycle Respiratory chain disorders Multiple carboxylase deficiency	Blood and CSF lactate Plasma and CSF amino acid analysis Urine organic acid analysis Diagnostic muscle biopsy to include histology, enzyme analyses
SUBGROUP C			
Neurologic dysfunction Vomiting Dehydration Hypotonia Coma ± Hepatomegaly, liver dysfunction ± Dilated cardiomyopathy Triggered by fasting or intercurrent illness	Hypoglycemia No ketones in urine Acidosis ± Hyperammonemia ± Lactic acidosis	Fatty acid oxidation defects MCAD LCHAD VLCAD CPT-II CAT MACD Ketogenesis defects HMG-CoA lyase MCKAT	Urine organic acid analysis Plasma carnitine level Plasma acylcarnitine profile Diagnostic fasting challenge Fatty acid oxidation studies in cultured skin fibroblasts
SUBGROUP D			
Neurologic dysfunction triggered by short fast Hepatomegaly	Severe fasting hypoglycemia Lactic acidosis Normal ammonia ± Ketosis ± Elevated serum uric acid ± Hypophosphatemia	Glycogen storage Glycogenosis type I Glycogenosis type III Fructose 1,6-diphosphatase deficiency	Diagnostic fasting challenge Enzyme studies in liver

CAT, Carnitine acylcarnitine translocase; *CDG,* congenital disorders of glycosylation; *CPT-II,* carnitine palmitoyltransferase II; *CSF,* cerebrospinal fluid; *HMG-CoA,* 3-hydroxy-3-methylglutaryl-CoA; *LCHAD,* long-chain 3-hydroxyacyl-CoA dehydrogenase; *MACD,* multiple acyl-CoA dehydrogenase deficiency (also known as glutaric aciduria type II); *MCAD,* medium-chain acyl-CoA dehydrogenase; *MCKAT,* medium-chain ketoacyl-CoA thiolase; *VLCAD,* very-long-chain acyl-CoA dehydrogenase.

developmental arrest. The only ubiquitous laboratory finding is an elevated cerebrospinal fluid (CSF/plasma glycine ratio).[13] Sulfite oxidase deficiency, either as a primary genetic defect or secondary to generalized deficiency of its molybdenum-containing cofactor, is another rare but important cause of neonatal-onset seizures. Profound neurologic dysfunction with seizures is one of many possible clinical presentations of infants with peroxisomal or respiratory chain disorders. Some subtypes of a still expanding list of congenital disorders of glycosylation present with seizures,[22] as do disorders of sterol production such as Smith-Lemli-Opitz syndrome,[28] but these diagnoses are often associated with stereotypic dysmorphic features and anomalies. Finally, disorders of neurotransmitter synthesis should be considered in any infant with idiopathic seizures and neurologic dysfunction, especially if a movement disorder, most commonly dystonia, is also present. Abnormal CSF neurotransmitter levels (5-methyltetrahydrofolate, 5-hydroxyindoleacetic acid, homovanillic acid, 3-methyl-DOPA) are the only associated laboratory diagnostic clue in this latter category of disease.

Severe persistent lactic acidosis is the hallmark of the disorders in subgroup B of early-onset energy deficiency diseases. The presence of metabolic acidosis with an elevated anion gap suggests the possibility of lactic acidosis (subgroup B) or an organic acidemia (see group 3, intoxication types); these are differentiated by measurement of blood lactate and urine organic acid analysis. Blood lactate is most reliably measured on arterial blood or a free-flowing sample drawn from an indwelling central venous catheter. Artifactual elevation of lactate in peripheral venous blood samples is nearly ubiquitous and should be confirmed by lactate measurement in a more appropriate sample. Secondary lactic acidosis resulting from asphyxia, poor tissue perfusion, or tissue necrosis is much more common and may be difficult to differentiate from the congenital lactic acidoses. Occult cardiac disease, intracranial hemorrhage, or bowel necrosis must considered and ruled out in infants with severe lactic acidosis. Congenital lactic acidosis generally persists despite adequate life support measures, including fluid resuscitation and ventilatory assistance. In certain enzyme deficiencies, the blood lactate level may further increase with IV dextrose infusion. Simultaneous measurements of blood and CSF lactate and amino acids are useful for differentiating primary from secondary lactic acidoses. In congenital lactic acidosis, the CSF lactate level often is higher than the blood lactate level, while the CNS is relatively protected from systemic acidosis in secondary lactic acidemias. The blood pyruvate level is elevated in some congenital lactic acidoses such as pyruvate dehydrogenase deficiency. However, accurate measurement of blood pyruvate is difficult and fraught with false-positive elevations. Elevated plasma alanine (which is measured as part of a plasma amino acid analysis) is a more stable and reliable indicator of pyruvic acidosis, as alanine and pyruvate are in equilibrium. Enzymatic analysis in cultured skin fibroblasts or mitochondria isolated from a fresh muscle biopsy often is necessary to confirm a specific enzyme deficiency.

Children with subgroup C defects present with hypoketotic hypoglycemia, triggered by fasting, metabolic stress, or intercurrent illness. In these disorders, utilization of fatty acids as fuel is impaired. The most common of the fatty acid oxidation defects is MCADD, which occurs in up to 1:10,000 Caucasian births. Although fatty acid oxidation and ketogenesis defects may present in the newborn period, particularly in the setting of delayed maternal milk production for exclusively breast-fed infants, the first clinically significant episode may not occur for weeks to months or even years after birth. With extended fasting or intercurrent illness where metabolic demand exceeds available energy supply, severe lethargy acutely develops and then progresses to coma. Recurrent vomiting and consequent dehydration may be associated. Sudden infant death after an overnight fast is an all too frequent initial presentation in up to one third of infants with fatty acid oxidation defects. Infants who survive may suffer recurrent episodes of fasting or illness-induced coma, leading to progressive CNS damage and permanent disability. Metabolic acidosis (resulting from accumulation of partially oxidized fatty acids or secondary lactic acidosis), hyperammonemia, hepatomegaly and liver dysfunction, and hypertrophic cardiomyopathy may occur during acute metabolic decompensation episodes. Liver histology is typified by severe steatosis. Chronically affected children may exhibit recurrent vomiting, failure to thrive, developmental delay, and muscular hypotonia. Certain disorders that affect oxidation of long-chain fatty acids are frequently associated with recurrent rhabdomyolysis and myoglobinuria (long-chain 3-hydroxyacyl-CoA dehydrogenase [LCHAD] deficiency, trifunctional protein deficiency, very-long-chain acyl-CoA dehydrogenase [VLCAD] deficiency, or carnitine-palmitoyl transferase [CPT]-II deficiency) or pigmentary retinopathy and slowly progressive vision loss (LCHAD or trifunctional protein deficiency). Mothers of infants with fatty acid oxidation disorders (particularly LCHAD or trifunctional protein deficiency) may present with acute liver dysfunction during pregnancy with an affected fetus. This may manifest as acute fatty liver of pregnancy or maternal HELLP (hemolysis, elevated liver enzymes, low platelets) syndrome. In the affected infant, hypoglycemia (serum glucose <40 mg/dl) with inappropriately low or absent ketone production during a symptomatic episode is the key laboratory finding that leads to suspicion of a disorder in this subgroup. Differentiation of the specific defects requires analysis of urine organic acids and plasma acylcarnitine species. Between episodes, when the child is clinically well, the urine organic acid profile may be completely normal. Acylcarnitine profiles are more consistently abnormal, but both tests, if normal initially, should be repeated on samples obtained during a symptomatic period to absolutely rule out the possibility of a fatty acid oxidation defect. Carnitine is required for normal fatty acid oxidation; long-chain fatty acids are activated to fatty acyl-CoA, then esterified to carnitine by CPT-I on the outer mitochondrial membrane. These acylcarnitine esters are then transported into mitochondria to complete the oxidation process. In fatty acid oxidation defects, the metabolic block leads to accumulation of the fatty acyl-CoA substrate specific to the deficient enzyme; these species appear in blood as acylcarnitine esters. Analysis of plasma acylcarnitine profiles by tandem mass spectrometry often suggests a specific enzyme deficiency in children with suspected fatty acid oxidation disorders.[23] Diagnostic confirmation may require enzyme analysis in liver tissue or radiometric evaluation of fatty acid oxidation in cultured skin fibroblasts. For certain defects, molecular DNA analysis is clinically available. Two disorders, namely, MCADD[43] and LCHAD deficiency, [37] are associated with relatively common disease-causing mutations. Treatment of all disorders in this subgroup is based upon the provision of adequate nonfat calories and prevention of fasting. Generous IV glucose infusion is lifesaving and essential during acute episodes of metabolic decompensation. Chronic dietary therapy is tailored to the specific enzyme deficiency involved. Many practitioners prescribe carnitine supplementation, initially intravenously during an acute episode and later orally, but the efficacy of this intervention has not been formally investigated in any controlled clinical trial, and its use in disorders of long-chain fatty acid oxidation remains controversial.

Hypoglycemia following a short fast of only 4 to 6 hours is highly suggestive of a glycogen storage disease or disorder of gluconeogenesis such as fructose 1,6-bisphosphatase deficiency. These disorders of energy deficiency are classified in subgroup D. These infants appear healthy while fed but quickly become obtunded and hypotonic with fasting hypoglycemia. Hepatomegaly is a prominent physical feature. During acute hypoglycemia, other biochemical derangements, including lactic acidosis, hypophosphatemia, hyperuricemia, and hypertriglyceridemia, are frequently present. Confirmation of the diagnosis may require a provocative fast under controlled conditions with continuous monitoring and, ultimately, measurement of glycogen content or enzymatic analysis on a liver biopsy specimen.

Group 3 Inborn Errors of Metabolism

Infants with group 3 IEM display symptoms and a progressive clinical course suggestive of intoxication. In these infants, who appear completely healthy at birth and for the first few days of life, neurologic dysfunction appears as toxic metabolites accumulate with increasing food intake. Initial symptoms may include vomiting and lethargy that progress, perhaps over only a few hours, to complete coma or shock. This specific clinical presentation in particular suggests the possibility of bacterial or viral sepsis; evaluation for infectious disease is entirely appropriate. However, the clinician must remain alert to the possibility of an underlying IEM in a previously healthy infant suffering catastrophic illness within the first days of life. Group 3 IEMs can be subdivided into four subgroups (A–D) based upon specific clinical and laboratory findings (Table 69–9).

Maple syrup urine disease ([MSUD], branched-chain ketoacid dehydrogenase [BCKD] deficiency) affects the catabolism of the branched-chain amino acids leucine, isoleucine, and valine and is the only disorder in subgroup A. Affected infants present with coma; abnormal body movements including seizures; and, in contrast to many IEMs, hypertonia and opisthotonus. A severe burst-suppression pattern is the typical EEG abnormality. A sweet body odor, concentrated particularly in urine and cerumen, is often present. Mothers with previously affected children can often diagnose MSUD in a new infant by the presence of this odor. Routine laboratory studies may

TABLE 69–9

Features of Group 3 Inborn Errors of Metabolism

Clinical Features	Associated Laboratory Findings	Possible Diagnoses	Specialized Diagnostic Tests
SUBGROUP A			
Neurologic deterioration, coma Abnormal movements Hypertonia Sweet odor	Mild acidosis Normal lactate ± Ketonuria Normal ammonia ± Urine DNPH test	Maple syrup disease (branched-chain ketoacid dehydrogenase deficiency)	Plasma amino acid analysis Urine organic acid analysis
SUBGROUP B			
Neurologic deterioration, coma Dehydration	Severe acidosis Severe ketonuria ± Hyperammonemia ± Lactic acidosis ± Hypoglycemia ± Neutropenia ± Thrombocytopenia – Urine DNPH test	Organic acidemias Propionic acidemia Methylmalonic acidemia Isovaleric acidemia MCD deficiency Other	Urine organic acid analysis Plasma carnitine level Plasma acylcarnitine profile Urine acylglycine profile
SUBGROUP C			
Neurologic deterioration, coma Seizures Hypotonia ± Liver dysfunction	Severe hyperammonemia No acidosis ± Alkalosis Low BUN Normal glucose Normal lactate	Urea cycle disorders CPS, OTC, ASS, ASL, other Triple H syndrome (hyperornithinemia-hyperammonemia-homocitrullinuria)	Plasma amino acid analysis Urine organic acid analysis Urine orotic acid Enzyme studies in liver
SUBGROUP D			
Neurologic deterioration Hepatomegaly Liver dysfunction Cholestatic jaundice	Direct hyperbilirubinemia ± Hypoglycemia ± Acidosis ± Lactic acidosis ± Ketosis	Galactosemia Fructosemia Tyrosinemia type I Neonatal hemochromatosis Respiratory chain disorder	Urine reducing substances Plasma amino acid analysis Urine organic acid analysis Urine succinylacetone Enzyme studies

ASL, Argininosuccinate lyase; *ASS,* argininosuccinate synthetase; *BUN,* blood urea nitrogen; *CPS,* carbamyl phosphate synthetase; *DNPH,* dinitrophenylhydrazine; *MCD,* multiple carboxylase deficiency; *OTC,* ornithine transcarbamoylase.

document mild metabolic acidosis and mild ketosis, but normal lactate and ammonia. The branched-chain ketoacids that accumulate in MSUD react only slightly with the urine dipstick test for ketones but readily form a flocculent white precipitate with 2,4-dinitrophenylhydrazine (DNPH) in a urine metabolic screen. The presence and specific identities of branched-chain ketoacids in urine are confirmed by urine organic acid analysis. Plasma amino acid analysis reveals tremendous elevation of leucine with lesser accumulations of valine and isoleucine. The neurologic symptoms associated with MSUD result entirely from leucine intoxication. Valine and isoleucine, which do not cross the blood-brain barrier as readily as leucine, seem to contribute little to the neurologic phenotype. Reduction of leucine levels in the body is the goal of MSUD treatment.[24] Emergency therapy during the initial clinical episode includes dietary protein restriction and IV infusion of dextrose-containing fluids. Hyponatremia is a common associated feature; IV hydration with hypotonic fluids easily exacerbates this problem. Additionally, leucine accumulates in CSF and brain and is strongly osmotically active. Rapid IV infusion of hypotonic solutions in several instances has led to acute cerebral edema and death. Dextrose solutions containing a minimum of 0.45% saline (one-half normal saline) are essential, but 10% dextrose with normal saline is preferred if the serum sodium is <135 mEq/L. With administration of IV dextrose, mild hyperglycemia secondary to insulin resistance may occur; inclusion of regular insulin (often only 0.05 U/kg body weight/hour) by either IV infusion or subcutaneous injection promotes anabolism, suppresses endogenous protein catabolism, and accelerates leucine clearance. The vitamin thiamine is a cofactor for BCKD; some individuals with BCKD deficiency (usually with a late rather than neonatal presentation) may respond clinically to thiamine supplementation. Oral thiamine (100 mg/day) is often given empirically to determine whether there is any effect on leucine levels. Once the diagnosis of MSUD is confirmed by plasma amino acid analysis, enteral feedings with a medical food that is free of branched-chain amino acids should be initiated even if the infant is comatose and nasogastric feedings are necessary. Parenteral hydration should continue until results of urine ketone and DNPH tests are negative and full enteral feeds are reestablished. On this regimen, plasma valine and isoleucine levels plummet rapidly, but several days may be required before plasma leucine normalizes. Valine and isoleucine deficiencies that frequently develop on this regimen stimulate endogenous protein catabolism, which impairs reduction of blood leucine, prolongs neurologic impairment, and chronically may be associated with symptoms of protein insufficiency (hair loss, skin breakdown, growth failure). Therefore valine and isoleucine supplementation (50–100 mg/kg/day) is required. Chronic life-long therapy involves dietary protein restriction and provision of sufficient energy and amino acids in a leucine-free synthetic medical food. Despite this, infants who suffered prolonged severe leucinosis as neonates often exhibit significant developmental disability. Early diagnosis and appropriate therapy critically enhance neurodevelopmental outcome.

Severe ketoacidosis is the hallmark of IEMs in subgroup B, the organic acidemias. Methylmalonic, propionic, and isovaleric acidemias are the most common disorders in this subgroup. Infants with organic acidemia present with catastrophic episodes of vomiting, dehydration, and coma. Hypoglycemia, lactic acidosis, hyperammonemia, neutropenia, or pancytopenia may be associated findings depending upon the specific IEM. The urine dipstick test for ketones is strongly positive, but in contrast to MSUD, little precipitate forms following the addition of DNPH reagent to the urine. Identification of the specific offending organic acid is accomplished by urine organic acid analysis using GC-MS. Diagnostic confirmation may require enzymatic analysis in tissues such as leukocytes, liver, or cultured skin fibroblasts. Cessation of protein intake, vigorous rehydration with dextrose-containing fluid, and management of acidosis with sodium bicarbonate infusion are the mainstays of emergency management. In severely acidotic patients, especially with associated hyperammonemia, hemodialysis may be useful for quickly removing both ammonia and the offending organic acid with the goal of minimizing CNS damage. IV infusion of L-carnitine (100–300 mg/kg/day) assists with the removal of the offending organic acid and prevents secondary carnitine deficiency. Oral L-glycine supplementation has a similar role in certain IEMs, most notably isovaleric acidemia. Chronic therapy is tailored to the specific enzyme deficiency but often involves dietary protein restriction and provision of a synthetic medical food supplying sufficient energy and amino acids. Recurrent episodes of life-threatening ketoacidosis and coma, generally triggered by fasting or intercurrent illness, are often the greatest long-term clinical difficulties.

Advancing dietary protein intake and normal protein catabolism during the first few days of life lead to severe hyperammonemia in infants with urea cycle and allied disorders (subgroup C). The clinical presentation is nonspecific, with progressive vomiting and neurologic dysfunction. Routine laboratory studies are generally deceptively normal, although the BUN often is below the limits of detection in infants who are unable to synthesize urea. No acidosis is present unless the infant is apneic or hypoperfused and secondary lactic acidosis has developed. Most severely hyperammonemic infants demonstrate respiratory alkalosis secondary to Kussmaul-like hyperventilation triggered by cerebral edema. Detection of hyperammonemia is the critical diagnostic key. The blood ammonia level must be measured in any child with acute-onset obtundation without a clear etiology such as trauma. Determination of the specific IEM involved requires analysis of blood amino acids and urine organic acids. Enzyme analysis in liver or for a few defects in cultured skin fibroblasts is necessary for diagnostic confirmation. Provision of nonprotein energy and suppression of protein catabolism through IV dextrose infusion are essential, as in the organic acidemias, but emergency hemodialysis to rapidly decrease blood ammonia is absolutely required if any possibility of favorable neurodevelopmental outcome is to be preserved. Ammonia clearance by exchange transfusion or peritoneal dialysis is insufficient to accomplish this goal. Even with prompt hemodialysis, the metabolic derangement in some infants is so severe that little sustained decrease in blood ammonia is observed. Despite aggressive therapy, neonatal-onset urea cycle disorders are frequently lethal. The few infants exposed to hyperammonemia for a prolonged period who, because of extraordinary life support efforts, survive are often profoundly neurologically impaired. On the other hand, clinical outcome is favorable in cases where blood ammonia levels rapidly correct on hemodialysis. This dichotomy in outcome presents a considerable dilemma to the intensivist faced with these critical treatment decisions. In practice, hemodialysis should be attempted as soon as possible after the discovery of hyperammonemia unless clinical signs of severe permanent CNS damage are already present. Disorder-specific therapy should continue for infants whose blood ammonia levels immediately normalize with hemodialysis. Aggressive life support measures should be limited for those infants with recalcitrant hyperammonemia. Following dialysis, generous IV hydration and provision of nonprotein calories should continue. The amino acid arginine, normally synthesized through the urea cycle, becomes an essential amino acid that must be provided exogenously in urea cycle disorders. L-Arginine hydrochloride is available for IV administration as 10% solution and should be added to the IV fluid bag to give 0.66 g arginine HCl/m^2/day (6 ml/kg/day in infants). The ammonia scavenging agents sodium phenylacetate and sodium benzoate are available as a combined IV solution (Ucyclyd Pharmaceuticals) but only on an investigational basis. Administration of this solution dramatically improves ammonia clearance and is indicated for the acute management of most urea cycle disorders, but it is associated with severe adverse effects including metabolic acidosis and erosive gastritis if administered inappropriately. They should be used only in consultation with a provider experienced in their administration and with careful monitoring. Long-term therapy is based upon dietary protein restriction and oral L-arginine or L-citrulline supplementation. Oral administration of sodium benzoate or sodium phenylbutyrate (Ucyclyd) as ammonia scavengers is often prescribed. Episodes of fasting or illness induced hyperammonemic coma frequently recur. Management of recurrent hyperammonemia in a patient known to have a urea cycle disorder is similar to that outlined earlier but can be tailored to the specific defect. Liver transplantation is a viable treatment option for individuals suffering recurrent hyperammonemia and chronic clinical and developmental difficulties despite adequate nutritional and medical therapy.

Hepatomegaly, liver dysfunction, and cholestatic jaundice in association with neurologic deterioration are the central presenting features of IEM in subgroup D. For all of these disorders, the accumulating toxin is particularly damaging to hepatocellular function. Hypoglycemia, acidosis, and mild ketosis may be present. Bacterial infection, particularly urinary tract infection, bacteremia, or meningitis, often caused by *E. coli* or other gram-negative enteral flora, is a frequent occurrence in infants with galactosemia. The specific diagnosis is suggested by the clinical scenario and by the results of screening laboratory studies. Infants with this clinical presentation who are breast-fed or receiving cow's milk-based infant formula are at risk for symptoms of galactosemia, given that lactose (milk sugar) is a disaccharide of galactose and glucose. Infants receiving exclusively soy milk-based formula ingest little galactose. The predominant dietary carbohydrates in soy formula are fructose and glucose, so infants fed soy formula who have this clinical presentation are likely to have fructosemia rather than galactosemia. More typically, infants with fructosemia present clinically after the introduction of fruit to their diet. In either galactosemia or fructosemia, reducing sugars are detected in urine following ingestion of the offending sugar by the urine reducing substance test (Clinitest). Plasma tyrosine level is elevated, urine organic acid analysis displays metabolites from the tyrosine pathway, and succinylacetone is detected in the urine of children with tyrosinemia type I (fumarylacetoacetate hydrolase deficiency). Neonatal hemochromatosis can be diagnosed only on liver biopsy by staining for iron. Diagnostic confirmation differs for each disorder but may include further metabolite analyses, enzymatic analysis in tissue, or molecular DNA testing. Initial therapy is nonspecific: cessation of enteral feeding and IV infusion of dextrose-containing fluid. Once the exact diagnosis is known, a specific therapy plan can be developed. For the carbohydrate disorders, the offending sugar must be reduced or eliminated from the diet. Galactosemic infants are fed soy-milk based formulas only. After weaning, ingestion of dairy products, including baked goods prepared with dairy products, are strictly avoided. Similarly, fructosemic individuals must strenuously avoid any fructose-containing foods. In prior eras, cirrhosis and liver failure were the inevitable outcome in children with tyrosinemia type I unless they received a liver transplant. Effective therapy that prevents liver degeneration in tyrosinemia has now been developed. The oral drug 2-(2-nitro-4-trifluoro-methylbenzoyl)-1, 3-cyclohexanedione (NTBC) blocks tyrosine metabolism upstream from FAH and prevents accumulation of the intermediate metabolites that are toxic to hepatocytes.[12] This medication was highly successful in preventing cirrhosis in two separate clinical trials and has been approved by the U.S. Food and Drug Administration for general use. The long-term efficacy of NTBC therapy, particularly with regard to the incidence of hepatic adenoma, a common complication of tyrosinemia I, has yet to be proven.[21]

Summary

Most IEMs with symptom onset in the neonatal period emerge as one of the clinical presentations described. As mentioned previously, many of these IEMs have milder or late-onset forms that present with identical symptoms as described, but months or years after birth and often following the stress of fasting or intercurrent illness. These clinical scenarios provide a framework for the recognition, initial evaluation, and emergency treatment of infants with IEM. The remainder of this chapter focuses upon the differential diagnosis of select clinical situations encountered in the pediatric intensive care unit.

Metabolic Acidosis

The key to the differential diagnosis of metabolic acidosis is calculating the serum anion gap ($Na - [Cl + HCO_3]$). This figure, which normally is 10 to 15 mM, represents the unmeasured negative ions, predominantly albumin, in blood. Normal anion gap acidosis (low serum HCO_3 but normal anion gap) is caused by excess bicarbonate loss from either the gut (diarrhea) or kidney (renal tubular acidosis). An elevated or so-called *positive anion gap* suggests the presence of another unmeasured anion. Incidentally, a low serum anion gap may be seen in extreme hypoalbuminemia, as occurs in nephrotic syndrome (see Chapters 62 and 99).

The differential diagnosis of positive anion gap metabolic acidosis in children is similar to that of adults (use your favorite mnemonic, such as MUDPILES or KETONES), but with the addition of another class of acidoses, the IEMs. Poisoning with methanol, ethanol, paraldehyde, isoniazid, or salicylates can be readily ruled out by history or drug screen. Uremia is also easily discovered by laboratory evaluation. The most common etiologies of a positive anion gap acidosis in children are ketosis, lactic acidosis, or a combination of the two. Extreme dehydration can cause both ketosis and lactic acidosis; these abnormalities are readily corrected with vigorous parenteral rehydration with dextrose-containing fluids. Persistent lactic acidosis suggests ongoing tissue damage from hypoxemia, hypoperfusion, or, more rarely, an inborn error of mitochondrial metabolism. It should be remember that several organic acids, such as propionic and methylmalonic acids, react with the urinary ketones dipstick. These pathologic organic acids can be differentiated only from the more typical ketones, 3-hydroxybutyric and acetoacetic acids, by urine organic acid analysis. Severe positive anion gap metabolic acidosis that cannot be easily explained by the clinical context, especially if it occurs recurrently or is recalcitrant to parenteral fluid therapy, suggests an inborn error of organic acid metabolism and should be evaluated with a battery of screening metabolic studies including plasma amino acid analysis, urine organic acid analysis, and urine qualitative metabolic screen.

Hypoglycemia

Hypoglycemia can be defined as a blood glucose concentration less than 40 mg/dl.[16] Low blood glucose may be present within the first few hours after birth, especially in preterm or low-birth-weight infants, but the capacity for effective gluconeogenesis and fatty acid oxidation is induced within the first day after birth. Therefore blood glucose less than 40 mg/dl is distinctly unusual after the first 24 hours of life, particularly in infants who have started feeding, and should be thoroughly investigated (Fig. 69–2). A review of hypoglycemia in infants and children along with a useful diagnostic algorithm have been published.[20] A detailed medical history and careful physical examination are essential to discovering the cause of hypoglycemia. The timing of hypoglycemia relative to feeding is a critical item of historical information. Persistent or postprandial hypoglycemia suggests hyperinsulinism. Hypoglycemia after a short fast (3–6 hours) along with permanent hepatomegaly suggests a glycogen storage disorder. Hypoglycemia following a longer fast (8–12 hours) suggests a defect in gluconeogenesis or a problem with utilization of fatty acids. The presence of ketones in urine (as measured qualitatively by urine dipstick) or in serum (quantitative measurement of 3-hydroxybutyrate or acetoacetate) is an important clue to the etiology of hypoglycemia. Ketosis during hypoglycemia demonstrates that insulin secretion is appropriately suppressed and that fatty acid mobilization and oxidation are intact. Glycogen storage disorders, gluconeogenic defects, and defects of ketone utilization all are associated with ketosis. The absence of ketogenesis during hypoglycemia suggests that either insulin levels are inappropriately elevated or fatty acid oxidation is blocked. An important caveat to this rule is that infants younger than approximately 1 week cannot normally produce enough ketones during fasting to trigger a positive urine dipstick test for ketones. The absence of urine ketones in an infant younger than 1 week does not contribute to the differential diagnosis of hypoglycemia. On the other hand, serum ketones increase with fasting even in neonates, and this test provides a valuable result in the investigation of hypoglycemia. In hypoketotic hypoglycemia, measurement of total serum free fatty acids provides further useful diagnostic information. During fasting, insulin secretion normally is suppressed, free fatty acids are mobilized into circulation from peripheral adipose tissues, and ketones are produced by oxidation of fatty acids in liver. A low serum total free fatty acid level during hypoketotic hypoglycemia strongly suggests inappropriate insulin secretion, even if insulin levels do not appear to be dramatically elevated. Hypoketotic hypoglycemia in association with elevated serum total free fatty acids suggests a defect in fatty acid oxidation.

The importance of treating hypoglycemia cannot be overemphasized as affected individuals are at high risk for seizures and permanent brain damage.[8,39] After appropriate diagnostic studies are obtained, hypoglycemia should be treated with IV glucose administration at the rate of normal hepatic glucose production, approximately 10 mg glucose/kg body weight per minute or 150 ml/kg per day of a 10% solution until the underlying disorder is identified and more appropriate therapies can be initiated.[30]

Hypoketotic hypoglycemia with low serum total free fatty acids suggests hyperinsulinism. Hyperinsulinism presenting in the newborn period may be caused by intrauterine exposure to elevated glucose levels (maternal diabetes mellitus), familial hyperinsulinemic hypoglycemia (defect in the sulfonylurea receptor), or hyperammonemia/hyperinsulinism syndrome (abnormality in regulation of insulin secretion secondary to mutation in glutamate dehydrogenase). Infants with hyperinsulinism often are obese and require glucose infusions greater than 10 mg/kg/min to maintain normoglycemia. Glucagon administration (0.03 mg/kg, up to 1-mg total dose) reverses hypoglycemia in hyperinsulinism. Oral diazoxide has not been shown to be efficacious in most neonatal cases; however, it can be effective in normalizing blood glucose levels in patients who have infantile forms of hyperinsulinism, including hyperammonemia/hyperinsulinism syndrome. This usually is given at doses of 5 to 10 mg/kg/day divided into three doses. When initially administered, it is given along with glucose and glucagon. Efficacy of diazoxide is defined by demonstrating normal

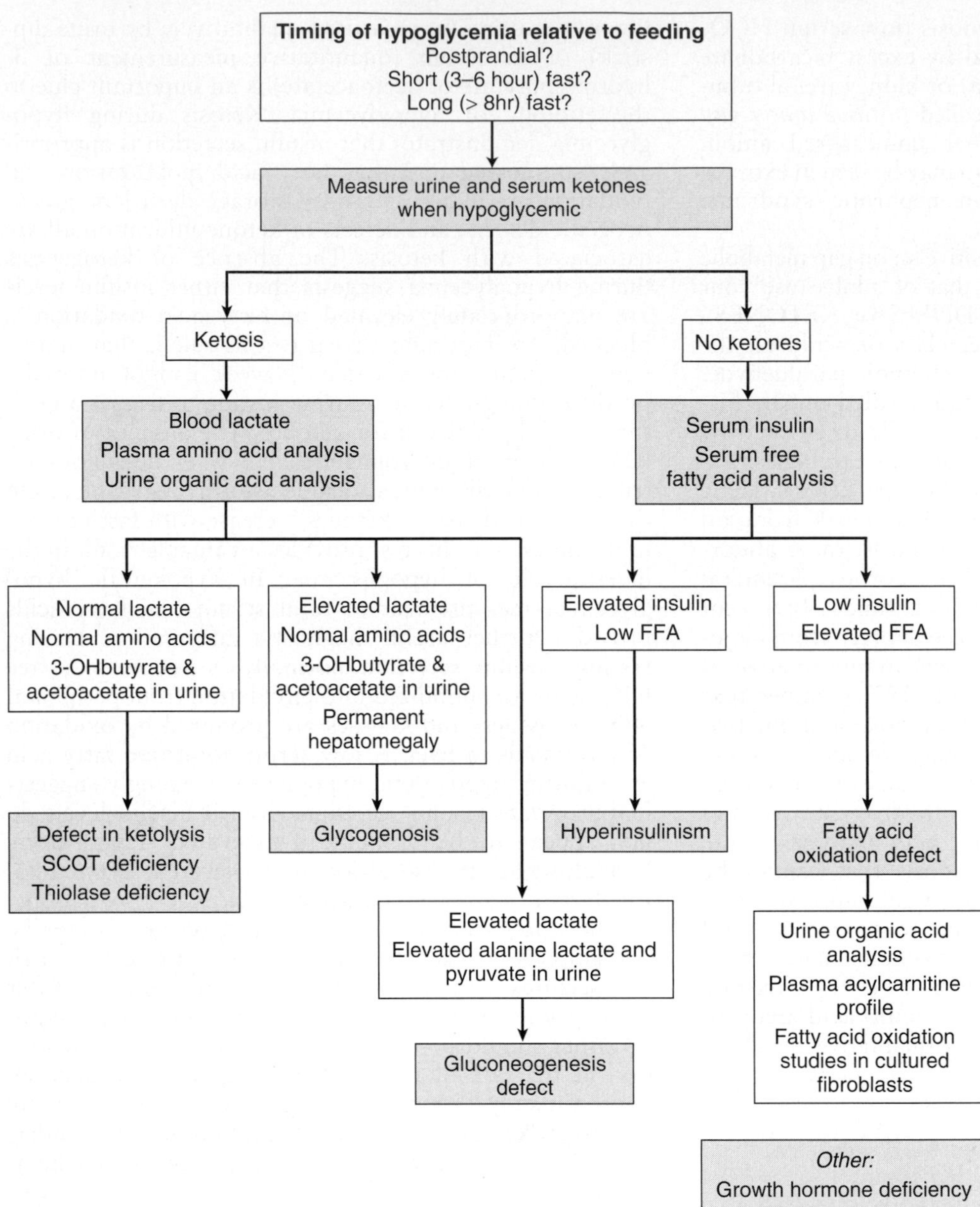

FIGURE 69–2 • Algorithm for evaluation of hypoglycemia in children. *FFA,* Free fatty acid; *SCOT,* succinyl-CoA oxoacid transferase.

preprandial and postprandial glucose concentrations after overnight fasting and after having stopped IV glucose and any other medications for 5 consecutive days.

Hypoketotic hypoglycemia with elevated serum total free fatty acids, usually occurring following an extended fast (8–12 hours) or in association with an intercurrent illness, suggests a defect in fatty acid oxidation. The clinical presentation of fatty acid oxidation disorders has been described. Although inherited deficiency of at least nine different enzymatic steps in the mitochondrial β-oxidation pathway has been described, the clinical presentation of infants and children with these diseases is stereotypically similar and can be differentiated only by appropriate metabolic testing. In all cases, vigorous hydration with dextrose-containing parenteral fluids is lifesaving. Fasting avoidance is key to long-term treatment and prevention of hypoglycemic episodes.

Infants and children with glycogen storage disorders present with hypoglycemia and permanent hepatomegaly. Hypoglycemia in these disorders is poorly responsive to glucagon administration. Enzymatic defects affecting glycogen synthesis, including glycogen synthase deficiency (GSD-0), as well as defects in glycogen breakdown, such as debranching enzyme deficiency (GSD-III), result in hypoglycemia. Glycogen synthase deficiency usually presents as severe morning hypoglycemia with hyperketonemia and low lactic acid and alanine. Debranching enzyme deficiency results in hypoglycemia secondary to limitation of glucose release from the outer branches of the glycogen molecule. Ketosis is present in GSD-III as the body attempts to generate fuel by increased fatty acid oxidation. Furthermore, the gluconeogenesis pathway is intact; thus hypoglycemia is much milder. In glucose 6-phosphatase deficiency (GSD-Ia) and glucose 6-phosphate translocase deficiency (GSD-Ib), hypoglycemia usually is apparent 2.5 to 3 hours postprandially as these disorders not only affect glucose release from glycogen but also disrupt gluconeogenesis. Individuals with these disorders have lactic acidosis, ketosis, and hyperuricemia in addition to hepatomegaly.

Hypoglycemia following a longer fast (8–12 hours) suggests a defect in gluconeogenesis, ketogenesis, ketolysis, or fatty acid oxidation. Fructose 1,6-bisphosphatase, a disorder of gluconeogenesis, presents as fasting hypoglycemia but also with metabolic decompensation following fructose ingestion. Ketonemia and lactic acidemia are major features, in addition to the hypoglycemia. The ketone synthesis defects that present with fasting hypoketotic hypoglycemia include 3-hydroxy-3-methylglutaryl-CoA synthase deficiency and 3-hydroxy-3-methylglutaryl CoA lyase deficiency. These patients have hypoglycemia in combination with normal blood lactate but no ketonuria. Infants with 3-hydroxy-3-methylglutaryl CoA lyase deficiency also are hyperammonemic. Defects in succinyl-CoA oxoacid transferase and methylacetoacetyl-CoA thiolase represent ketolysis defects. Although the consistent biochemical abnormality is severe ketoacidosis, hypoglycemia also can be seen. Blood lactic acid and ammonia concentrations usually are normal.

Cardiomyopathy and Inborn Errors of Metabolism

Cardiomyopathies, as a rule, are rare. Studies undertaken by the Pediatric Cardiomyopathy Registry have determined that the overall annual incidence is 11.8 per million patient-years and that the incidence was higher in children younger than 1 year than in those between 1 and 18 years old. In this regional study, 40% of cases were hypertrophic cardiomyopathies, 49% of cases were dilated cardiomyopathies, 3% of cases were restrictive or other types, and 8% were unspecified.[19] Further study revealed that of cases of hypertrophic cardiomyopathy, 16% had an identifiable IEM as the underlying cause. These causes included disorders of glycogen metabolism (5%), mucopolysaccharide metabolism (4%), oxidative phosphorylation (5%), and fatty acid metabolism (2%). In the cases of dilated cardiomyopathy, 5% were found to be of a metabolic etiology with disorders of glycogen metabolism (1%), mucopolysaccharide metabolism (2%), and oxidative phosphorylation (2%) as the recognizable underlying cause.[18] Thus it is important to consider IEM in the differential diagnosis of any child with dilated or hypertrophic cardiomyopathy. Because the prevalence of underlying metabolic disorders is so high, some authors have recommended that all children with cardiomyopathy undergo metabolic screening, including blood lactate, plasma amino acid analysis, urine organic acid analysis, urine metabolic screening (particularly for the detection of excessive urinary mucopolysaccharides), plasma carnitine levels, and plasma acylcarnitine profile (Box 69–3)[5]. Additionally, serum creatine kinase (CK) should be measured to exclude muscular dystrophy.

Autosomal dominant hypertrophic cardiomyopathy has an incidence of 1:500 but demonstrates extremely variable penetrance. Mutation in genes encoding structural sarcomeric proteins are frequent causes of dominant hypertrophic cardiomyopathy. More than 140 mutations in 15 different genes have been identified.[1]

Cardiomyopathy may be a complicating feature of several IEMs (Table 69–10), but with a few exceptions, other associated symptoms or physical examination findings at the time of presentation point toward the appropriate diagnosis. Very broadly, the pathogenesis of cardiomyopathy in IEMs is either myocardial energy deficiency, as occurs in the dilated cardiomyopathy associated with several organic acidemias, or excessive storage of complex molecules in the heart, as occurs in the hypertrophic cardiomyopathy of mucopolysaccharidoses such as Hurler syndrome. Cardiomyopathy occurs as the sole initial clinical manifestation in a relatively restricted list

BOX 69–3

Screening Laboratory Studies for Evaluation of Cardiomyopathy

- Blood lactate
- Serum creatine kinase
- Plasma amino acid analysis
- Urine organic acid analysis
- Urine metabolic screening
- Plasma carnitine levels
- Plasma acylcarnitine profile

TABLE 69–10

Cardiomyopathy and Inborn Errors of Metabolism

Cardiomyopathy as the sole or a key presenting feature	Carnitine transport defect
	Fatty acid oxidation defects
	  VLCAD deficiency
	  Mitochondrial trifunctional protein deficiency
	  Carnitine palmitoyltransferase deficiency
	Glycogen storage disease type II (Pompe disease)
	Glycogen storage disease type IX (phosphorylase B kinase deficiency)
	Disorders of oxidative phosphorylation (mitochondrial myopathy)

Cardiomyopathy as a secondary feature	Organic acidemias
	  Propionic acidemia
	  Methylmalonic acidemia
	  3-Methylglutaconic aciduria
	  D-2-Hydroxyglutaric aciduria
	  Biotinidase deficiency
	Glycogen storage disease type III
	Glycogen storage disease type IV
	Mucopolysaccharidoses
	Congenital disorders of glycosylation
	Congenital myotonic dystrophy
	Congenital muscular dystrophies

VLCAD, Very-long-chain acyl-CoA dehydrogenase.

BOX 69–4

Metabolic Causes of Cardiomyopathy

- Carnitine transporter deficiency
- Fatty acid oxidation disorders
- Glycogen storage diseases II and IX
- Disorders of mitochondrial oxidative phosphorylation

of metabolic diseases, including autosomal recessively inherited deficiency of the cellular carnitine transporter, fatty acid oxidation disorders, glycogenosis types II and IX, and disorders of oxidative phosphorylation (Box 69–4). The carnitine transporter defect is caused by deficiency of the sodium-dependent transporter OCTN2, which is responsible for transporting carnitine from the circulation into tissues including cardiac and skeletal muscle.[25] Dilated cardiomyopathy with symptoms of heart failure generally presents within the first years of life and is associated with severely low plasma total carnitine levels. Cardiac function improves dramatically after carnitine supplementation, and cardiomyopathy rarely recurs if carnitine is continued.

Hypertrophic cardiomyopathy resulting from myocardial steatosis may be an isolated presenting feature in several disorders of fatty acid oxidation, particularly those affecting long-chain fatty acid metabolism such as VLCAD or mitochondrial trifunctional protein deficiencies. Saudubray et al.[33] examined a series of 109 patients with fatty acid oxidation defects and found that cardiac involvement, including hypertrophic cardiomyopathy or arrhythmia, was apparent at presentation in 51% of cases. Fatty acid oxidation disorders are most reliably detected by analysis of plasma acylcarnitine profiles by tandem mass spectrometry. Long-chain fatty acids are activated to CoA derivatives and then esterified to carnitine prior to transport into mitochondria for β-oxidation. In fatty acid oxidation disorders, especially during acute metabolic decompensation, acylcarnitine species accumulate in plasma and provide a diagnostic profile that is specific to a given enzyme deficiency. Confirmation of the diagnosis may require enzymatic analysis in cultured fibroblasts or mutation analysis. Once the diagnosis of a long-chain fatty acid oxidation disorder has been established, restriction of dietary long-chain fat intake and provision of medium-chain triglyceride oil as an alternative fuel source for the myocardium often reverses cardiomyopathy. Cardiac support measures, including extracorporeal membrane oxygenation, may be necessary for as long as 1 to 2 weeks after presentation before heart function improves.

Glycogen storage disease type II (acid α-glucosidase deficiency; Pompe disease) is a disorder of lysosomal glycogen accumulation that frequently presents as hypertrophic cardiomyopathy, yielding the classic "boot-shaped" radiographic appearance of the cardiac silhouette. Skeletal myopathy manifesting as severe hypotonia may complicate the presentation. Confirmation of the diagnosis requires measurement of enzyme activity in skeletal or cardiac muscle or cultured fibroblasts. In the past, treatment has only been supportive, but clinical trials of IV enzyme replacement therapy have shown some early promise.[40]

Myocardial function is highly dependent upon mitochondrial oxidative phosphorylation; up to 30% of the total myocardial volume is composed of mitochondria.[29] Dilated or hypertrophic cardiomyopathy is a frequent presenting feature in infants with severe defects of mitochondrial oxidative phosphorylation. Skeletal muscle myopathy, liver dysfunction, renal tubulopathy, bone marrow failure, or CNS abnormalities may occur. Chronic lactic acidosis, if present, is an important indicator of mitochondrial dysfunction. Screening metabolic laboratory studies demonstrate nonspecific abnormalities associated with chronic lactic acidosis. Definitive diagnosis requires histologic evaluation of skeletal muscle and measurement of respiratory chain enzyme activities. Isolated deficiency of cytochrome *c* oxidase (COX or complex IV) and reduced nicotinamide adenine dinucleotide (NADH)-ubiquinone oxidoreductase (complex I) of the mitochondrial respiratory chain are the most common oxidative phosphorylation defects presenting with cardiomyopathy. Although some protein subunits of complexes I and IV are encoded by mtDNA, most infant-onset isolated complex deficiencies probably are the result of autosomal-recessively inherited deficiency of nuclear-encoded respiratory chain subunits or of chaperone proteins that ensure proper assembly of functional complexes. For instance, hypertrophic cardiomyopathy caused by functional COX deficiency has been associated with mutations in nuclear COX subunit genes[2,3] or nuclear genes for COX associated-proteins SCO1 and SCO2.[17]

Cardiomyopathy may be seen in several other IEMs, but in these disorders, other physical or biochemical features are generally apparent at initial clinical presentation. For instance, dilated cardiomyopathy may complicate propionic acidemia during acute metabolic decompensation, but features of severe metabolic acidosis, vomiting, dehydration, coma, and possibly hyperammonemia are part of the initial clinical presentation.

Metabolic Myopathies and Rhabdomyolysis

Rhabdomyolysis is a clinical syndrome resulting from skeletal muscle injury and release of potentially toxic substances into the circulatory system. Acute onset of severe muscle pain associated with increased serum CK levels is the hallmark of the disorder. In extreme cases, massive myoglobinuria may cause acute renal insufficiency. The threshold serum CK value that qualifies as clinically significant rhabdomyolysis is a matter of debate. Some institutions set CK levels five times greater than the laboratory upper limit as the marker for rhabdomyolysis,[11,41] whereas others use CK values greater than 1000 IU/L as the lower limit to make the diagnosis.[38] Although trauma and direct muscle injury are by far the most common causes of rhabdomyolysis, inborn errors of muscle metabolism should be considered in the differential diagnosis of rhabdomyolysis occurring at any age.

In the absence of a history of trauma, the differential diagnosis of acute rhabdomyolysis should include drug or toxin exposure, muscle hypoxia (often associated with seizures), temperature alterations, inflammatory diseases, and IEMs. Because muscle contraction depends upon adenosine triphosphate (ATP) generated by the mitochondrial electron transport chain, it follows that any process that impairs muscle ATP synthesis or that results in energy expenditure that surpasses ATP production could lead to rhabdomyolysis. The clinical history should lead toward the appropriate diagnosis. A family history that includes rhabdomyolysis or a history in which more than one episode of exercise-induced rhabdomyolysis has been observed should induce suspicion of a metabolic disorder. Along with muscular dystrophy and endocrine etiologies (hypothyroidism, hyperthyroidism, diabetic ketoacidosis, pheochromocytoma), glycolytic defects, fatty acid oxidation disorders, purine biosynthetic disorders, and disorders of mitochondrial oxidative phosphorylation should be considered if historical elements do not direct toward the more common etiologies. As described previously, the fatty acid oxidation disorders can be detected by urine organic acid analysis and plasma acylcarnitine profile. Chronic lactic acidosis may be a clue to a disorder of oxidative phosphorylation. Measurement of blood lactate level before and after an exercise treadmill protocol may help detect a respiratory chain defect if the postexercise lactate level is severely elevated. Definitive diagnosis of a mitochondrial disorder requires histologic and enzymatic analysis of a fresh muscle biopsy. The glycolytic defects of phosphofructokinase and phosphoglycerate mutase deficiencies along with myophosphorylase deficiency (glycogen storage disease type V or McArdle disease) cause severe recurrent rhabdomyolysis; their detection requires enzymatic analysis of muscle tissue. Likewise, myoadenylate deaminase deficiency, a defect in purine catabolism, and CPT-II deficiency are also diagnosed by measurement of the enzyme activities in muscle.

Neonatal Screening

Newborn screening for IEMs was first introduced in the 1960s, with screening for phenylketonuria. Technological advances, most significantly the introduction of tandem mass spectrometry, have greatly increased the number of disorders that can be identified by analysis of a dried blood spot on a filter paper card.[35] The trend in the United States and Europe is toward expanded newborn screening as several aminoacidopathies, fatty acid oxidation disorders, and organic acidurias now can be detected very early and appropriate therapies initiated. The cost versus benefits of expanded screening, whether to include specific very rare or poorly treatable disorders in the screening panel, and the availability of adequate follow-up resources have been debated,[42] but a general consensus is emerging that expanded newborn screening will be an effective tool for identifying IEM; early intervention; and, ultimately, preventing complications in disorders for which intervention is possible.[10] It must be remembered, however, that this expanded newborn screening is just that—a screen, and both false-positive and false-negative results are possible. Thus the astute clinician must remain cognizant of the fact that in an ill infant, a normal newborn screen is reassuring but should not be taken as absolute proof-positive that an IEM identifiable on NBS is not present. Appropriate screening laboratory evaluation and emergency treatment should be instituted if clinical signs and symptoms of an IEM are present in a sick child.

Conclusion

Inborn errors of metabolism are individually rare but collectively will make not-infrequent appearances in a busy pediatric intensive care unit. The signs and symptoms of IEM may be nonspecific and often overlap extensively with more common disorders. When clinical suspicion of an IEM arises, screening biochemical genetic laboratory studies must be ordered. Further confirmatory testing often is necessary if screening laboratory tests point toward a specific disease. Confirmatory testing and disease-specific therapy should be instituted following consultation with a biochemical genetics specialist. If detected and treated early, the clinical outcome for many IEMs can be favorable.

REFERENCES

1. Ackerman MJ, VanDriest SL, Ommen SR, et al: Prevalence and age-dependence of malignant mutations in the beta-myosin heavy chain and troponin T genes in hypertrophic cardiomyopathy: a comprehensive outpatient perspective, *J Am Coll Cardiol* 39: 2042-2048, 2002.
2. Antonicka H, Leary SC, Guercin GH, et al: Mutations in COX10 result in a defect in mitochondrial heme A biosynthesis and account for multiple, early-onset clinical phenotypes associated with isolated COX deficiency, *Hum Mol Genet* 12:2693-2702, 2003.
3. Antonicka H, Mattman A, Carlson CG, et al: Mutations in COX15 produce a defect in the mitochondrial heme biosynthetic pathway, causing early-onset fatal hypertrophic cardiomyopathy, *Am J Hum Genet* 72:101-114, 2003.
4. Baumgartner ER, Suormala T: Multiple carboxylase deficiency: inherited and acquired disorders of biotin metabolism, *Int J Vitam Nutr Res* 67:377-384, 1997.
5. Bonnet D, de Lonlay P, Gautier I, et al: Efficiency of metabolic screening in childhood cardiomyopathies. *Eur Heart J* 19:790-793, 1998.
6. Burton BK: Inborn errors of metabolism: the clinical diagnosis in early infancy, *Pediatrics* 79:359-369, 1987.
7. Clarke TA, Saunders BS, Feldman B: Pyridoxine-dependent seizures requiring high doses of pyridoxine for control, *Am J Dis Child* 133:963-965, 1979.
8. De Lonlay P, Giurgea I, Touati G, Saudubray JM: Neonatal hypoglycaemia: aetiologies, *Semin Neonatol* 9:49-58, 2004.
9. Eisensmith RC, Woo SL Population genetics of phenylketonuria, *Acta Paediatr Suppl* 407:19-26, 1994.
10. Fearing MK, Marsden DL: Expanded newborn screening, *Pediatr Ann* 32:509-515, 2003.
11. Gabow PA, Kaehny WD, Kelleher SP: The spectrum of rhabdomyolysis, *Medicine (Baltimore)* 61:141-152, 1982 .
12. Grompe M: The pathophysiology and treatment of hereditary tyrosinemia type 1, *Semin Liver Dis* 21:563-571, 2001 .
13. Hayasaka K, Tada K, Fueki N, et al: Nonketotic hyperglycinemia: analyses of glycine cleavage system in typical and atypical cases, *J Pediatr* 110:873-877, 1987.
14. Hoffmann GF, von Kries R, Klose D, et al: Frequencies of inherited organic acidurias and disorders of mitochondrial fatty acid transport and oxidation in Germany, *Eur J Pediatr* 163: 76-80, 2004.
15. Kleijer W: Inborn errors of metabolism. In Rodeck C, Whittle M, editors: *Fetal medicine: basic science and clinical practice.* London, 1999, Churchill Livingstone.
16. LaFranchi S: Hypoglycemia of infancy and childhood, *Pediatr Clin North Am* 34:961-982, 1987.
17. Leary SC, Kaufman BA, Pellecchia G, et al: Human SCO1 and SCO2 have independent, cooperative functions in copper delivery to cytochrome c oxidase, *Hum Mol Genet* 13:1839-1848, 2004.

18. Lipshultz SE, Sleeper LA, Towbin JA, et al: The incidence of pediatric cardiomyopathy in two regions of the United States, *N Engl J Med* 348:1647-1655, 2003.
19. Lipshultz SE, Sleeper LA, Towbin JA, et al: The incidence of pediatric cardiomyopathy: the prospective pediatric cardiomyopathy registry, *J Am Coll Cardiol Suppl* 37:1180-1196, 2001.
20. Lteif AN, Schwenk WF: Hypoglycemia in infants and children, *Endocrinol Metab Clin North Am* 28:619-646, vii, 1999.
21. Luijerink MC, Jacobs SM, van Beurden EA, et al: Extensive changes in liver gene expression induced by hereditary tyrosinemia type I are not normalized by treatment with 2-(2-nitro-4-trifluoromethylbenzoyl)-1,3-cyclohexanedione (NTBC), *J Hepatol* 39:901-909, 2003.
22. Marquardt T, Denecke J: Congenital disorders of glycosylation: review of their molecular bases, clinical presentations and specific therapies, *Eur J Pediatr* 162:359-379, 2003.
23. Millington DS, Kodo N, Norwood DL, Roe CR: Tandem mass spectrometry: a new method for acylcarnitine profiling with potential for neonatal screening for inborn errors of metabolism, *J Inherit Metab Dis* 13:321-324, 1990.
24. Morton DH, Strauss KA, Robinson DL, et al: Diagnosis and treatment of maple syrup disease: a study of 36 patients, *Pediatrics* 109:999-1008, 2002.
25. Nezu J, Tamai I, Oku A, et al: Primary systemic carnitine deficiency is caused by mutations in a gene encoding sodium ion-dependent carnitine transporter, *Nat Genet* 21:91-94, 1999.
26. NIH Consensus Statement Online. Phenylketonuria: screening and management. 17:1-27, 2000.
27. Nyhan WL, Ozand PT: *Atlas of metabolic diseases*. London, 1998, Chapman & Hall.
28. Opitz JM, Gilbert-Barness E, Ackerman J, Lowichik A: Cholesterol and development: the RSH (Smith-Lemli-Opitz) syndrome and related conditions, *Pediatr Pathol Mol Med* 21:153-181, 2002.
29. Page E, Polimeni PI, Zak R, et al: Myofibrillar mass in rat and rabbit heart muscle. Correlation of microchemical and stereological measurements in normal and hypertrophic hearts, *Circ Res* 30:430-439, 1972.
30. Prietsch et al: 2002.
31. Russo PA, Mitchell GA, Tanguay RM: Tyrosinemia: a review, *Pediatr Dev Pathol* 4:212-21, 2001.
32. Saudubray J-M, Charpentier C: Clinical phenotypes: diagnosis/algorithms. In Scriver CR, Beaudet AL, Sly WS, Valle D, editors: *The metabolic and molecular bases of inherited disease*. New York, 2001, McGraw-Hill.
33. Saudubray JM, Martin D, de Lonlay P, et al: Recognition and management of fatty acid oxidation defects: a series of 107 patients, *J Inherit Metab Dis* 22:488-502, 1999.
34. Saudubray JM, Narcy C, Lyonnet L, et al: Clinical approach to inherited metabolic disorders in neonates, *Biol Neonate* 58(suppl 1): 44-53, 1990.
35. Schulze A, Lindner M, Kohlmuller D, et al: Expanded newborn screening for inborn errors of metabolism by electrospray ionization-tandem mass spectrometry: results, outcome, and implications, *Pediatrics* 111(6 pt 1):1399-1406, 2003.
36. Scriver CR, Beaudet AL, Sly WS, Valle D, editors: *The metabolic and molecular bases of inherited disease*. New York, 2001, McGraw-Hill.
37. Sims HF, Brackett KC, Powell CK, et al: The molecular basis of pediatric long chain 3-hydroxyacyl-CoA dehydrogenase deficiency associated with maternal acute fatty liver of pregnancy, *Proc Natl Acad Sci U S A* 92:841-845, 1995.
38. Singhal PC, Kumar A, Desroches L, et al: Prevalence and predictors of rhabdomyolysis in patients with hypophosphatemia, *Am J Med* 92:458-464, 1992.
39. Stanley CA: Hyperinsulinism in infants and children, *Pediatr Clin North Am* 44:363-374, 1997.
40. Van den Hout JM, Kamphoven JH, Winkel LP, et al: Long-term intravenous treatment of Pompe disease with recombinant human alpha-glucosidase from milk, *Pediatrics* 113:e448-57, 2004.
41. Welch RD, Todd K, Krause GS: Incidence of cocaine-associated rhabdomyolysis, *Ann Emerg Med* 20:154-157, 1991.
42. Wilcken B: 2003 Ethical issues in newborn screening and the impact of new technologies, *Eur J Pediatr* 162(suppl 1): S62-S66.
43. Yokota I, Indo Y, Coates PM, Tanaka K: Molecular basis of medium chain acyl-coenzyme A dehydrogenase deficiency. An A to G transition at position 985 that causes a lysine-304 to glutamate substitution in the mature protein is the single prevalent mutation, *J Clin Invest* 86:1000-1003, 1990.

CHAPTER

70

Disorders of the Endocrine System Relevant to Pediatric Critical Illness

David B. Allen, Scott A. Hagen, and Aaron L. Carrel

PEARLS

- Hypertension that is responsive to α-blockade and much less responsive to alternative hypertensive therapy (e.g., sodium nitroprusside) strongly suggests the diagnosis of pheochromocytoma. Effective α-receptor blockade should always be achieved before β-blockade is attempted because a compromise in inotropy and chronotropy in the face of increased systemic vascular resistance risks cardiac failure.
- The prominent role of thyroid hormones in regulating energy metabolism and modulating catecholamine effects justifies the importance of thyroid physiology to intensive care medicine. It is clear from many invasive and noninvasive measurements in patients with thyroid disease that cardiac functions such as heart rate, cardiac output, and systemic vascular resistance are closely linked to thyroid status.
- Hypothermia increases thyrotropin-releasing hormone (TRH)-mediated thyroid-stimulating hormone (TSH) release. Factors that inhibit TSH release include dopamine, somatostatin, hyperthermia, glucocorticoids, and triiodothyronine (T_3). Norepinephrine and adrenergic agonists stimulate TSH release.
- Binding of T_3 to specific nuclear receptors modulates gene transcription and synthesis of messenger ribonucleic acid and cytoplasmic proteins.
- Tissue functions stimulated by this interaction include oxygen consumption, thermogenesis, amino acid and lipid metabolism, water and ion transport, and growth and development of tissues such as the central nervous system and skeleton. Thyroid hormone accelerates metabolism of various hormones (e.g., insulin and cortisol) and is needed for other endocrine functions (e.g., growth hormone and parathormone activity). Normal respiratory responses to hypoxia and hypercapnia are dependent on thyroid hormone.
- A marked decrease in serum thyroxine (T_4) is associated with increased mortality. When the serum T_4 level decreases to less than 4 μg/dl, mortality increases to 50%; when the serum T_4 level decreases to less than 2 μg/dl, mortality increases to 80%.
- Although hypothyroidism is infrequently seen in critical illness during childhood, undetected hypothyroidism may impair vital functions and further compromise serious illness.
- Detection of an exaggerated TSH response to TRH administration strongly suggests hypothyroidism; however, drugs commonly used in the intensive care setting (e.g., dopamine and glucocorticoids) inhibit TSH release and may confound this test.

- The intensivist frequently has the opportunity to perform a diagnostic-therapeutic evaluation of the hypoglycemic child at the time of hypoglycemia. This often yields a prompt diagnosis of a complex metabolic disorder and obviates the need for cumbersome and potentially hazardous fasting studies.
- Extracellular Ca^{2+} concentration is monitored by Ca^{2+}-sensing receptors.
- These receptors are plentiful on the surface of the chief cells of the parathyroid glands, in numerous kidney sites (juxtaglomerular apparatus, luminal surface of the proximal convoluted tubule, basolateral surface of the cortical thick ascending limb of the loop of Henle, apical and luminal membrane of the inner medullary collecting duct in the kidneys), the intestine, parts of the brain, thyroid C cells, breast, and adrenal glands. Acting in classic hormonal negative feedback fashion, binding of Ca^{2+} to this receptor activates phospholipase C and accumulation of inositol triphosphate, which secondarily leads to inhibition of the secretion and synthesis of parathyroid hormone, and activation of its proteolysis.
- Reduced amount of growth hormone released in pulses is related to low circulating levels of insulin-like growth factor (IGF)-1, IGF binding protein (IGFBP)-3, and acid-labile subunit, which suggests that a relative hyposomatotropism may participate in the pathogenesis of the wasting syndrome distinctively in the chronic phase of critical illness.
- Maintenance of normoglycemia with insulin reduces mortality and morbidity of critically ill adult patients.
- It appears that metabolic control as reflected by normoglycemia, rather than the infused insulin dose per se, is most closely related to the beneficial effects of intensive insulin therapy.

Normal growth and metabolism depend on the complex interplay of hormonal messengers. An effective response to serious illness or injury is also mediated by hormones. Therefore endocrine disorders can both cause and dramatically alter the response to critical illness. Prompt recognition of hormonal deficiency or excess as a cause of critical illness leads to specific therapy for what often appears to be a nonspecific clinical syndrome. In addition, awareness of physiologic, possibly adaptive alterations in endocrine function that occur in response to critical illness is needed to interpret hormonal studies properly in the intensive care setting. This chapter reviews the pathophysiology, physical and laboratory diagnosis, life-threatening complications, and treatment of childhood endocrine disorders likely to present with critical illness. Emphasis is placed on hormonal responses to nonendocrine illness of greatest importance in the pediatric intensive care unit. Disorders of water metabolism (see Chapter 60) and diabetic ketoacidosis (see Chapter 71) are discussed elsewhere. For additional information about nonacute aspects of pediatric endocrine disease, a current text is recommended.[1]

Adrenal Cortical Insufficiency

Pathophysiology

The adrenal cortex synthesizes three classes of steroids—glucocorticoids, androgens, and mineralocorticoids—in response to the trophic stimuli of adrenocorticotropin (adrenocorticotrophic hormone [ACTH]) and angiotensin-II (A-II). ACTH is a cleavage product of a larger precursor (pro-opiomelanocortin) synthesized in the anterior and intermediate lobes of the pituitary. Release of ACTH from the pituitary is modulated by hypothalamic corticotropin-releasing factor (CRF). Whereas binding of ACTH to specific adrenal cortex receptors promotes synthesis and secretion of all adrenal steroids, negative feedback control of ACTH is exerted by free cortisol alone at both the pituitary and hypothalamic levels. Impaired cortisol production because of enzyme deficiencies or gland failure is accompanied by chronic elevations of ACTH.

Although ACTH is clearly the primary stimulus for cortisol synthesis, mineralocorticoid synthesis by the adrenal zona glomerulosa is responsive primarily to A-II and the serum potassium concentration. Renin secretion is increased by (1) a decline in renal perfusion pressure, (2) an increase in renal adrenergic activity, and (3) a decline in distal tubular sodium load. Renin binds specifically to and cleaves angiotensinogen to create angiotensin-I, a decapeptide that is converted to A-II by angiotensin-converting enzyme predominantly in the pulmonary vascular bed. Angiotensin-II binds to specific receptors in the zona glomerulosa to stimulate early steps in steroid synthesis and increases renal perfusion pressure through its vasopressor properties. Elevations in serum K concentrations directly stimulate aldosterone secretion.

Serum ACTH levels are helpful in discerning the cause of adrenal failure (Table 70–1). Chronic or progressive primary adrenal insufficiency (Addison disease) is associated with hypersecretion of ACTH and is most often attributed to autoimmune phenomena. Antiadrenal antibodies, as well as autoantibodies to other organ systems (e.g., thyroiditis, diabetes, pernicious anemia, ovarian failure), can frequently be detected. Hemorrhage into the gland (Waterhouse-Friderichsen syndrome) is associated with severe septicemia (especially meningococcal or *Pseudomonas*) (see Chapter 96). Fungal infections, tuberculosis, metastatic cancer, and the acquired immune deficiency syndrome (AIDS) are rare causes of adrenal failure during childhood.

Salt-losing forms of congenital adrenal hyperplasia present early in life are suggested by ambiguous genitalia

TABLE 70–1

Causes of Adrenal Insufficiency in Childhood

Associated with low ACTH levels
CNS infection, hemorrhage, or infarction
Congenital hypopituitarism
Iatrogenic chronic adrenal suppression
Associated with high ACTH levels
Addison disease (autoimmune, infectious)
Congenital adrenal hypoplasia
Adrenal hemorrhage
Familial unresponsiveness to ACTH
Congenital adrenal hyperplasia
Adrenoleukodystrophy
Wolman disease (acid lipase deficiency)

ACTH, Adrenocorticotrophic hormone; *CNS,* central nervous system.

in the female infant and usually are not associated with cortisol deficiency unless the deficient enzyme is early in the metabolic pathway of cortisol synthesis (e.g., desmolase deficiency). Congenital adrenal hypoplasia and Wolman disease (acid lipase deficiency) present early in infancy with combined glucocorticoid and mineralocorticoid deficiency. Adrenoleukodystrophy, a rare X-linked recessive disorder, usually is characterized by neurologic degeneration (blindness and dementia) associated with panadrenal failure but occasionally occurs with isolated adrenal insufficiency as the presenting finding.

Failure of ACTH secretion and resulting (secondary) adrenal insufficiency can follow infection, hemorrhage, or infarction of the central nervous system (CNS) or pituitary. Multiple anterior pituitary hormone deficiencies are often present, and isolated ACTH deficiency is rare. The most common cause of secondary adrenal insufficiency is prolonged (i.e., >2 weeks) administration of supraphysiologic doses of glucocorticoids with resulting suppression of the hypothalamic-pituitary-adrenal (HPA) axis. Such therapy should be tapered gradually to allow for adrenal recovery, which can be documented by morning cortisol determinations or synthetic ACTH stimulation tests. Relative adrenal insufficiency and/or inadequate adrenal reserve are commonly reported in critically ill patients.

Glucocorticoid and adrenal androgen production are impaired in both primary and secondary adrenal insufficiency. Given the trophic effects of non-ACTH stimuli on the zona glomerulosa, an important distinction between primary (destruction of the adrenal gland) and secondary (ACTH deficiency) adrenal insufficiency is the preservation of mineralocorticoid synthesis in the latter. Rarely, isolated cortisol deficiency is seen in the syndrome of familial unresponsiveness to ACTH.[2] Individuals with these disorders may have adequate glucocorticoid production for ordinary metabolic demands but may be unable to increase plasma cortisol to levels typically observed after injury or acute infectious illness. Normally, a dramatic stress-induced increase in cortisol production (up to six times normal) accelerates glycogenolysis and mobilizes precursors for gluconeogenesis (protein catabolism and lipolysis), resulting in elevations in blood glucose (i.e., the so-called *stress response*) (see Chapter 68). Weak mineralocorticoid effects of cortisol are exaggerated by high serum concentrations and, in combination with aldosterone, promote sodium retention, kaliuresis, and restoration of blood volume after hypovolemia. Glucocorticoids must also be present, however, for excretion of a water load. The cardiovascular system, possibly through potentiation of catecholamine effects, responds to cortisol by increasing cardiac output and systemic vascular resistance. Cortisol is also necessary for maintaining the speed of synaptic transmission, particularly in multisynaptic regions such as the reticular-activating system.

Whether glucocorticoids play a "permissive" or "regulatory" role in the stress state is debated. During mild or moderate stress, basal cortisol levels may be sufficient to allow the full manifestation of homeostatic responses. More severe stress, by contrast, may require exaggerated fuel mobilization regulated by cortisol in a dose-dependent fashion. A role for accelerated release of glucocorticoids in limiting potentially detrimental host responses to stress has also been proposed.[3]

Physical and Laboratory Diagnosis

Manifestations of adrenal insufficiency are diverse and may have a gradual or sudden onset. Findings reflect the relative contributions of glucocorticoid and, in cases of panadrenal failure (Addison disease), mineralocorticoid deficiency. Symptoms of progressive glucocorticoid deficiency include weakness and fatigue, anorexia, weight loss, vomiting, and mental status deterioration, which may indicate symptomatic hypoglycemia. Mineralocorticoid deficiency and the resulting loss of extracellular fluid (ECF) volume lead to dehydration; hypotension; salt craving; and, rarely, quadriplegia as a result of severe hyperkalemia.

The most striking physical finding in the child with primary adrenal insufficiency and chronic ACTH elevation is increased pigmentation, most pronounced at the lip borders, on the buccal mucosa, nipples, scarred areas, pressure points, and the palmar, axillary, and groin creases. This progressive melanin deposition more likely is related to the direct effect of β-lipotropin or ACTH rather than melanocyte-stimulating hormone, although each is elevated in the patient with Addison disease. Vitiligo can be seen in association with hyperpigmentation and is ascribed to autoimmune destruction of melanocytes. The degree of hypotension and decrease in heart size depend on the degree of mineralocorticoid deficiency and may be late findings. In female patients of pubertal age, decreased body hair indicates impaired adrenal androgen production.[4]

Laboratory findings depend on whether glucocorticoids, mineralocorticoids, or both are deficient and on the completeness of the deficiency. A combined, severe deficit leads to reduced serum sodium, elevated serum potassium, metabolic acidosis, and hypoglycemia in response to fasting. Because termination of antidiuretic hormone (ADH) release is impaired by glucocorticoid deficiency, hyponatremia is exacerbated by persistent ADH secretion. Patients with secondary adrenal insufficiency (with ACTH deficiency or suppression and isolated glucocorticoid deficiency) do not have hyperpigmentation, have intact mineralocorticoid function and normal ECF volume, but typically have mild hyponatremia as a result of free water retention. Impaired gluconeogenesis and lipolysis may lead to hypoglycemia. Eosinophilia (>300 cells/μL) is often present. Suggestive historical or physical features and a discernible cause for precipitous decline are frequently absent in the child with acute adrenal insufficiency. When shock and unresponsiveness to volume expansion and pressor agents occur, pituitary or adrenal failure should be suspected. In a critically ill child, a cortisol level less than 20 μg/dl, particularly when accompanied by hyponatremia and hyperkalemia, suggests adrenal hypofunction. To further substantiate cortisol deficiency, the rapid ACTH stimulation test (Cortrosyn ≈ 150 μg/m^2 intravenous [IV] bolus, with serum samples obtained at 0 and 60 minutes; normal response is an increase in serum cortisol >20 μg/dl) can assess adrenal reserve during the early treatment period. However, patients with partial pituitary ACTH deficiency may respond normally to standard doses (i.e., 125–250 μg) exogenous ACTH. The "low-dose" ACTH test (IV administration of 0.05–0.1 μg synthetic ACTH followed by cortisol sampling at 30 minutes) has been shown to detect milder degrees of adrenal gland suppression; however, the utility of this test in the critical setting is unresolved.[5] When feasible, metyrapone, insulin-induced hypoglycemia, or prolonged ACTH testing can be used to further evaluate the HPA axis. Endogenous plasma ACTH levels greater than 200 pg/ml suggest primary adrenal failure; lower ACTH levels (inappropriate when compared with cortisol levels) indicate pituitary suppression or failure.

Therapy of Acute Adrenal Insufficiency

Adrenal crisis, manifested by hypotension, dehydration, shock, hypoglycemia, hyponatremia, and hyperkalemia, may be the initial presentation of adrenal insufficiency. Immediate therapy includes fluid resuscitation, glucocorticoid replacement, and attention to the precipitating condition (e.g., infection) if identified. Shock is treated with colloid or normal saline solution (10–20 ml/kg) during the first hour. Isotonic fluids containing dextrose (e.g., D_5NS) are administered at 1.5 to 2 times maintenance to restore intravascular volume and normoglycemia. Hypertonic saline solution may worsen dehydration and mental status and should be avoided. When adrenal insufficiency is suspected but not documented, initial glucocorticoid replacement should include dexamethasone (0.2 mg/kg up to a maximum of 1 mg every 6 hours), which does not interfere with quantitation of plasma cortisol by radioimmunoassay. The rapid ACTH stimulation test can be performed immediately thereafter. When the diagnosis is known, hydrocortisone (50 mg for small children; 100–150 mg for larger children and adolescents) is administered initially and is followed by 100 mg/m^2/day added to the IV fluids. The significant mineralocorticoid activity of large doses of hydrocortisone, in contrast to dexamethasone, obviates the need for additional mineralocorticoid replacement.

When the patient's condition is stable, the hydrocortisone dose is tapered by approximately one third each day toward maintenance oral cortisol replacement (20 mg/m^2/day given in a two-times-per-day or three-times-per-day regimen). Mineralocorticoid replacement (e.g., 0.1–0.2 mg 9-α-fludrocortisone) is added for the patient with primary adrenal insufficiency when the hydrocortisone dose is reduced to less than 100 mg/day. A MedicAlert tag must be issued to identify the child's cortisol dependency, and the family should be educated about the risk of acute episodes. Cortisol replacement should be doubled or tripled in response to febrile illnesses, trauma, or other significant stress in proportion to its severity. When oral medication cannot be taken or in situations of severe trauma or stress, injectable hydrocortisone (100-mg vial) should be promptly administered.

Adrenal Medullary Hyperfunction: Pheochromocytoma

Pathophysiology

The adrenal medulla develops from neuroectodermal-derived chromaffin cells that migrate into the developing adrenal cortex. Extraadrenal chromaffin tissue (e.g., organ of Zuckerkandl) predominates during fetal life and infancy but involutes before age 3 years, at which time the fully developed adrenal medulla comprises 10% of the weight of each adrenal gland. Whereas sympathetic nerve terminals synthesize and release the neurotransmitter norepinephrine (NE), the primary medullary catecholamine is epinephrine (EPI), the synthesis of which is localized to the adrenal by the dependence of the enzyme phenylethanolamine-N-methyltransferase on glucocorticoids. Splanchnic nerve impulses stimulate the release of stored epinephrine. Both NE (not inactivated by sympathetic nerve reuptake) and EPI are metabolized by catechol-o-methyl-transferase and monoamine oxidase to vanillylmandelic acid (VMA). However, the relative contributions of each can be determined by urinary measurement of the intermediates normetanephrine and metanephrine. Dopamine, a CNS transmitter and precursor for NE and EPI, is metabolized principally to homovanillic acid.

The physiologic effects of catecholamines are mediated by adrenergic receptors on target cell surfaces. NE is mainly an α-receptor stimulator, whereas EPI induces both α- and β-activity (see Chapter 23). Elevations of a specific catecholamine are often predicted by clinical manifestations. Both EPI and NE, through stimulation of both α-receptor subtypes, cause vasoconstriction, increases in systolic and diastolic blood pressure, glycogenolysis, lipolysis, and inhibition of insulin release. However, the additional effect of EPI on α_1 (inotropic and chronotropic) and, in particular, α_2 (vasodilatory) receptors causes cardiac stimulation to dominate the clinical picture of EPI excess, and marked vasoconstriction out of proportion to cardiac effects suggests NE excess.

Disorders of the adrenal medulla and sympathetic nervous system in children are primarily related to neoplasms. Undifferentiated and aggressive neuroblastomas and more mature ganglioneuroblastomas are tumors of intraadrenal or extraadrenal sympathetic nervous tissue. Although elevations in plasma catecholamine levels and metabolites are typical for these neoplasms and can serve as tumor markers, their clinical effects rarely require intensive care. Pheochromocytomas, by contrast, are rare (and rarely malignant), catecholamine-secreting tumors of chromaffin tissue origin that can produce dramatic, life-threatening manifestations of catecholamine excess. They usually arise in the adrenal medulla (right side more common) but may occur in the abdominal sympathetic chain, neck, thorax, and urinary bladder wall. Multiple tumors can occur in children. Boys are affected more often than girls, with a peak incidence at 9 to 12 years. Familial pheochromocytomas may occur as part of the multiple endocrine neoplasia (MEN) syndromes.[6]

Physical and Laboratory Diagnosis

The physiologic effects of markedly elevated NE and EPI levels produce variable clinical syndromes that can mimic essential hypertension, renal disease, hyperthyroidism, drug-induced states (e.g., amphetamines, cocaine), and psychiatric disorders, and diagnosis is often delayed when suspicion for pheochromocytoma is low. In most cases, secretion of NE predominates with lesser amounts of EPI. The resulting hypertension, which is often dramatic (e.g., systolic blood pressure levels of 250 mmHg), more often is sustained in children, rather than paroxysmal as seen in adults. Hypertensive encephalopathy, retinopathy, and cardiac failure may occur in association with a catecholamine-induced cardiomyopathy.

When paroxysms of catecholamine release occur, the patient experiences diaphoresis, headache, palpitations, flushing, emotional lability, and a sense of impending doom. Chronic vasoconstriction may produce a red-brown discoloration, swelling of the fingers (acrocyanosis), and orthostatic hypotension because of reduced plasma volume and inability to activate sympathetic reflexes. Episodic abdominal pain, constipation, polyuria (possibly from glycosuria), and polydipsia may confound early diagnosis. These symptoms in a child with neurofibromatosis, cerebellar hemangioblastoma, Cushing syndrome, or a family history of a MEN syndrome should lead to prompt evaluation for pheochromocytoma.

Urinary analysis for catecholamines and their metabolites (normetanephrine, metanephrine, VMA) provide the most specific diagnostic approach. Although 24-hour collections are desirable, simultaneous measurement of creatinine excretion allows extrapolation from truncated collections using age-appropriate control data. Although a pheochromocytoma can be reliably excluded by normal excretion of catecholamine metabolites, assessment of urinary NE and EPI provides important information about tumor location and expected clinical course. High levels of epinephrine usually indicate an adrenal medulla or organ of Zuckerkandl origin and predict an increased risk (compared with NE-secreting tumor) of α-adrenergic–mediated tachyarrhythmias and hypermetabolic syndromes. Use of urinary dopamine and homovanillic acid (HVA) excretion to distinguish malignant from benign disease has relatively poor sensitivity. When the episodes are paroxysmal, urine collections for NE and EPI, which reflect short-term changes in catecholamine production more accurately than metabolite screening, should coincide with the presence of symptoms.

To date, measurement of plasma catecholamine levels has been less useful in the diagnosis of pheochromocytoma in children. Levels may be normal during asymptomatic periods and may overlap with patients with essential hypertension. The "normal" range varies widely depending on position and emotional state, and numerous medications confound plasma NE and EPI analysis. Thus urine catecholamine determination remains the preferred diagnostic tool. However, when the diagnosis remains in doubt, evaluation of either suppression of plasma catecholamines by oral clonidine or provocation of catecholamine release by IV glucagon may be useful.

When an adrenal site is suspected, localization of the tumor can be attempted with equal likelihood of success with a computed tomographic scan, which detects masses larger than 1 cm, or magnetic resonance imaging. Uptake and storage of the compound metaiodobenzylguanidine (MIBG), labeled with either iodine 123 or iodine 131, simulates NE. MIBG scintigraphy is useful in identifying extraadrenal, recurrent, or metastatic disease requiring whole-body imaging. Approximately 10% of scans yield false-negative results, and misinterpretation of normal adrenal uptake accounts for most false-positive scans. Invasive diagnostic procedures, such as selective venous sampling and arteriography, have been virtually supplanted by these three imaging techniques. When attempted, attention should be paid to preprocedural sympathetic blockage as described in the next section.[7]

Treatment

Although definitive therapy for pheochromocytoma is surgical, medical therapy before and after the procedure is crucial for safe tumor resection. Acute correction of life-threatening hypertension requires effective α-blockade. Hypertension that is responsive to α-blockade and much less responsive to alternative hypertensive therapy (e.g., sodium nitroprusside) strongly suggests the diagnosis of pheochromocytoma. Effective α-receptor blockade should always be achieved before β-blockade is attempted because a compromise in inotropy and chronotropy in the face of increased systemic vascular resistance risks cardiac failure. Phentolamine (Regitine), a short-acting α-adrenergic blocking agent, given parenterally at 1 mg/dose, is effective initial treatment for a child. Subsequent titration of the drug can be accomplished by continuous IV infusion to control symptoms. When large amounts of EPI are present, β-adrenergic blockade is indicated to prevent or treat tachyarrhythmias. As mentioned, extreme care is required in the administration of β-blocking drugs, particularly when evidence of cardiomyopathy is present. Esmolol given intravenously or propranolol given enterally for control of dysrhythmia or for chronic control of β-adrenergic effects is effective for children with pheochromocytomas. Initial doses of propranolol are 5 to 10 mg given every 6 to 8 hours orally. Alternately, esmolol, a β-blocker with a short half-life, may be used as an IV drip to titrate treatment. Other therapies (for which there is limited experience in children) include combined α- and β-adrenergic blockade with labetalol and calcium channel blockade with nifedipine, which may interfere with exocytotic release of NE from storage vesicles of the tumor.

After stabilization and diagnostic evaluation, 2 weeks of preoperative adrenergic blockade is recommended (1) to blunt the physiologic consequences of excess NE or EPI release during the procedure and (2) to relieve vasoconstriction, allow restoration of ECF volume, and reduce the risk of intraoperative hypotension. Oral phenoxybenzamine hydrochloride (Dibenzyline, 0.25 mg/kg/day starting dose to 1 mg/kg/day given every 12 hours) is an effective α-adrenergic blocking agent usually well tolerated by children. The dose of medication is gradually increased twice weekly until normotension is achieved or until side effects, such as nasal congestion, gastrointestinal irritation, and hypotension, appear. Other useful α-adrenergic blocking agents are prazosin (Minipress), terazosin (Hytrin), and doxazosin (Cardura). If adjunct therapy is needed to control catecholamine effects, α-methyl-tyrosine (Demser), an inhibitor of tyrosine hydroxylase, blocks the conversion of tyrosine to dopa and thus reduces levels of NE, EPI, and dopamine. The drug is started orally at a dose of 5 to 10 mg/kg/day administered every 6 hours, with titration upward as needed. At recommended doses, sedation is usually the only side effect.[8]

During surgical removal of the pheochromocytoma, meticulous monitoring of blood pressure and cardiac function is required. An arterial line, Foley catheter, and pulmonary arterial catheter are standard care. Atropine-like drugs and halothane should be avoided as anesthetic agents. Intravenous phentolamine or sodium nitroprusside are useful for control of hypertension, and cardiac rhythm disturbances usually respond to β-blockers or lidocaine. If the volume deficit is not adequately replaced preoperatively, hypotension requiring treatment with NE may occur when the tumor is removed. Particularly for children, in whom bilateral adrenal or concurrent intra-adrenal and extraadrenal tumors are more common, hydrocortisone for parenteral administration should be available in the event bilateral adrenalectomy is required.

Postoperative fluctuations in blood pressure are common and reflect variable ECF volume status relative to the newly increased vascular capacity and decreased vascular tone. Hypotension is best managed with fluid and blood products. Avoidance of pressor agents is desirable. Persistent hypertension after surgery suggests residual tumor or coexisting renal vascular disease. Successful treatment with phentolamine provides a diagnostic-therapeutic test that suggests another tumor is present. An increase in insulin production by hyperresponsive β-cells may cause transient hypoglycemia. Postoperative analysis of urinary catecholamine levels is performed to ensure normalization of levels.[9]

Thyroid Disorders and Responses to Critical Illness

The prominent role of thyroid hormones in regulating energy metabolism and modulating catecholamine effects justifies the importance of thyroid physiology to intensive care medicine. It is clear from many invasive and noninvasive measurements in patients with thyroid disease that cardiac functions such as heart rate, cardiac output, and systemic vascular resistance are closely linked to thyroid status. However, disorders of the thyroid, although relatively common during childhood, rarely result in critical illness in children. Alterations in thyroid hormone metabolism, by contrast, occur frequently in seriously ill children. Whether such changes represent an adaptive response to stress or a factor contributing to illness is debated; thus interpretation of thyroid function studies remains a challenge in the intensive care setting.

Physiologic Principles

The thyroid gland concentrates iodide from the blood (the rate-limiting step in thyroid hormone synthesis), oxidizes it through the action of thyroid peroxidase to an active intermediate, and iodinates thyroglobulin-bound tyrosyl residues to form monoiodotyrosine and diiodotyrosine. Thyroid peroxidase catalyzes the coupling of iodotyrosines to form triiodothyronine (T_3) and thyroxine (T_4). Thyrotropin (thyroid-stimulating hormone [TSH])-stimulated hydrolysis of thyroglobulin (TG), an iodinated glycoprotein that provides tyrosyl residues for iodotyrosine synthesis, releases iodothyronines into the blood. Free iodide released by hydrolysis of TG is efficiently captured and reused for new hormone synthesis. Circulating TG concentrations, normally less than 80 mg/ml, decrease with age through childhood and, when elevated, reflect thyroidal hyperactivity from various causes or papillary-follicular carcinoma.

Thyrotropin stimulates multiple steps in thyroid hormone synthesis, the intrathyroidal monodeiodination of T_4 to form T_3, and thyroid growth. Pathologic thyroid-stimulating immunoglobulins (e.g., in Graves disease) may interact with (types of) TSH receptors to cause all or some of these effects. Low plasma iodide levels stimulate iodide uptake, whereas pharmacologic doses of iodide inhibit cyclic adenine monophosphate (cAMP) formation by TSH, thyroid peroxidase activity, and organification (Wolff-Chaikoff effect).

The tripeptide thyrotropin-releasing hormone (TRH), found in the hypothalamus and other tissues, modulates pituitary TSH secretion. Hypothermia increases TRH-mediated TSH release. Factors that inhibit TSH release include dopamine, somatostatin, hyperthermia, glucocorticoids, and T_3. Norepinephrine and adrenergic agonists stimulate TSH release. Feedback of thyroid hormone on TSH release occurs at both the pituitary and hypothalamic levels, with local pituitary conversion of free T_4 to free T_3 content probably having the most important effect.

Thyroxine is synthesized exclusively by the thyroid gland, whereas T_3 is predominantly (70%–90%) derived from monodeiodination of T_4 in nonglandular tissues. Only 0.03% of T_4 and 0.3% of T_3 circulate unbound by thyroxine-binding globulin, thyroxine-binding prealbumin, and albumin. The unbound fraction is capable of traversing membranes, binding nuclear receptors, and increasing protein synthesis. Thus binding proteins, which bind greater than 95% of circulating thyroid hormone, provide transport, buffering, and extrathyroidal storage of thyroid hormone reservoir. Nuclear receptor affinity is 10 times greater for T_3 than for T_4, accounting for threefold to fourfold increased metabolic potency of T_3. Because T_3 is also less tightly bound to binding proteins than is T_4, virtually all thyroid hormone activity is attributable to T_3 alone and may not be accurately reflected in the serum T_4 concentration. Pituitary conversion of T_4 to T_3 accounts for approximately 50% of the local pituitary T_3; the remainder is derived from circulating T_3 that is transported to the pituitary.

Metabolism of T_4 occurs by conversion to either metabolically active T_3 (5′-monodeiodination by either type I or type II outer ring monodeiodinase enzymes) or metabolically inactive reverse T_3 (rT_3; 5′-monodeiodination). This process can be dramatically altered by critical illness or malnutrition. The type I outer ring monodeiodinase enzyme is located predominantly in the liver and kidney and is responsible for peripheral conversion of T_4 to T_3 throughout postnatal life. The type II enzyme is found in brown adipose tissue, the pituitary thyrotropes, and the brain and is responsible for control of energy metabolism in brown adipose tissue and in the regulation of TSH secretion. Thyroid hormones and their deiodinated metabolites are excreted in urine and stool in both free and conjugated forms. Binding of T_3 to specific nuclear receptors modulates gene transcription and synthesis of messenger ribonucleic acid (mRNA) and cytoplasmic proteins. The T_3 receptor, which is similar to oncogene protein c-*erb* A, has mutations resulting in altered T_3 binding and rare clinical states of relative resistance to thyroid hormone action. Tissue functions stimulated by this interaction include oxygen consumption, thermogenesis, amino acid and lipid metabolism, water and ion transport, and growth and development of tissues such as the CNS and skeleton. Thyroid hormone accelerates metabolism of various hormones (e.g., insulin and cortisol) and is needed for other endocrine functions (e.g., growth hormone and parathormone activity). Normal respiratory responses to hypoxia and hypercapnia are also dependent on thyroid hormone.

Thyroid hormones increase the affinity and responsiveness of β-adrenergic receptors to catecholamines. Accentuated catecholamine effects seen in the hyperthyroid state reflect this "up-regulation" of receptor activity and occur with normal or lowered serum catecholamine concentrations. Although tachycardia and tremor can be diminished with β-receptor blockade, the underlying levels of cellular metabolic activity and thyroid function remain unchanged.

Thyrotoxic Crisis (Thyroid Storm)

Pathophysiology

Childhood hyperthyroidism usually is caused by Graves disease, an autoimmune disorder that occurs in a genetically predisposed population. Multisystem involvement gives rise to eye manifestations and dermopathy in addition to thyroid abnormalities. Immunoglobulin subclass G1 antibodies with thyroid-stimulating activity (TSA), capable of stimulating cAMP production in a TSH-like manner, cause the hyperthyroid state. Other autoantibodies, such as collagen-stimulating antibodies (associated with ophthalmopathy), thyroid growth-stimulating antibody (associated with large goiter), and antimicrosomal and antithyroglobulin antibodies may also be present.[10] Patients with autoimmune (Hashimoto) thyroiditis, in whom the thyroid gland is still responsive to coexisting TSA, may develop hyperthyroidism similar to Graves disease but usually of shorter duration. Other causes of hyperthyroidism observed in adults (toxic multinodular goiter, toxic nodular goiter, thyroid hormone ingestion, and neoplasia) are rare in children. Neonatal thyrotoxicosis can occur as a result of transplacental passage of TSA from a mother with active or inactive Graves disease and high TSA levels. The incidence of neonatal Graves disease is approximately 1% of infants born to mothers with Graves disease, including women treated in the past with thyroid ablation who continue to have high circulating immunoglobulin levels.[11] The onset of clinical hyperthyroidism is variable (usually between 2 and 9 days), depending on maternal antithyroid medication, degree of TSA stimulation, and presence of other transplacentally acquired autoantibodies. When TSH-blocking antibodies are simultaneously present, the onset of hyperthyroidism can be delayed for 4 to 6 weeks. Thyrotoxic infants manifest goiter, tachycardia, irritability, flushing, hypertension, and exophthalmos. Dysrhythmias, cardiac failure, and death can occur, and mortality has approached 25% in diagnosed cases. Aggressive antithyroid drug and supportive treatment are frequently required during the period of maximal TSA stimulation. The disease resolves as the maternal TSA is degraded (half-life ≈ 12 days) with an average clinical course of 3 to 12 weeks.[12]

Clinical and Laboratory Diagnosis

Manifestations of hyperthyroidism in childhood have been well described; critical illness is rare. Nervousness, palpitations, hyperphagia, and weakness reflect the hyperactivity of the sympathetic nervous system. Symptoms attributed to sympathetic activity improve with antithyroid therapy, whereas signs reflecting other autoantibody effects (e.g., goiter size and exophthalmos) do not predictably resolve when euthyroidism is achieved. Thyroid storm is an exaggerated thyrotoxicosis that usually follows an acute stress or illness, has an abrupt onset, and is marked by fever, cutaneous flushing, tachycardia, dysrhythmias, anxiety, anorexia, abdominal pain, and diaphoresis. Progression to extreme hyperpyrexia, coma, cardiovascular collapse, and death has been observed in untreated cases.

Differentiation of thyroid storm from sepsis, malignant hyperthermia, transfusion reaction, and adrenal crisis may not be obvious. Detection of a diffusely enlarged thyroid gland, especially when accompanied by palpable thyroid bruit or audible thyroid "murmur," is highly suggestive. Prior history or family history of thyroid disease or recognition of a disorder associated with hyperthyroidism (e.g., diabetes mellitus, Down syndrome, McCune-Albright syndrome) should alert the physician. Elevated levels of serum T_4, serum T_3 (usually increased more markedly than T_4), free T_4, free T_3, and depression of TSH below the normal range support the diagnosis. An absent or depressed TSH response to TRH and measurement of TSA may help confirm the diagnosis; however, treatment of the critically ill child may, of necessity, precede definitive diagnosis.

Treatment

Therapy of thyrotoxic crisis entails both supportive and specific aspects. Appropriate supportive measures include correction of hypovolemia and electrolyte/glucose disturbances and control of fever. Continuous electrocardiographic and arterial blood pressure monitoring are invariably necessary, and in situations requiring aggressive β-receptor blockade, a pulmonary arterial catheter for measurement of cardiac index and oxygen consumption is valuable. Specific therapy includes administration by oral or nasogastric tube of an antithyroid drug (e.g., propylthiouracil [PTU] 20 mg/kg/day in four divided doses) that inhibits both iodide organification and peripheral conversion of T_4 to T_3. Immediate therapy designed to diminish symptoms of thyrotoxicosis includes large doses of iodide (>0.1 mg/kg/day) given orally (Lugol solution, 5–10 drops every 8 hours) or intravenously (10% sodium iodide, 0.5–1.0 g every 8 hours), if necessary, which inhibit thyroid iodide transport, iodothyronine synthesis, and thyroid hormone release. Life-threatening reactions to iodide, including angioedema and laryngeal edema, can rarely occur. Nonspecific β-receptor blockade with esmolol infusion and subsequently with enteral propranolol is useful for controlling sympathetic hyperactivity and decreases conversion of T_4 to T_3. Although more specific blockade of cardiac β receptors (e.g., in a patient with asthma) may be obtained with atenolol or metoprolol, β-receptor blockade should be considered potentially hazardous in patients with cardiac failure or dysrhythmias.[13,14]

Neonatal thyrotoxicosis is treated in similar fashion with appropriate adjustment in drug dosages: PTU 5 to 10 mg/kg/day; Lugols solution one drop every 8 hours; and oral propranolol 1 to 2 mg/kg/day. Digitalis may be required to treat cardiac failure. Corticosteroids and the radiographic contrast agent sodium ipodate are useful adjunctive treatments in refractory cases.

With adequate thyroid-suppressive therapy and sympathetic blockade, clinical improvement should occur within 24 hours. Oral administration of propranolol (4 mg/kg/day in four divided doses) may be required for 1 week. Continuous medical antithyroid therapy, surgical resection, and radioiodine treatment are options for long-term management of autoimmune hyperthyroidism.

Euthyroid Sick Syndrome and Hypothyroidism

Pathophysiology

Metabolism of thyroxine by deiodination is a regulated process that generates metabolites of variable thyromimetic activity. Alterations in thyroid hormone metabolism occur in premature infants and children experiencing nonthyroid illness, caloric deprivation, and surgery. The euthyroid sick syndrome is the most commonly observed constellation: reduced serum T_3 concentrations, increased serum (relatively inactive) rT_3 concentrations, normal TSH levels, normal to increased free T_4 levels, and normal to decreased total T_4 concentrations. Reduced peripheral activity of the type II enzyme 5′-deiodinase is thought to account for these phenomena through decreased peripheral conversion of T_4 to T_3, coupled with reduced clearance of rT_3. Conservation of energy expenditure, particularly during carbohydrate deprivation and critical illness, results from this preferential deiodination of T_4 to rT_3. A similar syndrome of selective T_3 deficiency can be caused by drugs such as dexamethasone, radiographic contrast agents, PTU, propranolol, and amiodarone. Alterations in thyroid hormone binding also occur in nonthyroid illness, contributing to changes in T_3 and rT_3 levels independent of deiodinase enzyme activity. In mild illness, this involves only a decrease in T_3 levels; however, as the severity of illness increases, levels of both T_3 and T_4 drop. A thyroid hormone pattern of low T_3 and T_4 levels with normal or high free T_4 occurs in premorbid patients as a result of release of a thyroid hormone protein-binding inhibitor. Less commonly, a high T_4 level with normal free T_4 level is seen because of increased thyroid hormone-binding proteins as a result of liver disease, iodine dyes, or the antiarrhythmic agent amiodarone. The high iodine content in amiodarone may cause either hypothyroidism or hyperthyroidism in susceptible individuals.

The failure of TSH to increase given reduced T_3 concentrations most likely reflects preservation of intrapituitary 5′-deiodinase activity and T_4 to T_3 conversion and may reflect an adaptive response of the body to minimize catabolism and oxygen consumption during stress. This is supported by the observation that administration of synthetic T_3 to the patient with euthyroid sick syndrome increases catabolism, reflected by increased urinary nitrogen and 3-methyl-histidine excretion. A detrimental effect of rT_3 is suggested by experimental studies but is not confirmed by clinical observations. Understanding this syndrome is important to clinical outcomes. A marked decrease in serum T_4 is associated with increased mortality. When the serum T_4 level decreases to less than 4 μg/dl, mortality increases to 50%; when the serum T_4 decreases to less than 2 μg/dl, mortality increases to 80%.[15]

Although hypothyroidism is infrequently seen in critical illness during childhood, undetected hypothyroidism may impair vital functions and further compromise serious illness. Pulmonary function (maximum breathing capacity and lung compliance) and the ventilatory response to hypoxia are diminished. Congestive heart failure is very unusual, but cardiac output, heart rate, and stroke volume are diminished given reduced metabolic demands and normal peripheral arteriovenous oxygen differences. Pleural, pericardial, and peritoneal effusions may compromise function. Unexplained hypothermia and hyponatremia (as a result of impaired suppression of vasopressin by a water load) occur commonly in the hypothyroid patient. Recognition and treatment of thyroid hormone deficiency reverses each of these abnormalities. An important exception is the critically ill newborn who does not undergo newborn screening because of attention to life-threatening complications. Failure to complete the screening process for congenital hypothyroidism and delay in thyroxine replacement are likely to result in permanent CNS damage.

Diagnosis

Distinguishing the euthyroid sick syndrome from true hypothyroidism usually can be accomplished by determination of serum T_4, T_3, and TSH levels and resin T_3 uptake (T_3U), which is commonly ordered as free thyroxine index (Table 70–2). An elevation in serum TSH level is a sensitive indicator of *primary* hypothyroidism (thyroid gland failure). In ill or malnourished patients in whom a decrease in serum T_3 and T_4 levels may not elicit an increase in TSH, determination of free T_3 and T_4 levels provides a more accurate picture of metabolically active thyroid hormone status. Detection of an exaggerated TSH response to TRH administration strongly suggests hypothyroidism; however, drugs commonly used in the intensive care setting (e.g., dopamine and glucocorticoids) inhibit TSH release and may confound this test. Indicators of thyroid hormone binding, such as T_3U, are useful discriminators. A clearly elevated T_3U level suggests the euthyroid sick syndrome, whereas critical illness in a hypothyroid child (which alone leads to depressed T_3U) increases the T_3U into the normal range but not above it. Determinations of free T_4, T_3, and rT_3 levels, which tend to be low in hypothyroidism and elevated in euthyroid sick syndrome, by radioimmunoassay are useful in certain difficult cases, but values vary widely in patients with euthyroid sick syndrome.[16]

Treatment

Although clinical data are far from conclusive, thyroid hormone supplementation does not appear to be beneficial for patients with euthyroid sick syndrome. Administration of T_4 usually results in further increase in rT_3 levels without elevation of serum T_3 level. In a prospective randomized study of adult patients undergoing cardiopulmonary bypass,[17] patients given T_3 intravenously immediately after surgery had higher cardiac output and lower systemic resistance during the first 24 hours after surgery compared with placebo. However, postoperative mortality was not altered. Further administration of T_3 had no adverse effects in the studies.[18] Although a detrimental effect of direct T_3 administration might be expected, oral T_3 therapy in burn patients showed no adverse metabolic effects but also no reduction in mortality. Overall, therapy with T_4 appears to have no beneficial effects and may even delay normalization of TSH secretion and therefore thyroid function during recovery.

In contrast, thyroid hormone replacement in the hypothyroid child is critical to restoration of normal metabolic and neurologic function. Thyroxine can be administered intravenously in a daily dose equivalent to the oral dose (100 $\mu g/m^2$/day). In severely ill patients with an established diagnosis of hypothyroidism, T_3 administration may more quickly reverse impaired water excretion and the blunted ventilatory response to hypoxia because of its more rapid transport across the blood-brain barrier. Careful monitoring is imperative to avoid hyperthyroidism, however, because T_3 therapy bypasses the normally tightly regulated generation of thyroxine metabolites of variable thyromimetic activity.[19]

Glucose Homeostasis: Initial Evaluation and Treatment of Hypoglycemia

Hypoglycemia may present as critical illness and is a potential metabolic problem in any critically ill child. Depression of the whole blood glucose level (<40 mg/dl [plasma glucose ≈ 45 mg/dl] is a useful criterion during infancy and childhood) usually results from either (1) overutilization of glucose (e.g., excessive insulin effect) or (2) underproduction of glucose via glycogenolysis or conversion of gluconeogenic precursors. Analysis of metabolic control mechanisms governing glucose utilization and production during the hypoglycemic episode allows for a logical, algorithmic diagnostic evaluation of the hypoglycemic child.

TABLE 70–2

Thyroid Function Test Values in Patients with Euthyroid Sick Syndrome, Primary Hypothyroidism, and Primary Hypothyroidism and Concomitant Illness

Thyroid Function Test	Euthyroid Sick Syndrome	Primary Hypothyroidism	Primary Hypothyroidism and Concomitant Illness
Thyroxine (T_4)	Normal or ↑	↓	↓
Triiodothyronine (T_3) uptake	↑	↓	—
T_3	↓	Normal or ↓	↓
Thyrotropin (TSH)	Normal	↑	↑ (or normal*)
Free T_4 (by dialysis)	↑ Normal ↓	↓	↓
Reverse T_3	↑	↓	↓ Normal ↑
TSH release in response to thyrotropin-releasing hormone	Normal or ↓	↑	↑

*Particularly when dopamine is being administered.
From Morley JE, Slag MF, Elsaon MK, et al: *JAMA* 249:2378, 1983.

The intensivist frequently has the opportunity to perform a diagnostic-therapeutic evaluation of the hypoglycemic child. This often yields a prompt diagnosis of a complex metabolic disorder and obviates the need for cumbersome and potentially hazardous fasting studies. This section briefly addresses normal glucose homeostasis, a diagnostic approach to hypoglycemia based on categorizing fundamental impairments in glucose homeostasis, and the treatment options appropriate for each impairment. For a more detailed discussion of specific disorders, the reader is referred to a review publication.[20]

Pathophysiology

Maintenance of normoglycemia during fasting reflects the carefully orchestrated effects of glucose-lowering insulin and glucose-raising counterregulatory hormones (glucagon, EPI, NE, growth hormone, cortisol). Compared with adults, infants and children have smaller glycogen reserves (depleted in <12 hours in early infancy and 24 hours in late childhood and adulthood) and larger obligatory glucose requirements (8 mg/kg/min in the infant compared with 2–3 mg/kg/min in the adult). The latter is related to the larger percentage of total body mass comprised by the (glucose-requiring) brain, particularly in the infant.

Glycogen depletion prompts mobilization (from muscle and fat), hepatic uptake, and conversion of gluconeogenic substrates (predominantly alanine, lactate, and glycerol) to glucose. In the postabsorptive state, glucagon protects against hypoglycemia by enhancing glycogenolysis and promoting hepatic uptake of amino acids for gluconeogenesis. Epinephrine, which normally promotes release of gluconeogenic precursors (pyruvate and lactate from muscle, glycerol from fat) in response to glycogen depletion, activates glycolysis primarily when glucagon is deficient.[21] Marked increases in one or both of these counterregulatory hormones is essential for recovery from acute hypoglycemia. Epinephrine also decreases glucose utilization in insulin-dependent tissues through inhibition of peripheral glucose uptake and insulin secretion. Permissive levels of cortisol and growth hormone allow sustained mobilization of amino acids and glycerol, but further increases in their concentrations are not necessary for recovery from hypoglycemia.[22]

The normal term infant, in the fed state, shows a decline in blood glucose from maternal levels to 50 mg/dl at 2 hours of age, rising to approximately 70 mg/dl by the third day of life. A slowed glycogenolytic response to glucagon, delayed maturation of gluconeogenic enzymes, impaired generation of ketone bodies from free fatty acids, limited glycogen and intestinal nutrient stores, and a relatively large glucose-consuming CNS all predispose the small infant to hypoglycemia. Although these factors may explain frequent blood sugar levels lower than 40 mg/dl in growth-retarded or premature infants, prevention of deleterious effects of hypoglycemia is best achieved by intervening at a level of 40 mg/dl rather than relying on weight-adjusted criteria (e.g., 25–30 mg/dl for an infant <2500 g). Studies of CNS abnormalities after neonatal hypoglycemia indicate that early diagnosis and treatment are critical to preventing long-term sequelae.

During the past decade, understanding of the regulation of insulin secretion and strategies for treating disordered insulin release has increased substantially. Nutritional, hormonal, metabolic, and autonomic nervous system signals are transduced by a complex system that involves intracellular glucose metabolism, depolarization of the cell membrane, regulation of free intracellular cytosolic calcium concentration, and movement of insulin-containing secretory granules to fuse with the plasma membrane to release their contents. Adenosine triphosphate (ATP)-sensitive potassium channels in the plasma membrane, which contain both a high-affinity sulfonylurea receptor (SUR1) and an inward-rectifier Kir6.2, have a pivotal role in regulating insulin release. Mutations that alter the function of K_{ATP} channels can lead to continued membrane depolarization, resulting in uncoupling of insulin secretion from glucose metabolism and the clinical syndrome of hyperinsulinemia. More than 50 SUR1 mutations and three Kir6.2 mutations have been described. Other mutation abnormalities, such as constitutive activation of glucokinase or glutamate dehydrogenase, can result in hyperinsulinemia, the latter characteristically accompanied by hyperammonemia.[23]

Clinical and Laboratory Evaluation

The symptoms of hypoglycemia are not specific, particularly in the newborn. Although CNS dysfunction, manifested by seizures and coma, dominates the picture of profound hypoglycemia, subtle symptoms such as poor feeding, weakness, headache, confusion, irritability, and hunger are more common in infants and young children. These symptoms may not be accompanied by the classic autonomic response (tachycardia, diaphoresis, and nervousness) to a decreasing glucose level. Because of the nonspecific nature of these symptoms, a simultaneous blood glucose value is needed for definitive diagnosis of hypoglycemia.

A vigorous search for the cause of recurrent hypoglycemia should begin immediately upon its discovery. Diagnostic possibilities cover a broad spectrum but are narrowed significantly by the age at presentation and the specific response of glucose homeostatic mechanisms to the hypoglycemic episode. Neonatal hypoglycemia usually is transient, occurring with or as a result of maternal diabetes, polycythemia, respiratory distress syndrome, intrauterine growth retardation, or other problems. Recurrent severe hypoglycemia during the first year of life, with few exceptions, results from hyperinsulinism, hypopituitarism, or inborn errors of metabolism (e.g., glycogen storage disorders). During the toddler years, when children are first exposed to prolonged fasting, ketotic hypoglycemia and disorders of ketogenesis appear. Thereafter the onset of recurrent hypoglycemia usually indicates insulin excess (e.g., islet cell adenoma) or, rarely, counterregulatory hormone deficiency.

Most childhood hypoglycemia results from abnormal or inefficient adaptation to fasting. Laboratory studies comprising a "critical blood sample" (10–15 ml in appropriate collection tubes), obtained *at the time of documented hypoglycemia,* provide a snapshot of the child's metabolic status and usually identify the abnormality in fasting adaptation (Fig. 70–1). This opportunity to collect valuable diagnostic information is frequently overlooked in the haste to increase the blood glucose level and prevent the neurologic sequelae of prolonged hypoglycemia.

Analysis of the critical blood sample categorizes the causes of hypoglycemia according to the fundamental defect in glucose homeostasis (Table 70–3). A blood glucose level determined from a capillary blood sample by reflectance meters (which frequently is erroneous, especially at blood glucose concentrations <50 mg/dl) is first verified by a "stat" laboratory glucose or is repeated on a free-flowing sample with a blood glucose meter with meticulous technique. Serum electrolytes, with determination of the "anion gap," reliably determine the presence or absence of metabolic acidosis in the midst of hypoglycemia. Lactic acidosis indicates that substrate for gluconeogenesis is available but that utilization of this substrate is defective. This finding is the hallmark of various enzymatic impairments in glycogenolysis or gluconeogenesis resulting in underproduction of glucose (see Chapter 69). Hypoglycemia accompanied by a predominant ketoacidosis (and ketonuria) results from insufficient substrate supply for (intact) gluconeogenesis coupled with the inability of brain and muscle to meet acute energy needs through ketone utilization. For example, relatively common childhood "ketotic hypoglycemia" is associated with hypoalaninemia, although the exact pathogenesis is unresolved. Deficient substrate mobilization also results from genetic disturbances of amino acid metabolism (e.g., maple syrup urine disease) or lack of counterregulatory hormones (e.g., growth hormone or cortisol).

A normal anion gap in the midst of hypoglycemia indicates that production of potentially energy-yielding metabolic acids (lactate and ketoacids) is inhibited in spite of ongoing energy needs. Defects in fatty acid oxidation or ketogenesis result from specific enzymatic defects or carnitine deficiency and are characterized by intolerance to fasting, Reye syndrome-like vomiting and obtundation, dicarboxylic (organic) aciduria, and marked elevation in free fatty acids during hypoketotic hypoglycemia. Hyperinsulinemia causes overutilization of glucose and suppression of pathways of glucose production and mobilization. Hypoketosis, a high exogenous glucose requirement to maintain normoglycemia (>12 mg/kg/min), rapid development of hypoglycemia with fasting, an insulin level greater than 10 μU/ml or insulin/glucose ratio greater than 0.3 at the time of hypoglycemia, and a glycemic response to glucagon administration strongly suggest excess insulin effect. Even levels of insulin less than 10 μU/ml should be viewed with suspicion if documented during severe hypoglycemia. Failure to taper administration of highly concentrated dextrose solutions (e.g., total parenteral nutrition) and rapid delivery of concentrated nutrients to the small intestine (e.g., dumping syndrome) are preventable causes of hyperinsulinemia in critically ill children.

Treatment

After collection of blood and urine for diagnostic studies, correction of hypoglycemia can be accomplished through (1) administration of exogenous glucose, (2) release of inappropriately stored endogenous glycogen (hyperinsulinemic states), (3) provision of deficient counterregulatory hormones, or (4) reduction in serum insulin concentrations. Recognizing both the diagnostic and therapeutic

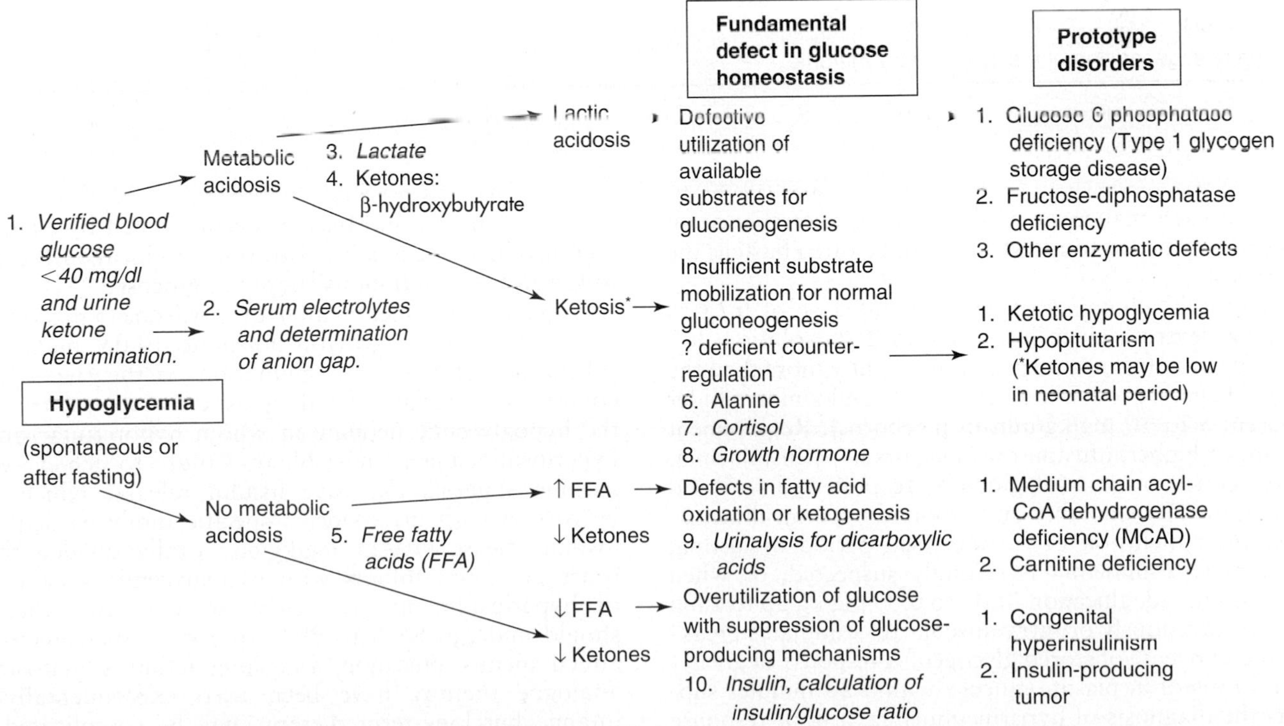

FIGURE 70–1 • Critical blood sample evaluation of hypoglycemia in infancy and childhood. *Words in italics* are components of the critical blood sample. *FFA*, Free fatty acid.

TABLE 70–3

Causes of Persistent Hypoglycemia During Infancy and Childhood

DEFICIENT SUBSTRATE FOR GLUCONEOGENESIS	DEFICIENT FATTY ACID OXIDATION OR KETOGENESIS
Ketotic hypoglycemia	Carnitine actyl transferase deficiency
Growth hormone deficiency	Long-chain fatty acid acyl-CoA dehydrogenase deficiency
Cortisol deficiency	Medium-chain fatty acid acyl-CoA dehydrogenase deficiency
Hypothyroidism	Short-chain fatty acid acyl-CoA dehydrogenase deficiency
Panhypopituitarism	Hydroxymethylglutaryl CoA lyase deficiency
Catecholamine deficiency	INCREASED PERIPHERAL GLUCOSE UTILIZATION
Glucagon deficiency	Hyperinsulinism
Inborn errors of amino acid metabolism	Insulin reaction in diabetic patient
Maple syrup urine disease	Infants of diabetic mothers
Propionic academia	Infants with erythroblastosis
Tyrosinosis	Beckwith syndrome
Methylmalonic aciduria	Congenital hyperinsulinism
Isovaleric acidemia	β-Cell hyperplasia, idiopathic
DEFECTIVE HEPATIC GLUCOSE RELEASE AND/OR UTILIZATION OF AVAILABLE GLUCONEOGENIC SUBSTRATE	Leucine-sensitive hypoglycemia
Enzymatic defects	Islet cell adenoma
Glycogen synthesis deficiency	Subclinical diabetes mellitus
Glycogen storage diseases	Abrupt cessation of intravenous hypertonic glucose solutions
Type I (glucose-6-phosphatase deficiency)	Oral hypoglycemic agents (biguanides, sulfonylureas)
Type III (amylo-1,6-glucosidase or debranching enzyme-deficiency)	Surreptitious insulin
Type IV (hepatophosphorylase deficiency)	Extrapancreatic tumors
Galactosemia (galactose-1-phosphate uridyltransferase deficiency)	TOXIC
Hereditary fructose intolerance (fructose-1-phosphate aldolase deficiency)	Salicylate
Fructose-1, 6-diphosphatase deficiency	Alcohol
Liver disease	Unripe ackees (hypoglycin) (Jamaican vomiting sickness)
Hepatitis	
Cirrhosis	
Fatty degeneration of the liver (Reye syndrome)	

utility of each maneuver while avoiding overreliance on exogenous glucose administration alone often hastens the diagnosis.

Glucose is administered as an initial dose of 0.25 to 0.5 g/kg dextrose given in a 10% to 25% solution, followed by an infusion rate providing slightly more than the normal hepatic production rate (3 to 5 mg/kg/min in older children, 5 to 10 mg/kg/min in newborns). Requirement of a much higher infusion rate suggests hyperinsulinemia. Lower concentrations of glucose are preferred to avoid fluctuations in osmolality and rebound hyperinsulinemia.

At the conclusion of a supervised period of fasting, when hyperinsulinemia is strongly suspected, or when access is limited, glucagon (0.01 to 0.03 mg/kg up to 1 mg given intravenously or intramuscularly) stimulates breakdown and release of stored glycogen. A response of greater than 30 mg/dl in plasma glucose within 20 minutes supports the diagnosis of hyperinsulinemia; a poor response is expected when glycogen is absent, glycogen storage or lysis is abnormal, or liver disease is present. Because its effect is transient and may be accompanied by exaggerated insulin release, administration of glucagon must be followed by a continuous supply of glucose.

Sequential treatment with hydrocortisone (5 mg/kg/day) or its equivalent, growth hormone (0.05 mg/kg/day subcutaneously), or a combination of the two agents comprises an initial 3-day diagnostic-therapeutic trial for the hypoglycemic neonate in whom hypopituitarism or hyperinsulinemia is most likely. Failure to achieve euglycemia suggests excessive insulin release, which can be treated with diazoxide, a specific inhibitor of β-cell insulin release (10–25 mg/kg/day orally divided three times per day). Infants with hypoglycemia as a result of hyperinsulinemia refractory to diazoxide therapy should undergo 85% to 90% subtotal pancreatectomy. Subcutaneous glucagon and long-acting somatostatin analogue therapy have been used experimentally in infants, but long-term therapy may be complicated by simultaneous suppression of growth hormone and other hormones.

Disorders of Calcium Homeostasis

The extracellular ionized calcium (Ca^{2+}) concentration must be maintained within narrow limits for its vital and ubiquitous role in normal metabolism. In cardiac pacemaker cells, a slow influx of Ca^{2+} initiates the action potential. Entry of Ca^{2+} into myocardial cells, facilitated by membrane depolarization and β-adrenergic stimulation, causes further release of Ca^{2+} from the sarcoplasmic reticulum, binding of Ca^{2+} to troponin, and muscle contraction. Cardiac contraction is enhanced by increased intracellular Ca^{2+} concentrations (resulting from infused calcium, β-adrenergic agonists, and other factors) and impaired by Ca^{2+}-lowering factors (hypocalcemia, calcium channel blockers). In skeletal muscle, the force of contraction is determined primarily by repetitive Ca^{2+}-facilitated release of acetylcholine from the neuromuscular junction. Several enzyme systems within the CNS (e.g., adenylate cyclase, phosphodiesterase, and protein kinases) appear to be regulated by the interaction of Ca^{2+} with calmodulin, a Ca^{2}-binding protein. This Ca^{2+}–calmodulin complex also stimulates myosin kinase in vascular smooth muscle so that Ca^{2} influx (enhanced by α-adrenergic and inhibited by β-adrenergic stimuli) causes vasoconstriction. In addition to its vital role in neuromuscular and neurologic function, the concentration of Ca^{2} plays a critical role in the clotting system and other membrane transport systems. Not surprisingly, alterations in calcium homeostasis frequently have important consequences in critically ill patients.

The extracellular Ca^{2+} concentration is monitored by Ca^{2+}-sensing receptors (CaRs).[24] This receptor is encoded by the 1078-amino-acid CaR gene in chromosome 3q13. The receptor consists of three structural regions: a large amino-terminal extracellular domain that contains clusters of acidic amino acids involved in the binding of Ca^{2+}, seven transmembrane helices characteristic of G protein-coupled receptors, and a cytoplasmic carboxy-terminal domain. These receptors are plentiful on the surface of the chief cells of the parathyroid glands, in numerous kidney sites (juxtaglomerular apparatus, luminal surface of the proximal convoluted tubule, basolateral surface of the cortical thick ascending limb of the loop of Henle, and apical and luminal membrane of the inner medullary collecting duct in the kidneys), intestine, parts of the brain, thyroid C cells, breast, and adrenal glands. Acting in classic hormonal negative feedback fashion, binding of Ca^{2+} to this receptor activates phospholipase C and accumulation of inositol triphosphate, which secondarily leads to inhibition of the secretion and synthesis of parathyroid hormone (PTH) and activation of its proteolysis. Importantly, the receptor lacks specificity, also binding and being stimulated by other divalent cations, particularly Mg^{2+}.

Regulation of Extracellular Calcium

Derangements in calcium homeostasis result from (1) changes in protein binding and chelation (with phosphate [PO_4] or other anions) that alter availability of Ca^{2} and (2) excessive or deficient hormonal action. The former is more common in the intensive care unit. More than half of the total serum calcium is bound to proteins, and this binding is pH dependent. An acidic pH decreases binding and increases ionized calcium (Ca^{2}), whereas alkalosis increases binding and reduces Ca^{2}. Thus estimation of Ca^{2+} from a total serum Ca level must take into account changes in serum proteins and pH and even then can be erroneous. Direct measurement of Ca^{2+} is desirable and now readily available.

Hormonal control of calcium homeostasis involves PTH, vitamin D, and calcitonin. Secretion of PTH by the parathyroid chief cell varies inversely with the serum Ca^{2+} level and is inhibited by hypomagnesemia and $1,25(OH)_2$-vitamin D. Rapid degradation of PTH yields a physiologically inactive C-terminal fragment (slowly cleared by the kidney) and an active NH_2-terminal fragment. PTH binds to cell surface receptors in bone (osteoblasts, but not mature osteoclasts) and kidney and exerts its effects through binding of the α subunit of a membrane-associated heterotrimeric protein (Gs protein), which mediates increased formation of cAMP. In bone, resultant increases in metabolic activity and H ion concentration lead to dissolution of bone mineral and release of Ca^{2+} and PO_4 into the ECF.

At the renal level, PTH inhibits proximal tubular PO_4 reabsorption and promotes phosphaturia. This loss of PO_4 inhibits bone mineralization and tends to shift the flow of calcium from bone to the ECF. Distal tubular reabsorption of filtered calcium is also increased by PTH. A third renal effect of PTH is stimulation of 1α-hydroxylation of 25(OH)-vitamin D. Metabolically active $1,25(OH)_2$-vitamin D stimulates intestinal absorption of calcium and PO_4. The overall effect of PTH is to raise serum calcium levels and lower serum PO_4 levels. This characteristic reciprocal relationship is helpful in distinguishing PTH disorders from those involving vitamin D alone.[25]

Hyperphosphatemia lowers Ca^{2+} by shifting the equilibrium in calcium flux from ECF toward bone and by inhibiting 1α-hydroxylation activity. Calcitonin is a 32-amino-acid, calcium-lowering hormone elaborated by C cells of the thyroid in response to rising Ca^{2+} levels. Although it rapidly reduces the bone resorptive function of osteoclasts and promotes calciuria and phosphaturia, its excess or absence causes no discernible disorder.

Hypocalcemia

Clinical and Laboratory Diagnosis

Hypocalcemia is frequently associated with critical illness in children. In some cases, hypocalcemia is associated with PTH deficiency, whereas in others hypercalcitoninemia or hypermagnesemia is cited. Children with severe burns may develop hypocalcemia, Mg^{2+} depletion, hypoparathyroidism, and renal resistance to PTH infusion. In this particular situation, a reduced set point for Ca^{2+} suppression of PTH secretion, rather than Mg^{2+} depletion, is thought to be the primary cause of low PTH production.[26]

Reduced Ca^{2+} levels inhibit acetylcholine release and impair effective muscular contraction in both sensory and motor nerves. Consequently, a variety of peripheral and CNS effects (tetany, convulsions [grand mal, petit mal, or focal], carpopedal spasms, muscle cramps and twitching, paresthesias, laryngeal stridor, and apnea in the newborn) are characteristic overt features of hypocalcemia. Latent tetany is manifested by Chvostek (provoked facial muscle twitching) and Trousseau (provoked carpopedal spasm) signs. Cardiovascular manifestations include hypotension, myocardial depression, congestive heart failure, and dysrhythmias. Somatic changes accompanying prolonged hypocalcemia include dry, coarse skin, eczematous dermatitis, brittle hair with areas of alopecia, brittle nails with smooth transverse grooves, and dental enamel hypoplasia.

Determination of the free ionized Ca^{2+} level is diagnostic, although the rate of decline also contributes to the development of symptoms. Estimations of Ca^{2+} correcting for protein binding (i.e., for every 1 g/dl reduction of serum albumin, the protein-bound calcium fraction is reduced by 0.8 mg/dl) and pH must be interpreted cautiously. Prolongation of the QT interval may be helpful in confirming reduced ionized calcium levels, although the correlation is not strong.

The causes of hypocalcemia are best recalled by reviewing the mediators of normal calcium homeostasis (Table 70–4). Reduced PTH effect can result from parathyroid gland failure (e.g., autoimmune or postsurgical hypo-parathyroidism), insensitivity to PTH (e.g., pseudohypoparathyroidism [PHP]), or suppression of PTH release (e.g., hypomagnesemia, maternal hypercalcemia, burns). Hyperphosphatemia is frequently present, and accompanying features (e.g., short stature, mental retardation, shortened metacarpals in PHP; moniliasis of the nails in hypoparathyroidism) should be sought. Measurement of immunoreactive PTH (iPTH) levels distinguishes hormonal deficiency from resistance to hormone action. Reduced vitamin D effect results from vitamin D deficiency (e.g., malabsorption, best detected by low 25(OH)-vitamin D levels), impaired activation of vitamin D [e.g., renal disease, requires determination of $1,25(OH)_2$-vitamin D levels], or exaggerated losses or metabolism (e.g., phenytoin). Acute changes in Ca^{2+} binding equilibrium or chelation are perhaps the most frequent causes of hypocalcemia in the intensive care setting. Respiratory alkalosis or hyperphosphatemia may dramatically reduce total and ionized calcium. Infusion of large amounts of citrate-preserved blood and acute phosphorus overload or retention (e.g., acute renal failure) rapidly deplete ECF calcium levels. Various drugs also contribute to development of hypocalcemia.

Treatment

Correction of hypocalcemia should be preceded by consideration of readily treated (acute respiratory alkalosis)

TABLE 70–4

Causes of Hypocalcemia

REDUCED PTH EFFECT

PARATHYROID GLAND FAILURE
- Hypoparathyroidism—idiopathic or autoimmune
- Trauma
- Postsurgery
- Post–^{131}I therapy
- Infarction
- Infiltration (e.g., sarcoid hemosiderosis)

INSENSITIVITY TO PTH
- Pseudohypoparathyroidism
- Hypomagnesemia

SUPPRESSION OF PTH RELEASE
- Hypomagnesemia
- Neonatal, resulting from maternal hypercalcemia
- Burns
- Sepsis
- Drugs
  - Aminoglycosides
  - Cimetidine
  - Cisplatin
  - β-adrenergic blockers

REDUCED VITAMIN D EFFECT

VITAMIN D DEFICIENCY
- Dietary insufficiency
- Increased losses related to
  - Malabsorption
  - Nephrotic syndrome
  - Phenytoin, phenobarbital

IMPAIRED ACTIVATION OF VITAMIN D
- Renal disease
- Hypoparathyroidism
- Liver failure
- Rhabdomyolysis

CHANGES IN Ca^{2+} BINDING OR CHELATION

ALKALOSIS
- Respiratory alkalosis
- Bicarbonate infusion

HYPERPHOSPHATEMIA
- Renal failure
- Phosphate administration (e.g., high-phosphate formulas, enemas)
- Chemotherapy
- Rhabdomyolysis
- Malignancy
- Pancreatitis
- Fat embolism
- Transfusion with citrate-preserved blood

DRUG/TOXINS
- Glucagon
- Mithramycin
- Calcitonin
- EDTA
- Protamine
- Sodium fluoride
- Colchicine
- Theophylline
- Ethylene glycol

Modified from Chernow B, Zaloga GP: SCCM, Ions for society members. In Shoemaker WC, editor: *Critical care: state of the art,* vol 5. Fullerton, CA, 1984, Society of Critical Care Medicine.

or confounding factors. Rapid development of hyperphosphatemia suggests acute renal failure, cell lysis, or excessive supply (see Chapter 74, Brecher). Efforts should be made to reduce serum phosphate levels because intravenous calcium therapy may cause metastatic deposition of calcium-phosphate salts. Hypomagnesemia impairs PTH release; response to PTH; and, consequently, correction of hypocalcemia. Critically ill patients may develop hypomagnesemia by several mechanisms involving excessive gastrointestinal or renal losses of Mg^{2+} or inadequate supplementation. Urgency of therapy is determined by the child's clinical status. Asymptomatic hypocalcemia is appropriately treated with oral calcium salts. For the seriously ill patient with evolving hypocalcemia, replacement therapy is accomplished with infusion of intravenous calcium gluconate (10% solution; 90 mg elemental calcium per 10 ml) at 75 to 150 mg of elemental calcium per kilogram per day. For impending cardiovascular or neuromuscular collapse, when a prompt and predictable rise in Ca^{2+} is required, 10 to 20 mg/kg of calcium chloride is administered intravenously over 5 to 10 minutes. The possibility of bradycardia and asystole with infusion of calcium should be anticipated, with cardiac monitoring and atropine readily available. Care is required to prevent tissue damage by extravasation, precipitation with concomitantly administered bicarbonate, and untoward cardiac rhythm disturbances in digitalized patients.

Oral administration of calcium salts is efficient for control of persistent hypocalcemia and is preferable to prolonged infusion. Liberal amounts can be given orally (e.g., 50 mg calcium per kilogram per day in 4–5 divided doses), with attention paid to the differing Ca content of various oral preparations. An exception is cases associated with fat malabsorption, where the effect of oral therapy is blunted. In appropriate cases, supplementation of calcium therapy with magnesium or vitamin D (ergocalciferol for vitamin D deficiency or calcitriol for hypocalcemia associated with lack of PTH effect) will be needed for maintenance of normocalcemia. In hypoparathyroidism secondary to Mg depletion, initial therapy consists of intravenous Mg chloride or gluconate (1–2 mmol/1.7 m^2/h) until normal Mg plasma level is achieved. Persistent Mg deficiency should be treated with oral administration of magnesium chloride, citrate, or lactate (2 mmol/kg/day), which may need to be continuous. Synthetic PTH has become available for use in highly selected situations and experimental trials. No information regarding its use in the intensive care setting is available.

Hypercalcemia

Clinical and Laboratory Diagnosis

In contrast to dramatic neuromuscular manifestations of hypocalcemia, the physical effects of hypercalcemia may be subtle and nonspecific. Nevertheless, a serum calcium level greater than 15 mg/dl is a medical emergency. Effects on the renal, cardiovascular, and central nervous systems predominate and reflect both the degree of calcium elevation and its duration. The increased filtered load of calcium creates hypercalciuria and accompanying polyuria, reduced urine-concentrating ability, dehydration, and eventual kidney stone formation. Hypertension is common, possibly mediated through increased renin production or direct effects on peripheral vasoconstriction and inotropy. Alterations in the cardiac conduction system include a shortened QT interval and a tendency to dysrhythmias. Impaired nerve conduction resulting from excess calcium creates hypotonia, hyporeflexia, and paresis in severe cases. Alterations in CNS function, including lethargy, confusion, and even coma, can occur. Constipation, anorexia, and abdominal pain resulting from reduced intestinal motility are frequent symptoms. Promotion of gastrin release by calcium may account for an increased incidence of peptic ulcer disease. Soft tissue deposition of calcium, usually facilitated by associated serum PO_4 elevation, can impair function of the lungs, kidneys, blood vessels, and joints.

In the absence of hyperproteinemia, determination of elevated serum calcium levels reliably indicates increased Ca^2 concentrations. Because common causes of hypercalcemia in adults (hyperparathyroidism and malignancies) are less common in children, hypercalcemia is encountered less frequently than hypocalcemia by the intensivist. Diagnostic possibilities are best approached by considering the predominant underlying mechanism of hypercalcemia (Table 70–5). Increased bone resorption reflects excess PTH effect (e.g., hyperparathyroidism, ectopic PTH), immobilization, or bone lysis by metastatic malignancy (e.g., neuroblastoma). PTH-mediated hypercalcemia is distinguished by a depressed serum phosphate concentration, decreased renal tubular reabsorption of phosphate (Tm_{PO4}/GFR) [$TmPO_4$/GFR], and an iPTH level inappropriately elevated for the simultaneous serum Ca^{2+} level. A search for MEN syndromes is warranted in the child with hyperparathyroidism. Heightened vitamin D effect is manifested by increased intestinal calcium absorption and can be related to vitamin D intoxication, increased sensitivity to vitamin D (proposed for hypercalcemia of infancy), or ectopically produced 1,25$(OH)_2$-vitamin D (sarcoidosis). Serum PO_4 levels and Tm_{PO4}/GFR) [Tm PO_4/GFR] ratios are normal or increased, and iPTH levels are suppressed in these disorders. Detection of an elevated 25(OH)-vitamin D level (nutritional excess) or 1,25$(OH)_2$-vitamin D level (sarcoidosis, hyperparathyroidism) may be helpful. Decreased excretion of calcium occurs with dehydration or treatment with thiazide diuretics and frequently aggravates the severity of hypercalcemia in patients with unrecognized hyperparathyroidism. Familial hypocalciuric hypercalcemia, an autosomal dominant disorder resulting from partially deactivating mutations in the CaR, is characterized by normal to slightly elevated iPTH levels and decreased urinary calcium excretion.[21] Thus determination of (a logical combination of) serum Ca^{2+}, PO_4, iPTH, (occasional) vitamin D metabolites, and urinary calcium and PO_4 excretion allows differentiation of most hypercalcemic disorders.

Treatment

A serum calcium level greater than 15 mg/dl may be life threatening and requires direct Ca-lowering therapy in

TABLE 70–5

Differential Diagnosis and Biochemical Findings in Childhood Hypercalcemia

		Serum					Urine	
Predominant Mechanism of Hypercalcemia	**Disorder**	**Ca**	**PO_4**	**25(OH)-Vitamin D**	**1,25(OH)-Vitamin D**	**iPTH**	**Ca**	**Tm_{PO_4}/GFR**
Increased bone reabsorption	1. Hyperparathyroidism	H	L	N	H	H	H	L
	2. Malignancy-ectopic PTH	H	L	N	N or L	L	H	L
	3. Immobilization, thyrotoxicosis, or bone lysis	H	N or H	N	L	L	H	H
Increased intestinal calcium absorption	1. Vitamin D intoxication	H	N or H	H	N or H	L	H	H
	2. Sarcoidosis	H	N or H	N	H	L	H	H
	3. ? Idiopathic infantile hypercalcemia or Williams syndrome	H	N	N	L, N or H	L	H	N or H
	4. Abrupt glucocorticoid withdrawal or deficiency	H	N or H	N	N	L	H	N or H
Decreased renal excretion of calcium	1. Familial hypocalciuric hypercalcemia	H	N or L	N	N or H	N or H	L	L

H, High; *L*, low; *N*, normal.

addition to attention to the underlying disorder. Hydration with isotonic saline solution (200–250 ml/kg/day) and furosemide diuresis (1 mg/kg every 6 hours) results in calciuresis and amelioration of hypercalcemia in the majority of cases. Excessive losses of sodium, potassium, magnesium, and PO_4 may occur. Thiazide diuretics should not be used because of their hypercalcemic effects.

Adjunct therapy is directed at the specific cause of hypercalcemia. Drugs that inhibit excessive bone resorption include calcitonin (10 U/kg given IV every 4–6 hours), mithramycin (25 mg/kg IV for 4 hours), and indomethacin (1 mg/kg/day). Calcitonin, now available in human (recombinant DNA) form, blocks PTH-induced bone resorption, facilitates calciuria, is relatively nontoxic, and has a prompt (but transient) peak effect at 1 hour. Mithramycin is a toxic antibiotic that inhibits osteoclastic activity within 24 hours but has potential side effects, including thrombocytopenia and hepatic and renal toxicity. Indomethacin (or aspirin) is useful when excessive prostaglandin E_2 production is suspected (e.g., some tumor-related hypercalcemic syndromes). More recently, bone-stabilizing bisphosphonates (e.g., pamidronate, etidronate) have been used successfully for treatment of persistent hypercalcemia.[27] Intestinal calcium absorption is reduced by corticosteroids (hydrocortisone 1 mg/kg every 6 hours or equivalent). Consequently, glucocorticoids are especially useful for treatment of vitamin D-related hypercalcemia. Their delayed onset of action, however, limits their use in the acute setting. Phosphates are not recommended because of the likelihood of soft tissue deposition of calcium-phosphate salts.

Vasopressin Deficiency in Critical Illness

Pathophysiology

The hormone vasopressin has complex physiologic properties that affect water and cardiovascular homeostasis. Its role in diabetes insipidus and water homeostasis is discussed in more detail in Chapter 60. The use of vasopressin in refractory vasodilatory shock states after fluid resuscitation and conventional catecholamine infusion has received increased attention in the past few years. The use of vasopressin under these conditions warrants a review of vasopressin deficiency related to shock states in the critically ill patient. The interested reader is referred to several excellent articles that review the physiology of vasopressin and the pathophysiology of vasodilatory shock.[28,29]

Vasopressin is produced in the paraventricular and supraoptic nuclei of the hypothalamus and is transported to the posterior pituitary gland, where it is stored (Fig. 70–2). Its release from the posterior pituitary is primarily regulated by plasma osmolality, intravascular volume, and intravascular pressure, but it also can be released in response to pain or hypoxia. Regulation of vasopressin release in response to changes in extracellular osmolality is a result of central and peripheral feedback from osmoreceptors that serve to maintain water homeostasis. Hypovolemia and hypotension are conditions that stimulate vasopressin release through vagal afferents from atrial, aortic arch, and carotid baroreceptors. Although under normal conditions vasopressin has little

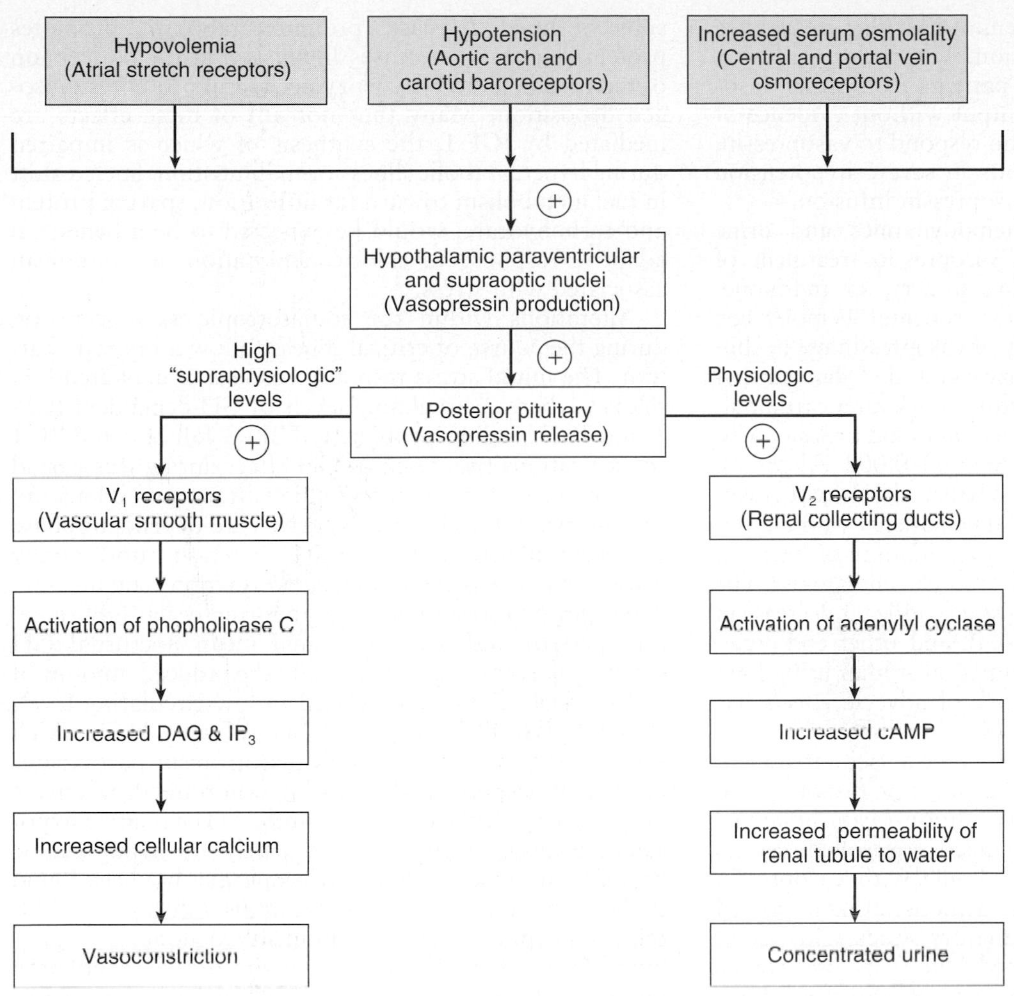

FIGURE 70–2 • Regulation of vasopressin release and its major sites of action in peripheral tissues. *cAMP,* Cyclic adenosine monophosphate; *DAG,* diacylglycerol; *IP_3,* inositol triphosphate.

influence on blood pressure, in early phases of shock levels increase in response to a decrease in intravascular volume and arterial pressures. Vasopressin's effect on blood pressure is mediated through V1 receptors located in the membrane of peripheral vascular smooth muscle. The V1 receptor is a G protein-coupled receptor that activates phospholipase C with a subsequent increase in intracellular Ca^{2+} and vasoconstriction.

Increased vasopressin levels occur in response to cardiogenic, hemorrhagic, and septic shock in both animal models and human studies. Its importance in the maintenance of cardiovascular stability in early endotoxin-induced shock is demonstrated by the dramatic decrease in blood pressure in response to endotoxin injection in vasopressin-deficient animals. A decrease in vasopressin levels may occur in the late phase of hemorrhagic, septic, and vasodilatory shock after cardiopulmonary bypass. This state of relative vasopressin deficiency may contribute to shock that is refractory to infusions of catecholamines such as dopamine, epinephrine, and norepinephrine. It appears that the etiology of vasopressin deficiency in late-phase vasodilatory shock is a decrease in the release of vasopressin hormone from the posterior pituitary gland.[30] Low-dose infusion of vasopressin in vasodilatory shock increases plasma levels, indicating that increased metabolism is not responsible for the decrease in vasopressin levels.[31]

Although the cause of vasopressin deficiency is unknown, evidence in septic patients indicates decreased vasopressin stores in the posterior pituitary or inhibition of vasopressin release mediated by an increased production of nitric oxide.

The specific mechanism by which vasopressin improves hemodynamics in shock has not been identified, but some possible actions of vasopressin on peripheral vascular smooth muscle include direct stimulation of available V1 receptors, inhibition of outward K-ATP channels, enhancing the effect of catecholamine pressors, and inhibition of the production of nitric oxide in vascular smooth muscle.

Treatment of Vasodilatory Shock with Vasopressin

Use of vasopressin for treatment of vasodilatory shock resistant to infusions of other vasopressor drugs has been studied in patients with septic and hemorrhagic shock and with shock after cardiopulmonary bypass. Only a few of these studies, however, have been randomized controlled studies and have included a small number of subjects.[32,33] In adult septic patients with vasodilatory shock refractory to catecholamine infusion, a low-dose infusion of vasopressin results in significant improvement in blood pressure and systemic vascular resistance without altering cardiac function. Vasopressin infusion resulted in the ability to wean patients from other vasopressors and increased urine output without evidence of end-organ injury. In patients who respond to vasopressin, its abrupt discontinuation results in severe hypotension requiring reinstitution of the vasopressin infusion.

Similar improvements in hemodynamics and urine output are demonstrated with vasopressin treatment of vasodilatory shock after cardiac surgery, in milrinone-induced hypotension, and in experimental hemorrhagic shock in animals. Only one study of vasopressin use in children has been published. Rosenzweig et al.[34] showed that children with refractory vasodilatory shock after cardiopulmonary bypass had an improvement in blood pressure with low-dose vasopressin infusions (0.0003–0.002 U/kg/min). In this study, treatment of vasodilatory shock with vasopressin resulted in survival of all nine patients who did not have cardiac dysfunction prior to initiation of therapy, despite their unresponsiveness to other catecholamines. The concern that vasopressin may cause a significant decrease in cardiac output, coronary perfusion, and other end-organ perfusion has not been demonstrated in studies using low-dose vasopressin infusion, but risk of adverse effects has been reported at higher infusion rates in adults.

In summary, vasopressin may become a useful treatment for vasodilatory shock states that are not responsive to adequate fluid resuscitation and traditional catecholamine infusions. However, no randomized controlled studies showing an improvement in outcome with vasopressin use have been performed. Studies demonstrating improved outcome in children with vasodilatory shock with use of vasopressin should be performed before its use can be recommended as a standard therapy for vasodilatory shock states.

Anabolic Hormone Therapy: Human Growth Hormone, Insulin-Like Growth Factor 1, and Insulin

Human growth hormone (hGH) is a 191-amino-acid protein secreted in pulsatile fashion by the anterior pituitary in response to two hypothalamic hormones: stimulatory growth hormone-releasing hormone (GHRH) and inhibitory somatostatin (somatotropin-release inhibiting hormone [SRIH]). A variety of physiologic (e.g., hypoglycemia, exercise, stress) and metabolic (e.g., arginine) factors influence GHRH and SRIH release and thereby indirectly stimulate release of hGH. Recombinant DNA technology made previously scarce hGH readily available not only for treatment of patients with hGH deficiency but also for treatment of other growth-impaired children (e.g., those with chronic renal failure, Turner syndrome) and for investigation of its potential use as an anabolic agent. In addition to its central role in the regulation of childhood linear growth, hGH and other hGH-related peptides (e.g., insulin-like growth factor 1 [IGF-1]) have important metabolic effects, including anabolic, immunomodulatory, and lipolytic properties that may prove therapeutically beneficial in the intensive care setting. In healthy subjects, hGH decreases protein catabolism, promotes protein synthesis, increases lipolysis and the conversion of fatty acids to acetyl-coenzyme A, and promotes glycogen deposition. Many (but not all) of these effects are mediated by IGF-1, the synthesis of which is impaired during hypercatabolic illness or malnutrition. Such a shift in fuel metabolism toward fat utilization, sparing protein and carbohydrate, would be expected to be a beneficial adaptive response to caloric deprivation or catabolism associated with stress.[35]

Alterations within the somatotropic axis occurring during the course of critical illness follow a biphasic pattern. The initial stress response consists of activated GH release, whereas circulating levels of GH-dependent IGF-1 and IGF binding protein (IGFBP)-3 fall and IGFBP-1 concentrations rise. Lack of GH effect during this period appears to result from peripheral resistance to GH action. In contrast, in the chronic intensive care-dependent phase of severe illness, pulsatile GH secretion substantially decreases whereas the nonpulsatile fraction remains relatively elevated, resulting in an abnormally flat GH secretory pattern and low to normal mean nocturnal GH serum concentrations. Specifically the reduced amount of GH released in pulses is related to low circulating levels of IGF-1, IGFBP-3, and acid-labile subunit (ALS), which suggests that a relative hyposomatotropism participates in the pathogenesis of the wasting syndrome distinctively in the chronic phase of critical illness.[36] The relative hyposomatotropism seems at least partly of hypothalamic origin because the whole somatotropic axis has been found to be very responsive to continuous infusion of GH-releasing peptide (GHRP), administered alone or in combination with GHRH, as evidenced by reactivated pulsatile GH secretion followed by substantial increases in circulating levels of IGF-I, IGFBP-3, and ALS.[37]

These observations have led to investigations of the therapeutic uses of hGH as an anabolic agent. In the setting of hypercatabolism associated with injury or severe illness, nutritional therapies blunt but do not overcome the gradual loss of organ mass and function. In experimental normal subjects, hGH improves nitrogen balance during hypocaloric (50% recommended) total parenteral nutrition feeding when adequate protein is supplied. Elderly patients demonstrate improved nitrogen retention with hGH therapy, as do obese individuals during caloric restriction. Preliminary studies of postoperative patients treated with hGH have shown similar improvement in nitrogen balance. Body composition analyses suggest that weight loss in surgery patients who receive hGH is predominantly confined to the fat compartment, preserving lean body mass. Studies of burn patients have generally yielded similar hGH-mediated improvements in nitrogen balance, provided adequate nutritional support accompanies hGH therapy.[38]

Improved wound healing after surgery and burns has been noted in experimental animals treated with hGH, although higher than conventional doses of hGH appear to be required, particularly for burn injury. However, at least one randomized trial failed to show significant differences in nitrogen retention, protein oxidation, and other metabolic parameters between placebo-treated and hGH-treated burn patients. Further, a prospective, multicenter, double-blind, randomized, placebo-controlled trial of high-dose GH therapy (mean ± SD daily dose, 0.10 ± 0.02 mg per kilogram of body weight or placebo for 21 days) in 247 Finnish and 285 other European intensive care patients revealed higher mortality in the patients who received GH hormone than in those who did not ($p < 0.001$).[39]

Interest has also focused on restoration of endogenous GH release in critically ill patients initially using GHRH and more recently GHRPs. Growth hormone-releasing hormone alone is unable to exert a significant GH-releasing and anabolic effect, which may point to an underlying reduced availability of the endogenous ligand for the GHRP receptor. GHRPs, on the other hand, have been shown to elicit responsiveness to restored endogenous pulsatile GH secretion during the chronic phase of critical illness but not in the acute phase (thought to be primarily a condition of GH resistance). In one study, coadministration of GHRP-2, TRH, and gonadotropin releasing hormone (GnRH) reactivated the GH, TSH, and luteinizing hormone (LH) axes in prolonged critically ill men and evoked beneficial metabolic effects that were absent with GHRP-2 infusion alone and only partially present with GHRP-2 + TRH.[40] These data underline the importance of correcting multiple hormonal deficits in patients with prolonged critical illness to counteract the hypercatabolic state. This novel strategy of restoring endogenous GH and other hormonal levels blunted by critical illness may lead to significant metabolic improvement related to the balanced endocrine responses. Whether GH secretagogues also enhance clinical recovery of protracted critically ill patients remains to be elucidated.

In attempts to circumvent the suppression of hGH-induced IGF-1 production during severe illness, therapy with recombinant IGF-1 has been investigated. Preliminary studies suggest that significant sparing of body protein requires very high serum IGF-1 concentrations.[41] Hypoglycemia, related to insulin-like effects of high levels of IGF-1, may be problematic and requires concurrent administration of glucose. Studies examining the role of IGF-1, the importance of its binding proteins, and concurrent administration of hGH in catabolic patients are under way.

Insulin, another important anabolic hormone, has been investigated for use in the intensive care setting. Maintenance of normoglycemia with insulin reduces mortality and morbidity of critically ill adult patients. In one large study of 1548 surgical intensive care patients, strict glycemic control (80–110 mg/dl) with insulin infusion substantially reduced overall mortality from 20% to 10% among patients requiring more than 5 days of intensive care.[42] This effect could result from lessening of the adverse metabolic effects of hyperglycemia, direct anabolic effects of insulin, or both. It appears that metabolic control as reflected by normoglycemia, rather than the infused insulin dose per se, is most closely related to the beneficial effects of intensive insulin therapy.

In summary, administration of exogenous GH (and possibly IGF-1 or insulin) or GHRP-induced restoration of endogenous GH secretion and action to stimulate protein synthesis, reduce protein breakdown, and promote fat utilization may be useful for supporting and hastening the healing of patients after surgery or burns and of other critically ill patients. However, available data do not support recommendations for use of GH or GHRP until further randomized, controlled studies of the clinical value and cost effectiveness of these agents on wound healing and recovery from illness are completed. In particular, more investigation of various dosages of recombinant GH in the intensive care setting is needed. On the other hand, data supporting the finding that maintenance of normoglycemia with insulin infusion reduces mortality and can be safely undertaken is fairly compelling.

REFERENCES

1. Kappy MS, Allen DB, Geffner ME, editors: *Principles and practice of pediatric endocrinology*. Springfield, 2005, CC Thomas.
2. Allen DB, Hendricks SA, Perloff WH, et al: Simultaneous presentation of Reye-like syndrome in two male siblings. (Familial unresponsiveness to ACTH), *Am J Med Genet* 32:52-59, 1989.
3. Munck A, Guyre PM, Holbrook NJ: Physiological functions of glucocorticoids in stress and their relation to pharmacological actions, *Endocr Rev* 5:25, 1984.
4. Winter WE: Autoimmune endocrinopathies. In Kappy MS, Blizzard RM, Migeon CJ, editors: *Diagnosis and treatment of endocrine disorders in childhood and adolescence*. Springfield, 1994, CC Thomas.
5. Nye E, Grice JE, Hockings GI, et al: Comparison of ACTH stimulation test and insulin hypoglycemia in normal humans, *J Clin Endocrinol Metab* 84:3648-3655,1999.
6. Bravo E: Evolving concepts in the pathophysiology, diagnosis, and treatment of pheochromocytoma, *Endocr Rev* 15:356-368, 1994.
7. Pacak K, Pacak K, Linehan WM, et al: Recent advances in genetics, diagnosis, localization, and treatment of pheochromocytoma, *Ann Intern Med* 134:315-329, 2001.
8. Ciftci AO: Pheochromocytoma in children, *J Pediatr Surg* 36: 447-452, 2001.
9. Hack HA: The perioperative management of children with pheochromocytoma, *Paediatr Anaesth* 10:463-476, 2000.
10. Weetman AP: Graves' disease, *N Engl J Med* 343:1236, 2000.
11. Momotani N: Thyroid function in breast feeding infants whose mothers take high doses of PTU, *Clin Endocrinol* 53:177, 2000.
12. Zakarija M, McDenzie JM, Hoffman WH: Prediction and therapy of intrauterine and late onset neonatal hyperthyroidism, *J Clin Endocrinol Metab* 62:368, 1986.
13. Raza J, Hindmarsh PC, Brook CGD: Thyrotoxicosis in children: thirty years' experience, *Acta Paediatr* 88:937, 1999.
14. Rivkees SA, Sklar C, Freemark M: The management of Graves' disease in children, *J Clin Endocrinol Metab* 83:3767,1998.
15. Moldonado LS: Do thyroid function tests independently predict survival in the critically ill? *Thyroid* 2:119, 1992.
16. Ross OC, Petros A: The sick euthyroid syndrome in paediatric cardiac surgery patients, *Intensive Care Med* 27:1124-1132, 2001.
17. Klemperer JD, Klein I, Gomez M, et al: Thyroid hormone treatment in cardiopulmonary bypass surgery, *N Engl J Med* 333: 1522-1527, 1995.
18. Klein I, Ojamaa K: Thyroid hormone and the cardiovascular system, *N Engl J Med* 344;501-509, 2001.
19. De Groot LJ: Dangerous dogmas in medicine: the nonthyroidal illness syndrome, *J Clin Endocrinol Metab* 84:151, 1999.
20. Lteif AN, Schwenk WF: Hypoglycemia in infants and children, *Endocrinol Metab Clin North Am* 28:619, 1999.
21. Pearce SH: Clinical disorders of extracellular calcium-sensing and the molecular biology of the calcium-sensing receptor, *Ann Med* 34:201, 2002.
22. Haymond MW, Sundhag G: Controlling the sugar bowl: regulation of glucose homeostasis in children, *Endocrinol Metab Clin North Am* 28:663, 1999.
23. Stanley CA: Advances in diagnosis and treatment of hyperinsulinism in infants and children, *J Clin Endocrinol Metab* 87: 4857-4859, 2002.
24. DeLuca F, Baron J: Molecular biology and clinical importance of the Ca2+-sensing receptor, *Curr Opin Pediatr* 10:435, 1998.
25. Marx SJ: Hyperparathyroid and hypoparathyroid disorders, *N Engl J Med* 343:1863, 2000.

26. Klein GL, Langman CB, Herndon DN: Persistent hypoparathyroidism following magnesium repletion in burn-injured children, *Pediatr Nephrol* 14:301-304, 2000.
27. Lteif AN, Zimmerman D: Bisphosphonates for treatment of childhood hypercalcemia, *Pediatrics* 102(4 pt 1):990, 1998.
28. Holmes CL, Patel BM, Russell JA, et al: Physiology of vasopressin relevant to management of septic shock. *Chest* 120:989, 2001.
29. Landry DW, Oliver JA: The pathogenesis of vasodilatory shock. *N Engl J Med* 345:588, 2001.
30. Landry DW, Levin HR, Gallant EM, et al: Vasopressin deficiency contributes to the vasodilation of septic shock, *Circulation* 95:1122, 1997.
31. Tsuneyoshi I, Yamada H, Kakihana Y, et al: Hemodynamic and metabolic effects of low-dose vasopressin infusions in vasodilatory septic shock, *Crit Care Med* 29:487, 2001.
32. Malay MB, Ashton RC, Landry DW, et al: Low-dose vasopressin in the treatment of vasodilatory septic shock, *J Trauma* 47:699, 1999.
33. Patel BM, Chittock DR, Russell JA, et al: Beneficial effects of short-term vasopressin infusion during severe septic shock, *Anesthesiology* 96:576, 2002.
34. Rosenzweig EB, Starc TJ, Chen JM, et al: Intravenous arginine-vasopressin in children with vasodilatory shock after cardiac surgery, *Circulation* 100(suppl II):II-182, 1999.
35. Carrel AL, Allen DB: Effects of growth hormone on body composition and bone metabolism, *Endocrine* 12:163,2000.
36. Balcells J, Moreno A, Audi L, et al: Growth hormone/insulin-like growth factors axis in children undergoing cardiac surgery, *Crit Care Med* 2001;29:1234.
37. Van den Berghe G, Wouters P, Weekers F, et al: Reactivation of the pituitary hormone release and metabolic improvement by infusion of growth hormone-releasing peptide and thyrotropin-releasing hormone in patients with protracted critical illness, *J Clin Endocrinol Metab* 84:1311,1999.
38. Jeschke MG, Barrow RE, Herndon DN: Recombinant human growth hormone treatment in pediatric burn patients and its role during the hepatic acute phase response, *Critical Care Medicine* 28:1578, 2000. IL: Charles C. Thomas, 1994:383-455.
39. Takala J, Ruokonen E, Webster NR, et al: Increased mortality associated with growth hormone treatment in critically ill adults, *N Engl J Med* 341:785-792, 1999.
40. Van den Berghe G: Neuroendocrine pathobiology of chronic critical illness, *Crit Care Clin* 8:509-528, 2002.
41. Clemmons DR: Role of insulin-like growth factor-1 in reversing catabolism, *J Clin Endocrinol Metab* 75:1183, 1992 (editorial).
42. Van Den Berghe G, Wouters P, Weekers F, et al: Intensive insulin therapy in critically ill patients, *N Engl J Med* 345: 1359-1367, 2001.

CHAPTER

71

Diabetic Ketoacidosis

Gail E. Richards

PEARLS

- Diabetic ketoacidosis (DKA) is the most common endocrine condition that a practitioner in a critical care setting likely will see.
- Diabetic ketoacidosis occurs under two general sets of circumstances:
  1. In patients who are known to have diabetes
  2. In patients in whom DKA is the precipitating event leading to diagnosis
- General principles of diagnosis and treatment in the acute phase are similar for both situations.
- DKA in a child not previously known to have diabetes results from lack of recognition of the importance of early symptoms of hyperglycemia, such as polydipsia, polyuria, and weight loss, symptoms more likely to be overlooked if the patient has no family members or friends with diabetes and has limited access to medical care.
- The goals of treatment of DKA are multiple:
  1. Replenish fluid and electrolyte losses
  2. Prevent further lipolysis and additional formation of ketoacids
  3. Facilitate elimination of ketoacids and restore normal acid-base equilibrium
  4. Normalize blood glucose and provide adequate carbohydrates to meet cellular energy needs
  5. Address and treat the underlying illnesses or other precipitating factors
- Education of the patient is the most effective prevention.

Diabetic ketoacidosis (DKA) is the most common endocrine condition that a practitioner in a critical care setting likely will see. Approximately 13,000 new cases of type I diabetes mellitus are diagnosed each year, with an overall prevalence of approximately 1:2500 by age 5 years and 1:300 by age 20 years. The likelihood of a significant complication from an episode of ketoacidosis is on the order of 1% to 3%, underscoring the importance of timely and effective management of this potentially life-threatening situation. Diabetic ketoacidosis occurs under two general sets of circumstances: in patients known to have diabetes and in patients in whom DKA is the precipitating event leading to diagnosis. General principles of diagnosis and treatment in the acute phase are similar for both situations. However, the longer-term considerations are different (see Appendix A).

Precipitating Factors

Diabetic ketoacidosis in a child not previously known to have diabetes results from lack of recognition of the importance of early symptoms of hyperglycemia, such as polydipsia, polyuria, and weight loss. These symptoms are more likely to be overlooked if the patient has no family members or friends with diabetes and has limited access to medical care. It is easy to presume that early symptoms are attributable to an intercurrent illness, especially in very young children.

In the majority of patients with type I diabetes, pancreatic β cells are destroyed by an autoimmune process that is significantly influenced by genetics. Genetic susceptibility does not explain all of the risks for diabetes, however, and there are undoubtedly other contributing and precipitating factors, such as exposure to viral antigens (e.g., rubella, mumps, cytomegalovirus). Exposure to cow's milk (but not commercial infant formula containing cow's milk protein) and soy protein also have been implicated but not rigorously proven. In addition, an extensive number of syndromes and medications have been associated with type I diabetes (Table 71-1). These factors should be considered at the time the patient presents with signs and symptoms of diabetes. In addition, diabetes is a component of specific syndromes, such as Wolfram syndrome. The role of emotional and physical stressors as precipitating events at the onset of DKA is difficult to prove, but clearly an anecdotal association exists.

In children known to have diabetes, a number of circumstances can lead to provision of inadequate insulin to meet energy needs. The most common scenario is omission of necessary insulin doses through forgetfulness or subconscious denial, or failure to adjust insulin appropriately for changing circumstances such as intercurrent illness. The role of psychological factors in precipitating DKA is controversial. Acute psychological stress or upset, such as extreme anger, appears to be capable of triggering DKA in some patients. This phenomenon may be more common than documented by the literature, especially during the teenage years.

In theory, all DKA is preventable through education. The general public, as well as health providers, can be made more aware of the increasing incidence of diabetes and the nonspecific nature of early symptoms to allow diagnosis of new-onset diabetes before DKA occurs. Patients who already have been diagnosed with diabetes almost always can be managed at home to prevent DKA, but access to such intensive services and advice that can prevent hospitalizations or emergency department visits is not universally available.

Definition and Diagnosis

There is no universal agreement on the exact blood pH or serum bicarbonate concentration or blood ketone measurement that defines patients with DKA. It is perhaps more useful to think of DKA as a spectrum ranging from early events with the potential to deteriorate into frank DKA (such as intercurrent illness, omission of an insulin injection, or early polyuria and polydipsia of a patient with new-onset diabetes) to severe metabolic decompensation that may be associated with loss of consciousness and shock. Pathophysiology in these situations is the same, and the general principles of treatment are the same. Accordingly, the broadest and most useful definition might be presence of ketoacids in the blood and/or urine in the face of relative insulin insufficiency.

In an emergency department setting, approximately 4% of children with various illnesses, including but not limited to fever and dehydration, have blood glucose concentrations greater than 150 mg/dl, leading to the suspicion of diabetes. Only about 2% of these children go on to develop diabetes, so it is important to be clear about diagnostic criteria. Current diagnostic criteria are plasma glucose >126 mg/dl after at least an 8-hour fast, random plasma glucose >200 mg/dl with classic signs and symptoms of diabetes (polyuria, polydipsia, weight loss, fatigue), or abnormal oral glucose tolerance with a 2-hour plasma glucose >200 mg/dl. Any one of these criteria should be confirmed on two separate days unless there is unequivocal hyperglycemia of metabolic decompensation.

Pathophysiology

Diabetic ketoacidosis occurs when cellular energy needs cannot be met by glucose supplied by an insulin-requiring transport mechanism. The body then must use fat stores as energy. The two major components of DKA are (1) hyperglycemia caused by inability of glucose to cross the cellular membrane when insulin is inadequate and (2) acidosis caused by the metabolic products of fat oxidation as the body is forced to change its energy source. Thus it follows that not all hyperglycemia results in ketoacidosis if the relative amount of insulin available is sufficient to meet cellular energy needs but is insufficient to

TABLE 71–1

Conditions Associated with Diabetes Mellitus in Childhood

Syndromes	Infections	Drugs	Endocrinopathies
Down syndrome	Congenital rubella	Diuretics	Acromegaly
Klinefelter syndrome	Cytomegalovirus	Diazoxide	Cushing syndrome
Turner syndrome	Coxsackie B virus	β adrenergic antagonists	Glucagonoma
Friedreich ataxia	Adenovirus	Diphenylhydantoin	Pheochromocytoma
Huntington chorea	Mumps	Glucocorticoids	Hyperthyroidism
Laurence-Moon Biedl syndrome		Oral contraceptives	Somatostatinoma
Myotonic dystrophy		Pentamidine	aldosteronoma
Porphyria		Cyclosporine	
Prader-Willi syndrome		FK506	
Rabson-Mendenhall syndrome		Opiates	
Lipoatrophic syndromes		asparaginase	

Modified from Gitelman SE: Diabetes mellitus. In: *Rudolph's pediatrics,* New York, 2003, McGraw-Hill Companies.

facilitate cellular uptake of enough glucose from the plasma and tissue compartments to achieve normoglycemia. Ketoacidosis without hyperglycemia is possible if the body uses fat as an energy source in the face of relatively little glucose delivered to the plasma and tissue compartments. This can occur under circumstances of nausea, vomiting, and reduced intake. In general, however, counterregulatory hormones (cortisol, growth hormone, glucagons, catecholamines) produce hyperglycemia even with relatively limited intake if insulin is inadequate.

Table 71-2 lists the mechanism of action on blood glucose of hormones that are believed to contribute to metabolic decompensation in DKA. It is important to note that the effects of all these hormones together is greater than the sum of individual effects in the experimental situation. The relative contributions of each of these hormones to the metabolic decompensation of DKA under facilitative precipitating conditions cannot be determined with any accuracy by measuring the hormones. Counterregulatory hormonal contribution to emotionally or psychologically precipitated DKA is poorly understood.

Figure 71-1 depicts the metabolism of glucose and pathway leading to ketoacid production (Chapter 67). The most relevant ketones produced are β-hydroxybutyrate, acetoacetate, and acetone. Under fasting conditions and under conditions of acidosis, formation of β-hydroxybutyrate is favored over acetoacetate causing significant increases in the ratio between the two compounds. Because the common urinary test for ketones measures primarily acetoacetate, this test can significantly underestimate the ketoacid burden. Although urine test may be useful for monitoring, serum ketones are more helpful for quantitative purposes.

Figure 71-2 shows the basic pathophysiology of DKA through effects of insulin deficiency on tissue metabolism that result in the observed signs and symptoms of DKA.

In addition to ketoacidosis, lactic acidosis may be present if there is significant dehydration and resultant poor tissue perfusion. If acidosis is present, there is often a compensatory respiratory alkalosis accompanied by the classic deep respirations through pursed lips described as Kussmaul respirations.

The absolute and relative fluid and electrolyte deficits of patients with DKA can be calculated in a number of standard ways. Table 71-3 lists the ranges of expected fluid and electrolyte deficits. It is important to recognize that observed hyponatremia in patients with DKA reflects not only sodium deficits but factitious measurement caused by hyperglycemia and hyperlipidemia. The observed sodium can be corrected for this artifact by the following formula:

$$Na^{+corrected} = Na^{+observed} + [(\text{Glucose in mg/dl} - 100)/100] \times 1.6$$

or

$$Na^{+corrected} = Na^{+observed} + [(\text{Glucose in mmol/L} - 5.6)/5.6] \times 1.6.$$

Treatment

The goals of treatment of DKA are multiple: to replenish fluid and electrolyte losses, to prevent further lipolysis and additional formation of ketoacids, to facilitate elimination of ketoacids and restore normal acid base equilibrium, to normalize blood glucose and provide adequate carbohydrate to meet cellular energy needs, and to address and treat the underlying illnesses or other precipitating factors.

Fluid and Electrolyte Therapy

To replenish fluid and electrolyte losses, the magnitude of the losses must first be estimated. This can be judged by comparison of present weight to previous weight (if known), presence of dry mucous membranes, poor skin turgor, low blood pressure, and tachycardia as in other types of dehydration. Empiric use of normal saline (0.9%) 10 to

TABLE 71–2

Effect of Stress-Related Hormones on Secretion of Islet Cell Hormones and on Metabolism of Adipocytes, Muscle, and Liver

	Islets		*Extrapancreatic Tissues*		
Hormone	**Insulin Secretion**	**Glucagon Secretion**	**Adipocytes; Lipolysis**	**Muscle: Glucose Utilization**	**Liver: Glucose Production**
Catecholamines	↓	↑	↑	↓	↑
Corticotropin	—	—	↑	—	—
Cortisol	↑	↑	↑	↓	↑
Growth hormone	↑	↑	↑	↓	↑
β Endorphin	—	↑	—	—	—
Vasopressin	—	↑	—	—	↓

↑, Increase; ↓, decrease; —, no effect or not known.
From Wilson JD, Foster DW, Kronenberg HM, Larson PR, editors: *Williams textbook of endocrinology,* ed 9, Philadelphia, 1998, WB Saunders.

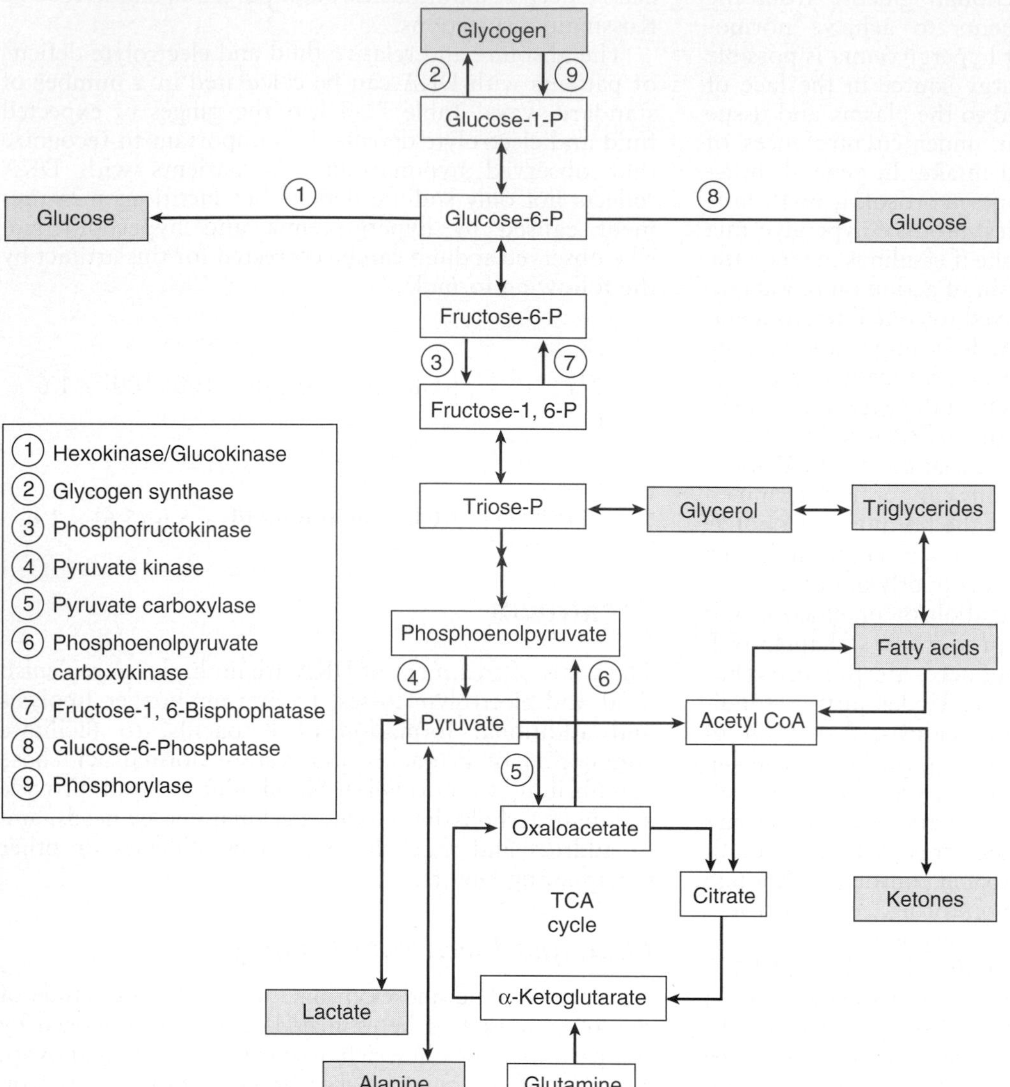

FIGURE 71–1 • Schematic representation of glucose metabolism. *CoA*, Coenzyme A; *TCA*, tricarboxylic acid (From Kronenberg HM, Melmed S, Polonsky KS, editors: *Williams textbook of endocrinology*, ed 10, Philadelphia, 2003, WB Saunders.)

20 ml/kg over the first hour is generally effective for restoring volume if losses are mild. Continuation of the initial volume expansion for another hour at the same rate may be needed if dehydration is in the range of 10%.

After the initial volume expansion, replacement of remaining fluid and electrolyte deficits and provision for maintenance and ongoing losses usually can be accomplished with 0.45% saline. Insulin therapy drives potassium that has moved from the intracellular to extracellular compartment, because of acidosis, back into the cells. This action of insulin has the potential to create potentially dangerous hypokalemia by unmasking total body potassium deficits. Thus it is important to provide generous potassium replacement. The most common method of replacement is to provide a total of 40 mEq/L of potassium, half as the chloride salt and half as phosphate. Phosphate has the theoretical advantage of improving adenosine triphosphate stores to aid cellular metabolism. The disadvantage of phosphate is that it can drive calcium down during the fluid repletion phase of treatment. Potassium should be replaced only after urination has been documented and renal function assessed. Generally, fluid administration rate during the rehydration phase should be calculated to account for maintenance plus replacement of estimated dehydration and ongoing losses. Usually only ongoing losses from vomiting, nasogastric drainage, diarrhea, or extremely high fever requires replacement. Ongoing urinary losses usually are adequately accounted for if maintenance therapy is provided. It often is helpful to formally calculate sodium deficit, especially if serum sodium is abnormal. If sodium losses are unusually large, it may be necessary to continue 0.9% saline for a time during the rehydration phase. Replacement should occur relatively slowly over approximately 48 hours. This correction can be skewed so that approximately 50% of the deficits of both fluid and sodium are corrected over about the first 12 hours. As with any fluid therapy, frequent reassessment of electrolytes every 4 hours or so and reassessment of detailed intake and output can guide adjustments in the rate and content of fluid therapy.

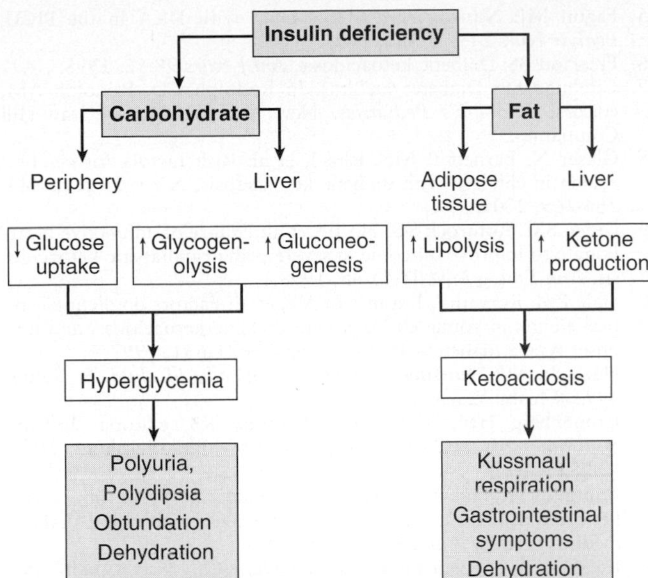

FIGURE 71–2 • Pathophysiologic mechanism underlying diabetic ketoacidosis with the consequent clinical signs and symptoms. Insulin effects on fat are approximately 10 times more potent than those on carbohydrate metabolism. Patients with both type I and type II diabetes mellitus have derangements in carbohydrate metabolism, but primarily those with type I diabetes mellitus and more severe insulin deficiency have lipolysis and diabetic ketoacidosis. (From Siperstein MD: *Endocrinol Metab Clin North Am* 21:415-432 ,1992.)

Often after the first several hours oral intake is possible. Patients can rehydrate well with oral therapy, but the amount and content of oral fluids must be calculated and adjustments made in intravenous therapy to prevent overhydration.

Use of bicarbonate to correct acidosis is not generally recommended, as the combination of insulin and fluid therapy is virtually always sufficient to correct metabolic acidosis. In general, more time is required for urine and plasma ketones to correct than for plasma glucose to return to an acceptable range. Indeed, if quantitative plasma ketones are being measured, there may even be an increase in ketones as rehydration expands the plasma compartment and the relative ratio of β-hydroxybutyrate to acetoacetate decreases, thus increasing acetoacetate, which is measured in common urinary tests for ketones. The theoretical argument against bicarbonate treatment is that it may worsen acidosis within the central nervous system and cause potassium shifts that can provoke arrhythmias. Additional empiric evidence documents that the practical outcome for patients with DKA is not improved by bicarbonate administration. If, however, persistent low pH is believed to be compromising cardiovascular function despite adequate fluid and insulin therapy, 1 to 2 mEq/kg of bicarbonate can be given slowly over about 2 hours. This therapy should be discontinued at the earliest possible moment when pH and plasma bicarbonate begin to increase. Large-volume DKA normal saline resuscitation may be associated with a nonanion gap, hyperchloremic metabolic acidosis.

TABLE 71–3

Fluid and Electrolyte Requirements in Diabetic Ketoacidosis

Element	Maintenance Requirement	Losses
Water	1500 ml/m^2	60–100 mL/kg
Sodium	45 mEq/m^2	5–13 mEq/kg
Potassium	35 mEq/m^2	4–6 mEq/kg
Chloride	30 mEq/m^2	3–9 mEq/kg
Phosphate	10 mEq/m^2	2–5 mEq/kg

Modified from Sperling MA: Diabetes mellitus. In Sperling MA, editor: *Pediatric endocrinology,* Philadelphia, 2002, WB Saunders.

Insulin Therapy

Insulin should be provided as soon as the diagnosis is determined. In some selected situations, treatment can be given with subcutaneous short-acting insulin. Subcutaneous therapy should be reserved for situations where acidosis and dehydration are minimal and intensive follow-up is certain. At the other end of the spectrum of severity, subcutaneous lispro or intramuscular regular insulin can be used as a temporary measure in a severely ill patient when establishing intravenous access likely will require some time. The more usually appropriate method for providing insulin in DKA is via continuous infusion or regular insulin. The usual starting dose is 0.1 U/kg/hour. This dosage sometimes can be decreased to 0.05 U/kg/hour if the patient is very young or is particularly insulin sensitive. The rate of insulin drip should be adjusted to decrease plasma glucose by approximately 100 mg/dl/hour until blood glucose reaches approximately 200 to 300 mg/dl. At that point, adding 5% glucose to the rehydration fluids is appropriate. Addition of glucose is more appropriate than decreasing the rate of insulin infusion because relative insulin deficiency is the primary problem and because glucose is needed to meet intracellular energy needs. The glucose infusion rate should be adjusted to maintain plasma glucose in the 100 to 150 mg/dl range.

Often the initial volume expansion decreases plasma glucose considerably. This decrease, which results from dilution of plasma glucose, should not impact provision of adequate insulin replacement therapy.

Cerebral Edema

This potentially life-threatening complication of DKA occurs in approximately 1% of children. Symptoms include headache, lethargy, and behavioral changes in the early phases, followed by pupillary abnormalities, seizures, and the hypertension and bradycardia commonly seen with increased intracranial pressure. Left untreated, these symptoms can lead to tentorial herniation, respiratory and cardiac arrest, and death. The pathophysiology leading to cerebral edema is not entirely clear. The most recent comprehensive analysis comparing children with DKA and cerebral edema with a control group with DKA but no cerebral edema showed a statistical correlation of cerebral edema only with initial serum urea nitrogen and initial partial pressure of arterial carbon dioxide. These statistical correlations suggest that cerebral edema tends to occur in children with more severe DKA. Controversy exists over the role of fluid administration in precipitating cerebral edema in DKA. Studies evaluating variables associated with cerebral edema implicated rate of fluid administration as a possible contributing cause, but the subsequent comprehensive analysis did not confirm a role for rate of fluid administration but did implicate bicarbonate treatment. This study provides further reason for great caution in bicarbonate administration to children with DKA.

All children with DKA should be carefully monitored for early signs of cerebral edema and should be evaluated with neuroimaging if suggestive signs or symptoms occur. Prompt treatment to decrease intracerebral pressure with mannitol, fluid restriction, and hyperventilation can prevent adverse outcomes in approximately half the patients who develop cerebral edema (Chapter 52).)

Nonketotic Hyperosmolar Coma

Nonketotic hyperosmolar coma is characterized by extremely high plasma glucose without acidosis. Glucose values can exceed 1000 mg/dl, which constitutes sufficient osmolar load to produce significant changes in water compartmentalization. Symptoms generally include polyuria and polydipsia with obtundation or lethargy. Acidosis is not present. Therapy is similar to therapy for DKA. Because there may be a greater sensitivity to insulin in the absence of acidosis, it may be advisable to begin therapy with a lower rate of insulin infusion than for DKA, for example, 0.05 U/kg/hour. The aim should be to decrease glucose slowly, certainly no more than 100 mg/dl/hour, and to rehydrate slowly over 48 hours.

Additional Issues

In every episode of DKA, a search should be made for the conditions or issues responsible for triggering the DKA. There should be education and support aimed at preventing recurrence of DKA. In the case of patients who have DKA at the onset of diabetes, the education required is extensive. A sample care pathway used for diabetes with DKA, sample admitting orders, and educational record are shown Appendixes B, C, and D.

Suggested Readings

1. Adrogue HJ, Madias NE: Medical progress: management of life-threatening acid-base disorders, part I, *N Engl J Med* 338:26-34, 1998.
2. American Diabetes Association Position Statement. Hyperglycemic crises in patients with diabetes mellitus, *Diabetes Care* 24(suppl 1): S83-S90, 2001.
3. Brink SJ: Diabetic ketoacidosis. *Acta Paediatr Suppl* 427:14-24, 1999.
4. Eisenbarth GE, Polonsky KS, Buse JB: Type 1 diabetes mellitus. In Wilson JD, Foster DW, Kronenberg HM, Larson PR, editors: *Williams Textbook of Endocrinology,* ed 9, Philadelphia, 1998, WB Saunders.
5. Fagon MJ: Nursing care of the child with DKA in the PICU, *Pediatr Nurs* 21:375-380, 1995.
6. Freeland BS: Diabetic ketoacidosis, *Am J Nurs* 98:52, 1998.
7. Gitelman SE: Diabetes mellitus. In Rudolph CD, Rudolph AM, editors: *Rudolph's Pediatrics,* New York, 2003, McGraw-Hill Companies.
8. Glaser N, Barnett P, McCaslin I, et al: Risk factors for cerebral edema in children with diabetic ketoacidosis, *N Engl J Med* 344: 264-269, 2001.
9. Green SM, Rothrock SG, Ho JD, et al: Failure of adjunctive bicarbonate to improve outcome in severe pediatric diabetic ketoacidosis, *Ann Emerg Med* 31:41-48, 1998.
10. Hale PM, Rezvani I, Braunstein AW, et al: Factors predicting cerebral edema in young children with diabetic ketoacidosis and new onset type 1 diabetes, *Acta Paediatr* 86:621-631, 1997.
11. Hazinski MF: *Nursing care of the critically ill child,* St. Louis, 1992, Mosby Yearbook.
12. Kronenberg HM, Melmed S, Polonsky KS, editors: *Williams textbook of endocrinology,* ed 10, Philadelphia, 2003, WB Saunders.
13. Kaufman FR, Halvorson M: The treatment and prevention of diabetic ketoacidosis in children and adolescents with type 1 diabetes mellitus, *Pediatr Ann* 28:576-582, 1999.
14. Kecskes SA: Diabetic ketoacidosis, *Pediatr Clin North Am* 40:355-363, 1993.
15. Keiss W, et al: Pediatric aspects of managing preschool children with type 1 diabetes, *Acta Pediatr* 425(suppl):67-41, 1998.
16. Levetan CS, Passaro MD, Jablonski KA, Ratner RE: Effect of physician specialty on outcomes in diabetic ketoacidosis, *Diabetes Care* 22:1790-1795, 1999.
17. Glaser N, Barnett P, McCaslin I, et al: Pediatric Emergency Medicine Collaborative Research Committee of the American Academy of Pediatrics: Risk factors for cerebral edema in children with ketoacidosis, *N Engl J Med* 344:264-269, 2001.
18. Sperling MA: Diabetes mellitus. In Sperling MA, editor: *Pediatric endocrinology,* ed 2. Philadelphia, 2002, WB Saunders.
19. White NH: Acute complications of diabetes. Diabetic ketoacidosis in children, *Endocrinol Metab Clin North Am* 29:657-682, 2000.

Appendix A

GUIDELINES OF CARE DIABETES KETOACIDOSIS (EMERGENCY DEPARTMENT AND CRITICAL CARE)

I. Description

Diabetic ketoacidosis (DKA) is a life-threatening manifestation of severe insulin deficiency characterized by a constellation of metabolic complications, including hyperglycemia, metabolic acidosis, ketosis, dehydration, total body potassium depletion, and hypophosphatemia. It can be precipitated by any major physiologic stress, such as infection, trauma, or omission of insulin dosing.

The following protocol is intended as a set of guidelines. It is expected that clinical decisions will be made based on the individual's evaluation, patient's response to initial management, and resources available.

II. Important Considerations

Note: Before admitting any patient with either known or new diabetes who is in DKA, it is advisable to contact the endocrinologist on call if the patient is either new or attends Children's Diabetes Clinic. If the patient receives diabetes care through another practitioner, it is appropriate to contact that practitioner. It is important to be aware that some practitioners on the staff at Children's are not part of the endocrine call system but do manage their own diabetic patients.

A. The most serious complication of DKA is cerebral edema, which may develop as the patient is being treated.
B. Decreasing glucose levels rapidly in DKA is not a priority and should be avoided.
C. Insulin adheres to the plastic IV tubing, so flush with 50 ml of insulin solution before administration.
D. After discussion with the endocrinologist, PICU admission may be considered for DKA patients with
   1. pH <7.2
   2. ≥10%–15% dehydration
   3. Hemodynamic instability
   4. Obtundation or other abnormal neurologic finding
   5. Marked hypersmolarity
   6. Young child (<5 years old) with DKA
   7. Additional factors that may affect status, such as substance use or pregnancy

III. Assessment

A. Obtain history
   1. Infection
   2. Previous insulin therapy last insulin dose
   3. Duration of symptoms
   4. Pregnancy
   5. GI status (vomiting, most recent oral intake)
B. Physical examination
   1. Assessment of cardiovascular status, respiratory status, state of hydration, ketosis, sites of infection, and mental status
   2. Vital signs monitored at a minimum frequency of q^{2h} and, as needed, with neuro checks q^{1h}
C. Neurologic
   1. Assess for signs of diabetic coma q^{1h} (secondary to hyperosmolar state)
      a. Decreased LOC
      b. Neuro checks q^{1h} as noted earlier.
   2. Assess for signs of cerebral edema q^{1h}
      a. Headache
      b. Decreased LOC, disorientation, agitation
      c. Hypertension/bradycardia
      d. Pupil anisocoria, impared reactivity to light.
      e. Polyuria secondary to DI (rare)
      f. Vomiting
      g. Seizures
      h. Any neurologic examination asymmetry
D. Respiratory
   1. Monitor for hyperpnea
   2. Assess for hypoventilation (most common cause is coma)
      a. Decreased O_2 saturation (monitor with continuous pulse oximetry)
      b. Alteration in blood gas with hypercapnia
   3. Assess for signs and symptoms of pulmonary edema continuously (rare complication of DKA)
      a. Respiratory distress as evidenced by
         (i) Tachypnea
         (ii) Nasal flaring
         (iii) Retractions
         (iv) Grunting
         (v) Decreased O_2 saturation
         (vi) Abnormal or diminished breath sounds
      b. Copious frothy sputum
      c. Deteriorating blood gases
E. Circulation/hydration
   1. Estimate degree of dehydration on presentation and during treatment
      a. Compare reference and admission weight if reference weight is recent and available.
      b. Assume at least 10% dehydration.
      c. Use physical examination and findings to estimate severity of dehydration as indicated in the following table.

Severity of Dehydration	Signs/Symptoms	Fluid Deficit %	Fluid Deficit ml/kg
Minimal	Few or none, thirst	3	30
Mild	Dry mucous membranes	3–5	30–50
Moderate	Sunken eyes, soft globe, sunken fontanel	5–7	50–70
Moderate–severe	Tenting of skin	7–12	70–120
Severe	Hypovolemic shock	>12	>120

   2. Monitor urine output hourly
   3. Strict hourly intake and output measurement until stable.
   4. Assess for signs of hypovolemic shock at least q^{1h} and as needed:
      a. Alteration in LOC
      b. Tachycardia
      c. Hypotension
      d. Weak peripheral pulses
      e. Prolonged capillary refill
      f. Cool extremities
      g. Pallor
      h. Decreased urinary output may not be present secondary to osmotic diuresis
      i. Acidosis (in DKA, degree of lactic acidosis may be obscured by ketoacidosis)
   5. If patient has evidence of hypovolemic shock.
F. Glucose/electrolytes/osmolarity
   1. Monitor glucose at least hourly until stable, and for duration of continuous insulin infusion.
   2. Measure and assess electrolytes as ordered (usually $q^{2\text{-}4h}$ until stable).
      a. Total body potassium depletion exists regardless of serum potassium
         (i) Potassium value may be initially elevated due to acidosis (potassium has shifted from intracellular to extracellular)
         (ii) Potassium will decrease rapidly with correction of acidosis (returning to intracellular compartment)
      b. Chloride usually high

c. Sodium usually low secondary to urinary losses
d. Phosphate usually low secondary to urinary losses
e. Magnesium may decrease as a result of phosphate replacement
f. Calcium may decrease if phosphate and bicarbonate are given

3. Assess direction of sodium and glucose levels. Serum sodium should be increasing as glucose is decreasing. If both are decreasing, it is likely serum osmolarity is decreasing too rapidly, placing the patient at increased risk for cerebral edema.
4. Monitor ECG for signs of electrolyte imbalance.
   a. Hyperkalemic
      (i) Prolonged PR interval
      (ii) Widened QRS
      (iii) Tenting of T waves
      (iv) Evolution of sine wave rhythm
   b. Hypokalemia
      (i) Flattened T waves
      (ii) ST-segment depression
      (iii) Presence of U waves
   c. Hypocalcemia
      (i) Prolonged QT interval
5. Monitor measured or calculated serum osmolarity (normal 270-295). For patients in a very hyperosmolar state (>330–360 mOsm/L) or very hypernatremic (corrected sodium >150mmol/L) at presentation, or for those more ill in general, replace fluids over at least 48 hours.
6. Hb A^{Ic} C-peptide, insulin antibodies and islet cell antibodies, T^4, TSH, and lipid panel should be checked after blood gases and electrolytes normalize.

IV. INTERVENTIONS

A. Comfort
   1. See ICU GOC, "Comfort."
   2. If patient does not require arterial line, place a large peripheral IV line that will draw blood for frequent oratory laboratory draws and glucose checks rather than frequent finger sticks whenever possible.

B. Neurologic
   1. Report any changes (even minor) to MD immediately.
   2. If clinical signs/symptoms of cerebral edema develop:
      a. With intubation and initial hyperventilation. Page anesthesia or intensivist to perform or assist with intubation.
      b. Administer osmotic diuretic (mannitol 0.25–1g/kg) as ordered.
      c. Extend glucose/rehydration correction time (48–72 hours).

C. Respiratory
   1. Be prepared to intubate for deteriorating LOC.
   2. Avoid drugs that may aggravate hypovolemic shock state (e.g., narcotics, barbiturates).
   3. Anticipate drugs needed to avoid increased ICP during intubation if cerebral edema is suspected (e.g., thiopental, lidocaine, neuromuscular blocking agent).

D. Hydration
   1. Rapid replacement of volume is necessary to stabilize if patient is truly in shock.
      a. Use 10–20 ml/kg of NS or LR as rapidly as possible until hypotension and perfusion are improved. If patient is not in shock, use 10–20 ml/kg once.
      b. Continually assess results of fluid boluses and stop once circulatory failure is reversed (to avoid too rapid correction of hyperosmolar state).
      c. Be sure to take into account fluids administered prior to transfer (e.g., from referring center or ED) and reduce calculated needs by that amount.
   2. Correct remaining fluid deficit over 36–48 hours.
      a. Maintenance fluids must also be provided during this period.
      b. It is usually not necessary to replace urine output, monitor output, and follow hydration status. There are hidden sources of water in DKA from oxidation of glucose and ketones, and ADH is elevated. Osmotic diuresis should subside once glucose is normalized (<180 mg/dl).
      c. Although factors precipitating cerebral edema remain unclear, the risk of acute cerebral edema is less if rate of hydration is kept <50 ml/kg/4 hours (even in the initial 4 hours) and <4 L/m^2/day.

E. Glucose/electrolyte/correction
   1. Use of bicarbonate is only indicated for patients in shock, unresponsive to fluid resuscitation, or hyperalkemia with ECG changes (1–3 mEq/kg to raise pH to >7.2). Bicarbonate should be administered only when perfusion and ventilation can be assured.
   2. Electrolyte replacement
      a. Total body potassium depletion exists regardless of serum potassium.
         (i) Potassium value may be initially elevated due to acidosis, secondary to cellular H^+/K^+ shifts.
         (ii) Potassium value will decrease rapidly with correction of acidosis, returning to intracellular compartment.
         (iii) Potassium may be carefully replaced as ordered (usually added to maintenance fluids often split between KCl and Kphos).
      b. Hyperchloremia is rarely treated. However, note that in the setting of very large volume NS resuscitation, a hyperchloremic (non anion gap) metabolic acidosis may ensue.
      c. Hyponatremia results from urinary losses of sodium during diuresis.
         (i) Administer fluid boluses of NS as ordered.
      d. Hypophosphatemia results from osmotic diuresis.

(i) KPO_4 may be supplied in IV fluids along with KCl
(ii) Replace phosphate carefully
- Watch for hypocalcemia
- Watch for hypomagnesemia

e. Hypomagnesemia may be a result of phosphate replacement.
(i) Watch for signs similar to hypocalcemia (see below)
(ii) Treat if indicated; may be difficult to correct with concomitant hypokalemia.
(iii) In the setting of hypomagnesemia, hypokalemia will be difficult to correct.

f. Hypocalcemia may result when phosphate and bicarbonate are given.
(i) Monitor for muscle cramps, spasms, seizures, decreased cardiac contractility, prolonged QT interval.
(ii) Treat as indicated.

F. Insulin administration
1. Initial insulin therapy is usually 0.05–0.1U/kg/hour IV continuous drip (up to 7 U/hour).
a. Insulin should be infused through a separate line if possible. Insulin adheres to plastic tubing, so flush line with 50 ml of solution before administration.
b. Standard solution is 50 U regular insulin in 250 ml NS so that 0.1 U/kg/hour = 0.2 ml/kg/hour.
c. Monitor serum glucose every 30–60 minutes as ordered.
d. Serum glucose should not fall faster than 100 mg/dl/hour.
2. Typically, when blood sugar reaches <200–300, rather than reducing or discontinuing the insulin infusion, dextrose is added to maintenance fluids until metabolic acidosis and ketonuria are resolved.
3. Conversion from IV to subcutaneous insulin
a. Subcutaneous insulin may be considered when
(i) Serum glucose falls below 250 mg/dl
(ii) Acidosis is resolved (HCO_3 >20)
(iii) Ketones are absent
(iv) ADA PO diet is initiated
(v) There should be a 1-hour overlap between administration of first dose of subcutaneous regular insulin (15–30 minutes if lispro insulin will be given) and discontinuing insulin infusion.
b. For a child with previously diagnosed diabetes, return to the child's previous insulin regimen, with supplemental rapid-acting insulin for hyperglycemia and/or ketonuria. Due to the patient's inactivity and possibly the precipitating cause of DKA (e.g., acute infection), insulin requirements may be higher during the first day post DKA.
c. If patient was not on subcutaneous insulin previously, a typical conversion pattern would be
(i) Daily requirement of 0.5–1 U/kg/day (usually 0.9–1 U/kg/day when presenting in moderate to severe DKA).
(ii) Divide ²/₃ of the dose for AM and ¹/₃ of the dose for PM
(iii) Each dose may be split ²/₃ intermediate-acting (NPH or lente) and ¹/₃ short-acting (regular or lispro). Supplemental doses of short-acting insulin (generally 10% of total daily dose) may also be used to help stabilize the patient's blood sugar and calculate permanent insulin dose.
d. Remember that food intake greatly affects blood glucose response to any insulin. Thus do not treat aggressively during the night or when child is not eating during the day. Treat only very high blood glucose readings (>350 mg/dl) or when moderate or large ketonuria during the night.
e. Supplemental doses should be approximately 10% to 15% of total daily dose (or 0.1–0.2 U/kg/dose). Thus for a 65-kg adolescent taking 60 U/day, 6-9 U would be an appropriate supplemental dose range. Humalog insulin, because of its rapid action (within 15 minutes) and short duration (2–3 hours), is recommended in this situation.

V. Outcomes

A. Gradual rehydration
B. Restoration and maintenance of electrolyte and acid-base balance
C. Gradual restoration of normal and stable blood glucose
D. Prevention or early detection of complications such as cerebral edema, prerenal failure, hypoglycemia, and hypokalemia

VI Patient/Family Education and Follow-up

A. The endocrinologist on call should be contacted prior to admission to be involved in the care plan:
1. To decide where to admit the patient (PICU vs. medical floor)
2. To give input to therapy during the PICU stay at the request of the PICU attending
3. To arrange hospital care once PICU level care is no longer needed
4. To arrange appropriate education, nutritional assessment and plan, and psychosocial assessment and plan while the patient is on a medical floor
5. To arrange posthospitalization care

B. The goals of the overall hospitalization to be achieved before discharge are as follows:
1. Clear ketones from blood and urine and achieve adequate control of blood glucose to be safe at home.
2. Patient/family understand the basic pathophysiology of diabetes and ketoacidosis, its complications, and treatment.
3. Patient/family are able to demonstrate adequate skill at the following:
a. Testing blood glucose, urine ketones
b. Mixing and administering insulin
c. Recognizing and treating hypoglycemia

4. Understand and indicate willingness and ability to implement diet plan
5. Provide adequate psychosocial support to implement treatment plan
6. Have adequate supplies to implement treatment plan
7. Arrange adequate follow-up
8. Be sure patient/family are able to access the appropriate telephone follow-up with the endocrine division in the immediate posthospitalization period

---

ADH, antidiuretic hormone; DI, diabetes insipidus; ECG, electrocardiogram; ED, emergency department; GI, gastrointestinal; IV, intravenous; LOC, loss of consciousness; LR, lactated ringers; NS, normal saline; PICU, pediatric intensive care unit; T_4, thyroxine; TSH, thyroid-stimulating hormone.

DIABETES

	PHASE 1: ADMIT/INITIATE TREATMENT DATE: / / TIME: _____:_______	PHASE 2: STABILIZE/MONITOR DATE: / / TIME: ____:____	PHASE 3: DISCHARGE TEACHING and DISCHARGE CRITERIA DATE: / / TIME: ____:____
CRITERIA FOR ADMISSION/ DISCHARGE	CRITERIA FOR ADMISSION: • New onset diabetic • Known diabetic with DKA Type 1 diabetes Type 2 Diabetes NON DKA MOVE TO PHASE 2 PICU admission may be considered for any DKA patient with: • pH<7.2 • ≥10%-15% dehydration • Hemodynamic instability • Obtundation or other abnormal neurological finding • Young child (≤ 5yo) with DKA	Phase Two: Monitor and stabilize patient moving from IV insulin gtt to SQ insulin. Monitor patient as SQ insulin routine for home management is established.	CRITERIA FOR DISCHARGE: • Stable insulin regimen • PO intake adequate to balance insulin regimen • D/C supplies at bedside • D/C teaching complete • PCP identified and contacted ☐ Met within 72 hrs of resolution of acidosis
HYDRATION Maintain rate of hydration <50ml/kg/4hr Replace fluid deficit over 48 hrs	Initial bolus: NS 10 20ml/kg over 1 hr Maintenance IV Fluids: 0.45 NS-0.9 NS + 20 meq/L KCL + 20 meq/L KPO4 Change to D5.45 ns + 20 meq/L KCL + 20 meq/L KPO4 once BG is <250	IV heplocked Adequate po intake to meet maintenance needs	IV Dc'd
IV INSULIN THERAPY Goal is blood glucose decreasing no faster than 50-100 mg/dl/hr DKA should be treated with IV insulin unless very mild acidosis	Standard solution: 50 u insulin in 250ml NS Start insulin gtt at 0.1unit/kg/hr = 0.5cc/kg/hr When blood glucose < 250, add D5 to maintenance fluids If blood glucose continues to decline with D5 in maintenance fluid, consider change to D10 ☐ No IV insulin—move to Phase 2	Criteria for conversion to SQ insulin: • Acidosis is resolved and blood glucose is <250 mg/dl • D/C IV insulin AFTER the start of SQ Insulin Overlap regular insulin by 1 hour Overlap Humalog® insulin by 15 minutes Known diabetic: return to home regimen. Adjust insulin as needed for hypoglycemia, hyperglycemia or ketonuria Pt may need to have injections observed by nurses	Evaluate effectiveness of insulin regimen: Document on insulin and glucose flowsheet in MAR book

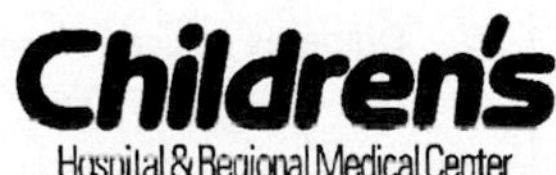

DIABETES: CLINICAL PATH
PAGE 1 OF 4

(addressograph)

PATIENT NAME:
MR#:
BIRTH DATE:

DIABETES CLINICAL PATH
52068 4/02

DIABETES

	PHASE 1: ADMIT/INITIATE TREATMENT DATE: / / TIME: _____:_______	PHASE 2: STABILIZE/MONITOR DATE: / / TIME: ____:____	PHASE 3: DISCHARGE TEACHING and DISCHARGE CRITERIA DATE: / / TIME: ____:____
IV INSULIN TO SQ INSULIN Rapid acting insulin [Humalog ®(lispro)]; onset 15 minutes, peak 1–2 hrs, duration 3–4 hrs. Fast acting insulin (regular): onset 15–30 minutes, peak 2–4 hrs, duration 6–8 hrs. Intermediate acting insulin (NPH): onset 2 hrs, peak 6–8 hrs, duration 10–12 hrs Long acting insulin (ultralente): onset 8 hrs, peak 12–18 hrs, duration 24–36 hrs. Long acting basal insulin [Lantus® (glargine)]: onset 1–2 hrs, no peak, duration 24 hrs. Will need fast-acting insulin at each meal.		☐ New diabetic regimen from IV to SQ insulin once acidosis is resolved Total daily dose 0.5–1.0 u/kg/d Regular 35% before breakfast 30% before lunch 25% before dinner 10% at 2300 OR NPH + Regular or Humalog® Split total daily dose between pre breakfast and pre dinner (2/3 and 1/3 respectively) NPH 2/3 of total daily dose Short acting is 1/3 of total daily dose D/C IV insulin after the start of SQ insulin following the recommended guidelines	Discharge Insulin Regimen: ______________________ ______________________ ______________________
ASSESSMENT/ EDUCATION	Vital signs q 2 hrs until on stable IV insulin regimen I&O Dipstick urine q 2 hrs until ketones negative x2 Daily weight Neuro checks Q 1–2 hrs until stable glucose level and normal neurological status Assess for signs & symptoms of hyper/hypoglycemia Fill out insulin glucose flowsheet (attached to clinical path) and keep in MAR	Routine viatal signs I&O Dipstick urine Q void until ketones negative x2 Daily weight Assess for signs & symptoms of hyper/hypoglycemia Psychosocial assessment ongoing with recommendations noted in teaching plan and plan of care ☐ Diabetes education initiated within 24 hrs of resolution of acidosis	Document ongoing education on education record at end of clinical path Weight at time of discharge __________kg ☐ Diabetes education completed

DIABETES: CLINICAL PATH
PAGE 2 OF 4

DIABETES CLINICAL PATH
52068 4/02

DIABETES

PHASE	INDICATORS	VARIANCE/REASON
1 Admit	☐ No IV insulin–move to Phase 2 ☐ Nutrition referral within 24 hrs of admission ☐ Child Life Specialist referral within 24 hrs of admit ☐ Social work/psychology referral within 24 hrs of admit	
2 Therapy	☐ IV insulin to SQ insulin once acidosis resolved ☐ Diabetes education initiated within 24 hrs of admit	
3 Discharge	☐ Meets discharge criteria within 72 hrs of acidosis resolved ☐ Diabetes ducation completed ☐ F/U appointment to endocrinology clinic made	

VARIANCE CODES AND REASONS

CODE	REASON	CODE	REASON
Patient and Family		**Clinician**	
110	Patient/Family decision	311	Clinician not available - PT/OT response delay
120	Patient not cooperative.	312	Clinician not available - Social work response delay
130	Family not available	313	Clinician not available - RT response delay
Patient condition		314	Clinician not available - Other
210	No response to standard treatment	320	Inadequate discharge planning
220	Post-Operative Infection	330	MD ordered, no reason documented
230	Post-Operative Hemorrhage	**Internal Systems**	
240	Post-Operative Pulmonary complication	341	Internal delay - Lab response delay
250	Other Post-Op complication	342	Internal delay - Pharmacy response delay
260	Medication intolerance	343	Internal delay - Consultation ordered, but did not occur
271	Complicated course - Pre-existing co-morbid medical condition	344	Internal delay - MD rounds too late to permit same day discharge
272	Complicated course - Other new onset medical complication	345	Internal delay - Other
273	Complicated course - Other	**External Systems**	
		410	External care provider delay

DATE	HRS	SIGNATURE	DATE	HRS	SIGNATURE	DATE	HRS	SIGNATURE

DIABETES: CLINICAL PATH

Page 4 of 4

DIABETES CLINICAL PATH

52068 4/02

DIABETES

	PHASE 1: ADMIT/INITIATE TREATMENT DATE: / / TIME:	PHASE 2: STABILIZE/MONITOR DATE: / / TIME:____:____	PHASE 3: DISCHARGE TEACHING and DISCHARGE CRITERIA DATE: / / TIME: ____:____
LABS	In ED or on admission pt must have the following checked: • Lytes, glucose, VBG, UA, HbgA1C, • C-peptide, TSH, T4 • VBG + Lytes q 2 hr while on insulin gtt • Blood glucose q 1-2 hrs while on insulin gtt Endocrine research team may obtain additional labs for studies as needed if consent completed on IRB approved protocol.	Daily lytes, glucose until stable Blood glucose tests before meals, HS and 0300 Children with new onset diabetes and their parents may use glucometer given to them by the team for home use. Requires training and MD order. Diabetics readmitted for DKA must use hospital-approved glucometer unless MD order on chart.	See education record
NUTRITIONAL MANAGEMENT	☐ Nutritional referral	Nutrition assessment to determine nutritional status, caloric needs, and establish a meal plan with recommended carbohydrate portions and snacks Family receives education in meal planning and carbohydrate counting	Nutrition portion of diabetes education completed
CONSULTS	☐ Child Life Specialist referral (3245) within 24 hrs of admission Date: / / Time: ☐ Social work/psychology referral (call intake office at 2760) within 24 hrs of admission Date: / / Time:	Family conference with endocrinologist or ARNP to discuss diabetes, insulin, blood glucose overview and to answer questions. Date: / / Time:	Primary MD called and aware of ongoing care planning needs Date: / / Time: ______________________ Discharge form and care plan faxed to office. Other consults or referrals: ☐ F/U appointment to Endocrinology Clinic made

(addressograph)

PATIENT NAME:
MR#:
BIRTH DATE:

DIABETES: CLINICAL PATH
Page 3 of 4

DIABETES CLINICAL PATH
52068 4/02

ACUTE CARE DIABETES PATHWAY
ADMITTING ORDERS

Date:______________ Time: ___________ Estimated LOS _______________

Medical Team _______ Sr. Resident____________________Intern _______________

Beeper _____________________ Beeper _______________

Attending MD: ____

Primary Diagnosis: ☐ DKA ☐ NEW ONSET DIABETES ☐ Type 1 ☐ Type 2

Secondary Diagnosis: ____

Weight ______kg Height/Length ______cm Allergies_____________________________

Diet: ____

Daily weight

Condition: ☐ Critical ☐ serious ☐ stable

Activity: ☐ ad lib ☐ may attend pool therapy when IV dc'd ☐ ☐ other ___________________

Isolation: ☐ none ☐ other __________________

Vital signs:☐q 2 hr with neuro checks until stable blood glucose, then q 4 hr ☐ q 4 hr

Strict I&O: ☐

Monitor:☐ none ☐ CR monitor until stable on q 4 hr vital signs

IV fluids: ☐ 0.45 NS + 20 meq/L KCL + 20 meq/L KPO4 @ _______________ cc/hr

☐ D5W + 20 meq/L KCL + 20 meq/L Kphos

☐ Other ____

☐ Keep D10 at bedside for pts on D5 maintenance fluid

Medications:

☐ Insulin drip (50u insulin in 250cc NS) Start at 0.1u/kg/hr=0.5cc/kg/hr _______________

☐ SQ insulin (circle) THESE ARE ONE-TIME ORDERS ONLY AND MUST BE REWRITTEN FOR EACH DOSE

Insulin	Lispro	Aspart	Regular	NPH	Lente	Ultralente	Other
Dose							
AM							
PM							

☐ Sliding scale insulin

Labs:

☐ In ED or on admission: lytes, glucose, VBG, UA, HbgA1c, TSH, T4, C-Peptid

☐ Lytes q ____ hrs while on insulin drip

☐ Chemstrip q 2 hrs while on insulin drip

☐ Chemstrip before meals, HS, and 0300 when on SQ insulin

☐ Urine ketone checks q 2 hr until negative x2

Call House Officer for:

☐ K <3.0 >5.5

☐ Glucose <200

Signature:_______________________________Beeper ________________ Date_____________

Printed Name: ________________________________

DIABETES PATHWAY Admitting Orders

(52068) 10/01 Page 1 of 1

ACUTE CARE DIABETIC KETOACIDOSIS

Patient/Family Education Record

Factors that impact teaching:
Communication/language ____________ Physical ____________ Cognitive ____________

Emotional ____________ Cultural ____________

Motivation ____________ Other ____________

No barriers____________

All primary caretakers will need to attend diabetic education. Who else do you think needs to know your child's careplan and/or attend diabetic education?
childcare provider ____________ School nurse ____________

Other____________

In what ways do you learn best? (circle 1 or more)

reading listening seeing pictures watching demonstrations doing

Learner needs and expected outcomes	
The patient and family will express understanding of or demonstrate the following: **Diabetes pathophysiology**	Learner: Parent, Child, Other Teaching methods: Verbal instruction, Written instruction, Demonstration, Audio Visual, Class, Other Level of understanding — Date Time ❑ Initial teaching, needs reinforcement ❑ Partial understanding/demonstrates with help ❑ Independent understanding/demonstrates skill
The patient and family will express understanding of or demonstrate the following: **Effects of insulin, diet, and exercise on blood sugar**	Learner: Parent, Child, Other Teaching methods: Verbal instruction, Written instruction, Demonstration, Audio Visual, Class, Other Level of understanding — Date Time ❑ Initial teaching, needs reinforcement ❑ Partial understanding/demonstrates with help ❑ Independent understanding/demonstrates skill
The patient and family will express understanding of or demonstrate the following: **Signs of ketoacidosis** **(includes demonstration of urine ketone testing)**	Learner: Parent, Child, Other Teaching methods: Verbal instruction, Written instruction, Demonstration, Audio Visual, Class, Other Level of understanding — Date Time ❑ Initial teaching, needs reinforcement ❑ Partial understanding/demonstrates with help ❑ Independent understanding/demonstrates skill

ACUTE CARE DIABETIC KETOACIDOSIS

The patient and family will express understanding of or demonstrate the following: **Demonstrate blood glucose meter and able to state goal for gycemic control**	<u>Learner</u> <u>Teaching methods</u> Parent Verbal instruction Audio Visual Child Written instruction Class Other Demonstration Other <u>Level of understanding</u> <u>Date Time</u> ❑ Initial teaching, needs reinforcement ❑ Partial understanding/demonstrates with help ❑ Independent understanding/demonstrates skill
The patient and family will express understanding of or demonstrate the following: **Insulin actions, insulin storage, insulin expiration, and needle disposal**	<u>Learner</u> <u>Teaching methods</u> Parent Verbal instruction Audio Visual Child Written instruction Class Other Demonstration Other <u>Level of understanding</u> <u>Date Time</u> ❑ Initial teaching, needs reinforcement ❑ Partial understanding/demonstrates with help ❑ Independent understanding/demonstrates skill
The patient and family will express understanding of or demonstrate the following: **Administration of insulin**	<u>Learner</u> <u>Teaching methods</u> Parent Verbal instruction Audio Visual Child Written instruction Class Other Demonstration Other <u>Level of understanding</u> <u>Date Time</u> ❑ Initial teaching, needs reinforcement ❑ Partial understanding/demonstrates with help ❑ Independent understanding/demonstrates skill
The patient and family will express understanding of or demonstrate the following: **Signs, symptoms, and treatment of hypoglycemia**	<u>Learner</u> <u>Teaching methods</u> Parent Verbal instruction Audio Visual Child Written instruction Class Other Demonstration Other <u>Level of understanding</u> <u>Date Time</u> ❑ Initial teaching, needs reinforcement ❑ Partial understanding/demonstrates with help ❑ Independent understanding/demonstrates skill
The patient and family will express understanding of or demonstrate the following: **Signs, symptoms, and treatment of hyperglycemia**	<u>Learner</u> <u>Teaching methods</u> Parent Verbal instruction Audio Visual Child Written instruction Class Other Demonstration Other <u>Level of understanding</u> <u>Date Time</u> ❑ Initial teaching, needs reinforcement ❑ Partial understanding/demonstrates with help ❑ Independent understanding/demonstrates skill
The patient and family will express understanding of or demonstrate the following: **Complications: signs, prevention, and treatment**	<u>Learner</u> <u>Teaching methods</u> Parent Verbal instruction Audio Visual Child Written instruction Class Other Demonstration Other <u>Level of understanding</u> <u>Date Time</u> ❑ Initial teaching, needs reinforcement ❑ Partial understanding/demonstrates with help ❑ Independent understanding/demonstrates skill

Patient/Family Education Record
Diabetic Pathway
00000 (6/01)
Page 2 of 5

ACUTE CARE DIABETIC KETOACIDOSIS

The patient and family will express understanding of or demonstrate the following: **Nutrition goals**	Learner Parent Child Other Level of understanding ❑ Initial teaching, needs reinforcement ❑ Partial understanding/demonstrates with help ❑ Independent understanding/demonstrates skill Teaching methods Verbal instruction Audio Visual Written instruction Class Demonstration Other Date Time
The patient and family will express understanding of or demonstrate the following: **Meal and snack planning**	Learner Parent Child Other Level of understanding ❑ Initial teaching, needs reinforcement ❑ Partial understanding/demonstrates with help ❑ Independent understanding/demonstrates skill Teaching methods Verbal instruction Audio Visual Written instruction Class Demonstration Other Date Time
The patient and family will express understanding of or demonstrate the following: **Grocery shopping**	Learner Parent Child Other Level of understanding ❑ Initial teaching, needs reinforcement ❑ Partial understanding/demonstrates with help ❑ Independent understanding/demonstrates skill Teaching methods Verbal instruction Audio Visual Written instruction Class Demonstration Other Date Time
The patient and family will express understanding of or demonstrate the following: **Coping strategies (family and child)**	Learner Parent Child Other Level of understanding ❑ Initial teaching, needs reinforcement ❑ Partial understanding/demonstrates with help ❑ Independent understanding/demonstrates skill Teaching methods Verbal instruction Audio Visual Written instruction Class Demonstration Other Date Time
The patient and family will express understanding of or demonstrate the following: **Parenting and developmental issues**	Learner Parent Child Other Level of understanding ❑ Initial teaching, needs reinforcement ❑ Partial understanding/demonstrates with help ❑ Independent understanding/demonstrates skill Teaching methods Verbal instruction Audio Visual Written instruction Class Demonstration Other Date Time

Patient/Family Education Record
Diabetic Pathway
00000 (6/01)
Page 3 of 5

ACUTE CARE DIABETIC KETOACIDOSIS

PATIENT AND FAMILY EDUCATION SUMMARY NOTES

DATE/TIME	NOTES	DATE/SIGNATURE

Patient/Family Education Record
Diabetic Pathway
00000 (6/01)
Page 4 of 5

ACUTE CARE DIABETIC KETOACIDOSIS

INSULIN DOSAGE AND BLOOD GLUCOSE TEST RESULTS
(please keep in MAR)

DATE	BREAKFAST		LUNCH		DINNER		BEDTIME		0300	
	Insulin	Glucose	Insulin	Glucose	Insulin	Glucose	Insulin	Glucose	Insulin	Glucose

Patient/Family Education Record
Diabetic Pathway
00000 (6/01)
Page 5 of 5

CHAPTER 72

Structure and Function of Hematopoietic Organs

Seth J. Corey and Julie Blatt

PEARLS

- Hematologic intervention is one of the most frequently used therapeutic modalities in the intensive care unit (ICU) setting.
- The variation in degree of hematopoiesis in a given bone with age is an important consideration when selecting a site for bone marrow aspiration or biopsy.
- The hematologic system is frequently affected by severe illnesses and often must be treated in the ICU setting.
- For major invasive procedures such as surgery or placement of arterial lines or endotracheal tubes, the platelet count should be maintained at a level of at least 50,000/μl.

With the extensive use of red blood cell (RBC) and platelet transfusions and the common occurrence of life-threatening infection in the presence of white blood cell (WBC) abnormalities, hematologic intervention is one of the most frequently used therapeutic modalities in the intensive care unit (ICU) setting. This chapter reviews the anatomy and physiology of the hematopoietic system to provide a basis for understanding the repercussions of primary hematologic abnormalities as well as its normal function in nonhematologic disease states. Aspects that are of practical importance to the intensivist are emphasized. The structure and function of the immune system (particularly B and T lymphocytes and macrophages) are discussed in Chapter 83.

Structure and Function of the Bone Marrow

During embryogenesis and fetal development, hematopoiesis shifts from the yolk sac to the liver and, at 28 weeks of gestation, to the bone marrow. Although hepatic erythropoiesis may persist for several weeks after birth, in the term infant hematopoiesis takes place almost entirely in the bone marrow. A defining feature of hematopoietic stem cells is their ability to home to the bone marrow. This homing occurs via chemoattractants such as stromal cell-derived factor-1 (SDF-1) and its cognate chemokine receptor on the stem cell, and via interaction between a variety of stem cell adhesion molecules and their ligands on stromal and endothelial cells. The hematopoietic stem cell may be identified by the presence of cell surface markers, such as CD34, or by the ability to exclude dyes, such as Hoechst 33342, via a drug transporter.

Grossly, two types of bone marrow can be recognized in normal individuals: yellow marrow, so called because of the predominance of fat cells, and red marrow, in which blood cells predominate. White marrow, consisting predominantly of stromal cells and intercellular matrix, may result from atrophy or starvation. As shown in Figure 72–1,[10] red marrow proportionately is a much greater component of body weight and volume in the infant than in the adult. Early in life, it is contained in the medullary cavities of the long bones, which gradually fill with fat such that, by late puberty, the adult distribution of hematopoiesis (sternum, pelvis, vertebrae, cranium, ribs, epiphyses of long bones) is achieved. The variation in the degree of hematopoiesis in a given bone with age is an important consideration when selecting a site for bone marrow

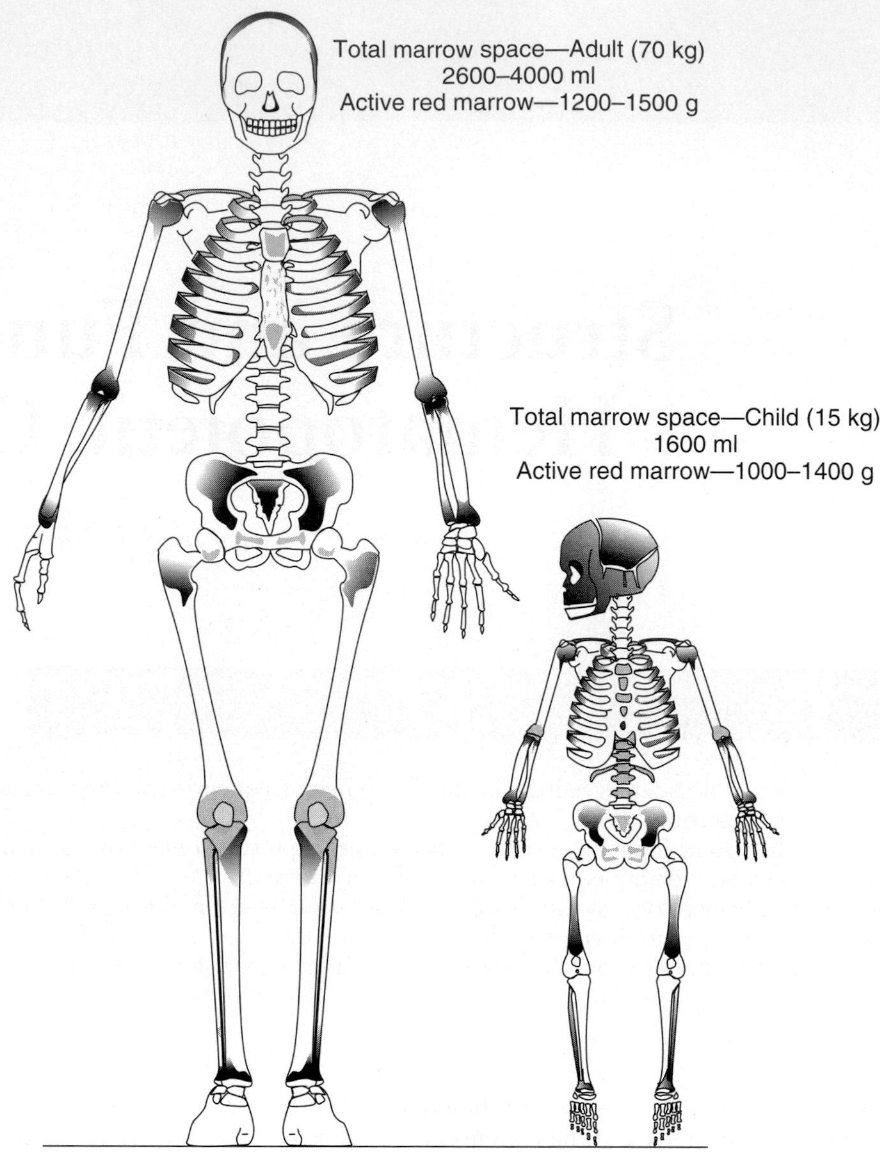

FIGURE 72–1 • Comparison of active red marrow-bearing areas in the child and the adult. Note the almost identical amount of active red marrow in the child and adult despite a fivefold discrepancy in body weight. (From MacFarlane RC, Robb-Smith AHT: *Functions of the blood.* Oxford, 1961, Blackwell.)

aspiration or biopsy. For example, although the anterior and posterior iliac crests can be used at any age, the tibia can be used only until age 2 years. In disease states characterized by excessive destruction of blood cells, such as some severe hemolytic anemias, hematopoiesis may increase twofold to eightfold. Active sites of hematopoiesis may expand, and extramedullary hematopoiesis may be found, particularly in the liver and spleen.

Microscopically, the marrow is a network of vascular channels (sinuses) separating islands of fat, hematopoietic cells, and rare osteoblasts and osteoclasts (which are important for bone remodeling.[16] The vasculature and cells are joined by a reticulin (fiber) network or scaffolding. By light microscopy, bone marrow aspirate specimens demonstrate hematopoietic elements; however, a bone marrow biopsy provides a more accurate measure of cellularity. Reticulin can be seen by light microscopy when special histochemical stains are used.

The blood vessels that feed the marrow are branches of vessels that feed the surrounding bone. Large central arteries run longitudinally within the marrow and send radial branches that penetrate the endosteum and form capillaries in the haversian and Volkmann canals of the bony cortex. These capillary systems drain into the bone marrow sinuses, which in turn drain into a central sinus or vein. Because the marrow circulation interconnects with the general circulation in this fashion, fluids and medication in bone marrow are absorbed as rapidly as through intravenous routes (see Chapter 18). Unlike peripheral veins, intramedullary vessels supported by their bony shell do not collapse in shock; therefore intraosseous infusion is appropriate when standard intravenous access is not available. It is noteworthy that the interconnection between the marrow and general circulation provides the mechanism by which bone marrow may embolize to the lung after osseous trauma or fracture. This has not been demonstrated to be of clinical significance in the case of intraosseous infusion.

The concept of the stem cell has expanded, and its ex vivo manipulation has raised much interest by a wide group of physicians and scientists studying nonhematologic systems. One essential feature of the stem cell is its plasticity.

Provocative studies have shown that stem cells isolated from the bone marrow can be driven to differentiate to muscle, liver, cardiac, or neuronal tissue. This raises the possibility that the marrow may be a convenient and ethically less challenging source of stem cells for stem cell engineering and tissue replacement. Although the clinical applications to nonhematologic tissues remain distant, use of hematopoietic stem cells to replace diseased marrow is a common practice. Alternative sources of hematopoietic stem cells have been found in peripheral blood following growth factor-induced mobilization or in umbilical cord blood.

Hematopoiesis

Cells within the hematopoietic island include the red blood cells, granulocytes (neutrophils, eosinophils, basophils), monocytes and macrophages, platelets, lymphocytes, and their precursors. The earliest precursors, or stem cells, are thought to look like small lymphocytes and usually are not distinguishable from them by microscopy. Their existence is best confirmed by in vitro culture assays in which nucleated cells from bone marrow aspirate specimens are plated onto tissue culture dishes layered with methylcellulose generate colonies (aggregates of cells) of one or more lineages. The first morphologically identifiable precursor cells are the proerythroblast, myeloblast, monoblast, megakaryoblast, and lymphoblast. These committed precursors and their terminally differentiated counterparts sit within the hematopoietic islands. Megakaryocytes (which make up <1% of hematopoietic cells) generally are located next to marrow sinusoids and shed platelets (fragments of megakaryocyte cytoplasm) directly into the lumen. Erythroblasts also are produced near the walls of the vascular sinuses in clusters with macrophages called *erythroblast islets*. As the erythroblasts develop, they extrude their nuclei, which are phagocytosed by the macrophages. In contrast, the granulocytes (most numerous of the hematopoietic cells), monocytes, and lymphocytes are produced throughout the marrow away from vascular sinuses. The mature WBCs are motile and migrate to the sinuses.

Within the peripheral circulation, the number of cells of each type is maintained in a narrow range in the normal individual. Adults and postpubertal adolescents have approximately 5000 granulocytes, 2000 lymphocytes, 500 monocytes, 5×10^6 RBCs, and 15,000 to 300,000 platelets per microliter of whole blood. Age-dependent values for younger children are listed in Table 72–1.[6] To a lesser extent, values also are a function of race and sex, so black males may have granulocyte counts less than 1500/μl. As summarized elsewhere, under normal conditions the rate of production of each cell type equals the rate of destruction. Because the lifespan of mature RBCs in adults is 100 to 120 days, 5×10^4 plateaus/μl are produced daily. The average platelet lifespan is 7 to 10 days so that approximately 2×10^4 plateaus/μl are produced daily. With less than a 12-hour lifespan, granulocytes production occurs at a rate of 10^4 cells/μl. The very slow rate of production of lymphocytes reflects their long lifespan.

The mechanisms that regulate this steady state are incompletely understood. However, evidence strongly suggests the existence of a pluripotent stem cell that is capable of self-renewal, from which progenitor cells committed to hematopoiesis (RBCs, granulocytes, megakaryocytes, and monocytes) and to lymphopoiesis develop (Fig. 72–2). The "trilineage myeloid" stem cell has been designated *colony-forming unit stem* (CFU-S) based on bone marrow culture assays and experiments in which the spleens of lethally irradiated mice infused with donor marrow cells are found to contain colonies each consisting of precursors of RBCs, granulocytes, monocytes, and megakaryocytes.[15] The existence of CFU-S in humans is further deduced from chromosomal studies in myeloproliferative disorders. In patients with chronic myeloid leukemia, the abnormal Philadelphia chromosome encoding Bcr-Abl is found in monocytes, megakaryocytes, and erythroid precursors (but not lymphoid precursors), in addition to granulocytes, which suggests that all these cells derive from the same clone. Lymphoid development appears to arise from a separate progenitor. Although CFU-S is found predominantly in the bone marrow, there probably are small numbers of circulating pluripotent stem cells because marrow of lethally irradiated animals can be reconstituted by using peripheral blood.[3]

The number of committed progenitor cells that differentiate in any time period is dependent on feedback from regulators that are produced within the marrow microenvironment and by extramedullary sources, including T cells, macrophages, endothelial cells, and fibroblasts. These hematopoietic growth factors (HGFs) are glycoproteins that are known by a variety of names. Crude supernatants (colony-stimulating activities) stimulate progenitor cells of different cell lineages to form discrete colonies of recognizable mature blood cells in bone marrow culture assays. Once the factor has been purified to homogeneity, its complementary deoxyribonucleic acid (DNA) cloned, and its in vitro properties better defined, it may be known as a *colony-stimulating factor* or interleukin (IL). Popular acceptance of an original descriptive property may become entrenched (e.g., leukemia inhibitory factor or stem cell factor), yet it may obscure its physiologic role. Generally, the HGFs fall under the rubric of cytokines. Many of the cytokines have overlapping functions. However, gene targeting in the mouse ("knockout mouse") of cytokines or their receptors has identified the essential nonredundant functions for several HGFs. Mice deficient in erythropoietin (EPO), thrombopoietin, and granulocyte colony-stimulating factor (G-CSF) suffer from severe anemia, thrombocytopenia, or neutropenia, respectively. Although the list of cytokines that regulate hematopoiesis continues to grow, clinical application remains limited to EPO, G-CSF, and IL-2. Screening of synthetic peptides has identified a novel erythroid-stimulating protein (darbepoetin alpha), and chemical modification of G-CSF (pegfilgastrim) has extended the half-life to permit administration once per chemotherapy cycle. Both are HGFs newly approved by the U.S. Food and Drug Administration. Their primary advantage is longer half-lives. Characteristics of specific HGFs, discussed in the following sections, are summarized in Table 72–2.

Erythropoiesis

On its way toward RBC maturation (see Fig. 72–2), the CFU-S sequentially differentiates into burst-forming

TABLE 72–1

Normal Values for Hematology

Age	Hemoglobin (g%)	Hematocrit (%)	Mean Corpuscular Volume (R)	Mean Corpuscular Hemoglobin Count (MCHC) (g/% RBC)	Reticulocytes (%)	WBC/μl × 100 range (avg)	% Neutrophils	Platelet (10^3/μl)
28-week gestation	14.5	45	120	31	5–10	—	—	275 ± 60
32-week gestation	15.0	47	118	32	3–10	—	—	290 ± 70
1 Day*	16.8–21.2	57–68	110–128	29.7–33.5	1.8–4.6	7–35 (18)	45–85	310 ± 68
1 Week*	15.0–19.6	46–62	107–129	30.4–33.6	0.1–0.9	4–20 (10)	30–50	
1 Month*	11.1–14.3	31–41	93–109	33.3–36.5	0.1–1.7	6–18 (10)	30–50	
3–5 Months	10.4–12.2	33	80–96	31.8–36.2	0.4–1.0	6–17 (10)	30–50	300 ± 50
6–11 Months	11.8	35	77	33	0.7–2.3	6–16 (10)	30–50	
1 Year	11.2	35	78	32	0.6–1.7	6–15 (10)	30–50	
2–10 Years	12.8	37	80	34	0.5–1.0	7–13 (9)	35–60	
11–15 Years	13.4	39	82	34	0.5–1.0	5–12 (8.5)	40–60	
Adult								300 ± 50
Male	16.0 ± 2.0	47 ± 7	91	34	0.8–2.5	4.3–10 (7)	25–62	
Female	14.0 ± 2.0	42 ± 5	(82–101)	(31.5–36)	0.8–4.1			

Absolute eosinophil count: average 250/μl (100–600/μl).
*Under 1 month of age, capillary hemoglobin exceeds venous: 1 hour—3.6 g difference
5 days—2.2 g difference
3 weeks—1.1 g difference
Data from Guest GM, Brown EW: *Am J Dis Child* 93:483, 1957; Matoth Y, et al; *Acta Paediatr Scandtr* 60:317, 1971; Wintrobe MN: *Clinical hematology*, ed 7, Philadelphia, 1974, Lea & Febiger; Mauer AM: *Pediatric hematology*, New York, 1961, McGraw-Hill; Oski FA, Naiman JL: *Hematologic problems in the newborn infant*, Philadelphia, 1972, WB Saunders; Nathan D, Oski F: *Hematology of infancy and childhood*, Philadelphia, 1981, WB Saunders.

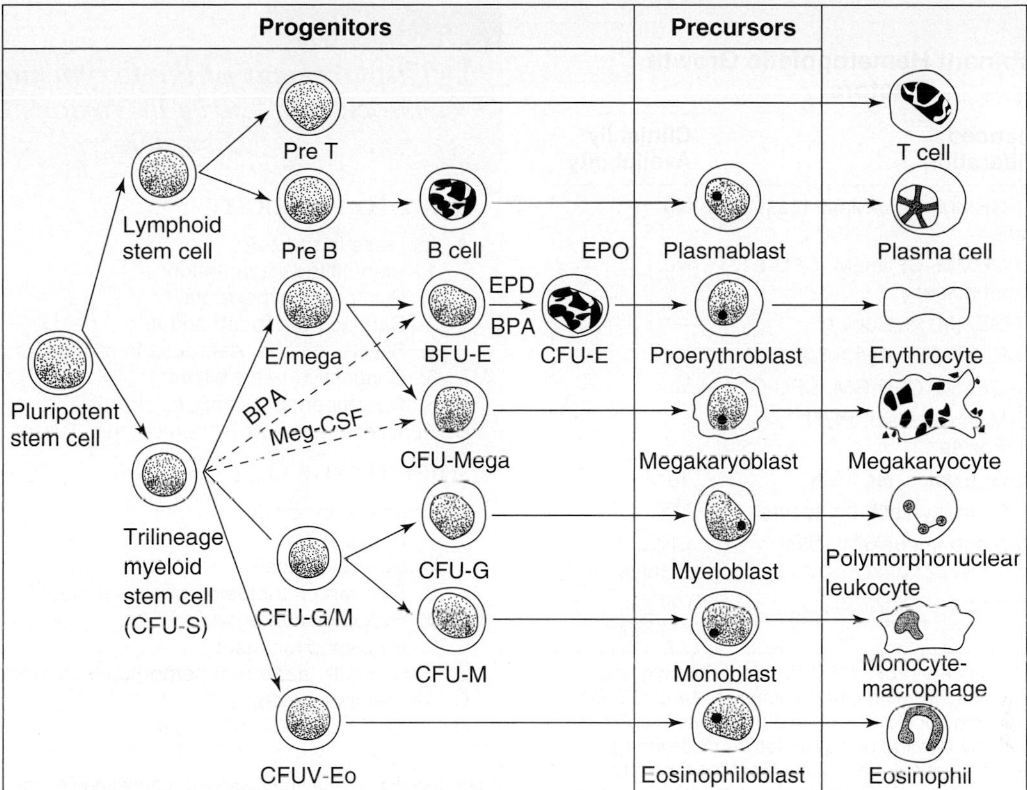

FIGURE 72–2 • Schematic outline of the progenitor basis of hematopoiesis. Not shown in this outline is the process of self-renewal of fractions of the progenitor cell populations, particularly the immature progenitors. Also not shown is the progressive amplification of progenitors and precursors as they mature and differentiate. The bipotential erythroid-megakaryocyte progenitor shown in this drawing has been demonstrated in the mouse but not definitively in man. *Dotted arrows* indicate an alternative scheme. (Modified from Nathan DG: Introduction: hematologic diseases. In Wyngaarden JB, Smith JH, editors: *Cecil's textbook of medicine,* Philadelphia, 1988, WB Saunders.[13])

unit-erythroid (BFU-E) and colony-forming unit erythroid (CFU-E), which are identifiable experimentally based on growth characteristics in culture. These phases of development, which involve amplification of cell number, are extensively reviewed elsewhere.[11,13] As noted earlier, the proerythroblast is the earliest morphologically identifiable precursor and presumably is the successor to the CFU-E. The subsequent sequence of RBC production normally takes 3 to 4 days in the marrow and involves multiple cell divisions with increasing differentiation, characterized chiefly by globin messenger ribonucleic acid (RNA), cytoplasmic synthesis of hemoglobin (Hb), and ultimately extrusion of the RBC nucleus. The enucleated cell is large and, because it contains residual RNA, stains deeply by the Wright-Giemsa technique (i.e., polychromatophilic macrocyte). Normally at this stage the erythrocyte is released into the circulation, where it can be demonstrated as a reticulocyte. In the newborn younger than 1 week, reticulocytes in the blood can compose more than 5% of the total RBCs. At any older age, the normal reticulocyte count is less than 2%. From this uncorrected reticulocyte count, the absolute reticulocyte count can be calculated by multiplying by the RBC count. The normal absolute reticulocyte count would be $0.02 \times 5 \times 10^6$ RBC/μl $= 10^5$/μl. This number can in turn be corrected for hematocrit by multiplying by the observed hematocrit divided by the normal hematocrit. Because the reticulocytes lose their RNA within 24 to 30 hours, their quantitation provides a rough estimate of the rate of erythropoiesis during the past 24 hours. This can be more accurately measured by ferrokinetic studies, which are not readily available. The proportion of erythroid precursors in a bone marrow aspirate also provides a more convenient estimate of total erythropoiesis that is valid if a cellular specimen is obtained and if granulopoiesis is normal. In the older child or adult, erythroid precursors normally are one third as plentiful as myeloid precursors (i.e., the myeloid/erythroid [M/E] ratio is approximately 3:1). Approximately 10% of erythroid precursors do not produce circulating RBCs (ineffective erythropoiesis).

Maturation of precursors is regulated by a number of nutritional factors. Erythropoietin appears to act predominantly by increasing proliferation of CFU-E (see Table 72–2 and Fig. 72–2). Its production is stimulated by hypoxemia or acute hemorrhage. During fetal development, it is mainly produced in the liver, but this site later shifts to the juxtamedullary region in the kidneys. Humoral factors less well characterized than EPO that are derived from multiple sources (spleen cells, peripheral blood monocytes, and mononuclear bone marrow cells) appear to act at an earlier stage of differentiation to amplify the number of progenitors committed to EPO responsiveness. Among these are burst-promoting activity (BPA), which enhances production and proliferation of BFU-E.

TABLE 72–2

Recombinant Hematopoietic Growth Factors

CSF	Enhanced proliferation	Clinically Availability
SCF	CFU-GEMM, CFU-Mast, mast cells	No
IL-3	CFU-GEMM, CFU-GM, CFU-E lymphoblast	No
Flt/flk	CFU-GEMM, myeloblast	—
EPO	CFU-E, BFU-E, erythroblast	Yes
GM-CSF	CFU-GEMM, CFU-GM, CFU-G CFU-M, myeloblast, PMN, monocyte	Yes
G-CSF	CFU-G, myeloblast, PMN	Yes
M-CSF	CFU-M, monoblast, monocyte	No
TPO	CFU-Mega, megakaryoblast	Clinical trials
IL-11	CFU-Mega	Clinical trials

BFU-E, Burst-forming unit erythroid; *CFU-E,* colony-forming unit erythroid; *CFU-G,* colony-forming unit granulocyte; *CFU-GEMM,* colony-forming unit granulocyte erythrocyte monocyte megakaryocyte; *CFU-GM,* colony-forming unit granulocyte macrophage; *CFU-Mast,* colony-forming unit mast cell; *CFU-Mega,* colony-forming unit megakaryocyte; *EPO,* erythropoietin; *Flt/flk,* fms-like tyrosine kinase/fetal liver kinase; *G-CSF,* granulocyte colony-stimulating factor; *IL,* interleukin; *M-CSF,* macrophage colony-stimulating factor; *PMN,* polymorphonuclear neutrophil; *SCF,* stem cell factor; *TPO,* thrombopoietin.

BOX 72–1

*Displacement of the Oxyhemoglobin Dissociation Curve in Various Clinical Disorders**

SHIFT TO THE RIGHT

A. Increase in red cell
   1. High-altitude adaptation
   2. Pulmonary hypoxemia
   3. Cardiac right-to-left shunt
   4. Severe anemia, decrease in red cell mass
   5. Congestive heart failure
   6. Decompensated hepatic cirrhosis
B. Functionally abnormal hemoglobin variants

SHIFT TO THE LEFT

A. Decrease in red cell
   1. Septic shock
   2. Severe acidosis
   3. Following transfusion of stored blood
   4. Hypophosphatemia
   5. Panhypopituitarism
B. Functionally abnormal hemoglobin variants
C. Methemoglobinemia
D. Carbon monoxide intoxication

From Bunn HF: Human hemoglobins: normal and abnormal. In Nathan DG, Oski FA, editors: Hematology of infancy and childhood. Philadelphia, 1987, WB Saunders.
*Corrected to pH 7.4.

Within the marrow, normal RBC maturation requires both folate and vitamin B_{12}. A deficiency of either results in abnormal nucleic acid synthesis and production of an abnormal precursor, the megaloblast. Iron is required for Hb synthesis, and deficiency results in poorly hemoglobinized, small (hypochromic, microcytic) RBCs.

Once in the peripheral blood, the lifespan of the normal RBC in the adult or older child is 100 to 120 days. In the term newborn the lifespan is approximately 60 days and grows progressively shorter with increasing prematurity.[13] Presumably these differences in age-dependent RBC longevity reflect differences in membrane stability and oxidative metabolism. Removal of RBCs from the circulation is not a random process. Senescent RBCs produced are removed selectively from the circulation by the macrophages of the reticuloendothelial system. Although this is primarily a function of the spleen (see later in this chapter), asplenic patients with normal RBCs accomplish this process in the liver and other sites and do not exhibit an increased RBC lifespan.

The primary function of circulating RBCs is to carry O_2 from the lungs to the tissues. Hemoglobin must be packaged within the RBC membrane to prolong its plasma half-life. Interference with the reversible binding of O_2 by Hb can occur by several mechanisms (Box 72–1),[11] including (1) methemoglobinemia, the inability to maintain ionic iron within the Hb molecule in the reduced state; (2) the presence of abnormal Hbs, among which are the methemoglobins that have an abnormal affinity for O_2; (3) age-or disease-related differences in the percentage of structurally normal HbF, which has a high affinity for oxygen; and (4) changes in the microenvironment that alter the intracellular concentration of 2,3-diphosphoglycerate (2,3-DPG). Oxyhemoglobin interaction also is complicated by the Bohr effect (↓pH →↓ O_2 affinity) independent of 2,3-DPG concentration. Thus as described by Bunn,[2] "patients with severe acidosis have low concentrations of 2,3-DPG, which results in an oxygen dissociation curve that shifts to the left. However, the in vivo curve may be normally placed because the Bohr effect counterbalances the reduction in red cell 2,3-DPG. If metabolic acidosis is rapidly corrected, the prompt rise in blood pH is reflected in a proportional increase in oxygen affinity (the Bohr effect). However, there is a lag of several hours before the red cell 2,3-DPG increases to normal. During this time, there is a shift to the left in *both* the in vivo and the in vitro oxygen dissociation curves. This phenomenon may compromise tissue oxygenation in patients who have diminished cardiovascular reserves."

Premature infants with respiratory failure may have a left-shifted O_2 affinity curve because of the high levels of HbF and because of an acidosis-induced decrease in 2,3-DPG levels. Exchange transfusions with adult blood have been found to reduce mortality, perhaps by providing blood with "normal" O_2 affinity. Other reasons for impaired O_2 delivery are decreased RBC mass (anemia, which leads to a compensatory increase in 2,3-DPG) and decreased blood flow, either because of vascular anatomic abnormalities or because of increased blood viscosity (e.g., in sickle cell disease). In addition to Hb-bound O_2, the oxygen dissolved in plasma (which normally amounts to < 2% of the total oxygen carried in the blood) increases linearly with increases in PO_2. For this reason, very anemic patients, although they have insufficient Hb with which to carry O_2, benefit from administration of O_2. Extensive research into the design of artificial blood has focused on both "red blood" (repackaged Hb from senescent or of Hb produced with genetic engineering) and "white blood" or perfluorocarbons (emulsions that dissolve large amounts of O_2). For now, red blood cell transfusions ameliorate anemia acutely, otherwise, EPO can be used to elevate Hb over several weeks.

Granulopoiesis

As shown in Figure 72–2, in addition to BFU-E, CFU-S gives rise to several other distinct cell populations. The best characterized of these are the colony-forming unit granulocyte-macrophage (CFU-GM, which in turn generates both colony-forming unit granulocyte [CFU-G] and colony-forming unit monocyte/macrophage [CFU-M]) and the colony-forming unit eosinophil (CFU-Eos). Like the CFU-E, these are not morphologically recognizable and probably masquerade in the bone marrow as small lymphocytes. They are identified on the basis of growth characteristics in in vitro bone marrow culture assays.

In contrast, subsequent stages of granulocytic (neutrophilic, eosinophilic, and basophilic) and monocytic differentiation can be visualized by routine histochemical stains of bone marrow aspirates. In the neutrophilic granulocyte (polymorphonuclear neutrophil [PMN]) series, the transition myeloblast to mature PMN involves an overall decrease in cell size; coarsening, indentation, and ultimately separation of nuclear chromatin, with loss of nucleoli; and replacement of azurophilic granules (whose contents include myeloperoxidase [MPO]), prominent in promyelocytes, by the specific granules (containing a number of secretory factors important for neutrophil function, but not MPO) in mature PMNs. Other structural changes during the course of PMN maturation include the disappearance of certain surface antigens, which can be identified by specific monoclonal antibodies and the appearance of receptor sites for complement (C3) and for the Fc portion of the immunoglobulin molecule. These stages in development are accompanied by functional changes, including increases in cell motility, responsiveness to chemoattractants, deformability, and phagocytic capabilities.

Parallel morphologic and functional changes occur with eosinophilic granulocyte differentiation. It is noteworthy that the peroxidase in eosinophil granules is different from that in neutrophils or monocytes so that congenital deficiencies of myeloperoxidase in the latter cells leave eosinophil function intact. The blood basophil (which histologically is similar to the tissue mast cell) also is presumed to arise in the bone marrow from the CFU-GM. In contrast to the CFU-Eos, there is no evidence for a separate basophil CFU. DNA labeling studies have demonstrated the kinetics of neutrophil development within the bone marrow. As shown in Figure 72–3,[17] there is a mitotic pool (myeloblast → myelocyte) that allows for amplification of cell number and a storage or reserve pool (metamyelocyte → segmented PMN) that in older children and adults contains roughly 100 times the number of granulocytes normally found in the peripheral blood. This reserve is mobilized and leads to mature neutrophilia at times of stress (e.g., sepsis, exercise, tachycardia, and pregnancy) or upon administration of pharmacologic doses of corticosteroids or exposure to endotoxin. In neonates, the storage pool is only two to three times the circulating pool of PMNs and can be depleted, for example, by overwhelming sepsis.[4]

Eosinophilic granulocytes also have mitotic and storage pools in the marrow that are approximately 300 times that seen in the periphery.[1] After less than 1 week, they are

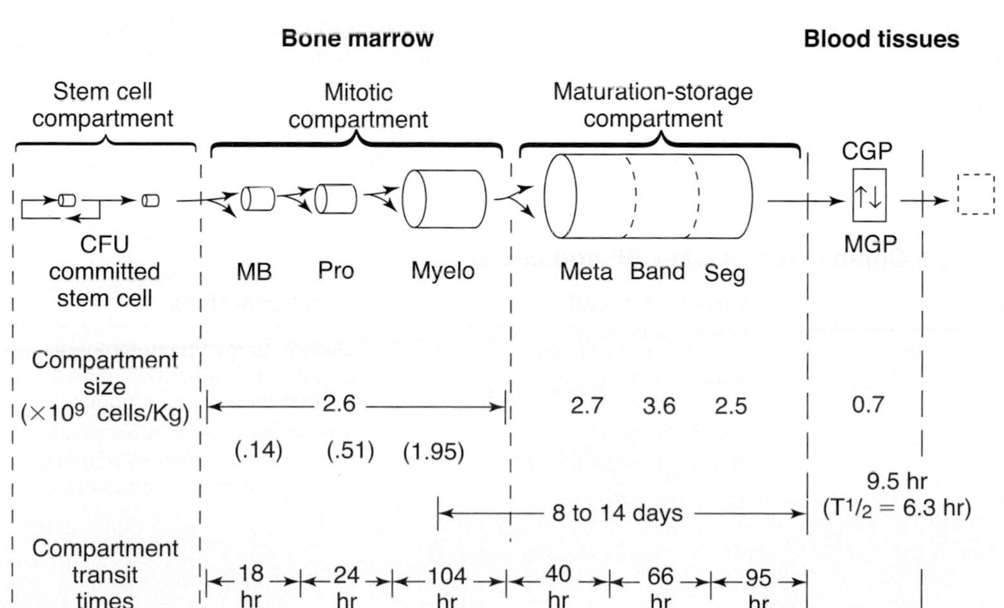

FIGURE 72–3 • Model of the production and kinetics of neutrophils in humans. The marrow and blood compartments have been drawn to show their relative sizes. The compartment transit times are shown on the *next to last line.* Values derived from tritiated thymidine studies are shown on the *last line.* (From Wintrobe MN, Lee RG, Boggs DR, et al: *Clinical hematology,* ed 8. Philadelphia, 1981, Lea & Febiger.)

released from the marrow in response to hypoxia and eosinophilic factors (e.g., heparin or histamine). In contrast to their effects on neutrophils, corticosteroids and epinephrine block mobilization of eosinophils from the marrow. The effect of epinephrine can be blocked by propranolol, suggesting mediation by β-adrenergic receptors. Little is known about basophil development in the bone marrow. Monocyte development, which, as previously suggested, is closely related to myelopoiesis, is poorly understood. However, there does not appear to be a storage pool.

The mature neutrophil escapes the marrow into the circulation by migration through reversible gaps between the endothelial cells lining the sinuses and capillaries. Factors known to influence this process include chemoattractants, such as products of the serum complement system. Those factors previously noted to mobilize the storage pool may cause egress of less mature granulocytes with a resultant "shift to the left" in the peripheral blood. Once in the periphery, approximately half of the polymorphs adhere to the blood vessels as the marginating pool while the other half actually circulate. Stress and epinephrine release the marginating cells and therefore double the absolute granulocyte count. Eosinophils have a similar arrangement of circulating and marginating cells, whereas the marginating pool of monocytes is three times that of the circulating pool.

The lifespan of the neutrophil once it is in the periphery is 6 to 12 hours and can be less in the presence of inflammation, fever, or infection. Neutrophils are irreversibly removed from the circulation into the liver, lungs, bowel, or bladder, back to the bone marrow, or to sites of infection where they contribute to the acute inflammatory response. Their extravascular half-life also is on the order of hours. Although the circulating half-life of eosinophils is comparable to that of neutrophils, eosinophils can persist in the tissues for many days. Under pathologic conditions, eosinophils may cycle back and forth between the tissues and circulation. Monocytes also have a circulating half-life measured in hours. Once in the tissues, however, they can persist for months or years and undergo the histologic (larger), biochemical (increased lysozymes and ectozymes), and functional (enhanced endocytosis) changes associated with tissue macrophages. The precise changes depend on the organ of residence; for example, in the liver they are identified as Kupffer cells and in the lung as alveolar macrophages.

The colony-stimulating factors that regulate myelopoiesis are diverse, and their biologic specificities may overlap.[5] Cytokines such as IL-1, tumor necrosis factor (TNF), granulocyte-macrophage colony-stimulating factor (GM-CSF), and G-CSF expand the PMF precursor compartment and mobilize them by promoting their diapedesis from the marrow and from vascular endothelium. Endotoxin promotes the host inflammatory response by stimulating endothelial cells, macrophages, and fibroblasts to produce cytokines.

Two cytokines have been approved for use in the treatment or prevention of myeloid suppression: GM-CSF (sargramostim) and G-CSF (filgrastim). A chemically modified version of G-CSF (pegfilgastrim) recently was approved for clinical use. With its longer half-life, it can be given once per course of chemotherapy. Both GM-CSF and G-CSF prime PMNs for enhanced phagocytosis and superoxide production in vitro, modulate cell surface expression of adhesion receptors, inhibit apoptosis, and promote antibody-dependent cellular cytotoxicity. However, GM-CSF inhibits chemotaxis, whereas G-CSF promotes it. G-CSF acts only on the granulocytic lineage. GM-CSF affects macrophages and eosinophils, which accounts for its side effects of eosinophilia and, at high doses, capillary leakiness. Because of stickiness and margination along vascular endothelium, a transient drop in O_2 saturation may occur minutes after administration. When given in recommended dosages, both drugs result in transient fever. Bone pain may occur with administration of either drug. WBCs must be monitored, and the drug is discontinued when the absolute neutrophil count exceeds 10,000/μl. When it is discontinued, the number of circulating PMNs decreases. Clinical uses of GM-CSF and G-CSF are listed in Table 72–3. Although nonhematopoietic tumor cell lines can display receptors for GM-CSF or G-CSF, administration of these drugs has not led to an increase in relapse or progressive disease in patients with solid tumors. Furthermore, these agents can be given to patients with myeloid leukemias or myelodysplastic syndromes without adverse effects. Multiple trials have demonstrated their efficacy in decreasing duration of profound neutropenia

TABLE 72–3

Comparison of GM-CSF and G-CSF

Factor	Source	Approved Indication	Additional Uses
G-CSF	*Escherichia coli*	Chemotherapy-induced suppression	Severe congenital neutropenia peripheral stem cell harvest, drug-induced neutropenia
GM-CSF	Yeast	Autologous bone marrow transplantation	Enhanced antigen presentation, peripheral stem cell harvest, drug-induced neutropenia
Starting dosage 5 μg/kg/day SQ or IV (G-CSF) 250 μg/m²/day SQ or IV			

or length of antibiotic coverage and hospitalization; their use has not changed the overall survival of patients receiving chemotherapy.

As in the case of RBC and platelet development, normal myelopoiesis requires the presence of vitamin and mineral growth factors. One hallmark of megaloblastic anemia (B_{12} and folate deficiencies) is the hypersegmented PMN. The hypochromic microcytic anemia of copper deficiency is characteristically associated with neutropenia.

Among the nonlymphoid WBCs, clinical sequelae of quantitative or qualitative deficiencies of neutrophils have been particularly well studied. Systemic or mucocutaneous bacterial infections (gram-positive and gram-negative organisms) are frequent. They occur with an incidence that increases with the degree and duration of neutropenia and in the presence of indwelling catheters, intravascular lines, and endotracheal tubes (see Chapter 85).

Recommendations for preventing infections in neutropenia include strict handwashing, changing sites of percutaneous lines as often as every 48 hours, and use of recombinant colony-stimulating factors in limited situations (as noted previously). Use of prophylactic antibiotics and reverse isolation (see Chapter 75) is controversial. Indications for granulocyte transfusions are discussed with regard to function both as a source of colony-stimulating factor for stimulation of granulocyte production and in an independent role in host defense against bacteria and fungi. However, the value of monocyte transfusions for treatment of fungal sepsis is unproved.

Megakaryocyte and Platelet Production

CFU-S gives rise to the committed megakaryocyte progenitor CFU-Mega (see Fig. 72–2), identifiable in in vitro clonogenic assays and by the presence of platelet glycoprotein surface antigens. Unlike RBC and granulocyte differentiation, in which cell division keeps up with mitosis, the next phase of development of megakaryocytes is characterized by endoreduplication, a process of mitosis without cell division that leads to increased DNA content up to a ploidy of 32N (where 2N is a diploid cell). With increasing ploidy comes increased cell volume, degree of nuclear lobulation, and granules containing factors that influence platelet function. A system of "demarcation membranes" identified by electron microscopy separates the megakaryocyte cytoplasm into several thousand anucleate platelets, which are shed into the lumens of the marrow sinusoids. The entire process takes approximately 5 days. Although megakaryocytes can be visualized on bone marrow aspirates and biopsy specimens, their quantitation by these techniques is approximate and correlates only loosely with platelet production. Factors controlling platelet shedding have not been studied extensively. With exceptions, however, large platelets or megathrombocytes (increased mean platelet volume) are seen in thrombocytopenia caused by increased platelet destruction. Normal platelet volume occurs more frequently in thrombocytopenia resulting from decreased platelet production.

Some platelets go directly from the marrow to the blood, where they remain; others go temporarily to the spleen, which possibly contributes to their further maturation. Normally one third of the total body platelet mass is sequestered there, although the number can go as high as 90% in pathologic states. Once in the peripheral blood, platelets have a lifespan of approximately 10 days. Chromium studies, useful for assessing platelet lifespan, have severe limitations in estimating the extent of organ-specific uptake of platelets and response to splenectomy.

Several HGFs influence megakaryopoiesis, but identification of the major megakaryocyte growth factor remained elusive until the purification and complementary DNA cloning of thromboprotein.[8,9] Whereas IL-3, GM-CSF, EPO, IL-11, and IL-6 stimulate CFU-Mega growth in vitro, none of these factors has proved to be highly effective in increasing platelet counts in clinical trials. Thrombopoietin potently stimulates the expression of CFU-Mega, resulting in increased platelet mass. Because mice that lack the gene for the thrombopoietin receptor but still produce some platelets have been created, other cytokines must contribute to platelet production. These factors, such as IL-3 and IL-11, most likely synergize with thrombopoietin, so clinical trials with combination cytokines may be effective. Whether EPO itself has thrombopoietic activity is controversial. Although iron deficiency anemia is often associated with thrombocytosis, increases in EPO may not be the immediate mechanism, and not all disease states associated with elevated EPO levels are characterized by increased platelet number. As with the other cell lines, megakaryopoiesis is also dependent on vitamins. Severe megaloblastic anemia may be associated with thrombopenia and bizarre platelet and megakaryocyte morphology.

Spontaneous bleeding is unlikely unless there are fewer than 20,000 normally functioning platelets/μl. However, for major invasive procedures such as surgery or placement of arterial lines or endotracheal tubes, the platelet count should be maintained at a level of at least 50,000/μl or even more than 100,000/μl. Other indications for platelet transfusions are discussed in Chapter 75. In the rare patient with idiopathic thrombocytopenic purpura and intracranial hemorrhage, optimum control of bleeding requires cooperation between neurosurgery, general surgery, hematology, and intensive care clinicians and some combination of splenectomy, dose intravenous immunoglobulin, steroid therapy, and platelet transfusions.

Structure and Function of the Secondary Lymphoreticular System

The bone marrow and thymus (see Chapter 82) are the primary lymphoid organs, the site of lymphocyte production. The secondary lymphoid organs, to which the B and T cells migrate, include the spleen, lymph nodes, and gut-associated lymphoid tissue (tonsils, appendix, and Peyer patches of the small intestine).

Spleen

The spleen is enclosed in a thick, fibromuscular capsule. Numerous trabeculae spring from the capsule to divide the interior pulp into lobules, within which is a scaffolding of reticular cells and fibers. Unlike the thymus, the spleen has a hilum through which the splenic artery and its branches enter and then branch further to course along the trabeculae. Collaterals from the gastric artery enter through the splenic capsule so that splenic artery ligation does not result in infarction. The branches of the splenic artery pass into the parenchyma to form central arteries that are surrounded for much of their length by a dense sheath of T lymphocytes and macrophages. Lymphoid follicles, some with germinal centers containing B cells from the bone narrow (as noted previously), are present in the periarterial lymphatic sheath. Together the B-cell– and T-cell–dependent areas compose the white pulp of the spleen. The rest of the splenic parenchyma is the red pulp. It contains radial branches of the central arteries that carry hemoconcentrated blood (plasma is skimmed off and runs in other arterial branches); well-defined endothelial lined venous sinuses that ultimately drain into the splenic vein; and an anatomically separate reticulin network, the splenic vein, which functions as endothelial lined blood vessels. Most of the circulation runs from the arterial system into the cords and then into the venous system, probably by squeezing through gaps in the endothelium. After the neonatal period, a marginal zone of the red pulp that abuts the white pulp becomes more prominent. It contains antigen-processing macrophages that are needed for B-cell function. It is believed to be the initial site of interactions between antigen and lymphocytes. Small numbers of efferent lymphatic vessels lie at the proximal end of the central arteries and leave the spleen through the trabeculae.

Normally the spleen is found in the left-upper quadrant of the abdomen. Its weight increases linearly with body weight until puberty, after which it shrinks somewhat. A spleen tip is palpable in 10% of normal children. Based on data from splenectomy cases, small accessory spleens occur in almost 20% of individuals. Generally they are located near the hilum of the main spleen, with which they share their vascular supply.

The spleen has many functions. The red pulp filters damaged (abnormal and old) RBCs from the systemic circulation by several mechanisms. (1) The cells are distorted and disrupted as they pass through the small lumens of the arterial capillaries or between the endothelial cells of the sinuses. In particular, cells with HbS undergo increased sickling, and cells with abnormalities of glycolytic metabolism or senescent cells become increasingly fragile in the face of decreased O_2 tension with lactic acidosis and decreased adenosine triphosphate production. (2) Cells are entrapped in the viscous blood within the fine mesh. (3) Cells undergo antibody (especially immunoglobulin G)-meditated hemolysis or phagocytosis, as seen in some autoimmune hemolytic anemias. Damaged cells or their debris produced by any of these mechanisms are removed by macrophages of the red pulp or may escape back into the circulation. Rigid inclusions such as Howell-Jolly (HJ) bodies may be pitted without destroying the parent RBC on passage through the sinus endothelium. Therefore the presence of even small numbers of HJ bodies is a subtle indicator of impaired splenic function, except in the term and especially in the premature neonate, in whom they also are seen and thought to be a normal developmental stage.

As mentioned earlier, the spleen is a temporary reservoir for platelets and to a small extent for WBCs. Thus after splenectomy there is a usually transient thrombocytosis that resolves within 3 to 6 months. In children it does not appear to carry a predisposition to thrombosis even with platelet counts as high as 10^9/μl.

In the presence of antiplatelet or antibody WBC (some synthesized by the spleen) and in hypersplenism without antibody, the spleen may function as a filter and result in thrombopenia and neutropenia, which may be reversible by splenectomy, steroids, or intravenous immunoglobulin (see section on platelet production).

The spleen, predominantly the white pulp and marginal zone, plays a number of roles in host defense, elegantly and elaborately discussed elsewhere.[7,14] In short, splenectomy has been associated with an increased incidence of serious infections with encapsulated bacteria, parasites, and possibly leukemia in patients who have splenectomy as part of the management of Hodgkin disease. Most clinicians recommend using *Haemophilus Influenzae* type b, meningococcal, and pneumococcal vaccines 1 to 2 weeks before splenectomy, with at least one booster against pneumococcal disease every 5 years and prophylactic antibiotics at least through adolescence. Although it is not a site of hematopoiesis beyond fetal life under normal conditions, in certain disease states the spleen can reactivate its hematopoietic potential. These states include some congenital hemolytic anemias and acquired diseases, such as myeloid metaplasia. All are associated with splenomegaly and usually with hepatomegaly, signifying a more general expansion of hematopoiesis. The liver can fulfill some of these functions so that in functionally or literally asplenic patients, RBC lifespan, for example, is not increased. However, the liver is less effective at other functions, including pitting and host defense.

Lymph Nodes

Like most of the rest of the lymphoreticular system, lymph nodes or thymus are surrounded by capsules and have architecturally distinct cortices and medullary zones, functionally distinct B-cell– and T-cell–dependent areas, and macrophages, all compartmentalized by a reticular meshwork. Many of the small lymphocytes, especially the T cells, continually are recycled through the systemic circulation by the thoracic duct. They function primarily as a site of interaction between the system and invading antigens. Mediastinal lymph node enlargement as a result of invasion by lymphoid or nonlymphoid tumors or from endogenous antigenic stimulation may compromise the airway and present anesthetic risks.

REFERENCES

1. Baehner RL: Disorders of granulopoiesis. In Miller DR, Baehner RL, editors: *Blood diseases of infancy and childhood*, ed 6, St. Louis, 1990, Mosby.
2. Bunn HF: Human hemoglobins: normal and abnormal. In Nathan DG, Oski FA, editors: *Hematology of infancy and childhood*, Philadelphia, 1987, WB Saunders.
3. Calvo W, Fliedner TM, Herbst E, et al: Regeneration of blood-forming organs after autologous leukocyte transfusion in lethally irradiated dogs. II. Distribution and cellularity of bone marrow in irradiated and transfused animals, *Blood* 47:593, 1976.
4. Christensen RD, Rothstein G: Exhaustion of mature marrow neutrophils in neonates with sepsis, *J Pediatr* 96:316, 1980.
5. Clark SC, Kamen R: The human hematopoietic colony-stimulating factors, *Science* 236:1229, 1987.

6. Cole CH, editor: *Harriet Lane handbook*, ed 10, Chicago, 1989, Year Book.
7. Ladish S, Miller DR: The spleen and disorders involving the monocyte-macrophage system. In Miller DR, Baehner RL, eds: *Blood diseases of infancy and childhood*, ed 6, St. Louis, 1990, Mosby.
8. DeSauvage FJ, Haas PE, Spender SD, et al: Stimulation of megakaryocytopoiesis and thrombopoiesis by the c-Mpl ligand. *Nature* 369:533, 1994.
9. Bartley TD, Bogenberger J, Hunt P, et al: Identification and cloning of a megakaryocyte growth and development factor that is a ligand for the cytokine receptor Mpl, *Cell* 77:1117, 1994.
10. MacFarlane RC, Robb-Smith AHT, editors: *Functions of the blood,* Oxford, England, 1961, Blackwell.
11. Miller DR: Erythropoiesis, hypoplastic anemias and disorders of heme synthesis. In Miller DR, Baechner RL, editors: *Blood diseases of infancy and childhood,* ed 6, St Louis, 1990, Mosby.
12. Nathan DG: Introduction: hematologic diseases. In Wyngaarden JB, Smith JH, editors: *Cecil's textbook of medicine*. Philadelphia, 1988, WB Saunders.
13. Oski FA, Naiman JL: *Hematologic problems in the newborn.* Philadelphia, 1966, WB Saunders.
14. Pearson HA: The spleen and disturbances of splenic function. In Nathan DG, Oski FA, editors: *Hematology of infancy and childhood.* Philadelphia, 1987, WB Saunders.
15. Till JE, McCulloch EA: A direct measurement of the radiation sensitivity of normal mouse bone marrow cells, *Radiat Res* 14:213, 1961.
16. Weiss L: The hematopoietic microenvironment of the bone marrow: an ultrastructural study of the stroma in rats, *Anat Rec* 186:161, 1976.
17. Wintrobe MN, Lee RG, Boggs DR, et al, editors: *Clinical hematology,* ed 8. Philadelphia, 1981, Lea & Febiger.

CHAPTER

73

Thromboembolism in Pediatric Critical Care Patients

Mary Jane F. Petruzzi

Although venous thromboembolism (VTE) is less common in children than in adults, there is increasing recognition of thrombosis in systemic and cerebral vessels, especially in pediatric tertiary care centers. VTEs are increasingly common in children as a result of therapeutic advances used to improve survival of patients at risk for complications. The development of microassays in the early 1980s enabled researchers to delineate age-dependent features of coagulant and anticoagulant levels.[1–3] Table 73–1 lists the published ranges for coagulation factor levels.

The hemostatic system of the young is evolving but functional. The coagulation system is highlighted as a cell-based model in the context of some key developmental aspects. Ultimately the interplay between coagulation and anticoagulation, moderated by endothelium—the "master regulator"—creates a hemostatic balance.

Endothelial cells are competent from infancy throughout childhood. They express procoagulant factors, such as tissue factor (TF), thrombin receptors, von Willebrand factor, and plasminogen activator inhibitor-1 (PAI-1), and anticoagulant factors, such as thrombomodulin (TM), tissue-type plasminogen activator (tPA), tissue factor pathway inhibitor (TFPI), and heparin sulfate.[4,5]

Cell-Based Model of Coagulation

The TF pathway drives initial thrombin generation and fibrin deposition. Initiation of hemostasis centrally involves exposure of a tissue-factor-bearing cell to blood flow. The resulting TF–factor VIIa (FVIIa) complex generates small amounts of thrombin complexed with factor X and its cofactor (factor Va). The generated thrombin serves as a potent activator of platelets and factor VIII, which primes for the amplification phase of coagulation. During amplification, circulating platelets bind to the injury site and become highly activated. These platelets have surface-bound activated factors V and VIII that are set up for massive thrombin generation. A "burst" of thrombin is generated on the activated platelets during the propagation phase of coagulation. Thrombin is the key serine protease in the regulation of coagulation. It augments its own generation, cleaves fibrinopeptides A and B from fibrinogen to form fibrin, and activates factor XIII to stabilize fibrin.[6] For a diagrammatic representation of the coagulation cell-based model see Figure 73–1.

Natural Anticoagulant System

The anticoagulation system prevents unwanted extension of thrombus beyond the site of vascular injury. Several important control mechanisms are in effect, including the TM/activated protein C/protein S system that inactivates factor Va and factor VIIIa.

Antithrombin (AT) inhibits thrombin, factor Xa, and factor IXa. AT inhibitory actions are greatly potentiated at high doses by endogenous glycosaminoglycans, exogenous heparin, and low-molecular-weight heparin (LMWH) derivatives. α_2-Macroglobulin is a direct thrombin inhibitor, and heparin cofactor II inhibits both surface-bound thrombin and unbound thrombin. TFPI exerts its inhibitory coagulation effect by binding and inactivating factor Xa and the TF–FVIIa complex.[7]

Fibrinolysis

Once the fibrin clot is stabilized, plasmin is the most important lytic agent. Plasmin is generated when plasminogen is activated by tPA and urokinase plasminogen activator (uPA). Fibrinolytic inhibitors include PAI-1, α_2-antiplasmin, and thrombin activatable fibrinolysis inhibitor (TAFI). The net effect of age-dependent decreased concentrations of vitamin K-dependent procoagulants, short-lived decreases in the inhibitors protein C, protein S,

TABLE 73–1

Coagulation Screening Tests and Coagulation Factor Levels in Fetuses, Full-Term Newborns, and Adults

	Fetuses (weeks gestation)				
Parameter	19–23 (n = 20)	24–29 (n = 22)	30–38 (n = 22)	Newborns (n = 60)	Adults (n = 40)
PT (s)	32.5 (19–45)	32.2 (19–44)†	22.6 (16–30)†	16.7 (12.0–23.5)*	13.5 (11.4–14.0)
PT (INR)	6.4 (1.7–11.1)	6.2 (2.1–10.6)†	3.0 (1.5–5.0)*	1.7 (0.9–2.7)*	1.1 (0.8–1.2)
aPTT (s)	168.8 (83–250)	154.0 (87–210)†	104.8 (76–128)†	44.3 (35–52)*	33.0 (25–39)
TCT (s)	34.2 (24–44)*	26.2 (24–28)	21.4 (17.0–23.3)	20.4 (15.2–25.0)†	14.0 (12–16)
Factor					
I (g/L, Von Clauss)	0.85 (0.57–1.50)	1.12 (0.65–1.65)	1.35 (1.25–1.65)	1.68 (0.95–2.45)†	3.0 (1.78–4.50)
I Ag (g/L)	1.08 (0.75–1.50)	1.93 (1.56–2.40)	1.94 (1.30–2.40)	2.65 (1.68–3.60)†	3.5 (2.50–5.20)
IIc (%)	16.9 (10–24)	19.9 (11–30)*	27.9 (15–50)†	43.5 (27–64)†	98.7 (70–125)
VIIc (%)	27.4 (17–37)	33.8 (18–48)*	45.9 (31–62)	52.5 (28–78)†	101.3 (68–130)
IXc (%)	10.1 (6–14)	9.9 (5–15)	12.3 (5–24)†	31.8 (15–50)†	104.8 (70–142)
Xc (%)	20.5 (14–29)	24.9 (16–35)	28.0 (16–36)†	39.6 (21–65)†	99.2 (75–125)
Vc (%)	32.1 (21–44)	36.8 (25–50)	48.9 (23–70)†	89.9 (50–140)	99.8 (65–140)
VIIIc (%)	34.5 (18–50)	35.5 (20–52)	50.1 (27–78)†	94.3 (38–150)	101.8 (55–170)
XIc (%)	13.2 (8–19)	12.1 (6–22)	14.8 (6–26)†	37.2 (13–62)†	100.2 (70–135)
XIIc (%)	14.9 (6–25)	22.7 (6–40)	25.8 (11–50)†	69.8 (25–105)†	101.4 (65–144)
PK (%)	12.8 (8–19)	15.4 (8–26)	18.1 (8–28)†	35.4 (21–53)†	99.8 (65–135)
HMWK (%)	15.4 (10–22)	19.3 (10–26)	23.6 (12–34)†	38.9 (28–53)†	98.8 (68–135)

From Reverdiau-Moalic P, Delahousse B, Body G, et al: *Blood* 88:900-906, 1996.
Values are given mean (lower and upper boundaries including 95% of the population). Ag, Antigenic value; c, coagulant activity.
*$P < .05$
†$P < .01$

and AT, and the persistent increase in the thrombin inhibitor α_2-macroglobulin is reduced thrombin generation capacity to 80% of adult values throughout childhood into adolescence. The age-dependent concentrations of fibrinolytic proteins (i.e., decreased plasminogen and increased PAI-1) cause diminished fibrinolytic capacity throughout childhood into adolescence.[8,9] Figures 73–2 and 73–3 show schematic representations of the anticoagulant and fibrinolytic systems, respectively.

Venous Thromboembolic Disease in Childhood

Incidence

In prospective Canadian and Dutch registries, the annual incidence of venous thrombotic events was estimated to be 0.07 to 0.14 per 10,000 children, or 5.3 per 10,000 pediatric hospital admissions and 24 per 10,000 admissions of neonates to neonatal intensive care units (ICUs). A neonatal survey in Germany estimated the incidence of symptomatic neonatal venous and arterial thromboembolism (TE) was 0.51 per 10,000 births.[10–12] A decreased index of clinical suspicion for pulmonary emboli (PE) in children and the absence of standardized diagnostic techniques lead to a very low estimate of the incidence of PE. A number of retrospective pediatric autopsy studies have estimated the overall incidence of PE in children to vary significantly from 0.5% to 4.2%, depending on whether microscopic studies were included.[13,14] Children aged 1 month to 10 years account for 50% of all cases of pediatric thrombosis, most occurring in the first year of life. No single year between ages 3 and 10 years accounts for more than 5% of pediatric thrombosis. After neonates, children aged 11 to 18 years represent the next largest cohort of children with venous thrombosis. The increase in the adolescent years reflects a coagulation profile in transition to the adult state, with a gradual increase in the ability to generate thrombin and continued decreased fibrinolytic capacity.[15]

Acquired Risk Factors in Pediatric Venous Thromboembolism

Thrombosis in pediatric patients usually represents a combination of underlying genetic predisposition and acquired precipitating events. Table 73–2 summarizes clinical risk factors for pediatric TE. Idiopathic VTE is less common in children than in adults. The majority of pediatric patients have a serious underlying illness that is transient or ongoing. The most common acquired risk factor for pediatric VTE, usually superimposed upon an underlying illness, is the presence of a central venous line (CVL). The high frequency of thrombosis in the upper venous system in pediatric patients reflects the typical location for CVL placement. Underlying illnesses most commonly associated with high risk of complicating VTE in children include surgery, trauma, and infection

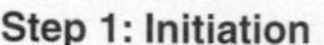

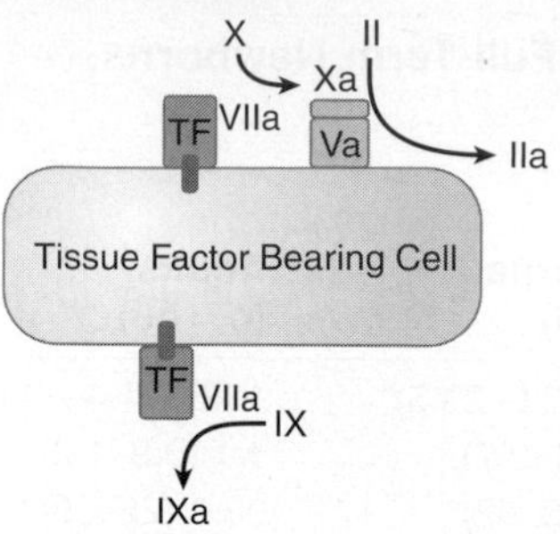

Step 2: Amplification

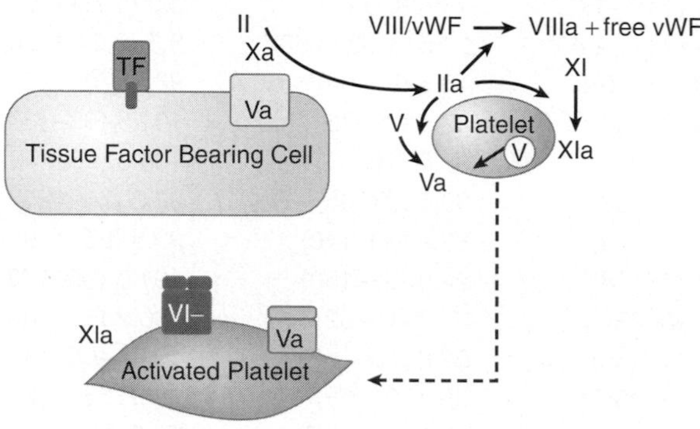

Step 3: Propagation

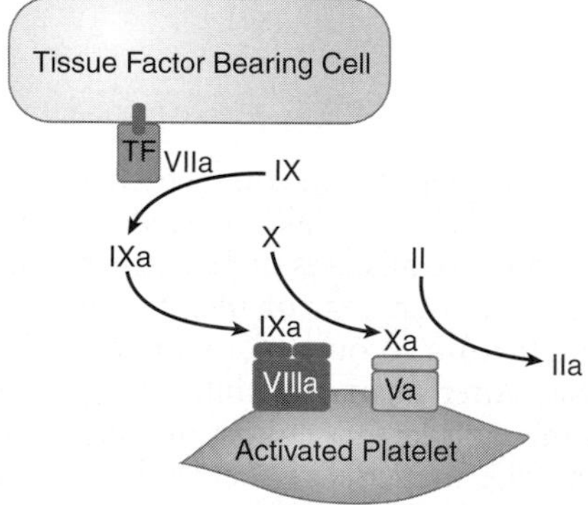

FIGURE 73–1 • Cell-based model of hemostasis. Three overlapping stages of coagulation occurring on two cell surfaces: tissue-factor-bearing cells and platelets. Step 1 *(initiation)* occurs on a tissue-factor-bearing cell. In step 2 *(amplification)*, platelets and cofactors are activated to set the stage for large-scale thrombin generation. In step 3 *(propagation)*, large amounts of thrombin are generated on the platelet surface. (Modified from Veldman A, Hoffman M, Ehrenforth S: *Curr Med Chem* 10:797-811, 2003.)

(especially in the context of disseminated intravascular coagulation [DIC]).[16–18]

A historical review of large studies of children with acute lymphoblastic leukemia who received the common induction drug L-asparaginase demonstrated the median incidence of TE in this patient subgroup was 2.5% (range 1.1% to 14.3%).[19] Although likely multifactorial, the AT deficiency caused by L-asparaginase is a key associated risk factor. A severe acquired protein S deficiency secondary to autoantibody development occurs in a group of children after varicella infection and results in TE or purpura fulminans. Renal disease, especially active nephrotic syndrome, leads to increased thromboembolic events that correlate with the degree of hypoalbuminemia, especially AT deficiency.[20–23]

Acquired risk factors, such as the occurrence of antiphospholipid antibodies (APLAs) and autoimmune disorders, use of estrogen-containing oral contraceptives, and smoking, increase in the adolescent age group. Adolescent sports-related injuries (muscle and joints) and overuse syndromes involving repetitive motion serve as thromboembolic triggers, often accompanied by an anatomic and/or prothrombotic predisposition. APLAs are classified either as lupus anticoagulants, which prolong phospholipid-dependent clotting assays such as the activated partial thromboplastin time (aPTT), or as anticardiolipin antibodies, which are detected by enzyme-linked immunosorbent assay. One hypothesis of the mechanism by which the APLAs predispose to thrombosis is their formation directed against phospholipid components of the endothelial membrane following endothelial injury.[24,25]

Congenital heart disease probably is one of the most common settings for the development of thromboembolic events in pediatric patients. Almost 50% of infants younger than 6 months and 30% of older children who present with thromboembolic stroke have underlying cardiac defects.[26]

Congenital Risk Factors in Pediatric Venous Thromboembolism

The role of congenital risk factors in the etiology of pediatric VTE is under investigation. Inherited prothrombotic disorders usually are suspected in children with an unexplained cause for thrombosis, a positive family history, a history of recurrent TE, or thrombosis in unusual locations. Spontaneous thrombosis secondary to an inherited prothrombotic disorder may present initially during infancy or childhood and therefore must be considered in otherwise healthy infants and children.

Inherited prothrombotic risk factors that play a role in pediatric VTEs include deficiencies of the anticoagulant proteins AT, protein C, and protein S. Factor V Leiden is the most common inherited disorder linked to TE. A single G→A mutation within the factor V gene makes activated factor V resistant to protein C inactivation. The prothrombin gene mutation at position 20210A results in high prothrombin levels that probably contribute to thrombotic risk by increasing thrombin generation.[27–31] Excessive plasma levels of homocysteine resulting from homozygous deficiencies of enzymes such as cystathione B synthase or methylene tetrahydrofolate reductase are associated with an increased risk for VTE. Increased levels of lipoprotein (a) are reported to increase VTE risk in a subgroup of pediatric patients. Several other possible prothrombotic risk factors being studied in pediatric VTE include high levels of factors VII, VIII, IX, and XI and high levels of the fibrinolysis inhibitor TAFI.[32–40]

To identify prothrombotic risk factors and the underlying illnesses responsible for pediatric thrombosis, a comprehensive personal and family history and a reasonable laboratory workup should be completed. Table 73–3 summarizes the laboratory evaluation. Genotyping can be performed at the onset of thrombosis. To prevent results

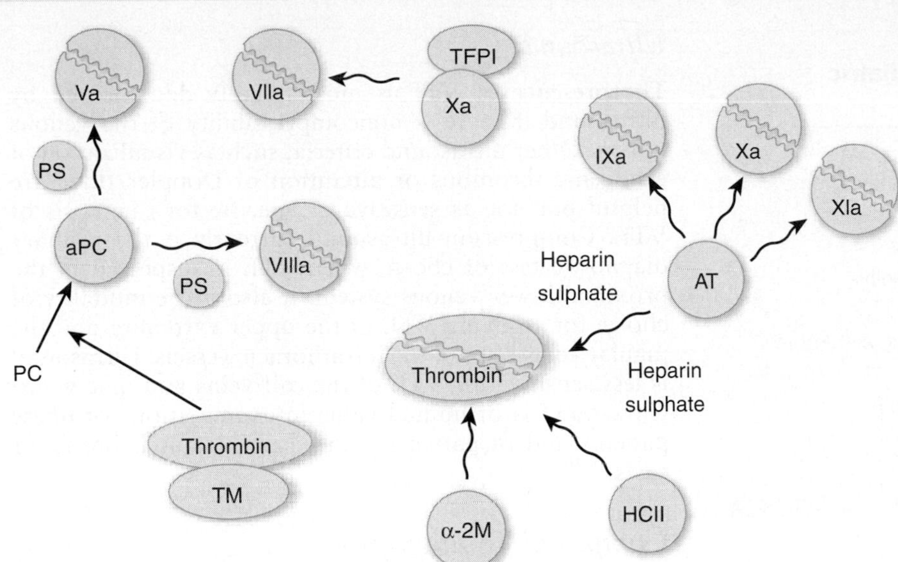

FIGURE 73–2 • Scheme of the anticoagulant system. *aPC,* Activated protein C; *α_2-M,* α_2-macroglobulin; *AT,* antithrombin; *HCII,* heparin cofactor II; *PC,* protein C; *TFPI,* tissue factor pathway inhibitor; *TM,* thrombomodulin. *Straight arrows* indicate promotion of the reaction. *Curly arrows* indicate inhibition. (Modified from Kuhle S, Male C, Mitchell L: *Semin Thromb Hemost* 29:329-338, 2003.)

of protein-based assays from being affected by the acute thrombotic onset, plasma levels can be determined at the onset but must be repeated at least 3 to 6 months after the thrombotic event or at least 14 to 30 days after withdrawal of oral anticoagulants.[41]

Several studies have shown that children with one congenital prothrombotic risk factor and especially children with two risk factors have an increased risk for recurrence. This may have an impact on the duration and intensity of anticoagulation given for acute events but also should make available effective prophylactic anticoagulation for high-risk events such as surgery.[42]

Principles of Diagnosis of Venous Thromboembolism

Clinical Diagnosis of Venous Thrombosis

The clinical diagnosis of non–CVL-related thrombosis is both insensitive and nonspecific. Diagnosis relies on symptoms such as swelling, erythema, skin discoloration, increased warmth, pain, tenderness, presence of subcutaneous collateral veins, or loss of CVL patency. Factors such as location, acuteness, and complexity of the underlying disease may mask symptoms.[43]

The main problem with clinical diagnosis of CVL-related VTE is poor sensitivity.[44–46] The majority of CVL-related VTEs usually are located in the central venous system, where obstruction may not result in limb swelling. Development of CVL-related VTE usually is gradual, permitting collateral vessels to form and minimizing the symptoms of acute VTE. Objective radiographic tests are necessary to establish or rule out the presence of VTE.

Radiographic Diagnosis of Venous Thrombosis

Venography

Venography is recognized as the reference standard for diagnosis of VTE in the lower and upper extremities.

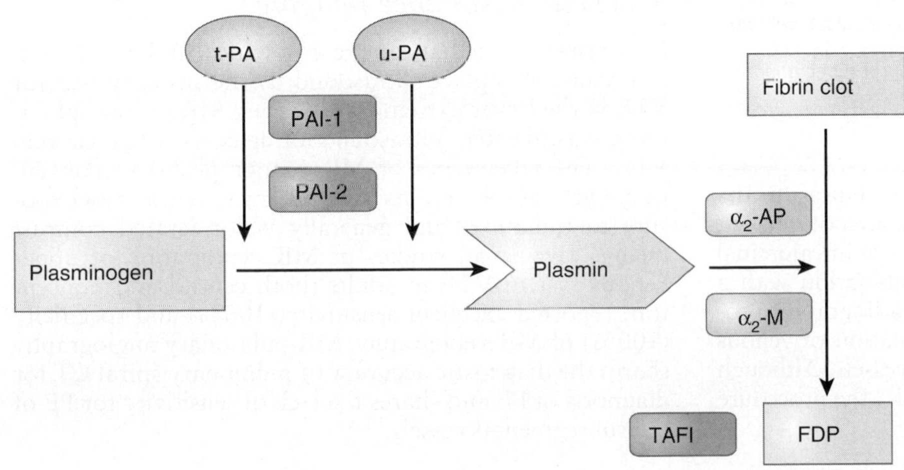

FIGURE 73–3 • Schematic representation of the fibrinolytic system. *α_2-AP,* α_2-Antiplasmin; *α_2-M,* α_2-macroglobulin; *FDP,* fibrin degradation product; *PAI-1,* plasminogen activator inhibitor-1; *PAI-2,* plasminogen activator inhibitor-2; *TAFI,* thrombin activatable fibrinolysis inhibitor; *tPA,* tissue-type plasminogen activator; *uPA,* urokinase-type plasminogen activator. (Modified from Albisetti M: *Semin Thromb Hemost* 29:339-348, 2003.)

TABLE 73–2

Clinical Risk Factors for Pediatric Thromboembolism

Perinatal Diseases	Birth asphyxia
	Respiratory distress syndrome
	Infants of diabetic mothers
	Neonatal infections
	Necrotizing enterocolitis
	Dehydration
	Congenital nephrotic syndrome
	Polycythemia
	Demise of a fetal twin
Medical Interventions	Central lines
	Operations
	Transplantation (kidney, heart, bone marrow)
	Immobilization
	Plaster casts
	Extracorporeal membrane oxygenation
Acute Diseases	Trauma
	Sepsis
	Dehydration
	Acute rheumatic diseases
	Nephrotic syndrome
	HUS/TTP
	Acute lymphoblastic leukemia
Chronic Diseases	Malignancies
	Renal diseases
	Cardiac malformations
	Chronic rheumatic diseases
	Sickle cell disease
	Inflammatory bowel disease
Drugs	*Escherichia coli* asparaginase
	Prednisone
	Activated coagulation factor concentrates
	Coagulation factor replacement: excessive levels
	Heparins
	Antifibrinolytic agents
	Oral contraceptives

From Nowak-Gottl U, Kosch A, Schlegel N, et al: *Curr Opin Hematol* 9:448–453, 2002.
HUS/TTP, Hemolytic uremic syndrome/thrombotic thrombocytopenic purpura.

Direct venography is performed by injecting contrast media into a subcutaneous vein peripheral to the area of interest. Diagnosis of VTE is based on visualization of intraluminal filling defects or nonvisualization in combination with a sudden cutoff of a deep vein seen on two radiographic projections. Venography does allow quantification of venous occlusion and identification of collateral vessels. Although venography is considered a "gold standard," the procedure is invasive and technically demanding.[47]

Ultrasound

The presence of VTE is most reliably documented by ultrasound if there is noncompressibility of the venous lumen. Other ultrasound criteria, such as visualization of echogenic thrombus or alteration of Doppler flow, are helpful but not as sensitive or specific for diagnosis of VTE. Compression ultrasound currently is the primary diagnostic test of choice when VTE is suspected in the proximal lower venous system. It also is the modality of choice for studying VTE of the upper extremity and the jugular veins but not the intrathoracic vessels. Ultrasound is less sensitive for VTE of the calf veins and iliac veins. Ultrasound is of limited value in examinations of obese patients and of patients with edema, trauma, burns, or casts.[48,49]

Computed Tomography

Spiral computed tomography (CT) allows for short examination times. CT venography compares well with ultrasound for detection of proximal lower extremity VTE.[50] It also identifies VTE in pelvic veins and the inferior vena cava that are not detected by ultrasound. Spiral CT pulmonary angiography is also used as a noninvasive imaging modality for PE. It allows pulmonary vessel visualization and assessment of the lung parenchyma. CT pulmonary angiography has a sensitivity and specificity of 94% for central PE. However, it has decreased sensitivity for subsegmental PE. Spiral CT has superior diagnostic accuracy compared with ventilation/perfusion (V/Q) scanning of the lung and now is the recommended initial test for suspected PE at many centers. V/Q scans still are used frequently as the initial study for suspected PE in pediatric and adult patients. Unfortunately, the majority of V/Q scans are neither high probability nor normal, making the predictive value poor.[51] Pulmonary angiography is the accepted "gold standard" for diagnosis of PE. However, pulmonary angiography is invasive and requires performer expertise for use in pediatric patients in whom technical difficulties are increased and interpretation is complicated, especially in children with complex congenital heart disease or pulmonary disease.[52]

Magnetic Resonance Imaging

Contrast-enhanced magnetic resonance (MR) venography will not replace ultrasound as the primary test for VTE in the lower extremity. However, MR venography is more sensitive than ultrasound for detection of pelvic vein VTE. The advantages of MR venography over conventional venography are its minimal invasiveness, nonexposure to radiation, and generally well-tolerated contrast media. Two small studies of MR venography of upper venous system VTE in adults (both central and noncentral) reported excellent sensitivity (100%) and specificity (100%) of MR venography. MR pulmonary angiography shares the diagnostic accuracy of pulmonary spiral CT for diagnosis of PE and shares the lack of sensitivity for PE of the subsegmental vessels.[53–56]

TABLE 73–3

Recommendations for Laboratory Testing of Children with Thrombosis as Recommended by the Subcommittee for Perinatal and Pediatric Thrombosis of the Scientific and Standardization Committee of the ISTH

Level I (should be performed after diagnosis of VTE)	Level II (should be performed if results of level I tests are negative and patient has strong positive family history for VTE, recurrent VTE, or life-threatening VTE)
Antithrombin	Euglobulin clot lysis time
Protein C activity	Plasminogen
Protein S antigen (free and total)	Fibrinogen activity and antigen
Factor V G1691A	Thrombin time
Factor II G20210A	Reptilase time
MTHFR T677T and/or fasting homocysteine level	Fibrin degradation products
Lipoprotein (a)	Plasminogen activator inhibitor
Lupus anticoagulant	Heparin cofactor II
Anticardiolipin antibodies	Paroxysmal nocturnal hemoglobinuria

From Manco-Johnson MJ, Grabowski EF, Hellgreen M, et al: *Thromb Haemost* 88:155–156, 2002.

Echocardiography

Echocardiography may be a helpful adjunct for visualizing clots at the junction of the brachiocephalic veins or the superior vena cava with the right atrium. Echocardiography is useful for assessing the severity of cardiac compromise associated with PE.[57]

Lineograms

Lineograms involve injection of contrast media into a CVL. Lineograms are primarily used to confirm the CVL location in the venous system and to identify some causes of CVL obstruction. Lineograms visualize fibrin sheets and clots that adhere to the CVL tip. Lineograms have poor sensitivity in detecting large-vessel thrombi that usually are located peripheral to the tip along the course of the catheter.[58]

Anticoagulants Used to Treat Pediatric Venous Thromboembolism in Children

Current standard therapy for the management of venous thromboembolic events in pediatric patients is suboptimally extracted from adult clinical trials. Treatment most commonly consists of initial therapy with unfractionated or low–molecular-weight heparin followed by oral anticoagulants, usually vitamin K antagonists such as coumadin. Before recommending therapy for specific pediatric thromboembolic complications, we must discuss how the developmental aspects of coagulation affect dosing, monitoring, efficacy, and complications of anticoagulation therapy in children.

Unfractionated Heparin

Commercial preparations of unfractionated heparin (UFH) contain fragments with an average molecular weight of 15,000 Da. UFH contains a penta accharide sequence that binds AT through lysine sites. This causes a conformational change at the reactive site that converts AT into a rapid inhibitor of serine proteases, especially factor IIa (thrombin) and factor Xa.[59]

The anticoagulant activities of heparin, which are mediated by catalysis of AT, can be impaired given acquired or age-appropriate decreased plasma levels of AT. We have discussed physiologically low AT concentrations in newborns (0.50 U/ml) and premature neonates (<0.30 U/ml). The capacity of children to generate thrombin is approximately 25% less than that of adults. Both an increased sensitivity and a resistance to the anticoagulant properties of UFH make dosing extrapolation from adults to infants and young children inadequate.[60]

The recommended therapeutic range for treatment of VTE in adults is an aPTT that reflects an anti-Xa level of 0.3 to 0.7 U/ml. In pediatric patients, the aPTT values correctly predict therapeutic heparin concentrations approximately 70% of the time. If aPTT values do not accurately reflect UFH concentrations, UFH levels should be preferentially used because they more accurately reflect the in vivo antithrombotic efficacy of UFH.[59]

Bolus doses of 75 to 100 U/kg result in therapeutic aPTT values in 90% of children. The maintenance heparin doses are age dependent. Infants younger than 1 year require an average of 28 U/kg/h and children older than 1 year of age require an average of 20 U/kg/h. Doses of UFH required for older children and adolescents are similar to the weight-adjusted requirement of 18 units/kg/h for adults. Oral anticoagulants can be initiated on day 1 of heparin therapy, except in the presence of extensive deep venous thrombosis (DVT) or PE when oral anticoagulation can be delayed. A validated nomogram for adjusting UFH dosing in pediatrics now is available (Table 73–4).[61,62]

Adverse Effects of Heparin

Bleeding is the most common complication of UFH. Because heparin clears rapidly, termination of heparin

TABLE 73–4

Protocol for Systemic Heparin Administration and Adjustment for Pediatric Patients

I. Loading dose: heparin 75 U/kg IV over 10 min
II. Initial maintenance dose: 28 U/kg/h for infants <1yr
III. Initial maintenance dose: 20 U/kg/h for children >1yr
IV. Adjust heparin to maintain aPTT 60 to 85 s (assuming this reflects an anti-factor Xa level of 0.30–0.70):

aPTT (s)	Bolus (U/kg)	Hold (min)	Rate Change (%)	Repeat aPTT
<50	50	0	+10	4 h
50–59	0	0	+10	4 h
60–85	0	0	0	Next day
86–95	0	0	−10	4 h
96–120	0	30	−10	4 h
>120	0	60	−15	4 h

V. Obtain blood for aPTT 4 hr after administration of the heparin loading dose and 4 hr after every change in the infusion rate
VI. When aPTT values are therapeutic, a daily CBC and aPTT.

From Michelson AD, Bovill E, Andrew M: *Chest* 108(4 suppl):506S–522S, 1995.

infusion is enough to control bleeding in most cases. If a more immediate effect is required, intravenous (IV) protamine sulfate rapidly neutralizes heparin based on the amount of heparin received in the previous 2 hours. Protamine sulfate can be administered at a concentration of 10 mg/ml at a rate not exceeding 5 mg/min. Hypersensitivity reactions to protamine can occur in patients with known reactions to fish or in patients who have been exposed to protamine-containing insulin.[59,63] Table 73–5 gives the protocol for reversal of heparin therapy.

Heparin-induced osteoporosis (HIO) is a true entity described in the adult literature. Data on the correlation of HIO with the UFH dose used or duration of therapy in children are inconclusive. There are only three case reports of HIO in pediatric patients, two involving concurrent steroid use.[64]

Heparin-Induced Thrombocytopenia. Heparin-induced thrombocytopenia (HIT) is a serious and potentially life-threatening complication of UFH. In the pediatric literature, HIT is reported in patients ranging in age from 3 months to 15 years. A bimodal frequency is observed in children, with a higher number of cases reported in neonates and infants up to age 2 years and in puberty. Heparin exposure leading to HIT ranges from low exposure from heparin flushes to supratherapeutic doses during cardiopulmonary bypass and hemodialysis. The majority of children with HIT are diagnosed during pediatric ICU admissions at a frequency of 2.3%. Mortality from HIT in children across reported cases is 14.5%.[65]

Pathophysiology of Heparin-Induced Thrombocytopenia. Unlike other drug-induced thrombocytopenias, HIT usually does not cause bleeding; instead it causes thrombosis (both venous and arterial). HIT is mediated by an antibody that recognizes new epitopes revealed by the platelet factor-4 (PF4)–heparin complex. The antibody–PF4–heparin complex binds to Fc R11 platelet receptors and cross-links them. This cross-linking of receptors induces intense platelet activation and aggregation.[66] Figure 73–4 illustrates the pathophysiology of HIT.[66]

Type I Heparin-Induced Thrombocytopenia. Type I HIT is not immune mediated. The thrombocytopenia usually is mild (80×10^9/L) and generally occurs within a few days of starting heparin therapy. Patients remain asymptomatic, and the thrombocytopenia resolves spontaneously within a few days even with continuation of heparin.[67]

Type II Heparin-Induced Thrombocytopenia. Unlike type I, type II HIT is immune mediated. Generally the thrombocytopenia occurs within 5 to 10 days of heparin exposure. In 30% of patients, HIT is diagnosed only when a rapid drop in platelet count follows reinstitution of heparin therapy. Only recent heparin therapy (usually within the preceding 100 days) is associated with rapid-onset HIT. There is generally a 50% drop in the baseline platelet count to a mean platelet nadir of 50×10^9/L. However, if the baseline platelet count is elevated, it may drop by 50% or greater and still be within the "normal range," necessitating close platelet monitoring and a high index of clinical suspicion.[68,69]

TABLE 73–5

Reversal of Heparin Therapy*

Time Since Last Dose of Heparin (min)	Protamine Dose
<30	1.0 mg/100 U heparin received
30–60	0.5–0.75 mg/100 U heparin received
60–120	0.375–0.5 mg/100 U heparin received
>120	0.25–0.375 mg/100 U heparin received
Maximum dose	50 mg
Infusion rate	10 mg/ml, solution should not exceed 5 mg/min

From Monagle P, Chan A, Massicotte P, et al: *Chest* 126(3 suppl): 645S–687S, 2004.

*Hypersensitivity reactions to protamine sulfate may occur in patients with known hypersensitivity reactions to fish or in those previously exposed to protamine therapy or protamine-containing insulin therapy.

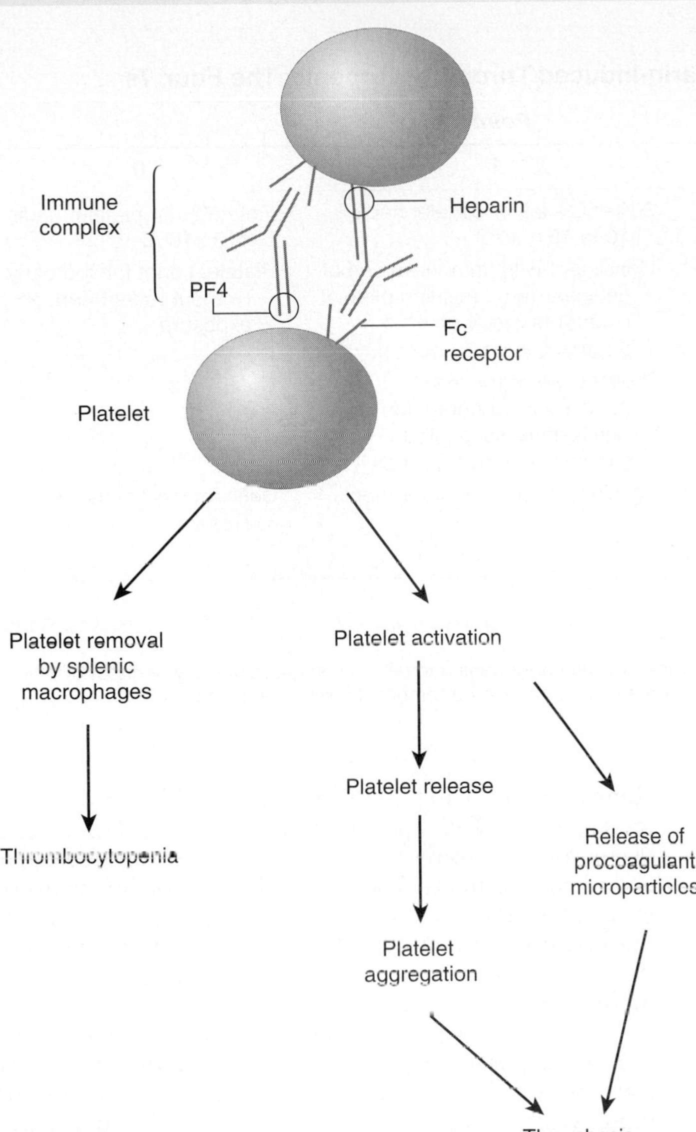

FIGURE 73–4 • Pathogenesis of heparin-induced thrombocytopenia. PF4, Platelet factor-4. (Adapted from Chong BH: *Br J Haematol* 1995;89:431-439.)

Heparin resistance may occur with development of HIT. Systemic symptoms such as fever, tachycardia, flushing, headache, chest pain, and dyspnea may occur in HIT patients following an intravenous bolus of heparin. Acute amnesia, cardiac arrest, and pulmonary arrest are reported.[69]

Warkentin et al. reported a catastrophic syndrome of venous gangrene associated with HIT generally in patients with proximal DVTs of the lower limb and concomitant heparin and coumadin therapy. Administration of coumadin resulted in a precipitous decrease in levels of anticoagulant protein C and a paradoxical worsening of symptoms. Arterial thrombosis leading to stroke, myocardial infarction, microvascular thrombosis, and DIC are reported in patients with HIT.[69]

The clinical diagnosis can be challenging in the ICU setting, and confirmatory laboratory results often are delayed. Daily monitoring of platelet counts of patients receiving heparin and a high index of suspicion are helpful. Warkentin and Heddle[70] suggest a score to estimate pretest probability of HIT (Table 73–6), but this method has not been validated in pediatric patients.

In most cases, diagnosis of HIT requires a combination of clinical suspicion and the presence of confirmatory or supporting laboratory tests. Laboratory tests for HIT include functional tests (platelet aggregation test, 14 serotonin release assay, heparin-induced platelet aggregation test, and flow cytometry microparticle release) or immunoassays that detect anti-PF4 antibodies. The immunoassays are more widely available, easier to perform, and more sensitive than many functional assays.[70]

Management of Heparin-Induced Thrombocytopenia. Even in the presence of isolated thrombocytopenia without thrombosis, discontinuation of heparin alone

TABLE 73–6

Estimating the Pretest Probability of Heparin-Induced Thrombocytopenia: The Four *Ts*

	Point		
	2	1	0
Thrombocytopenia	>50% fall or nadir 20–100	30%–50% fall or platelet nadir 10 to 19 × 10^9/L	Fall <30% or platelet nadir <10 ×10^9/L
Timing of platelet count fall or other sequelae	Clear onset between days 5 to 10 or <1 day (if recent heparin exposure [past 100 days])	Consistent with immunization but not clear (e.g., missing platelet counts) or onset of thrombocytopenia after day 10	Platelet count fall too early (without recent heparin exposure)
Thrombosis or other sequelae (e.g., skin lesions)	New thrombosis; skin necrosis; post-heparin bolus ASR	Progressive or recurrent thrombosis; erythematous skin lesions; suspected thrombosis not yet proven	None
Other cause for thrombocytopenia	No other cause for platelet count fall is evident	Possible other cause is evident	Definite other cause is present
Pretest probability score: 6–8 = high; 4–5 = intermediate; 0–3 = low.			

From Warkentin TE, Heddle NM: *Curr Hematol Rep* 2:148–157, 2003.
ASR, acute systemic reaction.
*Points 0, 1, or 2 for each of four categories; maximum score possible is 8.
†First day of immunizing heparin exposure considered day zero the day the platelet count begins to fall is considered the day of onset of thrombocytopenia (it generally takes 1–3 more days until an arbitrary threshold that defines thrombocytopenia is passed).

is not optimal. Heparin must be discontinued, but an alternative non–cross-reacting anticoagulant should be started. Although LMWH is associated with a significantly decreased incidence of HIT, it is contraindicated once HIT is diagnosed. As discussed, coumadin should initially be withheld. The alternative anticoagulants, lepirudin and argatroban, are acceptable anticoagulants. They both are direct thrombin inhibitors[71] that are not associated with development of heparin–PF4 immune complexes. Argatroban (metabolized hepatically) or lepirudin (excreted renally) should be continued for a minimum of 5 to 7 days or until thrombosis is controlled and a steady rise in the platelet count, ideally to >100 × 10^9/L, is observed. Initiation of coumadin should be delayed for several days and should overlap with argatroban or lepirudin administration until the desired coumadin international normalized ratio (INR) is achieved on 3 consecutive days.[71,72]

Low-Molecular-Weight Heparin

Use of LMWH therapy for both initial and long-term treatment of pediatric TE is increasing. Pharmacokinetic limitations of UFH include unpredictable anticoagulant response, which is magnified in children with developing hemostatic mechanisms, and neutralization of UFH activity by PF4 released from activated platelets. The pharmacokinetic and other limitations of UFH are overcome to a significant extent by LMWH preparations. Other advantages of LMWH include subcutaneous administration instead of the long-term inpatient intravenous administration needed for UFH, lack of interference with coadministered drugs, plasma proteins, or diets, probable reduced risk of osteoporosis, and reduced risk for HIT development.[73]

LMWH results from various chemical and enzymatic cleavage processes of UFH. The resulting LMWHs have decreased molecular weight distributions (3500–6700 Da) compared with UFH (5000–30,000 Da). The smaller size increases LMWH specificity for anticoagulation and decreases the reactivity with other plasma and vascular endothelial proteins. Like UFH, the anticoagulant properties of LMWH are mediated through catalysis of AT, but because of the decreased capacity of LMWH to bind AT and thrombin simultaneously, LMWH preferentially inhibits factor Xa.[74,75]

Age- and weight-adjusted doses of LMWH preparations (e.g., enoxaparin, reviparin, dalteparin, and tinzaparin) are listed in Table 73–7. Infants younger than 2 to 3 months or those weighing less than 5 kg require increased doses secondary to their larger volume of distribution. The therapeutic range for LMWH currently is extrapolated from adult data and is based on an anti-Xa level of 0.5 to 1 U/ml in a sample taken 4 hours after a subcutaneous injection.[76–80] Table 73–8 provides a nomogram for monitoring and dose adjustment of LMWH in pediatric patients.

In a single-institution pediatric cohort study of 146 courses of therapeutic enoxaparin, major bleeding occurred in 4.8% of patients (95% confidence interval [CI] 2% to 9.6%).[78] For episodes of minor bleeding, discontinuation of LMWH usually is adequate. For major bleeds, protamine sulfate can be used. The protamine sulfate dose is dependent on the dose of LMWH used. Although protamine sulfate completely neutralizes anti-IIa activity and only partly neutralizes anti-FXa activity, bleeding secondary to LMWH is completely reversed in animal models.[81]

Oral Anticoagulants

The most commonly used long-term anticoagulant in children is the vitamin K antagonist coumadin. Little information on the efficacy and safety of oral anticoagulant use in neonates is available. Information and therapy guidelines for coumadin are available for children older

TABLE 73–7

Protocols for Low-Molecular-Weight Heparin Administration and Adjustment for Pediatric Patients

	Weight-Dependent Dose of Reviparin	
	<5 kg	**<5 kg**
Initial treatment dose	150 U/kg/dose q12h	100 U/kg/dose q12h
Initial prophylactic dose	50 U/kg/dose q12h	30 U/kg/dose q12h
	Age-Dependent Dose of Enoxaparin	
	<2 months	**<2 months**
Initial treatment dose	1.5 mg/kg/dose q12h	1.0 mg/kg/dose q12h
Initial prophylactic dose	0.75 mg/kg/dose q12h	0.5 mg/kg/dose q12h
	Age-Dependent Dose of Tinzaparin	
	<3 months	**<3 months**
Initial treatment dose	250 anti-FXa IU/mL q24h	175 anti-Fxa IU/mL q24h
	Dose of Dalteparin*	
Initial treatment dose	129 ± 43 anti-Fxa IU/kg SC q24h	
Initial prophylactic dose	92 ± 52 anti-Fxa IU/kg SC q24h	

From Revel-Vilk S, Chan AK: *Semin Thromb Hemost* 29:425–432, 2003.
FXa, factor Xa.
*Dose is inversely related to age.

than 3 months. Vitamin K oral anticoagulants function by reducing plasma concentrations of the vitamin K-dependent proteins (FII, FVII, FIX, FX, protein C, and protein S).[82] Note, however, that protein C and protein S levels also are lowered by coumadin. Initially, coumadin can cause a paradoxical procoagulant state so that at least 5 days of overlap is needed when converting from heparin (UFH or LMWH) to coumadin. In North America, the prothrombin time (PT), reported as the INR, is the test most commonly used for monitoring oral anticoagulants. Currently, therapeutic INR ranges are extrapolated from adult recommendations. The target INR range for DVT/PE is 2 to 3 and for prosthetic heart valves is 2.5 to 3.5.[83] Anecdotal evidence indicates that lower INRs may be efficacious in children, but currently no confirmatory data are available. A prospective cohort study has resulted in a nomogram based on an initial loading dose of 0.2 mg/kg coumadin with dose adjustments based on INR values. Maintenance doses for oral anticoagulants are age dependent, with infants requiring the highest doses (0.32 mg/kg) and adolescents requiring the lowest doses (0.09 mg/kg).[84] Table 73–9 provides the pediatric therapeutic protocol for oral anticoagulation with coumadin.

Children taking oral anticoagulants require frequent dose adjustments. Breast-fed infants are very sensitive to oral anticoagulants because of lower concentrations of vitamin K in breast milk. Infants fed with nutrient formulas are resistant to oral anticoagulants because of higher concentrations of vitamin K found in most nutrient formulas.[85] Medications influence dose requirements for oral anticoagulants in a fashion similar to adults (Table 73–10).[86]

Bleeding is the main complication of vitamin K antagonists. Nonhemorrhagic complications include rare tracheal calcification and possible reduced bone density in children who receive coumadin for more than 1 year.[87] Table 73–11 lists therapies for reversing the effects of coumadin.[87] Newer oral anticoagulants are being developed that may overcome some of the limitations of coumadin. Ximalgatran, a prodrug of melgatran, is a direct thrombin inhibitor

TABLE 73–8

Nomogram for Monitoring of Low-Molecular-Weight Heparin

Anti-FXa (U/ml)	Hold	Dose Change (%)	Repeat Anti-FXa
<0.35	No	+25%	4 h after next dose
0.35–0.49	No	+10%	4 h after next dose
0.5–1.0	No	No	Next day, then 1 wk later and monthly thereafter (at 4 h after AM dose)
1.1–1.5	No	−20%	Before next dose
1.6–2.0	3h	−30%	Before next dose then 4 h after next dose
>2.0	Until ant-FXa 0.5 U/mL	−40%	Before next dose, if not 0.5 U/mL, repeat q12h

From Monagle P, Michelson AD, Bovill E, Andrew M: *Chest* 119:S344–S370, 2001.

TABLE 73–9

Protocol for Oral Anticoagulation Therapy to Maintain an INR between 2 and 3 for Pediatric Patients

I. Day 1: if the baseline INR is 1.0–1.3: dose 5 0.2 mg/kg orally

II. Loading days 2–4: If the INR is:

INR	Action
1.1–1.3	Repeat initial loading dose
1.4–1.9	50% of initial loading dose
2.0–3.0	50% of initial loading dose
3.1–3.5	25% of loading dose
>3.5	Hold until INR 3.5, then restart at 50% less than previous dose

III. Maintenance oral anticoagulation dose guidelines:

INR	Action
1.1–1.4	Increase by 20% of dose
1.5–1.9	Increase by 10% of dose
2.0–3.0	No change
3.1–3.5	Decrease by 10% of dose
>3.5	Hold until INR 3.5, then restart at 20% less than previous dose

From Michelson AD, Bovill E, Andrew M: *Chest* 108:506S-522S, 1995.

that shows promise for long-term anticoagulant use in adults.[88]

Thrombolytic Agents as Treatment for Thromboembolism in Children

Anticoagulation alone limits the rate of thrombus propagation but does not actively reduce thrombus size. Blood flow is restored by endogenous fibrinolysis and by the formation of collateral vessels.

TABLE 73–10

Drugs Commonly Used in Children That Affect Their INR Value

Drug	Effect on INR
Amiodarone	Increase
Aspirin	Increase or no change
Amoxicillin (Amoxil)	Slight increase
Cefaclor (Ceclor)	Increase
Carbamazepine (Tegretol)	Decrease
Phenytoin (Dilantin)	Decrease
Phenobarbital	Decrease
Cloxacillin	Increase
Prednisone	Increase
Trimethoprim-sulfamethoxazole	Increase
Ranitidine	Increase

From Michelson AD, Bovill E, Andrew M: *Chest* 108:506S-522S, 1995.

TABLE 73–11

Reversal of Oral Anticoagulation Therapy

1. No bleeding
   A. Rapid reversal of oral anticoagulants is necessary and the patient will require oral anticoagulants again in the near future: give vitamin K, 0.5–2 mg subcutaneously or IV (not intramuscularly), depending on the patient's size.
   B. Rapid reversal of oral anticoagulants is necessary and the patient will not require oral anticoagulants again: vitamin K1 2–5 mg subcutaneously or IV (not intramuscularly).
2. Significant bleeding
   A. Significant bleeding that is not life threatening and will not cause morbidity: treat with vitamin K1 as in step 1A plus FFP (20 ml/kg IV).
   B. Significant bleeding that is life threatening and will cause morbidity: treat with vitamin K1 IV (5 mg) by slow infusion over 10–20 min because of the risk of anaphylactic shock. Consider giving prothrombin concentrate (containing factors II, VII, IX, X) 50 U/kg IV rather than FFP (20 ml/kg IV).

From Michelson AD, Bovill E, Andrew M: *Chest* 108:506S-522S, 1995.

Thrombolytic agents include streptokinase, urokinase, and recombinant tPA, which lyse clots by converting endogenous plasminogen to plasmin. Streptokinase is not recommended for pediatric use because of this population's high prevalence of neutralizing antistreptococcal antibodies. Urokinase is no longer approved by the U.S. Food and Drug Administration (FDA) as a thrombolytic agent because of safety concerns. Therefore recombinant tPA is the thrombolytic agent used most often in children. However, there are no tPA dose finding studies in infants and children and no randomized, prospective studies comparing tPA to other therapies.[89]

Thrombolytic agents most commonly are indicated as low-dose therapy for restoring catheter potency and higher doses for lysing venous or arterial thrombi that are life threatening or limb threatening or thrombi that threaten organ function. Success rates for tPA use in pediatric patients vary in the literature. Zenz et al. reported using a dose of 0.5 mg/kg/h for the first hour followed by 0.25 mg/kg/h until clot lysis occurred or treatment had to be stopped because of bleeding complications. Complete clot lysis was achieved in 16 of 17 patients within 4 to 11 hours after the start of treatment. After complete lysis, new thrombosis developed in one patient 1.5 hours after the end of treatment.[90]

A variety of tPA dosing regimens have been used. Although many reports described tPA infusion rates of up to 0.5mg/kg/h, a report described rates of 0.01 mg/kg/h for catheter-directed local therapy to 0.03 mg/kg/h for systemic therapy. Both rates were safe and efficacious. Finding the lowest effective dose is important to improve the tPA profile, especially in neonates and younger children. A common practice is to use concomitant low-dose heparin (10 μg/kg/h) with tPA to allow for lysis and to prevent clot progression. This practice does not appear to be associated with an increased incidence of serious bleeding.[91]

Use of tPA in newborns and young children is influenced by their developing hemostatic system. Plasminogen levels often are decreased, so the efficacy of thrombolysis may be decreased. Supplementation with plasmas containing plasminogen (10 ml/kg prior to each tPA infusion) may be necessary.[92]

The therapeutic range is narrow, and tPA monitoring is difficult. The correlation between hemostatic parameters and the efficacy and safety of thrombolytic therapy is weak and therefore not used clinically. Measurements of fibrinogen degradation products and/or D-dimers can help determine whether a fibrinolytic effect is being achieved.[92]

At this time, no evidence suggests there is an advantage of local over systemic thrombolytic therapy in children. In fact, the small vessel size in children may increase the risk of local vessel injury causing new thrombus formation and vascular endothelial injury. Local therapy may be appropriate for treatment of catheter-related TE when the catheter is already in situ.[92]

Thrombolytic therapy has been reported to be associated with significant bleeding complications requiring transfusion is 39% of children. More recent reports document bleeding requiring transfusion in 10% of children. Protocol recommendations include the following:

1. Concurrent heparin therapy (10 μg/kg/h)
2. Fixed tPA infusions at 0.5 mg/kg/h for 6 hours with no extensions beyond 6 hours
3. FFP (10–15 ml/kg) given 30 minutes before each tPA infusion in neonates

Before thrombolytic therapy is initiated, correction of other concurrent hemostatic problems, such as thrombocytopenia or vitamin K deficiency, is strongly advised.[92]

The International Society of Thrombosis and Haemostasis recommends the following guidelines for tPA use in children[91]:

1. Primary use of tPA thrombolysis for vascular thrombosis in children should be in the conduct of clinical trials.
2. Concomitant heparin, when used, should be administered in prophylactic doses.
3. Standard contraindications to thrombolysis should be observed in pediatric patients so as to decrease hemorrhagic complications. These include major surgery or hemorrhage within 10 days of therapy, a severe asphyxial event within 7 days of therapy, invasive procedure within 3 days of therapy, seizures within 48 hours of therapy, prematurity of <32 weeks of gestation, septicemia, active bleeding at the time of therapy, or inability to maintain platelets >50 to 100,000/μl or fibrinogen >100 mg/dl.

Treatment of Venous Catheter-Associated Venous Thromboembolism

Central venous lines are associated with up to 60% of pediatric and 90% of neonatal thrombosis cases.[93] Currently, primary anticoagulant prophylaxis cannot be recommended. One exception is for CVL use in children on long-term total parenteral nutrition. Prophylaxis with coumadin (INR range 2–2.5) is recommended until the CVL is removed. Alternatively, coumadin or LMWH heparin can be used for the first 3 months after CVL placement.[94] Prophylaxis for pediatric CVL-related VTE involves avoiding known risk factors, if possible, including left-sided CVL insertion, subclavian vein insertion, percutaneous insertion technique, large-bore catheters relative to vessel size, and use of external, as opposed to implantable, catheters.[95] Prophylactic flushes with heparin, saline, or thrombolytic agents are standard catheter maintenance techniques, although efficacy is unknown.[96]

In the ICU setting, even in the presence of symptomatic CVL-associated DVT, catheters can remain in situ if they are functional and venous access is necessary. Anticoagulation with a therapeutic dose of LMWH or UFH is recommended for 5 to 10 days. Anticoagulation can be continued with either LMWH or coumadin for 3 months. If CVL remains in place, prophylactic doses of coumadin (INR 1.5–1.8) or LMWH (anti-Xa level range 0.1–0.3) is recommended until the CVL is removed. A nonfunctioning CVL should be removed after 3 to 5 days of anticoagulation therapy if clinically possible. If thrombus recurs during prophylactic therapy, acute anticoagulation followed by coumadin or LMWH at therapeutic doses can be continued until the CVL is removed or until at least 3-month period has passed.[92]

Systemic Venous Thromboembolism Treatment

Systemic VTE occurs in children in the absence of CVL. The principles of anticoagulation are similar but do not require catheter management. Anticoagulation recommendations still are based mostly on adult data. LMWH is at least as efficacious and safe as UFH. However, UFH has the advantage of easy and complete reversal, which may be important when invasive procedures or surgery is anticipated. A therapeutic dose of UFH or LMWH usually is continued for 5 to 10 days unless extensive DVT or massive PE is present. In these circumstances, longer initial therapy is recommended. Coumadin can be started on the first day of anticoagulation. From day 6, if the INR is in the therapeutic range for 2 consecutive days (target range 2.0–3.0), UFH or LMWH can be stopped safely. The duration of continued anticoagulation depends on the presence or absence of temporary or ongoing acquired risk factors and the presence or absence of congenital prothrombotic risk factors (single or multiple). For secondary TE in the absence of ongoing risk factors, coumadin or LMWH is generally continued for 3 months. In the presence of ongoing acquired risk factors, anticoagulants are continued beyond 3 months at therapeutic or prophylactic doses until the risk factor(s) has resolved. First idiopathic thrombotic events, especially in the absence of concomitant prothrombotic risk factors, can be treated with coumadin (INR 2.0–3.0) or therapeutic LMWH for at least 6 months. Making the commitment to life-long anticoagulation with coumadin in patients with first idiopathic TE in the presence of one or more congenital prothrombotic risk factors is difficult.

Thrombolytic therapy should not be routinely used for venous TE in children. It may be considered in massive PE with hemodynamic compromise or in extensive venous TE that is not organ, limb, or life threatening.[92]

Arterial Thromboembolism

The most common cause of arterial TE in children is iatrogenic complications associated with arterial catheterization. Insertion of the arterial catheter itself may cause direct vascular injury resulting in arterial occlusion and loss of arterial line patency. Ischemic injury to surrounding tissue can lead to TE at remote sites. To prevent catheter-associated arterial TE, prophylaxis with continuous heparin infusion (at least 1 U/ml) is effective. Intermittent heparin flushes are not effective. When arterial TE occurs, the catheter should be removed immediately. Depending on the clinical situation, subsequent anticoagulation therapy, with or without thrombolysis, is often required to quickly restore limb perfusion.

Vascular compromise is the most common complication of cardiac catheterization with access through the superficial femoral artery and rarely the brachial artery. Increased incidence of arterial occlusion in younger patients during cardiac catheterization is influenced by increased catheter/diameter, balloon dilatation, larger sheath size for given weight and body surface area, and repeated catheter manipulations. Use of a prophylactic heparin bolus (usually 100–150 U/kg) has significantly decreased the incidence of arterial thrombosis during cardiac catheterization. If femoral artery thrombosis occurs following cardiac catheterization, at least 5 to 7 days of intravenous UFH is recommended. The optimal duration is unknown. Children with limb- or organ-threatening femoral artery thrombosis who do not respond to initial heparin therapy should undergo thrombolytic therapy in the absence of contraindications. If thrombolysis is contraindicated or organ or limb loss is imminent, surgical intervention may be necessary.[92,97,98]

Non–Catheter-Related Arterial Thromboembolism Complications

Congenital disorders causing arterial TE include familial hyperlipidemia and hyperhomocystinemia. Acquired disorders include Takayasu arteritis, Kawasaki disease, complications of congenital heart disease, and arterial occlusion of transplanted organs, such as hepatic artery thrombosis and renal artery thrombosis.

Therapeutic options for treatment of acute arterial occlusion include anticoagulants, thrombolytic therapy, embolectomy, and reconstructive surgery. Most centers initiate therapy with UFH because 70% of arterial TEs resolve without thrombolytic therapy. LMWH in therapeutic doses also can be used. If anticoagulation fails, thrombolysis is preferred over embolectomy. Reconstructive surgery of an ischemic but viable limb in a small child usually is deferred, if possible, because future definitive surgery in larger vessels is more successful.[92]

Disseminated Intravascular Coagulation

Disseminated intravascular coagulation is the extreme expression of coagulation activation. It is characterized by widespread, uncontrolled activation of coagulation that results in vascular and microvascular fibrin deposition. This process leads to decreased levels of procoagulant and anticoagulant proteins, fibrinogen, and platelets so that thrombosis and bleeding occur simultaneously. Hemorrhagic tissue necrosis, small-vessel microthrombi, midsize and larger artery and vein thrombi, and organ fibrin deposition lead to the multiorgan failure often seen in DIC.[99]

It now is apparent that thrombin generation in DIC is mediated primarily by the interaction of TF and factor VII. In fact, TF is the primary mediator of coagulation activation in sepsis. Endotoxin and proinflammatory cytokines induce TF expression on circulating monocytes in septic patients. Fibrin deposition is amplified by dysregulation of endogenous anticoagulation systems. AT and protein C are continuously consumed by ongoing thrombin generation. Impaired hepatic synthesis and vascular leakage result in low circulating levels of both AT and protein C. AT is degraded by elastase released from activated neutrophils. High levels of tumor necrosis factor-α down-regulate TM, which in turn further decreases anticoagulant (protein C and protein S) levels. Propagation of fibrin deposition in DIC is favored by sustained release of PAI-1 and a secondary decrease in fibrinolysis. Very high levels of PAI-1 are associated with poor prognosis in sepsis.[100,101]

In clinical practice, diagnosis of DIC is based upon a decreased platelet count, increased global clotting times (aPTT, PT), at least two low procoagulant levels including factor VIII (acute phase reactant), a low anticoagulant level such as AT, and detection of fibrin degradation products. The measurement of soluble fibrin in plasma is very sensitive for the presence of DIC but is not very specific. Fibrinogen is widely used as a marker for DIC but it is not very beneficial.[102]

In some patients with sepsis and an intense systemic inflammatory response, DIC continues for a period after appropriate treatment of the underlying disorder has started. The recommendation for support with plasma, cryoprecipitate, or platelets in DIC is not based on randomized, controlled trials but appears to be rational therapy for bleeding patients or patients at risk for bleeding because of significant depletion of hemostatic factors. The suggestion that we have all heard—that administering blood components in DIC adds "fuel to the fire"—has never been proven in clinical or experimental studies. In fact, there are no absolute numbers to target with hemostatic support. Transfusion discussions should be primarily driven by clinical status, that is, the need for an invasive procedure, the actual presence of bleeding, or a perceived high risk for bleeding.[103]

Other therapy for DIC has included anticoagulants such as heparin. However, a beneficial effect of heparin on clinical outcomes has never been shown in controlled clinical trials. Also, the safety of heparin therapy for DIC is debatable because patients often have a high concomitant risk of bleeding. Theoretically, the most logical anticoagulant agent to use is directed against TF activity. Such agents (TFPI, nematode anticoagulant protein c2 [NAPc2]) currently are being studied in phase II/III clinical trials. The anticoagulant with proven efficacy in DIC and sepsis is protein C concentrate. A phase III trial of activated protein C concentrate in patients with sepsis reduced mortality at 28 days after inclusion to 24.7% in the activated protein C group versus 30.8% in the control group (19.4% relative risk reduction). Administration of activated protein C not only improves coagulation abnormalities but also down-regulates proinflammatory pathways by its interaction with the endothelial protein C receptor.[104]

New Anticoagulants

Heparin and coumadin are the cornerstones of treatment of pediatric thrombosis. Both drugs have pharmacokinetic and biophysical drawbacks. New anticoagulants are being developed to overcome some of these limitations. An ideal anticoagulant should have the following characteristics: efficacy at the site of thrombus formation, safety, oral bioavailability, a wide therapeutic window, no need for monitoring, and easy reversibility. The search for an ideal anticoagulant goes on. Table 73–12 reviews newer anticoagulants.

Treatment of Acute Pulmonary Embolism

Optimal therapy of acute PE remains a question for both adult and pediatric populations. Most current data originate from adult studies, and extrapolation to pediatric patients may not be efficacious. Treatment regimens for DVT and PE are similar because the two conditions are manifestations of the same disease process. When patients with proximal VTE are carefully studied, a majority also has PE. In acute nonmassive PE, initial treatment with LMWH or UFH for at least 5 days is recommended. In a systematic review of nine adult trials of patients with acute PE, thrombolytic therapy led to more rapid resolution of the

TABLE 73–12

Newer Anticoagulants

Anticoagulant	Coagulation Target	Route of Administration	Indication	Half-life	Reversibility & Monitoring
Inhibitors of coagulation Initiation					
TFPI (tissue factor pathway inhibitor)	FVIIa–tissue factor complex	IV: continuous infusion (25–50 μ/kg/h) × 4 days	Sepsis?	?	?
rNAP c2 (nematode anticoagulant peptide)	FVIIa–tissue factor complex	SQ	Orthopedic thromboprophylaxis, coronary syndromes	50 h	VIIa reversal agent
Inhibitors of coagulation propagation					
DX-9065a	Direct Xa inhibitor	IV: continuous infusion	Coronary syndromes	?	?
DP-C906	Direct Xa inhibitor	PO	Orthopedic thromboprophylaxis (elective knee arthroplasty)	?	?
Fondaparinux	Indirect Xa inhibitor	SQ	Orthopedic thromboprophylaxis VTE treatment, coronary syndromes	17–21 h	?
Idraparinux	Indirect Xa inhibitor	SQ	VTE treatment	80–130 h	?
Inhibitors of anticoagulation amplification					
Argatroban	Direct thrombin inhibitor	IV: 2 μg/kg/h	HIT	45 min	Monitor aPTT
Lepirudin (r-hirudin)	Direct thrombin inhibitor	IV: 0.4 mg/kg bolus 0.1–0.15 mg/kg/h	HIT	60–80 min IV 120 min SQ	Monitor aPTT
Bivalirudin	Direct thrombin inhibitor	IV: 1 mg/kg bolus 2.5 mg/kg/h × 4 h 0.2 mg/kg/h to 20 h	Percutaneous coronary intevention	25–45 min	Monitor aPTT
Ximelgartran	Direct thrombin inhibitor	PO DVT prophylaxis: 24 or 36 mg bid DVT/PE treatment: 24–60 mg bid atrial fibrillation: 36 mg bid	Orthopedic thromboprophylaxis VTE treatment, prophylaxis in nonvalvular atrial fibrillation	3–4 h	None

radiographic and hemodynamic abnormalities than did anticoagulant therapy alone. However, benefits were short-lived. No differences in outcomes were detected, including death rate or resolution of symptoms. The risk of intracranial hemorrhage in adults who receive thrombolytic therapy for treatment of PE is 1% to 2%. Systemic thrombolytic therapy is not recommended for most patients with PE but may be useful for hemodynamically unstable patients with PE. Local administration of thrombolytic therapy via a catheter is also recommended. If thrombolytic therapy is used for treatment of PE, a short infusion time is preferred over a prolonged infusion time. For adults, tPA is given as a 100-mg infusion over 2 hours. Concurrent UFH use is optional.[105,106]

REFERENCES

1. Andrew M, Paes B, Milner R, et al: Development of the human coagulation system in the full-term infant, *Blood* 70:165-172, 1987.
2. Andrew M, Paes B, Milner R, et al: Development of the human coagulation system in the healthy premature infant, *Blood* 72: 1651-1657, 1988.
3. Andrew M, Vegh P, Johnston M, et al: Maturation of the hemostatic system during childhood, *Blood* 80:1998-2005, 1992.
4. Gross PL, Aird WC: The endothelium and thrombosis, *Semin Thromb Hemost* 26:463-478, 2000.
5. Bombeli T, Mueller M, Haeberli A: Anticoagulant properties of the vascular endothelium, *Thromb Haemost* 77:408-423, 1997.
6. Hoffman M, Monroe DM 3rd: A cell-based model of hemostasis, *Thromb Haemost* 85:958-965, 2001.
7. Kuhle S, Male C, Mitchell L: Developmental hemostasis: pro- and anticoagulant systems during childhood, *Semin Thromb Hemost* 29:329-338, 2003.
8. Albisetti M: The fibrinolytic system in children, *Semin Thromb Hemost* 29:339-348, 2003.
9. Lijnen HR: Pathophysiology of the plasminogen/plasmin system, *Int Journal Clin Lab Res* 26:1-6, 1996.
10. Andrew M, David M, Adams M, et al: Venous thromboembolic complications (VTE) in children: first analyses of the Canadian Registry of VTE, *Blood* 83:1251-1257, 1994.
11. van Ommen CH, Heijboer H, Buller HR, et al: Venous thromboembolism in childhood: a prospective two-year registry in The Netherlands, *J Pediatr* 139:676-681, 2001.
12. Nowak-Gottl U, von Kries R, Gobel U: Neonatal symptomatic thromboembolism in Germany: two year survey, *Arch Dis Child Fetal Neonat Ed* 76:F163-F167, 1997.
13. Byard RW, Cutz E: Sudden and unexpected death in infancy and childhood due to pulmonary thromboembolism. An autopsy study, *Arch Pathol Lab Med* 114:142-144, 1990.
14. Jones RH, Sabiston DC Jr: Pulmonary embolism in childhood, *Monogr Surg Sci* 3:35-51, 1966.
15. Monagle P, Adams M, Mahoney M, et al: Outcome of pediatric thromboembolic disease: a report from the Canadian Childhood Thrombophilia Registry, *Pediatr Res* 47:763-766, 2000.
16. Hoppe C, Matsunaga A: Pediatric thrombosis, *Pediatr Clin North Am* 49:1257-1283, 2002.
17. Massicotte MP, Dix D, Monagle P, et al: Central venous catheter related thrombosis in children: analysis of the Canadian Registry of Venous Thromboembolic Complications, *J Pediatr* 133:770-776, 1998.
18. Prandoni P, Polistena P, Bernardi E, et al: Upper-extremity deep vein thrombosis. Risk factors, diagnosis, and complications, *Arch Intern Med* 157:57-62, 1997.
19. Athale UH, Chan AK: Thrombosis in children with acute lymphoblastic leukemia: part I. Epidemiology of thrombosis in children with acute lymphoblastic leukemia, *Thromb Res* 111:125-131, 2003.
20. Andrew M: Congenital prothrombotic disorders: presentation during infancy and childhood. In Andrew M, Brooker L, editors: *Thromboembolic complications during infancy and childhood.* Hamilton, Ontario, 2000, BC Dekker.
21. Dahlback B: Inherited thrombophilia: resistance to activated protein C as a pathogenic factor of venous thromboembolism, *Blood* 85:607-614, 1995.
22. Citak A, Emre S, Sairin A, et al: Hemostatic problems and thromboembolic complications in nephrotic children, *Pediatr Nephrol* 14:138-142, 2000.
23. Andrew M, Brooker LA: Hemostatic complications in renal disorders of the young, *Pediatr Nephrol* 10:88-99, 1996.
24. Lee T, von Scheven E, Sandborg C: Systemic lupus erythematosus and antiphospholipid syndrome in children and adolescents, *Curr Opin Rheumatol* 13:415-421, 2001.
25. Hansen KE, Kong DF, Moore KD, Ortel TL: Risk factors associated with thrombosis in patients with antiphospholipid antibodies, *J Rheumatol* 28:2018-2024, 2001.
26. Monagle P. Thrombosis in pediatric cardiac patients, *Semin Thromb Hemost* 29:547-555, 2003.
27. Chan AK, Deveber G, Monagle P, et al: Venous thrombosis in children, *J Thromb Haemost* 1:1443-1455, 2003.
28. Lane DA, Mannucci PM, Bauer KA, et al: Inherited thrombophilia: part 1, *Thromb Haemost* 76:651-662, 1996.
29. Rosendaal FR: Risk factors for venous thrombotic disease, *Thromb Haemost* 82:610-619, 1999.
30. Poort SR, Rosendaal FR, Reitsma PH, Bertina RM: A common genetic variation in the 3′-untranslated region of the prothrombin gene is associated with elevated plasma prothrombin levels and an increase in venous thrombosis, *Blood* 88:3698-3703, 1996.
31. Lawson SE, Butler D, Enayat MS, Williams MD: Congenital thrombophilia and thrombosis: a study in a single centre, *Arch Dis Child* 81:176-178, 1999.
32. Cattaneo M: Hyperhomocysteinemia and thrombosis, *Lipids* 36(suppl):S13-S26, 2001.
33. Libourel EJ, Bank I, Meinardi JR, et al: Co-segregation of thrombophilic disorders in factor V Leiden carriers; the contributions of factor VIII, factor XI, thrombin activatable fibrinolysis inhibitor and lipoprotein(a) to the absolute risk of venous thromboembolism, *Haematologica* 87:1068-1073, 2002.
34. Meijers JC, Tekelenburg WL, Bouma BN, et al: High levels of coagulation factor XI as a risk factor for venous thrombosis, *N Engl J Med* 342:696-701, 2000.
35. Nowak-Gottl U, Junker R, Hartmeier M, et al: Increased lipoprotein(a) is an important risk factor for venous thromboembolism in childhood, *Circulation* 100:743-748, 1999.
36. van Hylckama Vlieg A, van der Linden IK, et al: High levels of factor IX increase the risk of venous thrombosis, *Blood* 95:3678-3682, 2000.
37. Kosch A, Koch HG, Heinecke A, et al: Childhood Thrombophilia Study Group. Increased fasting total homocysteine plasma levels as a risk factor for thromboembolism in children, *Thromb Haemost* 91:308-314, 2004.
38. Nowak-Gottl U, Kosch A: Factor VIII, D-Dimer, and thromboembolism in children, *N Engl J Med* 351:1051-1053, 2004.
40. von Depka M, Nowak-Gottl U, Eisert R, et al: Increased lipoprotein (a) levels as an independent risk factor for venous thromboembolism, *Blood* 96:3364-3368, 2000.
41. Manco-Johnson MJ, Grabowski EF, Hellgreen M, et al: Laboratory testing for thrombophilia in pediatric patients. On behalf of the Subcommittee for Perinatal and Pediatric Thrombosis of the Scientific and Standardization Committee of the International Society of Thrombosis and Haemostasis (ISTH), *Thromb Haemost* 88:155-156, 2002.
42. Nowak-Gottl U, Junker R, Kreuz W, et al: Risk of recurrent venous thrombosis in children with combined prothrombotic risk factors, *Blood* 97:858-862, 2001.
43. Lensing AWA, Hirsch J, Buller HR: Diagnosis of venous thrombosis. In Colman RW, Hirsch J, Marder VJ, Salzman EW, editors: *Hemostasis and thrombosis: basic principles and clinical practice,* ed 2. Philadelphia, 1994, JB Lippincott.
44. Barnes RW, Wu KK, Hoak JC: Fallibility of the clinical diagnosis of venous thrombosis, *JAMA* 234:605-607, 1975.
45. Wells PS, Anderson DR, Bormanis J, et al: Value of assessment of pretest probability of deep-vein thrombosis in clinical management, *Lancet* 350:1795-1798, 1997.
46. Lee AY, Ginsberg JS: The role of D-dimer in the diagnosis of venous thromboembolism, *Curr Opin Pulm Med* 3:275-279, 1997.
47. Lensing AW, Buller HR, Prandoni P, et al: Contrast venography, the gold standard for the diagnosis of deep-vein thrombosis: improvement in observer agreement, *Thromb Haemost* 67:8-12, 1992.
48. Baarslag HJ, van Beek EJ, Koopman MM, Reekers JA: Prospective study of color duplex ultrasonography compared with contrast

venography in patients suspected of having deep venous thrombosis of the upper extremities, *Ann Intern Med* 136:865-872, 2002.
49. Perrier A, Bounameaux H, Morabia A, et al: Diagnosis of pulmonary embolism by a decision analysis-based strategy including clinical probability, D-dimer levels, and ultrasonography: a management study, *Arch Intern Med* 156:531-536, 1996.
50. Baldt MM, Zontsich T, Stumpflen A, et al: Deep venous thrombosis of the lower extremity: efficacy of spiral CT venography compared with conventional venography in diagnosis, *Radiology* 200:423-428, 1996.
51. Anonymous: Value of the ventilation/perfusion scan in acute pulmonary embolism. Results of the prospective investigation of pulmonary embolism diagnosis (PIOPED). The PIOPED Investigators, *JAMA* 263:2753-279, 1990.
52. van Rossum AB, Pattynama PM, Ton ER, et al: Pulmonary embolism: validation of spiral CT angiography in 149 patients, *Radiology* 201:467-470, 1996.
53. Thornton MJ, Ryan R, Varghese JC, et al: A three-dimensional gadolinium-enhanced MR venography technique for imaging central veins, *AJR Am J Roentgenol* 173:999-1003, 1999.
54. Kroencke TJ, Taupitz M, Arnold R, et al: Three-dimensional gadolinium-enhanced magnetic resonance venography in suspected thrombo-occlusive disease of the central chest veins, *Chest* 120:1570-1576, 2001.
55. Talbott GA, Winters WD, Bratton SL, O'Rourke PP: A prospective study of femoral catheter-related thrombosis in children, *Arch Pediatr Adolesc Med* 149:288-291, 1995.
56. Kearon C, Julian JA, Newman TE, Ginsberg JS: Noninvasive diagnosis of deep venous thrombosis. McMaster Diagnostic Imaging Practice Guidelines Initiative, [published erratum appears in Ann Intern Med 129:425, 1998] *Ann Intern Med* 128:663-677, 1998.
57. Marsh D, Wilkerson SA, Cook LN, Pietsch JB: Right atrial thrombus formation screening using two-dimensional echocardiograms in neonates with central venous catheters, *Pediatrics* 81:284-286, 1988.
58. Kuhle S, Male C, Mitchell L: Developmental hemostasis: pro- and anticoagulant systems during childhood, *Semin Thromb Hemost* 29:329-338, 2003.
59. Andrew M, Marzinotto V, Massicotte P, et al: Heparin therapy in pediatric patients: a prospective cohort study, *Pediatr Res* 35:78-83, 1994.
60. Andrew M, Mitchell L, Vegh P, Ofosu F: Thrombin regulation in children differs from adults in the absence and presence of heparin, *Thromb Haemost* 72:836-842, 1994.
61. Raschke RA, Reilly BM, Guidry JR, et al: The weight-based heparin dosing nomogram compared with a "standard care" nomogram. A randomized controlled trial, *Ann Intern Med* 119:874-881, 1993.
62. Michelson AD, Bovill E, Andrew M: Antithrombotic therapy in children, *Chest* 108(4 suppl):506S-522S, 1995.
63. Monagle P, Chan A, Massicotte P, et al: Antithrombotic therapy in children: the Seventh ACCP Conference on Antithrombotic and Thrombolytic Therapy, *Chest* 126(3 suppl):645S-687S, 2004.
64. Avioli LV: Heparin-induced osteopenia: an appraisal, *Adv Exp Med Biol* 52:375-387, 1975.
65. Warkentin TE: Heparin-induced thrombocytopenia, *Curr Hematol Rep* 1:63-72, 2002.
66. Suh JS, Aster RH, Visentin GP: Antibodies from patients with heparin-induced thrombocytopenia/thrombosis recognize different epitopes on heparin: platelet factor 4, *Blood* 91:916-922, 1998.
67. Horne MK: *Non-immune heparin-platelet interactions, implications for the pathogenesis of heparin-induced thrombocytopenia,* ed 1. New York, Marcel Dekker, 2000.
68. Warkentin TE, Levine MN, Hirsh J, et al: Heparin-induced thrombocytopenia in patients treated with low-molecular-weight heparin or unfractionated heparin, *N Engl J Med* 332:1330-1335, 1995.
69. Warkentin TE: Clinical picture of heparin-induced thrombocytopenia. In Warkentin TE, Greiner A, editors: *Heparin-induced thrombocytopenia,* ed 2. New York, Dekker.
70. Warkentin TE, Heddle NM: Laboratory diagnosis of immune heparin-induced thrombocytopenia, *Curr Hematol Rep* 2:148-157, 2003.
71. Risch L, Fischer JE, Herklotz R, Huber AR: Heparin-induced thrombocytopenia in paediatrics: clinical characteristics, therapy and outcomes, *Intensive Care Med* 30:1615-1624, 2004.
72. Hirsh J, Heddle N, Kelton JG: Treatment of heparin-induced thrombocytopenia: a critical review, *Arch Intern Med* 164:361-369, 2004.
73. Hirsh J, Warkentin TE, Shaughnessy SG, et al: Heparin and low-molecular-weight heparin: mechanisms of action, pharmacokinetics, dosing, monitoring, efficacy, and safety, *Chest* 119(1 suppl): 64S-694S, 2001.
74. Linker A, Hovingh P: Isolation and characterization of oligosaccharides obtained from heparin by the action of heparinase, *Biochemistry* 11:563-568, 1972.
75. Cade JF, Buchanan MR, Boneu B, et al: A comparison of the antithrombotic and haemorrhagic effects of low molecular weight heparin fractions: the influence of the method of preparation, *Thromb Res* 35:613-625, 1984.
76. Revel-Vilk S, Chan AK: Anticoagulation therapy in children, *Semin Thromb Hemost* 29:425-432, 2003.
77. Massicotte P, Adams M, Marzinotto V, et al: Low-molecular-weight heparin in pediatric patients with thrombotic disease: a dose finding study, *J Pediatr* 128:313-318, 1996.
78. Hofmann S, Knoefler R, Lorenz N, et al: Clinical experiences with low-molecular weight heparins in pediatric patients, *Thromb Res* 103:345-353, 2001.
79. Monagle P, Michelson AD, Bovill E, Andrew M: Antithrombotic therapy in children, *Chest* 119(1 suppl):344S-370S, 2001.
80. Weitz JI: Low-molecular-weight heparins, *N Engl J Med* 337:688-698, 1997.
81. Van Ryn-McKenna J, Cai L, Ofosu FA, et al: Neutralization of enoxaparine-induced bleeding by protamine sulfate, *Thromb Haemost* 63:271-274, 1990.
82. Hirsh J, Dalen J, Anderson DR, et al: Oral anticoagulants: mechanism of action, clinical effectiveness, and optimal therapeutic range, *Chest* 119(1 suppl):8S-21S, 2001.
83. Andrew M, Brooker LA, Ginsberg J: Clinical problems in anticoagulant therapy: antithrombotic therapy for pediatric patients-new indications and therapies. American Society of Hematology Education Book. 2000. 8-15.
84. Marzinotto V, Leaker M, Massicotte P, Andrew M: Childhood Thrombophilia programs: an approach to the prevention and treatment of thromboembolic disease in pediatric patients. In: Ansell JE, Oertil LB, Wittkowsky AK, editors. *Managing oral anticoagulation.* Gaithersburg, MD, 1996, Aspen Publishing.
85. Shearer MJ, Rahim S, Barkhan P, Stimmler L: Plasma vitamin K1 in mothers and their newborn babies, *Lancet* 2:460-463, 1982.
86. Michelson AD, Bovill E, Monagle P, Andrew M: Antithrombotic therapy in children, *Chest* 114(5 suppl):748S-769S, 1998.
87. Richardson MW, Allen GA, Monahan PE: Thrombosis in children: current perspective and distinct challenges, *Thromb Haemost* 88:900-911, 2002.
88. Kaplan KL, Francis CW: Direct thrombin inhibitors, *Semin Hematol* 39:187-196, 2002.
89. Monagle P, Chan A, Massicotte P, et al: Antithrombotic therapy in children: the Seventh ACCP Conference on Antithrombotic and Thrombolytic Therapy, *Chest* 126(3 suppl):645S-687S, 2004.
90. Browne M, Newall F, Campbell J, et al: Thrombolytic therapy with tissue plasminogen activator (tPA): analysis of safety and outcomes in children, *J Thromb Haemost* 1(suppl):1488 (abstract).
91. Manco-Johnson MJ, Grabowski EF, Hellgreen M, et al: Recommendations for tPA thrombolysis in children. On behalf of the Scientific Subcommittee on Perinatal and Pediatric Thrombosis of the Scientific and Standardization Committee of the International Society of Thrombosis and Haemostasis, *Thromb Haemost* 88:157-158, 2002.
92. Monagle P, Chan A, Massicotte P, et al: Antithrombotic therapy in children: the Seventh ACCP Conference on Antithrombotic and Thrombolytic Therapy, *Chest* 126(3 suppl):645S-687S, 2004.
93. David M, Andrew M: Venous thromboembolic complications in children, *J Pediatr* 123:337-346, 1993.
94. Andrew M, Marzinotto V, Pencharz P, et al: A cross-sectional study of catheter-related thrombosis in children receiving total parenteral nutrition at home, *J Pediatr* 126:358-363, 1995.
95. Male C, Chait P, Andrew M, et al: Central venous line-related thrombosis in children: association with central venous line location and insertion technique, *Blood* 101:4273-4278, 2003.
96. Journeycake JM, Buchanan GR: Thrombotic complications of central venous catheters in children, *Curr Opin Hematol* 10:369-374, 2003.
97. Price V, Massicotte MP: Arterial thromboembolism in the pediatric population, *Semin Thromb Hemost* 29:557-565, 2003.
98. Streif W, Monagle P, South M, et al: Spontaneous arterial thrombosis in children, *J Pediatr* 134:110-112, 1999.

99. Levi M, Ten Cate H: Disseminated intravascular coagulation, *N Engl J Med* 341:586-592, 1999.
100. Levi M, de Jonge E, van der Poll T, ten Cate H: Disseminated intravascular coagulation, *Thromb Haemost* 82:695-705, 1999.
101. Hermans PW, Hibberd ML, Booy R, et al: 4G/5G promoter polymorphism in the plasminogen-activator-inhibitor-1 gene and outcome of meningococcal disease. Meningococcal Research Group, *Lancet* 354:556-660, 1999.
102. Baglin T: Disseminated intravascular coagulation: diagnosis and treatment, *BMJ* 312:683-687, 1996.
103. Levi M, van der Poll T, ten Cate H, van Deventer SJ: The cytokine-mediated imbalance between coagulant and anticoagulant mechanisms in sepsis and endotoxaemia, *Eur J Clin Investig* 27: 3-9, 1997.
104. Bernard GR, Vincent JL, Laterre PF, et al: Recombinant human protein C Worldwide Evaluation in Severe Sepsis (PROWESS) study group. Efficacy and safety of recombinant human activated protein C for severe sepsis, *N Engl J Med* 344:699-709, 2001.
105. Anderson DR, Levine MN: Thrombolytic therapy for the treatment of acute pulmonary embolism, *CMAJ* 146:1317-1324, 1992.
106. Buller HR, Agnelli G, Hull RD, et al: Antithrombotic therapy for venous thromboembolic disease: the Seventh ACCP Conference on Antithrombotic and Thrombolytic Therapy, *Chest* 126 (3 suppl):401S-428S, 2004.

CHAPTER

74

Hematology and Oncology Problems in the Intensive Care Unit

Martin L. Brecher and Joan Roberts

PEARLS

- Proactive measures for tumor lysis syndrome include hydration with hypotonic or isotonic saline solution, alkalinization, use of allopurinol, avoidance of exogenous potassium, close monitoring of fluid status, and frequent monitoring of serum potassium, sodium, chloride, bicarbonate, calcium, phosphorus, uric acid, blood urea nitrogen, and creatinine concentrations.
- Clinically significant hyperleukocytosis occurs with white blood cell count greater than 200,000/µl in acute myeloid leukemia, greater than 300,000/µl in acute lymphocytic leukemia, and greater than 600,000/µl in chronic myeloid leukemia.
- Concurrent thrombocytopenia and hyperleukocytosis increase risk of death. Aggressive therapy to correct coagulopathy with fresh-frozen plasma and vitamin K and to maintain platelet count greater than 20,000/µl is critical.
- Oxygen consumption becomes delivery dependent when the hemoglobin concentration decreases to approximately 5g/dl or less.
- Signs of significant cardiovascular compromise may not become evident until the child has lost at least 25% of total blood volume.
- Antifungal therapy should be instituted in febrile, neutropenic patients whose fever fails to defervesce within 3 to 5 days of treatment with broad-spectrum antibiotics.
- In the absence of other hemorrhagic risks, platelet counts greater than or equal to 10,000/µl are associated with little risk of serious bleeding.
- Gastrointestinal bleeding is an important cause of morbidity and mortality in patients with end stage renal disease.
- Intravenous administration of desmopressin acetate at a dosage of 0.3 µg/kg over 30 minutes improves platelet dysfunction caused by uremia within 1 hour, and the effect is maintained for 4 to 8 hours.
- Treatment of babies with severe neonatal ISO-immune thrombocytopenia consists of platelet transfusion of antigen-compatible platelets from unrelated donors or from the mother.

A variety of hematologic and oncologic disorders may cause critical illness resulting in admission of a child to the intensive care unit (ICU). Hematologic abnormalities arising from other conditions or their treatment may pose a challenge to physicians caring for the critically ill child. This chapter addresses the more frequently encountered problems. Chapter 77 addresses the complications of sickle cell anemia. Chapter 76 addresses the complications related to hematopoietic stem cell transplantation.

Hematologic Emergencies

Anemia

Anemia results from a deficiency in the number of red blood cells (RBCs), the RBC hemoglobin concentration, or both. The primary function of erythrocytes is to deliver oxygen to the body tissues. Any impairment of that function may have profound effects on a variety of organ systems.

Oxygen (O_2) delivery is a function of cardiac output and arterial O_2 content. The latter is dependent upon the hemoglobin concentration and the percentage of O_2 carried by the hemoglobin molecule, or O_2 saturation. Oxygen dissolved in the plasma contributes a negligible amount to overall O_2 delivery. Cardiac output is a product of stroke volume and heart rate. Abnormalities in any of these parameters may impair tissue oxygenation.

Oxygen consumption remains constant and is independent of delivery until the critical level, which varies for each organ system, is reached. The critical level is approached when the hemoglobin concentration decreases to approximately 5g/dl or less, assuming all other parameters remain constant.[1] Below this level, O_2 consumption becomes delivery dependent. The primary response to acute, normovolemic anemia is increased cardiac output, through an increase in stroke volume, an increase in heart rate, or both. As the hematocrit falls, blood becomes less viscous, increasing venous return and thus augmenting preload. In the patient with chronic anemia, increases in cardiac output are supplemented by increased levels of 2,3-diphosphoglycerate. This shifts the oxyhemoglobin curve to the right, increasing O_2 offload and, therefore, delivery to the tissues.

Anemias generally are classified either by the mechanism resulting in the hemoglobin deficit—decreased production, accelerated destruction, or loss of erythrocytes—or by the morphologic appearance of the erythrocyte (Table 74–1).[2] Decreased RBC production may result from a variety of causes, including congenital defects, such as Fanconi anemia and Diamond-Blackfan anemia, or from postnatal causes, including acquired aplastic anemia, erythropoietin deficiency associated with renal disease, bone marrow suppression secondary to drugs or infectious agents, nutritional deficiencies, and bone marrow infiltration.

Increased RBC destruction may be seen with erythrocyte membrane defects, as in hereditary spherocytosis;

TABLE 74–1

Physiologic Classification of Anemia[2]

A. Disorders of red cell production in which the rate of red cell production is less than expected for the degree of anemia
   1. Marrow failure
      a. Aplastic anemia
         Congenital
         Acquired
      b. Pure red cell aplasia
         Congenital
            Diamond-Blackfan syndrome
            Aase syndrome
         Acquired
            Transient erythroblastopenia of childhood
            Other
      c. Marrow replacement
         Malignancies
         Osteopetrosis
         Myelofibrosis
            Chronic renal disease
            Vitamin D deficiency
      d. Pancreatic insufficiency–marrow hypoplasia syndrome
   2. Impaired erythropoietin production
      a. Chronic renal disease
      b. Hypothyroidism, hypopituitarism
      c. Chronic inflammation
      d. Protein malnutrition
      e. Hemoglobin mutants with decreased affinity for oxygen

B. Disorders of erythroid maturation and ineffective erythropoiesis
   1. Abnormalities of cytoplasmic maturation
      a. Iron deficiency
      b. Thalassemia syndromes
      c. Sideroblastic anemias
      d. Lead poisoning
   2. Abnormalities of nuclear maturation
      a. Vitamin B_{12} deficiency
      b. Folic acid deficiency
      c. Thiamine-responsive megaloblastic anemia
      d. Hereditary abnormalities in folate metabolism
      e. Orotic aciduria
   3. Primary dyserythropoietic anemias (types I, II, III, IV)
   4. Erythropoietic protoporphyria
   5. Refractory sideroblastic anemia with vacuolization of marrow precursors and pancreatic dysfunction deficiency

C. Hemolytic anemias
   1. Defects of hemoglobin
      a. Structured mutants
      b. Synthetic mutants (thalassemia syndromes)
   2. Defects of the red cell membrane
   3. Defects of red cell metabolism
   4. Antibody mediated
   5. Mechanical injury to the erythrocyte
   6. Thermal injury to the erythrocyte
   7. Oxidant-induced red cell injury
   8. Infectious agent-induced red cell injury
   9. Paroxysmal nocturnal hemoglobinuria
   10. Plasma lipid-induced abnormalities of the red cell membrane

deficits in RBC enzymes such as glucose 6-phosphate dehydrogenase (G6PD); and in microangiopathic processes, including hemolytic uremic syndrome, thrombotic thrombocytopenic purpura, and disseminated intravascular coagulation (DIC). Antibody-mediated red cell destruction, whether autoimmune, alloimmune, or drug related, may result in profound anemia. Blood loss secondary to trauma, surgery, hemorrhage, or even frequent phlebotomy may lead to severe anemia.

Morphologic classifications of anemia are based on either erythrocyte size, as defined by mean corpuscular volume (MCV) and mean corpuscular hemoglobin concentration (MCHC), or by abnormalities in the erythrocyte shape (Table 74–2).[2] The normal values for MCV and MCHC vary with the child's age. A wide variety of conditions, some intrinsic to the erythrocyte and others related to extrinsic factors, may result in abnormal RBC morphology.

The following is a brief review of some of the more common causes of profound anemia that may be encountered in the pediatric intensive care setting. These causes include hemorrhagic anemia, decreased RBC production, and hemolytic anemia. Chapter 78 provides a discussion of sickle cell anemia and its complications, and other hemoglobinopathies.

TABLE 74–2

Classification of Anemias Based on Red Cell Size[2]

A. MICROCYTIC ANEMIAS
  1. Iron deficiency (nutritional, chronic blood loss)
  2. Chronic lead poisoning
  3. Thalassemia syndromes
  4. Sideroblastic anemias
  5. Chronic inflammation
  6. Some congenital hemolytic anemias with unstable hemoglobin

B. MACROCYTIC ANEMIAS
  1. With megaloblastic bone marrow
     a. Vitamin B_{12} deficiency
     b. Folic acid deficiency
     c. Hereditary orotic aciduria
     d. Thiamine-responsive anemia
  2. Without megaloblastic bone marrow
     a. Aplastic anemia
     b. Diamond-Blackfan syndrome
     c. Hypothyroidism
     d. Liver disease
     e. Bone marrow infiltration
     f. Dyserythropoietic anemias

C. NORMOCYTIC ANEMIAS
  1. Congenital hemolytic anemias
     a. Hemoglobin mutants
     b. Red cell enzyme defects
     c. Disorders of the red cell membrane
  2. Acquired hemolytic anemias
     a. Antibody mediated
     b. Microangiopathic hemolytic anemias
     c. Secondary to acute infections
  3. Acute blood loss
  4. Splenic pooling
  5. Chronic renal disease (usually)

Hemorrhagic Anemia

Anemia may result from either acute or chronic blood loss. Chronic bleeding generally causes anemia through depletion of iron stores.[3] The absence of accompanying hypovolemia and the development of other mechanisms to increase O_2 delivery in patients with chronic blood loss allow the patient to tolerate hemoglobin levels well below the normal range, with relatively mild symptomatology. Signs and symptoms of acute hemorrhage result from poor end-organ perfusion, with consequent diminished O_2 delivery. However, diagnosis of the presence and degree of blood loss may be difficult in an otherwise healthy child. Signs of impending shock, such as pallor, anxiety, and tachypnea, may be subtle.[4] Signs of significant cardiovascular compromise may not become evident until the child has lost at least 25% of total blood volume. Patients who have lost >25% of blood volume usually manifest age-related systolic hypotension.[4] Initial management should include the establishment of a secure airway, maintenance of ventilation, and initiation of rapid volume replacement via an adequate intravenous catheter.[5] Either crystalloid or colloid solutions are effective in restoring circulating volume. RBC transfusion should be given if O_2 delivery to the end organ is impaired.[6] Either whole blood or packed RBCs can be used. Because most collection facilities routinely separate blood units into components, whole blood often is not available.

If packed RBCs or plasma-poor red cells are used to correct O_2-carrying capacity during massive blood loss, deficits of coagulation factors develop earlier than during transfusion of whole blood. Hypofibrinogenemia generally develops first, followed by deficits in other clotting factors and later by thrombocytopenia. Fresh-frozen plasma (FFP) should be used to treat coagulopathy that develops during replacement of massive blood loss with RBCs. Transfusion of platelets should be guided by serial platelet counts.[7]

Central venous pressure should be monitored to allow for rapid administration of RBCs and volume replacement while decreasing the risks of hypervolemia. Blood and other fluids may be administered very rapidly until central venous pressure rises to between 6 and 7 mmHg. Chapter 27 discusses the diagnosis and management of shock.

Anemia Secondary to Bone Marrow Failure

A variety of hematologic diseases are associated with markedly decreased blood cell production. Acquired aplastic anemia is characterized by pancytopenia and by hypocellular or acellular bone marrow. By definition, severe aplastic anemia includes at least two of the three following blood counts: granulocytes <500/μl, platelets <20,000/μl, and anemia with a corrected reticulocyte count <1%, in conjunction with markedly hypocellular bone marrow.[8] Some cases are associated with chemical or drug exposure. Posthepatitis aplastic anemia typically occurs in young males, with pancytopenia presenting several weeks after severe liver inflammation.[9] Serologic testing is generally negative for known hepatitis viruses.[10] However, the majority of cases of acquired aplastic anemia are idiopathic. The pathophysiology now is believed to be immune mediated, with active destruction of blood-forming cells by lymphocytes. Excessive production of interferon-γ, tumor necrosis factor, and interleukin-2 have been noted.[11] Altered immunity results in CD34 cell death and in intracellular pathways leading to cell cycle arrest.[12]

Acquired aplastic anemia can be distinguished from bone marrow failure related to Fanconi anemia by specific assays for chromosomal susceptibility to chemical cross-linking agents that characterize Fanconi anemia.[13] Other constitutional syndromes may be suspected based on the presence of a pedigree of typical physical stigmata. Cytogenetic studies usually are normal in aplastic anemia, whereas aneuploidy or structural abnormalities are relatively common in myelodysplasia.[12] Myelodysplasia may evolve in patients treated for aplastic anemia. Some patients with paroxysmal nocturnal hemoglobinuria (PNH) develop bone marrow failure; conversely, PNH may evolve years after aplastic anemia is diagnosed.[12] The diagnosis of PNH can be made by demonstrating a deficiency of CD59 on erythrocytes and leukocytes by flow cytometry.

Regardless of the etiology of bone marrow failure, life-threatening complications may arise from blood cytopenias. The most common causes of death are bacterial sepsis and fungal infection secondary to refractory granulocytopenia.[14] Broad-spectrum antibiotics should be used to treat suspected infection in the granulocytopenic patient. In the past, gram-negative organisms were the most frequent cause of fulminant infection in this patient population. With the increased use of central venous catheters, gram-positive organisms now predominate.[15] Antifungal therapy should be instituted for patients whose fever fails to defervesce within 3 to 5 days of treatment with broad-spectrum antibiotics. Persistent, unexplained fever may require radiologic evaluation to look for evidence of invasive fungal infection.

Platelet transfusions should be used judiciously in an effort to avoid alloimmunization to platelet antigens. They generally should be reserved for episodes of active bleeding. Likewise, RBC transfusions should be reserved for patients whose cardiopulmonary function may be compromised as a result of profound anemia. The patient should not receive blood products donated by family members to avoid sensitization of the patient to leukocyte and platelet antigens of potential bone marrow donors. All blood products should be irradiated and leukodepleted to decrease the risk of posttransfusion graft-versus-host disease in the immunocompromised patient.[15]

Treatment of severe acquired aplastic anemia involves either replacement of bone marrow through stem cell transplantation or use of immunosuppressive therapy. The patient and immediate family members should undergo human leukocyte antigen (HLA) typing. Bone marrow or peripheral blood stem cell transplantation from a histocompatible sibling produces long-term survival rates of 75% to 80%.[16] This is the treatment of choice in the pediatric population. Chapter 76 provides details on the role of stem cell transplantation in aplastic anemia.

As many as 70% of patients may lack a suitably matched sibling donor. Less promising results are seen when the source of stem cells is a matched unrelated donor, or umbilical cord blood, because of the higher rate of graft-versus-host disease. For these patients, immunomodulation, which usually includes a combination of antithymocyte globulin, cyclosporin, and corticosteroids, often with use of hematopoietic growth factors, has resulted in response rates of 70% to 80%.[17,18] Not all responders achieve a complete remission; late relapses, as well as evolution to myelodysplasia and leukemia, are reported.[19]

Hemolytic Anemia

Hemolysis is defined as the destruction of RBCs with liberation of hemoglobin. Hemolysis may occur within either the blood vessels (intravascular hemolysis) or the reticuloendothelial system (extravascular hemolysis). Anemia results when the rate of RBC destruction exceeds the capacity for new RBC production in the bone marrow.[20]

Laboratory findings in patients with hemolytic anemia usually include increased reticulocyte count and elevated serum concentrations of unconjugated bilirubin and lactate dehydrogenase. Intravascular hemolysis usually results in decreased serum haptoglobin concentrations. Premature destruction of RBCs may result from intrinsic RBC abnormalities, such as hemoglobinopathies or red cell membrane defects, or from a variety of extrinsic factors (Figure 74-1)[2]. Numerous hemoglobin variants that can result in shortened RBC survival have been identified. Individuals with sickling hemoglobinopathies are prone to a variety of complications that may require treatment in a critical care unit. Chapter 77 provides details on the management of sickle

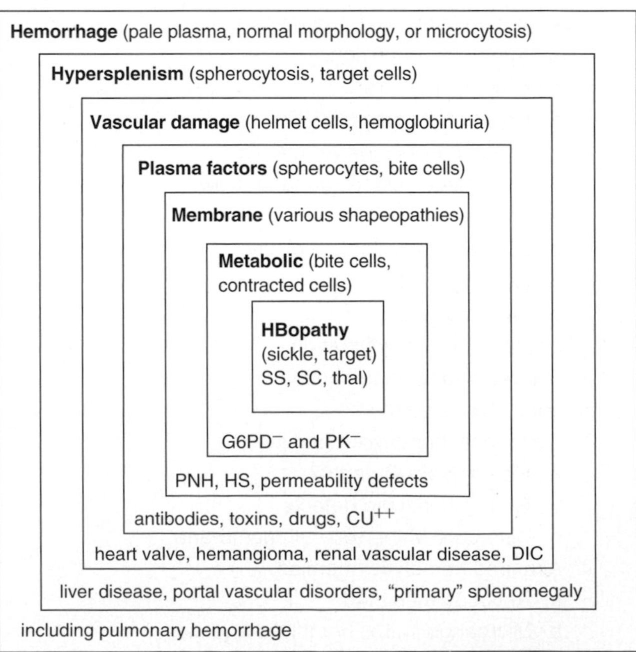

FIGURE 74–1 • Causes of premature destruction of the red blood cell.[21] *CU,* copper; *DIC,* disseminated intravascular coagulation; *G6PD,* glucose 6-phosphate dehydrogenase; *HS,* hereditary spherocytosis; *PK,* pyruvate kinase; PNH, paroxysmal nocturnal hemoglobinuria.

cell disease. Abnormalities in the structure of the RBC membrane, as in hereditary spherocytosis, or decreased quantities of RBC enzymes, as in G6PD deficiency, also result in shortened red cell survival. Hemolysis in these settings is primarily extravascular.

Mechanical disruption of the red cell membrane secondary to factors extrinsic to the RBC may lead to macroangiopathic hemolytic anemia, as with turbulent flow around a prosthetic heart valve, or microangiopathic hemolytic anemia, caused by fibrin deposition in the microvasculature. The latter process is seen in consumptive disorders, including DIC, hemolytic uremic syndrome, and thrombotic thrombocytopenic purpura.[21] In these entities, hemolysis is primarily intravascular. Schistocytes are characteristically seen on the blood film.

The hemolytic processes that result from abnormal interactions between erythrocytes and the immune system are known collectively as *autoimmune hemolytic anemia* (AIHA).[2] AIHA can be classified as either *primary,* in which there is no identifiable systemic illness other than a history of a recent viral-like illness in many cases, or *secondary,* in which the hemolytic anemia is present in the context of another illness. AIHA has been reported as a manifestation of systemic autoimmune disorders (e.g., lupus erythematosus), immunodeficiency disorders, malignancies, and specific infections, or it may be drug-induced (Table 74-3).[21]

AIHA also can be classified by the thermal sensitivity of the autoantibodies. The most common form is the result of warm-reactive immunoglobulin IgG autoantibodies directed against RBC membrane proteins. Hemolysis is extravascular, with sensitized erythrocytes cleared primarily in the spleen. Cold-agglutinin disease, the second most common form of AIHA, is most frequently associated with *Mycoplasma pneumoniae* infections, but it also is associated with other infectious agents, including Epstein-Barr virus, cytomegalovirus, and mumps virus. In this disorder, IgM autoantibody binds to the red cell and fixes complement. The erythrocytes may undergo intravascular hemolysis, or they may be cleared by the reticuloendothelial system, primarily in the liver. Paroxysmal cold hemoglobinuria is a rare variant of AIHA in which an IgG autoantibody that binds at cold temperature to the P-antigen of the erythrocyte and fixes complement efficiently (the Donath-Landsteiner antibody) causes intravascular hemolysis. It usually follows a viral-like illness.[21]

TABLE 74–3

Classification of Autoimmune Hemolytic Anemia in Children[21]

PRIMARY AIHA*
Warm-reactive autoantibodies, usually IgG
Paroxysmal cold hemoglobinuria, usually IgG
Cold-agglutinin disease, usually IgM
SECONDARY AIHA†
Systemic autoimmune disease (e.g., lupus)
Malignancy (Hodgkin and non-Hodgkin lymphoma)
Immunodeficiency
Infection (Mycoplasma, viruses)
Drug induced

AIHA, autoimmune hemolytic anemia; *IgG,* immunoglobulin G.
*Occurs in the majority of affected children and often follows a nonspecific viral-like syndrome, but in the absence of another systemic illness.
†Occurs in association with another systemic process.

Although drug-induced autoantibodies are not common in children, they are reported with a variety of antibiotics, including penicillins[22] and cephalosporins.[23] Mechanisms of drug-induced hemolysis may include autoantibody formation and adsorption of the drug onto the red cell membrane, with immune complex formation with IgG or IgM.[24]

Patients with AIHA usually present with pallor, jaundice, and splenomegaly on physical examination. The reticulocyte count is generally elevated, although initially it may be low or normal. Spherocytes and polychromasia are present on the peripheral blood film, and nucleated RBCs are frequently seen. RBC agglutination may be present in cold-reactive AIHA. The direct antiglobulin test (Coombs test) demonstrates the presence of antibodies or complement on the red cells. The indirect antiglobulin test measures the presence of unbound antierythrocyte antibodies in the patient's serum.

Therapy is determined by the type of AIHA and the severity of clinical symptoms. Profound anemia, usually with a hemoglobin level of less than 5 g/dl, may result in cardiovascular compromise and requires erythrocyte transfusion to increase O_2-carrying capacity. The presence of autoantibodies may make cross-matching blood difficult, and the patient may require transfusion with "least incompatible" blood.[25] Significant hemolytic transfusion reactions are infrequent.[25] However, severe hemolysis occurs on rare occasions, with hemoglobinemia and hemoglobinuria resulting in renal failure. Therefore transfusion should be started at a slow rate, and both plasma and urine samples should be checked periodically for free hemoglobin.[21] Patients with cold-reactive antibodies should be kept warm, and a blood warmer should be used for the transfused blood.[26] Even in the absence of transfusion, significant intravascular hemolysis may occur in patients with cold-reactive antibodies. Maintaining good renal blood flow and careful monitoring of urine output in this setting are important.[27]

Corticosteroids are useful in slowing the hemolytic process, particularly in patients with IgG autoantibodies, in whom they appear to inhibit Fc receptor-mediated clearance of sensitized erythrocytes.[28] The usual dosage is 1 to 2 mg/kg methylprednisolone given intravenously every 6 hours until the patient is clinically stable. The patient then can be switched to oral prednisone at a dosage of 2 mg/kg/day for 2 to 4 weeks, followed by a slow taper over 1 to 3 months.[21] Corticosteroids may also be effective in cold agglutinin disease, although the response is less predictable.[29] High-dose intravenous γ-globulin (IVIG), given on a schedule of 1 g/kg/day for 5 days, produces response in approximately one third of patients with warm-reactive disease.[30] Plasmapheresis and plasma exchange may be beneficial, particularly in patients with IgM autoantibodies.[31]

The overall prognosis for children with AIHA is good. Cold-reactive AIHA generally resolves completely.

Some patients with warm-reactive antibodies have a chronic course, marked by remissions and exacerbations.[21]

Thrombocytopenia

When the endothelium of blood vessels is interrupted, platelets bind to the newly exposed adhesive proteins, beginning a complex process that results in formation of a platelet plug. Thrombocytopenia or platelet dysfunction results in excessive bleeding, most commonly involving the skin and mucous membranes. Clinical manifestations include petechiae and purpura, epistaxis, gastrointestinal bleeding, hematuria, and menorrhagia. Intracranial hemorrhage is an infrequent manifestation of thrombocytopenia.

Thrombocytopenia may be secondary to either decreased platelet production or increased platelet destruction. Decreased platelet production may result from primary bone marrow failure states or from bone marrow infiltration by malignant cells, as in leukemia, lymphoma, and metastatic solid tumors. Bone marrow suppression is a common side effect of antineoplastic therapy, including both chemotherapy and radiotherapy, and frequently leads to periods of significant thrombocytopenia.

Indications for platelet transfusion in these settings vary with the underlying cause of decreased platelet production and the patient's clinical status. Patients with primary bone marrow failure, who likely will experience prolonged thrombocytopenia, are generally transfused only for active bleeding because of the risk of alloimmunization, which can decrease responsiveness to future transfusions. In addition, exposure to multiple platelet donors may jeopardize the success of bone marrow transplantation by increasing the risk of graft rejection.[32]

In the absence of other hemorrhagic risks, platelet counts of greater than or equal to 10,000/dl are associated with very little risk of bleeding.[33] The threshold for transfusion may need to be set higher in patients with sepsis, decreased humoral coagulants, or other risk factors. Transfusion of platelets is generally recommended for platelet counts less than 50,000/dl in the perioperative setting and for platelet counts less than 100,000/dl for neurologic or ophthalmologic surgery.[34] The risk of platelet alloimmunization can be reduced by using ABO-compatible donors and by leukoreducing blood products.[33] Use of single-donor apheresis units rather than pooled platelet concentrates can reduce donor exposure, but whether such usage reduces the incidence of platelet alloimmunization is unclear.[35]

Shortened platelet survival, with resultant thrombocytopenia, may be the result of either immune or nonimmune mechanisms.

Immune Thrombocytopenia

Immune platelet destruction may be caused by autoantibodies, drug-dependent antibodies, or alloantibodies. Alloantibodies result from exposure to polymorphic epitopes expressed on foreign platelets to which the patient has been exposed (see previous section). Drug-induced thrombocytopenia may be suggested by the patient's medication history. Laboratory tests for specific drug-associated antiplatelet antibodies are available. In immune thrombocytopenia purpura (ITP), autoantibodies to platelets may be associated with other autoimmune disorders or immune deficiency states, or following viral illness or immunization.[36] Frequently, no predisposing condition is identified (idiopathic thrombocytopenia purpura). Regardless of cause, antibody-coated platelets are rapidly removed in the reticuloendothelial system, with the bulk of the destruction occurring in the spleen. These children typically present with petechiae, purpura, and bleeding from mucous membranes. There is an isolated thrombocytopenia. The bone marrow responds with increased platelet production. The rapid turnover in platelets results in younger, somewhat larger, platelets entering the blood. Because these platelets are more hemostatically effective, serious bleeding rarely occurs.[37]

The primary goal of therapy in children with ITP is preventing central nervous system (CNS) bleeding and reducing the risk of blood loss from gastrointestinal bleeding, prolonged epistasis, menorrhagia, or hematuria. The need for intervention in the absence of significant hemorrhage remains the subject of debate.[38] The goals of therapy are to slow the clearance of sensitized thrombocytes in the spleen and to reduce antibody production. When therapy is warranted, initial medical management usually involves the use of corticosteroids or IVIG.[39,40] The usual steroid prescribed is prednisone at a dose of 2 mg/kg/day. High-dose methyl-prednisolone, given at a dose of 30 mg/kg/day intravenously for 3 days, also is effective.[41] Bone marrow should be evaluated to rule out malignancy before corticosteroid therapy is started. IVIG usually is given at a dose of 1 g/kg/day for 1 to 2 days. Intravenous infusion of anti-Rh(D) immunoglobulin, in doses of 50 to 75 μg/kg to individuals who have Rh(D)-positive RBCs, prolongs survival of antibody-coated platelets in patients with ITP. As with IVIG, the major mechanism is thought to be blockage of Fc receptors on reticuloendothelial cells.[42] Use of these agents usually halts bleeding and raises platelet counts to safe levels within a few days, although evidence indicating they affect the overall course of the disease is lacking.

Although intracranial hemorrhage is a rare complication of ITP, patients with headaches, persistent vomiting, or neurologic symptoms should be evaluated by computed tomographic scan of the head. Intracranial hemorrhage requires immediate intervention, usually including IVIG, corticosteroids, and emergency splenectomy.[43] A splenectomy should be performed if a craniotomy is required, to maximize the perioperative platelet count.[44] Platelet transfusions are of little benefit in ITP and generally do not result in an increase in the platelet count because of the rapid consumption of transfused platelets. Nevertheless, intermittent (2–4 U/m^2 every 6–8 hours) or continuous (0.5–1 U/m^2/hour) platelet transfusions have been given for life-threatening hemorrhage, with some decrease in bleeding reported.[44,45] Plasmapheresis may be beneficial in patients who do not respond to these interventions.[46]

Nonimmune Thrombocytopenia

Increased platelet consumption with resultant thrombocytopenia occurs in diseases associated with extensive vascular endothelial damage, including hemolytic uremic syndrome and thrombotic thrombocytopenic purpura.[47,48] Aggregates of activated platelets become trapped in small blood vessels, causing a microangiopathic hemolytic anemia. Schistocytes usually are present on the peripheral blood film. Platelet transfusions should be given only for life-threatening bleeding because they may worsen the thrombotic process.[49]

Endothelial activation may result in rapid platelet consumption in premature infants with necrotizing enterocolitis. In this setting, aggressive use of platelet transfusions may be required because of the high incidence of gastrointestinal bleeding and the risk of CNS hemorrhage in the preterm infant.

DIC is a process characterized by generalized activation of the plasma coagulation pathways within small blood vessels, with formation of fibrin and depletion of circulating levels of both humeral clotting factors and platelets. DIC is secondary to a systemic insult, most often sepsis or shock. Treatment should be directed to the underlying cause. Hemorrhage frequently occurs at platelet counts greater than 10,000/μl because of concomitant depletion of clotting factors. Platelet transfusions may be necessary to control the bleeding. DIC had been thought to be the etiology of much of the multiorgan system failure (MOF) in ICU patients, with formation of a large number of microthrombotic foci leading to organ microcirculation failure and subsequent failure of the organ itself.[50] More recently, some studies have suggested that vascular endothelial damage induced by humeral mediators is the primary cause of thrombocytopenic MOF.[51] In these instances, thrombocytopenia may be a marker of poor prognosis rather than a cause of ICU mortality.[52]

Bleeding in Uremia

Hemorrhagic manifestations in patients with renal failure are characterized by purpura and prolonged bleeding from puncture sites and mucous membranes. Gastrointestinal bleeding is an important cause of morbidity and mortality in patients with end-stage renal disease.[53] Concurrent hypertension increases the risk of subdural hematoma. The hemostatic defect in uremia is multifactorial and results in part from altered metabolism of platelets and vascular endothelial cells and from abnormal interactions between platelets and vascular endothelium.[54]

When uremia is present, clinical bleeding may be increased relative to the degree of thrombocytopenia resulting from secondary platelet dysfunction. Intravenous administration of desmopressin acetate (DDAVP) at a dosage of 0.3 μg/kg over 30 minutes improves platelet dysfunction caused by uremia within 1 hour, and the effect is maintained for 4 to 8 hours.[55] Tachyphylaxis may occur after two to three doses. Intravenous conjugated estrogens or oral estrogens cause slower but more sustained improvements in bleeding time.[53]

When severe anemia is present, platelets travel closer to the midstream and are less likely to interact with the vascular endothelium. In addition, RBCs exert metabolic effects on platelets by enhancing adenosine diphosphate (ADP) and thromboxane A_2 release. Therefore use of red cell transfusions or erythropoietin to increase the hematocrit to 30% helps to correct the bleeding time.[56] Further increase in hematocrit increases the risk of thrombosis, particularly of arteriovenous shunts and the extracorporeal hemodialysis circuit. Dialysis results in improved platelet function through reduction of azotemia.

Thrombocytopenia in Neonates

The major mechanism underlying neonatal thrombocytopenia, particularly in preterm babies in whom thrombocytopenia develops within 72 hours of birth, is reduced platelet production secondary to impairment of megakaryopoiesis.[57] In most cases, the pregnancy has been complicated by placental insufficiency and/or fetal hypoxia. Severe thrombocytopenia, with platelet nadir less than 50,000/μl, is unusual, and recovery generally occurs by 7 to 10 days of life. Treatment is rarely necessary. Late thrombocytopenia (presenting older than 72 hours of age) in preterm babies is most often associated with bacterial sepsis with or without DIC and often requires treatment. The most important aspect of therapy is treatment of the underlying sepsis, including removal of indwelling vascular access lines, if evidence of catheter-related sepsis is seen.[57] Platelet transfusions are recommended to maintain a platelet count greater than 50,000/dl, especially in the first week of life, because of the risk of intraventricular hemorrhage.[58]

In otherwise well full-term babies, the most common condition leading to severe thrombocytopenia with a high risk of hemorrhage is neonatal alloimmune thrombocytopenia, which usually is the result of anti-human platelet antigen 1 (anti-HPA1). In severe untreated cases, intracranial hemorrhage occurs in 10% to 30% of affected fetuses and babies. The diagnosis can be made from HPA-1 genotyping of the baby and the mother. Treatment of babies with significant thrombocytopenia consists of platelet transfusion of antigen-compatible platelets from unrelated donors or from the mother.[59]

The most appropriate platelet product for transfusion to neonates is leukodepleted and cytomegalovirus negative. Whenever possible, the plasma should be ABO compatible with the baby's RBCs. Response to platelet transfusion should be monitored by measuring the 1-hour posttransfusion platelet increment.[57]

Platelet transfusions are of little value in newborns with severe thrombocytopenia secondary to maternal ITP. In this setting, either corticosteroids or IVIG should be given for a platelet count less than 50,000/μl or for signs of bleeding.[57]

Oncologic Emergencies

Tumor Lysis Syndrome

Tumor lysis syndrome refers to any of a number of metabolic abnormalities that occur as a result of tumor cell death, either spontaneously or related to treatment interventions. Typically, initiation of chemotherapy for rapidly growing tumors that are sensitive to antineoplastic drugs results in release of the intracellular contents into the circulation. The release of intracellular potassium and organic and inorganic phosphates results in hyperkalemia and hyperphosphatemia. Hyperphosphatemia in turn leads to hypocalcemia. Hyperuricemia is caused by the rapid breakdown of nucleic acids, particularly because many chemotherapeutic regimens target deoxyribonucleic acid.

Hematologic malignancies, including acute leukemias and lymphomas, particularly Burkitt lymphoma, where tumor burden is large and growth fraction is high, have been the most frequently associated with tumor lysis syndrome. Laboratory criteria for tumor lysis syndrome, including abnormal serum levels of uric acid, electrolytes, and creatinine, have been reported in 70% of children with hematologic malignancies, with clinical tumor lysis syndrome (association of acute renal failure and/or hyperkalemia) present in 3%.[60] As more active and targeted chemotherapeutic regimens have become available, tumor lysis syndrome with solid tumors also has been recognized. The development of tumor lysis syndrome may be associated with radiation, corticosteroids, hormonal agents, and other agents given prior to the diagnosis of malignancy. In addition to type of malignancy, other risk factors for the development of tumor lysis syndrome include preexisting renal insufficiency, dehydration, and exposure to nephrotoxic drugs. Finally, elevated lactic dehydrogenase levels associated with tumor lysis syndrome are indicative of likely progression to renal failure.[61]

Hyperkalemia represents the most life-threatening derangement of tumor lysis syndrome. At plasma potassium concentrations of greater than 6.5 mmol/L, cardiac arrhythmias such as asystole, ventricular tachycardia, and ventricular fibrillation may occur. Other manifestations of hyperkalemia include weakness, paresthesias, muscle cramps, nausea, vomiting, and diarrhea. Hyperphosphatemia usually results in renal insufficiency after precipitation with calcium in the renal tubules. The serum calcium concentration rapidly decreases as precipitation with phosphate occurs. Hypocalcemia secondary to tumor lysis syndrome has been associated with the development of severe muscle cramping, tetany, and cardiac arrhythmias. In addition to occurring in the kidney, precipitation of calcium and phosphorus may occur in other tissues, such as muscle. Patients with hyperuricemia may experience nausea, vomiting, diarrhea, or hematuria. As urate crystal deposition occurs in the distal renal tubule, other symptoms of renal failure ensue, including edema, oliguria, anuria, flank pain, and lethargy.

Recognition of patients at risk for tumor lysis syndrome allows preventative measures to prevent its progression. Proactive therapies include admission to an ICU, establishment of adequate venous access, close observation of fluid status, and frequent laboratory monitoring of serum potassium, sodium, chloride, bicarbonate, calcium, phosphorus, uric acid, blood urea nitrogen, and creatinine concentrations. Hydration therapy, including hypotonic or isotonic saline, should begin as soon as possible to allow 24 to 48 hours prior to initiation of chemotherapy if possible and should continue 48 to 72 hours after completion of chemotherapy. A hypotonic saline solution should be used when the urinary sodium concentration is less than 150 mEq/L to reduce the risk of uric acid supersaturation.

Mannitol may be considered if sufficient diuresis cannot be achieved with intravenous hydration alone. Other preemptive measures include avoidance of oral or exogenous potassium, potassium-sparing diuretics, angiotensin-converting enzyme inhibitors, angiotensin II receptor blockers, heparin, and agents that block tubular reabsorption of uric acid. Finally, delay or reduction in chemotherapy must be considered, depending on the clinical circumstance.

Hyperkalemia

Hyperkalemia therapy includes cation exchange resins given either orally or rectally to bind potassium for elimination through the bowel, intravenous calcium gluconate to antagonize the action of potassium on cardiac myocytes, sodium bicarbonate to correct acidosis, shifting potassium into cells, insulin and glucose (which also shift potassium intracellularly), diuretic therapy to enhance excretion, and dialysis. Although temporizing measures to reduce hyperkalemia can be used, hyperkalemia associated with tumor lysis syndrome should be treated immediately with dialysis.

Hyperphosphatemia and Hypocalcemia

Phosphate binders such as aluminum antacids decrease the gut absorption of phosphate. Usually, treatment of hyperphosphatemia corrects any hypocalcemia. Calcium itself should not be administered (except for cases of hyperkalemia) because it may increase the calcium × phosphate solubility product, resulting in metastatic tissue calcification and nephrocalcinosis.

Hyperuricemia

Alkalinization with sodium bicarbonate favors ionization of uric acid to maximize its solubility. Generally, urine pH greater than 7 is sought, but caution should be exercised not to overly alkalinize patients. In such a case, elevated urinary pH may decrease the solubility of phosphate complexes, leading to massive phosphate crystalluria and precipitation of phosphate. The production of uric acid, the final product in the oxidation of purine nucleotides, is dependent on the enzyme xanthine oxidase. Allopurinol, an inhibitor of xanthine oxidase, should be administered at doses depending on renal clearance. Allopurinol has been the mainstay of treatment for many years but has several drawbacks. First, because it blocks production of new uric acid, accumulated uric acid still must be excreted, usually requiring 2 to 3 days before a reduction in uric acid concentration is observed. Second, levels of uric acid precursors such as xanthine are increased and may result in nephropathy. Third, allopurinol impairs metabolism of chemotherapeutic reagents. Urate oxidase is a nonhuman proteolytic enzyme that oxidizes human uric acid to allantoins. Allantoins are highly soluble at urinary pH and are readily excreted in the urine, with less potential for precipitation. Rapid reduction in uric acid levels occurs with no precursor buildup. Recombinant urate oxidase (Rasburicase), developed to avoid anaphylaxis, has been studied in pediatric patients, with reduction of mean uric acid level from 15.1 to 0.4 mg/dl in 24 to 48 hours in hyperuricemic patients.[62] Efficacy of Rasburicase compared with allopurinol in reducing exposure to plasma uric acid in children at high risk for developing tumor lysis syndrome has been suggested,[63] but Rasburicase remains much more expensive. Rasburicase is indicated for patients with very high levels of uric acid or renal failure, and prevention of ICU interventions have been shown to be cost effective.[64] Rasburicase is contraindicated in patients with G6PD deficiency who are unable to break down hydrogen peroxide, an endproduct of the urate oxidase reaction.

Hyperleukocytosis

The pathophysiology of hyperleukocytosis relates to marked elevation in blood viscosity, affected by both the sum of erythrocyte and leukocyte volumes and the deformability of cells. The normal serum viscosity relative to water is approximately 1.5, and the clinical manifestations of hyperviscosity become most apparent when the serum viscosity relative to water is greater than 4. Significantly elevated numbers of leukocytes result in aggregation of leukocytes and obstruction of small vessels, reduced perfusion of the microcirculation, and vascular stasis. Extreme elevation of blasts is associated with increased risk of intracranial parenchymal hemorrhage, typically in multiple lesions in the white matter. These may rupture into the ventricles or subarachnoid space. The disputed mechanisms of hemorrhage are leukostasis (plugging of small cerebral vessels by blasts) resulting in local hypoxia and vessel destruction or invasion of the blood vessels by growth of leukemia cells (leukemic nodules). It is becoming increasingly evident that leukostasis results from the adhesive interactions between leukemic blasts and the endothelium, likely mediated by cytokines in the vascular microenvironment, with subsequent migration of leukemic blasts in the perivascular space. The adhesion molecules displayed by the leukemic blasts and their chemotactic response to cytokines may be as important as cell number in causing leukostasis.[65] This may explain the variability in clinical presentation among patients with a range of peripheral blast counts and why some patients but not others develop leukostasis.

In adults the most prevalent causes of hyperviscosity syndrome include a variety of dysproteinemias, whereas in children malignancies are the most common diagnoses. Hyperleukocytosis, defined as a leukocyte (white blood cell [WBC]) count greater than 100,000/μl, is seen in 5% to 20% of children diagnosed with leukemia and is more often observed in patients with acute lymphocytic leukemia (ALL).[66] Clinically significant hyperleukocytosis occurs with WBC count greater than 200,000/μl in acute myeloid leukemia, greater than 300,000/μl in ALL, and greater than 600,000/μl in chronic myeloid leukemia.[67] Myeloblasts and monoblasts, which tend to be larger and more rigid than lymphoblasts and granulocytes, are more likely to obstruct vessels, even in smaller numbers. Other benign causes of hyperviscosity include leukemoid reaction, polycythemia vera, and accumulation of abnormal hemoglobins in sickle cell disease.

Although all organs are susceptible to the effects of hyperviscosity, the intracerebral and pulmonary circulations are most often affected. Symptoms may include headache, mental status changes, seizures, visual disturbance, respiratory distress, and hypoxemia. Subsequent adult respiratory distress syndrome with right ventricular failure may ensue.

Although elevated WBC count is diagnostic of hyperleukocytosis, additional studies may be helpful, depending on clinical circumstances. Arterial measurement of oxygenation should be promptly obtained rather than relying on pulse oximetry because elevated met-hemoglobin concentration may be present.[68] Immediate cytoreduction is indicated when excessive O_2 metabolism of leukocytes causes tissue hypoxemia. Elevated serum lactate levels have been described as an early sign of microcirculatory failure.[69] Chest x-ray findings of pulmonary leukostasis may be normal or reveal diffuse interstitial infiltrates.

The therapies for hyperleukocytosis have not undergone controlled study. Diuretic therapy and packed red cell transfusion both increase viscosity and should be avoided. Periods of concurrent thrombocytopenia and hyperleukocytosis increase risk of death. Aggressive therapy with FFP and vitamin K to correct coagulopathy and maintain platelet count greater than 20,000/μl is critical.[70] Hydration, alkalinization, and allopurinol have been used in patients with ALL and WBC greater than 100,000/μl, with 81% reduction of WBC within 36 hours without pulmonary or neurologic complications.[71] More aggressive therapies must be considered for patients who are symptomatic, those with laboratory evidence of hypoxia or ischemia, or in certain patients depending on malignancy type and WBC. Both exchange transfusion and leukapheresis can be used to rapidly lower WBC. Leukapheresis involves withdrawal of anticoagulated blood via a vascular catheter, separation of different blood components by either centrifugation or membrane filtration, removal of the undesired component, and reinfusion of the remaining components with replacement fluid into the patient. No randomized trials of cytoreduction have been performed, and although a reduced incidence of electrolyte abnormalities has been shown, no improvement in pulmonary status, CNS outcome, or mortality has been demonstrated. Despite the use of cytoreduction, hyperleukocytosis remains a clinicobiologic feature of high-risk disease. Complications of leukapheresis include difficulty with vascular access, rapid rebound of WBC count, and need for anticoagulation. No beneficial role has been demonstrated for use of steroids or emergency cranial radiation.[72]

Spinal Cord Compression

Spinal cord compression by malignancy is uncommon but not rare in children, affecting 2.7% to 5% of children with cancer and 4% of children at diagnosis of cancer.[67] Of 2259 children with solid malignant tumors treated from 1962 to 1987, 5% developed spinal epidural metastasis with spinal cord compression during the course of their disease.[73] Metastatic epidural spinal cord compression is more common than are primary spinal cord tumors. It is most frequent with Ewing sarcoma, neuroblastoma, and primitive neuroectodermal tumors and is less frequent with Hodgkin lymphoma, nephroblastoma, and germ cell tumors.[73,74]

Most cord compression in children with cancer results from epidural compression due to extension of paravertebral tumor through the intervertebral foramina or, less commonly, extension of the tumor in the vertebral column. Compression of the vertebral venous plexus by epidural tumor causes vasogenic cord edema, venous hemorrhage, myelin loss, and ischemia.[75]

Spinal cord compression is localized mainly to the dorsal and lumbosacral regions (42% each) and is the initial manifestation of the disease in 25% to 67% of patients who develop spinal cord compression.[74,76] Back pain, motor dysfunction, sphincter dysfunction, and alterations in sensation are common initial symptoms and should prompt thorough neurologic examination. Any evidence of neurologic deficit warrants further evaluation, and magnetic resonance imaging (MRI) is the first-line imaging modality. Myelography and cerebrospinal fluid examination both pose the risk of neurologic deterioration from lumbar puncture, and radiographs are abnormal in only 30% to 35% of pediatric patients with spinal cord compression.[67]

Spinal cord compression as a result of malignant disease is a medical emergency. The manifestations of spinal cord compression are difficult to diagnose at an early phase, particularly in the youngest patients. Unequivocally, the patient with a history of progressive spinal cord dysfunction and focal deficit or percussion tenderness of the spine requires 1 mg/kg dexamethasone intravenously over 30 minutes. A lower dose of dexamethasone 0.25 to 0.5 mg/kg orally every 6 hours has been suggested for cases without neurologic deficit, followed by MRI within the next 24 hours. Treatment of a cord-compressing lesion next mandates a decision between immediate surgical decompression, radiation therapy, or chemotherapy. This decision is influenced by a number of factors, including presence of a histologic diagnosis, likelihood of response to chemotherapy or radiotherapy, degree and rate of progression of neurologic deficit, and underlying chance of survival. Although controversy exists, decompressive laminectomy is indicated for tumors without a diagnosis, patients with small cell tumors with very rapid neurologic deterioration or complete loss of motor function, and sarcoma, with the exception of osteogenic sarcoma.[73] Preventing decompressive laminectomy in a child when possible is important because surgery often leads to scoliosis, kyphosis, and anterior subluxation. Most long-term survivors who are treated with surgery require subsequent treatment for orthopedic sequelae.[77] Although adults with complete sensory and motor loss below the level of spinal cord compression rarely recover neurologic function, 30% to 60% of treated children experience neurologic recovery.[73,74,78]

Superior Vena Cava Syndrome

Superior vena cava syndrome encompasses the signs and symptoms related to compression or obstruction of the superior vena cava (SVC), which in childhood most commonly results from anterior mediastinal mass, middle mediastinal lymph nodes, or occlusion of the SVC itself. Although SVC obstruction is uniformly present in the syndrome, compression of the other mediastinal structures, including trachea, large airways, pulmonary vessels, and aorta, may contribute to the pathologic consequences. SVC syndrome is most often caused by lymphoid malignancy, including non-Hodgkin lymphoma, acute lymphocytic leukemia, and Hodgkin disease. Indwelling catheters, previous cardiac surgery,[79] previous extracorporeal life support,[80] right-sided congenital diaphragmatic hernia,[81] and ventriculoperitoneal shunts are other causes of SVC syndrome in pediatric patients.

In children, respiratory symptoms predominate; air hunger, dyspnea, wheezing, and anxiety occur, particularly with position change. The gradual development of SVC syndrome may manifest with periorbital edema, conjunctival suffusion, facial swelling, dizziness, syncope, and cough. SVC syndrome can occur in conjunction with spinal cord compression (Rubin syndrome), where significant venous obstruction usually develops before the spinal cord compression. Patients with SVC syndrome and back pain should be evaluated with MRI of the vertebral spine when their condition is stable.

Evaluation of anterior mediastinal mass must be approached quickly and cautiously. Inappropriate delay, investigations, or management may be catastrophic. Posteroanterior and lateral chest x-ray films show widening of the mediastinum, often with tracheal compression or deviation. Further imaging, including computed tomography, should be pursued only without sedation and may require prone positioning because compression of the great vessels may occur despite a patent airway, resulting in profound hypoxia and reduced cardiac output. Complete blood count and α-fetoprotein, β-human chorionic gonadotropin, and lactate dehydrogenase levels should be obtained. Bone marrow aspiration, pleural or pericardial aspirate, or lymph node biopsy may be possible with use of local anesthetic only. If the diagnosis still is not clear after these procedures (27% of cases in one large series), either more invasive testing or empiric therapy can be considered.[82] Because treatment protocols are cell-type specific and incorporate risk stratification assignments, the correct diagnosis is preferable. Several modalities have been used to determine risk of induction of general anesthesia. First, echocardiography can evaluate cardiac motility and the degree of venous return. Second, pulmonary function tests showing peak expiratory flow rates greater than 50% predicted and tracheal cross-sectional area measuring greater than 50% are predictive of safe general anesthesia.[83] In a study designed to assess risk of general anesthesia in patients with SVC syndrome, 163 consecutive children with anterior mediastinal masses were reviewed, among whom 44 underwent general anesthesia prior to treatment.[82] Seven patients (16%) developed potentially life-threatening airway compromise, although all survived without sequelae. Three required chemotherapy or radiotherapy prior to successful extubation. The authors conclude that general anesthesia should be performed only when spontaneous ventilation can be preserved. Whenever possible, induction should proceed with the patient in the sitting position, intravenous access should be secured in the lower extremity, the patient's position must be readily changed if necessary, a rigid bronchoscope should be used by a skilled bronchoscopist, and extracorporeal support should be available. If these conditions are not feasible and empiric therapy is required for suspected hematologic malignancies, chemotherapy, including steroids, often is rapidly effective. Radiotherapy has been another mainstay of empiric therapy. Diagnosis should be established with the least invasive means available, with empiric anticancer therapy required if no histologic sample can be obtained safely. Tissue for definitive diagnosis should be obtained as soon as the patient's clinical status allows, to decrease the likelihood that empiric therapy will permanently obscure the diagnosis.

REFERENCES

1. Spence RK: Anemia in the patient undergoing surgery and the transfusion decision: a review, *Clin Orthop Rel Res* 357:19, 1998.

2. Oski FA, Brugnaro C, Nathan DG: A diagnostic approach to the anemic patient. In Nathan DG, Osk SH, editors: *Nathan and Oski's hematology of infancy and childhood,* ed 5, Philadelphia, 1998, WB Saunders.
3. Hillman RS: Acute blood loss anemia. In Williams EJ, Beuther E, Erslev AJ, et al, editors: *Hematology,* New York, 1990, McGraw Hill.
4. Kevy SV, Gorlin JB: Red cell transfusion. In Nathan DG, Osk SH, editors: *Nathan and Oski's hematology of infancy and childhood,* ed 5, Philadelphia, 1998, WB Saunders.
5. Morgan WM, O'Neill JA Jr: Hemorrhagic and obstructive shock in pediatric patients, *New Horizons* 6:150, 1998.
6. Huestis DW, Bove JR, Case J: *Practical blood transfusion,* ed 4, Boston, 1988, Little Brown.
7. Hippala S: Replacement of massive blood loss, *Vox Sang* 74:399-407, 1998.
8. Kirkpatrick DV: Aplastic anemia: pathogenesis, complications and treatment, *Cancer Bull* 37:221, 1985.
9. Brown KE, Tisdale J, Barrett AJ, et al: Hepatitis-associated aplastic anemia, *N Engl J Med* 336:1059, 1997.
10. Safadi R, Or R, Ilan Y, et al: Lack of known hepatitis virus in hepatitis-associated aplastic anemia and outcome after bone marrow transplantation, *Bone Marrow Transplant* 27:183, 2001.
11. Sloan EM, Maciejewski JP, Kirby M, et al: Bone marrow and peripheral blood lymphocytes of patients with severe aplastic anemia containing IFN-[gamma] detectable by flow cytometric analysis, *Blood* 90:20b, 1997.
12. Young NS: Acquired aplastic anemia, *Ann Intern Med* 136:534, 2002.
13. Sieff Ca, Nisbet-Brown E, Nathan DG: Congenital bone marrow failure syndromes, *Br J Haematol* III.30, 2000.
14. Zinner SH: Changing epidemiology of infections in patients with neutropenia and cancer: emphasis on gram-positive, *Clin Infect Dis* 29:490, 1999.
15. Leitman SF, Holland PV: Irradiation of blood products, indications and guidelines, *Transfusion* 25:293, 1985.
16. Deeg HJ, Leisenring W, Storb R, et al: Long-term outcome after marrow transplantation for severe aplastic anemia, *Blood* 91:3637, 1998.
17. Cacigalupo A, Broccia G, Corda G, et al: Antilymphocyte globulin, cyclosporin, and granulocyte colony-stimulating factor in patients with acquired severe aplastic anemia (SAA): a pilot study of the EBMT SAA Working Party, *Blood* 85:1348, 1995.
18. Rosenfeld SJ, Kimball J, Vining D, et al: Intensive immunosuppression with antithymocyte globulin and cyclosporine as treatment for severe acquired aplastic anemia, *Blood* 85:3058, 1995.
19. Miller DR: Hemolytic anemias. General considerations. In Miller DR, Baehne RL, editors: *Blood diseases of infancy and childhood,* St. Louis, 1989, Mosby.
20. Ware RE, Rosse WF: Autoimmune hemolytic anemia. In Nathan DG, Osk SH, editors: *Nathan and Oski's hematology of infancy and childhood,* ed 5, Philadelphia, 1998, WB Saunders.
21. Payne LG, Haywood CPM, Kelton JG: Destruction of red cells by the vasculature and reticuloendothelial system. In Nathan DG, Osk SH, editors: *Nathan and Oski's hematology of infancy and childhood,* ed 5, Philadelphia, 1998, WB Saunders.
22. Petz LD, Freidenberg HH: Coombs-positive hemolytic anemia caused by penicillin administration, *N Engl J Med* 274:171, 1966.
23. Branch Dr, Berkowitz LR, Becker RL, et al: Extravascular hemolysis following the administration of cefamandole, *Am J Hematol* 18:213, 1985.
24. Salama A, Mueller-Eckhard C: On the mechanisms of sensitization and attachment of antibodies to RBC in drug-induced immune hemolytic anemia, *Blood* 69:1006, 1987.
25. Sokol RJ, Hewitt S, Booker DJ, et al: Patients with red cell antibodies: Selection of blood for transfusion, *Clin Lab Haematol* 10:257, 1988.
26. Salama A, Berhofer H, Mueller-Eckhardt C: Red blood cell transfusion in warm-type autoimmune hemolytic anemia, *Lancet* 340:1515, 1992.
27. Warren RW, Collins ML: Immune hemolytic anemia in children, *Crit Rev Oncol Hematol* 8:65, 1988.
28. Fries LF, Brickman CM, Frank MM: Monocyte receptors for the Fc portion of IgG increase in number in autoimmune hemolytic anemia and other hemolytic states and are decreased by glucocorticoid therapy, *J Immunol* 131:1240, 1983.
29. Meytes D, Adler M, Viraq I, et al: High dose methylprednisolone in acute immune cold hemolysis, *N Engl J Med* 312:318, 1985.
30. Hilgartner MW, Bussel J: Use of intravenous gamma globulin for the treatment of autoimmune neutropenia of childhood and autoimmune hemolytic anemia, *Am J Med* 83:25, 1987.
31. Silberstein LE, Berkman EM: Plasma exchange in autoimmune hemolytic anemia (AIHA), *J Clin Apheresis* 1:238, 1983.
32. Storb R, Thomas ED, Bruckner CD, et al: Marrow transplantation in thirty "untransfused" patients with severe aplastic anemia, *Ann Intern Med* 92:30, 1980.
33. Slichter SJ: Optimizing platelet transfusions, *Semin Hematol* 35:269, 1998.
34. Practice parameter for the use of fresh frozen plasma, cryoprecipitate, and platelets, *JAMA* 271:777, 1994.
35. Anonymous: Leucocyte reduction and ultraviolet B irradation of platlets to prevent allo immunization and refractoriness to platelet transfusions. The Trial to Reduce Alloimmunization to Platelets Study Group, *N Engl J Med* 337:1861, 1997.
36. Nieminen U, Peltola H, Syrjala, MT: Acute thrombocytopenic purpura following measles, mumps and rubella vaccination, *Acta Paediatr* 82:267, 1993.
37. Kurtzberg J, Stockman JA III: Idiopathic autoimmune thrombocytopenic purpura, *Adv Paediatr* 41:111, 1994.
38. George JN, Woolf SH, Raskob GE, et al: Idiopathic thrombocytopenic purpura: A practical guideline developed by explicit methods for the American Society of Hematology, *Blood* 88:3, 1996.
39. Imbach P, Wagner HP, Berchtold W, et al: Intravenous gamma globulin versus oral corticosteroids in acute thrombocytopenic purpura in childhood, *Lancet* 2:464, 1985.
40. Buchanan GR, Holtkemp CA: Prednisone therapy for children with newly diagnosed idiopathic thrombocytopenic purpura. A randomized clinical trial, *Am J Pediatr Hematol Oncol* 6:355, 1984.
41. Ozsoylu S: Anti-platelet antibodies in chidlhood idiopathic thrombocytopenic purpura, *Am J Hematol* 51:328, 1996.
42. Bussel JB, Graziano JN, Kimberly RP, et al: Intravenous anti-D treatment of immune thrombocytopenic purpura: analysis of efficacy, toxicity and mechanism of effect, *Blood* 77:1884, 1991.
43. Beardsley DS, Nathan DG: Platelet abnormalities in infancy and childhood. In Nathan DG, Osk SH, editors: *Nathan and Oski's hematology of infancy and childhood,* ed 5, vol 2. Philadelphia, 1998, WB Saunders.
44. Lightsey AL, McMillen R, Koenig HM, et al: Childhood idiopathic thrombocytopenic purpura: aggressive management of life-threatening complications, *JAMA* 232:734, 1975.
45. Carr JM, Kruskall MS, Keye JA, et al: Efficacy of platelet transfusions in immune thrombocytopenia, *Am J Med* 80(b):1051, 1986.
46. Woerner SJ, Abildgaard CF, French BN: Intracranial hemorrhage in children with idiopathic thrombocytopenic purpura, *Pediatrics* 67:453, 1981.
47. Ruggenenti P, Remuzzo G: The pathophysiology and management of thrombotic thrombocytopenic purpura, *Eur J Haematol* 74:240, 1996.
48. Forsyth KD, Simpson AC, Fitzpatrick MM, et al: Neutrophil-mediated endothelial injury in haemolytic uraemic syndrome, *Lancet* 2:411, 1989.
49. Gordon LI, Kwaan HC, Ross EC: Deleterious effects of platelet transfusions and recovery thrombocytosis in patients with thrombotic microangiopathy, *Semin Hematol* 24:194, 1987.
50. Veruloet MG, Thijs LG, Hack CE: Derangements of coagulation and fibrinolysis in critically ill patients with sepsis and septic shock, *Semin Thromb Hemost* 24:33, 1998.
51. Uneo H, Hirasawa H, Oda S, et al: Coagulation/fibrinolysis abnormality and vascular endothelial damage in the pathogenesis of thrombocytopenic multiple organ failure, *Crit Care Med* 30:2242, 2002.
52. Parker RI: Thrombocytopenia and intensive care unit outcome: a sticky issue, *Crit Care Med* 30:1917, 2002.
53. Weigert AL, Shafer AI: Uremia bleeding: pathogenesis and therapy, *Am J Med Sci* 316:94, 1998.
54. Shafer AI: Acquired disorders of platelet function. In Loscalzo J, Schafer AI, editors: *Thrombosis and hemorrhage.* Oxford, 1994, Blackwell Scientific.
55. Mannucci PM, Remuzzi G, Pusineri G, et al: Deamino-8-D-arginine vasopression shortens the bleeding time in uremia, *N Engl J Med* 308:8, 1983.

56. Fernandez F, Goudable C, Sie P, et al: Low hematocrit and prolonged bleeding time in uraemic patients: effect of red cell transfusions, *Br J Haematol* 59:139, 1985.
57. Roberts IAG, Murray NA: Management of thrombocytopenia in neonates, *Br J Haematol* 105:864, 1999.
58. Blanchette VS, Kuhne T, Hume F, Hellman J: Platelet transfusion therapy in newborn infants, *Transfus Med Rev* 9:215, 1995.
59. Bussel JB, Zabusky MR, Berkowitz RL, McFarland JG: Fetal alloimmune thrombocytopenia, *N Engl J Med* 337:22, 1997.
60. Kedar A, Grow W, Neiberger RE: Clinical versus laboratory tumor lysis syndrome in children with leukemia, *Pediatr Hematol Oncol* 12:129, 1995.
61. Saccente SL, Kohaut EC, Berkow RL: Prevention of tumor lysis syndrome using continuous veno-venous hemofiltration, *Pediat Nephrol* 9:569, 1995.
62. Bosly A, Sonet A, Pinkerton CR, et al: Rasburicase (recombinant urate oxidase) for the management of hyperuricemia in patients with cancer, *Cancer* 98:1048, 2003.
63. Goldman SC, Holcenberg JS, Finklestein JZ, et al: A randomized comparison between rasburicase and allopurinol in children with lymphoma or leukemia at high risk for tumor lysis, *Blood* 97:2998, 2001.
64. Annemans L, Moeremans K, Lamotte M, et al: Incidence, medical resource utilisation and costs of hyperuricemia and tumour lysis syndrome in patients with acute leukemia and non-Hodgkin's lymphoma in four European countries, *Leuk Lymphoma* 44:77, 2003.
65. Porcu P, Farag S, Marcucci G, et al: Leukocytoreduction for acute leukemia, *Ther Apher* 6:15, 2002.
66. Lichtman MA, Rowe JM: Hyperleukocytic leukemias: rheological, clinical, and therapeutic considerations, *Blood* 60:279, 1982.
67. Kelly KM, Lange B: Oncologic emergencies, *Pediatr Clin North Am* 44:809, 1997.
68. Gartrell K, Rosenstrauch W: Hypoxaemia in patients with hyperleukocytosis: true or spurious and clinical implications, *Leuk Res* 17:915, 1993.
69. Stemmler J, Wittmann GW, Hacker U, et al: Leukapharesis in chronic myelomonocytic leukemia with leukostasis syndrome: elevated serum lactate levels as an early sign of microcirculation failure, *Leuk Lymphoma* 43:1427, 2002.
70. Nowacki P, Zdziarska B, Fryze C, et al: Co-existence of thrombocytopenia and hyperleukocytosis as a risk factor of haemorrhage into the central nervous system in patients with acute leukaemias, *Haematologia* 31:347, 2002.
71. Basade M, Dhar AK, Kulkarni SS, et al: Rapid cytoreduction in childhood leukemic hyperleukocytosis by conservative therapy, *Med Pediatr Oncol* 25:204, 1995.
72. Maurer HS, Steinherz PG, Gaynon PS, et al: The effect of initial management of hyperleukocytosis on early complications and outcome of children with acute lymphoblastic leukemia, *J Clin Oncol* 6:1425, 1988.
73. Klein SL, Sanford RA, Muhlbauer MS: Pediatric spinal epidural metastases, *J Neurosurg* 74:70, 1991.
74. Pollono D, Tomarchia S, Drut R, et al: Spinal cord compression: a review of 70 pediatric patients, *Pediatr Hematol Oncol* 20:457, 2003.
75. Kato A, Ushio Y, Hayakawa T, et al: Circulatory disturbance of the spinal cord with epidural neoplasm in rats, *J Neurosurg* 63:260, 1985.
76. Nicolin G: Emergencies and their management, *Eur J Cancer* 38:1365, 2002.
77. Mayfield JK, Riseborough EJ, Jaffe N, et al: Spinal deformity in children treated for neuroblastoma, *J Bone Joint Surg* 63:183, 1981.
78. DeBernardi C, Pianca G, Pistamiglio P, et al: Neuroblastoma with symptomatic spinal cord compression at diagnosis. Treatment and results with 76 cases, *J Clin Oncol* 19:183, 2001.
79. Karamazyn B, Dagan O, Vidne B, et al: Neuroimaging findings in neonates and infants from superior vena cava obstruction after cardiac operation, *Pediatr Radiol* 32:806, 2002.
80. Zreik H, Bengur AR, Meliones JN, et al: Superior vena cava obstruction after extracorpeal membrane oxygenation, *J Pediatr* 127:314, 1995.
81. Giacoia GP: Right-sided diaphragmatic hernia associated with superior vena cava syndrome, *Am J Perinatol* 11:129, 1994.
82. Ferrari LR, Bedford RF: General anesthesia prior to treatment of anterior mediastinal masses in pediatric cancer patients, *Anesthesiology* 72:991, 1990.
83. Shamberger RC, Holzmann RS, Griscom NT, et al: CT quantitation of tracheal cross-sectional area as a guide to the surgical and anesthetic management of children with anterior mediastinal masses, *J Pediatr Surg* 26:138, 1991.

CHAPTER

75

Basics of Transfusion Medicine

Naomi L.C. Luban

PEARLS

- One unit of whole blood contains approximately 450 ml of blood collected from a healthy adult donor into a plastic bag containing 63 ml of anticoagulant solution.
- In the setting of massive transfusion, use of fresh-packed red blood cells anticoagulated and preserved with high concentrations of glucose, mannitol, and adenine may pose some risk, especially to the tiny infant; however, data suggest that, in small volume transfusions, additive red blood cells are well tolerated in premature infants.
- By age 3 months, an infant's blood volume is 70 to 75 ml/kg, and the hemoglobin concentrations for packed red blood cells collected in CPDA-1 and preservative solutions are approximately 22 and 18 g/dl, respectively.
- Most transfusion formulas have been developed for adults. The effective posttransfusion platelet count depends on the patient's size, number of platelets per unit, and complicating clinical factors.
- Transfusion-acquired graft-versus-host disease occurs when an immunosuppressed or immunodeficient transfusion recipient receives immunologically competent donor lymphocytes; it is fatal in 90% of reported cases in children.

The first description of saving a bleeding patient from overwhelming blood loss dates to the 1800s, when James Blundell administered human blood to a woman dying of postpartum hemorrhage. Modern blood transfusion practice did not develop until blood could be anticoagulated and stored for future use. Technologic advances in blood collection and separation have resulted in component preparation, that is, separation of whole blood into red blood cells (RBCs), white blood cells (WBCs), platelets, and plasma. Transfusion practices today use these specially separated and prepared components, which are superior to whole blood.

Anticoagulants and the Storage Lesion

One unit of whole blood contains approximately 450 ml of blood collected from a healthy adult donor into a plastic bag containing 63 ml of anticoagulant solution. If RBCs are stored for transfusion, several basic prerequisites must be met. The transfused product must be sterile, the cellular components must remain viable during storage, and their in vivo survival after storage must remain at least 75% for 24 hours after transfusion. For components to be made, the anticoagulant-preservative must not be detrimental to the desired component, and the bag system must be adapted to permit sterile removal of individual components. Viability of RBCs and functional activity, however, require that the RBCs be preserved with solutions that maintain the energy needs of the RBC. Loss of RBC viability, poor in vivo survival, and inadequate oxygen delivery are collectively referred to as the *storage lesion.*

Red blood cells metabolize glucose through the glycolytic and hexose-monophosphate shunt pathways. Accordingly, lactate, which is the endproduct of these metabolic pathways, progressively accumulates during blood storage. As lactate increases, pH falls, inhibiting further glycolytic enzyme activity and decreasing adenosine triphosphate (ATP) and 2,3-diphosphoglycerate (2,3-DPG). As intraerythrocytic ATP concentrations decrease, membrane lipid is altered, and sodium/potassium ATPase-dependent ion pumps are inhibited. This results in rigid, spherocytic red cells; some of these cells have increased osmotic fragility and undergo spontaneous lysis, and some lyse in vivo. Intraerythrocyte 2,3-DPG is an important determinant of oxygen affinity and delivery. During storage, 2,3-DPG falls, and the oxygen dissociation curve shifts leftward. This shift reflects an increase in the oxygen affinity of hemoglobin, which results in poor oxygen offloading unless tissue oxygen tension is lower than normal.

Additional biochemical changes are associated with the storage lesion. They result from the utilization of glucose and its metabolism to lactic and other organic acids, production of ammonia, and release of lactic dehydrogenase, potassium, and plasma hemoglobin. Higher concentrations of these constituents are found with longer storage (Table 75–1). Advances in the development of anticoagulant-preservative solutions have focused on the use of nutrient cocktails designed to maintain 2,3-DPG and ATP, stabilize the RBC membrane, and maintain the 75% posttransfusion viability standard. Table 75–2 lists the anticoagulant-preservatives currently in use. The use of adenine was prompted by the studies of Nakao et al., who noted that exogenous adenine and inosine are rapidly taken up by the RBC and become part of the nucleotide pool. Mannitol is a component of some of the anticoagulant-preservative solutions because it stabilizes the RBC membrane. Others use very high concentrations of glucose and saline solution, which are added back into the packed red blood cell (PRBC) preparation after the plasma and platelets have been separated into satellite bags. Although citrate, phosphate, dextrose, and adenine (CPDA-1) preserve RBCs for 35 days, the newer nutrient solutions permit 42-day storage. Also, because additional fluid is added to the newer nutrient solutions, these units have lower hematocrits and more rapid flow characteristics compared with RBCs stored in CPDA-1. In the setting of massive transfusion, use of fresh-packed RBCs anticoagulated and preserved with high concentrations of glucose, mannitol, and adenine may pose some risk, especially to the tiny infant.[1,2] However, data suggest that additive RBCs (containing the above constituents) are well tolerated in premature infants given small volume transfusions.[3]

Components and Derivatives

Use of components is preferable to that of whole blood for several reasons. Most importantly, they conserve blood resources while providing specific therapy for specific deficiencies. If whole blood were used in place of specific products, platelet concentrates, plasma, albumin, and other blood derivatives could not be manufactured. Platelet function in whole blood stored for 24 hours is poor, and plasma coagulation factors, especially factors V and VIII, decrease throughout storage. Whole blood should be reserved for patients with brisk bleeding who require volume expansion, oxygen-carrying capacity, and stable coagulation factors. Whole blood or reconstituted whole blood is also indicated for manual exchange transfusions and for "priming" of extracorporeal circuits (e.g., infant cardiovascular bypass, extracorporeal membrane oxygenation, apheresis in small patients). Table 75–3 lists the volume, average total white blood cell content, and expiration of different blood components.

Red Blood Cell Products

Red blood cells, commonly referred to as *PRBCs*, are prepared from whole blood after centrifugation or sedimentation. PRBCs collected in CPDA-1 anticoagulant have a volume of approximately 250 ml with a hematocrit of 70% to 80%. They consist of 150 to 180 ml of pure red cells or 60 g of hemoglobin and 20 to 80 ml of plasma.

TABLE 75–1

Biochemical Changes in Blood Stored in CPDA-1

Variable	Day 0		Day 35	
	Whole Blood	**Red Blood Cells**	**Whole Blood**	**Red Blood Cells**
Percent viable cells (24 hours posttransfusion)	100.0	100.0	79.0	71.0
pH (measured at 37°C)	7.6	7.55	6.98	6.71
ATP (% of initial value)	100.0	100.0	56.0±16	45.0±12
2,3-DPG (% of initial value)	100.0	100.0	<10.0	<10.0
Plasma K^+ (mmol/L)	4.2	5.1	27.3	78.5*
Plasma Na^+ (mmol/L)	169.0	169.0	155.0	111.0
Plasma hemoglobin (mg/L)	82	78	461	658*

Modified from *Technical manual of the American Association of Blood Banks,* Arlington, Va, 1993, American Association of Blood Banks, p 53.
ATP, Adenosine triphosphate; 2,3-*DPG,* 2,3-diphosphoglycerate.
*Values for plasma hemoglobin and potassium concentrations may appear somewhat high in 35-day stored red blood cell units; the total plasma in these units is only about 70 ml.

TABLE 75–2

Anticoagulants and Their Shelf Life

Anticoagulant	Shelf Life (days)
CPD (PRBC, whole blood)	21
CPDA-1 (PRBC, whole blood)	35
Adsol, Nutricell, Optisol	42

PRBC, packed red blood cells.

Removal of much of the plasma during preparation reduces the anticoagulant solution and isoagglutinins A and B present in the plasma. When PRBCs are supplemented with additive preservative solutions, the volume of the PRBC unit is increased to approximately 350 ml and the hematocrit is reduced to 50% to 60%. Because PRBCs collected in additive preservative solutions have a longer expiration dating period, lower viscosity, and hence more rapid flow, this type of PRBC product is commonly used. Other RBC preparations include leukocyte-reduced, washed, and frozen deglycerolized RBCs. Leukocyte-reduced PRBCs may be prepared by a number of different techniques. The average total leukocyte content in 1 U of PRBCs cells is 2 to 5×10^9. According to Standards of the American Association of Blood Banks, a blood product leukocyte content should be reduced to less than 5×10^6 to be labeled as leukoreduced. In Europe, a value of less than 1×10^6 WBC per unit is used. Leukocyte reduction and the biologic effects of transfused leukocytes have been reviewed.[4] Leukocyte reduction by modern filtration technology reduces leukocyte content of RBCs by a factor of 10^3 to 10^4 and is often performed immediately after collection and prior to refrigerated storage. Cells may be washed in either an automated cell washer or by manual techniques. Washing removes 70% to 90% of leukocytes, plasma, platelets, anticoagulant, and microaggregates. Red cells may be cryopreserved by use of glycerol as a cryoprotectant. Deglycerolization requires defrosting and washing with automated cell washers. Cryopreserved and deglycerolized red cells are reduced in leukocyte content by approximately 100-fold. Frozen, deglycerolized RBCs are also free of platelets, plasma, anticoagulant solution, and microaggregates. If frozen within hours of collection, deglycerolized RBCs have high levels of 2,3-DPG and ATP. As with washed RBCs, deglycerolized cells have the disadvantage of 24-hour expiration once they have been manipulated by washing. Deglycerolized, washed cells of rare RBC phenotype can be refrozen for future use, but with loss of red cell number and decreased in vivo survival.

Occasionally a recipient of a massive transfusion may receive group O RBCs during an acute resuscitation. When the group and type of the individual are known, it is advantageous to switch to group- and type-matched products to conserve group O blood resources. However, if more than half of the patient's blood volume of group

TABLE 75–3

Volume, WBC Content, and Expiration of Different Blood Components

Component	Storage (°C)	Volume (ml)	Average Total WBC Content	Expiration
Whole blood	1–6	500	10^9	21–35 d†
RBCs (CPDA-1)	1–6	250	10^8	35 days*
RBCs (preservative solution)	1–6	350	10^8	42 days*
Washed RBCs	1–6	Variable	10^7	24 h
Deglycerolized RBCs	Frozen: <–65 or <–120 Deglycerolized:1–6	250	10^6–10^7	Frozen: 10 y Deglycerolized: 24 h
Platelet concentrate	20–24 with agitation	50–75	10^7	5 days (4 h after pooling)
Plateletpheresis unit	20–24 with agitation	200–500	10^6–10^8	5 days
Cryoprecipitate	Frozen: <–18 Thawed: 20–24	10–15	0	Frozen: 12 mo Thawed: 6 or 4 h after pooling
Fresh-frozen plasma	Frozen: <–18 Thawed: 1–6	200 (standard) 400–600 (large units)	0	Frozen: 12 mo Thawed: 24 h
Pediatric fresh-frozen plasma	Frozen: <–18 Thawed: 1–6	Variable	0	Frozen: 12 mo Thawed: 24 h
Liquid plasma	1–6	200	10^5	5 days after whole blood expiration
Single-donor plasma	Frozen: <–18 Thawed: 1–6	200	0	Frozen: 5 y Thawed: 24 h
Granulocyte concentrate	20–24, no agitation	200–300	10^{10}	24 h‡

RBC, Red blood cell; *WBC,* white blood cell.
*All components should be transfused within 4 hours of spiking blood product.
†Expiration depends on type of anticoagulant.
‡Should be transfused within 8 hours of collection if possible; may also contain up to 10^{11} platelets.

O RBCs has been transfused, it is wise to choose a maintenance regimen of group O RBC and plasma products compatible with the patient's original blood type until passively acquired anti-A and anti-B are no longer detectable. This may be determined by cross-matching the patient's serum with the group-specific cells.

Red blood cells are indicated to increase oxygen-carrying capacity. However, it is not clear that an increase in blood oxygen content always results in clinical benefit. One group has shown that an increase of oxygen delivery mediated by RBC transfusion did not necessarily correlate with increased oxygen consumption in pediatric patients with septic shock.[5] Hypovolemia without significant RBC mass deficit is best treated with other volume expanders. Red blood cells can be used with crystalloid in surgical patients to replace operative losses. Leukocyte-reduced PRBCs are indicated for patients who have febrile transfusion reactions as a result of repeated transfusions, to avoid the development of antileukocyte antibodies, or in patients with anti-human leukocyte antigen (HLA) antibodies. These specially prepared RBC products have several characteristics in common: they require more time to prepare, are more costly, and result in some RBC loss. Frozen deglycerolized PRBCs are indicated for patients with RBC alloantibodies who require blood of rare phenotype, those who have IgA deficiency with circulating anti-IgA antibody to avoid anaphylaxis from IgA in plasma (see Chapter 83), and those with recurrent febrile reactions to transfusion despite leukoreduction by more common methods.

Red Blood Cell Transfusion Formulas

Several formulas can be used to predict hemoglobin increments in transfusion recipients (Box 75-1).

By age 3 months, an infant's blood volume is 70 to 75 ml/kg, and the hemoglobin concentrations for PRBCs collected in CPDA-1 and preservative solutions are approximately 22 and 18 g/dl, respectively.

Platelets

A unit of random donor platelets is prepared by slow centrifugation of a whole blood unit within 8 hours of collection. The supernatant platelet-rich plasma is centrifuged again to produce a cell-free plasma used for plasma component manufacture. When the platelet pellet is resuspended in 50 to 75 ml of residual plasma, it is called a *platelet concentrate*. Each platelet concentrate contains 7.5×10^{10} platelets (minimum 5.5×10^{10}) in 50 to 75 ml of plasma. Platelets are stored at 22° C on a mechanical rotator to ensure their viability and may be stored for up to 5 days. Single-donor platelets are obtained by plateletpheresis with any one of several automated blood cell processors. Depending on the number of blood volumes passed through the machine, the equivalent of 6 to 12 U of platelet concentrate in 250 ml of plasma may be collected. Each plateletpheresis product contains 4.5×10^{11} platelets (minimum 3×10^{11}). They are collected in sterile systems that permit 5-day storage; they are stored at 22° C on a mechanical rotator. The degree of RBC and WBC contamination varies according to the technique and the machine used. Platelets have an in vivo lifespan of 9 to 10 days and are hemostatically effective for 3 to 5 days.

Platelets are indicated for quantitative and qualitative platelet disorders. They are used to prevent hemorrhage and to stop or attenuate ongoing bleeding. Clinical factors to be considered before platelet transfusion include the primary diagnosis, bone marrow function, and the probability for marrow recovery, presence of fever, splenomegaly, sepsis, ongoing oozing or bleeding that would increase consumption of platelets, and use of drugs that might induce platelet dysfunction (Fig. 75-1). The decision to use platelets must be based on an assessment of these factors because no prospective studies to guide the pediatric intensivist are available.

Like RBCs, platelets may undergo a storage lesion. This occurs because of decreases in plasma oxygen tension and anaerobic metabolism that result in a decrease in pH, increase in lactate, and subsequent loss of platelet viability and clinical efficacy. Advances in platelet storage methods ensure aerobic metabolism and decrease platelet activation. These improvements have included the development of oxygen-permeable bags, specifying the number of platelets per bag, and reducing the WBCs to decrease proinflammatory cytokines.

A platelet count of 50,000/µl is adequate for hemostasis, as has been supported by the adult oncologic literature. Even major abdominal surgery can be performed with platelet counts in this range if there is no other coagulopathy.[6] Patients with platelet counts less than 20,000/µl who have limited physiologic reserve can be treated with platelet transfusion, although some patients with platelets in this range do not bleed, especially if the marrow is recovering with young, large, "sticky" platelets. However, clinical judgment must be used, especially in patients with additional factors that might predispose to hemorrhage and who are to undergo invasive neurosurgical or general surgical procedures, and in those with sepsis or who have rapidly declining platelet counts. Such individuals may require transfusion to bring their counts above 50,000/µl. There are similarly no guidelines that help establish platelet counts above which it is safe to perform less invasive procedures such as bone marrow aspiration, lumbar puncture, venous or arterial catheterization, or intubation (American Society of Clinical Ontology guidelines).

BOX 75-1

Red Blood Cell Transfusion Formulas

6 ml of whole blood/kg of body weight increases the hemoglobin by 1 g/dl

3 ml of PRBCs (CPDA-1)/kg of body weight increases the hemoglobin by 1 g/dl

4 ml of PRBCs (preservative solution added)/kg of body weight increases the hemoglobin by 1 g/dl

Volume of blood to be transfused (in ml) = Blood volume (in ml) (Desired hemoglobin − Actual hemoglobin)/ Hemoglobin concentration of PRBCs

Clinical judgment and knowledge of the cause of both the thrombocytopenia and the bleeding are essential. For example, antibody-mediated idiopathic thrombocytopenic purpura is frequently associated with profound thrombocytopenia (platelet count <10,000/μl). Such patients do not benefit from platelet transfusions because the transfused platelets form a complex with antibody and are rapidly removed from the circulation by the reticuloendothelial system. This may occur within minutes of transfusion. Platelet transfusion in this circumstance should be reserved for life-threatening hemorrhage only, along with other therapy aimed to treat the primary clinical condition.

Use of prophylactic platelet transfusions is controversial, and few studies have been performed in children. Their use is limited to patients in otherwise stable condition who have leukemia or oncologic malignancies or bone marrow transplant recipients with severe thrombocytopenia (<10,000–20,000/μl) who are expected to remain aplastic because of their therapy. However, some studies have shown that the platelet transfusion threshold of 10,000/μl does not predispose to mortality or morbidity.[7] If platelet counts are decreasing rapidly or if there is an increased risk of hemorrhage from concomitant illness, then prophylactic transfusions might be indicated for a limited period of time.

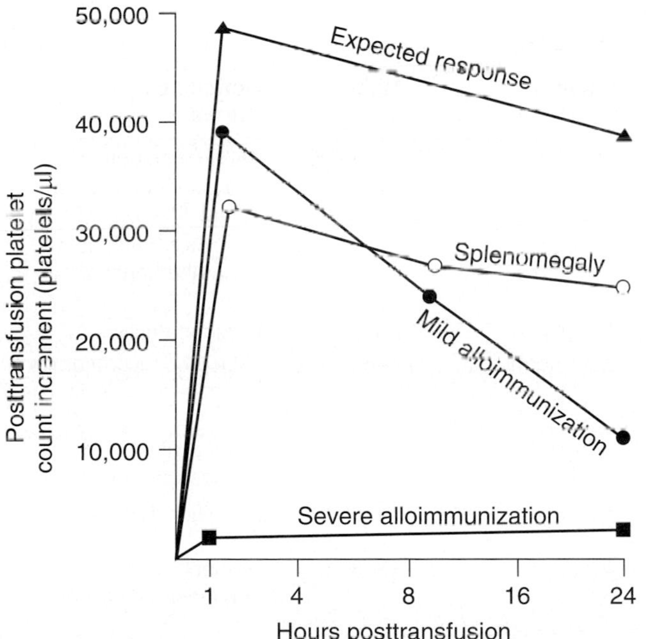

FIGURE 75–1 • Typical results after transfusion of 0.1 U of platelets/kg to a severely thrombocytopenic patient in various clinical settings. The *upper curve* is the expected response in a nonimmunized recipient. There is a posttransfusion platelet count increment of about 45,000 to 50,000 μl with an approximately 20% decrease in 24 hours. In patients with mild alloimmunization, the 1-hour posttransfusion platelet count increment may be adequate, but there is decreased survival of the platelets in subsequent hours. In patients with splenomegaly, there may be decreased recovery but with essentially normal subsequent survival. In patients with sepsis, disseminated intravascular coagulation, or fever with a temperature greater than 38.5° C, the response often is similar to that with mild alloimmunization, although in some patients the response is similar to that with severe alloimmunization. (From Tomosulo PA, Petz LD: Platelet transfusion. In Petz LD, Swisher SA, editors: *Clinical practice of transfusion medicine,* New York, 1989, Churchill Livingstone.)

Patients who have received massive transfusions and in whom more than one blood volume has been replaced in a relatively short time may develop thrombocytopenia. Such patients have a combination of loss of endogenous platelets and dilution from use of banked blood devoid of functioning platelets, as well as crystalloid or colloid. Studies in both adults and children demonstrate an inverse relationship between platelet counts and the blood volume transfused, but the decrease in platelet count is less than predicted from washout formulas. These studies suggest mobilization of platelets from endogenous sources, most likely the spleen. Some trauma transfusion algorithms recommend routine prophylactic use of platelets. Use of platelet concentrates based on number of units of transfused RBCs is not indicated because many patients do not bleed despite low platelet counts. Use of formulas may be helpful, however, in determining when platelet transfusion will be necessary based on the initial platelet count of the patient who has undergone massive transfusion.

Cardiopulmonary bypass induces platelet dysfunction and is associated with thrombocytopenia. The combined hemostatic defect may develop because of platelet adhesion to the membrane oxygenator and circuit, prosthetic materials, disrupted endothelial surfaces, consumption at the surgical site, and exposure to drugs and circulating cytokines. Platelet counts rarely fall below the number considered hemostatic; bleeding not considered to be "surgical" bleeding is more likely related to a functional defect or fibrinolysis. After bypass, the relationship between platelet count and bleeding time has been shown to be loose. Prolonged bleeding times at platelet counts greater than 100,000/μl likely are the result of release of α granules and dense bodies from the platelet. However, routine platelet transfusion to improve platelet counts and function after cardiopulmonary bypass was not helpful in a controlled trial. Platelet transfusion in this situation should be reserved for unexplained bleeding, where platelet dysfunction has been proved or is suspected after bypass surgery. Antifibrinolytic agents such as aprotinin and ε-amino-caproic acid may be useful in controlling bleeding associated with cardiopulmonary bypass (see Chapter 47).

Platelet Transfusion Formulas

Most transfusion formulas have been developed for adults. The effective posttransfusion platelet count depends on the patient's size, number of platelets per unit, and complicating clinical factors. A formula of 1 U of platelets per 10 kg that is sometimes used should increase the patient's count by 10,000 μL. For these reasons, the corrected count increment (CCI) is more helpful in assessing posttransfusion effectiveness than is the platelet count alone.

$$\text{CCI} = \frac{(\text{Posttransfusion platelet count} - \text{Pretransfusion platelet count}) \times \text{BSA}}{\text{No. of platelets (in units of } 10^{11})}$$

For example, assume a patient has a body surface area (BSA) of 0.75 m^2. The posttransfusion and pretransfusion

transfusion platelet counts are 40,000 and 5000/µl, respectively, and 4 U of platelets are administered, with each unit of platelets containing 5.5×10^{10} platelets. The CCI then is calculated as follows:

$$\frac{(40{,}000 - 5000) \times 0.75}{.55 \times 4} = 11{,}932$$

The CCI should be measured 1 or 24 hours after platelet transfusion; see Table 75–4 for CCI results that define refractoriness.

Other Considerations in Platelet Transfusion Therapy

Elevated levels of the cytokines (interleukin-1β and interleukin-6) have been demonstrated in the plasma supernatant of platelets following storage, probably secondary to secretion from contaminating leukocytes. These cytokines are responsible for febrile transfusion reactions that are relatively frequent following platelet transfusions.[8] Removal of these leukocytes before platelet storage prevents such reactions.

ABO antigens are present on platelets. There are conflicting data concerning the survival of ABO-incompatible platelets. ABO matching can improve response to platelet transfusions.[9,10] Another particular concern in infants and young children is the transfusion of isoagglutinins A and B in the plasma of the platelet concentrate. Sufficient anti-A, anti-B, or both may be present in plasma to produce a positive direct antiglobulin test result or hemolysis of recipient RBCs. Rh antigens are not present on the platelet membrane, so anti-Rh antibody should not affect platelet survival. Red blood cells are present in platelet concentrates as a "contaminant" of the manufacturing of platelets and have caused Rh sensitization. This is of particular concern in Rh-negative female patients. Platelets prepared by pheresis methods have very low numbers of RBCs. Rarely, antiplatelet antibody may be passively acquired after transfusion.

Whenever possible, ABO-compatible platelets should be administered. If ABO-incompatible platelets are to be administered and large volumes of incompatible plasma will be transfused, the platelets should be pooled, volume

TABLE 75–4

Coagulation Factor Facts

Name (Factor)	Molecular Weight	Site of Synthesis	Plasma Concentration	Half-life	Deficiency States
Fibrinogen (I)	340,000	Liver	200–400 mg/dl	3–5 days	Afibrinogenemia, dysfibrinogenemia, hypofibrinogenemia
Prothrombin (II)	68,000	Liver Vitamin K dependent	10 mg/dl	3–4.5 days	Hypoprothrombinemia, parahemophilia
Proaccelerin (V)	330,000	Liver	1 mg/dl	20 h	Parahemophilia
Proconvertin (VII)	48,000	Liver Vitamin K dependent	8–16 µg/ml	2–6 h	Hypoproconvertinemia
Antihemophilic (VIII:C)	50,000–100,000	Liver	50 µg/ml	6–12 h	Hemophilia A (classical hemophilia)
Von Willebrand(VIII:vWF)	200,000 (subunits)	Endothelial cells Megakaryocytes	–	16–24 h	Von Willebrand disease
Plasma thromboplastin component (PTC) (IX)	55,000	Liver Vitamin K dependent	4 µg/ml	18–30 h	Hemophilia B (Christmas disease)
Stuart-Prower (X)	55,000	Liver Vitamin K dependent	1 mg/dl	32–48 h	Stuart-Prower deficiency
Plasma thromboplastin antecedent (XI)	160,000	Liver	7–9 µg/ml	40–84 h	Hemophilia C (Rosenthal disease)
Hageman (XII)	80,000	Liver	29 µg/ml	48–52 h	Hageman trait
Fibrin-stabilizing (XIII)	156,000	Liver	1 mg/dl	3–5 days	Factor XIII deficiency
Prekallikrein (Fletcher)	85,000	Liver	33–66 µg/ml	–	Fletcher deficiency
High-molecular-weight kininogen (Fitzgerald)	160,000	Liver	47–122 µg/ml	–	Fitzgerald deficiency
Plasminogen	90,000	Liver	10–20 mg/dl	48–60 h	Thrombosis

From Goldsmith JC: Plasma component therapy. In Luban NLC, editor: *Transfusion theory in infants and children,* Baltimore, 1990, Johns Hopkins University Press.

BOX 75–2

Quantity of RBCs in Platelet Products

- Whole blood derived platelets ≈ 0.3–0.5 ml
- Apheresis 0.005–3 ml
- Apheresis by leukoreduction system method 0.0003–0.004 ml

reduced, and resuspended in an extra small volume of plasma or saline. However, the product must be transfused as soon as possible after plasma reduction because platelet viability deteriorates after storage at high platelet counts.

If Rh-positive platelets with RBC contamination are to be administered to Rh-negative female patients, Rh immunoglobulin should be used to prevent alloimmunization. The dose necessary can be calculated as shown in Box 75–2. Two different Rh immune globulin products are available in the United States. The standard product is for intramuscular use; the newer product can be administered by either an intravenous or intramuscular route for prevention of Rh immunization (Table 75–5).

Plasma and Plasma Products

Plasma for transfusion is prepared from whole blood during the preparation of either RBCs or platelet concentrates. To be labeled as fresh frozen plasma (FFP), plasma must be separated from the RBCs and stored at −18°C within 8 hours of collection. It also may be collected by apheresis methods. It can be stored frozen for 1 year, but once thawed it must be transfused within 24 hours. Some blood banks stock frozen plasma that has been frozen up to 24 hours after collection. Preliminary studies indicate there is no appreciable difference in coagulation factors in plasma held before freezing for either 8 or 24 hours. Once thawed, it can be refrigerated and transfused within 24 hours of thawing.

TABLE 75–5

Calculation for Recombinant Human Immunoglobulin G after D + Transfusions

	WinRho SDF™ Dose	
Route of Administration	**If Exposed to Rh_o (D)-Positive Whole Blood**	**If Exposed to Rh_o (D)-Positive Red Blood Cells**
Intravenous	9 µg (45 IU)/ml blood	18 µg (90 IU)/ml cells
Intramuscular	12 µg (60 IU)/ml blood	24 µg (120 IU)ml cells

Administer 600 µg (3000 IU) every 8 hours via the intravenous route, until the total dose, calculated from the table, is administered.
Administer 1200 µg (6000 IU) every 12 hours via the intravenous route, until the total dose, calculated from the table, is administered.

Fresh-frozen plasma is one of the most overused plasma products. Fresh-frozen plasma is indicated for plasma coagulation deficiencies when no alternative product is available. Examples include the rare single congenital deficiencies of factors II, V, VII, X, XI, and XIII. Adequate replacement of factors II and XI may be difficult with the volumes of plasma necessary to achieve greater than 50% concentration in homozygous deficiencies. Fresh-frozen plasma is most commonly used to treat multiple coagulation deficiencies, such as in patients with liver disease, fat-soluble vitamin K deficiency related to malabsorption, biliary disease, for bleeding or urgent surgery in patients on warfarin anticoagulants, or with disseminated intravascular coagulation. Other less common indications include replacement of C1 esterase inhibitor in patients with hereditary angioedema and use in patients with thrombotic thrombocytopenic purpura as a simple transfusion or as part of a therapeutic plasma exchange.[11] Fresh-frozen plasma should not be used as a volume expander because the risk from some transfusion-transmitted disease is as significant as with cellular products. Crystalloid, which has no viral transmission risks, or albumin, which has a markedly reduced viral transmission risk, is preferable to FFP. Vitamin K is the treatment of choice for coagulation factor replacement in vitamin K deficiency, unless there is an acute clinical indication for rapid replacement, in which case FFP may be used.

The appropriate volumes of FFP for treatment of single coagulation deficiencies are easy to calculate. Calculations are based on the assumption that there is 1 ml of factor activity for each milliliter of FFP. For most factor deficiencies, 30% of factor activity is sufficient for hemostasis, but a higher percentage of factor activity is required for invasive surgical procedures. Factor VIII and IX deficiencies are most often treated with recombinant or plasma-derived factor concentrates.

Those factor concentrates that are plasma derived now undergo several processes to destroy viral infectivity. These processes may include heat treatment, solvent-detergent treatment, preparation by monoclonal antibody affinity chromatography, and nanofiltration. Recombinant factor VIII and IX are prepared with little or no albumin stabilization and are essentially plasma free. They are used preferentially in hemophilia A and B, especially in infants and non–plasma-exposed children.

The amount of factor V required for replacement in a factor V-deficient patient with 5% factor V who requires surgery at 30% can be calculated as follows:

$$\text{Weight (in kg)} \times 70 \text{ ml (per kg)} = \text{Blood volume (in ml)} \quad (1)$$

$$\text{Blood volume (in ml)} \times (1.0 - \text{Hematocrit}) = \text{Plasma volume (in ml)} \quad (2)$$

$$\text{Plasma volume (in ml)} \times (\text{Desired factor V [U/ml]} - \text{Initial factor V [U/ml]}) = \text{Units factor V} \quad (3)$$

For example:

$$(35\text{-kg child}) \times (70 \text{ ml/kg}) = 2450 \text{ ml blood volume}$$

$$2450 \times (1.0 - 0.4) = 1470 \text{ ml plasma volume}$$

$$1470 \times (0.3 - 0.05) = 367.5 \text{ U of factor V}$$

Therefore 370 ml of FFP should be infused because the activity of coagulation factors in FFP is assumed to be 1 U/ml.

Knowledge of the half-life of the transfused factor is essential in planning the dosage schedule[12] (see Table 75–4). Measurement of the specific factor is helpful to monitor transfusion frequency. Active consumption or ongoing blood loss decreases the expected increment and mandates further laboratory study and additional treatment.

Cryoprecipitate

Cryoprecipitated antihemophilic factor is the cold-insoluble portion of plasma remaining after FFP has been thawed between 1° C and 6° C and refrozen; it usually is termed *cryoprecipitate.* Each bag of 10 to 15 ml contains 80 U of factor VIII and at least 150 mg of fibrinogen. These bags frequently are referred to as "units" of cryoprecipitate, which may be confusing to individuals trying to order units of factor VIII activity. Cryoprecipitate also contains factor VIII/von Willebrand factor (vWF) and fibronectin, an opsonic protein that aids in phagocytosis. There are no standards for the quantity of proteins other than factor VIII and fibrinogen in the manufacture of cryoprecipitate. Once thawed, cryoprecipitate should be transfused within 4 hours.

Cryoprecipitate can be used for treatment of von Willebrand disease. A therapeutic challenge with intravenous desmopressin (DDAVP) should generally be attempted before using blood products because DDAVP may be sufficient for types I and IIA von Willebrand disease. The U.S. Food and Drug Administration (FDA) has licensed detergent-treated, plasma-derived factor concentrates for use in von Willebrand disease with specific dosing guidelines, making the use of these products much less subjective than with cryoprecipitate. Quantitative or qualitative deficiencies of fibrinogen can be treated with cryoprecipitate. The most likely causes of an acquired deficiency are disseminated intravascular coagulation (DIC) or severe liver disease; dilutional hypofibrinogenemia may respond to cryoprecipitate treatment.

Quantitative deficiencies of fibronectin are associated with massive trauma. Fibronectin replacement in the form of cryoprecipitate has been recommended by some intensivists, although randomized, controlled therapeutic trials are lacking. Fibronectin depletion may develop during malnutrition or sepsis, with burn injuries, and in fulminant hepatic failure,[13] but even fewer studies have correlated administration of fibronectin in these settings with survival advantage.

For quantitative fibrinogen deficiency, the same replacement formulas can be applied as for any factor deficiency, except that the normal fibrinogen should be estimated at 250 mg/dl in the child, with quantitatively lower estimates in premature infants (150-200 mg/dl). For von Willebrand disease, calculations usually are not used because vWF is not quantitated in cryoprecipitate. Replacement for major hemorrhage usually is based on increasing the factor VIII coagulant activity to between 80% and 100% and the bleeding time to normal. In practice, one to two bags of cryoprecipitate per 5 kg of body weight are administered, with additional doses at 8- or 12-hour intervals, based on quantitative factor VIII levels and the clinical status of the patient. The newly licensed lyophilized pooled products make dosing much more accurate for von Willebrand disease when DDAVP is contraindicated.

Other Issues

Fresh-frozen plasma and cryoprecipitate should be ABO compatible with the recipient's RBCs. Because there are no RBCs in the product, the Rh type is not considered. Compatibility testing (cross-match) is not required. When large volumes of ABO-incompatible FFP or cryoprecipitate are administered, the isoagglutinins A and B in the product may produce a positive result on antiglobulin test and, rarely, hemolysis. Plasma product complications are the same as for cellular components, but there are disproportionately more allergic and anaphylactic reactions and fluid overload. Large doses of cryoprecipitate in a patient with normal fibrinogen may produce elevations of fibrinogen and precipitate acute thrombosis and DIC.

For complex coagulation factor deficiency, FFP can be administered in combination with cryoprecipitate. No controlled studies support these practices. Therapy for DIC should be directed at correcting the underlying disease. In the face of clinically apparent bleeding, 5 to 20 ml/kg of FFP can be administered every 12 to 24 hours with one bag of cryoprecipitate per 5 kg if quantitative fibrinogen is low. If the platelet count is less than 20,000/μl, platelet concentrates also would be indicated. Repeated measurements of coagulation tests are necessary to ensure that the component therapy is appropriate. Component therapy should not be used prophylactically. Conditions in which use of FFP is questionable include treatment of capillary leak syndromes, massive loss of lymph fluid, and nonbleeding patients with prolonged coagulation times who are not candidates for invasive procedures. Fresh-frozen plasma is not indicated prophylactically for coagulation factor replacement in the setting of massive transfusion.

Specialized Blood Products

Within the setting of the pediatric intensive care unit (PICU), use of specialized blood products may be indicated. Such products should be used after consultation with a transfusion medicine physician and in consultation with the child's primary care physician.

Blood Products Prepared to Reduce Risk of Cytomegalovirus Disease

Cytomegalovirus (CMV) is a ubiquitous virus of the herpes family that is harbored in WBCs.[14,15] A significant proportion of blood donors (30%–70%) are CMV seropositive, although regional differences may be related in part to different donor demographics such as age, sex, race, and socioeconomic status. Older age, female sex, and lower socioeconomic strata predispose to higher seroprevalence rates.

Three types of CMV infections are seen in the transfusion recipient: primary infection, reactivation infection, and reinfection. *Primary infection* occurs in a seronegative recipient of blood from a donor who is actively or latently infected. It is frequently symptomatic with a mononucleosis-like syndrome that is heterophile antibody negative. Viremia, viruria, and immunoglobulin (Ig)M-specific and then an IgG-specific anti-CMV antibody response can be demonstrated.

Reactivation occurs when a CMV-seropositive recipient receives blood from either a CMV-seropositive or CMV-seronegative donor. Donor dendritic leukocytes presumably present peptide–major histocompatibility complex (MHC) class II complexes to the recipient T lymphocytes, thereby triggering release of multiple cytokines and activation of latent CMV infection. An increase in IgG antibody titer and viral shedding may be observed. Most of these infections are asymptomatic, except in an immunocompromised host.[16] *Reinfection* or *coinfection* occurs in a CMV-seropositive blood recipient with a strain of CMV that differs from the strain that initially infected the recipient. An IgM and IgG response and viral shedding may be seen. The only way to distinguish reinfection from reactivation is to use molecular markers specific for different strains.

Both prospective and retrospective studies have demonstrated that IgG-seronegative blood and blood products have a low to nonexistent risk of transmitting CMV. Donors with IgM-specific CMV antibody or CMV viral antigen may be more able to transmit CMV because they are more likely to have acute viral infection and replication.[17] However, neither IgM antibody assays nor rapid polymerase chain reaction (PCR)-based testing for CMV viremia are standardized. Hence use of IgG-seronegative blood is considered to be gold standard, despite the fact that most IgG-seropositive units are not infectious.

Several different methods can be used to prevent or ameliorate posttransfusion CMV. Because the virus is harbored in WBCs, manipulations that can reduce or attenuate leukocyte cell number should reduce the risk of transmission. Historically these methods have included washing, freezing followed by washing, and filtration. However, filtration has clearly become the procedure of choice for removing leukocytes from RBC and platelet products, being capable of 10^3- to 10^4-fold (3–4 log) removal of WBCs.[18] In an often cited clinical trial, leukocyte-reduced blood products compared favorably with non–leukocyte-reduced blood products from seronegative donors in patients who had received bone marrow transplants.[19] That conclusion has been questioned based on a later study of more than 80 CMV-seronegative stem cell recipients; multivariant analysis did not support equivalency for RBCs.[20] Many patients undergoing chemotherapy with or without transplantation receive irradiated blood for prevention of graft-versus-host disease (GVHD). However, irradiation of blood to inhibit deoxyribonucleic acid replication (see later) does not prevent CMV infection.

There is a wide clinical spectrum associated with posttransfusion CMV. CMV infection may be asymptomatic and discovered only because of serial serologic or PCR-based tests, or it may produce significant morbidity and mortality. CMV pneumonia may develop in 10% of transplant recipients, and 60% to 80% of these cases may be fatal. The pediatric intensivist must be cognizant of certain patient groups at risk for pneumonia, cytopenia, hepatopathy, graft rejection, unexplained fever, and increased risk of bacterial and fungal infections associated with posttransfusion CMV. These groups include certain neonates, specifically those who weigh less than 1250 g who are seronegative and who require large amounts of blood, hematopoietic stem cell and some solid organ transplant recipients, infants receiving intrauterine transfusions, and congenitally immunodeficient patients. Other immunocompromised patients (e.g., cancer patients receiving chemotherapy), whether seronegative or seropositive, are at less risk of mortality and morbidity from CMV compared with transplant patients.

CMV infection develops in many patients infected with human immunodeficiency virus (HIV). In a retrospective study of patients infected with HIV, Sloand et al.[21] reported that the frequency of CMV infection was significantly increased in patients who had previously received transfusion compared with those who had received no transfusions. In vitro evidence suggests that the cellular elements of allogeneic blood transfusions may contribute to activation and dissemination of HIV or reactivation of latent CMV in this patient population.[22] CMV immediate early gene products have been shown to transactivate transcription of the HIV-1 genome in vitro, raising the possibility that CMV infection of HIV-infected patients hastens disease progression. The Viral Activation Transfusion Study (VATS) failed to support those theoretical models in HIV-infected patients.[23,24]

Some oncologists argue that patients who *may* undergo bone marrow transplantation should receive blood products manipulated to prevent CMV infection or reactivation, regardless of the marrow donor's serologic status. In support of this argument, in one study of patients receiving intensive chemotherapy for hematologic malignancy before allogeneic bone marrow transplantation, the proportion of seropositive patients among those actually receiving marrow transplantation increased from 36% to 48%.[25] This finding supports the practice of supplying products at reduced risk of transmitting CMV to potential recipients of marrow transplants who are CMV seronegative.

Many patients receiving blood that is CMV seronegative or leukodepleted receive CMV hyperimmune globulin or intravenous immunoglobulin with variable titers to CMV antibody and, in addition, may be receiving FFP. It may be difficult to assess the serostatus of these individuals because of passive acquisition of CMV antibody. Tests for CMV by direct culture or molecular techniques, such as PCR, are necessary to establish posttransfusion CMV infection in these individuals.

Irradiated Blood Products

Transfusion-acquired (TA) GVHD occurs when an immunosuppressed or immunodeficient transfusion recipient receives immunologically competent donor lymphocytes. The transfused histoincompatible T lymphocytes proliferate and engraft in the immunocompromised host, who is incapable of rejecting foreign cells. The degree of similarity between the HLA antigens of the blood donor and the recipient aids in engraftment. In the rare situation where the donor is homozygous for one of the recipient HLA haplotypes, then donor leukocytes will not be recognized as foreign, even in an immunocompetent host, and severe TA GVHD may occur. This situation is most likely to occur when family members serve as directed donors, although TA GVHD from unrelated donors has been reported, especially in populations with limited HLA phenotypes.[26]

Clinical symptoms of TA GVHD usually begin 4 to 30 days after transfusion and include fever, erythematous rash, anorexia, nausea, vomiting, and profuse watery diarrhea. The erythematous rash may progress to bullae and desquamation. Liver dysfunction, from simple liver enzyme elevations to fulminant hepatic coma, can occur. Severe cytopenias may develop and help differentiate TA GVHD from that occurring in bone marrow transplant recipients. In TA GVHD, the bone marrow hematopoietic progenitors are particularly affected. TA GVHD is fatal in 90% of reported pediatric cases. Diagnosis usually is made postmortem but can be made premortem with biopsy of the skin or gastrointestinal tract and molecular testing for the presence of donor HLA genes.[27,28]

Patient groups at risk for TA GVHD include bone marrow transplant recipients of any age, premature infants, and infants who have received in utero transfusions. Infants and children with unsuspected congenital immunodeficiency disease may develop TA GVHD, as may older children with immunodeficiency acquired congenitally or through chemotherapy.[27–29]

The incidence of TA GVHD is not known. Estimates for patients with leukemia range from 0.1% to 1% and 2% for lymphoma, but such rates are impossible to verify. Some neonatal centers use irradiated blood for all premature infants based on the known cellular and humoral immune dysfunction in these infants. However, this practice is not agreed upon by all.[30] It is likely that only the severest cases of TA GVHD are reported or, alternatively, that many are missed because of the similarities between the clinical manifestations of TA GVHD and chemotherapeutic and radiation-induced toxicities.

It is probable that there is a dose threshold for the number of viable lymphocytes that must be transfused to cause TA GVHD. Although the minimum number of leukocytes that may transmit TA GVHD is not precisely known, TA GVHD has been reported after transfusion of as few as 8×10^4 lymphocytes/kg body weight.[31] The greater the degree of immunosuppression of a transfusion recipient, the more likely that a given number of lymphocytes will cause TA GVHD. Therefore certain malignancies or stages of a given malignancy are not associated with TA GVHD because the attendant immunosuppression may be less intense. Other factors that may attenuate TA GVHD are the type of chemotherapy, concomitant use of radiotherapy, and other immunosuppressive regimens. The type of blood product is critical. Although TA GVHD has been associated with whole blood, PRBC, frozen deglycerolized RBCs, WBCs, platelets, and fresh plasma, it has not been associated with frozen thawed plasma or frozen thawed cryoprecipitate.

Because the lymphocyte is the most likely initiator of TA GVHD, the disease can be prevented by reducing the number of lymphocytes or by rendering them mitotically inactive. Because TA GVHD has been reported after leukocyte reduction by filtration,[32] γ irradiation currently is the only adequate method for preventing TA GVHD. The dose used should abrogate a mitogen or mixed lymphocyte culture response while producing no harm to the cellular components. With a sensitive limiting dilution assay of T-cell function, Pelszynski et al.[33] found that 2500 cGy was required to completely inactivate T cells in RBC units. Irradiation of platelet bags at 3000 cGy followed by storage does not alter platelet function. Irradiation of RBCs may not be benign; plasma potassium and hemoglobin concentrations in irradiated RBC units are higher (compared with nonirradiated units) after irradiation and storage.[31] In another study, when RBCs were irradiated with 3000 cGy and stored for 42 days, the in vivo survival was decreased compared with control, untreated cells.[34] The FDA recommends a 28-day expiration for irradiated RBCs. Red blood cell products transfused to fetuses or neonates or to children unable to tolerate potassium loads should be irradiated immediately before use and not stored.[31] Washed RBCs should be considered in certain patients who will receive products that have been stored for an extended period. Studies on the effect of irradiation of granulocyte products have produced variable results. Although chemotaxis and bactericidal killing remain intact at 5000 cGy, superoxide production was adversely affected at 2500 and 5000 cGy.[35] However, most authorities recommend irradiation of granulocyte products before administration.

Granulocyte Concentrates

Granulocyte concentrates are obtained by apheresis and contain 1×10^{10} cells in 200 to 400 ml. There is evidence that granulocyte yield and clinical outcomes may be increased by pretreatment of granulocyte donors with granulocyte colony-stimulating factor.[36]

Granulocyte concentrates are indicated in severely neutropenic patients with bacterial infections who have a chance of marrow recovery and who have not responded to antibiotic therapy. Their efficacy in fungal and yeast infections in similar patients is less certain. They usually are administered at a dose greater than 1×10^{10} granulocytes per day for 4 to 6 days. Because they have a hematocrit of 0.15%, they should be ABO and, if possible, Rh compatible with the recipient. Many adverse reactions to granulocyte transfusion have been reported, such as fever, rigors, and pulmonary reactions, including respiratory distress syndrome, deoxygenation, transmission of CMV, and GVHD. Previously HLA-alloimmunized recipients are at greatest risk for pulmonary toxicity. Their use in infants, although rare, has been advocated at 1×10^9/kg. Products should be CMV negative and irradiated to prevent posttransfusion CMV and GVHD. The collection, storage, and indications for granulocyte concentrates have been reviewed.[37]

Risks of Transfusion-Transmitted Diseases

Most blood donated in the United States is collected from voluntary donors who were screened before donation for high-risk activities, past medical history, use of medications, and travel history. In addition, donors are provided with the opportunity to self-exclude their donation at any point during or after the donation process. Blood is tested for a number of transmissible agents, including hepatitis B (hepatitis B surface antigen and core antibody), hepatitis C (hepatitis C antibody), acquired immunodeficiency syndrome (AIDS; HIV-1/2 antibody and p24 antigen), human T-lymphocyte virus (HTLV type I/II), and syphilis. Despite these safeguards and the introduction of nucleic acid testing for HIV and hepatitis C virus viral antigen, blood and blood products still may transmit disease. Hence *every* transfusion should be clearly indicated and documented; specific informed consent must be obtained from the patient or the patient's parent or guardian.

The current risks for transmission of viral disease are difficult to estimate because the rates now are so low that classic approaches such as investigations of clinically identified posttransfusion cases are no longer feasible. Most cases of viral infection are acquired during the donor "window period," that period of time between which the donor becomes infectious and the laboratory screening test result becomes positive. Both the American Red Cross and the Retrovirus Epidemiology Donor Study have calculated the risk of acquiring HIV, HTLV, hepatitis C, and hepatitis B with data from donor seroconversions and made estimates of window periods of the respective infections in the setting of nucleic acid testing for HIV and HCV (Tables 75–6 and 75–7) for current risks.[38,39]

Choice of Resuscitation Fluids

The primary treatment for a hemorrhaging patient should be a nonsanguineous fluid. Such solutions are more readily available, more rapidly administered, and effective even at low hematocrits at improving microvascular flow. As volume is restored, assessment of the extent of RBC loss can be made and RBCs requested. In the emergency situation, O-positive or O-negative packed cells can be provided without compatibility testing, which must be completed at a later time. Type-specific blood can be available in 5 to 10 minutes, whereas full compatibility testing of donor and recipient requires 45 minutes to 1 hour. Only normal saline solution (0.9% sodium chloride) should be used in the same infusion line as blood. Ringer's lactate contains calcium that chelates with the citrate anticoagulant and causes blood to clot in the container, whereas 5% dextrose is hypotonic and causes lysis of RBCs.

When RBCs are transfused rapidly, several adverse reactions may occur, including hypothermia as a result of the cold blood, and metabolic adverse effects such as hypocalcemia, hyperkalemia, hypokalemia, hypernatremia, hypoglycemia, and hyperglycemia. Hypertension as a result of rapid expansion of the intravascular space may occur.

Hypocalcemia is one of the most critical metabolic abnormalities because of its association with depressed myocardial contractility. Studies on the extent of this problem are contradictory, but the liver transplantation patient serves as the best model. Most transplant recipients are anhepatic for part of the procedure and therefore cannot metabolize citrate; they also receive large volumes of blood during a relatively short time. In such patients,

TABLE 75–6

Blood Products Used During Massive Transfusion

Blood Product	Availability*	Testing Required	Comments
O, uncross-matched PRBC†	5 min	None	Emergency use
ABO type-specific, uncross-matched PRBC†	10–15 min	ABO grouping	Emergency use
Cross-matched PRBC (negative screen)	30–60 min	ABO, RH, antibody screen	Blood compatible by cross-match
Cross-matched PRBC (positive screen)	90 min to several hours or longer	ABO, RH, antibody screen; ± special serologic studies	Good communication essential to prevent excessive delays
Platelets	20 min	No special testing‡	Pooled concentrates§ or apheresis product
Fresh-frozen plasma	45 min	No special testing¶	Thawing time required
Cryoprecipitate	15–20 min	No special testing	Thawing time required

*Does not include transportation time.
†Rh-negative units generally reserved for females of childbearing potential; Rh-positive units commonly used for males and older females.
‡ABO-compatible platelets generally provided, when available; Rh-negative platelets provided to Rh-negative females of childbearing potential.
§Refers to a pool of platelet concentrates derived from multiple whole-blood donations.
¶ABO-compatible plasma generally provided and routinely available.

TABLE 75–7

Infectious risks of transfusion in the United States, Canada, and other countries

Infectious agent	Source of estimate: United States and other countries	Canada
HIV (with NAT)	1:2.1 million U.S.—repeat donors 1:1 million U.S.—first-time donors	1:4.7 million
HCV (with NAT) 100	1:1.9 million U.S.—repeat donors 1:791,000 million U.S.—first-time donors	1:3.1 million
HTLV	1:641,000	1:1.9 million
HBV	1:30,000 to 250,000 U.S. 1:470,000 France	1:31,000
Syphilis	Virtually nonexistent	
HAV	1:10 million	
Malaria	1:4 million	
Chagas' disease	Extremely low	
CMV	Unknown	
WNV	Unknown	
Bacterial contamination		
Platelets*	1:1000 to 1:3000 U.S.	1:14,000 to 1:38,000 France
Platelet fatality*	1:140,000	
RBCs	1:500,000 U.S.	1:172,000 France 1:66,000 New Zealand
RBC fatality	1:8 million U.S.	1:1 million France

*Without pretransfusion culture of component, now routine in USA.

rapid blood product infusion is associated with decreased cardiac index, decreased ventricular function, and hypotension. Calcium infusion may be indicated in these patients. Other patients who receive massive transfusions should be monitored closely but should not receive prophylactic calcium infusions.

Hyperkalemia related to massive transfusion may depress myocardial contractility and should be monitored. Because banked blood is acidic as a result of the anticoagulant and the production of lactic acid during storage, a metabolic acidosis is expected in recipients and may further aggravate hypokalemia and hyperkalemia in massive transfusions. However, it is likely that hypoxemia and poor tissue perfusion play the most significant role in the development of this acidosis. Prophylactic administration of bicarbonate is not indicated, but pH should be monitored and metabolic defects treated as they are discovered.

Erythropoietin

Recombinant erythropoietin is efficacious in the treatment of the anemia associated with chronic renal failure and chemotherapy-induced anemia. Its use has been proposed for many other anemic conditions. With increased concern about the adverse effects of blood transfusion, critical care practitioners have looked toward this recombinant protein as a possible alternative to transfusion. Krafte-Jacobs et al.[40] examined endogenous erythropoietin levels in different groups of patients in a PICU. They compared acutely anemic critically ill patients, nonanemic critically ill patients, and patients with chronic anemia. The serum erythropoietin concentrations in the critically ill groups were significantly lower than erythropoietin values in the chronic anemia group. This held true even though the hemoglobin levels of the chronically ill and anemic critically ill patients were equivalent. They concluded that the erythropoietin response to known physiologic stimuli is blunted in critically ill children.[40] Conversely, there have been preliminary reports of elevated endogenous erythropoietin blood concentrations in children with sepsis and severe injuries.[41,42]

Severe anemia frequently occurs after extensive burns and may be related to many factors, including hemolysis, surgical blood loss, disturbed metabolism, infection, and possibly hormonal factors. There is controversy as to whether endogenous erythropoietin levels are high or inappropriately low in burn patients.[43] However, a report by Deitch and Sittig[44] indicates the erythropoietin response to anemia is appropriate in burn victims. Several investigators have evaluated the activity of recombinant erythropoietin in treating the anemia associated with thermal injury. Poletes et al.[45] described five burn patients with lowest hematocrit values ranging from 17% to 30% who were successfully treated without blood product transfusion by use of recombinant erythropoietin. In a retrospective study, Fleming et al.[46] compared a group of burn patients receiving recombinant erythropoietin and iron with a control group of patients receiving iron alone. The erythropoietin-treated patients showed increased reticulocytosis compared with the control patients, but there were no significant differences in the transfusion requirements between the two groups.[46] Furthermore, in a double-blind, prospective study of recombinant erythropoietin in patients with acute burns, other investigators found that this product did not prevent the development of postburn anemia or decrease transfusion requirements.[47]

Although there is evidence that recombinant erythropoietin may not be efficacious in patients with thermal injury, other groups of patients have not been thoroughly studied. Neonates, especially premature infants, have been studied extensively. Meta-analysis of 21 controlled clinical trials in infants with the anemia of prematurity failed to support its use[48] and was further supported by the results of the U.S. Neonatal Network trial,[49] where early institution of recombinant human erythropoietin plus iron had no impact on decreasing the transfusion requirements of this placebo-controlled trial of 290 infants. Clinical trials are needed to define which patient populations are most likely to benefit from this expensive form of therapy. In the interim it may be wise to restrict use of recombinant erythropoietin to those patients with known or suspected inappropriately low endogenous erythropoietin levels.

Alternative Products: Restricting Transfusion

With increased awareness of the adverse effects of transfusion, intensivists have sought other alternatives to blood product transfusion. One approach to decreasing these adverse effects is to adopt more restrictive transfusion criteria. In one small study, two groups of critically ill patients were randomly assigned to liberal and restrictive transfusion groups. These investigators found no differences in mortality or measurements of organ dysfunction between the two groups of patients.[50] The TRICC (Transfusion Requirements In Critical Care) trial provided data on more than 800 ICU patients randomized to either a restrictive approach (transfuse only if hemoglobin less than 7 g/dl and to hemoglobin between 7–9 g/dl) or liberal approach (transfuse at hemoglobin less than 10 g/dl and to range of 10–12 g/dl). Inpatient mortality was lower in the restrictive transfusion group, and subgroup analysis of patients younger than 55 years or those with Acute Physiology and Chronic Health Evaluations (APACHE II) scores less than or equal to 20 supported a restrictive approach.[51] This study and a smaller study on hip, abdominal, aortic, and coronary bypass surgery support lower triggers. Debate continues, however, on whether critically ill patients with impaired oxygen utilization, regional ischemia, and oxygen "debt," variably defined and measured, benefit from transfusion. Physiologic measurements, such as oxygen extraction ratio and oxygen consumption, have been used as surrogate markers for oxygen debt but lack specificity. They have not been used with any pediatric randomized clinical transfusion trials to date. Goodman et al.[52] evaluated 240 children in five PICUs in a retrospective cohort analysis to evaluate transfusion and mortality/morbidity. After controlling for effects of other variables, they found that transfusion was associated with increase of oxygen, days of mechanical ventilation, vasoactive agent infusions, and PICU and hospital length of stay.[52] These data on children support the findings of Hebert et al.[51] on restrictive transfusion policies improving outcomes in adult critical care.

Many of the complications of RBC transfusion, specifically the metabolic derangements, could be prevented if oxygen could be transported without human RBCs using hemoglobin-based oxygen carriers (HBOCs). To this end, two very different kinds of products have been developed: stroma-free hemoglobin (SFH) and perfluorochemical (PFC) emulsions. SFH can be prepared from outdated human blood, bovine, recombinant, or transgenic animal sources. The hemoglobin is extracted, treated with polymerization or other chemical modification, and may be crystallized or lyophilized. The advantages of HBOCs include no cross-matching, low viscosity and oncotic activity, and lack of antigenicity and disease transmission. However, these solutions have increased oxygen affinity, which limits their peripheral oxygen off-loading capability. Attempts have been made to package the hemoglobin in liposomes with 2,3-DPG and to encapsulate them with lecithin and cholesterol. This process should result in a more prolonged intravascular half-life, decreased renal excretion, and better oxygen off-loading. A polymerized, pyridoxylated hemoglobin having a relatively high P_{50} has been developed. The polymerization allows for a higher oxygen-carrying capacity at a relatively lower oncotic pressure compared with earlier SFH products. Therefore the hemoglobin concentration in this product may safely be as high as that of normal blood. Polymerized, pyridoxylated SFH has entered clinical trials.[53]

PFC emulsions have been under development since the 1960s. PFCs contain 8 to 10 carbon-fluorinated molecules that act as solvents for oxygen. When PFCs are transfused, oxygen is transported in three compartments: bound to hemoglobin, dissolved in plasma, and dissolved in PFC. Although results of in vitro studies were promising, in clinical studies the oxygen-transporting capacity of PFCs has been limited; patients required high inspired oxygen concentrations and had complement activation and reticuloendothelial blockade. One PFC emulsion has been licensed by the FDA for clinical use as an adjunct during angioplasty to protect myocardium from ischemic and postperfusion injury.

It is unlikely that either artificial platelets or granulocytes will be developed because of the complexity of their function. A more probable development is the use of mixtures of recombinant growth factors to promote hematopoietic differentiation of marrow stem cells. Studies for thrombopoietic stimulators are ongoing.

REFERENCES

1. Luban NLC: Massive transfusion in the neonate, *Transfusion Med Rev* 9:200, 1995.
2. Luban NLC, Strauss RG, Hume HA: Commentary on the safety of red blood cells preserved in extended storage media for neonatal transfusions, *Transfusion* 31:229, 1991.
3. Strauss RG, Burmeister LF, Johnson K, et al: Feasibility and safety of AS-3 red blood cells for neonatal transfusions, *J Pediatr* 136:215-219, 2000.
4. Blajchman MA, Dzik S, Vamvakas EC, et al: Clinical and molecular basis of transfusion-induced immunomodulation: summary of the proceedings of a state-of-the-are conference, *Transfus Med Rev* 15:108-135, 2001.
5. Mink RB, Pollack MM: Effect of blood transfusion on oxygen consumption in pediatric septic shock, *Crit Care Med* 18:1087, 1990.

6. Simpson MB: Platelet transfusion in selected clinical situations. In Smith DM, Summers SH, editors: *Platelets,* Arlington, Va, 1988, American Association of Blood Banks.
7. Gmur J, et al: Safety of stringent prophylactic platelet transfusion policy for patients with acute leukaemia, *Lancet* 338:1223, 1991.
8. Heddle NM, Blajchman MA, Meyer RM, et al: A randomized controlled trial comparing the frequency of acute reactions to plasma-removed platelets and prestorage WBC-reduced platelets, *Transfusion* 42:556-566, 2002.
9. Murphy S: ABO blood groups and platelet transfusion, *Transfusion* 28:401, 1988.
10. Skogen B, et al: Minimal expression of blood group A antigen on thrombocytes from A2 individuals, *Transfusion* 28:456, 1988.
11. Moak JL: Thrombotic thrombocytopenic purpura and the hemolytic uremic syndrome, *Arch Pathol Lab Med* 126:1430-1433, 2002.
12. Goldsmith JC: Plasma component therapy. In Luban NLC, editor: *Pediatric transfusion medicine,* Baltimore, 1990, Johns Hopkins University Press.
13. Schena FP, Pertosa G: Fibronectin and the kidney, *Nephron* 48:177, 1988.
14. Gerna G, et al: Human cytomegalovirus infection of the major leukocyte subpopulations and evidence for initial viral replication in polymorphonuclear leukocytes from viremic patients, *J Infect Dis* 166:1236, 1992.
15. Minton EJ, et al: Human-cytomegalovirus infection of the monocyte/macrophage lineage in bone marrow, *J Virol* 68:4017, 1994.
16. Hillyer CD, et al: The role of cytomegalovirus infection in solid organ and bone marrow transplant recipients: transfusion of blood product, *Transfusion* 30:659, 1990.
17. Lamberson HV, et al: Prevention of transfusion-associated cytomegalovirus (CMV) infection in neonates by screening donors for IgM for CMV, *J Infect Dis* 157:820, 1988.
18. *Technical manual of the American Association of Blood Banks,* ed 13, Bethesda, Md, 1999, American Association of Blood Banks.
18a. Wong ECC, Luban NLC: Cytomegalovirus and parvovirus transmission by transfusion. In Rossi EC, et al, editors: *Principles of transfusion medicine,* ed 3, Philadelphia, 2002, Lippincott, Williams & Wilkens.
19. Bowden RA, et al: A comparison of filtered leukocyte-reduced and cytomegalovirus (CMV) seronegative blood products for the prevention of transfusion-associated CMV infection after marrow transplant, *Blood* 86:3598, 1995.
20. Nichols WG, Price TH, Gooley T, et al: Transfusion-transmitted cytomegalovirus infection after receipt of leukoreduced blood products, *Blood* 101:4195-220, 2003.
21. Sloand E, et al: Transfusion of blood components to persons infected with human immunodeficiency virus type 1: relationship to opportunistic infection, *Transfusion* 34:48, 1994.
22. Busch MP, Lee TH, Heitman J: Allogeneic leukocytes but not therapeutic blood elements induce reactivation and dissemination of latent human immunodeficiency virus type 1 infection: implications for transfusion support of infected patients, *Blood* 80:2128, 1992.
23. Kruskall MS, Lee TH, Assmann SF, et al: Survival of transfused donor white blood cells in HIV-infected recipients, *Blood* 98: 272-279, 2001.
24. Collier AC, Kalish LA, Busch MP, et al: Leukocyte-reduced red blood cell transfusions in patients with anemia and human immunodeficiency virus infection: the Viral Activation Transfusion Study: a randomized controlled trial, *JAMA* 285:1592-1601, 2001.
25. Kelsey SM, Newland AC: Cytomegalovirus seroconversion in patients receiving intensive induction therapy prior to allogeneic bone marrow transplantation, *Bone Marrow Transplant* 4:543, 1989.
26. Shivdasani RA, et al: Graft-versus-host disease associated with transfusion of blood from unrelated HLA-homozygous donors, *N Engl J Med* 328:776, 1993.
27. Greenbaum BH: Transfusion-associated graft-versus-host disease: historical perspectives, incidence, and current use of irradiated blood products, *J Clin Oncol* 9:1889, 1991.
28. McMilin KD, Johnson RL: HLA homozygosity and the risk of related-donor transfusion-associated graft-versus-host disease, *Transfusion Med Rev* 7:37, 1993.
29. Ohto H, Anderson KC: Post-transfusion graft-versus-host disease in Japanese newborns, *Transfusion* 36:117, 1996.
30. Strauss RG: Data-driven blood banking practices for neonatal RBC transfusions, *Transfusion* 40:1528-1540, 2000.
31. Roberts GT, Sacher RA: Transfusion-associated graft versus host disease. In Rossi EC et al, editors: *Principles of transfusion medicine,* ed 2, Baltimore, 1996, Williams & Wilkins.
32. Akahoshi M, et al: A case of transfusion-associated graft-versus-host disease not prevented by white cell-reduction filters, *Transfusion* 32: 169, 1992.
33. Pelszynski MM, et al: Effect of gamma irradiation of red blood cell units on T-cell inactivation as assessed by limiting dilution analysis: implications for preventing transfusion-associated graft-versus-host disease, *Blood* 83:1683, 1994.
34. Davey RJ, et al: The effect of pre-storage irradiation on post-transfusion red cell survival, *Transfusion* 32:525, 1992.
35. Eastlund DT, Charbonneau TT: Superoxide generation and cytotoxic response of irradiated neutrophils, *Transfusion* 28:368, 1988.
36. Heuft HG, Goudeva L, Sel S, et al: Equivalent mobilization and collection of granulocytes for transfusion after administration of glycosylated G-CSF (3 microg/kg) plus dexamethasone versus glycosylated G-CSF (12 microg/kg) alone, *Transfusion* 42:928-934, 2002.
37. Price TH: Granulocyte transfusion in the G-CSF era, *Int J Hematol* 76(Suppl 2):77-80, 2002.
38. Dodd RY, Notari EP 4th, Stramer SL: Current prevalence and incidence of infectious disease markers and estimated window-period risk in the American Red Cross blood donor population, *Transfusion* 42:975-979, 2002.
39. Busch MP, Klineman SH, Nemo GJ: Current and emerging infectious risks of blood transfusions, *JAMA* 289:959-926, 2003.
40. Krafte-Jacobs B, et al: Erythropoietin response to critical illness, *Crit Care Med* 22:821, 1994.
41. Hawkins ML, Cue JI, DiPiro JT: Erythropoietin response to anemia of severe injury, *Crit Care Med* 22:A63, 1994 (abstract).
42. Krafte-Jacobs B, Bock GH: The relationship of erythropoietin and interleukin-6 in children with sepsis, *Crit Care Med* 24:1455-1459, 1996.
43. Vasko SD, et al: Evaluation of erythropoietin levels in the anemia of thermal injury, *J Burn Care Rehabil* 12:437, 1991.
44. Deitch EA, Sittig KM: A serial study of the erythropoietic response to thermal injury, *Ann Surg* 217:293, 1993.
45. Poletes GP, et al: Blood use in the burn unit: a possible role for erythropoietin, *J Burn Care Rehabil* 15:37, 1994.
46. Fleming RYD, et al: The effect of erythropoietin in normal healthy volunteers and pediatric patients with burn injuries, *Surgery* 112: 424, 1992.
47. Still JM, et al: A double-blinded prospective evaluation of recombinant human erythropoietin in acutely burned patients, *J Trauma* 38:233, 1995.
48. Vamvakas EC, Strauss RG: Meta-analysis of controlled clinical trials studying the efficacy of rHuEPO in reducing blood transfusions in the anemia of prematurity, *Transfusion* 41:406-415, 2001.
49. Ohls RK, Ehrenkranz RA, Wright LL, et al: Effects of early erythropoietin therapy on the transfusion requirements of preterm infants below 1250 grams birth weight: a multicenter, randomized, controlled trial, *Pediatrics* 108:934-942, 2001.
50. Hebert PC, et al: Transfusion requirements in critical care, *JAMA* 273:1439, 1995.
51. Hebert PC, Wells G, Blajchman MA, et al: A multicenter, randomized controlled clinical trial of transfusion requirements in critical care. Transfusion Requirements in Critical Care Investigators, Canadian Critical Care Trials Group, *N Engl J Med* 340:409-417, 1999.
52. Goodman AM, Pollack MM, Patel KM, et al: Pediatric red blood cell transfusions increase resource use, *J Pediatr* 142:123-127, 2003.
53. Gould SA, Moore EE, Hoyt DB, et al: The life-sustaining capacity of human polymerized hemoglobin when red cells might be unavailable, *J Am Coll Surg* 195:445-452, 2002.

CHAPTER

76

Hematopoietic Stem Cell Transplantation

Barbara Bambach

PEARLS

- Patients undergoing hematopoietic stem cell transplantation are severely immunocompromised for an extended length of time and are at high risk for opportunistic infections.
- Gastrointestinal symptoms in recipients of allogeneic stem cell transplants can be due to graft-versus-host disease or infections, and patients should undergo endoscopy with biopsies to determine the etiology.
- Recipients of allogeneic transplants who experience respiratory symptoms such as cough, tachypnea, or hypoxia should undergo bronchoalveolar lavage to determine the etiology. If the result is nondiagnostic and symptoms persist, open lung biopsy should be pursued.

Overview

Despite accomplishments of marrow grafting in mice after lethal irradiation, initial attempts in humans in the 1950s were unsuccessful. However, a decade later, upon recognition of the human histocompatibility system, successful transplantation in humans occurred for immunodeficiencies and malignancies.[1–3] The field of hematopoietic stem cell transplantation (HSCT) has grown to increase our knowledge regarding histocompatibility, use of alternative stem cell sources and donors, improved treatment of infectious complications, and identification of newer agents for treatment of graft-versus-host disease (GVHD).

Sources of Stem Cells and Identification of Donors

Hematopoietic stem cell transplantation involves transplanting pluripotent hematopoietic stem cells from a donor source into a recipient. These stem cells are capable of self-renewal and terminal differentiation and ultimately give rise to myeloid cells, lymphocytes, erythrocytes, and platelets (Fig. 76–1). The donor source of these stem cells can be from the patient or recipient themselves (autologous) or from another individual (allogeneic). A syngeneic transplant is an allogeneic transplant using a monozygotic twin as the source of stem cells. The source of the donor (autologous vs. allogeneic) is generally dependent upon the indication for which the transplant is being performed. Autologous transplants can be used for treatment of nonhematologic malignant diseases, whereas allogeneic transplants are used for hematologic malignancies and marrow failures or dysfunction.

Traditionally, HSCT has been performed using stem cells obtained from bone marrow. However, stem cells can be mobilized into the peripheral blood by the use of cytokines (e.g., granulocyte-colony stimulating factor [G-CSF]) or upon recovery from chemotherapy. These peripheral blood stem cells (PBSCs) allow for faster hematopoietic recovery and possibly less tumor contamination than bone marrow for autologous transplantation.[4,5] Umbilical cord blood has also been shown to have large numbers of stem cells capable of reconstituting hematopoiesis.[6,7] The first HSCT using cord blood was performed in 1988 on a 5-year-old child with Fanconi anemia using the patient's human leukocyte antigen (HLA)-identical sibling.[8] Since then, unrelated cord

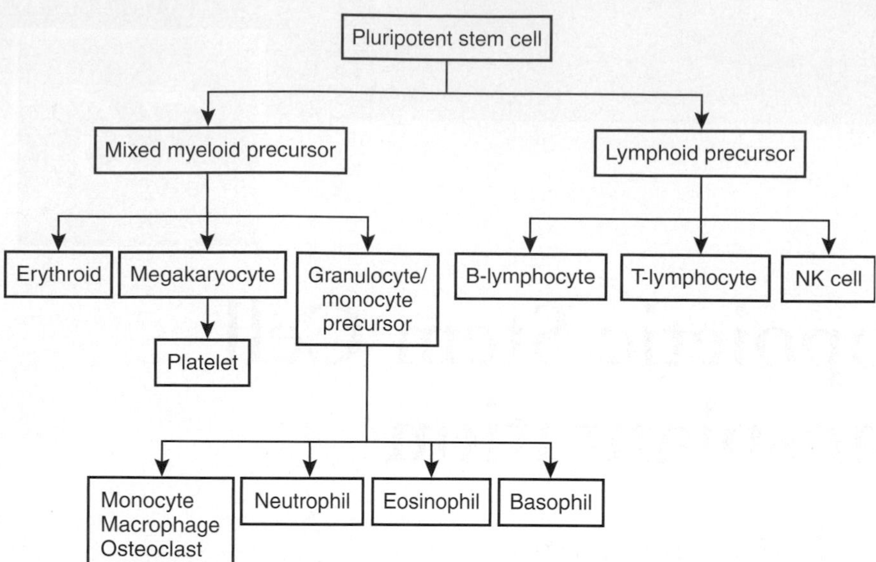

FIGURE 76–1 • Stem cell ontogeny. Differentiation and maturation of the pluripotent hematopoietic stem cell. *NK,* Natural killer.

blood stem cells have been used and numerous public cord blood banks have been established worldwide.

The major histocompatibility complex (MHC) is found on the short arm of chromosome 6 and has polymorphic closely related genes that encode for HLAs. These HLA antigens are involved in regulating immune recognition.[9] HLA class I antigens (A, B, C) are expressed on most nucleated cells, whereas class II antigens (DP, DQ, DR) are primarily on B lymphocytes, endothelial cells, and activated T cells. Each parent contributes an HLA allele to the child, and expression of HLA types is codominant. The patient undergoing allogeneic transplantation is HLA typed, as are the siblings, to determine if there is a genotypically matched sibling.

Allogeneic transplants are most successful when the recipient and donor are HLA identical. In the absence of a syngeneic donor, a genotypically HLA-matched sibling is the best donor. However, each sibling has only a 25% chance of being an HLA match to the patient. Therefore alternative donors may be sought, from either mismatched family members or phenotypically HLA-matched unrelated bone marrow or cord blood donors. Complications such as GVHD (see p. 1208, Graft-versus-host disease) and graft rejection are higher when these alternative donors are used. Despite the availabilities of unrelated bone marrow donor registries, many patients are unable to find a phenotypically HLA-matched donor. This is particularly true for the minority populations, which tend to be underrepresented in volunteer donor registries. Additionally, sophisticated immunologic and molecular techniques now routinely performed for HLA typing have narrowed the availability of bone marrow donors. Donors once thought to be matched by serologic techniques in fact may be mismatched by molecular techniques. Umbilical cord blood transplants appear to allow a greater degree of HLA mismatching without increasing the risk of GVHD, thereby allowing for a greater selection of donors.[10]

Indications and Outcomes

Allogeneic HSCT can be used as a mechanism to replace dysfunctional bone marrow such as in aplastic anemia or Fanconi anemia. It also can be used to provide a source of stem cells to replace abnormally functioning cells derived from stem cells (e.g., severe combined immunodeficiency) or deficient enzymes as seen in metabolic disorders (e.g., Hurler syndrome). The other role for HSCT is in the treatment of malignancies that either are at high risk for recurrence at diagnosis or have not responded to more conventional chemotherapy doses. As a general rule, patients with hematologic malignancies undergo allogeneic transplants, whereas patients with solid tumors would undergo autologous transplant in this setting. An area currently under investigation is the use of autologous HSCT for treatment of autoimmune diseases such as rheumatoid arthritis and systemic lupus.[11,12] Box 76–1 provides an overview of diseases for which HSCT has been successful or is under study. Outcomes from HSCT have improved with the development of broad-spectrum antibiotics and preventive treatments for GVHD. Survival results for HSCT are highly variable and are influenced by factors such as underlying disease (e.g., malignancy vs. bone marrow failure syndrome), remission status, and source of stem cells (e.g., related sibling vs. unrelated donor). Allogeneic transplants for aplastic anemia have survival rates of 48% to 100%.[13] Event-free survival for chronic myeloid leukemia is 50% to 90%,[14] 46% to 82% for acute myeloid leukemia,[15] and 27% to 84% for acute lymphoblastic leukemia.[16]

Transplant Procedure

Conditioning Regimen

Patients undergoing HSCT are subjected to a treatment regimen referred to as a *conditioning regimen* or *preparative regimen* prior to infusion of the hematopoietic stem cells. The purpose of this preparative regimen is multifold. In cases of malignant disorders, it provides cytoreduction and/or eradication of disease. In addition, the preparative regimen must be immunosuppressive in allogeneic transplantation to allow donor cells infused to establish themselves in the marrow cavity and overcome host rejection. The precise conditioning regimens can

BOX 76–1

Diseases Treated by Hematopoietic Stem Cell Transplantation

SOLID TUMORS

Neuroblastoma
Brain tumors
Lymphoma
Ewing sarcoma
Peripheral neuro-epithelial tumor
Germ cell tumors

LEUKEMIA

Acute lymphoblastic leukemia
Acute myeloblastic leukemia
Chronic myelogenous syndrome
Juvenile myelomono-cytic leukemia

ENZYME DEFICIENCIES/ METABOLIC DISORDERS

Lysosomal disorders
- Gaucher disease
- Niemann-Pick disease
- Wolman disease

Glycoprotein disorders
Leukodystrophies
- Childhood-onset X-linked ALD
- Globoid cell leukodystrophy
- Metachromatic leuko-dystrophy

Mucopolysaccharidase disorders
- Hurler syndrome
- Maroteaux-Lamy syndrome

BONE MARROW FAILURE/ DYSFUNCTION

Aplastic anemia
Fanconi anemia
Congenital immuno-deficiencies
Thalassemia
Sickle cell anemia
Osteopetrosis
Myelodysplastic syndrome
Kostmann syndrome
Thrombocytopenia absent radius syndrome
Schwachman-Diamond syndrome
Blackfan-Diamond syndrome
Glanzmann thromb-asthenia

AUTOIMMUNE DISEASES

Multiple sclerosis
Systemic lupus erythe-matosus
Rheumatoid arthritis
Scleroderma

include chemotherapy alone or in combination with radiation. Numerous regimens have been explored and are dependent upon the disease for which the transplant is required and the research interests of the institution performing the transplant.

Stem Cell Harvesting/Collection/ Cryopreservation

Stem cells can be collected or harvested from either bone marrow or peripheral blood. For patients or donors undergoing bone marrow harvest, general anesthesia or regional anesthesia is given in the prone position. Bone marrow is generally aspirated using special bone marrow harvest needles percutaneously from the posterior iliac crests using numerous passes. The amount of marrow taken is based upon the size of the recipient. If there is a significant size discrepancy between the donor and the recipient (recipient larger than the donor), the donor may lose a significant amount of blood because bone marrow is well perfused with blood. Donors can be placed on iron therapy after harvest, or they can electively store autologous blood ahead of time. A newer technique allows for the collected marrow to be processed with removal of red blood cells (particularly necessary in cases of major ABO incompatibility between donor and recipient), and these red blood cells can be given back to the donor postoperatively.

Peripheral blood stem cells can be mobilized in patients recovering from chemotherapy (autologous) or by giving allogeneic donors cytokines such as G-CSF. Their stem cells then can be collected using an apheresis machine in an outpatient setting. Collection of sufficient cells for transplantation may require several apheresis procedures.

Stem cells for allogeneic transplantation usually are collected on the day they are anticipated to be reinfused into the patient. Autologous collection of stem cells requires cryopreservation of the cells until the day of reinfusion. dimethyl sulfoxide (DMSO) is added to the collection product to ensure cell viability, and the cells are frozen in liquid nitrogen until needed.

Stem cells can be collected from umbilical cord blood. After delivery of the infant, sterile umbilical venous access is obtained and the blood is collected into anticoagulated tubes. This can be done either before or after delivery of the placenta. A sample of this cord blood is used for HLA typing and infectious disease testing; the remainder is cryopreserved.

Reinfusion

The day of stem cell reinfusion is referred to as day 0 for the transplant period. Cryopreserved stem cells are thawed in a water bath under sterile conditions and may be washed to remove the DMSO cryopreservant. Stem cells then are infused into the patient though the indwelling central venous catheter. These cells are capable of migrating into the bone marrow on their own. Blood transfusion-like complications can occur with reinfusion of stem cells, and patients are generally placed on cardiac monitors with emergency medications available at the bedside during the infusion. The infusion procedure is generally short, lasting anywhere from approximately 10 minutes to 1 hour, depending upon the volume of cells collected.

Recovery Period

Following the reinfusion of stem cells, patients wait for count recovery to occur and receive treatment for any toxicities they have developed (see p. 1202, Complications). Allogeneic transplant patients receive immunosuppressive medicines to prevent GVHD. Most patients are hospitalized for the entire transplant procedure, starting with the conditioning regimen. However, there is a trend toward outpatient HSCT, particularly in the autologous setting. A typical hospitalization for HSCT is 4 to 6 weeks, but it may be prolonged if umbilical cord blood is used or shortened for autologous transplants.

Complications

Hematopoietic stem cell transplantation is a therapy associated with significant morbidity and mortality. Complications can be acute during the immediate transplant period while the patient is still hospitalized, sub-acute for several months afterward, or chronic with late effects.

Myelosuppression and Hematologic Complications

The conditioning regimens used for HSCT result in myelosuppression with subsequent periods of profound neutropenia, anemia, and thrombocytopenia. The length of myelosuppression depends upon such variables as the source of stem cells, purging of the stem cells prior to transplant (to remove contaminating malignant cells), HLA disparity between donor and recipient, and dose of stem cells infused. Growth factors (i.e., G-CSF, granulocyte-macrophage [GM]-CSF) are often used to shorten the period of neutropenia and decrease the occurrence of infections. The median time to neutrophil recovery (absolute neutrophil count ≥500/μl) is 22 days for cord blood recipients[17] compared with allogeneic marrow or PBSC, which may require only 9 days for neutrophil recovery.[18]

Transplant patients require transfusion support with platelet and red cell products until they have adequate hematopoietic recovery. As a general rule, in the absence of comorbidities, platelet counts less than $20,000 \times 10^9$/L and hemoglobin less than 8 g/dl are thresholds for transfusions. All cellular blood products transfused should be leukofiltered and irradiated. Leukofiltration effectively prevents transmission of cytomegalovirus (CMV) and can prevent alloimmunization. γ-Irradiation of cellular blood products is used to prevent transfusion-associated GVHD. The dose of irradiation used results in a 5 log reduction in T-cell proliferation while preserving function of red blood cells, platelets, and granulocytes.[19–25]

Because ABO blood grouping and HLA genes are independently inherited, many patients undergo transplantation with ABO/Rh mismatched donors. ABO matching between recipient and donor may be (1) identical, (2) minor ABO incompatibility, (3) major ABO incompatibility, or (4) minor and major incompatibility. To minimize the hemolytic reactions that occur with ABO incompatibility, the appropriate blood component should be selected (Table 76–1). Minor ABO incompatibility occurs when recipient erythrocytes are incompatible with donor plasma (e.g., donor O, recipient A). Acute immune-mediated hemolysis can occur during stem cell reinfusion as a result of donor isohemagglutinins in the plasma. Donor plasma can be removed prior to stem cell reinfusion. Delayed hemolysis can occur 1 to 3 weeks after stem cell infusion because of donor lymphocytes infused with the stem cell product, which then produce isohemagglutinins. A positive direct antiglobulin test with clinical evidence of hemolysis

TABLE 76–1

Blood Product Selection in ABO-Incompatible Hematopoietic Stem Cell Transplantation

Donor	Recipient	Red Blood Cells	White Blood Cells	Plasma Platelets	*Platelets* First Choice	*Platelets* Second Choice*
A	A	A	A	A, AB	A, AB	B, O
B	B	B	B	B, AB	B, AB	A, O
O	O	O	O	O	O	A, B, AB
AB	AB	AB	AB	AB	AB	A, B, O
MINOR ABO INCOMPATIBILITY						
O	A	O	O	A, AB	A, AB	B, O
O	B	O	O	B, AB	B, AB	A, O
A	AB	A	A	AB	AB	A, B, O
B	AB	B	B	AB	AB	A, B, O
O	AB	O	O	AB	AB	A, B, O
MAJOR ABO INCOMPATIBILITY						
A	O	O	O	A, AB	A, AB	B, O
B	O	O	O	B, AB	B, AB	A, O
AB	O	O	O	AB	AB	A, B, O
AB	A	A	A	AB	AB	A, B, O
AB	B	B	B	AB	AB	A, B, O
MAJOR AND MINOR ABO INCOMPATIBILITY						
A	B	O	O	AB	AB	A, B, O
B	A	O	O	AB	AB	A, B, O

From Lopez-Plaza I, Triulzi D: Transfusion support in hematopoietic stem cell transplantation. In Ball E, Lister J, Law P, editors: *Hematopoietic stem cell therapy,* Philadelphia, 2000, Churchill Livingstone.

*Second-choice platelets must be concentrated to remove incompatible plasma.

is found in this situation. Donor-derived isohemagglutinins can be found in up to 50% of transplant patients, although only half of these will result in hemolysis.[26] When donor erythrocytes are incompatible with recipient plasma (i.e., donor A, recipient O), major ABO incompatibility exists, which can result in acute or delayed hemolysis and delayed red cell engraftment. The most frequently used technique to prevent this is processing of the stem cell product to remove donor red blood cells prior to reinfusion.[27–29] When recipient isohemagglutinin titers are ≥1:128, they can be depleted by intensive plasma exchange or extracorporeal immunoadsorption.[30] Delayed hemolysis in this setting can occur at the time of red blood cell engraftment in the presence of persistent recipient isohemagglutinin.[27,31] Transfusion with red blood cells compatible with recipient and donor isohemagglutinins is all that is necessary, although these patients have increased transfusion needs.[27,28]

Thrombotic microangiopathy can occur in the transplant patient, either clinically insignificant with schistocytic red cell fragments or as the full pentad of thrombotic thrombocytopenia purpura-hemolytic uremia syndrome (TTP-HUS) with anemia, thrombocytopenia, fever, uremia, and neurologic dysfunction. Endothelial injury is believed to be the initial event, and possible responsible factors include the specific conditioning regimen, use of cyclosporine A (CSA) or tacrolimus (FK506) for GVHD prophylaxis, presence of infection, or GVHD.[32–35] Clinically significant TTP has been reported in 6% to 10% of allogeneic stem cell transplants,[36] whereas red cell fragmentation only has been seen in up to 98% of HSCT recipients.[37] In one study that analyzed the natural history of TTP/HUS in bone marrow transplantation (BMT) recipients, 50% died within 3 months of diagnosis.[38] Either CSA or FK506 toxicity can result in an increase in fragmentation hemolysis, an increase in unconjugated bilirubin, and reticulocytosis. The hemolysis and red cell abnormalities that may occur resolve with a reduction in CSA or FK506 levels to normal. Both CSA and FK506 may be associated with central nervous system dysfunction (see neurologic complications), which can be confused with TTP-HUS. Treatment for TTP has included plasma exchange,[39] plasma exchange with protein A immunoadsorption,[40,41] or plasma exchange with vincristine.[42]

Immune Dysregulation

Immune dysfunction posttransplantation occurs for numerous reasons, including a quantitative decrease in neutrophils and lymphocytes, and altered cellular and humoral immunity functions. The rate of immune reconstitution is variable and is influenced by the type of donor and stem cell source (autologous, matched related allogeneic, unrelated allogeneic, bone marrow, PBSC, cord blood), presence of infections, and presence and treatment of GVHD. Immune recovery posttransplantation generally begins with basic phagocytic and nonspecific cytotoxic defenses.[43] Immunoglobulin (Ig) levels (IgM, IgG) are often suppressed for 3 to 4 months.[43,44] The normal CD4+/CD8+ T-cell ratio is inverted for as long as 9 to 12 months.[43,44] Neoantigen stimulation of immunoglobulin production is impaired during this time because this process is dependent upon T-cell and B-cell interaction. Secretory IgA production may be inhibited for many years later.[43,44] Immunosuppressive therapy and T-cell depletion of donor marrow as mechanisms for treatment or prevention of GVHD further dysregulate T-cell functions and lengthen the period of immune dysregulation. Additionally, patients with chronic GVHD have impairment of antigen-specific T lymphocyte response and ability to produce specific antibodies.[45]

Infection

Patients undergoing HSCT have increased susceptibility to many infections because of a combination of (1) neutropenia, (2) breakdown of physical barriers (mucositis, indwelling venous catheters), and (3) defects in cellular and humoral immunity as a result of the conditioning regimen and immunosuppressive therapy needed. The susceptibility to any particular organism varies over the course of the transplant period (Fig. 76–2).

During the first 2 to 4 weeks of the transplant, while the patient is neutropenic, bacterial infections account for approximately 90% of the infections. Enteric gram-negative

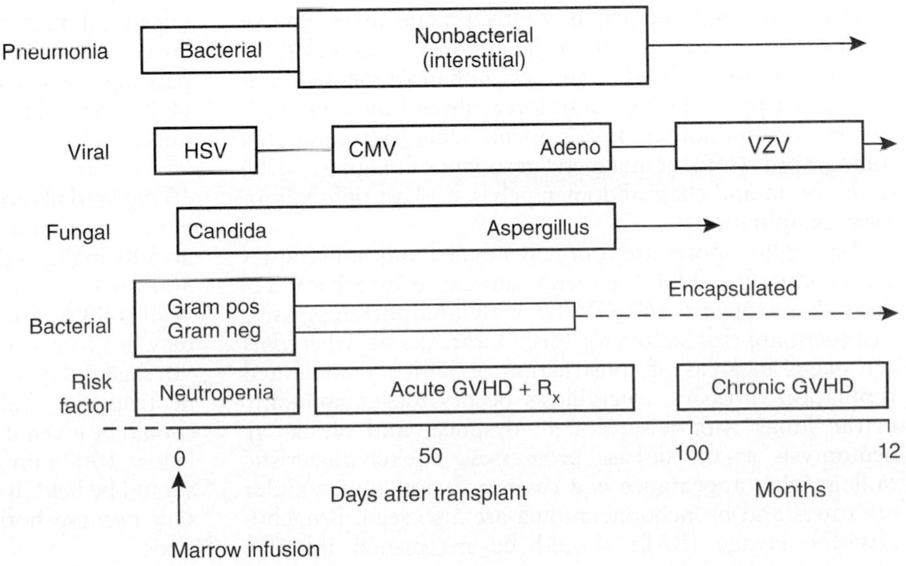

FIGURE 76–2 • Infectious syndromes at various times after bone marrow transplantation. *CMV,* Cytomegalovirus; *GVHD,* graft-versus-host disease; *HSV,* herpes simplex virus; *VZV,* varicella zoster virus.

bacilli (e.g., *Escherichia coli, Klebsiella, Enterobacter, Pseudomonas aeruginosa*) can cause rapid hemodynamic instability. The gram-positive infections (*Staphylococcus* and *Streptococcus*) are frequent causes of infections, due to the presence of central venous catheters. Therefore empiric antibiotic coverage for fevers during this time must be broad spectrum and provide adequate coverage for these organisms. Monotherapy with ceftazidime or imipenem is effective, simple, and has little toxicity.[46–48] Empiric use of vancomycin should be tempered by the emergence of vancomycin-resistant organisms. Because gram-positive infections are not immediately life threatening in most cases, vancomycin should be reserved for documented infections or the severely ill patient. Persistent or recurrent fevers during this time likely are caused by resistant organisms and should be aggressively sought and appropriately treated. Once neutropenia and mucositis have resolved, bacterial infections usually are acquired from the catheter, unless gastrointestinal (GI) or chronic GVHD is present.

Fungal infections are increasing in frequency with better treatment and prophylaxis of bacterial and viral infections, particularly after allogeneic transplantation. Fungal pathogens in HSCT patients include the yeasts (e.g., *Candida* species, *Cryptococcus neoformans*), molds (*Aspergillus, Fusarium, Mucormycosis*), and dimorphic fungi (*Coccidioides, Histoplasma, Blastomyces*). Of these, *Candida* and *Aspergillus* are most common. *Candida* species colonize the GI tract in more than half of healthy people,[49] but they become opportunistic infections in HSCT patients. *Candida albicans* and *Candida tropicalis* are sensitive to fluconazole. However, other resistant *Candida* organisms, such as *C. krausei, C. glabrata,* and *C. parapsilosis,* are emerging with widespread use of fluconazole prophylaxis.[50,51] Candidal infections can occur as superficial mucosal infections (e.g., thrush) or deeply invasive (hepatosplenic candidiasis). Esophageal candidiasis is associated with dysphagia and retrosternal pain. This may be difficult to distinguish from chemotherapy or radiation-induced mucositis or herpetic mucositis. Endoscopy may be necessary to diagnose and appropriately treat. Candidemia may present with fever and systemic symptoms and is frequently not associated with tissue involvement. Because most HSCT patients receive fluconazole prophylaxis, candidemia should be treated with amphotericin B. Many practitioners remove the indwelling catheter only if the cultures remain positive for more than 48 hours. Patients with documented candidemia or persistent/recurrent fevers should undergo evaluation for multiorgan involvement, including computed tomography (CT) or magnetic resonance imaging (MRI) of the brain and chest abdomen/pelvis, and an ophthalmologic examination.

Aspergillus spores are routinely inhaled and in immunocompromised or HSCT patients can cause invasive infections. Neutropenia and GVHD with immunosuppressive treatment are risk factors for this. Outbreaks of *Aspergillus* can occur in areas of construction or with contaminated ventilation. Invasive aspergillosis occurs most commonly in the lungs with fever, cough, dyspnea, and ultimately hemoptysis as the disease progresses. The characteristic radiographic appearance is a cavitary lesion, but nodular infiltrates and bronchopneumonia are also seen. Bronchoalveolar lavage (BAL) should be performed initially. However, up to 50% of patients have a negative BAL and should proceed to open lung biopsy.[52] The sinonasal area also can be infected with *Aspergillus*. Amphotericin formulations have been the standard therapy in the past. Newer and promising antifungal agents now are available and include the lipid formulations of amphotericin, such as AmBisome (liposomal formulation), Abelcet (complexed with lipid in ribbonlike structure), and Amphotec (complexed with lipid in a disklike structure). They appear to have equivalent or better efficacy and reduced nephrotoxicity,[53,54] Itraconazole, a newer triazole, is active against *Candida* and *Aspergillus*. Its use was limited in the past because of the lack of a parenteral preparation, erratic absorption of the oral preparation, and drug interactions with CSA or FK506. A new oral product with improved absorption is available. Although there are no randomized prospective studies with active fungal disease, itraconazole has shown clinical activity against *Aspergillus*.[55] Voriconazole, a new triazole, and Caspofungin, an echinocandin antifungal agent, also have activity against Aspergillosis.[56,57] In a published randomized trial comparing amphotericin B and voriconazole for invasive aspergillosis, voriconazole had a better response rate, improved survival, and fewer side effects.[58]

The herpes family of viral pathogens is the most problematic for HSCT patients post transplant. Herpes simplex can occur in autologous or allogeneic transplant patients within the first month after transplant. Cytomegalovirus (CMV) emerges in the allogeneic patient between 1 and 3 months posttransplantation if either the patient or donor were CMV positive pretransplantation. Varicella zoster can occur in the late transplant period, after day 100.

CMV lays dormant after the initial clinical infection. However, in immunosuppressed patients, this virus can reactivate and result in interstitial pneumonitis, enteritis, or bone marrow suppression. *CMV infection* is defined as the identification of CMV from any site or the seroconversion to CMV positivity. *CMV disease* is defined as the clinical manifestations seen in the presence of CMV infection. The use of CMV-negative blood products and leukofiltration of blood products has helped reduce the risk of CMV infections in patients undergoing transplant. Interstitial pneumonitis from CMV presents with hypoxia and fever and an interstitial pattern on chest x-ray film. Bronchoalveolar lavage should be performed immediately in any transplant patient experiencing these symptoms. Untreated, there is an 80% mortality rate.[59] Ganciclovir and intravenous immunoglobin (IVIG) is the recommended treatment for CMV interstitial pneumonitis.[60] Ganciclovir is given at 10 mg/kg daily for 21 days followed by 5 mg/kg/day 5 days per week until day 180 posttransplantation. IVIG is given at 500 mg/kg every other day for 21 days, followed by 500 mg/kg weekly until day 180. With this regimen, survival is 80%. For patients resistant to ganciclovir, foscarnet may be given at 60 mg/kg three times daily for 7 days, then 90 mg/kg/day until day 180.[61,62] Ganciclovir can cause neutropenia, and growth factor (e.g., G-CSF, GM-CSF) should be given if the absolute neutrophil count (ANC) falls below 1000/mm^3. If ANC is less than 500/mm^3, the drug should be held. In addition, renal adjustment may be necessary because both ganciclovir and foscarnet can be renal toxic.

Cytomegalovirus enteropathy presents with dysphagia, abdominal pain, nausea, vomiting, diarrhea, or GI bleeding. These symptoms can be seen with GVHD as well, and endoscopy should be performed to aid in the diagnosis. Treatment is similar to that of CMV pneumonia.

Prophylaxis of CMV with ganciclovir is prohibited by its marrow-suppressive effects. However, monitoring of CMV now is available with improved antigenemia testing and polymerase chain reaction, allowing for preemptive therapy if results of these tests become positive before onset of CMV disease. Ganciclovir then is given at 5 mg/kg twice daily for 7 to 14 days, then 5 mg/kg/day until day 120 posttransplantation.[63]

Prophylactic acyclovir is very effective at preventing herpes simplex infections in seropositive patients.[64]

As many as 50% of HSCT patients may develop varicella zoster reactivation posttransplantation.[65] Localized zoster is seen most often, although cutaneous dissemination or visceral involvement can occur. Intravenous acyclovir (500 mg/m^2 every 8 hours for 7 days, or until crusted) is given to patients with zoster or varicella posttransplantation to prevent this dissemination.

Mucositis and Nutritional Support

The GI tract can be affected by a direct toxic effect from the conditioning regimen, GVHD, or infections. Consequently, nutritional support can become extremely important during the posttransplant period.

Chemotherapy and radiation can individually and synergistically result in mucosal damage to the GI tract, which generally occurs within the first week or two of transplant. This mucositis may occur anywhere throughout the GI tract. In the oral and esophageal mucosa, ulcerative lesions can be visualized and result in pain. Supportive care during this period includes pain management with narcotics and aggressive nutritional support with hyperalimentation if necessary. Exquisite oral care is needed to prevent superinfection of ulcerative lesions. The exact regimen for oral care varies across institutions but can include rinses with saline, 0.12% chlorhexidine digluconate, sodium bicarbonate, or hydrogen peroxide. Topical anesthetic agents such as viscous lidocaine can help with pain control in the oral cavity. Numerous treatments for reducing or preventing mucositis are under investigation.

Graft-versus-host disease is discussed in detail on page 1208, in the section discussing Graft-versus-host disease. However, gut manifestations of GVHD can occur once engraftment has begun. Symptoms may include crampy abdominal pain, profuse diarrhea, nausea, vomiting, and anorexia. The diarrhea is secretory and induces a protein-losing enteropathy. Diagnosis must be established with endoscopy and biopsy. Hyperalimentation is needed until there is a response to immunosuppressive treatment.

Infections in the GI tract can occur at any point during the transplant process and involve any part of the GI tract. Thrush can be seen in the oral cavity while patients are neutropenic or taking steroids for prevention or treatment of GVHD. Candida esophagitis causes dysphagia and odynophagia. Diagnosis is established by endoscopy, and treatment usually is with fluconazole. Herpes simplex can cause ulcerative or vesicular lesions in the oral cavity or esophagus. Treatment is with high-dose acyclovir. Cytomegalovirus causes esophageal lesions, gastric lesions, or duodenal or colonic lesions. Inclusion bodies are evident histologically from the lesions. *Clostridium difficile* is common in transplant patients because of altered intestinal flora and use of broad-spectrum antibiotics. This should always be evaluated for and treated with metronidazole (Flagyl; intravenous or oral) or oral vancomycin.

Liver Complications and Veno-occlusive Disease

Hepatic complications of HSCT include infectious hepatitides (viral, fungal, bacterial), cholestasis, drug toxicity, veno-occlusive disease (VOD), and GVHD.

Viral hepatitis can be caused by any viral pathogen, including hepatitis C, CMV, Epstein-Barr virus (EBV), hepatitis B, *Adenovirus,* herpes simplex, and varicella zoster. The diagnosis of these pathogens is based upon clinical manifestations, with identification of the virus determined (1) histologically, (2) by culture of blood or tissue, or (3) by the presence of viral antigen or deoxyribonucleic acid within serum or liver tissue. Treatment is dependent upon identification of the viral pathogen. Herpes simplex and varicella zoster are treated with acyclovir, whereas CMV is treated with ganciclovir or foscarnet. EBV-induced donor lymphocytes have been used for EBV.[66]

Fungal involvement of the liver is often seen in conjunction with widespread dissemination. There may be granulomas, abscesses, cysts, fungus in biliary ducts, or infarcts from vascular occlusion. Typically, *Candida* species are seen; however, any fungal pathogen can occur. Ultrasound or CT scan may help identify a lesion. Ultrasound-guided fine-needle aspiration can confirm the diagnosis. Bacterial infections of the liver occur less commonly but present similarly.

Gallbladder stones from poor oral intake, cytoreductive therapy causing exfoliation of gallbladder mucous-containing cells, and increased biliary excretion of precipitable material (CSA, antibiotics) all contribute to a 70% incidence of gallbladder sludge.[67,68] Numerous medications required for HSCT can have direct toxicity on the liver, including antibiotics, fluconazole, and CSA. Histologically, drug effect should be suspected when there is significant hepatocellular necrosis and minimal inflammation.

Veno-occlusive disease following allogeneic HSCT was first reported in 1979[69] and now is recognized as a major cause of morbidity and mortality in the first 100 days of transplant. The pathogenesis is believed to result from hepatic venule and sinusoidal endothelial injury. Histologically, subendothelial edema, endothelial cell damage with microthrombosis, fibrin deposition, and expression of factor VIII and von Willebrand factor within venular walls is seen.[70] Hepatic necrosis occurs, and collagen deposition in the sinusoids, venular wall sclerosis, and collagen deposition in the venular lumen is seen as the disease progresses.[71] Risk factors can include elevated transaminases prior to the conditioning regimen,[72–74] use of methotrexate for GVHD prophylaxis,[75] presence of oral mucositis,[76] or interstitial pneumonitis.[77] Certain preparative regimens have also been found to have a higher incidence of

VOD, including those with high doses of total body irradiation, higher doses of cyclophosphamide, or the combination of busulfan and cyclophosphamide.[73,74] In patients who had VOD after busulfan and cyclophosphamide, a higher area under the curve was seen for busulfan than in those who did not develop VOD.[78] A subsequent study by the same group recommended routine busulfan pharmacokinetic measurement during busulfan administration to guide dosing.[79] This is commonly used today.

Clinically, VOD presents with hyperbilirubinemia, painful hepatomegaly, and fluid retention. The incidence varies based upon risk factors and the criteria used but reportedly is as high as 55%,[72] with mortality ranging from 3% to 67%.[80] Significant variability in mortality results from differing conditioning regimens and definitions of VOD. Two sets of criteria have been used for VOD. Jones et al.[73] first described VOD and modified this criteria as hyperbilirubinemia greater than 2 mg/dl with at least two of three other findings: hepatomegaly, ascites, or greather than or equal to 5% weight gain.[73] McDonald et al.[72] in Seattle defined VOD in their series as two of the following criteria occurring within 20 days of transplant: hyperbilirubinemia greather than 2 mg/dl, hepatomegaly or right upper quadrant pain, or sudden weight gain greater than 2% of body weight. Clinically, most patients with VOD develop symptoms between day 6 and 7 posttransplantation; peak around 10 days after onset; and return to baseline, if they are going to recover, 10 days later.[73] Multiorgan failure is seen more frequently in patients with VOD.[72,74] Pulmonary dysfunction, pleural effusions, hepatorenal syndrome, sodium retention with subsequent edema, and congestive heart failure all can occur and contribute to the high mortality rate. Bearman et al.[81] reported a model for predicting outcome in patients with VOD based upon preparative regimen used and level of bilirubin at certain time points. However, a retrospective study by Reiss et al.[82] involving only children did not find this model to be predictive. Transvenous liver biopsy and hepatic venous pressure gradient (HVPG) measurement has been found in a limited setting to have predictive value, with HVPG greater than 30 Hg associated with poor outcome,[83] and can be performed safely.[84] HVPG levels greater than 10 mmHg have been shown to be highly specific for diagnosis of VOD.[85,86]

Given that the pathogenesis is thought to involve endothelial injury and coagulation factor deposition, attempts have been made to reduce the hypercoaguable state with several agents, including heparin, prostaglandin, and bile salts. Use of heparin as a continuous infusion has been explored most extensively with conflicting results, although randomized studies to date have not shown any benefit.[87–89] Low-molecular-weight heparins are under investigation. Prostaglandin E administration was associated with severe toxicity and is not in use.[90] Ursodiol in historical studies and randomized trials has been shown to cause mild to moderate reduction in VOD occurrence.[91,92]

No agent for treatment of VOD has been evaluated in a prospective randomized trial. Thrombolytic therapy with recombinant tissue plasminogen activator (r-tPA) has been used successfully.[93,94] Pediatric dosing has been with low-dose r-tPA at 0.25 to 0.5 mg/kg for 4 days.[94] Careful monitoring for bleeding complications is required because these patients already are at high risk with thrombocytopenia and hepatic dysfunction. Defibrotide appears safe and is under investigation.[95] N-acetylcysteine, a thiol antioxidant, and nitric oxide have been tried in anecdotal reports.[96,97]

Hepatic GVHD usually occurs when GI GVHD is present. Clinically, cholestatic jaundice with increased serum alkaline phosphatase and hyperbilirubinemia occur. Hepatocellular dysfunction with ascites and coagulopathy are unusual unless there is multiorgan end-stage disease. Histologically, portal inflammation is the hallmark feature. Treatment is an increase or change in immunosuppressant medications, although normalization of liver test results may take weeks or months.

Neurologic Complications

Neurologic complications occur less often in autologous HSCT patients compared with allogeneic patients.[98,99] Most complications in allogeneic transplant patients are related to GVHD and the medications required to treat or prevent GVHD.

Metabolic encephalopathy probably is the most common neurologic complication with an incidence estimated to be as high as 37%.[100] Etiologically, this may be caused by hypoxia, ischemia, hepatic failure, electrolyte imbalance or renal failure. Clinically, patients are delirious or have a depressed mental status and no focal neurologic signs. Idiopathic hyperammonemia can occur in patients after high-dose chemotherapy, as in the transplant conditioning regimen. Altered mental status and respiratory alkalosis with elevated plasma ammonia occur acutely. Treatment involves holding intravenous nutrition and enhancing nitrogen excretion with continuous arteriovenous hemofiltration and using sodium benzoate or phenylacetate.[101] Left untreated, irreversible cerebral edema results.

Several chemotherapy agents that can be used in the conditioning regimen can have neurotoxicity. High-dose carmustine (BCNU), frequently used for autologous transplants for Hodgkin disease or lymphomas, has been associated with seizures. Busulfan, usually used in allogeneic transplants, can also cause seizures and epileptiform activity on electroencephalogram. Phenytoin is given prophylactically during busulfan administration.

Neurotoxicity from CSA or tacrolimus, used for GVHD prophylaxis or treatment, can include tremor, seizures, headaches, cortical blindness, neuropathy, or mental status changes. Frequently, these symptoms are observed with levels above the therapeutic range, but this is not always the case. These effects usually are reversible with elimination of the drug. As many as 5% to 6% of HSCT patients taking CSA may experience seizures.[102,103] Hypomagnesemia from renal wasting induced by CSA or tacrolimus may lower the seizure threshold and should be monitored. Phenytoin, phenobarbital, or carbamazepine, which may be used to treat seizures, can alter cytochrome P-450 and interfere with CSA or tacrolimus levels. Valproic acid may be a better alternative in this situation.[104]

Glucocorticoids used for immunosuppression can be associated with mood swings, dysphoria, agitation, or frank psychosis. Patients may experience steroid-induced myopathy that results in symmetrical weakness of proximal muscles.

Central nervous system infections are a consequence of neutropenia and immunosuppression. Depending upon the time period after transplant, patients may develop bacterial meningitis, aspergilloma invasion of brain parenchyma and vessels, or cerebral toxoplasmosis.

Peripheral nervous system neurotoxicity as an immune-mediated complication can be seen posttransplantation. Inflammatory degenerating polyneuropathy, myasthenia gravis, and polymyositis have been seen.[105–107] They present with muscle flaccidity, hypoactive deep tendon reflexes, and absence of extensor plantar reflexes.

Leukoencephalopathy occurs mostly in patients who received cranial radiation and/or intrathecal chemotherapy before and after transplantation.[108] This manifests days to months after transplantation and may present with dysarthria, ataxia, dysphasia, confusion, or decreased sensorium in severe cases. Either CT or MRI of the brain demonstrates white matter changes.

Pulmonary Complications

Almost half of all HSCT patients develop respiratory complications, which account for 40% of transplant deaths.[109,110] Mortality rates for transplant patients requiring mechanical ventilation are almost 95%.[111,112] Pulmonary complications can include parenchymal disease (idiopathic pneumonia, diffuse alveolar hemorrhage (DAH), pulmonary edema, pulmonary alveolar proteinosis), vascular disease (pulmonary VOD), or infections. Pulmonary infections are discussed elsewhere in this chapter; see Infection, page 1204.

Idiopathic pneumonia syndrome (IPS), once known as idiopathic interstitial pneumonia, is seen more commonly in patients receiving allogeneic transplants for hematologic malignancies.[113] This syndrome usually occurs before 100 days; the median time to onset is approximately 50 days posttransplantation.[114] Patients develop a nonproductive cough, fever, dyspnea, and hypoxia. Radiographic imaging shows diffuse or multilobar interstitial alveolar infiltrates. Bronchoscopy and/or lung biopsy should be performed to exclude infectious etiologies. Histologic results are variable, and interstitial inflammation, fibrosis, or diffuse alveolar damage may be seen. Causative factors are not known. However, there are associations of IPS with an increase in total dose or dose rate of radiation[115,116] or use of cyclophosphamide or carmustine in the conditioning regimen.[117,118] There is also an association between IPS incidence and severity of GVHD.[116,119,120] Data suggest that latent CMV or human herpes virus 6 in lung tissue may occur.[121,122] In the presence of GVHD, activated donor T lymphocytes and the cytokine cascade that occurs may result in acute lung injury.[122,123] Therapy for IPS is supportive, although anecdotal reports of corticosteroids exist.[113,114,116]

Diffuse alveolar hemorrhage occurs earlier than IPS, with a median onset at 12 days.[124] The clinical symptoms are similar to those of IPS, although hemoptysis may also be present. Radiographically, bilateral interstitial infiltrates, particularly centrally, and lower lung infiltrates are seen initially, then rapid progression to a diffuse bilateral alveolar pattern. Histologically, intraalveolar hemorrhage is seen. The usefulness of hemosiderin in alveolar macrophages obtained from BAL is limited because this finding is nonspecific, and there is no validated scoring system. There is no sensitivity or specificity to the correlation of bloody lavage fluid and histologic evidence of DAH. Additionally, alveolar hemorrhage can be present with infiltrative pneumonias.[125,126] Lung biopsy is the only definitive diagnostic test. The mortality rate from DAH can be as high as 75% to 100%,[127,128] although high-dose methylprednisolone (1.0 g/day) may improve this rate.[127]

Few studies exist regarding the incidence or pathogenesis of pulmonary edema in HSCT patients. In one study, 63% of patients developed pulmonary edema, all within the first 2 weeks.[129] These patients had developed weight gain, and echocardiography showed an increase in left ventricular end-diastolic volume. Vigorous diuresis resulted in resolution in 24 to 48 hours. This finding indicates that pulmonary edema posttransplantation is associated with volume overload. This can occur with the hydration necessary for the conditioning regimen, transfusions, antibiotics, and hyperalimentation. Other causative factors for pulmonary edema can include decreased serum oncotic pressure by protein losses and malnutrition posttransplantation, or increased capillary permeability by radiation or chemotherapy.[117] A capillary leak syndrome with noncardiogenic pulmonary edema, fever, renal failure, and hepatic dysfunction posttransplantation has been described.[130–132] This occurs within several days of engraftment and is hypothesized to be related to cytokine release of donor leukocytes and subsequent capillary endothelial injury. This form of pulmonary edema is associated with respiratory failure and high mortality.

Pulmonary alveolar proteinosis is a rare complication after transplantation.[133] Patients present with dyspnea, hypoxia, and diffuse alveolar infiltrates on radiography. The diagnosis is made by seeing abundant periodic acid–Schiff-positive proteinaceous material in BAL or lung tissue.

Pulmonary VOD is another rare pulmonary complication posttransplantation.[134,135] Cases occur between 40 and 60 days posttransplantation. Clinically, patients develop dyspnea, hypoxia, pulmonary hypertension, and right ventricular failure. Diagnosis is by lung biopsy, which shows occlusion of pulmonary venules and veins by intimal fibrosis. High-dose steroids are anecdotally successful.[135]

Because pulmonary complications posttransplantation can have many etiologies, transplant patients who develop respiratory symptoms (cough, dyspnea, hypoxia) should begin empirical therapy (broad-spectrum antibiotics, antifungal therapy) and immediately undergo bronchoscopy with BAL to further direct therapy. If no diagnosis is made and no clinical improvement is seen, lung biopsy should be performed.

Cardiac Complications

Cardiac complications following HSCT can occur acutely during the immediate transplant period or as a late sequela in survivors. Late effects of transplantation are discussed on page 1209, in the Late Effects section. Studies of acute cardiotoxicity primarily involve adults, and no specific pediatric studies for HSCT exist. Cardiac insufficiency can occur in the setting of septic shock, pneumonitis, or multiorgan failure. Myocardial ischemia, dysrhythmias, and severe myopericarditis have been described after high-dose cyclophosphamide therapy as used for transplantation.[136,137] A study from the University of Minnesota examined serious cardiac complications in BMT of adults and children.[138] Approximately 1% of their patients suffered major or fatal cardiotoxicity, which included rapid progressive heart failure, pericardial tamponade, acute ventricular fibrillation, and other cardiac arrhythmias. Thus it seems that cardiac toxicity is an uncommon, albeit serious, complication following transplantation.

Graft-versus-Host Disease

Graft-versus-host disease is a significant factor limiting use of allogeneic BMT. Donor T lymphocytes become alloreactive to host antigens or antigen-presenting cells. Activation of donor T lymphocytes, monocytes, and macrophages results in cytokine production with inflammatory manifestations leading to GVHD. Graft-versus-host disease can be acute or chronic, and target organs are predominantly skin, liver, and intestinal tract. Prevention of GVHD is best accomplished by HLA matching of donor and recipient. Despite this step, however, acute GVHD still occurs in 30% to 70% of HLA-genotypically matched recipients. There appears to be a correlation of GVHD with a graft versus leukemia/tumor effect, with a lower relapse rate seen in patients with higher GVHD grades.[139] Despite this finding, however, severe GVHD (grades III and IV) is associated with higher day 100 mortality rates and lower survival rates.[139]

Acute GVHD occurs at any point after engraftment until approximately 100 days posttransplantation. Clinically, fever, rash, diarrhea, and abnormal liver functions (elevation of bilirubin and/or alkaline phosphatase) can be seen. The rash is classically erythematous and maculopapular. It may be present on the palms and soles or become more widespread. Confirmation of GVHD should be sought prior to escalation of immunosuppressive therapy by biopsy of an affected area. Histologically, lymphocytic infiltration and apoptosis are seen with subsequent tissue destruction. Acute GVHD is given a clinical score based upon staging each affected organ and then assigning an overall grade dependent upon the stages of the affected organ systems (Table 76–2).

Onset of chronic GVHD can begin from approximately day 100 posttransplantation until 2 years after HSCT. Acute GVHD can evolve into chronic GVHD, or chronic GVHD can occur de novo. Patients with acute GVHD have an increased risk of developing chronic GVHD. Clinically, chronic GVHD is similar to autoimmune disorders, such as scleroderma. Skin changes can include hyperpigmentation, dermal atrophy, ulcers, and lichenoid patches, and the fibrosis present can cause contractures. The intestinal tract involvement can cause abdominal pain, strictures, vomiting, anorexia, diarrhea, or malabsorption. Liver manifestations show a cholestatic picture with jaundice and decreased protein synthesis. Other manifestations of chronic GVHD can include bronchiolitis obliterans and sicca syndrome with dry eyes and mouth. Patients may develop corneal abrasions and poor dental condition as a result of the sicca syndrome. Incomplete recovery of T-cell immunity and severe immunodeficiency are also seen with chronic GVHD.

Most institutions use cyclosporine or tacrolimus (FK506) either alone or in combination with short-course methotrexate and/or steroids as prophylaxis against GVHD. T-cell depletion of donor stem cells by various methods can reduce the risk of GVHD but is associated with higher rates of graft failure[140,141] and risk of a posttransplantation lymphoproliferative disorder. Cyclosporine is a cyclic undecapeptide that inhibits calcineurin, preventing transcription of the earlier activation genes in T lymphocytes. T cells already activated are not affected by cyclosporine. The major toxicity of cyclosporine is renal,

TABLE 76–2

Consensus Criteria for Clinical Staging and Grading of Acute Graft-versus-Host Disease

	Skin	Liver	Gut
STAGE			
1	Rash <25%* or persistent nausea§	Bilirubin 2–3 mg/dl†	Diarrhea >500 ml/day‡
2	Rash 25%–50%	Bilirubin 3–6 mg/dl	Diarrhea >1000 ml/day
3	Rash >50%	Bilirubin 6–15 mg/dl	Diarrhea >1500 ml/day
4	Generalized erythroderma with bullae	Bilirubin >15 mg/dl	Severe abdominal pain with or without ileus
GRADE¶			
I	Stage 1–2	None	None
II	Stage 3 or	Stage 1 or	Stage 1
III	—	Stage 2–3 or	Stage 2—4
IV	Stage 4 or	Stage 4 or	Stage 4‖

From Przepiorka D, Weisdorf D, Martin P, et al: *Bone Marrow Transplant* 15:825-828, 1995.
*Use "rule of nines" or burn chart to determine extent of rash.
†Range given as total bilirubin. Downgrade one stage if an additional cause of elevated bilirubin can be documented.
‡Volume of diarrhea applies to adults. For pediatric patients, the volume of diarrhea should be based on body surface area. Downgrade one stage if an additional cause of diarrhea has been documented.
§Persistent nausea with histologic evidence of graft-versus-host disease in the stomach or duodenum.
¶Criteria for grading given as degree of organ involvement required to confer that grade.
‖Grade IV may include lesser organ involvement with Karnofsky performance status <50%, so patients with stage 4 gut GVHD usually are grade IV.

which usually is reversible. Other side effects include magnesium wasting, gingival hyperplasia, hirsutism, hypertension, seizures, and cortical blindness. Cyclosporine usually is started at day −1 or −2 and started at 3 to 5 mg/kg/day as a continuous infusion. Oral preparations are available but are not bioequivalent, and conversion of intravenous dosing to oral depends upon the formulation used. Cyclosporine absorption is erratic and dependent upon numerous factors, such as certain foods and medications. The target level for cyclosporine varies depending upon the assay used (whole blood vs. plasma vs. serum, polyclonal antibody vs. monoclonal antibody vs. high-pressure liquid chromatography). Additionally, there is no evident correlation among dose, blood level, and risk of GVHD.

Tacrolimus is a macrolide antibiotic that also inhibits calcineurin and prevents activation of T cells. Tacrolimus has a similar toxicity profile to cyclosporine, although it does not cause hirsutism or gingival hyperplasia. Tacrolimus dosing typically starts at 0.03 mg/kg/day as a continuous infusion and has a conversion factor of 1:4 intravenous/oral, divided twice daily. Whole-blood trough levels of tacrolimus are monitored and therapeutic levels are 5 to 15 ng/ml, or up to 20 ng/ml.

If GVHD develops despite prophylaxis, front-line therapy is steroids. In stage I or II cutaneous GVHD, topical steroids may be used. In higher-stage or higher-risk patients, systemic steroids are used with a typical dose of methylprednisolone 2 mg/kg/day. Once a response occurs, tapering every 3 to 7 days by 20% to 50% should begin. Numerous therapies are emerging for treatment of steroid-refractory GVHD (Table 76–3). However, no good clinical trials are available to show superior efficacy of any particular therapy. Therefore second-line treatment of GVHD usually is institution dependent. These newer therapies are directed at interrupting the inflammatory response and inhibiting T-cell reactivity.

Patients with acute GVHD are at high risk for infectious complications, including bacterial, fungal, and CMV. These patients should receive fungal prophylaxis, and attentive skin care is necessary to prevent superinfection of denuded or desquamated areas.

Late Effects

As survival among patients undergoing HSCT improves, more information on late effects of transplantation is becoming available. These can include growth and development, reproductive issues, late cardiac effects, osteoporosis, and other endocrinologic complications. A discussion of these issues is beyond the scope of this chapter, and the reader is referred elsewhere for further detail.[142–144]

Conclusion

Hematopoietic stem cell transplantation can be curative for malignant and nonmalignant diseases. Advancements in this field have included (1) more precise HLA typing, allowing for better identification of donors and perhaps

TABLE 76–3

Agents for Treating Steroid-Refractory Acute Graft-versus-Host Disease

Mechanism of Action Drug	Drug Name (Trade Name)	Pediatric Dose
Inhibitor of T-cell activation	Sirolimus, Rapamycin (Rapamune)	>40 kg: 6 mg PO × 1, then 2 mg PO qd <40 kg: 3 mg/m^2 (6 mg max) PO × 1, then 1 mg/m^2/day (2 mg max)
Antimetabolite	Mycophenolate mofetil (CellCept)	600 mg/m^2/dose IV or PO bid
Antilymphocyte antibody	Antithymocyte globulin, ATG (Atgam)	15 mg/kg IV qod × 6 10 mg/kg IV qd × 14 30–40 mg/kg IV qd × 4
	Anti-CD52, alemtuzumab (Campath-1H)	No pediatric dosing
Anti-T-cell receptor antibody	Muromonab-CD3 (OKT3)	30 kg: 5 mg/d IV × 10–14 days < 30 kg: 2.5 mg/d IV × 10–14 days
Antibodies against T-cell activation antigens (IL-2 receptor blockade)	Anti-CD25, Daclizumab (Zenapax)	1 mg/kg IV q14d × 5 doses 1 mg/kg IV on days 1, 4, 8, 15, 22
Antibodies against T-cell costimulatory and adhesion molecules	Anti-CD5 immunotoxin, Xomazyme (Zolimomab, Aritox)	0.05–0.33 mg/kg/day IV × 14 days 0.1 mg/m^2/d IV × 7 days
	*Anti-LFA	
	*Anti-CD2	
Cytokine antagonists	Anti–TNF-α, Infliximab (Remicade)	5 or 10 mg/kg IV q week
	Anti-TNF R:Fc (Etanercept, Enbrel)	0.4 mg/kg (25 mg max) SQ 2 ×/week
	*Recombinant human IL-1 receptor antagonist	
	*Soluble recombinant human IL-1 receptor	

*Denotes an investigational agent.

decreased risk of GVHD; (2) utilization of other stem cell sources, including mobilized peripheral blood and umbilical cord blood; (3) identification and research into new immunosuppressant medications that may help treat or prevent GVHD; and (4) new antifungal agents for treating refractory or aggressive infections. Nonmyeloablative transplants are currently being evaluated in an attempt to decrease the toxicity from a fully ablative conditioning regimen. Mixed chimerism usually results from this treatment. Unanswered questions are (1) how chimerism changes over time, (2) how we can improve the chimerism, and (3) how much chimerism is needed. The answer to this last question likely is dependent on the underlying disease being treated, and what impact this will have on the cure of malignant diseases remains to be determined. Conceivably, nonmyeloablative transplants with mixed chimerism may allow for treatment of more patients with thalassemia, sickle cell disease, autoimmune diseases, or metabolic dysfunctions.

As HSCT proceeds over the next 30 years, the questions regarding nonmyeloablative transplants will be answered, with better knowledge of the immune system obtained with improvement in prevention and treatment of GVHD and improvement in graft-versus-tumor effect. These and other yet unpredicted discoveries hopefully will continue to improve the availability and effectiveness of HSCT.

REFERENCES

1. Gatti R, Meuwissen H, Allen H, et al: Immunological reconstitution of sex-linked lymphopenic immunological deficiency, *Lancet* 2:1366-1369, 1968.
2. Bach F, Albertini R, Joo P, et al: Bone marrow transplantation in a patient with the Wiskott-Aldrich syndrome, *Lancet* 2:1364-1366, 1968.
3. de Koning J, van Bekkum D, Dicke K, et al: Transplantation of bone-marrow cells and fetal thymus in an infant with lymphopenic immunological deficiency, *Lancet* 1223-1227, 1969.
4. Shpall E: Transplantation of enriched CD34-positive autologous marrow into breast cancer patients following high-dose chemotherapy: influence of CD34-positive peripheral blood progenitors and growth factors on engraftment, *J Clin Oncol* 12:28-36, 1995.
5. Bensinger W, Clift R, Martin P: Allogeneic peripheral blood stem cell transplantation in patients with advanced hematologic malignancies: a retrospective comparison with marrow transplantation, *Blood* 88:2794-2800, 1996.
6. Broxmeyer H, Douglas G, Hangoe G: Human umbilical cord blood as a potential source of transplantable hematopoietic stem/progenitor cells, *Proc Natl Acad Sci U S A* 86:3828-3832, 1989.
7. Broxmeyer H, Kurtzberg J, Gluckman E: Umbilical cord blood hematopoietic stem and repopulating cells in human clinical transplantation, *Blood Cells* 17:313-329, 1991.
8. Gluckman E, Broxmeyer H, Auerbach A: Hematopoietic reconstitution in a patient with Fanconi's anemia by means of umbilical cord blood from an HLA-identical sibling, *N Engl J Med* 321:174-178, 1989.
9. Filipovich A: The histocompatability barrier in bone marrow transplantation. In Johnson FL PC, Pochedly C, editors: *Bone marrow transplantation in children,* New York, 1990, Raven Press.
10. Kurtzberg J, Laughlin M, Graham M: Placental blood as a source of hematopoietic stem cells for transplantation into unrelated recipients, *N Engl J Med* 335:157-166, 1996.
11. Joske D, Ma D, Langlands D, et al: Autologous bone marrow transplantation for rheumatoid arthritis, *Lancet* 350:337-338, 1997.
12. Burt R, Traynor A, Ramsey-Goldman R: Hematopoietic stem-cell transplantation for systemic lupus erythematosus, *N Engl J Med* 337:1777-1778, 1997.
13. Wagner J, Storb R: Allogeneic transplantation for aplastic anemia. In Thomas ED, Blume KG, Forman SJ, editors: *Hematopoietic cell transplantation,* Malden, Mass, 1999, Blackwell Science.
14. Thomas E, Clift R: Allogeneic transplantation for chronic myeloid leukemia. In Thomas ED, Blume KG, Forman SJ, editors: *Hematopoietic cell transplantation,* Malden, Mass, 1999, Blackwell Science.
15. Margolis D, Casper J: Allogeneic transplantation for acute myeloid leukemia in children. In Thomas ED, Blume KG, Forman SJ, editors: *Hematopoietic cell transplantation,* Malden, Mass, 1999, Blackwell Science.
16. Davies S, Ramsay NKersey J: Allogeneic transplantation for acute lymphoblastic leukemia in children. In Thomas ED, Blume KG, Forman SJ, editors: *Hematopoietic cell transplantation,* Malden, Mass, 1999, Blackwell Science.
17. Wagner J, Kurtzberg J: Allogeneic umbilical cord blood transplantation. In Broxmeyer HE, editor: *Cellular characteristics of cord blood and cord blood transplantation,* Bethesda, Md, 1995, AABB Press.
18. Przepiorka D, Anderlini P, Ippoliti C, et al: Allogeneic blood stem cell transplantation in advanced hematologic cancers, *Bone Marrow Transplant* 19:455-460, 1997.
19. Pelszynski M, Moroff G, Luban N, et al: Effect of γ irradiation of red blood cell units on T-cell inactivation as assessed by limiting dilution analysis: implications for preventing transfusion-associated graft-versus-host disease, *Blood* 83:1683-1689, 1994.
20. Moore G, Ledford M: Effect of 400 rad irradiation on the in vitro storage properties of packed red cells, *Transfusion* 25:583-585, 1985.
21. Brugnara C, Churchill W: Effect of irradiation on red cell cation content and transport, *Transfusion* 32:246-252, 1992.
22. Read E, Kodis C, Carter C, et al: Viability of platelets following storage in the irradiated state: a pair controlled study, *Transfusion* 28:446-450, 1988.
23. Rock G, Adams A, Labow R: The effects of irradiation on platelet function, *Transfusion* 28:451-455, 1988.
24. Moroff G, George V, Siegl A, et al: The influence of irradiation on stored platelets, *Transfusion* 26:453-456, 1986.
25. Valerius N, Johansen K, Nielsen O, et al: Effect of in vitro X-irradiation on lymphocyte and granulocyte function, *Scand J Haematol* 27:9-18, 1981.
26. Robertson V, Henslee P, Jennings C, et al: Early appearance of anti-A isohemagglutinin after allogeneic, ABO minor incompatible, T cell depleted bone marrow transplant, *Transplant Proc* 19:4612-4617, 1987.
27. Sniecinsky I, Petz L, Oien L, et al: Immunohematologic problems arisisng from ABO incompatible bone marrow transplantation, *Transplant Proc* 19:4609-4611, 1987.
28. Lasky L, Warkenin P, Kersey J, et al: Hemotherapy in patients undergoing blood group incompatible bone marrow transplantation, *Transfusion* 23:277-285, 1983.
29. Blacklock H, Gilmore M, Prentice H, et al: ABO-incompatible bone-marrow transplantation: removal of red blood cells from donor marrow avoiding recipient antibody depletion, *Lancet* 2:1061-1064, 1982.
30. Bensinger W, Buckner C, Clift R, et al: Comparison of techniques for dealing with major ABO-incompatible marrow transplants, *Transplantation* 19:4605-4608, 1987.
31. Braine H, Sensenbrenner L, Wright S, et al: Bone marrow transplantation with major ABO blood group incompatibility using erythrocyte depletion of marrow prior to infusion, *Blood* 60:420-425, 1982.
32. Chappell M, Keeling D, Prentice H, et al: Haemolytic uraemic syndrome after bone marrow transplantation: an adverse effect of total body irradiation? *Bone Marrow Transplant* 3:339-347, 1988.
33. Guinan E, Tarbell N, Niemeyer C, et al: Intravascular hemolysis and renal insufficiency after bone marrow transplantation, *Blood* 72:451-455, 1988.
34. Rabinowe S, Soiffer R, Tarbel N, et al: Hemolytic-uremic syndrome following bone marrow transplantation in adults for hematologic malignancies, *Blood* 77:1837-1844, 1991.
35. Juckett M, Perry E, Daniels B, et al: Hemolytic uremic syndrome following bone marrow transplantation, *Bone Marrow Transplant* 7:405-409, 1991.
36. Gharpure V, Devine S, Holland H, et al: Thrombotic thrombocytopenic purpura associated with FK506 following bone marrow transplantation, *Bone Marrow Transplant* 16:715-716, 1995.
37. Valilis P, Zeigler Z, Shadduck R, et al: A prospective study of bone marrow transplant-associated thrombotic microangiopathy (BMT-TM) in autologous (Auto) and allogeneic (Allo) BMT, *Blood* 86:970a, 1995 (abstract).

38. Schriber J, Herzig G: Transplantation-associated thrombotic thrombocytopenia purpura and hemolytic uremic syndrome, *Semin Hematol* 34:126-133, 1997.
39. Sarode R, McFarland J, Flomenberg N, et al: Therapeutic plasma exchange does not appear to be effective in the management of thrombotic thrombocytopenic purpura/hemolytic uremic syndrome following bone marrow transplantation, *Bone Marrow Transplant* 16:271-275, 1995.
40. Zeigler Z, Shadduck R, Nath R, et al: Pilot study of combined cryosupernatant and protein A immunoadsorption exchange in the treatment of grade 3-4 bone marrow transplant-associated thrombotic microangiopathy, *Bone Marrow Transplant* 17:81-86, 1996.
41. Dua A, Zeigler Z, Shadduck R, et al: Apheresis in grade 4 bone marrow transplant associated thrombotic microangiopathy: a case series, *J Clin Apheresis* 11:176-184, 1996.
42. Silva V, Frei-Lahr D, Brown R, et al: Plasma exchange and vincristine in the treatment of hemolytic uremic syndrome/thrombotic thrombocytopenic purpura associated with bone marrow transplantation, *J Clin Apheresis* 6:16-20, 1991.
43. Lum L: The kinetics of immune reconstitution after human marrow transplantation, *Blood* 69:369-380, 1987.
44. Atkinson K: Reconstruction of the haemopoetic and immune systems after marrow transplantation, *Bone Marrow Transplant* 5:209-226, 1990.
45. Grazc P, Gale R: Chronic graft versus host disease: A syndrome of disordered immunity, *Am J Med* 66:611-620, 1979.
46. Pizzo P, Hathorn J, Hiemenez J, et al: A randomized trial comparing ceftazidime alone with combination antibiotic therapy in cancer patients with fever and neutropenia, *N Engl J Med* 315:552-558, 1986.
47. De Pauw B, Deresinski S, Feld R, et al: Ceftazidime compared with piperacillin and tobramycin for the empiric treatment of fever in neutropenic patients with cancer: a multicenter randomized trial. The Intercontinental Antimicrobial Study Group, *Ann Intern Med* 120:834-844, 1994.
48. Winston D, Ho W, Bruckner D, et al: Beta-lactam antibiotic therapy in febrile granulocytopenic patients: a randomized trial comparing cefoperazone plus piperacillin, ceftazidime plus piperacillin, and imipenem alone, *Ann Intern Med* 115:849 859, 1991.
49. Slavin M, Osborne B, Adams R, et al: Efficacy and safety of fluconazole prophylaxis for fungal infections after marrow transplantation: a prospective, randomized, double-blind study, *J Infect Dis* 171:1545-1552, 1995.
50. Abi-Said D, Anaisse E, Uzun O, et al: The epidemiology of hematogenous candidiasis caused by different *Candida* species, *Clin Infect Dis* 24:1122-1128, 1997.
51. Wingard J: Importance of *Candida* species other than *C. albicans* as pathogens in oncology patients, *Clin Infect Dis* 20:115-125, 1995.
52. Wald A, Leisenring W, van Burik J, et al: Epidemiology of *Aspergillus* infections in a large cohort of patients undergoing bone marrow transplantation, *J Infect Dis* 175:1459-1466, 1997.
53. Prentice H, Hann I, Herbrecht R, et al: A randomized comparison of liposomal versus conventional amphotericin B for the treatment of pyrexia of unknown origin in neutropenic patients, *Br J Haematol* 98:711-718, 1997.
54. Walsh T, Finberg R, Arndt C, et al: Liposomal amphotericin B for empirical therapy in patients with persistent fever and neutropenia: National Institute of Allergy and Infectious Diseases Mycoses Study Group, *N Engl J Med* 340:764-771, 1999.
55. Stevens D, Lee J: Analysis of compassionate use itraconazole therapy for invasive aspergillosis by the NIAID Mycoses Study Group criteria, *Arch Intern Med* 157:1857-1862, 1997.
56. Anonymous: Caspofungin: new preparation. A last resort in invasive aspergillosis, *Prescrire Int* 11:142-143, 2002.
57. Koss T, Bagheri B, Zeana C, et al: Amphotericin B-resistant Aspergillus flavus infection successfully treated with caspofungin, a novel antifungal agent, *J Am Acad Dermatol* 46:945-947, 2002.
58. Herbrecht R, Denning D, Patterson T, et al: Voriconazole versus amphotericin B for primary therapy of invasive aspergillosis, *N Engl J Med* 347:408-415, 2002.
59. Meyers J, Flournoy NED T: Risk factors for cytomegalovirus infection after human marrow transplantation, *J Infect Dis* 153:478-488, 1986.
60. Schmidt G, Kovacs A, Zaia J, et al: Ganciclovir/immunoglobulin combination therapy for the treatment of human cytomegalovirus-associated interstitial pneumonia in bone marrow allograft recipients, *Transplantation* 46:905-907, 1988.
61. Aschen J, Ringden O, Ljungman P, et al: Foscarnet for treatment of cytomegalovirus infections in bone marrow transplant recipients, *Scand J Infect Dis* 24:143-150, 1992.
62. Bacigalupo A, van Lint M, Tedone E, et al: Early treatment of CMV infections in allogeneic bone marrow transplant recipients with foscarnet or ganciclovir, *Bone Marrow Transplant* 13:753-758, 1994.
63. Goodrich J, Mori M, Gleaves C, et al: Early treatment with ganciclovir to prevent cytomegalovirus disease after allogeneic bone marrow transplantation, *N Engl J Med* 325:1601-1607, 1991.
64. Saral R, Burns W, Laskin O, et al: Acyclovir prophylaxis of herpes-simplex-virus infections, *N Engl J Med* 305:63-67, 1981.
65. Locksley R, Flournoy N, Sullivan K, et al: Infection with varicella-zoster virus after marrow transplantation, *J Infect Dis* 152:1172-1181, 1985.
66. Papadopoulos E, Ladanyi M, Emanuel D, et al: Infusions of donor leukocytes to treat Epstein-Barr virus-associated lymphoproliferative disorders after allogeneic bone marrow transplantation, *N Engl J Med* 330:1185-1191, 1994.
67. Schulman H, McDonald G: Liver disease after marrow transplantation. In Sale G, Schulman H, editors: *The pathology of bone marrow transplantation*. New York, 1984, Masson.
68. Frick M, Snover D, Feinberg S, et al: Sonography of the gallbladder in bone marrow transplant patients, *Am J Gastroenterol* 79:122-127, 1984.
69. Jacobs P, Miller J, Uys C, et al: Fatal veno-occlusive disease of the liver after chemotherapy, whole body radiation and bone marrow transplantation in refractory acute leukemia, *S Afr Med J* 55:5-10, 1979.
70. Shulman H, McDonald G, Matthews D, et al: An analysis of hepatic veno-occlusive disease and centrilobular hepatic degeneration following bone marrow transplantation, *Gastroenterology* 79:1178-1191, 1980.
71. Shulman H, Gown A, Nugent D: Hepatic veno-occlusive disease after bone marrow transplantation: immunohistochemical identification of the material within occluded central venules, *Am J Pathol* 127:549-558, 1987.
72. McDonald G, Sharma P, Matthews D, et al: Veno-occlusive disease of the liver after bone marrow transplantation: diagnosis, incidence and predisposing factors, *Hepatology* 4:116-122, 1984.
73. Jones R, Lee K, Beschorner W, et al: Veno-occlusive disease of the liver following bone marrow transplantation, *Transplantation* 44:778-783, 1987.
74. McDonald G, Hinds M, Fisher L, et al: Veno-occlusive disease of the liver and multiorgan failure after bone marrow transplantation: a cohort study, *Ann Intern Med* 118:255-267, 1993.
75. Essell J, Thompson J, Harman G, et al: Marked increase in veno-occlusive disease of the liver associated with methotrexate use for graft-versus-host disease prophylaxis in patients receiving busulfan/cyclophosphamide, *Blood* 79:2834-2840, 1992.
76. Wingard J, Niehaus C, Peterson D, et al: Oral mucositis after bone marrow transplantation: a marker of treatment toxicity and predictor of hepatic veno-occlusive disease, *Oral Surg Oral Med Oral Pathol* 72:419-424, 1991.
77. Wingard J, Mellitis E, Jones R, et al: Association of hepatic veno-occlusive disease with interstitial pneumonitis in bone marrow transplant recipients, *Bone Marrow Transplant* 4:685-689, 1989.
78. Grochow L, Jones R, Brundrett R, et al: Pharmacokinetics of busulfan: correlation with veno-occlusive disease in patients undergoing bone marrow transplantation, *Cancer Chemother Pharmacol* 25:55-61, 1989.
79. Grochow L, Piantodosi S, Santos G, et al: Busulfan dose adjustment decreases the risk of hepatic veno-occlusive disease in patients undergoing bone marrow transplantation, *Proc AACR* 33:1197, 1992.
80. Vinayek R, Demetris J, Rakela J: Liver disease in hematopoietic stem cell transplant recipients. In Ball E, Lister J, Ping L, editors: *Hematopoietic stem cell therapy*. Philadelphia, 2000, Churchill Livingstone.
81. Bearman S, Anderson G, Mori M, et al: Venoocclusive disease of the liver: development of a model for predicting fatal outcome after marrow transplantation, *J Clin Oncol* 11:1729-1736, 1993.
82. Reiss U, Cowan M, McMillan A, et al: Hepatic venoocclusive disease in blood and bone marrow transplantation in children

and young adults: incidence, risk factors, and outcome in a cohort of 241 patients, *J Pediatr Hematol Oncol* 24:746-749, 2002.
83. Shulman H, Gooley T, Dudley M, et al: Utility of transvenous liver biopsies and wedged hepatic venous pressure measurements in sixty marrow transplant recipients, *Transplantation* 59:1015-1022, 1995.
84. Bearman S: The syndrome of hepatic veno-occlusive disease after marrow transplantation, *Blood* 85:3005-3020, 1995.
85. Carreras E, Granena A, Navasa M, et al: Transjugular liver biopsy in BMT, *Bone Marrow Transplant* 11:21-26, 1993.
86. Shulman H, McDonald G: Transvenous liver biopsies and pressure measurements in bone marrow transplant recipients, *Hepatology* 16:148, 1992.
87. Marsa-Vila L, Gorin N, Laporte J, et al: Prophylactic heparin does not prevent liver veno-occlusive disease following autologous bone marrow transplantation, *Eur J Haematol* 47:346-354, 1991.
88. Attal M, Huguet F, Rubie H, et al: Prevention of hepatic veno-occlusive disease of the liver by continuous infusion of low-dose heparin: a prospective, randomized trial, *Blood* 79:2834-2840, 1992.
89. Bearman S, Hinds M, Wolford J: A pilot study of continuous infusion heparin for the prevention of hepatic veno-occlusive disease after bone marrow transplantation, *Bone Marrow Transplant* 5:407-411, 1990.
90. Bearman S, Shen D, Hinds M, et al: A phase I/II study of prostaglandin E1 for the prevention of hepatic venoocclusive disease after bone marrow transplantation, *Br J Haematol* 84:724-730, 1993.
91. Essell J, Schroeder M, Harman G, et al: Ursodiol prophylaxis against hepatic complications of allogeneic bone marrow transplantation. A randomized, double-blind, placebo-controlled trial, *Ann Intern Med* 128:975-981, 1998.
92. Ohashi K, Tanabe J, Watanabe R, et al: The Japanese multicenter open randomized trial of ursodeoxycholic acid prophylaxis for hepatic veno-occlusive disease after stem cell transplantation, *Am J Hematol* 64:32-38, 2000.
93. Bearman S, Shuhart M, Hinds M, et al: Recombinant human tissue plasminogen activator for the treatment of established severe venoocclusive disease of the liver after bone marrow transplantation, *Blood* 80:2458-2462, 1992.
94. Yu L, Malkani I, Regueira O, et al: Recombinant tissue plasminogen activator (rt-PA) for veno-occlusive liver disease in pediatric autologous bone marrow transplant patients, *Am J Hematol* 46:194-198, 1994.
95. Richardson PM, Warren D, Jin ZM, et al: Multi-institutional emergency use of defibrotide (DF) in 75 patients post-SCT with severe VOD and multisystem organ failure (MOF): response without significant toxicity in a high risk population, *Blood* 96:585a, 2000.
96. Ringden O, Remberger M, Lehmann S, et al: N-acetylcysteine for hepatic veno-occlusive disease after allogeneic stem cell transplantation, *Bone Marrow Transplant* 25:993-996, 2000.
97. Kajiume T, Yoshimi S, Nagita A, et al: Application of nitric oxide for a case of veno-occlusive disease after peripheral blood stem cell transplantation, *Pediatr Hematol Oncol* 17:601-604, 2000.
98. Graus F, Saiz A, Sierra J, et al: Neurologic complications of autologous and allogeneic bone marrow transplantation in patients with leukemia: a comparative study, *Neurology* 46:1004-1009, 1996.
99. Guerrero A, Perez-Simon J, Guitierrez N, et al: Neurologic complications after autologous stem cell transplantation, *Eur Neurol* 41:48-50, 1999.
100. Patchell R, White C, Clark A, et al: Neurologic complications of bone marrow transplantation, *Neurology* 35:300-306, 1985.
101. Rosario D, Werlin S, Laurer S: Hyperammonemic encephalopathy after chemotherapy: survival after treatment with sodium benzoate and sodium phenylacetate, *J Clin Gastroenterol* 25:682-684, 1997.
102. O'Sullivan D: Convulsions associated with cyclosporin A, *BMJ Clin Res Ed* 290:858, 1985.
103. Appleton R, Farrell K, Teal P, et al: Complex partial status epilepticus associated with cyclosporin A therapy, *J Neurosurg Psychiatry* 52:1068-1071, 1989.
104. Fischman M, Hull D, Bartus S, et al: Valproate for epilepsy in renal transplant recipients receiving cyclosporin (comment), *Transplantation* 48:542, 1989.
105. Eliashiv S, Brenner T, Abramsky O, et al: Acute inflammatory demyelinating polyneuropathy following bone marrow transplantation, *Bone Marrow Transplant* 8:315-317, 1991.
106. Zaja F, Barillari G, Russo D: Myasthenia gravis after allogeneic bone marrow transplantation: a case report, *Bone Marrow Transplant* 15:649-650, 1997.
107. Anderson B, Young P, Kean W, et al: Polymyositis in chronic graft versus host disease, *Arch Neurol* 39:188-190, 1982.
108. Thompson C, Sanders J, LFluornoy N, et al: The risks of central nervous system relapse and leukoencephalopathy in patients receiving marrow, *Blood* 67:195-199, 1986.
109. Cordonnier C, Bernaudin J, Bierling P, et al: Pulmonary complications occurring after allogeneic bone marrow transplantation. A study of 130 consecutive transplanted patients, *Cancer* 58:1047-1054, 1986.
110. Quabeck K: The lung as a critical organ in marrow transplantation, *Bone Marrow Transplant* 14:S19-28, 1994.
111. Afessa B, Tefferi A, Hoagland H, et al: Outcome of recipients of bone marrow transplants who require intensive care unit support, *Mayo Clin Proc* 67:117-122, 1992.
112. Paz H, Crilley P, Weinar M, et al: Outcome of patients requiring medical ICU admission following bone marrow transplantation, *Chest* 104:527-531, 1993.
113. Wingard J, Mellits E, Sostrin M, et al: Interstitial pneumonitis after allogeneic bone marrow transplantation, *Medicine* 67: 175-186, 1988.
114. Crawford S, Hackman R: Clinical course of idiopathic pneumonia after bone marrow transplantation, *Am Rev Respir Dis* 147: 1393-1400, 1993.
115. Keane T, Van Dyk J, Rider W: Idiopathic interstitial pneumonia following bone marrow transplantation: the relationship with total body irradiation, *Int J Radiat Oncol Biol Phys* 7:1365-1370, 1981.
116. Weiner R, Bortin M, Gale R, et al: Interstitial pneumonitis after bone marrow transplantation. *Ann Intern Med* 104:168-175, 1986.
117. Cooper J, White D, Matthay R: Drug-induced pulmonary disease, *Am Rev Respir Dis* 133:321-340, 1986.
118. Seiden M, Elias A, Ayash L, et al: Pulmonary toxicity associated with high dose chemotherapy in the treatment of solid tumors with autologous marrow transplant: an analysis of four chemotherapy regimens, *Bone Marrow Transplant* 10:57-63, 1992.
119. Clark J, Hansen J, Hertz M, et al: Idiopathic pneumonia syndrome after bone marrow transplantation, *Am Rev Respir Dis* 147:1601-1606, 1993.
120. Pino y Torres J, Bross D, W-C L, et al: Risk factors in interstitial pneumonitis following allogeneic bone marrow transplantation, *Int J Radiat Oncol Biol Phys* 8:1301-1307, 1982.
121. Cone R, Hackman R, Huang M-L: Human herpesvirus 6 in lung tissue from patients with pneumonitis after bone marrow transplantation, *N Engl J Med* 329:156-161, 1993.
122. Barbera J, Martin-Campos J, Ribalta T, et al: Undetected viral infection in diffuse alveolar damage associated with bone marrow transplantation, *Eur Respir J* 9:1195, 1996.
123. Muller C, Hebart H, Roos A, et al: Correlation of interstitial pneumonia with human cytomegalovirus-induced lung infection and graft-vs-host disease after bone marrow transplantation, *Med Microbiol Immunol* 184:115-121, 1995.
124. Robbins R, Linder J, Stahl M, et al: Diffuse alveolar hemorrhage in autologous bone marrow transplant recipients, *Am J Med* 87:511-518, 1989.
125. Agusti C, Ramirez J, Picado C, et al: Diffuse alveolar hemorrhage in allogeneic bone marrow transplantation, *Am J Respir Crit Care Med* 151:1006-1010, 1995.
126. de Lassence A, Fleury-Feith J, Escudier E, et al: Alveolar hemorrhage: diagnostic criteria and results in 194 immunocompromised hosts, *Am J Respir Crit Care Med* 151:157-163, 1995.
127. Metcalf J, Rennard S, Reed E, et al: Corticosteroids as adjunctive therapy for diffuse alveolar hemorrhage associated with bone marrow transplantation, *Am J Med* 96:327-334, 1994.
128. Jules-Elysee K, Stover D, Yahalom J, et al: Pulmonary complications in lymphoma patients treated with high dose therapy and autologous bone marrow transplantation, *Am Rev Respir Dis* 146:485-491, 1992.
129. Dickout W, Chan C, Hyland R, et al: Prevention of acute pulmonary edema after bone marrow transplantation, *Chest* 92:303-309, 1987.
130. Lee C, Gingrich R, Hohl R, et al: Engraftment syndrome in autologous bone marrow and peripheral stem cell transplantation, *Bone Marrow Transplant* 16:175-182, 1995.

131. Haire W, Ruby E, Gordon B, et al: Multiple organ dysfunction syndrome in bone marrow transplantation, *JAMA* 274:1289-1295, 1995.
132. Cahill R, Spitzer T, Mazumder A: Marrow engraftment and clinical manifestations of capillary leak syndrome, *Bone Marrow Transplant* 18:177-184, 1996.
133. Cordonnier C, Fleury-Feith J, Escudier E, et al: Secondary alveolar proteinosis is a reversible cause of respiratory failure in leukemic patients, *Am J Respir Crit Care Med* 149:788-794, 1994.
134. Troussard X, Bernaudin J, Cordonnier C, et al: Pulmonary veno-occlusive disease after bone marrow transplantation, *Thorax* 39:956-957, 1984.
135. Hackman R, Madtes D, Petersen F, et al: Pulmonary venoocclusive disease following bone marrow transplantation, *Transplantation* 47:989-992, 1989.
136. Gottdiener J, Appelbaum F, Ferrans V, et al: Cardiotoxicity associated with high-dose cyclophosphamide therapy, *Arch Intern Med* 141:758-763, 1981.
137. Buja L, Ferrans V, Graw R: Cardiac pathologic findings in patients treated with bone marrow transplantation, *Hum Pathol* 7:17-45, 1976.
138. Murdych T, Weisdorf D: Serious cardiac complications during bone marrow transplantation at the University of Minnesota, 1977-1997, *Bone Marrow Transplant* 28:283-287, 2001.
139. Gratwohl A, Hermans J, Apperley J, et al: Acute graft-versus-host disease: grade and outcome in patients with chronic myelogenous leukemia. Working Party Chronic Leukemia of the European Group for Blood and Marrow Transplantation, *Blood* 86:813-818, 1995.
140. Ash R, Herowitz M, Gale R, et al: Bone marrow transplantation from related donors other than HLA-identical siblings: effect of T cell depletion, *Bone Marrow Transplant* 7:443-452, 1991.
141. Quinones R, et al: Extended cycle elutriation to adjust T cell content in HLA disparate bone marrow transplantation, *Blood* 82:307-317, 1993.
142. Winters S, Syed M: Endocrine and metabolic complications. In Ball E, Lister J, Law P, editors: *Hematopoietic stem cell therapy.* Philadelphia, 2000, Churchill Livingstone.
143. Sanders J: Growth and development after hematopoietic cell transplantation. In Thomas E, Blume K, Forman S, editors: *Hematopoietic cell transplantation,* Oxford, 1999, Blackwell Science.
144. Deeg J: Delayed complications after hematopoietic cell transplantation. In Ball E, Blume K, Forman S, editors: *Hematopoietic cell transplantation,* Oxford, 1999, Blackwell Science.

CHAPTER 77

Hemoglobinopathy

Mauro Grossi

PEARLS

- The most useful laboratory tests in the diagnosis of hemoglobinopathies include a complete blood count with reticulocyte count and evaluation of red cell morphology.
- The majority of screening programs for sickle cell disease use isoelectric focusing of an eluate from dried blood spots that also are used to screen for hypothyroidism, phenylketonuria, and other disorders.
- Hemolysis is the major cause of anemia in patients with sickle cell hemoglobinopathies.
- Infection is a very serious complication among patients with sickle cell disease, with *Streptococcus pneumoniae* the single most common cause.
- The acute chest syndrome (ACS) is the number one cause of death and hospitalization among patients with sickle cell disease.
- Treatment for acute chest syndrome includes adequate pain control, rehydration, and oxygen administration for patients with low pulse oxymetry measurements, broad-spectrum antibiotics, bronchodilators, transfusion, bronchoscopy for patients not responding to initial therapy, aggressive ventilatory support, and corticosteroids and nitric oxide for patients not responding to conventional therapy.
- The most common sites of pain in patients with sickle cell disease are the bones and joints, including the spine, pelvis, and long bones.
- Chronic transfusion patients are at increased risk for complications of infection that may lead to chronic liver failure and hepatocellular carcinoma.

Definition

Hemoglobinopathies are a group of hereditary disorders characterized by abnormal hemoglobin structure. Hemoglobin is produced by genes that control expression of the hemoglobin protein; consequently defects of those genes produce abnormal hemoglobin. Since the early work from Linus Pauling, who introduced the concept of molecular disease, and Vernon Ingram, who studied the hemoglobin molecule by electrophoresis and chromatography, hundreds of abnormal hemoglobin variants with corresponding deoxyribonucleic acid (DNA) mutations have been discovered. Interestingly, most of these hemoglobin variants have minimal or no clinical manifestations.

Genetic mutations may alter the production of one of the two subunits of the hemoglobin molecule, as in thalassemia, or they may produce genetic alterations of the hemoglobin structure and produce an abnormal hemoglobin, as in sickle cell disease.

Molecular abnormalities have been found to affect the α, β, γ, and δ chains of the hemoglobin molecule. Genetic abnormalities include a single amino acid substitution, a two amino acid substitution (C-Harlem), fusion (Lepore), and deletion and elongation (Constant Spring). Functional abnormalities include aggregation (S, C), unstable hemoglobins (Köln), methemoglobins (M), and hemoglobins with abnormal oxygen affinity (Gun Hill, Kansas).

The most useful laboratory tests used in the diagnosis of hemoglobinopathies include a complete blood count (CBC) with reticulocyte count and evaluation of red cell morphology. Hemoglobin electrophoresis using cellulose acetate and citrate agar is required for detection of abnormal hemoglobins. Quantitation of hemoglobin F and A_2 and screening for Heinz bodies help to diagnose other hemoglobin abnormalities. Other laboratory studies including isoelectric focusing and globin chain electrophoresis should help identify other less common hemoglobin abnormalities.

This chapter reviews the most severe complications of hemoglobinopathies, including sickle cell disease and its variants, thalassemia major and intermediate, and the combinations of thalassemia with other hemoglobin mutations such as hemoglobin E.

Sickle Cell Disease

The term *sickle cell disease* includes many different conditions resulting from the inheritance of sickle hemoglobin. It can present as a homozygous state (HbSS) or a heterozygous state in combination with other abnormal hemoglobins, such as hemoglobin C, α and β thalassemia, and hemoglobin (D Punjab, O Arab. and Lepore Boston).

The molecular genetic defect in sickle cell disease is a single point mutation in the gene for β hemoglobin. The substitution in codon 6 of an adenine (A) for thymine (T) specifies the insertion of valine in place of glutamic acid in the β-globin chain (β6 glu-val).[1] Hemoglobin C results from a substitution in the first codon at the same site as hemoglobin S, with an insertion of lysine (β6 glu-lys).

Geographic Distribution

The association between the sickle cell mutation and a survival advantage against malaria determines the primary distribution of the sickle cell gene. Equatorial Africa is highly malarial, and the sickle cell mutation appears to have arisen on at least three or four separate occasions on the African continent. The mutations have been designated Benin, Senegal, Bantu, and Cameroon. The disease is seen in North and South America, the Caribbean, and southern Mediterranean countries such as Italy, Greece, and Turkey. In the eastern province of Saudi Arabia and in central India, there is a separate independent occurrence of the HbS gene or Asian haplotype, which is associated with a higher frequency of α thalassemia and high levels of fetal hemoglobin.[2]

Pathophysiology

The most prominent features in the pathophysiology of sickle cell disease can be summarized as processes activated by deoxygenation that trigger hemolysis, vasculopathy, anemia, and organ damage.

Polymerization

Hemoglobin S is a soluble compound when oxygenated. However, when oxygen tension decreases at the tissue level, oxygen is released from the hemoglobin molecule, causing polymerization or aggregation of the molecule and production of gels or crystals inside the cell.[3–5]

The mechanism involves the formation of 14 stranded fibers from hemoglobin molecules that have assumed a deoxy structure.[6] This formation subsequently produces cell rigidity, irreversible sickle cell formation, vaso-occlusion, and more hypoxia and organ damage. If reoxygenated, these polymers dissolve and the erythrocyte returns to normal. Hemoglobins F and A_2 are potent inhibitors of hemoglobin S polymerization.

Blood Viscosity

Increased blood viscosity slows blood flow in the microcirculation, initiating a cycle of increased oxygen extraction, additional sickling, and further rise in viscosity. The viscosity of deoxygenated sickled blood is influenced by the rate and extent of deoxygenation.[7] Membrane viscosity and deformability are markedly altered in sickle cell disease, even when the cell is fully oxygenated. The internal viscosity of these red cells is increased even in the basal state and is markedly increased when the hemoglobin becomes deoxygenated.[8]

Cellular Dehydration

Cellular dehydration is one of the pathologic features of sickle cell disease. Desiccation or formation of dense cells increases the polymerization process. The densest sickle cells, including irreversibly sickled cells, exhibit the most pronounced membrane abnormalities and the greatest adhesiveness to vascular endothelium.[9]

Dehydration of sickle red blood cells (RBCs) has pathophysiologic consequences, including increased RBC rigidity[10] and reduced cell lifespan.[11]

Oxygen saturation of hemoglobin, mean corpuscular hemoglobin concentration (MCHC),[4] pH,[12] temperature, and presence of other hemoglobins (HbF, HbC)[13] affect hemoglobin S polymerization. It is believed that factors influencing polymer formation and production of vaso-occlusive crisis include hypoxia, acidosis, and dehydration. Several mechanisms have been implicated in the process of cell dehydration and formation of dense cells, and three transport pathways may play an important role.[9] These pathways include the deoxygenation-induced pathway,[14–17] which permits passive K^+ losses and entry of Na^+ and Ca^{2+} into the cell; the K^+Cl^- cotransport pathway (KCC) activated by acidification or cell swelling[18–20]; and the Ca^{2+}-activated K^+ channel, or Gardos pathway,[21,22] which also can be induced by endothelin-1, platelet activato-facto (PAF), and interleukin-10.[23]

Cation transport and K-Cl cotransport also play important roles in determining RBC MCHC. The K-Cl cotransport is cell age dependent and is very active in young red cells.[24] Lower pH favors polymer formation and triggers K-Cl cotransport and an increase in MCHC.[20]

Endothelial Damage

Evidence that perturbation of vascular wall endothelium contributes to the vascular abnormalities of sickle cell anemia includes findings of histopathologic changes in splenic and cerebral vasculatures.[25,26] Sickle RBCs exhibit increased adherence to cultured endothelial cells under both static and flow conditions.[27–29] Membrane damage to the erythrocyte results from repeated cycles of RBC sickling and generation of oxygen radicals.[30] The production of oxidants is greater in sickle erythrocytes than in normal red cells.[31,32]

During a sickle cell vaso-occlusive episode, endothelial cell activators are generated and endothelial surfaces are altered.[33,34] There is increased production of vasoconstrictors[35,36] and vasodilators, an increase in the number of activated circulating endothelial cells, and expression of vascular cell adhesion molecule-1 (CD106), intracellular adhesion molecule 1 (CD54) (ICAM-1), E-selectin, and P-selectin reflecting endothelial injury.[37–41] It is likely that endothelial cell activation increases the risk of vaso-occlusion.[42] Cellular damage enables interaction between sickle cells, endothelial cells, and leukocytes.[28,43–45] Chronic activation of endothelial cells could be a risk factor for vaso-occlusion, and fluctuations in the activation of these cells might account for the apparently random attacks of vaso-occlusive crisis.[37]

Adherent leukocytes play a direct role in the pathogenesis of vaso-occlusion and influence disease prognosis.[46]

Vaso-occlusion can be described as a four-step process starting with (1) endothelial activation, which can be triggered by several processes including generation of oxygen radicals, adhesion, and infection. These various activating factors can induce expression of endothelial adhesion molecules and (2) promote the recruitment of adherent leukocytes. (3) Sickle erythrocytes interact with adherent leukocytes and (4) cause vascular clogging.[30,47]

At the same time, the phagocytic system destroys abnormally shaped red cells, producing hemolysis and anemia.

Hemolysis creates a population of red cells that is very young. These young cells have the tendency to adhere in the microcirculation and elevate the activity of transport proteins, which may lead to cell dehydration.[41]

Diagnosis

Neonatal Screening

Forty-four states, the District of Columbia, Puerto Rico, and the Virgin Islands currently provide universal screening for sickle cell disease. In the other six states, screening is available by request. The majority of screening programs use isoelectric focusing of an eluate from dried blood spots that are also used to screen for hypothyroidism, phenylketonuria, and other disorders.[48,49]

The sensitivity and specificity of current screening methodology are excellent[50] but not foolproof. There is a risk of failing to identify children who are born prematurely or who received blood transfusions prior to screening.[51,52]

The laboratory tests recommended to diagnose sickle cell disease include a CBC and evaluation of red cell morphology. A solubility test is available to screen for sickling hemoglobinopathies; the test gives rapid results and is inexpensive and accurate, but it is not specific for hemoglobin S.[53] The solubility test should be used only for screening purposes. Positive results should always be confirmed by hemoglobin electrophoresis, and no blood from infants younger than 6 months should be tested by this method.

Hemoglobin electrophoresis is the only way to confirm sickle cell disease or its variants. Cellulose acetate hemoglobin electrophoresis is a simple method for detecting abnormal hemoglobins.[54,55] Interpretations of results are based on known migration patterns and normal controls. Abnormal hemoglobins require confirmation by other methods, including citrate agar electrophoresis,[56] globin chain electrophoresis,[57] and isoelectric focusing.[58] Alkali denaturation test for fetal hemoglobin[59] and determination of hemoglobin A_2 by column chromatography are additional tests that help establish the presence of elevated hemoglobin F or hemoglobin A_2 in certain heterozygous combinations.

Clinical Features

Anemia

Anemia in sickle cell disease is primarily the consequence of dramatically shortened red cell survival. Factors known to determine the level of anemia are (1) intravascular and extravascular red cell destruction, (2) red cell production, (3) hemodilution, and (4) extent of the rightward shift of the hemoglobin-oxygen equilibrium curve.[60]

Although less impressive than in thalassemia major, there is an increase in extramedullary production of red cells among patients with sickle cell disease, with expanded bone marrow that replaces the fat from the marrow in long bones.[61–63] Renal damage has been postulated to decrease erythropoietin production.[64] Other factors that may influence anemia in sickle cell patients are erythrophagocytosis, hemodilution, and hemoconcentration.[60]

Dactylitis

Dactylitis, or hand-foot syndrome, is a limited avascular necrosis of marrow affecting the small bones or the juxtaarticular areas of long bones.[65] Dactylitis is manifested as painful acute swelling of the fingers, toes, or dorsum of the hands or feet. It affects both genders equally, and by age 2 years it affects 50% of patients. Recurrences occur in 40% of patients. Fever and other minor illness are frequently associated with dactylitis.

Splenic Sequestration

Splenic sequestration is defined as acute enlargement of the spleen with a decrease in hemoglobin concentration of at least 2 g/dl in a patient with normal bone marrow function. Most cases are mild. However, in severe episodes the spleen can be quite enlarged, filling the abdominal cavity, and the hemoglobin can drop to very low levels. Acute sequestration of cells and plasma may cause hypovolemic shock. Splenic sequestration is a life-threatening complication that requires immediate diagnosis and treatment. Splenic sequestration occurs in patients whose spleens have not undergone fibrosis. The majority of cases occur in patients who are younger than 2 years. Adult cases have been reported.[66,67] Most patients have hemoglobin SS disease, although patients with hemoglobin SC disease have been reported.

Treatment of splenic sequestration is immediate correction of the hypovolemia by packed RBC transfusion, which releases red cells trapped in the sinuses of the spleen, causes regression of spleen size, and increases the blood hemoglobin concentration. Recurrence of the sequestration process occurs in 50% of cases, with a mortality rate of 20%.[68] Most investigators recommend splenectomy following the second episode of sequestration. Despite concern for increased susceptibility to overwhelming infections, reports have shown minimal complications in sickle cell patients following splenectomy.[69] Educating the parents, teaching spleen palpation, and emphasizing the importance of seeking immediate medical attention when pallor or spleen enlargement occurs are fundamental to preventing this complication.

Aplastic Crisis

Hemolysis is the major cause of anemia in patients with sickle cell hemoglobinopathies. Aplastic crises are transient episodes caused by reduced production of red cells. Although the duration of these episodes is short, the degree of anemia can be severe because of the continuing process of hemolysis. Several viruses and bacteria have been associated with transient aplasia.[70,71] The agent identified most frequently has been human parvovirus (HPV) B19, which attacks erythroid precursors, depleting the bone marrow of precursors and reticulocytes. Most of the infection episodes related to parvovirus B19 are associated with fever, pain, splenic sequestration, or ACS.[72] Management of an aplastic crisis depends on the degree of anemia. It is recommended that patients with a decrease of 25% or greater from baseline hemoglobin and with associated reticulocytopenia should be transfused. Precautions should be taken to avoid hypertransfusion and increased blood viscosity and its complications.[73] New strategies to prevent parvovirus B19 infection and its complications have been suggested, including documentation of serotype. An effective vaccine is necessary.[72]

Infections

Infection remains a serious complication among patients with sickle cell disease, and *Streptococcus pneumoniae* is the single most common cause.[74,75] Other important pathogenic agents includes *Haemophilus influenzae, Neisseria meningitides,* viral influenza, *Salmonella, Mycoplasma pneumoniae, Chlamydia pneumoniae,* and parvovirus B19. Prevention of infection is the most significant defense. All patients with sickle cell disease should receive prophylactic penicillin.[76] Febrile patients should be evaluated by physical examination, blood count, and blood, urine, and throat cultures before they are given parenteral antibiotics. Some centers treat selected patients with antibiotics on an outpatient basis if they are stable and do not appear to have toxic symptoms.[77,78] Although preventive measures are most consistently recommended for patients with hemoglobin SS disease, health care personnel should be aware that splenic hypofunction and failure to make specific IgG antibodies to polysaccharide antigens also are seen in patients with other sickle cell hemoglobinopathies such as hemoglobin SC[79] and hemoglobin S B^+ thalassemia. Although it is often recommended that prophylactic penicillin be discontinued after age 5 years,[80] cases of septicemia with *S. pneumoniae* in older patients have been reported.

Pulmonary Complications

Acute Chest Syndrome

ACS is the number one cause of death and hospitalization among patients with sickle cell disease.[81] It is defined as fever, cough, wheezing, chest pain, tachypnea in the presence of a new pulmonary infiltrate involving at least one complete lung segment, and no atelectasis on chest radiograph. Several triggers in the pathophysiology of ACS have been identified, including atelectasis, fat embolism, true thromboembolism, and infection (Table 77–1). In 2000, Vichinsky et al.[82] reported the results of a prospective, multicenter study of ACS designed to determine the causes, incidence, and outcome of this complication. The study reported the results of 670 evaluable episodes of ACS. Fifty-eight percent were males and 82% had hemoglobin SS disease. Fifty-two percent were admitted with a diagnosis of ACS. Fever was present in 80% and cough in 62%. The mean number of lobes involved at diagnosis was 1.7, and 36% presented with a pleural effusion. The causes of the ACS are summarized in Table 77–1. Table 77–2 summarizes the infectious pathogens isolated in the 671 episodes of ACS.

The study concluded that there is generally a delay in making the diagnosis of ACS, the optimal treatment is unknown, and the cause usually is not determined. Patients may require more than one radiograph before the diagnosis is made, and serial blood work is required to monitor the disease.

Seventy-two of the patients who received either simple or exchange transfusion showed clear improvement in oxygenation. The rate of alloimmunization improved to 1% when phenotypically matched RBCs were used compared with 7% for regular transfusions. Bronchodilator therapy also was beneficial.

Recommendations for treatment of patients diagnosed with ACS include general management as adequate pain control, rehydration, and oxygen administration for

TABLE 77–1

Causes of Acute Chest Syndrome

Cause	All Episodes (N = 670)
Fat embolism	59 (8.8%)
Chlamydia	48 (7.2%)
Mycoplasma	44 (6.6%)
Virus	43 (6.4%)
Bacteria	30 (4.5%)
Mixed infections	25 (3.7 %)
Legionella	4 (0.6%)
Miscellaneous infections	3 (0.4 %)
Infarction	108 (16.1 %)
Unknown	306 (45.7%)

TABLE 77–2

Pathogens Associated with Acute Chest Syndrome

Pathogen	No. of Episodes
Chlamydia pneumoniae	71
Mycoplasma pneumoniae	51
Respiratory syncytial virus	26
Coagulase-positive *Staphylococcus aureus*	12
Streptococcus pneumoniae	11
Mycoplasma hominis	10
Parvovirus	10
Other	58
Total	249

Modified from Vichinsky EP et al: *N Engl J Med* 342:1855-1865, 2000.

patients with pulse oxymetry measurements less than 97% or 2% to 3% below baseline. More specific management of ACS includes (1) use of broad-spectrum antibiotics including a macrolide, (2) bronchodilators even if no wheezing is present, (3) transfusion, (4) bronchoscopy for patients who do not respond to initial therapy, and (5) aggressive ventilatory support including mechanical ventilation and/or extracorporeal membrane oxygenation (ECMO). New evidence suggests that use of corticosteroids and nitric oxide may be beneficial for severely ill patients who do not respond to conventional therapy.[83,84] For patients who are admitted to the hospital with severe pain, incentive spirometry should be considered, as well as daily monitoring for pulmonary disease. Use of hydroxyurea, chronic transfusion therapy, and bone marrow transplant should be considered for patients who suffer recurrent episodes of ACS.

Neurologic complications are frequently associated with ACS in patients with severe disease who require endotracheal intubation, ventilatory support, and transfusion. In a multicenter study,[82] neurologic complications developed in 22% of adults and 8% of children. Altered mental status, seizures, headaches, visual changes, and neuromuscular abnormalities are the most common events. The nonneurologic risk factor most highly predictive of stroke is a recent history of a pulmonary event.[85] In a group of children with ACS who developed neurologic complications, Henderson et al.[86] reported two seizures, three silent infarcts, two instances of cerebral hemorrhage, and three patients with reversible posterior leukoencephalopathy syndrome. They recommend magnetic resonance imaging (MRI) evaluation of the brain for all children with severe ACS who require endotracheal intubation and transfusion.

Pulmonary Hypertension

Pulmonary hypertension is increasingly recognized as a complication of sickle cell disease[87] associated with significantly increased mortality.[87–89] Aboubakr et al.[90] reported a 30% prevalence of pulmonary hypertension and a 2-month mortality rate of 30%.

Echocardiographic screening for pulmonary hypertension in patients with sickle cell disease[89] and efforts to identify reversible causes such as asthma, hypoxemia, and thromboembolism have been suggested. Hydroxyurea has been recommended for sickle cell patients with pulmonary hypertension.[91] Trials of oxygen, warfarin, transfusion, pulmonary vasodilators, and remodeling medications require further evaluation.[89]

Renal Complications

Renal pathology is prevalent among sickle cell patients, including patients with sickle cell trait. Acidosis, hypertonicity, and hypoxia are common in the renal medulla. Vaso-occlusion at the level of the vasa recta is the principal mechanism invoked to explain the physiopathology of renal complications.

Inability of the distal nephron to concentrate urine maximally or hyposthenuria (which in early years is manifested as enuresis) makes sickle cell patients more susceptible to dehydration, elevation of effective renal plasma flow, increased glomerular filtration rate, tubular dysfunction manifest as incomplete distal renal tubular acidosis, increased secretion of uric acid and creatinine, and glomerular abnormalities including proteinuria that may progress to nephrotic syndrome. Forty percent of patients with hemoglobin SS and nephrotic syndrome will develop end-stage renal disease.[92] Hematuria is one of the most common renal abnormalities in patients with sickle cell disease sickle cell trait. The bleeding originates from the left kidney in 80% of cases.[93] Management should be conservative, including bed rest, iron replacement, and/or transfusion. Vasopressin and ε-aminocaproic acid have been used successfully.[94,95] Papillary necrosis is also associated with both sickle cell disease and sickle cell trait. Acute renal failure has been associated with exertion-induced and nontraumatic rhabdomyolysis. Finally, renal medullary carcinoma, which is a highly aggressive malignancy of the kidney, should be ruled out in young sickle cell and trait patients who develop hematuria.[96]

Stroke and Central Nervous System Complications

Cerebrovascular accidents (CVAs) are severe complications of sickle cell disease and the leading cause of death in both children and adults.[85] The Cooperative Study of Sickle Cell Disease reported the prevalence of CVAs among 4082 patients was 3.75%.[85] The greatest age-adjusted prevalence estimate (4.01%) occurs in patients with hemoglobin SS disease, followed in decreasing order by 2.43% for hemoglobin S B° thalassemia, 1.29% for hemoglobin S B^+ thalassemia, and 0.84% for patients with hemoglobin SC disease.[85] The chance of having a first CVA by age 20 years was estimated to be 11% for patients with hemoglobin SS disease and 2% for patients with hemoglobin SC disease. Infarctive CVA predominates among patients younger than 20 years with hemoglobin SS disease, whereas hemorrhagic stroke predominates in patients age 20 to 29 years.[85] In untreated patients with CVA, repeat strokes occur in two thirds of the patients.[97] Transient ischemic attacks have been defined as ischemic events in which symptoms resolve in less than 24 hours. Several studies have sought to identify risk factors associated with CVA in neurologically asymptomatic hemoglobin SS patients. A compilation of those risks can be found in a review by Powars.[98] Patients should begin neuroimaging surveillance by age 4 years. Among the recommended neuroimaging studies are transcranial Doppler or duplex color Doppler ultrasonography, MRI and angiography, magnetic resonance spectroscopy, and positron emission tomography.

The clinical diagnosis of CVA is based on findings of hemiparetic and hemisensory focal deficits, including visual and language disturbances, or development of seizures, altered sensation, mentation, or alertness, severe headache, vomiting, stupor, or coma. The ideal treatment of stroke is prevention, and for that reason identifying the predictive risk factors for cerebral ischemia in young children is important so that counseling can be offered. Intracranial hemorrhage can present as a subarachnoid hemorrhage where the usual cause is rupture of a berry aneurysm or intraparenchymal hemorrhage usually associated with large vessel vasculopathy. Intraventricular hemorrhage is unusual but may be seen in patients with moyamoya vasculopathy.

Bone marrow transplantation from a histocompatible human leukocyte antigen donor is curative, but only 18% of patients with sickle cell disease in the United States have a compatible donor. Overall survival is 93% and event-free survival is 79%.[99] Chimeric, cord blood, and stem cell transplantation have the potential for a lower complication rate and more available donors, but randomized studies are not yet available.

Transfusion therapy remains the only treatment modality that is efficacious for sickle cell disease and CVA[100] despite the long-term morbidity, which includes alloimmunization and iron overload.

Erythrocytapheresis is well tolerated, does not increase alloimmunization, and reduces the iron overload, but it is more expensive and is not readily available.[101]

Although when to discontinue the chronic transfusion program after a patient has suffered a stroke is not clear, some suggest discontinuing transfusions after 10 to 15 years.[102] Ware et al.[103] present data on 16 pediatric patients in whom transfusions were discontinued because of erythrocyte alloantibodies or autoantibodies, recurrent stroke on transfusion, iron overload, noncompliance, or deferoxamine allergy. Patients were given hydroxyurea and underwent phlebotomies to reduce the iron overload. Three patients had neurologic events 3 to 4 months after discontinuing transfusions but before maximal hydroxyurea effects. These data suggest a new alternative to discontinuation of transfusion therapy.[103]

Neuroprotective therapy such as hypothermia and hyperventilation can be harmful to the patient. Steroids and mannitol are not useful. Studies evaluating calcium channel antagonists have been disappointing. Ongoing studies using magnesium sulfate are under way. Anticoagulation therapy carries the risk of intracranial bleeding, especially in patients with moyamoya vasculopathy. No studies have proved the benefit of low-dose aspirin. In the acute stage of CVA, treatment in adults without sickle cell disease includes administration of recombinant tissue plasminogen activator (t-PA) within 3 hours of onset. Data are available for children with sickle cell disease. Surgery may benefit patients with moyamoya vasculopathy using newly developed surgical techniques such as encephaloduroarteriosynagiosis and encephalomyosynangiosis.[104]

Cardiovascular Abnormalities

Most sickle cell patients have some signs or symptoms of cardiovascular abnormalities. Cardiomegaly and functional heart murmurs are prevalent. Physical work capacity is reduced in 60% to 70% of children and is related to the degree of anemia. Fluid overload is the most frequent cause of heart failure. Electrocardiographic findings are nonspecific. Echocardiograms usually show left and right ventricular dilatation inversely related to the degree of anemia.[105] Patients with sickle cell disease have a "relative" hypertension when their blood pressure is indexed to the severity of their anemia.[106] An association between decreased survival, stroke, and hypertension has been reported even when strokes occurred in patients with blood pressures lower than expected in normal population.[106] Renal disease and high-caloric, high-salt diets contribute to the prevalence of hypertension in sickle cell patients.

Sudden unexpected death and autonomic nervous system dysfunction have been reported among sickle cell patients.[107,108]

Gallbladder and Liver Diseases

Among the complications in patients with sickle cell disease, gallbladder and liver diseases are common.

Liver complications include hepatic sequestration, cholestasis, vascular occlusion, complication of transfusion such as hemosiderosis and hemochromatosis, autoimmune hepatitis, and viral hepatitis including hepatitis B and C. Gallbladder complications include biliary sludge, cholelithiasis, and acute and chronic cholecystitis. By age 18 years, 30% of sickle cell patients develop cholelithiasis. For that reason it is recommended that patients undergo serial gallbladder ultrasound examinations starting at approximately age 5 years. Once a diagnosis of cholelithiasis has been made, patients should undergo elective laparoscopic cholecystectomy with endoscopic retrograde cholangiopancreatography (ERCP). Hepatic crisis as a result of vaso-occlusion is a syndrome consisting of fever, elevated liver enzyme levels, right upper quadrant pain, and hepatomegaly. Hepatic sequestration is a complication similar to splenic sequestration. The crisis is characterized by a rapidly enlarging liver and decreased hemoglobin, elevated reticulocyte, and increased alkaline phosphatase levels.[109,110] Simple or exchange transfusion, coupled with conservative treatment, will resolve the condition. Cholestasis is a syndrome that may present as a benign condition with modest elevation of bilirubin, transaminases, and alkaline phosphatase in patients who have only jaundice and pruritus. Resolution occurs without therapy.[111] Progressive cholestasis is characterized by right upper quadrant pain, extreme elevation of bilirubin, and alkaline phosphatase, accompanied by renal failure, thrombocytopenia, and abnormal coagulation. Mortality resulting from hepatic failure is common. Exchange transfusion and supportive care aimed at correction of coagulopathy; stabilization of the acute liver disease; and, perhaps most important, avoidance of surgical intervention are the keys to successful outcome.[112]

Eye Disease

Patients with sickle cell disease should undergo annual eye examinations beginning in childhood and continuing through adulthood.[113] Examination includes visual acuity, pupillary reactivity, evaluation of the anterior structures of the eye, and thorough examination of the posterior and peripheral retina, including fluorescein angiography. The goal is to find and prevent the proliferation of new blood vessels in the retina that will progress to vitreous hemorrhage and retinal detachment.[113]

Techniques such as diathermy, cryotherapy, and laser photocoagulation have been used for the prevention. If retinal detachment occurs, surgical intervention such as vitrectomy and vitreoretinal microsurgery have been advocated. Any sickle cell patient who suffers eye trauma or experiences changes in vision should seek an emergent ophthalmology consultation.

Priapism

Priapism is a painful, persistent erection resulting from vaso-occlusive obstruction of the venous drainage of the penis. Priapism can occur as a brief episode that lasts less than 1 hour. It can occur frequently ("stuttering") or be prolonged, with duration of 1 hour to several days. Both stuttering and prolonged priapism lead to extensive infarction and fibrosis of penile tissue, with the subsequent complication of irreversible erectile dysfunction and psychosocial problems. Priapism is a common complication in sickle cell disease, with a reported incidence between 42% and 89% by age 20 years.[114,115]

Prolonged priapism is considered a medical emergency requiring immediate intervention in order to prevent more serious and permanent sequelae. Through the years many medical and surgical interventions have been used to treat patients with prolonged priapism, including hydration and pain control, alkalinization, frequent urination, transfusions[116] and exchange transfusions,[117] and more recently the use of vasodilators and hormone therapy.

Vasoactive agents such as the selective β-agonist terbutaline have been shown to be effective for treatment of severe episodes.[114,118]

Treatment available for prevention of priapism includes use of hormones that decrease testosterone production[119] and use of estrogens such as stilboestrol.[120] Other medications such as oral pseudoephedrine and oral or subcutaneous terbutaline have been used as preventive medications for treatment of stuttering and prolonged episodes.

Sayer and Parsons[121] in 1988 and Molina et al.[122] in 1989 reported successful treatment of priapism with intracorporeal epinephrine, using a penile injection of a diluted solution of 1:1,000,000 epinephrine. Similar results have been reported with phenylephrine injections.[123] In 2000 Mantadakis et al.[115] reported use of the procedure with a solution of 1:1,000,000 epinephrine in 15 pediatric patients (4–18 years) who underwent 39 aspirations and irrigation procedures. They reported no complications other than two penile hematomas. Long-term follow-up demonstrated normal potency and no other urologic complications, thus demonstrating the safety and efficacy of this method.

Exchange transfusion should be considered for patients who do not respond to penile irrigation, but one should be aware of potential complications ranging from headaches to seizures to obtundation that requires mechanic ventilation.[113] An *a*ssociation of *s*ickle cell disease, *p*riapism, *e*xchange transfusion, and *n*eurologic events is called *ASPEN syndrome.*[124] A shunt between the glans penis and the distal corpora cavernosa called the *Winter procedure* can be performed in order to allow blood to drain into the corpus spongiosa.[125] Finally, future episodes can be prevented with medications as pseudoephedrine, leuprolide, stilbestrol, and hydroxyurea, but further evaluation of these medications is warranted.

Bone and Joints

The most common sites of pain in patients with sickle cell disease are the bones and joints, including the spine, pelvis, and long bones. Infarction and collapse of the endplates of the vertebral bodies are called *codfish vertebra.*[113] Humerus, tibia, and femur are the most common sites in the long bones.[126] Dactylitis or hand-foot syndrome is a limited avascular necrosis of marrow affecting the small bones or the juxtaarticular areas of long bones.[65] Dactylitis is a painful acute swelling of the fingers, toes, or dorsum of hands or feet. It affects both genders equally, and by age 2 years it affects 50% of patients. Recurrences occur in 40% of cases. Fever and other minor illness are frequently associated with dactylitis. Pain and swelling can involve one to four extremities, involving the metacarpal, metatarsals, and phalanges. Symptoms last from 1 to 4 weeks with treatment that includes hydration and pain medication. Although this condition results in no serious long-term sequelae,[127] one study suggests that one episode of dactylitis associated with leukocytosis and severe anemia can predict severe complication later in life.[128]

Osteonecrosis is defined as the ischemic necrosis of juxtaarticular bone resulting from thrombosis of the endarterial vessels that leads to destruction of the adjacent joint. Sickle cell disease is the most common cause of avascular necrosis of the hip in children.[129] Osteonecrosis is more prevalent in patients with the combination of hemoglobin SS and α thalassemia.[130]

By age 35 years, almost 50% of hemoglobin SS patients have developed avascular necrosis, which usually results in serious morbidity, chronic progressive pain, and limitation of activity despite physical therapy or medical treatments such as transfusion. Collapse of the femoral head has been documented in 80% of hips with clinical avascular necrosis.[131]

Osteomyelitis and septic arthritis may arise from hematogenous spread of bacteria. Pain, swelling, and local warmth are common symptoms that can be confused with bone infarctions. Fever and white blood cell count elevation may help differentiate the conditions. Radiographs and radionuclide bone scans are of limited use. Positive blood cultures from aspirations of local bone or the joint may confirm the diagnosis.

Leg Ulcers

Between 10% and 20% of patients with hemoglobin SS disease develop painful, disfiguring, indolent leg ulcers. The etiology is unclear. Trauma, infection, severe anemia, and warmer temperatures may predispose to ulcer formation. Lesions begin as small elevated sores in the lower third of the leg or over the medial or lateral malleolus of the ankle. They can be single or multiple. There has been no well-controlled trial for treatment of leg ulcers. Recommendations for management include good pain control, bed rest and leg elevation, wet-to-dry dressings, oral zinc sulfate (200 mg three times per day), infection control with dressings soaked with diluted acetic acid or silver sulfadiazine cream, systemic antibiotics if required, and use of Unna boots. Use of blood transfusion remains controversial, and skin graft is not always successful.[113]

Anesthesia and Surgery

Anesthesia and surgery carry a high risk of complications and mortality due to severe anemia, chronic organ damage, hypoxia, and asplenia. Patients with hemoglobin SS disease and hemoglobin S B° thalassemia are at greatest risk. Vichinsky et al.[132] reported in 1995 the results of a multicenter randomized study that compared an aggressive arm having the goal of a hemoglobin S of less than 30% with a simple transfusion arm. No differences were found among 604 surgical episodes in the number of preoperative or postoperative complications other than those that were transfusion related. Standard guidelines for preoperative care include preoperative transfusion and hydration and operative monitoring of temperature, blood pressure, and oxygenation that should continue through the postoperative period.[113]

Extracorporeal Membrane Oxygenation

Extracorporeal membrane oxygenation is an accepted therapy for critically ill newborn infants with reversible pulmonary diseases who are refractory to conventional therapy.[133] Reports of successful ECMO treatment of sickle cell patients who developed ACS describe excellent recovery and no long-term side effects.[133,134]

Arginine and Nitric Oxide

The relationship of arginine and nitric oxide (NO) to the pathophysiology of sickle cell disease has become a topic of interest because it may play a role in vaso-occlusive complications of the disease.[135–137] Interest in developing specific, disease-targeted treatment of vaso-occlusive crisis has been growing. It has been suggested that reduced production of NO or defective NO-dependent mechanisms in sickle cell disease play a role in the pathophysiology of vaso-occlusion.[135] Nitric oxide is synthesized endogenously in the conversion of L-arginine to L-citrulline by NO synthase isozymes in a variety of cells and tissues, including vascular endothelium.[138] Nitric oxide is a central regulator of vascular tone, cellular endothelial adhesion, platelet aggregation, and thrombosis. Levels of NO metabolites and arginine are low during vaso-occlusive crisis and are inversely related to pain severity. Morris et al.[139] reported that low arginine levels during a vaso-occlusive crisis could reflect a state of acute substrate depletion and decreased NO production. The same authors suggest that, although arginine alone does not increase serum NO_x production, it does when given with hydroxturea.[140] Weiner et al.[141] designed a prospective double-blind, placebo-controlled study to explore the efficacy and safety of inhaled NO for treatment of vaso-occlusive crisis in pediatric patients. They concluded that inhaled NO may be beneficial for acute crisis.[141] Arginine therapy may also have a role in the treatment of pulmonary hypertension, which has high mortality and limited treatment options.[137]

Transfusion

Sickle cell disease patient are at risk for many complications that may require use of episodic transfusion or chronic transfusion therapy. Several methods of transfusion are used, including simple transfusion, partial exchange transfusion, and erythrocytapheresis. In general and when available, phenotypically matched blood for ABO, Rh, Kell, Duffy, Kidd, Lewis, Lutheran, P, and MNS groups would be ideal, although limited match to E, C, and Kell antigens usually is performed, unless patients have antibodies.[142] Sickle-negative, leukodepleted packed cells are the blood product of choice.[113] Transfusions are used to increase the oxygen-carrying capacity and decrease the proportion of sickle red cells, improving microvascular perfusion of tissues.[113] Because hyperviscosity is a potentially severe complication in patients with sickle cell disease, it is recommended that a posttransfusion hematocrit not higher than 36% be achieved.

Calculations for simple RBC transfusion include the following formulas[143]:

1. Total blood volume (TBV) = 70 – 75 cc/kg
2. Transfusions = Volume of RBCs = TBV × (Hgb desired – Hgb observed)/Hgb donor unit or
3. TBV × (Hct desired – Hct observed)/Hct donor unit
4. Packed Red Blood Cells have Hgb (22–24 g/dl) and Hct (65% – 80%).

The most common indications for simple transfusion in sickle cell disease include acute splenic sequestration, transient red cell aplasia, ACS, stroke, multiorgan failure, and preparation for surgery. Controversy remains over the use of transfusion for treatment of priapism, leg ulcers, and pregnancy. Inappropriate indications includes chronic steady-state anemia, uncomplicated pain episodes, infections, minor surgery, aseptic necrosis, and uncomplicated pregnancy.[113]

The most frequent transfusion complications include alloimmunization, hyperviscosity, and hypertension.

Other complications include production of alloantibodies to white cells, platelets, and serum proteins, which can be prevented by removal of leukocytes by filtration. Allergic reactions can be prevented with use of antihistaminics such as diphenhydramine (Benadryl). Infectious complications such as hepatitis and other transfusion-transmitted viral diseases are frequent in sickle cell patients, as in other patients receiving transfusions.

Hemolytic Transfusion Reactions

Hemolytic transfusion reactions (HTRs) are of concern in patients with sickle cell disease, not only because of the potential complications of hemolysis and severe anemia but because they may pose life-threatening problems.[144,145] This complication now is recognized as the sickle cell HTR syndrome.[146] Components of the HTR syndrome include acute or delayed HTR, painful crisis,[147] marked reticulocytopenia, severe anemia, exacerbation of anemia by subsequent transfusion, development of multiple alloantibodies,[148] recovery and improvement after withholding further transfusions, improvement with administration of corticosteroids, and chances of recurrence after subsequent transfusion. Sickle cell complications and therapies are summarized in Table 77–3.

Thalassemias

Thalassemias are hereditary disorders in which the rate of globin chain synthesis is reduced. Thomas B. Cooley first described the condition in 1927.[149] The main abnormality is impaired production of either α- or β-globin chains. α Thalassemia occurs when one or more of the α-chain genes fail to produce the α protein. Loss of one gene called a *silent carrier* has no clinical impact other than a slightly decreased production of α chains. Loss of two genes gives the clinical picture of mild microcytic anemia that can be confused with iron deficiency, although the patient remains asymptomatic. Patient with a three-gene deletion will have severe anemia that requires chronic transfusion. Such patients produce abnormal hemoglobin called *hemoglobin H* composed of four β chains (β4). Hemoglobin H does not carry oxygen well and produces hemolysis, causing a life-threatening anemia that, left untreated, is lethal in early life. An unusual but more severe form of the disease is the combination of hemoglobin H with the hemoglobin Constant Spring mutation ($\alpha^{cs}\alpha/\alpha\alpha$) or ($\alpha\alpha^{cs}/\alpha\alpha$), a four α gene deletion that is generally incompatible with life. Such patients produce only hemoglobin Barts (γ4), H (β4), or Portland (δ2γ2). In some patients, the disease was detected in utero and treated by in utero transfusion and subsequent chronic transfusion.

β Thalassemia is impaired production of β chains located on chromosome 11. When one gene fails, the condition is called *β thalassemia trait* or *minor.* Excess production of α chains stimulates the production of δ chains (hemoglobin A_2) and γ chains for production of hemoglobin F. Patients who have impaired production of both β chains have thalassemia major. Very little hemoglobin A is produced, with increased production of hemoglobins F and A_2. Even with increased production of hemoglobins F and A_2, the excessively produced α chains precipitate in the normoblast, producing intramedullary hemolysis.

Hemoglobin E/Thal^{+}

Hemoglobin E is a β-chain variant in which lysine is substituted for glutamic acid in position 26. It probably is the most common hemoglobinopathy in the world, occurring in southeast Asia, especially in Cambodia, Laos, and Thailand. Hemoglobin E trait or homozygous E does not produce any clinical manifestation other than mild microcytic anemia. However, when it is combined with other abnormal hemoglobin it can produce mild to severe anemia that may require chronic transfusion. Other hemoglobin combinations such as hemoglobins S and E or hemoglobin Lepore with β-thalassemia trait can produce similar pictures of moderate or severe anemia.

TABLE 77–3

Sickle Cell Suggested Therapies

	Intravenous Fluids	Antibiotics	Pain Control	Transfusion	Oxygen	Surgery
Fever	+	+		–	–	
Pain	+		+	±	–	±
Osteomyelitis	+	±	+		–	±
Splenic sequestration			+	+	–	
Acute anemia				+	±	
Acute chest syndrome	+	+	+	+	+	
Stroke		±		+		
Surgery	+			+	±	
Pregnancy				±	–	
Hepatobiliary	±	±	+	–	–	±
Avascular necrosis	–	–	+	–	–	±
Leg ulcers		±	±	±	±	

Chronic Transfusions

Chronic transfusion regimens strive to maintain hemoglobin levels of approximately 12 g/dl. Patients should be transfused with phenotypically matched, leukodepleted RBCs, if possible.

Treatment of chronic transfusion patients requires the efforts of a multidisciplinary team that includes the pediatrician, hematologist, endocrinologist, gastroenterologist, cardiologist, genetic counselor, and nutritionist, among other specialists. The most frequent complications include iron overload, endocrine failure, and cardiac and hepatic complications. The rate of iron load is dependent of the amount of blood transfused per year and the level of gastrointestinal absorption of iron. It is estimated that a patient who receives a pure red cell volume of 100 to 200 ml/kg/year will retain 5.8 to 11.6 g of iron per year, just from transfusion. Even though iron overload occurs equally in transfused patients with thalassemia and sickle cell disease, the organ dysfunction that frequently occurs in patients with thalassemia has not been reported in patients with sickle cell disease.[150] Complications of iron overload in thalassemia major patients are seen in the second decade and include fatal cardiac complications,[151] pituitary dysfunction, hypogonadism, osteopenia, osteoporosis, thyroid problems, diabetes, gallstones, hepatitis, liver fibrosis, and cirrhosis.

Chronic transfusion patients are at increased risk for complications of infection, including hepatitis that may lead to chronic liver failure and hepatocellular carcinoma. Other serious infection problems include tuberculosis and human immunodeficiency virus infection.

Comprehensive annual evaluation of chronically transfused patients, especially those with thalassemia major, include cardiac, liver, endocrine, ophthalmologic, and audiologic examinations.

REFERENCES

1. Marotta CA, et al: Human beta-globin messenger RNA. III. Nucleotide sequences derived from complementary DNA. *J Biol Chem* 252:5040-53, 1977.
2. Serjeant GR: The emerging understanding of sickle cell disease. *Br J Haematol* 112:3-18, 2001.
3. Noguchi CT, Schechter AN: The intracellular polymerization of sickle hemoglobin and its relevance to sickle cell disease. *Blood* 58: 1057-1068, 1981.
4. Eaton WA, Hofrichter J: Hemoglobin S gelation and sickle cell disease. *Blood* 70:1245-1266, 1987.
5. Ferrone FA, Hofrichter J, Eaton WA: Kinetics of sickle hemoglobin polymerization. II. A double nucleation mechanism. *J Mol Biol* 183:611-631, 1985.
6. Ferrone FA: The polymerization of sickle hemoglobin in solutions and cells. *Experientia* 49:110-117, 1993.
7. Mozzarelli A, Hofrichter J, Eaton WA: Delay time of hemoglobin S polymerization prevents most cells from sickling in vivo. *Science* 237:500-506, 1987.
8. Nash GB, Johnson CS, Meiselman HJ: Influence of oxygen tension on the viscoelastic behavior of red blood cells in sickle cell disease. *Blood* 67:110-118, 1986.
9. Bookchin RM, et al: Identification and characterization of a newly recognized population of high-Na+, low-K+, low-density sickle and normal red cells. *Proc Natl Acad Sci U S A* 97:8045-8050, 2000.
10. Evans E, Mohandas N, Leung A: Static and dynamic rigidities of normal and sickle erythrocytes. Major influence of cell hemoglobin concentration. *J Clin Invest* 73:477-488, 1984.
11. McCurdy PR, Sherman AS: Irreversibly sickled cells and red cell survival in sickle cell anemia: a study with both DF32P and 51CR. *Am J Med* 64:253-258, 1978.
12. Brugnara C, Van Ha T, Tosteson DC: Acid pH induces formation of dense cells in sickle erythrocytes. *Blood* 74:487-495, 1989.
13. Sunshine HR, Hofrichter J, Eaton WA: Requirement for therapeutic inhibition of sickle haemoglobin gelation. *Nature* 275:238-240, 1978.
14. Tosteson DC: Membrane transport of Na and K: a synopsis of contemporary concepts and experiments. *Physiologist* 9:89-96, 1966.
15. Tosteson DC, Shea E: Potassium and sodium of red blood cells in sickle cell anemia. *J Clin Invest* 31:406-411, 1952.
16. Tosteson DC: The effects of sickling on ion transport. II. The effects of sickling on sodium and cesium transport. *J Gen Physiol* 39:55-67, 1955.
17. Tosteson DC: The effects of sickling on ion transport. Effect of sickling on potassium transport. *J Gen Physiol* 39:31-53, 1955.
18. Joiner CH: Cation transport and volume regulation in sickle red blood cells. *Am J Physiol* 264(2 pt 1):C251-C270, 1993.
19. Brugnara C, Bunn HF, Tosteson DC: Regulation of erythrocyte cation and water content in sickle cell anemia. *Science* 232(4748): 388-390, 1986.
20. Canessa M, Spalvins A, Nagel RL: Volume-dependent and NEM-stimulated K+, Cl– transport is elevated in oxygenated SS, SC and CC human red cells. *FEBS Lett* 200:197-202, 1986.
21. Sarkadi B, et al: The function and regulation of the calcium pump in the erythrocyte membrane. *Ann N Y Acad Sci* 402:329-348, 1982.
22. Gardos G: The function of calcium in the potassium permeability of human erythrocytes. *Biochim Biophys Acta* 30:653-654, 1958.
23. Rivera A, Jarolim P, Brugnara C: Modulation of Gardos channel activity by cytokines in sickle erythrocytes. *Blood* 99:357 603, 2002.
24. Canessa M, et al: Volume-stimulated, Cl(–)-dependent K+ efflux is highly expressed in young human red cells containing normal hemoglobin or HbS. *J Membr Biol* 97:97-105, 1987.
25. Klug PP, Kaye N, Jensen WN: Endothelial cell and vascular damage in the sickle cell disorders. *Blood Cells* 8:175-184, 1982.
26. Rothman SM, Fulling KH, Nelson JS: Sickle cell anemia and central nervous system infarction: a neuropathological study. *Ann Neurol* 20:684-690, 1986.
27. Hebbel RP, et al: Abnormal adherence of sickle erythrocytes to cultured vascular endothelium: possible mechanism for microvascular occlusion in sickle cell disease. *J Clin Invest* 65:154-160, 1980.
28. Mohanda N, Hebbel RP: Sickle cell adherence. In HR Embury SH, Mohanda N, Steinberg MH, editors: *Sickle cell disease: basic principles and clinical practice*. New York, 1994, Raven Press.
29. Kaul DK, Fabry ME, Nagel RL: Microvascular sites and characteristics of sickle cell adhesion to vascular endothelium in shear flow conditions: pathophysiological implications. *Proc Natl Acad Sci U S A* 86:3356-3360, 1989.
30. Frenette PS: Sickle cell vaso-occlusion: multistep and multicellular paradigm. *Curr Opin Hematol* 9:101-106, 2002.
31. Hebbel RP, et al: Spontaneous oxygen radical generation by sickle erythrocytes. *J Clin Invest* 70:1253-1259, 1982.
32. Matsui NM, et al: P-selectin mediates the adhesion of sickle erythrocytes to the endothelium. *Blood* 98:1955-1962, 2001.
33. Pober JS, Cotran RS: Cytokines and endothelial cell biology. *Physiol Rev* 70:427-451, 1990.
34. Pober JS, Cotran RS: The role of endothelial cells in inflammation. *Transplantation* 50:537-544, 1990.
35. Jia L, et al: S-nitrosohaemoglobin: a dynamic activity of blood involved in vascular control. *Nature* 380:221-226, 1996.
36. Setty BN, Chen D, Stuart MJ: Sickle cell vaso-occlusive crisis is associated with abnormalities in the ratio of vasoconstrictor to vasodilator prostanoids. *Pediatr Res* 38:95-102, 1995.
37. Solovey A, et al: Circulating activated endothelial cells in sickle cell anemia. *N Engl J Med* 337:1584-1590, 1997.
38. Sowemimo-Coker SO, Meiselman HJ, Francis RB Jr: Increased circulating endothelial cells in sickle cell crisis. *Am J Hematol* 31: 263-265, 1989.
39. Sultana C, et al: Interaction of sickle erythrocytes with endothelial cells in the presence of endothelial cell conditioned medium induces oxidant stress leading to transendothelial migration of monocytes. *Blood* 92:3924-3935, 1998.

40. Spring FA, et al: Intercellular adhesion molecule-4 binds alphabeta and alpha(V)-family integrins through novel integrin-binding mechanisms. *Blood* 98:458-466, 2001.
41. Gee BE, Platt OS: Sickle reticulocytes adhere to VCAM-1. *Blood* 85:268-274, 1995.
42. Embury SH, Hebbel RR, Steinberg MH, Mohandas N: Pathogenesis of vasoocclusion. In HR Embury SH, Mohanda N, Steinberg MH, editors. *Sickle cell disease: basic principles and clinical practice.* New York, 1994, Raven Press.
43. Hebbel RP, et al: Erythrocyte adherence to endothelium as a determinant of vasocclusive severity in sickle cell disease. *Trans Assoc Am Physicians* 93:94-99, 1980.
44. Hebbel RP: Adhesive interactions of sickle erythrocytes with endothelium. *J Clin Invest* 100(11 Suppl):S83-S86, 1997.
45. Mohandas N, Evans E: Sickle erythrocyte adherence to vascular endothelium. Morphologic correlates and the requirement for divalent cations and collagen-binding plasma proteins. *J Clin Invest* 76: 1605-612, 1985.
46. Turhan A, et al: Primary role for adherent leukocytes in sickle cell vascular occlusion: a new paradigm. *Proc Natl Acad Sci U S A* 99:3047-3051, 2002.
47. Hofstra TC, et al: Sickle erythrocytes adhere to polymorphonuclear neutrophils and activate the neutrophil respiratory burst. *Blood* 87:4440-4447, 1996.
48. Newborn Screening Committee, The Council of Regional Networks for Genetic Services (CORN): *National Newborn Screening Report-1992.* Atlanta, 1995, CORN.
49. Pass KA, et al: US newborn screening system guidelines II: follow-up of children, diagnosis, management, and evaluation. Statement of the Council of Regional Networks for Genetic Services (CORN). *J Pediatr* 137(4 Suppl):S1-S46, 2000.
50. Sickle Cell Disease Guideline Panel: *Sickle cell disease: screening, diagnosis, management, and counseling in newborns and infants.* Clinical practice guideline no. 6. Rockville, Md., 1993, Agency for Health Care Policy and Research, Public Health Service, U.S. Department of Health and Human Services, AHCPR publication no. 93-0562.
51. Miller ST, et al: Newborn screening for sickle cell disease. When is an infant "lost to follow-up"? *Am J Dis Child* 144:1343-1345, 1990.
52. Reed W, et al: Sickle-cell disease not identified by newborn screening because of prior transfusion. *J Pediatr* 136:248-250, 2000.
53. National Committee for Clinical Laboratory Standards (NCCLS): *Solubility test to confirm the presence of sickling hemoglobins; approved standard.* Villanova, Pa, 1986, NCCLS, document H10-A.
54. Briere RO, Golias T, Batsakis JG: Rapid qualitative and quantitative hemoglobin fractionation. Cellulose acetate electrophoresis. *Am J Clin Pathol* 44:695-701, 1965.
55. National Committee for Clinical Laboratory Standards (NCCLS): *Detection of abnormal hemoglobin using cellulose acetate electrophoresis, approved standard,* ed 2. Villanova, Pa, 1994, NCCLS, document H8-A2.
56. National Committee for Clinical Laboratory Standards (NCCLS): *Citrate agar electrophoresis for confirming the identification of variant hemoglobins; tentative guidelines.* Villanova, Pa, 1988, NCCLS, document H23-T.
57. Schneider RG: Differentiation of electrophoretically similar hemoglobins—such as S, D, G, and P; or A2, C, E, and O—by electrophoresis of the globin chains. *Clin Chem* 20:1111-1115, 1974.
58. Newborn Screening Committee, The Council of Regional Networks for Genetic Services (CORN): *National Newborn Screening Report—1991.* Atlanta, 1994, CORN.
59. National Committee for Clinical Laboratory Standards (NCCLS): *Quantitative measurements of fetal hemoglobin by the alkali denaturation method; approved guideline.* Villanova, Pa, 1989, NCCLS, document H13-A.
60. Nagel RL, Platt OS, Orah S: General pathophysiology of sickle cell anemia. In MH Steinberg, Forget BG, Higgs DR, Nagel RL, editors: *Disorders of hemoglobin.* 2001, Cambridge, England, 2001, Cambridge University Press.
61. Milner PF, Brown M: Bone marrow infarction in sickle cell anemia: correlation with hematologic profiles. *Blood* 60:1411-1419, 1982.
62. Rao VM, et al: Painful sickle cell crisis: bone marrow patterns observed with MR imaging. *Radiology* 161:211-215, 1986.
63. Mankad VN, et al: Magnetic resonance imaging of bone marrow in sickle cell disease: clinical, hematologic, and pathologic correlations. *Blood* 75:274-283, 1990.
64. Cazzola M, et al: Red blood cell precursor mass as an independent determinant of serum erythropoietin level. *Blood* 91:2139-2145, 1998.
65. Stevens MC, Padwick M, Serjeant GR: Observations on the natural history of dactylitis in homozygous sickle cell disease. *Clin Pediatr (Phila)* 20:311-317, 1981.
66. Orringer EP, et al: Case report: splenic infarction and acute splenic sequestration in adults with hemoglobin SC disease. *Am J Med Sci* 302:374-379, 1991.
67. Bowcock SJ, et al: Fatal splenic sequestration in adult sickle cell disease. *Clin Lab Haematol* 10:95-99, 1988.
68. Topley JM, et al: Acute splenic sequestration and hypersplenism in the first five years in homozygous sickle cell disease. *Arch Dis Child* 56:765-769, 1981.
69. Kinney TR, et al: Long-term management of splenic sequestration in children with sickle cell disease. *J Pediatr* 117(2 Pt 1):194-199, 1990.
70. Glader B: Anemia. In Embury SH, Hebbel RP, Mohanda N, Steinberg M, editors: *Sickle cell disease: basic principles and clinical practice.* New York, 1994, Lippincott-Raven.
71. Serjeant GR, et al: Outbreak of aplastic crises in sickle cell anaemia associated with parvovirus-like agent. *Lancet* 2:595-597, 1981.
72. Smith-Whitley K, et al: Epidemiology of human parvovirus B19 in children with sickle cell disease. *Blood* 103:422-427, 2004.
73. Wayne AS, Kevy SV, Nathan DG: Transfusion management of sickle cell disease. *Blood* 81:1109-1123, 1993.
74. Gill FM, et al: Clinical events in the first decade in a cohort of infants with sickle cell disease. Cooperative Study of Sickle Cell Disease. *Blood* 86:776-783, 1995.
75. Leikin SL, et al: Mortality in children and adolescents with sickle cell disease. Cooperative Study of Sickle Cell Disease. *Pediatrics* 84:500-508, 1989.
76. Gaston MH, et al: Prophylaxis with oral penicillin in children with sickle cell anemia. A randomized trial. *N Engl J Med* 314: 1593-1599, 1986.
77. Williams LL, et al: Outpatient therapy with ceftriaxone and oral cefixime for selected febrile children with sickle cell disease. *J Pediatr Hematol Oncol* 18:257-261, 1996.
78. Rogers ZR, et al: Outpatient management of febrile illness in infants and young children with sickle cell anemia. *J Pediatr* 117: 736-739, 1990.
79. Lane PA, et al: Fatal pneumococcal septicemia in hemoglobin SC disease. *J Pediatr* 124:859-862, 1994.
80. Falletta JM, et al: Discontinuing penicillin prophylaxis in children with sickle cell anemia. Prophylactic Penicillin Study II. *J Pediatr* 127:685-690, 1995.
81. Platt OS, et al: Mortality in sickle cell disease. Life expectancy and risk factors for early death. *N Engl J Med* 330:1639-644, 1994.
82. Vichinsky EP, et al: Causes and outcomes of the acute chest syndrome in sickle cell disease. National Acute Chest Syndrome Study Group. *N Engl J Med* 342:1855-1865, 2000.
83. Gladwin MT, et al: The acute chest syndrome in sickle cell disease. Possible role of nitric oxide in its pathophysiology and treatment. *Am J Respir Crit Care Med* 159(5 Pt 1):1368-1376, 1999.
84. Bernini JC, et al: Beneficial effect of intravenous dexamethasone in children with mild to moderately severe acute chest syndrome complicating sickle cell disease. *Blood* 92:3082-3089, 1998.
85. Ohene-Frempong K, et al: Cerebrovascular accidents in sickle cell disease: rates and risk factors. *Blood* 91:288-294, 1998.
86. Henderson JN, et al: Reversible posterior leukoencephalopathy syndrome and silent cerebral infarcts are associated with severe acute chest syndrome in children with sickle cell disease. *Blood* 101:415-419, 2003.
87. Sutton LL, et al: Pulmonary hypertension in sickle cell disease. *Am J Cardiol* 74:626-628, 1994.
88. Powars D, et al: Sickle cell chronic lung disease: prior morbidity and the risk of pulmonary failure. *Medicine (Baltimore)* 67:66-76, 1988.
89. Gladwin MT, et al: Pulmonary hypertension as a risk factor for death in patients with sickle cell disease. *N Engl J Med* 350: 886-895, 2004.
90. Aboubakr SE, Girgis R, Swerdlow P: Pulmonary hypertension in sickle cell disease. *Am J Respir Crit Care Med* 160: A144(abstract), 1999.
91. Minter KR, Gladwin MT: Pulmonary complications of sickle cell anemia. A need for increased recognition, treatment, and research. *Am J Respir Crit Care Med* 164:2016-2019, 2001.

92. Powars DR, et al: Chronic renal failure in sickle cell disease: risk factors, clinical course, and mortality. *Ann Intern Med* 115: 614-620, 1991.
93. Ataga KI, Orringer EP: Renal abnormalities in sickle cell disease. *Am J Hematol* 63:205-211, 2000.
94. John EG, et al: Effectiveness of triglycyl vasopressin in persistent hematuria associated with sickle cell hemoglobin. *Arch Intern Med* 140:1589-1593, 1980.
95. Immergut MA, Stevenson T: The use of epsilon amino caproic acid in the control of hematuria associated with hemoglobinopathies. *J Urol* 93:110-111, 1965.
96. Davis CJ Jr, Mostofi FK, Sesterhenn IA: Renal medullary carcinoma. The seventh sickle cell nephropathy. *Am J Surg Pathol* 19: 1-11, 1995.
97. Powars D, et al: The natural history of stroke in sickle cell disease. *Am J Med* 65:461-471, 1978.
98. Powars DR: Management of cerebral vasculopathy in children with sickle cell anaemia. *Br J Haematol* 108:666-678, 2000.
99. Walters MC, et al: Collaborative multicenter investigation of marrow transplantation for sickle cell disease: current results and future directions. *Biol Blood Marrow Transplant* 3:310-315, 1997.
100. Russell MO, et al: Effect of transfusion therapy on arteriographic abnormalities and on recurrence of stroke in sickle cell disease. *Blood* 63:162-169, 1984.
101. Adams DM, et al: Erythrocytapheresis can reduce iron overload and prevent the need for chelation therapy in chronically transfused pediatric patients. *J Pediatr Hematol Oncol* 18:46-50, 1996.
102. Ware RE, Zimmerman SA, Schultz WH: Hydroxyurea as an alternative to blood transfusions for the prevention of recurrent stroke in children with sickle cell disease. *Blood* 94:3022-3026, 1999.
103. Ware RE, et al: Prevention of secondary stroke and resolution of transfusional iron overload in children with sickle cell anemia using hydroxyurea and phlebotomy. *J Pediatr* 145:346-352, 2004.
104. Vernet O, et al: Encephaloduroarterio-synangiosis in a child with sickle cell anemia and moyamoya disease. *Pediatr Neurol* 14:226-230, 1996.
105. Covitz W, et al: The heart in sickle cell anemia. The Cooperative Study of Sickle Cell Disease (CSSCD). *Chest* 108:1214-1219, 1995.
106. Rodgers GP, Walker EC, Podgor MJ: Is "relative" hypertension a risk factor for vaso-occlusive complications in sickle cell disease? *Am J Med Sci* 305:150-156, 1993.
107. Romero Mestre JC, et al: Cardiovascular autonomic dysfunction in sickle cell anemia: a possible risk factor for sudden death? *Clin Auton Res* 7:121-125, 1997.
108. James TN, Riddick L, Massing GK: Sickle cells and sudden death: morphologic abnormalities of the cardiac conduction system. *J Lab Clin Med* 124:507-520, 1994.
109. Hernandez P, et al: Clinical features of hepatic sequestration in sickle cell anaemia. *Haematologia (Budap)* 22:169-174, 1989.
110. Hatton CS, Bunch C, Weatherall DJ: Hepatic sequestration in sickle cell anaemia. *Br Med J (Clin Res Ed)* 290:744-745, 1985.
111. Buchanan GR, Glader BE: Benign course of extreme hyperbilirubinemia in sickle cell anemia: analysis of six cases. *J Pediatr* 91: 21-24, 1977.
112. Shao SH, Orringer EP: Sickle cell intrahepatic cholestasis: approach to a difficult problem. *Am J Gastroenterol* 90:2048-2050, 1995.
113. National Institutes of Health: *The management of sickle cell disease.* Bethesda, Md., 2002, National Institutes of Health.
114. Virag R, et al: Preventive treatment of priapism in sickle cell disease with oral and self-administered intracavernous injection of etilefrine. *Urology* 47:777-781, 1996; discussion 781.
115. Mantadakis E, et al: Outpatient penile aspiration and epinephrine irrigation for young patients with sickle cell anemia and prolonged priapism. *Blood* 95:78-82, 2000.
116. Seeler RA: Intensive transfusion therapy for priapism in boys with sickle cell anemia. *J Urol* 110:360-363, 1973.
117. Rifkind S, et al: RBC exchange pheresis for priapism in sickle cell disease. *JAMA* 242:2317-2318, 1979.
118. Lowe FC, Jarow JP: Placebo-controlled study of oral terbutaline and pseudoephedrine in management of prostaglandin E1-induced prolonged erections. *Urology* 42:51-53, 1993; discussion 53-54.
119. Levine LA, Guss SP: Gonadotropin-releasing hormone analogues in the treatment of sickle cell anemia-associated priapism. *J Urol* 150(2 Pt 1):475-477, 1993.
120. Serjeant GR, de Ceulaer K, Maude GH: Stilboestrol and stuttering priapism in homozygous sickle-cell disease. *Lancet* 2:1274-1276, 1985.
121. Sayer J, Parsons CL: Successful treatment of priapism with intracorporeal epinephrine. *J Urol* 140:827, 1988.
122. Molina L, et al: Diluted epinephrine solution for the treatment of priapism. *J Urol* 141:1127-1128, 1989.
123. Dittrich A, et al: Treatment of pharmacological priapism with phenylephrine. *J Urol* 146:323-324, 1991.
124. Rackoff WR, et al: Neurologic events after partial exchange transfusion for priapism in sickle cell disease. *J Pediatr* 120: 882-885, 1992.
125. Winter CC: Priapism cured by creation of fistulas between glans penis and corpora cavernosa. *J Urol* 119:227-228, 1978.
126. Keeley K, Buchanan GR: Acute infarction of long bones in children with sickle cell anemia. *J Pediatr* 101:170-175, 1982.
127. Worrall VT, Butera V: Sickle-cell dactylitis. *J Bone Joint Surg Am* 58:1161-1163, 1976.
128. Miller ST, et al: Prediction of adverse outcomes in children with sickle cell disease. *N Engl J Med* 342:83-89, 2000.
129. Man S, Koren A: Avascular necrosis of bones in children with sickle cell anemia. *Pediatr Hematol Oncol* 10:385-387, 1993.
130. Milner PF, et al: Sickle cell disease as a cause of osteonecrosis of the femoral head. *N Engl J Med* 325:1476-481, 1991.
131. Steinberg ME, et al: Core decompression with bone grafting for osteonecrosis of the femoral head. *Clin Orthop* 386:71-78, 2001.
132. Vichinsky EP, et al: A comparison of conservative and aggressive transfusion regimens in the perioperative management of sickle cell disease. The Preoperative Transfusion in Sickle Cell Disease Study Group. *N Engl J Med* 333:206-213, 1995.
133. Pelidis MA, et al: Successful treatment of life-threatening acute chest syndrome of sickle cell disease with venovenous extracorporeal membrane oxygenation. *J Pediatr Hematol Oncol* 19:459-461, 1997.
134. Zahraa JN, et al: Venovenous versus venoarterial extracorporeal life support for pediatric respiratory failure: are there differences in survival and acute complications? *Crit Care Med* 28:521-525, 2000.
135. Gladwin MT, Schechter AN: Nitric oxide therapy in sickle cell disease. *Semin Hematol* 38:333-342, 2001.
136. Morris CR, et al: Arginine therapy: a novel strategy to induce nitric oxide production in sickle cell disease. *Br J Haematol* 111:498-500, 2000.
137. Morris CR, et al: Arginine therapy: a new treatment for pulmonary hypertension in sickle cell disease? *Am J Respir Crit Care Med* 168:63-69, 2003.
138. Moncada S, Higgs A: The L-arginine-nitric oxide pathway. *N Engl J Med* 329:2002-2012, 1993.
139. Morris CR, et al: Patterns of arginine and nitric oxide in patients with sickle cell disease with vaso-occlusive crisis and acute chest syndrome. *J Pediatr Hematol Oncol* 22:515-520, 2000.
140. Morris CR, et al: Hydroxyurea and arginine therapy: impact on nitric oxide production in sickle cell disease. *J Pediatr Hematol Oncol* 25:629-634, 2003.
141. Weiner DL, et al: Preliminary assessment of inhaled nitric oxide for acute vaso-occlusive crisis in pediatric patients with sickle cell disease. *JAMA* 289:1136-1142, 2003.
142. Sosler SD, et al: A simple, practical model for reducing alloimmunization in patients with sickle cell disease. *Am J Hematol* 43: 103-106, 1993.
143. Kasprisin DO, Luban NLC: *Pediatric transfusion medicine,* vol II. 1987, CRC Press.
144. Milner PF, et al: Posttransfusion crises in sickle cell anemia: role of delayed hemolytic reactions to transfusion. *South Med J* 78: 1462-1469, 1985.
145. King KE, et al: Delayed hemolytic transfusion reactions in sickle cell disease: simultaneous destruction of recipients' red cells. *Transfusion* 37:376-381, 1997.
146. Petz LD, et al: The sickle cell hemolytic transfusion reaction syndrome. *Transfusion* 37:382-392, 1997.
147. Fabron A Jr, Moreira G Jr, Bordin JO: Delayed hemolytic transfusion reaction presenting as a painful crisis in a patient with sickle cell anemia. *Rev Paul Med* 117:38-39, 1999.

148. Cox JV, et al: Risk of alloimmunization and delayed hemolytic transfusion reactions in patients with sickle cell disease. *Arch Intern Med* 148:2485-2489, 1988.
149. Cooley T, Witwer E, Lee P: Anemia in children with splenomegaly and peculiar changes in bones; report of cases. *Am J Dis Child* 34:347-363, 1927.
150. Fung EB, et al: Progression of organ dysfunction in iron overload patients with β thalassemia and sickle cell disease. In: Forty-sixth Annual Meeting of American Society of Hematology. 2004, San Diego Calif, American Society of Hematology.
151. Zurlo MG, et al: Survival and causes of death in thalassaemia major. *Lancet* 2:27-30, 1989.

CHAPTER 78

Gastrointestinal Structure and Function

Timothy A. Sentongo and David M. Steinhorn

PEARLS

- Hepatobiliary system
- Synthesis of numerous plasma proteins
- Coagulation factors, acute phase proteins, albumin
- Hormonal counterregulation (see Table 78–3 within the chapter)
- Maintenance glucose homeostasis
- Elimination of drugs, toxins, ammonia
- Storage of nutrients
- Glycogen and vitamins A, D, and B_{12}
- Hepatocytes possess specialized function depending on their location in the hepatic acinus (see Fig. 78–1 within the chapter)
- Activation of Kupffer's cells and sinusoidal inflammation that contributes to pulmonary, renal, and systemic dysfunction in multiple organ dysfunction syndrome

Abnormalities in gastrointestinal (GI) and hepatobiliary function occur frequently in the pediatric intensive care unit (ICU) from primary GI disease, from complications of systemic disease, or after surgery. The pediatric intensivist is called on for expertise in the preoperative and postoperative management of numerous GI tract and hepatobiliary diseases, as well as secondary dysfunction that may complicate diseases involving other organ systems. The GI tract subserves a wide range of functions beyond simple digestion that have an impact on systemic immunological, endocrinological, and microbiological functions.[1,2] The importance of intact gut function beyond its digestive function is of vital importance for the maintenance of health. Recent attention to alterations in GI function and the interactions between liver and lung and between liver and kidneys has led to the view that the gut plays a role as an engine of multiple organ dysfunction (see Chapter 97).[3] Recent information has shed further light on genetic differences in the response to life-threatening illness. Thus a practical working knowledge of the GI system and its integrated function is essential for the management of critically ill patients.

Intestinal Structure, Digestion, Absorption of Nutrients, Water, and Electrolytes

A primary task of the alimentary tract involves the mechanical and enzymatic degradation of nutrients, absorption of biochemical substrates, hormonal regulation of substrate flow, separation of the external from the internal environments, and excretion of waste. The process of digestion must alter nutrients to be compatible with the internal aqueous environment of the body.

The basic functional unit of the small intestine consists of villi and crypts (Table 78–1). The cells (enterocytes) of

TABLE 78–1

Functional Unit of Intestine

Structure	Function
Enterocyte	Formed in crypts, migrate to villus over 2 to 3 days; life span: 6 days
Villi	Absorption
Crypts	Secretion
Microvilli	Amplifies surface area, contains enzymes and transport systems

the small intestine are separated from one another by specialized junctions that serve as gaskets to prevent the back-diffusion of material into the intestinal lumen. A layer of mucus secreted by the goblet cells residing in the crypts separates the enterocytes from direct contact with the luminal contents. Stem cells in the crypts produce enterocytes and other specialized epithelial cells that migrate up the crypt-villous axis as they become differentiated. The migratory process from crypts to villous apex takes 48 to 72 hours. Mature villi cells (typical life span 6 days) have microvilli (brush border) that contain digestive enzymes and membrane-bound transport systems for nutrients and electrolytes. The villous tip has a predominantly absorptive function, in contrast to crypt cells that are primarily secretory. Conditions such as rotavirus infection cause villous loss resulting in a small intestinal mucosa composed largely of crypts and immature villi. A net secretory state arises, leading to malabsorption and osmotic diarrhea. Other clinical manifestations of villous injury include malabsorption of nutrients.

A major determinant of water and solute flux across the epithelium is the surface area and the integrity of the intercellular junctions. The transport of solute and water across the epithelium occurs by active or passive transport or by facilitated diffusion as outlined in Table 78–2.[4] In the small and large bowel, the surface area is greatly amplified through the mucosal folds that form the villi and microvilli. Loss of mucosal surface area through disease or surgical resection greatly alters the net flux of solute and water in the GI tract. In addition, the loss of specialized absorptive function may occur after the loss of specific areas of the gut (e.g., *short bowel syndrome*), which results from resection of the terminal ileum (see the section on enterohepatic circulation).

The gut also must conserve large volumes of endogenously secreted material associated with digestion. Up to 5 L of fluid per square meter of body surface area enters the GI tract daily with a loss of only 100 ml/m^2 in the feces under normal conditions. Thus the reserve capacity for handling solute and fluid loads to the gut is enormous. On the other hand, malfunction of the absorptive mechanisms may lead to life-threatening loss of fluid and electrolytes.

Nutrients may be divided into macronutrients, which consist of carbohydrates, protein, and lipids, and micronutrients, which consist of minerals, electrolytes, trace elements, vitamins, and other metabolic cofactors such as biotin and carnitine. Critical illness leads to a reduced

TABLE 78–2

Intestinal Transport Mechanisms

Active	Against electrochemical gradient
	Saturable kinetics
	Requires ATP
Passive	Ionic specificity
	May be associated with transport of a nonelectrolyte
	Proceeds down electrochemical gradient
	Steady-state based upon concentration differences
	Displays first-order kinetics
	May occur by convection via osmotic or hydrostatic gradient
Facilitated diffusion	Saturable kinetics
	Substrate specific
	Depends on carrier molecules (glucose, amino acid)

ATP, Adenosine triphosphate.

intake of all nutrients and important alterations in substrate requirements and utilization (see also Chapter 68). It is useful to contrast the responses seen during fasting in a healthy person with those seen during periods of increased physiological stress. During prolonged fasting or starvation in otherwise healthy individuals, compensatory responses lead to a decrease in overall metabolic rate, a decrease in gluconeogenesis from amino acids, and an increased reliance on ketone bodies for energy as the body attempts to conserve energy and protein stores. This state is characterized by depressed levels of insulin, glucagon, cortisol, and catecholamines[5] and leads gradually to chronic malnutrition.

In contrast to the simple fasting state, prolonged physiological stress as seen during critical illness leads to an increased metabolic rate, gluconeogenesis in excess of that needed to maintain serum glucose, proteolysis, and peripheral oxidation of amino acids with increased ureagenesis.[5] This state leads rapidly to malnutrition as a result of so-called autocannibalism and is characterized by levels of glucagon higher than insulin levels and by elevated catecholamines and cortisol that drive the relentless breakdown of peripheral tissues. The understanding of the pathogenesis of the stress state remains incomplete, although the biologic mediators include cytokines such as tumor necrosis factor (TNF), interleukin-1 (IL-1), free radicals derived from superoxide anion and nitric oxide,[6,7] activation of the vascular endothelium, leukocytes, platelets, and tissue macrophages. These responses are detailed in Chapters 68, 84, 93, and 97.

During periods of high physiological stress, the mixture of fuels delivered to the patient must be changed to allow for the decreased reliance on fat and carbohydrates for energy production. Proteins are relied on increasingly for energy production and must be replaced with additional amino acids to support the ongoing synthesis of acute phase reactants and immunoglobulins by the liver and immune system. Depressed plasma levels of the branched-chain amino acids have been found in many critically ill children, paralleling those seen in critically ill adults. Unfortunately, it has been difficult to demonstrate a convincing benefit of specialized feeding formulations in critically ill children despite the tremendous enthusiasm for their use in the 1990s. Recent work in critically ill adults has demonstrated benefit from dramatically modified enteral feeding regimens.[8,9] As this edition of the text is being written, a multicenter study is under way in critically ill children to evaluate formulas containing modified fatty acids and antioxidants.

Digestions of Carbohydrates

The following are conditions that impair dietary carbohydrate uptake:

- Disaccharidase deficiency (acquired or congenital)
- Pancreatic insufficiency
- Membrane-associated transported defect

Dietary carbohydrates are classified as monosaccharides and disaccharides (simple sugars), polysaccharides (complex sugars), and fiber. Glucose and fructose are the principal dietary monosaccharides and are abundantly present in fruits, sweet corn, corn syrup, and honey. The disaccharides include lactose (glucose + galactose), the principal mammalian sugar, sucrose (glucose + fructose), and maltose (glucose + glucose). Polysaccharides are polymers of glucose (e.g., starch), which is a complex carbohydrate of plant origin abundantly present in wheat, grains, potatoes, dried peas, beans, and vegetables. Fiber consists of nondigestible complex polysaccharides of plant origin. Fiber may be further classified as water insoluble (celluloses, hemicelluloses, and lignins [e.g. in bran cereal made from wheat, rye, and rice]) or water soluble (pectins, gums, and mucilages [e.g., pectins from fruits and vegetables, β-glucan from oats and barley, gums from vegetables, mucilages from outer surface of plants such as sea weeds]), with the average American diet having a soluble to insoluble fiber ratio of 3:1. Conceptually, insoluble fibers affect fecal bulk, whereas soluble fibers have viscous effects in the upper GI tract that result in delayed gastric emptying, decreased postprandial glycemic response, and a constipating effect. Carbohydrates are a major source of calories in healthy children. The metabolic fate of carbohydrates in healthy persons is generally by means of the glycolytic (Embden-Meyerhof) and tricarboxylic acid (Krebs cycle) pathways (see also Chapter 67). Carbohydrates may be stored as glycogen and lipids when ingested beyond momentary energy needs or converted to structural materials. In general, a person's requirement for energy is highly dependent on activity level or, in the case of hospitalized patients, the degree of hypermetabolism accompanying illness. In addition, the maximal ability to use carbohydrates may be limited during periods of high physiological stress as a result of the complex effects of hormonal mediators of the stress response.

Digestion of carbohydrates starts with the process of chewing, which decreases the size of food particles, thereby increasing the total surface area for subsequent action by digestive juices. Salivary secretion is necessary for lubrication and also contains salivary amylase (ptyalin), an endoenzyme that cleaves the α-1-4 links of the polysaccharide chain, resulting in short, linear oligosaccharides with maltotriose and maltose. Salivary amylase is rapidly inactivated by gastric acid; most starch digestion occurs in the duodenum under the action of pancreatic amylase and the intestinal brush border disaccharidase enzymes. Amylase contained in human milk facilitates starch digestion in breast-fed infants who are relatively deficient in endogenous salivary and pancreatic amylase. Pancreatic amylase is the major enzyme of starch digestion, which results in short oligosaccharides, maltotriose, maltose, and α-limit dextrins; however, the enterocyte is incapable of absorbing carbohydrates larger than monosaccharides. Therefore further hydrolysis to monosaccharides is performed by the intestinal *brush-border disaccharidases,* which include lactase (lactose → glucose and galactose), glucoamylase (hydrolysis of 1-4 linked oligosaccharides liberating glucose monomers), sucrase (sucrose → glucose and fructose), and isomaltase ("debrancher enzyme"; it hydrolyzes the 1-6 glycosidic linkage in α-limit dextrins). These enzymes are synthesized in the rough endoplasmic reticulum of the enterocyte and are subsequently inserted into the apical brush border membrane. With the exception of lactase and occasionally sucrase, the disaccharidases are rarely rate limiting for complete carbohydrate digestion. Deficiencies (acquired or hereditary) of any of the disaccharidase enzymes may result in carbohydrate malabsorption and may lead to osmotic diarrhea (with elevated fecal reducing sugars), abdominal distension, and flatulence resulting from fermentation of undigested oligosaccharides by colonic bacteria.

Although simple diffusion of monosaccharides occurs during periods of high luminal carbohydrate concentration, two transport mechanisms exist in the brush border for the absorption of monosaccharides.[1] Glucose, galactose, and xylitol are transported with sodium by the Na^+/ glucose cotransporter. A low intracellular sodium concentration is created by the sodium-potassium-adenosine triphosphatase (Na^+/K^+-ATPase) pump located on the basolateral membrane. The concentration gradient leads to movement of luminal sodium across the apical membrane, bringing with it glucose or galactose in a one-to-one molar ratio. The second mechanism is a non–energy-dependent facilitated transport system for fructose. The intestinal transport mechanisms are summarized in Table 78–2.

Clinical conditions that lead to loss of the epithelium and brush border system such as rotaviral gastroenteritis, inflammatory bowel disease, celiac disease, sprue, ischemia/ hypoxia, bacterial overgrowth of the proximal gut as a result of stasis or use of antacids, and malnutrition may lead to symptoms of carbohydrate malabsorption (osmotic diarrhea, abdominal pain, gaseous discomfort, flatus). Severe mucosal damage requires 7 to 10 days for recovery of brush border function. Several infant and enteral formulas rely on starch as a carbohydrate source to minimize reliance on lactase. The digestion of carbohydrates is generally efficient, ranging from almost complete absorption of rice starch to an 80% absorption of starch from beans. Bacterial fermentation of fiber and undigested carbohydrates produces short-chain fatty acids, which are used as fuel by the enterocytes, as well as gaseous hydrogen and methane contributing to the flatulence associated with increased dietary fiber and malabsorption syndromes.

Digestion of Proteins

The following conditions impair dietary protein uptake:

- Ineffective pancreatic protease secretion
- Abnormal epithelial transport (Hartnup and lysinuric protein intolerance)

The GI tract has developed efficient mechanisms for processing exogenous peptides and complex proteins. It is also efficient at recycling endogenous proteins such as digestive enzymes, mucus, sloughed cells, and plasma proteins that leak into the alimentary tract. The recommended dietary protein intakes in healthy children range from 2.5 to 3.5 g/kg/day in early infancy to 1.2 g/kg/day during childhood, and 0.8 to 0.9 g/kg/day in adolescence.[10] The enteral processing of proteins may be divided into digestive and transport phases. Gastric acid secretion initiates denaturation of complex proteins and makes them more susceptible to the actions of proteolytic enzymes. The chief cells of the stomach release pepsinogens that are converted to active pepsins under the influence of gastric acid. In addition to initiating protein digestion in the mature subject, pepsins act as milk clotting factors, which are important in the neonate for curd formation and provide bulk to the infant's stools. The pepsins are endopeptidases that release relatively large peptides and are inactivated when the pH rises above 4 as the food enters the duodenum. Patients who have achlorhydria or those receiving antacids, histamine-2 (H_2) blockers, or both agents have no evidence of impaired protein digestion ability.

Luminal digestion proceeds in the small intestine mediated by five pancreatic peptidases that are secreted by the pancreatic acinar cells as proenzymes and are activated by enterokinase and trypsin. Each peptidase possesses proteolytic activity at specific internal or external peptide bonds. Proteins are degraded typically into mixtures of one-third free amino acids and two-thirds peptides containing two to six amino acid residues,[11] which are suitable substrates for the brush border peptidases. The brush border peptidases convert the oligopeptides into monopeptides, dipeptides, and tripeptides suitable for transport into the enterocyte.

Specific membrane-associated transport mechanisms exist for the uptake of amino acids and dipeptides.[12] They involve *simple diffusion, facilitated transport,* and *carrier-mediated active transport* (see Table 78–2). Na^+-coupled active transport is an energy-dependent process associated with the uptake of luminal Na^+ and an amino acid (or glucose) and exchange of the sodium and associated molecule for K^+ through the basolateral membrane on the serosal side.[13] An important characteristic of these transporters is that many amino acids are absorbed more rapidly as dipeptides than as free amino acids. This fact has been capitalized on in the development of enteral nutritional formulas because oligopeptide mixtures have a lower osmolarity and are more efficiently absorbed than single amino acid solutions of equal nitrogen content. Because of the efficient GI absorption of dipeptides, patients with specific amino acid transport defects (e.g., Hartnup disease [defective tryptophan transport] and lysinuric protein intolerance [defect in dibasic amino acid {lysine, arginine} transport]) infrequently have GI symptoms related to dietary protein malabsorption and instead more commonly have nongastrointestinal symptoms (e.g., aminoaciduria). Once inside the enterocyte, peptides are quickly degraded into their constituent amino acids by cytoplasmic peptidases that complement the activity of the brush border peptidases. Only minute quantities of intact peptide and protein gain access to the systemic circulation. The cytoplasmic amino acids derived from digested proteins are a major source of free amino acids used directly by the enterocyte. When absorbed beyond cellular needs, the free amino acids are released to the portal venous circulation for hepatic and systemic use. Only 23% of absorbed amino acid nitrogen passes to the periphery without modification.[14] Of the remaining nitrogen, 57% is converted to urea with the carbon skeleton salvaged for synthesizing other substances, and 20% of the total ingested amino acids is used directly for hepatic protein synthesis. During periods of fasting, the enterocyte derives most of its nourishment from the mesenteric arterial vascular supply, whereas during digestion, the enterocyte derives a significant part of its nutrient requirements from the luminal contents. Experience with mucosal recovery and adaptation after injury reveals that an enteral route of nutrition permits optimal recovery.

In the premature infant and neonate, the small intestine is capable of absorbing intact milk proteins by pinocytosis. These proteins may include secretory immunoglobulins from breast milk and food antigens.[15] Peptidase inhibitors have been shown in colostrum and breast milk, and this partially explains the failure of normal digestive mechanisms to degrade some of these complex dietary proteins. Both antibodies and antigens ingested with maternal milk create an important part of the immune repertory developed during early infancy.[16] Although the exact time of "closure" of the intestinal mucosa to the uptake of macromolecules has not been defined in human infants, other mammals show marked intestinal impermeability to foreign proteins by the time of weaning[17] from breastfeeding.

Digestion of Lipids

The following are conditions that impair dietary lipid uptake:

- Decreased bile salt pool in gut (biliary obstruction, short bowel syndrome)
- Impaired pancreatic secretions (pancreatic insufficiency, pancreatitis)
- Suboptimal pH in gut (gastric hypersecretion)
- Rapid transit time (short gut syndrome, diarrheal states)
- Mucosal diseases (celiac disease, inflammatory bowel disease, bacterial overgrowth)
- Impaired enterocyte function (abetalipoproteinemia)

Dietary fat accounts for approximately 50% to 70% of the nonprotein calories consumed by infants and approximately 34% of nonprotein calories consumed after age 2 years.[18] Dietary fat is ingested principally in the form of triglycerides that contain the fatty acids palmitate and oleate (C16:0 and C18:1, respectively). Dietary triglycerides of animal origin predominantly contain long-chain (i.e., longer than C14 chain length) saturated fatty acids. Polyunsaturated fatty acids are mostly of vegetable origin and include linoleic and linolenic acid, also referred to as essential fatty acids because of absent de novo synthesis in humans. Other dietary lipids include fat-soluble vitamins, cholesterol, prostaglandins, waxes, and phospholipids. In healthy adults, digestion and absorption of fat is complete with only 5% to 7% of ingested fat escaping absorption. Under normal physiological conditions healthy infants up to age 9 to 12 months fail to absorb 15% to 35% of dietary fat. Digestion and absorption of dietary fat is generally completed by the middle third of jejunum; however, the presence of dietary fiber may reduce the rate and extent of absorption. Loss of dietary fat places children at significant risk for calorie and fat-soluble vitamin malnutrition.

Fat digestion begins with formation of emulsions, which increase the surface area for enzyme interaction. Emulsification begins with the release of fat by mastication and gastric "milling" of chyme. Coating by phospholipid derived from the diet and bile salts results in a stable emulsion droplet with a hydrophobic center consisting of triglyceride, cholesterol esters, and diglyceride in a hydrophilic envelope. Mammary, lingual, and gastric lipases play an important role in direct lipolysis of long- and medium-chain triglycerides (MCTs) that are present in maternal milk.[19] Lingual and gastric lipases are active at pH less than 5 and begin digestion of fat in the stomach; however, overall they only play a limited role in the digestion of lipids. Most of the enzymatic degradation of dietary lipids to fatty acids and monoglyceride is by the action of pancreatic lipase and colipase and requires an alkaline environment (pH 6 to 8). Colipase is an essential cofactor for lipase action. Colipase's role is to displace the bile salt-triglyceride interaction in emulsion droplets and micelles to facilitate lipase hydrolysis of the triglyceride. Triglyceride hydrolysis occurs at the interface between the emulsion droplet and aqueous phase within the lumen. It involves two major steps: the first is the enzymatic hydrolysis of long-chain triglycerides and liberation of fatty acids from the glycerol backbone, and the second is formation of fatty acid micelles with the aid of bile salts, which traffic the fatty acids across the unstirred water layer to the mucosa for absorption.

When not limited by bile salt concentration or pancreatic insufficiency, the transit through the unstirred layer adjacent to the epithelial surface is considered the rate-limiting step in lipid absorption; however, there are intrinsic gut brush border lipase enzymes as well. The milieu of the unstirred water layer is acidic (pH 5 to 6) owing to activity of the brush border membrane sodium-hydrogen (Na^+/H^+) exchanger. The acid environment facilitates dissociation of fatty acids from micelles, and the result is a high concentration of fatty acids necessary for diffusion across the mucosal membrane.[20] Once inside the enterocyte, long-chain fatty acids and monoglycerides are resynthesized into triglycerides and packaged as chylomicrons. Lipoproteins (e.g., apo-A, apo-B) and cholesterol are attached to the intestinal chylomicrons and confer important properties for the subsequent systemic uptake and metabolism of the chylomicrons. They are exported into the intercellular space and transported through the intestinal lacteals to become part of the intestinal lymph. On entering the bloodstream through the thoracic duct, the chylomicrons are associated with other apolipoproteins that allow them to be recognized by specific peripheral tissues.

Dietary lipids containing short- and medium-chain (C6 - C12) triglycerides (MCTs) are handled differently from those of long-chain triglycerides. As much as 30% of MCTs may be absorbed intact by enterocytes by passive diffusion and enter the portal venous blood directly. In addition, MCTs are hydrolyzed by pancreatic and mammary lipases to fatty acids and monoglycerides and rapidly enter the enterocytes, where they emerge into the portal venous system without reesterification as occurs with long-chain fatty acids.

Intestinal Lymphatics

The intestinal lymph *chyle* is composed of chylomicrons and lipoproteins[21] that are secreted by the intestinal epithelium in the postprandial state together with nonresorbed interstitial fluid. Chyle follows the intestinal lymphatic channels along the mesentery and enters regional lymph nodes from which it flows cephalad through the thoracic duct and ultimately enters the central circulation. In the fasting state, intestinal lymph production is relatively low. It increases twentyfold during the active absorption of a typical meal. The intestinal chyle is joined by lymphatic drainage from other tissues including liver and pancreas. The protein content of chyle is 2.2 to 5.9 g/dl with a triglyceride content of 0.4 to 6 g/dl and 400 to 6800 lymphocytes per microliter. During digestion of a meal containing long-chain fats, chyle has a typical milky white appearance because of the presence of chylomicrons. The rate of formation of chyle depends on several factors such as the state of nutrient absorption, portal venous pressure, and the rate of lymphatic uptake. Factors that increase portal pressure (e.g., cirrhosis, congestive heart failure) or impair the flow of lymph back to the central circulation (e.g., increased central venous pressure, superior vena cava syndrome) predispose to the collection of chylous ascites in the abdomen.

Regulation of Electrolyte and Water Movement

The movement of water is closely linked to the movement of solute in the form of electrolytes and nutrients. A three-compartment model has been proposed for the absorption of fluid in the GI tract. In this model, the luminal contents are isolated from the vascular space by three compartments separated by two semipermeable membranes of differing porosities.[2,22,23] Electrolytes are taken up by the enterocytes and extruded through the basolateral membrane into the paracellular space. The relatively hypertonic paracellular fluid pulls water into this space and increases the hydrostatic pressure locally. Because the tight junction between enterocytes is more impermeable to fluid flux than the capillary membranes, fluid and electrolytes are preferentially driven in the direction of the vascular space.

Systemic and Endocrine Effects on Intestinal Fluid and Electrolyte Handling

To coordinate the digestive, transport, and motility functions of the gut, a system of regulation has evolved involving both systemic and local stimuli.[24] Numerous substances have been identified such as muscarinic receptor agonists, serotonin, substance P, and similar agents that probably work through increased adenyl cyclase activity or increased cytosolic Ca^{++} concentration to induce active chloride secretion. Systemic acidosis increases Na^+ and Cl^- absorption in the ileum and colon, whereas alkalosis has the opposite effect. As seen in other epithelial tissues, aldosterone increases ileal and colonic absorption of Na^+, and spironolactone blocks this effect. The terminal ileum and colon are particularly important in this respect, and the presence of an ileostomy increases the risk of excessive sodium losses, dehydration, and electrolyte abnormalities. Glucocorticoids play a role in intestinal maturation[25] and increase sodium and water absorption in the distal colon. Opiate receptor stimulation increases active sodium and chloride absorption in the ileum, and opiate antagonists decrease basal absorption of water and electrolytes. The primary antidiarrheal effect of opiates, however, is mediated through a slowing of transit time. Vasoactive intestinal peptide (VIP) mediates increased secretion of electrolytes and water by increased cyclic adenosine monophosphate production that stimulates active chloride secretion and inhibits sodium-chloride absorption. Certain arachidonic acid metabolites, especially prostaglandins (e.g., prostaglandin E_1), have been shown to increase active chloride secretion, leading to increased loss of electrolytes and fluid.

Many laxatives and antacids may affect fluid and electrolyte balance by stimulating active electrolyte and fluid secretion in the terminal ileum. In addition, these agents may increase mucosal permeability and stimulate motility. Hyperosmolality of the ileal and colonic contents leads to an osmotic diarrhea. This state is seen when unabsorbed nutrients enter the distal alimentary tract and are broken down by enteric bacteria; the results are increased luminal osmotic activity and osmotic diarrhea.

Gastrointestinal Neuroendocrine Control

Control over secretion and motility depends on a complex series of neurohormonal mechanisms frequently referred to as PINES (*p*aracrine *i*mmuno*n*euro*e*ndocrine *s*ystem of the gut). Its detailed discussion is beyond the scope of this text, and interested readers should consult one of the standard textbooks of gastroenterology for greater detail (see also Chapter 95).[2,24]

Secretion and motility are mediated through typical agonist membrane receptor mechanisms or by local autocrine and paracrine action, or they may demonstrate remote endocrine and neurocrine actions. The peptides are secreted by endocrine or nerve cells of the gut and influence a wide range of functions throughout the gut including control of cell proliferation, motility, secretion, and mesenteric perfusion.[25] Regulation of intestinal motility is critical for keeping the chyme in contact with the epithelial surface long enough for efficient absorption of nutrients and yet permitting removal of unusable material and bacteria from the alimentary tract on a regular basis. GI smooth muscle demonstrates phasic and tonic patterns of contraction. The frequency of contractions may be affected by (1) changes in autonomic tone, (2) stimulation of the gut by neurohormonal peptides and pharmacologic agents, or (3) noxious stimuli associated with infectious or inflammatory processes. Hypoxia and ischemia decrease motility and frequently lead to paralytic ileus.

Electrolyte Transport

Several basic mechanisms have evolved for the transport of electrolytes by the epithelia. Sodium is transported by (1) a Na^+-H^+ exchange mechanism present throughout the intestine resulting in 1:1 exchange of luminal sodium for protons (a critical system for maintaining intracellular pH, cell volume and sodium content), (2) coupled sodium-chloride absorption, (3) sodium-chloride cotransport, and (4) sodium-potassium-chloride cotransport and (5) down its electrochemical gradient. The Na^+-H^+ exchanger plays a role in regulation of intracellular pH, regulation of cell volume, initiation of cell growth in response to various trophic factors, and metabolic response to insulin. To maintain electrical neutrality, the epithelium simultaneously exchanges Na^+ for H^+ and Cl^- for HCO_3^-. In the colon, active absorption and secretion of K^+ occurs in a manner consistent with K^+-H^+ exchange. It is electroneutral and independent of Na^+-Cl^- exchange. The presence of glucose in the lumen of the small intestine stimulates increased sodium absorption through coupled transport. The uptake of glucose is carrier mediated; however, the coupled transport of glucose with sodium is electrogenically driven by the Na^+ gradient across the cell membrane.[26] After the ion has entered the enterocyte at the luminal surface, extrusion occurs through the basolateral membrane into the paracellular spaces. It is generally agreed that the process of sodium extrusion depends on Na^+/K^+-ATPase pumping function located at the basolateral membranes. Extrusion of Cl^- is probably along an electrochemical potential difference.[27] The intraluminal secretion of water and other electrolytes appears to follow active secretion of Cl^- from the crypt cells of the jejunum, ileum, and colon. This physiological pattern (i.e., water following the secretion of an osmotically active molecule) is a common theme in the liver (e.g., bile salt-dependent bile flow), pancreas, and kidney.

Because a major task for the GI tract is sodium conservation, backflow of sodium into the lumen is generally only a passive process. Disruption of normal Na^+/K^+ ATPase activity results in the net secretion of fluid and electrolytes. This mechanism is the final common pathway in a number of secretory diarrheal states such as cholera, enterotoxigenic *Escherichia coli*, *Salmonella*, *Campylobacter jejuni*, and *Clostridium perfringens*.[28] In addition, the effects of various paracrine and endocrine mediators alter intestinal adenyl cyclase activity and lead to changes in electrolyte and water balance.[27]

Zinc

Zinc is an important cofactor with increased requirements seen during wound healing. Zinc deficiency in critically ill patients may occur secondary to increased requirements in young children,[28a] intestinal fluid losses through GI stomas and fistulae, and urinary losses patients on hemofiltration[28b] or in association with continous therapy with sedatives containing disodium ethylenediaminetetraacetic acid [EDTA]).[28c] Zinc levels should be checked periodically in critically ill patients who fail to respond to nutritional support.

Hydrogen Ion

Hydrochloric acid secretion by the gastric parietal cell is necessary for pepsinogen activation (pH<5) and for the reduction of bacterial colonization. The main stimulants of gastric acid secretion are histamine, gastrin, and acetylcholine.[29] Pituitary adenyl cyclase-activating polypeptide also plays a major role in nocturnal acid secretion through the stimulation of histamine.[30] Histamine release by gastric enterochromaffin-like cells is the dominant physiological stimulus for acid secretion by the gastric parietal cells. Gastric distension, dietary amino acids, and amines stimulate gastrin hormone secretion by G-cells located in the gastric antrum. Gastrin hormone stimulates the enterochromaffin-like cells, in proximity to parietal cells to release histamine. Histamine then binds to H_2 receptors on parietal cells leading to acid secretion along with chloride (170 mEq/L) and potassium (8 to 20 mEq/L). The carbon dioxide derived from this process is converted to blood bicarbonate, producing a transient postprandial metabolic alkalosis. Prostaglandins and somatostatin have an inhibitory effect on gastric acid secretion through specific receptors located on the parietal cell.[31] H_2 receptor antagonists (e.g., ranitidine, famotidine, cimetidine) block histamine-mediated gastric acid secretion (e.g., postprandial acid secretion, Zollinger-Ellison syndrome, other disorders associated with hypergastrinemia). Proton pump inhibitors (PPIs) (e.g., omeprazole, lansoprazole, and pantoprazole) block H_2-, gastrin-, and cholinergic-mediated gastric acid secretion by inhibiting the parietal cell H^+/K^+ adenosine triphosphatase enzyme (the proton pump), which is the final common pathway for gastric acid secretion. Furthermore, because PPIs bind irreversibly to adenosine triphosphatase, subsequent secretion of acid can occur only with the synthesis of a new proton pump enzyme, a process that takes more than 12 to 24 hours. For these reasons, PPIs have revolutionized gastric acid suppression therapy.[32,33]

The Pancreas

The pancreas has both endocrine and exocrine functions. Through the endocrine function, the pancreas, together with the liver, serves as a major regulator of blood glucose levels. Endocrine-secreting cells of the pancreas are aggregated in the islets of Langerhans. Four distinct cell types that serve the endocrine function include B cells that secrete insulin, A cells that secrete glucagon, D cells that secrete somatostatin, and PP cells that secrete pancreatic polypeptide.[34] Functional ectopic pancreatic tissue may be found commonly throughout the upper GI tract. The blood supply to the pancreas derives from branches of the celiac, superior mesenteric, and splenic arteries. The venous drainage from the pancreas is via the pancreaticoduodenal veins, the splenic veins, and ultimately the portal vein, which provides direct hormonal influence over hepatic metabolism. Both parasympathetic and sympathetic innervation of the pancreas occurs by means of the vagi and abdominal plexuses, respectively. The vagal innervation of acini, islets, and ducts facilitates secretory function, whereas sympathetic innervation occurs primarily to vascular structures.

Pancreatic Exocrine Secretory Function

The exocrine function is derived from specialized cells that contain secretory granules and arranged in acini that drain into ductules, which coalesce to form the pancreatic duct. Ultimately, the pancreatic duct joins with the common bile duct and drains into the duodenum through the ampulla of Vater. Each acinar cell is capable of secreting all the pancreatic digestive enzymes in contrast to the pancreatic endocrine cells that demonstrate specialized function. Pancreatic juice is characteristically an isotonic, aqueous fluid containing Na^+, K^+, and Ca^{++} in concentrations similar to extracellular fluid along with traces of Mg^{++}, Zn^{++}, $HPO^=$, and HCO_3^- and is approximately 150 mEq/L. The contribution of each anion varies reciprocally, depending on the rate of secretory flow. Secretion of bicarbonate and water is mediated through the actions of the gut hormones, secretin, cholecystokinin, and VIP. Stimulation of the vagus nerves or the administration of acetylcholine induces digestive enzyme secretion, whereas these effects may be blocked with atropine.

There are four phases of pancreatic secretion:[35]

1. Basal secretion
2. Cephalic
3. Gastric
4. Intestinal

Basal secretion represents approximately 2% of the potential maximum HCO_3^- output. The *cephalic phase* is mediated by the vagal nerves in response to the sight and smell of food. Distention of the stomach either artificially or after the ingestion of food evokes a *gastric phase* that consists of secretion of a protein-rich pancreatic juice of low volume and HCO_3^-. The *intestinal phase* is characterized by marked output of digestive enzymes, fluid, and HCO_3^-. The presence of bicarbonate is essential to achieve an optimal pH (pH>5) for pancreatic digestive enzyme activity and to ensure solubility of bile salts. In addition to bicarbonate, the primary secretory products of the exocrine pancreas are amylase, lipase, and the proteases. The secondary digestive enzymes consist of nucleases, colipase, and lecithinase. The roles of the pancreatic digestive enzymes are discussed in the sections on carbohydrate digestion (amylase), lipid digestion (lipase), and protein digestion (proteases).

Inhibitors of exocrine pancreatic secretion include somatostatin, pancreatic polypeptide, and peptide YY. Somatostatin inhibits release of secretin from duodenal mucosa and is also a competitor at secretin receptor sites resulting in decreased pancreatic secretion of both bicarbonate and enzymes.[36] The pancreatic polypeptide hormone present in the islets of Langerhans also has an inhibitory effect on pancreatic secretion of water, bicarbonate, and enzymes. Peptide YY, released from the distal ileum and colon in response to intraluminal fat, exerts its inhibitory effect by decreasing pancreatic responses to cholecystokinin and secretin. Octreotide, a somatostatin analogue, has been used for its antisecretory effect in clinical management of pancreatic pseudocysts and fistulae.[37] Inflammation of the pancreas both from infectious and noninfectious causes can produce a dramatic systemic inflammatory response resulting in generalized permeability changes and acute lung injury. The inflammatory and healing response of the pancreas documented in a recent review by Bentrem and Joehl.[38]

Hepatobiliary System

Examination

A complete physical examination of all children admitted to an ICU should include inspection, palpation, and auscultation of the abdomen with particular attention to hepatic or splenic enlargement, distended superficial venous channels, abdominal masses, the characteristics of the bowel sounds, and finally visual inspection of the perianal region for signs of trauma, fistulae, and venous distension. Palpation of the liver provides information not only concerning the hepatobiliary tract but also about function of the right side of the heart. Normally, the liver is palpable no more than 1 to 3 cm below the right costal margin in the midclavicular line; however, assessment of liver *span*, and not palpation alone, is the only reliable nonradiological method for the determination of liver size. Liver span is determined by percussion, palpation, and auscultation along the right midclavicular line with the patient supine and breathing quietly. The dullness of the upper border is determined by percussion and palpation or auscultation used to establish the lower border.[39] The average liver span is 4 to 5 cm in preterm infants; 5 to 6.5 cm in healthy term infants; 6 to 7 cm between ages 1 and 5 years; 7 to 9 cm between ages 5 and 10 years; and 8 to 10 cm between ages 10 and 16 years.[40] Conditions associated with downward displacement of a normal liver include hyperinflated lungs, pneumothorax, retroperitoneal mass, and subdiaphragmatic abscess. Tenderness over the liver suggests inflammation or stretching of the fibrous capsule through rapid enlargement. End-stage liver disease and cirrhosis are associated with a reduced liver span corresponding to decreased hepatic cell mass. The spleen tip may be palpable normally in children, especially during inspiration. Enlargement of the spleen generally represents elevated portal venous pressures or invasive processes such as sequestration, malignancies, extramedullary hematopoiesis, or hyperplasia of the reticuloendothelial system.[41]

Anatomy

Microanatomy, Structure, and Function

The liver is the largest organ in the body and is composed of 60% hepatocytes, approximately 17% to 20% endothelial cells and Kupffer cells (reticuloendothelial cells), 3% to 5% bile ducts, and 1% Ito cells and oval cells. The liver has a dual vascular supply derived from the hepatic artery branches of the celiac axis and the portal vein. Innervation of the liver is by the parasympathetic branches derived from both vagi and sympathetic branches, which also carry afferent fibers deriving from thoracic segments.

The functional unit of the liver is the "liver lobule," which is composed of interconnected hepatocytes (hepatic plates) 1 to 2 cells thick and 20 to 25 cells in length separated by a venous sinusoidal space and radiating around the central vein like spokes in wheel (Fig. 78–1). Endothelial cells form a porous lining between the venous sinusoidal space and hepatic plates. Macrophage-derived Kupffer cells that have a phagocytic function, as well as mediation of the hepatic inflammatory response, also line the sinusoidal space. The narrow tissue space between the endothelial cells and hepatic plates is called the space of Disse, which in turn connects with lymphatic vessels in the interlobular septa. Ito cells, also known as *stellate cells,* also lie within the space of Disse. Ito cells serve as the hepatic storage site of vitamin A, are effectors of fibrogenesis, and play a role in extracellular matrix remodeling after recovery from injury. Chronic activation and proliferation of Ito cells may lead to noncirrhotic portal hypertension, fibrosis, and cirrhosis.[42,43] The endothelial lining has large pores that facilitate bidirectional exchange of solutes into the sinusoidal space (e.g., bilirubin, bile salts, and other protein-bound solutes can easily transfer from the sinusoid to the space of Disse and subsequently to the hepatocyte). Likewise, movement of products secreted by the hepatocytes (e.g., lipoproteins) is facilitated from the space of Disse to the sinusoid. In between adjacent hepatocytes are bile canaliculi that drain into small terminal bile ducts, which successively drain into larger bile ductules, intralobular bile ducts, and eventually the extrahepatic bile ducts. In addition to passive diffusion, several different carriers, receptors, and transport proteins facilitate movement of compounds across the sinusoidal, hepatocyte, and canalicular membranes. ATP-binding cassette (ABC) proteins are expressed in the canalicular membrane and play an important role in transportation of organic ions. The ABC proteins of interest include the multidrug resistance, or MDR 1 gene product, which plays a role in canalicular secretion of organic cations; MDR 2, which is thought to play a role in secretion of biliary phospholipids; and a multispecific organic anion transporter (MOAT) gene product that is important in secretion of bilirubin. The cystic fibrosis transmembrane regulator (CFTR) gene product is also expressed in biliary cells and appears to be an important determinant of biliary secretion and bile flow.[44] Alkaline phosphatase, leucine aminopeptidase, and γ-glutamyl transpeptidase are transaminase enzymes selectively localized in the bile canaliculi.

The microcirculatory "path" within the lobules leads along a declining hydrostatic pressure gradient from the terminal hepatic arterioles and portal venules toward the terminal branch of the hepatic vein resulting in three hepatocyte functional zones (see Fig. 78–1). Zone 1 hepatocytes closest to the portal tract are exposed to sinusoidal blood containing the highest concentration of solutes

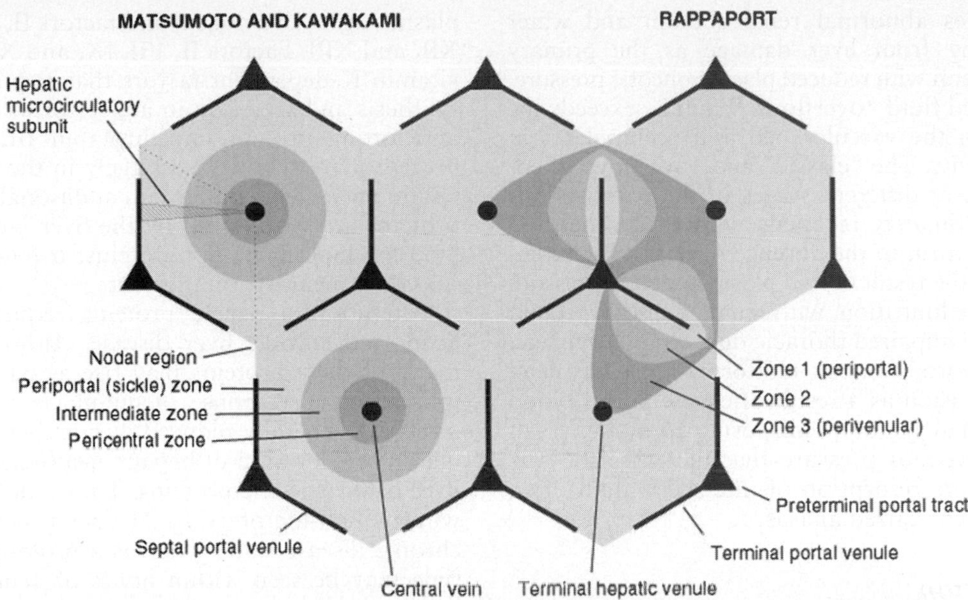

FIGURE 78–1 • Microanatomy of the liver depicting the hepatic acinus and microcirculatory subunits. Arrangement of simple liver acinus forms zones centered about portal triads; preterminal portal tract contains terminal afferent vascular branches, bile ductules, lymph vessels, and nerves. Zone 3 forms the microcirculatory periphery because its cells are the farthest from afferent vessels. Cell damage in the area surrounding the terminal hepatic venule, which extends into zone 3, produces a typical stellate pattern of fibrosis. Extensive fibrosis in zone 3 leads to "bridging necrosis." (From Wanless IR: Anatomy, histology, embryology, and developmental anomalies of the liver. In Feldman M, Friedman LS, Slesinger MH, editor: *Slesinger and Fordtran's gastrointestinal and liver disease,* ed 7, Philadelphia, 2002, Saunders/Elsevier.)

and oxygen. In contrast zones 2 and 3 represent hepatocytes more distant from the portal blood supply and therefore exposed to a declining oxygen and solute gradient. In addition, zone 3 hepatocytes actively participate in drug metabolism and disposition. As a result, centrizonal hepatocyte injury and necrosis are more commonly associated with ischemic and drug hepatotoxicity insults.

Kupffer cells represent the intrahepatic portion of the reticuloendothelial system. Their role along with the hepatocytes in setting the stage for the multiple organ dysfunction syndrome (MODS) has become apparent in recent years.[45–47] Both the intestine and the hepatic-based macrophages can serve as a major source of nitric oxide after injury or stimulation.[48–50] The recently recognized role of nitric oxide on immune function further emphasizes the role of the GI tract in systemic responses.[51] The frequent association of hepatic dysfunction with the acute respiratory distress syndrome has led to intensive investigation of the lung-liver axis during critical illness.[45,49] A major unifying theme in these organ interactions is the regional activation of macrophages and platelets and damage to the endothelium after injury leading to both localized and remote organ function disturbance.[46,49,52] For the pediatric intensivists, observations made in mature human or animal subjects provide only partial insights into the effects of life-threatening illness in very young children. As previously mentioned, in vitro work with isolated hepatocyte and Kupffer cell cocultures showed decreased responsiveness of the newborn cocultures to lipopolysaccharide stimulation compared with mature cells, suggesting a greater reserve capacity against inflammatory stimuli.[53]

Portal Circulation

The portal venous system drains the intestines, pancreas, and spleen with numerous collateral anastomoses to other venous beds of the abdomen. The portal vein delivers approximately 70% of the hepatic blood flow. There is a mixing of portal and systemic blood circulation within the sinusoids, and all the blood eventually drains from the liver via the hepatic veins to the inferior vena cava. The liver has a high blood flow (~27% of the resting cardiac output) and low vascular resistance with an average portal venous pressure of 9 mmHg, and hepatic vein pressure of 0 mmHg. A rise in hepatic venous pressure of up to 3 to 7 mmHg results in increased hepatic vascular pressure and ultimately a transcapsular fluid transudate containing a protein level of 80% to 90% as much as plasma protein. Obstruction of the portal venous drainage at any level leads to portal hypertension. Inferior vena caval pressures of 10 to 15 mmHg result in gross ascites.[54] Ascites may be classified as prehepatic, intrahepatic, or posthepatic, according to the level at which the obstruction to flow occurs. The determination of the location of obstruction is critical for instituting appropriate therapy. The "classic theory" of ascites formation implicates an increased resistance to blood flow through the liver resulting from cirrhosis. Impaired portal drainage leads to a decrease in circulating blood volume, which stimulates the renin-angiotensin-aldosterone system and releases antidiuretic hormone. This process induces sodium and water retention leading to plasma volume expansion and further portal hypertension. The "overflow theory" of ascites formation invokes abnormal renal sodium and water retention resulting from liver damage as the primary defect. In association with reduced plasma oncotic pressure, the excess retained fluid "overflows," that is, exceeds the Starling forces in the vascular bed and accumulates in the peritoneal cavity. The "classic" and "overflow" theories both operate at different stages in the pathogenesis of ascites and ultimately reconcile with each other.[55–57] Ascites may also form in the absence of portal hypertension primarily as the result of low plasma oncotic pressure associated with malnutrition, with renal or enteral protein losses, or through impaired thoracic duct lymph drainage. Rarely, arterial-portal venous malformations may lead to portal hypertension as a result of excess portal blood flow. An additional factor predisposing to ascites is an elevated central venous pressure that increases the formation and impairs resorption of interstitial fluid often associated with generalized anasarca.

Hepatic Function

The function of the liver may be broadly characterized in terms of (1) production of substances uniquely made in the liver; (2) the degradation, elimination, and detoxification of biological materials; (3) the maintenance of biochemical homeostasis; and (4) storage of nutritional materials.

The liver occupies an ideal place in the scheme of digestion. Hepatocytes are exposed to large quantities of absorbed nutrients after ingestion of a meal with 20% of the total absorbed nitrogen used for hepatic protein synthesis. Of the large number of plasma proteins synthesized by the liver, several are of major significance in the ICU and deserve particular attention. Albumin has a half-life of approximately 20 days and is the most significant contributor to colloid oncotic pressure. Therefore decreased serum levels may predispose to edema formation and decreased binding of bilirubin, calcium, xenobiotics, and other highly protein bound molecules. Low serum albumin levels may occur as a result of impaired synthesis from protein-calorie malnutrition, chronic liver disease, cachexia cytokines[58] or increased losses from proteinuria, protein-losing enteropathy, burns, and other iatrogenic losses including paracentesis. Prealbumin, also known as *transthyretin,* is a visceral protein with a short half-life of 1.9 days. Because hepatic synthesis is exquisitely sensitive to both the adequacy and levels of protein and energy intakes,[59] it may be used a nutritional marker and for monitoring short-term response to nutritional intervention. α_1-Antitrypsin is an important antiprotease with regulatory activity for elastase and other proteases.[60] α_1-Antitrypsin may be important in regulating elastase-induced tissue injury in certain lung diseases with its absence leading to uncontrolled proteolytic activity in the lung.[61] Because α_1-antitrypsin is an endogenous protein that is relatively resistant to hydrolysis by enteric bacteria, elevated levels detected in feces suggest protein losing enteropathy.[62] Hepatic synthesis of transferrin facilitates iron transport in the plasma by binding two molecules of iron. Storage of iron is accomplished primarily as ferritin with each molecule storing up to 4500 atoms of iron. Many coagulation factors are synthesized in the liver. They include plasminogen; fibrinogen; and factors II, V, VII, IX, X, XI, XII, and XIII. Factors II, VII, IX, and X are the so-called vitamin K–dependent factors that require vitamin K for synthesis and secretion in active form.[63] In addition, the anticlotting proteins antithrombin III, protein C, and protein S are synthesized largely in the liver and may be vitamin K dependent. Several additional common plasma proteins are synthesized by the liver including haptoglobin, ceruloplasmin, lipoproteins, α-fetoprotein, and the C3 component of complement.

Alterations in plasma proteins frequently occur during acute and chronic liver disease. Although the levels of many of these proteins may rise as part of the systemic inflammatory response (acute-phase reactants), plasma levels are generally reduced during liver disease, depending on the duration of hepatic insufficiency and the half-lives of the specific proteins. Thus a decrease in albumin with its half-life of 16 to 21 days generally represents a chronic disease state, whereas a prolonged prothrombin time may be seen within hours of acute hepatic failure because of the short half-life of factor VII (approximately 6 hours).[63]

Detoxification and catabolism of ammonia, bilirubin, and xenobiotics are essential to life. Ammonia arises through bacterial degradation of nitrogenous compounds in the intestine, as well as from other physiological sources including the kidneys and peripheral tissues such as skeletal muscle and the brain. High levels of ammonia are incompatible with life; therefore the liver is endowed with a large capacity for urea synthesis from ammonia. During hepatic failure, hyperammonemia represents a life-threatening aspect of liver disease. Bilirubin elimination is another critical excretory function of the liver. The largest source of bilirubin is heme that is derived from hemoglobin as a result of hemolysis with smaller amounts liberated through the breakdown of cytochromes and myoglobin. Heme is broken down into bilirubin in the reticuloendothelial system. Hepatic metabolism of bilirubin involves several steps, including transport to the hepatocyte and cellular uptake, cytosolic transport within the hepatocyte, conjugation, active cellular export, and elimination. Impairment at any juncture becomes manifest as hyperbilirubinemia and ultimately clinical jaundice. Bilirubin has a high affinity for elastin- and collagen-containing tissue, thus explaining the presence of noticeable scleral and palatal icterus in patients with jaundice.

Enterohepatic Circulation

Bile acids represent a family of steroid molecules derived from cholesterol. Their primary functions are the elimination of cholesterol from the body and the solubilization of dietary fats through a detergent-like action. Because a minimum concentration of bile acids is required for micelle formation, an efficient mechanism was evolved in the form of the enterohepatic circulation for the conservation of bile acids. Bile salts are secreted into the duodenum with reuptake of 97% in the terminal ileum, undergoing recycling 4 to 12 times per day. The distal and terminal ileum have specialized transport mechanisms for absorption of bile salts and vitamin B_{12}, which are adversely affected by terminal ileal resection, jejunostomies, inflammatory bowel disease, or other acquired lesions in this anatomical region (e.g. necrotizing enterocolitis). Functional loss of the distal and terminal ileum results in malabsorption of vitamin B_{12}, bile salt deficiency, and impaired digestion and absorption of fat soluble vitamins and long-chain fats. Furthermore, unresorbed bile acids have a detergent effect on the colonic epithelium, resulting in secretory diarrhea.[2]

The elimination of many drugs is affected by hepatic insufficiency either from immaturity or as a result of disease. A large number of commonly used drugs of all classes including aminophylline preparations, narcotics, barbiturates, H_2 blockers, vasodilators, antidysrhythmics, and others demonstrate significant hepatic elimination. The hepatic P-450 system refers to membrane bound internal enzymes that play a central role in many of the mixed-function oxidative reactions responsible for converting lipophilic compounds into more water-soluble ones. In addition, the liver may conjugate drug metabolites with sugars, amino acids, sulfates, or acetate to form products that can be more easily eliminated in bile or through the kidney. Additional hepatic enzymes—esterases, deaminases, hydrolases, and reductases—play an important role in the biotransformation of endogenous substances and xenobiotics.[64] The half-life of many drugs may be prolonged during hepatic insufficiency as a result of a decrease in the total number of functioning hepatocytes. In addition, the apparent half-life of many drugs may be prolonged through competitive inhibition by the presence of other drugs, or, in fact, may be shortened by induction of elimination. For example, phenobarbital decreases the half-life of xanthines and may increase the toxicity of acetaminophen. Adjustment of medication dosage and schedule must be considered for those drugs with significant hepatic elimination when impaired liver function exists.[64]

Hepatic regulatory function involves (1) interconversion of amino acids to maintain physiological plasma levels, (2) gluconeogenesis to maintain adequate serum levels for glucose-dependent tissues, and (3) regulation of numerous plasma hormones (Table 78–3). The direct secretion of insulin and glucagon into the portal circulation exposes the liver to much higher concentrations of these hormones than peripheral tissues. This relationship amplifies the hepatic influence over carbohydrate metabolism. Approximately 50% of secreted insulin is degraded on a first-pass basis by the liver with a large first-pass uptake of glucagon as well. Both of these hormones are known to have hepatotropic effects and are thought to be important for differentiation and regeneration of hepatocytes. The trophic effect of insulin on hepatocytes may be yet another benefit of the current move toward insulin supplementation in critically patients.[65,66]

The last category of hepatic function involves storage of glycogen, triglycerides, folic acid, vitamin B_{12}, and vitamins A and D. Hepatic glycogen stores provide the most immediate source of glucose to maintain serum levels by glycogenolysis. Pathological conditions associated with retention of excess storage material are familiar to pediatricians and include the glycogenoses and the mucopolysaccharidoses. Synthesis of vitamin D_3 (cholecalciferol) occurs in the skin with subsequent accumulation of D_3 in the liver. Hydroxylation in the 25-position that occurs in the liver results in a large pool of circulating 25-(OH)D_3, the precursor of the active 1, 25-(di OH)D_3. Defective storage and absorption of dietary vitamin D and 25 hydroxylation may be present in chronic liver failure.

TABLE 78–3

Hepatic Endocrine Regulation

Catabolized Primarily in the Liver	Catabolized in the Liver and Other Tissues
Insulin	Thyroid hormone
Glucagon	Luteinizing hormone
Growth hormone	Antidiuretic hormone
Glucocorticoids	Testosterone
Estrogens	Aldosterone
Progesterone	Oxytocin
Parathyroid hormone	Adrenocorticotropic hormone
Some gut hormones	Thyroid-stimulating hormone
	Thyroid-releasing hormone

From Johnston DG, Alberti KGMM: The liver and the endocrine system. In Wright R, Millward-Sadler GH, Alberti KGMM et al, editors: *Liver and biliary disease,* ed 2, Philadelphia, 1985, WB Saunders.

Host-Defense Mechanisms of the Gut: Immunology and Microbiology

The gut has become one of the important focuses in our evolving understanding of the syndrome of multiple organ dysfunction (MODS) (see also Chapter 97).[3,67] Integrity of the intestinal epithelium is vital to maintaining the separation between the environment outside the body and the "intèrieur" milieu. The epithelium of the small bowel possesses immunological and nonimmunological defense mechanisms serving to separate the host from the numerous microbes, antigens, and toxins present in the external environment. The normal microflora consists of more than 400 bacterial species. The average bacterial count is lowest in the stomach (10^3/g) and ileum (10^4/ml) because of the effects of gastric acid, and in the ileum rapid transit, biliary, and pancreatic secretions. The colon is the most densely colonized region of the GI tract with microbial counts ranging from 10^{11} to 10^{12}/g. The microflora of the mouth and upper alimentary tract consists predominantly of gram-positive organisms, whereas in the distal ileum and colon, gram-negative and anaerobic organisms predominate with bifidobacteria and bacteroides genera accounting for 25% and 30% of the total anaerobic counts.[68] Normal colonization of the alimentary tract proceeds rapidly after birth by means of oral inoculation.[69] Both oral and parenteral antibiotics profoundly reduce the number of anaerobic and coliform bacteria in the alimentary tract with recolonization taking 4 to 6 days after cessation of antibiotics.[70] In addition, pancreatic and biliary secretions have been shown to play a role in inhibiting bacterial proliferation and colonization of the small intestine in infants; however, this process does not appear to be as significant in older children and adults. Finally, protease and lipase activity lead to the destruction of antigens and viable bacteria providing control of the number and species of flora in the gut.

Nonimmunological Mechanisms

The nonimmunological defense mechanisms consist of gastric acid, proteolytic enzymes, gut motility, mucus, and glycocalyx barriers over the epithelium and the microvillus membrane.[71] In the healthy neonate, the infant's saliva and ingested breast milk provide both immunological and nonimmunological factors that protect the gut from infectious pathogens and intact dietary antigens. Gastric acid secretion provides a mechanism for reducing the bacterial load reaching the small intestine. Considerable attention has been directed toward the routine clinical practice of H_2-blocker therapy for stress-ulcer prophylaxis in critically ill patients, following reports in adults associating alkaline gastric pH with higher rates of gastric and upper airway colonization by gram-negative organisms and nosocomial pneumonia. A meta-analysis suggested that patients receiving an H_2 antagonist were at increased risk for nosocomial pneumonia compared with those receiving sucralfate,[72] although a large, randomized controlled trial subsequently rebuffed this assertion. Although the issue continues to be debated, it is necessary to be aware of potential iatrogenic problems resulting from changes in flora when treating low gastric pH. The need to prevent GI bleeding in critically ill patients will necessitate the ongoing use of H_2 antagonists or PPIs to control gastric pH.

Intestinal motility is a critical factor for clearing antigens and bacteria from the gut lumen and thus reducing bacterial overgrowth with its resultant malabsorption of nutrients. Decreased motility leading to bacterial overgrowth may be seen in premature infants and may be associated with many disorders seen in older children, including the use of narcotics and some neuromuscular blockers (e.g., pancuronium bromide). A physical barrier composed of mucin and the glycocalyx is formed over the intestinal epithelium by secretions from the goblet cells. It forms a gel that can change from a semisolid to a semifluid state under varying intraluminal conditions and thus provides either a relatively impervious barrier protecting the epithelium from osmolar forces or a fluid medium helping to propel bacteria and antigens aborally.[2]

Mucosal blood flow appears to be an important mechanism for maintaining mucosal integrity in both the stomach and the small intestine. Inadequate microcirculation in the gastric mucosa, which provides cytoprotection, appears to be a major factor contributing to stress ulceration in critically ill patients. As submucosal and mucosal blood flow diminishes, the buffering ability for acid that back diffuses into the tissues is reduced and leads to tissue necrosis. Hypoxia, hypotension, and states of high circulating catecholamines are commonly associated with altered mucosal circulation and stress ulceration. Finally, the small intestine, especially the terminal ileum, of neonates and infants is more sensitive to hypoxia and ischemia than that of adults; thus neonates and infants are predisposed to mucosal injury and necrotizing enterocolitis.

Bacterial Translocation

Considerable interest has been focused on the passage of live bacteria, their products, or both across the intestinal barrier to the mesenteric lymph nodes, general circulation, liver, spleen, or other organs. Known as translocation, this process is increasingly being recognized as potential source of pathogens producing bacteremia and sepsis in a variety of premorbid conditions.[73,74] Translocation may occur directly through the M cells that cover the Peyer's patches, or it may occur by ingestion of viable pathogenic material by the mobile phagocytic system with transport into the host bypassing the previously outlined barrier mechanisms. The three main mechanisms predisposing a host to bacterial translocation are (1) disruption of the ecological equilibrium allowing intestinal bacterial overgrowth, (2) deficiencies in the host immune defenses, and (3) damage to the intestinal mucosa and vasculature that causes increased permeability.[73] Certain aerobic enteric bacteria including *E. coli, Proteus mirabilis and Klebsiella pneumoniae* appear to be more commonly associated with translocation from the GI tract, presumably because oxygen in the blood may exert an inhibitory effect on anaerobic organisms. Intraabdominal inflammatory foci are susceptible to invasion by translocating bacteria, and this invasion suggests one mechanism for abdominal abscess formation. Attempts to prophylactically decontaminate the gut in critically ill but otherwise immunocompetent adult patients have not shown an improved outcome for the MODS.

Immunological Mechanisms

Of central importance to the immune function of the gut are the gut-associated lymphoid tissues (GALTs) consisting of Peyer's patches and single lymphoid nodules of the intestinal mucosa and appendix.[75] Migration of lymphocytes from one compartment to another provides communication of immunological information. In addition, migration of lymphocytes to extraintestinal tissues including the mammary gland, female genital tract, and bronchus-associated lymphoid tissue may mediate immune responses in those tissues. Peyer's patches consist of mononuclear cells, plasma cells, macrophages, and other antigen-presenting cells. B cells are the predominant lymphocyte. Peyer's patches are covered by a specialized epithelium containing M cells, which transport luminal antigen into the patches.

Penetration of the mucosal barrier by antigenic material occurs because the epithelial barrier is not totally impermeable to macromolecules. It may be accelerated by inflammation or mucosal damage. Increased permeability and tissue damage occur with such diverse disease entities as infectious enterocolitis, idiopathic inflammatory bowel disease, intestinal graft rejection enteropathies such as celiac disease, sprue, food allergies, and gut ischemia or hypoxia. As barrier mechanisms fail in the injured gut, bacterial penetration is more likely to occur, producing portal and systemic bacteremia. Cell-mediated cytotoxic reactions and antibody-dependent cell-mediated cytotoxicity represent two responses of the GALT to encounters with antigens. These processes involve the cooperative interaction of other lymphoid cells such as killer, lymphokine-activated killer, and natural killer cells. Infected or necrotic cells and noncellular antigenic material are targeted for ultimate lysis by phagocytic cells in the circulation and reticuloendothelial system.

Kupffer cells, which account for the largest pool of mononuclear phagocytes with direct access to the blood, play a major role in clearing portal bacteria. In addition, Kupffer cells are key participants in response to tissue injury or organ invasion through the elaboration of cytokine mediators, such as TNF and IL-1 and the release of nitric oxide, leading to many of the systemic responses seen in sepsis. Through their intimate proximity to the hepatocyte, Kupffer cells interact directly with hepatocytes by means of cell–cell and paracrine interactions. In response to TNF and IL-1, well-documented alterations in hepatic function occur including the inhibition of albumin synthesis, gluconeogenesis, and P-450-mediated detoxification. Acute-phase reactant synthesis is also induced by TNF and IL-1.[76]

Gastrointestinal and Hepatobiliary Testing in the Intensive Care Unit

Diagnostic testing in the ICU permits the identification of organ system injury and dysfunction. In addition, it assists in monitoring the course of a disease and the response to therapies.

Laboratory testing is helpful in detecting and monitoring hepatocellular injury and dysfunction, which represents the common final pathway resulting from a variety of both immunological and nonimmunological mechanisms. In the ICU setting, impaired synthetic function is the hallmark of liver failure, which is of more immediate concern than hepatocellular injury alone. Decreased synthesis of the liver-dependent clotting factors I (fibrinogen), II (prothrombin), V, VII, IX and X results in a prolonged prothrombin time (PT), which, in the absence of vitamin K deficiency or related inhibitors, represents liver failure.[63] Furthermore, because factor VII has the shortest half-life (2 to 6 hours) compared with the other factors, it becomes the rate-limiting step for conversion of prothrombin to thrombin (PT). For this reason, certain ICU settings such as management of intractable coagulopathy in fulminant liver failure, specific replacement therapy with recombinant factor VII may be required.[77] Other less specific measures of liver dysfunction include decreased serum albumin, as well as elevation or depression of serum cholesterol and triglycerides in association with their respective carrier lipoproteins. Liver failure may also be associated with life-threatening hypoglycemia from a variety of mechanisms including decreased hepatic synthesis and release of glucose, hyperinsulinemia (from impaired hepatic degradation), and increased glucose utilization that results from anaerobic metabolism.[78] A frequent finding in advanced liver failure is elevated serum ammonia, which reflects impaired deamination, clearance of ammonia, or both. Ammonia elevation results primarily from urea cycle defects, portal-systemic shunting, and events such as large GI bleeds that are substrate for increased ammonia production by enteric bacteria, which in the setting of impaired liver function leads to hyperammonemia.[78]

The biochemical tests commonly used to detect cholestasis (impaired bile flow) and hepatocellular injury are serum bilirubin and aminotransferase activities (ALT [alanine aminotransferase] and AST [aspartate aminiotransferase]). Liver disease can be broadly categorized into hepatocellular, cholestatic, and infiltrative processes. Preferential elevations in serum conjugated bilirubin, bile acids, alkaline phosphatase (ALK), γ-glutamyltransferase (GGT), or 5'-nucleotidase (5-NT) represents cholestasis, reduced bile excretion, transport, or obstruction in the canalicular or large biliary ducts. Conjugated bilirubinemia is assessed by the direct (van den Bergh) reaction, whereas the unconjugated (indirect) fraction represents the difference between the total bilirubin and the direct fraction. Elevated levels of predominantly indirect hyperbilirubinemia result from (1) increased bilirubin load to the liver (e.g., hemolysis), (2) diminished uptake and intracellular transport, and (3) reduced conjugation (e.g., immaturity, fulminant necrosis). In children, elevations in ALK may be seen with rickets or during periods of rapid skeletal growth, necessitating the determination of isoenzymes to distinguish between bone and biliary sources. Alanine transaminase (ALT or SGPT [serum glutamate pyruvate transaminase]) and aspartate transaminase (AST or SGOT [serum glutamate oxaloacetate transaminase]) are hepatic cytosolic enzymes that catalyze the reversible transfer of the α-amino group of the amino acids alanine and aspartic acids to the α-keto group of α-ketoglutaric acid producing pyruvic and oxaloacetic acids, respectively, plus glutamate. Elevations in serum activities of ALT and AST suggest hepatocellular injury (Table 78–4). AST is also present in myocardial tissue, skeletal muscle, the kidney, the pancreas, and erythrocytes; therefore increased serum activity is not specific for hepatocellular injury. Fortunately for the hepatologist, ALT is present in only relatively low concentrations in tissues other than liver, thus providing greater specificity for hepatocellular injury than AST. Elevated serum lactate dehydrogenase activity (LDH) lacks specificity and may be seen in association with hepatocellular injury, hemolysis, and myopathy; however, when in association with elevated serum creatinine phosphokinase (CPK), aldolase indicates myopathy or a rhabdomyolysis injury. In general biochemical tests have limited discriminative value for differentiating between primarily hepatocellular and cholestatic or infiltrative liver injury; nonetheless the differential diagnosis may be narrowed down (see Table 78–4).

Imaging of the hepatobiliary system has become easier, safer, and more reliable in the past decade. Ultrasonography is particularly useful in the ICU and allows rapid, safe, bedside evaluation of (1) hepatic vascular structures and patterns of blood flow; (2) structural abnormalities such as tumors, abscess, hematoma, or dilated intrahepatic bile ducts; (3) the gallbladder, extrahepatic, pancreatic, and common biliary system; (4) the pancreas; (5) the genitourinary system; and (6) the abdomen and retroperitoneum.

TABLE 78–4

Pattern of Biochemical Tests According to the Category of Liver Disease

Biochemical Test	Hepatocellular Necrosis	Cholestasis	Infiltrative Process
ALT, AST	++ to +++	0 to +	0 to +
ALK, GGT	0 to +	++ to +++	+
Total/conjugated bilirubin	0 to +++	0 to +++	0 to +
PT	Prolonged	Prolonged; responsive to vitamin K	0
Albumin	Decreased in chronic disorders	0	0
Cholesterol	0	0 to +++	0
Bile acids	+ to +++	+ to +++	0

ALK, Alkaline phosphatase; *ALT,* alanine aminotransferase; *AST,* aspartate aminotransferase; *GGT,* γ-glutamyltransferase; *PT,* prothrombin time; *0,* normal; + to +++, degrees of elevation.

In addition, ultrasound can provide guidance for therapeutic interventions such as drainage of abscesses. Computed tomographic (CT) scan with and without contrast and magnetic resonance imaging (MRI) provide additional methods for evaluation of the abdominal and retroperitoneal organs for masses, abscess, fluid collections, and so on; however, both modalities usually require a prolonged period away from the ICU, which may lead to instability in a tenuous, critically ill patient. Many of the radioisotope studies can be performed in the ICU and provide a wide range of diagnostic possibilities in critically ill patients. Technetium-99m (^{99m}Tc) IDA compounds are handled by the hepatobiliary system much like bilirubin and provide a qualitative and semiquantitative image of function and structure. These compounds may be used diagnostically to evaluate infants with persistent jaundice and may also be used in follow-up after Kasai procedure or liver transplantation.

Of the available biochemical markers of pancreatic disease, serum amylase and lipase determinations are the most widely available. Serum lipase is elevated in about 87% of patients with acute pancreatitis and shows fewer false-positive results than amylase testing. Transient hypocalcemia (<8.0 mg/dl) occurs in about 30% of patients with pancreatitis. Mild to moderate hyperglycemia as a result of islet cell damage is seen in up to 25% of patients; the administration of exogenous insulin is often necessary.

Evaluation of the alimentary tract consists of examining gastric aspirates and stool samples for gross bleeding or occult blood with the guaiac test (Hemoccult). A positive result mandates further evaluation and surveillance to determine the source and severity of GI tract blood loss. ^{99m}Tc sulfur colloid or red blood cells labeled with ^{99m}Tc may provide information regarding the site of active mucosal bleeding and are less invasive than arteriography. Esophageal pH probe recording to detect occult gastroesophageal reflux is indicated in the evaluation of unexplained apnea, recurrent pulmonary infections or wheezing, and unusual neck or body posturing. Multiple-site monitoring of pH in the esophagus, pharynx, and stomach is indicated when there is recurrent, unexplained

TABLE 78–5

Diagnosis of Selected Hepatobiliary Disorders

Form of Liver Injury	Supportive History/ Laboratory Data
PREDOMINANTLY HEPATOCELLULAR	
Viral hepatitis	Viral serology: hepatitis A, B, C, and E and EBV
Drug-induced hepatitis	History of toxic/excess ingestion, elevated eosinophil count
Ischemia	Shock, after cardiac operation
Autoimmune hepatitis	Increased globulin ratio, antinuclear antibody, antismooth muscle antibody, antiliver kidney microsomal antibody
Wilson's disease	Serum ceruloplasmin
α-Antitrypsin deficiency	Pi type
CHOLESTATIC	
Bacterial sepsis	Proteus, *Escherichia coli*, UTI
Galactosemia	Urine succinyl choline
Biliary atresia	Intraoperative cholangiogram
Structural anomalies/disease: choledochal cysts, biliary stricture, cholelithiasis, congential hepatic fibrosis, Caroli's disease, Sclerosing cholangitis	Ultrasonography, cholangiogram
Alagille's syndrome, cystic fibrosis	
GVHD, veno-occlusive disease	History of bone marrow transplant, high-dose busulfan
Ischemia	ECMO
INFILTRATIVE	
Hepatocellular carcinoma	α-Fetoprotein
PREDOMINANTLY COAGULOPATHY	
Neonatal hematochromatosis	Serum iron and ferritin

EBV, Epstein-Barr virus; *ECMO,* extracorporeal membrane oxygenation; *GVDH,* graft-versus-host disease; *UTI,* urinary tract infection.

cough or laryngeal symptoms; there is suspected bile reflux; and the efficacy of gastric acid suppression therapy needs to be monitored. The frequency and duration of episodes, during which the probe pH is less than 4 or greater than 8, correspond with acid and bile exposure, respectively, and the final interpretation is based on correlation with the clinical symptoms in question.

Imaging studies are of primary importance in acutely ill patients in a number of circumstances. Plain radiographs can be reliably used to locate radiopaque objects and to diagnose intestinal ileus, mechanical obstruction, and perforated viscus, whereas contrast studies are required to diagnose organ and soft tissue inflammation including appendicitis, pancreatitis and its complications, mesenteric and retroperitoneal masses, abscesses/fluid collections, intus susceptions, and anatomical anomalies.

GI bleeding from sites inaccessible to video endoscopy (e.g., distal to the ligament of Treitz and proximal to the terminal ileum, Meckel's diverticulum, vascular malformations, and altered anatomy after a GI operation) is best assessed with radionuclide scans, angiography, or capsule endoscopy.[79] Because of the need to perform the more sophisticated imaging studies away from the controlled environment of the ICU, the studies must be tailored to the patient's diagnostic needs according to the priorities of the initial stabilization of life-threatening illness and subsequent treatment of the underlying pathological condition.

Video or fiberoptic endoscopy in the hands of operators skilled in managing small children has found a place in ICU management to diagnose the source of upper GI tract bleeding, to control and sclerose bleeding varices, to place percutaneous gastrostomy tubes for feeding, and to place stents for the maintenance of the patency of the distal biliary and pancreatic tract.

Refer to Table 78–5 for suggested diagnostic tests for selected hepatobiliary disorders.

REFERENCES

1. Nagler-Anderson C, Terhoust C, Ghan AK et al: Mucosal antigen presentation and the control of tolerance and immunity, *Trends Immunol* 22:1200122, 2001.
2. Thomson A, Keelan M, Thiesen A et al: Small bowel review: normal physiology part 2, *Dig Dis Sci* 2001 46: 2588-2607, 2001.
3. Deitch E: Role of the gut lymphatic system in multiple organ failure, *Curr Opin Crit Care* 2001 7:92-98, 2001.
4. Ganong W: The general and cellular basis of medical physiology. *Review of medical physiology,* New York, 2003, McGraw-Hill.
5. Shronts E, Beilman G, Cerra F: The inflammatory response, immune dysfunction, and immunonutrition. In Irwin R, Cerra F, Rippe J, editors: *Irwin and Rippe's intensive care medicine*, Philadelphia, 1999, Lippincott-Raven.
6. Das U: Critical advances in septicemia and septic shock, *Crit Care* 4:290-296, 2000.
7. Szabo G, Romics L, G. Frendl F: Liver in sepsis and systemic inflammatory response syndrome, *Clin Liver Dis* 6:1045-1066, 2002.
8. Gadek J, DeMichele SJ, Karlstad MD et al: Effect of enteral feeding with eicosapentaenoic acid, gamma-linolenic acid, and antioxidants in patients with acute respiratory distress syndrome. Enteral Nutrition in ARDS Study Group, *Crit Care Med* 27: 1409-1420, 1999.
9. Pacht E, DeMichele SJ, Nelson JL et al: Enteral nutrition with eicosapentaenoic acid, gamma-linolenic acid, and antioxidants reduces alveolar inflammatory mediators and protein influx in patients with acute respiratory distress syndrome, *Crit Care Med* 31:491-500, 2003.
10. *Energy and protein requirements*, ed. J.F.W.U.E. Consultation. 1985, Geneva: WHO.
11. Silk D, Gimble G, Rees R: Protein digestion and amino acid and peptide absorption, *Proc Nutr Soc* 44: 63, 1985.
12. Leibach F, Ganapathy V: Peptide transporters in the intestine and the kidney, *Annu Rev Nutr* 16: 99, 1996.
13. Kekuda R., Torres-Zamorano V, Fei Y: Molecular and functional characterization of intestinal Na(+)-dependent neutral amino acid transporter, *Am J Physiol* 272:G1463, 1997.
14. Elwyn D: The role of the liver in regulation of amino acid and protein metabolism. In Munro H, editor: *Mammalian protein metabolism,* New York, 1970, Academic Press.
15. Jalonen T: Increased beta-lactoglobulin absoprtion during rotavirus enteritis in infants: relationship to intestinal permeability, *Pediatr Res* 30:290-298, 1991.
16. Holsapple M, West L, Landreth K: Species comparison of anatomical and functional immune system development, *Birth Defects Res B Dev Reprod Toxicol* 68:321-334, 2003.
17. Udall J, Walker W: The physiologic and pathologic basis for the transport of macromolecules across the intestinal tract, *J Ped Gastroenterol Nutr* 1: 295-302, 1982.
18. From the Centers for Disease Control and Prevention. Daily dietary fat and total food-energy intakes–NHANES III, Phase 1, 1988-91, *JAMA* 271:1309 1994.
19. Hamosh M: The milky way: from mammary gland to milk to newborn-Macy-Gyorgy Award presentation, *Adv Exp Med Biol* 503:17-25, 2002.
20. Shiau Y: Mechanism of intestinal fatty acid uptake in the rat: the role of an acidic microclimate, *J Physiol* 421:463-474, 1990.
21. Rodriguez M, Kalogenis TJ, Wang XL et al: Rapid synthesis and secretion of intestinal apolipoprotein A-IV after gastric fat loading in rats, *Am J Physiol* 272(4 Pt 2):R1170-R1177, 1997.
22. Madara J, Trier J: The functional morphology of the mucosa of the small intestine. In Johnson L, editor: *Physiology of the gastrointestinal tract*, New York, 1994, Raven Press.
23. Lencer W, Desjeux J: Transport of water and ions. In Walker W, Durie P, Hamilton JR et al, editors: *Pediatric gastrointestinal disease*, St Louis, 1996, Mosby.
24. Sellin J: Intestinal electrolyte absorption and secretion. In Feldman M, Friedman L, Slesinger M, editors: *Slesinger and Fordtran's gastrointestinal and liver disease*, Philadelphia, 2002, Saunders/Elsevier.
25. Murphy M, A.-G. A: Regulatory peptides of the gastrointestinal tract in early life. In Walker W, Durie P, Hamilton J et al, editors: *Pediatric gastrointestinal disease*, St Louis, 1996, Mosby.
26. Wright E, Loo D, Coupling between Na+, sugar, and water transport across the intestine, *Ann N Y Acad Sci* 915:54-66, 2000.
27. Holtug K, Hansen M, Skadhauge E: Experimental studies of intestinal ion and water transport, *Scand J Gastroenterol* 216: 95-110, 1996.
28. Field M: Intestinal ion transport and the pathophysiology of diarrhea, *J Clin Invest* 111:931-943, 2003.
28a. Thorp JW, Boeckx RL, Robbins S, et al: A prospective study of infant zinc nutrition during intensive care. *Am J Clin Nutr* 34(6):1056-1060, 1981.
28b. Story DA, Ronco C, Bellomo R: Trace element and vitamin concentration and losses in critically ill patients being treated with continous venovenous hemofiltration. *Crit Care Med* 27(1): 220-223, 1999.
28c. Higgins TL, Murray M, Kett DH, et al: Trace element homeostasis during continous sedation with propofol containing EDTA versus other sedatives in critically ill patients. *Intensive Care Med* 26 Suppl 4:S413-421, 2000.
29. Wolfe M., Soll A: The physiology of gastric acid secretion, *N Engl J Med* 319:1707-1715, 1988.
30. Zeng N, Athmann C, Kang T et al: PACAP type I receptor activation regulates ECL cells and gastric acid secretion, *J Clin Invest* 104:1383-1391, 1999.
31. DelVale J, Lucey M, Yamada TL: Gastric secretion. In Yamada T, Alpers DH, Owyang C et al, editors: *Textbook of gastroenterology*, Philadelphia, 1995, JB Lippincott.
32. Wolfe M, Sachs G: Acid suppression: optimizing therapy for gastroduodenal ulcer healing, gastroesophageal reflux disease, and stress-related erosive syndrome, *Gastroenterology* 118:S9-S31, 2000.
33. Pisegna J: Pharmacology of acid suppression in the hospital setting: focus on proton pump inhibition, *Crit Care Med* 30:S356-S361, 2002.

34. Kemp D, Thomas M, Habener J: Developmental aspects of the endocrine pancreas, *Rev Endocr Metab Disord* 4:5-17, 2003.
35. Yeo C, Cameron J: Exocrine pancreas. In Townsend CM, Beauchamp RD, Evers BM et al, editors: *Sabiston textbook of surgery: the biological basis of modern surgical practice*, Philadelphia, 2001, WB Saunders.
36. Henderson J: Pancreatitis. In Henderson J, editor: *Gastrointestinal pathophysiology*, Philadelphia, 1996, Lippincott-Raven.
37. Uhl W, Anghelacopoulos SE, Friess H et al: The role of octreotide and somatostatin in acute and chronic pancreatitis, *Digestion* 60: S23-S31, 1999.
38. Bentrem D, Joehl R: Pancreas: healing response in critical illness, *Crit Care Med* 31:S582-S589, 2003.
39. Boyle J: Hepatomegaly. In Kliegman R, Nieder ML, Super DM, editors: *Practical strategies in pediatric diagnosis and therapy*, Philadelphia, 1996, WB Saunders.
40. Naveh Y, Berant M: Assessment of liver size in normal infants and children, *J Ped Gastroenterol Nutr* 3:346-348, 1984.
41. Shurin S: Splenomegaly. In Kliegman R, editor: *Practical strategies in pediatric diagnosis and therapy*, Philadelphia, 1996, WB Saunders.
42. Hautekeete M, Geerts A: The hepatic stellate (Ito) cell: its role in human liver disease, *Virchows Arch* 430:195-207, 1997.
43. Davis B, Kresina T: Hepatic fibrogenesis, *Clin Lab Med* 16: 361-375, 1996.
44. Feranchak A, Sokol R: Cholangiocyte biology and cystic firbosis liver disease, *Semin Liver Dis* 21:471-488, 2001.
45. Matuschak G: Liver-lung interactions in critical illness, *New Horiz* 2:488-459, 1994.
46. Hauser C: Regional macrophage activation after injury and the compartmentalization of inflammation in trauma, *New Horiz* 4:235-251, 1996.
47. Xu D, Lu Q, Adams CA et al: Trauma-hemorrhagic shock-induced up-regulation of endothelial cell adhesion molecules is blunted by mesenteric lymph duct ligation, *Crit Care Med* 32:760-765, 2004.
48. Salzman A: Nitric oxide in the gut, *New Horiz* 33:33-44, 1995.
49. Rolla G: Hepatopulmonary syndrome: role of nitric oxide and clinical aspects, *Dig Liver Dis* 36:303-308, 2004.
50. Grange J, Amiot X: Nitric oxide and renal function in cirrhotic patients with ascites: from physiopathology to practice, *Eur J Gastroenterol Hepatol* 16:567-570, 2004.
51. Tritto I, Ambrosio G: The multi-faceted *Cardiovasc Res* behavior of nitric oxide in vascular "inflammation": catchy terminology or true phenomenon? 63:1-4, 2004.
52. Yegenaga I, Hoste E, Van Biesen W et al: Clinical characteristics of patients developing ARF due to sepsis/systemic inflammatory response syndrome: results of a prospective study, *Am J Kidney Dis* 43:817-824, 2004.
53. Steinhorn D, Cerra F: Comparative effects of lipopolysaccharide on newborn versus adult rat hepatocyte and nonparenchymal cell cocultures, *Crit Care Med* 25:121-127, 1997.
54. The liver as an organ. In Guyton A, Hall J, editors: *Textbook of medical physiology*, Philadelphia, 2000, Saunders.
55. Schrier R, Arroyo V, Bernardi M et al: Peripheral arterial vasodilation hypothesis: a proposal for the initiation of renal sodium and water retention in cirrhosis, *Hepatology* 8:1151-1157, 1988.
56. Cardenas A, Arroyo V: Mechanisms of water and sodium retention in cirrhosis and the pathogenesis of ascites, *Best Pract Res Clin Endocrinol Metab* 17:607-622, 2003.
57. Sivayokan T, Dillon J: Cirrhotic ascites: a review of management, *Hosp Med* 65:22-26, 2004.
58. Tisdale M: Biomedicine. Protein loss in cancer cachexia, *Science* 29:2293-2294, 2000.
59. Bernstein L, Ingenbleek Y: Transthyretin: its response to malnutrition and stress injury. clinical usefulness and economic implications, *Clin Chem Lab Med* 40:1344-348, 2002.
60. Stockley R: Proteases and antiproteases, *Novartis Found Symp* 234:189-199, 2001.
61. Needham M, Stockley R: Alpha 1-antitrypsin deficiency. 3: clinical manifestations and natural history, *Thorax* 59:441-445, 2004.
62. van der Sluys Veer A, Biemond I, Verspaget HW et al: Faecal parameters in the assessment of activity in inflammatory bowel disease, *Scand J Gastroenterol Suppl* 230:106-110, 1999.
63. Hedner U, Erhardtsen E: Hemostatic disorders in liver disease. In Schiff E, Sorrell M, Maddrey W, editors: *Schiff's diseases of the liver*, Philadelphia, 2003, Lippincott Williams & Wilkins.
64. Arns P, Wedlund P, Branch R: Adjustment of medications in liver failure. In Chernow B, editor: *The pharmacologic approach to the critically ill patient*, Baltimore, 1988, Williams & Wilkins.
65. van den Berghe G, Wouters P, Weekers F et al: Intensive insulin therapy in the critically ill patients. *N Engl J Med* 345:1359-1367, 2001.
66. Jeschke MG, Klein D, Bolder U, et al: Insulin attenuates the systemic inflammatory response in endotoxemic rats, *Endocrinology* 145:4084-93, 2004; Epub 2004 Jun 10.
67. Villar J, Maca-Meyer N, Perez-Mendez L et al: Bench-to-bedside review: understanding genetic predisposition to sepsis, *Crit Care* 8:180-189, 2004.
68. Hao W, Lee Y: Microflora of the gastrointestinal tract: a review, *Methods Mol Biol* 268:491-502, 2004.
69. Fanaro S, Chierici R, Guerrini P et al: Intestinal microflora in early infancy: composition and development, *Acta Paediatr Suppl* 91: 48-55, 2003.
70. Fry D, Schermer C: The consequences of suppression of anaerobic bacteria, *Surg Infect* 1:49-56, 2000.
71. Israel E, Walker W: Host defense development in gut and related disorders, *Pediatr Clin N Am* 35:-15, 1988.
72. Messori A, Trippoli S, Vaiani M et al: Bleeding and pneumonia in intensive care patients given ranitidine and sucralfate for prevention of stress ulcer: meta-analysis of randomised controlled trials, *BMJ* 321:1103-1106, 2000.
73. Lichtman S: Bacterial translocation in humans, *J Pediatr Gastroenterol Nutr* 33:1-10, 2001.
74. Steinberg S: Bacterial translocation: what it is and what it is not, *Am J Surg* 186:301-305, 2003.
75. Spahn T, Kucharzik T: Modulating the intestinal immune system: the role of lymphotoxin and GALT organs, *Gut* 53:456-465, 2004.
76. Pannen B, Robotham J: The acute phase response, *New Horiz* 3:183-197, 1995.
77. Brown JB, Emerick KM, Brown DL et al: Recombinant factor VIIa improves coagulopathy caused by liver failure, *J Pediatr Gastroenterol Nutr* 37:268-272, 2003.
78. Whitington P: Fulminant liver failure in children. In Suchy F, editor: *Liver disease in children*, St Louis, 1994, Mosby.
79. Jones BH, Fleischer DE, Sharma VK, et al: Yield of repeat wireless video capsule endoscopy in patients with obscure gastrointestional bleeding. *Am J Gastroenterol* 100(5):1058-1064, 2005.

CHAPTER

79

Disorders and Diseases of the Gastrointestinal Tract and Liver

Samuel A. Kocoshis

PEARLS

- So much reliance is placed on electronic monitoring of patients that physicians are often tempted to perform only a cursory examination or to go days without laying hands on the patient. Regrettably, adopting such an approach deprives the clinician of an adequate perspective on the patient's day-to-day condition and deprives the patient of optimal care.
- When compared with a scintiscan of the lungs after administration of a radiolabeled meal or with the discovery of lipid-laden macrophages after bronchoalveolar lavage, the use of colorants is notoriously inaccurate.
- Several antireflux barriers exist in the region of the lower esophageal sphincter. Beyond intrinsic myogenic tone, barriers such as the cardioesophageal angle, the abdominal esophagus (which acts as flutter valve), the mucosal rosette of the sphincter (which acts as a choke valve), and the diaphragmatic crura themselves act to prevent reflux of gastric contents.
- The association between *Helicobacter pylori* infection and both chronic gastritis and duodenal ulcer is well established, but the role of *H. pylori* in the pathogenesis of gastric ulceration remains somewhat speculative.
- Intravenous administration of somatostatin or its synthetic analogue, the active octreotide moiety, has been effective in stemming variceal hemorrhage and may work for other causes of bleeding. In addition to their hemodynamic effects, they inhibit gastric acid production.
- Crohn's disease and ulcerative colitis are chronic, relapsing disorders without known causes. The transmural inflammation of Crohn's disease may affect any portion of the alimentary tract in a patchy distribution, whereas the inflammation of ulcerative colitis is confined to the mucosa of the colon.
- The diagnosis of necrotizing enterocolitis may be confirmed by an abdominal plain film showing pneumatosis intestinalis, hepatic portal air, or both. A random breath histamine/carbon dioxide ratio greater than 8 ppm/mmHg strongly suggests the diagnosis. Because the pathogenesis is unknown, treatment must be symptomatic. In most centers, feedings are discontinued for 48 hours to 2 weeks depending on the severity of symptoms. Fluid resuscitation and broad-spectrum parenteral antibiotics are the basis of medical therapy. Surgical resection is reserved for severe cases when medical management fails and gangrenous bowel develops.

Gastrointestinal Evaluation of the Critically Ill Child

Dramatic advances in pediatric critical care have resulted in improved outcomes for children admitted to pediatric intensive care units (ICUs). Indeed, the improved technology available today has resulted in improved management strategies for a variety of conditions. So much reliance is placed on electronic monitoring of patients that physicians are often tempted to perform only a cursory examination or to go days without laying hands on the patient. Regrettably, adopting such an approach deprives the clinician of an adequate perspective on the patient's day-to-day condition and deprives the patient of optimal care. Daily physical examination is of paramount importance in the assessment of children with either life-threatening gastrointestinal disease or gastrointestinal manifestations of multisystem disease. Thus not only is the current approach to gastroenterological diagnosis and therapy reviewed in this chapter, but so too are the basic principles of gastroenterological physical examination.

Abdominal Examination

Astute clinicians recognize that the abdomen extends from "the neck to the knees." A thorough examination of the head, neck, and chest is essential when patients with abdominal symptoms are evaluated. For example, pneumonia may be discovered by chest auscultation in the child who experiences abdominal pain. All too often, a child whose abdominal symptoms are due to pneumonia undergoes exploratory laparotomy for a purportedly "surgical" abdomen.

The abdominal examination, which can be difficult to perform on young children without life-threatening illness, is made more difficult in the ICU setting. Pain and fear limit cooperation. Patients who are obtunded by narcotics, sedatives, or an underlying central nervous system (CNS) disorder display inconsistent responses to abdominal palpation. Neuromuscular blockade abolishes abdominal guarding. Children with multisystem trauma may not localize pain. These impediments notwithstanding, the observant clinician can glean a great deal of information from a carefully performed examination. Simple inspection of the child's abdomen can reveal generalized distention; abnormally prominent abdominal wall veins (which signify portal hypertension); or anterior and lateral abdominal wall ecchymoses, such as Cullen's sign or Grey Turner's sign (which herald acute pancreatitis). In addition, because of the child's relatively undeveloped abdominal musculature, visceromegaly or abdominal masses may be apparent on inspection.

Auscultation will ascertain the frequency and quality of peristaltic sounds. They normally occur every 10 to 30 seconds and are low pitched. High-pitched, frequent bowel sounds suggest enteritis or obstruction. In obstruction, bowel sounds characteristically reverberate and seem to originate "deep from a well." Bowel sounds are absent in paralytic ileus or peritonitis. Ancillary findings include venous hums, which suggest portal obstruction, or bruits, which denote arteriovenous malformations.

In pediatric patients, palpation should generally precede percussion because it is less threatening. The child should be in the supine position, and when possible the hips and knees should be comfortably flexed to enhance abdominal wall relaxation. The abdomen should be palpated through all phases of respiration in all four quadrants. The examiner should lightly palpate to judge guarding and tenderness and should use gentle ballottement. Deeper palpation better localizes organomegaly or masses.

Percussion permits estimation of visceral size and helps to diagnose obstruction, peritonitis, or ascites. Excessive tympany implies that bowel loops are distended with air, whereas dullness suggests that excessive fluid or a solid mass is present. Shifting dullness is relatively easy to detect in cooperative children with percussion of the abdomen with the child in the supine, left lateral, and right lateral positions. When the child with ascites is in the supine position, dullness is found primarily over the flanks. The dullness moves to a new level nearer the midline when the child is moved to each lateral position. It is essential to perform a digital examination of the rectum in children with gastrointestinal dysfunction. Inspection of the perineum may reveal perianal or perirectal abscesses, which may be the first sign of acute leukemia, chronic granulomatous disease of childhood, or Crohn's disease. Similarly, deep fissures or sentinel piles suggest ulcerative colitis or Crohn's disease, and hemorrhoids can be found in portal hypertension. The digital examination should be performed in the alert, older child only after its purpose is explained. Any material that returns on the examining finger should be evaluated for occult blood. Absence of stool in the vault can corroborate Hirschsprung's disease in an infant with abdominal distention and a history of obstipation. Rectal masses related to pelvic abscesses or tumors may be digitally palpated. Rectal tenderness signifies mural or extramural inflammation or infection.

Gastrointestinal Endoscopy

The development of flexible fiberoptic endoscopes appropriately sized for use in infants and children has greatly expanded the value of endoscopy in diagnosing and treating a variety of gastroenterological disorders in critically ill pediatric patients. For example, pediatric endoscopes with an outside diameter of 6.5 mm can now be used for diagnostic purposes in newborn infants. Electrocautery or injection therapy of gastrointestinal bleeding sites can also be performed with electrocautery probes or needles that now fit within the biopsy channels of a standard 9.4-mm pediatric endoscopy.

Upper gastrointestinal endoscopy (esophagogastroduodenoscopy [EGD]) is performed most often with the child under deep sedation or general anesthesia, although some clinicians report successful unsedated upper endoscopy in very young infants. Many pediatric endoscopists in North America use a combination of narcotic sedative and benzodiazepine to achieve acceptable sedation analgesia.[1] Other agents commonly used for sedation are propofol and ketamine. General anesthesia with endotracheal intubation is appropriate when the side effects of sedation or the endoscopy pose an undue risk of respiratory compromise (e.g., when underlying pulmonary disease, upper airway disease, or disorders of respiratory control are present) or if the patient is at risk for aspiration of gastric contents (e.g., when massive upper gastrointestinal hemorrhage is present or when an emergency foreign body extraction is performed on a child with a full stomach). In an ICU setting, patients supported by ventilators should receive additional sedation and neuromuscular blockade if the endoscopist anticipates that the procedure will be lengthy or excessively difficult.

Advantages of elective endotracheal intubation for EGD also include control of both the airway and ventilation during the procedure. In very small patients, the relatively large endoscope may partially obstruct the glottis, or distention of the gut with air may interfere with diaphragmatic movement. The risk of inadvertent extubation during EGD, however, mandates careful fixation of the endotracheal tube and careful monitoring of ventilation during the procedure by a physician from the critical care team.

Because bacteremia may occur during both upper and lower gastrointestinal endoscopy, some endoscopists routinely use perioperative antibiotics for endoscopy in patients with a central venous line or ventriculoperitoneal shunt. In recent years, therapeutic endoscopy has complemented diagnostic endoscopy. Gastrointestinal tract hemorrhage from varices, peptic ulceration, and angiodysplasia may be controlled by injection therapy or photocoagulation, electrocoagulation, and thermocoagulation. Band ligation of esophageal varices is also a proven therapy for variceal hemorrhage. Percutaneous endoscopic gastrostomy has become a popular alternative to surgical gastrostomy for patients in the ICU who cannot take oral alimentation on a long-term basis.

Gastroesophageal Reflux Monitoring

Like gastrointestinal endoscopy, esophageal reflux monitoring has benefited from technical advances that permit insertion of miniature, flexible electrodes into the esophagus of the smallest children.

Esophageal pH monitoring has been in use since the late 1970s. Esophageal pH is continuously recorded for 24 hours, and the duration of esophageal acidification, defined as decreases in pH less than 4, is quantified. Additional variables including the quantity of reflux in the 2 hours after a feeding and during fasting are determined. Detection of alkaline reflux episodes, which commonly occur in the postprandial period when food buffers gastric acid, is not possible with this technique. The administration of apple juice (pH < 4) rather than formula for feedings during the monitored period has been proposed to circumvent this limitation; however, it is an imperfect strategy insofar as normative data are scarce for older children whose esophageal pH is measured during apple juice feedings. Furthermore, the technique is unreliable for children who have been maintained with histamine 2 (H_2) antagonists or proton pump inhibitors. For reliable pH monitoring of such children, proton pump inhibitors must have been discontinued for at least 72 hours and H_2 antagonists for at least 48 hours. Critical care physicians may not have the luxury of stopping these agents temporarily in critically ill patients who are at risk for stress ulceration of the gastrointestinal tract.

Esophageal impedance monitoring[2] is the preferred means of measuring gastroesophageal reflux among patients who are receiving acid suppression or in whom alkaline reflux is suspected. The intraesophageal impedance device measures total opposition to current flow between two electrodes and expresses the value in ohms. Because air and fluid have different conductivities, the contents of the esophagus can be differentiated at any point in time. Thus when the esophagus is devoid of fluid, a baseline impedance is measured. When a bolus of fluid enters the esophagus from refluxed material or from a swallowed bolus, the impedance changes. These changes in intraluminal impedance thus permit the continuous monitoring of pH neutral or alkaline reflux episodes.

In addition to detecting pathological quantities of reflux in children who have symptoms suggestive of reflux disease, reflux monitoring is also useful in determining whether a temporal correlation exists between gastroesophageal reflux and pathological events such as cough, bronchospasm, or apnea. Because it does not determine the cause of vomiting, reflux monitoring adds little to the evaluation of vomiting children.

Use of Colorants to Identify Aspiration in the Intensive Care Unit

Patients who are obtunded or who have been ventilator dependent for an extended time are at significant risk of pulmonary aspiration. A deceptively simple way of documenting aspiration in patients receiving gavage or gastrostomy feedings was to add a coloring agent such as blue dye number one or methylene blue to formula. The rationale for this strategy was that quantities sufficient to tint formula should be readily apparent when suctioned from the lungs. The fallacy of the technique is that when compared with scintiscanning of the lungs after administration of a radiolabeled meal or with the discovery of lipid-laden macrophages after bronchoalveolar lavage, the use of colorants is notoriously inaccurate. Furthermore, all colorants are dangerous when instilled into the gastrointestinal tract. They are customarily absorbed in minimal quantities, but among critically ill patients, the gastrointestinal tract becomes porous to all macromolecules, and appreciable quantities of dye are absorbed. Once absorbed, even minimal quantities function as metabolic poisons, uncoupling oxidative metabolism, thereby resulting in life-threatening metabolic acidosis among susceptible patients.[3]

Radiological Procedures

Plain Films

The abdominal x-ray film provides valuable assistance to the clinician evaluating children with abdominal distention, guarding, or tenderness. Dilated, gas-filled bowel loops, with or without air-fluid levels, can signify obstruction or ileus. Air-fluid levels in a "stepladder" configuration along the length of small bowel suggest obstruction, whereas levels that appear in a parallel configuration suggest ileus. Pneumatosis intestinalis and mucosal "thumbprinting" are signs of bowel wall ischemia and can often be appreciated on the plain film. Pneumoperitoneum can be evaluated with the inspection for air in the lesser sack, air between bowel loops, or a visible falciform ligament. Even though an upright film is optimal for visualizing peritoneal air, lateral decubitus or cross-table lateral films are acceptable substitutes in bedridden patients. Air in an abscess cavity or air in liver parenchyma, biliary tree, or portal venous system should be acknowledged as signs of serious intraabdominal infection.

Abnormal densities such as abdominal masses, ascites, or calcifications can often be identified on plain film. Calcifications in the region of the gallbladder, pancreas, or appendix suggest cholelithiasis, pancreatitis, or appendicitis, respectively. The abdominal contour and the contour of extraperitoneal structures such as lung bases, pelvic organs, and kidneys should always be assessed.

Contrast Radiography

Although endoscopy is more sensitive than single-contrast radiography for identifying mucosal ulceration, contrast radiography remains a valuable procedure in the critical care setting. In general, the upper gastrointestinal tract series and small bowel series are indicated when partial small bowel obstruction is suspected. A contrast enema will document (and possibly treat) intussusception and document Hirschsprung's disease. The type of contrast agent for a particular examination depends on the clinical condition of the patient undergoing the examination. Although barium sulfate is superior to water-soluble contrast agents for outlining mucosa, its use in typical patients in the ICU is riskier because barium may form a concretion in a patient with ileus and because barium leaking into the peritoneum from a perforated hollow viscus can cause serious peritoneal injury. Hyperosmolar, water-soluble contrast agents are usually out of favor because they pose the risk of dehydration. Currently, isosmolar agents are more commonly used for studies on the critically ill patient.

Ultrasonography, Computed Tomography Scanning, and Magnetic Resonance Scanning

Ultrasonography, computed tomography (CT) scanning, and magnetic resonance imaging (MRI) each have advantages and disadvantages. For example, in the slim child with little mesenteric fat, ultrasonography is sometimes better than CT scanning of abdominal viscera. Conversely, CT scanning is superior for abdominal imaging of obese individuals.[4] MRI is limited by its inability to distinguish bowel loops from adjacent structures and by blurring caused by motion. It is helpful, though, in identifying vascular tumors, which are seen as low-intensity masses on T_1-weighted images and high-intensity masses on T_2-weighted images. Ultrasonography or CT is used when an intraabdominal abscess, cystic lesion, hepatobiliary disease, tumor, ascites, or pancreatitis is suspected. In the identification of pancreatic lesions, dynamic CT scanning is a most helpful imaging technique. CT also best identifies enlarged periaortic nodes. Ultrasonography of the liver and biliary tract identifies hepatic parenchymal disease, biliary stones, or congenital abnormalities such as choledochal cyst. Intussusception, pyloric stenosis, and acute appendicitis are particularly amenable to ultrasonographic diagnosis. In addition, Doppler flow analysis has significantly aided the preoperative and postoperative evaluation of liver transplant recipients by identifying congenital vascular anomalies and postoperative vascular thromboses.

Radionuclide Scanning

Radionuclide scanning is helpful when patients in the ICU have pulmonary aspiration, gastrointestinal bleeding, intraabdominal abscesses, or cholestasis.

Gastroesophageal reflux and the rate of gastric emptying can be measured with liquid-phase gastroesophageal scintigraphy.[5] Technetium 99-sulfur colloid is mixed with formula or another enterally administered liquid. When there is a scan above and below the diaphragm in 30- to 60-second windows during the first postprandial hour after isotope administration, the number of reflux episodes, the height of the reflux column, and the rate of gastric emptying are quantitated. A 4- to 6-hour delayed scan of the lungs determines whether pulmonary aspiration of that meal has occurred.[6]

Three techniques are used to aid in the diagnosis of gastrointestinal bleeding. Technetium 99-sulfur colloid and ^{99}Tc-labeled red cells are used in patients with continuous or intermittent bleeding. The advantage of sulfur colloid is that less than 0.1 ml of blood per minute will be shown. Bleeding in a spot near the liver or spleen, however, may be obscured by high levels of activity in those organs. Tagged red blood cell scans detect intermittent bleeding by means of delayed scans, but migration of blood down the gastrointestinal tract over time may preclude exact localization. ^{99}Technetium pertechnetate (Meckel's) scanning does not require active bleeding to localize a Meckel's diverticulum. Isotope is concentrated by gastric mucosa, and if a scan reveals an ectopic focus a Meckel's diverticulum can be suspected. Scan results are negative in the 15% of diverticula not containing gastric mucosa. A variety of non-Meckel's lesions (most of which require surgical correction) cause false-positive results on pertechnetate scans.

Resolution of hepatobiliary scans has improved dramatically since the introduction of derivatives of ^{99}Tc iminodiacetic acid. Scanning can now document cholecystitis when there is no gallbladder uptake or biliary obstruction when there is no excretion into the bowel. Other entities such as biliary leaks or cystic lesions of the biliary tree can also be documented. Furthermore, delayed or reduced hepatocyte uptake can confirm impaired hepatocellular function.

Intraabdominal abscesses and inflammatory intestinal lesions can be localized with radioscintigraphy.[7] Leukocytes are extracted from the patient, tagged with a radioisotope in vitro, and are reinjected. Scanning of the area in question is then performed. Technetium hexamethyl propyleneamine oxime (HMPAO) has replaced indium because of improved resolution of HMPAO scans and because HMPAO scans can be completed within 4 hours rather than 72 hours.

Testing for Occult Blood Loss

Occult blood loss is generally determined with the Hemoccult or Gastroccult test; these are modifications of the guaiac test.[8] They work because hemoglobin oxidizes the reagent to a blue product. The recently marketed Hemoccult Sensa slide detects as little as 2 to 3 ml of blood loss per day. This slide is virtually 100% sensitive when blood loss equals 10 ml/day.[8]

In the stomach, blood can be denatured, and this can lead to false-negative results. Gastroccult, which contains borate-buffered reagent, significantly improves the sensitivity for testing gastric contents. (Urine test tapes should never be used for gastrointestinal occult blood testing because they are too sensitive.) Therefore even physiological quantities of enteric blood loss (<1 ml of blood per day) will yield positive results.

Stool pH and Reducing Substances

Excessive enteral carbohydrate loads may worsen preexisting diarrhea in critically ill children. Carbohydrate malabsorption can be assessed with the measurement of reducing sugars and pH of stool. *The two tests should always be used in conjunction because colonic transit time and quantity or type of colonic flora* affect either of these tests. Malabsorbed sugars appear in feces when colonic transit is sufficiently rapid and are detected by Clinitest tablets or reagent strips; more than 0.5 mg of sugar per 100 ml of stool water suggests malabsorption. If the malabsorbed dietary sugar is primarily sucrose, a nonreducing sugar, the Clinitest result is negative unless the stool is first hydrolyzed with hydrochloric acid. Stools can be negative for reducing sugars despite carbohydrate malabsorption if colonic transit is slow enough to permit complete bacterial fermentation. In such an event, pH of fresh stool (measured by nitrazine paper) is consistently below 5.5. The pH of samples not tested for several hours, however, tends to rise over time as short-chain fatty acids generated from sugar fermentation are further metabolized.

The Intensive Care Unit as a Satellite Laboratory Facility

Regulations of the Joint Commission on Hospital Accreditation prohibit testing for occult blood loss or stool testing by anyone other than an individual certified in accordance with the Clinical Laboratory Improvement Act (CLIA). Thus for many pediatric critical care units, "bedside" testing has moved from the bedside to the clinical laboratory. Turnaround time for measuring occult blood in stool has risen from seconds to hours. Furthermore, when fecal samples are sent to the clinical laboratory for measurement of reducing sugars and pH, results are meaningless insofar as bacterial metabolism of sugars continues ex vivo in these samples between the times of collection to the time of testing. Critical care units wishing to perform reliable fecal testing on site must train a cohort of staff in common bedside tests and obtain CLIA certification for each staff member. Furthermore, just as many ICUs have chosen to comply with CLIA regulations and have established approved satellite laboratory facilities, to measure blood gases or serum electrolytes, they can extend the scope of their laboratory activities to include bedside gastroenterological testing.

Breath Hydrogen Testing

Breath hydrogen testing confirms monosaccharide or disaccharide malabsorption and small bowel bacterial overgrowth. The technique documents intestinal bacterial fermentation of carbohydrates; their byproduct is hydrogen gas. Fasting alveolar hydrogen concentrations greater than 40 ppm suggest bacterial overgrowth. A rise in concentration of 20 ppm occurring beyond 90 minutes after an enteral carbohydrate challenge suggests carbohydrate malabsorption. A peak less than 60 minutes after the challenge is consistent with bacterial overgrowth.

Because of difficulties in consistent alveolar air sampling, some investigators internally standardize by measuring both H_2 and carbon dioxide (CO_2) and expressing their results as a ratio.

Perhaps breath hydrogen testing is most valuable in the ICU as a screening test for neonatal necrotizing enterocolitis. Cheu, Brown, and Rowe[9] showed that randomly obtained breath H_2/CO_2 ratios greater than 8 ppm/mmHg strongly suggest necrotizing enterocolitis.

Life-Threatening Complications of Gastrointestinal Disorders

Esophagus

Congenital Esophageal Anomalies

Esophageal atresia and tracheoesophageal fistula are true neonatal emergencies. With an incidence of 1 in 3000 live births, they are among the most common congenital anomalies of the esophagus. Five anatomical varieties exist in the following descending order of frequency: (1) blind proximal esophageal pouch with distal esophagus originating at the tracheobronchial junction (80%), (2) blind proximal esophageal pouch with blind distal esophageal pouch (8%), (3) uninterrupted esophagus with H type tracheoesophageal fistula (4%), (4) proximal esophagus fistulizing into trachea with blind distal esophageal pouch (2%), and (5) interrupted esophagus with both proximal and distal esophagus communicating with trachea (1%).

The embryogenesis of this disorder is unknown, but other cardiovascular, gastrointestinal, skeletal, or urogenital anomalies are present in 50% of cases.

Infants with a blind proximal esophagus have excessive salivation, respiratory distress, and cyanosis. Diagnosis of blind proximal esophagus can be made by the failure to pass a nasogastric tube into the stomach. Complete atresia leads to a gasless lower gastrointestinal tract. An H-type fistula is sometimes seen on contrast radiography or esophagoscopy, but bronchoscopy is usually the most sensitive diagnostic tool.

Treatment is surgical. A simple fistula can be ligated, and a short atresia can be repaired primarily. Long atresia, however, may require staged treatment with initial esophagostomy and gastrostomy and subsequent definitive repair after internal or external traction is applied. Circular myotomy of the esophagus reduces anastomotic tension. Occasionally a "gastric tube" procedure or colonic interposition is required.

Caustic Injury to the Esophagus

Despite widespread efforts by poison control centers to publicize the dangers of household caustics, thousands of inadvertent ingestions occur annually; most occur in children younger than 5 years. Crystalline products produce greater damage to the hypopharynx and upper airway because of prolonged mouth contact and a smaller volume reaching the esophagus. In recent years most household cleaners have been reformulated to contain less lye, but pure liquid lye can be purchased if desired. Its resemblance to milk leads to numerous inadvertent ingestions by children.

Tissue damage can be caused by either strong alkali or acid. Deep esophageal burns are more common after alkali ingestion.[10] Alkalis produce rapid liquefaction of esophageal tissue, and burns can range from first to third degree in depth.[10] An intense inflammatory infiltrate develops, and blood vessels thrombose to produce ischemic necrosis. Perforation may occur within hours or days. Strictures can occur weeks to years after ingestion.[11] Esophageal burns occur infrequently after acid ingestion, but gastric or duodenal erosions have been reported.

Symptoms that predominate are chest pain and the inability to swallow secretions. Children with upper airway damage often exhibit stridor. When mouth burns are present, the chances of esophageal injury are 75%.[10] Conversely, 25% of patients with significant esophageal burns have no pharyngeal or mouth involvement.[10]

Treatment of severe stridor should be directed toward establishing an airway, and emergency tracheostomy should be contemplated. Upper endoscopy within 24 hours is advisable. If burns are minor, no further therapy is necessary, and patients are at low risk of sequelae. Third-degree burns require ongoing intensive care, though. The role of antibiotics and steroids remains controversial.[12] Although steroids reduce tissue damage when given before experimental injury, recent double-blind clinical trials show no efficacy of steroids in preventing sequelae.[12] When third-degree burns are endoscopically evident, a nasogastric tube should be positioned with endoscopic guidance. This tube will enable early feeding and serve as a guide for future dilations if they become necessary. Some surgeons have advocated early placement of gastrostomies and esophageal stents in patients with third-degree burns (see also Chapter 99).[13]

Esophageal Foreign Bodies

A variety of metallic, wooden, or plastic foreign bodies in a myriad of shapes and sizes can be swallowed by children. All that are lodged in the esophagus require urgent removal (within 24 hours). Even more urgent endoscopic retrieval is required for button batteries or pennies minted after 1983 that are lodged in the esophagus because both are caustic to esophageal mucosa and may cause damage within 1 to 4 hours. The preponderance of evidence suggests that once a battery has escaped the esophagus, complications from an unretrieved battery are rare.[14] Similarly, pennies, minted after 1983 are predominantly zinc based and can be nearly as caustic within the esophagus as button batteries. No published epidemiological studies are available on which to base the approach to zinc-based pennies within the stomach or small intestine.

Gastroesophageal Reflux

Several antireflux barriers exist in the region of the lower esophageal sphincter. Beyond intrinsic myogenic tone, barriers such as the cardioesophageal angle, the abdominal esophagus (which acts as flutter valve), the mucosal rosette of the sphincter (which acts as a choke valve), and the diaphragmatic crura themselves act to prevent reflux of gastric contents. A complex set of factors including hormonal changes, anatomical relationships, increased or decreased sensitivity to neurotransmitters, and CNS derangements act to produce inappropriate sphincter relaxation (usually transient), which leads to most episodes of gastroesophageal reflux.

Life-threatening events such as apnea and pulmonary aspiration can sometimes be attributed to reflux. The relationship between infantile apnea and reflux remains in question,[15] but both human and animal data suggest that reflux can occasionally be associated with obstructive breathing patterns. Severe pulmonary aspiration of refluxed material can also take place. A number of protective mechanisms such as an active gag reflex, cough reflex, and laryngospasm protect against aspiration,[16] but these reflexes may be lost under special circumstances such as obtundation.

Symptoms of obstructive apnea often include a brief episode of stridor accompanied by a struggle to breathe, a change in skin color to red or purple, and finally cyanosis and cessation of respiratory effort. Patients who have aspirated massive amounts of fluid become tachypneic and dyspneic shortly after the meal. Food or formula is often found in the nares or mouth. Cough may occur.

The diagnostic modality most helpful in documenting a temporal relationship between apnea and acid reflux is 24-hour esophageal reflux monitoring combined with simultaneous electrocardiography, pneumography by chest wall impedance, pneumography by nasal thermistor, pulse oximetry, and end-tidal CO_2 measurement. Aspiration is often difficult to document, but the presence of a new infiltrate on chest x-ray films and a consistent clinical history provide strong circumstantial evidence. If repeated aspiration is suspected, an upper gastrointestinal tract series may reveal gastroesophageal reflux and immediate aspiration of barium; however, aspiration of gastroesophageal refluxate that occurs minutes or hours after a feeding may be missed with contrast radiography. A milk scan may be more sensitive than radiography for documenting this type of aspiration. Children who are not fed orally may nevertheless aspirate oral secretions. The scintigraphic "salivagram" is performed with the placement of a drop of saline-containing ^{99m}Tc-sulfur colloid on the tongue.[17] Subsequent imaging permits observation of its handling. Appearance of isotope in the trachea and bronchi confirms aspiration.

When recurrent aspiration is suspected but not confirmed noninvasively, bronchoscopy with bronchoalveolar lavage may support the diagnosis by returning fluid-containing lipid-laden alveolar macrophages.[18] Aspiration during swallowing and aspiration of refluxed gastric contents cannot be distinguished by this method in patients who are fed orally.

Although some clinicians view one episode of reflux-induced aspiration or apnea as an absolute indication for fundoplication, the decision to perform fundoplication should be based on the severity of the initial episode, underlying conditions that predisposed the child to the episode, risk for recurrence, and the expected natural history of reflux for a particular patient. In other words, some patients may be successfully managed with pharmacotherapy (a proton pump inhibitor with or without a prokinetic agent such as metoclopramide or erythromycin).

Stomach and Duodenum

Gastric Volvulus

Acute gastric volvulus may be of two types. When the whole stomach revolves about its long axis, organoaxial volvulus has occurred. When the fundus and pylorus exchange positions, the volvulus is mesenteroaxial. Predisposing factors include paraesophageal hernias or eventration of the diaphragm.

Because a closed obstruction has occurred, the patient is unable to vomit despite severe pain, distention, and retching. Plain radiographs reveal a markedly distended stomach with air-fluid levels, and contrast radiography may reveal cardioesophageal junction obstruction. An immediate operation is indicated.

Gastric Ulcer

Whereas some authors suggest that duodenal ulcers outnumber gastric ulcers in childhood,[1] others have reported that young children are more likely to have gastric ulcers. Most gastric ulcers lie at the junction of gastric fundus and body. Those high in the fundus are usually related to stress. Antral ulcers are often the result of use of nonsteroidal antiinflammatory drugs (NSAIDs).

A well-recognized complication of severe illness requiring admission to the ICU is stress ulceration of the stomach. Bleeding becomes an important source of morbidity and mortality in patients with burns and trauma, as well as in those who have undergone major operations or have systemic disease. Prophylaxis against bleeding is common in the ICU setting. Antacids, H_2-receptor antagonists (H_2RA), or sucralfate are most often used. Unfortunately, elevation of gastric pH by antacids and H_2RA removes one barrier against bacterial colonization and may increase the risk of pneumonia with organisms colonizing the stomach.[19] Large controlled trials, however, have failed to confirm this concern. Sucralfate is equally effective as prophylaxis against bleeding but does not affect gastric pH. If sucralfate is given concurrently with antacids or acid-suppressing medications, its efficacy will be reduced because it requires an acidic environment for optimal effect.

Most patients with gastric ulcers are hypochlorhydric rather than hyperchlorhydric because exposure to detergents or toxins such as NSAIDs, pepsin, bile salts, or ethanol erodes the gastric barrier to back-diffusion. A second consistent finding among patients with gastric ulcers is delayed gastric emptying, which may be an epiphenomenon or central to the pathogenesis of ulcers.

The association between *Helicobacter pylori* infection and both chronic gastritis and duodenal ulcer is well established, but the role of *H. pylori* in the pathogenesis of gastric ulceration remains somewhat speculative.[20]

Clinical features of gastric ulcer resemble those of duodenal ulcer. Pain predominates and is epigastric in location but usually follows eating more closely. Nausea and vomiting may occur. Milk or antacids relieve the pain. The two complications of gastric or duodenal ulceration most commonly requiring intensive care are perforation and bleeding. Perforation, requiring immediate surgical intervention, produces exquisite pain and rapid development of peritoneal signs in patients without immunosuppression.

Hematemesis heralds gastric ulcer bleeding, which may be as massive as that of duodenal ulcer. Careful, repeated assessment of vital signs and prompt restoration of circulating blood volume by large-bore venous catheters are essential. Saline solution or epinephrine gastric lavage through a large sump tube is mandatory. "Iced" saline lavage offers no advantage and excessively depresses core temperature.

Efforts should also focus on reducing gastric acid production with a parenteral proton pump inhibitor.[21] Continuous intravenous vasopressin infusion, commonly used for control of variceal hemorrhage, reduces arterial flow through the splanchnic bed. Selective intraarterial infusion appears to be unnecessary. Intravenous administration of somatostatin or its synthetic, active octreotide moiety, has been effective in stemming variceal hemorrhage and may work for other causes of bleeding. In addition to their hemodynamic effects, they inhibit gastric acid production.

When the patient's condition is stable, endoscopy may be performed to localize the ulcer. Endoscopic therapy may then be performed on actively bleeding ulcers or those with visible vessels (which tend to rebleed). Ulcer beds may be photocoagulated, electrocoagulated, or thermocoagulated. They may also be injected with hemostatic agents such as epinephrine. If nonsurgical techniques fail to stop the bleeding, one of several surgical options (which include ulcer oversewing or resection, variations of gastric drainage procedures, and vagotomy) must be performed. Fortunately, successful pharmacological and endoscopic therapies have precluded the need for these surgical therapies in all but the rarest circumstances.

Duodenal Ulcers

The incidence of duodenal ulcer in childhood is unknown. A large series completed before the popularization of endoscopy suggested an incidence of 4.4 cases per 10,000 pediatric patients per year, which is no doubt an underestimation.[22] The male predominance seen among adults is present only among postpubertile children. The risk for patients with blood group O is 1.3 times that expected.

A number of factors have been implicated in the pathogenesis of duodenal ulcers. Unquestionably, excessive acid production plays a major role. Some factors leading to hypersecretion include excessive gastrin or histamine production and increased vagal tone. Approximately half of patients with ulcers are also hyperpepsinogenemic, and their mucosal integrity may therefore be suboptimal.[23] Infection with *H. pylori* reduces the ulcer healing rate and increases the recurrence rate.[24] Although approximately 90% of adult duodenal ulcers are associated with *H. pylori* infection, only about 50% of pediatric duodenal ulcers are related to *H. pylori*.[25] The effects of diet and stress have been minimized in the recent literature.

Symptoms are similar to those of adults. Epigastric pain occurs after meals and often awakens the child from sleep. Vomiting occurs in 40% of patients.

The major life-threatening complications are perforation and hemorrhage, which lead to a "surgical" abdomen and shock, respectively. Abdominal plain films reveal free air if perforation has occurred. Hemorrhage presents as hematemesis, hematochezia, or melena. Endoscopy is the most sensitive tool to localize the ulcer and to characterize the risk for rebleeding. Ulcers with visible vessels in the crater are at greatest risk of recurrent hemorrhage and may require endoscopic coagulation. Principles of management are identical to those for gastric ulcer. Obviously, antibiotics such as clarithromycin, amoxicillin, and metronidazole should be used for the first 14 days of a 1-month course of acid suppression when ulcers are associated with *H. pylori* infections.

Small Intestine and Colon

Malrotation

In embryonic life the cecum and ascending colon are located on the left side of the abdomen and the small bowel is on the right. During gestation the midgut transiently protrudes into the umbilicus and rotates 270 degrees, and the cecum is moved to the right lower quadrant and the duodenojejunal junction to the left upper quadrant. Incomplete rotation is of little consequence unless midgut volvulus, which can be a catastrophic event, occurs.

Some patients with malrotation experience partial duodenal obstruction because of extrinsic compression by mesenteric bands. Chronic diarrhea and protein-losing enteropathy may be seen among others without complete obstruction.

Clinical features of obstructing volvulus include severe abdominal pain, bilious vomiting, and abdominal distention. Surgical treatment requires a Ladd procedure, in which mesenteric bands are divided and the bowel is returned to its fetal position. Failure to promptly relieve the volvulus leads to ischemic necrosis of all of the gut supplied by the superior mesenteric artery (proximal jejunum to midtransverse colon). Short gut syndrome results from resection of the affected intestine.

Necrotizing Enterocolitis

Necrotizing enterocolitis is primarily a disorder of premature infants, affecting 2.5% of neonatal patients in the ICU but only 0.2% of all infants. The most common areas involved are the ileum and proximal colon, but any part of the intestinal tract may be affected. Its pathogenesis is unknown, but bowel ischemia, feeding of hyperosmolar formula, rapid advancement of feeding,[26] reduced immune surveillance, and population of the bowel by excessive quantities of enterotoxin-producing bacteria[27] may all play a role.

The classic clinical features are abdominal distention, bilious vomiting, and bloody stools, but symptoms are more subtle in some infants. If left unrecognized, necrotizing enterocolitis may become fulminant, leading to shock, disseminated intravascular coagulation (DIC), and apnea.

The diagnosis of necrotizing enterocolitis may be confirmed by an abdominal plain film showing pneumatosis intestinalis, hepatic portal air, or both. A random breath H_2/CO_2 ratio greater than 8 ppm/mmHg strongly suggests the diagnosis.[9] Because the pathogenesis is unknown, treatment must be symptomatic. In most centers, feedings are discontinued for 48 hours to 2 weeks depending on the severity of symptoms. Fluid resuscitation and broad-spectrum parenteral antibiotics are the basis of medical therapy. Surgical resection is reserved for severe cases when medical management fails and gangrenous bowel develops. Perforation may sometimes be managed successfully in infants with very low birth weight with simple peritoneal drainage performed with the infant under local anesthesia,[28] and a multicenter study is currently being conducted to compare the outcomes of simple drainage and resection in such high-risk infants.

Food Allergy

Food allergy can be defined as a reproducible, immunologically mediated reaction to an ingested food protein. Pathogenic events can be classified according to the schema of Gell and Coombs as type I (reagenic, immediate hypersensitivity reaction), type II (cytotoxic reaction), type III (immune-complex reaction), or type IV (delayed hypersensitivity reaction).

Manifestations may be systemic[29] or confined to the gastrointestinal tract.[30] Life-threatening systemic manifestations include acute urticaria and anaphylaxis.[29] Gastrointestinal reactions, which are sometimes severe, include allergic enteritis, allergic colitis, and celiac crisis.[30]

Acute urticaria is usually easily recognized by the classic wheal and flare cutaneous lesions often accompanied by laryngeal edema and angioedema. Anaphylaxis is an antigen-triggered immune reaction that leads to vascular collapse and bronchospasm.[31]

Food protein–induced enteropathy is characteristically a disorder of the infant and toddler.[30] The small bowel develops patchy villous atrophy. Symptoms and signs range from those of malabsorption and enteric protein loss to those of profound diarrhea and shock. Colitis caused by food protein sensitivity is seen most commonly among infants younger than 6 months.[30] Bloody, mucoid diarrhea develops several days or weeks after their first oral antigen challenge. Even though this colitis usually takes a benign course, it may be severe enough to mimic necrotizing enterocolitis.

Although some do not categorize gluten enteropathy as true food allergy, it shares enough features with allergy to justify inclusion with this category of disorders.[30] Celiac crisis is a rare, life-threatening complication that may occur among untreated patients with a large gluten load or in treated patients as a result of dietary indiscretion. Massive fluid and electrolyte loss leads to shock.

The cornerstone of long-term therapy is elimination of the offending food,[30] but emergency measures are also required. Immediate administration of epinephrine and corticosteroids is essential in the treatment of anaphylaxis.[31] Urticaria may require the administration of antihistamines, corticosteroids, and epinephrine.[31] Steroid use also seems to benefit patients in celiac crisis. Rapid administration of crystalloid or colloid is crucial in the management of any of these reactions.

Hemolytic-Uremic Syndrome

The hemolytic-uremic syndrome may occur in epidemic or sporadic forms. It is frequently preceded by enteric infection with bacterial[32] or viral pathogens. Infection with *Escherichia coli* O157:H7 has preceded an inordinately high number of cases.[32,33] Some instigating factors such as bacterial verotoxin cause endothelial damage in the kidney, liver, heart, brain, adrenal glands, and gastrointestinal tract.

Clinical features include a prodrome of abdominal pain, vomiting, and diarrhea, which may be bloody. Patients may have endoscopic, radiographic, or histological evidence of ischemic bowel disease. As gastrointestinal symptoms improve, anemia and thrombocytopenia rapidly appear and produce pallor, petechiae, and ecchymoses. Subsequently, patients become oliguric, hypertensive, and azotemic. The clinical course may be complicated further by pancreatitis. Seizures may occur.

The intensivist caring for children with acute, hemorrhagic colitis must pay exceptional attention to fluid balance, hemogram, and renal function tests. Any sudden change in hemoglobin, platelet count, blood urea nitrogen, or urine output should be considered a potential sign of the hemolytic-uremic syndrome. In the absence of hypovolemic shock, fluid intake should be curtailed if hemolytic-uremic syndrome is documented. In the event of severe renal insufficiency, dialysis is necessary. Plasma exchange and anticoagulants are probably not beneficial.[34] High-dose vitamin E has been suggested as a nonspecific adjunct to therapy (see also Chapter 64).

Inflammatory Bowel Disease

Crohn's disease and ulcerative colitis are chronic, relapsing disorders without known causes. The transmural inflammation of Crohn's disease may affect any portion of the alimentary tract in a patchy distribution, whereas the inflammation of ulcerative colitis is confined to the mucosa of the colon. The latter always involves distal colon, and its contiguous inflammation extends for varying distances from the rectum. The two entities are different enough to usually permit accurate categorization, but there is sufficient overlap in symptoms and distribution that the diagnosis is indeterminate in 15% of cases. Table 79–1 summarizes the clinical, radiographic, endoscopic, and histological differences between the two.

The cause of these disorders remains speculative. Clearly, genetic factors predispose patients to one or the other, but environmental factors also appear to play a role.[35] Etiological factors considered important over the years have included psychogenic predisposition, food allergies, infectious processes, immunological deficiency, and immunological hyperreactivity.

Presenting signs and symptoms include abdominal pain; bloody or nonbloody diarrhea; anorexia; abdominal mass; and extraintestinal manifestations such as weight loss, fever, arthritis, or erythema nodosum. Patients are often anemic and hypoproteinemic, and they may show hematological or biochemical signs of acute-phase response. The radiographic and histological features are typical (Table 79–1).

The cornerstone of medical management has long been the use of corticosteroids, but 5-aminosalicylic acid (5-ASA) is effective for mild to moderate ulcerative colitis and Crohn's colitis. Evidence is less compelling that 5-ASA is effective in small intestinal Crohn's disease. Immunosuppressants, such as 6-mercaptopurine and methotrexate, have been used for Crohn's disease, and 6-mercaptopurine also seems effective in the treatment of ulcerative colitis. Biologic therapy has revolutionized the therapy of Crohn's disease.[36] Infliximab, a monoclonal antibody against tumor necrosis factor, has shown dramatic efficacy against Crohn's disease in up to 75% of patients. Other biologic agents such as antibodies against proinflammatory cytokines and antisense molecules blocking white cell adhesion molecules are currently in development. Probiotics such as nonpathogenic helminths and anaerobic lactobacillus species are also under study.

Complications most likely to require an intensivist's attention are perforation, toxic dilation of the colon, and fulminant colitis. A patient whose bowel has perforated exhibits decreased bowel sounds and abdominal rigidity. Point and rebound tenderness may be present. Abdominal x-ray films may reveal free intraperitoneal air. Most perforations in Crohn's disease produce intraabdominal abscesses, but peritonitis does not. Some abscesses, however, can contaminate the peritoneum. Free colonic perforation tends to occur among patients with ulcerative colitis. Toxic dilation and fulminant colitis are also more common with ulcerative colitis but may occasionally occur in Crohn's colitis. Because management of severe inflammatory bowel disease frequently includes immunosuppression with high-dose corticosteroids, cyclosporine, or azathioprine, some of the signs and symptoms of perforation may be masked in the population most likely to have such complications. Factors such as patient immobility, antiperistaltic drugs, rigorous cathartic use, and electrolyte imbalance are frequently associated with toxic dilation of the colon. Patients initially have massive abdominal distention and pain. X-ray films reveal an increased transverse colonic diameter. The patient's status is observed through careful monitoring of vital signs, physical examination, and repeated abdominal radiographs. Management includes giving nothing by mouth during nasogastric tube suction and inserting a rectal tube for decompression. Frequent position changes may aid in redistributing air distally. Fluid and electrolyte balance is aggressively maintained, and broad-spectrum parenteral antibiotics are given. Efforts at medical management should not exceed a few hours because of the extreme risk of perforation. Clinical decompensation or

TABLE 79–1

Differential Diagnosis between Ulcerative Colitis and Crohn's Disease

Feature	Ulcerative Colitis	Crohn's Disease
RELATIVE INCIDENCE OF SYMPTOMS		
Rectal bleeding (gross)	Common	Rare
Diarrhea	Often severe	Moderate or even absent
Pain	Less frequent	Almost always
Anorexia	Mild or moderate	Can be severe
Weight loss	Moderate	Severe
Growth retardation	Usually mild	Often pronounced
Extraintestinal manifestations	Common	Common
INVOLVEMENT		
Small bowel involvement		
Extensive	—	10%
Lower ileum	5%-10%	90%
Colon	100%	75%
Rectum	95%	50%
Anus	5%	85%
DISTRIBUTION OF LESIONS	Continuous	Segmental
RADIOLOGICAL FEATURES	Superficial ulcers, loss of haustration, no skip areas, shortening	Serpiginous ulcers, thumbprinting, skip areas, string sign
PATHOLOGICAL CHANGES	Diffuse mucosal disease	Focal transmural disease, granulomas
RESPONSE TO TREATMENT		
Steroids and sulfasalazine	75%	25%-75%
Parenteral nutrition and elemental diets	Poor	Very good for small bowel
Azathioprine and 6-mercaptopurine	Good in selected cases	Good in selected cases
Surgery	Excellent	Fair or poor
COURSE		
Remissions	Common	Common
Relapse after surgery	Rare	5%-100%
Cancer risk	High in pancolitis	Slight

Modified from Silverman A, Roy CC, editors: *Pediatric clinical gastroenterology,* ed 3, St Louis, 1983, Mosby, p 354.

perforation is an indication for urgent surgical resection of the colon.

Fulminant colitis is characterized by fever, shock, severe abdominal pain, 10 or more bloody stools per day, and abdominal tenderness. Broad-spectrum antibiotics, intravenous steroids, immunosuppressants such as cyclosporine,[37] red blood cell transfusion, and fluid replacement are the mainstays of treatment for fulminant colitis. Small, uncontrolled series have also suggested that infliximab may be beneficial for fulminant colitis.[38] Failure to respond within a few days, however, warrants colectomy.

Hirschsprung's Disease

Hirschsprung's disease occurs in 1 in 5000 live births. It may be the result of incomplete craniocaudal migration of neural crest elements, but some investigators believe that ganglion cells degenerate after migration. Aganglionosis may involve as little as a few centimeters or the entire colon and small bowel (in rare cases). Total colonic Hirschsprung's disease occurs in clusters in some families with the risk being 21% in those families.[39] The inheritance of familial Hirschsprung's disease appears to be polygenic, with mutations in several loci of the RET proto-oncogene being associated with autosomal dominant Hirschsprung's disease that is most commonly the short-segment type. Mutations of the endothelin receptor type B gene are more likely to be observed in long-segment, autosomal recessively transmitted Hirschsprung's disease. Other gene mutations may also modify the expression of the disease.[39]

The most common feature of Hirschsprung's disease is the failure to pass meconium in a timely fashion after birth; 94% of infants with Hirschsprung's disease pass their first stool beyond 24 hours of life. Most patients with Hirschsprung's disease are constipated but cannot pass flatus. If their condition is undiagnosed during the first months of life, they may fail to thrive.

Physical findings include abdominal distention and an empty rectum on digital examination. Barium enema often reveals a narrow-caliber aganglionic distal colon; a transition zone; and a dilated, ganglionic proximal colon. It is essential that the barium enema be performed without prior enema preparation to preserve the transition zone. Absence of the anal-inhibitory reflex on anorectal manometry is suggestive. The diagnosis is confirmed histologically by rectal biopsy of the distal rectal mucosa where hypertrophic nerve trunks but no ganglion cells are found. Acetylcholinesterase staining of the specimen improves the diagnostic yield by enhancement of the abnormal nerve trunks.

In some children the course of Hirschsprung's disease is punctuated by episodic, severe enterocolitis, which leads to copious, bloody diarrhea, fever, and shock.

The intensive care of patients with enterocolitis should emphasize reconstitution of circulating blood volume with crystalloid, colloid, and red blood cells. Broad-spectrum parenteral antibiotics are advisable. After the patient's condition is stabilized, urgent decompressive enterostomy is indicated. Pull-through operations are usually performed after several months. Enterocolitis in the remaining ganglionated intestine may occur even in some patients who have undergone a pull-through operation.

Acute Colonic Pseudo-obstruction

First described by Oglivie,[40] acute colonic pseudo-obstruction is occasionally observed among critically ill adults and children who are immobilized in an ICU setting. It is characterized by massive cecal dilation of 5 to 10 cm on abdominal plain film. The mechanism is uncertain, but it appears to occur among patients given neuromuscular blockade and antimotility drugs such as narcotics. If left untreated, it may result in colonic perforation at the cecal level. Therapy should involve decompression of the gastrointestinal tract by nasogastric and rectal intubation and suction. Placing the patient in the prone position also seems to be effective initial therapy. None of these measures, though, seem to be as effective as is parenteral administration of neostigmine.[40] Adverse effects of neostigmine such as excessive salivation or abdominal cramping are self-limiting, but bradycardia that occasionally occurs must be managed with atropine.

Acute Pancreatitis

Even though gallstone pancreatitis and ethanolic pancreatitis are uncommon in children, numerous structural, toxic metabolic, and infectious diseases are associated with acute childhood pancreatitis (Box 79–1). Appropriate radiographic or biochemical evaluation for pancreatitis should be performed on all children admitted to the ICU with "acute abdomen."

Acute pancreatitis is preceded by intrapancreatic activation of proteases. The triggering mechanism remains obscure, but once protease inhibitors are overcome and trypsinogen is converted to trypsin, a cascade of steps produces active proteases, lipase, and amylase. The enzymes induce local and distant organ damage, which includes edema, increased vascular permeability, cytolysis, and fat necrosis.

The clinical hallmark of acute pancreatitis is severe, boring epigastric or left upper quadrant pain that radiates through to the back. Serum amylase and lipase levels are greatly elevated, and radiographic imaging studies reveal pancreatic enlargement, sonolucency, or irregularity of the margin. Ultrasonography is a satisfactory screening technique, but CT scanning should be used when the course is severe. If CT scanning is performed with a dynamic, contrast-enhanced technique, interstitial pancreatitis can be differentiated from the more ominous necrotic pancreatitis, which often requires surgical debridement.

Because serum lipase is almost exclusively pancreatic in origin and amylase comes from a number of organs, the serum lipase concentration may be a better indicator of pancreatitis. Use of both measures to follow the course of pancreatitis is preferable to using either one alone.

Several nonspecific laboratory derangements such as anemia, hypoglycemia, hypocalcemia, and hypoproteinemia may occur. Intensive support may be required for severe, acute attacks. Severe, hemorrhagic necrosis of the pancreas carries a poor prognosis. Extraordinarily large third-space fluid and electrolyte losses must be replaced. If significant hyperglycemia occurs, insulin must be given. Calcium infusions may also be necessary. Physicians should be able to minimize pancreatic stimulation by giving the patient *nothing by mouth* and using nasogastric suction, although the efficacy of suction has been questioned for patients without ileus. Use of protease inhibitors, H_2 antagonists, somatostatin, 5-fluorouracil, and glucagon has not found much support in the literature. Antibiotics are not indicated unless an abscess is suspected. Some studies support the use of free-radical scavengers such as selenium, methionine, vitamin E, and vitamin C.[41]

Several complications may be catastrophic. Rupture of a pancreatic duct or leakage of a pseudocyst must be suspected if ascites develops. Gastrointestinal hemorrhage during pancreatitis may originate from a variety of sources. Discovery of gastric varices suggests splenic vein thrombosis. Gastritis may also appear. Pseudoaneurysms of the hepatic or splenic artery may bleed into the pancreas. Small bowel or colonic ischemia caused by fat necrosis may produce gastrointestinal hemorrhage. Infected pancreatic necrosis is uniformly fatal unless the patient undergoes an emergency operation to debride the necrotic tissue.

Time to recovery from pancreatitis is variable and may be prolonged (weeks to months). Nutritional management during that interval is affected by the desire to avoid stimulation of the pancreas by enteral administration of nutrients. Although total parenteral nutrition (TPN) is indicated during the initial phase of severe pancreatitis,[42] enteral administration of elemental formulas by nasojejunal tube phase has been successfully implemented[43,44] early in the course of the illness. If such a nutritional strategy does not exacerbate the pancreatitis, it is preferable to using TPN because of its relative safety when compared with TPN.

Acute and Chronic Liver Failure

The term *liver failure* refers to the constellation of symptoms, signs, and biochemical aberrations that appear when hepatic synthetic capacity is severely compromised. Liver failure is categorized as fulminant when encephalopathy

BOX 79–1

Causes of Pancreatitis

INFECTIOUS

Mycoplasma pneumoniae
Viral infection
- Mumps
- Epstein-Barr virus
- Coxsackievirus B
- Rubella
- Hepatitis A
- Influenza A

SYSTEMIC DISEASES

Systemic lupus erythematosus
Hyperparathyroidism
Sarcoid disease
Henoch-Schönlein purpura
Crohn's disease
Reye's syndrome
Cystic fibrosis
Diabetes
Uremia

OBSTRUCTION

Biliary tract
- Choledochal cyst
- Choledochocele
- Gallstones

Duplication cyst (duodenum, gastropancreatic)
Peptic ulcer (penetrating posterior)
Ascariasis
Trauma
- Accidental
- Nonaccidental

Postsurgical (for peptic ulcer disease)
Duodenal obstruction
- Tumor (lymphoma)
- Stricture
- Annular pancreas

METABOLIC

Hyperlipidemia (types I and IV)
Hereditary pancreatitis
a_1-Antitrypsin deficiency
Malnutrition (kwashiorkor)
Rapid refeeding of the malnourished child

DRUGS, CHEMICALS, OR TOXIC AGENTS

Valproic acid
Alcohol
Steroids
Sulfasalazine
Tetracycline
Chlorothiazide
Furosemide
Borates
Oral contraceptives (estrogen)
Azathioprine
Sulfonamides
Hyperalimentation
Scorpion bites

IDIOPATHIC

Modified from Silverman A, Roy CC, editors: *Pediatric clinical gastroenterology,* ed 3, St Louis, 1983, Mosby, pp 844-845.

appears within the first 2 months of the illness, as late onset when it appears within 6 months, and as chronic when it appears beyond the sixth month of liver dysfunction. Infectious, metabolic, and toxic liver diseases, as well as biliary obstruction, may lead to liver failure (Box 79–2). Obviously, it is advisable to establish a cause of liver disease before the onset of liver failure. It is beyond the scope of this chapter to outline a diagnostic approach to childhood liver disease, but several reviews are available (see also Chapter 81).[45,46]

Elucidating the cause of fulminant hepatic failure is often made more difficult by the rapid development of coagulopathy and ascites, which preclude percutaneous liver biopsy. Laparotomy with surgical wedge biopsy may be necessary. More recently, techniques for transjugular liver biopsy have been developed.[47] A core of liver tissue is obtained by passing the biopsy forceps retrograde through the superior vena cava and hepatic vein after introduction via the jugular vein. The biopsy site then bleeds directly into the liver parenchyma, minimizing extravasation.

Hepatic encephalopathy is a consistent finding in adult liver failure, although it occurs inconsistently and relatively late in pediatric cases.[48] Virtually all pathogenic theories for hepatic encephalopathy assign a central role to ammonia in the development of coma, but the hypothesis that ammonia acts alone has fallen out of favor. Similarly, the theory that phenols and short-chain fatty acids interfere with ureagenesis provides only a partial explanation for encephalopathy. Elevation of serum aromatic amino acids and depression in branched-chain amino acids favor the hypothesis that octopamine and serotonin (products of aromatic amino acid metabolism) act as inhibitory false neurotransmitters. Their CNS levels, however, are generally not high enough to alter consciousness. The GABA (γ-aminobutyric acid) theory seems most consistent with observed biochemical changes that occur in liver failure. This theory proposes that GABA, an inhibitory transmitter, increases in the brain and acts as an agonist for other inhibitory transmitters and benzodiazepines.

Encephalopathy is generally treated by administration of ammonia-lowering agents. Neomycin, by qualitatively and quantitatively altering gut flora, reduces the enteral contribution to the ammonia load. Byproducts of the fermentation of lactulose by colonic bacteria reduce luminal pH to trap ammonia as ammonium for excretion in

BOX 79-2

Diseases that Cause Liver Failure

HEPATOCELLULAR

- Hepatitis A, B, C, or D
- Neonatal diseases
  - Rubella
  - Cytomegalic inclusion disease
  - Syphilis
  - Herpes simplex
  - Toxoplasmosis
  - Enterovirus infection
- Chronic active hepatitis
- Genetic diseases and metabolic disorders
  - a_1-Antitrypsin deficiency
  - Wilson's disease
  - Galactosemia
  - Tyrosinemia
  - Cystinosis
  - Porphyria hepatica
  - Fructose intolerance
  - Hemochromatosis—primary or secondary
  - Histiocytosis X
  - Lipid storage diseases
  - Glycogen storage disease (type IV)
  - Gangliosidosis
  - Hurler's disease
  - Zellweger's syndrome
- Jamaican vomiting sickness
- Indian childhood cirrhosis
- Drugs and toxins

OBSTRUCTIVE

- Intrahepatic and extrahepatic atresias
- Familial intrahepatic cholestasis
- Choledochal cyst
- Cystic fibrosis
- Cholangitis
  - Sclerosing cholangitis
  - Bacterial

Modified from Gryboski J, Walker WA, editors: *Gastrointestinal problems in the infant*, ed 2, Philadelphia, 1983, WB Saunders. p. 344.

stool. Cathartics can speed transit of protein through the gastrointestinal tract. Dietary protein can be limited and the quality altered to include less aromatic amino acid and more branched-chain amino acid. Progressive hepatic encephalopathy culminates in coma. When patients have entered coma, CNS resuscitation becomes necessary. Patients should undergo elective endotracheal intubation, and they should be hyperventilated. Administration of narcotics and benzodiazepines should be avoided. Benzodiazepine antagonists provide temporary improvement in consciousness among patients with hepatic encephalopathy.[49] Beyond CNS metabolic derangements, cytotoxic cerebral edema often complicates hepatic failure. Osmotic diuresis with mannitol and furosemide should be initiated, and fluid intake should be restricted. Placement of an intracranial monitoring device should be contemplated; the risk of instrumentation in patients with coagulopathy should be weighed against the benefit of continuous CNS pressure monitoring (see also Chapter 52).

The non-CNS manifestations of liver failure are protean. Hepatosplenomegaly is common in the early stages of fulminant failure, but the liver may shrink rapidly. In end-stage liver disease caused by cirrhosis, the liver is shrunken, firm, and nodular. Most patients with liver failure have jaundice. Spider angiomas, palmar erythema, ascites, and peripheral edema are common features of chronic liver disease. Fetor hepaticus (mercaptan breath) may be present.

The biochemical features of liver failure are variable depending on its cause, duration, and severity. Hypoglycemia should be corrected when present. Serum bilirubin levels may be elevated or normal. Liver aminotransferase concentrations are increased in acute liver disease but decrease as hepatocytes are lost and therefore may be only mildly elevated or normal in cirrhosis and in the terminal stages of failure. Decreasing aminotransferase levels and albumin in the face of rising bilirubin, prothrombin time, and partial thromboplastin time denotes a failing liver. Serum globulin and ammonia levels are usually elevated. The serum aminogram reveals an elevated aromatic/branched-chain amino acid ratio. Renal insufficiency may appear because of prerenal azotemia, acute tubular necrosis, or hepatorenal syndrome.[50]

Patients with late-onset or chronic liver failure are likely to have portal hypertension. Ascites may develop as plasma oncotic pressure decreases or portal pressure increases. Patients who are hyponatremic usually have total-body sodium overload,[50] and they should be treated with salt and fluid restriction, colloid administration, and diuretic therapy.

Spontaneous engorgement of esophageal, gastric, and rectal veins leads to varices. Similar prominent veins in the abdominal wall and around the umbilicus (caput medusa) may develop. Splenic congestion from impaired venous flow into the portal system results in splenomegaly and hypersplenism so that patients are classically anemic or pancytopenic. Less commonly, unknown factors lead to intrapulmonary arteriovenous shunting, which characteristically causes hypoxemia.

Coagulopathy and bleeding are frequent in patients with liver failure. Thrombocytopenia, which may be profound, is a common component of hypersplenism. Fat-soluble vitamin malabsorption in patients with cholestasis leads to vitamin K deficiency, which prevents hepatic production of clotting factors II, VII, IX, and X. Ultimately, failed synthesis of all liver-dependent clotting factors results in prolonged prothrombin time (unresponsive to vitamin K administration) and partial thromboplastin time.

The sites of bleeding are predictable. Bleeding from incisions, needle puncture sites, nose, and gingiva are common but are usually not life threatening. Persistent bleeding may require packed red blood cell transfusion. In contrast, intracranial and variceal bleeding may be fatal and demand immediate attention. Esophageal varices bleed because of acute changes in variceal pressure or because of gastric hyperacidity. Platelets should be given to patients with thrombocytopenia. Patients with coagulopathy may receive fresh frozen plasma if their coagulopathy is mild; however, those whose prothrombin time is markedly deranged (international normalized ratio [INR] >2) may have pulmonary edema if attempts are made to correct the coagulopathy by administration of plasma alone. Acceptable alternatives include plasmapheresis[51] or the administration of factor 7 concentrate[52] as a bridge to transplantation.

Mechanical means of hemorrhage control include direct compression, creation of portosystemic shunts, and surgical transection/reanastomosis of the esophagus. Endoscopic control of bleeding from varices involves sclerotherapy in infants too small to tolerate a banding device or endoscopic banding in toddlers and older children.[53] Balloon tamponade by Sengstaken-Blakemore tube carries substantial risk and has largely been abandoned. It should not be used to manage persistent bleeding after sclerotherapy because of the risk of esophageal perforation.

Complications of portal hypertension can be managed with surgical shunting procedures that decompress the portal system by creating a venous anastomosis between the portal and systemic circulations. Several surgical varieties exist. Central vascular shunts, such as portocaval or mesocaval shunts, carry substantial risk. Transjugular intrahepatic portosystemic shunts are frequently used in children who weigh more than 10 kg as a bridge to transplantation.[49] In the past, shunt thrombosis was sometimes treated with surgical esophageal transaction, but urgent liver transplantation with either a cadaveric or living related donor is the preferred therapeutic strategy under such conditions (see also Chapter 81).

Before liver transplantation became a reality, children with liver failure underwent benign neglect and died. In contrast, today's intensivist usually uses heroic measures to give children a chance for transplantation. Unfortunately, the absence of an available liver donor may prolong the need for intensive care of the patient with near-complete liver failure. In some cases, the use of prostaglandin E_2 as a cytoprotective agent[55] and performance of charcoal hemoperfusion to permit liver regeneration have shown promise. Other extracorporeal liver assist devices, analogous to dialysis for renal failure, remain investigational a decade after their inception.[56] In any event, the basic principles of therapy must be directed toward CNS resuscitation, minimization of gastrointestinal bleeding, normalization of metabolic state, and correction of coagulation profile. Ultimately, orthotopic transplantation holds the greatest promise for saving patients with end-stage liver disease.[57-60]

REFERENCES

1. Figueroa-Colon R, Gruen JE: Randomized study of premedications for esophagogastroduodenoscopy in children and adolescents, *J Pediatr Gastroenterol Nutr* 7:359, 1988.
2. Zintilin P, Dulbecco P, Savarino E et al: Combined multichannel intraluminal impedance and pH-metry: a novel technique to improve detection of gastroesophageal reflux literature review, *Dig Liver Dis* 36:565, 2004.
3. Maloney JP, Ryan TA: Detection of aspiration in enterally fed patients: a requiem for bedside monitoring of aspiration, *J Parenter Enteral Nutr* 26:S34, 2002.
4. Siegel MJ: Practical CT techniques. In Seigel MJ, editor: *Pediatric body CT*, New York, 1988, Churchill Livingstone.
5. Rosenthal MS, Klein HA, Orenstein SR: Simultaneous acquisition of physiological data and nuclear medicine images, *J Nucl Med* 29:1848, 1988.
6. McVeagh P, Howman-Giles R, Kemp A: Pulmonary aspiration studied by radionuclide milk scanning and barium swallow roentgenography, *Am J Dis Child* 141:917-921, 1987.
7. Bhargava S, Orenstein SR, Charron M: Technetium-99m hexamethylpropyleneamine-oxime-labelled scintigraphy in inflammatory bowel disease in children, *J Pediatr* 125:213, 1994.
8. Baker J, Carlson D, Ly P et al: Readability and sensitivity of two guaiac-based fecal occult blood tests, *Gastroenterology* 94:A18, 1988 (abstract).
9. Cheu HW, Brown DR, Rowe MI: Breath hydrogen excretion as a screening test for the early diagnosis of necrotizing enterocolitis, *Am J Dis Child* 143:156, 1989.
10. Moazam F, Talbert JL, Miller D et al: Caustic ingestion and its sequelae in children, *South Med J* 80:187, 1987.
11. Anderson KD, Rouse TM, Randolph JG: A controlled trial of corticosteroids in children with corrosive injury of the esophagus, *N Engl* J Med 323:637, 1990.
12. Wijburg FA, Heymans HS, Urbanus NA: Caustic esophageal lesions in childhood: prevention of stricture formation, *J Pediatr Surg* 24:171, 1989.
13. Sellars SL, Spence RA: Chemical burns of the oesophagus, *J Laryngol Otol* 101:1211, 1987.
14. Litovitz T, Schmitz BF: Ingestion of cylindrical and button batteries: an analysis of 2382 cases. *Pediatrics* 89:747, 1992.
15. Sacre L, Vandenplas Y: Gastroesophageal reflux associated with respiratory abnormalities during sleep, *J Pediatr Gastroenterol Nutr* 9:28, 1989.
16. Shaker R, Dodds WJ, Ren J et al: Esophageal closure reflex: a mechanism of airway protection, *Gastroenterology* 102:857, 1992.
17. Bar-Sever Z, Connolly LP, Treves ST: The radionuclide salivagram in children with pulmonary disease and high risk of aspiration, *Pediatr Radiol* 25:S180, 1995.
18. Nussbaum E, Maggi JC, Mathis R et al: Association of lipid-laden alveolar macrophages and gastroesophageal reflux in children, *J Pediatr* 110:190, 1987.
19. Cook DJ, Reeve BK, Guyatt GH et al: Stress ulcer prophylaxis in critically ill patients: resolving discordant meta-analyses, *JAMA* 275:308, 1996.
20. Blazer MJ: Gastric *Campylobacter*-like organisms, gastritis, and peptic ulcer disease, *Gastroenterology* 93:371, 1987.
21. Pisegna JR: Treating patients with acute gastrointestinal bleeding or rebleeding, *Pharmacotherapy* 23:81S,2003.
22. Drumm B, Rhoads JM, Stringer DA et al: Peptic ulcer disease in children: etiology, clinical findings and clinical course, *Pediatrics* 82:410, 1988.
23. Tam PKH: Serum pepsinogen I in childhood duodenal ulcer, *J Pediatr Gastroenterol Nutr* 6:904, 1987.
24. Coughlan G, Gilligan D, Humphries H et al: *Campylobacter pylori* and recurrence of duodenal ulcers: a 12 month follow-up study, *Lancet* 2:1109, 1987.
25. Blecker U, Gold BD: Gastritis and peptic ulcer disease in childhood, *Eur J Pediatr* 158:541,1999.
26. Berseth CL, Bisquiera JA, Paje VU: Prolonging small feeding volumes early in life decreases the incidence of necrotizing enterocolitis in very low birthweight infants, *Pediatrics* 111:529, 2003.
27. Scheifele DW, Bjornson GL, Dyer RA et al: Delta-like toxin produced by coagulase negative staphylococci is associated with neonatal necrotizing enterocolitis, *Infect Immun* 55:2268, 1987.
28. Ein SH, Shandling B, Wesson D et al: A 13-year experience with peritoneal drainage under local anesthesia for necrotizing enterocolitis perforation, *J Pediatr Surg* 25:1034, 1990.
29. Sampson HA: IgE-mediated food intolerance, *J Allergy Clin Immunol* 81:495, 1988.
30. Proujansky R, Winter H, Walker WA: Gastrointestinal syndromes associated with food sensitivity, *Adv Pediatr* 35:219, 1988.
31. Fisher M: Anaphylaxis, *Dis Mon* 33:441, 1987.
32. Neill MA, Tarr PI, Clausen CR et al: *Escherichia coli* O157:H7 as a predominant pathogen associated with the hemolytic uremic syndrome: a prospective study in the Pacific Northwest, *Pediatrics* 80:37, 1987.
33. Tarr PI: *Escherichia coli* O157:H7: clinical, diagnostic, and epidemiological aspects of human infection, *Clin Infect Dis* 20:1, 1995.

34. Siegler RL: Management of hemolytic-uremic syndrome, *J Pediatr* 112:1014, 1988.
35. Duerr RH: Update on the genetics of inflammatory bowel disease, *J Clin Gastroenterol* 37:166, 2004.
36. Rutgeerts PJ: An historical overview of the treatment of Crohn's disease: why do we need biological therapies? *Rev Gastroenterol Dis* 4(suppl 3):S3-S9, 2004.
37. Hyams JS, Treem WR: Cyclosporine treatment of fulminant colitis, *J Pediatr Gastroenterol Nutr* 9:383, 1989.
38. Russell GH, Katz AJ: Infliximab is effective in acute but not chronic ulcerative colitis, *J Pediatric Gastroenterol Nutr* 39:166, 2004.
39. Passarge E: Dissecting Hirschsprung's disease, *Nature Genetics* 31:11, 2002.
40. Ponec RJ, Saunders MD, Kimmey MB: Neostigmine for the treatment of acute colonic pseudo-obstruction, *N Engl J Med* 340:1655, 1999.
41. Uden S, Bilton D, Guyan PM et al: Rationale for antioxidant therapy in pancreatitis and cystic fibrosis, *Adv Exp Med Biol* 264:555, 1990.
42. Havala T, Shronts E, Cerra F: Nutritional support in acute pancreatitis, *Gastroenterol Clin N Am* 18:525, 1989
43. Latifi R, McIntosh JK, Dudrick SJ: Nutritional management of acute and chronic pancreatitis, *Surg Clin North Am* 71:579, 1991.
44. Marulendra S, Kirby DF: Nutrition support in pancreatitis, *Nutr Clin Pract* 10:45, 1995.
45. Balistreri WF: Viral hepatitis, *Pediatr Clin North Am* 35:375, 1988.
46. Fitzgerald JF: Cholestatic disorders of infancy, *Pediatr Clin North Am* 35:357, 1988.
47. McAfee JH, Keeffe EB, Lee RG: Transjugular liver biopsy, *Hepatology* 15:726, 1992.
48. Rivera-Pienera, Moreno J, Shaff C et al: Delayed encephalopathy in fulminant hepatic failure in the pediatric population and the role of liver transplantation, *J Pediatr Gastroenteerol Nutr* 24:128, 1997.
49. Als-Nielson B, Gluud LL, Gluud C: Benzodiazepine receptor antagonists for hepatic encephalopathy, *Cochrane Database Syst Rev* 4:CD002718, 2001.
50. Arroyo V, Bernardi M, Epstein M et al: Pathophysiology of ascites and functional renal failure in cirrhosis, *J Hepatol* 6:239, 1988.
51. Singer AL, Olthoff KM, Kim H et al: Role of plasmapheresis in the management of acute hepatic failure in children, *Ann Surg* 234: 418, 2001.
52. Brown JB, Emerich KM, Brown DL, et al: Recombinant factor VIIa improves coagulopathy caused by liver failure, *J Pediatr Gastroenterol Nutr* 37:268, 2003.
53. Hall RJ, Lilly JR, Stiegmann GV: Endoscopic esophageal varix ligation: technique and preliminary results in children, *J Pediatr Surg* 23:1222, 1988.
54. McCormick PA, Dick R, Burroughs AK: Review article: the transjugular intrahepatic portosytemic shunt (TIPS) in the treatment of portal hypertension, *Aliment Pharmacol Ther* 8:273, 1994.
55. Abecassis M, Falk JA, Makowka L et al: 16,16 Dimethyl prostaglandin E2 prevents the development of fulminant hepatitis and blocks the induction of monocyte/macrophage procoagulant activity after murine virus type 3 infection, *J Clin Invest* 80:881, 1987.
56. Sussman NL, Gislason GT, Kelly JH: Extracorporeal liver support: application to fulminant hepatic failure, *J Clin Gastroenterol* 18: 320, 1994.
57. Starzl TE, Demetris AJ: Liver transplantation: a 31-year perspective, part I, *Curr Probl Surg* 27:49, 1990.
58. Starzl TE, Demetris AJ: Liver transplantation: a 31-year perspective, part II, *Curr Probl Surg* 27:117, 1990.
60. Starzl TE, Demetris AJ: Liver transplantation: a 31-year perspective, part III, *Curr Probl Surg* 27:181, 1990.

CHAPTER

80

Gastrointestinal Pharmacology

Michael A. Cimino, Kristin K. Johnson, and Kelly A. Michienzi

PEARLS

- Medications that frequently cause nausea and vomiting include the following:
  - Antineoplastic agents with varying degrees of emetogenicity
  - Anesthetics (e.g., thiopental, halothane)
  - Antimicrobials (e.g., imipenem-cilastatin, erythromycin, metronidazole)
  - Contrast media
  - Opiates
- Nausea and vomiting can be both debilitating and life threatening, depending on the cause and severity.
- Severe or protracted vomiting can lead to aspiration of gastric contents and disruption of a surgical site.
- Vomiting and retching, in the presence of increased intracranial pressure, can be life threatening.
- Considering efficacy and safety profiles, the serotonin receptor antagonists appear to be the most effective and safest agents for the treatment or prevention of acute nausea and vomiting in children.
- Diarrhea in the critical care patient has multiple causes, including infections with viruses or bacteria or as a consequence of drug therapy.
- Constipation is a decrease in the normal frequency of defecation and in the pediatric critical care unit is most often a result of a neuromuscular handicap, a metabolic disorder, an endocrine disease, or narcotic use.
- Acute liver failure may occur as a result of infection, toxin exposure, drug therapy, or response to one's own immune system.

Nausea and Vomiting

Cause

Nausea and vomiting frequently occur in hospitalized patients because of numerous disease and treatment-related causes.[1] Common causes within the pediatric critical care setting include increased intracranial pressure that results from mass lesion or trauma; meningitis; bowel obstruction; ileus; hepatobiliary disease; diabetic ketoacidosis; hepatitis; pancreatitis; peritonitis; gastrointestinal bleeding; medications; and surgery, in particular neurosurgical and craniofacial operations. Medications frequently causing nausea and vomiting include antineoplastic agents with varying degrees of emetogenicity, anesthetics (e.g., thiopental, halothane), antimicrobials (e.g., imipenem-cilastatin, erythromycin, metronidazole), contrast media, and opiates. Nausea and vomiting can be both debilitating and life threatening, depending on the cause and severity. Severe or protracted vomiting can lead to aspiration of gastric contents and disruption of the surgical site. Vomiting and retching, in the presence of increased intracranial pressure, can be life threatening.

An understanding of chemotherapy-induced nausea and vomiting provides the clearest insight into the neurotransmitters, receptors, and pathways mediating these adverse reactions.[1] Both serotonin type 3 and tachykinin-neurokinin type 1 receptors in the gastrointestinal (GI) tract mediate the transmission of impulses to the nucleus tractus solitarius and vomiting center, where dopamine type 2, histamine type 1, muscarinic, serotonin type 3 and tachykinin-neurokinin type 1 receptors are stimulated to induce nausea and vomiting. With the exception of histamine type 1, the chemoreceptor trigger zone initiates impulses to the vomiting center through similar receptors in response to emetogenic substances in the blood. The cerebral cortex also influences the vomiting center in the overall process.

Treatment

When the group of medications with antiemetic effects is considered (see Table 80–1), the serotonin antagonist group, which includes ondansetron, granisetron, and dolasetron, has the potential to affect most pathways; this explains, in part, their relative high rate of efficacy. Aprepitant, the first of the neurokinin type 1 receptor antagonists marketed in the United States, is unique in its mechanism of action among these antiemetics.[2,3] Given the effectiveness of the serotonin receptor antagonists and neurokinin type 1 receptor antagonists, the other agents listed in Table 80–1 can be considered adjuvant medications. Adjuvant medications can be used in combination with the serotonin receptor antagonists to optimize control of emesis when effectiveness is less than desired. Within the pediatric population, several of these medications are avoided because of their adverse effect profile. Most notably, agitation, sedation, and extrapyramidal reactions are seen among the phenothiazines and metoclopramide; oculogyric crisis is seen, in particular.[1,4] Similar effects can be expected in children from agents in the butyrophenone and benzamide groups on the basis of their pharmacological properties and established side effect profiles. One case report suggests metoclopramide possesses the potential to increase intracranial pressure in patients experiencing head injury[5]; this further limits the use of this agent in the pediatric population. Therefore the antihistamines, benzodiazepines, corticosteroids, and serotonin antagonists remain the agents most appropriate in pediatrics.[6] Although not approved for use in the pediatric population, aprepitant may offer relief for patients who are difficult to manage,[2] particularly patients receiving chemotherapy. For example, after high-dose cisplatin chemotherapy, the addition of aprepitant to the antiemetic regimen improved efficacy by approximately 20% to 45%, with the greatest impact on delayed nausea and vomiting, which occurred on days 2 to 5 following chemotherapy.[3]

TABLE 80–1

Commonly Used Antiemetic Agents

Antiemetic Group	Specific Agents
Serotonin receptor antagonists	Ondansetron Granisetron Dolasetron
Dopamine receptor antagonists	Phenothiazines Prochlorperazine Promethazine Chlorpromazine Butyrophenones Droperidol Haloperidol Benzamides Metoclopramide Trimethobenzamide
Neurokinin type 1 receptor antagonists	Aprepitant
Antihistamine compounds	Diphenhydramine Hydroxyzine
Antimuscarini Agents	Scopolamine
Corticosteroids	Dexamethasone Methylprednisolone
Benzodiazepines	Lorazepam
Cannabinoids	Dronabinol

Ondansetron, granisetron, and dolasetron have been studied in the pediatric population for the prevention and treatment of chemotherapy-induced nausea and vomiting with comparable efficacy.[7-12] Reported efficacy rates range from approximately 60% to more than 90% during the first 24 hours of treatment, depending on the emetogenicity of the chemotherapy and concurrently administered antiemetics. Some evidence exists suggesting the antiemetic efficacy of an alternate serotonin antagonist when emesis is refractory to other agents in this group.[13] These agents appear to be most effective for nausea and emesis occurring within the first 24 hours of chemotherapy administration. Use of dexamethasone in combination with the serotonin receptor antagonists improves overall response, in particular for delayed emesis, which is defined as occurring after the first 24-hour period.[14-16]

The serotonin receptor antagonists have also been studied in the pediatric population for the prevention and treatment of postoperative nausea and vomiting,[14,17-29] and they show similar efficacy. All have been studied after strabismus operations with comparable efficacy.[22,26,27] Ondansetron has been compared with the antihistamine group of antiemetics, with conflicting results.[19,20] The addition of dexamethasone before an operation appears to prolong the antiemetic effect when compared with the serotonin antagonists alone.[28] In patients pretreated with dexamethasone, dolasetron and ondansetron provide equivalent postoperative vomiting control.[29] The addition of droperidol to granisetron also appears to improve antiemetic efficacy[22,30]; however, the use of droperidol in pediatric patients has been discouraged because of the potential for adverse effects, including QT prolongation, torsades de pointes, hypotension, dysphoria, drowsiness, hyperactivity, extrapyramidal effects, and anxiety.

Ondansetron has been shown to be effective after neurosurgical procedures such as craniotomy[31,32] and posterior fossa neurosurgical procedures.[33] Its role has been defined in craniofacial operations in children, with a single dose of 0.15 mg/kg[34] (Table 80-2). Ondansetron has been used successfully in controlling projectile vomiting in patients with neurosurgical trauma,[35] in children receiving radiation therapy for treatment of brain tumors,[36] and in children and adolescents undergoing radiofrequency catheter ablation

TABLE 80–2

Indications and Doses of Select Antiemetic Agents

Drug	Chemotherapy-Induced Nausea & Vomiting	Postoperative Nausea & Vomiting
Ondansetron	Children > 3 years of age: 0.15 mg/kg IV starting 30 min before chemotherapy then every 4 hr for 2 doses Maximum dose = 32 mg 4 to 11 years of age: 4 mg PO q 8 hr for 1 to 2 days starting 30 min before chemotherapy administration > 12 years of age: 8 mg PO q 8 hr for 1 to 2 days, starting 30 min before chemotherapy administration	Children 2 to 12 years of age: 0.1 mg/kg IV before anesthesia in patients weighing < 40 kg Dose may be repeated if nausea and vomiting occur Patients weighing > 40 kg: 4 mg IV × 1
Granisetron	Children > 2 years of age and adults: 10 µg/kg IV daily, starting 30 min before chemotherapy (maximum dose = 3 mg) Doses up to 20 to 40 µg/kg IV have been used	Children > 4 years of age: 20 to 40 µg/kg IV 1 (maximum dose = 1 mg) Adults: 1 mg IV × 1
Dolasetron	Children 2 to 16 years of age: 1.8 mg/kg IV (maximum = 100 mg) 30 min before chemotherapy The oral dose is the same but is given 1 hr before chemotherapy administration Adults: 100 mg IV as a single dose starting 30 min before chemotherapy administration or PO starting 1 hr before chemotherapy administration	Children 2 to 16 years of age: 0.35 mg/kg IV × 1, 15 min before the end of anesthesia (12.5 mg maximum dose) or 1.2 mg/kg PO within 2 hr before surgery (100 mg maximum dose) Adults: 12.5 mg IV × 1, 15 min before the end of anesthesia or 100 mg PO × 1, within 2 hr before surgery
Metoclopramide	Adults and children: 1 to 2 mg/kg/dose IV q 2 to 4 hr Dose adjustment is necessary for renal dysfunction	Children: 0.1 to 0.2 mg/kg/dose IV q 6 to 8 hr (10 mg maximum per dose) Children > 14 years of age and adults:10 mg IV q 6 to 8 hr
Aprepitant	Adults: 125 mg with a serotonin receptor antagonist and dexamethasone 12 mg PO on first day, then 80 mg daily × 2 days with dexamethasone 8 mg PO	

under general anesthesia with either propofol or isoflurane.[37] The addition of antiemetics, including ondansetron and droperidol, to the patient-controlled analgesia morphine solution does not appear to control postoperative nausea and vomiting after appendectomy in children.[38]

The serotonin receptor antagonists also appear optimal in treating the nausea and vomiting associated with acetaminophen poisoning (see also Chapters 98 and 99).[39] Although treatment with N-acetylcysteine (NAC) via the intravenous route is considerably less emetogenic than oral NAC, the use of serotonin receptor antagonists will likely continue to be necessary because vomiting frequently occurs as a result of toxic acetaminophen serum levels.[40]

Ondansetron, granisetron, and dolasetron are approved for the prevention and treatment of chemotherapy-induced nausea and vomiting in both adults and children. The dosage of ondansetron for this indication is 0.15 mg/kg (32 mg maximum), beginning 30 minutes before administration of chemotherapy and repeated at 4 and 8 hours after the first dose (see Table 79–2).[41] Ondansetron may be administered orally, when possible. For nausea and vomiting occurring or persisting beyond 24 hours after the first dose of chemotherapy, dexamethasone may be added for improved efficacy. The intravenous dosage commonly used for this indication is 10 mg/m^2 (20 mg maximum) as a first dose, then 5 mg/m^2 (10 mg maximum) every 6 hours. Despite the greater likelihood of adverse effects, metoclopramide continues to be used in some centers. The incidence of extrapyramidal side effects can be decreased, or the severity lessened, with the combined use of diphenhydramine. Diphenhydramine may be administered intravenously (IV) or orally, at a dosage of 5 mg/kg/day or 150 mg/m^2/day, divided every 6 to 8 hours in children, with a maximum dosage equivalent to the adult dose of 50 mg every 4 hours. Dexamethasone may be added to this combination for increased efficacy.

Both ondansetron and dolasetron are indicated for the prevention and treatment of postoperative nausea and vomiting in children. Granisetron is approved for this indication in adults. The dosage of ondansetron in children weighing less than 40 kg is 0.1 mg/kg IV as a single dose before anesthesia is initiated or after anesthesia if nausea or vomiting occurs. In children and adults weighing greater than 40 kg, a dose of 4 mg is recommended.

Lorazepam can be used adjunctively in patients with anticipatory nausea and vomiting, in those with a significant contribution to emesis arising from the cerebral pathway, and as a rescue medication when other antiemetics demonstrate an insufficient response. The recommended dosage of lorazepam for this indication is 0.04 to 0.08 mg/kg per dose (maximum of 4 mg), administered IV every 6 hours as needed.

Adverse Effects

Adverse effects related to metoclopramide include extrapyramidal reactions, which occur more frequently in children than in adults.[1] These most commonly include tardive dyskinesia and dystonic reactions. Other less common side effects include neuroleptic syndrome and supraventricular tachycardia. As a group, the serotonin receptor antagonists are well tolerated and associated with fewer adverse reactions, in particular, less extrapyramidal effects. These agents, however, may cause electrocardiographic interval changes (PR, QTc, and ST prolongation with QRS widening). Side effects associated with dexamethasone include those common to other corticosteroids such as gastrointestinal upset, anxiety, insomnia, euphoria, and hyperglycemia. The benzodiazepine medications, as a group, commonly cause sedation; amnesia; and rarely, respiratory depression and paradoxical emotional reactions.

Summary

When the efficacy and safety profiles of the various medications used in adults and children are considered, the serotonin receptor antagonists appear to be the most effective and safest agents for the treatment or prevention of acute nausea and vomiting in children. Most studies of these medications have primarily addressed chemotherapy-induced and postoperative nausea and vomiting. They are likely to be as effective and safe when used to treat these symptoms resulting from a variety of other causes. The duration of symptoms, however, may play a role in their effectiveness. Patients with nausea and vomiting resulting from head trauma or following a surgical procedure—in particular, those involving the central nervous system—generally appear in the critical care setting within the first 24 hours after the initiating event. During this time frame, the serotonin receptor antagonists are maximally effective; however, prevention and treatment of nausea and vomiting after the acute period may be less efficacious and may require the addition of other antiemetics such as dexamethasone and lorazepam. These medications are frequently administered concurrently in the critical care setting for other indications, including cerebral edema and sedation. In most cases, patients who have received chemotherapy do not require admission to a critical care unit. If admission is necessary, however, the time frame is generally during the period of delayed emesis. In these cases, dexamethasone, lorazepam, and the antihistamines may be useful adjunctively to control nausea and vomiting.

Diarrhea

Cause

Diarrhea in the critical care patient has multiple causes, including infections with viruses or bacteria or as a consequence of drug therapy. At birth the gastrointestinal tract is without intestinal flora; it is considered sterile. Organisms are acquired starting at the time of delivery by ingesting maternal flora (vaginal and fecal) or through the environment in cesarean-delivered infants. This acquired enteric flora may be modified by antibiotic use. Antibiotic-associated diarrhea, or diarrhea caused by the use of antibiotic therapy, is one well-known cause of diarrhea in the hospitalized patient. In fact, it is estimated that 20% to 40% of all children receiving broad-spectrum antibiotics have diarrhea.[42] Most antibiotic-associated diarrhea is thought to be due to disturbances in bacterial metabolism that affect short chain fatty acid production in the large intestine. Specifically, antibiotics kill the organisms responsible for producing the short chain fatty acids that are normally absorbed in the colon. Larger molecules therefore accumulate and exert an osmotic effect in the colon, resulting in diarrhea.[43] Rehydration is crucial and effective treatment for diarrheal diseases, and other therapies may be considered as determined appropriate.[44]

Clostridium Difficile

Clostridium difficile is an organism responsible for about one third of antibiotic-associated diarrhea cases. In these cases, the antibiotic causing the *C. difficile* disease should be discontinued if possible. Metronidazole is the treatment of choice for this diagnosis, with oral vancomycin as a second-line agent.[45] For those cases of antibiotic-associated diarrhea in which *C. difficile* is not isolated, there are few effective treatments in the pediatric population.

Treatment

Probiotics

Probiotics are defined as live organisms that result in health benefits, including prevention or elimination of a certain disease state. *Lactobacillus GG*, (previously classified as *Lactobacillus casei* and most recently classified as *Lactobacillus rhamnosus* GG), is one probiotic that when ingested has been shown to colonize the gastrointestinal tract with effective binding to intestinal epithelial cells while not being affected by gastric and bile secretions.[46] As a result of such colonization, *Lactobacillus GG* has been found to reduce the incidence of antibiotic-associated diarrhea in children treated with oral antibiotics.[42,47] Use of this agent may be helpful in the intensive care unit (ICU) setting when the patient has been treated for an extended time with antibiotics and has severe diarrhea or as a preventative measure to avoid the development of diarrhea. It has also been shown that infant formula supplemented with *Bifidobacterium bifidum* and *Streptococcus thermophilus* reduced the incidence of acute diarrhea and rotavirus shedding in hospitalized infants.[48] There are several other probiotics available such as *Saccharomyces boulardii and Bifidobacterium longum* that have also shown to reduce diarrhea in patients who were treated with antibiotics.[49,50] With an increasing number of probiotic options, it is most important to recognize that to be an effective and beneficial probiotic, the agent must have a sufficiently high live organism content.

Octreotide

Octreotide is a synthetic analogue of the naturally occurring somatostatin, an agent used to treat secretory diarrhea. It acts by inhibiting gastrointestinal hormone secretion, which leads to a decrease in chloride secretion and an increase in sodium absorption, ultimately resulting in decreased fluid losses. It also may prolong intestinal transit time. Octreotide has been used in many secretory diarrheal diseases with most pediatric experience described in case reports. It can be given through the intravenous or subcutaneous route, although it requires a longer time to reach maximum plasma concentration when given subcutaneously. Gastrointestinal absorption is poor, and therefore it should not be given orally. Side effects may include abdominal pain, sinus bradycardia, nausea, pain at the site of injection, elevation of liver enzymes, chest pain, emesis, headache, dizziness, fatigue, flushing, and diarrhea.[51]

Loperamide

Loperamide is a nonnarcotic antiperistaltic synthetic agent chemically related to meperidine and exhibits dose-related inhibition of intestinal motility. It slows intestinal motility through a direct effect on the nerve endings and the intramural ganglia of the intestinal wall. It prolongs transit time of intestinal contents and therefore reduces fecal volume, increases fecal viscosity and bulk density, and diminishes loss of fluid and electrolytes. Loperamide should not be used in the treatment of diarrhea resulting from any infectious cause; in patients with pseudomembranous colitis; or in patients in whom inhibiting intestinal motility could induce toxic megacolon, such as in acute ulcerative colitis. Side effects have been reported as unacceptably high, especially in infants, and include lethargy, ileus, respiratory depression and coma.[44]

Constipation

Cause

Constipation is a decrease in the normal frequency of defecation, and in the pediatric critical care unit it most often results from a neuromuscular handicap, a metabolic disorder, an endocrine disease, or narcotic use. It may be difficult to diagnose because bowel patterns vary among individuals according to age and diet.[52]

Narcotics are commonly used in the pediatric ICU to achieve sedation and pain control. Gastrointestinal hypomotility is an adverse effect to narcotic treatment, and constipation may result.[53] Illegal narcotic use may also cause constipation and may be noticed in a patient relatively soon after admission. Heroin use by American teenagers has been increasing year to year. Heroin is a potent semisynthetic analgesic produced by anhydrous acetylation of morphine. Approximately 40% of heroin users will initially experience adverse effects such as mild nausea and vomiting. Severe constipation may subsequently result and does not subside with continued use. As with most narcotics, withdrawal symptoms include vomiting and diarrhea, among other influenza-like symptoms. With heroin, this begins approximately 8 hours after the last dose taken.[54]

Treatment

Relief of constipation may be considered a two-step process consisting of disimpaction followed by maintenance therapy. If drug-induced, the offending agent should be discontinued and one or both of the steps of treatment may then be completed. Disimpaction may be pharmacologically achieved with oral or rectal medication. The oral approach is less invasive but the rectal route is quicker. Oral medications include high doses of mineral oil, polyethylene glycol electrolyte solutions, or both. High-dose magnesium hydroxide, magnesium citrate, lactulose, sorbitol, senna, and bisacodyl are laxatives that have been used successfully for initial disimpaction. Rectal disimpaction may be pharmacologically accomplished with phosphate soda enemas, saline enemas, or mineral oil enemas followed by a phosphate enema. Glycerin suppositories in infants and bisacodyl suppositories in older children have been effective. The use of soapsuds, tap water, and magnesium enemas is not recommended because of the potential for toxicity.[52,55]

If maintenance therapy is required after successful disimpaction, a lubricant such as mineral oil, or an osmotic laxative such as magnesium hydroxide, lactulose, or sorbitol, or a combination of a lubricant and an osmotic laxative are appropriate options. Results from long-term studies with mineral oil, magnesium hydroxide, and lactulose or sorbitol indicate that these are effective and safe with chronic use. Lactulose is commonly prescribed in the pediatric ICU for bowel therapy maintenance. Lactulose is metabolized in the colon by bacteria to acidic metabolites. The acidic pH stimulates peristalsis and decreases stool transit time. The decreased stool transit time leads to decreased water absorption, which results in softer stools. In addition, it also draws fluid into the gut by osmotic action softening stool and stimulating peristalsis. Consequently, it may cause significant abdominal cramping and flatulence.[55] A stimulant laxative such as bisacodyl may be necessary intermittently but is not recommended for prolonged use.[52]

Motility Disorders: Prokinetic Agents

In children, as in adults, the primary use of prokinetic agents has been to treat gastroesophageal reflux disease (GERD). The options of available prokinetic agents are unfortunately rather limited, and efficacy and safety data involving pediatric patients are lacking. Useful motility agents include metoclopramide, cisapride, and erythromycin.

Metoclopramide and Cisapride

Metoclopramide promotes gastric emptying by acting as an antagonist to the inhibitory actions of dopamine in the gut. It also sensitizes the gut to acetylcholine and increases lower esophageal sphincter tone.[56] Cisapride is a prokinetic agent that at one time was widely used not only for GERD but also for a variety of adult and pediatric motility disorders, including constipation and gastroparesis. It was prescribed more frequently than metoclopramide in children most likely because of its broader range of action and decreased risk of neurological side effects. Prolongation of the QTc interval with potential life-threatening ventricular arrhythmias was reported when cisapride was used concomitantly with drugs that inhibit the hepatic cytochrome P450-3A4 system. This uncommon yet potentially fatal adverse effect led Janssen Pharmaceutica to place it under a controlled access program, making it no longer available in the U.S.

market. It is available through the limited access protocol with close supervision by a pediatric gastroenterologist through contacting Janssen. The use of metoclopramide and cisapride is discussed further in the GERD section.

Erythromycin

Erythromycin is a macrolide antibiotic and motilin agonist. It increases motility in the proximal gastrointestinal tract. It is most commonly used in the treatment of diabetic gastroparesis.[57] Erythromycin is a prokinetic agent with the most frequent adverse effects being abdominal cramping, nausea, vomiting, diarrhea, cardiac dysrhythmias with interacting medications, and risk of bacterial overgrowth. Before this agent is ordered to treat constipation, the benefits for using this agent should greatly outweigh the severe adverse effects that may result.

Gastroesophageal Reflux Disease

Treatment of GERD should alleviate symptoms and prevent or heal esophageal damage. Although researchers of many pediatric studies have used varying doses, multiple drug therapies, and nonpharmacological therapies, guidelines do exist for the treatment of GERD in infants and children.[58]

Histamine 2–Receptor Antagonists

Histamine 2 (H_2)–receptor antagonists inhibit gastric acid secretion by means of competitive inhibition of H_2 receptors of the gastric parietal cells. H_2-receptor antagonists are generally well tolerated. Common adverse effects include nausea and headache. Although thrombocytopenia may occur, it is often difficult to determine as the sole cause in critically ill patients. Ranitidine should be avoided in patients with acute porphyria. All of the currently available H_2-receptor blockers require dosage adjustment for renal impairment. Although fewer pediatric studies exist for ranitidine and famotidine, these agents are frequently used and may be preferred over cimetidine because of fewer drug interactions and adverse effects on the central nervous system. Availability of both oral and intravenous formulations allow for easy continuation of therapy when patients are admitted to the ICU.

Proton Pump Inhibitors

By covalently bonding to the hydrogen potassium-ATPase of parietal cells, proton pump inhibitors suppress gastric acid secretion for the life of the parietal cell. Ideally, therapy should be given 30 minutes before feeding so that peak plasma concentrations coincide with parietal cell stimulation.[58] Although their serum half-lives are relatively short, the pharmacological effect persists until new parietal cells are generated. Proton pump inhibitors are also well tolerated. Both omeprazole and lansoprazole have been approved for use in pediatrics. Extemporaneously compounded suspensions of omeprazole and lansoprazole are frequently used, even in patients with various types of feeding tubes. Although intravenous lansoprazole has been approved, this formulation has not been widely tested in pediatric patients. Until sufficient pediatric dosing information becomes available, intravenous proton pump inhibitors are likely to be reserved for patients with active GI bleeding or contraindication to alternative therapies.

Antacids

Both aluminum hydroxide and magnesium hydroxide are effective treatments of GERD. In infants, however, aluminum hydroxide formulations can increase plasma levels of aluminum to those reported to cause osteopenia, microcytic anemia, and neurotoxicity. Aluminum-based antacids should be avoided in patients with renal impairment. Efficacy of calcium carbonate antacids has not been demonstrated in pediatric patients. Depending on the antacid formulation chosen, adverse effects may include electrolyte disturbances, nausea, flatulence, diarrhea, or constipation. Because alternative therapies are available and generally well tolerated, antacids should be reserved for intermittent symptom management rather than chronic treatment of GERD.[58]

Surface Agents

Sucralfate, an aluminum salt of sulfated sucrose, forms a protective barrier by binding to damaged mucosa in an acidic environment. Although it has demonstrated effectiveness in the treatment of esophagitis, it is not recommended for treatment of GERD in children because of a lack of efficacy data and safety concerns associated with aluminum.[58]

Prokinetic Therapy

Prokinetic agents are of interest in GERD because of their ability to enhance esophageal peristalsis and accelerate gastric emptying. These agents include cisapride, metoclopramide, and bethanechol. In pediatric patients whose regurgitation or vomiting is the primary symptom of GERD, cisapride has modestly alleviated symptoms. In addition cisapride has been shown to decrease esophageal acid exposure, duration of reflux episodes, and number of episodes lasting longer than 5 minutes.[58] Because of cardiac adverse effects, however, cisapride is restricted to a limited access program as previously described. Metoclopramide blocks dopamine receptors in the chemoreceptor trigger zone and accelerates gastric emptying and intestinal transit time without stimulating gastric, biliary, or pancreatic secretions.[41] Clinical studies in both adults and pediatrics have failed to consistently show efficacy in GERD treatment.[58] In addition, adverse effects are common; are dose dependent; and can include extrapyramidal effects, tardive dyskinesia, seizures, and Parkinsonian reactions, which may be irreversible.[41, 58]

Stress-Induced Mucosal Damage: Ulcer Prophylaxis

Prospective studies reveal similar incidence of gastrointestinal hemorrhage between adult and pediatric ICUs. Of 1006 patients admitted to a pediatric ICU, 10.2% had upper GI hemorrhage; however, only 1.6% of the admissions were viewed as clinically significant. Respiratory failure, coagulopathy, and a PRISM (Pediatric Risk of Mortality) score greater than or equal to 10 were identified as independent risk factors for GI hemorrhage.[59] Other studies also identified pneumonia, multitrauma, an operation longer than 3 hours, and circulatory shock in patients as high-risk factors.[60,61] Mechanical ventilation and coagulopathy are recognized as independent risk factors in adult patients.[62] Because of the low incidence of clinically significant hemorrhage, prophylaxis may only be warranted in those patients with risk factors.[63]

Sucralfate, H_2-receptor antagonists, antacids, and proton pump inhibitors have been used for prophylaxis of stress-induced mucosal damage in pediatric critical care patients. Individual trials including comparative studies and case series have shown each agent to be effective. With the low incidence of clinically significant bleeds, studies intending to demonstrate superiority of one drug class or agent over another would require an extremely large sample size.

One study included 165 patients treated with ranitidine, antacid, sucralfate, or placebo. There were no differences among the treatment groups, and all treatment groups had a lower incidence of bleeding than the placebo group.[64] Another study compared ranitidine, omeprazole, sucralfate, or placebo for stress ulcer prophylaxis and also compared adverse events. No differences were found among groups with regard to macroscopic stress ulcer bleeding, mortality, or ventilator-associated pneumonia.[65] Because multiple agents appear to be effective for stress ulcer prophylaxis, selecting an appropriate agent may be patient specific. Critical care patients do present challenges with regard to drug administration for antacids and sucralfate. Both agents require multiple doses per day, lack intravenous formulations, and may chelate or inhibit other drugs. In addition, aluminum toxicity may be of greater concern in critical care patients because of the potential for renal impairment. H_2-receptor antagonists are commonly used because of the availability of intravenous formulations. Adverse effects of the central nervous system, particularly in patients with renal impairment who have not been dose adjusted; thrombocytopenia; and drug interactions remain a concern. Most of these adverse events, however, can be prevented or at least monitored for early detection. Proton pump inhibitors may also be used orally, IV, or off label through feeding tubes.

Gastrointestinal Hemorrhage

Clinical guidelines for treatment of nonvariceal upper GI bleeding in adults include recommendations for pharmacotherapy.[66] Unfortunately this body of evidence does not exist in the pediatric population. H_2-receptor antagonist use is discouraged as primary treatment for patients with acute bleeding. Although octreotide and somatostatin are more effective than H_2-receptor antagonists, these agents are also not recommended for routine management. Proton pump inhibitors are cited as the drugs of choice for treatment of acute nonvariceal upper gastrointestinal bleeding.[66] High-dose intravenous proton pump inhibitor therapy (80 mg pantoprazole bolus followed by 8 mg/hr for 72 hours after endoscopic therapy) is preferred over H_2-receptor antagonists alone, or in combination with octreotide, to prevent rebleeding in adult patients. As more data become available regarding the use of intravenous proton pump inhibitors in pediatric patients, parallels may be seen between the treatment of adult and pediatric nonvariceal upper GI bleeding.

Proton Pump Inhibitors

Multiple oral proton pump inhibitors are approved for pediatric use. Both pantoprazole and lansoprazole are available IV in the United States; however, neither product's intravenous formulation has been well studied in pediatric patients. Doses have been extrapolated from the adult high-dose intravenous pantoprazole recommendations for use in clinical practice in pediatric patients with nonvariceal upper GI bleeding. Although it is not yet specified in the literature, many pediatric sites reportedly use a pantoprazole loading dose of 2 mg/kg IV, followed by 0.2 mg/kg/hr for 72 hours (neither the loading dose nor continuous infusion should exceed the adult dose).

Octreotide and Somatostatin

Octreotide is a somatostatin analogue. Its pharmacologic actions include inhibition of gastric acid secretion and decreased splanchnic blood flow. Although its 1.7-hour half-life is approximately 30 times longer than that of somatostatin, octreotide is usually administered through continuous infusion for GI hemorrhage. Adverse effects include abdominal pain and sinus bradycardia, as well as those effects previously mentioned. Long-term use (longer than 1 month) has been associated with changes in thyroid function, gallstone formation, and cholecystitis.[51]

In adults octreotide has been shown to decrease the duration of hemorrhage and prevent recurrence of peptic disease more so than cimetidine or ranitidine. A Cochrane Review showed improved initial hemostasis and decreased transfusion requirements; however, no change was evident in rebleeding or secondary outcomes when octreotide was used to treat variceal bleeding.[51] Few researchers have evaluated octreotide for GI hemorrhage in pediatric patients. In one study, continuous infusion of octreotide in seven patients was evaluated. Bleeding ceased in six of the seven patients. The duration of infusion ranged from 24 to 234 hours. Although bleeding stopped within 24 hours in nearly half of the patients, on average, bleeding stopped after 40 hours. The most notable adverse effect was hyperglycemia.[67] Subcutaneous octreotide has also been used for severe chronic GI hemorrhage for periods of 24 to 50 months.[68]

Vasopressin

Generally vasopressin has been used for treatment of variceal bleeding more frequently than for nonvariceal upper GI bleeding. In fact, adult guidelines do not address the use of vasopressin for nonvariceal bleeding.[66] Vasopressin acts by mechanisms similar to octreotide; however, its effects on blood pressure make it a less desirable option in many patients.[69]

Helicobacter Pylori Infection

Patients who have GI bleeding of unknown etiology should be tested for *Helicobacter pylori*. At minimum, therapy requires three different medications administered twice daily for 1 to 2 weeks. Three different regimens are recommended for first-line treatment in pediatrics. Each consists of a proton pump inhibitor in combination with amoxicillin and clarithromycin, amoxicillin and metronidazole, or metronidazole and clarithromycin. Second-line options incorporate bismuth subsalicylate or ranitidine, and tetracycline as one of the antibiotic choices.[70] Tetracycline is contraindicated in patients younger than 8 years because of permanent discoloration of teeth, enamel hypoplasia, and retardation of skeletal development and bone growth.[41] Noncompliance with *H. pylori* regimens is the most commonly cited reason for treatment failure.[70]

Drug-Induced Liver Injury

Cause

Acute liver failure may occur as a result of infection, toxin exposure, drug therapy, or response to one's own immune system (see also Chapter 81). The two most commonly used scales for determination of drug-induced liver injury (DILI) are the Roussel UCLAF Causality Assessment Method (RUCAM) and the Clinical Diagnostic Scale. Both methods take into account temporal relationship, course, exclusion of alternative causes, and rechallenge. The RUCAM also considers risk factors, exclusion of nondrug factors, and likelihood on the basis of product labeling. The Clinical Diagnostic Scale, developed more recently, evaluates extra hepatic manifestations and previous literature reports. Neither system addresses how the scores should affect clinical decision making or reporting to supervising agencies. The Acute Liver Failure Study Group is funded by the National Institutes of Health to collect data from 21 adult and 19 pediatric sites throughout the United States. Unlike the two previously mentioned causality assessment methods, this group collects data on a prospective basis for causality, pathophysiology, and treatment.[71] Table 80–3 highlights agents that are common causes of DILI, as well as those named in case reports in either adult or pediatric patients. For further review of the type of injury associated with each agent or a summary of the case report, please see the cited references.

Treatment

Several pharmacological interventions may be initiated to compensate for the various complications that occur during liver failure, either acutely or prophylactically.

Cerebral Edema and Hepatic Encephalopathy (see also Chapter 53)

Fluid restriction, intravenous mannitol, glucose control, and continuous infusion furosemide may be used to treat cerebral edema.[72] Bacterial consumption of lactulose acidifies the colon, which transforms free ammonia to ammonium ions, allowing the ions to become trapped in the colon. Serum ammonia levels are in turn decreased.[73] In a review of nonabsorbable disaccharides for adult hepatic encephalopathy, lactulose was found to reduce the risk of no improvement of encephalopathy when compared with placebo. Antibiotics decreased ammonia levels and reduced the risk of no improvement to a greater degree than lactulose.[74] Other references, however, recommend lactulose as first line over oral antibiotics, such as neomycin, for both acute and chronic encephalopathy in adults.[75] In pediatric patients, lactulose is more commonly used.[72] Adverse effects include diarrhea, flatulence, nausea, and vomiting.

Ascites

The lowest effective diuretic dose should be used to decrease ascites. Spironolactone, furosemide, and thiazides have been used most commonly. Spironolactone selectively inhibits the effects of aldosterone on the distal renal tubule and collecting systems, which may be advantageous in hepatogenous ascites because it is usually associated with secondary hyperaldosteronism.[76] Spironolactone may be used in combination with thiazide or loop diuretics, particularly if therapeutic endpoints are still not achieved after spironolactone dose escalation. Addition of a thiazide or loop diuretic increases the likelihood of adverse effects such as hypokalemia and metabolic alkalosis, which may precipitate hepatic encephalopathy by creating an environment that increases ammonia reabsorption.[76] Therefore serum electrolytes and acid base status should be closely monitored and appropriately treated. In patients with low albumin levels, albumin infusion followed by furosemide may also be used to treat ascites.

Coagulopathy and Hemorrhagic Complications

Effective management of coagulopathy may prevent or decrease bleeding episodes in hepatic failure. Prevention of GI bleeding can be achieved with H_2-receptor blockers and sucralfate. Although pediatric data are limited, beta-blockers have been used in primary and secondary prevention of variceal bleeding in adult patients with hepatic failure. Beta-blockers constrict splanchnic blood vessels, and this constriction decreases portal blood flow. In one small pediatric study beta-blockers prevented variceal bleeding. Failure to prevent bleeding was associated with nonadherence to therapy.[77] In general, because of the limited data in pediatrics, beta-blocker use in the prevention of variceal bleeding is considered adjunctive therapy to nonpharmacological treatments such as sclerotherapy or endoscopic variceal band ligation.[69] Both intravenous octreotide and vasopressin have been used in acute treatment of variceal bleeding.[51, 72] As previously mentioned, though, octreotide may be preferred over vasopressin to avoid undesired blood pressure effects. In a Cochrane Review of octreotide use in the treatment of variceal hemorrhage in adults, octreotide was associated with improved initial hemostasis and reduced need for transfusion.[51] In the small number of case series in which the use of vasopressin or octreotide in pediatric patients was evaluated, variceal bleeding ceased more than 50% of the time.[69]

TABLE 80–3

Drug-Induced Liver Injury[82-85]

Drug Class or Group	Specific Agents & Reaction	Comments
Analgesics	Acetaminophen — necrosis Aspirin — Reye's syndrome, hepatitis Bromfenac* — acute liver failure Sulindac, indomethacin — cholestasis, hepatitis Celecoxib — hepatocellular Diclofenac, meloxicam — hepatitis Etodolac — fulminant hepatic failure Ibuprofen (rare) — hepatitis, vanishing bile duct syndrome Oxaprozin — hepatocellular, hepatitis Piroxicam — hepatocellular, cholestasis, Necrosis	Although all drugs may not be hepatotoxic, NSAID use in patients with liver failure may worsen GI bleeding
Cardiovascular agents	Amiodarone — fatty liver Methyldopa — hepatitis, cirrhosis, granulomas, cholestasis Quinidine — granulomas *Beta blockers* (metoprolol, propranolol, acebutolol, atenolol, labetalol) — hepatocellular, cholestasis, (labetalol) — necrosis, hepatitis *Calcium channel blockers* (diltiazem, nifedipine, verapamil) — hepatitis, cholestasis Hydralazine — hepatitis, granulomas, cholestasis *Diuretics* (hydrochlorothiazide, chlorothiazide, chlorthalidone) — hepatitis, cholestasis *ACE inhibitors* (captopril, enalapril) — cholestasis,hepatitis	Labetalol considered most hepatotoxic beta-blocker
Drugs used in the treatment of diabetes mellitus	*Glucosidase inhibitors* (acarbose) — hepatitis, cholestasis Metformin — cholestasis, hepatitis Human insulin — hepatocellular *Sulfonylureas* (chlorpropamide, glimepiride, glipizide, tolbutamide) — hepatitis, cholestasis, vanishing bile duct syndrome *Thiazolidinediones* (troglitazone*) — fulminant liver failure	For thiazolidinediones, monitor baseline ALT & every 2 mo thereafter for first year of therapy
Lipid lowering agents	*HMG-CoA reductase inhibitors* (statins) (atorvastatin, cerivastatin*, fluvastatin, lovastatin, pravastatin, simvastatin) — cholestasis, hepatitis, acute liver failure *Fibrates* (gemfibrozil, fenofibrate, nicotinic acid) — hepatitis, necrosis, acute liver failure, cholestasis	For statins, monitor liver tests at baseline, 12 wk, and every 6 mo thereafter
Anticonvulsants	Phenytoin — hepatitis (rare) Carbamazepine — hepatitis, cholestasis, vanishing bile duct syndrome, granulomas Valproic acid — reversible increase in aminotransferases, necrosis, fatty liver (high-risk patients: < 3 years of age, personal or family history of mitochondrial enzyme deficiency, Reye's syndrome, Friedreich's ataxia, history of sibling with valproic acid toxicity, multiple drug therapy) Lamotrigine — hepatitis Felbamate — hepatitis, acute liver failure (reserve for refractory patients or Lennox-Gastaut syndrome) Topiramate — acute liver failure, hepatocellular	Often seen in conjunction with hypersensitivity syndromes (reactive metabolite syndrome)
Psychotropic & antidepressant drugs	Amitriptyline — hepatitis Haloperidol — cholestasis Imipramine — hepatitis Chlorpromazine — cholestasis Prochlorperazine — cholestasis Sertraline — hepatitis (rare) Clozapine — hepatocellular, fulminant hepatic failure Risperidone — hepatocellular Olanzapine — hepatitis, hypersensitivity syndrome Nefazodone — liver failure	

continued

TABLE 80–3—Cont'd

Drug-Induced Liver Injury[82-85]		
Drug Class or Group	**Specific Agents & Reaction**	**Comments**
Immunosuppressant and chemotherapy	Asparaginase — fatty liver Azathioprine — cholestatic hepatitis Busulfan — cholestasis Cyclosporine — cholestasis Gemcitabine — cholestatic, hepatitis Methotrexate — fatty liver Leflunomide — severe hepatic injury Infliximab — cholestasis, hepatitis Tamoxifen — cholestasis	
Anesthetics	Halothane, isoflurane — necrosis, hepatitis	
Antiinfectives	*Antibiotics* Erythromycin — cholestasis Dapsone — hepatitis Nitrofurantoin — hepatitis Rifampin — hepatitis Sulfonamides — granulomas Tetracycline fatty liver Sulfamethoxazole and trimethoprim — hepatitis, cholestasis *Antifungal agents* (ketoconazole, fluconazole, itraconazole) — hepatitis *Antiretroviral agents* Indinavir — fatty liver Nevirapine — hepatitis Ritonavir — fatty liver *nucleoside reverse transcriptase inhibitors* (abacavir, didanosine, lamivudine, stavudine, zalcitabine, zidovudine) — hepatic steatosis with lactic acidosis *Tuberculosis regimens* rifampin + pyrazinamide — hepatocellular, liver failure isoniazid — hepatitis	(Rifampin in combination with pyrazinamide use is discouraged by CDC because of adverse hepatic events)
Miscellaneous	Alcohol cirrhosis Various herbal supplements flutamide— hepatitis Methyl testosterone — cholestasis Norethynodrel/mestranol — cholestasis Tolcapone — liver failure (withdrawn from use in Europe, restricted use in United States) Zafirlucast — acute liver failure (evident in clinical trials and ostmarketing surveillance)	

Modified from Chitturi S, George J: Hepatotoxicity of commonly used drugs: nonsteroidal anti-inflammatory drugs, antihypertensives, antidiabetic agents, anticonvulsants, lipid-lowering agents, psychotropic drugs, *Sem Liv Dis* 22:169-183, 2002; Pishvaian AC, Trope BW, Lewis JH: Drug-induced liver disease in 2003, *Curr Opin Gastroenterol* 20:208-219, 2004; Harrison's Online; Chapter 296: Toxic and Drug-Induced Hepatitis. July 6, 2004; Timbrell JA: Drug hepatotoxicity, *Br J Clin Pharmac* 15:3-14, 1983.

*Withdrawn from market.

ACE, angiotensin-converting enzyme; *ALT*, alanine aminotransferase; *CDC*, Centers for Disease Control; *GI*, gastrointestinal; *HMG-CoA*, 3-hydroxy-3-methylglutaryl coenzyme A; *NSAID*, nonsteroidal antiinflammatory drug.

Intravenous vitamin K can treat cases of severe coagulopathy, whereas oral vitamin K is administered on a long-term basis along with other fat-soluble vitamins.[72] Recombinant factor VIIa has also been shown to improve coagulopathy in adult and pediatric patients with liver failure. It offers an alternative to those patients who either are overloaded with fluid or are refractory to correction of coagulopathy with blood products. Recombinant factor VIIa is generally well tolerated, absent of thrombotic complications, and corrects prothrombin time within 1 hour of infusion, but it is extremely expensive.[78]

Pruritus

Cholestyramine, rifampin, ondansetron, ursodiol, and naltrexone have been used to treat pruritus. Combination therapy is usually required for successful treatment.[72]

Cholangitis

Amoxicillin, cephalosporins, or trimethoprim may be used to prevent cholangitis. Trimethoprim is usually not used in patients who are younger than 2 months because of concern of bone marrow suppression. Although prophylactic antibiotic use may lead to antibiotic resistance, many think that the benefits outweigh the risks because biliary atresia, which may be worsened by cholangitis, remains the most common cause of liver failure in children.[72]

Miscellaneous

Acetaminophen is the most commonly occurring and most notorious cause of DILI.[72] Fortunately an antidote exists that decreases the degree of hepatic injury. NAC enhances levels of glutathione in the liver and plasma and may combine with the toxic acetaminophen metabolite (see also Chapter 99). Both intravenous and oral NAC are now available in the United States. The intravenous regimen offers a shorter course of therapy, as well as an alternative to those patients who do not tolerate the oral formulation because of its pungent odor.

NAC has also been used to treat neonatal hemochromatosis either alone or in combination with prostaglandin E_1, deferoxamine, selenium, and vitamin E.[72] Rapid initiation of combination therapy appears to be the most effective pharmacotherapy available.[72,79]

It has been proposed that NAC may be useful therapy in other types of liver failure because of its ability to enhance hepatosplanchnic perfusion and improve oxygen supply and demand[80] and its presumed cytoprotective and antioxidant effect.[81] Limited data are available at this time for either adult or pediatric populations.

Dose-Adjusting for Hepatic Dysfunction

The liver is the major location of most drug-metabolizing enzymes in the body. The enzymes are widely known as the cytochrome P-450 enzyme system and are composed of subfamilies and isoforms. The CYP450 enzyme system is the most important system involved in phase I drug metabolism. It appears that the CYP450 isoforms are affected to a greater extent by liver disease than are those that catalyze phase II reactions such as glucuronosyltransferases.[86]

In general, the severity of liver damage determines the extent of reduced drug metabolism. Unfortunately, the laboratory tests commonly used to assess liver function do not adequately assess the severity of disease relative to drug metabolism. Fortunately, most dose adjustments are not necessary until almost complete hepatic function is lost. In fact, even in severe cirrhosis, the extent of impairment is only to about 30% to 50% of the activity in patients without liver disease. For agents that undergo extensive first-pass metabolism, oral bioavailability may be increased two to four times in liver disease, potentially increasing the risk of exaggerated pharmacological responses and adverse effects.[87]

The Child-Turcotte-Pugh score is widely used to clinically classify liver disease and is used as an indicator of a patient's ability to metabolize drugs that are eliminated by the liver.[88] This classification has been primarily used in adult patients with liver cirrhosis to assess the degree of liver dysfunction and is easy to use as a bedside test. This assessment divides patients into low-risk (class A), intermediate-risk (class B), and high-risk (class C) hepatic dysfunction (Table 80–4). This useful tool is used to determine when an adult patient should be listed for transplantation (score 7 or higher).[89] In the absence of specific dosing guidelines for a medication, a Child-Pugh score equal to 8 to 9 (Class B) warrants a moderate decrease (approximately 25%) in the initial daily drug dose for agents that are 60% or more hepatically metabolized. A score of 10 or higher (Class C) indicates that a significant decrease in the initial daily dose (approximately 50%) is required for drugs mostly metabolized by the liver.[90]

Most studies on the influence of liver disease on drug dosing have been conducted in adults. As a result, these guidelines may not be extrapolated uniformly to pediatric patients. In general, less formal recommendations exist for dosing in hepatic failure compared with the guidelines available for dose-adjustments in renal failure. Similar to those in the adult population, general recommendations based on the proportion of the drug that is hepatically metabolized are followed for dose-adjusting agents in pediatric patients with liver disease.[90]

Rectal Administration of Medications

Many drugs intended for administration by the orogastric or parenteral routes have been administered rectally. The value of this route of administration lies primarily with the need to avoid the parenteral route in specific clinical situations, or the lack of availability of parenteral dosage forms. In addition, the rectal route of administration has been used under circumstances in which oral administration is not possible or when a high concentration of medication is desired locally. For example, rectal administration can provide locally effective concentrations within the lower

TABLE 80–4

Child-Pugh Classification[88]

Total Points:
- 5 to 6: Child-Pugh Class A
- 7 to 9: Child-Pugh Class B
- 10 to 15: Child-Pugh Class C

CLINICAL AND BIOCHEMICAL PARAMETERS			
	1	2	3
Bilirubin (mg/dl)	<2	2-3	>3
Albumin (g/dl)	>3.5	2.8-3.5	2.8
Ascites	Absent	Moderate	Tense
Encephalopathy	Absent	Moderate (stage I-II)	Severe (stage III-IV)
Prothrombin time	<4	4-6	>6
Seconds	>60	40-60	<40
prolonged %	<1.7	1.7-2.3	>2.3
INR			
IN CASE OF PRIMARY BILIARY CIRRHOSIS			
	1	2	3
Bilirubin (mg/dl)	<4	4-10	>10

Data from Pugh RNH, Murray-Lyon IM et al: Transection of the oesophagus for bleeding oesophageal varices, *Br J Surg* 60: 646-649, 1973.

INR, international normalized ratio.

GI tract while avoiding significant systemic drug exposure. Rectal administration may also serve as a cost-effective means of administering medications for which the parenteral dosage formulation is significantly more expensive. Commercially available formulations for rectal administration, however, are typically more expensive than the extemporaneously prepared dosage forms.

Transcellular absorption across the epithelial cells and paracellular absorption through tight junctions of mucosal cells lining the rectum represent the passive transport mechanisms accounting for drug absorption after rectal administration; no carrier-mediated drug transport process has been documented.[91-93] Absorption of drugs via the rectal mucosa is affected by a number of factors. These mainly include the liquefaction of solid dosage forms and dispersion of the drug-vehicle within the rectum and possibly the colon, the release of the drug from the vehicle making up the dosage form, the dissolution of released drug in a limited volume of rectal fluid, the volume of liquid instilled into the rectum, drug degradation within the rectal environment, high-drug concentration and potential for local irritation, the pH of the rectal contents, drug adherence to rectal contents, the defecation of rectal contents, and differences in bioavailability due to variable venous drainage pathways within the rectosigmoid region. The superior rectal vein perfuses the upper part of the rectum and drains into the portal vein, which then passes through the liver. The middle and inferior rectal veins drain the lower part of the rectum, which drain into the inferior vena cava, thus bypassing the liver. Bioavailability can be enhanced following absorption in the GI tract for drugs undergoing significant first-pass metabolism if absorption primarily occurs through the lower portion of the rectum.[92] Absorption solely through this portion of the rectum cannot be uniformly guaranteed, however.

The clinical application of this route of administration has centered on anticonvulsants,[94-97] in particular, lorazepam and diazepam, narcotic and nonnarcotic analgesics for postoperative pain control,[98,99] pain control in the palliative care setting,[100-102] local treatment of inflammatory bowel disease,[103,104] or pseudomembranous colitis with vancomycin when other therapies have failed.[105] The rectal route of administration has also been studied in the delivery of antiemetics, antibacterial agents, xanthine compounds, and cardiovascular agents.[92,93] Given the variability in drug absorption in critically ill patients, the role for rectal administration of drugs is somewhat limited in the pediatric critical care setting.

The most likely circumstances in which rectal administration may be useful in pediatric critical care patients include instances where placement of intravenous access is unnecessary or has been met with difficulty and drug administration cannot be delayed. As such, the rectal route of administration is often used to treat mild to moderate pain or fever in patients who require acetaminophen therapy yet cannot take this medication via the orogastric route. In addition, the rectal route of administration is often used for local management of inflammatory bowel disease and treatment of constipation, as discussed earlier in this chapter. This route may play a useful role in patients with status epilepticus if intravenous access cannot rapidly be achieved. A diazepam gel formulation is commercially available for rectal administration in fixed unit doses of 5, 10, 15, and 20 mg.[41] The recommended pediatric dosing is based on age and weight: ages 2 to 5 years, 0.5 mg/kg; 6 to 11 years, 0.3 mg/kg; and 12 years and older, 0.2 mg/kg. Doses are rounded upward to the next available unit dose (see also Chapter 55).

REFERENCES

1. ASHP Therapeutic Guidelines on the Pharmacologic Management of Nausea and Vomiting in Adult and Pediatric Patients Receiving Chemotherapy or Radiation Therapy or Undergoing Surgery, *Am J Health Syst Pharm* 56: 729-764, 1999.
2. Cada DJ, Levien T, Baker DE: Aprepitant, *Hosp Pharm* 38: 763-774, 2003.
3. F Poli-Bigelli S, Rodrigues-Pereira J, Carides AD et al; Aprepitant Protocol 054 Study Group: Addition of the neurokinin 1 receptor antagonist aprepitant to standard antiemetic therapy improves control of chemotherapy-induced nausea and vomiting. Results form a randomized, double-blind, Placebo-controlled trial in Latin America, *Cancer* 97:3090-3098, 2003.
4. Lifshitz M, Gavrilov V: Adverse reactions to metoclopramide in young children: a 6 year retrospective study and review of the literature, *J Pharm Technol* 18:125-127, 2002.
5. Deehan S, Dobb GJ: Metoclopramide-induced raised intracranial pressure after head injury, *J Neurosurg Anesthesiol* 14:157-160, 2002.
6. Roila F, Aapro M, Stewart A: Optimal selection of antiemetics in children receiving cancer chemotherapy, *Support Care Cancer* 6:215-220, 1998.
7. Matera MG, Di Tullio M, Lucarelli C et al: Ondansetron, an antagonist of 5-HT_3 receptors, in the treatment of antineoplastic drug-induced nausea and vomiting in children, *J Med* 24:161-170, 1993.
8. Miyajima Y, Numata S, Katayama I et al: Prevention of chemotherapy-induced emesis with granisetron in children with malignant diseases, *Am J Pediatr Hematol Oncol* 16:236-241, 1994.
9. Craft AW, Price L, Eden OB et al: Granisetron as antiemetic therapy in children with cancer, *Med Pediatr Oncol* 25:28-32, 1995.
10. Dick GS, Meller ST, Pinkerton GR: Randomized comparison of ondansetron and metoclopramide plus dexamethasone for chemotherapy induced emesis, *Arch Dis Child* 73:243 245, 1995.
11. Leclerc JM, Greenberg M, Lau R et al: Open label IV dolasetron mesylate in pediatric patients receiving moderately to highly emetogenic chemotherapy: pharmacokinetics, efficacy and safety, *Support Care Cancer* 3:343, 1995.
12. Tsuchida Y, Hayashi Y, Asami K et al: Effects of granisetron in children undergoing high-dose chemotherapy: a multi-institutional, cross-over study, *Int J Oncol* 14:673-679, 1999.
13. Carmichael J, Keizer HJ, Cupissol D et al: Use of granisetron in patients refractory to previous treatment with antiemetics, *Anti-Cancer Drugs* 9:381-385, 1998.
14. Culy CR, Bhana N, Plosker GL: Ondansetron: a review of its use as an antiemetic in children, *Paediatr Drugs* 3;441-479, 2001.
15. Kris MG, Pendergrass KB, Navari TH et al: Prevention of acute emesis in cancer patients following high-dose cisplatin with the combination of oral dolasetron and dexamethasone, *J Clin Oncol* 15:2135-2138, 1997.
16. Heron JF, Goedhals L, Jordaan JP et al: Oral granisetron alone and in combination with dexamethasone: a double-blind randomized comparison against high-dose metoclopramide plus dexamethasone in prevention of cisplatin-induced emesis, *Ann Oncol* 5:579-584, 1994.
17. Lawhorn CD, Kymer PJ, Stewart FC et al: Ondansetron dose response curve in high-risk pediatric patients, *J Clin Anesth* 9: 637-642, 1997.
18. Chen LK, Fan SZ, Huang CH et al: Effects of ondansetron on post-operative emesis in Chinese children, *Acta Anaesth Sin* 36:87-91, 1998.
19. O'Brien CM, Titley G, Whitehurst P: A comparison of cyclizine ondansetron and placebo as prophylaxis against postoperative nausea and vomiting in children, *Anaesthesia* 58:707-711, 2003.
20. McCall JE, Stubbs K, Saylors S et al: The search for cost-effective prevention of postoperative nausea and vomiting in the child undergoing reconstructive burn surgery: ondansetron versus dimenhydrinate, *J Burn Care Rehabil* 20:309-315, 1999.

21. Karamanlioglu B, Turan A, Memis D et al: Comparison of oral dolasetron and ondansetron in the prophylaxis of postoperative nausea and vomiting in children, *Eur J Anaesthesiol* 20:831-835, 2003.
22. Fujii Y, Saitoh Y, Tanaka H et al: Combination of granisetron and droperidol for the prevention of vomiting after paediatric strabismus surgery, *Paediatr Anaesth* 9:329-333, 1999.
23. Fujii Y, Saitoh Y, Tanaka H et al: Anti-emetic efficacy of prophylactic granisetron compared with perphenazine for the prevention of post-operative vomiting in children, *Eur J Anaesthesiol* 16:304-307, 1999.
24. Figueredo ED, Canosa LG: Ondansetron in the prophylaxis of postoperative vomiting: a meta-analysis, *J Clin Anesth* 10:211-221, 1998.
25. Fujii Y, Tanaka H: Prophylactic therapy with granisetron in the prevention of vomiting after paediatric surgery. A randomized, double-blind comparison with droperidol and metoclopramide. *Paediatr Anaesth* 8:149-153, 1998.
26. Caron E, Bussieres JF, Lebel D et al: Ondansetron for the prevention and treatment of nausea and vomiting following pediatric strabismus surgery, *Can J Ophthalmol* 38:214-222, 2003.
27. Wagner D, Pandit U, Voepel-Lewis T et al: Dolasetron for the prevention of postoperative vomiting in children undergoing strabismus surgery, *Paediatr Anaesth* 13:522-552, 2003.
28. Henzi I, Walder B, Tramer MR: Dexamethasone for the prevention of postoperative nausea and vomiting: a quantitative systematic review, *Anesth Analg* 90:186-194, 2000.
29. Sukhani R, Pappas AL, Lurie J et al: Ondansetron and dolasetron provide equivalent postoperative vomiting control after ambulatory tonsillectomy in dexamethasone-pretreated children, *Anesth Analg* 95:1230-1235, 2002.
30. Fujii Y, Toyooka H, Tanaka H: A granisetron-droperidol combination prevents postoperative vomiting in children, *Anesth Analg* 87:761-765, 1998.
31. Furst SR, Sullivan LJ, Soriano SG et al: Effects of ondansetron on emesis in the first 24 hours after craniotomy in children, *Anesth Analg* 83:325-328, 1996.
32. Kathirvel S, Dash HH, Bhatia A et al: Effect of prophylactic ondansetron on postoperative nausea and vomiting after elective craniotomy, *J Neurosurg Anesthesiol* 13:207-212, 2001.
33. Neufeld S: Pharmacology review: the role of ondansetron in the management of children's nausea and vomiting following posterior fossa neurosurgical procedures, *Axone* 23:24-29, 2002.
34. Gurler T, Celik N, Totan S et al: Prophylactic use of ondansetron for emesis after craniofacial operations in children, *J Craniofac Surg* 10:45-48, 1999.
35. Kleinerman KB, Deppe SA, Sargent AI: Use of ondansetron for control of projectile vomiting in patients with neurosurgical trauma: two case reports, *Ann Pharmacother* 27:566-568, 1993.
36. Lippens RJ, Broeders GR: Ondansetron in radiation therapy of brain tumor in children, *Pediatr Hematol Oncol* 13:247-252, 1996.
37. Erb TO, Hall JM, Ing RJ et al: Postoperative nausea and vomiting in children and adolescents undergoing radiofrequency catheter ablation: a randomized comparison of propofol- and isoflurane-based anesthetics, *Anesth Analg* 95:1577-1581, 2002.
38. Munro FJ, Fisher S, Dickson U et al: The addition of antiemetics to the morphine solution in patient controlled analgesia syringes used by children after an appendectomy does not reduce the incidence of postoperative nausea and vomiting, *Paediatr Anesth* 12:600-603, 2002.
39. Clark RF, Chen R, Williams SR et al: The use of ondansetron in the treatment of nausea and vomiting associated with acetaminophen poisoning, *J Toxicol Clin Toxicol* 34:163-167, 1996.
40. Scharman EJ: Use of Ondansetron and other antiemetics in the management of toxic acetaminophen ingestions, *J Toxicol Clin Toxicol* 36:19-25, 1998.
41. Taketomo CK, Hodding JH, Kraus DM: *Lexi-Comp's pediatric dosing handbook,* ed 10, Hudson, OH, 2003-2004, Lexi Comp.
42. Elstner CL, Lindsay AN, Book LS, Matsen JM: Lack of relationship of *Clostridium difficile* to antibiotic-associated diarrhea in children. Pediatr Inf Dis 1983; 2:364-366.
43. Vanderhoof JA, Young RJ: Use of probiotics in childhood gastrointestinal disorders, *J Pediatr Gastroenterol Nutr* 27:323-332, 1998.
44. Practice parameter: the management of acute gastroenteritis in young children. American Academy of Pediatrics, Provisional Committee on Quality Improvement, Subcommittee on Acute Gastroenteritis, *Pediatrics* 97:424-435, 1996.
45. McFarland LV, Brandmarker SA, Guandalini S. Pediatric *Clostridium difficile:* a phantom menace or clinical reality? *J Pediatr Gastroenterol Nutr* 31:220-231, 2000.
46. Goldin BR, Gorbach SL, Saxelin M et al: Survival of *Lactobacillus* species (strain GG) in human gastrointestinal tract, *Dig Dis Sci* 37:121-128, 1992.
47. Vanderhoof JA, Whitney DB, Antonson DL et al: *Lactobacillus GG* in the prevention of antibiotic-associated diarrhea in children, *J Pediatr* 135:564-568, 1999.
48. Saavedra JM, Bauman NA, Oung I et al: Feeding *Bifidobacterium bifidum* and *Streptococcus thermophilus* to infants in hospital for prevention of diarrhea and shedding of rotavirus, *Lancet* 344: 1046-1049, 1994.
49. Surawicz CM, Elmer GW, Speelman P et al: Prevention of antibiotic-associated diarrhea by *Saccharomyces boulardii* compared with placebo, *Am J Gastroenterol* 90:439-48, 1995.
50. Colombel JF, Cortot A, Newt C et al: Yogurt with *Bifidobacterium longum* reduces erythromycin-induced gastrointestinal effects, *Lancet* 2:43, 1987.
51. Heikenen JB, Pohl JF, Werlin SL et al: Octreotide in pediatric patients, *J Pediatr Gastroenterol Nutr* 35:600-609, 2002.
52. Baker SS, Liptak GS, Colletti RB et al: Constipation in infants and children: evaluation and treatment. A medical position statement of the North American Society for Pediatric Gastroenterology and Nutrition, *J Pediatr Gastroenterol Nutr* 29:612-626, 1999.
53. Heyland DK, Tougas C, King D et al: Impaired gastric emptying in mechanically ventilated, critically ill patients, *Intensive Care Med* 22:1339-1344, 1996.
54. Schwartz RH: Adolescent heroin use: a review, *Pediatrics* 102: 1461-1466, 1998.
55. Bulloch B, Tenenbein M: Constipation: diagonsis and management in the pediatric emergency department, *Pediatr Emerg Care* 18:254-258, 2002.
56. Booth CM, Heyland DK, Paterson WG: Gastrointestinal promotility drugs in the critical care setting: a systematic review of the evidence, *Crit Care Med* 30:1429-1435, 2002.
57. Horn JR: Use of prokinetic agents in special populations, *Am J Health Syst Pharm* 53(suppl 3): S27-29, 1996.
58. Rudolph CD, Mazur LJ, Liptak GS et al: Guidelines for evaluation and treatment of gastroesophageal reflux in infants and children: recommendations of the North American Society for Pediatric Gastroenterology and Nutrition: J Pediatr Gastroenterol Nutr 32 (suppl 2): S1-S31, 2001.
59. Chaibou M, Tucci M, Dugas MA et al: Clinically significant upper gastrointestinal bleeding acquired in a pediatric intensive care unit: a prospective study, *Pediatrics* 102(4 Pt 1):933-938, 1998.
60. Cochran EB, Phelps SJ, Tolley EA et al: Prevalence of, and risk factors for, upper gastrointestinal tract bleeding in critically ill pediatric patients, *Crit Care Med* 20:1519-1523, 1992.
61. Lacroix J, Nadeau D, Laberge S et al: Frequency of upper gastrointestinal bleeding in a pediatric intensive care unit, *Crit Care Med* 20:35-42, 1992.
62. Cook DJ, Fuller HD, Guyatt GH et al: Risk factors for gastrointestinal bleeding in critically ill patients, *N Engl J Med* 300:377-381, 1994.
63. Lacroix J, Gauthier M, Farrell CA et al: Prophylaxis of gastroduodenal hemorrhage caused by stress during pediatric intensive care, *Pediatrie* 46:393-403, 1991.
64. Lopez-Herce J, Dorao P, Elola P et al: Frequency and prophylaxis of upper gastrointestinal hemorrhage in critically ill children: a prospective study comparing the efficacy of almagate, ranitidine, and sucralfate. The Gastrointestinal Hemorrhage Study Group, *Crit Care Med* 20:1082-1089, 1992.
65. Yildizdas D, Yapicioglu H, Yilmaz HL: Occurrence of ventilator-associated pneumonia in mechanically ventilated pediatric intensive care patients during stress ulcer prophylaxis with sucralfate, ranitidine, and omeprazole, *J Crit Care* 17:240-245, 2002.
66. Barkun A, Bardou M, Marshall JK: Consensus recommendations for managing patients with nonvariceal upper gastrointestinal bleeding, *Ann Intern Med* 139:843-857, 2003.
67. Siafakas C, Fox VL, Nurko S: Use of octreotide for the treatment of severe gastrointestinal bleeding in children, *J Pediatr Gastroenterol Nutr* 26:356-359, 1998.
68. Zellos A, Schwarz KB: Efficacy of octreotide in children with chronic gastrointestinal bleeding, *J Pediatr Gastroenterol Nutr* 30:442-446, 2000.

69. Molleston JP: Variceal bleeding in children, *J Pediatr Gastroenterol Nutr* 37:538-545, 2003.
70. Gold BD, Colletti RB, Abbott M et al: *Helicobacter pylori* infection in children: recommendations for diagnosis and treatment, *J Pediatr Gastroenterol Nutr* 31:490-497, 2000.
71. Lee WM: Assessing causality in drug-induced liver injury, *J Hepatol* 33:1003-1005, 2000.
72. Kelly DA: Managing liver failure, *Postgrad Med J* 78:660-667, 2002.
73. MicroMedex Healthcare Series. Lactulose monograph, July 2, 2004.
74. Als-Nielsen B, Gluud LL, Gluud C: Non-absorbable disaccharides for hepatic encephalopathy: systematic review of randomised trials, *BMJ*, 328:1046, 2004.
75. Blei AT, Cordoba J, Practice Parameters Committee of the American College of Gastroenterology: Hepatic encephalopathy: *Am J Gastroenterol* 96:1968-1976, 2001.
76. Wyllie R, Arasu TS, Fitzgerald JF: Ascites: pathophysiology and management, *J Pediatr* 97:167-176, 1980.
77. Shashidhar H, Langhans N, Grand RJ: Propranolol in prevention of portal hypertensive hemorrhage in children: a pilot study. *J Pediatr Gastroenterol Nutr* 29:12-17, 1999.
78. Brown JB, Emerick KM, Brown DL et al: Recombinant factor VIIa improves coagulopathy caused by liver failure, *J Pediatr Gastroenterol Nutr* 37:268-272, 2003.
79. Flynn DM, Mohan N, McKiernan P et al: Progress in treatment and outcome for children with neonatal haemochromatosis, *Arch Dis Child Fetal Neonatal* Ed 88:F124-F127, 2003.
80. Devlin J, Ellis AE, McPeake J et al: N-acetylcysteine improves indocyanine green extraction and oxygen transport during hepatic dysfunction, *Crit Care Med* 25:236-242, 1997.
81. MicroMedex Healthcare Series. Acetylcysteine monograph, July 2, 2004.
82. Chitturi S, George J: Hepatotoxicity of commonly used drugs: non-steroidal anti-inflammatory drugs, antihypertensives, antidiabetic agents, anticonvulsants, lipid-lowering agents, psychotropic drugs, *Semin Liver Dis* 22:169-183, 2002.
83. Pishvaian AC, Trope BW, Lewis JH: Drug-induced liver disease in 2003, *Curr Opin Gastroenterol* 20:208-219, 2004.
84. Harrison's Online; Chapter 296: Toxic and Drug-Induced Hepatitis. http://www.accessmedicine.com/content.aspx?aID=91681&searchStr=hepatitis%2c+drug-induced#91681. July 6, 2004.
85. Timbrell JA: Drug hepatotoxicity, *Br J Clin Pharmac* 15:3-14, 1983.
86. Buratti S, Lavine JE: Drugs and the liver: advances in metabolism, toxicity, and therapeutics, *Curr Opin Pediatr* 14:601-607, 2002.
87. Gilman AG, Hardman JG, Limbard LE, editors: *Goodman & Gilman's the pharmacological basis of therapeutics,* ed 10, New York, 2001, McGraw-Hill.
88. Pugh RNH, Murray-Lyon IM, Dawson JL et al: Transection of the oesophagus for bleeding oesophageal varices, *Br J Surg* 60:646-649, 1973.
89. Carithers RL Jr: Liver transplantation. American Association for the Study of Liver Diseases, *Liver Transpl* 6:122-135, 2000.
90. Dipiro JT, Talbert RL, Yee GC et al, editors: *Pharmacotherapy: a pathophysiologic approach*, ed 5, New York, 2002, McGraw-Hill.
91. Alternative routes of drug administration—advantages and disadvantages (subject review). American Academy of Pediatrics. Committee on Drugs, *Pediatrics* 100:143-152, 1997.
92. Van Hoogdalem EJ, De Boer AG, Breimer DE: Pharmacokinetics of rectal drug administration, Part I: general considerations and clinical applications of centrally acting drugs, *Clin Pharmacokinet* 21:12-26, 1991.
93. Van Hoogdalem EJ, De Boer AG, Breimer DEL: Pharmacokinetics of rectal drug administration, Part II: clinical application of peripherally acting drugs, and conclusions, *Clin Pharmacokinet* 21:110-128, 1991.
94. Appleton R, Martland T, Phillips B: Drug management for acute tonic-clonic convulsions including convulsive status epilepticus in children, *Cochrane Database Syst Rev* (4):CD001905, 2002.
95. Dodson WE: Special pharmacokinetic considerations in children, *Epilepsia* 28(suppl 1):S56-S70, 1987.
96. Graves NM, Kriel RL: Rectal administration of antiepileptic drugs in children, *Pediatr Neurol* 3:321-326, 1987.
97. Seigler RS: The administration of rectal diazepam for acute management of seizures, *J Emerg Med* 8:205, 1990.
98. Kokinsky E, Thornberg E: Postoperative pain control in children: a guide to drug choice, *Pediatr Drugs* 5:751-762, 2003.
99. Romsing J, Moiniche S, Dahl JB: Rectal and parenteral paracetamol, and paracetamol in combination on NSAIDs, for postoperative analgesia, *Br J Anaesth* 88:215-226, 2002.
100. Warren DE: Practical use of rectal medications in palliative care, *J Pain Symptom Manage* 11:378-387, 1996.
101. Fine PG: Analgesic issues in palliative care gastroesophageal reflux pain and chronic non-cancer pain management, *J Pain Palliative Care Pharmacother* 16:87-89, 2002.
102. Kronenberg RH: Ketamine as an analgesic: parenteral, oral, rectal, subcutaneous, transdermal and intranasal administration, *J Pain Palliative Care Pharmacother* 16:27-35, 2002.
103. Williams CN. Role of rectal formulations: suppositories, *Scand J Gastroenterol* 25(suppl 172):60-62, 1990.
104. Wikberg M, Ulmius J, Ragnarsson G: Review article: targeted drug delivery in treatment of intestinal diseases, *Aliment Pharmacol Ther* 11(suppl 3):109-115, 1997.
105. Bublin JG: Rectal use of vancomycin, *Ann Pharmacother* 28:1357, 1994.

CHAPTER

81

Acute Liver Failure, Liver Transplantation, and Extracorporeal Liver Support

David M. Steinhorn, Estella M. Alonso, and Timothy E. Bunchman

PEARLS

- The cause of acute liver failure (ALF) in children is age dependent with viral hepatitis probably the most common cause of ALF in all age groups.
- There is no specific therapy for acute and end-stage liver failure except hepatic replacement.
- Management of coagulopathy and hemorrhage is a major part of the overall care of the child with ALF. Profound disturbances in hemostasis develop as a result of the failure of hepatic synthesis of clotting factors and fibrinolytic factors, the reduction in platelet numbers and function, or intravascular coagulation.
- The level of factor VIII may help differentiate between disseminated intravascular coagulation and ALF because it is synthesized by vascular endothelium and therefore is normal or increased in ALF, possibly as an acute-phase response or because of decreased utilization.
- Brain death associated with cerebral edema is the most frequent cause of death in ALF and contributes to reduced survival after liver transplantation.
- Laboratory evidence for citrate lock is a rising total of calcium with a dropping total of ionized calcium when it is measured in the patient's blood instead of it being a sample drawn from the hemofiltration circuit.
- Liver transplantation should be considered in all children who have stage II or IV hepatic coma because mortality in this group exceeds 70%.
- During the first 30 days after transplant, vascular complications are a major cause of graft failure. Forty-three percent of liver graft loss in children is directly attributable to either hepatic arterial or portal vein thrombosis.
- Liver biopsy is important to confirm the diagnosis of acute rejection and distinguish patients with viral infection, biliary obstruction or graft ischemia who may have a similar clinical presentation. Early detection of rejection is critical to allow the initiation of intensified immunosuppression to reverse the process and minimize graft loss.

Acute liver failure (ALF) is a relatively rare but often fatal disease. It is a heterogeneous condition with many different causes; because the functional changes are unclear, they prevent substantial advances in specific therapy. Recognized causes include infections, toxins, metabolic disorders, infiltrative diseases, autoimmune hepatitis, ischemic, or irradiation damage although a proportion of cases are cryptogenic.[1] For the pediatric intensivist, the mainstay of therapy consists of supportive measures, with a focus on prevention or treatment of complications and early consideration for liver transplantation.[2-8] With the onset of cerebral edema in children with ALF, the risk for permanent disability increases dramatically [9,10] Thus the timely intervention to prevent the metabolic derangements associated with ALF are pivotal in the prevention of the progression and the morbidity associated with this condition.[11] The rewards of bridging children with end-stage liver failure to transplant are reflected in the recent United Network for Organ Sharing (UNOS) statistics with 3-year survival approaching 77% and 83% for children younger than or older than age 1 year, respectively (www.unos.org).

Definition

Liver failure is defined as the loss of vital functions of the normal liver, which encompass synthesis of serum proteins including clotting factors and albumin, bile production and excretion, detoxification of organic anions, metabolism and storage of glucose and fatty acids, and elimination of ammonia and other byproducts of energy utilization. The significant compromise of these functions implies loss of a critical mass of hepatocytes, and the clinical manifestations of liver failure depend on the extent and time course of liver cell death.

The clinical syndrome of *acute* or *"fulminant" liver failure* is defined as the onset of hepatic encephalopathy and coagulopathy *within* 8 weeks of the onset of liver disease in the absence of preexisting liver disease in any form.[1,12] This narrow definition does not adequately address children with new-onset liver disease who have encephalopathy more than 8 weeks after presentation or children with subclinical chronic liver disease such as autoimmune hepatitis or Wilson's disease who appear initially with liver failure. The management principles of children are similar for most causes of liver failure, even though the prognosis can be remarkably different.

Cause

The cause of ALF in children is age dependent,[1,13] with viral hepatitis probably the most common cause of ALF in all age groups. Severe hepatitis due to echovirus and adenovirus is seen almost exclusively in the neonatal population. Liver failure can be one of the manifestations of overwhelming herpes infection in the neonate or immunocompromised patient. Metabolic liver disease and familial erythrophagocytosis are most commonly found in infants. Acute hepatitis A and B infections are the most common cause in most large published series of school-aged children. Nevertheless, there is a distinct geographic impact on the frequency and type of viral hepatitis. Many of the cases of presumed viral hepatitis in the United States cannot be linked to a known viral pathogen. These cases, often referred to as *sporadic nontypable* or *indeterminate hepatitis,* are thought to result from a yet unknown virus.[6] Drug-induced liver disease is more common in older children, especially disease that results from intentional acetaminophen overdose (see also Chapters 98 and 99).

The incidence of ALF in childhood is not well described but has been estimated to be 2000 cases per year in adults in the United States. A recently established multicenter database, including 24 pediatric liver centers in the United States, Canada, and England, has collected demographics and outcome data from 230 pediatric cases of ALF over a 3-year period. A specific cause could not be determined in 51% of the cases. Overall survival in this group was 81% at 3 weeks after presentation with 32% requiring liver transplantation. (R Squires, personal communication). Considering the infrequency of this diagnosis and the frequent associated morbidity and mortality, it is not unexpected that few pediatric subspecialists are comfortable managing patients with this diagnosis.

Clinical Presentation by Cause

The clinical presentation varies with etiology but, in most cases admitted to the pediatric intensive care unit (PICU), there is hepatic dysfunction with hypoglycemia, coagulopathy, and encephalopathy. Jaundice may be a late feature, particularly in metabolic disease. The clinical onset may be within hours or weeks. Most pediatric patients who have ALF were previously healthy, with no history of major medical problems and no clear exposure to hepatitis or toxins.

Beyond the acute stabilization and attempts at detoxification of children with ALF, subsequent diagnosis and management of these patients must occur at a center familiar with the needs of this subset of critically ill children and with the resources (e.g., blood banking, continuous renal replacement therapy) necessary to provide optimal care until either recovery or transplantation occurs. The decision to transfer a patient with evolving signs of progressive liver failure must be made in a timely manner because the risks of transporting patients in a deteriorating condition with advanced hepatic encephalopathy or uncontrolled bleeding can be monumental. When liver transplantation is not possible because of geography or other considerations, it may be a futile effort and a disruptive experience to transfer a terminal patient with advanced liver failure to a distant center.

Family Support

Families of children with ALF are naturally devastated by the development of potentially fatal acute organ failure in their child. Such families require a considerable amount of psychological support and counseling, particularly because many families will not be able to grasp the seriousness of their child's condition and the implications of liver transplantation. Living donor transplantation is a reasonable option for families who are able to quickly assimilate the broad implications of ALF. The family's ability to comply with long-term care and medication regimens, should liver transplantation be necessary, is critical to the ultimate success of the process. The particular problems of suicide attempts and gestures in adolescents may require additional psychiatric help.

Management

Initial Assessment and Care

There is no specific therapy for acute and end-stage liver failure except hepatic replacement. Therefore management is directed toward early consideration for liver transplantation, hepatic support, treatment of acquired infections, and prevention and treatment of complications while the patient is awaiting recovery or a suitable donor for liver transplantation.[14-18] The key elements in managing patients before transplantation are meticulous medical support in the setting of an intensive care unit and rapid referral to a transplant center. It is essential to obtain a full history from the parents, which would include establishing appropriate risk factors such as information on intravenous (IV) injections, infusions of blood products, foreign travel, or contact with jaundice. It is important to establish the medications the child has taken, including over-the-counter preparations, folk remedies and herbal supplements and the medications in the household, and to ask adolescents about the use of elicit drugs and sexual contact. Until a diagnosis is made, it is assumed that all children are infectious and that all blood, excretions, and secretions are potentially capable of transmitting viral hepatitis. Enteric isolation procedures must be enforced (Box 81–1) until an infectious cause has been ruled out.

The initial physical examination should establish hepatic, cerebral, cardiovascular, respiratory, renal, and acid-base status. The patient's level of consciousness and degree of hepatic coma (Table 81–1) should be established with a reliable scale,[19] and a complete central nervous system (CNS) examination should be performed. Progression of coma may be assessed through serial examinations (see also Chapter 54). Evidence of chronic liver disease or other signs that may suggest a cause, such as Kayser-Fleischer rings, caput succedaneum, cataracts, and needle marks, should be established. Liver size and consistency should be determined and documented. The presence of impaired CNS function with acute liver disease is an indication for immediate hospitalization independent of any other clinical or biochemical findings.

A central venous catheter is useful for assessment of right heart function and volume status but must be placed with care in patients with significant coagulopathy or thrombocytopenia. Use of a multilumen catheter, which enables simultaneous administration of blood products, dextrose solutions to maintain normal serum glucose levels, IV fluids, and drugs, is helpful and may be replaced if needed to facilitate exchange blood transfusions or renal replacement therapy when required. An indwelling arterial line for continuous measurement of blood pressure and for biochemical and acid-base monitoring is frequently helpful, especially in patients with evolving cardiopulmonary instability. A nasogastric tube is passed and placed to gravity, with regular gentle saline lavage to detect upper gastrointestinal hemorrhage. The urinary bladder is catheterized and strict output measured to help in the evaluation of fluid status and renal function. Ideally, the patient is placed on a bed that permits the body weight to be recorded frequently.

Baseline biochemical and other investigations should be performed (see Box 81–1), and management should be initiated as listed in Box 81–2. The frequency of biochemical monitoring will depend on the severity of illness, ranging from daily in mild cases to every 4 to 6 hours in

BOX 81–1

Investigations in Fulminant Hepatic Failure

Baseline essential investigations
Biochemistry
- Bilirubin, transaminases
- Alkaline phosphatase
- Albumin
- Urea and electrolytes
- Creatinine
- Calcium, phosphate
- Ammonia
- Acid-base, lactate
- Glucose

Hematology
- Full blood count, platelets
- PT, PTT
- Factors V or VII
- Blood group cross-match

Septic screen
- Omitting lumbar puncture

Radiology
- Chest x-ray
- Abdominal ultrasound
- Head CT scan or MRI

Neurophysiology
- EEG

Diagnostic investigations
Serum
- Paracetamol levels
- Cu, caeruloplasmin (>3 years)
- Autoantibodies
- Immunoglobulins
- Amino acids
- Hepatitis A, B, C, E
- EBV, CMV, HSV
- Leptospira (if clinically relevant)
- Other viruses

Urine
- Toxic metabolites
- Amino acids, succinylacetone
- Organic acids
- Reducing sugars

CMV, cytomegalovirus; *CT,* computed tomography; *Cu,* copper; *EBV,* Epstein-Barr virus; *EEG,* electroencephalogram; *HSV,* herpes simplex virus; *MRI,* magnetic resonance imaging; *PT,* prothrombin time; *PTT,* partial thromboplastin time.

TABLE 81–1

Clinical Stages of Hepatic Encephalopathy[22,66]

Stage	Asterixis	EEG Changes	Clinical Manifestations
I (prodrome)	Slight	Minimal	Mild intellectual impairment, disturbed sleep-awake cycle
II (impending)	Easily elicited	Usually generalized	Drowsiness, confusion, coma-inappropriate behavior, disorientation, mood swings
III (stupor)	Present if patient cooperative	Grossly abnormal slowing of rhythm	Drowsy, unresponsive to verbal commands, markedly confused, delirious, hyperreflexia (+) Babinski sign
IV (coma)	Usually absent	Appearance of delta waves, decreased amplitudes	Unconscious, decerebrate or decorticate response to pain present (IVA) or absent (IVB)

patients in stage III and IV coma, and should include monitoring of the complete blood cell count, blood gases, electrolytes, aminotransferases, and prothrombin time; plus plasma creatinine, bilirubin, and ammonia should be monitored daily. A baseline chest x-ray image is useful to diagnose cardiac dysfunction or aspiration. An abdominal ultrasound may indicate liver size and patency of hepatic and portal veins, particularly if liver transplantation is being considered.

BOX 81–2

Management of Fulminant Hepatic Failure

- No sedation except for procedures
- Minimal handling
- Enteric precautions until infection ruled out
- Monitor:
  - Heart and respiratory rate
  - Arterial BP, CVP
  - Core/toe temperature
  - Neurological observations
  - Gastric pH (>5.0)
  - Blood glucose level (>4 mmol/L)
  - Acid-base
  - Electrolytes
  - PT, PTT
- Fluid balance
  - 75% maintenance
  - Dextrose 10% to 50% (provide 6-10 mg/kg/min)
  - Sodium (0.5-1 mEq/kg/day)
  - Potassium (2-4 mEq/kg/day)
- Maintain circulating volume with colloid/FFP
- Coagulation support only if required
- Drugs
  - Vitamin K
  - H_2-antagonist
  - Antacids
  - Lactulose
  - *N*-acetylcysteine for acetaminophen toxicity
  - Broad-spectrum antibiotics
  - Antifungals
- Nutrition
  - Enteral feeding (1-2 g protein/kg/day)
  - PN if ventilated

BP, blood pressure; *CVP,* central venous pressure; *FFP,* fresh frozen plasma; *H_2,* histamine 2; *PN,* parenteral nutrition; *PT,* prothrombin time; *PTT,* partial thromboplastin time.

Fluid Balance

The aim of fluid balance is to maintain hydration and renal function while not provoking cerebral edema. Maintenance fluids consist of 10% dextrose in 0.25N saline, and intake should be 75% of normal maintenance requirements unless cerebral edema develops. A total sodium intake of 0.5 to 1 mEq/kg/day is usually adequate. Potassium requirements may be large, 3 to 6 mEq/kg/day, as guided by the serum concentration. Because patients may have hypophosphatemia, IV phosphate may be given as potassium phosphate.

Attempts should be made to maintain urinary output with loop diuretics in large doses (furosemide [1 to 3 mg/kg every 6 hours], dopamine [2 to 5 μg/kg/min], and colloid/fresh frozen plasma [FFP]) to maintain adequate preload and renal perfusion. Should profound oliguria occur, consideration should be given to hemofiltration or dialysis (see following section on hemofiltration).

Anemia should be corrected, and the hemoglobin concentration should be maintained above 10 g/dl to provide optimal oxygen delivery to tissues. Coagulopathy should be managed conservatively; the massive requirements for FFP may result in fluid overload, requiring the institution of renal replacement therapy.

Nonspecific Adjunctive Therapy

It is usual to prescribe vitamin K (2-10 mg IV), although it is not usually effective. Histamine 2 (H_2)–antagonists and antacids (see later) should be administered prophylactically to prevent gastrointestinal hemorrhage from stress erosions. The role of *N*-acetylcysteine (70 mg/kg every 4 hours) in the management of ALF other than acetaminophen poisoning has been investigated with promising results.[20]

Antibiotic Therapy

The results of surveillance cultures can be used to guide antibiotic therapy in the event of suspected infection, but broad-spectrum antibiotics (amoxicillin, cefuroxime, metronidazole, and prophylactic fluconazole) are only prescribed if sepsis is suspected or liver transplantation is anticipated.

Nutritional Support

The role of parenteral nutrition in the management of patients with ALF is controversial. The main aims of therapy are the following:

1. Maintain blood glucose level (>40 mg/dl) and ensure sufficient carbohydrates for energy metabolism
2. Reduce protein intake to 1 to 2 g/kg/day, either enterally or parenterally
3. Provide sufficient energy intake to reverse catabolism, either enterally or parenterally

Children who are connected to a mechanical ventilator should receive parenteral nutrition because it may be 7 to 10 days before a full normal diet is resumed after transplantation.

Central Nervous System Monitoring

A baseline electroencephalogram (EEG) may be helpful to stage coma; however, the findings are typically nonspecific. Computed tomography (CT) scans are probably not useful early in encephalopathy but may provide information on cerebral edema or irreversible brain damage later in the disease. Frequent evaluation of neurological function with serial examinations and blood ammonia is essential to follow the progress of hepatic encephalopathy. Continuous or frequent electroencephalography may show abnormal electrical activity predisposing to convulsions, particularly in infants, but it is not generally necessary. The role of intracranial pressure (ICP) monitoring remains controversial (see the sections Encephalopathy and Cerebral Edema later). The choice of ICP monitoring system depends on the standards of the individual institution and neurosurgeon consulting on the case. All forms of intracranial monitoring are potentially hazardous in patients with severe coagulopathy, but they may provide helpful information on changes in ICP and improve selection for liver transplantation.

Prevention and Management of Complications

The clinical course before transplantation of patients with advanced hepatic failure is dominated by the myriad complications affecting a wide range of organ systems. Monitoring for evidence of those complications and their skillful and timely management should be the focus of the intensivist in the preoperative period. The following sections cover the most common organ system dysfunctions seen in this critically ill patient population.

Hypoglycemia

Hypoglycemia (blood glucose level <40 mg/L) develops in most children. It may contribute to CNS impairment and other organ dysfunction.

Factors contributing to hypoglycemia include (1) failure of hepatic glucose synthesis and release; (2) hyperinsulinemia (due to failure of hepatic degradation); (3) increased glucose use (due to anaerobic metabolism); and (4) secondary bacterial infection.[21-24]

Frequent bedside monitoring of blood glucose concentrations (every 2 to 4 hours) and the IV administration of glucose (10% to 50% dextrose) are required to prevent this complication. Patients may typically require 5 to 8 mg/kg/min of dextrose infused to meet these goals; however, clinicians should avoid excessively high rates of glucose infusion. Increased insulin production, resulting from excess glucose infusion, leads to increased glucose need and net lipogenesis, which can be avoided if the blood glucose level remains between 40 and 60 mg/L. Profound refractory hypoglycemia carries a grave prognostic implication and often heralds the imminent death of the patient.

Coagulopathy and Hemorrhage

The management of coagulopathy and hemorrhage is a major part of the overall care of the child with ALF. Profound disturbances in hemostasis develop as a result of the failure of hepatic synthesis of clotting factors and fibrinolytic factors, the reduction in platelet numbers and function, or intravascular coagulation.[25] The coagulation factors synthesized by hepatocytes include factors I (fibrinogen), II (prothrombin), V, VII, IX, and X, and a reduction in synthesis leads to the prolongation of prothrombin and partial thromboplastin time.

The prothrombin time is the most clinically useful measure of hepatic synthesis of clotting factors. Prolongation of the prothrombin time often precedes other clinical evidence of hepatic failure, such as encephalopathy, and may alert the clinician to the severity of acute hepatitis; it is a guide to the urgency of liver transplantation. Administering vitamin K parenterally (2 to 10 mg IV) ensures the sufficiency of this essential cofactor but rarely improves coagulation in ALF.

The prothrombin time depends on the availability of factor VII, which has a shorter half-life (≈4 to 7 hours) than other factors and decreases more rapidly than other liver-derived clotting factors. As a result, measurement of factor VII may be a more sensitive indicator than the prothrombin time. Fibrinogen concentrations are usually normal unless there is also disseminated intravascular coagulation (DIC). The level of factor VIII may help differentiate between DIC and ALF because it is synthesized by vascular endothelium and therefore is normal or increased in ALF, possibly as an acute-phase response or as a result of decreased use. Decreased levels of factor XIII may contribute to poor clot stabilization.

A reduction in platelet numbers (80×10^9/L) occurs in up to half of adult patients, although thrombocytopenia is less of a problem in pediatric patients. Severe thrombocytopenia, requiring platelet transfusion, suggests hypersplenism, intravascular coagulation, or aplastic anemia. The use of extracorporeal support devices may also contribute.

Intravascular coagulation as detected by abnormal concentrations of fibrin degradation products is present in almost all patients, indicating ongoing clot deposition and dissolution, most probably as a consequence of tissue necrosis in the liver. DIC is rarely significant but can contribute to organ damage. The administration of commercial concentrates that contain activated clotting factors may precipitate DIC.

Oozing from needle puncture sites and line insertion is common, whereas pulmonary or intracranial hemorrhage may be terminal events. Petechiae reflect decreased platelet function, disturbed vascular integrity, or DIC.

Although in the early stages of assessment prolongation of prothrombin time is a sensitive guide to prognosis and the need for liver transplantation, life-threatening coagulopathy should be corrected with FFP, cryoprecipitate, and platelets as needed. In the very small infant, recombinant factor VIIa may provide significant hemostasis with less volume loading. It is not necessary to maintain coagulation parameters (prothrombin time) in the normal range. In general, mild to moderate coagulopathy (prothrombin time <25 seconds) requires no therapy except support for procedures. Marked coagulopathy (prothrombin time >40 seconds) should be corrected (10 ml/kg of FFP every 6 hours) to prevent the risk of bleeding, particularly intracranial hemorrhage. If major bleeding occurs, additional attempts should be made to correct coagulation with 15 to 20 ml/kg FFP every 6 hours or continuous infusions at a rate of 3 to 5 ml/kg/hr.

Administration of recombinant factor VIIa (80 μg/kg) reliably corrects the coagulation defect in patients with ALF for a period of 6 to 12 hours and may be useful in preparation for invasive procedures.[26] Double-volume exchange transfusion may temporarily improve coagulation and DIC and may control hemorrhage. Hemofiltration may be necessary to control fluid balance and provide fluid "space" if much coagulation support is required. Platelet counts should be maintained above 50×10^9/L by infusion of platelets. DIC is rarely severe enough to require heparin infusion.

Prevention of Gastrointestinal Hemorrhage

Gastrointestinal tract hemorrhage may be life threatening because of gastritis or stress ulceration. High-dose H_2-antagonists (ranitidine 1 to 3 mg/kg every 8 hours) or proton-pump inhibitors (omeprazole 10 to 20 mg/kg/day) should be administered intravenously, and sucralfate (1 to 2 g every 4 hours) may be given through a nasogastric tube to reduce upper gastrointestinal tract bleeding. Prevention of gastrointestinal hemorrhage may also avert further hyperammonemia because of a large protein load to the intestines.

Encephalopathy

Clinically, *acute hepatic encephalopathy* is defined as any brain dysfunction that occurs as a result of acute hepatic dysfunction[27] and may be exacerbated by sepsis, gastrointestinal bleeding, electrolyte disturbances or sedation, particularly benzodiazepine administration. Clinical manifestations and progression are highly variable, but acute hepatic encephalopathy usually evolves over days through definable stages. In rare cases, it may progress rapidly with coma and fatal cerebral edema, developing within hours of the earliest detectable signs.

A scale for grading clinical encephalopathy is presented in Table 81–1.[28,29] This scale is useful for assessing encephalopathy in older patients but has less value in assessing neonates and infants, particularly in the early stages of encephalopathy.

The earliest abnormalities may not be detectable by clinical assessment but are apparent to family members. Personality changes that are reflective of forebrain dysfunction include regression, irritability, apathy, and occasionally euphoria. Younger children are more likely to be irritable and apathetic. Sleep disturbances, such as insomnia or sleep inversion, are often observed.

Intellectual deterioration, observed in stage I of chronic hepatic encephalopathy, is usually not evident in acute encephalopathy. Constructional apraxia related to disturbed spatial recognition may be present. Simple age-related tasks may be clinically useful tools for the day-to-day assessment of inattentiveness and apraxia. Subtraction of serial sevens, recall of events (such as recently viewed videos), handwriting, and figure drawing are appropriate tasks that older children can be asked to repeat daily to assess early encephalopathy. When asked to color a figure in a simple coloring book, younger children may not complete the task (inattentiveness) or scribble far outside the lines (constructional apraxia).

As the patient progresses into stage II hepatic encephalopathy, drowsiness and lethargy are readily apparent. Mental deterioration is clearly evident—the personality changes and behavior becomes inappropriate, with outbursts of anger or crying. Infants exhibit increasing irritability and often produce high-pitched screams. They may refuse to take feedings. Asterixis develops and is a useful sign, but it cannot be elicited with regularity in children younger than age 8 to 10 years. Motor impairment becomes evident, including ataxia, dysarthria, and apraxia. Other neuromotor disturbances that can be detected at this stage include hyperreflexia, sustained clonus, rigidity, extensor posturing, and bizarre facial expressions. EEG abnormalities are detectable at this stage.

Stage III hepatic encephalopathy is characterized by deepening somnolence and stupor. The patient is aroused by vigorous physical stimuli but does not respond to commands. Patients are disoriented and often do not recognize family members. School-aged children and teenagers in deepening stage II and stage III coma often exhibit extreme agitation and rage. Biting may be a problem, and individuals caring for such children must be aware of the potential health risks involved. Seizures may develop. Neurological findings are more profound (see Table 81–1).

Progression into stage IV hepatic encephalopathy is heralded by the onset of coma. The patient responds only to painful stimuli. At first, the patient is flaccid, but in deeper stage IV the patient will assume decerebrate posturing and brainstem reflexes are lost. Respirations may become ineffective requiring mechanical support to prevent death.

Acute hepatic encephalopathy is completely reversible after resolution of the hepatic dysfunction as long as neuronal death has not developed because of the consequences of cerebral edema.

Management of Hepatic Encephalopathy

Although the role played by ammonia in the development of encephalopathy is controversial, therapy to reduce ammonia production or accumulation is indicated. The essential components of therapy are (1) restriction of dietary protein, (2) enteral antibiotics, (3) enteral lactulose, (4) continuous hemofiltration, and (5) control of the complications of ALF that contribute to ammonia accumulation.

In the early stages of hepatic encephalopathy, conventional measures are taken to minimize the formation of nitrogenous substances by the intestine. Some units give enemas with a high magnesium sulphate content to evacuate colonic contents and cleanse the large bowel periodically with a solution such as 1% dextrose. A cathartic, such as sodium-free magnesium sulphate or a nonabsorbable disaccharide (lactulose 1 to 2 ml/kg every 4 to 6 hours), may be administered orally or through the nasogastric tube. Neomycin (50 to 100 mg/kg/day) may also be used to prevent ammonia production if diarrhea resulting from lactulose is a problem. Protein intake should be limited to 0.5 to 1 g/kg/day in this phase and may be administered enterally or parenterally to limit the production of ammonia. Caloric intake is maintained in the early stages with glucose polymers and supplemented by infusion of 10% dextrose solution, while the blood glucose level is frequently monitored.

The older patient with aggressive delirium is a particular risk to care providers. Sedation is not usually necessary, except in violent patients to prevent self-injury. Elective ventilation should be considered if the encephalopathy progresses and compromises the airway or if respiratory distress occurs. If sedation is required, either for restraint or during procedures, short-acting barbiturates or opiates can be safely used, but benzodiazepines should be avoided. If chemical paralysis is required, the role of hepatic metabolism (or lack thereof) should be considered (see also Chapter 115). There are potential therapeutic implications related to the GABA (γ-aminobutyric acid) receptor, which has been implicated in encephalopathy. Flumazenil, a benzodiazepine antagonist, may produce temporary reversal of hepatic encephalopathy.[30] Administration is followed within minutes by a clinical response, which may last for several hours, and it has been suggested that a lack of response to flumazenil may indicate a poor prognosis. Flumazenil holds significant potential for improving the diagnosis and establishing the prognosis in children with hepatic encephalopathy. It may also facilitate the management of ALF by rendering patients more responsive and thereby extending the time before protective airway management and other invasive interventions are required.

Cerebral Edema

Cerebral edema may develop between stage III and stage IV encephalopathy and present within hours of the onset of coma. Brain death associated with cerebral edema is the most frequent cause of death in ALF and contributes to reduced survival after liver transplantation.[31-33] Every effort should be made to prevent cerebral edema because the prognosis is poor once it is evident.

The diagnosis and management of cerebral edema associated with hepatic failure is analogous to those used for other forms of cytotoxic cerebral edema.[33] The reader is referred to detailed discussion of this topic contained elsewhere (see also Chapter 52).

Renal Dysfunction

Renal insufficiency complicates the course in 75% of children[34,35] and may be due to prerenal azotemia, acute tubular necrosis, and functional renal failure (see also Chapter 64).

Prerenal azotemia may be due to dehydration or gastrointestinal bleeding caused by absorption of nitrogenous substances from the gut. A marked increase in blood creatinine concentration may develop from decreased glomerular filtration, increased muscle breakdown, or both.

Acute tubular necrosis is seen in a minority of patients and may occur because of hypovolemia or dehydration related to mannitol infusion or diuretic therapy. Features include abnormal urinary sediment, a urinary sodium concentration greater than 20 mmol/L, a reduction in creatinine clearance (urine/plasma creatinine ratio <10), and oliguria (urine output <0.5 ml/kg/hr).

Functional renal failure (hepatorenal syndrome) is the most common cause of renal insufficiency. Features include sodium retention (urinary sodium concentration <20 mmol/L), normal urinary sediment, and reduced urinary output (<1 ml/kg/hr). The cause is multifactorial, and electrolyte imbalance, sepsis and hypovolemia all play a part. Endotoxemia may contribute to renal injury.

The aim of management is to maintain circulating volume to prevent hypovolemia and ensure that urine output is more than 0.5 ml/kg/hr. A fluid challenge with isotonic volume expander (10 ml/kg) may be successful unless central venous pressure indicates fluid overload (>8 to 10 cm H_2O), in which case the use of furosemide (1 to 2 mg/kg IV) or (0.25 mg/kg/hr by infusion) may be effective. Established renal failure requires hemodialysis or continuous renal replacement therapy as detailed later (see also Chapter 65).

Although functional renal failure recovers quickly after liver transplantation, acute tubular necrosis may severely complicate the postoperative management.[36] Although 50% of patients require hemodialysis or continuous renal replacement therapy, renal function returns to normal after successful liver transplantation.

Ascites

The use of ultrasound in the pretransplant assessment has shown excessive peritoneal fluid in most patients, probably due to acute portal hypertension from lobular collapse, vasodilatation, poor vascular integrity, and reduced oncotic pressure. Clinically evident ascites occurs in less than half the patients but may be a site for secondary bacterial or fungal infection, indicating the necessity for paracentesis in patients who have sepsis without an obvious focus of infection. Therapy is not indicated, other than the correction of oncotic pressure with albumin infusion and general fluid management. Paracentesis may be indicated if peritonitis is suspected or if the intra-abdominal pressure leads to impaired renal perfusion (see also Chapter 15). Paracentesis, however, is frequently associated with dramatic intravascular volume shifts as ascites reaccumulates and may predispose to peritonitis.

Secondary Bacterial and Fungal Infections

Most adults and 50% of children will have significant infection,[37] which may be related to impairment of cellular and humoral immune systems. The organisms most often implicated are gram-positive (*Staphylococcus aureus*, *Staphylococcus epidermidis*, and streptococci), presumably of skin origin. Occasionally gram-negative bacteria or fungal infection are observed. Urinary tract infections, from indwelling catheters, and pulmonary infection, particularly in children receiving ventilatory support, are common.

Management includes surveillance cultures from the endotracheal tube, indwelling catheters, and urine. Broad-spectrum antibiotics should be started at the first suspicion of sepsis because the signs may be subtle. If there is a suspicion of anaerobic infection, cefuroxime (75 to 150 mg/kg/day divided every 8 hours), piperacillin/tazobactam (270 mg/kg/day, piperacillin component divided every 8 hours), and metronidazole (30 mg/kg/day divided every 6 hours) are reasonable first-line medications. Prophylactic antifungals such as amphotericin (1.5 mg/kg/day) or fluconazole (3 to 6 mg/kg/day) may be effective, although potentially nephrotoxic. Cultures positive for infection in the absence of clinical infection should result in the removal or replacement of the infected catheter and administration of the appropriate antimicrobials, with close attention to the possibility of additional, perhaps opportunistic, infection. Aminoglycoside antibiotics should be avoided, if possible, because they can contribute to renal failure.

Hemofiltration for Hepatic Support

Although the definitive therapy for irreversible hepatic failure is organ transplant, transplantation may not be available in a short enough time to prevent irreversible complications (e.g., cerebral edema, fatal hemorrhage) because of limited organ availability. Therefore therapies have been developed over the past decade intended to temporize and support adult patients with acute fulminant hepatic failure or so-called acute-on-chronic hepatic failure. These therapies have been used in the adult population, and they use a single vascular access with a clearance against a charcoal filter of toxins resulting from hepatic failure.[38] Such techniques have been used less frequently in pediatric patients, and to date there is no pediatric literature to support these therapies. Attempts to create extracorporeal artificial liver systems with living hepatocytes in various configurations have shown promise[39,40]; however, as yet unsolved technical problems have limited the utility and widespread availability of this approach to research centers only.[40,41]

Alternately, many programs have used continuous hemofiltration as a way to support electrolyte, ammonia, and requirements and to permit the administration of large quantities of FFP in patients with hepatic failure. This has been used in patients either with or without concurrent renal failure. This therapy is continued until either the patient recovers or progresses on to irreversible loss of hepatic function with subsequent hepatic transplant or death. The specific techniques of continuous hemofiltration will depend on the capability of the given PICU, but all such approaches depend on optimizing clearance of medium and small molecular weight compounds and maximizing nutritional and anticoagulation support.

To date, data have shown that small molecular weight solute (e.g., urea) can be equally and effectively cleared by convective (continuous veno-venous hemofiltration [CVVH]) and diffusive (continual veno-venous hemodiafiltration [CVVHD]) methods (see also Chapter 65).[42] Personal experience has also shown that ammonia, which is a byproduct of acute hepatic failure, can be equally cleared by CVVH and CVVHD. Furthermore, supplied amino acids (i.e., total parenteral nutrition [TPN]), can be equally cleared with both the modalities with the potential of a preference in convective methods.

Therefore the choice of CVVH or CVVHD is based on the preferences and experience of each center. Using this therapy requires controlled anticoagulation, despite the prolonged clotting times associated with liver failure. Because of the underlying coagulopathy, such patients may require little to no anticoagulation.[43] It should be remembered that the prolonged clotting times resulting from liver failure are due to decreased factor levels rather than to direct antagonism of clotting mechanisms (i.e., anticoagulation). Thus some patients may have a paradoxical coagulation status in which they appear "anticoagulated" because of clotting times yet have a tendency to be hypercoagulable partially because of depressed levels of anticlotting factors. Most programs have used heparin or no therapy for this population for anticoagulation. Recent experience has shown citrate to be an alternative anticoagulation therapy for pediatric patients.[44] The use of citrate is essentially used as a way to bind calcium within the hemofiltration circuit decreasing the availability of calcium for clotting function. Calcium then is infused back to the patient independent of the hemofiltration circuit to rescue the patient from potential risk of citrate toxicity. Citrate is cleared through both the dialysis membrane and hepatic function. Hepatic citrate metabolism results in bicarbonate production, which usually results in metabolic alkalosis. In patients with failing hepatic function, citrate is poorly metabolized and may accumulate over time. This condition may result in so-called citrate lock, which represents residual citrate in the patient as the delivery of citrate exceeds its clearance. This can be accentuated by the citrate that patients receive in banked blood products such as FFP. Citrate can easily be used in this population with minimization of citrate infusion and close observation of the signs and symptoms of citrate lock. Laboratory evidence for citrate lock is a rising total of calcium with a decrease in ionized calcium when measured in the patient's blood rather than a sample drawn from the hemofiltration circuit. The decision to use no anticoagulation, heparin anticoagulation, or citrate anticoagulation is based on local experience. In the hands of an experienced physician in a hemofiltration program, any of these approaches can be successfully used.

If one is going to use either replacement therapy (CVVH) or dialysis therapy (CVVHD), then one needs to use solutions to provide for either convective or diffusive clearance. To date there are no solutions approved by the

U. S. Food and Drug Administration (FDA) for convective clearance; thus many programs use saline, lactated Ringer's solution, or custom pharmacy-compounded solutions for replacement therapy. Although the first two solutions are generally reasonable approaches, use of a custom-mixed solution increases the risk for human error. Personal experience and inquiries from other programs made us aware of pharmacy errors resulting in electrolyte disturbance from the dialysate bath that led to life-threatening complications.

If one is going to use a diffusive method (CVVHD), three solutions are available. One is a lactate-based solution (Baxter Hemofiltration Solution; Deerfield, Ill.), and the others are Normocarb, a bicarbonate-based solution (Dialysis Solutions, Inc., Richmond Hills, Ontario, Canada) and PrismaSate-L (Gambro; Lakewood, Colo.). Recent work with Normocarb as a replacement solution allows for options of bicarbonate-based solutions for either convective or diffusive clearance.[45] Lactate is normally hepatically metabolized, but in this population lactate from the dialysis solution will rise because of diminished hepatic clearance. Although lactate is not thought to be directly toxic, rising lactate levels may be a sign to investigate for conditions such as sepsis and bowel necrosis. It is well recognized that patients with lactate-based solutions (either lactated Ringer's solution as replacement or the Baxter Hemofiltration Solution for dialysis) will have levels of lactate that are detectable[46] with conventional clinical lactate assays. One can easily discriminate lactate derived between patient and dialysis solution by measuring the dextro-portion and levo-portion of lactate. Unfortunately, this test is not widely available and often will take an average of 4 to 6 weeks for an answer. Data by Barenbrock et al[47] have demonstrated that bicarbonate-based convective solutions result in improved hemodynamics when compared with lactate-based solutions. Therefore many programs prefer bicarbonate-based solution. Clinicians can choose solutions compounded by the hospital pharmacy or the recent FDA-approved solution Normocarb, which is now available for dialysis and continuous therapy. The latter eliminates the risk for pharmacy error and is less expensive.[48]

Once one has instituted continuous hemofiltration, the goals for hepatic support are several; the *first* is fluid management of the patient. A patient with edema at the time of liver transplant will have difficulty with closure of the abdomen and subsequent wound healing. Therefore preoperative maintenance of euvolemia and minimizing tissue edema is desirable. The *second goal* is the correction of electrolyte disturbances. Often patients with fulminant hepatic failure have sodium perturbations, metabolic acidemia, and other electrolyte disturbances. CVVHD with Normocarb can maintain normal electrolytes and minimize the adverse effects of electrolyte changes on the CNS. The *third goal* is to optimize nutrition and minimize the loss of visceral and somatic protein pools. The provision of nutrition in these patients not only benefits their postoperative care, but also helps support them during the period of organ failure before transplantation. Providing protein beyond what the body can use risks generating additional ammonia and may worsen hepatic encephalopathy. By balancing nutrition with the clearance of amino acids and ammonia through continuous hemofiltration, one optimizes nutrition support, which benefits both the pretransplant and posttransplant status of the patient. The *fourth goal* is to maintain a balanced state of anticoagulation while not predisposing the patient to bleeding. Many programs use frequent or continuous FFP therapy to reduce the risk of spontaneous bleeding from the underlying coagulopathy and to improve the response to anticoagulation therapy. The use of continuous or frequent dosing of FFP will provide not only colloid, but also citrate. Through the use of CVVHD, one can minimize the excess of fluid retention by removing the crystalloid and the citrate contained in FFP. The last benefit of continuous therapy is control of ammonia levels and removal of potentially toxic substances not eliminated by the failed liver. Although hyperammonemia is not the sole cause of hepatic encephalopathy, the use of continuous hemofiltration is an effective adjunct in controlling the ammonia level in patients with hepatic failure.

If the condition of the patient necessitates ongoing continuous hemofiltration preoperatively, one may need to consider its intraoperative use as well. Intraoperative fluid flux with blood products, as well as other fluid managements, may need to be dealt with during the time of the operation. Blood transfusion can expose the patient to large potassium loads that are not tolerated well by patients with oliguria. Experience has shown that the use of intraoperative hemofiltration during the time of liver transplantation can be safely and effectively undertaken.[49] The use of hemofiltration without anticoagulation provides optimal intraoperative support while continuing to infuse calcium to offset the risk of hypocalcemia associated with intraoperative FFP and blood administration.

Continuous hemofiltration represents an important adjunctive support modality for patients with advanced hepatic failure and multiorgan dysfunction. By virtue of its ability to both provide a modicum detoxification and create a more desirable fluid balance, continuous hemofiltration may be a life-sustaining bridge to transplant for patients.

Liver Transplantation

Liver transplantation should be considered in all children who have a stage III or IV hepatic coma because mortality in this group exceeds 70%.[1,50,51] Transplantation is indicated for all forms of ALF, namely, viral hepatitis (including hepatitis B), acetaminophen overdose, halothane hepatitis, and mushroom poisoning. It is also appropriate for certain forms of inborn errors of metabolism, for example, Wilson's disease and tyrosinemia type I, although it is contraindicated for some children with multisystem disease or mitochondrial deletions.[52] Because a successful outcome after liver transplantation is less likely than with other forms of liver disease,[53,54] selection is critical[55] and is based on previous experience of mortality in the pretransplant era.[50] Transplantation with a living donor can accelerate the process and is associated with better outcome in the setting of AFL.[56-58]

The cause of ALF is an important factor in determining whether transplantation is appropriate. The highest mortality is seen in children with indeterminate hepatitis, particularly those with a rapid onset of coma and progression to stage III or IV hepatic coma, a shrinking liver, falling transaminases associated with an increase in bilirubin, and coagulopathy. Such children should be immediately considered for transplantation. Children with fulminant Wilson's disease are unlikely to recover with medical treatment and require transplantation.

In contrast, children with hepatitis A and children with drug-induced liver disease, particularly acetaminophen poisoning, may make a complete recovery with intensive medical therapy. Thus careful monitoring for poor prognostic factors is required before selection.

In practical terms, it is appropriate to list for emergency liver transplantation all children who have reached stage III hepatic coma. The shortage of donor organs may mean a considerable wait for transplantation, or death, on the waiting list.

Because the development of irreversible brain damage is a major contraindication to transplantation, it is essential to be certain that brain damage has not occurred before the operation. Current diagnostic techniques are inadequate, but they include ICP observation; identification of cerebral infarction or intracranial hemorrhage by cerebral CT or magnetic resonance imaging (MRI) scans; and demonstration of midbrain herniation, such as fixed, dilated pupils.

Auxiliary transplantation, in which the recipient liver is left in situ to regenerate, is a controversial treatment for ALF, but its benefit may be that the graft may be removed if the original liver regenerates.[59,60] It is not suitable for transplantation for ALF caused by metabolic liver disease because there is no potential for these livers to recover and there may be a risk of hepatoma in the cirrhotic liver.

Relative contraindications for transplantation include untreated sepsis, human immunodeficiency virus (HIV) infection, and the presence of vascular thrombosis.[61] Absolute contraindications include progressive terminal extrahepatic disease, irreversible or rapidly degenerative CNS disease, intestinal failure, or untreatable metastatic diseases.

Technical Aspects of Liver Transplantation

A detailed discussion of the techniques of liver transplantation is beyond the scope of this chapter. Several aspects of intraoperative management, however, are pertinent to the intensivist in managing the patient postoperatively.

First and foremost, reducing intraoperative and postoperative morbidity involves sending the patient for transplantation in the best condition possible. This means that (1) infections have been treated, (2) excess edema has been avoided or corrected, (3) cardiopulmonary and renal systems are functioning well, and (4) the brain has been spared irreversible damage.

The availability of donor organs has led to the development of techniques for the use of technical variant grafts (reduced-size, living donors, and split liver) to expand the donor pool and reduce waiting time. The ability to provide a reduced segment allows smaller children to receive grafts from larger donors; thus the availability of organs for younger patients is increased. Although technical variant grafts may reduce waiting-list mortality in the setting of ALF, they are associated with a higher rate of postoperative complications. Patient survival for recipients of technical variant grafts, however, is similar to that seen in patients who receive whole liver transplants. The result is a favorable risk-benefit ratio for selection of these types of grafts.

Intraoperative issues affecting the postoperative course are listed in Table 81–2. In general, these issues can be managed with conventional approaches, while two critical, postoperative principles are adhered to: (1) maintain patency of vascular anastomoses and (2) maintain normal to slightly supraphysiological arterial pressure to provide adequate perfusion of the graft. Avoiding excessive hemoconcentration and rapidly correcting all clotting parameters are key to successful care.

Immune Suppression

Currently, the use of calcineurin inhibitors (e.g., cyclosporine [Neoral] or tacrolimus [Prograf]) is the initial approach to immunosuppression. Tacrolimus is usually combined with low-dose steroids. Cyclosporine-based protocols may incorporate steroids and a third agent, such as azathioprine or mycophenolate (CellCept).[51]

Most centers have tended to reduce the use of corticosteroids because of the poor growth and infectious risks associated with their use. The practice of steroid withdrawal varies between centers with weaning often started at 3 to 12 months after transplantation. The exception to this rule pertains to children who underwent transplantation for autoimmune hepatitis who have a high incidence of recurrence.

Postoperative Management Issues of Concern to the Intensivist

The postoperative period is critical because of the need to anticipate predictable complications and to detect unexpected issues as early as possible. The intensivist must be aware of the risk for early complications including primary nonfunction, bleeding, hepatic artery or portal vein thrombosis, and bile leak. Later complications include infections,

TABLE 81–2

Common Postoperative Issues after Liver Transplantation

Postoperative Condition	Intraoperative Cause
Fluid overload	Intraoperative crystalloid, fluid shifts
Capillary leak syndrome	Altered perfusion state, multiple blood products, venous congestion
Hypoxemia	Atelectasis, edema, mucus plugging, distended abdomen impairing ventilation
Renal dysfunction	Altered perfusion, impaired venous return, renal vasoconstriction resulting from calcineurin inhibitor exposure
Coagulopathy	Inadequate FFP/platelets transfusion, small for size graft, primary poor graft function

FFP, fresh frozen plasma.

rejection, hypertension, renal dysfunction, and lymphoproliferative disease.

As in all other organs, prolonged ischemia due to vascular compromise will potentially lead to the loss of graft function. It is impossible to overly stress the need for *close and rapid communication* between the PICU team caring for the transplant patient postoperatively and the surgical and hepatology teams responsible for the operative interventions and management of the immunosuppression after transplantation. Joint rounding in the immediate postoperative period of *at least* once a day with all teams caring for the patient will facilitate the best communication during the critical postoperative period.

Primary Nonfunction. Primary nonfunction of the graft is a disastrous complication necessitating immediate retransplantation. Of children with graft failure within 30 days, primary graft dysfunction accounted for 25.6%.[51] Evidence of primary nonfunction includes worsening coagulopathy, acidemia, rising liver enzymes, and cholestasis. All measures used to support a patient with minimal liver function must be considered and instituted because the condition will become rapidly fatal in the absence of retransplantation.[61]

Bleeding. Postoperative bleeding occurs because of the profound coagulopathy and thrombocytopenia many patients have going into liver transplantation, as well as the dilutional coagulopathy and thrombocytopenia that can occur intraoperatively. Bleeding should abate as function of the graft returns postoperatively. In addition, patients may return to the PICU on heparin infusions in an attempt to maintain patency of the hepatic artery and portal vein anastomoses. Monitoring drainage devices for trends in the amount and the characteristics of the drainage is critical to detect postoperative bleeding at the surgical site. Additionally, monitoring of the hemoglobin level is important; it is an indirect sign of bleeding and can ensure adequate oxygen-carrying capacity, optimally 9 to 12 g/dl. Platelet count should be followed and maintained in a suitable postoperative range as agreed on by both surgical and medical teams. Attempts to achieve perfect clotting function are generally avoided because of the high potential to promote thrombosis of the vascular anastomoses. Worsening coagulopathy suggests hepatic dysfunction, sepsis with DIC, or unrecognized internal bleeding and requires rapid, aggressive diagnosis with treatment of the underlying cause.

Monitoring Vascular Anastomotic Patency. Progress in microsurgical techniques has led to improvements in maintaining vascular patency. During the first 30 days after transplant, vascular complications are a major cause of graft failure. Forty-three percent of liver graft loss in children is directly attributable to either hepatic arterial or portal vein thrombosis.[51] Of the vascular complications, hepatic artery thrombosis occurs most commonly, 10% overall, and is probably the most important because it can lead to biliary leaks, strictures, and intraabdominal infection.[62] Routine assessment of patency with color Doppler ultrasonography at the bedside is critical during this period. MR-angiography or CT-angiography can be helpful in defining the status of vascular structures but can be technically difficult to perform in critically ill patients. Attempts at revascularization may be successful, if performed early. The intensivist should work closely with the surgical and radiology team to detect early signs of vascular occlusion. Avoidance of excess hemoglobin (hyperviscosity) and overzealous transfusion of platelets and clotting factor replacement in the immediate postoperative period is essential. Once again, detailed discussion with the other members of the transplant team will achieve consensus and minimize risks.

Infection. Sepsis continues to be the most frequent final pathway leading to death in recipients of liver transplants. The presence of arterial thrombosis or biliary leak significantly increases the risk of infection and abscess formation. Patients who underwent previous abdominal operations (e.g., Kasai procedure) are also at increased risk for postoperative infection, which increases the potential for bowel perforation. Percutaneous drainage of intraabdominal abscesses can be an effective method to treat these infections provided there is no evidence of an enteric leak. A high index of suspicion for postoperative infection in the immunosuppressed patient must be maintained with early culture and institution of antibiotic treatment, including antifungal and anticytomegalovirus (anti-CMV) as indicated by the patient and donor status. Children are at particular risk for CMV and Epstein-Barr virus (EBV) infections because many are naive to these viruses at the time of transplantation. Passenger donor lymphocytes in the graft are a frequent source of primary infection. Prophylactic therapy with antiviral medication can delay infection, and monitoring active viral replication by polymerase chain reaction (PCR) can be a useful tool to assist in the adjustment of immunosuppressive medications in patients with early, acute infection.[51]

Biliary Complications. Biliary complications include biliary anastomosis dehiscence and bile leaks from the cut surface of the liver. Approximately 15% of patients experience biliary complications within the first 30 days, and 25% or more will experience this complication in long-term follow-up.[51,62] Early bile leaks may be diagnosed by the appearance of bile in the abdominal cavity drains and by nuclear scan or transhepatic contrast studies. Cut surface leaks from minor biliary radicals may resolve spontaneously, but leaks from the biliary anastomosis or from larger cut surface ducts require operative management. Bile duct ischemia caused by hepatic artery thrombosis, which results in a stricture or leak, will likely require retransplantation. Bile leaks increase the risk of postoperative infections that require aggressive attempts to diagnose and treat with targeted antibiotic therapy when possible.

Rejection. The median time to first rejection after transplant in one series was 16 days with 40% to 70% of children experiencing a first episode of rejection 7 to 10 days after successful transplantation.[63] Laboratory findings included elevations in aspartate aminotransferase (AST) and γ-glutamyl transpeptidase (GTP) followed by elevations in bilirubin. Liver biopsy is important to confirm the diagnosis of acute rejection and distinguish patients with viral infection, biliary obstruction, or graft ischemia who may have a similar clinical presentation. Early detection of rejection is critical to allow the initiation of intensified immunosuppression to reverse the process and minimize graft loss.

Complications of Immune-Suppressive Medications. Each of the immune-suppressant agents in common use has

TABLE 81–3

Adverse Effects of Immunosuppressants

Agent	Adverse Effect
Tacrolimus	Hypertension, headache, infection, seizures, hyperglycemia, insulin resistance/diabetes, renal failure, posttransplant lymphoproliferative disorder (PTLD), cardiomyopathy
Cyclosporine	Hypertension, infection, seizures, hyperglycemia, renal failure, hirsutism, gingival hyperplasia, PTLD
Sirolimus	Hypercholesterolemia, infection, edema, PTLD
Corticosteroids	Hypertension, increased appetite, Cushing's syndrome, acne, gastritis, poor wound healing, osteoporosis, poor linear growth
Mycophenolate	Intestinal hypermotility, cramping, diarrhea, infection, leucopenia, thrombocytopenia

potential undesirable side effects. The most common issues are listed in Table 81–3. Most patients will receive a calcineurin inhibitor and corticosteroids; thus the stage is set for postoperative hypertension with or without deterioration in biochemical renal function. Hypertension is treated with conventional pharmacological agents and may remain a persistent problem. Diabetes is also relatively common in patients receiving tacrolimus with a prevalence of 25% at 3 months after transplantation. Hyperglycemia in the immediate postoperative period can be controlled by insulin infusion and should not limit the clinician's ability to deliver adequate caloric intake.[64] Cyclosporin- and tacrolimus-related encephalopathy and seizures occur in 11% and 8% of patients, respectively, with the most common onset in the first 2 weeks after transplantation. Both can be managed by reduction or elimination of the calcineurin inhibitor exposure. Seizure control will frequently require short-term treatment with antiepileptic medications.[65]

REFERENCES

1. Pineiro-Carrero V, Pineiro E: Liver, *Pediatrics* 113:1097-1106, 2004.
2. Lee WM: Acute liver failure, *N Engl J Med* 329:1862-1872, 1993.
3. Bhaduri BR, Mieli-Vergani G: Fulminant hepatic failure: pediatric aspects, *Sem Liv Dis* 16:349-355, 1996.
4. Lee WM, Schiodt FV: Fulminant hepatic failure. In Schiff ER, Sorrell MF, Maddrey WC, editors: *Schiff's diseases of the liver*, Philadelphia, 1999, Lippincott-Raven.
5. Cox K, Berquist W, Castillo R: Paediatric liver transplantation: indications, timing and medical complications, *J Gastroenterol Hepatol* 14:S61-S6, 1999.
6. Whitington PF, Alonso EM: Fulminant hepatitis in children: evidence for an unidentified hepatitis virus, *J Pediatr Gastroenterol Nutr* 33:529-536, 2001.
7. Sanyal AJ, Stravitz RT: Acute liver failure. In Zakim D, Boyer TD, editors: *Hepatology*, Philadelphia, 2003, Saunders.
8. Wirklund R: Peroperative preparation of patients with advanced liver disease, *Crit Care Med* 32:S106-S115, 2004.
9. Alper G, Jarjour I, Reyes J et al: Outcome of children with cerebral edema caused by fulminant hepatic failure, *Pediatr Neurol* 18: 299-304, 1998.
10. Ee L, Shepherd R, Cleghorn G et al: Acute liver failure in children: a regional experience, *J Paediatr Child Health* 39:107-110, 2003.
11. Kobayashi S, Ochiai T, Hori S, et al: Complete recovery from fulminant hepatic failure with severe coma by living donor liver transplantation, *Hepatogastroenterology* 50:515-518, 2003.
12. Trey C: The critically ill child: acute hepatic failure, *Pediatrics* 45:93-98, 1970.
13. Sokol RJ: Fulminant hepatic failure In Balistreri WF, Stocker JT, editors: *Pediatric hepatology*, New York, 1990, Hemisphere Publishing.
14. Devictor D, Tahiri C, Rousset A, et al: Management of fulminant hepatic failure in children-an analysis of 56 cases, *Crit Care Med* 21(suppl 9):S348-S349, 1993.
15. Kucharski SA: Fulminant hepatic failure, *Crit Care Nurs Clin North Am* 5:141-151, 1993.
16. Munoz SJ: Difficult management problems in fulminant hepatic failure, *Sem Liv Dis* 13:395-413, 1993.
17. Herrera JL: Management of acute liver failure, *Dig Dis* 16: 274-283, 1998.
18. Singer AL, Olthoff KM, Kim H et al: Role of plasmapheresis in the management of acute hepatic failure in children, *Ann Surg* 234:418-424, 2001.
19. Duncan C, Ment L, Shaywitz B: Evaluation of level of consciousness by the Glasgow coma scale in children with Reye's syndrome, *Neurosurgery* 13:650-653, 1983.
20. Sklar G, Subramaniam M: Acetylcysteine treatment for non-acetaminophen-induced acute liver failure, *Ann Pharmacother* 38:498-500, 2004.
21. Vilstrup H, Iversen J, Tygstrup N: Glucoregulation in acute liver failure, *Eur J Clin Invest* 16:193-197, 1986.
22. Harry R, Auzinger G, Wendon J: The clinical importance of adrenal insufficiency in acute hepatic dysfunction, *Hepatology* 36: 395-402, 2002.
23. Clark SJ, Shojaee-Moradie F, Croos P et al: Temporal changes in insulin sensitivity following the development of acute liver failure secondary to acetaminophen, *Hepatology* 34:109-115, 2001.
24. Walsh TS, Wigmore SJ, Hopton P et al: Energy expenditure in acetaminophen-induced fulminant hepatic failure, *Crit Care Med* 28:649-654, 2000.
25. O'Grady JG, Langley PG, Isola LM et al: Coagulopathy of fulminant hepatic failure, *Sem Liver Dis* 6:159-163, 1986.
26. Brown J, Emerick K, Brown D et al: Recombinant factor VIIa improves coagulopathy caused by liver failure, *J Pediatr Gastroenterol Nutr* 37:268-272, 2003.
27. Ferenci P, Lockwood A, Mullen K, et al: Hepatic encephalopathy—definition, nomenclature, diagnosis, and quantification: final report of the working party at the 11th World Congresses of Gastroenterology, Vienna, 1998, *Hepatology* 35:716-721, 1998.
28. Trey C, Davidson CS: The management of fulminant hepatic failure, *Prog Liver Dis* 2:282-298, 1970.
29. Teasdale G, Jennett B: Assessment of coma and impaired consciousness. A practical scale, *Lancet* 2:81-83, 1974.
30. Bansky G, Meier PJ, Riederer E et al: Effects of the benzodiazepine receptor antagonist flumazenil in hepatic encephalopathy in humans, *Gastroenterology* 97:744-750, 1989.
31. O'Brien CJ, Wise RJS, O'Grady JG: Neurological sequelae in patients recovered from fulminant hepatic failure, *Gut* 28:93-95, 1987.
32. Blei A: Hypothermia for fulminant hepatic failure: a cool approach to a burning problem, *Liver Transpl* 6:245-247, 2000.
33. Jalan R: Intracranial hypertension in acute liver failure: pathophysiological basis of rational management. *Semin Liver Dis* 23: 271-282, 2003.
34. Wilkinson SP, Hurst D, Portmann B et al: Pathogenesis of renal failure in cirrhosis and fulminant hepatic failure, *Postgrad Med J* 51:503-505, 1975.
35. Bihari DJ, Gimson AE, Williams R: Cardiovascular, pulmonary and renal complications of fulminant hepatic failure, *Sem Liver Dis* 6:119-128, 1986.
36. Brown RS Jr, Lombardero M, Lake JR: Outcome of patients with renal insufficiency undergoing liver or liver-kidney transplantation, *Transplantation* 62:1788-1798, 1996.
37. Rolando N, Harvey F, Brahm J, et al: Prospective study of bacterial infection in acute liver failure: an analysis of fifty patients, *Hepatology* 11: 49-53, 1990.

38. Sauer I, Goetz M, Steffen J, et al: In vitro comparison of the molecular adsorbent recirculation system (MARS) and single-pass albumin dialysis (SPAD), *Hepatology* 39:1408-1414, 2004.
39. Mitzner S, Stange J, Peszunski P, et al: Extracorporeal support of the failing liver, *Cur Opin Crit Care* 8:171-177, 2002.
40. Chamuleau R: Artificial liver support in the third millennium, *Artif Cells Blood Substit Immobil Biotechnol* 21:117-126, 2003.
41. Tiles A, Berthiaume F, Yarmush M, et al: Bioengineering of liver assist devices, *J Hepatobiliary Pancreat Surg* 9:686-696, 2002.
42. Maxvold N, Smoyer W, Custer J et al: Amino acid loss and nitrogen balance in critically ill children with acute renal failure: a prospective comparison between classic hemofiltration and hemofiltration with dialysis.Amino acid loss and nitrogen balance in critically ill children with acute renal failure: a prospective comparison between classic hemofiltration and hemofiltration with dialysis, *Crit Care Med* 28:1161-1165, 2000.
43. Bunchman T, McBryde K, Mottes T et al: Pediatric acute renal failure: outcome by modality and disease, *Pediatr Nephrol* 16: 1067-1071, 2001.
44. Bunchman T, Maxvold N, Barnett J et al: Pediatric hemofiltration: Normocarb dialysate solution with citrate anticoagulation, *Pediatr Nephrol* 17:150-154, 2002.
45. Bunchman T, Maxvold N, Brophy P: Normocarb replacement fluid and citrate anticoagulation, *Am J Kidney Dis* 42:1248-1252, 2003.
46. Maxvold N, Flynn J, Smoyer W, et al: Prospective, crossover comparison of bicarbonate vs lactate-based dialysate for pediatric CVVHD, *Blood Purif* 17:27, 1999 (abstract).
47. Barenbrock M, Hausberg M, Matskies F et al: Effects of bicarbonate- and lactate-buffered replacement fluids on cardiovascular outcome in CVVH patients, *Kidney Int* 58:1751-1757, 2000.
48. Bunchman T, Rhodes R, Maxvold N: Normocarb vs. hemofiltration solution vs. pharmacy produced: Costs and liability, *Blood Purif* 2004 (in press).
49. Brophy P, McBryde K, Mottes T et al: Characteristics of interoperative continuous veno-venous hemofiltration in the pediatric intensive care unit, *Blood Purif* 18:33, 2000 (abstract).
50. O'Grady JG, Alexander GJM, Hayllar KM et al: Early indicators of prognosis in fulminant hepatic failure, *Gastroenterology* 97: 439-445, 1989.
51. McDiarmid S: Current status of liver transplantation in children, Pediatr Clin North Am 50:1335-1374, 2003.
52. Thomson M, McKiernan P, Buckels J, et al: Generalised mitochondrial cytopathy is an absolute contraindication to orthotopic liver transplant in childhood, *J Pediatr Gastroenterol Nutr* 26:478-481, 1998.
53. Superina RA, Pearl RH, Roberts EA et al: Liver transplantation in children: the initial Toronto experience, *J Pediatr Surg* 24:1013-1019, 1989.
54. Brems JJ, Hiatt JR, Ramming KP et al: Fulminant hepatic failure: the role of liver transplantation as primary therapy, *Am J Surg* 154:37-141, 1987.
55. Emond JC, Aran PP, Whitington PF et al: Liver transplantation in the management of fulminant hepatic failure, *Gastroenterology* 96:1583-1588, 1989.
56. Mack CL, Ferrario M, Abecassis M, et al: Living donor liver transplantation for children with liver failure and concurrent multiple organ system failure, *Liver Transpl* 7:890-895, 2001.
57. Miwa S, Hashikura Y, Mita A et al: Living-related liver transplantation for patients with fulminant and subfulminant hepatic failure, *Hepatology* 30:1521-1526, 1999.
58. Emre S, Schwartz ME, Shneider B et al: Living related liver transplantation for acute liver failure in children, *Liver Transpl Surg* 5:161-165, 1999.
59. Azoulay D, Samuel D, Ichai P, et al: Auxiliary partial orthotopic versus standard orthotopic whole liver transplantation for acute liver failure: a reappraisal from a single center by a case-control study, *Ann Surg* 234:723-7331, 2001.
60. Otte JB: Auxiliary partial orthotopic liver transplantation for acute liver failure in children, *Pediatr Transplant* 3:252-256, 1999.
61. Rand E, Olthoff K:Overview of pediatric liver transplantation, *Gastroenterol Clin* 32:913-929, 2003.
62. SPLIT Research Group:Studies of Pediatric Liver Transplantation (SPLIT): year 2000 outcomes, *Transplantation* 72:463-476, 2001.
63. A comparison of tacrolimus (FK506) and cyclosporine for immunosuppression in liver transplantation. The U.S. Multicenter FK506 Liver Study Group, *N Engl J Med* 331:1110-1118, 1994.
64. Jain A, Reyes J, Kashyap R et al: Liver transplantation under tacrolimus in infants, children, adults, and seniors: long-term results, survival and adverse events in 1000 consecutive patients, *Transplant Proc* 30:1403-1404, 1998.
65. Bronster D, Emre S, Boccagni P, et al: Central nervous system complications in liver transplant recipients-incidence, timing, and long-term follow-up, *Clin Transplant* 14:1-7, 2000.
66. Sussman NB: Fulminant hepatic failure. In Zakim D, Boyer TD, editors: *Hepatology*, Philadelphia, 1996, WB Saunders.

CHAPTER 82

Acute Abdomen

Yi-Horng Lee and Guy F. Brisseau

PEARLS

- The assessment of a child with an acute abdomen requires a thorough medical history and physical examination.
- Adjunct studies, especially diagnostic imaging, are often necessary to aid in the diagnosis. Ultrasonography and computerized tomography (CT) scanning are important and complimentary imaging modalities.
- Management decisions require good communication among all members of the health care team, especially the surgeon and intensivist. Aggressive resuscitation and antibiotic therapy are often required. Operative management, if necessary, must be individualized.
- Sir Zachary Cope first wrote a concise treatise on this topic in *Cope's Early Diagnosis of the Acute Abdomen* in 1921. In this treatise, he delineated the principles of evaluating "acute abdomen" that have remained the cornerstone of today's algorithm. Improvements in the understanding of the disease processes and as technical advances in laboratory and diagnostic imaging have improved diagnostic acumen. Nevertheless, CT scanning and ultrasonography can never replace an accurate history and a physical examination, as well as the ensuing decisions made by thoughtful physicians and surgeons.
- The decision on which management to pursue requires a thoughtful discussion between the pediatric intensivist and the surgeon. It is critical that a diagnosis be as clearly defined as possible before that decision is made. Finally, a decision is sometimes necessary to do a diagnostic procedure such as a laparotomy or laparoscopy to fully assess and potentially treat the critically ill patient with the acute abdomen.

Overview

Acute abdomen refers to a constellation of diseases with a wide spectrum of severity that requires methodical and systematic evaluation to optimize the outcome. The term *acute abdomen* has been used loosely to include a variety of illnesses that may cause acute abdominal pain from ischemia, infectious or inflammation. The primary goal in the evaluation of a patient with acute abdomen is the establishment of a diagnosis. This requires clinical acumen that can only be gained through arduous study of each disease process and versatile utility of diagnostic modalities. Sir Zachary Cope first wrote a concise treatise on this topic in *Cope's Early Diagnosis of the Acute Abdomen* in 1921. In this treatise, he delineated the principles of evaluating "acute abdomen" that have remained the cornerstone of today's algorithm. Improvements in the understanding of the disease processes and technical advances in laboratory and diagnostic imaging have improved diagnostic acumen. Nevertheless, computed tomography (CT) scanning and ultrasonography can never replace an accurate history and a physical examination, as well as the ensuing decisions made by thoughtful physicians and surgeons.[1]

Much of the literature on the evaluation and treatment of acute abdomen has been written about adult patients, but many of the same principles apply to infants and children. The differential diagnosis, however, must be modified to reflect the diseases that are more frequently inflicting young patients. Once the diagnosis is established, a correct treatment regimen can be individualized to the patient.

History

Age

Age is a much more important factor in the evaluation of a pediatric patient with acute abdomen than it is in adults. Although congenital conditions such as complicated meconium ileus, intestinal atresia, Hirschsprung's disease, or imperforate anus are diagnosed more commonly or exclusively in neonates, intussusception may be diagnosed in slightly older infants. If the patient is a premature infant, the likelihood of necrotizing enterocolitis increases. Peptic ulcer disease, appendicitis, and cholecystitis are more commonly found in older children.

When a neonatal patient or a young infant is evaluated, a history of not only the patient but also of the mother, including pregnancy and delivery, should be obtained. There are hints in the prenatal history that may suggest the cause of the patient's problem. For example, polyhydramnios may suggest a high intestinal atresia, whereas maternal diabetes may suggest a small left colon syndrome. The history of delivery is also important to assess for possible trauma.

Pain

Abdominal pain is a common denominator for most patients with acute abdomen. Pain becomes more useful as a diagnostic tool when the patient is old enough to vocalize such a complaint.

When it is reliably obtained through history or inference, the character of the pain is often useful. Unfortunately as the child's age decreases this becomes less helpful. Pain that is sharp and severe and constant suggests peritonitis, either diffuse or localized. The child can often describe every bump on the drive to the hospital. Pain that is crescendo-decrescendo in nature suggests pain of bowel distention. Often the pain is described as vague. This is less helpful.

The timing of the pain is also important. Sudden onset of pain is more in keeping with an acute event such as a perforated viscus from an ulcer or trauma. A ruptured ovarian cyst can also present this way. Parents often report a history of having to pick up their child from school because of sudden severe abdominal pain. On careful questioning, however, the pain was often less severe for a while before the child reported it. It is common for appendicitis to present in this manner. When the child cannot provide an accurate account for the onset of pain, it is sometimes useful to rely on the description from a school teacher or nurse.

When the onset of pain is more insidious, the patient often describes it as nagging and vague. This is more consistent with gastritis, inflammatory bowel disease, irritable bowel syndrome, or early appendicitis. Some diseases have a classic pain pattern that if present is useful. In a case of intussusception, the patient may be writhing in pain with intervening periods of lethargy. The presence of this pattern is helpful; however, the lack of the specific pattern does not exclude the diagnosis.[2]

The history of antecedent trauma should be noted. Liver or spleen lacerations are often preceded by trauma from contact sports, falls, or vehicular accidents. Sometimes the pain is not so severe at the beginning, but it worsens as the subcapsular hematoma enlarges. Diffuse abdominal pain ensues if the hepatic or splenic capsules rupture and the patient ends up with hemoperitoneum.

The location of pain is also important to note. Pain arising from the upper gastrointestinal (GI) tract, pancreas, gallbladder, and biliary tree is often felt first in the epigastrium. The pain of large intestine, either from colitis or constipation, is mostly felt in the hypogastrium. Pain arising from the lower abdomen in a young female may raise concerns regarding ruptured ovarian cyst, ectopic pregnancy, or pelvic inflammatory disease. Change of pain over time in location and character is also important. The classic shifting of the pain in appendicitis, when pain can shift from epigastric or periumbilical region to the right lower quadrant when present, is diagnostic of acute abdomen. Unfortunately, this can also be seen in other inflammatory conditions such as Crohn's disease, Meckel's diverticulitis, and mesenteric adenitis.

Radiation of the pain can also be helpful in arriving at a diagnosis. Gallbladder and biliary tract disease such as acute cholecystitis often radiates from the epigastrium/right upper quadrant (RUQ) around the right costal margin and may continue to the right scapula to the right shoulder. Pain in acute pancreatitis is usually epigastric in origin with subsequent radiation to the back. Ureteral calculi present as an acute onset of back pain that radiates to the unilateral groin region.

Aggravating or relieving factors should be noted. Pain from gastritis and peptic ulcer disease usually improves after food intake, whereas pain from biliary colic, acute cholecystitis, or pancreatitis worsens with food intake. This is especially true for fatty foods in the case of gallbladder disease. Vomiting can sometimes provide temporary relief from pain for the patient with intestinal obstruction; the distension improves on the expulsion of the stomach contents. Practically nothing can relieve the pain from intestinal obstruction if there is an element of ischemia involved, such as closed loop obstruction or strangulated hernia.

Feeding Intolerance

Feeding intolerance is more pertinent in younger children or infants. Before these patients can vocalize their complaints, feeding intolerance in the form of vomiting or irritability during feeds can herald signs of intraabdominal disease. Although feeding intolerance is frequently seen in nonemergency conditions such as hypertrophic pyloric stenosis or gastroesophageal reflux disease, its acute onset in a child who was thought to be previously healthy can indicate the presence of an abdominal catastrophe, such as midgut volvulus from undiagnosed malrotation or perforated appendicitis.

Vomiting

All babies spit up, but all parents know their babies' pattern. One must pay attention to parents who complain of excessive "spitting up" or "vomiting." If the patient is older, additional information may be obtained regarding the nature of vomiting (e.g., whether the vomiting is accompanied by cramping abdominal pain and whether such pain is relieved after vomiting).

The character of the vomited material is useful in diagnosis. The presence of bile suggests a problem distal to the ampulla of Vater. In a pediatric patient, especially an infant, the presence of bilious vomiting without a reason is considered malrotation until proven otherwise. Other obstructions are possible, but malrotation is the most dangerous given the potential for midgut volvulus and significant loss of bowel. Because the site of obstruction moves distally in the GI tract, the vomitus progressively becomes more brown and feculent.

Conditions that cause proximal nonbilious vomiting that result in acute abdomen, such as acute gastric volvulus, are rare but do exist. Vomiting can also occur in the absence of a mechanical obstruction. Such an obstruction includes the presence of a paralytic ileus from any source such as peritonitis from a perforated appendix. Finally, vomiting may occur as result of severe pain alone, as with renal colic.

Bowel Habits

Any history of constipation, diarrhea, and a recent change in bowel habits can aid in the diagnosis of acute abdomen. Although constipation itself can cause severe abdominal pain, it is a diagnosis of exclusion. In a patient who has chronic constipation, it is important to rule out Hirschsprung's disease or Hirschsprung-associated enterocolitis. These conditions can be ruled out with the obtainment of a thorough history[3]; however, if doubt remains, a rectal biopsy may be necessary.

Diarrhea can occur in many contexts, including inflammatory bowel disease and infectious enteritis. Many of these conditions are self-limiting; however, they occasionally cause profound systemic disease and require an emergency colectomy. Besides primary colonic diseases, any process that inflames the colon can cause diarrhea. An example of this is the diarrhea associated with an intra-abdominal abscess.

The character of stool should be noted. Blood in the stool can be helpful in diagnosis. In a premature infant, bloody stools may be the first sign of necrotizing enterocolitis. Older infants with intussusception often have currant jelly stools. Children with inflammatory bowel disease may have rectal bleeding.

Menstruation

Pediatric physicians care for young female patients who are menstruating. The regularity and the date of last period are essential in the evaluation of a young woman with abdominal pain. The timing of a ruptured follicular or corpus luteum cyst in relation to menses is obvious at 14 days after the first day of the last period. Discussion regarding sexual activities may not be fruitful because the patient may not be forthcoming with such information, especially in the presence of parents. Therefore determining the pregnancy status of all female patients of reproductive age is important. Abdominal pain from a ruptured ectopic pregnancy can have potentially life-threatening consequences.

Pain accompanying menstruation in a patient who has no previous history of dysmenorrhea may indicate a threatened early abortion, an ectopic pregnancy, or a pelvic inflammatory disease. Even for patients who have nonpregnancy-related abdominal diseases, physicians should determine the pregnancy status of the patient before embarking on a series of diagnostic imaging studies and deciding on a treatment plan that may be harmful to the fetus.[4-6]

Comorbid Conditions

Knowing the medical and surgical history of the patient will provide invaluable insight to the current disease process. Specific operations have late complications that are both common to all operations and unique to others. Patients who underwent abdominal operations have adhesions. Small bowel obstructions that result from adhesions are much more likely in this population. In a patient who has previous gastric fundoplication, gastric bloat syndrome must be suspected. Mononucleosis may lead to splenomegaly with an increased chance for splenic trauma. Patients with spherocytosis and other red cell disorders may have abdominal pain from symptomatic cholelithiasis, such as cholecystitis, cholangitis, or gallstone pancreatitis. Patients with sickle cell disease may have abdominal crisis or autoinfarction of the spleen.[7] Patients with portal hypertension and ascites may have spontaneous bacterial peritonitis. A patient with neutropenia may have neutropenic enterocolitis, also known as typhlitis.[8]

Patients in pediatric intensive care units often have a myriad of medical problems. Many of these require vasopressive support or had profound hypotension or arrest prior to admission. In these patients a suspicion for mesenteric ischemia is often raised and can be difficult to diagnose.

The medication history is also important because many medications may cause diseases such as pancreatitis.[9-12] Steroids that mask the inflammatory process make the interpretation of the physical examination difficult. Also, some medications such as narcotics and paralytic agents make the physical examinations less reliable.

Physical Examination

Although physical examination of critically ill patients can be difficult to interpret at times, a good amount of data to help with the care of the patient can be obtained from this time-honored process. One must be able to understand the findings in the context of the patient's overall condition. Sedation, chemical paralysis, and capillary leak syndrome with peripheral edema can make the physical examination much more difficult.

General Appearance

The general appearance of the patient with acute abdomen is enlightening. The patient who is happy and talking with his parents is different from the intubated and paralyzed child with multiple intravenous (IV) drips. Although this may seem obvious, it is important that the astute clinician be able to recognize a sick patient and be able to modify the technique and interpretation of the physical examination.

Vital Signs

The vital signs are the next step in a physical examination for determination of acute abdomen. The presence of a fever is helpful in suggesting an inflammatory condition. The lack of a fever, however, does not rule this out. The pulse and blood pressure are important indicators of the hemodynamic status of the patient; however, they need to be placed in the context of the patient's overall condition. The presence of hypotension is a worrisome sign because blood pressure is normally maintained and is the last parameter to be affected in otherwise healthy pediatric patients. The respiratory rate is also important. Unexplained tachypnea may need to be assessed and treated quickly. Pediatric patients with acute abdomens may be tachypneic from abdominal pain or a metabolic acidosis due to underresuscitation or dead bowel. These vital signs not only will help with the diagnosis of the patient but will also be useful in guiding resuscitative therapy.

Chest Examination

Examination of the chest is an important part in assessment of the patient with acute abdomen. Decreased breath sounds at the base of the lungs suggest the possibility of pneumonia, which can mimic acute abdomen. Bowel sounds in the chest may represent a diaphragmatic hernia that causes obstruction from incarcerated bowel. Absent breath sounds may be a pneumothorax or hemothorax after trauma. The nature of the decreased breath sounds can be sorted out with percussion.

Abdominal Examination

The most important part of the physical examination for acute abdomen is the abdominal examination. The order of the steps used in the abdominal examination is up to each physician. We start with inspection. This ensures that the entire abdomen is exposed from the xiphisternum to the groins, including the flanks. In thin abdominal walls, such as those that exist in neonates, intraabdominal disease is often reflected with abdominal wall findings. These include erythema, either localized or diffuse. Similarly, abdominal wall edema may occur. If stool has leaked from the bowel, this may also be seen through a thin abdominal wall. In older children, pancreatitis can present with bluish discoloration in the flank (Grey Turner's sign) or in the periumbilical area (Cullen's sign). Inspection may also suggest hernias of the abdominal wall, including the groins.

After inspection, we use palpation. Palpation starts lightly and then increases in pressure. In the acute abdomen we feel for the presence of peritoneal irritation, either diffuse or localized, and for masses. Accurate palpation for peritonitis is as much art as science, and unfortunately there is little substitute for experience. The signs of peritoneal irritation include involuntary guarding and rigidity. Involuntary guarding is present when the abdominal wall tenses on gentle palpation. This is often localized over the area of intraabdominal disease. Rigidity is present when the abdominal wall is hard without palpation, and this is often diffuse. This condition suggests a free intraabdominal process that has irritated the entire peritoneum such as a visceral perforation. Masses are also palpated to help with the diagnosis of acute abdomen. Intraabdominal abscesses and tumors often present with masses and may suggest the cause of the patient's problem.

Auscultation follows the palpation stage and serves two purposes. First, when placing the stethoscope on the abdomen in all quadrants, one can confirm that the guarding felt on palpation is truly involuntary because the wakeful patient is distracted. Second, the presence of bowel sounds is useful. Most inflammatory processes lead to an ileus with the absence of bowel sounds, whereas high-pitched bowel sounds may suggest a bowel obstruction.

We use percussion last. Again, this can reconfirm the true nature of the local peritoneal findings in the wakeful child. Percussion is also used to assess the nature of the distension such as tympanic air compared with more dull-sounding liquids, such as ascites.

Ancillary Studies

Despite the complete medical history and physical examination of a patient, the exact cause of acute abdomen is often not clear. Ancillary studies are helpful, and the history and physical examination should be used to guide these studies.

Laboratory Evaluation

Although the prudent use of hospital resources is appropriate, a relatively complete hematological and biochemical work-up is indicated in the patient with the acute abdomen. Hematologic evaluation is useful to ensure that the patient does not have an undiagnosed neutropenic state such as in leukemia with neuropenic enterocolitis.[17] In the acute abdomen patient a drop in the hemoglobin after resuscitation suggests intraabdominal bleeding. Biochemical evaluation is also important to assess the liver and pancreas as etiology to the acute abdomen. The acid-base status is useful in management and evaluation of the patient. With an unexplained lactic acidosis the possibility of dead bowel must be entertained.[2,12,15]

Diagnostic Imaging Evaluation

Diagnostic imaging has become a crucial part of the evaluation of these patients with a difficult condition. It often will lead to the diagnosis and may indicate that an operation is unnecessary, or it can help in preoperative planning and parental consent.

Plain X-ray Film

Plain films of the chest and abdomen are a good start toward diagnosis. They may help assess alternative diagnosis such as the presence of pneumonia on chest x-ray film. If possible, an upright chest x-ray film is best to also assess for free air. The abdominal films will reveal many details of the abdomen. Distended bowel loops with collapsed distal bowel suggest an obstruction, whereas distension throughout the GI tract suggests an ileus. A gasless abdomen may have a high-grade obstruction or ascites. The lateral decubitus film is important, especially in the sick patient. This film will show free air in the abdomen and air-fluid levels within the bowel. Despite a gasless abdomen on supine films there often will be air-fluid levels on lateral decubitus films (Figure 82–1).

Abdominal Ultrasonography

Abdominal ultrasonography (US) is useful in the study of a patient with an acute abdomen.[16-20] It has many advantages for the patient in the ICU. Ultrasound is portable so the patient does not have to be moved from the ICU. The study is in real time and is easily repeatable to assess changes over time. Finally, no ionizing radiation is used.

A variety of uses of ultrasound in the patients with acute abdomen have been studied. Ultrasound can assess the viability of bowel by assessing the blood flow in the bowel wall (Figure 82–2) and the presence of bowel wall movement. The character of intraperitoneal fluid can be assessed to differentiate simple ascites from particulate matter that is more in keeping with perforated bowel.[13] The presence of abscesses can also be assessed. Finally, individual organs can be assessed. These include the liver, gallbladder, biliary tree, pancreas, spleen, kidneys, and pelvic organs. In fact, ultrasound gives better detail to many of these organs than a CT scan.

Given the physics of sound waves there are certain limitations to US technology. An adequate study can be difficult to obtain in the obese patient. Furthermore, an abdomen full of bowel gas or free air may obscure the structures behind because gas is to ultrasound as metal is to x-ray films. Finally, US is the most user-dependent

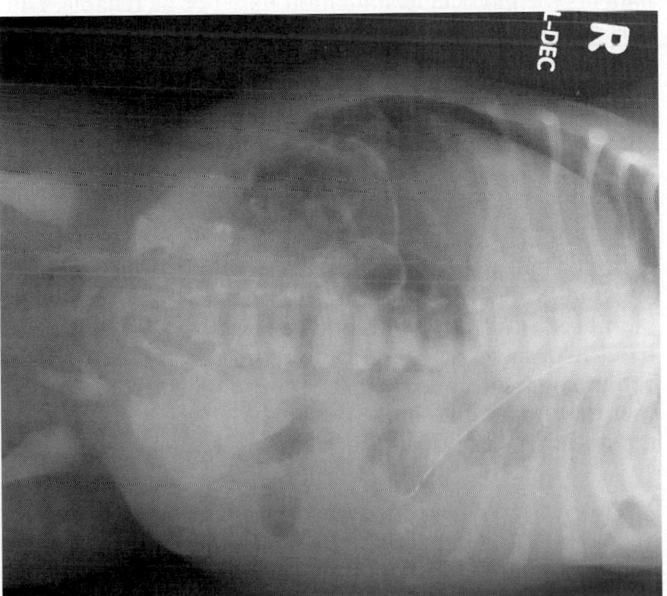

FIGURE 82–1 • A lateral decubitus abdominal film with right side up showing free air over the liver.

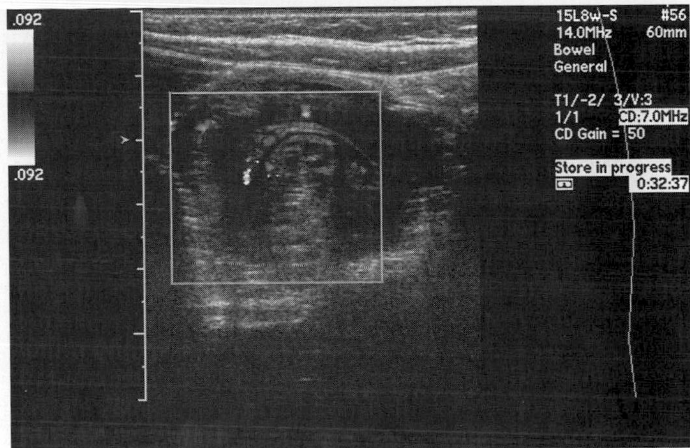

FIGURE 82–2 • An abdominal sonogram of intussuscepted bowel showing good blood flow (blue and red signals) in the intussusceptum.

technique in diagnostic imaging. Despite these limits US is an ever-increasing diagnostic modality in the ICU.

The use of ultrasound by nonradiology clinicians is increasing. This trend started in the trauma room with the Focused Abdominal Sonography for Trauma (FAST).[21] Current indications and utilization are increasing.[22,23] Despite this trend, without expertise in the interpretation of abdominal US in these complex patients, consultation with an experienced ultrasonographer is imperative.

Computerized Tomography Scanning

Computerized tomography (CT) scanning has revolutionized the way physicians are able to care for the patient with the acute abdomen.[24] Current CT imaging is fast, and the image quality has improved significantly over the past 15 years. CT allows visualization of all of the peritoneal and retroperitoneal organs. It is also not limited by air as US is, given the difference in technology (radiation compared with sound waves). IV contrast allows for sharper visualization because of the increased visual contrast seen when the dye flows to the organs. GI contrast is preferred to help compare fluid that may be extraluminal. Bladder contrast is useful to assess the potential for rupture. In the absence of a clinical suspicion of bladder rupture the bladder is adequately seen on delayed images with clearance of the IV contrast by the kidneys.

CT scanning is useful in the diagnosis of many causes of the acute abdomen. The solid organs are well visualized (Figure 82–3). Hollow viscus organs are also well seen with intraluminal contrast. The size and thickness of the bowel is well seen, and this is useful in the assessment of bowel obstructions or inflammatory processes. Extraluminal leakage of contrast suggests a perforation; however, failure to show leakage of contrast does not rule out a perforation.[25]

Extraluminal fluid is clearly seen (see Figure 82–3). This fluid can be free fluid or a loculated collection. A suggestion of the complexity of the fluid can be assessed as well (Figure 82–4). CT scanning is exquisitely sensitive at detecting free air.

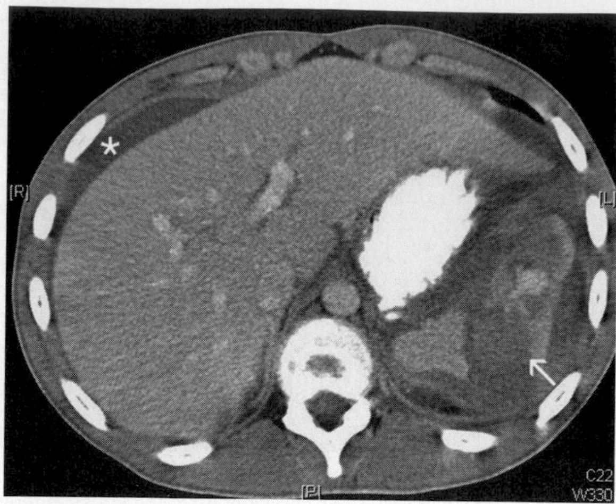

FIGURE 82–3 • An abdominal computerized tomography scan showing a fractured spleen (*arrow*) and free intraabdominal fluid, which is blood (*).

The correct interpretation of the CT scan can only be made within the clinical setting. The presence of a small amount of free air may be important in a patient with trauma who has diffuse abdominal pain, rigidity, and free fluid in the abdomen with no solid organ injury. This patient has the classic signs for a small bowel perforation. The same patient with few abdominal symptoms and a traumatic pneumothorax, however, may just have a little air tracing from the chest.[26]

The disadvantages of CT scanning must be appreciated before this technology is used for patients. The first hurdle is that the patient must be able to be transported to the scanning facility, and this is undesirable for patients who are unstable in the ICU. Optimal scanning requires both GI and IV contrasts. A patient with ileus may not tolerate GI contrast; the risk of aspiration may ensue as GI contrast is given. An IV contrast agent is nephrotoxic, and it can precipitate acute renal failure, especially in the poorly perfused patient who is critically ill. The final point of CT scanning is the potential long-term negative impact of this technology. Recent data have suggested that diagnostic CT imaging increases the lifetime risk of death from radiation-induced malignancy.[27–29] This risk, although real, must be balanced against the risk of not doing the study in the patient.

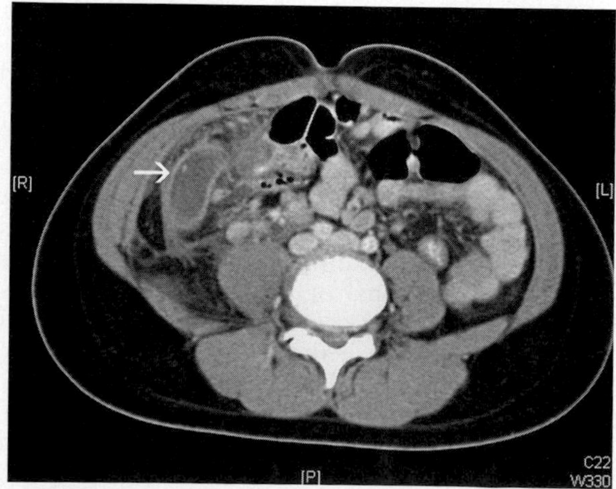

FIGURE 82–4 • An abdominal computerized tomography scan showing an intraperitoneal abscess with an appendicolith within it (*arrow*).

Magnetic Resonance Imaging

In the past several years the technology of magnetic resonance (MR) scanning has improved greatly. Newer machines are able to do faster scans. To address the issues of ionizing radiation, researchers have recently attempted to use MR to assess patients with acute abdomen in several small studies. These small studies have shown good results and show promise for this technology.[30,31] Currently limits remain when this technology is applied to the critically ill patient. As with CT scanning, the patient must be transferred to the MR suite. There is increased time in the MR scanner, and given the configuration of the MR suite, monitoring of the patient during the procedure can be difficult.

Other Diagnostic Imaging

In unusual circumstances a GI contrast study may be useful in the patient with acute abdomen. These include an upper GI study, which is a contrast study from the esophagus to the ligament of Trietz or a contrast enema. When a perforation is considered, barium is not normally used and rather a water-soluble media is used (see Table 82–1).

Nuclear medicine scans have little use in the acute abdomen given the time to perform these studies.

Other Diagnostic Tests

Diagnostic Peritoneal Lavage

Diagnostic peritoneal lavage (DPL) is a useful technique to assess the abdomen when one is unsure of the integrity of the bowel. This is most useful in the very sick patient in the ICU who is systemically ill, requires ventilation, has paralysis, and is not suitable for transport to CT scan. In these patients the physical examination may not be reliable. DPL was developed more than three decades ago for assessment of the adult patient with abdomen trauma. Today DPL has been almost completely replaced by FAST ultrasound in patients with trauma.[23,32] DPL can also be used in settings where ultrasound findings are equivocal or ultrasound technology is not available.

DPL involves surgically placing a small catheter in the abdomen. The fluid is aspirated. If no fluid is aspirated, then normal saline is instilled at 10 ml/kg, allowed to sit, and then retrieved. The fluid is then assessed for white blood cells (WBCs), red blood cells (RBCs), amylase, and bile. Aspiration of enteric contents or elevated WBC count suggests a bowel perforation. This technique is user dependent but can be invaluable in the assessment of the critically ill patient with acute abdomen.[33,34]

Diagnostic Minilaparoscopy

All of the techniques presented cannot directly visualize the abdomen. Before the advent of minimally invasive technology, laparotomies were required. Currently, however, a minilaparoscopy without anesthesia is available.[15,35]

TABLE 82–1

Diagnostic Imaging Modality	Pros	Cons
Plain films	Portable Easy Good screen	
Ultrasound	Portable Sensitive and specific Repeatable Real-time and dynamic No ionizing radiation	Requires expertise Limited in obese Limited by bowel air
CT scan	Visualize entire abdomen Sensitive and specific Readily available Less user dependent	Must transport patient Ionizing radiation? Cancer risk
MR scan	Early studies suggest good results	Must transport patient Longer scan Utility not fully defined
GI contrast studies	Useful in specific indications	Must transport patient Limited indications

CT, computerized tomography; *GI,* gastrointestinal; *MR,* magnetic resonance.

This procedure allows for direct visualization of the bowel to aid in the diagnosis of patients with the most difficult conditions.

Differential Diagnosis

The differential diagnosis for acute abdominal pain represents a complete list of most problems with all of the intraabdominal, retroperitoneal and pelvic organs. A useful differential diagnosis list is included in Table 82–2.

Management of the Acute Abdomen

Resuscitation

Most patients with an intraabdominal inflammatory response have a large fluid shift. These fluids may be intraluminal, as with a bowel obstruction, or intraperitoneal, as with a perforation. This shift is exacerbated by a systemic inflammatory response and a third space of fluid from the intravascular to the extravascular space. Patients with acute abdomen generally need an aggressive fluid resuscitation. Although the use of inotropes may be indicated, the first line of therapy remains fluid resuscitation.

Antibiotic Therapy

When an infective process may be contributing to acute abdomen, antibiotic therapy is generally recommended. Initial therapy is directed at the broad range of GI bacteria contaminants. The exact antibiotics to be used are institution dependent, but one should ensure adequate coverage

TABLE 82–2

Differential Diagnosis of Acute Abdomen

System	Diagnoses
GI tract	Gastritis/peptic ulcer disease Infectious enteritis Small/large bowel obstruction (all type) Meckel's diverticulitis Inflammatory bowel disease Intestinal perforation Intestinal ischemia Incarcerated hernia Omental infarction or cyst Constipation
Solid organs and biliary tract	Hepatitis Cholangitis Cholecystitis Pancreatitis Ruptured choledochal cyst
Urinary system	Pyelonephritis Renal colic
Reproductive system	Pelvic inflammatory disease Ectopic pregnancy Ruptured ovarian cyst Ovarian torsion Testicular torsion
Abdominal wall	Abscess Trauma
Other	Retroperitoneal hematoma Spontaneous bacterial peritonitis Sickle cell crisis Acute porphyria Hypercalcemia SLE

GI, gastrointestinal; *SLE,* systemic lupus erythematosus.

for anaerobic bacteria, gram-negative bacilli, and gram-positive enterococcus.

Definitive Management

Each diagnosis in the differential of acute abdomen has its unique management. Many diagnoses require urgent operations after resuscitation. Others require purely nonoperative management. A final group requires conservative management with an operation for failure of conservative management. The decision on which management to pursue requires a thoughtful discussion between the pediatric intensivist and the surgeon. It is critical that a diagnosis be as clearly defined as possible before that decision is made. Finally, a decision is sometimes necessary to do a diagnostic procedure such as a laparotomy or laparoscopy to fully assess and potentially treat the critically ill patient with acute abdomen. With current diagnostic techniques this has become less prevalent.

Summary

The diagnosis of the pediatric patient with acute abdomen takes the skill of an astute clinician. This clinician must be able to integrate the data of a well-obtained history and physical examination and be able to obtain the needed diagnostic studies to develop the diagnosis or at least a correct differential diagnosis. Once the diagnosis is established, acute abdomen becomes another diagnosis that has a unique therapeutic course. Active dialog between the intensivist and the surgeon is paramount to have a successful outcome in these children with a difficult condition.

REFERENCES

1. William Silen, editor: *Cope's early diagnosis of the acute abdomen*, ed 20, New York, 2000, Oxford University Press.
2. Stringer DA, Ein SH: Pneumatic reduction: advantages, risks and indications, *Pediatr Radiol* 20:475-477, 1990.
3. Lewis NA, Levitt MA, Zallen GS et al: Diagnosing Hirschsprung's disease: increasing the odds of a positive rectal biopsy result, *J Pediatr Surg* 38:412-416; discussion 412-416, 2003.
4. Friedman JM: Teratogen update: anesthetic agents, *Teratology* 37:69-77, 1988.
5. Kuczkowski KM: Nonobstetric surgery during pregnancy: what are the risks of anesthesia? *Obstet Gynecol Surv* 59:52-56, 2004.
6. Ratnapalan S, Bona N, Chandra K et al: Physicians' perceptions of teratogenic risk associated with radiography and CT during early pregnancy, *AJR Am J Roentgenol* 182:1107-1109, 2004.
7. Bonadio WA: Clinical features of abdominal painful crisis in sickle cell anemia, *J Pediatr Surg* 25:301-302, 1990.
8. Habek D, Cerkez Habek J, Galic J et al: Acute abdomen as first symptom of acute leukemia, *Arch Gynecol Obstet* 270:122-123, 2004.
9. Fisher AA, Bassett ML: Acute pancreatitis associated with angiotensin II receptor antagonists, *Ann Pharmacother* 36:1883-1886, 2002.
10. Grauso-Eby NL, Goldfarb O, Feldman-Winter LB et al: Acute pancreatitis in children from Valproic acid: case series and review, *Pediatr Neurol* 28:145-148, 2003.
11. Herrlinger KR, Kreisel W, Schwab M et al: 6-thioguanine–efficacy and safety in chronic active Crohn's disease, *Aliment Pharmacol Ther* 17:503-508, 2003.
12. Kasi VS, Estrada CA, Wiese W: Association of pancreatitis with administration of contrast medium and intravenous lipid emulsion in a patient with the acquired immunodeficiency syndrome, *South Med J* 96:66-69, 2003.
13. Azarow K, Connolly B, Babyn P et al: Multidisciplinary evaluation of the distended abdomen in critically ill infants and children: the role of bedside sonography, *Pediatr Surg Int* 13:355-359, 1998.
14. Ein SH, Superina R, Bagwell C et al: Ischemic bowel after primary closure for gastroschisis, *J Pediatr Surg* 23:728-730, 1988.
15. Gagne DJ, Malay MB, Hogle NJ et al: Bedside diagnostic minilaparoscopy in the intensive care patient, *Surgery* 131:491-496, 2002.
16. Bachar GN, Shafir G, Postnikov V et al: Sonographic diagnosis of right segmental omental infarction, *J Clin Ultrasound* 33:76-79, 2005.
17. Byrne AT, Goeghegan T, Govender P et al: The imaging of intussusception, *Clin Radiol* 60:39-46, 2005.
18. Patino MO, Munden MM: Utility of the sonographic whirlpool sign in diagnosing midgut volvulus in patients with atypical clinical presentations, *J Ultrasound Med* 23:397-401, 2004.
19. Puylaert JB: Ultrasonography of the acute abdomen: gastrointestinal conditions, *Radiol Clin North Am* 41:1227-1242, vii, 2003.
20. Vasavada P: Ultrasound evaluation of acute abdominal emergencies in infants and children, *Radiol Clin North Am* 42:445-456, 2004.
21. Rozycki GS, Feliciano DV, Schmidt JA et al: The role of surgeon-performed ultrasound in patients with possible cardiac wounds, *Ann Surg* 223:737-744; discussion 744-746, 1996.
22. Ashley DW, Gamblin TC, McCampbell BL et al: Bedside insertion of vena cava filters in the intensive care unit using intravascular ultrasound to locate renal veins, *J Trauma* 57:26-31, 2004.
23. Knudtson JL, Dort JM, Helmer SD et al: Surgeon-performed ultrasound for pneumothorax in the trauma suite, *J Trauma* 56:527-530, 2004.
24. Taourel P, Baron MP, Pradel J et al: Acute abdomen of unknown origin: impact of CT on diagnosis and management, *Gastrointest Radiol* 17:287-291, 1992.
25. Cox TD, Kuhn JP: CT scan of bowel trauma in the pediatric patient, *Radiol Clin North Am* 34:807-818, 1996.
26. Hamilton P, Rizoli S, McLellan B et al: Significance of intra-abdominal extraluminal air detected by CT scan in blunt abdominal trauma, *J Trauma* 39:331-333, 1995.
27. Berdon WE, Slovis TL: Where we are since ALARA and the series of articles on CT dose in children and risk of long-term cancers: what has changed? *Pediatr Radiol* 32:699, 2002.
28. Brenner D, Elliston C, Hall E et al: Estimated risks of radiation-induced fatal cancer from pediatric CT, *AJR Am J Roentgenol* 176: 289-296, 2001.
29. Brenner DJ, Elliston CD, Hall EJ et al: Estimates of the cancer risks from pediatric CT radiation are not merely theoretical: comment on "point/counterpoint: in x-ray computed tomography, technique factors should be selected appropriate to patient size. against the proposition," *Med Phys* 28:2387-2388, 2001.
30. Birchard KR, Brown MA, Hyslop WB et al: MRI of acute abdominal and pelvic pain in pregnant patients, *AJR Am J Roentgenol* 184: 452-8, 2005.
31. Pedrosa I, Rofsky NM: MR imaging in abdominal emergencies, *Radiol Clin North Am* 41:1243-1273, 2003.
32. Brooks A, Davies B, Smethhurst M et al: Prospective evaluation of non-radiologist performed emergency abdominal ultrasound for haemoperitoneum, *Emerg Med J* 21:e5, 2004.
33. Kumar A, Saltzman D, Shukula M et al: Diagnostic peritoneal lavage for assessing acute abdomen in pediatric oncology and stem cell transplantation patients, *J Pediatr Hematol Oncol* 26:824-826, 2004.
34. Naidu VV, Kate V, Koner BC et al: Diagnostic peritoneal lavage (DPL)–is it useful decision making process for management of the equivocal acute abdomen? *Trop Gastroenterol* 24:140-143, 2003.
35. Rosser JC Jr, Palter SF, Rodas EB et al: Minilaparoscopy without general anesthesia for the diagnosis of acute appendicitis, *JSLS* 2:79-82, 1998.

CHAPTER 83

The Innate Immune System

Brett P. Giroir

PEARLS

- *Innate immunity* represents an ancient, evolutionarily conserved system that provides the host with an immediate defense against a wide variety of pathogens. The innate immune system does not require previous exposure to the pathogen.
- The innate immune system did not evolve to contend with overwhelming bacteremia, multiple trauma, massive transfusion, and other major insults of modern civilization.
- The innate immune system is activated in nearly every patient admitted to the pediatric intensive care unit, due to an infection, a tissue injury, or an ongoing isolated organ inflammation such as what occurs during chronic heart failure.
- Whether a robust immune response occurs depends largely on the patient's innate immune genetic program and the interaction of these genes with a multitude of environmental stressors (e.g., malnutrition, barrier breeches, drugs).
- Current therapeutic strategies aimed at modifying the innate immune response include the blockade of toll-like receptor recognition with molecules such as bactericidal/permeability increasing protein; modulation of the coagulation response with recombinant activated protein C, pooled plasma protein C, or specific inhibitors such as tissue factor pathway inhibitor; and blockade of specific effectors such as platelet-activating factor.
- The optimization of these therapies may only occur when individuals' genetic predispositions are understood.

Adaptive immunity is the biological process in which exquisitely specific immune effector mechanisms are generated in response to pathogen (or vaccine) exposure. Adaptive immunity requires days or weeks for development and often involves somatic gene rearrangements. Components of the adaptive immune system include immunoglobulins and specific T- and B- cell recognition molecules and their responses.

In contrast, *innate immunity* represents an ancient, evolutionarily conserved system that provides the host with an immediate defense against a wide variety of pathogens.[1] The innate immune system does not require previous exposure to the pathogen.[2,3] Cells of the innate immune system are monocytes, neutrophils, endothelial cells, and dendritic cells but are also non–bone marrow–derived cells; organs such as the liver, heart, and lungs are composed of these latter cells. Once activated, the innate immune system launches potent cellular and humoral effectors to kill or contain the invading microbe. Simultaneously, the innate immune system is modulated by numerous inputs, including products secreted from innate immune cells; catecholamines; hormones; and perhaps most interesting, direct innervation from the central nervous system.

Whereas the adaptive immune system is associated with immunologists, the innate immune system should be associated with the intensivist. Septic shock, for example, is the result of coordinated activation of the innate immune response throughout the host. Pathogenesis of the acute respiratory response syndrome and multiorgan failure also involve activation and propagation of the innate immune response. Furthermore, recent data indicate that even the pathogenesis of cardiac dysfunction in neonates after cardiopulmonary bypass reflects, at least in part, activation of innate immune responses in the heart, which directly depress cardiac contractility. Some therapies targeting the innate immune system are currently in clinical trials; other therapies, such as recombinant activated protein C, have already been approved for selected adult populations. Therefore the purpose of this chapter is to provide the intensivist a comprehensive understanding of the role of innate immune activation in critically ill and injured children and to provide a conceptual framework for which new therapeutics can be developed and tested.

Pathogen Recognition

Cells of the innate immune system use two systems for recognizing invading microorganisms. The first mechanism relies on the identification of *pathogen associated molecular patterns* (PAMPs), which are microbial molecules primarily composed of lipids or carbohydrates that are essential to pathogen survival. PAMPs, by definition, have no homologue in humans. The recognition of a microbial PAMP is coupled to prostimulatory signals that activate the innate immune response. The second mechanism used to detect microbes has been termed *recognition of missing self.* Normal uninfected host cells (but not microbial cells) express surface molecules, such as major histocompatibility complex (MHC) class-I molecules. Recognition of *self* molecules such as MHC-I triggers inhibitory signals in cells that prevent innate immune activation.[4,5]

The prototypical PAMP of gram-negative bacteria is lipopolysaccharide (LPS) or endotoxin, which, when administered to animals or humans, can mimic the pathophysiology of septic shock. Discovery of the LPS recognition system elucidated the mechanism of PAMP recognition by the innate immune system.

During the course of an infection with gram-negative bacteria, LPS is present on the bacterial surface and is also spontaneously shed into the plasma. During certain infections, such as meningococcal sepsis, bacterial membrane blebbing results in the extremely high levels of spontaneously shed endotoxin, yielding plasma levels of endotoxin at least 100-fold greater than in other gram-negative infections. Endotoxin may also be shed rapidly from the bacterial membrane after treatment with antibiotics. In all cases, LPS is first bound to LPS-binding protein (LBP), a 60-kD acute phase glycoprotein synthesized in the liver and present in the plasma. LBP facilitates transfer of LPS to a cell surface complex consisting of the CD14 molecule and the recently discovered toll-like receptor 4 (TLR-4) molecule.

TLRs appear to be the primary recognition receptors for microbial molecules (PAMPs). Thus far, 10 TLRs have been identified in humans.[6] These receptors are strikingly homologous to receptors in *Drosophila* species, in which the toll molecule is essential for antipathogen responses. For example, deficiency of the toll protein in *Drosophila* species results in overwhelming *Aspergillus* infection and death from the fly equivalent of fungal sepsis. In 1998 Beutler[7] discovered that TLR-4 is responsible for recognition of endotoxin in mammals. Deficiency of TLR-4 results in complete protection from LPS challenge yet complete lethality from challenge with even a few gram-negative organisms.

The functions of other TLRs have also been elucidated. TLR-2 recognizes essential components of gram-positive bacteria such as peptidoglycans and lipoteichoic acids and also recognizes cell wall components of yeast and mycobacteria. It also appears that TLR-2 may recognize an atypical LPS molecule produced by *Leptospira interrogans*. TLR-5 is known to recognize flagellin, a monomeric constituent of flagella on bacteria such as *Listeria* and *Salmonella* organisms. Another receptor in this family, TLR-9, recognizes DNA sequences that are found in viruses, bacteria, parasites, and other potential pathogens (so-called CpG DNA) but are not found in mammals (Table 83–1).[8,9]

The function of the other TLRs is yet to be discovered; however, additional principles are already emerging.

TABLE 83–1

Components of the Innate Immune System

Pathogen Molecules	Innate Immune Receptors	Innate Immune Effectors
LPS (gram-negative bacteria) → RSV Hsp 60	TLR 4	Cells Neutrophils Monocytes Macrophages NK cells
Lipopeptides → Lipoteichoic acids Peptidoglycans (gram-positive bacteria) (Mycobacteria) (*Borrelia burgdorferi*)	TLR 2	Sentinel cytokines TNF-α IL-1 Chemokines NO
Yeast		Late response cytokines HMG-1 MIF
		Innate immunoproteins
CpG DNA →	TLR 9	MBL Complement
Flagellin →	TLR 5	BPI Defensins Lactoferrin CRP
		Procoagulants/antifibrinolytic tissue factors PAI-1 TAFI

BPI, bactericidal/permeability increasing protein; *CRP,* C-reactive protein; *HMG-1,* high mobility group-1 protein; *Hsp,* heat shock protein; *IL-1,* interleukin-1; *LPS,* lipopolysaccharide; *MBL,* mannose-binding lectin; *MIF,* macrophage migration-inhibitory factor; *NK,* natural killer; *NO,* nitric oxide; *PAI-1,* plasminogen-activator inhibitor-1; *RSV,* respiratory syncytial virus; *TAFI,* thrombin-activated fibrinolysis inhibitor; *TLR,* toll-like receptor; *TNF-α,* tumor necrosis factor α.

TLR-1 and TLR-6 may be involved in the enhancement of responses of other TLRs. Data now suggest that TLRs may associate both as homodimers or heterodimers (i.e., one molecule of TLR-4 closely associated with TLR-1). If the existence of such a combinatorial system proves to be correct, the recognition repertoire of the innate immune system may be exponentially greater than originally envisioned (2^9 potential specificities), providing even more certainty that newly emerging PAMPs would also be recognized by the innate immune system.

Of particular interest is that TLR-4 may also be involved in nonbacterial signaling, in that respiratory syncytial virus triggers an innate immune response through TLR-4. In addition, heat shock protein 60 (Hsp 60) has also been shown to be a TLR-4 ligand, providing a direct explanation for why a variety of insults, including trauma and ischemia-reperfusion, trigger a systemic inflammatory response syndrome (SIRS) similar to that due to infection. It is clear based on this discussion that the phenotype of systemic inflammation caused by innate immune activation represents a general response to injury and invasion with a common set of molecular effectors.

Signaling

TLR recognition likely occurs in the phagosome after ingestion of pathogens by cells of the innate immune system. For TLR-4, there is an additional requirement that the TLR-4 extracellular domain must be complexed to myeloid differentiation protein 2 (MD-2), a soluble protein required for TLR-4 interaction with endotoxin. Binding of TLR-2 or TLR-4 to their pathogen substrates results in dimerization, recruitment of the adapter protein myeloid differentiation primary response gene (88) (MyD88), and subsequently a critical serine threonine kinase named IL-1 (interleukin 1) receptor–associated kinase (IRAK). Once recruited, IRAK undergoes autophosphorylation and then binds to tumor necrosis factor receptor-associated factor 6 (TRAF6), an additional adaptor molecule. This complex in turn activates the IκB kinase (IKK) complex, which phosphorylates IκB. Once phosphorylated, IκB is degraded in the proteosome, and this allows nuclear factor-κB (NF-κB) to translate to the nucleus and modulate gene transcription.[4]

Although TLR activation of NF-κB via a MyD88 pathway is currently the most clearly understood, there are many other pathways, including the p38, that are also activated in response to TLR activation. Recent evidence also indicates that other molecules (e.g., RP105, Nod1, and Nod2), which are structurally related to TLRs, may share or contribute to PAMP recognition function in specific cellular subsets, such as in mature peripheral B cells.

Pathogen Killing

Recognition of pathogens by TLRs signals for production of cytokines (e.g., tumor necrosis factor α [TNF-α], IL-1, and chemokines) by macrophages and other sentinel cells. These cytokines, through enhanced expression of adhesion molecules on phagocytic and endothelial cells, facilitate homing of neutrophils to the site of infection. Recognition of pathogen also stimulates neutrophil production of reactive oxygen intermediates, which are essential for microbial killing. In addition to these "rapid response" cytokines, at least one additional cytokine (high mobility group-1 protein [HMG-1]) is induced many hours after initial pathogen identification and signaling; in early animal studies, HMG-1 mediates, at least in part, delayed mortality and multiple system organ failure after LPS challenge.[10]

In addition to cytokine biosynthesis and secretion, the alternative complement pathway is activated by LPS and other PAMPs. Complement activation is facilitated by circulating plasma mannose-binding lectin (MBL), which binds to carbohydrate structures on the surface of bacteria, viruses, and fungi. Activated complement contributes to plasma microbiocidal activity along with other antimicrobial proteins such as bactericidal/permeability increasing protein (BPI), defensins, and lactoferrin.

Localization of Infection by Coagulation

Compelling data now indicate that the extrinsic pathway of coagulation is a central, critical component of the innate immune system.[11] Endotoxin, peptidoglycan, and other PAMPs stimulate the expression of *tissue factor* on monocytes, and possibly on endothelial cells, via the induction of TNF-α and IL-1. The surface expression and release of tissue factor activates factor VII, which initiates the extrinsic coagulation cascade leading to activation of factor X to factor Xa, which in the presence of factor Va converts prothrombin to thrombin, resulting in the cleavage of fibrinogen to fibrin.[12] The deposition of fibrin at the site of pathogen recognition can serve to localize microorganisms and thereby limit systemic dissemination. This tendency toward thrombosis is coupled with an inhibition of fibrinolysis. Specifically, the innate immune response is associated with an increase in plasminogen-activator inhibitor-1 (PAI-1) and the thrombin-activated fibrinolysis inhibitor (TAFI), both of which diminish the system's ability to degrade fibrin. In addition to thrombin's essential role in fibrin deposition, thrombin is also potentially proinflammatory, thereby creating a local positive feedback cycle designed to enhance inflammation at the site of pathogen sequestration.

Modulators of Innate Immune Inflammation

Although a comprehensive understanding of innate immune regulation is lacking, it appears that the profound enhancement of inflammation at a local tissue site of infection is coupled with an effort to insulate noninfected tissues from proinflammatory events. As such, a complex and partially redundant set of antiinflammatory systems has coevolved with the proinflammatory components of the innate immune network.[13-15]

Coupled with the secretion of proinflammatory cytokines are potent antiinflammatory proteins such as the IL-1 receptor antagonist (IL-1Ra), IL-10, and soluble

TNF receptors. Stress hormones (including cortisol and epinephrine), other hormones (α-melanocyte-stimulating hormone [α-MSH]), and vasoactive intestinal peptide potently inhibit transcription and translation of cytokine genes. Indeed, it has been clearly demonstrated that infusion of humans with typical doses of epinephrine used to treat shock markedly blunts the production of TNF in response to endotoxin challenge. Indeed, β agonists in general have substantial antiinflammatory effects on a number of cells and tissues.

Perhaps the most important, yet until recently unappreciated, mechanism of regulation is *direct neural control*. Specifically, Tracey et al[16] have demonstrated that afferent vagus nerve fibers, likely via specific cytokine receptors, instruct the central nervous system that an innate immune response has been triggered. Subsequently, efferent vagus nerve fibers release acetylcholine that inhibits proinflammatory, but not antiinflammatory, cytokine production by the liver and gut (the primary sources of TNF-α during sepsis). The proximal mediator of this effect is acetylcholine acting via nicotinic cholinergic receptors residing on macrophages and other immune cells. In experimental models, division of the vagus nerves leads to markedly increased systemic TNF levels after endotoxin challenge, whereas division of the vagus nerve followed by hyperstimulation of efferent vagus fibers with a nerve stimulator not only decreases cytokine production but also preserves systemic arterial pressure and improves survival. Because the vagus nerve innervates a number of organs, including the spleen and heart, it is possible that modulation of this "cholinergic antiinflammatory pathway" could become a therapeutic target in clinical trials for diverse diseases including sepsis, inflammatory bowel disease, and myocarditis. It also raises the possibility that new classes of antiinflammatory compounds that act centrally but have systemic effects could be developed.

Clinical Manifestations of the Innate Immune Response

The human innate immune response developed in an evolutionary context of *recognizing*, *containing*, and *killing* a small number of pathogens that breached a single tissue barrier. The innate immune system did not evolve, however, to contend with overwhelming bacteremia, multiple trauma, massive transfusion, and other major insults of modern civilization. In these circumstances, the coordinated activation of the innate immune response throughout the host results in a progressive phenotype of SIRS; severe SIRS; and ultimately, SIRS with shock and multiple organ failure.

Because there is significant sharing of signal transduction pathways (including IRAK and NF-κB) among TLRs, the innate immune response is stereotyped, at least to a degree. This stereotyped response partially explains the clinical similarities of sepsis and SIRS caused by a wide range of microbial pathogens. Perhaps as important, TLR-4 has also been reported to be a specific receptor for Hsp 60, which may be induced by a variety of infectious and noninfectious stimuli, such as trauma, heat stress, and hypoxia. This finding suggests a potential molecular mechanism explaining how noninfectious insults can also cause SIRS that is clinically indistinguishable from SIRS caused by infection.

Coordinated activation of innate immune responses leads to high tissue and circulating levels of TNF-α and IL-1, which depress cardiac contractility and result in myocardial failure through several mechanisms. The anaphylotoxins, C3a and C5a, produced as a result of activation of complement, contribute directly to vasodilation and vascular permeability. In addition, activation of the contact system of coagulation results in the generation of kallikrein, which in turn releases the potently vasoactive bradykinin molecule from high-molecular-weight kininogen. TNF-α and IL-1 also cause transcription and translation of the inducible form of nitric oxide synthase (iNOS), and these result in markedly enhanced nitric oxide (NO) production. Although NO participates in microbial killing, particularly of intracellular pathogens, high levels of NO activate myosin phosphatase, thereby dephosphorylating myosin and inducing vasodilation. In addition, NO has been shown to uncouple cardiac β-adrenergic receptors from adenyl cyclase, and the effects of β-receptor–dependent inotropes are thereby limited. Lactic acidosis that results from tissue hypoxia or other causes worsens vasodilation and hypotension by activating K_{ATP} channels, hyperpolarizing cell membranes, and thereby inactivating voltage-gated calcium channels that are required to increase intracellular calcium in response to vasoconstrictors.

Transmigration of neutrophils, evolutionarily intended to occur only at an infected site, occurs diffusely into organs because of systemic innate immune activation. Neutrophils, already primed through TLR-dependent mechanisms, release free radicals and proteases, which are important for pathogen killing, but also contribute to lung injury. High levels of NO react with released superoxides to form the highly reactive free radical peroxynitrite. Peroxynitrite has numerous deleterious effects, including lipid peroxidation of cell membranes, S-nitrosylation of proteins, and inhibition of heme-containing enzymes responsible for mitochondrial respiration. In addition, peroxynitrite induces strand breaks in DNA, with subsequent NAD+ depletion that results from continuous activation of poly-ADP ribose synthase.

High levels of TNF-α, IL-1, IL-6, and other cytokines enhance tissue factor expression on circulating monocytes and possibly on endothelial cells. This enhancement leads to disseminated intravascular coagulation (DIC). Removal of fibrin (fibrinolysis) is impeded by exaggerated release of PAI-1 from platelets and endothelial cells. Ongoing consumption of the coagulation regulators *antithrombin*, *protein S*, and *protein C* cause unmodulated coagulopathy.[17-20] This dysregulation is worsened because *thrombomodulin*, which is absolutely required to activate protein C, is itself profoundly down-regulated on the endothelium through cytokine-dependent mechanisms.[21]

The human sepsis phenotype is *procoagulant* and *antifibrinolytic*. As a result, disseminated microthromboses occur, further exacerbating endothelial injury and tissue ischemia. This self-perpetuating spiral of further capillary injury, inflammation, and coagulation has the potential to result in vasomotor collapse, multiple organ dysfunction, and death (see also Chapter 97).

Genetic Polymorphisms, Innate Immunity, and Individual Manifestations of Disease

In their classic adoptee study published in 1988, Sorensen et al reported that the genetic component contributing to premature death in adults was higher for infections than for either cardiac disease or cancer.[22] There is currently sufficient evidence to conclude that polymorphisms in innate immune genes significantly contribute to this genetic risk.[23] For example, structural variants of MBL are a major cause for susceptibility to invasive meningococcal disease and may account for as many as one third of all meningococcal cases. Polymorphisms in the TNF locus, which govern the amount of TNF induced, may contribute as much as a threefold risk of death in meningococcal disease and a sevenfold risk of death or serious neurologic sequelae in cerebral malaria.[24] Polymorphisms in the coagulation system have also been studied. Children with a polymorphism in the PAI-1 gene, which promotes increased gene transcription, have a sixfold higher risk of having a septic shock phenotype, rather than a simple meningitic phenotype, during the course of invasive *Neisseria meningitidis* infections.[25] Polymorphisms in the TLR system have already been discovered in humans. Preliminary data suggest that a polymorphism in TLR-2, the receptor for gram-positive lipoproteins, may predispose to staphylococcal septic shock.[26] In addition, common mutations in the TLR-4 extracellular domain are associated with endotoxin hyporesponsiveness in humans. These TLR-4 mutations may be present in upto 6% to 12% of humans.[27] One might predict that humans with endotoxin hyporesponsiveness might have a higher risk of invasive gram-negative infections, yet during the course of these infections manifest less collateral damage such as organ dysfunction. To date, the human health implications of TLR-4 mutations are not known. Also, there have been no published studies on TLR polymorphisms in children.

Innate Immunotherapeutics in Pediatric Critical Care

Until recently, large clinical trials conducted with adults with sepsis that were designed to block endotoxin, TNF-α, IL-1, PAF, or NO either showed no benefit or actually caused harm. Recent evidence, however, suggests that the failure of these early trials may have stemmed from inadequate study design, experimental agents, or both. Modulation of the innate immune response in critically ill adults and children remains a viable target for the development of novel therapeutics.

As the prototypical PAMP, LPS is a potential therapeutic target in severe gram-negative sepsis and in other conditions in which there is significant endotoxemia (e.g., burns, hemorrhage, polytrauma, cardiopulmonary bypass). Meningococcemia is characterized by fulminant septic shock, coagulopathy, multiple organ failure and death, the pathogenesis of which is highly linked to the robust shedding of endotoxin-containing blebs from the etiologic bacteria *N. meningitidis*.

The first large-scale randomized trial of immune modulation in meningococcemia was designed to enhance endotoxin clearance through the administration of HA-1A, a monoclonal antibody, which did bind, but did not neutralize, endotoxin. Although this trial failed to show a statistically significant benefit, there was a strong trend toward survival advantage in the group treated with HA-1A. Unfortunately, HA-1A treatment was also associated with a trend toward enhanced morbidity in survivors.

In a larger trial, published in 2000, the researchers determined whether pharmacological administration of a recombinant form of BPI, a normal human protein secreted by neutrophils after microbial provocation, would improve the outcome of children with the most severe forms of meningococcal sepsis. BPI binds endotoxin and facilitates its removal from the circulation. Moreover, unlike HA-1A, BPI completely neutralizes endotoxin by blocking interaction of LPS with LBP and therefore CD14:TLR-4. BPI is also bactericidal and can kill (in clinically achievable plasma concentrations) both smooth and rough forms of gram-negative bacteria, including *N. meningitidis*. Data from the phase III randomized placebo-controlled trial ($n = 393$ children) indicated that treatment with a recombinant N-terminal fragment of BPI ($rBPI_{21}$) reduced clinically significant morbidities (including severe amputations; $p = 0.06$) and enhanced overall functional outcome as measured by the Pediatric Overall Performance Category score ($p = 0.019$).[28] Although there was a numerical mortality advantage in the BPI-treated group, the study was underpowered to statistically prove a survival benefit. The data from this trial were insufficient to gain Food and Drug Administration (FDA) approval for this indication; however, the data did strongly indicate a powerful biological effect that could serve as the basis for additional confirmatory trials either in meningococcal sepsis or a more general severe sepsis population.

An innovative trial of innate immunomodulation targeted the coagulation-inflammation network directly. Protein C is a primary modulator of coagulation, fibrinolysis, and coagulation-induced inflammation. In both children and adults, acquired deficiencies in protein C (due to consumption in DIC) and deficits in protein C activation (due to decreased thrombomodulin expression) are directly correlated with morbidity and mortality in septic shock. Protein C deficiency arises during sepsis as a result of multiple causes because diverse pathogens all stimulate the extrinsic pathway of coagulation through cytokine enhancement of tissue factor expression.[29,30]

In a randomized, placebo-controlled trial with 1690 patients, the administration of recombinant human activated protein C (rhAPC) to adults with sepsis and organ failure resulted in a 19.6% relative risk reduction in mortality ($p = 0.005$).[31] The survival benefit occurred irrespective of underlying cause (gram-negative, gram-positive, or no bacteria isolated). Administration of rhAPC significantly reduced the plasma levels of D-dimers, compared with placebo-treated patients, and also reduced serum IL-6 levels. rhAPC is currently approved for the treatment of adults with severe sepsis who have a high risk of mortality.

Hundreds of children have been treated in open-label, non–placebo-controlled studies. Preliminary data suggest that the dosing of rhAPC will be similar in children and adults. Currently, a large, placebo-controlled trial of rhAPC in children who have severe sepsis, are connected to a ventilator, and receive inotropes is under way. This study will require approximately 3 years for completion.

Conclusions

The innate immune system is activated in nearly every patient admitted to the pediatric intensive care unit because of an infection, a tissue injury, or ongoing isolated organ inflammation such as what occurs during chronic heart failure. Whether a robust immune response occurs depends largely on the patient's innate immune genetic program and the interaction of these genes with a multitude of environmental stressors (e.g., malnutrition, barrier breeches, drugs). Current therapeutic strategies aimed at modifying the innate immune response include the blockade of TLR recognition with molecules such as BPI; the modulation of the coagulation response with rhAPC, pooled plasma protein C, or specific inhibitors such as tissue factor pathway inhibitor; and the blockade of specific effectors such as PAF. The first generation of pharmacologic agents, such as CNI-1493, which act centrally to increase vagal efferent antiinflammatory signals, is also in clinical trials.[32, 33]

Although it is likely that one or more of these strategies will prove beneficial, the optimization of these therapies can only occur when the individual's genetic predispositions are understood. For example, a high producer of TNF might potentially benefit from TNF blockade, whereas a genetic low producer of TNF might experience harm. The same can be hypothesized for children with genetic susceptibility for enhanced clotting (PAI-1 polymorphs) or hyporesponders to endotoxin (TLR-4 polymorphs). Within the next several years, the technology to rapidly ascertain these genotypes will become available and will allow understanding of the innate immune system at the level of the individual patient.

REFERENCES

1. Mushegian A, Medzhitov R: Evolutionary perspective on innate immune recognition, *J Cell Biol* 155:705-710, 2001.
2. Hoffmann JA, Kafatos KC, Janeway CA et al: Phylogenetic perspectives in innate immunity, *Science* 284:1313-1318, 1999.
3. Janeway CA, Medzhitov R: Introduction: the role of innate immunity in the adaptive immune response, *Semin Immunol* 10:349-350, 1998.
4. Vasselon T, Detmers PA: Toll receptors: a central element in innate immune responses, *Infect Immun* 70:1033-1041, 2002.
5. Takeda K, Akira S: Roles of Toll-like receptors in innate immune responses, *Genes Cells* 6:733-742, 2001.
6. Anderson KV: Toll signaling pathways in the innate immune response, *Curr Opin Immunol* 12:13-19, 2002.
7. Beutler B: Endotoxin, toll-like receptor 4, and the afferent limb of innate immunity, *Curr Opin Microbiol* 1:23-28, 2000.
8. Häcker G, Redecke V, Häcker H: Activation of the immune system by bacterial CpG-DNA, *Immunology* 105:245-251, 2002.
9. Hallman M, Rämet M, Ezekowitz RA: Toll-like receptors as sensors of pathogens, *Pediatr Res* 50:315-321, 2001.
10. Wang H, Bloom O, Zhang M et al: HMG-1 as a late mediator of endotoxin lethality in mice, *Science* 285:248-251, 1999.
11. Esmon CT, Fukudome K, Mather T et al: Inflammation, sepsis, and coagulation, *Haematologica* 84:254-259, 1999.
12. Esmon CT: Regulation of blood coagulation, *Biochim Biophys Acta* 1477:349-360, 1999.
13. Strieter RM, Belperio JA, Keane MP: Cytokines in innate host defense in the lung, *J Clin Invest* 109:699-705, 2002.
14. Knuefermann P, Nemoto S, Baumgarten G et al: Cardiac inflammation and innate immunity in septic shock, *Chest* 121:1329-1336, 2002.
15. Chen G, Goeddel DV: TNF-R1 signaling: a beautiful pathway, *Science* 296:1634-1635, 2000.
16. Tracey KJ, Czura CJ, Ivanova S: Mind over immunity, *FASEB J* 15:1575-1576, 2001.
17. Fijnvandraat K, Derkx B, Peters M et al: Coagulation activation and tissue necrosis in meningococcal septic shock: severely reduced protein C levels predict a high mortality, *Thromb Haemost* 73: 15-20, 1995.
18. Sorensen TI, Nielsen GG, Andersen PK et al: Genetic and environmental influences on premature death in adult adoptees, *N Engl J Med* 318:727-732, 1988.
19. Kornelisse RF, Hazelzet JA, Savelkoul HF et al: The relationship between plasminogen activator inhibitor-1 and proinflammatory and counterinflammatory mediators in children with meningococcal septic shock, *J Infect Dis* 173:1148-1156, 1996.
20. Yan SB, Helterbrand JD, Hartman DL et al: Low levels of protein C are associated with poor outcome in severe sepsis, *Chest* 120: 915-922, 2001.
21. Faust SN, Levin M, Harrison OB et al: Dysfunction of endothelial protein C activation in severe meningococcal sepsis, *N Engl J Med* 345:408-416, 2001.
22. Rosenberg RD, Aird WC: Vascular-bed-specific hemostasis and hypercoagulable states, *N Engl J Med* 340:1555-1564, 1999.
23. van Deventer SJH: Cytokine and cytokine receptor polymorphisms in infectious disease, *Intensive Care Med* 2000; 26(suppl 1): S98-S102, 2000.
24. Nadel S, Newport MJ, Booy R et al: Variation in the tumor necrosis factor-alpha gene promoter region may be associated with death from meningococcal disease, *J Infect Dis* 4:878-880, 1996.
25. Westendorp RGJ, Hottenga JJ, Slagboom PE: Variation in plasminogen-activator-inhibitor-1 gene and risk of meningococcal septic shock, *Lancet* 354:561-563, 1999.
26. Lorenz E, Mira JP, Cornish KL et al: A novel polymorphism in the toll-like receptor 2 gene and its potential association with staphylococcal infection, *Infect Immun* 68:6398-6401, 2000.
27. Arbour NC, Lorenz E, Schutte BC et al: TLR4 mutations are associated with endotoxin hyporesponsiveness in humans, *Nat Genet* 25:187-191, 2000.
28. Levin M, Quint PA, Goldstein B et al: Recombinant bactericidal/permeability-increasing protein (rBPI21) as adjunctive treatment for children with severe meningococcal sepsis: a randomized trial, *Lancet* 356:961-967, 2000.
29. White B, Livingstone W, Murphy C et al: An open-label study of the role of adjuvant hemostatic support with protein C replacement therapy in purpura fulminans-associated meningococcemia, *Blood* 96:3719-3724, 2000.
30. White B, Schmidt M, Murphy C et al: Activated protein C inhibits lipopolysaccharide-induced nuclear translocation of nuclear factor κB (NF-κB) and tumor necrosis factor α (TNF-α) production in the THP-1 monocytic cell line, *Br J Haematol* 110:130-134, 2000.
31. Bernard GR, Vincent JL, Laterre PF, et al: Efficacy and safety of recombinant human activated protein C for severe sepsis, *N Engl J Med* 344:759-762, 2001.
32. Bernik TR, Friedman SG, Ochani M et al: Pharmacological stimulation of the cholinergic antiinflammatory pathway, *J Exp Med* 195:781-788, 2000.
33. Blalock JE: Harnessing a neural-immune circuit to control inflammation and shock, *J Exp Med* 195:F25-F28, 2002.

CHAPTER 84

Infection and the Host Response

Mary Michele Mariscalco

PEARLS

- Innate immune recognition is genetically predetermined. These receptors have evolved by natural selection and have defined specificities for infectious organisms.
- In the adaptive immune system, in contrast to the innate system, the T-cell and B-cell receptors are somatically generated in a way that gives each lymphocyte a unique structural receptor.
- Pattern recognition receptor (PRR) molecules recognize sugar residues that are rich on microbial surfaces and can function directly as opsonins, promoting phagocytosis.
- Interleukin 6 (IL-6) is the factor most directly responsible for the production of acute phase reactants.
- Exposure to granulocyte colony-stimulating factor (G-CSF) or granulocyte-macrophage colony stimulating factor (GM-CSF) decreases apoptosis, leading to prolonged survival of circulating neutrophils and those that have emigrated to a site of infection. Removal of these cytokines, as occurs in the resolution phase of inflammation, leads to induction of apoptosis and increased clearance of neutrophils.
- Nitric oxide (NO) is a stable, free radical gas. It is the major messenger molecule regulating immune function and blood vessel dilation and serving as neurotransmitter.
- The CD4+ naive cells—those never exposed to antigen—can differentiate into effector cells expressing specific patterns of cytokines that have been described as Th1 and Th2.
- Interferon (IFN)–γ is the "signature" cytokine produced by Th1 cells, but the Th1 cells also produce substantial amounts of IL-2, tumor necrosis factor α (TNF-α), and TNF-β. The Th1 response is considered "proinflammatory."
- IL-4, in contrast to IFN-γ, is the "signature" cytokine produced by Th2 cells, along with IL-5, IL-9, and IL-13.
- IL-4 and IL-13 are considered "antiinflammatory" or immunosuppressive.

Historical Perspectives

Rubor et tumor cum calore et dolore—redness and swelling with heat and pain—were recognized as the four cardinal signs of inflammation by Cornelius Celsus (30 BC-AD 38). It was not established until the late 1800s and early 1900s that the body used both cellular and humoral components to identify and destroy microbes. Through the work of such pioneers as Elie Metchnikoff, Paul Ehrlich, and Almoth Roth, certain humoral factors called *opsonins,* which were later identified as serum antibodies and complement products, were shown to render bacteria more susceptible to ingestion and destruction by phagocytic cells. Antibodies, together with complement, could also directly destroy bacteria.

Traditionally the immune system has been divided into innate and adaptive components. Clonal expansion of lymphocytes in response to infection is absolutely critical to the development of the immune response. It takes 3 to 5 days, however, for clonal expansion to produce sufficient numbers of "effector" cells. Clearly, this is more than enough time for a pathogen to damage the host.

The innate immune system is fundamental in eliminating the infection or controlling it until the adaptive immune responses eliminate it. If the innate and adaptive immune responses are adequate, the infection remains localized. If not, then the systemic response to infection or sepsis results (see also Chapter 83). What has become increasingly clear is that the adaptive immune system can affect the functioning of the innate immune system and vice versa.[1]

In the past 20 years new concepts that are fundamental to the care of the critically ill patient have arisen directly from an understanding of the host's response to infection; namely, (1) Inflammatory reactions first characterized as a response to infection are the foundation of a number of other pathogenic mechanisms, such as ischemia/reperfusion injury, direct trauma, drug-induced injury, inhalational injury, and multiple-system organ dysfunction (see also Chapter 97). (2) The response to infection may lead to further injury of the host. Alternatively, an exuberant antiinflammatory response may likewise be deleterious and may result in immune suppression and fibrosis (see also Chapters 93, 94, and 96). (3) There is a direct interaction between the neuroendocrine axis and inflammation (see also Chapter 95). (4) There is a fundamental interrelationship between endothelium, inflammation, and coagulation, and efforts to intervene in one will likely have effects in others (see also Chapters 94, 96, and 97).

Comparison of Innate Immune and Adaptive Immune Responses

The innate immune system is phylogenetically ancient. Innate immune recognition is genetically predetermined (i.e., by germline-encoded receptors). Thus these receptors have evolved by natural selection and have defined specificities for infectious organisms (see also Chapter 83). In contrast, in the adaptive immune system, the T-cell and B-cell receptors are somatically generated in a way that gives each lymphocyte a unique structural receptor. Because the T- and B-cell receptors are not encoded in a germline, they are not predetermined to recognize any particular antigen. No matter how useful these "receptors" become, they cannot be passed down to the next generation. Although there are potentially a large number of variants of germline-encoded receptors (perhaps in the hundreds), there are 10^{14} and 10^{18} different somatically generated immunoglobulin (Ig) receptors and T-cell receptors, respectively.[1] Microbes are heterogenous and can mutate at high rates that can be handled by the adaptive immune system. This heterogeneity represents more of a challenge for the innate immune system. Because such a different strategy has evolved, the innate immune system has developed receptors that recognize pathogen-associated molecular patterns (PAMPs). PAMPs are highly conserved structures present in a large group of microorganisms. The following are common features: (1) PAMPs are only produced by microbial pathogens, not hosts. (2) Structures recognized by the innate immune system are usually essential for survival or pathogenicity of the microorganism. (3) PAMPs are usually invariant structures shared by an entire class of pathogen. The best known examples of PAMPs are bacterial lipopolysaccharide (LPS), peptidoglycan, lipoteichoic acid (LTA), mannans, bacterial DNA, double-stranded RNA, and glucans.[2]

Pattern Recognition Receptors

In the innate immune system, pathogen recognition molecules are called *pattern recognition receptors* (PRRs) and belong structurally to several families of proteins: leucine-rich repeat domains, calcium-dependent lectin domains, and scavenger receptors domains. Functionally, PRRs can be divided into three classes: secreted, endocytic, and signaling. Secreted PRRs function as opsonins. They bind to microbial cell walls, flagging them for recognition by the complement system and by phagocytes. Members of the secreted PRRs include C-reactive protein (CRP), mannose-binding lectin, and the ficolins.[3-5] These molecules (PRRs) recognize sugar residues that are rich on microbial surfaces and can function directly as opsonins, promoting phagocytosis. Alternatively, they can also function indirectly by activating the classic complement pathway (CRP) or the lectin-dependent pathway (ficolins and mannose-binding lectin).[5]

Endocytic pattern-recognition receptors occur on phagocytes and can mediate the uptake and delivery of pathogens into lysosomes. Once in the lysosomes, the microbe can be destroyed. The macrophage mannose receptor recognizes carbohydrates with large numbers of mannoses (characteristic of microorganisms) and mediates their phagocytosis by macrophages. The macrophage scavenger receptor binds to bacterial cell walls and effectively clears them from the circulation. In addition to recognizing microbes opsonized with complement, complement receptor 3 (also known as Mac-1 and CD11b/CD18) can function by binding mannose molecules directly. It can also function as an endocytic PRR.[1]

Toll-like Receptors

Work done by Janeway[6] and Medzhitov[2] revolutionized the understanding of the critical role of the innate immune system as the first step in adaptive immunity. They identified the human counterpart of a protein found in fruit flies (*Drosophila melanogaster*) known as Toll. The Toll protein in fruit flies is responsible for infectious susceptibility to fungi. This protein in humans, human toll-like receptor 4 (TLR-4), recognizes LPS and is located on antigen-presenting cells (APCs) such as dendritic cells (DCs), macrophages, and monocytes. Through a complex signaling cascade, TLR-4 results in activation of cytoplasmic nuclear factor-κB (NF-κB) that can then move into the nucleus and induce the transcriptional activation of a wide variety of inflammatory and immune responses.[1] These responses include the induction of cytokines such as tumor necrosis factor α (TNF-α), interleukin-1 (IL-1), IL-6, IL-12, and the induction of costimulatory molecules such as CD80 and CD86. The presentation of antigen by the major histocompatibility complex (MHC) II molecule on the APC is insufficient to induce the activation of the T-cell receptor and thus the T cell. There must also be expression of CD80 or CD86 by the APC, which is required for full T-cell receptor activation (discussed later in this chapter) (see Fig. 84–7). Thus only normally pathogen-specific T cells, not self-antigen, should be activated.

Currently, there are 13 mammalian TLR paralogs (11 in humans and 12 in mice).[7,8] What is clear is that the TLRs recognize pathogens ranging from protozoa to bacteria to fungi and to viruses[7] (see also Chapter 83) (Table 84–1). According to a number of reports endogenous proteins such as heat shock proteins, surfactant protein A, high mobility group 1 (HMGB1), and fibrinogen may also function as ligands for TLRs. These studies are problematic, however, because of concerns for contamination of reagents by LPS and other bacterial products.[9] For the purposes of this review, we only focus on the pathogen ligands of the TLR. The TLRs are single membrane spanning proteins and are thought to be mostly homodimers, though heterodimers, such as TLR2:TLR1 and TLR2:TLR6, exist.[7]

It had been recognized for a number of years that CD14, present on monocytes and neutrophils, blood-derived macrophages, and LPS-binding protein (LBP) found in plasma were critical for an LPS response. CD14, however, is a glycosylphosphatidylinositol-anchored protein, lacking transmembrane and intracellular domains, and is unable to signal intracellular processes. CD14 is present on blood-derived monocytes, macrophages, and, to a limited extent, neutrophils.[10] In addition, a soluble form of CD14 could substitute for a membrane-bound form of CD14 in

TABLE 84–1

Biological Properties of the Immunoglobulin Classes and Immunoglobulin G Subclasses

Property	IgG1	IgG2	IgG3	IgG4	IgM	IgA	IgE	Secretory IgA
First detectable antibody	–	–	–	–	+	–	–	–
Major part of secondary response	+	+	+	+	–	–	–	–
Placental transport	++	+	++	++	–	–	–	–
Complement activation								
Classic pathway	++	+	++	–	–	–	–	–
Alternate pathway	–	–	–	–	–	++	+	+
Agglutination	+	+	+	+	++	–	–	–
Opsonization	+	+	+1	+	++	–	–	–
Virus neutralization	+	+	+	+	+	–	–	+
Anaphylaxis	–	–	–	–			++	–
Present in exocrine secretions (gastrointestinal system and lung)	+	+	+	+	+	+	+	++
Binds to receptors on								
Macrophages	++	±	++	±	–	–	+	–
Lymphocytes	+	±	+	±	–	–	–	–
Neutrophils	+	+	+	+	+	+	±	+
Platelets	+	+	+	+	–	–	–	–
Mast cells	–	–	–	–	–	–	+	–
Binding to Fc receptors								
FcγRI (CD64)	++	±	++	+	–	–	–	–
FcγRII (CD 32)	++	+	++	±	–	–	–	–
FcγRIII (CD 16)	++	±	++	±	–	–	–	+
FcαR	–	–	–	–	–	+	–	+
FcμR	–	–	–	–	+	–	–	–
FcεRI and FcεRII	–	–	–	–	–	–	+	–

Ig, immunogobulin; ++, very strong; +, strong; ±, equivocal; –, absent.

LPS-mediated signaling. Thus it was clear that at least one other molecule present on the cell surface would be needed to elicit an LPS-dependent response. TLR-4 knockout mice and human TLR-4 mutations conferred such a role for this receptor for LPS-induced responses in humans and mice. TLR-4 requires an additional molecule, MD-2, which is part of the complex on the cell surface. LBP is an acute phase reactant.[1,11] It catalyzes the transfer of LPS to CD14, which is then able to interact with TLR-4 and MD-2. The result is intracellular signaling through the Toll/IL-1 receptor homologous region (TIR) adaptor molecules (MYD88/MAL-TRIP, TRAM, and TRIF), the protein kinases associated with them, and downstream signaling events (Fig. 84–1).[7] Downstream signaling events result in release of transcriptional activating factors including NF-κB and signal transducer and activator of transcription 1 (STAT-1) and activator protein 1 (AP-1), which guide gene transcription of many genes including TNF and interferon-β (IFN-β). TNF is discussed at greater length later in this chapter; however, it is a central mediator in innate immune response pathway. IFN-β is critical in the adaptive antiviral immune response.

Endogenous Antimicrobials

The epithelial surface of the skin, gastrointestinal (GI) tract, and bronchial tree produces a number of antibacterial peptides and other proteins.[12] In addition, leukocytes are a rich source of these same, or similar, proteins, which can be secreted into the phagolysosome or can be alternatively secreted into biofilms that protect the mouth and GI tract.[13,14] These antimicrobial proteins include the defensins, cathelicidin, lactoferrin, and bacterial/permeability increasing protein (BPI).[15] As the antimicrobial peptides are heavily positively charged (because of cationic amino acids), they specifically target bacterial cell membranes whose outermost leaflet of lipid bilayer is heavily populated with negatively charged phospholipid head groups.[12] Thus they act as PRRs. Plant and animal cell membranes have their negatively charged lipids on the inner leaflet; thus they are resistant to the antimicrobials' effects. It is still unclear exactly how these antimicrobial peptides actually kill microbes. Possibilities include the creation of physical holes that cause cell contents to "leak out," disturbances of cell membrane function by "scrambling" the lipid bilayer, or fatal depolarization of the normally energized bacterial membrane.[12]

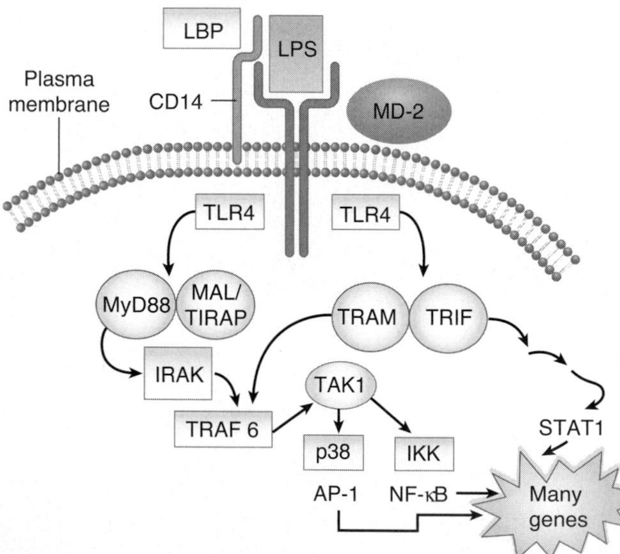

FIGURE 84–1 • Signaling through TLR4 receptor. LPS is a pathogen-associated molecular pattern (PAMP) for TLR4. The LPS/CD14/LBP complex binds to TLR4 receptor-MD-2. Note that the TLR4 is a homodimer. This interaction signals the cell through the TIR (Toll/interleukin-1 receptor homologous region) adaptor proteins MYD88, MAL/TRIP, TRAM, and TRIF, which associate with one another. Through a series of signaling events, transcription factors are released that guide gene transcription. *LBP,* lipopolysaccharide-binding protein; *LPS,* lipopolysaccharide; *MyD88,* myeloid differentiation factor 88; *MAL/TIRAP,* MyD88-adaptor-like/TIR-associated protein; *TRAM,* Toll-receptor-associated-molecule; *TRIF,* Toll-receptor-associated activator of interferon; *IRAK,* IL-1R-associated kinase; *TRAF6,* TNF receptor-associated factor 6; *TAK1,* transforming growth factor β-activated-kinase1; *AP-1,* activator protein-1; *IKK,* inhibitor of κB kinase; *STAT-1,* signal transducer and activator of transcription 1.

The α defensins are stored in the granules of neutrophils, monocytes, and macrophages, and are released extracellularly. The β defensins are produced by Paneth's cells, reproductive tissues, epithelial cells, and keratinocytes; some are produced constitutively and some in response to LPS and proinflammatory products such as TNF and IL-1. Cathelicidin LL37 is stored in neutrophil granules but is also produced by keratinocytes and epithelial cells in response to inflammatory stimuli. In addition to the antimicrobial effect of the defensins and cathelicidin, they are chemotactic for CD4 and CD8 T cells, phagocytes, and immature DCs. They also enhance antigen-specific immunity and regulate complement activation.[15] Patients with Kostmann's syndrome (congenital neutropenia) have severe periodontal disease even when neutrophil counts are restored with granulocyte colony-stimulating factor (G-CSF).[13] This appears to be due to deficiencies of neutrophil cathelicidin LL37 and to a lesser extent α defensins with resulting diminished levels of these antimicrobial peptides in the saliva and blood.[13]

Lactoferrin and BPI are found in secondary and primary granules of the neutrophils, respectively, but they are also secreted or presented on epithelial surfaces. Lactoferrin is found in milk; tears; saliva; and other secretions such as bile, pancreatic juice, and small intestinal secretions. Lactoferrin is structurally similar to transferrin, although its affinity for iron is about 300 times higher. Thus it can retain iron at low pH.[16] Both lactoferrin and BPI have cationic-rich regions that are critical to binding and neutralizing LPS. Lactoferrin also has direct antimicrobial actions. Lactoferrin can potentiate the cytotoxic effects of monocytes and T cells.[16] BPI was initially identified in neutrophil primary granules. Because of its high affinity for the lipid A region of LPS, it is particularly cytotoxic for gram-negative bacteria, and its antibacterial activities are synergistically enhanced by defensins and cathelicidin.[17] In addition, BPI can function as an opsonin, enhancing phagocytosis.

Antimicrobial peptides have been used in a number of conditions, and although they were initially promising, their potential has not been completely realized. In the largest study to date, recombinant fragment of BPI, $rBPI_{21}$, was tested in 400 children with severe meningococcal sepsis.[18] Although $rBPI_{21}$ had no effect on survival, fewer patients had multiple severe amputations, and by day 60 they had a more functional outcome compared with those who did not receive $rBPI_{21}$ (see Chapter 96).[18] A mammalian cathelicidin, protegrin, had no effect on the development or reduction of mucositis in those patients who received stomatotoxic chemotherapy.[19] Results from several smaller studies indicate that lactoferrin may be useful in adjunctive treatment of *Helicobacter pylori* and indomethacin-induced enteropathy.[20,21]

Soluble Components of Immunity

C-reactive Protein

CRP is phylogenetically ancient and is highly conserved in evolution. It is a member of the pentraxin family of calcium-dependent ligand-binding plasma proteins, the only other member of which is serum amyloid P (SAP). Although CRP is an acute phase reactant in humans, SAP is not. In mice the major acute phase reactant is SAP, with a minor fraction being CRP. In humans plasma CRP is produced only by hepatocytes and is predominantly under the transcriptional control of IL-6. It is greatly elevated in infections, allergic complications of infection, inflammatory diseases, necrosis, trauma, and malignancy. It is modestly elevated or absent in systemic lupus erythematosus, scleroderma, dermatomyositis, ulcerative colitis, leukemia, and graft-versus-host disease. CRP binds to glycan and phospholipids of bacteria, fungi, and parasites. When aggregated or bound to macromolecular ligands, CRP is recognized by C1q and activates the classic complement pathway; thus it initiates direct microbial toxicity. Because it also recognizes phospholipids, in particular phosphocholine, it may be involved in handling apoptotic and necrotic cells.[4]

Complement System

The complement system is critically positioned to participate in both the innate and adaptive immune response.[22] It is also critical for the disposal of immune complexes from tissues and clearance of apoptotic cells.[5] The three pathways in which complement may become activated are the classical, alternative, and mannose-binding lectin pathway. Although complement activation initiates differently in each, all three converge at the cleavage of C3 (Fig. 84–2). The classical pathway is initiated by the binding of the C1 complex, which consists of C1q, C1r, and C1s, to antibodies bound to antigen on the cell wall. The mannose-binding lectin pathway is initiated by binding of

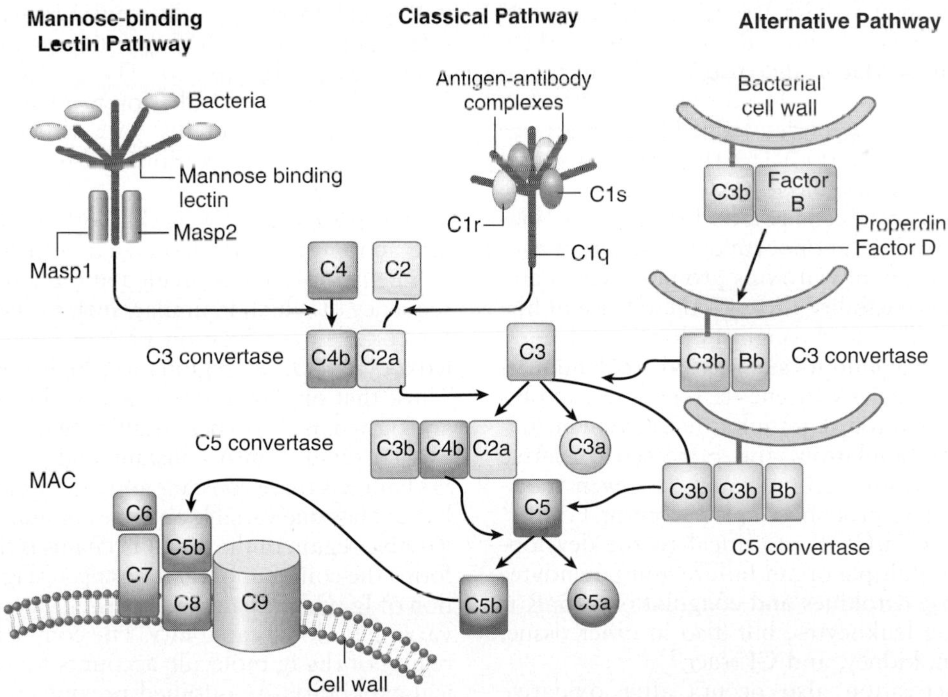

FIGURE 84–2 • The three activation pathways of complement: the mannose-binding lectin (MBL), the classical, and alternative pathways. The three pathways converge at the point of cleavage of C3. The MBL pathway is initiated by binding of the complex of the MBL and MBL-associated proteases 1 and 2 (MASP1, MASP2) to arrays of mannose on the bacterial cell wall. MASP2 then activates first C4, then C2 to form the C3 convertase, C4b2a. The classical pathway is initiated by the binding of the C1 complex (which consists of C1q, two molecules of C1r, and two molecules of C1s) to antibodies bound to antigen on the surface of bacterial cell wall. C1s, similar to MASP2, then activates C4 followed by C2 to form C4b2a (the C3 convertase). The alternative pathway is initiated by covalent binding of a small amount of C3b to hydroxyl groups on the cell-surface carbohydrates and is activated by low-grade C3 in plasma. This C3b binds factor B to form C3bB, which is then activated by factor D to form C3bBb, the alternative pathway C3 convertase. Properdin stabilizes this activation step. The C3 convertase then cleaves many molecules of C3 to C3b and C3a (an anaphylatoxin). C3b binds covalently around the site of complement activation, some of which binds to the C4b and C3b of the classical and alternative pathway C3 convertase, respectively, to form the C5 convertase. The C5 convertase cleaves C5 to C5a (an anaphylatoxin) and C5b, which initiates the formation of the membrane attack complex (MAC). (Modified from Walport MJ: *N Engl J Med* 344:1058, 2001).

the complex of mannose-binding lectin and the mannose-binding lectin-associated proteases 1 and 2 (MASP1 and MASP2) to arrays of mannose groups on the surface of the cell bacterial cell wall. Both MASP2 and C1q then function similarly in forming the C4bC2a complex, which is the convertase for C3. Bacterial products, LPS, yeast cell wall particles, and aggregated antibody including IgA and IgE can activate the alternative pathway. The alternative pathway is initiated through low-grade cleavage of C3 in plasma to C3b. C3b binds to the hydroxyl groups on cell surface carbohydrates. C3b binds factor B to form a C3bB complex, which is activated by factor D, forming C3bBb and stabilized with properdin. C3bBb then functions as an alternative convertase for C3, which cleaves many molecules of C3 to C3b. C3b binds to hydroxyl groups on the microorganism around the area of complement activation. C3a, an anaphylatoxin, is released by the C3 convertase. C3b can also bind to the C3 convertase to form C5 convertase. The C5 convertase releases the anaphylatoxin C5a and initiates the formation of the membrane attack complex (MAC), C5b6789.[5] The MAC created inserts into the cell membrane, creates large pores, and leads to osmotic lysis of the target.

Thus the complement system amplifies the initial response to the organism. In addition to lysis of the target organism, opsonization with complement fragments C3b/C4b and C3bi (fragment C3b) occurs. The result is phagocytosis by neutrophils, monocytes, and macrophages. Binding occurs through specific complement receptors, CR1 for C3b/C4b (CD35) and CR3 for C3bi (CD11b/CD18, also known as Mac-1 and $\alpha_M\beta2$). The anaphylatoxins C3a, C4a, and C5a produced are low-molecular-weight, biologically active peptides defined by their actions on small blood vessels, smooth muscle, mast cells, and peripheral blood leukocytes. Blood vessels, smooth muscle cells, basophils, and mast cells respond to all three anaphylatoxins. Neutrophils, monocytes, and macrophages respond to C5a. The anaphylatoxins promote edema and increase vascular permeability through the release of histamine from mast cells and through the local production of vasodilatory prostaglandins such as prostaglandin E_2 (PGE_2) and edemogenic leukotrienes (LTs) C_4, D_4, and E_4. C5a is a powerful activator of granulocyte function including chemotaxis, degranulation, and increased oxidative metabolism. C5a actions occur through its seven transmembrane-spanning, G-protein–coupled receptor, C5aR.[23] In animal models, C5a/C5aR is critical to the development of sepsis and multiple organ failure and potentiates many early response cytokines and coagulation. C5aR is present not only on leukocytes, but also in other tissue, including the brain, kidney, and GI tract.[23,24]

Complement activation also occurs after oxidative stress such as with ischemia/reperfusion, although the exact molecular mechanism has not been fully elucidated. Nonetheless, complement activation is an early event, and the inhibition of complement activation or its components offer tissue protection after reperfusion.[25] Finally, complement proteins or cell fragments transduce various cell signals. Complement can activate B and T cells. It can regulate apoptosis of various cell types (see also Chapter 93). Receptor-dependent and receptor-independent signals are transduced.[22,26]

Immunoglobulin

The different Igs secreted by B cells (IgG, IgA, IgM, IgD, and IgE) are known as *isotopes*. IgD plays a little role, if any, in containment of microorganisms. Ig isotypes can be divided into subclasses, variants that show slight structural differences but are sufficiently alike structurally to be essentially identical to other members of the isotype class. There are four IgG subclasses: IgG1, IgG2, IgG3, and IgG4. As seen in Table 84–1, isotype subclasses have specialized roles in the immune response. For example, IgG2 has a major role in the formation of carbohydrate antibodies but has poor complement fixation characteristics. The antibody system consists of that present in serum, protecting the blood and tissue spaces; that present in the secretory system, lining the GI and respiratory tracts; and that present in tears. The serum component is mostly IgG (85%), with lesser amounts of IgA and IgM. The secretory system consists mostly of secretory IgA (85%), which is structurally different than serum IgA, and lesser amounts of IgG and IgM. All Igs have a basic four-chain structure composed of an identical pair of heavy (H) and light (L) chains. The H-L pairs are held together by interchain disulfide bonds and noncovalent forces. The binding site for antigen is formed by one H and one L chain. IgM is a polymer of 5 four-chain units, and secretory IgA is a dimer. Polymeric forms (see Fig. 84–3) possess a J chain that is synthesized with the H and L chains and stabilizes the sulfhydryl groups during polymerization. At regular intervals along the peptide chain a disulfide bond forms an intrachain loop, known as the *Ig domain.* This motif is repeated among Igs, T-cell receptors, adhesion proteins, and histocompatibility antigens. Proteins with these Ig domains share close homology structurally and functionally and suggest a common evolutionary origin. They are termed *members of the Ig superfamily* (IgSF), and all are involved in cell interaction processes associated with recognition.

The Ig molecule is divided into regions, the amino acid sequence of which is similar, such as those regions needed for complement fixation or attachment to receptors on leukocytes. Other regions are highly variable, however. Those that bind to antigen have the highest divergence and are known as the hypervariable region. Thus each Ig chain can be divided into constant and variable regions. The H chain has three constant and one variable region, and the L chain has one variable and one constant region. The hypervariable region of the L and H chains is tightly apposed and forms the combining site for antigen (Fig. 84–3). The digestion of Ig with papain and pepsin generates fragments with varying biologic capability. The complement fixation (Fc) region of the Ig molecule accounts for its isotypic biological capability. As outlined previously, this is the region critical for complement fixation and recognition by Fc receptors on the leukocytes. The Fab region provides for specific unique antigen-antibody interactions. The $F(ab)_2$ fragment is formed with pepsin cleavage; the affinity for antigen is twice as great as Fab alone.

Contact Activation System

There are four major plasma protein systems that contribute to the host's defense and participate in the

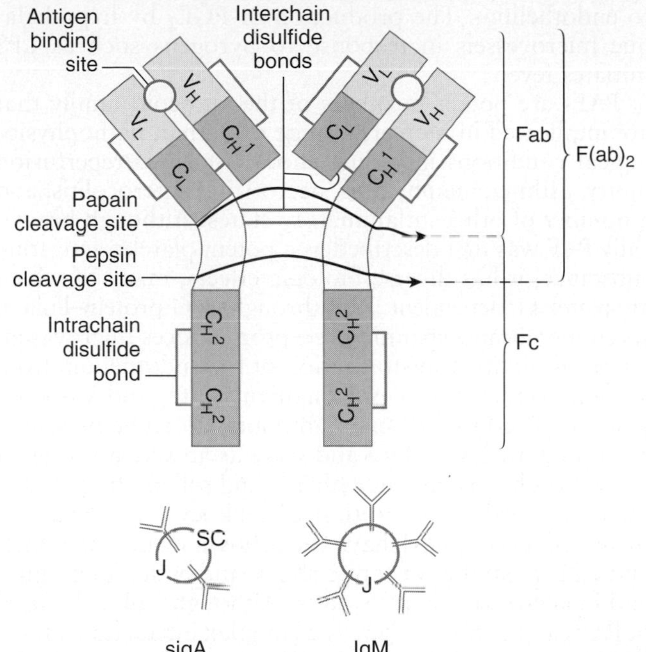

FIGURE 84–3 • Basic immunoglobulin (Ig) structure. Sites of cleavage for papain or pepsin are shown with resulting fragments. The intrachain disulfide bond forms the region of the Ig domain. Insets show polymeric Igs, secretory IgA (*left*) and IgM (*right*). J chain is common to all polymeric forms. *SC*, secretory component; V_L, variable domain of light chain; C_L, constant domain of light chain; V_H, variable domain of heavy chain; C_H, constant domains of heavy chain.

development of inflammatory tissue injury. The complement system has been previously reviewed. The others include the contact activation system (also known as *Hageman factor* or *intrinsic coagulation system*), the extrinsic coagulation, and the fibrinolytic system (see also Chapters 74, 75, and 96). The contact activation system is critical to host defense and control of local blood flow at sites of injury. Hageman factor (factor XII) is activated spontaneously (XIIa) on contact with negatively charged surfaces, such as lipid A of LPS and vascular basement membranes (Fig. 84–4). High-molecular-weight kininogen (HMWK), prekallikrein, and factor XI circulate in the plasma as complexes. XIIa will activate factor XI and cleave prekallikrein to kallikrein. Kallikrein will then cleave HMWK to bradykinin. The kallikrein-kinin system also encompasses the tissue (or glandular) kallikrein-kinin system (Fig. 84–4). Tissue kallikrein is immunologically distinct from plasma kallikrein and present throughout the body as an inactive "pro" substance. In the presence of intracellular enzymes, plasmin, or plasma kallikrein, tissue kallikrein is produced, secreted, and active in the tissue where it is made. Tissue kallikrein can then cleave HMWK to bradykinin directly or it can cleave low-molecular-weight kininogen (LMWK) or tissue kininogen (T-kininogen) to kallidin, which is then directly converted to bradykinin. In the plasma, 80% of kininogen is low molecular weight.

Bradykinin is an exceedingly potent vasoactive peptide. It can cause venular dilation, increased vascular permeability, hypotension, bronchoconstriction, and activation of phospholipase A_2. Phospholipase A_2 releases arachidonic acid (AA) from cell membrane and initiates the production of both proinflammatory and antiinflammatory phospholipids-derived products (see subsequent section and Fig. 84–4). Bradykinin is metabolized by angiotensin-converting enzyme (ACE) to inactive peptides. Bradykinin, along with prostanoids, stimulates the pain response through polymodal receptors and C-fibers (capsaicin-sensitive).[27] In animal models, bradykinin has been shown to be responsible for the four signs of inflammation: *heat, redness, swelling,* and *pain.* The bradykinin effect is enhanced by simultaneous production of prostanoids. The prostanoids, along with in particular the low

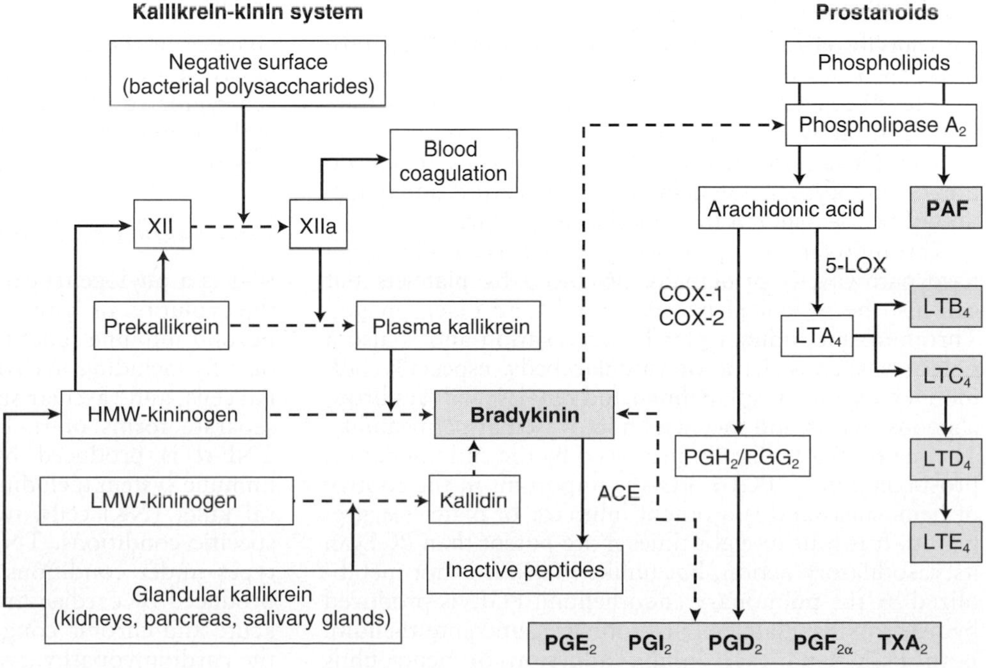

FIGURE 84–4 • Contact activation system and prostanoid production. Bradykinin can be produced by either the plasma kallikrein (*top left*) or tissue (glandular) kallikrein system (*bottom left*). Once formed, bradykinin can activate phospholipase A_2 and thus drive prostanoid production. In addition it can potentiate the effects of the prostaglandins and vice versa. Bradykinin is metabolized into inactive peptides through several steps; in the last, it is enzymatically driven by angiotensin-converting enzyme *(ACE). HMW,* high molecular weight; *LMW,* low molecular weight; *PAF,* platelet-activating factor; *COX-1,* cyclooxygenase-1; *COX-2,* cyclooxygenase-2; *5-LOX,* 5-lipoxygenase; *LT,* leukotriene; TXA_2, thromboxane A_2; *PG,* prostaglandin. (Modified from Ueno A, Oh-ishi S: *J Pharmacol Sci* 93:1, 2003).

pH of exudates, inhibit the activity of kininases such as ACE. These activities occur through the bradykinin-2 receptor.

Lipid-Derived Mediators of Inflammation

Although lipid-derived mediators of inflammation are not soluble components of immunity per se, their production has both proinflammatory and antiinflammatory effects, and they are discussed here because of their production as a result of the contact activation syndrome (see Fig. 84-4). These mediators are not stored preformed but are rapidly generated after cell stimulation. AA (or eicosapentaenoic acid) is a 20-carbon fatty acid. Its metabolites are termed *eicosanoids*. The eicosanoids are produced by a variety of cell type-, tissue-, and species-specific biosynthetic pathways. Prostanoids are a specific class of mediators generated through initial actions of cyclooxygenase. The eicosanoid family includes the thromboxanes, prostacyclins, leukotrienes (LTs), hydroxyeicosatetraenoic acids (HETEs), epoxyeicosatrienoic acids (EETs), lipoxins, and isoprostanes. The release of AA and the 1-alkyl-2-acetyl analogs of phosphatidyl choline (platelet-activating factors [PAFs]) occurs through the action of phospholipase A_2 and phospholipase C on cell membrane phospholipids (see Fig. 84-4). Phospholipases are stored in lysozymes or are in the cytoplasm. Through cell activation, they translocate to the inner cell membrane where they can hydrolyze the cell membrane phospholipids. The major routes of AA metabolism for proinflammatory effects are the 5-lipoxygenase pathway (production of the LTs) and the cyclooxygenase pathway (production of prostaglandins and thromboxane [i.e., prostanoids]). Of particular interest is a new class of prostanoids derived from polyunsaturated fatty acids and eicosapentanoic acid through the cyclooxygenase pathway that appear to have antiinflammatory effects.[28]

The 5-lipoxygenase pathway is prominent in leukocytes and mast cells (see Fig. 84-4). LTs C_4, D_4, and E_4 were first described as the "slow-reacting substances of anaphylaxis." They are potent vasoconstrictors and bronchoconstrictors with specific effects on the peripheral airways. LTB_4 is produced by neutrophils, monocytes, and macrophages within minutes of cell activation. LTB_4 is a powerful chemoattractant and activator of other leukocytes, resulting in enhanced leukocyte-endothelial cell interactions, sequestration of leukocytes in the pulmonary vasculature, and induction of permeability at the endothelial interface.

Thromboxane A_2, produced through the cyclooxygenase pathway, is principally produced by platelets but can also be produced by neutrophils and macrophages. Thromboxane induces platelet aggregation and is also a potent vasoconstrictor of vascular beds, especially pulmonary, coronary, splanchnic, and renal. It induces bronchoconstriction and increases microvascular permeability. The major prostaglandin produced by the endothelium is prostaglandin I_2 (PGI_2). PGI_2 is important in the control of hemostasis and is a potent inhibitor of platelet aggregation. It is four to eight times more potent than PGE_2 in its vasodilatory action, but unlike PGE_2, it is not metabolized by the pulmonary endothelium. PGE_2 is produced by neutrophils, platelets, macrophages, and endothelium. Both PGE_2 and PGI_2 inhibit adhesion of neutrophils to endothelium. The production of PGE_2 by hypothalamic microvessels in response to pyrogens such as LPS initiates fever.

PAFs are potent members of the autocoid family that are implicated in a diverse range of human pathophysiological conditions including shock, ischemia/reperfusion injury, asthma, anaphylaxis, necrotizing enterocolitis, and a number of other inflammatory states. Although historically PAF was first described as a potent platelet-activating substance, it has diverse biologic effects, many of which are platelet independent. PAF, through its G-protein–linked, seven membrane–spanning receptor, induces microvascular permeability, transformation of the endothelium from an anticoagulant to a procoagulant state, and vasoconstriction. Produced in small amounts, it can be presented at the endothelial surface and serve as an activating agent for neutrophils as they are tethered and roll on the endothelium (see further description of leukocyte localization). Increased levels of PAF have been shown in animal models and clinical studies of septic shock and acute lung injury and in necrotizing enterocolitis. Although isolated effects of PAF can be shown, there is a complex interaction among PAF, prostaglandins, and cytokines in the pathophysiological changes associated with sepsis, shock, trauma, and ischemia/reperfusion injury.[29,30]

Cytokines

Cytokines are signaling proteins secreted by cells that affect the functional properties of other cells of the same organism. The cytokine family includes the lymphokines, chemokines, ILs, and IFNs. Unlike circulating hormones, cytokines travel short extracellular distances before interacting with target cell surface receptors in a paracrine or autocrine manner. Cytokines can be detected in serum samples, particularly during times of maximal production, as with sepsis. Cytokines as a group are low-molecular-weight (<80 kDa) proteins. They interact with high-affinity cell surface receptors specific for each cytokine. Their cell surface binding ultimately leads to changes in the pattern of protein synthesis, altered cell behavior, or both. They often have multiple-overlapping cell regulatory functions. Many cytokines are produced early in infection, whereas others are produced at later stages.

Interleukin 1 and Tumor Necrosis Factor

IL-1 is a phylogenetically ancient molecule that predates the evolution of lymphocytes and Ig. Its activity extends beyond immune function. IL-1 is produced by a variety of cells including macrophages, endothelial cells, epithelial cells, and vascular smooth muscle cells. There are two separate forms of IL-1, IL-1α, and IL-1β. In contrast TNF-α is produced by cells primarily of the innate immune system including monocytes/macrophages, natural killer (NK) cells, mast cells, and neutrophils under specific conditions. TNF is also produced by other cell types under conditions of stress. For example, TNF is produced by cardiac myocytes and is implicated in both acute and chronic congestive heart failure, as well as in the cardiomyopathy associated with sepsis. TNF-β (also known as *lymphokine*) is produced by T lymphocytes, but occasionally antigen-activated T cells may also produce TNF-α. Both TNF and IL-1 are produced as small precursor molecules or "pro" molecules that are cleaved by IL-1β converting enzyme (ICE) (but now known as caspase 1) and TNF-α converting enzyme (TACE) (but now known as ADAM17 [*A Disintegrin And Metalloproteinase*]). Once cleaved these proteins are then excreted. Note that caspase 1 and ADAM 17 are multifunctional proteinases and have activity on other ILs and inflammatory molecules. IL-1 is the only cytokine with a natural inhibitor, IL-1 receptor antagonist (IL-1 RA), which is produced by the same cells that produce IL-1. IL-1 RA functions to down-regulate the proinflammatory effects of IL-1. IL-1 and TNF-α are the early major mediators of gram-negative endotoxin shock (see also Chapter 96). As outlined earlier in this chapter, signaling of cells by TNF and IL-1 occurs at least in part through NF-κB and consequently shares a similarity in receptor function and signaling molecules.

For routine infection and injury, IL-1β and TNF-α are transiently expressed and secreted. Their activities are modulated by coproduction of naturally occurring antiinflammatory cytokines, such as IL-10 and IL-1 RA. The levels of production fall off rapidly; thus it is tightly regulated. Dysregulated cytokine production, the kind that occurs in chronic diseases such as rheumatoid arthritis and inflammatory bowel disease, has led to the development of novel anticytokine therapy such as human recombinant IL-1 RA (anakinra), human/murine chimeric monoclonal antibody against TNF-α (infliximab), and recombinant fusion protein composed of the extracellular binding domain of TNF receptor II and human IgG1 (etanercept). With the development of these products, there is increasing evidence that neutralization of TNF-α is associated with increased risk of opportunistic infections, including mycobacterial diseases. Currently, blockade of IL-1 with IL-RA appears to be safe.[31] When such blocking agents are used in animal models, neutralization or gene deletion of TNF-α appears to be associated with the reduction of host defense in models of live gram-positive or gram-negative infections and infection by intracellular microbes such as *Salmonella* and *Listeria*. Absence of IL-RA can also result in decreased resistance to *Listeria* or gram-positive bacteria. TNF and IFN-γ (discussed in the following paragraphs) are required for defense against infection caused by *Mycobacterium tuberculosis*.[31]

Interleukin 18

IL-18 is a member of the IL-1 family of ligands. It has unique characteristics in that only in conjunction with IL-12 is IFN-γ produced by activated T cells and by LPS-stimulated macrophages. IL-18 is implicated in the development of endotoxic shock and in the myocardial depression that occurs in these models.[32] As a key mediator of IFN-γ production, IL-18 serves an important role in controlling infections due to *Salmonella*, *Cryptococcus*, *Toxoplasma*, *Candida*, and *Mycobacterium* organisms, often through its modulation of the production of nitric oxide (NO).[32,33]

Interleukin 12

IL-12 is produced by monocytes, macrophages, DCs, neutrophils, and to a lesser extent B cells. IL-12 effects are primarily on T and NK cells. The responses by T cells and NK cells include increased proliferation, increased IFN-γ production, increased cytotoxic activity (cytotoxic T lymphocytes and NK cells), and polarization toward a Th1 phenotype (T cells only) (see following discussion). Patients with defects in IL-12 or IL-12 receptor have increased susceptibility to mycobacterial and *Salmonella* infections. Neonates have diminished IL-18 and IL-12 production, which contribute to inadequate IFN-γ production and increased susceptibility to infections.[34,35]

Interleukin 6

IL-6 is one member of the IL-6 family of cytokines. It is produced by many cell types including the cardiac and skeletal myocytes, but it is mainly produced by macrophages and monocytes, adipose cells, endothelial cells, T lymphocytes, mast cells, and osteoclasts. Many cell types respond to IL-6, including hepatocytes. IL-6 is the factor most directly responsible for the production of acute phase reactants. Its production is somewhat delayed compared with IL-1 and TNF, and its levels remain elevated for a longer period. Animals with an IL-6 deficiency have an increased susceptibility to *Listeria monocytogenes*, *Streptococcus pneumoniae*, *Escherichia coli*, *Candida albicans*, and mycobacterial infections.[31,36]

Interleukin 10

IL-10, like IL-6, is a pleiotropic cytokine that exerts both immunosuppressive and immunostimulatory effects. It is produced primarily by CD4+ T cells, B cells, macrophages, and DCs. Its predominant suppressive effect is to inhibit Th1 (IFN-γ and IL-2) cytokine production. It down-regulates MHC Class II expression, thus limiting its interaction with T cells and NK cells. It also inhibits cytokines involved in inflammatory responses including PGE_2, TNF-α, IL-1, IL-6, and IL-8. IL-10 induces the production of IL-1 RA. IL-10's up-regulation of FCRγI on monocytes, macrophages, and NK cells enhances antibody-mediated cellular cytotoxicity.

Interleukin 2

IL-2 is produced by CD4 T cells when they encounter their foreign peptide-MHC complex. This cytokine is critical for adaptive immune response in that it has both an autocrine and a paracrine function, triggering T cells to undergo multiple rounds of proliferation and differentiate into effector T cells.

Interferons

IFN-α and IFN-β are known as type I IFNs. IFN-α is produced by monocytes and macrophages, whereas IFN-β is produced by fibroblasts. The major stimuli for type I IFN are viral infections and T-cell derived factors in adaptive immune responses. Type I IFNs inhibit viral replication, and patients with insufficient production have severe progressive or fulminant viral disease. These IFNs inhibit cell proliferation, enhance the lytic potential of NK cells, and increase class I human leukocyte antigen (HLA), while decreasing class II HLA. IFN-γ is a type II IFN and is produced primarily by CD4+, CD8+, and NK cells (Fig. 84–5). IFN-γ has antiviral and antiproliferative activity. It up-regulates class I and II HLA expression, thus enhancing cellular toxicity and antigen presentation, respectively. IFN-γ's activation of monocytes, macrophages, and neutrophils results in enhanced killing of intracellular organisms, including mycobacteria and *Listeria*. In addition, IFN-γ induces inducible NO synthase in macrophages; the result is the generation of NO, a critical component for bactericidal function. Animals with a deficiency of IFN-γ have decreased survival in response to *Salmonella* and mycobacterial infections. Patients with complete loss of IFN-γ receptors have severe infections early in life with salmonella and viruses (including respiratory syncytial virus [RSV], parainfluenza, herpes simplex virus [HSV], and cytomegalovirus [CMV]). These are associated with a high mortality rate.[31,35,37] IFN-γ is a critical cytokine at the interface of the adaptive and innate immune system because of its function on NK cells and ultimately monocytes/macrophages.

Macrophage Migration Inhibitory Factor

Macrophage migration inhibitory factor (MIF) has been identified for more than 40 years, although its function has only been well-defined in the past 15 years with the cloning of human MIF cDNA. Although T cells were initially thought to be the main source, monocytes, eosinophils, basophils, DCs, B cells, mast cells, and neutrophils all express MIF. In contrast to other cytokines, MIF is secreted and stored in intracellular pools and therefore does not require de novo protein synthesis before secretion. MIF has a broad tissue distribution and is expressed by cells and tissues that are in direct contact with the host's natural environment, as well as by organs involved in the stress response (hypothalamus, pituitary, and adrenal glands). MIF is implicated in both gram-negative and gram-positive infections. MIF-deficient animals have increased susceptibility to low-dose inoculum of *Salmonella* and *E. coli*. In contrast blockade of MIF results in improved survival in animals treated with high doses of *E. coli*, after cecal ligation and puncture or after bacterial superantigen challenge.[38]

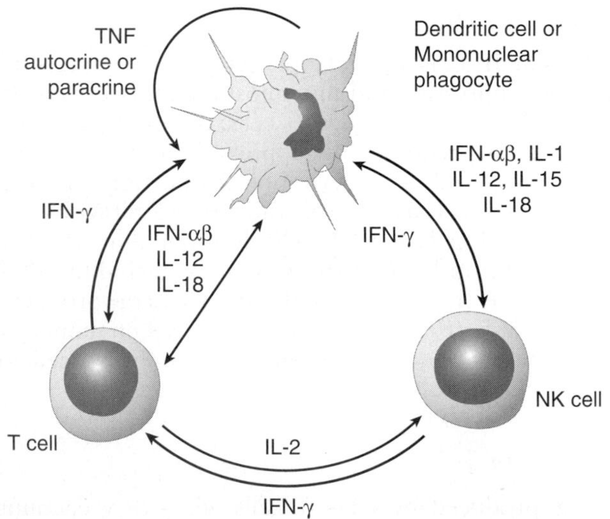

FIGURE 84–5 • Secreted cytokines and effects on adaptive (T cell) and innate (dendritic cell/mononuclear phagocyte) and NK cells. NK cells activate mononuclear phagocytes and dendritic cells through IFN-γ secretion. With activation, mononuclear phagocytes have increased phagocytic and antimicrobial actions against intracellular pathogens. The phagocytes secrete cytokines that activate the NK cells, inducing IFN-γ production. IFN-γ from NK cells and IFN αβ, IL12, and IL-18 from the mononuclear phagocytes/dendritic cells in turn activate the T cell along the Th1 pathway. Activation of the T cell produces IL-2 and IFN-γ, which affect the mononuclear phagocyte/dendritic cell, NK cell, and other T cells. Note that activation of the mononuclear phagocyte/dendritic cell results in production of TNF, which has both autocrine and paracrine effects. (Modified from Douglas S, Kapur R, Merrill JD et al: The mononuclear phagocytic, dendritic cell and natural killer systems. In Stiehm ER, Ochs HD, Winkelstein JA, editors: Immunologic disorders of infants and children, Philadelphia, 2004, Elsevier Saunders.)

High Mobility Group Box 1

HMGB1 has been recently identified to be a late mediator of sepsis. As with MIF, antibodies to HMGB1 can be given many hours after the induction of sepsis and improve survival in animal models.[38,39] Also similar to MIF, HMGB1 is released from the cytoplasmic pool. Intracellular HMGB1 has diverse functions, including nucleosomal structure and function, as well as binding of transcription factors to their cognate DNA sequences. In systemic concentrations, however, it has diverse proinflammatory responses mirroring the "late" effects of systemic inflammation, including loss of gut epithelial barrier function; bacterial translocation; release of liver enzymes; activation of neutrophils, monocytes, macrophages, and endothelium; and acute lung injury.[39] Macrophages and neutrophils, when stimulated with LPS and C5a, respectively, release large amounts of HMGB1 into the culture medium. Systemic HMGB1 accumulation occurs in mice 8 hours after LPS administration, long after TNF and IL-1β levels have decreased. Humans with sepsis have elevated levels of HMGB1, and those whose levels were most elevated were at highest risk of dying.[40] In a mouse model of cecal ligation and puncture in which mortality was 75%, treatment with anti-HMGB1 monoclonal antibody 24 hours after injury decreased mortality to 25%. It had no effect on recovery of bacterial counts from the spleens on these animals and thus did not appear to affect bacterial clearance.[41]

Chemokines

Chemokines are structurally and functionally related inflammatory cytokines with the ability to stimulate the chemotactic migration of distinct sets of cells, including neutrophils, monocytes, lymphocytes, DCs, macrophages, fibroblasts, stem cells, and smooth muscle cells. The chemokine family is the largest family of cytokines, and although their main function is characterized as "chemotaxis" or directing migration through a concentration gradient, they also have a number of other functions including cell activation, signaling, effects on angiogenesis and tumorigenesis, and immune cell polarization. To date there are 40+ identified chemokines.[42] They are small (approximately 8-14 kDa), mostly basic molecules. They function through unique receptors that are G-protein coupled and are seven-membrane spanning (i.e., have seven transmembrane domains).[43] The cytoplasmic domains of the receptors are critical for cell signaling and function. Chemokines may use more than one receptor for function. Chemokines are central to the process of extravasation of leukocytes, which includes multiple steps involving interactions of adhesion molecules and the chemoattractant function of these proteins. Chemokines are defined by structure, not function, and can be divided into two large and two small subgroups depending on the number and arrangement of conserved cysteines. The subgroups are CC, CXC, C, and CX3C. Note that in the past 5 years, chemokines are designated by their subgroup followed by a ligand number; for example, IL-8 is CXCL8. Most chemokines are classified into two main groups according to function: (1) those concerned with hemostasis, which are constitutively expressed and coordinate leukocyte trafficking during hematopoiesis and those with lymphocyte recirculation, and (2) those concerned with inflammation and tissue injury. Chemokines are produced by hematopoietic cells themselves as well as by endothelial cells, epithelial cells, and cells arising from the mesoderm including fibroblasts, myocytes, hepatocytes, and lymphatic cells. Table 84–2 lists a select group of chemokines that are involved in infection and inflammation.

Granulocyte Colony-Stimulating Factor and Granulocyte-Macrophage Colony-Stimulating Factor

Granulocyte colony-stimulating factor (G-CSF) and granulocyte-macrophage colony-stimulating factor (GM-CSF) were initially identified by their ability to induce granulocytopoiesis and monocytopoiesis; however, they have marked effects on neutrophil and monocyte function. Although both G-CSF and GM-CSF are produced by bone marrow stromal cells, they are also produced by activated monocytes/macrophages and fibroblasts. G-CSF is also produced by epithelial cells of the gut and lung in response to inflammation. GM-CSF is also produced by T lymphocytes and NK cells. G-CSF enhances the physiological activation of mature neutrophils, whereas GM-CSF stimulates the functional activity of neutrophils, eosinophils, and monocytes/macrophages.[44,45] GM-CSF is also critically involved in the normal surfactant turnover, and alveolar proteinosis is an autoimmune disease targeting GM-CSF.[46] Critical to the immune response is that production of G-CSF and GM-CSF results in increased neutrophil survival. Neutrophils usually have a half-life of less than 12 hours before removal from the circulation and undergo apoptosis. Exposure to G-CSF or GM-CSF, however, decreases apoptosis; this leads to prolonged survival of circulating neutrophils and those that have emigrated to a site of infection. Removal of these cytokines, as in the resolution phase of inflammation, leads to induction of apoptosis and increased clearance of neutrophils. G-CSF and GM-CSF are approved for use in a variety of hematological diseases.[45] G-CSF and GM-CSF have been proposed to be used in the nonneutropenic critically ill adult and neonatal population. To date, however, studies do not support their routine use as either a treatment of established systemic infection or as a prophylaxis to prevent systemic infection in high-risk individuals.[47-49]

Nitric Oxide

NO• is a stable, free radical gas. Extensive work over the past 20 years has converged to establish NO as a major messenger molecule regulating immune function and blood vessel dilation and serving as a neurotransmitter. NO is formed from arginine by the enzyme nitric oxide synthase (NOS). NOS-2 or inducible NOS (iNOS) is present in many tissues, whereas NOS-1 and NOS-3 are primarily present in neuronal and endothelial cells, respectively. NOS-1 and NOS-3 are present in low amounts and generate NO• for neurotransmission and vasodilation. In contrast, NOS-2 is induced by microbial peptides and inflammatory cytokines and serves as a major bactericidal and tumoricidal agent. NO• is critical in adaptive immunity to intracellular pathogens such as *M. tuberculosis* and *L. monocytogenes*. NO• enhances the activity of NK cells, γδ T cells, and macrophages. The interaction of intracellular NO• and the reactive oxygen superoxide, O_2^-, results in the production of peroxynitrite ($OHNOO^-$), which decays to the highly reactive hydroxyl radical (OH•) and nitrogen dioxide. These agents contribute in part to the killing of the microorganisms in tightly regulated structurally "isolated" areas of phagocytes, the phagolysosomes, discussed in the subsequent section (see also Chapter 97).

Cellular Components of Immunity

The cellular components of immunity have traditionally been divided into innate and adaptive immunity, but such distinctions have become increasingly blurred and critical overlap occurs. For example, the DCs and other APCs, such as the macrophage and monocytes, are part of the innate immune system; nonetheless, they directly drive adaptive immunity (see also Chapter 85).

The cells of the immune system can be defined by the surface antigens they display. These surface antigens are denoted by the CD nomenclature and refer to cluster designation. These antigens denote the lineage and often the functional capacity of a cell. Surface antigens are revealed with monoclonal antibodies, most commonly with a technique known as *flow cytometry.*

Lymphocytes include the T cells, B cells, NK cells, and the natural kill T cells (NKTs), which have features of both NK and T cells. T cells are called such because most of them arise from the thymus. They mediate antigen-specific cellular immunity and play a critical role in facilitating antigen-specific, B-cell–dependent humoral immunity. B cells are the subset of lymphocytes that synthesize, express Ig on their surface, and differentiate to plasma cells that produce Ig. B cells arise from the *b*one marrow in humans and other mammals or *b*ursa in birds.[50]

The major T cell subsets are the $CD4^+$ helper/inducer and the $CD8^+$ suppressor/killer cells. Most T cells

TABLE 84–2

Chemokine/Receptor Families (partial list)

	Name	Original Ligand Name*	Chemokine Receptor
CXC CHEMOKINE/RECEPTOR FAMILY	CXCL1	GRO-α/MGSA-α	CXCR2 > CXCR1
	CXCL2	GRO-β/MGSA-β	CXCR2
	CXCL3	GRO-γβ/MGSA-γ	CXCR2
	CXCL5	ENA-78	CXCR2
	CXCL7	NAP-2	CXCR2
	CXCL8	IL-8	CXCR1, CXCR2
	CXCL9	Mig	CXCR3
	CXCL10	IP-10	CXCR3
	CXCL12	SDF-1	CXCR4
C CHEMOKINE/RECEPTOR FAMILY	XCL-1	Lymphotactin	XCR1
CX3C CHEMOKINE/RECEPTOR FAMILY	CX3CL1	Fractalkine	CX3CR1
CC CHEMOKINE/RECEPTOR FAMILY	CCL2	MCP-1	CCR2
	CCL3	MIP-1α	CCR1, CCR5
	CCL4	MIP-1β	CCR5
	CCL5	RANTES	CCR1, CCR3, CCR5
	CCL8	MCP-2	CCR3
	CCL11	Eotaxin	CCR3
	CCL19	MIP-3β	CCR7
	CCL21	6Ckine	CCR7
	Receptor Name	**Original Ligand Name***	**Cellular Distribution**
CHEMOKINE RECEPTORS AND CELLULAR DISTRIBUTION	XCR1	Lymphotactin	T, B, NK
	CXCR1	IL-8, GRO-α	N, M, T, NK, En, Ms, Bs
	CXCR2	IL-8, GRO-α,-β-γ, NAP-2, ENA-78	N,M,T,NK,Ms,As, Nn, En
	CXCR3	IP-10, Mig	Activated T
	CXCR4	SDF-1	Myeloid, T, B, Ep,En, DC
	CX3CR1	Fractalkine	NK, M, T
	CCR1	RANTES, MIP-1α, MCP-2, MCP-3	N, M, T, NK, B, Ms, As, Nn
	CCR2	MCP-1	M, T, B, Bs
	CCR3	RANTES, eotaxin	Eo, Bs, T
	CCR5	RANTES, MIP-1α, MIP-1β, MCP-2	T, M, Mφ
	CCR7	MIP-3β, 6Ckine	T, B, DC

Modified from Murdoch C, Finn A: *Blood* 95:3032, 2000 and Zlotnik A, Yoshie O: *Immunity* 12:121, 2000.

*The ligand names are human chemokines.

GRO, growth regulating peptide; *MGSA,* melanocyte growth stimulating activity; *ENA,* epithelial-derived neutrophil attractant; *NAP,* neutrophil activating peptide; *IL-8,* interleukin-8; *IP-10,* γ interferon-induced peptide 10; *SDF,* stroma derived factor; *MCP,* monocytes chemotactic peptide; *MIP,* macrophage inflammatory peptide; *RANTES,* regulated on activation, normal T cell expressed and secreted; *T,* T cell; *B,* B cell; *NK,* NK cell; *M,* monocytes/macrophage; *N,* neutrophil; *Ms,* mast cell; *Bs,* basophil; *As,* astrocyte; *Nn,* neuron; *En,* endothelium; *Eo,* eosinophil; *DC,* dendritic cell; *Ep,* epithelial cell; *Mφ,* macrophage.

bear a T cell receptor composed of an α- and β-chain; they also express CD4 or CD8 coreceptors. Almost all the αβ T cells recognize protein antigen in the form of peptide fragments bound to classic MHC molecules (class I or class II). The CD4 molecule augments binding to antigens presented in association with MHC II antigens, whereas CD 8 molecules are necessary for antigen binding to MHC I. The immunological synapse is the highly ordered junction that forms between the APCs such as the DCs or tissue macrophages and the T cell during antigenic stimulation. The structure resembles a doughnut in which the T cell receptor-peptide-MHC, CD3, CD4, or CD8 are in the center of the synapse. The costimulatory molecules CD2, CD28, CD, and CD54 (intercellular adhesion molecule-1 [ICAM-1]) on the T cell bind to their respective ligands LFA-3 (CD 58), CD80-CD86, and LFA-1(CD11a/CD18) on the APC on the perimeter of synapse (Fig. 84–6).[51]

The CD4$^+$ naïve cells (i.e., those never exposed to antigen) can differentiate into effector cells expressing specific patterns of cytokines, which have been described as Th1 and Th2. Most of these cytokines are secreted but

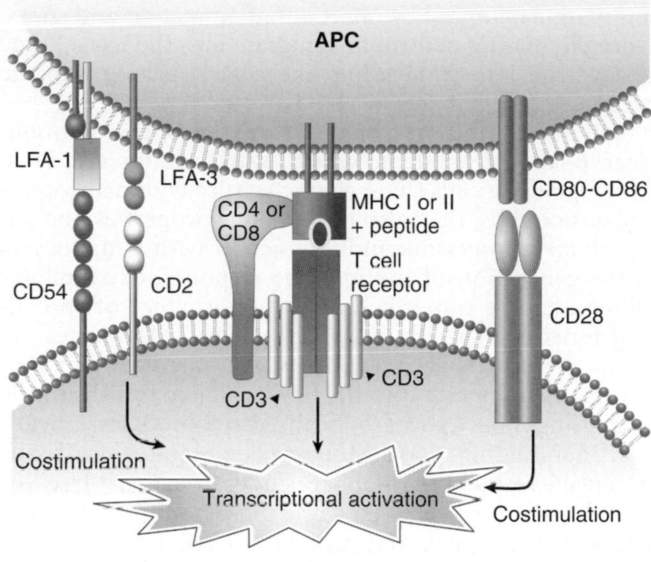

FIGURE 84–6 • Immunological synapse. Protein antigen bound to the major histocompatibility complex I or II (MHC I or II) is presented by the antigen-presenting cell (APC) to the T cell receptor on the T cell. The T cell receptor/CD3 complex is composed of the two chains of the T cell receptor (α and β) and the six subunits of the CD3 (a γ and a δ subunit , 2 each of the ε and ζ subunits). CD8 or CD4 interacts with the MHC I or MHC II/antigen complex, respectively. Engagement of the T-cell receptor can then signal the T cell to activate a number of activities, including transcription. For activation to occur, however, there must be additional signals through costimulatory molecules on the T cell and APC. Note that the T cell receptor/CD3/CD4 (or CD8) complex is centered in the middle of the immunological synapse, whereas the costimulatory molecules are in the periphery (see text for additional details).

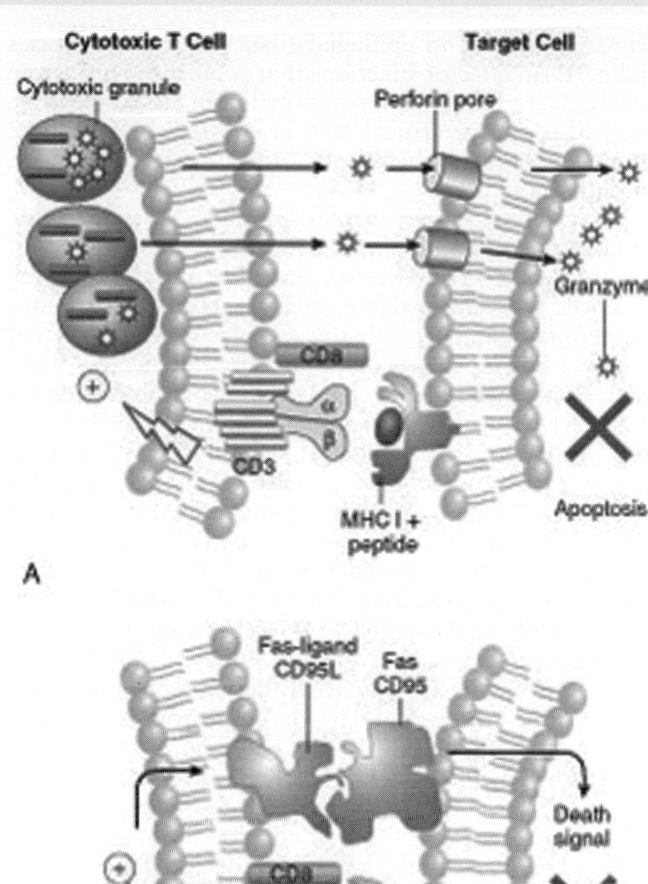

FIGURE 84–7 • Mechanisms of antigen-specific, MHC I–restricted, T cell–mediated cytotoxicity. The engagement of the αβ T cell receptor (TCR) in the CD3/CD8 complex of the T cell by antigenic peptide bound to MHC I on the target cell leads to T cell activation and target cell death. **A,** Cytotoxicity occurs through the release of the contents of the cytotoxic granules from the T cell, including perforin and granzyme. A perforin pore is introduced into the target cell membrane through which granzymes can enter the target cell. This leads to the triggering of apoptosis and cell death. **B,** The activation of the T cells leads to up-regulation of the Fas-ligand (CD95L), which engages Fas (CD95) on the target cell, resulting in the delivery of a death signal culminating in apoptosis. Both of these mechanisms are also used by NK (natural killer) T cells and NK cells. (Modified with permission from Lewis DB, Wenwei T: The physiologic immunodeficiency of immaturity. In Stiehm ER, Ochs HD, Winkelstein JA, editors: Immunologic disorders of infants and children, Philadelphia, 2004, Elsevier Saunders.)

can be expressed on the cell surface. IFN-γ is the signature cytokine produced by Th1 cells, but the Th1 cells also produce substantial amounts of IL-2, TNF-α, and TNF-β. The Th1 response is considered proinflammatory. In contrast IL-4 is the signature cytokine produced by Th2 cells, along with IL-5, IL-9, and IL-13. IL-4 and IL-13 (along with IL-10 discussed previously and produced by monocytes/macrophages) are considered antiinflammatory or immunosuppressive. The Th2 response is critical for eosinophil function and is important in the development of IgE responses and the killing of parasites.

Naive $CD8^+$ cells are not effective killer cells, but following activation with antigen in the context of MHC class I by APCs in the presence of IL-2 and IL-12 they differentiate quickly into CD8+ cytotoxic cells. These cells express perforin, granzymes, and Fas ligand and produce effector cytokines including TNF-α and IFN-γ. Perforins introduce pores into the target cell through which granzymes can enter into the target cell, leading to the triggering of apoptosis and cell death. Alternatively the cytotoxic T cell up-regulates the Fas ligand (CD95L), which engages Fas (CD95) on the target cell, resulting in delivery of death signal culminating in apoptosis (Fig. 84–7).

A small proportion of T cells in the circulation have γδ T-cell receptors that are not restricted to antigen recognition bound to either MHC class I or MHC class II. Thus γδ T cells do not have either CD4 or CD8 molecules on their surface. The γδ T cell recognize either stress-induced or nonclassic MHC molecules directly, or nonpeptide antigens, such as host or pathogen-derived lipids bound to these nonclassic MHC molecules. The γδ T cells are primarily located in epithelial tissues in certain species and perform effector functions that protect the host from infections and malignancy and maintain tissue integrity. They also play a critical role in the regulation of the immune response, which leads to resolution of infection and inflammation.[52]

NK cells are large granular lymphocytes with innate immune function that play a critical role in the early host defense against viral, bacterial, and other infections, as well as cancer. NK cells recognize their targets through unique NK receptors and are able to recognize self-MHC class I or class I-like molecules that inhibit or enhance NK function. Their phenotype is characterized by the expression of the CD56 surface antigen and the lack of CD3. NK cells produce IFN-γ, TNF-α, IL-10, and GM-CSF. They have spontaneous cytotoxic activity against virus-infected cells and mediated antibody-dependent cell cytotoxicity through FCRγIII (CD16). Cytotoxicity is the major effector function of NK cells. They bridge the innate and adaptive immune response (see Fig. 84–5).[53,54] The NKT cells express both CD56 and CD3–T-cell receptor and thus share receptor structures of both conventional NK and T cells. NKT cells are potentially capable of rapid secretion of large amounts of Th1 or Th2 cytokines but also contain perforin. Both NK and NKT cells use the same mechanisms as the cytotoxic $CD8^+$ T cell for killing (i.e., perforin/granzyme cytotoxicity and Fas-ligand/fas cytotoxicity) (see Fig. 84–7). The control and resolution of viral infections require the elimination of the source of the virus and thus the destruction of the virus-infected cell before progeny virus is produced. This is mediated during the innate phase of the immune response by NK cells, but in most cases resolution of active viral infection ultimately requires the development of antigen-specific T lymphocytes, most of which are MHC class I–restricted $CD8^+$ T cells, although MHC class II $CD4^+$ cells and γδ T cells may also mediate cytotoxicity.

Phagocytic cells include neutrophils, eosinophils, monocytes/macrophages, and DCs. They have in common a number of different properties that are of prime importance to the host inflammatory response. Neutrophils, eosinophils, and monocytes/macrophages share the ability to phagocytose foreign material, release granule constituents, secrete inflammatory mediators and regulators, and form reactive oxygen products through a unique system of reduced nicotinamide adenine dinucleotide phosphate (NADPH) oxidase enzyme that is present on the cell membrane. Neutrophils, eosinophils, and basophils are all polymorphonuclear leukocytes (PMNLs). Neutrophils and eosinophils share similar mechanisms of cell migration, phagocytosis, and pathogen killing. All three cell types have segmented nuclei and contain granules, although their granule content varies. Neutrophils are the host's main defense against bacterial and fungal infections. Eosinophils are important for the control of parasitic infections. Neutrophils may remain in the storage pool of the bone marrow for up to 5 days. Released from the bone marrow into the blood, about half the neutrophils circulate for about 10 hours; the other half remains in a marginated pool, so it is not accessible to phlebotomy. This marginated pool is thought to be in the spleen, along vessel walls, and in the lung. Cells can be mobilized from this marginated pool by infection/inflammation and stress. Once circulating neutrophils migrate into the tissue, they survive for 1 to 2 days but likely survive longer in the presence of G-CSF and GM-CSF.

Monocytes and macrophages are part of the mononuclear phagocyte system, which also includes the DCs. Although these cells share characteristics with neutrophils and eosinophils, they also have unique properties, including antigen processing and interaction with lymphocytes in the generation of the immune response, extracellular killing of some tumor cells, and performance of specialized functions specific for macrophages. Monocytes are released from the bone marrow and circulate for 1 to 4 days, then migrate into the tissues. Three fourths of the circulating monocytes are localized to blood vessel walls in a marginating pool. Monocytes emigrate into tissue to replace resident macrophages and are either "free" or "fixed." Free macrophages are those found in pleural, synovial, peritoneal, and alveolar spaces and in inflammatory sites. Fixed macrophages are generally less motile and include those in the splenic sinusoids, Kupffer's cells (liver), bone marrow reticulum, lamina propria of the GI tract, and lymph node reticulum. They also include those as osteoclasts (in the bone) and as microglia (in the central nervous system).[54] These macrophages are heterogenous in their phenotype and function. It has been hypothesized that macrophages have functional patterns such as seen with T cells (i.e., Th1- or Th2-driven phenotypes). Recent work, however, supports that monocytes and tissue macrophages develop their phenotypic function in response to changes in the microenvironment in which they are located rather than representing particular populations of monocytes that have been recruited there.[10]

Localization of phagocytes to a site of infection is discussed in a subsequent section. Once localization occurs, however, recognition of the pathogen by the phagocyte occurs through FcRs and complement receptor or other PRRs present on the phagocyte. Once a particle/pathogen is encountered, the appropriate receptors are activated, and the phagocyte membrane ruffles. The phagocyte then assumes a bipolar configuration, with the formation of a "head" or pseudopod and "tail" or uropod. The pseudopod surrounds a particle and fuses at its distal end to form a phagolysosome, thus internalizing the particle and a portion of the plasma membrane. The pseudopodia only advance over the portion of the particle or pathogen that is opsonized or where there are molecular patterns that fit the appropriate receptor on the phagocyte. Granules present in the phagocyte then join this newly formed vacuole and discharge their contents within seconds. Neutrophils have at least three types of granules containing microbial enzymes, myeloperoxidase and lysozyme, proteases, cationic proteins, BPI and defensins, and acid hydrolases. They also contain molecules critical for adhesion and locomotion, such as Mac-1 (CD11b/CD18). Release of myeloperoxidase from primary granules is important in oxygen-dependent microbial killing. Release of other granule constituents, such as lysozyme, lactoferrin, defensins, and BPI, is of critical importance in the decrease of the pH of the phagolysosome and in oxygen-independent microbial killing. Phagocytes are responsive to environmental cytokines such as TNF-α, IFN-γ, and chemokines that can prime the phagocyte for increased killing. Phagocytes also produce a large number of products in response to bacterial challenge. Monocytes/macrophages are a rich source of TNFα and IL-1; neutrophils can also produce TNF-α. Both monocytes/macrophages and neutrophils produce chemokines that attract other neutrophils, macrophages, and lymphocytes to the inflammatory focus. Phagocytes can also produce a number of lipid mediators that further stimulate the innate immune response.

The respiratory burst refers to the coordinated consumption of oxygen and production of metabolites that occur when phagocytes are exposed to appropriate stimuli. These events underlie all oxygen-dependent killing by phagocytes. Defects in the respiratory burst mechanisms result in chronic granulomatous disease (CGD). The NADPH oxidase system is a transmembrane electron transport system in which NADPH, the primary electron donor on the cytoplasmic side of the membrane, reduces oxygen in the extracellular fluid or within the phagolysosome to form $O_2^{\bullet}$. In turn two molecules of $O_2^{\bullet}$ spontaneously generate hydrogen peroxide (H_2O_2). Although both $O_2^{\bullet}$ and H_2O_2 can directly injure bacteria, it is the oxidants that are formed from them that are primarily responsible for the microbicidal action. Myeloperoxidase released into the phagolysosome in the presence of halide ion will enzymatically form hypohalous acids from $O_2^{\bullet}$. Hypohalous acids like hypochlorous acid (HOCl) are extremely potent antimicrobials. Alternatively, hypohalous acids can react with ambient amines (RNH_2) to form N-chloramines (RNHCl). RNHCl are lipophilic oxidizing and chlorinating agents that readily penetrate cellular membranes. The toxic effects of HOCl and RNHCl include sulfhydryl oxidation; hemeprotein inactivation; protein, amino acid, and DNA degradation, and inactivation of essential metabolic cofactors. Oxyradicals, in particular hydroxyl radical ($HO^{\bullet}$), are some of the most powerful oxidizing substances known. In the presence of Fe^{3+}, $O_2^{\bullet}$ and H_2O_2 combine to form $HO^{\bullet}$. The presence of NOS-2 in phagocytes, in particular the macrophages, provides a source of NO, which can react with $O_2^{\bullet}$, producing a peroxynitrite (ONOO—), another toxic and powerful oxidant.[55]

Neutrophils from patients with CGD retain some of the antimicrobial activity of normal neutrophils. It is due to the presence of many endogenous antimicrobials present in the granules that are critical to the killing of microbes. These antimicrobials include defensins, BPI, lactoferrin, and lysozyme, which were discussed earlier in this chapter. A number of other proteases, hydrolases, and nucleases in the granules of phagocytes, although not directly microbicidal, act synergistically with the antimicrobial agents to contribute to killing but can also result in cell injury if released from the neutrophil. Neutrophil elastase, collagenase, and gelatinase can hydrolyze key components of the extracellular matrix. Neutrophil elastase not only can degrade almost all components of the extracellular matrix, but also can cleave a variety of key plasma proteins such as Igs, complement proteins, and clotting factors. The activity of the elastase outside the cells is regulated primarily by α1-proteinase inhibitor. Neutrophil elastase can mediate injury outside the neutrophil when α1-proteinase inhibitor is inactivated by oxidants.[56]

Dendritic cells (DCs) are a distinct lineage of migratory leukocytes. They serve to initiate the primary immune response yet are part of the innate immune system. DCs exist in most tissues of the reticuloendothelial system. They are prominent in tissues exposed to the external environment with frequent exposure to foreign antigen. DCs from different tissues have varying cell membrane markers and functions and include thymic DCs, interstitial DCs (heart, lung, kidney, and intestine), interdigitating DCs (lymph nodes), and Langerhans' cells (epidermis). The features these DCs have in common are that they originate from bone marrow $CD34^+$ stem cells and migrate through the bloodstream to other tissues and become immature DCs. Immature DCs take up antigen or respond to environmental cues through PRRs and other receptor and nonreceptor mechanisms. This then results in maturation of the DCs and production of unique sets of cytokines and receptors. Depending on the specific environmental signal, DCs will mature into different clones. Mature DCs lose the ability to phagocytose and attain the ability to migrate to local lymphoid tissue. Having up-regulated the production of receptors, cytokines, and chemokines, DCs are able to stimulate naive $CD4^+$ and $CD8^+$ cells.[69]

Immature DCs migrate to and remain in the periphery, where they express low levels of MCH class I and II. These immature DCs will then mature either after phagocytosis of foreign antigen or by activation of one of its receptors (such as TLR). The mature DCs will then migrate to the local lymphoid organ. As they do, they increase cell surface expression of MHC and T costimulatory molecules (i.e., CD80 CD86) and begin to secrete specific cytokines. Mature DCs loose the ability to phagocytose. In the lymphold organ, the DC will present antigen to the $CD4^+$ or $CD8^+$ T cell receptor via MHC II or I, respectively. The DC costimulatory molecules, CD80 or CD86, must engage their ligand, CD28, on the T cell for full activation (see Fig. 84–6). Note that for the initial immune response, the DC (or APC) must be in geographic proximity of the $CD8^+$ and CD4+ cell. Alternatively, the DC or APC may be preconditioned by an activated $CD4^+$ cell, which is then able to activate naive $CD8^+$ cells to become cytotoxic T cells.[69] Not all macrophages function well as APCs. Although elicited peritoneal macrophages do, alveolar macrophages and Kupffer's cells do not.[10]

As previously described, in the contact activation system, hemostasis and inflammation overlap. The endothelial surface, which is usually anticoagulant, becomes procoagulant in infection and inflammation. *Platelets* themselves have inflammatory, antimicrobial, and immune modulating factors. In a platelet thrombus, neutrophils and to a lesser extent monocytes are recruited to the developing thrombus through adhesion receptors (discussed later). In addition, leukocytes and platelets that are adherent to endothelial surface can attract the other cell type. Platelets secrete a number of stored chemokines that activate neutrophils and monocytes, T cells, and NK cells. These include the neutrophil-activating chemokines NAP2 (CXCL7), PR4 (CXCL4), GRO-α, (CXCL1), and ENA-78 (CXCL5) and the monocyte-activating chemokines RANTES (CCL5), MIP-1α (CCL3), and MCP-3 (CCL7).

Platelets also contain antimicrobial peptides such as thrombocidins and HMGB1. They can synthesize IL-1β. Platelet interactions with neutrophils alter the production of LTB_4, which may be important for T-cell homing. Platelets can also convert arachidonate metabolites supplied by neutrophils to LT C_4 and lipoxins, providing additional modulatory signals in cell–cell interactions.[57]

Leukocyte Localization

In response to infection and in normal immune surveillance all leukocytes must travel from their sites of production to the point at which their function is required. There is a multistep process for localization to occur. Permutations in this process exist in specialized vascular beds such as the lung, liver, and kidney.[58]

In general the multistep process begins by activation of the postcapillary venular endothelial surface by inflammatory cytokines such as IL-1, TNF, IL-4, and IFNγ. The surface transforms from a nonadhesive surface to one that is proadhesive through the expression of specific ligands. These ligands will recognize their cognate receptors on the circulating effector leukocytes (i.e., neutrophils, eosinophils, monocytes, NK cells, and activated T cells). Endothelial ligands that are up-regulated include members of the selectin family (Table 84–3). Selectins are responsible for the initial capture of the leukocyte from the free-flowing stream, and rolling on the endothelial surface. Members of the IgSF are critical for leukocyte slowing, arrest, and migration on the cell surface (Fig. 84–8). The leukocyte receptors for the IgSF are the β_2 integrins, in particular Mac-1 (CD11b/CD18), LFA-1 (CD11a/CD18), and the β_1 integrin VLA-4 (CD49d/CD29). The leukocyte integrins are heterodimers composed of an α and a β subunit. The β subunit may be shared by multiple members of a subfamily, whereas the α subunit confers specificity. Mac-1 functions not only in leukocyte recruitment, but also as a receptor for complement fragment C3bi, thus its alternative name of complement receptor 3. Note also that LFA-1 functions as a coinducer of the immune response in the immunological synapse, as discussed earlier. The leukocyte ligand for E- and P-selectin is PSGL-1 (CD162, P-selectin glycoprotein ligand 1) (Table 84–3). The endothelial surface also secretes a number of chemokines and other activating substances, such as PAF, which activate the leukocyte and mediate the transition from rolling to arrest. Once the leukocyte has arrested, it polarizes, then "crawls" and emigrates through the endothelial lining of the vessel. This emigration, known as *diapedesis,* is in response to activating agents (chemokines, LTB_4) released by cells present in the subendothelial matrix, to released bacterial products (N-formyl peptides), or through complement activation (C5a). This process also depends on leukocyte integrins that recognize the IgSF on the endothelial cells necessary for transendothelial migration (Fig. 84–8). Locomotion through the subendothelial matrix requires additional leukocyte integrins (VLA-1, VLA-2, VLA-3, VLA-5, and VLA-6) that recognize matrix proteins including fibronectin, collagen, vitronectin, and vimentin. Which effector cell is recruited and the tissue to which it is recruited depends on the adhesion molecules present on the endothelial surface, the effector cells, and the "signals" released or presented at the endothelial surface and in the subendothelial region.[58-60]

This multistep paradigm is also critical for the homing of lymphocytes to the high endothelial venules, a specialized endothelium of the secondary lymphoid organs. Here naive lymphocytes (rather than activated cells) tether, roll, arrest, and emigrate through the endothelial surface. The naive lymphocytes migrate toward DCs or APCs that secrete cytokines and chemokines necessary for activation of the T cell through the T cell receptor.[60] One critical chemokine is SDF-1 (CXCL12). Its receptor, which is present on almost all lymphocytes and many monocytes, is CXCR4.

The multistep paradigm, however, is not operative in all vascular beds. In lungs the inflammatory cells do not "roll" but instead are physically trapped in the pulmonary capillary bed and emigrate from this area rather than in the postcapillary venules.[61] In the liver, leukocytes are physically trapped in the sinusoids. Because the sinusoidal endothelia has large pores, the leukocytes can easily interact with the underlying hepatocytes.[62] The platelet can also function as a surface to which a leukocyte can bind by the activated release from the Weibel-Palade body of P-selectin at sites of injury or inflammation (Fig. 84–8).

An increasing number of genetic defects in leukocyte localization have been identified. Those that involve adhesion receptors critical for neutrophil recruitment result in neutrophilia and severe, recurrent skin abscesses. In patients with leukocyte adhesion deficiency type 1 (LAD-1) there is a selective defect in the expression or functional activation of β_2 (CD18) integrins. In patients with the rarer defect, LAD 2, there is defective rolling of leukocytes on inflamed endothelium because of a lack of fucosylated glycoconjugates on the selectins. Finally, patients with LAD-3 have a functional defect in the activation of β_1- and β_2-integrin avidity, leading to defective leukocyte arrest on vascular endothelium.[58,63,64]

Summary

There is a coordinated and highly regulated response by the body to microbial infection. As outlined in Figure 84–9 the first defense is local immunity. The epithelial surface functions as a physical barrier. Through the release of antimicrobial peptides from the epithelium and secretory IgA from submucosal plasma cells, microbial burden is decreased. The epithelial cells at the site of infection will produce cytokines and chemokines that regulate the invasion of the area by leukocytes. These cytokines, however, will also modulate the submucosal macrophages and plasma cells that are constitutively present. The presence of soluble agents critical for opsonization (including Ig and complement components) permits the efficient phagocytosis of organisms by recruited neutrophils, monocytes, and resident macrophages. The presence of T cells and plasma cells early in the infection depends on a previous encounter with the organism. If the host has "immunological memory" for the microbe, then there will be fairly rapid (i.e., within 1 day) expansion of the memory T cells to effector cells (i.e., cytotoxic T cells) and expansion of memory

TABLE 84–3

Adhesion Molecules in Inflammation and Hemostasis

Name	CD Classification	Primary Cell Expression	Ligand
INTEGRIN FAMILY			
β1 Integrins			
a1β1 (VLA-1)	CD49a/CD29	T- and B-cell subsets, mono	COL I, COL IV, LN
a2β1 (VLA-2)	CD49b/CD29	T-cell subsets, mono, PLT, PMN	COL I, COL IV, LN
a3β1 (VLA-3)	CD49c/CD29	T-cell subsets, mono	FN, COL I, LN
a4β1 (VLA-4)	CD49d/CD29	T-cell, B-cell, Eos, mono, PMN, baso	FN, VCAM, Tsp, JAM2
a5β1 (VLA-5)	CD49e/CD29	T-cells, PMN, PLT	FN, Tsp
a6β1 (VLA-6)	CD49f/CD29	T-cells, PMN, PLT, EC	LN
α9β1		PMN, mono	VCAM-1, OSP, tenascin
β2 Integrins			
aLβ2 (LFA-1)	CD11a/CD18	PMNS, T- and B-cell, Eos, mono, NK, macro	ICAM-1, ICAM-2, ICAM-3, JAM-1
aMβ2 (Mac-1)	CD11b/CD18	PMNS, mono, Eos, NK, macro, Lymph subset	ICAM-1, iC_3b, Fg, FN, Factor X, JAM-3,
aXβ2 (p150, 95)	CD11c/CD18	PMN, mono, Eos, lymph subset	GPIb- IX-V
β3 Integrins			
aIIbβ3 (GPIIbIIIa)	CD41/CD61	PLTS	VWf, FN, Fg, VN, Tsp, COL
aVβ3 (Vitronectin Receptor)	CD51/CD61	Macro, mono, T-cell, PLT, EC, PMN	VWf, VN, FN, Fg, PECAM-1, Tsp, LN, OSP, tenascin, COL
β7 Integrins			
a4β7	CD49d/β 7	Gut-associated lymphocyte	VCAM, MAdCAM-1, FN
aEβ7	CD103/β7	Gut-associated lymphocytes	E-CAD
IMMUNOGLOBULIN SUPERFAMILY (IGSF)			
ICAM-1	CD54	T-cell, mono, EC, pneumocyto, hepatocyte, epithelial cells, fibroblasts	LFA-1, Mac-1
ICAM-2	CD102	EC	LFA-1
ICAM-3	CD50	Lymph, PMN, Mono	LFA-1, aDβ2
VCAM-1	CD106	EC	a4β1,a4β7
JAM-1		EC, epithelial cells, PMNs, mono, lymph, RBC	LFA-1, JAM-1
JAM-2		HEV, EC	JAM-2, JAM-3, α4β1
JAM-3		Lymph	Mac-1, JAM3
MAdCAM-1		Peyer's patch HEV, mesenteric LN	a4β7, L-selectin
PECAM-1*			
SELECTINS			
L-selectin	CD62-L	Lymph, mono, Eos, baso, PMN	CD34, GlyCAM-1, MAdCAM-1, unknown EC ligand, PSGL-1, PNAD, sLe^x-bearing ligands
P-selectin	CD62-P	EC, PLTS	PSGL-1, E-selectin, GPIb- IX-V
E-selectin	D62-E	EC	PSGL-1, sLe^X-bearing ligand(s), CLA
SELECTIN LIGANDS			
PSGL-1	CD162	PMN, Eos, mono, lymph	P-selectin, L-selection, E-selectin
GlyCAM-1		Lymph node + lung EC	L-selectin
CD34	CD34	Peripheral LN HEV, leukocyte precursors	L-selectin
OTHER			
CD99	CD99	T cells, endothelial cells, monocytes	CD99, ?
PECAM-1*	CD31	EC, PMN, PLT, mono, lymphocyte subsets	PECAM-1, aVβ3

*Although PECAM-1 is now considered a member of the ITIM family, by convention it is still listed in the "IGSF" and "Other" categories.

VLA, very late antigen; *mono,* monocytes; *PLT,* platelet; *Eos,* eosinophils; *PMNL,* polymorphonuclear leukocyte; *baso,* basophil; *EC,* endothelial cell; *COL I,* collagen type I; *COL IV,* collagen type IV; *LN,* laminin; *FN,* fibronectin; *VCAM,* vascular cell adhesion molecule; *Tsp,* thrombospondin; *NK,* natural killer cells; *macro,* macrophages; *ICAM,* intercellular adhesion molecule; *JAM,* junctional adhesion molecule; *lymph,* lymphocyte; *iC3b,* inactivated form of complement component C3b; *Fg,* fibrinogen; *PECAM-1,* platelet endothelial adhesion molecule-1; *OSP,* osteopontin; *MAdCAM-1,* mucosal addressin cell adhesion molecule-1; *E-CAD,* E-cadherin; *GlyCAM-1,* glycosylation-dependent cell adhesion molecule-1; *PSGL-1,* P-selectin glycoprotein ligand-1; *sLe^x,* sialylated Lewis X antigen; *CLA,* cutaneous lymphocyte-associated antigen; *VWf,* von Willebrand Factor, *VN,* vitronectin; *PNAD,* peripheral node addressin; *GP1b-IX-V,* glycoprotein complex present on the surface of platelets.

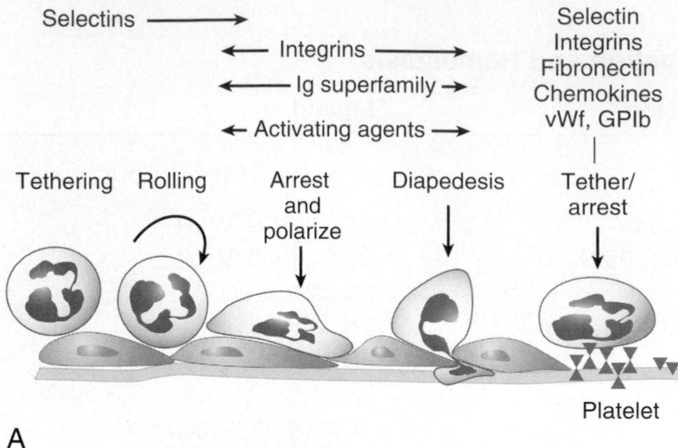

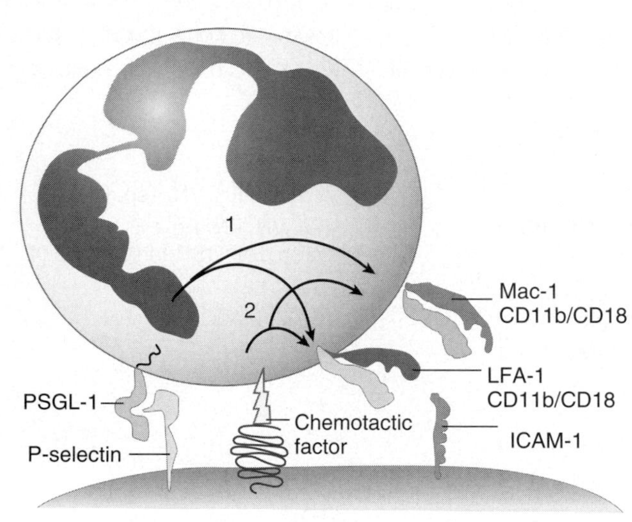

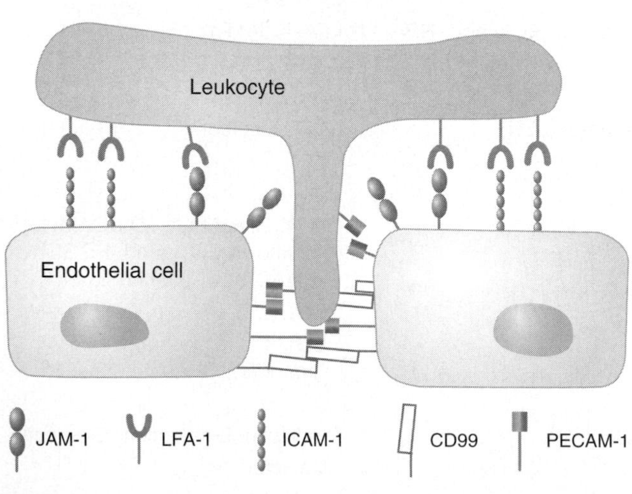

FIGURE 84–8 • Leukocyte localization. **A,** Leukocytes are captured from the free-flowing stream (tether) and roll on the endothelial lining of the blood vessel. This interaction is mediated by all three members of the selectin family. The leukocyte slows, arrests, and changes shape (polarizes). Integrins and their ligands, the Ig superfamily (IgSF), mediate these steps. The cells then crawl or "diapedese" over the surface of the endothelium until they migrate through the endothelium. The integrins, members of the IgSF and CD99, all have a role in this response. A leukocyte also may be tethered by adherent platelets or adherent leukocytes. Platelets through β3 integrins and GPIb-IX-V can bind directly to collagen or fibronectin on exposed basement membrane or alternatively to von Willebrand factor bound to the endothelium or basement membrane. Platelets can release cytokines that activate leukocytes directly once tethered. Leukocytes can bind to platelets directly through integrins or to fibrinogen that is bound to platelets. *Ig,* immunoglobulin; *vWF,* von Willebrand factor. **B,** Model of leukocyte activation leading to arrest. Leukocytes tether to the endothelium expressing P-selectin through P-selectin-glycoprotein-ligand 1 (PSGL-1). In the presence of shear, PSGL-1 can activate the leukocyte integrins, LFA-1 and Mac-1 (*arrow 1*). Chemotactic factors expressed on the endothelial surface can also directly activate LFA-1 and Mac-1 (*arrow 2*). Both LFA-1 and Mac-1 can bind to endothelial ICAM-1 at domains 1 and 3, respectively. **C,** Proposed mechanisms for transendothelial migration. With stimulation of the endothelial cell, ICAM-1 is up-regulated. JAM-1, which is localized at the interendothelial cleft, is mobilized away from the cleft. With activation of the leukocytes, migration across the vascular endothelial can then occur through LFA-1, PECAM-1, JAM-1, and CD99. Leukocyte LFA-1 can bind to JAM-1 and ICAM-1 on the endothelial surface. Leukocytes can then traverse the interendothelial cleft through sequential transhomophilic interactions of PECAM-1 and CD99. *JAM,* junctional adhesion molecule; *PECAM,* platelet endothelial adhesion molecule. (With permission from Mariscalco M: Integrins and cell adhesion molecules. In Polin RA, Fox WW, Abman SH, editors: Fetal and neonatal physiology, Philadelphia, 2004, Elsevier, Saunders.)

B cells and differentiation to plasma cells to produce IgG. Note that at each step of the process, the number of bacteria decreases.[62,65]

If the host must mount a primary immune response to control and eliminate the infection, it may take 3 to 5 days for microbial or viral elimination to occur if local mechanisms or innate immune systems response is inadequate. As outlined in Figure 84–10, the initiation of adaptive immunity for a typical viral infection occurs within 2 days. Between 3 and 4 days there is the establishment of the adaptive immune response with clonal expansion of $CD8^+$ and $CD4^+$ effector cells, and eradication of the infection occurs. After eradication of the infection there is contraction of the clonal response, but the continued presence of antibody, residual effector cells, and immunologic memory provides lasting protection against reinfection.

Apoptosis is the process of programmed cell death necessary for the resolution of the inflammatory response. As cells begin to die they express ligands on their surfaces that signal resident tissue macrophages for removal through phagocytosis. During apoptosis the cell's nucleus and cytoplasm condense, nuclear DNA is degraded into small dense pieces, and marked cytoplasmic vesiculation and blebbing of the plasma membrane occur. In the final stages the cell collapses into multiple fragments (apoptic bodies). Apoptosis can be triggered by external forces such as interaction of CD95 ligand (Fas ligand) on cytotoxic T lymphocytes or NK cells with CD95 on a target cell such as a virally infected cell (see Fig. 84–5). Apoptosis can also be initiated by signals arising from DNA or mitochondrial damage.[66,67] The signals converge on activation of a family of proteases called *caspases,* which cleave to multiple substrates to induce destruction of the cell from within. This process is central to peripheral deletion of excess T and B lymphocytes as the immune response wanes, infected cells are cleared, and inflammation resolves with the removal of emigrated leukocytes.[68] The final step of apoptosis is the removal through the

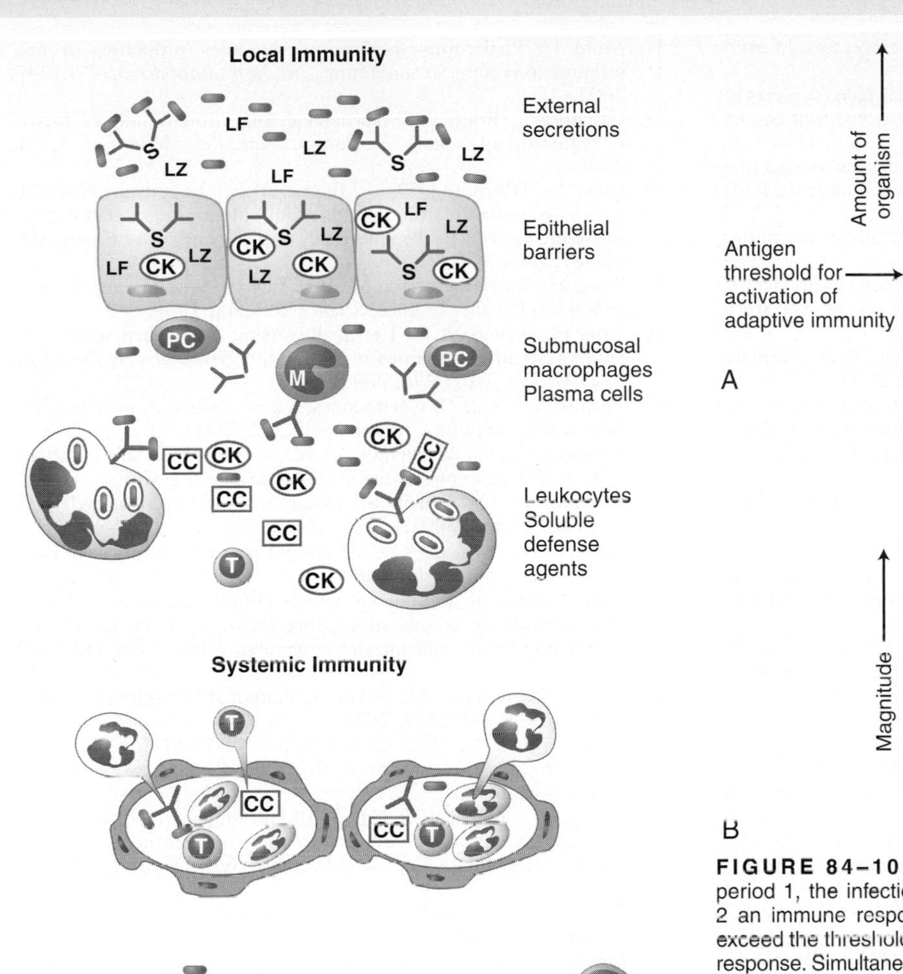

FIGURE 84–9 • An overview of defenses at a mucosal site to a bacterial infection. In this example, the host has been previously exposed to the bacterial pathogen. Thus there is a rapid innate immune response, specific antibody, and T cell response. The number of bacteria decreases as each level of defense is encountered. See text for further details. (Modified with permission from Goldman AS: *Pediatr Rev* 21: 342, 2000.)

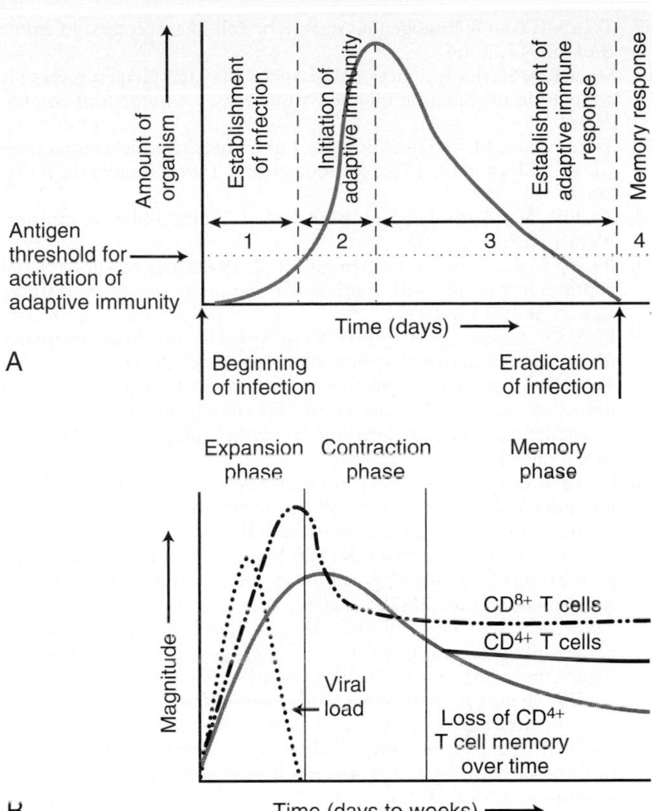

FIGURE 84–10 • Time course of a typical acute infection. **A,** During period 1, the infectious agent (bacterial or viral) replicates. In period 2 an immune response is initiated when the numbers of pathogen exceed the threshold dose of antigen required for an adaptive immune response. Simultaneously the pathogen continues to replicate, retarded only by the innate and nonadaptive responses. Immunologic memory is thought to be initiated during this stage. During period 3, after 4 to 5 days, effector arms of the immune response begin to clear the infection. In period 4 the clearance of the infectious agent and the decrease in the antigen dose below the response threshold result in the cessation of the response. The presence of antibody, residual effector cells, and immunologic memory provides lasting protection against reinfection. **B,** During a viral infection, antigen-specific T cells clonally expand during the first phase in the presence of antigen. Soon after the virus is cleared, the contraction phase follows, and the number of antigen-specific T cells decreases because of apoptosis. After the contraction phase, the number of virus-specific T cells stabilizes and can be maintained for great lengths of time (memory phase). Note that the magnitude of the CD4+ T cell response is less than that of the CD8+ cells, and the contraction phase can be less pronounced. The number of memory CD4+ T cells may decline slowly over time. (Modified with permission from Huang AYC, Rigby MR: The immune response: generation, regulation, and maintenance. In, Stiehm ER, Ochs HD, Winkelstein JA, editors: *Immunologic disorders of infants and children,* Philadelphia, 2004, Elsevier Saunders.)

tissue macrophage.[69] In the process of eliminating apoptotic cells, the macrophage produces immunosuppressive cytokines such as transforming growth factor-β (TGF-β) and other cytokines that down-regulate the inflammatory response such as IL-10 (see also Chapter 93).

REFERENCES

1. Medzhitov R, Janeway C Jr: Innate immunity, *N Engl J Med* 343:338, 2000.
2. Janeway CA Jr, Medzhitov R: Innate immune recognition, *Annu Rev Immunol* 20:197, 2002.
3. Lu J, Teh C, Kishore U et al: Collectins and ficolins: sugar pattern recognition molecules of the mammalian innate immune system, *Biochim Biophys Acta* 1572:387, 2002.
4. Pepys MB, Hirschfield GM: C-reactive protein: a critical update, *J Clin Invest* 111:1805, 2003.
5. Walport MJ: Complement. First of two parts, *N Engl J Med* 344:1058, 2001.
6. Janeway CA Jr: A trip through my life with an immunological theme, *Annu Rev Immunol* 20:1, 2002.
7. Beutler B: Inferences, questions and possibilities in Toll-like receptor signalling, *Nature* 430:257, 2004.
8. Mukhopadhyay S, Herre J, Brown GD et al: The potential for Toll-like receptors to collaborate with other innate immune receptors, *Immunology* 112:521, 2004.

9. Tsan MF, Gao B: Endogenous ligands of Toll-like receptors, *J Leukoc Biol* 76:514, 2004.
10. Stout RD, Suttles J: Functional plasticity of macrophages: reversible adaptation to changing microenvironments, *J Leukoc Biol* 76:509, 2004.
11. Triantafilou M, Triantafilou K: Lipopolysaccharide recognition: CD14, TLRs and the LPS-activation cluster, *Trends Immunol* 23:301, 2002.
12. Zasloff M: Antimicrobial peptides of multicellular organisms, *Nature* 415:389, 2002.
13. Putsep K, Carlsson G, Boman HG et al: Deficiency of antibacterial peptides in patients with morbus Kostmann: an observation study, *Lancet* 360:1144, 2002.
14. Levy O: Antimicrobial proteins and peptides of blood: templates for novel antimicrobial agents, Blood 96:2664, 2000.
15. Yang D, Chertov O, Oppenheim JJ: Participation of mammalian defensins and cathelicidins in anti-microbial immunity: receptors and activities of human defensins and cathelicidin (LL-37), *J Leukoc Biol* 69:691, 2001.
16. Caccavo D, Pellegrino NM, Altamura M et al: Antimicrobial and immunoregulatory functions of lactoferrin and its potential therapeutic application, *J Endotoxin Res* 8:403, 2002.
17. Levy O, Canny G, Serhan CN et al: Expression of BPI (bactericidal/permeability-increasing protein) in human mucosal epithelia, *Biochem Soc Trans* 31:795, 2003.
18. Levin M, Quint PA, Goldstein B et al: Recombinant bactericidal/permeability-increasing protein (rBPI21) as adjunctive treatment for children with severe meningococcal sepsis: a randomised trial. rBPI21 Meningococcal Sepsis Study Group, *Lancet* 356:961, 2000.
19. Giles FJ, Rodriguez R, Weisdorf D et al: A phase III, randomized, double-blind, placebo-controlled, study of iseganan for the reduction of stomatitis in patients receiving stomatotoxic chemotherapy, *Leuk Res* 28:559, 2004.
20. Troost FJ, Saris WH, Brummer RJ: Recombinant human lactoferrin ingestion attenuates indomethacin-induced enteropathy in vivo in healthy volunteers, *Eur J Clin Nutr* 57:1579, 2003.
21. Di Mario F, Aragona G, Dal Bo N et al: Use of bovine lactoferrin for *Helicobacter pylori* eradication, *Dig Liver Dis* 35:706, 2003.
22. Carroll MC: The complement system in regulation of adaptive immunity, *Nat Immunol* 5:981, 2004.
23. Riedemann NC, Guo RF, Ward PA: A key role of C5a/C5aR activation for the development of sepsis, *J Leukoc Biol* 74:966, 2003.
24. Huber-Lang M, Sarma VJ, Lu KT, et al: Role of C5a in multiorgan failure during sepsis, *J Immunol* 166:1193, 2001.
25. Hart ML, Walsh MC, Stahl GL: Initiation of complement activation following oxidative stress. In vitro and in vivo observations, *Mol Immunol* 41:165, 2004.
26. Bohana-Kashtan O, Ziporen L, Donin N, et al: Cell signals transduced by complement, *Mol Immunol* 41:583, 2004.
27. Ueno A, Oh-ishi S: Roles for the kallikrein-kinin system in inflammatory exudation and pain: lessons from studies on kininogen-deficient rats, *J Pharmacol Sci* 93:1, 2003.
28. Serhan CN, Oliw E: Unorthodox routes to prostanoid formation: new twists in cyclooxygenase-initiated pathways, *J Clin Invest* 107:1481, 2001.
29. Lee JS, Polin RA: Treatment and prevention of necrotizing enterocolitis, *Semin Neonatol* 8:449, 2003.
30. Zimmerman GA, McIntyre TM, Prescott SM et al: The platelet-activating factor signaling system and its regulators in syndromes of inflammation and thrombosis, *Crit Care Med* 30:S294-S301, 2002.
31. Dinarello CA: Anti-cytokine therapeutics and infections, *Vaccine* 21(suppl 2):S24-S34, 2003.
32. Dinarello CA, Fantuzzi G: Interleukin-18 and host defense against infection, *J Infect Dis* 187(suppl 2):S370-S384, 2003.
33. Gracie JA, Robertson SE, McInnes IB: Interleukin-18, *J Leukoc Biol* 73:213, 2003.
34. Watford WT, Moriguchi M, Morinobu A et al: The biology of IL-12: coordinating innate and adaptive immune responses, *Cytokine Growth Factor Rev* 14:361, 2003.
35. Rosenzweig SD, Holland SM: Phagocyte immunodeficiencies and their infections, *J Allergy Clin Immunol* 113:620, 2004.
36. Kerr R, Stirling D, Ludlam CA: Interleukin 6 and haemostasis, *Br J Haematol* 115:3, 2001.
37. Muhl H, Pfeilschifter J: Anti-inflammatory properties of pro-inflammatory interferon-gamma, *Int Immunopharmacol* 3:1247, 2003.
38. Calandra T, Roger T: Macrophage migration inhibitory factor: a regulator of innate immunity, *Nat Rev Immunol* 3:791, 2003.
39. Sama AE, D'Amore J, Ward MF et al: Bench to bedside: HMGB1-a novel proinflammatory cytokine and potential therapeutic target for septic patients in the emergency department, *Acad Emerg Med* 11:867, 2004.
40. Wang H, Bloom O, Zhang M, et al: HMG-1 as a late mediator of endotoxin lethality in mice, *Science* 285:248, 1999.
41. Yang H, Ochani M, Li J et al: Reversing established sepsis with antagonists of endogenous high-mobility group box 1, *Proc Natl Acad Sci U S A* 101:296, 2004.
42. Zlotnik A, Yoshie O: Chemokines: a new classification system and their role in immunity, *Immunity* 12:121, 2000.
43. Murdoch C, Finn A: Chemokine receptors and their role in inflammation and infectious diseases, *Blood* 95:3032, 2000.
44. Hamilton JA: GM-CSF in inflammation and autoimmunity, *Trends Immunol* 23:403, 2002.
45. Hubel K, Dale DC, Liles WC: Therapeutic use of cytokines to modulate phagocyte function for the treatment of infectious diseases: current status of granulocyte colony-stimulating factor, granulocyte-macrophage colony-stimulating factor, macrophage colony-stimulating factor, and interferon-gamma, *J Infect Dis* 185:1490, 2002.
46. Trapnell BC, Whitsett JA, Nakata K: Pulmonary alveolar proteinosis, *N Engl J Med* 349:2527, 2003.
47. Carr R, Modi N, Dore C: G-CSF and GM-CSF for treating or preventing neonatal infections, *Cochrane Database Syst Rev* (3): CD003066, 2003.
48. Cheng AC, Stephens DP, Currie BJ: Granulocyte colony stimulating factor (G-CSF) as an adjunct to antibiotics in the treatment of pneumonia in adults, *Cochrane Database Syst Rev* (3): CD004400, 2003.
49. Azoulay E, Delclaux C: Is there a place for granulocyte colony-stimulating factor in non-neutropenic critically ill patients? *Intensive Care Med* 30:10, 2004.
50. Insel RA, Looney RJ: The B-lymphocyte system: fundamental immunology. In Stiehm ER, Ochs HD, Winkelstein JA, editors: *Immunologic disorders in infants and children,* Philadelphia, 2004, Elsevier Saunders.
51. Wilson CB, Edelman KH: The T lymphocyte system. In Stiehm ER, Ochs HD, Winkelstein JA, editors: *Immunologic disorders in infants and children,* Philadelphia, 2004, Elsevier Saunders.
52. Jameson J, Witherden D, Havran WL: T-cell effector mechanisms: gammadelta and CD1d-restricted subsets, *Curr Opin Immunol* 15:349, 2003.
53. Papamichail M, Perez SA, Gritzapis AD et al: Natural killer lymphocytes: biology, development, and function, *Cancer Immunol Immunother* 53:176, 2004.
54. Douglas SD, Kapur R, Merrill JD et al: The mononuclear phagocytic, dendritic cell, and natural killer cell systems. In Stiehm ER, Ochs HD, Winkelstein JA, editors: *Immunologic disorders in infants and children,* Philadelphia, 2004, Elsevier Saunders.
55. Hampton MB, Kettle AJ, Winterbourn CC: Inside the neutrophil phagosome: oxidants, myeloperoxidase, and bacterial killing, *Blood* 92:3007, 1998.
56. Weiss SJ: Tissue destruction by neutrophils, *N Engl J Med* 320:365, 1989.
57. Weyrich AS, Zimmerman GA: Platelets: signaling cells in the immune continuum, *Trends Immunol* 25:489, 2004.
58. Mariscalco MM: Integrins and cell adhesion molecules. In Polin RA, Fox WW, Abman SH, editors: *Fetal and neonatal physiology,* Philadelphia, 2004, Elsevier Saunders.
59. Salazar-Mather TP, Hokeness KL: Calling in the troops: regulation of inflammatory cell trafficking through innate cytokine/chemokine networks, *Viral Immunol* 16:291, 2003.
60. Springer TA: Traffic signals on endothelium for lymphocyte recirculation and leukocyte emigration, *Annu Rev Physiol* 57:827, 1995.
61. Burns AR, Smith CW, Walker DC: Unique structural features that influence neutrophil emigration into the lung, *Physiol Rev* 83:309, 2003.

62. Kaech SM, Wherry EJ, Ahmed R: Effector and memory T-cell differentiation: implications for vaccine development, *Nat Rev Immunol* 2:251, 2002.
63. Badolato R: Leukocyte circulation: one-way or round-trip? Lessons from primary immunodeficiency patients, *J Leukoc Biol* 76:1, 2004.
64. Etzioni A, Doerschuk CM, Harlan JM: Of man and mouse: leukocyte and endothelial adhesion molecule deficiencies, *Blood* 94:3281, 1999.
65. Goldman AS: Back to basics: host responses to infection, *Pediatr Rev* 21:342, 2000.
66. Green DR, Kroemer G: The pathophysiology of mitochondrial cell death, *Science* 305:626, 2004.
67. Nelson DA, White E: Exploiting different ways to die, *Genes Dev* 18:1223, 2004.
68. Simon HU: Neutrophil apoptosis pathways and their modifications in inflammation, *Immunol Rev* 193:101, 2003.
69. Lauber K, Blumenthal SG, Waibel M et al: Clearance of apoptotic cells: getting rid of the corpses, *Mol Cell* 14:277, 2004.

CHAPTER

85

Congenital Immunodeficiency

Marianne T. Sweetser

PEARLS

- Children with underlying immunodeficiency disorders are likely to be seen by pediatric intensivists when they are first seen with an overwhelming infection (e.g., acute *Pneumocystis carinii* pneumonia) and during hospitalizations for serious infections or noninfectious complications (e.g., cancer, autoimmune disease) of their immunodeficiency disease.
- Patients with complete immunoglobulin A (IgA) deficiency are at risk for anti-IgA antibodies and may have a severe reaction after infusion of IgA-containing blood products.
- Most patients with primary immunodeficiency will have recurrent serious infections or infections with unusual pathogens. The type of infection may offer clues as to the component of the immune system affected.

Children with defects of their immune systems usually present with recurrent serious infections or infections with unusual pathogens. The type of infection the patient has provides clues about the cause of the problem (Table 85–1). Infections with low-grade pathogens (i.e., opportunistic infections) suggest T-cell deficiency. Recurrent bacterial sinopulmonary infections may herald an underlying antibody problem. Repeated episodes of bacterial sepsis or meningitis may be due to antibody or complement deficiency. Frequent abscesses (superficial or deep-seated), especially those due to *Staphylococcus aureus,* may indicate a phagocyte deficiency (Table 85–2). Children with underlying immunodeficiency disorders are likely to be seen by pediatric intensivists when they are first seen with an overwhelming infection (e.g., acute *Pneumocystis carinii* pneumonia) and during hospitalizations for serious infections or noninfectious complications (e.g., cancer, autoimmune disease) of their immunodeficiency disease.

Antibody Deficiencies

Antibody deficiencies are the most common types of primary immunodeficiencies and were recently reviewed in detail.[1] Patients are usually healthy until 6 to 12 months of age when maternal antibodies have waned. Children with antibody deficiency usually have recurrent or chronic respiratory tract infections including otitis media, sinusitis, and pneumonia due to encapsulated bacterial organisms such as *Haemophilus influenzae* and *Streptococcus pneumoniae*. Occasionally, they may have more serious infections such as bacterial sepsis or meningitis. Patients with antibody deficiency have difficulty handling enteroviral infections. Paralytic polio resulting from live polio vaccine infection, chronic meningoencephalitis due to echovirus, and a dermatomyositis-like illness caused by echovirus have been described. Patients also have a greater susceptibility to protozoa and may be seen with chronic *Giardia* infections.

Defects resulting in antibody deficiencies can be intrinsic to the B cell, occurring throughout B cell development and differentiation, or can be extrinsic to the B cell, such as lack of a costimulatory signal required for B cell function. Defects occurring early in the pathway can lead to severe hypogammaglobulinemia with an absence of B cells, whereas those that occur later may result in defects in class switching or production of specific antibodies. Patients with combined immunodeficiencies, such as

Wiskott-Aldrich syndrome (WAS), X-linked hyper immunoglobulin M (IgM) syndrome, ataxia telangiectasia, and severe combined immunodeficiency, also have defects in humoral immune function.

Hypogammaglobulinemia with Absent B Cells

There are at least five known genetic lesions that block early B-cell development in the bone marrow at the pre–B-cell stage. Signaling from the pre–B-cell receptor is required for transition to an immature B cell, and these mutations affect individual components of the pre–B-cell receptor or signal transducing molecules associated with the receptor. Most patients with hypogammaglobulinemia and absent B cells (80% to 90% of cases) are males with X-linked agammaglobulinemia (XLA) that results from mutations in Bruton's tyrosine kinase (BTK). The other known disorders are due to mutations of the IgM heavy chain, the surrogate light chain (λ5 or 14.1, CD179b), the Ig-α component of the B cell receptor (CD79a), and the signal-transducing molecule B-cell linker protein (BLNK or SLP-65).

Hyper Immunoglobulin M Syndrome

Patients with hyper-IgM syndrome (HIM) have normal to elevated serum IgM levels but low IgG, IgA, and IgE levels. This deficiency results from an inability of B cells to switch from IgM to IgG, IgA, and IgE production. In patients with an autosomal recessive form of HIM, mutations have been found in the RNA-editing enzyme, activation-induced cytidine deaminase (AID), and in uracil–DNA glycosylase (UNG), which are required for class switching and somatic hypermutation of immunoglobulin genes. Patients with autosomal recessive HIM have marked lymphoid hyperplasia with adenopathy, characterized by large germinal centers, which are detected during histological examination. In these patients, T-cell function is intact, and complications with opportunistic infections such as *P. carinii* are not observed.

Common Variable Immunodeficiency

Common variable immunodeficiency (CVID) is a heterogenous group of disorders for which the molecular defects have not been defined. Patients can have defects in both B- and T-cell function and are predominantly seen with hypogammaglobulinemia (usually low IgG and variable levels of IgA and IgM) and abnormal antibody responses to antigenic challenge. Patients can present in early childhood, in adolescence, or as young adults. Approximately 20% to 25% of patients have autoimmune disorders, including seronegative arthritis, autoimmune cytopenias, vasculitis, autoimmune endocrinopathies (especially those involving the thyroid), and autoimmune neurological disorders. Approximately one third of patients have a benign lymphoproliferative disease and an increased incidence of lymphoma, especially later in life.

Immunoglobulin A Deficiency

Other forms of antibody deficiency include selective IgA deficiency, defined as a serum IgA concentration of less than 7 mg/dl, with normal IgG and IgM levels. Most patients are asymptomatic, but a subset of patients has an increased number of sinopulmonary infections. An increased incidence of autoimmune disorders, CVID, and atopy have been observed in patients with selective IgA deficiency. Patients with complete IgA deficiency are at risk for anti-IgA antibodies and may have a severe reaction after infusion of IgA-containing blood products.

Immunoglobulin G Subclass Deficiencies

There are four subclasses of IgG (IgG1, IgG2, IgG3, and IgG4), and each IgG subclass has different biological properties. For example, IgG1 and IgG3 play an important role in the response to protein antigens, whereas IgG2 plays a key role in the response to polysaccharide antigens. Similar to patients with selective IgA deficiency, most patients with deficiencies in one or more IgG subclass are asymptomatic; however, a subset may have frequent and severe bacterial infections of the upper and lower respiratory tracts, as well as viral infections. In particular, patients with IgG2 deficiency may be more prone to infection with pneumococcal organisms.

Combined Deficiencies

Children with T-cell deficiency present primarily with opportunistic and viral infections. They experience interstitial pneumonia (usually due to *P. carinii* or cytomegalo virus [CMV]), chronic diarrhea (due to viruses, *Giardia, Isospora,* or *Cryptosporidium*), localized *Candida* infection, disseminated fungal infection (e.g., *Aspergillus*) infection, atypical mycobacterium infection, and overwhelming viral infections (e.g., chickenpox, measles, adenovirus). Patients with T-cell deficiency may also develop autoimmune disease, cancer (primarily of the lymphoid system), and severe chronic dermatitis (e.g., eczema, seborrhea). Graft-vs-host disease (GVHD), which is characterized by skin rash, diarrhea, and liver disease, occurs when T-cell–deficient children receive foreign immunocompetent T cells (e.g., bone marrow transplant, blood transfusion, exposure to maternal T cells in utero). Children with profound T-cell deficiency or combined immunodeficiency also have antibody deficiency and are susceptible to bacterial infections (e.g., sinusitis, pneumonia, sepsis, meningitis) and opportunistic infections.

Severe Combined Immunodeficiency

Severe combined immunodeficiency (SCID) is a large group of diverse genetic disorders characterized by profound defects in immunity. The most common symptoms include chronic diarrhea with failure to thrive, pneumonia, otitis, sepsis, and cutaneous infections. Infections with opportunistic agents, such *as P. carinii, Candida albicans*, varicella-zoster virus, CMV, Epstein-Barr virus (EBV), respiratory syncytial virus, adenovirus, and bacille Calmette-Guérin

(BCG), can be severe and result in death. The most common form of SCID (~44% of cases) is X-linked SCID due to mutations of the common γ chain (γ_c), which forms a component of the receptor for multiple cytokines (interleukin-2 [IL-2], IL-4, IL-7, IL-9, IL-15, and IL-21). Patients with SCID can be classified according to phenotypes depending on their defect.

Patients with absent T cells and normal or elevated numbers of B cells are called T–B+SCID. These patients have defective signaling through the IL-2 receptor, which is required for T-cell growth and differentiation. Mutations in the γ_c chain (previously described), the α chain of the IL-7 receptor, and the tyrosine kinase Jak3 (Janus kinase 3) all result in marked decreases of circulating T cells.

Patients with absent T and B cells are called T–B–SCID. Approximately half of these patients have mutations in the recombinase-activating genes 1 and 2 (RAG1/2), which are required for rearrangement of the T and B cell receptor genes. Patients with Omenn's syndrome have missense of the RAG1 and RAG2 genes, which lead to partial function. Mutations in Artemis, a novel variable diversity joining (VDJ) recombination/DNA repair factor, prevent DNA repair during RAG1/2-mediated rearrangement of the antigen receptors. These patients also have increased sensitivity to radiation.

The most common form of autosomal recessive SCID is adenosine deaminase (ADA) deficiency, which is a defect in a purine salvage enzyme. Patients with ADA deficiency have a buildup of toxic metabolites (e.g., 2'-deoxyadenosine 5'-triphosphate [dATP], *S*-adenosylhomocysteine) in their T and B cells that results in severe lymphopenia. Patients with defects in purine nucleoside phosphorylase (PNP), a second purine salvage enzyme in this pathway, have a similar phenotype.

A subset of patients has T cells that appear normal but fail to respond to stimulation of the T-cell antigen receptor. These patients can have mutations in components of the T-cell receptor complex (e.g., CD3γ, CD3δ, CD3ε) or in associated tyrosine kinases such as zeta chain-associated protein (ZAP-70), which results in the absence of CD8 T cells.

Other T Lymphocyte–Related Immunodeficiency Diseases

Wiskott-Aldrich Syndrome

WAS is an X-linked disorder characterized by eczema, bleeding, thrombocytopenia, and recurrent infections (primarily bacterial respiratory tract infections). This disorder is caused by mutations in the WAS protein (WASP), which is a gene involved in cytoskeletal reorganization in all hematopoietic stem cell–derived lineages. Mutations in the WASP have also been found in X-linked thrombocytopenia (without immunodeficiency) and X-linked neutropenia.

Children with WAS have slightly decreased IgM, increased IgA and IgE, and normal to low IgG levels and are unable to make an antibody response to polysaccharide and other antigens. Circulating T cells progressively decrease with age, and lymphocyte responses to mitogens are reduced. The thrombocytopenia seen in WAS is unique because the platelets are very small. With time, children with WAS may develop serious problems with central nervous system bleeding, recurrent infections, malignancy (primarily lymphoreticular), and autoimmune disease.

Hyper Immunoglobulin M Syndrome

Patients with X-linked HIM syndrome (XHIM) have recurrent bacterial infection. At presentation, opportunistic infections, especially those due to *P. carinii*, are seen in up to 40% of patients; neutropenia also is seen. Lymphoid hyperplasia is milder than in autosomal recessive HIM; however, lymph nodes in patients with HIM1 lack germinal centers. Patients are at increased risk for neoplasms, especially lymphomas, but liver and biliary tract tumors are also observed. XHIM results from mutations in CD40 ligand (CD154), which is expressed on activated T cells and interacts with CD40 on B cells. The interaction between CD40 ligand and CD40 are required for optimal stimulation of the T cell and induction of B-cell class switching. Patients with mutations in the CD40 gene have an identical phenotype, but the inheritance is autosomal recessive.

Ataxia-Telangiectasia

Ataxia-telangiectasia is an autosomal recessive disorder characterized by cerebellar ataxia, oculocutaneous telangiectasia, recurrent sinopulmonary infections, and increased incidence of malignancy. Severe neurological impairment may develop as the disease progresses with the patient's confinement to a wheelchair by the second decade of life. Most patients with ataxia-telangiectasia have variable degrees of antibody deficiency (e.g., deficiency of IgA, IgE, IgG2, IgG4) and T-cell deficiency. The genetic cause is mutations of the ataxia-telangiectasia mutated (ATM) gene, which is a DNA-dependent protein kinase involved in detecting double-strand breaks in DNA. Deficiency of ATM leads to increased sensitivity to ionizing radiation, defective DNA repair, and accumulation of chromosomal abnormalities. Approximately 95% of patients with ataxia-telangiectasia have elevated serum α-fetoprotein, a useful marker when an attempt is made to establish the diagnosis. Similar disorders include Nijmegen breakage syndrome, which results from mutation of Nibrin (NBS1), which is part of the ATM DNA-damage sensing pathway, and an ataxia-telangiectasia-like syndrome, which results from mutations in the Mre11A gene.

Thymic Hypoplasia (DiGeorge Syndrome)

DiGeorge syndrome is an example of a T-cell deficiency that results from a thymus defect. In these children, a genetic defect is associated with abnormal development of the third and fourth pharyngeal pouches during early embryogenesis that may lead to an absent or small thymus (T-cell deficiency), absent parathyroid glands (hypocalcemia), cardiac abnormalities, and facial abnormalities (e.g., hypertelorism, short philtrum, low-set ears, and hypoplastic mandible). The degree of thymic hypoplasia varies, and in most cases, patients have mild immunological impairment. In cases of total thymic aplasia, patients are susceptible to opportunistic infections and GVHD. DiGeorge syndrome maps to microdeletions of specific DNA sequences from chromosome 22q11.2 in most cases and chromosome 10p in a small number of cases.

Phagocytic Defects

Phagocytes (neutrophils and macrophages) are a key component of the body's response to infection. Any defect in phagocyte number, function, or both can predispose patients to recurrent infections of the skin and soft tissue, deep-seated abscesses (e.g., liver, lung, bone, spleen), lung infections, recurrent osteomyelitis (primarily of small bones), and periodontal disease. The main organisms involved are *Staphylococcus aureus*; gram-negative rods (*Escherichia coli, Klebsiella, Serratia,* and *Pseudomonas* spp.); and *Aspergillus, Candida,* and *Nocardia* spp. Many advances in the identification of and knowledge about the molecular basis of phagocytic defects have been made in the past few years.[2]

Chronic Granulomatous Disease

The classic form of phagocyte defect is chronic granulomatous disease (CGD), which results from mutations in nicotinamide adenine dinucleotide phosphate (NADPH) oxidase, the enzyme complex required for the production of hydrogen peroxide and superoxide radicals. Within the phagocytic vacuole, metabolites of superoxide activate neutrophil elastase and cathepsin G and result in microbial killing.[3] The X-linked form of CGD, which accounts for most cases (70%), involves mutations in $gp91^{phox}$, and the remainder are autosomal recessive forms involving the three other structural genes of the NADPH oxidase complex ($p22^{phox}$, $p47^{phox}$, and $p67^{phox}$). Patients are extremely susceptible to infection with *S. aureus* and *Aspergillus*, with *Nocardia, Serratia,* and *Burkholderia cepacia* accounting for most of the remaining infections. The most frequent sites of infection are the lung, skin, lymph nodes, and liver. A variant of CGD is caused by mutations of Rac2 guanosine triphosphatase (GTPase), which interacts with NADPH oxidase.

Leukocyte Adhesion Defect

Leukocyte adhesion to the endothelium and migration into the tissue toward sites of inflammation and infections are mediated through interactions with selectins and integrins. Defects in these pathways prevent recruitment of neutrophils into infected or inflamed sites. Leukocyte adhesion deficiency type 1 (LAD-1) is an autosomal recessive disorder caused by mutations in the gene encoding CD18 or β_2 integrin. The β_2 integrins are heterodimers, and CD18, which is required for normal expression, noncovalently binds to three individual α chains (CD11a, CD11b, or CD11c). CD11a/CD18 forms leukocyte function–associated molecule 1 (LFA-1). CD11b/CD18 forms macrophage antigen 1 (Mac-1) or complement receptor 3 (CR3), and CD11c/CD18 forms complement receptor 4 (CR4). LFA-3 binds to intercellular adhesion molecule-1 (ICAM-1) and mediates tight adhesion of leukocytes to the endothelium before diapedesis. Without LFA-1, leukocytes are trapped in the circulation and cannot migrate to sites of infection. Patients with LAD-1 are prone to recurrent infections of the skin, airways, bowel, and perirectal area, which are necrotic and ulcerating without pus formation. The most common organisms are *S. aureus* or gram-negative bacteria. Patients have delayed umbilical stump separation (>30 days), omphalitis, persistent leukocytosis, severe gingivitis, and periodontitis. Wound healing is poor, and aggressive medical management, including debridement and grafting, may be necessary.

LAD-2 is an autosomal recessive disorder caused by mutations in a guanosine diphosphate (GDP)-fucose transporter, which is required for the expression of sialyl-Lewis X (CD15s) that binds to E-selectin. Without this interaction, leukocytes cannot make the initial binding to the endothelium and therefore cannot role along the vascular wall. Other rare causes of LAD include abnormal E-selectin expression; mutations in Rac2, which is required for regulation of the actin cytoskeleton; and mutations in Rap1, which is involved in integrin activation and signaling.

Interferon-γ Interleukin-12 Pathway Defects

Defects in components of the interferon-γ (IFN-γ)/IL-12 axis result in defective IFN-γ binding or signaling and susceptibility to intracellular organisms, especially nontuberculous *Mycobacteria* and *Salmonella*. Mononuclear phagocytes play a key role in the immune response against intracellular microorganisms. During phagocytosis of an organism, macrophages produce IL-12, which stimulates IFN-γ production by T helper cells and NK cells. Mutations have been found in the p40 subunit of IL-12; the β1 chain of the IL-12 receptor; both the α and β chains of the IFN-γ receptor; and the signal transducer and activator of transcription 1 (STAT-1) molecule, which is required for signaling of the IFN-γ receptor. The patients with mutations in the IFN-γ receptor have the most severe phenotype and are seen early in life with disseminated severe infections, including BCG if the patient was previously immunized.

Congenital and Cyclic Neutropenias

Severe neutropenia (neutrophil count less than 500/μL) can predispose the patient to life-threatening bacterial infections. The neutropenia may be due to impaired neutrophil production (e.g., disorders of proliferation and maturation of myeloid cells), infection, drugs, autoimmunity, hypersplenism, or bone marrow replacement. Cyclic neutropenia presents with regular cycles (every 2 to 5 weeks) of neutropenia that are sometimes associated with fever, mouth ulcers, and skin infections. Cyclic neutropenia is an autosomal dominant disorder caused by mutations in the elastase gene. A related disorder, congenital agranulocytosis (Kostmann's syndrome), is an autosomal dominant disorder caused by mutations in the receptor for granulocyte colony-stimulating factor (G-CSF).

Chédiak-Higashi Syndrome

Chédiak-Higashi syndrome is associated with hypopigmentation or albinism, severe immunodeficiency, mild bleeding tendency, and neurological symptoms. The syndrome is caused by mutations in a lysosomal transport protein (LYST) that prevent normal formation of phagolysosomes and melanosomes. On routine blood smears, giant granules are seen in leukocytes. Patients are susceptible to recurrent severe pyogenic infections, often with *S. aureus*, and often develop a fatal lymphoproliferative syndrome with lymphohistiocytic infiltrates, fever, jaundice, hepatosplenomegaly, lymphadenopathy, pancytopenia, and bleeding.

Complement Defects

Complement is a key component of the immune system. Activation of complement via the classical or alternative pathway enhances clearance of infectious agents by promoting chemotaxis, opsonization, and phagocytosis. Activation of the complement cascade also leads to generation of the terminal membrane attack complex (C5-C9) that directly lyses organisms. For most bacteria, clearance is primarily by phagocytosis, which is promoted by the binding of activated C3 to the organism's surface. Some bacteria (e.g., *Neisseria* species), however, require lysis by terminal complement components for optimal clearance.

With the exception of factor B, deficiencies of all components of both the classical and alternative complement cascades have been described. Patients with deficiencies of the early complement components (C1q, C1r, C2, and C4) usually have autoimmune diseases (e.g., systemic lupus erythematosus, dermatomyositis, chronic glomerulonephritis), and deficiency of these components results in faulty dissolution of immune complexes. Recurrent bacterial infections (e.g., sepsis, meningitis, pneumonia) due to encapsulated bacteria are occasionally seen with these early complement deficiencies. Patients with deficiencies of the terminal complement components (C5-C8) have recurrent neisserial infections and rheumatic disease. Recurrent neisserial infections are seen in patients who lack the alternative pathway components factor D and properdin and in some patients who have C9 deficiency.

C3 is a pivotal component of both the classical and alternative complement pathways. Absence of C3 is associated with recurrent pyogenic bacterial infections, similar to those seen in the antibody deficiencies. Lack of C3 can result from a genetic defect of C3 or from deficiency of the regulatory proteins factor I or factor H, which results in spontaneous activation of the alternative pathway with consumption of C3.

A third pathway of complement activation, the lectin pathway, is mediated by mannose-binding lectin. Deficiency of mannose-binding lectin or its associated serine protease is often associated with recurrent pyogenic infections.

Deficiency of C1 esterase inhibitor presents as attacks of recurrent angioedema and not immunodeficiency. This autosomal dominant disorder usually begins in childhood with episodes of angioedema (involving the face, extremities, trunk, or mucous membranes) and abdominal pain. Life-threatening upper airway obstruction may develop. The angioedema is circumscribed, nonpruritic, and nonpainful. Approximately 85% of patients with hereditary angioedema lack C1 inhibitor, and 15% have a nonfunctional form of C1 inhibitor.

Clinical Approach To Suspected Immunodeficiency

Most patients with primary immunodeficiency will have recurrent serious infections or infections with unusual pathogens. The type of infection may offer clues as to the component of the immune system affected (Table 85–1); however, a considerable amount of overlap in the type of infections and specific immunodeficiencies exists. If a child has an infection that is severe, invasive, or unusual,

TABLE 85–1

Infections Associated with Primary Immunodeficiencies

Antibody Deficiency	Combined Immunodeficiency	Phagocytic Defect	Complement Defect
Recurrent sinopulmonary with or without gastrointestinal infections Chronic enteroviral and rotaviral infections Recurrent/severe bacterial infections: (*Streptococcus pneumoniae, Staphylococcus aureus, Haemophilus influenzae, Pseudomonas aeruginosa, Neisseria meningitidis, Mycoplasma hominis, Ureaplasma ureolyticum*) Protozoa (*Giardia*)	Intracellular organisms: Bacteria (*Mycobacteria, Listeria, Legionella, Salmonella typhi*) Viruses (especially herpes, CMV, EBV) Fungi: invasive (*Aspergillus, Cryptococcus*), mucocutaneous (*Candida*) Protozoa (*Giardia, P. carinii, Toxoplasma, Cryptosporidium*) Recurrent sinopulmonary infections occur in most patients because of associated deficits in antibody production	Invasive infections with *Staphylococcus*, opportunistic gram-negative organisms (enteric flora, *Pseudomonas aeruginosa, Salmonella typhi, N. asteroids, Serratia*) and fungi (*Aspergillus, Candida*). IFN-γ/IL-12 deficiencies: *Mycobacteria* (nontuberculous and TB), *Salmonella*	Recurrent infections with *Neisseria* species and *S. pneumoniae* Recurrent/recalcitrant skin infections

CMV, cytomegalovirus; *EBV*, Epstein-Barr virus; *IFN*, interferon; *IL*, interleukin.

the underlying infection should be treated appropriately, and an immunologist should be consulted to arrange further testing. Secondary testing is often performed in special reference laboratories, and some specimens need to be drawn, prepared, and handled in a specific manner to prevent artifacts. Interpretation of tests can be complicated on the basis of the patient's age, medical condition, and prior therapies. Depending on the therapy received, conclusive diagnostic testing may need to be deferred.

Medical and Physical Examination

The first step in the evaluation of a child with recurrent infections is to obtain a thorough history and perform a complete physical examination. Particular attention should be made to determine the types, frequency, and severity of the infections and the response to treatment. The family history should be examined for infections or early deaths in other family members, and the possibility of consanguinity should be explored. During a physical examination, the presence and absence of lymphoid tissue may give important clues.

Laboratory Evaluation

Some screening tests may be helpful in the determination of which portion of the immune system is abnormal (Table 85–3). A complete blood count with differential provides a good starting point to determine whether there are any abnormalities in the absolute numbers and percentages of myeloid and lymphoid cells, as well as platelet number and size. Abnormal inclusions or granules in the neutrophils may suggest a disorder such as Chédiak-Higashi syndrome. Immunoglobulin levels (IgG, IgM, and IgA) and determination of hemolytic complement activity (CH50) can provide an overview of humoral immunity. The patient's history, type of infection, and screening results can then tailor the evaluation for assessment of the portion of the immune system most likely to be abnormal and to rule out other causes.

If a primary antibody deficiency is suspected, initial screening includes immunoglobulin levels, measurement of isoagglutinins, and measurement of antibodies to previously administered vaccines (e.g., diphtheria, tetanus). Immunoglobulin levels vary with age and should

TABLE 85–2

Specific Immunodeficiencies

Antibody Deficiency	Combined Immunodeficiency/ T Cell Deficiencies	Phagocytic Defects	Complement Defects
Agammaglobulinemias: X-lined Autosomal recessive HIM (autosomal recessive) Common Variable Immunodeficiency Selective IgA deficiency IgG subclass deficiencies Specific antibody deficiency with normal immunoglobulins (impaired antibody response to polysaccharides)	Severe combined immunodeficiency (SCID) Defective cytokine signaling (common gamma chain, Jak3, IL-2Rα, IL-7Rα) Defective T-cell receptor signaling (ZAP-70, CD3ε, CD3γ) Defective receptor gene recombination (RAG1, RAG2) Defective MHC class I expression (TAP1, TAP2) Defective MHC class II transcription (Bare lymphocyte syndrome) Adenosine deaminase deficiency Purine nucleoside phosphorylase deficiency Other HIM (X-linked) Wiskott-Aldrich syndrome DiGeorge syndrome Ataxia-telangiectasia Other DNA repair defects: Nijmegen breakage syndrome, Artemis deficiency Ataxia-like syndrome X-linked lymphoproliferative syndrome Nuclear factor κB essential modifier (NEMO) deficiency	Cyclic neutropenia Congenital agranulocytosis Chronic granulomatous disease: X-linked and autosomal recessive Leukocyte adhesion deficiency: CD18, FUCT1, Rap-1, Rac2 Chédiak-Higashi syndrome Myeloperoxidase deficiency Glucose-6-phosphate dehydrogenase deficiency (complete) IFN-γ/IL-12 defects: IL-12/IL-23 receptor, IL-12p40, IFN-γ receptor, STAT-1 deficiency Defective NK function: CD16 deficiency	Hereditary angioedema: C1 esterase inhibitor deficiency Specific deficiencies in proximal, alternative, and terminal complement components: C1q, C1r, C4, C2, C3, C5, C6, c7, C8a, C8b, C9, factor I, factor H, factor D, properidin Deficiencies in lectin pathway complement activation: MBP, MASP2

HIM, hyper-IgM syndrome; *Ig,* immunoglobulin; *IFN,* interferon; *IL,* interleukin; *Jak3,* Janus kinase 3; *MASP2,* mannose-associated serine protease; *MBP,* mannose-binding protein; *MHC,* major histocompatibility complex; *NK,* natural killer; *RAG,* recombinase-activating gene; *STAT-1* signal transducer and activator of transcription 1.

be compared with age-matched control subjects.[4] IgG levels reach their nadir between 4 and 6 months when passively acquired maternal antibody is waning and reach adult levels by age 6 years. IgM levels increase steadily from birth and reach adult levels around ages 6 to 8 years. IgA levels are low in the blood and absent from mucosal secretions at birth. They rise slowly and reach adult concentrations at ages 6 to 8 years. An immunoglobulin level within two standard deviations of the mean for age is considered normal. For example, infants with HIM may have an IgM level within the upper limits of normal for an adult and be overlooked. Because isoagglutinins measure IgM function, they may provide a useful measurement of B-cell function in infants. Secondary evaluation for antibody deficiency, if indicated, includes assessing antibody responses to specific challenge with booster diphtheria/tetanus and nonconjugated pneumococcal vaccines (e.g., Pneumovax). Assessment of the polysaccharide response to pneumococcal antigens should only be performed in patients older than 2 years because it is unreliable before then. Additional testing may include IgG subclasses and analysis of B- and T-cell numbers and function in vitro. IgG subclasses show wide variation in concentration. IgG2 and IgG4 subclasses are relatively delayed in development, and healthy children younger than 2 years often have low concentrations. Thus a diagnosis of IgG subclass deficiency is not reliable in this age group. Isolated IgG4 deficiency is usually not clinically significant because 10% of the healthy population has absent IgG4 levels.

Deficiencies in cell-mediated immunity often present with severe and unusual infections with intracellular and cell-associated microbes (see Table 85–1), failure to thrive, and chronic diarrhea. The initial screening evaluation for suspected T cell and combined immunodeficiency includes lymphocyte counts and testing for human immunodeficiency virus (HIV) infection. HIV testing can be difficult because passive maternal antibody to HIV can persist for up to 18 months after birth. Tests to detect antibodies to HIV (e.g., enzyme-linked immunosorbent assay [ELISA], or Western blot) may be falsely negative if the infection was too recent to induce an antibody response or if appropriate antibody responses are lost because of overwhelming infection. More reliable tests for HIV include polymerase chain reaction (PCR) to detect viral DNA or RNA, culture of the virus, or detection of specific viral protein antigens. Testing for HIV should be performed more than once by a combination of methods (see also Chapter 86). Delayed-type hypersensitivity (DTH) skin testing and chest radiography to look for a thymic shadow are often not useful. DTH testing requires adequate previous exposure to antigen. Most infants younger than 6 to 12 months will not respond because of a lack of exposure to the antigen. The thymus may also shrink in response to stress such as infection or surgery. Secondary testing for defects in cell-mediated immunity includes assessment of T-cell numbers and function in vitro. Enumeration of T cell subsets, NK cells, and B cells is performed by flow cytometry on a fluorescence-activated cell sorter (FACS). T-cell subsets should be adjusted for age-matched controls.[5] General T-cell function is tested by proliferation to mitogens (e.g., phytohemagglutinin, concanavalin A), to anti-CD3 antibody, or to specific antigens (e.g., tetanus toxoid, *Candida*).

TABLE 85–3

Evaluation

Screening Test	Advanced Testings	Advanced Specialized Testing
History and physical examination (including family history)	IgG subclasses, IgE levels	Biochemical testing
Complete blood count with differential, platelet count and volume, and peripheral smear	Enumeration of B and T cell numbers by FACS analysis	Adenosine deaminase, purine nucleoside phosphorylase
Hemolytic complement (CH50)	T cell in vitro proliferation:	Myeloperoxidase, glucose-6-phosphate dehydrogenase
Immunoglobulin concentrations (IgG, IgM, IgA)	To antigens (tetanus, *Candida*)	Cytogenic studies
Isoagglutinin (anti-A and anti-B) titers	To mitogens (phytohemagglutinin, concanavalin A, pokeweed, anti-CD3 receptor antibody)	Karyotyping
Antibody titer to previous vaccines (tetanus, diphtheria, hepatitis)	T cell lymphokine production	FISH (e.g., chr 22 deletion, DiGeorge syndrome)
Delayed-type hypersensitivity (DTH) testing if older than 2 yr	Antibody response to new vaccines or special antigens (e.g., pneumococcal or *Haemophilus influenzae* polysaccharides, bacteriophage)	XY chromosomal analysis
Other tests of exclusion:	Levels of specific complement components	DNA and RNA based techniques
HIV, sweat test, α1-antitrypsin	Immune complexes	Restriction fragment length polymorphisms (RFLPs)
	NBT dye reduction or FACS analysis or respiratory burst	Short tandem repeat (STR) polymorphisms
	Bacterial killing assays (*Staphylococcus aureus, Escherichia coli*)	Southern blotting
		Northern blotting
		Reverse transcriptase polymerase chain reaction (RT-PCR)
		X chromosome inactivation
		Single strand conformational polymorphism (SSCP)
		Dideoxy fingerprinting (ddF)

FACS, fluorescence-activated cell sorter; FISH, fluorescence in situ hybridization; *HIV,* human immunodeficiency virus; *NBT,* nitroblue tetrazolium.

Phagocyte deficiencies can be suspected if there is an alteration of neutrophil numbers in a complete blood cell count (CBC). Decreased numbers may indicate iatrogenic, autoimmune, or genetic causes. Cyclic neutropenia was traditionally assessed through obtainment of CBCs three times a week for a month. Recently, the genetic basis of cyclic neutropenia has been elucidated and attributed to a deficiency of elastase.[6] LAD often presents with invasive tissue infections, usually associated with persistent neutrophilia. The diagnosis is confirmed by flow cytometry for CD18, Mac-1, and LFA-1; CD18 is absent in this disease and is required for Mac-1 and LFA-1 expression. CGD was previously assessed by the nitroblue tetrazolium (NBT) test, which has now been replaced with a flow cytometry method that measures hydrogen peroxide reduction after stimulation of neutrophils (often called the *respiratory burst test*). The most current sensitive version of this test uses dihydrorodamine dye and can distinguish the X-linked from the autosomal forms of CGD on the basis of the amount of shift.[7,8]

Recurrent infections with encapsulated organisms or *Neisseria* suggest a complement deficiency. Approximately 5% of patients with an initial invasive meningococcal infection have a complement deficiency. Individuals who are older, who are infected with an unusual serotype, or who have more than one invasive infection with *Neisseria meningitidis* or *Neisseria gonorrhoeae* are at even greater risk and should be evaluated for complement deficiencies. A hemolytic complement (CH50) is useful for screening purposes and recognizes deficiencies of all components of the classical complement pathway. The alternative pathway can be analyzed with an AH50, which is particularly important in the evaluation of male patients because the only X linked complement component (properdin) is part of the alternative pathway. Homozygous complement component deficiency will reduce the CH50 or AH50 markedly, generally to values less than 10% of normal with the exception of C9 and properdin deficiency, in which values are usually reduced to approximately 50% of normal. If reductions of this magnitude are identified and confirmed, specialized testing to measure the individual complement components can be done by a reference laboratory. Complement levels are sensitive to heat inactivation, and the samples should be processed immediately by the hospital laboratory and frozen. In the setting of severe sepsis or disseminated intravascular coagulation, alterations in complement levels may be uninterpretable with respect to diagnosis of an immunodeficiency and may need to be performed after the event has resolved.

Therapeutic Considerations in Primary Immunodeficiencies

Antibiotics, Antifungals, and Antivirals

Because patients with primary immunodeficiency or suspected immunodeficiency are at risk for life-threatening infections, patients with fevers or other manifestations of infection should be started immediately antibiotics. On the basis of clinical symptoms, blood, throat, and other cultures should be obtained, as appropriate, before therapy if possible. If a patient does not respond promptly to antibiotics, a search for other possible infections, including fungal, mycobacterial, viral, or protozoal, should be undertaken.

In patients with known primary immunodeficiency, continuous prophylactic antibiotics are often beneficial. Patients with significant cellular immunodeficiency should be placed on *P. carinii* prophylaxis (trimethoprim-sulfamethoxazole [TMP/SMX]), 160 mg/m^2/day of TMP and 750 mg/m^2/day of SMX given in divided doses [bid] three times per week). In patients with CGD, TMP/SMX prophylaxis (5 mg/kg/day divided bid) reduces the frequency of staphylococcal and other bacterial infections. In patients with CGD, antifungal prophylaxis with itraconazole (100 mg/day for <50 kg and 200 mg/day for ≥ 50 kg) has been shown to reduce the risk of fungal infections.[9]

Blood Products

Children with T-cell deficiency or combined immunodeficiency can develop life-threatening GVHD after the transfusion of viable T cells. Therefore all blood products that these children receive must be irradiated and preferably leukoreduced. This will prevent proliferation of the T cells from the blood product and avoid GVHD. For the potential reactivation of transmitted viral agents to be prevented, the blood products must be CMV negative. Transfusions of granulocytes immediately after harvest by leukophoresis can be used in patients with LAD or other immunodeficiencies with severe life-threatening infections. The use of granulocyte infusions, however, is limited because of potential concerns of transmitting infections (hepatitis, CMV, and HIV) and the development of antigranulocyte antibodies.

Immunoglobulin Preparations

Patients with antibody deficiencies and those with T-cell deficiencies are unable to make specific antibodies following antigenic challenge. This has important implications both in the identification of infectious pathogens and in the need for antibody replacement. Diagnostic tests based on the detection of antibodies to infectious pathogens (e.g., hepatitis C antibodies) will give false-negative results, and tests based on the detection of specific antigens or genetic material (PCR based) should be used.

Replacement therapy with intravenous infusions of human intravenous immunoglobulin (IVIG) is the most widely used treatment in patients with primary immunodeficiencies, especially in those with agammaglobulinemia, CVID, SCID, WAS, HIM, or ataxia-telangiectasia. IVIG is usually dosed at 400 to 600 mg/kg/mo. In the intensive care unit (ICU) setting, patients with newly diagnosed primary immunodeficiency may require extra loading doses of IVIG to more rapidly attain therapeutic IgG trough levels of at least 500 mg/dl. Similarly, patients with known primary immunodeficiency may require increased doses of IVIG because of increased catabolism or third spacing in the setting of stress and infection.

Special uses of IVIG may also be considered. Patients with XLA are prone to chronic meningoencephalitis due to enteroviral infection. Treatment with high-dose IVIG or intraventricular immunoglobulin may modify the infection. Oral immunoglobulin may be given to treat severe diarrhea from rotavirus, *Campylobacter, Cryptosporidium,* or other pathogens.

Enzyme Replacement Therapy

In SCID caused by ADA deficiency, enzyme replacement with polyethylene glycol-modified bovine ADA (PEG-ADA) has resulted in clinical and immunological improvement[10,11]; however, the immune reconstitution is less than what is normally seen with bone marrow transplant. The usual dose of PEG-ADA is 30 U/kg, given subcutaneously once or twice weekly.

Cytokines

In a large, multicenter, randomized, placebo-controlled study, recombinant human IFN-γ (50 μg/m^2 subcutaneously three times a week) has been shown to reduce the severity and frequency of infections in patients with CGD.[12] Recombinant IFN-γ may also be used in some patients with defects of IL-12 or the IL-12 receptor, or with partial deficiency of the IFN-γ receptor.[13] Recombinant G-CSF can be used in patients who have neutropenia such as HIM, congenital agranulocytosis, and cyclic neutropenia, and in patients who have undergone recent bone marrow transplantation for their immunodeficiency. Recombinant IL-2 may be used in select patients with severe combined immunodeficiency due to defective IL-2 synthesis.

Bone Marrow Transplantation

Bone marrow transplantation is the optimal treatment for patients with combined immunodeficiency and WAS and has been used in a number of other primary immunodeficiencies.[14,15] The primary goal of bone marrow transplantation is to provide normal hematopoietic stem cells to correct the underlying genetic defects in the immune system. The preferred bone marrow donors are human leukocyte antigen (HLA)-matched siblings. If an HLA-identical donor is unavailable, a haploidentical, T cell–depleted bone marrow transplant can be performed in patients with SCID. In patients with other forms of primary immunodeficiency, stem cells from matched unrelated marrow donors can be used. Recently, umbilical cord blood from HLA-identical siblings and matched unrelated cord blood have been used. In patients who have a complete lack of cellular immunity, a conditioning regimen may not be required. In patients with intact or slightly decreased T-cell immunodeficiency, such as WAS, immunosuppression before transplantation is necessary to ensure engraftment. The major risks associated with bone marrow transplant are death resulting from infection, GVHD, and veno-occlusive disease (see also Chapter 76).

Gene Therapy

Gene therapy is an exciting new option on the horizon that will provide the opportunity to correct primary immunodeficiencies due to defects in single genes expressed in blood cells in patients who lack suitable HLA-matched donors for bone marrow transplant. A correct copy of the gene can be inserted into the patient's own hematopoietic stem cells, which one then reintroduces into the patient without the risk of GVHD or graft rejection. The successes and risks of gene therapy have been recently reviewed.[16] Successful immune reconstitution has been shown in both X-linked SCID and ADA deficiency; however, clonal leukemic proliferation of transduced T cells occurred in 3 of the 10 patients with X-linked SCID who underwent gene therapy. Additional research is under way to improve the safety of the integrating gene vectors.

Summary

Children with underlying immunodeficiency are usually first seen with recurrent serious infections or infections with unusual pathogens. The kind of infection(s) that the patient experiences suggests which component of the immune system, if any, is faulty. When a patient with a known or suspected primary immunodeficiency disorder is treated, it is prudent to consult with a trained immunologist as soon as possible during the course of therapy. Infections should be treated aggressively with broad-spectrum coverage until a pathogen is identified. Alternative methods of identification of pathogens may be required. In patients with known immunodeficiency, standard treatment regiments such as replacement therapy with IVIG may need to be reevaluated and optimized.

REFERENCES

1. Ballow M: Primary immunodeficiency disorders: Antibody deficiency, *J Allergy Clin Immunol* 109:581, 2002.
2. Rosenzweig SD, Holland SM: Phagocyte immunodeficiencies and their infections, *J Allergy Clin Immunol* 113:620, 2004.
3. Reeves EP, Lu H, Jacobs HL et al: Killing activity of neutrophils is mediated through activation of proteases by K+ flux, *Nature* 416:291, 2002.
4. Stiehm ER, Fudenberg HH: Serum levels of immune globulins in health and disease: a survey, *Pediatrics* 37:715, 1966.
5. Ochs HD, Winkelstein Y, Stiehm ER: Immunodeficiency disorders: general considerations. In Stiehm ER, Ochs HD, Winkelstein Y, editors: *Immunologic disorders in infants and children,* ed 5, Philadelphia, 2004, WB Saunders.
6. Dale DC, Bolyard AA, Aprikyan A: Cyclic neutropenia, *Semin Hematol* 39:89, 2002.
7. Vowells SJ, Sekhsaria S, Malech HL et al: Flow cytometric analysis of the granulocyte respiratory burst: a comparison study of fluorescent probes, *J Immunol Methods* 178:89, 1995.
8. Vowells SJ, Fleisher TA, Sekhsaria S, et al: Genotype-dependent variability in flow cytometric evaluation of reduced nicotinamide adenine dinucleotide phosphate oxidase function in patients with chronic granulomatous disease, *J Pediatr* 128:104, 1996.
9. Gallin JI, Alling DW, Malech HL et al: Itraconazole to prevent fungal infections in chronic granulomatous disease, *N Engl J Med* 248:2416, 2003.
10. Hershfield MS, Buckley RH, Greenberg ML et al: Treatment of adenosine deaminase deficiency with polyethylene glycol-modified adenosine deaminase, *N Engl J Med* 316:589, 1987.
11. Hershfield MS: PEG-ADA replacement therapy for adenosine deaminase deficiency: an update after 8.5 years, *Clin Immunol Immunopathol* 76:S228, 1995.
12. International Chronic Granulomatous Disease Cooperative Study Group: A controlled trial of interferon-gamma to prevent infection in chronic granulomatous disease, *N Engl J Med* 324:509, 1991.

13. Holland SM: Treatment of infections in the patient with Mendelian susceptibility to mycobacterial infection, *Microbes Infect* 2:1579, 2000.
14. Buckley RH: A historical review of bone marrow transplantation for immunodeficiencies, *J Allergy Clin Immunol* 113:793, 2004.
15. Buckley RH, Fischer A: Bone marrow transplantation for primary immunodeficiency diseases. In Ochs HD, Smith CIE, Puck JM, editors: *Primary immunodeficiency diseases: a molecular and genetic approach*, New York, 1999, Oxford University Press.
16. Chinen J, Puck JM: Successes and risks of gene therapy in primary immunodeficiencies, *J Allergy Clin Immunol* 113:594, 2004.

CHAPTER

86

Acquired Immune Dysfunction

Gwenn E. McLaughlin and Andrew Argent

PEARLS

- Most patients admitted to the pediatric intensive care unit (ICU) are immunosuppressed.
- The release of interleukin 10 (IL-10) is associated with down-regulation of major histocompatibility complex class II molecule expression on the surface of monocytes, but not B cells. This limits the ability of monocytes to elicit antigen specific T-cell responses.
- The long-term effects of transfusions on the immune system and disease susceptibility are unknown, but even 19 years after a blood transfusion, recipients have fewer peripheral T-cells, particularly helper T cells, than patients who did not undergo transfusion.
- As of December 2003, 2.5 million children lived with human immunodeficiency virus/acquired immune deficiency syndrome (HIV/AIDS) worldwide, of which 700,000 were infected and 500,000 died annually.
- Worldwide, approximately one third of the human population is infected with the *Mycobacterium* bacillus. Most of these individuals live in developing countries where the prevalence of HIV infection is high.
- The chest radiograph generally shows diffuse interstitial infiltrates with decreased lung volume. Pulmonary infiltrates can be variable in children, in part because infants have a greater propensity for atelectasis. Hypoxemia is likely to be out of proportion to clinical and radiographic examination. A selectively elevated serum lactate dehydrogenase level is suggestive, although not diagnostic, of *Pneumocystis carinii* pneumonia (PCP). To confirm the diagnosis of PCP bronchoalveolar lavage should be performed.
- Malignancies account for 2% of AIDS-defining illnesses in pediatric patients. As in the other patients with congenital and acquired immunodeficiencies, the loss of the body's surveillance system against tumors appears to contribute to this increase.
- Lymphomas are generally of B-cell type and often arise in the central nervous system (CNS).
- Several of these malignancies are associated with chronic viral infection. Epstein-Barr virus (EBV) DNA has been identified in most CNS tumors and in soft tissue tumors.
- The history of respiratory failure due to PCP in HIV-infected patients provides a vignette that shows many of the dilemmas surrounding the care of patients with AIDS.
- Zidovudine (ZDV) is the only agent proven to prevent transmission of HIV in humans and is therefore the first drug of choice in postexposure prophylaxis.

Acquired immune dysfunction is by definition a secondary phenomenon following another disease process, such as infection or trauma, or an intended or unintended effect of therapy. Protein calorie malnutrition probably accounts for the greatest number of immunodeficient patients in intensive care units (ICUs) worldwide, whereas human immunodeficiency virus (HIV) infection is the most widely recognized cause of acquired immune deficiency.[1] Impairments in humoral and cellular immunity occur as a consequence of immaturity, malignancy, transfusion, sepsis, shock, viral infections, tuberculosis (TB), and malaria.[1-3] Iatrogenic immunosuppression occurs most frequently with medications given to either inactivate or kill lymphocyte populations, particularly those used in cancer chemotherapy and autoimmune disease, and to control transplant rejection.[4] When all these precipitants of immunodeficiency are taken into account, it becomes apparent that most patients admitted to the pediatric ICU are immunosuppressed. Understanding patterns of disease that are specific to each type of immune dysfunction can lead to earlier appropriate empiric therapy and diagnostic tests (Table 86–1).

Immune Function and Critical Illness

Endotoxin tolerance was the first description of what is increasingly understood as the body's immunological response to stress.[5] Endotoxin tolerance, which is a temporary insensitivity to repeated lipopolysaccharide challenge that was first described in animals, is associated with monocyte reprogramming such that the proinflammatory cytokines tumor necrosis factor α (TNF α), interferon; and interleukin1 (IL-1), IL-6, and IL-12 are produced. Simultaneously, antiinflammatory agents such as IL-10 and TNF receptor are also produced. The release of IL-10 is associated with down-regulation of major histocompatibility complex class II molecule expression on the surface of monocytes, but not B cells. This limits the ability of monocytes to elicit antigen specific T-cell responses.[5,6] Activated T cells are important sources of interferons, which in turn control infection by stimulating nicotinamide adenine dinucleotide phosphate oxidase (NADPH oxidase) and nitric oxide production and by increasing adhesion molecule expression.[7] This down-regulation of human leukocyte antigen–DR (HLA-DR) expression on monocytes is known as immunoparalysis and has been shown in patients after trauma, neurosurgical procedures, and cardiopulmonary bypass operation.[8-10] This phenomenon may in part explain the increased incidence of life-threatening nosocomial infections in these patients.[8,11-13]

Up-regulation of the immune response with granulocyte colony-stimulating factor (G-CSF) or granulocyte macrophage colony-stimulating factor (GM-CSF) or interferon has been proposed as treatment for immunoparalysis.[14-16] In neutropenic patients with sepsis, G-CSF reduces the likelihood of death; however, in nonneutropenic patients only one clinical trial has yet shown benefit.[17] Adults with severe community-acquired pneumonia treated with G-CSF plus antibiotics had less sepsis-related organ failure than those treated with antibiotics alone.[17] Similarly, GM-CSF given to septic patients with acute respiratory distress syndrome (ARDS) was associated with improved gas exchange and increased neutrophil respiratory burst.[18] Interferon gamma-1b therapy administered to 10 consecutively admitted patients with less than 30% HLA-DR

TABLE 86–1

Infections Seen with Various Types of Immune Deficiency

	Common	Less Common
GRANULOCYTOPENIA		
Bacteria	*Staphylococcus aureus, Staphylococcus pneumonia, Klebsiella, Pseudomonas*	*Enterobacter, Acinetobacter, Stenotrophomonas*
Fungi/molds	*Candida, Aspergillosis, Zygomycosis*	
Parasites		
Viruses		HSV1 or 2, VZV
CELLULAR DEFECTS		
Bacteria	*Legionella, Nocardia*	*Mycobacterium tuberculosis*
Fungi/molds	*Pneumocystis, Cryptococcus, Mucormycosis*	
Parasites	*Toxoplasma*	
Viruses	CMV, EBV, adenovirus, VZV	
HUMORAL DEFECTS		
Bacteria	*S. pneumonia, Haemophilus influenzae*	
Fungi/molds		*Pneumocystis*
Parasites		*Giardia lamblia*
Viruses		VZV
COMBINED DEFECTS		
Bacteria	*S. aureus, S. pneumonia, Klebsiella, Pseudomonas*	*M. tuberculosis, Listeria monocytogenes, Legionella*
Fungi/molds	*Pneumocystis*, aspergillosis, *Cryptococcus*	Zygomycosis, murcomycosis
Parasites	Toxoplasmosis	
Viruses	CMV, VZV, influenza, parainfluenza, RSV, adenovirus	HSV 1 or 2

Modified from Safdar A, Armstrong D: Infectious morbidity in critically ill patients with cancer, *Crit Care Clin* 17:531, 2001.
CMV, cytomegalovirus, *EBV,* Epstein-Barr virus; *HSV,* herpes simplex virus; *VZV,* varicella-zoster virus.

expression restored both HLA-DR expression and production of IL-6 and TNF-α.[19] Aerosolized interferon-α administered to trauma patients with immunoparalysis was associated with a lower incidence of ventilator-associated pneumonia.[20]

Critically ill patients frequently receive blood transfusions that are known to modify the immune response. Patients with cancer who receive transfusion at the time of resection have greater risk of dying than those who do not.[21] In contrast, certain patients who receive blood transfusion before transplant have a lower incidence of rejection[21]; however, transplant recipients who receive an HLA-DR mismatched transfusion have accelerated graft rejection.[22] The long-term effects of transfusions on the immune system and disease susceptibility are unknown, but even 19 years after transfusion blood recipients have fewer peripheral T cells, particularly helper T cells, than patients who did not undergo transfusion.[23] Blood transfusions after trauma or cardiopulmonary bypass are associated with increased infection; however, in major surgery or trauma it is difficult to sort out the effect of transfusion compared with the effect of critical illness.[24,25] The use of autologous transfusion in elective surgery may reduce the risk of immunosuppression.[26]

In addition to HIV, viruses such as measles, influenza, and human T-cell lymphotrophic virus-1 can suppress the immune response.[2,27,28] The neutrophils of patients infected with measles are not activated and therefore are unable to phagocytize and kill bacteria.[3] Chronic malaria also leads to depressed T-cell function.[29,30]

Malnutrition and Immune Deficiency

Epidemiological studies confirm a frequent historical observation that famine and pestilence, malnutrition, and infectious diseases aggregate and aggravate each other.[31] TB is a classic example of this phenomenon: the epidemiological distribution of TB worldwide matches that of malnutrition.[32] Immune system dysfunction occurs so early in the course of malnutrition that measures of immune competence such as anergy and total T-cell numbers are sensitive indicators of a patient's nutritional status.[31] Nutrition influences the course of HIV, susceptibility to infection in older patients, the body's ability to respond to vaccines, and many other aspects of immune function.[31-33]

Protein or protein-calorie malnutrition is generally only studied in humans in its most severe form. Because of interspecies variability in immunoglobulin synthesis and cytokine regulation, extrapolation of animal data to humans may be inappropriate.[34] Protein malnutrition alters production of epithelial cell membrane glycoprotein receptors, immunoglobulin A, and mucus, increasing the risk of bacterial colonization.[34] Mobilization of neutrophils is delayed, natural killer cell lytic activity is reduced, and imbalances in critical T-cell subsets occur. All contribute to increased susceptibility to infection. Severe malnutrition attenuates the acute phase response and interferon-γ production, but other proinflammatory compounds and T-cell subsets are up-regulated. The common tautology that protein deficiency reduces all protein synthesis is not supported by available data.[34] In the human condition, selective protein deficiency without concomitant essential fatty acid and micronutrient deficiency is unlikely.

By definition, essential fatty acids, linoleic and alpha-linoleic acids, cannot be synthesized by mammalian cells and must be obtained through the diet.[35] Linoleic acid is found in plant oils and animal fats, alpha-linolenic acid in plant oils.[35,36] For children in many parts of the world access to fat other than cow's milk is severely limited.[37] The n-3 polyunsaturated fatty acids (PUFAs), eicosopentaenoic acid and docosahexaenoic acid (DHA), synthesized from alpha-linolenic acid or obtained from a diet of fish, suppress lymphocyte responses to mitogen stimulation.[34] Accumulating evidence suggests that dietary supplementation with n-3 PUFAs is a "natural" immunosuppressant that may be useful in autoimmune diseases such as lupus erythematosus, rheumatoid arthritis, and diabetes mellitus.[35] Moderate n-3 PUFA intake can enhance the immune response. For example, supplementation of infant formula with a small amount of DHA accelerates development of T-cell responsiveness in preterm infants (see also Chapter 68).[36]

There are many specific nutrients now identified as vital to immune function. Vitamin A has essential functions in immune cells and indirectly contributes to protection from infection through maintenance of vital epithelial cell differentiation and barrier function of the lung and intestine.[38] Vitamin A deficiency occurs in an estimated 100 million children worldwide[38] and is a risk factor for increased death from pneumonia and diarrhea.[31] A survey of hospitalized children in Malawi showed that one third had severe vitamin A deficiency and one third had moderate deficiency.[39] Paradoxically, these children had higher TNF-α–producing than IL-10–producing monocytes. This shift was perhaps triggered by the underlying disease that prompted hospitalization. Results of several randomized, double-blinded, placebo-controlled trials conducted in malnourished children have shown improved antibody response to vaccines and fewer diseases of the gastrointestinal and respiratory systems after vitamin A supplementation.[31,38,39] Vitamin A supplementation in individuals who are not deficient has no benefit, whereas high retinal levels are associated with an increased diarrhea and pneumonia.[40] Vitamin C (ascorbic acid) is highly concentrated in leukocytes, and low leukocyte vitamin C concentrations are associated with reduced immune function.[36] Epidemiological data suggest that higher vitamin C consumption lowers the risk of cancer and cardiovascular disease, but despite numerous clinical trials with participants of both sexes and varying ages, no definitive evidence that vitamin C supplementation reduces the frequency or symptoms of upper respiratory infections exists. High-dose vitamin C does improve several measures of immune function and does not appear to have any side effects.[36] Vitamin D receptors are found on numerous immune cell types.[41] Vitamin D deficiency is associated with depressed macrophage function and impaired delayed hypersensitivity.[41] Vitamin E (α-tocopherol) is a potent lipid-soluble antioxidant. Study results of vitamin E supplementation ranging from 200 to 800 mg/day in healthy adults showed increasing CD4/CD8 ratios, mitogen responsiveness, antibody production, and decreasing free radical production; however, a dosage of 300 mg/day for 3 weeks resulted in suppressed bactericidal activity in humans.[36] Optimal daily requirements of these nutrients in health and disease remain to be determined.

Of the trace elements that may affect the immune system, selenium, zinc, and iron have been the most widely studied. Selenium balances redox states and suppresses inflammation through its vital role in several antioxidant enzymes and intranuclear factors, including glucocorticoid receptor, activator protein-1, and nuclear factor-κB.[36] In HIV infection, selenium supplementation modifies cytokine release, decreasing TNF-α and IL-8 while increasing IL-2. Selenium improves T-cell proliferation and differentiation. Selenium deficiency in the host enhances the mutation rate of Coxsackie and influenza viruses, but excessive selenium intake is toxic to the immune system and other organs.[36] Zinc, like selenium, is required for the activity of more than 100 enzymes.[42] Zinc supplementation increases the number of CD4+ T cells; thus the CD4/CD8 T-cell ratio is improved. Zinc deficiency has been documented in alcoholics and in patients with burns and gastrointestinal disorders.[43] Zinc supplementation reduces bacteremia, hospitalization rates, and vaso-occlusive crises in patients with sickle cell anemia.[36] In young children, zinc supplementation reduced the duration of diarrhea and frequency of respiratory infections.[36] Worldwide, 20% to 25% of the population has iron deficiency, which results in impaired cell mediated immunity, particularly in neutrophil and natural killer cell function.[42] Although an association between iron availability and susceptibility to certain bacterial infections exists, there is little evidence that iron supplementation in deficient individuals inhibits immune responses or increases susceptibility to infections.[36]

Human Immunodeficiency Virus Infection and Acquired Immune Deficiency Syndrome

Acquired immune deficiency syndrome (AIDS) is a clinical syndrome resulting from infection by HIV-1 (and very rarely HIV-2), an RNA retrovirus dependent on a reverse transcriptase for replication.[44] Surrounding the RNA and its reverse transcriptase are core proteins p24 and p18. An envelope made up of the host cell membrane is studded with glycoproteins gp120 and gp40. Entry of HIV into cells is mediated by the binding of gp120 to the host cell's CD4 membrane protein in the presence of a host coreceptor of the chemokine family, either CCR5 on macrophages or CXCR4 on other cell lines. After HIV replication, the host cell undergoes apoptosis. The resultant loss of T helper cells results in severe deficiency of both cell-mediated and humoral immunity. Suppressed monocyte/macrophage function causes reduced clearance of immune complexes, impaired antigen-presenting capabilities, and decreased natural killer cell function. Because pediatric HIV infection is most commonly transmitted from mother to infant, the acquired immunodeficiency is occurring in a host whose immune system, unlike the adult's immune system, is relatively naive and has developed little natural immunity.[45,46] This may in part explain the shorter time required for progression of HIV infection to AIDS in perinatally infected children when compared with children infected after the age of 2 years.[47]

The diagnosis of HIV-1 infection in adults and children older than 18 months is accomplished by identification of antibodies specific to viral proteins: first through a rapid enzyme-linked immunosorbent assay and then confirmed by the more time-consuming Western blot analysis. Because infants carry transplacentally acquired maternal antibodies, HIV infection in infants younger than 18 months must be documented by HIV DNA polymerase chain reaction (PCR) or culture.[48] Generally DNA PCR is repeated three times (at birth, at 2 weeks, and at 6 months) with sensitivity increasing from 38% to 96% over time.[19] If positive, the child's HIV enzyme-linked immunosorbent assay (ELISA) can be repeated at 1 year to document seroconversion.[48]

The diagnosis of AIDS requires confirmation of both HIV infection and an AIDS-defining illness. AIDS-defining illnesses include nonspecific findings such as fever; weight loss; lymphadenopathy or diarrhea for more than 2 months; and specific findings such as encephalopathy, lymphoid interstitial pneumonitis (LIP), opportunistic infections, recurrent infections, and associated malignancies.[50] In 1994 the United States Centers for Disease Control and Prevention (CDC) modified an earlier classification system for HIV infection ranging from indeterminate to asymptomatic to severely symptomatic (i.e., AIDS) in an effort to stratify the severity or progression of the disease, by adding age specific CD4+ T cell counts and percentages.[50] These categories aside, there appear to be at least two patterns of response to HIV infection in untreated children.[51,52] Children younger than 4 years, especially those aged 1 year or younger, are more likely to have *Pneumocystis carinii* pneumonia (PCP); have severe progressive encephalopathy, wasting, or both; and die earlier. Older children tend to have a less serious course, which is characterized by recurrent bacterial infections, LIP, nephropathy, and thrombocytopenia. The time course for vertically transmitted HIV infection to progress to AIDS in children is variable and may be more than 10 years; however, in children, AIDS is most commonly seen between 5 and 8 months.[53,54] The density of CCR5 receptor on nonactivated T cells correlates with the decline of CD4+ T cells and prognosis.[55]

Epidemiology

In the United States the prevalence of HIV is increasing because more people are living with HIV infection because of access to antiretroviral treatment.[56] An increase in all sexually transmitted diseases between homosexual partners suggests complacency about the risks of HIV/AIDS and poor compliance with safe sex practices. Fifty-five percent of new infections occur in African Americans. Infections in women appear to be related to their unknowingly having sex with bisexual or drug-injecting men.[49] Sub-Saharan Africa had the highest incidence of HIV infection with young women two and a half times more likely than men to be infected. Because of cultural, economic, and political factors, HIV prevention and treatment have been only slowly introduced in this region. East Africa and Central Africa have reduced the prevalence of HIV infection through educational programs. In Western Europe many new cases of HIV/AIDS are reported from persons who emigrated from or traveled to countries with a high HIV prevalence.[57]

As of December 2003, 2.5 million children lived with HIV/AIDS worldwide, of which 700,000 were infected and 500,000 died annually.[57] Vertical transmission of HIV infection from untreated mother to fetus occurs at a rate of 20% to 35% but is reduced by 66% when antiretroviral therapy monotherapy (zidovudine [ZDV]) is taken during pregnancy, delivery, and the neonatal period.[58,59] When used in combination with elective cesarean delivery and formula feeding, perinatal antiretroviral therapy has reduced the vertical transmission of HIV to less than 2% in the United States. Even simple inexpensive monotherapy can reduce vertical transmission by 40% to 50%, but it is available in only a few developing countries.[58,59] In South Africa in 2002, 25% of pregnant women tested positive for HIV. Seventy percent of African countries have no programs to reduce perinatal HIV transmission.[57] In Malawi, without antiretroviral therapy, the mortality rate at 3 years of age for HIV-infected children reached 89%.[60] This high mortality rate may be related to the burdens of infectious diseases and malnutrition. In contrast, 75% of HIV-infected children in the United States are alive at age 5 years.[60]

TABLE 86–2

Adverse Effects of Antiretroviral Agents

NUCLEOSIDE ANALOGUE REVERSE TRANSCRIPTASE INHIBITORS	
Almost all produce headache, GI distress, fever; less frequently peripheral neuropathy, pancreatitis, and lactic acidosis with hepatomegaly occur	
Abacavir	5% severe hypersensitivity reaction
Didanosine (ddl)	
Lamivudine	
Stavudine	
Zalcitabine	
Zidovudine	Bone marrow suppression, myopathy, mitochondrial dysfunction, liver toxicity
NONNUCLEOSIDE REVERSE TRANSCRIPTASE INHIBITORS	
Almost all produce headache, fatigue, GI distress and rash sometimes progressing to Stevens-Johnson syndrome	
Delavirdine	
Efavirenz	CNS alterations: somnolence, delirium
Nevirapine	Hepatitis, hypersensitivity reaction
PROTEINASE INHIBITORS	
Almost all produce headache, GI distress, paresthesias, rash; less frequently pancreatitis, hyperglycemia	
Amprenavir	Rash including Stevens-Johnson syndrome, diabetes mellitus
Indinavir	Asymptomatic hyperbilirubinemia, nephrolithiasis, elevated lipids
Lopinavir/ritonavir	
Nelfinavir	
Ritonavir	Increased liver transaminases
Saquinavir	Exacerbation of chronic liver disease

Modified from Van Rossum AM, Fraaij PL, de Groot R: Efficacy of highly active anti-retroviral therapy in HIV-1 infected children, *Lancet Infect Disease* 2:93, 2002.

CNS, central nervous system; *GI,* gastrointestinal.

Antiretroviral Therapy

In the United States, antiretroviral therapy for HIV-infected children was initiated in 1985 with ZDV, a reverse transcriptase inhibitor, as monotherapy.[61] As of February 2000, 14 antiretroviral agents were approved for use in the United States.[62] Because resistance develops with monotherapy, multiple drug regimens known as *highly active antiretroviral therapy* (HAART) are used in children and adults.[62] Measurement of both HIV-1 viral load (by RNA PCR) and the number of CD4+ T cells[48,62] is performed to monitor the effectiveness of HAART. Fifty percent to 70% of adults have a significant reduction in viral load in response to current HAART regimens; however, baseline viral loads are higher in children than in adults and have a slower decay rate after the introduction of HAART.[63] Pediatric studies in which dosage adjustments were directed by pharmacokinetics resulted in superior decreases in viral loads compared with fixed dosages based on weight.[63] Each antiretroviral therapy has its own toxicity and potential for drug interactions (Table 86–2).

Ninety percent of HIV-infected children live in sub-Saharan Africa and underdeveloped countries of Asia.[57] The care of these children is complicated by overcrowding, limited access to clean water, and malnutrition, which contributes to the high frequency of TB, cytomegalovirus (CMV), hepatitis, and gastroenteritis seen in this population. In Durban, South Africa, for example, patients with symptoms who have the ability to pay have access to four antiretroviral agents; monitoring consists of blood counts with differentials and liver function tests.[60] Because of a lack of funding and infrastructure, more than 95% of patients in sub-Saharan Africa are not receiving antiretroviral therapy, and few other interventions, such as prophylaxis, are provided.[57]

Most data regarding outcome and survival of HIV-infected children presented in this chapter are drawn from patients who did not receive antiretroviral therapy from the time of birth and may have never received it. Such data are likely still applicable to underdeveloped countries. Additionally, in countries with a high incidence of HIV infection, such as South Africa, the contribution of HIV infection to hospitalization rates from other common pediatric diseases such as respiratory syncytial virus (RSV), parainfluenza, TB, and bacteremia is difficult to assess.[64]

Pulmonary Complications and Respiratory Failure

Pulmonary complications remain the most frequent indication for admission of children with AIDS to an ICU.[64] Bacterial pneumonia is common in this population, but it is not likely to cause serious respiratory obstruction unless superimposed on already compromised lung function.[65,66]

Along with the usual pathogens frequently seen in childhood, such as *Streptococcus pneumoniae* and mycoplasma, immunodeficient children are also susceptible to pseudomonal and staphylococcal infections.[66,67] The incidence of *Hemophilus influenzae* infection is declining where vaccination is available. Empiric therapy for pneumonia in such children should cover the most common pathogens and be based on hospital-specific susceptibility profiles.

Pneumocystis Carinii Pneumonia

Although increased emphasis on early prophylaxis has reduced its incidence, PCP is still the most common AIDS-defining illness in pediatrics.[37,64,66,67] Children not previously recognized to be infected with HIV have symptoms of this complication between 4 and 6 months of age, which coincides with the timing of a natural decline in maternal antibodies. In children known to be infected with HIV, PCP prophylaxis is indicated from birth as CD4+ T cell counts obtained before the development of infection are not predictive of infection and can drop precipitously.[54,68-70] PCP generally presents with cough, fever, tachypnea, and dyspnea of several days' duration. Physical examination typically reveals retractions and grunting. Auscultation of the chest may reveal normal examination findings or rales, rhonchi, and wheezing. The chest radiograph generally shows diffuse interstitial infiltrates with decreased lung volume. Pulmonary infiltrates can be variable in children, in part because infants have a greater propensity for atelectasis.[71] Hypoxemia is likely to be out of proportion during clinical and radiographic examinations. A selectively elevated serum lactate dehydrogenase level is suggestive, although not diagnostic of PCP.[71] For a confirmation of a PCP diagnosis, bronchoalveolar lavage should be performed. Flexible fiberoptic bronchoscopy has a diagnostic yield of 90% to 97% and allows one to look for other pathogens as well.[72,73] Nonbronchoscopic bronchoalveolar lavage and sputum induction can also be used.[74-76] Patients in whom no diagnosis is obtained from bronchoalveolar lavage should undergo an open lung biopsy. This procedure has a diagnostic yield for PCP of 97%.[77]

The preferred antiprotozoal therapy for PCP is the combination of trimethoprim and sulfamethoxazole (TMP-SMX) (20 mg/kg/day trimethoprim).[48,78] Patients in whom this combination agent fails have not been shown to respond to a change in antiprotozoal therapy. In fact, higher doses of both components may be required to achieve therapeutic levels in critically ill patients.[41] Sulfa allergy as manifested by severe drug eruptions including Stevens-Johnson syndrome is less frequent in children than in adults; however, this complication may prompt a change to therapy with pentamidine isethionate (4 mg/kg/day).[48,79] When adverse events such as pancreatitis and renal failure occur as a result of pentamidine, atovaquone (40 mg/kg/day) is an alternative treatment.[80] Twenty-one days of therapy are followed by prophylactic therapy for which TMP-SMX is also the agent of choice. For patients allergic to sulfa, PCP prophylaxis can be achieved with pentamidine, dapsone, or atovaquone, although these agents have not been rigorously studied in children.

Several adult randomized controlled trials showed efficacy of high-dose steroids in adults with moderate PCP.[81] Although no controlled studies have been performed in children, improved outcomes in children who received corticosteroids have been described in several case studies.[82,83] Even in the face of respiratory failure, the survival rates reported with adjunctive corticosteroids therapy are 91% to 100% in a limited number of children.[84,85] Because PCP mimics other diseases such as miliary TB and CMV pneumonitis, PCP should be confirmed and other coinfections excluded before corticosteroid administration. Before the use of corticosteroid therapy, CMV coinfection did not increase the likelihood of death from PCP,[86] but corticosteroids may provide additional immunosuppression allowing invasive CMV disease to develop.[87,88] Adults who have respiratory failure despite adjunctive corticosteroids have a high risk of death. Failure to improve after 5 days of mechanical ventilation and the development of pneumothorax were strongly predictive of death in adults.[89]

Because the alveoli of patients infected with pneumocystis are filled with protozoal and inflammatory cells, PCP is associated with a reduced functional residual capacity. A ventilator management strategy that increases functional residual capacity while avoiding barotrauma is optimal. Because many of these patients are small infants in whom the second inflection point of the lung's pressure-volume curve is reached at relatively low peak and mean airway pressures, early institution of high frequency oscillatory ventilation may be warranted.

Cytomegalovirus Pneumonitis

Children at risk for vertical transmission of HIV are also at risk for CMV infection. The presentation of CMV pneumonitis can closely mimic that of PCP with diffuse interstitial infiltrates and hypoxemia, but there is generally a more insidious onset; however, some reports of a more fulminant course exist.[87,90] Failure of PCP to respond to conventional therapy may be evidence of concomitant CMV infection. Signs of retinitis, hepatitis, or colitis should be evaluated in patients with pneumonia because they may indicate CMV disease.

The definitive diagnosis of CMV pneumonitis must be made by identification of characteristic intracellular viral inclusion bodies in pulmonary macrophages or biopsy specimen because recovery of CMV from bronchoalveolar lavage by culture may represent viral shedding rather than invasive disease.[91] Detection of viral antigen by immunofluorescence is a second confirmatory test.[91] Serological markers of CMV are not useful in HIV-infected adults.[92] The treatment for CMV disease, in addition to HAART, is ganciclovir 5 mg/kg given twice daily followed by long-term suppressive therapy.[66] Foscarnet and cidofovir have been used in other immunosuppressed patients, but these drugs have significant nephrotoxicity.[93,94] The use of CMV immunoglobulin has not been studied in patients with AIDS.

Several authors reported life-threatening CMV of infection when corticosteroids were given to children with AIDS.[83,85,88] Although the numbers of patients reported are inadequate to allow control group comparisons, the possible increase in invasive CMV disease seen in children treated with corticosteroids may reflect the higher incidence of primary infection rather than reactivation of a preexisting infection in this age group. Although solid organ transplant recipients receive prophylaxis against CMV disease with ganciclovir either with or without high anti-CMV titer immunoglobulin, this approach has not been applied to patients with AIDS. The exclusive use of CMV-negative blood products in seronegative patients may reduce the risk of primary infection.

Other Viral Pathogens

Children with AIDS are more likely to experience lower tract disease and pneumonia when contracting RSV and influenza.[95,96] For RSV, the estimated incidence of lower tract disease was twofold greater in HIV-infected children. It is not clear that HIV-infection increases the likelihood of death.[96,97] The American Academy of Pediatrics Committee of Infectious Diseases stated that aerosolized ribavirin should be considered in severe cases of RSV.[98] The decision to use ribavirin therapy and the duration of therapy must be individualized. The incidence of lower respiratory tract disease requiring hospitalization in influenza was eightfold higher in children with HIV infection.[95] HIV-infected children with influenza pneumonia were older and more likely to have another underlying disease or concurrent infection. Despite these comorbidities there was no difference in clinical outcome. Two M2 blockers (effective against influenza A only) and two neuraminidase inhibitors are licensed for use in children but are most effective when given in the first 48 hours of illness.[99] Adenovirus also causes serious respiratory infection in patients with AIDS.[100-102] Ribavirin and cidofovir have been effectively used against this infection.[103-106] Other pathogenic viruses recovered from pediatric patients with AIDS include parainfluenza, herpes simplex, and measles. In vitro data suggest ribavirin and cidofovir may be effective against some of these viral pathogens; however, evidence of in vivo efficacy is limited to anecdotal reports in immunosuppressed patients.[94,107]

Mycobacterial Pathogens

Worldwide, approximately one third of the human population is infected with the *Mycobacterium* bacillus.[108] Most of these individuals live in developing countries where the prevalence of HIV infection is high.[109] The incidence of *Mycobacterium tuberculosis* (TB) appeared to level off in the United States by 1985 but began rising steadily in 1988—an increase attributed to the AIDS epidemic.[110] The increased incidence of pediatric TB is likely due to increased exposure to adults with active infection.[110] HIV-infected children with TB have higher CD4+ T-cell counts than those observed with other classic opportunistic infections.[54] Although adults generally acquire HIV infection after acquiring TB, the opposite is true in children. Thus the HIV-infected child never has a chance to mount an immunological response to *M. tuberculosis.*

In contrast to adults who have apical, cavitary lesions, children have more peripheral disease.[108] Most pediatric patients with AIDS have diffuse infiltrates consistent with LIP or PCP.[111] These children also have a high incidence of extrapulmonary manifestations such as hepatosplenomegaly and meningitis.

Aggressive efforts to confirm mycobacterium infection by culture are required because anergy obscures Mantoux testing, as well as the development of pleural effusions and localized lymphadenopathy. Use of PCR to identify *M. tuberculosis* nucleic acids in bronchoalveolar lavage and cerebrospinal fluid (CSF) specimens can accelerate the ability to diagnose this infection.[112] Recovery of mycobacterium by sputum induction has been reported in infants and very young children.[74] In some regions, organism recovery is necessary for antimicrobial susceptibility determination; 25% of isolates are resistant.[61] In countries where the diagnostic approaches are not readily available, it is useful to have radiographs of family members.[113]

Pending sensitivity reports, treatment of TB is initiated with a five-drug regimen.[114] The presence of multidrug resistance increases the likelihood of death. These patients should simultaneously be treated with antiretroviral therapy; however, rifampin is contraindicated with protease inhibitors and nonnucleoside reverse transcriptase inhibitors.[114] During HAART, reconstitution of the immune system may increase the inflammatory response to pulmonary TB. Children with TB and HIV infection who are not treated with HAART have a higher mortality rate than children not infected with HIV.[115] They must be treated for a longer time, perhaps because of poor drug absorption and a weakened immune system.[116]

Mycobacterium avium-intracellulare complex (MAC) can also be recovered from the lungs of children with pneumonia.[66] Colonization is difficult to differentiate from invasive disease. Treatment options include coverage with clarithromycin in combination with ethambutol, rifabutin, or amikacin. Primary prophylaxis once a week with azithromycin is recommended in children older than 2 years and younger than 1 year with CD4 counts persistently below 75. Children aged between 1 and 2 years should receive prophylaxis for CD4 counts less than 50.[66]

Fungal Infections

Pulmonary *Candida* infections are difficult to document. *Candida* is frequently recovered from sputum and bronchoalveolar lavage samples in children with AIDS, but whether it is a true pathogen is questionable. Documentation of pulmonary parenchymal involvement must be done with an open lung biopsy in a small child.[116] In adults in whom a biopsy specimen can be obtained by bronchoscopy, *Candida* is thought to be a rare cause of pulmonary disease but a more frequent cause of bronchitis.[117]

Aspergillosis has also been reported in adult patients with AIDS who are severely debilitated.[117] This complication is seen in older children with multiple opportunistic infections, prolonged hospitalization, neutropenia, and corticosteroid use.[116] Unlike *Candida,* recovery of aspergillosis from the respiratory tract is indicative of invasive disease. Both *Candida* and aspergillosis are treated with amphotericin. For the reduction of renal toxicity, liposomal amphotericin products may be used, and higher doses may be tolerated. Caspofungin is indicated when amphotericin is poorly tolerated. Itraconazole can be used as consolidation therapy (5 to 12 mg/kg/day orally), but the incidence of drug–drug interactions is high.

Cryptococcosis occurs in 5% to 15% of adults but in only 0.6% to 1% of children.[116] This ubiquitous organism enters the body through the respiratory tract. Therefore initial symptoms are generally both pulmonary and nonspecific. Bronchoalveolar lavage fluid should be examined by India ink stain and culture. Blood culture and latex agglutination are also necessary. There have been no therapeutic trials in children. Recommended therapy is amphotericin B in combination with 5-flucytosine (100 mg/kg/day) for 2 weeks followed by fluconazole (12 mg/kg/day divided in two doses) for 8 additional weeks.[116] Lifelong prophylaxis with fluconazole at 6 mg/kg/day is recommended. Cryptococcal antigen titers are useful in the evaluation of possible relapse. Prophylaxis for the prevention of cryptococcal disease is not recommended in children.

Fusariosis has been reported in neutropenic patients with AIDS. Other fungal infections such as histoplasmosis, cryptococcosis, coccidiomycosis, and disseminated *Penicillium marneffei* are reported in patients with AIDS who are living in or traveling through endemic areas.[66,118]

Lymphoid Interstitial Pneumonitis

LIP is a lymphoproliferative disorder associated with viral infections. In children LIP is almost exclusively seen with Epstein-Barr virus (EBV) and HIV.[119] LIP occurs in 30% to 50% of pediatric patients with AIDS, presenting in the second year of life in that patient population with high antibody titers and recurrent bacterial infections. Generally the children also have diffuse lymphadenopathy and hepatosplenomegaly. Children with LIP may have mild pulmonary symptoms such as dry cough but generally are admitted to the pediatric ICU only when an acute infection is superimposed on their chronic condition. When such is the case, maximal therapy of the acute exacerbation is indicated, including mechanical ventilation. On chest radiograph hilar adenopathy and reticulonodular infiltrates are seen. Pulmonary function tests reveal reduced lung volumes and diffusing capacity. Histologically, peribronchial lymphoid nodules containing plasma cells and lymphocytes are observed. Most specimens show predominantly CD8-positive T cells.

Spontaneous radiographic resolution was reported in 65% of children with LIP.[120] Patients with hypoxemia are treated with steroids, and resolution is seen in most patients in 2 to 4 weeks. If the patient is persistently febrile, MAC infection should be ruled out before steroid administration.[66]

Upper Airway Obstruction

Young children and infants have upper airway obstruction with greater frequency than adults. Whereas classic viral laryngotracheitis is the most common cause in the immunocompetent patient, immunocompromised patients are susceptible to a greater variety of infectious entities, including bacterial tracheitis, CMV-related ulceration of the trachea, and *Candida* infections of the airway oropharynx.[121-123] Although in the general population *Staphylococcus aureus* is the most commonly reported cause of bacterial tracheitis, *Pseudomonas* species are a frequent cause of tracheitis in patients with AIDS. There are multiple reports of Kaposi's sarcoma causing airway obstruction in adult patients with AIDS.[124-127] Given the complexity of the differential diagnosis of stridor in this population, early laryngoscopy and bronchoscopy are indicated. Recurrent tracheitis may be an indication for tracheostomy. Length of stay and outcome are not affected by the presence of HIV infection.[122]

Cardiovascular Complications

Septic Shock (see also Chapter 96)

In the era of PCP prophylaxis, severe sepsis is becoming the most common reason for ICU admission in patients with AIDS.[128] Of bacteremia episodes with an identified organism identified in the Pediatric AIDS Clinical Trials Group, 69% were pneumococcal.[54] In this study there was a low incidence of *H. influenzae* probably because of vaccination. HIV-infected patients do appear to be more susceptible to *S. aureus* and *Pseudomonas* infections. In one series of pediatric patients with AIDS, 10% of patients had gram-negative bacillary bacteremia with a risk of death that was greater than 40%.[129] *Pseudomonas* sepsis accounted for 26% of these episodes.[129] *Pseudomonas* infection is frequently associated with neutropenia, which may be the cause or effect of *Pseudomonas* sepsis.[128,129]

Candidaemia leading to disseminated candidiasis is a common complication of prolonged hospitalization and indwelling catheters.[130] Fifty percent of isolates may be non–*Candida albicans*; thus amphotericin is necessary as first-line therapy. These infections require a high index of suspicion. Thrombocytopenia is suggestive of candidal infection and should prompt empiric antifungal therapy if the patient is deteriorating. Catheter removal is mandatory if the catheter is infected.

Vasculitis

Vasculitis has been reported in patients with HIV infection, but it is not clear if HIV causes the condition or is merely an association.[131-134] Many infections reported in HIV-infected patients, including herpes viruses and mycobacterium, can cause inflammation by direct infection or an immune-mediated response. The most frequently involved organs are skin, peripheral nerve or muscle, and the central nervous system (CNS).[132] Several cases of polyarteritis nodosa have been reported.[132] When vasculitis is noted, an infectious agent should be sought. We have observed an increased incidence of arterial catheter complications in HIV-infected children.

Myocardial Dysfunction

Cardiac dysfunction develops in 19% to 25% of HIV-infected children and is the presenting sign in a minority of children.[135,136] About 10% of the survey population had chronic congestive heart failure, whereas another 10% had transiently decreased ventricular function.[112] Cardiac complications appear to occur more frequently in rapidly progressing patients with encephalitis and other AIDS-defining illnesses. Because tachycardia and hepatomegaly are so common in pediatric AIDS patients with fever, pulmonary infection, and anemia, a clinical diagnosis of cardiac involvement is difficult to make. Enlargement of the cardiac silhouette may not be appreciable even in patients with significant muscle hypertrophy or pericardial effusion. Given these inherent difficulties in the detection of cardiac disease, assessment of a critically ill child with AIDS should include echocardiography. When assessment is prospectively followed by echocardiography, the earliest sign of cardiac involvement is diastolic dysfunction.[136] Progressive left ventricular dilatation is sometimes accompanied by hypertrophy, but hypertrophy is insufficient to reduce peak systolic wall stress.[137] At autopsy, aside from the biventricular dilatation, macroscopic evidence of cardiac dysfunction has been difficult to find in adults or children. Microscopically, in a limited number of cases, lymphocytic infiltrates are observed, but actual myocyte necrosis is rare.[138] Mild foci of lacy interstitial fibrosis also occur.[138,139] True myocyte inflammation or myocarditis is rare in children.

HIV cardiomyopathy likely has several causes. Direct evidence of myocardial infection by HIV-1 has been documented by culture, Southern blot test, and in situ hybridization,[140-142] but it is unclear if the myocytes, which contain no CD4 receptors, harbor HIV. Coxsackie B3 virus, CMV, adenovirus, EBV, and *Toxoplasmosis gondii* have been identified as pathogens.[140,141] Of 32 HIV-infected children who died, 7 had evidence of CMV infection and 10 had evidence of adenovirus infection by PCR performed on myocardial tissue.[140] Selenium deficiency has been documented in severely malnourished children with AIDS whose cardiac function improved after selenium supplementation.[143] In additional case reports, ZDV is indicated as a cause of cardiac failure.[141]

In the ICU, patients with severe cardiac dysfunction respond to management of preload, increasing contractility, and afterload reduction. Endocarditis, myocardial ischemia, and other potentially treatable causes of cardiac dysfunction should be ruled out with electrocardiography and echocardiography. Pharmacological afterload reduction should be considered as first-line therapy, with digitalization and diuretic therapy as appropriate. Other than selenium supplementation there is no direct therapy available for HIV-related cardiomyopathy.[143] Agents that are associated with myocardial dysfunction, such as pentamidine, foscarnet, and dideoxyinosine (ddI), should be avoided.[141,144] A small population of patients has been noted to have transient cardiac dysfunction manifested by tachycardia and poor peripheral perfusion despite adequate filling pressures. This has been noted during PCP infection and may be related to cytokine release. Survival data following clinically evident congestive heart failure in children undergoing HAART have not been reported.

Dysrhythmias

In a survey of 81 HIV-infected children, dysrhythmias occurred in 35% of children, including atrial and ventricular ectopy, ventricular tachycardia, and ventricular fibrillation.[135] A syndrome of autonomic dysfunction has been reported in adult patients with AIDS, and similar lability in blood pressure and heart rate has been noted in a number of children. Catecholamine surges have been described in adults. Additionally peripheral neuropathy may contribute to altered vascular regulation and a propensity for cardiac arrhythmias.

Pericardial Disease

Pericardial disease is reported in approximately 30% of children undergoing echocardiography or autopsy.[135,139] In five pediatric patients in whom fluid was cultured, no pathogens were identified. In 14 adult patients in whom fluid was obtained, atypical mesothelial cells were identified. One patient had lymphoma, one had histoplasmosis, and a third had CMV identified by a pericardial biopsy specimen. A pericardial effusion greater than 5 mm in diameter was detected in 5.4% of prospectively evaluated HIV-infected children, but no episodes of tamponade were reported.[136,145] Cardiac arrest due to tamponade has been reported in five adult patients with AIDS.[146]

Renal Failure

HIV nephropathy was first reported in 1983 and may often be the first manifestation of AIDS.[147-149] This complication generally arises between ages 2.5 and 4.9 years. It appears to be more prevalent in children of African or Afro-Caribbean descent. The usual presentation of renal dysfunction is severe proteinuria (>3.5 g/day) with hypoalbuminemia and anasarca. This may be associated with renal tubular acidosis. Creatinine clearance is usually normal. Proteinuria may be accompanied by hematuria. Immunoglobulins are usually elevated while complement is normal. On ultrasound, the kidneys are enlarged. Biopsy specimens show focal and segmental glomerulosclerosis.[148] Atypical hemolytic uremic syndrome is also described in pediatric patients with AIDS.[150]

The course of the disease before HAART was usually fulminant, with end-stage renal disease developing in 8 to 9 months. Uncontrolled studies indicate that antiretroviral therapy slows or reverses the course of HIV nephropathy.[151] Corticosteroids and other immunosuppressant therapies have not been studied systematically in HIV nephropathy for fear of infectious complications.

Potentially nephrotoxic drugs to which the HIV-infected patient may be exposed are legion. Pentamidine-induced renal toxicity usually occurs in the second week of therapy. Proteinuria and particularly hematuria, which may be falsely attributed to HIV nephropathy or catheter-induced trauma, are hallmarks of pentamidine toxicity. Early recognition of this complication and cessation of pentamidine are key to recovery; rechallenge with the drug will prompt early return of proteinuria and hematuria. Toxicity from sulfadiazine during the treatment of toxoplasmosis is also reported and can be reduced by hydration.[152] Amphotericin-induced nephrotoxicity is particularly problematic when the drug is used in combination with aminoglycosides. Liposomal-encapsulated amphotericin B allows for higher doses with less toxicity.

In critically ill patients with AIDS, acute tubular necrosis may be precipitated by sepsis, hypovolemia, or hypoperfusion, and as in non–HIV-infected patients, it is reversible. Thus the same principles for management and support of a patient with reversible acute renal failure apply to the HIV-infected population. For patients who are seen in the ICU with end-stage renal disease due to HIV nephropathy, the indications for dialysis are the same as in other patient populations, but the decision to undertake dialysis must be made on an individual basis. Peritonitis during ambulatory peritoneal dialysis in pediatric patients with AIDS does not occur with any apparent greater frequency than in immunocompetent patients.[153]

Typically in patients with renal failure, interstitial infiltrates and hypoxemia suggest pulmonary edema due to fluid overload. Management of the immunocompromised patient should include assessment of cardiac filling pressures and diagnostic bronchoalveolar lavage because it is impossible to clinically distinguish between infectious and noninfectious causes of ARDS.

Abdominal Complications

Patients with AIDS have multiple gastrointestinal complaints including dysphagia, abdominal pain, and chronic diarrhea, but these are generally not important in the ICU except that they affect nutritional status. Other more life-threatening complications include severe dehydration, intraabdominal sepsis, pancreatitis, and hepatic failure (Table 86–3).

Gastroenteritis

Diarrhea occurs in 40% to 60% of children with AIDS and may produce severe dehydration in children.[53,154] Worldwide, acute diarrhea is the most common cause of death in children with AIDS.[154] In underdeveloped countries where poor sanitation increases the risk of diarrheal diseases, HIV-related hypovolemic shock is a common indication for pediatric ICU admission. Copious diarrhea is suggestive of small intestine involvement, whereas tenesmus suggests infection involving the distal colon and rectum. Diffuse enterocolitis produces a secretory diarrhea with profound volume losses. Patients with AIDS may have typical infectious enteritis and enterocolitis caused by salmonella, shigella, *Giardia, Campylobacter,* and rotavirus, but may also have an atypical, more prolonged course.[155] The frequent use of systemic antibiotics in HIV-infected children results in *Clostridium difficile* colitis. MAC, *Cryptosporidium, Giardia* and *Isospora belli*, CMV, and adenovirus may all induce opportunistic small bowel enteropathy.[121,154,156-158] Patients with MAC, CMV, and *Candida* infection typically also have extragastrointestinal infection.[154] A nonspecific enteropathy may arise as a result of the overgrowth of normal gut flora due to the effects of local immunodeficiency and antibiotic use. It is not uncommon to find heavy growth of *C. albicans* or *Pseudomonas aeruginosa* in stool cultures.

If findings from stool culture and analysis are negative, a flexible sigmoidoscopy with a rectal biopsy should be considered in the child with rectal bleeding, tenesmus, or both.

TABLE 86–3

Gastrointestinal Complications in Immunodeficient Patients

- Diarrhea
  - Bacteria
    - *Salmonella*
    - *Shigella*
    - *Clostridium difficile*
  - Fungi
    - *Candida*
    - *Pneumocystis*
    - Viruses
    - CMV
    - Herpes
    - Varicella
    - Adenovirus
    - Rotavirus
  - Parasites
    - *Cryptosporidium*
    - *Microsporidium*
    - *Entamoeba histolytica*
    - *Giardia intestinalis*
    - *Blastocystis hominis*
  - Medications
    - Atovaquone
    - Antiretrovirals
- Pancreatitis
  - Infections
    - CMV
    - Adenovirus
  - Medications
    - Protease inhibitors
    - Pentamidine
    - Foscarnet

A rectal biopsy combined with microbiological analysis of stool has been described as the most sensitive and specific diagnostic approach.[159] Aspiration of duodenal secretions is particularly helpful in evaluation of patients from underdeveloped countries in that the aspirate may reveal infection with *I. belli*, *Cryptosporidium parvum,* or helminthic species. Additional evaluation may be desirable, including small bowel radiography or abdominal computed tomography (CT) scanning. If results of all diagnostic studies are negative, diarrhea may be due to HIV therapy because most antiretroviral agents are associated with diarrhea.

MAC may be isolated from the blood in the presence of invasive disease. If indicated, percutaneous needle aspiration with CT guidance may be useful in the biopsy of enlarged intraabdominal nodes.[160,161] Antimicrobial therapy of disseminated MAC infection before HAART was unrewarding, and disseminated MAC was rapidly fatal. Current antimicrobial therapy is a double drug regimen of clarithromycin and ethambutol with the possible addition of a third agent, including rifabutin, ciprofloxacin, or azithromycin. Prophylaxis against MAC with azithromycin is indicated in children with CD4 counts less than 75/mm^3 and in infants with counts less than 100/mm^3.[162]

The Acute Abdomen (see also Chapter 82)

The evaluation and management of acute abdominal pain in HIV-infected children is complicated by their immunosuppressed state. Localized signs of infection can be masked by immunosuppression, debilitation, and previous or current use of antibiotics. In fact, a significant intraabdominal abscess may result in minor symptoms, with unremarkable elevations in white blood cell count or temperature. Thus diagnostic imaging with abdominal CT scan is invaluable for evaluation in this population.[163,164] Although morbidity after surgical intervention is somewhat higher in patients with AIDS, there is still a significant survival when such intervention is undertaken promptly.[165-167] Gastric and proximal small bowel symptoms such as pain or bleeding may arise from stress gastritis and infiltrative processes caused by viruses, particularly CMV and adenovirus, *Giardia lamblia*, and lymphoma. Supportive management of these conditions is the same as that for immunocompetent patients, although the appropriate antimicrobial therapy may be different.

Pancreatitis

Pancreatitis in the AIDS population results from both the disease and its treatment. Pancreatitis presents as acute or persistent midepigastric pain and elevation of serum amylase, lipase, and triglyceride levels. Infectious causative entities include CMV; adenovirus; mycobacterium; fungal infections; *Cryptococcus;* herpes simplex virus (HSV); and protozoal infections such as toxoplasmosis, pneumocystis, and cryptosporidium.[21] The list of drugs known to cause pancreatitis is extensive and includes the antiretroviral agent zalcitibine and the antiprotozoal agent pentamidine.[168-171] The mechanism by which drugs induce pancreatitis is unknown.

Pancreatitis often goes undiagnosed. Autopsy findings reveal significant pancreatic lesions in approximately 10% of patients with AIDS, yet pancreatic lesions are rarely recognized during life.[172] Nine of 53 children (17%) seen at one institution had pancreatitis.[173] Four of five of these carried CMV. In one of these patients CMV was cultured from pancreatic duct fluid. Six of nine had serological evidence of EBV. Five children were receiving pentamidine at the time of presentation. Maintaining a high index of suspicion for pancreatitis is important because vomiting, abdominal distension, and malabsorption are common complaints in the HIV-infected child. Evaluation of these patients should include both serum lipase and amylase determinations because parotid inflammation seen in HIV infection can cause isolated elevations of serum amylase concentrations. Abdominal ultrasound is only useful in the detection of a large edematous pancreas and in follow-up assessment for pancreatic pseudocyst.

Treatment includes bowel rest and hyperalimentation along with removal of the offending agent as in the case of drug-induced pancreatitis.[21,173] In infectious pancreatitis, treatment of the underlying cause, while indicated, may not change the course of the disease.[21,173] Despite intervention, seven of eight reported children with pancreatitis had active or recurrent disease at the time of death. The mean survival time from onset to death was 8 months (range, 0.5 to 13 months).[173] In this patient population anatomical abnormality is rarely the cause of pancreatitis, and there is little role for surgical intervention.

Hepatobiliary Failure

The cause of hepatic failure in HIV-infected patients differs from that of adults and is affected by the patient's degree of immunosuppression.[174] In early stages, hepatic disease is usually a result of drug toxicity or hepatotropic virus infection. Drug-induced hepatotoxicity has been reported with sulfa drugs, isoniazid, rifampin, rifabutin, and ddI.[174,175] As HIV progresses to AIDS the liver manifests systemic involvement of opportunistic infections.[174,176] Reviews of hepatic tissue disease in HIV-infected children document that CMV and mycobacterial disease are common in children, whereas classic viral hepatitis is relatively rare.[174,177,178]

Liver biopsy is only indicated when mycobacterial disease is expected or jaundice is present.[174] Drug toxicity has no specific disease. Other diseases can be diagnosed by serological testing or PCR. The HIV virus itself can cause a giant cell hepatitis. Dense lymphoid infiltrates, similar to those in the lung in LIP, are also described. Adenovirus and HSV can cause acute jaundice and hepatitis with fever.[174,179] Hepatitis B and C can occur in patients with AIDS.[180] Chronic hepatitis becomes clinically significant as survival increases in patients receiving HAART. Biopsy may be useful in those patients who progress to severe liver disease to direct therapy.[174]

Treatment of hepatic failure is supportive and aimed at reducing encephalopathy and hemorrhage. Because drug-induced hepatotoxicity may be reversible, aggressive support for this cause of hepatic failure is indicated. Hepatitis B can be treated with the antiretroviral agent lamivudine.[174] Hepatitis C can be treated with ribavirin and interferon.[180] In most cases HAART is suspended to hepatitis C therapy. Liver transplantation, once contraindicated, is now controversial.[181]

Cholangitis and cholecystitis are well described in adult patients with AIDS and will undoubtedly be seen more frequently in children as survival becomes more prolonged. Biliary tract infections have been attributed to CMV, adenovirus, *Cryptosporidium,* and *Microsporidia.*[182-184] Ultrasonography may be useful in evaluation of the hepatobiliary system; in limited cases, retrograde cholangiograms may prove helpful.

Hematologic Complications

Hematologic abnormalities are common in patients with HIV/AIDS. Isolated thrombocytopenia is likely mediated by antiplatelet antibodies and should prompt HIV testing.[185-187] As with other forms of antibody-mediated thrombocytopenia, this may respond to immunoglobulin.

In a case of chronic refractory thrombocytopenia, subtotal splenectomy was reported effective.[188] Neutropenia may be antibody mediated, drug related, or secondary to sepsis. Granulocyte colony growth factors have reduced the incidence of sepsis in this setting.[189,190]

Anemia occurs in 20% to 73% of HIV-infected children[191,192] and is an independent predictor of death from AIDS.[191,193] This may reflect anemia's role as a marker of inflammatory activity resulting in anemia of chronic disease or an indicator of opportunistic infections such as MAC that suppresses bone marrow erythropoiesis. Transfusion may accelerate the progression of AIDS.[193]

Most HIV-infected patients have normal erythrocyte size and shape but inadequate reticulocytosis. Iron deficiency, possibly related to malabsorption, accounts for 10% to 45% of anemia in HIV-infected children. Nutritional deficiencies of folate and vitamin B_{12} may also contribute to anemia. Many medications that are given to patients with AIDS cause anemia, including ZDV, acyclovir, TMP-SMX, and pentamidine. Anemia of chronic disease, mediated by inflammatory cytokines, likely accounts for additional cases. Rarely, antierythrocyte and antierythropoietin antibodies have been reported in patients with AIDS.[193] Pediatric patients with AIDS who have renal failure may lack erythropoietin.

Malignancies

Malignancies account for 2% of AIDS-defining illnesses in pediatric patients.[194] As in the other patients with congenital and acquired immunodeficiencies, the loss of the body's surveillance system against tumors appears to contribute to this increase.[195] Of 162 pediatric AIDS patients with malignancy reported to the CDC, 134 had non-Hodgkin's lymphoma and 28 had Kaposi's sarcoma.[195] Lymphomas are generally of the B-cell type and often arise in the CNS.[196] Other reported conditions include B-cell leukemia, hepatoblastoma, leiomyomas or leiomyosarcomas, and cervical carcinoma.[194,195]

Several of these malignancies are associated with chronic viral infection. Epstein-Barr virus DNA has been identified in most CNS tumors and in soft tissue tumors such as leiomyosarcomas or rhabdomyosarcomas reported in patients with AIDS.[196] EBV infection has also been associated with a polyclonal, polymorphic B-cell lymphoproliferative disorder similar to that seen in transplant patients receiving immunosuppression. In addition, in body cavity based lymphoma, infection with human herpes virus type 8 (HHV-8) has been implicated. HSV itself is associated with invasive cervical cancer.[197] Hepatitis B infection is associated with the development of hepatocellular carcinoma.

Kaposi's sarcoma is a malignancy unique to acquired immunodeficiencies seen in transplant and AIDS patients. Its true incidence in the pediatric AIDS population is unknown because many tumors are intraabdominal and intrathoracic; thus they are only noted on autopsy. Cutaneous manifestations are uncommon in the pediatric age group. This tumor has also been associated with chronic infection with HHV-8.[198]

Neurological Complications

CNS involvement occurs in 20% to 60% of HIV-infected children.[199] The clinical manifestations of CNS involvement are many, but generally it is the comatose patient with AIDS in the ICU who is a diagnostic dilemma. In this situation, treatable conditions must be ruled out before the diagnosis of AIDS encephalopathy can be made. Acute neurological manifestations include seizure disorders, cerebral vascular accidents, CNS lymphoma, and aseptic meningitis.[200] Evaluation of these patients generally requires a series of biochemical and radiological tests. Biochemical tests can reveal hyponatremia, hypoglycemia, and hyperammonemia, which can arise from severe malnutrition, hepatic dysfunction, and pancreatitis. A toxicology screen can rule out ingestion. Imaging studies such as CT and magnetic resonance imaging (MRI) can reveal mass-occupying lesions such as intracranial hemorrhage, malignancies, or calcifications consistent with infection.[201] Lumbar puncture is necessary to rule out infection and should be routinely cultured and investigated for specific pathogens.

Human Immunodeficiency Virus Encephalopathy

Primary HIV infection of the CNS probably occurs in 4% of HIV-infected children by the age of 12 months.[202] This entity is termed *HIV encephalopathy* and can generally be divided into two types: static with developmental delay or progressive similar to AIDS dementia in adults with progressive decline in neurologic functioning.[203] Direct HIV infection of the macrophages and microglia of the CNS is thought to cause release of inflammatory neurotoxins such as TNF or platelet-activating factor. Pathologically gliosis, microglial nodules, demyelination, and multinucleate giant cells are seen. Diffuse atrophy is noted on CT. Bifrontal white matter abnormalities are commonly seen on MRI.[201] In more severe cases periventricular and centrum semiovale hypodense areas may occur. One third of infected children may show calcifications of the basal ganglia. Calcifications observed before age 10 months are more likely due to an infection other than HIV, such as toxoplasmosis or CMV.[204]

Spinal cord examination similarly shows degeneration of corticospinal tracts, which clinically present as spastic diplegia.[205] Vacuolar myelopathy involving the lateral and posterior columns, which presents as progressive muscle wasting and sensory loss, has also been observed in children.[205,206]

AIDS encephalopathy is a diagnosis of exclusion. Other pathogens must be ruled out. Therefore evaluation includes imaging of the brain by CT or MRI and blood and CSF studies in search of specific pathogens such as *Cryptococcus*, mycobacterium, CMV, HSV, varicella-zoster virus, and *Treponema pallidum*. If no alternative pathogen is identified, then therapy is directed at reducing the HIV RNA viral load.[207] The antiretroviral agents with the best CNS penetration are ZDV, stavudine, and nevirapine.[48]

Cerebrovascular Disease

Vascular complications involving the CNS in HIV-infected patients are many.[208] A cerebral vasculopathy was reported to occur in 25% of patients who underwent an autopsy and is thought to account for the incidence of 1.3 strokes per year in HIV-infected children.[203] Although infarctions were first thought to be a consequence of direct HIV injury to the vascular endothelium, others now argue that the vascular injury results from other infections.[209,210] Cerebral vasculitis has been reported in CMV, HSV, neurosyphilis, and other infections of the CNS, even when they occur in non–HIV-infected patients. A hypercoagulable state associated with elevated levels of anticardiolipid antibody and antiphospholipid antibody, decreased levels of protein S, and a clinical condition similar to thrombotic thrombocytopenic purpura has also been described in association with HIV infection.[211] Although stroke is common in patients with AIDS, intracranial hemorrhage is relatively rare. Autoimmune-mediated thrombocytopenia, diffuse intravascular coagulation, and CMV infection have been reported to lead to intracranial hemorrhage in patients with AIDS.[201,205,208,212,213]

Central Nervous System Malignancy

High-grade B-cell lymphoma is found in 4% of HIV-infected children and is the most common mass lesion found in the CNS of children with AIDS.[199] It generally presents between ages 5 and 10 years. Lymphoma can be distinguished from toxoplasmosis by increased uptake of tracer on single photon emission computed tomography (SPECT) or positron emission tomography (PET) imaging. It most frequently arises in periventricular white matter and is associated with EBV infection. Metastatic lymphoma can also occur.

Infections of the Central Nervous System

CNS infection by usual and opportunistic organisms in childhood AIDS accounts for only 13% of neurologic complications.[214-216] Primary CNS infections in HIV-infected children are caused by the usual etiologic bacterial organisms and *M. tuberculosis*. The usual presenting signs and symptoms are seen. Opportunistic infections such as CMV and aspergillosis are frequently observed at autopsy and generally result from disseminated disease.[216] Reactivated infections such as toxoplasmosis, herpes zoster, and progressive multifocal leukoencephalopathy caused by Jacob-Creutzfeldt virus infection also occur but are rare when compared with those in the adult population.[199,216]

The protozoal infection toxoplasmic encephalitis occurs in 30% of adult patients with AIDS but is generally seen in only older children. The incidence of maternal-fetal transmission does not appear to be affected by maternal HIV infection. Combination therapy with sulfadiazine and pyrimethamine is generally effective if initiated early. Clindamycin is an appropriate alternative in patients with sulfa allergy.[217] Corticosteroids are sometimes used in addition to first-line therapy to reduce edema. Relapse is common after treatment is stopped and maintenance therapy is necessary. Primary prophylaxis is offered to adults with serological findings that are positive for *Toxoplasma* and a CD4 count of less than 200.

Progressive multifocal leukoencephalopathy presents with ataxia, aphasia, weakness, and lethargy.[214,218] CT may be relatively unremarkable with one or two nonenhancing hypodense areas of demyelination generally in subcortical white matter. MRI is more sensitive than CT for detection of these lesions. Presumptive diagnosis can be confirmed by stereotactic biopsy and identification of virus by DNA probes. There is no treatment for this condition, and death usually results from apnea.

Although not considered a reactivated infection, cryptococcal meningitis is typically seen in older children.[199,216] Cryptococcus spreads via the bloodstream to the CNS. Classic presentation includes fever, headache, and preceding alterations in mental status. Focal signs and meningeal signs are minimal. CSF counts may be normal, although intracranial pressure (ICP) is typically elevated. Wet mounts stained with India ink, cultures, CSF-antigen detection assays, and serum latex agglutination. CT findings are nonspecific.

Treatment of coma in the HIV-positive patient is directed at the underlying cause. Supportive care follows the principles of therapy for all comatose patients, including airway protection, control of ICP where appropriate, and nutritional support. Specific therapy for the underlying condition must be applied. In situations in which no explanation for an acute neurologic deterioration is readily available, we have initiated antiviral therapy with ganciclovir, acyclovir, or both and awaited clinical improvement. This decision was based on evidence that CMV coinfection may be responsible for neurologic deterioration.[210,216] Some improvement has been reported in patients with HIV encephalopathy who were treated with ZDV or ganciclovir therapy, but the waxing and waning nature of the condition even without therapy makes any intervention difficult to evaluate.

Ethical Issues

The history of respiratory failure due to PCP pneumonia in HIV-infected patients provides a vignette that shows many of the dilemmas surrounding the care of patients with AIDS. When the death rate was first reported as greater than 90% for these patients, many physicians refused to institute mechanical ventilation for this condition. Meanwhile, other physicians who would not concede that mechanical ventilation was hopeless eventually reported that the death rate for PCP-related respiratory failure was possibly only 50%, thereby stressing that such therapy was not futile. Physicians who were willing to try new therapies for PCP subsequently reported that the death rate could be reduced to 10% if corticosteroids were given. This story confirms that it is impossible to determine a therapy's efficacy at the outset of an individual patient's illness and a refusal to intervene only perpetuates the myth of futility. Only by continuing to care for these patients can physicians increase their clinical skills and obtain an opportunity to ultimately improve the survival of these patients.

Thus intervention and a trial of therapy appear indicated in all cases, bearing in mind that if the patient does not respond, care can be withdrawn. If time permits, before the therapy is instituted it is preferable to discuss with the patient or the patient's family the possibility of futility and the option to withdraw care should the therapy fail in the patient. Without these discussions both the parent and the physician may feel obligated to continue with ineffective therapy. Although a physician cannot determine quality of life for the patient or the patient's family, it is reasonable to discuss quality of life as a factor in the decision process. When a patient has multiple complications for which no other treatment is available, continuation of aggressive intervention for the immediately life-threatening illness is not indicated.

Because HIV-infected children are frequently orphaned, especially in underdeveloped countries, multiple ethical problems are created, including obtaining procedural consent, receiving permission to withdraw care, and planning follow-up care at discharge. Identification of the patient's guardian or health care surrogate should be made before emergencies arise. If no guardian is identified, the courts can appoint a guardian ad litem to make decisions for the child. The appointment of a surrogate who actually observes the child in the ICU setting helps counterbalance the urge to maintain life at all costs with an understanding suffering and futility.

Occupational Human Immunodeficiency Virus Exposure

Serious exposure to HIV in the health care setting is most likely to occur in the emergency department or ICU. The risk of exposure after a percutaneous exposure is 0.3%. This risk increases with exposure to a large bore needle previously inserted in an infected patient's vein or artery and in proportion to the source patient's viral load.[219] If both risk criteria are present, a three-drug prophylaxis regimen is recommended for 4 weeks. If only one is present, then a two-drug regimen is recommended. For smaller exposure, such as a skin puncture with suture needle, a two-drug regimen is also recommended. For mucous membrane and skin exposure to blood and blood-containing fluids, the risk of exposure is 0.1% and less than 0.1%, respectively, and therefore antiviral therapy is offered but not recommended. No prophylaxis is recommended for mucous membrane or skin exposure to body fluids other than blood. ZDV is the only agent proven to prevent transmission of HIV in humans and is therefore the first drug of choice in postexposure prophylaxis. Indinavir and nelfinavir used in prophylaxis regimens have been associated with hepatitis, nephrolithiasis, and pancytopenia and therefore should only be used in high-risk settings.

In summary, a critically ill child with a life-threatening infection or trauma should be presumed to be immunodeficient. The approach to such patients requires selective surveillance and a low threshold for empiric therapy. Through experience, patterns of infections characteristic of specific immunodeficient states can be recognized, but the unusual presentation is always possible. In the future, immune stimulants may also be part of the physician's armamentarium, in addition to antimicrobial therapy.

REFERENCES

1. Abbas AK, Lichtman AH, Pober JS: Congenital and acquired immune deficiency. *Cellular and molecular immunology,* ed 2, Philadelphia, 1994, WB Saunders.
2. South MA, Montgomery JR, Rawls WE: Immune deficiency in congenital rubella and other viral infections, *Birth Defects Orig Artic Ser* 11:234-238, 1975.
3. Thatte UM, Gangal PS, Kulkarni MR et al: Polymorphonuclear and monocyte functions in measles, *J Trop Pediatr* 37:67, 1991.
4. Safdar A, Armstrong D: Infectious morbidity in critically ill patients with cancer, *Crit Care Clin* 17:531, 2001.
5. Wolk K, Döcke WD, von Baehr V et al: Impaired antigen presentation by human monocytes during endotoxin tolerance, *Blood* 96: 218, 2000.
6. Volk HD, Reinke P, Krausch D et al: Monocyte deactivation-rationale for a new therapeutic strategy in sepsis, *Intensive Care Med* 22:S474, 1996.
7. Yadavelli GK, Auletta JJ, Gould M et al: Deactivation of the innate cellular immune response following endotoxic and surgical injury, *Exp Molecul Pathol* 71:209, 2001.
8. Asadallah K, Woiciechowsky C, Docke WD et al: Immunodepression following neurosurgical procedures, *Crit Care Med* 23:1976, 1995.
9. Napolitano LM, Fiast E, Wichmann MW et al: Immune dysfunction in trauma. *Surg Clin N Am* 79:1385, 1999.
10. Peters M, Petros A, Dixon G et al: Acquired immunoparalysis in pediatric intensive care: a prospective observational study, *BMJ* 319:609, 1999.
11. Reinke P, Volk HD: Diagnostic and predictive value of an immune monitoring program for complications after kidney transplantation, *Urol Int* 49:69, 1992.
12. Van den Burke JMM, Oldenberger RHJ, Van den Berg AP et al: Low HLA-DR expression on monocytes as a prognostic marker for bacterial sepsis after liver transplantation, *Transplantation* 63.1846, 1997.
13. Wakefield CH, Carey PD, Foulds S et al: Changes in major histocompatibility complex class II expression in monocytes and T cells of patients developing infection after surgery, *Br J Surg* 80:205, 1993.
14. Caulfield JJ, Fernandez MH, Sousa AR et al: Regulation of major histocompatibility complex class II antigens on human alveolar macrophages by granulocyte-macrophage colony-stimulating factor in the presence of glucocorticoids, *Immunology* 98:104-110, 1999.
15. DeMetz J, Sprangers F, Endert E et al: Interferon-γ has immunomodulatory effects with minor endocrine and metabolic effects in humans, *J Appl Physiol* 86: 517, 1999.
16. Wolk K, Döcke WD, von Baehr V et al: Comparison of monocyte function after LPS- or IL-10-induced reorientation: importance in clinical immunoparalysis, *Pathobiology* 67:253-256, 1999.
17. Hubel K, Dale DC, Liles WC: Therapeutic use of cytokines to modulate phagocyte function for the treatment of infectious diseases: current status of granulocyte colony stimulating factor, granulocyte-macrophage colony stimulating factor, macrophage- colony stimulating factor, and interferon gamma, *J Infect Dis* 185:1490, 2002.
18. Presneill JI, Harris T, Stewart AG et al: A randomized Phase II trial of granulocyte-macrophage colony stimulating factor therapy in severe sepsis with respiratory dysfunction, *Am J Resp Crit Care Med* 166:138-143, 2002.
19. Kox WJ, Bone RC, Krausch RC et al: Interferon gamma 1b in the treatment of compensatory anti-inflammatory response syndrome. A new approach: proof of principle, *Arch Intern Med* 157:389, 1997.
20. Nakos G, Malamou-Mitsi VD, Lachana A, et al: Immunoparalysis in patients with severe trauma and the effect of inhaled interferon-γ, *Crit Care Med* 30:1488, 2002.
21. Blumberg N, Heal JM: Effects of transfusion on immune function. Cancer recurrence and infection, Arch Pathol Lab Med 118:371, 1994.
22. Lagaaij EL, Riugrok MB, Van Rood JJ et al: Blood transfusion induced changes in cell-mediated lympholysis: to immunize or not to immunize, *J Immunol* 147:3348, 1991.
23. Tartter PI: Immunologic effects of blood transfusion, *Immunol Invest* 24;277, 1995.
24. Chelemer SB, Prato BS, Cox PM et al: Association of bacterial infection and red blood cell transfusion after bypass surgery, *Ann Thorac Surg* 73:138-142, 2002.

25. Offner PJ, Moore EE, Biffl WL et al: Increased rate of infection associated with transfusion of old blood after severe injury, *Arch Surg* 137:711-717, 2002.
26. Kirkley SA, Cowles J, Pelligrini VD et al: Blood transfusion and total joint replacement surgery: T helper 2 (TH2) cytokine secretion and clinical outcome, *Transfusion Med* 8:195, 1998.
27. Griffin MD, Xing N, Kumar R: Vitamin D and its analogs as regulators of immune activation and antigen presentation, *Annu Rev Nutr* 23:17, 2003.
28. Skoner DP, Angelini BL, Jones A et al: Suppression of in vivo cell-mediated immunity during experimental influenza A virus infection of adults, *Int J Pediatr Otorhinolaryngol* 38:143, 1996.
29. Piessens WF, Hoffman SL, Ratiwayanto S et al: Opposing effects of filariasis and chronic malaria on immunoregulatory T lymphocytes, *Diagn Immunol* 1:257, 1983.
30. Wedderburn N, Dracott BN: The immune response to type III pneumococcal polysaccharide in mice with malaria, *Clin Exp Immunol* 28:130, 1977.
31. Chandra RK: Nutrition and immunology: from the clinic to cellular biology and back again, Proc Nutr Soc 58:681, 1999.
32. Schwenk A, Macallan DC: Tuberculosis, malnutrition and wasting, *Curr Opin Clin Nutr Metab Care* 3:285, 2000.
33. Ball CS: Global issues in pediatric nutrition: AIDS, *Nutrition* 14(10): 767-770, 1998.
34. Woodward B: Protein, calories and immune defenses, *Nutr Rev* 56:S84, 1998.
35. Uauy R, Mena P, Valenzuela A: Essential fatty acids as determinants of lipid requirements in infants, children and adults, *Eur J Clin Nutr* 53:S66, 1999.
36. Field CJ, Johnson IR, Schley PD: Nutrients and their role in host resistance to infection, *J Leukocyte Biol* 72:16-32, 2002.
37. Bye MR, Bernstein LJ, Glaser J et al: Pneumocystis carinii pneumonia in young children with AIDS, *Pediatr Pathol* 9:251, 1990.
38. Jason J, Archibald LK, Nwanyanwu OC et al: Vitamin A levels and immunity in humans, *Clin Diagn Lab Immunol* 9:616, 2002.
39. Rosales FJ: Vitamin A supplementation of vitamin A deficient measles patients lowers the risk of measles related pneumonia in Zambian children, *J Nutr* 132:3700, 2002.
40. Stephensen CB: Vitamin A, infection, and immune function, *Annu Rev Nutr* 21:167, 2001.
41. Griffin DE: Immunologic abnormalities accompanying acute and chronic viral infections. *Rev Infect Dis* 13(suppl 1):S129, 1991.
42. Oken E, Duggan C: Update on micronutrients: iron and zinc, *Curr Opin Pediatr* 14:350, 2002.
43. Erikson KL, Medine EA, Hubbard NE: Micronutrients and innate immunity, *J Infect Dis* 182:S5, 2000.
44. Hirsch MS, D'Aquila RT: Therapy for immunodeficiency virus infection, *N Engl J Med* 328:1686, 1994.
45. Goulder P JR, Jeena P, Tudor-Williams G et al: Paediatric HIV infection: correlates of protective immunity and global perspectives in prevention and management, *Br Med Bull* 58: 89-108, 2001.
46. Walker AR: HIV infections in children, *Emerg Med Clin North Am* 13:147, 1995.
47. Krasinski K, Borkowsky W, Holzman RS: Prognosis of human immunodeficiency virus infection in children and adolescents, *Pediatr Infect Dis J* 8:216, 1989.
48. Laufer M, Scott GB: Medical management of HIV disease in children, *Pediatr Clin North Am* 47:127-153, 2000.
49. Mofenson LM: Technical report: perinatal human immunodeficiency virus testing and prevention of transmission. Committee on Pediatric AIDS, *Pediatrics* 106:E88, 2000.
50. Anonymous: 1994 revised classification system for immunodeficiency virus infection in children less than 13 years of age, *MMWR Morb Mortal Wkly Rep* 43:1, 1994.
51. Tovo PA, De Martino M, Gabiano C et al: Prognostic factors and survival in children with perinatal HIV infection, *Lancet* 339:1249, 1992.
52. Willoughby A: Epidemiology of human immunodeficiency virus infection in children, *Ann Allergy* 72:185, 1994.
53. Chui DW, Owen RL: AIDS and the gut, *J Gastroenterol Hepatol* 9:291, 1994.
54. Danker WM, Lindsey JC, Levin MJ et al: Correlates of opportunistic infections in children infected with the human immunodeficiency virus managed before highly active antiretroviral therapy, *Pediatr Infect Dis* J 20:40-48, 2001.
55. Gervaix A, Nicolas J, Portales P et al: Response to treatment and disease progression linked to CD4? T cell surface CC chemokine receptor density in human immunodeficiency virus type 1 vertical infection, *J Infect Dis* 185:1055-1061, 2002.
56. Centers for Disease Control and Prevention (CDC): Diagnosis and reporting of HIV and AIDS in states with HIV/AIDS surveillance—United States, 1994-2000, *MMWR Morb Mortal Wkly Rep* 51:595, 2002.
57. UNAIDS: Global summary of the HIV/AIDS epidemic: December 2003. Available at http://www.unaids.org/wad/2003/Epiupdate2003. Accessed ???.
58. Anonymous: Prevention of mother-to-child transmission of HIV: challenges for the current decade, *Bull World Health Org* 79:1138, 2001.
59. Anonymous: The global HIV and AIDS epidemic, *MMWR Morb Mortal Wkly Rep* 50:434, 2001.
60. Taha, TE, Graham SM, Kumwenda NI et al: Morbidity among human immunodeficiency virus-1-infected and uninfected African children, *Pediatrics* 106:6, 2000. Available at http://www.pediatrics/org/cgi/contents/full/106/6/e77. Accessed ???.
61. Krasinski K: Antiretroviral therapy for children, *Acta Pediatr* 400S:63, 1994.
62. Anonymous: Guidelines for the use of antiretroviral agents in HIV-infected adults and adolescents, *MMWR Morb Mortal Wkly Rep* 47: 43, 1998.
63. Van Rossum AM, Fraaij PLA, de Groot R: Efficacy of highly active anti-retroviral therapy in HIV-1 infected children, *Lancet Infect Disease* 2:93, 2002.
64. Zar HJ, Hanslo D, Tannenbaum E et al: Etiology and outcome of pneumonia in human immunodeficiency virus-infected children hospitalized in South Africa, *Acta Paediatr* 90:119, 2001.
65. Klein M, Zar H: ICU outcome in HIV-associated childhood pneumonia, *S Afr Med J* 88:1438, 1998.
66. Perez Mato S, Van Dyke RB: Pulmonary infections in children with HIV infection, *Semin Respir Infect* 17:33, 2002.
67. Nicholas SW: The opportunistic and bacterial infections associated with pediatric human immunodeficiency virus disease, *Acta Paediatr Suppl* 400:46, 1994.
68. CD4 T cell count predictor of *Pneumocystis carinii* pneumonia in children born to mothers infected with HIV. European Collaborative Study Group, *BMJ* 308:437, 1994.
69. Saunders-Laufer D, DeBruin W, Edelson P: *Pneumocystis carinii* infection in HIV-infected children, *Pediatr Clin North Am* 38:69, 1991.
70. Simonds RJ, Lindegren ML, Thomas P et al: Prophylaxis against *Pneumocystis carinii* pneumonia among children with perinatally acquired human immunodeficiency virus infection in the United States, *N Engl J Med* 332:786, 1995.
71. Zar HJ, Dechaboon A, Hanslo D et al: *Pneumocystis carinii* pneumonia in South African children infected with human immunodeficiency virus, *Pediatr Inf Dis J* 19:603, 2000.
72. Abadco DL, Amaro-Galvez R, Rao M et al: Experience with flexible fiberoptic bronchoscopy with bronchoalveolar lavage as a diagnostic tool in children with AIDS, *Am J Dis Child* 146:1056, 1992.
73. Golden JA, Hollander H, Stubarg MS et al: Bronchoalveolar lavage as the exclusive diagnostic modality for *Pnuemocystis carinii* pneumonia: a prospective study among patients with acquired immunodeficiency syndrome, *Chest* 90:18, 1986.
74. Zar HJ, Tannenbaum E, Apolles P et al: Sputum induction for the diagnosis of pulmonary tuberculosis in infants and young children in an urban setting in South Africa. *Arch Dis Child* 82:305, 2000.
75. Dargaville PA, South M, McDougall PN: Comparison of two methods of diagnostic lung lavage in ventilated infants with lung disease, *Am J Resp Crit Care Med* 160:771, 1999.
76. Morrow B, Argent A: Risks and complication of nonbronchoscopic bronchoalveolar lavage in a pediatric intensive care unit, *Pediatr Pulmonol* 32:378, 2001.
77. Mason WH, Seigel SE, Tacker BL: Diagnostic open lung biopsy for diffuse pulmonary disease in immunocompromised pediatric patients, *Am J Pediatr Hematol Oncol* 4:355, 1992.
78. Wharton JM, Coleman DL, Wofsky CB et al: Trimethoprim sulfamethoxazole or pentamidine for *Pneumocystis carinii* pneumonia in the acquired immunodeficiency syndrome, *Ann Int Med* 105:37, 1996.
79. Goa KL, Campoli-Richards DM: Pentamidine isethionate: a review of its antiprotozoal activity, pharmacokinetic properties and therapeutic use in *Pneumocystis carinii* pneumonia, *Drugs* 33:242, 1987.

80. White A, Lafon S, Rogers M et al: Clinical experience with atovaquone on a treatment investigation protocol for Pneumocystis carinii pneumonia, *J Acquir Immune Def Syndr Hum Retroviral* 9:2800, 1995.
81. Amundson GE, Murray KM, Brodine S et al: High-dose corticosteroids therapy for *Pneumocystis carinii* pneumonia in patients with acquired immunodeficiency syndrome, *South Med J* 82:711, 1989.
82. Bye MR, Cairns-Bazarian AM, Ewig JM: Markedly reduced mortality associated with corticosteroid therapy of *Pneumocystis carinii* pneumonia in children with acquired immunodeficiency syndrome, *Arch Pediatr Adolesc Med* 148:638, 1994.
83. Marriage SC, Nadel S, Kampmann B: Corticosteroid therapy for *Pneumocystis carinii* pneumonia, *J Pediatr* 127:1007, 1995.
84. McLaughlin GE, Virdee S, Schleien CL et al: Effect of corticosteroid on survival of children with acquired immunodeficiency syndrome and *Pneumocystis carinii*-related respiratory failure, *J Pediatr* 126:821, 1995.
85. Sleasman JW, Hemenway C, Klein AS et al: Corticosteroids improve survival of children with AIDS and *Pneumocystis carinii* pneumonia, *Am J Dis Child* 147:30, 1993.
86. Bozzettte SA, Arcia J, Bartok AE et al: Impact of concomitant viral pathogens on the course of *Pneumocystis carinii* pneumonia, *J Protozool* 38:183S, 1991.
87. Aukrust P, Farstad IN, Froland SS et al: Cytomegalovirus (CMV) pneumonitis in AIDS patients: the result of intensive CMV replication? *Eur Respir J* 5:362, 1992.
88. Nelson MR, Erskine D, Hawkins DA et al: Treatment with corticosteroids—a risk factor for the development of clinical cytomegalovirus disease in AIDS, *AIDS* 7:375, 1993.
89. Bedos JP, Dumoulin JL, Gachot B et al: *Pneumocystis carinii* pneumonia requiring intensive care management: survival and prognostic study in 110 patients with human immunodeficiency, *Crit Care Med* 27: 1109, 1999.
90. Beck JM, Rosen MJ, Peavy HH: Pulmonary complications of HIV infection. Report of the Fourth NHLBI workshop, *Am J Respir Crit Care Med* 164:2120, 2001.
91. Paradis IL, Grurich WF, Dummer JS et al: Rapid detection of cytomegalovirus pneumonia from lung lavage cells, *Am Rev Respir Dis* 138:697, 1988.
92. Lazzarato T, Dal Monte P, Boccuni MC et al: Lack of correlation between virus detection and serologic test for diagnosis of active cytomegalovirus infection in patients with AIDS, *J Clin Microbiol* 30:1027, 1992.
93. Morbidity and toxic effects assisted with ganciclovir or foscarnet therapy in a randomized cytomegalovirus retinitis trial. Studies of ocular complications of AIDS Research Group, in collaboration with the AIDS Clinical Trials Group, *Arch Intern Med* 155: 65, 1995.
94. Safrin S, Cherrington J, Jaffe HS, et al: Clinical uses of cidofovir, *Rev Med Virol* 7:145,1997.
95. Madhi SA, Ramasamy N, Bessellar TG et al: Lower respiratory tract infections associated with influenza A and B viruses in an area with a high prevalence of pediatric human immunodeficiency type 1 infection, *Pediatr Infect Dis* 21:291, 2000.
96. Madhi SA, Venter M, Madhi A et al: Differing manifestations of respiratory syncytial virus-associated severe lower tract infections in human immunodeficiency virus type-1-infected and uninfected children, *Pediatr Infect Dis* 20:164, 2001.
97. Chandwani S, Borkowsky W, Krasinski K et al: respiratory syncytial virus infection in human immunodeficiency virus-infected children, *J Pediatr* 117:251, 1990.
98. Reassessment of the indications for Ribavirin therapy in respiratory syncytial virus. American Academy of Pediatrics Committee on Infectious Diseases, *Pediatrics* 97:137, 1996.
99. Englund JA: Antiviral therapy of influenza, *Semin Pediatr Infect Dis* 13:120, 2002.
100. Bhanthumkosol D: Fatal adenovirus infections in infants probably infected with HIV, *J Med Assoc Thailand* 81:214, 1998.
101. Janner D, Petru AM, Belchis D et al: Fatal adenovirus infection in a child with acquired immunodeficiency syndrome, *Pediatr Infect Dis J* 9:434, 1990.
102. Koopman J, Dombrowski F, Rockstroh JK et al: Fatal pneumonia in an AIDS patient coinfected with adenovirus and pneumocystis carinii, *Infection* 28:323, 2000.
103. Legrand F, Berrebi D, Houhou N et al. Early diagnosis of adenovirus infection and treatment with cidofovir after bone marrow transplantation in children, *Bone Marrow Transplant* 27:621, 2001.
104. Maslo C, Girard PM, Urban T et al: Ribavirin therapy for adenovirus pneumonia in an AIDS patient, *Am J Resp Crit Care Med* 1556:1263, 1997.
105. Ribaud P, Scieux C, Freymouth F et al: Successful treatment of adenovirus disease with intravenous cidofovir in an unrelated stem-cell transplant recipient, *Clin Infect Dis* 28:690-691, 1999.
106. Shetty AK, Gans HA, So S et al: Intravenous ribavirin therapy for adenovirus pneumonia, *Pediatr Pulmonol* 29:96, 2000.
107. Gururangan S, Stevens RF, Morris DJ: Ribavirin response in measles pneumonia, *J Infect* 20:219, 1990.
108. Datta M, Swaminathan S: Global aspects of tuberculosis in children, *Pediatr Respir Rev* 2:91, 2001.
109. Bakshi SS, Alvarez D, Hilfer CL et al: Tuberculosis in human immunodeficiency virus-infected children, *Am J Dis Child* 147:320, 1993.
110. Jones DS, Malecki JM, Bigler WJ et al: Pediatric tuberculosis and human immunodeficiency virus infection in Palm Beach County FL, *Am J Dis Child* 146:166,1992.
111. Haller JO, Ginsburg KJ: Tuberculosis in children with acquired immunodeficiency syndrome, *Pediatr Radiol* 27:186, 1997.
112. Miller N, Hernandez SG, Cleary TJ: Evaluation of Gen-probe amplified Mycobacterium tuberculosis direct test and PCR for detection of Mycobacterium tuberculosis in clinical specimens, *J Clin Microbiol* 32:393, 1994.
113. Schaaf HS, Donald PR, Scott F: Maternal chest radiography as supporting evidence for the diagnosis of tuberculosis in childhood, *J Tropical Pediatr* 37:223, 1991.
114. Prevention and treatment of tuberculosis among patients infected with human immunodeficiency virus: principles of therapy and revised recommendations. Centers for Disease Control and Prevention, *MMWR Recomm Rep* 47:1, 1998.
115. Blusse Van Oud-Alblas HJ, Van Vliet ME, Kimpen JL et al: Human immunodeficiency virus infection in children hospitalized with tuberculosis, *Ann Trop Paediatr* 22:115, 2002.
116. Muller FM, Groll AH, Walsh TJ: Current approaches to diagnosis and treatment of fungal infections in children with human immunodeficiency virus, *Eur J Pediatr* 158:187, 1999.
117. American Thoracic Society: Fungal infection in HIV-infected persons, *Am J Respir Crit Care Med* 152:816, 1995.
118. Hajjeh RA, Pappas PG, Henderson H et al. Multi-center case-control study of risk factors for histoplasmosis in human immunodeficiency virus infected persons, *Clin Infect Dis* 32:1215, 2001.
119. Fishback N, Koss M: Update on lymphoid interstitial pneumonitis, *Curr Opin Pulmon Med* 2: 429, 1996.
120. Lynch JL, Blickman J, ter Meulen DC et al: Radiographic resolution of lymphocytic interstitial pneumonia (LIP) in children with human immunodeficiency virus (HIV): not a sign of clinical deterioration, *Pediatr Radiol* 31; 299-303, 2002.
121. Imoto E, Stein RM, Shellito JE et al: Central airway obstruction due to cytomegalovirus induced necrotizing tracheitis in a patient with AIDS, *Am Rev Resp Dis* 142:884, 1990.
122. Jeena PM, Bobat R, Kindra G et al: The impact of human immunodeficiency virus 1 on laryngeal airway obstruction in children, *Arch Dis Child* 87:212, 2002.
123. Valor RR, Polintsky CA, Tanis DJ et al: Bacterial tracheitis with upper airway obstruction in a patient with acquired immunodeficiency syndrome, *Am Rev Resp Dis* 146:1590,1992.
124. Bullingham A, McKenzie S: Laryngeal obstruction in HIV infection, *Anesthesia* 44:1003, 1989.
125. Chin R II, Jones DF, Pegram PS et al: Complete endobronchial occlusion by Kaposi's sarcoma the absence of cutaneous involvement, *Chest* 105:1581, 1994.
126. Greenberg JE, Fischl MA, Berger JR: Upper airway obstruction secondary to acquired immunodeficiency syndrome related Kaposi's sarcoma, *Chest* 88: 638, 1985.
127. Roy TM, Dow FT, Puthuff DL: Upper airway obstruction from AIDS related Kaposi's sarcoma, *J Emerg Med* 9(1-2):23, 1991.
128. Rosenberg AL, Seneff MG, Atiyeh L et al: The importance of bacterial sepsis in intensive care units with acquired immunodeficiency syndrome: implications for future care in the age of increasing antiretroviral resistance, *Crit Care Med* 29:683, 2001.
129. Rongkavilit C, Rodriquez ZM, Gomez-Marin O et al: Gram-negative bacillary bacteremia in human immunodeficiency virus type 1-infected children, *Pediatr Inf Dis J* 19:122-128, 2000.

130. Leibovitz E, Rigaud M, Chandwani S et al: Disseminated fungal infection in children with human immunodeficiency virus, *Pediatr Infect Dis* 10:888, 1991.
131. Cebrian M, Miro O, Font C et al: HIV-related vasculitis, *AIDS Patient Care STDS* 11:245, 1997.
132. Chetty R: Vasculitides associated with HIV infection, *J Clin Pathol* 54:275, 2001.
133. Gisselbrecht M, Cohen P, Lortholary O et al: Human immunodeficiency virus-related vasculitis. Clinical presentation of and therapeutic approach to eight cases, *Ann Med Interne* (Paris) 149:398, 1998.
134. Nair R, Robbs JV, Naidoo NG et al: Occlusive arterial disease in HIV-infected patients: a preliminary report, *Eur J Vasc Endovasc Surg* 20:353, 2000.
135. Luginbuhl LM, Orav J, McIntosh K et al: Cardiac morbidity and related mortality in children with HIV infection, *JAMA* 269: 2869, 1993.
136. Starc TJ, Lipshultz SE, Easley KA et al: Incidence of cardiac abnormalities in children with human immunodeficiency virus infection: the prospective P^2C^2 HIV study, *J Pediatr* 141:327, 2002.
137. Lipshultz SE, Chanuck S, Sanders SP et al: Cardiovascular manifestations of human immunodeficiency virus infection in infants and children, *Am J Cardiol* 63:1489, 1989.
138. Hansen BF: Pathology of the heart in AIDS, *APMIS* 100:273, 1992.
139. Joshi VV, Gadol C, Connor E at al: Dilated cardiomyopathy in children with acquired immunodeficiency syndrome: pathologic study of five cases, *Hum Pathol* 19:69, 1988.
140. Barbaro G. Lipshultz S: Pathogenesis of HIV-associated cardiomyopathy, Ann N Y Acad Sci 946:57, 2001.
141. Bowles NE, Kearney DL, Ni J et al: Detection of viral genomes by polymerase chain reaction in the myocardium of pediatric patients with advanced HIV disease, *J Am Coll Cardiol* 34:857, 1999.
142. Lipshultz SE, Fox CH, Perez-Atayde AR et al: Identification of human immunodeficiency virus-1 RNA and DNA in the heart of a child with cardiovascular abnormalities and congenital acquired immunodeficiency syndrome, *Am J Cardiol* 66:246, 1990.
143. Kavanaugh-McHugh AL, Ruff A, Perlman E at al: Selenium deficiency and cardiomyopathy in acquired immunodeficiency syndrome, *J Parenteral Ent Nutr* 15:347, 1991.
144. Brown DL, Sather S, Cheitlin M: Reversible cardiac dysfunction associated with foscarnet therapy for cytomegalovirus esophagitis in AIDS patients, *Am Heart J* 125:1439, 1993.
145. Mast HL, Haller JO, Schiller MS et al: Pericardial effusion and its relationship to cardiac disease in children with acquired immunodeficiency syndrome, *Pediatr Radiol* 22:540, 1992.
146. Zakowski MF, Ianuale-Shanerman A: Cytology of pericardial effusions in AIDS patients, *Diagn Cytopathol* 9:266, 1993.
147. Ingulli E, Tejani A, Fikrig S et al: Nephrotic syndrome associated with acquired immunodeficiency syndrome in children, *J Pediatr* 119:710, 1991.
148. Rao KS: A decade of human immunodeficiency virus associate nephropathy (HIVAN), *Transplant Proc* 25:243, 1993.
149. Strauss J, Abitbol C, Zilleruelo G et al: Renal disease in children with the acquired immunodeficiency syndrome, *N Engl J Med* 321:625, 1989.
150. Turner ME, Kher K, Rakusan T et al: Atypical hemolytic uremic syndrome in human immunodeficiency virus-1-infected children, *Pediatr Nephrol* 11161, 1997.
151. Brook MG, Miller RF: HIV-associated nephropathy: a treatable condition, *Sex Transm Infect* 77:97, 2001.
152. Molina JA, Belenfant X, Doco-Lecompte T et al: Sulfadiazine-induced crystalluria in AIDS patients with toxoplasma encephalitis, *AIDS* 5:587, 1991.
153. Kimmel PL, Umana WO, Simmens SJ et al: Continuous ambulatory peritoneal dialysis and survival of HIV-infected patients with end stage renal disease, *Kidney Int* 44:373, 1993.
154. Kahn E: Gastrointestinal manifestations in pediatric AIDS, *Pediatr Pathol Lab Med* 17:171, 1997.
155. Haller JO, Cohen HL: Gastrointestinal manifestations of AIDS in children, *Am J Roentgenol* 162:387, 1994.
156. Janoff EN, Orenstein JM, Manischewitz JF et al: Adenovirus colitis in the acquired immunodeficiency syndrome, *Gastroenterology* 100:976, 1991.
157. Maddox A, Francis N, Moss J et al: Adenovirus infection of the large bowel and HIV-positive patients, *J Clin Pathol* 45:684, 1992.
158. Pollok R: Viruses causing diarrhea in AIDS, *Novartis Found Symp* 238:276, 2001.
159. Connolly GM, Forbes A, Gazzard BG: Investigation of seemingly pathogen-negative diarrhea in patients infected with HIV-1, *Gut* 31:886, 1990.
160. Nyberg DA, Federle MP, Jeffrey RB et al: Abdominal CT findings of disseminated mycobacterium avium intracellulare in AIDS, *AJR Am J Roentgenol* 145:297, 1985.
161. Pursner M, Haller JO, Berdon WE: Imaging features of mycobacterium avium intracellular complex (MAC) in children with AIDS, *Pediatric Radiol* 30:426-429, 2000.
162. Anonymous: 2001 U.S. public health service guidelines for the prevention of opportunistic infections in persons infected with human immunodeficiency virus. Available at www.aidsinfo.nih.gov/guidelines/op_infections. Accessed ???.
163. Wall SD, Jones B: Gastrointestinal tract in the immunocompromised host: opportunistic infections and other complications, *Radiology* 185: 327, 1992.
164. Wyatt SH, Fishman EK: The acute abdomen in individuals with AIDS, *Radiol Clin North Am* 32:1023, 1994.
165. Bizer LS, Pettorino R, Ashikari A: Emergency abdominal operations in patients with acquired immunodeficiency syndrome, *J Am Coll Surg* 1800:205, 1995.
166. Gerst PH, Pandya G, Nirmul DD: Abdominal pathology at emergency laparatomy for AIDS-related complications, *Contemporary Surg* 46:69, 1995.
167. Whitney TM, Brunel W, Russell TR et al: Emergent abdominal surgery in AIDS: experience in San Francisco, *Am J Surg* 168:239, 1994.
168. Daniels M: Pancreatitis in AIDS patients treated with didanosine, *Am J Gastroenterol* 88: 459, 1993.
169. Pais JR, Cazorla c, Novo E et al: Massive hemorrhage from rupture of a pancreatic pseudocyst after pentamidine-associated pancreatitis, *Eur J Med* 1:251, 1992.
170. Seidlin M, Lambert JS, Dolin R et al: Pancreatitis and pancreatic dysfunction in patients taking dideoxyinosine, *AIDS* 6:831, 1992.
171. Villamil A, Hammer RA, Rodriguez FH: Edematous pancreatitis associate with intravenous pentamidine, *South Med J* 84:796,1991.
172. Dowell SF, Murre W, Hutchins GM: The spectrum of pf pancreatic pathology in patients with AIDS, *Mod Pathol* 3:49, 1990.
173. Miller TL, Winter SH, Luginbuhl LM et al: Pancreatitis in pediatric human immunodeficiency virus infection, *J Pediatr* 120:223, 1992.
174. Lacaille F, Fournet JC, Blanche S: Clinical utility of liver biopsy in children with acquired immunodeficiency syndrome, *Pediatr Infect Dis J* 18:143-147, 1999.
175. Lai KK, Gand DL, Zawacki JK et al: Fulminant hepatic failure associated with 2', 3'dideoxyinosine (ddI), *Ann Intern Med* 115: 283, 1991.
176. Prufer-Kramer L, Kramer A, Weigel R et al: Hepatic involvement in patients with human immunodeficiency virus infection: discrepancies between AIDS patients and those with earlier stages of infection, *J Infect Dis* 163:866, 1991.
177. Kahn E, Breco MA, Davin F et al: Hepatic pathology in pediatric acquired immunodeficiency syndrome, *Hum Pathol* 22:11, 1991.
178. Nigro G, Taliani G, Krzysztofiak A et al: Multiple viral infections in HIV-infected children with chronically-evolving hepatitis, *Arch Virol* 8S: 237, 1993.
179. Dombrowski F, Eis-Hubinger AM, Ackermann T et al: Adenovirus induced liver necrosis in a case of AIDS, *Virchows Arch* 431:469, 1997.
180. Resti M, Azzari C, Bortolotti F: Hepatitis C virus infection in children co-infected with HIV: epidemiology and management, *Pediatric Drugs* 4:571, 2002.
181. Halkic N, Bally F, Gillet M: Organ transplantation in HIV-infected patients. *N Engl J Med* 347:1801, 2002.
182. Hedderwick SA, Greenson JK, McGaughy VR et al: Adenovirus cholecystitis in the patient with AIDS, *Clin Infect Dis* 26:997, 1998.
183. Kavin H, Jonas RB, Chowdhury L et al: Acalculous cholecystitis and cytomegalovirus infection in the acquired immunodeficiency syndrome, *Ann Intern Med* 104:53, 1986.
184. Pol S, Romano CA, Richard S et al: Microsporidia infection in patients with the human immunodeficiency virus and unexplained cholangitis, *N Engl J Med* 328:95, 1993.
185. Beattie RM, Trounce JQ, Lyall EG et al: Early thrombocytopenia in HIV infection, *Arch Dis Child* 67:1093, 1992.

186. Forsyth KP, Sharp RA, Ghosh S: Thrombocytopenia as the presenting feature of persistent generalized lymphadenopathy in a one year old, *Scott Med J* 32:21, 1987.
187. Roux W, Pieper C, Cotton M: Thrombocytopenia as marker for HIV exposure in the neonate, *J Tropical Pediatr* 47:208, 2001.
188. Monpoux F, Kurzenne JY, Sirvent N et al: Partial splenectomy in a child with human immunodeficiency virus-related immune thrombocytopenia, *J Pediatr Hematol Oncol* 21:441, 1999.
189. Hermans P: Haematopoietic growth factors as supportive therapy in HIV-infected patients, *AIDS* 9(suppl 2):S9, 1995.
190. Kuritzkes DR, Parent D, Ward DJ et al: Filgastrim prevents severe neutropenia and reduces infective morbidity in patients with advanced HIV-infection: results of a randomized, multicenter, controlled trial. G-CSF 930101 Study Group, *AIDS* 12:65, 1998.
191. Clark TD, Mmiro F, Ndugwa C et al: Risk factors and cumulative incidence of anemia among human immunodeficiency virus-infected children in Uganda, *Ann Tropical Pediatr* 22:11, 2002.
192. Eley BS, Sive AA, Shuttleworth M et al: A prospective, cross-sectional study of anaemia and peripheral iron status in antiretroviral naive, HIV-1 infected children in Cape Town, South Africa, *BMC Infect Dis* 2:3, 2002.
193. Kreuzer KA, Rockstroh JK: Pathogenesis and pathophysiology of anemia in HIV infection, *Ann Hematol* 75:179, 1997.
194. McClain KL, Joshi V, Murphy S: Cancers in children with HIV infection, *Hematol Oncol Clin North Am* 10:1189-2001, 1996.
195. Mueller BU: Cancers in children infected with the immunodeficiency virus, *Oncologist* 4:309, 1999.
196. McClain KL, Leach CT, Jenson HB et al: Association of Epstein-Barr virus leiomyosarcomas in young children with AIDS, *New Engl J Med* 332:12, 1995.
197. Cesarman E, Chang Y, Moore PS et al: Kaposi's sarcoma-associated herpes virus-like DNA sequences and AIDS-related body-cavity-based lymphomas, *N Engl J Med* 332:1186,1995.
198. Moore PS, Chang Y: Detection of herpes virus–like DNA sequences in Kaposi's sarcoma in patients with and those without HIV infection, *N Engl J Med* 332:1181, 1995.
199. Gavin P, Yogev R: Central nervous system abnormalities in pediatric human immunodeficiency virus infection, *Pediatr Neurosurg* 31.115, 1999.
200. Zuckerman G, Metrov M, Bernstein LJ et al: Neurologic disorders and dermatologic manifestations in HIV-infected children, *Pediatr Emerg Care* 7:99, 1991.
201. Kauffman WM, Sivit CJ, Fitz CR et al: MRI evaluation of intracranial involvement in pediatric HIV infection: a clinical imaging correlation, *AJNR Am J Neuroradiol* 13:949, 1992.
202. Labato MN, Caldwell MP, Paulus NG et al: Encephalopathy in children with perinatally acquired human immunodeficiency virus infection, *J Pediatr* 126:710, 1995.
203. Pavlakis SG, Frank Y, Nocyze M et al: Acquired immunodeficiency syndrome in the developing nervous system, *Adv Pediatr* 41:427, 1994.
204. Safriel YI, Haller JO, Lefton DR, et al: Imaging of the brain in the HIV-positive child, *Pediatric Radiol* 30:725, 2000.
205. Keohane C, Gray F: Central nervous system pathology in children with AIDS. A review, *Ir J Med Sci* 160:277, 1991.
206. Joshi VV: Pathology of childhood AIDS, *Pediatr Clin North Am* 38:97,1991.
207. Exhenry C, Nadal D: Vertical human immunodeficiency virus-1 infection: involvement of the central nervous system and treatment, *Eur J Pediatr* 155:839-850, 1996.
208. Brannagan TH: Retro-viral associated vasculitis of the nervous system, *Neurological Clinics* 15:927, 1997.
209. Fulmer BB, Dillard SC, Musulman EM et al: Two cases of cerebral aneurysms in HIV? children, *Pediatr Neurosurg* 28:31-34, 1998.
210. Giang DW: Central nervous system vasculitis secondary to infections, toxins and neoplasm, *Semin Neurol* 14:313, 1994.
211. Charasse C, Michelet C, Le Tulzo Y et al: Thrombotic thrombocytopenic purpura with the acquired immunodeficiency syndrome: a pathologically documented case report, *Am J Kid Dis* 17:80, 1991.
212. Garavelli PL: Cerebral hemorrhage during AIDS, *Acta Neurol* 15:151, 1993.
213. Rodriguez-Mahou M, Lopez-Longo J, Lapointe N et al: Autoimmune phenomenon in children with human immunodeficiency virus infection and acquired immunodeficiency syndrome, *Acta Paediatr Suppl* 400:5, 1994.
214. Berger JR, Scott G, Albrecht J et al: Progressive multifocal leukoencephalopathy in HIV-infected children, *AIDS* 6:837, 1992.
215. Dickson DW, Llena JF, Nelson SJ et al: Central nervous system pathology in pediatric AIDS, *Ann N Y Acad Sci* 693:93, 1993.
216. Wrzolek MA, Brudkowski J, Kozlowski PB et al: Opportunistic infections of the central nervous system in children with HIV infection: report of nine autopsy cases and review the literature, *Clin Neuropath* 14:187, 1995.
217. Fung HB, Kirschenbaum HL: Treatment regimens for patients with toxoplasmic of encephalitis, *Clin Ther* 18:1037, 1996.
218. Vandersteenhoven JJ, Dbaibo G, Boyko OB et al: Progressive multifocal leukoencephalopathy in pediatric acquired immunodeficiency syndrome, *Pediatr Infect Dis J* 11:232,1992.
219. U.S. Public Health Service: Updated U.S. Public Health Service Guidelines for the Management of Occupational Exposures to HBV, HCV, and HIV and Recommendations for Postexposure Prophylaxis, *MMWR Recomm Rep* 50:1, 2001.

CHAPTER

87

Bacterial Infection, Antimicrobial Use, and Antibiotic-Resistant Organisms in the Pediatric Intensive Care Unit

John S. Bradley, Alice Pong, Deborah Franzon, and Susan Duthie

PEARLS

- Although it is important to treat infections aggressively to obtain the best clinical and microbiological outcomes, judicious use of antibiotics is also important to reduce antibiotic pressure on pathogens and reduce the creation of antibiotic resistance.
- In general, both clarithromycin and azithromycin are better tolerated than erythromycin because of the lack of degradation products seen with erythromycin that stimulate motilin receptors and lead to nausea, vomiting, and abdominal cramps.
- The basic mechanisms of resistance include (1) alteration of the antibiotic structure by bacterial enzymes; (2) alteration of the antibiotic's target site within the pathogen (by mutation at the binding site or enzymatic alterations of the binding site); (3) extrusion of the antibiotic from within the organism by efflux pumps; and (4) changes in the cell wall that prevent movement of the antibiotic into the organism.
- *Acinetobacter baumannii* has caused recent outbreaks reported primarily from Asia and Europe. The most critical aspect of *Acinetobacter* for the clinician is the ability of the organism to acquire resistance to all classes of antibiotics.
- Broad-spectrum antibiotics should be administered empirically on the basis of susceptibility patterns of nosocomial pathogens in the child's hospital. The more severely ill the child, the more broad-spectrum antibiotics should be applied because the physician may have only one chance for cure.

Overview

Antibiotics are important tools for the pediatric intensivist. A bacterial infection may be the primary cause for admission into the pediatric intensive care unit (PICU) or may represent a complication for a child admitted for another reason. Because of the severity of illness of children in the PICU, there is little room for error in selecting the appropriate agent or combination of agents to treat bacterial infections. Antibiotic resistance has been increasing for both community-acquired pathogens and nosocomial pathogens, and the task of antibiotic selection has been made increasingly difficult. The understanding of the mechanisms of the development and spread of antibiotic resistance has increased and has allowed better prediction of which pathogens are most likely to cause infections in any particular PICU. Each PICU will have access to the susceptibility patterns of both community-acquired and nosocomial pathogens from the institution's microbiology laboratory, which tracks antibiotic resistance of isolated pathogens and distributes these data within the hospital as the *antibiogram*. These data will provide the clinician with the percentage of each pathogen that is susceptible to each antibiotic. For highly resistant organisms for which no routinely tested antibiotic is active, reference laboratories can test for susceptibility to investigational agents.

With the extensive use of older antibiotics and the creation and use of newer agents comes the significant selective pressure on pathogens for an ever increasingly complex set of mechanisms of antibiotic resistance. Although it is important to treat infections aggressively to obtain the best clinical and microbiological outcomes, judicious use of antibiotics is also important to reduce antibiotic pressure on pathogens and reduce the creation of antibiotic resistance. This chapter reviews the most clinically important classes of antibiotics, including those currently under investigation and not approved by the U.S. Food and Drug Administration (FDA) for use in children. Many textbooks about infectious diseases have excellent in-depth reviews of antibiotic characteristics,[1-3] and an annually updated review of all available, FDA-approved antiinfectives is published by the American Society of Health-System Pharmacists.[4] Mechanisms of antibiotic resistance are reviewed, particularly because they are relevant to practice in the PICU. Antibiotic therapy designed to meet the challenge of currently isolated antibiotic-resistant organisms is discussed.

As with the treatment of any infection in a child, the clinical presentation, physical findings, and supporting laboratory and imaging studies help determine the site(s) of infection and the likely pathogens. Empiric therapy is begun after appropriate cultures have been obtained. The more life-threatening the infection, the more important it is that the empiric therapy be accurate. No antibiotic is without some degree of toxicity; it is common practice to use the least toxic antibiotic possible to prevent complications of therapy and any additive toxicity consequent to other therapy the patient in the PICU may be receiving. Tissue-penetration characteristics and dosing of the antibiotic are critical; pharmacodynamic characteristics of different classes of antibiotics against different types of pathogens often help determine the dosing regimen required for microbiological and clinical cure.[5,6] Inadequate dosing of antibiotics may actually facilitate the development of antibiotic resistance.[7] Timing of the first dose of antibiotics is also critical, and delay may increase morbidity and mortality.[8-10]

Once culture results are available and the child's clinical response to empiric therapy can be evaluated, selection of definitive antibiotic therapy should occur. At this point, the most narrow spectrum, least toxic antibiotic therapy should be used in appropriate doses for a defined period to cure the infection. Prolonged, unfocused broad-spectrum antibiotic therapy is hazardous: antibiotic toxicities may develop; altered patient bacterial flora will result, allowing antibiotic-resistant bacteria and yeast to more easily be colonized in the child; and prolonged exposure of certain pathogens to antibiotics will lead to the development of antibiotic resistance.

Antibiotic Classes

β-*Lactam Antibiotics*

β-Lactam antibiotics are a diverse group of relatively nontoxic antibiotics with extensive use in infants and children. The β-lactam ring that characterizes these compounds is usually attached to a ring structure that defines the class of antibiotic agents as penicillins, cephalosporins, carbapenems, or monobactams (Fig. 87–1). The β lactam structure is thought to interfere with cell wall synthesis and repair by preventing transpeptidation and transglycosylation of the pentapeptide precursors in the formation of peptidoglycan in the creation of the cell wall.[11] The target transpeptidase enzymes, also known as *penicillin-binding proteins* (PCPs), are vital for creating cell wall integrity to maintain the osmotic gradient between the organism and the external environment. The PBPs carried by different bacterial species have different structures, leading to differences in the binding affinity for various β-lactam agents. Each organism may actually produce several PBPs, each with a specific structure and function within the cell. Mutations in the PBP binding site of the β-lactam antibiotic in any one of the PBPs may decrease the affinity of the antibiotic for the PBP and lead

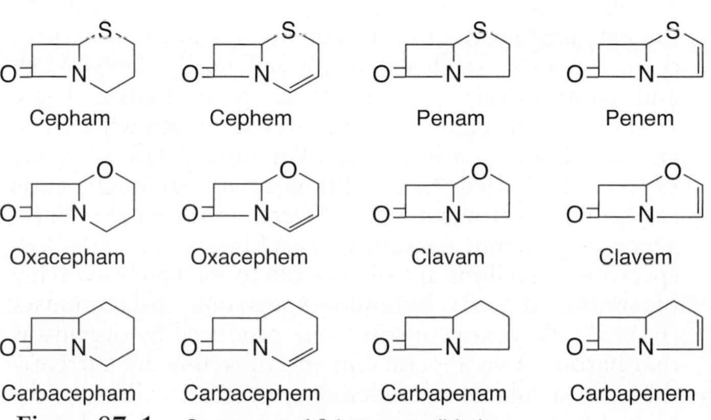

Figure 87–1 • Structures of β-lactam antibiotics.

to a decrease in the ability of the antibiotic to inhibit the growth of the organism. As a class of antibiotics, β-lactams are bactericidal at concentrations up to 2 to 4 times the minimum inhibitory concentration (MIC) of the agent.

Penicillins

Penicillins were the first agents of the β-lactam class to be developed and can be divided into groups that are based largely on spectrum of activity and chemistry: the natural penicillins (penicillin G, penicillin V); the aminopenicillins (ampicillin and amoxicillin), the penicillinase-resistant penicillins, that is, the penicillinase of *Staphylococcus aureus* (methicillin, oxacillin, nafcillin); and the extended-spectrum penicillins (carbenicillin, mezlocillin, ticarcillin, piperacillin). Crystalline penicillin G was discovered by Alexander Fleming more than a half century ago and is primarily active against gram-positive organisms, both aerobic and anaerobic. The aminopenicillins, ampicillin and amoxicillin, are more active against gram-negative organisms such as *Escherichia coli* and *Haemophilus influenzae* than penicillin G. Penicillinase-resistant penicillins were developed to meet the challenge of the rapid development of penicillinase-mediated resistance in *S. aureus*. The β-lactamase of *S. aureus*, however, is distinct from the β-lactamases of the gram-negative bacilli, against which these antibiotics are ineffective. These penicillinase-resistant penicillins are all active against *S. aureus*, except methicillin-resistant *S. aureus* (MRSA) strains that have an entirely different mechanism of resistance. They are also active against streptococci (except *Enterococcus* spp.). Nafcillin differs pharmacologically from the others in being excreted primarily by the liver rather than by the kidneys. Nafcillin displays a relative lack of nephrotoxicity compared with methicillin. Oxacillin also has a better renal safety profile than methicillin. Long-term, high-dose use of all β-lactam agents may be associated with reversible neutropenia.

The extended-spectrum penicillins all display enhanced gram-negative activity, compared with the aminopenicillins. Based on the specific modifications of the side chains with each agent, there are some variations in the activity demonstrated against *Klebsiella, Enterobacter, Serratia, Citrobacter,* and *Pseudomonas*. All of the agents in this class, however, are susceptible to the type I, chromosomal β-lactamases that are inducible or constitutively produced in strains of *Enterobacter, Serratia, Citrobacter,* and *Pseudomonas*. Exposure to the extended-spectrum β-lactams will select out in vitro, or in a patient, strains that are genetically derepressed, and constitutively produce these β-lactamases. These strains are considered antibiotic-resistant and when present, will result in a high rate of treatment failure. Some experts think that the addition of an aminoglycoside to the β-lactam agent will prevent or retard the emergence of β-lactam resistance. In addition, the extended-spectrum penicillins are susceptible to the newly evolving plasmid-mediated extended-spectrum β-lactamases (ESBLs), which are constitutively produced by organisms that harbor them. Piperacillin and ticarcillin are currently the only available extended-spectrum penicillins in the United States.

β-Lactam plus β-Lactamase Inhibitor Combination

Timentin, (ticarcillin/clavulanate), Zosyn (piperacillin/tazobactam), and Unasyn (ampicillin/sulbactam) are all combinations of two β-lactam drugs. The first β-lactam drug has poor intrinsic activity as an antibiotic but still displays high affinity to and may bind irreversibly to and neutralize the β-lactamase enzyme the organism has produced. This agent is also known as a β-lactamase inhibitor. The second β-lactam drug, the true antibiotic, effectively binds to the target site in the bacteria resulting in death of the organism, assuming that the first β-lactam drug neutralizes the organism's β-lactamase. Thus the combination only adds to the spectrum of the original antibiotic when the mechanism of resistance is a β-lactamase enzyme, and only when the β-lactamase inhibitor is capable of binding to that β-lactamase. Similar to the variability in a β-lactam antibiotic's ability to bind to the different PBPs, not all β-lactamase inhibitors have an equal ability to inhibit all β-lactamases; some β-lactamase inhibitors are "narrow spectrum" and can only inhibit the enzymes produced by a few pathogens. Timentin and Zosyn have no significant activity against *Pseudomonas* beyond that of ticarcillin or piperacillin because their β-lactamase inhibitors do not effectively inhibit the β-lactamases of *Pseudomonas*. In general, the β-lactamase inhibitors present in the antibiotics Timentin, Zosyn, and Unasyn do not inhibit the adenosine monophosphate 3′5′ (AmpC), type 1 chromosomal β-lactamases present in *Enterobacter, Serratia,* and *Citrobacter.* They do, however, inhibit enzymes present in a number of other pathogens, including the β-lactamases often present in strains of *H. influenzae, Bacteroides fragilis,* and *S. aureus*.

Cephalosporins

Cephalosporins can be distinguished on the basis of activity against gram-negative pathogens and stability of the antibiotic to a number of the gram-negative β-lactamases. The cephalosporins fall roughly into four categories ("generations") on the basis of these characteristics. First-generation cephalosporins (cephalothin, cefazolin) are active against most strains of *E. coli* but are not entirely stable to the β-lactamases produced by some strains of *E. coli* and *H. influenzae*. The activity of these antibiotics against gram-positive pathogens such as *S. aureus* is close to that of the β-lactamase–stable penicillins, oxacillin and nafcillin; however, none of the current cephalosporin antibiotics of any generation display reasonable activity against the enterococci. Clinically relevant activity against *B. fragilis* does not exist for the first-generation cephalosporins.

The second-generation cephalosporins (cefamandole, cefuroxime) have chemical additions to the cephem ring structure to increase the intrinsic activity against gram-negative organisms, including *E. coli* and *Klebsiella*. The chemical modifications also provide some stability against the principal β-lactamases of *E. coli* and *H. influenzae*. Intrinsic in vitro activity against *S aureus* is significantly decreased compared with the first-generation cephalosporins but is sufficient to achieve clinical success in many situations and to warrant FDA approval for treatment of these organisms. A slightly different group of antibiotics, the cephamycins (cefoxitin, cefotetan), have activity against the gram-negative enteric bacilli similar to the second-generation cephalosporins but display enhanced anaerobic activity against *B. fragilis* and may play a role in the treatment of intraabdominal infections. Their activity against *B. fragilis,* however, is inferior to metronidazole, clindamycin, or the carbapenems.

The third-generation cephalosporins, cefotaxime and ceftriaxone, have enhanced stability against the most prevalent β-lactamases of *H. influenzae, E. coli,* and *Klebsiella* and enhanced activity against many of the Enterobacteriaceae but are, unfortunately, not stable to the inducible chromosomal β-lactamases (AmpC, type I) of *Enterobacter, Serratia,* or *Citrobacter,* particularly when they are constitutively produced in derepressed mutant strains. Ceftazidime, another third-generation cephalosporin, has far greater intrinsic activity against *Pseudomonas aeruginosa* than previous cephalosporins, but it too is degraded by the inducible chromosomal β-lactamases of *Enterobacter, Serratia,* and *Citrobacter,* as well as the chromosomal β-lactamases of *Pseudomonas.* None of the third-generation cephalosporins are as active against *S. aureus* as the first- or second-generation antibiotics are. All the first-, second-, and third-generation cephalosporins are susceptible to the newly emerging ESBLs. Cefepime, a fourth-generation cephalosporin, has the best overall activity against both gram-negative and gram-positive pathogens, with activity against *P. aeruginosa* equivalent to ceftazidime and activity against *S. aureus* equivalent to second-generation cephalosporins. It is also the most stable to β-lactamase degradation by all but some of the ESBL class of β-lactamases.

Carbapenems

Two carbapenems, imipenem (combined with an inhibitor of a renal tubular dehydropeptidase enzyme, which degrades imipenem into toxic metabolites) and meropenem, are currently FDA approved in pediatric patients. Pediatric clinical investigation of ertapenem, a third carbapenem recently FDA approved for adults, is currently nearing completion. The carbapenems have a β-lactam ring structure that differs slightly from the penicillins and cephalosporins (see Fig. 87–1), with chemical modifications to enhance activity and stability, similar to those of cephalosporins. The broad antimicrobial spectrum of activity of imipenem and meropenem is similar and includes gram-negative, gram-positive, and anaerobic organisms. Relevant gram-negative pathogens include enteric bacilli such as E. *coli, Klebsiella, Enterobacter,* and *Citrobacter*, in addition to *P. aeruginosa.* These carbapenems are stable to the β-lactamases of *E. coli* and *H. influenzae;* are stable to the chromosomal β-lactamases of *Enterobacter, Serratia, Citrobacter,* and *P. aeruginosa;* and are stable to the ESBLs primarily found in *Klebsiella* and *E. coli.* They are active against gram-positive organisms including *S. aureus* and streptococci, although activity against the enterococci is substantially less than penicillin G or ampicillin. Meropenem is slightly more active against gram-negative pathogens, and imipenem is slightly more active against gram-positive pathogens, although there is probably no clinical significance in these differences for most infections being treated. Both agents are active against anaerobes, including β-lactamase–positive strains of *B. fragilis.*

With respect to toxicity, the carbapenems are well tolerated, although imipenem displays more interference with central nervous system (CNS) γ-aminobutyric acid inhibition of neuron activity and was shown to be associated with an increase in seizure activity in children treated for bacterial meningitis, compared with historical controls.[12] On the basis of these observations, meropenem is the preferred carbapenem for children with CNS infections or for children in the PICU with underlying CNS inflammation (e.g., CNS trauma, ruptured arteriovenous [AV] malformation, underlying seizure disorder) who require carbapenem therapy for both CNS and non-CNS infections.

Ertapenem has a similar spectrum of activity to the other carbapenems, although intrinsic activity against *P. aeruginosa* is less than that of the other carbapenems. Nevertheless, it has a prolonged serum elimination half-life compared with the other agents, allowing for once- or twice-daily therapy, compared with three or four times daily.

Monobactams

Aztreonam, the only monobactam currently available, has a unique chemical structure in which the β-lactam ring is not attached to an adjacent 5- or 6-membered ring but does have chemical additions to the β-lactam ring that enhance activity and stability to β-lactamases. It only displays aerobic, gram-negative activity, including activity against many strains of *P. aeruginosa.*

Aminoglycosides

Aminoglycoside antibiotics are bactericidal in a concentration-dependent fashion against a wide range of aerobic pathogens. The first antibiotic in this class, streptomycin, was isolated from *Streptomyces griseus* and was first available in 1944. Subsequently, other aminoglycosides have been isolated from fungi, and chemical modifications to enhance activity and decrease toxicity have been made to older agents. These agents inhibit protein synthesis by irreversible binding to the 30S ribosomal subunit. The gram-negative spectrum of activity is extensive, including enteric bacilli (*E. coli, Klebsiella, Enterobacter, Serratia*), *P. aeruginosa,* and many free-living gram-negative bacilli that may only be pathogenic for immune-compromised children or those with trauma in which environmental contamination of deep tissues has occurred. These antibiotics have no clinically relevant anaerobic activity.

Although the first aminoglycosides exhibited substantial renal toxicity and ototoxicity, subsequent agents are significantly safer. With serum concentrations present within the therapeutic range, renal toxicity and ototoxicity are unusual. The most widely available parenteral agents are gentamicin, tobramycin, and amikacin. Because of the relatively low serum concentrations necessary to prevent toxicity and penetration into spinal fluid of approximately

10% to 20%, these agents are not used as primary therapy of CNS infections. Direct intrathecal instillation should also not be considered routinely for CNS infections because data collected during a prospective study of aminoglycosides as adjunctive therapy in neonatal gram-negative meningitis revealed higher rates of morbidity.[13] Streptomycin, the most toxic of the aminoglycosides, continues to be used infrequently in the treatment of tuberculosis, plague, and tularemia in children. Neomycin continues to be used as a topical agent.

Caution should be exercised in the use of these agents in undrained abscess infections, including intraabdominal infections. The acidic and anaerobic conditions present in abscesses produce, in vitro, MICs against aerobic gram-negative organisms that are 10 times higher than those documented under ideal laboratory conditions.[14]

Aminoglycosides have demonstrated excellent clinical efficacy against susceptible organisms. Nevertheless, the toxicity of the antibiotics precludes the attainment of serum and tissue concentrations that are severalfold higher than the MICs of the pathogens, often achievable with β-lactam agents. Synergy between a β-lactam agent and an aminoglycoside in bacterial killing can be demonstrated against many gram-negative pathogens. For the critically ill or immune-compromised child, a combination of agents is often used to obtain the maximal antibiotic killing. In addition, some experts believe that the combination will retard the emergence of antibiotic resistance in gram-negative organisms containing inducible AmpC, chromosomal β-lactamases.

Glycopeptides

Vancomycin is currently the only available glycopeptide in the United States, although teichoplanin is available in other areas of the world, and a new generation of glycopeptides is presently in clinical trials in adults. The glycopeptides are primarily active against gram-positive organisms, both aerobic and anaerobic. This class of antibiotic is cell wall active, like the penicillins, but has a different mechanism of action in prevention of pentapeptide cross-linking in the formation of cell wall peptidoglycan. The large glycopeptide molecules interact with the two terminal peptides of the pentapeptide, physically interfering with transpeptidation. Activity against gram-positive transpeptidases is possible because of the extracellular location of these enzymes. In gram-negative organisms, however, the transpeptidases are located inside the cell wall's outer membrane, a structure through which the glycopeptides cannot pass.

Vancomycin is bactericidal against virtually all strains of staphylococci and against most strains of streptococci, although it is bacteriostatic against the enterococci. Resistance to vancomycin is noted to occur in strains of *Enterococcus faecium* (vancomycin-resistant enterococcus [VRE])[15] and has now been described in *S. aureus*.[16]

The tissue distribution of vancomycin is extensive, with elimination of unchanged antibiotic by the kidney. Dosage adjustment is required in renal insufficiency. Penetration into the cerebrospinal fluid (CSF) is not well studied and is erratic. Serum concentrations of approximately 40 μg/ml are thought to be necessary to achieve CSF concentrations sufficiently high enough to achieve a reliable microbiological cure in meningitis or ventriculitis. The toxicities of vancomycin are primarily nephrotoxicity and ototoxicity. As with the aminoglycosides, close attention to serum antibiotic concentrations will avoid clinically significant toxicity.

Macrolides

Although erythromycin and related macrolides have been primarily used in the outpatient arena, they may be required in the PICU for children with severe pertussis or atypical pneumonia, or in children with extensive drug allergy precluding the use of standard antiinfective agents. The macrolides bind to the 50S ribosomal subunit of susceptible bacteria to prevent the formation of peptide chains, thereby inhibiting protein synthesis. These large, 14-member lactone ring structures are primarily bacteriostatic at achievable tissue concentrations. Erythromycin is available for parenteral use as a lactobionate salt, whereas clarithromycin is only available as an oral agent. Azithromycin is composed of a 15-member ring structure and is considered an azalide. It is available in both oral and parenteral forms. In general, both clarithromycin and azithromycin are better tolerated than erythromycin because of the lack of degradation products seen with erythromycin that stimulate motilin receptors and lead to nausea, vomiting, and abdominal cramps. The macrolides have traditionally been used in the treatment of nonserious infections caused by group A streptococci, *S. aureus,* and *Streptococcus pneumoniae.* Both clarithromycin and azithromycin exhibit enhanced activity against respiratory gram-negative pathogens (e.g., *H. influenzae*). Ketolides, which are currently under investigation, have enhanced activity against some macrolide-resistant strains of *S. pneumoniae* and group A streptococcus, with the same degree of activity against gram-negative organisms as clarithromycin.

All the macrolides demonstrate activity against *Mycoplasma pneumoniae, Chlamydia, Legionella,* and *Bordetella pertussis.* Macrolides are metabolized by cytochrome P450 enzymes, which cause potential drug-drug interactions (see also Chapter 112). These interactions have been well documented with erythromycin and clarithromycin but appear to be absent with azithromycin. Clarithromycin and azithromycin achieve high intracellular concentrations, with demonstrated efficacy against intracellular pathogens such as *Mycoplasma, Chlamydia,* and *Legionella.* Clarithromycin and azithromycin also demonstrate activity against a number of nontuberculous mycobacteria.

Fluoroquinolones

This class of broad-spectrum agents has been extremely successful in adults over the past 20 years. Because of concerns regarding cartilage toxicity in weight-bearing joints of experimental animals, however, pediatric studies were not undertaken. With the emergence of resistance to β-lactam agents in *S. pneumoniae,* increasing resistance in gram-negative pathogens, and the need for an oral agent in the treatment of *P. aeruginosa* and other resistant gram-negative pathogens, pediatric studies began in earnest in 1998 after the FDA acknowledged the need for these agents for serious and refractory infections in pediatric patients. Ciprofloxacin, the first of the agents approved for use in adults, shows outstanding activity against *P. aeruginosa,* as well as many enteric bacilli causing both nosocomial infections (*E. coli, Klebsiella, Enterobacter, Serratia, Citrobacter*) and gastrointestinal infections (*Salmonella, Shigella, Campylobacter, Yersinia,* and *Aeromonas*). Although resistance to ciprofloxacin in *P. aeruginosa* and other bacilli has been increasing, susceptibility in pediatric inpatient units has remained reasonable. Subsequent chemical modifications of fluoroquinolones have resulted in a set of agents with good to excellent activity against gram-positive cocci, including group A streptococcus, *S. pneumoniae,* and *S. aureus.* These newer agents—levofloxacin, gatifloxacin, trovafloxacin, and moxifloxacin—are effective in both gram-positive and gram-negative infections. Successful pediatric investigations have been performed in pediatric bacterial meningitis (trovafloxacin), community-acquired pneumonia (levofloxacin), and otitis media (gatifloxacin and levofloxacin). Because of concerns for possible hepatotoxicity, trovafloxacin is used for serious infections only. No documented case of cartilage toxicity unequivocally caused by fluoroquinolones in children has been reported to date to the FDA or has been published in any prospective study.[17] Safety of this class of drugs, however, remains under long-term investigation, but the risks and benefits of possible toxicity need to be compared with the risks of infections improperly treated because of the reluctance to use this class of agents.

The mechanism of action of quinolones involves inhibition of DNA synthesis by interference with two bacterial enzymes: DNA gyrase and topoisomerase IV, both of which inhibit supercoiling during DNA replication, leading to breakage of the nucleic acid strands. The activity of each specific quinolone and the rapidity of the development of resistance to the specific quinolone depend on the relative activity of the quinolone against these enzymes.[18]

These antibiotics have been effective in the therapy of a wide range of infections in adults, most of which are respiratory tract, gastrointestinal, skin and skin structure, and urinary tract. They have not been widely used for therapy of CNS infections.

Miscellaneous

Clindamycin

A member of the lincosamide family, clindamycin, like erythromycin, inhibits the growth of bacteria by binding to the 50S subunit of the ribosome. Enzymatic methylation of the binding pocket for clindamycin on the ribosome leads to resistance not only to clindamycin, but also to the macrolides and the streptogramins. Clindamycin is active against gram-positive organisms and many anaerobes, including most strains of *B. fragilis.* Activity against β-lactam–resistant strains of *S. pneumoniae* and *S. aureus* (MRSA) has led to the successful increased use of clindamycin in children.[19]

For children in the intensive care unit, strains of *S. aureus* or group A streptococcus that are suspected to produce toxin-mediated disease (e.g., toxic-shock syndrome, necrotizing fasciitis), clindamycin is often used (in conjunction with a β-lactam agent) to stop toxin production as quickly as possible. Retrospectively collected data suggest improved outcomes in patients treated with the combination.[20] Although diarrhea is relatively common with clindamycin (10% to 20%), *Clostridium difficile*–mediated pseudomembranous colitis occurs infrequently (approximately 0.1%) in children. Clindamycin comes in both an intravenous and a rather poor-tasting oral formulation.

Oxazolidinones

Linezolid is the first in a class of new antibiotics, the oxazolidinones. These antibiotics are protein synthesis inhibitors that interfere with mRNA binding at the 30S ribosome subunit, thereby preventing the formation of a functional initiation complex. With a unique mechanism of action, this bacteriostatic agent has been useful in the treatment of infections caused by gram-positive organisms, including MRSA and coagulase-negative staphylococci, and vancomycin-resistant enterococcus (VRE), in addition to β-lactam and macrolide-resistant strains of *S. pneumoniae.* Linezolid has been studied and has received FDA approval for use in pediatric patients, including the neonatal age group.

Linezolid is excreted by nonrenal mechanisms, although the oxidative metabolites are eliminated by the kidney. No dosage adjustment is currently recommended in renal insufficiency or in mild to moderate hepatic insufficiency. A theoretical concern, which appears to have little clinical relevance in relatively healthy children treated under controlled conditions, is the drug's nonselective, reversible inhibition of monamine oxidase. Nevertheless, this drug interaction profile has potential impact on the patient in the PICU who is receiving adrenergic or serotonergic drugs. According to published clinical studies linezolid has been well tolerated, with clinical and laboratory adverse events occurring at the same frequency between children treated with linezolid and controls treated with antibiotics.

Metronidazole

A nitroimidazole derivative first available in 1957, metronidazole has remained a safe and effective antibiotic for parasitic and anaerobic bacterial infections. The primary use of metronidazole in the PICU includes infections caused by β-lactamase–positive strains of *B. fragilis* (intraabdominal infections) and those caused by *C. difficile* (pseudomembranous colitis). Resistance to metronidazole has not been a clinical problem, despite significant clinical use. Unfortunately, little is known about the mechanism of action. The distribution of drug in tissues is extensive, including CNS penetration. It has been a standard component of therapy for anaerobic deep tissue space infections and has been used in the treatment of anaerobic brain abscesses. It is the agent of choice (by the oral route, if possible) for the therapy of *C. difficile* colitis.

It is metabolized by hepatic mechanisms and eliminated by renal pathways; therefore some dosing adjustments are required in patients with hepatic insufficiency. Less is known about dosing adjustments required in renal insufficiency. The antibiotic comes in both parenteral and oral tablet formulations. The oral formulation is particularly poorly tolerated by children who cannot swallow tablets. Suspension formulations are not commercially available in the United States.

Colistin

During antibiotic drug development in the 1960s, the polymyxins were studied and approved for use in adults. Because of significant clinical toxicity, however, these agents were largely abandoned for systemic use and became agents for topical therapy. Unfortunately, with antibiotic resistance increasing dramatically in gram-negative pathogens present in critical care units, colistin has returned to clinical use and now represents therapy of last resort for organisms resistant to all other available antibiotic therapy.[21] Colistin (colistimethate), or polymixin E, has broad-spectrum bactericidal activity against gram-negative organisms by acting as a cationic detergent, destroying the bacterial cytoplasmic membrane. In the PICU, this agent may have a role in treatment of infections caused by gram-negative pathogens (e.g., *P. aeruginosa, Acinetobacter, Enterobacter, Klebsiella*) that are resistant to all other agents, including the fluoroquinolones. Colistin has no activity against gram-positive organisms or against *B. fragilis*. The renal toxicity may manifest as decreased urine output, increasing blood urea nitrogen (BUN) and serum creatinine, proteinuria, hematuria, and acute tubular necrosis. Neurotoxicity may also be problematic, with peripheral neuropathy, confusion, coma, and seizures. The drug is renally eliminated, and dosage adjustment is required for renal failure to avoid further toxicity from drug accumulation in serum. No published data exist on colistin toxicity in the current literature for children receiving state-of-the-art critical care; data from current adult series suggest less toxicity than reported at the time colistin was originally made available for clinical use in 1970.

Antibiotic Resistance

In the PICU, the clinician will encounter both community-acquired and hospital-acquired infections. Community-acquired infections caused by *S. aureus* and *S. pneumoniae* are increasingly problematic because of antibiotic resistance. Nosocomial infections may be caused by antibiotic-resistant gram-positive cocci (*Staphylococcus* spp., *Enterococcus* spp.) or gram-negative bacilli (enteric bacilli, *P. aeruginosa, Acinetobacter* spp. and other nonfermenting gram-negative rods). Infections caused by these organisms include bloodstream infections related to intravenous and intraarterial catheters, ventilator-associated pneumonia, urinary tract infections, surgical wound infections, and infections related to implanted foreign devices. Antibiotic resistance may lead to increased morbidity and mortality, as well as to increased health care costs.[22]

Antibiotic Resistance Mechanisms

In the intensive care unit, antibiotic use is extensive, resulting in selective pressure for antibiotic-resistant pathogens. Antibiotic resistance is certainly not a new phenomenon, with bacteria having developed resistance mechanisms long before humans were using antibiotics therapeutically. Bacteria are capable of surviving in an environment containing antibiotics by the expression of one or more of many different potential antibiotic-resistance mechanisms. The basic mechanisms of resistance include (1) alteration of the antibiotic structure by bacterial enzymes; (2) alteration of the antibiotic's target site within the pathogen (by mutation at the binding site or enzymatic alterations of the binding site); (3) extrusion of the antibiotic from within the organism by efflux pumps; or (4) changes in the cell wall that prevent movement of the antibiotic into the organism. Although community-acquired pathogens most often express only one mechanism of resistance, nosocomial pathogens may express many of these mechanisms simultaneously, and the result is a high degree of antibiotic resistance. In addition, the regulation of resistance gene expression may be altered to allow increased production of the gene product that leads to resistance.

Genes encoding antibiotic resistance may be shared between organisms within a species, or between species. The transfer of antibiotic resistance genes by plasmids is a common method by which resistance is shared between bacteria. The description of mobile genetic elements helps explain the rapid development and spread of antibiotic resistance within the pathogens responsible for nosocomial infections.[23] Antibiotic resistance gene cassettes have the ability to assemble on integrons, which in turn may be associated with transposons, which are capable of "jumping" from plasmids to chromosomes, or vice versa, and from one segment of nucleic acid to another.[24] Antibiotic resistant mutants normally exist at low frequencies in any given population of bacteria. Antibiotic exposure is often the selection pressure allowing these otherwise silent mutants to achieve significant numbers, leading to treatment failure.

Enzymatic Antibiotic Inactivation

The best known of the enzymes that inactivate antibiotics are the β-lactamases that hydrolyze the β-lactam ring of penicillins, cephalosporins, carbapenems, and monobactams. The structure and substrate specificity of β-lactamases are varied and continue to evolve under antibiotic pressure.[25,26] A certain number of the β-lactamases are active against only penicillins, others are active against cephalosporins, and still others are active against a wide variety of β-lactam antibiotics. An organism may carry plasmid-mediated β-lactamases, chromosomally encoded β-lactamases, or a combination of the two. Each of several enzymes, which may be carried by an organism, may prefer a different β-lactam substrate, increasing the spectrum of β-lactam resistance for that organism. Although chromosomal β-lactamases are generally not transmissible, transposon-mediated movement of these enzymes into plasmids facilitate their spread among bacteria.

Although some of the earlier characterized β-lactamases demonstrated activity against ampicillin (the "TEM" β-lactamase in *E. coli* and *H. influenzae*, and the "SHV" β-lactamase in *Klebsiella*), the chromosomal β-lactamases (class I, or AmpC β-lactamases) found in many enteric bacilli and *Pseudomonas* are capable of hydrolyzing the extended-spectrum penicillins, as well as the second- and third-generation cephalosporins. Presumably with the selective pressure exerted from extensive use of broad-spectrum antibiotics, a number of mutations in the plasmid-carried TEM and SHV enzymes have occurred that now confer resistance to extended-spectrum penicillins; to second- and third-generation cephalosporins; and to some extent, against cefepime, a fourth-generation cephalosporin.[26-28] More than 100 of these new, more potent β-lactamases have been described and sequenced. These newly emergent TEM- and SHV-related enzymes, designated as ESBLs, have spread rapidly through many parts of the world, including the United States; thus treatment of infections caused by strains of *E. coli* and *Klebsiella* that harbor these enzymes is ineffective with extended-spectrum penicillins and third-generation cephalosporins.

Metallo-β-lactamases, which are active against the carbapenems, are present as constitutively produced chromosomal enzymes in *Stenotrophomonas maltophilia*, a nosocomial pathogen present in many PICUs. This organism is intrinsically resistant to imipenem, meropenem, and ertapenem, limiting their usefulness for empiric therapy of infection in the PICU, which is "colonized" by these organisms. These potent metallo-β-lactamases may now be found in antibiotic resistance cassettes within integrons on plasmids in *P. aeruginosa* and a variety of enteric bacilli.

Regulation of the production of chromosomal β-lactamases may also become altered, giving rise to constitutive hyperproduction of AmpC chromosomal enzymes, which are found primarily in species of *Enterobacter, Citrobacter, Serratia*, and *Pseudomonas*. The location of these enzymes in the periplasmic space allows these pathogens to display resistance to extended-spectrum penicillins and third-generation cephalosporins.[29]

Aminoglycoside-Modifying Enzymes

Enzymes capable of inactivating the aminoglycosides by adenylation, acetylation, or phosphorylation may be found in several species of bacteria, both gram-negative and gram-positive.[30] These resistance determinants are generally present on plasmids and transposons and can be shared between organisms. As with β-lactamases, there exists variation in substrate specificity of these enzymes for the various aminoglycoside antibiotics.

Target Binding Site Modification

As noted at the beginning of this chapter, many antibiotics effectively inhibit the growth of bacteria by binding to essential structures and interfering with cell metabolism. For the β-lactam antibiotics, a mutation in the β-lactam binding site on the transpeptidase (penicillin-binding-protein [PBP]) leads to decreased affinity of antibiotic binding, which will in turn decrease the ability of the antibiotic to inhibit transpeptidase function and cell metabolism. This decrease in binding results in an increase of some degree in the MIC of the antibiotic against the organism and will lead to clinical failure in treatment if the increase in the MIC is substantial.

Because bacteria may contain several different transpeptidases, mutations at each transpeptidase binding site will lead to additive resistance. Some of the mutations may lead to small decreases in the binding affinity by the antibiotic and relatively little change in the inhibition of enzyme function; however, some changes will cause dramatic alterations in binding, effectively resulting in antibiotic resistance and treatment failure. MRSA strains have developed resistance to semisynthetic penicillins by using a different PBP for cell wall synthesis than that used by methicillin-susceptible *S. aureus* (MSSA) strains. The alternate PBP has a lower affinity to the β-lactam drugs, making them functionally resistant to this entire class of agents.[31] Enterococci use a similar low affinity PBP. The results are a decreased susceptibility to penicillin and ampicillin, and a complete resistance to cephalosporin antibiotics.[32]

As previously noted, macrolides and clindamycin bind to the identical 50S ribosomal subunit. An alteration of the binding site by methylation of an adenine residue prevents the association of the antibiotic with the binding site and yields an organism that is resistant to all of the macrolides (erythromycin, azithromycin, and clarithromycin) and clindamycin.[33]

Vancomycin resistance in some gram-positive pathogens is based on a resistance gene that produces an altered substrate for vancomycin binding at the level of the cell wall precursors. Resistance is found in some strains of *E. faecium* and *Enterococcus faecalis*.

More recently, strains of *S. aureus* have been found with resistance to glycopeptides.[16] Also, fluoroquinolone resistance occurs by alteration in the binding site of fluoroquinolones to one or both of the two target enzymes, DNA gyrase, or topoisomerase IV.[34]

Efflux Pumps

One mechanism of bacterial survival in an environment containing lethal factors is the efflux pump, designed to transport specific types of molecules from the intracellular to the extracellular environment.[35] Although some of the best-studied transport systems are involved in β-lactam antibiotic transport out of the bacteria, fluoroquinolone and macrolide efflux pumps are also clinically relevant causes of antibiotic resistance. Multidrug efflux pumps that bind multiple classes of antibiotics have recently been described, along with alterations in the genetic regulation of pump expression leading to increased antibiotic efflux. Multiple efflux pumps of various types may coexist within gram-negative and gram-positive organisms, and the observed in vitro antibiotic resistance may be increased.[36]

Cell Wall Porin-Deficient Mutants

For an antibiotic to enter the cytoplasm of a gram-negative bacillus, it must pass through a complex cell wall, characterized by an outer membrane, a periplasmic space, and a cytoplasmic membrane. As previously noted, this requirement prevents the movement of large molecules (e.g., vancomycin, macrolides) through the outer membrane; however, many smaller antibiotic molecules cannot diffuse directly into the periplasmic space but must enter through the porins of the outer cell membrane. Gram-negative pathogens, most notably *P. aeruginosa* and the enteric bacilli, may display resistance to antibiotics because of a deficiency of specific porins in the outer cell wall membrane.[37] Some porins are known to be part of an efflux mechanism responsible for capturing an antibiotic in the cytoplasm, transporting it through the periplasmic space, and extruding it through a porin of the outer membrane into the extracellular environment. Imipenem-resistant *P. aeruginosa* has been recognized for the past 20 years, with resistance linked to mutants demonstrating a deficiency of OprD porins. In up to 20% of all patients treated for *Pseudomonas* infection with imipenem, antibiotic-resistant mutants can be isolated after therapy.[38] The same phenomenon may also occur with other carbapenems.

Genetic Regulation Mutations

As mentioned in the preceding sections, genes regulating production of β-lactamases or efflux pumps may undergo a mutational change. This can lead to excess production of these proteins and subsequent highly antibiotic-resistant phenotypes. Organisms with altered regulation of production of resistance factors may have a survival advantage in an environment of high antibiotic pressure. Many strains of enteric gram-negative bacteria have derepressed regulation of chromosomal AmpC class β-lactamase genes. This leads to hyperproduction of β-lactamase, resulting in resistance to extended-spectrum penicillins and third-generation cephalosporins. In gram-positive organisms such as *S. pneumoniae,* some strains are constitutive producers of ribosomal methylase; the result is observed macrolide resistance.[33]

Multiple Simultaneous Resistance Mechanisms

The clinical expression of antibiotic resistance may involve several different mechanisms operating simultaneously within a pathogen, with each mechanism expressed to a different degree, on the basis of the regulation of resistance at a molecular level. For example, an organism with a weak β-lactamase that appears susceptible to an antibiotic in vitro may acquire an efflux pump, may develop porin deficiency, or both. Either of these additional mechanisms will lead to a much lower concentration of antibiotic intracellularly, allowing the weak β-lactamase the opportunity to degrade the antibiotic before significant cell injury can occur. Most often, when a laboratory tests for susceptibility of a pathogen to an antibiotic, the sum of all resistance mechanisms (except those that may require induction) leads to an in vitro determination of susceptibility, which the clinician must use in determining the best agent(s) for treatment.

Antibiotic Resistance and Infections in the Pediatric Intensive Care Unit

Current clinical challenges relate to pathogens that display newer resistance patterns. The ESBL-producing gram-negative pathogens are resistant to extended-spectrum penicillins, third-generation, and some fourth-generation cephalosporins, with a proportion of these organisms also demonstrating decreased susceptibility to aminoglycosides, carbapenems, and fluoroquinolones. Some of these organisms are susceptible to β-lactam/β-lactamase inhibitor combinations. Outbreaks caused by ESBL-producing *Klebsiella* and *E. coli* have been widely reported.[39] Outbreaks by enteric gram-negative bacilli that carry chromosomal AmpC β-lactamases (present in *Enterobacter, Serratia,* and *Citrobacter*) have been occurring for several years and continue to present challenges.[40] *Acinetobacter baumannii* has caused recent outbreaks reported primarily from Asia and Europe. The most critical aspect of *Acinetobacter* for the clinician is the ability of the organism to acquire resistance to all classes of antibiotics. *P. aeruginosa* has always been a nosocomial problem in neonatal and pediatric intensive care units.[41] The nonfermenting gram-negative bacteria, including *Stenotrophomonas, Comamonas, Chryseobacteria* spp. (previously known as strains of *Flavobacteria*), and *Acinetobacter* spp., may also cause antibiotic-resistant organism infections, particularly in the immunocompromised child.

Although the prevalence of MRSA in pediatric institutions is lower than in adult hospitals and nursing homes, community-acquired MRSA is increasingly a significant pathogen in children.[42] VRE strains have been reported in pediatric hospitals, particularly in neonatal intensive care units, in oncology wards, and in patients with gastrointestinal disease.[15,43]

An Approach to Therapy in the Pediatric Intensive Care Unit

General Considerations for Antibiotic Therapy

Once an infection is suspected, on the basis of the clinical, laboratory, and imaging characteristics of the child, appropriate cultures should be obtained. Broad-spectrum antibiotics should be administered empirically, according to the susceptibility patterns of nosocomial pathogens in the child's hospital. The more severely ill the child, the more broad-spectrum the antibiotics should be because the physician may have only one chance for cure. As previously noted, data suggest that using active antibiotics in the appropriate dose without delay will decrease the morbidity and mortality of the infection, decrease the overall costs of treating the infection, and decrease the emergence of resistance. The relative activity of antimicrobial agents against gram-negative (Table 87–1) and gram-positive pathogens (Table 87–2) is provided, although clinicians should consult the local antibiogram for the susceptibility pattern of the pathogens isolated in their institutions. Published data on resistance patterns comes from a variety of sources, including databases from both

TABLE 87–1

Antibiotic Activity for Gram-Negative Pathogens (0 to –++++)*

Organism	Ceftazidime	Ceftriaxone	Cefepime	Tobramycin	Ticarcillin-clavulanate	Piperacillin-tazobactam	Ciprofloxacin	Meropenem
E. coli	++++	++++	++++	++++	++++	++++	++++	+++++
Klebsiella spp.	++++	++++	++++	++++	++++	++++	++++	+++++
Enterobacter spp.	+++	+++	++++	++++	++	+++	++++	+++++
Pseudomonas aeruginosa†	+++	+	++++	++++	+++	++++	+++	++++
Acinetobacter spp.‡	++	++	+++	+++	+++	++	++	++++
Stenotrophomonas‡	+++	+	++	+	+++	++	++	+

*Susceptibility data are averaged,[44-46,48,49] with local hospital data potentially much different than these values.
†Colistin may be effective in vitro against organisms resistant to all available agents, with limited data on efficacy and significant toxicities.[21]
‡Trimethoprim-sulfamethoxazole is the most active antibiotic against *Stenotrophomonas* in vitro.

TABLE 87–2

Antibiotic Activity for Gram-Negative Pathogens (0 to +++++)*

	Antibiotic				
Organism	**Ampicillin**	**Oxacillin**	**Cefazolin**	**Vancomycin**	**Linezolid**
Methicillin-susceptible *Staphylococcus* spp. (*Staphylococcus aureus* or coagulase-negative staphylococci)	0	+++++	+++++	+++++	++++
Methicillin-resistant *Staphylococcus* spp.	0	0	0	+++++	++++
Enterococcus faecalis†	++++	0	0	++++	++++
Enterococcus faecium†	++	0	0	++++	++++

*Susceptibility data are averaged,[40,44,50] with local hospital data potentially much different than these values.
†For vancomycin-susceptible strains.

government (Centers for Disease Control and Prevention) and industry-based sources (MYSTIC, The Surveillance Network, TRUST, SENTRY, Alexander Project). Each collection of isolates on which resistance is reported may include information for different geographic regions, different population groups (mostly adult based), different patient comorbidities, different tissue sites of infection, and different previous antibiotic exposures.[44-46] Because few published data collections have specific information on children, it is critical that the conclusions reached in these reports be taken with caution when they are applied to pediatric patients.

Once bacterial culture results are available, a decision regarding the role of the isolated organisms must be made. Contamination and colonization must be considered in the interpretation of positive culture results. On the basis of the overall clinical assessment, supported by laboratory and imaging data and the response (or lack of response) to empiric therapy, the physician needs to decide whether to continue therapy for a complete treatment course or to stop the antibiotics if data do not support an infection as the cause of the child's clinical state.

Once empiric therapy is started, the culture results will fortunately allow more appropriate antibiotic agents to be used for completion of therapy. An *E. coli* infection that is susceptible to first-generation cephalosporins should not require therapy with second-, third-, or fourth-generation agents, or with carbapenems. If the organism is resistant to all cephalosporins on the basis of ESBL production, however, then an aminoglycoside, a carbapenem, or a fluoroquinolone may be required. For gram-negative pathogens resistant to all antibiotics, colistin should be considered as a last option. The risk-benefit analysis for selecting antibiotic therapy of critically ill children may well favor the use of antibiotics that do not have a favorable safety profile, if no other alternatives exist.

Antibiotic Therapy for Specific Pathogens

Children with infections caused by enteric gram-negative bacilli that carry chromosomal AmpC β-lactamases (*Enterobacter, Serratia,* and *Citrobacter*), which may test as susceptible to extended-spectrum penicillins or third-generation cephalosporins at the time the organisms are initially cultured, are at risk for treatment failure if these antibiotics are used as sole therapy. Definitive therapy of these pathogens should take into account the selection of organisms that constitutively produce AmpC β-lactamase and may include the addition of an aminoglycoside to the third-generation cephalosporin or extended-spectrum penicillin, the use of cefepime (a fourth-generation cephalosporin), or the use of a carbapenem (meropenem, imipenem, or ertapenem). For gram-negative pathogens, including *Acinetobacter,* for which no other options are available, colistin may be used as intravenous therapy.

For *P. aeruginosa,* ceftazidime (or an extended-spectrum penicillin) and an aminoglycoside (tobramycin or amikacin) represent effective therapy in most institutions to achieve synergy and to retard the development of β-lactam resistance. Alternatives for ceftazidime and extended-spectrum penicillin-resistant strains include cefepime (with or without an added aminoglycoside), meropenem or imipenem (with or without an added aminoglycoside), or a fluoroquinolone such as ciprofloxacin if resistance is present for β-lactams and aminoglycosides.

For MRSA infection, vancomycin remains the mainstay for treatment for serious infections. For hospitals and communities in which MRSA is present, the child admitted to the PICU with a serious infection potentially caused by *S. aureus* should be treated empirically with vancomycin until culture results are known. Fortunately, clindamycin exhibits greater activity against "community acquired" MRSA strains than against strains previously documented to cause hospital-acquired infections and may represent alternative effective therapy. Strains of MRSA may also be susceptible to trimethoprim-sulfamethoxazole, selected fluoroquinolones, and linezolid.

Treatment of VRE infection can be problematic. Penicillin and ampicillin may be effective with certain strains of VRE that remain susceptible to these agents, although higher doses than required for therapy of other pathogens may be necessary. As previously noted, a promising agent with activity against VRE is linezolid. Development of resistance to linezolid occurs far less rapidly than resistance to dalfopristin/quinupristin (Synercid). Unfortunately, *E. faecium* with resistance to linezolid has already been reported.

S. pneumoniae has developed increasing resistance to β-lactam antibiotics, macrolides, and trimethoprim-sulfamethoxazole over the past decade.[47] For children with suspected pneumococcal meningitis or other life-threatening pneumococcal infections, the addition of vancomycin to either ceftriaxone or cefotaxime has been the standard of care. Treatment failures with ceftriaxone and cefotaxime in nonmeningitis infections, however, have not been reported to date. Ceftriaxone and cefotaxime are more active in vitro than penicillin against most penicillin-resistant strains and achieve higher and more prolonged tissue concentrations than penicillin, which may explain the observed clinical success with these agents. In CNS infections, however, with the blood-brain barrier effectively preventing high cerebrospinal fluid concentrations of these antibiotics from being achieved, vancomycin is used in combination. Once susceptibility data are reported, if the organisms are documented to be susceptible to ceftriaxone or cefotaxime, vancomycin may be discontinued. Other options for therapy of non-CNS infections caused by ceftriaxone and cefotaxime-resistant strains include the fluoroquinolones gatifloxacin and levofloxacin, or linezolid.

Summary

As medical care becomes more sophisticated and children are hospitalized for longer periods, the risk of development of complicated infections caused by multidrug resistant pathogens increases. The physician is constantly being challenged to deliver effective antibiotic therapy, while at the same time preventing the selection of antibiotic resistance. Knowledge of the pathogens most likely to be present and the potential resistance mechanisms in these organisms is important in selecting empiric antibiotic therapy. An appropriate collection of cultures to obtain susceptibility information on the pathogens is crucial to optimize subsequent therapy and minimize antibiotic resistance.

REFERENCES

1. Feigin RD, Cherry JD: Antibacterial therapeutic agents. *Textbook of pediatric infectious diseases*, ed 4, Philadelphia, 1998, WB Saunders.
2. Jensen HB, Baltimore RS: Anti-infective therapy. *Pediatric infectious diseases: principles and practice*, rev. ed. Philadelphia, 2002, WB Saunders.
3. Long SS, Pickering LK, Prober CG: Antimicrobial agents. *Principles and practice of pediatric infectious diseases*, ed 2, Philadelphia, 2003, Elsevier Science (USA).
4. McEvoy GK: AHFS Drug Information. Bethesda, Md, 2003, American Society of Health-System Pharmacists, Inc.
5. Craig WA: Pharmacokinetic/pharmacodynamic parameters: rationale for antibacterial dosing of mice and men, *Clin Infect Dis* 26:1, 1998.
6. Dudley MN, Ambrose PG: Pharmacodynamics in the study of drug resistance and establishing in vitro susceptibility breakpoints: ready for prime time, *Curr Opin Microb* 3:515, 2000
7. Drusano GL: Prevention of resistance: a goal for dose selection for antimicrobial agents, *Clin Infect Dis* 36:S42, 2003.
8. Ibrahim EH, Sherman G, Ward S et al: The influence of inadequate antimicrobial treatment of bloodstream infections on patient outcomes in the ICU setting, *Chest* 118:146, 2000.
9. Iregui M, Ward S, Sherman G et al: Clinical importance of delays in the initiation of appropriate antibiotic treatment for ventilator-associated pneumonia, *Chest* 122:262, 2002.
10. Kollef MH: An empirical approach to the treatment of multi–drug-resistant ventilator-associated pneumonia, *Clin Infect Dis* 36:1119, 2003.
11. Koch AL: Penicillin binding proteins, ß-lactams, and lactamases: offensives, attacks, and defensive countermeasures, *Crit Rev Microbiol* 26:205, 2000.
12. Wong VK, Wright HT, Ross LA et al: Imipenem/cilastatin treatment of bacterial meningitis in children, *Pediatr Infect Dis J* 10:122, 1991.
13. McCracken GH Jr, Mize SG, Threlkeld N: Intraventricular gentamicin therapy in gram-negative bacillary meningitis of infancy. Report of the Second Neonatal Meningitis Cooperative Study Group, *Lancet* 1:787, 1980.
14. Bryant RE, Fox K, Oh G et al: Beta-lactam enhancement of aminoglycoside activity under conditions of reduced pH and oxygen tension that may exist in infected tissues, *J Infect Dis* 165: 676, 1992.
15. Gray JW, George RH: Experience of vancomycin-resistant enterococci in a children's hospital, *J Hosp Infect* 45:11, 2000.
16. Chang S, Sievert DM, Hageman JC et al: Vancomycin-Resistant *Staphylococcus aureus* Investigative Team. Infection with vancomycin-resistant *Staphylococcus aureus* containing the vanA resistance gene, *N Engl J Med* 348:1342, 2003.
17. Burkhardt JE, Walterspiel JN, Schaad UB: Quinolone arthropathy in animals versus children, *Clin Infect Dis* 25:1196, 1997.
18. Jafri HS, McCracken GH Jr: Fluoroquinolones in paediatrics, *Drugs* 58:43, 1999.
19. Marcinak JF, Frank AL. Treatment of community acquired methicillin-resistant *Staphylococcus aureus* in children, *Curr Opin Infect Dis* 16:265, 2003.
20. Russell NE, Pachorek RE: Clindamycin in the treatment of streptococcal and staphylococcal toxic shock syndromes, *Ann Pharmacother* 34:936, 2000.
21. Garnacho-Montero J, Ortiz-Leyba C, Jiménez-Jiménez FJ et al: Treatment of multidrug-resistant *Acinetobacter baumannii* ventilator associated pneumonia (VAP) with intravenous colistin: a comparison with imipenem-susceptible VAP, *Clin Infect Dis* 36:1111, 2003.
22. Howard DH, Scott II RD, Packard R et al: The global impact of drug resistance, *Clin Infect Dis* 36:4, 2003.
23. Recchia GD, Hall RM: Origins of the mobile gene cassettes found in integrons, *Trends Microbiol* 5:389, 1997.
24. Leibert CA, Hall RM, Summers AO: Transposon Tn21, flagship of the floating genome, *Microbiol Mol Rev* 63:507, 1999.
25. Bush K, Jacoby GA, Medeiros AA: A functional classification scheme for ß-lactamases and its correlation with molecular structure, *Antimicrob Agents Chemother* 39:1211, 1995.
26. Bush K: New ß-lactamases in gram-negative bacteria: diversity and impact on the selection of antimicrobial therapy, *Clin Infect Dis* 32:1085, 2001.
27. Bradford PA: Extended-spectrum ß-lactamases in the 21st century: characterization, epidemiology, and detection of this important resistance threat, *Clin Microbiol Rev* 14:933, 2001.
28. Livermore DM: Bacterial resistance: origins, epidemiology, and impact, *Clin Infect Dis* 36:11, 2003.
29. Livermore DM: ß-lactamases in laboratory and clinical resistance, *Clin Microbiol Rev* 8:557, 1995.
30. Wright GD: Aminoglycoside-odifying enzymes, *Curr Opin Microbiol* 2:499, 1999.
31. Livermore DM: Antibiotic resistance in staphylococci, *Int J Antimicrob Agents* 16:S3, 2000.
32. Cetinkaya Y, Falk P, Mayhall CG: Vancomycin-resistant enterococci, *Clin Microbiol Rev* 13:686, 2000.
33. Leclercq R: Mechanisms of resistance to macrolides and lincosamides: nature of the resistance elements and their clinical implications, *Clin Infect Dis* 34:482, 2002.
34. Hooper DC: Emerging mechanisms of fluoroquinolone resistance, *Emerg Infect Dis* 7:337, 2001.
35. Poole K: Multidrug efflux pumps and antimicrobial resistance in Pseudomonas aeruginosa and related organisms, *J Mol Microbiol Biotechnol* 3:255, 2001.

36. Lee A, Mao W, Warren MS et al: Interplay between efflux pumps may provide either additive or multiplicative effects on drug resistance, *J Bacteriol* 182:3142, 2000.
37. Hancock RE, Brinkman FS: Function of *Pseudomonas porins* in uptake and efflux, *Annu Rev Microbiol* 56:17, 2002.
38. Calandra GB, Hesney M, Brown KR: Imipenem/cilastatin therapy of serious infections: a U.S. multicenter noncomparative trial, *Clin Ther* 7:225, 1985.
39. Kim YK, Pai H, Lee HJ et al: Bloodstream infections by extended-spectrum ß-lactamase-producing *Escherichia coli* and *Klebsiella pneumoniae* in children: epidemiology and clinical outcome, *Antimicrob Agents Chemother* 46:1481, 2002.
40. Manning ML, Archibald LK, Bell LM et al: Serratia marcescens transmission in a pediatric intensive care unit: a multifactorial occurrence, *Am J Infect Control* 29:115, 2001.
41. Foca M, Jakob K, Whittier S et al: Endemic *Pseudomonas aeruginosa* infection in a neonatal intensive care unit, *N Engl J Med* 343: 695, 2000.
42. Hussain FM, Boyle-Vavra S, Bethel CD et al: Current trends in community-acquired methicillin-resistant *Staphylococcus aureus* at a tertiary care pediatric facility, *Pediatr Infect Dis J* 19:1163, 2000.
43. Malik RK, Montecalvo MA, Reale MR et al: Epidemiology and control of vancomycin-resistant enterococci in a regional neonatal intensive care unit, *Pediatr Infect Dis J* 18:352, 1999.
44. Hoban DJ, Biedenbach DJ, Mutnick AH et al: Pathogen of occurrence and susceptibility patterns associated with pneumonia in hospitalized patients in North America: results of the SENTRY antimicrobial surveillance study (2000), *Diagn Microbiol Infect Dis* 45:279, 2003.
45. Mathai D, Lewis MT, Kugler KC et al: Antibacterial activity of 41 antimicrobials tested against over 2773 bacterial isolates from hospitalized patients with pneumonia: I - results from the SENTRY antimicrobial surveillance program (North America, 1998), *Diagn Microbiol Infect Dis* 39: 105, 2001.
46. Mathai D, Jones RN, Pfaller MA et al: Epidemiology and frequency of resistance among pathogens causing urinary tract infections in 1,510 hospitalized patients: a report from the SENTRY antimicrobial surveillance program (North America), *Diagn Microbiol Infect Dis* 40:129, 2001.
47. Kaplan SL, Mason EO Jr, Barson WJ et al: Six-year multicenter surveillance of systemic pneumococcal infections in children, *Pediatrics,* 2003 (in press).
48. Gales AC, Jones RN, Forward KR et al: Emerging importance of multidrug-resistant *Acinetobacter* species and *Stenotrophomonas maltophilia* as pathogens in seriously ill patients: geographic patterns, epidemiological features, and trends in the SENTRY antimicrobial surveillance program (1997-1999), *Clin Infect Dis* 32:104, 2001.
49. Karlowsky JA, Draghi DC, Jones ME et al: Surveillance for antimicrobial susceptibility among clinical isolates of *Pseudomonas aeruginosa* and *Acinetobacter baumannii* from hospitalized patients in the United States, 1998 to 2001, *Antimicrob Agents Chemother* 47: 1681, 2003.
50. Birmingham MC, Rayner CR, Meagher AK et al: Linezolid for the treatment of multidrug-resistant, gram-positive infections: experience from a compassionate-use program, *Clin Infect Dis* 36:159, 2003.

CHAPTER

88

Life-Threatening Viral Disease and Its Treatment

Danielle M. Zerr, Nicole H. Tobin, and Ann J. Melvin

PEARLS

- Obtain serum to store for future serological testing when viral pathogens are considered as the potential cause of a critical illness.
- Diagnostic sensitivity is generally enhanced when samples for viral culture and staining are sent as early as possible in the course of illness.
- Samples that are obtained for fluorescent antibody, whether for a herpes virus or a respiratory pathogen, should contain adequate cells.
- Initiate empiric treatment with acyclovir rapidly when herpes simplex virus encephalitis or neonatal disease is suspected.
- Initiate appropriate infection control precautions early to prevent spread of infection to staff and other patients when viral pathogens are suspected.

Viral infections are a frequent cause of disease in individuals of all ages. In general, the spectrum of illness is varied; however, young children and those with suppressed or deficient immune systems are at higher risk of having severe disease. This chapter covers viral causes of entities commonly seen in the intensive care unit: myocarditis, hepatitis, pneumonitis, and meningitis/encephalitis. The content is focused on cause, diagnosis, and treatment, in an attempt to provide the reader with guidance on the initial management of patients with serious viral diseases in terms of diagnosis and specific antiviral therapy.

Myocarditis

Background

Although many infectious and noninfectious causes have been identified, viruses account for most cases of myocarditis.[1] The spectrum of disease ranges from asymptomatic, with only minimal changes on the electrocardiogram (ECG), to fulminant, with rapid onset of severe disease. Most patients have an indolent illness, which may progress to dilated cardiomyopathy. Because of the varied presentations and the difficulty in the establishment of a definitive diagnosis, the true incidence of myocarditis is unknown. In a large series from Sweden, 1% of myocardial biopsies from autopsies conducted over a 10-year period fulfilled the Dallas criteria for myocarditis.[2]

Pathogenesis

Although the pathogenesis of viral myocarditis is not well understood, myocardial damage is thought to occur at least in part as a direct result of viral infection, with active viral replication leading to myocardial necrosis.[3] Coxsackie virus protease 2A cleaves dystrophin in cultured myocytes and in infected mouse hearts. The results are impaired dystrophin function and poor myocyte contractility.[4] In addition, both humoral and cellular immune responses contribute to the pathogenesis of myocarditis,[5,6] through postinfectious autoimmune processes,[6] cytotoxic T lymphocytes, and antibody-dependent cell-mediated cytotoxicity.[7] Cytokines may also cause direct myocardial injury and affect cardiac function.

Cause

The viruses most frequently associated with myocarditis are enteroviruses, particularly Coxsackie virus B, and adenoviruses (serotypes 2 and 5). Many other viruses have caused myocarditis in children, including influenza A, herpes simplex virus (HSV); human immunodeficiency virus (HIV); cytomegalovirus (CMV); respiratory syncytial virus (RSV); and the mumps and measles viruses, before the widespread use of the measles-mumps-rubella (MMR) vaccine (Table 88–1). Polymerase chain reaction (PCR) of cardiac tissue from endomyocardial biopsy specimens in 34 children with a clinical diagnosis of myocarditis identified adenovirus in 44%, enterovirus in 24%, and HSV in 6%.[8] In addition to enteroviruses, adenovirus and CMV are increasingly recognized as important causes of myocarditis in adolescents and adults. Adenoviruses and enteroviruses are the viruses most frequently identified in patients with dilated cardiomyopathy.

Clinical Presentation

Infants with myocarditis usually have symptoms that include poor feeding, fever, irritability, and listlessness. Physical findings are consistent with congestive heart failure. Enteroviral myocarditis in infancy frequently occurs in conjunction with severe hepatitis, pneumonitis, or both and can be difficult to distinguish from bacterial sepsis.[9] The death rate may be as high as 75%. Severe dysrhythmias have been described in infants with myocardial involvement from RSV,[10] and viral myocarditis has been implicated in some cases of sudden infant death.[11]

Older children and adolescents are more likely to appear for examination after a prodromal viral illness. Early symptoms include lethargy, low-grade temperature, and decreased appetite. They may have diaphoresis, dyspnea on exertion, malaise, and palpitations. Chest pain was a frequent symptom in series of adult patients.[12] Resting tachycardia disproportionate to the amount of fever is common, and an apical systolic murmur may be heard. A subset of children and adults have fulminant myocarditis, characterized by rapid onset of symptoms, severe hemodynamic compromise, and fever.[13]

Laboratory abnormalities may include elevated white blood cell count and erythrocyte sedimentation rate.[14] Serum aspartate aminotransferase levels are often elevated,[15] as are creatinine kinase—MB levels. Cardiac troponin I (cTnI) may be a more sensitive measure of cardiac muscle injury in myocarditis.[16]

Electrocardiographic abnormalities are almost always present in acute myocarditis, with findings of low-voltage QRS complexes and nonspecific ST and T wave changes. Both atrial and ventricular arrhythmias may be present, including supraventricular and ventricular tachycardia, as well as conduction abnormalities. Echocardiography reveals left ventricular dysfunction either with segmental wall motion abnormalities or global hypokinesis in most cases. Pericardial effusions are common. In one series, nondilated, thickened, and hypocontractile left ventricles (LVs) were seen in subjects with fulminant myocarditis compared with significant LV dilatation and normal LV thickness in subjects with a more insidious onset. The subjects with fulminant myocarditis had more evidence of inflammation on endomyocardial biopsy and were more likely to recover ventricular function.[17] Pulmonary edema, enlarged cardiac silhouette, and prominent pulmonary vasculature may be seen on a chest radiograph.

Fulminant Hepatitis

Background:

Fulminant hepatic failure (FHF) is a rare condition, which, before the availability of orthotopic liver transplant, carried a death rate of more than 80%. FHF is defined as the rapid development of jaundice and hepatic encephalopathy in a person without a history of liver disease. Because there is a relationship between the time course of symptoms and prognosis, a classification scheme has been suggested (hyperacute, acute, and subacute liver failure) with an interval of 1 week, 1 to 4 weeks, and 5 to 12 weeks between the appearance of jaundice and encephalopathy.[18] There is significant overlap between causes and prognoses of the different classes. Approximately 30% to 50% of cases of hepatic failure are caused by viral infections.

Cause

Although less than 1% of infections with these viruses results in FHF, the hepatotropic viruses, hepatitis A and B, cause most cases of FHF with a definitive viral diagnosis. Studies in adults with FHF have found hepatitis A to be the cause in 4% to 10% and hepatitis B in 10% to 45% of the reported cases.[19] A greater percentage of cases of FHF in children may be due to hepatitis A.[20] Many other viruses have been implicated in fulminant hepatitis including hepatitis C, D, E, and G, as well as HSV. Infants with perinatally acquired hepatitis B and C rarely have symptoms, and fulminant hepatitis in infants is more likely to be associated with systemic illness due to enteroviruses, HSV, human herpesvirus 6 (HHV-6), or CMV.[21] Infants born to women with both HBsAg (hepatitis B surface antigen) and anti-HBeAb (hepatitis B e-antibody) appear to be at greater risk for fulminant hepatitis due to perinatally acquired hepatitis B.[22]

Infection with hepatitis C rarely causes FHF; however, there are case reports of fulminant hepatitis both with postnatally and perinatally acquired hepatitis C in children.[23,24] The prevalence of hepatitis C virus (HCV) infection as a cause of FHF appears to have geographic variability. Most studies from the United States and Europe have failed to show the presence of HCV-RNA in patients with non-A, non-B FHF[25]; however, in several Japanese series, HCV-RNA has been shown in a significant number of patients with non-A, non-B FHF.[26] Coinfection with hepatitis B virus (HBV) and HCV has been associated with a worse prognosis.[19] HSV should be considered as a cause of FHF, particularly in patients with minimally elevated bilirubin levels. Risk factors for HSV hepatitis include pregnancy

TABLE 88–1

Viral Causes of Myocarditis, Fulminant Hepatitis, Pneumonia, Meningitis, Encephalitis, and Myelitis

	Myocarditis	Hepatitis	Pneumonia	Meningitis	Encephalitis	Myelitis
Adenovirus	XXX	X	XX	X	X	X
Arboviruses (arthropod-borne viruses):				XX	XX	
• Western equine encephalitis virus				X	X	
• Eastern equine encephalitis virus					X	
• St Louis encephalitis virus				X	X	
• California encephalitis virus (La Crosse)				X	X	
• Colorado tick fever				X	X	
• West Nile encephalitis virus					X	
Enteroviruses	XXX	X	X	XXX	XX	XX
Hantavirus			X			
Hepatitis A		XXX				X
Hepatitis B		XXX				
Hepatitis C		X				
Hepatitis D		X				
Hepatitis E		X				
Hepatitis G		X				
Herpesviruses:						
• HSV 1 and 2	X	X		XX	XX	X
• VZV			XX*	X	X	X
• EBV				X	X	XX
• CMV	X	X	XXX*		X	XX
• HHV-6		X			X	
HIV	X				X	
HTLV					X	
Influenza A	X		XXX		X	X
Influenza B			X			
JC virus					X*	
Lymphocytic choriomeningitis virus				X	X	X
Mumps	X			X	X	X
Measles	X			X	X	X
Parainfluenza virus types 1, 2, 3			XXX			
Rabies					X	
Respiratory syncytial virus	X		XXX			
Rhinovirus			X			
Rubella					X	X

*Primarily in immunocompromised hosts.
XXX = most frequent, XX = frequent, and X = less common or rare.
CMV, cytomegalovirus; *EBV,* Epstein-Barr virus; *HHV-6,* human herpes virus 6; *HIV,* human immunodeficiency virus; *HSV,* herpes simplex virus; *HTLV,* human T-lymphotropic virus; *VZV,* varicella-zoster virus.

and immune suppression.[27] Hepatitis E virus (HEV) is an enterically transmitted virus that causes epidemic hepatitis in many areas of the world, particularly the Indian subcontinent and Southeast Asia. It is not endemic in Western countries.

Clinical Presentation

Symptoms of acute hepatitis include jaundice, anorexia, fatigue, nausea, and vomiting.[28] In fulminant disease there is rapid progression to hepatic failure and encephalopathy. Physical examination may reveal fever, hepatosplenomegaly with liver tenderness, scleral or cutaneous icterus, and mucosal bleeding. Patients with severe vomiting may have significant dehydration. Laboratory studies include elevated hepatic enzymes (tenfold to 100-fold increases in serum aspartate aminotransferase [AST] and alanine aminotransferase [ALT]), hyperbilirubinemia, prolonged prothrombin time, and elevated ammonia levels. As hepatocyte necrosis progresses, hepatic enzyme levels and liver size may decrease. Cerebral edema is common in patients with severe encephalopathy, and renal failure occurs in more than 50% of patients with FHF.[28]

Viral Pneumonia/Pneumonitis

Background

Influenza and pneumonia combined are a leading cause of death of children in developing countries and the seventh leading cause of death in the United States for patients of all ages. A greater burden of disease is present in infants, young children, and older individuals.[29] Although only 10% of pneumonias in adults are attributed to viral pathogens, viral pathogens account for most of the 200,000 pneumonia hospitalizations each year for children younger than 15 years. Peak seasons are from midwinter to early spring.

Cause

The etiological agents of viral pneumonia are varied (Table 88–1) and are identified in approximately 50% of cases. RSV is responsible for most severe viral respiratory illness, accounting for approximately 90,000 to 100,000 hospitalizations and 4500 deaths each year in both infants and young children.[30] Usually primary RSV infection is more symptomatic than repeat infection, involving the lower respiratory tract approximately 90% of the time. Repeat infections are common, and in the healthy host, they are localized in the upper respiratory tract. Infection of infants may be more severe when coinfected with a newly discovered virus, human metapneumovirus.[31]

Influenza epidemics occur annually with significant morbidity and death in young children and older individuals. Infected infants younger than 2 months may have symptoms mimicking bacterial sepsis, commonly including apnea. In children younger than 5 years, influenza can cause symptoms of laryngotracheobronchitis, whereas pneumonia occurs in 10% to 15% of those younger than 3 years. Finally, older children generally have the classic flulike symptoms of fever, headache, myalgia, and malaise with upper respiratory tract symptoms. Bacterial superinfection is a common and potentially severe complication of influenza.

Parainfluenza 1, 2, and 3 are the most common agents of acute laryngotracheitis in children aged 6 months to 3 years and are also a common cause of upper respiratory tract infection. In infants and immunocompromised hosts, however, parainfluenza can cause bronchiolitis and pneumonia. In immunocompromised hosts, parainfluenza pneumonia (proven lower tract disease) has a death rate of 30% to 35%.[32,33] Unlike RSV lower tract disease, in which RSV is usually the single pathogen, copathogens are identified with parainfluenza pneumonia more than 50% of the time,[34] and treatment for parainfluenza pneumonia should include coverage for copathogens. Additional information about RSV, parainfluenza, influenza, measles, and adenovirus is available in Chapter 42.

Although CMV usually causes relatively benign disease in immunocompetent hosts, it is frequently severe and often fatal in immunocompromised hosts. The large DNA virus infects epithelial cells and leukocytes. Cellular damage is caused directly by the viral lytic infection or indirectly by the immune response of the host. Risk factors for CMV disease include seropositivity of donor, allogeneic transplant, human leukocyte antigen (HLA) mismatch, age older than 10 years, and development of graft-versus-host disease. CMV occurs at a median time of 40 to 50 days after transplant and is rare before engraftment. The pneumonitis is severe with diffuse interstitial infiltrates. Death rates from CMV pneumonitis are greater than 50%, even when ganciclovir and CMV immunoglobulin are administered.[35]

Hantaviruses are known for causing hemorrhagic fevers and acute severe respiratory infection in young adults. Hantaviruses can spread from mammal to mammal, including humans, by exposure to aerosolized feces, infected urine, or other secretions. In the United States, the Sin Nombre virus, which causes the pulmonary syndrome, is found in 10% to 80% of deer mice in rural areas of North America. Hantaviruses cause disease by creating leakage of plasma and erythrocytes through the vascular endothelium in the lung (hantavirus pulmonary syndrome [HPS]) or the kidneys (hemorrhagic fever syndrome). The differential diagnosis includes influenza A, *Legionella, Chlamydia pneumoniae,* and *Pneumocystis carinii.* Despite current therapy, HPS is fatal in 40% to 70% of clinical cases.[36,37] Hantavirus pulmonary syndrome is also discussed in Chapter 89.

Severe acute respiratory syndrome (SARS) results in a life-threatening, atypical pneumonia caused by a novel coronavirus, now named the SARS virus.[38-40] The virus, thought to be derived from animal reservoirs, potentially palm civets, or raccoon dogs,[41] crossed into humans in the Guangdong Province in China in fall 2002. SARS is spread by close contact with infected humans, mostly to household contacts and health care workers. The incubation period is 2 to 7 days. The case definition of SARS is continuously evolving (see www.cdc.gov/SARS for update) but should be suspected in individuals who meet the clinical criteria for moderate or severe respiratory illness of unknown cause and epidemiologic criteria for exposure. *Moderate respiratory illness* is defined as a temperature greater than 100.4° F (>38 °C) and one or more clinical findings of respiratory illness (e.g., cough, shortness of breath, difficulty breathing, or hypoxia), and *severe respiratory illness* is defined as moderate respiratory illness plus radiographic evidence of pneumonia, or respiratory distress syndrome, or autopsy findings consistent with pneumonia or respiratory distress syndrome. Epidemiologic criteria include travel (including transit in an airport) within 10 days of onset of symptoms to an area with current or previously documented or suspected community transmission of SARS or close contact within 10 days of onset of symptoms with a person known or suspected to have SARS. Death from progressive respiratory failure occurs in approximately 3% to 10% of adult patients; in children, morbidity is less and death rarely occurs.[42,43]

Clinical Presentation

The clinical presentation of viral pneumonia/pneumonitis usually consists of fever; increased respiratory rate; cough; and increased work of breathing with grunting, flaring, retracting, and use of accessory muscles in infants and young children. Decreased oral intake with increased insensible loss due to the increased respiratory rate is often present and may lead to dehydration. Some patients have centrally mediated apnea, and other patients have an overwhelming sepsislike syndrome with increased peripheral pulses, decreased central blood pressure, and lethargy. A history or examination findings of certain symptoms, including rhinorrhea, conjunctivitis, otitis media, and previous exposure to an ill child or adult, should immediately raise suspicion of a viral cause. Radiographic findings generally include evidence of hyperinflation and peribronchial cuffing, and a focal or diffuse infiltrate may or may not be present.

Clinical features of HPS, a noncardiogenic pulmonary edema, include a prodrome of fever, headache, and myalgia usually with nausea and diarrhea for 4 to 5 days before the onset of cough and dyspnea. Tachycardia and tachypnea with hypotension then develop and rapidly progress to acute respiratory distress syndrome (ARDS). Laboratory findings include leukocytosis, abnormal or increased lymphocytes, thrombocytopenia, and prolonged partial thromboplastin time (PTT) in severe cases. Rapidly evolving diffuse, bilateral, interstitial infiltrates are seen on chest radiograph.

SARS in adolescents and adults has a similar presentation to HPS with initial infection characterized by fever (99% of patients), chills or rigor (78%), and development of a dry, nonproductive cough (60%) and dyspnea (30%) a few days later. Other associated symptoms include malaise, headache, dizziness chest pain, sore throat, vomiting, and diarrhea. Oxygen saturation is less than 95% in only 10% of patients at presentation, with severe hypoxemia developing as the disease progresses.[38,44-47] Children are more frequently seen with cough and rhinorrhea rather than chills and rigor.[42] Laboratory findings in children include lymphopenia (68%) rather than lymphocytosis, thrombocytopenia (33% to 44%), anemia (78%), and leukopenia (26%). Elevations in lactate dehydrogenase creatine kinase and ALT may also be seen. Early in the disease, chest radiographs are often normal or have a peripheral/pleural-based opacity as the only abnormality.

Central Nervous System Infections

Background

Aseptic meningitis, encephalitis, and myelitis are inflammatory conditions of the central nervous system (CNS) (meninges, brain, and spinal cord, respectively). Disease is caused by a variety of infectious pathogens, but viruses cause most disease. Viruses gain entry to the CNS via the bloodstream (enteroviruses and arboviruses) or by direct neuronal spread (HSV and rabies). Pathogenesis may involve direct viral invasion or a vigorous virus-specific immune response resulting in damage to the neurons and supporting cells. Alternatively, infection may trigger activation of an immune response specific for the oligodendroglia or the myelin components themselves. In the latter case, disease may follow an upper respiratory tract or other infection and primarily take the form of a demyelinating process. This disease is commonly termed *postinfectious encephalomyelitis* or *acute disseminated encephalomyelitis*.

Individuals of all ages are at risk for CNS viral infections. Neonates, older individuals, and those with immune deficiencies are prone to more frequent and more serious CNS viral infections, though.

Cause

The potential viral causes are multiple; however, enteroviruses, herpesviruses, and arboviruses are responsible for most disease (Table 88–1). Enteroviruses account for up to 99% of cases of aseptic meningitis when a cause is identified.[48] Enterovirus meningitis in older children and adults is typically self-limited and associated with few complications. In contrast, enteroviral infections in neonates may mimic bacterial sepsis, and CNS involvement is often manifested as encephalitis.

HSV is a common cause of CNS infection in individuals of all ages. During the neonatal period, type 2, and to a lesser extent type 1 causes encephalitis because of the vertical transmission of the virus.[49] In contrast, in older children and adults, most HSV encephalitis is caused by type 1. HSV 2, however, can cause benign aseptic meningitis in association with primary and recurrent genital infections.[50] Other members of the herpesvirus family (CMV, Epstein-Barr virus [EBV], varicella-zoster virus [VZV], and HHV-6) can also cause aseptic meningitis and encephalitis, though they are less common. CMV encephalitis occurs mostly in immunosuppressed individuals but may occasionally appear in otherwise healthy individuals.[51,52] EBV aseptic meningitis and encephalitis presents with or without the classic findings of infectious mononucleosis.[53] Acute cerebellar ataxia is a common and usually benign complication of chickenpox. VZV encephalitis can sometimes occur in immunocompetent individuals,[54,55] but more frequently occurs in immunocompromised individuals following days, weeks, or months after varicella or zoster. Zoster encephalitis can be complicated by small or large vessel vasculitis (granulomatous arteritis), which carries the potentially serious consequences of infarction.[54,56] HHV-6 has only rarely been reported to cause encephalitis in healthy children during primary infection,[57] whereas it appears to be a more common problem for immunosuppressed patients, such as those receiving stem cell transplants.[58,126]

Arboviruses (arthropod-spread viruses) are important causes of aseptic meningitis and encephalitis. The specific arbovirus determines the epidemiology, morbidity, and risk of death of associated disease. The La Crosse and St. Louis encephalitis viruses account for most arboviral CNS infections in the United States. The La Crosse virus is found mainly in the Midwest, typically occurs in the summer and early fall, and is associated with a relatively low death rate. The St. Louis encephalitis virus occurs in every state but is more common in the Midwest, Florida, and Texas and has been responsible for large urban outbreaks.[59,60] Eastern equine virus occurs less frequently, mainly in the Northeast and Southeast, but carries a high rate of morbidity (70% to 80%) and death (20% to 80%).[61,62] West Nile virus encephalitis first appeared in the United States in the summer of 1999 in New York State.[63] Over the following summers, the West Nile virus moved southward and westward across the United States, infecting both animals and humans. Most individuals infected with the West Nile virus are symptom free or experience flulike illness; however, older individuals and those with underlying immune deficiency can experience encephalitis that may result in death. In addition to the more typical presentation of encephalitis, an acute flaccid paralysis has also been associated with West Nile virus infection.[64]

A number of viruses are infrequent causes of encephalitis, including mumps, influenza, and lymphocytic choriomeningitis viruses (LCMVs). Historically, mumps virus accounted for a large proportion of aseptic meningitis and encephalitis cases in the United States.[65] Currently, because of the widespread use of the trivalent MMR vaccine, meningitis and encephalitis due to mumps are extremely rare.[66] Influenza has been associated with encephalitis/encephalopathy, especially in Japan. In a national survey representing the 1998-1999 season, 142 cases, most occurring in children younger than 5 years, are reported.[67] LCMV is an infrequently recognized cause of meningoencephalitis. This virus is found in the urine, droppings, and saliva of infected mice, guinea pigs, and hamsters, and disease in humans arises after exposure to these substances.

Postinfectious encephalomyelitis refers to an acute self-limited demyelinating process most commonly following viral respiratory infections and varicella. In contrast, subacute sclerosing panencephalitis (SSPE) and progressive multifocal leukoencephalopathy (PML) are two chronic, usually fatal, demyelinating diseases due to measles and JC virus, respectively. SSPE most commonly follows 5 to 10 years after natural measles infection. SSPE is extremely rare in the United States; however, it may occur as often as one case per a population of 10,000 in areas of the world where MMR vaccine is not widely used.[68] PML is also rare, usually affecting those with acquired immune deficiency syndrome (AIDS) or, rarely, those with other serious immunodeficiencies.

Transverse myelitis has been most frequently associated with enteroviruses; however, VZV,[69,70] CMV, influenza A,[71] and hepatitis A[72] have been reported causes. even in immunologically normal individuals.

Clinical Presentation

Historical clues and physical findings can be helpful in focusing the search for an etiological agent. Travel or residence in areas where arboviruses are endemic during the appropriate season for arthropod transmission (typically summer months) and a history or evidence of insect bites should raise suspicion for arboviruses. Seasonality also plays a role in enteroviral diseases because in temperate climates enteroviruses are more prevalent during summer and fall months. History of a mother with recent symptoms consistent with viral illness (fever, sore throat, gastroenteritis, rash) should raise suspicion of enterovirus in a neonate with encephalitis or sepsislike illness. VZV encephalitis and myelitis typically follow chickenpox or zoster by weeks to months and commonly occur in older individuals or those with immunosuppression, such as transplant recipients.[73] VZV encephalitis may be complicated by CNS vasculopathy and resulting infarctions. Chronic encephalitis/meningitis due to enteroviruses occur in individuals with agammaglobulinemia. Chronic or relapsing encephalitis may also be due to VZV, measles (SSPE), or rubella (progressive rubella panencephalitis), though the latter two are extremely rare with the current widespread use of the MMR vaccine. HIV itself may cause encephalopathy/encephalitis or may also be associated with certain opportunistic infections such as PML. Significant exposure to rodent droppings should raise concern for LCMV. Finally, history of exposure to a bat should raise the concern for rabies.

The classic clinical presentation of viral meningitis is characterized by acute onset of fever, headache, photophobia, vomiting, and nuchal rigidity. A more chronic presentation might indicate enteroviral disease in an immunosuppressed host, whereas recurrent aseptic meningitis can be associated with HSV 2. Encephalitis is characterized by acute onset of fever, signs of encephalopathy such as depressed consciousness, focal neurologic findings, and seizures. A chronic progressive presentation might indicate more unusual causes, such as PML and SSPE. Transverse myelitis is characterized by an abrupt onset of weakness of the limbs progressing to flaccid paralysis. Diminished deep tendon reflexes progress to nonexistent, and there is associated sensory deficit. VZV myelitis usually follows varicella or zoster by 1 to 2 weeks.

Cerebrospinal fluid (CSF) findings in aseptic meningitis typically include a normal glucose level, a normal to slightly elevated protein level, and a pleocytosis of up to 1000 cells/mm^3. The pleocytosis is classically monocytic (>80%); however, there can be an initial predominance of polymorphonuclear cells in the first 48 hours of illness.[74] CSF findings in encephalitis can be normal or there may be pleocytosis and elevated protein levels.

The results of brain computed tomography (CT) and magnetic resonance imaging (MRI) studies are usually normal in viral meningitis, whereas disease is often seen in the setting of viral encephalitides. In general, CT scan is relatively insensitive for detecting acute encephalitis. MRI is the more sensitive study for detecting disease because of its ability to detect altered water content.[75] In acute viral encephalitis early findings include edema with minimal contrast enhancement. As disease progresses, edema and enhancement become more obvious and may be accompanied by mass effect, hemorrhagic changes, and necrosis. As the inflammation resolves, atrophy may become prominent. In HSV, imaging studies may reveal edema and enhancement, often times first involving the temporal lobes with subsequent spread to other areas of the brain. Changes can ultimately progress to atrophy, multicystic encephalomalacia, and gyriform high attenuation, especially in children.[76,77] In postinfectious encephalomyelitis, the lesions may be seen throughout the CNS. The lesions are more readily elucidated by MRI and primarily involve the white matter, although gray matter may also be involved.

Exotic Viral Diseases

With both the increase in foreign travel and the threat of bioterrorism, the potential to treat a child with an exotic viral disease exists. Although discussion of these infections, which include Andes virus, B virus, monkeypox, and the hemorrhagic fever viruses (Ebola virus, Marburg virus, Lassa virus, Crimean-Congo hemorrhagic fever virus, Argentine hemorrhagic fever virus, and Bolivian hemorrhagic fever virus) is beyond the scope of this chapter, these infections should be kept in mind. If one of these agents is suspected, then the patient and patient garments should be contained in a single room, and infection control, infectious diseases, or the public health department should be called immediately.[78-81]

Diagnosis

The key to diagnosis of viral pathogens is high-quality specimens obtained early in the course of disease. There are five main ways to diagnose a viral infection: (1) identification of the virus in cell culture through observation of characteristic cytopathic effect; (2) identification of the virus by assays that link specific antibodies to the viral antigens (complement fixation, neutralization, immunofluorescence assays, enzyme-linked immunosorbent assay [ELISA]); (3) microscopic identification of characteristic viral inclusion bodies; (4) serological procedures that show either an early antibody (immunoglobulin M [IgM]) or a fourfold or higher rise in IgG antibody titers between an acute phase and convalescent phase (at least 10 to 14 days later) serum; and (5) molecular techniques that amplify target viral DNA or RNA.

If a viral cause is suspected, a few diagnostic studies can be performed immediately. Acute-phase serum should be held for later interpretation. It is critical that this specimen is drawn before administration of intravenous immunoglobulin (IVIG) or blood products. Viral cultures should be collected from the appropriate sites with Dacron swabs with plastic shafts (both cotton and wood inhibit viral growth). The virology laboratory should be informed of the diagnosis or suspected pathogens because the cell lines chosen for inoculation vary by what virus is suspected. Nasal washes and swabs of the base of a vesicle or ulcer (for VZV, HSV) should include good cellular content because fluorescent antibody assays stain cells and the more cells available, the more sensitive the assay. Table 88–2 outlines appropriate samples and testing for a number of specific viral pathogens.

Myocarditis

Isolation of virus from the myocardium provides a definite viral diagnosis of myocarditis; however, recovery of viruses from the myocardium by culture is rarely possible, even in cases of histologically proven myocarditis. Viral culture of peripheral specimens such as stool and nasopharyngeal secretions or the demonstration of a fourfold rise in specific viral antibody titers provides an indirect determination of causality; however, the sensitivity is also low, 16% to 26%[8,12] and 30% to 40%, respectively.

Molecular biologic techniques such as PCR and in situ hybridization have expanded the number of viruses implicated in the etiology of myocarditis. In addition, because of the increased sensitivity of PCR, the application of PCR for viral nucleic acid in myocardial tissue provides a virologic diagnosis in up to 60% of cases.[8]

Hepatitis

Viral diagnosis relies on serological testings, the detection of viral nucleic acid in serum, and the detection of viral antigens or nucleic acids in tissue obtained from a liver biopsy specimen. Hepatitis A virus (HAV) infection is confirmed with the detection of anti-HAV IgM antibodies. In patients with acute hepatitis A, anti-HAV IgM antibodies are detectable in the serum at the onset of symptoms, peak 1 week after onset of symptoms, and become undetectable by 3 to 6 months after infection. The presence of HBsAg in serum indicates active HBV replication and is present in acute and chronic HBV infection. Because of the destruction of actively infected hepatocytes, HBsAg may be absent in FHF, and the only marker of acute HBV infection may be anti-hepatitis B core antibody (anti-HBcAb) (anti-HBV core) IgM antibodies. Hepatitis B DNA can also be detected in serum and liver tissue by PCR. Absence of HBsAg or HBV-DNA in the serum does not rule out HBV as the cause of FHF because HBV DNA has been shown in liver tissue of patients with non-A and non-B FHF in whom serologic markers did not suggest HBV infection.[82] Hepatitis D, a hepatotropic virus that causes infection only in the presence of active hepatitis B infection, should be looked for in patients with acute HBV hepatitis because coinfection or superinfection with HDV may result in more severe disease.[83] Hepatitis D coinfection can be determined with anti-HDV antibodies or HDV-RNA in serum.[84]

Although the newer generation antibody assays for hepatitis C are more sensitive than past assays, anti-HBcAbs may not be detectable early in disease. Therefore when the epidemiologic findings suggest possible infection with HCV, serum and liver tissue should be analyzed for HCV-RNA by PCR. Detection of HEV-RNA in blood or liver confirms acute infection with HEV. HSV hepatitis is frequently a result of newly acquired infection; thus serologic testing may not be helpful. Ulcerative mucosal lesions, if present, should be cultured for HSV. Liver tissue should be sent for viral culture and PCR for HSV. PCR may also determine HSV in blood.

Pneumonia/Pneumonitis

Fluorescence assays on nasal wash specimens are the diagnostic test of choice because most of these pathogens are concentrated in the nasopharynx. The sensitivity of indirect immunofluorescence assays is greater than 90% to 95% sensitive for RSV; parainfluenza 1,2,3; and influenza

TABLE 88–2

Diagnostic Tests and the Specimens Used for Various Viral Agents

Viral Agent	Diagnostic Tests	Specimens Used
Adenovirus	FA, PCR, culture, shell vial	NP, BAL fluid, tissue
Arboviruses (California encephalitis, Colorado tick fever, EEE, SLE, WEE, West Nile)	Serology, PCR, and immunohistochemistry for some	Serum (acute and convalescent), CSF
Enteroviruses (echoviruses, Coxsackie viruses, enteroviruses)	PCR, culture, serology available for some	CSF, pharynx, stool,* serum (acute and convalescent)
Hantavirus	Culture, PCR, serology	BAL fluid, serum
Hepatitis viruses	Serology for all	Serum
• HAV	Anti-HAV IgM	Serum
• HBV	HBsAg, anti-HBcAb IgM, PCR	Serum, liver
• HCV	Anti-HCV, PCR	Serum, liver
• HDV	Anti-HDV, PCR	Serum, liver
• HEV	Anti-HEV IgM, PCR	Serum, liver
• HGV	PCR (not widely available)	Serum
Herpes viruses		
• CMV	FA, PCR, culture, shell vial, serology, buffy coat antigen	NP, BAL, blood, tissue, urine, plasma
• EBV	PCR, serology, in situ hybridization	Serum, tissue, CSF
• HHV-6	PCR	Plasma or serum, CSF
• HSV 1 and 2	PCR, FA, culture	CSF, base of lesion, tissue, NP, conjunctiva, stool (neonates)
• VZV	Culture, FA	Base of lesion, tissue
Influenza A and B	FA, culture, IA (rapid)	NP, BAL fluid, tissue
JC Virus	Brain biopsy†, PCR	Brain, CSF
LCMV	Serology	Serum
Measles (rubeola)	Serology, culture (rarely grows)	Serum
• SSPE	Oligoclonal bands, IgG, measles titer	CSF
Mumps	Serology, culture (rarely grows)	Serum, pharynx, urine, CSF
Parainfluenza	FA, cultures	NP, tissue, BAL fluid
Parvovirus	PCR, serology	Blood, serum
Rabies virus	CSF antibody, virus isolation/culture (rarely helpful), fluorescent microscopy (consult ID)	Punch biopsy (nape of neck), brain, saliva, CSF, urine
Retroviruses		
• HIV	PCR, serology	Serum, plasma, blood, CSF,
• HTLV	PCR, serology	Serum, tissue
Rotavirus	EIA	Stool
RSV	FA, culture, shell vial, IA (rapid)	NP, BAL, tissue
Rubella	Serology, culture	Serum, NP, pharynx, CSF, blood, urine

*Enteroviruses are shed in the stool for weeks and may not be diagnostic.
†Gold standard.
BAL, bronchoalveolar lavage; *CSF,* cerebrospinal fluid; *CMV,* cytomegalovirus; *EEE,* eastern equine encephalitis; *EBV,* Epstein-Barr virus; *EIA,* enzyme immunoassay; *FA,* fluorescence assay; *HAV,* hepatitis A virus; *HBcAb,* hepatitis B core antibody; *HBsAg,* hepatitis B surface antigen; *HBV,* hepatitis B virus; *HCV,* hepatitis C virus; *HDV,* hepatitis D virus; *HEV,* hepatitis E virus; *HGV,* hepatitis G virus; *HHV-6,* human herpesvirus 6; *HIV,* human immunodeficiency virus; *HSV,* herpes simplex virus; *HTLV,* human T-lymphotropic virus; *IA,* immunoassay; *ID,* infectious disease; *IgM,* immunoglobulin M; *JCV,* JC virus; *LCMV,* lymphocytic choriomeningitis virus; *NP,* nasopharyngeal; *PCR,* polymerase chain reaction; *RSV,* respiratory syncytial virus; *SLE,* St. Louis encephalitis; *SSPE,* subacute sclerosing panencephalitis; *VZV,* varicella-zoster virus; *WEE,* western equine encephalitis.

A and B. A rapid immunoassay for RSV and influenza is also available. Adenovirus immunofluorescence assays are available in some laboratories, but sensitivity is generally lower (around 70%). Shell vial assays can increase sensitivity, and although they are usually performed for CMV, they can also be performed for adenovirus. The same samples can be sent for culture in addition to immunofluorescence studies, and this should be done for immunocompromised and severely ill children. The diagnosis of Hantavirus can be made by culture of the virus (which is difficult), PCR for Hantavirus RNA, or serologic testing. The SARS virus can be identified by PCR amplification, culture of the virus in respiratory secretions, or serologic testing. These tests can be performed through each state's health department in association with the Centers for Disease Control (CDC) (Table 88–2) (ref:www.cdc.gov/SARS).

Meningitis/Encephalitis

CSF, blood, and throat swabs should be collected for evaluation. One can make a diagnosis of enterovirus by culturing the virus from CSF or by detecting virus in CSF using reverse transcriptase-PCR. Because of the greater sensitivity of PCR, compared with culture,[85,86] it should be used whenever possible. Viral culture of a throat swab may also reveal enterovirus and is indicative of a current or recent infection. Rectal or stool viral cultures are less helpful because enteroviruses may be shed in the stool for weeks after infection. DNA PCR of CSF offers relatively sensitive and specific diagnosis of herpesviruses.[52] Detection of viral specific antibodies in the CSF can add supporting evidence. Additionally, the detection of HHV-6 DNA in plasma or serum by PCR confirms active systemic viral replication. Arboviruses are typically diagnosed through detection of antibodies in acute and convalescent serum specimens. CSF may also be tested for antibodies. PCR and immunohistochemistry have also been used to diagnose arboviral infections and are available in some settings. Diagnosis of LCMV is made through serologic testing. The JC virus can be detected in CSF with PCR, and this appears to be a relatively sensitive and specific method for diagnosing PML.[87,88] Definitive diagnosis, however, is usually made with brain biopsy. Diagnosis of SSPE is made with the evaluation of CSF for oligoclonal bands, IgG level, and specific measles antibody titer.

Treatment

In general, for most life-threatening viral infections the primary treatment is supportive. Because of improvements in intensive medical care, death from these illnesses has decreased even without the availability of specific antiviral therapy. Despite recent advances, there are no effective antiviral medications for many viral infections. There are, however, antivirals for most of the herpes group viruses and many of the respiratory viruses. For most infections, efficacy of antiviral therapy is decreased if therapy is delayed, so early diagnosis and rapid initiation of therapy are essential. Consultation with an infectious disease specialist is recommended because some antiviral agents are not commercially available and new treatment modalities continue to be identified. A listing of antiviral agents, indications, and dosages is provided in Table 88–3.

Myocarditis

Mechanical circulatory support should be considered for children with fulminant myocarditis unresponsive to standard management. Aggressive therapy is warranted because both adults and children who survive their illness have a good prognosis for return to normal ventricular function.[89,90] Cardiac transplantation may be necessary for those children refractory to other management.

Current recommendations do not support the use of immunosuppressive therapy[14,91] or nonsteroidal anti-inflammatory agents,[92] particularly early in the course of myocarditis.

Treatment with high-dose IVIG has been associated with improved left ventricular function in several small studies in children and adults.[93,94] IVIG is generally well tolerated and warrants investigation in larger, controlled studies. Several immune modulators such as interferon-α and interleukin-2 are being investigated for use in treatment of myocarditis.[92] Specific antiviral therapy is indicated when the inciting viral agent has been identified.

Hepatitis

The role of antiviral therapy in FHF is limited. Acyclovir should be initiated if HSV is suspected or confirmed, and pleconaril has shown some benefit in enteroviral sepsis.[95]

Controlled trials with plasma exchange and plasmapheresis have shown improved hemodynamic parameters, decreased intracranial pressure, and improved survival.[96] Experimental therapies such as hepatocyte transplantation and artificial hepatic support systems are in development and have shown promise in early studies.[97] Currently, orthotopic liver transplantation provides the primary treatment modality. For a detailed discussion of the management of FHF see Chapter 79 and reference 90.

Pneumonitis

The cornerstone of treatment remains supportive with oxygen, fluids, bronchodilators, and mechanical ventilation. Corticosteroids are generally of no proven benefit in viral mediated pneumonia, and the data to suggest benefit in bronchiolitis remain controversial.[98-101]

Generally treatment of RSV with ribavirin in immunocompetent hosts has not shown clinical benefit,[102] despite initial studies that had suggested a modest clinical benefit and led to the licensing of ribavirin.[103-105] Evidence is developing, however, that a combination of inhaled ribavirin with either intravenous RSV immunoglobulin or monoclonal antibody may substantially decrease the high death rate of RSV pneumonia in bone marrow transplant subjects from 50% to 70% with ribavirin alone to 9% to 42% in combination.[106-109]

Patients whose symptoms are suggestive of SARS should be immediately isolated in a negative pressure room with the use of airborne precautions (N95 respirator or PAPR [powered air purifying respirator]) and contact precautions (gowns and gloves).[67,101,109a] Both hospital infection control and the local public health department need to be contacted immediately. Treatment of SARS remains controversial. The CDC website (www.cdc.gov) and infectious diseases consultation should be accessed for up-to-date diagnostics, treatment, and isolation guidelines.

Encephalitis

Untreated, HSV encephalitis carries a death rate in excess of 70%[110] and even treated, death and complications for

TABLE 88–3

Antiviral Agents and Indications for Use

Virus	Drug of Choice/Dose	Alternate Agents
Adenovirus	There is no currently approved therapy for the treatment of adenoviral infections.	Both ribavirin and cidofovir have in vitro activity against adenovirus. Small case series in immunocompromised children have suggested potential efficacy with intravenous ribavirin (25 mg/kg loading dose then 10 mg/kg/daily—available on compassionate use basis) or cidofovir (5 mg/kg once weekly)[115,116]
Enterovirus	There is no currently approved therapy for the treatment of enteroviral infections	Pleconoril (VP63843) (5 mg/kg po or per nanogram tid, maximum dose 400 mg) has not yet been approved by the FDA but is available on a compassionate-use basis for neonatal enteroviral sepsis, myocarditis, chronic meningocephalitis, severe infections in patients with bone marrow transplants, and vaccine-associated paralytic polio
Hantavirus	Intravenous ribavirin has shown benefit in hantavirus renal syndrome,[117] but not in hantavirus pulmonary syndrome[112]	
Herpesvirus		
CMV	Ganciclovir (5 mg/kg q 12 hr × 2-3 wk, then 5 mg/kg q 24 hr) is primary therapy for CMV disease; IVIG (500 mg/kg qod × 2 wk then once weekly) or CMV-IG (150 mg/kg, same schedule) should be given concurrently for CMV pneumonia in immunocompromised patients	Foscarnet (90 mg/kg q 12 hr × 2-3 wk, then 90 mg/kg q 24 hr), cidofovir (5 mg/kg/wk—high risk of renal toxicity, use with probenecid and saline hydration); increased efficacy of cidofovir suggested in allogeneic stem cell transplant recipients with CMV pneumonia in one small study[113]
HSV	Acyclovir (20 mg/kg/dose IV q 8 hr) for encephalitis in neonates and children younger than 12 yr and for neonates with disseminated disease	No specific dosing recommendations are available for HSV-associated hepatitis and pneumonitis; at least 10 mg/kg/dose should be considered outside of the neonatal period
HHV-6	Foscarnet and ganciclovir have in vitro activity; case reports and series show variable clinical response with one or both drugs in combination	
VZV	Acyclovir (10-12 mg/kg/dose q 8 hr) High dose (20 mg/kg/dose) should be used for VZV encephalitis or for disease in immunocompromised children	
Influenza A/B	Oseltamivir (2 mg/kg bid × 5 days—max, 75 mg bid)	Rimantadine or amantidine (5 mg/kg/day div bid—max, 75 mg bid)—influenza A only
JC Virus	No effective therapy	In HIV infection, treatment with combination antiretroviral therapy may improve survival; potential role for cidofovir[114]
Parainfluenza		Treatment for parainfluenza pneumonia should include coverage for copathogens; ribavirin and IVIG remain controversial, with a recent review showing no benefit[34]
RSV	Aerosolized ribavirin (6 g reconstituted in 100 ml tid × 5 days) has been used with modest efficacy in patients with severe RSV pneumonia and in immunocompromised patients—not recommended for uncomplicated disease	Combination therapy with ribavirin and palivizumab (RSV monoclonal antibody) or ribavirin and RSV-IG may improve outcome of RSV pneumonia in immunocompromised patients—under investigation

CMV, cytomegalovirus; *div*, divided; *HHV-6*, human herpesvirus 6; *HIV*, human immunodeficiency virus; *HSV*, herpes simplex virus; *IG*, immunoglobulin; *IV*, intravenous; *IVIG*, intravenous immunoglobulin; *JCV*, JC virus; *max*, maximum; *RSV*, respiratory syncytial virus.

those who survive remain on the order of 15% and 20%, respectively.[111] Similarly, despite treatment, neonatal HSV CNS disease carries significant risk of death and morbidity, ranging from 0% to 15% and 43% to 68%, respectively.[49] Early identification of patients and rapid initiation of acyclovir have been associated with better outcome.[110,111] Unless an alternative cause is clear, high-dose acyclovir should be initiated in all children with encephalitis until HSV can be ruled out. Other specific antiviral therapy may be directed as outlined in Table 88–3.

REFERENCES

1. Pisani B, Taylor DO, Mason JW: Inflammatory myocardial diseases and cardiomyopathies, *Am J Med* 102:459-469, 1997.
2. Gravanis MB, Sternby NH: Incidence of myocarditis. A 10-year autopsy study from Malmo, Sweden, *Arch Pathol Lab Med* 115: 390-392, 1991.
3. Khatib R, Chason JL, Lerner AM: A mouse model of transmural myocardial necrosis due to coxsackievirus B4: observations over 12 months, *Intervirology* 18:197-202, 1982.
4. Badorff C, Lee GH, Lamphear BJ, et al: Enteroviral protease 2A cleaves dystrophin: evidence of cytoskeletal disruption in an acquired cardiomyopathy, *Nat Med* 5:320-326, 1999.
5. Liu PP, Mason JW: Advances in the understanding of myocarditis, *Circulation* 104:1076-1082, 2001.
6. Maisch B, Ristic AD, Hufnagel G, et al: Pathophysiology of viral myocarditis: the role of humoral immune response, *Cardiovasc Pathol* 11:112-122, 2002.
7. Wong CY, Woodruff JJ, Woodruff JF: Generation of cytotoxic T lymphocytes during coxsackievirus tb-3 infection. II. Characterization of effector cells and demonstration cytotoxicity against viral-infected myofibers1, *J Immunol* 118:1165-1169, 1977.
8. Martin AB, Webber S, Fricker FJ, et al: Acute myocarditis. Rapid diagnosis by PCR in children, *Circulation* 90:330-339, 1994.
9. Kaplan MH, Klein SW, McPhee J, et al: Group B coxsackievirus infections in infants younger than three months of age: a serious childhood illness, *Rev Infect Dis* 5:1019-1032, 1983.
10. Thomas JA, Raroque S, Scott WA, et al: Successful treatment of severe dysrhythmias in infants with respiratory syncytial virus infections: two cases and a literature review, *Crit Care Med* 25: 880-886, 1997.
11. Dancea A, Cote A, Rohlicek C, et al: Cardiac pathology in sudden unexpected infant death, *J Pediatr* 141:336-324, 2002.
12. Sainani GS, Dekate MP, Rao CP: Heart disease caused by Coxsackie virus B infection, *Br Heart J* 37:819-823, 1975.
13. Lieberman EB, Hutchins GM, Herskowitz A, et al: Clinicopathologic description of myocarditis, *J Am Coll Cardiol* 18: 1617-1626, 1991.
14. Mason JW, O'Connell JB, Herskowitz A, et al: A clinical trial of immunosuppressive therapy for myocarditis. The Myocarditis Treatment Trial Investigators, *N Engl J Med* 333:269-275, 1995.
15. Helin M, Savola J, Lapinleimu K: Cardiac manifestations during a Coxsackie B5 epidemic, *Br Med J* 3:97-99, 1968.
16. Smith SC, Ladenson JH, Mason JW, et al: Elevations of cardiac troponin I associated with myocarditis. Experimental and clinical correlates, *Circulation* 95:163-168, 1997.
17. Felker GM, Boehmer JP, Hruban RH, et al: Echocardiographic findings in fulminant and acute myocarditis, *J Am Coll Cardiol* 36:227-232, 2000.
18. O'Grady JG, Schalm SW, Williams R: Acute liver failure: redefining the syndromes, *Lancet* 342:273-275, 1993.
19. Tibbs C, Williams R: Viral causes and management of acute liver failure, *J Hepatol* 22:68-73, 1995.
20. Ciocca M: Clinical course and consequences of hepatitis A infection, *Vaccine* 18:S71-S74, 2000.
21. Durand P, Debray D, Mandel R, et al: Acute liver failure in infancy: a 14-year experience of a pediatric liver transplantation center, *J Pediatr* 139:871-876, 2001.
22. Beath SV, Boxall EH, Watson RM, et al: Fulminant hepatitis B in infants born to anti-HBe hepatitis B carrier mothers, *BMJ* 304: 1169-1170, 1992.
23. Kong MS, Chung JL: Fatal hepatitis C in an infant born to a hepatitis C positive mother, *J Pediatr Gastroenterol Nutr* 19: 460-463, 1994.
24. Taga T, Ikeda M, Suzuki K, et al: Fulminant hepatitis caused by hepatitis C virus, *Pediatr Infect Dis J* 17:1174-1176, 1998.
25. Feray C, Gigou M, Samuel D, et al: Hepatitis C virus RNA and hepatitis B virus DNA in serum and liver of patients with fulminant hepatitis, *Gastroenterology* 104:549-555, 1993.
26. Yoshiba M, Sekiyama K, Sugata F, et al: Diagnosis of type C fulminant hepatitis by the detection of antibodies to the putative core proteins of hepatitis C virus, *Gastroenterol Jpn* 26:234, 1991.
27. Peters DJ, Greene WH, Ruggiero F, et al: Herpes simplex-induced fulminant hepatitis in adults: a call for empiric therapy, *Dig Dis Sci* 45:2399-2404, 2000.
28. Shakil AO, Kramer D, Mazariegos GV, et al: Acute liver failure: clinical features, outcome analysis, and applicability of prognostic criteria, *Liver Transpl* 6:163-169, 2000.
29. National Vital Statistics Report, Vol 49, No. 11. Hyattsville (MD): National Center for Health Statistics, Centers for Disease Control and Prevention. U.S. Department of Health and Human Services; October 12, 2001.
30. Glezen WP, Taber LH, Frank AL, et al: Risk of primary infection and reinfection with respiratory syncytial virus, *Am J Dis Child* 140:543-546, 1986.
31. Greensill J, McNamara PS, Dove W, et al: Human metapneumovirus in severe respiratory syncytial virus bronchiolitis, *Emerg Infect Dis* 9:372-375, 2003.
32. Lewis VA, Champlin R, Englund J, et al: Respiratory disease due to parainfluenza virus in adult bone marrow transplant recipients, *Clin Infect Dis* 23:1033-1037, 1996.
33. Wendt CH, Weisdorf DJ, Fordan MC, et al: Parainfluenza virus respiratory infection after bone marrow transplantation, *N Engl J Med* 326:921-926, 1992.
34. Nichols WG, Corey L, Gooley T, et al: Parainfluenza virus infections after hematopoiectic stem cell transplantation: risk factors, response to antiviral therapy, and effect on transplant outcome, *Blood* 98:573-578, 2001.
35. Reed EC, Bowden RA, Dandliker PS, et al: Treatment of cytomegalovirus pneumonia with fanciclovir and intravenous cytomegalovirus immunoglobulin in patients with bone marrow transplants, *Ann Intern Med* 109:783-788, 1988.
36. Duchin JS, Koster FT, Peters CJ, et al: Hantavirus pulmonary syndrome: a clinical description of 17 patients with a newly recognized disease. The Hantavirus Study Group, *N Engl J Med* 330: 949-955, 1994.
37. Levy H, Simpson SQ: Hantavirus pulmonary syndrome, *Am J Respir Crit Care Med* 149:1710-1713, 1994.
38. Peiris JSM, Lai ST, Poon LLM, et al: Coronavirus as a possible cause of severe acute respiratory syndrome, *Lancet* 361:1319-1325, 2003.
39. Ksiazek TG, Erdman D, Goldsmith C, et al: A novel coronavirus associated with severe acute respiratory syndrome, *N Engl J Med* 348:1953-1966, 2003. Epub 2003 Apr 10.
40. Drosten C, Gunther S, Preiser W, et al: Identification of a novel coronavirus in patients with severe acute respiratory syndrome, *N Engl J Med* 348:1967-76, 2003. Epub 2003 Apr 10.
41. Cyranoski D, Abbott A: Virus detectives seek source of SARS in China's wild animals, *Nature* 423:467, 2003.
42. Hon KLE, Leung CW, Cheng WTF, et al: Clinical presentations and outcome of severe acute respiratory syndrome in children, *Lancet* 361:1701-1703, 2003.
43. Maskalyk J, Hoey J: SARS update, *CMAJ* 168:1294-1295, 2003.
44. Booth CM, Matukas LM, Tomlinson GA, et al: Clinical features and short-term outcomes of 144 patients with SARS in the greater Toronto area, *JAMA* 289:2801-2809, 2003.
45. Tsang KW, Ho PL, Ooi GC, et al: A cluster of cases of severe acute respiratory syndrome in Hong Kong, *N Engl J Med* 348: 1977-1985, 2003. Epub 2003 Mar 31.
46. Lee N, Hui D, Wu A, et al: A major outbreak of severe acute respiratory syndrome in Hong Kong, *N Engl J Med* 348:1986-1994, 2003. Epub 2003 Apr 7.
47. Poutanen SM, Low DE, Henry B, et al: Identification of severe acute respiratory syndrome in Canada, *N Engl J Med* 348: 1995-2005, 2003. Epub 2003 Mar 31.
48. Berlin LE, Rorabaugh M, Heldrich F, et al: Aseptic meningitis in infants <2 years of age: diagnosis and etiology, *J Infect Dis* 168: 888-892, 1993.
49. Kimberlin DW, Lin C, Jacobs RF, et al: Natural history of neonatal herpes simplex virus infections in the acyclovir era, *Pediatrics* 108:223-229, 2001.
50. Tedder DG, Ashley R, Tyler KL, et al: Herpes simplex virus infection as a cause of benign recurrent lymphocytic meningitis, *Ann Intern Med* 121:334-338, 1994.
51. Arribas JR., Storch GA, Clifford DB, et al: Cytomegalovirus encephalitis, Ann Intern Med 125: 577-587, 1996.
52. Prosch S, Schielke E, Reip A, et al: Human cytomegalovirus (HCMV) encephalitis in an immunocompetent young person and diagnostic reliability of HCMV DNA PCR using cerebrospinal fluid of nonimmunosuppressed patients, *J Clin Microbiol* 36:3636-3640, 1998.

53. Domachowske JB, Cunningham CK, Cummings DA, et al: Acute manifestations and neurologic sequelae of Epstein-Barr virus encephalitis in children, *Pediatr Infect Dis J* 15:871-875,1996.
54. Caruso JT, Tung GA, Brown WD: Central nervous system and renal vasculitis associated with primary varicella infection in a child, *Pediatrics* 107:E9, 2001.
55. Hausler M, Schaade L, Kemeny S, et al: Encephalitis related to primary varicella-zoster virus infection in immunocompetent children, *J Neurol Sci* 195:111-116, 2002.
56. Kuroiwa Y, Furukawa T: Hemispheric infarction after herpes zoster ophthalmicus: computed tomography and angiography, *Neurology* 31:1030-1032, 1981.
57. Ahtiluoto S, Mannonen L, Paetau A, et al: In situ hybridization detection of human herpesvirus 6 in brain tissue from fatal encephalitis, *Pediatrics* 105:431-433, 2000.
58. Tiacci E, Luppi M, Barozzi P, et al: Fatal herpesvirus-6 encephalitis in a recipient of a T-cell depleted peripheral blood stem cell transplant from a 3-loci mismatched related donor, *Haematologica* 85:94-97, 2000.
59. Centers for Disease Control (CDC: Arboviral disease-United States, 1994, *MMWR Morb Mortal Wkly Rep* 44:641-644, 1995.
60. Centers for Disease Control (CDC): Arboviral infections of the central nervous system-United States, 1996-1997, *MMWR Morb Mortal Wkly Rep* 47:517-522, 1998.
61. Lowry PW: Arbovirus encephalitis in the United States and Asia, *J Lab Clin Med* 129:405-411, 1997.
62. Whitley RJ: Viral encephalitis, *N Engl J Med* 323:242-250, 1990.
63. Nash D, Mostashari F, Fine A, et al: The outbreak of West Nile virus infection in the New York area in 1999, *N Engl J Med* 344:1807-1814, 2001.
64. Centers for Disease Control (CDC): Acute flaccid paralysis syndrome associated with West Nile Virus infection-Mississippi and Louisiana, July-August 2002, *MMWR Morb Mortal Wkly Rep* 51: 825-828, 2002.
65. Forsey T: Mumps vaccines-current status, *J Med Microbiol* 41:1-2, 1994
66. Centers for Disease Control (CDC): Mumps prevention, *MMWR Morb Mortal Wkly Rep* 38;388-400, 1989.
67. Morishima T, Togashi T, Yokota S, et al: Encephalitis and encephalopathy associated with an influenza epidemic in Japan, *Clin Infect Dis* 35:512-517, 2001.
68. Kondo K, Takasu T, Ahmed A: Neurological diseases in Karachi, Pakistan-elevated occurrence of subacute sclerosing panencephalitis, *Neuroepidemiology* 7:66-80, 1988.
69. Celik Y, Tabak F, Mert A, et al: Transverse myelitis caused by varicella, *Clin Neurol Neurosurg* 103:260-261, 2001.
70. Gilden DH, Beinlich BR, Rubinstien EM, et al: Varicella-zoster virus myelitis: an expanding spectrum, *Neurology* 44:1818-1823, 1994.
71. Salonen O, Koshkiniemi M, Saari A, et al: Myelitis associated with influenza A virus infection, *J Neurovirol* 3:83-85, 1997.
72. Tyler KL, Gross RA, Cascino GD, et al: Unusual viral causes of transverse myelitis: hepatitis A virus and cytomegalovirus, *Neurology* 36:855-858, 1986.
73. Koc Y, Miller KB, Schenkein DP, et al: Varicella zoster virus infections following allogenic bone marrow transplantation: frequency, risk factors, and clinical outcome, *Biol Blood Marrow Transplant* 6:44-49, 2000.
74. Feigin RD, Shackelford PG: Value of repeat lumbar puncture in the differential diagnosis of meningitis, *N Engl J Med* 289:571-574, 1973.
75. Tarr RW, Edwards KM, Kessler RM, et al: MRI of mumps encephalitis: comparison with CT evaluation, *Pediatr Radiol* 17: 59-62, 1987.
76. Noorbehesht B, Enzmann DR, Sullender W, et al: Neonatal herpes simplex encephalitis: correlation of clinical and CT findings, *Radiology* 162:813-819, 1987.
77. Shaw DW, Cohen WA: Viral infections of the CNS in children: imaging features, *AJR Am J Roentgenol* 160:125-133, 1993.
78. Campbell BA, Pequegnat MD, Clayton AJ: A hospital contingency plan for exotic communicable diseases, *Infect Control* 5:565-569, 1984.
79. Centers for Disease Control (CDC): Update: management of patients with suspected viral hemorrhagic fever-United States, *MMWR Morb Motal Wkly Rep* 44:475-479, 1995.
80. Centers for Disease Control (CDC): Management of patients with suspected viral hemorrhagic fever, *MMWR Morb Mortal Wkly Rep* 37(suppl 3):1-16, 1988.
81. Weber DJ, Rutala WA: Risks and prevention of nosocomial transmission of rare zoonotic diseases, *Clin Infect Dis* 32:446-456, 2001.
82. Fukai K, Yokosuka O, Fujiwara K, et al: Etiologic considerations of fulminant non-A, non-B viral hepatitis in Japan: analyses by nucleic acid amplification method, *J Infect Dis* 178:325-333, 1998.
83. Hoofnagle JH: Type D (delta) hepatitis, *JAMA* 261:1321-1325, 1989.
84. Tang JR, Cova L, Lamelin JP, et al: Clinical relevance of the detection of hepatitis delta virus RNA in serum by RNA hybridization and polymerase chain reaction, *J Hepatol* 21:953-960, 1994.
85. Carroll KC, Taggart B, Robison J, et al: Evaluation of the Roche AMPLICOR enterovirus PCR assay in the diagnosis of enteroviral central nervous system infections, *J Clin Virol* 19:149-156, 2000.
86. Sawyer MH, Holland D, Aintablian N, et al: Diagnosis of enteroviral central nervous system infection by polymerase chain reaction during a large community outbreak, *Pediatric Infect Dis J* 13: 177-182, 1994.
87. Bogdanovic G, Priftakis P, Hammarin AL, et al: Detection of JC virus in cerebrospinal fluid (CSF) samples from patients with progressive multifoccal leukoencephalopathy but not in CSF samples from patients with herpes simples encephalitis, enteroviral meningitis, or multiple sclerosis, *J Clin Microbiol* 36:157-163, 1998.
88. Koralnik I J, Boden D, Mai VX, et al: JC virus DNA load in patients with and without progressive multifocal leukoencephalopathy, *Neurology* 52:253-260, 1999.
89. Duncan BW, Bohn DJ, Atz AM, et al: Mechanical circulatory support for the treatment of children with acute fulminant myocarditis, *J Thorac Cardiovasc Surg* 122:440-448, 2001.
90. McCarthy RE III, Boehmer JP, Hruban RH, et al: Long-term outcome of fulminant myocarditis as compared with acute (nonfulminant) myocarditis, *N Engl J Med* 342:690-695, 2000.
91. O'Connell JB, Reap EA, Robinson JA: The effects of cyclosporine on acute murine Coxsackie B3 myocarditis, *Circulation* 73:353-359, 1986.
92. Frishman WH, O'Brien M, Naseer N, et al: Innovative drug treatments for viral and autoimmune myocarditis, *Heart Dis* 4:171-183, 2002.
93. Drucker NA, Colan SD, Lewis AB, et al: Gamma-globulin treatment of acute myocarditis in the pediatric population, *Circulation* 89:252-257, 1994.
94. McNamara DM, Holubkov R, Starling RC, et al: Controlled trial of intravenous immune globulin in recent-onset dilated cardiomyopathy, *Circulation* 103:2254-2259, 2001.
95. Rotbart HA, Webster AD, Pleconaril Treatment Registry Group: Treatment of potentially life-threatening enterovirus infections with pleconaril, *Clin Infect Dis* 32:228-235, 2001.
96. Kondrup J, Almdal T, Vilstrup H, et al: High volume plasma exchange in fulminant hepatic failure, *Int J Artif Organs* 15:669-676, 1992.
97. Rahman T, Hodgson H: Clinical management of acute hepatic failure, *Intensive Care Med* 27:467-476, 2001.
98. KlassenTP, Sutcliffe T, Watters LK, et al: Dexamethasone in salbutamol-treated inpatients with acute bronchiolitis: a randomized, controlled trial, *J Pediatr* 130:170-172, 1997.
99. McBride JT: Dexamethasone and bronchiolitis: a new look at an old therapy? *J Pediatr* 140:8-9, 2002.
100. Roosevelt G, Sheehan K, Grupp-Phelan J, et al: Dexamethasone in bronchiolitis: a randomized controlled trial, *Lancet* 348: 292-295, 1996.
101. Schuh S, Coates AL, Binnie R, et al: Efficacy of oral dexamethasone in outpatients with acute bronchiolitis, *J Pediatr* 140:27-32, 2002.
102. Wheeler JG, Wofford J, Turner RB: Historical cohort evaluation of ribavirin efficacy in respiratory syncytial virus infection, *Pediatr Infect Dis* J 12:209-213, 1993.
103. Hall CB, McBride JT, Gala CL, et al: Ribavirin treatment of respiratory syncytial virus infection in infants with underlying cardiopulmonary disease, *JAMA* 254:3047-3051, 1985.
104. Hall CB, McBride JT, Walsh EE, et al: Aerosolized ribavirin treatment of infants with respiratory syncytial infection. A randomized double-blind study, *N Engl J Med* 308:1443-1447, 1983.

105. Taber LH, Knight V, Gilbert BE, et al: Ribavirin aerosol treatment of bronchiolitis associated with respiratory syncytial virus infection in infants, *Pediatrics* 72:613-618, 1983.
106. Boeckh M, Verrey MM, Bowden RA, et al: Phase 1 evaluation of the respiratory syncytial virus-specific monoclonal antibody palivizumab in recipients of hematopoietic stem cell transplants, *J Infect Dis* 184:350-354, 2001.
107. DeVincenzo JP, Hirsch RL, Fuentes RJ, et al: Respiratory syncytial virus immune globulin treatment of lower respiratory tract infection in pediatric patients undergoing bone marrow transplantation—a compassionate use experience, *Bone Marrow Transplant* 25:161-165, 2000.
108. Ljungman P, Ward KN, Crooks BN, et al: Respiratory virus infections after stem cell transplantation: a prospective study from the Infectious Diseases Working Party of the European Group for Blood and Marrow Transplantation, *Bone Marrow Transplant* 28:479-484, 2001.
109. Whimbey E, Champlin RE, Englund JA, et al: Combination therapy with aerosolized ribavirin and intravenous immunoglobulin for respiratory syncytial virus disease in adult bone marrow transplant recipients, *Bone Marrow Transplant* 16:393-399, 1995.
109a. Centers for Disease Control SARS Investigative Team. Severe acute respiratory syndrome (SARS) and Coronavirus Testing - United States, 2003. MMWR 52:297-302, 2003 and reprinted in JAMA 289:2203-2206, 2003.
110. Whitley RJ, Corey L, Arvin AM, et al: Changing presentation of herpes simplex virus infection in neonates, *J Infect Dis* 158: 109-116, 1988.
111. Raschilas F, Wolff M, Delatour F, et al: Outcome of and prognostic factors for herpes simplex encephalitis in adult patients: results of a multicenter study, *Clin Infect Dis* 35: 254-260, 2002.
112. Chapman LE, Mertz GJ, Peters CJ, et al: Intravenous ribavirin for hantavirus pulmonary syndrome: safety and tolerance during 1 year of open-label experience. Ribavirin Study Group, *Antivir Ther* 4:211-219, 1999.
113. Ljungman P, Deliliers GL, Platzbecker U, et al: Cidofovir for cytomegalovirus infection and disease in allogeneic stem cell transplant recipients. The Infectious Diseases Working Party of the European Group for Blood and Marrow Transplantation, *Blood* 97:388-392, 2001.
114. De Luca A, Giancola ML, Ammassari A, et al: Potent antiviral therapy with or without cidofovir for AIDS-associated progressive multifocal leukoencephalopathy: extended follow-up of an observational study, J Neurovirol 7:364-368, 2001.
115. Gavin PJ, Katz BZ: Intravenous ribavirin treatment for severe adenovirus disease in immunocompromised children, Pediatrics 110:e9, 2002
116. Hoffman JA, Shah AJ, Ross LA, Kapoor N: Adenoviral infections and a prospective trial of cidofovir in pediatric hematopoietic stem cell transplantation, Biol Blood Marrow Transplant 7: 388-394,2001.
117. Huggins JW, Hsiang CM, Cosgriff TM, et al: Prospective, double-blind, concurrent, placebo-controlled clinical trial of intravenous ribavirin therapy of hemorrhagic fever with renal syndrome, J Infect Dis 164:1119-1127, 1991.

CHAPTER

89

Infectious Syndromes in the Pediatric Intensive Care Unit

Sonny Dhanani and Peter N. Cox

PEARLS

- Because of the rapid progression of septicemia from meningococcus and variability of markers of infection such as white blood cell count and C-reactive protein, clinical diagnosis is imperative.
- Negative blood cultures do not rule out staphylococcus; accordingly, clinical suspicion must often be relied upon.
- *Streptococcus pneumoniae* is the most common cause of otitis media and is a frequent cause of sinusitis. With regard to invasive disease in the critical care setting, pneumococcus most commonly presents as bacteremia, pneumonia, arthritis, and meningitis.
- The differential diagnosis for tuberculosis includes *Staphylococcus aureus, Streptococcus pneumonia, Infectious mononucleosis,* human immunodeficiency virus, and cat scratch disease. Leukemia and lymphoma also must be ruled out.
- Relying on serologic tests alone rather that clinical suspicion of Lyme disease can lead to missed diagnoses and overtreatment; markers should be ordered only to confirm objective clinical signs.
- Empiric therapy for Rocky Mountain spotted fever is essential early in the course of illness because fatal outcomes have been linked to missed or delayed diagnosis and treatment.
- West Nile virus presents as an influenza-like illness. Cases are characterized by abrupt onset of fever, headache, backache, and myalgias lasting for 3 to 6 days.

The pediatric critical care unit is the epicenter of severe infection in most children's hospitals. Many of these infectious processes are nosocomial and are associated with either patient (e.g., immunocompromised) or procedural issues. Other infectious processes affect specific organs (bronchiolitis and meningitis). These specific infections and the general principles of sepsis management are described in Chapters 57 and 96. In this chapter, we describe some of the infections that may precipitate a systemic response and multiorgan involvement requiring intensive care unit admission. We highlight the salient and identifying features and, where appropriate, comment on specific therapeutic strategies.

Meningococcus

Etiology and Epidemiology

Neisseria meningitidis is a gram-negative diplococcus that is a common cause of bacterial meningitis. It also is responsible for 500,000 cases of a severe sepsis syndrome reported worldwide annually.[190] It was estimated that 1.6 cases occurred per 100,000 population, with 3437 cases reported in 1996 in the United States.[50] Of the 13 serogroups, strains A, B, C, Y, and W-135 are implicated most often. Most cases are isolated or sporadic, with less than 5% associated with outbreaks.[7] In the United States, serogroup B accounts for 30% to 70% of sporadic cases, whereas serogroup C is much less common but is often associated with small outbreaks.[158] Serogroup A is a common cause of cyclic epidemics in Africa and Asia.[198]

The disease most often occurs in children younger than 5 years, with the peak attack rate between the ages of 3 and 5 months. Children with complement C5-9 deficiency and asplenia are at increased risk.[7] Asymptomatic carriage state has been recognized, and pathogenesis is thought to begin on the nasopharyngeal surface.[18] Patients are considered capable of transmitting the organism for up to 24 hours after treatment.[2,3,8]

Clinical Presentation

Most invasive meningococcal infections present as meningitis, whereas approximately 10% present as sepsis alone and approximately 40% present as both systemic and central nervous system (CNS) disease.[113] Since the use of *Haemophilus influenzae* vaccine, *N. meningitidis* has become the second most common cause of bacterial meningitis in North America after pneumococcus.[151] With meningitis alone, the classic signs of headache and meningismus are present but their severity can be variable. Onset of septicemia often is abrupt, with fever, chills, malaise, and rash. Rash is the hallmark sign presenting in up to 80% of cases.[125] Although petechial rash appearing in clusters at pressure sites is classic, urticarial or maculopapular rashes also may present[50] (Figure 89–1). The shock state is mediated by endotoxin (lipopolysaccharide) release with subsequent complement activation and release of numerous inflammatory mediators.[18,28,29,113] Subsequently, rapid endothelial cell injury occurs, leading to capillary leakage, microvascular thrombosis, refractory peripheral vasoconstriction, and acute myocardial failure.[27] Septicemia can rapidly progress within hours to disseminated intravascular coagulopathy (DIC), shock, and death. Invasive disease can be complicated by an immune-mediated arthritis, pancarditis, endophthalmitis, pneumonia, and adrenal insufficiency from Waterhouse-Friderichsen syndrome.[7,88,135]

Diagnosis

Because of the rapid progression of septicemia and the variability of markers of infection such as white blood cell count and C-reactive protein, clinical diagnosis is imperative. Clinical suspicion should be based on the characteristic rash and symptoms and signs of hypoperfusion, such as tachycardia, cool peripheral extremities, decreased urine output, and altered mental state. Aggressive treatment should be instituted prior to the onset of overt hypotension, which usually occurs before culture results are available.[134,150]

Confirmation may be difficult, particularly when patients have received early antibiotics. Positive cerebrospinal fluid (CSF) and blood cultures range from 50% to 80% in various series.[149] Nevertheless, cultures from blood and CSF are indicated. Lumbar puncture should be delayed if evidence of increased intracranial pressure, coagulopathy, or cardiovascular instability is present. Cultures from petechial scrapings and other body fluids such as synovial fluid can be helpful.[113] Because *N. meningitidis* may be a part of normal flora, nasopharyngeal cultures are not helpful.[7] Latex agglutination is helpful for CSF but unreliable for urine and blood specimens. Polymerase chain reaction (PCR) for bacterial protein now is being used in various centers, with sensitivity and specificity near 90%.[138]

Management

Conventional Therapy

Experience and epidemiologic data support rapid early intervention in the peripheral center and aggressive treatment in a tertiary care pediatric intensive care unit.[148] Rapid administration of antibiotics prior to transfer has been shown to improve prognosis.[39] Ceftriaxone 100 mg/kg/day divided once or twice daily is recommended as initial empiric therapy. Once *N. meningitidis* is confirmed, then penicillin G 500,000 U/kg/day divided in six doses can be used based on sensitivities. Chloramphenicol is an alternative if the patient is allergic to penicillin.[7,113]

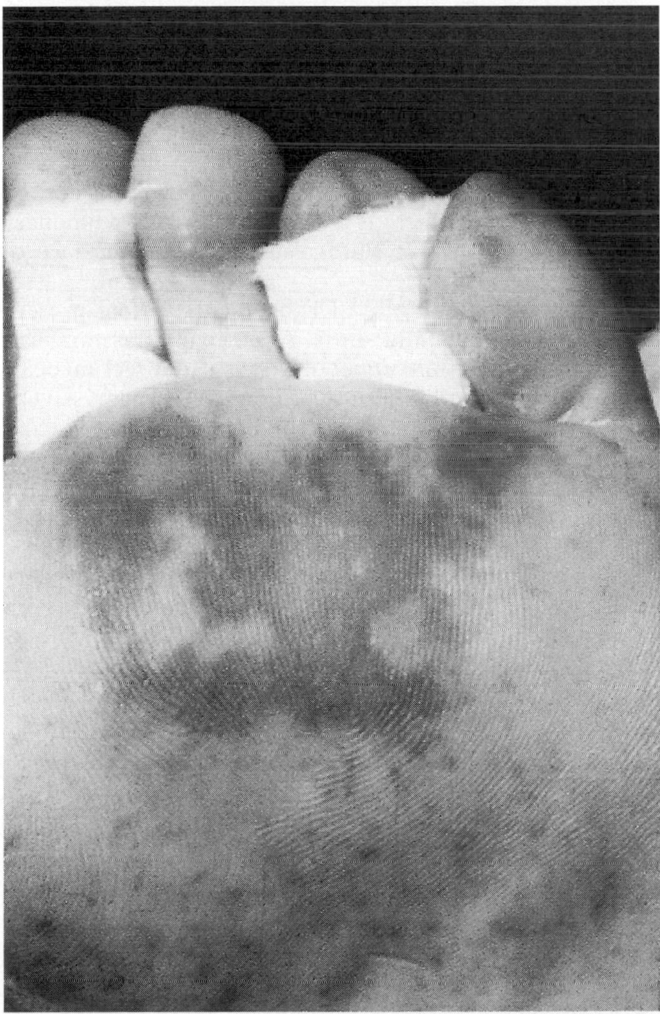

FIGURE 89–1 • Ecchymosis of a sole with meningococcal sepsis. (See also Color Insert.) (From Apicella MA: Neisseria meningitides. In Mandell GL, Bennett JE, Dolin R, editors: *Mandell: Principles and Practice of Infectious Diseases,* ed 5. New York, 2000, Churchill Livingstone.)

Significant capillary leakage is the hallmark feature in meningococcal sepsis. Thus the prominent problem faced in the early stages is maintenance of adequate circulating volume. Early and aggressive volume resuscitation is vital and has been shown to improve outcome.[38,134] Normal saline or 5% albumin solutions have been the standard; no evidence indicates that other colloids, such as blood, change outcome. Ongoing need for continued volume resuscitation should be based on clinical signs of shock and may be as high as twice the child's circulating volume (e.g., 120 ml/kg).[113,149] Myocardial depression should be assumed and inotropes such as dopamine should be used early concomitantly with fluid to ensure adequate cardiac output. Epinephrine, norepinephrine, or vasopressin may be necessary. However, the need for high-dose α-adrenergic agents and vasopressin to maintain blood pressure may need to be balanced against the risk for distal extremity ischemia and necrosis. To ensure appropriate and rapid volume and inotropic delivery, central venous access should be established as soon as meningococcal sepsis is suspected; however, volume resuscitation should not be delayed and should be started with peripheral or intraosseous access if central access is not yet available.[149]

Respiratory support often is necessary when fluid requirements greater than 40 ml/kg are required. Even if the patient is alert and oriented, intubate and ventilate early for resuscitation and transport when meningococcus is suspected in order to ensure adequate oxygenation, reduce the patient's work of breathing, theoretically decrease metabolic demands, and maintain stability for transport.[113] More importantly, there is a significant risk of pulmonary edema after aggressive fluid resuscitation in the face of myocardial depression.[149]

Numerous metabolic derangements often present because of cellular fluid shifts. Abnormal potassium, calcium, and magnesium concentrations can affect myocardial function and should be managed aggressively. Hypoglycemia is a common finding, so serum glucose concentration should be monitored closely. Metabolic acidosis is common and usually corrects with adequate perfusion and lactate clearance. Replacement of bicarbonate is reserved for pH less than 7.2.[135]

DIC is common because of factor loss from capillary leak and clotting factor consumption. Derangements are treated with fresh-frozen plasma and cryoprecipitate as needed to prevent life-threatening bleeds. This process is associated with anemia and thrombocytopenia, for which packed red blood cells and platelet transfusions may be necessary, especially if spontaneous bleeding from mucus membranes and venipuncture sites occurs.

Plastic surgical interventions may be necessary for amputations and skin grafting. Consultation with other services may be necessary for renal failure, secondary infections, and neurologic complications.

Novel Therapy

In addition to standard cardiovascular and respiratory support, multiple new treatment strategies have been proposed. They have been aimed at altering the inflammatory cascade, treating hemostatic abnormalities, and inducing vasodilation and perfusion.

The role of steroid therapy remains unclear. Cortisol in the septic setting has been thought to enhance up-regulation of adrenergic receptors and improve the response to catecholamines, such as exogenous inotropes. No evidence supports the routine use of steroids in meningococcemia; however, adrenal replacement doses of hydrocortisone 1 to 2 mg/kg have been suggested for fluid and vasopressor recalcitrant septic shock.[113]

Immunotherapy, such as antiserum to *Escherichia coli,* which was thought to halt the immune cascade if given early enough, has not been shown to be beneficial in several trials.[102] Likewise, anti-endotoxin HA-1A, a human monoclonal immunoglobulin (Ig)M antibody, had no significant benefit.[69] The overall limitation of anti-endotoxin therapy is that it must be given very early in the disease process in order to halt the inflammatory response. An alternative to anti-endotoxins may be bacteriocidal/permeability increasing proteins (BPI). BPI are found in neutrophils and neutralize endotoxins after their release. The results of a large multicenter trial are promising but preliminary.[85] Plasmapheresis to remove cytokines and other mediators are being studied, but no difference in plasma concentrations or overall outcomes has been reported.[75,80] Anticytokine therapy such as interleukin-1 receptor antagonists and anti-tumor necrosis factor antibodies are being studied for sepsis but not specifically for meningococcus. Hemofiltration and plasma exchange to remove inflammatory mediators have been performed safely. However, the results are mixed, so they are not currently standard therapy.[22,129,155] As mentioned, several hemostatic abnormalities are related to meningococcal disease, and it is postulated they are key to pathogenesis and severity of disease. Potential therapies to combat DIC include antithrombin-III (AT-III), tissue plasminogen activator (tPA), activated protein C, and heparin, as reviewed by Leclerc et al.[115] Case reports are encouraging, but adequate trials are pending. AT-III infusion may promote return of peripheral perfusion and salvage of limbs.[59] Tissue plasminogen activator was associated with an improvement in shock and a decrease in amputations.[4] Activated protein C has been shown to reverse end-organ dysfunction but has not yet been demonstrated to prevent other morbidity, such as significant loss of limbs.[156] Many case reports have supported heparin infusions, but the benefits have not been reproduced in controlled studies.[114] Because of the significant risk of intracerebral bleeding, cost of therapy, and lack of prospective randomized studies, the impact of these adjunct therapies on morbidity and mortality are still being debated and investigated.[116]

Vasodilators to improve peripheral and end-organ perfusion have been studied in small populations, and results are variable. Prostacyclin has been reported to improve distal perfusion, whereas nitroprusside infusions and topical nitroglycerin also have been attempted, with some anecdotal success.[61,116]

Prognosis

Morbidity and mortality with meningococcus has been difficult to estimate because of multiple serotypes, regional differences, and seasonal variations. Mortality of meningococcal disease is reported between 7% and 19% in review of multiple centers, with some studies reporting mortality rates as high as 53% worldwide.[113] Morbidity is less well reported but ranges between 11% and 19% and includes complications such as need for skin grafting, loss of limbs/digits, and neurologic disability.[113] Several prognostic scores have been developed using multiple clinical and laboratory values. A widely used and validated system is the Glasgow Meningococcal Septicemia Prognostic Score developed by Sinclair and validated by Thomson et al.[113,185] Data suggests that early recognition, aggressive resuscitation, and transfer to a pediatric intensive care unit can reduce mortality of severely ill children to less than 35%.[117,148]

Staphylococcus Toxic Shock Syndrome

Etiology and Epidemiology

Staphylococcus aureus is a gram-positive coccus grouped typically in clusters. It is responsible for a wide spectrum of clinical manifestations, including sepsis, pneumonia, cellulitis, arthritis, meningitis, and endocarditis. Staphylococcal toxic shock syndrome (TSS) came into prominence in the early 1980s with the use of superabsorbent tampons and was named *menstrual-associated toxic shock*.[121] Thus this form of TSS has a particular predilection for adolescents and young women.[10] Nonmenstrual cases have been associated with localized infections, surgery, or insect bites and now account for about one third to half of TSS cases.[41,45,57]

Staphylococci produce various toxins. In particular, TSS is linked to an enterotoxin named *toxic shock syndrome toxin-1* (TSST-1). TSST-1 accounts for approximately 90% of cases of menstrual toxic shock. Other enterotoxins are responsible for up to 50% of nonmenstrual cases.[121] TSST-1 is a superantigen that acts as a stimulating factor for the release of inflammatory mediators such as interleukin-1β, tumor necrosis factor-α, interleukin-2, and γ-interferon from macrophages and lymphocytes. This massive inflammatory mediator release causes generalized lymphocytic perivasculitis and interstitial edema. This capillary leak syndrome is characteristic of TSS and results in multiorgan dysfunction, including heart, lung, kidney, and brain involvement.[14]

Clinical Presentation

The Centers for Disease Control and Prevention (CDC) has defined toxic shock syndrome as fever, rash, hypotension, multiorgan involvement, and desquamation with specific criteria (Box 89-1). Onset usually is abrupt, with fever, chills, malaise, and diffuse macular erythroderma. Fever often is remarkably high and resistant, occurring with intense myalgias, vomiting, and diarrhea. The rash is described as a generalized erythematous, deep-red "sunburn" and can be accompanied by conjunctival erythema. Within 24 hours, cardiovascular depression becomes prominent, with hypotension and decreasing systemic perfusion leading to severe shock and multiorgan dysfunction. Progressive liver and renal failure are common. The patient may manifest symptoms of diffuse encephalopathy, usually without meningeal signs. Renal failure can be oliguric or nonoliguric. Scaling and desquamation, which are included in the diagnostic criteria, occur with resolution of fever and usually are prominent on the palms and soles.[66,94,104,194]

BOX 89–1

Staphylococcus Toxic Shock Syndrome Case Definition

- Fever: temperature ≥ 38.9°C
- Rash: diffuse macular erythroderma
- Desquamation: 1–2 weeks after onset of illness; involvement of palms, soles, fingers, and toes
- Hypotension: systolic blood pressure ≤ 90 for adults; ≤ 5th percentile for age in children; or orthostatic syncope
  AND
- Involvement of ≥ 3 of the following organ systems:
  - Central nervous system: disorientation or alteration in consciousness, without focal neurologic signs, when fever and hypotension are absent
  - Gastrointestinal: vomiting or diarrhea at onset of illness
  - Hematological: platelets ≤ 100,000
  - Hepatic: total bilirubin or transaminase concentrations greater than twice the upper limit of normal
  - Muscular: severe myalgia or CPK level greater than twice the upper limit of normal
  - Mucus membrane: vaginal, oropharyngeal, or conjunctival hyperemia
  - Renal: blood urea nitrogen or creatinine concentration greater than twice the upper limit of normal or at least five white blood cells per high-power field in the absence of urinary tract infection
  AND
- Negative results on the following test:
  - Blood, throat, or cerebrospinal fluid cultures for other organisms
  - Serologic tests for Rocky Mountain spotted fever, leptospirosis, or measles

Modified from Centers for Disease Control and Prevention: *MMWR* 32:201, 1982.

Diagnosis

Differential diagnosis for syndromes that include fever, rash, and multiorgan involvement are numerous and are summarized in Box 89–2.

Diagnosis is mainly clinical but can be supported with inflammatory markers associated with sepsis. However, the degree of leukocytosis often is not impressive but the percentage of immature cells usually is markedly high.[57] Metabolic derangements can support the diagnosis; for example, hypocalcemia and hypophosphatemia can be profound.[58] Liver function abnormalities are common. Elevated urea and creatinine concentrations result from prerenal causes initially but also may involve acute tubular necrosis. Persistent lactic acidosis even with restoration of hemodynamics may reflect decreased tissue perfusion and end organ ischemia.[104]

Negative blood cultures do not rule out staphylococcus; accordingly, clinical suspicion often must be relied on. Lumbar puncture is not warranted because CSF usually is benign in TSS. Swabs of the primary infection site, such as the postsurgical site, or vaginal swabs can be helpful.

BOX 89-2

Differential Diagnosis of Staphylococcus Toxic Shock Syndrome

- Bacterial
  - Meningococcemia
  - Invasive group A β-hemolytic streptococcus toxic shock
  - Group A β-hemolytic streptococcus scarlet fever
  - Staphylococcus scalded skin syndrome
  - Salmonella infection
- Viral
  - Measles
  - Enterovirus syndrome with myocarditis
- Tick-borne
  - Rocky Mountain spotted fever
  - Leptospirosis
  - Ehrlichiosis
- Other
  - Stevens-Johnson syndrome and toxic epidermal necrolysis (drug reaction)
  - Kawasaki disease
  - Systemic lupus erythematosus

Modified from Chesney PJ: Pediatric infectious disease-associated syndromes. In Fuhrman BP, Zimmerman JJ, editors: *Pediatric critical care.* St. Louis, 1992, Mosby.

TSST-1 antibody assays have been developed but are not recommended, especially because many of the nonmenstrual cases may have other causative endotoxins.[194]

Management

Because the course can be variable and unpredictable, close monitoring and observation are essential when TSS is suspected. Rapid and aggressive fluid administration is required because the severity of end-organ involvement is related to the degree of hypotension and duration of decreased perfusion. Volume requirements may be exceptionally high because of the massive capillary leak characteristic of TSS.[117,148] As a result, acute respiratory distress syndrome (ARDS), myocardial failure, and generalized edema are common. Fluid administration should be guided by close monitoring of blood pressure, central venous pressure, perfusion, and urine output.

Two premises to antibiotic therapy for TSS exist. The first is to kill the organism with a bacteriocidal antistaphylococcal β-lactamase–resistant agent such as cloxacillin or vancomycin. The second is to stop enzyme, toxin, and cytokine production with a protein synthesis inhibitor such as clindamycin.[121] Vancomycin is less effective against *Staphylococcus* and should be limited to resistant organisms or allergic patients.[118]

Vaginal examination should be performed as soon as possible and foreign bodies removed and sent for cultures. Other possible foci for infection should be drained and irrigated, especially postsurgical sites.

Intravenous γ-globulin (IVIG) has been shown to prevent T-cell stimulation by enterotoxin and may have a role in modulating the inflammatory response.[181] No systematically studied trials in humans have described benefits of IVIG, but numerous animal models exist.[131] There are anecdotal examples of its effectiveness, especially in refractory cases.[14,160] Doses of 150 to 600 mg/kg/day for 5 days or a single dose of 1 to 2 g/kg have been used. In theory, the drug must be given early in the course of illness because its role is to prevent rather than treat the systemic inflammatory response.[10]

Corticosteroids have been used after retrospective studies reported beneficial effects on severity and duration of illness.[191] However, no further prospective studies have shown specific benefits against the TSST-1 enterotoxin. Therefore steroids usually are reserved for refractory cases where hypotension does not respond to fluids and inotropes.

Other management issues include correction of acid-base abnormalities, electrolyte disorders including hypocalcemia, coagulopathies, renal failure, and fluid overload. Aggressive ventilation strategies may be necessary in the presence of ARDS.

Prognosis

With aggressive therapy, prognosis is good, with a mortality rate of 5%. Death usually is related to ARDS or refractory arrhythmias.[33] Mortality is higher in nonmenstrual cases. Other specific risk factors for higher mortality have not been identified, although increasing age has been linked to poorer outcome.[33] Recurrent cases have been noted for both menstrual and nonmenstrual causation.[14,104]

Invasive Pneumococcus

Etiology and Epidemiology

Streptococcus pneumoniae is the most common cause of otitis media and a frequent cause of sinusitis. With regard to invasive disease in the critical care setting, pneumococcus most commonly presents as bacteremia, pneumonia, arthritis, and meningitis. Meningitis is discussed in Chapter 57. This chapter focuses on bacteremia and pneumonia. Other less common pneumococcal infections include endocarditis, soft tissue cellulitis, pericarditis, peritonitis, and salpingitis.

S. pneumoniae is an encapsulated gram-positive diplococcus organized in chains. It is a nasopharyngeal colonizer and is found in up to 40% of healthy children.[133] Transmission via secretions and respiratory droplets increase in environments of close contacts, such as day care centers.[74] Infection from *S. pneumoniae* may be secondary to mucosal barrier changes from other viral infections. In one study, invasive disease in children was more prevalent between September and May and was associated with other viral illnesses such as influenza.[109] There are more than 90 serotypes of *S. pneumoniae,* with only a few identified as causing invasive disease.[182] Once cells are invaded, the organism is resistant to phagocytosis because of its capsule and subsequently causes tissue damage. Most other streptococcal species cause damage via toxin-mediated mechanisms.[182] The incidence is higher and the severity of invasive illness greater in children with congenital or acquired humoral immunodeficiencies, including human immunodeficiency virus (HIV) (see Chapters 86 and 87).

Patients with deficient splenic function are susceptible (Box 89–3).

The overall rate of invasive disease is 23 per 100,000 persons per year in the United States.[157] It is relatively more common in newborns and infants up to age 2 years and much less in older children and teenagers.[36] Most younger cases result from bacteremia, with up to 160 per 100,000 infants younger than 12 months.[32,157] Older children are more likely to develop pneumonia. Per annum, an estimated 500,000 cases of pneumonia, 60,000 cases of bacteremia, and 3,000 cases of meningitis related to streptococcus occur in the United States.[46] Meningitis occurs most commonly between the ages of 6 and 18 months, bacteremia occurs between 6 and 36 months, and pneumonia presents between 3 and 60 months.[205] Of the many children in the third world who die of lower respiratory tract infection, streptococcus is the primary agent.[77] Globally, *S. pneumoniae* is the most common cause of bacterial pneumonia, accounting for up to 70% of cases.[40]

Clinical Presentation

Invasive pneumococcal disease is defined as the isolation of *S. pneumoniae* from normally sterile sites such as blood, pleural fluid, joint fluid, and CSF. Approximately 3% to 5% of febrile children between 3 and 36 months old are at risk for occult or asymptomatic bacteremia, of which 90% are caused by *S. pneumoniae*.[20] In most cases, occult bacteremia resolves without sequelae. However, persistent bacteremia may lead to septic shock with hypotension and end-organ involvement, spreading to the meninges, pleura, bones, and joints.

Pneumococcal pneumonia is associated with bacteremia in 40% of cases.[127,182] Presentation can be quite nonspecific, especially in infants. Symptoms range from those managed as an outpatient to those requiring mechanical ventilatory support. Most commonly, symptoms include fever, cough, tachypnea, malaise, and emesis.[126] On physical examination, hypoxia is associated with localized crepitations and decreased breath sounds that correlate with lobar infiltration on chest radiographs. Almost 50% of cases present with multilobar involvement and 40% with pleural effusions.[182] Although rare, necrotizing pneumonia, pneumatoceles, and lung abscesses can be seen. Pleural empyema occurs in up to 14% of pneumococcal pneumonia.[183] Interestingly, lower lobe pneumonia may present with abdominal symptoms and signs, whereas upper lobe pneumonia may be associated with nuchal rigidity.[182]

BOX 89–3

Risk Factors for Invasive Pneumococcal Disease

ORGANISM FACTORS

- Invasive properties of the pneumococcal serotype

HOST FACTORS

- Serotype-specific humoral immunity
- Age ≤2 years
- Specific ethnic background:
  - African American
  - Native American
  - Alaskan Eskimo
  - Micronesian
  - Aboriginal (Australia and New Zealand)
- Presence of viral respiratory infection
- Lack of breast-feeding
- Underlying illness:
  - Congenital or acquired antibody deficiency
  - HIV infection
  - Complement deficiency
  - Congenital or acquired splenic dysfunction:
    - Sickle cell disease
    - Other hemoglobinopathies
    - Surgical splenectomy
  - Malignancy
  - Nephrotic syndrome

ENVIRONMENTAL FACTORS

- Day care attendance
- Recent antibiotic use
- Season of year
- Smoke exposure
- Overcrowding

Modified from Tan TQ: *Pediatr Ann* 31:242, 2002.

Diagnosis

Diagnosis depends mostly on clinical suspicion. Initially, *S. pneumoniae* bacteremia should be suspected when the white blood cell count (WBC) is greater than 15,000 and absolute neutrophil count is greater than 10,000.[20] Isolation from blood or sterile fluid confirms the diagnosis but should not delay treatment if pneumococcus is suspected. Pneumococcal rapid antigen testing and PCR can aid in making the diagnosis, especially if antibiotics have already been started.[144] Sputum samples are rarely helpful in children; nasopharyngeal cultures may reflect only colonization rather than infection. However, if intubated, samples obtained via bronchioalveolar lavage are beneficial. Ultrasound or computed tomography (CT) can help identify effusions or empyema, which subsequently can be aspirated.[126]

Management

For critically ill patients potentially infected with invasive *S. pneumoniae,* a third-generation cephalosporin such as ceftriaxone or cefotaxime 25 mg/kg/dose every 8 hours is recommended. Cefuroxime, a second-generation agent, is also an appropriate choice.[8,105] If the patient is toxic, immunodeficient, or antibiotic resistance is suspected, then vancomycin 10 mg/kg/dose every 6 hours should be added. However, even when nonsusceptible strains were identified, complications, recovery, and mortality were no different than when penicillin alone was used.[67,79,132] Thus vancomycin should not be used routinely but is suggested when severe multilobar pneumonia, carditis, meningitis, or hypoxia and hypotension are present. When pneumococcus is confirmed and sensitivities are determined, then antibiotics should be reevaluated and penicillin G 400,000 U every 4 to 6 hours started if susceptible.

Clindamycin can be used for patients with penicillin hypersensitivity.[8,105]

During the past two decades, antibiotic resistance among pneumococcal strains has continued to increase and has complicated the management of invasive infections. Resistance stems from the alteration of penicillin-binding proteins, which are enzymes that are important in the production of bacterial cell walls. As a result of these alterations, there is a decreased affinity for β-lactam antibiotics and thus decreased susceptibility.[105] In the United States, 34% of strains were nonsusceptible to β-lactams, with 21% showing full resistance and 13% showing intermediate resistance. Similarly, full resistance to ceftriaxone also increased to 14%.[72] Resistance to other classes of antibiotics occurs by other mechanisms and is summarized by Kaplan.[105] Although resistance to vancomycin is not yet described, tolerance such that *S. pneumoniae* is inhibited but not killed has been reported.[93]

Treatment should continue for 7 days for bacteremia and 10 to 14 days for pneumonia. Symptoms such as fever and tachypnea may persist for 3 to 4 days after initiation of treatment. If fever persists, then further investigations for infectious collections or resistance are necessary.[133]

If empyema is suspected, then the etiology should be established definitively with immediate thoracocentesis and empyema drainage. These procedures have been shown to decrease the severity and duration of illness. If only effusions are present, then draining is not imperative unless loculations develop or symptoms persist.[127]

BOX 89–4

Case Definition for Streptococcal Toxic Shock Syndrome

Isolation of group A β-hemolytic streptococci:
- From a normally sterile site: blood, cerebrospinal fluid, peritoneal fluid, tissue biopsy, etc.*
  AND
  Clinical signs of severity:
  Hypotension:
  - Systolic blood pressure ≤ 90 for adults; ≤ 5th percentile for age in children
  AND
- Multiorgan involvement with ≥ 2 of the following:
  - Acute respiratory distress syndrome
  - Coagulopathy: platelets ≤ 100,000 or disseminated intravascular coagulopathy
  - Hepatic: total bilirubin or transaminases greater than twice the upper limit of normal
  - Rash: generalized macular erythroderma that may desquamate
  - Renal: creatinine twice the upper limit for age
  - Soft tissue necrosis: necrotizing fasciitis, myositis, or gangrene

*If group A β-hemolytic streptococcus is isolated from a *nonsterile* site but other criteria are still fulfilled, then defined as a *probable* case.

Modified from The Working Group on Severe Streptococcal Infections: *JAMA* 209:390-391, 1993.

Prognosis

In most children, occult pneumococcal bacteremia resolves spontaneously without apparent sequelae.[59] Overall mortality from documented bacteremia was reported to be 0.4% in one review.[106] The possibility of persistent bacteremia and spread to sterile site results in significant morbidity. The case/fatality rate for pneumococcal pneumonia is 1% in children but up to 20% in adults.[123] Pleural empyema and chronic lung changes may occur in up to 14%.[183] The impact of penicillin resistance on the clinical presentation and outcome of invasive pneumococcus is still unclear. The role of new heptavalent conjugate vaccines on morbidity and mortality is evolving.

Invasive Group A β-Hemolytic Streptococcus

Etiology and Epidemiology

Invasive group A β-hemolytic streptococcus (GABHS) is a gram-positive coccus often grouped as chains. Infections resulting from GABHS have become more common, presenting with the two overlapping syndromes of TSS and necrotizing fasciitis.[95,176,185] The CDC has defined TSS caused by GABHS as having prominent features of shock and multiorgan failure (Box 89–4). TSS caused by GABHS is similar to the clinical entity described for staphylococcus TSS. However, GABHS TSS is more commonly associated with bacteremia and underlying soft tissue infection compared with staphylococcal TSS. Necrotizing fasciitis is characterized by extensive local necrosis of soft tissue and skin. GABHS TSS is associated with necrotizing fasciitis in 50% of cases.[24] Apart from these two entities, invasive GABHS can present with more localized infections such as meningitis, pneumonia, osteomyelitis, septic arthritis, and surgical wound infections. It is important to note that severe invasive GABHS rarely occurs following isolated pharyngitis; rather, most infections reflect the skin or soft tissue as the portal of entry.[176]

The CDC estimates the incidence is 4 to 5 cases per 100,000, with approximately 10,000 cases occurring yearly.[141] Overall mortality in the pediatric population is approximately 5% to 10% but is much higher in adults.[64] Approximately 10% of cases are hospital-acquired infections. Infections in clusters or outbreaks, even with close contacts, are uncommon.[65] Streptococcal necrotizing fasciitis can occur in otherwise healthy people at any age, but the incidence is higher in young children and the elderly. Risk factors include diabetes mellitus, chronic cardiac or pulmonary disease, immunodeficiency syndromes, intravenous drug use, and alcoholism.[95] In children, varicella seems to be an increasing risk factor in recent years. GABHS should be suspected as a secondary infection in children with recurrence of fever especially after day 3 of varicella illness or when lesions are more painful.[71,202] Several reports have implicated nonsteroidal antiinflammatory drug agents as a risk factor for GABHS infection; however, a causal relationship has not been established.[5,175]

The pathogenic mechanism is unknown but is thought to be associated with streptococcal pyrogenic exotoxin, which may act as a superantigen. This stimulates intense activation and proliferation of T lymphocytes and macrophages, resulting in a massive production of cytokines that in turn mediate tissue injury and shock.[161]

Clinical Presentation

With TSS, most cases present initially with nonspecific "flu"-like symptoms that include fever, chills, and myalgias. Half of the patients develop hypotension within the first 4 hours.[173] Multiorgan failure including ARDS and acute renal failure occurs in up to 55% of patients. Mechanical ventilation is necessary in 90% of patients. Otherwise, presentation includes myositis, perihepatitis, peritonitis, myocarditis, and generalized sepsis.[65]

With fasciitis, pain is the most common initial symptom, usually without correlating physical signs.[176] It usually is an acute process with rapid progression. The legs are the most common site, but the abdominal wall, groin, and perianal areas also are frequently affected. In newborns, the site most commonly affected is the umbilicus. Approximately 80% of infants eventually develop obvious signs of soft tissue infection, and of these 70% develop into deeper infections requiring surgical debridement. Initially over 24 to 48 hours, the area becomes erythematous and swollen without sharp margins. Skin vesicles and bullae may be bluish and may appear by days 4 to 5, heralding fasciitis. By this time, the area often becomes anesthetic and gangrenous secondary to thrombosis of small blood vessels. Marked swelling and edema may lead to compartment syndrome requiring urgent fasciotomies.

Diagnosis

Signs and symptoms may not be specific for group A streptococcus; thus treatment is initiated before diagnosis is confirmed. Invasive GABHS should be suspected especially when a risk factor such as varicella or diabetes mellitus is present. Swab Gram stain and cultures taken from focal lesions probably are the most useful diagnostic tool. Bacteremia is present in 60%, but pending blood culture results should not delay treatment. Often only mild leukocytosis is present, but a left shift is striking.[31] Rising serum creatinine kinase concentration has correlated well to deeper soft tissue infections. When necrotizing fasciitis is suspected, magnetic resonance imaging can be helpful in confirming the diagnosis by identifying muscle and underlying fascia inflammation and necrosis.[206] GABHS was identified in 71% of necrotizing fasciitis cases.[173] However, one study in children found GABHS as a single organism in only 25% of the cases; the rest were polymicrobial.[103] Other organisms include *Bacteroides, Peptostreptococcus, Enterococcus, Staphylococcus* species, *Clostridium,* and *E. coli.* Approximately half of necrotizing fasciitis cases involve mixed aerobic and anaerobic flora[62] (Table 89–1).

Management

When invasive GABHS is suspected, aggressive hemodynamic support and specific antibiotic therapy are essential. In addition, prompt surgical intervention is necessary with necrotizing fasciitis. Aggressive debridement is necessary to remove infected and necrotic tissue to prevent progression of inflammation and necrosis. Fasciotomies often are needed in the presence of compartment syndrome in order to facilitate adequate perfusion. Frequently, massive amounts of intravenous fluids are required because of the extensive capillary leak. Inotropic agents such as dopamine usually are needed early in order to support adequate cardiac output. Vasoconstrictors such as epinephrine, norepinephrine, and vasopressin should be used with caution because impaired perfusion to necrotic areas may lead to loss of limbs. Milrinone may be a useful adjunct when vasodilation is necessary.[5,11]

With TSS, both GABHS and *S. aureus* should be covered with broad-spectrum antibiotics. With a microbiologic diagnosis, the antibiotics can be tailored later. Group A streptococci in general are extremely sensitive to β-lactams, but invasive GABHS infections seem to respond less well to penicillins alone.[174,177] With GABHS identified, penicillin G 200,000 to 400,000 U/kg/day in 4 to 6 divided doses can be administered. Clindamycin as an adjunct has proved effective at doses of 25 to 40 mg/kg/day in 3 to 4 divided doses.[51,178] Clindamycin works by inhibiting protein synthesis, thus suppressing bacterial toxin production and decreasing penicillin-binding protein synthesis. Clindamycin also has been shown to modulate the immune response.[178] However, no controlled clinical trials have demonstrated improved outcome with the addition of clindamycin.[5]

With necrotizing fasciitis, prompt surgical exploration and aggressive debridement are critical, with involvement

TABLE 89–1

List of Common Organisms Causing Necrotizing Fasciitis

Gram-Positive Organisms	Percent	Gram-Negative Organisms	Percent
Group A streptococci	18–46	*Escherichia coli*	8–28
Enterococci	16–34	*Enterobacter*	2–12
Coagulase-negative *Staphylococcus*	15–37	*Pseudomonas*	9–20
Staphylococcus aureus	9–37	*Proteus*	6–12
Staphylococcus epidermidis	18	*Serratia*	2–6
Clostridia	5–21	*Bacteroides*	18–48
Mixed Gram positives	10	Mixed gram negatives	16

Modified from Cunningham JD, Silver L, Rudikoff D: *Mt Sinai J Med* 68:258, 2001.

of both general and plastic surgeons. By the time clinical signs are present, saving viable tissue may not be possible, but debridement is necessary to prevent the progression of tissue destruction. The patient often is returned to the operating room daily for inspection until the infection is adequately controlled. Amputation may be necessary and should be undertaken early if necessary. Then, daily dressing changes can continue with close monitoring of surgical margins.[62]

Antibodies specific for the toxin do not exist, but use of IVIG 1 to 2 g/kg in a single dose has been effective in case reports.[21,115] The possible mechanism may involve prevention of T-cell proliferation and reduction of cytokine release. Some anecdotal reports of the benefits of hyperbaric oxygen also exist but are inconclusive.[189] No controlled trials have demonstrated the efficacy of either of these therapies.

Prognosis

Mortality rates for TSS vary from 30% to 70%.[65,68] For necrotizing fasciitis, morality rates range from 6% to 33%.[62] Morbidity is high, including surgical intervention in greater than 50% of suspected fasciitis cases.[176] Irreversible renal impairment is seen in up to 10%. Unfavorable outcome has been shown to be affected by delayed diagnosis and by the presence of organ failure at the time of admission.[78]

BOX 89-5

High-Risk Groups for Tuberculosis Infection

GROUPS AT HIGH-RISK OF EXPOSURE OR INFECTION:

- Close contacts of person with TB
- Foreign-born persons from high-risk countries:
  - Asia, Africa, Eastern Europe, Latin America, Russia
- Residents and employees of high-risk congregate settings:
  - Correctional institutions, nursing homes, homeless shelters, hospitals, drug treatment centers
- Medically underserviced, low-income populations
- High-risk racial or ethnic minority populations
- Injection drug users
- Children exposed to adults in high-risk categories

GROUPS AT HIGHER RISK OF DEVELOPING ACTIVE DISEASE ONCE INFECTED:

- Recent TB infection (within past 2 years)
- History of inadequately TB treatment
- Persons with underlying medical conditions:
  - Diabetes mellitus, malignancy, malnutrition, renal disease
- Immunosuppressed patients:
  - Congenital or acquired, including HIV
- Children <4 years, especially infants

Modified from Centers for Disease Control and Prevention: *Core curriculum on tuberculosis,* ed 4, Atlanta, 2000, US Department of Health and Human Services.

Tuberculosis

Etiology and Epidemiology

Tuberculosis is one of the leading causes of death from infectious disease throughout the world. There has been a resurgence of disease since the 1980s, especially in the developed world. Many factors have contributed to increasing rates in North America, including the HIV/acquired immunodeficiency epidemic, economic decline, deterioration in public health, and, most significantly, increased immigration from third world countries. The World Health Organization estimates approximately eight million new cases and three million deaths each year.[204] Greater than 90% of these cases occur in the developing world. The rates in the United States have been decreasing since public health efforts have increased, but an estimated 5% or approximately 15 million people still are infected with tuberculosis (TB).[47,128] TB is more common in ethnic and minority groups by percentage, but the Caucasian population still accounts for more cases overall. Risk factors include lower socioeconomic class, HIV infection, immunocompromised state, drug use, homelessness, travel to endemic areas, incarceration, and health care professions[49] (Box 89-5).

TB is caused by *Mycobacterium tuberculosis,* which is an acid-fast bacillus. It is an unusually hardy microorganism that can remain in a dormant state for many years until it becomes active. Transmission is via respiratory droplets during active disease. It is estimated that 4 to 8 hours of contact is required for transmission. Most children become infected through contact with a close family member in their household.[166] However, children younger than 12 years are generally not contagious even when they have active pulmonary disease.[25,166]

Exposure does not necessarily lead to infection, and the organism can remain dormant in a latent phase where the patient is not ill and not contagious. The highest risk of progression to active disease is within the first 2 years. Young children, especially those younger than 1 year, have a higher risk of progression.[166]

Clinical Presentation

Active TB disease may be pulmonary, extrapulmonary, or both. TB may often present as ARDS in the intensive care unit. Pulmonary disease accounts for 75% of cases in children. Approximately 80% of infants present with symptoms, whereas only 44% of older children have symptoms even in the face of extensive pulmonary involvement. Thus children often are asymptomatic initially but may have cough (80%), fever (64%), weight loss (15%), decreased appetite (43%), lymphadenopathy, seizures (11%), or meningismus. Infants may have failure to thrive and recurrent fevers. Hemoptysis is rarely seen in children.[106] Often these cases are diagnosed by routine screening of infected contacts. Primary infection is more common in children as opposed to reactivation in adults.

Extrapulmonary disease is more common in children. Involvement of the lymphatics accounts for 70%, but other sites include the CNS, renal, and musculoskeletal systems. Lymphadenitis usually involves the cervical nodes, putting

TB in the differential of other infections and malignancies. TB meningitis occurs in 13% of pediatric cases and is most common in younger infants.[47] Neurologic symptoms are similar to other forms of bacterial meningitis but often are more insidious, progressing over days and weeks. Meningitis is often associated with miliary TB.[170] Cerebral infarcts may present in advanced cases, and later stages may be complicated by hydrocephalus, SIADH, intracranial tuberculomas, cranial nerve palsies, seizures, and even death.[170]

The differential diagnosis for TB includes *S. aureus, S. pneumonia,* infectious mononucleosis, HIV, and cat scratch disease. Leukemia and lymphoma must be ruled out.

The incubation period varies with site of TB disease, where disseminated disease such as miliary TB and meningitis can present as early as 1 month after infection. Pulmonary TB can develop within 6 to 24 months. Renal disease may develop years later.[166]

Diagnosis

The Mantoux subdermal skin test is the standard method of diagnosis. Sensitivity and specificity depend on the prevalence of disease. In the United States, where the incidence is 5% to 10%, the positive predictive value is approximately 90%. Positive reactions can vary among individuals, depending on their underlying risk factors (Box 89-6). False-negative reaction may occur because of inaccurate administration, recent or overwhelming TB infection, anergy, or age younger than 6 months. In fact, up to 25% of patients with active TB may not react to the tuberculin skin test initially, especially with disseminated disease.[87,96] False-positive results may occur because of previous BCG vaccination.

The acid-fast bacilli (AFB) smear and TB cultures should be taken from sputum if possible. The AFB smear is available within a few hours but is rarely positive in children because of the low number of organisms in samples. In addition, sputum samples are not practical in young children. Because of low bacterial load, approximately 95% have negative AFB smears and 60% have negative culture even with active disease.[30] Early-morning gastric aspirates have been shown to be the best method of diagnosis for young children. Collection on three consecutive mornings increases sensitivity.[152] Collection by bronchioalveolar lavage can be as sensitive as gastric aspiration. The overall yield with gastric aspirates or bronchoalveolar lavage is approximately 40%.[193] PCR also can be used and is approximately 95% specific but only 50% sensitive.[167]

Because of the low yield and number of false-positive reactions, a negative Mantoux test does not rule out TB. Even in the absence of a positive Mantoux test and negative cultures, clinical findings consistent with TB and adult contact with TB should be considered diagnostic.

Elevations in WBC count can be variable without specific left shift or neutrophilia. CSF findings in meningeal disease reveal elevated WBC counts usually between 10 and 500 cells, with lymphocytic predominance, very high protein, and low glucose. Acid-fast bacilli are rarely seen in CSF. PCR can be helpful but often is not sensitive. Head CT scan may show meningeal enhancement with calcification, especially at the base of the brain and basal ganglia.

BOX 89-6

Definitions of Positive Tuberculin (Mantoux) Skin Test Results in Infants, Children, and Adolescents

Tuberculin skin test read 48–72 hours after placement*

INDURATION 5 MM:

- Children in close contact with known or suspected contagious cases of tuberculosis disease:
  - Households with active or previously active cases if treatment cannot be verified as adequate before exposure
  - Treatment was initiated after the child's contact
  - Suspected reactivation of latent tuberculosis infection
- Children suspected to have tuberculosis disease:
  - Chest radiograph consistent with active or previously active tuberculosis
  - Clinical evidence of tuberculosis disease
  - Children receiving immunosuppressive therapy
  - Children with immunosuppressive illnesses, including HIV

INDURATION 10 MM:

- Children at increased risk for disseminated disease:
  - Young age: <4 years
  - Underlying disease:
    - Malignancy, chronic renal failure, malnutrition
- Children with increased exposure to tuberculosis disease:
  - Children or their parents born in high-prevalence regions of the world
  - Children frequently exposed to adults who are infected with HIV or are homeless, drug users, residents of nursing homes, incarcerated, or migrant farm workers
  - Travel and exposure to high-prevalence regions of the world

INDURATION 15 MM:

- Children >4 years without any risk factors

*Definitions apply regardless of previous exposure to bacilli Calmette-Guerin immunization.

Modified from American Academy of Pediatrics: Tuberculosis. In Pickering LK, editor: *2000 Red Book: Report of the Committee on Infectious Diseases,* ed 25, Elk Grove Village, IL, 2000, American Academy of Pediatrics.

Chest radiograph is recommended in children with positive skin test because as many as 50% are asymptomatic with primary disease. Pulmonary TB in children can present in all lobes. Apical cavitary lesions as seen in adults are not seen in children, but hilar and paratracheal infiltrates and pleural effusion are more common. Miliary pulmonary TB, which is associated with disseminated disease, presents as evenly distributed micronodular infiltrates.

Management

The recommended therapy for TB involves multidrug therapy because of the high incidence of resistance[12]

(Table 89–2). Six months of therapy is recommended for pulmonary and lymphatic TB, whereas 12 months is necessary for disseminated miliary or meningitic TB. Medications are generally well tolerated in children, and their effects have been summarized by Smith.[166] Isoniazid (INH) is well tolerated and has only rare side effects, such as hepatitis and peripheral neuritis, in children. Rifampin causes body fluids to turn orange because of an excreted metabolite and can cause hepatotoxicity, thrombocytopenia, and leukopenia. Pyrazinamide can cause hepatotoxicity and hyperuricemia.

Steroids are recommended for TB meningitis to reduce the inflammatory reaction, and they have been shown to decrease the incidence of neurologic sequelae and mortality.[84] Steroids have been shown to be beneficial in patients with pleural or pericardial effusions.[73]

In the United States, approximately 10% of TB cases are resistant to at least one drug.[25,42] A number of factors contribute to drug resistance, including a history of TB treatment, travel or exposure to areas with high resistance, nonadherence to therapy, and physician error in appropriate prescribing and dosing.[122]

Prophylactic INH for children younger than 5 years for exposure to active TB, along with evaluation including physical examination, tuberculin skin test, and chest radiograph, has been highly successful in preventing infection.[97,137]

Prognosis

Even with appropriate treatment, symptoms may persist for weeks to months, with resolution by 1 year.[12] Radiologic changes may take 2 to 3 years to resolve, and some children develop calcified areas in the lungs. Children with TB meningitis may develop significant morbidity related to hydrocephalus, cerebral infarcts, SIADH, cranial nerve palsies, and increased intracranial pressure. TB meningitis has been associated with more severe neurologic sequelae and death, especially when the initial presentation is severe and delayed.[179]

Lyme Disease

Etiology and Epidemiology

Lyme disease is a multiorgan system disease caused by the spirochete *Borrelia burgdorferi*. Endemic to many parts of the United States, Lyme disease is transmitted by deer tick bites.[51,54] It has become the most common reported tick-borne disease in the United States, with almost 18,000 cases reported by the CDC in 2000. The number of cases has been increasing yearly since 1992*s24* (Figure 89–2). Incidence is greatest in the northeastern, mid-Atlantic, and north-central regions of the United States,

TABLE 89–2

Recommended Treatment Regimens for Drug-Susceptible Tuberculosis in Infants, Children, and Adolescents

Infection or Disease Category	Regimen	Remarks
Latent TB (positive TST, no clinical disease)	INH daily for 9 months	If daily therapy is not possible.Twice per week. Directly observed therapy for 9 months
INH resistant	Rifampin daily for 6 months	
INH and rifampin resistant	Consult specialist	
Pulmonary TB	INH, rifampin, pyrazinamide daily for 2 months, then INH and rifampin daily for 4 months	Ethambutol or streptomycin added for 2 months if resistance is suspected
	OR	
	INH and rifampin daily for 9 months	For hilar adenopathy only
	OR	
	INH and rifampin for 1 month, then INH and rifampin twice per week for 8 months	
Extrapulmonary TB (meningitis, miliary, bone/joint, renal disease)	INH, rifampin, pyrazinamide, and streptomycin for 2 months, then INH and rifampin daily for 7–10 months	Streptomycin stopped if not resistant organism
	OR	
	INH, rifampin, pyrazinamide, and streptomycin daily for 2 months, then INH and rifampin twice per week for 7–10 months	
Other cervical lymphadenopathy	Same as for pulmonary disease	
	Same as for pulmonary disease	

Modified from American Academy of Pediatrics: Tuberculosis. In Pickering LK, editor: *2000 Red Book: Report of the Committee on Infectious Diseases,* ed 25. Elk Grove Village, IL, 2000, American Academy of Pediatrics.
INH, isoniazid; *TB,* tuberculosis; *TST,* tuberculin skin test.

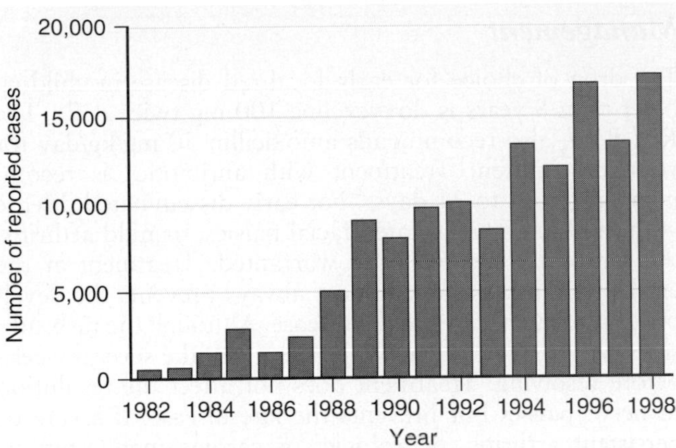

FIGURE 89–2 • Number of reported cases of Lyme disease-United States, 1982-1998. (From Orloski KA: Surveillance for Lyme disease, 1982–1998. *MMWR* 49(SS3), 2000.)

although the incidence is rising in the northwest[54,172] (Figure 89–3). Numerous reports have commented on the overdiagnosis of Lyme disease as a result of misinterpretation of serologic tests, which may account for the inflated numbers.[154]

Clinical Presentation

The classic infection was well described by Steere[171] in 1989 and outlined by the CDC in 1995.[44] The clinical manifestations are divided into three stages: early localized, early disseminated, and late disease. In 80% of patients, Lyme disease in so-called stage 1 starts as a slowly expanding erythema migrans rash with central clearing. The lesion begins as a red macule or papule at the site of the bite, which usually is in the head and neck region. The rash expands over days to a diameter greater than 5 cm. Only one third of cases presents with the classic central clearing rash. This characteristic "bull's-eye" or "target" rash often is accompanied by nonspecific, intermittent "flu-like" symptoms such as fever, malaise, fatigue, headache, myalgias, and arthralgias. The incubation period from infection to onset of erythema migrans typically is 7 to 14 days but may be as short as 3 days and as long as 30 days.[81,169,171] Gerber et al. described initial presentations in children with a single migrans lesion in 66%, multiple lesions in 23%, arthritis in 7%, meningitis in 1%, and carditis in 0.5%. In 1990 Williams[200] found similar results but an almost 60% incidence of joint symptoms in children and seventh nerve palsy in 14%. Fever in 24%, fatigue in 58%, arthralgias in 33%, and headache in 42% also were described.[82,201] Some infected individuals have no recognized illness and have only serologic evidence of infection. The initial rash usually fades within 3 weeks.[172]

After a few weeks the disease enters stage 2 and becomes disseminated. The first sign often is multiple smaller erythema migrans lesions and frank arthritis in up to 80% of cases. Approximately 15% of untreated patients develop

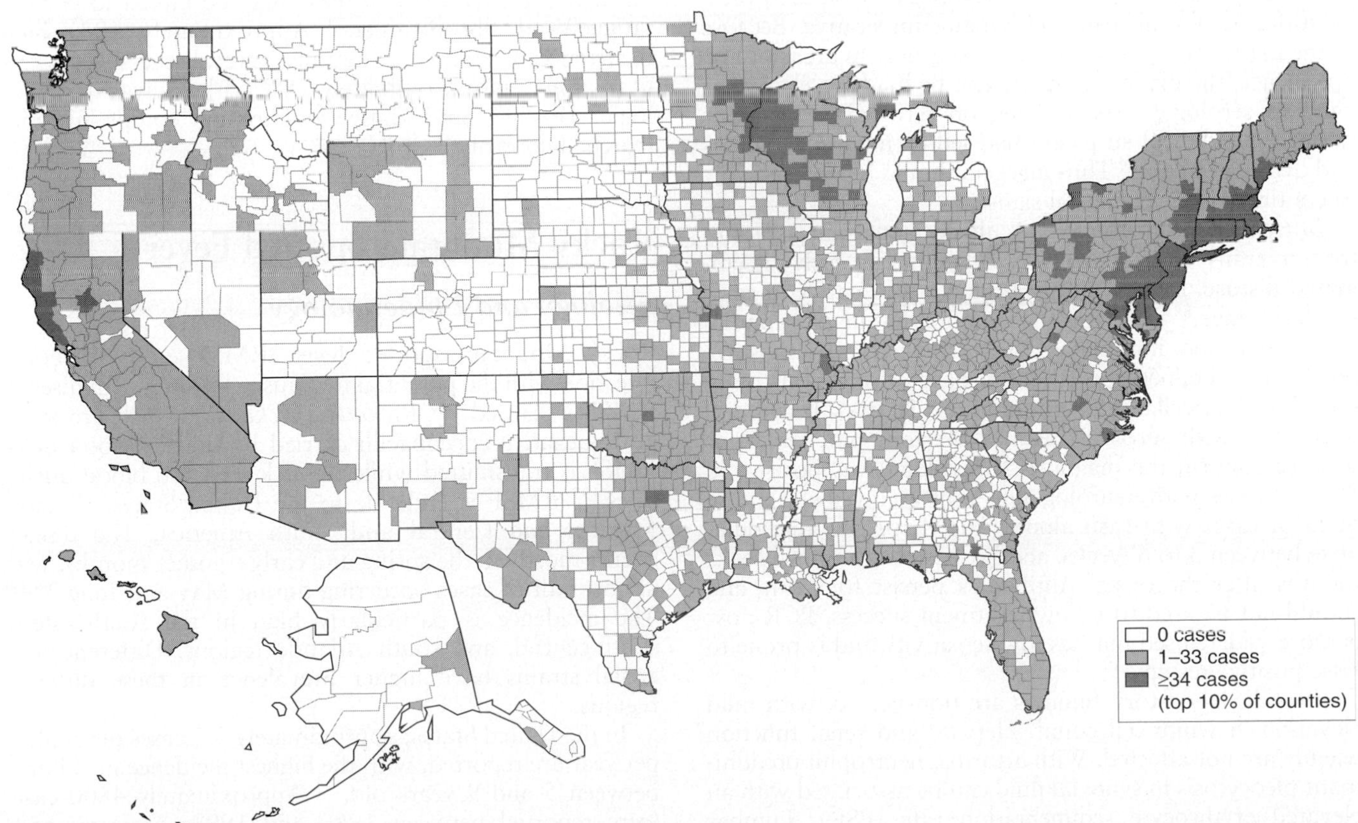

*Includes Pennsylvania cases for 1994-1998 and Oregon cases for 1993-1998.

FIGURE 89–3 • Number of reported cases of Lyme disease by county–United States, 1982–1998. (From Orloski KA: Surveillance for Lyme disease, 1982–1998. *MMWR* 49(SS3), 2000.)

neurologic symptoms such as a lymphocytic meningitis, encephalitis, pseudotumor cerebri, cerebellar ataxia, radiculoneuritis, and focal neuropathies, particularly seventh nerve facial palsies and optic nerve deficits.[23,142] The neurologic abnormalities typically improve even without treatment. Approximately 5% of patients develop acute cardiac manifestations, most commonly atrioventricular block of varying degrees but also myocarditis and dilated cardiomyopathy. Carditis from Lyme disease is rare in children and usually is transient.[19,203] Arthritis of the knee and hip is the most common late presentation of Lyme disease, especially in children.[201] However, the diagnosis often is missed because of assumption of septic arthritis from other bacterial etiologies.[19]

In stage 3, late manifestations of damage to major organ systems may persist, particularly to joints and the neurologic system. In 5%, chronic symptoms of encephalitis, polyneuropathy, and cognitive impairment may persist. However, late neurologic disease is rare in children.[35,120] In 90% of patients, the arthritis is single joint and involves the knee; it can last up to 2 years.[180] Typically, the arthritis involves swelling rather than pain and redness; thus it presents as a less "septic" picture. Chronic arthritis now is rare with antibiotic treatment, but arthralgia symptoms persist in up to 33%.[143,169,171]

Diagnosis

Although the diagnosis usually is based on clinical suspicion, serologic assays can help confirm the diagnosis. However, patients frequently are seronegative on early presentation, so clinical suspicion remains imperative. Because of the many false-positive results, especially in areas of low prevalence, the diagnosis should not be made solely on the basis of serologic tests. Relying on serologic tests alone rather than clinical suspicion had led to missed diagnoses and overtreatment.[154] Thus markers should be ordered only to confirm objective clinical signs.

Borrelia is often found on culture from skin aspirates from migrans lesions or from blood culture in early disseminated disease. Blood cultures usually are negative in early localized stage.[86] Serologic confirmation has improved with use of enzyme immunoassays, but again false-positive results are obtained for other spirochetal infections, viral infections (varicella), and autoimmune diseases. Because of difficulties with serologic assays, Western blot testing is used to confirm the diagnosis.[44] Serology was positive in 80% of cases with neurologic or joint involvement and in 50% of cases with rash alone.[201] IgM-specific antibodies arise between 3 to 6 weeks, and IgG rises slowly and peaks months after the onset. Antibodies persist for years and should not be used to follow treatment success. PCR now is more widely used but has low sensitivity and is prone to false-positive results.[140]

Overall, laboratory findings are nonspecific, with mild elevation in white cell count. Hepatic and renal function usually are not affected. With arthritis, neutrophil predominant pleocytosis in synovial fluid can be associated with an elevated erythrocyte sedimentation rate (ESR). Lumbar puncture is recommended if neurologic symptoms are present. However, the need for lumbar puncture is controversial when facial palsies present in isolation.

Management

The drug of choice for early localized disease in children older than 8 years is doxycycline 100 mg twice daily. The *Red Book* also recommends amoxicillin 50 mg/kg/day for younger children. Treatment with antibiotics is recommended for 14 to 21 days.[6] For early disseminated disease with mild migrans, isolated facial palsies, or mild arthritis, the same oral regimens are warranted. Treatment at the erythema migrans stage almost always prevents the development of later stages of the disease. Although the rash subsides within days, other symptoms may take several weeks before resolving. Treatment does not affect the resolution of nerve palsies but prevents the late disease. If severe or persistent arthritis, neurologic, or cardiac manifestations occur, then ceftriaxone 100 mg/kg/day intravenously for 21 days is recommended. Corticosteroids are not a proven effective therapy. Nonsteroidal antiinflammatory agents are helpful.[6,140,169,172]

Prognosis

Although Lyme disease is rarely fatal, the morbidity, especially related to neurocognitive effects, can be severe if untreated. Behavioral and sleep changes and auditory and visual deficits have been identified.[26] However, children treated appropriately have shown no cognitive deficits on long-term neuropsychological testing in prospective studies.[3] Almost half of children report recurrence of symptoms, usually arthralgias, but almost none have residual true arthritis. Lyme disease may be linked to chronic fatigue and fibromyalgia.[70] Approximately 10% have recurrence of erythema migrans. Overall the success rate of treatment is approximately 95% with equivalent neurologic, cardiac, and daily functioning compared with matched controls.[83,159,162,163,199]

Rocky Mountain Spotted Fever

Etiology and Epidemiology

Rocky Mountain spotted fever (RMSF) is a tick-borne infection with the potential for causing multisystem disease. RMSF is caused by *Rickettsia rickettsii,* which are small gram-negative coccobacilli carried by dog or wood ticks. RMSF is transmitted while the tick feeds on blood during bites.[197] RMSF is endemic to the United States, Canada, Mexico, and Central and South America. The disease occurs mostly in the spring and early summer months, with almost half of cases occurring during May and June.[164,188] The incidence is particularly high in the southeastern, south-central, and south Atlantic regions. Different rickettsial strains have higher prevalence in these different regions.

In the United States, approximately 3.3 cases per million per year are reported, with the highest incidence in children between 5 and 9 years old.[192] Approximately 4800 cases were reported between 1990 and 1998. Approximately 20% of these cases and almost 15% of the deaths were in children younger than 10 years.[1] Serologic infection with rickettsii is much more common than indicated by disease incidence reports, suggesting the existence of subclinical disease.[184]

Clinical Presentation

The incubation period after a tick bite is 2 to 14 days (mean 7 days).[195] The classic triad consists of fever, rash, and headache with a history of a tick bite. The classic triad is present in only 60% and in less than 20% during the first 3 days.[92] Approximately 30% to 40% of patients do not recall having a tick bite.[164] Initial symptoms often are nonspecific, with malaise and myalgias.[2,34] The fever is observed in two thirds of patients by day 3. Other common presenting symptoms are nausea, vomiting, and abdominal pain, especially in younger children.[34,188] The rash often begins by day 4, with blanching maculopapules classically starting at the wrists and ankles and then appearing on the palms, soles, and trunk (Figure 89–4). Later, in up to 50% of patients the rash may become petechial, purpuric, or even gangrenous.[1,92] Younger patients tend to develop the rash earlier.[63] Importantly, the absence of the pathognomonic rash does not exclude RMSF; an estimated 10% of cases are "spotless."[101] The headache is present in almost all adults and in most older children.[164] Encephalitis, focal neurologic deficits, and meningismus have been described in some patients.[112]

Rickettsiae invade and multiply in the endothelial cells of the vasculature, resulting in cytopathic vascular injury that is responsible for morbidity and mortality. The endothelial damage results in activation of the clotting cascade, extravasation of fluid, and reduced perfusion.[188,197] The increased vascular permeability leads to the major complications of edema, hypovolemia, and hypotension, with end-organ failure such as shock, coma, myocarditis, liver dysfunction, and renal failure.[1,92,188] Renal insufficiency on presentation is secondary to glomerular and tubular damage and has been shown to have prognostic implications with increased fatal outcomes.[60] On autopsy, rickettsial vasculitis has been found in the brain, spinal cord, cardiac tissue, and lungs.[196] Other complications include cardiac arrhythmias, gastrointestinal bleeding, and skin necrosis.[1]

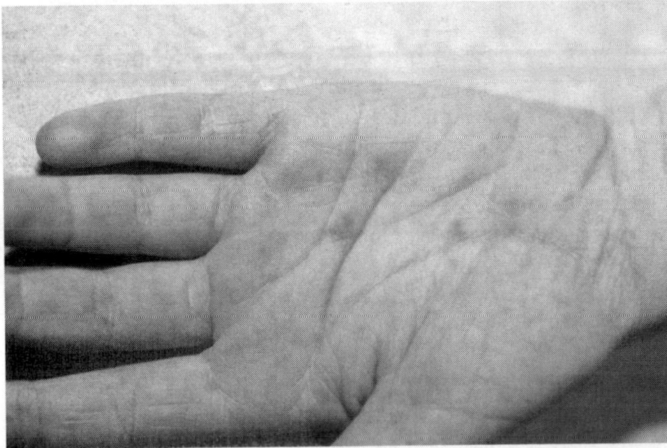

FIGURE 89–4 • Palmar rash associated with Rocky Mountain spotted fever. (See also Color Insert.) (From Walker DH, Raoult D: Rickettsia rickettsii and other spotted fever group rickettsiae (Rocky Mountain spotted fever and other spotted fevers). In Mandell GL, Bennett JE, Dolin R, editors: *Mandell: principles and practice of infectious diseases,* ed 5, New York, 2000, Churchill Livingstone.)

Diagnosis

The WBC count often is quite variable and usually is not helpful. Most patients, however, develop thrombocytopenia as the disease progresses. Approximately 30% of patients also are anemic. Liver and renal function abnormalities are common.[9,92,110,164,197] Approximately 20% of patients have hyponatremia and hypoalbuminemia resulting from massive capillary leak and fluid shift. CSF shows mononuclear pleocytosis in one third of samples, with an elevated protein concentration in 20%.[90]

Because *R. rickettsii* often is not cultured, the diagnosis usually is clinical. For confirming the diagnosis, direct immunofluorescence and immunoperoxidase staining are up to 90% sensitive and 100% specific on skin biopsies if a rash is present.[153] If available, PCR can reliably confirm the diagnosis early in blood or biopsy.[9] Serum antibodies using indirect immunofluorescence, complement fixation, and latex agglutination can be obtained but do not become positive until 7 to 10 days into the illness.[192] Thus these tests are impractical in the acute setting, and pending results should not delay treatment.

A differential diagnosis of enterovirus, measles, Epstein-Barr virus, cytomegalovirus, mycoplasma, scarlet fever, TSS, meningococcus, ehrlichiosis, and Kawasaki disease should be considered.[2,34]

Management

Empiric therapy is essential early in the course of illness because fatal outcomes have been linked to missed or delayed diagnosis and treatment.[2,56,111] The drug of choice for treatment of RMSF is doxycycline. Until recently, chloramphenicol was recommended by the American Academy of Pediatrics (AAP) and CDC for children younger than 9 years because of the risk of teeth staining with tetracycline usage.[9] However, because of the risk of aplastic anemia and retrospective evidence of higher case/fatality rates with chloramphenicol, doxycycline now is first-choice therapy even in young patients. In fact, the risk of staining is limited with a short course of therapy.[63,119] The fluoroquinolones also have activity against rickettsiae but have not been well studied in humans.[89]

Doxycycline can be administered orally but should be used intravenously in the critical care setting when the patients are vomiting, obtunded, or have multiorgan involvement. Doses of 2 to 4 mg/kg/day divided every 12 hours are given for a minimum of 5 to 7 days and until the patient has been afebrile for at least 2 days.[9,188] Because initial therapy is empiric, other broad-spectrum antibiotics such as third-generation cephalosporins also should be started to cover other infections in the differential diagnosis.

Along with antibiotic therapy, aggressive supportive measures must be instituted. Restoration of massive fluid imbalances and cardiovascular support may be necessary. Correction of electrolyte imbalance and coagulopathy are essential, and close monitoring of liver and renal dysfunction is indicated.[34,188]

Prognosis

Prior to antirickettsial therapy and aggressive supportive care, case/fatality rates were higher than 30%, and approximately 13% of children with RMSF died. Even with treatment and the supportive care now available, the case/fatality ratio is 2% to 3%.[1,192] Delayed diagnosis and late initiation of specific therapy, especially after day 5 of illness, have the most significant association with higher mortality, emphasizing the need for empiric doxycycline as soon as RMSF is suspected.[164] Other risk factors for fatal outcomes include nonwhite, male, age older than 40 years, absence of headache, no history of tick bite, gastrointestinal symptoms, and renal dysfunction.[63,89,112]

Hantavirus

Etiology and Epidemiology

Hantavirus was first recognized in 1993 in the southwest United States and subsequently was named *hantavirus pulmonary syndrome* (HPS).[76,107,139] In Europe and Asia, hantavirus species have been linked to a group of diseases with varying severity of hemorrhagic fever with renal syndrome (HFRS).[76,108] Since then, HPS has been recorded throughout North and South America.[147] A total of 318 cases with 20 to 50 new cases annually have been identified in 31 states.[53] Average age was 35 years, with the youngest 11 years (eight patients younger than 16 years).[108] Ten cases in adolescents and five cases younger than 12 years (youngest 5 years) were reported in Argentina.[147] Hantavirus has been linked to mice and rat species endemic to many areas in both urban and rural environments. The deer mouse is the main vector in rural areas throughout the United States and Canada. Infection occurs most commonly via inhalation of aerosolized saliva or excreta of infected rodents. The virus subsequently invades the pulmonary mucosa, causing direct cellular damage that leads to increased vascular permeability.

Clinical Presentation

HPS initially presents with a nonspecific illness manifested as fever, myalgia, headache, and gastrointestinal symptoms. When reviewed by Duchin et al.[76] in 1994, myalgia seemed to be the most frequently observed initial symptom. Shortness of breath and cough occurred in 76%. Gastrointestinal symptoms varied from abdominal pain, nausea, vomiting, and diarrhea in up to 76%. The hallmark feature is rapidly progressive, noncardiogenic, pulmonary edema and ARDS. The most common physical findings were tachypnea, tachycardia, and significant hypoxemia but otherwise were nonspecific (i.e., fever, malaise, anorexia).[76]

Hallmarks of the hemorrhagic fever with renal syndrome (HFRS) are prominent vascular permeability with subsequent petechiae and frank hemorrhages as well as severe renal involvement. Usually five stages are present, including febrile, hypotensive, oliguric, diuretic, and convalescent phases. Up to 30% present with moderate-to-severe disease. Most often patients have severe abdominal and back pain. Pulmonary involvement does not seem to be a feature in Europe and Asia.[15,17] Although this serotype has been found, the HFRS clinical picture is rare in the United States, for reasons that are still unclear.

Diagnosis

Almost all patients had an elevated WBC count, with significant left shift, neutrophilia, myeloid precursors, and sometimes atypical lymphocytes.[76] PTT was elevated in two thirds of patients with elevated D-dimers and abnormal fibrinogen levels. On urinalysis, 40% had proteinuria and almost 60% had hematuria, although renal function abnormalities were uncommon in cases occurring in the United States.[76] The diagnosis is confirmed by PCR or by serology using enzyme-linked immunosorbent assay (ELISA) techniques.[107]

Chest radiographs show mostly rapidly progressive bilateral, diffuse infiltrates and developing pleural effusions.

Differential diagnosis includes other sepsis syndromes such as meningococcus and other infectious causes of acute respiratory failure, such as pneumonic plague, leptospirosis, rickettsial infections, legionellosis, and atypical viral or bacterial pneumonias.

Management

Treatment is mainly supportive, especially of the respiratory system. Early intensive care management with prompt correction of pulmonary, cardiovascular, and electrolyte abnormalities is critical.[177,169] Cardiovascular support for hypotension and subsequent arrhythmias may be necessary, especially with hemorrhagic fever with renal insufficiency. However, fluid administration for hypotension must be balanced in the face of massive vascular leakage and significant pulmonary edema. Thus early use of vasopressors is recommended.[108] Intravenous ribavirin has been used but has not shown a benefit in reducing mortality in HPS.[100]

Prognosis

Mortality is high with hantavirus infection and usually is secondary to severe hypotension and arrhythmias secondary to vascular leakage and progressive hypoxemia. The CDC reports the case/fatality rate is 37% but was as high as 76% in some reviews of HPS.[53,76] Case/fatality rates in adolescents were up to 60% in patients younger than 12 years in an Argentinian review.[147]

West Nile Virus

Etiology and Epidemiology

West Nile virus (WNV) was first isolated in 1937 in Uganda. Since then it has spread across the world, with outbreaks reported in other parts of Africa, Asia, Middle East, and Europe.[124,130,168] The first reported cases in North America occurred in late 1999 with cases of fatal meningoencephalitis in New York.[136] Cases across North America have since increased. In 2001 the CDC reported 66 cases of documented WNV meningoencephalitis in 10 states, mostly along the East Coast. Actual incidence of WNV infection may be vastly underreported because surveillance has focused on neurologic disease only. Since 1999, WNV has been found in birds, mosquitoes, and horses in 27 states, with dramatic spread into the mid-west, southward into Florida, as well as northward into Canada.[55,91]

WNV is a member of the genus *Flavivirus,* which includes other encephalitic pathogens such as the St. Louis encephalitis virus.[48] Bird-feeding mosquitoes are the main vector. Transcontinental transmission is thought to have been introduced by migrating birds.[181] Although humans may become infected via the bite of an infected mosquito, they rarely experience infectious level viremia. The incubation period is 5 to 15 days.[130]

Clinical Presentation

WNV presents as an influenza-like illness. Cases are characterized by an abrupt onset of fever, headache, backache, and myalgias lasting for 3 to 6 days. Some cases involved gastrointestinal and respiratory symptoms. A maculopapular or roseola-like rash has been described. Generalized lymphadenopathy is common.[99,124,130] Severe neurologic manifestations are rare and occur in approximately 1% of infected patients, mostly in the elderly and occasionally in children. An encephalitic picture is most commonly reported, but aseptic meningitis, meningoencephalitis, myelitis, optic neuritis, or polyradiculitis can be present.[98,145] Surveys from the New York epidemic in 1999 estimate that 1 in 5 infected people develop a febrile illness, and approximately 1 in 150 infections result in neurologic symptoms.[16,52,145] Severe muscle weakness, particularly in the setting of encephalitis, may provide a clinical clue to the presence of WNV. Almost 10% of hospitalized patients with neurologic symptoms had flaccid paralysis in the New York outbreak.[200] The most common cause of death is cerebral edema after neuronal death and degeneration with severe encephalitis.[124] Myocarditis, pancreatitis, and fulminant hepatitis have been described in cases outside of North America prior to 1990.[145]

Diagnosis

Laboratory findings may include leukopenia and an elevated ESR. CSF pleocytosis and elevated protein may occur in patients with neurologic sequelae. However, virus is rarely isolated from CSF of meningoencephalitic patients. Confirmation is made with serologic testing mainly with ELISA methods testing for WNV-specific IgM antibodies. The sensitivity approaches 100%. However, the antibody usually is not detectable until about day 4 of illness. The test should be repeated at day 10 of illness, with a fourfold rise in titers confirming an acute viremia. Confirmation of the diagnosis also can be made by viral isolation on cell culture.[37,124]

Other causes of neurologic syndromes should be ruled out, including herpes and enterovirus infection, bacterial meningoencephalitides, Guillain-Barré syndrome, and lupus cerebritis.

Management

Treatment of uncomplicated WNV infections is symptomatic. All patients with suspected meningoencephalitis should be hospitalized for observation and supportive care. Particular attention should be paid to progressive neurologic dysfunction, cerebral edema, and respiratory compromise. Of the 19 cases admitted to the hospital in New York in 2000, five patients were admitted to the intensive care unit and two patients required mechanical ventilation.[200] No specific therapy is available, and no controlled studies on the prophylactic use of corticosteroids, anticonvulsants, or mannitol have been performed. However, steroids and osmotic agents have been shown to control brain swelling in other viral encephalitides. The benefits of a short course of steroids must be weighed against the risk of potentiating the WNV infection.[37,124] Acyclovir and third-generation cephalosporins should be started to cover other potential pathogens. Ribavirin and interferon-α have been proven *in vitro* to inhibit the replication and cytopathogenicity of WNV in human and rat neuronal cells. Despite the potential clinical usefulness of these agents, only anecdotal support for their use exists. IVIG also has been attempted, with anecdotal success.[13,165]

Prognosis

Case/fatality rates worldwide among hospitalized patients range from 4% to 14%.[146] In 2001, 14% of cases in the United States were fatal.[55] Advanced age is the most important risk factor for meningoencephalitis and death. Limited data on long-term morbidity are available. Follow-up surveys after the New York outbreak found significant persistent symptoms such as fatigue (67%), memory loss (50%), and muscle weakness (44%).[16]

REFERENCES

1. Abrahamian FM: Consequences of delayed diagnosis of Rocky Mountain spotted fever in children—West Virginia, Michigan, Tennessee, and Oklahoma, May-July 2000. *Ann Emerg Med* 37: 537, 2001.
2. Abramson JS, Givner LB: Rocky Mountain spotted fever. *Pediatr Infect Dis J* 18:539, 1999.
3. Adams WV, Rose CD, Eppes SC, et al: Cognitive effects of Lyme disease in children: a 4 year followup study. *J Rheumatol* 26:1190, 1999.
4. Aiuto LT, Barone SR, Cohen PS, et al: Recombinant tissue plasminogen activator restores perfusion in meningococcal purpura fulminans. *Crit Care Med* 25:1079, 1997.
5. American Academy of Pediatrics: Lyme disease. In Pickering LK, editor: *2000 Red Book: Report of the Committee on Infectious Diseases.* Elk Grove Village, IL, 2000, American Academy of Pediatrics.
6. American Academy of Pediatrics: Meningococcal infections. In Pickering LK, editor: *2000 Red Book: Report of the Committee on Infectious Diseases.* Elk Grove Village, IL, 2000, American Academy of Pediatrics.
7. American Academy of Pediatrics: Pneumococcal infections. In Pickering LK, editor: *2000 Red Book: Report of the Committee on Infectious Diseases.* Elk Grove Village, IL, 2000, American Academy of Pediatrics.

8. American Academy of Pediatrics: Rocky Mountain Spotted Fever. In Pickering LK, editor: *2000 Red Book: Report of the Committee on Infectious Diseases.* Elk Grove Village, IL, 2000, American Academy of Pediatrics.
9. American Academy of Pediatrics: Severe invasive group A streptococcal infections: a subject review. *Pediatrics* 101:136, 1998.
10. American Academy of Pediatrics: Staphylococcus aureus infection. 25:514, 2000.
11. American Academy of Pediatrics: Streptococcal group A infections. In Pickering LK, editor: *2000 Red Book: Report of the Committee on Infectious Diseases.* Elk Grove Village, IL, 2000, American Academy of Pediatrics
12. American Academy of Pediatrics: Tuberculosis. In Pickering LK, editor: *2000 Red Book: Report of the Committee on Infectious Diseases.* Elk Grove Village, IL, 2000, American Academy of Pediatrics.
13. Anderson JF, Rahal JJ: Efficacy of interferon alpha-2b and ribavirin against West Nile virus in vitro. *Emerg Infect Dis* 8:107, 2002.
14. Andrews MM: Recurrent nonmenstrual toxic shock syndrome: clinical manifestations, diagnosis, and treatment. *Clin Infect Dis* 32:1470, 2001.
15. Anonymous: New York Department of Health: West Nile virus surveillance and control: an update for healthcare providers in New York City. *City Health Information* 20, 2001.
16. Anonymous: Haemorrhagic fever with renal syndrome; memorandum from a WHO meeting. *Bull World Health Organ* 61:269, 1993.
17. Antoniadis A, Le Duc JW, Daniel-Alexiou S: Clinical and epidemiological aspects of hemorrhagic fever with renal syndrome (HFRS) in Greece. *Eur J Epidemiol* 3:295, 1987.
18. Apicella MA: Neisseria meningitidis. In Mandell GL, Bennett JE, Dolin R, editors: *Mandell: principles and practice of infectious diseases.* New York, 2000, Churchill Livingstone.
19. Bachman DT, Srivastava G: Emergency department presentations of Lyme disease in children. *Pediatr Emerg Care* 14:356, 1998.
20. Baraff LJ, Bass JW, Fleisher GR, et al: Practice guideline for the management of infants and children 0 to 36 months of age with fever without source. *Ann Emerg Med* 22:1198, 1993.
21. Barry W, Hudgins L, Donta ST, et al: Intravenous immunoglobulin therapy for toxic shock syndrome. *JAMA* 267:3315, 1992.
22. Best C, Walsh J, Sinclair J, et al: Early haemo-diafiltration in meningococcal septicaemia. *Lancet* 347:202, 1996.
23. Bingham PM, Galetta SL, Athreya B, et al: Neurologic manifestations in children with Lyme disease. *Pediatrics* 96:1053, 1995.
24. Bisno AL, Stevens DL: Streptococcal infections of skin and soft tissues. *N Engl J Med* 334:240, 1996.
25. Bloch AB, Cauthen GM, Onorato IM, et al: Nationwide survey of drug-resistant tuberculosis in the United States. *JAMA* 271:665, 1994.
26. Bloom BJ, Wyckoff PM, Meissner HC, et al: Neurocognitive abnormalities in children after classic manifestations of Lyme disease. *Pediatr Infect Dis J* 17:189, 1998.
27. Boucek MM, Boerth RC, Artman M, et al: Myocardial dysfunction in children with acute meningococcemia. *J Pediatr* 105:538, 1984.
28. Brandtzaeg P, Halstensen A, Kierulf P, et al: Molecular mechanisms in the compartmentalized inflammatory response presenting as meningococcal meningitis or septic shock. *Microb Pathog* 13:423, 1992.
29. Brandtzaeg P, Mollnes TE, Kierulf P: Complement activation and endotoxin levels in systemic meningococcal disease. *J Infect Dis* 160:58, 1989.
30. Braun M: Pediatric tuberculosis, bacilli Calmette-Guerin immunization and acquired immunodeficiency syndrome. *Semin Infect Dis* 4:261, 1993.
31. Braunstein H: Characteristics of group A streptococcal bacteremia in patients at the San Bernardino County Medical Center. *Rev Infect Dis* 13:8, 1991.
32. Breiman RF, Spika JS, Navarro VJ, et al: Pneumococcal bacteremia in Charleston County, South Carolina: a decade later. *Arch Intern Med* 150:1401, 1990.
33. Broome CV: Epidemiology of toxic shock syndrome in the United States: overview. *Rev Infect Dis* 11(suppl 1):S14, 1989.
34. Buckingham SC: Rocky Mountain spotted fever: a review for the pediatrician. *Pediatr Ann* 31:163, 2002.
35. Bujak DI, Weinstein A, Dornbush RL: Clinical and neurocognitive features of the post Lyme syndrome. *J Rheumatol* 23:1392, 1996.
36. Burman LA, Norrby R, Trollfors B: Invasive pneumococcal infections: incidence, predisposing factors, and prognosis. *Rev Infect Dis* 7:133, 1985.
37. Campbell GL, Marfin AA, Lanciotti RS, et al: West Nile virus. *Lancet Infect Dis* 2:519, 2002.
38. Carcillo JA, Davis AL, Zaritsky A: Role of early fluid resuscitation in pediatric septic shock. *JAMA* 266:1242, 1991.
39. Cartwright K, Strang J, Gossain S, et al: Early treatment of meningococcal disease. *BMJ* 305:774, 1992.
40. Catterall JR: Streptococcus pneumoniae. *Thorax* 54:929, 1999.
41. Centers for Disease Control and Prevention: Consequences of delayed diagnosis of Rocky Mountain Spotted fever in children-West Virginia, Michigan, Tennessee, and Oklahoma, May-July 2000. *JAMA* 284:2049, 2000.
42. Centers for Disease Control and Prevention: Active Bacterial Core Surveillance (ABCs) Report, Emerging Infections Program Network (EIP), Streptococcus pneumoniae, 1998. Available at www.cdc.gov. Last accessed 1999.
43. Centers for Disease Control and Prevention: *Core curriculum on tuberculosis: what a clinician should know,* ed 4, Atlanta, 2000, US Department of Health and Human Services.
44. Centers for Disease Control and Prevention: Epidemiologic notes and reports toxic-shock syndrome-United States. *MMWR* 46:492, 1997.
45. Centers for Disease Control and Prevention: Hantavirus pulmonary syndrome-United States: updated recommendations for risk reduction. *MMWR* 51:1, 2002.
46. Centers for Disease Control and Prevention: Hantavirus pulmonary syndrome-northeastern United States 1994. *MMWR* 43:548, 1994.
47. Centers for Disease Control and Prevention: Lyme disease-United States, 2000. *MMWR* 51:29, 2002.
48. Centers for Disease Control and Prevention: National action plan to combat multidrug-resistant tuberculosis. *MMWR* 41:5, 1992.
49. Centers for Disease Control and Prevention: Outbreak of West Nile-like viral encephalitis-New York, 1999. *MMWR* 48:849, 1999.
50. Centers for Disease Control and Prevention: Prevention and control of meningococcal disease. *MMWR* 49:1, 2000.
51. Centers for Disease Control and Prevention: Recommendations for test performance and interpretation from the second National Conference on Serologic Diagnosis of Lyme Disease. *MMWR* 44:590, 1995.
52. Centers for Disease Control and Prevention: Reduced incidence of menstrual toxic-shock syndrome: United States, 1980-1990. *MMWR* 39:421, 1990.
53. Centers for Disease Control and Prevention: Reported tuberculosis in the United States, 1998. Available at www.cdc.gov. Last accessed 1999.
54. Centers for Disease Control and Prevention: Serosurveys for West Nile virus infection—New York and Connecticut counties, 2000. *MMWR* 50:39, 2001.
55. Centers for Disease Control and Prevention: Surveillance for Lyme disease-United States, 1992-1998. *MMWR* 49:1, 2000.
56. Centers for Disease Control and Prevention: West Nile virus activity-United States, 2001. *MMWR* 51:497, 2002.
57. Chesney PJ, Davis JP, Purdy WK, et al: Clinical manifestations of toxic shock syndrome. *JAMA* 246:741, 1981.
58. Chesney RW, McCarron DM, Haddad JG, et al: Pathogenic mechanisms of the hypocalcemia of the staphylococcal toxic-shock syndrome. *J Lab Clin Med* 101:576, 1983.
59. Cobcroft R, Henderson A, Solano C, et al: Meningococcal purpura fulminans treated with antithrombin III concentrate: what is the optimal replacement therapy? *Aust N Z J Med* 24:575, 1994.
60. Conlon PJ, Procop GW, Fowler V, et al: Predictors of prognosis and risk of acute renal failure in patients with Rocky Mountain spotted fever. *Am J Med* 101:621, 1996.
61. Cremer R, Leclerc F, Jude B, et al: Are there specific haemostatic abnormalities in children surviving septic shock with purpura and having skin necrosis or limb ischaemia that need skin grafts or limb amputations? *Eur J Pediatr* 158:127, 1999.
62. Cunningham JD, Silver L, Rudikoff D: Necrotizing fasciitis: a plea for early diagnosis and treatment. *Mt Sinai J Med* 68:253, 2001.
63. Dalton MJ, Clarke MJ, Holman RC, et al: National surveillance for Rocky Mountain spotted fever, 1981-1992: epidemiologic summary and evaluation of risk factors for fatal outcome. *Am J Trop Med Hyg* 52:405, 1995.
64. Davies HD, Matlow A, Scriver SR, et al: Apparent lower rates of streptococcal toxic shock syndrome and lower mortality in

children with invasive group A streptococcal infections compared with adults. *Pediatr Infect Dis J* 13:49, 1994.
65. Davies HD, McGeer A, Schwartz B, et al: Invasive group A streptococcal infections in Ontario, Canada. Ontario Group A Streptococcal Study Group. *N Engl J Med* 335:547, 1996.
66. Davis JP, Chesney PJ, Wand PJ, et al: Toxic-shock syndrome: epidemiologic features, recurrence, risk factors, and prevention. *N Engl J Med* 303:1429, 1980.
67. Deeks SL, Palacio R, Ruvinsky R, et al: Risk factors and course of illness among children with invasive penicillin-resistant Streptococcus pneumoniae. The Streptococcus pneumoniae Working Group. *Pediatrics* 103:409, 1999.
68. Demers B, Simor AE, Vellend H, et al: Severe invasive group A streptococcal infections in Ontario, Canada: 1987-1991. *Clin Infect Dis* 16:792, 1993.
69. Derkx B, Wittes J, McCloskey R: Randomized, placebo-controlled trial of HA-1A, a human monoclonal antibody to endotoxin, in children with meningococcal septic shock. European Pediatric Meningococcal Septic Shock Trial Study Group. *Clin Infect Dis* 28:770, 1999.
70. Dinerman H, Steere AC: Lyme disease associated with fibromyalgia. *Ann Intern Med* 117:281, 1992.
71. Doctor A, Harper MB, Fleisher GR: Group A beta-hemolytic streptococcal bacteremia: historical overview, changing incidence, and recent association with varicella. *Pediatrics* 96(3 pt 1):428, 1995.
72. Doern GV, Heilmann KP, Huynh HK, et al: Antimicrobial resistance among clinical isolates of Streptococcus pneumoniae in the United States during 1999-2000, including a comparison of resistance rates since 1994-1995. *Antimicrob Agents Chemother* 45:1721, 2001.
73. Dooley DP, Carpenter JL, Rademacher S: Adjunctive corticosteroid therapy for tuberculosis: a critical reappraisal of the literature. *Clin Infect Dis* 25:872, 1997.
74. Doyle MG, Morrow AL, Van R, et al: Intermediate resistance of Streptococcus pneumoniae to penicillin in children in day-care centers. *Pediatr Infect Dis J* 11:831, 1992.
75. Drapkin MS, Wisch JS, Gelfand JA, et al: Plasmapheresis for fulminant meningococcemia. *Pediatr Infect Dis J* 8:399, 1989.
76. Duchin JS, Koster FT, Peters CJ, et al: Hantavirus pulmonary syndrome: a clinical description of 17 patients with a newly recognized disease. The Hantavirus Study Group. *N Engl J Med* 330: 949, 1994.
77. Editorial: Acute respiratory infections in under-fives: 15 million deaths a year. *Lancet* ii:699, 1985.
78. Elliott DC, Kufera JA, Myers RA: Necrotizing soft tissue infections. Risk factors for mortality and strategies for management. *Ann Surg* 224:672, 1996.
79. Friedland IR: Comparison of the response to antimicrobial therapy of penicillin-resistant and penicillin-susceptible pneumococcal disease. *Pediatr Infect Dis J* 14:885, 1995.
80. Garlund B, Sjolin J, Nilsson A, et al: Plasma levels of cytokines in primary septic shock in humans: correlations with disease severity. *J Infect Dis* 172:296, 1995.
81. Gerber MA, Shapiro ED, Burke GS, et al: Lyme disease in children in southeastern Connecticut. Pediatric Lyme Disease Study Group. *N Engl J Med* 335:1270, 1996.
82. Gerber MA, Shapiro ED: Diagnosis of Lyme disease in children. *J Pediatr* 121:157, 1992.
83. Gerber MA, Zemel LS, Shapiro ED: Lyme arthritis in children: clinical epidemiology and long-term outcomes. *Pediatrics* 102(4 pt 1): 905, 1998.
84. Girgis NI, Farid Z, Kilpatrick ME, et al: Dexamethasone adjunctive treatment for tuberculous meningitis. *Pediatr Infect Dis J* 10:179, 1991.
85. Giroir BP, Quint PA, Barton P, et al: Preliminary evaluation of recombinant amino-terminal fragment of human bactericidal/permeability-increasing protein in children with severe meningococcal sepsis. *Lancet* 350:1439, 1997.
86. Goodman JL, Bradley JF, Ross AE, et al: Bloodstream invasion in early Lyme disease: results from a prospective, controlled, blinded study using the polymerase chain reaction. *Am J Med* 99:6, 1995.
87. Gurkan F, Bosnak M, Dikici B, et al: Miliary tuberculosis in children: a clinical review. *Scand J Infect Dis* 30:359, 1998.
88. Harrison LH, Pass MA, Mendelsohn AB, et al: Invasive meningococcal disease in adolescents and young adults. *JAMA* 286:694, 2001.
89. Hattwick MA, Retailliau H, O'Brien RJ, et al: Fatal Rocky Mountain spotted fever. JAMA 240:1499, 1978.
90. Haynes RE, Sanders DY, Cramblett HG: Rocky Mountain spotted fever in children. *J Pediatr* 76:685, 1970.
91. Health Canada: West Nile virus surveillance 2002: Canada. Infectious diseases news brief. Centre for Infectious Disease Prevention and Control, Population and Public Health Branch, 2002.
92. Helmick CG, Bernard KW, D'Angelo LJ: Rocky Mountain spotted fever: clinical, laboratory, and epidemiological features of 262 cases. *J Infect Dis* 150:480, 1984.
93. Henriques NB, Novak R, Ortqvist A, et al: Clinical isolates of Streptococcus pneumoniae that exhibit tolerance of vancomycin. *Clin Infect Dis* 32:552, 2001.
94. Hodes DS, Barzilai A: Invasive and toxin-mediated Staphylococcus aureus diseases in children. *Adv Pediatr Infect Dis* 5:35, 1990.
95. Hoge CW, Schwartz B, Talkington DF, et al: The changing epidemiology of invasive group A streptococcal infections and the emergence of streptococcal toxic shock-like syndrome: A retrospective population based study. *JAMA* 269:384, 1993.
96. Holden M, Dubin MR, Diamond PH: Frequency of negative intermediate-strength tuberculin sensitivity in patients with active tuberculosis. *N Engl J Med* 285:1506, 1971.
97. Hsu KK, Starke JR: Diagnosis and treatment of tuberculosis infection. *Semin Pediatr Infect Dis* 4:283, 1993.
98. Hubalek Z: Comparative symptomatology of West Nile fever. *Lancet* 358:254, 2001.
99. Huggins JW, Hsiang CM, Cosgriff TM, et al: Prospective, double-blind, concurrent, placebo-controlled clinical trial of intravenous ribavirin therapy of hemorrhagic fever with renal syndrome. *J Infect Dis* 164:1119, 1991.
100. Hughes C: Rocky Mountain "spotless" fever with an erythema migrans-like skin lesion. *Clin Infect Dis* 21:1328, 1995.
101. J5 Sudy Group: Treatment of severe infectious purpura in children with human plasma from donors immunized with Escherichia coli J5: a prospective double-blind study. *J Infect Dis* 165:695, 1992.
102. Jarrett P, Rademaker M, Duffill M: The clinical spectrum of necrotising fasciitis: a review of 15 cases. *Aust N Z J Med* 27:29, 1997.
103. Kain KC, Schulzer M, Chow AW: Clinical spectrum of nonmenstrual toxic shock syndrome (TSS): comparison with menstrual TSS by multivariate discriminant analyses. *Clin Infect Dis* 16:100, 1993.
104. Kaplan SL, Mason EO Jr, Barson WJ, et al: Three-year multicenter surveillance of systemic pneumococcal infections in children. *Pediatrics* 102(3 pt 1):538, 1998.
105. Kaplan SL, Mason EO, Jr: Mechanisms of pneumococcal antibiotic resistance and treatment of pneumococcal infections in 2002. *Pediatr Ann* 31:250, 2002.
106. Khan AS, Khabbaz RF, Armstrong LR, et al: Hantavirus pulmonary syndrome: the first 100 US cases. *J Infect Dis* 173:1297, 1996.
107. Khan AS, Ksiazek TG, Peters CJ: Hantavirus pulmonary syndrome. *Lancet* 347:739, 1996.
108. Kim PE, Musher DM, Glezen WP, et al: Association of invasive pneumococcal disease with season, atmospheric conditions, air pollution, and the isolation of respiratory viruses. *Clin Infect Dis* 22:100, 1996.
109. Kirk JL, Fine DP, Sexton DJ, et al: Rocky Mountain spotted fever. A clinical review based on 48 confirmed cases, 1943-1986. *Medicine (Baltimore)* 69:35, 1990.
110. Kirkland KB, Marcom PK, Sexton DJ, et al: Rocky Mountain spotted fever complicated by gangrene: report of six cases and review. *Clin Infect Dis* 16:629, 1993.
111. Kirkland KB, Wilkinson WE, Sexton DJ: Therapeutic delay and mortality in cases of Rocky Mountain spotted fever. *Clin Infect Dis* 20:1118, 1995.
112. Kirsch EA, Barton RP, Kitchen L, et al: Pathophysiology, treatment and outcome of meningococcemia: a review and recent experience. *Pediatr Infect Dis J* 15:967, 1996.
113. Kuppermann N, Inkelis SH, Saladino R: The role of heparin in the prevention of extremity and digit necrosis in meningococcal purpura fulminans. *Pediatr Infect Dis J* 13:867, 1994.
114. Lamothe F, D'Amico P, Ghosn P, et al: Clinical usefulness of intravenous human immunoglobulins in invasive group A Streptococcal infections: case report and review. *Clin Infect Dis* 21:1469, 1995.

115. Leclerc F, Leteurtre S, Cremer R, et al: Do new strategies in meningococcemia produce better outcomes? *Crit Care Med* 28 (9 Suppl):S60, 2000.
116. Levin M, Galassini R, de Munter C, et al: Improved survival in children admitted to intensive care with meningococcal disease. 1998.
117. Levine DP, Fromm BS, Reddy BR: Slow response to vancomycin or vancomycin plus rifampin in methicillin-resistant *Staphylococcus aureus* endocarditis. *Ann Intern Med* 115:674, 1991.
118. Lockary ME, Lockhard PB, Williams JT: Doxycycline and staining of permanent teeth. *Pediatr Infect Dis J* 17:429, 1998.
119. Logigian EL, Kaplan RF, Steere AC: Chronic neurologic manifestations of Lyme disease. *N Engl J Med* 323:1438, 1990.
120. Lowy FD: *Staphylococcus aureus* infections. *N Engl J Med* 339: 520, 1998.
121. Mahmoudi A, Iseman MD: Pitfalls in the care of patients with tuberculosis: Common errors and their association with the acquisition of drug resistance. *JAMA* 270:65, 1993.
122. Malley R, Ambrosino D: Pneumococcal diseases in children: morbidity, mortality, and resistance. University of Chicago Children's Hospital Reports on Current Concepts in the Use of Pediatric Vaccines. 1:1, 1998.
123. Marfin AA, Gubler DJ: West Nile encephalitis: an emerging disease in the United States. *Clin Infect Dis* 33:1713, 2001.
124. Marzouk O, Thomson AP, Sills JA, et al: Features and outcome in meningococcal disease presenting with maculopapular rash. *Arch Dis Child* 66:485, 1991.
125. McCracken GH Jr: Diagnosis and management of pneumonia in children. *Pediatr Infect Dis J* 19:924, 2000.
126. McCracken GH Jr: Etiology and treatment of pneumonia. *Pediatr Infect Dis J* 19:373, 2000.
127. McKenna MT, McCray E, Onorato I: The epidemiology of tuberculosis among foreign-born persons in the United States, 1986 to 1993. *N Engl J Med* 332:1071, 1995.
128. Mcmaster P, Shann F: The use of extracorporeal techniques to remove humoral factors in sepsis. *Pediatr Crit Care Med* 4:2, 2003.
129. Meek J: West Nile virus in the United States. *Curr Opin Pediatr* 14:72, 2002.
130. Melish ME, Murata S, Fukunaga C, et al: Endotoxin is not an essential mediator in toxic shock syndrome. *Rev Infect Dis* 11(suppl 1):S219, 1989.
131. Mufson MA, Stanek RJ: Bacteremic pneumococcal pneumonia in one American City: a 20-year longitudinal study, 1978-1997. *Am J Med* 107(1A):34S, 1999.
132. Musher DM: Pneumococcus. In Mandell GL, Bennett JE, Dolin R, editors: *Mandell: principles and practice of infectious diseases.* New York, 2000, Churchill Livingstone.
133. Nadel S, Britto J, Booy R, et al: Avoidable deficiencies in the delivery of health care to children with meningococcal disease. *J Accid Emerg Med* 15:298, 1998.
134. Nadel S, Levin M, Habibi P: Treatment of meningococcal disease in childhood. In Cartwright K, editor: *Meningoccal disease.* Chichester, 1995, John Wiley and Sons.
135. Nash D, Mostashari F, Fine A, et al: The outbreak of West Nile virus infection in the New York City area in 1999. *N Engl J Med* 344:1807, 2001.
136. Nemir RL, O'Hare D: Tuberculosis in children 10 years of age and younger: three decades of experience during the chemotherapeutic era. *Pediatrics* 88:236, 1991.
137. Newcombe J, Dyer S, Blackman L, et al: PCR-single-stranded confirmational polymorphism analysis for non-culture-based subtyping of meningococcal strains in clinical specimens. *J Clin Microbiol* 35:1809, 1997.
138. Nichol ST, Spiropoulou CF, Morzunov S, et al: Genetic identification of a hantavirus associated with an outbreak of acute respiratory illness. *Science* 262:914, 1993.
139. Nocton JJ, Dressler F, Rutledge BJ, et al: Detection of Borrelia burgdorferi DNA by polymerase chain reaction in synovial fluid from patients with Lyme arthritis. *N Engl J Med* 330:229, 1994.
140. O'Brien KL, Levine OS, Schwartz B: The changing epidemiology of group A streptococcus infections. *Semin Pediar Infect Dis* 8:1, 1997.
141. Oschmann P, Dorndorf W, Hornig C, et al: Stages and syndromes of neuroborreliosis. *J Neurol* 245:262, 1998.
142. Ostrov BE, Athreya BH: Lyme disease: Difficulties in diagnosis and management. *Pediatr Clin North Am* 38:535, 1991.
143. Peter G: The child with pneumonia: diagnostic and therapeutic considerations. *Pediatr Infect Dis J* 7:453, 1988.
144. Petersen LR, Marfin AA: West Nile virus: a primer for the clinician. *Ann Intern Med* 137:173, 2002.
145. Petersen LR, Roehrig JT: West Nile virus: a reemerging global pathogen. *Emerg Infect Dis* 7:611, 2001.
146. Pini NC, Resa A, del Jesus LG, et al: Hantavirus infection in children in Argentina. *Emerg Infect Dis* 4:85, 1998.
147. Pollack MM, Alexander SR, Clarke N, et al: Improved outcomes from tertiary center pediatric intensive care: a statewide comparison of tertiary and nontertiary care facilities. *Crit Care Med* 19:150, 1991.
148. Pollard AJ, Britto J, Nadel S, et al: Emergency management of meningococcal disease. *Arch Dis Child* 80:290, 1999.
149. Pollard AJ, DeMunter C, Nadel S, et al: Abandoning empirical antibiotics for febrile children. *Lancet* 350:811, 1997.
150. Pollard AJ, Moxon ER: The meningococcus tamed? *Arch Dis Child* 87:13, 2002.
151. Pomputius WF, III, Rost J, Dennehy PH, et al: Standardization of gastric aspirate technique improves yield in the diagnosis of tuberculosis in children. *Pediatr Infect Dis J* 16:222, 1997.
152. Procop GW, Burchette JL Jr, Howell DN, et al: Immunoperoxidase and immunofluorescent staining of Rickettsia rickettsii in skin biopsies: a comparative study. *Arch Pathol Lab Med* 121:894, 1997.
153. Qureshi MZ, New D, Zulqarni NJ, et al: Overdiagnosis and overtreatment of Lyme disease in children. *Pediatr Infect Dis J* 21:12, 2002.
154. Reeves JH, Butt WW: Blood filtration in children with severe sepsis: safe adjunctive therapy. *Intensive Care Med* 21:500, 1995.
155. Rivard GE, David M, Farrell C, et al: Treatment of purpura fulminans in meningococcemia with protein C concentrate. *J Pediatr* 126:646, 1995.
156. Robinson KA, Baughman W, Rothrock G, et al: Epidemiology of invasive Streptococcus pneumoniae infections in the United States, 1995-1998: opportunities for prevention in the conjugate vaccine era. *JAMA* 285:1729, 2001.
157. Rosenstein NE, Perkins BA, Stephens DS, et al: The changing epidemiology of meningococcal disease in the United States, 1992-1996. *J Infect Dis* 180:1894, 1999.
158. Salazar JC, Gerber MA, Goff CW: Long-term outcome of Lyme disease in children given early treatment. *J Pediatr* 122:591, 1993.
159. Schlievert PM, Assimacopoulos AP, Cleary PP: Severe invasive group A streptococcal disease: clinical description and mechanisms of pathogenesis. *J Lab Clin Med* 127:13, 1996.
160. Schlievert PM: Use of intravenous immunoglobulin in the treatment of staphylococcal and streptococcal toxic shock syndromes and related illnesses. *J Allergy Clin Immunol* 108(4 suppl):S107, 2001.
161. Seltzer EG, Gerber MA, Cartter ML, et al: Long-term outcomes of persons with Lyme disease. *JAMA* 283:609, 2000.
162. Seltzer EG, Shapiro ED, Gerber MA: Long-term outcomes of Lyme disease. *JAMA* 283:3068, 2000.
163. Sexton DJ, Kaye KS: Rocky mountain spotted fever. *Med Clin North Am* 86:351, 2002.
164. Shimoni Z, Niven MJ, Pitlick S, et al: Treatment of West Nile virus encephalitis with intravenous immunoglobulin. *Emerg Infect Dis* 7:759, 2001.
165. Smith KC, Starke JR, Eisenach K, et al: Detection of Mycobacterium tuberculosis in clinical specimens from children using a polymerase chain reaction. *Pediatrics* 97:155, 1996.
166. Smith KC: Tuberculosis in children. *Curr Probl Pediatr* 31:1, 2001.
167. Smithburn KC, Hughes TP, Burke AW, et al: A neurotropic virus isolated from the blood of a native of Uganda. *Am J Trop Med Hyg* 20:471, 1940.
168. Sood SK: Lyme disease. *Pediatr Infect Dis J* 18:913, 1999.
169. Starke JR: Tuberculosis of the central nervous system in children. *Semin Pediatr Neurol* 6:318, 1999.
170. Steere AC: Lyme disease. *N Engl J Med* 321:586, 1989.
171. Steere AC: Lyme disease. *N Engl J Med* 345:115, 2001.
172. Stevens DL, Bryant AE, Hackett SP: Antibiotic effects on bacterial viability, toxin production, and host response. *Clin Infect Dis* 20(suppl 2):S154, 1995.

173. Stevens DL, Gibbons AE, Bergstrom R, et al: The Eagle effect revisited: efficacy of clindamycin, erythromycin, and penicillin in the treatment of streptococcal myositis. *J Infect Dis* 158:23, 1988.
174. Stevens DL: Could nonsteroidal antiinflammatory drugs (NSAIDs) enhance the progression of bacterial infections to toxic shock syndrome? *Clin Infect Dis* 21:977, 1995.
175. Stevens DL: Invasive group A streptococcal infections: the past, present and future. *Pediatr Infect Dis J* 13:561, 1994.
176. Stevens DL: Invasive group A streptococcus infections. *Clin Infect Dis* 14:2, 1992.
177. Stevens DL: Streptococcal toxic-shock syndrome: spectrum of disease, pathogenesis, and new concepts in treatment. *Emerg Infect Dis* 1:69, 1995.
178. Sumaya CV, Simek M, Smith MH, et al: Tuberculous meningitis in children during the isoniazid era. *J Pediatr* 87:43, 1975.
179. Szer IS, Taylor E, Steere AC: The long-term course of Lyme arthritis in children. *N Engl J Med* 325:159, 1991.
180. Takei S, Arora YK, Walker SM: Intravenous immunoglobulin contains specific antibodies inhibitory to activation of T cells by staphylococcal toxin superantigens. *J Clin Invest* 91:602, 1993.
181. Tan TQ, Mason EO Jr, Barson WJ, et al: Clinical characteristics and outcome of children with pneumonia attributable to penicillin-susceptible and penicillin-nonsusceptible Streptococcus pneumoniae. *Pediatrics* 102:1369, 1998.
182. Tan TQ: Pneumococcal infections in children. *Pediatr Ann* 31:241, 2002.
183. Taylor JP, Tanner WB, Rawlings JA, et al: Serological evidence of subclinical Rocky Mountain spotted fever infections in Texas. *J Infect Dis* 151:367, 1985.
184. The Working Group on Severe Streptococcal Infections: Defining the group A streptococcal toxic shock syndrome: rationale and consensus definition. *JAMA* 269:390, 1993.
185. Thomson AP, Sills JA, Hart CA: Validation of the Glasgow meningococcal septicemia prognostic score: a 10-year retrospective survey. *Crit Care Med* 19:26, 1991.
186. Thorburn K, Baines P, Thomson A, et al: Mortality in severe meningococcal disease. *Arch Dis Child* 85:382, 2001.
187. Thorner AR, Walker DH, Petri WA Jr: Rocky mountain spotted fever. *Clin Infect Dis* 27:1353, 1998.
188. Tibbles PM, Edelsberg JS: Hyperbaric oxygen therapy. *N Engl J Med* 334:1642, 1996.
189. Tikhomirov E, Santamaria M, Esteves K: Meningococcal disease: public health burden and control. *World Health Stat Q* 50:170, 1997.
190. Todd JK, Ressman M, Caston SA, et al: Corticosteroid therapy for patients with toxic shock syndrome. *JAMA* 252:3399, 1984.
191. Treadwell TA, Holman RC, Clarke MJ, et al: Rocky Mountain spotted fever in the United States, 1993-1996. *Am J Trop Med Hyg* 63:21, 2000.
192. Vallejo JG, Ong LT, Starke JR: Clinical features, diagnosis, and treatment of tuberculosis in infants. *Pediatrics* 94:1, 1994.
193. Waldvogal FA: *Staphylococcus aureus*. In Mandell GL, Bennett JE, Dolin R, editors: *Mandell: principles and practice of infectious diseases*. New York, 2000, Churchill Livingstone.
194. Walker DH, Lane TW: Rocky Mountain spotted fever: clinical signs, symptoms, and pathophysiology. In Walker DH, editor: *Biology of rickettsial diseases*. Boca Raton, 1998, CRC Press.
195. Walker DH, Matern WD: Rickettsial vasculitis. *Am Heart J* 100:896, 1980.
196. Walker DH, Raoult D: Rickettsia rickettsii and other spotted fever group rickettsiae (Rocky Mountain spotted fever and other spotted fevers). In Mandell GL, Bennett JE, Dolin R, editors: *Mandell: principles and practice of infectious diseases*. New York, 2000, Churchill Livingstone.
197. Wang JF, Caugant DA, Li X, et al: Clonal and antigenic analysis of serogroup A Neisseria meningitidis with particular reference to epidemiological features of epidemic meningitis in the People's Republic of China. *Infect Immun* 60:5267, 1992.
198. Wang TJ, Sangha O, Phillips CB, et al: Outcomes of children treated for Lyme disease. *J Rheumatol* 25:2249, 1998.
199. Weiss D, Carr D, Kellachan J, et al: Clinical findings of West Nile virus infection in hospitalized patients, New York and New Jersey, 2000. *Emerg Infect Dis* 7:654, 2001.
200. Williams CL, Strobino B, Lee A, et al: Lyme disease in childhood: clinical and epidemiologic features of ninety cases. *Pediatr Infect Dis J* 9:10, 1990.
201. Wilson GJ, Talkington DF, Gruber W, et al: Group A streptococcal necrotizing fasciitis following varicella in children: case reports and review. *Clin Infect Dis* 20:1333, 1995.
202. Woolf PK, Lorsung EM, Edwards KS, et al: Electrocardiographic findings in children with Lyme disease. *Pediatr Emerg Care* 7:334, 1991.
203. World Health Organization: *Groups at risk: WHO report on the tuberculosis epidemic*. 1996. Geneva, 1996, World Health Organization.
204. Zangwill KM, Vadheim CM, Vannier AM, et al: Epidemiology of invasive pneumococcal disease in southern California: implications for the design and conduct of a pneumococcal conjugate vaccine efficacy trial. *J Infect Dis* 174:752, 1996.
205. Zittergruen M, Grose C: Magnetic resonance imaging for early diagnosis of necrotizing fasciitis. *Pediatr Emerg Care* 9:26, 1993.

CHAPTER

90

Nosocomial Infections in the Pediatric Intensive Care Unit: Epidemiology and Control

Jacques Lacroix, France Gauvin, Peter Skippen, Peter Cox, Joanne M. Langley, and Anne G. Matlow

PEARLS

- Regardless of cause, the more severe the underlying illness or the greater the number of comorbidities, the higher the risk of acquiring a nosocomial infection.
- Systemic inflammatory response syndrome and multiple organ dysfunction syndrome are risk factors of nosocomial infections in critically ill patients.
- Underlying disease is the strongest predictor of death from a nosocomial infection. Handwashing is the single most important means of preventing nosocomial infection, yet 66% of persons in contact with pediatric intensive care unit (PICU) patients or their equipment are not compliant.
- A single positive culture of blood drawn through a catheter can indicate either intraluminal catheter colonization or hub contamination rather than a bloodstream infection.
- It is estimated that at least 400,000 catheter-related bloodstream infections occur each year in the United States. We suggest using clinical and radiologic data to detect possible cases of nosocomial pneumonia in critically ill children. However, cultures of respiratory secretions are necessary to validate the diagnosis. We do not recommend using invasive techniques to diagnose nosocomial pneumonia in a mandatory fashion, but they can be helpful in specific cases. Cultures of endotracheal secretions are safe and, if negative, almost with certainty exclude the diagnosis.
- Nosocomial pneumonia, tracheitis, and sinusitis have a similar pathogenesis. Colonization of the buccal oropharyngeal mucosa and alteration of the endogenous microflora appear to be crucial antecedents to endotracheal colonization and nosocomial respiratory tract infections in both children and adults.
- Costs associated with and attributable to nosocomial pneumonia are significant. In adults, nosocomial pneumonia accounts for an increase in mean hospital ICU stay of 4 to 9 days, which is a major increase in hospital cost ($24,000 per case in 1986).
- Most nosocomial skin infections observed in ICU are wounded infections.
- Prophylactic postoperative antibiotics are almost universally used but unfortunately tend to be abused in this setting.

General Considerations

Patients acquire infections after admission to the hospital. These infections are referred to as *cross-infection, hospital-acquired infection,* or *nosocomial infection.* The first breakthrough with respect to these infections occurred in 1847 when the obstetrician Semmelweis discovered that handwashing controlled childbed fever (group A streptococcal sepsis). Lister and Altmeier then identified ways of controlling surgical and other infections. By the early 1900s, strict control measures were initiated when children were admitted to the hospital; these measures included restricting visitors and instituting lengthy routine handwashes. Introduction of antibiotics in the 1940s and 1950s stimulated a premature wave of optimism that nosocomial infections (then caused by group A *Streptococcus*) would disappear; therefore aseptic practices were loosened. Instead, the prevalence of organisms causing these infections has changed, first to *Staphylococcus aureus* and now to coagulase-negative staphylococci, methicillin-resistant *S. aureus*, and other antibiotic-resistant organisms. Viruses and fungi have emerged as important pathogens. Opportunities for introducing infection have increased with the development of new diagnostic and therapeutic maneuvers. Many patients, such as survivors of transplantation or cancer, are more susceptible to contracting a nosocomial infection.

Nosocomial infections increase both morbidity and mortality. Many of these infections are preventable: data suggest that 35% of nosocomial bloodstream infections, 22% of pneumonias, 33% of urinary tract infections, and 35% of surgical wound infections could be prevented if hospitals had an effective infection control program.[111] This chapter addresses the problem of nosocomial infections acquired in the pediatric intensive care unit (PICU). The chapter is divided in two parts. In the first part, we discuss the following points: definitions, diagnosis, incidence, pathophysiology (pathogenesis, mode of bacterial entry, modes of transmission, causative agents), risk factors (host-, device-, procedure- and environmental-related factors), morbidity and mortality, management, and prevention. The second part of the chapter discusses the same points, with comments specific for each type of nosocomial infection (bloodstream, respiratory, etc.).

EPIDEMIOLOGY

Incidence

Reports of nosocomial infection rates in the PICU have varied widely, ranging from 3% to 24.1% (median 11%).[32,70,130,186,211,256] Richards et al.[233] reported a cumulative incidence rate of 5.7% nosocomial infections among 110,709 critically ill children in 61 American PICUs. A point-prevalence survey published in 2002 reported that a nosocomial infection occurred among 61 (11.9%) patients.[109]

In 1989 the most common type of nosocomial infection in the PICU was bacteremia (35.9%), followed by skin (24.6%), respiratory tract (14.8%), eye (9.8%), digestive tract (9.2%), and urinary tract infection (2.6%).[94] In 1999 the most prevalent nosocomial infections were bloodstream (41%), lower respiratory tract (23%), urinary tract (13%), and skin or soft tissue (8%).[109] These proportions changed with age (Figure 90–1). For example, urinary tract infections are the most frequent in adults.[232] A significant proportion of critically ill patients (8%–62%) present two or more concomitant nosocomial infections.[181,256,267]

Early studies reported the frequency of infection by rates, that is, by number of infections (the numerator) per admissions in the ICU (the denominator). However, density of incidence rather than cumulative incidence rates should be used. As Jarvis et al.[130] wrote, the use of patient-days or device-days (e.g., catheter-days, ventilator-days) in the denominator helps to control for variation in the average length of patient ICU stay or to take into account possible exposure to a risk factor over time. Stover et al.[271] reported an overall nosocomial infection rate of 13.9 per 1000 patient-days in 24 American PICUs.[271]

Concomitant nosocomial infections are a frequent observation in adults. It more likely occurs with nasal sinusitis (100%), catheter-related infections (93%), and pneumonia (74%).[181] Data in PICUs are lacking, but the possibility that a child simultaneously presents many nosocomial infections should be considered.

Pathophysiology

Pathogenesis

Bacteria can enter the circulation from various sources: from contamination at the time of injury, from endogenous

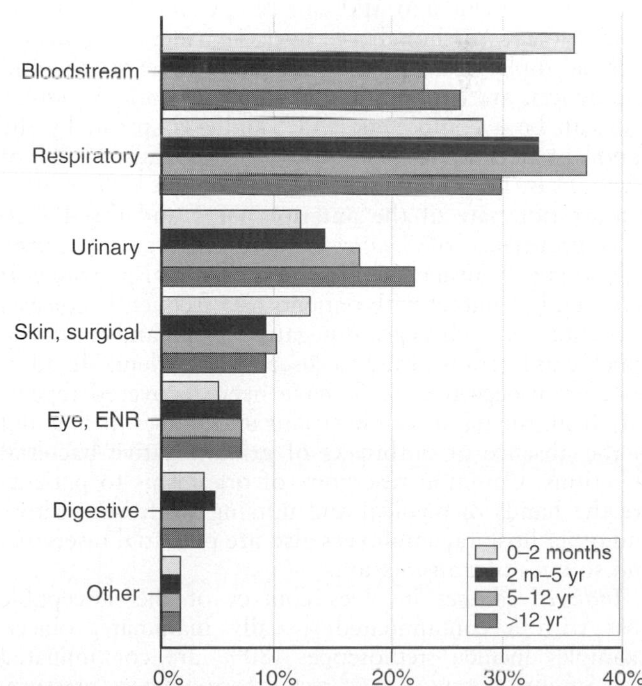

FIGURE 90–1 • Frequency of different types of nosocomial infections observed in 61 American pediatric intensive care units. Cases of sinusitis are included in ear, nose, and throat (ENR) infections. (Modified from Richards MJ, Edwards JR, Culver DH, Gaynes RP, the National Nosocomial Infections Surveillance System: *Pediatrics* 103(e39):1-7, 1999.)

reservoirs, during performance of procedures, from the local environment, and from cross-transmission. Nosocomial infections are generally associated with some type of intravascular monitoring device or life support system, the implication being that many can be prevented. The chief barrier against infection is intact normal integument. Invasive and operative procedures, both diagnostic and therapeutic, are hazardous if skin antisepsis is inadequate, if devices are not maintained aseptically, or if devices are left in place too long. Handwashing and careful skin preparation are essential.

Some organisms are more hazardous than others, perhaps because of factors related to virulence, bacterial antibiotic sensitivity, or patient health status. Bacteria adhere more easily to the host (e.g., buccal or respiratory mucosa) if the patient has a severe underlying illness and is malnourished. Resident bacterial flora most likely is altered in patients with a prolonged hospital or ICU course who received broad-spectrum antibiotics.

Modes of Transmission

Acquisition of microorganisms and resulting infection usually occurs by one or more of the following major routes.

Contact. Contact is a frequent mode of transmission of nosocomial pathogens. Contact transmission is subdivided as follows:

Direct contact involves physical transmission of microorganisms from an infected or colonized person to a susceptible host, such as via the intermediary of hospital personnel or between two patients. The microbial flora of skin consists of both resident and transient flora. In contrast to transient flora, resident flora survives and multiplies on the skin and can be recovered repeatedly from carriers. Although relatively avirulent organisms, such as diphtheroids, *Staphylococcus epidermidis,* and micrococci, are common in the resident flora, *S. aureus* also can be a component and usually is spread by the hands of personnel. The potential for transmission of *S. aureus* by hospital staff is reflected by the 30% to 50% colonization rate of the anterior nares and the 4% to 47% prevalence of *S. aureus* hand carriage in healthy individuals. Transient hand flora of hospital personnel is acquired by contact with patients and frequently consists of pathogens, such as gram-negative bacilli and *S. aureus,* which can be transmitted to susceptible patients. In addition, gram-negative bacilli have been recovered repeatedly from the hands of physicians and nurses during and in the absence of outbreaks of gram-negative bacterial infections. Common reservoirs of organisms to patients are the hands of medical and nursing staff, but visitors and other hospital employees also are potential reservoirs and sources of transmission.

Indirect contact involves contact of the susceptible host with a contaminated, usually inanimate, object. Examples include stethoscopes (80% are contaminated with *Staphylococcus* spp),[264] rectal thermometers, pressure-monitoring transducers, handwashing brushes, and resuscitation equipment. All wet areas in a hospital, such as sinks and taps, are generally contaminated. Water is a well-known reservoir for "water bugs," such as *Pseudomonas, Serratia,* and *Legionella.*[6]

Droplet contact involves transmission of microorganisms from the conjunctivae, nose, and/or mouth of an infected person to the patient, as the result of coughing or sneezing. In contrast to airborne transmission, infected droplets travel less than 3 feet, so transmission by this route requires close contact. Although this route has been an infrequent cause of epidemics, it has occasionally been implicated in outbreaks. Important agents transmitted in this manner are respiratory syncytial virus and rhinoviruses.

Contaminated Vehicle. Nosocomial infection can result from transmission through administration of contaminated items, such as water, intravenous fluids, lipid emulsion, total parenteral nutrition, and blood products.

Airborne Route. Airborne transmission occurs by dissemination, either of nuclei (residue of evaporated droplet nuclei that remain suspended in the air for long periods) from patients or personnel or of dust particles containing the infectious agent. Organisms transmitted in this manner can be widely dispersed by air currents before they are acquired by the susceptible host. True airborne transmission of nosocomial infections has been reported with pertussis, *Varicella zoster,* influenza A, influenza B, parainfluenza, and measles virus. Mumps, rubella, echovirus, and adenoviruses also have been implicated. Only a few bacteria have been incriminated in transmission by the airborne route. *Mycobacterium tuberculosis* is most widely known, but *Neisseria meningitidis, Nocardia asteroides, Yersinia pestis, Bordetella pertussis*, and *Chlamydia psittaci* have been reported. *S. aureus* and *Streptococcus pyogenes* have caused surgical wound infections by an airborne route. *Pneumocystis carinii* may be a potential source of airborne nosocomial infection.[89] The hospital air supply may be contaminated with fungi from dust during renovations, outside construction with a malfunctioning hospital ventilation system, contaminated fireproofing and insulation, pigeon droppings in the air vents, and contaminated air filters and air conditioning coils. The fungi involved in previous outbreaks have been *Aspergillus* and *Rhizopus.*[122] Hospital waste, laundry chutes, elevators, and tube systems are potential airborne distributors.

Vectorborne Route. Although this route of transmission has not occurred in North America, it is a theoretical risk in tropical countries, where open windows could result in mosquito-transmitted infections (e.g., malaria, yellow fever).

Causative Agents

Causative agents of nosocomial infections observed in PICU vary by site and procedure. The proportional frequency of pathogens by site is listed in the second part of this chapter and in Tables 90–1 and 90–2. PICU staff must become familiar with the microorganisms observed in their own institution because those pathogens probably will be involved if their patients contract a nosocomial infection.

Gram-positive pathogens are more common than gram-negative pathogens (42% vs. 35%, respectively).[210] Multiple-resistant bacteria are an increasing problem. Although methicillin-resistant *S. aureus,* when treated, is not more pathogenic than methicillin-sensitive *S. aureus,* units that do not have this organism should make every effort to prevent its entry and transmission. One PICU outbreak occurred when the PICU was consolidated with

TABLE 90–1

Most Commonly Reported Causative Pathogens in Cases of Nosocomial Infections Observed in 61 American Pediatric Intensive Care Units

	Bloodstream	Urinary Tract	Surgical Site
Gram-negative bacteria	n = 1887 (%)	n = 1045 (%)	n = 544 (%)
Haemophilus influenzae	0.1	0	0.9
Enterococcus spp.	11.2	10.0	8.1
Klebsiella pneumoniae	4.1	7.3	3.7
Pseudomonas aeruginosa	4.9	13.1	14.5
Serratia marcescens	2.0	1.2	2.8
Enterobacter spp.	6.2	10.3	8.1
Escherichia coli	2.9	19.0	5.1
Acinetobacter spp.	2.0	0.4	0.7
Citrobacter spp.	0.5	4.3	1.8
Total	33.9	65.6	45.5
Gram-positive bacteria			
Staphylococcus aureus	9.3	1.5	20.2
Staphylococcus epidermidis	37.0	1.3	14.0
Streptococcus group B	0.1	0.1	0.4
Streptococcus pneumoniae	0.6	0	0.6
Total	47.8	4.9	35.2
Other pathogens			
Candida spp.	9.3	21.1	7.0
Aspergillus spp.	0.1	0	0.7
Other fungi	0.2	1.6	0.2
Viruses	0.1	0.2	0
Total	9.7	22.9	7.9

Richards MJ, Edwards JR, Culver DH, et al: *Pediatrics* 103(e39):1, 1999.
Data on respiratory infections are detailed in Table 90-2.

an adult surgical unit and ended when the units were separated.[231] Intestinal decontamination can help to control an outbreak of intestinal colonization and infection with multiresistant gram-negative bacteria but should not be recommended for routine prevention.[31]

The proportional frequency of fungal infections appears to be increasing, amounting to 20% of the total.[109,210] This increase is perplexing; data gathered through use of new molecular epidemiologic tools suggests that exogenous acquisition via hands is likely and infection from endogenous sources is not necessarily the rule.[36]

Viral disease appears to occur at a far lower rate in the PICU than in parts of the hospital where viral respiratory and diarrheal diseases are more common.[94] Unmeasured differences that might explain this finding are less exposure (through 1:1 nursing ratios), less cross-coverage with infected patients, fewer visitors (including siblings), personalized equipment, absence of child–child contact, and lack of hand-to-mouth contact.

Risk Factors

Host-Related Factors

Regardless of cause, the more severe the underlying illness or the greater the number of comorbidities, the higher the risk of acquiring a nosocomial infection.

Severity of Cases. The severity of cases can be evaluated by the Pediatric Risk of Mortality (PRISM) score. Patients with PRISM scores greater than 10 on admission are significantly more likely to become infected than those with scores less than 10 (10.8% vs. 3.4%; $p < 0.001$), an association that held true for age, service, and length of stay. The sensitivity, specificity, and positive and negative predictive values of a PRISM score >10 for nosocomial infections were 75%, 53%, 11%, and 97%, respectively.[186,210]

Immune Dysfunction. Meduri et al.[181] wrote that nosocomial infections might indicate changes in host defenses more than change in the colonization of the host. Dysfunction of the immune system is indeed a risk factor of nosocomial infections (see Chapters 85 and 86). Among pediatric patients, the range of potential causes of immune system deficiency or dysfunction is extremely wide. Immunodeficiency can be transient or chronic, congenital or acquired. Alternatively, it may have an iatrogenic etiology or may occur as a result of several investigational and therapeutic maneuvers that interfere with normal immune defense barriers.

The inflammatory process observed in severe cases of systemic inflammatory response syndrome and multiple organ dysfunction syndrome is so important that the response of the immune system to infection is jeopardized. Not surprisingly, systemic inflammatory response syndrome and multiple organ dysfunction syndrome are

TABLE 90–2

Most Commonly Reported Causative Pathogens in Cases of Nosocomial Respiratory Infections Observed in 61 American Pediatric Intensive Care Units

	Lower Respiratory Tract Infections	Pneumonia
Gram-negative bacteria	n = 935 (%)	n = 1459 (%)
Haemophilus influenzae	5.8	10.2
Enterococcus I	1.2	1.0
Klebsiella pneumoniae	3.5	5.3
Pseudomonas aeruginosa	15.1	21.8
Serratia marcescens	3.6	3.6
Enterobacter spp.	12.2	9.3
Escherichia coli	3.2	3.6
Acinetobacter spp.	3.1	3.1
Citrobacter spp.	1.1	0.5
Total	48.8	58.3
Gram-positive bacteria		
Staphylococcus aureus	18.8	16.9
Staphylococcus epidermidis	1.5	0.9
Streptococcus group B	0	0.2
Streptococcus pneumoniae	2.6	3.4
Total	22.9	21.4
Other pathogens		
Candida spp.	4.7	2.0
Aspergillus spp.	0.1	0.5
Other fungi	0.1	0.7
Viruses	10.1	2.5
Total	15.0	5.7

From Richards MJ, Edwards JR, Culver DH, et al: *Pediatrics* 103(e39):1, 1999.

risk factors of nosocomial infections in critically ill patients.[66,87] Many other diseases and treatments, such as cancer, chemotherapy, and transplantation, can disturb the immune system.

Trauma. Adult studies reveal that patients who survive the initial insult of multiple trauma have a 20% to 60% risk of developing a nosocomial infection.[270] After neurologic death, sepsis becomes the leading cause of mortality in these patients.[106] The risk of infectious complications after trauma is related to the severity of injury, multiple integumentary breakdown, catabolic state, aspiration, multiple interventions by medical teams (invasive vascular access, tubes, transfusions, medications, surgery), environmental contamination (e.g., exposure to multiresistant organisms), and degree of depression of the immune state.[215] It is clear that the overall immune response is nonspecific in trauma, and that almost all aspects of the immune system are involved, including the inflammatory response, reticuloendothelial function, and humoral and cellular immunity.[200] The premorbid health status of the victim with a possibly impaired immune system also must be considered. Much research has been directed toward isolating a postulated circulating immunosuppressive factor released as a consequence of the injury, whether multitrauma or a burn. A myriad of possible immunosuppressives have been found, including endotoxin, tumor necrosis factor, interleukin-1, interleukin 2, complement, and many other mediators.

Acute Viral Infections. Up to one of every six children admitted to a pediatric ward acquires a nosocomial viral infection, depending on the season and the prevalence in the children admitted from the community. The effects of viruses on the immune system are protean. They can affect the humoral or cellular components of immunomodulation. The end result is increased susceptibility to secondary infections, especially bacteria.[241] Moreover, human immunodeficiency virus (HIV) infection is becoming an important causative agent that predisposes children to both opportunistic and nosocomial infections.

Malnutrition. Chronic illness and/or malnutrition both are implicated in causing immune defects. Worldwide, malnutrition is the most frequent cause of immunodeficiency. It is associated with increased surgical mortality (at least in adult studies), poor wound healing, and prolonged hospital stay. Malnutrition affects all facets of the immune system. The resultant defects can be corrected by restoring normal nutritional status.[2]

Malignancy. Patients with malignancy may be immunocompromised as a result of both the underlying cancer and the therapeutic modalities (drug, radiotherapy, bone marrow transplantation). Neutropenia and aplastic or blastic crises are the greatest risk factors for acquiring a nosocomial infection.

Organ Transplantation. Increasing numbers of patients are being admitted to ICUs following organ transplantation. These patients are immunosuppressed and often have lengthy PICU stays. In addition to prolonged surgery, they have many invasive lines, undergo several procedures, and invariably receive large-volume transfusions, with all of the attendant risks. Their nutritional state often is suboptimal preoperatively. Postoperatively, sepsis or rejection is common and may require treatment with many immunosuppressive drugs, such as steroids, azathioprine, cyclosporine, antilymphocyte globulins, or OKT_3, resulting in further immunosuppression.

Device and Procedure-Related Factors

The duration of exposure to any risk factor, such as length of insertion of an invasive device, greatly influences the risk of nosocomial infection. This holds true for all invasive devices used in critically ill patients, including central venous catheters, endotracheal tubes, and bladder catheters. The relationship between duration of exposure and risk of nosocomial infection is discussed in details in the section on catheter-related bloodstream infection.

Devices. Iatrogenic dysfunction of the intact integument is common in the PICU and results from the need to penetrate the natural defense barriers of the skin, mucous membranes, and upper airway. Problems arise because these devices are inserted into the most critically ill patients, often under less than ideal aseptic conditions and frequently during emergencies.

Some materials facilitate the adherence of microorganisms. Anticipated developments intended to minimize this adherence include nonthrombogenic and colonization-resistant polymers, heparin bonding of catheter, incorporation of unique antimicrobial, and addition of nontoxic biodegradable antiseptics.

Surgery and Anesthesia. Surgery and anesthesia have been widely believed to contribute to impaired or delayed immune responsiveness.[184] However, it is difficult to isolate the effects of surgery and anesthesia in the critically ill patient who already is suffering from a degree of immunosuppression. There are confounding factors such as breach of barriers, multiple transfusions and drug administration, and complications such as systemic inflammatory response syndrome and multiple organ dysfunction syndrome, which themselves predispose to infection. Surgery per se has been implicated as a factor in the reduced immune responsiveness of the postoperative period, a condition that generally falls under the category of "nonspecific operative stress."[23]

All anesthetic agents, both general (intravenous and inhalational) and local, have been implicated in various types of altered immune response. However, most of the effects are transient and fully reversible. It is difficult to attribute postoperative infection to a particular anesthetic in either a previously healthy or a critically ill patient.[269]

Cardiac Surgery. Hypothermia and cardiopulmonary bypass are frequently used during cardiac surgery. Hypothermic patients are predisposed to infections.[160] Cardiopulmonary bypass can disturb both the inflammatory and the coagulation systems.[282]

Transfusions. Blood transfusion can increase the risk for nosocomial infections by several mechanisms.[275] Blood transfusion is a well-known medium of nosocomial infection, including viral hepatitis and more exotic organisms such as malaria.[125,261] Blood transfusion can impair the immune system. Evidence indicates that transfused red blood cells (RBCs) may result in clinically important immune suppression in the recipient.[138] Viruses known to suppress cellular immunity (e.g., cytomegalovirus, HIV) can be transmitted.[125] The altered immune responses following RBC transfusions may predispose critically ill transfusion recipients to nosocomial infections.[184,191,274] Use of leukocyte-depleted packed RBC units may decrease the risk of infection,[131] but this technique remains to be proven in critically ill children.

Drugs. Many drugs have known adverse effects on the host immune function. These drugs include antibiotics (antibacterials to antiparasitics), topical antiseptics (mafenide, silver sulfadiazine), immunosuppressive agents (including steroids, antineoplastic drugs, cyclosporine, and high-dose thiopental), sedatives, and muscle relaxants.[87]

Environmental Factors

Patients may acquire an infection from two major sources: (1) endogenous and (2) exogenous, in the hospital environment. For example, tap water from faucets contaminated with *Pseudomonas aeruginosa* can propagate this pathogen in critically ill patients.[230] Virtually every device or structure in the ICU or hospital, including respiratory equipment and catheters, has been implicated in the transmission of infection.

Design of an ICU sometimes affects the incidence of nosocomial infections.[124] Of particular importance are the amount of space between patients, convenient and plentiful handwashing sinks, an appropriate number of nurses, and isolation facilities.[76] However, whether units are open or isolated probably does not decrease the colonization or infection rate.[212] No evidence indicates that single rooms do more than decrease the number of patient contacts, unless they are equipped with an anteroom and they are provided with negative or positive airflow to prevent airborne transmission and protect the immunocompromised. Nevertheless, segregating children with viral disease or those colonized with multiple drug-resistant organisms appears to have merit.

Risk Factors: Conclusion

Many risk factors for nosocomial infections have been characterized in critically ill children. Singh-Naz et al.[256] created a multivariate logistic regression model that retained operative status, PRISM score, device utilization ratio, antimicrobial therapy, parenteral nutrition, and length of stay in PICU as the most important risk factors. They later validated this model. Three factors remained as independent risk factors: invasive device use (risk ratio 2), parenteral nutrition (risk ratio 6), and the interaction between severity of illness-modified PRISM III-24 score and postoperative status (risk ratio 1.5; area under the receiver operating characteristic curve 0.764).[257]

Morbidity and Mortality

Systemic inflammatory response syndrome and multiple organ dysfunction syndrome are risk factors of nosocomial infection. Vice versa, nosocomial infections can cause or worsen these syndromes.[66] Bloodstream and respiratory nosocomial infections are deadlier than nosocomial skin, urinary tract, and eye infections in critically ill patients. However, underlying disease is the strongest predictor of death from a nosocomial infection.[31]

Economic costs attributable to nosocomial infections are huge. In the United States, it was estimated that the economic burden associated with hospital-wide nosocomial infections in 1989 was $4 billion annually.[185]

Management

A treatment regimen consisting of antibiotics is required for bacterial nosocomial infections. Wunderink[291] summarized fallacies of antibiotic therapy or prophylaxis: "broader is better; failure to respond is failure to cover; when in doubt, change drugs or add another; more disease(s), more drugs; sickness requires immediate treatment; response implies diagnosis; bigger disease, bigger drugs; bigger disease, newer drugs; antibiotics are nontoxic." Evidence indicates that inappropriate use of antibiotics can increase the risk of death in critically ill patients.[33,80,145,256] Therefore antibiotics should be used only when a nosocomial infection is suspected or evidence indicates that a given antibioprophylaxis is useful. When a nosocomial infection is suspected, the choice of antibiotics must be adapted to the infection site and the germs that are prevalent at this site in a given unit.

Specific antibiotic regimens are discussed in the sections on nosocomial bloodstream, respiratory, skin/surgical, and urinary infections.

Prevention

Hand Hygiene

Resident flora are firmly attached and multiplying. They include *S. epidermidis, Propionibacter,* and, occasionally, gram-negative organisms. Approximately 10% to 20% inhabit deep epidermal layers. Although many skin flora are not virulent, they may cause infection in patients during surgery or other invasive procedures, in those who are immunocompromised, or in patients with abnormal heart valves. Personnel with dermatitis often carry increased numbers of pathogenic bacteria. They should be treated, wear gloves, and possibly be removed from patient care until the dermatitis is improved.

Transient organisms can be removed by applying soap and washing with water. Transient carriage of organisms is common among staff members who do not stop at a sink after patient contact. Vigorous rinsing with running water for 3 to 10 seconds is sufficient to remove viruses.

Handwashing is the single most important means of preventing nosocomial infection, yet 66% of persons in contact with PICU patients or their equipment are not compliant.[114] Antiseptic handwashes decrease skin bacterial counts more effectively than do soap and water.[92] Chlorhexidine and alcohol are frequently used as antiseptics. Alcohol-based hand rubs are convenient (require less time to use), safe (less irritating to the skin), and cost-effective (decrease hand contamination and material costs).[155] Use of nonsterile gloves over unwashed hands and antiseptic handwashing confer similar reduction in the number of microorganisms.[237]

Skin Antisepsis

A two-step procedure (alcohol followed by antiseptic) effectively reduces skin germ counts. The antiseptic can be removed, after at least 30 seconds, to improve visualization of the area.

Antibioprophylaxis

Perioperative antibiotics are worthwhile to prevent wound infections, but antibioprophylaxis does not seem to be effective preventing nosocomial bloodstream, respiratory, and urinary tract infections.[57] A single intravenous dose of antibiotics at induction of anesthesia is recommended for clean nonimplant neurosurgical operations. A few additional doses might be useful if the procedure was contaminated and insufficient data are available to make any recommendations after shunt surgery.[127]

Antibiotics Restriction or Cycling

High-risk organisms, such as *Pseudomonas, Acinetobacter,* methicillin-resistant *S. aureus,* and many other antibiotic-resistant bacteria are selected by prior antibiotics.[108,278] Therefore some investigators suggest a restrictive antibiotic policy[41,110] and/or scheduled change of antibiotic class.[110,146,190] The usefulness of such a strategy in the PICU remains to be determined.

Gown, Gloves, and Mask

In a controlled study in a PICU, routine use of gowns did not result in improved rates of handwashing, nosocomial infection, or intravascular catheter colonization and so is not recommended on a routine basis.[69] The same observation was made in a neonatal ICU (NICU).[204] However, wearing of gowns could be useful in specific cases, such as children with solid organ transplantation.[263]

Use of clean nonsterile latex gloves over unwashed hands confers similar reduction in contamination, as does handwashing with an antiseptic solution.[237]

When gowns and gloves are used as means of protective isolation, a decreased infection rate and longer intervals before nosocomial colonization were documented in critically ill children in whom mechanical ventilation is required. Wearing gowns and gloves decreases the rate of nosocomial infections in children with solid organ transplantation.[263]

Wearing a surgical mask decreases the risk of contracting some infections, such as meningococcemia. Submicron surgical masks can be useful for highly contagious respiratory disease such as tuberculosis. On the other hand, disposable particulate respirators and submicron surgical masks may not offer greater protection than standard surgical mask in nonoutbreak situations.[96] Gowns, gloves, and masks must be used when a central catheter is inserted.

Other Devices

All devices used with critically ill patients must be disinfected. Dedicating devices to a given patient may be useful. Stethoscopes used only for a given patient are less frequently contaminated than those belonging to individual caregivers.[264] Therefore it can be beneficial to use one stethoscope per patient. This should be true for other devices, such as thermometers, ventilatory bags, blood pressure cuffs, and pulse oximeter sensors.

Isolation

The underlying premise in adapting an isolation system to the PICU is that all pediatric patients are a potential source of infection. Preventing transmission of pathogens to or from patients depends on the interaction between staff and patients. Patients may be the source of multiple-resistant organisms even if the patients are asymptomatic. To prevent serious infections or outbreaks, it is critical to apply infection control principles to all interactions with patients at all times. This means that transport of critically ill patients should be limited as much as possible. Moreover, specific isolation technique may be useful in specific cases. The Centers for Disease Control (CDC) recommends four isolation categories[290]:

- *Standard Precautions:* Wash hands, gloves, and gown in specific situations (contact with blood, body fluids,

or secretions), mask and goggles/glasses when splashes of body fluid are anticipated.
- *Airborne Precautions:* Standard precautions, plus negative pressure room, highly protective mask (not only surgical mask).
- *Droplet Precautions:* Standard precautions, plus private room with door closed, mask.
- *Contact Precautions:* Standard precautions, plus private room or placing patients with identical infection (e.g., bronchiolitis caused by respiratory syncytial virus) in the same room, gown and gloves, dedicated equipment (stethoscope, thermometer), handwashing before leaving the room.
- Patients with airborne diseases (e.g., varicella, measles, pertussis, influenza, early meningococcal, *Haemophilus influenzae* disease, extensive infected dermatitis) should be in single negative pressure rooms with anteroom to minimize the risk of transmission to others.

Making Infection Control Work

PICU staff may profit from forming their own infection-control committee composed of key unit personnel and hospital infection-control staff. In this forum, all infection-control issues can be addressed, including those related not only to surveillance but also to exposures, outbreaks, occupational health, education, policies and procedures, and environmental management. The need to initiate further investigations can be reviewed and findings that might lead to recriminations discussed.[93,95]

Conclusion

Nosocomial infections are a significant problem in the PICU. In the following sections we discuss the nosocomial infections in their order of frequency, beginning with bloodstream infections. Recommendations for applying evidence-based medicine are included in the sections on management and prevention. Three types of recommendation are considered: recommended, not recommended, and indeterminate.

Specific Infections

Bloodstream and Catheter-Related Nosocomial Infections

Definitions

Bloodstream infection can be primary or secondary. In *primary bacteremia,* a bacteria is recovered from the blood but without an identified source of infection. A *secondary bacteremia* comes from a defined source. The bloodstream infection can originate either from a remote focus of infection, such as an abscess or a nosocomial pneumonia, or from a catheter.

Catheter-related infectious complications include colonization and infection of the catheter site, catheter tip, and blood. Diagnosis of the different types of bloodstream infections and catheter-related infections can be tricky. For example, a single positive culture of blood drawn through a catheter can indicate either intraluminal catheter colonization or hub contamination rather than a bloodstream infection. This situation explains why culture of the catheter tip or paired blood cultures should be used to diagnose bloodstream infections and catheter-related infections in critically ill patients. Criteria of nosocomial bloodstream infections and catheter-related infectious complications vary widely, but the following definitions fairly represent the trends in the literature.

Catheter Site Inflammation. Catheter site inflammation can be diagnosed on the basis of the presence of lymphangitis, purulence, or at least two signs of inflammation (erythema, tenderness, increased warmth, or induration).

Catheter-Related Infection. Infection from contamination of skin or colonization of catheter-tip can be discriminated by semi-quantitative culturing of segments of withdrawn catheter. The cutoff point is still a matter of debate, but the most commonly used threshold is ≥15 colony-forming units (CFUs) on semi-quantitative culture.[168,223] Semi-quantitative cultures are performed by rolling 5 to 7 cm of the catheter tip on agar. Quantitative culture can be performed by submerging the catheter segment in broth so that the intraluminal organisms can grow. A catheter infection is diagnosed if ≥100 CFUs are present on quantitative culture.[223,251] If the catheter is not withdrawn, simultaneous collection of peripheral and central blood can be cultured quantitatively and higher counts in the cannula specimen used for diagnostic purposes.

Catheter-Related Bloodstream Infection. The two kinds of catheter-related bloodstream infection are catheter-related bacteremia and catheter-related sepsis. *Catheter-related bacteremia* is present if blood cultures obtained peripherally and centrally and a catheter segment culture are positive for the same organism.[223] *Catheter-related sepsis* is considered in the presence of clinical features consistent with bloodstream infection.

Other bloodstream infections include septic thrombophlebitis, right-sided endocarditis, cellulitis, and exit-site and tunnel infections.

Diagnosis

As suggested in the definitions, the diagnosis of nosocomial bloodstream and catheter-related infections is based on clinical data (e.g., fever, pus at insertion site) and results of laboratory investigation (e.g., blood cultures, catheter tip culture). Routine culture of the catheter tip is not routinely recommended[199] but can be useful if a catheter-related infection is suspected. The negative predictive value of a negative culture of blood drawn from a catheter is very good.[174] However, the predictive value of a positive culture is more difficult to interpret because the positive result can be caused by contamination or colonization rather than by a bacteremia.

If a bloodstream infection is suspected, collecting blood from at least two different sites is suggested. A central to peripheral blood culture CFU ratio of more than 8:1 is indicative of a catheter-related bloodstream infection (sensitivity 92.8%, specificity 98.8%).[216] This diagnostic marker requires quantitative blood culture on a standard basis, which is not the protocol at all hospitals.

Blot et al.[25] suggested that differential time to positivity for cultures of blood collected from a catheter hub and from a peripheral site might be a good diagnostic marker. The sensitivity of the measure was 90% and specificity was 96% when the hub-blood culture became positive at least 120 minutes earlier than the peripheral-blood culture, and a catheter-related infection could be excluded almost with certainty if the time to positivity was 24 hours or more. However, the results of another study did not support this concept.[235] This technique is labor intensive, and more studies are required before it can be considered accurate and useful.

Many other tests have been promoted for the diagnosis of catheter-related bloodstream infection, such as endoluminal brushing of catheter[277] and Gram stain of blood drawn from a catheter,[142] but the accuracy and cost-effectiveness of these tests remain to be determined.[85]

To conclude, we suggest drawing blood from two different sites when a catheter-related bloodstream infection is suspected. Qualitative cultures are sufficiently predictive in most cases.

Incidence

Bloodstream nosocomial infections can be primary, secondary to a focus of infection, or secondary to a catheter (Figure 90–2). Laupland et al.[156] studied a cohort of 1158 admissions in an ICU for more than 48 hours. Bacteremia was detected in 4.4% of adults (5.2/1000 patient-ICU days). In the cohort study of Renaud et al.,[228] bloodstream nosocomial infections were primary in 29% of cases, secondary to a remote nidus of infection in 26%, and catheter related in 45%; bacteremia occurred after a median of 10 days.

Because most bloodstream infections observed in ICU are catheter related, they should be of major concern to intensivists. It is estimated that at least 400,000 catheter-related bloodstream infections occur each year in the United States.[218] Renaud et al.[228] reported that the incidence rate of catheter-related infections in an adult ICU was 1.8% (39/2201). The incidence changed with the site of catheter insertion and catheter type. Stover et al[271] reported 6.5 bloodstream nosocomial infections per 1000 device-days in 23 PICUs.

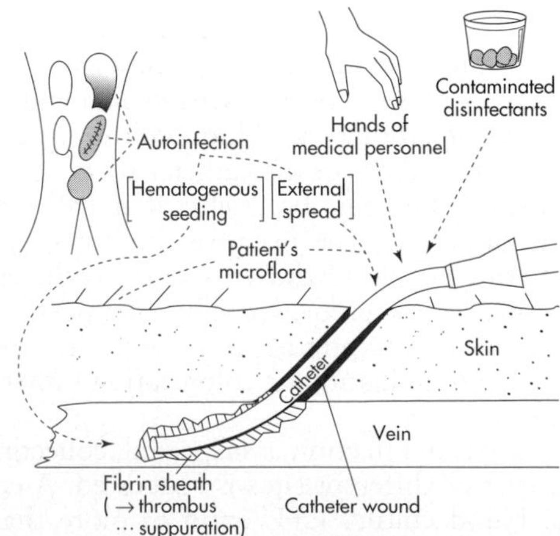

FIGURE 90–2 • Sources of vascular cannula-related infection. (Redrawn from Phillips I, Meers PO, D'Arcy PF, editors: *Microbiologic hazards of intravenous therapy.* Lancaster, England, 1977, MTP Press.)

Nontunneled central line provides a direct passage into major vessels. The rate of systemic sepsis for nontunneled central venous lines is 23 infections per 1000 catheter-days of line use.[43] The incidence of catheter-related infections frequently is stated to be lower with tunneled central lines, in which a few centimeters of subcutaneous tunneling and cuff provide protection from skin flora. The infection rate for tunneled central lines is 2 to 4 infections per 1000 patient-days of line use.[260] Jarvis et al.[130] reported 11.4 nosocomial bloodstream infections per 1000 central line-days in PICU, but the proportion of nontunneled central line was not stated. On the other hand, peripheral venous catheter seems safe. Collignon[43] reported a 64-fold lower risk of catheter-related sepsis associated with the latter compared with central venous catheter. No epidemiologic data on peripherally inserted central catheters (PICC lines) are available.

Myers et al.[192] prospectively studied 170 pulmonary artery catheter (PAC) insertions in 113 patients. Using a semi-quantitative culture technique, they found a 5.8% incidence of positive cultures (10 patients). Six of the 10 patients had concurrent positive blood cultures, but the isolate corresponded to the organism grown from the catheter tip in only three of the patients. In a much larger prospective analysis of the complications of 1400 catheterizations in patients undergoing cardiac surgery, Damen et al.[59] found a colonization rate of 2.3%. All patients in the study were given prophylactic antibiotics. There were no clinical diagnoses of endocarditis. Examination of the temporal relationship between presence of catheter and infection showed a significantly greater colonization rate for catheters in place longer than 72 hours than for those in place less than 72 hours (7.2% vs. 1.72%). Kac et al.[136] reported a cutoff of 4 days rather than 3 days. It must be emphasized that no studies reported that the density of incidence of infection related to PAC increased with time. The risk of infection with PAC sometimes is stated to be higher than with central venous catheters. This statement is not supported by the available evidence, which suggests that the relative risk of infection is similar with both catheters (2.6 vs 2.3 per 1000 catheter-days).[199]

Arterial line colonization ranges from 0.85% to 25.4%,[1,159,255] and arterial line–related septicemia ranges from 0% to 4%.[75,196,276] However, use of small catheters, inserted percutaneously in units with strictly enforced protocols for insertion and maintenance, has reduced the risk of colonization and infection diagnosed by semi-quantitative culturing. A study of 304 arterial lines in the PICU at Sainte-Justine Hospital, Montreal, Canada, reported a 2.3% incidence of catheter-related local infection and a 0.6% incidence of possible catheter-related septicemia. The density of incidence stabilized 4 days after insertion, ranging from 4.4 to 6 catheter-related infectious complications per 10,000 hours of insertion (Figure 90–3).[98] The risk of catheter-related infections is low with arterial lines, and evidence indicates that the risk is lower with arterial than with central venous catheters.

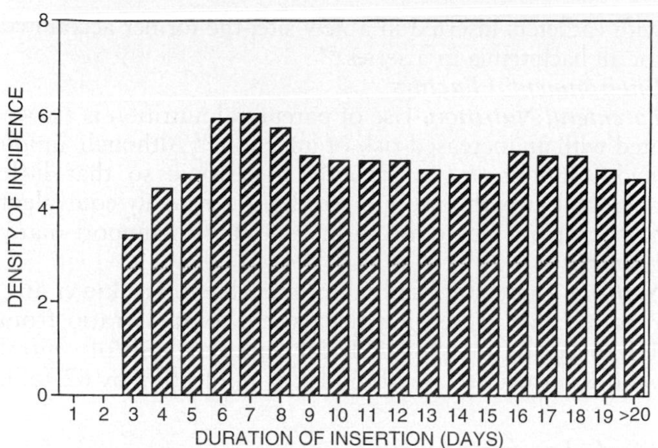

FIGURE 90–3 • Density of incidence of arterial catheter-related infectious complications. The daily probability of infectious complications per 10,000 hours of insertion is represented for days 1 through 20. (Redrawn from Furfaro S, Gauthier M, Lacroix J, Lafleur L, Mathews S: *Am J Dis Child* 13:1037, 1991.)

Pathophysiology

Pathogenesis. Bacteremia can occur at insertion or thereafter. Catheter insertion in the bladder through the urethra causes bacteremia in 8% of recipients.[272] How often catheter insertion in an artery or central vein causes bacteremia is unknown, but it should be significant. Most catheter-related bloodstream infection occurs a few days after insertion. In such instances, infection originates at the catheter-cutaneous junction where microorganisms migrate from the puncture site to the catheter tip. Contamination occurs at insertion or shortly thereafter. Two major routes of bacterial seeding of indwelling catheters are well established. A catheter can become infected by either an extraluminal or an endoluminal route. In the former, catheter-related infection originates from the cutaneous insertion site of the catheter, and the bacteria migrate along the external surface of the catheter. In the latter, bacteria obtain access to the endoluminal surface of the catheter through hub contamination.

Evidence of the importance of the endoluminal route includes correlation of organisms on the skin with organisms subsequently shown to cause septicemia, semiquantitative cultures, and Gram stains of external surfaces of catheter segments, which also correlate with positive blood cultures. The time lag between catheter insertion and catheter tip infection also can be accounted for by the time required for the pathogens to migrate from the skin to the catheter tip. Skin colonization at the insertion site (odds ratio 56.5, 95% confidence interval [CI] 10.8–296), is the most frequent source of catheter-related infections.[189]

Catheter hubs are frequently manipulated in critically ill patients, and strong evidence indicates that hub colonization is a frequent source of catheter-related infections (odds ratio 17.9, 95% CI 2.4–132).[189,259]

The pressure monitoring system, flush solutions, and even the ice used for chilling syringes can be sources of infection. The CDC reported that, from 1977 to 1987, 33% of nosocomial bloodstream infections were derived from arterial infusion used for pressure monitoring.[20] One can ask if pressure monitoring systems must be changed routinely every 2 or 3 days. Transducer chamber domes are frequently contaminated,[167] but these chambers are completely isolated from the patient, which might explain why contamination of a patient from such a chamber does not occur, regardless of their duration of use.[252] This holds true for disposable modular systems incorporating a continuous-flow device, chamber dome, and electronic transducer.[163] The latest evidence questioned the routine change of tubing, infusion fluid, and continuous-flow device.[98,163] Routine replacement of pressure monitoring systems probably is unnecessary.

Infusates, flush solutions, and parenteral nutrition are recognized sources of infection. Collecting and culturing such solutions is advised in some cases.

Causative Agents. In the PICU of the Hospital for Sick Children, Toronto, Canada, 71.5% of bacteremia cases were caused by gram-positive organisms, predominantly coagulase-negative *Staphylococci,* and 12.7% by gram-negative bacilli.[94] Most catheter-related infections are caused by skin microflora, but other germs can be involved (*Enterococci,* Enterobacteriaceae). A significant proportion of nosocomial bloodstream infections are polymicrobial in the adult ICU (10.8%[228]) and in the PICU (13%[121]). However, increasingly more cases are caused by fungi. Catheter colonization with *Candida* is frequently associated with systemic infections.[189] No agreement exists in the literature regarding the best method for assessing such colonization of skin and hubs. Sampling with swabs or Rodac plates are the two most commonly used methods. These methods are useful for isolating pathogens, but there is no consensus on the cutoff points that differentiate positive from negative cultures.[189]

Risk Factors

Host-Related Factors. In a large cohort study, cases of trauma had the highest incidence of nosocomial bloodstream infection.[228] Skin colonization at the insertion site is a significant risk factor (odds ratio 56.5, 95% CI 10.8–296).[189]

Device and Procedure-Related Factors. The duration of exposure to any risk factor, such as length of stay in the PICU or duration of insertion of an invasive device, greatly influences the risk of nosocomial infection. All invasive devices must be withdrawn from critically ill patients as soon as the devices are not required. However, the best practice when a device is still required is not clearly delineated. Because length of insertion is so important, some authorities recommend routine scheduled replacement of devices, such as arterial and central venous catheters, in order to decrease infection risk, but routine replacement of invasive device is still a matter of debate. A large controlled trial showed that routine central venous catheters change every 3 days does not prevent infection and that replacement of catheters is associated with increased mechanical complications, such as pneumothorax or bloodstream infections.[42] Data in Figure 90–3 do not support routine scheduled replacement because the density of incidence of catheter-related infectious complications remains stable after the fourth day, indicating that the risk of acquiring a catheter-related infection does not increase thereafter when the device is kept in place. The risk of thrombosis also must be considered. A prospective descriptive cohort study reported that insertion of a central venous catheter itself is a risk factor for venous thrombosis.[19]

To conclude, data reporting the frequency rates of catheter-related infections show that each day carries a risk of acquiring a catheter-related infection if a central venous line is kept in place. On the other hand, data reporting the density of the incidence of catheter-related infections suggest that the risk is similar from one day to the next. Moreover, some data suggest that catheter replacement carries its own risk of mechanical complications and thrombosis. Accordingly, it is clear that unnecessary devices should be removed at once, but routine replacement of invasive device probably is not required. Increasingly more experts believe a catheter should not be removed if the catheter is still necessary and no sign of infection is present.

A few more points related to specific types of catheter must be addressed.

Multilumen Central Venous Lines. Pemberton et al.[205] prospectively studied the sepsis rate of single-lumen versus triple-lumen catheters in patients receiving parenteral nutrition. The rate of catheter-related infection was 3.5% in the former group and 15% in the latter group. McCarthy et al.[177] found similar rates and concluded that triple-lumen catheters should not be used for long-term parenteral nutrition. Hilton et al.[119] prospectively studied 502 catheters (126 single-lumen catheters and 93 triple-lumen catheters) in 362 patients. There was a marked difference between the two groups: 8% of patients with single-lumen catheters developed catheter-related infection as opposed to 32% of patients with triple-lumen catheters (mean duration of insertion 6.01 and 4.76 days, respectively). Reasons for the possible increased risk of infection remain unclear, although they may be related to increased catheter size with concomitant tissue and vascular trauma and more manipulations. However, increased rates of infection were not recognized by Gil et al.[104] who classified patients according to severity of illness using the APACHE score. Studies of the infectious risk of multilumen catheters have yielded conflicting results, probably because of the failure to control for the sicker baseline state of the patients in whom triple-lumen catheters are used. Despite the conflicting evidence, triple-lumen catheters have the advantage of offering what otherwise would require three independent, single-lumen catheters.

PICC Lines. Use of PICC lines increases when a central catheter may be required for a significant length of time.[74] The diameter of these catheters usually is smaller than that of standard central venous catheters, which should decrease the risk of thrombosis and infection. However, the incidence rates of thrombosis and infection associated with PICC lines is not known.

Arterial Lines. Factors associated with increased risk of sepsis include duration of cannulation, cutdown versus percutaneous insertion, and local inflammation. The risk of infection by site (radial vs. femoral artery) remains controversial.[276] The risk of infection with catheters placed over a guidewire at an old site is considerably higher than with catheters inserted in a new site; the former accounted for all bacteremia in a series.[196]

Environmental Factors

Parenteral Nutrition. Use of parenteral nutrition is associated with an increased risk of infection.[97] Although amino acid solutions are sufficiently hypertonic so that little microbial growth is supported, lipid is roughly equivalent to microbial culture media in its ability to support many bacteria.

Staffing. Understaffing may be a problem. Fridkin et al.[97] reported that increasing the patient-to-nurse ratio from 1:1 to 2:1 in an adult ICU increases the risk of central venous catheter-related bloodstream infection by 62-fold.

Morbidity and Mortality

Catheter-related infectious complications include not only infections of the catheter site, catheter tip, and blood, but also septic thrombophlebitis, right-sided endocarditis, cellulitis, and death.

Indwelling catheters can cause a local thrombosis,[19] which is a significant risk factor for bloodborne infection; the opposite is true, that is, catheter-tip colonization is a risk factor for thrombosis.[220] A septic thrombophlebitis can cause a right-sided endocarditis if it is related to a central venous catheter and a left-sided endocarditis if it is related to a PAC.

The unique positioning of PACs may cause trauma to both the right-sided endocardium and right heart valves. Rowley et al.[242] examined 55 patients who had undergone pulmonary artery catheterization within 1 month of death; 4 patients (7%) had infective endocarditis, 3 had vegetations on the pulmonary valve, and 1 had vegetations in the right atrium. In a postmortem analysis of 20 patients who had a PAC prior to death,[91] one had infective endocarditis on the tricuspid valve. Although the endocardial lesions may be incidental autopsy findings, endocardial damage may act as a nidus for infection.

Patients commonly die with a catheter in place, but mortality attributable to a catheter seems rare. Rello et al.[226] were unable to detect any cause-and-effect relationship between central venous catheter and death in critically ill patients. On the other hand, Renaud et al.[228] reported an excess mortality of 11.5% with catheter-related bloodstream infections.

Rello et al.[226] reported that catheter-related infections increased the length of ICU stay by 20 days. Slonim et al.[262] reported in 2001 that the excess radiology, pharmacy, and laboratory costs attributable to a nosocomial bloodstream infection were $12,211 per catheter-related bloodstream infection in critically ill children.

Management

Treatment of a nosocomial bloodstream infection includes antibiotics and catheter removal. Empirical antibiotics should be active against usual skin flora, and vancomycin can be a good choice. However, another antibiotic should be added to the regimen if a remote focus such as a nosocomial pneumonia is suspected. The choice of antibiotics must be adapted as soon as the causative organism(s) is recognized. A 2-week course is recommended in most instances, but septic thrombosis and endocarditis require at least a 4-week course.[217] Amphotericin or fluconazole should be given if a fungus is the causative agent.

All unnecessary catheters must be removed when a patient contracts a nosocomial bloodstream infection. However, most critically ill patients require such catheters. In such instances, removing the catheter(s) is not essential; antibiotics can be given for a while, but a catheter must be considered again if the bacteremia persists or recurs a few days later.[217]

Prevention

General Preventive Strategies. An education program decreased the incidence rate of catheter-related bloodstream infections in critically ill patients by 66%.[53] Such a program must be implemented in ICUs, and it must be updated regularly.[199] Many other preventive measures also are effective.

Insertion Technique. In the case of central venous catheters, a sterile gown, mask, cap, gloves, and sterile drapes should be used at insertion because the practice decreases the risk of sepsis by sixfold[219] (see Chapter 15).

The risk of bloodstream infection is lower when the catheter is inserted into a subclavian or femoral vein than into an internal jugular vein.[199] The risk of mechanical complications in children is lower when the femoral vein is used.[199]

The skin must be well prepared. If available, 2% chlorhexidine applied for a minimum of 30 seconds is preferable to povidone-iodine or 70% alcohol in preparation of an intravascular site. Contact time with the antiseptic is vitally important; only incineration kills microbes on contact. Antiseptics can be compared in several ways, including immediate, cumulative, or persistent effect. Chlorhexidine distinguishes itself by persistent action and activity in the presence of organic material.[199,246]

The environment where the central catheter is inserted could be important. In a prospective (nonrandomized) study of PACs, central catheters inserted in the operating room with full barrier precautions resulted in lower infection rates than with those inserted under less stringent conditions in the PICU.[178] Colonization of the introducer and external catheter beneath the sheath were more likely to occur in the PICU. However, this study did not look at adverse events occurring during transport from the PICU to the operating room. The costs versus the benefits of such a practice require further study before the practice of inserting central catheters in the operating room rather than the PICU can be recommended.

The risk of catheter-related infections frequently is stated to be lower with tunneled central lines, in which a few centimeters of subcutaneous tunneling and cuff provide protection from skin flora. Meta-analysis of 12 randomized clinical trials showed that tunneling decreased bacterial colonization of the catheter by 39% and catheter-related sepsis by 44% compared with a standard catheter, but the reduction in risk was not statistically significant.[222] Current evidence does not support routine tunneling, but this technique should be considered when a central venous catheter is expected to be necessary for many weeks.

Site Care. The site-care regimen, including antiseptic preparation, dressing, and follow-up care, strongly influences rates of catheter-related infections. Good aseptic technique should include handwashing and application of an antiseptic. Two randomized clinical trials showed that chlorhexidine is more effective than povidone-iodine for insertion site care,[99,187] but the risk of local dermitis with chlorhexidine limits its use in neonates.[99] Dressings should be as dry as possible. Meta-analysis showed that the risk of catheter-tip infection is significantly increased with use of transparent compared with gauze dressings (risk ratio 1.78, 95% CI 1.38–2.3).[120] Changing dressings on a steady basis may be good practice, but no strong evidence supports such a recommendation.

Scheduled Replacement of Infusion Sets. Infusion sets should be replaced no more frequently than at 72-hour intervals, unless a catheter infection is suspected.[199]

Scheduled Replacement of Catheter. A systematic review of 12 randomized clinical trials showed that "Exchanging catheters over guidewires or at new sites every 3 days is not beneficial in reducing infections, compared with catheter replacement on an as-needed basis."[51] Therefore as others,[189,223] we do not recommend routine catheter replacement.[199] However, the catheter must be removed immediately when it no longer functions, when the catheter insertion site becomes purulent, and when catheter sepsis is diagnosed. In neonates, a central catheter should be removed if three blood cultures are positive for coagulase-negative *Staphylococcus*.[21] If a catheter must be removed, it can be changed either by using a guidewire or by changing the site.[119]

Changes Over a Guidewire. A catheter can be replaced over a guidewire or at a new site. Which is the best strategy remains controversial. Change over a guidewire obviates a second puncture, thereby avoiding some mechanical problems and decreasing the risk of thrombosis, but indications for its use remain controversial. Risk of infection correlates with the number of attempts to insert the line. On the other hand, changing a colonized catheter over a guidewire has been shown to cause colonization of the new catheter.[107] In 1996, the U.S. Hospital Infection Control Practices Advisory Committee supported new site replacement.[203] In 1997, meta-analysis showed that guidewire exchange is associated with a trend toward more catheter colonization (relative risk 1.26, 95% CI 0.87–1.84), but it was associated with fewer mechanical complications (relative risk 0.48, 95% CI 0.12–1.91) relative to replacement at a new site.[51] Therefore the best strategy is unclear, and physicians can choose either. If a catheter is changed over a guidewire, a prudent policy is to send both the guidewire and removed catheter for microbiologic culture and to remove the newly inserted cannula if culture is positive.

Antibiotic- or Antiseptic-Impregnated Catheter and Heparin-Bonded Catheter. Colonization of catheter can be prevented by antibiotic- or antiseptic-impregnated catheter, which can kill bacteria, or by heparin-bonded catheter, which can prevent adherence of bacteria to catheter or thrombus.

A first meta-analysis involving 12 randomized clinical trials compared chlorhexidine-silver sulfadiazine–impregnated central venous catheters with standard catheters: the odds ratio for catheter colonization was

0.44 (95% CI 0.36–0.54), and the odds ratio for catheter-related bloodstream infection was 0.56 (95% CI 0.37–0.84).[284] Another systematic review involving 11 studies showed that catheters protected with antibiotics and heparin-bonded catheters decrease catheter-related infection rate by 2.32% (95% CI 1.04%–3.61%).[171] Despite these data, the usefulness of antibiotic- or antiseptic-impregnated catheters should be estimated and the development of antimicrobial resistance must be addressed before their use is routinely implemented in clinical practice.

Fibrin sheath enhances bacteria growth and adherence to a catheter, which significantly increases the risk of contracting a nosocomial catheter-related infection.[182] Only two randomized clinical trials on the efficacy of heparin-bonded catheter in preventing catheter-related infections have been completed.[5,207] Even though both trials were positive, more data are required before the use of such catheters should be considered mandatory.

In 2000 the cost of a catheter impregnated with antibiotics was $36 greater than a standard catheter, whereas the accrual of cost was approximately $6 for a heparin-bonded catheter.[171] Actually, antibiotic-impregnated and heparin-bonded central venous catheters may be useful, but their cost-usefulness remains to be determined.[171,284] Moreover, insufficient data are available to determine if heparin-bonded catheters are better than antibiotic- or antiseptic-impregnated catheters.

Catheter Hub. Catheter hub can be a source of infection. León et al.[158] undertook a randomized clinical trial to estimate the efficacy of a new antiseptic chamber-containing hub (Segur-Lock). Antiseptic (3% iodinated alcohol) was incorporated in the chamber of the new hub model. The incidence rate of catheter-related bloodstream infection originating from the catheter hub was significantly different in 230 critically ill adults (Luer-Lok vs. new hub: 7% vs. 1.7%, $p < 0.049$; relative risk 4.1, 95% CI 0.8–19). More data are required before the use of this device can be considered mandatory, but this new hub probably is cost-effective if its use is reserved for patients who require a central venous line for 6 or more days.[150]

Respiratory Infections

Definitions

A nosocomial respiratory infection can be defined as an infection of the lung parenchyma, airways, or sinus that was neither present nor incubating at the time of hospital admission.[129] Bacterial pneumonia, viral bronchiolitis, bacterial tracheitis, bacterial sinusitis, and otitis media are the nosocomial respiratory tract infections most frequently encountered in PICU.

Diagnosis

Diagnosis of Nosocomial Respiratory Infections. As defined by the CDC, bacterial nosocomial respiratory tract infections can be considered only after 48 hours of hospital stay, which takes into account the incubation period of most bacterial diseases.[37] A more prolonged length of hospital stay must be considered for diseases with a longer incubations period, such as tuberculosis and many viral diseases.

Diagnosis of Nosocomial Pneumonia. Ongoing debate is considerable with regard to the best diagnostic method to use when a nosocomial pneumonia is suspected.[63]

Clinical criteria are useful for detecting possible cases of pneumonia; they include fever, cough, purulent respiratory secretions, leukocytosis, rales, tachypnea, and apnea in newborn. X-ray films usually show an infiltrate. These criteria are of limited value as diagnostic markers because they lack specificity. A study on histopathologic and clinical diagnosis in a group of adults with acute respiratory distress syndrome (ARDS) who died reported that 30% of nosocomial bacterial pneumonia cases were misdiagnosed by bedside clinical criteria.[4] In the critically ill patient, pneumonia can be mimicked by a number of noninfectious conditions. Classic clinical findings of pneumonia may be absent. There is also a problem differentiating contamination, colonization, and respiratory infection in the mechanically ventilated patient. The diagnosis demands that the clinical state of the child be considered before responding to isolated bacteriology results or presence of lung infiltrates.

The definitive diagnostic procedure is autopsy: "Pneumonia is defined as the presence of foci of bronchopneumonia, characterized by an intense polymorphonuclear leukocyte accumulation within bronchioles and adjacent alveoli and disseminated within large zones of non specific alveolar damage" (Figure 90–4).[240] Obviously, biopsies are more appropriate in the clinical setting. However, transthoracic needle aspiration, transbronchial biopsy, and open lung biopsy are neither perfectly sensitive nor perfectly specific. For example, Rouby et al.[240] reported false results with open lung biopsy in 25% of cases. Nosocomial pneumonia is disseminated throughout all pulmonary segments, but the infectious process is focal,[81,239] and most pneumonic nidi are less than 2 mm in diameter,[238] which could explain the lack of reliability of lung biopsy. In addition, these techniques are associated with significant morbidity and mortality in the mechanically ventilated critically ill patient.[11] The reported incidence of severe adverse events (death, pneumothorax) when an open lung biopsy is performed

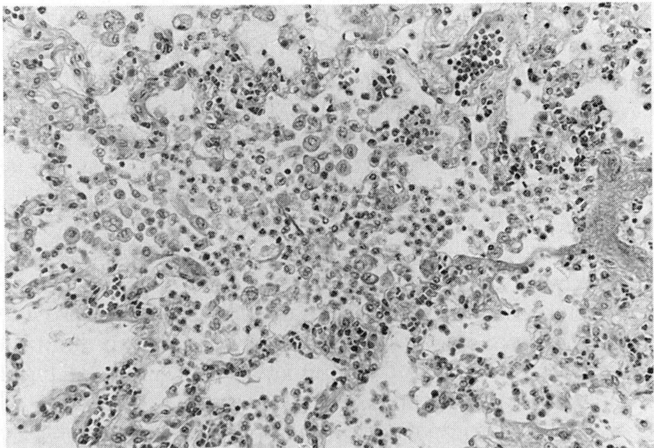

FIGURE 90–4 • Lung biopsy specimen of a focal nosocomial bronchopneumonia. Most alveolar spaces are filled with neutrophils and macrophages (original magnification ×40). (Courtesy Dr. Pierre Russo, Sainte-Justine Hospital.)

in children with respiratory failure ranges from 45% to 65%.[60,148] A bleeding diathesis, inability to oxygenate the patient, and hemodynamic instability are contraindications to all kinds of lung biopsy.[198] Although there are restrictions, some indications for open lung biopsy exist. For example, a critically ill child who will not tolerate bronchoscopy or suctioning because of inability to maintain oxygenation is an obvious candidate for biopsy if a rapid diagnosis is imperative to management.[179] However, a diagnostic test safer than lung biopsy would be a better choice if available. For this reason, less invasive techniques using microbiologic criteria have been evaluated. Most were studied in adult ICUs.

Isolation of a germ from pus sampled in a lung abscess or an empyema is considered a reliable diagnostic criterion for nosocomial respiratory infection but is rarely available.

Positive blood cultures associated with clinical and radiologic signs of pneumonia are considered quite suggestive of a pneumonia, but such findings occur in only 8% to 25% of cases.[14] Also, remember that a significant proportion of critically ill patients present many concomitant nosocomial infections; therefore the germ found in a blood culture can originate from elsewhere than the lungs, even given clinical and radiologic evidence of a nosocomial pneumonia.[181]

Cultures of transtracheal aspirates are considered quite reliable, but presently this technique is not recommended because it has the potential for serious complications[11] and because it is inappropriate in intubated patients.[10]

Cultures of endotracheal aspirates are frequently used. However, there is a problem differentiating contamination and colonization from infection in the intubated, mechanically ventilated patient. The suction catheter becomes contaminated as it passes through the endotracheal tube. Cultures of endotracheal aspirates and sputum specimens do not reliably identify pathogens in the distal lung causing pneumonia. The sensitivity of endotracheal aspirates is quite good (75%–100%), [169,279] but its specificity is low (1%–57%).[279,280] Therefore culture of endotracheal aspirates can be considered a good screening test for detecting cases of nosocomial pneumonia, but it is not sufficiently reliable to diagnose such pneumonia. However, some data suggest that semi-quantitative cultures of endotracheal aspirates can be as reliable as cultures of respiratory secretions collected by a protected brush specimen or a bronchoalveolar lavage.[173,247] Further studies are necessary to support this point of view.

Bronchial washing (as opposed to bronchoalveolar lavage) via a flexible fiberoptic bronchoscope suffers from problems similar to those of catheter suction, but it is useful for cytology.[12] Similarly, routine bronchial brushings are of no added benefit.

Use of a double-lumen protected brush catheter theoretically is an improvement, but contamination of the inner brush still occurs during bronchoscopy. Reported sensitivities and specificities range from 59% to 90%.[28,40,285] It is especially useful if semi-quantitative culture techniques are used.[82] The experience in NICU or PICU is limited. All pediatric studies were performed with blinded protected brush specimen; 10^3 CFU/ml seemed to be the best cutoff point.[77,149,234]

Bronchoalveolar lavage is becoming increasingly important as a safe, rapid, and reliable method of collecting bacteriologic and cytologic specimens.[62,197] An isolated lung segment is lavaged after a variable amount of saline is instilled via the wedged fiberoptic bronchoscope. The centrifuged fluid can be immediately examined for *Pneumocystis*, bacteria, fungus, mycobacteria, and *Legionella*.[101] Semi-quantitative cultures also are performed (cutoff point usually used to diagnose a pneumonia in adults is 10^4 or 10^5 CFU/ml).[39,46,134] A meta-analysis, which considered simultaneously both sensitivity and specificity, found that the global performance of bronchoalveolar lavage was either identical or better than that of protected brush specimen; it also showed that antibiotic use prior to sampling decreased the global performance of protected brush specimen more than that of bronchoalveolar lavage.[63] Another benefit of bronchoalveolar lavage may be the microscopic examination of lavage fluids: a pneumonia should be immediately suspected if the proportion of neutrophils with intracellular bacteria is 1% or more.[101,265] The intubated infant in whom a fiberoptic bronchoscope cannot be used for obtaining specimens still presents a problem. The situation may be obviated by two described modifications of the bronchoalveolar lavage technique not requiring use of a bronchoscope. One technique uses a styletted intracath wedged blindly via the endotracheal tube.[17] The other involves blind wedging of a double-catheter system.[101,240] In adults, the sensitivity of blinded bronchoalveolar lavage performed with a simple lumen catheter is 53%[214] to 76%,[208] and its specificity is nearly 100%.[208] The sensitivity of blinded lavage performed with a protected double lumen catheter is 70% to 91%, and its specificity is 65% to 75%.[206,239,240]

The experience with brush and lavage is limited in critically ill children.[17,77,101,149,234,236,248] Protected methods, namely, protected specimen brush or bronchoalveolar lavage with a double-lumen catheter, have decreased contamination and improved specificity. A prospective study showed that the reproducibility of blinded protected bronchoalveolar lavage with a double-lumen protected catheter is good in critically ill children when three passages of 0.5 ml/kg (minimum 2 ml; maximum 50 ml) of nonbacteriostatic sterile normal saline 0.9% are used.[101] Reproducibility with other techniques has not been evaluated. Therefore we recommend blinded bronchoalveolar lavage with a double-catheter system, even though the cutoff point for semi-quantitative cultures is not clearly established in children. Further studies are necessary to define the best cutoff points of blinded protected bronchoalveolar lavage in mechanically ventilated infants.

The accuracy of techniques such as protected specimen brush and bronchoalveolar lavage (blinded or not) in diagnosing nosocomial pneumonia is better than clinical data alone. However, their usefulness—more than their reliability—is still a matter of debate.[38,195] Two randomized clinical trials[26,84] and one cohort study[117] showed that invasive diagnostic techniques can result in less antibiotics use. However, only one randomized clinical trial reported improvement in clinically significant outcomes such as organ dysfunction and death.[84] Intense controversy still surrounds the usefulness of invasive techniques for diagnosing nosocomial pneumonia in critically ill patients. Some authors claimed improved outcome of ventilator-associated pneumonia,[84,268] whereas others considered the outcome was not influenced by invasive diagnostic techniques.[245] Other studies are required to better estimate the benefits and cost-effectiveness of these techniques. Meanwhile, they can be used in specific cases, but their use as a standard practice cannot yet be recommended.

Other tests have been suggested, such as detection of elastin fiber[78,250] or endotoxin[213] in respiratory secretions, and detection of neutrophil CD64 expression in blood.[193] None of these test have been well validated.

To conclude, we suggest using clinical and radiologic data to detect possible cases of nosocomial pneumonia in critically ill children. However, cultures of respiratory secretions are necessary to validate the diagnosis. We do not recommend use of invasive techniques to diagnose nosocomial pneumonia in a mandatory fashion, but they can be of help in specific cases. Cultures of endotracheal secretions are safe, and they exclude almost with certainty the diagnosis if negative. Isolation of germs that do not colonize airways, such as *Pneumocystis,* mycobacteria, and *Legionella,* is definitive proof of a nosocomial pneumonia if the length of hospital stay is sufficiently long. Heavy growth of other bacteria supports the diagnosis, more so if respiratory secretions were collected by a protected bronchoalveolar lavage.

Diagnosis of Nosocomial Tracheitis. Screening for a nosocomial tracheitis is easy in intubated patients. Endotracheal secretions become purulent and sticky, and their color is yellow or green.[87] It is more difficult to adjudicate the diagnosis. The diagnostic criteria of bacterial tracheitis or bronchitis are mainly clinical. The CDC[37] suggests the following criteria: (1) no clinical or radiologic evidence of pneumonia; (2) at least two symptoms detected by physical examination (fever >38°C, cough, increased amount of tracheal or purulent secretions, rhonchi, wheezing); and (3) recovery of at least one species of bacteria from tracheal secretions or positive bacterial antigens in tracheal aspirate. Three other symptoms are considered in children younger than 1 year: dyspnea, apnea, and bradycardia.

To differentiate colonization and infection of the trachea is not always easy. The former is characterized by less than 25 neutrophils per field, and few bacteria are recovered from tracheal secretions; in bacterial tracheitis, the neutrophils count usually is greater than 25 per field, and bacterial growth is heavy.

To differentiate tracheitis and pneumonia may be even more difficult. Both frequently occur together. A pneumonia can be excluded if a patient with a tracheitis does not show any abnormality on chest x-ray films. A negative bronchoalveolar lavage or protected brush specimen also is quite suggestive.

Diagnosis of Nosocomial Sinusitis. Sinus drainage of infected secretions from a sinus remains the reference standard for diagnosing a sinusitis, but many intensivists consider this test too invasive in critically ill patients. The value of radiography, echography, scanner, and magnetic resonance in diagnosing maxillary and frontal sinusitis is fair in adults,[9,229] even though all of these tests are far from being perfect.

The diagnosis of sinusitis is difficult in children. Glasier et al.[105] showed that radiographic sinus opacification in infants younger than 1 year is of uncertain significance and is not diagnostic of sinusitis. Therefore in this age group, only isolation of a pathogen from culture of purulent material obtained from sinus cavity can demonstrate bacterial sinusitis. However, bacterial sinusitis is likely in children older than 1 year who have upper respiratory tract symptoms and abnormal sinus radiograph.[286]

Incidence

A degree of caution is required in quoting prevalence statistics because of the variance in diagnostic methods used. Many studies did not include surveillance of viral agents; thus the reported incidence may be lower than the actual incidence. In a study performed at the PICU of Sainte-Justine Hospital, the rate of nosocomial bacterial pneumonia among critically ill children who were not in brain death was 1.2% (95% CI 0.7%-1.9%).[87] In the same PICU, the rate of nosocomial bacterial pneumonia among 19 organ donors was 40%.[175] Elward et al.[79] reported that the frequency rate of nosocomial pneumonia was 3.3% in 911 critically ill children (5.1% mechanically ventilated patients). Similar frequency rates of nosocomial pneumonia were reported in cases of pediatric trauma (5.5%[202]) and cases of pediatric surgery (2.3%[211]). These figures demonstrate that the incidence of pneumonia in the PICU is low, unlike the data available for adult ICU where a cumulative incidence rate as high as 28% is reported in mechanically ventilated adults.[116]

In the PICU, a density of incidence of 2.6 nosocomial pneumonia per 1000 patient-days[87] and of 4.7 ventilator-associated pneumonia per 1000 ventilator-days are reported.[130] In adults, density of incidence of 12.5 nosocomial pneumonia per 1000 patient-days and of 20.5 cases per 1000 ventilator-days are reported.[103]

Only one study prospectively estimated the incidence of nosocomial bacterial tracheitis in PICU: the rate was 1.8% (95% CI 0.8%–2.6%),[87] and the density of incidence was 3.9 nosocomial tracheitis per 1000 patient-days.[87] The rate of nosocomial tracheitis seems to be higher among organ donors (50%[175]).

Acute otitis media and sinusitis should be considered in the septic critically ill patient without an obvious septic focus.[65,67] The incidence of acute otitis media and sinusitis in PICUs is unknown.[65,67]

Pathophysiology

Pathogenesis. The pathogenesis of nosocomial pneumonia, tracheitis, and sinusitis is quite similar. Colonization of the buccal oropharyngeal mucosa and alteration of the endogenous microflora appear to be crucial antecedents to endotracheal colonization and nosocomial respiratory tract infections in both children and adults.[243] Colonization of upper airways is frequent in critically ill patients. It has been demonstrated that after 10 days in an ICU, 86% of patients are colonized with gram-negative bacilli and 70% with yeast.[141] Any patient who has been ill for some time or recently hospitalized likely has altered endogenous pharyngeal microflora, associated with prolonged hospitalization (especially in an ICU), serious underlying illness, recent antimicrobial therapy, and immunosuppression.[132] Once the buccal oropharyngeal mucosa is colonized, the risk of lower respiratory tract colonization is greater, frequently resulting in pneumonia. An early study that examined the relative predictive value of positive surveillance cultures of the upper airways in high-risk patients found that 45% of the patients became colonized with aerobic gram-negative bacilli by the end of the first week. Lower airway colonization is followed by infection with the same germ(s) and preceded ventilator-associated pneumonia in two thirds of episodes.[64] The incidence of nosocomial respiratory infections in colonized patients was 23%, in contrast to only 3.3% in noncolonized patients.[133] Oral colonization with *Acinetobacter baumannii* yielded a 7.45-fold increased risk of pneumonia with the same germ.[100]

The stomach-oral route may be a significant source of organisms colonizing the oropharynx.[8] However, tracheal colonization preceded ventilator-associated pneumonia in 93.5% versus gastric colonization in only 13%.[103] Thus an infectious agent most commonly gains entry to the lower respiratory tract by aspiration of secretions from the upper respiratory tract. Less common routes include inhalation of contaminated aerosolized fluids or medications and hematogenous seeding (e.g., right-sided bacterial endocarditis).

Physicians have long been aware of increased adherence of microorganisms to the epithelial cells of the oropharynx in the ill patient.[135] Adherence of *P. aeruginosa* to tracheal cells exceeds that in normal patients if the ill patient has a recent respiratory viral infection.[221] Patients with chronic tracheostomies also exhibit greater tracheal cell adherence, which may not reflect buccal cell adherence. Poor nutrition aggravates this condition.[194] The mechanism by which bacteria colonize the oropharynx and the tracheobronchial tree is under investigation.

Once the organisms gain entry to the lower respiratory tract, the normal defenses usually are sufficient to prevent infection. However, under certain conditions, the function of the alveolar macrophage is disturbed. For example, in patients with ARDS or preexisting pneumonia, secretion of cytokines such as interleukin-1 increases.[128] The recruited granulocytes likewise function abnormally. Pulmonary edema impairs bacterial clearance from the lung.[151] These abnormalities may help explain the high incidence of pneumonia in patients who develop ARDS.[64,172]

Modes of Transmission. The predominant reservoirs for nosocomial respiratory tract infections are the patient's oropharynx and the digestive tract. The predominant mode of inoculation is aspiration, although translocation through the gut mucosa is possible. Colonization with Enterobacteriaceae originates primarily from the patient's endogenous flora.[132] Water bugs *(P. aeruginosa, Serratia marcescens, Legionella* spp) can be transmitted by a contaminated ventilator circuit.

Viral respiratory infections are transmitted from infected patients via the hands of staff and directly from the hands of infected staff. Infected children and staff shed very large amounts of virus with symptoms (e.g., 10^5 virions/ml of respiratory secretions). In fact, shedding may precede symptoms by as much as 1 week. The virus lasts for hours on nonporous surfaces and for shorter periods on porous surfaces, such as cloth, paper, and hands. Virus in very small numbers (e.g., rhinovirus) can induce infection when introduced through the eye or nasal mucosa. Repeated infections on exposure are the rule, at least in the first 3 years of life in patients and in staff with fewer than 3 years of experience.

Causative Agents. A pathogen should be recovered from blood, pleural fluid, lung abscess, or lung biopsy to show with certainty that the pathogen is the cause of the pneumonia. Detection in respiratory secretions of a recognized pathogen that does not colonize the respiratory tract, such as *P. carinii, Legionella, Mycoplasma pneumoniae, M. tuberculosis,* influenza virus, and respiratory syncytial virus, also is diagnostic.[13]

Bacterial Diseases. The majority of nosocomial pneumonias are caused by aerobic gram-negative organisms (Table 90–2).[55] They account for up to 60% of these infections, with *P. aeruginosa* the most frequent organism implicated.[55] Few data from PICUs report the causative agents of pneumonia, but *S. aureus, H. influenzae, P. aeruginosa,* and *Klebsiella pneumoniae* are frequently found.[87] Additional bacteria of concern are *Meningococcus, M. tuberculosis, B. pertussis,* and *Legionella pneumoniae.* Anaerobic organisms are found more frequently following aspiration. *Moraxella (Branhamella) catarrhalis* requires special isolation techniques and is increasingly recognized in PICUs. Although gram-negative organisms remain the most common cause of nosocomial pneumonias in the immunosuppressed patient, other organisms that must be considered include fungal infections, *P. carinii,* and *Neisseria asteroides.* Although anaerobic organisms are frequently found following aspiration, they are rarely isolated in cases of ventilator-associated pneumonia. Marik and Careau[170] reported finding no such organisms among 56 cases despite "painstaking efforts."

Pathogens of ventilator-associated pneumonia differ in patients who received prior antimicrobial therapy, and this factor determines higher mortality rates. For example, Rello et al.[224] reported that, in patients who had received antibiotics, the rate of infection caused by *H. influenzae* was statistically lower ($p < 0.05$), whereas the rate of *P. aeruginosa* was statistically higher ($p < 0.01$).

Causative agents are different with early-onset (≤4 days) nosocomial pneumonia, representing 54.2% of nosocomial pneumonia in ICU, and late-onset (> 4 days) nosocomial pneumonia.[90,153] In adults, as well as in children, germs such as *H. influenzae* and *Streptococcus pneumoniae* are more frequent with early-onset pneumonia, whereas *P. aeruginosa, Escherichia coli, Enterobacter* spp, *Acinetobacter* spp, *K. pneumoniae, Serratia marcescens, S. aureus,* and *Legionella pneumophila* are more frequent with late-onset pneumonia.[90,202]

Remember that a significant proportion of nosocomial pneumonias are polymicrobial. This proportion is unknown in the PICU but is between 26% and 50% in adults.[14,55,102,103]

Most nosocomial tracheitis are caused by *S. aureus, M. catarrhalis, H. influenzae, P. aeruginosa,* and *K. pneumoniae.*[87]

Pathogens involved in nosocomial sinusitis acquired in PICU are unknown. However, in adults, nosocomial pneumonia and sinusitis have been noted to occur together, often with the same bacteria at both sites.[181] One can speculate that the situation should be the same in children.

Viral Respiratory Disease. Most viral infections are community acquired. On pediatric wards, viral bronchiolitis and pneumonia are frequent nosocomial infections, some of which will require intensive care admission. Respiratory syncytial virus, the predominant pathogen, is implicated in numerous hospital outbreaks of respiratory infection. Parainfluenza virus and influenza virus are other major causes. At the PICU of the Hospital for Sick Children, 45.9% of all respiratory infections were of viral origin.[94] Viral infections may predispose to bacterial superinfections, especially in children younger than 12 months. Other less common viral agents implicated in nosocomial respiratory infections include chickenpox and rhinovirus. *Herpes simplex,* cytomegalovirus, and *Varicella zoster* can cause pneumonia, especially in hospitalized immunosuppressed patients.

Risk Factors

Host-Related Factors. Risk factors for nosocomial pneumonia, tracheitis, and sinusitis are similar (Figure 90–5).

Immune deficiency is a very significant risk factor of nosocomial pneumonia (relative risk 14.3, 95% CI 3.5–58.8).[86] Not surprisingly, conditions that are harmful to the immune system, such as multiple organ dysfunction, shock, severe polytraumatism, severe head trauma, burns, and cancer, are also risk factors.[7,52,86,202]

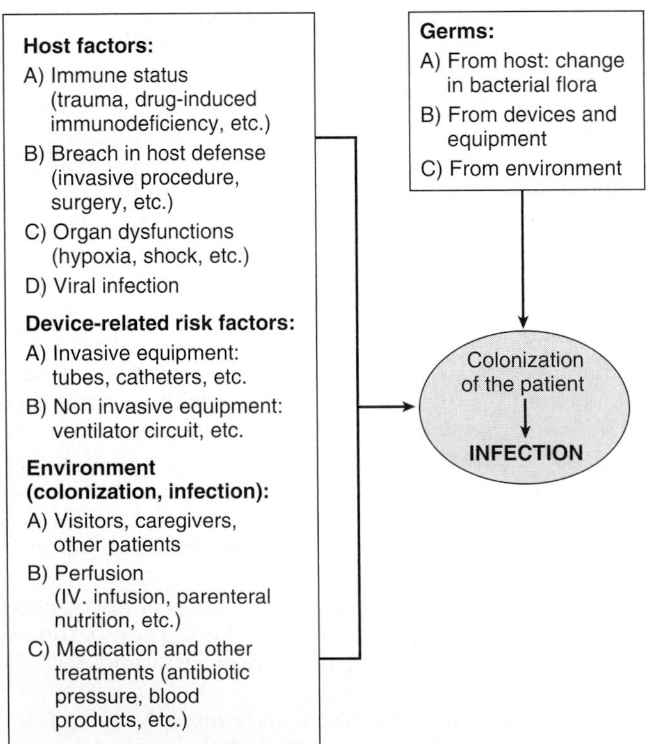

FIGURE 90–5 • Risk factors of nosocomial respiratory tract infections in critically ill patients.

Huxley et al.[126] found that 45% of normal subjects and 70% of patients with depressed levels of consciousness aspirate during sleep. The numbers may approach 100% for the intubated patient who is lying supine. This becomes important if the aspirated material contains potentially pathogenic microorganisms. Patients with paralytic ileus on ventilatory support are prone to gastric colonization with gram-negative bacilli, which increases the risk of nosocomial respiratory tract infections.

Previous viral respiratory illness predisposes patients to the development of staphylococcal pneumonia, especially in young children.

Device, Procedure-Related, and Environmental Factors. Endotracheal intubation is frequently considered a risk factor of nosocomial respiratory tract infections. Suction catheters cause mucosal denudation and suppress mucociliary transport.[152] Almost all intubated patients aspirate some oropharyngeal secretions.[126] A dense bacterial polysaccharide biofilm has been shown to coat endotracheal tubes.[249] Detachment and aspiration of aggregates during tracheal suctioning could constitute a large pulmonary inoculum, which may be poorly handled by an impaired lower respiratory defense. Nasogastric tubes allow a direct route from the upper gastrointestinal tract to the nasopharynx. Tracheostomies likewise have been associated with increased risk of nosocomial pneumonia.[30] Not surprisingly, the length of respiratory assistance and endotracheal intubation and therefore the device-related risk are frequently reported as significant risk factors of nosocomial pneumonia.[154] However, a large prospective epidemiologic study reported that neuromuscular blocking agents (relative risk 17.5, 95% CI 5.4–57.1) were far more predictive of nosocomial pneumonia than mechanical ventilation (relative risk 6.6, 95% CI 1.4–28.5) or endotracheal intubation (relative risk 7.5, 95% CI 2.0–27.5).[87]

Nasotracheal tubes, nasogastric tubes, and facial trauma can obstruct drainage of the eustachian tubes and paranasal sinuses, and they are risk factors of middle ear infection and sinusitis.[65,67]

Colonized hands of medical personnel, especially staff with concurrent dermatitis, are obvious avenues of contamination of the respiratory tract.[68] Viral respiratory infections are transmitted via the hands of hospital staff or visitors.

Risk Factors: Conclusion. In a large prospective epidemiologic study completed in the PICU of Sainte-Justine Hospital, multivariate analysis retained only three independent risk factors or risk markers for pneumonia (immunodepressant drugs, immunodeficiency, and use of neuromuscular blockade agent) and two for tracheitis (respiratory failure and head trauma). Colinearity between neuromuscular blockade, mechanical ventilation, and endotracheal intubation explained why neuromuscular blockade picked up most of the risk associated with nosocomial pneumonia. Age and PRISM score were found to be confounding variables for both pneumonia and tracheitis. The cutoff points for pneumonia were PRISM score ≥16 (relative risk 7.0, 95% CI 2.3–21.6) and ≤2 months of age (4.0; 1.3–12.3). The cutoff points for tracheitis were PRISM score ≥12 (relative risk 4.1, 95% CI 1.6–10.4) and ≤28 months of age (relative risk 4.1, 95% CI 1.3–12.4).[87]

Morbidity and Mortality

In a cohort study of 1114 consecutive admissions in the PICU of Sainte-Justine Hospital, multiple organ system failure resulted from pneumonia in 8% of cases but never from tracheitis. On the other hand, the reintubation rate was 24% in tracheitis cases.[87]

Pneumonia is the most common fatal nosocomial infection in critically ill adults; associated mortalities range from 20% to 70%, depending on the causative organism.[55] However, dying with pneumonia does not mean dying of pneumonia; actually, it is estimated that the mortality attributable to nosocomial pneumonia in adult ICUs is 7% to 27%.[22,55,83] In PICUs, the mortality attributable to a nosocomial pneumonia or tracheitis is less than 1%.[87] Prognosis associated with gram-negative bacillary pneumonias, especially *P. aeruginosa,* is considerably worse than that with gram-positive or viral agents, which appears to increase mortality only in specific population subsets.[115,227] The risk of death is higher with late-onset than with early-onset pneumonia.[145]

Costs associated with and attributable to nosocomial pneumonia are significant. In adults, nosocomial pneumonia accounts for an increased mean hospital ICU stay of 4 to 9 days, which is a major increase in hospital cost ($24,000 per case in 1986).[22,54,118] Prescription of antibiotics frequently is attributable to nosocomial pneumonia.[87] The exact costs of nosocomial respiratory infections in PICUs remain to be determined.

Most nosocomial viral bronchiolitis is caused by respiratory syncytial virus, although adenovirus and parainfluenza virus are not so rare. Respiratory syncytial virus infection increases morbidity and mortality in young children who have congenital heart disease,[70] are immunosuppressed,[113] or suffer from bronchopulmonary dysplasia, chronic lung disease, or asthma.[32] The mortality rate of respiratory syncytial virus in patients with congenital heart disease is 37%, compared with 1.5% in those without underlying heart disease.[70,164]

The morbidity and mortality of acute otitis media and sinusitis in PICUs are unknown.[65,67]

Management

Aggressive and prompt treatment is required when a nosocomial pneumonia is suspected in a critically ill patient. A good approach is to begin with large-spectrum antibiotics and then change to antibiotics with a narrower spectrum as soon as the causative germ(s) and its sensitivity are known. Such a strategy allows rapid protection of the patient, without increasing the risk of multiresistant bacteria. We suggest the following management strategy.

- *Step 1: Empirical Therapy.* The outcome of critically ill patients who contract nosocomial pneumonia is better if they are treated sooner with an appropriate treatment. Therefore antibiotics must be prescribed as soon as a nosocomial pneumonia is suspected. Moreover, it is critical that this early empirical antibiotic therapy be appropriate.[225] Guiding initial antibiotic selection on the basis of the results of microbiologic specimens already available for a given patient is of limited value unless the germs were isolated from the respiratory secretions.[116] The best strategy probably is to select initially one or many antibiotics able to treat germs that are prevalent in the PICU and then widen the spectrum of activity of the antibiotics prescribed if germs with specific resistance are identified later in the patient. The initial selection of antibiotics must take into account the time when the nosocomial respiratory tract infection appears. Germs observed in community-acquired pneumonia are more frequent when the nosocomial pneumonia appears 4 or fewer days after entry to the ICU (early-onset pneumonia), whereas germs such as *Pseudomonas* and *Staphylococcus* are predominant in late-onset pneumonia.
    - *Early-onset pneumonia and no prior antibiotic (≤4 days).* We suggest giving an antibiotic such as cefuroxime or cloxacillin. Vancomycin must be considered in ICUs where methicillin resistant *Staphylococcus* is prevalent.[35] Erythromycin should be given if *Mycoplasma, Legionella,* or *Bordetella* is the possible causative germ.
    - *Late-onset pneumonia or patient was already receiving antibiotics.* Monotherapy with one antibiotic should not be used in such a case because it significantly increases the risk of selecting multiresistant bacteria (19% with a cephalosporin, 11% with imipenem, 9% with ciprofloxacin).[291] The American Thoracic Society[3] suggested a combination of at least two wide-spectrum antibiotics: (1) a β-lactamine (e.g., ceftazidime, cefotaxime, imipenem) or piperacillin; and (2) an aminoglycoside (e.g., tobramycin). A combination of clindamycin or meropenem plus tobramycin is another good choice.[253,287] Combined antibiotics, such as ticarcillin–clavulanic acid (Timentin) or tazobactam–piperacillin (Tazocin), also can be used instead of a β lactamine. Vancomycin must be added to the regimen in ICUs where methicillin-resistant *Staphylococcus* is prevalent.[3]
- *Step 2: Adjust Therapy a Few Days Later.* Antimicrobial resistance and superinfections develop more frequently if the course of empirical antibiotic therapy is prolonged rather than short term.[254] Prolonged use of wide-spectrum antibiotics increases the risk of death when antibiotics are given to patients who received empirical antibiotherapy because a pneumonia was suspected but for whom the diagnosis was not supported 2 or 3 days later. Wide-spectrum antibiotics must be stopped as soon as possible unless they are required to treat specific germ(s). On the other hand, antibiotics must be given for 10 to 14 days if the diagnosis of nosocomial pneumonia is supported by new clinical and laboratory evidence.[3]

Nosocomial tracheitis and sinusitis should be treated with the same antibiotics that can be used to treat pneumonia. Moreover, frequent endotracheal suctioning is warranted in cases of tracheitis, more so if the pus is abundant and/or sticky. The utility of sinus drainage as a treatment measure of nosocomial sinusitis in the PICU remains to be determined.

Prevention

Strategies Specific to Respiratory Devices. Nosocomial pneumonia, tracheitis, and sinusitis follow acquisition of potential bacterial pathogens in the upper airways, originating predominantly as an endogenous source but also transmitted from the environment. Attention to the environment is the first step in prevention, especially with regard to handwashing practices and to contamination and handling of respiratory equipment. Routine respiratory care should not be overlooked, such as posture, physiotherapy, sterile endotracheal suctioning, adequate analgesia, and early mobilization if conditions allow. Manual ventilation bags should be disinfected.[243]

The risk of contracting nosocomial sinusitis in critically ill adults is lower with oral than with nasal intubation.[47] However, no evidence indicates that this factor is important in critically ill children. Routine periodic changes of endotracheal tubes is strongly discouraged,[18] even though they are rapidly contaminated.[243] The latter recommendation is supported by the fact that the daily hazard of contracting a nosocomial pneumonia decreases after day 5 (3.3% at day 5, 2.3% at day 10, and 1.3% at day 15).[52]

No hard data support the point of view that closed endotracheal suctioning system (e.g., Trach-Care) decreases the incidence of nosocomial pneumonia. However, it decreases significantly the cost of suctioning, and suctioning may be safer with such a system when a patient requires a high level of positive end-expiratory pressure.

Results of two randomized clinical trials suggested that subglottic secretion drainage may be effective in preventing nosocomial pneumonia in mechanically ventilated adults.[165,283] However, we believe, as do Cook et al.,[48] that more data are required before such preventive strategy is considered mandatory.

Up to the 1990s, contamination of respiratory support equipment was considered a frequent source of nosocomial respiratory tract infection.[56] It now is clear that changes of the ventilatory circuit are not necessary, and that the ventilatory circuit should not be changed routinely in neonatal[166] or in adult ICUs.[72,144] We recommend not changing the ventilator circuit unless evidence indicates they are contaminating a patient.[47]

The modern humidifiers of the cascade or servocontrolled wick variety, and use of sterile water in these devices, are safe from bacterial contamination, mainly because pathogens cannot survive in the reservoir where the temperature is 50° C.[18] We recommend not changing humidifiers unless there is a specific reason to do so.[47]

Noninvasive ventilation may be associated with a lower risk of nosocomial pneumonia, but more evidence is required to support strongly this association.

General Preventive Strategies. Patients with resistant organisms should be isolated.

Use of prophylactic aerosolized polymyxin B sulfate or prophylactic endotracheal gentamicin has produced either no improvement in outcome or emergence of resistant organisms.[88,143] We do not recommend routine aerosolized antibioprophylaxis to mechanically ventilated children.

Use of prophylactic intravenous antibiotics is a matter of debate. Increasingly more evidence indicates that prophylaxis with wide-spectrum antibiotics increases the mortality of critically ill patients. The only known exception to this observation is cases of severe head trauma where two single doses of cefuroxime (1500 mg intravenously 12 hours apart in adults) given soon after entry to the ICU prevent early-onset nosocomial pneumonia.[258] However, some evidence indicates that such practice may increase the risk of contracting a late-onset pneumonia.[80]

In adults, attempts have been made to reduce the rates of nosocomial pneumonia by "selective digestive decontamination." The concept is that selective digestive decontamination can prevent lower respiratory tract infection by modulating carriage of aggressive bacteria in the oropharynx, stomach, and gut. It is clear that oropharyngeal colonization is of paramount importance in the genesis of ventilator-associated pneumonia.[24] The role of the stomach and gut remains to be determined. Topical oropharyngeal and gastric-instilled antibiotics are used to reduce the aerobic gram-negative intestinal load while minimizing the effects on the anaerobic population, with or without systemic antibiotics. More than 40 studies and at least four meta-analyses on the effectiveness of different regimens of selective digestive decontamination (with or without intravenous antibiotics, with different kind of antibiotics) in preventing nosocomial pneumonia in critically ill patients have been published.[27] These regimens have been successful in reducing oropharyngeal and tracheal colonization. The incidence of pneumonia also was reduced, but the overall mortality rate was affected only with the regimen that included both topical and intravenous prophylaxis.[57,161] To date, resistant organisms have not been a problem, but many investigators are concerned by the possibility that selective digestive decontamination can increase the emergence of multiresistant germs.[27,209] Presently, selective digestive decontamination is not recommended as a routine regimen to prevent nosocomial respiratory infections in critically ill patients.

On the other hand, scheduled change of antibiotic classes used for empirical treatment of suspected cases of nosocomial respiratory tract infection in the ICU seems to reduce the incidence of resistant bacteria.[146] Kollef et al.[147] reported that such a strategy reduces the occurrence of inadequate empirical antibiotic administration for nosocomial infections in critically ill adults. This factor has not been studied in PICU.

Concern has been expressed about gastric alkalinization. H_2 antagonists and antacids have been shown to increase gastric colonization with the patient's endogenous flora.[244] A higher incidence of nosocomial pneumonias has been reported when antacids and H_2 antagonists were compared with sucralfate, a nonalkalinizing agent used to prevent stress ulceration.[54,73] However, a meta-analysis by Cook et al.[49] did not find such association. A large randomized clinical trial showed that H_2 antagonists were more effective than sucralfate in preventing clinically significant upper gastrointestinal bleeding acquired in ICU (difference statistically significant), but the incidence rate of nosocomial pneumonia was lower in patients who received sucralfate (difference not statistically significant).[45] We recommend not using antacids to prevent stress ulcer in critically ill patients, but H_2 antagonists or sucralfate could be a good choice.

The effect of gastric volume and gastric pH on the incidence of nosocomial respiratory infections must be considered because gastric volume seems to be an important risk factor for aspiration. H_2 antagonists decreased gastric volume. Gastric feeding given by bolus increases gastric volume and gastric pH. Continuous gastric feeding, rather than bolus feeds, decreases the volume in the stomach but increases gastric pH. Turning such feeding off overnight allows gastric pH to fall under 3.5, which could decrease the risk for nosocomial respiratory infections.[18] Another method for decreasing gastric volume is to administer small intestinal rather than gastric feeding; however, a randomized clinical trial showed no difference with respect to the incidence of ventilator-associated pneumonia in patients fed through duodenum.[140]

Placing patients in a semi-recumbent position (30°–45° head elevation) significantly decreases the incidence of nosocomial pneumonia.[71] Gastroesophageal reflux is greater in the supine than in the semi-recumbent position, which might explain the observation.[281] Semi-recumbent position is recommended if there is no contraindication to its implementation in a given patient.[50,273]

At present it is impossible to prevent all viral respiratory infections, regardless of the strategy used. Although a study has shown that use of gloves and gowns can reduce nosocomial spread of respiratory syncytial virus,[157] studies of effectiveness have not been performed . Compliance may be a problem. Evidence suggests, however, that nosocomial viral outbreaks can be controlled by handwashing and by isolating and grouping of infected patients and staff,[112] and that awareness of deaths from respiratory disease and regular review of infection surveillance results motivate staff to comply with readily available precautions.[273] Passive immunization with specific immunoglobulins to *V. zoster* is recommended if an immunodeficient patient has significant contact with an infected person. Respiratory syncytial virus immunoglobulin may be cost saving and useful if it is used in high-risk patients, such as infants with severe cardiopathy or transplant recipients having close contact with the virus.[15,294] On the other hand, the role of antiviral drugs (e.g., amantadine, ganciclovir), revaccination to *S. pneumoniae*, or vaccination for influenza or varicella remains to be determined. The role of passive immunization with nonspecific immunoglobulin also remains to be determined.[289,294]

Zach et al.[293] reported that implementation of an education program decreased the density of incidence of nosocomial pneumonia in an adult ICU by 57.6%. Such a program must be used; how frequently it must be repeated is unknown.

Urinary Tract Infections

Diagnosis

Stark and Maki[266] showed that low-level bacteriuria (<10^5 organisms/ml) almost always results in high-level bacteriuria (occurs 96% of the time within 3 days of initial culture). Thus one can consider a nosocomial urinary tract infection if some bacteria is present in urine collected from the bladder of a patient with a catheter.

Incidence

The risk of infection increases with duration of catheterization and is estimated at 5.8 per 1000 catheter-days in the PICU.[130] The cumulative risk of acquiring a urinary tract infection related to an indwelling urinary catheter in PICU patients is 29.1%.[139] Higher rates are observed in children younger than 1 year.[139]

Pathophysiology

Nosocomial urinary tract infections can be contracted from blood or from an indwelling catheter. The latter is significantly more frequent than the former.

Most nosocomial urinary tract infections are caused by the germs found in community-acquired infections, such as *E. coli* and *K. pneumoniae*. However, Enterobacteriaceae such as *Pseudomonas* spp. and opportunistic germs such as *S. aureus, S. epidermidis,* and *Candida* spp. also can be involved.

Risk Factors

Catheterization and periurethral colonization with potential pathogens are the major risk factors. In a study of pediatric patients, including those in the PICU, 92% of infections occurred in catheterized patients.[162]

Morbidity and Mortality

Catheter-related urinary tract infection may be complicated by bacteremia in 3% of children.[162,288] Secondary infections are well documented and include bacteremia and wound infection. Nosocomial urinary tract infections affect the cost of hospitalization (each episode costs an additional US $676[246]), patient morbidity, and, in extreme cases, mortality. Mortality associated with nosocomial urinary tract infection is high (12.5%–50%),[162,288] but death actually attributed to a nosocomial urinary tract infection seems to be rare in the PICU.[139]

Management

The bladder catheter must be removed if possible. Antibiotics are required to treat a nosocomial urinary tract infection. A third-generation cephalosporin and an aminoside can be a good choice. An antibiotic active against *S. aureus* and *S. epidermidis*, such as vancomycin, can be added in some instances. Fluconazole is a good choice if the urinary tract infection is caused by fungi; if the infection is widespread, then amphotericin is necessary.

Prevention

The impetus for prevention is strong. As with other invasive devices, urinary catheters should not be inserted if they are not required. The risk of infection associated with a single in-and-out catheterization in children is not well defined but is 0.5% to 8% in adults. Only a closed urinary catheter drainage system should be used, and it should be manipulated as infrequently as possible.[246] Urinary catheters should be removed as soon as possible.

Studies showed the presence of bacterium in the tubing or bag before colonization of the bladder. The success of the Foley catheter results from several factors: it is an intact closed system, it is maintained aseptically, and it is inserted only after careful disinfection. The ease with which bacteria migrate along tubing when a system is broken must be understood.

Antibiotics do not protect against urinary tract infections in catheterized patients. Kasian et al.[139] reported that 11% of critically ill children receiving antibiotics contracted a urinary tract infection versus 3.8% of children not receiving antibiotics. Moreover, the occurrence of more resistant organisms is reported if antibiotics are used.[139] Therefore antibiotics should not be given to prevent urinary tract infections in PICU patients.

Nosocomial Skin Infections

Diagnosis

Diagnosis depends on regular wound inspection and the usual signs of inflammation, with or without pus. Culture of the apparent skin infection frequently is helpful, although differentiating colonization and infection in some cases may be difficult. Diagnostic tests for deep infection, such as nuclear radiology, are also used.

Incidence

Skin infections are the second most frequent nosocomial infection in the PICU.[94] Skin infections accounted for 6.9% of nosocomial infections in the NICU and 24.6% in the PICU.[94]

Most nosocomial skin infections observed in ICU are wound infections. Donowitz[70] reported a postoperative wound infection rate of 1.4% in PICU patients compared with 0.5% for ward admissions. Brown et al.[31] reported an incidence of 2.3% in the PICU compared with 5.1% in the adult medical/surgical ICU.

Pathophysiology

Pathogenesis. The determinants of a surgical wound infection are a complex interplay of three factors: amount and type of wound contamination, surgical technique, and host resistance. Wound contamination, although most often endogenous, can occur by direct inoculation and by airborne or hematogenous-lymphatic seeding. Methods of prevention are directed toward each of these causative factors.

Causative Agents. Postoperative wound infections often are polymicrobial. *S. aureus* is the chief culprit. Mehta et al.[183] reported that the causative agents for sternal wound infection were *S. aureus* (6), *P. aeruginosa* (1), and *H. influenzae* non-type b (1). Gram-negative organisms may be involved, with *E. coli* and *P. aeruginosa* the most common.[201] In the Hospital for Sick Children in Toronto, postoperative wound infections following cardiovascular surgery were more likely to be *P. aeruginosa* and *Candida* spp. if the sternum was left open. In procedures in which the sternum can be closed, staphylococcal species were more common.[211] Nonbacterial pathogens, such as fungi, are rare causes of nosocomial postoperative wound infections.[292] Of growing importance are infections caused by multiple-resistant organisms, chiefly methicillin-resistant *S. aureus*, methicillin- and cephalosporin-resistant coagulase-negative *Staphylococcus* (MR-CNS), cephalosporin- and gentamicin-resistant gram-negative rods, and fungi.[16,123,201]

Risk Factors

Studies on the influence of age on the incidence of nosocomial wound infections have yielded varied results. Davis et al.[61] found that age was not a risk factor, whereas others did.[180,183] Multiple trauma is a risk factor for skin infection in the ICU.[29] Untreated infection at any site before surgery increases the risk of postoperative wound infection.

Cardiac surgery and a high PRISM score might be risk factors. A study of 310 cardiovascular surgery patients admitted to the PICU at the Hospital for Sick Children was performed to examine the causes of wound infection. Patients were characterized by surgical procedure and PRISM score on admission to the PICU. Of these patients, 22 (6.9%) developed wound infections within 2 months of surgery. Early wound infection followed 8% of closed, nonpump cases and 6.7% of open, pump cases. Wound infection was more likely if the sternum was open on the ward (electively or emergency) (27.6% open vs. 5% closed, $p = 0.0003$) or if the PRISM score was ≥10 on admission to the PICU (10.7% if ≥10 vs. 2.3% if <10; $p = 0.003$). Mehta et al.[183] reported that sternal wound infection developed in 10 (5%) of 202 children after median sternotomy. The infection was superficial in 6 (3%) children and deep in 4 (2%). Lower age, higher American Society of Anesthesiologist score, and longer length of PICU stay were risk factors.

Morbidity and Mortality

Surgical wound infections are an important cause of morbidity, mortality, and increased health care expenditure. From 60% to 80% of infections are incisional; the remainder occur at adjacent deeper sites. Complications can be local or systemic.

Management

Skin cleaning, wound care, and antibiotics are the main components of treatment.

Prevention

Prevention of a perioperative wound infection depends on a combination of prophylactic perioperative management, perioperative antibiotic prophylaxis, and prospective surgical wound infection surveillance with provision of feedback to individual surgeons.

Postoperative Care. The basic aims of postoperative care are to (1) optimize the physiologic condition of the patient through good nutrition and treatment of intercurrent illnesses or infections, (2) minimize the risk of postoperative colonization of the patient's skin with multiresistant flora, (3) minimize contamination of the surgical wound after the operation, and (4) maintain adequate tissue perfusion and oxygenation.

Antibiotic Prophylaxis. Prophylactic postoperative antibiotics are almost universally administered but unfortunately tend to be abused in this setting. The three important basic principles are as follows: (1) the selected antibiotic should be active against the predominant contaminating organisms; (2) the spectrum of the antibiotic must be as narrow as possible; and (3) antibiotic use must be as short as possible. Although the duration of administration is controversial, antibiotics probably do not need to be continued beyond the actual surgery, even though they frequently are used during the 24 hours after the surgery. The American Heart Association considers that the prophylaxis should be stopped 24 hours after surgery.[58]

Indications for antibiotic prophylaxis include the following: surgery associated with a high risk of postoperative wound infection; patients with a high risk of postoperative wound infection (immunosuppressed patients); or cases where the risk of infection is low but the consequences are extreme.[188]

The antibiotics most commonly used are the first- or second-generation cephalosporins. They have a broad spectrum of activity and a low incidence of allergic side effects. However, the emergence of multiple-resistant organisms and the failure of cephalosporins to prevent infections from such organisms necessitate a reappraisal of current practices. The choice and duration of antibiotic prophylaxis depends on the surgical procedure, degree of wound contamination, emergency or elective surgery, patient allergy, and surgeon's preference.[137]

Prospective Surgical Wound Infection Surveillance. Use of a prospective program of wound surveillance, with provision of feedback on infection rates to surgeons, helps reduce surgical wound infection rates. It should form part of every hospital's infection control program.[44]

Other Nosocomial Infections

Conjunctivitis

Eye infections occur frequently in critically ill patients.[94] Manipulations about the eye that lead to splattering of respiratory secretions (including suctioning) have been associated with *Pseudomonas* spp., *M. catarrhalis*, and *Candida* spp. conjunctivitis and, in some cases, corneal opacification. Preventive strategies include covering the eyes and preventing tracking of secretions into the eye.

Ventriculotomy-Related Infections

Risk factors for ventriculotomy-related infection include placement longer than 5 days, trauma, intracerebral hemorrhage with intraventricular hemorrhage, neurosurgical operations, intracranial pressure of 20 mmHg or more, and irrigation.[176]

SUGGESTED READINGS

Anonymous: Guidelines for prevention of nosocomial pneumonia. Centers for Disease Control and Prevention. *MMWR* 46(RR-1): 1-79, 1997

Jarvis WR: *Nosocomial pneumonia.* New York, 2000, Marcel Dekker.

O'Grady NP, Alexander M, Dellinger EP, Gerberding JL, Heard SO, Maki DG, Masur H, McCormick RD, Mermel LA, Pearson ML, Raad II, Randolph A, Weinstein RA: Guidelines for the prevention of intravascular catheter-related infections. *MMWR* 51(RR-10):1-29, 2002.

REFERENCES

1. Adams JM, Speer ME, Rudolph AJ: Bacterial colonization of radial artery catheters, *Pediatrics* 65:94, 1980.
2. Alexander JW, Gottschlich MM: Nutritional immunomodulation in burn patients, *Crit Care Med* 18:S149, 1990.
3. American Thoracic Society: Hospital-acquired pneumonia in adults: diagnosis, assessment of severity, initial antimicrobial therapy, and preventive strategies. *Am J Respir Crit Care Med* 153:1711, 1995.
4. Andrews CP, Coalson JJ, Smith JD, et al: Diagnosis of nosocomial bacterial pneumonia in acute, diffuse lung injury. *Chest* 80:254, 1981.
5. Appelgren P, Ransjo U, Bindsley L, et al: Surface heparinization of central venous catheters reduces microbial colonization in vitro and in vivo: results from a prospective, randomized trial. *Crit Care Med* 24:1482, 1996.
6. Arnow PM, Chou T, Weil D, et al: Nosocomial legionnaires disease caused by aerosolized tap water from respiratory devices. *J Infect Dis* 146:460, 1982.
7. Artigas AT, Dronda SB, Vallès EC, et al: Risk factors for nosocomial pneumonia in critically ill trauma patients. *Crit Care Med* 29:304, 2001.
8. Atherton ST, White DJ: Stomach as source of bacteria colonizing respiratory tract during artificial ventilation. *Lancet* 2:968, 1978.
9. Auboyer C, Caudemont L, Jospé R, et al: Diagnostic échographique des comblements sinusiens chez les patients intubés. *Réanim Urg* 3:719, 1994.
10. Bartlett JG: Diagnostic accuracy of transtracheal aspiration bacteriologic studies. *Am Rev Respir Dis* 115:777, 1977.
11. Bartlett JG: Diagnosis of bacterial infections of the lung. *Clin Chest Med* 8:119, 1987.
12. Bartlett JG, Alexander J, Mayhew J, et al: Should fiberoptic bronchoscopy aspirate be cultured? *Am Rev Respir Dis* 114:74, 1976.
13. Bartlett JG, Mundy LM: Community-acquired pneumonia. *N Engl J Med* 333:1618, 1995.
14. Bartlett JG, O'Keefe P, Tally FP, et al: Bacteriology of hospital-acquired pneumonia. *Arch Intern Med* 146:868, 1986.
15. Barton LL, Grant KL, Lemen RJ: Respiratory syncytial virus immune globulin: decisions and costs. *Pediatr Pulmonol* 32:20, 2001.
16. Bartzokas CA, Raine CH, Stoll PM, et al. Bacteriological assessment of patients undergoing major head and neck surgery. *Clin Otolaryngol* 9:99, 1984.
17. Barzilay Z, Mandel M, Keren G, et al: Nosocomial bacterial pneumonia in ventilated children: clinical significance of culture-positive peripheral bronchial aspirates. *J Pediatr* 112:421, 1988.
18. Bassin AS, Niederman MS: Prevention of ventilator-associated pneumonia. *Clin Chest Med* 16:195, 1995.
19. Beck C, Dubois J, Grignon A, et al: Incidence and risk factors of catheter-related deep venous thrombosis in a pediatric intensive care unit. A prospective study. *J Pediatr* 133:237, 1998.
20. Beck-Sague C, Jarvis WR: Epidemic bloodstream infections associated with pressure transducers: a persistent problem. *Infect Control Hosp Epidemiol* 10:54, 1989.
21. Benjamin DK, Miller W, Garges H, et al: Bacteremia, central catheters, and neonates: when to pull the line. *Pediatrics* 107:1272, 2001.
22. Bercault N, Boulain T: Mortality rate attributable to ventilator-associated nosocomial pneumonia in an adult intensive care unit: a prospective case-control study. *Crit Care Med* 29:2303, 2001.
23. Berenbaum MC, Fluck PA, Hurst NP: Depression of lymphocyte responses after surgical trauma. *Br J Exp Pathol* 54:597, 1973.
24. Bergmans DCJJ, Bonten MJM, Gaillard CA, et al: Prevention of ventilator-associated pneumonia by oral decontamination. *Am J Respir Crit Care Med* 164:382, 2001.
25. Blot F, Nitenberg G, Chachaty E, et al: Diagnosis of catheter-related bacteraemia: a prospective comparison of the time to positivity of hub-blood versus peripheral cultures. *Lancet* 354:1071, 1999.
26. Bonten MJ, Bergmans DCJJ, Stobberingh EE, et al: Implementation of bronchoscopic techniques in the diagnosis of ventilator-associated pneumonia to reduce antibiotic use. *Am J Respir Crit Care Med* 156:1820, 1997.
27. Bonten MJM, Weinstein RA: Selective decontamination of the digestive tract. In Jarvis WR, editor: *Nosocomial pneumonia.* New York, 2000, Marcel Dekker.

28. Bordelon JY, Legrand P, Gewin WC, et al: The telescoping plugged catheter in suspected anaerobic infections. *Am Rev Respir Dis* 128:465, 1983.
29. Brachman PS, Dan BB, Haley RW, et al: Nosocomial surgical infections: incidence and cost. *Surg Clin North Am* 60:15, 1980.
30. Brook I: Bacterial colonization, tracheobronchitis and pneumonia following tracheostomy and long-term intubation in pediatric patients. *Chest* 76:420, 1979.
31. Brown RB, Hosmer D, Chen HC: A comparison of infections in different ICUs within the same hospital. *Crit Care Med* 13:472, 1985.
32. Brown RB, Stechenberg B, Sands M, et al: Infections in a pediatric intensive care unit. *Am J Dis Child* 141:267, 1987.
33. Brun-Buisson C: Could invasive diagnostic techniques for ventilator-associated pneumonia be associated with reduced antibiotic usage in the ICU? *New Horizons* 4:345, 1996.
34. Brun-Buisson C, Legrand P, Rauss A, et al: Intestinal decontamination for control of nosocomial multiresistant gram-negative bacilli. Study of an outbreak in an intensive care unit. *Ann Intern Med* 110:873, 1989.
35. Bryan CS, Reynolds KL: Bacteremic nosocomial pneumonia: analysis of 172 episodes from a single metropolitan area. *Am Rev Respir Dis* 129:668, 1984.
36. Burnie JP, Odds FC, Lee W, et al: Outbreak of systemic Candida albicans in intensive care unit caused by cross infection. *Br Med J* 290:746, 1985.
37. Centers for Disease Control: CDC definitions for nosocomial infections, 1988. *Am Rev Respir Dis* 139:1058, 1989.
38. Chastre J, Fagon JY: Invasive diagnostic testing should be routinely used to manage ventilated patients with suspected pneumonia. *Am J Respir Crit Care Med* 150:570, 1994.
39. Chastre J, Fagon JY, Soler P, et al: Diagnosis of nosocomial pneumonia in intubated patients undergoing ventilation: comparison of the usefulness of bronchoalveolar lavage and the protected specimen brush. *Am J Med* 85:499, 1988.
40. Chastre J, Viau F, Brun P, et al: Prospective evaluation of the protected specimen brush for the diagnosis of pulmonary infections in ventilated patients. *Am Rev Respir Dis* 130:924, 1984.
41. Climo MW, Israel DS, Wong ES, et al: Hospital-wide restriction of clindamycin: effect on the incidence of *Clostridium difficile*-associated diarrhea and cost. *Ann Intern Med* 128:989, 1998.
42. Cobb DK, High KP, Sawyers RG, et al: A controlled trial of scheduled replacement of central venous and pulmonary artery catheters. *N Engl J Med* 327:1062, 1992.
43. Collignon PJ: Intravascular catheter associated sepsis: a common problem. The Australian study on intravascular catheter associated sepsis. *Med J Aust* 161:374, 1994.
44. Condon RE, Haley RW, Lee JTJ, et al: Does infection control control infection? *Arch Surg* 123:250, 1988.
45. Cook D, Guyatt G, Marshall J, et al: Comparison of sucralfate and ranitidine for the prevention of upper gastrointestinal bleeding in patients requiring mechanical ventilation. *N Engl J Med* 338:791, 1998.
46. Cook DJ, Brun-Buisson C, Guyatt GH, et al: Evaluation of new diagnostic technologies: bronchoalveolar lavage and the diagnosis of ventilator-associated pneumonia. *Crit Care Med* 22:1314, 1994.
47. Cook DJ, De Jonghe B, Brochard L, et al: Influence of airway management on ventilator-associated pneumonia. *JAMA* 279:781, 1998.
48. Cook DJ, HÈbert PC, Heyland DK, et al: How to use an article on therapy or prevention: pneumonia prevention using subglottic secretion drainage. *Crit Care Med* 25:1502, 1997.
49. Cook DJ, Laine LA, Guyatt GH, et al: Nosocomial pneumonia and the role of gastric pH. A meta-analysis. *Chest* 100:7, 1991.
50. Cook DJ, Meade MO, Hand LE, et al: Toward understanding evidence uptake: semirecumbency for pneumonia prevention. *Crit Care Med* 30:1472, 2002.
51. Cook DJ, Randolph A, Kerneman P, et al: Central venous catheter replacement strategies: a systematic review of the literature. *Crit Care Med* 25:1417, 1997.
52. Cook DJ, Walter SD, Cook RJ, et al: Incidence of and risk factors for ventilator-associated pneumonia in critically ill patients. *Ann Intern Med* 129:433, 1998.
53. Coopersmith CM, Rebman TL, Zack JE, et al: Effect of an education program on decreasing catheter-related bloodstream infections in the surgical intensive care unit. *Crit Care Med* 30:59, 2002.
54. Craven DE, Kunches LM, Kilinsky V, et al: Risk factors for pneumonia and fatality in patients receiving continuous mechanical ventilation. *Am Rev Respir Dis* 133:792, 1986.
55. Craven DE, Kunches LM, Lichtenberg DA, et al: Nosocomial infection and fatality in medical and surgical intensive care unit patients. *Arch Intern Med* 148:1161, 1988.
56. Cross AS, Roupe B: Role of respiratory assistance devices in endemic nosocomial pneumonia. *Am J Med* 70:681, 1981.
57. D'Amico R, Pifferi S, Leonetti C, et al: Effectiveness of antibiotic prophylaxis in critically ill adult patients: systematic review of randomised controlled trials. *BMJ* 316:1275, 1998.
58. Dajani AS, Bisno AL, Chung KJ: Prevention of bacterial endocarditis. Recommendations by the American Heart Association. *JAMA* 264:2919, 1990.
59. Damen J, Bolton D: A prospective analysis of 1,400 pulmonary artery catheterizations in patients undergoing cardiac surgery. *Acta Anaesthesiol Scand* 30:386, 1986.
60. Davies L, Dolgin S, Kattan M: Morbidity and mortality of open lung biopsy in children. *Pediatrics* 99:660, 1997.
61. Davis SD, Sobocinski K, Hoffmann RG, et al: Postoperative wound infections in a children's hospital. *Pediatr Infect Dis J* 3:114, 1984.
62. de Blic J, Midulla F, Barbato A, et al: Bronchoalveolar lavage in children. *Eur Respir J* 15:217, 2000.
63. de Jaeger A, Litalien C, Lacroix J, et al: A meta-analysis evaluating the diagnostic accuracy of protected specimen brush and of bronchoalveolar lavage to diagnose bacterial nosocomial pneumonia. *Crit Care Med* 27:2548, 1999.
64. Delclaux C, Roupie E, Blot F, et al: Lower respiratory tract colonization and infection during severe acute respiratory distress syndrome. *Am J Respir Crit Care Med* 156:1092, 1997.
65. Derkay CS, Bluestone CD, Thompson AE, et al: Otitis media in the pediatric intensive care unit: a prospective study. *Otolaryngol Head Neck Surg* 100:292, 1989.
66. Despond O, Proulx F, Carcillo J, et al: Pediatric sepsis and multiple organ dysfunction syndrome. *Curr Opin Pediatr* 13:247, 2001.
67. Deutschman CS, Wilton P, Sinow J, et al: Paranasal sinusitis associated with nasotracheal intubation: a frequently unrecognized and treatable source of sepsis. *Crit Care Med* 14:111, 1986.
68. Dixon RE: Effect of infections on hospital care. *Ann Intern Med* 89:749, 1978.
69. Donowitz LG: Failure of the overgown to prevent nosocomial infection in a pediatric intensive care unit. *Pediatrics* 77:35, 1986.
70. Donowitz LG: High risk of nosocomial infection in the pediatric critical care patient. *Crit Care Med* 14:26, 1986.
71. Drakulovic MB, Torres A, Bauer TT, et al: Supine position as a risk factor for nosocomial pneumonia in mechanically ventilated patients: a randomized trial. *Lancet* 354:1851, 1999.
72. Dreyfuss D, DjedaÔni K, Weber P, et al: Prospective study of nosocomial pneumonia and of patient and circuit colonization during mechanical ventilation with circuit changes every 48 hours versus no change. *Am Rev Respir Dis* 143:738, 1991.
73. Driks MR, Craven DE, Celli BR, et al: Nosocomial pneumonia in intubated patients given sucralfate as compared with antacids or histamine type 2 blockers. *N Engl J Med* 317:1376, 1987.
74. Dubois J, Garel L, Tapiero B, et al: Peripherally inserted central catheters in infants and children. *Radiology* 204:622, 1997.
75. Ducharme FM, Gauthier M, Lacroix J, et al: Incidence of infection related to arterial catheterization in children: a prospective study. *Crit Care Med* 16:272, 1988.
76. duMoulin G: Minimizing the potential for nosocomial pneumonia: architectural engineering and environmental considerations for the intensive care unit. *Eur J Clin Microbiol Infect Dis* 8:69, 1989.
77. Durand P, Coseron-Zerbib M, Costa Y, et al: Évaluation du prélèvement distal protégé pour le diagnostic de pneumopathie nosocomiale chez l'enfant ventilé mécaniquement. *Réanim Urg* 3:649, 1994.
78. El-Ebiary M, Torres A, Gonz·lez J, et al: Use of elastin fibre detection in the diagnosis of ventilator associated pneumonia. *Thorax* 50:14, 1995.
79. Elward AM, Warren DK, Fraser VJ: Ventilator-associated pneumonia in pediatric intensive care unit patients: risk factors and outcomes. *Pediatrics* 109:758, 2002.
80. Ewig S, Torres A, El-Ebiary M, et al: Bacterial colonization patterns in mechanically ventilated patients with traumatic and medical head injury. *Am J Respir Crit Care Med* 159:188, 1999.

81. Fàbregas N, Torres A, El-Ebiary M, et al: Histopathologic and microbiologic aspects of ventilator-associated pneumonia. *Anesthesiology* 84:760, 1996.
82. Fagon JY, Chastre J, Hance AJ, et al: Detection of nosocomial lung infection in ventilated patients: use of a protected specimen brush and quantitative culture techniques in 147 patients. *Am Rev Respir Dis* 138:110, 1988.
83. Fagon JY, Chastre J, Hance AJ, et al: Nosocomial pneumonia in ventilated patients: a cohort study evaluating attributable mortality and hospital stay. *Am J Med* 94:281, 1993.
84. Fagon JY, Chastre J, Wolf M, et al: Invasive and noninvasive strategies for management of suspected ventilator-associated pneumonia: a randomized trial. *Ann Intern Med* 132:621, 2000.
85. Farr BM: Accuracy and cost-effectiveness of new tests for diagnosis of catheter-related bloodstream infections. *Lancet* 354:1487, 1999.
86. Fayon M, Lacroix J, Champagne G, et al: Plasma malondialdehyde, gastric intramucosal pH and serum lactate in children undergoing cardiopulmonary bypass. *J Intensive Care Med* 13: 44, 1998.
87. Fayon M, Tucci M, Lacroix J, et al: Nosocomial bacterial pneumonia and tracheitis in pediatric intensive care: a prospective study. *Am J Respir Crit Care Med* 155:162, 1997.
88. Feely TW, DuMoulin GC, Hedley-Whyte J, et al: Aerosol polymyxin and pneumonia in seriously ill patients. *N Engl J Med* 293:471, 1975.
89. Fenelon LE, Keane CT, Bakir M, et al: A cluster of *Pneumocystis carinii* infections in children. *Br Med J* 291:1683, 1985.
90. Fleming CA, Steger KA, Craven DE: Host- and device-associated risk factors for nosocomial pneumonia. In Jarvis WR, editor: *Nosocomial pneumonia,* New York, 2000, Marcel Dekker.
91. Ford SE, Manley PN: Indwelling cardiac catheters. An autopsy study of associated endocardial lesions. *Arch Pathol Lab Med* 106:314, 1982.
92. Ford-Jones EL: Antiseptics. In Koren A, Prober CA, Grold R, editors: *Antimicrobial therapy: infants and children,* New York, 1988, Marcel Dekker.
93. Ford-Jones EL, Mindorff CM, Gold K: Satellite infection control committees within the hospital: decentralizing for action. *Infect Cont Hosp Epidemiol* 10:368, 1989.
94. Ford-Jones EL, Mindorff CM, Langley JM, et al: Epidemiologic study of 4684 hospital-acquired infections in pediatric patients. *Pediatr Infect Dis J* 8:668, 1989.
95. Ford-Jones EL, Mindorff CM, Pollock E, et al: Evaluation of a new method of detection of nosocomial infection in the pediatric intensive care unit-the Infection Control Sentinel Sheet System. *Infect Cont Hosp Epidemiol* 10:515, 1989.
96. Fridkin SK, Manangan L, Boylard E, et al: SHEA-CDC TB survey, Part II: efficacy of TB infection control programs at member hospitals, 1992. *Infect Control Hosp Epidemiol* 16:135, 1995.
97. Fridkin SK, Pear SM, Williamson TH, et al: The role of understaffing in central venous catheter-associated bloodstream infections. *Infect Control Hosp Epidemiol* 17:150, 1996.
98. Furfaro S, Gauthier M, Lacroix J, et al: Arterial catheter-related infections in children: a one-year cohort analysis. *Am J Dis Child* 145:1037, 1991.
99. Garland JS, Alex CP, Mueller CD, et al: A randomized trial comparing povidone-iodine to a chlorhexidine gluconate-impregnated dressing for prevention of central venous catheter infections in neonates. *Pediatrics* 107:1431, 2001.
100. Garrouste-Orgeas M, Chevret S, Arlet G, et al: Oropharyngeal or gastric colonization and nosocomial pneumonia in adult intensive care units patients. *Am J Respir Crit Care Med* 156:1647, 1997.
101. Gauvin F, Lacroix J, Guertin MC, et al: Reproducibility of blind protected bronchoalveolar lavage in mechanically-ventilated children. *Am J Respir Crit Care Med* 165:1618, 2002.
102. George DL: Epidemiology of nosocomial ventilator-associated pneumonia. *Infect Control Hosp Epidemiol* 14:163, 1993.
103. George DL, Falk PS, Wunderink RG, et al: Epidemiology of ventilator-acquired pneumonia based on protected bronchoscopic sampling. *Am J Respir Crit Care Med* 158:1839, 1998.
104. Gil RT, Kruse JA, Thill-Baharozian MC, et al: Triple vs. single lumen catheters: a prospective study in a critically ill population. *Arch Intern Med* 149:1139, 1989.
105. Glasier CM, Mallory GB, Steele RW: Significance of opacification of the maxillary and ethmoid sinuses in infants. *J Pediatr* 114:45, 1989.
106. Goris RJ, Gimbrere JS, van Niekerk JL, et al: Improved survival of multiply injured patients by early internal fixation and prophylactic mechanical ventilation. *Injury* 14:39, 1982.
107. Graeve AH, Carpenter CM, Schille WR: Management of central venous catheters using a wire introducer. *Am J Surg* 142:752, 1981.
108. Griswold J, Hamood A, Duhan C: Length of antibiotic treatment influences risk of repeated Pseudomonas infections. *Crit Care Med* 23:A166, 1995.
109. Grobskopf LA, Sinkowitz-Cochran RL, Garrett DO, et al: A national point-prevalence survey of pediatric intensive care unit-acquired infections in the United States. *J Pediatr* 140:432, 2002.
110. Gruson D, Hilbert G, Vargas F, et al: Rotation, restricted use of antibiotics in a medical intensive care unit. *Am J Respir Crit Care Med* 162:837, 2000.
111. Haley RW, Culver DH, White JW, et al: The efficacy of infection surveillance and control programs in preventing nosocomial infections in U.S. hospitals. *Am J Epidemiol* 12:182, 1985.
112. Hall CB, Geiman JM, Douglas RGJ, et al: Control of nosocomial respiratory syncytial viral infections. *Pediatrics* 62:728, 1978.
113. Hall CB, Powell KR, MacDonald NE, et al: Respiratory syncytial virus infection in children with compromised immune function. *N Engl J Med* 315:77, 1986.
114. Harbarth S, Pittet D, Grady L, et al: Compliance with hand hygiene practice in pediatric intensive care. *Pediatr Crit Care Med* 2:311, 2001.
115. Hauser AR, Cobb E, Bodì M, et al: Type III protein secretion is associated with poor clinical outcomes in patients with ventilator associated pneumonia by *Pseudomonas aeruginosa*. *Crit Care Med* 30:521, 2002.
116. Hayon J, Figliolini C, Combes A, et al: Role of serial routine microbiologic culture results in the initial management of ventilator associated pneumonia. *Am J Respir Crit Care Med* 165:41, 2002.
117. Heyland DK, Cook D, Marshall J, et al: The clinical utility of invasive diagnostic techniques in the setting of ventilator-associated pneumonia. *Chest* 115:1076, 1999.
118. Heyland DK, Cook DJ, Griffith L, et al: The attributable morbidity and mortality of ventilator-associated pneumonia in the critically ill patient. *Am J Respir Crit Care Med* 159:1249, 1999.
119. Hilton E, Haslett TM, Borenstein MT, et al: Central catheter infections: single- versus triple-lumen catheters. Influence of guide wires on infection rates when used for replacement of catheters. *Am J Med* 84:667, 1988.
120. Hoffmann KK, Weber DJ, Samsa GP, et al: Transparent polyurethane film as an intravenous catheter dressing. A meta-analysis of the infection risks. *JAMA* 267:2072, 1992.
121. Holzel H, de Saxe M: Septicaemia in paediatric intensive-care patients at the Hospital for Sick Children, Great Ormond Street. *J Hosp Infect* 22:185, 1992.
122. Hopkins CC, Weber DJ, Rubin RH: Invasive aspergillus infection: possible non-ward common source within the hospital environment. i13:19, 1989.
123. Houang ET, Marples RR, Weir I, et al: Problems in the investigation of an apparent outbreak of coagulase-negative staphylococcal septicaemia following cardiac surgery. *J Hosp Infect* 8:224, 1986.
124. Huebner J, Frank U, Kappstein I, et al: Influence of architectural design on nosocomial infection in intensive care units. *Intensive Care Med* 15:179, 1989.
125. Hume HA, Kronick JB, Blanchette VS: Review of the literature on allogeneic red blood cell and plasma transfusions in children. *Can Med Assoc J* 156(suppl 11):S41, 1997.
126. Huxley EJ, Viroslav J, Gray WR, et al: Pharyngeal aspiration in normal adults and patients with depressed consciousness. *Am J Med* 64:564, 1978.
127. Infection in Neurosurgery Working Party of the British Society for Antimicrobial Chemotherapy: antimicrobial prophylaxis in neurosurgery and after head injury. *Lancet* 344:1547, 1994.
128. Jacobs RF, Tabor DR, Burks AW, et al: Elevated interleukin-1 release by human alveolar macrophages during ARDS. *Am Rev Respir Dis* 140:1686, 1989.
129. Jarvis WR: *Nosocomial pneumonia,* New York, 2000, Marcel Dekker.

130. Jarvis WR, Edwards JR, Culver DH, et al: Nosocomial infection rates in adult and pediatric intensive care units in the United States. *Am J Med* 191(suppl 3B):185, 1991.
131. Jensen LS, Kissmeyer P, Wolff B, et al: Randomised comparison of leucocyte-depleted versus buffy-coat-poor blood transfusion and complications after colorectal surgery. *Lancet* 348:841, 1996.
132. Johanson WG, Pierce AK, Sanford JP: Changing pharyngeal bacterial flora of hospitalized patients: emergence of gram-negative bacilli. *N Engl J Med* 281:1137, 1969.
133. Johanson WG, Pierce AK, Sanford JP, et al: Nosocomial respiratory infections with Gram negative bacilli: the significance of colonization of the respiratory tract. *Ann Intern Med* 77:701, 1972.
134. Johanson WG, Seidenfeld JJ, Gomez P, et al: Bacteriologic diagnosis of nosocomial pneumonia following prolonged mechanical ventilation. *Am Rev Respir Dis* 137:259, 1988.
135. Johanson WGJ, Woods DE, Chandhuri T: Association of respiratory tract colonization with adherence of gram-negative bacilli to epithelial cells. *J Infect Dis* 139:667, 1979.
136. Kac G, Durain E, Amrain C, et al: Colonization and infection of pulmonary artery catheter in cardiac surgery patients: epidemiology and multivariate analysis of risk factors. *Crit Care Med* 29:971, 2001.
137. Kaiser AB: Antimicrobial prophylaxis in surgery. *N Engl J Med* 315:1129, 1986.
138. Kaplan J, Sarnaik S, Gitlin J, et al: Diminished helper/suppressor lymphocyte ratios and natural killer activity in recipients of repeated blood transfusions. *Blood* 64:308, 1984.
139. Kasian GF, Elash JH, Tan LK: Bacteriologic surveillance at indwelling urinary catheters in PICU patients. *Crit Care Med* 16:679, 1988.
140. Kearns PJ, Chin D, Mueller L, et al: The incidence of ventilator-associated pneumonia and success in nutrient delivery with gastric versus small intestinal feeding: a randomized clinical trial. *Crit Care Med* 28:1742, 2000.
141. Kerver AJ, Rommes JH, Merissen-Verhage EA, et al: Colonization and infection in surgical intensive care patients—a prospective study. *Intensive Care Med* 13:347, 1987.
142. Kite P, Dobbins BM, Wilcox MH, et al: Rapid diagnosis of central-venous-catheter-related bloodstream infection without catheter removal. *Lancet* 354:1504, 1999.
143. Klastersky J, Huysmans E, Weerts D, et al: Endotracheally administered gentamicin for the prevention of infections of the respiratory tract in patients with tracheostomy: a double-blind study. *Chest* 6:650, 1974.
144. Kollef MH, Shapiro SD, Fraser VJ, et al: Mechanical ventilation with and without 7-day circuit changes. *Ann Intern Med* 123: 168, 1995.
145. Kollef MH, Silver P, Murphy DM, et al: The effect of late-onset ventilator-associated pneumonia in determining patients mortality. *Chest* 108:1655, 1995.
146. Kollef MH, Vlasnik J, Sharpless L, et al: Scheduled change of antibiotic classes. *Am J Respir Crit Care Med* 156:1040, 1997.
147. Kollef MH, Ward S, Sherman G, et al: Inadequate treatment of nosocomial infections is associated with certain empiric antibiotic choices. *Crit Care Med* 28:3456, 2000.
148. Kornecki A, Shemie SD: Open lung biopsy in children with respiratory failure. *Crit Care Med* 29:1247, 2001.
149. Labenne M, Poyart C, Rambaud C, et al: Blind protected specimen brush and bronchoalveolar lavage in ventilated children. *Crit Care Med* 27:2537, 1999.
150. Lacroix J, Gauvin F: The habit and the hub. *Crit Care Med* 31:1583, 2003.
151. LaForce FM, Mullane JF, Boehme RF, et al: The effect of pulmonary edema on antibacterial defenses of the lung. *J Lab Clin Med* 82:634, 1973.
152. Landa JF, Kwoka MA, Chapman GA, et al: Effects of suctioning on mucociliary transport. *Chest* 77:202, 1980.
153. Langer M, Cigada M, Mandelli M, et al: Early onset pneumonia: a multicenter study in intensive care units. *Intensive Care Med* 13:342, 1987.
154. Langer M, Mosconi P, Cigada M, et al: Long-term respiratory support and risk of pneumonia in critically ill patients. *Am Rev Respir Dis* 140:302, 1989.
155. Larson EL, Aiello AE, Bastyr J, et al: Assessment of two hand hygiene regimens for intensive care unit personnel. *Crit Care Med* 29:944, 2001.
156. Laupland KB, Zygun DA, Favies D, et al: Population-based assessment of intensive care unit-acquired bloodstream infections in adults: incidence, risk factors, and associated mortality rate. *Crit Care Med* 30:2462, 2002.
157. Leclair JM, Freeman J, Sullivan BF, et al: Prevention of nosocomial respiratory syncytial virus infections through compliance with glove and gown isolation precautions. *N Engl J Med* 317:329, 1989.
158. León C, Álvarez-Lerma F, Ruiz-Santana S, et al: An antiseptic chamber-containing hub reduces central venous catheter-related infection: a prospective, randomized study. *Crit Care Med* 31:1318, 2003.
159. Leroy O, Billiau V, Beuscart C, et al: Nosocomial infections associated with long-term radial artery cannulation. *Intensive Care Med* 15:241, 1989.
160. Lewin S, Brettman LR, Holzman RS: Infections in hypothermic patients. *Arch Intern Med* 141:920, 1981.
161. Liberati A, D'Amico R, Pifferi S, et al: *Antibiotics for preventing respiratory tract infections in adults receiving intensive care (Cochrane Review)*. Update software. Issue 3. The Cochrane Library, 2001, Oxford.
162. Lohr JA, Donowitz LG, Sadler JEI: Hospital-acquired urinary tract infection. *Pediatrics* 82:193, 1989.
163. Luskin RL, Weinstein RA, Nathan C, et al: Extended use of disposable pressure transducers. A bacteriologic evaluation. *JAMA* 255:916, 1986.
164. MacDonald NE, Hall CB, Suffin SC, et al: Respiratory syncytial viral infection in infants with congenital heart disease. *N Engl J Med* 307:397, 1982.
165. Mahul P, Auboyer C, Jospe R, et al: Prevention of nosocomial pneumonia in intubated patients: respective role of mechanical subglottic secretions drainage and stress ulcer prophylaxis. *Intensive Care Med* 18:20, 1992.
166. Makhoul IR, Kassis I, Berant M, et al: Frequency of change of ventilator circuit in premature infants: impact on ventilator-associated pneumonia. *Pediatr Crit Care Med* 2:127, 2001.
167. Maki DG, Hassemer CA: Endemic rate of fluid contamination and related septicemia in arterial pressure monitoring. *Am J Med* 70:733, 1981.
168. Maki DG, Weise CE, Sarafin HW: A semiquantitative culture method for identifying intravenous-catheter-related infection. *N Engl J Med* 296:1305, 1977.
169. Marchand S, Borderon J, Borderon JC, et al: Diagnostic des infections broncho-pulmonaires chez l'enfant en unitÈ de soins intensifs. *Ann PÈdiatr (Paris)* 32:593, 1985.
170. Marik PE, Careau P: The incidence of anaerobes in ICU patients with ventilator-associated pneumonia and aspiration pneumonia. *Crit Care Med* 26:A106, 1998.
171. Marin MG, Lee JC, Skurnick JH: Prevention of nosocomial bloodstream infections: effectiveness of antimicrobial-impregnated and heparin-bonded central venous catheters. *Crit Care Med* 28: 3332, 2000.
172. Markowicz P, Wolff M, DjadaÔni K, et al: Multicenter prospective study of ventilator-associated pneumonia during acute respiratory distress syndrome. *Am J Respir Crit Care Med* 161:1942, 2000.
173. Marquette CH, Georges H, Wallet F, et al: Diagnostic efficiency of endotracheal aspirates with quantitative bacterial cultures in intubated patients with suspected pneumonia: comparison with the protected brush specimen. *Am Rev Respir Dis* 148:138, 1993.
174. Martinez JA, DesJardin JA, Aronoff M, et al: Clinical utility of blood cultures drawn from central venous or arterial catheters in critically ill surgical patients. *Crit Care Med* 30:7, 2002.
175. Masri C, Farrell CA, Gauvin F, et al: Potential infectious risk of pediatric organ donors. *Pediatr Crit Care Med* 1:S47, 2000.
176. Mayhall CG, Archer NH, Lamb A, et al: Ventriculostomy-related infections. *N Engl J Med* 310:553, 1984.
177. McCarthy MC, Shires JK, Robison RJ, et al: Prospective evaluation of single and triple lumen catheters in total parenteral nutrition. *J Parenter Enteral Nutr* 11:259, 1987.
178. McCormick R, Maki DG: The importance of maximal sterile barriers during insertion of central venous catheters: a prospective study. 29th Interscience Conference on Antimicrobial Agents and Chemotherapy, Houston, September 17–20, 1989.

179. McElvein RB: Open lung biopsy versus empirical antibiotic therapy in the immunosuppressed patient. *Ann Thorac Surg* 40: 419, 1985.
180. Mead PB, Pories SE, Hall P, et al: Decreasing the incidence of surgical wound infections. Validation of a surveillance notification program. *Arch Surg* 121:458, 1986.
181. Meduri GU, Mauldin GL, Wunderink RG, et al: Causes of fever and pulmonary densities in patients with clinical manifestations of ventilator-associated pneumonia. *Chest* 106:221, 1994.
182. Mehall JR, Saltzman DA, Jackson RJ, et al: Fibrin sheath enhances central venous catheter infection. *Crit Care Med* 30:908, 2002.
183. Mehta PA, Cunningham CK, Colella CB, et al: Risk factors for sternal wound and other infections in pediatric cardiac surgery patients. *Pediatr Infect Dis J* 19:1000, 2000.
184. Mezrow CK, Bergstein I, Tartter PI: Postoperative infections following autologous and homologous blood transfusions. *Transfusion* 32:27, 1992.
185. Miller PJ, Farr BM, Gwaltney JMJ: Economic benefits of an effective infection control program: case study and proposal. *Rev Infect Dis* 11:284, 1989.
186. Milliken J, Tait GA, Ford-Jones EL, et al: Nosocomial infection in a pediatric intensive care unit. *Crit Care Med* 16:233, 1988.
187. Mimoz O, Pieroni L, Lawrence C, et al: Prospective, randomized trial of two antiseptic solutions for prevention of central venous arterial catheter colonization and infection in intensive care unit patients. *Crit Care Med* 24:1818, 1996.
188. Mollitt DL: Pediatric surgical infection and antibiotic usage. *Pediatr Infect Dis J* 4:326, 1985.
189. Moro ML, ViganÚ EF, Lepri AC, et al: Risk factors for central venous catheter-related infections in surgical and intensive care units. *Infect Control Hosp Epidemiol* 15:253, 1994.
190. Moss WJ, Beers C, Johnson E, et al: Pilot study of antibiotic cycling in a pediatric intensive care unit. *Crit Care Med* 30:1877, 2002.
191. Murphy PJ, Connery C, Hicks GL, et al: Homologous blood transfusion as a risk factor for postoperative infection after coronary artery bypass graft operations. *J Thorac Cardiovasc Surg* 104:1092, 1992.
192. Myers ML, Austin TW, Sibbald WJ: Pulmonary artery catheter infections. A prospective study. *Ann Surg* 201:237, 1985.
193. NG PC, Raymond KL, Wong PO, et al: Neutrophil CD64 expression: a sensitive diagnostic marker for late-onset nosocomial infection in very low birthweight infants. *Pediatr Res* 51:296, 2002.
194. Niederman MS, Merrill WM, Ferranti RD, et al: Nutritional status and bacterial binding in the lower respiratory tract in patients with chronic tracheostomy. *Ann Intern Med* 100:795, 1984.
195. Niederman MS, Torres A, Summer W: Invasive diagnostic testing is not needed routinely to manage suspected ventilator-associated pneumonia. *Am J Respir Crit Care Med* 150:565, 1994.
196. Norwood SH, Cormier B, McMahon NG, et al: Prospective study of catheter-related infection during prolonged arterial catheterization. *Crit Care Med* 16:836, 1988.
197. Nussbaum E: Pediatric fiberoptic bronchoscopy: clinical experience with 2,836 bronchoscopies. *Pediatr Crit Care Med* 3:171, 2002.
198. O'Brien JD, Ettinger NA, Shevlin D, et al: Safety and yield of transbronchial biopsy in mechanically ventilated patients. *Crit Care Med* 25:440, 1997.
199. O'Grady NP, Alexander M, Dellinger EP, et al: Guidelines for the prevention of intravascular catheter-related infections. *MMWR* 51(RR-10):1, 2002.
200. O'Mahony JB, Palder SB, Wood JJ, et al: Depression of cellular immunity after multiple injury in the absence of sepsis. *J Trauma* 24:869, 1984.
201. Palmer DL, Kuritsky JN, Lapham SC, et al: Enterobacter mediastinitis following cardiac surgery. *Infect Control Hosp Epidemiol* 6:115, 1985.
202. Patel JC, Mollitt DL, Pieper P, et al: Nosocomial pneumonia in the pediatric trauma patient: a single center's perspective. *Crit Care Med* 28:3530, 2000.
203. Pearson ML, Hierholzer WJ, Garner JS, et al: Guideline for prevention of intravascular-device-related infections. *Infect Contr Hosp Epidemiol* 17:438, 1996.
204. Pelke S, Ching D, Easa D, et al: Gowning does not affect colonization or infection rates in a neonatal intensive care unit. *Arch Pediatr Adolesc Med* 148:1016, 1994.
205. Pemberton LB, Lyman B, Lander V, et al: Sepsis from triple- vs single-lumen catheters during total parenteral nutrition in surgical or critically ill patients. *Arch Surg* 121:591, 1986.
206. Phillips JO, Metzler MH, Huckfeldt RE, et al: A prospective study of non-bronchoscopic bronchoalveolar lavage compared to protected specimen brush in the diagnosis of nosocomial pneumonia in the ventilated ICU patient. *Crit Care Med* 27:A142, 1999.
207. Pierce CM, Wade A, Mok Q: Heparin-bonded central venous lines reduce thrombotic and infective complications in critically ill children. *Intensive Care Med* 26:967, 2000.
208. Piperno D, Gaussorgues P, Valon B, et al: IntÈrÎt diagnostique du lavage broncho-alvÈolaire non fibroscopique dans les pneumopathies en ventilation mÈcanique. *Rev Mal Respir* 4:17, 1987.
209. Pittet D, Eggimann P, Rubinovitch B: Prevention of ventilator-associated pneumonia by oral decontamination. *Am J Respir Crit Care Med* 164:338, 2001.
210. Pollock E, Ford-Jones EL, Corey M, et al: Use of the Pediatric Risk of Mortality score to predict nosocomial infection in a pediatric intensive care unit. *Crit Care Med* 19:160, 1991.
211. Pollock EMM, Ford-Jones EL, Rebeyka I, et al: Early nosocomial infections in a pediatric cardiovascular surgery patients. *Crit Care Med* 18:378, 1990.
212. Preston GA, Larson EL, Stamm WE: The effect of private isolation rooms on patient care practices, colonization and infection in an intensive care unit. *Am J Med* 70:641, 1981.
213. Pugin J, Auckenthaler R, Delaspre O, et al: Rapid diagnosis of Gram negative pneumonia by assay of endotoxin in bronchoalveolar lavage fluid. *Thorax* 47:547, 1992.
214. Pugin J, Auckenthaler R, Mili N, et al: Diagnosis of ventilator-associated pneumonia by bacteriologic analysis of bronchoscopic and nonbronchoscopic "blind" bronchoalveolar lavage fluid. *Am Rev Respir Dis* 143:1121, 1991.
215. Quattrocchi KB, Miller CH, Wagner FC, et al: Cell mediated immunity in severely head-injured patients: the role of suppressor lymphocytes and serum factors. *J Neurosurg* 77:694, 1992.
216. Quilici N, Audibert G, Conroy MC, et al: Differential quantitative blood cultures in the diagnosis of catheter-related sepsis in intensive care units. *Clin Infect Dis* 25:1066, 1997.
217. Raad II: Intravascular-catheter-related infections. *Lancet* 351: 893, 1998.
218. Raad II, Darouiche RO: Catheter-related septicemia: risk reduction. *Infect Med* 13:807, 1996.
219. Raad II, Hohn DC, Gilbreath BJ, et al: Prevention of central venous catheter-related infections by using maximal sterile barrier precautions during insertion. *Infect Control Hosp Epidemiol* 15:231, 1994.
220. Raad II, Luna M, Khalil SA, et al: The relationship between the thrombotic and infectious complications of central venous catheters. *JAMA* 271:1014, 1994.
221. Ramphal R, Small PM, Shands JWJ, et al: Adherence of Pseudomonas aeruginosa to tracheal cells injured by influenza infection or by endotracheal intubation. *Infect Immunol* 27:614, 1980.
222. Randolph A, Cook DJ, Gonzales CA, et al: Tunneling short-term central venous catheters to prevent catheter-related infection: a meta-analysis of randomized, controlled trials. *Crit Care Med* 26:1452, 1998.
223. Reed CR, Sessler CN, Glauser FL, et al: Central venous catheter infections: concepts and controversies. *Intensive Care Med* 21:177, 1995.
224. Rello J, Ausina V, Ricart M, et al: Impact of previous antimicrobial therapy on the etiology and outcome of ventilator-associated pneumonia. *Chest* 104:1230, 1993.
225. Rello J, Gallego M, Mariscal D, et al: The value of routine microbial investigation in ventilator-associated pneumonia. *Am J Respir Crit Care Med* 156:196, 1997.
226. Rello J, Ochagavia A, Sabanes E, et al: Evaluation of outcome of intravenous catheter-related infections in critically ill patients. *Am J Respir Crit Care Med* 162:1027, 2000.
227. Rello J, Rué M, Jubert P, et al: Survival in patients with nosocomial pneumonia: impact of the severity of illness and the etiologic agent. *Crit Care Med* 25:1862, 1997.

228. Renaud B, Brun-Buisson C, for the ICU-Bacteremia Study Group: Outcomes of primary and catheter-related bacteremia. *Am J Respir Crit Care Med* 163:1584, 2001.
229. Renault A, Kaczmarek R, Quinio P, et al: Sinusites en réanimation: intérêt et validité de la radiographie standard au lit du patient, incidence de Blondeau modifiée. *Réanim Urg* 4:760, 1995.
230. Reuter S, Sigge A, Wiedeck H, et al: Analysis of transmission pathways of Pseudomonas aeruginosa between patients and tap water outlets. *Crit Care Med* 30:2222, 2002.
231. Ribner BS, Landry MN, Kidd K, et al: Outbreak of multiply resistant *Staphylococcus aureus* in a pediatric intensive care unit after consolidation with a surgical intensive care unit. *Am J Infect Control* 17:244, 1989.
232. Richards MJ, Edwards JR, Culver DH, et al: Nosocomial infections in medical intensive care units in the United States. *Crit Care Med* 27:887, 1999.
233. Richards MJ, Edwards JR, Culver DH, et al: Nosocomial infections in pediatric intensive care units in the United States. *Pediatrics* 103(e39):1, 1999.
234. Rigal E, Roze JC, Villers D, et al: Prospective evaluation of the protected specimen brush for the diagnosis of pulmonary infections in ventilated newborns. *Pediatr Pulmonol* 8:268, 1990.
235. Rijnders BJ, Verwaest C, Peetermans WE, et al: Differences in time to positivity of hub-blood versus nonhub-blood cultures is not useful for the diagnosis of catheter-related bloodstream infection in critically ill patients. *Crit Care Med* 29:1399, 2001.
236. Rock MJ: The diagnostic utility of bronchoalveolar lavage in immunocompetent children with unexplained infiltrates on chest radiograph. *Pediatrics* 95:373, 1995.
237. Rossoff LJ, Borenstein M, Isenberg HD: Is hand washing really needed in an intensive care unit? *Crit Care Med* 23:1211, 1995.
238. Rouby JJ: Bacteriology of ventilator-associated pneumonia. *Am Rev Respir Dis* 147:1321, 1993.
239. Rouby JJ, de Lassale EM, Poete P, et al: Nosocomial bronchopneumonia in the critically ill: histologic and bacteriologic aspects. *Am Rev Respir Dis* 146:1059, 1992.
240. Rouby JJ, Rossignon MD, Nicolas MH, et al: A prospective study of protected bronchoalveolar lavage in the diagnosis of nosocomial pneumonia. *Anesthesiology* 71:679, 1989.
241. Rouse BT, Horahov DW: Immunosuppression in viral infections. *Rev Infect Dis* 8:850, 1986.
242. Rowley KM, Clubb KS, Smith GJ, et al: Right-sided infective endocarditis as a consequence of flow-directed pulmonary-artery catheterization. A clinicopathological study of 55 autopsied patients. *N Engl J Med* 311:1152, 1984.
243. Rubenstein JS, Kabat K, Shulman ST, et al: Bacterial and fungal colonization of endotracheal tubes in children: a prospective study. *Crit Care Med* 20:1544, 1992.
244. Ruddell WS, Axon AT, Findley JM, et al: Effect of cimetidine on the gastric bacterial flora. *Lancet* 1:672, 1980.
245. Ruiz M, Torres A, Ewig S, et al: Noninvasive versus invasive microbiological investigation in ventilator-associated pneumonia. *Am J Respir Crit Care Med* 162:119, 2000.
246. Saint S, Savel RH, Matthay MA: Enhancing the safety of critically ill patients by reducing urinary and central venous catheter-related infections. *Am J Respir Crit Care Med* 165:1475, 2002.
247. Sauaia A, Moore FA, Moore EE, et al: Diagnosing pneumonia in mechanically ventilated patients: endotracheal aspirate versus bronchoalveolar lavage. *J Trauma* 35:512, 1993.
248. Schindler MB, Cox PN: A simple method of bronchoalveolar lavage. *Anaesth Intensive Care* 22:66, 1994.
249. Scottile FD, Marie TJ, Prough DS, et al: Nosocomial pulmonary infection: possible etiologic significance of bacterial adhesion to endotracheal tubes. *Crit Care Med* 14:265, 1986.
250. Shepherd KE, Lynch KE, Wain JC, et al: Elastin fibers and the diagnosis of bacterial pneumonia in the adult respiratory distress syndrome. *Crit Care Med* 23:1829, 1995.
251. Sherertz RJ, Raad II, Belani A, et al: Three-year experience with sonicated vascular catheter cultures in a clinical microbiology laboratory. *J Clin Microbiol* 28:76, 1990.
252. Shinozaki T, Deane RS, Mazuzan JEJ, et al: Bacterial contamination of arterial lines. A prospective study. *JAMA* 249:223, 1983.
253. Sieger B, Berman SJ, Geckler RW, et al: Empiric treatment of hospital-acquired lower respiratory tract infections with meropenem or ceftazidime with tobramycin: a randomized study. *Crit Care Med* 25:1663, 1997.
254. Singh N, Rogers P, Atwood CW, et al: Short-course empiric antibiotic therapy for patients with pulmonary infiltrates in the intensive care unit. *Am J Respir Crit Care Med* 162:505, 2000.
255. Singh S, Nelson N, Acosta I, et al: Catheter colonization and bacteremia with pulmonary and arterial catheters. *Crit Care Med* 10:736, 1982.
256. Singh-Naz N, Sprague BM, Patel KM, et al: Risk factors for nosocomial infection in critically ill children: a prospective cohort study. *Crit Care Med* 24:857, 1996.
257. Singh-Naz N, Sprague BM, Patel KM, et al: Risk assessment and standardized infection rate in critically ill children. *Crit Care Med* 28:2069, 2000.
258. Sirvent JM, Torres A, El-Ebiary M, et al: Protective effect of intravenously administered cefuroxime against nosocomial pneumonia in patients with structural coma. *Am J Respir Crit Care Med* 155:1729, 1997.
259. Sitges-Serra A, Linares J, Perez JL, et al: A randomized trial on the effect of tubing changes on hub contamination and catheter sepsis during parenteral nutrition. *J Parenter Enteral Nutr* 9:322, 1985.
260. Sitzmann JV, Townsend TR, Siler MC, et al: Septic and technical complications of central venous catheterization. A prospective study of 200 consecutive patients. *Ann Surg* 202:766, 1985.
261. Slinger R, Giulivi A: Bacterial contamination of blood components: is it in the bag? *Can Med Assoc J* 160:535, 1999.
262. Slonim AD, Kurtines HC, Sprague BM, et al: The costs associated with nosocomial bloodstream infections in the pediatric intensive care unit. *Pediatr Crit Care Med* 2:170, 2001.
263. Slota M, Green M, Farley A, et al: The role of gown and glove isolation and strict handwashing in the reduction of nosocomial infection in children with solid organ transplantation. *Crit Care Med* 29:405, 2001.
264. Smith MA, Mathewson JJ, Ulert IA, et al: Contaminated stethoscopes revisited. *Arch Intern Med* 156:82, 1996.
265. SolÈ-Viol·n J, RodrÌguez de Castro F, Rey A, et al: Usefulness of microscopic examination of intracellular organisms in lavage fluid in ventilator-associated pneumonia. *Chest* 106:889, 1994.
266. Stark RP, Maki DG: Bacteriuria in the catheterized patient. *N Engl J Med* 311:560, 1984.
267. Stein F, Trevino R: Nosocomial infections in the pediatric intensive care unit. *Pediatr Clin North Am* 41:1245, 1994.
268. Sterling TR, Ho EJ, Brehm WT, et al: Diagnosis and treatment of ventilator-associated pneumonia-Impact on survival. *Chest* 110:1025, 1996.
269. Stevenson GW, Hall SC, Rudnick S, et al: The effect of anesthetic agents on the human immune response. *Anesthesiology* 72:542, 1990.
270. Stillwell M, Caplan ES: The septic multiple trauma patient. *Infect Dis Clin North Am* 3:155, 1989.
271. Stover BH, for the Pediatric Prevention Network: Nosocomial infection rates in US children's hospitals neonatal and pediatric intensive care units. *Am J Infect Control* 29:152, 2001.
272. Sullivan NM, Sutter VL, Mims MM, et al: Clinical aspects of bacteremia after manipulation of the genitourinary tract. *J Infect Dis* 127:49, 1973.
273. Tablan OC, Anderson LJ, Arden NH, et al: Guideline for prevention of nosocomial pneumonia. *Infect Contr Hosp Epidemiol* 15:588, 1994.
274. Tartter PI: Blood transfusion and postoperative infections. *Transfusion* 29:456, 1989.
275. Taylor RW, Manganaro L, O'Brien J, et al: Impact of allogenic packed red blood cell transfusion on nosocomial infection rates in the critically ill patient. *Crit Care Med* 30:2249, 2002.
276. Thomas F, Burke JP, Parker J, et al: The risk of infection related to radial vs femoral sites for arterial catheterization. *Crit Care Med* 11:807, 1983.
277. Tighe MJ, Kite P, Fawley WN, et al: An endoluminal brush to detect the infected central venous catheter in situ: a pilot study. *BMJ* 313:1528, 1996.
278. Tolzis P, Hoyen C, Spinner-Block S, et al: Factors that predict preexisting colonization with antibiotic-resistant gram-negative bacilli in patients admitted to a pediatric intensive care unit. *Pediatrics* 103:719, 1999.
279. Torres A, Puig de la Bellacasa J, RodrÌguez-Roisin R, et al: Diagnostic value of telescoping plugged catheters in mechanically ventilated patients with bacterial pneumonia using the Metras catheter. *Am Rev Respir Dis* 138:117, 1988.

280. Torres A, Puig de la Bellacasa J, Xaubet A, et al: Diagnostic value of quantitative cultures of bronchoalveolar lavage and telescoping plugged catheters in mechanically ventilated patients with bacterial pneumonia. *Am Rev Respir Dis* 140:306, 1989.
281. Torres A, Serra-Batlles J, Ros E, et al: Pulmonary aspiration of gastric contents in patients receiving mechanical ventilation: the effect of body position. *Ann Intern Med* 116:540, 1992.
282. Utley JR, Stephens DB, Wachtel C, et al: Effect of albumin and mannitol on organ blood flow, oxygen delivery, water content, and renal function during hypothermic hemodilution cardiopulmonary bypass. *Ann Thorac Surg* 33:250, 1982.
283. Valles J, Artigas A, Rello J, et al: Continuous aspiration of subglottic secretions in preventing ventilator associated pneumonia. *Ann Intern Med* 12:179, 1995.
284. Veenstra DL, Saint S, Saha S, et al: Efficacy of antiseptic-impregnated central venous catheters in preventing catheter-related bloodstream infection. *JAMA* 271:261, 1999.
285. Villers D, Derriennic M, Germaud P, et al: Reliability of the bronchoscopic protected catheter brush in intubated and ventilated patients. *Chest* 88:527, 1985.
286. Wald ER, Milmoe GJ, Bowen AD, et al: Acute maxillary sinusitis in children. *N Engl J Med* 304:749, 1981.
287. Weiland DE, Bay C, Csontos L: Using decision tree analysis of antibiogram data to determine efficacious empiric antibiotic treatment of early nosocomial pneumonia in ICU's. *Crit Care Med* 24:A48, 1996.
288. Welliver RC, McLaughlin S: Unique epidemiology of nosocomial infection in a children's hospital. *Am J Dis Child* 138:131, 1984.
289. Williams WW, Arden NH, Butler JC: Immunoprophylaxis and immunomodulation for prevention of nosocomial pneumonia. In Jarvis WR, editor: *Nosocomial pneumonia*. New York, 2000, Marcel Dekker.
290. Woeltje KF, Fraser VJ: Preventing nosocomial infections in the intensive care unit—Lessons learned from outcomes research. *New Horizons* 6:84, 1998.
291. Wunderink RG: Ventilator-associated pneumonia. *Clin Chest Med* 16:173, 1995.
292. Yau YC, de Nanassy J, Summerbell RC, et al: Fungal sternal wound infection due to *Curvularia lunata* in a neonate with congenital heart disease: case report and review. *Clin Infect Dis* 19:735, 1994.
293. Zach JE, Garrison T, Trovillion E, et al: Effect of an education program aimed at reducing the occurrence of ventilator-associated pneumonia. *Crit Care Med* 30:2407, 2002.
294. Zamora MR: Use of cytomegalovirus immune globulin and ganciclovir for the prevention of cytomegalovirus disease in lung transplantation. *Transpl Infect Dis* 3(suppl 2):49, 2001.

CHAPTER

91

Rheumatic Diseases and Their Treatment

Victoria W. Cartwright and Laurie O. Beitz

PEARLS

- Diagnosis of a rheumatic illness should be considered in the setting of multiorgan involvement, presence of fever and other constitutional symptoms, and laboratory studies suggestive of a systemic inflammatory response such as elevated acute-phase reactants. Infection and malignancy are great mimickers and should be justifiably excluded if possible.
- A patient with a known rheumatologic diagnosis and prior use of immunosuppressives is at high risk for a significant infection. The patient taking steroids may not mount the expected inflammatory response, such as fever or elevated white blood cell count, to an infection because of the immunosuppressive effects of the steroids. Treatment should be directed, but empiric antimicrobial therapy pending culture results may help prevent associated mortality from infection in this special population.
- A patient who used steroids chronically for 6 and even up to 12 months earlier may be predisposed to adrenal insufficiency in the stressful setting of an acute illness or surgery and should be treated accordingly.
- The clinical picture of isolated central nervous system vasculitis is rare, as most systemic connective tissue diseases or vasculitides have characteristic multisystem involvement. Other diagnoses such as infection or vascular abnormalities should be sought.
- Rheumatologic laboratory studies are rarely confirmatory of vasculitis. They are helpful in confirming clinical suspicion based on signs and symptoms, especially if they cluster in typical patterns, such as high-titer antinuclear antibody with low complements and positive double-stranded deoxyribonucleic acid. Pathologic examination of a biopsy sample from an affected organ, such as skin, kidney, or even brain, can help confirm a rheumatologic diagnosis in many cases.

Multiple inflammatory diseases can manifest with severe or life-threatening complications. They include diseases complicated by vasculity such as the vasculitides systemic lupus erythematosus (SLE) and juvenile dermatomyositis, and vasculopathies such as scleroderma. Other conditions that have significant morbidity and mortality include thrombotic thrombocytopenic purpura (TTP), antiphospholipid (APL) syndrome, and macrophage activation syndrome (MAS) that is associated with a variety of connective tissue diseases but most commonly in pediatric patients with systemic onset type of juvenile arthritis. This chapter discusses several clinical scenarios that require high-level monitoring, such as complications of pharmacotherapeutics and anaphylaxis.

Rheumatic illnesses include systemic connective diseases and systemic vasculitides. Life-threatening complications result from both the illness and its treatment. Vasculitides as a group share the pathophysiology of inflammation of blood vessels. Few diagnostic tests are confirmatory and few clinical features are pathognomonic for rheumatic diseases. A high clinical suspicion is necessary for any patient who has multiorgan involvement to help make the diagnosis and consequently institute appropriate management. The exact etiology of each of these diseases remains elusive and is beyond the scope of this chapter. However, animal models suggest for some rheumatic illnesses the theory of environmental trigger(s) in a genetically susceptible host initiating immune system dysregulation or inflammation and resultant organ damage.[1–3] Several diseases that may require intensive care are outlined, and typical clinical features, an initial approach to management, and common associations are discussed.

Life-Threatening Rheumatic Diseases

Sytemic Lupus Erythematosus

SLE is the prototypic multiorgan inflammatory disease. Onset may be insidious or dramatic. Initial manifestations of the disease include nephritis, rash, pericarditis, pleuritis, hepatosplenomegaly, central nervous system (CNS) involvement, or cytopenias (leukopenia, lymphopenia, anemia, thrombocytopenia)[4a] (Table 91–1).

The diagnosis of SLE is dependent on clinical and laboratory criteria. Laboratory studies that are helpful in diagnosing SLE include antinuclear antibody titer (commonly 1:640 or greater) and low complement components (C3 and C4). Other autoantibodies may be detected, including antibodies against double-stranded deoxyribonucleic acid and Smith antigens. Pathologic examination of a biopsy sample from an affected organ, such as skin or kidney, may aid in diagnosing SLE. Secondary diagnoses may include APL syndrome or TTP (discussed on page 1428). The primary differential diagnosis is mixed connective tissue disease, which also is characterized by multiorgan involvement but has high titers of antibody against ribonuclear protein (anti-RNP) combined with clinical findings found in other inflammatory diseases such as scleroderma or dermatomyositis.

Kidney disease may be quite severe in SLE. SLE nephritis may be associated with hypertension, nephrotic range proteinuria and associated sequelae, and renal insufficiency severe enough to require dialysis. Biopsy of the kidney in a stable patient may help to characterize the extent of disease and to rule out concomitant microangiopathic disease. Pathologic features of the kidney biopsy sample may direct treatment options for the acutely ill patient with SLE.

Associated morbidity may result from neurologic, pulmonary, cardiac, and gastrointestinal (GI) involvement. Specific neurologic manifestations of SLE include coma, headaches, seizures, psychosis, stroke, neuropathies, and retinopathy. Ophthalmologic examination may show the presence of cotton wool spots or direct visualization of vasculitis of the retina. No definitive study confirms neurologic SLE. Magnetic resonance imaging (Figure 91–1) and cerebrospinal fluid studies may be useful adjuncts, but neither is tremendously sensitive nor specific for neurologic SLE.

Pulmonary manifestations of SLE include pleuritis, pneumonitis, hemorrhage, and, rarely, bronchiolitis obliterans. Pleuritic chest pain and pleuritis may be associated with effusion of varying degrees. Pneumonitis may be associated (Figure 91–2). Severe pulmonary complications include pulmonary hemorrhage, thought to result from the underlying vasculitis but possibly from concomitant infection, and pulmonary hypertension, also resulting from either the underlying vasculitis or thrombosis of the pulmonary vasculature. Pulmonary hemorrhage can occur without preceding hemoptysis.[5]

Cardiac complications of SLE include pericarditis, myocarditis, and endocarditis. Pericarditis affects 12% to 48% of patients with SLE at some time during the course of their illness[6] but may not be clinically serious in a majority of patients. Chronic pericarditis may lead to constrictive disease, whereas acute disease may result in tamponade.[7] Symptoms of pericarditis include precordial chest pain that may be relieved with positioning, and associated fever, tachycardia, and decreased heart sounds on auscultation. Pericardial tamponade is associated with progressive dyspnea, increased jugular venous pulsations, decreased heart sounds, or a friction rub. Infectious pericarditis has been reported in SLE patients. Therefore pericardiocentesis is indicated for large fluid collections and when infection is considered (see Chapter 15). Myocarditis causes heart failure in patients with SLE.

TABLE 91–1

Selected Systemic Inflammatory Conditions and Associated Clinical Characteristics

Disease	Characteristics
SLE	Neutropenia, thrombocytopenia, anemia (may be hemolytic), malar rash, naso-oral ulcers, serositis, nephritis with associated renal insufficiency, nephrotic range proteinuria, seizures or psychosis, arthritis, high-titer ANA in conjunction with dsDNA and/or anti-Smith antibodies, antiphospholipid syndrome, hypocomplementemia
JDMS	Proximal muscle weakness, characteristic rash on knuckles and extensor surfaces, heliotrope rash, nailfold capillary inflammation, elevated muscle enzymes (creatine kinase, aldolase, lactate dehydrogenase, AST, ALT), inflammation of muscles and subcutaneous tissue on muscle biopsy or on magnetic resonance imaging with STIR sequences, dysphonia, dysphagia, and respiratory compromise if severe muscle weakness present
Systemic sclerosis	Characteristic skin changes, pulmonary involvement with ground-glass appearance on high-resolution chest computed tomography, esophageal achalasia, antibody to scl-70 or ANA with centromere pattern may be positive
MCTD	Can include any combination of the manifestations of disease in SLE, JDMS, scleroderma, or juvenile arthritis and typically has high-titer antibody against ribonuclear protein
SoJRA	One of three types of juvenile arthritis characterized by high daily spiking fevers > 101°F with acutely ill-appearing child having evanescent salmon-colored rash on trunk and extremities, leukocytosis, thrombocytosis, pericarditis, hepatosplenomegaly, and absence of infection or malignancy; arthritis may develop late in course

ANA, Antinuclear antibody; *JDMS,* juvenile dermatomyositis; *MCTD,* mixed connective tissue disease; *SLE,* systemic lupus erythematosus; *SoJRA,* systemic onset type of juvenile rheumatoid.

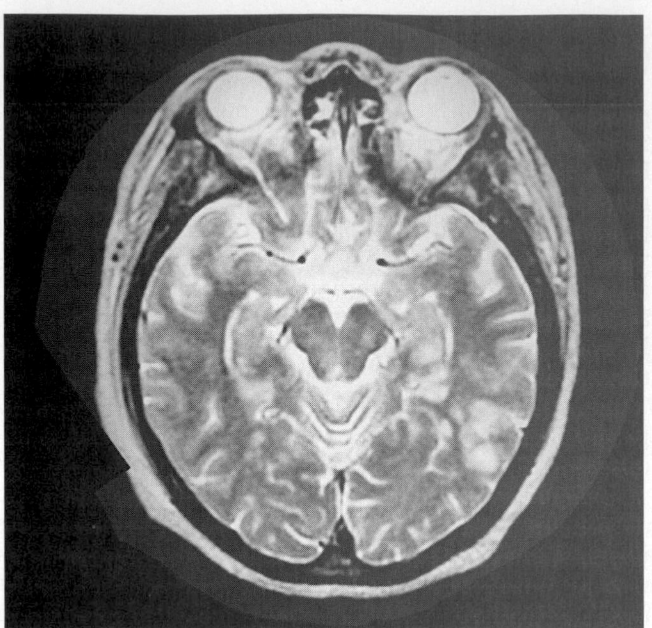

FIGURE 91–1 • Magnetic resonance image of the brain of a 16-year-old female patient with systemic lupus erythematosus. This image was obtained after the patient was stabilized. Multiple areas of increased signal are scattered throughout both cerebral hemispheres, consistent with ischemic infarctions resulting from lupus cerebritis. Other views demonstrated similar infarcts in the brainstem and cerebellar hemisphere. Magnetic resonance angiography obtained at the same time revealed normal vasculature, suggesting pathologic involvement of brain tissue but sparing of vessels. The patient responded well to pulse intravenous methylprednisolone and cyclophosphamide, with no residual neurologic deficit.

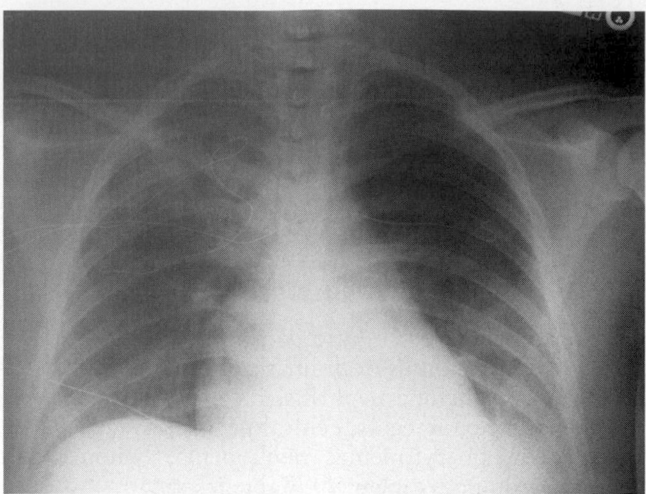

FIGURE 91–2 • Portable chest radiograph of the same patient shown in Figure 91–1. Lupus pneumonitis is reflected by infiltrate in the right upper lobe and bilateral diffuse interstitial changes. Pleural fluid suggested by haziness over the left lower lobe, as well as blunted left costophrenic angle (not shown), was confirmed by bilateral decubitus films.

Endocarditis may result in valve destruction and conduction abnormalities. Patients with SLE are at increased risk for premature coronary artery disease.[8] Myocardial infarction must be considered in patients with acute chest pain.

GI manifestations of SLE include pancreatitis, vasculitis of the mesenteric bed, hepatitis, and Arnold-Chiari syndrome. Neurologic, pulmonary, cardiac, or GI system involvement can prompt serious illness and require careful monitoring and possibly intensive care support.

Treatment of SLE is directed at the underlying vasculitis and specifically at affected organ systems.[4b] The mainstay of therapy is corticosteroids. These drugs can be given orally, topically for skin rashes, or systemically (large doses are required). In the very ill patient, typically parenteral administration of methylprednisolone 30 mg/kg/dose up to maximum dose of 1 g/day can be given sequentially for a total of 3 days. Some clinicians divide this daily dose to provide corticosteroids 2 to 4 times per day to increase potency. Treatment also includes intravenous cyclophosphamide for disease control. Cyclophosphamide has been shown to improve survival with renal disease.[9,10] It also is indicated in the patient with CNS disease. The dose and duration varies depending on the clinical course; typically 0.5 to 1 g/m^2 intravenous pulses are used at 1-month intervals for seven doses and then the interval lengthened depending on patient response.[11] If the etiology is unclear, combining immunosuppression with anticoagulation for concomitant antiphospholipid syndrome is a treatment consideration for special clinical cases with severe or so-called catastrophic neurologic disease.[12] Treatment for pericarditis typically consists of corticosteroids with additional nonsteroidal antiinflammatory drugs. Interventions in addition to corticosteroids or immunosuppression include plasmapheresis, particularly in the setting of comorbid microangiopathic disease of TTP.[13] Appropriate antifungal and antibiotic therapy, including *Pneumocystis carinii* coverage in the setting of respiratory symptoms, should be considered in any ill patient with SLE undergoing immunosuppressive therapy who develops new headache, seizures, change in mentation, chest pain, prolonged cough, tachypnea, rash, or abdominal pain. This is important in patients with fever and increased C-reactive protein. Therapy should continue until the etiology of the new clinical finding has been identified.

Juvenile Dermatomyositis

Juvenile dermatomyositis (JDMS) is an inflammatory disease characterized by muscle and skin inflammation. Proximal muscle weakness can be profound. Physical findings include a Gower sign, head lag because of lack of spinal support, inability to dress oneself, shortness of breath, and difficulty swallowing. Pathognomonic skin manifestations include Gottron papules, facial erythema, and heliotrope discoloration of the upper eyelids. Nailfold capillary abnormalities are commonly present. Complications of this illness can be life-threatening and require intensive monitoring and supportive care.

Life-threatening complications of JDMS encompass several organ systems, including the GI, respiratory, and cardiac systems. GI complications include bleeding, infarction, perforation, and dysmotility. Visceral vasculitis can present with nonspecific abdominal pain and may result in massive GI bleeding, pneumatosis intestinalis, or bowel wall perforation. Patients may have severe palatal and pharyngeal weakness resulting in dysphonia and dysphagia, which predispose these patients to aspiration.

Patients with JDMS are at risk of developing spontaneous pneumothorax and, rarely, interstitial lung disease and pulmonary hypertension. Cardiovascular complications of JDMS include arrhythmias with or without heart block, myocarditis, and severe hypertension.

Treatment of JDMS initially involves rapid recognition of the underlying disease and any associated complications that may require supportive care. Immunomodulatory agents include corticosteroids, methotrexate, intravenous immunoglobulin, and cyclosporine A.[14–16] Cyclophosphamide is also a consideration for treatment of the severely ill child,[17] particularly with GI vasculitis. Care should be taken when administering medications to a gut mucosa that may be inflamed because of underlying disease. Parenteral administration may be necessary in severely affected JDMS patients until the clinical course improves significantly.

Scleroderma

Scleroderma may be localized (morphea, linear scleroderma) or diffuse and associated with internal organ involvement (systemic sclerosis; *c*alcinosis cutis, *R*aynaud phenomenon, *e*sophageal dysfunction, *s*clerodactyly, *t*elangiectasia [CREST] syndrome). The incidence is 0.2 to 1 per 100,000 for the local form and is even rarer for systemic sclerosis.[18,19] The etiology is unclear, but microvasculature changes may lead to disease pathogenesis given that histology shows endothelial cell necrosis[20] and sequentially edema, vascularity, sclerosis, collagen deposition, and atrophy.[19]

Three stages of scleroderma disease are generally recognized. In the initial stage, the skin appears indurated or puffy. The second stage is defined by fibrosis and hardening. In the third stage, softening occurs as the disease is "burnt out." Calcinosis may occur, especially with CREST syndrome. Raynaud phenomenon is common, typically in more than 90% of patients with the diagnosis of systemic sclerosis, and often is one of the presenting symptoms. The characteristic pulmonary involvement is alveolitis followed by fibrosis. Scleroderma can have severe manifestations of disease, including renal crisis or cardiac manifestations that may require ICU management.[21]

The heart and kidney are the primary foci of life-threatening complications of scleroderma. Cardiac complications include congestive heart failure, arrhythmias, and pulmonary hypertension and have been shown to correlate with morbidity in this patient population. Pericardial effusion may occur (Figure 91–3) but is not typical. Echocardiography is a sensitive and noninvasive diagnostic modality that helps in the diagnosis of pulmonary hypertension. Pulmonary hypertension may require treatment with epoprostenol infusion. If severe, sildenafil[22] and new oral therapy with the endothelin-1 antagonist bosentan currently is under investigation, but preliminary data are encouraging.[23]

Renal crisis may be precipitated by various factors, including high-dose corticosteroid therapy within the prior 6 months,[24] hypovolemia, or vasospasm similar to that seen in Raynaud phenomenon. Clinicians should be suspicious of impending renal crisis in any patient with decreasing creatinine clearance or increasing proteinuria or blood pressure measurements. If malignant hypertension develops, renal insufficiency and associated morbidity can follow rapidly if angiotensin-converting enzyme inhibitors are not started quickly. Also, judicious lowering of blood pressure in patients with malignant hypertension is important to preserve renal blood flow and prevent further renal crisis. Patients with scleroderma should be monitored closely and frequently with serial blood pressure measurements, determination of serum creatinine concentration, and urinalyses to facilitate rapid recognition and management of renal crisis. A patient with scleroderma requires close attention to renal, cardiac, and lung functions to help prevent complications and associated mortality.

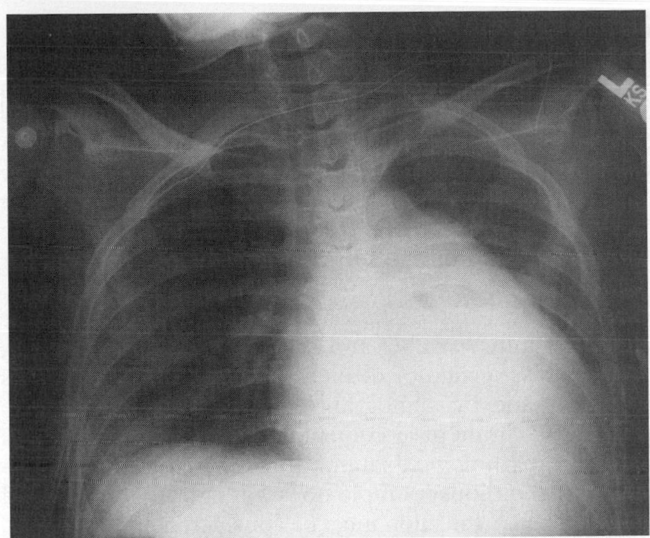

FIGURE 91–3 • Portable chest radiograph of a 12-year-old female patient with scleroderma. The patient arrived at the intensive care unit with sudden onset of orthopnea and thrombocytopenia. Cardiomegaly was observed. As in Figure 91–4, echocardiography revealed pericardial effusion. However, pulmonary vascularity is normal in this patient. Physical examination revealed sclerodactyly. The patient eventually developed cor pulmonale as a result of pulmonary hypertension. Inflammatory changes suggestive of other collagen vascular diseases may be seen in the early course of scleroderma. Use of pulse intravenous methylprednisolone reduced these early inflammatory changes, although as an outpatient the patient maintained stable right-sided heart disease that was not responsive to immunosuppressive medication, consistent with scleroderma.

Vasculitis

Vasculitis is a general term that refers to inflammation of blood vessels that may be systemic or organ specific. The systemic vasculitides are generally characterized by vessel size. Large-vessel disease includes Takayasu arteritis, medium-vessel disease encompasses polyarteritis nodosa and Kawasaki disease, and small-vessel vasculitis describes Wegener granulomatosus (WG), microscopic polyangiitis, serum sickness, and Henoch-Schönlein purpura (HSP). All of the vasculitides can have serious complications or manifestations of disease (discussed on page 1421).

Primary Vasculitis of the Central Nervous System

Primary vasculitis or angiitis of the CNS is characterized by inflammation of vessels within the CNS and by exclusion of vasculitis in other organ systems.[25] Inflammatory vessel changes may be apparent at angiography, but biopsy may be necessary for diagnosis. It is quite rare in children and has been described primarily in case reports.[26]

The clinical manifestations of primary angiitis of the CNS are quite variable and include seizures, headache, hemiparesis, vertigo or dizziness, and aphasia. Diagnosis may be made by angiography, but small-vessel disease may require brain or leptomeningeal biopsy for diagnosis. However, pathologic examination is prone to lower sensitivity if the biopsy sample does not capture an affected vessel area.[25,27] Infection must be considered and excluded, similar to other acute manifestations of vasculitis discussed on page 1424. Cerebrospinal fluid is not diagnostic because it can be normal, especially in the pediatric age group. Imaging or biopsy of the CNS that demonstrates vasculitis in the absence of other organ involvement characterizes primary angiitis of the CNS.

Because primary CNS angiitis is rare, treatment trials are sparse. However, corticosteroids and cyclophosphamide have been shown to improve survival.[27a] The severity of disease and the potential of primary angiitis of the CNS for mortality and morbidity suggest aggressive treatment at the outset. Continuation of therapy for up to 6 to 12 months arguably can be justifiable given reports of relapse or deterioration after termination of immunosuppression.[25,26]

Wegener's Granulomatosus

Wegener granulomatosus (WG) is a systemic vasculitis characterized by granulomas in the kidneys, lungs including airways and parenchyma, ears, and sinuses. Serious sequelae of this disease include pulmonary hemorrhage and renal failure. Table 91–2 lists the clinical syndromes that involve both renal failure and hemoptysis. Neurologic manifestations can occur in a significant portion of patients with WG and include peripheral nervous system disease, mononeuritis multiplex, CNS disease, infarct, hemorrhage, stroke, mass lesions, and transverse myelitis.[28] Serious complications of WG include tracheal stenosis with symptoms of shortness of breath and stridor, pulmonary insufficiency, and renal insufficiency.

Diagnosis of WG can be made by typical granulomatous features on biopsy sample from an affected site. WG is strongly suggested by the presence of antineutrophil cytoplasmic antibody (ANCA), specifically antibodies against proteinase-3. Goodpasture syndrome may mimic WG with regard to renal and pulmonary involvement, but antibasement membrane antibodies are specific for Goodpasture syndrome.

Treatment of WG includes immunosuppression with cyclophosphamide and corticosteroids, a combination that has been shown to decrease mortality and to induce remission in the majority of patients. The typical daily dose of cyclophosphamide 2 mg/kg/day can be escalated or even given as a higher pulse dose in the setting of serious, life-threatening disease. Pulse dosing of corticosteroids may be given in conjunction with this regimen until the inflammation and clinical setting improve. Daily antibiotic therapy has been used as adjunctive therapy for patients with WG.[29,30]

Henoch-Schönlein Purpura

Henoch-Schönlein purpura (HSP) is a small-vessel vasculitis and, along with Kawasaki disease, one of the most frequently occurring vasculitis of childhood. The typical course is self-resolving with few sequelae; severe disease warrants appropriate intensive care management. The classic clinical features include palpable purpura and abdominal pain. Arthritis or arthralgias, periarticular swelling, and colicky abdominal pain associated with nausea typically are present. Significant morbidity results from affected GI and renal systems. Varying degrees of GI edema and hemorrhage may occur, and infrequently intussusception results. Rapidly progressive glomerulonephritis may occur, but most patients with renal involvement have only microscopic hematuria. Rare but potentially fatal complications of HSP include pulmonary hemorrhage and CNS involvement such as encephalopathy, hemorrhage, seizures, or infarcts.

Diagnosis of HSP is primarily clinical, with laboratory studies helping to exclude other vasculitic diseases. Treatment is primarily supportive if the disease is mild. For aggressive disease with significant organ involvement, high-dose corticosteroids are the most studied. They show some beneficial effects on renal involvement in small observational studies.[31] Immunosuppression with cyclophosphamide, azathioprine, cyclosporine, intravenous immunoglobulin, and plasmapheresis have been described.[32]

Polyarteritis Nodosa

Polyarteritis nodosa (PAN) is a rare disease in childhood but should be considered in any patient who has a combination of hypertension, GI or musculoskeletal involvement, rash, and fever. Diagnosis is difficult because of clinical variability. Constitutional symptoms include fever and weight loss. Muscle tenderness, arthritis, or arthralgia may occur. Nervous system involvement is possible, with psychosis, seizures, strokes, or neuropathy. Skin manifestations can be varied, with painful nodules, purpura, petechiae, or edema. Abdominal pain is nonspecific but can result from infarcts in various GI organs. Cardiac involvement is possible. Diagnosis is aided by pathologic findings on excisional biopsy of affected skin, biopsy of nerve or muscle, or angiography demonstrating aneurysms. Treatment mainstays include high-dose corticosteroids frequently requiring the addition of cyclophosphamide or azathioprine. Streptococcus-associated disease has been described and should receive appropriate antibiotic therapy and antibiotic prophylaxis in some cases.[33]

Microscopic Polyangiitis

Microscopic polyangiitis (MP), like PAN, may involve vessels supplying the kidneys, peripheral nerves, skin, GI tract, and muscles. It characteristically also affects the pulmonary vasculature. Typically the patient has constitutional symptoms such as fever, fatigue, weight loss, and associated symptoms of affected organs. Serious illness may result from pulmonary hemorrhage, GI bleeding or infarction, heart failure, or kidney failure.

Diagnosis of MP is primarily clinical, because most laboratory tests reflect the inflammatory process and are not specific for diagnostic purposes. ANCA typically is positive in patients with MP, especially for the neutrophil component myeloperoxidase. However, antibody testing is neither sensitive nor specific. ANCA was positive in 60% of patients with renal disease, 75% of patients with alveolar hemorrhage, and 75% overall.[34] It can be positive in other diseases such as SLE and rheumatoid arthritis. Biopsy of affected vessels, if positive, helps with the diagnosis but may be negative in almost half of cases.

Management includes supportive care and use of corticosteroids to control the inflammation of MP. If escalation of therapy is necessary, a cytotoxic agent such as cyclophosphamide is associated with a lower mortality rate.[34] Some cases with pulmonary hemorrhage require extracorporeal membrane oxygenation treatment in addition to management of the underlying vasculitis. Plasmapheresis may be helpful in severe cases or in the setting of pulmonary hemorrhage.[34,35] Review Table 91–2 for clinical characteristics of pulmonary manifestations of systemic disease.

Kawasaki Disease

Kawasaki disease (KD) is a childhood illness characterized by acute onset of fever at least 5 days, conjunctivitis, cervical lymphadenopathy, enanthem, exanthem, and extremity changes with redness, edema, and later desquamation. The predominant morbidity results from coronary artery aneurysm development. Other peripheral arteries infrequently develop aneurysms. Not all patients fulfill the classic clinical criteria, and so-called atypical or incomplete Kawasaki disease can have significant coronary artery involvement.[36] The aneurysms of KD are at greater risk for stenosis or obstruction than are unaffected vessels and are prone to thrombosis and resultant morbidity.

Management for KD depends on prompt initial diagnosis and treatment with intravenous immunoglobulin and aspirin. This treatment helps prevent aneurysm formation and resultant associated complications.[37] For cases refractory to standard treatment, use of parenteral steroids has been advocated and is undergoing further investigation.[37,38] Anticoagulants should be considered in the setting of a large aneurysm to prevent further cardiovascular sequelae. In the clinical scenario with concomitant myocarditis, supportive care including inotropes, fluid management to include diuretics, and/or pacemaking may be necessary. KD is a self-limited vasculitis, and attention to prompt recognition and effective treatment helps prevent the cardiac sequelae. A high clinical suspicion of aneurysm and associated thrombus in a patient known to have KD helps prevent any further complications of this illness.

Takayasu Arteritis

Takayasu arteritis is an inflammatory disease that affects the aorta and major branches. It typically occurs in young women. Symptoms include fever, fatigue, and weight loss. Patients may develop absent pulses, visual difficulties, syncope, or stroke. Cardiac features include symptoms of angina and congestive heart failure. Diagnosis is made by arteriography of the entire aorta, although ultrasound, magnetic resonance imaging, or computed tomography may be useful adjunctive diagnostic procedures. Again, corticosteroids are the primary treatment modality, augmented by immune modulation with cyclophosphamide, methotrexate, azathioprine, or in some cases anti-tumor necrosis factor (TNF)-α therapy.[39,40]

TABLE 91–2

Clinical Syndromes That Involve Both Renal Failure and Pulmonary Disease

Pulmonary Manifestations	Disease	Clinical Characteristics
Pulmonary hemorrhage	SLE	Facial rash, cytopenias, renal disease, hypocomplementemia, arthritis, carditis
	Wegener granulomatosus	Granulomatous lesions in sinuses, renal disease, ANCA (PR3)
		Claudication, renal disease, gastrointestinal involvement, rash, fever
	PAN	
	HSP	Classic palpable purpura, arthritis or swelling, colicky abdominal pain, intussusception
	RPGN	Can include Goodpasture syndrome, renal disease
	MP	Renal insufficiency, pulmonary disease, ANCA (MPO)
Pulmonary hypertension	Systemic sclerosis	Tight skin, tapered fingers, pulmonary interstitial disease "ground-glass" changes on radiography, renal disease
Respiratory failure	JDMS	Proximal muscle weakness, classic rash over knuckles (Gottron papules) and eyelids (heliotrope)
		Respiratory complications due to weakness of diaphragm and accessory muscles
		May have aspiration pneumonia

ANCA, Antineutrophil cytoplasmic antibody; *HSP,* Henoch-Schönlein purpura; *JDMS,* juvenile dermatomyositis; *MP,* microscopic polyangiitis; *PAN,* polyarteritis nodosum; *RPGN,* rapidly progressive glomerulonephritis; *SLE,* systemic lupus erythematosus.

TABLE 91–3

Immune Modulating Agents for Inflammatory Diseases

Medication	Doses to Consider
Methylprednisolone	1–2 mg/kg/dose daily or divided twice daily, or pulse dose of 30 mg/kg up to 1 g maximum dose daily up to 3 days
Cyclophosphamide	1–2 mg/kg/dose daily or divided twice daily, or pulse dose of 750–1000 mg/m^2 depending on total lymphocyte count
Intravenous immunoglobulin	1–2 g/kg/dose; repeat doses if clinically indicated
Hydrocortisone	"Stress dose" may vary; consider hydrocortisone 25–40 mg/m^2/day (3× maintenance) or 1 mg/kg/day continuous infusion or divided 4–6 times per day

Complications of Inflammatory Diseases

Systemic inflammatory illnesses sometimes are accompanied by life-threatening secondary complications, including prothrombotic states (thrombotic thrombocytopenic purpura, antiphospholipid antibody syndrome), overwhelming cytokine storm (MAS, Castleman disease), and infection secondary to immunosuppressive treatment of the primary disease (Table 91–3). Common complications of inflammatory diseases are discussed in this section.

Thrombotic syndromes include antiphospholipid (APL) antibody syndrome, which can be primary, or secondary with SLE or mixed connective tissue disease. The syndrome is defined by the presence of antibodies to phospholipids and associated proteins measured by either functional coagulation assays (lupus anticoagulant) or antibody titers (anticardiolipin and β_2-glycoprotein), and a clinical event such as recurrent arterial or venous thrombosis, thrombocytopenia, or recurrent fetal loss.

Antiphospholipid (APL) syndrome is important to consider in the setting of severe neurologic manifestations such as stroke, transverse myelitis, seizures, or mononeuritis multiplex. If thrombosis is present, the definitive treatment is anticoagulation. If APL is present with an additional diagnosis such as vasculitis, additional therapy with immunosuppression is warranted.[41]

Thrombotic thrombocytopenic purpura (TTP) is characterized by microangiopathic hemolytic anemia, thrombocytopenia, and abnormalities of the renal system and CNS. Clinical features include fever, headaches, change in mental status, coma, rash, and gross hematuria. Laboratory studies may show hemolytic anemia, schistocytes and nucleated red blood cells, hematuria, proteinuria, and azotemia.

The presence of TTP may be underdiagnosed because of the overlapping symptoms of both SLE and TTP, so clinical suspicion is key to differentiating the two entities. Microangiopathic changes such as schistocytes or gross hematuria suggest the presence of TTP. This is an important diagnosis to confirm because treatment with corticosteroids and immune suppression such as cyclophosphamide may be beneficial for both TTP and SLE, but treatment with plasmapheresis with plasma exchange greatly improves survival in patients with TTP.[41] If both diagnoses coexist, treatment with both immunosuppression and plasmapheresis is indicated. If a patient has TTP with associated nephrotic-range proteinuria at the time of diagnosis, subsequent development of SLE is significantly associated.[42]

MAS is a life-threatening condition that can result from acute or chronic illness. MAS may be the presenting manifestation of systemic disease. It typically is associated with systemic-onset juvenile arthritis but also is described with other illnesses such as SLE. A patient with macrophage activation syndrome may display high fever, vomiting, hemorrhage, neurologic symptoms such as coma or seizures, hepatomegaly, splenomegaly, lymphadenopathy, or cytopenias.[43] MAS may be idiopathic or associated with Epstein-Barr virus infection, medication use, or previous viral illness.[44] Note that the medication associations have not been shown to be definitively causal.

Laboratory findings in MAS include transaminitis and coagulation disorders, typically with features of disseminated intravascular coagulation (DIC) syndrome. A clue to the diagnosis in a patient with inflammation because of juvenile arthritis with associated inflammatory markers of leukocytosis and thrombocytosis and elevated erythrocyte sedimentation rate is that the acutely ill child will have a paradoxical drop or normalization in all three laboratory parameters yet increasing C-reactive protein concentration. Other associated findings include elevated triglycerides, elevated ferritin, and low albumin concentration. Diagnosis of MAS can be confirmed using bone marrow examination, but false-negative test results have been described.

Treatment is dependent on rapid diagnosis of MAS and institution of supportive care. Clinical suspicion should remain high in a seriously ill patient with known SLE or systemic-onset juvenile arthritis. Laboratory studies such as D-dimer[45] or ferritin[46] serially can be used to screen for MAS. Treatment typically involves use of high-dose steroids,[43,47,48] but cyclosporine A may be a useful adjunct.[43,49] Early recognition of MAS and appropriate therapy helps prevent the high mortality often reported with this disease.

Critical Care Issues for Patients with Arthritis

Systemic onset–type juvenile arthritis can have serious organ involvement that may require intensive care. It is one of three types of juvenile rheumatoid arthritis characterized by high daily spiking fevers, hepatosplenomegaly,

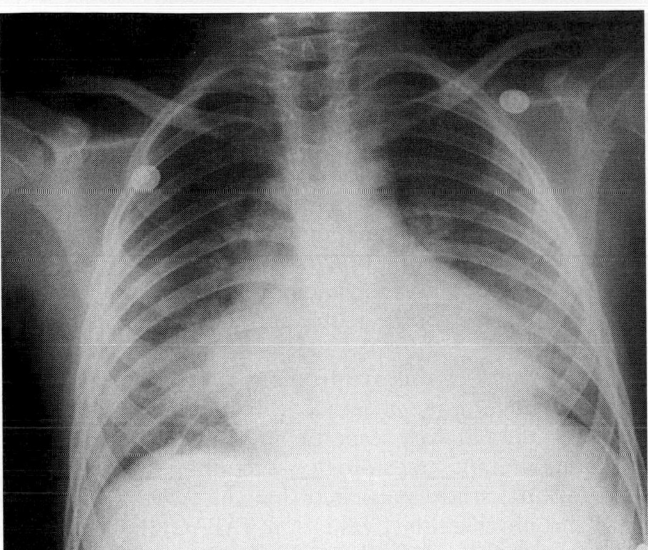

FIGURE 91–4 • Portable chest radiograph of a 7-year-old male patient with systemic juvenile rheumatoid arthritis who had pericarditis and severe myocarditis, with S3 gallop on examination. Although the cardiomegaly is mild, there is diffuse bilateral perihilar consolidation consistent with pulmonary edema. Echocardiography revealed mild pericardial effusion but severe left ventricular dysfunction consistent with the diffuse bilateral perihilar consolidation on radiograph resulting from pulmonary edema. The patient responded to digoxin, furosemide, and pulse intravenous methylprednisolone at a dose of 7.5 mg/kg every 6 hours.

thrombocytosis, leukocytosis, and a classic evanescent salmon-colored rash on the trunk. Arthritis may occur later in the disease course, which can make initial diagnosis difficult. Patients with the systemic subtype of juvenile arthritis should be monitored for cardiac changes such as pericarditis and associated tamponade (Figure 91–4). Note that pericarditis may precede the arthritis, making the definitive diagnosis of this type of childhood arthritis difficult initially, or the pericarditis may progress insidiously. Reassuringly, tamponade occurs rarely in the child with arthritis. Myocarditis and endocarditis have been reported. Congestive heart failure, pleural effusions, or valvular insufficiency may result from systemic juvenile arthritis.

Arthritis may effect either the cricoarytenoid region or the cervical spine. Both of these may have life threatening complications. Cricoarytenoid arthritis may directly compromise a child's airway. Inflammation at C1 and C2 may allow subluxation due to damage and resultant ligament laxity. Compression of the anterior spinal cord is possible with hyperextension of the neck, resulting in neurologic damage such as quadriplegia. Extension with intubation for placement of a definitive airway in an acute care setting should be cautious. If imaging is not available and time allows, use of nasotracheal or visually guided fiberoptic endotracheal intubation is the most conservative course.[50] Careful planning in conjunction with a careful medical history helps prevent neurologic complications for which a child with arthritis may have higher risk.

Infection and Inflammatory Illnesses

Overwhelming sepsis is a complication of the underlying inflammatory disease, immunosuppressive therapy to treat the disease, and the newer biologic therapies targeted at specific inflammatory cytokines involved with rheumatic illnesses. Infection has become the most common cause of mortality in patients with SLE, surpassing renal failure in recent years.[51,52] Infection was the cause of death in 29% of patients in a series of microscopic polyangiitis.[53] Diagnosing infective illnesses in these individuals is difficult because fever and leukocytosis may not be present secondary to immunosuppression.

Risk for infection with *Pneumocystis carinii* pneumonia is higher in patients with rheumatic illnesses and should be considered in any patient with acute pulmonary symptoms. The underlying inflammatory process may predispose certain patients to infection, such as those with WG. Use of corticosteroids and immunosuppressives places the patient at much greater risk for development of infection. Some patients receive antibiotic prophylaxis against this organism, but no set standard exists because the level of immune suppression for therapy is so varied. As noted on page 1424, acute pulmonary disease may necessitate treatment with antimicrobials combined with immunosuppressives pending confirmation of the etiology of the disease.

Biologic therapies such as anti–TNF-α have greatly advanced the rheumatologist's ability to fight disease; however, these targeted therapies can predispose the patient to a higher risk of infection. Tuberculosis is the most commonly reported infection associated with biologic therapy, but histoplasmosis and latent infections may become manifest.[54–56] Use of anti-CD20 monoclonal antibody (rituximab) is associated with various life-threatening infections, including visceral varicella-zoster, parvovirus B19 resulting in pure red cell aplasia, enteroviral meningitis, and cytomegalovirus, as well as increased risk of bacterial infections. Caution dictates the early judicious use of antimicrobials in an ill rheumatic patient who has been exposed to any form of immunosuppression because clinical signs and symptoms may not be as revealing as in an immunocompetent individual.

Corticosteroid Supplementation in Adrenal Insufficiency

Patients with rheumatic illnesses have likely received high doses of corticosteroids over a long duration, predisposing them to adrenal insufficiency. Corticosteroids given daily at greater than endogenous production (approximately 0.3 mg/kg/day hydrocortisone) may suppress the hypothalamic pituitary adrenal axis, but data suggesting the dosage amounts or duration of therapy that may predispose a patient are inadequate. Caution suggests that any patient who has received supraphysiologic doses of steroid for an extended period in the past year, or during the current hospitalization, should be covered with so-called stress doses of steroids if they are severely ill or undergoing surgery. The dosage may be 100 mg hydrocortisone intravenously every 8 hours for an adult, or 1 mg/kg/day as continuous infusion or divided 4 to 6 times daily. Local protocols may vary these dosages. Once the severe illness resolves or surgery is complete, the hydrocortisone can be tapered and discontinued. Careful management of the patient with underlying inflammatory disease includes supporting or assisting normal physiologic functions, such as the adrenal gland's response to stressful situations.

Summary Comments

Some patients with multiorgan involvement may not have a clear unifying diagnosis when treatment is necessary to prevent impending morbidity or mortality. Empirical therapy is appropriate, yet the following points should be considered carefully.[57] The differential diagnosis of inflammatory diseases such as vasculitis includes both infection and malignancy. Medications commonly used to treat rheumatic diseases (e.g., corticosteroids or immunosuppressive medications such as cyclophosphamide) may complicate both the diagnosis and treatment of these two differential diagnoses. Hence treatment should aim to improve the clinical course of the patient but also should allow for any future therapies if the real diagnosis is determined. Immunodeficiency, either inherited (complement defects, other) or acquired (medication, infection), should be included during the development of differential diagnoses of an intensely ill child. Failure to pursue appropriate diagnostic studies may delay appropriate therapies for an immunodeficient patient. Additionally, the clinician should establish a working diagnosis and select clinical outcomes to monitor for any treatment effects *a priori*. Such practice will help to modify any treatments and will ensure baseline measurements of any useful laboratory or imaging studies are obtained prior to the start of therapy. It also will help to delineate an appropriate time course for a therapeutic trial in case further therapies are necessary if the diagnosis remains unclear.

Drug Reactions Requiring Intensive Care

Some medications used to treat rheumatic diseases are associated with serious adverse reactions. The increased risk for sepsis or overwhelming infection with use of immunosuppressive agents or biologic therapies was discussed on page 1429. Other medications considered for treatment of serious illness in the special population of patients with inflammatory diseases are discussed here (see Chapter 112).

Various rheumatic agents have been reported to be associated with significant clinical scenarios. D-Penicillamine, useful for scleroderma, has been associated with several severe illnesses, including myasthenia gravis and Goodpasture disease.[4] Sulfasalazine, commonly used for treatment of spondyloarthropathies, can cause Stevens-Johnson syndrome. Aplastic anemia may complicate gold therapy (historical treatment of juvenile arthritis) or cyclosporine use. Rarely, nonsteroidal antiinflammatory drugs may cause enough gastric irritation to prompt a silent GI hemorrhage. Reassuringly, most drug reactions are rare.

Polyneuropathy/Myopathy of Critical Illness

One clinical entity associated with neuromuscular blockade is critical illness polyneuropathy and myopathy. This condition is characterized by flaccid paralysis of sudden onset, muscle atrophy, rhabdomyolysis, sensorimotor polyneuropathy, deficiency of deep tendon reflexes, and inability to decrease supplemental respiratory support, muscle wasting, and biopsy findings demonstrating atrophic muscle fibers in both acute and chronic denervation states.[58,59]

The etiology of this syndrome is thought to be multifactorial, including pharmacotherapeutics, underlying illness or inflammatory response, nutritional factors, sepsis, and concomitant physiologic reactions. A prospective observational study suggested that the Acute Physiology and Chronic Health Evaluation (APACHE) III score, presence of systemic inflammatory response syndrome, and aminoglycoside exposure were the only significant factors on univariate analysis of 98 cases.[60] Other factors such as vecuronium, midazolam, steroids, or sepsis severity score were not found to be significant. Other prospective studies suggest a role of steroids in the development of this syndrome in the ICU setting.[61] There are no proven treatments for this syndrome; however, supportive care for multiorgan failure and sepsis may decrease the development of the syndrome initially. Immune modulating therapies have some role based on the hypothesized pathogenic model of disease of immune dysregulation.[60] Table 91–3 lists some immune modulating agents used for inflammatory disease.

Finally, some treatments for rheumatic illnesses require a critical care approach during therapy. These clinical situations likely are rare but may necessitate the same careful attention to the patient in the intensive care setting as required by any of the rheumatic illnesses of childhood (Tables 91–4 and 91–5).

Anaphylaxis, Hypersensitivity, and Angioedema

Anaphylaxis

Anaphylaxis results from immunoglobulin E (IgE)-mediated massive mast cell chemokine release. Mast cells and basophils are activated by cross-linking of the high-affinity IgE receptor or by other less specific interactions (Figure 91–5). Basophils and mast cells degranulate, releasing histamine, leukotrienes, prostaglandins, and platelet-activating factor. These, in turn, result in activation of inflammatory pathways, including kinin, complement cascade, and coagulation factors for both clot formation and degradation.

Anaphylaxis typically occurs in a sensitized individual upon rechallenge with the inciting antigen. Another term, *anaphylactoid reaction,* has a similar clinical picture but has an absence of prior sensitization and does not have associated IgE effects.

Drugs that are most commonly associated with anaphylaxis include nonsteroidal antiinflammatory drugs

TABLE 91–4

Complications of Rheumatology Diagnoses or Drugs That May Be Used in the Intensive Care Unit

Complication	Associated Rheumatology Diagnoses
Sepsis	History of immunosuppressive therapy
Pneumocystis carinii infection	History of immunosuppressive therapy
Renal crisis	Scleroderma
Gastrointestinal hemorrhage	NSAID use
	HSP
Gut perforation or infarction	JDMS
Hemoptysis	SLE
	Wegener granulomatosus
	PAN
	HSP
	RPGN
	Microscopic polyangiitis
Myocardial infarction	Coronary aneurysm, Kawasaki disease
	SLE
	PAN
Pericardial tamponade	Systemic-onset juvenile arthritis
	SLE
	MCTD
Macrophage activation syndrome	Systemic-onset juvenile arthritis
	SLE
	Other
Aplastic anemia	Use of cyclosporine, gold, other
Goodpasture syndrome	Use of D-penicillamine
Stevens-Johnson syndrome	Use of sulfasalazine, other
Myasthenia gravis	Use of D-penicillamine

HSP, Henoch-Schönlein purpura; *JDMS,* juvenile dermatomyositis; *MCTD,* mixed connective tissue disease; *NSAID,* nonsteroidal antiinflammatory drug; *PAN,* polyarteritis nodosum; *RPGN,* rapidly progressive glomerulonephritis; *SLE,* systemic lupus erythematosus.

and antibiotics. Foods can cause episodes; classically peanuts and shellfish are causal agents. Radiocontrast agents are less frequently involved because of improvements in the agents used. Exposure to stress, exercise, cold ambient temperature, sunlight, or therapeutics such as γ globulin, dextran, and albumin may cause an anaphylactoid reaction.[62]

The patient may describe symptoms such as hoarseness, cough, bronchospasm, and a sense of impending doom. Dyspnea and rhinitis are common. Skin findings may include flushing, pruritus, diaphoresis, urticaria, and angioedema. GI manifestations vary from nausea and vomiting to diarrhea. Hypotension, arrhythmias, myocardial ischemia, and cardiovascular collapse may ensue in severe cases.

Treatment of anaphylaxis is supportive. Maintaining an airway and adequate ventilation are of paramount importance, as is maintaining adequate blood pressure with intravenous fluids, positioning, and pressor infusions. Antihistamines such as diphenhydramine 1 mg/kg up to a maximum dose of 400 mg/day intravenously and ranitidine help antagonize histamine effects. Corticosteroids are instituted to prevent symptom onset hours after the initial attack.

Hypersensitivity Vasculitis

Another disease entity resulting from an exaggerated immune response is hypersensitivity vasculitis or serum sickness. Serum sickness is the prototypic immune complex disease. It has various inciting agents, including medications and infections. Disease occurs 1 to 2 weeks after initial antigen exposure and includes fever, rash, arthralgia or arthritis, and lymphadenopathy. The rash varies from urticaria to purpura. Diagnosis is primarily clinical, although skin biopsy showing presence of leukocytoclastic vasculitis of the small vessels and positive staining for immune complexes may be helpful. Treatment is supportive, and antihistamine or corticosteroids are useful adjunctive therapies.

Hereditary Angioedema

Hereditary angioedema is an autosomal dominant absence of any functioning complement component C1 inhibitor (C1INH). It is characterized by recurrent swelling of various body parts, but it can have life-threatening complications because of development of laryngeal edema. Acute abdominal pain with vomiting and guarding appears worrisome for an acute abdomen, but fever and leukocytosis are absent. The easiest laboratory test that

TABLE 91–5

Therapies for Rheumatic Diagnoses That Require Intensive Monitoring

Medication	Diagnosis
Epoprostenol	Pulmonary hypertension
Autologous stem cell transplant	Juvenile arthritis, systemic lupus erythematosus
Sodium nitroprusside drip[65-67]	Erythromelalgia
Plasmapheresis	Thrombotic thrombocytopenic purpura; other diagnoses have less definite response

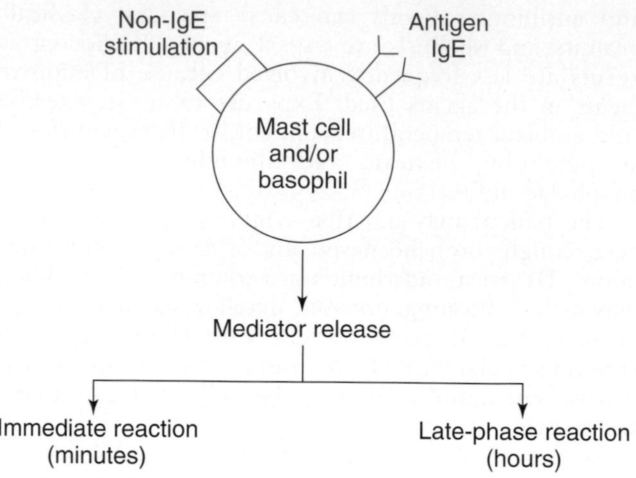

FIGURE 91–5 • Mast cell or basophil activation can occur after the binding of two immunoglobulin E (IgE) molecules by antigen or through non-IgE stimulation. The consequence of this mediator release depends on the target organ involved and can occur within minutes (immediate reaction) or over a period of hours (late-phase reaction).

helps with diagnosis is C4, which is low even if the patient does not have symptoms. Combining C1INH levels with C4 measurement improves diagnostic accuracy.[63,64] Treatment of hereditary angioedema includes use of epinephrine and airway support if required.

Summary

The patient with autoimmune or inflammatory diseases may have life-threatening complications of the disease, their treatment, or a combination of both. Vasculitis may present initially in the critical care setting and should be considered in any patient with multiorgan involvement, especially if fever and inflammatory markers are present and infection and malignancy have been ruled out. Few pathognomonic signs or laboratory studies confirm the diagnosis of rheumatic illness, requiring the clinician to have a high clinical suspicion at the outset. Recognition of the pulmonary, cardiac, nervous system, and GI complications of rheumatic diseases help institute appropriate therapy in a timely manner, improving outcomes for patients with these serious diseases. Infection should be sought and treated as indicated. Immune dysregulation can occur in any patient, and attention to supportive care of the airway and circulation has a significant role in the treatment plan. Patients with known inflammatory diseases are prone to morbidity and mortality, but rapid recognition and directed aggressive therapy may improve clinical outcomes in this special population.

REFERENCES

1. Hammer R, Maika S, Richardson J, et al: Spontaneous inflammatory disease in transgenic rats expressing HLA-B27 and human beta 2m: an animal model of HLA-B27 associated with human disorders, *Cell* 63:1099-1112, 1990.
2. Reumaux D, Duthilleal P, Roos D: Pathogenesis of diseases associated with antineutrophil cytoplasm autoantibodies, *Hum Immunol* 65: 1-12, 2004.
3. Steere A, Malwista S, Snydman D, et al: Lyme arthritis: an epidemic of oligoarticular arthritis in children and adults in three Connecticut communities, *Arthritis Rheum* 20:7-17, 1977.

4a. Cassidy JT, Petty RE: Systemic lupus erythematosus. Laxer RM, Gazarian M: Pharmacology and drug therapy. In Cassidy JT, Petty RE, editors: *Textbook of pediatric rheumatology,* ed 4, Philadelphia, 2001, WB Saunders.

4b. Laxer RM, Gazarian M: Pharmacology and drug therapy. In Cassidy JT, Petty RE, editors: *Textbook of pediatric rheumatology,* ed 4, Philadelphia, 2001, WB Saunders.

5. Miller RW, Salcedo JR, Fink RJ, et al: Pulmonary hemorrhage in pediatric patients with systemic lupus erythematosus, *J Pediatr* 108:576-579, 1986.
6. Moder KG, DT Miller, Tazelaar HD: Cardiac involvement in systemic lupus erythematosus, *Mayo Clin Proc* 74:275-284, 1999.
7. Oshiro AC, Derbes SJ, Stopa AR, Gedalia A: Anti-Ro/SS-A and anti-La/SS-B antibodies associated with cardiac involvement in childhood systemic lupus erythematosus, *Ann Rheum Dis* 56: 272-274, 1997.
8. Rahman P, Urowitz RM, Gladman DD, et al: Contribution of traditional risk factors to coronary artery disease in patients with systemic lupus erythematosus, *J Rheumatol* 26:2363-2368, 1999.
9. Bansal VK, Beto JA: Treatment of lupus nephritis: a meta-analysis of clinical trials, *Am J Kidney Dis* 29:193-199,1997.
10. Boumpas DT, Austin HA III, Vaughn EM, et al: Controlled trial of pulse methylprednisolone versus two regimens of pulse cyclophosphamide in severe lupus nephritis, *Lancet* 340:741-745, 1992.
11. Klippel J: Systemic lupus erythematosus. In Klippel J, Dieppe P, editors: *Rheumatology,* ed 2, St Louis, 2001, Mosby.
12. Wallace DJ, Hahn BH: *Dubois' lupus erythematosus,* Philadelphia, 2002, Lippincott Williams & Wilkins.
13. Musio F, Bohen EM, Yuan CM, Welch PG: Review of thrombotic thrombocytopenic purpura in the setting of systemic lupus erythematosus, *Semin Arthritis Rheum* 28:1-19, 1998.
14. Al-Mayouf S, Al-Mayyed A, Bahabri S: Efficacy of early treatment of severe juvenile dermatomyositis with intravenous methylprednisolone and methotrexate, *Clin Rheumatol* 19:138-141, 2000.
15. Al-Mayouf SM, Laxer RM, Schnieder R, et al: Intravenous immunoglobulin therapy for juvenile dermatomyositis: efficacy and safety, *J Rheumatol* 27:2498-2503, 2000.
16. Reiff A, Rawlings DJ, Shaham B, et al: Preliminary evidence for cyclosporine A as an alternative in the treatment of recalcitrant juvenile rheumatoid arthritis and juvenile dermatomyositis, *J Rheumatol* 24:2436-2443, 1997.
17. Riley P, Maillard SM, Wedderburn LR, et al: Intravenous cyclophosphamide pulse therapy in juvenile dermatomyositis. A review of efficacy and safety, *Rheumatology* 43:491-496, 2004.
18. Foeldvari I, Wulffraat N: Recognition and management of scleroderma in children, *Paediatr Drugs* 3:575-583, 2001.
19. Murray KJ, Laxer RM: Scleroderma in children and adolescents, *Rheum Dis Clin North Am* 28:603-24, 2002.
20. Fleishmajer R, Perlish JS: Capillary alterations in scleroderma, *J Am Acad Dermatol* 2:161-70, 1980.
21. Uziel Y, Miller ML, Laxer RM: Scleroderma in children, *Pediatr Clin North Am* 42:1171-1203, 1995.
22. Sastry BKS, Narasimhan C, Reddy NK, Raju BS: Clinical efficacy of sildenafil in primary pulmonary hypertension, *J Am Coll Cardiol* 43:1149-1153, 2004.
23. Sitbon O, Badesch DB, Channick RN, et al: Effects of the dual endothelin receptor antagonist bosentan in patients with arterial hypertension: a 1-year follow-up study, *Chest* 124:247-54, 2003.
24. Steen VD, Medsger TA: Case-control study of corticosteroids and other drugs that either precipitate or protect from the development of scleroderma renal crisis, *Arthritis Rheum* 41:1613-1619, 1998.
25. Calabrese LH, Duna GF, Lie JT: Vasculitis in the central nervous system, *Arthritis Rheum* 40:1189-1201, 1997.
26. Gallagher KT, Shaham B, Reiff A, et al: Primary angiitis of the central nervous system in children: 5 cases, *J Rheumatol* 28: 616-623, 2001.
27. Younger DS: Vasculitis of the nervous system, *Curr Opin Neurol* 17:317-336, 2004.

27a. Calabrese LH, Mallek JA: Primary angiitis of the central nervous system. Report of 8 new cases, review of the literature, and proposal for diagnostic criteria, *Medicine* 67:20-39, 1987.

28. de Groot K, Schmidt DK, Arlt AC, et al: Standardized neurologic evaluations of 128 patients with Wegener granulomatosus, *Arch Neurol* 58:1215-1221, 2001.
29. Abdou NI, Kullman GJ, Hoffman GS, et al: Wegener's granulomatosis: survey of 701 patients in North America. Changes in outcome in the 1990s, *J Rheumatol* 29:309-16. 2002.
30. Regan MJ, Hellmann DB, Stone JH: Treatment of Wegener's granulomatosus, *Rheum Dis Clin North Am* 27:863-886, 2001.
31. Mollica F, Li Volti S, Garozzo R, Russo G: Effectiveness of early prednisone treatment in preventing the development of nephropathy in anaphylactoid purpura, *Eur J Pediatr* 151:140-144, 1992.
32. Szer IS: Henoch-Schonlein purpura: when and how to treat, *J Rheumatol* 23:1661-1665, 1996.
33. Falcini F: Vascular and connective tissue diseases in the pediatric world, *Lupus* 13:77-84, 2004
34. Guillevin L, Durand-Gasselin B, Cevallos R, et al: Microscopic polyangiitis. Clinical and laboratory findings in eighty-five patients, *Arthritis Rheum* 42:421-430, 1999.
35. Jennette JC, Falk RJ: Small-vessel vasculitis, *N Engl J Med* 337: 1512-1523, 1997.
36. Rowley AH, Gonzolez-Crussi F, Gidding SS, et al: Incomplete Kawasaki disease with coronary artery involvement, *J Pediatr* 110: 401-413, 1987.
37. Barron KS, Shulman ST, Rowley A, et al: Report of the National Institutes of Health workshop on Kawasaki disease, *J Rheumatol* 26:170-190, 1999.
38. Sundel RP, Baker AL, Fulton DR, Newburger JW: Corticosteroids in the initial treatment of Kawasaki disease: report of a randomized trial, *J Pediatr* 142:611-6, 2003.
39. Sabbadini MG, Bozzolo E, Baldisera E, Bellone M: Takayasu's arteritis: therapeutic strategies, *J Nephrol* 14:525-531, 2001.
40. Hoffman GS, Merkel PA, Brasington RD, et al: Anti-tumor necrosis factor therapy in patients with difficult to treat Takayasu arteritis, *Arthritis Rheum* 50:2296-2304, 2004
41. Fessler BJ: Life threatening complications of autoimmune disease: thrombotic syndromes and autoimmune diseases, *Rheum Dis Clin North Am* 23:463-479, 1997.
42. Brunner HI, Freedman M, Silverman ED: Close relationship between systemic lupus erythematosus and thrombotic thrombocytopenic purpura in childhood, *Arthritis Rheum* 42:2346-2355, 1999.
43. Ravelli A: Macrophage activation syndrome, *Curr Opin Rheumatol* 14:548-552, 2002.
44. Stephan JL, Kone-Paut I, Galambrum C, et al: Reactive haemophagocytic syndrome in children with inflammatory disorders. A retrospective study of 24 patients, *Rheumatology* 40:1285-1292, 2001.
45. Bloom BJ, Tucker LB, Miller LC, Schaller JG: Fibrin d-dimer as a marker of disease activity in systemic onset juvenile rheumatoid arthritis, *J Rheum* 25:1620-1625, 1998.
46. Emmenegger U, Reimers A, Frey U, et al: Reactive macrophage activation syndrome: a simple screening strategy and its potential in early treatment initiation, *Swiss Med Wkly* 132:230-236, 2002.
47. Hadchouel J, Prieur A-M Griscelli C: Acute hemorraghic, hepatic, and neurologic manifestations in juvenile rheumatoid arthritis: possible relationships to drugs or infection, *J Pediatr* 106:561-566, 1985.
48. Mukamel M, Bernstein BH, Brik R, Lehman TJA: The prevalence of coagulation abnormalities in juvenile rheumatoid arthritis, *J Rheumatol* 14:1147-1149, 1987.
49. Mouy R, Stephan JL, Pilet P, et al: Efficacy of cyclosporine A in the treatment of macrophage activation syndrome in juvenile arthritis: report of five cases, *J Pediatr* 129:750-754, 1996.
50. Popat MT, Chippa JH, Russell R: Awake fibreoptic intubation following failed regional anaesthesia for Caesarean section in a parturient with Still's disease, *Eur J Anaesthesiol* 17:211-214, 2000.
51. Wang LC, Yang YH, Lu MY, Chiang BL: Retrospective analysis of mortality and morbidity of pediatric systemic lupus erythematosus in the past two decades, *J Microbiol Immunol Infect* 36:203-208, 2003.
52. Thong BY, Tai DY, Goh SK, Johan A: An audit of patients with rheumatic disease requiring medical intensive care, *Ann Acad Med Singapore* 30:254-250, 2001.
53. Guillevin L, Durand-Gasselin B, Cevallos R, et al: Microscopic polyangiitis. Clinical and laboratory findings in eighty-five patients, *Arthritis Rheum* 42:421-430, 1999.
54. Hamilton CD: Infectious complications of treatment with biologic agents, *Curr Opin Rheumatol* 16:393-398, 2004.
55. Breshnihan B, Cunnane G: Infection complications associated with the use of biologic agents, *Rheum Dis Clin North Am* 29:185-202, 2003.
56. Quartier P, Brethon B, Phillippet P, et al: Treatment of childhood autoimmune haemolytic anaemia with rituximab, *Lancet* 358:1511-1513, 2001.
57. Barr WG, Robinson JA: Rheumatology in the ICU. In Hall JB, Schmidt GA, Wood LDH, editors: *Principles of critical care,* ed 2, New York, 1998, McGraw-Hill.
58. Hansen-Flashen J: Neuromuscular disorders of critical illness, *Up To Date.* Last updated November 2003.
59. Hudson LD, Lee CM: Neuromuscular sequelae of critical illness, *N Engl J Med* 348:745-747, 2003.
60. deLetter M-ACJ, Schmitz PIM, Visser LH, et al: Risk factors for the development of polyneuropathy and myopathy in critically ill patients, *Crit Care Med* 29:2281-2286, 2001.
61. De Jonghe B , Sharshar T, Lefaucheur J-P, et al: Paresis acquired in the intensive care unit. A prospective multicenter study, *JAMA* 288:2859-2867, 2002.
62. Lieberman PL: Anaphylaxis and anaphylactoid reactions. In: *Middleton's Allergy Principles and Practice,* ed 6, Adkmson NF, Yuninger JW, Busse WW, et al, editors. Philadelphia, 2003, Mosby.
63. Gompels MM, Lock RJ, Morgan JE, et al: A multicentre evaluation of the diagnostic accuracy of serological investigations for C1 inhibitor deficiency, *J Clin Pathol* 55:145-147, 2002.
64. Karim Y, Griffiths H, Deacock S: Normal complement C4 values do not exclude hereditary angioedema, *J Clin Pathol* 57:213-214, 2004.
65. Chan MKH, Tucker AI, S Madden, et al: Erythromelalgia: an endothelial disorder responsive to sodium nitroprusside. *Arch Dis Child* 87:229-230, 2002.
66. Ozsoylu S, Caner H, Gokalp A: Successful treatment of erythromelalgia with sodium nitroprusside. *J Pediatr* 94:619-621, 1979.
67. Drenth JPH, Nichiels, Ozsoylu S: Acute secondary erythermalgia and hypertension in children. *Eur J Pediatr* 154:882-885, 1995.

CHAPTER

92

Genomic and Proteomic Medicine in Critical Care

David Jardine

PEARLS

- When contemplating the great diversity among humans, it is somewhat surprising to realize that the deoxyribonucleic acid (DNA) of two unrelated humans is more than 99.9% identical.
- One single nucleotide polymorphism (SNP) is believed to occur in every 100 to 300 bases. Although most of the SNPs in the human genome remain to be identified, if this figure holds true for the entire genome, then more than 20 million SNPs exist in our genome, which constitutes an enormous source of variation.
- Although high-throughput screening technology has not yet been implemented for individual patients, almost certainly in the near future high-throughput technologies will be used to provide information on an individual patient's disease or response to therapy.
- Most examples of medical applications for genomic and proteomic technologies come from the fields of cancer and pharmacology. Genomic technologies have great promise for critical care medicine. In the future, these technologies may help us to diagnose disease and to select appropriate medications and doses for our patients.
- Genomic medicine will provide us with tremendous benefits and challenges. Perhaps one of the greatest benefits will be the understanding that human similarities and differences transcend the racial and ethnic categories that have proved so contentious in the past.

The recently developed disciplines of genomics and proteomics are producing significant change in the biologic sciences. In the next decade, these disciplines are projected to have a major effect on clinical medicine, both in speeding the development of new therapies and in helping to create individualized therapy that is specifically tailored to the disease and drug metabolism characteristics of each patient.

A hallmark of these new technologies is their production of massive quantities of data, so they often are described as "high-throughput" technologies. They force us to simultaneously consider many components of a biologic system rather than focusing on a single pathway or product. To meet the challenge of extracting meaningful information from overwhelming quantities of data, the new discipline of systems biology is being developed. The goals of systems biology are to integrate information from a variety of sources and to develop a comprehensive picture of the relationships and interactions between the components of a biologic system.

From the Discovery of the Double Helix to the Human Genome Project

In 1953, in a manuscript that scarcely exceeded one page,[1] the double helical structure of deoxyribonucleic acid (DNA) was described. This brief report opened the door for a new understanding of heredity and gene function. In this new era, the field of molecular biology emerged and deciphering the genetic code began. For the first 40 years, elucidating the structure and sequence of genes proceeded slowly, depending mostly on methodical detective work and a certain measure of luck. Thirty years passed before the gene for Huntington disease was mapped to a region on the short arm of chromosome 4, marking the first time that a disease-causing gene was mapped to a region of an apparently normal chromosome (Figure 92–1). Because the methods for isolating and sequencing genes were in their infancy, another 10 years would elapse before the sequence of the gene was known and the abnormality causing Huntington disease was identified. The cystic fibrosis gene was among the earliest disease-causing genes to be sequenced. Among the insights gained was that the disease was genetically heterogenous. Only 70% of patients with this illness had the most common mutation (δF508); the remaining patients could have any of hundreds of mutations in the chloride channel protein encoded by this gene. Knowledge of the gene's structure helped to explain the tremendous diversity in the clinical manifestations of this disease.

By 1990, a handful of genes had been identified and sequenced. Although the efforts of scientists around the world were gradually yielding results, progress was slow. A long time elapsed before a large proportion of human genes were identified and sequenced. A solution to this problem came from two complementary advances in seemingly unrelated scientific fields. High-throughput automated DNA sequencing was developed, allowing rapid determination of long DNA sequences. This development was a mixed blessing because managing the large volumes of sequence information could have overwhelmed investigators and slowed progress. Fortunately, the rapid increase in computing power in mainframe and desktop computers and the availability of the Internet to link investigators to public databases provided a solution to this problem. A skillful fusion of these technologies greatly accelerated the pace of gene sequencing.

In the late 1980s and early 1990, leaders from the National Institutes of Health and the Department of Energy began to create the infrastructure necessary for large-scale sequencing of the human genome. Although the Human Genome Project began in the early 1990s, the international effort to sequence the entire genome did not begin until 1998.[2] Remarkably, this massive project was completed just 5 years later.[3] In what must be one of the more significant acts of placing the greater good before prestige and personal gain, scientists throughout the world contributed DNA sequence data to public databases so that the entire sequence of the human genome is freely available to any investigator with a computer and Internet access.

In the early 1990s, as the DNA sequence of an increasing number of genes became available, a small number of investigators began to experiment with gene microarrays. These investigators printed slides with a series of spots, in which each spot contained the DNA from a single gene. As the technology improved, the investigators were able to examine the expression of an increasingly larger number of genes in a single experiment. In the earliest published experiments, the investigators examined expression patterns of 45 yeast genes.[4] Less than a decade later, commercially produced microarrays are available with more than 30,000 human genes on each array.[5] These powerful tools are readily available to laboratory investigators and are beginning to find their way into clinical practice. Clearly, microarrays and other high-throughput technologies will have a profound effect on clinical medicine in the future.

How Microarrays Work

DNA microarray use has increased exponentially since 1995 when the first DNA microarray publications appeared in the literature (Figure 92–2). This technology

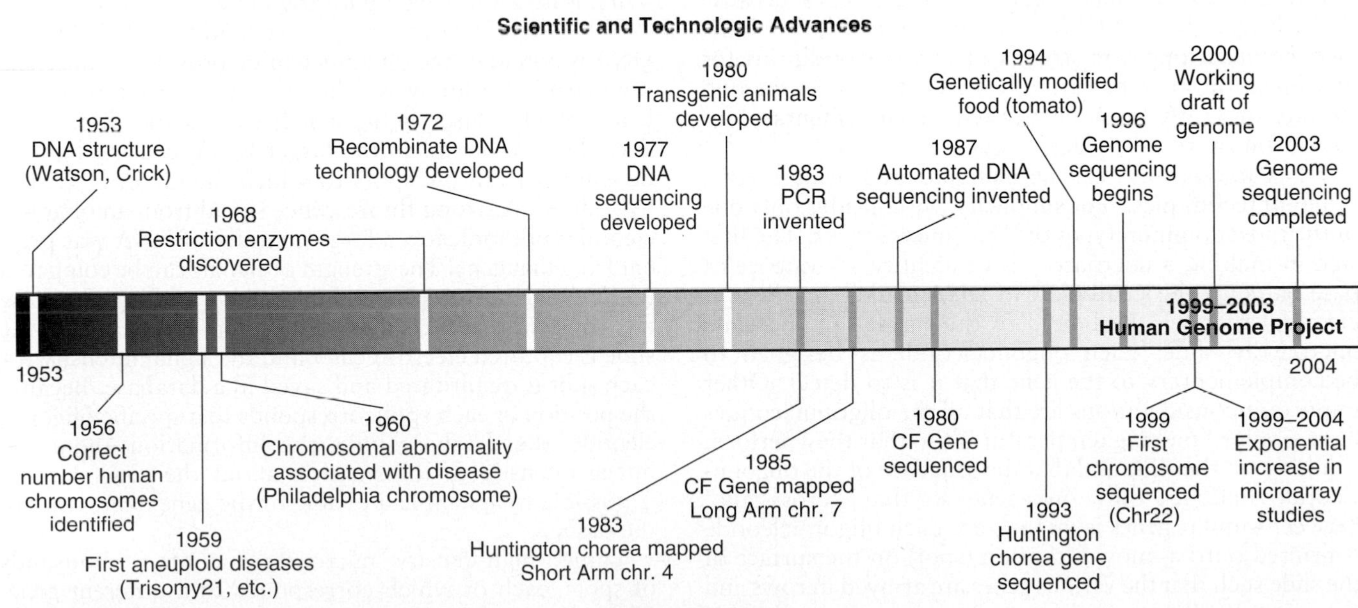

FIGURE 92–1 • Milestones in molecular biology and sequencing of the human genome.

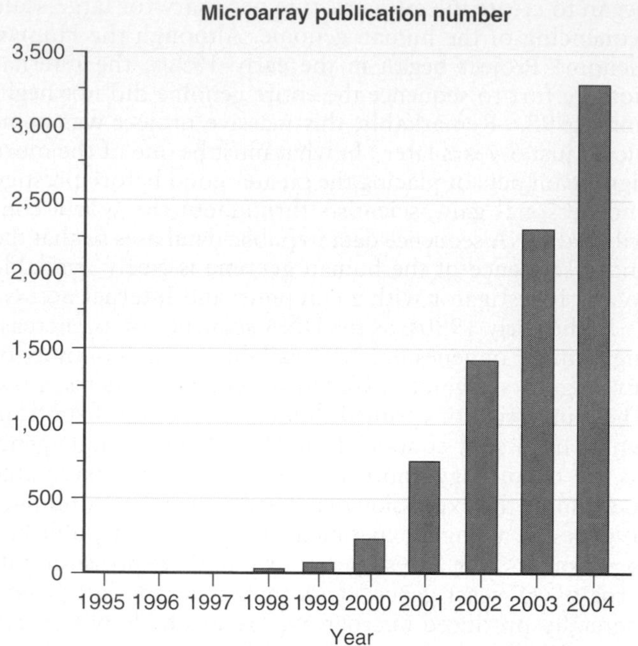

FIGURE 92–2 • Exponential increase in publications discussing or using microarray technology.

is a major new tool that will continue to produce biologic insights for many years to come.

All DNA microarrays start with known gene sequences. This information is taken from public databases. As new information about the sequence and function of genes becomes available, it is added to the database so that the latest information is readily available to investigators who are using microarrays. DNA microarrays depend on the property of a single strand of DNA in solution to hybridize with a complementary strand of DNA that is bound to the microarray slide. Hybridization occurs because of hydrogen bonding between purine and pyrimidine base pairs on opposite strands of DNA. Conditions for hybridization must be carefully selected because the two strands of DNA must be perfectly complementary for hybridization to take place.

DNA microarrays can be manufactured using several different techniques.[6] For simplicity, we consider only one of the most common types of DNA microarrays. The first step in making a microarray is to identify a sequence of base pairs for the small piece of DNA (called an *oligonucleotide)* that will be bound to the surface of the glass microarray slide. Each oligonucleotide is designed to be complementary to the gene that it is to detect. Other important considerations are that all the oligonucleotides have similar "melting temperatures" so that they perform similarly on the slide and that the sequence of the oligonucleotide matches only one gene so that "cross-talk" between similar genes is minimized. Each oligonucleotide is printed onto a known location (spot) on the surface of the slide such that the various genes are arrayed in rows and columns. Each spot contains a unique oligonucleotide designed to hybridize with a single gene. The oligonucleotides bound to the slide are called *probes*.

Quantifying Gene Expression

When a gene is expressed in a cell, the DNA from that gene is transcribed into ribonucleic acid (RNA). This is transported out of the nucleus and then used as a template to guide the synthesis of proteins in the cell. At any given time, the RNA content of a cell represents a snapshot of the genes being expressed and the proteins being made in the cell.

To learn about the metabolic activity of a tissue, the RNA must be extracted from the cells. If a gene is turned on (up-regulated), more RNA will be produced from that gene. Conversely, if a gene is turned off (down-regulated), less RNA will be produced from that gene. RNA does not hybridize well to DNA,[1] so the RNA is reverse transcribed to make DNA. Because this DNA is complementary to RNA, it is called *complementary DNA* (cDNA). During reverse transcription, the cDNA is labeled with a fluorescent dye so that it can be detected once it is hybridized (bound) to an oligonucleotide on the microarray.

Once the labeled cDNA is made, the solution containing the labeled cDNA is placed on the microarray and the conditions are carefully adjusted so that the oligonucleotides will hybridize only with strands of cDNA that are exactly complementary (Figure 92-3). At the end of the hybridization, the amount of labeled cDNA hybridized to each oligonucleotide spot will be proportional to the quantity of RNA that was expressed from the target gene. Microarray experiments usually are designed so that gene expression from two tissue samples can be directly compared. This allows investigators to learn how different conditions can alter gene expression. (Note: Although most microarrays operate by the principle described here, one of the most popular types of microarrays, which is manufactured by the Affymetrix Corporation, works on the principle of hybridizing very short segments of labeled RNA to the oligonucleotide probes. Because the length of the RNA is limited to approximately 20 base pairs, it hybridizes well with the DNA.)

When hybridization is complete and the labeled target DNA is bound to the oligonucleotide probes, the microarray is ready for analysis. The microarray is exposed to a beam of blue laser light, which excites the fluorescent dyes that are bound to the target DNA, causing light to be emitted from the spots to which the target DNA has hybridized. A strong fluorescence signal from an oligonucleotide spot indicates a large quantity of RNA was present from that gene. The strength of signals can be compared under different experimental conditions to determine how the conditions affect gene regulation. An image of the slide is captured electronically and the signal intensity for each spot is quantitated and saved in a database. Because the position of each spot corresponds to a specific oligonucleotide, the database links the information about the image intensity to information about the gene. It now is possible to assemble a profile of the gene expression in the tissue.

Large, high-density microarrays contain thousands of spots, each of which corresponds to a different gene. Managing and analyzing this data would be nearly impossible if not for the substantial power available from desktop computers and the use of specialized software

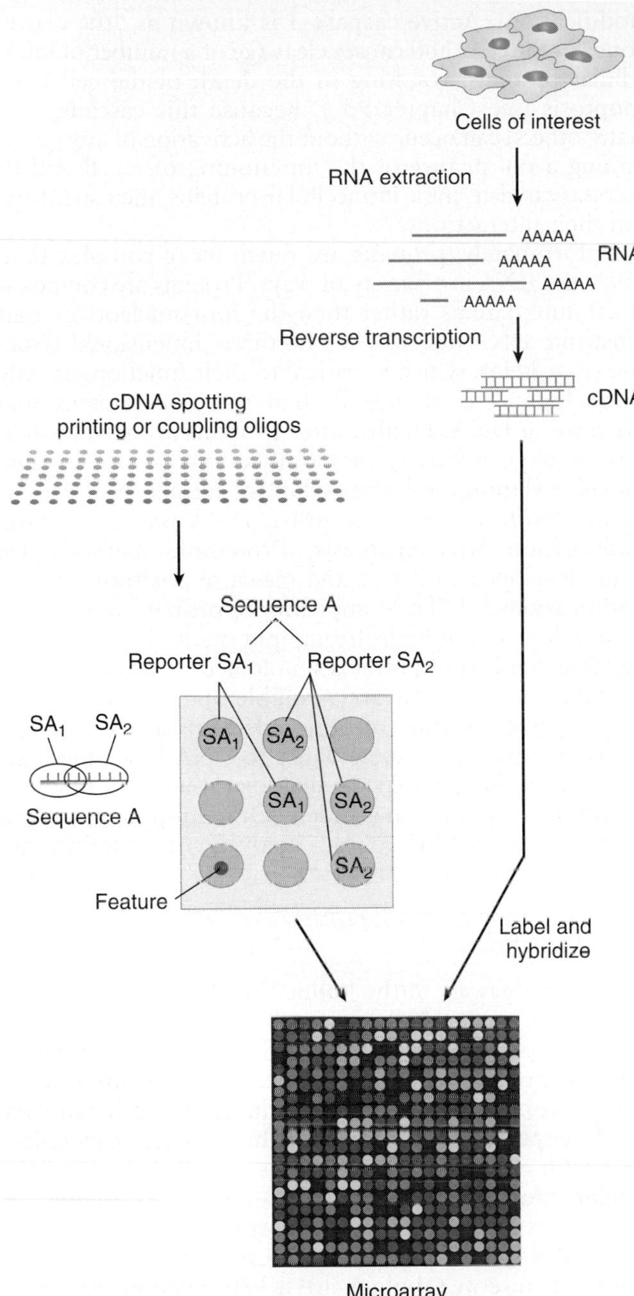

FIGURE 92–3 • Making of a microarray. Ribonucleic acid (RNA) is isolated from a cell and reverse transcribed into labeled complementary deoxyribonucleic acid (cDNA). This is placed on the surface of a slide, which is covered with spots of oligonucleotides that are complementary to the cDNA. Under carefully regulated conditions, the labeled cDNA specifically hybridizes with a complementary oligonucleotide. Under a fluorescent laser, the brightness of each oligonucleotide spot is proportional to the quantity of cDNA bound to it. The brightness is measured to determine the relative amounts of RNA from each gene in the cells.

packages designed for microarray data analysis. Using this technology, it is possible to track the expression patterns of sets of genes and observe how these patterns change under different conditions. Analysis of gene expression patterns can provide new insights into how tissues and organs respond to a disease or a therapy.

One of the most important aspects of information gained from gene expression analysis is determining how gene expression is altered by different situations. At the cellular level, maintenance of homeostasis often means altering gene expression to compensate for changes in a cell's environment. Learning which genes are activated or suppressed by changes caused by disease can suggest new targets for therapies directed specifically at correcting the molecular changes created by a disease state. The study of gene expression and gene function is termed *functional genomics.*

Genes, Human Variation, and Single Nucleotide Polymorphisms

It is an accepted axiom that two people differ because of differences between their DNA. When contemplating the great diversity among humans, it is somewhat surprising to realize that the DNA of two unrelated humans is more than 99.9% identical.[7] Most of the crucial differences in our genes can be attributed to the substitution of one nucleotide for another. The single nucleotide substitutions are called *single nucleotide polymorphisms* (SNPs). For example, the sequences GATCACA and GATTACA differ because the cytosine (C) in the first sequence has been replaced by a thymine (T) in the second sequence. This example represents the most common human SNP, which involves the substitution of T for C.

Although such substitutions may occur spontaneously and represent a new mutation, the vast majority of substitutions are stable variations in the human gene pool. If a substitution at a given site occurs in more than 1% of the population, it is deemed to be a *polymorphism.*[8] SNPs are the most common type of polymorphism, accounting for approximately 90% of human variation.[9] One SNP is believed to occur in every 100 to 300 bases. Although most of the SNPs in the human genome remain to be identified, if this figure holds true for the entire genome, then more than 20 million SNPs exist in our genome, which constitutes an enormous source of variation.

SNPs may alter function in several ways. For example, altering a single base can alter an amino acid in a protein, leading to a change in protein function. SNPs can also have significant effects without altering proteins. An SNP occurring in a promoter region, which controls protein synthesis, may lead to increased or decreased synthesis of that protein, which may have significant effects. Although SNPs are still being mapped and the function of most SNPs is still being defined, clearly these substitutions are responsible for the vast majority of human phenotypes, from differences in hair color to differences in response to medications.

DNA microarrays have been designed for SNP genotyping. These microarrays are similar to those used for gene expression studies, but the oligonucleotides on SNP arrays have each been designed to selectively hybridize with one form of an SNP. These microarrays can quickly reveal the SNP genotype of a research subject. The ability to define the genetic components of variation with speed and precision is more than a valuable research tool.

In the near future, this information will be used to help select therapies for illness, taking into consideration the individual variations that can be predicted on the basis of a patient's SNP genotype. As more SNPs are identified and their function understood, this technology likely will become an integral part of clinical practice. In the future, SNP technology likely will permit physicians to plan highly individualized therapy for each patient, taking into account issues such as individual disease susceptibility and variations in drug metabolism.

Beyond DNA Microarrays

Although DNA microarrays are the best known and most widely used high-throughput technology to emerge from the genomic revolution, other important technologies are being increasingly used as research tools and show promise as future clinical tools. Although our genes carry the blueprint for an organism, proteins form much of the structure and perform most of the mechanical work. Seeking to achieve an integrated view of the proteins in an organism (the proteome), investigators are developing methods that permit simultaneous analysis of large numbers of proteins, in much the same way that DNA microarrays permit simultaneous analysis of large numbers of genes. This new field is termed *proteomics.* Similar developments are taking place in the area of metabolism (termed *metabolomics).* Finally, the field of systems biology is being developed as investigators attempt to integrate the information from the fields of genomics, proteomics, and metabolomics.

Proteomics

Genes are the main sites of biologic information, but proteins are the main centers of biologic activity, which gives proteins a unique importance. The discipline of proteomics encompasses the study of all the proteins encoded by the genome and includes the study of the modifications that occur after protein synthesis. Because the protein complement within a cell can vary widely over time in response to intracellular and extracellular influences, any picture of the proteome must consider these influences. Knowing which genes are expressed or suppressed by a given disease state is important but is only part of the picture. After proteins are synthesized, they can be modified in a number of ways that can dramatically alter their function. For example, the tumor necrosis factor (TNF) signaling pathway can induce apoptosis (programmed cell death) through a series of protein modifications that do not require activation of any genes. After TNF binds to its receptor, a group of signaling proteins forms an active multimer (association is the first of protein modification in this cascade). This multimer cleaves caspase-8, converting one of the fragments into the active form (second protein modification). Activated caspase-8 damages the mitochondrion, causing leakage of cytochrome C into the cytoplasm. The presence of cytochrome C results in the association of several proteins into a structure called an *apoptosome* (third protein modification). The apoptosome cleaves procaspase-3 to the active form (fourth protein modification). Active caspase-3 is known as "the executioner of the cell" and causes cleavage of a number of intracellular proteins, resulting in the death of the cell from apoptosis (see Chapter 93). Because this cascade (and many others) can occur without the activation of any genes, gaining a full picture of the functioning of a cell will be necessary to determine intracellular proteins, their structure, and their interactions.

Unfortunately, proteins are much more complex than DNA and RNA in a variety of ways. Proteins are composed of 20 amino acids rather than the four nucleotides that constitute DNA and RNA. The three-dimensional structure of proteins, which is critical to their function, usually is much more complicated than the three-dimensional structure of DNA. Finally, after proteins are synthesized, they undergo a variety of modifications (e.g., cleavage, phosphorylation, and glycosylation) termed *posttranslational modifications.* In contrast, DNA undergoes little modification after synthesis. Proteomic methods are being developed to detect and measure posttranslational modifications.[10,11] The complexity of proteins has slowed the development of high-throughput methods for examining large numbers of proteins simultaneously. Nevertheless, several techniques now are available that permit simultaneous characterization of hundreds of proteins. Some of the techniques bear a resemblance to DNA-based microarrays, except that proteins or ligands rather than oligonucleotides are spotted on a slide.[12] Other approaches, such as mass spectrometry-based analysis of proteins, are showing considerable promise.[13]

Metabolomics

Perhaps the newest of the "omic" fields is metabolomics, which is the study of all the metabolites within a cell. The goal is to provide a comprehensive picture of the metabolic state of a cell or tissue by measuring the full suite of metabolites. The metabolites produced in a cell can vary widely depending on external influences and can reflect the health of the cell. Metabolites are at the end of the cellular information chain (DNA → RNA → proteins → metabolites), but the metabolic state of the cell often drives RNA and protein synthesis through feedback loops. Because metabolites are a heterogenous group of small molecules, many of which are structurally unrelated, this field presents great challenges. Substantial progress is being made in measuring the metabolic state of a cell using the technologies of gas and liquid chromatography coupled to mass spectrometry.[14,15] At present, most efforts are directed at developing a comprehensive understanding of metabolic interactions in simple organisms (microbes and yeast), which are less complex than higher organisms. Undoubtedly, metabolomic investigations in higher organisms will follow.

Systems Biology

Together, the fields of genomics, proteomics, and metabolomics characterize biologic processes at a level of detail that was almost unimaginable 20 years ago. However, amalgamating these details into a meaningful narrative is one of the greatest challenges facing scientists (the genomic data alone can have more than 30,000 data points per experiment). The ambitious goal of systems biologists is to integrate data from all the "omic" disciplines, identify important components, and assemble the knowledge into a meaningful whole that can be validated (Figure 92–4).[16] Because of the obvious technical challenges in such an undertaking, this field is still relatively new. As techniques advance, systems information should provide scientists with opportunities to model system behavior.[17] Hopefully this undertaking will provide a more integrated understanding of the behavior of biologic organisms and enhance our ability to predict outcomes and develop new therapies.[18] Ultimately, to realize the tremendous potential that is inherent in genomics, proteomics, and metabolomics, we will require an understanding of the interactions of these systems to help us determine the interactions between these systems.

Systems biology is not the only approach being used by investigators to integrate information from genomics and proteomics. Metabolic control analysis is another discipline dedicated to the development of an integrated overview of genetic, enzymatic, and substrate control mechanisms in biologic systems. When a metabolic control analysis is fully developed, a control coefficient is assigned to each step in an enzymatic pathway.[19] These coefficients reflect the magnitude of change that is induced in a pathway compared with the change in the state or level of an enzyme. Enzymes with high coefficients are logical targets for therapeutic intervention (drug design). Identification of important regulatory points also can help with the understanding of carcinogenesis and can provide new insights into genetic disorders.

Clinical Applications of Genomic Technologies

These new technologies offer great promise for clinical medicine. At the research level, new biologic insights already are becoming available as a result of high-throughput technologies. Clearly, genomic screening of tumors can aid in diagnostic classification, and SNP analysis of enzymes involved in drug metabolism can characterize an individual's response to some drugs. Although high-throughput screening technology has not yet been implemented for individual patients, almost certainly in the near future high-throughput technologies will provide information about an individual patient's disease or response to therapy.

Almost every human disease has a genetic component.[7] For monogenic diseases with an easily detectable phenotype and strong penetrance, the genetic component is easily recognized (e.g., cystic fibrosis, Huntington chorea). For many such monogenic diseases, the gene has been isolated and cloned, and the abnormal, disease-causing sequence has been identified. Progress from recognition of a monogenic disease through identifying the gene occurs far more rapidly now that the human genome has been sequenced.

Unfortunately, for other common diseases, such as type II diabetes and atherosclerotic cardiovascular disease, the story likely is far more complex. Many diseases appear to result from interactions among several genes. Such polygenic diseases will be far more difficult to understand because a polymorphism of one gene may be pathogenic only when it occurs in the presence of disease-causing

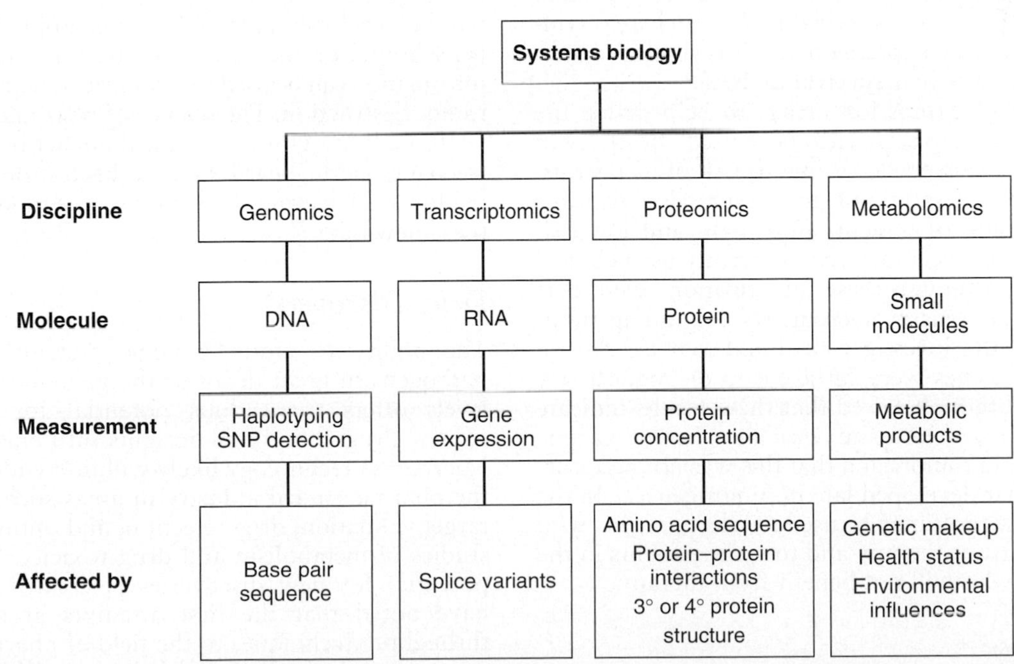

FIGURE 92–4 • The goal of systems biology is to provide an integrated picture of all cellular functions. Each of the "omic" fields provides a comprehensive picture of one aspect of cellular function. (Modified from Minie ME: 2004. Expression resources. Module 7. In: *NCBI Advanced Workshop for Bioinformatics Information Specialists.* Geer RC, Messersmith DJ, Alpi K, Bhagwat M, Chattopadhyay A, Gaedeke N, Lyon J, Minie ME, Morris RC, Ohles JA, Osterbur DL, Tennant MR. Available at http://www.ncbi.nlm.nih.gov/Class/NAWBIS/. March 31, 2005.)

polymorphisms in other genes. To add to the complexity, environmental factors influence the development of disease, so these effects also must be considered. Although monogenic diseases are far easier to understand, only a minority of diseases appear to be monogenic. A complete understanding of the cause of many diseases will not be determined by a simple one gene–one disease approach. Instead, it will depend on understanding the complex interactions of polymorphisms of a group of genes and the effect of the environment on these polymorphisms. Nevertheless, the knowledge gained from genomics almost certainly will be widely utilized in clinical medicine. In particular, SNP analysis likely will be used to help determine a patient's disease susceptibility, prognosis, and response to therapy.

Cancer

Oncologists have made extensive use of gene expression profiling to revise and more accurately classify the prognostic categories of malignancies.[20-23] One of the earliest uses of microarray technology for prognostic purposes was to study lymphomas using a specialized microarray, the "Lymphochip." Using this microarray, investigators were able to identify different histologic classes of lymphoma by their gene expression patterns, indicating that histologically distinguishable tumors differ in their gene expression, so these tumors can be distinguished at a molecular level. More importantly, the investigators found patients with gene expression patterns that permitted them to separate B-cell lymphomas into two groups: one group that resembled germinal center B cells and another that resembled activated B lymphocytes. Although these subgroups had identical histology, patient survival was significantly altered by the gene expression patterns. The lymphomas that had gene expression patterns similar to germinal center B cells had a 5-year survival of 76%, whereas lymphomas that had gene expression patterns similar to activated B cells had a 5-year survival of 16%.

The promise of expression arrays to help define the prognosis of tumor types has also been used effectively in classifying breast cancers according to risk of metastasis. Use of microarray analysis of gene expression patterns permitted grouping of patients into high- and low-risk groups with greater accuracy than currently used clinical parameters.[24,25] Although these investigations were performed with high-density microarrays containing thousands of genes, the investigators found that expression levels of just 70 genes were sufficient to distinguish risk groups.[24] The authors believed that these results indicate the propensity to metastasize was an inherent genetic property of certain tumors and that this was not necessarily something that developed late in tumorigenesis. In the near future, these tools may be used to select patients who will require adjuvant therapy and to spare patients in the low-risk group who will not benefit from therapy.

Pharmacology

High-throughput genomic and proteomic technologies already are being used in the field of pharmacology to speed the discovery of new drug targets, learn more about the mechanisms of drug action, and identify genetic polymorphisms that alter efficacy and increase risk of toxicity[26] (see Chapter 110). Genes that are differentially regulated in disease may be targets for drug therapy, or they may provide clues about possible pathways to be targeted.[27,28] The combination of genomic technology with pharmacology has led to the new field of *pharmacogenomics*.[29] The goal of this new discipline is to tailor therapy according to individual genetic markers that will help determine a patient's course and response to therapy.[30] When this approach is ready for use in clinical medicine, we will move beyond the paradigm in which a therapy is selected because it does the greatest good for the greatest number of patients. The new paradigm will allow complete individualization of therapy on the basis of a patient's genetic profile.

One of the most important tools in pharmacogenomics is SNP analysis. For years, the goal of pharmaco*genetics* has been individualization of drug therapy to optimize therapeutic effect and minimize toxicity. Attaining these goals has been difficult because it often was impossible to predict an individual's response to therapy before treatment was initiated. Instead, using pharmacodynamic data (drug levels), optimization was attempted after therapy was started. It was clear that inheritance played an important role in individual responses to drug therapy; however, until recently it has been impossible to easily identify variations in an individual's genetic makeup that would determine therapeutic responses.

A number of polymorphisms that are responsible for variations in drug metabolism or drug response because of target alterations such as receptor polymorphisms have been identified. SNPs in certain genes can be used to predict the toxicity of some chemotherapeutic agents, whereas other SNPs can predict tumor sensitivity to chemotherapy.[31,32] As the effect of SNPs in groups of critical genes becomes more thoroughly characterized, microarrays will be developed that will permit rapid characterization (<24 hours) of an individual's response to therapy. This information can be used to minimize toxicity and maximize tumor destruction. The science of pharmacogenomics has yet to make a significant clinical impact but is anticipated to change in the near future as this testing becomes more readily available and clinicians become more adept at using these new data.[29]

Drug Discovery

The ability to study biologic systems of hosts and pathogens in great detail at the genomic and proteomic levels offers tremendous potential for the discovery of new drugs[33] and new insights into existing therapies. Microarray technology likely will find wide acceptance in the pharmaceutical industry in areas such as therapeutic target validation, drug selection, and optimization and in studies of metabolism and drug toxicity.[28] Although the potential for new discoveries is great,[18] some authors have noted that the first attempts at applying high-throughput techniques to the field of pharmacology have not yet accelerated drug development.[34] They speculate that the large number of targets discovered by this technology may have a paradoxical effect and temporarily slow drug development because of the large number of targets to be validated. Fortunately, new high-throughput validation techniques using tissue microarrays may help with this problem.[35,36]

Biomarkers

A *biomarker* is a biologically derived indicator of the presence or progression of a process or condition such as an illness. Genomic and proteomic technologies should accelerate the discovery of new biomarkers for a variety of illnesses. These markers should enable physicians to better understand the presence and progression of various conditions. In turn, this should help in identifying the optimal time point for delivery of therapy during the course of an illness. In breast cancer treatment, the application of microarray technology has led to the identification of new prognostic indicators, given novel insights into the biology of the tumors, and suggested new therapeutic targets.[37] A similar approach has been used to identify new potential biomarkers for hepatocellular carcinoma[23] and bladder cancer.[38] Investigators seeking to identify novel biomarkers for low doses of radiation have used microarray technology to identify a set of genes whose regulation is altered by exposure to sublethal levels of radiation.[39]

In addition to single biomarkers, genomic and proteomic technologies open the possibility of using multiple biomarkers as a "molecular signature." An example of such an application is the development of pathogen chips, which are microarrays containing genes from viral or bacterial pathogens. These chips can be used to identify genes and gene expression patterns that will identify a pathogen and tell us about the drug sensitivity of the organism.[40] Microarray-based technologies are being used to search for unique markers for biologic conditions, such as radiation exposure, for which no markers are known.[39] Because proteins are obvious candidates for biomarkers, a substantial body of research is focusing on disease-related functional proteomics in the hopes of developing new protein biomarkers.[10]

Predict Diagnosis

By the year 2010, predictive genetic tests may be available for a dozen or more common diseases.[7] This number will continue to grow. Using genomic, proteomic, and metabolomic markers of disease, physicians will have a powerful set of tools to identify who is at risk for developing an illness long before clinical signs become apparent. Individuals identified through such screening will be counseled by their physicians about the options available to them to minimize the disease burden or to delay the onset of clinical symptoms. Unfortunately, therapeutic options may not be available for some diseases. At present, no treatment exists for Huntington chorea, so susceptible individuals face a difficult choice when deciding whether to undergo screening. As we gain the ability to screen for a larger number of illnesses, no doubt we will face the problem that some of illnesses will be untreatable.

Critical Care

Most examples of medical applications for genomic and proteomic technologies come from the fields of cancer and pharmacology. Genomic technologies have great promise for critical care medicine. In the future, these technologies may help us to diagnose disease and to select appropriate medications and doses for our patients. Some of the earliest benefits to critical care patients likely will come from a systems biology approach to understanding inflammation. As the effects of genomic and proteomic components of the inflammatory cascade are understood in an integrated fashion, we should be able to identify critical points in selected pathways that will permit us to favorably alter the inflammatory response. Multigene studies should provide new insights into the mechanisms and prognosis of diseases such as sepsis, acute respiratory distress syndrome, and hypoxic injury. Intriguing examples of potential applications of this technology to the field of critical care are already appearing.

A variety of polymorphisms have been identified in certain key genes in the inflammatory process, such as TNF, various interleukins, and toll-like receptors.[8] These variations may help explain some of the well-recognized susceptibility to infectious diseases that is observed in certain families and ethnic groups. An animal study showed that mononuclear cells from the blood of animals suffering neurologic injury expressed different genes than those of healthy animals.[41,42] A new area that offers great potential for application in critical care research is the field of nutrigenomics, in which microarray technology is used to examine the complex interactions of nutrition in health and illness.[43]

Patients in critical care units are extensively monitored. In the future, this monitoring probably will include genomic and proteomic monitoring of responses to therapy as well as the previously mentioned pharmacogenomic monitoring.[44] Managing the volumes of information that will result from these tests will be a challenge to physicians, but these challenges will provide us with an opportunity to optimize our patients' therapies in ways that could not have been imagined one decade ago.

Ethical Issues

The benefits of genomic technologies are often touted, but there may also be risks. In the near future, it will be possible to completely genotype patients. Such information will permit a physician to assess a patient's risk of disease with a far greater level of certainty than has ever been possible. For some diseases, such as coronary artery disease, patients can be counseled to avoid risk factors. For other diseases, physicians may elect to preemptively initiate therapy in order to stave off the ravages of illness. A troubling problem arises when genomic testing reveals a serious illness for which no effective therapy exists. Whether patients will wish to be told of a problem for which there is no treatment is not clear. Geneticists have already encountered this situation with patients who are at risk for Huntington disease. Through genetic testing, we can identify which patients at risk for the illness actually carry the gene that will sentence them to an early death. Although patients may be relieved to know they do not carry this gene, they often do not want to know the results of testing because they will be burdened with awareness of an early, unpleasant death. As genomic testing becomes integrated into clinical medicine, general physicians may find themselves having to consider how to approach patients about similar issues.

Detailed information about a patient's genome will have implications for future health care costs. Patients who are identified as having genes that put them at risk for expensive illnesses might be denied insurance coverage, even while they are healthy. Patients and insurance companies will be very interested in this information, but they may have opposing ideas about how this information should be used. National policies governing the use of this information almost certainly will need to be formulated.

Genetic determinism refers to the concept that our genes govern health and disease. Although it is far too early to predict, the possibility exists that certain behavioral traits will be found to be associated with certain genotypes. Investigators in psychiatry are using genomic technology in the hopes of identifying genes that determine a patient's risk for schizophrenia.[45] Although many consider schizophrenia to be a polygenic disease that also is influenced by environmental factors, when the genes contributing to the risk of this illness have been identified and the contribution of each gene to the risk of illness has been identified, it will greatly aid in the diagnosis and treatment of this disorder. These benefits come at a price: what should be done with the information that indicates an individual may be at risk for schizophrenia or other psychiatric disorders? If the confidentiality of this information is not protected, the consequences might be devastating for an individual who might never develop this disorder.

An even more difficult issue concerns the rights of society to this information. If a patient is found to have a high risk of stroke, seizures, sudden cardiac death, or schizophrenia (to name just a few illnesses), should restrictions be placed on the types of employment that can be undertaken by the patient? For example, would it be appropriate for such an individual to pilot a large commercial aircraft if he or she appears otherwise healthy? These are difficult questions, but they will require answers as we enter the era of genomic medicine. To grapple with these issues, 3% to 5% of the budget for the Human Genome Project was set aside for research to explore the ethical, legal, and social implications that might arise once the sequence of the human genome was known.[7]

Genomic medicine will provide us with tremendous benefits and challenges. Perhaps one of the greatest benefits will be the understanding that human similarities and differences transcend the racial and ethnic categories that have proved so contentious in the past.[46]

REFERENCES

1. Watson JD, Crick FH: Molecular structure of nucleic acids; a structure for deoxyribose nucleic acid. *Nature* 171:737-738, 1953.
2. Thomas G, Cann H: Irruption of genomics in the search for disease related genes. *Gut* 52(suppl 2):ii1-5, 2003.
3. Pennisi E: Human genome. Reaching their goal early, sequencing labs celebrate. *Science* 300:409, 2003.
4. Schena M, Shalon D, Davis RW, Brown PO: Quantitative monitoring of gene expression patterns with a complementary DNA microarray. *Science* 270:467-470, 1995.
5. Tefferi A, Bolander ME, Ansell SM, et al: Primer on medical genomics. Part III: microarray experiments and data analysis. *Mayo Clin Proc* 77:927-940, 2002.
6. Heller MJ: DNA microarray technology: devices, systems, and applications. *Annu Rev Biomed Eng* 4:129-153, 2002.
7. Collins FS, McKusick VA: Implications of the Human Genome Project for medical science. JAMA 285:540-544, 2001.
8. Cariou A, Chiche JD, Charpentier J, et al: The era of genomics: impact on sepsis clinical trial design. *Crit Care Med* 30(5 suppl):S341-S348, 2002.
9. SNP Fact Sheet 2004. Cited November 30, 2004. Available at http://www.ornl.gov/sci/techresources/Human_Genome/faq/snps.shtml.
10. Hanash S: Disease proteomics. *Nature* 422:226-232, 2003.
11. de Hoog CL, Mann M: Proteomics. *Annu Rev Genomics Hum Genet* 5:267-293, 2004.
12. Phizicky E, Bastiaens PI, Zhu H, et al: Protein analysis on a proteomic scale. *Nature* 422:208-215, 2003.
13. Aebersold R, Mann M: Mass spectrometry-based proteomics. *Nature* 422:198-207, 2003.
14. Kell DB: Metabolomics and systems biology: making sense of the soup. *Curr Opin Microbiol* 7:296-307, 2004.
15. Weckwerth W: Metabolomics in systems biology. *Annu Rev Plant Biol* 54:669-689, 2003.
16. Morel NM, Holland JM, van der Greef J, et al: Primer on medical genomics. Part XIV: introduction to systems biology-a new approach to understanding disease and treatment. *Mayo Clin Proc* 79: 651-658, 2004.
17. Ishii N, Robert M, Nakayama Y, et al: Toward large-scale modeling of the microbial cell for computer simulation. *J Biotechnol* 113: 281-294, 2004.
18. Davidov E, Holland J, Marple E, Naylor S: Advancing drug discovery through systems biology. *Drug Discov Today* 8:175-183, 2003.
19. Cascante M, Boros LG, Comin-Anduix B, et al: Metabolic control analysis in drug discovery and disease. *Nat Biotechnol* 20:243-249, 2002.
20. Chung CH, Bernard PS, Perou CM: Molecular portraits and the family tree of cancer. *Nat Genet* 32(suppl):533-540, 2002.
21. Staudt LM: Molecular diagnosis of the hematologic cancers. *N Engl J Med* 48:1777-1785, 2003.
22. MacGregor JT: Biomarkers of cancer risk and therapeutic benefit: new technologies, new opportunities, and some challenges. *Toxicol Pathol* 32(suppl 1):99-105, 2004.
23. Neo SY, Leow CK, Vega VB, et al: Identification of discriminators of hepatoma by gene expression profiling using a minimal dataset approach. *Hepatology* 39:944-953, 2004.
24. van de Vijver MJ, He YD, van't Veer LJ, et al: A gene-expression signature as a predictor of survival in breast cancer. *N Engl J Med* 347:1999-2009, 2002.
25. van 't Veer LJ, Dai H, van de Vijver MJ, et al: Gene expression profiling predicts clinical outcome of breast cancer. *Nature* 415:530-536, 2002.
26. Nees M, Woodworth CD: Microarrays: spotlight on gene function and pharmacogenomics. *Curr Cancer Drug Targets* 1:155-175, 2001.
27. Lee RT: Functional genomics and cardiovascular drug discovery. *Circulation* 104:1441-1446, 2001.
28. Gerhold DL, Jensen RV, Gullans SR: Better therapeutics through microarrays. *Nat Genet* 32(suppl):547-551, 2002.
29. Weinshilboum R, Wang L: Pharmacogenomics: bench to bedside. *Nat Rev Drug Discov* 3:739-748, 2004.
30. Emilien G, Ponchon M, Caldas C, et al: Impact of genomics on drug discovery and clinical medicine. QJM 93:391-423, 2000.
31. Iqbal S, Lenz HJ: Targeted therapy and pharmacogenomic programs. *Cancer* 97(8 suppl):2076-2082, 2003.
32. McLeod HL, Yu J: Cancer pharmacogenomics: SNPs, chips, and the individual patient. *Cancer Invest* 21:630-640, 2003.
33. Chanda SK, Caldwell JS: Fulfilling the promise: drug discovery in the post-genomic era. *Drug Discov Today* 8:168-174, 2003.
34. Basik M, Mousses S, Trent J: Integration of genomic technologies for accelerated cancer drug development. *Biotechniques* 35:580-582, 584, 586, 2003.
35. Mobasheri A, Airley R, Foster CS, et al: Post-genomic applications of tissue microarrays: basic research, prognostic oncology, clinical genomics and drug discovery. *Histol Histopathol* 19:325-335, 2004.
36. van de Rijn M, Gilks CB: Applications of microarrays to histopathology. *Histopathology* 44:97-108, 2004.
37. Bertucci F, Viens P, Hingamp P, et al: Breast cancer revisited using DNA array-based gene expression profiling. *Int J Cancer* 103:565-571, 2003.
38. S·nchez-Carbayo M: Use of high-throughput DNA microarrays to identify biomarkers for bladder cancer. *Clin Chem* 49:23-31, 2003.

39. Kang CM, Park KP, Song JE, et al: Possible biomarkers for ionizing radiation exposure in human peripheral blood lymphocytes. *Radiat Res* 159:312-319, 2003.
40. Campbell CJ, Ghazal P: Molecular signatures for diagnosis of infection: application of microarray technology. *J Appl Microbiol* 96: 18-23, 2004.
41. Tang Y, Lu A, Aronow BJ, Sharp FR: Blood genomic responses differ after stroke, seizures, hypoglycemia, and hypoxia: blood genomic fingerprints of disease. *Ann Neurol* 50:699-707, 2001.
42. Tang Y, Nee AC, Lu A, et al: Blood genomic expression profile for neuronal injury. *J Cereb Blood Flow Metab* 23:310-319, 2003.
43. Müller M, Kersten S: Nutrigenomics: goals and strategies. *Nat Rev Genet* 4:315-322, 2003.
44. Hopf HW: Molecular diagnostics of injury and repair responses in critical illness: what is the future of "monitoring" in the intensive care unit? *Crit Care Med* 31(8 suppl):S518-S523, 2003.
45. Sklar P, Pato MT, Kirby A, et al: Genome-wide scan in Portuguese Island families identifies 5q31-5q35 as a susceptibility locus for schizophrenia and psychosis. *Mol Psychiatry* 9:213-218, 2004.
46. Foster MW, Sharp RR: Beyond race: towards a whole-genome perspective on human populations and genetic variation. *Nat Rev Genet* 5:790-796, 2004.

CHAPTER 93

Molecular Foundations of Cellular Injury: Apoptosis and Necrosis

Craig M. Coopersmith

PEARLS

- As an "accidental" form of death, necrosis is an uncontrolled process.
- Apoptosis is a controlled, evolutionarily conserved process.
- Alterations in the balance between cellular proliferation and death can lead to disease. Altered apoptosis is estimated to play a role in half of all medical illness for which prevention is lacking.
- Apoptosis appears to play a role in critical illness, both in septic and noninfectious inflammatory states.
- Traumatic head injury results in both necrotic and apoptotic responses in affected brain tissue.

Cell Death

Each day, the human body produces and eradicates 60×10^9 cells, a rate of cell death of nearly one million per second.[1] Cells die by one of two mechanistically distinct processes: apoptosis or necrosis (Table 93–1).[2] Both forms of cell death can be distinguished by both morphologic and molecular biologic criteria.

In necrosis, an overwhelming acute injury is followed by cell and organelle swelling, with early dissolution of the plasma membrane and subsequent cell lysis. As the cell bursts, its contents enter the interstitial space, leading to an accompanying inflammatory response to the toxic enzymes and proteases released. Morphologically, cells undergoing necrosis show swelling of the entire cell and its internal organelles. Deoxyribonucleic acid (DNA) fragmentation has no characteristic pattern, and electrophoretic gels demonstrate a random pattern. As an "accidental" form of death, necrosis is an uncontrolled process.

In contrast, apoptosis (also known as *programmed cell death* or *"cell suicide"*) is a controlled, evolutionarily conserved process.[3,4] Following an appropriate trigger, a cell's apoptotic machinery leads to orderly death of the cell. This is characterized by cell and organelle shrinkage (pyknosis), nuclear fragmentation (karyorrhexis), and cytoplasmic blebbing with retention of plasma membrane integrity. Ultimately, there is fragmentation of the cell into small apoptotic bodies that are phagocytosed by neighboring cells. Orderly DNA fragmentation is identifiable on electrophoretic gels as a characteristic "ladder" pattern. Because cytosolic contents are not released into the interstitial space, there is no accompanying inflammatory response.

Apoptosis is critical to the existence of virtually all multicellular organisms and is involved in widely divergent physiologic processes, including embryonic development, maturation, immunity, repair, and cellular homeostasis. However, alterations in the balance between cellular proliferation and death can lead to disease. Altered apoptosis is estimated to play a role in half of all medical illness for which prevention is lacking.[5,6] Inadequate levels of apoptosis have been implicated in the etiology of cancer and autoimmunity, whereas excessive apoptosis has been noted in the origins of neurodegenerative disease, osteoarthritis,

TABLE 93–1

Differences between Necrosis and Apoptosis

Necrosis	Apoptosis
Cell and organelle swelling	Cell and organelle shrinkage (pyknosis)
Early loss of membrane integrity	Preservation of membrane integrity until late in process
Random DNA breakdown-smear	DNA broken down in "ladder" pattern on electrophoresis
Accompanied by inflammation	No accompanying inflammation
	Nuclear fragmentation

(From Hotchkiss RS, Tinsley KW, Swanson PE, Karl IE: *Crit Care Med* 30[5 suppl]:S225-S228, 2002.)

allograft infection and graft-versus-host disease, type I diabetes, and heart failure.[1,7] Importantly, apoptosis is increasingly recognized as playing a role in critical illness, both in septic and noninfectious inflammatory states. Because of the importance of apoptosis in multiple disease states, a number of ongoing phase II and phase III trials targeting apoptotic pathways are ongoing.[1,8]

Pathways of Apoptosis

Apoptosis is initiated by two main pathways: a receptor-mediated pathway and a mitochondrial-mediated pathway (Figure 93–1).[9–12] The receptor-mediated pathway can be activated by a number of ligands, including Fas and tumor necrosis factor (TNF)-α. The mitochondrial pathway can be activated by a number of different stimuli following DNA damage, including reactive oxygen species, radiation therapy, and chemotherapy, and appears to be the dominant pathway in sepsis-induced apoptosis.

Within the mitochondrial pathway, the Bcl-2 family plays a critical role. This group of proteins includes more than 20 proapoptotic and antiapoptotic molecules, many of which physically interact with each other.[1,11,13] Their primary function appears to be regulation of cytochrome *c* release from the mitochondria, with proapoptotic family members promoting and apoptotic family members suppressing its release. The prototypical antiapoptotic protein is Bcl-2, whereas the prototypical proapoptotic family member is Bax.

Both receptor-mediated and mitochondrial-mediated pathways activate specific members of the cysteine aspartyl-specific protease (caspase) family.[14] Produced as inactive precursors, caspases are triggered by proteolytic processing as part of a cascade into their active counterparts. Depending on their location in the apoptosis cascade, caspases can be either upstream "initiators" or downstream "effectors" of cell death. Although several pathways for inducing these molecules exist, the receptor-mediated pathway acts by inducing caspase-8. In the mitochondrial pathway, cytochrome *c* binds to apoptotic protease-activating factor-1 (APAF-1), which in turn induces caspase-9. Both caspase-8 and caspase-9 converge on the final common pathway of apoptosis via induction of the death effector caspase-3, leading to the ultimate death of the cell.

Human Studies

Several human studies showed apoptosis and necrosis both were altered in critical illness. The potential functional importance of these alterations has been recognized, with the development of agents aimed at manipulating cell death for therapeutic benefit currently undergoing preclinical and clinical trials.[1,8]

Sepsis

A prospective analysis by Hotchkiss et al.[15] of 37 patients who died in a surgical intensive care unit and underwent immediate autopsy demonstrated increased lymphocytic and gut epithelial apoptosis in approximately 50% of septic patients with multiple organ dysfunction syndrome compared with essentially no alterations in cell death in critically ill, nonseptic patients (Figure 93–2). In contrast, necrosis was detectable in 35% of patient livers but was minimal or absent in all other tissues examined (see Chapters 96 and 97).

Increased apoptosis in septic patients was associated with an increase in active caspase-3 activity. Further studies from this same group indicated that B and CD4+ T lymphocytes are disproportionately lost in septic patients.[16] The B and CD4+ T lymphocyte apoptosis is caspase-9 dependent, and the degree of cell death is greater the longer the patient is septic. Antigen-presenting dendritic cells are also decreased in spleens of septic patients.[17]

Apoptosis is significantly decreased, however, in macrophages obtained by bronchoalveolar lavage (BAL) in septic patients compared with nonseptic controls.[18] This decrease in apoptosis is associated with lower levels of Bcl-2 than in control patients. An inverse correlation was found between the severity of sepsis and the percentage of apoptotic alveolar macrophages. Minimal macrophage necrosis was present in BAL fluid.

Apoptosis is also decreased in neutrophils in patients who become septic after an initial traumatic insult through up-regulation of tyrosine phosphorylation by circulating mediators.[19] This appears to be related to the septic insult, as neutrophil apoptosis is not significantly different between noninfected trauma patients and healthy volunteers.[19] In addition, circulating neutrophil apoptosis is decreased in infected patients with the systemic inflammatory response syndrome compared with controls. The decrease in neutrophil death is not associated with alterations in caspase-3 levels. Of note, however, levels of apoptosis are similar to those seen in patients who underwent elective abdominal aortic aneurysmectomy.[20]

Noninfectious Inflammation

Similar to sepsis, tissue lymphocyte and intestinal epithelial apoptosis are increased in patients who have been subjected to shock and trauma. Intestinal specimens resected from 10 patients following motor vehicle collisions or gunshot

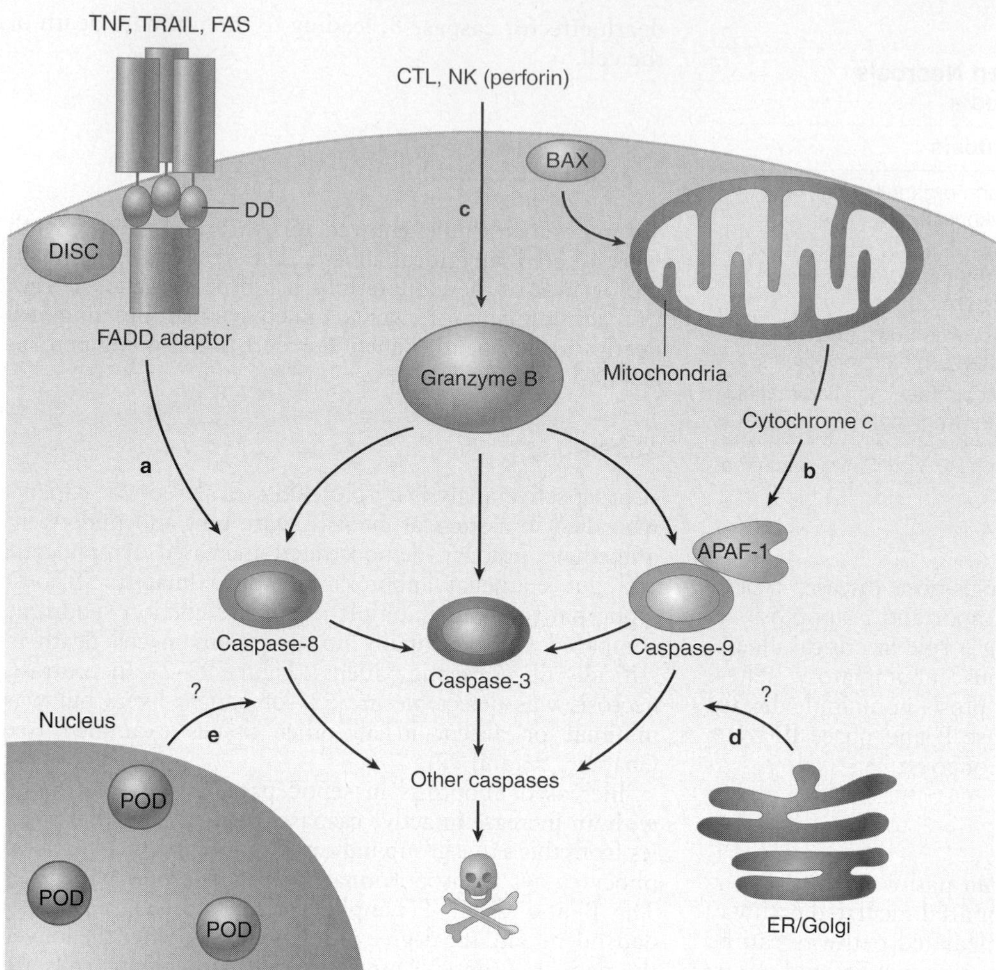

FIGURE 93–1 • Schematic representation of major pathways of apoptosis and their convergence in a final common pathway leading to cellular death. *APAF-1,* Apoptotic protease-activating factor-1; (From Reed JC: *Nat Rev Drug Discov* 1:111-121, 2002.)

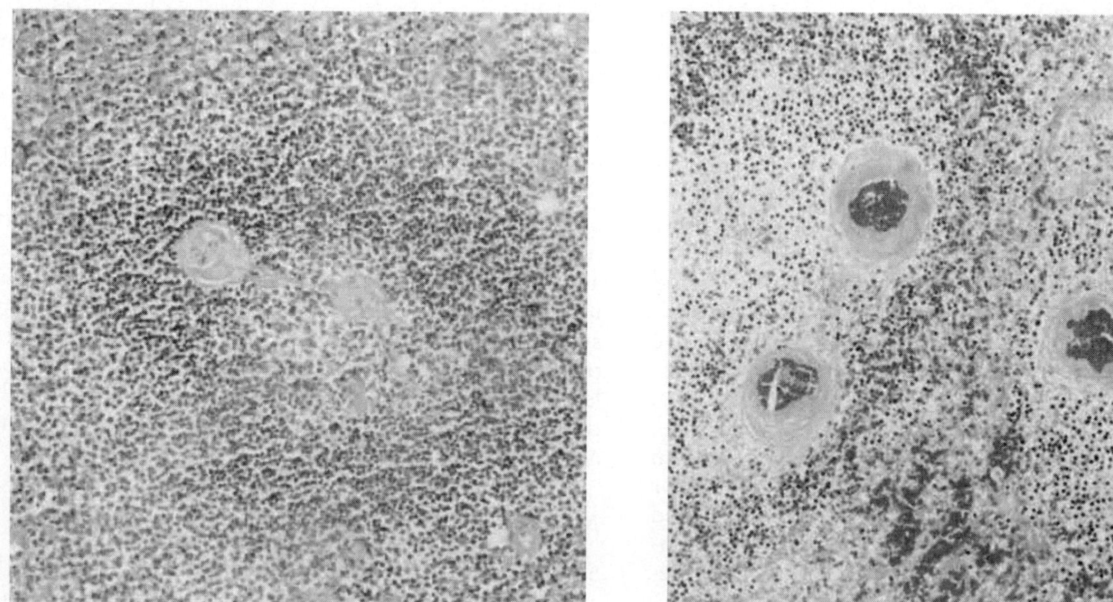

FIGURE 93–2 • Spleen from a control patient **(A)** demonstrating a normal lymphoid follicle and from a septic patient **(B)** with substantial depletion in the lymphoid follicle. (From Hotchkiss RS, Swanson PE, Freeman BD, et al: *Crit Care Med* 27:1230-1251, 1999.)

wounds revealed extensive crypt epithelial and gut lymphocytic apoptosis, whereas control patients who underwent elective bowel resections had no obvious change in levels of cell death.[21] Apoptosis was detectable within 2 hours of traumatic injury, and patients with the highest injury severity score had the most severe apoptosis. Importantly, patients with high apoptosis on initial evaluation following trauma had no evidence of increased cell death at follow-up elective laparotomy.

Increased apoptosis is present in circulating T lymphocytes of patients who sustained blunt trauma or burn injury.[22,23] Although increased apoptosis of lymphocytes in the bloodstream was not directly associated with a negative outcome in the 30 individuals studied, patients with very high levels of apoptosis prior to complete activation and expansion of the T-cell response appear to be predisposed to anergy and organ failure.

The apoptotic response of polymorphonuclear leukocytes to trauma has not been fully elucidated. Ogura et al.[24] reported that apoptosis is decreased in this cell type for as long as 3 weeks following trauma. This contrasts with data showing that neutrophil apoptosis is decreased in septic trauma patients but is not significantly different between patients 24 hours after traumatic injury and control volunteers.[19]

Neutrophil apoptosis is low in BAL fluid from patients with the acute respiratory distress syndrome (ARDS) and those at risk for ARDS.[25,26] Levels of apoptosis did not correlate with patient survival. Interestingly, BAL fluid from ARDS victims resulted in a lower proportion of apoptosis when incubated with human polymorphonuclear leukocytes from ARDS victims than BAL fluid from healthy volunteers. The antiapoptotic effect of BAL fluid on normal neutrophils is highest during early ARDS, decreases during late ARDS, and correlates with levels of granulocyte colony-stimulating factor and granulocyte-macrophage colony-stimulating factor.[27]

Soluble Fas ligand is present in BAL fluid before and after onset of ARDS.[28] However, its concentration is higher at the onset of ARDS in patients who eventually die. Importantly, BAL fluid from patients with ARDS induces a Fas dependent apoptosis in distal lung epithelial cells, whereas BAL fluid from patients at risk for ARDS but without the disease does not have an effect on distal lung epithelial cell death. BAL fluid also has elevation in concentrations of apoptosis-related molecules perforin, granzyme A, and granzyme B in critically ill patients with early ARDS compared with those not having lung injury or late ARDS.[29]

Brain Injury

Traumatic head injury results in both necrotic and apoptotic responses in affected brain tissue (see Chapters 58 and 107). Although necrosis is the main finding in cerebral contusion, apoptosis has been identified in more than one third of brain specimens in patients who underwent emergency craniotomy for evacuation of contusions associated with mass effect.[30] Bax expression was detected in all patients with apoptosis. Bcl-2 was detected in only half the patients with both cerebral contusion and apoptosis and was associated with improved survival. Although the site of injury is the main location of apoptosis following traumatic brain injury, apoptosis has been identified in remote neurons days to weeks following cerebral contusion, as well as in oligodendrocytes and astrocytes.[31]

The mechanisms underlying apoptosis in traumatic brain injury have been examined by studying the cerebral spinal fluid (CSF) of head-injured patients. Soluble Fas was detected in 118 of 120 CSF samples for up to 2 weeks postinjury in 10 patients with isolated head trauma compared with no detectable levels in CSF obtained from healthy volunteers.[32] Fas also was detected in the blood in half of patients with brain injury but was absent in all controls. Caspase-3 also was identified in the CSF of 30% of patients after traumatic brain injury (compared with no detectable levels in controls), with peak levels seen 2 to 5 days postinjury.[33]

Animal Studies

Although human studies demonstrate that apoptosis and necrosis both are altered in critical illness, the functional importance of these descriptive associations has not been studied in patients. Animal models of sepsis and noninfectious inflammation can help determine whether altered cell death is harmful in critical illness and offer mechanistic insights into the pathways underlying changes in cell death.

Sepsis

Similar to human autopsy studies, apoptosis is primarily localized in lymphocytes and the gut epithelium in animal models of sepsis. In both cecal ligation and puncture (CLP), a murine model of ruptured appendicitis, and overwhelming infection from *Pseudomonas aeruginosa* pneumonia, sampling of multiple cell and tissue types yielded maximal lymphocytic and intestinal apoptosis 24 hours after onset of septic insult without substantial necrosis reported (Figure 93–3).[34–39]

Molecular pathways involved in lymphocytic apoptosis appear to be dependent to some degree upon where the lymphocyte resides. Studies in LPS responder (C3H/HeN) and hyporesponder (C3H/HeJ) mice subjected to CLP demonstrate the majority of sepsis-induced lymphocytic apoptosis occurs via an endotoxin-independent, TNF-independent pathway in both thymus and spleen, although thymic apoptosis also occurs via a separate pathway that is driven by endotoxin activation.[35] Thymic apoptosis is also Fas independent, but is related to release of endogenous steroids, potentially acting via Bcl-2 expression.[40] Splenocyte apoptosis in CLP also occurs via an endotoxin-independent pathway, but unlike thymocytes this process is Fas ligand dependent.[41] Similarly, intestinal epithelial lymphocytes and lamina B lymphocytes undergo Fas ligand-dependent, endotoxin-independent apoptosis.[42,43]

Lymphocyte apoptosis can be blocked by either selective caspase-3 inhibitors or polycaspase inhibitors.[44,45] Programmed cell death also can occur independent of this common effector, as caspase-3 knockout mice continue to exhibit, albeit diminished, lymphocyte apoptosis.[45] In addition, sepsis-induced apoptosis is not dependent upon the presence of mature lymphocytes as evidenced

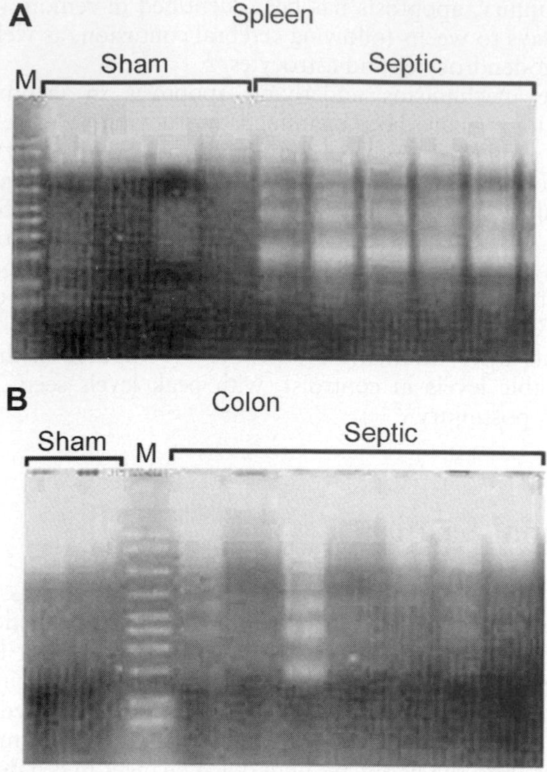

FIGURE 93–3 • DNA agarose gel showering characteristic "laddering" pattern in spleen **(A)** and colon **(B)** in septic but not sham mice. (From Hotchkiss RS, Swanson PE, Cobb JP, Jacobson A, Buckman TG, Karl IE: *Crit Care Med* 25:1298-1307, 1997.)

by extensive programmed cell death in Rag-1 mice lacking this cell type.[34]

Increased lymphocytic apoptosis appears to be detrimental to survival in sepsis. Overexpression of Bcl-2 in transgenic mice overexpressing either T lymphocytes or B lymphocytes improves survival twofold to fourfold in three different strains of inbred mice subjected to CLP.[45,46] Administration of the polycaspase inhibitor N-benynzyloxycarbonyl-Val-Ala-Asp(O-methyl) fluoromethyl ketone (z-VAD) or the caspase-3 specific inhibitor M-971 causes similar improvements in outcome.[44,45] The beneficial effects of caspase inhibitors on survival in murine sepsis require the presence of lymphocytes; there is no survival benefit conferred to Rag-1 mice treated with caspase inhibitors. Adoptive transfer of T lymphocytes that overexpress Bcl-2 into Rag-1 animals improves survival similar to that seen in transgenic mice that overexpress Bcl-2 in their lymphocytes.[45]

The mechanisms that account for worse outcomes with increasing lymphocytic apoptosis appear to involve immunosuppression. T cells contained in splenic suspensions stimulated *in vitro* have increased interleukin (IL)-2 and interferon-γ levels 6 hours after stimulation with CD3 and anti-CD28. Potentially, these cytokines activate macrophages and other cells in the innate immune system, an interaction that would be decreased with increasing lymphocytic death.[45]

Gut epithelial apoptosis is increased in CLP, *P. aeruginosa* pneumonia,[37] and *in vitro* after infection with invasive enteric pathogens *Salmonella dublin* and *Escherichia coli*.[47] Intestinal cell death appears to be detrimental in sepsis of polymicrobial or monomicrobial sepsis originating in the intestine or the lungs, as overexpression of Bcl-2 in the gut epithelium of transgenic mice confers a twofold survival advantage in CLP[39] and a tenfold survival advantage in *P. aeruginosa* pneumonia (Figures 93-4 and 93-5).[37] The mechanism underlying the improvement in survival caused by decreasing gut epithelial apoptosis is unclear. Bacterial translocation is similar between transgenic and nontransgenic animals with sepsis-induced pneumonia despite widely varying survival, and there are no statistically significant differences in cytokine levels.

The role of lung apoptosis in sepsis is controversial. Respiratory epithelial cells are highly resistant to apoptosis when treated with *P. aeruginosa,* undergoing cell death *in vitro* only under specific epithelial conditions when treated with virulent bacteria capable of expressing both adhesins and cytotoxins.[48] In addition, lung epithelial apoptosis reportedly is absent in *P. aeruginosa* pneumonia in mice.[36] However, Grassme et al.[49] reported that *P. aeruginosa* pneumonia induces respiratory epithelial apoptosis in mice through activation of the Fas/Fas ligand system. Respiratory apoptosis appeared to be essential for survival in this study, with rapid sepsis-induced mortality in Fas or Fas ligand-deficient mice that lacked bronchial apoptosis.

Alveolar and bronchiolar apoptosis are present in rats 8 hours after pneumonia is induced with *Streptococcus sanguis* (which resolves after 1 week) or *Streptococcus pneumoniae* type 25 (which progresses to pulmonary fibrosis).[50,51] Apoptosis is widespread for the first 4 days following either type of pneumonia. Eight days following *S. sanguis* pneumonia, apoptosis is localized to lung abscesses, implying a role for cell death in the resolution of injury.[50] By contrast, apoptosis remains widespread and actually increases in intensity after *S. pneumoniae* type 25 pneumonia. Lung apoptosis is also induced following CLP in multiple mouse strains.[34,35]

Few animal studies demonstrate sepsis-induced apoptosis in other cell types. One exception is an increase in murine hepatocyte apoptosis following infection with *Listeria monocytogenes*.[52] Liver apoptosis is greatest at the edge of microabscesses and is independent of endotoxin, Fas, and nitric oxide. Apoptosis is also increased in murine granulocytes after CLP through a pathway that can be suppressed by a TNF inhibitor.[53] In contrast, blood leukocyte apoptosis is decreased in mice 24 hours following the same insult.[53]

Noninfectious Inflammation

Although lymphocyte and intestinal epithelial apoptosis are present extensively in human and animal studies of noninfectious inflammation, cell death is elevated in a higher variety of organs in inflammatory models compared with that seen in animal models of sepsis. Both thymocyte apoptosis[54,55] and B-cell Peyer patch apoptosis[56] are increased following either trauma/hemorrhage or hemorrhage alone. Thymocyte IL-3 release is decreased following

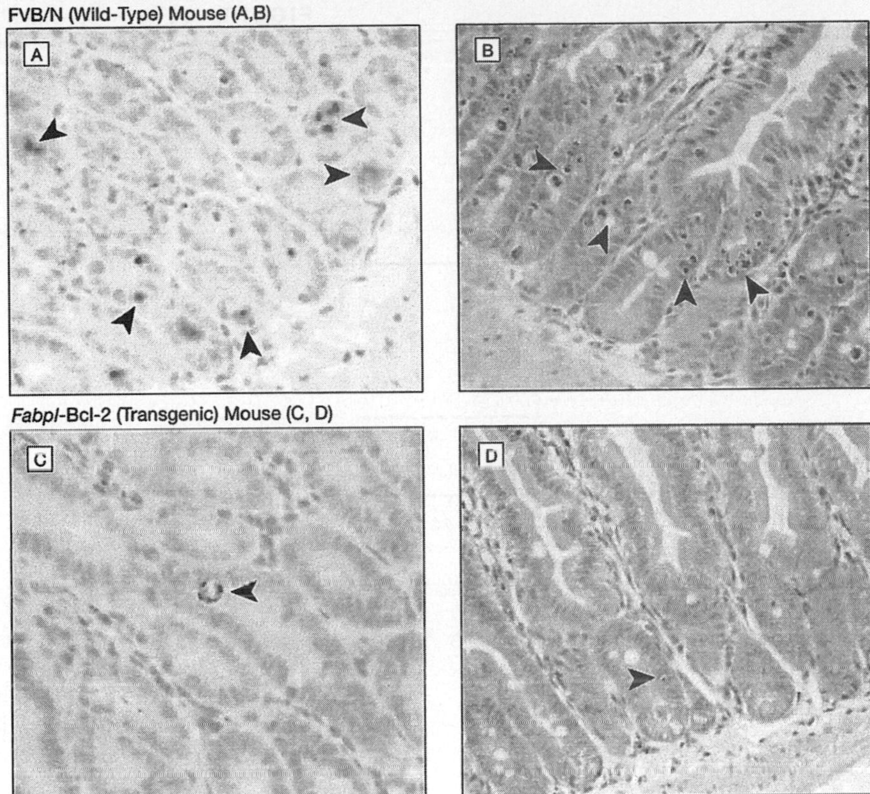

FIGURE 93–4 • Intestinal epithelial sections from wild-type (**A, B**) and Bcl-2 transgenic mice (**C, D**) with sepsis from *Pseudomonas aeruginosa* pneumonia. Bcl-2 decreases apoptosis when assessed by active caspase 3 (**A, C**) or hematoxylin and eosin (**B, D**). (From Coopersmith CM, Stromberg PE, Dunne WM, et al: *JAMA* 287:1716-1721, 2002.)

either insult,[54] whereas thymus-derived granulocyte-macrophage colony-stimulating factor is increased following trauma/hemorrhage but not following hemorrhage alone. The increase in thymic apoptosis following trauma/hemorrhage is associated with a gender dimorphism, in that cell death levels of predominantly CD8$^+$ thymocytes are higher in males and are associated with greater suppression of IL-3.[55] Lymphocyte apoptosis in Peyer patches also occurs following either trauma/hemorrhage or hemorrhage alone and is associated with elevated Fas expression.[56]

Thymocyte, splenocyte, Peyer patch, and intraepithelial lymphocyte apoptosis all are increased following thermal injury.[57–62] Thymocyte and splenocyte apoptosis are associated with increased levels of active caspase-3 but are independent of endotoxin.[58,59] Cell death is also dependent upon corticosteroids, as pretreatment with the glucocorticoid receptor antagonist mifepristone significantly reduced both apoptosis and active caspase 3 activity following burn injury.[59] Mifepristone also reduces apoptosis in intraepithelial lymphocytes.[61] The roles of both TNF-α and Fas ligand in burn-induced lymphocyte apoptosis are more complicated. Thymus and spleen apoptosis both are elevated in TNF$^{\%}$ mice.[58] Whereas TNF-α levels are elevated following thermal injury in both thymus and spleen in C57BLKS/J mice, TNF-α protein levels are disproportionately elevated in thymus tissue, which is associated with elevated thymic and not splenic apoptosis.[62] Thymocyte, splenocyte, and CD8$^+$ T-cell Peyer patch apoptosis all are Fas ligand independent,[59,61] whereas B-cell Peyer patch cell death is dependent on the presence of this molecule, as burn-induced apoptosis is eliminated in C3H/HeJ-FasL(gld) mice that lack functional Fas ligand.[61]

As in human studies, gut epithelial apoptosis is increased in animal models of ischemial reperfusion[63–68] and thermal injury.[69–72] Apoptosis is suppressible in murine ischemia reperfusion by overexpression of Bcl-2[63] or IL-11[67] but is independent of ornithine decarboxylase despite its effect of repairing damaged intestinal mucosa.[66]

Acute lung injury (ALI) causes increased death in multiple cells within the lung.[51,73] Intratracheal injection of LPS induces apoptosis in alveolar wall cells, neutrophils, and macrophages.[73] This process is associated with upregulation of Fas in alveolar and inflammatory cells, and lung injury can be blocked by administration of an anti-Fas antibody. Respiratory apoptosis is also increased in a diffuse fashion in a hyperoxia model of ALI and in a patchy distribution in ALI caused by intravenous injection of oleic acid.[51]

Whether endothelial apoptosis occurs with inflammation is unclear. Numerous *in vitro* studies have examined this question, with mixed results.[74] A single murine study demonstrated that LPS induces endothelial apoptosis after generation of the proapoptotic lipid ceramid.[75] This finding conflicts with studies showing no evidence of

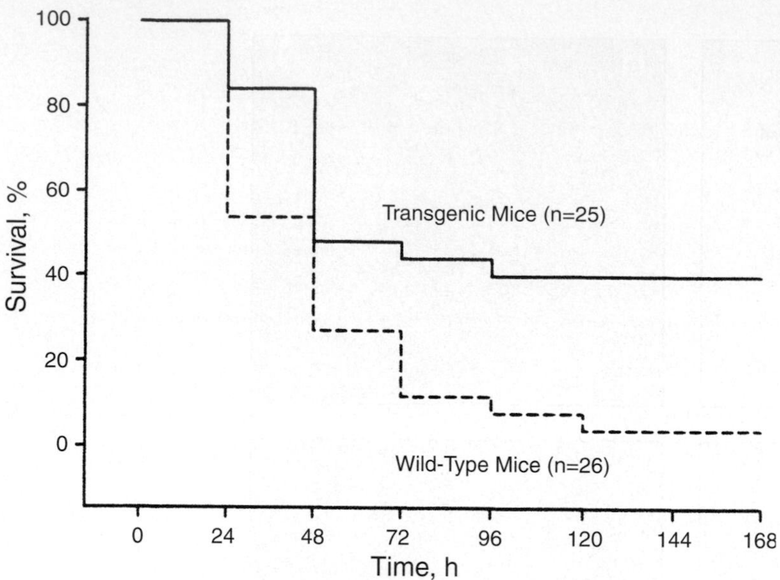

FIGURE 93–5 • Survival 7 days after sepsis from *Pseudomonas aeruginosa* pneumonia in transgenic mice that overexpress Bcl-2 in their intestinal epithelium and wild-type mice. (From Coopersmith CM, Stromberg PE, Dunne WM, et al: *JAMA* 287:1716-1721, 2002.)

endothelial apoptosis in rat thoracic aortas following CLP and extremely rare endothelial cell death in lungs from mice with *P. aeruginosa* pneumonia.[74]

The endothelium plays a role, however, in influencing neutrophil apoptosis.[76] Rat lung neutrophil apoptosis shows a significant delay following intratracheal LPS instillation. The mechanism underlying the delay is unrelated to LPS, as a similar delay is seen following the addition of the potent apoptosis-inducer TNF-α. The process of endothelial transmigration appears to play a major regulatory role in regulating neutrophil apoptosis. Adhesion molecules from the integrin and selectin families also have a role in modulating neutrophil cell death.[76]

Preliminary reports show that bums increase apoptosis in a variety of tissues. Thermal injury induces cardiac apoptosis, predominantly in the subendocardial region of the left ventricle,[70] liver apoptosis and proliferation,[77] and skeletal muscle apoptosis with alterations in levels of caspase 1, caspase 3, and caspase 9.[78]

Brain Injury

Similar to human studies, animal models of traumatic head injury result in both necrosis and apoptosis, with the relative levels and mechanisms dependent upon the model used. A murine model using a device that produces controlled cortical impact that causes reproducible deficits in sensory or motor function induces increasing neuronal apoptosis with increasing injury severity.[79] In contrast, a rotational head acceleration model in rabbits that causes subarachnoid hemorrhage leads to increased glutamate, glycine, and c-Jun within a few hours and brain edema within 24 hours. This, in turn, leads to a combination of neuronal apoptosis and necrosis 10 days following the insult in the cerebral cortex, hippocampus, and cerebellum.[80] Finally, although both forms of cell death may occur after controlled severe brain injury, the massive mitochondrial cytochrome *c* release that accompanies traumatic brain injury is a predictor of necrotic but not apoptotic cell death, as mice deficient in manganese superoxide dismutase have increased loss of cytochrome *c* following trauma, with increased cortical lesions and increased levels of necrosis but decreased apoptosis.[81]

REFERENCES

1. Reed JC: Apoptosis-based therapies. *Nat Rev Drug Discov* 111-121, 2002.
2. Columbano A: Cell death: current difficulties in discriminating apoptosis from necrosis in the context of pathological processes in vivo. *J Cell Biochem* 58:181-190, 1995.
3. Kerr JF, Wyllie AH, Currie AR: Apoptosis: a basic biological phenomenon with wide-ranging implications in tissue kinetics. *Br J Cancer* 26:239-257, 1972.
4. Raff M: Cell suicide for beginners. *Nature* 396:119-122, 1998.
5. Reed JC: Mechanisms of apoptosis. *Am J Pathol* 157:1415-1430, 2000.
6. Thompson CB: Apoptosis in the pathogenesis and treatment of disease. *Science* 267:1456-1462, 1995.
7. Hetts SW: To die or not to die: an overview of apoptosis and its role in disease. *JAMA* 279:300-307, 1998.
8. Nicholson DW: From bench to clinic with apoptosis-based therapeutic agents. *Nature* 407:810-6, 2000.
9. Roy S, Nicholson DW: Cross-talk in cell death signaling. 192: F21-F25, 2000.
10. Krammer PH: CD95's deadly mission in the immune system. *Nature* 407:789-795, 2000.
11. Adams JM, Cory S: The Bcl-2 protein family: arbiters of cell survival. *Science* 281:1322-1326, 1998.
12. Rich T, Allen RL, Wyllie AH: Defying death after DNA damage. *Nature* 407:777-783, 2000.
13. Ranger AM, Maylnn BA, Korsmeyer SJ: Mouse models of cell death. *Nat Genet* 28:113-118, 2001.
14. Thornberry NA, Lazebnik Y: Caspases: enemies within. *Science* 281:1312-1316, 1998.
15. Hotchkiss RS, Swanson PE, Freeman BD, et al: Apoptotic cell death in patients with sepsis, shock, and multiple organ dysfunction. *Crit Care Med* 27:1230-1251, 1999.
16. Hotchkiss RS, Tinsley KW, Swanson PE, et al: Sepsis induced apoptosis causes progressive profound depletion of B and CD4+ T lymphocytes in humans. *J Immunol* 166:6952-6963, 2001.
17. Hotchkiss RS, Tinsley KW, Swanson PE, et al: Depletion of dendritic cells, but not macrophages, in patients with sepsis. *J Immunol* 168:2493-2500, 2002.

18. Liacos C, Katsaragakis S, Konstadoulakis MM, et al: Apoptosis in cells of bronchoalveolar lavage: a cellular reaction in patients who die with sepsis and respiratory failure. *Crit Care Med* 29:2310-2317, 2001.
19. Ertel W, Keel M, Infanger M, et al: Circulating mediators in serum of injured patients with septic complications inhibit neutrophil apoptosis through up-regulation of protein-tyrosine phosphorylation. *J Trauma* 44:767-775, 1998.
20. Jimenez MF, Watson RW, Parodo J, et al: Dysregulated expression of neutrophil apoptosis in the systemic inflammatory response syndrome. *Arch Surg* 132:1263-1269, 1997.
21. Hotchkiss RS, Schmieg RE Jr, Swanson PE, et al: Rapid onset of intestinal epithelial and lymphocyte apoptotic cell death in patients with trauma and shock. *Crit Care Med* 28:3207-3217, 2000.
22. Pellegrini JD, De AK, Kodys K, et al: Relationships between T lymphocyte apoptosis and anergy following trauma. *J Surg Res* 88: 200-206, 2000.
23. Lebedev MJ, Ptitsina JS, Vilkov SA, et al: Membrane and soluble forms of Fas (CD95) in peripheral blood lymphocytes and in serum from burns patients. *Burns* 27:669-673, 2001.
24. Ogura H, Tanaka H, Koh T, et al: Priming, second-hit priming, and apoptosis in leukocytes from trauma patients. *J Trauma* 46: 774-781, 1999.
25. Matute-Bello G, Liles WC, Radella F, et al: Neutrophil apoptosis in the acute respiratory distress syndrome. *Am J Respir Crit Care Med* 156:1969-1977, 1997.
26. Lesur O, Kokis A, Hermans C, et al: Interleukin-2 involvement in early acute respiratory distress syndrome: relationship with polymorphonuclear neutrophil apoptosis and patient survival. *Crit Care Med* 28:3814-3822, 2000.
27. Matute-Bello G, Liles WC, Radella F, et al: Modulation of neutrophil apoptosis by granulocyte stimulating factor and colony-stimulating factor during the course of acute respiratory distress syndrome. *Crit Care Med* 28:1-7, 2000.
28. Matute-Bello G, Liles WC, Steinberg KP, et al: Soluble Fas ligand induces epithelial cell apoptosis in humans with acute lung injury (ARDS). *J Immunol* 163:2217-2225, 1999.
29. Hashimoto S, Kobayashi A, Kooguchi K, et al: Upregulation of two death pathways of perforin/granzyme and FasL/Fas in septic acute respiratory distress syndrome. *Am J Respir Crit Care Med* 161:237-243, 2000.
30. Ng I, Yeo TT, Tang WY, et al: Apoptosis occurs after cerebral contusions in humans. *Neurosurgery* 46:949-956, 2000.
31. Raghupathi R, Graham DI, McIntosh TK: Apoptosis after traumatic brain injury. *J Neurotrauma* 17:927-938, 2001.
32. Lenzlinger PM, Marx A, Trentz O, et al: Prolonged intrathecal release of soluble fas following severe traumatic brain injury in humans. *J Neuroimmunol*;122:167-174, 2002.
33. Harter L, Keel M, Hentze H, et al: Capase-3 activity is present in cerebrospinal fluid from patients with traumatic brain injury. *J Neuroimmunol* 121:76-78, 2001.
34. Hotchkiss RS, Swanson PE, Cobb JP, et al: Apoptosis in lymphoid and parenchymal cells during sepsis: findings in normal and T-and B-cell-deficient mice. *Crit Care Med* 25:1298-1307, 1997.
35. Hirarnatsu M, Hotchkiss RS, Karl IE, Buchman TG: Cecal ligation and puncture (CLP) induces apoptosis in thymus, spleen, lung, and gut by an endotoxin and TNF-independent pathway. Shock 7: 247-253, 1997.
36. Hotchkiss RS, Dunne WM, Swanson PE, et al: Role of apoptosis in *Pseudomonas aeruginosa* pneumonia. *Science* 294:1783, 2001.
37. Coopersmith CM, Stromberg PE, Dunne WM, et al: Inhibition of intestinal epithelial apoptosis and survival in a murine model of pneumonia-induced sepsis. *JAMA* 287:1716-1721, 2002.
38. Ayala A, Herdon CD, Lehman DL, et al: Differential induction of apoptosis in lymphoid tissues during sepsis: variation in onset, frequency, and the nature of the mediators. *Blood* 87:4261-4275, 1996.
39. Coopersmith CM, Chang KC, Swanson PE, et al: Overexpression of Bcl-2 in the intestinal epithelium improves survival in septic mice. *Crit Care Med* 30:195-201, 2002.
40. Ayala A, Xu YX, Chung CS, Chaudry IH: Does Fas ligand or endotoxin contribute to thymic apoptosis during polymicrobial sepsis? *Shock* 11:211-217, 1999.
41. Ayala A, Chung CS, Xu YX, et al: Increased inducible apoptosis in CD4+ T lymphocytes during polymicrobrial sepsis is mediated by Fas ligand and not endotoxin. *Immunology* 97:45-55, 1999.
42. Chung CS, Wang W, Chaundry IH, Ayala A: Increased apoptosis in lamina propria B cells during polymicrobial sepsis is FasL but not endotoxin mediated. *Am J Physiol Gastrointest Liver Physiol* 280:G812-G818, 2001.
43. Chung CS, Xu YX, Wang W, et al: Is Fas ligand or endotoxin responsible for mucosal lymphocyte apoptosis in sepsis? *Arch Surg* 133:1213-1220, 1998.
44. Hotchkiss RS, Tinsley KW, Swanson PE, et al: Prevention of lymphocyte cell death in sepsis improves survival in mice. *Proc Natl Acad U S A* 96:14541-14546, 1999.
45. Hotchkiss RS, Chank KC, Swanson PE, et al: Caspase inhibitors improve survival in sepsis: a critical role of the lymphocyte. *Nat Immunol* 1:496-501, 2000.
46. Hotchkiss RS, Swanson PE, Knudson CM, et al: Overexpression of Bcl-2 in transgenic mice decreases apoptosis and improves survival in sepsis. *J Immunol* 162;4148-4156, 1999.
47. Kim JM, Eckmann L, Savidge TC, et al: Apoptosis of human intestinal epithelial cells after bacterial invasion. *J Clin Invest* 102:1815-1823, 1998.
48. Rajan S, Cacalano G, Bryan R, et al: Pseudomonas Aeruginosa induction of apoptosis in respiratory epithelial cells: analysis of the effects of cystic fibrosis transmembrane conductance regulator dysfunction and bacterial virulence factors. *Am J Respir Cell Mol Biol* 23:304-312, 2000.
49. Grassme H, Kirschnek S, Riethmueller JA, et al: CD95/CD95 ligand interactions on epithelial cells in host defense to Pseudomonas aeruginosa. *Science* 290:527-530, 2000.
50. Kazzaz JA, Horowitz S, Xu J, et al: Differential patterns of apoptosis in resolving and nonresolving bacterial pneumonia. *Am J Respir Crit Care Med* 161:2043-2050, 2000.
51. Mantell LL, Kazzaz JA, Xu J, et al: Unscheduled apoptosis during acute inflammatory lung injury. *Cell Death Differ* 4:600-607, 1997.
52. Rogers HW, Callery MP, Deck B, Unanue ER: Listeria monocytogenes induces apoptosis of infected hepatocytes. *J Immunol* 156:679-684, 1996.
53. Ayala A, Karr SM, Evans TA, Chaudry IH: Factors responsible for peritoneal granulocyte apoptosis during sepsis. *J Surg Res* 69: 67-75, 1997.
54. Xu YX, Wichmann MW, Ayala A, et al: Trauma hemorrhage induces increased thymic apoptosis while decreasing IL-3 release and increasing GM-CSF. *J Surg Res* 68:24-30, 1997.
55. Angele MK, Xu YX, Ayala A, et al: Gender dimorphism in trauma-hemorrhage-induced thymocyte apoptosis. *Shock* 12:316-322, 1999.
56. Xu YX, Ayala A, Monfils B, et al: Mechanism of intestinal mucosal immune dysfunction following trauma-hemorrhage: increased apoptosis associated with elevated Fas expression in Peyer's patches. *J Surg Res* 70:55-60, 1997.
57. Nakanishi T, Nishi Y, Sato EF, et al: Thermal injury induces thymocyte apoptosis in the rat. *J Trauma* 44:143-148, 1998.
58. Fukuzuka K, Rosenberg JJ, Gaines GC, et al: Caspase-3-dependent organ apoptosis early after burn injury. *Ann Surg* 229:851-858, 1999.
59. Fukuzuka K, Edwards CK III, Clare-Salzler M, et al: Glucocorticoid-induced, caspase-dependent organ apoptosis early after burn injury. *Am J Physiol Regul Integr Comp Physiol* 278:R1005-R1018, 2000.
60. Nishimura T, Nishiura T, deSerres S, et al: Transforming growth factor-beta1 and splenocyte apoptotic cell death after burn injuries. *J Burn Care Rehabil* 21:128-134, 2000.
61. Fukuzuka K, Edwards CK III, Clare-Salzer M, et al: Glucocorticoid and Fas ligand induced mucosal lymphocyte apoptosis after burn injury. *J Trauma* 49:710-716, 2000.
62. Cho K, Adamson LK, Greenhalgh DG. Parallel self-induction of TNF-alpha and apoptosis in the thymus of mice after burn injury. *J Surg Res* 98:9-15, 2001.
63. Coopersmith CM, O'Donnell D, Gordon JI: Bcl-2 inhibits ischemia-reperfusion-induced apoptosis in the intestinal epithelium of transgenic mice. *Am J Physiol* 276(3 pt 1):G677-G686, 1999.
64. Sun Z, Wang X, Deng X, et al: The influence of intestinal ischemia and reperfusion on bidirectional intestinal barrier permeability, cellular membrane integrity, proteinase inhibitors, and cell death in rats. *Shock* 10:203-212, 1998.
65. Shah KA, Shurey S, Green CJ: Apoptosis after intestinal ischemia-injury: a morphological study. *Transplantation* 64:1393-1397, 1997.

66. Noda T, Iwakiri R, Fujimoto K, et al: Programmed cell death induced by ischemia-reperfusion in rat intestinal mucosa. *Am J Physiol* 274(2 pt 1):G270-G276, 1998.
67. Du X, Liu Q, Yang Z, et al: Protective effects of interleukin-11 in an murine model of ischemic bowel necrosis. *Am J Physiol* 272 (3 pt 1):G545-G552, 1997.
68. Ikeda H, Suzuki M, Koike M, et al: Apoptosis is a major mode of cell death caused by ischaemia and ischaemia/reperfusion injury to the rat intestinal epithelium. *Gut* 42:530-537, 1998.
69. Wolf SE, Ikeda H, Martin S, et al: Cutaneous burn increases apoptosis in the gut epithelium of mice. *J Am Coll Surg* 188:10-16, 1999.
70. Lightfoot E Jr, Horton JW, Maass DL, et al: Major burn trauma in rats promotes cardiac and gastrointestinal apoptosis. *Shock* 11:29-34, 1999.
71. Ramzy PI, Wolf SE, Irtun O, et al: Gut epithelial apoptosis after severe effects of gut hypoperfusion. *J Am Coll Surg* 190:281-287, 2000.
72. Jeschke MG, Debroy MA, Wolf SE, et al: Burn and starvation increase programmed cell death in small bowel epithelial cells. *Dig Dis Sci* 45:415-420, 2000.
73. Kitamura Y, Hashimoto S, Mizuta N, et al: Fas/FasL-dependent apoptosis of alveolar cells after lipopolysaccharide-induced lung injury in mice. *Am J Respir Crit Care Med* 163 (3 pt 1);762-769, 2001.
74. Hotchkiss RS, Tinsley KW, Swanson PE, Karl IE: Endothelial cell apoptosis in sepsis. *Crit Care Med* 30(5 suppl):S225-S228, 2002.
75. Haimovitz-Friedman A, Cordon-Cardo C, Bayoumy S, et al: Lipopolysaccharide induces disseminated endothelial apoptosis requiring ceramide generation. *J Exp Med* 186:1831-1841, 1997.
76. Watson RW, Rotstein OD, Nathens AB, et al: Neutrophil apoptosis is modulated by endothelial transmigration and adhesion molecule engagement. *J Immunol* 158:945-953, 1997.
77. Jeschke MG, Low JF, Spies M, et al: Cell proliferation, apoptosis, expression, enzyme, protein, and weight changes in livers of burned rats. *Am J Physiol Gastrointest Liver Physiol* 280:G1314-G1320, 2001.
78. Yasuhara S, Kanakubo E, Perez ME, et al: The 1999 Moyer Award. Burn injury induces skeletal muscle apoptosis and the activation of caspase pathways in rats. *J Burn Care Rehabil* 20:462-470, 1999.
79. Fox GB, Fan L, Levasseur RA, Faden AI: Sustained sensory/motor and cognitive deficits with neuronal apoptosis following controlled cortical impact brain injury in the mouse. *J Neurotrauma* 15: 599-614, 1998.
80. Runnerstam M, Bao F, Huang Y, et al: A new model for diffuse brain injury by rotational acceleration: II. Effects on extracellular glutamate, intracranial pressure, and neuronal apoptosis. *J Neurotrauma* 18:259-273, 2001.
81. Lewen A, Fujimura M, Sugawara T, et al: Oxidative stress-dependent release of mitochondria1 cytochrome c after traumatic brain injury. *J Cereb Blood Flow Metab* 21:914-920, 2001.

CHAPTER 94

Endotheliopathy

Yves Ouellette

PEARLS

- The vascular architecture provides endothelial cells the ability to interact with blood components, such as flow, soluble factors, and other cells, and to integrate these signals into a cohesive regulation of vascular responses.
- The endothelium controls the vascular tone of the underlying smooth muscle cells through the production of vasodilator and vasoconstrictor mediators.
- Endothelial cell activation in response to inflammation changes endothelial cell regulatory function and results in altered vascular function.

Until recently, scientists and clinicians considered the endothelium, the cell layer that lines the blood vessels, an inert barrier separating the various components of blood and the surrounding tissues. The vascular endothelium now is recognized as a highly specialized and metabolically active organ performing a number of critical physiologic, immunologic, and synthetic functions. These functions include regulation of vascular permeability, vascular tone, cell adhesion, homeostasis, and vasculogenesis.[1]

The normal vascular endothelium is only one cell layer thick, separating the blood and vascular smooth muscle. The endothelium responds to physical and biochemical stimuli by releasing regulatory substances affecting vascular tone and growth, thrombosis and thrombolysis, and platelet and leukocyte interactions with the endothelium. Normal endothelial functions include control over thrombosis and thrombolysis, platelet and leukocyte interactions with the vessel wall, and regulation of vascular tone and growth. Of particular interest to intensivists is the fact that the endothelium secretes both powerful vasorelaxing (e.g., nitric oxide [NO]) and vasoconstricting substances (e.g., endothelin-1 [ET-1]). Because normal endothelial function plays a central role in vascular homeostasis, it is logical to conclude that endothelial dysfunction contributes to disease states characterized by vasomotor dysfunction, abnormal thrombosis, or abnormal vascular proliferation.

The endothelium lies between the lumen and the vascular smooth muscle, where it is uniquely positioned to "sense" changes in hemodynamic forces or blood-borne signals by membrane receptor mechanisms. The endothelial cells can respond to physical and chemical stimuli by synthesizing or releasing a variety of vasoactive and thromboregulatory molecules and growth factors. Substances released by the endothelium include prostacyclin, NO, endothelins, endothelial cell growth factors, interleukins, plasminogen inhibitors, and von Willebrand factor (vWF). The vascular endothelium possesses numerous enzymes, receptors, and transduction molecules. It interacts with other vessel wall constituents and circulating blood cells. In addition to these universal functions, the endothelium may have organ-specific roles that are differentiated for various parts of the body, such as gas exchange in the lungs, control of myocardial function in the heart, and phagocytosis in the liver and spleen.

Studies of endothelial structure and function have been accomplished by a variety of techniques, including ultrastructural studies, in vitro experiments for endothelial cell isolation and culture, physiologic studies in animals, and, most recently, clinical studies in humans. This knowledge has facilitated the development of treatment strategies based on administration of endothelial products, such as prostacyclin and NO, or their antagonists.

Normal Endothelial Function

Endothelial Cell Heterogeneity

Many vascular diseases appear to be restricted to specific vascular beds. For example, thrombotic events often are localized to single vessels. Commonly, certain vasculitides specifically affect particular arteries, veins, or capillaries to affect specific organs. Tumor cells often metastasize, more commonly within particular vascular beds. The basis for this variability in vascular disease is poorly understood but may be explained by the heterogeneity of endothelial cells. Knowledge of how endothelial cell heterogeneity may contribute to the maintenance of organ-specific function and the development of disorders restricted to specific vascular beds has increased.[2,3]

The morphology of capillary endothelium from different vascular beds may explain differences in tissue function. For example, the brain microcirculation is lined by endothelial cells connected by tight junctions that maintain the blood-brain barrier. In contrast, sinusoids in the liver, spleen, and bone marrow are lined by endothelial cells that allow transcellular trafficking between intercellular gaps. Similarly, fenestrated endothelial cells in the intestinal villi, endocrine glands, and kidneys facilitate selective permeability, which is required for efficient absorption, secretion, and filtering.[4]

Another example of endothelial cell heterogeneity lies in the expression of cell surface receptors involved in cell-to-cell signaling and cell trafficking. For example, in mice, lung-specific endothelial cell adhesion molecule is expressed exclusively by pulmonary postcapillary endothelial cells and some splenic venules. Similarly, specific mucosal cell adhesion molecules are expressed primarily on endothelial venules in Peyer patches of the small intestine.[5,6] Tumor cells may show clear preferential adhesion to the endothelium of specific organs paralleling their in vivo metastatic propensities.[7] Distinct subsets of endothelial cells often exist within a single organ. Two distinct sinusoidal endothelial cell phenotypes can be recognized in the adult human liver: hepatic periportal vessels express specific cell surface molecules such as platelet endothelial cell adhesion molecule (PECAM)-1 and CD34, whereas sinusoidal intrahepatic endothelial cells do not.

Cultured microvascular endothelial cells express surface markers, protein transporters, and intracellular enzymes specific to their tissue of origin, such as brain, liver, and other organs. These tissue-specific phenotypic differences can be maintained for some time under identical tissue culture conditions. Endothelial phenotype can be manipulated by changing the microenvironment, a phenomenon referred to as *transdifferentiation*. For example, aortic endothelial cells cultured on lung-derived extracellular matrix are induced to express lung-specific endothelial cell adhesion molecule, whereas the same cells develop fenestrae when they are cultured on matrix derived from kidney-derived MDCK cells. Similarly, endothelial cells grown on extracts of basement membrane from different organs develop preferential adhesivity for tumor cells prone to metastasize to that organ.

Coagulation and Fibrinolysis

A normal physiologic function of the endothelium is to provide an antithrombotic surface that inhibits platelet adhesion and clotting, thus facilitating normal blood flow. Under pathophysiologic conditions, the endothelium transforms into a prothrombotic surface. A dynamic equilibrium exists between the two states that permits rapid response to an insult and rapid recovery.[8]

Anticoagulant Mechanisms

The endothelium has anticoagulant, antiplatelet, and fibrinolytic properties.[9] Endothelial cells are the major site for anticoagulant reactions involving thrombin. Thrombin plays a key role in coagulation, including activation of platelets, activation of several coagulation enzymes and cofactors, and stimulation of procoagulation pathways on the endothelial cell surface. In the normal state, there is little thrombin enzyme activity. The surrounding endothelial cell matrix contains heparin sulfate and related glycosaminoglycans that activate antithrombin III. The subendothelial cell matrix contains dermatan sulfate, which promotes the antithrombin activity of heparin cofactor II. Microvascular endothelial cells release tissue factor pathway inhibitor, which inhibits the factor VIIa–tissue factor complex and further contributes to anticoagulation (Figure 94–1).

Thrombin activity is also modulated by endothelial cell synthesis of thrombomodulin.[10,11] Binding of thrombin to thrombomodulin facilitates the enzyme's activation of the anticoagulant protein C. Activated protein C activity is enhanced by cofactor C, which is synthesized by endothelial cells and by other cells. Thrombomodulin also inhibits prothrombinase activity indirectly by binding factor Xa.

Platelet adhesion to endothelial cells is markedly inhibited by endothelium-derived prostacyclin.[12] The same stimuli that activate platelets, such as thrombin, adenosine diphosphate, and adenosine triphosphate (ATP), also act to release prostacyclin from the endothelium, which allows the endothelium to limit the extent of platelet plug formation. The interactions between platelets and endothelium regulate platelet function, coagulation cascades, and local vascular tone.

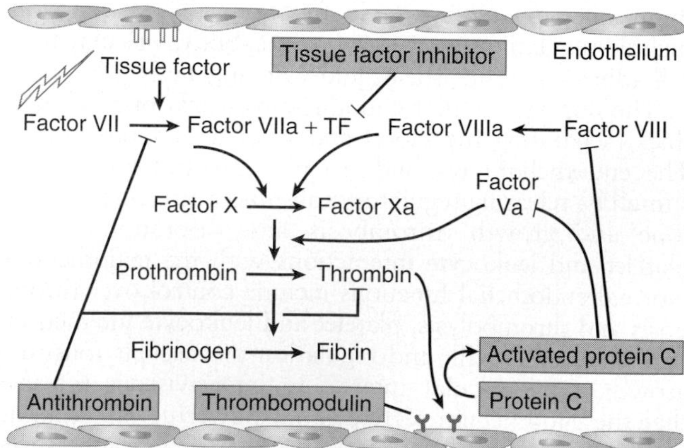

FIGURE 94–1 • Endothelium control of the coagulation cascade. An inflammatory stimulus up-regulates the interaction of tissue factor *(TF)* with factor VII, which generates activated factor VII (factor VIIa). The TF–factor VIIa complex then leads to conversion of factor X to factor Xa. Interaction of factors Xa and Va results in conversion of prothrombin to thrombin and of fibrinogen to fibrin. Three key anticoagulant pathways can inhibit this process. Protein C is activated through its interaction with cell surface thrombomodulin and inhibits the activities of factors Va and VIII. Antithrombin blocks the activation of multiples factors, including factor X and thrombin. Tissue factor pathway inhibitor interferes directly with the tissue factor–factor VIIa complex.

Microvascular endothelial cells may secrete tissue-type plasminogen activator (tPA), the powerful thrombolytic agent in frequent clinical use for treatment of coronary thrombotic occlusion.[13] tPA release is stimulated in vivo by norepinephrine, vasopressin, or stasis within the vessel lumen. Thrombin also may stimulate tPA release, providing another endothelium-mediated safeguard against uncontrolled coagulation.

Procoagulant Mechanisms

The expression and release of tissue factor is the pivotal step in transforming the endothelium from an anticoagulant to a procoagulant surface.[14,15] Tissue factor accelerates factor VIIa-dependent activation of factors X and IX (Figure 94–1). Synthesis of tissue factor is induced by a number of agonists, including thrombin, endotoxin, several cytokines, shear stress, hypoxia, oxidized lipoproteins, and other endothelial insults. Once endothelial cells expressing tissue factor are exposed to plasma, prothrombinase activity is generated and fibrin is formed on the surface of the cells.

Endothelium-Derived Vasodilators

The important role of endothelium in controlling vascular tone has only recently been appreciated. As clinicians and researchers, we have come to appreciate that the endothelium controls underlying smooth muscle tone in response to certain pharmacologic and physiologic stimuli. This response involves a number of luminal membrane receptors and complex intracellular pathways and the synthesis and release of a variety of relaxing and constricting substances, described in the following sections.

Nitric Oxide

Furchgott and Zawadzki[16] first postulated the existence of an endothelium-derived relaxing factor (EDRF) in 1980, when they noted that the presence of endothelium was essential for rabbit aortic rings to relax in response to acetylcholine. The biologic effects of EDRF later were determined to be mediated by NO.[17]

NO is generated from the conversion of L-arginine to NO and L-citrulline by the enzyme nitric oxide synthase (NOS).[18] The two general forms of NOS are constitutive and inducible. In the unstimulated state, NO is continuously produced by constitutive NO synthase (cNOS). The activity of cNOS is modulated by calcium, which is released from endoplasmic stores in response to activation of certain receptors. Substances such as acetylcholine, bradykinin, histamine, insulin, and substance P stimulate NO production through this mechanism. Shearing forces acting on the endothelium are another important mechanism regulating NO release. The inducible form of NOS (iNOS) is not calcium dependent. Instead it is stimulated by the actions of cytokines (e.g., tumor necrosis factor [TNF]-α, interleukins) and/or bacterial endotoxins (e.g., lipopolysaccharide). Induction of iNOS occurs over several hours and results in NO production that may be more than a 1,000-fold greater than that produced by cNOS. This is an important mechanism in the pathogenesis of inflammation (Figure 94–2). Inhibition of NOS using competitive analogues of L-arginine drastically reduces endothelium-dependent relaxations in vitro, particularly in large conduit arteries, thereby evoking vasoconstriction. Chronic treatment of animals with NOS inhibitors or suppression of the cNOS gene reportedly induces hypertension.[19–21]

Once NO is formed by an endothelial cell, it readily diffuses out of the cell and into adjacent smooth muscle cells, where it binds and activates the soluble form of guanylyl cyclase. This process results in the production of cyclic guanosine monophosphate (cGMP) from guanosine triphosphate.[22] cGMP in turn activates a number of cGMP-modulated enzymes (Figure 94–2). Increased cGMP activates a kinase that leads to inhibition of calcium influx into the smooth muscle cell and decreased calcium-calmodulin stimulation of myosin light-chain kinase. This in turn decreases the phosphorylation of myosin light chains, thereby decreasing smooth muscle tension development and causing vasodilation. Some evidence indicates that increases in cGMP can lead to myosin light-chain dephosphorylation by activating the myosin light-chain phosphatase. In addition, cGMP-dependent protein kinase phosphorylates K^+ channels to induce hyperpolarization and thereby inhibits vasoconstriction.[23,24] Interestingly, NO inhibition of platelet aggregation also is related to the increase in cGMP. Drugs that inhibit cGMP breakdown, such as inhibitors of cGMP-dependent phosphodiesterase (e.g., sildenafil), potentiate the effects of NO-mediated actions on the target cell.

NO therefore contributes to the balance between vasodilator and vasoconstrictor influences that determine vascular tone.[25] The exogenous nitrovasodilators sodium nitroprusside and nitroglycerin use the same pathways. Generation of NO from L-arginine can be specificaly blocked by arginine analogues, such as N^G-monomethyl-L-arginine (L-NMMA), which has proved to be a useful tool

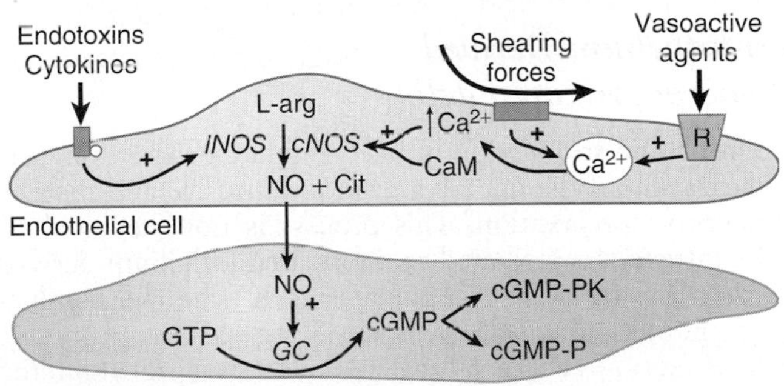

FIGURE 94–2 • Nitric oxide *(NO)* is generated from L-arginine *(L-arg)* by the action of nitric oxide synthase *(NOS)*. In the resting state, constitutive NOS *(cNOS)* is modulated by intracellular Ca^{2+} and calmodulin *(CaM)*. Stored Ca^{2+} is released in response to vasoactive agents (e.g., acetylcholine and bradykinin) and other external stimuli, such as shearing forces. Cytokine and endotoxin activation of endothelial cells results in increased expression of inducible NOS *(iNOS)*. Citrulline *(Cit)* is a byproduct of NO production. NO has a half-life of only a few seconds in vivo and quickly diffuses to surrounding cells, such as smooth muscle cells. NO stimulates the production of the intracellular mediator cyclic guanosine monophosphate *(cGMP)*. Increased cGMP activates a series of cGMP-dependent protein kinases *(cGMP-PK)* and cGMP-dependent phosphatases *(cGMP-P)*.

in clinical research, allowing investigation of the biologic distribution and role of NO.

Prostacyclin

Another major endothelium-derived vasodilator is the prostaglandin prostacyclin, a derivative of arachidonic acids through the action of the enzyme cyclooxygenase. Endothelial cells are capable of producing a variety of vasoactive substances that are products of arachidonic acid metabolism. Among these are prostaglandins, prostacyclin (PGI_2), leukotrienes, and thromboxanes. These substances act as either vasodilators or vasoconstrictors, among their other biologic activities. Prostacyclin is a potent vasodilator and is active in both the pulmonary and systemic circulations. In addition to its vasodilatory effects, prostacyclin has antithrombotic and antiplatelet activity. Its release may be stimulated by bradykinin and adenine nucleotides. Like NO, it is chemically unstable with a short half-life.[26] However, unlike NO, prostacyclin activity in arterial beds depends on its ability to bind to specific receptors in vascular smooth muscle. Therefore its vasodilator activity is determined by the expression of such receptors. Prostacyclin receptors are coupled to adenylate cyclase to elevate cyclic adenosine monophosphate (cAMP) levels in vascular smooth muscle.[27] The increase in cAMP results in (1) stimulation of ATP-sensitive K^+ channels resulting in hyperpolarization of the cell membrane and inhibition of the development of contraction; and (2) increase efflux of Ca^{2+} from the smooth muscle cell and inhibition of the contractile machinery.

In addition, prostacyclin facilitates the release of NO by endothelial cells, and the action of prostacyclin in vascular smooth muscle is potentiated by NO. Interestingly, NO may also potentiate the effects of prostacyclin. The NO-mediated increase in cGMP in smooth muscle cells inhibits a phosphodiesterase that breaks down cAMP, indirectly prolonging the half-life of the second messenger of prostacyclin.[28]

Endothelium-Derived Hyperpolarizing Factor

Endothelium stimulation by acetylcholine produces hyperpolarization of the underlying smooth muscle and thereby induces vasorelaxation. This process is not mediated by NO; instead it is mediated by another endothelium-derived factor. This factor acts by increasing K^+ channel conductance in smooth muscle cells, resulting in smooth muscle cell relaxation. The resulting vasodilation is not inhibited by L-NMMA, the specific antagonist of NO, but is inhibited by ouabain, an Na^+/K^+-ATPase inhibitor. In addition, in most medium- to resistance-sized arteries, electrophysiologic studies have established that endothelium-dependent hyperpolarization of vascular smooth muscle is resistant to the combined inhibition of both NOS and cyclooxygenases. Accordingly, a component of the endothelium-dependent relaxation in these arteries is mediated by a substance different from NO and prostacyclin. This component of endothelium-dependent vasodilatation has been attributed to a yet unidentified diffusible endothelium-derived hyperpolarizing factor (EDHF).[29]

EDHF acts by opening K^+ channels in vascular smooth muscle. Hyperpolarization inhibits vasoconstriction by closing voltage-sensitive Ca^{2+} channels, impairing the receptor-dependent activation of phospholipase C and the subsequent release of Ca^{2+} from intracellular stores and reducing the Ca^{2+} sensitivity of the contractile proteins. Of significant clinical importance is the fact that the EDHF-mediated effect increases as arterial diameter decreases, as in resistance arteries. EDHF likely plays a significant role in the regulation of peripheral vascular resistance and local hemodynamics. Unfortunately, in the absence of selective inhibitors of the EDHF pathway, evaluation of the relevance of EDHF in vivo is not possible.[29]

Endothelium-Derived Vasoconstrictors

Endothelins (Endothelium-Derived Contracting Factors)

Endothelin is a 21-amino-acid peptide and is one of the most potent vasoconstrictors yet identified. Endothelial cells synthesize the prohormone bigendothelin and express endothelin-converting enzymes to generate endothelin. Endothelin exists in three isoforms, but only one (ET-1) has been shown to be released from human endothelial cells. ET-1 is synthesized in the endothelial cells, and its release is mediated by a variety of stimuli. ET-1 release is stimulated by angiotensin II, antidiuretic hormone, thrombin, cytokines, reactive oxygen species, and shearing forces acting on the vascular endothelium. ET-1 release is inhibited by NO, prostacyclin, and atrial natriuretic peptide.[30,31]

ET-1 has a short half-life, which suggests that, similar to NO, ET-1 is mainly a locally active vasoregulator. Once released by endothelial cells, ET-1 binds to the ET_A membrane receptor found on adjacent vascular smooth muscle cells. This binding leads to calcium mobilization and smooth muscle contraction. The ET_A receptor is coupled with a G protein linked to phospholipase C, resulting in the formation of inositol 1,4,5-triphosphate (IP_3). Interestingly, ET-1 can also bind to an ET_B receptor located on the vascular endothelium, which stimulates the formation of NO by the endothelium. This release of NO appears to modulate the ET_A receptor-mediated contraction of the vascular smooth muscle. Its physiologic role includes maintenance of basal vascular resistance, and it is present in low concentrations in healthy subjects. Elevated endothelin levels have been found in patients with systemic and pulmonary hypertension, coronary artery disease, and heart failure. The role of ET-1 in the pathophysiology of these conditions is postulated but not proven.[30,31]

Reactive Oxygen Species

Endothelial cells secrete oxygen-derived free radicals and hydrogen peroxide in response to shear stress and endothelial agonists such as bradykinin. Such reactive oxygen species reportedly inactivate NO, resulting in vasoconstriction. Reactive oxygen species may facilitate mobilization of cytosolic Ca^{2+} in vascular smooth muscle cells and promote Ca^{2+} sensitization of the contractile elements. Because endothelium-derived superoxide anion is primarily a chemical antagonist of NO, this scavenger of the free-radical superoxide anion dismutase reportedly potentiates endothelium-dependent vasodilatation.[32]

Vasoconstrictor Prostaglandins

Metabolism of arachidonic acid by cyclooxygenase in endothelial cells may lead to secretion of precursors of thromboxanes and leukotrienes. These prostaglandins act on receptors in vascular smooth muscle to induce vasoconstriction. Prostacyclin, however, is the major endothelial metabolite of arachidonic acid, which is generated through the cyclooxygenase pathway. Thus under normal circumstances, the influence of the small amounts of vasoconstrictor prostanoids released by endothelial cells is masked by the production of prostacyclin, NO, and EDHF.[33,34]

Endothelium and Blood Cell Interactions

In addition to the interactions of endothelium with blood coagulation factors, endothelial cells express cell surface molecules that orchestrate the trafficking of circulating blood cells. These cell-associated molecules help direct the migration of leukocytes into specific organs under physiologic conditions and accelerate migration toward sites of inflammation. They also have been implicated in the adhesion of platelets and erythrocytes in several common disorders associated with homeostasis.

Interactions of Leukocytes with the Vessel Wall

It is well established that flowing leukocytes adhere to specific regions of the endothelium in response to tissue injury or infection. These multicellular interactions are essential precursors of physiologic inflammation. Leukocytes interact with vessel surfaces through a multistep process that includes: (1) initial formation of usually reversible attachments; (2) activation of the attached cells; (3) development of stronger, shear-resistant adhesion; and (4) spreading, emigration, and other sequelae (Figure 94–3).[35]

Selectins are key molecules in the interaction of leukocytes and endothelial cells. They are transmembrane glycoproteins that recognize cell surface carbohydrate ligands found on leukocytes and initiate and mediate tethering and rolling of leukocytes on the endothelial cell surface. Selectins constitute a family of three known molecules. L-selectin is expressed on most leukocytes and binds to ligands constitutively expressed on endothelial cells found in venules of lymphoid tissues. Its expression is induced on endothelium at sites of inflammation. E-selectin is expressed on activated endothelial cells and leukocytes. P-selectin is rapidly redistributed from secretory granules to the surface of platelets and endothelial cells stimulated with thrombin. Endothelial cell E-selectin and P-selectin both bind to ligands on leukocytes.[36]

With stimulation, leukocytes usually attach to postcapillary venule endothelial cells, where shear stresses are lowest. Leukocytes adherent to the endothelium can make contact with flowing leukocytes through the L-selectin

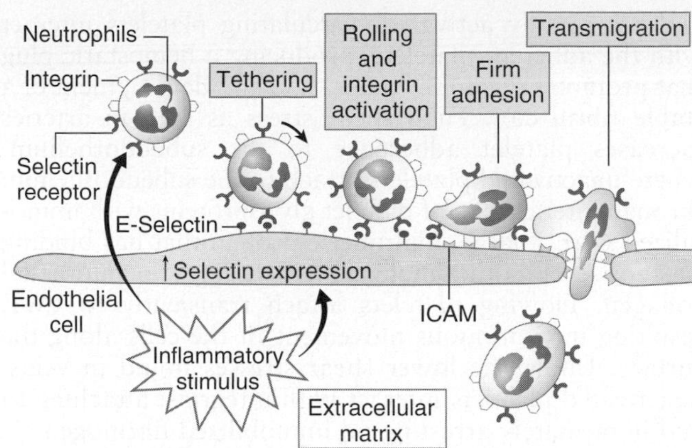

FIGURE 94–3 • Leukocyte recruitment process and transmigration. The multistep model for leukocyte recruitment at sites of inflammation begins with activation of neutrophils and endothelial cells. Once activated, endothelial cells express selectins whose binding to neutrophils initiates rolling and adhesion of neutrophils to the endothelium. Activated integrins on the surface of neutrophils bind to endothelial cell ICAMs, facilitating a firm adhesion. Transmigration through the endothelium further involves interactions with other molecules, such as platelet endothelial cell adhesion molecules and cadherins on the surface of endothelial cells.

molecule, resulting in amplification of leukocyte recruitment to sites of inflammation. It is generally understood that selectins initiate inflammatory, immune, and hemostatic responses by promoting transient multicellular interactions.[37]

Proinflammatory molecules presented on the surface of the endothelium proceed to activate a second family of adhesion molecules, the integrins, and cause cells to firmly adhere. After the initial tethering of leukocytes to endothelial cells, leukocytes then must roll prior to transmigrating through the endothelium. Inhibition of leukocyte adhesion does not reduce leukocyte rolling, suggesting that rolling and adhesion are distinct molecular events. In addition, inhibiting rolling reduces adhesion, suggesting that rolling is a prerequisite of leukocyte adhesion/recruitment and ultimately the inflammatory response.

Leukocytes subsequently migrate between endothelial cells into tissues by mechanisms that are not completely understood but which we know are affected by gradients of chemokines, integrins activation states, and interactions with PECAM-1, an immunoglobulin-like receptor. This migration requires disruption of endothelial cell to endothelial cell interaction of cadherins at tight junctions. Leukocyte recruitment to lymphoid tissues or inflammatory sites requires the coordinated expression of specific combinations of adhesion and signaling molecules. Diversity at each step of the cascade ensures that the appropriate leukocytes accumulate for a restricted period in response to a specific challenge.[4,37]

Platelet Adhesion

Endothelial cells and circulating platelets normally do not interact because of the release of PGI_2, the release of NO, and the expression of a CD39 on the surface of endothelial cells.[38] During vascular injury and inflammation, platelets adhere to exposed subendothelial components and are rapidly activated. Circulating platelets interact with the adherent platelets, producing a hemostatic plug that promotes thrombin generation and development of a stable fibrin clot. High shear stress as seen in arteries increases platelet adherence to the subendothelium, where unactivated platelets attach to the subendothelium through interactions of platelet glycoproteins with immobilized vWF, a large, multimeric protein that has binding sites for several other molecules, including subendothelial collagen. Flowing platelets attach transiently to vWF, resulting in continuous movement of the cells along the surface. Under the lower shear stresses found in veins, unactivated platelets interact with integrins, attaching to and immediately arresting on immobilized fibrinogen.[39]

Once platelets adhere to either vWF or fibrinogen, they are activated by secreted products such as adenosine diphosphate or epinephrine, or by surface molecules such as collagen, which cross-link the integrins and other platelet receptors. The activated platelets spread and adhere more avidly to the subendothelial surface, which recruits additional platelets into aggregates. Shear-resistant adhesion may be further enhanced by interactions of other integrins or receptors with laminin, fibronectin, and thrombospondin. As thrombin is generated, converting bound fibrinogen to fibrin, the aggregated platelets contract to strengthen the clot.[39]

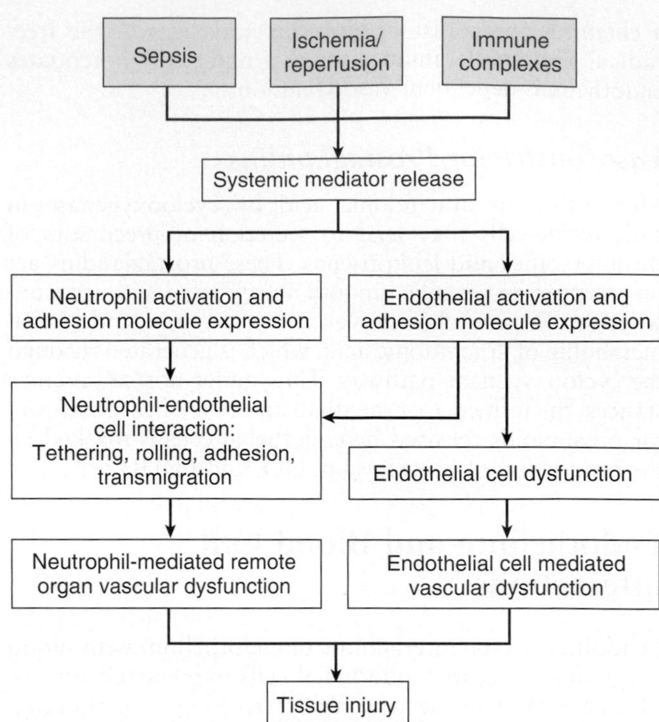

FIGURE 94–4 • Schematic illustration of the mechanisms that underlie the development of local and remote organ injury following an initial inflammatory event. Activation of endothelial cells and circulating neutrophils lead to expression and activation of adhesion molecules that facilitate neutrophil invasion of vascular beds and result in local and remote organ dysfunction.

Endothelial Cell Dysfunction

Ischemia/Reperfusion Injury

Reperfusion of previously ischemic tissues can place organs at risk for further cellular injury, thereby limiting recovery of function. The microvasculature, particularly the endothelial cells, is vulnerable to the deleterious consequences of ischemia and reperfusion (I/R). I/R is recognized as a potentially serious problem that is encountered during a variety of standard medical and surgical procedures, such as thrombolytic therapy, organ transplantation, and cardiopulmonary bypass.[40]

The molecular and biochemical changes in the vascular wall that occur during I/R are characteristic of an acute inflammatory response (Figure 94–4). The intensity of this inflammatory response can be so severe that the injury response to reperfusion also manifests in susceptible organs such as the lungs and cardiovascular system. The resulting systemic inflammatory response syndrome (SIRS) and multiple organ dysfunction syndrome (MODS) are associated with significantly increased mortality and morbidity.[41]

Microvascular dysfunction associated with I/R is manifested as impaired endothelium-dependent dilation in arterioles, enhanced fluid filtration, leukocyte plugging in capillaries, and trafficking of leukocytes and plasma protein extravasation in postcapillary venules. During the initial period following reperfusion, activated endothelial cells in the microcirculation produce more oxygen radicals and less NO. The resulting imbalance between superoxide and NO in endothelial cells leads to production and release of inflammatory mediators (e.g., platelet-activating factor, TNF-α) and enhances biosynthesis of adhesion molecules that mediate leukocyte–endothelial cell adhesion.[42]

The inflammatory mediators released as a consequence of reperfusion appear to activate endothelial cells in remote organs that are not exposed to the initial ischemic insult. Oxidants and activated leukocytes have been implicated as mediators of remote organ injury in I/R. This distant response to I/R can result in leukocyte-dependent microvascular injury that is characteristic of SIRS and MODS. The pulmonary damage associated with MODS can range from mild dysfunction, as seen in acute lung injury, to severe failure, as seen in acute respiratory distress syndrome. The pulmonary injuries associated with acute lung injury and acute respiratory distress syndrome include increased pulmonary microvascular permeability and accumulation of neutrophil-rich alveolar fluid. Respiratory failure often is associated with cardiovascular, hepatic, gastrointestinal, and renal dysfunction, as well as central nervous system involvement. MODS is associated with dysfunction of the coagulation cascade and the immune system, resulting in thrombosis, disseminated intravascular coagulation, and immunocompromise. Initiation of MODS may lead to additional tissue ischemia, resulting in further insult[43] (see Chapter 97).

Sepsis

Sepsis is a generalized systemic response to an infectious insult and manifests as SIRS. The clinical syndrome is characterized by a series of circulatory disturbances, including decreased vascular resistance and maldistribution of blood flow in association with impaired oxygen utilization.

As a consequence, focal tissue hypoxia and cell injury soon follow the onset of sepsis. Despite aggressive volume resuscitation, systemic administration of antibiotics, vasopressors, and other sophisticated intensive care measures, sepsis is frequently associated with multiple organ dysfunction and patient death (see Chapter 96).

Although the pathophysiologic process of multiple organ dysfunction is multifactorial, one common feature is the dysfunction of the microcirculation, including the resistance arteries, capillaries, and postcapillary venules. The microcirculation cannot be considered a simple passive conduit. Rather, it is a functionally active system of interactions between the vascular wall, circulating and tissue-associated cells such as leukocytes, platelets, and mast cells, and extracellular mediators that contribute to the regulation of local, downstream, and upstream vascular tone (Figure 94–4). Sepsis is particularly associated with microvascular endothelial cell dysfunction leading to: (1) breakdown of endothelial barrier function, leading to tissue edema and uncontrolled inflammatory cell infiltration; (2) vasomotor dysfunction, leading to the formation of arteriovenous shunts in association with loss of peripheral resistance; and (3) disturbance of oxygen transport and utilization by tissue cells.[44]

Septic shock is often associated with loss of fluid from the intravascular into the extravascular space, with potential progressive loss of circulating blood that eventually leads to depression of cardiac output. Similarly, loss of fluid into the extravascular space can lead to life-threatening edema in the lungs, kidney, and brain of septic patients. The loss of fluid is not believed to be associated with changes in hydrostatic and/or osmotic pressures within the vascular compartment but rather to the breakdown of endothelial barrier function. This breakdown allows migration of water and macromolecules, including proteins, into the extravascular space. The pathophysiologic mechanisms proposed include the separation of tight junctions between endothelial cells rather than destructive changes of endothelial cells leading to defects in the endothelium.[45]

In animal models of sepsis, a loss of vasoconstrictor response of resistance arterioles to catecholamines is observed, and the vasorelaxing response to the microcirculatory segment is blunted. Although in vitro experiments demonstrate decreased biosynthesis of NO by endotoxin-exposed cultured endothelial cells, the overriding reaction with respect to NO synthesis is up-regulation of smooth muscle NO synthase. The ensuing overproduction of NO is the essential factor in the massive peripheral vasodilatation characteristic of the septic state. However, another suggestion is that endotoxin-induced NO synthesis and consequently increased levels of NO in the septic organism decrease the sensitivity to the relaxing effect of acetylcholine. In septic rats, the vasoconstrictor response to a variety of vasopressor agents (vasopressin, endothelin, angiotensin) was attenuated. The microvascular response could be partially or completely restored by administration of inhibitors of NO, suggesting that NO plays a key role in mediating vasomotor dysfunction in sepsis.[46]

Studies on microcirculation of the gut have shown the development of a gap between microvascular and venous oxygen tension, suggesting enhanced shunting of the microcirculation. Defects in distributing blood to regional vascular beds or the microcirculation could be responsible for tissue hypoxia and limited oxygen extraction (see Chapter 67). Clinical evidence of decreased microvessel density in the sublingual microcirculation of fluid-resuscitated septic patients is consistent with findings of decreased functional capillary flow in the gut, liver, and skeletal muscle microcirculation in animal models of sepsis. This clinical finding raises the possibility that abnormal microvascular O_2 transport develops in multiple organs despite fluid resuscitation, leading to heterogeneous microvascular dysfunction and local tissue hypoxia in severe cases of sepsis.

Hemolytic Uremic Syndrome

Thrombotic thrombocytopenic purpura (TTP) and the hemolytic uremic syndrome (HUS) are related disorders characterized clinically by microangiopathic hemolytic anemia and thrombocytopenia. Pathologically, both conditions include the development of platelet microthrombi that occlude small arterioles and capillaries. Endothelial dysfunction plays a prominent role in the pathogenesis of the two disorders. HUS commonly occurs in early childhood (approximately 90% of cases). It often follows an episode of bloody diarrhea caused by enteropathic strains of *Escherichia coli* that release the exotoxin verotoxin-1 (VT-1). VT-1 binds with high affinity to receptors expressed in high density on renal glomerular endothelial cells. VT-1 is directly cytotoxic to endothelial cells, where it promotes neutrophil-mediated endothelial cell injury. VT-1 induces production of TNF-α by monocytes and cells within the kidney. TNF-α, in synergy with interleukin-1, increases VT-1 receptor expression and exacerbates the sensitivity of the endothelium to toxin-mediated and antibody-mediated cytotoxicity. It also promotes vWF release and impairs fibrinolytic activity.[47]

Considerable evidence suggests that endothelial cell injury plays a role in the pathogenesis of TTP. Platelet microthrombi in patients with TTP contain abundant vWF but little fibrinogen, in contrast to those seen in disseminated intravascular coagulopathy. In a subgroup of patients who suffer from chronic relapsing TTP, the plasma continues to contain elevated levels of unusually large vWF multimers (ULvWF) between relapses. ULvWFs may exacerbate microvascular thrombosis through their ability to aggregate platelets at high levels of shear stress. The secretion of ULvWF by cultured endothelial cells is stimulated by many agonists, including Shiga toxin. However, elevated vWF levels occur in other thrombotic microangiopathies, and their exact role in TTP/HUS requires further study. Endothelial damage plays a pivotal role in the pathogenesis of the disease. The events that initiate TTP are unknown. Plasma from patients with TTP and HUS has been reported to induce apoptosis in microvascular endothelial cells. Interestingly, cells from dermal, renal, and cerebral origin were most susceptible, whereas pulmonary and coronary arterial cells were less susceptible.[48]

Vasculitic Disorders

Vasculitis is a disease that targets all levels of the arterial tree from aorta to capillaries; it also affect venules, with leukocyte infiltration and necrosis. Different forms of vasculitis attack different vessels and are classified accordingly (see Chapter 91). The inflammatory process may target vessels of any type throughout the vascular system, although distinct clinicopathologic entities preferentially involve vessels of particular sizes and locations. Small vessels anywhere in the body may be affected by focal necrotizing lesions, where extravasation of leukocytes drives the inflammatory responses and results in vasculitis. Leukocyte adhesion molecules that participate in interactions with endothelial cells belong to three major families: selectins, sialomucins, and integrins. Interestingly, these interactions participate in tissue specificity in various vasculitic conditions. For instance, specific selectin interactions mediate cutaneous tropism in several inflammatory disorders, including graft-versus-host disease and dermatomyositis.[49]

Conclusion

The endothelium can no longer be viewed as a static physical barrier that simply separates the blood from tissue. We now recognize that the endothelium coordinates key functions of different tissues in normal and pathophysiologic conditions. These functions are accomplished by the interaction of endothelial cells with circulating factors and cells and the ability of endothelial cells to transmit biochemical and biophysical signals to surrounding tissues. Our increasing understanding of endothelial physiology can lead to novel therapeutic approaches to complex clinical conditions.

REFERENCES

1. Rubanyi GM: The role of endothelium in cardiovascular homeostasis and diseases. *J Cardiovasc Pharmacol* 22: S1-S14, 1993.
2. Aird WC: Endothelial cell heterogeneity. *Crit Care Med* 31:S221-S230, 2003.
3. Kumar S, West DC, Ager A: Heterogeneity in endothelial cells from large vessels and microvessels. *Differentiation* 36:57-70, 1987.
4. Dejana E: Endothelial adherens junctions: implications in the control of vascular permeability and angiogenesis. *J Clin Invest* 98:1949-1953, 1996.
5. Butcher EC, Picker LJ: Lymphocyte homing and homeostasis. *Science* 272:-66, 1996.
6. Zhu DZ, Cheng CF, Pauli BU: Mediation of lung metastasis of murine melanomas by a lung-specific endothelial cell adhesion molecule. *Proc Natl Acad Sci U S A* 88:9568-9572, 1991.
7. McCarthy SA, Kuzu I, Gatter KC, et al: Heterogeneity of the endothelial cell and its role in organ preference of tumour metastasis. *Trends Pharmacol Sci* 12:462-467, 1991.
8. Bombeli T, Mueller M, Haeberli A: Anticoagulant properties of the vascular endothelium. *Thromb Haemost* 77:408-423, 1997.
9. Rosenberg RD, Rosenberg JS: Natural anticoagulant mechanisms. *J Clin Invest* 74:1-6, 1984.
10. Esmon CT, Fukudome K. Cellular regulation of the protein C pathway. *Semin Cell Biol* 6:259-268, 1995.
11. Esmon NL: Thrombomodulin. *Semin Thromb Hemost* 13:454-463, 1987.
12. Majerus PW: Arachidonate metabolism in vascular disorders. *J Clin Invest* 72:1521-1525, 1983.
13. Levin EG, Santell L, Osborn KG: The expression of endothelial tissue plasminogen activator in vivo: a function defined by vessel size and anatomic location. *J Cell Sci* 110(pt 2):139-148, 1997.
14. Nemerson Y: Tissue factor: then and now. *Thromb Haemost* 74:180-184, 1995.
15. Rapaport SI, Rao LV: The tissue factor pathway: how it has become a "prima ballerina." *Thromb Haemost* 74:7-17, 1995.
16. Furchgott RF, Zawadzki JV: The obligatory role of endothelial cells in the relaxation of arterial smooth muscle by acetylcholine. *Nature* 288:373-376, 1980.
17. Garland CJ, Plane F, Kemp BK, et al: Endothelium-dependent hyperpolarization: a role in the control of vascular tone. *Trends Pharmacol Sci* 16:23-30, 1995.
18. Stamler JS, Singel DJ, Loscalzo J: Biochemistry of nitric oxide and its redox-activated forms. *Science* 258:1898-1902, 1992.
19. Forstermann U, Closs EI, Pollock JS, et al: Nitric oxide synthase isozymes. Characterization, purification, molecular cloning, and functions. *Hypertension* 23:1121-1131, 1994.
20. Forstermann U: Biochemistry and molecular biology of nitric oxide synthases. *Arzneimittelforschung* 44:402-407, 1994.
21. Moncada S, Palmer RM, Higgs EA: Nitric oxide: physiology, pathophysiology, and pharmacology. *Pharmacol Rev* 43:109-142, 1991.
22. Rapoport RM, Murad F: Agonist-induced endothelium-dependent relaxation in rat thoracic aorta may be mediated through cGMP. *Circ Res* 52:352-357, 1983.
23. Bolotina VM, Najibi S, Palacino JJ, et al: Nitric oxide directly activates calcium-dependent potassium channels in vascular smooth muscle. *Nature* 368:850-853, 1994.
24. Lincoln TM, Komalavilas P, Cornwell TL: Pleiotropic regulation of vascular smooth muscle tone by cyclic GMP-dependent protein kinase. *Hypertension* 23:1141-1147, 1994.
25. Stamler JS, Loh E, Roddy MA, et al: Nitric oxide regulates basal systemic and pulmonary vascular resistance in healthy humans. *Circulation* 89:2035-2040, 1994.
26. Moncada S, Vane JR: The role of prostacyclin in vascular tissue. *Fed Proc* 38:66-71, 1979.
27. Kukovetz WR, Holzmann S, Wurm A, et al: Prostacyclin increases cAMP in coronary arteries. *J Cyclic Nucleotide Res* 5:469-476, 1979.
28. Delpy E, Coste H, Gouville AC: Effects of cyclic GMP elevation on isoprenaline-induced increase in cyclic AMP and relaxation in rat aortic smooth muscle: role of phosphodiesterase 3. *Br J Pharmacol* 119:471-478, 1996.
29. Feletou M, Vanhoutte PM. Endothelium-derived hyperpolarizing factor. *Clin Exp Pharmacol Physiol* 23:1082-1090, 1996.
30. Masaki T: The discovery, the present state, and the future prospects of endothelin. *J Cardiovasc Pharmacol* 13(suppl 5):S1-S4, 1989.
31. Yanagisawa M, Kurihara H, Kimura S, et al: A novel peptide vasoconstrictor, endothelin, is produced by vascular endothelium and modulates smooth muscle Ca2+ channels. *J Hypertens* (suppl 6): S188-S191, 1988.
32. Rubanyi GM, Vanhoutte PM: Superoxide anions and hyperoxia inactivate endothelium-derived relaxing factor. *Am J Physiol* 250:H822-H827, 1986.
33. Coleman RA, Smith WL, Narumiya S: International Union of Pharmacology classification of prostanoid receptors: properties, distribution, and structure of the receptors and their subtypes. *Pharmacol Rev* 46:205-229, 1994.
34. Halushka PV, Mais DE, Mayeux PR, et al: Thromboxane, prostaglandin and leukotriene receptors. *Annu Rev Pharmacol Toxicol* 29:213-239, 1989.
35. Kubes P, Kerfoot SM: Leukocyte recruitment in the microcirculation: the rolling paradigm revisited. *News Physiol Sci* 16:76-80, 2001.
36. McEver RP, Moore KL, Cummings RD: Leukocyte trafficking mediated by selectin-carbohydrate interactions. *J Biol Chem* 270: 11025-11028, 1995.
37. Springer TA: Traffic signals on endothelium for lymphocyte recirculation and leukocyte emigration. *Annu Rev Physiol* 57:827-872, 1995.
38. Schafer AI: Vascular endothelium: in defense of blood fluidity. *J Clin Invest* 99:1143-1144, 1997.
39. Roth GJ: Platelets and blood vessels: the adhesion event. *Immunol Today* 13:100-105, 1992.
40. Grace PA, Mathie RT: *Ischemia-reperfusion injury.* London, 1999, Blackwell Science.
41. Neary P, Redmond HP: Ischemia-reperfusion injury and the systemic inflammatory response syndrome. In Grace PA, Mathie RT, editors: *Ischemia-reperfusion injury.* London, 1999, Blackwell Science, 1999.
42. Granger DN: Ischemia-reperfusion: mechanisms of microvascular dysfunction and the influence of risk factors for cardiovascular disease. *Microcirculation* 6:167-178, 1999.

43. Orfanos SE, Mavrommati I, Korovesi I, et al: Pulmonary endothelium in acute lung injury: from basic science to the critically ill. *Intensive Care Med* 30:1702-1714, 2004.
44. Lehr HA, Arfors KE: Mechanisms of tissue damage by leukocytes. *Curr Opin Hematol* 1:92-99, 1994.
45. Diaz NL, Finol HJ, Torres SH, et al: Histochemical and ultrastructural study of skeletal muscle in patients with sepsis and multiple organ failure syndrome (MOFS). *Histol Histopathol* 13:121-128, 1998.
46. Li H, Forstermann U: Nitric oxide in the pathogenesis of vascular disease. *J Pathol* 190:244-254, 2000.
47. Moake JL: Haemolytic-uraemic syndrome: basic science. *Lancet* 343:393-397, 1994.
48. Mitra D, Jaffe EA, Weksler B, et al: Thrombotic thrombocytopenic purpura and sporadic hemolytic-uremic syndrome plasmas induce apoptosis in restricted lineages of human microvascular endothelial cells. *Blood* 89:1224-1234, 1997.
49. Savage CO: The evolving pathogenesis of systemic vasculitis. *Clin Med* 2:458-464, 2002.

CHAPTER

95

Neuroendocrine–Immune Mediator Coordination and Disarray in Critical Illness

Kathryn Felmet and Joseph Carcillo

PEARLS

- Activation of the hypothalamic-pituitary-adrenal (HPA) axis is normal during stress. Lack of activation in the acute setting causes many of the signs and symptoms of critical illness.
- Relative adrenal insufficiency should be suspected in any patient with catecholamine-resistant shock and in patients with prolonged critical illness.
- Lymphopenia and monocyte dysfunction occurs commonly in the intensive care unit and may result from unopposed immune-suppressive stress hormones.
- Dopamine use suppresses prolactin and growth hormone release and may suppress the immune system and anabolic pathways.
- Opioids used for analgesia may have immune-suppressive effects.
- The neuroendocrine state in prolonged critical illness differs from acute stress and may be dysfunctional.

Clinically relevant cross-talk occurs among the central nervous system, the endocrine system, and the immune system. For example, psychological stress leads to release of cortisol, a potent inhibitor of immune function, whereas immune activation initiates central nervous system pathways generating fever, pain sensation, and behaviors associated with recovery. These neuroendocrine—immune (NEI) interactions are relevant in critical illness. A normally functioning hypothalamic-pituitary-adrenal (HPA) axis, the primary efferent limb of the NEI system, is essential to surviving critical illness. Certain disease states such as septic shock are strongly associated with dysfunction of the NEI system. Drugs used to resuscitate shock, including catecholamines, vasopressin, and glucocorticoids, are mediators for the efferent limb of this system. Dopamine infusion profoundly effects release of the neuroendocrine products growth hormone and prolactin. Molecules of the afferent limb of the NEI system, primarily cytokines, have been targets for adjuvant therapies for severe sepsis.

This chapter distills a broad range of data from the fields of immunology, endocrinology, and neuroscience into clinically useful concepts. We provide a conceptual framework, building on the concept of the stress response and focusing on the best-understood aspects of neuroendocrine mediators and their relevance to critical care. We describe situations in which breakdown of the NEI system plays a role in the development of critical illness. We discuss situations in which physicians, using common intensive care unit (ICU) therapies, may inadvertently interfere with NEI function.

Organization of the Stress Response

The stress response has been considered an extension of the fight or flight response, which halts growth, digestion, and other daily activities in order to ready the body for immediate action. These signals, namely, activation of the sympathetic nervous system, the HPA axis, and endogenous opioids, primarily are antiinflammatory. If this were the whole of the stress response, then humans, after fleeing their aggressor or delivering their babies, would be left with disrupted epithelial barriers and a suppressed immune system. Modern science has shown that the stress response is a complex dynamic process that can be initiated by the immune system or the central nervous system.

Stress can be understood as any threat to an organism's homeostatic internal milieu. An organism must defend itself against two types of threats. *Macroscopic threats,* such as an encounter with a predator, an episode of hypotension, or a traumatic hemorrhage, threaten the whole organism at once. *Microscopic threats* attack epithelial and endothelial barriers, which are essential to organ function. To maintain integrity against microscopic threats, the organism must be vigilant against microbial invasion in the face of the wear and tear of daily activities such as digestion, excretion, and procreation. The central stress response to macroscopic threats puts housekeeping on hold as the vital functions are marshaled against an assault. The response to microscopic threats is a matter of day-to-day housekeeping and is primarily the responsibility of the immune system. They are equally important and must balance each other: they are the yin and the yang of the response to stress.

Central Stress Response

All types of stress—physical, emotional, or immune—cause stimulation of the sympathetic nervous system, activation of the HPA axis, and release of hypothalamic hormones, including vasopressin, prolactin, and growth hormone (Figure 95–1). The HPA system is the major coordinator of the central stress response (see Chapter 68). Hypothalamic release of corticotropin-releasing hormone occurs in response to cortical signals generated by fear, pain, or hypotension, as well as in response to immune-derived signal molecules, especially interleukin (IL)-1β, tumor necrosis factor (TNF)-α and IL-6.[1] Corticotropin-releasing hormone in the brain stimulates sympathetic outflow and causes release of adrenocorticotropic hormone (ACTH) by the pituitary. Vasopressin, which is also released in response to immune signals and stress, is powerfully synergistic with corticotropin-releasing hormone in promoting ACTH secretion.[2] Circulating ACTH reaches the adrenal cortex, where it stimulates conversion of cholesterol to the steroid hormone cortisol. Cortisol release suppresses further ACTH secretion within minutes and more slowly feeds back to suppress secretion of corticotropin-releasing hormone.[3] Cortisol and its synthetic analogues, the glucocorticoids, act in tandem with the sympathetic nervous system to prepare a body for action by putting growth and housekeeping functions on hold, making fuel substrates available, and supporting blood pressure and intravascular volume. Failure of this normal stress response leads to cardiovascular collapse.

Cortisol inhibits growth in all tissues, decreases deoxyribonucleic acid and ribonucleic acid synthesis, and increases protein catabolism except in the liver, where protein synthesis is enhanced. Cortisol increases the availability of glucose, amino acids, and free fatty acids for immediate use. Cortisol increases vascular tone and increases expression of adrenergic receptors, potentiating the vasoconstrictive action of catecholamines. Cortisol also regulates the distribution of total body water. It activates the renin-angiotensin system, causing hypertension, and is necessary for secretion of a water load.[3] In suppressing the body's maintenance functions, cortisol suppresses immune responses. Cortisol reduces circulating numbers of lymphocytes, monocytes, and eosinophils by stimulating apoptosis. It stabilizes lysosomal membranes, decreases capillary permeability, impairs demargination of white blood cells and phagocytosis, and decreases release of IL-1, preventing fever. Cortisol supports a T_H2 (humoral immunity) over a T_H1 (cellular immunity) phenotype.[3]

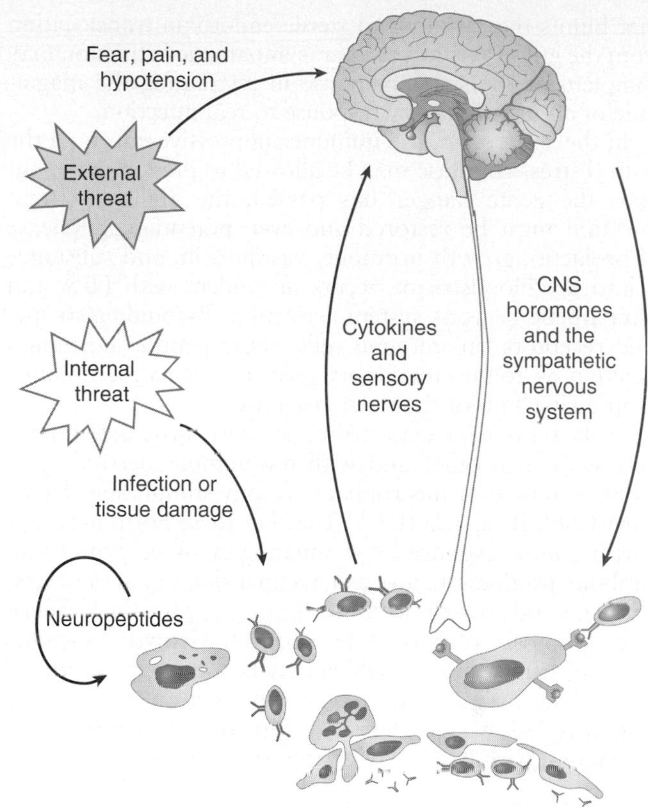

FIGURE 95–1 • Neuroendocrine immune loop. Stimulation of the central stress axis generates immune suppressive signals (activation of the hypothalamic-pituitary-adrenal axis, sympathetic nervous system, endogenous opioids) and immune supportive signals (release of proinflammatory peptides, e.g., vasopressin and prolactin.) A threat to the homeostatic milieu, in the form of trauma or infection, activates the immune system. Activated immune cells produce cytokines such as tumor necrosis factor-α, interleukin-1, and interleukin-6, which in turn activate the central stress response. Some immune cells produce neuropeptide hormones for autocrine or paracrine action. *CNS,* Central nervous system.

As the counterpoint to the parasympathetic nervous system, which generally promotes maintenance functions, activation of the sympathetic nervous system complements the actions of cortisol. The impact of sympathetic nervous system stimulation on the immune system is complex and imperfectly understood and is discussed later in this chapter. The parasympathetic limb of the autonomic nervous system also plays a role in regulating the immune response. Fibers from the vagus nerve innervate liver macrophages, called *Kupffer cells,* and in these cells parasympathetic tone dramatically attenuates cytokine secretion in response to endotoxin. This pathway may be a protective mechanism that blunts the response to sterile endotoxin translocation from the gut. Alternatively, parasympathetic activation may complement the stress response in restraining the magnitude of an inflammatory response to real infection.

In the short term, the immune suppressive effects of the central stress response may be allowed to predominate, but once the acute danger has passed, the ability to fight infection must be restored and even potentiated. Release of prolactin, growth hormone, vasopressin, and substance P into the bloodstream occurs in tandem with HPA and sympathetic nervous system activation. By binding to specific receptors on immune cells, these peptide hormones function as counterregulatory mechanisms to the immune suppressive limb of the stress response.

Prolactin and growth hormone share structural homology with each other and with the immune-derived cytokines granulocyte-macrophage colony-stimulating factor (GM-CSF), IL-2, and IL7.[4,5] Together these hormones support immune response by stimulating cytokine expression, antibody production, and clonal expansion of lymphocytes. Prolactin and growth hormone directly oppose the lymphocyte apoptosis promoted by cortisol. Growth hormone also affects metabolism, which may be important in critical illness. The overall impact of vasopressin on the immune system is less well understood, but its function in direct interaction with lymphocytes appears to be supportive.

Immune Response to Microscopic Threats

The immune system is a sensory organ that allows early recognition of, and response to, microscopic threats. Day-to-day activities result in wear and tear on epithelial barriers, leading to microbial and other non-self invasion. These peripheral stressors initiate a cascade of molecules and activated cells that amplify the initial signal and stimulate the central stress response. The central stress response, in turn, down-regulates and eventually terminates the immune response.

Inflammation and phagocytic cells comprise the first line of defense and recognition. Tissue damage caused by microbial invasion or trauma initiates the nonspecific cascade called the *inflammatory response* (see Chapter 83). It leads to vasodilatation, increased capillary permeability, and an influx of phagocytes. Histamine and kinins are important mediators of the inflammatory response. Phagocytic cells may be blood monocytes, neutrophils, or tissue macrophages. Macrophages engulf foreign matter and bacteria, break them down into large molecules, and present these as antigens to T lymphocytes, thus activating the specific adaptive immune response.

Phagocytic cells also produce proinflammatory cytokines, primarily IL-1, IL-6, and TNF-α, which amplify the immune response locally. Cytokines help determine whether the specific immune response takes on a T_H1 or T_H2 phenotype. Cytokines carry messages between different cell types within the immune system and between the immune system and other organ systems. In the latter role, they comprise the most important afferent limb of the NEI system. Cytokines circulating in the bloodstream reach the central nervous system, where receptors for IL-1α and IL-1β, IL-2, IL-4, IL-6, TNF-α, and interferon (IFN)-γ are found. Afferent nerves also carry inflammatory signals to the brain. When stimulated by cytokines and endotoxin, signals from the vagus lead to HPA axis activation.[6]

Binding of cytokines to their specific receptors in the brain can activate the full spectrum of the central stress response, including release of corticotropin-releasing hormone and other hypothalamic hormones, activation of the sympathetic nervous system, and release of endogenous opioids from the hindbrain and spinal cord. Hypothalamic hormones lead to release of effector molecules such as cortisol and insulin-like growth factor. In general, hypothalamic hormones such as prolactin and growth hormone support the immune response, whereas corticotropin-releasing hormone, ACTH, and cortisol suppress immune response. NEI mediators also may play a role in determining the predominance of a T_H1 or T_H2 phenotype.

Interestingly, neuroendocrine mediators that trigger the antiinflammatory cascade in the central nervous system, such as vasopressin and corticotropin-releasing hormone, may have the opposite effect when they are released in tissues. Both corticotropin-releasing hormone and vasopressin are clearly immune supportive in peripheral tissues. Corticotropin-releasing hormone is found in high concentrations at inflammatory sites, although plasma levels may be undetectable.[7,8] Corticotropin-releasing hormone augments T-lymphocyte proliferation and IL-2 expression in vitro, augments cytokine expression by macrophages, and triggers mast cell degranulation.[7,9] Immunoneutralization of corticotropin-releasing hormone decreases inflammation as effectively as neutralizing antibodies to TNF-α.

The normal pathways that lead to increased local concentrations of hypothalamic hormones and their clinical relevance in peripheral tissues are not completely understood. Corticotropin-releasing hormone is a neurotransmitter of postganglionic sympathetic nerves, some of which innervate lymphoid organs and may be a mediator of autonomic control of inflammation. In some cases, immune cells actually secrete neuropeptides for autocrine or paracrine action. Immune cell secretion of neurotransmitters may affect peripheral nerve activity and may represent a second method by which the immune system alerts the central nervous system to the presence of microbial invasion.

Acute Versus Chronic Stress

The body's response to stress has been studied mostly as an acute event occurring in normal healthy people. Through the use of advanced therapies and machines, we have created in the modern ICU a state of prolonged critical illness that does not exist in nature and to which the neuroendocrine system must adapt. The state of prolonged stress is not well understood, but the hormonal milieu that exists and which we intentionally create in the acute phase of resuscitation—that of catecholamine and cortisol excess—likely will not be appropriate later. Like healthy people, critically ill patients need a balance between immune suppressive and immune supportive signals, between a short-term improvement in blood pressure and long-term growth and repair. The neuroendocrine system in critically ill patients cannot be judged by reference to established norms. It may not be possible to know what levels of these hormones are "natural." In studying the NEI system in critical illness, the appropriate hormone level is that associated with the best outcome. In the future, dysfunction of the NEI system that occurs in prolonged critical illness may be recognizable as an organ failure and part of the multiple organ dysfunction complex.

Neuroendocrine–Immune Dysfunction Causing Critical Illness

Some categories of critical illness are caused by dysfunction of the NEI system. Breakdown of the central stress response leads to a shock state. The most obvious example is the autonomic instability associated with spinal shock. Complete adrenal failure with breakdown of the HPA axis causes shock, but this phenomenon is relatively rare. More important to critical care is the syndrome of relative adrenal insufficiency. An acquired, reversible adrenal insufficiency can occur in any critically ill patient but is particularly associated with sepsis and septic shock. A syndrome of inadequate circulating vasopressin also has been implicated in the pathogenesis of shock, particularly vasodilatory or warm shock.

Hypothalamic-Pituitary-Adrenal Axis

In general, critically ill patients have elevated cortisol levels, which correspond to the severity of illness. In the acute phase of critical illness, adequate cortisol is necessary for maintenance of vascular tone and normal catecholamine responsiveness.[10] In some critically ill patients, the HPA axis seems to fail. These patients have cortisol levels that are inadequate for their degree of illness or inadequate relative to the ACTH levels measured in their blood. The incidence of relative adrenal insufficiency varies according to author and definition criteria. The reported incidence ranges from 0% to 75%. Relative adrenal insufficiency is associated with poor outcomes in adults and children.[11–13]

During the prolonged phase of critical illness, the normal association between ACTH and cortisol often is strikingly reversed. In the face of ongoing stress, cortisol levels in critically ill patients tend to remain elevated despite a decline in ACTH levels.[14] Sustained cortisol production may result from direct autonomic innervation of steroidogenic cells, paracrine action of the products of the adrenal medulla, or the action of cytokines, which can directly stimulate cortisol production.[15–17] Decreased cortisol clearance by the liver may contribute to elevated cortisol levels in prolonged critical illness.[14]

Adrenal insufficiency should be suspected in any patient with catecholamine-resistant shock and in patients with prolonged critical illness. Pathologic scenarios that may produce relative or absolute adrenal insufficiency include suppression of corticotropin-releasing hormone or ACTH secretion, adrenal unresponsiveness, increased cortisol clearance, or end organ unresponsiveness to cortisol (Table 95–1). For a thorough discussion of causes of relative adrenal insufficiency, see the excellent review by Beishuizen and Thijs.[18]

How can we identify the syndrome of relative adrenal insufficiency? Defining what constitutes a normal cortisol response to critical illness is difficult because the range of cortisol levels observed in critically ill patients is so broad, varying from the healthy normal level to 20 times normal. Additionally, measured cortisol levels may overestimate biologically active free cortisol in the acute phase of critical illness because levels of cortisol-binding globulin are low.[19,20] Most authors agree that a "normal" level in the face of acute illness probably is inadequate.[18]

The ACTH stimulation test can be used to identify absolute adrenal failure but may fail to identify a clinically significant adrenal insufficiency. The ACTH dose used in the standard test (250 μg for adults and children older than 2 years, 125 μg for children younger than 2 years) produces plasma ACTH levels 100 to 200 times the physiologic maximum stress levels of ACTH. A 1 μg-test has been suggested but has not been standardized for adults or children.[21] Beishuizen et al.[21] demonstrated that patients with a normal response to the standard test but an

TABLE 95–1

Causes of Adrenal Insufficiency

		Notes
Central	Hypothalamic or pituitary disease	
	Brain injury	
	Recent steroid use	Follows the "rule of ones": 1 day of steroid use may suppress adrenal function for 1 week; 1 week for 1 month; 1 month for 1 year
Peripheral	Preexisting adrenal failure	Associated with increased pigmentation, hypoglycemia, mild hyponatremia, and hyperkalemia
	Acute adrenal failure	Adrenal hemorrhage or autoimmune adrenalitis
	Inadequate substrate	Low cholesterol[48]
	P450 impairment	From ketoconazole, etomidate, sepsis, prematurity, or age <6 months[77–79]
	Increased clearance	Occurs with rifampin, phenytoin, and phenobarbital[80]
	End-organ unresponsiveness	Cytokines can change glucocorticoid receptor sensitivity[19,80]
Other	Sepsis/inflammation	Circulating inflammatory mediators can cause hypothalamic-pituitary-adrenal axis suppression, particularly in patients with fungal infection or human immunodeficiency virus[18]

inadequate response to the 1-μg test improved clinically with decreased pressor requirement in response to hydrocortisone treatment. More recently, a study of diagnostic criteria for relative adrenal insufficiency in adult patients with septic shock compared the 1-μg ACTH stimulation test, the 250-μg ACTH stimulation test, and random cortisol level. A random cortisol level less than 25 was the best predictor of a hemodynamic response to hydrocortisone, defined as the ability to discontinue pressor agents within 24 hours of the first dose.[22]

Standard reference ranges for normal healthy subjects accept minimum peak values after ACTH stimulation of 18 to 22 μg/dl (500–600 nmol/L) or a minimum change in cortisol level of 7 to 9 μg/dl (200–250 nmol/L). Failure according to these requirements is associated with a high 28-day mortality in adults.[4] ACTH stimulation tests should be interpreted in light of the basal cortisol level because the change in serum cortisol after ACTH stimulation is a measure of adrenal reserve.

It may be impossible to rely on results of an ACTH stimulation test in the acute setting of severe catecholamine-unresponsive shock, when time is of the essence. Because the criteria for diagnosis of relative adrenal insufficiency in the critical care setting is imprecise, some authors believe a negative or inconclusive result should not prohibit use of glucocorticoids. Instead, a rapid hemodynamic response to glucocorticoids may be the best clue to the diagnosis of relative adrenal insufficiency. One author suggests that, at present, we have no choice but to rely on clinical assessment of the severity of stress and make "an educated guess of the adequacy of the measured serum cortisol concentration."[20]

Although several studies on administration of pure glucocorticoids to septic shock patients have failed to demonstrate a survival advantage, more recently the use of steroids with both glucocorticoid and mineralocorticoid activity has shown some benefit.[23–25] Annane et al.[23] reported a large prospective, placebo-controlled randomized clinical trial in adults with septic shock, demonstrating that treatment with hydrocortisone (50 mg every 6 hours) and fludrocortisone (50 μg/day) decreased 28-day mortality in all patients. Most of the survival benefit was seen in patients in whom relative adrenal insufficiency was identified by standard-dose corticotropin stimulation test with change in stimulated minus baseline cortisol response of less than 9 μg/dl. In this group, ICU and hospital mortality and time to vasopressor withdrawal were significantly reduced.[23]

At present, the American College of Critical Care Medicine clinical practice parameters for the hemodynamic support of pediatric and neonatal septic shock recommend the use of hydrocortisone in patients with catecholamine resistance and suspected adrenal insufficiency. Risk factors that should alert the clinician to high risk for adrenal insufficiency include physical examination findings suggestive of absolute adrenal insufficiency, disseminated intravascular coagulation or purpura fulminans, and history of steroid use. The authors would add to this list a history of prolonged stress (i.e., decompensation in a patient during a long ICU stay), severe septic shock, risk of P450 impairment as a result of drugs, and extreme youth.

The physiologic replacement dose of hydrocortisone is 12.5 mg/m²/day. In critical illness, dosing ranges from 50 mg/m²/day in stress states to 50 mg/kg/day in severe shock. Hydrocortisone has a short half-life and should be given as a bolus, followed by continuous infusion. Although critically ill patients may receive steroids for a variety of indications, steroids that lack mineralocorticoid activity may not be sufficient for adrenal replacement in shock. Table 95–2 gives a comparison of the relative glucocorticoid and mineralocorticoid potency of steroids commonly used in the ICU. Glucocorticoids given over a prolonged period are associated with an increased risk for superinfection, gastrointestinal bleeding, hyperglycemia, polyneuropathy of critical illness, and prolonged adrenal insufficiency. Exogenous hydrocortisone should be tapered or discontinued as soon as hemodynamics allow.

Vasopressin

Vasopressin is a hormone of the posterior pituitary that is secreted in response to high serum osmolarity. Excitation of atrial stretch receptors inhibits vasopressin secretion. Vasopressin is also released in response to stress, inflammatory signals, and some medications. Hypotension, morphine, nicotine, angiotensin II, glucocorticoids, and IL-6 all stimulate release of vasopressin.[2] Inadequate levels of circulating vasopressin may contribute to critical illness and have

TABLE 95–2

Comparison of Common Corticosteroids

	Glucocorticoid Potency (as Hydrocortisone Equivalent Dose)	Mineralocorticoid Potency
Stress dose hydrocortisone: 50 mg/m²/day	Approximately 2 mg/kg/day	++
Shock dose hydrocortisone: 50 mg/kg/day	50 mg/kg/day	++
Annane study[3]: hydrocortisone 50 mg q6h and fludrocortisone 50 μg/day	Approximately 3 mg/kg/day	+++++
Dexamethasone for postextubation stridor: 0.5 mg/kg q8h	35 mg/kg/day	0
Methylprednisolone in severe asthma: 1 mg/kg q6h	20 mg/kg/day	0
Methylprednisolone in spinal cord injury: 30 mg/kg load, followed by 5.4 mg/kg/h over 23 hours	770 mg/kg/day	0

been proposed as a mechanism in the pathogenesis of vasodilatory shock. Circulating vasopressin levels usually are high in the early phase of septic shock but normalize later. The level of vasopressin that is normal in the late phase of sepsis is unclear.[26]

In general, vasopressin decreases water excretion by the kidneys by increasing water reabsorption in the collecting ducts, hence its other name antidiuretic hormone. Vasopressin also has a potent constricting effect on arterioles throughout the body.[5] Vasopressin potentiates ACTH release leading to cortisol release, which may contribute to its salutary effects in cardiac arrest and vasodilatory shock.[2]

Vasopressin has been proposed as a replacement or adjunct to epinephrine in the resuscitation of cardiac arrest and of catecholamine-unresponsive shock. The interest in vasopressin for resuscitation is based on the fact that vasopressin may increase coronary perfusion without increasing myocardial oxygen demand and without the arrhythmogenic effects of epinephrine. Also, repeated doses of vasopressin tend to support blood pressure after the epinephrine response wanes.[27] When given as the first drug in cardiac arrest, vasopressin has been shown to confer a survival advantage in out-of-hospital arrest but not in arrests occurring in stressed, hospitalized patients.[28,29] Vasopressin's effects on NEI mediators may explain this discrepancy. In a person with normal adrenal reserves of cortisol, exogenous vasopressin may cause a surge of endogenous cortisol, which should improve catecholamine responsiveness. Hospitalized patients with decreased adrenal reserves may not experience this benefit of vasopressin.

Some evidence indicates that low-dose vasopressin (restoring high–normal levels) may be beneficial in vasodilatory shock. High doses of vasopressin are associated with unacceptable side effects, such as gut and digital ischemia and decreased urine output. However, several small clinical studies have suggested that these problems do not occur at physiologic doses. Doses given to adults range from 0.01 to 0.1 U/min.[27–29] Two case series totaling 16 pediatric patients reported that doses of 0.0003 to 0.008 units/kg/min were not associated with negative side effects, resulted in increased blood pressure, and allowed a decrease in the doses of catecholamine vasopressors.[56] Randomized clinical trials evaluating the safety and efficacy of vasopressin in septic shock are ongoing.

Vasopressin has effects on the immune system independent of its effect in stimulating the HPA axis. When given intraventricularly to rats, vasopressin decreases the T-cell response to mitogen independently of the HPA axis, probably via the sympathetic nervous system.[31] Like CRH, vasopressin stimulates immune responses in peripheral tissues. Circulating or local vasopressin enhances lymphocyte reactions and potentiates primary antibody responses.[32] Elevated vasopressin levels are found in a mouse model of autoimmune disease, and antibody neutralization ameliorates the inflammatory response in these mice.[2] Vasopressin can potentiate the release of prolactin, a proinflammatory peptide hormone.[33]

Because vasopressin has immune suppressive effects when present in the central nervous system and immune supportive effects when present in peripheral tissues, predicting which effect would predominate during vasopressin infusion in the ICU is difficult.

Intensive Care Unit Therapies That Interfere with the Neuroendocrine–Immune System

The NEI system is so crucial in the maintenance of blood pressure that the most powerful therapies available to resuscitate shock are analogues of naturally occurring NEI mediators. Catecholamines, glucocorticoids, vasopressin, and somatostatin are all hormonal therapies. These molecules are often used without a full understanding of the role they play in the balance between promoting and suppressing immune responses. The incidental effect of most of these therapies is immune suppression (Figure 95–2 and Table 95–3). Prolactin and growth hormone, the NEI mediators that counterbalance the immune suppressive effect, are particularly subject to suppression by catecholamines, especially dopamine. A prolonged imbalance between the immune suppressive and immune supportive elements of the NEI system can lead to development of lymphopenia, which in turn is associated with considerable morbidity and mortality.[34]

Catecholamines and the Sympathetic Nervous System

Catecholamines are the most important immediate effector molecules of the fight or flight response. These drugs

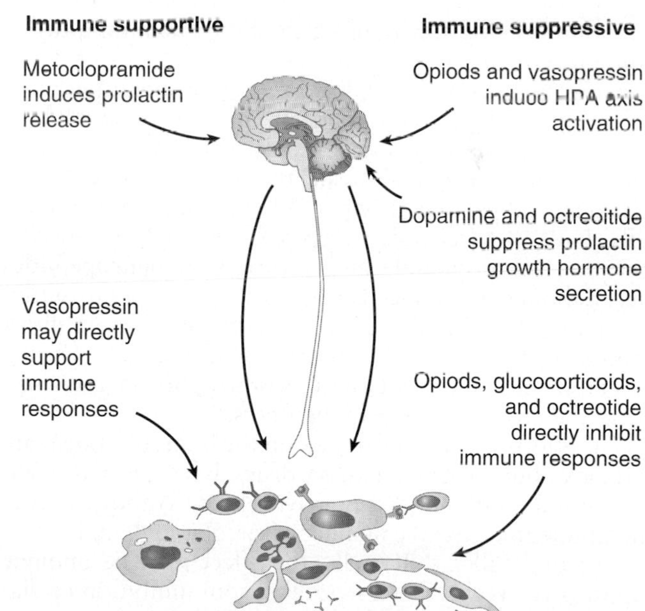
Immune supportive
Immune suppressive
Metoclopramide induces prolactin release
Opiods and vasopressin induce HPA axis activation
Dopamine and octreotide suppress prolactin growth hormone secretion
Vasopressin may directly support immune responses
Opiods, glucocorticoids, and octreotide directly inhibit immune responses

FIGURE 95–2 • Neuroendocrine-immune impact of commonly used intensive care unit (ICU) therapies. Common drugs infusions in the ICU influence immune function by altering neuroendocrine secretory activity and by binding to immune cells directly. Opioids and vasopressin activate the hypothalamic-pituitary-adrenal *(HPA)* axis, leading to cortisol release. Dopamine and octreotide block the release of the immune supportive hormones prolactin and growth hormone. Opioids and octreotide have direct effects on immune cells, decreasing lymphocyte proliferation, primary antibody responses, and monocyte and macrophage function. All of these effects are immune suppressive. Only vasopressin in the periphery, which supports lymphocyte function, and metoclopramide, which induces prolactin release, are immune supportive.

TABLE 95–3

Summary of the Effects of Neuroendocrine–Immune Mediators on Immune Cell Types

	T-Cell Proliferation and Cytokine Release	B-Cell Antibody Production	Monocyte Activation	Natural Killer Cell Function	Macrophage Function and Cytokine Release	Neutrophil Chemotaxis
Circulating catecholamines	–	–	+/–			
Dopamine	–	–	–	–	–	
Prolactin	+	+	+	+	+	?
Opioids	–	–	–		–	
Somatostatin	–	?	?			
Hypothalamic-pituitary-adrenal axis/cortisol	–	–	–		–	–
Vasopressin peripheral	+	+				
CRH peripheral	+				+	

impact the NEI system by directly influencing immune responses and by altering the release of other NEI mediators. Norepinephrine is the primary effector molecule for the sympathetic nervous system. Epinephrine is secreted into the bloodstream by the adrenal gland in response to sympathetic nervous system activation. Together they regulate cardiovascular and respiratory function, smooth muscle contraction, and secretions. Like cortisol, they put the housekeeping functions of the body, including digestion, growth, and reproduction, on hold in favor of blood pressure support and mobilization of fuel substrates.[5]

The sympathetic nervous system innervates the immune system. Bone marrow, thymus, spleen, lymph nodes, and gut-associated lymphoid tissue receive adrenergic, dopaminergic, and peptidergic input.[34] T cells and other immune cells have β-adrenergic receptors, as well as specific receptors for dopamine and a variety of neuropeptides (acetylcholine, substance P, neuropeptide Y, somatostatin, prolactin).[34] Sympathetic nerve terminals are in direct apposition to T cells, B cells, and dendritic cells. During development, immune-derived neurotrophic factors may direct the growth of innervating fibers.[35]

The effects of catecholamines on the immune system are complex, but in general these drugs have been thought to exert an immune suppressive effect. Although catecholamines increase the number of circulating lymphocytes and natural killer (NK) cells, the effect may be immune suppressive, as this increase results from inhibition of diapedesis and homing to the spleen.[36] Adrenergic receptor activation decreases mitogen-induced T-cell proliferation and decreases both IL-2 production and IL-2R expression on T cells. More recent evidence suggests that the effects of β-adrenergic receptor stimulation depend on the activation state of the lymphocyte or on the tissue in which immune cells are found. For instance, catecholamines have been shown to increase the expression of TNF-α, IL-1, and IL-8 by lung mononuclear cells.[37]

The overall impact of sympathetic nervous system activation on immune responses may depend on its inhibitory effect on parasympathetic output. Tissue macrophages, especially in the liver and gut, receive vagal innervation. Stimulation of the vagus nerve inhibits endotoxin-stimulated TNF-α production by Kupffer cells in the liver. Acetylcholine, the principal neurotransmitter of the vagus nerve, decreases cytokine production by cultured macrophages.[6]

The degree to which circulating catecholamines given in the ICU can mimic the effects of sympathetic outflow is unclear. Of more certainty is that catecholamines in pharmacologic dose impact the release of other NEI mediators in vivo. Dopamine has a powerful inhibitory effect on release of the proinflammatory mediator prolactin and has been shown to decrease lymphocyte proliferation.[38,39] Dopamine inhibits pulsatile release of growth hormone, thus contributing to the catabolic state observed in critical illness.[39] Other catecholamines have similar effects, albeit to a much lesser degree.

Growth and Lactogenic Hormone Family

Prolactin

Prolactin is a hormone produced by anterior pituitary cells and lymphocytes that has been shown to have immunoregulatory function. It is best known for its role in promoting milk secretion. Although it is produced in both sexes, prolactin levels are highest in lactating mothers and newborns. Prolactin release is stimulated by suckling, IL-1β, IL-2, IL-6, oxytocin, serotonin, and thyrotropin-releasing hormone. A prolactin secretory response to psychological and physical stress is reported.[4,40,41] In the normal state, prolactin secretion is tonically inhibited by hypothalamic dopamine.

Prolactin may be the most important counterbalance to the immune suppressive effects of the central stress response. Prolactin supports circulating lymphocyte numbers as a necessary cofactor for IL-2 and mitogen-stimulated proliferation[4] and by opposing glucocorticoid-induced apoptosis. [42] Prolactin increases IL-2 production by T cells and is necessary for expression of the

IL-2 receptor. Prolactin increases antibody production by B cells and increases cytokine release capacity of macrophages and NK cells.[4]

Disturbances of prolactin have clinically significant effects on immune function. Prolactin levels are increased in some autoimmune diseases and in association with episodes of organ rejection.[43] The immune suppressive drug cyclosporine exerts its effect through the prolactin receptor on lymphocytes.[44] Bromocriptine, an oral agent that prevents prolactin release, has shown promise in the treatment of autoimmune disease and in animal models of organ transplantation.[45] Prolactin levels are suppressed in critically ill patients in response to hemorrhage.[46,47] Hemorrhage has been associated with lymphopenia, decreased T-cell proliferative response, and increased risk of sepsis and multiple organ failure.[46] Prolactin administration has been shown to improve cytokine release and survival in posthemorrhage mice subjected to the cecal ligation and puncture experimental model of sepsis.

Pituitary prolactin production is strongly inhibited by exogenous dopamine at doses as low as 1 μg/kg/min. Dopamine-associated hypoprolactinemia has been associated with decreased T-cell response to mitogen ex vivo, decreased circulating lymphocyte numbers, and increased risk of secondary infection in the ICU.[38,48] Adrenergic agents other than dopamine have a similar, albeit much less potent, effect on prolactin release. Prolactin release may be inadvertently inhibited by somatostatin, serotonin, corticosteroids, and histamine (H_1) blockers. Metoclopramide and vasopressin increase pituitary prolactin release.[40]

Given that prolactin is one of the few antagonists to the overwhelmingly immune-suppressive effects of the stress response, use of therapies that inhibit its release, particularly dopamine, should be carefully considered. Recombinant human prolactin may have therapeutic potential to reverse lymphopenia observed in the ICU and to speed hematopoietic reconstitution after bone marrow transplant.[49]

Growth Hormone and Insulin-like Growth Factor

Growth hormone is a large peptide hormone produced by the anterior pituitary. It is structurally similar to prolactin. Like prolactin, growth hormone has immune stimulatory effects and is suppressed by catecholamines.[50] In states of health, growth hormone increases protein synthesis, gene transcription, and the size and mitosis of somatic cells. It decreases glucose uptake and utilization and promotes differentiation. Growth hormone induces liver production of insulin-like growth factor-1, which mediates many of the effects of growth hormone.[5]

Growth hormone supports the immune response. Animal models suggest an important role for growth hormone in the development of the immune system. In growth hormone–deficient humans, growth hormone increases the differentiation of B-cell and NK-cell activity. Growth hormone increases IL-2 production by lymphocytes and increases IL-1, TNF-α, and superoxide production by monocytes in animal models and in growth hormone-deficient subjects.[43,50] Growth hormone also improves phagocytic cell function. Like prolactin, growth hormone is produced by cells throughout the immune system.[50]

The hypercatabolic state seen in critically ill patients has been attributed in part to growth hormone dysfunction. Trauma, sepsis, and surgery are thought to induce a state of growth hormone resistance.[49,52] Dopamine infusion and prolonged critical illness are associated with lower mean levels of growth hormone and a pronounced flattening in the normal pattern of pulsatile growth hormone release[39,51] (Figure 95–3). The hyperglycemic catabolic state induced by growth hormone depletion and resistance is compounded by the normal stress response, the effects of immune-derived cytokines, and inadequate calorie delivery in the ICU.[52] Use of exogenous growth hormone to preserve muscle and improve healing has received some interest. Administering growth hormone perioperatively improves nitrogen balance, increases liver protein synthesis, increases muscle strength and lean body mass, and decreases postoperative fatigue over controls.[13] Growth hormone also increases the rate of healing in burn patients and increases the rate of protein synthesis in sepsis and trauma patients.[53]

Unfortunately, an elevated growth hormone level in critically ill patients is associated with increased mortality. In two large European studies of growth hormone use in critically ill adults, patients treated with growth hormone had a 1.9- to 2.4-fold relative risk of mortality, mostly due to multiple organ dysfunction syndrome,

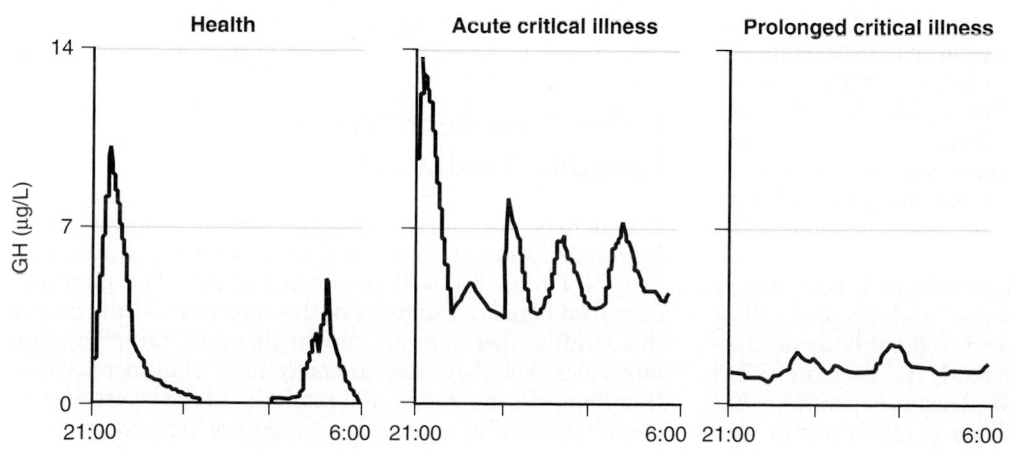

FIGURE 95–3 • Secretion profile of growth hormone in health and illness. A healthy person has robust, predictable nocturnal growth hormone release. In the acute phase of critical illness, both peak levels and interpulse levels are significantly elevated. In prolonged critical illness, growth hormone secretion becomes chaotic, and the mean growth hormone levels are decreased. (Modified from Van den Berghe G: *Best Pract Res Clin Endocrinol Metab* 15:407, 2001.[81])

shock, or uncontrolled infection. Growth hormone–treated patients also had increased morbidity as measured by prolonged mechanical ventilation and longer ICU stay.[54] Increased endogenous growth hormone is associated with increased mortality in children with meningococcemia.[55] A consensus statement from the Growth Hormone Research Society recommends against use of growth hormone in the acute phase of critical illness.[56]

The reasons behind this association between elevated growth hormone and increased morbidity and mortality are not clearly understood. Growth hormone treatment is associated with an increase in blood glucose concentration, which may support bacterial growth.[52] This hypothesis is supported by evidence that tight glycemic control is associated with a decreased risk of death from sepsis in adult surgical patients.[51] Growth hormone's effects on the immune system may play a role. At very high levels, growth hormone binds in significant quantities to the prolactin receptor. Both of these hormones, at 10 to 20 times physiologic levels, may mediate immune-suppressive effects in vitro.[4,5] At more moderate doses, excessive growth hormone may cause overshoot of the immune/inflammatory response, which could be detrimental.

For more information on growth hormone and insulin-like growth factor in the ICU, see the excellent reviews by Carroll[52] and G. Van den Berghe.[19]

Morphine and Other Opioids

Almost every pediatric ICU patient is given morphine or one of its relatives. The negative hypotensive effects of exogenous opioids are well known. Endogenous opioids or endorphins are released in response to stress and play a role in the development of shock. The opiate antagonist naloxone attenuates the hypotensive response to endotoxin in animal models. Endorphins decrease sympathetic outflow, whereas exogenous opiates injected intraventricularly result in sympathetic nervous system activation.[57,58]

Opioids have immune-suppressive effects. Opioid abusers and their animal model counterparts have increased susceptibility to infection. In animal models, this effect is blocked by naloxone.[59] Opioid use increases metastases and decreases survival in tumor-bearing animals.[60,61] Acutely, centrally acting morphine activates the sympathetic nervous system, which in turn innervates immune tissue. Good evidence indicates that most of the observed immune-suppressive effects of morphine occur via this pathway.[62,63] Morphine also activates the HPA axis, which may lead to cortisol-mediated immune suppression, particularly during chronic administration. Opioids induce immune suppression at analgesic doses by binding to classic, naloxone-sensitive opioid receptors in the brain. In addition, both classic and nonclassic opioid receptors are present on immune cells, but the extent to which morphine interacts directly with these cells to cause immune suppression in vivo is unclear.[64,66]

Morphine reduces the T-cell proliferative response to mitogen, increases T-cell apoptosis, and decreases IL-6 levels in vitro. Morphine decreases B-cell antibody production. In vitro, morphine acts directly to decrease T-cell responsiveness by suppressing IL-2 gene expression, but the extent to which this mechanism is important in vivo is unclear.[64,66] Acute and chronic exposure to morphine decreases splenic and peripheral NK cell activity.[65] NK cells have significant tumoricidal activity, and decreased NK cell function may be associated with an increase in tumor cell dissemination and growth of micrometastases.[61]

Treatment with morphine for as little as 36 to 72 hours impairs macrophage response to macrophage colony-stimulating factor in mice and may affect phagocytosis and superoxide production ex vivo. Macrophages from morphine-treated animals are still sensitive to GM-CSF, a recombinant form of which is available for clinical use. This may represent one of the few methods by which clinicians might antagonize the immune suppressive effects of morphine.[65]

Opioid use is ubiquitous in critical care and may contribute to lymphocyte depletion observed in the ICU. Because many of the effects of opioids on the immune system occur via the μ receptor, morphine derivatives such as fentanyl likely have the same effect. Unfortunately, there is no known analgesic with efficacy comparable to the opioids. When the desired effect is anxiolytic, nonopioid alternatives should be considered. More research on this topic is necessary before therapy can be changed. Patients who are dependent on morphine for pain control may someday be candidates for immune stimulants.

Somatostatin

Somatostatin was first discovered as a potent inhibitor of growth hormone release, but it now is known to also inhibit insulin release, decrease secretion and absorption in the gastrointestinal tract, and decrease splanchnic blood flow.[5] Somatostatin analogues (octreotide) are used for treatment of gastrointestinal hemorrhage.

Somatostatin has direct immune suppressive effects in vitro. Somatostatin receptors are expressed on peripheral T and B lymphocytes, on activated monocytes, and in hematopoietic precursors.[67] In the bone marrow, somatostatin inhibits proliferation, particularly in response to granulocyte colony-stimulating factor (G-CSF).[68] Somatostatin strongly inhibits IFN-γ production by T cells, thereby decreasing macrophage activation and antigen presentation.[13] Local concentrations of substance P antagonize the effects of somatostatin on IFN-γ production.[69] Somatostatin also decreases prolactin release by the pituitary, and some of its immune suppressive effects may occur via this mechanism.[40] The effect of octreotide infusions on immune function in critically ill patients has not been studied.

Other Neuroendocrine–Immune Mediators

Researchers are still discovering new neurotransmitters, hormones, and cytokines, and they continue to recognize new NEI roles for well-known molecules. The molecules described here are examples of this interface. At the time of this writing, there are no known therapies targeting these molecules, but they may someday have clinical relevance. If nothing else, they serve as a reminder of the layers of complexity to the NEI system that we do not yet understand.

Macrophage Migration Inhibitory Factor

Macrophage migration inhibitory factor (MIF) was discovered in the 1950s on the basis of its ability to inhibit the migration of macrophages in capillary tubes. More recently, MIF has been recognized as the unique protein hormone released by the anterior pituitary and the adrenal gland in tandem with HPA axis activation. It also is produced by activated macrophages in response to levels of bacterial lipopolysaccharide that are lower than the levels that stimulate TNF-α production, making it a very early mediator of inflammation.[70]

Like prolactin and substance P, MIF antagonizes some of the peripheral effects of glucocorticoids. It appears to play a major role in the amplification of the immune response. MIF promotes cytokine expression by macrophages and T cells. MIF up-regulates the expression of toll-like receptors, which are cell surface receptors involved in recognition of bacterial endotoxin by the innate immune system. MIF levels are elevated in septic shock patients compared with nonseptic critically ill patients, and MIF levels increase with the development of ARDS.[71]

No therapies for modulating the expression or actions of MIF are available. Drugs that oppose MIF may someday play a role in inflammatory conditions such as ARDS and asthma.

Substance P, Neuropeptide Y, and Calcitonin Gene-Related Peptide

Substance P, a neuropeptide present in afferent nerves in the dorsal horn of the spinal column, originally was discovered to be a mediator of pain sensation. Substance P plays a role in inducing inflammation in response to a variety of irritants and may be part of the CNS pathways involved in psychological stress.[52] Immune cells contain receptors for substance P in addition to other neuropeptides. The actions of substance P in the immune system appear to be proinflammatory and immune supportive. It induces mast cell degranulation, stimulates lymphocyte proliferation and cytokine release, and may play a role in chronic inflammation.[72,73] In vitro and in vivo, substance P counteracts glucocorticoid-mediated apoptosis.[72]

Substance P is one of a growing group of neuropeptides that have been shown to have immune regulatory function. Others include calcitonin gene-related peptide, neuropeptide Y, vasoactive intestinal peptide, pro-opiomelanocortin-related peptides, and β endorphins.[50] Whether the actions of neuropeptides on immune cells is stimulatory or inhibitory may depend on the activation state of the cells and the T-cell phenotypes.[74] At the time of this writing, little is known about their function in the normal state or the stress response. Currently, there are no known therapeutic agents directed at them. Further research may prove the importance of these molecules.

Clinical Relevance

The acute phase of critical illness is characterized by supranormal release of neuroendocrine mediators from the hypothalamus and pituitary. As a consequence of this secretory activity, short-term goals of blood pressure support and mobilization of fuel substrates are met at the expense of neglecting homeostatic mechanisms, immune function, growth, and repair. When a patient's own fight or flight response is insufficient to maintain perfusion, shock ensues. For intensivists, the NEI system represents a set of tools for influencing the hemodynamic, metabolic, and immune/inflammatory state of the patient. In the first hours to days of critical illness, replacement of an inadequate neuroendocrine response with catecholamines, vasopressin, and/or steroids is lifesaving.

During the acute phase of critical illness, the antiinflammatory effect of steroids and catecholamines may be beneficial in many patients. Although clinical trials of anti-inflammatory therapies in sepsis have generally been disappointing, most authors agree there is a subset of patients whose robust inflammatory response puts them at increased risk for early death from septic shock. During the prolonged phase of critical illness, the effects of fight-or-flight mediators, whether endogenous or exogenous, may be harmful.

Decreased levels of anterior pituitary hormones and loss of the normal pattern of pulsatile release of these hormones characterize the prolonged phase of critical illness (Figure 95–3). ACTH, growth hormone, thyroid-stimulating hormone, prolactin, and luteinizing hormone are all similarly affected. Cortisol levels remain elevated in chronic critical illness despite a decrease in ACTH release. The metabolic consequence of this neuroendocrine milieu is an impaired ability to use fatty acids as fuel substrates and a tendency to store fat and to waste protein from muscle and organs. The immune consequences are impaired lymphocyte and monocyte function and increased lymphocyte apoptosis. In patients who fail to recover but go on to develop multiple organ dysfunction, the state of catabolism and immune suppression persists even in the absence of dopamine, glucocorticoids, or other well-known suppressors of the somatotropic axis.

Because dysfunction of normal homeostatic mechanisms may occur independently of ICU therapies, it may be tempting to label the neuroendocrine profile of chronically critically ill patients "normal." In fact, prolonged critical illness does not occur without medical intervention, and in the natural state these patients would not survive. In some chronically critically ill patients, the neuroendocrine system may fail as other organ systems fail. Investigators must ask what neuroendocrine milieu is associated with the best outcomes, including recovery of organ function, effective wound healing, and freedom from nosocomial infection.

Prolonged use of steroids, opioids, or hemodynamic support likely plays a role in the immune suppression and the suppression of anabolic pathways seen in chronic critical illness. Duration of immune suppression correlates strongly with the incidence of related infection, so even a low-grade immune suppression may become clinically significant over time. Lymphopenia and monocyte deactivation are associated with increased risk for poor outcomes, including nosocomial infection, prolonged hospital stay and mechanical ventilation, multiple organ dysfunction, and death.[75,76] In a review of autopsies of children who died of multiple organ failure, among those who were admitted with a diagnosis of sepsis, 75% had persistent infection at autopsy, suggesting that some patients with multiple organ failure have clinically significant immune depression.[9]

After the first week of ICU care, as patients move into the chronic phase of critical illness, it is important to begin to think about restoring the capacity to grow, heal wounds, build muscle, and fight infection. Steroids should be tapered as soon as hemodynamics or underlying conditions allow. Morphine and other opioids should be used no more than necessary to control the patient's pain. In situations where catecholamines have no proven benefit, as in the case of "renal dose" dopamine, it may be appropriate to consider whether the negative effects on the immune system and on metabolism outweigh the potential benefits of the drug.

Clinicians should be vigilant for the acquired immune deficiency that occurs in prolonged critical illness. When lymphopenia is persistent, indicators of T- and B-cell function should be measured. Patients with low CD4 counts may benefit from early prophylaxis against fungus or *Pneumocystis carinii* pneumonia. Patients with low immunoglobulin levels may benefit from intravenous immunoglobulin. In the prolonged phase of critical illness, patients may be candidates for immune stimulants, including G-CSF or GM-CSF. Investigational therapies targeting lymphopenia may be available in the near future.

REFERENCES

1. Zaloga GP, Marik P: Hypothalamic-pituitary-adrenal insufficiency. *Crit Care Clin* 17:25-41, 2001.
2. Chikanza IC, Grossman AS: Hypothalamic-pituitary mediated immunomodulation: arginine vasopressin is a neuroendocrine immune mediator. *J Rheumatol* 37:131-136, 1998.
3. Greenspan FS, Strewler GJ, editors: *Basic and clinical endocrinology*, ed 2, Stamford, CT, 1997, Appleton and Lange.
4. Chicanza IC: Prolactin and immunomodulation: in vitro and in vivo observations. *Ann N Y Acad Sci* 876:119-130, 1999.
5. Guyton AC, Hall JH: Textbook of medical physiology. Philadelphia, 1996, WB Saunders.
6. Borovikova LV, Ivanova S, Zhang M, et al: Vagus nerve stimulation attenuates the systemic inflammatory response to endotoxin. *Nature* 405:458-462, 2000.
7. Crofford LJ, Sano H, Karalis K, et al: Corticotropin releasing hormone in synovial fluids and tissues of patients with rheumatoid arthritis and osteoarthritis. *J Immunol* 151:1587-1596, 1993.
8. Karalis K, Sano H, Redwine J, et al: Autocrine or paracrine inflammatory actions of corticotropin releasing hormone in vivo. *Science* 25:421-423, 1991.
9. Amoo-Lamptey A, Dickman P, Carcillo JA: Comparative pathology of children with sepsis and MOF, pneumonia without MOF, and MOF without infection. *Pediatr Res* 2001 (abstract).
10. Vermes I, Beishuizen, A: The hypothalamic-pituitary-adrenal response to critical illness. *Best Pract Res Clin Endocrinol Metab* 15:494-507, 2001.
14. Vermes I, Beishuizen A, Hampsink RM, et al: Dissociation of plasma adrenocorticotropin and cortisol levels in critically ill patients: possible role of endothelin and atrial natriuretic hormone. *J Clin Endocrinol Metab* 80:1238-1242, 1995.
15. Ehrhart-Bornstein M, Hinson JP, Bornstein SR, et al: Intraadrenal interactions in the regulation of adrenocortical steroidogenesis. *Endocr Rev* 19:101-143, 1998.
16. Marx C, Ehrhart-Bornstein M, Scherbaum WA, et al: Regulation of adrenocortical function by cytokines—relevance for immune-endocrine interactions. *Horm Metab Res* 30:416-420, 1998
17. Toth IE, Hinson JP: Neuropeptides in the adrenal gland: distribution, localization of receptors, and effects of steroid hormone synthesis. *Endocr Res* 21:39-51, 1995.
18. Beishuizen A, Thijs LG: Relative adrenal failure in intensive care: an identifiable problem requiring treatment? *Best Pract Res Clinical Endocrinol Metab* 15:513-531, 2001
19. Beishuizen A, Bonte HA, Vermes I: Patterns of corticosteroid binding globulin and free cortisol index during severe sepsis and multi trauma. *Intensive Care Med* 25:S62, 1999.
20. Hammond GL, Smith CL, Paterson NA, et al: A role for corticosteroid binding globulin in the delivery of cortisol to activated neutrophils. *J Clin Endocriniol Metab* 71:34-39, 1990.
21. Beishuizen A, van Lijf JH, Lekkerkerker JF, et al: The low dose (1 microgram) ACTH stimulation test for assessment of the hypothalamic-pituitary adrenal axis. *Neth J Med* 56:91-99, 2000.
22. Marik PE, Zaloga GP: Adrenal insufficiency during septic shock. *Crit Care Med* 31:141-145, 2003.
23. Annane D, Sebillle V, Charpentier C, et al: Effect of treatment with low dose hydrocortisone and fludrocortisone on mortality in patients with septic shock. *JAMA* 288:862-887, 2002.
24. Briegel J, Forst H, Haller M, et al: Stress doses of hydrocortisone reverse hyperdynamic septic shock: a prospective randomized double blind, single center study. *Crit Care Med* 27:723-32, 1999.
25. Cronin L, Cook DJ, Carlet J, et al: Corticosteroid treatment for sepsis: a critical appraisal and meta analysis of the literature. Crit Care Med 23:1430-39, 1995.
26. Sharshar T, Carlier R, Blanchard A, et al: Depletion of neurohypophyseal content of vasopressin in septic shock. *Crit Care Med* 30:497-500, 2002.
27. Krismer AC, Wenzel V, Mayr VD, et al: Arginine vasopressin during cardiopulmonary resuscitation and vasodilatory shock: current experience and future perspectives. *Curr Opin Crit Care* 7:157-169, 2001.
28. Linder KH, Dirks B, Strohmenger HU, et al: Randomised comparison of epinephrine and vasopressin in patients with out-hospital ventricular fibrillation. *Lancet* 349:535-537, 1997.
29. Stiell IG, Hebert PC, Wells GA, et al: Vasopressin versus epinephrine for inhospital cardiac arrest: a randomized controlled trial. *Lancet* 359:105-109, 2001.
30. Liedel JL, Meadow W, Nachman J, et al: Use of vasopressin in refractory hypotension in children with vasodilatory shock: five cases and review of the literature. *Pediatr Crit Care Med* 3:15-18, 2002.
31. Shibasaki T, Hotta S, Wakabayashi I: Brain vasopressin is involved in the stress induced suppression of immune function in the rat. *Brain Res* 808:84-92, 1998.
32. Bell J, Adler MW, Greenstein JI: The effect of arginine vasopressin on autologous mixed lymphocyte reactions. *Int Immunopharmacol* 14:93-103, 1992.
33. Chikanza IC, Petrou P, Chrousos G: Perterbations of arginine vasopressin secretion during inflammatory stress, pathophysiologic implications. *Ann N Y Acad Sci* 917:825-834, 2000.
34. Besedovsky HO, Del Rey A: Immune-neuro-endocrine Interactions: facts and hypotheses. *Endocr Rev* 17:64-102, 1996.
35. Yang H, Wang L, Huang CS, et al: Plasticity of GAP-43 innervation of the spleen during immune response in the mouse: evidence for axonal sprouting and redistribution of the nerve fibers. *Neuroimmunomodulation* 5:53-60, 1998.
36. Kohm AP, Sanders VM: Norepinephrine and beta 2 adrenergic receptor stimulation regulate CD4+ T and B lymphocyte function in vitro and in vivo. *Pharmacol Rev* 53:487-525, 2001.
37. Kohm AP, Sanders VM: Norepinephrine, a messenger from the brain to the immune system. *Immunol Today* 21:539-542, 2000.
38. Devins SS, Miller A, Herndon BL, et al: Effects of dopamine on t-lymphocyte proliferative responses and serum prolactin concentration in critically ill patients. *Crit Care Med* 20:1644-49, 1992.
39. Van den Berghe G, de Zegher F: Anterior pituitary function during critical illness and dopamine treatment. *Crit Care Med* 24: 1580-1590, 1996.
40. Freeman ME, Kanycska B, Lerany A, et al: Prolactin: structure, function and regulation of secretion. *Physiol Rev* 80:1523-1631, 2000.
41. Noel GL, Suh HK, Stone JG, et al: Human prolactin and growth hormone release during surgery and other conditions of stress. *J Clin Endocrinol Metab* 35:840-851, 1972.
42. Fletcher-Chiappini SE, Compton MM, La Voie HA, et al: Glucocorticoid-prolactin interactions in NB2 lymphoma cells: antiproliferative versus anticytolytic effects. *Proc Soc Exp Biol Med* 202:345-352, 1993.

43. Velkeniers B, Dogusan Z, Naessens F, et al: Prolactin, growth hormone, and the immune system in humans. *Cell Mol Life Sci* 54: 1102-1108, 1998.
44. Russell DH, Kibler R, Matrisian L, et al: Prolactin receptors on human T and B lymphocytes: antagonism of prolactin binding by cyclosporine. *J Immunol* 134:3027-3031, 1985.
45. Jorgensen C, Sany J: Prospects and advances in hormonal immunomodulatory therapy. *Ballieres Best Pract Res Clin Rheumatol* 10:379-392, 1996.
46. Chaudry IH, Ayala A, Ertel W, et al: Hemorrhage and resuscitation: immunological aspects. *Am J Physiol* 259(4 pt 2):R663-R678, 1990.
47. Kayne RD, Burrow GN: Anterior pituitary function in women with postpartum hemorrhage. *Yale J Biol Med* 51:151-156, 1978.
48. Felmet K, Hall MA, Carcillo JA, et al: Unpublished manuscript. 2003.
49. Richards SM, Murphy WJ: Use of human prolactin as a therapeutic protein to potentiate immunohematopoietic function. *J Neuroimmunol* 109:56-62, 2000.
50. Berczi I, Chalmers IM, Nagy E, et al: Immune effects of neuropeptides. *Baillieres Best Pract Res Clin Rheumatol* 10:227-259, 1996.
51. Van den Berghe G, Wouters P, Weekers F, et al: Intensive insulin therapy in critically ill patients. *N Engl J Med* 345:1359-1367, 2001.
52. Carroll P: Treatment with growth Hormone and insulin-like growth factor-1 in critical illness. *Best Pract Res Clin Endocrinol Metab* 15:435-451, 2001.
53. Gilpin DA, Barrow RE, Rutan RL, et al: Recombinant human growth hormone accelerates wound healing in children with large cutaneous burns. *Ann Surg* 220:19-24, 1994.
54. Takala J, Ruokonen E, Webster NR, et al: Increased mortality associated with growth hormone treatment in critically ill adults. *N Engl J Med* 341:785-792, 1999.
55. de Groof F, Joosten KF, Janssen JA, et al: Acute stress response in children with meningococcal sepsis: important differences in the growth hormone/insulin-like growth factor I axis between non-survivors and survivors. *J Clin Endocrinol Metab* 87:3118-3124, 2002.
56. Critical evaluation of the safety of recombinant human growth hormone administration: statement from the Growth Hormone Research Society. *J Clin Endocrinol Metab* 86:1868-1870, 2001.
57. Holaday JW, D'Amato RJ, Ruvio BA, et al: Adrenalectomy unlocks pressor responses to naloxone in endotoxic shock: evidence for sympathomedullary involvement. *Circ Shock* 11: 201-210, 1983.
58. Long JB, Lake CR, Reid AA, et al: Effects of naloxone and thyrotropin releasing hormone on plasma catecholamines, corticosterone, and arterial pressure in normal and endotoxemic rats. *Circ Shock* 18:1-10 1986.
60. Lewis JW, Shavit Y, Terman GW, et al: Stress and morphine affect survival of rats challenged with a mammary ascites tumor (MAT13762B). *Nat Immune Cell Growth Regul* 3:43-50, 1983.
61. Yeager MP, Collacchiop TA: Effect of morphine on growth of metastatic colon cancer in vivo. *Arch Surg* 126:454-456, 1991.
62. Carr DJ, France CP: Immune alterations in chronic morphine treated rhesus monkeys. *Adv Exp Med Biol* 335:35-39, 1993.
63. Hall DM, Suo JL, Weber RJ: Opioid mediated effects on the immune system: sympathetic nervous system involvement. *J Neuroimmunol* 83:29-35, 1998.
64. Houghtling RA, Mellon RD, Tan RJ, et al: Acute effects of morphine on blood lymphocyte proliferation and plasma IL-6 levels. *Ann N Y Acad Sci* 917:771-777, 2000.
65. Roy S, Loh HH: Effects of opioids on the immune system. *Neurochem Res* 11:1375-1386, 1996.
66. Madden JJ, Whaley WL, Ketelsen D: Opiate binding sites in the cellular immune system: expression and regulation. *J Neuroimmunol* 83:57-62, 1998.
67. Lichtenauer-Kaligis EG, van Hagen PM, Lamberts SW, et al: Somatostatin receptor subtypes in human immune cells. *Eur J Endocrinol* 143:S21-S25, 2000.
68. Oomen SP, Hofland LJ, van Hagen PM, et al: Somatostatin receptors in the haematopoietic system. *Eur J Endocrinol* 143:S9-S14, 2000.
69. Weinstock JV, Elliot, D: The somatostatin immunoregulatory circuit present at sites of chronic inflammation. *Eur J Endocrinol* 143:S15-S19, 2000.
70. Baughn JA, Bucala R. Macrophage migration inhibitory factor. *Crit Care Med* 30:S27-S35, 2002.
71. Beishuizen A, Thijs LG, Haanen C, et al. Macrophage migration inhibitory factor and hypothalamic pituitary adrenal function during critical illness. *J Clin Endocrinol Metab* 107:13-20, 2001.
72. Dimri R, Sharabi Y, Shoham J: Specific inhibition of glucocorticoid-induced thymocyte apoptosis by substance P. *J Immunol* 164: 2479-2486, 2000.
73. Harrion S, Geppetti P: Substance P. *Int J Biochem Cell Biol* 33: 555-576, 2001.
74. Levite M: Nerve driven immunity: the direct effects of neurotransmitters on T-cell function. *Ann N Y Acad Sci* 917:307-321, 2000.
75. Volk HD, Reinke P, Krausch D, et al: Monocyte deactivation—rationale for a new therapeutic strategy in sepsis. *Intensive Care Med Suppl* 4:S474-S481, 1996.
77. Ledingham IM, Watt I: Influence of sedation on mortality in critically ill multiple trauma patients. *Lancet* 1:1270 1983.
78. Absalom A, Pledger D, Kong A: Adrenocortical function in critically ill patients 24 hours after a single dose of etomidate. *Anaesthesia* 54:861-867, 1999.
79. Catalano RD, Parameswaran V, Ramachandran J, et al: Mechanisms of adrenocortical depression during *Escherichia* coli shock. *Arch Surg* 119:145-150, 1984.
80. Bamberger CM, Schulte HM, Chrousos GP. Molecular determinants of glucocorticoid receptor function and tissue sensitivity. *Endocr Rev* 17:221-244, 1996.
81. Van den Berghe G: The neuroendocrine response to stress is a dynamic process. *Best Pract Res Clin Endocrinol Metab* 15: 405-419, 2001.

CHAPTER

96

Sepsis

Thomas P. Shanley, Craig Hallstrom, and Hector R. Wong

PEARLS

- The typical patient with septic shock has simultaneous derangements of cardiovascular function, intravascular volume status, respiratory function, immune/inflammatory regulation, renal function, coagulation, hepatic function, and/or metabolic function.
- The complexity of septic shock warrants a systematic and multifaceted approach on the part of the pediatric intensivist.
- Although some overlap exists among some of the terms for shock (systemic inflammatory response syndrome, sepsis, septic shock, severe sepsis), particularly between septic shock and severe sepsis, each is intended to define a particular patient population.
- Sepsis now is seen as a dysregulation of immunologic pathways directed toward pathogen eradication and restoration of homeostasis.
- From a clinical standpoint, the treatment of sepsis entails four important goals: initial resuscitation, elimination of pathogen, maintenance of oxygen delivery, and carefully directed regulation of the inflammatory response.

Management of a patient with septic shock embodies the discipline of pediatric critical care medicine. The typical patient with septic shock has simultaneous derangements of cardiovascular function, intravascular volume status, respiratory function, immune/inflammatory regulation, renal function, coagulation, hepatic function, and/or metabolic function. The degree to which any of these derangements manifests in a given patient is highly variable and influenced by multiple host and nonhost factors, including developmental stage, presence or absence of comorbidities, causative agent of septic shock, host's immune/inflammatory state, and host's genetic background. These factors combine to profoundly influence the ultimate outcome of septic shock.

The complexity of septic shock warrants a systematic and multifaceted approach on the part of the pediatric intensivist. Optimal management requires a strong working knowledge not just of cardiovascular physiology and infectious diseases but also of multiple organ function/dysfunction, inflammation-related biology, immunity, coagulation, pharmacology, and molecular biology. The pediatric intensivist also needs a working knowledge of genetics for the future management of patients with septic shock. This chapter provides a comprehensive description of the many aspects that influence the development and outcome of septic shock, pathophysiology at the physiologic and molecular levels, contemporary management of septic shock, and what we believe to be the next important future directions in the field. Ultimately, this information must be integrated with the bedside experience, which cannot be supplanted by a book chapter.

Epidemiology

A true picture of the epidemiology of septic shock is clouded by the lack of a reliable case definition. This is true for both the adult population and the pediatric population.[1] A few pediatric-specific studies, however, illustrate the importance of septic shock in today's modern intensive care unit. Proulx et al.[2] analyzed the incidence and outcome of the systemic inflammatory response syndrome (SIRS), sepsis, severe sepsis, and septic shock (see next section for definitions) in a single institution. A total of 1058 admissions were analyzed over a 1-year period. SIRS was present in 82% of patients, while 23% had sepsis, 4% had severe sepsis, and 2% had septic shock. The overall mortality rate for this patient population was 6%, with the majority of deaths occurring in patients with multiple organ dysfunction syndrome (MODS). Among the patients with MODS, distinct mortality rates were associated with SIRS (40%), sepsis (22%), severe sepsis (25%) and septic shock (52%).

Later studies by Watson et al.[3] at the University of Pittsburgh provide perhaps the most comprehensive and current epidemiologic surveys of pediatric septic shock. By linking 1995 hospital records from seven large states (representing 24% of the United States population) with census data, they estimated an incidence of 42,371 cases of severe sepsis in individuals younger than 20 years (0.6 cases/1000 population). The highest incidence was in neonates (5.2 cases/1000 population), compared with children ages 5 to 14 years who had an incidence of 0.2 cases/1000 population. The overall mortality rate in this population was 10.3% (4364 deaths nationally). In addition, patients younger than 1 year and patients with comorbidities had higher mortality rates than patients between 5 and 14 years old and patients without comorbidities, respectively. Their study also estimated an annual national health care cost of $1.7 billion associated with severe sepsis.

In a follow-up study, Watson et al.[4] compared the epidemiology of severe sepsis between 1995 and 1999. Using a similar survey strategy as described for their earlier study, they found a 13% increase in the absolute number of cases of severe sepsis during this time period. The majority of the increase was accounted for by severe sepsis in children younger than 1 year. In contrast, the mortality rate for severe sepsis decreased from 10.3% to 9.0% during this time period.

Collectively, these data illustrate that septic shock continues to present a major health problem in terms of incidence, mortality, and health care costs. Nevertheless, there is a great need for additional quality epidemiologic studies of septic shock in children. One major issue that must be addressed is the development of more meaningful and consistent case definitions. These types of future studies are necessary for our understanding not only of incidence but also of the impact of new knowledge and therapies and for the design of more effective interventional trials specific to the pediatric population.

Definitions

Intuitively, the experienced pediatric intensivist knows when he or she encounters a patient with septic shock. Thus definitions of sepsis and septic shock could be viewed as being of limited value in daily practice. Despite this common perception, there is a clear need for standard definitions of sepsis and septic shock for several reasons. First, with the development of standard definitions, we will be able to more accurately characterize the epidemiologic features of septic shock in the pediatric population. Second, as novel, expensive, and potentially higher-risk therapies are developed, it will be important to accurately identify and stratify patients early in the course of septic shock if we are to realize a favorable benefit/risk ratio in a given patient. Finally, standard definitions are crucial to the design of much needed, pediatric-specific interventional trials.

The most widely used definition of pediatric septic shock is based on the 1992 American College of Chest Physicians/Society of Critical Care Medicine Consensus Conference, with adaptations for the pediatric population.[2,5] The following four terms are widely used in the literature: *SIRS*, *sepsis*, *septic shock*, and *severe sepsis*. Although some overlap exists among some of these terms (particularly between septic shock and severe sepsis), each is intended to define a particular patient population.

SIRS is intended to represent a state of relative inflammatory/immune activation in a given patient and is said to be present when a patient has at least any two of the four criteria listed in Box 96–1. Importantly, the physiologic changes must occur as an acute change from baseline and not be explained by other causes. Thus patients with diverse clinical conditions, such as sepsis, pancreatitis, burns, or hypermetabolism following major trauma, can meet criteria for SIRS. Because of its relative nonspecific qualities and the broad range of patients who can be classified as having SIRS, the validity and usefulness of SIRS criteria have been debated in the literature.[6,7] Nevertheless, the criteria have been widely used in both descriptive and interventional studies and, if anything, are of important historical interest.

Sepsis is defined as SIRS secondary to a systemic infection, either documented by microbiology cultures or in the presence of other clinical evidence of infection. *Severe sepsis* is defined by sepsis criteria plus evidence of insufficient end-organ perfusion (Box 96–2). *Septic shock* is defined by sepsis criteria plus hypotension (two distinct measurements <3rd percentile for age) after the administration of 20 ml/kg crystalloid or colloid, plus the criteria listed in Box 96–3.

These criteria have been used extensively for conducting clinical investigations and are of proven value. Nevertheless, they have been criticized for lack of both sensitivity and specificity.[1] Updated consensus definitions with contemporary guidelines for management of severe sepsis and septic shock as an aspect of the surviving sepsis campaign have been published by an international consortium of organizations interested in sepsis intensive care.[8] The revisions are primarily targeted to the adult population and require further tailoring to the pediatric population. Refinement of pediatric-specific criteria for septic shock is imperative for future clinical trials and epidemiologic investigations.

BOX 96–1

*Criteria for SIRS**

1. Temperature >38° C rectal (37.8° C oral, 37.2° C axillary) or <36° C rectal (35.8° C oral, 35.2° C axillary)
2. Heart rate >90th percentile for age
3. Respiratory rate >90th percentile for age or hyperventilation to $Paco_2$ <32 torr (4.3 kPa)
4. White blood cell count >12,000 cells/mm^3 or <4000 cells/mm^3

*Presence of at least two criteria, representing an acute change from baseline, and in the absence of other known causes for these changes.

BOX 96–2

Criteria for Severe Sepsis

Sepsis plus any *one* of the following:

- Glasgow coma scale score < 15 in the absence of CNS disease
- Arterial blood lactate > 1.6 mmol/L or venous blood lactate > 2.2 mmol/L
- Urine output < 1 ml/kg/hour for 2 consecutive hours with a urinary catheter in place

Clinical Presentation

As a disease entity that affects the entire body, sepsis can present initially with a variety of symptoms. The most common clinical manifestations of sepsis include fever or hypothermia, tachypnea, tachycardia, leukocytosis or leukopenia, thrombocytopenia, and change in mental status. One of the earliest signs that alerts caregivers to the possibility of infection is fever. A number of the cytokines elicited in response to infection are pyrogens, particularly interleukin (IL)-1β and tumor necrosis factor (TNF)-α. The development of a fever may be beneficial because it stimulates the body to produce heat shock proteins.[9] Patients also can have hypothermia, which is more common in infants than older children. Adults patients who do not develop a temperature higher than 99.6° F in the first 24 hours of infection have an increased risk for mortality.[10,11]

In the traditional classifications of shock states, four broad categories are defined: hypovolemic, cardiogenic, obstructive, and distributive shock (see Chapter 27). Septic shock is unique in that all four forms may be involved simultaneously. The patient may have hypovolemic shock resulting from capillary leak, increased insensible losses, and decreased effective blood volume secondary to venodilation; cardiogenic shock related to myocardial-depressant effects of bacterial toxins and inflammatory cytokines (as reviewed later); obstructive shock from diffuse small vessel thrombosis; and distributive shock from decreased systemic vascular resistance and cytopathic hypoxia. The degree to which an individual patient manifests these physiologic perturbations varies. In some cases, patients display increased cardiac output with diminished systemic vascular resistance. The presenting symptoms are tachycardia and bounding pulses characteristic of the distributive mode of shock or the so-called "warm" shock state. Despite this appearance, the perfusion of major organs during this shock state may remain compromised. Alternatively, a patient with depressed cardiac output and elevated systemic vascular resistance appears cool with diminished pulses and poor capillary refill characteristic of the "cold" shock state. Data suggest this presentation is common in pediatric septic shock.[12] Although it is important to recognize that patients may transition from one state to another, the presence of hypotension, or shock, often is a late and particularly ominous sign that requires prompt intervention because its presence is associated with increased mortality.[13]

BOX 96–3

Criteria for Septic Shock

Sepsis with hypotension (two distinct measurements of blood pressure < 3rd percentile for age) after administration of 20 ml/kg crystalloid or colloid, plus any *one* of the following:

- Requirement for inotropic or vasopressor support (excluding dopamine ≤ 5 μg/kg/min)
- Any of the diagnostic criteria for severe sepsis listed in Box 96–2

Patients with sepsis often have presenting symptoms of respiratory abnormalities, notably tachypnea that reflects a compensatory, respiratory alkalosis aimed at counteracting a metabolic acidosis. Chest x-ray film often reveals a small heart in the presence of hypovolemia with few vascular markings. However, in the face of capillary leak and decreased myocardial function, patients with septic shock usually develop pulmonary edema as fluid resuscitation proceeds, so progression to acute respiratory failure or acute respiratory distress syndrome (ARDS) is not uncommon.[14] Endotracheal intubation and mechanical ventilatory support may be necessary because of increasing respiratory effort and often decreasing neurologic status. Care should be taken after tracheal intubation to ensure that the patient is provided minute ventilation to a similar degree as was present prior to removal of their respiratory drive.

All of the body's systems are affected by poor perfusion and decreased oxygen delivery resulting from perturbations in cardiac and respiratory function and impairment of oxygen utilization at the cellular level. In addition, they are injured by direct effects of bacterial toxins and circulating cytokines. The mental status of a child with sepsis frequently is altered, ranging from agitation to obtundation. Depressed mental status can be present even in the absence of meningitis. The skin frequently is hypoperfused with decreased capillary refill and mottling. Petechiae and purpura may be present and, although helpful in diagnosis, can be ominous signs.

Pathogenesis

Both clinical and basic science studies by many critical care investigators have focused on the mechanisms underlying the development of the clinical responses to sepsis in humans outlined previously. Over the past decade, at least three major hypotheses have been proposed to explain the development of sepsis and its sequelae. The first hypothesis proposed that bacteria and/or their products cause the tissue injury and organ dysfunction associated with sepsis. Although some evidence supports this concept, the recognition that noninfectious triggers of the sepsis response, combined with the observation that there is no correlation between sepsis and the presence of infections, led to additional hypotheses. A second common hypothesis attributes the development of sepsis to an excessive host inflammatory response. For consistency with the historical literature, this whole-body reaction has been coined as the systemic inflammatory response syndrome (SIRS). Again, much of the basic and preclinical research data support this hypothesis and are reviewed later. However, in light of several failed attempts at providing clinical benefit with strategies aimed at blocking this excessive proinflammation, combined with the identification of a pronounced counterregulatory, antiinflammatory response, investigators have proposed a third hypothesis. They hypothesize that sepsis reflects an inadequate compensatory, antiinflammatory response (or syndrome, coined CARS), which results in dysregulated and excessive proinflammation in the host. The section reviews the data supporting each of these hypotheses, as the clinically heterogeneous populations of septic patients likely reflect evidence of each of these pathophysiologic processes. It is important to consider the likelihood that these pathophysiologic processes are not mutually exclusive and that facets of each likely contribute to the clinical complexity in any given patient.

The human species is subject to infectious challenges from a variety of pathogens, including bacteria, viruses, fungi, and protozoa. In some cases, overwhelming spread of a pathogen (e.g., bacteria) and significant release of toxins (e.g., exotoxin) can result in direct host injury and organ dysfunction. In order to survive, higher-order organisms developed an immune system designed to eradicate pathogens. Immunity to microorganisms has evolved to include two systems: the *innate,* or natural, immune system and the *acquired,* or adoptive, immune system.[15] The innate immune system has been highly conserved and presumably exists in most organisms. The mechanisms by which these systems recognize pathogens and mount their effector responses are important evolved features of the immune response[16] (see Chapter 83). First, host recognition molecules, so-called pattern recognition receptors (PRRs), must identify highly conserved structures that exist on a broad array of microorganisms. Second, these molecular structures, termed *pathogen-associated molecular patterns,* must be conserved on several microorganisms. Examples of such molecular patterns include lipopolysaccharide (LPS) on gram-negative bacteria, lipoteichoic acid on gram-positive bacteria, mannans on yeast cells, double-stranded ribonucleic acid (RNA) of RNA viruses, and CpG DNA from bacteria. Additionally, host PRRs must be able to differentiate self from non-self.[17] Furthermore, the effector mechanisms that are activated in the innate immune system (e.g., phagocytes, complement) are activated immediately upon infection and serve to rapidly control replication of the microorganism and explain the rapid kinetics of this response.

The PRR initiating the effector mechanisms of the innate immune system are ubiquitously expressed on antigen-presenting cells of the innate immune system. Structurally, they represent a diverse series of proteins. Only recently has the group of Toll-like receptors (TLRs) been identified as perhaps the most critical pathogen recognition receptor family in the context of sepsis (see section on LPS recognition). Other well-characterized families of PRR include the collagenous (C type) lectins that bind to a variety of carbohydrate moieties on cells, bacteria, and viruses. Members of this family, which include the collectins, are expressed on antigen-presenting macrophages and natural killer cells. Many of these proteins share structural homology to the complement protein C1q and functionally can substitute for C1q in activating the complement cascade.[18] A second family of proteins possesses leucine-rich regions, which facilitates protein–protein interactions necessary for immune recognition. Examples include CD14, a protein that exists on the cell surface of macrophages and binds to LPS to initiate intracellular signal events resulting in proinflammatory gene expression (reviewed later). Scavenger receptors, such as the macrophage scavenger receptor, can bind to bacterial cell walls.[19] Finally, integrins, which are ubiquitously expressed on several types of leukocytes, can mediate not only cell–cell communication, but they also bind to LPS. Other PRRs exist as serum proteins, such as pentraxins, which are acute-phase reactants synthesized by the liver (e.g., C-reactive protein) and lipid transferases (e.g., lipopolysaccharide-binding protein [LBP], which binds to LPS and facilitates binding of LPS to CD14–TLR cellular complex).[20]

The complement system is a complex cascade of proteins possessing a series of protease activities. Broad immune functions can be attributed to complement proteins, including opsonization (C3), neutrophil chemotaxis (C5a), and perforating cytotoxicity (C6-9, MAC complex). As a result, complement proteins possess a variety of antipathogen activities, including the ability of complement protein C1 to bind to and directly lyse viruses.[21] Furthermore, viral infection of cells can directly activate the alternative complement pathway, resulting in activation of the chemoattractant components C3a and C5a. In summary, there exists a diverse set of pathogen recognition proteins aimed at protecting the host from infectious challenges.

Once a pathogen is recognized by the innate immune system, a series of effector mechanisms are initiated. These include (1) production of proinflammatory mediators such as cytokines and chemokines, (2) recruitment of cellular components of the immune system, (3) costimulatory activation of the adaptive immune response, and (4) regulation of the acute immune response to control host tissue injury. The observation that this essential immune response can become dysregulated and result in host autodestruction led to the second hypothesis discussed earlier in the pathogenesis section. Description of the host inflammatory response to infection in patients with sepsis-related organ dysfunction and the observation that noninfectious triggers of this response (e.g., trauma, pancreatitis, cardiopulmonary bypass) led to an explosion of clinical and basic science data supporting this observation.

Lipopolysaccharide Recognition

Activation of pathogen-recognizing cells, particularly the tissue macrophage and blood monocyte, results in their activation with subsequent expression of a series of potentially deleterious mediators. As reviewed previously,[22] sepsis research began several hundred years ago when Ernest von Bergmann introduced the term *sepsin* in describing the pus-derived toxin from infected patients. In time, Richard Pfeiffer coined the term *endotoxin* for the highly pyrogenic product of *Vibrio cholerae* with which he was working. By the middle of the twentieth century, the structure of endotoxin, or LPS, from gram-negative bacteria was determined. The structure of endotoxin reveals three principal domains: an outer hydrophilic chain, a central acidic core region, and a lipid-rich region (Figure 96–1). The hydrophilic,

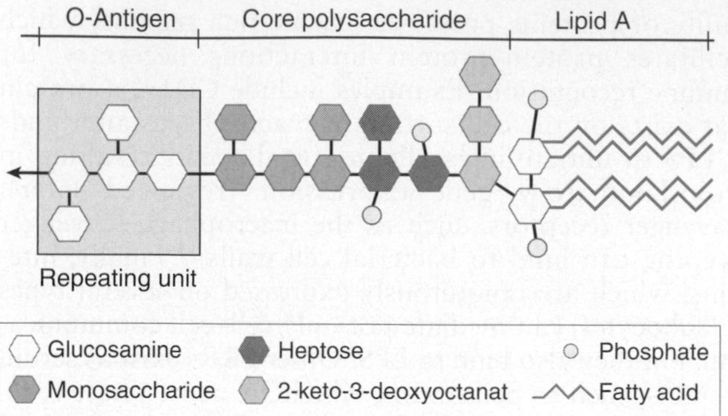

FIGURE 96–1 • Structure of endotoxin.

polysaccharide chain determines the O-antigenicity of each LPS. Variable repeats of monopolysaccharides and heteropolysaccharides with complex side chain structure provide a complexity that forms the basis of the distinct antigenic characteristics of each endotoxin.[23] This O-region is linked to the lipid A region via an acidic core oligosaccharide composed of glucose, galactose, heptose, and ketodeoxyoctonic acid with phosphoethanolamine residues.[23] The lipid A region is highly conserved among endotoxins and possesses much of the toxic activity attributed to intact LPS.[24] Despite this structural knowledge, how LPS triggered the inflammatory responses characteristic of sepsis remained incompletely understood.

A series of seminal observations helped elucidate the molecular pathophysiologic mechanisms by which LPS activates inflammation. The first involved the observation of an LPS-resistant strain of mice, the C3H/HeJ strain, and the subsequent determination that this phenotype was linked to a single genetic mutation.[25,26] A second important observation was that the lethal effects of endotoxin were conferred by hematopoietic cells.[27] In a series of elegant cell transfer studies, endotoxin-tolerant mice could be sensitized to LPS after reconstitution with hematopoietic cells from the LPS-sensitive strain, ultimately shown to be cells derived from the monocyte/macrophage lineage. Third was the observation that endotoxin treatment of monocyte-derived cells resulted in production of several cytokines and chemokines critical to the systemic inflammatory response. Among these, TNF and IL-1 were shown to be key proximal initiators of the septic response and could partly substitute for endotoxin in mediating experimental sepsis responses.[28–30] Finally, identification of the previously elusive LPS receptor(s) began to clarify the signal transduction mechanisms by which endotoxin triggered its selective inflammatory gene expression. Initially CD-14 was shown to be required for LPS signaling[31]; however, the realization that this receptor possessed no cytoplasmic domain made investigators skeptical that CD14 comprised the entire receptor complex.

Parallel to the search for the "complete" LPS receptor, investigators working with *Drosophila* had identified genes responsible for the dorsoventral polarization in embryonic development.[32] In the course of these studies, a plasma membrane receptor termed *Toll* was shown to signal through the rel family (homologous to the nuclear factor [NF]-κB family) of proteins to transcribe those genes required for polarization.[33] Subsequent studies in which Toll was functionally mutated showed the receptor played a role in host defense against *Aspergillus fumigatus*,[34] thus making the important connection between Toll receptors and innate immune defense. The additional observation of homology between the TLRs and the mammalian IL-1 family of receptors provided evidence that this family was crucial to the human innate immune response.[35] Subsequently the endotoxin tolerant mouse strain, C3H/HeJ, was determined to possess mutations in Toll-like receptor-4 (TLR-4), proving it was absolutely necessary for LPS signaling.[36] At present, 10 mammalian TLRs have been identified, each with a relatively specific set of ligands.[35,37,38]

In humans, TLR-4 is a necessary component of the LPS–receptor complex that is responsible for transmitting the cell surface binding of endotoxin to intracellular signaling pathways that result in downstream inflammatory gene production. Other members of the LPS–receptor complex include CD14,[31] MD-2,[39] and MyD88[40] (Figure 96–2). In addition, LPS binding to its receptor complex is facilitated by the presence of LBP.[20] A conserved Toll/IL-1 receptor (TIR) homology domain is necessary for propagating the signal from the cell membrane to additional intracellular signaling domains, such as the IL-1 receptor-activating kinase (IRAK) (Figure 96–2).[41] Subsequently, activation of downstream domains, such as the TNF receptor-associated factor (TRAF)-6, results in further activation of downstream pathways such as the mitogen-activated protein

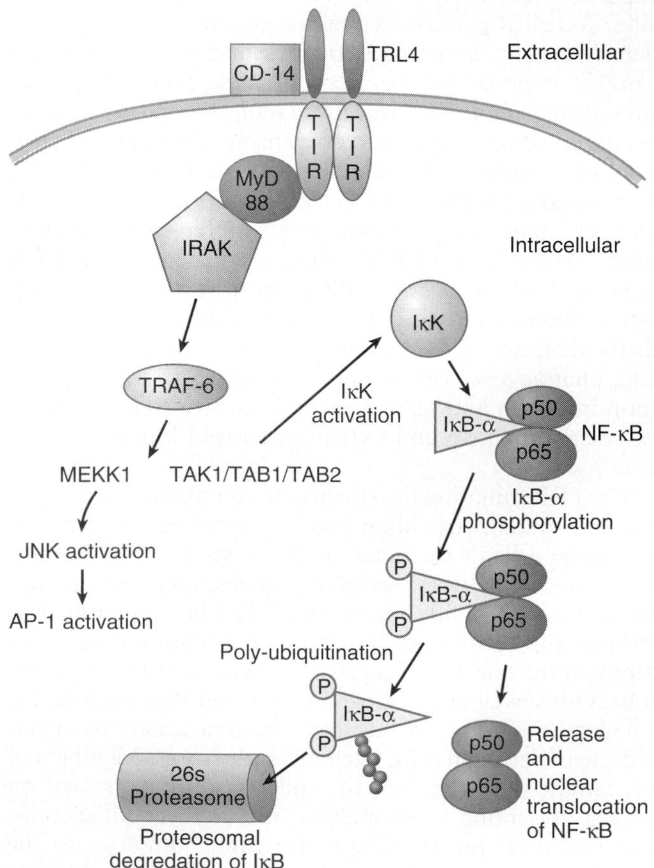

FIGURE 96–2 • Lipopolysaccharide–receptor complex.

kinase (MAPK) or IκK/NF-κB pathways of transcriptional activation (Figure 96–2). Although initially thought to play a role in LPS signaling, later studies support the concept that TLR-2 initiates signaling after binding to products of gram-positive bacteria, notably lipoteichoic acid.[42] More recently, TLR-9 has been shown to be a signaling receptor for bacterial CpG DNA.[43,44] Ongoing basic science research efforts are focusing on these and additional mammalian TLRs and their activation by pathogen ligands in the hopes of identifying potential therapeutic targets.

Inflammatory Cell Signaling

After engagement of cell surface receptors, several kinases are activated, resulting in the eventual activation of transcriptional factors. Among the many activated signaling pathways, the NF-κB and the MAPK pathways appear to play prominent roles in propagating the sepsis response.

Nuclear Factor-κB Signaling

NF-κB is a family of transcriptionally activating proteins that regulate the expression of a number of inflammatory gene products. For a complete review, the reader is referred to excellent summaries of this transcriptional factor.[45–47] Activation of the TLR-4 receptor causes phosphorylation and activation of the inhibitor of κB kinases (IKK), which causes phosphorylation of the intracellular inhibitor of NF-κB (IκB) (Figure 96–2). Once phosphorylated, IκB becomes poly-ubiquinated and subsequently degraded via the 26S proteasome pathway. This release unmasks the nuclear translocation sequences of the canonical NF-κB complex, the p50/p65 heterodimer, allowing it to move into the nucleus, where it binds to NF κB elements on the promoter regions of multiple genes critical to the inflammatory response, including cytokines (e.g., TNF), chemokines (e.g., IL-8), adhesion molecules (e.g., E-selectin), and others (e.g., inducible form of nitric oxide synthase [iNOS] and granulocyte-macrophage colony-stimulating factor).[45] A growing body of clinical data supports the concept that NF-κB is activated in the cells of patients succumbing to sepsis and acute lung injury, a common sequela. Bohrer et al.[48] distinguished survivors from nonsurvivors on the basis of NF-κB binding activity in peripheral blood mononuclear cells and showed it was as predictive as Acute Physiology and Chronic Health Evaluation (APACHE)-II scores. Similarly, Schwartz et al.[49] found increased activation of NF-κB in alveolar macrophages obtained by bronchoalveolar lavage in patients with ARDS compared with controls. Thus molecular signaling through NF-κB likely plays a critical role in propagating the sepsis response as a critical transcriptional activator of numerous inflammatory gene products.

AP-1 Signaling

The AP-1 family of transcription activating proteins consists of various homodimers and heterodimers of the Jun, Fos, or activating transcription factor protein.[45,50,51] Several combinations of these proteins are described; however, the heterodimer complex composed of c-fos and c-jun might be described as the canonical AP-1 complex that is also capable of directing transcription of a number of "early" activation genes similar to NF-κB. Activation of the AP-1 transcriptional complex family results from signaling that proceeds through a series of MAPKs. In humans, three MAPK pathways are identified: p38 protein kinase,[52] extracellular-regulated protein kinase (ERK),[52] and c-Jun NH_2-terminal kinase (JNK)[54,55] (Figure 96–3). Each of these signaling pathways is implicated by experimental evidence as playing a role in inflammatory disease states. For example, TNF production by both neutrophils and macrophages is dependent on p38 activation. In experimental endotoxemia in human volunteers, a p38 MAPK inhibitor decreases monocyte expression of inflammatory cytokines and lessens the clinical signs attributed to endotoxin.[56,57] As a result, the p38 MAPK pathway remains a therapeutic target in sepsis. Similarly, LPS stimulation of monocytes activates JNK with downstream activation of AP-1 and subsequent IL-1β production; however, its role in sepsis is not fully defined. Finally, LPS induction of TNF is dependent on activation of the ERK pathway,[58,59] although its role in acute inflammatory states is less understood. Together, the two major transcriptional activating family of proteins NF-κB and AP-1 are crucial to the propagation of signals from the cell surface to eventual expression of key inflammatory gene products, such as cytokines, chemokines, and adhesion molecules reviewed later. As such, these pathways mark potential sites for future therapeutic intervention in sepsis.

Role of Cytokines as Principal Mediators of the Sepsis Response

Much of the work reviewed has resulted in a better understanding of the mediators of sepsis that cause the cellular and organ dysfunction associated with it. Although numerous proteins play a role in sepsis, this section highlights principal mediators in this cascade. Among the most important of these mediators are cytokines that are intracellular and extracellular small-molecular-weight peptides that mediate an extraordinary number of cellular functions.

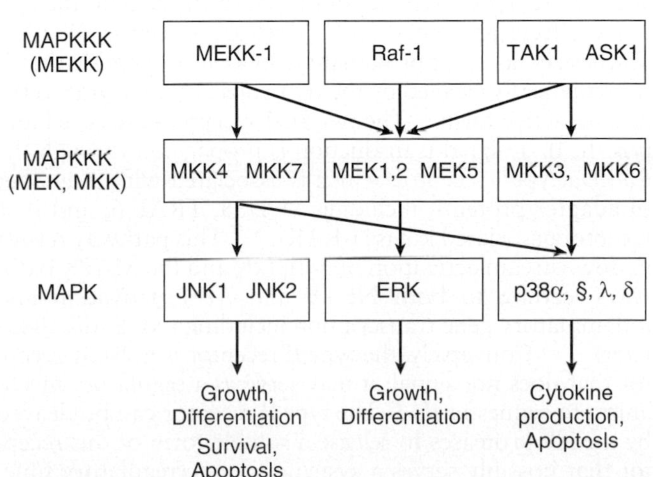

FIGURE 96–3 • Three mitogen-activated protein kinase (MAPK) pathways.

Tumor Necrosis Factor-α

Perhaps the most well-studied cytokine that is causally linked to sepsis is TNF-α. Evidence for TNF mediation of sepsis includes the observation that TNF is produced by hematopoietic cells, its expression is temporally related to the development of shock, it can induce experimental septic shock in animals, and passive immunization against TNF blunts the endotoxin-induced sepsis response.[60–62] TNF functions as a trimeric protein that binds to either the p55 or p75 TNF receptor through which it mediates a signaling cascade that ultimately is responsible for a number of inflammatory effects. These effects include leukocyte–endothelial cell adhesion (via increased adhesion molecule and chemokine expression), transformation to a procoagulant vascular phenotype (via up-regulation of tissue factor and inhibition of protein C), induction of iNOS, and action as a principal "early" cytokine in the subsequent cascade of mediators promulgating the septic response.[63] A number of clinical studies support the seminal preclinical work that identified these multiple effects of TNF.[64] Investigators correlated serum levels of TNF to mortality,[65] development of shock and purpura fulminans,[66] and the incidence of sepsis-induced ARDS and shock.[67] Furthermore, in a well-defined model of endotoxemia in human volunteers, TNF was identified as a proximal cytokine with kinetics of expression approximating the onset of tachycardia, tachypnea, and fever[68] and could substitute for the endotoxin effect in this model.[69] Thus clinical investigators enthusiastically proceeded with therapeutic trials aimed at blocking TNF via a variety of strategies. Results of these studies have been disappointing and likely relate to a number of factors.[70] However, these results indicate that additional cytokines possess independent, redundant, or even synergistic effects with TNF.

Interleukin-1β

In addition to TNF, IL-1 is one of the cytokines identified as contributing to sepsis. IL-1 now is described as a family of proteins consisting of two agonists (IL-1α and IL-1β) and one antagonist, the IL-1 receptor antagonist (IL-1Ra) protein.[71,72] IL-1α is predominantly membrane bound, whereas IL-1β is secreted and believed to mediate the systemic effects attributed to IL-1 release in sepsis. IL-1β is synthesized as an approximately 30-kDa propeptide that is proteolytically cleaved by the IL-1 converting enzyme to the mature active form.[73] The two IL-1 receptors are type I and type II. IL-1 signal transduction is propagated through the 80-kDa type I receptor, which is associated with a number of adapter proteins, including MyD88, TRAF-6, and IL-1 receptor associated kinase (IRAK).[74,75] This pathway results in downstream activation of both IκK and the MAPK pathways leading to both NF-κB and AP-1 activation and inflammatory gene transcription including iNOS (discussed later).[76–78] Conversely, the type II receptor is a decoy receptor that does not signal; it may serve as a regulatory mechanism to sequester IL-1. The type II receptor can be cleaved by metalloproteases to release a soluble form of this receptor that possibly serves a systemic counterregulatory function. IL-1Ra is a circulating inhibitor of IL-1 activity in that it can bind to the type I receptor without initiating a signaling cascade.[79] Because expression of IL-1Ra follows peak expression of IL-1, IL-1Ra is hypothesized to modulate IL-1 activity by competitively blocking the IL-1 receptor. Although preclinical data supported this hypothesis, IL-1Ra in clinical sepsis trials failed to improve mortality.[80–82]

Despite the failure of IL-1Ra trials, similar data support the role of IL-1 in sepsis, as reviewed for TNF. For example, in animal models, IL-1β can elicit fever, hypotension, and leukocytic infiltration to the lungs.[83] Similar to TNF, IL-1 stimulates mononuclear cell activation and phagocytosis,[84] increases endothelial cell adhesion molecule expression,[85] and activates a procoagulant state via tissue factor activation and inhibiting thrombomodulin secretion.[86] In the human endotoxemia model, IL-1β peaks at 4 hours in association with clinical signs.[87] Finally, when detected in the circulation of septic patients, IL-1 levels correlate with mortality.[88] Thus the failure of clinical trials aimed at neutralizing the effect of IL-1 more likely reflects inadequate testing of the concept that IL-1 is a key sepsis mediator rather than a confirmatory exclusion of this possibility.

Of note, a number of preclinical and clinical studies support the concept of synergy among redundant inflammatory cytokines. For example, concomitant administration of TNF and IL-1 at doses that singularly produced no physiologic changes synergistically mediated severe lung injury and hypotension.[83] Furthermore, in a cecal ligation and puncture model of sepsis in mice, concurrent and prolonged (3-day) administration of the type I soluble TNF receptor and IL-1Ra significantly improved mortality.[89] Thus future clinical studies designed to block proximal cytokine-mediated effects must consider the presence of multiple, synergistic cytokines.

Interleukin-6

As proximal mediators in the sepsis cytokine cascade, TNF and IL-1 are responsible for the subsequent induction of a host of other mediators. Among them, IL-6 has been consistently found to be elevated during the course of sepsis[90,91] and is the cytokine for which levels at admission are most closely correlated to death.[92] IL-6 is a pleiotropic cytokine possessing a number of functions, including driving the acute-phase response in hepatocytes, differentiating myeloid cells, stimulating immunoglobulin production, and activating T-cell proliferation.[93,94] On the basis of subsequent structural analysis and signaling studies, IL-6 was identified as a member of a family of proteins that served as gp130 receptor ligands.[93] Further studies aimed at defining the role of IL-6 in sepsis failed to provide convincing evidence that IL-6 mediates any of the inflammatory pathophysiology associated with sepsis. Rather, IL-6 has been recognized as a potential useful marker in stratifying patients with sepsis[95] or as a component of a broader scoring model incorporating demographics, physiologic variables, and serum cytokine levels.[96]

Interleukin-8

IL-8 is a member of a diverse family of chemoattractant cytokines, termed *chemokines,* that are separated into four classes on the basis of the positioning of conserved cysteine motifs in their amino acid structure.[97,98] IL-8 falls into the CXC (X denoting a nonconserved amino acid) family of chemokines that are principally neutrophil chemoattractants and activators. Both TNF and IL-1 can induce IL-8 production from a variety of cells, including endothelial cells, macrophages, neutrophils, and epithelial cells. Although the role of IL-8 in mediating systemic inflammation is incompletely defined, it appears to play a critical role in the recruitment of neutrophils to the lungs in patients with sepsis-induced acute lung injury.[99] Bronchoalveolar lavage fluid levels of IL-8 have been suggested to be an important predictor of the development and outcome in ARDS.[100–103] However, additional chemokines (e.g., monocyte chemoattractant protein [MCP]-1) that recruit other leukocyte cell populations likely are important mediators of this important sequela of sepsis.[104]

Adhesion Molecules

An important breakthrough in the molecular understanding of sepsis-induced organ dysfunction came with the identification of the process responsible for the characteristic infiltration of leukocytes into the organs of patients with sepsis. This so-called "leukocyte–endothelial cell adhesion cascade" (Figure 96–4) was the experimental target of numerous groups during the 1990s and resulted in an improved understanding of the role of the endothelium and adhesion molecules in sepsis.[105,106] This cascade is characterized by early cytokine-mediated activation of the selectin family of endothelial cell adhesion molecules that can mediate a process of neutrophil "rolling" whereby sialyated moieties constitutively present on neutrophils interact with selectins (e.g., E-selectin). In the second phase, activation of the "rolling" neutrophil causes increased expression and activation of the integrin family of adhesion molecules that interact with the similarly up-regulated intercellular adhesion molecule (ICAM)-1 on the endothelial cell surface. This ligand interaction facilitates firm adhesion of the neutrophil to the endothelium. Subsequently, in response to a variety of chemotactic molecules, neutrophils migrate through the endothelium to the site of inflammation responsible for release of chemotactic molecules. Release of a variety of radical species, both oxygen and nitrogen based, and proteases by the neutrophils are believed to contribute to subsequent endothelial and organ dysfunction.

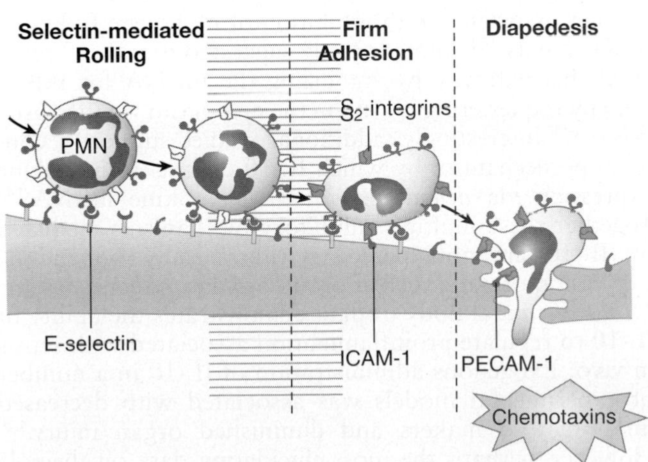

FIGURE 96–4 • Leukocyte-endothelial cell adhesion cascade.

Nitric Oxide

Nitric oxide (NO) received tremendous attention in the 1980s and was named the "Molecule of the Year" by *Science* in 1992. Seminal work in the field showed NO is responsible for endothelial-derived relaxation of blood vessels[107] and thus crucial to regulating vascular tone.[108,109] During an explosion of research in the field, three isoforms of NO synthase were determined to be responsible for production of NO from oxidative deamination of L-arginine to L-citrulline. The three isoforms are *type I,* a neuronal isoform (nNOS); *type II,* an inducible isoform (iNOS), and *type III,* a constitutive, endothelial isoform (eNOS).[111] A mitochondrial NOS isoform is proposed (see Chapter 99). Relevant to sepsis research, the cytokines TNF and IL-1β were determined to be important inducers of iNOS[111] and resulted in significant elevations of this isoform in vivo, with correlative elevations in the amount of NO produced in experimental animal models.[112,113] Given the finding of increased levels of circulating, stable byproducts of NO (nitrite/nitrate) in both septic adults[114–116] and children[117] who simultaneously displayed decreased systemic vascular tone, NO was hypothesized to play a principal role in the pathophysiology of septic shock. In addition, substantial release of circulating NO was believed to mediate direct myocardial depressant effects.[118] Later research suggests that the proinflammatory cytokines TNF and IL-1β are the so-called "myocardial depressant factors" and that they mediate this effect through induction of iNOS.[119] Whether NO is the exclusive mediator of these effects or contributes to this pathophysiology in combination with other oxygen- and nitrogen-based radicals is questioned.[120] However, in light of the evidence supporting the role of NO in septic shock and encouraged by the resistance to endotoxin-induced shock displayed by the iNOS knockout mouse,[121] investigators proceeded with clinical trials using NO synthesis inhibitors in septic shock. Several early clinical reports and small studies reported that NOS inhibitors were associated with significant increases in both systemic and pulmonary vascular resistances and improved blood pressures, although often at the expense of decreased cardiac output secondary to increased afterload.[110,111] Consequently, results from larger, randomized trials failed to show any benefit of NOS inhibition. A later trial was abandoned because of increased mortality observed in the treatment group, despite improvements in hemodynamics.[121] Thus the potential benefit of NOS inhibition in sepsis has not been realized and may await the development of more selective NOS inhibitors.

Although substantial data suggest that the direct myocardial and vascular effects of NO are its principal contribution to sepsis pathophysiology, NO may contribute to the septic state via other mechanisms. NO can rapidly combine with the superoxide anion to form the highly reactive species peroxynitrite, which can have several toxic effects.[123] The peroxynitrite anion directly reacts with sulfhydryl groups to form disulfides, which can result in inactivation of an affected protein.[124] Peroxynitrite can also nitrate tyrosine residues to alter protein function, as in the case of surfactant protein A.[125] Finally, peroxynitrite impairs mitochondrial respiration and activates the poly-ADP ribose synthase enzyme, which decreases nicotinamide adenine dinucleotide (NAD) levels and impairs adenosine triphosphate (ATP) synthesis.[126] Additionally, NO may suppress vasopressin release by the central nervous system and could provide an additional explanation for the shock state often associated with sepsis.[127] Despite these harmful effects, NO provides several beneficial effects as a signaling molecule, an antibacterial agent, an antitumor agent, an inhibitor of platelet aggregation, and a regulator of tonic vascular tone. Thus it is imperative to identify strategies that inhibit the pathologic effects of excessive NO production, without interfering with its basal, constitutive functions that appear critical to maintaining physiologic homeostasis.

Putative Role of "Late" Mediators in the Pathogenesis of Sepsis

Despite the experimental and clinical evidence supporting the role of these "early" cytokines in the pathogenesis of sepsis, therapies directed against these mediators have been mostly ineffectual in large adult trials. This finding has led some investigators to examine the possibility that additional molecules with delayed kinetics of expression influence the outcome in sepsis. Mice treated with LPS often die long after peak expressions of TNF and IL-1β, supporting the concept that late-acting, therapeutically accessible proteins mediate delayed endotoxin-induced death.[128] In testing this hypothesis, Tracey and colleagues[128] observed the presence of a member of the high mobility group (HMG)-1 family in conditioned media 16 hours after LPS stimulation of murine macrophage-like cells. Discovered nearly 30 years earlier as a nonhistone, chromosomal protein with multiple cellular functions, including determining nuclear structure and stability, this protein, renamed *HMGB1,* was shown to be a ligand for the receptor for advanced glycation endproducts (RAGE).[129,130] This receptor is expressed on monocytes and vascular smooth muscle, and ligation by HMGB1 activates both the NF-κB and MAPK pathways.[128] Importantly, significant elevations of HMGB1 were found in mice subjected to endotoxic shock and in critically ill patients having surgical sepsis or sepsis-induced organ dysfunction, with increased levels correlating to nonsurvival.[131] The biologic role of HMGB1 was confirmed by delayed passive immunization of mice with anti-HMGB1, which ameliorated the inflammation and mortality associated with endotoxemia,[131] cecal ligation and puncture,[128] and LPS-triggered acute lung injury.[132] It is hoped that identification of HMGB1 and similar "late" mediators will widen the therapeutic window available for successful immune-modulating therapy in sepsis.

Role of Host Mediators in the Resolution of Sepsis

Although the multiple mechanisms at play in the initiation and propagation of the sepsis response have become increasingly clear, the mechanism(s) responsible for its resolution is less well understood. One hypothesis suggests that resolution of sepsis results from an eventual down-regulation, or turnoff, of initiating mediators such as TNF and IL-6. Data suggest that the failure of these mediators to decrease over the course of sepsis provides a major risk factor for mortality from sepsis.[92,133] However, as alluded to earlier, multiple attempts at neutralizing these early mediators have met with clinical failure at the bedside.[134] Thus an alternative hypothesis is that a separate signaling or counterregulatory pathway is present and responsible for resolution of the septic response. Activation of monocytes with endotoxin results not only in production of proinflammatory cytokines but also in expression of a number of naturally occurring cytokine antagonists, including soluble TNF receptors, IL-1Ra, and a host of potent antiinflammatory, regulatory cytokines.[135] Notable among these regulatory cytokines are IL-10 and transforming growth factor-β.

Interleukin-10

IL-10 is perhaps the best studied of the antiinflammatory cytokines. It is an 18-kDa protein initially identified from T_H2 helper T cells on the basis of its ability to inhibit interferon-γ production from T_H1 T cells.[136] Upon successful recombinant expression, IL-10 was demonstrated to be a potent inhibitor of cytokine production from activated monocytes.[137] Since this observation, a number of antiinflammatory properties have been attributed to IL-10.[138,139] The mechanism by which IL-10 modulates proinflammation is multifactorial. In vitro, IL-10 inhibits expression of cytokines known to contribute to sepsis, such as TNF and IL-1, and important chemokines, including IL-8. IL-10 can down-regulate expression of a variety of cell surface receptors important to host defense, such as MHC class II molecules, CD-14, and the costimulatory molecule B7, thereby "deactivating" the monocyte and blunting its ability to respond to antigenic challenges.[140] Conversely, IL-10 up-regulates additional antiinflammatory molecules such as IL-1Ra[141] and soluble TNF receptors.[142] Because of the inhibitory effects of IL-10 on cytokine expression, its effect on signal transduction pathways regulating gene expression has been examined. Multiple investigations have shown that pretreatment with IL-10 abrogates NF-κB activation via a variety of mechanisms. Phosphorylation and subsequent degradation of the inhibitory protein IκB-α was impaired by IL-10 in a manner associated with inhibition of monocyte Iκ kinase (IκK) activity.[143] Another study suggested that IL-10 regulated this pathway by stabilizing the mRNA for IκB-α, thereby sequestering NF-κB in the cytoplasm via increased IκB-α.[144] Interestingly, additional studies support a contrasting mechanism by which IL-10 decreases chemokine expression via *de*stabilization of chemokine mRNA.[145] Together these multiple inhibitory mechanisms mediated by IL-10 are anticipated to substantially impair the expression of a number of proinflammatory genes.

A substantial body of data demonstrates the ability of IL-10 to regulate proinflammation associated with sepsis in vivo. Exogenous administration of IL-10 in a number of experimental models was associated with decreased inflammatory makers and diminished organ injury.[139] However, perhaps the most elucidating data on the role of IL-10 in modulating inflammation was derived from experiments using the IL-10 null mutant mouse (IL-$10^{-/-}$). Importantly, immunologic characterization of IL-$10^{-/-}$ mice revealed that otherwise sublethal doses of endotoxin resulted in 100% mortality and were associated with substantially increased levels of proinflammatory cytokines.[146] Thus IL-10 is believed to be a key endogenous antiinflammatory molecule serving to regulate production of proinflammatory mediators. Corroborative data in humans was shown by Donnelly et al.,[147] who reported that patients with higher mortality rates from ARDS had lower levels of IL-10 in their bronchoalveolar lavage fluid.[147] Furthermore, the inability to increase IL-10 in response to meningococcal infection was associated with increased mortality.[148] In summary, IL-10 possesses a number of antiinflammatory properties: inhibition of cytokine synthesis, inhibition of adhesion of leukocytes to activated endothelial cells, inhibition of key signal transduction pathways associated with activation of the proinflammatory response, and up-regulation of naturally occurring cytokine antagonists. In light of the multiple mechanisms by which IL-10 regulates inflammation, exogenous administration of IL-10 appears promising and is being studied in clinical trials. Enthusiasm for this therapeutic approach is tempered by the evidence that IL-10 limits the host immune response directed at pathogen eradication in several in vivo models of infection and in human studies.[138] Thus titrating IL-10 to strike a balance between protection against dysregulated proinflammation and pathogen clearance remains a substantial clinical challenge.

Role of the Coagulation Cascade in Sepsis

Clinical investigations have continued to link the inflammatory cascade with the coagulation cascade.[149] The coagulation cascade is activated in sepsis, as reflected by consumption of clotting factors, increases in activation markers, alterations in fibrinolysis, and reduced anticoagulant activity.[149–151] This activation of the coagulation cascade in association with the endothelial cell dysfunction results in the hemostatic changes characterized by a procoagulant endothelium.

Principal among the hematologic observations in sepsis is the development of disseminated intravascular coagulation (DIC), which is broadly defined as an acquired syndrome of activation of coagulation and intravascular fibrin formation resulting in vascular thrombosis.[152] Additionally, consumption of coagulation factors and secondary fibrinolysis can lead to bleeding episodes (see Chapter 74). Although proinflammatory cytokines appear capable of activating the coagulation cascade, monocyte tissue factor (TF) activation also appears to play a prominent role in the pathophysiology of DIC.[153] In addition to the enhanced production of fibrin is coexisting dysregulation of the anticoagulant pathway characterized by decreased fibrinolysis from increased plasminogen activator inhibitor type 1 (PAI-1) and dysfunction/depletion of antithrombin (AT)-III, protein C, protein S, and tissue factor pathway inhibitor (TFPI).

The role of TF in sepsis has been elucidated in both animal and human studies.[154] Normally TF is unexposed to circulating leukocytes. However, when the endothelium is disrupted as in sepsis, TF becomes activated and initiates fibrin formation. In addition to endotoxin, both activated complement and cytokines (e.g., IL-1) can induce TF expression on monocytes and endothelial cells, further activating the extrinsic pathway of the coagulation cascade.[155–157] Importantly, inhibition of TF activity with TFPI has resulted in reduced mortality in preclinical trials of sepsis. Thus TFPI, which is a glycoprotein that forms a quaternary complex with TF, factor VIIa, and factor Xa and blocks the generation of thrombin from prothrombin, is a potential therapeutic option in patients with sepsis.[158–161]

During the course of sepsis, depletion and/or dysfunction of the natural anticoagulants AT-III, protein C, and protein S contribute to impaired fibrinolysis and excessive fibrin generation. AT-III inhibits thrombin by forming thrombin–antithrombin (TAT) complexes. The activity of AT-III is augmented by heparan sulfates produced endogenously by endothelial cells, but this production is inhibited by endotoxin.[162] Multiple etiologies for decreased AT-III in sepsis are reported, including consumption from ongoing thrombin generation, degradation by elastases from activated neutrophils,[163] dilution secondary to volume resuscitation, and impaired hepatic synthesis.[164] Despite the documentation of low AT-III levels in patients with sepsis and its correlation to poor outcome and death,[165] replacement trials of AT-III have failed to consistently demonstrate a benefit as measured by improved mortality.[164]

In addition to AT-III, depletion of protein C is consistently reported in patients with sepsis and septic shock and plays a key role in the pathogenesis of sepsis.[166,167] Regulation of activation of protein C in the coagulation cascade is mediated in a complex manner. Activation of the clotting cascade results in conversion of prothrombin to thrombin, which is bound at high affinity by thrombomodulin that is highly expressed on the endothelial cells of the microcirculation. Binding of thrombomodulin to thrombin blocks its ability to activate platelets and the endothelium and substantially increases activation of protein C.[168] The protein C receptor on endothelium binds APC, concentrating it near TAT complexes and facilitating its activation.[169] APC then dissociates from its receptor and binds to the necessary cofactor protein S, subsequently inactivating factor Va or VIIIa and thus playing a key role in regulating coagulation.

A more recent observation is that APC possesses antiinflammatory activity. For example, in both baboon and rodent models of endotoxemia, APC decreased cytokine production and attenuated neutrophil activation.[170,171] Multiple molecular mechanisms have been identified to explain these antiinflammatory effects, which appear independent of APC's anticoagulant effect. First, APC binds to a specific site on mononuclear cells, decreasing an endotoxin-mediated calcium influx and impairing TNF production.[172] APC also inhibits nuclear translocation of NF-κB and impairs cytokine secretion.[171] APC can inhibit TF expression from monocytes in a manner dependent on binding to the protein C receptor.[173] In light of these encouraging preclinical findings, clinical trials examining the effect of APC on mortality from sepsis were initiated. The trend toward successful reduction of morbidity and 28-day mortality that was observed in early, small clinical trials prompted a larger phase III trial. Results from the recombinant human activated Protein C Worldwide

Evaluation in Severe Sepsis (PROWESS) trial were reported by Bernard et al.[174] Use of APC demonstrated for the first time a statistically significant reduction in 28-day mortality in sepsis in adults. Although encouraging for the pediatric population, the observation that older, sicker patients appeared to derive the most benefit from APC and the noted risk of hemorrhage have tempered unabashed enthusiasm for use of APC in pediatric sepsis (Table 96–1). A phase III trial of activated protein C in severe pediatric sepsis will provide definitive data.

Genetic Regulation of the Sepsis Response

One common experience among pediatric intensivists is the observation that patients with seemingly similar pathologic insults display strikingly different pathophysiology and outcomes. A hypothesis explaining this variability is that genetic differences among hosts are responsible for altered gene expression to similar insults (see Chapter 92). Several lines of investigation support the evolution of this concept. As referenced previously, varying sensitivities to endotoxin among different strains of mice were mediated by a mutation in the coding sequence for TLR-4.[175–177] Subsequently, similar findings of an attenuated response to endotoxin were reported in patients with mutations in the TLR-4 gene.[178] A novel polymorphism in TLR-2, the cell surface receptor for gram-positive bacterial cell wall components, has been suggested to predispose patients to severe gram-positive bacterial infections.[179] More recently, a polymorphism within the CD14 promoter gene (C→T transition at base pair −159) was identified.[180] Both the CT and TT genotypes were significantly overrepresented among septic shock patients compared with healthy controls having the TT phenotype displaying a significantly higher mortality rate (71% vs. 48% for other genotypes) and independently associated with an increased relative risk of death.[180] Together these studies suggest that genetic alteration in the receptors that signal activation of innate immune responses significantly alters the host response.

TABLE 96–1

Common Pathogens in Pediatric Sepsis

Patient Group	Likely Infectious Agent
Neonates	Group B β-hemolytic *Streptococcus*
	Enterobacter species
	Listeria monocytogenes
	Staphylococcus aureus
	Neisseria meningitidis
Children	*Streptococcus pneumoniae*
	Neisseria meningitidis
	Staphylococcus aureus
	Enterobacter species
	Haemophilus influenzae (prior to immunization)
Children, immunocompromised	*Enterobacter* species
	Staphylococcus aureus
	Pseudomonas species
	Candida albicans

As suggested previously, the degree of the patient's inflammatory response appears to influence outcome. For example, an association between TNF and fatal outcome was found in the setting of meningococcemia.[65] Importantly, differences in expression of these mediators are thought to reflect polymorphisms in the genes encoding them. In the example of TNF, a single base pair mutation in the promoter region that results in the so-called TNF2 allele was associated with increased TNF production and was found more commonly in patients with septic shock and in those who died.[181] Additional polymorphisms in the TNF locus have been identified and correlate with TNF levels and outcome.[182] In these studies, the TNFB2 allele in the homozygous form was associated with increased expression of TNF and a higher mortality in sepsis compared with patients homozygous for the TNF B1 allele or heterozygous for the alleles.[182] An association has been found between the TNFB2 allele and increased mortality in children with bacteremia.[183] Other genetic alterations in the complement pathway place the host at risk for severe and recurrent meningococcal disease.[184,185] Furthermore, a polymorphism in the IL-1 family, so-called IL-1ra RN2, was significantly increased in septic patients and associated with nonsurvival,[186] whereas patients with additional alleles in the IL-1 family showed lower mortality rates in a separate study.[187]

Thus it has become increasingly clear that genetic influences on the expression of multiple sepsis mediators may influence outcome, as dysregulation of the regulatory relationship between antiinflammatory IL-10 and proinflammatory TNF may also contribute to sepsis pathophysiology. As an example, families with the phenotype characterized by both increased TNF expression and decreased IL-10 production carried an increased risk for death secondary to sepsis.[148] In a similar manner, decreased expression of IL-10 in bronchoalveolar lavage fluids of patients with ARDS portended a worse prognosis.[147] The difference in the level of IL-10 expression may be a result of polymorphisms in the promoter region of its gene.[188,189] Although the vast majority of these data are derived from adult studies, pediatric studies supporting the hypothesis of genetic control of outcome in critical illness remain limited to the disease entities of meningococcemia and cerebral malaria. It is anticipated that the successful establishment of a multi-institutional project examining the genomic expression of more than 30,000 human genes in children with sepsis and septic shock using microarray technology will shed greater light on the degree to which genetic influences regulate the sepsis response and affect therapeutic responses and outcome. However, at present therapeutic options remain mostly limited to supportive care directed at maintaining oxygen delivery and eradication of infections as reviewed later.

Treatment Strategies

Overview

As the cellular response to sepsis becomes better understood, the approach to treatment of sepsis becomes broader. Sepsis no longer is viewed as merely an insult by an overwhelming pathogen wherein the sepsis is resolved if the pathogen is killed. Rather, it is seen as a dysregulation of immunologic pathways directed toward pathogen eradication and restoration of homeostasis. From a clinical standpoint, treatment of sepsis entails four important goals: initial resuscitation, elimination of pathogen, maintenance of oxygen delivery, and carefully directed regulation of the inflammatory response.

Initial Resuscitation

As in any disease process, the first step in treatment of sepsis is the initial stabilization of the patient. In this regard, children present many of the same challenges as adult patients, including respiratory and cardiovascular stabilization. The primary goals of therapy in the first hours are to maintain oxygenation and ventilation, achieve normal perfusion and blood pressure, and reestablish appropriate urine output for age.

Children with signs of sepsis may have significantly decreased mental status, raising concern about the ability to protect their airway. Also, in septic shock the work of breathing can represent a significant portion of oxygen consumption (as much as 15%–30%). Because these children also receive large amounts of fluid to restore intervascular volume in the face of capillary leak, they are at increased risk for developing pulmonary edema. Lung compliance decreases, and work of breathing can increase substantially. Together, these respiratory abnormalities often necessitate tracheal intubation and mechanical ventilatory support. Arterial blood gas analysis often reveals hypoxemia and metabolic acidosis. However, the decision to provide mechanical ventilatory support should not wait on laboratory findings; rather, it should be based on clinical findings of increased work of breathing, hypoventilation, impaired mental status, or obtundation. Mechanical ventilatory support provides the added benefit of reducing work of breathing, therefore decreasing the overall oxygen consumption, especially when combined with sedation and paralysis. If early tracheal intubation is chosen, sedative agents for induction should be selected to maintain hemodynamic stability (e.g., etomidate or ketamine) (see Chapter 119).

For a variety of reasons, patients with sepsis almost universally have decreased effective intravascular volume. Many had poor oral intake of fluid for a period of time prior to developing sepsis. With the development of increased vascular permeability, intravascular volume has been lost because of third spacing. Finally, the vasodilation related to excessive NO production (see earlier) results in abnormally increased vascular capacitance decreasing the effective volume. When sepsis is suspected, vascular access should be obtained and 20 ml/kg isotonic fluid administered as quickly as possible. While following clinical examination for signs of overly aggressive volume resuscitation (new onset of rales, increased work of breathing, development of a gallop, or hepatomegaly), fluid should be administered quickly with the goal of improving blood pressure and tissue perfusion. Data from pediatric patients suggest that administering more than 60 ml/kg isotonic fluid in the first hour of resuscitation is associated with improved survival.[190] The American College of Critical Care Medicine (ACCM) Clinical Practice Parameters for Hemodynamic Support of Pediatric and Neonatal Septic Shock reports that volumes up to 200 ml/kg may be required during the first hour.[12] Despite very large volumes of fluid in the initial resuscitation, the incidences of ARDS and/or cerebral edema remain low in children.[190–192] The importance of vigorous, goal-directed therapy (central venous pressure [CVP] 8–12, SvO_2 ≥70%, MAP >65, urine output >0.5 ml/kg/hour) in significantly reducing sepsis mortality in adults is convincingly demonstrated.[122,193]

Once fluid resuscitation starts, initiation of inotropes and vasopressors often is necessary. In children, vasoactive medicines should be considered second-line agents to fluid. The most common initial agent selected for vasoactive support is dopamine, which provides both inotropic support at lower concentrations and vasomotor tone at higher concentrations. Often it is necessary to escalate the dopamine dosage to high levels (up to 20 µg/kg/min) or to add agents to maintain adequate tissue perfusion. The decision of which second agent to start often is based on the following determinations: whether the cardiovascular compromise is related to inadequate cardiac output from direct cardiodepressant effects, which requires increased inotropy; decreased vascular tone, which requires vasopressors (e.g., α agonist); or increased afterload from vasoconstriction, which requires peripheral vasodilators (see Chapter 23). In this regard, the clinician often can be assisted by garnering additional data on the basis of invasive monitoring.

Invasive Monitoring

The final step in the initial resuscitation of a child with sepsis is placement of appropriate and necessary access and monitors. However, attention to the clinical examination as part of the ongoing assessment is imperative. In sepsis, the primary endpoints to assess are changes in level of consciousness, decreased urine output, and poor peripheral perfusion characterized by delayed capillary refill and diminished distal pulses. Unfortunately, children with sepsis are difficult to examine because they often are tracheally intubated and sedated and may not have produced any initial urine because of severe hypovolemia. Also, they frequently are receiving vasopressors, which can make examination of the skin for assessment of perfusion less reliable. For these reasons, invasive monitoring often is necessary and helpful.

Central venous access is a necessity for the child in septic shock. The decision to place a central venous catheter in the internal jugular, subclavian, or femoral position is dictated by a number of factors, such as the experience level of the operator and the presence of coagulopathy (see Chapter 15). Central venous catheters provide access for delivery of vasoactive medicines and large volumes of fluid. However, they also can be used to obtain a measurement of CVP and, depending on location, may provide an approximate measurement of the mixed venous oxygen saturation.[193] Although use of CVP for estimating left ventricular end-diastolic volume is controversial, CVP minimally can be used to trend an estimate of the intravascular fluid status. Femoral catheters, in the absence of abdominal pathology, can be used to estimate CVP with good correlation.[194] CVP must be assessed critically because a low CVP can be a reliable indicator of hypovolemia. However, a normal or high CVP does not necessarily exclude the presence of hypovolemia. Factors that can elevate CVP even in the presence of hypovolemia include pulmonary hypertension, right ventricular dysfunction, tricuspid regurgitation, cardiac tamponade, and intracardiac left-to-right shunts. Accurate determination of the true mixed venous saturation in the pulmonary artery requires a pulmonary arterial catheter (PAC), but approximations of the saturation can be provided by a line resting near the right atrium. A superior vena cava oxygen saturation greater than 70% is associated with improved outcome during the first 6 hours of septic shock in adults.[193] Because of significant differences in oxygen extraction between the upper extremities, abdomen, and lower extremities, mixed venous saturations from a femoral line do not accurately correlate with those measured in the pulmonary artery.

In the face of severe sepsis and septic shock, an intraarterial cannula becomes necessary. This line becomes both a source of clinical information on blood pressure, pulse pressure, and hemodynamic variation with respiration and an access for frequent blood draws. Whereas blood pressure alone does not always equate to tissue perfusion because of differences in regional perfusion and vasoconstriction supporting blood pressure, a fluid-resuscitated child with normal or high systolic blood pressure will be more tolerant of manipulations to increase perfusion (i.e., afterload reduction) than children with lower blood pressures. This condition occurs in children who have poor ventricular ejection and high systemic vascular resistance. The arterial blood also provides the best information on arterial oxygen content that can be used to both assess the function of the lungs and to maximize oxygen delivery.

Use of PACs to optimize left ventricular preload, monitor changes in cardiac index, and provide accurate measurements of oxygen delivery and consumption is controversial. Interpretation of PAC data requires the absence of intracardiac shunting, and the presence of normal mitral valve function as either shunting or mitral regurgitation alters cardiac index determination and pulmonary capillary wedge pressure measurements. Because data from adults showed no benefit of PAC use,[195] a consensus statement regarding PAC use stated that the role of PAC was unclear.[196] In light of studies showing that the information obtained from PACs is important in identifying cardiovascular conditions different from those previously suspected in septic patients but which directly impact on patient care,[197] a consensus panel concluded that PAC use is potentially beneficial in improving the management of pediatric patients.[196,198] PAC placement should be considered for pediatric patients who remain in shock after resuscitation and initiation of the usual vasoactive agents and whose fluid status and cardiac function remain unclear.

Elimination of Pathogens

Early identification of the source of a possible offending organism in septic shock dictates the choice of antimicrobial coverage and is important to long-term outcome. In a study of more than 1100 patients, providing appropriate antimicrobial coverage at least 1 day prior to identification of the organism was associated with improved survival.[199] The offending organism also affects prognosis. For example, fungal infections are associated with the lowest survival rate (approximately 17%), followed by bacteria (52% gram-positive bacteria, 57% gram-negative bacteria). The highest survival rate was reported in patients who had no identified pathogen (73%).[200] The specific antibiotic selected plays a role in the quantity of endotoxin released from its action. Antibiotics that inhibit protein production cause less release of endotoxin in gram-negative sepsis.[201]

Because of the importance of appropriate antimicrobial therapy, the decision regarding which agents to empirically start must balance potential side effects against maximizing coverage. In this respect it is important to consider the likely pathogens. Initially, broad antibiotic coverage is initiated. Neonates should be given ampicillin and either gentamicin or a third-generation cephalosporin such as cefotaxime. In infants and children older than 4 to 6 weeks, the decision to begin vancomycin therapy empirically should be considered in light of the increasing antibiotic resistance of *Streptococcus pneumoniae*. Nosocomial infections require additional coverage for the possibility of *Pseudomonas* species and other resistant organisms. Acyclovir should be given if there is a clinical presentation or suspicion of an overwhelming viral (herpetic) infection. Starting antifungal medicines initially in an immunocompetent child usually is not necessary. However, this decision should be reconsidered if the child does not improve over the first 2 days or in case of higher risk for fungal infection (presence of indwelling devices, immunosuppression, or other significant comorbidities). The ability to limit treatment once the organism is known can reduce the number of potential side effects from broad-spectrum antibiotics.

Maintenance of Oxygen Delivery

The current mainstay for treatment of sepsis is supportive, with the ultimate goal of maintaining adequate oxygen delivery in the face of direct insult from bacterial toxins, myocardial depression, capillary leak, acidosis, and massive cytokine release. A number of studies suggest improved outcomes when supranormal levels of oxygen delivery are achieved,[202,203] but whether this process improves outcome in children has not been demonstrated. The ultimate lack of benefit from this approach is suggested by the observation that septic patients may have a perturbed ability to extract oxygen. For these reasons, the best assessment of adequate oxygen delivery and uptake includes measures of perfusion such as lactate level and urine output, along with blood pressure and mixed venous oxygen saturation.

Although most children with sepsis begin in the hypovolemic state, they may remain so even after adequate fluid resuscitation because of ongoing, increased, insensible fluid loss and capillary leak with third spacing. Providing adequate preload to the patient in septic shock may require increased fluid administration for several days. The choice of fluid to be used in resuscitation is controversial. The three choices of fluids are crystalloid, nonblood colloid, and blood. As evident when calculating the arterial content of oxygen, maintaining an adequate hemoglobin level is an important factor in providing adequate oxygen delivery.

Although there is no recommended hemoglobin level for children, the most recent consensus recommendations indicated a hemoglobin concentration of 10 g/dl for adults with cardiopulmonary compromise on the basis of improved emergency outcomes when this goal was achieved.[122,193] Despite possible development of total body fluid overload, administration of diuretics to eliminate extra fluid should be avoided until hemodynamic stability is achieved.

Provision of adequate tissue oxygenation requires maintenance of adequate tissue perfusion. Factors regulating tissue perfusion include cardiac output and peripheral vascular tone. In addition to fluid replacement, many patients require inotropic and/or vasopressor agents to achieve optimal blood pressure and perfusion. Pediatric septic shock patients with decreased vascular tone require initiation of a vasopressor agent in the form of an α-receptor agonist such as epinephrine or norepinephrine. Remember that blood pressure alone as a goal may not correlate with optimal tissue perfusion. For this reason, additional assessments of adequate oxygen delivery to the organs, such as mixed venous oxygen saturation, lactic acid levels, and urine output, can be simultaneously followed.[193] When examining these additional parameters along with determinations of cardiac output and systemic and pulmonary vascular resistances from a PAC, it may be apparent that the optimal blood pressure at which the best oxygen delivery is achieved differs from previous estimations. Examples of this possibility are reported with use of milrinone, which increases inotropy and decreases afterload as mechanisms for increasing cardiac output in pediatric patients with shock related to significant peripheral vasoconstriction.[204] Risks of starting milrinone include hypotension and a longer duration of action than is typical for intravenous vasoactive agents. Finally, a small group of patients may be aided by initiation of pure afterload reduction with NO-donating agents such as sodium nitroprusside. Regardless of the vasoactive regimen chosen, close monitoring of oxygen delivery as assessed by end-organ function, mixed venous oxygen saturation, and falling lactate levels is necessary to tailor ongoing treatment.

Patients with sepsis may have poor nutrition prior to presentation and often are not fed during the first few days of illness. Because of an increased metabolic rate and poor nutrition, septic patients frequently are catabolic and at risk for development of protein calorie malnutrition.[205] Intestinal ischemia in association with loss of the mucosal barrier from malnutrition is associated with translocation of bacteria and endotoxin from the intestine into the bloodstream.[206,207] Use of enteral feeding in critically ill patients has been shown to improve survival and decrease hospital stay.[208] The benefit of enteral feeding should be balanced with the risk of stressing the intestinal function in the face of poor splanchnic perfusion, especially in the presence of vasopressors such as epinephrine and norepinephrine.[209,210] Regardless of the feeding mode, adequate nutrition and nitrogen balance are important for maintaining adequate host immune function and achieving homeostasis. Malnutrition may adversely affect immune function and the ability to generate an appropriate immune response (see Chapter 68).[211] Finally, in the absence of enteral feedings, protection from stress-related gastrointestinal bleeding is advised.

Immune Modulation

Children with sepsis may have a dysregulated, proinflammatory cytokine response. Steroids have long been proposed as a general antiinflammatory medicine to ameliorate the magnitude of this inflammatory response. In many clinical settings, septic patients treated with antibiotics developed worsening of their shock prior to improvement in a time frame consistent with onset of antibiotic activity.[212] The massive release of bacterial toxins resulting from the death of high numbers of bacteria has been proposed to cause an inappropriately exuberant immune response. Animals treated with antiinflammatory drugs (ibuprofen or methylprednisolone) prior to receiving antibiotics were noted to have a less severe response to bacterial lysis.[213,214] Similar studies in children have not been adequately performed. However, prior studies using high-dose steroids early during sepsis in adults showed no improvement in mortality and perhaps a worsening of patient condition.[215,216] Despite the earlier data, subsequent studies have suggested a possible benefit of using lower doses of steroids over a longer period of time. Later studies in adults showed a benefit to this approach, including reduced time to cessation of vasopressor therapy.[217–219] Adrenal insufficiency frequently may be unrecognized in children with septic shock.[220] Low basal cortisol levels, especially in association with an abnormal corticotropin stimulation test, are associated with high mortality rates,[221,222] and such patients may benefit from administration of exogenous steroids. This concept is supported by a study by Annane et al.,[223] who observed that treatment with stress-dose hydrocortisone and fludrocortisone for 7 days in adult patients with septic shock who were classified as "nonresponders" to the corticotropin test significantly reduced the risk of death. Thus any patient who appears refractory to resuscitative measures, has a known history of adrenal insufficiency, has already received exogenous steroids, or has an abnormal corticotropin stimulation test result should be considered for physiologic steroid replacement with hydrocortisone (Annane et al. used 50 mg intravenously [IV] every 6 hours, $\approx$30 mg/m^2 IV every 6 hours for a child).

NO is implicated as a mediator in the myocardial depression, vasodilation, and subsequent hypotension observed in septic shock.[223,224] However, attempts to improve mortality by nonspecific inhibition of NO synthase have been unsuccessful.[122,226,227] As a result, although use of nonspecific NO synthase inhibitors shows some promise, it remains theoretical in pediatric patients.

Because the host response to sepsis may be partly related to endotoxin and circulating inflammatory mediators, removal of these molecules via hemofiltration or exchange transfusion has been hypothesized to improve outcome. A number of studies show that oxygenation and hemodynamics can be improved with use of hemofiltration during sepsis and multiple organ failure.[228–230] While promising, hemofiltration and hemodialysis are associated with significant risks that must be considered before beginning therapy. Problems include difficult vascular access in smaller children, fluid and electrolyte imbalance, hypothermia, anticoagulation requirements because of extracorporeal circuits, and acutely altered hemodynamics when connecting the vascular access to the extracorporeal circuit. In addition, beneficial proteins such as albumin, immunoglobulins, clotting factors, and counterregulatory cytokines may be removed to the detriment of the patient. To date the experience with hemofiltration in children with sepsis shows the process can be performed safely, but whether it will improve outcome is unclear.[231,232]

Part of the inflammatory response involves cytokines that cause widespread activation of the coagulation cascade with suppression of fibrinolysis. This procoagulation DIC has been implicated in the etiology of multiple organ injury leading to MODS. Many septic patients are deficient in AT-III, and abnormal levels of activated protein C are noted.[233,234] Low levels of AT-III and activated protein C are associated with increased mortality.[165,235,236] At least one large meta-analysis supports improved outcome in septic patients who receive AT-III,[237] but a large, randomized, placebo-controlled trial failed to demonstrate any beneficial effect on 28-day mortality.[238] More promising is a report that administration of activated protein C is associated with a significant decrease in 28-day mortality.[174] Although activated protein C is not routinely used and pediatric dosing is not fully established, activated protein C may become more widely used after appropriate clinical testing in pediatric sepsis.

Multiple other potential therapeutic agents have been identified and are being investigated. Many antiinflammatory agents have been attempted, but large, randomized clinical studies have not shown them to be of any benefit.[70] These agents include anti–IL-1, antibradykinin, antiendotoxin, anti–TNF-α, soluble TNF receptor, and antiplatelet-activating factor. It is hoped that better designed studies that carefully stratify patients, consider the presence or absence of an offending pathogen, and possibly identify genetic factors influencing outcome will provide insight into the appropriate immunomodulating agents that will be clinically beneficial to pediatric patients with septic shock.

Concluding Perspectives

Sepsis is and will continue to be an important challenge to the pediatric intensivist. Indeed, sepsis is one of the few disease processes for which the pediatric intensivist can claim "ownership." Although much is known about the biologic and molecular mechanisms involved in sepsis, this knowledge has not directly translated to improved bedside care. At present, most of the therapeutic modalities for sepsis are supportive and founded on the fundamental principles that define the discipline of critical care medicine. Although this approach has directly improved the outcome of sepsis in children, the fact that more than 4000 children per year continue to die in association with severe sepsis warrants further advances. Realization of this goal is feasible but requires further mechanistic insights at the physiologic, molecular, and genetic levels and the design of large-scale, pediatric-specific interventional trials. As "owners" of pediatric septic shock, pediatric intensivists are well positioned to lead this effort on all fronts.

REFERENCES

1. Angus DC, Wax RS: Epidemiology of sepsis: an update. *Crit Care Med* 29:S109-116, 2001.
2. Proulx F, Fayon M, Farrell CA, et al: Epidemiology of sepsis and multiple organ dysfunction syndrome in children. *Chest* 109: 1033-1037, 1996.
3. Watson RS, Linde-Zwirble WT, Carcillo JA, Angus DC: Severe sepsis in children: a U.S. Epidemiologic Survey. *Crit Care Med* 28: A46, 2001.
4. Watson RS, Linde-Zwirble WT, Lidicker J, et al: The increasing burden of severe sepsis in U.S. children. *Crit Care Med* 29:A8, 2002.
5. Bone RC, Sibbald WJ, Sprung CL: The ACCP-SCCM consensus conference on sepsis and organ failure. *Chest* 101:1481-1483, 1992.
6. Marshall JC: SIRS and MODS: what is their relevance to the science and practice of intensive care? *Shock* 14:586-589, 2000.
7. Baue AE: A debate on the subject "Are SIRS and MODS important entities in the clinical evaluation of patients?" The con position. *Shock* 14:590-593, 2000.
8. Dellinger RP, Carlet JM, Maser H, et al: Surviving Sepsis Campaign guidelines for management of severe sepsis and septic shock. *Crit Care Med* 32:858-872, 2004.
9. Dinarello CA: Proinflammatory and anti-inflammatory cytokines as mediators in the pathogenesis of septic shock. *Chest* 112:321S-329S, 1997.
10. Kreger BE, Craven DE, McCabe WR: Gram-negative bacteremia. IV. Re-evaluation of clinical features and treatment in 612 patients. *Am J Med* 68:344-355, 1980.
11. Kreger BE, Craven DE, Carling PC, et al: Gram-negative bacteremia. III. Reassessment of etiology, epidemiology and ecology in 612 patients. *Am J Med* 68:332-343, 1980.
12. Carcillo JA, Fields AI: Clinical practice parameters for hemodynamic support of pediatric and neonatal patients in septic shock. *Crit Care Med* 30:1365-1378, 2002.
13. Bone RC, Fisher CJ Jr, Clemmer TP, et al: Sepsis syndrome: a valid clinical entity. Methylprednisolone Severe Sepsis Study Group. *Crit Care Med* 17:389-393, 1989.
14. Dorinsky PM, Gadek JE: Mechanisms of multiple nonpulmonary organ failure in ARDS, *Chest* 96:885-892, 1989.
15. Janeway CA Jr, Medzhitov R: Introduction: the role of innate immunity in the adaptive immune response. *Semin Immunol* 10:349-350, 1998.
16. Medzhitov R, Janeway C Jr: Innate immune recognition: mechanisms and pathways. *Immunol Rev* 173:89-97, 2000.
17. Medzhitov R, Janeway C Jr: Innate immunity. *N Engl J Med* 343:338-344, 2000.
18. Haurum JS, Thiel S, Jones IM, et al: Complement activation upon binding of mannan-binding protein to HIV envelope glycoproteins. *AIDS* 7:1307-1313, 1993.
19. Kraal G, van der Laan LJ, Elomaa O, et al: The macrophage receptor MARCO. *Microbes Infect* 2:313-316, 2000.
20. Tobias PS, Ulevitch RJ: Lipopolysaccharide binding protein and CD14 in LPS dependent macrophage activation. *Immunobiology* 187:227-232, 1993.
21. Cooper NR, Jensen FC, Welsh RM Jr, et al: Lysis of RNA tumor viruses by human serum: direct antibody-independent triggering of the classical complement pathway. *J Exp Med* 144:970-984, 1976.
22. Beutler B: Signal transduction during innate and adaptive immunity. *Biochem Soc Trans* 29:853-859, 2001.
23. Westphal O, Jann K, Himmelspach K: Chemistry and immunochemistry of bacterial lipopolysaccharides as cell wall antigens and endotoxins. *Prog Allergy* 33:9-39, 1983.
24. Rietschel ET, Schade U, Jensen M, et al: Bacterial endotoxins: chemical structure, biological activity and role in septicaemia. *Scand J Infect Dis Suppl* 31:8-21, 1982.
25. Watson J, Kelly K, Largen M, et al: The genetic mapping of a defective LPS response gene in C3H/HeJ mice. *J Immunol* 120:422-424, 1978.
26. Watson J, Riblet R, Taylor BA: The response of recombinant inbred strains of mice to bacterial lipopolysaccharides. *J Immunol* 118:2088-2093, 1977.
27. Michalek SM, Moore RN, McGhee JR, et al: The primary role of lymphoreticular cells in the mediation of host responses to bacterial endotoxin. *J Infect Dis* 141:55-63, 1980.

28. Mahoney JR Jr, Beutler BA, Le Trang N, et al: Lipopolysaccharide-treated RAW 264.7 cells produce a mediator that inhibits lipoprotein lipase in 3T3-L1 cells. *J Immunol* 134:1673-1675, 1985.
29. Beutler B, Greenwald D, Hulmes JD, et al: Identity of tumour necrosis factor and the macrophage-secreted factor cachectin. *Nature* 316:552-554, 1985.
30. Beutler B, Milsark IW, Cerami AC: Passive immunization against cachectin/tumor necrosis factor protects mice from lethal effect of endotoxin. *Science* 229:869-871, 1985.
31. Wright SD, Ramos RA, Tobias PS, et al: CD14, a receptor for complexes of lipopolysaccharide (LPS) and LPS binding protein. *Science* 249:1431-1433, 1990.
32. Belvin MP, Anderson KV: A conserved signaling pathway: the Drosophila toll-dorsal pathway. *Annu Rev Cell Dev Biol* 12: 393-416, 1996.
33. Anderson KV, Bokla L, Nusslein-Volhard C: Establishment of dorsal-ventral polarity in the Drosophila embryo: the induction of polarity by the Toll gene product. *Cell* 42:791-798, 1985.
34. Lemaitre B, Nicolas E, Michaut L, et al: The dorsoventral regulatory gene cassette spatzle/Toll/cactus controls the potent antifungal response in Drosophila adults. *Cell* 86:973-983, 1996.
35. Brightbill HD, Modlin RL: Toll-like receptors: molecular mechanisms of the mammalian immune response. *Immunology* 101:1-10, 2000.
36. Poltorak A, He X, Smirnova I, et al: Defective LPS signaling in C3H/HeJ and C57BL/10ScCr mice: mutations in Tlr4 gene. *Science* 282:2085-2088, 1998.
37. Read RC, Wyllie DH: Toll receptors and sepsis. *Curr Opin Crit Care* 7:371-375, 2001.
38. Medzhitov R, Janeway C Jr: The Toll receptor family and microbial recognition. *Trends Microbiol* 8:452-456, 2000.
39. Shimazu R, Akashi S, Ogata H, et al: MD-2, a molecule that confers lipopolysaccharide responsiveness on Toll-like receptor 4. *J Exp Med* 189:1777-1782, 1999.
40. Medzhitov R, Preston-Hurlburt P, Kopp E, et al: MyD88 is an adaptor protein in the hToll/IL-1 receptor family signaling pathways. *Mol Cell* 2:253-258, 1998.
41. Jefferies C, O'Neill LA: Signal transduction pathway activated by Toll-like receptors. *Mod Asp Immunobiol* 2:169-175, 2002.
42. Schwandner R, Dziarski R, Wesche H, et al: Peptidoglycan- and lipoteichoic acid-induced cell activation is mediated by toll-like receptor 2. *J Biol Chem* 274:17406-17409, 1999.
43. Medzhitov R: CpG DNA: security code for host defense. *Nat Immunol* 2:15-16, 2001.
44. Hemmi H, Takeuchi O, Kawai T, et al: A Toll-like receptor recognizes bacterial DNA. *Nature* 408:740-745, 2000.
45. Wong HR, Shanley TP: Signal transduction pathways in acute lung injury: NF-κB and AP-1. In H. R. a. S. Wong, T.P., editors: *Molecular biology of acute lung injury*. Norwell, MA, 2001, Kluwer Academic Publishers.
46. Karin M, Delhase M: The I kappa B kinase (IKK) and NF-kappa B: key elements of proinflammatory signalling. *Semin Immunol* 12:85-98, 2000.
47. Karin M, Ben-Neriah Y: Phosphorylation meets ubiquitination: the control of NF-[kappa]B activity. *Annu Rev Immunol* 18:621-663, 2000.
48. Bohrer H, Qiu F, Zimmermann T, et al: Role of NFkappaB in the mortality of sepsis. *J Clin Invest* 100:972-985, 1997.
49. Schwartz MD, Moore EE, Moore FA, et al: Nuclear factor-kappa B is activated in alveolar macrophages from patients with acute respiratory distress syndrome. *Crit Care Med* 24:1285-1292, 1996.
50. Karin M: The regulation of AP-1 activity by mitogen-activated protein kinases. *J Biol Chem* 270:16483-16486, 1995.
51. Karin M, Liu Z, Zandi E: AP-1 function and regulation. *Curr Opin Cell Biol* 9:240-246, 1997.
52. Herlaar E, Brown Z: p38 MAPK signalling cascades in inflammatory disease. *Mol Med Today* 5:439-447, 1999.
53. Garrington TP, Johnson GL: Organization and regulation of mitogen-activated protein kinase signaling pathways. *Curr Opin Cell Biol* 11:211-218, 1999.
54. Davis RJ: Signal transduction by the JNK group of MAP kinases. *Cell* 103:239-252, 2000.
55. Ip YT, Davis RJ: Signal transduction by the c-Jun N-terminal kinase (JNK)–from inflammation to development. *Curr Opin Cell Biol* 10:205-219, 1998.
56. Fijen JW, Zijlstra JG, De Boer P, et al: Suppression of the clinical and cytokine response to endotoxin by RWJ-67657, a p38 mitogen-activated protein-kinase inhibitor, in healthy human volunteers. *Clin Exp Immunol* 124:16-20, 2001.
57. Faas MM, Moes H, Fijen JW, et al: Monocyte intracellular cytokine production during human endotoxaemia with or without a second in vitro LPS challenge: effect of RWJ-67657, a p38 MAP-kinase inhibitor, on LPS-hyporesponsiveness. *Clin Exp Immunol* 127:337-343, 2002.
58. Guha M, Mackman N: LPS induction of gene expression in human monocytes. *Cell Signal* 13:85-94, 2001.
59. van der Bruggen T, Nijenhuis S, van Raaij E, et al: Lipopolysaccharide-induced tumor necrosis factor alpha production by human monocytes involves the raf-1/MEK1-MEK2/ERK1-ERK2 pathway. *Infect Immun* 67:3824-3829, 1999.
60. Cerami A, Beutler B: The role of cachectin/TNF in endotoxic shock and cachexia. *Immunol Today* 9:28-31, 1988.
61. Tracey KJ, Lowry SF, Cerami A: Cachetin/TNF-alpha in septic shock and septic adult respiratory distress syndrome. *Am Rev Respir Dis* 138:1377-1379, 1988.
62. Mannel DN, Echtenacher B: TNF in the inflammatory response. *Chem Immunol* 74:141-161, 2000.
63. Strieter RM, Belperio JA, Kelley D, Sakkour A, Keane MP: Innate immune mechanisms triggering lung injury. In H. R. a. S. Wong, T.P., editors: *Molecular biology of acute lung injury*. Norwell, MA, 2001, Kluwer Academic Publishers.
64. Beutler B, Cerami A: The biology of cachectin/TNF—a primary mediator of the host response. *Annu Rev Immunol* 7:625-655, 1989.
65. Waage A, Halstensen A, Espevik T: Association between tumour necrosis factor in serum and fatal outcome in patients with meningococcal disease. *Lancet* 1:355-357, 1987.
66. Girardin E, Grau GE, Dayer JM, et al: Tumor necrosis factor and interleukin-1 in the serum of children with severe infectious purpura. *N Engl J Med* 319:397-400, 1988.
67. Marks JD, Marks CB, Luce JM, et al: Plasma tumor necrosis factor in patients with septic shock. Mortality rate, incidence of adult respiratory distress syndrome, and effects of methylprednisolone administration. *Am Rev Respir Dis* 141:94-97, 1990.
68. Michie HR, Manogue KR, Spriggs DR, et al: Detection of circulating tumor necrosis factor after endotoxin administration. *N Engl J Med* 318:1481-1486, 1988.
69. Michie HR, Spriggs DR, Manogue KR, et al: Tumor necrosis factor and endotoxin induce similar metabolic responses in human beings. *Surgery* 104:280-286, 1988.
70. Bone RC: Why sepsis trials fail. *JAMA* 276:565-566, 1996.
71. Dinarello CA: Interleukin-1. *Cytokine Growth Factor Rev* 8: 253-265, 1997.
72. Dinarello CA: Biologic basis for interleukin-1 in disease. *Blood* 87:2095-2147, 1996.
73. Shanley TP, Peters JL, Jones ML, et al: Regulatory effects of endogenous interleukin-1 receptor antagonist protein in immunoglobulin G immune complex-induced lung injury. *J Clin Invest* 97:963-970, 1996.
74. Auron PE: The interleukin 1 receptor: ligand interactions and signal transduction. *Cytokine Growth Factor Rev* 9:221-237, 1998.
75. O'Neill LA, Greene C: Signal transduction pathways activated by the IL-1 receptor family: ancient signaling machinery in mammals, insects, and plants. *J Leukoc Biol* 63:650-657, 1998.
76. Suzuki N, Suzuki S, Duncan GS, et al: Severe impairment of interleukin-1 and Toll-like receptor signalling in mice lacking IRAK-4. *Nature* 416:750-756, 2002.
77. Qian Y, Commane M, Ninomiya-Tsuji J, et al: IRAK-mediated translocation of TRAF6 and TAB2 in the interleukin-1-induced activation of NFkappa B. *J Biol Chem* 276:41661-41667, 2001.
78. Guo F, Wu S: Antisense IRAK-1 oligonucleotide blocks activation of NF-kappa B and AP-1 induced by IL-18. *Immunopharmacology* 49:241-246, 2000.
79. Arend WP, Malyak M, Guthridge CJ, et al: Interleukin-1 receptor antagonist: role in biology. *Annu Rev Immunol* 16:27-55, 1998.
80. Fisher CJ Jr, Opal SM, Lowry SF, et al: Role of interleukin-1 and the therapeutic potential of interleukin-1 receptor antagonist in sepsis. *Circ Shock* 44:1-8, 1994.
81. Fisher CJ Jr, Dhainaut JF, Opal SM, et al: Recombinant human interleukin 1 receptor antagonist in the treatment of patients with sepsis syndrome. Results from a randomized, double-blind, placebo-controlled trial. Phase III rhIL-1ra Sepsis Syndrome Study Group. *JAMA* 271:1836-1843, 1994.

82. Fisher CJ Jr, Slotman GJ, Opal SM, et al: Initial evaluation of human recombinant interleukin-1 receptor antagonist in the treatment of sepsis syndrome: a randomized, open-label, placebo-controlled multicenter trial. The IL-1RA Sepsis Syndrome Study Group. *Crit Care Med* 22:12-21, 1994.
83. Okusawa S, Gelfand JA, Ikejima T, et al: Interleukin 1 induces a shock-like state in rabbits. Synergism with tumor necrosis factor and the effect of cyclooxygenase inhibition. *J Clin Invest* 81:1162-1172, 1988.
84. Bone RC: Sepsis syndrome. New insights into its pathogenesis and treatment. *Infect Dis Clin North Am* 5:793-805, 1991.
85. Mulligan MS, Ward PA: Immune complex-induced lung and dermal vascular injury. Differing requirements for tumor necrosis factor-alpha and IL-1. *J Immunol* 149:331-339, 1992.
86. Salgado A, Boveda JL, Monasterio J, et al: Inflammatory mediators and their influence on haemostasis. *Haemostasis* 24:132-138, 1994.
87. Burrell R: Human responses to bacterial endotoxin. *Circ Shock* 43:137-153, 1994.
88. Casey LC, Balk RA, Bone RC: Plasma cytokine and endotoxin levels correlate with survival in patients with the sepsis syndrome. *Ann Intern Med* 119:771-778, 1993.
89. Remick DG, Call DR, Ebong SJ, et al: Combination immunotherapy with soluble tumor necrosis factor receptors plus interleukin 1 receptor antagonist decreases sepsis mortality. *Crit Care Med* 29:473-481, 2001.
90. Calandra T, Gerain J, Heumann D, et al: High circulating levels of interleukin-6 in patients with septic shock: evolution during sepsis, prognostic value, and interplay with other cytokines. The Swiss-Dutch J5 Immunoglobulin Study Group. *Am J Med* 91:23-29, 1991.
91. Damas P, Ledoux D, Nys M, et al: Cytokine serum level during severe sepsis in human IL-6 as a marker of severity. *Ann Surg* 215:356-362, 1992.
92. Calandra T, Baumgartner JD, Grau GE, et al: Prognostic values of tumor necrosis factor/cachectin, interleukin-1, interferon-alpha, and interferon-gamma in the serum of patients with septic shock. Swiss-Dutch J5 Immunoglobulin Study Group. *J Infect Dis* 161:982-987, 1990.
93. Gadient RA, Patterson PH: Leukemia inhibitory factor, Interleukin 6, and other cytokines using the GP130 transducing receptor: roles in inflammation and injury. *Stem Cells* 17:127-137, 1999.
94. Kishimoto T, Akira S, Taga T: Interleukin-6 and its receptor: a paradigm for cytokines. *Science* 258:593-597, 1992.
95. Abraham E, Glauser MP, Butler T, et al: p55 Tumor necrosis factor receptor fusion protein in the treatment of patients with severe sepsis and septic shock. A randomized controlled multicenter trial. Ro 45-2081 Study Group. *JAMA* 277:1531-1538, 1997.
96. Slotman GJ: Prospectively validated prediction of physiologic variables and organ failure in septic patients: the Systemic Mediator Associated Response Test (SMART). *Crit Care Med* 30:1035-1045, 2002.
97. Rossi D, Zlotnik A: The biology of chemokines and their receptors. *Annu Rev Immunol* 18:217-242, 2000.
98. Zlotnik A, Yoshie O: Chemokines: a new classification system and their role in immunity. *Immunity* 12:121-127, 2000.
99. Strieter RM, Kunkel SL, Keane MP, et al: Chemokines in lung injury: Thomas A. Neff Lecture. *Chest* 116:103S-110S, 1999.
100. Meduri GU, Kohler G, Headley S, et al: Inflammatory cytokines in the BAL of patients with ARDS. Persistent elevation over time predicts poor outcome. *Chest* 108:1303-1314, 1995.
101. Chollet-Martin S, Montravers P, Gibert C, et al: High levels of interleukin-8 in the blood and alveolar spaces of patients with pneumonia and adult respiratory distress syndrome. *Infect Immun* 61:4553-4559, 1993.
102. Donnelly SC, Strieter RM, Kunkel SL, et al: Interleukin-8 and development of adult respiratory distress syndrome in at-risk patient groups. *Lancet* 341:643-647, 1993.
103. Jorens PG, Van Damme J, De Backer W, et al: Interleukin 8 (IL-8) in the bronchoalveolar lavage fluid from patients with the adult respiratory distress syndrome (ARDS) and patients at risk for ARDS. *Cytokine* 4:592-597, 1992.
104. Rosseau S, Hammerl P, Maus U, et al: Phenotypic characterization of alveolar monocyte recruitment in acute respiratory distress syndrome. *Am J Physiol Lung Cell Mol Physiol* 279: L25-35, 2000.
105. Hack CE, Zeerleder S: The endothelium in sepsis: source of and a target for inflammation. *Crit Care Med* 29:S21-27, 2001.
106. Zimmerman GA, Prescott SM, McIntyre TM: Endothelial cell interactions with granulocytes: tethering and signaling molecules. *Immunol Today* 13:93-100, 1992.
107. Furchgott RF, Cherry PD, Zawadzki JV, et al: Endothelial cells as mediators of vasodilation of arteries. *J Cardiovasc Pharmacol* 6:S336-S343, 1984.
108. Palmer RM, Ferrige AG, Moncada S: Nitric oxide release accounts for the biological activity of endothelium-derived relaxing factor. *Nature* 327:524-526, 1987.
109. Ignarro LJ, Buga GM, Wood KS, et al: Endothelium-derived relaxing factor produced and released from artery and vein is nitric oxide. *Proc Natl Acad Sci U S A* 84:9265-9269, 1987.
110. Lorente JA, Landin L, Esteban A: Nitric oxide biology in sepsis and shock states. In Fein AM, et al, editors: *Sepsis and multiorgan failure,* Baltimore, 1997, Williams & Wilkins.
111. Vincent JL, Zhang H, Szabo C, et al: Effects of nitric oxide in septic shock. *Am J Respir Crit Care Med* 161:1781-1785, 2000.
112. Liu S, Adcock IM, Old RW, et al: Lipopolysaccharide treatment in vivo induces widespread tissue expression of inducible nitric oxide synthase mRNA. *Biochem Biophys Res Commun* 196:1208-1213, 1993.
113. Zhang H, Rogiers P, Smail N, et al: Effects of nitric oxide on blood flow distribution and O2 extraction capabilities during endotoxic shock. *J Appl Physiol* 83:1164-1173, 1997.
114. van Dissel JT, Groeneveld PH, Maes B, et al: Nitric oxide: a predictor of morbidity in postoperative patients? *Lancet* 343: 1579-1580, 1994.
115. Ochoa JB, Udekwu AO, Billiar TR, et al: Nitrogen oxide levels in patients after trauma and during sepsis. *Ann Surg* 214:621-626, 1991.
116. Gomez-Jimenez J, Salgado A, Mourelle M, et al: L-arginine: nitric oxide pathway in endotoxemia and human septic shock. *Crit Care Med* 23:253-258, 1995.
117. Wong HR, Carcillo JA, Burckart G, et al: Increased serum nitrite and nitrate concentrations in children with the sepsis syndrome. *Crit Care Med* 23:835-842, 1995.
118. Finkel MS, Oddis CV, Jacob TD, et al: Negative inotropic effects of cytokines on the heart mediated by nitric oxide. *Science* 257:387-389, 1992.
119. Kumar A, Krieger A, Symeoneides S, et al: Myocardial dysfunction in septic shock: Part II. Role of cytokines and nitric oxide. *J Cardiothorac Vasc Anesth* 15:485-511, 2001.
120. Iqbal M, Cohen RI, Marzouk K, et al: Time course of nitric oxide, peroxynitrite, and antioxidants in the endotoxemic heart. *Crit Care Med* 30:1291-1296, 2002.
121. Wei XQ, Charles IG, Smith A, et al: Altered immune responses in mice lacking inducible nitric oxide synthase. *Nature* 375: 408-411, 1995.
122. Watson D, Grover R, Anzueto A, et al: Cardiovascular effects of the nitric oxide synthase inhibitor N^G-ethyl-L-arginine hydrochloride (S46C88) in patients with septic shock: results of a randomized, double blind, placebo-controlled multicenter study (study no. 144-002). *Crit Care Med* 32:13-20, 2004.
123. Beckman JS, Beckman TW, Chen J, et al: Apparent hydroxyl radical production by peroxynitrite: implications for endothelial injury from nitric oxide and superoxide. *Proc Natl Acad Sci U S A* 87:1620-1624, 1990.
124. Radi R, Beckman JS, Bush KM, et al: Peroxynitrite oxidation of sulfhydryls. The cytotoxic potential of superoxide and nitric oxide. *J Biol Chem* 266:4244-4250, 1991.
125. Haddad IY, Ischiropoulos H, Holm BA, et al: Mechanisms of peroxynitrite-induced injury to pulmonary surfactants. *Am J Physiol* 265:L555-564, 1993.
126. Szabo C, Cuzzocrea S, Zingarelli B, et al: Endothelial dysfunction in a rat model of endotoxic shock. Importance of the activation of poly (ADP-ribose) synthetase by peroxynitrite. *J Clin Invest* 100:723-735, 1997.
127. Giusti-Paiva A, De Castro M, Antunes-Rodrigues J, et al: Inducible nitric oxide synthase pathway in the central nervous system and vasopressin release during experimental septic shock. *Crit Care Med* 30:1306-1310, 2002.
128. Wang H, Yang H, Czura CJ, et al: HMGB1 as a late mediator of lethal systemic inflammation. *Am J Respir Crit Care Med* 164:1768-1773, 2001.

129. Bustin M: Regulation of DNA-dependent activities by the functional motifs of the high-mobility-group chromosomal proteins. *Mol Cell Biol* 19:5237-5246, 1999.
130. Hori O, Brett J, Slattery T, et al: The receptor for advanced glycation end products (RAGE) is a cellular binding site for amphoterin. Mediation of neurite outgrowth and co-expression of rage and amphoterin in the developing nervous system. *J Biol Chem* 270: 25752-25761, 1995.
131. Wang H, Bloom O, Zhang M, et al: HMG-1 as a late mediator of endotoxin lethality in mice. *Science* 285:248-251, 1999.
132. Abraham E, Arcaroli J, Carmody A, et al: HMG-1 as a mediator of acute lung inflammation. *J Immunol* 165:2950-2954, 2000.
133. Pinsky MR, Vincent JL, Deviere J, et al: Serum cytokine levels in human septic shock. Relation to multiple-system organ failure and mortality. *Chest* 103:565-575, 1993.
134. Arndt P, Abraham E: Immunological therapy of sepsis: experimental therapies. *Intensive Care Med* 27:S104-S115, 2001.
135. Opal SM, DePalo VA: Anti-inflammatory cytokines. *Chest* 117: 1162-1172, 2000.
136. Fiorentino DF, Bond MW, Mosmann TR: Two types of mouse T helper cell. IV. Th2 clones secrete a factor that inhibits cytokine production by Th1 clones. *J Exp Med* 170:2081-2095, 1989.
137. de Waal Malefyt R, Abrams J, Bennett B, et al: Interleukin 10(IL-10) inhibits cytokine synthesis by human monocytes: an autoregulatory role of IL-10 produced by monocytes. *J Exp Med* 174: 1209-1220, 1991.
138. Moore KW, de Waal Malefyt R, Coffman RL, et al: Interleukin-10 and the interleukin-10 receptor. *Annu Rev Immunol* 19:683-765, 2001.
139. Oberholzer A, Oberholzer C, Moldawer LL: Interleukin-10: a complex role in the pathogenesis of sepsis syndromes and its potential as an anti-inflammatory drug. *Crit Care Med* 30:S58-S63, 2002.
140. Shanley TP: Anti-inflammatory cytokines: Role in regulation of acute lung injury. In H. R. a. S. Wong, T.P., editors: *Molecular biology of acute lung injury,* Norwell, MA, 2001, Kluwer Academic Publishers.
141. Cassatella MA, Meda L, Gasperini S, et al: Interleukin 10 (IL-10) upregulates IL-1 receptor antagonist production from lipopolysaccharide-stimulated human polymorphonuclear leukocytes by delaying mRNA degradation. *J Exp Med* 179:1695-1699, 1994.
142. Dickensheets HL, Freeman SL, Smith MF, et al: Interleukin-10 upregulates tumor necrosis factor receptor type-II (p75) gene expression in endotoxin-stimulated human monocytes. *Blood* 90: 4162-4171, 1997.
143. Schottelius AJ, Mayo MW, Sartor RB, et al: Interleukin-10 signaling blocks inhibitor of kappaB kinase activity and nuclear factor kappaB DNA binding. *J Biol Chem* 274:31868-31874, 1999.
144. Shames BD, Selzman CH, Meldrum DR, et al: Interleukin-10 stabilizes inhibitory kappaB-alpha in human monocytes. *Shock* 10: 389-394, 1998.
145. Shanley TP, Vasi N, Denenberg A: Regulation of chemokine expression by IL-10 in lung inflammation. *Cytokine* 12:1054-1064, 2000.
146. Berg DJ, Kuhn R, Rajewsky K, et al: Interleukin-10 is a central regulator of the response to LPS in murine models of endotoxic shock and the Shwartzman reaction but not endotoxin tolerance. *J Clin Invest* 96:2339-2347, 1995.
147. Donnelly SC, Strieter RM, Reid PT, et al: The association between mortality rates and decreased concentrations of interleukin-10 and interleukin-1 receptor antagonist in the lung fluids of patients with the adult respiratory distress syndrome. *Ann Intern Med* 125:191-196, 1996.
148. Westendorp RG, Langermans JA, de Bel CE, et al: Release of tumor necrosis factor: an innate host characteristic that may contribute to the outcome of meningococcal disease. *J Infect Dis* 171:1057-1060, 1995.
149. Aird WC: Vascular bed-specific hemostasis: role of endothelium in sepsis pathogenesis. *Crit Care Med* 29:S28-S34; discussion S34-S25, 2001.
150. McGilvray ID, Rotstein OD: Role of the coagulation system in the local and systemic inflammatory response. *World J Surg* 22:179-186, 1998.
151. Vervloet MG, Thijs LG, Hack CE: Derangements of coagulation and fibrinolysis in critically ill patients with sepsis and septic shock. *Semin Thromb Hemost* 24:33-44, 1998.
152. Muller-Berghaus G, Madlener K, Blomback M, et al: *DIC: pathogenesis, diagnosis and therapy of disseminated intravascular fibrin formation,* Amsterdam, 1993, Elsevier Science Publishers BV.
153. Doshi SN, Marmur JD: Evolving role of tissue factor and its pathway inhibitor. *Crit Care Med* 30:S241-S250, 2002.
154. Levi M, van der Poll T, ten Cate H, et al: The cytokine-mediated imbalance between coagulant and anticoagulant mechanisms in sepsis and endotoxaemia. *Eur J Clin Invest* 27:3-9, 1997.
155. Osterud B: Tissue factor expression by monocytes: regulation and pathophysiological roles. *Blood Coagul Fibrinolysis* 9(suppl 1): S9-S14, 1998.
156. Saadi S, Holzknecht RA, Patte CP, et al: Complement-mediated regulation of tissue factor activity in endothelium. *J Exp Med* 182:1807-1814, 1995.
157. Nawroth PP, Handley DA, Esmon CT, et al: Interleukin 1 induces endothelial cell procoagulant while suppressing cell-surface anticoagulant activity. *Proc Natl Acad Sci U S A* 83:3460-3464, 1986.
158. Kaiser B, Hoppensteadt DA, Fareed J: Tissue factor pathway inhibitor: an update of potential implications in the treatment of cardiovascular disorders. *Expert Opin Investig Drugs* 10: 1925-1935, 2001.
159. Bajaj MS, Bajaj SP: Tissue factor pathway inhibitor: potential therapeutic applications. *Thromb Haemost* 78:471-477, 1997.
160. Abraham E, Reinhart K, Svoboda P, et al: Assessment of the safety of recombinant tissue factor pathway inhibitor in patients with severe sepsis: a multicenter, randomized, placebo-controlled, single-blind, dose escalation study. *Crit Care Med* 29:2081-2089, 2001.
161. Creasey AA, Reinhart K: Tissue factor pathway inhibitor activity in severe sepsis, *Crit Care Med* 29:S126-S129, 2001.
162. Mesters RM, Mannucci PM, Coppola R, et al: Factor VIIa and antithrombin III activity during severe sepsis and septic shock in neutropenic patients. *Blood* 88:881-886, 1996.
163. Seitz R, Wolf M, Egbring R, et al: The disturbance of hemostasis in septic shock: role of neutrophil elastase and thrombin, effects of antithrombin III and plasma substitution. *Eur J Haematol* 43:22-28, 1989.
164. Levi M, de Jonge E, van der Poll T: Rationale for restoration of physiological anticoagulant pathways in patients with sepsis and disseminated intravascular coagulation. *Crit Care Med* 29: S90-S94, 2001.
165. Fourrier F, Chopin C, Goudemand J, et al: Septic shock, multiple organ failure, and disseminated intravascular coagulation. Compared patterns of antithrombin III, protein C, and protein S deficiencies. *Chest* 101:816-823, 1992.
166. Esmon CT: Protein C anticoagulant pathway and its role in controlling microvascular thrombosis and inflammation. *Crit Care Med* 29:S48-S51; discussion S51-S42, 2001.
167. Faust SN, Heyderman RS, Levin M: Coagulation in severe sepsis: a central role for thrombomodulin and activated protein C. *Crit Care Med* 29:S62-S67; discussion S67-S68, 2001.
168. Esmon CT: The roles of protein C and thrombomodulin in the regulation of blood coagulation. *J Biol Chem* 264:4743-4746, 1989.
169. Esmon CT, Xu J, Gu JM, et al: Endothelial protein C receptor. *Thromb Haemost* 82:251-258, 1999.
170. Taylor FB Jr, Chang A, Esmon CT, et al: Protein C prevents the coagulopathic and lethal effects of Escherichia coli infusion in the baboon. *J Clin Invest* 79:918-925, 1987.
171. Murakami K, Okajima K, Uchiba M, et al: Activated protein C prevents LPS-induced pulmonary vascular injury by inhibiting cytokine production. *Am J Physiol* 272:L197-L202, 1997.
172. Hancock WW, Tsuchida A, Hau H, et al: The anticoagulants protein C and protein S display potent antiinflammatory and immunosuppressive effects relevant to transplant biology and therapy. *Transplant Proc* 24:2302-2303, 1992.
173. Shua F, Kobayashia H, Fukudomeb K, et al: Activated protein C suppresses tissue factor expression on U937 cells in the endothelial protein C receptor-dependent manner. *FEBS Lett* 477: 208-212, 2000.
174. Bernard GR, Vincent JL, Laterre PF, et al: Efficacy and safety of recombinant human activated protein C for severe sepsis. *N Engl J Med* 344:699-709, 2001.
175. Poltorak A, Smirnova I, He X, et al: Genetic and physical mapping of the Lps locus: identification of the toll-4 receptor as a candidate gene in the critical region. *Blood Cells Mol Dis* 24: 340-355, 1998.

176. Qureshi ST, Lariviere L, Leveque G, et al: Endotoxin-tolerant mice have mutations in Toll-like receptor 4 (Tlr4). *J Exp Med* 189:615-625, 1999.
177. Qureshi ST, Gros P, Malo D: Host resistance to infection: genetic control of lipopolysaccharide responsiveness by TOLL-like receptor genes. *Trends Genet* 15:291-294, 1999.
178. Arbour NC, Lorenz E, Schutte BC, et al: TLR4 mutations are associated with endotoxin hyporesponsiveness in humans. *Nat Genet* 25:187-191, 2000.
179. Lorenz E, Mira JP, Cornish KL, et al: A novel polymorphism in the toll-like receptor 2 gene and its potential association with staphylococcal infection. *Infect Immun* 68:6398-6401, 2000.
180. Gibot S, Cariou A, Drouet L, et al: Association between a genomic polymorphism within the CD14 locus and septic shock susceptibility and mortality rate. *Crit Care Med* 30:969-973, 2002.
181. Mira JP, Cariou A, Grall F, et al: Association of TNF2, a TNF-alpha promoter polymorphism, with septic shock susceptibility and mortality: a multicenter study. *JAMA* 282:561-568, 1999.
182. Stuber F, Petersen M, Bokelmann F, et al: A genomic polymorphism within the tumor necrosis factor locus influences plasma tumor necrosis factor-alpha concentrations and outcome of patients with severe sepsis. *Crit Care Med* 24:381-384, 1996.
183. McArthur JA, Zhang Q, Quasney MW: Association between the A/A genotype at the lymphotoxin-alpha+250 site and increased mortality in children with positive blood cultures. *Pediatr Crit Care Med* 3:341-344, 2002.
184. Nusinow SR, Zuraw BL, and Curd JG: The hereditary and acquired deficiencies of complement. *Med Clin North Am* 69: 487-504, 1985.
185. Lee TJ, Snyderman R, Patterson J, et al: Neisseria meningitidis bacteremia in association with deficiency of the sixth component of complement. *Infect Immun* 24:656-660, 1979.
186. Fang XM, Schroder S, Hoeft A, et al: Comparison of two polymorphisms of the interleukin-1 gene family: interleukin-1 receptor antagonist polymorphism contributes to susceptibility to severe sepsis. *Crit Care Med* 27:1330-1334, 1999.
187. Ma P, Chen D, Pan J, et al: Genomic polymorphism within interleukin-1 family cytokines influences the outcome of septic patients. *Crit Care Med* 30:1046-1050, 2002.
188. Eskdale J, Gallagher G: A polymorphic dinucleotide repeat in the human IL-10 promoter. *Immunogenetics* 42:444-445, 1995.
189. Eskdale J, Gallagher G, Verweij CL, et al: Interleukin 10 secretion in relation to human IL-10 locus haplotypes. *Proc Natl Acad Sci U S A* 95:9465-9470, 1998.
190. Carcillo JA, Davis AL, Zaritsky A: Role of early fluid resuscitation in pediatric septic shock. *JAMA* 266:1242-1245, 1991.
191. Zadrobilek E, Hackl W, Sporn P, et al: Effect of large volume replacement with balanced electrolyte solutions on extravascular lung water in surgical patients with sepsis syndrome. *Intensive Care Med* 15:505-510, 1989.
192. Powell KR, Sugarman LI, Eskenazi AE, et al: Normalization of plasma arginine vasopressin concentrations when children with meningitis are given maintenance plus replacement fluid therapy. *J Pediatr* 117:515-522, 1990.
193. Rivers E, Nguyen B, Havstad S, et al: Early goal-directed therapy in the treatment of severe sepsis and septic shock. *N Engl J Med* 345:1368-1377, 2001.
194. Yung M, Butt W: Inferior vena cava pressure as an estimate of central venous pressure. *J Paediatr Child Health* 31:399-402, 1995.
195. Connors AF Jr, Speroff T, Dawson NV, et al: The effectiveness of right heart catheterization in the initial care of critically ill patients. SUPPORT Investigators. *JAMA* 276:889-897, 1996.
196. Pulmonary Artery Catheter Consensus conference: consensus statement. *Crit Care Med* 25:910-925, 1997.
197. Ceneviva G, Paschall JA, Maffei F, et al: Hemodynamic support in fluid-refractory pediatric septic shock. *Pediatrics* 102:e19, 1998.
198. Pulmonary artery catheter consensus conference. Chicago, December 6–8, 1996. *New Horiz* 5:173-296, 1997.
199. Bryan CS, Reynolds KL, Brenner ER: Analysis of 1,186 episodes of gram-negative bacteremia in non-university hospitals: the effects of antimicrobial therapy. *Rev Infect Dis* 5:629-638, 1983.
200. Glauser MP, Zanetti G, Baumgartner JD, et al: Septic shock: pathogenesis. *Lancet* 338:732-736, 1991.
201. Shenep JL, Barton RP, Mogan KA: Role of antibiotic class in the rate of liberation of endotoxin during therapy for experimental gram-negative bacterial sepsis. *J Infect Dis* 151:1012-1018, 1985.
202. Kern JW, Shoemaker WC: Meta-analysis of hemodynamic optimization in high-risk patients. *Crit Care Med* 30:1686-1692, 2002.
203. Gattinoni L, Brazzi L, Pelosi P, et al: A trial of goal-oriented hemodynamic therapy in critically ill patients. SvO2 Collaborative Group. *N Engl J Med* 333:1025-1032, 1995.
204. Barton P, Garcia J, Kouatli A, et al: Hemodynamic effects of i.v. milrinone lactate in pediatric patients with septic shock. A prospective, double-blinded, randomized, placebo-controlled, interventional study. *Chest* 109:1302-1312, 1996.
205. Atkinson S, Sieffert E, Bihari D: A prospective, randomized, double-blind, controlled clinical trial of enteral immunonutrition in the critically ill. Guy's Hospital Intensive Care Group. *Crit Care Med* 26:1164-1172, 1998.
206. Crouser ED, Dorinsky PM: Gastrointestinal tract dysfunction in critical illness: pathophysiology and interaction with acute lung injury in adult respiratory distress syndrome/multiple organ dysfunction syndrome. *New Horiz* 2:476-487, 1994.
207. Swank GM, Deitch EA: Role of the gut in multiple organ failure: bacterial translocation and permeability changes. *World J Surg* 20:411-417, 1996.
208. Marik PE, Zaloga GP: Early enteral nutrition in acutely ill patients: a systematic review. *Crit Care Med* 29:2264-2270, 2001.
209. Marik PE, Mohedin M: The contrasting effects of dopamine and norepinephrine on systemic and splanchnic oxygen utilization in hyperdynamic sepsis. *JAMA* 272:1354-1357, 1994.
210. Meier-Hellmann A, Reinhart K, Bredle DL, et al: Epinephrine impairs splanchnic perfusion in septic shock. *Crit Care Med* 25:399-404, 1997.
211. Balk RA: Pathogenesis and management of multiple organ dysfunction or failure in severe sepsis and septic shock. *Crit Care Clin* 16:337-352, vii, 2000.
212. Hurley JC: Antibiotic-induced release of endotoxin: a reappraisal. *Clin Infect Dis* 15:840-854, 1992.
213. Jansen NJ, van Oeveren W, Hoiting BH, et al: Methylprednisolone prophylaxis protects against endotoxin-induced death in rabbits. *Inflammation* 15:91-101, 1991.
214. Jenkins JK, Carey PD, Byrne K, et al: Sepsis-induced lung injury and the effects of ibuprofen pretreatment. Analysis of early alveolar events via repetitive bronchoalveolar lavage. *Am Rev Respir Dis* 143:155-161, 1991.
215. Bone RC, Fisher CJ Jr, Clemmer TP, et al: Early methylprednisolone treatment for septic syndrome and the adult respiratory distress syndrome. *Chest* 92:1032-1036, 1987.
216. Sprung CL, Caralis PV, Marcial EH, et al: The effects of high-dose corticosteroids in patients with septic shock. A prospective, controlled study. *N Engl J Med* 311:1137-1143, 1984.
217. Meduri GU: New rationale for glucocorticoid treatment in septic shock. *J Chemother* 11:541-550, 1999.
218. Briegel J, Forst H, Haller M, et al: Stress doses of hydrocortisone reverse hyperdynamic septic shock: a prospective, randomized, double-blind, single-center study. *Crit Care Med* 27:723-732, 1999.
219. Bollaert PE, Charpentier C, Levy B, et al: Reversal of late septic shock with supraphysiologic doses of hydrocortisone. *Crit Care Med* 26:645-650, 1998.
220. Hatherill M, Tibby SM, Hilliard T, et al: Adrenal insufficiency in septic shock. *Arch Dis Child* 80:51-55, 1999.
221. Rothwell PM, Udwadia ZF, Lawler PG: Cortisol response to corticotropin and survival in septic shock. *Lancet* 337:582-583, 1991.
222. Soni A, Pepper GM, Wyrwinski PM, et al: Adrenal insufficiency occurring during septic shock: incidence, outcome, and relationship to peripheral cytokine levels. *Am J Med* 98:266-271, 1995.
223. Annane D, Sebille V, Charpentier C, et al: Effect of treatment with low doses of hydrocortisone and fludrocortisone on mortality in patients with septic shock. *JAMA* 288:862-871, 2002.
224. Walley KR: Many roles of nitric oxide in regulating cardiac function in sepsis. *Crit Care Med* 28:2135-2137, 2000.
225. Hollenberg SM, Cunnion RE, and Zimmerberg J: Nitric oxide synthase inhibition reverses arteriolar hyporesponsiveness to catecholamines in septic rats. *Am J Physiol* 264:H660-H663, 1993.

226. Lorente JA, Landin L, De Pablo R, et al: L-arginine pathway in the sepsis syndrome. *Crit Care Med* 21:1287-1295, 1993.
227. Petros A, Lamb G, Leone A, et al: Effects of a nitric oxide synthase inhibitor in humans with septic shock. *Cardiovasc Res* 28: 34-39, 1994.
228. Pearson G, Khandelwal PC, and Naqvi N: Early filtration and mortality in meningococcal septic shock? *Arch Dis Child* 83: 508-509, 2000.
229. Manns M, Sigler MH, Teehan BP: Hemodynamic changes during continuous veno-venous hemodialysis in septic patients. *Blood Purif* 13:395-402, 1995.
230. Hoffmann JN, Hartl WH, Deppisch R, et al: Effect of hemofiltration on hemodynamics and systemic concentrations of anaphylatoxins and cytokines in human sepsis. *Intensive Care Med* 22:1360-1367, 1996.
231. Kornecki A, Tauman R, Lubetzky R, et al: Continuous renal replacement therapy for non-renal indications: experience in children. *Isr Med Assoc J* 4:345-348, 2002.
232. Reeves JH, Butt WW, Shann F, et al: Continuous plasmafiltration in sepsis syndrome. Plasmafiltration in Sepsis Study Group. *Crit Care Med* 27:2096-2104, 1999.
233. Mesters RM, Helterbrand J, Utterback BG, et al: Prognostic value of protein C concentrations in neutropenic patients at high risk of severe septic complications. *Crit Care Med* 28:2209-2216, 2000.
234. Inthorn D, Hoffmann JN, Hartl WH, et al: Antithrombin III supplementation in severe sepsis: beneficial effects on organ dysfunction. *Shock* 8:328-334, 1997.
235. Hellgren M, Egberg N, Eklund J: Blood coagulation and fibrinolytic factors and their inhibitors in critically ill patients. *Intensive Care Med* 10:23-28, 1984.
236. Yan SB, Helterbrand JD, Hartman DL, et al: Low levels of protein C are associated with poor outcome in severe sepsis. *Chest* 120:915-922, 2001.
237. Eisele B, Lamy M, Thijs LG, et al: Antithrombin III in patients with severe sepsis. A randomized, placebo-controlled, double-blind multicenter trial plus a meta-analysis on all randomized, placebo-controlled, double-blind trials with antithrombin III in severe sepsis. *Intensive Care Med* 24:663-672, 1998.
238. Warren BL, Eid A, Singer P, et al: Caring for the critically ill patient. High-dose antithrombin III in severe sepsis: a randomized controlled trial. *JAMA* 286:1869-1878, 2001.

CHAPTER

97

Pediatric Multiple Organ Dysfunction Syndrome

Pelin Cengiz and Jerry J. Zimmerman

PEARLS

- Multiple organ dysfunction syndrome (MODS) represents the ultimate complication of trauma, illness, and critical illness.
- MODS can be defined as simultaneous occurrence of two or more organ dysfunctions. Organ systems typically included in the diagnostic criteria of pediatric MODS are cardiovascular, pulmonary, neurologic, hematologic, renal, hepatic, and gastrointestinal.
- In one study the maximum number of organ failures occurred within 72 hours of admission to the pediatric intensive care unit (PICU) in 87% of patients, and diagnostic criteria for MODS were met on the day of admission in 86% of patients. Unlike adults, occurrence of sequential MODS in children is rare.
- Primary MODS is considered the direct result of a well-defined insult in which organ dysfunctions occur early and can be attributed to the insult itself. However, secondary MODS may be the consequence of the host's response and is defined in the context of systemic inflammatory response syndrome (SIRS).
- In adults, organ failures typically occur sequentially over days to weeks, leading to late onset of maximum organ failure number. The higher incidence of secondary MODS in adults compared with children may account for the differences in mortality.
- Incidence of MODS (11%–27%) is much more frequent than death in PICUs. Accordingly, a score that can be used to estimate the severity of MODS would be an additional key outcome measure in critically ill children.
- Pediatric Logistic Organ Dysfunction (PELOD) and daily PELOD (dPELOD) scores are valid outcome measures of the severity of MODS in critically ill children.
- Surviving MODS likely involves reestablishing a balance between SIRS (associated with inflammatory autoinjury) and compensatory antiinflammatory response syndrome (associated with secondary infection from acquired immunodeficiency).
- Neural, endocrine, and inflammatory mediator servocommunications promote oscillator variability in healthy biologic systems. Uncoupling, loss of variability, and decomplexification are associated with increasing illness severity and the downward spiral of MODS.
- Although numerous unifying hypotheses for the pathophysiology of MODS are proposed, one that appears to encompass most of the associated research is the vicious reciprocal cycle of ischemia/reperfusion and inflammation: literally, "one thing leads to another."
- Characteristics of the endothelial activated phenotype include expression of intercellular adhesion molecules (e.g., intercellular adhesion molecule-1), production of proinflammatory cytokines (e.g., interleukin-8), polymerization of actin stress fiber cytoskeleton, and switch to a procoagulant cell surface.
- Mechanisms for cytopathic hypoxia may involve alterations in pyruvate dehydrogenase, activation of poly ADP-ribose synthase, competition of nitric oxide with oxygen for cytochrome oxidase, oxidation of mitochondrial DNA proteins, and increased mitochondrial permeability transition.

- Virchow's classic tissue infarction triad includes low blood flow, a hypercoagulable state, and endothelial cell activation and injury, and it essentially is very early recognition of the critical relationship between ischemia/reperfusion and inflammation.
- In the absence of evidence-based medicine approaches to reduce MODS for pediatric patients, at least four commonsense PICU approaches exist to limit inflammation and ischemia/reperfusion. These measures include: (1) ensure adequate cardiac output and treat shock states early and aggressively; (2) treat infections early with appropriate antibiotics and resect foci of infected/necrotic tissue as appropriate; (3) resolve/prevent metabolic acidosis; and (4) eliminate medical errors.

". . . all of the vital mechanisms, varied as they are, have only one object: that of preserving constant the conditions of life in the milieu interieur. . .."

Claude Bernard, 1878

Epidemiology

Multiple organ dysfunction syndrome (MODS), systemic inflammatory response syndrome (SIRS), and sepsis are major clinical issues in pediatric intensive care units (PICUs). MODS represents the ultimate complication of trauma, illness, and critical illness. Despite advances in medical technology and innovative treatment strategies, 97% to 100% of deaths in PICUs are attributed to MODS. In fact, prehospital and hospital technical advances in critical care have fostered the emergence of this modern-day malady. Although the mortality rate for sepsis has decreased from 97% in 1963 (infants with gram-negative sepsis and septic shock)[1] down to 5% in 1999 (children with meningococcal septic shock),[2] reports indicate that the vast majority of children who die of septic shock have MODS.[3]

Although sepsis appears to be an important primary insult leading to MODS, MODS develops in the absence of sepsis in more than half of critically ill pediatric patients.[4] Interestingly, in developed countries, high identical mortality rates are seen in MODS with or without associated sepsis.[4] This finding indicates that many conditions other than sepsis are associated with MODS in critically ill children. An initial epidemiologic study examined the mortality rates associated with sepsis and MODS in children in the United States. Surprisingly, an association of MODS and sepsis in pediatric patients,[4] unlike adults,[5] was found to have no impact on mortality rates. Mortality rates for MODS patients with and without sepsis were 46% and 47%, respectively.[4] Mortality rates for early (53%) and late (33%) sepsis subgroups were different but not statistically. Sepsis did not significantly increase mortality rates in the groups with organ system failure, indicating the importance of other underlying pathophysiologic mechanisms operative in MODS in critically ill pediatric patients.[4] On the other hand, pediatric intensivists from Lima, Peru, reported an epidemiologic study and described experience with pediatric MODS in their 16-bed PICU.[6] Fewer PICU resources, different pathophysiologies, and different socioeconomic, nutritional, and immunization status of patients likely affected the presentation and outcome of pediatric MODS patients in their study. The authors from Peru reported that sepsis was associated with increased mortality in their study population (odds ratio [OR] 2.33; 95% confidence interval [CI] 1.18–4.59).[6] The mortality rate of children with MODS plus sepsis was significantly higher than in those who did not demonstrate this association (51.7% vs. 28.9%, $p < 0.001$). National statistics from Peru indicated that 16% of children in urban areas and 33% of children in the PICU at Instituto de Salud del Nino in Lima were malnourished. Because malnutrition impairs all aspects of the immune system,[7,8] perhaps it was not surprising that 87% of patients with MODS also had sepsis. Besides malnutrition, late presentation of most patients to the PICU resulted in an overall mortality rate of 25.7% (vs. 6%–11% in developed countries) (Table 97–1). A retrospective review of 2,346 children (age 1 month to 21 years) admitted to a single PICU from 1998 to 1999 revealed that MODS was associated with 73% of sepsis cases and 100% of sepsis-associated mortality.[9] Most of the patients in the 147-patient sepsis cohort carried some oncologic diagnosis. No deaths occurred in previously healthy patients, but sepsis in children with bone marrow transplantation was associated with 38% mortality. For all patients, sepsis mortality was 0% and 19% without and with MODS, respectively. Other pediatric investigations have also established a clear link between sepsis mortality and the presence of MODS.[10,11]

Diagnostic criteria for sepsis, severe sepsis, septic shock, and SIRS were suggested by the American College of Chest Physicians/Society of Critical Care Medicine Consensus Conference in 1992 (Table 97–2).[12] Today, pediatric intensivists are using modifications of these definitions, particularly in terms of enrolling appropriate patients into certain clinical trials.[13,14] Although the modified criteria currently are widely used in children admitted to PICUs, definitions likely will evolve concomitant with the introduction of new concepts in sepsis, which most probably will include consideration of proinflammatory and anti-inflammatory mediators involved in SIRS.[15] In 2001, the *PIRO* approach was proposed as a hypothetical model to describe sepsis: *P* represents patient predisposition, which is based on genetics; *I* represents infection, the infecting organism, and the extent of infection; *R* represents the host biochemical and physiologic response in terms of specific mediators and genetic markers; and *O* represents

TABLE 97–1

Summary of Epidemiologic Studies of Pediatric Multiple Organ Dysfunction Syndrome

Author	Wilkinson et al.[19]	Wilkinson et al.[4]	Proulx et al.[17]	Proulx et al.[18]	Kutco et al.[9]	Tantalean et al.[6]
Year of publication	1986	1987	1994	1996	2003	2003
No. of admissions	831	726	777	1058	2346	276
Median age of patients (months)	32.5	NA	42.6	35.0	NA	19.5
Median age of patients with MODS (months)	17	22	23	NA	NA	NA
Incidence of:						
MODS	226 (27%)	177 (24%)	85 (10.9%)	191 (18%)	NA	156 (56.5%)
MODS + sepsis	NA	47%	22%	38%	3%	56%
1 OD n (%)	241 (52%)	NA	NA	NA	NA	85 (75%)
2 OD n (%)	142 (30%)	NA	NA	86 (45%)	NA	78 (50%)
3 OD n (%)	72 (15%)	NA	NA	59 (31%)	NA	54 (34.6%)
4 OD n (%)	12 (3%)	NA	NA	24 (13%)	NA	19 (12%)
5 OD n (%)	NA	NA	NA	6 (3%)	NA	4 (2.5%)
6 OD n (%)	NA	NA	NA	3 (1%)	NA	1 (0.6%)
Mortality from:						
MODS	54%	47%	50.6%	36%	NA	41.6%
MODS + sepsis	NA	46%	NA	22%	18.6%	51.7%
1 OD	0.8%	NA	NA	NA	NA	NA
2 OD	11%	26%	6%	NA	NA	29.4%
3 OD	50%	62%	80%	NA	NA	38.8%
4 OD	75%	88%	78%	NA	NA	84.2%
5 OD	NA	NA	83%	NA	NA	100
PRISM score of survivors (mean ± SD)	NA	NA	10 ± 6	NA	9 ± 6	16
PRISM score of nonsurvivors (mean ± SD)	NA	NA	22 ± 11	NA	24 ± 16	22

MODS, Multiple organ dysfunction syndrome; *NA,* not available; *OD,* organ dysfunction; *PRISM,* Pediatric Risk of Mortality.

quantification of organ dysfunction.[16] However, this model must be tested for at least 5 to 10 years as an approach before determination of which factors predict death and which patients would benefit from certain therapies provided in ICUs.

Other than sepsis, admitting medical diagnoses of patients who develop MODS include acute asphyxia, inborn errors of metabolism, acute respiratory failure, acute renal failure, intracranial hemorrhage, and degenerative neurologic disease. Admitting surgical diagnoses include

TABLE 97–2

Diagnostic Criteria of Pediatric Systemic Inflammatory Response Syndrome, Sepsis, Severe Sepsis, and Septic Shock[12,25,48]

Pediatric SIRS is characterized by the presence of at least two of the following criteria:

1. *Temperature* > 38°C rectal (37.8°C oral, 37.2°C axillary) or < 35°C rectal (35.8°C oral, 35.2°C axillary)
2. *Heart rate* > 90th percentile for age
3. *Tachypnea* with respiratory rate > 90th percentile for age or hyperventilation as indicated by $PaCO_2$ < 32 mmHg (< 4.3kPa)
4. *White blood cell count* (WBC) > 12 × 10^9/L (> 12,000 cells/μL) or < 4 × 10^9/L (< 4000 cells/μL) or > 10% immature (band) form

Sepsis is SIRS caused by a documented or strongly suspected infection (any positive culture obtained immediately prior to or during admission to pediatric intensive care unit, showing bacterial, viral, or fungal pathogen and/or clinical evidence of infection, e.g., chickenpox or purpura fulminans).

Severe sepsis is characterized by the occurrence of sepsis plus one or more of the following criteria:

1. Decreased level of consciousness (Glasgow Coma Score < 15 without central nervous system disease
2. Arterial blood lactate level > 1.6 mmol/L (> 1.6 mEq/L) or venous blood lactate level > 2.2 mmol/L (> 2.2 mEq/L)
3. Urine output < 1 ml/kg/hour for 2 consecutive hours measured by urinary catheter

Septic shock is defined by the presence of hypotension (with two distinct measurements of blood pressure) < 3rd percentile for age after administration of 20 ml/kg or more of crystalloid or colloid plus

1. Requirement of inotropic or vasopressor support (dopamine or dobutamine ≥ 5 μg/kg/min) or
2. Any of the previously defined diagnostic criteria for severe sepsis

SIRS, systemic inflammatory response syndrome.

postoperative cardiac surgery, trauma (burns), orthotropic liver transplantation, and intussusception.[17] Postoperative cardiac patients and other children with MODS have similar mortality rates over time.[17]

Epidemiology of MODS in children has been detailed in seven studies.[4,6,9,17–20] Wilkinson et al.[19] first reported in 1986 the incidence and mortality of MODS were 27% and 54%, respectively, in 831 consecutive children admitted to a single PICU. Prior to this investigation, only data on adult MODS were available in the literature. Reported incidences for SIRS (82%), sepsis (21%–23%), MODS (11%–27%), severe sepsis (4%), and septic shock (2%) indicate that SIRS occurs more frequently than any other diagnostic category in PICUs.[4,6,9,17–20] In addition, mortality rates of pediatric patients with MODS and a specific diagnostic category reveal interesting findings. Reported mortality rates are 52% for patients with MODS and septic shock, 40% for patients with MODS and severe sepsis, 25% for MODS and SIRS, and 12% for MODS without SIRS.[17] Table 97–1 provides comparisons of the different epidemiologic studies in children with MODS.

MODS can be defined as simultaneous occurrence of two or more organ dysfunctions.[21] Organ systems typically included in the diagnostic criteria of pediatric MODS are cardiovascular, pulmonary, neurologic, hematologic, renal, hepatic, and gastrointestinal. Among all reports on pediatric MODS, two did not include hepatic and gastrointestinal organ system failures in the diagnostic criteria.[17,19] However, hepatic and gastrointestinal organ system failures were included in subsequent reports defining organ dysfunction in children. Currently used diagnostic criteria for pediatric MODS are displayed in Table 97–3.[21] Most commonly noted organ dysfunctions in children are dysfunctions involving respiratory, cardiovascular, and neurologic systems.[6,19] Hepatic and gastrointestinal dysfunctions were reported least frequently.[6] A very low frequency of gastrointestinal hemorrhage, which is one of the criteria for gastrointestinal system failure in MODS diagnostic criteria, was reported in children admitted to PICUs.[22] However, involvement of hepatic and gastrointestinal organ dysfunction was associated with greater mortality. Unfortunately, among existing MODS diagnostic criteria, none defines immune system dysfunction, although acquired immunodeficiency and/or immunologic dissonance[23] likely play a major role in the development and progression of MODS.

Proulx et al.[17] reported timing of onset of organ failure, MODS diagnosis, and subsequent death in children. Maximum number of organ failures occurred within 72 hours of admission to the PICU in 87% of patients, and diagnostic criteria for MODS were met on the day of admission in 86% of patients. Unlike adults, occurrence of sequential MODS in children is rare (1%).[24] These data suggest that the insult leading to MODS occurs mainly before PICU admission. Most MODS-associated deaths (88.4%) occurred within 7 days after diagnosis of MODS. Multivariate analysis identified three independent risk factors for death in pediatric MODS: maximum number of simultaneous organ system failures during PICU stay (OR55.9); age 12 months or younger (OR17.1), and Pediatric Risk of Mortality (PRISM) score on day of admission (OR1.25).[17]

TABLE 97–3

Diagnostic Criteria for Pediatric Multiple Organ Dysfunction Syndrome (MODS)[21]

CARDIOVASCULAR SYSTEM

1. Systolic BP < 40 mmHg (if age < 1 year) or < 50 mmHg (if age ≥ 1 year)
2. HR < 50 beats/min or > 220 beats/min (if age < 1 year) or < 40 beats/min or > 200 beats/min (if age ≥ 1 year)
3. Cardiac arrest
4. Serum pH < 7.2 with a normal PaO_2 value
5. Intravenous infusion of inotropic agents (excluding dopamine ≤ 5 mg/kg/min)

RESPIRATORY SYSTEM

1. RR > 90 breaths/minute (if age < 1 year) or > 70 breaths/min (if age =1 year)
2. $PaCO_2$ > 65 mmHg (8.7 kPa)
3. $PaCO_2$ < 40 mmHg (5.3 kPa) in the absence of cyanotic congenital heart disease
4. Mechanical ventilation (for > 24 hours in a postoperative patient)
5. PaO_2/FIO_2 < 200 in the absence of cyanotic congenital heart disease

NEUROLOGIC SYSTEM

1. Glasgow coma score < 5
2. Fixed dilated pupils

HEMATOLOGIC SYSTEM

1. Hemoglobin level < 50 g/L (< 5 g/dl)
2. White blood cell count < 3 × 10^9/L (< 3000 cells/μl)
3. Platelet count < 20 × 10^9/L (< 20,000 platelets/μl)
4. D-Dimer > 0.5 mg/ml with prothrombin time > 20 seconds or thromboplastin time > 60 seconds

RENAL SYSTEM

1. Serum urea nitrogen ≥ 36 mmol/L (≥ 100 mg/dl)
2. Serum creatinine ≥ 177 mmol/L (> 2.0 mg/dl) without preexisting renal disease
3. Dialysis

HEPATIC SYSTEM

1. Total bilirubin > 60 mmol/L (> 3 mg/dl)

GASTROINTESTINAL SYSTEM

1. Gastroduodenal bleeding and one of the following criteria:
   - A. Drop in hemoglobin level ≥ 20 g/L (≥ 2 g/dl), or
   - B. Blood transfusion, or
   - C. Hypotension with blood pressure < 3rd percentile for age, or
   - D. Gastric or duodenal surgery, or
   - E. Death

BP, blood pressure; *HR,* heart rate; *RR,* respiratory rate.

Discussion of pediatric primary versus secondary MODS was first reported in 1996.[18] *Primary MODS* was defined as the occurrence of two simultaneous organ dysfunctions within the first week after PICU admission, without subsequent evidence of sequential organ dysfunction. *Secondary MODS* was defined as one of the following: (1) appearance of MODS more than 7 days after admission to PICU, or (2) diagnosis of MODS 7 days or less after PICU admission, with subsequent sequential organ dysfunctions defined as an interval longer than 72 hours between time of MODS diagnosis onset and attainment of maximum number of simultaneous organ dysfunctions. Interestingly, patients having secondary MODS had higher mortality rates (74% vs. 30%), longer duration of MODS (10.9 ± 11.6 days vs. 3.6 ± 3.7 days), longer duration of PICU stay (24.6 ± 24.0 days vs. 7.9 ± 14.2 days), and worse PRISM scores (26.1 ± 14.7 vs. 20.1 ± 13) compared with patients having primary MODS.[18] Incidence of secondary MODS was lower than primary MODS (12% vs. 88%), and the risk of mortality was 6.5 times higher among children with secondary MODS. Primary MODS is considered the direct result of a well-defined insult in which organ dysfunctions occur early and can be attributed to the insult itself. However, secondary MODS may be the consequence of the host's response and is defined in the context of SIRS.[23,25]

Mortality rates for pediatric patients with MODS increase with increasing number of organ system failures.[4,6,9,17,18] Reported mortality rates for two, three, or four or more organ system failures are outlined in Table 97–1. As noted in Wilkinson's original report on pediatric MODS (but not substantiated in several subsequent studies), mortality rates for MODS patients who had two, three, or four or more organ failures were not related to the presence or absence of sepsis.[19] Similarly, there was no significant difference in mortality between medical and surgical patients in one-, two-, or four-organ system failure groups; however, there was a significant difference in the three-organ system failure groups.[19] Most children simultaneously developed the maximum number of organ system failures.

MODS was first described almost 20 years ago in adults admitted to ICUs with ruptured aortic aneurisms.[26] Incidence of MODS in adults reportedly ranges from 8% to 38%.[27,28] Unlike children, sepsis was the reported predominant trigger for adult MODS and was associated with high mortality rates.[5,29] Incidence of MODS is higher in adults with sepsis (70%)[30] than in children (47%).[4] Adult trauma and surgical patients with sepsis and extensive tissue damage (burns) or who have undergone emergency laparotomies for peritonitis or abscess drainage had the highest mortality. Infections sites are different in adult versus pediatric MODS. Less than 5% of pediatric patients admitted to PICUs had emergency abdominal surgeries or multiple trauma.[4] Typically respiratory and central nervous system infections are associated with pediatric MODS. Overall mortality in adult MODS patients ranges from 56% in young polytrauma victims to 98% in patients with extensive burns.[5,31] These numbers indicate that adults die more frequently with MODS compared with children. Interestingly, organ failures in adults typically occur sequentially over days to weeks, leading to late onset of maximum organ failure number.[32] The higher incidence of secondary MODS in adults compared with children may account for the differences in mortality. In addition, investigations examining adult MODS suggest that the mechanisms causing MODS differ fundamentally from those involved in pediatric MODS.

Illness Severity versus Organ Dysfunction Scoring Systems

Two main types of scoring systems have been developed for use in the ICU: those primarily focusing on survival (single endpoint) and those focusing on morbidity (organ dysfunction scores) (see Chapter 7). In order to provide accurate information, these scoring systems must be validated for use among different patient populations, and the scores must demonstrate good calibration, discrimination, reproducibility, and transportability across geographic, time, and methodologic boundaries.[33]

Illness severity scoring systems have been developed for quantifying severity of illness (in neonatal, pediatric, and adult populations) at the time of ICU admission or within the first 24 hours after admission. These scores are used to estimate the probability of mortality.[34–36] They generally have not been developed for repeated use at subsequent time points during a patient's ICU stay. ICU admission scoring systems are used to measure performance (risk-adjusted mortality and risk-adjusted length of stay), to study ICU resource utilization and management, and to control for severity of illness in clinical trials[34–37] (see Chapter 7). An objective approach to defining and quantifying severity of illness uses development of probability models predicting mortality risk. One of the most commonly used tools of illness severity in children is the Pediatric Risk of Mortality score III (PRISM III), which is a third-generation illness severity score developed by Pollack et al.[35–37] This score was developed and initially validated on a sample of 11,165 (543 deaths) admissions to 32 PICUs and used 17 physiologic variables subdivided into 26 ranges on the basis of the first 24 hours of care. The variables most predictive of mortality were stupor/coma, abnormal pupillary reflexes, and minimum systolic blood pressure.[35] Illness severity scores used in adults include acute physiology and chronic health evaluation (Acute Physiology and Chronic Health Evaluation [APACHE]),[34] Simplified Acute Physiology Score (SAPS),[38] and Mortality Probability Models (MPM).[39]

However, mortality alone is considered insufficient for assessing ICU efficiency or conducting clinical trials. Hence analysis of morbidity is important.[40,41] This notion is especially relevant for children because the death rate in PICUs is substantially lower than the rate in adult ICUs (≈6% vs. 20%).[34,35,42] Thus the low death rate in PICUs enormously increases the sample size required for clinical trials using mortality as an endpoint. Incidence of MODS (11%–27%) is much more frequent than death in PICUs. Accordingly, a score that estimates the severity of MODS would be an additional key outcome measure in critically ill children.

Alternative scoring systems have been developed, not to predict outcome but to describe complications in ICU patients. Such systems quantify organ dysfunction (OD) on the basis of objective criteria of severity.[43,44] As mortality is tightly linked to MODS,[4,9,18,19,43–45] and prevalence of MODS in PICUs ranges from 11% to 27%,[4,17–19,21] MODS scores may represent a good alternative outcome as a surrogate for death in clinical trials. These scores may allow evaluation of efficacy of innovative ICU therapies with smaller sample sizes compared with investigations where survival is used as the primary outcome.[21,44,45] MODS scoring systems were developed as outcome measures rather than predictive indexes. In developing organ function scores, three important principles deserve consideration.[43] First, organ dysfunction reflects a spectrum, which may range from mild altered function to overt organ failure. Second, the degree of organ dysfunction may vary with time during the course of the disease, and scores need to be calculated longitudinally in order to evaluate patients in a timely manner. Third, objective, simple, reliable, and readily available variables must be chosen that are specific to the organ in question and are independent of other patient variables. Scores ideally should be independent of therapeutic variables, but this is practically impossible to achieve. For instance, oxygenation assessed by the PaO_2/FIO_2 ratio is dependent on mean airway pressure. Similarly, hematocrit level may be influenced by erythrocyte transfusions.

In 1995 a scoring system for MODS that could be used either on the first day of admission to the ICU or daily afterward was developed by a literature review of clinical studies of multiple organ failure from 1969 to 1993. The system was validated by Marshall et al.[45] in critically ill adults. Best possible descriptors of organ dysfunction were identified and validated against a clinical database. Six organ systems were chosen, and a score from 0 to 4 was selected for each organ according to function (where 0 is normal function and 4 is most severe dysfunction), with a maximum score of 24. This score is termed the *Multiple Organ Dysfunction Scoring System*. When applied on the first day of ICU admission as a prognostic indicator, and when calculated over the subsequent ICU stay as an outcome measure, the score correlated with the ICU mortality rate. In addition, it showed excellent discrimination, as reflected in the area under the receiver operating characteristic (ROC) curve of 0.936 in the development set and 0.928 in the validation set.

Logistic Organ Dysfunction System

The *Logistic Organ Dysfunction System* (LODS) score was developed in 1996 by Le Gall et al.[44] using logistic regression techniques to determine severity levels and relative weights for LODS score and for conversion of the LODS score to a probability of mortality. To calculate the score, each organ system received points according to the worst value for any variable for that system on that day. Organ dysfunction severity was scored from 0 to 5 (where 0 is no organ dysfunction and 5 is maximum organ dysfunction). Resulting LODS scores ranged from 0 to 22. This score was designed to be used during the first 24 hours of ICU admission rather than as a repeated assessment measure. Model calibration was very good in the developmental and validation samples ($p = 0.021$ and $p = 0.050$, respectively), as was model discrimination (area under the ROC curves of 0.843 and 0.850, respectively).

In 1999 Leteurtre et al.[46] used the aforementioned adult strategies to develop two MODS scoring systems for children. The *Pediatric Multiple Organ Dysfunction* (PEMOD) system was derived using the method developed by Marshall et al.[45] All variables were identified from published clinical studies of MODS and evaluated against a set of criteria established to describe the ideal descriptor of organ dysfunction. The *Pediatric Logistic Organ Dysfunction* (PELOD) system was derived from the approach developed by Le Gall et al.[44] For each of the six organ systems, the PEMOD system included one variable and the PELOD system included several variables. Severity levels and relative weights or organ dysfunctions were determined according to the mortality rate (PEMOD) or logistic regression (PELOD). For this study, 594 pediatric admissions, including 51 deaths (9%), were analyzed.[46] The PELOD system was more discriminant than the PEMOD system (areas under the ROC curves 0.98 and 0.92, respectively, $p < 0.05$). Moreover, with the PEMOD system, four organ dysfunctions did not contribute significantly to prediction of PICU outcome. The PELOD system was more discriminant and had the advantage of taking into account both the relative severities among all organ dysfunctions and the degree of severity of each organ dysfunction.

With the purpose of validating the PELOD system (Table 97–4), 1806 consecutive patients (median age 24 months) from seven multidisciplinary tertiary-care PICUs were enrolled into a prospective, observational, multicenter cohort study.[47] The PELOD score, which includes six organ systems (excluding gastrointestinal system) and 12 variables, was recorded daily. For each variable, the most abnormal value recorded each day and during the whole stay was used to calculate the daily Pediatric Logistic Organ Dysfunction (dPELOD) score and the PELOD score, respectively. Results indicated that the PELOD score was significantly higher in nonsurvivors than survivors (mean 31 vs. 9.4, $p < 0.0001$). Calibration and discrimination (area under the ROC curve) scores were good. Accordingly, PELOD and dPELOD scores are valid outcome measures of the severity of MODS in critically ill children. Use of these scores as primary outcome measures could significantly reduce the sample size required to complete clinical trials in critically ill children. Currently the PELOD score is the only validated MODS scoring system used in children.

Pathophysiology

Because MODS represents the most common cause of death in ICUs, considerable research effort is directed toward understanding its complex pathophysiology. Classic views of MODS pathophysiology originated in the mediator hypothesis (uncontrolled inflammation from macrophage activation), the gut origin hypothesis (loss of gut barrier function resulting in bacterial and toxin translocation), and the ischemia/reperfusion hypothesis (microcirculatory alterations associated with widespread endotheliopathy).[48,49] A two-hit model involving multiple, modest sequential insults was suggested. More recently the importance of inflammation-driven (e.g., interleukin [IL]-6, IL-1) protein catabolism and cytopathic hypoxia in MODS has been invoked.[50]

Surviving MODS likely involves reestablishing a balance between SIRS (associated with inflammatory autoinjury) and compensatory antiinflammatory response syndrome (associated with secondary infection from acquired immunodeficiency)[23] (Figure 97–1). Interactions involved in this balance are complex, redundant, networked, dynamic, and increasingly recognized to be genetically influenced.[51,52] Rather than the two-dimensional "teeter-totter" interplay model, elements of the inflammation/immunology system are better described as a resonating community of steel balls and springs, all interconnected.[53] Neural, endocrine, and inflammatory mediator servocommunications promote oscillator variability in healthy biologic systems. Uncoupling, loss of variability, and decomplexification are

TABLE 97–4

Pediatric Logistic Organ Dysfunction (PELOD) Scoring System[46,47]

Organ Dysfunction and Variable	Scoring values 0	1	10	20
Neurologic*				
Glasgow coma score	12–15	7–11	4–6	3
	and		**or**	
Pupillary reactions	Both reactive	NA	Both fixed	NA
Cardiovascular†				
Heart rate (beats/min)				
< 12 years	≤ 195	NA	> 195	NA
≥ 12 years	≤ 150	NA	> 150	NA
	and		**or**	
Systolic blood pressure (mmHg)				
< 1 month	> 65	NA	35–65	<35
1 month–1 year‡	> 75	NA	35–75	<35
1–12 years‡	> 85	NA	45–85	<45
≥ 12 years	> 95	NA	55–95	<55
Renal				
Creatinine (μmol/L)				
< 7 days	< 140	NA	≥ 140	NA
7 days–1 year‡	< 55	NA	≥ 55	NA
1–12 years‡	< 100	NA	≥ 100	NA
≥ 12 years	< 140	NA	≥ 140	NA
Respiratory§				
PaO_2 (kPa)/FIO_2	> 9.3	NA	≥ 9.3	NA
	and		**or**	
$PaCO_2$ (kPa)	≤ 11.7	NA	> 11.7	NA
	and			
Mechanical ventilation§	No	ventilation	NA	NA
Hematologic				
White blood cell count (×10⁹/L)	≥ 4.5	1.5–4.4	< 1.5	NA
	and			
Platelets (×10⁹/L)	≥ 35	< 35	NA	NA
Hepatic				
Aspartate transaminase (IU/L)	< 950	≥ 950	NA	NA
	and		**or**	
Prothrombin time¶ (IU/L)	> 60%	≥ 60%	NA	NA

FIO_2, Fraction of inspired oxygen; *PaO_2*, partial pressure of arterial oxygen; *$PaCO_2$*, partial pressure of arterial carbon dioxide.

*Glasgow coma score (GCS): Use lowest value. If patient is sedated, record estimated GCS before sedation. Assess patient only with known or suspected acute central nervous system disease. Pupillary reactions: Nonreactive pupils must be > 3 mm. Do not assess after iatrogenic pupillary dilation.

†Heart rate and systolic blood pressure: Do not assess during crying or iatrogenic agitation.

‡Strictly less than age indicate. PaO_2: Use arterial measurement only.

¶Percentage of activity.

§PaO_2/FIO_2 ratio, which cannot be assessed in patients with intracardiac shunts, is considered normal in children with cyanotic heart disease. $PaCO_2$ can be measured from arterial, capillary, or venous samples. Mechanical ventilation: Use of mask ventilation is not counted as mechanical ventilation.

associated with increasing illness severity and the downward spiral of MODS.[54–57]

Although numerous unifying hypotheses for the pathophysiology of MODS are proposed, one that appears to encompass most of the associated research is the vicious reciprocal cycle of ischemia/reperfusion and inflammation: literally, "one thing leads to another" (Figure 97–2). Contributing to this vicious cycle of MODS, which mediates so-called *collateral damage* associated with critical illness, is endothelial activation/injury, enhanced oxidant stress, altered apoptosis, and dysregulated coagulopathy. Each of these pathogenic processes contributes to, and is affected by, both ischemia/reperfusion and inflammation.

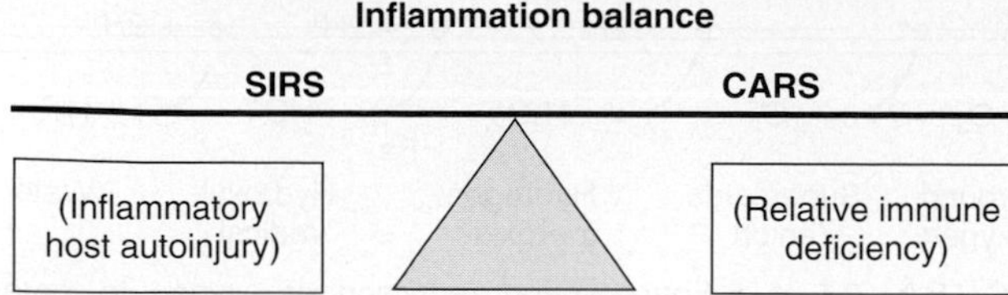

FIGURE 97–1 • Schematic concept of a balanced inflammatory response involving the systemic inflammatory response syndrome (SIRS) and the compensatory antiinflammatory response syndrome (CARS).

Endothelial Activation/Injury

In adults, the endothelial system comprises roughly 10^{13} cells and represents ≈1 kg of tissue and 4000 to 7000 m^2 of surface area. The interface between the circulating blood and various tissues is responsive to other cells, the extracellular matrix, hypoxemia, various mediators, as well as mechanical stress. Endothelia regulate vasomotor tone, cellular trafficking, angiogenesis, coagulation, and capillary permeability and in general act as a multifunctional biosensor as noted previously.[58]

A variety of insults, including decreased cardiac output, enhanced capillary leak, constricted arterioles, generalized vasoplegia, impaired erythrocyte, and leukocyte deformability, as well as an activated, procoagulant endothelial phenotype, can impair microcirculatory flow and accordingly affect endothelial behavior.[59] Inflammation is activated with ischemia through at least two distinct endothelial cellular signaling pathways. Decreased shear stress in the setting of ischemia leads to endothelial plasmalemma depolarization via a potassium adenosine triphosphatase (ATPase) channel. This event is subsequently associated with activation of endothelial NADPH oxidase, resulting in a shift toward a more oxidized intracellular environment that leads to activation of nuclear transcription factors such as nuclear factor NF-κB. In addition, cellular depolarization leads to activation of a voltage-dependent calcium channel that results in increased cellular calcium influx with resultant activation of nitric oxide synthase.[60] Impaired microcellular circulatory flow is further compromised in the postischemic state by intravascular hemoconcentration and thrombosis, swelling of endothelial cells, leukocyte and platelet aggregation, interstitial edema, impaired erythrocyte deformability, and enhanced expression of endothelial adherence proteins.[61] In summary, the endothelial response to ischemia/reperfusion is characterized by four major activities: vasomotor, coagulation, permeability, and inflammation.[62] Activation of the endothelial network results in altered barrier function involving cellular rounding, interendothelial gap formation, and enhanced vesicle-mediated transport[63] characterized clinically as diffuse capillary leak. Characteristics of the endothelial activated phenotype include expression of intercellular adhesion molecules (e.g., intercellular adhesion molecule-1), production of proinflammatory cytokines (e.g., IL-8), polymerization of actin stress fiber cytoskeleton, and switch to a procoagulant cell surface. Vascular endothelial damage associated with dysregulated coagulation and fibrinolysis is linked to thrombocytopenic MODS.[64]

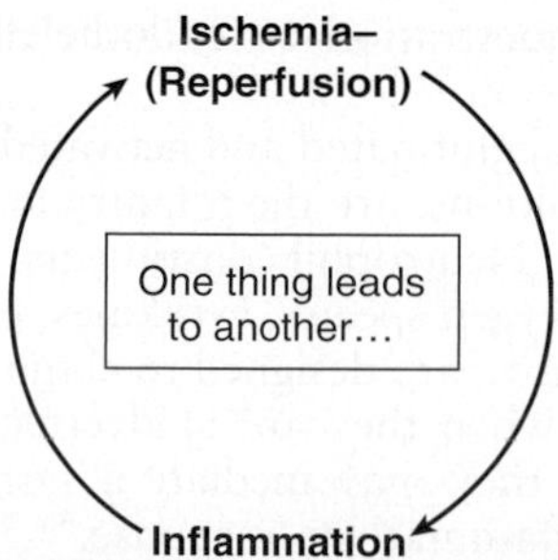

FIGURE 97–2 • Vicious reciprocal cycle of ischemia/reperfusion and inflammation as a unifying pathophysiology for multiple organ dysfunction syndrome.

An example of a clinical correlation relating ischemia with activation of inflammation has been ascertained with gastric tonometry examining the relationship between gastric mucosal acidosis and cytokine release in patients with septic shock. As the P_{CO_2} gap increased (a relative measure of gastric endothelial ischemia), local production of tumor necrosis factor (TNF)-α correspondingly increased (Spearman correlation coefficient 0.94).[65]

Enhanced Oxidant Stress

Enhanced oxidative stress induces multiple alterations of cellular physiology, including inhibition of cell membrane Na/K-ATPase, mobilization of intracellular calcium, alteration of cellular shape, modification of cellular differentiation, oxidation of macromolecules (i.e., many enzymes are inactivated by enhanced oxidant stress), and promotion of cellular necrosis and apoptosis.[66] Sources for increased production of the parent oxy-radical species, superoxide anion are multiple, but four primary sources are electron bleed from the mitochondrial electron transport chain, xanthine oxidase, eicosanoid metabolism, and respiratory burst of activated phagocytes. NAD(P)H oxidases responsible for generation of superoxide anion have been identified in endothelial cells, platelets, and phagocytes.[67–70] For example, platelet-derived microparticles isolated from septic patients contain NADPH oxidase cytochrome b_{558}, generate superoxide anion, and promote induction of vascular endothelial and smooth muscle apoptosis.[70]

In addition to superoxide anion, the other parent oxidative species is nitric oxide. At least four nitric oxide synthases (NOS) have been identified. They are constitutive NOS, which is found in endothelial cells and associated with beat-to-beat regulation of blood pressure; neuronal NOS, which is responsible for synthesis of nitric oxide as a central nervous system signaling molecule; inducible NOS, which is prominent in inflammatory states such as severe sepsis; and a mitochondrial NOS, which may be important in regulation of respiration, including cytopathic hypoxia.[71,72] Nitric oxide is synthesized from arginine and oxygen with NADPH, tetrahydrobioptrim, and FMN/FAD as cofactors for the oxidoreductase enzyme. Nitric oxide and superoxide may condense with diffusion-limited kinetics (≈2×10^{10} M^{-1} s^{-1}) to form peroxynitrite. Peroxynitrite is an extremely reactive oxidant compound[73,74] that likely plays a role in activating the polyadenosine diphosphate (ADP)-ribose synthase pathway, leading to polyadenylation of injured deoxyribonucleic acid (DNA) with the potential for depletion of cellular NADH and ATP.[75,76]

In general, enhanced oxidant stress with nitric oxide leads to a vasodilated state. On the other hand, enhanced oxidant stress with superoxide as the parent species generally results in vasoconstriction mediated by inactivation of nitric oxide, inhibition of prostacyclin synthesis, oxidative injury of endothelial cells, and induction of chemokine synthesis.[77] Accordingly, enhanced superoxide production in the setting of inflammation is expected to facilitate ischemia.

Particularly in the setting of ischemia/reperfusion, xanthine oxidase is an important source of increased superoxide anion production (Figure 97–3).[78] During ischemia, high-energy phosphate bonds are successively hydrolyzed, with resultant accumulation of adenosine, inosine, and hypoxanthine. Simultaneously, during ischemia, cellular xanthine dehydrogenase is converted to xanthine oxidase. The resultant enzyme preferentially utilizes oxygen as an electron acceptor instead of NAD. With reintroduction of oxygen into the system with reperfusion, the stage is set for a burst of superoxide anion production because of accumulation of hypoxanthine substrate. More recently, xanthine oxidase has been established to be a peroxynitrite synthase with nitric oxide generated at the molybdenum site of the enzyme from nitrite, whereas superoxide is generated at the FAD prosthetic site of the enzyme.[79] Xanthine oxidase is widely distributed in the endothelial network, particularly along the splanchnic circulation, which is at particular risk for ischemia (and hence xanthine oxidase activation) during systemic low-flow states. Release of xanthine oxidase from splanchnic endothelia has been demonstrated to mediate distal pulmonary injury.[80]

Nitric oxide induces the transcription of heme oxygenase, which enhances metabolism of heme to free iron, biliverdin, and carbon monoxide. Free iron induces the transcription of ferritin to sequester iron; bilirubin acts as an antioxidant; and carbon monoxide mediates vasodilation in a manner analogous to nitric oxide.[81]

Mitochondria permit controlled four-electron reduction of ground state oxygen to water (Figure 97–4) (see Chapter 67). Under normal circumstances, approximately 1% to 2% of this electron flow terminates in

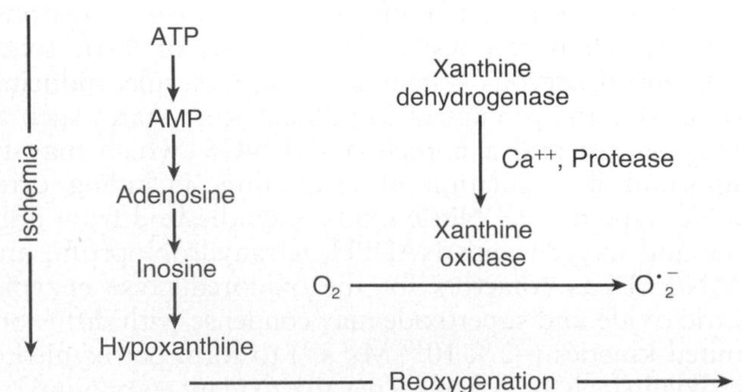

FIGURE 97–3 • Generation of superoxide anion from xanthine oxidase during ischemia reperfusion.

$$O_2 \xrightarrow{e^-} O_2^{\cdot -} \xrightarrow{e^- + 2H^+} H_2O_2 \xrightarrow[Fe]{e^- + 2H^+} HO^{\cdot} \xrightarrow{e^- + 2H^+} H_2O$$

Ground oxygen — Superoxide anion — Hydrogen peroxide — Hydroxyl radical — Water

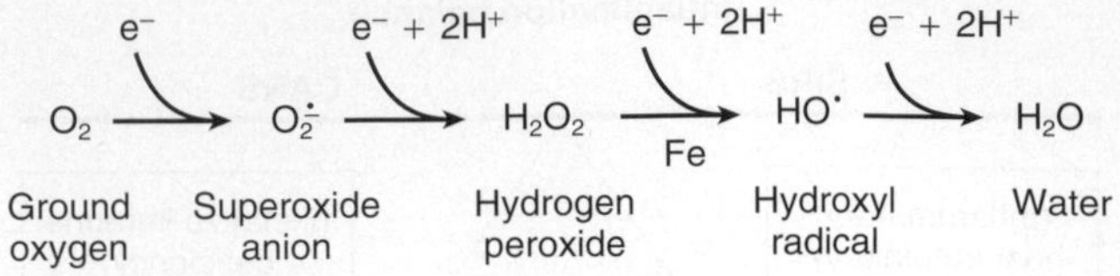

FIGURE 97–4 • Four-electron reduction of oxygen to water. Incomplete reduction leads to generation of incompletely reduced, toxic oxygen species.

superoxide anion. However, under severe cellular stress states such as sepsis, the proportion of incompletely reduced oxygen can increase significantly, resulting in increased mitochondrial oxidant stress, with the potential for impaired respiration.[82,83] Cellular dysoxia may occur through stagnant (low blood flow), hypoxic (low hemoglobin saturation), anemic (low hemoglobin level), or cytopathic mechanisms. Haldane elegantly noted that tissue hypoxia, resulting from any of these mechanisms, not only stops the mitochondrial machine (i.e., impaired use of oxygen) but also destroys the mitochondrial machinery (i.e., subsequent impairment of phosphorylation). Mechanisms for cytopathic hypoxia may involve alterations in pyruvate dehydrogenase, activation of poly ADP-ribose synthase, competition of nitric oxide with oxygen for cytochrome oxidase, oxidation of mitochondrial DNA proteins, and increased mitochondrial permeability transition.[84] Abnormal permeability of the inner and outer mitochondrial membrane has been demonstrated during endotoxemia. Accordingly, in experimental models mimicking severe sepsis, enhanced high-amplitude mitochondrial swelling, altered respiratory function, increased mitochondrial permeability transition, elevated mitochondrial Bax and ceramides, and increased outer membrane permeability to cytochrome *c* have been demonstrated.[85,86]

Another important source of enhanced oxidant stress associated with MODS is the activated phagocyte, particularly neutrophils.[87] In the setting of ischemia/reperfusion, enhanced oxidant production (e.g., by xanthine oxidase) leads to subsequent increased production of inflammatory mediators, which result in increased production of neutrophil adhesion molecules.[80,88] As noted previously, enhanced endothelial oxidants are also associated with increased nuclear transcription factor translocation, such as NF-κB and AP-1, which facilitate increased endothelial adhesion molecule expression. In combination, such events lead to leukosequestration on endothelial cells following ischemia/reperfusion.[89]

Neutrophils, agglutinated and activated under ischemia/reperfusion conditions, are the infantry arm of the inflammatory response. Neutrophil constituents, including a variety of reactive oxygen species, cytokines, proteases, lipases, and phospholipases, are designed to eliminate foreign antigens. However, when they are inadvertently released into the host milieu, they may mediate a systemic, as well as a localized, inflammatory response.[90,91] The activated neutrophil generates increased production of superoxide anion[87] (via NADPH oxidoreductase) and hydrogen peroxide and releases myeloperoxidase. This latter heme-containing enzyme, which comprises approximately 5%

of the dry weight of neutrophils, catalyzes the production of hypochlorous acid (HClO) from hydrogen peroxide and chloride.[92] Hypochlorous acid, essentially chlorine bleach, is highly effective as a bactericidal agent, but it also can mediate host autoinjury. For example, hypochlorous acid can inactivate a critical methionine on α_1 anti-protease. Without adequate inhibition from α_1 anti-protease, elastase also released by the activated neutrophil can mediate unmitigated proteolytic damage. Accordingly, neutrophil oxidative stress can be associated with localized enhanced proteolytic stress.[93] Activity of platelet-activating factor acetylhydrolase, another neutrophil enzyme, is decreased in postinjury-associated MODS,[94] which tends to promote and perpetuate a proinflammatory state.

A key example of neutrophil involvement in MODS is reflected in the pathophysiology of acute respiratory distress syndrome (ARDS).[95,96] In this clinical scenario, inflammation in the lung generated by activated neutrophils can drive a systemic inflammatory response. Conversely, a systemic inflammatory response such as bacterial peritonitis can facilitate the onset of ARDS. In addition to its direct role in mediating necrotic cell death (with oxidants, proteases, and lipases), neutrophils can direct apoptosis within the lung during ARDS. Inflammatory mediators, such as IL-8, thromboxane A_2, and endotoxin, may activate neutrophils to increase production and release of Fas ligand. Subsequently, Fas ligand may bind to both endothelial and epithelial receptors in the lung to increase Fas-mediated apoptosis.[97] Moreover, constitutive neutrophil apoptosis can be inhibited by microbial products, IL-1β, granulocyte macrophage colony-stimulating factor, TNF-α, and IL-8.[98–101]

Altered Apoptosis

Enhanced oxidant stress has been clearly shown to initiate apoptosis. In cell culture models, pulmonary artery endothelial cells exposed to 0.25 μm hydrogen peroxide for 24 hours increase their level of apoptosis eightfold compared with control cells exposed to culture media only.[102] A variety of investigations implicate the importance of altered apoptosis in clinical illness. Early lymphocyte apoptosis is associated with poor outcome in human sepsis.[103–105] Enhanced soluble Fas and soluble Fas ligand are correlated with adult and pediatric sepsis-induced MODS.[106,107] Elevated nucleosome levels reflecting an endproduct of apoptosis have been demonstrated in human systemic inflammation in sepsis.[108] Regulation of Fas ligand expression has been described during systemic inflammation.[109] In addition, the perforin/granzyme apoptotic pathway appears to be operative.[110] Although evidence indicates enhanced lymphocyte apoptosis is associated with MODS, delayed constitutive neutrophil[98–101] and macrophage[111] apoptosis are described and, as noted previously, may be mediated by microbial products, host-derived mediators, common inhibitor of apoptosis proteins, and various physiologic processes.[112]

Altered Coagulation

Virchow's classic tissue infarction triad includes low blood flow, a hypercoagulable state, and endothelial cell activation and injury, and it essentially is very early recognition of the critical relationship between ischemia/reperfusion and inflammation. The activated endothelium exhibits a procoagulant state relative to the anticoagulant phenotype of the quiescent endothelial cell[113] (Table 97–5). Abnormal microvascular blood flow was elegantly demonstrated using orthogonal polarization spectral imaging in patients with sepsis.[114] This clinical investigation indicated decreased vascular density, particularly among small vessels, increased nonperfused and intermittently perfused small vessels, and marked heterogeneity in vessel perfusion in septic patients compared with normal volunteers. Moreover, the alterations were more severe in nonsurvivors. The abnormalities were reversible with topical acetylcholine. In addition to low blood flow facilitating coagulation, impaired erythrocyte deformability is operative. In patients with sepsis, this physical/chemical alteration of the erythrocyte membrane is thought to occur as a result of oxidant injury of membrane lipid and intracellular proteins and direct binding and incorporation of endotoxin into the erythrocyte membrane.[115] Although thrombin plays a paramount role in catalyzing formation of the fibrin clot (to stop bleeding and sequester/contain infection but enhance ischemia), thrombin also displays a number of proinflammatory activities, such as binding to protease-activated receptors, up-regulating tissue factor expression, increasing expression of IL-6 and IL-8, enhancing production of E-selectin and P-selectin, and inducing platelet-activating factor expression. Activated protein C exhibits a number of actions along the coagulation cascade, including inactivation of tissue factor VIIa, tissue factor Va, and plasminogen activator inhibitor-1, stimulation of fibrinolysis, and prevention of tissue-associated factor inhibitor (TAFI) activation. However, protein C also reduces neutrophil rolling, and hence endothelial adherence, to modulate of NF-κB activity and inhibit apoptosis.[116]

For children with MODS, the importance of uncontrolled, persistent inflammation from unrecognized infection in promoting thrombosis, thrombocytopenia, and bleeding (thrombotic microangiopathy) has been emphasized.[117] In general, abnormal coagulation regulation in patients with MODS fosters a persistent procoagulant/antifibrinolytic state that

TABLE 97–5

Quiescent versus Activated Endothelium

Anticoagulant	→	Procoagulant
• Thrombomodulin		• Adhesion molecules
• Proteins S and C		• Inflammatory mediators
• Proteoglycans		• Endothelin
• Tissue plasminogen activator		• Tissue factor
• Prostacyclin, nitric oxide		• Protease-activated receptors
• Adenosine diphosphatase		• Phospholipid microparticles
• Antithrombin–III		• Plasminogen activator inhibitor (type 1) (PAI-1)

Hack CE, Zeeleder S: *Crit Care Med* 29(suppl):S21-S27, 2001.

results in microvascular thrombosis, tissue ischemia, and organ hypoperfusion.[118]

Practical Treatment Guidelines for Multiple Organ Dysfunction Syndrome

On the basis of the complex pathophysiology of MODS, no "magic bullet" interventions are available to prevent or treat MODS. However, practice of currently available evidence-based critical care medicine suggests several practical approaches to interrupt the vicious cycle of ischemia/reperfusion and inflammation that is central to the genesis and propagation of MODS. In terms of maneuvers for limiting ischemia/reperfusion activation of inflammation, early resuscitation of shock is essential in both pediatric and adult populations.[119–122] Worse outcome for pediatric patients is demonstrated with inadequate, untimely resuscitation from septic shock.[119,121] On the other hand, goal-directed therapy to normalize oxygen delivery and consumption provides a strong survival benefit in adult patients with early sepsis.[122] Although erythrocyte transfusion may play a key role in goal-directed therapy to restore oxygen delivery, the ideal transfusion threshold is uncertain, as blood transfusion is an independent risk factor for MODS and mortality.[123]

In terms of reducing the stimulus of inflammation that perpetuates ischemia/reperfusion, pediatric MODS is associated with evidence of systemic inflammation.[124–127] However, a number of critical interventions now are available to the intensivists to address this MODS-associated proinflammatory state. Activated protein C (Xigris) reduces relative mortality in adult sepsis by 19.4%,[128] an effect associated with reduced organ dysfunction.[129] As noted previously, activated protein C has a multitude of antiinflammatory actions in addition to its propensity to decrease ischemia. Similarly, stress dose steroids provide a survival benefit in adult patients with septic shock.[130] Such intervention decreases length of hemodynamic support, mechanical ventilation support, and ICU and hospital stay. Steroids modulate virtually every aspect of the inflammatory response,[131,132] and these antiinflammatory effects are documented in septic patients demonstrating a clinical benefit from stress dose steroids.[133] By using lower tidal volumes that result in less alveolar stretch and accordingly less induction of a proinflammatory pulmonary response (biotrauma), mortality associated with ARDS is reduced.[134] Strict glycemic control in adult patients significantly improved outcome in a large cohort of adult surgical patients, with the main benefit related to a decreased incidence of sepsis and MODS in the strict glycemic control group.[135] Hyperglycemia is associated with mortality in adult medical ICU patients (OR 2.6, $p = 0.009$) and is correlated to elevated serum IL-6 levels.[136] Insulin mediates a number of antiinflammatory activities.[137]

In the absence of evidence-based medicine approaches to reduce SIRS in pediatric patients with MODS, at least four PICU commonsense approaches limit inflammation and ischemia/reperfusion. These measures include (1) ensure adequate cardiac output and treat shock states early and aggressively; (2) treat infections early with appropriate antibiotics and resect foci of infected/necrotic tissue as appropriate; (3) resolve/avoid metabolic acidosis, and (4) eliminate medical errors. Several clinical "red flags" should alert the intensivist to the risk for development and/or progression of MODS (Table 97–6).[138,139] In the usual tradition of pediatric medicine, prevention strategies for MODS are the best treatment approach (Table 97–7).[138,139]

Poets and philosophers have noted that all things are connected. This includes not only stars of the universe but also molecules in an individual. Therefore it is not

TABLE 97–6

Clinical "Red Flags" Suggesting Risk for Development and/or Progression of Multiple Organ Dysfunction Syndrome (MODS)

- Extremes of age
- Chronic disease
- Malnutrition
- Head injury
- Coma
- Immunodeficiency
- Fever of undetermined origin
- Ongoing hemorrhage, shock
- Sepsis
- Transfusion
- High illness severity score
- Persistent lactic acidosis
- Prolonged cardiac arrest circulatory arrest, aortic cross-clamp
- Infected or necrotic tissue

TABLE 97–7

Prevention Strategies to Prevent, Minimize, or Resolve Multiple Organ Dysfunction Syndrome (MODS)

- Promote trauma centers, other centers of excellence
- Prescribe stress bleeding prophylaxis
- Use open lung and permissive hypercapnia approach to mechanical ventilation
- Practice vigorous (goal-directed) initial resuscitation
- Prescribe deep venous thrombosis prophylaxis
- Provide early (enteral) nutrition
- Monitor for complications
- Minimize pain and anxiety
- Treat the underlying disease
- Support gun control, auto safety, smoking cessation
- Expect zero deficit/definitive surgery
- Prescribe early, appropriate antimicrobials
- Maintain strict glycemic control
- Excise infected/necrotic tissue
- Eliminate iatrogenic complications

surprising that events favoring ischemia/reperfusion foster inflammation and vice versa. Using any intervention to interrupt the vicious cycle of this MODS vortex seemingly would be beneficial for the critically ill patient.

REFERENCES

1. DuPont HL SW: Infections due to gram-negative organism: an analysis of 860 patients with bacteremia at University of Minnesota Medical Center. *Medicine (Baltimore)* 48:307, 1968.
2. Pollard AJ, Britto J, Nadel S, et al: Emergency management of meningococcal disease. *Arch Dis Child* 80:290-296, 1999.
3. Carcillo JA: Pediatric septic shock and multiple organ failure. *Crit Care Clin* 19:413-440, 2003.
4. Wilkinson JD, Pollack MM, Glass NL, et al: Mortality associated with multiple organ system failure and sepsis in pediatric intensive care unit. *J Pediatr* 111:324-328, 1987.
5. Bell RC, Coalson JJ, Smith JD, et al: Multiple organ system failure and infection in adult respiratory distress syndrome. *Ann Intern Med* 99:293-298, 1983.
6. Tantalean JA, Leon RJ, Santos AA, et al: Multiple organ dysfunction syndrome in children. *Pediatr Crit Care Med* 4:181-185, 2003.
7. Chandra RK: Nutrition and immunology: from the clinic to cellular biology and back again. *Proc Nutr Soc* 58:681-683, 1999.
8. Scrimshaw NS, San Giovanni JP: Synergism of nutrition, infection, and immunity: an overview. *Am J Clin Nutr* 66:464S-477S, 1997.
9. Kutko MC, Calarco MP, Flaherty MB, et al: Mortality rates in pediatric septic shock with and without multiple organ system failure. *Pediatr Crit Care Med* 4:333-337, 2003.
10. Duke TD, Butt W, South M: Predictors of mortality and multiple organ failure in children with sepsis. *Intensive Care Med* 23:684-692, 1997.
11. Watson RS, Carcillo JA, Linde-Zwirble WT, et al: The epidemiology of severe sepsis in children in the United States. *Am J Respir Crit Care Med* 167:695-701, 2003.
12. Bone RC, Balk RA, Cerra FB, et al: Definitions for sepsis and organ system failure and guidelines for the use of innovative therapies in sepsis. The ACCP/SCCM Consensus Conference Committee. American College of Chest Physicians/Society of Critical Care Medicine. *Chest* 101:1644-1655, 1992.
13. Hayden WR: Sepsis and organ failure definitions and guidelines. *Crit Care Med* 21:1612-1613, 1993 (letter).
14. Goldstein B, Giroir B, Randolph A: International Consensus Conference Panel. International pediatric severe sepsis consensus conference: definitions for sepsis and organ dysfunction in pediatrics. *Pediatr Crit Care Med* 6:2-8, 2005.
15. Dellinger RP, Carlet JM, Masur H, et al: Surviving Sepsis Campaign guidelines for management of severe sepsis and septic shock. *Crit Care Med* 32:858-871, 2004.
16. Levy MM, Fink MP, Marshall JC, et al: SCCM/ESICM/ACCP/ATS/SIS International Sepsis Definitions Conference. *Crit Care Med* 31:1250-1256, 2003.
17. Proulx F, Gauthier M, Nadeau D, et al: Timing and predictors of death in pediatric patients with multiple organ system failure. *Crit Care Med* 22:1025-1031, 1994.
18. Proulx F, Fayon M, Farrell CA, et al: Epidemiology of sepsis and multiple organ dysfunction syndrome in children. *Chest* 109:1033-1037, 1996.
19. Wilkinson JD, Pollack MM, Ruttiman UE, et al: Outcome of pediatric patients with multiple organ system failure. *Crit Care Med* 14:271-274, 1986.
20. Duke TD, Butt W, South M. Predictors of mortality and multiple organ failure in children with sepsis. *Intensive Care Med* 23:684-692, 1997.
21. Proulx F, BB, Lacroix J: Paediatric multiple organ dysfunction syndrome. *Intensive Care World* 14:78-82, 1997.
22. Lacroix J, Nadeau D, Laberge S, et al: frequency of upper gastrointestinal bleeding in a pediatric intensive care unit. *Crit Care Med* 20:35-42, 1992.
23. Bone RC: Sir Isaac Newton, sepsis, SIRS, and CARS. *Crit Care Med* 24:1125-1128, 1996.
24. Nichter MA, S-FJ, Costarino AT: Pediatric multiple organ failure syndrome. *Crit Care Med* 19:S78, 1991 (abstract).
25. American College of Chest Physicians/Society of Critical Care Medicine Consensus Conference: definitions for sepsis and organ failure and guidelines for the use of innovative therapies in sepsis. *Crit Care Med* 20:864-874, 1992.
26. Tilney NL, Bailey GL, Morgan AP: Sequential system failure after rupture of abdominal aortic aneurysms: an unsolved problem in postoperative care. *Ann Surg* 178:117-122, 1973.
27. Darling GE, Duff JH, Mustard RA, et al: Multi-organ failure in critically ill patients. *Can J Surg* 31:172-176, 1988.
28. Tran DD, Groeneveld AB, van der Meulen J, et al: Age, chronic disease, sepsis, organ system failure, and mortality in a medical intensive care unit. *Crit Care Med* 18:474-479, 1990.
29. Marshall WG Jr, Dimick AR: The natural history of major burns with multiple subsystem failure. *J Trauma* 23:102-105, 1983.
30. Fry DE, Pearlstein L, Fulton RL, et al: Multiple system organ failure. The role of uncontrolled infection. *Arch Surg* 115:136-140, 1980.
31. Faist E, Baue AE, Dittmer H, et al: Multiple organ failure in polytrauma patients. *J Trauma* 23:775-787, 1983.
32. Fry D: *Multiple system organ failure,* St. Louis, 1992, Mosby.
33. Vincent JL, Ferreira F, Moreno R: Scoring systems for assessing organ dysfunction and survival. *Crit Care Clin* 16:353-366, 2000.
34. Knaus WA, Wagner DP, Draper EA, et al: The APACHE III prognostic system. Risk prediction of hospital mortality for critically ill hospitalized adults. *Chest* 100:1619-1636, 1991.
35. Pollack MM, Patel KM, Ruttimann UE: PRISM III: an updated Pediatric Risk of Mortality score. *Crit Care Med* 24:743-752, 1996.
36. Pollack MM, Ruttimann UE, Getson PR: Pediatric risk of mortality (PRISM) score. *Crit Care Med* 16:1110-1116, 1988.
37. Pollack MM, Cuerdon TT, Patel KM, et al: Impact of quality-of-care factors on pediatric intensive care unit mortality. *JAMA* 272:941-946, 1994.
38. Le Gall JR, Loirat P, Alperovitch A, et al: A simplified acute physiology score for ICU patients. *Crit Care Med* 12:975-977, 1984.
39. Lemeshow S, Klar J, Teres D: Outcome prediction for individual intensive care patients: useful, misused, or abused? *Intensive Care Med* 21:770-776, 1995.
40. Predicting outcome in ICU patients. 2nd European Consensus Conference in Intensive Care Medicine. *Intensive Care Med* 20:390-397, 1994.
41. Petros AJ, Marshall JC, van Saene HK: Should morbidity replace mortality as an endpoint for clinical trials in intensive care. *Lancet* 345:369-371, 1995.
42. Le Gall JR, Lemeshow S, Saulnier F: A new Simplified Acute Physiology Score (SAPS II) based on a European/North American multicenter study. *JAMA* 270:2957-2963, 1993.
43. Vincent JL, Moreno R, Takala J, et al: The SOFA (Sepsis-related Organ Failure Assessment) score to describe organ dysfunction/failure. On behalf of the Working Group on Sepsis Related Problems of the European Society of Intensive Care Medicine. *Intensive Care Med* 22:707-710, 1996.
44. Le Gall JR, Klar J, Lemeshow S, et al: The Logistic Organ Dysfunction system. A new way to assess organ dysfunction in the intensive care unit, ICU Scoring Group. *JAMA* 276:802-810, 1996.
45. Marshall JC, Cook DJ, Christou NV, et al: Multiple organ dysfunction score: a reliable descriptor of a complex clinical outcome. *Crit Care Med* 23:1638-1652, 1995.
46. Leteurtre S, Martinot A, Duhamel A, et al: Development of a pediatric multiple organ dysfunction score: use of two strategies. *Med Decision Making* 19:399-410, 1999.
47. Leteurtre S, Martinot A, Duhamel A, et al: Validation of the paediatric logistic organ dysfunction (PELOD) score, prospective, observational, multicenter study. *Lancet* 362:192-197, 2003.
48. Despond O, Proulx F, Carcillo JA, et al: Pediatric sepsis and multiple organ dysfunction syndrome. *Curr Opin Pediatr* 13:247-253, 2001.
49. Livingston DH, Mosenthal AC, Deitch EA: Sepsis and multiple organ dysfunction syndrome: a clinical-mechanistic overview. *New Horiz* 3:257-266, 1995.
50. Balk RA: Pathogenesis and management of multiple organ dysfunction or failure in severe sepsis and septic shock. *Crit Care Clin* 16:337-352, 2000.
51. Reid CL, Perrey C, Pravica V, et al: Genetic variation in proinflammatory and anti-inflammatory cytokine production in multiple organ dysfunction syndrome. *Crit Care Med* 30:2216-2221, 2002.

52. Schroder O, Alexander L, Held B, et al: Association of interleukin-10 promotor polymorphism with the incidence of multiple organ dysfunction following major trauma: results of a prospective pilot study. *Shock* 21:306-310, 2004.
53. Zimmerman JJ: A question of balance. *Crit Care Med* 27:7-8, 1999.
54. Godin PJ, Buchman TG: Uncoupling of biological oscillators: a complementary hypothesis concerning the pathogenesis of multiple organ dysfunction syndrome. *Crit Care Med* 24:1107-1116, 1996.
55. Goldstein B, Fiser DH, Kelly MM, et al: Decomplexification in critical illness and injury: relationship between heart rate variability, severity of illness, and outcome. *Crit Care Med* 26:352-357, 1998.
56. Buchman TG, Cobb JP, Lapedes AS, Kepler TB: Complex systems analysis: a tool for shock research. *Shock* 16:248-251, 2001.
57. Tibby SM, Frndova H, Durward A, Cox P: Novel method to quantify loss of heart rate variability in pediatric multiple organ failure. *Crit Care Med* 31:2059-2067, 2003.
58. Aird WC: Endothelium as an organ system. *Crit Care Med* 32(suppl):S271-S279, 2004.
59. Hinshaw LB: Sepsis/septic shock. Participation of the microcirculation. *Crit Care Med* 24:1072-1078, 1996.
60. Fisher AB: Shear stress and endothelial cell activation. *Crit Care Med* 30(suppl):S192-S197, 2002.
61. Menger M: Capillary dysfunction in striated muscle ischemia-reperfusion: on the mechanism of capillary "no-reflow." *Shock* 8: 2-7, 1997.
62. Verrier E: The microvascular cell and ischemia-reperfusion injury. *J Cardiovasc Pharmacol* 27(suppl):S26-S30, 1996.
63. Lum H, Malik AB: Regulation of vascular endothelial barrier function. *Am J Physiol (Lung Cell Molec Physiol)* 267:L223-L241, 1994.
64. Ueno H, Hirasawa H, Oda S et al: Coagulation/fibrinolysis abnormality and vascular endothelial damage in the pathogenesis of thrombocytopenic multiple organ failure. *Crit Care Med* 30:3242-2248, 2002.
65. Tamion F, Richard V, Sauger F, et al: Gastric mucosal acidosis and cytokine release in patients with septic shock. *Crit Care Med* 31:2137-2143, 2003.
66. Zimmerman JJ: Oxyradical pathophysiology. In Barness LA, editor: *Advances in pediatrics*. St. Louis, 1994, Mosby-Yearbook.
67. Saran M: To what end does nature produce superoxide? NADPH oxidase as an autrine modifier of membrane phospholipids generating paracrine lipid messengers. *Free Radic Res* 37:1045-1059, 2003.
68. Lassegue B, Clempus RE: Vascular NAD(P)H oxidases: specific features, expression and regulation. *Am J Physiol Regul Integr Comp Physiol* 285:R277-R297, 2003.
69. Terada LS: Oxidative stress and endothelial activation. *Crit Care Med* 30(suppl):S186-S191, 2002.
70. Janiszewski M, do Carmo A, Pedro MA, et al: Platelet-derived exosomes of septic individuals possess proapoptotic NAD(P)H oxidase activity: a novel vascular redox pathway. *Crit Care Med* 32:818-825, 2004.
71. Giulivi C: Characterization and function of mitochondrial nitric-oxide synthase. *Free Radic Biol Med* 15:397-408, 2003.
72. Alderton WK, Cooper CE, Knowles RG: Nitric oxide syntheses: structure, function and inhibition. *Biochem J* 357:593-615, 2001.
73. Beckman JS, Koppenol WH: Nitric oxide, superoxide, and peroxynitrite: the good, the bad and the ugly. *Am J Physiol Cell Physiol* 271:C1424-C1437, 1996.
74. Radi R, Peluffo G, Alvarez MN, et al: Unraveling peroxynitrite formation in biological systems. *Free Radic Biol Med* 30:463-488, 2001.
75. Szabo C: Multiple pathways of peroxynitrite cytotoxicity. *Toxicol Lett* 11:140-141, 2003.
76. Szabo C: DNA strand breakage and activation of poly-ADP ribosyltransferase: a cytotoxic pathway triggered by peroxynitrite. *Free Radic Biol Med* 21:855-869, 1996.
77. Katusic ZS: Superoxide anion and regulation of arterial tone. *Free Radic Biol Med* 20:443-448, 1996.
78. McCord JM: Oxygen-derived free radicals in postischemic tissue injury. *N Engl J Med* 312:159-163, 1985.
79. Millar TM: Xanthine oxidase is a peroxynitrite synthase: newly identified roles for a very old enzyme. *Redox Report* 7:1-6, 2002.
80. Repine JE, Cheronis JC, Rodell TC, et al: Pulmonary oxygen toxicity and ischemia-reperfusion injury. *Am Rev Respir Dis* 136:483-485, 1987.
81. Otterbein L, Choi AMK: Hemoxygenase: colors of defense against cellular stress. *Am J Physiol* 279:L1029-L1037, 2000.
82. Taylor DE, Ghio AJ, Piantidosi CA: Reactive oxygen species produced by liver mitochondria of rats in sepsis. *Arch Biochem Biophys* 316:70-76, 1995.
83. Kowaltowski AJ, Vercesi AE: Mitochondrial damage induced by conditions of oxidative stress. *Free Radic Biol Med* 26:463-471, 1999.
84. Fink M: Cytopathic hypoxia: is oxygen use impaired in sepsis as a result of an acquired intrinsic derangement in cellular respiration? *Crit Care Clin* 18:165-175, 2002.
85. Crouser ED, Julian MW, Blaho OV, et al: Endotoxin-induced mitochondrial damage correlates with impaired respiratory activity. *Crit Care Med* 30:276-284, 2002.
86. Crouser ED, Julian MW, Huff JE, et al: Abnormal permeability of inner and outer mitochondrial membranes contributes independently to mitochondrial dysfunction in the liver during acute endotoxemia. *Crit Care Med* 32:478-488, 2004.
87. Babior BM, Lambeth JD, Nauseef W: The neutrophil NADPH oxidase. *Arch Biochem Biophys* 397:342-344, 2002.
88. Granger DN: Role of xanthine oxidase and granulocytes in ischemia-reperfusion injury. *Am J Physiol Heart Circ Physiol* 24: H1269-H1275, 1988.
89. Eppihimer MJ, Granger DN: Ischemia/reperfusion-induced leukocyte-endothelial interactions in post-capillary venules. *Shock* 8:16-25, 1997.
90. Downey GP, Fialkow L, Fukushima T: Initial interaction of leukocytes within the microvasculature: deformability, adhesion, and transmigration. *New Horiz* 3:219-228, 1995.
91. Weiss SJ: Tissue destruction by neutrophils. *N Engl J Med* 320: 365-376, 1989.
92. Kettle AJ, Winterbourn CC: Myeloperoxidase: a key regulator of neutrophil oxidant production. *Redox Report* 3:3-15, 1997.
93. Ossanna PJ, Test ST, Matheson NR, et al: Oxidative regulation of neutrophil elastase-alpha-1-proteinase inhibitor interactions. *J Clin Invest* 77:1939-1951, 1986.
94. Patrick DA, Moore EE, Moore FA, et al: Reduced PAF-acetylhydrolase activity is associated with post injury multiple organ failure. *Shock* 7:170-174, 1997.
95. Weiland JE, Davis WB, Holter JF, et al: Lung neutrophils in the adult respiratory distress syndrome. *Am Rev Respir Dis* 133:218-225, 1986.
96. Martin TR: Neutrophils and lung injury: getting it right. *J Clin Invest* 110:1603-1605, 2002.
97. Matute-Bello G, Liles WC, Steinberg KP, et al: Soluble Fas ligand induces epithelial cell apoptosis in humans with acute lung injury (ARDS). *J Immunol* 163:2217-2225, 1999.
98. Carlotta F, Re F, Polenatrutti N, et al: Modulation of granulocyte survival and programmed cell death by cytokines and bacterial products. *Blood* 80:2012-2020, 1992.
99. Ertel W, Kee LM, Infanger M, et al: Circulating mediators in serum of injured patients with septic complications inhibit neutrophil apoptosis through up-regulation of protein-tyrosine phosphorylation. *J Trauma* 44:767-775, 1998.
100. Jimenez MF, Watson RW, Parodo J, et al: Disregulated expression of neutrophil apoptosis in the systemic inflammatory response syndrome. *Arch Surg* 132:1263-1269, 1997.
101. Matute-Bello G, Martin TR: Science review: apoptosis in acute lung injury. 7:355-358, 2003.
102. Machino T, Hashimoto S, Maruoka S, et al: Apoptosis signal-regulating kinase 1-mediated signaling pathway regulates hydrogen peroxide-induced apoptosis in human pulmonary vascular endothelial cells. *Crit Care Med* 31:2776-2781, 2003.
103. Le Tulzo, YL, Pangault C, Gacouin A, et al: Early circulating lymphocyte apoptosis in human septic shock is associated with poor outcome. *Shock* 18:487-494, 2002.
104. Hotchkiss RS, Swanson PE, Freeman BD, et al: Apoptotic cell death in patients with septic shock and multiple organ dysfunction. *Crit Care Med* 27:1230-1251, 1999.
105. Hotchkiss RS, Tinsley KW, Swanson PE, et al: Sepsis-induced apoptosis causes progressive, profound depletion of B and CD4+ T lymphocytes in humans. *J Immunol* 166:6952-6963, 2001.
106. Papathanassoglou EDE, Moynihan JA, McDermott MP, et al: Expression of Fas (CD 95) and Fas ligand on peripheral blood mononuclear cells in critical illness and association with multi-organ dysfunction severity and survival. *Crit Care Med* 29: 709-718, 2001.

107. Doughty L, Clark RSB, Kaplan SS, et al: sFas and sFas ligand and pediatric sepsis-induced multiple organ failure syndrome. *Pediatr Res* 52:922-927, 2002.
108. Zeerleder S, Zwart B, Wuillemin WA et al: Elevated nucleosome levels in systemic inflammation and sepsis. *Crit Care Med* 31: 1947-1951, 2003.
109. Marsik C: Regulation of Fas (APO-1, CD 95) and Fas ligand expression during systemic inflammation. *Shock* 20:493-496, 2003.
110. Hashimoto S, Kobayashi A, Kooguchi K, et al: Upregulation of two death pathways of perforin/granzyme and FasL/Fas in septic acute respiratory distress syndrome. *Am J Respir Crit Care Med* 161:237-243, 2000.
111. Liacos C, Katsaragakis S, Konstadoulakis MM, et al: Apoptosis in cells of bronchoalveolar lavage: a cellular reaction in patients who die with sepsis and respiratory failure. *Crit Care Med* 29:2310-2317, 2001.
112. Watson WR, Rotstein OD, Parodo J, et al: The IL-1 beta-converting enzyme (caspase-1) inhibits apoptosis of inflammatory neutrophils through activation of IL-1 beta. *J Immunol* 161:957, 1998.
113. Hack CE, Zeeleder S: The endothelium in sepsis: source of and a target for inflammation. *Crit Care Med* 29(suppl):S21-S27, 2001.
114. DeBacker D: Microvascular blood flow is altered in patients with sepsis. *Am J Respir Crit Care Med* 166:98-104, 2002.
115. Poschi JMB: Endotoxin binding to erythrocyte membrane and erythrocyte deformability in human sepsis and *in vitro*. *Crit Care Med* 31:924-928, 2003.
116. Dhainaut J-F, Aird WC, Esmon CT, editors: Protein C pathways: bedside to bench. The Margaux V Conference on Critical Illness. *Crit Care Med* 32(suppl):S193-S341, 2004.
117. Nguyen T, Hall M, Han Y, et al: Microvascular thrombosis in pediatric multiple organ failure: is it a therapeutic target? *Pediatr Crit Care Med* 2:187-196, 2001.
118. Nimah M, Brilli RJ: Coagulation dysfunction in sepsis and multiple organ system failure. *Crit Care Clin* 19:441-448, 2003.
119. Carcillo JA, Davis AL, Zaritsky A: Role of early fluid resuscitation in pediatric septic shock. *JAMA* 266:1242-1245, 1991.
120. Carcillo JA, Fields AI, Task Force Members: Clinical practice parameters for hemodynamic support of pediatric and neonatal patients in septic shock. *Crit Care Med* 30:1365-1378, 2002.
121. Han YY, Carcillo JA, Dragotta MA, et al: Early reversal of pediatric-neonatal septic shock by community physicians is associated with improved outcome. *Pediatrics* 112:793-799, 2003.
122. Rivers E, Nguyen B, Havstad S, et al: Early goal-directed therapy in the treatment of severe sepsis and septic shock. *N Engl J Med* 345:1368-1377, 2001.
123. Silliman CC, Moore EE, Johnson JL, et al: Transfusion of the injured patient: proceed with caution. *Shock* 21:291-299, 2004.
124. Doughty LA, Kaplan SS, Carcillo JA: Inflammatory cytokine and nitric oxide responses in pediatric sepsis and organ failure. *Crit Care Med* 24:1137-1143, 1996.
125. Doughty L, Carcillo JA, Kaplan S, Janosky J: Plasma nitrite and nitrate concentrations and multiple organ failure in pediatric sepsis. *Crit Care Med* 26:157-162, 1998.
126. Hatherill M, Tibby SM, Turner C, et al: Procalcitonin and cytokine levels: relationship to organ failure and mortality in pediatric septic shock. *Crit Care Med* 28:2591-2594, 2000.
127. Whalen M, Doughty L, Carlos TM, et al: Intercellular adhesion molecule-1 and vascular cell adhesion molecule are increased in the plasma of children with sepsis-induced multiple organ failure. *Crit Care Med* 28:2600-2607, 2000.
128. Bernard GR, Vincent J-L, Laterre P-F, et al: Efficacy and safety of recombinant human activated protein c for severe sepsis. *N Engl J Med* 344:699-709, 2001.
129. Vincent J-L, Angus DC, Artigas A, et al: Effects of drotrecogin alfa (activated) on organ dysfunction in the PROWESS trial. *Crit Care Med* 31:834-840, 2003.
130. Annane D, Sebille V, Charpentier C, et al: Effect of treatment with low doses of hydrocortisone and fludrocortisone on mortality in patients with septic shock. *JAMA* 288:862-871, 2002.
131. Didonato JA, Saatcioglu F, Karin M: Molecular mechanisms of immunosuppression and anti-inflammatory activities by glucocorticoids. *Am J Respir Crit Care Med* 154:S11-S15, 1996.
132. Barnes PJ: Mechanism of action of glucocorticoids in asthma. *Am J Respir Crit Care Med* 154:S21-S27, 1996.
133. Keh D, Boehnke T, Weber-Cartens S, et al: Immunologic and hemodynamic effects of "low dose" hydrocortisone in septic shock. *Am J Respir Crit Care Med* 167:512-520, 2003.
134. Acute Respiratory Distress Syndrome Network: Ventilation with lower tidal volumes as compared to traditional tidal volumes for acute lung injury and the acute respiratory distress syndrome. *N Engl J Med* 342:1301-1308, 2000.
135. Van den Berghe G, Wouters P, Weekers F, et al: Intensive insulin therapy in critically ill patients. *N Engl J Med* 345:1359-1367, 2001.
136. Wasmuth HE, Kunz D, Graf J, et al: Hyperglycemia at admission to the intensive care unit is associated with elevated serum concentrations of interleukin-6 and reduced *ex vivo* secretion of tumor necrosis factor alpha. *Crit Care Med* 32:1109-1114, 2004.
137. Das UN: Insulin and the critically ill. Crit Care 6:262-263, 2002.
138. Baue AE: Multiple organ failure, multiple organ dysfunction syndrome, and the systemic inflammatory response syndrome—where do we stand? *Shock* 2:385-397, 1994.
139. Baue AE, Durham R, Faist E: Systemic inflammatory response syndrome (SIRS), multiple organ dysfunction syndrome (MODS), and multiple organ failure (MOF): are we winning the battle? *Shock* 10:79-89, 1998.

PART

III

Environmental Hazards

CHAPTER

98

Principles of Toxin Assessment and Screening

Alan D. Woolf

PEARLS

- The diagnosis of unknown poisoning still is based on obtaining a good history and thorough physical examination. Rarely does a laboratory finding reveal a totally unexpected diagnosis.
- Clinicians beware! Some toxins (e.g., acetaminophen, *Amanita* mushroom poisoning) are notable for the delay between the time of ingestion to the onset of symptoms. Other toxins, such as methadone, can have symptom recurrence hours after the initial onset.
- Often the clinician can predict the severity of medical outcome simply by noting the tempo of progression of the poisoned patient's symptoms and signs of toxicity over time.

Epidemiology

Despite progress in preventive measures during the past 3 decades, poisonings in children and adolescents continue to be common occurrences. More than 52% of 2.1 million poison center calls in the United States in 2003 involved children younger than 6 years.[1] Although many of these exposures are medically trivial, poisonings account for an important number of all pediatric hospital visits and hospitalizations. In one study of 638 pediatric hospitalizations for poisoning between 1992 and 1995 at a teaching hospital, the toxic agents implicated in the most serious cases included caustics, prescription medications (e.g., antidepressants), analgesics (e.g., acetaminophen), and heavy metals (e.g., lead).[2]

Not all children are equally at risk for serious poisoning. The incidence of poisoning is highest among children 1 to 3 years old. Boys slightly outnumber girls as victims of unintentional exposures. Children with developmental delays and pica, as occurs with autistic spectrum disorders, have an increased risk for self-poisoning. A second peak of serious poisonings occurs in adolescence, when a suicide attempt by poisoning (with females disproportionately overrepresented) or a misadventure involving substance abuse becomes the common circumstance underlying a poisoning episode. Adolescents with anorexia nervosa or psychiatric conditions such as clinical depression are especially vulnerable to self-poisoning.

Typically childhood poisoning occurs around mealtime, when parents are preoccupied with food preparation or are otherwise distracted.[3] Many poisonings involve medications or household products that are open and being used at the time of the poisoning. The second most common site of a poisoning other than the child's own home is that of the grandparents. Children in power struggles with parents, and those in socially isolated, stressed families, tend to suffer repeated poisoning events.[3]

Common Agents Involved

The most common agents involved in preschooler poisonings are medications (e.g., analgesics, cough and cold preparations, dermatological preparations), household products (e.g., cleaning agents, soaps, detergents), and plants. Table 98–1 lists those agents responsible for the most calls to poison control centers. The agents most frequently involved in serious pediatric poisonings (those requiring intensive care) are prescription medications (e.g., cyclic antidepressants, anticonvulsants, digitalis, opiates),

TABLE 98–1

Agents Most Frequently Involved in Childhood (<6 Years) Poisonings in the United States in 2001

Toxic Agent	No. Poison Center Calls	Percent
Cosmetics and personal care products	154,076	13.2
Cleaning substances	123,301	10.5
Analgesics	83,166	7.1
Foreign bodies	82,614	7.1
Topicals	76,795	6.6
Plants	73,287	6.3
Cough and cold preparations	59,949	5.1
Pesticides	46,929	4.0
Vitamins	42,150	3.6
Gastrointestinal preparations	35,633	3.0
Antimicrobials	33,033	2.8
Arts/crafts/office supplies	31,443	2.7
Antihistamines	30,968	2.6
Hormones and hormone antagonists	27,171	2.3
Hydrocarbons	22,319	1.9
Total	922,834	78.8%

Modified from Table 17B in Litovitz TL, Klein-Schwartz W, Rodgers GC, Cobaugh DJ, Youniss J, Omslaer JC, May ME, Woolf AD, Benson BE: *Am J Emerg Med* 20:4000, 2002.

Note: Percentages are based on the total number of exposures in children < 6 years (1,169,478) rather than the number of substances.

alcohol, and hydrocarbon-based household products. Lead poisoning and carbon monoxide poisoning related to house fires are less recognized but frequent causes of poisoning hospitalization in childhood.

Clinicians should ask caretakers about the types and doses of any medications, herbs, vitamins, or diet supplements being used to treat the child's other health problems. Such therapies may be interacting with the toxins responsible for the poisoning or otherwise contributing to the child's toxicity.

Resources for the Clinician

In making the diagnosis of an unknown poisoning, the physician must rely on powers of observation, history-taking abilities, and clinical skills. Laboratory analyses and radiographic findings sometimes are helpful. References such as *Drug Information* (available annually from the American Hospital Formulary Service [AHFS], American Society of Hospital Pharmacists, Bethesda, MD,) and the *Poisindex*© computer database (Micromedex™ Cooperation, Greenwood Village, CO,) can be helpful in identifying drugs and their actions and precautions. The regional poison control center (telephone: 1-800-222-1222) can provide helpful consultative services by toxicologists. Such services may include the following:

1. Assistance with differential diagnosis toxins known to cause a particular constellation of symptoms and signs
2. Information about drug–drug, drug–chemical, or drug–herb interactions
3. Expected clinical course of the patient, give known kinetics of the agents involved
4. Help with locating laboratories that can assay tissue samples for exotic drugs and chemicals
5. Advice about current management techniques for specific poisoning
6. Help in locating supplies of particular antidotes or antisera
7. Surveillance for clusters of poisoning in a community representing a public health hazard
8. Assistance in reporting adverse drug or dietary supplement reactions or medical errors to appropriate public health authorities

General Assessment of the Poisoned Patient

History

An accurate history is vitally important in the diagnosis of unknown poisoning. Surprisingly, the physician in the intensive care unit (ICU) may be the first health professional who can sit with parents and carefully review the possible circumstances of the exposure(s). Poisonings may occur by various routes, including ingestion, inhalation, ocular exposure, dermal exposure, mucous membrane involvement, or parenteral exposure. Once the child's condition has been stabilized, the pediatrician should query the family about the incident, with particular attention to the environmental, patient, and toxic agent factors listed in Table 98–2.

In acute accidental exposures in young children, the precise time and toxin involved frequently are accurately known. The importance of obtaining the precise ingredients in the suspected toxic agents cannot be overemphasized. Parents should bring the product containers or medication labels. For estimations of liquid toxins, the average swallow of a young child is approximately 5 to 10 ml, and that of the older child and adolescent is 10 to 15 ml. The clinician must appreciate the fact that parents frequently minimize the child's exposure to a toxin in an attempt to deny the

TABLE 98–2

History Taking and Unknown Poisoning in the Pediatric Patient

Environment	Patient	Toxin
Witnesses	Intentionality	Agent(s) involved
Time of ingestion	Past medical problems	Exact ingredients
Site of ingestion	Current medications	Dose (maximal estimated)
Illness of family members	Known drug allergies	Concentration
Medications of family members	Time of symptoms onset	Route of exposure
Open containers	Prior medical management	

threat of injury or to assuage their guilt that such an episode occurred. Therefore it is prudent to assume the worst possible scenario in calculating the maximum dose of a drug or household product a child could have swallowed in a poisoning and to treat the patient accordingly. Calculation of the dose the child might have received is sometimes helpful, using the maximum number of missing tablets or amount of liquid, the concentration of the drug or chemical, and the child's weight.

The latency between the time of ingestion and the onset of symptoms is important. Some toxins, such as acetaminophen, paraquat, diphenoxylate, and the *Amanita* mushroom toxin classically have an asymptomatic period of 12 hours or more. The tempo of progression of symptoms and signs also may help the clinician gauge the severity of the intoxication and the urgency with which intervention is necessary.

Adolescent poisonings are confounded by the intentionality of the episode and the frequent unreliability of the adolescent's history. Adolescents in distress may be evasive, misleading, or otherwise uncommunicative. Their ability to remember or provide a coherent account of what happened may be distorted by the effects of the drugs taken. The clinician cannot assume that the time of exposure, dose, or even the toxic agents themselves are accurately recounted.

Physical Examination

The physical examination is crucial for assessment of the patient's medical stability and for identification of the unknown poison. Specific changes in vital signs and symptoms are associated with likely toxins or groups of toxins. Such characteristic clinical patterns of illness are sometimes termed *toxidromes*. Table 98–3 lists some of the more common toxidromes important in pediatric poisoning (see Chapter 99). Families are using herbs and diet supplements with increasing frequency to treat their children's illnesses or simply to promote their general well-being. However, serious poisonings in which herbs and dietary supplements are implicated are appearing in the medical literature.[4] Table 98–4 lists some examples of toxicities associated with particular herbal remedies.

Many toxins affect the cardiovascular or neurologic system. Frequently the gastrointestinal tract is involved early in a poisoning. Nonspecific findings after a drug or chemical overdose include nausea, vomiting, abdominal pain, and loose stools. A variety of drugs can cause fever. Overdoses with cocaine, phenothiazines, atropine, or salicylates often are associated with an elevated temperature. For specific discussions of the effects of toxins on other selected organ systems, the reader is referred to the general reviews listed in the Additional Readings and to Chapter 99.

Cardiovascular System

Table 98–5 lists examples of drugs and toxic agents associated with specific effects on the cardiovascular system.

Blood Pressure

Toxins may cause hypertension/hypotension by direct effects on vascular smooth muscle, neurogenic effects on autonomic nervous centers governing vascular innervation, direct effects on the heart, or renal effects. Specific agents associated with hypertension include adrenergic stimulants: amphetamines, cocaine, phencyclidine, phenylpropanolamine, ephedrine, and phenylephrine. Although the hypertension caused by sympathomimetics frequently lasts only a few hours, it may be associated with acute encephalopathy and/or intracranial hemorrhage.

Acute hypotension frequently is associated with the following: opiates, cyclic antidepressants, phenothiazines, clonidine, beta-blockers, calcium channel blockers, antihypertensives, and antiarrhythmic overdose. Anaphylactic or allergic responses to many agents may result in hypotension.

TABLE 98–3

Common Toxidromes in Pediatric Poisoning

Symptoms and Signs	Agent
Miosis, salivation, diarrhea, bronchorrhea, lacrimation, seizures, respiratory failure, bradycardia	Organophosphate insecticides
Fever, tachypnea, hyperpnea, lethargy, metabolic acidosis	Salicylates
Seizures, metabolic acidosis, history of tuberculosus, hyperglycemia	Isoniazid
Dry mouth, flushed appearance, dilated pupils, fever, ileus, urinary retention, disorientation	Anticholinergic syndrome
Oculogyric crises, dystonia, opisthotonus	Phenothiazines
Severe metabolic acidosis, sluggish pupils, hyperemic retina, blurred vision	Methanol
Hypoglycemia, lethargy, ataxia, seizures, characteristic breath odor	Ethanol
Lethargy or coma, metabolic acidosis, active urinary sediment, crystalluria	Ethylene glycol
Headache, "influenza-like" syndrome, lethargy, dizziness, coma	Carbon monoxide
Pinpoint pupils, coma, respiratory depression	Opiate
Metabolic acidosis, prolonged QRS interval, coma, seizures, dilated pupils, dysrhythmias	Tricyclic antidepressants
Protracted vomiting, tremors, tachycardia, anxiety, seizures, hypotension	Theophylline
Feeling of impending doom, sudden coma, metabolic acidosis, hypotension, bitter almond odor	Cyanide
Rotatory nystagmus, delirium, combative, catatonia, convulsions, coma (4 *C*s)	Phencyclidine

TABLE 98–4

Herbs Associated with Toxicity

Herbal Product	Toxic Chemicals	Effect or Target Organ
Chamomile (*Matricaria chamomilla, Anthmis noblis)*	Allergens: *Compositae* Plant species	Anaphylaxis, contact dermatitis
Chapparal *(Larrea divericata, Larrea tridentata)*	Nordihydro-guaiaretic acid	Nausea, vomiting, lethargy, hepatitis
Cinnamon oil *Cinnamomum* spp	Cinnamaldehyde	Dermatitis, abuse syndrome
Coltsfoot *(Tussilago farfara)*	Pyrrolizidines	HVOD
Comfrey *(Symphytum officinale)*	Pyrrolizidines	HVOD
Crotalalaria spp	Pyrrolizidines	HVOD
Echinacea (*Echinacea augustifolia Compositae* spp)	Polysaccharides	Asthma, atopy, anaphylaxis, urticaria, angioedema
Eucalyptus *(Eucalyptus globulus)*	1,8-cineole	Drowsiness, ataxia, seizures, coma, nausea, vomiting, respiratory failure
Garlic *(Allium sativum)*	Allicin	Dermatitis, chemical burns, oxiziding agent
Germander *(Teucrium chamaedrys)*		Hepatotoxicity
Ginseng *(Panax ginseng)*	Ginsenoside	Ginseng abuse syndrome (insomnia, diarrhea, anxiety, hypertension)
Glycerated Asafetida	Oxidants	Methemoglobinemia
Grousel *(Senecio longilobus)*	Pyrrolizidine	HVOD
Heliotrope, turnsole *(Heliotropium* spp, *Crotalaria fulva, Cynoglossum officinale*)	Pyrrolizidiness	HVOD
Jin Bu Huan *(Stephania* spp, *Corydalis* spp*)*	L-Tetrahydropalmitine	Hepatitis, lethargy, coma
Kava kava *(Piper methysticum)*	Kawain, methysticide	Hepatic failure, "kavaism" neurotoxicity
Laetrile	Cyanide	Coma, seizures, death
Licorice *(Glycyrrhiza glabra)*	Glycyrrhetic acid	Hypertension, hypokalemia, cardiac arrhythmias
Ma Huang *(Ephedra sinica)*	Ephedrine	Cardiac arrhythmias, hypertension, seizures, stroke
Monkshood *(aconitum naplleus, Aconitum columbianum)*	Aconite	Cardiac arrhythmias, shock, seizures, weakness, coma, paresthesias, vomiting
Nutmeg *(Myristica fragrans)*	Myristacin, eurogenol	Hallucinations, emesis, headache
Nux vomica	Strychnine	Seizures, abdominal pain respiratory arrest
Pennyroyal *(Mentha pulegium or Hedeoma* spp*)*	Pulegone	Centrilobular liver necrosis, shock, fetotoxicity, seizures, abortion
Ragwort (golden) *(Senecio jacobaes [Senecio aureus or Echium])*	Pyrrolizidines	HVOD
Wormwood	Thujone	Seizures, dementia, tremors, headache

From *Children's Environmental Health*, ed 2. Elk Grove Village, IL, 2003, Committee on Injuries & Poison Prevention, American Academy of Pediatrics.
HVOD, hepatic venoocclusive disease.

Pulse

Tachycardia frequently is associated with ingestion of any of the sympathetic nervous system stimulants listed in Table 98–5. A notable exception is phenylpropanolamine, which, as a pure α-adrenoceptor agonist, causes peripheral vasoconstriction associated with reflex bradycardia or normal pulse. Tachycardia also is associated with exogenous thyroid preparation ingestion, the early phase of poisoning with tricyclic antidepressants, theophylline overdoses, and caffeine or nicotine intoxications.

Bradycardia may accompany exaggerated vagal responses to some compounds or direct negative chronotropic

TABLE 98–5

Toxins Associated with Cardiovascular Findings

Sign	Agents
Tachycardia	Amphetamines Antihistamines Anticholinergics Cocaine α-Adrenergic agonists (albuterol, terbutaline) Theophylline
Bradycardia	Antiarrhythmics β-Adrenergic blockers Calcium channel blockers Cardiac glycosides Clonidine Ergotamine Opiates Organophosphates Phenylpropanolamine Quinidine Sedative-hypnotics
Torsades de pointes	Amantadine Antiarrhythmics Amiodarone Arsenic Astemizole Chloral hydrate Chloroquine Cisapride Disopyramide Encainide Fluoride Lidocaine Mexiletine Organophosphates Terfenadine Quinidine Procainamide Pentamidine Phenothiazines Prenylamine Suxamethonium Cyclic antidepressants
Ventricular tachycardia	Amphetamines Antiarrhythmics (e.g., quinidine, flecainide) Carbamazepine Chloral hydrate Chlorinated hydrocarbons Cocaine Cyclic antidepressants Digitalis Theophylline Thioridazine

effects on the heart. Interference with the cardiac conduction system may cause a slowed pulse. Cardiac drugs associated with bradyarrhythmias include the calcium channel blockers, digitalis, and β-adrenergic blocking agents. Antiarrhythmics such as quinidine and procainamide can slow the pulse.

Neurologic System

Consciousness

Many drugs and chemicals depress a patient's consciousness either directly or by hypoxia resulting from decreased respiratory drive or simple asphyxia. Table 98–6 provides a suitable scoring system for determining the level of consciousness in the intoxicated patient. The dynamic nature of a poisoning injury mandates serial assessments of consciousness using this objective scoring system to gauge accurately whether the patient's overall condition is deteriorating or improving. The effects of therapies such as naloxone or oxygen also can be assessed. In many serious intoxications, such as carbon monoxide or cyanide poisoning, the state of consciousness may be the singular best guide to the patient's overall prognosis. Box 98–1 lists some of the agents that may cause coma in the pediatric patient. Box 98–2 lists some common causes of seizures.

Pupillary Changes

Pupil size depends on the balance between dilating and constricting fibers and is under complex autonomic nervous system control. Both sympathetic and parasympathetic nerves regulate the iris and can be affected by a variety of toxins. Anticholinergic drugs (e.g., tricyclic antidepressants, antihistamines, belladonna) paralyze the parasympathetic fibers leading to pupillary dilation. Conversely, agents that inactivate cholinesterase leading to accumulations of acetylcholine (e.g., organophosphate pesticides, physostigmine) constrict the pupil. Ethanol, phenothiazines, and barbiturates also constrict the pupils. Opiates act centrally to cause extreme pupillary constriction (miosis). Sympathomimetics, such as amphetamines and cocaine, cause extreme pupillary dilation (mydriasis). Pilocarpine directly stimulates the sphincter muscle of the iris, causing constriction.

TABLE 98–6

Reed Scale for Clinical Assessment of Consciousness

Grade	Description
0	Asleep Can be aroused Will answer questions
1	Comatose Withdraws from painful stimuli Intact reflexes
2	Comatose Does not withdraw from painful stimuli No respiratory or circulatory depression Intact reflexes
3	Comatose Reflexes absent No respiratory or circulatory depression
4	Comatose Reflexes absent Respiratory or circulatory problems

From Ellenhorn MJ, Barceloux DG: *Medical toxicology*, New York, 1988, Elsevier Publishers.

BOX 98–1

Agents Associated with Coma in the Pediatric Patient

Anticonvulsants
Aromatic hydrocarbons
Asphyxiant gases
Barbiturates
Benzodiazepines
Carbon monoxide
Clonidine
Cyanide
Cyclic antidepressants
Ethanol
Ethylene glycol
γ-Butyrolactone
γ-Hydroxybutyrate
Hypoglycemic agents
Ketamine
Lead (encephalopathy)
Lithium
Methanol
Nonbarbiturate sedative-hypnotics
Opiates
Organochlorine pesticides
Phenothiazines
Salicylates (Reye syndrome)

Toxins can be responsible for unequal pupil size. Local instillation of atropine to the eye causes ipsilateral pupillary dilation.

It is important to recognize that polydrug overdoses may include agents with opposite pupillary actions. Overreliance on pupillary size alone in deciding which poison is responsible for the patient's condition may lead to a misdiagnosis. Closed head trauma or central nervous system (CNS) hemorrhage, sometimes seen in the context of a poisoning with drugs such phenylpropanolamine[5] or ephedrine,[6,7] which both can cause hypertension, can themselves cause pupillary effects.

BOX 98–2

Agents Associated with Seizures at Presentation

Amphetamines
Camphor
Cocaine
Cyanide
Cyclic antidepressants
Ephedrine
Gyromitra (mushroom species)
Insecticides
Isoniazid
Methylene dioxymethamphetamine (MDMA)
Monoamine oxidase inhibitors
Nicotine
Phenylpropanolamine
Propoxyphene
Strychnine
Theophylline
Water hemlock (plant)

Altered Sensorium

When treating a disoriented, delirious pediatric patient, the clinician must consider which intoxications may be responsible. Because of their central anticholinergic effects and common availability, antihistamines (e.g., chlorpheniramine, diphenhydramine) must be considered. Alcohol-containing household products or liquor may be responsible. In the adolescent, drugs of abuse may cause delirium or hallucinations. Hallucinogens include lysergic acid diethylamide (LSD), psilocybin, mescaline, "magic mushrooms," and some amphetamine congeners ("designer drugs," e.g., 3-methoxy 4,5-methylenedioxyamphetamine [MMDA], 3,4-methylenedioxy-N-methamphetamine (MDMA, "ecstasy"), or 3,4-methylenedioxy-N-ethylamphetamine [MDEA]). Both cocaine and amphetamines can cause an acute psychosis. Newer, smokable forms of methamphetamine (known as "crystal" or "ice") and phencyclidine (PCP) cause symptoms of agitation, aggression, and combativeness.

Intensivists should be alert for abstinence syndromes in adolescents suffering from chronic substance abuse. Drug withdrawal from opiates, benzodiazepines, or alcohol (delirium tremens) often cause agitation, irritability, or even delusional thinking in affected patients. Withdrawal from chronic γ-hydroxybutyrate use (GHB, a popular "designer drug") is characterized by anxiety, insomnia, tremor, confusion, delirium, hallucinations, cardiovascular changes, nausea, vomiting, and diaphoresis.[8]

Other Neurologic Findings

Phenytoin and phencyclidine frequently cause nystagmus. Tinnitus is associated with ingestions of ergot, quinine, salicylates, and streptomycin. Changes in color vision may be seen in chronic digitalis overdose or cinchonism (quinidine).

Skin Examination

Many poisonings cause skin manifestations. Abusers of intravenous narcotics or other drugs may have needle tracks, characteristic tattoos, or scarring from "skin popping." Those suffering from inhalant abuse frequently have rashes around the nose and mouth as a result of defatting and irritative effects of inhaled solvents. Methemoglobinemia as a result of a variety of oxidizing agents causes acute cyanosis despite relatively normal blood gas values (Box 98–3). A variety of rashes can be seen with adverse drug reactions and allergic responses to drugs, plants, or chemicals. Typical chemical burns may result from dermal exposure to caustics. Alopecia is associated with exposures to antimetabolite medications and other antineoplastic agents and to overdoses of chemicals such as arsenic, thallium, and selenium. Jaundice may result from exposure to carbon tetrachloride, aniline dyes, quinacrine, or phenothiazines.

Breath Odors

The physician must be alert to characteristic odors in containers found at the scene of the exposure, of substances

BOX 98–3

Drugs, Chemicals, and Foods Causing Methemoglobinemia

DRUGS

Acetanilid
Amyl nitrite
Benzocaine
Cetacaine
Chloroquine
Chloroquinone
Clofazimine
Dapsone (sulfones)
Diaminodiphenylsulfone
Hydroxylamine
Lidocaine
Menadione
Methylene blue
Metoclopramide
Nitroglycerin
Nitrosobenzene
Para-aminobenzoic acid
Para-aminopropiophenone
Para-hydroxylaminopropiophenone
Phenacetin
Phenazopyridine hydrochloride (Pyridium)
Phenylhydroxylamine
Phenytoin
Potassium permanganate
Prilocaine
Primaquine
Procaine
Resorcinol
Silver nitrate
Sodium nitrate
Sodium nitrite
Sodium nitroprusside
Sulfamethoxazole
Sulfanilamide
Sulfapyridine
Sulfathiazide

CHEMICALS

Acetanilid
Alloxan
Ammonium nitrate
Aniline dyes
Antipyrine
Arsine
Benzene derivatives
Butyl nitrite
Chlorates
Chlorobenzene
Cobalt preparations
Dimethylaniline
Dinitrobenzene
Dinitrophenol
Dinitrotoluene
Hydroquinone
Inks/shoe polish
Isobutyl nitrite
Menthol
Naphthalene
Naphthylamines
Nitrates/nitrites
Nitric oxide
Nitroalkanes
Nitrobenzene
Nitrofuran
Nitrogen oxide
Nitrogen trifluoride
Nitroglycerin
Nitrophenol
Nitrous gases/nitric oxide
Ozone
Para-bromoaniline
Paraquat (or Monolinuron)
Para-toluidine
Phenazopyridine
Phenetidin
Phenols
Phenylhydrazine
Phenylhydroxylamine
Pyridine
Smoke (products of combustion)
Sulfones
Toluidine
Trinitrotoluene
Xylidine

FOODS

Beets
Cabbage
Nitrite/nitrate preservatives
Nitrogen-rich foods
Preserved meats
Spinach
Well water

spilled on the patient's skin or clothing, or on the patient's breath. Organophosphate insecticides or thallium impart the strong odor of garlic. Cyanide exposures have the characteristic aroma of bitter almond (although 50% of the population is of the genotype that cannot detect the odor of bitter almonds). Ethanol, kerosene, camphor, and gasoline impart their strong odors to the breath. Adolescents abusing volatile organic compounds by inhalation may have a solvent smell on their breath and on their clothes. Table 98–7 lists some of the typical intoxications that can be diagnosed by the patient's breath odors.

Laboratory Tests

Toxic Screens

Although laboratory testing of the blood or urine occasionally reveals an unanticipated toxin involved in an overdose, more frequently it confirms the physician's clinical diagnosis on the basis of a careful history and physical examination. The pediatric intensivist is well advised to know which compounds are included in the toxicology screen performed by the institution because the menu of substances detectable by a commercial laboratory is

TABLE 98–7

Toxins Associated with Characteristic Breath Odors

Toxin	Characteristic Odor
Acetone	Acetone
Arsenic	Garlic
Camphor	Mothballs
Chloroform	Sweet
Cyanide	Bitter almond
Ethanol	Ethanol
Hydrogen sulfide	Rotten eggs
Isopropanol	Acetone
Methyl salicylate	Wintergreen
Nicotine	Stale tobacco
Organophosphates	Garlic
N-Pyridylmethylnitrophenylurea (Vacor rat poison)	Peanuts
Paraldehyde, chloral hydrate	Pears (urine)
Phenol, cresol	Phenolic
Phosphorus	Garlic
Salicylates	Acetone
Thallium	Garlic
Turpentine	Violets

variable and frequently based on cost, ease of detection, available technical equipment, relative frequency of the overdose in the community, and other considerations. Most hospitals include the following compounds on a toxicology screen: acetaminophen, ethanol, barbiturates, opiates, anticonvulsants, some benzodiazepines, phenothiazines, and salicylates. Some toxicology screens may or may not include drugs of abuse (e.g., amphetamines, cocaine, tetrahydrocannabinol), older tricyclic antidepressants (e.g., amitriptyline, imipramine), and methanol. Many common toxic agents, including carbon monoxide, cyanide, methemoglobin, iron, lithium, heavy metals such as lead or arsenic, and ethylene glycol, are never included on a toxicology screen and must be ordered specifically.

A "negative" toxicology screen result does not rule out the diagnosis of a toxic exposure. For example, some enzyme multiplied immunoassay technique (EMIT) assays routinely used to screen for opiates do not necessarily detect dextromethorphan, a chemically related compound commonly used in cough preparations and also abused by adolescents to get "high."[9] An adolescent whose urine tests negative for opiates could, in fact, be suffering the adverse effects of dextromethorphan intoxication. The more specific a clinician is in communicating with laboratory personnel about which toxins are suspected clinically, the more directed laboratory personnel can be in seeking specific answers through laboratory methods. Because some toxins (e.g., cocaine, other drugs of abuse, some heavy metals) are detected more easily in urine than in blood, both specimens should be submitted when the toxicology screen is ordered. Gastric contents can be assessed when the patient is seen shortly after an ingestion, before absorption of the drug or chemical is likely.

Some toxicology screens include, as a first step, qualitative spot chromatography tests or thin-layer chromatography (TLC) in the analysis of an unknown sample of blood or urine. These tests are accurate for qualitative analysis of the presence of a toxin but are imprecise for quantitative analysis. For many compounds, TLC or spot test analyses may have unacceptable false-positive rates or cross-reactions within a class of chemicals. For a more quantitative confirmation of the presence of a drug or chemical, EMIT can be performed as a screening test. An immunoassay positive for a drug must be confirmed by a second technique before the drug is considered present in the blood or urine. For more precise assays, as "second" techniques to confirm the results of screening assays, and for detection of more exotic drugs or chemicals, high-pressure liquid chromatography (HPLC) or gas–liquid phase chromatography–mass spectrometry (GLC-MS) are used. For detecting heavy metals and many salts, flame ionization spectroscopy or atomic absorption spectroscopy is the quantitative assay of choice. Reliability in the screening for drugs or toxins requires not only a sound analytic technique but also adequate sample collection, chain of custody (in cases involving judicial prosecution), and timely reporting of the results. Sources of error include delay in the time between sample collection and assay, problems with sample collection (wrong tube, loss of fluid, poor labeling), natural chemical reactions (volatilization, enzymatic degradation), purposeful sample alteration, technical limits on the detection threshold of the assay used, and misinterpretation of the units in reporting the results.

Blood Levels

Quantitative assessments of some toxins correlate with the severity of intoxication. Serum concentrations of acetaminophen, aspirin, barbiturates, carbamazepine, carbon monoxide, digoxin, ethanol, ethylene glycol, iron, isopropanol, lead, lithium, methanol, phenytoin, and theophylline are useful in guiding patient management. Cooximetry can provide blood levels of abnormal hemoglobins caused by toxins, such as carboxyhemoglobin, sulfemoglobin, and methemoglobinemia. Box 98–3 lists drugs, chemicals, and foods capable of causing methemoglobinemia in susceptible individuals.

Serum Osmolality

Certain toxins (e.g., ethanol, ethylene glycol, isopropanol, methanol) introduce osmotically active particles into the serum. These particles increase serum osmolality, which can be measured by either vapor pressure or freezing point depression. However, vapor pressure techniques give falsely low values in the presence of volatiles (e.g., any of the alcohols).[10,11] The calculated serum osmolality is derived by the following equation: Calculated serum osmolality = 2 × Na (in mEq/L) + Blood urea nitrogen (in g/dL)/2.8 + Glucose (in mg/dL)/18 (see Chapter 62). Calculated osmolality then is subtracted from the measured osmolality: Measured osmolality − Calculated osmolality = Osmolar gap. A normal osmolar gap is between −3 and 10 mOsm/kg H_2O.

The presence of toxins listed in Table 98–8 is associated with an elevated osmolar gap (>10). An estimate of the serum toxin concentration can be derived using the serum osmolality as measured by the freezing point depression technique, calculating the osmolar gap, and applying the conversion factors listed in Table 98–8. Intensivists are cautioned that elevated osmolar gaps also are seen in patients with lipemic blood or in those receiving therapies such as mannitol, glycerol, sorbitol, propylene glycol, or some types of contrast agents in preparation for diagnostic imaging studies. Conversely, a falsely low osmolar gap can be seen in ethylene glycol or methanol poisoning if the vapor pressure method of serum osmolarity determination is erroneously used.

Serum Anion Gap

The principle of electroneutrality requires that positive and negative charged molecules in the serum must balance. The presence of toxins in the blood that cause a metabolic acidosis also frequently increase the gap between the total measured versus theoretical anions by the direct addition of organic acid anions, the indirect generation of such anions, or (rarely) the reduction of cations in the serum. The anion gap calculation is derived as follows:

$$\text{Anion gap} = Na^+ - (Cl^- + HCO_3),$$

where all components are expressed in milliequivalents per liter.

The "normal" anionic gap ranges from 3 to 16 mEq/L in older children and adults. Hypoalbuminemia or diluted blood both can cause misleadingly low anion gaps. The presence of elevated concentrations of unmeasured anions (e.g., as a result of dehydration or treatment with sodium salts of citrate, lactate, or acetate) or conditions associated with a decrease in unmeasured cations (e.g., as a result of hypomagnesemia, hypocalcemia, hypokalemia) can lead to an elevated anion gap.

Table 98–9 lists toxins associated with changes in the total serum anions (see Chapter 62).

Tests for Rhabdomyolysis

Many agents that cause seizures (e.g., isoniazid, organochlorine pesticides, theophylline, tricyclic antidepressants) or excessive muscular activity and hyperthermia (e.g., cocaine, amphetamines, phencyclidine, neuroleptic malignant syndrome, serotonin syndrome) may predispose the patient to rhabdomyolysis and subsequent myoglobin-induced acute renal failure. The overdose patient who is agitated or delirious and is held in physical restraints for long periods and the overdose comatose patient who has muscle necrosis from dependency position injury are at high risk for rhabdomyolysis. Laboratory parameters that may be useful in serial monitoring in such circumstances include serum lactic acid, creatine phosphokinase, aldolase, and myoglobin levels and urinary sediment, urine output, and myoglobin levels.

TABLE 98–8

Osmolar Gap Conversions to Calculate Serum Concentration: Alcohols and Glycols*

Toxin	Conversion Factor
Methanol	2.6
Ethanol	4.3
Ethylene glycol	5.0
Acetone	5.5
Isopropanol	5.9

*Serum concentration (mg/dl) of given toxin divided by corresponding conversion factor equals serum osmolality (mOsm/kg H_2O) attributable to that toxin.

TABLE 98–9

Anion Gap Changes Associated with Specific Toxin Exposures

Elevated Anion Gap	Depressed Anion Gap
Methanol	Bromide
Paraldehyde, phenformin	Lithium
Iron, isoniazid	
Ethylene glycol, ethanol	
Salicylate, strychnine	

Other Blood Tests

Frequently other baseline measures are included in the initial evaluation of the patient. Depending on the agent involved and the clinical course, the following tests often are clinically useful in the evaluation of the poisoned patient: arterial blood gases (acid-base assessment), blood count, platelet count, and leukocyte differential, blood clotting parameters, electrocardiogram, electroencephalogram, liver function tests, renal function tests, serum electrolytes and blood glucose, and urinalysis including urine pH.

Radiologic Examination

Radiographs can be helpful in locating swallowed foreign bodies having toxic potential. Patients who have ingested disc batteries should undergo serial chest/abdominal radiography to ensure that the battery has cleared the esophagus and is continuing movement down the gastrointestinal tract.

BOX 98–4

Drugs and Chemicals That May Be Radiopaque

- Bezoars, bags (filled with illegal drugs)
- Calcium carbonate
- Chloral hydrate
- Enteric-coated tablets
- Heavy metals
- Iodine
- Iron
- Phenothiazines
- Potassium compounds

TABLE 98–10

Useful Diagnostic Trials

Agent Detected	Agent Administered	Technique	Positive Results
Benzodiazepines	Flumazenil	0.2–0.3 mg/kg IV (maximum 3 mg)	Improved consciousness
Iron	Deferoxamine	40 mg/kg IM (maximum 2 g)	"Vin rose" urine color
Opiates	Naloxone hydrochloride	0.03 mg/kg (up to 4 mg)	Improved consciousness
Organophosphate	Atropine	0.1 mg/kg	Mydriasis, less secretions
Phenothiazine (dystonia)	Diphenhydramine	1–2 mg/kg IV (maximum 25 mg)	Resolution
Phenothiazine (neuroleptic malignant syndrome)	Dantrolene	1–3 mg/kg IV	Resolution
Insulin reaction	Dextrose	1 g/kg IV	Improved consciousness
Isoniazid	Pyridoxine	5 g IV	Seizures abate; improved consciousness

Drug smugglers who have swallowed quantities of heroin or cocaine-filled balloons, condoms, or other containers can be diagnosed as a "body packer" by x-ray examination. Chest and abdominal x-ray films are of variable value in locating pills or tablets. Sometimes agglutinated masses of pills (bezoars) can be detected in this manner or even highlighted by the use of small amounts of radiopaque contrast material. Box 98–4 lists some drugs and chemicals that may be visualized on x-ray films.

Diagnostic Trials

For a few suspected toxins, administration of an antidote not only initiates therapy but also assists in the diagnosis of the agent involved. Table 98–10 lists some of the diagnostic trials that may be appropriate in the pediatric ICU setting. For example, flumazenil, a specific benzodiazepine antagonist, can be used as a diagnostic agent administered to the comatose patient. At an intravenous dose of 1 to 2 mg, adults showed rapid improvements in consciousness (analogous to naloxone's effectiveness in reversing narcotic-induced CNS depression) after overdose involving a variety of benzodiazepines.

REFERENCES

1. Litovitz TL, Klein-Schwartz W, Rodgers GC, et al: 2001 annual report of the American Association of Poison Control Centers toxic exposure surveillance system. *Am J Emerg Med* 20:391, 2002
2. Woolf A, Wieler J, Greenes D: Costs of poison-related hospitalizations at an urban teaching hospital for children. *Arch Pediatr Adolesc Med* 151:719-723, 1997.
3. Woolf AD, Lovejoy FN: Epidemiology of drug overdose in children. *Drug Safety* 9:291, 1993.
4. Palmer ME, Haller C, McKinney PE, et al: Adverse events associated with dietary supplements: an observational study. *Lancet* 361: 101-106, 2003
5. Kernan WN, Viscoli CM, Brass LM, et al: Phenylpropanolamine and the risk of hemorrhagic stroke. *N Engl J Med* 343:1826-1832, 2000
6. Samenuk D, Link MS, Homoud MK, et al: Adverse cardiovascular events temporally associated with Ma Hung, an herbal source of ephedrine. *Mayo Clinic Proc* 77:12-16, 2000.
7. Haller CA, Benowitz NL: Adverse cardiovascular and central nervous system events associated with dietary supplements containing ephedra alkaloids. *N Engl J Med* 343:1833-1838, 2000
8. Dyer JE, Roth B, Hyma BA: Gamma-hydroxybutyrate withdrawal syndrome. *Ann Emerg Med* 37:147-153, 2001
9. Storrow AB, Magoon MR, Norton J: The dextromethorphan defense: dextromethorphan and the opioid screen. *Acad Emerg Med* 2:791-794, 1995
10. Jacobsen D, McMartin KE: Methanol and ethylene glycol poisonings. *Med Toxicol* 1:309, 1986.
11. Chabali R: Diagnostic use of anion and osmolal gaps in pediatric emergency medicine. *Pediatr Emerg Care* 13:204-210, 1997

ADDITIONAL READINGS

1. Bailey DN: Results of limited versus comprehensive toxicology screening in a university medical center. *Am J Clin Pathol* 105:572, 1996.
2. Bond GR: The poisoned child: evolving concepts in care. *Emerg Med Clin North Am* 13:343, 1995.
3. Boyer EW, Woolf A: What's new on the street? *Clin Pediatr Emerg Med* 1:180-185, 2000.
4. Cantrou PG, Khanzanie P: Limited toxicology screening: end of a controversy? *Am J Clin Pathol* 105:527, 1996.
5. Cox MN, Baum CR: Toxicology reviews: immunoassay in detecting drugs of abuse. *Pediatr Emerg Care* 14:372, 1998
6. Ellenhorn MJ: *Medical toxicology—diagnosis and treatment of human poisoning*, ed 2, Baltimore, 1997, Williams & Wilkins.
7. Mitchell AA, Lovejoy FH, Goldman P: Drug ingestions associated with miosis in comatose children. *J Pediatr* 89:30, 1976.
8. Olson KP, Pentel PR, Kelley MT: Physical assessment and differential diagnosis of the poisoned patient. *Med Toxicol* 2:52, 1987.
9. Sugarman JM, Rodgers GC, Paul RI: Utility of toxicology screening in pediatric emergency department. *Pediatr Emerg Care* 13:194, 1997.
10. Woolf AD: Poisoning by unknown agents. *Pediatr Rev* 20:166, 1999.
11. Woolf AD, Shannon MW: Clinical toxicology for the pediatrician. *Pediatr Clin North Am* 42:317-333, 1995.
12. Wright R, Woolf AD: Methemoglobin: etiology, pharmacology, and clinical management. *Ann Emerg Med* 34:646, 1999.
13. Wu AHB, McKay C, Broussard LA, et al: National Academy of Clinical Biochemistry laboratory medicine practice guidelines: recommendations for use of laboratory tests to support the poisoned patient who presents to the emergency department. *Clin Chem* 49:357-379, 2003.
14. Zweiner RJ, Ginsburg CM: Organophosphate and carbamate poisoning in infants and children. *Pediatrics* 81:121, 1988.

CHAPTER 99

Toxidromes and Their Treatment

Prashant Joshi, MD

PEARLS

- When given for a benzodiazepine overdose, flumazenil may precipitate acute withdrawal in the patient who habitually uses benzodiazepine or may unmask seizures caused by a coingested substance.
- Although rare, pulmonary edema may be a serious complication of reversal of opioids with naloxone.
- Beta-blockers, when used to lower blood pressure in a sympathomimetic overdose, may lead to unopposed alpha-receptor stimulation and therefore paradoxical worsening of hypertension.
- Physostigmine should be reserved for severe, life-threatening manifestations of anticholinergic toxicity because of the risk of asystole or seizures.
- Transcutaneous pulse oximetry is unreliable in methemoglobinemia and may show falsely increased or falsely decreased values depending on the methemoglobin concentration.
- Methylene blue should not be administered to individuals with known glucose-6-phosphate dehydrogenase (G6PD) deficiency because they lack adequate concentrations of reduced nicotinamide adenine dinucleotide phosphate (NADPH) to produce reductase activity and because methylene blue can trigger hemolysis or methemoglobinemia in those individuals.
- The skin is a distinguishing factor between sympathomimetic (pale, cool, and diaphoretic) and anticholinergic (flushed, warm, and dry) toxidromes.
- The toxic differential diagnosis of hyperthermia should include malignant hyperthermia, serotonin syndrome, neuroleptic malignant syndrome, sympathomimetic poisoning, and anticholinergic poisoning.
- An elevated osmolar gap suggests ingestion of a toxic alcohol; a normal result does not exclude it.
- Succinylcholine is contraindicated in cholinesterase-inhibitor toxicity.
- Nitrites should be used with extreme caution in patients with cyanide poisoning and concomitant carbon monoxide poisoning because of the risk of further decreasing oxygen-carrying capacity.
- Total iron-binding capacity (TIBC) may be falsely elevated in patients with acute iron overdose and is not a reliable marker in iron toxicity.
- In the United States, the local Regional Poison Center may be reached by calling 1-800-222-1222.

Every year more than 2 million exposures to toxic substances are reported to poison centers in the United States.[1] Of these, approximately 60% involve children younger than 12 years. Although three fourths of calls are managed without referral to a health care facility, of the 25% of patients who are seen in a health care facility, 1 in 8 is admitted to a critical care unit.

In most cases of poisoning, the agents involved are known, or at least circumstantial evidence points to a specific toxin or toxins. Even in those cases, however, in which the toxic exposure is unknown or in which the clinical presentation is inconsistent with the history, the intensivist can possibly find clues of the inciting agent and provide more targeted therapy.

The term *toxidrome,* a contraction of *toxic syndrome,* refers to a constellation of signs that is associated with certain substances or groups of substances. Several toxidromes have been described, and although their expression may not always be complete in every case, they may provide valuable information to guide investigation and treatment. A list of toxidromes appears in Chapter 98.

The patient should be examined carefully and thoroughly. Particular attention should be paid to vital signs, mental status, pupil size and reactivity, skin characteristics (color, temperature, moisture), and bowel sounds. Other important aspects of the physical examination include muscle tone, respiratory effort, presence of tremor, and features of the mucous membranes.

This chapter addresses some common presentations of toxic ingestions and their treatment. For more in-depth information the reader is referred to several comprehensive textbooks of medical toxicology.

Opiate

The classic triad of respiratory depression, coma, and miosis is seen with both naturally occurring opiates and synthetic opioids. Additional features include bradycardia, hypotension, and decreased gastrointestinal (GI) motility. A similar clinical picture may be encountered with ingestion of clonidine, a centrally acting a_2 agonist that decreases sympathetic tone. Naloxone is an opiate-receptor antagonist that reverses the toxic effects of opioids. For life-threatening opiate-induced depression, a starting dose of 0.1 mg/kg intravenously is recommended. If no intravenous access is available, it may also be given subcutaneously, intramuscularly, or via an endotracheal tube. It may precipitate acute withdrawal in opioid-dependent individuals; in such patients a lower starting dose, titrated upward to effect, may be warranted. Naloxone has been reported anecdotally to reverse clonidine overdose, although failure of naloxone to reverse clonidine has also been described. In patients with apnea, artificial ventilation should be provided promptly before the administration of naloxone. Because the duration of action of naloxone is shorter than that of many opiates, repeated doses or a continuous intravenous infusion may be necessary. Reversal of opioid toxicity has been associated with pulmonary edema, although it has also been described in the setting of opiate toxicity itself.[2,3]

Nalmefene is a newer long-acting opiate-receptor antagonist. Before it is used, a test dose of naloxone should be used to exclude the possibility of acute withdrawal. It probably offers no advantages over a continuous naloxone infusion.

Sympathomimetic

Symptoms and signs of sympathetic excess may be seen with a number of therapeutic and illicit agents. Drugs that produce the sympathomimetic toxidrome are listed in Box 99–1. Any or all of the manifestations in Box 99–2 may be observed, depending on the agent involved. For instance, agents with predominantly beta activity are more likely to produce tachycardia and even hypotension from peripheral vasodilation, whereas agents with predominantly alpha effect may produce severe hypertension with reflex bradycardia. Clinical effects may be produced by direct stimulation of adrenergic receptors or produced indirectly through the release of norepinephrine (e.g., cocaine). Increased metabolic activity may lead to hyperthermia, rhabdomyolysis, and myoglobinuria. Myocardial ischemia may occur, especially with cocaine. Ischemic or hemorrhagic stroke may be seen. The methylxanthines caffeine and theophylline are not sympathomimetics per se but may produce many of the same clinical features. Severe hypertension, tachycardia, agitation, and muscular overactivity should be treated with benzodiazepines as a first-line agent to reduce central nervous system (CNS) catecholamine release. Caution should be exercised when adrenergic antagonists are used to treat tachycardia and hypertension: beta-blocker use may result in unopposed alpha-receptor stimulation and cause a paradoxical worsening of hypertension. The use of labetalol, a beta-blocker with alpha-blocking activity, or concomitant administration of a vasodilator is recommended. Also, agents such as cocaine may cause depletion of norepinephrine and lead to cardiovascular collapse. Treatment of hypertension with a short-acting agent is therefore advisable.

This syndrome is not seen with centrally acting α agonists such as clonidine, which decrease sympathetic outflow and result in coma, bradycardia, and hypotension.

BOX 99–1

Agents That Cause Sympathomimetic Syndrome

Albuterol
Amphetamines
Caffeine
Catecholamines
Cocaine
Ephedrine
Ketamine
PCP (phencyclidine)
Phenylephrine
Phenylpropanolamine
Pseudoephedrine
Terbutaline
Theophylline

BOX 99–2

Sympathomimetic Toxidrome Features

Agitation
Seizures
Mydriasis
Tachycardia
Hypertension
Diaphoresis
Pallor
Cool skin
Fever

Anticholinergic

The anticholinergic toxidrome is produced by a number of agents that possess antimuscarinic properties as their primary effect or as a "side effect." Examples of such toxins are provided in Box 99–3. Muscarinic receptors are located in the CNS, in the target organs of the parasympathetic nervous system, and in the sweat glands (sympathetic nervous system). The syndrome may have features that are similar to those of the sympathomimetic toxidrome (Box 99–4). Examination of the skin usually provides clues to differentiate between the two. Hypertension and tachycardia are typically less severe than that seen with sympathomimetics. Also, the dilated pupils of the anticholinergic syndrome are nonreactive, and there is associated cycloplegia.

Treatment of agitation is important to prevent hyperthermia because sweating is inhibited in intoxicated patients. Benzodiazepines are the drug of choice. Physostigmine is a cholinesterase inhibitor that may be used to reverse the central and peripheral manifestations of anticholinergic toxicity. Because of case reports of convulsions[4] or asystole[5] associated with its administration, it should not be used to treat the anticholinergic manifestations of tricyclic antidepressant overdose.

BOX 99–4

Anticholinergic Toxidrome Features

Agitation
Delirium
Coma
Mydriasis
Dry mouth
Warm, dry, flushed skin
Tachycardia
Hypertension
Fever
Urinary retention
Decreased bowel sounds

Cholinergic

Cholinergic agents may be divided into three categories:

1. Muscarinic agents
2. Nicotinic agents
3. Cholinesterase inhibitors

Muscarinic agents act in the CNS, at postganglionic parasympathetic nerve endings, and in the sweat glands. Nicotinic agents act in the CNS, in the autonomic ganglia (sympathetic and parasympathetic). Cholinesterase inhibitors increase available acetylcholine in the cholinergic synapse and present with a combined picture. Agents with cholinergic activity are listed in Box 99–5. Signs and symptoms of cholinergic excess are produced by a number of chemical and medicinal agents listed in Box 99–6.

Direct-acting muscarinic agents produce typical features of excess parasympathetic activity. Atropine effectively reverses toxicity. Nicotine produces salivation, nausea, and vomiting. Hypotension, bradycardia, and respiratory depression may be preceded by tachycardia, hypertension, and tachypnea. Central features may include initial stimulation and then seizures, lethargy, and coma. Neuromuscular blockade may occur. Management of nicotine poisoning is entirely supportive.

Cholinesterase inhibitors such as organophosphate pesticides and nerve agents produce a mixed picture of toxicity, although parasympathetic manifestations tend to dominate the autonomic component of toxicity. Organophosphates bind to and inactivate acetylcholinesterase, preventing the normal termination of cholinergic stimulation of postsynaptic receptors. The end result is excessive nicotinic and muscarinic activity in the peripheral nervous system and CNS. At the neuromuscular junction, the product is depolarizing neuromuscular blockade. Over time the enzyme becomes phosphorylated, and cholinesterase activity is only restored by synthesis of a new enzyme. Carbamates bind reversibly to acetylcholinesterase, and the enzyme-chemical complex undergoes spontaneous hydrolysis, restoring cholinesterase function generally within hours.

BOX 99–3

Anticholinergic Agents

Antihistamines—diphenhydramine, hydroxyzine
Atropine
Benztropine mesylate
Carbamazepine
Cyclic antidepressants
Cyclobenzaprine
Hyoscyamine
Jimsonweed
Oxybutynin
Phenothiazines
Scopolamine
Trihexyphenidyl

BOX 99–5

Drugs Causing Cholinergic Excess

Inhibitors of acetylcholinesterase
- Organophosphate insecticides (malathion, parathion, diazinon)
- Carbamate insecticides (aldicarb, carbaryl, propoxur)
- Nerve agents (soman, sarin, tabun, Vx, cyclosarin)
- Drugs used for myasthenia gravis/reversal of neuromuscular blockade-physostigmine, pyridostigmine, neostigmine, edrophonium

Direct muscarinic agonists
- Bethanechol
- Carbachol
- Methacholine
- Pilocarpine
- Muscarinic mushrooms—*Clitocybe* spp., *Inocybe* spp.

Nicotinic agents
- Nicotine
- Water hemlock

BOX 99–6

Cholinergic Toxidrome Features

- Muscarinic effects (DUMBBELS)
  - Diarrhea
  - Urinary incontinence
  - Miosis
  - Bradycardia
  - Bronchorrhea
  - Emesis
  - Lacrimation
  - Salivation
- Nicotinic effects
  - Fasciculations
  - Weakness
  - Paralysis
  - Tachycardia
  - Hypertension
  - Agitation
- Central effects
  - Lethargy
  - Coma
  - Agitation
  - Seizures

Carbamates do not penetrate the CNS as well, so central manifestations tend to be less severe. Death results from respiratory failure because these agents cause bronchorrhea, bronchospasm, decreased respiratory drive, and paralysis of the muscles involved in breathing. The order of appearance of symptoms and signs depends on the route of administration. For example, with dermal exposure, the first manifestation may be local hyperhidrosis followed by systemic manifestations once the agent is absorbed through the skin. Inhalational exposure results in initial upper airway manifestations and respiratory distress. Ingestion presents with drooling and vomiting as the earliest expression of toxicity.

Treatment of organophosphates involves atropine to reverse the muscarinic effects, an oxime to reverse neuromuscular blockade, and benzodiazepines to treat seizures. Extremely large doses of atropine may be necessary, and the end point of therapy is the drying of secretions, *not* heart rate or pupil size. Depending on the agent involved, repeated doses or even a constant infusion may be necessary. Pralidoxime is the oxime that is available in North America. It works by reactivating acetylcholinesterase. Pralidoxime is generally not indicated in carbamate overdose, in which reversible binding of toxin to acetylcholinesterase limits the duration toxicity.

Methemoglobinemia

Methemoglobinemia is a condition in which the oxidization of the iron in hemoglobin from the ferrous (2+) form to the ferric (3+) form results in the inability to carry oxygen. Methemoglobinemia is associated with drugs and toxins that cause an oxidative stress (Box 99–7). Clinically the patient appears cyanotic, and the cyanosis does not respond to the administration of oxygen. The blood is chocolate colored, and exposure of the blood sample to oxygen does not restore a normal appearance. The diagnosis is confirmed by multiple-wavelength co-oximetry. Transcutaneous pulse oximetry, which uses only two wavelengths of light, cannot reliably be used to assess the degree of methemoglobinemia. It may overestimate or underestimate true oxygen saturation, depending on the methemoglobin level.[6,7] PaO_2 is normal.

BOX 99–7

Toxins That Cause Methemoglobinemia

- Benzocaine
- Dapsone
- Inhaled nitric oxide
- Lidocaine
- Naphthalene (found in certain mothballs)
- Nitrates
- Nitrites
- Nitroprusside
- Phenazopyridine
- Prilocaine
- Sulfonamides

Under normal conditions, the body produces a small amount of methemoglobin (typically <1%), which is reduced by a methemoglobin reductase that is dependent on reduced nicotinamide adenine dinucleotide (NADH). Because a large oxidative stress overwhelms the reducing capacity of this pathway, the result is clinically apparent methemoglobinemia. Also, a pathway that is dependent on reduced nicotinamide adenosine dinucleotide phosphate (NADPH) is only of minor significance at physiologic conditions.

Although patients may appear blue with methemoglobin concentrations as low as 15 g/L, treatment is not required in the absence of signs and symptoms of tissue hypoxia. Therapy, if required, begins with the administration of 100% oxygen (to maximize oxygen-carrying capacity with the certainty that unaffected hemoglobin is fully saturated). This is followed by intravenous methylene blue at a dose of 1 mg/kg. Methylene blue is reduced to leukomethylene blue with the NADPH-dependent methemoglobin reductase; methylene blue then reduces the heme iron to its normal state. Response is rapid and occurs within 30 minutes. Depending on the toxin involved, recrudescent methemoglobinemia may be seen and may require repeated doses of methylene blue. The total (cumulative) dose should not exceed 7 mg/kg because methylene blue is itself an oxidizing agent. Methylene blue may be ineffective in patients with glucose-6-phosphate dehydrogenase (G6PD), in whom it may cause hemolysis or methemoglobinemia.

Hyperthermia (see also Chapter 101)

There are several distinct hyperthermia syndromes described as being caused by drugs. In addition to the following syndromes described, the sympathomimetic and anticholinergic syndromes may also cause hyperpyrexia and are detailed separately. The differences between malignant hyperthermia, serotonin syndrome and neuroleptic malignant syndrome are provided in Table 99–1.

Malignant Hyperthermia

Malignant hyperthermia is a genetically determined condition that is triggered by exposure to depolarizing neuromuscular blocking agents and to inhalational anesthetics. It is life threatening and requires prompt intervention including treatment with dantrolene. Malignant hyperthermia is discussed in more detail in Chapter 117.

Serotonin Syndrome

Serotonin syndrome is a constellation of features resulting from excessive serotonergic activity in the CNS. It is most commonly associated with therapeutic regimens that include two or more drugs that increase CNS serotonin transmission (Box 99–8), although it may also be seen with single agents in overdose. The hallmark features are altered mental status, excessive muscle activity, and autonomic instability. Diagnostic criteria have been suggested by Sternbach.[8] The diagnosis requires history of exposure to a serotonergic agent(s) and the presence of three of the following: mental status change, agitation, myoclonus, hyperreflexia, diaphoresis, shivering, tremor, diarrhea, incoordination, fever. Symptoms typically start within hours of exposure to the offending agent and resolve within 24 hours. Most cases are mild and self-limiting; patients with severe toxicity may have severe hyperthermia and rhabdomyolysis with renal failure and cardiovascular collapse. Treatment is supportive with withdrawal of all serotonergic agents, benzodiazepines for muscle overactivity, and cooling. Cyproheptadine, a serotonin blocker, has been proposed for the treatment of serotonin syndrome, but its utility has not been established.[9]

BOX 99–8

Drugs Associated with Serotonin Syndrome

Amphetamines
Bupropion
Cocaine
Dextromethorphan
Fenfluramine
Lithium
LSD
L-tryptophan
Meperidine
Monoamine oxidase inhibitors
Selective serotonin reuptake inhibitors (SSRIs)
Trazodone
Tricyclic antidepressants
Venlafaxin

Neuroleptic Malignant Syndrome

Neuroleptic malignant syndrome (NMS) is a constellation of features triggered by exposure to neuroleptic drugs (phenothiazines, butyrophenones, atypical antipsychotics). It is most commonly associated with initiation of therapy or with dose escalation. The onset is insidious, occurring over several days. The diagnosis requires exposure to a neuroleptic drug, fever, muscular rigidity, and at least two of the following: mental status change, mutism, tachycardia, labile blood pressure, diaphoresis, dysphagia, tremor, incontinence, leukocytosis, or elevated creatine kinase (CK) level.[10] Distinguishing NMS from lethal catatonia may be difficult. NMS is thought to represent the extreme end of the spectrum of extrapyramidal (antidopaminergic) side effects of these medications. Unlike its milder counterparts, however, it is unresponsive to centrally acting anticholinergic agents. The treatment is supportive, including sedation, neuromuscular blockade, and active cooling if required. Hyperthermia does not respond to antipyretics. Myoglobinuria and renal failure may complicate the course. Bromocriptine, a dopamine-receptor antagonist, and dantrolene have been advocated in the treatment of NMS, but their value is debated.[11]

Metabolic Acidosis with Increased Anion Gap

Metabolic acidosis presents a substantial toxicological differential diagnosis. Common nontoxicologic causes of this disorder in children include diabetic ketoacidosis, uremia, lactic acidosis, and inborn errors of metabolism. The agents most commonly associated with metabolic acidosis are listed in Box 99–9 (see also Chapter 61). In addition, any agent that causes shock can cause a lactic acidosis with increased anion gap. Note that although metabolic acidosis from toxic agents is generally associated with an

TABLE 99–1

Differences between Drug-Induced Hyperthermia Syndromes

Syndrome	Causative Agent	Timing of Onset	Treatment
Malignant hyperthermia	Depolarizing neuromuscular blockers Inhalational anesthetics	Minutes	Dantrolene
Serotonin syndrome	Coadministration of two or more serotonergic agents	Hours	Supportive care, cyproheptadine
Neuroleptic malignant syndrome	Antipsychotic drugs	Days	Supportive care, bromocriptine

BOX 99–9

Agents That Cause Anion Gap Metabolic Acidosis

Carbon monoxide
Cyanide
Ethylene glycol
Iron
Isoniazid
Metformin
Methanol
Paraldehyde
Phenformin
Salicylates

increase in the anion gap, a nonanion gap acidosis may be seen with the therapeutic use of carbonic anhydrase inhibitors such as acetazolamide or topiramate, or with toxins such as toluene that cause renal tubulopathy with chronic use.

Methanol and Ethylene Glycol

Methanol and ethylene glycol are toxic alcohols that are found in various automotive antifreeze products and as chemical reagents. They are clear liquids at room temperature. Ethylene glycol has a sweet taste. Ethylene glycol–containing radiator antifreeze products contain fluorescein, and examination of the urine under a Wood's lamp has been advocated to screen for ingestion,[12] but urinary fluorescence was shown in most hospitalized pediatric patients in one study.[13] This finding called the usefulness of this simple test into question. Both compounds produce depression of the CNS but beyond that have little toxic effect in their parent form. Both substances are metabolized by alcohol dehydrogenase (ADH) to highly toxic metabolites. The end product of methanol metabolism is formic acid, and it causes severe metabolic acidosis and retinal toxicity. Ethylene glycol is converted to a number of intermediate toxic products and ultimately to oxalate; this conversion results in severe metabolic acidosis, renal failure, and hypocalcemia.

Ingestions greater than 0.5 ml/kg of either agent are potentially toxic, and ingestions of more than 1 ml/kg are potentially fatal. Because both substances are osmotically active, they will increase serum osmolality and will therefore raise the osmolal gap, the difference between calculated and actual osmolality as determined by freezing point depression. Caution should be exercised in interpreting this gap, however. Because the normal range is −8 to +12, significant levels of toxic alcohols may be present with a "normal" osmolal gap. In short, an elevated gap suggests toxic alcohol poisoning, whereas a normal result does not exclude it. Measured levels of ethylene glycol and methanol are the gold standard. An additional caveat applies to patients with late presentation: the parent compound may be completely metabolized, and therefore levels may be undetectable in the face of severe toxicity. Hemodialysis is still indicated in those patients to eliminate toxic metabolites and correct metabolic abnormalities.

Once the diagnosis of toxic alcohol poisoning is made and life-sustaining measures have been undertaken, initial therapy is targeted at blocking ADH to limit further generation of toxic metabolites. This may be achieved either with ethanol or with fomepizole. Ethanol infusion is difficult to titrate; requires frequent measurements; and carries the risks of inebriation, CNS depression, hypoglycemia, and hypotension. Fomepizole, a drug with known kinetics and with approval by the Food and Drug Administration (FDA) for the treatment of toxic alcohol poisoning, is the agent of choice. Once ADH is blocked, the parent alcohol is excreted through the kidneys with a half-life of 19.7 hours for ethylene glycol[14] and 54 hours for methanol.[15] Hemodialysis is then recommended in the presence of high levels of methanol or ethylene glycol, in the presence of significant acidosis or electrolyte disturbance, if there is renal impairment or visual impairment.

Carbon Monoxide

Carbon monoxide (CO) is the product of incomplete combustion of carbonaceous fuels. These include natural gas, fuel oil, gasoline, propane, and charcoal. CO causes tissue hypoxia through several mechanisms: it binds with high affinity to oxygen-binding sites of hemoglobin; it binds to myoglobin and disrupts the transfer of oxygen from erythrocytes to mitochondria; it binds to mitochondrial cytochrome oxidase; and it interferes with electron transport and adenosine triphosphate (ATP) production. CO also displaces nitric oxide from platelets leading to increased peroxynitrite generation. Transcutaneous pulse oximetry is unreliable at detecting CO poisoning and overestimates arterial oxygen saturation. The diagnosis is made with (four wavelength) co-oximetry on a blood sample. Correlation between symptoms and carboxyhemoglobin (COHb) level is poor, but levels are obtained to confirm the diagnosis. At low levels of CO symptoms are nonspecific and may include fatigue, malaise, nausea, and headache. Higher concentrations lead to impaired cognition and finally coma. CO poisoning may also cause hypotension and syncope. This may be explained in part by the effect of CO on nitric oxide. CO poisoning is also associated with delayed or persistent neurological sequelae, particularly in patients with loss of consciousness or syncope.

Treatment consists of accelerating the removal of CO from hemoglobin by providing as much oxygen as possible. The half-life of COHb under various oxygen concentrations is provided in Table 99–2. Hyperbaric oxygen (HBO), the administration of oxygen at supraatmospheric pressure, has been advocated in the treatment of severe CO poisoning. In addition to increasing the rate of resolution of COHb, it accelerates the removal of CO from cytochrome oxidase. A further effect is seen on leukocyte adhesion to endothelium, which is diminished. It is through this last mechanism that it is proposed to decrease the incidence of delayed neurologic sequelae, although two randomized trials led to conflicting results.[16,17] There are no clinical trials of HBO in children. Although its use remains controversial, it is recommended in children who

TABLE 99–2

Half-life of Carboxyhemoglobin

Oxygen Concentration	Half-life
21% (room air) 4	5 hr
100% (mask or endotracheal) 60	90 min
100% (hyperbaric molecular oxygen) 20	30 min

have a history of loss of consciousness or syncope or who have persistent neurologic findings on examination despite treatment with simple oxygen. Adverse reactions to HBO therapy include claustrophobia, barotrauma (pneumothorax, tympanic membrane rupture), and oxygen toxicity (seizures).

Fetal hemoglobin has a higher affinity for CO than does adult hemoglobin. As a result, neonates may have higher COHb levels than older children with the same exposure.

Cyanide

Cyanide is a highly toxic compound that may produce poisoning from a variety of sources. It is widely used as a reagent in industry. A number of plants, including the seeds of several edible fruits such as apples, cherries, peaches, and pears, contain cyanogenic glycosides that may be converted to cyanide in the GI tract. The unapproved substance Laetrile, sometimes used to treat cancer, is synthesized from amygdalin, a cyanogenic glycoside. Fires, particularly those in which plastics are combusted, can generate hydrogen cyanide (HCN). Finally, nitroprusside is metabolized to cyanide and can cause toxicity at high doses or in the presence of renal failure.

Cyanide produces toxicity rapidly, especially through the inhalational route (HCN). Cyanide salts (sodium cyanide [NaCN], potassium cyanide [KCN]), when ingested, are converted to HCN in the presence of gastric acid, which is then absorbed. Cyanide binds to heme iron in the cytochrome complex, and the result is the inhibition of oxidative phosphorylation. Consequently, the patient is unable to use oxygen to produce ATP, and the result is energy failure. Signs and symptoms are nonspecific and reflect tissue hypoxia. Death may occur within minutes. Venous oxygen levels are elevated because of the cell's inability to use oxygen. Because of this, patients are not cyanotic.

Treatment of cyanide poisoning involves immediate life support measures followed by administration of antidote. Sodium nitrite is administered intravenously. Nitrites induce methemoglobinemia. Although the mechanism of action of nitrites in cyanide poisoning is incompletely understood, methemoglobin has a higher affinity for cyanide than does cytochrome oxidase. Nitrites are potent vasodilators and can cause significant hypotension that may be avoided by slow administration. Excessive methemoglobinemia is also a potential risk, and levels should be monitored. Nitrites should not be routinely administered to fire victims, who may have significant CO poisoning. The induction of methemoglobin in these individuals may reduce oxygen-carrying capacity below critical levels. The second antidote is sodium thiosulfate. Thiosulfate reacts with cyanide in the presence of the mitochondrial enzyme rhodanese to produce the nontoxic thiocyanate that is then excreted in the urine. Hydroxocobalamin is an alternative antidote that is not available in the United States. It reacts with cyanide to produce cyanocobalamin (vitamin B_{12}).

Iron

Iron is available alone and in combination with other vitamins. There are several salts available, all of which have different proportions of elemental iron. Iron toxicity is generally divided into several phases. The first phase occurs early, usually within 30 minutes, and consists of GI manifestations of vomiting and diarrhea and may include both hematemesis and hematochezia. Fluid and electrolyte losses may be severe during this period, and aggressive resuscitation may be necessary. The second phase, or so-called latent period, is a quiescent period in which the GI phase has ceased but in which the patient continues to feel unwell. During this phase, the patient may remain tachycardic, and metabolic acidosis develops. The third phase, which begins after 12 hours, is the phase of cardiovascular collapse and shock. The fourth phase is liver failure. The corrosive effect of iron on the GI tract may also lead to the development of scarring or stricture. Doses higher than 20 mg/kg of elemental iron reliably produce GI irritation, although systemic toxicity is not generally seen until doses of greater than 60 mg/kg. Absence of a prodromal GI phase generally precludes the development of serious systemic iron toxicity.

Iron is not bound effectively to activated charcoal, and lavage of the stomach or whole bowel irrigation should be considered. Plain radiographs of the abdomen may help to visualize the location of pills and guide decontamination decisions. Serum iron levels should be determined within 6 hours of ingestion; after that time, significant redistribution to tissues may have occurred. TIBC, used in the evaluation of chronic iron overload, may be falsely elevated in acute iron ingestion and should not be used in treatment decisions.

Chelation with deferoxamine is indicated for serum levels higher than 500 μg/dl or for signs of circulatory failure. The dose is 15 mg/kg/hr intravenously. If the patient remains symptomatic beyond 24 hours, then the deferoxamine dose should be decreased because prolonged use is associated with the development of acute respiratory distress syndrome (ARDS).[18]

Isoniazid

Isoniazid (INH) is a relative of pyridoxine and of nicotinic acid used in the treatment of tuberculosis. It has a complex set of metabolic actions on several enzyme systems. It produces its acute toxicity primarily by interfering with pyridoxine metabolism.

After acute ingestion of a large quantity of isoniazid, early GI symptoms and drowsiness are followed by seizures, coma, and metabolic acidosis. The seizures are difficult to control with usual anticonvulsant therapy. The acidosis is lactic in nature and is produced by seizure activity and possibly by interference by INH in the conversion of lactate to pyruvate. Treatment of INH poisoning is with pyridoxine, which should be administered in a dose that is equal to the ingested dose of INH (by weight). If the dose ingested is unknown, then 5 g would be a reasonable starting dose. INH is effectively removed by hemodialysis, although the efficacy of pyridoxine should obviate the need for it in most cases.

Salicylates

There are several forms of salicylates, the most common of which is acetylsalicylic acid (ASA) or aspirin. The most potent form is wintergreen oil, which is made up of 98% methylsalicylate. Other forms include bismuth subsalicylate, sodium salicylate, and magnesium salicylate. Doses up to 100 mg/kg are likely to produce only minimal toxicity, whereas doses above 300 mg/kg may have serious consequences, including death.

Early signs of salicylate toxicity include an increase in minute ventilation (primary respiratory alkalosis) and tinnitus. Nausea and vomiting are also common. Salicylates also produce a metabolic acidosis through several mechanisms including uncoupling of oxidative phosphorylation and inhibition of the tricarboxylic acid cycle. Uncoupling of oxidative phosphorylation may also lead to hyperpyrexia. Cerebral edema and pulmonary edema are rare but potentially fatal complications of salicylate poisoning and are more common with chronic toxicity than with acute poisoning.

Enhancement of elimination of salicylates may be achieved through alkalinization of the urine. This is usually accomplished by administration of an infusion of sodium bicarbonate. The urine pH should be monitored frequently (every void in patients without a catheter) and the bicarbonate infusion rate adjusted accordingly to target a urine pH above 7.5. The goal is to maintain a normal urine output and not to perform *forced diuresis*. Serum pH should be monitored periodically to avoid serious alkalemia. Hemodialysis is also effective at clearing salicylate. Its use should be considered for very high serum levels; in the presence of renal impairment, volume overload, or pulmonary edema; and in the case of severe electrolyte or acid-base abnormalities.

Bradycardia, Hypotension, and Cardiac Conduction Abnormality

The most important cardiovascular agents that cause bradycardia and hypotension are calcium-channel antagonists, β-adrenergic antagonists, and digoxin. All of these agents may result in severe toxicity that requires specific therapy.

Calcium Channel Blockers

Calcium channel blockers exert their action on L-type calcium channels in the heart and vascular smooth muscle. Blockade of calcium channels in the heart results in negative inotropic, chronotropic, and dromotropic effects. Blockade of calcium channels in arteriolar smooth muscle causes vasodilation. Dihydropyridine calcium channel antagonists (e.g., nifedipine, amlodipine, felodipine, nicardipine) act primarily on the vascular smooth muscle. Verapamil also has potent cardiac calcium channel blocking activity and causes bradycardia, heart block, and myocardial depression. Diltiazem has similar effects to verapamil but is a less potent inhibitor of cardiac calcium channels. Calcium channel blockers also impair the release of insulin in overdose and may cause hyperglycemia.

Treatment depends on the agent involved and the severity of toxicity. Except in extremely large ingestions, dihydropyridines produce hypotension and reflex tachycardia. These patients may respond to volume expansion alone. Intravenous calcium and vasopressors are indicated if hypotension doesn't respond to intravenous fluids. Verapamil and diltiazem overdose is further complicated by pump failure. These patients may benefit from inotropes such as dobutamine or phosphodiesterase inhibitors (amrinone, milrinone). Glucagon, which acts at a specific receptor to increase cyclic adenosine monophosphate (cAMP), has been reported to reverse refractory hypotension in calcium channel overdose. The reported dose is 0.15 mg/kg intravenous bolus followed by an infusion of 0.05 to 0.1 mg/kg/hr.[19] High-dose insulin/euglycemia therapy has also been reported in several case reports and series to reverse cardiogenic shock associated with calcium channel blocker overdose.[20, 21] The dose used has ranged up to 1 U/kg/hr of insulin. Patients who are unresponsive to medical management should be considered for a left ventricular assist device (LVAD) or extracorporeal life support (ECLS) (see also Chapter 47).

Beta-Blockers

β-Adrenergic antagonists comprise a fairly extensive list of therapeutic agents that are distinguished from each other largely by their selectivity (or lack thereof) for the β_1 receptor. Atenolol, metoprolol, esmolol, and acebutolol are β_1-selective agents, whereas agents such as propranolol, nadolol, and pindolol act both at β_1 and β_2 receptors. In addition, certain agents have other activities. Propranolol has sodium channel–blocking activity and labetalol also possesses alpha-receptor-blocking activity. The β_1 receptor is found largely in the heart, and agonism causes positive inotropic and chronotropic effects. β_2 receptors are found in the airway smooth muscle where they cause bronchodilation, in the small blood vessels where they cause vasodilation, and in several other organs where they have a number of effects that are not important in the context of poisoning.

Acute overdose of beta-blockers results in bradycardia, hypotension, and conduction delay. Toxicity is generally much lower than with agents such as verapamil and diltiazem. Bronchospasm may occur in susceptible individuals. Propranolol, by virtue of its sodium channel–blocking activity, causes QRS widening, exaggerated negative inotropy, chronotropy, and conduction delay. It is also lipid soluble, and its crossing into the CNS results in coma and seizures. Labetalol may cause vasodilation in addition to β receptor blockade. Hypoglycemia may also be seen with these drugs.

Treatment beyond monitoring is not necessary if the only manifestation is asymptomatic bradycardia. Patients with bradycardia and hypotension may respond to atropine, although it is expected that such patients would have decreased vagal tone to start with, in response to bradycardia. β Agonists have variable effects in the presence of beta-blockade; in theory mixed agonists could worsen hypotension by causing β_2 receptor–mediated vasodilation. The phosphodiesterase inhibitors amrinone and milrinone have theoretical benefit in improving contractility by blocking the breakdown of cAMP. Glucagon acts via a nonadrenergic receptor to increase intracellular cAMP and improve cardiac contractility. The recommended dose is the same as that previously described for calcium channel blockers. Patients who do not respond to these measures, such as patients with calcium channel blocker overdose, should be considered for ECLS. Seizures should be treated with benzodiazepines as first-line therapy, and bronchospasm might respond to anticholinergic agents if inhaled β_2 agonists fail to overcome the beta-blockade.

Digoxin

Digoxin and related digitalis glycosides are used in the management of cardiac failure and tachydysrhythmias. Digoxin blocks Na/K-ATPase and ultimately leads to increased intracellular calcium concentration and improved contractility. It also increases vagal tone and causes sinoatrial (SA) and atrioventricular (AV) nodal depression. In overdose, sympathetic tone is increased and may lead to increased automaticity.

Overdose of digoxin presents with nausea, vomiting, lethargy or confusion, and cardiac dysrhythmias. Although virtually every rhythm has been described in digoxin toxicity, bidirectional ventricular tachycardia and atrial tachycardia with AV block are characteristic. Blockade of Na/K-ATPase causes hyperkalemia. The diagnosis is confirmed with measurement of the serum digoxin level.

Sinus bradycardia or heart block may respond to atropine alone. More serious arrhythmias are an indication for treatment with digoxin-specific Fab fragments (Digibind, DigiFab). Drugs that further depress the SA or AV node should be avoided. Hyperkalemia resolves with Fab fragment therapy because it restores function of the Na-K pump. Because digoxin causes intracellular hypercalcemia, calcium is best avoided because it could theoretically increase toxicity. Fab fragment therapy in children is indicated with known digoxin ingestion (strong history of ingestion of at least 0.1 mg/kg *or* digoxin level over 5 ng/ml) *and* signs and symptoms of digoxin toxicity (rapidly progressing signs and symptoms of digoxin toxicity *or* potentially life-threatening arrhythmias *or* serum potassium over 6 mEq/L).[22]

A clinical picture similar to digoxin poisoning may be seen with the ingestion of certain cardiac glycoside-containing plants such as oleander. Oleander poisoning may cause a false-positive result on digoxin immunoassay and may respond to Fab fragment therapy.[23]

Acetaminophen (Paracetamol)

Although it does not cause a toxidrome per se, acetaminophen is the most commonly ingested drug in intentional overdose, and it may cause fulminant hepatic failure leading to admission to the pediatric intensive care unit (PICU). The major route of elimination of acetaminophen is through conjugation and then excretion in the urine. A minor pathway is via CYP2E1 to produce a toxic metabolite N-acetyl-*p*-benzoquinone-imine (NAPQI), which can bind to hepatocytes and cause cell death. With therapeutic doses of acetaminophen, NAPQI is rapidly detoxified by glutathione. In overdose, larger amounts are formed and may overwhelm this mechanism and cause hepatic necrosis.

Patients may be seen initially with nausea and vomiting, but often patients have no symptoms or signs. Metabolic acidosis may occur in extremely large ingestions. Transaminases begin to be elevated at approximately 24 hours after ingestion and peak between 48 and 72 hours. Patients either progress to fulminant hepatic failure or recover completely (see also Chapter 81). Treatment with N-acetylcysteine (NAC) reduces the incidence of hepatotoxicity when administered in a timely fashion after overdose. It acts through several mechanisms including enhancing the synthesis of glutathione. It is most efficacious when administered within 10 hours of ingestion but may be beneficial when given up to 24 hours after ingestion. Decision to treat is based on plotting a single acetaminophen blood level at least 4 hours after ingestion on the Rumack-Matthew nomogram (Figure 99–1). In patients who are seen late, with established hepatic encephalopathy, NAC may also be beneficial, although its mechanism of action in this scenario is unclear. In one study, intravenous NAC decreased the risk of death from acetaminophen-induced fulminant hepatic failure.[21]

Tricyclic Antidepressants

Tricyclic antidepressants (TCAs) are a group of drugs with potentially serious toxicity that are used in the treatment of psychiatric disorders, enuresis, and pain syndromes. Although they have largely been supplanted as first-line agents by less toxic compounds in the treatment of depression, they still represent a significant cause of morbidity and death.

TCAs have multiple mechanisms of toxicity and produce a wide spectrum of clinical effects. Their anticholinergic properties may produce the anticholinergic toxidrome (Box 99–4). α-Adrenergic inhibition may cause sedation and hypotension. Blockade of cardiac sodium channels causes decreased myocardial contractility and is seen on the electrocardiogram (ECG) as widening of the QRS complex. QRS widening correlates with the development of seizures (QRS >100 ms) and arrhythmias (QRS >160 ms).[25] Potassium channel blockade leads to a prolonged QT interval. Seizures, which tend to be single and short-lived, occur and may be due to a combination of TCA effects on γ-aminobutyric acid (GABA) and on reuptake of biogenic amines in the CNS. This constellation of anticholinergic syndrome, seizures, hypotension, and widening of the QRS complex should create a high index of suspicion of TCA overdose. A similar picture may be seen with Type Ia antiarrhythmics.

Severe toxicity tends to occur early in the course of TCA poisoning. Patients who do not manifest QRS widening,

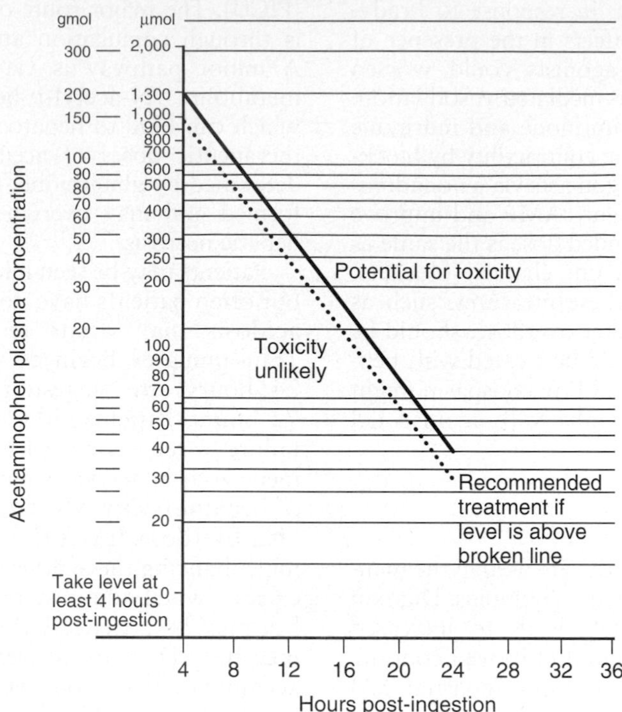
Use of Nomogram in Management of Acute Acetaminophen Overdose
An approach to management of acute acetaminophen overdose
1. Draw blood for acetaminophen plasma assay 4 or more hours post-ingestion.
2. PLOT ON NOMOGRAM.
3. If the acetaminophen level, determined at least 4 hours following an overdose, falls above the broken line, administer the entire course of acetylcysteine treatment.
4. If the acetaminophen level, determined at least 4 hours following an overdose, falls below the broken line, acetylcysteine treatment is not necessary or if already initiated may be discontinued.
5. Serum levels drawn before 4 hours may not represent peak levels.
gmol
µmol
Acetaminophen plasma concentration
Potential for toxicity
Toxicity unlikely
Recommended treatment if level is above broken line
Take level at least 4 hours post-ingestion
Hours post-ingestion

FIGURE 99–1 • Use of nomogram in management of acute acetaminophen overdose.

conduction abnormalities on ECG, altered mental status, seizures, or hypotension within the first 6 hours can be classified as low risk and no longer need PICU monitoring.[26] Anticholinergic manifestations should be treated supportively only. Seizures, if prolonged, should be treated with benzodiazepines. If benzodiazepines have been coingested by the patient, then flumazenil, a benzodiazepine receptor antagonist, should *not* be administered because it may unmask TCA-induced seizures. Widening of the QRS complex (>100 ms in adults) or ventricular arrhythmias should be treated with sodium bicarbonate to produce alkalinization of the serum. Bicarbonate should be given in boluses until ECG improvement is seen (narrowing of the QRS). Recurrence of QRS widening may be treated in the same manner. Alternatively, a bicarbonate infusion can be started after the initial bolus to maintain alkalemia (with monitoring to prevent overalkalinization [i.e., pH greater than 7.55]). If continuous infusion of bicarbonate is performed, then it may be stopped and the ECG monitored after approximately 6 hours of normal ECG tracings.

REFERENCES

1. Watson WA, Litovitz TL, Rodgers GC Jr et al: 2002 annual report of the American Association of Poison Control Centers Toxic Exposure Surveillance System, *Am J Emerg Med* 21:353-421, 2003.
2. Brimacombe J, Archdeacon J, Newell S et al: Two cases of naloxone-induced pulmonary oedema—the possible use of phentolamine in management, *Anaesth Intensive Care* 19:578-580, 1991.
3. Sterrett C, Brownfield J, Korn CS et al: Patterns of presentation in heroin overdose resulting in pulmonary edema, *Am J Emerg Med* 21:32-34, 2003.
4. Newton RW: Physostigmine salicylate in the treatment of tricyclic antidepressant overdosage, *JAMA* 231:941-943, 1975.
5. Pentel P, Peterson CD: Asystole complicating physostigmine treatment of tricyclic antidepressant overdose, *Ann Emerg Med* 9: 588-590, 1980.
6. Watcha MF, Connor MT, Hing AV: Pulse oximetry in methemoglobinemia, *Am J Dis Child* 143:845-847, 1989.
7. Ralston AC, Webb RK, Runciman WB: Potential errors in pulse oximetry. III: effects of interferences, dyes, dyshaemoglobins and other pigments, *Anaesthesia* 46:291-295, 1991.
8. Sternbach H: The serotonin syndrome, *Am J Psychiatry* 148: 705-713, 1991.
9. Graudins A, Stearman A, Chan B: Treatment of the serotonin syndrome with cyproheptadine, *J Emerg Med* 16:615-619, 1998.
10. American Psychiatric Association: *Diagnostic and statistical manual for mental disorders,* ed 4, Washington, DC, American Psychiatric Press.
11. Rosebush PI, Stewart T, Mazurek MF: The treatment of neuroleptic malignant syndrome. Are dantrolene and bromocriptine useful adjuncts to supportive care? *Br J Psychiatry* 159:709-712, 1991.
12. Winter ML, Ellis MD, Snodgrass WR: Urine fluorescence using a Wood's lamp to detect the antifreeze additive sodium fluorescein: a qualitative adjunctive test in suspected ethylene glycol ingestions, *Ann Emerg Med* 19:663-667, 1990.
13. Casavant MJ, Shah MN, Battels R: Does fluorescent urine indicate antifreeze ingestion by children? *Pediatrics* 107:113-114, 2001.
14. Sivilotti ML, Burns MJ, McMartin KE et al: Toxicokinetics of ethylene glycol during fomepizole therapy: implications for management. For the Methylpyrazole for Toxic Alcohols Study Group [see comment], *Ann Emerg Med* 36:114-125, 2000.
15. Brent J, McMartin K, Phillips S et al: Fomepizole for the treatment of methanol poisoning, *N Engl J Med* 344:424-429, 2001.
16. Scheinkestel CD, Bailey M, Myles PS et al: Hyperbaric or normobaric oxygen for acute carbon monoxide poisoning: a randomised controlled clinical trial, *Med J Aust* 170:203-210. 1999.
17. Weaver LK, Hopkins RO, Chan KJ et al: Hyperbaric oxygen for acute carbon monoxide poisoning, *N Engl J Med* 347:1057-1067, 2002.
18. Tenenbein M, Kowalski S, Sienko A et al: Pulmonary toxic effects of continuous desferrioxamine administration in acute iron poisoning [see comment], *Lancet* 339:699-701, 1992.
19. Bailey B: Glucagon in beta-blocker and calcium channel blocker overdoses: a systematic review. *J Toxicol Clin Toxicol* 41:595-602, 2003.

20. Yuan TH, Kerns WP II, Tomaszewski CA et al: Insulin-glucose as adjunctive therapy for severe calcium channel antagonist poisoning, *J Toxicol Clin Toxicol* 37:463-474, 1999.
21. Boyer EW, Duic PA, Evans A: Hyperinsulinemia/euglycemia therapy for calcium channel blocker poisoning, *Pediatr Emerg Care* 18:36-37, 2002.
22. Woolf AD, Wenger TL, Smith TW et al: Results of multicenter studies of digoxin-specific antibody fragments in managing digitalis intoxication in the pediatric population, *Am J Emerg Med* 9(2 suppl 1):16-20; discussion 33-34, 1991.
23. Gupta A, Joshi P, Jortani SA et al: A case of nondigitalis cardiac glycoside toxicity, *Ther Drug Monit* 19:711-714, 1997.
24. Keays R, Harrison PM, Wendon JA et al: Intravenous acetylcysteine in paracetamol induced fulminant hepatic failure: a prospective controlled trial, *BMJ* 303:1026-1029, 1991.
25. Boehnert MT, Lovejoy FH Jr: Value of the QRS duration versus the serum drug level in predicting seizures and ventricular arrhythmias after an acute overdose of tricyclic antidepressants, *N Engl J Med* 313:474-479, 1985.
26. Foulke GE: Identifying toxicity risk early after antidepressant overdose, *Am J Emerg Med* 13:123-126, 1995.

CHAPTER

100

Bites and Stings

Sean P. Bush

PEARLS

- Snakebite-related injury and death are reduced most by rapid transport, intensive care, and antivenom.
- Measures *not* recommended for snakebite first aid are incision, suction, tourniquets, electric shock, ice directly on wound, alcohol, or folk therapies.
- Antivenoms can induce immediate anaphylactic (type I hypersensitivity) or anaphylactoid reactions, which can be rapidly life threatening. Airway swelling, wheezing, shock, and urticaria characterize these reactions. Anaphylactic and anaphylactoid reactions are treated with antihistamines, histamine (H_2) blockers, epinephrine, steroids, and ventilatory/circulatory support as needed.
- All children with snake envenomations should be admitted to the hospital. Serious effects can be delayed and can recur even after treatment with antivenom.
- Typically, the bite site has a "target" appearance. There may be a central reddened, indurated area around fang puncture site(s) surrounded by an area of blanching and an outer halo of redness. The findings around the bite wound may be subtle.
- Any bee, wasp, or ant can cause toxic, even fatal, complications when they attack en masse. Sting removal following a honeybee sting should be done as quickly as possible, regardless of the method of removal.

The general principles of envenomation medicine are similar around the world, although the availability of resources varies widely. A comprehensive discussion of all available antivenoms is beyond the scope of this textbook.[1] On the basis of my experience and in consideration of space constraints, the scope of this textbook, and its audience, the chapter focuses on U.S. antivenoms. Readers are encouraged to become familiar with the prescribing information for the antivenom(s) available in their area(s) of practice for the envenomations they may encounter.

Snakebites

Snakebite is a particularly challenging clinical problem because of the wide variety of toxic effects. Children with snakebites may have little more than a fang puncture mark, or they may have multisystem failure and death.[2,3] Part of this is due to the extreme variability of snake venom, even within the same species.[4] Snake venom contains multiple enzymes, proteins, and peptides that can damage local tissues and have serious systemic effects. Unfortunately, it is difficult to predict at the time of the bite which patients will have relatively mild symptoms and which will have a rapidly progressive and potentially fatal envenomation syndrome.

Snakebite envenomation syndromes can be loosely associated with snake family. Viperidae includes old-world vipers and pit vipers (collectively referred to as *viperids*). Most snakebites in the United States are inflicted by pit vipers, which include rattlesnakes, cottonmouths (also known as water moccasins), and copperheads.[5] All pit vipers have a triangular head, elliptical pupils, and a heat-sensing pit between the eye and nostril (Fig. 100–1).[6] The pit organ has thermal receptors that can detect temperature differences of 6° C at 1.5 m in predatory interactions and 10° C at 1 m in defensive contexts (Krochman A: Personal communication, January 17, 2005). The family Elapidae ("elapids") includes cobras, coral snakes, kraits, and mambas.[7] Their venom effects can be as diverse as the

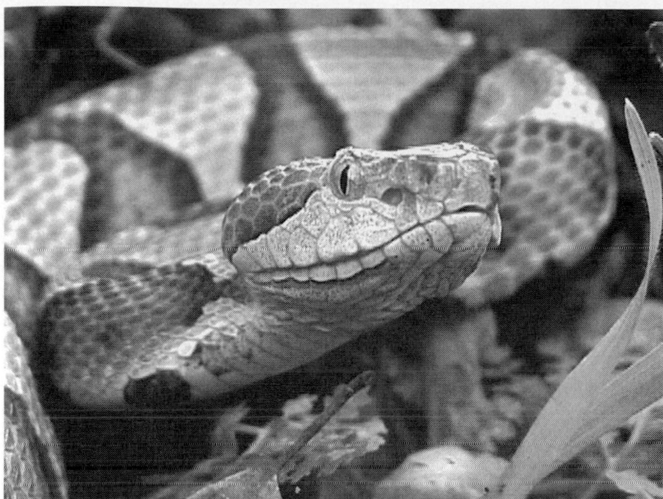

FIGURE 100–1 • Copperhead (*Agkistrodon contortrix*). (Photo by Sean Bush, MD.)

species that make up this family of snakes. Cobras are showy, hooded, high-profile snakes that inhabit Africa and southern Asia (Fig. 100–2). The coral snakes of the Americas and kraits of Asia and India are often small, shy, colorfully banded snakes (Fig.100–3). Mambas in Africa are long, lean, and very fast moving. Australian elapids can be large and nondescript. Sea snakes possess some of the world's most toxic snake venom, although few bites occur mostly because of the marine distribution and nonaggressive temperament of these snakes. Most snakes from the Colubridae family ("colubrids") are considered harmless, although several species possess venom and some have primitively specialized teeth to facilitate venom delivery. Some, such as the boomslang in Africa, are considered dangerous to humans, and antivenom is produced.

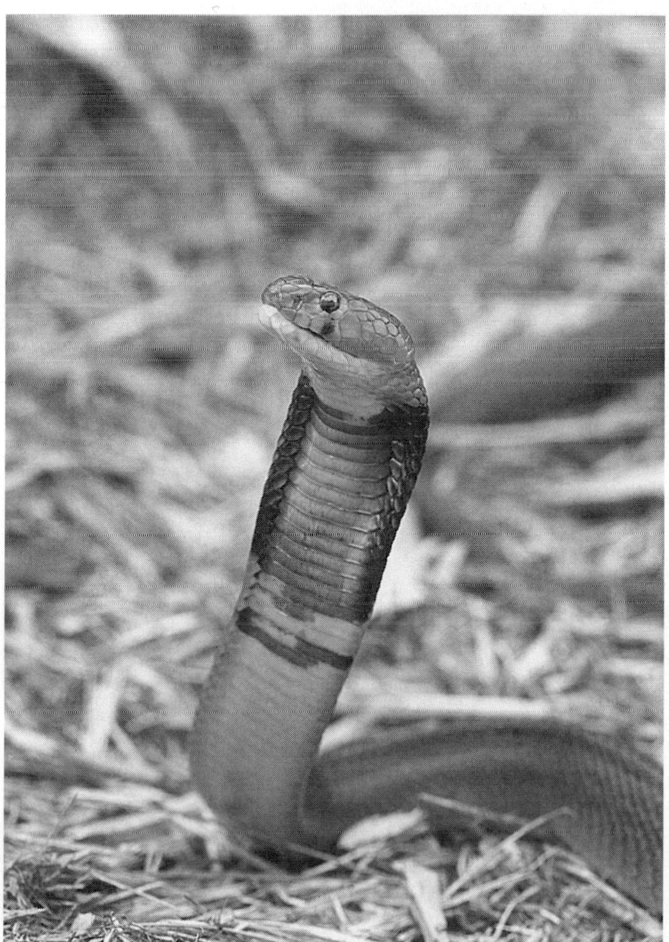

FIGURE 100–2 • Red spitting cobra (*Naja pallida*). Photo by Mike Cardwell.

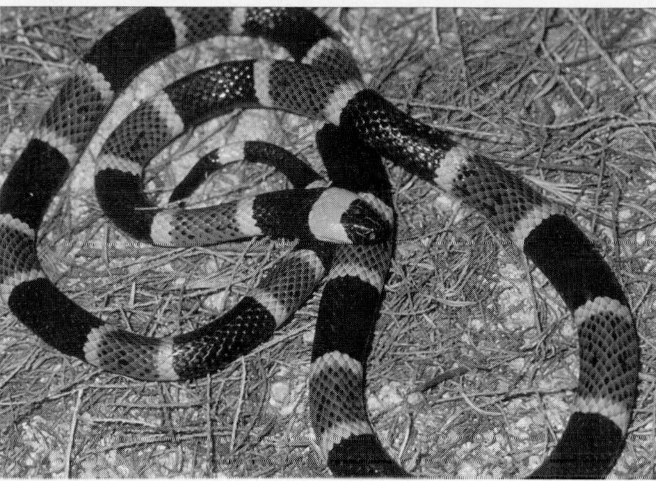

FIGURE 100–3 • Eastern coral snake (*Micrurus fulvius*). Photo by Mike Cardwell.

Epidemiology

It is often stated that children are more severely affected by snakebite than adults.[8] Indeed some preliminary data suggest that smaller patients present have increased severity. There is not much in terms of evidence, however, to support the assertion that outcomes for children are worse than adults. For example, of the 104,750 exposures and 23 deaths described by the American Association of Poison Control Centers (AAPCC) since its first report in 1983, there have only been two deaths described in pediatric patients.[9] In some respects, children are no different than adults when it comes to snakebite. For instance, antivenom dosing is not based on the patient's weight,[10, 11] yet there are a few concerns specific to pediatric patients. For example, because young children may not be able to give a good description of the snake or circumstances, it may be unclear whether a venomous snake has bitten them.

Pathophysiology

Although viper and pit viper venom composition varies from snake to snake, components can lead to capillary leak, abnormal clotting, inefficient muscle movement, or neurotoxicity. Capillary leak and abnormal clotting can lead to tachycardia, hypotension, or even hemorrhagic shock. Neurotoxicity or inefficient muscle movement can lead to respiratory difficulty or distress.[12] Meanwhile, proteolytic enzymes, predominant in viper and pit viper venoms, digest tissue. The longer enzymatic components of venom have time to work, the more tissue gets damaged. Thus "time is tissue."[13] The sooner that antivenom can be started, the sooner that irreversible injury can be prevented.[14] Once tissue is injured by way of digestion, however, antivenom will not reverse the damage; it will have to heal over time.[15] Myotoxicity and rhabdomyolysis can ensue.

Envenomation by most elapids is notable for severe neurological dysfunction, such as cranial nerve abnormalities, paralysis, and respiratory arrest. Some elapids, however, such as spitting and monocellate cobras, can also cause local necrosis. Most do not induce coagulopathy. Other symptoms and signs may include swelling, lethargy, vomiting, chest pain, and shock. Some cobras and cobralike species can "spit" venom toward the face of an antagonist, which can result in eye pain and visual impairment.

Sea snake envenomation can cause profound neurotoxicity and myotoxicity but generally does not induce coagulopathy or result in serious local injury. Sea snakes are found in waters around Southeast Asia and Australia.

Additionally, some individuals may experience anaphylactic or anaphylactoid reactions to venom.[16,17] Finally, some responses can be attributed to anxiety, although this should be a diagnosis of exclusion.[6]

Clinical Presentation

Immediately after a snakebite, the only apparent manifestation may be fang puncture wounds. If a patient is seen soon after a snakebite, an envenomation syndrome might not have developed yet. The onset of symptoms and signs can occur rapidly or it may be insidious. Generally the more severe an envenomation, the more rapidly it progresses; however, even a slowly progressing envenomation can lead to severe sequelae. If a patient is seen very late, the envenomation could have already run its course, and antivenom will not be as effective.[14]

Typically snakebites by pit vipers and vipers cause pain around the bite site as tissues distort with swelling. There may or may not be associated taste changes. Difficulty breathing can follow many types of venomous snakebites and can progress to respiratory distress or failure in some cases. Patients may experience nausea, vomiting, or diarrhea, and venom-induced coagulopathies (often associated with viper and pit viper envenomation) can lead to hematemesis, hematochezia, or both. Certain snakebites, such as those inflicted by most elapids and some populations of rattlesnakes, can also be associated with neurological symptoms, such as motor weakness or paresthesias. Syncope or lethargy can result from severe or prolonged hypotension.[6]

Vital signs may reflect tachycardia, hypotension or hypertension, tachypnea, or hypoventilation. On physical examination, there may be one, two, or more fang puncture wounds, or none may be discernable. There is usually tenderness and swelling surrounding the bite site, which expands as the venom spreads locally. Other local signs can include erythema, ecchymosis, and bullae after viperid envenomation (Fig. 100–4). Systemic evidence of viperid envenomation may manifest in many ways. There may be abnormal bleeding, such as prolonged bleeding from fang puncture wounds or intravenous (IV) start sites. Patients may have epistaxis or gingival bleeding. Serious and potentially life-threatening bleeding may manifest via the gastrointestinal tract or within the cranium. In extremely rare instances, snakebite can also cause hypercoagulability, which can lead to infarcts. Additionally, there may be neurological signs, such as ptosis (Fig. 100–5), and muscle fasciculations.[6]

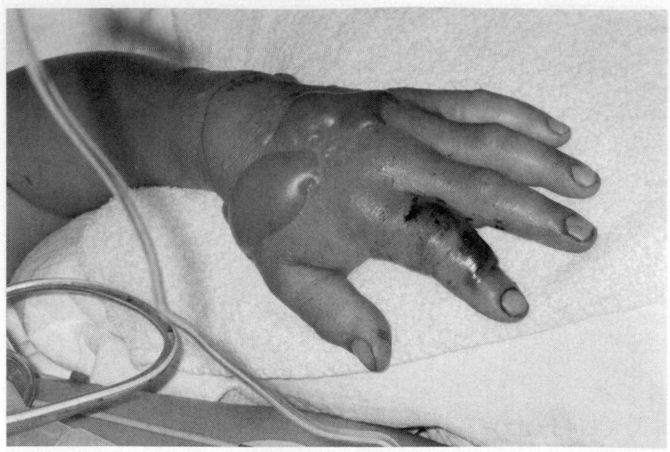

FIGURE 100–4 • Southern Pacific rattlesnake (*Crotalus helleri*) bite wounds.
Photo by Sean Bush, MD.

Diagnostic Studies

Initial laboratory tests after pit viper or viper envenomation should include a complete blood count (CBC), prothrombin time (PT), partial thromboplastin time (PTT), international normalized ratio (INR), fibrinogen, and a type and screen (T + S). Venom-induced coagulopathy is common after many types of viperid envenomations (although not after elapid or sea snake envenomations) and is most typically characterized by thrombocytopenia and hypofibrinogenemia. If coagulation values are *normal* on presentation, they may need to be rechecked, depending on the clinical scenario. Venom-induced coagulopathies can develop late,

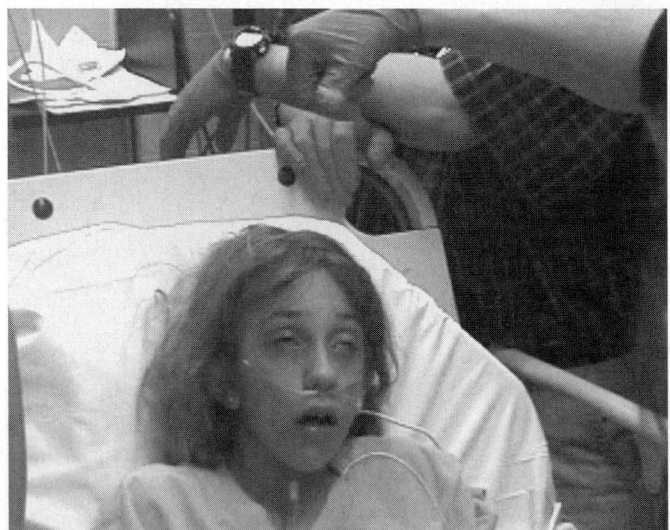

FIGURE 100–5 • Ptosis after Mohave rattlesnake (*Crotalus scutulatus*) envenomation.
Photo by Sean Bush, MD.

recur, or persist. If initial laboratory findings are *abnormal*, more frequent monitoring may be necessary depending on how severely abnormal they are and how they respond to treatment. If the findings are abnormal, repeating the CBC, PT, PTT, INR, and fibrinogen tests 1 hour after completion of an infusion of antivenom may be helpful to monitor treatment efficacy. When laboratory values are rechecked, order the same tests as initially drawn and add tests for creatine kinase (CK), electrolytes, blood urea nitrogen (BUN), and creatinine clearance. Patients with just about any kind of snakebite can have rhabdomyolysis, which usually responds to aggressive fluid hydration, but can require dialysis if myoglobinuric renal failure develops. In certain regions, such as Australia, venom detection kits (e.g., enzyme-linked immunosorbent assays [ELISAs]) may be available to help identify species and guide specific antivenom selection. Other diagnostic studies may be indicated on the basis of a patient's medical history or special circumstances.[6]

Pitfalls

It is possible that a snakebite might be mistaken for a puncture wound from another cause (e.g., from a plant thorn,) if the patient is seen very early, if the envenomation is mild, or if there are difficulties obtaining a reliable history. If there is any question about whether a patient has been bitten by a venomous snake, an observation period and diagnostic studies may help clarify the diagnosis. Snakebites usually progress if significant envenomation has occurred. Certain signs (e.g., ecchymosis), symptoms (e.g., local paresthesias), and laboratory data (e.g., thrombocytopenia or hypofibrinogenemia), if affected, are fairly consistent with viperid envenomation. If a bite by an elapid is suspected, envenomation should be assumed.

Prehospital Care

The factors that most reduce snakebite-related injury and death in the United States are rapid transport, intensive care, and antivenom.[18] All patients with snakebites should be transported to the hospital as expeditiously and safely as possible, preferably through a 911 call (where available). The following measures are not recommended for first aid: incision, suction, tourniquets, electric shock, ice directly on wound, alcohol, or folk therapies.[19-21] Insufficient evidence exists for splinting or positioning (e.g., above or below the level of the heart). Therefore the extremity should initially be maintained in a neutral position of comfort. The Australian technique of pressure immobilization resulted in significantly longer survival, but higher intracompartmental pressures after artificial, intramuscular western diamondback rattlesnake envenomation in a pig model.[22] This technique involves immediately wrapping the entire extremity that was bitten starting at the bite site and proceeding proximally with an elastic ACE wrap or crepe bandage as tightly a one would wrap for a sprain, then splinting and immobilizing the extremity. Although pressure immobilization is not recommended widely, certain scenarios may warrant its use. It is generally not recommended for most viper bites or for bites by spitting cobras, but it is recommended for most types of Australian fauna, cape cobras, kraits, coral snakes, mambas, and sea snakes. Once pressure immobilization is placed, it should not be removed until antivenom is ready to infuse (if asymptomatic) or infusing (if symptomatic) because of a potential bolus effect after its removal. Although it is difficult to predict snakebite severity at the time of the bite, certain factors may reflect increased likelihood of a more severe envenomation: large snake size, dangerous snake species, small patient size, prolonged fang contact, previous snakebites (treated or not) or exposures to snakes, or delays to medical care.

Emergency and Critical Care

All emergency personnel should be able to distinguish a venomous from a nonvenomous snake. If there is uncertainty about whether a particular snake is venomous, consider taking photographs of the snake from a safe distance of at least 6 feet away using a digital or Polaroid camera. These images can be seen immediately and may help make clinical decisions. Although it may be helpful to identify the species of snake,[15,23] transporting it (alive or dead) is discouraged because of inherent dangers. On scene, snakes should only be moved or contained if absolutely necessary. A snake hook or long shovel may be helpful to move the snake into a large, empty trash canister where it can be recovered by professionals, such as an animal control agent.

Airway support, advanced pediatric life support (APLS) protocol, or both should be provided as needed. Severe respiratory difficulty may require intubation and mechanical ventilation. Check vitals frequently, provide oxygen, and place monitors (cardiac, blood pressure, and pulse oximetry). Start two IV lines. Central venous or interosseous access may need to be obtained. Avoid placing a central line in a noncompressible site (e.g., internal jugular), however, after viperid envenomation because of the risk of bleeding from venom-induced coagulopathy. A normal saline fluid bolus of 20 ml/kg should be given. If there is evidence of shock, give a second fluid bolus. Because viperid envenomation can induce coagulopathy and bleeding, transfusion may be required after treatment with two fluid boluses. Give packed red blood cells of 10 ml/kg for acute, life-threatening blood loss. Persistent hypotension may require pressors. Urine output may be used as a measure of adequate hydration. The patient should take nothing by mouth until it has been determined that the patient will not need to be mechanically ventilated.

After pit viper or viper envenomation, remove rings, other constricting jewelry, and clothing in anticipation of severe swelling. The expanding area of swelling and tenderness can be used to follow the progression of viperid envenomations. Tenderness is more sensitive than swelling for detecting progression. Also, it is preferable to follow the advancing edge of tenderness or swelling than to follow serial measurements of circumference. Palpate until the edge of advancing tenderness is found. Mark this leading edge with a permanent marker and write the time alongside. Repeat this often enough to gauge progression. This may mean checking every 15 to 20 minutes initially.

Once antivenom is started, it should still be followed every 1 to 2 hours.

All hospitals should stock at least enough antivenom to treat one patient. This should be arranged ahead of time if possible, although sometimes there are antivenom shortages and other resource challenges. Two agents are available in the United States for treatment of pit viper envenomation: Crotalidae Polyvalent Immune Fab (Ovine), which goes by the trade name CroFab, and Antivenin Crotalidae Polyvalent (equine).[24] CroFab is manufactured by Protherics Inc. (Nashville, TN) and distributed by Fougera (Melville, NY [800-231-0206]). A similar formulation is produced for European vipers. Antivenin Crotalidae Polyvalent, manufactured by Wyeth-Ayerst (Madison, NJ), is still available on the shelves of many hospital pharmacies but is no longer being produced. Several manufacturers produce antivenom for elapid bites in Africa (e.g., South African Vaccine Producers in Johannesburg, http://www.savp.co.za/default.htm); Asia, Europe, and Australia (e.g., Commonwealth Serum Laboratories [CSL] in Melbourne, http://www.allergytest.com/index.cfm); and the Americas (e.g., Instituto Bioclon in Mexico, http://www.bioclon.com.mx; Instituto Clodomiro Picado in Costa Rica, http://www.icp.ucr.ac.cr/indice.shtml; and the Butantan Institute in Brazil, http://bernard.pitzer.edu/~lyamane/butantan.htm). A polyvalent sea snake antivenom (CSL) is the drug of choice for sea snake envenomation, but tiger snake antivenom may have adequate efficacy if sea snake antivenom is not available. Haffkine Institute in Bombay, India, produces an alternate sea snake antivenom.

Information on antivenom should be researched ahead of time, and practitioners should be familiar with sources and administration techniques for the antivenoms available for envenomations they may encounter. Each antivenom has varying specificity, efficacy, and safety. Some antivenoms developed for one species may have some efficacy against other closely related species. If an exotic envenomation is encountered in the United States, calling the AAPCC or consulting the Antivenom Index may help locate antivenom. Many zoos stock antivenoms for the exotic species they keep.

If antivenom is unavailable, a patient with an elapid or sea snake envenomation may need his or her airway secured and ventilatory support for days or even weeks. Meanwhile, hypotension should be treated with IV fluids and then vasopressors. Edrophonium may temporarily improve weakened muscles of respiration after elapid envenomation while awaiting antivenom. After pretreatment with atropine, Edrophonium (5 mg slow IV push if <35 kg or 10 mg if >35 kg) may be given. Edrophonium can cause cholinergic crisis, which is treated with additional atropine.

Determine the need for antivenom in your patient. Many grading scales are available, but it is better to treat a patient based on envenomation progression or potential. Grading scales should not be used for elapid or sea snake envenomations. Antivenom should be given promptly for best results, although it may have benefit for days to weeks after an envenomation. Anytime antivenom is given, allergic reactions should be anticipated. It may be helpful to know whether the patient has allergies or previous exposures to papain, papaya or animal serums, or other agents used to make antivenom. Obtain informed consent when possible. Many of the principles of antivenom administration are similar; thus the technique for administering CroFab is outlined as an example. A starting dose of CroFab is 4 to 6 vials,[25] which is the same for children as it is in adults. Each vial is reconstituted with 10 ml of sterile water. It can take anywhere from about 10 to 30 minutes to go into solution. It is best to swirl or roll the vials between the hands rather than to shake them. Once each vial goes into solution, it should be further diluted into a total volume of 250 ml of normal saline. No skin test is recommended for CroFab, although manufacturers of many other types of antivenom recommend skin testing. With CroFab, the infusion is started slowly, at a rate of 1 ml/min for the first 10 minutes. While the infusion is started, a physician skilled in resuscitation should be at bedside. Difficult airway equipment, epinephrine, diphenhydramine and a histamine (H_2) blocker (such as cimetidine) should be immediately available. If the infusion is tolerated for the first 10 minutes without evidence of an adverse reaction, the rate should be increased to complete the total volume of 250 ml in an hour. If there is a problem at any time, stop the infusion, treat the adverse reaction accordingly, and reassess the need to continue antivenom treatment. A physician should be nearby at all times during the remainder of the infusions. Repeat four- to six-vial increments until initial control is achieved. *Initial control* is defined as the arrest of progression of any and all components of the envenomation syndrome (i.e., no further advancement of swelling, improvement of systemic effects, and improving coagulopathy). Assess at up to 1 hour after each dose. After initial control is achieved, a maintenance dose of two vials of CroFab every 6 hours for three doses is recommended to reduce recurrence.[26] Read the package insert for additional details.[25] For pharmacokinetic reasons that are not entirely understood, recurrence phenomena are associated with antivenoms.[27-29] *Local recurrence* is the return of new progressive swelling after initial control. That is, the leading edge of tenderness or swelling begins to advance again. An additional two vials of CroFab should be given as soon as progressive swelling recurs, and more antivenom may be necessary to regain control. Patients with rattlesnake bites commonly have thrombocytopenia and hypofibrinogenemia, which can resolve with CroFab and then recur (*coagulopathy recurrence*). Indications for an additional two vials of CroFab are serious abnormal bleeding, fibrinogen less than 50 μg/ml, platelet count less than 25,000 mm^3, INR greater than 3, multicomponent coagulopathy, worsening trend in patient with prior severe coagulopathy, high-risk behavior for trauma, or comorbid conditions that increase bleeding risk. Coagulopathy can recur as late as 2 weeks or more after treatment.

Transfuse if antivenom does not correct coagulopathy or if there is an imminent risk of serious bleeding. Transfusion of the appropriate blood product is generally recommended for life-threatening bleeding, platelets less than 20,000 mm^3, or hemoglobin less than 7 g/dl. Additionally, fresh frozen plasma, platelets, or both may be required to treat venom-induced coagulopathy if antivenom does not promptly resolve. Consider computerized tomography of the brain if the patient has a severe headache or an altered level of consciousness with a severe coagulopathy.

Ocular exposure to venom necessitates prompt and copious irrigation and an ophthalmologist's evaluation.

Provide pain relief (e.g., morphine sulfate 0.1 mg/kg IV, titrated to relief of pain and maintaining a respiratory rate and blood pressure that is appropriate for age). Nonsteroidal antiinflammatory drugs (NSAIDs) are contraindicated for approximately 2 weeks after viper and pit viper envenomation because they can contribute to venom-induced coagulopathy and bleeding.

Prophylactic antibiotics are unnecessary. Empiric antibiotic therapy should only be started if an infection develops and once aerobic and anaerobic wound cultures have been obtained. If an abscess occurs, it should be drained in standard fashion. An infected snakebite should prompt a further examination of the wounds for potential retained teeth or fangs.[5]

Envenomations by vipers and pit vipers are remarkable for the amount of swelling they can produce. With prompt and adequate antivenom treatment, fasciotomy or digit dermotomy is rarely indicated, even after severe viperid envenomation.[30-33] Fasciotomy, however, may be indicated if measured compartment pressures remain persistently and severely elevated despite adequate antivenom. Antivenom has been shown to limit the decrease in perfusion pressure associated with compartment syndrome.[34] Compartment syndrome may manifest subjectively, with complaints of increasing pain, and objectively, with tenderness on passive muscle stretch, a rock hard feel to the compartment, or a diminished capillary refill. True compartment syndrome, however, is rare after snakebites, even in patients with severe swelling. It may be difficult to distinguish compartment syndrome from the effects of envenomation. Similar to compartment syndrome, viperid envenomation may cause a bluish discoloration of the skin or pallor (because of subcutaneous bruising), severe swelling, paresthesias, and pain. If effects are only caused by envenomation and the patient does not have compartment syndrome, capillary refill should be normal and compartmental pressures should not be elevated. If compartment pressures are elevated, Gold et al[31] recommend limb elevation, along with IV mannitol (1 to 2 mg/kg) administration and an additional four to six vials of CroFab over 1 hour. Consultation with a surgeon (e.g., general, orthopedic, or hand) should be initiated concurrently. Compartment pressures should be measured before surgical intervention.

Therapeutic Complications

Antivenoms can induce immediate anaphylactic (type I hypersensitivity) or anaphylactoid reactions, which can be rapidly life threatening. Airway swelling, wheezing, shock, and urticaria characterize these reactions. Anaphylactic and anaphylactoid reactions are treated with antihistamines, H_2 blockers, epinephrine, steroids, and ventilatory/circulatory support as needed.

Antivenoms can also cause serum sickness, a delayed (type III hypersensitivity) reaction characterized by fever, urticaria, lymphadenopathy, and polyarthralgias days to weeks after treatment. Although serum sickness can be an uncomfortable experience, it is usually benign and self-limited, and the patient is treated on an outpatient basis with antihistamines and steroids. Also, adverse reactions are much less common after treatment with Fab-based antivenoms than they are with whole immunoglobulin formulations.[14]

All commercially available antivenoms in the United States use mercury, in the form of thimerosal, as a preservative, which in high doses can cause nerve and kidney toxicities in small children.[25] The manufacturer of CroFab is investigating alternative preservatives and plans to remove thimerosal from its product sometime in 2005 or 2006.

Resources

The AAPCC can assist in the management of envenomations. Poison control may be contacted at (800) 222-1222.

Disposition

It is prudent to admit all children with snake envenomations to the hospital. Serious effects can be delayed and can recur even after treatment with antivenom. Therefore close observation with monitoring, frequent measurements of swelling/tenderness, and neurological checks for at least 24 hours are recommended. This degree of monitoring may require transfer and admission to a pediatric intensive care unit (ICU). On discharge, the patient should return immediately for further swelling or severe pain. Additionally, the patient should return immediately for any abnormal bleeding or bruising, dark tarry stools, petechiae, or severe headache. Also, patients should be given wound care instructions and told to return for signs of wound infection. Signs of serum sickness should be outlined, and the patient should return or follow up if these signs show up anytime in the few weeks after treatment with antivenom. The patient should be told not to take NSAIDs for 2 weeks after a pit viper or viper bite. Instead, acetaminophen with or without a combined opiate analgesic should be prescribed. The patient should not engage in contact sports or schedule any elective surgery or dental work for 2 weeks after viperid bites. Recommend that the patient drink plenty of liquids and advise that the patient return if decreased urination or cola-colored urine is noticed. Some patients may need referral to a physical therapist. Blisters, blebs, and bullae should be left in place but may need debridement along with necrotic tissue after several days, so surgical referral as appropriate is suggested.[30] Skin grafting is sometimes necessary. If the patient was bitten on the foot or leg, crutches and crutch training should be provided. The patient should be encouraged, however, to bear weight and mobilize the extremity as tolerated. In some cases, a next-day wound check may be appropriate. Otherwise, the patient should return or follow up in a few days.[28] At that time, laboratory tests may need to be repeated, depending on the clinical scenario. Retreat with antivenom as needed.

Prognosis

Most patients recover fully after snakebite. Viperid envenomation results, however, in tissue loss, deformity, or loss of function in a clinically significant percentage of patients.[8,35]

Prevention

Preventative measures should be explained to parents and children. Teach children to leave snakes alone. They should never touch, handle, or try to kill venomous snakes. Many people are bitten when they are intentionally interacting with the snake. Even after a snake is believed to be dead, fangs still can inject venom. Snakes that were presumed dead have bitten many people and delivered serious, even fatal, envenomations. Additionally, a snake can strike faster and farther than one might think—about half its body length. Children should stay at least two giant steps away from snakes. If a child finds a snake, he or she should tell an adult. Additionally, tell children not to reach or step into places that they cannot see. Wearing boots and jeans may prevent some (but not all) snakebites.

If your patients live in snake territory, let them know that there is no way to keep snakes completely off their property. There are a few things, however, that may make a property less appealing for snakes. For example, eliminate places where snakes can hide (e.g., log piles or heavy vegetation). Educate children about what to do if a snake bites them (i.e., it is important that they tell an adult right away).

Future Directions

Modifications of the antivenom molecule or formulations may reduce recurrence phenomena, and this is being investigated.

Widow Spider Bites

Widow spiders belong to the genus *Latrodectus* and are represented in the United States by the black widows (Fig. 100–6), the brown widow, and the red-legged widow.[36] The redback spider is endemic to Australia. Other species, such as the kara kurt and black button spider, are found in other parts of the world, including Europe, South America, and South Africa. The adult female black widow spider is approximately 2 cm in length and shiny black with a red-orange hourglass or spot on the ventral abdomen. The male is much smaller, brown, and much less commonly implicated in human envenoming. Juvenile females are also brown with yellow and white markings but have the general body shape of the adult. Males and juveniles have a pale hourglass shape, similar to adult females. Webs are irregular; low lying; and commonly seen in garages, barns, outhouses, and foliage. Other widow spiders around the world are generally black but may have red spots, such as the kara kurt, or a dorsal red stripe, such as the redback spider. The brown widow is brown with red and yellow markings. Similar species include the false black widow or cupboard spider, *Steatoda* sp., which can produce symptoms that are similar in character but milder in intensity than widow spiders.

Epidemiology

No deaths caused by widow spider envenomation have been reported to the AAPCC since its first annual report in 1983. A recent death was reported, however, after a black widow spider bite in Greece.[37,38]

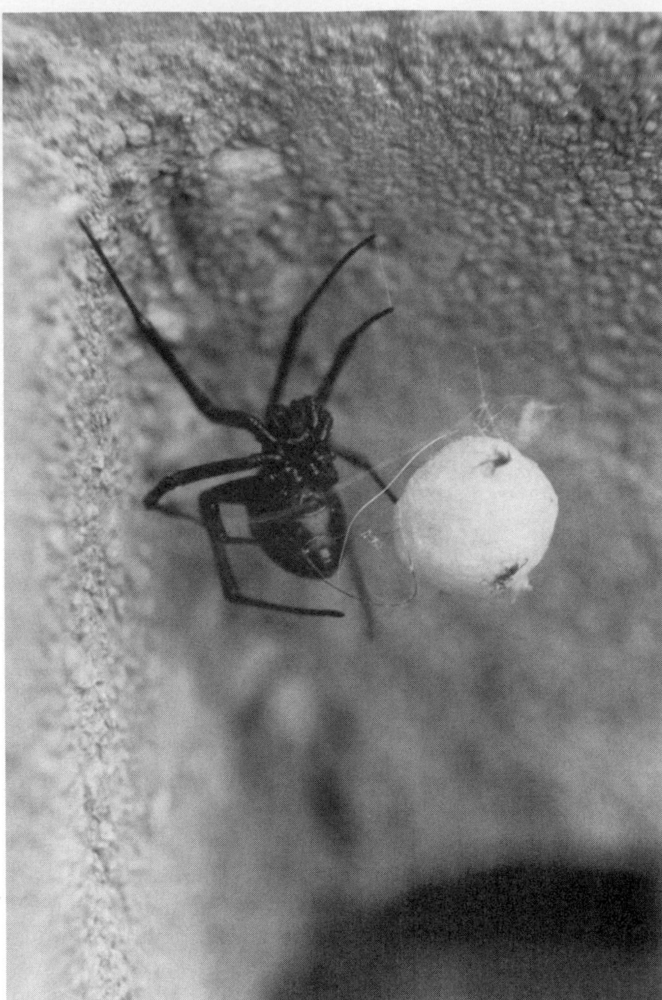

FIGURE 100–6 • Black widow spider (*Latrodectus hesperus*). Photo by Sean Bush, MD.

Pathophysiology

The envenomation syndrome caused by the various species of widow spiders around the world is similar.[39,40] The predominant clinical effects after widow spider envenomation are neurological and autonomic.

Clinical Presentation

Typically, the bite site has a "target" appearance. There may be a central reddened, indurated area around fang puncture site(s) surrounded by an area of blanching and an outer halo of redness (Fig. 100–7). The findings around the bite wound may be subtle, and the wound does not become necrotic. The predominant symptoms frequently involve painful muscle cramping. If a person is bitten on the lower extremity, pain usually progresses from the foot, up the leg, and into the back and abdomen. If a person is bitten on the upper extremity, pain usually progresses from the hand, up the arm, and into the chest and abdomen. Abdominal pain may be so severe as to mimic an acute

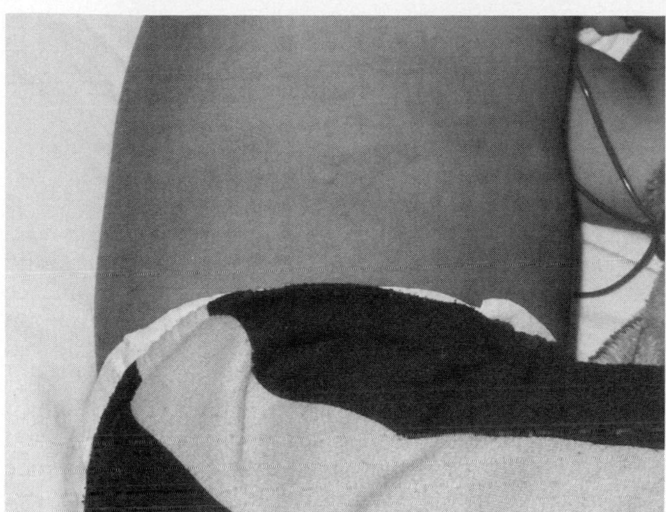

FIGURE 100–7 • Black widow spider bite site.
Photo by Sean Bush, MD.

abdomen, with tenderness and rigidity.[41] Diaphoresis locally around the bite site is distinctive for widow spider envenomation, although diaphoresis may be diffuse and profuse or it may manifest in unusual patterns remote from the bite site. Local piloerection is sometimes seen. Patients may exhibit "*Latrodectus* facies" (Fig.100–8), characterized by spasm of facial muscles; edematous eyelids; and lacrimation, which may be mistaken for an allergic reaction. Other common symptoms and signs include high blood pressure, rapid heart rate, nausea, vomiting, headache, and anxiety. In a typical progression, symptoms onset within an hour, reach maximum intensity by about 12 hours, and can last for days to weeks. Unusual presentations have been described following widow spider envenomation including pulmonary edema, myocarditis, and priapism.[37,42]

It has been suggested that there may be increased danger to pediatric patients with widow spider bites and that this population may require more aggressive treatment and hospitalization, although this assertion has been challenged.[43]

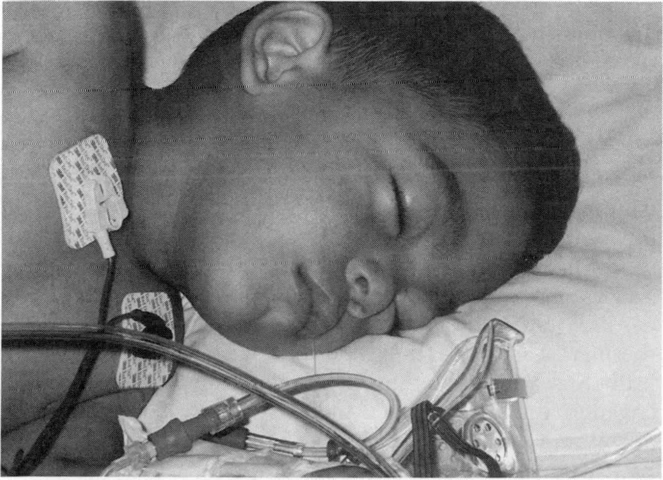

FIGURE 100–8 • *Latrodectus* facies.
Photo by Sean Bush, MD.

Little evidence supports either argument. The only recent documented fatality from widow spider envenomation involved a healthy 19-year-old woman.

Diagnostic Studies

Rhabdomyolysis has been reported after widow spider envenomation,[42] so a total CK test should be done if severe envenomation develops. If the patient has respiratory difficulty, get a chest radiograph. Electrocardiography (ECG) or echocardiography may detect that rare case of venom-induced myocarditis in a critically ill patient. Otherwise, diagnostics are not particularly helpful. If the diagnosis is uncertain, evaluation should be aimed uncovering other causes (such as appendicitis).

Pitfalls

Misdiagnosing an acute abdomen in a patient with a widow spider envenomation could lead to unnecessary surgery.

Emergency and Critical Care

There are two basic treatment options. Widow spider envenomation can be managed with antivenom or a combination of pain medications and sedatives. There are risks and benefits associated with each. Management with an opioid analgesic, such as morphine 0.1 mg/kg IV or intramuscular (IM), and a benzodiazepine such as lorazepam 0.01 mg/kg IV or IM, is generally considered safe. This treatment option, however, is purely palliative, and symptoms may persist for days or even weeks. The pain and discomfort associated with widow spider envenomation can be severe. In contrast, antivenom is remarkably effective. Unfortunately it can be associated with severe side effects and death.[44] Because death is so rare after widow spider envenomation, some would argue that the treatment is more dangerous than the bite itself. Historically, intravenous calcium was recommended, although it has now been found to be ineffective.[11] Several antivenoms have been manufactured including Black Widow Spider Antivenin (equine) in the United States, Australia Redback Spider Antivenom, USSR Monovalent (*Latrodectus tredecimguttatus*), and South Africa spider antivenom (button spider).[1] Indications for antivenom use and routes of administration vary around the world. According to the package insert of Black Widow Spider Antivenin, one vial should be reconstituted in 2.5 ml of the sterile diluent supplied. It is further diluted into a volume of 10 to 50 ml saline and administered intravenously over 15 minutes. Patients usually experience dramatic relief within an hour of treatment with one vial, although sometimes two and rarely three vials are necessary. It may be effective days, weeks, or possibly even months after the envenomation.[45] The risk of allergy to antivenom must be weighed against the benefit of relieving prolonged discomfort, avoiding hospitalization, and preventing complications. Although most widow spider envenomations can be managed with opioid analgesics and benzodiazepines, antivenom may be indicated for patients who have severe envenomations with pain refractory to these measures. Antivenom should be given if there is an imminent risk of a severe complication of envenomation. Factors that could increase the risk of antivenom include allergy or previous exposure to horse serum or a medical history of reactive airways.[46]

Antibiotics are not indicated for widow spider envenomation. Also, update tetanus prophylaxis as appropriate.

Therapeutic Complications

Serious, even fatal, adverse reactions have been documented after treatment with black widow spider antivenom. Anaphylactic and anaphylactoid reactions to antivenom can occur and may even be more life threatening than the envenomation itself. Skin testing, with the intradermal injection of 0.02 ml of the test material supplied and the observation for an urticarial wheal in 10 minutes, variably predicts immediate hypersensitivity to antivenom and may influence the decision regarding its administration. Increasing the volume of dilution and slowing the rate of infusion may reduce the chance that an allergic (anaphylactoid) reaction will occur. Additionally, premedication with antihistamines (H_1 and H_2 blockers) may reduce the likelihood that an acute allergic reaction will occur. Serum sickness, characterized by fever, urticaria, lymphadenopathy, and polyarthralgias, can occur days to weeks after treatment and is treated with antihistamines and steroids.

Resources

The AAPCC may be helpful with management of widow spider envenomations and can be contacted at (800) 222-1222.

Disposition

Because it so effectively resolves symptoms, antivenom has been shown to decrease the need for hospitalization after widow spider envenomation. Admission to the hospital and possibly the pediatric ICU is prudent for severely symptomatic children, those with intractable pain and contraindications to antivenom, those with unusual complications of envenomation, and those who have anaphylaxis to antivenom. Patients who experience relief with opioid analgesics, benzodiazepines, or antivenom may be discharged. On discharge, signs of serum sickness should be outlined, and the patient should return or follow up if these signs show up anytime in the few weeks after treatment with antivenom.

Prognosis

The envenomation syndrome usually resolves completely, with or without treatment, and does not leave the patient with long-term sequelae. Death is rare.

Prevention

Spider bites may be prevented by eliminating the spider's food and habitat; by shaking sheets, shoes, and clothing before donning; by keeping the child's bed away from the wall; and by brushing spiders off rather than crushing them.

Future Directions

Safer antivenoms are being developed and investigated.

Scorpion Stings

Most scorpion stings results in a simple, painful, local reaction that can be treated with analgesics, antihistamines, and symptomatic/supportive care. Some scorpions from the families Buthidae and genus *Hemiscorpius,* however, are potentially dangerous to humans and are considered medically important.[47] A triangular sternal plate helps distinguish Buthidae from other scorpion families in which the sternal plate is more pentagonal (Figs. 100–9 and 100–10). Medically important genera of scorpions include *Centruroides* in the southern United States, Mexico, Central America, and the Caribbean. The bark scorpion, *Centruroides exilicauda,* is found in Mexico and the southwestern United States, primarily Arizona and small parts of Texas, New Mexico, Nevada, and California; *Tityus* is found in Central and South America and the Caribbean; *Buthus* is found across the Mediterranean area, from Spain to the Middle East; *Mesobuthus* is found throughout Asia; *Parabuthus* is found in western and southern Africa; *Buthotus* (i.e., *Hottentotta*) is found across southern Africa to southeast Asia; *Leiurus* is found across northern Africa and the Middle East; and *Androctonus* is found from northern Africa to southeast Asia.[48] Scorpions may occasionally be found outside their natural range of distribution when inadvertently transported with items such as luggage.[49]

Epidemiology

In 2003 a total of 14,417 scorpion envenomations were reported to the AAPCC. Only one death from the Arizona bark scorpion (*C. exilicauda*) has been reported since 1964.[50] Global death rates estimates vary wildly.[48] Children are thought to have an increased risk of death.

Pathophysiology

The most important clinical effects of scorpion envenomations are neuromuscular, neuroautonomic, or local tissue effects.

Clinical Presentation

Patients with medically important scorpion stings often complain of pain, paresthesias, nausea, and vomiting. On physical examination, local tissue effects may vary. Most scorpions cause minimal local tissue injury, but some species can cause necrosis. Vital signs may reflect tachycardia, bradycardia, hypertension, hypotension, or hyperthermia. There can be respiratory difficulties, which can lead to death. Arrhythmias have been reported. Scorpion envenomation can affect the nervous system producing autonomic, somatic, or cranial nerve abnormalities. Patients may exhibit signs of sympathetic overdrive and parasympathetic signs, such as salivation, lacrimation, urination, defecation, and gastric emptying. Cranial nerve

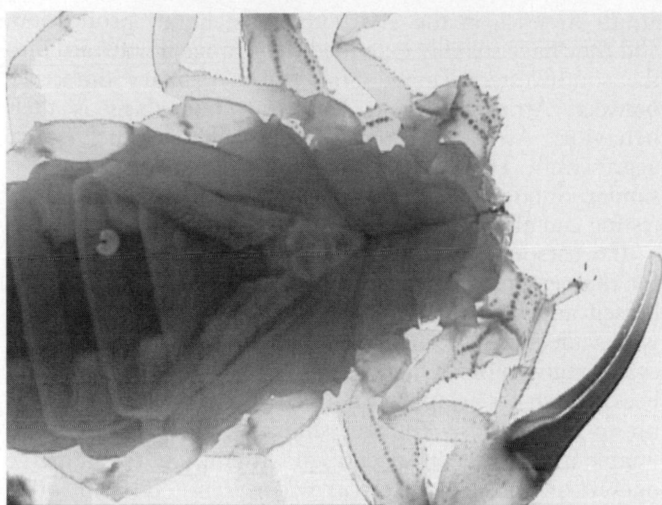

FIGURE 100–9 • A triangular sternal plate helps distinguish Buthidae from other scorpion families.
Photo by Sean Bush, MD.

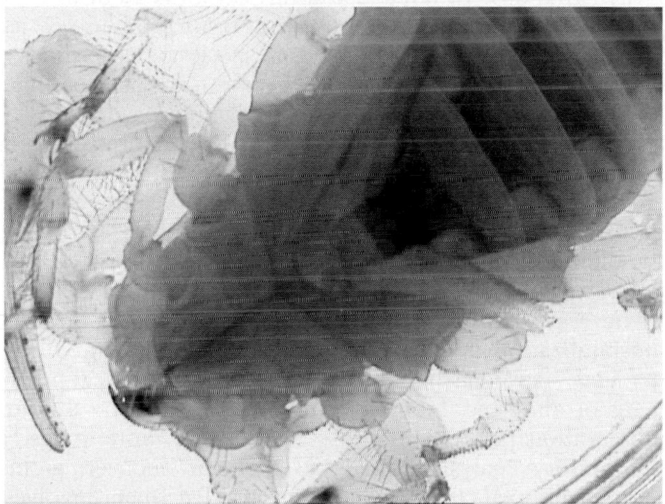

FIGURE 100–10 • Most scorpions have a pentagonal sternal plate.
Photo by Sean Bush, MD.

findings may include roving or rotary eye movements, tongue fasciculations, and difficulty swallowing. Somatic anomalies can involve restlessness and involuntary muscle jerking that can be mistaken for seizures. Cerebral infarction, cerebral thrombosis, and acute hypertensive encephalopathy have been described.

Diagnostic Studies

Laboratory tests will vary from case to case. In most situations, no laboratory tests are necessary; however, certain laboratory tests are suggested for specific scorpion stings. For example, hemolysis has been associated with *Hemiscorpius lepturus* stings, and defibrination has been reported following *Buthus tamulus* stings. Therefore a CBC and coagulation values are suggested following stings by these scorpions. Electrolytes, BUN, creatinine, and urinalysis should be checked as well. Renal failure may occur as a result of hemoglobinuria from hemolysis or myoglobinuria from rhabdomyolysis. A total CK test may reveal rhabdomyolysis after severe muscle hyperactivity. Because pancreatitis can occur after *Tityus trinitatis* envenomation, a lipase should be drawn. Respiratory difficulty may prompt arterial blood gas (ABG) measurements and a chest radiograph. Arrhythmias may necessitate an electrocardiogram.

Pitfalls

A skin test is recommended for many antivenoms, although the test may not be a reliable indication of immediate hypersensitivity. An urticarial wheal with surrounding erythema developing within 10 minutes is usually indicative of a positive result.

Use caution with opioid analgesia after severe scorpion envenomations because of possible synergistic effects on respiration between narcotics and venom. This concern is particularly pertinent for children and patients with unsecured airways who exhibit systemic signs of envenomation. Atropine is used to decrease respiratory secretions, but it could potentiate the sympathetic overdrive symptoms, which would be dangerous. It should be used, however, for symptomatic bradycardia. Also, obtain informed consent before giving antivenom when possible.

Emergency, Intensive Care Unit, and Hospital Care

Supportive care is the cornerstone of treatment for systemic symptoms. Analgesia should be given as needed with the aforementioned precautions in mind. Update tetanus prophylaxis as appropriate. Prophylactic antibiotic are unnecessary. Steroids have not been proved effective in treating venom toxicity. Hypertensive emergencies should be treated with standard antihypertensive therapy. Conversely, hypotension may necessitate fluid resuscitation, pressors, or both.

There are dozens of different types of scorpion antivenom.[1] They are available for a number of different species and have varied efficacy. Antivenom use remains a controversial issue. Many researchers report decreased morbidity, death, and hospital stay with its use. These researchers think that antivenom therapy cannot be matched by supportive care in severe Buthidae scorpion envenomations. Others suggest that adverse effects (e.g., anaphylactic reactions, serum sickness; see the following Therapeutic Complications section) limit or contraindicate its use.

Therapeutic Complications

Because anaphylaxis can occur whenever antivenom is given, appropriate therapeutic agents for treatment of anaphylaxis should be available for immediate use. Premedication, with antihistamines, for example, may reduce the severity and possibly the likelihood of adverse reactions to antivenom. Serum sickness can also develop and may be treated with steroids and antihistamines.

Resources

The AAPCC may be helpful with the management of scorpion stings and can be contacted at (800) 222-1222. The University of Arizona Poison and Drug Information Center

(520-626-6016 from outside Arizona or 800-362-0101 from Arizona only) has special experience in *Centruroides* envenomation. See also the eMedicine web page about scorpion envenomations (http://www.emedicine.com/emerg/topic524.htm). Specimen identification by an entomologist may also be helpful, if the scorpion can be captured safely.

Disposition

Patients with moderate to severe *Centruroides* stings and other severe Buthidae envenomations should be admitted to the ICU, treated with antivenom, or both. Some clinicians discharge patients from the emergency department (ED) safely after treatment with antivenom and complete resolution of their systemic symptoms.[51] Young children may not recover as quickly as adults after scorpion envenomation and are more likely to require observation. Patients with mild *Centruroides* envenomations may be discharged. Discharge of patients with other Buthidae envenomations is more problematic because onset of systemic symptoms may be delayed up to 24 hours. Instruct patient regarding progression. Discuss symptoms of delayed serum sickness with patients treated with antivenom.

Prognosis

Prognosis depends on many factors, including species of scorpion, patient health, and access to medical care. Most patients recover fully after scorpion envenomation.

Prevention

Protective clothing, such as shoes or gloves, may prevent some scorpion envenomations. Shoes and equipment left outside in areas with indigenous scorpions should be checked for arthropods before use.

Future Directions

Recently, the U.S. Food and Drug Administration gave preliminary approval for clinical trials to evaluate a Mexican antivenom for scorpion stings (Alacramyn; Laboratorios Silanes, Mexico City, Mexico) for use in the United States.

Hymenoptera Stings (Bees, Wasps, and Ants)

Stings by bees, wasps, and ants are less of a toxicological concern than they are an allergic one. Details on treatment of anaphylaxis are covered elsewhere in this text. The focus of this section will be mass envenomation.

Any bee, wasp, or ant can cause toxic, even fatal, complications when they attack en masse. Bee behavior, however, can vary, even within the same species. European honeybees tend to be docile and will tolerate approach of their hive to some degree but can become provoked. Africanized honeybees (*Apis mellifera scutellata*), however, are much more aggressive and will defend their hive much more proactively. Africanized honeybees were imported to South America in the 1950s to boost honey production, and they have steadily extended their range northward into the southwestern United States. The primary difference between Africanized and European honeybees is their behavior: Africanized honeybees behave much more aggressively. The effect of an individual stinging event is similar. Subtle wing morphological differences and DNA testing can also distinguish the bees.

If a person is swarmed by bees or wasps, the best thing for the person to do is create barriers between himself or herself and the bees. For example, getting behind a door will evade many bees and getting behind another door will evade many more. Older children may be able to outrun bees, which fly at approximately 4 mph and may pursue up to 150 yards. Younger children, however, may be unable to run fast or far enough. Attempting to submerge oneself or another person in water is not recommended because Africanized honeybees will wait until the person surfaces to continue delivering stings. This can result in multiple stings to the airway.

A lethal dose of honeybee stings is estimated at 500 to 1200, but serious envenomation can result from as few as 50 stings (or even fewer after certain species of wasp stings).

Sting removal should be done as quickly as possible, regardless of the method of removal. Even a delay of a second or two (to find a knife or credit card) results in a higher dose of venom injected. Contrary to conventional advice, it has been shown that grasping the stinger does not increase the venom dose.

Clinical complications can include hemolysis, coagulopathy, rhabdomyolysis, and liver dysfunction. Delayed toxic reactions have been documented, and so 24-hour hospitalization is recommended for pediatric and older patients, as well as patients with underlying medical problems or abnormal laboratory test results within a 6-hour observation period and those with 50 or more stings.[52] Laboratory analysis should be aimed at uncovering the aforementioned clinical complications. Treatment involves IV fluids, intensive care, and possibly dialysis and transfusion as needed.

For sensitive individuals, venom immunotherapy in children leads to a significantly lower risk of systemic reaction to stings even decades later.[53]

If an Africanized honeybee hive is suspected, local vector control authorities should be contacted. Avoiding perfume and brightly colored clothes may prevent some stings.

Similar to African honeybees, fire ants (*Solenopsis invicta*) are extending their range in the southeastern Untied States and can cause serious (even fatal) complications after massive envenomation, particularly in infants and small children. These ants typically bite and sting.

REFERENCES

1. Boyer DM: *Antivenom index*, Bethesda, 1999, American Zoo and Aquarium Association.
2. Bush SP, Jansen PW: Severe rattlesnake envenomation with anaphylaxis and rhabdomyolysis, *Ann Emerg Med* 25:845-848, 1995.
3. Bush SP, Thomas TL, Chin ES: Envenomations in children, *Pediatr Emerg Med Rep* 2:1-12, 1997.
4. French WJ, Hayes WK, Bush SP et al: Mojave toxin in venom of *Crotalus helleri* (southern Pacific rattlesnake): molecular and geographic characterization, *Toxicon* 44:781-791, 2004.

5. Norris RL Jr, Bush SP: North American venomous reptile bites. In Auerbach PS editor: *Wilderness medicine,* ed 4, St Louis, 2001, Mosby.
6. Gold BS, Dart RC, Barish RA: Bites of venomous snakes, *N Engl J Med* 347:347-356, 2002.
7. Norris RL Jr, Minton SA: Non-North American venomous reptile bites. In Auerbach PS, editor: *Wilderness medicine,* ed 4, St Louis, 2001, Mosby.
8. Dart RC, McNally JT, Spaite DW et al: The sequelae of pit viper poisoning in the United States. In Campbell JA, Brodie ED, editors: Biology of the pitvipers, Tyler, TX, 1992, Selva Press.
9. Watson WA, Litovitz TL, Klein-Schwartz W et al: 2003 annual report of the American Association of Poison Control Centers toxic exposure surveillance system, *Amer J Emerg Med* 22:335-404, 2004.
10. Behm MO, Kearns GL, Offerman S et al: Crotaline Fab antivenom for treatment of children with rattlesnake envenomation, *Pediatrics* 112:1458-1459, 2003 (letter).
11. Offerman SR, Bush SP, Moynihan JA et al: Crotaline fab antivenom for the treatment of children with rattlesnake envenomation, *Pediatrics* 110:968-971, 2002.
12. Bush SP, Siedenburg E: Neurotoxicity associated with suspected southern Pacific rattlesnake (*Crotalus viridis helleri*) envenomation, *Wilderness Environ Med J* 10:247-249, 1999.
13. Dart RC, Waeckerle JF: Introduction: "Advances in the management of snakebite" symposium, *Ann Emerg Med* 37:166-167, 2001.
14. Dart RC, McNally J: Efficacy, safety, and use of snake antivenoms in the United States, *Ann Emerg Med* 37:181-188, 2001.
15. Bush SP, Green SM, Moynihan JA et al: Crotalidae polyvalent immune Fab (ovine) antivenom is efficacious for envenomations by Southern Pacific rattlesnakes (*Crotalus helleri*), *Ann Emerg Med* 40:619-624, 2002.
16. Hinze JD, Barker JA, Jones TR et al: Life-threatening upper airway edema caused by a distal rattlesnake bite, *Ann Emerg Med* 38: 79-82, 2001.
17. Camilleri C, Offerman S: Anaphylaxis after rattlesnake bite, *Ann Emerg Med* 43:784-785, 2004 (letter).
18. Hardy DL: Fatal rattlesnake envenomation in Arizona: 1969-1984, *J Toxicol Clin Toxicol* 24:1-10, 1986.
19. Bush SP, Hegewald K, Green SM et al: Effects of a negative pressure venom extraction device (Extractor) on local tissue injury after artificial rattlesnake envenomation in a porcine model, *Wilderness Environ Med J* 11:180-188, 2000.
20. Bush SP: Snakebite suction devices don't remove venom—they just suck, *Ann Emerg Med* 43:187-188, 2004 (editorial).
21. Bush SP, Hardy DL Sr: Immediate removal of Extractor is recommended, *Ann Emerg Med* 38:607-608, 2001 (letter).
22. Bush SP, Green SM, Laack TA et al: Pressure-immobilization delays mortality and increases intra-compartmental pressure after artificial intramuscular rattlesnake envenomation in a porcine model, *Ann Emerg Med* 44:599-604, 2004.
23. Bush SP, Cardwell MD: Mojave rattlesnake (*Crotalus scutulatus scutulatus*) identification, *Wilderness Environ Med J* 10:6-9, 1999.
24. Dart RC, Seifert SA, Carroll L et al: Affinity-purified, mixed monospecific crotalid antivenom ovine Fab for treatment of crotalid venom poisoning, *Ann Emerg Med* 30:33-39, 1997.
25. CroFab [prescribing information], Nashville, TN, 2000 Protherics, Inc.
26. Dart RC, Seifert SA, Boyer LV et al: A randomized multicenter trial of crotaline polyvalent immune Fab (ovine) antivenom for the treatment for crotaline snakebite in the United States, *Arch Intern Med* 161:2030-2036, 2001.
27. Seifert SA, Boyer LV: Recurrence phenomena after immunoglobulin therapy for snake envenomations: part 1. Pharmacokinetics and pharmacodynamics of immunoglobulin antivenoms and related antibodies, *Ann Emerg Med* 37:189-195, 2001.
28. Boyer LV, Seifert SA, Cain JS: Recurrence phenomena after immunoglobulin therapy for snake envenomations: part 2. Guidelines for clinical management with crotaline Fab antivenom, *Ann Emerg Med* 37:196-201, 2001.
29. Bush SP, Wu VH, Corbett SW: Rattlesnake venom–induced thrombocytopenia response to Antivenin (Crotalidae) Polyvalent: a case series, *Acad Emerg Med* 7:181-185, 2000.
30. Hall EL: Role of surgical intervention in the management of Crotaline snake envenomation, *Ann Emerg Med* 37:175-180, 2001.
31. Gold BS, Barish RA, Dart RC: Resolution of compartment syndrome after rattlesnake envenomation utilizing non-invasive measures, *J Emerg Med* 24:285-288, 2003.
32. Rosen PB, Leiva J, Ross C: Delayed antivenom treatment for a patient after envenomation by *Crotalus atrox*, *Ann Emerg Med* 35:86-88, 2000.
33. Tanen DA, Ruha AM, Graeme KA et al: Epidemiology and hospital course of rattlesnake envenomations cared for at a tertiary referral center in central Arizona, *Acad Emerg Med* 8:177-182, 2001.
34. Tanen DA, Danish DC, Clark RF: Crotalidae polyvalent immune fab antivenom limits the decrease in perfusion pressure of the anterior leg compartment in a porcine crotaline envenomation model, *Ann Emerg Med* 41:384-390, 2003.
35. Lavonas EJ, Gerardo CJ, O'Malley G et al: Initial experience with crotaline fab antivenom in the treatment of copperhead snakebite, *Ann Emerg Med* 43:200-206, 2004.
36. Boyer LV, McNally JT, Binford GJ: Spider bites. In Auerbach PS, editor: *Wilderness medicine,* ed 4, St Louis, 2001, Mosby.
37. Pneumatikos IA, Galiatsou E, Goe D et al: Acute fatal toxic myocarditis after a black widow spider envenomation, *Ann Emerg Med* 41:58, 2003.
38. Bush SP: Why no antivenom? *Ann Emerg Med* 42:431-432, 2003 (letter).
39. Graudins A, Padula M, Broady K et al: Red-back spider (*Latrodectus hasselti*) antivenom prevents the toxicity of widow spider venoms, *Ann Emerg Med* 37:154-160, 2001.
40. Daly FFS, Hill RE, Bogdan GM et al: Neutralization of *Latrodectus hesperus* venom by antivenom raised against *L. hasselti* in a murine model, *Ann Emerg Med* 35: S57-S58, 2000 (abstract).
41. Bush SP: Black widow spider envenomation mimicking cholecystitis, *Am J Emerg Med* 17:315, 1999 (letter).
42. Cohen J, Bush SP: Case report: compartment syndrome after a suspected black widow spider bite, *Ann Emerg Med* 45:414-416, 2005.
43. Woestman R, Perkin R, Van Stralen D: The black widow: is she deadly to children? *Pediatr Emerg Care* 12:360-364, 1996.
44. Clark RF, Wethern-Kestner S, Vance MV: Clinical presentation and treatment of black widow spider envenomation: a review of 163 cases, *Ann Emerg Med* 21:782-787, 1992.
45. Allen RC, Norris RL: Delayed use of widow spider antivenin, *Ann Emerg Med* 26:393-394, 1995.
46. Bush SP, Naftel J, Farstad D: Injection of a whole black widow spider, *Ann Emerg Med* 27:532-533, 1996 (letter).
47. Keegan HL: *Scorpions of medical important, vol 1,* Jackson, MS, 1980, University Press of Mississippi.
48. Simard JM, Watt DD: Venoms and toxins. In Polis GA, editor: *The biology of scorpions,* Stanford, CA, 1990, Stanford University Press.
49. Bush SP: Envenomation by the scorpion *Centruroides limbatus* outside its natural range and recognition of medically important scorpions, *Wilderness Environ Med* 10:161-164, 1999.
50. Boyer L, Heubner K, McNally J et al: Death from Centruroides scorpion sting allergy, *J Toxicol Clin Toxicol* 39:561-562, 2001, (abstract).
51. Bond GR: Antivenin administration for Centruroides scorpion sting: risks and benefits, *Ann Emerg Med* 21:788-791, 1992.
52. Kolecki P: Delayed toxic reaction following massive bee envenomation, *Ann Emerg Med* 33:114-116, 1999.
53. Golden DB, Kagey-Sobotka A, Norman PS et al: Outcomes of allergy to insect stings in children, with and without venom immunotherapy, *N Engl J Med* 351:668-674, 2004.

CHAPTER 101

Heat Injury

Ofer Yanay and Eli Gilad

PEARLS

- According to the Centers for Disease Control and Prevention, from 1979 to 1999, excessive heat exposure caused 8015 deaths in the United States. During this period, more people died of extreme heat than as a result of hurricanes, lightning, tornadoes, floods, and earthquakes combined. Thus hot weather and heat waves became significant environmental issues.
- After the onset of heatstroke, the inflammatory response may continue despite adequate control of body temperature. Inflammation, coagulopathy, and progression to multiple organ failure may ensue. New approaches for modulation of the inflammatory response may play a role in treatment of heat-related injury in the future.
- With global warming and an increased occurrence of heat waves, even in temperate areas, the risk of heat-related illness is increasing rapidly.
- Thorough knowledge and understanding of these disorders may prevent the progression from heat stress to heatstroke.
- Maintaining organ perfusion and rapid cooling are the major treatment goals for patients with heatstroke.
- The central nervous system is particularly vulnerable to heat, with the cerebellum being most susceptible. Pyramidal dysfunction, dysphagia, mental changes, quadriparesis, extrapyramidal syndrome and neuropathy, have all been described.
- Neurological dysfunction is a cardinal feature of heatstroke. Brain dysfunction is usually severe but may be subtle, manifesting only as inappropriate behavior or impaired judgment; more often, however, patients have delirium or coma.

Interest in heat-related illnesses has grown enormously, largely because of predictions of global warming and an increased frequency of heat waves.[1,2] According to the Centers for Disease Control and Prevention, from 1979 to 1999, excessive heat exposure caused 8015 deaths in the United States.[3] During this period, more people died of extreme heat than as a result of hurricanes, lightning, tornadoes, floods, and earthquakes. Thus hot weather and heat waves became significant environmental issues.

Among the pediatric population, neonates and infants are at highest risk mainly because of poorly developed thermoregulatory mechanisms and total dependence on caregivers to provide adequate protection from excessive heat. Adolescents are also at increased risk because of drug abuse or poor judgment in extreme heat. Children with mental illness and chronic diseases are also at high risk. Over the past decade, the understanding of cellular and molecular responses to heat stress has improved dramatically. This is a multiorgan injury resulting from a complex interplay among the cytotoxic effect of the heat and the inflammatory and coagulation responses of the host.[4] Despite these advances in the understanding of the pathophysiology of heat injury, treatment remains supportive with emphasis on immediate cooling. Prevention and education are still the best tools available in the hands of health care providers to minimize heat-related morbidity and death. This chapter covers the epidemiology, pathophysiology, clinical manifestations, and treatment of nonexertional heat-related illness in the pediatric population.

Definitions

There are several heat-related illnesses that may take the form of heat syncope, heat cramps, heat exhaustion, or heatstroke. The following are key terms used in this chapter.

Heat syncope (fainting) is a mild form of heat illness, which results from physical exertion in a hot environment. In an effort to increase heat loss, the skin blood vessels dilate to such an extent that blood flow to the brain is reduced. This reduction results in symptoms of faintness, dizziness, headache, increased pulse rate, restlessness, nausea, vomiting, and possibly even a brief loss of consciousness. Inadequate fluid replacement, which leads to dehydration, contributes significantly to the problem.

Heat cramps are painful sustained muscle contractions, most often in the legs or abdominal wall, primarily due to inadequate circulation, dehydration, hyponatremia, and muscle fatigue. Body temperature is usually normal.[5,6]

Heat exhaustion is a mild to moderate illness due to water or salt depletion (excessive sweat) resulting from exposure to high environmental heat or strenuous physical exercise. The patient may have a headache, intense thirst, muscle weakness, dizziness, fainting, nausea, and visual disturbances. Core temperature may be normal or elevated but less than 40° C. Patient may have postural hypotension.

Heatstroke is a life-threatening emergency that occurs when core temperature exceeds 40° C and the patient is in hypovolemic shock and has central nervous system abnormalities such as delirium, convulsions, or coma. Exposure to environmental heat (classic heatstroke) or strenuous physical exercise (exertional heatstroke) could cause heatstroke. Alternatively it can be defined as a form of hyperthermia associated with a systemic inflammatory response leading to a syndrome of multiorgan dysfunction in which encephalopathy predominates.[1]

Exertional heatstroke is heatstroke that develops in a previously healthy patient in the setting of a recreational or occupational exercise. It results from heat production by muscular work, which exceeds the body ability to dissipate it.

Classic heatstroke is heatstroke that develops in the setting of high ambient temperature. The term *nonexertional heatstroke* has also been used to describe this condition.

Heat index is a measure of the effect of combined elements (e.g., heat, humidity) on the body.

Wet-bulb temperature is a standard created to reflect the combined influence of temperature and humidity.

Wet-bulb globe temperature (WBGT) is an index of heat stress that reflects the combined influence of temperature, humidity, and solar radiation.

A *heat wave* is 3 or more consecutive days of air temperatures greater than or equal to 90° F (≥ 32.2° C).

Heat-related death, according to the definition by the National Association of Medical Examiners (NAME), includes exposure to high ambient temperature either causing the death or substantially contributing to it; cases in which the body temperature at the time of collapse was greater than or equal to105° F (≥ 40.6° C); and a history of exposure to high ambient temperature and the reasonable exclusion of other causes of hyperthermia.[7] Because death rates from other causes (e.g., cardiovascular and respiratory disease) increase during heat waves, deaths classified as caused by hyperthermia represent only a portion of heat-related death.

Epidemiology

During 1979-1997, an annual average of 371 deaths in the United States was attributable to "excessive heat exposure."[8] This translates into a mean annual death rate of 1.5 per million. Persons aged 14 years and younger accounted for 4% of deaths within the group of deaths caused by weather conditions.[9] During heat waves there is a significant increase in the heat-related death rate. For example, in 1980, a year with a record heat wave, the death rate was more than three times higher than that for any other year during the 19-year period (1979-1997).[9] Data on heat-related death are imprecise because this condition is underdiagnosed, its definition varies,[4] and many cases of patients with near-fatal heatstroke who survive the acute hospitalization have a high 1-year death rate.[10] In Saudi Arabia, where the temperature is extremely hot, the incidence of heatstroke varies seasonally, from 22 to 250 cases per 100,000 population.[11] Heat-related illness is reported from subtropical and cold parts of the world as well. In Taiwan, a subtropical country without any history of heat waves, a cluster of heat shock cases was reported during periods of sustained hotter than average temperatures.[12] In an observational study in which cold and hot areas in Europe were compared, it was shown that heat-related death started at higher temperatures in hot regions than in cold ones.[13] High ambient temperature and humidity, lack of acclimatization, unavailability of air conditioning, and vigorous physical activity[14] are major predisposing factors for heat-related illness. Within the pediatric population, children younger than 2 years are at higher risk, with specific factors like diarrheal disease, sweat gland dysfunction, child neglect, and underlying chronic or febrile illness. Risk factors for adolescents include poor judgment that may lead to continuation of physical exertion despite warning symptoms. Alcohol and drug abuse and exposure to environmental toxins may put the adolescent at risk. Neuroleptic phenothiazines and tricyclic antidepressants, taken for medical indications; amphetamine and derivatives; marijuana and cocaine; or organophosphates, constituents of many pesticides, may all lead to heat-related illness.[15] Their effect may be due to impaired heat loss or increased heat production.[16] Lithium and fluoxetine (Prozac) may induce heat intolerance.[17]

Pathophysiology and Pathogenesis of Heat-Related Illnesses

Understanding the pathophysiology of heat-related illnesses, systemic and cellular, involves appreciation of thermoregulation, physiological alterations directly related to hyperthermia, acute phase response, and the production of heat shock proteins (Hsps). For normal enzymatic and cellular function, it is essential that body core temperature be maintained within a narrow range of about 37° C ± 0.5-0.9° C.[15,18] The thermoregulation system, controlled by the hypothalamus, receives input from thermosensitive receptors in the skin and body core, compares the data with a reference level (the "set point"), and responds to elevation of 0.3° C [15,19] with activation of heat loss mechanisms.[4 15,20]

Heat dissipation occurs by means of four mechanisms: (1) conduction to the adjacent air and objects, (2) convection through air or liquid, (3) radiation of heat energy, and (4) evaporation. Once activated by the hypothalamus, the efferent heat response is both autonomic and behavioral. Blood delivery to the body surface is increased by sympathetic discharge causing cutaneous vasodilatation. Blood flow may increase eightfold to sixteenfold, up to 8 L/min.[21] Thermal sweating, in response to parasympathetic discharge, can produce about 1 L/hr/m^2 of body surface of sweat. Evaporation of 1.7 ml of sweat will consume 1 kCal of heat energy; thus at maximal efficiency, sweating can dissipate 588 kCal of energy per hour. Secondary to cutaneous vasodilatation and sweating, blood is shunted toward the periphery, and visceral perfusion is reduced, especially to the liver, kidneys, and intestines.[22] Rising core temperature will also lead to tachycardia, high cardiac output state, and an increase in minute ventilation.

When ambient temperature equals or exceeds body temperature, conduction, convection and radiation cease to be effective. Losses of salt and water through sweating may lead to dehydration and salt depletion, resulting in impaired thermoregulation.[23] A combination of high ambient humidity and temperature creates a particularly dangerous situation. With ambient humidity of 90% to 95%, evaporation of sweat essentially stops, and if ambient temperature reaches body temperature, the body can no longer eliminate heat.

Acclimatization

Prolonged exposure to a hot environment results in adaptation and tolerance to higher temperature levels. Acclimatization to heat may take several weeks and involves multiple organs. Sweat glands develop increased capacity to secrete sweat, plasma volume is increased, and the renin-angiotensin-aldosterone axis is activated and leads to improved salt conservation. The adaptability of the cardiovascular system is probably the most important single determinant in one's ability to tolerate heat stress.[4,24] Even acclimatized people have definite limitations for heat tolerance. Once driven beyond a critical level, progression to a catastrophic condition may result.

Hyperthermia directly induces cellular injury. Severity of injury depends on the level and duration of exposure to high temperatures. In humans, a body temperature of 41.6° C to 42° C for 45 to 420 minutes will cause a lethal or near-lethal injury.[25]

Once extreme temperatures of 49° C to 50° C have been reached, full destruction and cell necrosis occur. At lower temperatures cell death is mainly due to apoptosis.[26]

Acute Phase Response

Heat stress will initiate cellular acute phase response aimed to protect against injury and promote tissue repair. A variety of cytokines are produced in response to heat stress. Cytokines mediate a wide range of cellular, systemic, and both proinflammatory and antiinflammatory acute phase protein productions. For example, interleukin-6 (IL-6) has a pivotal role in modulating inflammatory cytokines synthesis, both locally and systemically.[4,27] IL-6 also stimulates production of antiinflammatory cytokines, which inhibit production of reactive oxygen species (ROS) and proteolytic enzyme release from activated leukocytes.[27,28] Plasma levels of both proinflammatory (tumor necrosis factor α [TNF-α], IL-1β, and interferon-γ) and antiinflammatory cytokines (IL-6, IL-10, TNF receptors p55 and p75) are elevated in patients with heatstroke.[29-34] Soluble TNF, IL-2, and IL-6 receptors are also elevated in heatstroke.[35,36] Severity of symptoms during heatstroke correlated well with IL-1 and IL-6 levels.[29] Progression from heat stress to heatstroke depends on the time and extent of exposure to severe environmental conditions, but the acute phase response may continue even after the patient is cooled. Onset of inflammation may be local with systemic progression[4,34] that involves endothelial cell activation, release of endothelial vasoactive factors,[37] endothelial cell injury, and microvascular thrombosis.[37-40] The gastrointestinal tract may also play a role in the exaggeration of the inflammatory response. Decrease in blood flow may lead to ischemia and intestinal hyperpermiability.[22,41-44] Evidence for this phenomenon exists in animal models but much less in humans.[22, 41,43-47] Alterations in barrier function of the intestines may allow leakage of endotoxins that fuel the inflammatory response.

Part of the effect on endothelial cells involves activation of both the coagulation and the fibrinolysis systems.[39] Heat stress by itself is a procoagulation condition because it causes platelet clumping in small vessels. In addition, heat stress may mediate endotoxemia, elevated proinflammatory cytokines level, and macrophage activation (via factor VIIa), all of which are well-known inducers of coagulation. Injured endothelium, (e.g., heatstroke) plays an important role in producing and releasing both procoagulant and anticoagulant substances (e.g., von Willebrand factor antigen [vWF-Ag], tissue plasminogen activator, and plasminogen activator inhibitor).[37,38] Circulating vWF-Ag, thrombomodulin, endothelin-1 , nitric oxide (NO) metabolites, soluble E-selectin, and ICAM-1 (intercellular adhesion molecule 1) are elevated in heat-related illness, creating a clinical picture of disseminated intravascular coagulation (DIC).[37, 48-50] The cooling of patients with heatstroke reverses only part of these coagulation abnormalities.[39] Another aspect of the cellular response to stress involves the heat shock response.

Nearly all cells will respond to heat stress with increased production of Hsps. Expression of Hsp is controlled mainly at the gene transcription level. Increased intracellular Hsp levels facilitate tolerance to heat stress with better cell survival.[51,52] In animal models it was shown that preconditioning with heat or chemical stress conferred significant protection against heatstroke-induced hyperthermia, hypotension, and brain injury.[53-55] These effects were mediated mainly by Hsp 70 and 72.[54] Blocking the production of Hsp results in increased cellular sensitivity to even mild degrees of heat stress.[56] Conditions associated with low level of expression of Hsp such as lack of acclimatization or certain genetic polymorphism may make certain patients more vulnerable to heat stress or faster progression to heatstroke.

There appears to be a preferential expression of different families of Hsps in different cell populations. There are also distinct postinjury time frames of induction for each family of Hsp, emphasizing differences in cellular functional requirements for each family of Hsp.[57] It was suggested that Hsp 72 may be used as a semiquantitative diagnostic probe of heat stress.[58] In one human study, researchers found that levels of autoantibodies against Hsp 71 in heat-induced diseases correlated well with the severity of illness.[59]

Thus the individual response to heat stress depends on the direct thermal injury (including thermal cytotoxicity, cardiovascular failure, and hypoxia in the face of increased metabolic requirement) and the acute phase response of the host. Genetic factors likely play a significant role in determining response to heat stress. This complex interplay between leukocytes, endothelial and epithelial cells, and a variety of systemic changes may lead to the most extreme form of heat-related illness, heatstroke. A similar sequence of events has been shown to occur in sepsis.[60]

Systemic Clinical Features

Involvement of multiple organs may be seen, to a certain degree, in heat syncope, heat cramps, and exhaustion. Heatstroke is a true systemic disorder. Per definition, core temperature must exceed 40° C and the patient exhibits hypovolemic shock and central nervous system abnormalities such as delirium, convulsions, or coma. The heatstroke mediated systemic dysfunction was shown to be similar to exertional heatstroke in reported cases with adult patients.[10]

Neurological

Neurological dysfunction is a cardinal feature of heatstroke. Brain dysfunction is usually severe but may be subtle, manifesting only as inappropriate behavior or impaired judgment; more often, however, patients have delirium or coma.[20] Seizures may occur, especially during cooling. The central nervous system is particularly vulnerable to heat, the cerebellum being most susceptible.[61] Pyramidal dysfunction, dysphagia, mental changes, quadriparesis, extrapyramidal syndrome, and neuropathy have all been described.[20,62] No data regarding long-term neurologic outcome in children have been reported. In one adult series, 33% of the patients had moderate to severe impairment of neurologic function at discharge from the hospital.[10]

Pulmonary

The pulmonary system is not involved in early stages of heat-related illnesses. High incidence (23% to 25%) of acute respiratory distress syndrome (ARDS) was reported in adult patients with heatstroke.[63,64] Patients with ARDS have poor prognosis, with up to a 75% mortality rate.[63] Lung involvement is part of the systemic response, as indicated by the fact that all patients who had ARDS also had coagulopathy and DIC.[63]

Cardiovascular

The cardiovascular system is usually compromised in heat-related illness. Hypotension may result from dehydration, translocation of blood from central circulation to the periphery, or increased production of NO.[20] Usually, circulation is hyperdynamic in these patients with tachycardia and high cardiac output.[65] Electrocardiographic changes are common in patients with heatstroke, including rhythm disturbances, conduction defects, prolonged QT interval, and ST segment changes. These may subside with cooling or may require correction of potassium, magnesium, or calcium abnormalities.[66]

Renal

Elevated urea and creatinine levels are seen even in mild heat-related disease such as heat cramps.[67] Moderate to severe renal insufficiency is common in classic heatstroke (up to 53% in one series[10]). Direct thermal injury, hypoperfusion (due to dehydration, cardiac failure, or both), rhabdomyolysis with myoglobinuria, release of vasoactive mediators, and DIC may all contribute to renal injury.[4,20,68,69]

Gastroenterological

Involvement of the gastrointestinal system resulting from direct thermal injury combined with hypoxia due to splanchnic blood flow redistribution plays a role in the development of multiple organ dysfunction syndrome (MODS) in patients with heatstroke.[4,70] The importance of the gastrointestinal system in other forms of heat-related illnesses is not well studied.

Liver function tests with abnormal results may be seen during heat-related illnesses. Mild elevation of aspartate aminotransferase (AST), alanine aminotransferase (ALT), γ-glutamyl transpeptidase (γ-GT), lactate dehydrogenase (LDH), and total bilirubin have been described.[10,20,67] Severe liver damage is more common in exertional heatstroke. Fulminant liver failure is rare and usually carries grave prognosis even with liver transplant.[71]

Metabolic

Early in the course of heat injury, the most common acid-base abnormality is mixed nonanion gap metabolic acidosis and respiratory alkalosis. Hypokalemia resulting from the respiratory alkalosis, sweat losses, and renal wasting may change to hyperkalemia because of a cellular leak of cellular potassium. Several hours into the injury the clinical picture changes into predominantly metabolic acidosis that is caused by sustained tissue injury.[10,20,72]

Hematologic

Thrombocytopenia, prolonged clotting time, and DIC are well documented in patients with heatstroke.[4,10,20,40]

The pathophysiology of DIC in patients with heatstroke was previously discussed.

Infectious

In the early phase of heatstroke, blood culture findings are negative,[73] but within 24 hours from admission, up to 27% of patients had blood cultures with positive findings and 25% had urine cultures with positive findings in one study.[10] The existing data come from adult series. Incidence of positive findings in blood or urine cultures in the pediatric population with heatstroke is unknown.

Treatment

Despite the progress in the understanding of the pathophysiology of heatstroke and the connection with an exaggerated inflammatory response, treatment of these patients remains supportive. Maintenance of organ system perfusion and function and rapid cooling are the two major goals. Adherence to the basic resuscitative guidelines is required, with protection of the airway, management of breathing and monitoring for hypovolemia/shock, and appropriate response with fluids. The most severely affected children have altered mental status, rising body temperature, and hypovolemic shock. After the airway is secured, the child with heatstroke should be moved to a cool environment; clothes should be removed; IV access with one or two large bore lines should be started; and a normal saline or Ringer's lactate solution bolus of 20 ml/kg should be given. Fluid resuscitation, besides ensuring organ perfusion, increases heat dissipation and lowers core temperature[23] by improving skin blood flow. Cooling should be started with whatever method is available, and the patient should be transported to the nearest hospital appropriate for children. Decreasing body temperature below 38.9° C within 30 minutes of presentation was shown to improve survival.[20]

A variety of cooling methods have been used to promote heat loss, and controversy continues regarding the best cooling technique. Cold/ice-water immersion was twice as rapid in reducing the core temperature as the evaporative spray method in patients with both classic and exertional heatstroke in one study.[74] The mechanism for this rapid cooling relates to the high thermal gradient between skin and ice-water, leading to a faster heat loss by conductance as compared with evaporation.[75] Ice-water is easily available everywhere, does not require special equipment, and is suitable for both classic and exertional heatstroke. Critics of immersion point out that it may complicate resuscitation efforts of the comatose child who requires intubation, mechanical ventilation, and close observation. Also, it is uncomfortable to the conscious child and may cause shivering and cutaneous vasoconstriction, which is counterproductive. Sponging the patient with ice-water while massaging the body and using a fan may overcome some of these disadvantages, yet other studies have shown that keeping the skin relatively warm while allowing evaporation and convection to dissipate body heat is the most rapid way to decrease body core temperature.[76,77] This can be done with special cooling units,[76,78] but the concept of keeping the patient "wet and windy" can be easily achieved with application of tepid water to the skin while a fan is used to keep high air flow and to maintain cool ambient temperature.[79] Thus hospitals located in high-risk areas may consider buying special equipment, but most emergency departments and pediatric intensive care units (PICUs) may use this technique with readily available and cheap equipment.

Antipyretics such as acetaminophen or salicylates are considered noneffective in the lowering of the body temperature of patients with heatstroke. We could not find clinical studies in which that subject was evaluated, though.

Dantrolene, which has been used successfully in the treatment of malignant hyperthermia, was tried in cases of heat stress. Some studies claimed it may be effective in the treatment of heatstroke,[80,81] whereas in others, including a double-blind randomized study,[82] it was shown to be ineffective. Once body core temperature of 38.9° C has been achieved, active cooling should be stopped. All pediatric patients with heatstroke should be observed in the PICU, even if respiratory support is not required. Basic laboratory workup should include electrolytes (including sodium, potassium, magnesium, and calcium), renal and liver function tests, complete blood count, and coagulation studies. Urine output should be followed closely, and a urine sample should be sent for myoglobin analysis. As previously mentioned, patients with heatstroke may continue to deteriorate even after body temperature is normalized because of the inflammatory response. There are no specific guidelines for treating patients with MODS that results from heatstroke.

Prevention is still the best treatment for heat-related illness. Whenever possible, people should acclimatize themselves to hot weather. Physical activity should be undertaken during cooler hours, and water intake should be increased. Children should never be left unattended in a closed car during hot weather. Physicians' awareness and knowledge may promote diagnosis of early forms of heat-related illness, thus preventing progression to heat stroke. On a national level, a good weather forecasting system and air-conditioned shelters for vulnerable populations may decrease heat-related morbidity and death during heat waves.[83,84]

REFERENCES

1. Kalkstein LS, Greene JS: An evaluation of climate/mortality relationships in large U.S. cities and the possible impacts of a climate change, *Environ Health Perspect* 105:84-93, 1997.
2. McMichael AJ, Haines A: Global climate change: the potential effects on health, *BMJ* 315:805-809, 1997.
3. Centers for Disease Control and Prevention: Extreme heat. Available at http://www.cdc.gov/nceh/hsb/extremeheat/default.htm. Accessed August 4, 2003.
4. Bouchama A, Knochel JP: Heat stroke, *N Engl J Med* 346:1978-1988, 2002.
5. Eichner ER: Ttreatment of suspected heat illness, *Int J Sports Med* 19:S150-S153, 1998.
6. Squire DL: Heat illness. Fluid and electrolyte issues for pediatric and adolescent athletes, *Pediatr Clin North Am* 37:1085-1109, 1990.
7. Centers for Disease Control and Prevention (CDC): Heat-related deaths-United States, 1993, *MMWR Morb Mortal Wkly Rep* 42:558-560, 1993.
8. National Center for Health Statistics: Compressed mortality file. US Department of Health and Human Services, Centers for Disease Control and Prevention, 2000, Atlanta.

9. Centers for Disease Control and Prevention (CDC: Heat-related illnesses, deaths, and risk factors—Cincinnati and Dayton, Ohio, 1999, and United States, 1979-1997, *MMWR Morb Mortal Wkly Rep* 49 470-473, 2000.
10. Dematte JE, O'Mara K, Buescher J et al: Near-fatal heat stroke during the 1995 heat wave in Chicago, *Ann Intern Med* 129: 173-181, 1998.
11. Ghaznawi HI, Ibrahim MA: Heat stroke and heat exhaustion in pilgrims performing the Haj (annual pilgrimage)in Saudi Arabia, *Ann Saudi Med* 7:323-326, 1987.
12. How CK, Chern CH, Wang LM et al: Heat stroke in a subtropical country, *Am J Emerg Med* 18:474-477, 2000.
13. Keatinge WR, Donaldson GC, Cordioli E et al: Heat related mortality in warm and cold regions of Europe: observational study, *BMJ* 321:670-673, 2000.
14. Kilbourne EM, Choi K, Jones TS et al: Risk factors for heatstroke: a case-control study, *JAMA* 247:3332-3336, 1982.
15. Lomax P, Schonbaum E: The effects of drugs on thermoregulation during exposure to hot environments, *Prog Brain Res* 115: 193-204, 1998.
16. Clark WG, Lipton JM: Drug-related heatstroke, *Pharmacol Ther* 26:345-388, 1984.
17. Epstein Y, Albukrek D, Kalmovitc B et al: Heat intolerance induced by antidepressants, *Ann N Y Acad Sci* 813:553-558, 1997.
18. Cox B, Green MD, Lomax P: Behavioral thermoregulation in the study of drugs affecting body temperature, *Pharmacol Biochem Behav* 3:1051-1054, 1975.
19. Cox B, Ary M, Lomax P: Dopaminergic involvement in withdrawal hypothermia and thermoregulatory behavior in morphine dependent rats, *Pharmacol Biochem Behav* 4:259-262, 1976.
20. Grogan H, Hopkins PM: Heat stroke: implications for critical care and anaesthesia, *Br J Anaesth* 88:700-707, 2002.
21. Rowell LB: Cardiovascular aspects of human thermoregulation, *Circ Res* 52:367-379, 1983.
22. Hall DM, Buettner GR, Oberley LW et al: Mechanisms of circulatory and intestinal barrier dysfunction during whole body hyperthermia, *Am J Physiol Heart Circ Physiol* 280:H509 H521, 2001.
23. Deschamps A, Levy RD, Cosio MG et al: Effect of saline infusion on body temperature and endurance during heavy exercise, *J Appl Physiol* 66:2799-2804, 1989.
24. Knochel JP: Catastrophic medical events with exhaustive exercise: "white collar rhabdomyolysis," *Kidney Int* 8:709-719, 1990.
25. Bynum GD, Pandolf KB, Schuette WH et al: Induced hyperthermia in sedated humans and the concept of critical thermal maximum, *Am J Physiol* 235:R228-R236, 1978.
26. Sakaguchi Y, Stephens LC, Makino M et al: Apoptosis in tumors and normal tissues induced by whole body hyperthermia in rats, Cancer Res 55:5459-5464, 1995.
27. Gabay C, Kushner I: Acute-phase proteins and other systemic responses to inflammation, *N Engl J Med* 340:448-454, 1999.
28. Xing Z, Gauldie J , Cox G et al: IL-6 is an antiinflammatory cytokine required for controlling local or systemic acute inflammatory responses, *J Clin Invest* 101:311-320, 1998.
29. Bouchama A, Al Sedairy S, Siddiqui S et al: Elevated pyrogenic cytokines in heatstroke, *Chest* 104:1498-1502, 1993.
30. Bouchama A, Parhar RS, el-Yazigi A et al: Endotoxemia and release of tumor necrosis factor and interleukin 1 alpha in acute heatstroke, *J Appl Physiol* 70:2640-2644, 1991.
31. Camus G, Nys M, Poortmans JR et al: Endotoxaemia, production of tumour necrosis factor alpha and polymorphonuclear neutrophil activation following strenuous exercise in humans, *Eur J Appl Physiol* 79:62-68, 1998.
32. Chang DM: The role of cytokines in heat stroke, *Immunol Invest* 22:553-561, 1993.
33. Lu KC, Wang JY, Lin SH et al: Role of circulating cytokines and chemokines in exertional heatstroke, *Crit Care Med* 32:399-403, 2004.
34. Moldoveanu AI, Shephard RJ, Shek PN: Exercise elevates plasma levels but not gene expression of IL 1beta, IL 6, and TNF-alpha in blood mononuclear cells, *J Appl Physiol* 89:1499-1504, 2000.
35. Hammami MM, Bouchama A, Al-Sedairy S et al: Concentrations of soluble tumor necrosis factor and interleukin-6 receptors in heatstroke and heatstress, *Crit Care Med* 25:1314-1319, 1997.
36. Hammami MM, Bouchama A, Shail E et al: Elevated serum level of soluble interleukin-2 receptor in heatstroke, *Intensive Care Med* 24:988, 1998
37. Bouchama A, Hammami MM, Haq A et al: Evidence for endothelial cell activation/injury in heatstroke, *Crit Care Med* 24:1173-1178, 1996.
38. Ang C, Dawes J: The effects of hyperthermia on human endothelial monolayers: modulation of thrombotic potential and permeability, *Blood Coagul Fibrinolysis* 5:193-199, 1994.
39. Bouchama A, Bridey F, Hammami MM et al: Activation of coagulation and fibrinolysis in heatstroke, *Thromb Haemost* 76:909-915, 1996.
40. al-Mashhadani SA, Gader AG, al Harthi SS et al: The coagulopathy of heat stroke: alterations in coagulation and fibrinolysis in heat stroke patients during the pilgrimage (Haj) to Makkah, *Blood Coagul Fibrinolysis* 5:731-736, 1994.
41. Bosenberg AT, Brock-Utne JG, Gaffin SL et al: Strenuous exercise causes systemic endotoxemia, *J Appl Physiol* 65:106-108, 1988.
42. Eshel GM, Safar P, Stezoski W: The role of the gut in the pathogenesis of death due to hyperthermia, *Am J Forensic Med Pathol* 22:100-104, 2001.
43. Sakurada S, Hales JR: A role for gastrointestinal endotoxins in enhancement of heat tolerance by physical fitness, *J Appl Physiol* 84:207-214, 1998.
44. Shapiro Y, Alkan M, Epstein Y et al: Increase in rat intestinal permeability to endotoxin during hyperthermia, *Eur J Appl Physiol Occup Physiol* 55:410-412, 1986
45. Gathiram P, Wells MT, Brock-Utne JG et al: Antilipopolysaccharide improves survival in primates subjected to heat stroke, *Circ Shock* 23:157-164, 1987.
46. Gathiram P, Wells MT, Raidoo D et al: Portal and systemic plasma lipopolysaccharide concentrations in heat-stressed primates, *Circ Shock* 25:223-230, 1988
47. Graber CD, Reinhold RB, Breman JG et al: Fatal heat stroke. Circulating endotoxin and gram-negative sepsis as complications, *JAMA* 216:1195-1196, 1971.
48. Alzeer AH, Al-Arifi A, Warsy AS et al: Nitric oxide production is enhanced in patients with heat stroke, *Intensive Care Med* 25: 58-62, 1999.
49. Hammami MM, Bouchama A, Al Sedairy S: Levels of soluble L-selectin and E-selectin in heatstroke and heatstress, *Chest* 114: 949-950, 1998.
50. Shieh SD, Shiang JC, Lin YF et al: Circulating angiotensin-converting enzyme, von Willebrand factor antigen and thrombomodulin in exertional heat stroke, *Clin Sci* (Lond) 89:261-265, 1995.
51. Moseley PL: Heat shock proteins and heat adaptation of the whole organism, *J Appl Physiol* 83:1413-1417, 1997.
52. Polla BS, Bachelet M, Elia G et al: Stress proteins in inflammation, *Ann N Y Acad Sci* 851:75-85, 1998.
53. Chen J, Graham SH, Zhu RL et al: Stress proteins and tolerance to focal cerebral ischemia, *J Cereb Blood Flow Metab* 16:566-577, 1996.
54. Yang YL, Lin MT: Heat shock protein expression protects against cerebral ischemia and monoamine overload in rat heatstroke, *Am J Physiol Heart Circ Physiol* 276:H1961-H1967, 1999.
55. Yellon DM, Marber MS: Hsp70 in myocardial ischaemia, *Experientia* 50:1075-1084, 1994.
56. Riabowol KT, Mizzen LA, Welch WJ: Heat shock is lethal to fibroblasts microinjected with antibodies against hsp70, *Science* 242:433-436, 1988.
57. Reynolds LP, Allen GV: A review of heat shock protein induction following cerebellar injury, *Cerebellum* 2:171-177, 2003.
58. Bratton SL, Jardine DS, Mirkes PE: Constitutive synthesis of heat shock protein (72 kD) in human peripheral blood mononuclear cells: implications for use as a clinical test of recent thermal stress, *Int J Hyperthermia* 13:157-168, 1997.
59. Wu T, Chen S, Xiao C: Presence of antibody against the inducible Hsp71 in patients with acute heat-induced illness, *Cell Stress Chaperones* 6:113-120, 2001.
60. Despond O, Proulx F, Carcillo JA et al: Pediatric sepsis and multiple organ dysfunction syndrome, *Curr Opin Pediatr* 13:247-253, 2001.
61. Albukrek D, Bakon M, Moran DS et al: Heat-stroke-induced cerebellar atrophy: clinical course, CT and MRI findings, *Neuroradiology* 39:195-197, 1997.
62. Kalita J, Misra UK: Neurophysiological studies in a patient with heat stroke, *J Neurol* 248:993-995, 2001.
63. El-Kassimi FA, Al-Mashhadani S, Abdullah AK et al: Adult respiratory distress syndrome and disseminated intravascular coagulation complicating heat stroke, *Chest* 90:571-574, 1986.

64. Soliman SM, Abu-Taleb Z, Khogali M et al: Pulmonary aspiration and adult respiratory distress syndrome in 40 cases of heat stroke. In Khogali MK, Hales JRS, editors: *Heat stroke and temperature regulation,* Sydney, 1983, Academic Press.
65. Shahid MS, Hatle L, Mansour H et al: Echocardiographic and doppler study of patients with heat stroke and heat exhaustion, *Int J Cardiac Imaging* 15:279-285, 1999.
66. Akhtar MJ, Al-Nozha M, AL-harti S et al: Electrocardiographic abnormalities in patients with heat stroke, *Chest* 104:411-414, 1993.
67. Donoghue AM, Sinclair MJ, Bates GP: Heat exhaustion in a deep underground metalliferous mine, *Occup Environ Med* 57:165-174, 2000.
68. Lin YF, Wang JY, Chou TC et al: Vasoactive mediators and renal haemodynamics in exertional heat stroke complicated by acute renal failure, *QJM* 96:193-201, 2003.
69. Semenza JC: Acute renal failure during heat waves, *Am J Prev Med* 17:97, 1999.
70. Yoshitake S, Noguchi T, Hoasi S et al: Changes in intramucosal pH and gut blood flow during whole body heating in porcine model, *Int J Hyperthermia* 14:285-291, 1998.
71. Berger J, Hart J, Millis M et al: Fulminant hepatic failure from heat stroke requiring liver transplantation, *J Clin Gastroenterol* 30: 429-431, 2000.
72. Bouchama A, De Vol EB: Acid-base alterations in heatstroke, *Intensive Care Med* 27:680-685, 2001.
73. Bouchama A: Features and outcomes of classic heat stroke, *Ann Intern Med* 130:613, 1999.
74. Armstrong LE, Crago AE, Adams R et al: Whole-body cooling of hyperthermic runners: comparison of two field therapies, *Am J Emerg Med* 14:355-358, 1996.
75. Gaffin SL, Gardner JW, Flinn SD: Cooling methods for heatstroke victims, *Ann Intern Med* 132:678, 2000.
76. Weiner JS, Khogali M: A physiological body-cooling unit for treatment of heat stroke, *Lancet* 1:507-509, 1980.
77. Wyndham CH, Strydom NB, Cooke HM et al: Methods of cooling subjects with hyperpyrexia, *J Appl Physiol* 14:771-776, 1959.
78. Al-Aska AK, Abu-Aisha H, Yaqub B et al: Simplified cooling bed for heatstroke, *Lancet* 1:381, 1987.
79. Slovis CM: Features and outcomes of classic heat stroke, *Ann Intern Med* 130:614-615, 1999.
80. Channa AB, Seraj MA, Sadique AA et al: Is dantrolene effective in heat stroke patients? *Crit Care Med* 18:290-292, 1990.
81. Moran D, Epstein Y, Wiener M et al: Dantrolene and recovery from heat stroke, *Aviat Space Environ Med* 70:987-989, 1999.
82. Bouchama A, Cafege A, Devol EB et al: Ineffectiveness of dantrolene sodium in the treatment of heatstroke, *Crit Care Med* 19: 176-180, 1991.
83. Changnon SA, Easterling DR: Disaster management: U.S. policies pertaining to weather and climate extremes, *Science* 289:2053-2055, 2000.
84. Kalkstein LS: Saving lives during extreme weather in summer, *BMJ* 321:650-651, 2000.

CHAPTER 102

Cold Injury

Björn Gunnarsson and Christopher Heard

PEARLS

- Accidental hypothermia is a potentially lethal complication of exposure to cold. It can occur as a result of exposure to cold air, water immersion, or submersion (near-drowning).
- Risk factors include accidents, neglect, toxins, mental disorders, and violence.
- Information about the duration and severity of cold exposure, scene details, and any other associated injuries may help in the selection of the appropriate facility and rewarming methods.
- Many organ systems are affected by hypothermia. There is a marked depression of cerebral blood flow and oxygen use.
- Rescuers should initiate resuscitation on all patients with hypothermia unless a patient has a frozen chest or any other obvious nonsurvivable injury. The hallmark of rescue in all individuals with hypothermia is prevention of further heat loss, careful transport, and rewarming. Avoiding excess activity and rough movements of patients with hypothermia is important because this may precipitate cardiac dysrhythmias.
- Various techniques have been used for in-hospital resuscitation from deep hypothermia, but no controlled studies in which rewarming methods are compared exist and rigid treatment protocols cannot be recommended. Active external rewarming has been shown to be effective. Extracorporeal rewarming of blood is the preferred method, however, to resuscitate patients with severe hypothermia and cardiac arrest or cardiovascular instability.
- Prediction of patient outcome is difficult. Laboratory values may help identify those who had irreversible asphyxia before hypothermia commenced, but no chemical factor can predict with accuracy who will survive. Successful resuscitation will be rare, however, if drowning precedes the hypothermia. Cases of good outcome after submersion are generally associated with water temperatures at, or near, freezing and with the individual already hypothermic on admission to hospital. The decision to terminate resuscitative efforts must be based on the unique circumstances of each case.

Humans have a high capacity to dissipate heat and a relative poor capacity to increase heat production, and humans rely heavily on environmental regulation in the form of clothing and warm shelter to maintain normal body temperature. Thermoregulation is controlled by the hypothalamus. Heat production increases with movement; shivering increases the rate of heat production three to five times above resting levels but at the cost of great oxygen consumption. There are four primary means of heat loss: (1) conduction, (2) convection, (3) radiation, and (4) evaporation. Changes in the environment can radically increase heat loss (e.g., cold-water immersion can increase conductive heat loss 32 times).[1]

There is no uniformity in the definition of hypothermia. *The 2000 Guidelines for Cardiopulmonary Resuscitation and Emergency Cardiovascular Care* classify a core temperature of 34° C to 36° C as mild hypothermia, 30° C to 34° C as moderate hypothermia, and less than 30° C as severe hypothermia.[2] Hypothermia is further classified as accidental or intentional (as in cardiac bypass) and primary or secondary. Primary accidental hypothermia is due to environmental exposure, with no underlying medical condition causing disruption of temperature regulation. Susceptibility to heat loss is greater in children than in adults because of a large surface area relative to body mass and less subcutaneous tissue, but severe accidental hypothermia is uncommonly encountered in most pediatric intensive care units. Neonates have a capacity for nonshivering thermogenesis, primarily by metabolism of brown fat; however, this is at the cost of greatly increased oxygen consumption. Neonates are therefore extremely sensitive to relatively minor deviations from neutral thermal environment.

Pathophysiology

The body can compensate to a great degree for mild hypothermia. The hypothalamus sends signals that produce cutaneous vasoconstriction, increased muscle tone, and metabolic rate. When muscle tone reaches a certain level, shivering thermogenesis begins. The clinical manifestations depend on the severity, acuity, and duration of temperature reduction; the patient's age; premorbid conditions; and superimposed disease states. Each organ system may be affected.[3,4]

Central Nervous System

Central nervous system dysfunction is progressive. Cerebral oxygen consumption decreases in proportion to the reduction in metabolism. Cerebral blood flow decreases 6% to 7% for each 1° C decrease in temperature.[1] Mild hypothermia may be associated with confusion, dysarthria, and impaired judgment.[3-5] Deep tendon reflexes are depressed at core temperature below 32° C because of slowed peripheral nerve conduction. As body temperature drops, many patients no longer complain of cold. Shivering thermogenesis ceases at about 31° C. Pupillary responses decline and dilated unreactive pupils may be noted at temperatures below 30° C. Patients may experience hallucinations and sometimes paradoxically remove their clothes. The electroencephalogram shows abnormal activity at temperatures less than 32° C, and at 20° C the electroencephalogram may appear consistent with brain death.[1]

Cardiovascular

The initial cardiovascular responses are vasoconstriction, tachycardia, and increased cardiac output.[5] Further hypothermia results in decreased pacemaker and conduction velocity, causing bradycardia, heart block, and prolongation of PR, QRS, and QT intervals. Bradycardia becomes severe by 32° C. The myocardium becomes irritable and arrhythmias are common when core temperature reaches 30° C. The electrocardiogram may show characteristic J or Osborne wave following the QRS complex (Fig. 102–1).[1,6,7] The presence of this wave is not pathognomonic for hypothermia and has no prognostic implications.[8] Myocardial contractility, systemic blood pressure, and cardiac output are often decreased dramatically in patients who have severe hypothermia. These changes may be persistent during rewarming.[9] Patients with hypothermia generally are volume contracted because of cold-induced diuresis.[1,5,10]

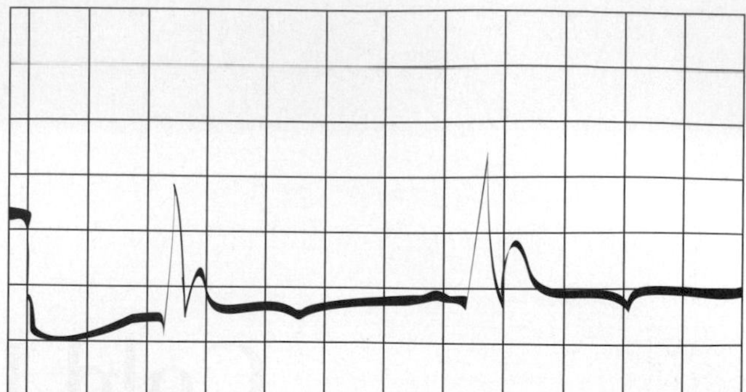

FIGURE 102–1 • Characteristic J or Osborne wave of hypothermia closely follows QRS. It may be mistaken for T wave with narrow QT interval if the true T wave is not appreciated. Slightly rounded peak distinguishes it from R` of bundle branch block. (From Welton D, Mattox K, Miller R et al: *JAMA* 240:2291, 1978.)

Respiratory

Hypothermia affects tissue oxygenation through several complex physiologic mechanisms. Initially, the respiratory rate may be increased. As hypothermia worsens, the respiratory center becomes depressed and hypoventilation causes carbon dioxide retention, although the carbon dioxide production decreases with increasing hypothermia. Respiratory arrest is a late occurrence. Suppression of cough and mucociliary reflexes leads to atelectasis and pneumonia.[5] Oxygen delivery to the tissues is further compromised through the shifting of the oxyhemoglobin dissociation curve to the left.[1] Blood gas analyzers warm blood to 37° C before analysis.[11] In patients with hypothermia, arterial blood gases show higher oxygen and carbon dioxide levels and a lower pH than a patient's actual values. The best approach to interpretation is to compare the uncorrected blood gas values with the normal values at 37° C (alpha-stat strategy).[12-14]

Renal

Renal injury may occur either because of hypothermia or during the rewarming process.[15] The mechanisms involved in cold diuresis may include peripheral vasoconstriction and blunted response to antidiuretic hormone. Renal vasoconstriction and ischemia to the kidney may lead to oliguria and acute tubular necrosis in those with severe hypothermia.[5] Progressive hypokalemia develops during hypothermia, probably because of the shifting of potassium from extracellular to intracellular compartment, and significant hyperkalemia may develop during rewarming.[2,16-18] Metabolic and respiratory acidoses are not uncommon findings in patients who have moderate and severe hypothermia.[11] Hemodialysis has been required for renal failure and may also be of use as an active rewarming strategy.[19]

Coagulation

Hypothermia inhibits the intrinsic and extrinsic pathways in the clotting process. The degree of coagulopathy, however, is often underestimated because dynamic coagulation tests are generally performed at 37° C in the laboratory. Thrombocytopenia, from bone marrow suppression and splenic sequestration, and platelet dysfunction are common.[1,12]

Treatment

The hallmark of rescue in all individuals with hypothermia is prevention of further heat loss, careful transport, and rewarming.[1] Wet clothes should be removed, and the individuals should be insulated and shielded from wind and cold. Paying special attention to the head and neck is important because radiant heat loss from those areas can be profound. Detecting signs of life in patients with deep hypothermia may be difficult, and the rescuer should therefore assess breathing and then pulse for 30 to 60 seconds to confirm respiratory arrest, cardiac arrest, or bradycardia. Chest compressions should be started immediately if the patient is pulseless with no detectable signs of circulation. Endotracheal intubation should be performed if the patient with hypothermia is unconscious or if ventilation inadequate. Anecdotal reports of sudden cardiac death associated with tracheal intubation appear to be exaggerated, particularly if the patient is adequately preoxygenated and the procedure is performed in a gentle manner. If cervical spine injury is suspected, the neutral position must be maintained with manual cervical stabilization. Care should be taken not to overventilate the patient's lungs because this can increase ventricular irritability.[20] Rewarming by the administration of warmed humidified oxygen (42° C to 46° C) and warmed saline (43° C) should begin as soon as possible. Ringer's lactate solution is not recommended because a hypothermic liver cannot metabolize lactate. Defibrillation can be tried up to three times for ventricular tachycardia or fibrillation. If arrhythmia is resistant to three shocks in a patient with deep hypothermia, then further defibrillation attempts should be deferred until core temperature is increased.[1,2] The hypothermic heart may also have a reduced response to cardioactive drugs and pacemaker stimulation.[1,2] There is concern that medications can accumulate to toxic levels if they are administered repeatedly in the patient with severe hypothermia.

No randomized controlled clinical trials in which rewarming methods are compared exist.[13] The rewarming of patients who are conscious and who have only mild or moderate hypothermia can be achieved with passive techniques (e.g., blankets, warm shelter). Management of severe hypothermia in the field is more controversial.[2] Active external rewarming with heat devices (e.g., forced air, radiant heat, warm bath, warm packs) requires careful monitoring and should therefore be used with caution. The concerns are core temperature afterdrop and rewarming shock.[1,4,12,13,21-23] The term *core temperature afterdrop* refers to a continued decrease in core temperature and associated clinical deterioration of a patient after rewarming has begun. Some researchers suggest that peripheral vasodilatation due to external rewarming leads to circulation of cold blood into the core of the body.[22] Simple equilibration of temperature between the periphery and the core is probably a far more important mechanism; heat flows from the core to the periphery during cooling and the opposite is true during external rewarming. There is a delay in the reversal of temperature flow in deeper tissues, however, and the core temperature may decrease for some time after rewarming has begun. It follows that the magnitude of core temperature afterdrop is greater if cooling is rapid because the temperature gradient between the surface and core is greater.[24] The hazard of afterdrop may be grossly overrated. It is not uncommon, though, for patients with hypothermia to have "rewarming shock" or "postrescue collapse." This has been attributed to afterdrop; cooling of the heart would cause arrhythmias or arrest.[1,23,25,26] The underlying pathophysiological condition behind this remains obscure, however, and several mechanisms may contribute, including myocardial dysfunction, decreased vascular tone, derangements of the microcirculation, and hypoxia or sudden changes in pH.[9,23,25] Depleted intravascular volume may also contribute to the development of shock, and most patients will benefit from volume expansion.[1,11] The patient should be kept horizontal to minimize hypotension and sympathetic discharge. Avoiding excess activity and rough movements of patients with hypothermia is important because this may precipitate cardiac dysrhythmias.

Techniques that can be used for in-hospital rewarming of hemodynamically stable patients include continued active external rewarming, and active core rewarming with lavage of body cavities or warming of blood with extracorporal circulation. Active external rewarming can be effective, and there are several reports of successful use of active external rewarming or minimally invasive techniques in children with severe hypothermia and cardiac arrest.[27-35] Cardiopulmonary bypass should be considered in patients without cardiac arrest with severe hypothermia and is the preferred method to resuscitate patients with severe hypothermia and cardiac arrest or cardiovascular instability.[1,2,36-46] In most reports, partial bypass from femoral artery to femoral vein is described in adult patients. Full bypass with a median sternotomy may be preferential in small children.[38,47]

Other methods of core rewarming that can be considered include peritoneal lavage with heated potassium-free dialysate, closed pleural irrigation with warm sterile saline, and the use of esophageal rewarming tubes.[48-50]

Outcome

Knowledge about outcome is mostly based on adult studies and isolated pediatric case reports. If rewarmed and resuscitated, patients with accidental hypothermia may recover neurologically intact after prolonged arrest. This was recently confirmed in a 16-year longitudinal review of profound hypothermia. In this series of 46 Swiss patients with deep hypothermia (temperature <28° C) and circulatory arrest, 32 underwent rewarming with cardiopulmonary bypass and 15 of those were long-term survivors, all with excellent functional outcome.[37] Recovery has occurred in an adult patient who sustained prolonged circulatory arrest with initial core temperature of 13.7° C, and there are many reports of successful resuscitation of children with severe hypothermia.[25,31-34,47,51]

If drowning precedes the hypothermia, successful resuscitation will be rare.[2] This notion was ascertained in a recent series of 26 Norwegian patients, with hypothermia and circulatory failure or cardiac arrest, who were resuscitated with the use of extracorporeal circulation. Of those who probably had asphyxia before and during cooling, only 1 of 15 survived, compared with 7 of 11 patients who did not have asphyxia.[38] Most cases in the asphyxia group were pediatric drowning accidents. There are many reports, however, of dramatic recovery after prolonged cold-water submersion of pediatric patients.[25,32,34,35,44,52,53] Cases of good outcome are generally associated with water temperatures at, or near, freezing and with the individual already having hypothermia on admission to hospital. It is therefore reasonable to assume that good outcome in these cases must be associated with cerebral hypothermia.[13,52,54] Rapid cooling of the body due to large surface area relative to body mass and little subcutaneous tissue may offer protection to pediatric patients. Furthermore, it is thought that rapid cooling of the brain may largely depend on repeated aspiration of cold water into the lungs.[23,44,54,55] Reviews from Finland and Canada, however, did not show a correlation between water temperature and age on outcome, so other factors must play a critical role.[52,56,57]

Severe coagulopathy, acidosis (venous pH ≤6.5), and hyperkalemia (>10 mmol/L) are among factors that have been associated with poor outcome.[40,58] These laboratory values may help identify those who had irreversible asphyxia before hypothermia commenced, but no chemical factor can predict with accuracy who will survive.[13,38,59] A good example of this is a 31-month-old girl who survived extreme hypothermia. Her rectal temperature on arrival to the hospital was 14.2° C, and her serum potassium level was 11.8 mmol/L.[47] Clinical judgment will have to be exercised, and it must be kept in mind that children with accidental hypothermia have tremendous potential for good outcome despite a catastrophic presentation. A reasonable approach, in most cases, is to resuscitate and warm the child aggressively until the core temperature reaches near normal. At that point, if no signs of life are present and the patient is not responding to aggressive life support measures, termination of resuscitation may be indicated.

REFERENCES

1. Reuler J: Hypothermia: pathophysiology, clinical settings and management, *Ann Intern Med* 89:519, 1978.
2. Guidelines 2000 for Cardiopulmonary Resuscitation and Emergency Cardiovascular Care. Part 8: advanced challenges in resuscitation: section 3: special challenges in ECC. The American Heart Association in collaboration with the International Liaison Committee on Resuscitation, *Circulation* 102(8 suppl):I229, 2000.
3. Hanania NA, Zimmerman JL: Accidental hypothermia, *Crit Care Clin* 15:235, 1999.
4. Bartley B, Crnkovich DJ, Usman AR et al: Techniques for managing severe hypothermia, *J Crit Illn* 11:123, 1996.
5. Bartley B, Crnkovich DJ, Usman AR, et al: How to recognize hypothermia in critically ill patients, *J Crit Illn* 11:118, 1996.
6. Welton D, Mattox K, Miller R et al: Treatment of profound hypothermia, *JAMA* 240:2291, 1978.
7. Cheng D: The EKG of hypothermia, *J Emerg Med* 22:87, 2002.
8. Gussak I, Bjerregaard P, Egan TM et al: ECG phenomenon called the J wave: history, pathophysiology, and clinical significance, *J Electrocardiology* 28:49, 1995.
9. Tveita T: Rewarming from hypothermia: newer aspects on the pathophysiology of rewarming shock, *Int J Circumpolar Health* 59: 260, 2000.
10. Olsen DH, Gothgen IH: Behandling af accidentel hypothermi [Treatment of accidental hypothermia], *Ugeskrift for Laeger* 162: 4790, 2000.
11. Delaney KA, Howland MA, Vassallo S et al: Assessment of acid-base disturbances in hypothermia and their physiologic consequences, *Ann Emerg Med* 18:72, 1989.
12. Danzl DF, Pozos RS: Accidental hypothermia, *N Engl J Med* 331: 1756, 1994.
13. Larach MG: Accidental hypothermia, *Lancet* 345:493, 1995.
14. Orlowski JP: Drowning, near-drowning and ice-water drowning, *JAMA* 260:390, 1988.
15. Yoshitomi Y, Kojima S, Ogi M et al: Acute renal failure in accidental hypothermia of cold water immersion, *Am J Kidney Dis* 31:856-9, 1998.
16. Kanter GS: Regulation of extracellular potassium in hypothermia, *Am J Physiol* 205:1285, 1963.
17. Koht A, Cane R, Cerullo LJ: Serum potassium levels during prolonged hypothermia, *Intensive Care Med* 9:257, 1983.
18. Zydlewski AW, Hasbargen JA: Hypothermia-induced hypokalemia, *Mil Med* 163:719, 1998.
19. Owda A, Osama S: Hemodialysis in management of hypothermia, *Am J Kidney Dis* 38:E8, 2001.
20. Danzl DF, Pozos RS, Hamlet MP: Accidental hypothermia. In Auerbach PS, editor: *Wilderness medicine: management of wilderness and environmental emergencies,* St Louis, 1995, Mosby.
21. Jolly BT, Ghezzi KT: Accidental hypothermia, *Emerg Med Clin North Am* 10:311, 1992.
22. Hayward JS, Eckerson JD, Kemna D: Thermal and cardiovascular changes during three methods of resuscitation from mild hypothermia, *Resuscitation* 11:21, 1984.
23. Giesbrecht GG: Cold stress, near drowning and accidental hypothermia: a review, *Aviat Space Environ Med* 71:733, 2000.
24. Webb P: Afterdrop of body temperature during rewarming: an alternative explanation, *J Appl Physiol* 60:385, 1986.
25. Lloyd EL: Accidental hypothermia, *Resuscitation* 32:111, 1996.
26. Giesbrecht GG: Emergency treatment of hypothermia, *Emerg Med* 13:9, 2001.
27. Steele MT, Nelson MJ, Sessler DI et al: Forced air speeds rewarming in accidental hypothermia, *Ann Emerg Med* 27:479, 1996.
28. Koller R, Schnider TW, Neidhart P: Deep accidental hypothermia and cardiac arrest—rewarming with forced air, *Acta Anaesthesiol Scand* 41:1359, 1997.
29. deCaen A: Management of profound hypothermia in children without the use of extracorporeal life support therapy, *Lancet* 360: 1394, 2002.
30. Thompson DA, Anderson N: Successful resuscitation of a severely hypothermic neonate, *Ann Emerg Med* 23:1390, 1994.
31. Anderson S, Herbring BG, Widman B: Accidental profound hypothermia, *Br J Anaesth* 42:653, 1970.
32. Kvittingen TD, Naess A: Recovery from drowning in fresh water, *Br Med J* 1:1315, 1963.
33. Balagna R, Abbo D, Ferrero F et al: Accidental hypothermia in a child, *Paediatr Anaesth* 9:342, 1999.
34. Siebke H, Breivik H, Rod T et al: Survival after 40 minutes' submersion without cerebral sequelae, *Lancet* 1:1275, 1975.
35. Orlowski JP: Drowning, near-drowning, and ice-water submersion, *Pediatr Clin North Am* 34:75, 1987.
36. Lazar HL: The treatment of hypothermia, *N Engl J Med* 337:1545, 1997.
37. Walpoth BH, Walpoth-Aslan BN, Mattle HP et al: Outcome of survivors of accidental deep hypothermia and circulatory arrest treated with extracorporeal blood warming, *N Engl J Med* 337: 1500, 1997.
38. Fastad M, Andersen KS, Koller ME et al: Rewarming from accidental hypothermia by extracorporeal circulation: a retrospective study, *Eur J Cardiothorac Surg* 20:58, 2001.
39. Bolgiano E, Sykes L, Barish RA et al: Accidental hypothermia with cardiac arrest: recovery following rewarming by cardiopulmonary bypass, *J Emerg Med* 10:427, 1992.
40. Hauty MG, Esrig BC, Hill JG et al: Prognostic factors in severe accidental hypothermia: experience from the Mt. Hood tragedy, *J Trauma* 27:1107, 1987.
41. Laub GW, Banaszak D, Kupferschmid J: Percutaneous cardiopulmonary bypass for the treatment of hypothermic circulatory collapse, *Ann Thorac Surg* 47:608, 1989.

42. Vretenar DF, Urschel JD, Parrott JC et al: Cardiopulmonary bypass resuscitation for accidental hypothermia, *Ann Thorac Surg* 58:895, 1994.
43. Waters DJ, Belz M, Lawse D et al: Portable cardiopulmonary bypass: resuscitation from prolonged icewater submersion and asystole, *Ann Thorac Surg* 57:1018, 1994.
44. Wollenek G, Honarwar N, Golej J et al: Cold water submersion and cardiac arrest in treatment of severe hypothermia with cardiopulmonary bypass, *Resuscitation* 52:255, 2002.
45. Gregory JS, Bergstein JM, Aprahamian C et al: Comparison of three methods of rewarming from hypothermia: advantages of extracorporeal blood warming, *J Trauma* 31:1247, 1991.
46. Gentilello LM, Cobean RA, Offner PJ et al: Continuous arteriovenous rewarming: rapid reversal of hypothermia in critically ill patients, *J Trauma* 32:316, 1992.
47. Dobson JA, Burgess JJ: Resuscitation of severe hypothermia by extracorporeal rewarming in a child, *J Trauma* 40:483, 1996.
48. Papenhausen M, Burke L, Antony A et al: Severe hypothermia with cardiac arrest: complete neurologic recovery in a 4-year-old child, *J Pediatr Surg* 36:1590, 2001.
49. Hall KN, Syverud SA: Closed thoracic cavity lavage in the treatment of severe hypothermia in human beings, *Ann Emerg Med* 19:204, 1990.
50. Kristensen G, Gravesen H, Benveniste D et al: An oesphageal thermal tube for rewarming in hypothermia, *Acta Anaesthesiol Scand* 29:846, 1985.
51. Gilbert M, Busund R, Skagseth A et al: Resuscitation from accidental hypothermia of 13.7° C with circulatory arrest, *Lancet* 355:375, 2000.
52. Biggart MJ, Bohn DJ: Effect of hypothermia and cardiac arrest on outcome of near-drowning accidents in children, *J Pediatr* 117:179, 1990.
53. Bolte RG, Black PG, Bowers RS: The use of extracorporeal rewarming in a child submerged for 66 minutes, *JAMA* 260:377, 1988.
54. Golden F: Mechanisms of body cooling in submersed victims, *Resuscitation* 35:107, 1997.
55. Golden F, Tipton MJ, Scott RC: Immersion, near-drowning and drowning, *Br J Anaesth* 79:214, 1997.
56. Suominen P, Baillie C, Korpela R et al: Impact of age, submersion time and water temperature on outcome in near-drowning, *Resuscitation* 52:247, 2002.
57. Suominen PK, Korpela RE, Silfvast TG et al: Does water temperature affect outcome of nearly drowned children? *Resuscitation* 35:111, 1997.
58. Schaller M-D, Fischer AP, Perret CH: Hyperkalemia: a prognostic factor during acute severe hypothermia, *JAMA* 264:1842, 1990.
59. Mair P, Kornberger E, Furtwaengler W et al: Prognostic markers in patients with severe accidental hypothermia and cardiocirculatory arrest, *Resuscitation* 27:47, 1994.

CHAPTER

103

Near-Drowning

Ashok P. Sarnaik and Mary W. Lieh-Lai

PEARLS

- More than 1600 drowning deaths occur each year in the United States in children younger than 19 years. Children younger than 5 years and boys aged 15 to 19 years are the two groups most at risk. Accidental drowning is the second most common cause of unintentional injury death in children, exceeded only by motor vehicular accidents.
- Acute respiratory distress syndrome (ARDS) is the hallmark of delayed pulmonary insufficiency resulting from aspiration in near-drowning and is sometimes referred to as *secondary drowning*. This is characterized by progression of alveolar-capillary block, increased capillary permeability, and pulmonary edema.
- The goal of mechanical ventilation is to provide adequate gas exchange to ensure tissue viability while minimizing the inevitable ventilator-associated injury from oxytrauma, barotrauma, volutrauma, and ineffective tracheobronchial toilet.
- Central nervous system (CNS) injury is by far the most important cause of death and long-term functional impairment among the immediate survivors of submersion accidents.
- The outcome of near-drowning victims depends largely on the success of resuscitative measures at the scene of injury. Patients who are successfully resuscitated and who are conscious on arrival at a hospital have an excellent chance of intact survival.
- Pulmonary edema encountered in children after near-drowning is due to ARDS and not from fluid overload. It should be treated with positive end-expiratory pressure and not diuretics. Such children are often hypovolemic and may require isotonic fluid resuscitation.
- In an unexplained near-drowning episode or with a similar history in familial members, an underlying predisposing disorder such as long QT syndrome should be suspected.

Of all the clinical entities encountered in a pediatric intensive care unit (PICU), drowning and near-drowning accidents are among the most tragic. Within minutes, previously healthy children with hopeful futures die or are left severely incapacitated with no chance of meaningful cognition. The parents, once full of dreams for their youngsters, are suddenly beset with tremendous grief and guilt because in most instances the accident could have been prevented by simple measures.

Definitions

Various terms used in relation to submersion accidents need clarification. *Drowning* is death from suffocation by submersion in water, whereas the term *near-drowning* refers to survival, even if a temporary one, after asphyxia from the submersion episode.[1] Approximately 10% to 15% of persons who drown die of asphyxia without ever aspirating water into their lungs. This entity is referred to as *dry drowning* or *drowning without aspiration*. The term *secondary drowning* refers to the delayed onset of pulmonary insufficiency from acute respiratory distress syndrome (ARDS) after a near-drowning episode. The temperature of the water where the submersion incident occurs is referred to as *warm* (≥20° C), *cold* (<20° C), or *very cold* (≤5° C).[2]

Epidemiology

More than 1600 drowning deaths occur each year in the United States in children younger than 19 years.[3,4] Children younger than 5 years and boys aged 15 to 19 years are the two groups most at risk. Accidental drowning is the second most common cause of unintentional injury death in children, exceeded only by motor vehicular accidents.[3,5] The drowning rate is twice as high for white as for African American children younger than 5 years, whereas African Americans are at a higher risk at all other ages.[6] Males are four times more likely to drown than females. The residential swimming pool is the most common accident site for children younger than 5 years, whereas older children and adults drown more frequently in canals, lakes, ponds, and oceans.[6] The frequency of submersion accidents is highest during the summer months.[7] Bathtub drownings mainly involve infants and people with a seizure disorder.[6,8,9] Child abuse should be suspected when bathtub drownings involving young children occur.[10] Over the past 25 years, drowning rates have declined in adolescents and toddlers but have increased in infants.[11] Nonetheless, in many states, drowning remains one of the three leading causes of death in children younger than 5 years. Morbidity from near-drowning is substantial. For every drowning death, there are almost 4 hospital admissions and 14 emergency department visits.[4] The risk factors for near-drowning are the same as they are for drowning.

A profile of the pediatric drowning victim has been well described.[12] The child at greatest risk is usually a preschool male nonswimmer who drowns in a home swimming pool while under the care of a responsible adult. There is often a breakdown in safety precautions with either an unlocked or a malfunctioning safety fence or a lapse in supervision. Alcohol is a significant risk factor in teenage and adult drownings.[13] Ethanol and other neurotropic agents can diminish manual dexterity, impair judgment, and increase risk-taking behavior. Additionally, recent alcohol consumption by supervising adults may contribute to submersion accidents involving children.[2]

Expert swimmers have been known to drown during underwater swimming. The practice of hyperventilation to prolong the duration of underwater swimming is particularly hazardous in this regard because significant hypoxemia may result in loss of consciousness before hypercarbia stimulates respiration.[14]

Pathophysiological Considerations

The sequence of events after submersion has been described by Karpovich[15] in animal studies. After the initial panic and violent struggle, automatic swimming movements are followed by breathholding and swallowing of large amounts of water. Subsequently, water is aspirated into the lungs as a result of attempts to breathe. Convulsions and spasmodic efforts precede death resulting from asphyxia. The single most important and prognostically significant consequence of submersion is a decreased oxygen delivery to the tissues. A number of clinical variables determine the magnitude of hypoxia and the subject's ability to withstand it. The pathophysiology of near-drowning is thus closely integrated with the genesis of hypoxemia and its effects on various organ functions. A working knowledge of these pathophysiological principles and multiorgan involvement is extremely helpful in directing therapeutic strategies for optimum survival.

Type of Aspirated Fluid

Freshwater, which is considerably hypotonic in comparison with plasma, is rapidly absorbed across the alveoli into the circulation. Aspiration of large amounts of freshwater may cause increased blood volume and hemodilution resulting in hypoelectrolytemia and hemolysis. The osmolality of seawater is three to four times greater than that of plasma. Presence of seawater in the lung draws water from the circulation into the alveoli with potential for hemoconcentration, hyperelectrolytemia, and decreased blood volume. The extent to which these changes occur, however, depends on the amount of aspirated fluid.

Aspiration of more than 11 ml of fluid per kilogram of body weight is required for blood volume to be altered, and aspiration of more than 22 ml/kg is necessary before significant electrolyte changes occur.[16,17] Most near-drowning victims aspirate less than 3 to 4 ml of fluid per kilogram of body weight. Although the differences between changes in electrolytes and blood volume after saltwater and freshwater aspiration have been emphasized in the past, they are of little clinical significance in patients who survive long enough to be transported to a medical facility.[18] Hypervolemia resulting from freshwater aspiration is rarely a problem. Most near-drowning victims are intravascularly hypovolemic regardless of the type of aspiration because of excessive capillary permeability resulting from asphyxia and the loss of protein-rich fluid into the alveoli.

Pulmonary Effects

Functional residual capacity (FRC) is the only source of gas exchange at the pulmonary capillary level in the submerged state. Increased metabolic demands from struggling, breathholding, a depletion of FRC from breathing efforts, and aspiration of fluid into the lungs all result in seriously compromised molecular oxygen (O_2) uptake and carbon dioxide (CO_2) elimination, with consequent hypoxia and hypercarbia. Between 10% and 15% of drowning victims have severe laryngospasm after submersion resulting in dry-drowning from fatal asphyxiation without aspiration of water into their lungs (Fig. 103–1). A combined respiratory and metabolic acidosis caused by hypercapnia and anaerobic metabolism is often encountered. Patients without significant fluid aspiration recover from asphyxia rapidly if they are successfully resuscitated before cardiac arrest or irreversible brain damage occurs. Aspiration of fluid,

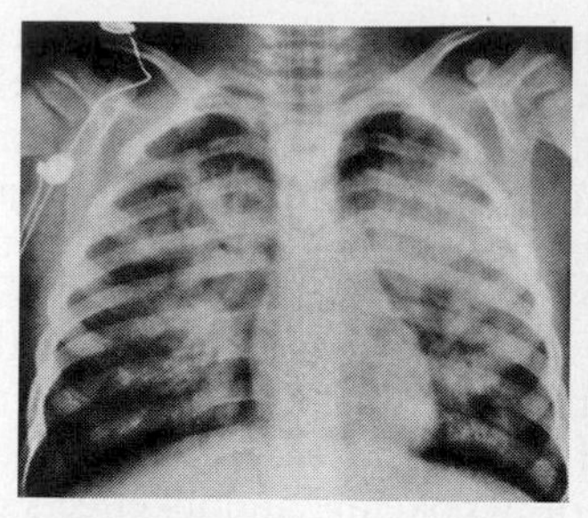

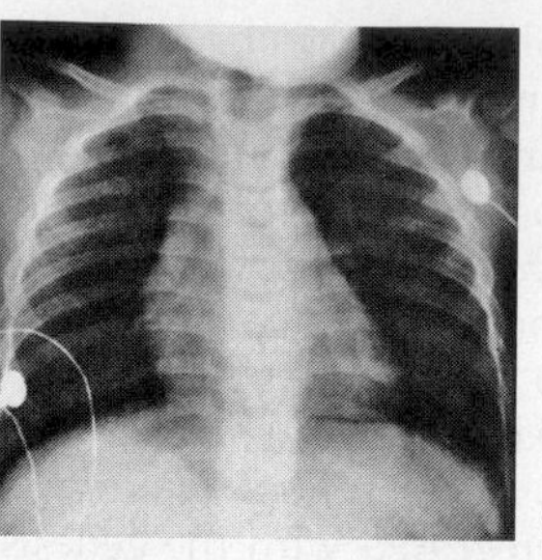

FIGURE 103–1 • Near-drowning with and without aspiration. Radiographs show a patient with severe pulmonary edema **(A)**, and another without significant fluid aspiration **(B)**. (From Ciullo JV: *Clinics in sports medicine,* Philadelphia, 1986, WB Saunders.)

however, results in persistently abnormal gas exchange. Aspiration of as little as 1 to 3 ml/kg body weight results in profound impairment of gas exchange.[17,19] Soon after the aspiration of fluid, there is an elevation of $Paco^2$ and a fall in Pao_2 as a result of airway obstruction, hypoventilation, and impaired gas exchange between alveoli and pulmonary capillary blood. With adequate resuscitation, normocapnia or even hypocapnia is usually achieved while hypoxemia persists. This indicates a significant ventilation/perfusion mismatch and diffusion defect leading to intrapulmonary shunting and venous admixture (see also Chapter 36).[20]

The surfactant system of the lung is affected differently in freshwater and seawater aspiration.[21] Freshwater aspiration results in marked disruption of the surfactant system of the lung resulting in alveolar instability and atelectasis. Seawater, because of its hypertonicity, draws water into the alveoli. Although the surfactant may be diluted by the presence of seawater in alveoli, its surface tension properties are not significantly altered. Karch[22] showed marked changes in the pulmonary vasculature in rabbits within 30 minutes of aspiration of both freshwater and saltwater. Mitochondrial swelling and disruption of pulmonary vascular endothelial cells were consistently observed in these experiments. Clinically, pulmonary abnormalities are encountered in both freshwater and seawater aspiration. These are consistent with pronounced injury to alveoli and pulmonary capillaries resulting in increased membrane permeability, exudation of proteinaceous material in alveoli, pulmonary edema, decreased lung compliance, and increased airway resistance. The extent of these abnormalities may not be manifested fully for several hours after the submersion episode and may be progressive in nature. ARDS is the hallmark of delayed pulmonary insufficiency resulting from aspiration in near-drowning and is sometimes referred to as *secondary drowning.* This is characterized by progression of alveolar-capillary block, increased capillary permeability, and pulmonary edema (see also Chapter 46). Reduced FRC and diffusion barrier resulting from accumulation of fluid and inflammatory cells in the alveoli and interstitium further accentuate hypoxemia. Aspiration of stomach contents and other debris such as sand, mud, and algae may also impair gas exchange. Bacterial pneumonia resulting from aspiration of contaminated water may further contribute to pulmonary insufficiency.

Understanding the alterations in pulmonary mechanics is important to provide the necessary support in the least injurious fashion. Predominant manifestations are those of ARDS complicating the near-drowning event. Although pulmonary involvement is often bilateral and diffuse, there is considerable inhomogeneity with some areas more affected than others. Overall, the lung compliance is reduced, necessitating higher inflation pressure to maintain adequate tidal volume (V_T). Low V_T at low FRC leads to a vicious cycle of atelectasis, decreased compliance, and further reduction in V_T. Critical opening pressure necessary to begin alveolar inflation is increased. Appropriate positive end-expiratory pressure (PEEP) needs to be administered to maintain the necessary FRC for adequate oxygenation and ventilation above the critical opening pressure. Airway resistance is relatively less affected or only minimally elevated unless there is airway obstruction from aspirated debris. Time constant, a product of compliance and resistance, reflects the time needed for pressure equilibration between proximal airway and alveoli to occur. In ARDS, time constant is decreased, allowing for quicker approximation of pressures at these sites during the inspiratory and expiratory phases of mechanical ventilation. Relatively large V_T (10 to 12 ml/kg) is associated with greater ventilator-induced lung injury in ARDS, whereas smaller V_T (6 ml/kg) is associated with less volutrauma. Because of the short time constant, prolongation of inspiratory time to improve oxygenation and increasing the respiratory rate for Co_2 elimination are often effective options during mechanical ventilation.

Cardiovascular Effects

Profound cardiovascular instability is often encountered after an episode of severe near-drowning, and it poses an immediate threat to survival after the initial rescue. Life-threatening dysrhythmias such as ventricular tachycardia or fibrillation and asystole are most often a result of hypoxemia rather than electrolyte abnormalities. The two integral components of oxygen delivery, namely arterial O_2 content and cardiac output, can be adversely affected by the immersion episode. A decrease in Pao_2, if sufficiently severe, decreases oxygen saturation and therefore arterial oxygen content. Cardiac output may similarly be affected by decreased stroke volume. Additionally, therapeutic application of PEEP may cause decreased venous return and therefore the preload. Cardiogenic shock may result from hypoxic damage to the myocardium. Metabolic acidosis may further impair myocardial performance. Pulmonary vasoconstriction from inflammatory mediators can cause increased right ventricular afterload and stroke work. If pulmonary hypertension is severe enough, right ventricular decompensation leads to decreased right ventricular stroke volume, left ventricular preload, and cardiac output. Smooth muscle contraction banding in the media of the major coronary arteries, local ventricular myocyte hypereosinophilia, ventricular myocyte contraction banding, and focal myocardial necrosis have been described after a submersion episode.[23,24] Cytosolic calcium overload and oxygen-derived free radicals have also been implicated in the mechanism of myocardial injury after resuscitation from cardiac arrest.[25] Structural microvascular damage and actions of various humoral mediators involved in ARDS result in pulmonary hypertension with a consequent increase in right ventricular afterload, increased right ventricular stroke work, and eventually right ventricular decompensation and failure.[26] Most patients have low left ventricular filling pressure after a serious episode of near-drowning either in freshwater or saltwater. This is due to excessive permeability of pulmonary and systemic capillaries resulting in hypovolemia. These alterations of oxygen delivery, namely oxygen content, myocardial contractility, left and right ventricular afterload, and preload, can potentially result in inadequate supply of oxygen to tissues to meet their metabolic demands.

Central Nervous System Effects

Hypoxia, sufficiently prolonged, causes profound disturbances of central nervous system (CNS) function. The severity of brain injury depends on the magnitude and duration of hypoxia. Progressive oxygen depletion and impaired neuronal metabolism result in loss of consciousness. During the early stages, however, even severe encephalopathy is still reversible if the victim is promptly rescued and successfully resuscitated.[27] The pathogenesis of hypoxic encephalopathy is poorly understood. Experimental evidence suggests that neuronal dysfunction may not be entirely due to the acute hypoxic episode. Neurons can survive and maintain normal metabolic functions despite prolonged anoxia.[28,29] Restoration of circulation after an ischemic-hypoxic insult may result in transient vasodilation followed by a marked decrease in cerebral blood flow.[30] Thus significant neuronal damage may continue to occur even after restoration of circulation and oxygenation.

Several pathogenetic mechanisms have been proposed to explain postresuscitation cerebral hypoperfusion and progressive CNS injury (see also Chapter 59). These include increased intracranial pressure (ICP), cytotoxic cerebral edema, excessive accumulation of cytosolic calcium, and oxygen-derived free radical damage. In our experience, significant intracranial hypertension is not encountered in the first 72 hours after the hypoxic event even in patients with profound impairment of cerebral function.[31] Cerebral arteriolar spasm that results from calcium entry into the vascular smooth muscle has been proposed as the mechanism of postresuscitation cerebral ischemia.[32] Increased intracellular calcium may also set off a complex chain of events resulting in the generation of free radicals during the reperfusion phase.[33] These free radicals can cause disintegration of cell membrane and neuronal death after circulation is reestablished. Intracellular acidosis triggering dissociation of protein-bound iron has also been indicated in free radical damage to membrane lipids and proteins.[34] With improved techniques of cardiopulmonary support, the extent of CNS injury has become the major determinant of survival and neurological morbidity in patients reaching the PICU after near-drowning.

Effects on Other Organ Systems

Multisystem failure resulting from prolonged ischemic-hypoxic state, sepsis, and therapeutic modalities used to manage these children may complicate the clinical course.[35] Renal and hepatic insufficiency, disseminated intravascular coagulation, gastrointestinal injury, and metabolic abnormalities are important management considerations. These complications rarely pose a threat to survival in an otherwise salvageable patient, however.

Mammalian Diving Reflex

A certain degree of protection against submersion hypoxia has been proposed to occur in the form of a response similar to the diving reflex observed in seals and other air-breathing diving mammals. The ability of these animals to remain submerged for periods of up to 20 minutes is due to a remarkable redistribution of blood flow that occurs after diving underwater. Although the heart, brain, and lungs remain adequately perfused, blood flow to tissues resistant to hypoxia (e.g., gastrointestinal tract, skin, muscle) is markedly reduced. Significant bradycardia occurs with a reduction in cardiac output. Such a response, albeit quantitatively less, is also observed in humans after total body immersion.[36] The mammalian diving reflex acts as an oxygen-conserving adaptation in response to submersion. It has been proposed that this reflex is most active in infancy and is potentiated by fear and low water temperature.[37] A combination of marked bradycardia and impalpable pulses resulting from vasoconstriction may make the victim appear dead at a time when mouth-to-mouth resuscitation could be lifesaving.[36] Clinical studies involving children and adults have failed to show an efficient diving reflex in response to cold-water submersion.[38,39] Young children had a significantly decreased breathhold duration and consequently a weaker dive response compared with older children and adults.[39] The role of the mammalian diving reflex in enabling children to withstand prolonged cold-water submersion thus remains controversial.

Preexisting Associated Conditions

An underlying etiological mechanism should be explored depending on a given clinical scenario involving an unexplained submersion episode. Children with a seizure disorder are at greater risk for submersion accidents. Similarly, an occurrence of vasovagal syncope or a hypoglycemic episode during swimming may be the underlying factor responsible for submersion. Occult cardiomyopathy or a cardiac arrhythmia should also be considered in an unexplained near-drowning event. An episode of near-drowning might be the first manifestation of long QT syndrome (LQTS). Ackerman et al[40] studied blood samples or archived autopsy tissue samples in 35 cases of autosomal dominant LQTS. Six of these patients had a history or extended family history of near-drowning. All of these patients were found to have LQTS causing mutations in *KVLQT1*, whereas such an abnormality was found in only 3 of remaining 29 patients who did not have a history of submersion episode. Thus swimming appears to be a gene-specific (*KVLQT1*) arrhythmogenic trigger for LQTS. Diagnosis of inherited LQTS allows for identification of other family members with similar affliction. Yoshinaga et al[41] showed that face immersion in cold water results in abnormal lengthening of the QT interval in children identified with nonfamilial LQTS, and such children could potentially be at risk of a life-threatening arrhythmia during swimming (see also Chapter 26).

Submersion Hypothermia

Cold-water submersion may significantly alter the pathophysiology of near-drowning.[42] Astonishingly good outcomes in isolated cases have been reported in children submerged in ice water (≤5° C) for prolonged periods.[16,43,44] It appears that for submersion hypothermia to be protective, rapid cooling in icy water (<5° C) is necessary.[44] A lesser degree of hypothermia in warmer water (>5° C) does not offer cerebral protection.[45] Furthermore, intact survival is more an exception than a rule in patients with prolonged submersion, even in ice water. The young and older individuals are most susceptible to hypothermia. Infants lose heat rapidly when subjected to a hypothermic environment because of their relatively large surface area. Because of its CNS depressant effects and vasodilatory properties, alcohol intoxication can contribute significantly to the development of immersion hypothermia and heat loss from environmental exposure.

The most important effect of severe hypothermia is a decrease in energy use, which is reduced to 50% of normal energy use at 28° C.[46] Hypothermia profoundly affects the cerebral metabolic rate. Cerebral blood flow decreases 6% to 7% per 1° C temperature drop, and this decrease results in significant depression of sensorium. The pupils are dilated below 30° C, and the electroencephalogram (EEG) becomes isoelectric below 20° C.[46] Its protective effects notwithstanding, hypothermia by itself poses a direct threat to survival (see Chapter 102).[16]

Management

Because the full extent of CNS injury cannot be adequately determined immediately after the rescue, all victims of near-drowning should receive aggressive basic and advanced life support at the site of the accident and in the emergency department. It cannot be overemphasized that the major determinant of survival and maximal brain salvage is prompt and effective management of hypoxemia and acidosis. In this context, the management in the immediate postimmersion period is paramount. The success or failure of cardiopulmonary resuscitation (CPR) at the site of the accident often determines the outcome.[27,47] The issue of the duration of submersion in relation to the success of resuscitation is often raised. Although asphyxia for longer than 5 minutes frequently results in significant brain injury, this should not be a consideration in the decision of whether to initiate the on-site resuscitation. The emotional excitement surrounding the accident makes it impossible to estimate accurately the duration of hypoxia.

Management at the Scene

Ensuring the adequacy of the airway, breathing, and circulation is the goal of basic life support after the initial rescue. In cases of inadequate airway and cardiopulmonary status, CPR must be instituted immediately. The fundamentals of basic life support are the same after near-drowning as for any other situation requiring CPR; however, some practical aspects are worth considering when a nearly drowned victim is managed. The aim of resuscitation at the scene is to prevent irreversible tissue injury from prolonged hypoxia and ischemia. The victim should be removed from the water as soon as possible. Mouth-to-mouth breathing should be performed even while in the water if it can be accomplished. Chest compressions should not be attempted in water because they are ineffective and waste valuable time.[48] Prolonged attempts to remove water from the lungs are futile and may hinder ongoing ventilatory support. Heimlich and Patrick[49] have recommended the use of subdiaphragmatic pressure in drowning victims to remove water from the airway. Fresh water aspirated into the lungs is quickly absorbed into the systemic circulation, whereas saltwater aspiration results in pulmonary edema. Furthermore, most nearly drowned victims aspirate relatively small amounts of water. There is no evidence to suggest that the Heimlich maneuver can remove aspirated fresh water or pulmonary edema fluid.[50,51] On the other hand, such patients frequently swallow large amounts of water. Consequently, increased abdominal pressure may result in regurgitation of gastric contents into the oropharynx and aspiration into the tracheobronchial tree.[27,51] Any debris observed in the oropharynx should be removed before initiation of mouth-to-mouth breathing. Presence of airway obstruction caused by a foreign body should be suspected if effective chest expansion cannot be accomplished with appropriate ventilatory technique. A subdiaphragmatic thrust in such a situation would be indicated. Pressure used during resuscitation to inflate the lungs of near-drowning victims may have to be higher than anticipated because of reduced compliance of the edematous lungs. Overinflation should be avoided, however, because this can lead to pulmonary barotrauma, air embolism, and overdistention of the stomach with regurgitation and aspiration of gastric contents. Supplemental oxygen should be administered as soon as it is available and continued in all patients during transport even if satisfactory oxygenation has been shown. Noninvasive assessment of oxygenation and ventilation with the use of pulse oximetry and transcutaneous O_2/CO_2 monitor provides valuable information, especially when such patients are transported to appropriate facilities.

Emergency Department Evaluation and Stabilization

As with any form of accidental injury, other forms of associated trauma must be considered. Children who slip and fall into the pool may sustain external head injury such as abrasions, lacerations, and contusions. Occasionally, profuse bleeding from scalp lacerations may be sufficient to aggravate hypovolemic shock. In bathtub drownings or in instances in which child abuse is suspected, fractures and other evidence of previous injury should be looked for. In adolescent victims, near-drowning is frequently associated with illicit drug or alcohol use. When appropriate, urine and blood toxicology tests should be performed. Spinal injuries associated with near-drowning are not uncommon, especially with diving accidents involving young adults.[50]

The need for hospitalization should be determined by the severity of the submersion episode and clinical evaluation. All patients with a history of near-drowning should be observed in the emergency department for 4 to 6 hours. Those with insignificant history and normal findings from physical examination may be safely treated as outpatients.[52] Patients with respiratory symptoms, decreased O_2 saturation indicated by pulse oximetry or blood gas determination, and altered sensorium should be hospitalized.

The extent of cerebral hypoxia can be quantified by Conn's criteria as category A (awake), category B (blunted consciousness), and category C (comatose). Category C is subclassified into C_1 (decorticate), C_2 (decerebrate), and C_3 (flaccid).[53] The Glasgow Coma Scale (GCS) has also been proposed to estimate severity of neurologic dysfunction.[54] Both the GCS and Conn's classification are helpful in determining management and judging response to therapy and for prognosticating.

Maintaining adequate airway, respirations, and peripheral perfusion with continued attention to oxygenation, ventilation, and cardiac performance should take priority. Electrocardiogram (ECG) monitoring and arterial blood gas determination should be performed as soon as possible. Ventricular dysrhythmias, asystole, and hypotension may result from the asphyxial episode and are commonly encountered during the early resuscitation phase. The standard CPR techniques also apply to the nearly drowned child. Patients who have respiratory acidosis and hypoxemia and those who are unconscious with significant respiratory distress or poor respiratory efforts require intubation and mechanical ventilation. Early use of PEEP is effective in reversing hypoxemia. Because pulmonary edema is not caused by hypervolemia in near-drowning, diuretics are not helpful and, in addition, may exacerbate the prevalent hypovolemia. Therefore pulmonary edema after near-drowning is best treated mechanically with positive pressure breathing and PEEP rather than diuretics. Hypovolemia is commonly encountered in the early resuscitation phase. Isotonic crystalloids (20 ml/kg) or colloids (10 ml/kg) infused over 15 to 20 minutes should be used for intravascular volume expansion. Additional volume expansion can be carried out on the basis of clinical and hemodynamic status. Administration of large amounts of hypotonic fluid is contraindicated because of the lack of effective volume expansion. Furthermore, the resultant decrease in serum osmolality may exacerbate cerebral edema. In the face of continued hypotension or impaired peripheral perfusion after appropriate intravascular volume expansion, inotropic support with dopamine or dobutamine may be necessary. Central venous pressure (CVP) monitoring is extremely helpful for ongoing assessment and management of intravascular volume. Mild-to-moderate metabolic acidosis may resolve, along with improvement of oxygenation and tissue perfusion. In more severe cases, sodium bicarbonate administration may be necessary on the basis of blood gas values. Radiological studies should include a chest radiograph to determine the presence or absence of pneumothorax or pneumomediastinum. Unless head injury is suspected, computed tomography scan of the head is usually not necessary because early findings are often normal even in the face of severe hypoxic damage.[55]

Severe bradycardia and intense vasoconstriction associated with marked hypothermia (<32° C) may make near-drowning victims appear dead. Resuscitative efforts should be continued, however, while body temperature is normalized. Treatment of hypothermia is discussed in Chapter 102.

Management in the Pediatric Intensive Care Unit

Continued attention to oxygenation and ventilation status and cardiac performance is essential. Pulse oximetry is readily available and provides a good indication of oxygen saturation and may especially be useful in continuous monitoring of patients who may have ARDS. Because of the nature of the oxygen-hemoglobin dissociation curve, however, pulse oximetry does not accurately reflect changes in PaO_2 greater than 70 mmHg. Arterial and CVP monitoring are necessary in most patients who require intensive care. Placement of a flow-directed pulmonary arterial catheter may provide useful information in those patients with myocardial failure and severe lung disease requiring high PEEP; however, its influence on improving outcome is debatable. A useful parameter to monitor is mixed venous oxygen saturation (Svo_2). Provided Cao_2 and Vo_2 (volume of oxygen utilization) remain constant, Svo_2 is a useful indicator of changes in cardiac output.

The need for endotracheal intubation and different ventilatory strategies should be determined on an individual basis and by clinical judgment. Patients with respiratory acidosis, Pao_2 less than 60 torr in Fio_2 greater than 0.5, clinical signs of impending respiratory fatigue, and depressed level of consciousness are the most common indications for mechanical ventilation. Early use of PEEP and supplemental oxygen is extremely effective in reversing hypoxemia.

The goal of mechanical ventilation is to provide adequate gas exchange to ensure tissue viability while minimizing the inevitable ventilator associated injury from oxytrauma, barotrauma, volutrauma, and ineffective tracheobronchial toilet. Ventilatory strategy should take into account the major alterations in pulmonary mechanics. As noted earlier, most children with near-drowning have decreased FRC, compliance, and time constant and increased critical opening pressure. Salutary effects of PEEP are from maintaining alveolar stability and alveolar recruitment and increasing FRC. It stabilizes the relatively softer chest wall of a child, thus minimizing chest wall recoil and further decrease in FRC. Because PEEP also displaces intraalveolar water into interstitial and perilymphatic spaces, the results are decreased venous admixture and improved compliance. On the other hand, excessive amounts of PEEP can result in decreased venous return and cardiac output, pulmonary overdistension and decreased compliance, and barotrauma. Maintenance of normovolemia is an important consideration in patients receiving PEEP.

It has been recently recognized that in patients with acute lung injury and ARDS, ventilation with lower V_T (6 ml/kg) results in improved survival compared with those ventilated with a larger V_T (12 ml/kg).[56] There are various ventilatory strategies that may be used to minimize barotrauma in a patient with ARDS while maintaining adequate gas exchange. The underlying principle is to recruit lung volume by application of optimum PEEP to maintain FRC above the critical opening pressure and ventilate with V_T approximating 6 to 7 ml/kg. Both pressure-controlled and volume-controlled strategies can be used with this principle. We recommend pressure-controlled ventilation with a relatively low peak airway pressure and prolonged inspiration while still allowing adequate time for complete exhalation. The level of PEEP can be optimized by gradual increments depending on its effects on increasing PaO_2/FIO_2 ratio. The ability of modern ventilators to display exhaled V_T and graphic display of flow, pressure, and volume waveforms has enabled the clinician to adjust mechanical ventilatory support according to individual alterations in pulmonary mechanics. Optimal PEEP, as evidenced by improvement in dynamic compliance, can be determined with the measurement of exhaled V_T at varying levels of PEEP. When PEEP exceeds critical opening pressure or the lower inflection point on the pressure/volume curve, dynamic compliance improves. Ventilatory rate, inspiratory/expiratory times, and peak airway pressures can also be adjusted according to their effects on dynamic compliance and ascertaining the return of expiratory flow to baseline. In patients without CNS injury and intracranial hypertension, the technique of permissive hypercapnia can be used to minimize barotrauma in a patient with ARDS. This involves using lower inflation pressures or V_T and accepting higher levels of PCO_2 as long as pH remains near normal (see also Chapter 44).

High-frequency ventilation is another strategy that can be used in the management of hypoxic respiratory failure. This mode of ventilation uses a relatively high mean airway pressure while minimizing excessive fluctuations in pressures during the respiratory cycle. High-frequency ventilation is a safe and effective modality in the treatment of severe acute respiratory failure that is unresponsive to conventional mechanical ventilation.[57,58]

Extracorporeal life support (ECLS) may be used in the treatment of severe lung injury in near-drowning. The presumed benefit of ECLS is the avoidance of barotrauma and oxygen toxicity in patients who do not improve despite maximum ventilatory support. The risks of carotid artery ligation for the purposes of ECLS cannulation in patients who may have hypoxic-ischemic CNS injury are unknown (see also Chapter 47).

Secondary bacterial infection resulting from aspiration or as a complication of endotracheal intubation and mechanical ventilation is sometimes observed. The routine use of antibiotics for "prophylaxis" has not been shown to be effective in preventing pneumonia. Nevertheless, fulminant *Streptococcus pneumoniae* bacterial sepsis and pneumonia have been described shortly after a severe submersion injury. It is therefore reasonable to institute empiric antibiotic therapy in patients with severe cardiopulmonary deterioration, especially when this occurs after a period of stability.[59] The use of steroids for aspiration pneumonia is probably of no benefit.[60]

Once the patient is successfully resuscitated, the severity of encephalopathy is the main determinant of death and morbidity from near-drowning. With improved techniques of cardiopulmonary support, delayed deaths resulting from pulmonary insufficiency are becoming less frequent. CNS injury is by far the most important cause of death and long-term functional impairment among the immediate survivors of submersion accidents. Measures for cerebral protection in the postimmersion period have been used by several investigators.[37,53] The emphasis of such modalities is on managing cerebral edema, controlling intracranial hypertension, and decreasing the cerebral metabolic requirements, with the use of fluid restriction, diuretics, mechanical ventilation, hypothermia, steroids, barbiturates, and muscle paralysis. Study results, however, have failed to show beneficial effects of such therapy in improving the outcome of hypoxic encephalopathy associated with near-drowning.[61] Furthermore, a significant increase in infections and pulmonary insufficiency was observed in association with therapeutic hypothermia. Pentobarbital has the theoretical advantage of decreasing cerebral oxygen demand. Nevertheless, induction of pentobarbital coma, although effective in controlling intracranial hypertension, has not improved the neurological outcome of comatose children.[61-63] The role of cerebral edema and intracranial hypertension in potentiating CNS injury in otherwise salvageable children is questionable. Our experience suggests that significant intracranial hypertension is not commonly encountered in the early postimmersion period, whereas late, uncontrollable intracranial hypertension carries an unfavorable prognosis.[31] Additionally, satisfactory control of intracranial hypertension is not necessarily associated with improved outcome.[31,61,62] It appears that the occurrence of cerebral edema and intracranial hypertension 2 to 3 days after a submersion accident is a reflection of the early hypoxic injury rather than a manifestation of a reversible process. Late, persistent intracranial hypertension associated with a comatose state is of ominous significance and is almost always associated with an unfavorable outcome.[31]

Currently, the routine use of ICP monitoring in children with hypoxic-ischemic encephalopathy after near-drowning is not recommended. The emphasis of management of a comatose child in the immediate postimmersion period should be on maintaining adequate oxygenation/ventilation and oxygen delivery, and avoiding hypotonic fluid overload. Pathophysiological changes from asphyxia and various therapies aimed at cerebral salvage such as barbiturates and osmotic diuresis adversely affect myocardial performance.[64] Cardiovascular support with maintenance of intravascular volume and the use of inotropic agents are often necessary to maintain optimum organ perfusion in patients who have a significant hypoxic-ischemic insult.

Prognosis

The outcome of near-drowning victims depends largely on the success of resuscitative measures at the scene of injury. Patients who are successfully resuscitated and who are conscious on arrival at a hospital have an excellent chance of intact survival.[47,65,66] With improved ventilatory techniques and aggressive management, pulmonary injury can be successfully managed in most patients. For those who continue to require resuscitation in the emergency department, a variety of prognostic factors have been evaluated. Variables such as age, length of submersion, serum pH, and body temperature, although previously thought to influence outcome,[67] have not been shown to be reliable prognostic indicators.[63] In addition, our experience suggests that the absence of cognitive function 72 hours after the hypoxic episode is strongly associated with either death or survival in a persistent vegetative state.[31] The need for continued CPR at the hospital, CPR greater than 25 minutes, fixed and dilated pupils, seizures, flaccidity, GCS of 5 or less, and decreased cerebral blood flow are of poor prognostic significance in the absence of hypothermia.[68-70] Severe hypothermia has been shown to influence the outcome favorably even after prolonged submersion; however, not all hypothermic near-drowning victims are fortunate enough to escape serious neuronal damage.[71]

REFERENCES

1. Modell JH: Drown versus near drown: a discussion of definitions, *Crit Care Med* 9:351, 1981.
2. Shaw KN, Briede CA: Submersion injuries: drowning and near-drowning, *Emerg Med Clin North Am* 7:355, 1989.
3. Center for Disease Control and Prevention. Compressed Mortality File, CDC WONDER website. Leading causes of unintentional injury deaths, United States, ages <1 to 18 years. Available at http://wonder.cdc.gov. Accessed February 3, 2003.
4. Wintemute GJ: Childhood drowning and near-drowning in the United States, *Am J Dis Child* 144:663, 1990.
5. Rosenberg ML, Rodriguez JG, Chorba TL: Childhood injuries: where are we? *Pediatrics* 86:1084, 1990.
6. Brenner RA, Trumble AC, Smith GS et al: Where children drown, United States, 1995, *Pediatrics* 108:85-89, 2001.
7. Gulaid JA, Sattin RW: Drowning in the United States, 1978-1984, *MMWR CDC Surveill Summ* 37:27, 1988.
8. Budnick LD, Ross DA: Bathtub-related drowning in the United States, 1979-81, *Am J Public Health* 75:630, 1985.
9. Pearn J: Why children drown, *Aust Pediatr J* 22:161, 1986.
10. Griest KJ, Zumwalt RE: Child abuse by drowning, *Pediatrics* 83:41, 1972.
11. Brenner RA, Smith GS, Overpeck MD: Divergent trends in childhood drowning rates, 1971 through 1988, *JAMA* 271:1606, 1994.
12. Rowe MI, Arango A, Allington G: Profile of pediatric drowning victims in a water-oriented society, *J Trauma* 17:587, 1977.
13. Howland J, Hingson R: Alcohol as a risk factor for drownings: a review of the literature (1950-1985), *Accid Anal Prev* 20:19, 1988.
14. Craig AP: Causes of loss of consciousness during underwater swimming, *J Appl Physiol* 16:583, 1961.
15. Karpovich PV: Water in the lungs of drowned animals, *Arch Pathol Lab Med* 15:828, 1933.
16. Martin TG: Near drowning and cold water immersion, *Ann Emerg Med* 13:263, 1984.
17. Modell JH, Moya F, Newby EJ et al: The effects of fluid volume in seawater drowning, *Ann Intern Med* 67:68, 1967.
18. Modell JH, Davis JH: Electrolyte changes in human drowning victims, *Anesthesiology* 30:414, 1969.
19. Model JH, Moya F: Effects of volume of aspirated fluid during chlorinated fresh water drowning, *Anesthesiology* 27:662, 1966.
20. Modell JH, Moya F, Williams HD et al: Changes in blood gases and A-aDO_2 during near-drowning, *Anesthesiology* 29:456, 1968.
21. Giammoma ST, Modell JH: Drowning by total immersion. Effects on pulmonary surfactant of distilled water, isotonic saline and sea water, *Am J Dis Child* 114:612, 1967.
22. Karch SB: Pathology of the lung in near-drowning, *Am J Emerg Med*, 4:4, 1986.
23. Karch SB: Pathology of the heart in drowning, *Arch Pathol Lab Med* 109:76, 1985.
24. Lunt DWR, Rose AG: Pathology of the human heart in drowning, *Arch Pathol Lab Med* 111:939, 1987.
25. Opie LH: Reperfusion injury and its pharmacology modification, *Circulation* 80:1049, 1989.
26. Sarnaik AP, Lieh-Lai MW: Adult respiratory distress syndrome in children, *Pediatr Clin North Am* 41:337, 1994.
27. Pearn J: Pathophysiology of drowning, *Med J Aust* 142:586, 1985.
28. Ames A III, Gurian BS: Effects of glucose deprivation on function of isolated mammalian retina, *J Neurophysiol* 26:617, 1963.
29. Hossman KA, Keihues P: Reversibility of ischemic brain damage, *Arch Neurol* 29:375, 1973.
30. Ames A 3rd, Wright RL, Kowada M et al: Cerebral ischemia II: the no reflow phenomenon, *Am J Pathol* 52:437, 1968.
31. Sarnaik AP, Preston G, Lieh-Lai M et al: Intracranial pressure and cerebral perfusion pressure in near-drowning, *Crit Care Med* 13: 224, 1985.
32. White BC, Gadzinski DS, Hoehner PJ et al: Effect of flunarizine on canine cerebral blood flow and vascular resistance postcardiac arrest, *Ann Emerg Med* 11:119, 1982.
33. Safar P: Resuscitation from clinical death: pathophysiologic limits and therapeutic potentials, *Crit Care Med* 16:923, 1988.
34. Siesjo BK: Mechanisms of ischemic brain damage, *Crit Care Med* 16:954, 1988.
35. Hoff BH: Multisystem failure: a review with special reference to drowning, *Crit Care Med* 7:310, 1979.
36. Gooden BA: Drowning and the diving reflex in man, *Med J Aust* 2:583, 1972.
37. Conn AW, Edmonds JF, Barker GA: Cerebral resuscitation in near-drowning, *Pediatr Clin North Am* 26:691, 1979.
38. Hayward JS, Hay C, Matthews BR et al: Temperature effect on the human dive response in relation to cold water near-drowning, *J Appl Physiol* 56:202, 1984.
39. Ramey CA, Ramey DN, Hayward JS: Dive response of children in relation to cold-water near-drowning, *J Appl Physiol* 63:665, 1987.
40. Ackerman MJ, Tester DJ, Porter CJ: Swimming, a gene-specific arrhythmogenic trigger for inherited long QT syndrome, *Mayo Clin Proc* 74:1088-1094, 1999.
41. Yoshinaga M, Kamimura J, Fukushige T et al: Face immersion in cold water induces prolongation of the QT interval and T-wave changes in children with nonfamilial long QT syndrome, *Am J Cardiol* 83:1494-1497, 1999.
42. Biggart MJ, Bohn DJ: Effect of hypothermia in cardiac arrest on outcome of near-drowning accidents in children, *J Pediatr* 117:179, 1990.
43. Bolte RG, Black PG, Bowers RS et al: The use of extracorporeal rewarming in a child submerged for 66 minutes, *JAMA* 260:377, 1988.
44. Orlowski JP: Drowning, near-drowning, and ice-water drowning, *JAMA* 260:390, 1988.
45. Quan L, Kinder D: Pediatric submersions: prehospital predictors of outcome, *Pediatrics* 90:909, 1992.
46. Reuler JB: Hypothermia: pathophysiology, clinical settings, and management, *Ann Intern Med* 89:519, 1978.
47. Fandel I, Bancalari E: Near-drowning in children: clinical aspects, *Pediatrics* 58:573, 1976.
48. American Heart Association: Standards and guidelines for cardiopulmonary resuscitation and emergency cardiac care. Available at http://circ.ahajournals.org. Accessed February 3, 2003.
49. Heimlich HJ, Patrick EA: Using the Heimlich maneuver to save near-drowning victims, *Postgrad Med* 84:62, 1988.
50. Ornato JP: The resuscitation of near-drowning victims, *JAMA* 256: 75, 1986.
51. International Life Saving Federation Medical Commission: Statement on the Use of Abdominal Thrusts in Near Drowning, September 26, 1998. Available at http://www.usla.org/PublicInfo/library/ILS_Med_State_AT.doc. Accessed on February 3, 2003.
52. Pratt FD, Haynes BH: Incidence of "secondary drowning" after saltwater submersion, *Ann Emerg Med* 15:1084, 1986.
53. Conn AW, Montes JE, Barker GA et al: Cerebral salvage in near-drowning following neurological classification by triage, *Can Anesth Soc J* 27:201, 1980.
54. Dean JN, Kaufman ND: Prognostic indicators in pediatric near-drowning: the Glasgow coma scale, *Crit Care Med* 9:5536, 1981.
55. Taylor SB, Quencer RM, Holzman BH et al: Central nervous system anoxic-ischemic insult in children due to near-drowning, *Radiology* 156:641, 1985.
56. The ARDS Network: Ventilation with lower tidal volumes as compared with traditional tidal volumes for acute lung injury and the Acute Respiratory Distress Syndrome, *N Engl J Med* 2000; 342:1301-1308.
57. Arnold JH, Hanson JH, Toro-Figuero LO et al: Prospective, randomized comparison of high-frequency oscillatory ventilation

and conventional mechanical ventilation in pediatric respiratory failure, *Crit Care Med* 22:1530, 1994.
58. Sarnaik AP et al: Efficacy of high frequency ventilation (HFV) in children with severe acute respiratory failure (SARF), *Crit Care Med* 21:S154, 1993.
59. Vernon DD, Banner W Jr, Cantwell GP et al: *Streptococcus pneumoniae* bacteremia associated with near-drowning, *Crit Care Med* 18:1175, 1990.
60. Oakes DD, Sherck JP, Maloney JR et al: Prognosis and management of victims of near-drowning, *J Trauma* 22:544, 1982.
61. Bohn DJ, Biggar WD, Smith CR et al: Influence of hypothermia, barbiturate therapy, and intracranial pressure monitoring on morbidity and mortality after near-drowning, *Crit Care Med* 14:529, 1986.
62. Frewen TC, Sumabat WO, Han VK et al: Cerebral resuscitation therapy in pediatric near-drowning, *J Pediatr* 106:615, 1985.
63. Nussbaum E: Prognostic variables in nearly drowned, comatose children, *Am J Dis Child* 139:1058, 1985.
64. Hildebrand CA, Hartmann AG, Arcinue EL et al: Cardiac performance in pediatric near-drowning, *Crit Care Med* 16:331, 1988.
65. Nussbaum E, Maggi JC: Pentobarbital therapy does not improve neurologic outcome in nearly-drowned, flaccid-comatose children, *Pediatrics* 81:630, 1988.
66. Peterson B: Morbidity of childhood near-drowning, *Pediatrics* 59:364, 1977.
67. Orlowski JP: Prognostic factors in pediatric cases of drowning and near-drowning, *JACEP* 8:176, 1979.
68. Ashwal S, Schneider S, Lawrence T et al: Prognostic implications of hypoglycemia and reduced cerebral blood flow in childhood near-drowning, *Neurology* 40:820, 1990.
69. Lavelle JM, Shaw KN: Near drowning: is emergency department cardiopulmonary resuscitation or intensive care unit resuscitation indicated? *Crit Care Med* 21:368, 1993.
70. Waugh JH, O'Callaghan MS, Pitt WR: Prognostic factors and long-term outcomes for children who have nearly drowned, *Med J Austral* 161:594, 1994.
71. Young RS, Salveraitis EL, Dooling EC: Neurological outcome in cold water drowning, *JAMA* 244:1233, 1980.
64. Spack L, Gedeit R, Splaingard M, Havens PL: Failure of aggressive therapy to alter outcome in pediatric near-drowning. *Ped Emerg Care,* 1997; 13:98-102.

CHAPTER 104

Burn and Inhalation Injuries

Hugo F. Carvajal and James A. Griffith

PEARLS

- The care of burned children is best delivered in the pediatric critical care unit rather than in the burn unit.
- In burned children obligatory oliguria resulting from excessive secretion of antidiuretic hormone is often confused with a dehydrated state.
- Urine output is not a reliable guide to fluid resuscitation in burned children.
- State of sensorium, hematocrit measure, and vital signs are considered the best guides to fluid resuscitation in burned children.
- Early excision and grafting of partial- and full-thickness burn injuries is the single most important contributor to burn survival.
- Smoke inhalation and heat injuries of the airway are major contributors to burn morbidity and must be addressed early and aggressively.
- Meticulous care of the burn wound minimizes conversion to deeper injuries and is associated with increased survival.
- Early diagnosis of burn sepsis and septicemia are paramount to successful outcomes in burned children.
- The use of body surface area rather than weight to estimate rehydration fluids and caloric requirements is preferred.
- A composite isotonic burn resuscitation solution containing 12.5 g of human serum albumin (HSA) per liter (1.25%) is ideal for resuscitation of burned children older than 1 year.
- In infants younger than 1 year, the concentration of sodium in resuscitation fluids must be lowered to prevent hypernatremia.
- Sedation and pain management are best achieved with narcotics (fentanyl citrate, morphine sulfate), anxiolytics (benzodiazepines or midazolam), and nonnarcotic analgesics such as ketorolac or "dissociative" anesthetics such as ketamine.

The care of the burned patient is complex and generally requires a multidisciplinary approach. When the burned patient happens to be a child, the challenges to the burn team are magnified. In children, but particularly in infants, the margin of safety is narrower and therapeutic errors tend to have greater consequences than for adults. Treatment programs must take into consideration not only differences in age and size but also the physiological makeup of the developing child.[1] Accepting the premise that "children are different" and not "merely little adults" is essential to the development of appropriate therapeutic strategies and curtailment of iatrogenic complications, which are seldom recognized as preventable. Although the care of burned children has traditionally taken place in burn units or general surgery wards, pediatric critical care units (PCCUs) are better suited for this purpose. The availability of physicians, nurses, and other health care professionals trained in the care of severely injured pediatric patients makes the PCCU the ideal setting for the initial management of the patient. In the PCCU the focus of attention is the child; the burn merely represents the affliction that prompted the admission. This is in contrast to "burn units" where patients of all ages are admitted and the burn, rather than the child, receives all of the attention.

The approach to patient care in the PCCU involves a cadre of doctors, nurses, and therapists whose training and expertise centers on the child as a whole. Consultants in burn care are then brought in, as would be the case for other injuries or illnesses. Likewise, the training of students, house staff, and fellows in the care of children with acute burns is best accomplished in the PCCU setting, where a comprehensive and physiologically oriented approach to the child is the norm.

Pathogenesis and Pathophysiology

Surface Burn

Burn injuries occur when thermal energy makes contact with skin and other tissues. Tissue damage begins at temperatures of 40° C and increases logarithmically as the temperature rises.[2] At 40° C, denaturation of tissue proteins ensues, and recovery is no longer possible. The exact mechanism by which injury develops is not entirely clear, but the noxious effects of heat and the inflammatory response that follows may last beyond 24 hours after injury.

Tissue damage is seldom homogenous and, in accordance with Jackson,[3] three consecutive zones of significant thermal injury can be identified: coagulation, stasis, and hyperemia. The zone of coagulation represents the area most intimately in contact with the heat source. Cells in this area undergo coagulative necrosis and do not recover. A concentric area of lesser tissue damage, termed the zone of stasis, extends in a three-dimensional fashion away from the zone of coagulation. Prevention of secondary microvascular changes and amelioration of the inflammatory response in the zone of stasis have been the focus of much investigation. The zone of hyperemia is immediately adjacent to the zone of stasis, and it borders unaffected tissues. Cells in this area sustain minimal injury and, in most cases, recover within 7 to 10 days.

Burn injuries are also classified according to the depth of tissue damage.[3] First-degree burns affect only the superficial layer of the skin. This injury manifests itself by pain and redness. Within a few days, the damaged epithelium peels away from the subjacent skin, which heals completely without residual scarring. In second-degree or partial-thickness burns, the dermis is damaged, but deep appendages and other skin structures from which reepithelialization may occur are preserved. These partial-thickness burns are further classified as either superficial or deep. Typical of the former are pain and blister formation, whereas the latter are characterized by a white, leathery, marblelike appearance. Most partial-thickness burns heal within 14 to 17 days.[4] Marginally viable tissue, as seen in the deeper burns, can still heal spontaneously but only when optimal conditions for preservation of these elements can be maintained. If conditions are not optimal (edema, ischemia, infection), conversion from partial- to full-thickness necrosis is commonly seen.[5,6] Third-degree or full-thickness burns are well-demarcated injuries that do not blister. These injuries can only heal from the margins and, by definition, require skin grafting. They have a black or brown leathery appearance, and because they are devoid of nerve endings, they are painless. Fourth-degree burns involve the entire thickness of the skin and subjacent structures (subcutaneous fat, fascia, muscle, or bone). In addition to grafting, reconstructive surgery is often neccessary for fourth-degree injuries, and severe disfigurement is the usual end result.

Burns are also classified according to the heat vector and mechanism of injury into the following categories:

1. Thermal burns
2. Electrical burns
3. Radiation burns
4. Chemical burns

Thermal, electrical, and radiation burns result in protein denaturation through the absorption of energy.[7] Chemical burns differ in that the injury occurs through chemical disruption and alteration of physical properties. This, plus the potential for local and systemic toxicity, increases the chance of morbidity and death associated with chemical burns.

Hemodynamic Changes

Major hemodynamic, autonomic cardiopulmonary, renal, and metabolic disturbances develop rapidly after severe burns. Within minutes of the injury and before significant hypovolemia develops, the cardiac output falls,[8,9] but the exact etiopathogenic mechanism remains elusive.[10,11] Myocardial contractility is not significantly affected at this time; however, a plasma factor (or factors) that depresses myocardial contractility has been isolated in animal studies during the latter stages of shock and is thought to be responsible for the development of persistent hypotension.[12]

In the face of a decreased cardiac output and a relative or absolute hypovolemia, arteriolar vasoconstriction takes place and the systemic vascular resistance increases. The mean arterial pressure is maintained, but the pulse pressure narrows and the peripheral pulses become feeble and difficult to palpate. Capillary refill time is prolonged (>3 seconds), and the noninjured skin turns pale, cold, and mottled. Tachycardia, tachypnea, severe oliguria, and lethargy develop, and the body temperature progressively declines.

Simultaneously, the permeability of the entire vascular tree increases, and water, electrolytes, and proteins are lost from the vascular compartment into the interstitium of injured and noninjured tissues.[12] Burn edema ensues, and the intravascular volume progressively declines. As tissue oxygen delivery decreases, anaerobic metabolic processes lead to increased lactic acid production, impairment of cellular functions, and eventually cell death. The increase in vascular permeability is maximal at 30 minutes after burn, but the capillary integrity is not restored until 8 to 12 hours after the injury.[13,14] These responses are comparable for partial- and full-thickness injuries.[15] In the noninjured tissues, transient extravasation of fluids and proteins only occurs when the total burn area exceeds 40% of the body surface.

Denuded skin offers no barrier to fluid evaporation, and a sixfold to sevenfold increase in evaporative fluid losses is the rule.[16] Fluid losses also occur in the form of burn exudates (blisters) and direct oozing from the burn wound.

Although insensible fluid loss is equivalent to electrolyte-free water, exudative fluid loss has an electrolyte content similar to plasma, and its protein concentration is equivalent to one half of that in plasma. Unless replaced, these losses lead to varying degrees of dehydration, electrolyte imbalance, and hypoalbuminemia.

Neuroendocrine Responses

Burn injuries are associated with severe alterations in metabolism and enhanced neuroendocrine responses that exceed those reported for any other illness or injury (see also Chapter 68). These were first described by Cuthbertson[17] as occurring in two distinct time periods: the "ebb" phase, encompassing the first 24 hours, and a subsequent "flow" phase, which may last several days.

The ebb phase begins with the sensory signal to the brain that tissue injury has occurred and the consequent release of corticotropin (ACTH) and antidiuretic hormone (ADH) in response to pain, fear, hypoxia, and hypovolemia. This phase is dominated by α-adrenergic receptor stimulation and catecholamine secretion and is characterized by redistribution of blood flow from skin to vital organs. Plasma cortisol, aldosterone, and growth hormone levels are markedly elevated, and insulin secretion is curtailed. Hyperglycemia resulting from increased sympathetic activity, secretion of epinephrine, inhibition of insulin release, and cortisol and glucagon release is common in adults, but hypoglycemia is frequently observed in children.[18] The child's reduced glycogen stores and proportionally higher basal energy expenditures may explain the different responses in serum glucose.

It has been postulated that ADH secretion stimulated by pain, fear, apprehension, narcotics, sedatives, and other drugs often leads to a state of antidiuresis, which persists beyond restoration of fluid deficits.[19,20] Under these circumstances urine production no longer reflects intravascular volume and the value of hourly urine measurement because a guide to hydration is lost. Trauma also stimulates the secretion of aldosterone,[10] which leads to kaliuresis and sodium retention and further contributes to oliguria and edema formation.

The flow phase generally begins 24 hours after injury, lasts several days; and is characterized by hypermetabolism, increased cardiac output, and increased oxygen consumption. Accelerated tissue catabolism, increased urinary nitrogen losses, and altered glucose metabolism are invariably present. The degree of hypermetabolism generally correlates with the extent of the injury and is associated with a moderate increase in body temperature.

After fluid resuscitation, the cardiac index increases to levels as high as 6 to 8 L/m^2 of body surface area (BSA). This is a compensatory response to increased oxygen demands. In some instances, tissue oxygen uptake may be compromised, and a dissociation between oxygen delivery and oxygen extraction occurs. Increased blood flow is directed to the surface wound, but oxygen use at the cellular level remains impaired. Splanchnic blood flow may be increased as well but in proportion to local oxygen demand. Also, the increased metabolic rate, often regarded as a primary effect of the injury, may be aggravated by cold exposure, anxiety, septicemia, or organ failure.

Insulin concentrations return to normal after 24 to 48 hours, but hyperglycemia persists. This is thought to occur from increased gluconeogenesis caused by cortisol secretion. Other studies have shown that the gut is transformed from an organ of glucose utilization to one of primary glucose release and that it interacts with the liver in the synthesis of new glucose.[21] Glutamine becomes the alternate fluid for the enterocyte, and the three carbon compounds that are produced are reused by the liver to form new glucose. The release of alanine by the gut is enhanced, and alanine becomes a key gluconeogenic precursor. Although fat remains the primary fuel for the resting skeletal muscle, injured tissues continue to metabolize glucose anaerobically and develop a large capacity for lactate production.[21] When fat stores are depleted, protein becomes a secondary fuel. Unless supplied with adequate quantities of fat and carbohydrates, the burned organism is bound to develop a severe protein-caloric malnutrition.

Inhalation Injury

The fire atmosphere is composed of heated air (approaching 1200° C), particulate matter, and gaseous products of combustion and heat degradation (pyrolysis). Inhalation of toxic materials, which may occur in the absence of cutaneous burns, is responsible for many immediate deaths. The death rate for patients with surface burns in excess of 20% total body surface area (TBSA) is increased by 35% to 40% when the child also has an inhalation injury.[22] Because children are involved in 2.5 times as many scald burns as flame burns, the percentage of children with respiratory system injury is less than that of adults.[23,24] The gaseous products vary dramatically depending on the changing conditions of temperature, oxygen concentration, and available fuel.

More than 50 chemicals, less than one half of which can be identified, have been extracted from blood and tissue samples of patients with inhalation injury. With the exception of carbon monoxide (CO), the products of complete combustion are generally less toxic than those produced by pyrolysis.

The toxicity of inhaled materials is determined by the compounds generated, the dose inhaled, and the duration of exposure. The child's greater minute ventilation accentuates the effects of closed space fires (dwellings, airplanes, automobiles), increasing exposure to the toxin. Conscious breathholding in response to irritants transiently reduces the inhaled toxin dose, but as consciousness is impaired, the rate and depth of respiration increase. In children, visual and perceptual disorientation delays escape from house fires and prolongs the duration of exposure to gaseous toxins.

Toxic inhalants can be classified as systemic toxins, irritants, or asphyxiants (CO and cyanide). Hydrocarbons, product of synthetic material combustion, can have anesthetic and narcotic-like systemic effects that may mimic asphyxia. Asphyxia may also occur as the fraction of oxygen in the fire atmosphere decreases to 10% to 15%. Cyanide is produced when such common materials as wool, silk, nylon, polystyrene, and polyurethane burn. Cyanide inhibits cellular respiration by complexing with cytochrome and disrupting mitochondrial oxygen utilization.

Carbon Monoxide

The final product of hydrocarbon oxidation is carbon dioxide and water. In fires, incomplete oxidation leads to the production of CO.

CO is a colorless, odorless gas that is rapidly absorbed from the lungs.[25] This is the most dangerous chemical in smoke and is responsible for up to 80% of inhalation fatalities. It has approximately 250 times the affinity for hemoglobin (Hb) iron, as does oxygen. This affinity is so strong that breathing 0.1% inspired CO (normal level 0.001%) generates greater than 60% carboxyhemoglobin (HbCO). With prolonged exposure, CO can also bind to other proteins, notably mitochondrial cytochrome oxidase and myoglobin, interfering with cellular oxygen utilization and energy production.

The displacement of oxygen from Hb diminishes the oxygen-carrying capacity of the blood, shifts the oxyhemoglobin dissociation curve to the left, and induces tissue hypoxia and metabolic acidosis. As the fraction of dissolved oxygen and PaO_2 remain normal, arterial blood gases do not reflect the degree of cellular hypoxia. The pulse oximeter is similarly fooled by the presence of Hb saturated with CO, dropping only 1% for each 10% HbCO present. Because calculated oxygen saturations do not reflect the presence of HbCO, direct measurements of both HbCO and oxyhemoglobin are necessary.

The severity of CO poisoning is proportional to the degree of induced hypoxia, which leads to cardiac and central nervous system dysfunction. Blood HbCO levels are only loosely correlated with the clinical condition of the patient and may be falsely lowered by oxygen administration before hospitalization. Extrapolation of HbCO levels to the time of rescue, by the use of nomograms, has greater prognostic value. Levels less than 20% are accompanied by minor symptoms of headache and irritability. Levels greater than 60% are frequently fatal. Studies in animals have shown that blood HbCO levels are not the only determining factor and that even when extrapolations to zero time are possible, the outcome cannot be accurately predicted.

Airway Burns

Inhalation of dry air heated to greater than 150° C can burn the face and upper respiratory system. Thermal injury is principally limited to the supraglottic airway and rarely extends below the vocal cords.[26] The large capacity for evaporative cooling in the upper airway was dramatically demonstrated by Moritz, Henriques, and McLean in 1945.[27] They subjected dogs to direct pharyngeal heated dry air exposure and measured gas temperature in the airway. Laryngeal gas temperatures of 300° C to 500° C fell to 50° C and 60° C at the tracheal bifurcation, and exhaled gas temperatures were normal. Additional protection to the distal airway is provided by reflex closure of the vocal cords. Inhaled steam, with 4000 times the heat capacity of dry air and little opportunity for heat transfer, routinely causes deep airway or parenchymal injuries.

The mechanism of injury is similar for the airways as it is for other tissues, but the progression from erythema to edema and ulceration in the airway mucosa is fastest. The local release of thromboxane A_2, histamine, serotonin, and oxygen-free radicals intensifies the phenomenon of increased microvascular permeability. The loose tissue of the supraglottic airway rapidly swells and can obstruct the airway. This is the reason early intubation may become life saving. Mucosal edema can be further aggravated by vigorous fluid resuscitation and loss of plasma protein.[28]

Particulate Matter

Most particulate matter in the fire atmosphere is simple carbon soot, which is relatively nontoxic. Visible particles greater than 5 kμ have little chance of reaching the alveoli but can cause focal burns and erosions in the distal airway. Toxins can be absorbed by soot and adhere to airway mucosa, increasing local exposure. Excess soot can physically plug the bronchi when mixed with irritating exudates. Commonly, soot is cleared within the first 1 to 2 days.

Chemical Toxins

Injury to the tracheobronchial tree occurs primarily as a result of inhaled chemical irritants. Rubber and plastic items release ammonia, oxides of sulfur, and chlorine gases, when burned. Garments treated with flame retardants release dangerous pyrolysates. Water-soluble irritants, such as ammonia, chlorine, hydrogen chloride, and oxides of sulfur, incite immediate symptoms because they dissolve on the moist mucosa of the upper airway and form strong alkalis and acids.[29] The degree of conjunctivitis, rhinorrhea, bronchospasm, and cough parallels the intensity of exposure. Lipid-soluble materials, such as oxides of nitrogen, aromatics, aldehydes, and phosgene, can cause direct cellular injury, impair ciliary function, and activate alveolar macrophages.[30]

Chemical irritation initiates a tenfold increase in bronchial blood flow and increased vascular permeability, producing tracheobronchial mucosal edema. The inflammatory cascade is stimulated, and leukocytes are recruited. The injured epithelium is shed, and an inflammatory exudate is formed. The resulting debris narrows the airway caliber and increases the airway resistance. The lack of an intact epidermal barrier and impaired ciliary activity promotes the development of pneumonia.

When the pulmonary parenchyma is injured by inhalants, it responds nonspecifically with a delayed permeability pulmonary edema and decreased lung compliance. The synthesis of surfactant is transiently disrupted by the inflammatory reaction.[31] In the absence of overwhelming smoke inhalation, however, alveolar edema is uncommon during the early stages.

Treatment

Initial Evaluation and Emergency Department Care

An orderly approach to the emergency care of the burned child is essential. It is recommended that emergency medical technicians (EMTs) in the field and health care teams in emergency departments rehearse the necessary steps and post their treatment plans in conspicuous areas.

Treatment priorities begin with the basics: airway, breathing, and circulation (Table 104–1). Airway patency may be impaired by edema and loss of protective reflexes. Unconscious individuals require immediate intubation and supportive ventilation.

TABLE 104–1

"Mini" Physical, the ABCs

*A*irway	Ensure patency Determine the need for artificial airway
*B*reathing	Ensure adequate air exchange Ensure optimal oxygenation Rule out inhalation injury
*C*irculation	Assess capillary refill Evaluate central and peripheral pulses Evaluate the state of sensorium
*D*epth	Determine depth of the injuries Note circumferential burns and determine the need for escharotomies
*E*xtend	Map partial- and full-thickness burns Rule out other injuries to skeleton or CNS

CNS, Central nervous system.

Simultaneously with the evaluation of the respiratory status, cardiac hemodynamics must be assessed, and the patient should be inspected for unrecognized injuries (secondary survey). Central and peripheral pulses are palpated, and capillary refill (preferably in an unburned extremity) is assessed. Hypotension is a late finding and often indicative of severe volume depletion; when present it should be treated aggressively.

Because fluid and electrolyte deficits develop rapidly, they must be corrected expediently. Isotonic salt solutions must be started as soon as a large-bore intravenous (IV) or intraosseous line is established (18 to 16 gauge). Line placement should avoid burned tissues, but in patients with extensive burns, the options are limited and cutdowns or intraosseous lines through burned skin may be necessary.

As would be the case in children with other forms of shock, the initial approach to the burned child entails isotonic fluid administration at a rate of 20 ml/kg or 600 ml/m^2 of body surface per hour. If signs of hypovolemia persist, additional fluid boluses may be given until all signs of "intravascular dehydration" subside. A nasogastric tube is inserted and the stomach is emptied simultaneously to minimize the effects of acute gastric dilatation and to prevent vomiting or aspiration of stomach contents. This is recommended in all patients with burns exceeding 20% of the body surface. A urinary catheter to empty the bladder and monitor urine production is inserted routinely in all children with burns in excess of 20% of their body surface. As soon as a "fresh" urine sample can be obtained, a urinalysis should be performed.

Because fluid requirements are proportional to the age and size of the child, as well as to the extent of the injury, particular attention must be directed to measurements of weight, height, BSA, and surface area burned. Accurate weight should be obtained before the wounds are dressed and bed clothing or restraints are applied, and afterward as well. The wounds are then cleansed and debrided, and their depth and extent are assessed with body surface charts corrected for age (Table 104–2). The wounds should be inspected and mapped by two independent observers. The method of Lund and Browder is preferred.[32]

When the extent of the injury is estimated, only second- and third-degree burns are considered. Burns in excess of 60% are more accurately and conveniently mapped with estimation of the nonburned areas.

TABLE 104–2

Body Proportions Corrected for Age (%)

	Age		
Body Area	**1-4 y**	**5-9 y**	**10-14 y**
Head and neck	19	15	13
Anterior trunk	16	17	17
Posterior trunk	16	17	17
Right arm	9	9	9
Left arm	9	9	9
Right leg	15	16	17
Left leg	15	16	17

Modified from Lund CL, Browder NC: The estimation of areas of burns, *Surg Gynecol Obstet* 79:352, 1944.

Circumferential deep second- or third-degree burns must be evaluated, and their tourniquet effect must be recognized to avoid limb ischemia or respiratory embarrassment resulting from chest wall involvement. When indicated, escharotomies should be performed early because as edema worsens, blood supply to viable tissues is further compromised.

Fluid Resuscitation: First 24 Hours

The ultimate goal of fluid resuscitation is restoration of body homeostasis (Box 104–1). For this to be achieved, existing deficits of fluid, electrolytes, and protein must be replenished, and concurrent losses must be anticipated and replaced.

Because excessive quantities of fluids can be as detrimental to burned patients as insufficient resuscitation, great care must be exercised in estimating fluid needs and monitoring the results of fluid therapy.[33] For preexisting deficits to be estimated, the severity of dehydration

BOX 104–1

Objectives of Fluid Resuscitation

GENERAL

Replace existing deficits of fluid, electrolytes, and proteins
Replace concurrent losses
Minimize organ dysfunction and edema formation

SPECIFIC

Restore body homeostasis in all fluid compartments
Correct acid-base imbalance
Preserve and restore organ function
Optimize the delivery of oxygen and other nutrients to tissue beds:
- Promote spontaneous healing
- Prevent wound conversion
- Minimize wound colonization
- Prepare injured tissues for early grafting

must be assessed. This can be accomplished clinically (Table 104–3). Unless the patient is in frank shock, "fluid pushes" should be avoided, and rehydration should proceed without overloading the circulation and preferably over a period of 24 hours. Attempts to replace deficits over shorter periods of time are fraught with multiple complications (including excessive edema formation) and should be discouraged. Errors in fluid therapy may have great consequences during the first 24 hours. Underhydration can prolong the state of shock, worsen the metabolic acidosis, and induce organ dysfunction; overhydration fosters edema formation, paralytic ileus, and pulmonary congestion.

Restoration of fluid and electrolyte balance and organ function does not mean a return of all physiological variables to normal. Oliguria resulting from hormonal secretion may persist for 48 to 72 hours or even longer after the burn.[19,20] Cardiac output may increase beyond preburn levels within 24 hours of the injury, and the hypercatabolic state may last several days. Physicians should take into consideration not only the physiological makeup of the child, which differs significantly from that of the adult, but also the specific responses of the various organs to the burn injury.[34]

For the accurate prediction of fluid requirements, burn formulas must allow for burn-related fluid losses and maintenance fluids separately. Estimates of maintenance fluid requirements must take into consideration the child's high rates of heat and water exchange in relation to body weight and the proportionally larger insensible fluid losses and urine output of children as compared with adults. The use of BSA area rather than weight corrects for these differences and offers greater accuracy, consistency, and simplicity. The scheme that we have developed and used extensively for many years has the following key features:

Fluid Formula

Total fluid allowance for the first 24 hours is based on BSA and TBSA burned in square meters. BSA is calculated from standard nomograms, and the extent of the injury is estimated with body proportions corrected for age (see Table 104–2). TBSA (m^2) is calculated by multiplying the percentage of the burn (as per the method of Lund and Browder previously noted) times the BSA.

Total fluid requirements for the first day are estimated as follows:

$$2000\ \text{ml/m}^2\ \text{BSA/24 h}$$
$$+$$
$$5000\ \text{ml/m}^2\ \text{TBSA/24 h}$$

Half of the 24-hour fluid allowance is administered during the first 8 hours, and the other half is administered during the subsequent 16 hours (Fig. 104–1). Fluids given during transportation or initial resuscitation (first 1 to 2 hours) can be disregarded, and replacement of fluids may start anew when the burns have been properly mapped, the wounds are dressed, and all estimates have been completed.

No ceilings for burn size or body surface are used and, except as already noted, fluids are administered intravenously at a constant hourly rate. Ranitidine may be offered orally or intravenously, and except for ice chips, the patient remains NPO (nothing by mouth) for the first 24 hours.

Composition of Resuscitation Fluids

Our program uses an isotonic glucose-containing composite solution, to which we add 12.5 g of human serum albumin (HSA) per liter. This solution is used exclusively for the first 24 hours and in combination with an appropriate enteral formula during the second 24 hours (Fig. 104–1). The burn solution is prepared by mixing 950 ml of 5% dextrose in lactated Ringer's injection with 50 ml of 25% HSA (12.5 g). The final electrolyte and protein composition of the mixture is the following: sodium, 132 mEq/L; chloride, 109 mEq/L; lactate, 26.6 mEq/L; potassium, 3.8 mEq/L; glucose, 47.5 g/L; and albumin, 12.5 g/L.

In infants, the concentration of sodium in the hydrating solution must be lowered to prevent hypernatremia, otherwise a common occurrence. For children younger than 12 months, a modified solution can be prepared by mixing 930 ml of 5% dextrose in 0.33% sodium chloride injection, 20 ml of sodium bicarbonate injection (1 mEq/ml), and 50 ml of 25% HSA. The final composition of this mixture is the following: sodium, 81 mEq/L; chloride, 61 mEq/L; HCO_3^-, 20 mEq/L; glucose, 46.5 g/L; and albumin, 12.5 g/L.

Because injured cells release potassium into extracellular fluids, no potassium is added to hydrating solutions during the first 24 hours after the burn. Thereafter, 20 to 30 mEq of potassium phosphate may be added to each liter of IV fluids.

Plasma and urine glucose levels are monitored at frequent intervals. If intolerance develops, glucose is omitted from hydrating fluids.[35]

A major advantage of using a composite solution is that fluids, electrolytes, and albumin can be simultaneously replaced in quantities that approximate the patient's losses. The rate of infusion then becomes the only adjustment needed. Furthermore, the total 24-hour infusate can be prepared in advance and kept refrigerated. This method also avoids the so-called piggy backs and allows more accurate control of fluid intake.

Monitoring the Adequacy of Hydration

Monitoring the results of fluid therapy is a difficult task in the burned patient. The reason is that no single criterion can be used to predict the state of hydration, consistently or accurately, and many indicators must be correlated before a decision to increase or decrease the quantities of fluid to be administered is made. The hourly urine volume is not a good predictor because the kidneys are under the influence of exaggerated hormonal responses, which correlate poorly with the state of hydration. Also, common but not easily explained are marked fluctuations in hourly urine production. Intermittent release of ADH and rapid degradation of the hormone, as well as reflex mediated changes in renal hemodynamics, are plausible but unconfirmed explanations for this phenomenon.

Although none of the many variables used to guide hydration are consistently accurate, when several variables are correlated together and trends instead of individual measurements are used, the state of hydration can be more precisely ascertained (Box 104–2). The child's general

TABLE 104–3

Physical Findings in Acute Dehydration

Severity of Dehydration	Mucous Mem-branes	Skin Turgor	Fontanelle	Heart Rate	Urine Output	Sensorium	Respirations	Body Temper-ature	Tears	Eyes	Blood Pressure	Peripheral Circulation
Mild (3%-5% acute weight loss)	*Dry	*Decreased	N	N	N	N	N	N	N	N	N	N
Moderate (6%-10% acute weight loss)	Dry	*Decreased	*Sunken	*Tachycardia	*Oliguria	*Lethargy	*Tachypnea	*Fever	N	N	N	N
Severe (11%-15% acute weight loss)	Parched	Poor	Sunken	Tachycardia	*Periods of anuria (6-12 h)	*Stupor and irritability	*Deep and pauseless (Kussmaul's respiration)	*Fever	*Absent	*Sunken	*Hypo-tension	*Decreased perfusion
Extreme (>15% acute weight loss)	Parched	Poor	Sunken	Rapid and thready pulse	Anuria for >12 h	*Coma moribund	*Slow and shallow	Fever or *hypo-thermia	Absent	Sunken	Shock	Mottling and cyanosis

*Overlapping signs and symptoms.

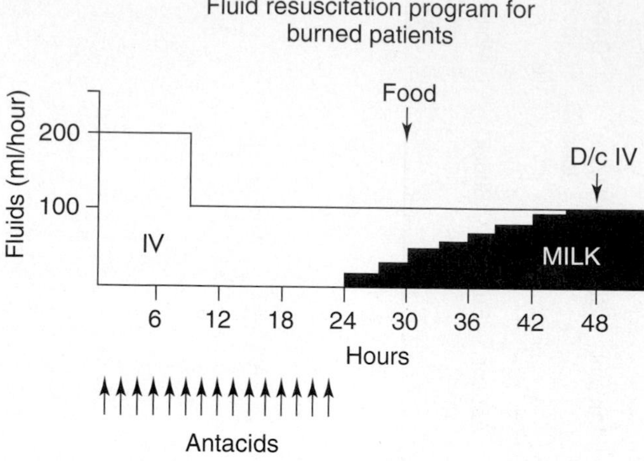

FIGURE 104–1 • Rate of fluid administration for the first 48 hours. Notice that fluids are given at a constant rate. On the second day, intravenous fluids are proportionally decreased as enteral feedings are progressively increased.

(From Carvajal HF: A physiologic approach to fluid therapy in severely burned children. *Surg Gynecol Obst* 150:379, 1980)

appearance and sensorium provide valuable information regarding fluid balance. For example, a conscious and alert child who is responsive to commands is usually well hydrated; the lethargic, thirsty, and anxious patient with decreased capillary filling or evidence of peripheral vascular insufficiency (cold, dry, discolored, and mottled skin) is obviously dehydrated. A rapid, thready pulse and a high respiratory rate would also be indicative of volume contraction. Although the mean arterial pressure does not change until the intravascular volume deficits exceed 11% to 12% of normal, a decreased pulse pressure may be seen during

BOX 104–2

Hydration Guides

PHYSICAL EXAMINATION

General appearance
Vital signs
Sensorium
Venous capillary filling
Weight
Urine output*

LABORATORY

Hematocrit (Hct)
Blood urea nitrogen (BUN)
Electrolytes and osmolality (serum and urine)
Arterial blood gases (ABGs)

INVASIVE MONITORING†

Cardiac output (CO)
Pulmonary capillary wedge pressure (PCWP)
Oxygen consumption (V_{O_2})
Oxygen extraction (O_2 ext)
Mixed venous oxygen saturation (Sv_{O_2})

*Expect marked fluctuations (15 to 45 ml/m²/h).
†Rarely necessary.

the early stages of dehydration. In the absence of renal failure, a moderate increase in blood urea nitrogen (BUN) indicates a reduction in renal blood flow and glomerular filtration rate (prerenal azotemia). A hypercatabolic state may be differentiated from renal insufficiency with measurement of urine urea nitrogen (UUN), urine and plasma osmolality, and urine electrolytes. In the presence of oliguria, a urinary sodium (UNa) level in excess of 30 mEq/L, coupled with isostenuria (urine osmolality ~ 300 mOsm/L and a UUN/BUN ratio of < 10) would suggest acute renal failure. A prerenal state would manifest itself by a low UNa level, a high urine osmolality, and a UUN/BUN ratio in excess of 20 (see also Chapter 62).

A rising hematocrit resulting from fluid, electrolyte, and protein losses and hemoconcentration are commonly seen during the immediate postburn period. As the intravascular volume is restored, the hematocrit progressively declines. Failure to demonstrate this change indicates persistent volume deficit.[33]

Certain variables can be misleading. For example, a rising specific gravity or urine osmolality may indicate secretion of ADH, but not necessarily volume contraction. If present, the latter can be confirmed with documentation of sodium retention (UNa <20 mEq/L).

Subsequent Fluid, Electrolyte, and Protein Replacement

By the end of the first 24 hours, most burned patients are hemodynamically stable and ready to begin enteral nutrition. In general, patients with serum albumin levels greater than 2 g/dl and colloid osmotic pressures (COPs) in excess of 15 mmHg can tolerate oral feedings beginning the second day. By the end of the first day, capillary permeability has been restored, and abnormal fluid losses are limited to exudative and evaporative losses. These correspond to approximately three fourths of the first day's requirements. Thus the quantity of fluids to be administered on the second and subsequent days may be estimated as follows:

$$1500 \text{ ml/m}^2 \text{ BSA/24 h} \\ + \\ 3750 \text{ m/m}^2 \text{ TBSA/24 h}$$

Evaporative fluid losses are electrolyte free, and they represent the major source of fluid loss beyond the first day. Sodium requirements at this time are markedly curtailed. Replacement of sodium losses can be easily accomplished with oral or IV solutions with concentrations of sodium of 50 mEq/L. Infants younger than 1 year require lower concentrations of sodium, usually in the range of 30 to 40 mEq/L. Because most enteral formulas have sodium concentrations below 30 mEq/L, supplementation of sodium is usually necessary.

Potassium losses during the first 24 hours and during the diuretic phase (third to fourteenth postburn days) may lead to significant total body potassium deficits. In the absence of renal dysfunction, major deficits can be averted by allowing 35 to 40 mEq of potassium for every liter of IV or enteral solutions. Potassium phosphate instead of potassium chloride is preferred because it allows the preparation of a more physiological fluid mixture (sodium/chloride ratio of 3:2), while simultaneously replacing exaggerated phosphate losses.

It should be possible to routinely start a suitable enteral formula by the twenty-fifth postburn hour. As the oral intake is increased, IV fluids (composite burn solution) are decreased so that the hourly fluid intake remains constant. In most cases, a soft diet is tolerated by the second to third day.

Topical Antimicrobial Therapy

Once the extent and depth of the injury are assessed, the wounds are covered with one layer of fine mesh gauze saturated with silver sulfadiazine in 1% soluble cream base. Precut elastic net is used to hold the impregnated gauze in place. The *in vitro* antimicrobial spectrum of silver sulfadiazine includes *Staphylococcus aureus*, *Enterobacteriaceae*, *Escherichia coli*, and *Candida albicans*. Its poor absorption through denuded skin, along with its low toxicity and wide antimicrobial spectrum, have made silver sulfadiazine the topical agent of choice for burned patients.[26] Used prophylactically on a once- or twice-daily basis, this agent can delay wound colonization by gram-negative bacilli for 10 to 14 days in extensive burns. After 2 weeks, the wounds invariably become colonized in moderate density. The addition of cerium nitrate to silver sulfadiazine has improved the *in vitro* antibacterial activity against gram-negative organisms, but a significant clinical advantage over silver sulfadiazine alone has not been demonstrated.[38]

Another useful topical agent that forms part of the burn armamentarium is 0.5% silver nitrate solution. Although an effective antimicrobial, silver nitrate is not popular because it stains bed clothing, equipment, and physical facilities and discolors the burn wounds, making them difficult to assess.[37]

Gentamicin or tobramycin cream is a suitable alternative for patients with superinfected wounds or allergies to sulfa preparations. Mafenide acetate, a methylated sulfonamide available commercially as a 10% preparation in a water-miscible hygroscopic cream base, has antibacterial activity against gram-positive and gram-negative organisms but limited antifungal activity. Mafenide acetate is limited by the fact that it is rapidly absorbed from the wounds and therapeutic wound concentrations are difficult to maintain. The drug is a strong carbonic anhydrase inhibitor, and metabolic acidosis commonly develops. Deaths from secondary pulmonary failure have been reported.

Management of the Burn Wounds

One of the most significant advances in burn care that has precipitously decreased morbidity and death is early excision and closure of the burn wound.[39] Partial excision of the burn wound had been attempted during the early 1960s, but it had met with only limited success. During the 1980s improvements in fluid resuscitation and infection control and better support of the hypercatabolic response made burn excision plausible. Renewed interest and research in the subject, together with the application of newer surgical techniques, made all the difference. Currently, serial wound excision and grafting represents the standard of care for the management of full-thickness injuries.[40] When the burn area exceeds the donor site supply, the wound can be covered with homograft allograft or skin substitutes. Total wound excision and grafting performed within 24 to 48 hours of the injury has also been advocated by many but has yet to receive widespread acceptance. The reason is that potentially viable tissue is usually sacrificed with this technique. In some centers, however, improved survival with total excision and grafting has been achieved.

Sedation and Pain Control

During the immediate postburn period, the pain associated with superficial and deep partial-thickness injuries can be ameliorated with the placement of a cover over the wounds and the reduction of exposure to air currents. The application of gauze impregnated with a topical antimicrobial has an analgesic effect and is soothing to the child. We routinely administer one or two doses of IV morphine during the first 2 to 3 hours after injury but withhold subsequent doses until the effect of dressing of the wounds is fully appreciated and a clear-cut indication for additional analgesics is demonstrated.

In patients with extensive burns or burns about the face or upper extremities, pain is often intensified by fear and anxiety. Under these circumstances, the drugs of choice are the benzodiazepines. Midazolam or lorazepam may be given intravenously every 3 to 4 hours to minimize anxiety and facilitate pain control.

Morphine or fentanyl citrate may be used alone or in combination with benzodiazepines to control pain and anxiety associated with dressing changes, hydrotherapy, debridement, escharotomies, or other painful procedures.[41] Patients requiring mechanical ventilatory support are best managed with light to moderate sedation with fentanyl because this drug can be rapidly reversed with naloxone. Nonnarcotic analgesics such as ketorolac may be used as well in between dressing changes.[41]

Ketamine, a "dissociative" anesthetic, has been used to provide short periods of anesthesia during hydrotherapy and dressing changes. Although adequate analgesia can be attained with low doses (0.2 to 0.3 mg/kg), hypertension, myocardial depression, and other cardiovascular and neurological sequelae have limited its widespread use.[42]

Nutritional Requirements

Most patients who sustain burn injuries are well nourished before the insult, but unless an aggressive nutritional program is instituted from the onset, upper catabolism rapidly leads to a state of protein-calorie malnutrition.[43]

Measurements of actual calorie needs by direct or indirect calorimetry are fraught with considerable difficulties, and despite monumental efforts, currently available equipment and methods do not permit accurate measurements of caloric expenditure in the spontaneously breathing patient.[44,45] Extrapolation from adult norms may not be appropriate because the available formulas are based on body weight[46] and caloric requirements are considerably greater in children. A "two figure" formula that takes into account BSA and the size of the burn was first proposed by Hildreth and Carvajal in 1980.[47] In children with burns in the range of 15% to 90% adherence to the formula has resulted in adequate weight gain and no evidence of malnutrition.

Caloric requirements for burned children are thus estimated as follows:

Maintenance requirements: 1800 kcal/m^2 of BSA/day
+
Burn requirements: 2200 kcal/m^2 of TBSA/day

A liquid diet with a caloric density not to exceed 27 calories per ounce plus regular food consumption has allowed 18% to 22% of the calories to be derived from proteins; 15% to 20% from fat; and the rest from carbohydrate. Vitamins and minerals are provided as recommended by the Committee on Dietary Allowances.[48] Unless a deficiency is documented, supplements should not exceed established guidelines for healthy individuals.

Optimal management beyond the second postburn day includes maintenance of fluid and electrolyte balance; albumin replacement to maintain COP levels above 15 mmHg; adequate nutrition to support the enhanced metabolic demands; daily irrigation and debridement of the wounds; topical antimicrobial therapy; splinting of affected parts; and various other surgical procedures. Anemia resulting from bone marrow depression, hemolysis, and oozing of blood from the wound sites must be detected and appropriately corrected. Except in the actively bleeding patient, packed red blood cells in quantities of 10 ml/kg are usually sufficient. With a "split" packed red blood cell approach, small children will be exposed to fewer donors. Mild anemia down to levels of 8.5 g of Hb is usually well tolerated, and unless the patient is anticipating a surgical intervention, may not need immediate correction.

Inhalation Injury

For an accurate prediction of morbidity and death associated with inhalation injuries, the following three factors must be assessed:

1. The degree of asphyxial injury (local hypoxemia, CO, and cyanide poisoning)
2. The degree of thermal injury to the upper airway
3. The degree of exposure and the type of inhaled chemical irritants

The complex interaction of these factors makes predicting those children who will have respiratory tract injury an inexact science. Most clinical scoring systems predict thermal or smoke exposure by tabulating various historical and clinical parameters present at the time of the initial examination, but they fail to gauge the degree of potential injury or provide a graded prognosis. A notable exception is the scoring system proposed by Clark et al,[51] which takes into account age and burn size, and has been shown to be highly accurate in predicting subsequent death.

Chest radiographs, electrocardiograms, arterial blood gases, and CO oximetry cannot differentiate reliably between exposure to smoke and true injury, although they may be helpful in evaluating asphyxial injury. Likewise, HbCO levels are not reliable when the patient has received oxygen before blood sampling.

Thermal and chemical injury to the upper airway can be assessed with direct laryngoscopy or fiberoptic laryngotracheoscopy.[52] Spirometry and flow-volume measurements of airflow can provide objective documentation of progressive airway edema.[53] These techniques are more valuable when performed serially during the first 24 to 48 hours, but they may be inaccurate in the presence of hypovolemia. Furthermore, they require a level of cooperation not often found in a burned, frightened child.

Injury to the smaller airways and pulmonary parenchyma can be detected with a xenon-133 scintiphotogram.[49,50] Delayed clearance of the ^{33}Xe from the lung or segmental retention indicates inhalation injury or small airway dysfunction. Serum immunoreactive calcitonin released from injured pulmonary neuroendocrine cells has been proposed as an accurate marker of pulmonary injury.[54]

The site of injury can also be approximated from the time of onset of symptoms. Immediate decompensation results from severe asphyxia due to environmental hypoxemia, unconsciousness, airway obstruction, and CO or hydrogen cyanide poisoning. In the absence of cutaneous burns, cyanide toxicity should be suspected when the patient fails to respond to oxygen therapy and the mental status remains clouded.

Deterioration during the first 12 hours is usually the result of progressive upper airway edema or bronchospasm. After 24 hours, further airway obstruction from bronchorrhea and mucosal shedding is evident, and fluid shifts and noncardiogenic pulmonary edema develop. Late decompensation (after 72 hours) results from secondary pneumonia; pulmonary emboli; or, rarely, bronchiolitis obliterans.

Supplemental oxygen should be administered to all victims of fires. Inhaled oxygen immediately begins to displace CO from HbCO. The half-life of HbCO can be decreased from 4 to 6 hours in room air to 40 to 60 minutes while the patient is breathing 100% oxygen at high flows.[10] Oxygen therapy should be continued until the concentration of HbCO is less than 15%, metabolic acidosis is corrected, and alterations in consciousness resolve.[55]

Hyperbaric oxygen (HBO) therapy at 2 to 3 atm can further reduce the half-life of HbCO to less than 30 minutes. HBO has the advantages of increasing dissolved molecular oxygen (O_2) availability to tissues and competitively displacing CO bound to mitochondrial cytochromes. Whether this approach changes the overall incidence of delayed neurological deterioration or late demyelination syndrome remains to be evaluated.[52] Delays in transport and initiation of treatment (averaging 4.5 to 7 hours),[52,53] patient instability, and lack of patient access make routine use of HBO therapy logistically difficult.

Thermal injury to the upper airway is best managed by elective early nasotracheal intubation. This is particularly true when patients have circumferential burns of the neck or lips, intraoral burns, swelling, stridor, or vocal cord dysfunction. Oral endotracheal (ET) tubes, while easier to place initially, are difficult to maintain in position. Primary tracheostomies, especially through burn tissue, are associated with many complications and increased risk of sepsis. Their use should be restricted to patients in whom ET intubation is impossible or those in whom timely extubation fails. Elevation of the head of the bed and methodical meticulous pulmonary toilet are particularly important because of mucosal shedding and increased risk of ET tube plugging and obstruction. Although significant swelling of the airways resolves within 2 to 6 days, vocal cord dysfunction may persist for 3 to 4 weeks.[52]

Although most tracheobronchial injuries related to heat and smoke are self-limited and resolve within 48 to 72 hours, full repair of the mucosa is delayed for 1 to 2 weeks. Supportive care, including adequate humidification and pulmonary toilet, is the hallmark of therapy. Mucorrhea and viscous intraluminal debris may cause airway obstruction at 48 to 72 hours. This may be prevented with mucolytics or repeated bronchial lavage. Bronchodilators occasionally improve airflow, but often the obstruction is purely mechanical. Intubation is occasionally necessary to manage secretions and maintain the patency of the tracheobronchial lumen.

Direct injury to the pulmonary parenchyma is infrequent and varies in severity. Treatment is nonspecific and may include supplemental O_2, positive pressure support (continuous positive airway pressure/positive end-expiratory pressure [CPAP/PEEP]), mechanical ventilatory support, pulmonary toilet, and judicious use of fluids. Bronchiolar lavage is of questionable efficacy once the injury cascade is triggered. Steroids have been shown to increase the risk of death from 13% to 53% and infectious complications from 31% to 82%.[55] Thus in the burn patient with inhalation injury, their use is proscribed.

REFERENCES

1. Scherer LR III: Critical care of the severely injured child, *Surg Clin North Am* 82:333-347, 2002.
2. Moritz AR, Henrique FC Jr.: Studies of thermal injury: the relative importance of time and surface temperature in the causation of cutaneous burns, *Am J Pathol* 23:695, 1947.
3. Jackson DM: The diagnosis of the depth of burning, *Br J Surg* 40:588, 1953.
4. Order SE, Moncrief JA: *The burn wound*, Springfield, IL, 1965, Charles C Thomas.
5. Hinshaw JR: Early changes in the depth of burns, *Ann N Y Acad Sci* 150:548, 1968.
6. Sevitt S: Inflammatory changes in burned skin: reversible and irreversible effects and their pathogenesis. In Sevitt S, editor: *Burns, pathology and therapeutic implications*, London, 1957, Butterworth & Co.
7. Koumbourlis AC: Electrical injuries, *Crit Care Med* 30:1, 2002.
8. Fozzard HA: Myocardial injury in burn shock, *Ann Surg* 154:113, 1961.
9. Michie DD, Goldsmith RS, Mason AD et al: Hemodynamics of the immediate postburn period, *J Trauma* 3:111, 1973.
10. Arturson G: Metabolic changes and nutrition in children with severe burns, *Prog Pediatr Surg* 14:81, 1981.
11. Turner R, Carvajal HF, Traber DL: Effects of ganglionic blockage upon the renal and cardiovascular dysfunction induced by thermal injury, *Circ Shock* 4:103, 1977.
12. Baxter CR, Moncrief JA, Prager MH et al: A circulating myocardial depression factor in burn shock. In Matter P, Barclay TL, Konickova Z, editors: *Research in burns. Transactions of the third International Congress in Research in Burns, Prague*, Bern, 1971, Hans Huber Publishers.
13. Carvajal HF, Linares HA: Effect of burn depth upon edema formation and albumin extravasation in rats, *Burns* 7:79, 1980.
14. Brouhard BH, Carvajal HF, Linares HA: Burn edema and protein leakage in the rat: 1. Relationship to time of injury, *Microvasc Res* 15:221, 1978.
15. Carvajal HF, Linares HA, Brouhard BH: Relationship of burn size to vascular permeability changes in rats, *Surg Gynecol Obstet* 149:193, 1979.
16. Lamke LO, Nilsson GE, Reithner HL: The evaporation water loss from burns and the water vapor permeability of grafts and artificial membranes used in the treatment of burns, *Burns* 3:159, 1977.
17. Cuthbertson DP: Observation on the disturbance of metabolism produced by injury to the limbs, *Q J Med* 25:233, 1932.
18. Weise K, Zaritsky A: Endocrine manifestations of critical illness in the child, *Pediatr Clin North Am* 34:119, 1987.
19. Carvajal HF: A physiologic approach to fluid therapy in severely burned children, *Surg Gynecol Obstet* 150:379, 1980.
20. Carvajal HF, Parks DH: Optimal composition of burn resuscitation fluids, *Crit Care Med* 16:695, 1988.
21. Souba WW, Smith RJ, Wilmore DW: Effects of glucocorticoids on glutamine metabolism in visceral organs, *Metabolism* 34:450, 1985.
22. Thompson PB, Herndon DN, Traber DL et al: Effect on mortality of inhalation injury, *J Trauma* 26:163, 1986.
23. Rossignol AM, Boyle CM, Locke JA et al: Hospitalized burn injuries in Massachusetts: an assessment of incidence and product involvement, *Am J Public Health* 76:1341, 1986.
24. Feller I, Jones CA, James MH: Burn epidemiology: focus on youngsters and the aged, *J Burn Care Rehabil* 3:285, 1982.
25. Peterson JE, Stewart RD: Absorption and elimination of carbon monoxide by young men, *Arch Environ Health* 21:165, 1970.
26. Pruitt BA, Erickson DR, Morris A: Progressive pulmonary in sufficiency and other pulmonary complications of thermal injury, *Trauma* 15:369, 1975.
27. Moritz AR, Henriques FC, McLean R: The effects of inhaled scat on the air passages and lungs, *Am J Pathol* 21:311, 1945.
28. Kramer GC, Herndon DN, Linares HA et al: Effects of inhalation on airway blood flow and edema formation, *J Burn Care Rehabil* 10:45, 1989.
29. Dyer RF, Esch VH: Polyvinyl chloride toxicity in fires: Hydrogen chloride toxicity in fire fighters, *JAMA* 235:393, 1976.
30. Miller K, Chang A: Acute inhalation injury, *Emerg Med Clin North Am* 21:533-557, 2003.
31. Nieman GF, Clark WR, Wax SD et al: The effect of smoke inhalation on pulmonary surfactant, *Ann Surg* 191:171, 1980.
32. Lund CL, Browder NC: The estimation of areas of burns, *Surg Gynecol Obstet* 79:352, 1944.
33. Carvajal HF: Resuscitation of the burned child. In Carvajal HF, Parks DH, editors: *Burns in children*, Chicago, 1988, Year Book Medical Publishers.
34. Metcoff J, Buchman H, Jacobson M et al: Losses and physiologic requirements for water and electrolyte after extensive burns in children, *N Engl J Med* 265:101, 1961.
35. Carvajal HF: A psychological approach to fluid therapy in severely burned children, *Surg Gynecol Obstet* 150:379, 1980.
36. Carvajal HF: Acute management of severely burned patients, *ER Rep* 1:45, 1980.
37. Monafo WW, Auyazaian WH: Topical therapy, *Surg Clin North Am* 58:1157, 1978.
38. Kaye ET: Topical antibacterial agents, *Infect Dis Clin North Am* 14:321-339, 2000.
39. Hansbrough JF, Hansbrough W: Pediatric burns, *Pediatr Rev* 20:117-123, 1999.
40. Heimbach D: What's new in general surgery: burns and metabolism, *J Am Coll Surg* 194:156, 2002.
41. Henry DB, Foster RL: Burn pain management in children, *Pediatr Clinic North Am* 47: 681-698, 2000.
42. Stoddard FJ: Treatment of pain in acutely burned children, *J Burn Care Rehabil* 23:135, 2002.
43. Souba WW, Schindler BA, Carvajal HF: Nutrition and metabolism. In Carvajal HF, Parks DH, editors: *Burns in children*, Chicago, 1988, Year Book Medical Publishers.
44. Weissman C, Damask MC, Askanazi J et al: Evaluation of a noninvasive method for the measurement of metabolic rate in humans, *Chin Sci* (Lond) 69:135, 1985.
45. Daly JM, Heymsfield SB, Head CA et al: Human energy requirements: overstimulation by widely used prediction equation, *Am J Clin Nutr* 42:1170, 1985.
46. Curreri PW: Supportive therapy in burn care. Nutritional replacement modalities, *J Trauma* 19(suppl 11):906, 1979.
47. Hildreth M, Carvajal HF: Caloric requirements in burned children. A simple formula to estimate daily caloric requirements, *J Burn Care Rehabil* 3:78, 1980.
48. Committee on Dietary Allowances: *Recommended dietary allowances*, ed 9, Washington DC, 1980, National Academy of Science.
49. Peirce EC: A registry for carbon monoxide poisoning in New York City, *Clin Toxicol* 26:419, 1988.

50. Agee RN, Long JM, Hunt JL et al: Use of xenon in early diagnosis of inhalation injury, *J Trauma* 16:218, 1976.
51. Clark CJ, Reid WH, Gilmour WH et al: Mortality probability in victims of fire trauma: revised equation to include inhalation injury, *Br Med J* 292:1303, 1986.
52. Hunt JL, Agee RN, Pruitt BA: Fiberoptic bronchoscopy in acute inhalation injury, *J Trauma* 15:641, 1975.
53. Haponik EF, Meyers DA, Munster AM et al: Acute upper airway injury in burn patients. Serial changes of flow-volume curves and nasopharyngoscopy, *Am Rev Respir Dis* 135:360, 1987.
54. Skolnick A: Medical news and perspectives—calcitonin assays may help identify burn patients at risk for respiratory distress, *JAMA* 264:565, 1990.
55. Rabinowitz PM, Siegel MD: Acute inhalation injury, *Clin Chest Med* 23:707-715, 2002.

PART

IV

TRAUMA

CHAPTER

105

Evaluation, Stabilization, and Initial Management after Multiple Trauma

Stanley T. Lau and Guy F. Brisseau

PEARLS

- Children are vulnerable to major abdominal injuries resulting from relatively minor forces. Motor vehicle injuries are the leading cause of death in children. The most common bicycle-related injury is head trauma.
- In children who die soon after injury, the primary mechanisms that cause death are airway compromise, hypovolemic shock, and central nervous system damage.
- The primary survey is always the first step in the care of the injured child. This is a quick survey to assess and treat immediate life-threatening injuries. This is often referred to by the mnemonic ABCDE (Airway, Breathing, Circulation, Disability, Exposure).
- After the primary survey is completed and before the secondary survey is started there is an opportunity to ensure that all of additional monitoring and adjunct testing has been done on the patient.
- The secondary survey is the point in the assessment at which the complete history is obtained and a physical examination takes place.

Background

Pediatric trauma remains one of the major sources of morbidity and death in children, with injury accounting for most deaths among children older than 1 year. In fact, injury exceeds all other causes of death in children combined. Each year, approximately 20,000 children and teenagers die as a result of injury, with 65% of all injury deaths in children younger than 19 years resulting from unintentional injury. Furthermore, for each child who dies of trauma, 40 other children are hospitalized, and 1120 are treated in emergency departments. In other words, each year in the United States more than 20 million children require medical attention for traumatic injury.

Most pediatric trauma involves blunt injury, with penetrating injuries accounting for only a small percentage of patients. Compared with adults, children are more vulnerable to major abdominal injuries resulting from relatively minor forces. Children have a more immature musculoskeletal system than adults, affording them less protection from external forces. Furthermore, because a child's intraabdominal organs are proportionally larger and closer together compared with those in adults, children are predisposed to multiple organ injury.[1,2]

Motor vehicle injuries are the leading cause of death in children. In 2002, 1543 children younger than 15 years were killed in the United States as a result of motor vehicle crashes, and approximately 227,000 were injured.[3] Half of the children who were killed in these motor vehicle crashes were unrestrained. A driver under the influence of alcohol was involved in 25% of the fatal injuries, with more than two thirds of these children riding in the car of the drunk driver.[4] Other mechanisms of injury are common in children. Pedestrian injuries are the leading cause of death in children ages 5 to 9 years, and bicycle injuries are also common as the children's ages increase.[5] The most common bicycle-related injury is head trauma.[6]

The physiologic differences between a child and an adult lead to different injury patterns because of the different biomechanics of a child's body. A child's head is proportionally larger when compared with the size of an adult's head. This leads to greater inertia, movement, and transfer of energy to the head and brain leading to a higher percentage of head injuries in children. There is less soft tissue and muscle, so a greater amount of energy is transferred to the internal organs. A child's center of gravity is also much higher than an adult's. An infant has a center of gravity slightly above the umbilicus; at age 1 year, it is at the umbilicus. It continues to descend until it is closer to the pubic symphysis in the adult. If a child is restrained in a two-point lap belt in a car, the center of gravity is still above the point of restraint, causing a jackknife effect during a forward collision and often leading to intestinal and spinal cord injuries.

In children who die soon after injury, the primary mechanisms that cause death are airway compromise, hypovolemic shock, and central nervous system (CNS) damage. Rapid evaluation and management of these children will decrease the chance of death and morbidity. Multiple algorithms have been developed to aid in the evaluation and management of the patient with trauma. The most widely recognized system used in North America is the Advanced Trauma Life Support (ATLS) program of the American College of Surgeons. The core of ATLS is a systematic approach to the care of the patient with trauma.[7] Although it is not the only system to exist, it allows trauma care providers to speak the same language and understand the process of care of the patient. We think that all providers of care to the child with trauma should be knowledgeable in the principles of ATLS.

The Big Picture

In the trauma center a rapid sequence of events occurs to rapidly assess, resuscitate, and definitively manage the patient. A logical order of events should be followed to first address the most life-threatening conditions and then move on to the next problem (Table 105–1). In a trauma center with a dedicated trauma team, many of the tasks that involve, for example, monitors, blood work, and tubes can happen simultaneously; however, addressing issues in an orderly manner before moving on is important. This sequence is not linear because patients can change rapidly and new circumstances, such as new airway insufficiency, may require that previously screened conditions be readdressed. The trauma team leader (TTL) does not necessarily need to be a surgeon, but he or she must be versed in the assessment and care of the child with trauma. The TTL must take responsibility for the patient from the time of entry into the trauma hospital or system until the ultimate disposition in the operating room or other definitive care site. Although each patient is unique, attempts should be made to facilitate and expedite the care of the patient, limiting the time in the trauma suite to less than 30 minutes. Other members of the trauma team include trauma nurses, surgeons, anesthesiologists, and intensivists. Each institution will individualize its trauma team on the basis of local needs and expertise. In centers that are less experienced with pediatric patients, a Broselow Pediatric Emergency Tape can be used to guide the size of tubes and doses of drugs.[7]

TABLE 105–1

Steps in a Trauma Evaluation
Primary survey
Adjuncts to primary survey
Secondary survey
Adjuncts to secondary survey (investigations)
Definitive management

The Primary Assessment

The primary assessment is always the first step in the care of the injured child. This is a quick survey to assess and treat immediate life-threatening injuries. It is often referred to by the mnemonic ABCDE.

Airway (A)

Without an airway, there is no chance for survival. Airway management in children is hampered by their anatomy. Compared with adults, children have a proportionally larger head and occiput. When children are supine, the head often bends forward and impinges on the posterior pharynx. This becomes particularly important because most injured children are placed on a conventional spine board in a cervical collar. The problem is addressed with the placement of one or more blankets on the spine board under the child's torso, allowing the child to go into the sniffing position. Specially designed pediatric spine boards have been developed to avoid this problem.

Maintaining the pediatric airway requires expertise in assessment and management. The relatively large oropharyngeal soft tissue makes visualization difficult. This is especially true when in-line cervical spine stabilization must be maintained. The short trachea in the pediatric patient leads to a greater incidence of main stem intubations. Oral pharyngeal tubes should not be used unless the patient is unconscious. A chin lift or jaw thrust with oral suctioning is often adequate to improve a partially obstructed airway. In the unconscious patient, once the airway is established, adequate oxygenation should be ensured before mechanical methods such as endotracheal intubation are used to further secure the airway. Orotracheal intubation under direct visualization is the preferred method of establishing an airway in the child with trauma. In-line stabilization of the cervical spine by an experienced assistant is imperative during this procedure. Nasotracheal intubation in children older than 9 years may be possible but is not preferred because the method requires blind intubation with potential damage to the cranial vault, nasopharynx, and oropharynx.

Some patients require sedation for adequate intubation. The choice of medication must have as little effect on the circulatory system as possible. With respect to sedation during intubation, all patients should be managed as if they are hypovolemic because sedation can often make a patient hypotensive because of unappreciated hypovolemia. The current ATLS recommendations include etomidate or midazolam for sedation. Cricoid pressure is recommended, and succinylcholine is used for paralysis if determined to be necessary and safe.[7]

Sometimes establishment of an airway is impossible because of anatomy or facial trauma. In this rare instance, a surgical airway is indicated. In children, the preferred method of establishing a surgical airway is a needle cricothyroidotomy. This jet ventilation system will temporarily secure the airway, allowing oxygenation but inadequate ventilation. A more definitive airway can follow quickly under more controlled settings. In children younger than 12 years, the cricoid cartilage is the main support structure to the airway. A surgical cricothyroidotomy is rarely indicated in children and, given the anatomy, should only be performed in children older than 12 years. In younger children, a formal tracheostomy is necessary, and the temporizing needle cricothyroidotomy will allow time to establish the definitive airway establishment.

Breathing and Ventilation (B)

Once the airway is established, the next step in the algorithm is to assess the breathing. Hypoxia remains the most common cause of pediatric cardiac arrests in trauma. Breathing and ventilation are assessed by inspection, percussion, and auscultation. Supplemental oxygen should be given to most patients with trauma. A chest radiograph will follow after a completed primary survey. As a quick assessment, if the child is screaming and pink, then the ventilation is fine; however, tachypnea, cyanosis, and decreased oxygen saturation can be indicators of ventilation difficulties. On auscultation, decreased air entry can be from a pneumothorax, which will be tympanitic on percussion, or a hemothorax, which will be dull on percussion. One pitfall that must be avoided is a mainstem intubation, which can lead to decreased air entry on the contralateral side, typically left.

A simple pneumothorax generally requires a chest tube placed in the anterior-mid axillary line at the fifth intercostal space. A tension pneumothorax is a clinical diagnosis and should be treated without an x-ray film. Signs include decreased air entry, altered hemodynamic status, and a shift in the midline of the trachea at the sternal notch. The ability to see distended neck veins is often limited by the cervical collar. A tension pneumothorax needs immediate decompression with a large bore catheter (Angiocath) (14 or 16 gauge) placed over the second rib in the midclavicular line. The air is released, converting a tension pneumothorax to an open pneumothorax. A standard chest tube can then be placed in a controlled fashion. In the setting of hemodynamic instability and decrease air entry, one should not hesitate to do this lifesaving maneuver. In patients with a traumatic open pneumothorax a chest tube can often be placed through the defect saving another incision.

A hemothorax is also treated with a chest tube. Most injuries are self-limited and do not need a thoracotomy. Large amounts of initial blood (one-third blood volume), ongoing bleeding (3 ml/kg/h for 2 to 4 hours), or both, however, are harbingers of a surgical source of bleeding.

Circulation (C)

Once airway and breathing are established the next life-threatening condition is shock. Pediatric patients have increased cardiovascular reserve and are able to maintain their physiologic status until they have lost at least 30% of their blood volume. In the trauma center, circulation is primarily assessed with the cardiovascular values (heart rate, blood pressure, and palpable pulses). Skin color, capillary refill, urine output, and CNS responses are useful adjuncts to aid in the assessment. Given the changes in cardiovascular norms with age, the clinician must be facile at interpreting the physiologic measurements at all ages. *Mild shock* is defined as less than 30% blood volume loss and manifests with tachycardia, normal blood pressure, and a decreased capillary refill. *Moderate shock* is defined as a 30% to 45% blood volume loss and presents with a marked tachycardia, little change in the blood pressure, lethargy, and cyanotic extremities. Severe shock greater than 45% blood volume loss will show hypotension, little CNS activity, and pale cold skin. Realizing that pediatric patients will protect their blood pressure until the end is important; hypotension is a worrisome sign that needs aggressive resuscitation.

Treatment of shock involves controlling ongoing hemorrhage and fluid administration. Controlling hemorrhage can be as simple as direct pressure to a bleeding laceration. Tourniquets are rarely required for extremity bleeding. Blind clamping of vessels in the wound should be avoided. Treatment to limit the bleeding from other specific causes can be addressed in the trauma center. These include splinting bilateral femur fractures and closing the volume of an open book pelvis fracture with an external fixator or a blanket.

Along with controlling ongoing loss, fluid resuscitation should be initiated. Fluid resuscitation in the pediatric patient is based on that of the adult, but there may be additional venous access problems. An algorithm of resuscitation is shown in Figure 105–1. A bolus of 20 cc/kg with crystalloid is started, and volume status is reassessed. This is repeated one to two times if necessary. After the repeat bolus of crystalloid, consideration should be given to packed red blood cell (PRBC) transfusion. This is ordered as cross-matched, type-specific, or O-negative blood. The dose is 10 ml/kg of PRBC. In response to fluids, patients are classified as responders, transient responders, and nonresponders. The management depends on which category the patient fits. The TTL will investigate the cause of the shock in responders with the expectation that many will not need therapeutic intervention. Transient and nonresponders need immediate investigation and determination of the cause of the shock with the expectation that a therapeutic intervention may be necessary. The hypovolemic shock may be due to intraabdominal, intrathoracic, pelvic, or extremity injuries (bilateral femur fractures). Also, in young children before cranial suture closure, intracranial hemorrhage can lead to shock.

Occasionally a patient may have a traumatic cardiac arrest. Emergency thoracotomy has been attempted to rescue these patients. Despite heroic attempts, little data

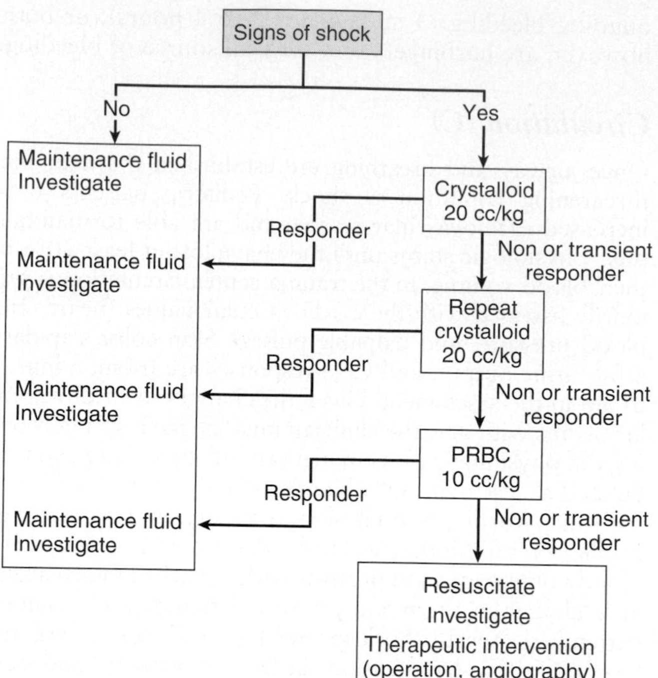

FIGURE 105–1 • This is a suggested algorithm to guide fluid resuscitation in a pediatric patient with trauma.

TABLE 105–2

Glasgow Coma Scale*

Domain		**Score**
EYE OPENING		
Spontaneous		4
To speech		3
To pain		2
None		1
BEST MOTOR RESPONSE		
Obeys command		6
Localized pain		5
Withdraws (from pain)		4
Decorticate (flexion)		3
Decerebrate (extension)		2
None		1
ADULT VERBAL RESPONSE	PEDIATRIC VERBAL RESPONSE	
Oriented	Appropriate words/gestures	5
Confused conversation	Consolable	4
Inappropriate words	Irritable	3
Unrecognized sounds	Agitated and restless	2
None	None	1

*Sum of best in each category (3-15) (only use one verbal response). Pick the appropriate verbal response according to age.

support this practice. The only patients to have a small chance of survival are those with a penetrating injury who have a witnessed arrest in the hospital/trauma room. These patients have a 15% chance of survival. All other groups, which include most pediatric patients with trauma, have case-reportable survival.

Venous access is one area that makes pediatric trauma unique. Ideally two large-bore catheters (14- or 16-gauge in adults) are placed in the antecubital fossa. This is not always possible in children because of their smaller size. Alternative techniques have been developed. These include percutaneous central venous lines, venous cutdowns (e.g., a saphenous vein cutdown), and intraosseous (IO) lines. The IO line can be particularly useful in the infant who has hypovolemia with poor venous filling.

Various fluid regimens have been investigated in adult patients for use in resuscitation. These include early colloid use and hypertonic saline. Although it is safe, colloid provides little advantage and is not recommended for acute trauma resuscitation.[8,9] Hypertonic saline is currently under investigation, but ongoing studies show promising results.[10-12] It appears to confer some benefit in patients with head injuries. The role of hypertonic saline in the resuscitation of the pediatric patient with trauma has yet to be defined.

Disability (D) and Exposure (E)

After resuscitation, a quick assessment of the neurologic status of the patient is important. The pediatric Glasgow Coma Scale (Table 105–2) should be assessed, as well as the patient's ability to move the extremities. This assessment will guide decisions further along in the investigative tree. Furthermore, a GCS of 8 or below warrants intubation for airway protection. The most important aspect in the resuscitation and management of the patient with a head injury is the maintenance of adequate oxygenation and systemic perfusion. The best outcomes are not possible without adequate oxygenation of the brain.

Exposure and environment are important in the assessment of the patient with trauma. Many injuries are missed by not fully exposing the patient. Thermoregulation, however, is an enormous problem in the pediatric patient with trauma. The increased ratio of surface area to body mass leads to increased heat loss. Aggressive and proactive methods to prevent hypothermia are often necessary. The room should be preheated, and overhead warmers should be used. Intravenous fluid should be warmed, and the patient should be covered as much as possible. Outside clothing, especially if wet, needs to be removed. With these maneuvers hypothermia can typically be avoided, and the outcome of the patient is improved.

Monitoring and Adjunct Measures

After the primary survey is completed and before the secondary survey is started, there is an opportunity to ensure that the patient has undergone all requisite, additional monitoring and adjunct testing. Other members of the trauma team will have already addressed many of these measures. The patient's electrocardiogram (ECG), molecular oxygen (O_2) saturation, and blood pressure should be monitored. Blood work and baseline radiographs (chest, lateral cervical spine, and pelvis) should be obtained. Recent data have suggested that some of these investigations may not be necessary in all pediatric patients with trauma, but exclusion is based on clinical decision by the TTL or the individual trauma program. Adequate venous access and supplemental oxygen should be ensured.

Secondary Survey

The secondary survey is the point in the assessment at which the complete history is obtained and a physical examination takes place. The history of the accident is noted, and any inconsistencies in the story are noted. Injuries that are not consistent with the history are also noted. Any suggestion of nonaccidental trauma should lead to a more extensive workup for injuries because the extent of trauma obtained through history and physical examination is often underestimated. The history may also suggest certain mechanisms of injury that may be useful in predicting injury patterns. Several examples include lap belt injuries of the duodenum, pancreas, and spine, as well as corneal abrasions associated with air bag deployment. After the history is obtained, the physical examination should be carried out. This is a complete head to toe examination; every system of the body should be checked. Every orifice must be examined, and a nasogastric and urinary catheter should be placed if indicated and safe. In the presence of facial or skull trauma, the gastric tube should be placed in an orogastric fashion. The urinary catheter should not be placed if there is a possibility of urethral trauma such as an open book pelvic fracture, a high-riding prostate, or blood at the urethral meatus. In this case a retrograde urethrogram will be necessary to assess the urethra before the catheter placement. The final part of the examination involves assessment of the spine by "logrolling" the patient. This is an ideal time to remove the hard spine board and place a thin sliding board for transferring the patient between bed and stretchers. Removing the board is not necessary at this point because some clinicians like to obtain computed tomography (CT) scans on the board. This is acceptable as long as every attempt is made to get the patient off of the hard spine board as soon as possible to prevent pressure ulcers. After the secondary survey, a plan for investigation and definitive management is made.

Investigations

Initial Plain Radiology

In the trauma center, as an adjunct to the primary survey, three standard radiographs are taken. They are images of (1) a lateral cervical spine, (2) a supine chest, and (3) an anteroposterior pelvis. The cervical spine film is important as a screen for a cervical spine injury; however, it is not sufficient to clear the spine radiographically. This will be addressed after the initial definitive management is done. The chest radiograph is completed as a screen for pulmonary or mediastinal injuries. The pelvis film is a screen to look for major pelvic disruption; however, it is inadequate to fully screen the pelvis. Recent data have suggested that not all patients with trauma need all three films and the choice of films used can be individualized.[13]

Ultrasound

Trauma ultrasound has revolutionized the assessment of intraabdominal bleeding in the adult patients.[14] With the use of the Focused Abdominal Sonography for Trauma (FAST) examination, many centers have essentially eliminated the need for diagnostic peritoneal lavage. FAST uses a bedside ultrasound to assess for intraabdominal fluid and pericardial fluid. It can reliably be done in less than 1 minute and has a high sensitivity (Fig. 105–2). The effectiveness of a FAST in adults cannot, however, be readily extrapolated to children. Conflicting results of the utility of the FAST in pediatric trauma have been reported in recent literature.[15-18] FAST provides the equivalent of a noninvasive peritoneal lavage. Few pediatric patients with trauma actually needed a peritoneal lavage, however, because the presence of blood in the peritoneal cavity does not mandate an operation. In selected patients FAST is a powerful tool. A nonresponding pediatric patient with hypotension can be a challenge to diagnose and treat. In such a patient, FAST can quickly and effectively assess the peritoneal and pericardial spaces. This is especially important in the pediatric population in which intracranial bleeding can also cause hypotension and require management vastly different from intraabdominal bleeding. Fortunately these patients are unusual, and therefore large studies have failed to show a major change in management with a broad application of this technology.

Computed Tomography Scan

The CT scan is the backbone of the workup for the pediatric patient with trauma. The CT scan can rapidly assess the head (Fig. 105–3), spine, chest, abdomen (Fig. 105–4), and pelvis. It gives anatomical detail that is pristine, and most children with trauma will require this imaging modality. Recent evidence has suggested that diagnostic CT scans increase the population-based risk of fatal cancers[19-21]; however, the risk of a missed injury or needless procedure far outweighs this real but hypothetical risk. Over time CT scanners have improved in both speed and precision, but they are often located in an isolated part of the hospital. The old rule of not taking an unstable patient to CT scan generally remains true today.

Patients with trauma are complex, and often the exact modality of scanning needs to be altered while the patient

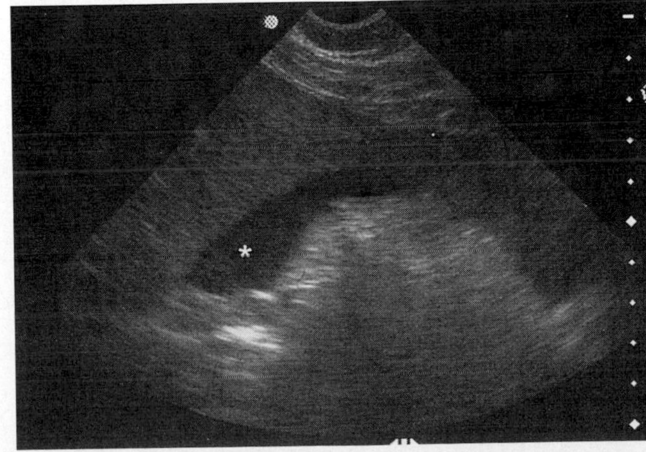

FIGURE 105–2 • A FAST ultrasound in an 8-year-old child who fell while tobogganing. Intraabdominal fluid (*asterisk*) is shown between the liver to the left and the kidney to the right.

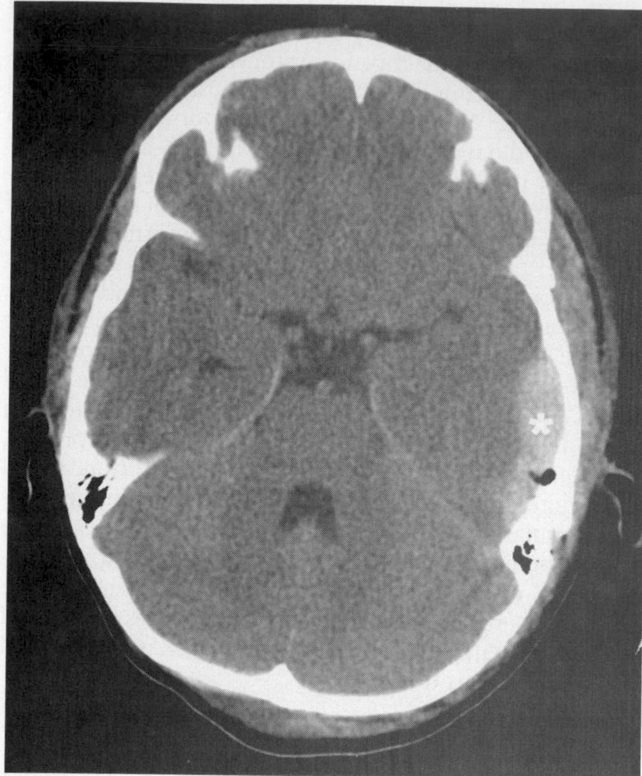

FIGURE 105–3 • A CT scan in an 8-year-old pedestrian struck by a car that shows an asymptomatic epidural hematoma (*asterisk*) and pneumocephalus just below the asterisk.

is in the scanner. Ideally, real-time feedback and decision making can be done in the scan room to avoid a second trip to the CT scanner. Later scans of the urinary system may be necessary, though, to assess the bladder, and thin slices of the pelvis may be necessary to evaluate its integrity.

Chest CT should be done with intravenous contrast to assess the mediastinum. This is a useful screen for an aortic injury and can avoid needless angiography. Abdominal CT traditionally uses oral and intravenous contrast. Often with a gastroparesis following trauma, the patient may vomit the high volume of oral contrast. Good data exist that challenge the need for oral contrast in children with trauma.

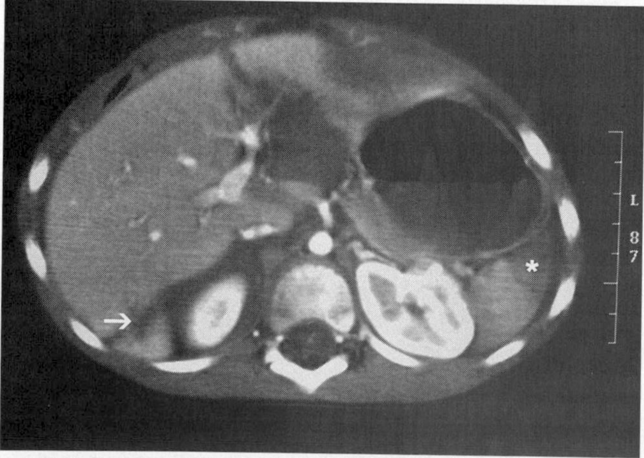

FIGURE 105–4 • A CT scan showing an ischemic spleen (*asterisk*) and a fractured liver (*arrow*) in a 4-year-old child run over by an all-terrain vehicle. This child was treated nonoperatively.

Angiography

Angiography has two functions. The first is diagnostic, and the second is therapeutic. Diagnostic angiography is rapidly being supplanted by CT angiography; however, this will not eliminate the need for angiography. Therapeutic angiography is an important method of controlling bleeding. This is especially important in areas that are difficult to access surgically, such as the pelvis. Ongoing bleeding from the pelvis, despite closure of the pelvic volume by a clamp or fixator, requires angiography to embolize the bleeding pelvic vessel, typically the superior gluteal artery. There has been an increasing trend in the adult population to embolize bleeding splenic vessels. The utility of this technique in the pediatric population is doubtful, however, because most pediatric splenic trauma stops bleeding spontaneously.

Extremity Radiographs

Extremity radiographs and completion spine films can be done after the life-threatening injuries have been assessed. Taking just a few extra images in the trauma room will needlessly delay the assessment of the patient and often leads to inferior films that must be repeated.

Echocardiography

Echocardiography has several purposes in patients with the trauma, particularly those with blunt chest trauma. In patients with myocardial contusions, transthoracic echocardiography is useful to assess the pericardium and cardiac function. The pericardium is assessed in the FAST examination,[22] but the detail is not sufficient to assess cardiac problems. Transesophageal echocardiography is a good method for visualizing the aorta in cases of suspected aortic injury when the CT scan cannot effectively rule it out.[23]

Definitive Management

The disposition of the patient depends on the disease process and the need for definitive management. Most patients do not need operative management of their injuries and are best managed in the pediatric intensive care unit with careful monitoring during the critical period after the injury. The decision not to operate on a specific injury must be made by the team responsible for operative management. This decision clearly needs to be in consultation with the entire team that cares for these complex patients. Occasionally, the decision to pursue a nonoperative management strategy must be reassessed because of changes in patient status. An example of this is the patient with a liver injury who continues to bleed and ultimately requires operative management.

The initial care of the child with trauma requires a systematic team approach that quickly assesses and treats the patient for life-threatening injuries. After resuscitation, definitive investigations and management of injuries are undertaken. Communication and coordination of patient care until disposition is the responsibility of the TTL. The TTL must be an expert at the assessment of resuscitation and investigation of the child with trauma. Definitive management decisions will be coordinated depending on the specific injuries of the patient.

REFERENCES

1. Gaines BA, Ford HR: Abdominal and pelvic trauma in children, *Crit Care Med* 30:S416-S423, 2002.
2. McAnena OJ, Moore EE, Marx JA: Initial evaluation of the patient with blunt abdominal trauma, *Surg Clin North Am* 70:495-515, 1990.
3. National Highway Traffic Safety Administration: Traffic safety facts 2002: children, Pub No DOT-HS-809-607, Washington, DC, 2004.
4. Shults RA, Sleet DA, Elder RW et al: Association between state level drinking and driving countermeasures and self reported alcohol impaired driving, *Inj Prev* 8:106-110, 2002.
5. Rivara FP: Child pedestrian injuries in the United States. Current status of the problem, potential interventions, and future research needs, *Am J Dis Child* 144:692-696, 1990.
6. Puranik S, Long J, Coffman S: Profile of pediatric bicycle injuries, *South Med J* 91:1033-1037, 1998.
7. Committee on Trauma, American College of Surgeons: *Advanced trauma life support for doctors, student course manual*, ed 7, Chicago, 2004, American College of Surgeons.
8. Fan E, Stewart TE: Albumin in critical care: SAFE, but worth its salt? *Crit Care* 8:297-299, 2004.
9. Finfer S, Bellomo R, Boyce N et al: SAFE Study Investigators: A comparison of albumin and saline for fluid resuscitation the intensive care unit, *N Engl J Med* 350:2247-2256, 2004.
10. Kramer GC: Hypertonic resuscitation: physiologic mechanisms and recommendations for trauma care, *J Trauma* 54:S89-S99, 2003.
11. Moore FA, McKinley BA, Moore EE: The next generation in shock resuscitation, *Lancet* 363:1988-1996, 2004.
12. Rocha ESR, Caneo LF, Lourenco Filho DD et al: First use of hypertonic saline dextran in children: a study in safety and effectiveness for atrial septal defect surgery, *Shock* 20:427-430, 2003.
13. Their ME, Bensch FV, Koskinen SK et al: Diagnostic value of pelvic radiography in the initial trauma series in blunt trauma, *Eur Radiol* 15:1533-1537, 2005.
14. Rozycki GS, Ochsner MG, Jaffin JH et al: Prospective evaluation of surgeons' use of ultrasound in the evaluation of trauma patients, *J Trauma* 34:516-526; discussion 526-527, 1993.
15. Coley BD, Mutabagani KH, Martin LC et al: Focused abdominal sonography for trauma (FAST) in children with blunt abdominal trauma, *J Trauma* 48:902-906, 2000.
16. Emery KH, McAneney CM, Racadio JM et al: Absent peritoneal fluid on screening trauma ultrasonography in children: a prospective comparison with computed tomography, *J Pediatr Surg* 36: 565-569, 2001.
17. Ong AW, McKenney MG, McKenney KA et al: Predicting the need for laparotomy in pediatric trauma patients on the basis of the ultrasound score, *J Trauma* 54:503-508, 2003.
18. Teitelbaum DH: Ultrasound is an effective triage tool to evaluate blunt abdominal trauma in the pediatric population, *J Trauma* 46:357-359, 1999.
19. Berdon WE, Slovis TL: Where we are since ALARA and the series of articles on CT dose in children and risk of long-term cancers: what has changed? *Pediatr Radiol* 32:699, 2002.
20. Brenner D, Elliston C, Hall E et al: Estimated risks of radiation-induced fatal cancer from pediatric CT, *AJR Am J Roentgenol* 176:289-296, 2001.
21. Brenner DJ, Elliston CD, Hall EJ et al: Estimates of the cancer risks from pediatric CT radiation are not merely theoretical: comment on "point/counterpoint: in x-ray computed tomography, technique factors should be selected appropriate to patient size against the proposition," *Med Phys* 28:2387-2388, 2001.
22. Rozycki GS, Feliciano DV, Schmidt JA et al: The role of surgeon-performed ultrasound in patients with possible cardiac wounds, *Ann Surg* 223:737-744; discussion 744-746, 1996.
23. Cinnella G, Dambrosio M, Brienza N et al: Transesophageal echocardiography for diagnosis of traumatic aortic injury: an appraisal of the evidence, *J Trauma* 57:1246-1255, 2004.

CHAPTER

106

Child Abuse and Neglect

Paula Mazur, James Woytash, and Lynn J. Hernan

PEARLS

- Accidental trauma differs from nonaccidental trauma in presentation, workup, treatment, and outcome. In child abuse, the history of trauma is absent or falsified, and if the presenting symptoms are vague and nonspecific, the diagnosis and treatment of injuries are delayed. This contributes to the increased death and long-term morbidity seen in abused children.
- Abusive head trauma is the most common injury seen in the pediatric intensive care unit (PICU) in the abused child. It is the most common cause of death in abused children. Abusive head trauma is more likely to be fatal and more likely to cause long-term morbidity in the survivors than accidental head trauma.
- The infant brain is more vulnerable to injury, especially shaken baby syndrome (SBS). The neck muscles are weaker and the head is proportionately larger compared with those of the adult. Large cerebrospinal fluid (CSF) spaces in the infant allow greater movement of the brain within the skull. The infant brain has greater water content, increasing deformability. Neurons and axons are less protected because of incomplete myelinization. Increased cerebral vasoreactivity predisposes the infant brain to cerebral edema.
- Accidental head trauma generates translational forces that result in focal damage. Nonaccidental trauma (e.g., shaking) generates rotational forces from rapid acceleration/deceleration of the head. Rotational forces tear cerebral bridging veins (creating subdural hematoma) and axons (creating diffuse axonal injury).
- Signs of SBS consist of subdural hemorrhage, retinal hemorrhage, and skeletal injury. A small number of cases will have all three signs. The presence of subdural hemorrhage and retinal hemorrhage, alone or in combination, in the appropriate clinical setting can suggest SBS.
- Posterior rib fractures, metaphyseal fractures, and spinous process fractures are highly specific for abuse because their proposed mechanisms of injury are unlikely to occur accidentally.
- Abdominal trauma is the second leading cause of fatal child abuse, with death rates approaching 40% to 50%. Inflicted abdominal injury is often occult, presenting without obvious signs or symptoms; thus recognition is delayed. Treatment may be delayed because of a delay to seek medical attention and failure to consider nonaccidental injury in the differential diagnosis.
- Two types of forces are generated in inflicted abdominal trauma. Compression forces crush viscera against the anterior spine, and this crush causes burst injuries of the solid viscera and perforation of air-filled viscera. Deceleration forces cause shear injuries at the site of fixed, ligamentous attachments, with tears and hematoma formation at the ligamentous attachments of the liver and small bowel. Children with inflicted abdominal injury have concomitant injuries commonly seen in child abuse (bruises, head trauma, long-bone and skull fractures).
- Abusive thermal burns are of uniform thickness and closely replicate the shape of the inflicting object. Accidental thermal burns have varying degrees of thickness and irregular shapes. Abusive scald burns have an immersion pattern with a burn that is circumferential, is of uniform depth with a well-defined edge, and spares body creases. Accidental scald burns have more random patterns, vary in depth, have poorly defined edges, and do not spare body creases.

- All cases of suspected child abuse must be reported to child protective services and law enforcement. All cases of fatal child abuse must be referred to the medical examiner (ME). Detailed, legible, medical documentation and good communication between the treating physician and the ME are essential to secure evidence needed for successful prosecution of the case.

Only a small percentage of physically abused children require hospitalization in the pediatric intensive care unit (PICU), but these children have been shown to have higher morbidity and death rates when compared with critically injured victims of accidental trauma.[1,2] The types of injuries resulting from nonaccidental injury, along with delays in diagnosis and management, account for the poorer outcome in abuse victims when compared with accident victims.

Diagnosis and timely management of inflicted, potentially life-threatening injuries are often delayed because a history of preceding trauma is absent, vague or so minor by description that the physician is led away from a possible traumatic cause for the patient's condition. The "golden hour" allotted for successful trauma resuscitation is spent considering an infectious, neurologic, or metabolic cause for the child's illness. In addition, there can be considerable delay in seeking medical care. Several hours to days may elapse between time of injury and time of presentation to a medical facility.

Head trauma is the most common type of inflicted injury seen in the PICU. Abdominal trauma is the second most common, followed by burns and thoracic trauma.

Child abuse victims should be approached as trauma patients. They can have multiple organ injury, some of which will be occult. The discovery of one injury demands a thorough evaluation for additional trauma. A meticulous investigation for injury has obvious medical utility, but it also becomes an essential part of the forensic investigation that ensues once a report of suspected child abuse is filed with child protective services and law enforcement.

The Recognition of Child Abuse

History of Injury

The history of an injury must account for the type and severity of injury that is seen during physical examination. Suspicion of abuse should arise when any of the following occur:

- The caretaker is unable to explain the injuries or gives a mechanism of injury that does not match the degree of injury seen. For example, a minor fall would not explain the presence of life-threatening cerebral edema.
- The timing of the injury does not fit with the time of presentation (e.g., a critical head injury cannot be attributed to a fall that occurred 1 week before presentation).
- The child's developmental stage is not in sync with the history (e.g., rolling off a changing table should raise suspicion if the child is younger than 4 months).
- The history of injury changes over time or from caretaker to caretaker. A careful review of all histories documented in the medical record may reveal discrepancies.

Patterns of Injury

Inflicted injury may be differentiated from accidental injury by its appearance, location, and distribution on the body (Table 106–1).

Bruising

Inflicted bruises are often bilateral, widely distributed, and located on soft tissue areas of the body that are unlikely to make surface contact during a fall. They may take the shape of the inflicting object (e.g., fingers, a hand print, linear whip marks from a belt, loop marks from a folded belt or cord). They are frequently found on the posterior trunk, buttocks, and the posterior side of the extremities because the victim would naturally be trying to run away from the perpetrator.

Bruise color is not a reliable indicator of the time an injury occurred. Bruises resolve and therefore change color at different rates depending on their location and the force with which they were inflicted.[3] Nevertheless, documenting bruise colors is important, particularly with the presence of bruises of markedly different colors at the same time, suggesting that the child may have been abused on more than one occasion. A simple gingerbread man drawing of the child's body, marked with the locations of all the child's injuries, is a concise descriptive tool, which will quickly jar a physician's memory before any legal proceeding.

Photographic documentation of the child's injuries is essential. Every effort should be made to obtain the best photographs; 35mm photographs taken by a medical or law enforcement photographer are the ideal. If a professional photographer is unavailable or if the attempt to

TABLE 106–1

Patterns of Injury

Accidental	Nonaccidental
Unilateral	Bilateral/symmetrical
Isolated injury	Multiple injuries
Amorphous shape	Well-defined shape
Prominent bone areas	Soft tissue areas
Posterior aspect of body	Anterior aspect of body
One age of injury	Multiple ages of injury

obtain a professional will delay documentation of rapidly resolving bruises (e.g., petechiae), any staff person familiar with the use of a 35mm camera should take photographs for the medical record. Polaroid photographs have been used in court, but they are inferior to 35mm photographs in both clarity and durability. Digital photographs are not used in court proceedings because they can be altered.

Burns

Numerous researchers have attempted to describe the profile of an abused burned child and to characterize inflicted burns. In general, the child is often from a single-parent family of lower socioeconomic status on which previous suspicions of child abuse or neglect may have been filed. Compared with accidental burns, abuse burns are more extensive in degree and distribution, and often require management in a PICU.[4,5]

Inflicted burns are of two types. Thermal injuries involve forced contact with a hot object, and scald injuries involve contact with a hot liquid, usually water. Abusive thermal burns are of uniform thickness and closely replicate the shape of the inflicting object.

Accidental thermal burns have varying degrees of thickness and irregular shapes. For example, an inflicted cigarette burn is approximately 8 mm round and uniform in depth. If a child accidentally brushes against a hot cigarette, the burn will be more linear and of varying depth along its length.[6]

Abusive scald burns have an immersion pattern. Part of the child's body, usually the buttocks or limbs, are forcefully immersed and held in hot water. The resulting burn is circumferential and of uniform depth with a well-defined edge called a *tide mark*. Body creases are spared (withdrawal sign) during inflicted scald injury because the child pulls and folds his arms and legs inward to avoid immersion in the hot water. Accidental scald burns have more random patterns, vary in depth, have poorly defined edges and do not spare body creases.

Ideally, photograph documentation should be done before the initial burn dressing. Additional photographs taken 24 to 48 hours later, when the burn has fully evolved in depth and distribution, can be valuable during litigation, though.

Fractures

Many of the characteristics used to recognize inflicted bruises and burns can be applied to fractures. The mechanism of injury described by the caretaker must remain consistent, be compatible with the child's developmental stage, and must account for enough force to break the child's bone. Inflicted fractures can be bilateral fractures of the same age or multiple fractures in different stages of healing. In his textbook *Diagnostic Imaging of Child Abuse,* Dr. Kleinman[7] divides fractures according to their degree of specificity for inflicted injury. Posterior rib fractures, metaphyseal fractures, and spinous process fractures are highly specific for abuse because their proposed mechanisms of injury are unlikely to occur accidentally. Scapula and sternum fractures are highly specific for abuse if the caretaker's history does not account for a tremendous amount of force having been applied to these bones. Fractures of low specificity for abuse are fractures commonly seen after bumps and falls (e.g., clavicle fractures, linear skull fractures, long-bone fractures in ambulatory toddlers). Between high and low specificity is acute, bilateral fractures, multiple fractures of different ages, widened (diastatic) or depressed skull fractures, and long-bone shaft fractures occurring in the young, nonambulatory infant.

It was long held that spiral fractures were highly suggestive of abuse because their spiral configuration implied that a forceful twisting motion had been applied along the length of the bone. Dalton et al[8] looked at femur fractures in children younger than 3 years, dividing the fractures into three types (oblique, transverse, spiral), and into three age categories (0 to 1 year, 1 to 2 years, 2 to 3 years). Their results showed that the incidence of spiral fractures increased significantly with increasing age, whereas the incidence of abuse was highest in the youngest age group regardless of fracture type. Spiral fractures can occur accidentally in vigorous, ambulatory toddlers. The age of the child holds more significance than fracture type when the possibility of inflicted injury is considered.[8,9]

Posterior Rib Fractures. Posterior rib fractures and metaphyseal fractures are frequently seen in shaken or battered infants. Posterior rib fractures occur when the child's chest is compressed. This compression causes the rib to rock back over its articulation with the transverse vertebral process. The transverse process acts as a fulcrum for the rib, and a fracture occurs on the rib's pleural surface. Although this fracture has been seen in pediatric patients with major, high-speed trauma, it does not occur accidentally in healthy children during mild to moderate thoracic trauma. Cardiopulmonary resuscitation (CPR) has not been shown to cause posterior rib fractures.[10] A detailed discussion of posterior rib fractures can be found in Kleinman's textbook, *Diagnostic Imaging of Child Abuse.*[7]

Acute rib fractures are difficult to see on a plain film. They may only first be visible 2 to 3 weeks after injury, when a callus has formed around the fracture site. Therefore finding a calloused fracture on x-ray film is discovering trauma that occurred at least 2 to 3 weeks before the radiograph.[10,11]

Metaphyseal Fractures. The periosteum of a pediatric long bone is loosely attached to its cortex. Any violent pull, tear, or twist on the shaft of a child's long bone displaces the periosteum. The results are subperiosteal hemorrhage and periosteal elevation that can be seen on x-ray film. Conversely, the periosteum is tightly attached at its point for origin, the metaphyseal plate. The metaphyseal plate, which is the most newly laid down bone above the growth plate, has delicate trabeculations. Violent forces applied to the midshaft periosteum are transferred to its point of origin, the metaphyseal plate, and an avulsion fracture occurs through the delicate trabeculae. Depending on the angle at which the radiograph is taken, a metaphyseal avulsion fracture can appear as a thin line through the metaphysis, as "corners" broken off the edges of the long bone, or as a "bucket handle" attached to the end of the long bone. Like posterior rib fractures, metaphyseal fractures are pathognomonic for abuse.[12] These corner fractures or bucket handle fractures are occult. There is no deformity or swelling, and they are not obviously tender to palpation. Like posterior rib fractures, metaphyseal fractures are usually found on a radiograph obtained for other reasons or on a skeletal survey done during the medical investigation of a suspected abuse case.

Spinous process fractures are the remaining type of fractures listed under "high specificity" in Dr. Kleinman's text. They are thought to occur during infant shaking, when the spine is in hyperflexion, causing sudden stress on the posterior spinous ligament as it articulates with the posterior spinous processes. Like posterior rib fractures, they are not easily seen until a callus has formed at the fracture site.[13]

Dating Fractures. The guidelines for dating fractures are broad. In general, periosteal elevation can occur acutely, within hours to days after injury. Callous formation is seen approximately 2 weeks after injury. Loss of the fracture line begins to occur 3 weeks after the injury, and remodeling of the fracture occurs anywhere from 3 months to a year after injury, depending on the child's age. Infants will heal and remodel faster than older children. Skull fractures and metaphyseal fractures are difficult to date because they do not show the same periosteal reactions that healing ribs and long bones do.[7]

Skeletal Survey

Finding one suggestive injury on a child necessitates a radiological evaluation of the entire skeleton. Skeletal survey is the most common screening tool used in child abuse investigation. Two views of every bone in the body, radiographed with orthopedic technique, is the gold standard. "Body-grams" or "baby-grams," in which the entire infant's skeleton is pictured on one x-ray plate, are unacceptable. We have been able to obtain adequate surveys at the bedside when the patient has been too unstable to move from the critical care area to the radiology department. We have also obtained postmortem skeletal survey's before transferring the child's body to the medical examiner (ME) because the quality of our surveys far surpasses radiographs performed in the morgue and therefore may serve to focus the ME on particular areas of the skeleton during autopsy.

The younger the child, the higher is the yield of a skeletal survey. Because smaller children are easier to lift, shake, throw, or pull, it is possible to generate the forces required to create the classic abuse fractures previously discussed. In general, skeletal surveys have the highest yield in children younger than 2 years and are obtained in children up to age 5 years, after which the yield becomes low.[6]

Bone Scan. Occult fractures can be detected by bone scan, but bone scan is not specific for fracture. The radioactive isotope used in bone scan will also enhance areas of infection, neoplasm, and growth. Therefore positive bone scans cannot be used as evidence of injury in court. A positive scan serves to focus attention on a particular area of the skeleton in need of closer study, but the area of injury must always be verified by subsequent plain film. Bone scans are most useful in detecting occult rib fractures. They are not as useful in verifying metaphyseal fractures because the metaphysis lies next to an area of vigorous bone growth, and growth areas are normally enhanced in pediatric scans.

Abusive Head Trauma

Abusive head trauma is the most common form of child abuse seen in the PICU and is the number one cause of death in child abuse victims overall. Roughly 50% of all trauma in children younger than 1 year is head trauma. When Bruce and Zimmerman[1] looked at their population of children younger than 2 years with head trauma, they found that 90% of the head injuries were accidental, and 10% were attributed to abuse. Eighty percent of the deaths from head trauma, however, occurred in the smaller percentage of abused children. Outcome studies on children who have survived accidental compared nonaccidental head trauma show a significantly higher morbidity rate in the nonaccidental victims. Clearly, abusive head injury vastly differs from accidental head injury.[14]

Characteristics of the Infant Brain

The infant brain is more vulnerable to injury than the adult brain for several reasons. The neck muscles inadequately support the infant's head, which is relatively large compared with the rest of the body. Consequently, the head is put through a broad range of random motion during a traumatic event like shaking. The cerebrospinal fluid (CSF) spaces are large. These spaces allow greater movement of the brain within the skull, and the brain has greater water content, increasing deformability. Open sutures increase skull flexibility so that an infant's skull can be pushed inward causing cortical damage without fracturing. Incomplete myelinization leaves neurons and their axons less protected, and increased cerebral vasoreactivity at the site of injured neurons predisposes the brain to cerebral edema.[15]

Mechanisms of Head Injury

Accidental head trauma, such as a fall from height, generates translational forces, which are applied directly to the site of impact resulting in focal damage to the cerebral cortex. We may see a focal contusion, coup-contre-coup injury, or an epidural hematoma. Nonaccidental trauma (e.g., shaking) generates rotational force as a consequence of rapid acceleration/deceleration movements of the head. Rotational force distorts both gross and microscopic cortical structure.[15] The tearing of cerebral bridging veins creates subdural hematoma. Axons that are torn at the microscopic level result in neuron death and global cerebral injury.[16] Although subdural hematomas are a hallmark of shaken baby syndrome (SBS), they are not usually life-threatening lesions. Diffuse axonal injury (DAI) is thought to be largely responsible for the increased death and morbidity of nonaccidental trauma. Furthermore, increased vasoreactivity at the site of damaged axons causes a rapid onset of diffuse cerebral edema, which increases intracranial pressure (ICP) and compromises blood flow to vital areas of the brain. Therefore the child is placed at risk for seizures, respiratory compromise, herniation, and death. Within hours of a shaking injury, computed tomography (CT) scan will begin to show a "black brain" with diffuse edema and a loss of gray-white matter differentiation.

Retinal Hemorrhages

It is widely hypothesized that the eye is subjected to the same acceleration/deceleration forces that the brain endures. Retinal vessels, coursing through the 11 layers of retina, will randomly tear, forming hemorrhages of multiple shapes (e.g., dots, blots, flame hemorrhages). Hemorrhage shape is determined by the cell orientation in the particular retinal layer where tearing occurs. Intraretinal hemorrhages of multiple shapes in various retinal layers are a classic finding in SBS.[2] Controversy still surrounds the mechanism of retinal hemorrhage formation,[2,17-19] and there have been scattered reports of scant retinal hemorrhage found after CPR, or in the face of increased ICP (Terson's syndrome) or increased thoracic pressure (Purtscher's retinopathy).[18] These retinal hemorrhages, however, often differ in appearance from the classic retinal hemorrhages of SBS.[18,20,21] A recent study of 75 shaken babies found no correlation between the presence of increased ICP or increased intrathoracic pressure.[22] Approximately 30% of healthy neonates will have retinal hemorrhages at birth, but these rapidly resolve by the third or fourth week of life.[23]

Shaken Baby Syndrome

The diagnosis of SBS is made in the presence of a constellation of signs (i.e., subdural hemorrhage, retinal hemorrhage, and skeletal injury).[24] The mechanisms of injury proposed to cause subdural hematoma and retinal hemorrhage have been previously discussed. Posterior rib fractures occur when the infant's chest is compressed during shaking. Metaphyseal fractures are thought to occur as the legs and arms are flailed back and forth.[12]

Only a small percentage of cases will have all three signs of SBS (i.e., subdural hematomas, retinal hemorrhages, and skeletal injury). More than half the cases will show both subdural hematoma and retinal hemorrhage, but the presence of subdural hemorrhage or retinal hemorrhage alone still suggests the diagnosis of SBS.

A proposed sequence of events in SBS would be as follows: The frustrated caretaker impulsively attempts to stop the infant's crying by violently shaking the infant. The infant immediately loses consciousness and becomes apneic, at which time the caretaker impacts the infant down onto the mattress or floor and leaves the child to recover on its own. The cerebral damage and ensuing edema lead to increased ICP, ischemia, seizures, and further respiratory compromise.[1] Eventually medical care is sought for the child.

The clinical history is vague. There is usually some history of altered mental status. The child has nonspecific symptoms such as lethargy, poor feeding, and irritability or may have had a seizurelike episode.[24] The differential diagnosis includes sepsis, meningitis, new onset seizure, or a metabolic disorder. These children commonly have no external evidence of trauma. Trauma may only become part of the differential when a CT scan done for other purposes reveals intracranial hemorrhage or when a bloody spinal tap fails to clear. Bloody taps that fail to clear should be spun down within 2 hours to look for xanthochromic CSF, which is indicative of a preexisting intracranial hemorrhage. CSF that has a clear supernatant suggests the presence of blood for less than 2 hours, supporting a diagnosis of bloody tap. For early diagnosis and management of a potentially lethal injury to be facilitated, trauma must always be included in the differential when a young child is seen with altered mental status, seizures, or apnea.

Jenny et al[25] reviewed 174 children with abusive head injury who were seen at the Denver Children's Hospital over a 5-year period and found that, in 31% of these children, the diagnosis of abusive head trauma was missed on first presentation for medical evaluation. The most frequent misdiagnoses made were gastroenteritis, followed by accidental head injury, sepsis, increasing head size, otitis media, and seizure disorder. Examiners were most likely to make the correct diagnosis if one of the following was present: severe respiratory symptoms, seizures, facial or scalp injuries, or single-parent household. Cases were often missed in the youngest patients, white infants, infants with less severe symptoms, and two-parent households.[25]

Inflicted Visceral Trauma

Abdominal Trauma

After head injury, abdominal trauma is the second leading cause of fatal child abuse. Death rates approach 40% to 50%.[26-28] Cooper et al[29] reviewed 10,000 pediatric patients with trauma who were admitted between 1972 and 1986, identifying approximately 4400 victims of inflicted injury. Of these, only 22, or 0.5%, had abdominal trauma, but the death rate for this small subgroup was 45%. Several factors probably contribute to these high death rates. Inflicted abdominal injury is often occult, presenting without obvious signs or symptoms; this delays recognition. There is usually a delay between time of inflicted injury and time of presentation to a medical facility. Parents may not bring the child to medical attention until the secondary effects of severe abdominal trauma, namely, hemorrhagic shock and peritonitis, manifest. Health care personnel further delay treatment by failing to consider nonaccidental injury in the differential diagnosis. In the study by Cooper et al[29] the mean time of delay between time of injury and time of presentation for medical care was 13 hours.

Of significance, all the children with inflicted abdominal injury in the study by Cooper et al[29] had concomitant injuries commonly seen in child abuse. Ninety-five percent had soft tissue injuries, 45% had head trauma, and 27% and 18% had long-bone fractures and skull fractures, respectively. Half of the families had been previously reported to child protective services for suspected abuse or neglect. The most recent abdominal injuries seemed to represent an escalation of abuse in the home. Therefore any suggestive injury should prompt physicians to look for occult abdominal trauma and to contact child protective services for investigation of the child's social situation.

Mechanism and Spectrum of Inflicted Abdominal Injury

Children with nonaccidental abdominal trauma tend to be older (>1 year) than children with abusive head trauma. Because they are larger and ambulatory, they are more difficult to grab, lift, and shake, but they are still vulnerable to physical blows. Inflicted abdominal trauma is blunt force applied to the abdominal wall, usually a punch, kick, or blow to the midepigastrium. Two types of force are generated. Compression forces crush viscera against the anterior spine, and deceleration forces cause shear injuries at the site of fixed, ligamentous attachments. We may find burst injuries of the solid viscera, perforation of the hollow, air-filled viscera, or tears and hematoma formation at the ligamentous attachments of the liver and small bowel.[29]

The spectrum of inflicted abdominal injuries varies from that seen in accidental abdominal injury because the force of an inflicted blow is more deeply concentrated in the midepigastrium. Most inflicted injury will involve the small bowel (duodenal hematoma), liver lacerations, and pancreatic injury. A wider array of injury is seen in accident victims, involving kidneys; spleen; liver; and, to a much lesser extent, small bowel and pancreas.[30] Pancreatitis is rare in childhood, and trauma is the primary cause. Unless there is a history of significant injury to the epigastrium, nonaccidental injury must be strongly considered when pancreatitis is found in young children. Given the occult nature of nonaccidental abdominal trauma, CT scan of the abdomen is the evaluation of choice when intraabdominal trauma is ruled out in child abuse victims.[27,31]

Thoracic Trauma

Beyond the pathognomonic rib fractures of child abuse, extensive thoracic trauma is rarely seen. A child's thoracic cage is so plastic and deformable, however, that, even in the absence of rib fractures, a child abuse victim could sustain compromising pulmonary injuries, namely, pneumothoraces, hemothoraces, or pulmonary contusions. As with abdominal trauma, the physician's index of suspicion must remain high to avoid delayed management of a life-threatening thoracic injury. The reader is referred to subsequent chapters of this text for detailed discussion of pediatric thoracic trauma.

Sexual Abuse

Physically abused children are also sexually abused. When a patient is examined for evidence of physical trauma, a careful genital examination is warranted. Any evidence of old or new genital trauma must be documented with photographs. Genital trauma is usually subtle, difficult to recognize, and difficult to photograph. When possible, consult a physician who specializes in sexual abuse and who may be able to perform a noninvasive colposcopic examination of the external genitalia. The best photo-documentation of genital injury is obtained with a colposcopy. If acute genital trauma is suspected or identified, a "rape kit" or forensic collection of evidence must be performed, and the police must be involved early. The forensic evidence becomes legal documentation of the sexual assault, and a chain of evidence must be carefully maintained between the hospital and the forensic laboratory. All cultures must be collected in culture medium or broth. DNA probes for gonorrhea and chlamydia cannot be used as evidence in court. Ideally, evidence collection should occur before any washing of the genitalia, including before the skin prep for insertion of a Foley catheter. Speculum and bimanual examination of sexually abused children is not warranted unless there is concern about internal lacerations in need of surgical repair. To avoid the need for repeat examinations, a sexual abuse expert or pediatric gynecologist should perform this examination with the patient under anesthesia.[6]

Protocol for the Medical Investigation of Child Abuse

To ensure complete and objective evidence collection during the medical investigation of child abuse, we have established an investigative protocol for our institution that is based on the current medical literature. This protocol has worked well across all pediatric subspecialty services in our institution and has provided consistency when communications occurs with law enforcement, legal services, child protective services, and our community pediatricians (Box 106–1).

Fatal Child Abuse

History

Fatal child abuse is not a phenomenon of the twentieth century. There have been reports of fatal child abuse

BOX 106–1

Protocol for Medical Investigation of Child Abuse

- Physical examination for skin and genital trauma
- Photography of all injury
- Skeletal survey for children younger than 5 years
- Bone scan (if skeletal survey negative—see text)
- CT head scan for children younger than 3 years
- Ophthalmology consultation to rule out retinal hemorrhage
- Abdominal trauma laboratory values
  - Serum amylase/lipase
  - Liver enzymes
    - Urine analysis
- CT abdomen scan
  - All nonverbal children
  - Positive findings from abdominal examination
  - Abnormal laboratory results

CT, Computed tomography.

throughout history. Caligula's daughter died of inflicted head trauma in AD 41. The French literature records the fatal whipping of a 4-year-old girl in the 1850s. In 1860, Professor Ambroise Tardieu published a paper describing fatal physical and sexual abuse inflicted on infants and children by parents. Tardieu's account listed thermal burns, fingernail imprints, contusions due to pinching, intracranial hemorrhages, and other injuries similar to those seen today. Likewise, these parents and caretakers offered explanations for the injuries, which were incompatible with the severity of injury, such as falls during play or by other minor accidents. Knight[32] concludes, in his historical review of child abuse, that fatal child abuse is nothing new.

Communicating with the Medical Examiner

Fatal Head Trauma

Eighty percent of fatal child abuse is caused by head injury. Because many of these children undergo surgical intervention before their death, the forensic pathologist/ME is often faced with an autopsy in which the injuries have been altered by surgical procedures. An exact description of the injuries' present treatment is essential, for example, the extent (amount), location, and radiological information (CT, magnetic resonance imaging [MRI], plain films) for all epidural, subdural, and subarachnoid hemorrhage. The chart must reference any biopsy specimens (usually blood clots) submitted to the pathology laboratory during surgical procedures. Documenting the extent and location of retinal hemorrhages may assist the forensic pathologist/ME during gross examination of the eyes. Although there are nontraumatic causes of retinal hemorrhage, CPR is not a common cause.

The location and size (in inches/centimeters) and a brief description of any abrasions, lacerations, and contusions should be stated. With respect to contusions, the color on admission and on successive days should be recorded. Likewise, any skin breakdown following medical procedures, notably on the posterior scalp and neck, needs documentation.[33]

Fatal Abdominal Trauma

As previously stated, visceral trauma is the second leading cause of death in child abuse. Abdominal injuries include liver, spleen, intestinal, mesenteric and renal contusions, lacerations, and rupture. There may be minimal external evidence of such catastrophic injuries. In the event that they are discovered during surgery, the amount of blood in the peritoneum and extent of organ damage should be carefully documented. Abdominal injuries resulting from CPR are extremely rare.[34]

Osseous Injury in Fatal Child Abuse

Fractures of bones in fatal child abuse are evidence. Documentation of the site of fracture (e.g., metaphyseal distal femur), type of fracture (e.g., transverse, spiral), and possible dating by x-ray analysis should be done on all cases. A head-to-toe approach with skeletal survey will aid the forensic pathologist/ME by locating injuries before the autopsy. During the autopsy, sections of these fractures are taken. Although some authorities consider histologic dating to be accurate, there are wide variations in the chronological healing of fractures. Only an approximate time frame can be assigned to a fracture.[35] Osseous injuries will also alert the staff to possible nontraumatic causes such as osteogenesis imperfecta.

Scene Investigation in Fatal Child Abuse

The scene is where the infant became unresponsive, became apneic, or sustained injuries that led to hospital admission. The scene typically belongs to and is secured by law enforcement officers, so the earlier they become involved, the more timely and accurate the scene investigation will be.

Emergency medical service (EMS) providers or firefighters are often the first to arrive on the scene. Their narrative description of the immediate circumstances and surroundings is a crucial part of scene investigation. They are encouraged to describe the place and position in which the child was found; the type of bed and bedding the child was found in; the presence of body fluids (blood, vomit, urine, feces) at the scene; the tidiness of the environment; and the presence of drugs, medications, drug paraphernalia, or alcohol at the scene. They often record the initial reactions of caretakers, identify potential witnesses to the preceding events, and discover other vulnerable children within the household. Talking to EMS providers on their arrival with the critically injured child can provide a wealth of information leading to early suggestions of child abuse/neglect, timely medical interventions, and early law enforcement and child protective services involvement.

Autopsy

The successful identification of tragic fatal child abuse cases depends on a team approach. Box 106–2 lists the minimal information desired by the forensic pathologist/ME before autopsy.[36] Clearly this list is best assembled as a collaborative effort of EMS, law enforcement, and physicians. Ideally, representatives of the pediatric team, law enforcement, and the district attorney's office would attend the autopsy examination. Although law enforcement attendance is routine in all fatal child abuse cases,

BOX 106–2

Scene Investigation Information

Law enforcement jurisdiction
Date, time, address of place of injury
Witnessed by whom (or unwitnessed)
First responders to scene
Field interventions (CPR, intubation, drugs)
Description of victim as found
Description of environment
Scene diagram (supplied by law enforcement)
Interviews with parents, caretakers, witnesses

CPR, Cardiopulmonary resuscitation.

numerous constraints usually interfere with pediatric representation at autopsy. Minimally, a phone conversation between the ME and the pediatric attending physician is strongly recommended.

Organ Procurement Organization and Fatal Child Abuse

The limited supply of organs for transplantation is well known. Although all age groups are represented, there is a lower organ donation percentage in the pediatric age group because this group has a lower relative death rate. Thus the use of organs from the pediatric age group is critical. When a child or infant sustains injuries leading to brain death, organ procurement is sought by organ procurement organizations (OPOs). Initially, some forensic pathologists/MEs may deny the use of organs on the basis that it may cause problems with judicial procedures.[37] This is not absolute. All three agencies must examine each individual case. The district attorney, forensic pathologist/ME, and the pediatrician must work with the OPO to see if organs not damaged by injury may be used in transplantation. If all parties are satisfied, then a representative of the ME's office (ideally the forensic pathologist/ME who will do the autopsy) should be present when the organs are retrieved for transplantation. The interacting groups are listed in Box 106–3.

Documentation and Testifying in Court

Testimony of medical personnel begins with thorough and legible documentation in the medical record. Complete, rather than brief, documentation is strongly recommended because trials may be delayed for months to years. Handwritten notes will become a memory lifeline during testimony.

Document information objectively. Be specific about where information is coming from. When recording conversations with caretakers, place their exact words in italics and write "per conversation with . . . ." Months to years later, one will not remember exactly who was interviewed or who actually said what is written in the chart. Written words may be misconstrued as opinion, and defense attorneys frequently make this an issue when witnesses testify to confuse or discredit testimony.

Testifying on behalf of a child who has been abused or murdered is emotional. Stick to the facts and remain objective. Remember that medical personnel are not the judge in this case. Stay calm, particularly when being cross-examined by the defense attorney, and remember that medical personnel and their work are not on trial.

There is no urgency in court. Take the time you need to formulate answers. Response should be brief and limited to the question asked, unless one is specifically told to elaborate further. If a question is not understood, ask that it be clarified before an answer is given. If a detail (e.g., a date, a time, a person's name) cannot be recalled, simply state so. One is allowed to refer to the medical records once they have been entered into medical evidence. If a witness does not think that he or she possesses the expertise to answer a question, then the witness should simply state so.

The more prepared one is, the less stressful the experience in court will be. It is the responsibility of medical personnel to review the medical records, laboratory reports, and radiological studies before trial. If the prosecuting attorney is properly preparing the case, the attorney will meet with each witness before testimony is given. This meeting gives both the attorney and the witness a chance to clarify specific issues that will be raised in court and to discuss the limits of the testimony. One may be asked to submit an updated curriculum vitae to establish credentials. If one is being called as a fact-finding witness, the court will not solicit opinions. During the trial, one may be qualified as an expert witness in his or her medical subspecialty. Then, one will be allowed to express opinions more freely. If one is called to testify again regarding the same case or if a deposition was given before trial, then previously recorded statements should be reviewed so that testimony remains consistent. It serves to keep the witness from becoming uncomfortably entangled in unintended contradiction and legal rhetoric when on the stand. Included in the following reference list are suggested readings that may be helpful in preparation for trial.[38-40]

BOX 106–3

Key Groups Needed for Tissue Procurement

Pediatrician representing family's request
Organ procurement organization representative
Medical examiner's office
District attorney's office

REFERENCES

1. Bruce D, Zimmerman RA: Shaken impact syndrome, *Ped Ann* 18:482, 1989.
2. Clark BJ, Adams GGW, Luthert PJ: Retinal hemorrhages in infant head injury, *Brain* 125:677, 2002.
3. Stephenson T: Ageing of bruising in children, *J R Soc Med* 90:312, 1997.
4. Andronicus M, Oates RK, Peat J et al: Non-accidental burns in children, *Burns* 24:552, 1998.
5. Bennett B, Gamelli R: Profile of an abused burned child, *J Burn Care Rehabil* 19:88, 1998.
6. Reese RM: *Child abuse: medical diagnosis and management,* ed 1, Malvern, PA, 1993, Lea & Febiger.
7. Kleinman PK: *Diagnostic imaging of child abuse,* ed 2, St Louis, 1998, Mosby.
8. Dalton HJ, Slovis T, Helfer RE et al: Undiagnosed abuse in children younger than 3 years with femoral fracture, *Am J Dis Child* 144:875, 1990.
9. Thomas SA, Rosenfield NS, Leventhal JM et al: Long-bone fractures in young children: distinguishing accidental injuries from child abuse, *Pediatrics* 88:471, 1991.
10. Kleinman PK, Schlesinger AE: Mechanical factors associated with posterior rib fractures: laboratory and case studies, *Ped Radiol* 27:87, 1997.
11. Kleinman PK, Marks SC, Adams VI et al: Factors affecting visualization of posterior rib fractures in abused infants, *Am J Radiol* 150:635, 1988.
12. Kleinman PK: Diagnostic imaging in infant abuse, *Am J Radiol* 155:703, 1990.
13. Kleinman PK: Avulsion of the spinous processes caused by infant abuse, *Radiology* 151:389, 1984.

14. Haviland J, Ross R: Outcome after severe non-accidental head injury, *Arch Dis Child* 77:504, 1997.
15. Merten DF, Osbourne DRS: Craniocerebral trauma in the child abuse syndrome, *Ped Ann* 12:882, 1983.
16. Caulder IM, Hill I, Scholtz CL: Primary brain trauma in non-accidental injury, *J Clin Pathol* 37:1095, 1984.
17. Geddes J, Whitwell H: Reply, *Brain* 125:678, 2002.
18. Gilliland MGF, Luckenbach MW: Are retinal hemorrhages found after resuscitation attempts, a study of the eyes of 169 children, *Am J Forensic Med Path* 14:187, 1993.
19. Morad Y, Kim YM, Armstrong DC et al: Correlation between retinal abnormalities and intracranial abnormalities in the shaken baby syndrome, *Ophthalmol* 134:354, 2002.
20. Parulekar MV, Elston JS: Neuropathology of inflicted head injury in children, *Brain* 125:676, 2002.
21. Weedn VW, Mansour AM, Nichols MM: Retinal hemorrhage in an infant after cardiopulmonary resuscitation, *Am J Forensic Med Pathol* 11:79, 1990.
22. Odom A, Christ E, Kerr N et al: Prevalence of retinal hemorrhages in pediatric patients after in hospital cardiopulmonary resuscitation: a prospective study, *Pediatrics* 99:1, 1997.
23. Bergen R, Margolis S: Retinal hemorrhages in the newborn, *Ann Ophthalmol* 8:53, 1976.
24. Duhaime AC, Gennerelli TA, Thibault LE et al: The shaken baby snydrome: a clinical, pathological and biochemical study, *J Neurosurg* 66:409, 1987.
25. Jenny C, Hymel KP, Ritzen A et al: Analysis of missed cases of abusive head trauma, *JAMA* 281:621, 1999.
26. Ng CS, Hall CM, Shaw DG: The range of visceral manifestations of non-accidental injury, *Arch Dis Child* 77:167, 1997.
27. Sivit CJ, Taylor GA, Eichelberger MR: Visceral injury in battered children: a changing perspective, *Radiology* 173: 659, 1989.
28. Touloukian RJ: Abdominal visceral injuries in battered children, *Pediatrics* 42:642, 1968.
29. Cooper A, Floyd T, Barlow B et al: Major blunt abdominal trauma due to child abuse, *J Trauma* 28:1483, 1988.
30. Gornall P, Ahmed S, Jolleys A et al: Intra-abdominal injuries in the battered baby syndrome, *Arch Dis Child* 47:211, 1872.
31. Kirks DR: Radiological evaluation of visceral injuries in the battered child syndrome, *Ped Ann* 12:888, 1983.
32. Knight B: The history of child abuse, *Forensic Sci Int* 30:35, 1986.
33. Case ME, Graham MA, Handy TC et al: Position paper on fatal abusive head injuries in infants and young children, *Am J Forensic Med* 22:112, 2001.
34. Price EA, Rush LR, Perper JA et al: Cardiopulmonary resuscitation related injuries and homicidal blunt abdominal trauma in children, *Am J Forensic Med Pathol* 21:307, 2000.
35. Zumwalt RE, Fanizza-Orphanos AM: Dating of healing rib fractures in fatal child abuse, *Adv Pathol* 3:193, 1990.
36. Centers for Disease Control and Prevention: Guidelines for death scene investigation of sudden unexplained infant deaths. Recommendations of the Interagency Panel on Sudden Infant Death Syndrome, *MMWR Mob Mortal Wkly Rep* 45(RR-10): 1-6, 1996.
37. Wetli CV, Kolovich RM, Dinhofer L: Modified cardiectomy, *Am J Forensic Med Pathol* 23:137, 2002.
38. Clayton EW: Potential liability in cases of child abuse and neglect, *Ped Ann* 26:173, 1997.
39. Hanes M, Mcauliff T: Preparation for child abuse litigation: perspectives of the prosecutor and the pediatrician, *Ped Ann* 26:288, 1997.
40. Wall N: Judicial attitudes to expert evidence in children's cases, *Arch Dis Child* 76:485, 1997.

CHAPTER 107

Severe Traumatic Brain Injury in Infants and Children

Patrick M. Kochanek, Michael L. Forbes, Randall Ruppel, Hülya Bayır, P. David Adelson, and Robert S.B. Clark

PEARLS

- Complete and rapid physiologic resuscitation is essential to the initial treatment of infants and children with severe traumatic brain injury.
- Monitoring and control of intracranial hypertension should begin with first-tier therapies and progress to less well-established second-tier therapies in refractory cases.
- The choice of second-tier therapy is based in part on an in-depth knowledge of the physiologic derangements involved and the preferences of the treating team.

The topic of severe traumatic brain injury (TBI) in infants and children has been the focus of many chapters and reviews but of few clinical reports and even fewer randomized controlled trials (RCTs). The overall lack of clinical trials in infants and children with severe TBI became apparent when a group of physicians and scientists (pediatric critical care medicine specialists, pediatric neurologic surgeons, pediatric emergency medicine specialists, and experts in the methodology of evidence-based medicine) met and published an evidence-based document outlining "Guidelines for the Management of Severe TBI in Infants, Children, and Adolescents" (henceforth referred to as "the pediatric guidelines" in this chapter).[1] The document focused on evidence from pediatric studies. Small controlled studies or even uncontrolled case series of specific therapies in the setting of severe pediatric TBI were scarce. Studies focused on the age-related effects of therapies within the pediatric population were largely absent. Similarly, therapeutic trials in important pediatric subgroups—such as victims of inflicted childhood neurotrauma (child abuse)—were rare. Based on the existing literature, strong recommendations at the guideline level could be made in only a few therapeutic categories. Despite these limitations, this chapter addresses a practical and contemporary approach to the management of these patients based on several sources of information: (1) the pediatric data presented in the pediatric guidelines, (2) data from studies in adults with severe TBI, and (3) accepted principles of the physiology and pathophysiology of the cerebral circulation and cranial vault.

This chapter focuses on severe TBI, specifically on management in the pediatric intensive care unit (PICU). The evolution of PICU management has progressed from exclusively supportive care to strategies attempting to (1) optimize substrate delivery and cerebral metabolism, (2) prevent herniation, and (3) target specific mechanisms involved in the evolution of secondary injury with novel therapies. The goal of contemporary neurointensive care is the prevention of secondary injury. The role of newer technologies and the differences between adults and children are highlighted. For information on mild or moderate TBI, outcomes, or rehabilitation of pediatric TBI, the reader is referred to materials on these topics.[2,3]

Epidemiology

Traumatic brain injury remains a significant pediatric health problem, with an estimated incidence of approximately 230 cases per 100,000.[4] Approximately 100,000 to 200,000 new cases of pediatric TBI are reported each year.[5] This corresponds to a frequency of approximately one case every 2 to 3 minutes.[6] Traumatic brain injury is the most important cause of death and disability in children.[6,7] Specifically, 3000 to 4000 pediatric deaths are reported annually.[8] Approximately 10% to 15% of TBI cases in infants and children are severe (Glasgow coma scale [GCS] score <8), and these cases contribute most of the observed death or permanent brain damage observed.[9] The incidence of pediatric TBI is distributed evenly within three age groups (0–4 years, 5–10 years, 11–15 years) based upon data from the Traumatic Coma Data Bank.[10] Although children 5 to 15 years of age generally have favorable outcomes relative to adults, children 4 years or younger have a worse outcome than older children and adults. Inflicted childhood neurotrauma is the leading cause of severe TBI in infants and is believed to be the key contributor to poor outcome in this young subgroup, although a variety of other factors may play some role.[10] Penetrating injuries such as gunshot wounds, although not as common as either motor vehicle accidents or child abuse, also inflict significant morbidity and mortality on the pediatric population.[11]

Pathophysiology

Traumatic brain injury involves a *primary injury,* which includes direct disruption of brain parenchyma, and *secondary injury,* characterized by a cascade of biochemical, cellular, and molecular events involved in the evolution of secondary damage. In this chapter we define only the key pathophysiologic factors. For detailed information on this topic, the reader is referred to other reviews.[12–14] Secondary injury includes the endogenous evolution of brain damage and the effects of secondary extracerebral insults (i.e., hypotension, hypoxemia) at the injury scene and in the PICU. Three basic categories of mechanisms can be defined (Figure 107–1): those associated with (1) ischemia, excitotoxicity, energy failure, and resultant cell death cascades; (2) secondary cerebral swelling; and (3) axonal injury. A constellation of mediators of secondary damage and repair are involved within each category. The contribution of each mediator to outcome and the interplay among them remain poorly defined. The biochemical and molecular responses to severe TBI resulting from child abuse often are unique and generally severe.[13]

Posttraumatic Ischemia

Since the seminal work of Pickels[14] and Bruce et al.,[15] study on cerebral blood flow (CBF) in pediatric TBI has focused on the role of hyperemia in secondary brain swelling. However, clinical studies in adults showed that CBF is

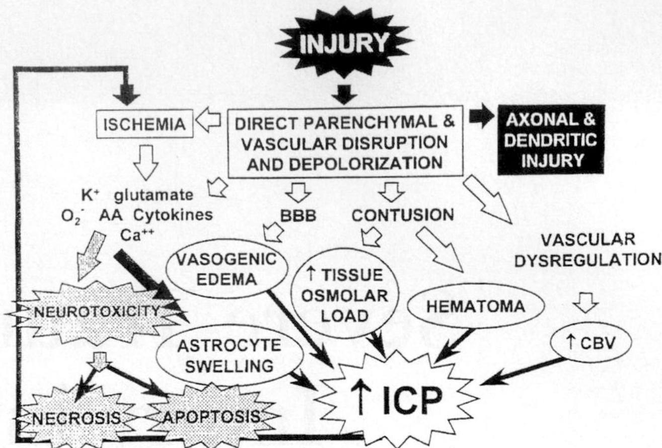

FIGURE 107–1 • Categories of mechanisms proposed to be involved in the evolution of secondary damage after severe traumatic brain injury in infants and children. Three major categories for these secondary mechanisms are (1) ischemia, excitotoxicity, energy failure, and cell death cascades, (2) cerebral swelling, and (3) axonal injury.

reduced early after injury and suggested that early posttraumatic ischemia might be of special importance.[16,17] The devastating consequences of secondary extracerebral insults (i.e., hypotension, hypoxemia) early after TBI are consistent with this possibility. Adelson et al.[18] assessed CBF in 30 infants and children after severe TBI. Early posttraumatic hypoperfusion was common, and a global CBF less than 20 ml/100 g/min was associated with poor outcome. After the initial 24 hours, CBF often recovered, in some cases to high levels. However, delayed increases in CBF were not associated with poor outcome. This work shifted the emphasis away from delayed hyperemia in children toward the recognition and possible treatment of hypoperfusion early after TBI. Numerous mechanisms may underlie early posttraumatic hypoperfusion, including (1) an attenuated vasodilatory response to nitric oxide (NO), cyclic guanosine monophosphate (cGMP), cyclic adenosine monophosphate (cAMP), and/or prostanoids; (2) loss of endothelial NO production; and (3) elaboration of endothelin-1.[13] Early after injury, increases in metabolic demands resulting from uptake of glutamate are reported.[19,20] Thus, reduced metabolic demands coupled with CBF reduction in severely injured brain regions are an unlikely explanation for hypoperfusion.

Excitotoxicity

Excitotoxicity is the process by which glutamate and other excitatory amino acids cause neuronal damage. Glutamate is the most abundant neurotransmitter in the brain, but exposure to toxic levels produces neuronal death.[21] Glutamate exposure produces neuronal injury in two phases. Sodium-dependent neuronal swelling quickly occurs,[22] followed by delayed, calcium-dependent degeneration. These effects are mediated through both ionophore-linked receptors, labeled according to specific agonists (*N*-methyl-D-aspartate [NMDA], kainate, and α-amino-3-hydroxy-5-methyl-4-isoxazolepropionic acid [AMPA]), and receptors linked to second messenger systems (i.e., metabotropic receptors). Activation of these receptors leads to calcium accumulation through receptor-gated or voltage-gated channels or through release of intracellular stores. Increased intracellular calcium concentration triggers a number of processes that can lead to cell death. One mechanism involves activation of constitutive NO synthase, leading to NO production, peroxynitrite formation, and resultant deoxyribonucleic acid (DNA) damage. Poly(ADP-ribose) polymerase (PARP) is an enzyme operative in DNA repair. In the face of excessive DNA damage, PARP activation leads to adenosine triphosphate (ATP) depletion, metabolic failure, and necrotic cell death.[23] In cerebrospinal fluid (CSF) from adults with TBI, glutamate concentrations were approximately 5–fold greater than in control patients (up to 7 μM).[24] These levels are sufficient to cause neuronal death in cell culture. Increased concentrations of glutamate also are seen in CSF of infants and children with TBI and correlate with poor outcome and child abuse as an injury mechanism.[25] Anti-excitotoxic therapies improve outcome after experimental TBI. Pretreatment with NMDA antagonists (e.g., MK-801) attenuate behavioral deficits after experimental TBI.[26] Other therapies that modify glutamate–NMDA receptor interaction and improve outcome after experimental TBI are magnesium, glycine site antagonists, hypothermia, and pentobarbital.[13] Despite these findings, clinical trials with anti-excitotoxic therapies have been unsuccessful in adults. The lack of result may result from side effects of these drugs, delayed treatment, or the antiexcitotoxic effects of many current therapies (e.g., barbiturates, hypothermia, sedatives).[27] Developing neurons are more susceptible to excitotoxic injury than mature cells; however, concerns have been raised about use of NMDA antagonists in children because these drugs may induce apoptotic neurodegeneration.[28] This is a key area for future research.

Apoptosis Cascades

Cells that die after TBI can be categorized on a morphologic continuum ranging from necrosis to apoptosis.[29,30] Apoptosis is a morphologic description of cell death defined by cell shrinkage and nuclear condensation, internucleosomal DNA fragmentation, and formation of apoptotic bodies.[31] In contrast, cells that die of necrosis display cellular and nuclear swelling with dissolution of membranes. Apoptosis requires a cascade of intracellular events for completion of cell death; thus "programmed cell death" is the currently accepted term for the process that leads to apoptosis. In diseases with complex and multiple mechanisms, such as TBI, distinguishing clinical apoptotic from necrotic cell death as classically defined may be difficult,[32] and some cells have mixed phenotypes. In mature tissues, programmed cell death requires initiation via either intracellular or extracellular signals (Figure 107–2). Intracellular signaling appears to be initiated in mitochondria, triggered by disturbances in cellular homeostasis such as ATP depletion, oxidative stress, or calcium fluxes.[33] Mitochondrial dysfunction leads to egress of cytochrome *c* into the cytosol. Cytochrome *c* release can be blocked by anti-apoptotic members of the Bcl-2 family (e.g., Bcl-2, Bcl-xL, Bcl-w, and Mcl-1) and promoted by pro-apoptotic members of the Bcl-2 family (e.g., Bax, Bcl-xS, Bad, and Bid).[34] Cytochrome *c* in the presence of dATP and a specific apoptotic-protease activating factor (APAF-1) in cytosol activates the initiator cysteine protease caspase-9.[35] Caspase-9 then activates the effector cysteine protease caspase-3, which cleaves cytoskeletal proteins, DNA repair proteins, and activators of endonucleases.[36] Extracellular signaling of apoptosis occurs through the tumor necrosis factor (TNF) superfamily of cell surface death receptors, which include TNFR-1 and Fas/Apo1/CD95.[37] Receptor-ligand binding of TNFR-1–TNF-α or Fas–FasL promotes formation of a trimeric complex of TNF- or Fas-associated death domains, respectively. These death domains contain caspase recruitment domains, ultimately leading to activation of caspase-3, where the mitochondrial and cell death receptor pathways converge (Figure 107–2). Both the intrinsic and extrinsic pathways may contribute to the evolution of cell death after severe TBI in infants and children. CSF levels of the anti-apoptotic protein Bcl-2 in pediatric patients after TBI were increased approximately fourfold in TBI versus controls.[38] Similarly, CSF levels of sFas receptor and sFas ligand are increased in TBI patients versus controls.[39] Apoptosis may be a particularly important therapeutic target for novel therapies in infants with severe TBI. Finally, current therapies likely attenuate both necrotic and apoptotic injury cascades.

Taken together, the currently available data strongly suggest that early after injury, severe TBI produces a state of hypoperfusion with simultaneous increased metabolic demands from excitotoxicity. This is a state of enhanced vulnerability to secondary insults (i.e., hypotension, hypoxemia). These processes are intimately linked with the evolution of neuronal death by either necrosis or apoptosis.

Cerebral Swelling

After the initial minutes to hours of posttraumatic hypoperfusion and hypermetabolism, a phase of metabolic depression occurs. Cerebral metabolic rate of oxygen ($CMRO_2$) decreases to approximately one third of normal[40,41] and is maintained at that level for the duration of coma. The exact etiology of this state remains to be defined; however, contributions from reduced synaptic activity and mitochondrial failure may be important.[42] Sustained increases in glycolytic metabolic demands are reported in some cases, possibly related to seizure activity or sustained increases in glutamate levels,[20] but these cases appear to be the exception, at least in adults in whom this finding is best characterized. During the PICU phase, cerebral swelling develops and generally peaks between 24 and 72 hours after injury, although sustained increases in intracranial pressure (ICP) for 1 week or longer occasionally are observed.

Cerebral Blood Volume

Several mechanisms may contribute to intracranial hypertension in infants and children after severe TBI (Figure 107–1). Brain swelling and accompanying intracranial hypertension contribute to secondary damage in two ways. Intracranial hypertension can compromise cerebral perfusion leading to secondary ischemia, and it can produce the devastating consequences of deformation through herniation syndromes. Bruce et al.[15] described the phenomenon of "malignant posttraumatic cerebral swelling" in children. Cerebral blood flow was measured in six children, and hyperemia was believed to be the major culprit. Muizelaar et al.[43] in a series of 32 children and Beyda et al.[44] suggested similar findings. However, Sharples et al.[45,46]

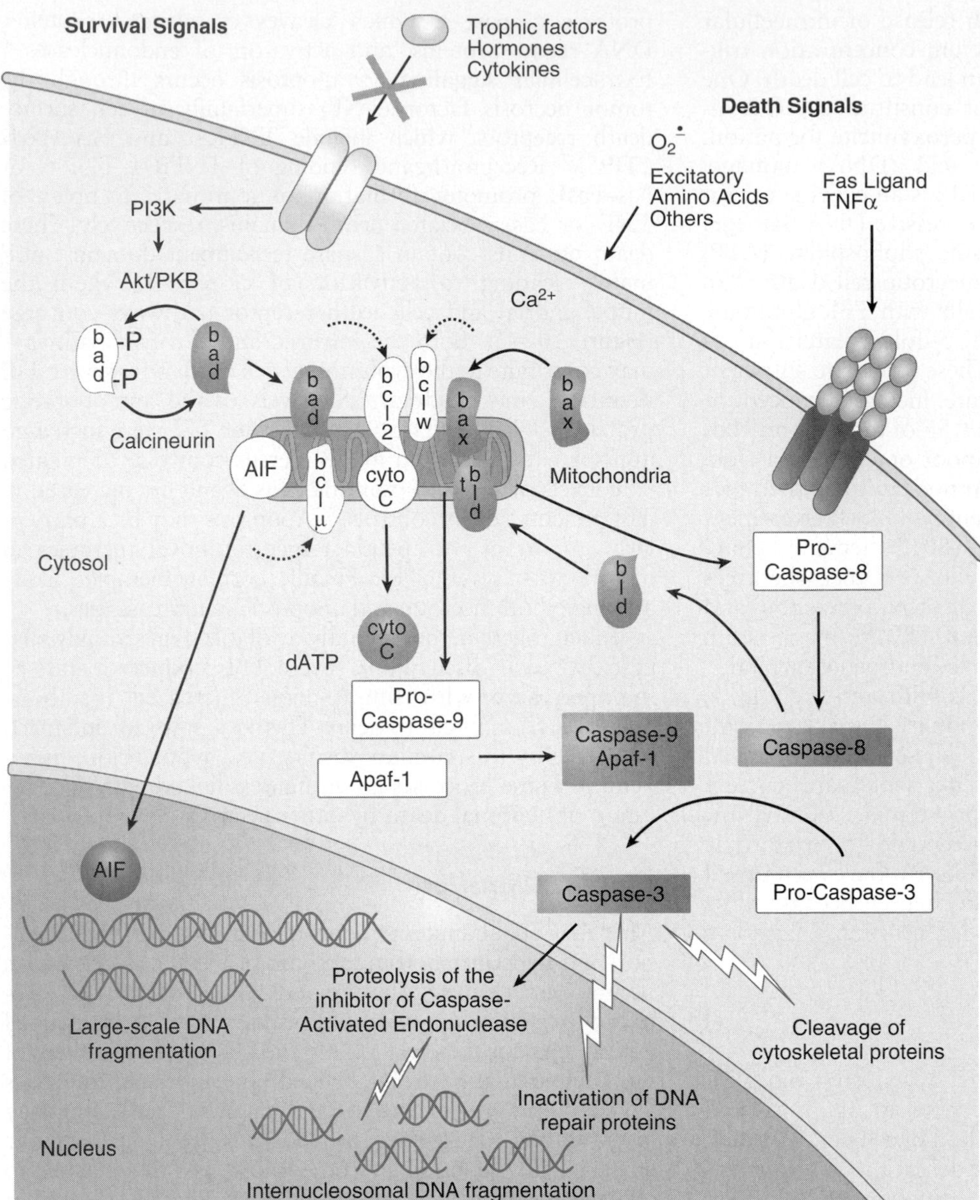

FIGURE 107–2 • Cell death cascades involved in delayed neuronal death after severe traumatic brain injury.

suggested that hyperemia was uncommon after severe TBI in children; rather, reduced $CMRO_2$ was associated with poor outcome. Suzuki[47] measured CBF in 80 unanesthetized normal children. They showed an age dependence of CBF, with remarkably high values in children ages 2 to 9 years, levels previously suggested to represent posttraumatic hyperemia. Nevertheless, after resolution of the early posttraumatic hypoperfusion, CBF may increase to levels greater than metabolic demands in some children, producing a state of relative hyperemia.[13] Bergsneider et al.[20] posed the alternative hypothesis of "hyperglycolysis" to explain the increases in CBF in patients with severe TBI whose CBF is uncoupled from $CMRO_2$. Cerebral glutamate uptake is coupled to glucose utilization by glycolysis in astrocytes. Thus in injured brain regions with reduced $CMRO_2$, increases in CBF may be coupled to local increases in glucose utilization by astrocytes even in the absence of ischemia. Local or global "hyperglycolysis" occurs in adults with severe TBI.[20] The incidence and/or importance of secondary "hyperemia" or hyperglycolysis in pediatric TBI remains to be determined. It may occur in select cases, but secondary increases in CBF probably are not the major culprit in the development of intracranial hypertension. Increases in CBF were not associated with intracranial hypertension in adults,[48] and hyperemia was not associated with poor outcome in children.[4] The contribution of hyperemia (increased cerebral blood volume [CBV]) to the development of intracranial hypertension has been studied in adults with TBI.[49] Increased CBV was seen in only a small number of patients. These studies suggest that the importance of posttraumatic hyperemia may have been overstated, and edema rather than hyperemia may be the predominant contributor to cerebral swelling after TBI.[50]

Edema

Both cytotoxic and vasogenic edema may play important roles in cerebral swelling (Figure 107–3). However, our

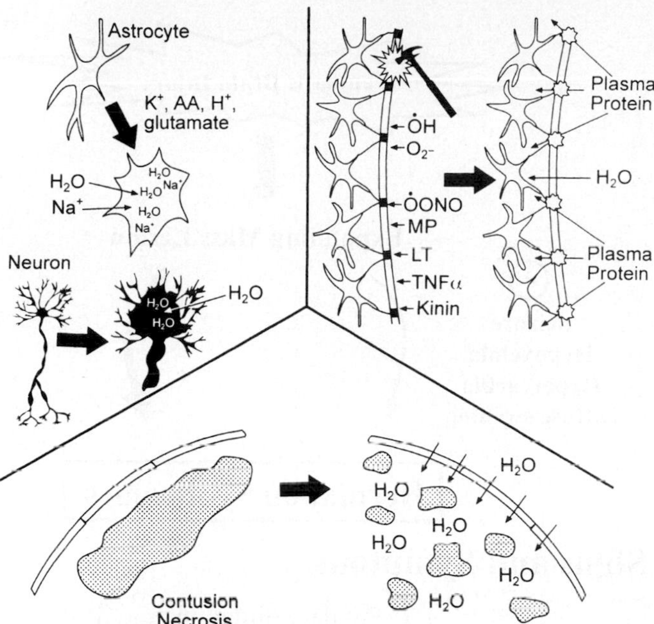

FIGURE 107–3 • Schematic of three cascades leading to cerebral edema. **Top left,** Cellular swelling is predominantly seen in astrocytes and is stimulated by potassium, acidosis, glutamate, arachidonic acid *(AA),* and other factors. This key pathway is less representative of a toxic process and more consistent with a homeostatic or mediator-driven process. Neuronal swelling from pump leak probably is less important. **Bottom:** Osmolar swelling from contusion necrosis. In the hours after injury, reconstitution of the blood-brain barrier (BBB) or development of an osmolar barrier around a contusion sets the stage for massive local swelling as the macromolecules in the contusion break down, increasing local osmolality. **Top right:** Vasogenic edema results from protein and water accumulation across the damaged BBB, which is formed by tight junctions (astrocyte foot processes). Direct vascular disruption by trauma, reactive oxygen species such as hydroxyl radical (•OH), superoxide anion (O_2^-), and peroxynitrite (•ONOO), metalloproteases (MP), kinins, leukotrienes (LT), cytokines, and other mediators contribute to BBB damage.

traditional concept of cytotoxic and vasogenic edema is evolving. There appear to be four putative mechanisms for edema formation in the injured brain. First, vasogenic edema may form in the extracellular space as a result of blood-brain barrier (BBB) disruption. Second, cellular swelling can be produced in two ways. Astrocyte swelling can occur as part of the homeostatic uptake of substances such as glutamate. Glutamate uptake is coupled to glucose utilization via a sodium/potassium ATPase, with sodium and water accumulation in astrocytes. Swelling of both neurons and other cells in the neuropil can result from ischemia- or trauma-induced ionic pump failure. Finally, osmolar swelling may contribute to edema formation in the extracellular space, particularly in contusions. Osmolar swelling actually is dependent on an intact BBB or an alternative solute barrier. Cellular swelling may be of greatest importance. Using a model of diffuse TBI in rats, Barzo et al.[51] applied diffusion-weighted magnetic resonance imaging (MRI) to localize the increase in brain water. A decrease in the apparent diffuse coefficient after injury suggested predominantly cellular swelling rather than vasogenic edema in the development of intracranial hypertension. Katayama et al.[52] also suggested that the role of BBB in the development of posttraumatic edema may have been overstated, even in the setting of cerebral contusion. An intriguing possibility is that as macromolecules are degraded within injured brain regions, the osmolar load in the contused tissue increases. As the BBB reconstitutes (or as other osmolar barriers form), a considerable osmolar driving force for local accumulation of water develops, resulting in the marked swelling so often seen in and around cerebral contusions. Thus in either diffuse injury or focal contusion, BBB permeability may play only a limited role in the development of cerebral swelling. If these results can be generalized, then hypertonic saline or mannitol seem to represent optimal therapies. This is in contrast to traditional recommendations, where hyperventilation (rather than mannitol) has been suggested.[53,54] Studies of the extent of BBB injury and the contribution of cellular swelling to intracranial hypertension in pediatric TBI are needed.

Axonal Injury

Traumatic axonal injury (TAI) encompasses the spectrum from mild to severe TBI.[55,56] The extent and distribution of TAI depend on injury severity and category (focal vs. diffuse). The incidence and nature of axonal injury appear to be age independent,[57] but the consequences may be particularly devastating in children.[58] The effects of TAI in children during a period of developmental axonal connectivity remain unknown but likely are considerable. During development, numerous signaling molecules can function as attractants or repellents.[59] To our knowledge, no clinical data on these molecules after pediatric TBI are available. Traumatic axonal injury appears to be even more prevalent in victims of child abuse.[60] The classic view that TAI occurs because of immediate physical shearing is represented primarily in severe injury where frank axonal tears occur. Experimental studies suggest that TAI occurs by a delayed process termed *secondary axotomy,* which results from either calcium accumulation or altered axoplasmic flow.[61] Traumatic axonal injury contributes to the morbidity after TBI.[61] Laboratory studies suggest that hypothermia and cyclosporine A can attenuate TAI, but clinical data are lacking.

History

Unlike adult TBI, where the history is generally straightforward, the special case of inflicted childhood neurotrauma contributes to increased importance of the history in pediatric TBI. For a discussion of the topic, the reader is referred to Duhaime.[62] In cases of severe TBI resulting from child abuse, a history that is incompatible with the observed injury is often given. In some cases of severe inflicted childhood neurotrauma, there is no history of trauma.[63] Occult presentations of inflicted childhood neurotrauma can be particularly important because they may be recognized as cases of severe TBI relatively late in their treatment course.[64] In this setting, brain edema already may have evolved to life-threatening levels, and other superimposed secondary insults (e.g., seizures, apnea) may complicate management and worsen outcome.

TABLE 107–1

Coma Scales

Glasgow Coma Scale	Modified Coma Scale for Infants	Point Value
Eye opening		
Spontaneous	Spontaneous	4
To speech	To speech	3
To pain	To pain	2
None	None	1
Verbal		
Oriented	Coos, babbles	5
Confused	Irritable	4
Inappropriate words	Cries to pain	3
Grunting	Moans to pain	2
None	None	1
Motor		
Follows commands	Normal spontaneous movements	6
Localizes pain	Withdraws to touch	5
Withdraws to pain	Withdraws to pain	4
Abnormal flexion	Abnormal flexion	3
Abnormal extension	Abnormal extension	2
Flaccid	Flaccid	1

Signs and Symptoms

The GCS score[65] (Table 107–1), first described in 1974, remains a valuable tool for grading and communicating severity of neurologic injury after TBI. The verbal and motor components of the GCS score have been modified for assessment of infants,[66] but this modification has not been validated in infants and young children. The motor score probably is the most important component of the GCS score. A rapid "mini-neuroassessment," which allows evaluation of the patient's level of consciousness, pupillary size and light response, the fundi, extraocular movements, response of extremities to pain, deep tendon reflexes, and brainstem reflexes, provides valuable information and should be part of the initial evaluation.[67] Until proven otherwise, an altered level of consciousness, pupillary dysfunction, and lateralizing extremity weakness in an infant or child should raise suspicion of a mass lesion that may require surgery.[68] These signs of impending herniation require an immediate response, as outlined in Figure 107–4.

Initial Resuscitation

The identification and correction of airway obstruction, inadequate ventilation, and shock take priority over a detailed neurologic assessment.[69] Thus the first step in managing the head-injured patient is complete, rapid physiologic resuscitation.[1] Although intracranial hypertension and cerebral herniation are the major complications of severe TBI, brain-specific interventions in the absence of signs of herniation or other neurologic deterioration currently are not recommended. Mannitol may be counterproductive for the management of malignant intracranial hypertension during initial resuscitative efforts. In the acute

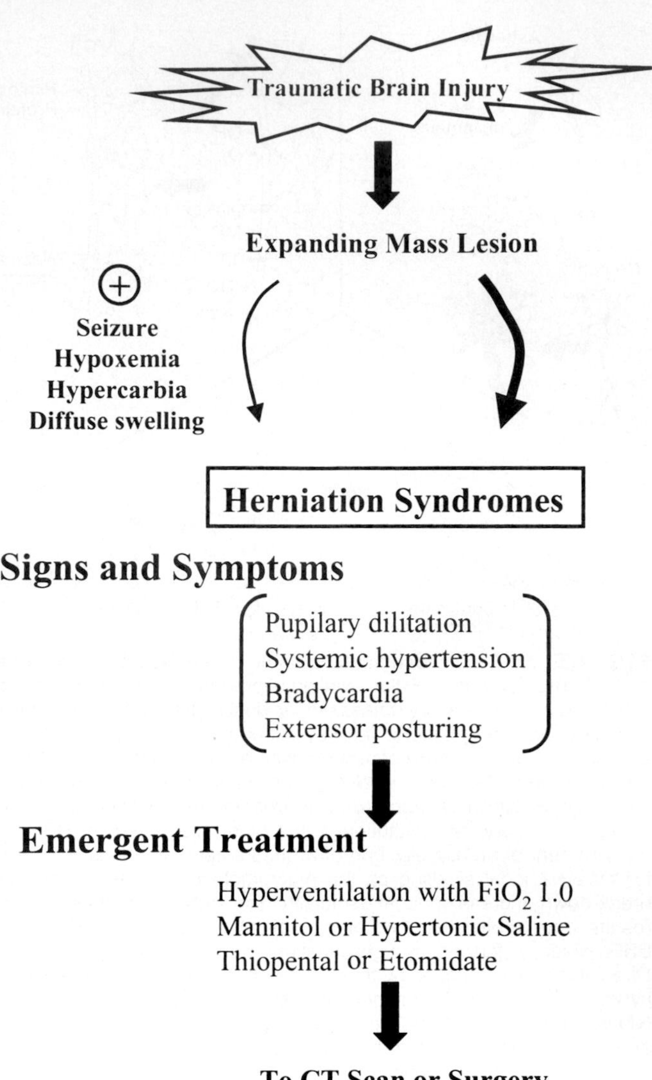

FIGURE 107–4 • Treatment paradigm for management of signs and symptoms of acute herniation after severe traumatic brain injury in infants and children.

TBI resuscitation setting, hypertonic saline may be a better alternative (discussed on page 1608). Studies have consistently shown increased morbidity and mortality associated with hypotension and hypoxemia.[70,71] Gentleman[71] reported that, during an 11-year period in England, the increased use of endotracheal intubation and ventilation from 11% to 82% produced a concomitant reduction in episodes of hypoxemia from 22% to 8%. This was accompanied by a reduction in the mortality rate from 45% to 32% and an increase in good outcome from 40% to 58%. Although the basis for this improvement may be multifactorial, early targeted intervention specifically directed at correcting hypoxemia and hypovolemia must be the objective of initial therapy. However, specific recommendations for intubation at the scene are complex and likely are influenced by the expertise of the paramedics or other caregivers in the field and by the transport distance, among other factors.[1]

All trauma patients with supraclavicular injury should be assumed to have cranial and cervical spine injuries until proven otherwise. The initial evaluation of a child after severe TBI begins by demonstrating the presence of a patent, maintainable airway—the patient must be conscious, alert, and breathing spontaneously. Unconscious patients must be assumed to have an obstructed airway requiring immediate airway evaluation. The relatively large head, occiput, and tongue and the short narrow epiglottis of the infant facilitate airway obstruction if the child's sensorium has been clouded. The rescuer must alleviate this situation immediately (while protecting the cervical spine) in order to minimize secondary injury from hypoxia.

We previously outlined the use of the mnemonic S-O-A-P to define the necessary components for optimal preparation for securing the airway in the case of severe TBI requiring intubation in either the emergency department or the PICU.[72] *S (suction):* For most patients, a flexible 10F catheter suffices. However, for school-age children (older than 5 years), we recommend the Yankauer rigid plastic suction catheter, which allows direct oropharyngeal suctioning. *O (oxygen):* Oxygen ($FIO_2 = 1$) should be delivered to the patient by face mask immediately prior to intubation. Optimal positioning of the patient requires immobilization of the neck to stabilize the cervical spine. Delivery of 100% oxygen facilitates washout of nitrogen from the functional residual capacity, allowing adequate alveolar oxygenation for safe intubation of the trachea. *A (airway):* Once the patient is properly positioned, ventilation and oxygenation are controlled, and an age-appropriate laryngoscope blade and endotracheal tube are selected. The endotracheal tube is secured with adhesive tape, which should not pass circumferentially around the neck because cerebral venous return may be compressed. *P (pharmacology):* The medications chosen must be potent and rapid in their onset of action. The goals of analgesia, amnesia, and neuromuscular blockade must be met rapidly. Ideally, the patient never receives a preintubation positive-pressure breath.

Optimal tracheal intubation of the child with severe TBI requires a cerebroprotective, rapid-sequence technique whenever possible. Bag-valve-mask positive-pressure ventilation should be avoided. However, in cases of hypoxemia or impending herniation, positive-pressure ventilation should be instituted immediately.[73] Bag-valve-mask technique may cause more unintentional cervical spine manipulation than previously appreciated, so great care is advised during manual ventilation.[74] If a victim of TBI meets any of the criteria given in Box 107–1, assisted ventilation is indicated with an orotracheal tube as the modality of choice.[73,75]

In children, the recommended route of initial airway control is "orotracheal intubation under direct vision."[76] Nasotracheal intubation should be avoided. Blind passage of the endotracheal tube around the acute nasopharyngeal angle makes this procedure an unnecessary obstacle to rapid, complete physiologic resuscitation. Orotracheal intubation can be accomplished using a two-person strategy that protects the cervical spine from injury. A normal lateral c-spine roentgenogram is reassuring but *does not rule out* cervical spine injury.[77] Spinal immobilization must be maintained.[78] This is accomplished via in-line cervical immobilization by one operator while the second intubates the trachea. Care must be taken to avoid pressing into the soft tissues of the submental region and strap muscles because inadvertent airway obstruction may ensue.

BOX 107–1

Criteria for Intubation of the Head-Injured Child

GCS score ≤ 10
Decrease in GCS of > 3, independent of the initial GCS
Anisocoria > 1 mm
Cervical spine injury compromising ventilation
Apnea
Hypercarbia ($PaCO_2$ > 45 mmHg)
Loss of pharyngeal reflex
Spontaneous hyperventilation causing $PaCO_2$ < 25 mmHg

Rapid-Sequence Induction and Intubation

Endotracheal intubation, although life saving, is a noxious stimulus. The technique of rapid-sequence induction and intubation secures the airway of an unprepared patient, who is at risk for aspiration of gastric contents, in an immediate and safe manner. There is no resistance to direct laryngoscopy, and the normal responses to intentional placement of a large foreign body into the trachea are eliminated. Rapid-sequence induction is documented to be a safer technique than either nasotracheal intubation or orotracheal intubation without neuromuscular blockade.[79,80] In the pediatric patient with TBI, a cerebroprotective rapid-sequence induction strategy should be used. The sequence involves preparation, preoxygenation, sedation, neuromuscular blockade, and orotracheal intubation. Pharmacologic adjuncts are used to prevent morbidity associated with hypotension, hypoxemia, intracranial hypertension, and gastric aspiration. The neurologic and hemodynamic status of the patient directs the choice of adjunctive pharmacologic strategy. For a victim in cardiac arrest, cardiopulmonary resuscitation should begin immediately, accompanied by direct orotracheal intubation. No pharmacologic adjuncts are necessary to secure the airway. For the hemodynamically unstable patient, the combination of etomidate, lidocaine, and rocuronium bromide is the first choice. An alternative is the combination of fentanyl, lidocaine, and vecuronium (Table 107–2). Either of these same sequences of drugs can be used in hemodynamically stable patients, for whom a rapidly acting benzodiazepine (midazolam) can be added. An alternative in the hemodynamically stable patient is thiopental. Both etomidate and thiopental are ultrafast acting and rapidly reduce cerebral metabolism.[81–84] This in turn attenuates the intracranial hypertension associated with direct laryngoscopy. The rapid cerebral uptake of these agents is matched by rapid washout. Therefore, these agents must be followed with another sedative/analgesic agent. The short-acting narcotic fentanyl, in combination with lidocaine, reduces the catecholamine surge associated with direct laryngoscopy.[73]

Circulatory Stabilization

Assessment of circulatory function after trauma involves the rapid determination of heart rate, blood pressure, central and peripheral pulse quality, capillary refill, and

TABLE 107–2

Drugs for Intubation of the Head-Injured Child

Situation	Drugs
Cardiopulmonary arrest	Resuscitation drugs
Hemodynamically unstable	Etomidate 0.2–0.6 mg/kg* Lidocaine 1 mg/kg Rocuronium 1 mg/kg or vecuronium 0.3 mg/kg *Or* Fentanyl 2–4 μg/kg Lidocaine 1 mg/kg Rocuronium 1 mg/kg or vecuronium 0.3 mg/kg
Hemodynamically stable	Etomidate 0.2–0.6 mg/kg* Lidocaine 1 mg/kg Midazolam 0.1–0.2 mg Rocuronium 1 mg/kg or vecuronium 0.3 mg/kg *Or* Fentanyl 2–4 μg/kg Lidocaine 1 mg/kg Midazolam 0.1–0.2 mg/kg Rocuronium 1 mg/kg or vecuronium 0.3 mg/kg *Or* Thiopental 4–5 mg/kg Lidocaine 1 mg/kg Rocuronium 1 mg/kg or vecuronium 0.3 mg/kg

*Use of etomidate in this setting in some centers is limited to children older than 1 year.

cerebral perfusion.[85] Posttraumatic hypoperfusion must be assumed to be hypovolemic (i.e., hemorrhagic) in nature, but it also may have a secondary component of myocardial depression resulting from cardiac contusion. However, cardiac contusion is less common in children than in adults. In severe TBI, fluid therapy for hypovolemic shock entails rapid replacement of vascular volume. The choice of resuscitation fluid is controversial. The current recommendation is 20 ml/kg isotonic crystalloid (0.9% NaCl solution) administered as soon as vascular access is obtained. Hypotonic fluid should not be used in the initial resuscitation of the brain-injured patient. Subsequent doses of fluid should be isotonic crystalloid, colloid, or packed red blood cells and titrated based on serial assessment of blood pressure, perfusion, and hematocrit. Although concerns exist regarding the relative hypotonicity of lactated Ringer solution,[86] evidence from studies in laboratory animals supports the safety of lactated Ringer solution use in patients with TBI.[87] Fisher et al.[88] reported the successful use of 3% saline as a maintenance fluid in pediatric TBI. Titration of 3% saline as an infusion to prevent development of intracranial hypertension is an acceptable first-tier strategy. Although not yet proved in a clinical trial, inclusion of hypertonic saline should be considered in the setting of volume resuscitation of the pediatric TBI victim with initial signs or symptoms of intracranial hypertension. Details of the approach to osmotherapy are discussed later.

Herniation

The need to simultaneously address airway control, cardiovascular assessment and stabilization, treatment of extracerebral insults (hemorrhage, multiple trauma), and initial trauma survey in the field and/or emergency department makes management particularly challenging. Although mass lesions are less common in children than in adults, they still occur in approximately 30% of children with severe TBI.[6] Some of these patients, particularly those with rapidly expanding mass lesions (e.g., epidural hematoma), can present with signs and symptoms of herniation (pupillary dilatation, systemic hypertension, bradycardia, extensor posturing). Because the devastating complications of herniation sometimes can be prevented or treated in the initial minutes of their progression, the importance of aggressively and presumptively treating signs and symptoms of herniation, which is a medical emergency, cannot be overemphasized until these signs and symptoms are proved not to represent herniation. Appropriately, there has been a move away from prophylactic application of aggressive hyperventilation for the management of adults or children with severe TBI. However, it is important to recognize that use of hyperventilation with $FIO_2 = 1.0$ is a therapy that can be immediately applied and can be life saving in the setting of impending herniation. Intubating doses of thiopental or etomidate and mannitol (0.25–1.0 g/kg) or hypertonic saline[88] also should be administered emergently in this setting. One must recognize that factors other than a focal mass lesion may lead to herniation, and that these situations may arise more commonly in children than in adults. Diffuse swelling is more common in infants and children than in adults, and in this setting, inadvertent hypercarbia or hypoxemia, iatrogenic excessive fluid administration, or status epilepticus can precipitate herniation. Although discussed in this chapter, early in the continuum of care, it must be recognized that herniation also can occur during PICU management, and this general approach to treatment also applies (Figure 107–4).

Transition from the Emergency Department to the Pediatric Intensive Care Unit: Computed Tomographic Scan and Intracranial Pressure Monitoring

The transition of patients with severe TBI from the emergency department to the PICU includes computed tomographic (CT) evaluation of the head (and other anatomic regions, when clinically indicated) followed by attachment to an ICP monitor, transport to the operating suite for surgical intervention, or both. In the initial resuscitation, sedation must be carefully titrated, maintaining the difficult balance that produces stability, analgesia, and anxiolysis during transport and scanning while allowing for rapid emergence for clinical assessment (as indicated) until a decision is made regarding surgery or ICP monitoring. Because the early period after injury generally reflects a state of increased vulnerability of the brain to secondary insults because of the brain's increased metabolic demands and compromised perfusion, adequate sedation and stable hemodynamics are particularly important. Clinical trials supporting definitive recommendations are not available. Nevertheless, the risks of intrahospital transport are well described[89]; therefore, a physician should accompany the infant or child on transport to the scanner and then to direct care because serial assessment to titrate therapy is needed during the acute phase of injury.

Diagnostic Studies and Monitoring Modalities

Computed Tomography

Since becoming commercially available in 1973, CT has been of enormous benefit to neurointensive care.[90] A three-dimensional anatomic map of the brain structure facilitates the diagnosis and management of children with severe TBI. Examples of classic findings in severe pediatric TBI are shown in Figure 107–5. Comprehensive classifications of CT findings in adults with severe TBI are reported. The Marshall classification is the most commonly used (Table 107–3).[91] A similar system specifically for pediatric TBI is not described, although several reviews characterize the spectrum of injury in infants and children as defined by CT.[92,93] Ewing-Cobbs et al.[92] compared acute CT findings in infants and children with inflicted and noninflicted injuries. Subdural interhemispheric and convexity hemorrhages and preexisting lesions were two to three times more common in the inflicted TBI group. Epidural hematomas were more common in the noninflicted TBI group. Timing of repeat cranial CT scans has been investigated, including studies in children. Routine reimaging at 24 or 48 hours after injury has been suggested.[94] However, Tabori et al.[95] evaluated the impact of routine reimaging on 67 children after severe TBI and noted that although some new lesions were identified, reimaging did not lead to surgical or medical changes in therapy in any patient. A decision to reimage based on changes in ICP or clinical examination was recommended. Such an approach also is recommended in published pediatric guidelines.[1] Studies in adults and children indicate that CT scans are not without limitations and must be used as only one, albeit important, piece of information. After severe TBI, approximately 15% of adults with a normal CT scan develop clinically significant intracranial hypertension. In contrast, in a study in 65 children, Hirsch et al.[96] reported CT scan had a high false-positive rate in defining increased ICP. Finally, patients with normal initial head CT scans who also have hypotension or abnormal posturing have the same propensity to develop intracranial hypertension as their counterparts with an abnormal scan.[30,31]

Magnetic Resonance Imaging

Magnetic resonance imaging may have future applications salient to acute management in TBI. The application of diffusion-weighted MRI for studying the evolution of cerebral edema[49] and the use of novel MRI methods for quantifying CBF[97] are being investigated. The potential ability to couple these techniques with MR spectroscopy and functional MRI should yield unprecedented advances in our understanding of the brain's response to injury. However, MRI suites in most institutions are remote from the emergency department and PICU, introducing the risk of intrahospital transport. Currently, hardware incompatibilities (ventilators, intravenous pumps) and long data acquisition times (relative to CT) limit the utility of this important tool.

Intracranial Pressure Monitoring

It has long been recognized that clinical signs such as pupillary size and light response and papilledema fail as early indicators of intracranial hypertension. Although the most reliable clinical signs are those associated with herniation, the introduction of ICP monitoring devices has allowed detection of intracranial hypertension before such changes are observed.[98,99] In the pediatric guidelines,[1] ICP monitoring was suggested as appropriate in children with an abnormal admission head CT scan and initial GCS between 3 and 8. In addition, ICP monitoring was suggested to be appropriate in adults with severe TBI and a normal head CT scan if the clinical course was complicated by hypotension or motor posturing. This modality is essential to implementation of a physiologically guided approach to management of cerebral perfusion pressure (CPP) in the infant or child with severe TBI.[100] ICP monitoring has not been studied in an RCT to establish its efficacy in altering outcome after severe TBI in either adults or children. Given that intracranial hypertension correlates with poor outcome, there is strong rationale for identifying and expeditiously treating this problem.[101,102] As discussed earlier, although CT is useful for identifying patients at high risk for developing intracranial hypertension (e.g., those with mass lesions), the finding of a "normal" cranial CT scan does not rule out the potential for intracranial hypertension.[103] Finally, consideration of risk versus benefit for ICP monitoring must be involved in the clinical decision in cases where the complication rate is high, such as patients with coagulopathy.

Currently, ICP monitoring by ventricular catheter is considered the most accurate, low-cost, reliable method.[1] The ventricular catheter also affords a key therapeutic option—CSF drainage. Other acceptable methods include parenchymal fiberoptic and microtransducer systems; subarachnoid, subdural, and epidural monitors of any type are less reliable.[104] The type of monitor (ventricular catheter or fiberoptic pressure transducer) used is dependent on the local preference of the neurosurgical staff.

Location of monitors in the hospital varies among centers and includes the emergency department/trauma bay, operating room, or PICU. Despite the flurry of activity that often surrounds the stabilization of a critically injured child with severe TBI, it is important to provide adequate anesthesia during attachment of the monitor to prevent pain-induced spikes in ICP and/or herniation.

Monitoring and treatment of ICP are essential to optimal contemporary management. Use of a ventricular catheter affords the added opportunity of CSF drainage as a therapeutic option. Adult victims of severe TBI with an ICP greater than 20 mmHg have a poorer outcome that those without

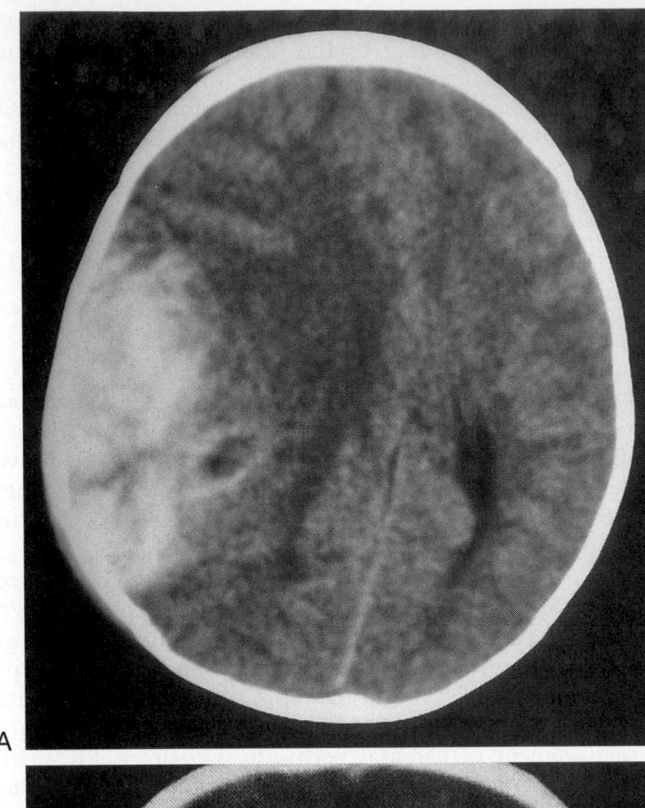

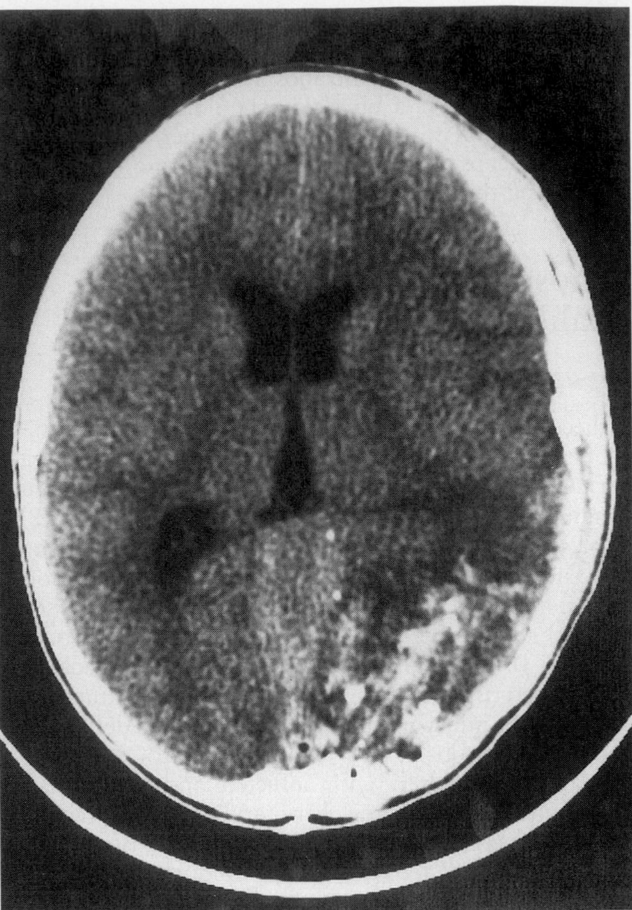

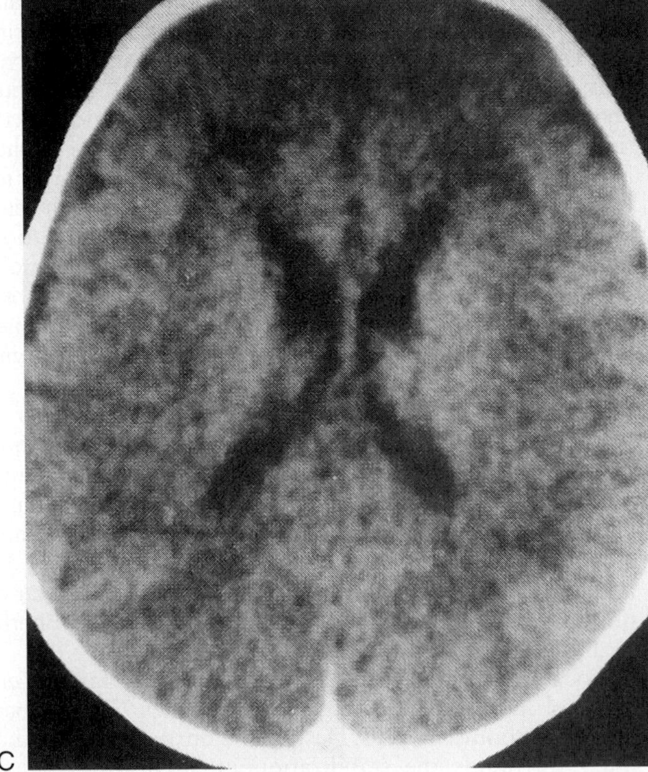

FIGURE 107–5 • Axial cranial computed tomographic (CT) images of important lesions in pediatric traumatic brain injury including **(A)** acute epidural hematoma, **(B)** penetrating brain injury resulting from a gunshot wound (with bullet fragments), and **(C)** inflicted childhood neurotrauma (shaken baby syndrome) with a subtle posterior subdural hematoma.

increased ICP.[104] Similarly, although a large prospective RCT of children with and without both ICP monitoring and CPP management has not been performed, a prospective cohort study suggested better outcome in adults monitored and treated with CSF drainage versus those without ICP monitoring.[105] Further study is needed.

Advanced Monitoring Techniques

Several techniques for assessing CBF or metabolism can provide additional insight into the occurrence of cerebral ischemia during the management of infants and children with severe TBI and thus help guide therapy. However, information on the use of these techniques and their impact

TABLE 107–3

Marshall Classification of Cranial Computed Tomographic Scans

Classification	Findings on Scan
Diffuse injury I (no visible pathologic change)	No visible intracranial pathologic change seen on CT
Diffuse injury II	Cisterns are present with shift 0–5 mm *and/or* Lesion densities present No high or mixed density lesion > 25 ml May include bone fragments and foreign bodies
Diffuse injury III (swelling)	Cisterns compressed or absent with shift 0–5 mm No high or mixed density lesion > 25 ml
Diffuse injury IV (shift)	Shift > 5 mm No high or mixed density lesion > 25 ml
Evacuated mass lesion	Any surgically evacuated lesion
Nonevacuated mass lesion	High or mixed density lesion > 25 ml, not surgically evacuated
Brain dead	No brainstem reflexes Flaccidity Fixed and nonreactive pupils No spontaneous respirations with a normal Pa_{CO_2} Spinal reflexes permitted

on outcome in infants and children with severe TBI is inadequate. In some cases, use of these methods is limited to clinical research or specialized trauma centers with particular interest in pediatric neurointensive care.

Techniques for measuring CBF after severe TBI include (1) stable xenon (Xe)-enhanced CT, (2) radioactive (inhaled or injected) ^{133}Xe methods, and (3) transcranial Doppler (TCD) methods. Stable Xe CT CBF measurement is a tool that can aid in clinical decision making during management of infants and children with severe TBI.[18,72,106,107] Although not a "monitor" in the sense that it does not provide minute-to-minute assessment of changes, stable Xe CT CBF measurement provides important information about regional CBF and its relationship to anatomic disturbances (Figure 107–6). This technique can be readily coupled to nearly all CT scans obtained in the evaluation and follow-up of severely brain-injured infants and children, including the initial scan.[18,72,106,107] The procedure can be completed in less than 30 minutes. It is complicated when F_{IO_2} or mean airway pressure is high (because of the need for inhalation of 50% Xe gas and the effect of its inherently increased density) or if ICP is markedly increased. In those settings, careful monitoring of the patient is needed during the study. Serial stable Xe CT CBF measurements can be coupled to a physiologic manipulation, such as alteration of mean arterial blood pressure or Pa_{CO_2} (Figure 107–7).[72,108,109] These dynamic "pre and post" studies often provide additional insight into the optimal titration of bedside interventions

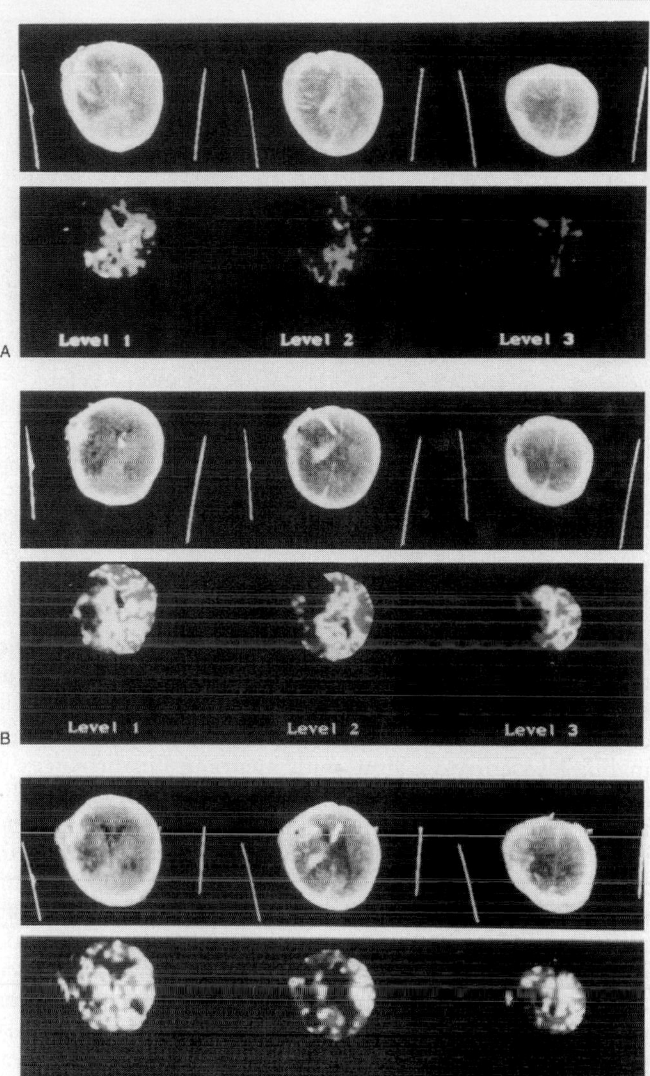

FIGURE 107–6 • Time course of cerebral blood flow (CBF) measured by xenon (Xe)-enhanced computed tomography (CT) in a 2-month-old infant after severe traumatic brain injury from a motor vehicle accident. Standard CT images **(upper row)** and Xe-enhanced CBF maps **(lower row)** are shown from studies performed on admission *(a)* and at 2 days *(b)* and 5 days *(c)* after injury. Cerebral blood flow is severely reduced *(black)* on admission. Some recovery of CBF is seen at 2 days and 5 days after injury. CBF ranges from lowest *(darkest image)* to highest *(brightest image)*.

such as CO_2 levels and additional prognostic information. Although titration of therapy to ICP or CPP is important, this technique demonstrates that the response of the brain to an intervention such as manipulation of blood pressure or Pa_{CO_2} or administration of a specific drug often is not homogeneous and may be unpredictable. The response often but not always is reflected by a change in ICP or CPP, as seen with focal losses of blood pressure autoregulation of CBF or reactivity to changes in Pa_{CO_2}. Currently, the stable Xe technique can be used as part of clinical care, but informed consent is required (Personal Communication, Howard Yonas). The ^{133}Xe method for assessment of patients with TBI was pioneered by Obrist et al.[110] By using multiple detectors, this method can provide information on regional CBF, and it can be used in dynamic studies. The advantage of the ^{133}Xe method over the stable Xe CT method is that the ^{133}Xe

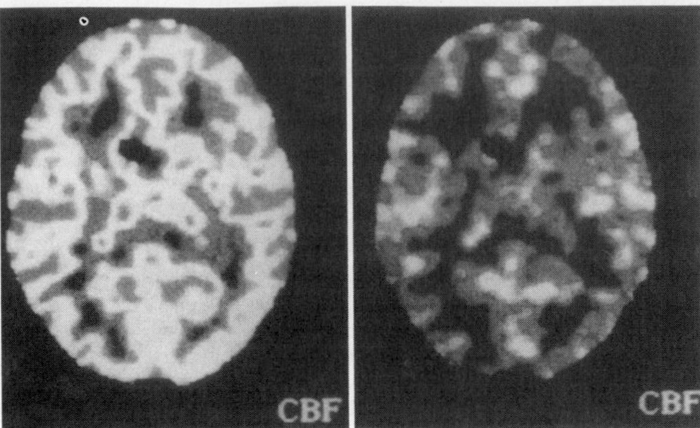

FIGURE 107–7 • Xenon-enhanced cerebral blood flow (CBF) maps from a child with severe traumatic brain injury before **(left)** and after **(right)** escalation of hyperventilation in the scanner. Intact reactivity of CBF to change in $Paco_2$ is demonstrated by an obvious reduction in flow. Cerebral blood flow ranges from lowest *(darkest image)* to highest *(brightest image)*.

method is a monitoring technique that can be repeated frequently at the bedside. This method has been used in children with TBI to define the time course and magnitude of changes in CBF and its regulation.[15,43–46] However, its inability to correlate flow with anatomic disturbances is an important limitation. At our institution, we prefer the stable Xe CT method. Transcranial Doppler, a method sometimes used in adult neurointensive care, has been of limited use in children.[111,112] Transcranial Doppler can serve as an early warning monitor of the development of an unfavorable trend in cerebral perfusion.[111,112] This method measures velocity rather than flow and usually is applied to assess the middle cerebral artery distribution. However, the ability to acquire regional information using Xe CT and MRI has limited the application of the TCD method in children.[113]

Monitoring Cerebral Metabolism

Jugular venous saturation has been used extensively to monitor cerebral oxygen delivery in adults; limited information on the utility of this technique in children is available.[43–46] Studies in adults suggest that therapies such as barbiturates and hyperventilation can be titrated according to jugular venous saturation.[113,114] Desaturations below the threshold value of 50% are associated with mortality in adults.[115] However, jugular venous desaturation below this level was rarely the sole indication that urgent intervention was necessary, and false desaturations occurred. Nevertheless, this tool can provide valuable information that can assist in clinical decision making. Several other modes of monitoring cerebral metabolic rate may aid in patient management after severe TBI. However, Coles et al.[116] suggest that jugular venous saturation monitoring failed to identify regional CBF reductions into the ischemic range in adults with severe TBI. Near-infrared spectroscopy (NIRS) has been used to track the oxidative state of cytochromes in brain. It reportedly aided in clinical decision making during treatment of brain-injured adults, warning of reduced cerebral oxygenation, sometimes with greater sensitivity than jugular venous saturation.[112] Near-infrared spectroscopy has been used for assessment of cerebral metabolic status in hypoxemic-ischemic neonates[117,118] and is beginning to be used in pediatric TBI.[119] Although its exact role remains to be defined, it may prove valuable as a trend monitor.[120] Limitations with topographic resolution and the dominance of the superficial brain tissue in generating the signal are remaining concerns. Monitoring Po_2 in brain parenchyma with a microelectrode implanted in the frontal lobe is feasible in adults.[121] A threshold value of approximately 8.5 mmHg was associated with a reduction in CPP below 60 mmHg. The major limitations of this technique are its invasiveness and provision of only focal information. However, coupled to cerebral microdialysis, this method can provide significant metabolic information, such as local glutamate, glucose, lactate, or ATP levels.[122,123] Finally, positron emission tomography (PET) has been used in adults with severe TBI.[20] Although this method is limited by long acquisition times and the risk of intrahospital transport of critically ill patients, the metabolic maps generated provide significant insight, particularly into cerebral glucose utilization after TBI. Diringer et al.[124] used PET to provide important insight into the effect of hyperventilation on $CMRo_2$ in adults with severe TBI (discussed later in this chapter). Positron emission tomography, along with advanced MRI, can provide critical insight into regional brain disturbances and the effect of therapy (Figure 107–8).

Treatment in the Pediatric Intensive Care Unit

Once the initial resuscitation is completed and evacuable intracranial masses have been addressed, maintenance of physiologic stability and recognition and management of intracranial hypertension are the priorities. A flow diagram illustrating a general approach to first-tier treatments of the child with severe TBI was provided in the pediatric guidelines (Figure 107–9). The injured brain has complex metabolic requirements that are poorly understood.[125]

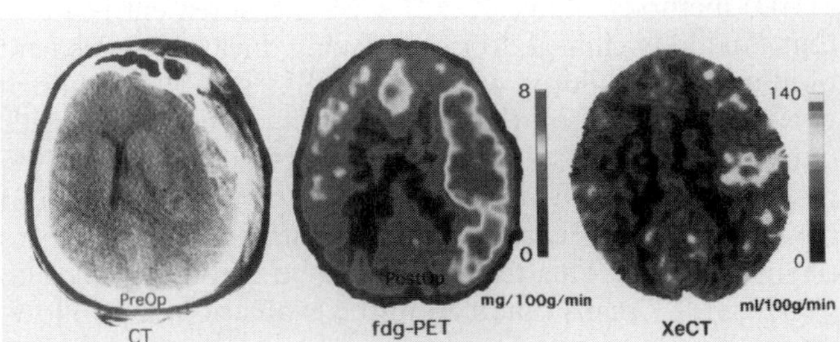

FIGURE 107–8 • Axial computed tomographic (CT) image **(left)** showing an acute subdural hematoma with mass effect that was treated with emergent surgical evacuation. ^{18}F-flurodexoyglucose positron emission tomographic map **(center)** obtained at 5 days after surgery showing marked local increases in cerebral glucose utilization in the brain regions underlying the hematoma. Stable xenon CT cerebral blood flow (CBF) map also obtained at 5 days after surgery shows increased CBF in the same brain region, indicating that the increase in glucose utilization is not the result of hypoperfusion. This phenomenon is termed *hyperglycolysis* and is suggested to represent increased glucose utilization by astrocytes coupled to glutamate uptake and other mediator-driven processes. This highlights the complex regional metabolic demands of the traumatically injured brain.

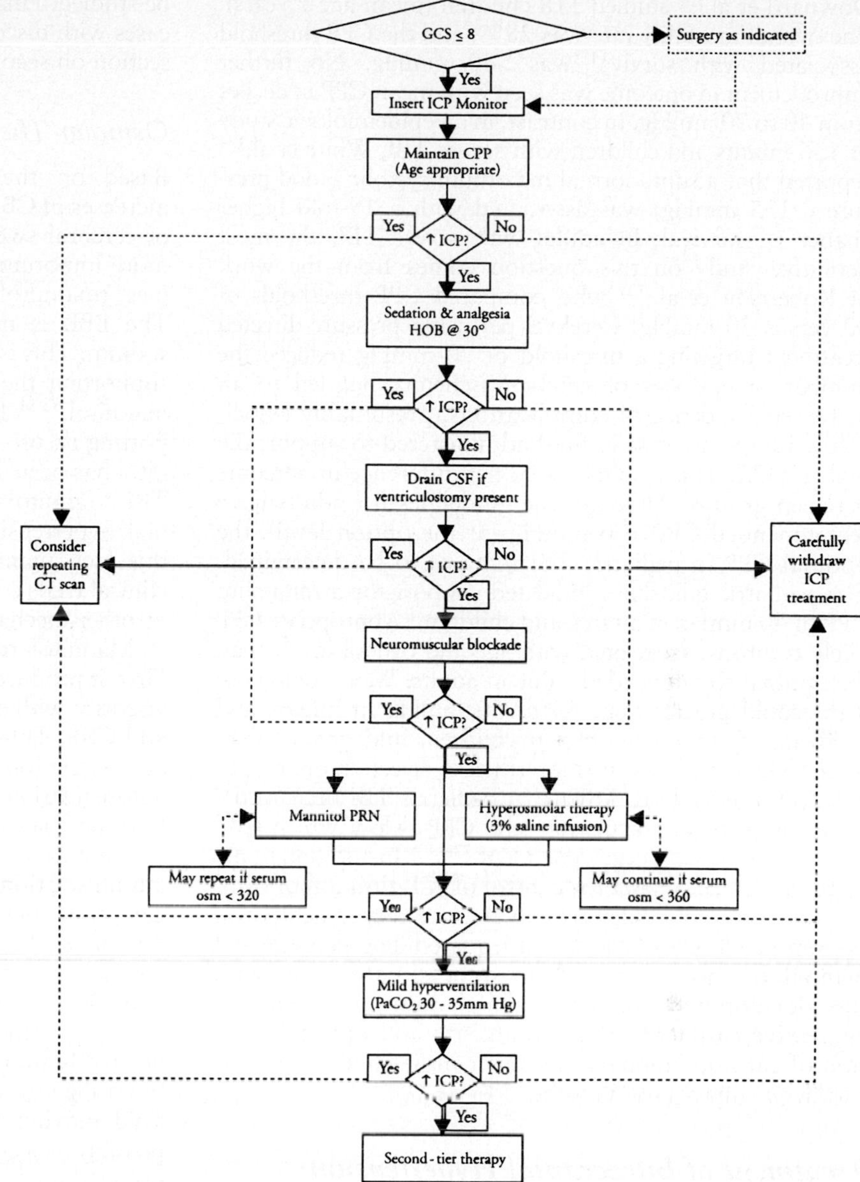

FIGURE 107–9 • First-tier management approach based on the "Guidelines for the Management of Severe TBI in Infants, Children, and Adolescents."[1]

Cerebral blood flow autoregulation may be disturbed, and metabolic demands may be either decreased or increased.[13,20,43–46,110] It is clear, however, that evidence of neuronal death from cerebral ischemia is a common finding on autopsy in patients who die after severe TBI. Control of ICP and maintenance of adequate CPP are central to minimizing the risk of developing secondary ischemia.[100–102]

Intracranial Pressure and Cerebral Perfusion Pressure Thresholds

Adult victims of severe TBI with ICP >20 mmHg have a poorer outcome that those without increased ICP.[100–102,126] Although a prospective RCT in patients with and without both ICP monitoring and targeted management has not been performed, a prospective cohort study by Ghajar et al.[105] suggested better outcome in adults monitored and treated with CSF drainage versus those without ICP monitoring. Several studies suggest that optimal outcome is achieved when even more modest levels of intracranial hypertension (i.e., ICP >15 mmHg) are the target.[105] Although no pediatric study has compared ICP thresholds and their effect on outcome using a specific treatment regimen, review of the pediatric literature provides clues on the optimal ICP threshold for treatment. Four of five major studies, including a total of more than 230 cases of severe pediatric TBI, reported that poor outcome was associated with ICP >20 mmHg.[45,127–130] Thus, the literature supports this value as a rational threshold in pediatric TBI. What remains to be determined is whether this threshold is lower for infants in whom physiologic mean arterial blood pressure (MAP) is lower than in adults.

As with ICP, no RCT has defined the optimal CPP for pediatric TBI, although its importance in patient management is well recognized. Reductions in CPP below specific threshold values are associated with poor outcome. In severe pediatric TBI, four studies defined the CPP associated with poor outcome as between 40 and 65 mmHg.[130–133]

Downard et al.[130] studied 118 children (mean age 7 years). The overall mortality rate was 28%, and the CPP threshold associated with survival was >40 mmHg. No further improvement in outcome was seen with mean CPP in deciles from 40 to 70 mmHg. In contrast, in an epidemiologic study of 136 infants and children with severe TBI, White et al.[134] reported that a supranormal maximum systolic blood pressure (≥135 mmHg) was associated with a 19-fold higher chance of survival. In adults with severe TBI, the most definitive study on this question comes from the work of Robertson et al.,[135] who compared CPP thresholds of 50 versus 70 mmHg. Cerebral perfusion pressure-directed treatment targeting a threshold of 70 mmHg reduced the number of episodes of cerebral ischemia but led to an increased incidence of complications, presumably associated with the increase in fluid administered to support the higher MAP. This resulted in no net difference in outcome between groups. Although the guidelines for adults have recommended CPP >70 mmHg (at the option level), the optimal CPP in pediatric TBI remains to be determined. The pediatric guidelines indicated support for a minimum CPP of 40 mmHg in infants and children.[1] Appropriate CPP likely is directly correlated with age and overall lower than the optimal recommended value in adults. We currently use a threshold greater than 40 to 50 mmHg in infants and toddlers, 50 to 60 mmHg in children, and greater than 60 mmHg in adolescents. Nevertheless, selection of an optimal CPP threshold is difficult in pediatric TBI because the lower limit of autoregulation (the CPP below which CBF begins to decrease) is age dependent.[136–139] In addition to the methods described later for control of ICP, titration of vasopressor or inotropic support may be necessary to achieve an appropriate level of CPP once adequate filling pressure and hemoglobin are confirmed. In some situations, as with the development of neurogenic pulmonary edema, aggressive cardiovascular monitoring and optimal titration of cardiopulmonary support can be challenging and key determinants of outcome.

Treatment of Intracranial Hypertension: First-Tier Therapies

Ventricular Cerebrospinal Fluid Drainage

Ventricular CSF drainage has been used for the management of intracranial hypertension in adults for more than 40 years. Cerebrospinal fluid drainage for treatment of intracranial hypertension in children was shown to improve CBF in 1971.[140] Fortune et al.[141] compared the effect of CSF drainage and mannitol in adults after severe TBI and observed similar effects on CBF and ICP. Cerebrospinal fluid drainage was associated with a greater increase in jugular venous saturation than mannitol administration. Cerebrospinal fluid can be drained intermittently or continuously, with threshold values for drainage determined based on the clinical indication. However, the efficacy of CSF drainage versus other treatments of intracranial hypertension remains unclear. Nevertheless, it is the first line of therapy that we recommend. Intermittent versus continuous drainage strategies have never been compared. It is our clinical impression that CSF drainage reduces requirements for other therapies targeting ICP. However, this remains to be studied. Finally, lumbar CSF drainage can reduce ICP in cases with discernible basal cisterns; this is discussed in the section on second-tier therapies.

Osmolar Therapy

Based on the hypothesis that BBB permeability and increases in CBV play only limited roles in the development of cerebral swelling and that tissue osmolar load may be more important, particularly in contusion, osmolar therapies (mannitol, hypertonic saline) seem to be logical. The BBB is nearly impermeable to both mannitol and sodium. This is in contrast to traditional recommendations supporting the use of hyperventilation and avoidance of mannitol.[53,54] Despite its ubiquitous use and studies supporting its use for the management of TBI in adults, mannitol has been subjected to limited investigation in pediatric TBI. Mannitol is a cornerstone for management of intracranial hypertension in pediatric and adult TBI.[1,104] Despite this fact, mannitol has not been subjected to controlled clinical trials compared with placebo, other osmolar agents, or other mechanism-based therapies in children.

Mannitol reduces ICP by two distinct mechanisms.[104] First, it produces a rapid reduction in ICP by reducing blood viscosity with a resultant decrease in blood vessel diameter and CBV. This mechanism is dependent on intact viscosity autoregulation of CBF that is linked to blood pressure autoregulation of CBF. The effect of mannitol administration on blood viscosity and CBV is transient (lasting ≈75 minutes). The second mechanism by which mannitol administration reduces ICP is via an osmotic effect. This effect develops more slowly (over approximately 15–30 minutes) and results from movement of water from parenchyma into the circulation. The effect persists between 1 and 6 hours and is dependent on an intact BBB. Changes in serum osmolality reduce brain water only in relatively normal brain regions. Mannitol may accumulate in injured brain regions and a reverse osmotic shift may occur—with fluid moving from the circulation to the parenchyma—possibly exacerbating intracranial hypertension. Mannitol is excreted unchanged in urine, and a risk for development of acute tubular necrosis and renal failure has been suggested for mannitol administration with serum osmolarity greater than 320 mOsm in adults. However, the literature supporting this finding dates from the late 1970s and early 1980s, an era when dehydration therapy in combination with mannitol use was common. Hyperosmolar euvolemia is targeted with contemporary mannitol use. High levels of serum osmolarity (365 mOsm) appear to be tolerated in children when induced with hypertonic saline.[142] Few data support the concomitant use of diuretics and mannitol to reduce ICP. James[143] performed a retrospective study of 60 patients (age 1–73 years) treated with intravenous mannitol for increased ICP. After bolus mannitol administration, ICP decreased after 116 of the 120 doses. In that study, the reduction in ICP in response to mannitol administration was dose dependent between 0.18 and 2.5. In contrast, Marshall et al.[144] reported equivalence for doses between 0.25 and 1 g/kg in adults. Despite a remarkable track record for controlling intracranial hypertension in the management of infants and children with severe TBI, clinical investigation of mannitol use in infants and children is lacking.

Surprisingly, an epidemiologic study suggested that mannitol administration was associated with prolonged PICU length of stay but no survival advantage.[134] Nevertheless, mannitol remains a first-tier therapy in severe pediatric TBI.

Use of hypertonic saline for treatment of intracranial hypertension was first described in 1919 but failed to gain clinical acceptance.[145] Interest in this treatment has undergone a recent resurgence. Penetration of sodium across the BBB is low. Sodium has a reflection coefficient higher than that of mannitol and shares with mannitol both the favorable rheologic effects on CBV and osmolar gradient effects. Hypertonic saline exhibits other theoretical benefits, such as restoration of cell resting membrane potential, stimulation of atrial natriuretic peptide release, inhibition of inflammation, and enhancement of cardiac performance. Hypertonic saline was studied in more than 130 pediatric patients with severe TBI. There are two types of studies: (1) treatment of refractory intracranial hypertension and (2) comparison of hypertonic saline to maintenance fluid as a continuous infusion. Fisher et al.[88] compared 3% saline and 0.9% saline in children with severe TBI. During the 2-hour trial, hypertonic saline was associated with a lower ICP. Serum sodium level increased approximately 7 mEq/L after 3% saline administration. Khanna et al.[146] reported a prospective study of 3% saline (514 mEq/L) given on a sliding scale to maintain ICP less than 20 mmHg in children with resistant intracranial hypertension. A reduction in ICP and an increase in CPP were noted with 3% saline. The mean highest serum sodium level and osmolarity were approximately 170 mEq/L and approximately 365 mOsm/L, respectively. Sustained hypernatremia and hyperosmolarity were generally tolerated. Two patients developed acute renal failure. Peterson et al.[142] reported a retrospective study on the use of 3% saline infusion titrated to reduce ICP to less than or equal to 20 mmHg in infants and children with TBI. The mean daily doses of hypertonic saline ranged between approximately 11 and 27 ml/kg/day. There was no control group, but only three patients died of uncontrolled ICP, and 73% of patients had good or moderate outcome. Rebound in ICP or other side effects were not seen. Theoretical concerns associated with use of hypertonic saline include development of extrapontine myelinolysis (EPM), rapid shrinking of the brain associated with mechanical tearing of bridging vessels leading to subarachnoid hemorrhage, renal failure, and rebound intracranial hypertension.[147] Extrapontine myelinolysis is related to central pontine myelinolysis (CPM) but occurs with hypernatremia and/or its correction. It is characterized by demyelination of the thalamus, basal ganglia, and cerebellum.[148] Neither EPM nor CPM has been reported in human trials of hypertonic saline for treatment of TBI. EPM has been reported in dehydrated children with serum sodium levels of 168 to 195 mEq/L, and CPM has been reported with rapid correction of chronic hyponatremia to serum sodium levels greater than 132 mEq/L.[140] Peterson et al.[142] performed MRI evaluations in 11 patients in their study, and none had evidence of CPM. However, rats with normal serum sodium subjected to sodium increases of 39 ± 8 mEq/L showed severe demyelinating lesions.[149] Similarly, subarachnoid hemorrhage has been reported with serum sodium concentrations from 149 to 206 mEq/L within 1 hour after injection of 9% hypertonic saline in normal kittens.[150] Renal failure is a concern with use of hyperosmolar therapies. Use of hypertonic saline (vs Lactated Ringer solution) in the resuscitation of burn patients is associated with a fourfold increase in renal failure,[151] but this complication has not been seen with hypertonic saline use in children after TBI.[142] Rebound intracranial hypertension has been described with use of hypertonic saline bolus therapy or after cessation of continuous infusion.[142,152] Patients may require a progressive increase in hypertonic saline infusion rates to control ICP. It is unclear whether this is a rebound effect or a natural evolution of the patient's brain injury. Hypertonic saline, mannitol, and CSF drainage are first-tier therapies for intracranial hypertension.

Sedation Analgesia and Neuromuscular Blockade

Sedation and neuromuscular blockade should be used as needed in the setting of intracranial hypertension once appropriate monitoring has been established and thus are integrated into first-tier treatment. Narcotics, benzodiazepines, or small doses of barbiturates are generally recommended for routine use. To our knowledge, no controlled trial of varying sedation regimen has been performed in pediatric patients with severe TBI. Hsiang et al.[153] reported on 514 adults with severe TBI and suggested that prophylactic neuromuscular blockade was associated with increased length of ICU stay and nosocomial pneumonia. However, the study was not prospective and should not preclude the use of neuromuscular blockade in pediatric TBI. As with most therapies in this setting, careful assessment of indication and titration of therapy are essential. Finally, intermittent doses of thiopental and/or lidocaine often are needed to blunt excessive rises in ICP secondary to routine patient care maneuvers such as suctioning.

Head Position

This is an area of controversy. Feldman et al.[154] conducted a prospective RCT of the effect of head position on ICP, CPP, and CBF in 22 adults after severe TBI. Both ICP and mean carotid pressure were reduced in the 30° position versus the 0° position. CPP and CBF did not change with this intervention. Thus, in general, the 30° head elevated position reduced ICP without deleterious effects on CPP and is preferred. Head elevation and midline position improve jugular venous and possibly CSF drainage and decrease the contributions of these components to ICP.

Treatment of Intracranial Hypertension: Second-Tier Therapies

Refractory intracranial hypertension occurs in 20% to 40% of cases of severe pediatric TBI and is associated with mortality rates between 30% and 100%.[127–129,130–135,155–157] A number of second-tier therapies are available for treatment of refractory intracranial hypertension. These were presented in the pediatric guidelines and are shown in Figure 107–10. Second-tier therapies include barbiturates, hyperventilation, hypothermia, decompressive craniectomy, and lumbar CSF drainage.

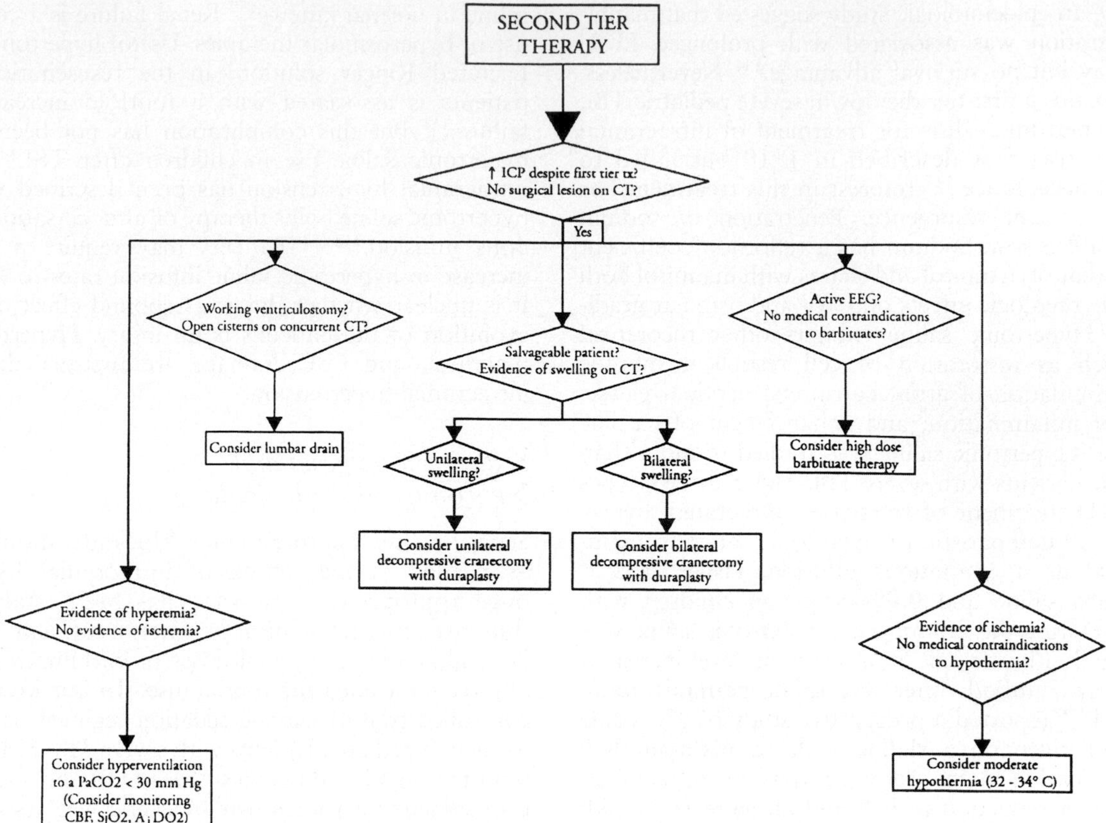

FIGURE 107–10 • Second-tier therapies for the management of refractory intracranial hypertension based on the "Guidelines for the Management of Severe TBI in Infants, Children, and Adolescents."[1]

Barbiturates

Barbiturates produce a reduction in ICP via a decrease in cerebral metabolic rate. Although an RCT of barbiturate therapy for treatment of severe TBI in adults did not demonstrate a beneficial effect on outcome,[158] barbiturates can be effective in the setting of refractory intracranial hypertension.[159] Goodman et al.[160] reported an improvement in brain interstitial concentration of lactate and glutamate accompanying a reduction of ICP in seven adults treated with barbiturates for refractory intracranial hypertension. In contrast, Cruz[113] reported that approximately one third of adults given barbiturates experience a deterioration (rather than improvement) in jugular venous saturation. If either frequent dosing or barbiturate infusion is used, an electroencephalogram (EEG) should be used to assess the cerebral metabolic response to treatment. The endpoint of barbiturate coma is generally burst suppression. Pentobarbital or thiopental often is infused to achieve a burst suppression response on EEG. However, that goal should only represent the maximal barbiturate dose used for ICP control because (1) smaller doses—those still associated with EEG activity—may be adequate to control ICP, and (2) indiscriminate use can be associated with undesirable side effects such as hypotension.[161] A lack of ICP response to barbiturates is associated with poor outcome. When barbiturates are used, hypotension should be avoided. Patients should be carefully monitored for reduced cardiac output or inadequate systemic perfusion, as clinically indicated. As the use of hyperventilation for the management of children with refractory intracranial hypertension has waned, alternative therapies such as barbiturates appear to be increasingly utilized.

Hyperventilation

Hyperventilation has been used for the management of pediatric patients with severe TBI since the late 1950s.[162] Bruce et al.[15] suggested that hyperemia was the predominant mechanism involved in the development of intracranial hypertension in children. Consequently, hyperventilation instead of mannitol or other therapies was recommended as first-line therapy. Until the mid-1980s, prophylactic hyperventilation was the standard of care. In addition to reducing postinjury hyperemia, hyperventilation was suggested to reduce brain acidosis and restore CBF autoregulation. Subsequently, studies in experimental models suggested hyperventilation had deleterious effects. Prophylactic hyperventilation depletes brain interstitial bicarbonate buffering capacity and is accompanied by gradual loss of local vasoconstrictor effects.[163] In an RCT in adults after severe TBI, prophylactic hyperventilation for 5 days to a Pa_{CO_2} of approximately 25 mmHg versus approximately 35 mmHg was associated with worse outcome.[164] Skippen et al.[165] reported that hyperventilation to Pa_{CO_2} approximately 25 mmHg reduced CBF to levels less than 18 ml/100 g/min in 73% of infants and children with severe TBI. Coles et al.[116] found similar results in adults. However, neither of these studies assessed the effect of hyperventilation on either regional cerebral metabolism or neurologic outcome. In experimental TBI in rats, aggressive hyperventilation ($PaCO_2$ = 20 mmHg) early after injury enhanced hippocampal cell death. The pediatric guidelines recommend that prophylactic hyperventilation not be used.[1] A $PaCO_2$ of approximately 35 mmHg was recommended. Supporting this approach in infants and children, early after severe TBI, hypoperfusion rather than hyperemia was shown to be associated with poor outcome.[18] Zwienenberg and Muizelaar[50] questioned the occurrence of hyperemia in children after severe TBI, suggesting instead that normal CBF values previously were underestimated and are higher in children than in adults. Again, however, the risk of hyperventilation is being challenged in clinical studies by Diringer et al.[124] Between 8 and 14 hours after severe TBI in adults, hyperventilation ($PaCO_2$ ≈30 mmHg) reduced CBF but did not further reduce cerebral metabolic rate for oxygen as assessed using PET. This finding suggests that in TBI, after the acute hypermetabolic phase, hypometabolism follows and hyperventilation may be a relatively safe means to reduce ICP in the PICU. This study did not evaluate outcome. Nevertheless, the study suggests that hyperventilation, if appropriately monitored and titrated, can be used as adjunct treatment of refractory intracranial hypertension, particularly during the delayed postinjury phase. Its use in this manner was supported as a second-tier therapy in the pediatric guidelines. Based on our current state of knowledge, when hyperventilation ($PaCO_2$ <30 mmHg) is used to manage refractory intracranial hypertension, assessment or monitoring of CBF or jugular venous or tissue O_2 is recommended to rule out iatrogenic ischemia. Finally, in the absence of signs and symptoms of herniation, there is no physiologic rationale for applying prophylactic hyperventilation.

Hypothermia

In models of TBI and in some clinical trials in adults after TBI, hypothermia improved outcome, presumably via multiple mechanisms.[166] Unfortunately, an RCT did not unequivocally benefit from application of hypothermia after TBI,[33] although a meta-analysis supports the use of hypothermia in adults with severe TBI.[167,168] In contrast, hypothermia clearly is useful for the management of increased ICP[171,172] in adults after severe TBI. Hypothermia can be used in the setting of refractory posttraumatic intracranial hypertension. Unlike studies showing benefit from transient (12–24 hours) use of mild hypothermia (33 °C) in adults after cardiac arrest,[169,170] a variety of temperature ranges are necessary to control ICP; thus a titrated approach to use of hypothermia in this setting is suggested.[171,172] Rewarming should be carried out carefully, at a rate no faster that 1 °C per hour, and great care should be taken to monitor and treat hypotension that can occur with peripheral vasodilation during rewarming. However, the meta-analysis in adults suggested that extremely slow rewarming (>24 hours) may be associated with complications, presumably from protracted hypothermia. RCTs of hypothermia in infants and children with severe TBI are ongoing in Canada and the United States. Finally, hyperthermia is extremely deleterious in experimental models of TBI, exacerbating neuronal death. This effect is seen even when a brief 3-hour period of clinically relevant hyperthermia (39 °C) is applied. Natale et al.[173] supported the clinical relevance of this work by showing that early hyperthermia (>38.5 °C within the first 24 hours of admission) occurred in 29.9% of pediatric TBI patients and was associated with poor outcome and increased length of stay. Care should be taken to treat or prevent hyperthermia after severe TBI.

Decompressive Craniectomy

Another controversial area in the management of both adults and children with refractory intracranial hypertension is the use of decompressive craniectomy. Controlled studies on this modality are limited. Cushing[174] initially described this modality in 1905. Several studies suggest that this procedure may exacerbate cerebral edema formation. However, there has been a resurgence of interest in this approach in laboratory studies, and several case reports suggest that this approach may result in decreased ICP and good outcome in selected cases with extremely refractory intracranial hypertension. The successful examples cited in these studies are generally children or young adults. Decompressive craniectomy is a controversial therapy that is based on the complex metabolic demands of the brain and the equally complex but poorly understood side effects of many of the therapies used to treat refractory intracranial hypertension (ischemia, hyperosmolality, metabolic suppression, hypotension). However, this simplistic approach may have merit. Three contemporary pediatric studies have been performed. Cho et al.[175] reported on the use of decompressive craniectomy versus medical management for treatment of infant victims of the shaken baby syndrome with refractory intracranial hypertension. Although the series was small, they reported an improved outcome compared with medical therapy, with some survivors showing good outcome. This study is one of the few specifically examining treatment of severe TBI victims in whom child abuse is the injury mechanism. Polin et al.[176] reported on the use of extensive bifrontal decompressive craniectomy for the management of 35 adults and children with severe TBI and either refractory intracranial hypertension or diffuse edema on CT scan. They reported a very favorable percentage of survivors with good or moderate disability (improved outcome vs. retrospectively matched cases from the Traumatic Coma Data Bank) and suggested a 48-hour time window for successful application. However, the patients in this report were generally not treated with either CSF drainage or barbiturates. Nevertheless, the best results were seen in the children in this study. Taylor et al.[177] reported on an RCT of early decompressive craniectomy versus standardized medical management alone. Although the sample size was limited (n = 27 children), strong trends toward reduction in ICP and improvement in long-term outcome were seen with decompressive craniectomy. Decompressive craniotomy is a second-tier therapy that is used with varying frequency depending on local experience and the discretion of the management team.

Lumbar Cerebrospinal Fluid Drainage

Lumbar CSF drainage is effective in treating refractory intracranial hypertension in children. Levy et al.[178] reported that controlled lumbar CSF draining was effective in reducing refractory ICP in 14 of 16 pediatric patients, and it eliminated the need for barbiturates in their series. In adults with severe TBI, Munch et al.[179] reported an immediate and lasting reduction in ICP in 23 patients with very refractory intracranial hypertension. This modality is an acceptable treatment option in this setting, but to avoid the risks of herniation, the patient must have open basal cisterns and no important mass effect or shift, and a functional ventriculostomy must already be in place.

Controlled Arterial Hypertension

Induced arterial hypertension is a controversial area in the management of refractory intracranial hypertension. Whether pressure autoregulation of CBF is intact or defective, arterial hypotension or inadequate CPP must be rigorously avoided. If pressure autoregulation is impaired, CBF is directly related to CPP and hypotension directly reduces flow. If pressure autoregulation is intact, then as CPP is reduced, reflex cerebral vasodilatation occurs (to maintain flow), which increases CBV and ICP.[180] This latter phenomenon occurs as CPP is reduced within the autoregulatory range. Based on the relationship among CPP, vessel diameter, CBV, and ICP, in selected adults with refractory intracranial hypertension, induced arterial hypertension (CPP increased to between 100 and 140 mmHg via infusion of phenylephrine) produced a reduction in ICP.[180] However, arterial hypertension reduces ICP only when pressure autoregulation of CBF is intact because hypertension-mediated reduction in vessel caliber produces the reduction in CBV (to maintain a constant flow) and resultant reduction in ICP. Use of this intervention is particularly complex in pediatric TBI because a single general threshold value of CPP is not applicable. Management must be tailored to each individual patient. In addition, the short-term and long-term effects of the greater hydrostatic pressure on the development of cerebral edema are unclear. Optimal management of blood pressure after severe TBI requires both extensive monitoring of the involved factors and an in-depth understanding of the mechanisms at work.[180] Induced hypertension is a controversial "last-ditch" therapy that is not addressed in the pediatric guidelines.[1]

Finally, a few groups managing adults with severe TBI have adopted a very different therapeutic approach to blood pressure and ICP management termed the *Lund Concept*. This approach includes aggressive control of ICP with the unusual combination of beta-blocker, ergotamine, and barbiturates, with avoidance of systemic hypertension.[181] In some sense, this represents a form of chemical hyperventilation, that is, pharmacologically controlled CBV. Remarkably, this approach has produced good outcome data and no exacerbation of cerebral ischemia, as assessed using intracerebral microdialysis in adults.[182] There is one report of this approach to ICP control in children with meningitis,[183] but no data in pediatric TBI.

Is Rigorous Intracranial Pressure Control the Common Denominator in Studies with Exceptionally Good Outcome?

Whatever approach is selected to control ICP after severe TBI, the devastating and sometimes preventable consequences of secondary ischemia and herniation must be meticulously addressed. Interestingly, some of the best outcomes reported in clinical series of either adults or children with severe TBI have come from extremely divergent, albeit aggressive and protocol-based, approaches, namely, aggressive hyperventilation as reported by Bruce et al.,[184] remarkably aggressive use of hyperosmolar therapy reported by Peterson et al.,[142] rigorous application of hypothermia with tightly controlled hemodynamics as reported by Marion et al.,[166] aggressive CPP management as described by Robertson et al.[135] and Rosner et al.,[185] and aggressive control of ICP using the Lund concept.[181] Perhaps the common denominator in these reports is the aggressive, meticulous, and protocol-driven control of ICP.

Miscellaneous

Seizures should be treated aggressively. However, the pediatric guidelines suggest prophylactic phenytoin only as a treatment option to prevent early posttraumatic seizures in severe TBI because prophylactic treatment has not been shown to improve outcome.[1] Additional anticonvulsants are given as needed to treat seizures.

Even if hypertonic saline is not used as a therapy, careful attention should be paid to the serum sodium level. It should be monitored at least twice daily in children with severe TBI. To prevent the development of hyponatremia, we recommend using 0.9% normal saline as the initial IV fluid for children with severe TBI. For infants, D_5 (5% dextrose) normal saline can be used. Serum glucose concentration should be maintained less than 250 mg/dl with an insulin infusion, as needed. Hyponatremia that develops while only isotonic fluids are being administered can generally be attributed to either syndrome of inappropriate antidiuretic hormone secretion (SIADH) or cerebral salt wasting.[186] Care should be taken to determine the correct cause of hyponatremia because the management of SIADH involves fluid restriction while that of cerebral salt wasting involves the administration of isotonic or hypertonic saline.

The provision of adequate calories and protein is essential during the catabolic response to critical illness, and beneficial effects of early feeding (either enteral or parenteral) in the critically ill or injured patient are well described. In critically ill adults, a cumulative deficit of 10,000 kcal was associated with increased mortality, and in the PICU this amount can be easily surpassed in less than 1 week.[187] In adults with severe TBI, Hadley et al.[188] reported that early jejunal feeding (within 36 hours of admission) reduced septic complications and ICU days by 50% compared with delayed feeding (when gastric atony had resolved). Care must be taken to prevent the complications of overfeeding (hyperglycemia with parenteral nutrition or hypoosmolality with enteral feedings). Frequent monitoring of blood glucose, electrolytes, and calorimetry may be useful.[189] Glutamate-containing hyperalimentation formulations have been shown to increase glutamate levels, possibly exacerbating excitotoxicity.[190] The optimal nutritional approach in severe TBI needs to be addressed.

Routine use of glucocorticoids for treatment of patients with severe TBI is not recommended.[1] However, hypotension in the setting of severe TBI in rare cases is associated with pituitary failure, possibly from vascular disruption.[191]

Outcomes

Outcome from severe TBI has generally been assessed as a function of age at the time of injury and in relationship to three diagnostic categories: noninflicted (accidental) closed head injuries, inflicted childhood neurotrauma (child abuse), and penetrating injury (predominantly gunshot wounds). Accurate assessment of long-term outcome has been somewhat hampered in infants and children by the lack of validated outcome assessment tools. Application of modifications of adult outcome tools (e.g., Glasgow outcome scale) have been the general approach; however, these tools have important limitations when applied across the pediatric age spectrum.[192] In the most important paper published to date on pediatric outcomes, citing the results of the National Institutes of Health Traumatic Coma Data Bank, Levin et al.[10] highlighted the dramatic effect of age on outcome. In that study, approximately two thirds of children between the ages of 5 and 10 years had good outcome (normal or moderate disability), whereas more than 60% of children age 4 years or younger died. Rates of good outcome as high as 73% have been reported in contemporary studies of clinical trials in pediatric TBI.[142] Specific studies of inflicted childhood neurotrauma and gunshot wounds have generally reported poorer outcome than results of series of accidental closed head injury. However, even within these two high-risk diagnostic categories, good outcome in contemporary series has been reported to be approximately 35% in severe TBI resulting from inflicted childhood neurotrauma and as high as 24% in severe TBI resulting from gunshot wounds.[175,193] Rehabilitation can have dramatic effects after severe TBI, particularly in the setting of focal injury. Successful rehabilitation may require prolonged periods of therapy (i.e., months or even years).[194]

Conclusion

Optimal care of the infant or child with severe TBI requires a multidisciplinary approach. Prompt and vigorous resuscitation, including stabilization and control of ventilation, is essential. After initial evaluation and surgical intervention, where appropriate, monitoring and carefully titrated management of intracranial hypertension is essential to reduce ICP, optimize cerebral perfusion, and facilitate metabolic homeostasis. Meticulous and optimal neurointensive care is the basis on which future targeted therapies will be delivered as additional information on the evolution of secondary neuronal damage becomes available. In the introduction, we stated that the goal of contemporary pediatric neurointensive care is the prevention of secondary injury. Much of that care focuses on preventing secondary insults. The goal of future pediatric neurointensive case will be to overlay, on this therapeutic plan, strategies manipulating tissue injury in the evolution of secondary damage at a cellular level, along with strategies to foster regeneration and rehabilitation.

REFERENCES

1. Division of Injury Control, Center for Environmental Health and Injury Control, Centers for Disease Control: Childhood injuries in the United States, *Am J Dis Child* 144:627-646, 1990.
2. Wilberger JE: Traumatic brain injuries in athletes. In Marion, DW editor: *Traumatic brain injury.* New York, 1999, Thieme.
3. Valko AS: Rehabilitation and disabilities. In Marion DW, editor: *Traumatic brain injury,* New York, 1999, Thieme.
4. Kraus JF, Fife D, Conroy C: Pediatric brain injuries: the nature, clinical course, and early outcomes in a defined United States population, *Pediatrics* 79:501-507, 1987.
5. *www.census.gov/population/estimates*
6. Anderson VA, Catroppa C, Hariton F, et al: Identifying factors contributing to child and family outcome 30 months after traumatic brain injury in children. *J Neurol Neurosurg Psychiatry* 76:401-408, 2005.
7. Ewing-Cobbs L, Levin HS, Fletcher JM, et al: The Children's Orientation and Amnesia Test: relationship to severity of acute head injury and to recovery of memory, *Neurosurgery* 27:683-691, 1990.
8. Walker M, Storrs B, Mayer T: Factors affecting the outcome in the pediatric patient with multiple trauma: further experience with the modified injury severity scale, *Childs Brain* 11:387-397, 1984.
9. Levin HS, Ewing-Cobbs L, Eisenberg HM: Neurobehavioral outcome of pediatric closed head injury. In Broman SH, Michel ME, editors: *Traumatic head injury in children.* New York, 1995, Oxford University Press.
10. Levin HS, Eisenberg HM, Wigg NR, Kobaashi K: Memory and intellectual ability after head injury in children and adolescents, *Neurosurgery* 11:668-673, 1982.
11. Maugans TA, McComb JG, Levy ML, et al: Penetrating craniocerebral injuries. In Albright A, Pollack IF, Adelson PD, editors: *Principles and practice of pediatric neurosurgery.* New York, 1999, Thieme.
12. Kochanek PM, Clark RSB, Ruppel, et al. Cerebral resuscitation after traumatic brain injury and cardiopulmonary arrest in infants and children in the new millennium. In: Orlowski JP, editor: *Pediatric clinics of North America.* Philadelphia, 2001, WB Saunders.
13. Kochanek PM, Clark RSB, Ruppel RA, et al: Biochemical, cellular, and molecular mechanisms in the evolution of secondary damage after severe traumatic brain injury in infants and children: lessons learned from the bedside, *Pediatr Crit Care Med* 1:4-19, 2000.
14. Pickles W: Acute general edema of the brain in children with head injuries, *N Engl J Med* 242:607-611, 1950.
15. Bruce DA, Alavi A, Bilaniuk L, et al: Diffuse cerebral swelling following head injuries in children: the syndrome of "malignant brain edema," *J Neurosurg* 54:170-178, 1981.
16. Marion DW, Darby J, Yonas H: Acute regional cerebral blood flow changes caused by severe head injuries, *J Neurosurg* 74:407-414, 1991.
17. Bouma GJ, Muizelaar JP, Stringer WA, et al: Ultra-early evaluation of regional cerebral blood flow in severely head-injured patients using xenon-enhanced computerized tomography, *J Neurosurg* 77:360-368, 1992.
18. Adelson PD, Clyde B, Kochanek PM, et al: Cerebrovascular response in infants and young children following severe traumatic brain injury: a preliminary report, *Pediatr Neurosurg* 26:200-207, 1997.
19. DeSalles AAF, Kontos HA, Becker DP, et al: Prognostic significance of ventricular CSF lactic acidosis in severe head injury, *J Neurosurg* 65:615-624, 1986.
20. Bergsneider M, Hovda DA, Shalmon E, et al: Cerebral hyperglycolysis following severe traumatic brain injury in humans: a positron emission tomography study, *J Neurosurg* 86:241-251, 1997.
21. Choi DW, Maulucci-Gedde M, Kriegstein AR: Glutamate neurotoxicity in cortical cell culture, *J Neurosci* 7:357-368, 1987.
22. Choi DW: Ionic dependence of glutamate neurotoxicity, *J Neurosci* 7:369-379, 1987.
23. Zhang J, Dawson VL, Dawson TM, et al: Nitric oxide activation of poly(ADP-ribose) synthetase in neurotoxicity, *Science* 263: 687-689, 1994.
24. Palmer AM, Marion DW, Botscheller ML, et al: Increased transmitter amino acid concentration in human ventricular CSF after brain trauma, *NeuroReport* 6:153, 1994.
25. Ruppel RA, Kochanek PM, Adelson PD, et al: Excitotoxicity amino acid concentrations in ventricular cerebrospinal fluid after severe traumatic brain injury in infants and children: the role of child abuse, *J Pediatr* 138:18-25, 2001.

26. Hayes R, Jenkins L, Lyeth B, et al: Pretreatment with phencyclidine, an N-methyl-D-aspartate receptor antagonist, attenuates long-term behavioral deficits in the rat produced by traumatic brain injury, *J Neurotrauma* 5:287-302, 1988.
27. Doppenberg EMR, Choi SC, Bullock R: Clinical trials in traumatic brain injury. What can we learn from previous studies? *Ann N Y Acad Sci* 825:305-322, 1997.
28. Ikonomidou C, Bosch F, Miksa M, et al: Blockade of NMDA receptors and apoptotic neurodegeneration in the developing brain, *Science* 283:70-74, 1999.
29. Rink A, Fung K-M, Trojanowski JQ, et al: Evidence of apoptotic cell death after experimental traumatic brain injury in the rat, *Am J Pathol* 147:1575-1583, 1995.
30. Clark RS, Kochanek PM, Chen M, et al: Increases in Bcl-2 and cleavage of Caspase-1 and Caspase-3 in human brain after head injury, *FASEB J* 13:813-821, 1999.
31. Kerr JF, Wyllie AH, Currie AR: Apoptosis: a basic biological phenomenon with wide-ranging implications in tissue kinetics, *Br J Cancer* 26:239-257, 1972.
32. Portera-Cailliau C, Price DL, Martin LJ: Excitotoxic neuronal death in the immature brain is an apoptosis-necrosis morphological continuum, *J Comp Neurol* 378:70-87, 1997.
33. Zamzami N, Susin SA, Marchetti P, et al: Mitochondrial control of nuclear apoptosis. *J Exp Med* 183:1533-1544, 1996.
34. Adams JM, Cory S: The Bcl-2 protein family: arbiters of cell survival, *Science* 281:1322-1326, 1998.
35. Li P, Nijhawan D, Budihardjo I, et al: Cytochrome c and dATP-dependent formation of Apaf-1/Caspase-9 complex initiates an apoptotic protease caspase, *Cell* 91:479-489, 1997.
36. Clark RSB, Kochanek PM, Watkins SC, et al: Caspase-3 mediated neuronal death after traumatic brain injury in rats, *J Neurochem* 74:740-753, 2000.
37. Ashkenazi A, Dixit VM: Death receptors: signaling and modulation, *Science* 281:1305-1308, 1998.
38. Clark RSB, Kochanek PM, Adelson PD, et al: Increases in bcl-2 protein in cerebrospinal fluid and evidence for programmed-cell death in infants and children following severe traumatic brain injury, *J Pediatr* 137:197-204, 2000.
39. Seidberg NA, Clark RSB, Kochanek PM, et al: Soluble fas is increased in CSF from infants and children after head injury, *Crit Care Med* 27:A38, 2000.
40. Lassen NA: The luxury-perfusion syndrome and its possible relation to acute metabolic acidosis localized within the brain, *Lancet* 19:1113-1115, 1966.
41. Obrist WD, Langfitt TW, Jaggi JL, et al: Cerebral blood flow and metabolism in comatose patients with acute head injury, *J Neurosurg* 61:241-253, 1984.
42. Verweij BH, Muizelaar JP, Vinas FC, et al: Impaired cerebral mitochondrial function after traumatic brain injury in humans, *J Neurosurg* 93:815-820, 2000.
43. Muizelaar JP, Marmarou A, DeSalles AAF, et al: Cerebral blood flow and metabolism in severely head-injured children. Part I: relationship with GCS score, outcome, ICP, and PVI, *J Neurosurg* 71:63-71, 1989.
44. Beyda DH: Time course of cerebral blood flow and metabolism in pediatric head trauma, *Crit Care Med* 24:134, 1996.
45. Sharples PM, Stuart AG, Matthews DSF, et al: Cerebral blood flow and metabolism in children with severe head injury. Part 1: relation to age, Glasgow coma score, outcome, intracranial pressure, and time after injury, *J Neurol Neurosurg Psychiatry* 58:145-152, 1995.
46. Sharples PM, Matthews DSF, Eyre JA: Cerebral blood flow and metabolism in children with severe head injuries: Part 2. Cerebrovascular resistance and its determinants, *J Neurol Neurosurg Psychiatry* 58:153-159, 1995.
47. Suzuki K: The changes of regional cerebral blood flow with advancing age in normal children, *Nagoya Med J* 34:159-170, 1990.
48. Kelly DF, Kordestani RK, Martin NA, et al: Hyperemia following traumatic brain injury: relationship to intracranial hypertension and outcome, *J Neurosurg* 85:762-771, 1996.
49. Marmarou A, Barzo P, Fatouros P, et al: Traumatic brain swelling in head injured patients: brain edema or vascular engorgement? *Acta Neurochir Suppl (Wien)* 70:68-70, 1997.
50. Zwienenberg M, Muizelaar JP: Severe pediatric head injury: the role of hyperemia revisited, *J Neurotrauma* 16:937-943, 1999.
51. Barzo P, Marmarou A, Fatouros P, et al: Contribution of vasogenic and cellular edema to traumatic brain swelling measured by diffusion-weighted imaging, *J Neurosurg* 87:900-907, 1997.
52. Katayama Y, Mori T, Maeda T, et al: Pathogenesis of the mass effect of cerebral contusions: rapid increase in osmolality within the contusion necrosis, *Acta Neurochir Suppl (Wien)* 71:289-292, 1998.
53. Bruce DA, Gennarelli TA, Langfitt TW: Resuscitation from coma due to head injury, *Crit Care Med* 6:254-269, 1978.
54. Bruce DA, Raphaely RC, Goldberg AI, et al: Pathophysiology, treatment and outcome following severe head injury in children. *Childs Brain* 5:174-191, 1979.
55. Adams JH, Doyle D, Ford I, et al: Diffuse axonal injury in head injury: definition, diagnosis, and grading, *Histopathology* 15: 49-59, 1989.
56. Gennarelli TA, Thibault LF, Adams TH, et al: Diffuse axonal injury and traumatic coma in the primate, *Ann Neurol* 12:564-574, 1982.
57. Graham DI, Lawrence AE, Adams JH, et al: Brain damage in fatal non-missile head injury without high intracranial pressure, *J Clin Pathol* 41:34-37, 1988.
58. Chiaretti A, Visocchi M, Viola L, et al: Diffuse axonal lesions in childhood, *Pediatr Med Chir* 20:393-397, 1998.
59. Tear G: Molecular cues that guide the development of neural connectivity. *Essays Biochem* 33:1-13, 1998.
60. Shannon P, Smith CR, Deck J, et al: Axonal injury and the neuropathology of shaken baby syndrome, *Acta Neuropathol (Berl)* 95:624-631, 1998.
61. Povlishock JT, Christman CW: The pathobiology of traumatically induced axonal injury in animals and humans: a review of current thoughts. In: Bandak FA, Eppinger RH, Ommaya AK, editors: *Traumatic brain injury: bioscience and mechanics*. New York, 1996, Mary Ann Liebert.
62. Duhaime AC: Acute care. In Marion DW, editor: *Traumatic brain injury*. New York, 1999, Thieme.
63. Duhaime AC, Christian CW, Rorke LB, Zimmerman RA: Nonaccidental head injury in infants—the "shaken-baby syndrome," *N Engl J Med* 338:1822-1829, 1998.
64. Jenny C, Hymel KP, Ritzen A, et al: Analysis of missed cases of abusive head trauma, *JAMA* 281:621-626, 1999.
65. Teasdale G, Jennett B: Assessment of coma and impaired consciousness: a practical scale, *Lancet* 2:81-84, 1974.
66. *Pediatric Field Reference*. Pittsburgh, Penn., 1994, Children's Hospital of Pittsburgh Communications Center, Children's Hospital of Pittsburgh.
67. Tullous M, Walker ML, Wright LC: Evaluation and treatment of head injuries in children. In Fuhrman B, Zimmerman J, editors: *Pediatric critical care*. St. Louis, 1992, Mosby-Yearbook.
68. Mendelow AD, Karmi MZ, Paul KS, et al: Extradural haematoma: effect of delayed treatment, *BMJ* I:1240-124, 1979.
69. American College of Surgeons Committee on Trauma: *Advanced Trauma Life Support*. Chicago, 1993, American College of Surgeons.
70. Chestnut RM, Marshall LF, Klauber MR, et al: The role of secondary brain injury in determining outcome from severe head injury, *J Trauma* 34:216-222, 1993.
71. Gentleman D: Causes and effects of systemic complications among severely head injured patients transferred to a neurosurgical unit, *Int Surg* 77:297-302, 1992.
72. Forbes ML, Kochanek PM, Adelson PD: Severe traumatic brain injury in children: critical care management. In Albright A, Pollack IF, Adelson Pd, editors: *Principles and practice of pediatric neurosurgery*. New York, 1999, Thieme.
73. Mansfield RT, Kochanek PM: Traumatic head or spinal injury. In McCloskey K, Orr R, editors: *Textbook of pediatric transport medicine*. Baltimore, 1995, Mosby.
74. Hauswald M, Sklar DP, Tandberg D, et al: Cervical spine movement during airway management. Cinefluoroscopic appraisal in human cadavers, *Ann Emerg Med* 20:450, 1991.
75. Gentleman D, Dearden M, Midgley S, et al: Guidelines for resuscitation and transfer of patients with serious head injury, *Br Med J* 307:547-552, 1993.
76. American College of Surgeons Committee on Trauma: Pediatric trauma. In: *Advanced trauma life support,* ed 5. Chicago, 1993, American College of Surgeons.
77. Pang D, Pollack IF: Spinal cord injury without radiographic abnormality in children—the SCIWORA syndrome, *J Trauma* 29:654-664, 1989.

78. American College of Surgeons Committee on Trauma: Airway and ventilatory management. In: *Advanced trauma life support.* Chicago, 1993, American College of Surgeons.
79. Yamamoto LG, Yim GK, Britten AG: Rapid sequence anesthesia induction for emergency intubation, *Pediatr Emerg Care* 6: 200-213, 1990.
80. Dronen SC, Merigan KS, Hedges JR, et al: A comparison of blind nasotracheal and succinylcholine-assisted intubation in the poisoned patient, *Ann Emerg Med* 16:650-652, 1987.
81. Modica PA, Tempelhoff R: Intracranial pressure during induction of anaesthesia and tracheal intubation with etomidate-induced EEG burst suppression, *Can J Anaesth* 39:236-241, 1992.
82. Marvez-Valls E, Houry D, Ernst AA, et al: Protocol for rapid sequence intubation in pediatric patients—a four-year study, *Med Sci Monit* 4:CR229-CR234, 2002.
83. Guldner G, Schultz J, Sexton P, et al: Etomidate for rapid-sequence intubation in young children: hemodynamic effects and adverse events, *Acad Emerg Med* 10:134-139, 2003.
84. Sokolove PE, Price DD, Okada P: The safety of etomidate for emergency rapid sequence intubation of pediatric patients, *Pediatr Emerg Care* 16:18-21, 2000.
85. Pediatric advanced life support study guide. In: Aehlert B, editor: *Textbook of pediatric advanced life support.* Baltimore, 1994, Mosby Year-Book.
86. Zornow MH, Todd MM, Moore SS: The acute cerebral effects of changes in plasma osmolality and oncotic pressure, *Anesthesiology* 67:936-941, 1987.
87. Feldman Z, Zachari S, Reichenthal E, et al: Brain edema and neurological status with rapid infusion of lactated Ringer's or 5% dextrose solution following head trauma, *J Neurosurg* 83:1060-1066, 1995.
88. Fisher B, Thomas D, Peterson B: Hypertonic saline lowers raised intracranial pressure in children after head trauma, *J Neurosurg Anesthesiol* 4:4-10, 1992.
89. Wallen E, Venkataraman ST, Grosso J, et al: Intrahospital transport of critically ill patients, *Crit Care Med* 23:1588-1595, 1995.
90. Valadka AB, Ward JD, Smoker WRK: Brain imaging in neurologic emergencies. In Prough DS, Traystman RJ, editors: *Critical care: state of the art.* Anaheim, Calif, 1993, Society of Critical Care Medicine.
91. Marshall LF, Marshall SB, Klauber MR, et al: The diagnosis of head injury requires a classification based on computed axial tomography, *J Neurotrauma* 9:S287-S291, 1992.
92. Ewing-Cobbs L, Prasad M, Kramer L, et al: Acute neuroradiologic findings in young children with inflicted or noninflicted traumatic brain injury, *Childs Nerv Syst* 16:25-34, 2000.
93. Prasad MR, Ewing-Cobbs L, Swank PR, Kramer L: Predictors of outcome following traumatic brain injury in young children, *Pediatr Neurosurg* 36:64-74, 2002.
94. Givner A, Gurney J, O'Connor D, et al: Reimaging in pediatric neurotrauma: factors associated with progression of intracranial injury, *J Pediatr Surg* 37:381-385, 2002.
95. Tabori U, Kornecki A, Sofer S, et al: Repeat computed tomographic scan within 24-48 hours of admission in children with moderate and severe head trauma, *Crit Care Med* 28:840-844, 2000.
96. Hirsch W, Beck R, Behrmann C, et al: Reliability of cranial CT versus intracerebral pressure measurement for the evaluation of generalized cerebral oedema in children, *Pediatr Radiol* 30: 439-443, 2000.
97. Forbes ML, Hendrich KS, Kochanek PM, et al: Assessment of CBF and CO_2 reactivity after controlled cortical impact by perfusion magnetic resonance imaging using arterial spin labeling in rats, *J Cereb Blood Flow Metab* 17:1263, 1997.
98. Lundberg N: Continuous recording and control of ventricular-fluid pressure in neurosurgical practice, *Acta Psychiatr Scand* 149:36, 1960.
99. Langfitt TW, Kumar VS, James HE, et al: Continuous recording of ICP in patients with hypoxic brain damage. In Brierley JB, Meldrum BS, editors: *Brain hypoxia.* Philadelphia, 1971, JB Lippincott.
100. Rosner MJ, Daughton S: CPP management in head injury, *J Trauma* 30:933-941, 1990.
101. Becker DP, Miller JD, Ward JD, et al: The outcome from severe head injury with early diagnosis and intensive management, *J Neurosurg* 47:491-502, 1977.
102. Marmarou A, Anderson RL, Ward JD, et al: Impact of ICP instability and hypotension on outcome in patients with severe head trauma, *J Neurosurg* 75:S59-S66, 1991.
103. O'Sullivan MG, Statham PF, Jones PA, et al: Role of ICP monitoring in severely head injured patients without signs of intracranial hypertension on initial computerized tomography, *J Neurosurg* 80:46-50, 1994.
104. Bullock MR, Povlishock JT: Guidelines for the management of severe head injury, *Neurotrauma* 13:653, 1996.
105. Ghajar JB, Hariri RJ, Patterson RH: Improved outcome from traumatic coma using only ventricular CSF drainage for ICP control, *Adv Neurosurg* 21:173-177, 1992.
106. Marion DW, Darby J, Yonas H: Acute regional CBF changes caused by severe head injuries, *J Neurosurgery* 74:407-414, 1991.
107. Gur D, Yonas H, Good WF: Local CBF by xenon-enhanced CT: current status, potential improvements, and future directions, *Cereb Brain Metab Rev* 1:68-86, 1989.
108. McLaughlin MR, Marion DW: CBF and vasoresponsivity within and around cerebral contusions, *J Neurosurg* 85:871-876, 1996.
109. Darby JM, Yonas H, Marion DW, et al: Local "inverse steal" induced by hyperventilation in head injury, *Neurosurgery* 23: 84-88, 1988.
110. Obrist WD, Langfitt TW, Jaggi JL, et al: CBF and metabolism in comatose patients with acute head injury: relationship to intracranial hypertension, *J Neurosurg* 61:241-253, 1984.
111. Chan K-H, Miller JD, Dearden NM, et al: The effect of changes in CPP upon middle cerebral artery blood flow velocity and jugular bulb venous oxygen saturation after severe brain injury, *J Neurosurg* 77:55-61, 1992.
112. Mandera M, Larysz D, Wojtacha M, et al: Changes in cerebral hemodynamics assessed by transcranial Doppler ultrasonography in children after head injury, *Childs Nerv Syst* 18: 124-128, 2002.
113. Cruz J: Adverse effects of pentobarbital on cerebral venous oxygenation of comatose patients with acute traumatic brain swelling: relationship to outcome, *J Neurosurg* 85:758-761, 1996.
114. Cruz J: An additional therapeutic effect of adequate hyperventilation in severe acute brain trauma: normalization of cerebral glucose uptake, *J Neurosurg* 82:379-385, 1995.
115. Gopinath SP, Robertson CS, Contant CF, et al: Jugular venous desaturation and outcome after head injury, *J Neurol Neurosurg Psychiatry* 57:717-723, 1994.
116. Coles JP, Minhas PS, Fryer TD, et al: Effect of hyperventilation on cerebral blood flow in traumatic head injury: clinical relevance and monitoring correlates, *Crit Care Med* 30:1950-59, 2002.
117. Cope M, Delpy DT: A system for long term measurement of cerebral blood and tissue oxygenation in newborn infants by near infrared transillumination, *Med Biol Eng Comput* 26:289-294, 1988.
118. Wyatt JS, Cope M, Delpy DT, et al: Quantification of cerebral oxygenation and haemodynamics in sick newborn infants by near infrared spectrophotometry, *Lancet* 2:1063-1066, 1986.
119. Adelson PD, Nemoto E, Colak A, et al: The use of near infrared spectroscopy (NIRS) in children after traumatic brain injury: a preliminary report, *Acta Neurochir* 71:250-254, 1998.
120. Gopinath SP, Robertson CS, Contant, CF, et al: Early detection of delayed traumatic intracranial hematomas using near-infrared spectroscopy, *J Neurosurg* 83:438-444, 1995.
121. Kiening KL, Unterberg AW, Bardt TF, et al: Monitoring of cerebral oxygenation in patients with severe head injuries: brain tissue PO_2 versus jugular vein oxygen saturation, *J Neurosurg* 85: 751-757, 1996.
122. Goodman JC, Valadka AB, Gopinpath SP, et al: Lactate and excitatory amino acids measured by microdialysis are decreased by pentobarbital coma in head-injured patients, *J Neurotrauma* 13:549-556, 1996.
123. Bullock R, Zauner A, Tsuji O, et al: Excitatory amino acid release after severe human head trauma: effect of ICP and CPP changes. In Nagai H, Kamiya K, Ishii S, editors: *ICP 9.* Tokyo, 1994, Springer-Verlag.
124. Diringer MN, Yundt K, Videen TO, et al: No reduction in cerebral metabolism as a result of early moderate hyperventilation following severe traumatic brain injury, *J Neurosurg* 92:7-13, 2000.
125. Hovda DA, Lee SM, Smith ML, et al: The neurochemical and metabolic cascade following brain injury: moving from animal models to man, *J Neurotrauma* 12:903-906, 1995.

126. Saul TG, Ducker TB: Effect of ICP monitoring and aggressive treatment on mortality in severe head injury, *J Neurosurg* 56: 498-503, 1982.
127. Pfenninger J, Kaiser G, Lutschg J, et al: Treatment and outcome of the severely head injured child, *Intensive Care Med* 9:13-16, 1983.
128. Esparza J, M-Portillo J, Sarabia M, et al: Outcome in children with severe head injuries, *Childs Nerv Syst* 1:109-114, 1985.
129. Shapiro K, Marmarou A: Clinical applications of the pressure-volume index in treatment of pediatric head injuries, *J Neurosurg* 56:819-825, 1982.
130. Downard C, Hulka F, Mullins RJ, et al: Relationship of cerebral perfusion pressure and survival in pediatric brain-injured patients, *J Trauma* 49:654-658, 2000.
131. Kaiser G, Pfenninger J: Effect of neurointensive care upon outcome following severe head injuries in childhood—a preliminary report, *Neuropediatrics* 15:68-75, 1984.
132. Barzilay Z, Augarten A, Sagy M, et al: Variables affecting outcome from severe brain injury in children, *Intensive Care Med* 14:417-442, 1988.
133. Elias-Jones AC, Punt JA, Turnbull AE, et al: Management and outcome of severe head injuries in the Trent region 1985-90, *Arch Dis Child* 67:1430-1435, 1992.
134. White JR, Farukhi Z, Bull C, et al: Predictors of outcome in severely head-injured children, *Crit Care Med* 29:534-540, 2001.
135. Robertson CS, Valadka AB, Hannay HJ, et al: Prevention of secondary ischemic insults after severe head injury, *Crit Care Med* 10:2086-2095, 1999.
136. Laptook AR, Stonestreet BS, Oh W: Brain blood flow and O_2 delivery during hemorrhagic hypotension in the piglet, *Pediatr Res* 17:77-80, 1983.
137. Szymonowicz W, Walker AM, Yu VYH, et al: Regional CBF after hemorrhagic hypotension in the preterm, near-term, and newborn lamb, *Pediatr Res* 28:361-366, 1990.
138. Raju TNK, Doshi UV, Vidyasagar D: CPP studies in healthy preterm and term newborn infants, *J Pediatr* 100:139-142, 1982.
139. Goitein KJ, Tamir I: CPP in central nervous system infections of infancy and childhood, *J Pediatr* 103:40-43, 1983.
140. Langfitt TW, Kumar VS, James HE, et al: Continuous recording of intracranial pressure in patients with hypoxic brain damage. In Brierley JB, Meldrum BS, editors: *Brain hypoxia*. Philadelphia, 1971, JB Lippincott.
141. Fortune JB, Feustel PJ, Graca L, et al: Effect of hyperventilation, mannitol, and ventriculostomy drainage on cerebral blood flow after head injury, *J Trauma* 39:1091-1099, 1995.
142. Peterson B, Khanna S, Fisher B, Marshall L: Prolonged hypernatremia controls elevated intracranial pressure in head-injured pediatric patients, *Crit Care Med* 28:1136-1143, 2000.
143. James HE: Methodology for the control of intracranial pressure with hypertonic mannitol. *Acta Neurochir* 51:161-172, 1980.
144. Marshall LF, Smith RW, Rauscher LA, Shapiro HM: Mannitol dose requirements in brain-injured patients, *J Neurosurg* 48: 169-172, 1978.
145. Kaieda R, Todd MM, Cook LN, Warner DS: Acute effects of changing plasma osmolality and colloid oncotic pressure on the formation of brain edema after cryogenic injury, *Neurosurgery* 24:671-677, 1989.
146. Khanna S, Davis D, Peterson B, et al: Use of hypertonic saline in the treatment of severe refractory posttraumatic intracranial hypertension in pediatric traumatic brain injury, *Crit Care Med* 28:1144-1151, 2000.
147. Bay1r H, Clark RSB, Kochanek PM: Promising strategies to minimize secondary brain injury after head trauma, *Crit Care Med* 31:S112-S117, 2003.
148. Sterns RH, Riggs JE, Schochet SS Jr: Osmotic demyelination syndrome following correction of hyponatremia, *N Engl J Med* 314:1535-1542, 1986.
149. Soupart A, Penninckx R, Namias B, et al: Brain myelinolysis following hypernatremia in rats, *J Neuropathol Exp Neurol* 55:1076-113, 1996.
150. Findberg L, Litrell C, Redd H: Pathogenesis of lesions in the nervous system in hypernatremic states. Part II: experimental studies of gross anatomic changes and alterations of chemical composition of the tissues, *Pediatrics* 23:46-53, 1959.
151. Huang PP, Stucky FS, Dimick AR, et al: Hypertonic sodium resuscitation is associated with renal failure and death, *Ann Surg* 221:543-554, 1995; discussion 554-547.
152. Qureshi AI, Suarez JI, Bhardwaj A: Malignant cerebral edema in patients with hypertensive intracerebral hemorrhage associated with hypertonic saline infusion: a rebound phenomenon? *J Neurosurg Anesthesiol* 10:188-192, 1998.
153. Hsiang JK, Chestnut RM, Crisp CB, et al: Early, routine paralysis for ICP control in severe head injury: is it necessary? *Crit Care Med* 22:1471-1476, 1994.
154. Feldman Z, Kanter MJ, Robertson CS, et al: Effect of head elevation on ICP, CPP, and CBF in head-injured patients, *J Neurosurg* 76:207-211, 1992.
155. Alberico AM, Ward JD, Choi SC, et al: Outcome after severe head injury. Relationship to mass lesions, diffuse injury, and ICP course in pediatric and adult patients, *J Neurosurg* 67:648-656, 1987.
156. Aldrich EF, Eisenberg HM, Saydjari C, et al: Diffuse brain swelling in severely head-injured children. A report from the NIH Traumatic Coma Data Bank, *J Neurosurg* 76:450-454, 1992.
157. Juul N, Morris GF, Marshall SB, et al: Intracranial hypertension and cerebral perfusion pressure: influence on neurological deterioration and outcome in severe head injury. The Executive Committee of the International Selfotel Trial, *J Neurosurg* 92: 1-6, 2000.
158. Ward JD, Becker DP, Miller DP, et al: Failure of prophylactic barbiturate coma in the treatment of severe head injury, *J Neurosurg* 62:383-388, 1985.
159. Pittman T, Bucholz R, Williams D: Efficacy of barbiturates in the treatment of resistant intracranial hypertension in severely head-injured children, *Pediatr Neurosci* 15:13-17, 1989.
160. Goodman JC, Valadka AB, Gopinpath SP, et al: Lactate and excitatory amino acids measured by microdialysis are decreased by pentobarbital coma in head-injured patients, *J Neurotrauma* 13:549-556, 1996.
161. Kasoff SS, Lansen TA, Holder D, et al: Aggressive physiologic monitoring of pediatric head trauma patients with elevated intracranial pressure, *Pediatr Neurosci* 14:241-249, 1988.
162. Lundberg N, Kjallquist A, Bien C: Reduction of increased intracranial pressure by hyperventilation, *Acta Psychiatr Scand* 34:4-64, 1959.
163. Muizelaar JP, van der Poel HG: Pial arteriolar vessel diameter and CO_2 reactivity during prolonged hyperventilation in the rabbit, *J Neurosurg* 69:923-927, 1988.
164. Muizelaar JP, Marmarou A, Ward JD, et al: Adverse effects of prolonged hyperventilation in patients with severe head injury: a randomized clinical trial, *J Neurosurg* 75:731-739, 1991.
165. Skippen P, Seear M, Poskitt K, et al: Effect of hypothermia on regional cerebral blood flow in head-injured children, *Crit Care Med* 25:1402-1409, 1997.
166. Marion DW, Penrod LE, Kelsey SF, et al: Treatment of traumatic brain injury with moderate hypothermia, *N Engl J Med* 336: 540-546, 1997.
167. McIntyre LA, Fergusson DA, Hebert PC, et al: Prolonged therapeutic hypothermia after traumatic brain injury in adults: a systematic review, *JAMA* 289:2992-2997, 2003.
168. Kochanek PM, Safar PJ: Therapeutic hypothermia for severe traumatic brain injury—"cool heads" will prevail, *JAMA* 289:3007-3009, 2003.
169. Mild therapeutic hypothermia to improve the neurologic outcome after cardiac arrest. Hypothermia after cardiac arrest study group, *N Engl J Med* 346:549-556, 2002.
170. Bernard SA, Gray TW, Buist MD, et al: Treatment of comatose survivors of out-of-hospital cardiac arrest with induced hypothermia, *N Engl J Med* 346:557-563, 2002.
171. Tateishi A, Soejima Y, Taira Y, et al: Feasibility of the titration method of mild hypothermia in severely head-injured patients with intracranial hypertension, *Neurosurgery* 42:1065-1070, 1998.
172. Tokutomi T, Morimoto K, Miyagi T, et al: Optimal temperature for the management of severe traumatic brain head injury: effect of hypothermia on intracranial pressure, systemic and intracranial hemodynamics, and metabolism, *Neurosurgery* 52:102-111, 2003.
173. Natale JE, Joseph JG, Helfaer MA, et al: Early hyperthermia after traumatic brain injury in children: risk factors, influence on length of stay, and effect on short-term neurologic status, *Crit Care Med* 28:2608-2615, 2000.
174. Cushing H: The establishment of cerebral hernia as a decompressive measure for inaccessible brain tumors: with the description of

intermuscular methods of making the bone defect in temporal and occipital regions. *Surg Gynecol Obstet* 1:297-314, 1905.
175. Cho DY, Wang YC, Chi CS: Decompressive craniotomy for acute shaken/impact baby syndrome, *Pediatr Neurosurg* 23:192-198, 1995.
176. Polin RS, Shaffrey ME, Bogaev CA, et al: Decompressive bifrontal craniectomy in the treatment of severe refractory posttraumatic cerebral edema, *Neurosurgery* 41:84-94, 1997.
177. Taylor A, Butt W, Rosenfeld J, et al: A randomized trial of very early decompressive craniectomy in children with traumatic brain injury and sustained intracranial hypertension, *Childs Nerv Syst* 17:154-162, 2001.
178. Levy DI, Rekate HL, Cherny WB, et al: Controlled lumbar drainage in pediatric head injury, *J Neurosurg* 83:453-460, 1995.
179. Munch E, Horn P, Schurer L, et al: Management of severe traumatic brain injury by decompressive craniectomy, *Neurosurgery* 47:315-322, 2000.
180. Bouma GJ, Muizelaar JP, Bandoh K, et al: Blood pressure and ICP-volume dynamics in severe head injury: relationship with CBF, *J Neurosurg* 77:15-19, 1992.
181. Asgeirsson B, Grande PO, Nordstrom CH: A new therapy of post-trauma brain oedema based on haemodynamic principles for brain volume regulation, *J Intensive Care Med* 20:260-267, 1994.
182. Stahl N, Ungerstedt U, Nordstrom CH: Brain energy metabolism during controlled reduction of cerebral perfusion pressure in severe head injuries, *Intensive Care Med* 27:1215-1223, 2001.
183. Grande PO, Myhre EB, Nordstrom CH, Schliamser S: Treatment of intracranial hypertension and aspects on lumbar dural puncture in severe bacterial meningitis, *Acta Anaesthesiol Scand* 46: 264-270, 2002.
184. Bruce DA, Schut L, Bruno LA, et al: Outcome following severe head injuries in children, *J Neurosurg* 48:679-688, 1978.
185. Rosner MJ, Rosner SD, Johnson AH: Cerebral perfusion pressure: management protocol and clinical results, *J Neurosurg* 83: 949-962, 1995.
186. Sivakumar V, Rajshekhar V, Chandy MJ: Management of neurosurgical patients with hyponatremia and natriuresis, *J Neurosurg* 34:269-274, 1994.
187. Blackburn GL, Kudsk KA: Enteral vs. parenteral nutrition. In: *Proceedings of the 23rd Educational and Scientific Symposium of the Society of Critical Care Medicine, Anaheim, California.* 1994, Society of Critical Care Medicine.
188. Hadley MN, Grahm TW, Harrington T, et al: Nutritional support in neurotrauma: a critical review of early nutrition in 45 acute head injury patients, *Neurosurgery* 19:367-373, 1986.
189. Sunderland PM, Heilbrun MP: Estimating energy expenditure in traumatic brain injury: comparison of indirect calorimetry with predictive formula, *Neurosurgery* 31:246-253, 1992.
190. Stover JF, Kempski OS: Glutamate-containing parenteral nutrition doubles plasma glutamate: a risk factor in neurosurgical patients with blood-brain barrier damage? *Crit Care Med* 27:2252-2256, 1999.
191. Kelly DF, Gonzalo IT, Coha P, et al: Hypopituitarism following traumatic brain injury and aneurysmal subarachnoid hemorrhage: a preliminary report, *J Neurosurg* 93:743-752, 2000.
192. Robertson CMT, Joffe AR, Moore AJ, et al: Neurodevelopmental outcome of young pediatric intensive care survivors of serious brain injury, *Pediatr Crit Care Med* 3:345-350, 2002.
193. Paret G, Barzilai A, Lahat, et al: Gunshot wounds in brains of children: prognostic variables in mortality, course, and outcome, *J Neurotrauma* 15:967-972, 1998.
194. Boyer MG, Edwards P: Outcome 1 to 3 years after severe traumatic brain injury in children and adolescents, *Injury* 22: 315-320, 1991.

CHAPTER

108

Thoracic Injuries in Children

Jorge R. Beltran, Guy F. Brisseau, and Michael G. Caty

PEARLS

- Thoracic injuries in children are uncommon but result in significant morbidity and mortality, mainly from the frequent association with head trauma and abdominal trauma.
- Most thoracic injuries in children result from blunt trauma. The most common modifications of thoracic trauma in children are rib fractures, pneumothoraces, hemothoraces, and pulmonary contusions.

Thoracic injuries in children are relatively uncommon but result in a disproportionate percent of morbidity and mortality compared with other traumatic injuries, mainly because thoracic injuries often are associated with life-threatening conditions. Children with significant thoracic injuries require intensive monitoring and hemodynamic and respiratory support. It is important to establish an accurate diagnosis. High-resolution imaging techniques such as helical computed tomography (CT) currently are indicated to detect intrathoracic lesions. This chapter discusses the epidemiology, diagnosis, and immediate approach to children with thoracic injuries and the current management of specific injuries to the thorax.

Epidemiology

The National Pediatric Trauma Registry (NPTR) was created in 1994 and has collected information from 94 trauma centers in the United States. From 1994 to 2001, 3721 patients with thoracic injuries were reported, which corresponds to 7.7% of all pediatric trauma.[1] Interestingly, isolated thoracic injuries account for only 0.7% of all pediatric trauma patients.

Thoracic trauma occurs more frequently in males, with a male/female ratio of approximately 2:1. No differences in age distribution are noted. Blunt, as opposed to penetrating, trauma is the most frequent cause of injury (92%).

Nakayama et al.[2] analyzed all consecutive patients in a level I trauma center and found that the most common thoracic injuries are pulmonary contusion (48%), pneumothorax/hemothorax (39%), and rib fractures (32%).

Most commonly, thoracic injuries present concomitantly with other injuries, and this observation is consistent.[1–3] From 60% to 85% of children with thoracic injuries have significant injury to at least one other organ system, most notably the central nervous system, the abdominal cavity, or the musculoskeletal system.[2,3] The most common mechanisms of injury are motor vehicle-related accidents (40.7%), children as pedestrians (19.2%), bicycle accidents (6.6%), and falls (5.8%). With the escalating use of firearms in society, the incidence of penetrating chest injury in urban areas is increasing, currently accounting for 8% of all thoracic injuries.[1]

The clinical importance of thoracic injuries is reflected in the greater severity of injury observed in children with thoracic injuries [Trauma Score (TS) 11, Injury Severity Scale (ISS) 27] compared with that seen in children without thoracic injuries [TS 15; ISS 7].[3] This observation is corroborated by data from the NPTR in which 42% of patients with thoracic trauma have an ISS greater than 20 and 30% have a Pediatric Trauma Score (PTS) less than 5 in 42% and 30%, respectively.[1]

According to the NPTR, the overall mortality for trauma in the pediatric population is 3%. Thoracic injuries are present in 33% of fatal cases.

The mortality rate for thoracic trauma is 12.2%. Central nervous system injuries are the major cause of death (63.1%), followed by uncontrollable hemorrhage in 13.5% of children.[1] The number and severity of associated injuries are important determining factors.[2–4] Stratification of mortality rates according to the number and type of associated injuries illustrates this point. Children with abdominal and thoracic injuries have a 20% mortality rate; children with chest and head injuries have a 35% mortality rate; and children with all three injuries have a 39% mortality.[3] Fortunately, immediately life-threatening chest injuries are infrequent; consequently, emergency thoracotomies are required in only 3% to 6% of all pediatric thoracic trauma.[5]

Diagnosis and Immediate Management of the Child with Chest Injuries

The initial evaluation of the child with known or suspected thoracic trauma conforms to the standard evaluation for all trauma.[50] First, the patency of the airway is established (Box 108–1). Inability to maintain an airway because of anatomic obstruction or depressed consciousness (Glasgow Coma Scale [GCS] ≤8) warrants endotracheal intubation. All patients with suspected cervical injuries should have manual in-line cervical stabilization maintained during intubation. If endotracheal intubation is not possible, an age-appropriate surgical or needle cricothyroidotomy should be performed.

After the airway is secured, breathing is assessed. Both hemithoraces are observed for symmetrical motion, and auscultation is performed to evaluate transmitted breath sounds. The position of the endotracheal tube should be checked in the intubated patient with asymmetric chest expansion or decreased breath sounds before any invasive procedures are performed. Arterial PO_2 analysis and pulse oximetry are useful for assessing oxygenation, whereas PCO_2 level and in-line capnography, where available, are extremely helpful for assessing ventilation.

The stable child with decreased breath sounds on one side should undergo immediate chest radiography. A chest tube should be placed if either a pneumothorax or hemothorax is demonstrated. In an unstable child, needle thoracentesis should be performed immediately on the side with decreased breath sounds (Figure 108–1).

Assessment of the circulation begins with recording the pulse rate and blood pressure. Observation of capillary refill provides an approximation of tissue perfusion. Appropriate intravenous access is established, and fluid resuscitation is initiated. Cardiac tamponade should be suspected in the child with equal breath sounds and a normal chest x-ray film but hemodynamic instability. Pulsus paradoxus and jugular venous distension are inconsistent findings, and their absence should not be used to rule out the presence of cardiac tamponade.

BOX 108–1

Acute Thoracic Conditions Requiring Immediate Correction

Airway obstruction
Tension pneumothorax
Massive hemothorax
Cardiac tamponade

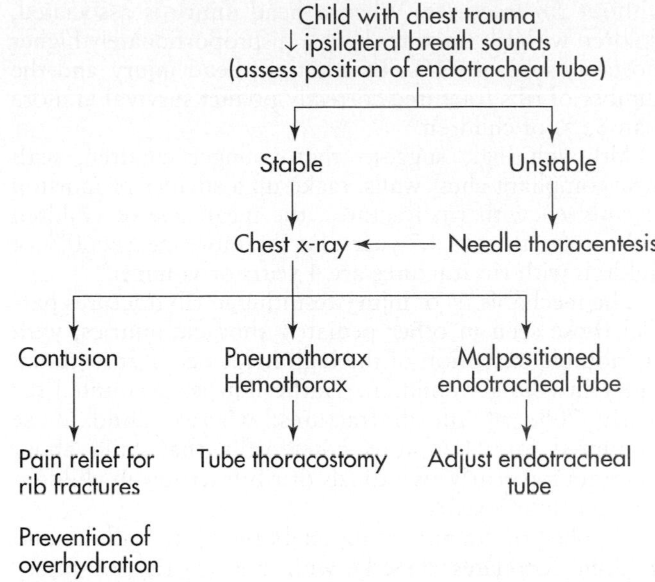

FIGURE 108–1 • Management of the child with decreased breath sounds.

Additional clues to the nature of injuries are obtained by observation and palpation. Specifically, look for patterns of abrasions and contusions that suggest the mechanism of injury and allow prediction of potential intrathoracic injuries. One example is the child with a sternal contusion who should be assessed for a cardiac contusion. The thoracic cage should be palpated from under the arms to the abdomen in a sequential fashion, looking for rib tenderness and/or flail segments. Chest radiography completes the initial evaluation. The physician checks the x-ray film for evidence of pneumothorax, hemothorax, pulmonary contusion, and rib fractures. First and second rib fractures do not seem to be reliable indicators of aortic injury in children.[27,51]

In general, approximately 60% of patients with a thoracic trauma diagnosis are admitted to the pediatric intensive care unit for further monitoring and management.[2,6]

Rib Fractures

Fractures of the bony thorax, specifically rib fractures, are more common than previously suspected.[2,4,7] In one large study, rib fractures were noted in 32% of all children with thoracic injuries.[3] However, in the context of all injured children admitted, rib fractures were infrequent and were observed in only 1.6% of injured children. Again, the pediatric experience stands in sharp contrast to the adult experience, in which rib fractures are frequently seen and are present in 33% of injured adult patients.[4]

The importance of rib fractures as a marker of severity has been emphasized.[27] In this study, rib fractures were noted in only 1.6% of children admitted. However, the mortality rate of children with rib fractures was 42%, compared with the 2.1% mortality rate noted in children without rib fractures. When a head injury is associated, children with rib fractures have a disproportionately higher mortality rate of 71%. In addition, head injury and the number of ribs fractured correctly predict survival in more than 85% of children.[6]

Although logic suggests that younger children, with their compliant chest walls, make up a smaller proportion of children with rib fractures, the mean age of children with rib fractures is 4.7 years. Furthermore, nearly 60% of children with rib fractures are 4 years or younger.[6]

The mechanisms of injury resulting in rib fractures parallel those seen in other pediatric thoracic injuries, with the notable exception of the high incidence of intentional injury in younger children. Traffic injuries accounted for nearly 70% of all rib fractures, whereas child abuse accounted for 21%. It is noteworthy that child abuse accounts for nearly two thirds of rib fractures in children younger than 3 years.[6]

Number of fractured ribs in both injured adults and children correlates directly with the severity of injury (assessed by the Revised Trauma Score [RTS] and the ISS), the likelihood of multisystem and intrathoracic injury, and higher mortality rates.[6,14]

Presence of three or more rib fractures in a child reliably identifies him or her as having a significant likelihood of intrathoracic, as well as other organ involvement, and a significantly higher probability of dying.[4]

Consistent with the literature on adults with rib fractures, first and second rib fractures in children do not correlate with the presence of concomitant injury to the great vessels and in isolation do not warrant aortography.[2,6,8] Additionally, neither posterior rib fractures nor scapular rib fractures were indicative of great vessel injury. However, evidence suggests that the presence of thoracic spine fractures should heighten the suspicion of great vessel injury.[9]

The key to successful management of chest wall injuries is adequate pain control to promote effective air exchange and to facilitate pulmonary toilet.[4,10,11] Regional anesthetic techniques, such as epidural and pleural catheters, and intercostal nerve blocks play an expanding role in pain control and are increasingly viewed as effective and safe adjuncts to traditional analgesia techniques.[10,11]

Finally, for flail chest injury patients, an ISS greater than 23, the need for blood transfusions within the first 24 hours, and the presence or development of shock on admission are suggested as factors that predict the need for ventilatory assistance.[10] These assertions stem from an analysis of adult patients. Their validity in the treatment of children awaits further evaluation. Fortunately, the majority of children with fractured ribs do not require ventilatory assistance and have a good overall prognosis.[6]

Pulmonary Contusion

Pulmonary contusion rivals pneumothorax/hemothorax as the most common childhood thoracic injury. It is present in as many as 48% of children with thoracic injuries.[2,3] Evidence suggestive of pulmonary contusion, such as external chest wall abrasions, tachypnea, and abnormal breath sounds, are frequently absent in children. Considering the disparity between the size of the average child and the magnitude of the force imparted by automobile crashes, which represent the most common mechanisms of injury, it is not surprising that pulmonary contusion usually is associated with other potentially more life-threatening conditions such as pneumothorax and hemothorax or other systemic injuries.[3,6,12–15] Rib fractures are present in up to 32% of children with intrathoracic injuries,[3,6,12–15] and the importance of such markers of internal injuries is enhanced because the radiographic manifestations of these intrathoracic injuries often are delayed. Up to 40% of cases of pulmonary contusion and other intrathoracic lesions were not radiographically evident until 48 hours after injury.[12] When pulmonary contusion is accompanied by rib fractures, serial chest radiographs should be performed during the initial 48 hours after injury to promptly identify other intrathoracic injuries.[12] Although most patients with pulmonary contusion are identified by sequentially obtained chest radiographs, CT scan may be of greater value in demonstrating posttraumatic intrathoracic pathology in patients requiring intubation and mechanical ventilation. For patients with an oxygenation index (PaO_2/FIO_2) less than 300, a CT scan may be helpful in defining the extent of pulmonary contusion and identifying those patients at higher risk for acute pulmonary failure or those with unsuspected or incompletely treated hemo/pneumothoraces.[16]

Management of pulmonary contusion centers on judicious fluid management, adequate pulmonary toilet, and respiratory support. Corticosteroids are ineffective and probably are harmful.[12] Prognosis for most children with pulmonary contusion is excellent because usually the majority of these injuries are mild to moderate in severity, and children recover without the need for ventilatory support.

For severe pulmonary contusions, differential lung ventilation may be valuable.[17–19] Early success of synchronized independent lung ventilation using a double-lumen endobronchial tube connected to two ventilators indicates a potentially lifesaving treatment option for the child with a significant pulmonary contusion.[13] Early institution of synchronized independent lung ventilation may increase survival in the severely injured patient with pulmonary contusion.[2,3,13,15,20]

Pneumothorax/Hemothorax

Pneumothorax and hemothorax collectively represent the second most common intrathoracic injuries seen in children.[2,3,12] Together, they account for 39% to 50% of childhood intrathoracic injuries.

The majority (76%) of chest injuries resulting in pneumothorax or hemothorax require only a tube thoracostomy for successful management (see Chapter 15).[2,3,22] One of the most common mistakes in managing a significant hemothorax is placing a chest tube that is not large enough to adequately evacuate the blood, thus predisposing the patient to the development of a fibrothorax and subsequent entrapment of the lung. Tube thoracostomy is best performed with the upper extremity fully abducted. This position elevates the ribs and widens the intercostal space, facilitating the placement of the chest tube, which may be at once diagnostic and therapeutic.

The chest tube is inserted more caudally and more posteriorly for a suspected hemothorax than for a pneumothorax. Ideally, the fifth intercostal space is used along the midaxillary line. At this level there is little danger to the long thoracic nerve and relatively little risk to the liver or spleen. More posterior placement of the tube can result in obstruction of the tube when the child lies in the supine position.

Because of the low arterial pressures in the pulmonary circulation, bleeding from tears in the lung parenchyma is slow, and homeostasis occurs early after the lung is reexpanded. Exsanguinating hemorrhage usually involves intercostal, hilar, or mediastinal vessels. Thoracotomy is indicated when the initial thoracotomy tube output is greater than or equal to 20% to 30% of blood volume, when the output is greater than 2 to 3 ml/kg/hour over the following 6 hours, or when significant rebleeding occurs.[23]

It is widely accepted that the erect chest x-ray film with posteroanterior and lateral projections is highly accurate in demonstrating major intrathoracic pathology. However, with the overriding concern for possible cervical spine injury, chest radiographs during trauma resuscitation usually are taken with the child in the supine position. In that position, small and even modest collections of air may not be readily demonstrated. Although the portable chest x-ray film has a well-defined role during assessment of thoracic injuries, its limitations must be borne in mind.[22]

Whenever possible, erect anteroposterior and lateral chest x-ray projections should be obtained as soon as clinical conditions allow. Some authorities, noting the lower sensitivity of chest radiographs, recommend that emergent chest CT scans be performed in stable patients with blunt, high-energy torso trauma, cross-body injury patterns, or mechanisms of injury suggestive of chest trauma.[14,15,24] The focused assessment sonography for trauma (FAST) in the setting of thoracic trauma is useful for detecting fluid in the pleural cavity and has 95% sensitivity in detecting pneumothoraces compared with chest x-ray films.[25]

The increased mobility of the child's mediastinum places the pediatric patient at increased risk for the physiologic consequences of a tension pneumothorax, which may occur in 25% of children presenting with a pneumothorax.[2] The approach to the unstable patient with a tension pneumothorax from a massive air leak is discussed in Chapters 15 and 105. Fortunately, in the majority of cases pneumothorax results from small disruptions of the lung parenchyma. These disruptions are associated with small to modest air leaks and are effectively treated with a tube thoracostomy.[3,26,27]

Persistent air leaks suggest disruption of a major airway. If ventilatory support is necessary and if the size of the child's airway allows, a double-lumen tube can be used for selective management of the uninjured and injured lungs, thus minimizing the severity of the air leak and optimizing ventilation.[3,26–28] Single-lung intubation is an efficient alternative maneuver if double-lumen ventilation cannot be accomplished.

Severe tracheobronchial disruptions usually are seen after high-energy impact injuries, most frequently motor vehicle crashes. Consequently, these injuries in children likely have associated multisystem injuries that may require emergent treatment. Because of the increased compliance of the child's chest wall, tracheobronchial injury may occur without the suggestive chest wall injuries anticipated in the adult patient with a similar mechanism of injury.

The most common presenting signs and symptoms are subcutaneous emphysema, dyspnea, sternal tenderness, and hemoptysis.[3,26–28] The typical radiographic findings are subcutaneous emphysema, pneumomediastinum, pneumothorax, air surrounding the bronchus, and an abnormal appearance of the endotracheal tube. These findings, in association with upper thoracic fractures, are highly suggestive of tracheobronchial disruption. An uncommon finding, but nonetheless highly specific for tracheobronchial injury, is collapse of the lung toward the chest wall.[27–30]

When the constellation of a likely mechanism of injury, a suggestive clinical picture, and x-ray findings are present, diagnostic bronchoscopy is a priority. In a stable patient, either flexible or rigid bronchoscopy should be performed to confirm the location and the extent of airway disruption. If possible, a flexible bronchoscope is passed through the endotracheal tube, with the tube withdrawn enough to inspect the entire trachea. If size disparities preclude passing the flexible bronchoscope through the endotracheal tube, the trachea should be examined with a ventilating bronchoscope.

Tracheobronchial injuries range from irregular tears to complete transections. Major sternal injuries have been associated with partial or complete horizontal transections of the trachea. An associated esophageal laceration must be promptly recognized to avoid esophageal fistula and fatal mediastinitis.

The site of the injury influences the choice of thoracotomy incision.[31] Injuries to the left main stem bronchus or parenchyma are managed best through a left thoracotomy. A right thoracotomy affords the best exposure for injuries to the right lateral or posterior aspect of the trachea or to the right bronchi or parenchyma. The anterior or left lateral aspect of the mediastinal trachea is approached best through a median sternotomy. Principles of bronchial surgery dictate conservative debridement of irregular ends; precise end-to-end approximation using interrupted, absorbable sutures; proportional placement of all sutures before tying; and layer coverage to provide an airtight seal and to prevent pleural bronchial fistulas.[32]

Primary reconstruction of the tracheobronchial tree should be performed as soon as possible to ensure the best results. Delayed operations have a high incidence of late scar formation, necessitating further operations.[28]

Rarely, pneumomediastinum without damage to the mediastinal organs is seen after blunt trauma to the torso.[33] The explanation offered for this phenomenon is that blunt trauma induces a sudden rise in intrapulmonary pressure, leading to passage of air from the perihilar alveoli into the mediastinum along the peribronchial and perivascular spaces. Nevertheless, the clinical priority when pneumomediastinum is recognized on x-ray examination is to exclude, by whatever means deemed appropriate, the presence of aerodigestive tract injury.

Finally, the emerging video-assisted thoracoscopic surgery (VATS) is suitable in cases of residual hemothorax, persistent air leaks, or posttraumatic empyema.[34,35]

Cardiac Injuries

Most cardiac injuries in children result from blunt trauma. These injuries have inconsistent manifestations, making diagnosis problematic. The incidence of trauma-related cardiac injuries in children is less than 3%.[24] For those who reach a hospital, cardiac injuries are discovered at autopsy in up to 15% of cases. Of these patients, 46% die at the scene of the accident; the rest die in the emergency department or later during hospitalization.[38]

Myocardial contusion is by far the most common cardiac injury.[36] In a multicenter review, 95% of cardiac trauma was caused by myocardial contusion in patients with a mean ISS of 27.[37] Cardiac contusion may resemble a myocardial infarction, with depressed myocardial function, or it may present as supraventricular and ventricular arrhythmias. Cardiac contusions are more common than previously appreciated in the pediatric population.[7] Associated injuries include pulmonary contusions (50.5%) and rib fractures (23%). Cardiac contusion is more commonly diagnosed in the context of severe multiple system trauma rather than an isolated event.[37]

Diagnosis of myocardial contusion depends on a high index of suspicion. Although the electrocardiogram (ECG) is generally accepted as a reliable screening tool, its sensitivity in children has been questioned.[37]

Other studies of varying utility in identifying cardiac contusion are serum creatinine kinase and its isoenzymes, troponin, radionuclide angiography, and echocardiography.[39–46]

Attempts to reliably identify patients at high risk for cardiac complications after blunt chest trauma have been challenging and have explored the predictive validity of a number of tests. One study identified an abnormal ECG and ISS greater than 10 as predictive of a myocardial contusion. However, this same study was unable to identify other factors predicting the development of complications of myocardial contusion.

Although a plethora of studies have addressed ways to diagnose myocardial contusion, it is important to recognize that, in most instances, cardiac contusion has limited clinical significance.[39–46] Indeed, the incidence of cardiac sequelae among patients with myocardial contusion is low.[42] Cardiac complications usually occur within 12 hours of injury and are forewarned by an abnormal ECG in most cases.[49] Patients with isolated chest wall contusions, a normal admission ECG, and normal rhythm 4 hours after injury rarely develop any cardiac-related complications during the course of their hospitalization.[43]

Other recognized trauma-related cardiac injuries are valvular dysfunction from papillary muscle or chordae tendineae rupture, cardiac rupture, pericardial effusion, and cardiac dysrhythmia.[7,36,43,47,49–58] Although of limited screening use, echocardiography is valuable for identifying pericardial effusions and global or segmental defects in heart wall motion (see Chapter 21). Conduction abnormalities noted on the admission ECG may be predictive of subsequent serious dysrhythmias, warranting close monitoring and possible treatment.[46] Echocardiography and isoenzyme levels, although frequently positive, do not predict cardiac-related morbidity. In considering the issue of cardiac injuries in pediatric trauma patients, it is important to bear in mind that because a standard is lacking for the various diagnostics test required for diagnosis of cardiac trauma, patients who develop life-threatening complications in most instances can be identified in the emergency department setting using modalities readily available in most hospitals (e.g., 12-lead ECG). [46]

The mortality rate among patients with cardiac injury is 13%, mainly as a result of head or intraabdominal injuries. Approximately 5% of survivors will have significant cardiac sequelae, most commonly valvular insufficiency and ventricular septal defects. Follow-up of children with cardiac injury should be ensured.[37]

Aortic and Great Vessel Injuries

The overall mortality rate observed in children with aortic and great vessel injuries is 75%.[3] Of these children, approximately 85% die at the scene and 15% die after arrival to the hospital. Fatal hemorrhage in the 25% of patients who survive is avoided because the surrounding tissue contains the bleeding. However, left undiagnosed and untreated, 30% of those who arrive alive at the hospital will exsanguinate within 24 hours after admission.[59] Fortunately, these injuries are uncommon in children and are seen in only approximately 1% to 3% of injured children.[2,3] The most common and lethal of these injuries is traumatic aortic disruption, characteristically seen in the older adolescent population.[2,3] The well-recognized signs and symptoms associated with traumatic aortic rupture are midscapular back pain, unexplained hypotension, upper extremity hypertension, bilateral femoral pulse deficits, and large initial chest tube outputs.[60–62] Early recognition of these signs can prevent tragic delays in diagnosis. However, acute traumatic aortic rupture remains a highly lethal injury, with no change in prognosis during the past 2 decades.[63]

The findings on chest x-ray examination are well recognized: widened mediastinum, deviation of the nasogastric tube or central venous lines, blurring of the aortic knob, abnormal paraspinous stripe, rightward tracheal deviation, or upward shift of the left main stem bronchus.[60–62] Transverse mediastinal width and mediastinal width/chest width (M/C) ratio on supine chest films have been touted as useful tools for identifying the patient with possible traumatic aortic rupture.[6] However, their clinical usefulness is limited by considerable overlap between normal and abnormal measurements as is seen in infants with an enlarged thymus. This has prompted others to suggest that subjective assessment of anatomical mediastinal abnormality is more reliable in determining the need for aortography.[6]

The role of CT scan and angiography in ruling out a potential intrathoracic vascular injury remains debatable. Traditionally, invasive aortography has been considered the test of choice to rule out such injuries. Authors in favor of this technique find aortography more accurate and expeditious, with high sensitivity (98%) in detecting aortic and major branch vessels injuries.[64–66] Both cut film arteriography and digital subtraction arteriography are used, with similar results and enhanced visualization.[67] On the other hand, helical CT scan is a noninvasive procedure that can be used as the initial diagnostic tool, with a sensitivity and negative predictive value of 100%, equivalent to that of aortography.[68] Helical CT scanning prevents unnecessary aortography, expedites patient care, and reduces costs. Some scanners are capable of performing CT aortography, which creates a three-dimensional reconstruction of the aorta. Using helical CT scan to exclude a mediastinal hematoma and to evaluate the cause of an abnormal aortic contour promotes more selective use of aortography.[68–70]

Another useful diagnostic tool is multiplane transesophageal echocardiography (TEE). In patients with severe blunt chest trauma, TEE and helical CT scan have similar diagnostic accuracy for identifying surgical acute traumatic aortic injury. Transesophageal echocardiography also allows functional and anatomic assessment of the heart and identifies intimal or medial lesions of the thoracic aorta more readily.[71,72] Additional randomized studies comparing these techniques are required.

The issue of treatment priorities in patients with traumatic aortic rupture is evolving. The most common cause of death is hemorrhage, and 95% of these patients have associated injuries requiring surgery. The most common associated injuries requiring emergent treatment are serious closed-head injuries and intraabdominal hemorrhage. The hemodynamically unstable patient with known intraabdominal hemorrhage should undergo laparotomy before any other procedure. The hemodynamically stable patient with intraabdominal hemorrhage should undergo aortography followed by laparotomy. Left hemothorax, pseudocoarctation, and/or supraclavicular hematoma can be found in patients at high risk for sudden free rupture and exsanguination. Patients demonstrating these characteristics may benefit from immediate thoracic exploration rather than waiting for aortography.[60] Repair of an aortic rupture using simple aortic cross-clamping alone is feasible in the majority of patients without increased mortality or spinal cord injury.[63]

Although the traditional therapy for blunt traumatic rupture of the thoracic aorta is immediate repair, in some patients with concomitant head trauma, respiratory failure, cardiac dysfunction, or sepsis, this injury can be managed conservatively with selective delayed operative repair without increasing the risk for exsanguinating hemorrhage.[73]

Other Injuries

Significant injury from thoracic trauma may occur in less common sites in the chest. Although infrequent, these injuries have equal capacity to result in morbidity and mortality. Among these injuries are diaphragmatic and esophageal rupture, posttraumatic lung cysts, and intercostal hernias. Diaphragmatic ruptures occur most commonly on the left side as a result of severe thoracoabdominal compression or by penetrating injury. A large diaphragmatic rupture can cause immediate respiratory compromise because of displacement of intraabdominal viscera into the chest. However, most diaphragmatic injuries initially are asymptomatic and cause problems later because of incarcerated viscera. The key to diagnosis is a high index of suspicion for any abnormal chest x-ray film.

Radiographic findings that suggest diaphragmatic rupture include displacement of the nasogastric tube tip into the chest, abnormal gas patterns in the chest, and haziness of the diaphragm.[74] Most diaphragmatic injuries are best repaired through the abdomen. The lacerated diaphragm is primary repaired and a chest tube is placed. If the injury results in loss of diaphragmatic tissue, a prosthetic patch may be necessary to close the defect.

Esophageal rupture rarely occurs after blunt trauma. It more likely occurs after penetrating trauma. It should be suspected in the patient with pneumomediastinum or hydrothorax after thoracic trauma. If the rupture is detected early, primary repair of the esophagus usually is possible.

Lung cysts may present immediately after blunt thoracic trauma. They are thought to occur as a result of lung laceration. Although there are exceptions, most undergo slow resolution without surgical intervention. Injury to the intercostal muscles during blunt trauma may create an area of weakness, leading to an intercostal hernia. The weakness in the thoracic wall can be detected soon after injury or late in the course, up to 4 years. When detected they should be closed with muscle or fascia from the adjacent thoracic cavity. A prosthetic mesh is required in some instances.[75,76]

Penetrating Trauma

Penetrating thoracic wounds are a challenge for the surgeon and often carry a high mortality rate. The vast majority of penetrating trauma occurs in patients older than 12 years old, mainly in males. In a review of an urban level I trauma center, 55% of penetrating injuries resulted from stab wounds; the remainder were caused by gunshot wounds. Isolated injuries were present in 69% of cases, whereas 31% incurred additional extrathoracic injuries.[77] Although most penetrating injuries are isolated, any chest injury at or below the nipple line anteriorly, or at or below the tip of the scapula posteriorly, is better classified as a thoracoabdominal injury. In children with penetrating injuries of this type, presence of intraabdominal injuries must be excluded. Diagnostic aids include peritoneal lavage, triple-contrast CT scan, and laparoscopy. The latter has been found to be effective in assessing disruption of the diaphragm in hemodynamically stable patients.[34] In patients with suspected penetrating cardiac injury, pericardial focused ultrasound has 100% sensitivity and 97% accuracy in detecting pericardial blood.[78]

Use of autotransfusion devices in children with significant hemothoraces may be beneficial. Patients with ISS greater than or equal to 25 and blood pH less than 7.3 at admission are more likely to require an operation. Also, these two parameters are good predictors for mortality in both gunshot wounds and stab wounds. Overall mortality rate for penetrating trauma is 17%, largely as a result of cardiac and intrathoracic great vessel injuries.[77] Almost all patients will require intensive monitoring after surgery.

Functional Outcome

Among all patients with pediatric thoracic trauma, more than 75% leave the hospital without serious disabilities, but approximately 15% will require some sort of rehabilitation. In terms of functional status, the assessment of the Functional Independence Measure (FIM) for children older than 7 years has shown that 68% will achieve complete independence, 7% will require minimal to moderate assistance, and 7% will be completely unable to recuperate their abilities. Most of these limitations are related to extrathoracic injuries, especially intracranial sequelae.[1]

Summary

Thoracic injuries are a rare but potentially lethal subset of childhood injuries. Because they are so uncommon, the timely implementation of diagnostic and therapeutic measures may be less than satisfactory. The framework for successful management of pediatric chest injuries includes the widely held principles of establishing and managing the patient's airway, assessing breathing, and monitoring the adequacy of circulation. A detailed primary and secondary survey for extent of thoracic and associated nonthoracic injuries is essential. Rapid resuscitation and institution of definitive therapy minimize morbidity and mortality.

REFERENCES

1. DiScala C: National Pediatric Trauma Registry biannual report. Memorandum to NPTR participants, December 2001.
2. Nakayama DK, Ramenofsky ML, Rowe MI: Chest injuries in childhood. *Ann Surg* 210:770-775, 1989.
3. Peclet MH, Newman KD, Eichelberger MR, et al: Thoracic trauma in children: an indicator of increased mortality. *J Pediatr Surg* 25:961-965, 1990; discussion 965-966.
4. Lee RB, Bass SM, Morris JA Jr, et al: Three or more rib fractures as an indicator for transfer to a Level I trauma center: a population-based study. *J Trauma* 30:689-694, 1990.
5. Langer JC, Hoffman MA, Pearl RH, et al: Survival after emergency department thoracotomy in a child with blunt multisystem trauma. *Pediatr Emerg Care* 5:255-256, 1989.
6. Garcia VF, Gotschall CS, Eichelberger MR, et al: Rib fractures in children: a marker of severe trauma. *J Trauma* 30:695-700, 1990.
7. Ildstad ST, Tollerud DJ, Weiss RG, et al: Cardiac contusion in pediatric patients with blunt thoracic trauma. *J Pediatr Surg* 25: 287-289, 1990.
8. Kram HB, Wohlmuth DA, Appel PL, et al: Clinical and radiographic indications for aortography in blunt chest trauma. *J Vasc Surg* 6:168-176, 1987.
9. Sturm JT, Hynes JT, Perry JF Jr, et al: Thoracic spinal fractures and aortic rupture: a significant and fatal association. *Ann Thorac Surg* 50:931-933, 1990.
10. Freedland M, Wilson RF, Bender JS, et al: The management of flail chest injury: factors affecting outcome. *J Trauma* 30:1460-1468, 1990.
11. Svennevig JL, Vaage J, Westheim A, et al: Late sequelae of lung contusion. *Injury* 20:253-256, 1989.
12. Bonadio WAHellmich T: Post-traumatic pulmonary contusion in children. *Ann Emerg Med* 18:1050-1052, 1989.
13. Frame SB, Marshall WJ, Clifford TG: Synchronized independent lung ventilation in the management of pediatric unilateral pulmonary contusion: case report. *J Trauma* 29:395-397, 1989.
14. Schild HH, Strunk H, Weber W, et al: Pulmonary contusion: CT vs plain radiograms. *J Comput Assist Tomogr* 13:417-420, 1989.
15. Wagner RB, Jamieson PM: Pulmonary contusion. Evaluation and classification by computed tomography. *Surg Clin North Am* 69:31-40, 1989.
16. Blostein PA, Hodgman CG: Computed tomography of the chest in blunt thoracic trauma: results of a prospective study. *J Trauma* 43:13-18, 1997.
17. Talbot AR, Fu CC: Clinical use of differential lung ventilation in the treatment of asymmetric lung injury: report of a case. *Ma Zui Xue Za Zhi* 27:67-73, 1989.
18. Zandstra DF, Stoutenbeek CP: Reflection of differential pulmonary perfusion in polytrauma patients on differential lung ventilation (DLV). A comparison of two CO_2-derived methods. *Intensive Care Med* 15:151-154, 1989.
19. Zandstra DF, Stoutenbeek CP, Bams JL: Monitoring lung mechanics and airway pressures during differential lung ventilation (DLV) with emphasis on weaning from DLV. *Intensive Care Med* 15: 458-463, 1989.
20. Lee MC, Wong SS, Chu JJ, et al: Traumatic asphyxia. *Ann Thorac Surg* 51:86-88, 1991.
21. Kerr TM, Sood R, Buckman RF Jr, et al: Prospective trial of the six hour rule in stab wounds of the chest. *Surg Gynecol Obstet* 169:223-225, 1989.
22. Helling TS, Gyles NR III, Eisenstein CL, et al: Complications following blunt and penetrating injuries in 216 victims of chest trauma requiring tube thoracostomy. *J Trauma* 29:1367-1370, 1989.
23. Eichelberger MR, Randolph JG: Progress in pediatric trauma. *World J Surg* 9:222-235, 1985.
24. Hehir MD, Hollands MJ, Deane SA: The accuracy of the first chest X-ray in the trauma patient. *Aust N Z J Surg* 60:529-532, 1990.
25. Dulchavsky SA, Schwarz KL, Kirkpatrick AW, et al: Prospective evaluation of thoracic ultrasound in the detection of pneumothorax. *J Trauma* 50:201-205, 2001.
26. Taskinen SO, Salo JA, Halttunen PE, et al: Tracheobronchial rupture due to blunt chest trauma: a follow-up study. *Ann Thorac Surg* 48:846-849, 1989.
27. Unger JM, Schuchmann GG, Grossman JE, et al: Tears of the trachea and main bronchi caused by blunt trauma: radiologic findings. *AJR Am J Roentgenol* 153:1175-1180, 1989.
28. Baumgartner F, Sheppard B, de Virgilio C, et al: Tracheal and main bronchial disruptions after blunt chest trauma: presentation and management. *Ann Thorac Surg* 50:569-574, 1990.
29. Flynn AE, Thomas AN, Schecter WP: Acute tracheobronchial injury. *J Trauma* 29:1326-1330, 1989.
30. Pate JW: Tracheobronchial and esophageal injuries. *Surg Clin North Am* 69:111-123, 1989.
31. Tam VKH CA, Buchman TG: Management of penetrating thoracic trauma. In Turney SZ, Rodriguez A, Cowley RA, editors: *Management of cardiothoracic trauma.* Baltimore, 1990, Williams & Wilkins.
32. Mathisen DJ, Grillo H: Laryngotracheal trauma. *Ann Thorac Surg* 43:254-262, 1987.
33. Capizzi FD, Bonora M, D'Alessandro M, et al: Pneumomediastinum not associated with lesion of mediastinal organs. *Acta Chir Scand* 155:159-161, 1989.
34. Villavicencio RT, Aucar JA: Analysis of laparoscopy in trauma. *J Am Coll Surg* 189:11-20, 1999.
35. Villavicencio RT, Aucar JA, Wall MJ Jr: Analysis of thoracoscopy in trauma. *Surg Endosc* 13:3-9, 1999.
36. Kulshrestha P, Das B, Iyer KS, et al: Cardiac injuries—a clinical and autopsy profile. *J Trauma* 30:203-207, 1990.
37. Dowd MD, Krug S: Pediatric blunt cardiac injury: epidemiology, clinical features, and diagnosis. Pediatric Emergency Medicine Collaborative Research Committee: Working Group on Blunt Cardiac Injury. *J Trauma* 40:61-67, 1996.
38. Scorpio RJ, Wesson DE, Smith CR, et al: Blunt cardiac injuries in children: a postmortem study. *J Trauma* 41:306-309, 1996.
39. Baxter BT, Moore EE, Moore FA, et al: A plea for sensible management of myocardial contusion. *Am J Surg* 158:557-61, 1989; discussion 561-562.
40. Bertinchant JP, Polge A, Mohty D, et al: Evaluation of incidence, clinical significance, and prognostic value of circulating cardiac troponin I and T elevation in hemodynamically stable patients with suspected myocardial contusion after blunt chest trauma. *J Trauma* 48:924-931, 2000.
41. Biffl WL, Moore FA, Moore EE, et al: Cardiac enzymes are irrelevant in the patient with suspected myocardial contusion. *Am J Surg* 168:523-527, 1994; discussion 527-528.
42. Dubrow TJ, Mihalka J, Eisenhauer DM, et al: Myocardial contusion in the stable patient: what level of care is appropriate? *Surgery* 106:267-273, 1989; discussion 273-274.

43. Foil MB, Mackersie RC, Furst SR, et al: The asymptomatic patient with suspected myocardial contusion. *Am J Surg* 160:638-642, 1990; discussion 642-643.
44. Holness R, Waxman K: Diagnosis of traumatic cardiac contusion utilizing single photon-emission computed tomography. *Crit Care Med* 18:1-3, 1990.
45. Miller FB, Shumate CR, Richardson JD: Myocardial contusion. When can the diagnosis be eliminated? *Arch Surg* 124:805-807, 1989; discussion 807-808.
46. Wisner DH, Reed WH, Riddick RS: Suspected myocardial contusion. Triage and indications for monitoring. *Ann Surg* 212:82-86, 1990.
47. Helling TS, Duke P, Beggs CW, et al: A prospective evaluation of 68 patients suffering blunt chest trauma for evidence of cardiac injury. *J Trauma* 29:961-965, 1989; discussion 965-966.
48. Reif J, Justice JL, Olsen WR, et al: Selective monitoring of patients with suspected blunt cardiac injury. *Ann Thorac Surg* 50:530-532, 1990; discussion 533.
49. Langer JC, Winthrop AL, Wesson DE, et al: Diagnosis and incidence of cardiac injury in children with blunt thoracic trauma. *J Pediatr Surg* 24:1091-1094, 1989.
50. Brathwaite CE, Rodriguez A, Turney SZ, et al: Blunt traumatic cardiac rupture. A 5-year experience. *Ann Surg* 212:701-704, 1990.
50. Westaby S, Brayley N: ABC of major trauma. Thoracic trauma—I. *BMJ* 300:1639, 1990.
51. Foussas SG, Athanasopoulos GDCokkinos DV: Myocardial infarction caused by blunt chest injury: possible mechanisms involved—case reports. *Angiology* 40:313-318, 1989.
52. Fulda G, Rodriguez A, Turney SZ, et al: Blunt traumatic pericardial rupture. A ten-year experience 1979 to 1989. *J Cardiovasc Surg (Torino)* 31:525-530, 1990.
53. Glock Y, Massabuau P, Puel P: Cardiac damage in nonpenetrating chest injuries. Report of 5 cases. *J Cardiovasc Surg (Torino)* 30: 27-33, 1989.
54. Mock CN, Campbell R, Burchard KW: Survival after blunt traumatic rupture of the left ventricle. *Am Surg* 56:561-565, 1990.
55. Moront M, Lefrak EA, Akl BF: Traumatic rupture of the interventricular septum and tricuspid valve: case report. *J Trauma* 31: 134-136, 1991.
56. Pevec WC, Udekwu AO, Peitzman AB: Blunt rupture of the myocardium. *Ann Thorac Surg* 48:139-142, 1989.
57. Pevec WC, el Hillel M, McArdle DQ, et al: Rupture of the left ventricle and interventricular septum by blunt trauma. *Crit Care Med* 17:837-838, 1989.
58. Van Roye S, Zienkowicz BS: Delayed isolated mitral incompetence after being kicked in the chest by a bull. *Thorac Cardiovasc Surg* 37:329-331, 1989.
59. Roe BB: Cardiac trauma including injury of great vessels. *Surg Clin North Am* 52:573-583, 1972.
60. Clark DE, Zeiger MA, Wallace KL, et al: Blunt aortic trauma: signs of high risk. *J Trauma* 30:701-705, 1990.
61. Kawada T, Mieda T, Abe H, et al: Surgical experience with traumatic rupture of the thoracic aorta. *J Cardiovasc Surg (Torino)* 31:359-363, 1990.
62. Kram HB, Appel PL, Wohlmuth DA, et al: Diagnosis of traumatic thoracic aortic rupture: a 10-year retrospective analysis. *Ann Thorac Surg* 47:282-286, 1989.
63. Razzouk AJ, Gundry SR, Wang N, et al: Repair of traumatic aortic rupture: a 25-year experience. *Arch Surg* 135:913-918, 2000; discussion 919.
64. Ahrar K, Smith DC, Bansal RC, et al: Angiography in blunt thoracic aortic injury. *J Trauma* 42:665-669, 1997.
65. Brasel KJ, Weigelt JA: Blunt thoracic aortic trauma. A cost-utility approach for injury detection. *Arch Surg* 131:619-625, 1996; discussion 625-626.
66. Chen MY, Regan JD, D'Amore MJ, et al: Role of angiography in the detection of aortic branch vessel injury after blunt thoracic trauma. *J Trauma* 51:1166-1171, 2001; discussion 1172.
67. Johnson MS, Shah H, Harris VJ, et al: Comparison of digital subtraction and cut film arteriography in the evaluation of suspected thoracic aortic injury. *J Vasc Interv Radiol* 8:799-807, 1997.
68. Parker MS, Matheson TL, Rao AV, et al: Making the transition: the role of helical CT in the evaluation of potentially acute thoracic aortic injuries. *AJR Am J Roentgenol* 176:1267-1272, 2001.
69. Downing SW, Sperling JS, Mirvis SE, et al: Experience with spiral computed tomography as the sole diagnostic method for traumatic aortic rupture. *Ann Thorac Surg* 72:495-501, 2001; discussion 501-502.
70. Gavant ML, Flick P, Menke P, et al: CT aortography of thoracic aortic rupture. *AJR Am J Roentgenol* 166:955-961, 1996.
71. Cohn SM, Burns GA, Jaffe C, et al: Exclusion of aortic tear in the unstable trauma patient: the utility of transesophageal echocardiography. *J Trauma* 39:1087-1090, 1995.
72. Pearson GD, Karr SS, Trachiotis GD, et al: A retrospective review of the role of transesophageal echocardiography in aortic and cardiac trauma in a level I Pediatric Trauma Center. *J Am Soc Echocardiogr* 10:946-955, 1997.
73. Maggisano R, Nathens A, Alexandrova NA, et al: Traumatic rupture of the thoracic aorta: should one always operate immediately? *Ann Vasc Surg* 9:44-52, 1995.
74. Brandt ML, Luks FI, Spigland NA, et al: Diaphragmatic injury in children. *J Trauma* 32:298-301, 1992.
75. Min SA, Gow KW, Blair GK. Traumatic intercostal hernia: presentation and diagnostic workup. *J Pediatr Surg* 34:1544-1545, 1999.
76. Othersen H: Cardiothoracic injuries. In R T, editor: *Pediatric trauma*. St. Louis, 1990, Mosby.
77. Reinhorn M, Kaufman HL, Hirsch EF, et al: Penetrating thoracic trauma in a pediatric population. *Ann Thorac Surg* 61:1501-1505, 1996.
78. Rozycki GS, Feliciano DV, Ochsner MG, et al: The role of ultrasound in patients with possible penetrating cardiac wounds: a prospective multicenter study. *J Trauma* 46:543-551, 1999; discussion 551-552.

CHAPTER

109

Abdominal Trauma in Pediatric Critical Care

James C. Gilbert and Christopher P. Coppola

PEARLS

- In the assessment and resuscitation of trauma victims, never forget to first secure the ABCs: *A*irway, *B*reathing, and *C*irculation.
- When in doubt, intubate the patient.
- Often the more conservative and safe route is exploration of the patient with abdominal trauma and unknown internal injuries. However, with the advances in intensive care and radiographic imaging in the past 25 years, only rarely are abdominal injuries in children not managed nonoperatively.
- Splenic preservation in particular is usually possible, and its importance increases with decreasing age.
- Vigilance and reexamination are necessary to avoid missing a small bowel injury. This injury, if overlooked, increases morbidity, especially after the first 24 hours.

Trauma is the leading cause of morbidity and mortality in the pediatric age group. An estimated 22 million pediatric injuries occur each year, resulting in 800,000 hospitalizations and 20,000 deaths.[1] Thus trauma exceeds all other causes of death combined. Trauma to the abdomen is particularly morbid. Blunt abdominal injuries to the abdomen in children are associated with a mortality rate of 9%.[2] Abdominal injuries are a marker of severe trauma, and evaluation of the child with an abdominal injury must include a thorough examination of the entire child. Failure to accurately assess the abdomen is the single most common error in all phases of the early treatment of the injured patient.[3] Management of pediatric trauma requires a multidisciplinary approach with emergency department physicians, intensivists, and surgeons working as a team to provide prompt stabilization, assessment, and treatment. Performing the primary and secondary survey, instituting fluid resuscitation, and arriving at a decision as to the most appropriate management plan are the principal goals of the trauma team leader.

The vast majority of abdominal injuries in children are preventable. Health care providers must work with governmental agencies to identify and alleviate causes of pediatric trauma. Education, public safety measures, and legislation will serve to eliminate many causes of pediatric injury. Intentional abdominal trauma to children must be considered in every evaluation and, if suspected, must be reported to the appropriate state or local agency. Developments in pediatric abdominal trauma include increased reliance on imaging modalities such as ultrasonography and computed tomography, which allows for increased utilization of nonoperative management. Alternate procedures such thoracoscopy, laparoscopy, and interventional radiology are being used in special situations.

Mechanisms and Patterns of Injury

The severity of the abdominal injury correlates with the mechanism of injury. Blunt injury accounts for 83% of abdominal trauma in children. The most common mechanisms are motor vehicle accidents, motor pedestrian accidents, falls from heights, bicycle accidents, and abuse.[4] In pediatric blunt abdominal trauma, solid viscus organs such as the liver, spleen, and kidney are more frequently injured than hollow viscus organs; however, children restrained with lap belts who were in motor vehicle accidents may present with small bowel perforations as a result of deceleration.[5] Motor pedestrian accidents may result in head injury, splenic fracture, and left femur fracture (Waddell triad). However, in one series this pattern occurred in only 2.4% of pedestrians struck.[6] In addition, urban violence and the high prevalence of firearms result in penetrating abdominal injuries in children. Regarding firearm-related injuries, homicides exceed unintentional injuries in the age group 1 to 9 years.[7] A national decrease in violent crime has reduced the incidence of penetrating trauma in the past decade. Specific recreational activities commonly practiced by children, such as bicycling, skating, skiing, snowboarding, and horseback riding, each results in common patterns of injury that will guide the clinician's evaluation. Although the mechanism of injury may correlate with the extent of injury, ongoing clinical assessment is a more sensitive indicator of the extent of blood loss and hemodynamic instability and determines the resuscitation and management of the child with an abdominal injury.

Evaluation and Resuscitation

Evaluation and resuscitation occur simultaneously when the trauma center is initially presented with a child with an abdominal injury (Figure 109–1). The Advanced Trauma Life Support protocols should be used. The initial assessment, or primary survey, includes stabilization of the cervical spine while evaluating airway patency, function of breathing, and adequacy of circulation. Prompt intubation should occur in any patient in whom the stability of these functions is in doubt. Obtaining intravenous access in the small child or infant can be particularly challenging, and personnel skilled in obtaining access should be used. Basic neurologic function is assessed. The patient must be completely exposed for examination and then covered with blankets and warmed to quickly achieve normal body temperature. Children and infants are more susceptible to heat loss and dehydration because of their greater surface area/mass ratio.

Abdominal examination includes observation of external signs of trauma, then palpation for tenderness and firmness. Children swallow a large amount of air when they cry, and gastric distension may present as abdominal distension requiring nasogastric tube decompression. Upper quadrant ecchymosis, tenderness, and associated rib fractures suggest the presence of liver or spleen injury. Midabdominal ecchymosis and tenderness suggest the possibility of a small bowel injury. The clinical evaluation is a more sensitive indicator of evolving intestinal injury than the presence of free air because the initial plain film may appear normal.[8] Stability of the pelvis is assessed with lateral and axial manual compression of the pelvic ring. The possibility of a bladder rupture in association with a pelvic fracture must be considered. Extraperitoneal bladder ruptures may have

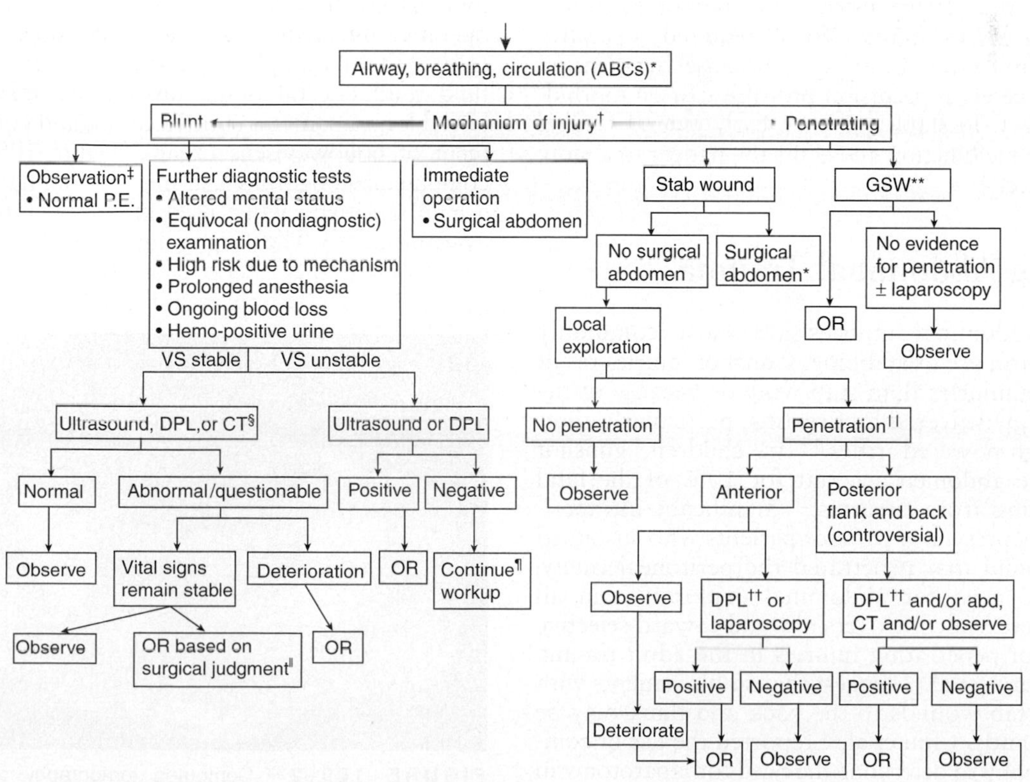

FIGURE 109–1 • Algorithm for evaluation of abdominal trauma.

localized suprapubic tenderness, whereas an intraperitoneal bladder rupture may present as generalized abdominal distension.

Laboratory examinations, including complete blood counts, serum chemistries, and urinalysis, should be obtained on all trauma patients. Additional studies, such as liver function tests and pancreatic enzymes, are indicated in certain injuries. Elevated transaminase levels suggest nonspecific parenchymal liver injury, elevated amylase and lipase levels suggest a pancreatic injury, and a base deficit of –6 or less is a strong indicator of intraabdominal injury in blunt trauma.[9,10] Hematuria is a sensitive indicator for the presence of intraabdominal injury and renal injury.[11,12] Urinalysis demonstrating more than five red blood cells per high-power field combined with clinical assessment accurately predicts intraabdominal injury.[13,14]

Prompt plain radiographs of the chest, lateral cervical spine, and pelvis should be obtained during initial assessment. Patients who are hemodynamically stable may undergo further radiographic workup, whereas patients with evidence of an abdominal injury who remain clinically unstable after resuscitation with 40 ml/kg of fluid should be taken to the operating room for exploration.

Children often demonstrate surprising hemodynamic stability in the face of significant hemorrhagic loss until their compensatory vasoconstriction is overcome. Although fluid resuscitation is the primary modality, children may require inotropic support after major trauma because myocardial depression may occur.[15] Hemoglobin concentrations less than or equal to 7g/dl are well tolerated in children after blunt abdominal injury, provided intravascular volume is repleted.[16,17] Frequent serial abdominal examinations are performed to determine the need for surgical exploration for progressive distension or peritonitis from a missed hollow viscus injury. When required, operative intervention should not be delayed because hypotension and decreased cerebral perfusion pressure worsen morbidity and mortality. In stable patients, early enteral feeding maintains immune function and shifts the patient to a more anabolic balance.[18]

Penetrating Abdominal Trauma

Penetrating abdominal injuries are most commonly caused by firearm use or stabbing. Gunshot injuries result in more severe injuries than stab wounds because of the increased energy delivered by firearms, particularly shotguns and high-powered rifles.[19] In children, gunshot wounds to the abdomen account for 10% of the fatal injuries resulting from firearms.[20] Significant intraperitoneal injury is present in 89% of patients who sustained a gunshot wound that penetrated the peritoneal cavity, suggesting the need for abdominal exploration in all patients.[21] There is a controversial trend toward selective management of penetrating injuries in the adult trauma literature.[22] Burns et al.[23] suggest that stable patients with gunshot and stab wounds to the back and flank may be treated expectantly. Chiu et al.[24] reported the use of computed tomography to determine the need for laparotomy in penetrating torso trauma. Although selective management of abdominal and right thoracoabdominal gunshot wounds has been suggested and demonstrated not to incur additional morbidity or mortality, the American College of Surgeons Committee on Trauma still suggests all gunshot wounds to the abdomen should be taken to the operating room for exploration.[25,26] Most trauma centers perform mandatory laparotomy on all patients with gunshot wounds to the abdomen, although some negative explorations resulting in postoperative complications will occur.[27] In a similar manner, abdominal stab wounds that penetrate the transversalis fascia should be explored in the operating room via laparotomy or laparoscopy for evidence of a bowel injury. Expectant observation of stab wounds in children is cautiously applied because the true extent of the injury is not always appreciated on local exploration.

Additional Assessment

Radiographic Assessment

Computed tomography is the procedure of choice for definitive radiographic assessment of blunt abdominal trauma in children. Clinical impression remains the most sensitive indicator of the need for computed tomography.[28] Computed tomography can be used to identify hepatic, splenic, intestinal, pancreatic, renal, and bladder injuries in children and can even detect intestinal and mesenteric injury with sensitivities of 94% and 96%, respectively.[29] Lap belt injury and abuse are two mechanisms associated with significant abdominal injuries documented by computed tomography. Serial clinical assessment must be made during the preparation for, and performance of, computed tomography. If evidence of deterioration is present, prompt operative intervention should be considered. Findings on computed tomography suggestive of injury are unexplained fluid solid visceral organ disruptions, misdistribution of bowel loops, contrast extravasation, and contrast enhancement of hollow viscus organs (Figure 109–2). Although computed tomography can miss abdominal injuries, it has a high sensitivity when used in combination with clinical assessment.[30,31] The Organ Injury Scaling Committee of

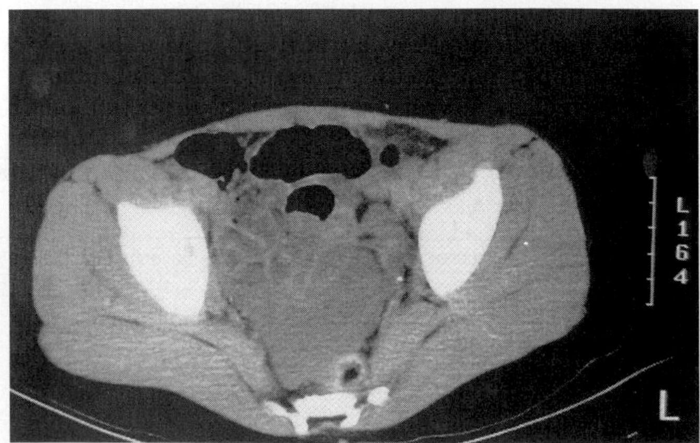

FIGURE 109–2 • Computed tomography of a patient with hepatic laceration demonstrating free intraperitoneal fluid in the pelvis.

the American Association for the Surgery of Trauma has developed a grading system to estimate the extent of abdominal injury.[32,33] Short of operative exploration, computed tomography is the method used to grade the extent of injury.

Ultrasound is also a modality used to further evaluate the abdomen of the injured child. Various reports note that ultrasonography for abdominal trauma has sensitivity of 55% to 86% and specificity of 95% to 98%.[34–37] Although ultrasound accurately identifies intraperitoneal free fluid and thus strongly suggests the presence of an abdominal injury, it does not accurately demonstrate the specific solid or hollow viscus injury.[38–41] Ultrasound is comparable to diagnostic peritoneal lavage (DPL) as a method for detecting free peritoneal fluid and is less invasive. However, it does not supplant computed tomography in its ability to define the specific nature and extent of abdominal injury.[42]

Diagnostic Peritoneal Lavage

Options that are used frequently in adults, such as DPL, are more difficult to apply to children. Initial studies suggested the use of DPL as a triage tool in selectively applying laparotomy for blunt abdominal trauma in children.[43] In one series, the cell count, amylase activity, and particulate matter in the DPL specimen were able to identify small bowel perforation with a sensitivity of 100%.[44] Refinements in the nonoperative management of many pediatric abdominal traumas make DPL noncontributory because the presence of free intraperitoneal blood is not an absolute indication for surgery in children.[45]

Diagnostic Laparoscopy

Diagnostic video-assisted laparoscopic evaluation has been suggested as a safe and effective modality for evaluating the abdomen in the stable patient after penetrating trauma.[46,47] However, Rossi et al.[48] cautioned that laparoscopy does not accurately evaluate the entire abdominal cavity and that further studies are warranted. Uribe et al.[49] reported that thoracoscopy in hemodynamically stable penetrating trauma patients resulted in a decrease in negative abdominal explorations and afforded identification of thoracic and diaphragmatic injuries. In our institution, we found laparoscopy to be highly effective in the evaluation of diaphragmatic injury after penetrating abdominal trauma. Meyer et al.[50] reported that diaphragmatic injuries could be diagnosed and repaired via the laparoscopic approach.

Nonoperative Management of Solid Organ Injuries

The standard of care in treating hemodynamically stable children with hepatic and splenic injuries is nonoperative observation. Mooney et al.[51] reported the management of these injuries varied widely between adult and pediatric facilities, and many splenectomies could be avoided if all children were treated with this nonoperative strategy. The American Pediatric Surgical Association Trauma Committee has proposed guidelines for care based on radiographic severity of injury (Table 109–1). Although this observation traditionally has taken place in the intensive care unit, evidence gathered to determine these recommendations suggests that observation on the patient ward is safe.[52]

TABLE 109–1

Proposed Guidelines for Resource Utilization in Children with Isolated Spleen or Liver Injury

	Computed Tomographic Grade			
	I	II	III	IV
Intensive care unit stay (days)	None	None	None	1
Hospital stay (days)	2	3	4	5
Predischarge imaging	None	None	None	None
Postdischarge imaging	None	None	None	None
Activity restriction (wk)*	3	4	5	6

*Return to full-contact, competitive sports (e.g., football, wrestling, hockey, lacrosse, mountain climbing) should be at the discretion of the individual pediatric trauma surgeon. The proposed guidelines for return to unrestricted activity include "normal" age-appropriate activities.

From Stylianos S, APSA Trauma Committee: *J Pediatr Surg* 35: 164-169, 2000.

Specific Organ Injuries and Management

Injury to the Spleen

The spleen can extend below the costal margin in children and is the most commonly injured intraabdominal organ following blunt trauma. Treatment of splenic injury has evolved from routine splenectomy to nonoperative management and splenic preservation.[53] Splenic injury most often is caused by a direct blow to the left upper quadrant resulting in localized tenderness, abrasion, or ecchymosis. Splenic injury is graded by computed tomography in stable patients (Figures 109–3 and 109–4 and Table 109–2).

Operative intervention for splenic trauma usually results in splenectomy. For this reason, nonoperative management should be attempted in patients with splenic injury, regardless of severity, if they are hemodynamically stable. However, if a stable patient with a splenic injury requires laparotomy for falling hematocrit or injury to another organ, splenorrhaphy and autotransfusion increase the rate of splenic salvage.[54] At pediatric trauma centers, operating on a child with an isolated splenic injury is very rare.[55] The indications for operative intervention are generally limited to (1) persistent hypotension or other evidence of continued hemorrhage, (2) greater than 50% blood volume replacement required, and (3) other life-threatening associated intraabdominal injuries.

Nonoperative management generally consists of large-bore venous access through which crystalloid resuscitation is administered, a nasogastric tube for gastric decompression,

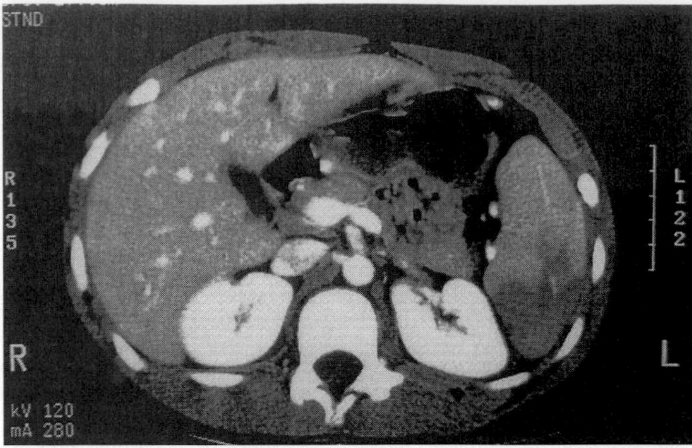

FIGURE 109–3 • Computed tomography of a patient with a grade IV splenic laceration.

intensive care unit monitoring, frequent hematocrit values, serial physical examinations, and up to 7 days of bed rest. Recommendations from the American Pediatric Surgery Association Trauma Committee indicate shorter periods of observation.[52] Lynch et al.[56] report that if transfusions are not required after 48 hours of observation, intensive care unit monitoring is unnecessary, and 7 days of bed rest is excessive.[56] Resolution of splenic injury is related to the grade of the initial insult, and the reported incidence of delayed splenic rupture is low.[57] Grade 1 and 2 injuries healed in 4 months as determined by computed tomography. Grade 3 and 4 injuries healed by 6 and 11 months, respectively.[58]

Injury to the Liver

The liver, which also extends below the costal margin in children, is the second most commonly injured organ in blunt abdominal trauma. Liver injuries are associated with the highest mortality and may require surgical correction of injuries to the hepatic veins or vena cava.[59] However, as with splenic injuries, liver injuries in stable patients can be

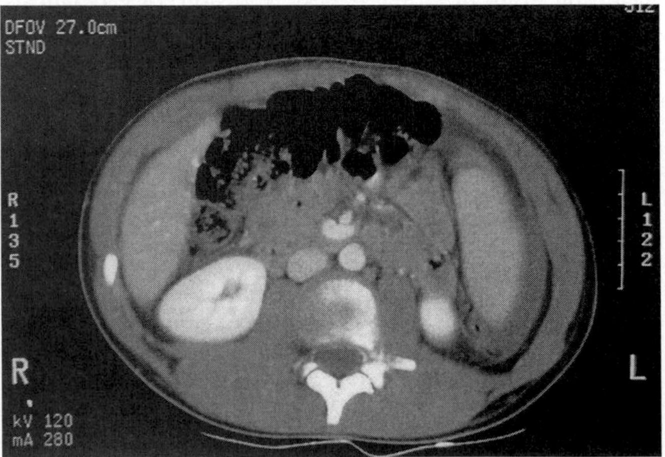

FIGURE 109–4 • Computed tomography of a patient with a grade IV splenic laceration demonstrating free fluid around the tip of the spleen.

TABLE 109–2

Grading of Splenic Injuries on Computed Tomography

Grade	Injury Description
I Hematoma	Subcapsular, <10% surface area
I Laceration	Capsular tear, <1 cm parenchymal depth
II Hematoma	Subcapsular, 10%–50% surface area; intraparenchymal, <5 cm in diameter
II Laceration	1–3 cm parenchymal depth that does not involve a trabecular vessel
III Hematoma	Subcapsular, >50% surface area or expanding; ruptured subcapsular or parenchymal hematoma; intraparenchymal hematoma >5 cm or expanding
III Laceration	>3 cm parenchymal depth or involving trabecular vessels
IV Laceration	Laceration involving segmental or hilar vessels producing major devascularization (>25% of spleen)
V Laceration	Completely shattered spleen
V Vascular	Hilar vascular injury that devascularizes spleen

From Moore EE, Cogbill TH, Jurkovich GJ, et al: *J Trauma* 38: 323-324, 1995.
Advance one grade for multiple injuries, up to grade III.

managed nonoperatively.[60] Ecchymosis, bruising, or abrasions over the right upper quadrant suggest significant injury. Major injuries, especially those involving the aforementioned venous injuries, may present with shock. Liver injury is graded by appearance on computed tomography in hemodynamically stable patients (Table 109–3). However, the clinical course of the patient, not the appearance on computed tomography, should determine treatment (Figures 109–5 and 109–6). Circumferential zones of low attenuation surrounding the intrahepatic portal veins on computed tomography are suggestive of hepatic injury and are associated with increased mortality.[61] Elevated serum transaminase concentrations are associated with liver trauma and other intraabdominal injury.[62] Nonoperative treatment of hepatic injuries was suggested by the finding that the majority of liver injuries had stopped bleeding at the time of operation.[63] The mortality associated with operative management of hepatic injuries is higher than in the nonoperative group. Late complications associated with nonoperative treatment of liver injuries include bile peritonitis, abscess formation, hemorrhage, and hematobilia.[64] Angiography is helpful in managing complications associated with bleeding, especially hematobilia.

Operative treatment is required for major hepatic trauma associated with hepatic vein or retrohepatic canal injuries. Often, definitive repair is not possible at the time of initial exploration, necessitating damage control surgery with packing, stabilization, resuscitation, and repeat laparotomy.[65] Early operative packing with planned reexploration is advocated as an alternative to selective hepatic arterial ligation.[66]

TABLE 109–3

Grading of Hepatic Injuries on Computed Tomography

Grade	Injury Description
I Hematoma	Subcapsular, <10% surface area
I Laceration	Capsular tear, <1 cm parenchymal depth
II Hematoma	Subcapsular, 10%–50% surface area; intraparenchymal, <10 cm in diameter
II Laceration	1–3 cm parenchymal depth, <10 cm in length
III Hematoma	Subcapsular, >50% surface area or expanding; ruptured subcapsular or parenchymal hematoma; intra-parenchymal hematoma >10 cm or expanding
III Laceration	>3 cm parenchymal depth
IV Laceration	Parenchymal disruption involving 25%–75% of hepatic lobe or 1–3 Couinaud segments within a single lobe
V Laceration	Parenchymal disruption involving >75% of hepatic lobe or >3 Couinaud segments within a single lobe
V Vascular	Juxtahepatic venous injuries, e.g., retrohepatic vena cava/central major hepatic veins
VI Vascular	Hepatic avulsion

From Moore EE, Cogbill TH, Jurkovich GJ, et al: *J Trauma* 38: 323-324, 1995.
Advance one grade for multiple injuries, up to grade III.

Injury to the Duodenum

Duodenal injuries are rare in children but occur more commonly than in adults after blunt trauma.[67] Children may present with localized right upper quadrant tenderness, but the presentation may be subtle and result in delayed diagnosis.[68] The majority of duodenal injuries in children result in a duodenal hematoma without disruption of the lumen, but duodenal disruption can occur. Computed tomography demonstrates extraluminal gas or oral contrast extravasation in the right anterior pararenal space. Thickening of the duodenal wall is appreciated when a duodenal hematoma is present.[69] In a multicenter study of duodenal injuries by Cogbill et al.,[70] associated injuries were present in 84% of the patients sustaining blunt injury to the duodenum. Duodenal injuries are classified from grade I to V based on severity (Table 109–4). The majority of pediatric duodenal injuries are grades I and II. Overall, mortality is 18% for patients with duodenal injuries. For grade I lesions, the mortality is 8%, with associated injuries as the proximate cause of death.

Observation and parenteral hyperalimentation constitute treatment for duodenal hematoma, and resolution occurs in 2 to 4 weeks. Repair of full-thickness duodenal injury may involve duodenorrhaphy, pyloric exclusion, duodenoduodenostomy, duodenojejunostomy, pancreatoduodenectomy, or simple drainage. The majority of injuries are treated with debridement and primary closure

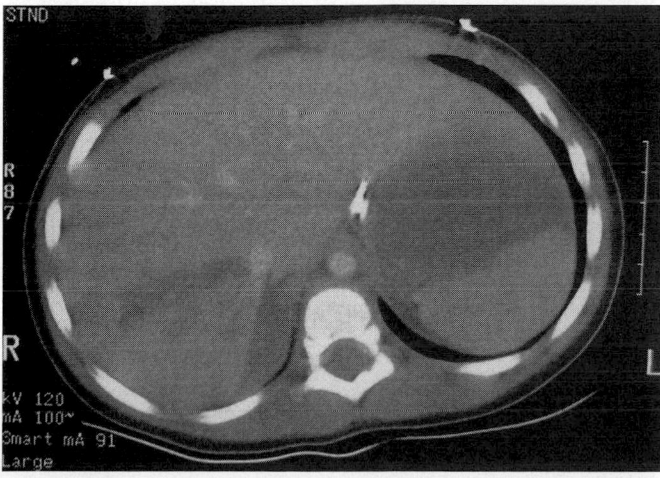

FIGURE 109–5 • Computed tomography of a patient with a grade II hepatic hematoma.

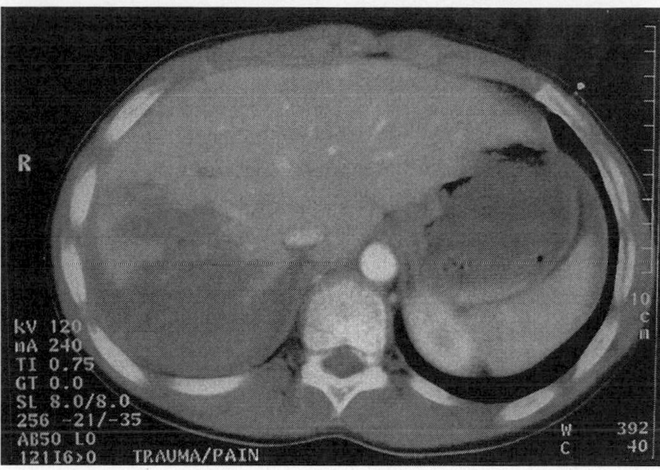

FIGURE 109–6 • Computed tomography of a patient with a grade IV hepatic laceration.

TABLE 109–4

Duodenum Injury Scale

Grade	Injury Description
I Hematoma	Involving single portion of duodenum
II Laceration	Partial thickness, no perforation
II Hematoma	Involving more than one portion
II Laceration	Disruption <50% of circumference
III Laceration	Disruption 50%–75% circumference of second portion
IV Laceration	Disruption >75% circumference of second portion; involving ampulla or distal common bile duct
V Laceration	Massive disruption of duodenopancreatic complex
V Vascular	Devascularization of duodenum

From Moore EE, Cogbill TH, Malangoni MA, et al: *J Trauma* 30:1427, 1990.
Advance one grade for multiple injuries, up to grade III.

with drainage. Pyloric exclusion is the procedure of choice for the majority of complex duodenal injuries; duodenostomy is generally not necessary. In children, pancreaticoduodenectomy is rarely required to treat a duodenal injury.

Injury to the Pancreas

Injuries to the pancreas may require operative intervention depending on the anatomy of the injury and the integrity of the main pancreatic duct (Table 109–5). Upper abdominal tenderness, elevated amylase level, edema of the gland, and unexplained fluid in the lesser sac on computed tomography suggest pancreatic injury. Suspicion for injury must be sustained because clinical evaluation, serum amylase level, and computed tomography may miss the initial signs of pancreatic injury. Bicycle handlebar accidents, direct blows to the abdomen, and motor vehicle accidents are the most common mechanisms of injury. The gland is usually fractured as it crosses the vertebral column (Figure 109–7). Complete transection of the gland requires distal pancreatectomy and drainage, which is best performed early. When the main pancreatic duct is intact, nonoperative treatment with an extended course of bowel rest and parenteral nutrition should be attempted. Devascularization of the pancreas and duodenum in blunt abdominal trauma is rare in children. However, in penetrating injuries, significant tissue loss and vascular compromise may occur, requiring debridement, drainage, and pyloric exclusion. After pancreatic injury, pseudocysts may develop and require internal or external drainage after maturation. Endoscopic retrograde cholangiopancreatography for both evaluation of injury and drainage with pancreatic duct stents is a promising alternative.[71]

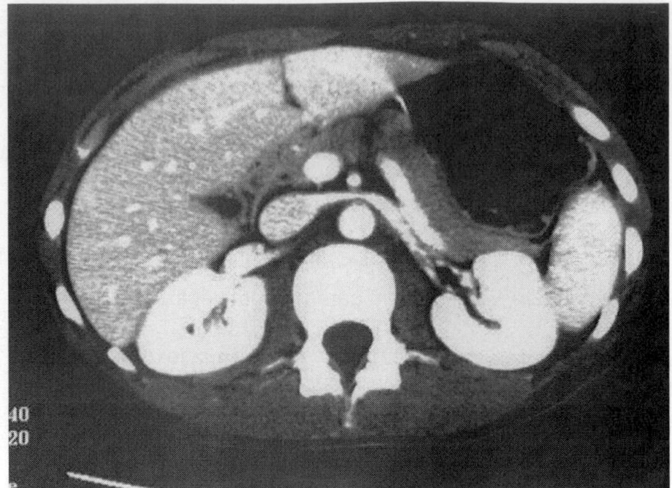

FIGURE 109–7 • Computed tomography of patient with a grade III pancreatic laceration. (Courtesy Martin Eichelberger, M.D., and Patrick Mclaughlin, B.S.)

Injury to Small Bowel

Bowel injuries resulting from blunt trauma are relatively rare; the reported incidence is approximately 1% in both pediatric and adult series.[67] However, a high index of suspicion must be maintained to avoid a delayed diagnosis, which is more common in children. Nance et al.[72] reported an increased incidence of small bowel injury associated with an increased number of other organs injured. The mechanisms of injury associated with blunt bowel trauma include motor vehicle/pedestrian accidents, handlebar injuries, lap belt injuries, and child abuse. Deceleration injuries in children restrained with a lap belt may occur as a constellation that includes intestinal injury, abdominal wall ecchymosis, and flexion distraction injury (Chance fracture) to the lumbar spine (Figure 109–8).

Intestinal injuries include bowel disruption, mesenteric avulsion, and bowel wall contusion. Areas of the small bowel particularly prone to injury are the points of

TABLE 109–5

Pancreas Injury Scale

Grade	Injury Description
I Hematoma	Minor contusion without duct injury
I Laceration	Superficial laceration without duct injury
II Hematoma	Major contusion without duct injury or tissue loss
II Laceration	Major laceration without duct injury or tissue loss
III Laceration	Distal transection or parenchymal/duct injury
IV Laceration	Proximal transection or parenchymal injury involving ampulla
V Laceration	Massive disruption of pancreatic head

From Moore EE, Cogbill TH, Malangoni MA, et al: *J Trauma* 30:1427, 1990.
Advance one grade for multiple injuries, up to grade III.

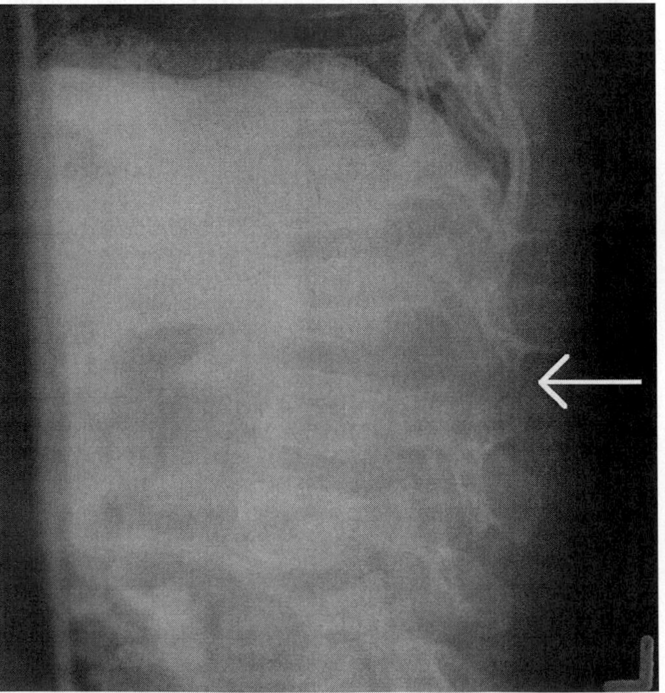

FIGURE 109–8 • Plain lateral lumbar spine radiograph. *Arrow* indicates distraction injury to posterior spine secondary to lap belt injury.

retroperitoneal fixation, such as the proximal jejunum at the ligament of Treitz or the terminal ileum near the junction with the cecum. A perforation may be present without free air or significant spillage of succus entericus on DPL.[73] Delayed perforations may occur as a result of mesenteric disruptions and subsequent segmented bowel necrosis. In some instances, a prolonged ileus that fails to resolve may be the only evidence of intestinal injury.

Diagnosis should be suspected given a sufficient mechanism of injury and abdominal wall ecchymosis. Signs of peritoneal irritation may be present on physical examination. Until spinal injuries are ruled out, a lateral decubitus film is preferred over an upright chest film for detection of free air. Findings on computed tomography consistent with small bowel injury are free air, contrast extravasation, focal bowel thickening, free fluid, and fat stranding or fluid in the mesentery.[74]

Once diagnosed, all bowel injuries are treated by laparotomy, exploration, and repair. Excision of injury and primary anastomosis usually are possible to reestablish gastrointestinal continuity. Morbidity and mortality are not increased if the delay in diagnosis is less than 24 hours.[44,73]

Renal Trauma

Renal trauma is commonly found in conjunction with injury to other organs. Physical findings suggestive of kidney injury include flank tenderness, mass, or ecchymosis. Hematuria, either gross or microscopic, is the best laboratory indicator of serious renal injury and is usually present when injury results from blunt trauma.[75] However, serious injury, especially renal pedicle injuries, may be present even in the absence of hematuria. In hemodynamically stable patients, computed tomography with intravenous contrast allows very accurate determination of the extent of injury and function (Figure 109–9). Ultrasonography also provides accurate diagnosis of injuries.[76] Emergent preoperative assessments of renal injuries are possible on an abdominal plain film obtained after bolus contrast injection, which provides a limited intravenous pyelogram.

Renal trauma usually consists of hematoma, laceration, or vascular injury (Table 109–6). Children who are hemodynamically stable and are found to have contusions, lacerations, or hematomas with or without urinary extravasation may be safely managed nonoperatively. Angiography with embolization can stop hemorrhage when active contrast extravasation is present.[77] Exploration is warranted in children who are hemodynamically unstable and have an expanding hematoma, an uncontained perirenal hematoma, or an associated intraabdominal injury necessitating exploration. Associated injuries are present in approximately 30% of children with renal injuries. Isolated urinary extravasation is not an indication for emergent exploration, but delayed operation or percutaneous drainage may be required for persistent extravasation or infection. If urinary extravasation is present, antibiotics should be administered to prevent secondary infection. Patients with extravasation and devascularized segments on initial computed tomography have a higher incidence of delayed complications. Observation and bed rest usually result in excellent outcome even with deep parenchymal lacerations associated with urinary extravasation. Patients with gross hematuria are kept on bed rest until the urine is grossly clear. Reevaluation is necessary for persistent hematuria, tenderness, or mass. All patients with renal injuries, regardless of severity, should be monitored and followed as outpatients for delayed onset of hypertension. A captopril-furosemide DTPA (technetium-99m diethylenetriamine pentaacetic acid) renal scan is used to follow function of the injured kidney (Figure 109–10).

Renal pedicle injuries are rare but are suggested by lack of renal contrast enhancement on computed tomography. Renal angiography definitively establishes the diagnosis and directs operative management. Ureteral injuries require operative repair. Because of the absence of clinical findings, diagnosis of ureteropelvic junction disruption as a result of blunt trauma may be delayed.[78]

TABLE 109–6

Kidney Injury Scale

Grade	Injury Description
I Contusion	Microscopic or gross hematuria
I Hematoma	Subcapsular, nonexpanding without parenchymal laceration
II Hematoma	Nonexpanding perirenal hematoma confined to renal retroperitoneum
II Laceration	<1 cm parenchymal depth of renal cortex without urinary extravasation
III Laceration	<1 cm parenchymal depth of renal cortex without collection system rupture or urinary extravasation
IV Laceration	Parenchymal laceration extending through the renal cortex, medulla, and collecting system
IV Vascular	Main renal artery or vein injury with contained hemorrhage
V Laceration	Completely shattered kidney
V Vascular	Avulsion of renal hilum, which devascularizes kidney

From Moore EE, Shackford SR, Pachter HL, et al: *J Trauma* 29:1664, 1989.
Advance one grade for multiple injuries, up to grade III.

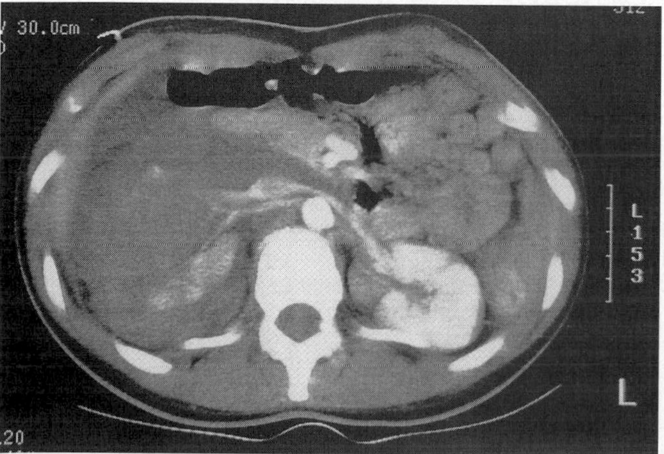

FIGURE 109–9 • Computed tomography of a patient with a grade IV renal laceration and vascular injury.

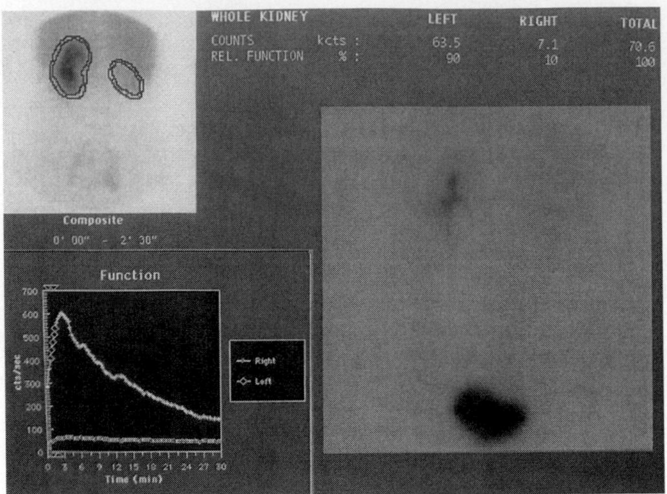

FIGURE 109–10 • Renal scan of a patient with grade IV renal laceration and vascular injury.

Blunt Abdominal Aortic Injury

Injury to the aorta resulting from blunt trauma is rare. The mechanism of injury is a direct blow to the abdomen. However, high-speed motor vehicle accidents with lap belt restraints may result in injury to the aorta. An aortogram is the diagnostic procedure of choice, although computed tomographic scan with intravenous contrast may suggest the presence of the injury. The aortic injury may vary from intimal dissection with contusion to complete disruption. The most frequent site of disruption is at the level of the inferior mesenteric artery or at the level of the kidneys. Patients present with diminished or absent distal lower extremity pulses. Neurologic deficits may result from aortic compromise. Associated injuries usually are present in 65% of cases. When blunt abdominal aortic injury is recognized early, surgical intervention may dramatically lower the mortality rate.[79] When operative intervention is delayed, a pseudoaneurysm is often identified at exploration. Major abdominal venous injuries resulting from blunt trauma are usually fatal.[80]

Bladder Injuries

Bladder injuries are most often associated with blunt mechanisms. The bladder is predominantly intraabdominal in children; therefore, burst injuries associated with lap belt restraints are not uncommon. Bladder rupture is commonly associated with pelvic fractures. The clinical presentation of a bladder rupture may be subtle with mild suprapubic tenderness. The severity of associated injuries may mask the clinical signs of a bladder injury. Hematuria is the most consistent finding suggesting the presence of a bladder injury. Recognizing the presence of injury and identifying the extent of injury as intraperitoneal or extraperitoneal are important.

Cystography is best for establishing the diagnosis. Lack of extravasation on computed tomography does not exclude a bladder injury. Peritoneal fluid located in the lateral perivesical recess, superior to the bladder, and in the pouch of Douglas is suggestive of an intraperitoneal bladder rupture. Extraperitoneal bladder rupture may be noted by fluid extending superiorly and anteriorly to the level of the umbilicus and by fluid in the retrorectal presacral space.[81]

The distinction between intraperitoneal and extraperitoneal bladder rupture is important for treatment purposes. Controlled extraperitoneal ruptures are treated nonoperatively with catheter drainage. Extensive extraperitoneal rupture or intraperitoneal injuries require operative intervention.

Pelvic Fractures

The most common mechanism resulting in pelvic fracture in children is a pedestrian struck by a motor vehicle. Early recognition is important so that resuscitation, stabilization, and evaluation of associated injuries can be accomplished. Single fractures of the pubic rami are rarely associated with significant abdominal injury. However, children with multiple fractures of the pelvic ramus are at significant risk for abdominal injury even if they are hemodynamically stable on admission (Table 109–7).

Pelvic fractures usually are evident on initial physical examination. Findings consistent with pelvic fractures include abrasions, bruising, hemorrhage, or swelling. Asymmetry of the bony structure, pain on palpation, instability, or crepitus can be present. After recognition, attention should be directed toward stabilization and assessment of hemodynamic status. Prehospital providers may use pneumatic antishock garments, but they should be replaced with another method of stabilization after arrival to the hospital. An anteroposterior radiograph of the pelvis is obtained in the trauma bay to determine the anatomy of

TABLE 109–7

Associated Injury by Location of Pelvic Fracture

Fracture Site	No. (%)	No. with Abdominal Injury (%)	No. with Genitourinary Injury (%)
Unifocal	44 (81.5)	5 (11)	0
Pubic ramus	32 (59.3)	2 (6)	0
Iliac/pelvic rim	9 (16.7)	3 (33)	0
Sacrum	3 (5.60)	0	0
Multiple	10 (18.5)	6 (60)	4 (40)
Total	54	11 (20)	4 (7.4)

From Bond SJ, Gotschall CS, Eichelberger MR: *J Trauma* 31:1169-1173, 1991.

the fracture. Opening of the pelvic ring, associated with fracture at two points, should be stabilized with a sheet wrapped around the pelvis, a C-clamp, or an external fixator. Vertical shear injuries usually are not amenable to this treatment. Hemodynamically unstable patients should be aggressively resuscitated. Early angiography and embolization of bleeding vessels should be considered.

Hemodynamically stable patients should undergo computed tomography to evaluate for associated injuries. Special attention should be directed toward the rectum and urethra, which are especially susceptible to injury by bony fragments. Unlike adults in whom mortality results from hemorrhage and sepsis, children are more at risk for complications secondary to associated head injuries.[82]

REFERENCES

1. Stylianos S: Late sequelae of major trauma in children, *Pediatr Clin North Am* 45:853-859, 1998.
2. Eichelberger MR, Managubat EA, Sacco WJ, et al: Outcome analysis of blunt injury in children, *J Trauma* 28:1109, 1988.
3. Davis JW, Hoyt DB, McArdle MS, et al: An analysis of errors causing morbidity and mortality in a trauma system: a guide for quality improvement, *J Trauma* 32:660-666, 1992.
4. Cooper A, Barlow B, DiScala C, String D: Mortality and truncal injury: the pediatric perspective, *J Pediatr Surg* 29:33-38, 1994.
5. Glassman SD, Johnson JR, Holt RT: Seatbelt injuries in children, *J Trauma* 33:882-886, 1992.
6. Orsborn R, Haley K, Hammond S, Falcone RE: Pediatric pedestrian versus motor vehicle patterns of injury: debunking the myth, *Air Med J* 18:107-110, 1999.
7. Christoffel KK: Pediatric firearm injuries: time to target a growing population, *Pediatr Ann* 21:430-436, 1992.
8. Cobb LM, Vinocur CD, Wagner CW, Weintraub WH: Intestinal perforation due to blunt trauma in children in an era of increased non-operative treatment, *J Trauma* 26:461-463, 1986.
9. Hennes HM, Smith DS, Schneider K, et al: Elevated liver transaminase levels in children with blunt abdominal trauma: a predictor of liver injury, *Pediatrics* 86:87-90, 1990.
10. Davis JW, Mackersie RC, Holbrook TL, Hoyt DB: Base deficit as an indicator of significant abdominal injury, *Ann Emer Med* 20:842-844, 1991.
11. Knudson MM, McAninch JW, Gomez R, et al: Hematuria as a predictor of abdominal injury after blunt trauma, *Am J Surg* 164: 482-486, 1992.
12. Stalker HP, Kaufman RA, Stedje K: The significance of hematuria in children after blunt abdominal trauma, *AJR Am J Roentgenol* 154:569-571, 1990.
13. Isaacman DJ, Scarfone RJ, Kost SI, et al: Utility of routine laboratory testing for detecting intra-abdominal injury in the pediatric trauma patient, *Pediatrics* 92:691-694, 1993.
14. Holmes JF, Sokolove PE, Land C, Kuppermann N: Identification of intra-abdominal injuries in children hospitalized following blunt torso trauma, *Acad Emerg Med* 6:799-806, 1999.
15. Abou-Khalil B, Scalea TM, Trooskin SZ, et al: Hemodynamic responses to shock in young trauma patients: need for invasive monitoring, *Crit Care Med* 22:633-639, 1994.
16. Cosentine CM, Luck SR, Barthel MJ, et al: Transfusion requirements in conservative non-operative management of blunt splenic and hepatic injuries during childhood, *J Pediatr Surg* 25:950-954, 1990.
17. Umali E, Andrews HG, White JJ: A critical analysis of blood transfusion requirements in children with blunt abdominal trauma, *Am Surg* 58:736-739, 1992.
18. Kudsk KA, Minard G, Wojtysiak SL, et al: Visceral protein response to enteral versus parenteral nutrition and sepsis in patients with trauma, *Surgery* 116:516-523, 1994.
19. Dokucu AI, Otcu S, Ozturk H, et al: Characteristics of penetrating abdominal firearm injuries in children, *Eur J Pediatr Surg* 10: 242-247, 2000.
20. Beaver BL, Moore VL, Peclet M, et al: Characteristic of pediatric firearm fatalities, *J Pediatr Surg* 25:97-100, 1990.
21. Muckart DJJ, Adool-Carrim ATO, King B: Selective conservative management of abdominal gunshot wounds: a prospective study, *Br J Surg* 77:652-655, 1990.
22. McCarthy MC, Lowdermilk GA, Canal DF, Broadie TA: Prediction of injury caused by penetrating wounds to the abdomen, flank, and back, *Arch Surg* 126:962-965, 1991.
23. Burns RK, Sariol HS, Ross SE: Penetrating posterior abdominal trauma, *Injury* 25:429-431, 1994.
24. Chiu WC, Shanmuganathan K, Mirvis SE, Scalea TM: Determining the need for laparotomy in penetrating torso trauma: a prospective study using triple-contrast enhanced abdominopelvic computed tomography, *J Trauma* 51:860-868, 2001.
25. Renz BM, Feliciano DV: Gunshot wounds to the right thoracoabdomen: a prospective study of non-operative management, *J Trauma* 37:737-744, 1994.
26. Maier RV: Evaluation of abdominal trauma, *Bull Am Coll Surg* 80:37-38, 1995.
27. Renz BM, Feliciano DV: Unnecessary laparotomies for trauma: a prospective study of morbidity, *J Trauma* 38:350-356, 1995.
28. Taylor GA, Eichelberger MR, O'Donnell R, Bowman L: Indications for computed tomography in children with blunt abdominal trauma, *Ann Surg* 213:212-218, 1991.
29. Killeen KL, Shanmuganathan K, Poletti PA, et al: Helical computed tomography of bowel and mesenteric injuries, *J Trauma* 51:26-36, 2001.
30. Meyer DM, Thal ER, Coln D, Weigelt JA: Computed tomography in the evaluation of children with blunt abdominal trauma, *Ann Surg* 217:272-276, 1993.
31. Sievers EM, Close BJ, Marshall KW, Cywes R: Abdominal computed tomography scan in pediatric blunt abdominal trauma, *Am Surg* 65:968-971, 1999.
32. Moore EE, Cogbill TH, Malangoni MA, et al: Organ injury scaling, II: pancreas, duodenum, small bowel, colon, and rectum, *J Trauma* 30:1427-1429, 1990.
33. Moore EE, Shackford SR, Pachter HL, et al: Organ injury scaling: spleen, liver, and kidney, *J Trauma* 29:1664-1666, 1989.
34. Luks FI, Lemire A, Dickens S, et al: Blunt abdominal trauma in children: the practical value of ultrasonography, *J Trauma* 34: 607-611, 1993.
35. Holmes JF, Brant WE, Bond WF, et al: Emergency department ultrasonography in the evaluation of hypotensive and normotensive children with blunt abdominal trauma, *J Pediatr Surg* 36:968-973, 2001.
36. Dolich MO, McKenney MG, Varela JE, et al: 2,576 ultrasounds for blunt abdominal trauma, *J Trauma* 50:108-112, 2001.
37. Coley BD, Mutabagani KH, Martin LC, et al: Focused abdominal sonography for trauma (FAST) in children with blunt abdominal trauma, *J Trauma* 48:902-906, 2000.
38. McKenney M, Lentz K, Nunew D, et al: Can ultrasound replace diagnostic peritoneal lavage in the assessment of blunt trauma? *J Trauma* 37:439-441, 1994.
39. Akgur FM, Tanyel FC, Akhan O, et al: The place of ultrasonographic examination in the initial evaluation of children sustaining blunt abdominal trauma, *J Pediatr Surg* 28:78-81, 1993.
40. Goletti O, Ghisell G, Lippolis PV, et al: The role of ultrasonography in blunt abdominal trauma: results in 250 consecutive cases, *J Trauma* 36:178-181, 1994.
41. Glaser K, Tschmelitsch J, Klingler P, et al: Ultrasonography in the management of blunt abdominal and thoracic trauma, *Arch Surg* 129:743-747, 1994.
42. Rossi D, deVille de Goyet J, Clement de Clety S, et al: Management of intra-abdominal organ injury following blunt abdominal trauma in children, *Intensive Care Med* 19:415-419, 1993.
43. Rothenberg S, Moore EE, Marx JA, et al: Selective management of blunt abdominal trauma in children: the triage of peritoneal lavage, *J Trauma* 27:1101-1106, 1987.
44. Fang JF, Chen RJ, Lin BC, et al: Small bowel perforation: is urgent surgery necessary? *J Trauma* 47:515-520, 1999.
45. Karp MP, Cooney DR, Pros GA, et al: The nonoperative management of pediatric hepatic trauma, *J Pediatr Surg* 18:512, 1983.
46. Sosa JL, Sims D, Martin L, Seppa R: Laparoscopic evaluation of tangential abdominal gunshot wounds, *Arch Surg* 127:109-110, 1992.
47. Fernando HC, Alle KM, Chen J, et al: Triage by laparoscopy in patients with penetrating abdominal trauma, *Br J Surg* 81:384-385, 1994.

48. Rossi P, Mullins D, Thal E: Role of laparoscopy in the evaluation of abdominal trauma, *Am J Surg* 166:707-710, 1993.
49. Uribe RA, Pachon CE, Frame SB, et al: A prospective evaluation of thoracoscopy for the diagnosis of penetrating thoracoabdominal trauma, *J Trauma* 37:650-654, 1994.
50. Meyer G, Huttl TP, Hatz RA, Schildberg FW: Laparoscopic repair of traumatic diaphragmatic hernias, *Surg Endosc* 14:1010-1014, 2000.
51. Mooney DP, Birkmeyer NJ, Udell JV, Shorter NA: Variation in the management of pediatric splenic injuries in New Hampshire, *J Pediatr Surg* 33:1076-1078, 1998.
52. Stylianos S, APSA Trauma Committee: Evidence-based guidelines for resource utilization in children with isolated spleen or liver injury, *J Pediatr Surg* 35:164-169, 2000.
53. Morse MA, Garcia VF: Selective non-operative management of pediatric blunt splenic trauma: risk for missed associated injuries, *J Pediatr Surg* 29:23-27, 1994.
54. White CL, Esser MJ, Rappaport WD: Updating the management of salvageable splenic injury, *Ann Surg* 215:261-265, 1992.
55. Cosentino CM, Luck SR, Barthel MJ, et al: Transfusion requirements in conservative nonoperative management of blunt splenic and hepatic injuries during childhood, *J Pediatr Surg* 25:950-954, 1990.
56. Lynch JM, Ford H, Gardner MJ, Weiner ES: Is early discharge following isolated splenic injury in the hemodynamically stable child possible? *J Pediatr Surg* 28:1403-1407, 1993.
57. Kluger Y, Paul DB, Raves JJ, et al: Delayed rupture of the spleen: myths, facts and their importance: case reports and literature review, *J Trauma* 36:568-571, 1994.
58. Benya EC, Bulas DI, Eichelberger MR, Sivit CJ: Splenic injury from blunt abdominal trauma in children: follow-up evaluation with CT, *Radiology* 195:685-688, 1995.
59. Trunkey DD, Shires GT, McClelland R: Management of liver trauma in 811 consecutive patients, *Ann Surg* 179:722-728, 1974.
60. CAPS: Trauma committee: Canadian Association of Pediatric Surgeons: liver trauma study, *J Pediatr Surg* 24:1035-1040, 1989.
61. Sivit CJ, Taylor GA, Eichelberger MR, et al: Significance of periportal low-attenuation zones following blunt trauma in children, *Pediatr Radiol* 23:338-390, 1993.
62. Holmes JF, Sokolove PE, Land C, Kuppermann N: Identification of intra-abdominal injuries in children hospitalized following blunt torso trauma, *Acad Emerg Med* 6:799-806, 1999.
63. Oldham KT, Guice KS, Ryckman F, et al: Blunt liver injury in children: evolution of therapy and current prospective, *Surgery* 100:542-549, 1986.
64. Gates JD: Delayed hemorrhage with free rupture complicating the non-surgical management of blunt hepatic trauma: a case report and review of the literature, *J Trauma* 36:572-575, 1994.
65. Moulton SL, Lynch FP, Hoyt D, et al: Operative intervention for pediatric liver injuries: avoiding delay in treatment, *J Pediatr Surg* 27:958-963, 1992.
66. Cue JI, Cryer HG, Miller FB, et al: Packing and planned reexploration for hepatic and retroperitoneal hemorrhage: critical refinements of a useful technique, *J Trauma* 30:1007-1013, 1990.
67. Allen GS, Moore FA, Cox CS Jr, et al: Hollow visceral injury and blunt trauma, *J Trauma* 45:69-75, 1998.
68. Pokorny WJ, Brandt ML, Harberg FJ: Major duodenal injuries in children: diagnosis, operative management, and outcome, *J Pediatr Surg* 21:613-616, 1986.
69. Kunin JR, Korobkin M, Ellis JH, et al: Duodenal injuries caused by blunt abdominal trauma: value of CT in differentiating perforation from hematoma, *AJR Am J Roentgenol* 160:1221-1223, 1993.
70. Cogbill TH, Moore EE, Feliciano DV, et al: Conservative management of duodenal trauma: a multicenter perspective, *J Trauma* 30:1469-1475, 1990.
71. Kim HS, Lee DK, Kim IW, et al: The role of endoscopic retrograde pancreatography in the treatment of traumatic pancreatic duct injury, *Gastrointest Endosc* 54:49-55, 2001.
72. Nance ML, Keller MS, Stafford PW: Predicting hollow visceral injury in the pediatric blunt trauma patient with solid visceral injury, *J Pediatr Surg* 35:1300-1303, 2000.
73. Fang JF, Chen RJ, Lin BC: Cell count ratio: new criterion of diagnostic peritoneal lavage for detection of hollow organ perforation, *J Trauma* 45:540-544, 1998.
74. Strouse PJ, Close BJ, Marshall KW, Cywes R: CT of bowel and mesenteric trauma in children, *Radiographics* 19:1237-1250, 1999.
75. Smith EM, Elder JS, Spirnak JP: Major blunt renal trauma in the pediatric population: Is a non-operative approach indicated? *J Urol* 149:546-548, 1993.
76. Wessel LM, Scholz S, Jester I, et al: Management of kidney injuries in children with blunt abdominal trauma, *J Pediatr Surg* 35:1326-1330, 2000.
77. Hagiwara A, Sakaki S, Goto H, et al: The role of interventional radiology in the management of blunt renal injury: a practical protocol, *J Trauma* 51:526-531, 2001.
78. Boone TB, Gillina PJ, Husmann DA: Ureteropelvic junction disruption following blunt abdominal trauma, *J Urol* 150:33-36, 1993.
79. Amin A, Alexander JB, O'Malley KF, Doolin E: Blunt abdominal aortic trauma in children: case report, *J Trauma* 34:293-296, 1993.
80. Fayiga YJ, Valentine RJ, Myers SI, et al: Blunt pediatric vascular trauma: analysis of forty-one consecutive patients undergoing operative intervention, *J Vasc Surg* 20:419-424, 1994.
81. Sivit CJ, Cutting JP, Eichelberger MR: CT diagnosis and localization of rupture of the bladder in children with blunt abdominal trauma, *AJR Am J Roentgenol* 164:1243-1246, 1995.
82. Bond SJ, Gotschall CS, Eichelberger MR: Predictors of abdominal injury in children with pelvic fracture, *J Trauma* 31:1169-1173, 1991.

PART

V

PHARMACOLOGY

CHAPTER

110

Principles of Drug Disposition in the Critically Ill Child

Lara Primak and Jeffrey L. Blumer

PEARLS

- Studies devoted to the disposition of drugs in critically ill patients and children are limited.
- *Therapeutics* is the branch of pharmacology concerned with the use of drugs for their therapeutic effects. It focuses on four fundamental questions that can serve as an outline for the clinician designing any pharmacotherapeutic plan: what drug, what dose, what route, and how long?
- Drug disposition is controlled by *pharmacokinetics* and *pharmacodynamics*. Pharmacokinetics is the discipline within clinical pharmacology that broadly describes the changes in the quantity of drug and/or drug metabolite in various body compartments over time. Whereas pharmacokinetics describes what the body does to the drug, pharmacodynamics encompasses the pharmacologic aspects that impact how the drug affects the body.
- Pharmacokinetic processes that influence drug disposition include absorption, distribution, metabolism, and excretion. Both ontogeny and critical illness may significantly impact any of these processes. Metabolism may be further affected by genetic differences in involved enzymes.
- Ontogeny and critical illness affect pharmacodynamics in infants and children, although formal study of these effects is limited.
- Pharmacotherapeutic strategies that can be used in the critically ill patient include the *target-concentration* and *target-effect* strategies. The target-concentration strategy relies on concentration of drug in blood or plasma (usually) to guide therapy; this approach is best applied to drugs used chronically for signs or symptoms that manifest intermittently. The target-effect strategy, the strategy most commonly used in the pediatric intensive care unit, relies upon an accepted clinical endpoint to determine drug dosing; clinical evidence of toxicity also impacts dosing. The latter strategy probably is the most reliable means by which to administer the "right amount" of drug to a highly variable patient population.

Pharmacology is the study of the interaction between chemical agents and biologic systems. When these chemical agents are used with the intent of palliating or curing disease, the agents are termed *drugs*. Perhaps nowhere is drug therapy more important than in critical care. In this setting, however, drug response often is difficult to predict. Physiologic aberrations and coincident pharmacologic and nonpharmacologic therapies may thwart intended drug effects. For the pediatric intensivist, pharmacotherapeutic decisions are further complicated by ontogenetic differences in drug processing and response. Finally, experience upon which to base pharmacotherapeutic expectations or prescription is sparse. Most drugs used in the intensive care setting have never been formally investigated in critically ill patients, let alone in children. As such, it is imperative that the pediatric intensivist have an understanding of the pharmacologic and related developmental constructs that influence drug response in patients.

The discipline of therapeutics provides a useful outline by which to design and monitor drug treatment. *Therapeutics* is the branch of pharmacology concerned with the use of drugs for their therapeutic effects. It focuses on four fundamental questions pertaining to drug therapy as it relates to patient care: what drug, what dose, what route, and how long? The task of answering these important questions is facilitated by an understanding of the general pharmacologic principles that dictate drug response and the factors that lead to variation among patients.

Drug Disposition in Infants and Children

It should come as no surprise that controversy exists regarding drug dosing in pediatric patients. Over the years, a number of dosing rules been developed with the intent that drugs be safely administered to young children. All these rules depend on the standard adult dose with a scale-down factor based on body weight or age. However, distinct differences in pharmacokinetics and pharmacodynamics (Box 110–1) distinguish the pediatric patient from the adult patient. Critical illness may further alter pharmacokinetics and pharmacodynamics in children. These differences must be recognized before providing safe and effective dosing and during the initial selection of the drug itself.

Determinants of Effective Therapy

Effective therapy results when the drug(s) selected for a given condition has both favorable pharmacokinetic and favorable pharmacodynamic properties (Box 110–1). Moreover, administration to the patient must be individualized based on (1) a realistic clinical endpoint determined before administration, (2) sound knowledge of the quantitative aspects of the disposition of the drug selected, and (3) an understanding of the impact on the patient's illness of both the dosing regimen to be used and the anticipated therapeutic effect.

BOX 110–1

Determinants of Effective Therapy

PHARMACOKINETICS

Absorption
Distribution
Metabolism
Excretion

PHARMACODYNAMICS

Drug–receptor interactions
Structure–activity relationships
Receptor–effector coupling
Safety profile

Pharmacokinetics

Pharmacokinetics is the discipline within clinical pharmacology that broadly describes the changes in the quantity of drug and/or drug metabolite in various body compartments over time. These changes can be described by four processes: absorption, distribution, metabolism, and excretion. Each of these processes can be affected by both development and disease. A clear understanding of pharmacokinetic processes and the factors affecting them will permit the clinician to design an effective treatment plan or troubleshoot when an undesired response to treatment occurs. In other words, an understanding of basic pharmacokinetic principles will increase the likelihood that any treatment goal will be successfully accomplished with minimal adverse effects.

Drug Absorption

Absorption refers to the translocation of a drug from its site of administration into the bloodstream. When drugs are administered intravenously, as often occurs in the intensive care unit (ICU), the need for absorption is bypassed. When intravenous administration is not possible or convenient, several other routes of administration can be effectively used. Physicochemical properties of the drug and specific factors related to each route determine the rate and magnitude of absorption. Knowledge of these factors increases the likelihood that the clinician will be able to predict, if not control, this component of drug disposition.

Enteral Absorption. Absorption of drugs from the gastrointestinal tract is affected by a number of factors (Box 110–2).[1,2] In general, enteral absorption depends upon gastric emptying, intestinal surface area and motility, and hepatic first pass. Ontogeny and critical illness may significantly affect these and other patient factors (Figure 110–1 and Box 110–3).

BOX 110–2

Factors Affecting Drug Absorption

PHYSICOCHEMICAL FACTORS

Disintegration of tablets or solid phase
Dissolution of the drug in gastric or intestinal fluids, and number of ionizable groups
Degree of lipid solubility of the lipid-soluble form
Molecular weight

PATIENT FACTORS

Surface area available for absorption
Gastric and duodenal pH
Gastric emptying time
Bile salt pool size
Bacterial colonization of the gastrointestinal tract
Underlying disease states

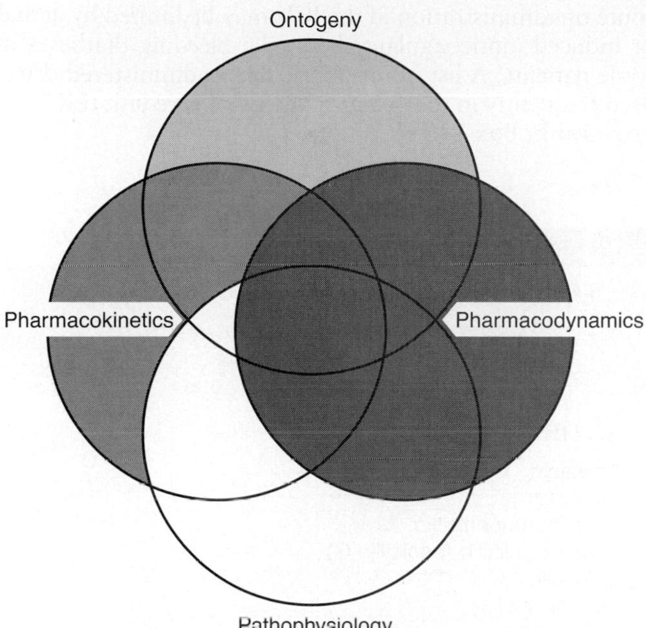

FIGURE 110–1 • Determinants of effective therapy.

Gastric Acidity. Gastric and duodenal pH affect drug solubility and ionization, as well as gastrointestinal motility.[3] Gastric absorption is facilitated by passive nonionic diffusion.[4] Therefore in the acidic gastric environment, only weak acids (low pK_a) will be appreciably absorbed because they will be in a unionized, more lipid-soluble form. In contrast, a relatively high pH (as in states of achlorhydria) will enhance the translocation of basic drugs and retard the absorption of acidic drugs. Although neonates, both premature and term, have demonstrated the ability to attain pH values around 2,[5] gastric pH is elevated (pH 6–7) after 24 hours of life and remains higher than adult values (pH 2–3) until age 20 to 30 months.[6]

BOX 110–3

Selected Disease States Affecting Gastrointestinal Absorption of Drugs

GASTRIC ACID SECRETION

- Proximal small bowel resection

DELAYED GASTRIC EMPTYING

- Pyloric stenosis
- Congestive heart failure
- Protein calorie malnutrition

INTESTINAL TRANSIT TIME

- Protein calorie malnutrition
- Thyroid disease
- Diarrheal disease

BILE SALT EXCRETION

- Cholestatic liver disease
- Extrahepatic biliary obstruction

DECREASED SURFACE AREA

- Short bowel syndrome
- Protein calorie malnutrition

Gastric Emptying. Because the primary site of absorption for drugs given enterally is the small intestine, the rate of gastric emptying is an important determinant of the rate and extent of drug absorption. If the rate of gastric emptying is slowed, the rate of intestinal drug absorption may be reduced, which in turn will reduce the peak serum drug concentrations. If the rate of gastric emptying is hastened, however, the extent of intestinal absorption may be reduced as a result of decreased contact time with the absorptive surface. Both of these effects presuppose that intestinal motility remains constant.

The rate of gastric emptying is variable during the neonatal period. Reduced gastric emptying commonly afflicts preterm infants.[5] The type of feed used impacts gastric emptying rates; for example, breast milk results in faster emptying than does formula.[5,7] There is an inverse relationship between the rate of gastric emptying and caloric density (not osmolality).[8] Additionally, the type of fat in feedings influences the rate of gastric emptying. Slower emptying is seen in feedings with long-chain fatty acids compared with medium-chain triglycerides.[8] By age 6 to 8 months, gastric emptying rates approach the rates seen in adults.[6,8]

Delayed gastric emptying may be associated with certain disease states in the neonate, including gastroesophageal reflux, respiratory distress syndrome, and congenital heart disease. In adults, delayed gastric emptying has been demonstrated in patients with closed head injury,[9,10] burns,[9] or sepsis and in those on mechanical ventilation.[9,11] Significant abdominal surgery, trauma, and any cause of compromised blood flow may affect gastric emptying. Certain drugs (e.g., opioids, dopamine, anticholinergics) and metabolic abnormalities (e.g., hypokalemia) may delay gastric emptying.[9]

The ontogeny of additional physiologic processes may influence gastrointestinal absorption of xenobiotics. Intestinal motility is generally increased in the infant, potentially reducing absorption because of more rapid transit past the primary site of absorption. Anatomic factors such as extensive resection may limit intestinal absorption and hence overall absorption of enterally administered drugs. The rate of synthesis and the pool size of bile salts are reduced in newborn infants compared with adults.[12] Clinically, this may manifest as a reduced rate and extent of absorption of lipid-soluble drugs or nutrients such as vitamins D and E. Also, the colonization of gastrointestinal tract bacterial flora differs, depending on gestational age, type of delivery, and type of feeding.[13] Changes in bacterial flora during the neonatal period may be important in the hydrolysis of drug conjugates that are excreted in bile. The clinical significance of these physiologic variables remains to be defined.

Bioavailability. Bioavailability (F) describes the fraction of a dose of drug that reaches the systemic circulation. Bioavailability of a single drug may vary significantly depending on the route of administration. By routes other than intravenous, absorption is a primary determinant of F. In enteral administration, an additional factor influences F. Excluding drugs primarily absorbed by the oral mucosa, drugs administered into the gastrointestinal tract may undergo metabolism by intestinal mucosal cells and/or metabolism and/or biliary excretion when they pass through the liver, before reaching the systemic circulation. This is known as the *first-pass effect.* With affected drugs, this phenomenon may significantly reduce F. This accounts for the fact that the enteral dose for many drugs is significantly greater than the intravenous dose. The susceptibility of a drug to hepatic first-pass metabolism may influence how the drug is administered; for example, nitroglycerin is given sublingually to circumvent a considerable first-pass effect in this drug.[4] Aside from the physicochemical nature of the drug itself, other factors may influence the extent of hepatic first-pass metabolism. Changes in hepatic blood flow may alter this action.[4] Age likely further influences the extent of hepatic first pass. As described later in the chapter, maturation of hepatic enzyme systems and transporters appears to occur postnatally.[14] Although the data dedicated to the ontogeny of metabolizing enzymes and transporters in the liver are limited, particularly as they relate to drug bioavailability, F likely decreases with age as these systems mature.[14]

Absorption of Drugs Administered Intramuscularly. The parenteral route of drug administration is important when a patient's disease state precludes oral therapy or when the bioavailability of an oral formulation is poor. The intravenous route for drug delivery is preferred over intramuscular (IM) injection. However, in children with poor intravenous access, IM injection is a viable and effective alternative for administration of many drugs.

Both physicochemical and physiologic factors affect the rate of drug absorption from the IM injection site.[15] Lipophilicity of a drug favors rapid diffusion into the capillaries; however, the drug must retain a degree of water solubility at physiologic pH to prevent precipitation at the injection site. For example, the sodium salt of phenytoin is principally an acid and thus is insoluble in the extracellular milieu of skeletal muscle. This explains the poor IM absorption of phenytoin. By contrast, phenobarbital and benzathine penicillin are well absorbed after IM administration. Both of these drugs are weak acids with pK_a values close to physiologic pH and are therefore unlikely to precipitate in muscle under most physiologic conditions. By having knowledge of the physicochemical properties of a drug preparation, the clinician can predict, even control to some extent, how the drug is absorbed. While aqueous preparations will undergo rapid absorption, drugs in a solution of oil or other repository vehicles will be absorbed at a slower and more continuous rate.[16]

Another important factor that influences absorption of drug from an IM injection site is local blood flow, which may be compromised in patients with poor peripheral perfusion.[17] Rate and extent of absorption from an IM injection site also are influenced by the total surface area of muscle in contact with the injected solution, similar to the dependency of oral absorption on the total available absorptive area in the intestines.[15]

A final consideration in IM absorption is muscle activity, which may affect the rate of absorption and therefore affect the peak serum concentration. Sick, immobile infants and children or those chemically paralyzed may show reduced absorption rates after IM drug administration. Use of this route of administration in the ICU may be limited by actual or induced (anticoagulant therapy[16]) bleeding diatheses in some patients. A list of intramuscularly administered drugs used frequently in the pediatric intensive care unit (PICU) is provided in Box 110–4.

BOX 110–4

Drugs Demonstrating Effective System Absorption After Intramuscular Administration

ANTIBACTERIAL

Amikacin
Ampicillin
Benzathine penicillin
Benzyl penicillin (penicillin G)
Cefazolin
Cefotaxime
Ceftazidime
Ceftriaxone
Clindamycin
Gentamicin
Kanamycin
Methicillin
Oxacillin
Nafcillin
Piperacillin
Ticarcillin ± clavulanate
Tobramycin
Antituberculous Agents
  Isoniazid
  Streptomycin

ANTICONVULSANTS

Diazepam ±
Midazolam
Phenobarbital

SEDATIVES/TRANQUILIZERS

Chlorpromazine
Promethazine
Cardiovascular Drugs
  Hydralazine
  Procainamide
  Pyridostigmine
Diuretics
  Acetazolamide
  Furosemide
  Bumetanide
Endocrine
  Corticotropin (ACTH)
  Cortisone
  Desoxycorticosterone
  Glucagon
Pituitary
  Vasopressin (tannate oil)

VITAMINS

D
K

From Blumer JL: Therapeutic agents. In Fanaroff AA, Martin RJ, editors: *Neonatal-perinatal medicine: diseases of the fetus,* ed 4. St. Louis, 1987, Mosby.

Subcutaneous Absorption. As with absorption of drugs from IM sites, absorption of subcutaneously administered drugs is influenced by local blood flow, as well as by proximal scarring or injury.[4] The pattern of absorption varies similarly to that following IM injection, depending on the physicochemical properties of the preparation. Frequently, drugs given by the subcutaneous route undergo slow and sustained absorption.[16] As such, the rate of absorption can be regulated by the drug formulation. For example, when drugs are administered in solid pellet form, absorption may occur over weeks to months.[16] Absorption can be slowed by the addition of a vasoconstrictor.[16] This route of administration is not appropriate for large volumes or drugs that are irritating to tissues.

Percutaneous Absorption. Percutaneous absorption is inversely related to the thickness of the stratum corneum and directly related to skin hydration.[18] The stratum corneum is generally assumed, but not proven, to be thinner in children than in adults. Integument of the full-term neonate possesses intact barrier function.[19] This is not assured in the case of the premature infant.[8] Another important factor dictating percutaneous absorption is the surface area/body weight ratio, which is much larger in the full-term neonate than in an adult. Theoretically, if a newborn receives the same percutaneous dose of a compound as an adult, the systemic availability per kilogram body weight is approximately 2.7 times greater in the neonate.

The percutaneous route of drug administration is taking on greater importance in the ICU setting. Historically, the most commonly used cutaneous preparation for systemic therapy is nitroglycerin.[20] More recently, advances in the technology associated with drug delivery systems has resulted in the common use of clonidine as a percutaneous preparation for treatment of hypertension and narcotic withdrawal. In addition, a number of narcotics exist as cutaneous preparations so that essentially "continuous infusions" of these drugs can be administered safely outside the ICU.[21] Finally, even drugs such as nitroglycerin ointment are finding potential new uses in the PICU, for example, treatment of the distal ischemia associated with purpuric injuries.

Rectal Absorption. Rectal administration of drugs is of potential therapeutic importance if a patient cannot take an agent orally and intravenous access for drug administration is impracticable. Because of the routes of the respective venous drainage systems, drugs administered into the superior aspect of the rectum are susceptible to hepatic first pass, whereas drugs administered lower into the rectum initially bypass the liver.[22] This may be an advantage for drugs such as lidocaine or propranolol, which demonstrate a significant hepatic first-pass effect. The predominant mechanism for drug absorption from the rectum probably is similar to that observed in the upper gastrointestinal tract (i.e., passive diffusion). Theoretically, the physicochemical and host factors discussed earlier with respect to oral drug absorption also influence rectal drug absorption. In general, absorption from aqueous or alcoholic solutions is more rapid than from suppositories.

Lipophilic drugs with pK_a between 7 and 8, such as barbiturates and benzodiazepines, seem to be ideally suited for rectal administration because they exist mostly in unionized form and readily cross cell membranes. Rectal use of drugs such as thiopental and diazepam may be effective when intravenous access is a problem and rapid induction of anesthesia is desired or when a child is convulsing. Dulac et al.[23] showed that rectal administration of 0.25 to 0.5 mg/kg of a diazepam solution to children age 2 weeks to 11 years produced serum concentrations comparable with those observed after intravenous administration. Additionally, peak serum concentrations occurred within minutes of administration. Potentially effective anticonvulsant serum concentrations were maintained for 1 to 3 hours in most of the study patients. Knudsen[24] demonstrated similar results in 20 infants age 1 to 2 years and further ascertained the clinical efficacy of rectal diazepam in preventing recurrent febrile seizures. In a similar fashion, Burckart et al.[25] reported rapid and effective sedation after rectal administration of thiopental suspension to 36 infants and children undergoing computed tomographic scanning.

Drug Distribution

Knowledge of drug distribution is important for selecting the appropriate drug and dose to be administered. Distribution of most drugs in the body is influenced by a variety of age-dependent factors, including protein binding, body compartment sizes, hemodynamic factors such as cardiac output and regional blood flow, and membrane permeability.[26,27] Any of these factors also can be altered by disease. This section briefly reviews the pharmacokinetic description of distribution and the effect of ontogeny and critical illness on several factors that determine drug distribution.

The primary pharmacokinetic parameter representative of drug distribution is the volume of distribution (V_d). V_d reflects the apparent space within the body available to contain drug and relates the amount of drug in the body to its concentration in a biologic fluid, usually blood or plasma.[16] V_d varies among drugs, based on the drug's extent of protein and tissue binding and partition coefficient in fat.[16] Additionally, for any given drug, V_d varies among patients because of differences in protein stores or binding and body composition as a result of age or illness. For example, in neonates and infants, a relatively increased extracellular fluid volume, decreased protein binding, and increased brain and liver size all contribute to increased weight-normalized V_d for most drugs.[28] An understanding of the factors influencing V_d is of paramount importance to the clinician caring for critically ill children. V_d relates the administered dose of drug to its plasma or blood concentration, which determines therapeutic effects, both favorable and adverse. Alterations in V_d produce reciprocal changes in drug concentration.[28] Familiarity with the concept of V_d and the ontogenic and other factors influencing its variation will assist the intensivist in understanding why a standard drug dose might be inappropriate for a given patient.

Developmental Aspects of Protein Binding. Plasma protein binding of drugs depends on the concentration of binding proteins available, the affinity constant of the drug for the protein(s), the number of available binding sites, and the presence of pathophysiologic conditions or endogenous compounds that may alter drug–protein interaction.[29]

The affinity of albumin for acidic drugs increases, as do total plasma protein levels, from birth to early infancy.[30] These values do not reach normal adult levels until age 10 to 12 months. In addition, although plasma albumin may reach adult levels shortly after birth, the neonatal albumin level in blood is directly proportional to gestational age, reflecting placental transport and fetal synthesis.[31] Binding of basic drugs by α_1-acid glycoprotein also is affected.[28,32] Studies in cord blood suggest that decreased levels of α_1-acid glycoprotein cause this decreased binding.[32]

Some of the drugs that have exhibited decreased protein binding in the infant include diazepam, furosemide, propranolol, thiopental, phenytoin, and some antibiotics.[28] The comparative binding of some of these drugs in neonates and adults is given in Table 110–1. The impact of decreased binding of many of these drugs on efficacy has not been determined.[28] For drugs that are highly protein bound and subject to therapeutic monitoring (e.g., phenytoin), however, any decrease in protein binding may result in a lower measured total drug concentration.[28] In such cases, monitoring of free drug concentration (if possible) will prove more clinically relevant.

Influence of Endogenous Substances on Protein Binding. A number of endogenous molecules may, as drugs do, bind to plasma proteins.[33] In the process, they may displace drugs from these binding sites and at least transiently increase the apparent volume of distribution of the displaced drug. More important, the increase in the fraction of free drug, which occurs because of the displacement reaction, may result in a transiently intensified pharmacologic response at a given drug dose or in serum total drug concentration.

A clinically significant protein binding displacement reaction will occur only if a drug is more than 80% to 90% protein bound[34] and, more specifically, if the drug's clearance is capacity limited and binding sensitive. Another prerequisite for a significant displacement reaction is that the V_d must be small, usually less than 0.15 L/kg.[34] Above this value, only a small percentage of total drug in the body is found in plasma.

Under these conditions, the following sequence of events may occur: the displacement reaction increases the amount of free drug, which may result in a heightened pharmacologic response if the concentration–effect relationship is reasonably steep. However, this intensified pharmacologic effect is only transient because the displacement reaction increases the amount of free drug available for metabolism or excretion. The net result, once steady state is achieved, is a decreased concentration of total drug in plasma accompanied by an unchanged free drug concentration and, hence, pharmacologic effect.[28]

TABLE 110–1

Comparative Protein Binding of Some Representative Drugs

Drug	% Bound	
	Newborn	Adult
Acetaminophen	37	48
Ampicillin	10	18
Diazepam	84	99
Lidocaine	20	70
Morphine	46	66
Phenobarbital	32	51
Phenytoin	80	90
Propranolol	60	93
Theophylline	36	56

Modified from Kurz H, Mauser-Ganshom A, Stickel HH: *Eur J Clin Pharmacol* 11:463, 1977.

Free Fatty Acids. Nonesterified fatty acids are reversibly bound to albumin and are present at relatively high concentrations in the plasma of newborn infants.[35] Significant reductions in albumin binding of salicylic acid, phenylbutazone, bishydroxycoumarin, and phenytoin at high serum levels of free fatty acids (FFAs) approximating 2000 μEq/L or an FFA/albumin molar ratio of 3.5 have been demonstrated.[36] Although these values are rarely attained, they have been observed under certain pathophysiologic conditions, such as gram-negative septicemia.[37] Interestingly, similar elevations in FFA levels have not been observed with gram-positive septicemia.

Hunninghake and Azarnoff[38] demonstrated a comparable rise in serum FFA concentrations in humans after apparent β-adrenergic stimulation. Fredholm et al.[39] reported a linear correlation between unbound plasma phenytoin concentrations and the ratio of serum FFA to albumin concentration in neonates.

Bilirubin. Bilirubin is noncovalently bound to albumin, and this association is freely reversible.[40] The bilirubin binding affinity of albumin at birth is independent of gestational age and is less in the newborn than in the adult. The binding affinity of albumin for bilirubin increases with age and reaches that of adult serum by approximately 5 months of age.[40] The lower bilirubin binding affinity of albumin in neonates is believed to be a contributing factor to their susceptibility to kernicterus.[40,41] Certain drugs that may compete for binding (e.g., phenytoin, sulfonamides) can augment this risk by displacing bilirubin.[16,42] Other factors that may contribute to increased risk include hypothermia, acidosis, hypoglycemia, hypoxemia, sepsis, birth asphyxia, and hypercapnia, any of which may alter the permeability of the blood-brain barrier and/or bilirubin-albumin binding, must be considered.[43]

Stutman et al.[44] evaluated the in vitro effect of several newer antimicrobial agents on bilirubin-albumin binding. Aztreonam (a monobactam), azlocillin (a ureidopenicillin), enoxacin and ciprofloxacin (oxyquinolones), and imipenem (a carbapenem) did not effectively compete with bilirubin for albumin-binding sites. Cefoperazone, a third-generation cephalosporin, resulted in an increase in the unbound bilirubin fraction at concentrations unlikely to be achieved in vivo.

Developmental Aspects of Fluid Compartment Sizes

Total Body Water. Alterations in body water compartment sizes affect the volume of distribution of a drug. Age-dependent changes in the various fluid compartments (Table 110–2) were reviewed in detail by Cheek et al.[45] and Friis-Hansen[46] (see Chapter 60). Regardless of age, critical illness and related therapies may alter total body water and other fluid compartment volumes.

Extracellular Fluid Volume. At 40 weeks of gestation, measurements of extracellular fluid volume have ranged

TABLE 110–2

Fluid Compartment Size as a Function of Age

Age	Total Body Water*	Extracellular Fluid*	Intracellular Fluid*
<3-month fetus	92	65	25
Term gestation	7560	35-44-23	3337
4–6 months			
12 months		26-30	
Puberty	**-6050-60**	20	40
Adult		20	40

*As a percentage of body weight.

from 350 to 440 ml/kg body weight. Cassady[47] demonstrated that the extracellular fluid volume of newborn infants correlated more closely with body weight than with gestational age. By age 1 year, extracellular fluid volume decreases to approximately 26% to 30% of body weight. After the first year, it decreases slowly and gradually approaches the adult value of 20% body weight by puberty.

Intracellular Fluid Volume. Intracellular fluid volume increases from 25% of body weight in the young fetus to 33% at birth to approximately 37% of body weight at age 4 months. Except for a sudden increase during early childhood, the intracellular fluid volume remains relatively constant thereafter, approximating 40% of body weight.

The clinical relevance of this gradual reduction in the size of extracellular body water compartments with age cannot be overemphasized. To achieve comparable plasma and tissue concentrations of drugs distributing into extracellular fluid, higher doses per kilogram body weight must be given to infants and children than to adults.[48]

Developmental Aspects of Body Composition. The percentage of body weight composed of adipose tissue approximately doubles over the first year of life.[28] Additionally, the liver and brain account for a higher percentage of body weight in the neonate than in the adult.[8,28] All of these factors may lead to significant differences in weight-normalized V_d between infants and adults, depending on the drug. Differences in the amount of adipose tissue may alter clearance of some drugs.

Critical Illness and Drug Distribution. Because of impaired production or increased losses, respectively, conditions such as liver disease and nephrotic syndrome reduce circulating albumin concentrations, resulting in an increase in apparent V_d. Diseases that induce an acute phase reaction (e.g., malignancy, myocardial infarction, inflammatory bowel disease) may provoke increased binding of basic drugs because of increased levels of α_1-acid glycoprotein.[16] Additionally, accumulation of extravascular fluid collections (e.g., pleural effusions and ascites) results in the development of a reservoir for drugs that are distributed into the total body water.[49]

Drug Clearance

Clearance reflects the removal of drug from the body. Clearance occurs by two processes: biotransformation (i.e., metabolism) and excretion. Metabolism occurs primarily in the liver. Excretion is predominately facilitated by the kidney, although excretion also can occur via exhalation, saliva, sweat, or the gastrointestinal tract.[8,16] Redistribution of drug can contribute to total clearance if the reference compartment is blood or plasma, as often is the case.[4] When reflected in the blood or plasma, clearance quantitatively describes the volume of blood or plasma from which all drug is removed per unit of time.[4,8] Clearance is an important pharmacokinetic parameter to consider when the goal is maintenance of steady-state drug concentration, which correlates with therapeutic efficacy. Once steady state is achieved, clearance of drug determines the quantity of drug that must be administered in order to maintain that concentration (i.e., Drug out = Drug in).[4,14] The clinically relevant pharmacokinetic concepts related to clearance are discussed later in this chapter.

The ontogeny of systemic clearance mechanisms probably accounts for a significant portion of the difference in pharmacologic response between infants and adults.[14] These developmental factors also produce variability among pediatric patients. Critical illness may have an additional profound impact on clearance mechanisms.

Hepatic Drug Metabolism

Hepatic xenobiotic metabolism assumes an extremely important role in determining the pharmacokinetic and pharmacodynamic properties of many drugs. Clearance of a drug (Cl) by an individual organ depends on blood flow to the organ (Q) and the organ's extraction ratio (E) and can be described as follows[50]:

$$Cl = Q \times E,$$

where E is the ratio of the arteriovenous concentration difference divided by the arterial concentration (extraction) as expressed by the following relationship:

$$E = (C_a - C_v)/C_a,$$

where C_a and C_v are the arterial and venous concentrations, respectively.

Organ clearance concepts are best described for the liver and kidneys. Hepatic clearance depends on hepatic blood flow, plasma free drug concentration, cellular uptake, hepatic metabolism, and biliary excretion. The hepatic clearance of a drug can be expressed by the following equation:

$$Cl_H = \frac{Q \times f_B \times Cl_{int}}{Q + (f_B \times Cl_{int})},$$

where Cl_H = hepatic clearance; Q = hepatic blood flow; f_B = fraction of free drug; and Cl_{int} = intrinsic clearance, which is a measure of hepatocellular metabolism. Drugs that are primarily cleared by the liver can be classified as flow limited or capacity limited.[51] If a drug displays a high Cl_{int} and E, then doubling the Cl_{int} will have little effect on Cl_H, whereas a change in blood flow will produce a proportional change in Cl_H. In other words, for drugs that are highly extracted (>80%) and metabolized by the liver, Cl_H reflects the amount and rate of drug delivered to the liver.[52] The considerable declines in hepatic blood flow and oxygen delivery that occur immediately following birth do not appear to translate to significantly reduced clearance of flow-limited drug in the newborn compared with the adult.[14] Drugs with high extraction ratios are subjected to the first-pass effect when administered enterally.

Capacity-limited drugs display low extraction ratios (<20%) and a low intrinsic metabolic clearance. Therefore hepatic clearance depends on the degree of hepatic uptake and metabolism of the drug and is independent of hepatic blood flow. Capacity-limited drugs can be further subdivided into binding-sensitive and binding-insensitive drugs. Binding-sensitive drugs, such as clindamycin, have extraction ratios that approach the free drug concentration ($E = f_B$). Therefore factors that increase f_B, such as decreased protein binding, increase hepatic clearance. In contrast, other drugs may display extraction ratios that are much less than the free drug concentration. In these cases, an increase in f_B does not enhance extraction of the drug, and therefore the hepatic clearance is a function of the intrinsic clearance and is independent of protein binding. These drugs are referred to as binding-insensitive (e.g., chloramphenicol).

Developmental Aspects of Hepatic Clearance. At every level, from the ontogenetic changes in hepatic blood and portal oxygen tension to the developmental alterations in protein binding and xenobiotic metabolizing enzyme activities, there is the potential for age to affect the processes associated with hepatic clearance. Very little investigative effort has been expended to elucidate these effects; however, some of the important available data are discussed further. For detailed reviews of this data, the reader is referred to articles by Alcorn and McNamara[14] and Leeder and Kearns.[53]

Drug Transport. The first step in drug metabolism is uptake of the drug by the metabolizing cell. Animal studies suggest that carrier-mediated hepatocellular uptake is limited in the infant.[14] Ligandin, or Y protein, is a basic protein that binds bilirubin and organic anions such as drugs. It is present in hepatocytes, proximal renal tubular cells, and nongoblet, small intestine mucosal cells.[54,55] The concentration of ligandin in the fetus and neonate is low but appears to approach adult values during the first 5 to 10 days of postnatal life.[48,54] Thus the hepatic clearance of capacity-limited drugs likely will be lower in neonates than in older infants and children.

Biliary excretion facilitates the elimination of certain drugs and drug conjugates.[14] Numerous studies in animals and humans demonstrate deficient biliary excretion in infants.[14]

Biotransformation: Phase I Reactions. Biotransformation of endogenous and exogenous substances occurs primarily in the liver, although the adrenal gland, placenta, kidney, gut, and skin also are capable of metabolizing compounds. Once a drug enters the hepatocyte, it may be transformed by one or more enzymatic reactions. These pathways, or phase I reactions, include oxidation, reduction, hydrolysis, and hydroxylation.[56,57] Generally, these reactions are responsible for transforming compounds into more polar, less lipid-soluble molecules that are more rapidly eliminated by the kidney, biliary system, or lung. However, parent compounds may be transformed into pharmacologically active intermediates, such as theophylline to caffeine, or into toxic metabolites, as occurs with oxidation of acetaminophen. Additionally, pharmacologically inactive parent compounds (prodrugs) may be converted to active moieties, as occurs with hydrolysis of chloramphenicol succinate to chloramphenicol.

The ontogeny of human enzyme systems differs dramatically from most animal species, especially for oxidation and glucuronidation pathways.[58] Therefore extrapolating data for enzyme system maturation from animals to humans is difficult. Of the enzyme systems capable of metabolizing drugs, the hepatic cytochrome P450 (CYP) mixed-function oxidase system has been studied in greatest detail. It is responsible for most of the phase I reactions catalyzed in the human liver.

Yaffe et al.[59] first demonstrated drug-oxidizing enzymes in the human fetal liver. During fetal life, these enzymes are present at 30% to 60% of adult activity in vitro.[60] Following birth, total CYP levels increase, approaching adult range by age 1 year.[14] Activity of all CYP enzymes is generally thought to be considerably lower in children, particularly neonates and infants, than in adults. In truth, the developmental aspects of expression and function vary among CYP enzyme families and isoforms. Although data delineating these variations are limited, particularly for specific families or isoforms, some insight into the ontogeny of select enzymes has been gleaned from immunochemical studies in hepatic microsomes and tissue, pharmacokinetic studies of known enzyme substrates, and studies evaluating the biotransformation of pharmacologic "probes" (e.g., carbamazepine in the case of CYP3A4). The ontogeny and the drugs affected by some of the important CYP isoforms are outlined in Table 110–3. A limited discussion of the most clinically relevant isoforms in pediatric patients follows.

CYP1A2. Cytochrome P450 1A2, the only CYP1A isoform found in human liver, is involved in the biotransformation of many drugs, including the methylxanthines.[53] Immunohistochemical studies have suggested that this protein is sparse, if present at all, in fetal liver.[61] These studies also demonstrate that levels of CYP1A2 do not appreciably increase until several weeks to months after birth, remaining below adult levels well into childhood. These findings are reflected in studies examining enzyme activity as assessed by biotransformation of theophylline. Nassif et al.[62] reported a significant correlation between a decreasing elimination half-life for enterally administered theophylline and increasing age. Decreased elimination was further suggested by a marked difference in dosage requirement, with patients younger than 4 months requiring approximately half the daily dose needed in patients age 8 to 13 months to maintain therapeutic levels. Tateishi et al.[63] evaluated biotransformation of intravenous theophylline, quantifying three metabolites (1-methyluric acid [IMU], 3-methylxanthine [3MX], and 1,3-dimethyluric acid [DMU]) in urine. The ratios of metabolites to theophylline in urine increased dramatically from the neonatal period to age 3, when they appeared to essentially plateau. However, a greater variation in these ratios was seen among patients older than 3 years. This study also established that the relative production of DMU, a product of reactions catalyzed by other CYP enzymes, including CYP2E1 and CYP3A4, was higher in the youngest patients compared

TABLE 110–3

Ontogeny of Select Hepatic Enzymes

Enzyme	Representative Substrates	Developmental Evolution
PHASE I		
CYP1A2	Acetaminophen, caffeine, theophylline, warfarin	Negligible in fetal liver. Adult levels of activity by approximately age 4 months. Activity exceeds that in adults after age 1 year; gradually declines to adult levels by end of puberty.
CYP2C9	Diazepam, phenytoin, NSAIDs, tolbutamide, S-warfarin	Undetectable to low in fetal liver. Adult levels of activity by age 1–6 months. Activity exceeds that in adults from age 3–10 years; gradually declines to adult levels by conclusion of puberty.
CYP2D6	Numerous, including captopril, codeine, dextromethorphan, haloperidol, metoprolol, propranolol, ondansetron, tricyclics	Undetectable in fetal liver. Expression and activity appear to be stimulated by parturition. Complete maturation may occur by age 1 year, although acquisition of adult activity levels has been reported to occur as late as age 5 years.
CYP3A4	Numerous, including acetaminophen, amiodarone, budesonide, carbamazepine, cyclosporin, erythromycin, lidocaine, nifedipine, tacrolimus, theophylline, verapamil, R-warfarin	Low in fetal liver; replaces CYP3A7 as the predominant isoform following birth. Based on pharmacokinetic and drug disposition studies, activity in children thought to be greater than that in adults. Decline toward adult levels begins at approximately age 4 years. Adult levels reached by end of puberty.
PHASE II		
Uridine 5′-diphosphate glucuronyltransferases (UGTs)	Numerous, including acetaminophen, benzodiazepines, bilirubin, chloramphenicol, dextromethorphan, morphine, naloxone, NSAIDs, propofol, thyroxine	Varies by isoform; difficult to characterize individual isoforms because of overlapping substrate specificities. As a group, activity appears to be deficient in the neonate and infant. Variably reported acquisition of adult levels of activity; anywhere from age 2–30 months, depending on the proposed isoforms involved.
N-acetyltransferase-2 (NAT2)	Caffeine, clonazepam, hydralazine, ioniazid, procainamide	Low activity in neonates and infants. Movement toward adult phenotypes (≈50% fast and 50% slow acetylators) after nearly 3 months of age.
Methyltransferase group (MT)	Catecholamines, captopril, serotonin, spironolactone	S-methylation capacity (TPMT) approximately 50% greater in infants than in adults. Limited studies evaluating maturation after this point; one Korean study demonstrated adult level activity by age 7–9 years.
Sulfotransferase group (ST)	Acetaminophen, bile acids, chloramphenicol, cholesterol, dopamine, polyethylene glycols, salicylates	At least some isoforms well developed in the infant; compensates for deficient glucuronidation of certain substrates (e.g., acetaminophen).

Substrate listings from Leeder JS, Kearns GL: *Pediatr Clin North Am* 44:55, 1997. Additional data related to substrates and all remaining data derived from references cited in the text.
NSAID, nonsteroidal antiinflammatory drug.

with those older than 3 years. The relative production of the other two metabolites, which result from CYP1A2 activity alone, is similar between the groups. After age 1 year into early childhood, rates of theophylline clearance appear to exceed the rates in adults, prompting the need for an increased dose to maintain therapeutic levels.[53]

CYP2C9. The CYP2C family comprises a substantial portion (≈20%) of CYP enzymes in the adult liver and has comparable importance in the metabolism of drugs.[14] CYP2C9 is the principal isoform in this family. Enzyme protein is undetectable[64] to low[53,61] in fetal liver. In vitro studies in fetal hepatic microsomes suggest comparably low enzyme activity. Demethylation of diazepam, which is mediated by the CPY2C family, occurs at a level less than 5% that in adult microsomes.[64] On the other hand, hydroxylation of tolbutamide, which is catalyzed specifically by CYP2C9, is not at all evident in fetal microsomes.[64] Several studies, both in vitro and in vivo, suggest an increase in enzyme expression and activity within the first month of life. Following sedation with diazepam, levels of desmethyl diazepam in urine are very low at age 1 to 2 days and increase within the first postnatal week.[64] CYP2C9 protein reaches adult levels in hepatic tissue after age 6 months.[61] Enzyme activity corresponds. By age 1 to 6 months, production of the phenytoin metabolite 5-(4-hydroxyphenyl)-5-phenylhydantoin is comparable to that seen in adults.[65] In fact, CYP2C9 activity appears to supersede that observed in adults by age 3 to 10 years, declining to adult range by the conclusion of puberty.[65] This explains the frequent need for a relatively increased dose of phenytoin in this age group.

CYP2D6. A number of drugs undergo biotransformation by CYP2D6, and some are more relevant to critically or chronically ill children than well children. Enzyme protein levels are undetectable in fetal liver except for those obtained from fetuses delivered by spontaneous or induced abortion. These specimens are far more likely to contain detectable enzyme, suggesting that parturition stimulates expression.[66] Enzyme activity, as evidenced by O-methylation of dextromethorphan, is negligible in fetal hepatic microsomes. Enzyme protein levels increase rapidly after birth, but the time at which they reach adult levels is variably reported in the literature. Levels in hepatic tissue from subjects age 1 month to 5 years reportedly were only approximately two thirds the adult levels,[14] but another study reported no difference in expression between patients younger than 1 year and those older than 1 year, suggesting that development of this isoform is complete by age 1 year.[67]

CYP3A4. The CYP3A family comprises the largest fraction of measurable CYP450 enzymes in adult liver.[14] In the fetal liver, CYP3A7 is the predominant isoform. After birth, there is a shift between CYP3A7 and CYP3A4, levels of which are negligible in fetal hepatic tissue. The mechanisms of this transition have not been elucidated. In infants and children, the activity of CYP3A4 is generally increased above that in adults. The biotransformation of carbamazepine demonstrates this developmental difference. Studies in children demonstrate that both clearance and production of the metabolite carbamazepine-10,11-epoxide significantly decrease with increasing age.[68–70] The role that other enzymes, particularly microsomal epoxide hydrolase, which further transforms carbamazepine-10,11-epoxide, play in these developmental differences is uncertain.[53] In addition, although these age-related differences have been described in pediatric patients on monotherapy, coadministration of anticonvulsants that are known to induce CYP3A4 are speculated to skew these findings. Nonetheless, these developmental differences in CYP3A4 activity have been suggested by study of other substrates, among them cyclosporin, which also exhibits increased clearance in children compared with adults.

The development of other phase I enzyme systems has been studied much less extensively. Alcohol dehydrogenase activity is detectable in 2-month fetuses at levels no greater than 3% to 4% of adult activity.[71] Moreover, the level of activity does not approach adult values until after age 5 years.

Aromatic nitroreductase activity is detectable in fetal livers by 7 to 8 weeks of gestation; however, the hepatic activity at midgestation remains low, and no specific postnatal pattern of development has been described. Also, few data exist on the ontogeny of hydrolytic enzymes. Echobichon and Stephens[72] found low levels of blood esterase activity in the fetus and neonate.

Biotransformation: Phase II Reactions. Conjugation reactions, or phase II reactions, synthesize more water-soluble compounds by combining a substance with an endogenous molecule to enhance excretion of that substance. Glucuronide, sulfate, and glycine are the common endogenous molecules to which drugs are bound. A drug must possess a specific functional group, such as a carboxyl, hydroxyl, amine, or sulfhydryl, in order to be conjugated. Alternatively, a drug must acquire one of these functional groups by undergoing phase I metabolism. Phase II enzyme groups have been studied far less than CYP450 enzymes; therefore the ontogeny of phase II enzymes remains relatively elusive.

Glucuronidation. Glucuronidation is the most common conjugation pathway because of the availability of glucuronic acid and the variety of functional groups with which it can combine. The uridine 5′-diphosphate glucuronyltransferases (UGTs) participate in the biotransformation of at least 100 drugs (e.g., acetaminophen, morphine, nonsteroidal antiinflammatory drugs [NSAIDs]) and endogenous compounds, including bilirubin and thyroxine. Ready elucidation of the ontogeny of UGT isoforms has been precluded by overlapping specificities. For a detailed summary of available information about the UGT enzyme family, the reader is referred to the review by de Wildt et al.[73]

The activity of a number of UGTs is decreased in the fetus and neonate, as assessed by in vitro studies.[73–75] In addition, there is ample in vivo evidence of deficient glucuronidation in infants and particularly neonates. A profound example of this is the association of "gray baby syndrome" with the drug chloramphenicol, which normally undergoes glucuronidation. Morphine glucuronidation serves as a "probe" for isoform UGT2B7 activity. Studies have demonstrated significantly decreased clearance[76,77] and biotransformation[76] of morphine in neonates. Depending on how values are standardized between pediatric and adult subjects, morphine clearance approximates adult levels anywhere from age 2 to 30 months.[14,77] Reduced UGT activity during infancy is also reflected in the biotransformation of acetaminophen. Levy et al.[78] demonstrated that 2- to 3-day-old term infants had a limited ability to conjugate acetaminophen with glucuronide, which is the major conjugation pathway in adults. However, this limitation in glucuronidation was compensated for by a well-developed sulfation pathway. This supports the findings of Alam et al.,[79] who showed that rates for glucuronidation are much lower and sulfation much higher with salicylamide and acetaminophen as substrates in children 7 to 10 years old compared with adults.

Studies evaluating bilirubin and chloramphenicol glucuronidation have reported low rates at birth, with adult rates achieved by age 3 years.[79] However, some evidence indicates that phenobarbital may induce glucuronidation in newborns and older children. Talafant et al.[80] administered phenobarbital 10 mg/kg/day to healthy full-term infants for their first 3 days of life. One group received phenobarbital intramuscularly and one group received phenobarbital orally; one group served as a control. These authors described significantly higher urinary glucaric acid concentrations on day 7 in the IM group than in the controls. This finding correlated well with a downward trend in serum bilirubin in the group receiving IM bilirubin.

The ontogeny and potential substrates of other phase II enzymes is summarized in Table 110–3.

Additional Factors Affecting Hepatic Biotransformation. Several factors in addition to those of a developmental nature may affect hepatic biotransformation. Although the impact of each on hepatic enzyme systems is incompletely characterized, factors such as genetics, concomitant drug therapy, and critical illness may alter drug biotransformation and, hence, patient response.

Genetic Polymorphisms. Genetic variation of a number of hepatic isoenzymes has been described, with corresponding variation in phenotype. For example, 7% to 8% of Caucasian children are characterized as "poor metabolizers" with reference to the enzyme CYP2D6, which may manifest as insufficient metabolism of several categories of drugs, including β-agonists, antidepressants, antipsychotics, antiarrhythmics, and derivatives of morphine.[53] Variants of CYP2C9 have been described, affecting metabolism of drugs such as tolbutamide, NSAIDs, warfarin, and phenytoin.[53] Polymorphism of the phase II enzyme N-acetyltransferase-2 (NAT2) affects half of the Caucasian and African-American populations in North American. In this case, "slow metabolizers" are at increased risk for several adverse drug responses, including drug-induced lupus erythematosus following procainamide or isoniazid therapy and Stevens-Johnson syndrome or toxic epidermal necrolysis following sulfonamide exposure.[53] Finally, several UGT isoforms are subject to genetic mutation. The best known of these genetic variations occur in UGT1 and UGT1A1, producing absent or reduced bilirubin glucuronidation in the case of the former isoenzyme and reduced bilirubin conjugation in the latter. Phenotypically, these mutations manifest as Crigler-Najjar and Gilbert syndrome, respectively. The effect of these UGT polymorphisms with respect to drug metabolism has not been substantially studied.[53] However, sparse data suggest that glucuronidation of drugs may also be affected in these patients.[53,81]

Inducers and Inhibitors. The frequent need for polytherapy in the ICU increases the possibility that hepatic biotransformative enzyme systems will be induced or inhibited, affecting the metabolism of any substrate of that system. A list of drugs known to induce or inhibit hepatic metabolic enzymes was compiled by Leeder and Kearns.[53]

Critical Illness. Even less is known about the effect of critical illness on hepatic enzyme function than that of development. Several factors may contribute to altered hepatic metabolism in critically ill patients. Decreases in cardiac output and, consequently, hepatic blood flow reduced clearance of lidocaine in adult patients; in these patients, treatment with dobutamine improved plasma clearance.[82] In vivo studies suggest that certain CYP isoforms, including those in the CYP3A family, are exquisitely vulnerable to hypoxia, demonstrating alteration of activity after as few as 8 hours of hypoxia.[82] The systemic inflammatory response appears to potentially alter CYP activity as well. Mice infected with *Listeria monocytogenes* experienced decreased expression of some CYP450 enzymes that returned to normal levels after 96 hours.[83] Many inflammatory mediators reduce expression of CYP isoforms, including CYP1A1, CYP2C, CYP2E1, and CYP3A in human hepatocytes.[84] Decreased metabolism of a number of known substrates of CYP450 has been demonstrated in patients with fever induced by infection and drugs and with hypothermia following cardiopulmonary bypass.[82] Of course, linking pharmacokinetic variations in the critically ill patient to impaired hepatic metabolism is difficult in the face of other pathophysiologic alterations.

Drug Elimination

The elimination half-life ($t_{1/2\beta}$) of a drug is commonly used to describe its disappearance from the blood and is measured as the time required for half the amount of drug present in the blood to disappear. As such, $t_{1/2\beta}$ can be used to reflect drug clearance, although changes in V_d also affect this parameter. This and related pharmacokinetic principles are discussed more thoroughly later in the chapter.

Renal Excretion. Most drugs and/or their metabolites are excreted from the body by the kidneys. Renal excretion depends on glomerular filtration, tubular reabsorption, and tubular secretion.[85] The amount of drug that is filtered per unit of time is influenced by the extent of protein binding and renal plasma flow. When the latter is constant, the greater the extent of protein binding, the smaller the fraction of circulating drug that is filtered. The degree of protein binding also influences drug elimination in patients undergoing dialysis in a similar manner; drugs that are highly protein bound are less easily dialyzed.[86,87] This section also examines developmental aspects of renal function and their influence on renal drug excretion (see Chapter 59).

Renal Blood Flow. Renal blood flow and renal plasma flow increase with age as a result of increased cardiac output and reduced peripheral vascular resistance.[88–90] The kidneys of neonates receive only 5% to 6% of the cardiac output compared with 15% to 25% in adults. Renal plasma flow averages 12 ml/min (0.72 L/hr) at birth and increases to 140 ml/min (8.4 L/hr) by age 1 year. If renal plasma flow is corrected for body surface area, adult values are reached before 30 weeks of extrauterine life. Using clearance of para-aminohippurate to estimate renal plasma flow, Calcagno and Rubin[91] demonstrated adult rates by age 5 months.

Glomerular Filtration Rate. At birth, glomerular filtration rate (GFR) is directly proportional to gestational age.[92] However, a linear relationship is not evident before 34 weeks of gestation. Inulin clearance rates below 10 ml/min have been described in newborns under 34 weeks of gestation, reflecting a significantly reduced GFR. This process must be considered when administering drugs or fluid to the premature newborn.[92]

At birth, GFR for full-term infants ranges from 2 to 4 ml/min. In the first 2 to 3 days of postnatal life, GFR in full-term babies increases markedly to rates between 8 and 20 ml/min. During the first several weeks of life, increases in GFR correlate with postconceptual age, not postnatal age.[92] Adult values for GFR (127 ml/min) are reached by age 2.5 to 5 months.[93] The postnatal increase in GFR most likely results from the combined effects of increased cardiac output, decreased peripheral vascular resistance, increased mean arterial blood pressure, increased surface area available for filtration, and increased membrane pore size.[94] In fact, the finding that increases in GFR correlate with postconceptual age suggests that maturational changes are an important factor in the observed increase in glomerular function.

The clinical implications for maturation of GFR become apparent when considering drugs that are primarily eliminated by glomerular filtration. Several studies have investigated the pharmacokinetics of aminoglycosides in preterm and term infants. Szefler et al.[95] demonstrated a decreasing $t_{1/2\beta}$ for gentamicin with increasing gestational age in infants younger than 7 days.

Development of Tubular Function. Proximal convoluted tubules in the normal kidney of a full-term infant are small in relation to their corresponding glomeruli. This glomerulotubular size imbalance is reflected by functional differences in the transport capacity (secretion) of the proximal tubular cells.[96] Therefore tubular function matures at a slower rate than does glomerular function. Reasons for this reduced functional capacity include not only the small size of the tubules but also a smaller mass of functioning tubular cells, reduced blood flow to the outer cortex, and immaturity of energy-supplying processes. This imbalance continues for the first year of life, after which function of both glomerular and tubular components is comparable to that in healthy, young adults.[6] Processes of both active absorption (i.e., secretion) and passive absorption (i.e., reabsorption) are impacted in the immature kidney.

Many drugs rely on either the organic anion or cation transport systems present in the proximal tubules for renal excretion. Penicillin is actively secreted. Results of pharmacokinetic studies of ampicillin, ticarcillin, benzylpenicillin, and methicillin show that the $t_{1/2\beta}$ for the penicillins varies inversely with gestational and postnatal age.[97–100] In all the studies cited here, $t_{1/2\beta}$ for penicillins was highly variable but generally decreased to 1 to 2 hours by 2 weeks postnatal age. These observations may be partially explained by findings in animals that the capacity of the pathways responsible for penicillin secretion may undergo substrate stimulation. Substrate stimulation has not been formally studied in human neonates, but evidence indicates that it does occur. Kaplan et al.[98] showed a reduction in $t_{1/2\beta}$ for ampicillin in both preterm and term infants after multiple doses compared with a single dose.

Furosemide is another drug secreted by the proximal tubules. In addition to being filtered, evidence for tubular secretion is inferred from adult data describing reduced rates of plasma clearance and urinary excretion after probenecid administration.[101] Aranda et al.[102] found an eightfold prolongation in $t_{1/2\beta}$ and an eightfold reduction in the elimination rate constant for furosemide in fluid-overloaded term and preterm neonates with normal renal function compared with adults. Peterson et al.[103] evaluated single-dose kinetics for furosemide in preterm and term infants and found a mean $t_{1/2\beta}$ of 19.9 and 7.7 hours, respectively. This is in contrast to a $t_{1/2\beta}$ of 30 minutes in healthy adults. These prolonged plasma half-lives correspond with the prolonged duration of diuretic and saluretic effect seen in infants,[104] although the response to furosemide most likely is dependent on its rate of urinary excretion.

Effects of Critical Illness on Renal Excretion. The sensitivity of the kidney to hypoxic and ischemic insult is well known. Because this is one of the most important final common pathways for serious illness in infants and children, it follows that renal functional impairment is relatively frequent in patients in the PICU. Kidney function may be further impeded by the frequent use of nephrotoxic drugs such as amphotericin B and aminoglycosides in PICU patients. Clearly, varying degrees of renal functional impairment seen in critically ill infants and children can seriously complicate drug therapy in this setting.[33,105]

Drug Delivery Systems

As discussed previously, the maintenance of steady-state drug concentration requires that the amount of drug being administered match the amount of drug being cleared from the body. Several factors determine how much of a drug can be administered to any given patient at any given time. Although uncommon in the ICU, the available routes of administration may limit bioavailability and, hence, ultimate drug concentration. In the patient who requires fluid restriction, limitations in the maximal concentration of drugs may prove problematic. In the smallest of patients, full delivery of intravenous drug doses contained in diminutive volumes of vehicle may not be assured. Administration of a drug as a bolus generally ensures that the patient has received the full dose, provided any tubing between the site where the drug is given and where it enters the vein is adequately flushed. In the case of drugs given over a discrete interval or by continuous infusion, the drug delivery system influences the amount of a given drug dose received by the patient. Regardless of the technology used, the amount of drug delivered by a system depends upon the designated flow rate and the amount of tubing between where the drug is introduced and the patient's bloodstream.[28] When a drug is added to a fluid reservoir, delivery also depends on the volume of drug added.[28] An example of the impact of these factors on drug delivery is as follows. If a drug is added to the reservoir in a system where the flow rate is 25 ml/hour, drug delivery may not begin for almost 2 hours and would require nearly 4 hours for completion.[28] Consequently, administering drug in this manner could result in delayed and/or incomplete drug delivery. Additionally, an inability to pin down the timing of drug delivery complicates interpretation of drug levels when monitored.[28]

Fortunately, considerable advances in drug delivery technology have been made over the past 20 years[106] and have been of particular benefit in the PICU. Infusion pumps that provide greater volumetric accuracy have facilitated full delivery of small volumes. In some cases, improvements in infusion continuity have enabled uninterrupted delivery of continuously administered drugs, a fact that is of particular importance for drugs with very short $t_{1/2\beta}$ values (e.g., nitroprusside).[106] It is important that the intensivist have some familiarity with the technology used in his or her unit; this knowledge may be helpful when an unintended response to pharmacotherapy occurs. For a comprehensive review of this technology, the reader is referred to the chapter by Kwan.[106]

Effect of Extracorporeal Therapies on Drug Disposition

Extracorporeal therapies, including hemofiltration, dialysis, and extracorporeal membrane oxygenation (ECMO), can alter drug disposition in affected critically ill patients. Although relatively little study has been devoted to drug disposition in patients on ECMO (see Chapters 47 and 65), evidence supports the idea that this treatment modality alters pharmacokinetics. In neonates and infants, the largest number of studies have looked at the disposition of gentamicin and vancomycin.[107] Increased V_d, increased $t_{1/2}$, and decreased clearance compared with control or post-ECMO values were demonstrated in the majority of these studies.[107–09] In one study investigating vancomycin, only an increased $t_{1/2}$ differentiated ECMO patients from non-ECMO controls.[110] Other drugs, including theophylline,[111] morphine,[112,113] tobramycin,[107] bumetanide,[107] and ranitidine[107] have been shown to increase V_d, decrease clearance, and/or increase $t_{1/2}$ in patients on ECMO. The addition of an extracorporeal reservoir contributes to the increase in V_d, and alterations in hepatic and renal function in ECMO patients impact clearance. Additionally, adhesion of some drugs to circuit hardware may alter serum or blood concentrations. The age of the circuit appears to influence this factor to some extent. Dagan et al.[113] evaluated the "elimination" of drugs following direct injection into two circuits: a new one and a circuit that had been used by a patient for 5 days. A relatively increased elimination of several drugs by the new circuit was described (vancomycin 36% vs. 11%; gentamicin 10% vs. 0%; phenobarbital 17% vs. 6%; phenytoin 43% vs. 0%; morphine 36% vs. 16% in the new vs. used circuit).[113] Several other drugs are subject to this phenomenon, including heparin, furosemide, fentanyl, benzodiazepines, propofol, and perhaps morphine.[107] Propofol appears particularly susceptible to this effect. In vitro studies using entire circuits and various individual components report recovery of propofol has been 10 percent or less.[107] In the in vitro studies, priming of the circuit with albumin appears to reduce adsorption of at least some of these drugs.[107] This method of priming may have contributed to the maintenance of serum morphine concentrations in an in vivo study as well.[114] Drug concentrations may be altered when a circuit containing some fraction of that drug is discarded and replaced.[107] Finally, pharmacokinetics may be altered by in-line hemofiltration, which is required in approximately 12% of neonates on ECMO, and by dialysis, which is required by approximately 3% to 4% of these patients.[107]

Pharmacodynamics

In contrast to pharmacokinetics, which operationally describes what the body does to the drug, pharmacodynamics deals with what the drug does to the body.[115] As such, this discipline within pharmacology deals with the mechanisms of action of drugs, their safety profile, drug–receptor interactions, and receptor–effector coupling phenomena.

Infants and children have been described to exhibit different clinical responses to several medications than do adults. One example of this difference is the hyperexcitability children may experience following exposure to antihistamines and barbiturates in contrast to the sedation normally observed in adults.[116] Children also have a greater incidence of dystonic reactions following the administration of dopamine antagonists (e.g., haloperidol, chlorpromazine, metoclopramide), which has been speculated to result from an increased concentration of DA-2 receptors in the young brain.[116] When no pharmacokinetic explanation for different drug responses between children and adults has been offered, a difference in "sensitivity" has been proclaimed. Variable sensitivity to drugs, including some of the nondepolarizing neuromuscular blocking agents (e.g., pancuronium) and the catecholamines, has been described in infants compared with adults. For example, a decreased sensitivity to dopamine has been observed in infants, manifested by an insignificant change in any physiologic variable (including heart rate) below a dose of 15 μg/kg/min.[116]

The formal study of ligand–receptor interactions and their consequences is covered comprehensively in Chapter 111 and in two referenced texts.[117,118] However, the translation of these principles into the practice of medicine is embodied in the discipline of therapeutics.

Just as important developmental changes determine the related absorption, distribution, metabolism, and excretion of drugs, ontogenetic changes in drug responsiveness account for both the qualitative and quantitative differences observed in efficacy and toxicity when drugs are used in infants and children. Unfortunately, the latter have not been evaluated with the same intensity that has characterized our assessment of developmental changes in pharmacokinetics.[119,120]

Actions of drugs in the immature individual may be altered for a variety of reasons, including altered numbers of receptor sites compared with mature individuals, altered affinity of the receptor for its primary ligand or agonists, and/or altered receptor–effector coupling resulting in altered drug responsiveness. Additional work is necessary to bring this level of sophistication to the clinical setting.

Effect of Disease on Drug Action

During serious illness, substantial changes may occur in receptor function, tissue architecture, and postreceptor function that ultimately are responsible for changes in drug action. These often result from vascular volume or electrolyte derangements and from the effects associated with derangements in acid-base status. Nevertheless, conditions such as pulmonary fibrosis and cardiomyopathy may be associated with diminished responsiveness to drugs acting on the affected organ. Infection with *Haemophilus influenzae* type B has been associated with decreased pulmonary β_2-receptor function with a resultant increase in airway resistance.[121,122] Protracted use of catecholamines may result in down-regulation of functional β receptors in target organs, requiring frequent dose increases to achieve the maintained desired pharmacologic effect.[123–125]

Finally, remember that most drugs used in the PICU are potent agents that have the potential to cause serious side effects.[126] Unfortunately, drug toxicity in a critically ill patient may be an amplified event. Such patients are the least likely to be able to tolerate such effects. Thus the therapeutic index for most of the drugs used commonly becomes increasingly narrow as the patient's condition warrants more aggressive therapy.[127]

Pharmacokinetic Principles

Evaluation of the Plasma Concentration–Time Curve

The application of pharmacokinetic principles to patient care should permit rational drug dosing and result in effective pharmacotherapy. Most of the drugs used in clinical medicine are metabolized via linear first-order kinetic processes (Figure 110–2). This means that a constant percentage of drug is removed from the body per unit of time. Virtually all of the pharmacokinetic parameters used on a routine basis can be derived from a plot of serum/plasma concentration versus time, which then is converted to a semilogarithmic display (Figure 110–3). The straight, terminal portion of the former represents the elimination phase for the drug, and its slope is the elimination rate constant K_e (Table 110–3 and Figure 110–4).

The elimination half-life for the drug $t_{1/2\beta}$ (see Figure 110–2) then can be determined directly by inspection of the semilogarithmic graph as the time required for the concentration to decrease by half, or it may be calculated from the exponential decay curve considerations once K_e is determined:

$$t_{1/2\beta} = \frac{0.693}{K_e}$$

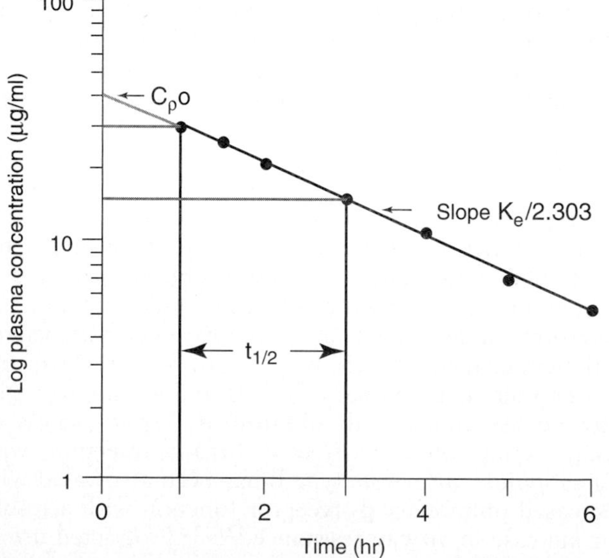

FIGURE 110–2 • First-order elimination. Plasma concentration versus time curve for a drug eliminated via first-order kinetics. Note the elimination half-life is depicted as the time required for the drug concentration to be reduced by half. Constant fraction of the drug in the body is eliminated in each equal interval of time.

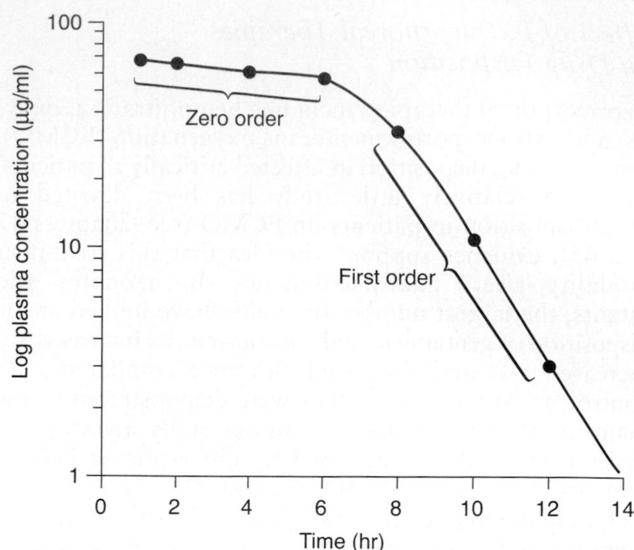

FIGURE 110–3 • Michaelis-Menten kinetics. Log plasma concentration versus time curve for a drug showing saturation of the elimination mechanism. Initially, a constant *amount* of drug is eliminated per unit time rather than a constant *fraction* of drug per unit time. This initial phase is said to show zero-order elimination. Later, the plasma concentration falls below the saturating level and the elimination process becomes first order.

The area under the serum concentration versus time curve (AUC) can be determined by applying an approximate integration formula, most commonly the trapezoidal rule.[128] This method involves the description of a given plasma concentration–time curve as a series of straight lines, which enables the curve to be divided into a number of trapezoids (Figure 110–5). The area of each trapezoid can be easily calculated, and the sum of all such areas equals the area under the AUC. The latter value is important in deriving two other values of clinical importance: bioavailability and clearance of the drug. Finally, by extrapolating the terminal elimination phase of the curve b to time 0, the intercept on the Y axis denotes the concentration that would have resulted if the total dose of the drug had instantaneously distributed throughout the body (Figure 110–6). This concentration, termed C_o, can be used to determine the apparent volume of distribution of the drug V_d, using the following equation:

$$V_d = \frac{D,}{C_o}$$

where D is the dose administered.

In children, a number of important compounds demonstrate saturation kinetics at clinically useful doses (Box 110–5). In this case, the drugs appear to have longer half-lives at higher concentrations. For these drugs, the relationship between serum concentration and time is better described by the values V_{max} and K_m than by V_d and Cl.[26,129] The most important drug demonstrating this type of biodisposition is phenytoin.[130] With this drug, a small increase in dose may result in a large increase in serum concentration. Disease states and drug interactions can pose particular problems for patients receiving drugs cleared by saturable processes. A patient with liver dysfunction may have decreased V_{max} for a given drug

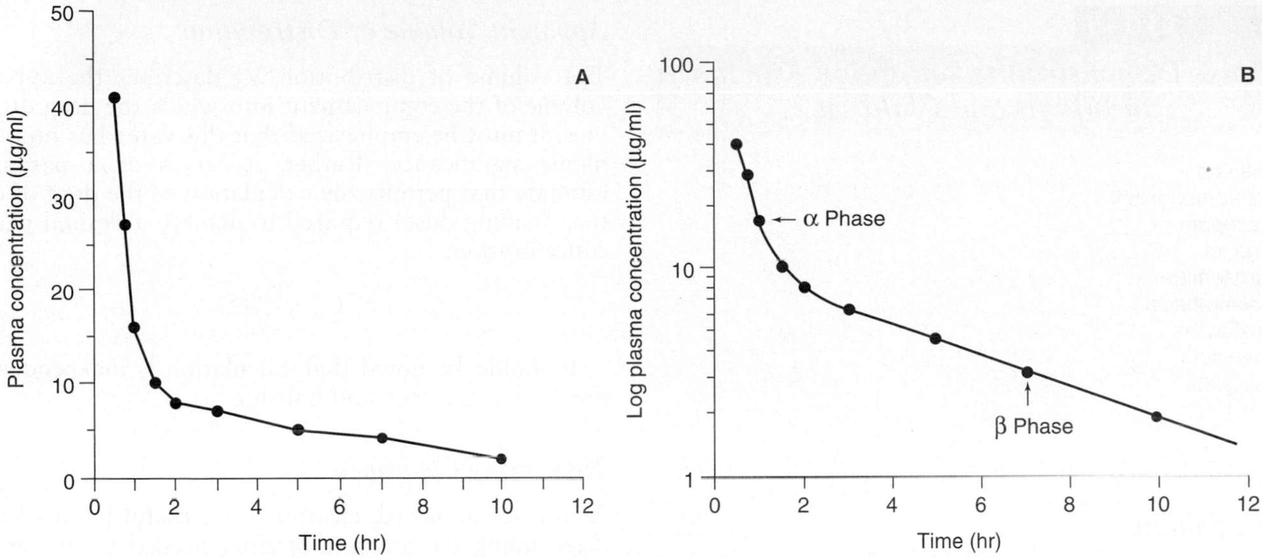

FIGURE 110–4 • Two-compartment model. **A,** Plasma concentration versus time curve presented using rectangular coordinates. **B,** Semilogarithmic transformation of the data shows a biphasic curve rather than a straight line. This is thought to represent the interaction between two compartments: plasma and extracellular fluid space. The *upper portion* of the curve is called α phase and is thought to represent drug distribution. The *lower portion* is termed the β phase and is thought to represent actual drug elimination. Slope of the β phase = –K/2.303.

compared with a healthy child. Consequently, saturation of metabolic elimination may occur at a lower concentration than normal.

Applied Pharmacokinetics

Use of pharmacokinetic parameter estimates is essential to the development of proper dosing regimens, the effective use of the drug analysis laboratory, and ultimately in optimization of drug therapy. Among the available parameters, the most important in the PICU are clearance (Cl), volume of distribution (V_d), and half-life ($t_{1/2\beta}$). In addition, if oral therapy is contemplated, bioavailability (F) must be considered. Each of these parameters can be used for mathematically describing the biodisposition of a drug under steady-state conditions.

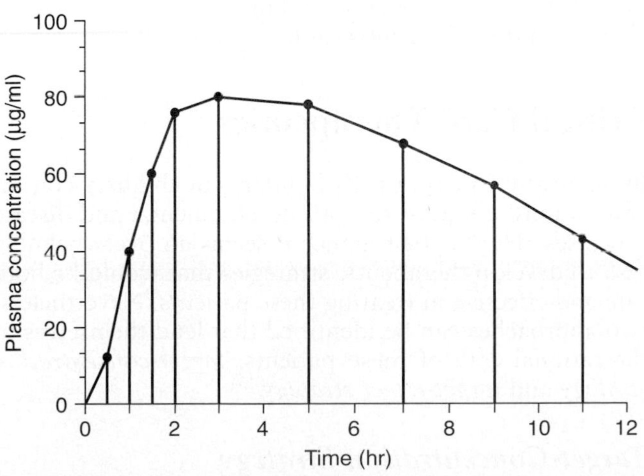

FIGURE 110–5 • Trapezoidal rule. Plasma concentration versus time curve for a drug after oral administration. The area under the curve (AUC) represents the total amount of an individual dose that is absorbed. This area can be calculated by dividing the curve into a series of trapezoids, calculating the area for each, and summing all of the areas.

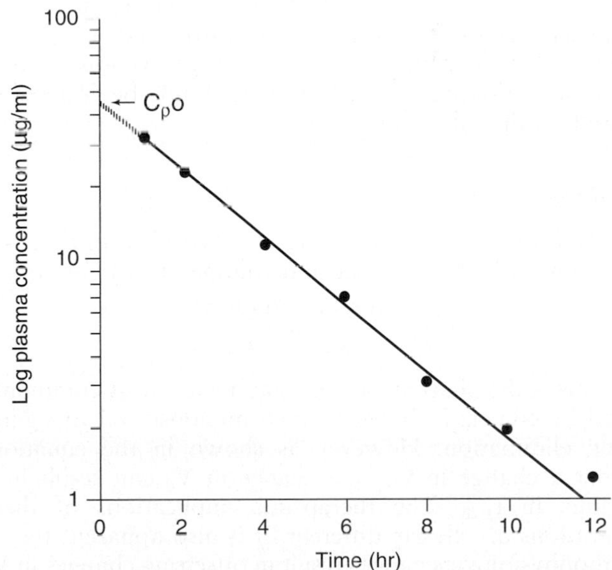

FIGURE 110–6 • Log plasma concentration versus time curve depicting C_po. This is a semilogarithmic plot of plasma drug concentration versus time after intravenous infusion of drug. This drug shows one-compartment, first-order elimination as indicated by the *single straight line.* Extrapolation of the line back to time zero yields an estimate of C_po or the drug concentration that would result if the total dose was administered and distributed immediately throughout the body. If the dose administered is known and the Co ascertained, the apparent volume of distribution V_d of the drug administered can be calculated.

BOX 110–5

Drugs Demonstrating Saturation Kinetics in Infants and Children

Caffeine
Chloramphenicol
Diazepam
Ethanol
Furosemide
Indomethacin
Mezlocillin
Phenytoin
Salicylate

Bioavailability

The concept of bioavailability was discussed extensively in the section related to drug absorption. For most drugs administered intravenously, the bioavailability is 100% and $F = 1$. In clinical terms, the "relative" bioavailability of a drug is most important. Bioavailability F is defined as the ratio of the AUC for the drug given by a nonintravenous route (AUC_{Oral}) to the AUC of the same drug administered intravenously (AUC_{IV}):

$$F = \frac{AUC_{Oral}}{AUC_{IV}}.$$

Relative bioavailability can be used to convert from one route of administration to another. For example, the relative bioavailability of theophylline is 1. Therefore in switching from intravenous to oral dosing, the same total daily dose of theophylline should be administered. In contrast, relative bioavailability of furosemide is approximately 0.5. Thus in switching from intravenous to oral administration, the dose of the drug should be doubled to maintain the same diuretic effect.

Half-life

Elimination half-life of a drug is a hybrid term that is a function of both clearance and volume of distribution:

$$t_{1/2\beta} = \frac{0.693}{K_e} = \frac{0.693V_d}{Cl}.$$

This is the pharmacokinetic parameter most commonly used by clinicians, but it is often misconstrued to signify drug elimination. However, as shown in the equation, either a change in Cl or a change in V_d can result in a change in $t_{1/2\beta}$. The therapeutic implications of these alterations are clearly different. It is also apparent that if pathophysiologic changes result in offsetting changes in V_d and Cl, the elimination half-life could remain unaffected in the face of significant disease.

The most important clinical application of half-life is as a determinant of drug dosing. Four to five half-lives are required for a drug to reach steady-state plasma concentration at any given dose. This is true whether therapy is being initiated or the dose is being changed.

Apparent Volume of Distribution

The volume of distribution V_d describes the apparent volume of the compartment into which the drug distributes. It must be emphasized that this value has no physiologic significance. Rather, it serves as a parameter estimate that permits the calculation of the dose of drug (i.e., loading dose) required to achieve a desired plasma concentration:

$$C_p = \frac{Dose}{V_d}.$$

It should be noted that calculation is independent of the drug's clearance and half-life.

Total Body Clearance

As previously noted, clearance is a useful parameter for determining the amount of drug needed to maintain a desired steady-state plasma concentration. Because by definition the rate of drug elimination at steady state is equal to the rate of drug administration, then[27,51,128]

$$\text{Elimination rate} = C_p \times Cl,$$

where C_p is the average steady-state plasma concentration:

$$\text{Administration rate} = \frac{F \times D}{\tau},$$

where D = dose and t = dosing interval.

At steady state:

$$C_p \times Cl = D, \tau,$$

or, rearranging:

$$C_p = F \times D,$$

where the solutions provide the average steady-state plasma concentration. It is obvious from the equation that to maintain a steady-state plasma concentration, disease-associated changes in Cl must be compensated by changes in dose D or interval t.

Critical Care Therapeutics

In the treatment of critically ill infants or children, consideration must be given to both developmental and disease processes. Thus at first glance it seems an overwhelming task to develop therapeutic strategies that would be both safe and effective in treating these patients. Nevertheless, two approaches can be identified that lend themselves to the rational care of these patients: *target-concentration strategy* and *target-effect strategy.*[131]

Target-Concentration Strategy

The target-concentration strategy can be considered for drugs that are used chronically to treat clinical problems that manifest themselves intermittently (Box 110–6). Such problems include reversible reactive airway disease,

BOX 110–6

Principles of the Target-Concentration Strategy in Drug Therapy

- Strategy may be effective for drugs used on a chronic basis to treat diseases that manifest signs and symptoms intermittently.
- Caregivers must have some knowledge of the pharmacokinetics of the drugs being used.
- A relationship between drug or metabolite concentration in the sampled biologic fluid and therapeutic efficacy or clinical toxicity must have been established.
- Appropriate sampling time must be known and a reliable assay must be available.
- Target concentrations must be used as guides; treat patients, not drug levels.

seizures, and cardiac dysrhythmias. Application of this therapeutic strategy requires recognition that certain target serum concentrations are associated with either the therapeutic or the toxic effects attributed to a given pharmacologic agent. It is important to remember that these target-concentration ranges are determined using population-based data rather than individual patient data. Therefore the so-called *therapeutic* or *toxic* ranges may not be strictly applicable to the patient currently being treated. However, they serve as useful guides for the initiation and ongoing monitoring of therapy. As part of this ongoing monitoring, effective use of the drug analysis laboratory is essential. To apply the target concentration strategy, physicians must have some knowledge of the pharmacokinetics of the drug being used (Box 110–7). Such knowledge includes an awareness of any active metabolites that may be involved in the expression of the drug's therapeutic activity.

The approach to treatment of the patient in whom the target-concentration strategy is to be used requires that the physician have an expectation regarding the clinical manifestations of drug efficacy and drug toxicity before any therapy is initiated. This should be accompanied by an awareness of the appropriate sampling times for the various drugs and an overall understanding that drug "levels" are guides to therapy rather than therapeutic endpoints themselves. Therapeutic drug monitoring does not substitute for other means of patient evaluation.

Effective drug dosing using the target-concentration strategy requires a familiarity with the pharmacokinetic parameters previously described and the effective use of the drug analysis laboratory. When a target plasma concentration is known, an initial dose can be chosen. Under some circumstances, it may be desirable to achieve the target concentration immediately. In these instances, the initial dose is termed a *loading dose* and calculated as:

$$\text{Loading dose} = \frac{C_p \times V_d}{F},$$

where C_p is the target concentration.

Use of a loading dose is not always appropriate. Under certain circumstances, the calculated loading dose can result in toxic plasma concentrations before tissue distribution. The alternative is to begin therapy with what is termed the *maintenance dose:*

$$\text{Maintenance dose} = \frac{C_p \times \tau \times V_d}{F}.$$

When therapy is initiated with a maintenance dose, dosing for a total of four to five half-lives will be required to reach the desired steady-state plasma concentration. In contrast, when used in conjunction with a loading dose, the maintenance dose should maintain the plasma concentration attained with the loading dose.

Effective use of therapeutic drug monitoring in the critical care setting requires integration of certain characteristics of the drugs to be used, the laboratory where drug analysis occurs, and physician behavior. The drug selected for therapeutic drug monitoring should be one from which a relatively sustained and constant effect is expected over a comparatively long period of time. Monitoring should be limited to drugs characterized by wide interindividual variation in pharmacokinetics, as well as those that manifest a narrow therapeutic index. Finally, it is imperative that a set of data exists to relate the clinical effects of the drug directly to its concentration in the serum.

For drugs fulfilling these criteria, sensitive and specific assays for determination of their concentrations in various types of biologic fluids must be available. Moreover, this service must be provided with a turnaround time that is appropriate to the type of therapy being rendered. Thus it may be appropriate to provide aminoglycoside serum concentration determinations with a 24-hour reporting schedule; however, the safe and effective adjustment of theophylline dosing requires that serum concentrations be available within 1 hour from the time the blood is drawn. In addition, the results provided by any laboratory must be internally consistent. Standard curves must be checked frequently, and this quality assurance information must be available to all physicians on request.

Use of the target-concentration strategy places heavy demands on the physician. Values for commonly used pharmacokinetic parameters describing absorption, distribution, and elimination should be known or readily available. The physician must be aware of conditions in which

BOX 110–7

Drugs Used in the Target-Concentration Strategy

Antiarrhythmic agents: amiodarone, procainamide, quinidine, lidocaine
Anticonvulsant agents: phenytoin, phenobarbital, valproic acid, carbamazepine, pentobarbital
Antibiotics: aminoglycosides, chloramphenicol, vancomycin (±)
Methotrexate
Cyclosporine
Antipyretics: acetaminophen, salicylate
Theophylline

these pharmacokinetic parameter estimates may be altered and the extent to which these alterations may affect therapy. The physician must have a working knowledge of the average steady-state concentrations of drug in serum associated with both drug effectiveness and drug toxicity. Moreover, the pathophysiologic conditions that may alter these concentration-response relationships must be understood. Finally, clinical experience and sound judgment must prevail. Therapy must consist of an ongoing commitment to treat patients and not to drug levels.

Target-Effect Strategy

The target-effect strategy embodies the therapeutic approach most commonly practiced in the PICU. In fact, the therapeutic strategy allows for rational application of most of the drug classes required in the intensive care setting to the pediatric patient (Box 110–8).

Application of the target-effect strategy requires that the clinician determine a therapeutic endpoint before initiating drug treatment and accept a commitment to monitor for both drug effectiveness and toxicity. In using this approach, the clinician must have a reasonable understanding of the pharmacodynamic actions of the drugs to be used, including their side effect profiles. Moreover, the impact of both ontogeny and disease on drug action must be considered.

Once therapy is started, the dose is increased until the desired effect is achieved unless the sequential increase in drug dose results in no increase in therapeutic benefit and the desired effect is not achieved or drug toxicity supervenes. The amount of time taken in dosage escalation is dictated by the clinical circumstance at hand. In some circumstances, days of adjustments may be acceptable, whereas in others minutes may be too long. Nevertheless, inherent in this strategy is a belief that responses to drugs are dose related and that any concept of a preexisting maximal dose is precluded. Thus if either lack of efficacy or toxicity becomes apparent, the mandated response is to *change* the drug.

In summary, rational therapeutics for the critically ill child must account for the impact of development and disease on drug action. The scenario suggests use of short-acting drugs with large therapeutic indexes and requires that expectations regarding drug effects be ascertained prospectively. This approach mandates rigorous attention to monitoring but ultimately ensures that the dosage used will be sufficient to achieve the desired response.

BOX 110–8

Classes of Drugs Used in the Target-Effect Strategy for Critically Ill Children

Anticoagulants
Catecholamines
β-Lactam antibiotics
Diuretics
Corticosteroids
Oxygen
Anxiolytics, sedatives
Neuromuscular blockers
Vasodilators
Antihypertensives
Inotropes: amrinone

REFERENCES

1. Parson RL: Drug absorption in gastrointestinal disease with particular reference to malabsorption syndromes. *Clin Pharmacokinet* 2:45, 1977.
2. Radde IC: Mechanisms of drug absorption and their development. In Macleod SM, Radde IC, editors: *Textbook of pediatric clinical pharmacology.* Littleton, Mass, 1985, PSG Publishing Co.
3. Welling PG: Influence of food and diet on gastrointestinal drug absorption: a review. *J Pharmacokinet Biopharm* 5:291, 1977.
4. Rudy AC, Brater DC: Pharmacokinetics. In Chernow B, editor: *The pharmacologic approach to the critically ill patient.* Baltimore, 1994, Williams & Wilkins.
5. Kelly EJ, Newell SJ: Gastric ontogeny: clinical implications. *Arch Dis Child* 71:F136, 1994.
6. Kearns GL: Impact of developmental pharmacology on pediatric study design: overcoming the challenges. *J Allergy Clin Immunol* 106:S128, 2000.
7. Ewer AK, Durbin GM, Morgan MEI, Booth IW: Gastric emptying in preterm infants: a comparison of breast milk and formula. *Arch Dis Child* 71:F24, 1994.
8. Reed MD, Besunder JB: Development pharmacology: ontogenic basis of drug disposition. *Pediatr Clin North Am* 36:1053, 1989.
9. Ritz MA, Fraser R, Tam W, Dent J: Impacts and patterns of disturbed gastrointestinal function in critically ill patients. *Am J Gastroenterol* 95:3044, 2000.
10. Kao CH, Chang Lai SP, Chieng PU, et al: Gastric emptying in head-injured patients. *Am J Gastroenterol* 93:1108, 1998.
11. Dive A, Moulart M, Jonard P, et al: Gastroduodenal motility in mechanically ventilated critically ill patients: a manometric study. *Crit Care Med* 22:441, 1994.
12. Watkins JB, Ingall D, Szczepanik P, et al: Bile salt metabolism in the newborn. *N Engl J Med* 288:431, 1973.
13. Yoshioka H, Iseki K, Fujita K: Development and differences of intestinal flora in the neonatal period in breast-fed and bottle-fed infants. *Pediatrics* 72:317, 1983.
14. Alcorn J, McNamara PJ: Ontogeny of hepatic and renal systemic clearance pathways in infants: part I. *Clin Pharmacokinet* 41:959, 2002.
15. Greenblatt DJ, Koch-Weser J: Intramuscular injection of drugs. *N Engl J Med* 195:542, 1976.
16. Wilkinson GR: Pharmacokinetics: the dynamics of drug absorption, distribution and elimination. In Hardman JG, Limbird LE, editors: *Goodman and Gilman's the pharmacological basis of therapeutics.* New York, 2001, McGraw-Hill.
17. Williams RL, Benet LZ: Drug pharmacokinetics in cardiac and hepatic disease. *Annu Rev Pharmacol Toxicol* 20:389, 1980.
18. Morselli PL: Clinical pharmacokinetics in neonates. *Clin Pharmacokinet* 1:81, 1976.
19. Cavell B: Gastric emptying in infants fed human milk or infant formula. *Acta Paediatr Scand* 70:639, 1981.
19. Lester RS: Topical formulary for the pediatrician. *Pediatr Clin North Am* 30:749, 1983.
20. Reichek N, Goldstein RE, Redwood DR: Sustained effects of nitroglycerin ointment in patients with angina pectoris. *Circulation* 50:348. 1974.
21. Langer R: Implantable controlled release systems. In Ihler GM, editor: *Methods of drug delivery: international encyclopedia of pharmacology and therapeutics.* Oxford, 1986, Pergamon Press.
22. de Boer AG, Moolenaar F, de Leede LGJ, et al: Rectal drug administration: clinical pharmacokinetic considerations. *Clin Phannacokinet* 7:285,1982.
23. Dulac O, Aicardi J, Rey E, et al: Blood levels of diazepam and single rectal administration in infants and children. *J Pediatr* 93:1039 1978.
24. Knudsen FU: Recurrence risk after first febrile seizure and effect of short-term diazepam prophylaxis. *Arch Dis Child* 60:1045, 1985.

25. Burckart GJ, White TJ, Siegle RL, et al: Rectal thiopental versus intramuscular cocktail for sedating children before computerized tomography. *Am J Hasp Pharm* 376:222, 1980.
26. Besunder JB, Reed MD, Blumer JL: Principles of drug biodisposition in the neonate: a critical evaluation of the pharmacokinetic-pharmacodynamic interface (part I). *Clin Pharmacokinet* 14:189, 1988.
27. Gibaldi M, Koup JR: Pharmacokinetic concepts—drug binding, apparent volume of distribution and clearance. *Eur J Clin Pharmacol* 20:299. 1981.
28. Notterman DA: Pediatric pharmacotherapy. In Chernow B, editor: *The pharmacologic approach to the critically ill patient.* Baltimore, 1994, Williams & Wilkins.
29. Piafsky KM: Disease-induced changes in the plasma binding of basic drugs. *Clin Pharmacokinet* 5:246, 1980.
30. Morselli PL, Franco-Morselli R, Bossi L: Clinical pharmacokinetics in newborns and infants: age related differences and therapeutic implications. *Clin Pharmacokinet* 5:485, 1980.
31. Hyvarinen M, Zeitzer P, Oh W, et al: Influence of gestational age on serum levels of alpha-, fetoprotein, IgG globulin, and albumin in newborn infants. *J Pediatr* 82:430, 1973.
32. Kurz H, Mauser-Ganshom A, Stickel HH: Differences in the binding of drugs to plasma proteins from newborn and adult man. I. *Eur J Clin Pharmacol* 11:463, 1977.
33. Rane A, Wilson JT: Clinical pharmacokinetics in infants and children. *Clin Pharmacokinet* 1:2, 1976.
34. Sjoqvist F, Borga O, Onne MLE: Fundamentals of clinical pharmacology. In Speight TM, editor: *Avery's drug treatment.* ed 3, Sydney.
35. Thiessen H, Jacobsen J, Brodersen R: Displacement of albumin bilirubin by fatty acids. *Acta Paediatr Scand* 61:285, 1972.
36. Rudman D, Bixler TJ, DelRio AE: Effect of free fatty acids on binding of drugs by bovine serum albumin by human serum albumin, and by rabbit serum. *J Pharmacol Exp Ther* 176:261, 1971.
37. Gallin JI, Kaye D, O'Leary WM: Serum lipids in infection. *N Engl J Med* 281:1081, 1969.
38 Hunninghake DB, Azamoff DL: Drug inhibition of catecholamine induced metabolic effects in humans. *Ann N Y Acad Sci* 129: 971,1967.
39 Fredholm BB, Rane A, Persson B: Diphenylhydantoin binding to proteins in plasma and its dependence on free fatty acid and bilirubin concentration in dogs and newborn infants. *Pediatr Res* 9:26, 1975.
40. McDonagh AF, Lightner DA: Life: a shriveled blood orange—bilirubin, jaundice, and phototherapy. *Pediatrics* 75:443, 1985.
41. Brodersen R: Bilirubin transport in the newborn infant, reviewed with relation to kernicterus. *J Pediatr* 96:349, 1980.
42. Rane A, Lunde PKM, Jailing B, et al. Plasma protein binding of diphenylhydantoin in normal and hyperbilirubinemic infants. *J Pediatr* 78:877, 1971.
43. Walker PC: Neonatal bilirubin toxicity: a review of kernicterus and the implications of drug-induced bilirubin displacement. *Clin Pharmacokinet* 13:26, 1987.
44. Stutman HR, Parker KM, Marks MI: Potential of moxalactam and other new antimicrobial agents for bilirubin-albumin displacement in neonates. *Pediatrics* 75:294, 1985.
45. Cheek DB, Mellits D, Elliott D: Body water, height, and weight during growth in normal children. *Am J Dis Child* 112:312, 1966.
46. Friis-Hansen B: Water distribution in the fetus and newborn infant. *Acta Paediatr Scand* 305(suppl):7, 1983.
47 Cassady G: Bromide space studies in infants of low birth weight. *Pediatr Res* 4:14, 1970.
48. Boreus LO: Principles of pediatric pharmacology. In Azamoff DL, editor: *Monographs in clinical pharmacology,* vol 6. New York, 1982, Churchill Livingstone.
49. Klotz U: Pathophysiological and disease-induced changes in drug distribution volume: pharmacokinetic implications. *Clin Pharmacokinet* 1:204, 1976.
50. Lesar TS, Zaske DE: Antibiotics and hepatic disease. *Med Clin North Am* 66:257, 1982.
51. Wilkinson GR, Shand DG: A physiologic approach to hepatic drug clearance. *Clin Pharmacol Ther* 18:377, 1975.
52. Wilkinson GR: Pharmacokinetics of drug disposition: hemodynamic considerations. *Annu Rev Pharmacol* 15:11, 1975.
53. Leeder JS, Kearns GL: Pharmacogenetics in pediatrics: implications for practice. *Pediatr Clin North Am* 44:55, 1997.
54. Fleischner GM, Arias IM: Structure and function of ligandin (Y protein, GSH transferase B) and Z protein in the liver: a progress report. In Popper H, Shaffner F, editors: *Progress in liver disease,* vol 5. New York, 1976, Grune & Stratton.
55. Levi AJ, Gatmaiton Z, Arias IM: Two hepatic cytoplasmic protein fractions, y and z, and their possible role in the hepatic uptake of bilirubin, sulfobromophthalein and other anions. *J Clin Invest* 48:2156, 1969.
56. Juchau MR: Fetal and neonatal drug biotransformation. In Kacew S, editor: *Drug toxicity and metabolism in pediatrics.* Boca Raton, Fla, 1990, CRC Press.
57. Roberts RJ: Pharmacologic principles in therapeutic in infants. In Roberts RJ, editor: *Drug therapy in infants.* Philadelphia, 1984, WB Saunders Co.
58. Rane AA, Tomson G: Prenatal and neonatal drug metabolism in man. *Eur J Clin Pharmacol* 18:9, 1980.
59. Yaffe SJ, Rane A, Sjogvist F, et al: The presence of a monooxygenase system in human fetal liver microsomes. *Life Sci* 9:1189, 1970.
60. Pelkonen O, Karki NT: Drug metabolism in human fetal tissues. *Life Sci* 13:1163, 1973.
61. Ratanasavanh D, Beaune P, Morel F, et al: Intralobular distribution and quantitation of cytochrome P-450 enzymes in human liver as a function of age. *Hepatology* 13:1142, 1991.
62. Nassif EG, Weinberger MM, Shannon D, et al: Theophylline disposition in infancy. *J Pediatr* 98:158, 1981.
63. Tateishi T, Asoh M, Yamaguchi A, et al: Developmental changes in urinary elimination of theophylline and its metabolites in pediatrics patients. *Pediatr Res* 45:55, 1999.
64. Treluyer JM, Gueret G, Cheron G, et al: Developmental expression of CYP2C and CYP2C-dependent activities in the human liver: in-vivo/in-vitro correlation and inducibility. *Pharmacogenetics* 7:441, 1997.
65. Dodson WE: Special pharmacokinetic considerations in children. *Epilepsia* 28(suppl 1):556, 1987.
66. Treluyer JM, Jacqz-Aigrain E, Alvarez F, Cresteil T: Expression of CYP2D6 in developing human liver. *Eur J Biochem* 202:583, 1991.
67. Tateishi T, Nakura H, Asoh M, et al: A comparison of hepatic cytochrome P450 expression between infancy and postinfancy. *Life Sci* 61.2567, 1997.
68. Furlanut M, Montanari G, Bonin P, Casara GL: Carbamazepine and carbamazepine 10,11 epoxide serum concentrations in epileptic children. *J Pediatr* 106:491, 1985.
69. Korinthenberg R, Haug C, Hannak D: The metabolism of carbamazepine to carbamazepine-10,11-epoxide in children from the newborn age to adolescence. *Neuropediatrics* 25:214, 1994.
70. Riva R, Contin M, Albani F, et al: Free and total serum concentrations of carbamazepine and carbamazepine-10,11-epoxide in infancy and childhood. *Epilepsia* 26:320, 1985.
71. Pikkarainen PH, Raiha NCR: Development of alcohol dehydrogenase activity in the human liver. *Pediatr Res* 1:165, 1967.
72. Echobichon DJ, Stephens DS: Perinatal development of human blood esterases. *Clin Pharmacol Ther* 14:41, 1973.
73. de Wildt SN, Kearns GL, Leeder JS, van den Anker JN: Glucuronidation in humans: pharmacogenetic and developmental aspects. *Clin Pharmacokinet* 36:439, 1999.
74. Pacifici GM, Kubrich M, Giuliani L, et al: Sulphation and glucuronidation of ritodrine in human fetal and adult tissues. *Eur J Clin Pharmacol* 44:259, 1993.
75. Coughtrie MW, Burchell B, Leakey JE, Hume R: The inadequacy of perinatal glucuronidation: immunoblot analysis of the developmental expression of individual UDP-glucuronyltransferase isoenzymes in rat and human liver microsomes. *Mol Pharmacol* 34:729, 1988.
76. Choonara IA, McKay P, Hain R, Rane A: Morphine metabolism in children. *Br J Clin Pharmacol* 28:599, 1989.
77. Anderson BJ, McKee AD, Holford NHG: Size, myths and the clinical pharmacokinetics of analgesia in paediatric patients. *Clin Pharmacokinet* 33:313, 1997.
78. Levy G, Khanna NN, Soda DM, et al: Pharmacokinetics of acetaminophen in the human neonate: formation of acetaminophen glucuronide and sulfate relation to plasma bilirubin concentration and D-glucaricacid excretion. *Pediatrics* 55:818, 1975.
79. Alam SN, Robert RJ, Fischer LJ: Age-related differences in salicylamide and acetaminophen conjugation in man. *J Pediatr* 90:130, 1977.

80. Talafant E, Hoskova A, Pojerova A: Glucaric acid excretion as index of hepatic glucuronidation in neonates after phenobarbital treatment. *Pediatr Res* 9:480, 1975.
81. Wasserman E, Myara A, Lokiec F: Severe CPT-11 toxicity in patients with Gilbert's syndrome: two case reports. *Ann Oncol* 8:1049, 1997.
82. Park GR: Molecular mechanisms of drug metabolism in the critically ill. *Br J Anaesth* 77:32, 1996.
83. Armstrong SG, Renton KW: Mechanism of hepatic cytochrome P450 modulation during *Listeria monocytogenes* infection in mice. *Mol Pharmacol* 43:542, 1993.
84. Abdel-Razzak Z, Loyer P, Fautrel A, et al: Cytokines down-regulate expression of major cytochrome P-450 enzymes in adult human hepatocytes in primary culture. *Mol Pharmacol* 44:707, 1993.
85. Brater DC: The pharmacological role of the kidney. *Drugs* 19:31,1980.
86. Brater DC, Vasko MR: Pharmacokinetics. In Chernow B, editor: *The pharmacologic approach to the critically ill patient,* ed 2, Baltimore, 1988, Williams & Wilkins.
87. Whelton A: Antibiotic pharmacokinetics and clinical application in renal insufficiency. *Med Clin North Am* 66:267, 1982.
88. Aschinberg LC, Goldsmith DI, Olbing H, et al: Neonatal changes in renal blood flow distribution in puppies. *Am J Physiol* 228:1453, 1975.
89. Hook JB, Bailie MD: Perinatal renal pharmacology. *Annu Rev Pharm Toxicol* 19:491, 1979.
90. West JR, Smith HW, Chasis H: Glomerular filtration rate, effect on renal blood flow, and maximal tubular excretory capacity in infancy. *J Pediatr* 32:10, 1948.
91. Calcagno PL, Rubin MI: Renal extraction of paraaminohippurate in infants and children. *J Clin Invest* 42:1632, 1963.
92. Leake RD, Trygstad CW, Oh W: Inulin clearance in the newborn infant: relationship to gestational and postnatal age. *Pediatr Res* 10:759, 1976.
93. Besunder JB, Reed MD, Blumer JL: Principles of drug biodisposition in the neonate: a critical evaluation of the pharmacokinetic-pharmacodynamic interface (part I). *Clin Pharmacokinet* 14:189, 1988.
94. Morselli PL: Clinical pharmacokinetics in neonates. *Clin Pharmacokinet* 1:81, 1976.
95. Szefler SJ, Wynn RJ, Clarke DF, et al: Relationship of gentamicin serum concentrations to gestational age in preterm and term neonates. *J Pediatr* 97:312, 1980.
96. Hook JB, Bailie MD: Perinatal renal pharmacology. *Annu Rev Pharm Toxicol* 19:491, 1979.
97. McCracken GH Jr, Ginsberg C, Chrane DP, et al: Clinical pharmacology of penicillin in newborn infants. *J Pediatr* 82:692, 1973.
98. Kaplan JM, McCracken GH, Horton LJ, et al: Pharmacologic studies in neonates given large doses of ampicillin. *J Pediatr* 84:571, 1974.
99. Nelson JD, Shelton S, Kusmiesz H: Clinical pharmacology of ticarcillin in the newborn infant: relation to age, gestational age, and weight. *J Pediatr* 87:474, 1975.
100. Sarff LD, McCracken GH Jr, Thomas ML, et al: Clinical pharmacology methicillin in neonates, *J Pediatr* 90:1005, 1977.
101. Odiind B, Beermann B: Renal tubular secretion and effects of furosemide. *Clin Pharmacol Ther* 27:784, 1980.
102. Aranda JV, Perez J, Sitar DS, et al: Pharmacokinetic disposition and protein binding of furosemide in newborn infants. *J Pediatr* 93:507,1978.
103. Peterson RG, Simmons MA, Rumanck BH, et al: Pharmacology of furosemide in the premature newborn infant. *J Pediatr* 97:139, 1980.
104. Witte MK, Stork JE, Blumer JL: Diuretic therapeutics in the pediatric patient. *Am J Cardiol* 57:44A, 1986.
105. Brater DC: *Drug use in renal disease.* Sydney, 1983, ADIS.
106. Kwan JW: Drug delivery systems. In Chernow B, editor: *The pharmacologic approach to the critically ill patient.* Baltimore, 1994, Williams & Wilkins.
107. Buck ML: Pharmacokinetic changes during extracorporeal membrane oxygenation: implications for drug therapy of neonates. *Clin Pharmacokinet* 42:403, 2003.
108. Cohen P, Collart L, Prober CG, et al: Gentamicin pharmacokinetics in neonates undergoing extracorporeal membrane oxygenation. *Pediatr Infect Dis J* 9:562, 1990.
109. Bhatt-Mehta V, Johnson CE, Schumacher RE: Gentamicin pharmacokinetics in term neonates receiving extracorporeal membrane oxygenation. *Pharmacotherapy* 12:28, 1992.
110. Buck ML: Vancomycin pharmacokinetics in neonates receiving extracorporeal membrane oxygenation. *Pharmacotherapy* 18:1082, 1998.
111. Mulla H, Nabi F, Nichani S, et al: Population pharmacokinetics of theophylline during paediatric extracorporeal membrane oxygenation. *Br J Clin Pharmacol* 55:23, 2003.
112. Dagan O, Klein J, Bohn D, Koren G: Effects of extracorporeal membrane oxygenation on morphine pharmacokinetics in infants. *Crit Care Med* 22:1099, 1994.
113. Dagan O, Klein J, Gruenwald C, et al: Preliminary studies of the effects of extracorporeal membrane oxygenator on the disposition of common pediatric drugs. *Ther Drug Monit* 15:263, 1993.
114. Geiduschek JM, Lynn AM, Bratton SL, et al: Morphine pharmacokinetics during continuous infusion of morphine sulfate for infants receiving extracorporeal membrane oxygenation. *Crit Care Med* 25:360, 1997.
115. Benet LZ, Mitchell JR, Sheiner LB: General principles. In Gilm AG, et al, editors: *The pharmacological basis of therapeutics,* ed 8. Elmsford, NY, 1990, Pergamon Press.
116. Nies AS: Principles of therapeutics. In Hardman JG, Limbird LE, editors: *Goodman and Gilman's the pharmacological basis of therapeutics.* New York, 2001, McGraw-Hill.
117. Pratt WB, Taylor P, editors: *Principles of drug action. The basis of pharmacology,* ed 3, New York, 1990, Churchill Livingstone.
118. Ross EM: *Pharmacodynamics: mechanisms of drug action and the relationship between drug concentration and effect in pharmacological basis of therapeutics,* ed 8, New York, 1990, Pergamon Press.
119. Radde 1C, Holland FJ: Receptors and drug action. In MacLeod SM, Radde IC, editors: *Textbook of pediatric clinical pharmacology.* Littleton, 1985, PSG Publishing Co.
120. Rane A: Basic principles of drug disposition in infants. In Yaffe, editor: *Pediatric pharmacology: therapeutic principles in practice.* New York, 1980, Grune & Stratton.
121. Schreurs A, Nijkamp F: *Haemophilus influenzae* induced loss of lung p-adrenoreceptor binding sites and modulation by changes in peripheral catecholaminergic input. *Eur J Pharmacol* 77:95, 1982.
122. Schreurs A, Terpstra G, Raaijmakers J, et al: The effects of *Haemophilus influenzae* vaccination on anaphylactic mediator release and isoprenaline-induced inhibition of mediator release. *Eur J Pharmacol* 62:261, 1980.
123. Aarons RD, Nies AS, Molinoff PB: Elevation of beta adrenergic receptor density in human lymphocytes after propranolol administration. *J Clin Invest* 65:949, 1980.
124. Hoffman BB, Lefkowitz RJ: Radioligand binding studies of adrenergic receptors: new insights into molecular and physiological regulation. *Annu Rev Pharmacol Toxicol* 20:581, 1980.
125. Nattel S, Rnagno R, Van Loon G: Mechanism of propranolol withdrawal phenomena. *Circulation* 59:1158, 1979.
126. Blumer JL, Bond GR, editor: Toxic effects of drugs in the ICU. *Care Clin* 7:489, 1991.
127. Watson CB: Complications of drug therapy. In Lumb PD, Bryan-Brown CW, editors: *Complications in critical care medicine.* Chicago, 1988, Yearbook Medical Publishers.
128. Gibaldi M, Perriex D: *Pharmacokinetics,* ed 2, New York, 1982, Marcel Dekker.
129. Jusko WJ: Pharmacokinetic principles in pediatric pharmacology. *Pediatr Clin North Am* 19:81, 1972.
130. Atkinson AJ, Shaw JM: Pharmacokinetic study of a patient with diphenylhydantoin toxicity. *Clin Pharmacol Ther* 14:521, 1973.
131. Sheiner LB, Tozer TN: Clinical pharmacokinetics: the use of plasma concentrations of drugs. In Melmon KL, Morrelli HF, editors: *Clinical pharmacology: basic principles in therapeutics.* New York, 1978, MacMillan Publishing.

CHAPTER

111

Molecular Aspects of Drug Actions: From Receptors to Effectors

Catherine Litalien and Pierre Beaulieu

PEARLS

- Receptors play a central role in determining the nature of the pharmacologic effects produced by a drug.
- Most drugs and endogenous compounds (e.g., hormones, neurotransmitters) exert their action by binding to a receptor or by modulating an ion channel.
- G proteins are a superfamily of propeller proteins that allow transduction between activated receptor (by an agonist) and different intracellular effectors, such as enzymes or ion channels, relaying signals from more than 1000 receptors.
- Continued exposure of a receptor to an agonist often results in progressive loss of receptor responsiveness, with a diminished receptor-mediated response over time. This is called *desensitization* or *tachyphylaxis*.
- Calcium exerts its control on cellular function through its ability to regulate the activity of many different proteins, such as channels, transporters, and transcription factors. In the majority of cases, a calcium binding protein serves as an intermediate between Ca^{2+} and the regulated functional protein.
- The role of inheritance in the individual variation of drug response is increasingly recognized with the identification of polymorphisms in genes encoding drug-metabolizing enzymes, drug targets, and proteins involved in signal transduction.

Optimizing drug response is a challenging task that clinicians confront daily. This is particularly true for clinicians caring for critically ill patients for whom many factors influencing drug response are increasingly being recognized. These factors include decreased metabolism and elimination and alterations in drugs receptors, signaling mechanisms, and effectors.[1–7] Advances in molecular pharmacology have shed more light on the processes that transduce extracellular signals into intracellular messages controlling cell function. This knowledge has led to the elucidation of multiple points at which modulation of signal transduction, either by drugs or diseases, can occur. In addition, the role of inheritance in the individual variation of drug response is being recognized, with the identification of polymorphisms in genes encoding drug-metabolizing enzymes, drug targets (e.g., receptors, enzymes), and proteins involved in signal transduction.[8–13] Finally, major developmental changes occurring during childhood can alter drug disposition and action.

This chapter aims to provide a thorough understanding of how drugs work at the molecular level and how this complex system is influenced by genetic factors, developmental characteristics, and disease processes (Figure 111–1). Ultimately, the objective is to help pediatric intensivists to better tailor the pharmacotherapy they use, that is, to choose the right drug (or combination

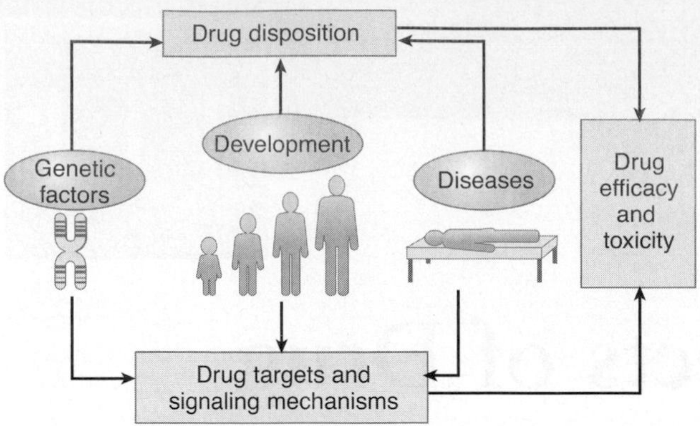

FIGURE 111–1 • Relationships between genetic factors, development, diseases, and drug efficacy and toxicity.

of drugs) for the right patient, in order to achieve maximal efficacy with no or minimal toxicity. This chapter does not address signaling pathways involved in diseases *per se*.

Targets for Drug Action

The initial step in the cascade of biochemical events resulting in drug action mostly consists of binding of drugs to specific cellular targets. The targets can be broadly divided into four categories: (1) receptors; (2) ion/receptor channels; (3) enzymes; and (4) transporters (or carrier molecules) (Figure 111–2). The vast majority of important drugs act on one of these types of proteins. Table 111–1 lists the targets of some pharmacologic agents commonly used in the pediatric intensive care unit (PICU).

Receptors

Receptors can be defined as the sensing elements in the system of chemical communication that coordinate the function of all different cells in the body, with various hormones, neurotransmitters, other mediators, or drugs as the chemical messengers.[14] Ligands (e.g., hormones, drugs) that bind with receptors are termed *agonists* if their binding results in the expected effect and are termed *antagonists* if binding stops or decreases an agonist-induced activity.[15] Administration of a receptor antagonist in the absence of agonist results in no effect because antagonists bind to receptors but do not activate them. An antagonist is said to be *surmountable* when maximal response to the agonist can be restored by raising the agonist concentration (parallel displacement of the agonist dose–response curve to the right). Likewise, an antagonist is said to be *insurmountable* when even high concentrations of the agonist cannot elicit the maximal expected agonist response (Figure 111–3, *A*).[16] The terms *competitive* and *noncompetitive* do not describe a pharmacologic behavior; rather, they refer to the receptor binding site of the antagonist with regard to that of the agonist. A competitive antagonist binds to the same site as the agonist on the receptor, whereas a noncompetitive antagonist has its own binding site separate from that of the agonist and makes the receptor refractory to the agonist. Both *competitive* and *noncompetitive* antagonists can be *insurmountable*.

The duration of action of an *insurmountable* antagonist is mostly dependent on synthesis of new receptors, which can take several days. This may have clinically important consequences. For example, phenoxybenzamine, an *insurmountable* α-adrenergic receptor antagonist, is sometimes used in stage I Norwood procedures to balance the pulmonary and systemic circulations.[17,18] Attenuation or reversal of the decrease in systemic vascular resistance produced may not be achieved with an α-adrenergic receptor agonist such as dopamine (high dose) or norepinephrine, depending on the dose of phenoxybenzamine given. In such circumstances, use of a pressor agent that does not act through the α-adrenergic receptor must be considered. The success of vasopressin, which acts on V_1 receptors of smooth muscle cells,[19] in reversing phenoxybenzamine-induced hypotension in one neonate who underwent a Norwood procedure is reported.[20]

Partial agonists are ligands that bind to the same receptor as full agonists but have less intrinsic capacity to produce a response as strong as full agonists, despite full receptor occupancy (Figure 111–3, *B*). The exact mechanism accounting for the blunted maximal response seen with partial agonists is unknown. Simultaneous administration of a partial agonist and a full agonist prevents the maximal response usually observed with the full agonist alone because partial agonists have the ability to occupy the receptor population (Figure 111–3, *C*). Finally, inverse agonists are ligands that reduce the level of constitutive activation encountered in some receptor systems (Figure 111–3, *D*).[21]

Receptors play a central role in determining the nature of the pharmacologic effects produced by a drug. First, receptors bind with only one or a limited number of structurally related ligands, ensuring that the final effect seen in a normal setting occurs only in response to defined stimuli. Second, for a given dose or concentration of a drug, the drug's affinity to bind to the receptor and the total number of available receptors directly influence the maximal effect a drug can produce. Third, drugs differ in their intrinsic activity with respect to their receptors (e.g., partial agonist vs. full agonist). Thus the magnitude of response to any drug is proportional to both the extent of receptor occupancy and the intrinsic activity of the receptor itself, resulting in different dose or concentration relationships for different agonists. The classification of receptors is discussed in greater detail in the following.

Ion/Receptor Channels

Ion channels are molecular machines that serve as principal integrating and regulatory devices for controlling cellular excitability. Different types of ion channels have been described: channels that respond to mechanical, electrical (voltage-dependent ion channels), or chemical stimuli (ligand-gated ion channels); ion channels that are controlled by phosphorylation/dephosphorylation mechanisms; and ion channels that are dependent on G proteins. Most ion channels are of the voltage-dependent type and consist mainly of sodium (Na^+), potassium (K^+), and calcium (Ca^{2+}) channels. Drugs can affect ion channel function directly by binding to the channel protein and altering its function or

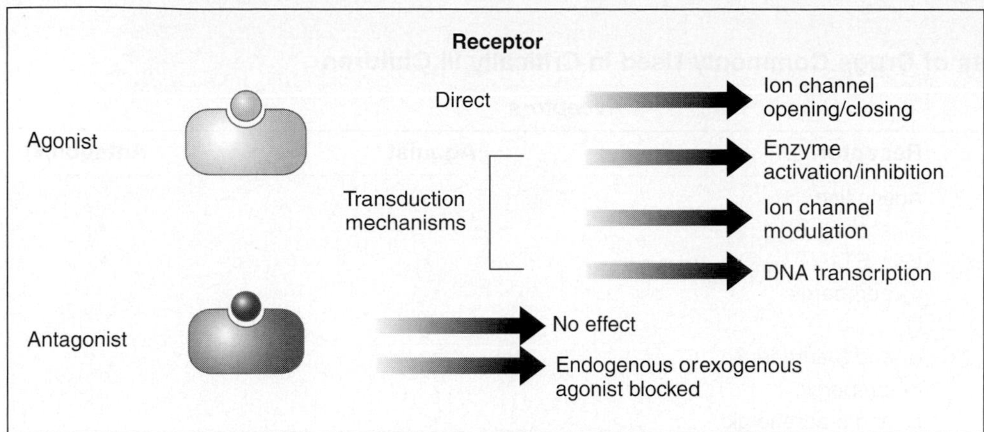

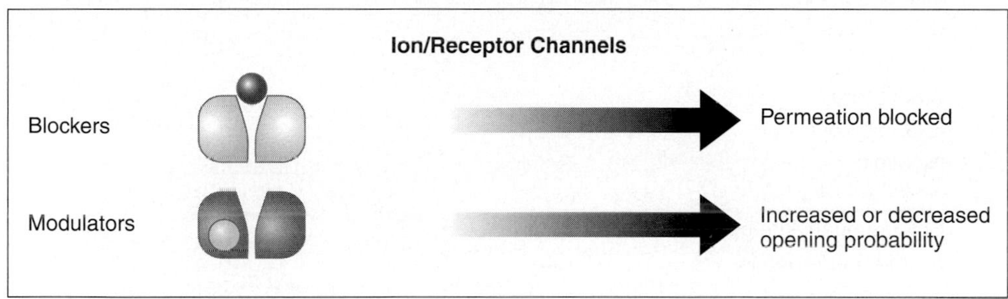

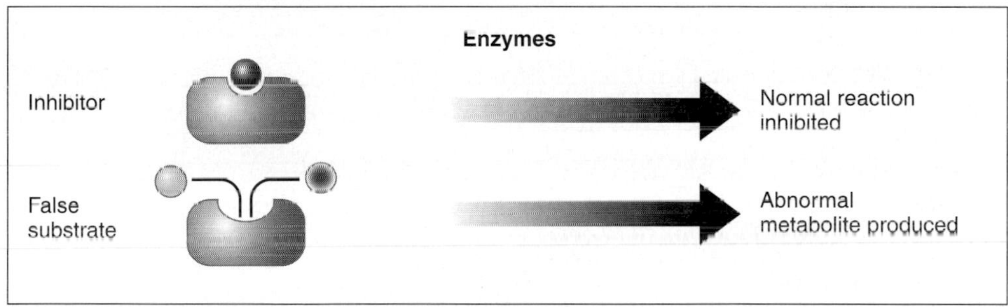

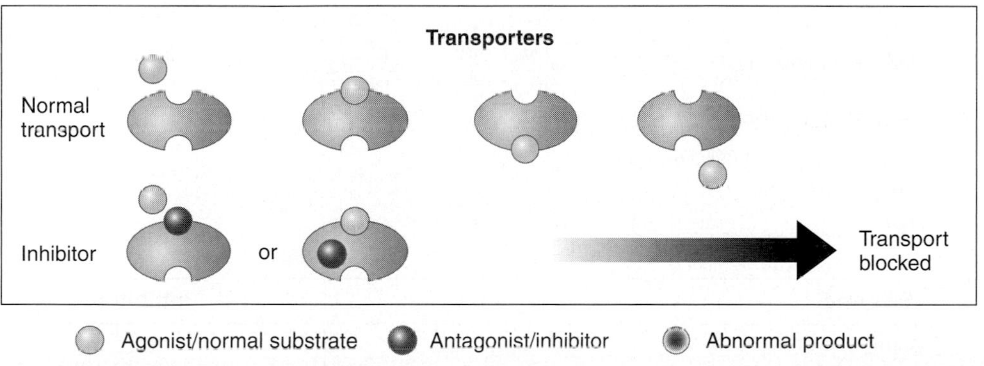

FIGURE 111–2 • Targets for drug action. (Modified from Rang HP, Dale MM, Ritter JM, Moore PK: *Pharmacology,* ed 5, London, 2003, Churchill Livingstone.)

indirectly through G proteins and other intermediates. Lidocaine is a good example of a drug that directly affects voltage-gated Na^+ channels by blocking the channel and thus Na^+ entry into the cell. Channel-linked receptors are discussed later.

Enzymes

Enzymes are a specialized class of proteins responsible for catalyzing chemical reactions within the cell and thus are ideal drug targets. Most drugs that alter enzymes activity are substrate analogues of enzymes that inhibit their activity either reversibly (e.g., angiotensin-converting enzyme inhibitors acting on peptidyl dipeptidase) or irreversibly (e.g., acetylsalicylic acid acting on cyclooxygenase). Drugs also may prevent the normal functioning of enzymes. Fluorouracil, an anticancer drug, is a good example of such drug. It is converted into an abnormal nucleotide that inhibits thymidylate synthetase, thus blocking deoxyribonucleic acid (DNA) synthesis.

TABLE 111–1

Targets of Drugs Commonly Used in Critically Ill Children

Receptors

Drug	Receptor	Agonist	Antagonist
Adenosine	Adenosine	•	
Atropine	Muscarinic		•
Bosentan	ET_A, ET_B		•
Clonidine	α_2-adrenergic	•	
Dopamine	D_1	•	
	α- and β-adrenergic	•	
Dobutamine	β-adrenergic	•	
Epinephrine	α- and β-adrenergic	•	
Glucocorticoids	Glucocorticoid	•	
Haloperidol	D_2		•
Insulin	Insulin	•	
Isoproterenol	β-adrenergic	•	
Naloxone	μ, δ, κ opioid		•
Neuromuscular blockers (depolarizing and nondepolarizing)	Nicotinic		•
Nitric oxide	Soluble guanylate cyclase	•	
Norepinephrine	α- and β-adrenergic	•	
Opioids	μ, δ, κ opioid	•	
Phenoxybenzamine	α-adrenergic		•
Phenylephrine	α-adrenergic	•	
Propranolol	β-adrenergic		•
Ranitidine	H_2		•
Vasopressin	V_1, V_2, V_3	•	
Salbutamol	β-adrenergic	•	
Spironolactone	Mineralocorticoid		•

Ion/Receptor Channels

Drug	Ion Channel(s)	Blocker	Modulator
Adenosine	Ca^{2+}	•	
Amiodarone	Na^+, K^+, Ca^{2+}	•	
Barbiturates	$GABA_A$-gated Cl^-		•
Benzodiazepines	$GABA_A$-gated Cl^-		•
Flumazenil	$GABA_A$-gated Cl^-	•	
Ketamine	Glutamate-gated (NMDA) cation	•	
Lidocaine	Na^+	•	
Propafenone	Na^+	•	

Enzymes

Drug	Enzyme	Inhibitor
Acetazolamide	Carbonic anhydrase	•
Captopril	Angiotensin-converting enzyme (peptidyl dipeptidase)	•
Milrinone	Phosphodiesterase III	•
Nonsteroidal anti-inflammatory drugs	Cyclooxygenase-1 and -2	•
Sildenafil	Phosphodiesterase V	•

Transporters

Drug	Transporter	Inhibitor
Digoxin	Na^+/K^+-ATPase pump	•
Loops diuretics	$Na^+/K^+/Cl^-$ cotransporter	•
Omeprazole	H^+/K^+ ATPase pump	•
Thiazides	Na^+/Cl^- cotransporter	•

D, dopaminergic; *ET*, endothelin; *GABA*, γ-aminobutyric acid; *H*, histamine; *NMDA*, N-methyl-D-aspartate; *V*, vasopressin.

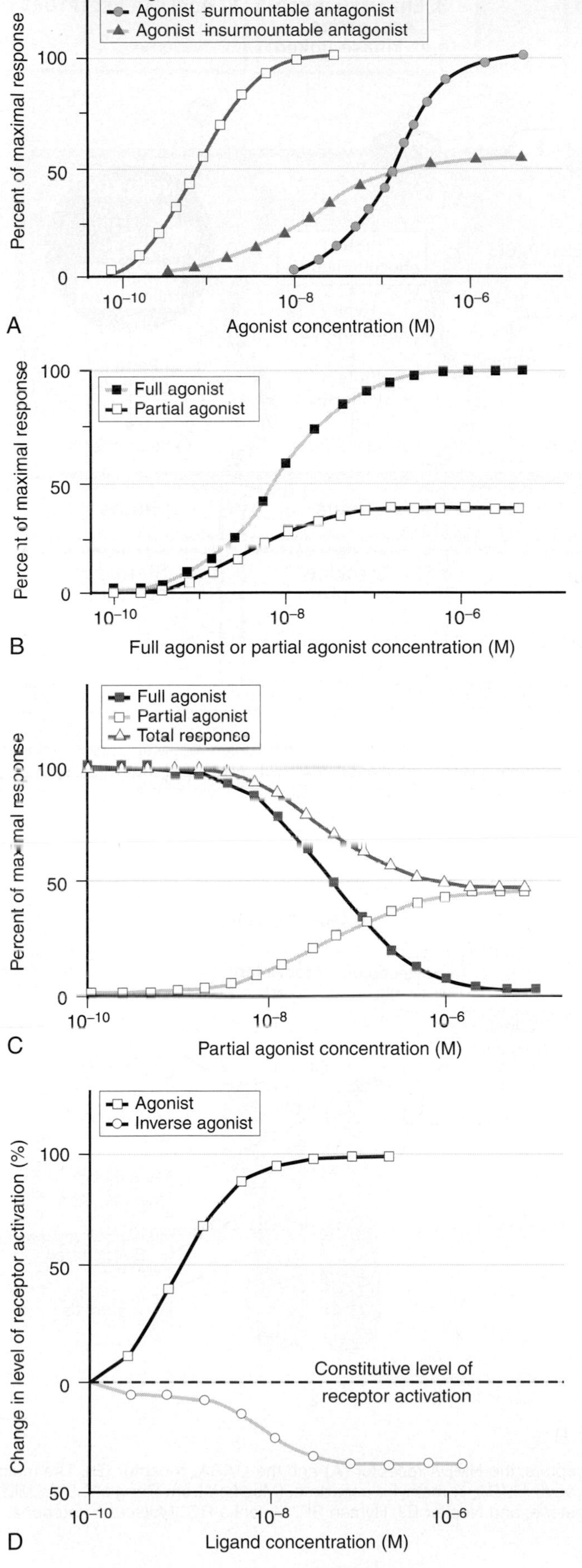

FIGURE 111–3 • **A,** Concentration–response curves for an agonist in the absence or presence of a surmountable or insurmountable antagonist. (Modified from Harman JG, Limbird LE: *Goodman & Gilman's the pharmacological basis of therapeutics,* ed 9, New York, 1996, McGraw-Hill.) **B,** At similar concentrations, a partial agonist produces a lower response than does a full agonist. (Modified from Katzung BG: *Basic & clinical pharmacology,* ed 8, New York, 2001, McGraw-Hill.) **C,** Response pattern observed during simultaneous treatment with a single concentration of a full agonist and increasing concentration of a partial agonist. (Modified from Katzung BG: *Basic & clinical pharmacology,* ed 8, New York, 2001, McGraw-Hill.) **D,** When an appreciable level of activation of a receptor exists in the absence of an agonist (constitutive activation), the presence of an inverse agonist decreases the degree of receptor activation. *M,* mol/L. (Modified from Rang HP, Dale MM, Ritter JM, Moore PK: *Pharmacology,* ed 5, London, 2003, Churchill Livingstone.)

Transporters

Several biologic signals, such as ions and organic molecules, are not sufficiently lipid soluble to be able to cross the plasma membrane; they require a carrier protein to be transported within or outside the cell. Some drugs bind to these carrier proteins and interfere with the transport system. Cardiac glycosides (e.g., digoxin) are a typical example of drugs that produce their effect via this mechanism, by blocking the transporter protein Na^+/K^+-ATPase pump.

Receptors and Signal Transduction Mechanisms

Most transmembrane signaling is accomplished by only a few molecular mechanisms, each of which is adapted to transduce many different signals. These protein families include cell surface receptors and receptors within the cell, as well as enzymes and other components that generate, amplify, coordinate, and terminate postreceptor signaling.[15] Receptors and their signal transduction mechanisms are discussed later.

Classification of Receptors

Most drugs and endogenous compounds (e.g., hormones, neurotransmitters) exert their action by binding to a receptor or by modulating an ion channel. Four families of receptors, three cell surface receptor types, and one nuclear receptor are described (Figure 111–4).

Channel-Linked Receptors

Channel-linked receptors, also known as *ligand-gated ion channels* or *ionotropic receptors,* mediate fast responses, affecting ion fluxes and membrane potential. Broadly speaking, two types are identified: receptors of excitatory mediators and receptors of inhibitory mediators.

Receptors of excitatory mediators (glutamate, aspartate, and acetylcholine), which comprise the N-methyl-D-aspartate (NMDA) receptor (Figure 111–5, *A*) and the nicotinic acetylcholine receptor, are receptors whose activation provokes depolarization of the cell, leading to propagation of the action potential and ultimately secretion of

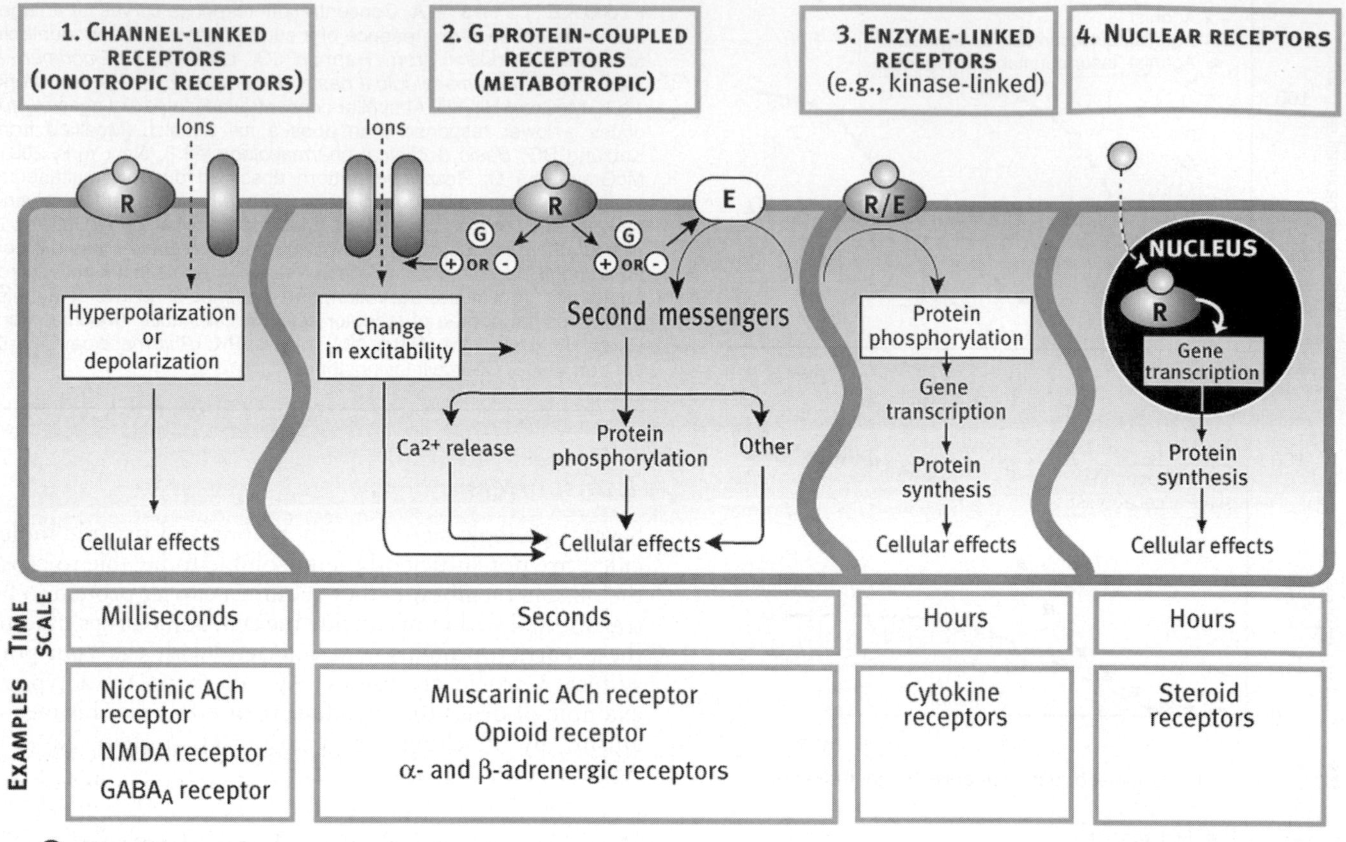

FIGURE 111–4 • Four families of receptors are classically described: channel-linked receptors, G protein-coupled receptors, enzyme-linked receptors, and nuclear receptors. *ACh,* Acetylcholine; *E,* enzyme; *G,* G protein; *GABA,* γ-aminobutyric acid; *NMDA,* N-methyl-D-aspartate; *R,* receptor. (Modified from Rang HP, Dale MM, Ritter JM, Moore PK: *Pharmacology,* ed 5, London, 2003, Churchill Livingstone.)

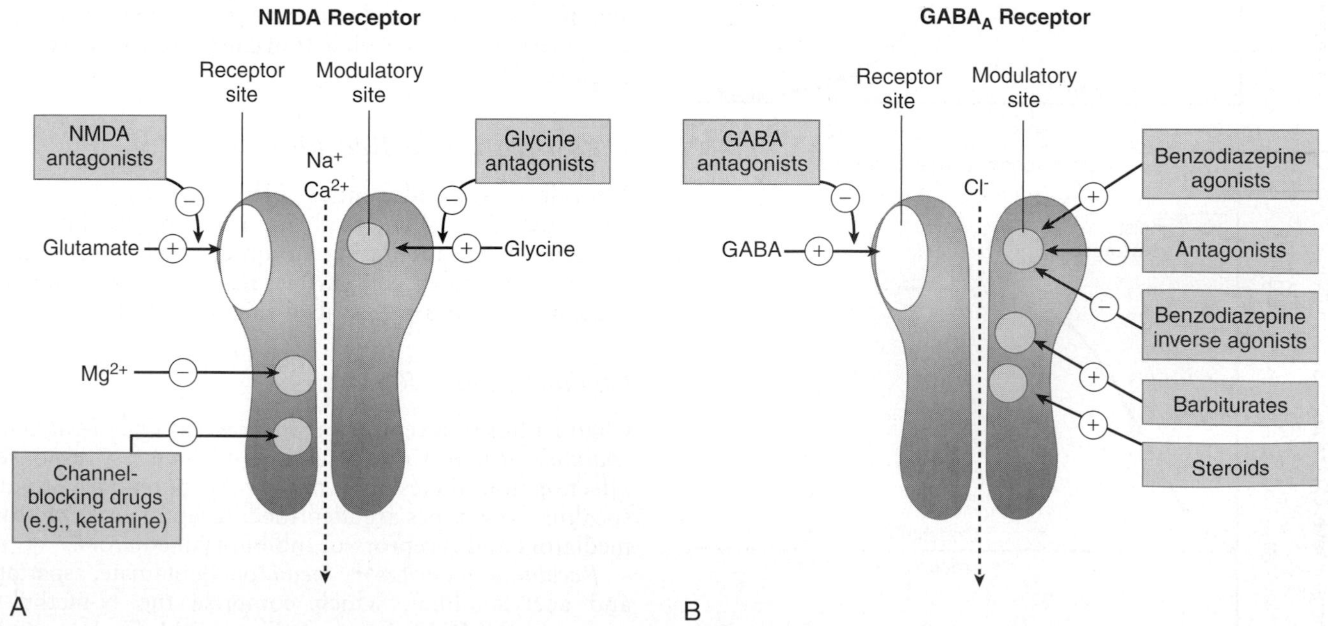

FIGURE 111–5 • Two important members of the channel-linked receptors: the NMDA receptor **(A)** and the GABA$_A$ receptor **(B).** The main sites of drug action on these receptors are shown. *GABA,* γ-aminobutyric acid; *NMDA,* N-methyl-D-aspartate. (Modified from Rang HP, Dale MM, Ritter JM, Moore PK: *Pharmacology,* ed 5, London, 2003, Churchill Livingstone; and Nestler EJ, Hyman SE, Malenka RC: *Molecular neuropharmacology,* New York, 2001, McGraw-Hill.)

a neuromediator and muscular contraction, for example. These receptors are permeable to monovalent and divalent cations, mainly Na^+, K^+, Ca^{2+}, and magnesium (Mg^{2+}). Ketamine, a dissociative anesthetic frequently used in PICU, is a noncompetitive surmountable NMDA receptor antagonist that acts by preventing the opening of ion channels by glutamate. In addition, the potential neuroprotective effects of ketamine appear to be mediated via NMDA receptor blockade.[22,23] Increasing evidence indicates that NMDA receptor activation by glutamate release during neuronal injury can cause further cellular injury and death (see Chapters 58 and 107). Some animal studies have shown that NMDA receptor blockade can attenuate the neuronal damage caused by hypoxia.[24–27] Furthermore, NMDA receptor activation is involved in the development of μ opioid receptor tolerance, with NMDA receptor antagonists preventing the development of opioid tolerance and withdrawal without affecting the analgesic effects of morphine.[28–30] To date, most of these data come from studies performed in rodents and few from human trials.

Receptors of inhibitory mediators, whose activation provokes hyperpolarization of the cell and therefore decreases cellular excitability, are a group that includes γ-aminobutyric acid $(GABA)_A$ (Figure 111–5, *B*) and glycine receptors. These ligand-gated ion channels are selective for anions such as chloride (Cl^-) or phosphate (PO_4^{3-}). GABA is the major inhibitory neurotransmitter in the central nervous system, and drugs that potentiate GABAergic inhibition in the brain (e.g., benzodiazepines and barbiturates) result in sedation and hypnosis.[15] Benzodiazepine agonists enhance Cl^- ion conductance induced by GABA by increasing the frequency of channel-opening events, whereas barbiturates seem to do so by increasing the duration of GABA-gated channel openings.[31] Both classes of agents bind to receptors on the $GABA_A$ molecule that are different from each other and from the GABA receptor.

G Protein-Coupled Receptors

In 1994, Alfred G. Gilman and Martin Rodbell were awarded the Nobel Prize in Physiology and Medicine for their discovery of G proteins and their role in signal transduction in cells.[32] G proteins are a superfamily of propeller proteins that allow transduction between the activated receptor (by an agonist) and different intracellular effectors such as enzymes or ion channels, relaying signals from more than 1000 receptors.[33] G protein-coupled receptors (GPCRs), also known as *metabotropic receptors*, are the first component in the cellular amplification cascade (Figure 111–6). Activation of target enzymes through GPCRs leads to synthesis of numerous second messengers that in turn activate other enzymes. The intervention of the second messenger system allows for the diversity of cellular targets (see later).

All GPCRs share a serpentine structure consisting of seven transmembrane domains including three extracellular and three intracellular loops. The extracellular regions are involved in ligand binding, whereas the intracellular regions are primarily involved in signaling.[34] The latter is coupled to a heterotrimeric guanine nucleotide-binding regulatory protein (G protein) located on the cytoplasmic portion of the cell membrane and made of three subunits. Each G protein is composed of an α subunit that is loosely bound to a tightly associated dimer made up of β and γ subunits. The activity of a trimeric G protein is regulated by the binding and hydrolysis of guanosine triphosphate (GTP) by the α subunit (Figure 111–7).

Each of the three subunits is encoded by a separate gene selected from at least 20 α, 6 β, and 12 γ genes, respectively. The α subunit is essential in "receptor–effector" coupling. Various α subunits define different G protein trimers (G_s = stimulatory G protein, G_i = inhibitory G protein, G_o = other G protein…), each of which regulates a distinctive set of downstream signaling pathways. Table 111–2 shows some examples of GPCRs with their trimeric G protein along with their target enzymes or ion channels and second messengers. Some receptors act via more than one type of G protein trimer (e.g., μ opioid receptor). Approximately 50% of the GPCRs couple to G_i/G_o proteins, approximately 25% couple to G_s, and approximately 25% couple to G_q proteins.[35] G_s proteins (made of α_s subunits) can activate adenylate cyclase and

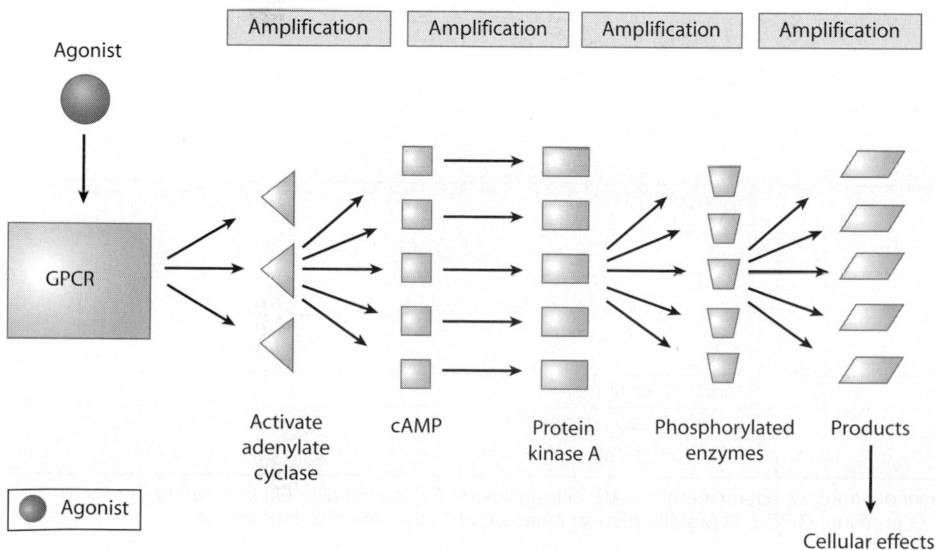

FIGURE 111–6 • Cellular amplification cascade. After binding to a G protein–coupled receptor *(GPCR)*, a ligand (agonist) activates a target enzyme (adenylate cyclase), which synthesizes the second messenger cyclic adenosine monophosphate *(cAMP)*. The latter then activates other enzymes (protein kinases), which phosphorylate proteins and mediate specific cellular effects.

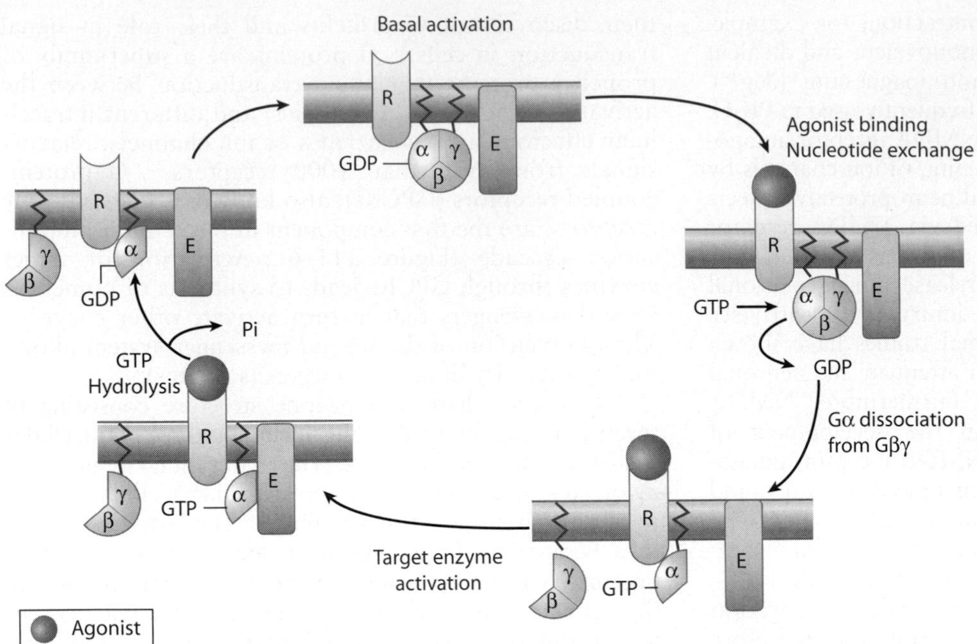

FIGURE 111–7 • Functional cycle of the G proteins. The receptor *(R)* becomes activated after binding an agonist. Guanosine diphosphate *(GDP)* bound to the G protein is replaced by guanosine triphosphate *(GTP)*, and the α subunit of the G protein dissociates from the βγ-subunit complex. The α subunit/GTP complex binds to the target enzyme *(E)* or ion channel. The GTPase activity of the α subunit is increased when the target enzyme or ion channel is bound, leading to hydrolysis of the bound GTP to GDP, whereupon the α subunit reunites with the βγ-subunit complex and the agonist dissociates from the receptor.

are inhibited by cholera toxin. In contrast, G_i proteins (made of α_i subunits) can inhibit adenylate cyclase and open K^+ channels and are inhibited by pertussis toxin. Agonists or antagonists of GPCRs, as well as agents that interfere with cellular pathways regulated by these receptors, are widely used in drug therapy.

Enzyme-Linked Receptors

This large and heterogeneous group of membrane receptors is mainly composed of kinase-linked receptors and guanylate cyclase-linked receptors. Enzyme-linked receptors have an extracellular ligand-binding domain linked to an intracellular domain that possesses intrinsic tyrosine kinase activity or

TABLE 111–2

Examples of Some G Protein–Coupled Receptors with Their Trimeric G Protein, Target Enzyme and/or Ion Channel, and Second Messengers

GPCRs	G Protein	Target Enzyme/Ion Channel	Second Messengers
α_1- and β_2- adrenergic D_1 H_2 V_2	G_s	↑ Adenylate cyclase	↑ cAMP
α_2-adrenergic M_2, M_4 μ opioid Chemokine AT_1	G_i	↓ Adenylate cyclase	↓ cAMP
α_1-adrenergic M_1, M_3, M_5 ET_A, ET_B AT_1 H_1 V_1	$G_{q/11}$	↑ Phospholipase C	↑ IP_3, DAG
μ opioid	$G_{i/o}$	Opens K^+ channels	
μ opioid	G_o	Closes voltage-dependent Ca^{2+} channels	↓ $[Ca^{2+}]_i$

AT, angiotensin; *cAMP*, cyclic adenosine monophosphate; *D*, dopaminergic; *DAG*, diacylglycerol; *ET*, endothelin; G_s, stimulatory G protein; G_i, inhibitory G protein; G_o, other G proteins; *GPCR*, G protein-coupled receptor; *H*, histamine; *IP3*, inositol 1,4,5-triphosphate; *M*, muscarinic; *V*, vasopressin.

guanylate cyclase activity. Cytosolic enzymes presenting an activity similar to that of enzyme-linked receptors also are considered to belong to this family of receptors (e.g., soluble guanylate cyclase receptors activated by nitric oxide [NO]).

Kinase-linked receptors include receptors for neurotrophin,[36] growth factors (epidermal growth factor, platelet-derived growth factor), certain cytokines, insulin, and many other trophic hormones. These receptors shift from an inactive monomeric state to an active dimeric state upon agonist binding (dimerization). This is followed by autophosphorylation of the intracellular domain of each receptor and binding of SH_2-domain proteins that themselves are phosphorylated. Depending on the receptor subtype, SH_2-domain proteins allow the phosphorylated receptor to activate other functional proteins, eventually resulting in stimulation of gene transcription, or are enzymes such as phospholipases, leading to the formation of second messengers (see later). Two important pathways involved in the transduction mechanisms of kinase-linked receptors are the Ras/Raf/MAP kinase pathway (Figure 111–8), which is important in cell division, growth, and differentiation, and the Jak/Stat pathway, which is activated by many cytokines and controls the synthesis and release of many inflammatory mediators. Unlike growth factor receptors, cytokine receptors usually do not possess intrinsic kinase activity. Instead, they associate with cytosolic kinases (Jaks) following the dimerization of receptors that occurs after cytokine binding. Then, Jak phosphorylates a family of transcription factors (stats) that, once phosphorylated, migrate in the nucleus and activate gene expression (see Chapters 83, 84, and 96).

Guanylate cyclase-linked receptors are particular because they synthesize their own second messengers upon agonist binding. The natriuretic peptide receptors, including atrial natriuretic peptide (ANP), brain natriuretic peptide (BNP), and C-type natriuretic peptide (CNP) receptors, belong to this family (Figure 111–9). The extracellular NH_2-terminal constitutes the binding domain. There is a short transmembrane segment whose role is to anchor the receptor protein to the membrane. The intracellular domain is made of two different entities: (1) a protein kinase homology domain whose function is to control and relay receptor activation to

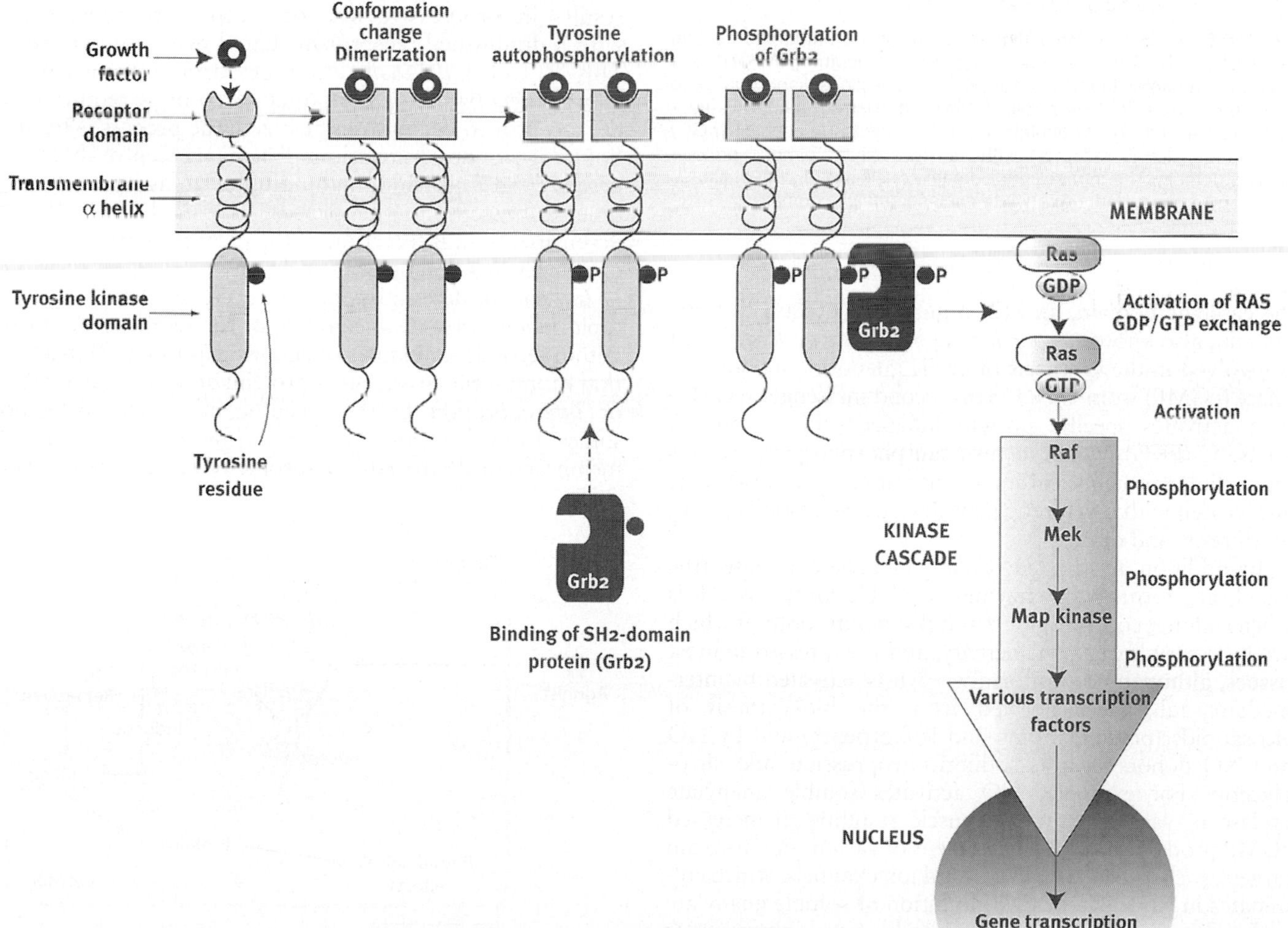

FIGURE 111–8 • Functioning of kinase-linked receptors. The main steps are dimerization of the receptor, autophosphorylation, and phosphorylation of targeted proteins. The growth factor pathway is shown with the kinase cascade involving the successive phosphorylation of many enzymes (Raf, Mek, Map kinase), eventually leading to gene transcription. *GDP,* Guanosine diphosphate; *GTP,* guanosine triphosphate. (Modified from Rang HP, Dale MM, Ritter JM, Moore PK: *Pharmacology,* ed 5, London, 2003, Churchill Livingstone.)

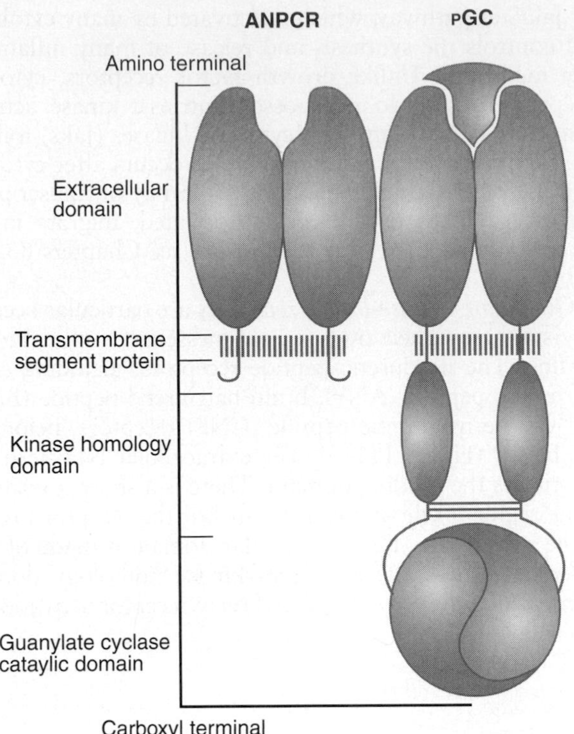

FIGURE 111–9 • Molecular structure of the natriuretic peptide receptors. **Left,** Atrial natriuretic peptide-C receptor *(ANPCR)* is a clearance receptor that does not possess the kinase and guanylate cyclase domains. It plays a role in the catabolism of natriuretic peptides. **Right,** Typical particulate guanylate cyclase receptor *(pGC)* (ANP-A or ANP-B receptor) with its extracellular dimeric protein-binding domain. The intracellular domain consists of a protein kinase homology domain and a guanylate cyclase catalytic domain.

the catalytic domain, and (2) a guanylate cyclase catalytic domain, also known as *particulate guanylate cyclase,* which is involved in the synthesis of cyclic guanosine monophosphate (cGMP) from GTP.[37] This second messenger (cGMP) then activates specific protein kinases, such as protein kinase G (PKG), which in turn can phosphorylate various intracellular proteins leading to the varieties of physiologic effects seen with natriuretic peptides such as vasodilatation, natriuresis, and diuresis.

In addition to the particulate guanylate cyclase (the membrane form of the enzyme), a soluble form exists. It is a heterodimer consisting of α and β subunits, both of which are necessary for enzyme activity, and is expressed in most tissues, although not uniformly.[38,39] It is activated by intermediate substances derived from the biosynthesis of eicosanoids (prostaglandins and leukotrienes) and by NO and NO donors such as sodium nitroprussiate and nitroglycerin. For example, NO activates soluble guanylate cyclase in vascular smooth muscle resulting in increased cGMP production with engagement of various downstream targets, such as protein kinases and ion channels, which culminates in vasodilatation.[40] Inhibition of soluble guanylate cyclase by agents such as methylene blue and intravascular destruction of NO by cell-free oxyhemoglobin (intravascular hemolysis) decrease cGMP production and promote vasoconstriction.[41]

Nuclear Receptors

Nuclear receptors belong to a family of functionally and structurally related proteins. They regulate gene expression and are not associated with a membrane. Their principal mechanism of action is shown in Figure 111–10. The agonist, which must be lipid soluble, diffuses into the cell and binds to the nuclear receptor, which becomes activated. The complex agonist-activated receptor then binds on high-affinity sites on DNA, the hormone response element (HRE), situated on the promoter region of genes whose transcription then can be induced or suppressed. Because gene transcription is at their origin, these effects are slow to develop.

Endogenous agonists for these receptors include steroid and thyroid hormones and agents such as retinoic acid and vitamin D. The most commonly used drugs that target these receptors include exogenous steroids and lipid-lowering agents. For many of these receptors, the corresponding hormone or vitamin has not been identified, so these receptors are referred to as *orphan nuclear receptors.*

Receptor Regulation

Continued exposure of a receptor to an agonist often results in progressive loss of receptor responsiveness, with a diminished receptor-mediated response over time. This is called *desensitization* or *tachyphylaxis.* When agonist occupancy of the target receptor is required for the receptor to become desensitized, the process is termed *homologous* desensitization. When a receptor becomes desensitized following the binding of an agonist to other types of receptors, the process is called *heterologous* desensitization. Interaction of the receptor with an antagonist prevents desensitization.

In general, desensitization can occur in three ways: (1) rapid *inactivation* or *uncoupling* of the receptor, occurring within seconds to minutes of agonist exposure; (2) inactivation of intracellular signaling protein; and (3) *sequestration* or *internalization* of the receptor in vesicles or endosomes; from there, the receptor can be recycled to the cell membrane or destroyed in lysosomes (Figure 111–11, *A*).[42]

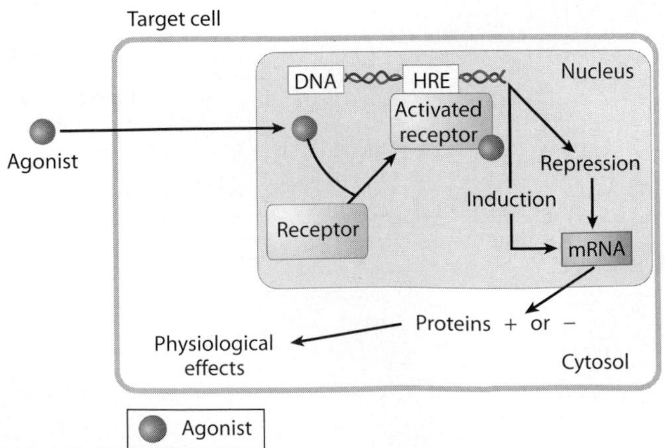

FIGURE 111–10 • Activation and action of nuclear receptors. *DNA,* deoxyribonucleic acid; *HRE,* hormone response element.

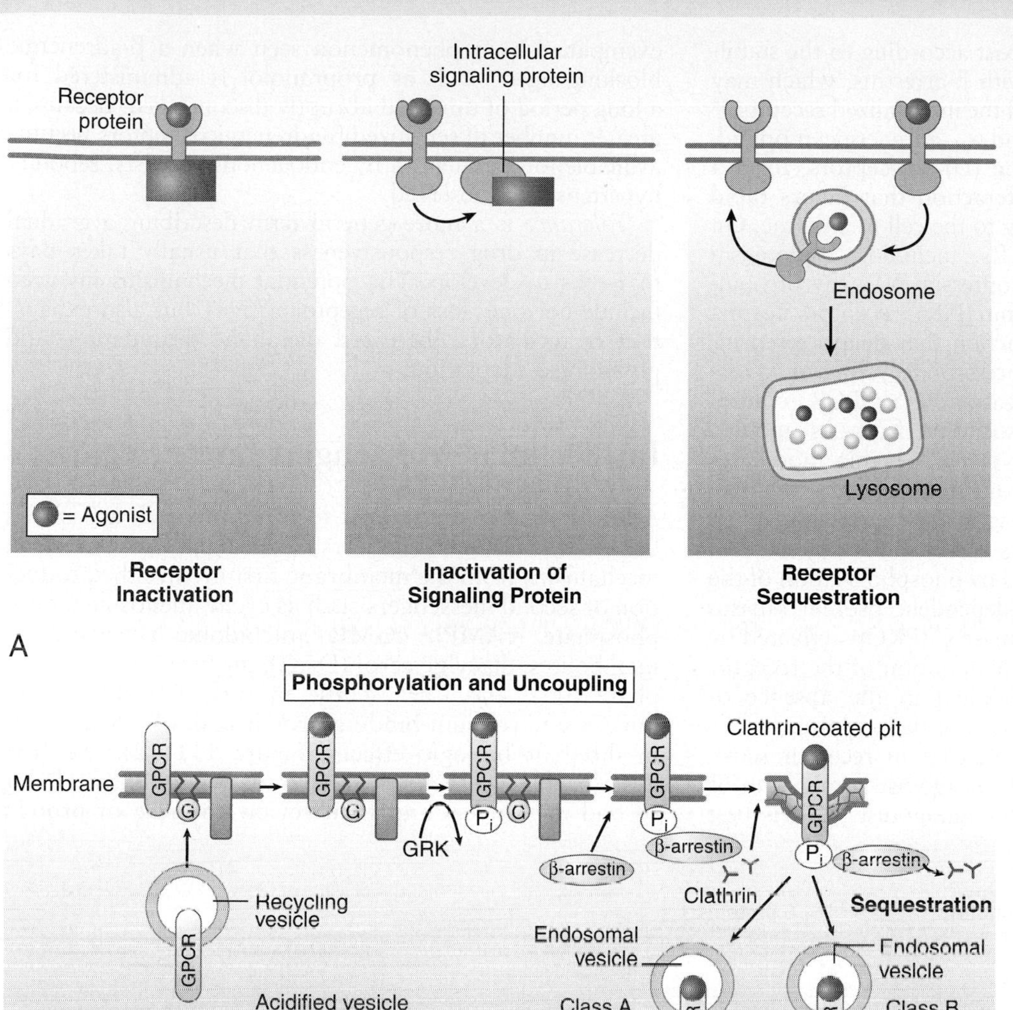

FIGURE 111–11 • Desensitization in response to an agonist. **A,** Ways in which receptors can become desensitized to an agonist. (Modified from Alberts B, Johnson A, Lewis J, Raff M, Roberts K, Walter P: *Molecular biology of the cell,* ed 4, 2002, New York, Garland Science.) **B,** Homologous desensitization of G protein-coupled-receptor *(GPCR).* See text for details. *E,* G protein effector; *G,* G protein; *GRK,* G protein-coupled receptor kinase. (Modified from Luttrell LM, Lefkowitz RJ. *J Cell Sci* 115:455-465, 2002.)

Down-regulation which takes hours to days, is characterized by a net loss of receptors at the cell membrane and develops more slowly than uncoupling. In addition to receptor degradation, decreased synthesis of the receptor contributes to this process.[43] Down-regulation is responsible for the decreased responsiveness to prolonged exogenous catecholamine infusion frequently seen in the critical care population.[44] Desensitization is usually reversible, within minutes (inactivation) to hours (sequestration/down-regulation) of removal of the agonist depending on the specific receptor and cell type, the concentration of the agonist, and the duration of exposure to the agonist.

The decreased responsiveness of GPCRs in the continued presence of an agonist results from three distinct and coordinated processes: receptor inactivation, sequestration, and down-regulation.[45] Desensitization of GPCRs begins within seconds of exposure to the agonist and is initiated by phosphorylation of the receptor. Homologous desensitization of GPCRs depends on phosphorylation of the receptor by specific kinases: G protein-coupled receptor kinases (GRKs) (Figure 111–11, *B*). Once phosphorylated, the receptor binds with high affinity to members of the arrestin gene family, the β-arrestins. The β-arrestin binding prevents receptor–G protein interaction, leading to termination of signaling by G protein effectors. The receptor-bound β-arrestin also can act as an adapter protein to couple the receptor to clathrin-coated pits, inducing receptor-mediated endocytosis or sequestration. Subsequently, the receptor is either recycled to the cell membrane or degraded (down-regulation of the receptor). Some evidence indicates that two distinct classes of GPCRs exist according to the stability of the complex they form with β-arrestins, which may play a role in dictating the fate of the internalized receptor.[46] Class A GPCRs, including β_2- and α_{1B}-adrenergic, μ opioid, endothelin $(ET)_A$, and dopamine $(D)_{1A}$ receptors, form a transient receptor–β-arrestin interaction that favors rapid dephosphorylation and recycling to the cell membrane. On the other hand, class B GPCRs, including angiotensin (AT_{1a}), neurotensin (NT_1) , vasopressin $(V)_2$, thyrotropin-releasing hormone, and neurokinin $(NK)_1$ receptors, form a stable receptor–β-arrestin interaction that delays resensitization and either slows the process of recycling or favors receptor degradation. Resensitization of a GPCR requires its dephosphorylation and dissociation from its agonist. Interestingly, data show that hypoxia/ischemia modulates GRK and β-arrestin in the neonatal rat brain and may contribute to hypoxia/ischemia–induced brain damage.[47]

In contrast to homologous desensitization, heterologous desensitization is initiated by phosphorylation of the receptor by second messenger-dependent protein kinases (protein kinase A and protein kinase C [PKC]) activated by any receptor system. Such phosphorylation of the receptor impairs receptor–G protein coupling in the absence of β-arrestins and leads to inactivation of the receptor.

Up-regulation refers to the increase in receptor sensitivity seen in the setting of lack of agonist stimulation or prolonged presence of a receptor antagonist. This is best exemplified by a phenomenon seen when a β-adrenergic blocking agent such as propranolol is administered for a long period of time and abruptly discontinued. Because a greater number of sensitized β-adrenergic receptors become available for stimulation by endogenous agonists, rebound hypertension is observed.

Tolerance is a more general term describing a gradual decrease in drug responsiveness that usually takes days to weeks to develop. The potential mechanisms involved include not only loss of receptor activity but also exhaustion of mediators, increased metabolic degradation, and physiologic adaptation.

Intracellular Messengers and Effectors

After binding of an agonist to receptors such as GPCRs or enzyme-linked receptors, the signal transduction mechanisms from the membrane first involve the production of second messengers such as cyclic adenosine monophosphate (cAMP), cGMP, arachidonic acid and its metabolites, diacylglycerol (DAG), inositol 1,4,5-triphosphate (IP_3), and Ca^{2+}. These in turn activate protein kinases and calcium-binding proteins, all of which result in different biologic effects (Figure 111–12). We first describe the synthesis and degradation of intracellular second messengers and then review the role of protein

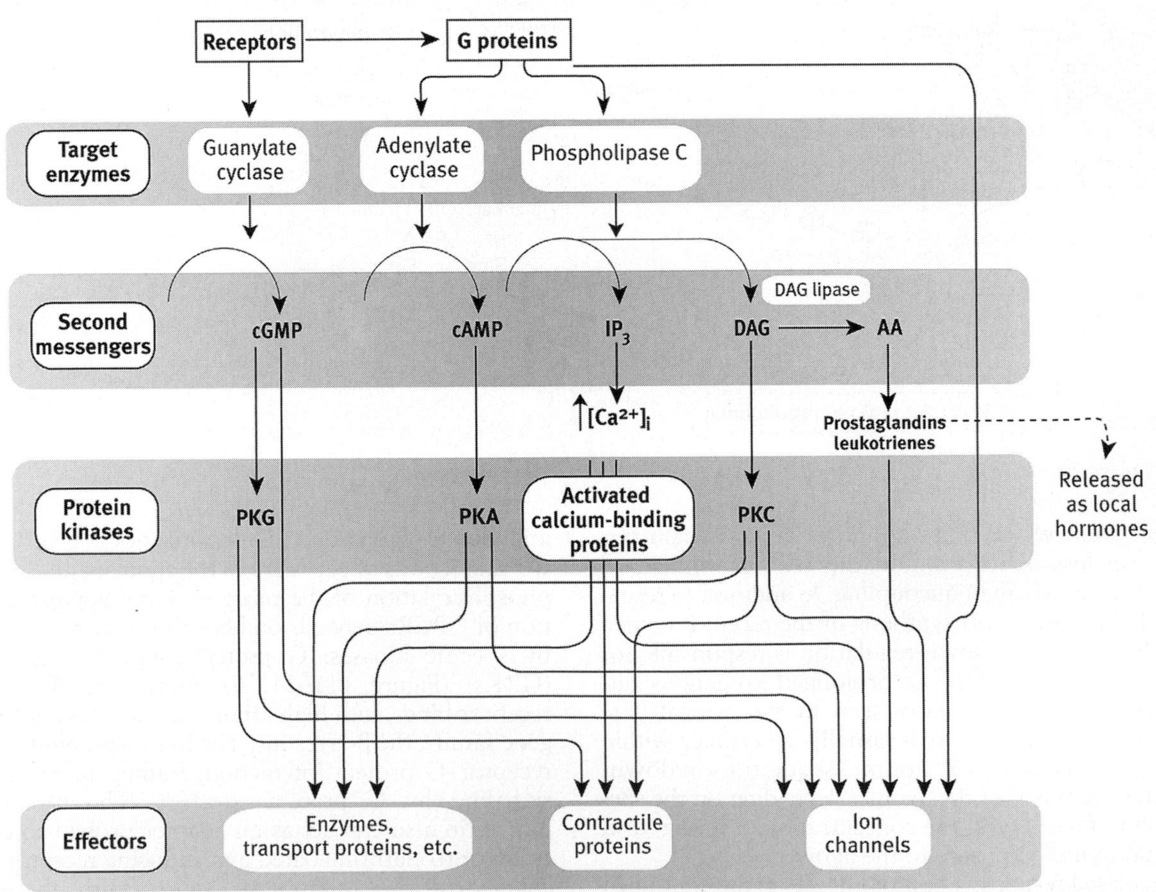

FIGURE 111–12 • Transduction mechanisms of membrane signaling. *AA,* Arachidonic acid; *cAMP,* cyclic adenosine monophosphate; *cGMP,* cyclic guanosine monophosphate; *DAG,* diacylglycerol; *IP_3,* inositol triphosphate; *PKA,* protein kinase A; *PKC,* protein kinase C; *PKG,* protein kinase G. (Modified from Rang HP, Dale MM, Ritter JM, Moore PK: *Pharmacology,* ed 5, London, 2003, Churchill Livingstone.)

kinases and calcium-binding proteins in the transduction mechanisms.

Second Messengers

Cyclic Adenosine Monophosphate

This pathway is involved in signal transduction initiated by binding of agonists to GPCRs. Cyclic AMP is synthesized from adenosine triphosphate (ATP) after the action of adenylate cyclase, which is a transmembrane glycoprotein of the cell membrane. Nine forms of adenylate cyclase (types I–IX) have been identified using molecular cloning, and several have described features that are hypothetical.[48] Cyclic AMP regulates many aspects of cellular function (cell division and differentiation, ion transport) by one common mechanism involving activation of protein kinases. These, in turn, regulate the function of many different cellular proteins by catalyzing the phosphorylation of serine and threonine residues. Phosphorylation can then either activate or inhibit target enzymes or ion channels.[14] As mentioned previously, receptors coupled with G_s proteins stimulate adenylate cyclase and produce an increase in cAMP, whereas receptors coupled with G_i proteins inhibit adenylate cyclase and reduce cAMP.

Degradation of cAMP is catalyzed by phosphodiesterases leading to production of 5′-AMP, an inactive product. Phosphodiesterases are a complex family of enzymes currently divided into 11 groups according to their mechanism of regulation, their selectivity for the substrate (cAMP and/or cGMP), their preferential localization, and their sensitivity to various inhibitors.[49] In critically ill children, amrinone and milrinone, used for their positive inotropic effect and vasodilating properties, are phosphodiesterase inhibitors selective for the type III isoenzyme.

Cyclic Guanosine Monophosphate

Guanylate cyclase is part of the cytosolic portion of some transmembrane receptors (membrane form) but also exists as a cytosolic enzyme (soluble form), activated by various molecules including NO. Stimulation of guanylate cyclase and the resultant accumulation of cGMP regulates complex signaling cascades through immediate downstream effectors, including cGMP-dependent protein kinases (PKG), cGMP-regulated phosphodiesterases (mainly type II and III), and cyclic nucleotide-gated ion channels (cells of the retina).[50] Guanylate cyclases and cGMP-mediated signaling cascades play a central role in the regulation of diverse pathophysiologic processes, including vascular smooth muscle motility, intestinal fluid and electrolyte homeostasis, and retinal phototransduction.

As with cAMP, degradation of cGMP into inactive GMP is catalyzed by phosphodiesterases. In vascular smooth muscle cells, phosphodiesterase type V is responsible for degradation of cGMP. Inhibition of this enzyme results in accumulation of cGMP in the cytosol with smooth muscle relaxation and vasodilatation. Phosphodiesterase type V inhibitors (e.g., sildenafil), widely recognized as efficacious for treatment of erectile dysfunction in men, induce pulmonary vasodilatation in both children and adults and are part of the new strategies available for treatment of pulmonary hypertension.[51–54]

Arachidonic Acid and Its Metabolites

Arachidonic acid and its metabolites (prostaglandins and leukotrienes) now are considered intracellular messengers.[55] Arachidonic acid is a component of membrane phospholipids released in either a one-step process, after phospholipase A_2 (PLA_2) action, or a two-step process, after phospholipase C and DAG lipase actions. Arachidonic acid then is metabolized by cyclooxygenase (COX) and 5-lipoxygenase, resulting in synthesis of prostaglandins and leukotrienes, respectively. These intracellular messengers play an important role in the regulation of signal transduction implicated in pain and inflammatory responses. Corticosteroids inhibit PLA_2 activity, whereas nonsteroidal antiinflammatory drugs inhibit COX activity.

Diacylglycerol and Inositol Triphosphate

Phospholipase C is the target enzyme for some GPCRs (phospholipase C-β) and for enzyme-linked receptors such as tyrosine kinase receptors (phospholipase C-γ). It splits phosphatidylinositol, a membrane-bound phospholipid, into DAG and IP_3, both of which function as second messengers. The most important function of DAG is to activate the membrane-bound PKC, which catalyzes the phosphorylation of a variety of intracellular proteins. IP_3 binds to and opens an IP_3-gated Ca^{2+}-release channel on the endoplasmic reticulum membrane, resulting in an increase in intracellular Ca^{2+} concentration ($[Ca^{2+}]_i$).

Calcium Ions

$[Ca^{2+}]_i$ is critically important as a regulator of cell function. An increase in $[Ca^{2+}]_i$ is the most important intracellular messenger signaling pathway known in biologic systems. When $[Ca^{2+}]_i$ is at its baseline value, few proteins have an affinity sufficient to bind to Ca^{2+}. Membrane signaling results in an increase in $[Ca^{2+}]_i$, derived from either the extracellular space or the lumen of the endoplasmic reticulum, which then allows binding of proteins to Ca^{2+}. Finally, this binding can trigger contraction, secretion, a modification in metabolism regulation, or several other effects, depending on the cell type involved. To maintain a low resting $[Ca^{2+}]_i$, Ca^{2+} is permanently expulsed from the cytosol into the extracellular compartment or into the endoplasmic reticulum, via a Ca^{2+}-ATPase and Na^+/Ca^{2+} exchanger.

Phosphorylation of Proteins

Many receptor-mediated signals produce variations in the concentration of second messengers, such as cAMP, cGMP, arachidonic acid, DAG, IP_3, and Ca^{2+}. These second messengers can modify the activity of other proteins, mainly protein kinases and calcium-binding proteins.

Protein Kinases

Protein kinases, which are located in the cytoplasm, are enzymes that phosphorylate proteins. The main protein kinases are PKA, PKG, PKC,[56] and tyrosyl protein kinases (part of tyrosine kinase receptors). They are distinguished from each other by the different intracellular second messengers involved in their regulation and by the selective substrates they use. They all have a binding site for Mg^{2+}-ATP (phosphate donor), substrate protein, and various regulatory sites. Phosphorylation of these proteins is short lived, as protein phosphatases rapidly dephosphorylate proteins previously phosphorylated by protein kinases, thus terminating the intracellular signal.

Calcium-Binding Proteins

Calcium exerts its control on cellular function by virtue of its ability to regulate the activity of many different proteins, such as channels, transporters, and transcription factors. In the majority of cases, a calcium-binding protein serves as an intermediate between Ca^{2+} and the regulated functional protein. Calcium-binding proteins represent a large group of cytosolic proteins and include the calmodulin and annexin (or lipocortin) families.

Drug Response and Genetic Polymorphisms

The same medication, at a given dose, frequently can produce different responses with respect to efficacy and toxicity in different patients. This is termed *interindividual variability.* It is estimated that genetic factors can account for 20% to 95% of variability in drug disposition and effects.[57] Pharmacogenetics is the field that studies the role of inheritance in the individual variation in drug response. Pharmacogenomics is the field that uses genome-wide approaches to elucidate the inherited basis of differences between individuals in their responses to various drugs. Most genetic variations involve single-nucleotide polymorphisms (SNPs), the exchange of a single nucleotide in the DNA sequence. Small insertions and deletions, variable-number tandem repeats, gene deletions, and gene duplications also occur. Depending on where SNPs occur, they can result in no change in the protein amino acid sequence (silent polymorphism or synonymous SNP), a change in the coded amino acid sequence (nonsynonymous SNP) that can have no functional consequence, or altered protein function. The latter can have significant clinical and/or therapeutic implications. In addition, given that genes often present many SNPs, it is increasingly recognized that single SNPs fail to predict drug responses, whereas combinations of SNPs on a given chromosome (specific haplotype) are clinically more significant and can better determine drug effects.[58]

Each person has two alleles for each gene, one from each parent. The dominant wild-type allele from one parent may be expressed more than the recessive mutant allele from the other parent. Two identical alleles result in a homozygous dominant or recessive trait of that gene, whereas a combination of two different alleles leads to a heterozygous trait. Thus a particular protein, such as an enzyme or a receptor, encoded by a gene with polymorphism may be expressed in different amounts. Therefore it is easy to comprehend that a drug response can be altered by genetic polymorphisms occurring in genes that encode drug-metabolizing enzymes, drug targets (e.g., receptors, enzymes), drug transporters, and/or proteins involved in signal transduction[59] (see Chapter 92).

Genetic Polymorphisms and Drug Disposition

Many major enzymes involved in phase I and II drug metabolism have known polymorphisms leading to phenotypic differences, that is, clinically significant alteration in drug-metabolizing enzyme activities.[60] For a specific drug-metabolizing enzyme (e.g., CYP2C19), homozygous individuals for the wild-type allele exhibit the greatest enzymatic activity (extensive metabolizers), heterozygous individuals have intermediate enzymatic activity (heterozygous extensive metabolizers), and homozygous individuals with the mutant allele have low enzymatic activity (poor metabolizers). The clinical consequences of such polymorphisms may be threefold: (1) in contrast to extensive metabolizers, poor metabolizers can have an enhanced drug effect than can be therapeutic or toxic as a result of higher plasma concentrations of a given drug; (2) diminished drug effect can be seen in extensive metabolizers who may have ultrarapid metabolism, which results in markedly lower plasma concentrations of a given drug and thus inadequate therapeutic response; and (3) diminished drug effect can be seen in poor metabolizers as a result of the inability of a prodrug to be converted into the active molecule because of low enzymatic activity. All these effects must be considered to appropriately adjust drug dosing.

Genetic Polymorphisms, Drug Targets, and Signaling Mechanisms

Genetic polymorphisms in signaling mechanisms involving GPCRs and enzymes have been identified.[61–63] These polymorphisms can result in either decreased or enhanced agonist efficacy and can influence drug response. Mutations in G proteins cause certain diseases.[64] The genetic variation occurring in the genes of β_1- and β_2-adrenergic receptors and the G protein β_3 subunit are good examples of how polymorphisms in drug target and signal transduction genes can alter drug effects. These polymorphisms can potentially affect the pharmacologic response of drugs commonly used in the PICU, such as epinephrine, norepinephrine, dobutamine, and salbutamol.

β_1-Adrenergic Receptor Polymorphisms

The β_1-adrenergic receptor is coupled to the stimulatory G protein G_s, which mediates chronotropic and inotropic responses to catecholamines via an increase in cAMP. Two nonsynonymous SNPs [serine (Ser) to glycine (Gly) substitution at codon 49 and arginine (Arg) to glycine (Gly) substitution at codon 389) occur in the gene encoding the β_1-adrenergic receptor.[65] *In vitro* studies suggest that both polymorphisms have functional consequences. The Gly49 form of the receptor results in greater agonist-promoted down-regulation than the Ser49 form,[66,67] and the Arg389 form of the receptor results in twofold to threefold higher basal and agonist-stimulated adenylate cyclase activity than form of the receptor results in twofold to threefold higher basal and agonist-stimulated adenylate cyclase activity than the Gly389 form.[68] In vivo studies demonstrate that these polymorphisms, either as single SNP or haplotype (the array of SNPs on a given chromosome), are important determinants of the antihypertensive response to β-adrenergic receptor blockade. Individuals homozygous for Arg at codon 389 experience a significantly larger decrease in blood pressure in response to atenolol and metoprolol compared with those who carry the variant allele.[69,70] The underlying hypothesis is that hypertensive patients who are homozygous for Arg389 have hypertension predominantly mediated through the adrenergic nervous system and thus have a greater antihypertensive response to β-adrenergic receptor blockers.

Of specific interest for the care of critically ill patients, an in vitro study using isolated human myocardial tissue expressing receptor variants of the Arg389Gly polymorphism showed significantly increased inotropic potency to norepinephrine in tissue from individuals homozygous for Arg at codon 389 compared with individuals homozygous for Gly at codon 389. Tissue cAMP levels also were greater in the former group, whereas cAMP-dependent protein kinase activity was the same in both variants.[71]

β_2-Adrenergic Receptor Polymorphisms

The β_2-adrenergic receptor is a GPCR of the stimulatory G_s subtype, which mediates bronchodilation and vasodilation upon agonist stimulation. Four nonsynonymous SNPs in its coding gene and one nonsynonymous SNP in the 5′ leader cistron sequence, which encodes a peptide modulating receptor translation, have been identified (Figure 111–13).[72,73] In addition, SNPs in the 5′ promoter region have been identified and appear to alter β_2-adrenergic receptor gene expression.[74]

Cell-based and transgenic mouse-based mechanistic studies evaluating the phenotypic consequences of a given SNP in isolation have shown that (1) a SNP at amino acid position 16 results in increased agonist-promoted downregulation of the β_2-adrenergic receptor, (2) a SNP at amino acid position 27 abolishes agonist-induced downregulation of the β_2-adrenergic receptor, (3) a SNP at amino acid position 164 results in a markedly dysfunctional β_2-adrenergic receptor with altered high-affinity binding and decreased coupling to the stimulatory G_s, and (4) a SNP at amino acid position 47 results in increased receptor expression.[73,75,76] Some in vivo studies showed a correlation between individual SNPs and the bronchodilatory response to β-adrenergic receptor agonists or the extent of tachyphylaxis with chronic use of these agents, whereas others failed to show any correlation or showed discordant results. Because more than one SNP on the β_2-adrenergic receptor gene may be present in a given individual and interactions between SNPs may occur, determination of the effect of haplotypes appears to provide the greatest amount of genetic information. Drysdale et al.[58] showed that complex promoter and coding region β_2-adrenergic receptor haplotypes alter receptor expression and predict in vivo responsiveness. They determined the relevance of the five most common β_2-adrenergic receptor haplotype pairs by assessing the bronchodilator response to β-adrenergic receptor agonists in asthmatics. Response was significantly related to haplotype pairs but not to individual SNPs, and mean responses by haplotype pairs varied by more than twofold.

G Protein β_3-Subunit Polymorphism

A SNP in the gene encoding the β_3 subunit of trimeric G proteins (GNB3) consisting of the exchange of cytidine for thymidine at position 825 (C825T) in the cDNA has been described.[77] This change was found to be associated with a shortened slice variant of the G protein β_3 subunit that gives rise to enhanced signal transduction via pertussis toxin-sensitive G proteins.[78] α_2-Adrenergic receptors are the prototype of receptors coupled to these G proteins.[79] At present, the recognized clinical consequences of this polymorphism are (1) positive associations with certain conditions, such as obesity, essential hypertension in Caucasians and Blacks, stroke, and myocardial infarction, and (2) alterations in drug response. Compared with 825CC homozygous individuals, 825T allele carriers have a more pronounced decrease in blood pressure upon administration of thiazide diuretics and clonidine, enhanced improvement

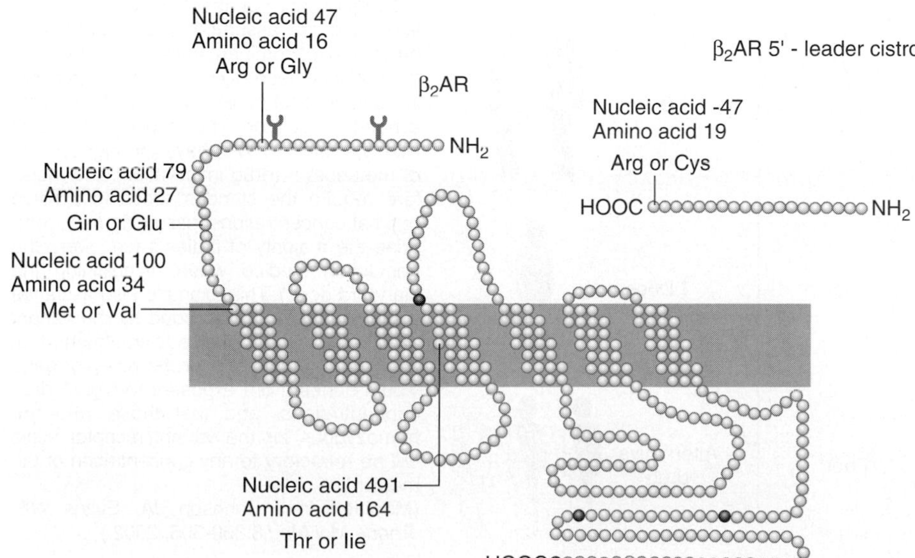

FIGURE 111–13 • Amino acid sequence of human β_2-adrenergic receptor and its 5′ leader cistron. Shown are the location of polymorphisms in the deoxyribonucleic acid (DNA) sequence that result in variation in amino acids at the indicated positions. *Darkened circles* indicate codons where the DNA sequence is variable but does not result in variation in the encoded amino acid. *Arg,* Arginine; *Cys,* cysteine; *Gln,* glutamine; *Glu,* glutamic acid; *Gly,* glycine; *Ile,* isoleucine; *Met,* methionine; *Thr,* threonine; *Val,* valine. (Modified from Liggett SB: *Am J Respir Crit Care Med* 161:S197-S201, 2000.)

of symptoms upon treatment with different antidepressants, and improved erectile response to sildenafil.[12,80,81] Many more SNPs have been identified in the gene encoding GNB3, and major haplotypes have been determined, but their functional consequences, if any exist, are not yet described.[82]

Summary

The future for predicting the impact of genetic variation on drug response most likely lies in a polygenic approach that considers the influence of variability in multiple genes rather than analysis of single genes alone (Figure 111–14). Studies evaluating the effects of SNPs for a given gene will need to consider specific haplotypes or combination of haplotypes because individual SNPs may have poor predictive power as pharmacogenetic loci.

Drug Response and Development

As Dr. Abraham Jacobi, the father of American pediatrics, once wrote, "Pediatrics does not deal with miniature men and women, with reduced doses and the same class of disease in smaller bodies, but . . . has its own independent range and horizon."[83] From birth through puberty, dramatic developmental changes occur that can have a profound impact on drug disposition and action.

Most studies have evaluated the effect of age on pharmacokinetics, revealing clinically important differences compared with adults.[84,85] The ontogenesis of important drug-metabolizing enzymes, the cytochrome P450 enzymes (Figure 111–15),[86–90] is a good example of how development affects drug disposition and how age is an important determinant in selecting appropriate doses.

Developmental changes are expected to affect the different players involved in pharmacodynamics. This area of research is in its "neonatal" period, and few data on the ontogenesis of specific drug targets, signal transduction mechanisms, and intracellular messengers are available. To date, human studies have mainly dealt with receptor expression (and not function), mostly in the brain, and have found age-related differences in terms of both receptor density and regions of the brain where receptors are expressed.[91–96] One study also evaluated postnatal ontogenesis of G proteins and GTP binding in the frontal cortex of postmortem human brains.[97] The study showed a steep increase in the amounts of G_o at approximately age 2 years and a similar tendency for G_s, G_i, and G_q. Moreover, GTP binding of G_s, G_i, and G_o also transiently increased at approximately age 2 years. The exact consequences of all these differences are unknown, but they are speculated to play a role in organ maturation and in the pathophysiology of diseases and drug response.

Drug Response and Disease

A vast literature exists on the effects of diseases on drug pharmacokinetics, but limited data are available on pharmacodynamic changes occurring as a consequence of illness. Of particular interest for the critically ill population is the association between myocardial hyporesponsiveness to

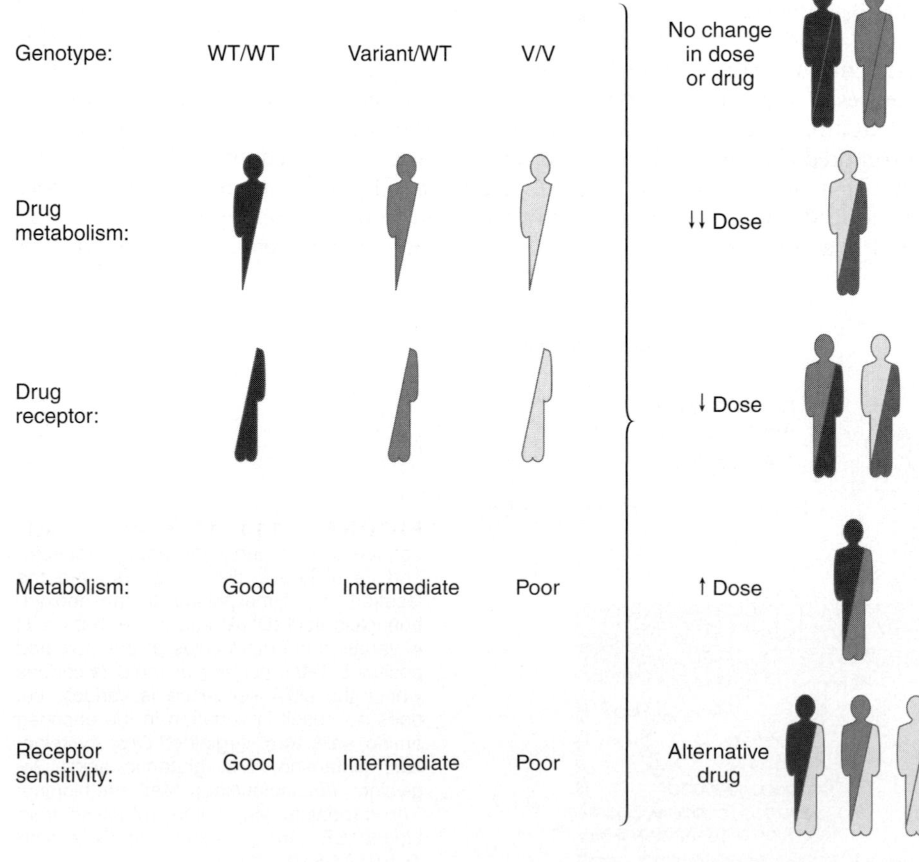

FIGURE 111–14 • Patient genotypes and treatment modifications. The simplest form of polygenic drug response is illustrated, where the genes encoding the predominant pathway for drug inactivation and the principal receptor for pharmacologic effects exhibit genetic polymorphism that has functional consequences. For the purpose of illustration, both are assumed to be inherited as autosomal codominant traits, with the variant form of each gene *(V)* encoding a protein that is nonfunctional or less sensitive to the prescribed medication. Thus those who inherit wild-type alleles *(WT)* have the highest rate of metabolism (drug inactivation) and therefore require the standard dose to achieve optimal concentrations, assuming they comprise the majority of patients (i.e., were the population studied when establishing the standard dose). This example also assumes that drug receptors encoded by the variant allele are less responsive to treatment, that patients heterozygous for the receptor gene would benefit from exposure to higher drug concentrations, and that those who are homozygous for the variant receptor allele will be refractory to any concentration of the medication.
(Modified from Johnson JA, Evans WE: *Trends Mol Med* 8:300-305, 2002.)

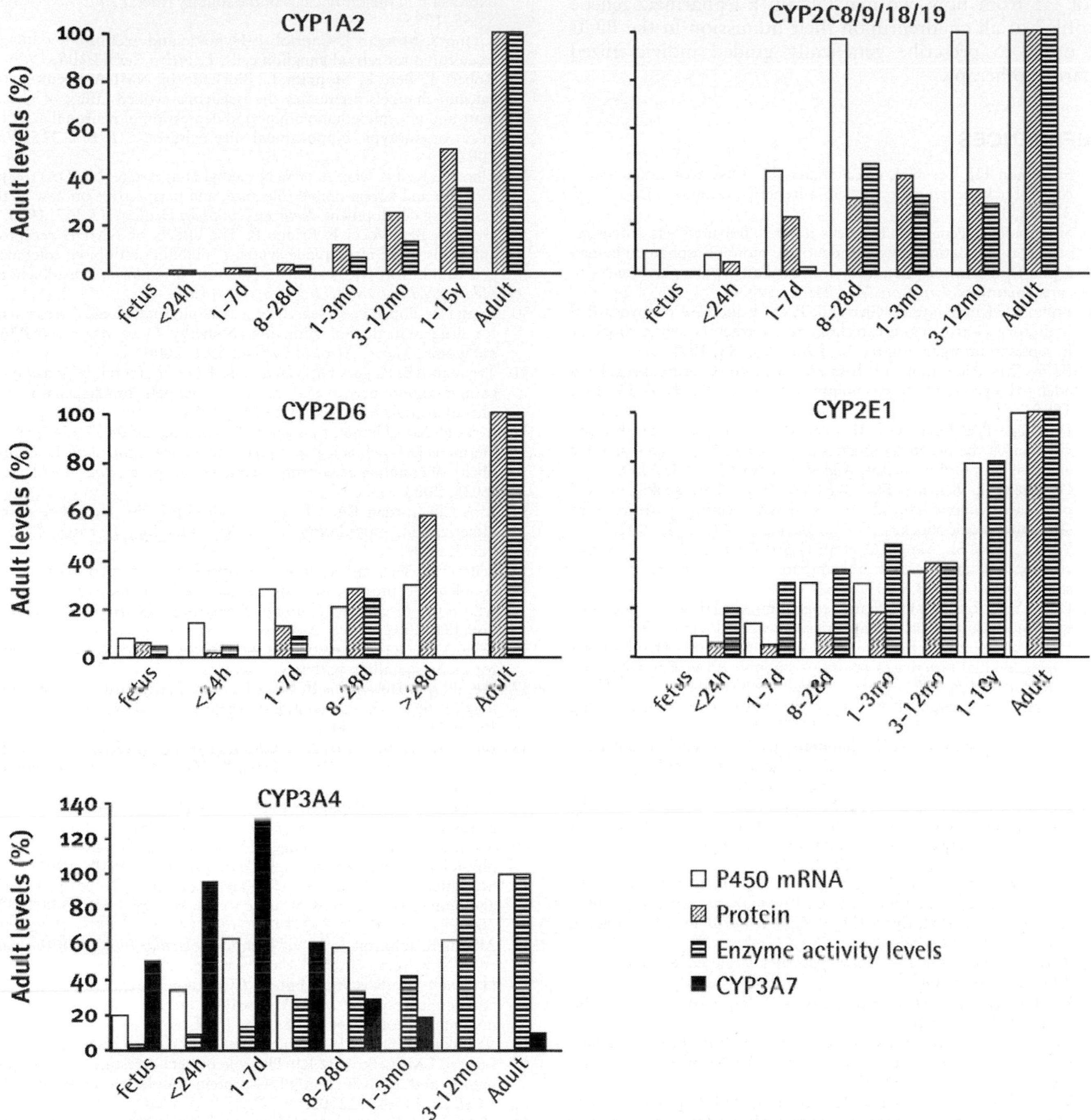

FIGURE 111–15 • Ontogenesis of cytochrome P450 *(CYP)* mRNA, protein, and enzyme activity levels in the human liver. All data are expressed as percentage of adult levels. *d,* Day; *h,* hour; *mo,* month; *y,* year. (Adapted from Alcorn J, McNamara PJ: *Clin Pharmacokinet* 41: 959-998, 2002.)

dobutamine during human septic shock and β-adrenergic receptor dysfunction.[2] One postulated mechanism is alterations distal to the β-adrenergic receptor (G protein or adenylate cyclase), possibly mediated by circulating cytokines.[98,99] An animal study supports the theory of postreceptor alterations. In the rat heart during the late hypodynamic phase of sepsis, myocardial G_i protein levels were increased with a reduction in adenylate cyclase activity.[7]

Conclusion

Even though our knowledge of how drugs work at a molecular level has grown tremendously over the past decade, continued elucidation of normal signal transduction physiology and of the effects of genetics, development, and disease states on the functional integrity of receptors, signaling pathways, and effectors should improve and refine pharmacologic interventions administered to critically ill children.

Not far from now, we may obtain a "pharmacogenetic profile" in all children upon their admission in the PICU in order to prescribe genetically guided individualized pharmacotherapy.

REFERENCES

1. Silverman HJ, Lee NH, el-Fakahany EE: Effects of canine endotoxin shock on lymphocytic beta-adrenergic receptors, *Circ Shock* 32:293, 1990.
2. Silverman HJ, Penaranda R, Orens JB, et al: Impaired beta-adrenergic receptor stimulation of cyclic adenosine monophosphate in human septic shock: association with myocardial hyporesponsiveness to catecholamines, *Crit Care Med* 21:31, 1993.
3. Bohm M, Kirchmayr R, Gierschik P, et al: Increase of myocardial inhibitory G-proteins in catecholamine-refractory septic shock or in septic multiorgan failure, *Am J Med* 98:183, 1995.
4. Bohm M: Alterations of beta-adrenoceptor-G-protein-regulated adenylyl cyclase in heart failure, *Mol Cell Biochem* 147:147, 1995.
5. De Paepe P, Belpaire FM, Rosseel MT, et al: Influence of hypovolemia on the pharmacokinetics and the electroencephalographic effect of propofol in the rat, *Anesthesiology* 93:1482, 2000.
6. De Paepe P, Belpaire FM, Buylaert WA: Pharmacokinetic and pharmacodynamic considerations when treating patients with sepsis and septic shock, *Clin Pharmacokinet* 41:1135, 2002.
7. Wu LL, Yang SL, Yang RC, et al: G protein and adenylate cyclase complex-mediated signal transduction in the rat heart during sepsis, *Shock* 19:533, 2003.
8. Evans WE, Relling MV: Pharmacogenomics: translating functional genomics into rational therapeutics, *Science* 286:487, 1999.
9. Evans WE, Johnson JA: Pharmacogenomics: the inherited basis for interindividual differences in drug response, *Annu Rev Genomics Hum Genet* 2:9, 2001.
10. Roden DM, George AL Jr: The genetic basis of variability in drug responses, *Nat Rev Drug Discov* 1:37, 2002.
11. Turner ST, Schwartz GL, Chapman AB, et al: C825T polymorphism of the G protein beta(3)-subunit and antihypertensive response to a thiazide diuretic, *Hypertension* 37:739, 2001.
12. Nurnberger J, Dammer S, Mitchell A, et al: Effect of the C825T polymorphism of the G protein beta 3 subunit on the systolic blood pressure-lowering effect of clonidine in young, healthy male subjects, *Clin Pharmacol Ther* 74:53, 2003.
13. Serretti A, Artioli P: Predicting response to lithium in mood disorders: role of genetic polymorphisms, *Am J Pharmacogenomics* 3:17, 2003.
14. Rang HP, Dale MM, Ritter JM, et al: *Pharmacology*, ed 5, London, 2003, Churchill Livingstone.
15. Katzung BG: *Basic & clinical pharmacology*, ed 8, New York, 2001, McGraw-Hill.
16. Kenakin TP: *Pharmacological analysis of drug-receptor interaction*, ed 2, 1993, Lippincott-Raven.
17. Tweddell JS, Hoffman GM, Fedderly RT, et al: Phenoxybenzamine improves systemic oxygen delivery after the Norwood procedure, *Ann Thorac Surg* 67:161, 1999.
18. Tweddell JS, Hoffman GM, Mussatto KA, et al: Improved survival of patients undergoing palliation of hypoplastic left heart syndrome: lessons learned from 115 consecutive patients, *Circulation* 106:I82, 2002.
19. Birnbaumer M: Vasopressin receptors, *Trends Endocrinol Metab* 11:406, 2000.
20. O'Blenes SB, Roy N, Konstantinov I, et al: Vasopressin reversal of phenoxybenzamine-induced hypotension after the Norwood procedure, *J Thorac Cardiovasc Surg* 123:1012, 2002.
21. Kenakin T: Inverse, protean, and ligand-selective agonism: matters of receptor conformation, *FASEB J* 15:598, 2001.
22. Jantzen JP: [Cerebral neuroprotection and ketamine], *Anaesthesist* 43(suppl 2):S41, 1994.
23. Fitzal S: [Ketamine and neuroprotection. Clinical outlook], Philadelphia, *Anaesthesist* 46(suppl 1):S65, 1997.
24. Yassin M, Scholfield CN: NMDA antagonists increase recovery of evoked potentials from slices of rat olfactory cortex after anoxia, *Br J Pharmacol* 111:1221, 1994.
25. Haxhiu MA, Strohl KP, Cherniack NS: The N-methyl-D-aspartate receptor pathway is involved in hypoxia-induced c-Fos protein expression in the rat nucleus of the solitary tract, *J Auton Nerv Syst* 55:65, 1995.
26. Kitano S, Morgan J, Caprioli J: Hypoxic and excitotoxic damage to cultured rat retinal ganglion cells, *Exp Eye Res* 63:105, 1996.
27. Robert F, Bert L, Stoppini L: Blockade of NMDA-receptors or calcium-channels attenuates the ischaemia-evoked efflux of glutamate and phosphoethanolamine and depression of neuronal activity in rat organotypic hippocampal slice cultures, *C R Biol* 325:495, 2002.
28. Elliott K, Kest B, Man A, et al: N-methyl-D-aspartate (NMDA) receptors, mu and kappa opioid tolerance, and perspectives on new analgesic drug development, *Neuropsychopharmacology* 13:347, 1995.
29. Herman BH, Vocci F, Bridge P: The effects of NMDA receptor antagonists and nitric oxide synthase inhibitors on opioid tolerance and withdrawal. Medication development issues for opiate addiction, *Neuropsychopharmacology* 13:269, 1995.
30. Bisaga A, Popik P: In search of a new pharmacological treatment for drug and alcohol addiction: N-methyl-D-aspartate (NMDA) antagonists, *Drug Alcohol Depend* 59:1, 2000.
31. Twyman RE, Rogers CJ, Macdonald RL: Differential regulation of gamma-aminobutyric acid receptor channels by diazepam and phenobarbital, *Ann Neurol* 25:213, 1989.
32. Coles H: Nobel honours pursuit of G proteins, *Nature* 371:547, 1994.
33. Hermans E: Biochemical and pharmacological control of the multiplicity of coupling at G-protein-coupled receptors, *Pharmacol Ther* 99:25, 2003.
34. Rios CD, Jordan BA, Gomes I, et al: G-protein-coupled receptor dimerization: modulation of receptor function, *Pharmacol Ther* 92:71, 2001.
35. Seifert R, Wenzel-Seifert K: Constitutive activity of G-protein-coupled receptors: cause of disease and common property of wild-type receptors, *Naunyn Schmiedebergs Arch Pharmacol* 366:381, 2002.
36. Chao MV: Neurotrophins and their receptors: a convergence point for many signalling pathways, *Nat Rev Neurosci* 4:299, 2003.
37. Tremblay J, Desjardins R, Hum D, et al: Biochemistry and physiology of the natriuretic peptide receptor guanylyl cyclases, *Mol Cell Biochem* 230:31, 2002.
38. Budworth J, Meillerais S, Charles I, et al: Tissue distribution of the human soluble guanylate cyclases, *Biochem Biophys Res Commun* 263:696, 1999.
39. Andreopoulos S, Papapetropoulos A: Molecular aspects of soluble guanylyl cyclase regulation, *Gen Pharmacol* 34:147, 2000.
40. Moncada S, Palmer RM, Higgs EA: Nitric oxide: physiology, pathophysiology, and pharmacology, *Pharmacol Rev* 43:109, 1991.
41. Schechter AN, Gladwin MT: Hemoglobin and the paracrine and endocrine functions of nitric oxide, *N Engl J Med* 348:1483, 2003.
42. Alberts B, Johnson A, Lewis J, et al: *Molecular biology of the cell*, ed 4, New York, 2002, Garland Science.
43. Hadcock JR, Ros M, Malbon CC: Agonist regulation of beta-adrenergic receptor mRNA. Analysis in S49 mouse lymphoma mutants, *J Biol Chem* 264:13956, 1989.
44. Wallukat G: The beta-adrenergic receptors, *Herz* 27:683, 2002.
45. Luttrell LM, Lefkowitz RJ: The role of beta-arrestins in the termination and transduction of G-protein-coupled receptor signals, *J Cell Sci* 115:455, 2002.
46. Oakley RH, Laporte SA, Holt JA, et al: Association of beta-arrestin with G protein-coupled receptors during clathrin-mediated endocytosis dictates the profile of receptor resensitization, *J Biol Chem* 274:32248, 1999.
47. Lombardi MS, van den Tweel E, Kavelaars A, et al: Hypoxia/ischemia modulates G protein-coupled receptor kinase 2 and beta-arrestin-1 levels in the neonatal rat brain, *Stroke* 35:981, 2004.
48. Hanoune J, Defer N: Regulation and role of adenylyl cyclase isoforms, *Annu Rev Pharmacol Toxicol* 41:145, 2001.
49. Essayan DM: Cyclic nucleotide phosphodiesterases, *J Allergy Clin Immunol* 108:671, 2001.
50. Lucas KA, Pitari GM, Kazerounian S, et al: Guanylyl cyclases and signaling by cyclic GMP, *Pharmacol Rev* 52:375, 2000.
51. Carroll WD, Dhillon R: Sildenafil as a treatment for pulmonary hypertension, *Arch Dis Child* 88:827, 2003.
52. Adatia I: Recent advances in pulmonary vascular disease, *Curr Opin Pediatr* 14:292, 2002.
53. Atz AM, Wessel DL: Sildenafil ameliorates effects of inhaled nitric oxide withdrawal, *Anesthesiology* 91:307, 1999.

54. Prasad S, Wilkinson J, Gatzoulis MA: Sildenafil in primary pulmonary hypertension, *N Engl J Med* 343:1342, 2000.
55. Toker A: Phosphoinositides and signal transduction, *Cell Mol Life Sci* 59:761, 2002.
56. Schenk PW, Snaar-Jagalska BE: Signal perception and transduction: the role of protein kinases, *Biochim Biophys Acta* 1449:1, 1999.
57. Kalow W, Tang BK, Endrenyi L: Hypothesis: comparisons of inter- and intra-individual variations can substitute for twin studies in drug research, *Pharmacogenetics* 8:283, 1998.
58. Drysdale CM, McGraw DW, Stack CB, et al: Complex promoter and coding region beta 2-adrenergic receptor haplotypes alter receptor expression and predict in vivo responsiveness, *Proc Natl Acad Sci U S A* 97:10483, 2000.
59. Evans WE, McLeod HL: Pharmacogenomics—drug disposition, drug targets, and side effects, *N Engl J Med* 348:538, 2003.
60. Weinshilboum R: Inheritance and drug response, *N Engl J Med* 348:529, 2003.
61. Sadee W, Hoeg E, Lucas J, et al: Genetic variations in human G protein-coupled receptors: implications for drug therapy, *AAPS PharmSci* 3:E22, 2001.
62. Marian AJ, Safavi F, Ferlic L, et al: Interactions between angiotensin-I converting enzyme insertion/deletion polymorphism and response of plasma lipids and coronary atherosclerosis to treatment with fluvastatin: the lipoprotein and coronary atherosclerosis study, *J Am Coll Cardiol* 35:89, 2000.
63. Drazen JM, Yandava CN, Dube L, et al: Pharmacogenetic association between ALOX5 promoter genotype and the response to anti-asthma treatment, *Nat Genet* 22:168, 1999.
64. Farfel Z, Bourne HR, Iiri T: The expanding spectrum of G protein diseases, *N Engl J Med* 340:1012, 1999.
65. Maqbool A, Hall AS, Ball SG, et al: Common polymorphisms of beta1-adrenoceptor: identification and rapid screening assay, *Lancet* 353:897, 1999.
66. Rathz DA, Brown KM, Kramer LA, et al: Amino acid 49 polymorphisms of the human beta1-adrenergic receptor affect agonist-promoted trafficking, *J Cardiovasc Pharmacol* 39:155, 2002.
67. Levin MC, Marullo S, Muntaner O, et al: The myocardium-protective Gly-49 variant of the beta 1-adrenergic receptor exhibits constitutive activity and increased desensitization and down-regulation, *J Biol Chem* 277:30429, 2002.
68. Mason DA, Moore JD, Green SA, et al: A gain-of-function polymorphism in a G-protein coupling domain of the human beta1 adrenergic receptor, *J Biol Chem* 274:12670, 1999.
69. Johnson JA, Zineh I, Puckett BJ, et al: Beta 1-adrenergic receptor polymorphisms and antihypertensive response to metoprolol, *Clin Pharmacol Ther* 74:44, 2003.
70. Sofowora GG, Dishy V, Muszkat M, et al: A common beta1-adrenergic receptor polymorphism (Arg389Gly) affects blood pressure response to beta-blockade, *Clin Pharmacol Ther* 73:366, 2003.
71. Sandilands AJ, O'Shaughnessy KM, Brown MJ: Greater inotropic and cyclic AMP responses evoked by noradrenaline through Arg389 beta 1-adrenoceptors versus Gly389 beta 1-adrenoceptors in isolated human atrial myocardium, *Br J Pharmacol* 138:386, 2003.
72. Reihsaus E, Innis M, MacIntyre N, et al: Mutations in the gene encoding for the beta 2-adrenergic receptor in normal and asthmatic subjects, *Am J Respir Cell Mol Biol* 8:334, 1993.
73. Parola AL, Kobilka BK: The peptide product of a 5′ leader cistron in the beta 2 adrenergic receptor mRNA inhibits receptor synthesis, *J Biol Chem* 269:4497, 1994.
74. Scott MG, Swan C, Wheatley AP, et al: Identification of novel polymorphisms within the promoter region of the human beta2 adrenergic receptor gene, *Br J Pharmacol* 126:841, 1999.
75. Green SA, Cole G, Jacinto M, et al: A polymorphism of the human beta 2-adrenergic receptor within the fourth transmembrane domain alters ligand binding and functional properties of the receptor, *J Biol Chem* 268:23116, 1993.
76. Green SA, Turki J, Innis M, et al: Amino-terminal polymorphisms of the human beta 2-adrenergic receptor impart distinct agonist-promoted regulatory properties, *Biochemistry* 33:9414, 1994.
77. Siffert W, Rosskopf D, Siffert G, et al: Association of a human G-protein beta3 subunit variant with hypertension, *Nat Genet* 18:45, 1998.
78. Rosskopf D, Busch S, Manthey I, et al: G protein beta 3 gene: structure, promoter, and additional polymorphisms, *Hypertension* 36:33, 2000.
79. Richardson M, Robishaw JD: The alpha2A-adrenergic receptor discriminates between Gi heterotrimers of different betagamma subunit composition in Sf9 insect cell membranes, *J Biol Chem* 274:13525, 1999.
80. Zill P, Baghai TC, Zwanzger P, et al: Evidence for an association between a G-protein beta3-gene variant with depression and response to antidepressant treatment, *Neuroreport* 11:1893, 2000.
81. Sperling H, Eisenhardt A, Virchow S, et al: Sildenafil response is influenced by the G protein beta 3 subunit GNB3 C825T polymorphism: a pilot study, *J Urol* 169:1048, 2003.
82. Rosskopf D, Manthey I, Siffert W: Identification and ethnic distribution of major haplotypes in the gene GNB3 encoding the G-protein beta3 subunit, *Pharmacogenetics* 12:209, 2002.
83. Halpern S: American pediatrics: the social dynamic of professionalism, 1880–1980. Berkeley, 1988, University of California Press.
84. Alcorn J, McNamara PJ: Ontogeny of hepatic and renal systemic clearance pathways in infants: part I, *Clin Pharmacokinet* 41:959, 2002.
85. Kearns GL, Abdel-Rahman SM, Alander SW, et al: Developmental pharmacology-drug disposition, action, and therapy in infants and children, *N Engl J Med* 349:1157, 2003.
86. Treluyer JM, Jacqz-Aigrain E, Alvarez F, et al: Expression of CYP2D6 in developing human liver, *Eur J Biochem* 202:583, 1991.
87. Vieira I, Sonnier M, Cresteil T: Developmental expression of CYP2E1 in the human liver. Hypermethylation control of gene expression during the neonatal period, *Eur J Biochem* 238:476, 1996.
88. Treluyer JM, Gueret G, Cheron G, et al: Developmental expression of CYP2C and CYP2C-dependent activities in the human liver: in-vivo/in-vitro correlation and inducibility, *Pharmacogenetics* 7:441, 1997.
89. Lacroix D, Sonnier M, Moncion A, et al: Expression of CYP3A in the human liver-evidence that the shift between CYP3A7 and CYP3A4 occurs immediately after birth, *Eur J Biochem* 247:625, 1997.
90. Sonnier M, Cresteil T: Delayed ontogenesis of CYP1A2 in the human liver, *Eur J Biochem* 251:893, 1998.
91. Kumar DV, Sastry PS: Dopamine receptors in human foetal brains: characterization, regulation and ontogeny of [3H]spiperone binding sites in striatum, *Neurochem Int* 20:559, 1992.
92. Laquerriere A, Leroux P, Gonzalez B, et al: Somatostatin receptors in the human cerebellum during development, *Brain Res* 573:251, 1992.
93. Watzka M, Bidlingmaier F, Beyenburg S, et al: Corticosteroid receptor mRNA expression in the brains of patients with epilepsy, *Steroids* 65:895, 2000.
94. Chugani DC, Muzik O, Juhasz C, et al: Postnatal maturation of human GABAA receptors measured with positron emission tomography, *Ann Neurol* 49:618, 2001.
95. Law AJ, Weickert CS, Webster MJ, et al: Expression of NMDA receptor NR1, NR2A and NR2B subunit mRNAs during development of the human hippocampal formation, *Eur J Neurosci* 18:1197, 2003.
96. Mato S, Del Olmo E, Pazos A: Ontogenetic development of cannabinoid receptor expression and signal transduction functionality in the human brain, *Eur J Neurosci* 17:1747, 2003.
97. Ozawa H, Ukai W, Kornhuber J, et al: Postnatal ontogeny of GTP binding protein in the human frontal cortex, *Life Sci* 65:2315, 1999.
98. Beckner SK, Farrar WL: Inhibition of adenylate cyclase by IL 2 in human T lymphocytes is mediated by protein kinase C, *Biochem Biophys Res Commun* 145:176, 1987.
99. Gulick T, Chung MK, Pieper SJ, et al: Interleukin 1 and tumor necrosis factor inhibit cardiac myocyte beta-adrenergic responsiveness, *Proc Natl Acad Sci U S A* 86:6753, 1989.

CHAPTER 112

Adverse Drug Reactions and Drug–Drug Interactions

Wade W. Benton, D. Michael Lindsay, Christopher M. Rubino, and Rapheus C.Q. Villanueva

PEARLS

- Although adverse drug events in ambulatory pediatric patients may be relatively uncommon, epidemiologic studies in inpatient settings confirm that the problem is just as important for children as it is for adults. Overall, the incidence of adverse events in pediatric inpatients can range from 5% to 21% of hospital admissions, which is higher than the estimated incidence of approximately 4% in adults.
- The pediatric intensivist is confronted daily with potentially hazardous drug–drug interactions in the critical care setting. The ability to recognize every potential drug–drug interaction in the pediatric critical care setting is nearly impossible; however, in most cases, drug–drug interactions are predictable and preventable, with appropriate dosage modifications or avoidance of combinations.
- Prescription medications are the most common cause of iatrogenic seizures. Drug-related factors that may contribute to seizures are the intrinsic epileptogenicity of the agent, factors that influence serum levels (dose, schedule, route), and factors that affect central nervous system drug levels (lipid solubility, molecular weight, ionization of the drug, protein binding, transport by endogenous systems).
- Parenteral administration of drug therapy poses a potential source of drug–drug interactions in the pediatric/neonatal intensive care unit. In this scenario, polypharmacy arising from an extensive problem list and limited intravenous access conspire to force the mixing of various drug solutions. However, disparate physicochemical properties and varying administration times preclude the indiscriminate admixing of numerous drugs into a single large or small volume parenteral.

Adverse Drug Reactions

The fields of clinical pharmacology and drug development have been shaped in part by adverse events in children. Two great tragedies promulgated changes in the drug regulatory process in the United States: (1) the death of 107 patients (mostly children) as a result of a sulfanilamide elixir that contained diethylene glycol prompted the first requirement for safety testing of new drug products and (2) birth defects in babies secondary to maternal use of thalidomide resulted in the requirement that drugs be deemed safe and effective and that safety and efficacy in one population did not infer safety and efficacy in another.[39,230] Ironically, the changes that arose from these events only further limited the testing of new drug products in children. Regulations have started to address this issue, and the resultant studies are beginning to close the information gap, helping to ensure the safety and efficacy of medications in children.[53]

Steps are now being taken to help alleviate adverse events caused by the lack of knowledge of the drug effects on children, but remaining issues still cause children to be more susceptible to adverse drug events. For example, the common practice of using weight-based dosing adds another layer of complexity to drug therapy in children.

In addition, many parenteral therapies require dilution of stock solutions, providing an opportunity for errors. Finally, sick infants and children may have reduced ability to survive iatrogenic events if and when they occur.

Publications have brought to light the importance of adverse drug events in adults and their impact on the health care system in general.[244] Although adverse drug events in ambulatory pediatric patients may be relatively uncommon, epidemiologic studies in inpatient settings confirm that the problem is just as important for children as it is for adults.[58,102,114,160,161,262] Overall, the incidence of adverse events in pediatric inpatients can range from 5% to 21% of hospital admissions,[97,102,114,262] which is higher than the estimated incidence of approximately 4% in adults.[27,130]

One of the difficulties in reviewing the literature on adverse drug reactions is how they are defined. There are many different examples of what constitutes an adverse drug reaction. Many professional organizations have tried to standardize exactly how an adverse drug reaction is defined. The World Health Organization (WHO)[265] defines an adverse drug reaction as any response to a drug that is noxious and unintended and that occurs at doses normally used in humans for prophylaxis, diagnosis, or therapy of disease or for modification of physiologic function. The Joint Commission on Accreditation of Healthcare Organizations (JCAHO)[107] defines an adverse drug reaction as an undesirable response associated with use of a drug that compromises therapeutic efficacy, enhances toxicity, or both.

For reporting purposes, the Food and Drug Administration (FDA)[115] categorizes a serious adverse event (events relating to drugs and devices) as one in which "the patient outcome is death, life threatening (real risk of death), hospitalization (initial or prolonged), disability (significant, persistent or permanent), congenital anomaly or required intervention to prevent permanent impairment or damage."

The American Society for Health-System Pharmacists (ASHP)[4] defines a significant adverse drug reaction as any unexpected, unintended, undesired, or excessive response to a drug that:

- Requires discontinuing the drug (therapeutic or diagnostic)
- Requires changing drug therapy
- Requires modifying the dose (except for minor dosage adjustments)
- Necessitates admission to a hospital
- Prolongs stay in a health care facility
- Necessitates supportive treatment
- Significantly complicates diagnosis
- Negatively affects prognosis, or
- Results in temporary or permanent harm, disability, or death

The ASHP also defines what is not an adverse drug reaction as follows:

- Side effects
- Drug withdrawal
- Drug abuse syndrome
- Accidental poisoning
- Drug overdose complications

The mechanisms by which adverse drug reactions occur can be divided into two main types: type A and type B. Type A mechanisms usually are thought of as preventable, predictable, and related to the pharmacologic action of the medication. Knowledge of the effects caused by the medication can predict the likelihood of an adverse drug reaction occurring. Appropriate monitoring of the medication can assist in preventing adverse drug reactions.[60,84,164] Type B mechanisms usually are considered to be unavoidable and not predictable. These reactions normally are uncommon and not related to the pharmacologic action of the medication. Idiosyncratic and hypersensitivity reactions are common type B reactions.[60,84,164]

A critical factor in assessing adverse drug reactions is establishing a causal relationship between the suspected drug and the adverse reaction.[111] Identification of adverse drug reactions can be arbitrary. Some of the confounding factors are the ambiguous characteristics of the reactions, the fact that patients usually are taking more than one medication at the time of the reaction, and the inability to perform definitive cause and effect tests.[111]

There have been numerous attempts to try and formalize the process.[108,111,124,164] Karch and Lasagna[111] designed decision tables that can identify a potential reaction, assess the certainty of a link between the drug and the event, and evaluate the underlying cause of the reaction. It provides a framework for systematic evaluation of potential adverse drug reactions and reduces the ambiguity that presently characterizes the assessment of adverse drug reactions.

Kramer et al.[124] devised an operational assessment using an algorithm with six axes to assess the probability of an adverse drug reaction occurrence. A scoring system for each axis and an overall score help delineate the likelihood that an adverse drug reaction has occurred. Similarly, Naranjo et al.[164] developed an adverse drug reaction probability scale using 10 questions answered positively (yes), negatively (no), or unknown to determine the likelihood that an adverse drug reaction had occurred. The Naranjo method has been shown to improve the reproducibility of adverse drug reactions assessments.

An FDA algorithm that assesses the characteristics of the event (temporal relationship, dechallenge, rechallenge, and relationship to disease) has been presented.[108] The algorithm contains four questions in order to assess the likelihood that an adverse drug reaction had occurred:

- Did the reaction follow a reasonable temporal sequence?
- Did the patient improve after stopping the drug?
- Did the reaction reappear on repeated experience (rechallenge)?
- Could the reaction be reasonably explained by known characteristics of the patient's clinical state?

The categories remote, possible, probable, and highly probable are used based on the answers to the four questions.

Comparisons of the different methods have been conducted. Michel and Knodel[154] compared the Kramer, Naranjo, and FDA methods. The Kramer method was considered to be the standard of practice at the time, and Naranjo and FDA methods both compared favorably. The Naranjo method was shown to be simpler and less time consuming. The lack of a numerical score in the FDA algorithm caused the authors to decide there was a need for more data to recommend its use over Naranjo method, even though the FDA algorithm was less time consuming than either method.[154] Busto et al.[32] compared the Kramer and Naranjo methods. The two methods were determined to be equal in terms of reproducibility, but the Kramer method was more complex.

Once an adverse drug reaction is identified, appropriate reporting is critical. Reporting can occur by several mechanisms. The event can be reported through the health care systems adverse drug reaction program as mandated by the JCAHO. This program usually is coordinated by the pharmacy department. Another avenue is to contact the drug manufacturer, as all companies have a mechanism for documenting adverse drug reactions. Finally, severe and significant reactions can be reported to the FDA through the MedWatch program.

Adverse Drug Reactions by Organ System

Renal (see Chapter 63)

Nephrotoxicity accounts for nearly 7% of all adverse drug reactions.[130] Several factors place the renal system at risk for adverse drug reactions. The renal system is responsible for elimination of many drugs and metabolites, of which several are known nephrotoxins. Additionally, the renal vascular system receives approximately 20% to 25% of resting cardiac output. Therefore the kidneys are exposed to high concentrations of drugs and diagnostics. Although the renal system is highly vulnerable to nephrotoxicity, there are only a few mechanisms by which nephrotoxins can induce injury. These mechanisms include hemodynamically mediated nephrotoxicity, tubular necrosis, interstitial nephritis, obstructive nephropathy, and vascular toxicity. Many nephrotoxins can injure the kidney through more than one mechanism.

A variety of drugs are associated with acute tubular necrosis, including aminoglycosides, cisplatin, amphotericin B, radiocontrast media, cyclosporine, and intravenous (IV) immunoglobulins.[136,142,226] Acute tubular necrosis is one of the most common renal disorders associated with drug therapy. Minimizing risk factors for nephrotoxicity with these agents is imperative (e.g., administering a saline load and repletion of volume have proved beneficial in reducing toxicity).[141] Table 112–1 provides a more complete list of medications associated with tubular necrosis.

Several drugs are implicated in alteration of renal blood flow. Some of the most common include angiotensin-converting enzyme inhibitors (ACEIs) (e.g., enalaprilat), nonsteroidal antiinflammatory drugs (NSAIDs) (e.g., ketorolac), β-blockers (e.g., propranolol), and calcineurin inhibitors (e.g., cyclosporine).[55,61,161,183,216,219,233,243,263] ACEIs can induce renal insufficiency in patients suffering from bilateral renal artery stenosis or unilateral stenosis with a single kidney.[99] The mechanism involves inhibiting the conversion of angiotensin I to angiotensin II, which results in dilation of the efferent arterioles, with resultant decreased glomerular capillary hydrostatic pressure and reduced glomerular filtration. Incidence of ACEI-induced renal failure in patients with renovascular hypertension ranges from 20% to 38%.[243] NSAIDs inhibit prostaglandin synthesis, which leads to reduced renal blood flow and reduced glomerular filtration. The incidence of renal insufficiency is most common in patients with chronic renal disease, hypovolemia, sepsis, and use of concomitant nephrotoxic drugs.[55,183,216,219,233,263] NSAID-induced renal toxicity is reversible if the toxic agent is discontinued immediately.[234] Table 112–1 provides a more complete list of drugs associated with hemodynamic renal failure.

Acute interstitial nephritis is another common source of drug-induced nephrotoxicity. It is reported to cause 3% to 8% of all cases of acute renal failure.[123] The clinical presentation of acute interstitial nephritis can appear anywhere between 2 and 44 days after initiation of offending therapy.[120,140] Typical clinical symptoms include fever, skin rash, and flank tenderness.[120,140] Common laboratory findings include hematuria, sterile pyuria, and eosinophilia.[123] Histologic findings of acute interstitial nephritis include interstitial infiltrate of lymphocytes, plasma cells, eosinophils, and neutrophils.[120,123,140] Prompt discontinuation of the offending drug from therapy is recommended, and administration of corticosteroids may improve recovery.[242] Table 112–1 lists some medications associated with acute interstitial nephritis.

TABLE 112–1

Drugs That Cause Nephrotoxicity

Tubular Necrosis	Interstitial Nephritis		Hemodynamic-Mediated Renal Failure
Aminoglycosides	Allopurinol	Penicillins	Angiotensin-converting enzyme inhibitors
Amphotericin	Amioglycosides	Phenobarbital	
Carboplatinum	Aztreonam	Phenytoin	
Cephalosporins	Captopril	Ranitidine	Cyclosporine
Cisplatin	Carbamazepine	Rifampin	Mannitol
Cyclosporine	Cephalosporins	Sulfonamides	NSAIDs
Mannitol	Cimetidine	Tacrolimus	Propranolol
Methoxyflurane anesthesia	Ciprofloxacin	Thiazide and loop diuretics	Radiologic contrast agents
NSAIDs	Cyclosporine		Tacrolimus
Pentamidine	Erythromycin	Valproic acid	
Radiologic contrast agents	Interferon-α	Vancomycin	
	NSAIDs	Warfarin	

NSAID, nonsteroidal antiinflammatory drug.

Renal tubular obstruction is associated with renotubular precipitation of endogenous products, drugs, and their metabolites. Formation of uric acid precipitates after chemotherapy can result in renal obstruction. Hydrating patients prior to chemotherapy, urinary alkalinization, and use of allopurinol or rasburicase can help prevent uric acid precipitation. Rhabdomyolysis can cause intratubular precipitation of myoglobin and lead to acute renal failure. Terbutaline overdose has resulted in rhabdomyolysis-induced renal failure.[23] Drugs associated with formation of crystals include acyclovir, sulfonamides, mannitol, pentobarbital, methotrexate, and dextran.[59,64,126,165]

Aminoglycosides are used frequently for treatment of gram-negative infections. All aminoglycosides have been shown to be toxic to the proximal renal tubules.[221] Aminoglycoside nephrotoxicity is related to dose, high trough concentrations, and prolonged therapy.[221] The drug-induced nephrotoxicity normally manifests as nonoliguric renal failure.[21] Several risk factors for developing aminoglycoside nephrotoxicity include the need for intensive care, decreased albumin, poor nutritional status, prolonged therapy, hypovolemia, pneumonia, shock, preexisting liver or kidney disease, and elevated initial steady-state drug concentrations.[21,80] Additionally, vancomycin, piperacillin, furosemide, amphotericin B, and cephalosporins when administered concomitantly with aminoglycosides are associated with an increased risk for developing nephrotoxicity.[21] Predicting nephrotoxicity based on the risk factors stated is an extremely complicated, inexact task.[21,129] Typically aminoglycoside nephrotoxicity is reversible upon discontinuation of the offending agent.[221,156a]

Drug-induced nephrotoxicity is a common serious adverse drug reaction that can lead to morbidity and lengthen hospital stays.[203] It is important to recognize potential nephrotoxins before initiating therapy and to evaluate therapeutic options. It is important to monitor therapy appropriately for signs of toxicity and to modify therapy as needed.

Hepatic (see Chapter 80)

A variety of medications cause drug-induced hepatotoxicity. It often is difficult to determine the source of unexplained liver injury, so detailed examination of past and current drug therapies is needed to rule out possible drug-related causes. The pathogenesis of drug-induced liver disease is mediated either through immune response or direct cell damage.[110,271] Elevations in alanine aminotransferase (ALT), aspartate aminotransferase (AST), and lactate dehydrogenase (LDH) reflect hepatocellular injury, although subclinical liver injury is common and has little clinical consequence.[106] In severe cases of drug-induced hepatic injury, jaundice and hepatic failure may ensue.[271] Typically drug-induced hepatic disease may occur expectedly as a result of high-dose therapy of a known hepatotoxin or unexpectedly as a result of an idiosyncratic reaction to a drug not associated with hepatotoxicity. Overall, children are less prone to drug-induced liver disease than are adults.[30] However, specific hepatotoxin have been shown to afflict children more than adults. Reye syndrome is a hepatocellular disease often associated with aspirin use in children.[79] Valproate hepatotoxicity occurs more frequently in children younger than 2 years who have preexisting neurologic or physical defects.[6]

Drug-induced hepatic disease can occur by a variety of mechanisms, including hepatocellular, cholestatic, and vascular. These injuries are associated with intrinsic or idiosyncratic hepatotoxins. Intrinsic hepatotoxins typically show a dose-related toxic effect. Idiosyncratic hepatic disease is an unpredictable reaction that can occur by immune-mediated hypersensitivity, metabolically or both. Hypersensitivity reactions in the liver can cause cell injury to hepatocytes. The reactions do not correlate with dosage and are difficult to anticipate. This immune-mediated reaction results from antigenic complexes that stimulate T lymphocytes, which can result in hepatic injury. These reactions can be accompanied by fever, skin rash, lymphadenopathy, and eosinophilia.[271] The reactions typically resolve upon discontinuation of therapy and resurface when therapy is rechallenged.[271] *Metabolic idiosyncrasy* occurs when a compound that is metabolized to nontoxic metabolites and eliminated in the majority of patients is metabolized to a toxic metabolite in a small number of patients because of genetic differences in metabolism (e.g., with isoniazid.)[81a] Box 112–1 lists a number of agents that are associated with drug-induced hepatotoxicity.

Cardiovascular (see Chapter 23)

Several drugs are associated with adverse effects on the cardiovascular system and the mechanisms are often thought to be related to the agents' pharmacologic action. Cardiovascular toxicities that have been observed with use of vasopressors stem from their receptor-mediated effects. The β agonism of the sympathomimetics produces palpitations, ectopic heartbeats, sinus tachycardia, and ventricular arrhythmias.[96] The direct effect on myocardial tissues may be manifested as electrocardiographic (ECG) changes, such as a reduction in T-wave amplitude, reported during epinephrine infusions in normal individuals. Increased myocardial oxygen demand may precipitate an infarction, especially in individuals with underlying cardiac disease. A dramatic rise in heart rate and peripheral vascular resistance may produce severe hypertension, which could lead to cerebral hemorrhage or hemiplegia. Excessive α-adrenergic stimulation may produce vasoconstriction so severe in the extremities, kidneys, or liver that tissues become ischemic

BOX 112–1

Drugs That Cause Hepatotoxicity

Acetaminophen	Phenobarbital
Amoxicillin-clavulanic acid	Phenytoin
Carbamazepine	Rifampin
Erythromycin	Sulfonamides
Isoniazid	Terbutaline
Ketoconazole	Tetracyclines
Labetalol	Trazodone
Nitrofurantoin	Valproate
NSAIDs	Voriconazole

or necrotic. Gangrene of the extremities is reported with high doses of dopamine in patients with underlying occlusive vascular disease. Extravasation of a sympathomimetic agent may lead to tissue necrosis.[149]

Another class of agents whose cardiovascular toxicities may be predicted from its pharmacologic effects on myocardial tissue is the cardiac glycosides. Digoxin can produce a large array of dysrhythmias; the most common in adults includes unifocal or multifocal ventricular premature complexes and nonparoxysmal atrioventricular junctional tachycardia.[186] Sinus bradycardia and a sick sinus syndromelike effect have been reported as digoxin-induced adverse effects.[150] The narrow therapeutic index of this drug class is of special concern in the pediatric population. Among infants and children, cardiac arrhythmias often are the most reliable indicator of digoxin-induced toxicity, preceding the incidence of gastrointestinal (anorexia, nausea, vomiting, diarrhea) and central nervous system ([CNS] headache, dizziness, mental disturbances) effects.

Ventricular arrhythmias in infants and children, unlike adults, are relatively uncommon. However, the clinician should be sensitive to the presence of sinus bradycardia in infants receiving digoxin. The most commonly reported arrhythmias in pediatric patients include conduction disturbances or supraventricular tachyarrhythmias (e.g., atrial tachycardia and junctional tachycardia).

Torsades de pointes is a life-threatening subset of arrhythmias and is characterized on electrocardiogram by lengthening of the QT interval and waxing/waning QRS amplitude. A number of agents have this alarming side effect (Box 112–2). It is important to be aware of factors that may increase the plasma concentration of these drugs via pathophysiologic alterations in elimination or pharmacokinetic interactions with other drugs. The antiarrhythmics, tricyclic antidepressants, and fluoroquinolones are general classes of agents that demonstrate the potential to prolong the QT interval.[91,92]

Anthracycline antineoplastic agents illustrate a specific pattern of direct toxicity to myocardial tissue. Drugs in this class include doxorubicin, epirubicin, and idarubicin. Acute cardiotoxicity may be manifested as arrhythmias, whereas long-term adverse effects are generally related to the magnitude of cumulative drug exposure, with cardiomyopathy being most common. Children who have endured anthracycline therapy may exhibit signs of abnormal cardiac function anywhere between 4 and 20 years after exposure.[68] These defects include abnormal right ventricular wall motion, impaired myocardial growth and contractility, conduction abnormalities such as QT prolongation, and congestive heart failure.[68] Severe anthracycline toxicity cannot be reversed, and such a diagnosis leads to a poor prognosis and high mortality. Heart transplantation may be the only option in such cases.[68] Due to the severity of anthracycline cardiac toxicity and the clear association with total cumulative dose received, anthracycline lifetime dosage should be documented for each patient so that cumulative dose thresholds are not exceeded.

BOX 112–2

Drugs That Can Prolong the QTc Interval

Amiodarone	Haloperidol
Amitriptyline	Levofloxacin
Cisapride	Moxifloxacin
Clarithromycin	Ondansetron
Clomipramine	Procainamide
Clozapine	Propafenone
Chlorpromazine	Quinidine
Desipramine	Sotalol
Dofetilide	Sparfloxacillin
Dolasetron	Sumatriptan
Droperidol	Thioridazine
Erythromycin	Ziprasidone
Gatifloxacin	Zolmitriptan
Halofantrine	

From Hansten PD, Horn JR: The top 100 drug interactions: a guide to patient management. Edmonds, WA, 2002, H&H Publications.

Central Nervous System

Prescription medications are the most common cause of iatrogenic seizures.[214] Drug-related factors that may contribute to seizures include the intrinsic epileptogenicity of the agent, factors that influence serum levels (dose, schedule, route), and factors that affect CNS drug levels (lipid solubility, molecular weight, ionization of the drug, protein binding, transport by endogenous systems).[2] Patient-related factors may influence the risk for drug-induced seizures, such as preexisting epilepsy, neurologic abnormality, decreased drug elimination capacity (renal, hepatic), and conditions that disrupt the blood-brain barrier.[2] Several classes of medications cause seizures. Theophylline and aminophylline can cause seizures and usually are related to increased serum concentrations (especially >25 mg/ml).[214] Phenothiazine tricyclic antidepressants (chlorpromazine, thioridazine) cause seizures.[214] Meperidine may induce seizures because of accumulation of the normeperidine metabolite, especially in patients with renal insufficiency.[214] Rapid administration of fentanyl can cause seizures.[214] Several antiinfective and immunosuppressive medications, such as β-lactams, imipenem, high-dose metronidazole, isoniazid, cyclosporine, and chlorambucil, induce seizures.[214] Antiepileptic drugs themselves are implicated in worsening seizure activity. This usually occurs when higher than normal concentrations are used. Seizures also may be precipitated by medication withdrawal.[2] Withdrawal of antiepileptic drugs may cause seizures because of either subtherapeutic levels or too rapid removal of the agent (see Chapter 55).

Drug-induced headache can be caused by many medications. Headaches can be acute or chronic. They may be caused by use and abuse of the agent.[134] Headache may occur during substance withdrawal. Many medications cause acute headaches, including NSAIDs (e.g., indomethacin), vasodilators (e.g., β-blockers, calcium channel blockers, ACEI), immunomodulators (e.g., cyclosporine, tacrolimus, antithymocyte globulin), cytotoxic agents (intrathecal methotrexate, interferon-β_1, interleukin-2), and antimicrobials (e.g., amphotericin-B, tetracycline, sulfonamides).[134,224] Chronic headaches may be caused by overuse and abuse of simple analgesics, narcotics, and combination analgesics with barbiturates/sedatives and ergotamine.[224]

Numerous drugs may cause sedation. Drug-induced sedation usually is an extension of the pharmacologic action of the medication. This effect frequently is transient and diminishes with continuation of therapy. Sedation can result from excessive dosage of the medication and can be managed by decreasing the dose of medication. Excessive sedation may occur with combination therapy.

Ototoxicity usually is iatrogenic.[10] The main sites of action of ototoxic drugs are the cochlea, vestibulum, and stria vascularis.[74] Several medications cause ototoxicity, with salicylates and aminoglycosides the most commonly implicated.[220,74] Other agents involved are cisplatin, loop diuretics, erythromycin, and vancomyin.[220,74] The effect usually is dose dependent.[10,220,74] High-dose and long-term therapy are common risk factors for aminoglycoside-induced ototoxicity.[220,74] For aminoglycosides, streptomycin is mostly vestibulotoxic and neomycin is more cochleotoxic.[220] Cisplatin is the most ototoxic of the antineoplastic agents.[220] Ethacrynic acid has the greatest potential for causing ototoxicity for the loop diuretics.[220] Appropriate dosing and monitoring of agents associated with ototoxicity are important for prevention and early detection.

Hematologic

The most common and serious adverse drug reaction resulting from chemotherapy with cytotoxic agents is bone marrow suppression. The decline in hematopoiesis results from injury to rapidly dividing stem cells and can lead to secondary morbidities. For example, neutropenia predisposes a patient to opportunistic infections and sepsis. Chemotherapy-induced thrombocytopenia may render a patient vulnerable to hemorrhage in the CNS or gastrointestinal (GI) tract. Severe anemia may lead to dizziness, fatigue, hypotension, and myocardial infarction.[81] In addition to bone marrow suppression, some antineoplastics may produce thrombotic and hemorrhagic coagulation toxicities. For example, L-asparaginase has been reported to induce changes in the von Willebrand factor multimer in children and thereby promote platelet aggregation.[68]

Respiratory

Drugs may cause central hypoventilation, motor neuropathy, neuromuscular blockade, or myopathies.[43] The long list of drugs suspected of causing or exacerbating bronchospastic reactions demonstrates the need to be aware of drug-induced causes of acute episodes, especially in asthmatic patients.[133] Analgesics and NSAIDs are two of the most common causes of drug-induced bronchospasms.[133] Other agents include antimicrobials (e.g., sulfonamides), cardiovascular agents (e.g., β-blockers and ACEI), and excipients (e.g., preservatives, coloring agents, antioxidants).[43,133] These reactions are more common in patients with asthma.

Virtually any drug can cause pulmonary infiltrates as part of a general hypersensitivity reaction. Azathioprine, 6-mercaptopurine, procarbazine, penicillamine, phenytoin, carbamazepine, and sulfasalazine are medications commonly involved in hypersensitivity pulmonary reactions.[43]

High concentrations of aspirin can lead to increased vascular permeability causing pulmonary edema. A syndrome of massive fluid retention and pulmonary edema may be seen with interleukin-2. All-*trans*-retinoic acid may cause acute lung disease secondary to massive, total body fluid accumulation. Opiates (e.g., methadone, codeine) may cause acute respiratory failure secondary to a noncardiogenic pulmonary edema.[43] Acute pulmonary disease manifesting as flulike symptoms is common for some antibiotics (e.g., rifampin, nitrofurantoin).[43]

Chronic pneumonitis/fibrosis is a relatively common syndrome associated with drug-induced pulmonary reactions and is manifested by slowly progressive symptoms of cough and dyspnea.[43] Nitrofurantoin is associated with pulmonary fibrosis most commonly in patients receiving chronic, high-dose therapy and/or patients with renal insufficiency.[46] A delayed presentation (months to years) is the most common form of fibrosis seen with amiodarone,[100] but it also may cause an acute fibrosis manifesting within the first few weeks of therapy.[46,100] Many cytotoxic agents cause pulmonary fibrosis, including bleomycin, carmustine (BCNU), mitomycin, mitomycin/vinca alkaloid combination therapy, and cyclophosphamide. Risk factors for this reaction to cytotoxic agents are cumulative dose, age at treatment, radiation therapy, multidrug regimens, and preexisting pulmonary disease.[46]

Endocrine and Metabolic

Several medications are associated with adverse drug reactions involving endocrine or metabolic systems. Although idiosyncratic reactions unrelated to the pharmacologic mechanism of an agent can occur, most endocrine and metabolic adverse drug reactions represent an extension of the drugs' pharmacologic effect.

Several pharmaceuticals are associated with hyperglycemia and hypoglycemia. Drugs that can cause hyperglycemia and hypoglycemia are listed in Table 112–2.[145,254] Glucocorticoid usage is commonly associated with hyperglycemia and glycosuria.[37] Corticosteroids increase blood glucose via hepatic gluconeogenesis and by increasing peripheral insulin resistance.[98] This adverse drug reaction appears to be dose dependent and usually is reversible upon discontinuation of therapy.[98] Patients on high-dose, long-term glucocorticoid therapy are at significant risk for suppression of the hypothalamic-pituitary-adrenal axis.[78,125] Symptoms of adrenal insufficiency include arthralgias, dizziness, hypotension, nausea, and weakness.[78]

Drug-induced electrolyte disturbances can occur with a variety of pharmaceutical agents. Several medications are associated with initial or worsening hypokalemia, hyperkalemia, and hyponatremia (Table 112–2).[38,156] Electrolyte disorders represent a common adverse drug reaction and can greatly complicate therapy. Accordingly, frequent monitoring of electrolytes is warranted for patients on multiple drug therapy.

Although uncommon, prolonged usage of nitroprusside can result in methemoglobinemia and cyanide or thiocyanate toxicity.[8,88] Thiocyanate or cyanide toxicity is uncommon but can occur in patients suffering from kidney or hepatic failure or in patients receiving high-dose prolonged infusion of nitroprusside.[209] An early indicator of thiocyanate or cyanide toxicity is metabolic acidosis.[194] Other medications associated with anion gap metabolic

TABLE 112–2

Drugs That Cause Endocrine/Metabolic Changes

Hypoglycemia	Hyperglycemia		Hypokalemia	
ACEIs	Acetazolamide	Liposome	Acetazolamide	Metolazone
Cotrimoxazole	Albuterol	Furosemide	Albuterol	Mycophenolate
Haloperidol	Amiodarone	Glycerin	Alprostadil	Nafcillin
Indomethacin	Amphotericin	Isoniazid	Amphotericin	Na Penicillin G
Insulins	B Liposome	Levalbuterol	Bumetanide	Na Phosphates
Lidocaine	Asparaginase	Loperamide	Caspofungin	Sirolimus
Metoprolol	Basiliximab	Metolazone	Corticosteroids	Sodium
Octreotide	Bumetanide	Mycophenolate	Corticotropin	Polystyrene
Pentamidine	Carvedilol	Octreotide	Dextrose	Sulfonate
Propranolol	Clonidine	Phenytoin	Foscarnet	Tacrolimus
Ranitidine	Corticosteroids	Rifampin (oral)	Furosemide	Terbutaline
Salicylic acid	Corticotropin	Rituximab	Gatifloxacin	Thiazide diuretics
	Cyclosporine	Somatropin	Itraconazole	
	Dapsone	Tacrolimus	Levalbuterol	
	Dextrose	Terbutaline		
	Diazoxide	Thiazide diuretics		
	Doxorubicin			

Hyperkalemia	Hyponatremia
ACEIs	ACEIs
Arginine	Antidepressants
Barbiturates	Antipsychotics
β-Blockers	Bumetanide
Cyclosporine	Carbamazepine
Digitalis	Carboplatin
Epinephrine	Cisplatin
Heparin	Clonidine
Indomethacin	Foscarnet
Potassium-sparing diuretics	Haloperidol
Potassium supplements	Indomethacin
Propofol	NSAIDs
Rituximab	Spironolactone
Spironolactone	Thiazide diuretics
Succinylcholine	Vasopressin

ACEI, Angiotensin-converting enzyme inhibitor; *NSAID*, nonsteroidal antiinflammatory drug.

acidosis include chloramphenicol, epinephrine, norepinephrine, papaverine, and salicylates.[76,159]

Some life-threatening adverse drug reactions with propofol use in pediatric critical care are reported. In 2001, the U.S. Food and Drug Administration (FDA) communicated a warning against off-label use of propofol for sedation in pediatric intensive care.[54,63] The FDA concern came from reviewing data of a randomized, controlled clinical trial evaluating the safety and efficacy of propofol versus standard sedation in pediatric intensive care. Approximately 10% of patients treated with propofol died compared with 4% of children receiving standard treatment. A 1992 published report described five children with croup or bronchiolitis in the pediatric intensive care unit who received propofol sedation and subsequently died of metabolic acidosis and myocardial failure.[181] Some pediatric patients receiving propofol have experienced metabolic acidosis during infusion, although whether this is related to the drug or the underlying disease is unclear.[206] Reed et al.,[206] however, evaluated the clinical course of more than 140 infants and children between the ages of 1 week and 15 years and reported no cases of serious metabolic acidosis or morbidity or mortality associated with propofol. The most common drug-related adverse event in this cohort was hypotension, which appears to be related to loading doses in patients with high sympathetic tone and relative intravascular volume depletion.[206] A plausible relationship between metabolic acidosis and propofol use in pediatrics patients is difficult to confirm because of the lack of a large, well-controlled trial of pediatric patients offering direct evidence.

Dermatologic

Erythema multiforme major, Stevens-Johnson syndrome, and toxic epidermal necrolysis are severe cutaneous reactions. They are characterized by the triad of symptoms of mucous membrane erosions, target lesions, and epidermal necrosis with skin detachment.[122] Drugs are frequently cited as the cause of these reactions. The more severe the reaction, the more likely it is drug induced.[122] Numerous medications are implicated as the cause of these reactions, such as antiepileptic agents, antibiotics (e.g., sulfonamides), allopurinol, and NSAIDs (e.g., piroxicam).[122,158] For most agents, the pathogenesis is unknown. However, with sulfonamides and antiepileptics, the cause can be linked to a toxic metabolite that, in predisposed patients with a genetic defect, can bind covalently to proteins and elicit an immune response that causes a cutaneous reaction.[122]

Hypersensitivity syndrome reaction is a multisystem idiosyncratic reaction that manifests as fever, rash, and symptomatic or asymptomatic involvement of internal organ systems (liver, kidney, lungs, spleen, muscles, pancreas, lymph nodes, and blood).[34,122] Reactions usually occur with first exposure to medication, with initial symptoms occurring 1 to 6 weeks after exposure.[122] Aromatic antiepileptic agents (carbamazepine, phenobarbital, phenytoin, primidone) form a toxic metabolite that causes a secondary immune or hypersensitivity reaction.[34,215] Lamotrigine, valproic acid, and ethosuximide are other antiepileptics that may cause reactions. Sulfa drugs (dapsone, sulfasalazine, sulfonamide), allopurinol, and diltiazem also are implicated in hypersensitivity reactions.[34]

Drug rashes are the cutaneous manifestation of drug hypersensitivity. Red-neck or red-man syndrome, associated with the rapid infusion of vancomycin, is a histamine reaction and not a true allergic reaction. Prolongation of the administration prevents this reaction. β-Lactams and sulfamethoxazole are other common agents that cause rash.[46]

β-Lactams (most commonly) and sulfamethoxazole are medications known to cause anaphylaxis. The signs and symptoms of this immunoglobulin E-mediated allergic reaction are pruritus, urticaria, cutaneous flushing, hives, angioedema, bronchospasm, nausea, vomiting, diarrhea, nasal congestion, rhinorrhea, laryngeal edema, and hypotension (see Chapter 91).

Several medications are associated with drug-induced lupuslike reactions. Procainamide, hydralazine, isoniazid, nitrofurantoin, and griseofulvin are some of the agents involved.[46,122] Determination of the reaction is based on symptom resolution with drug discontinuation, absence of idiopathic lupus, development of antibodies, and one clinical symptom of lupus.[122]

Drug–Drug Interactions

The pediatric intensivist is confronted daily with potentially hazardous drug–drug interactions in the critical care setting. A potential drug–drug interaction can be defined as the following: "the possibility that one drug may alter the intensity of pharmacological effects of another drug given concurrently. The net result may be enhanced or diminished effects of one or both of the drugs or the appearance of a new effect that is not seen with either drug alone."[167] The ability to recognize every potential drug interaction in the pediatric critical care setting is nearly impossible. Given the extent of polypharmacy that occurs, the potential risk is significant. Of the thousands of documented drug–drug interactions, only a small fraction are clinically significant.[90] The ability to differentiate between clinically significant and insignificant interactions requires an understanding of their mechanisms. In most cases, drug–drug interactions are predictable and preventable with appropriate dosage modifications or avoidance of combinations.

The magnitude of drug–drug interactions is measured by the intensity of the response. Drugs with narrow therapeutic indexes are especially susceptible to drug–drug interactions because small alterations in exposure can lead to large changes in response. Typically, drugs with large therapeutic indexes are at minimal risk for clinically significant drug–drug interactions.

Drug–drug interactions can occur by three different mechanisms of action: pharmacokinetic, pharmacodynamic, and pharmaceutical. *Pharmacokinetic drug–drug interactions* can be defined as "interactions which affect a target drug through alterations in their absorption, distribution, metabolism, or excretion; the result may be an increase or decrease in the concentration of drug at the site of action."[167] *Pharmacodynamic interactions* are defined as interactions at a common receptor site or that have additive or inhibitory effects as a result of actions at different sites.[167] Pharmaceutical interactions or incompatibilities "occur when drugs interact *in vitro* so that one or both are inactivated."[205]

The ability to distinguish significant drug–drug interactions in the critical care setting is vital to patient care. The following discussion emphasizes the mechanism underlying various drug–drug interactions and identifies clinically significant interactions among therapeutic classes.

Pharmacokinetic Drug–Drug Interactions

The most common and well-studied etiology of drug–drug interactions occurs through pharmacokinetic interactions. Pharmacokinetic interactions can occur throughout the entire pharmacologic spectrum and can potentially affect the absorption, distribution, metabolism, or elimination of the compound of interest. However, drug–drug interactions are only important when they impact the resulting drug exposure to such an extent that the patient experiences an alteration in the expected drug effect, either through diminution of drug effect (when drug exposure is decreased) or through predisposition to adverse effects (when drug exposure is increased). It is important to recognize that the dearth of pharmacokinetic information available for most drugs in children often makes recognition of drug–drug interactions difficult. However, a thorough understanding of the mechanisms behind these interactions can create an index of suspicion that is necessary to identify potential interactions clinically.

Interactions Affecting Drug Absorption

Enteral Absorption. Several factors determine the rate and extent of oral absorption of drug products. Drug–drug interactions affecting enteral absorption occur through several mechanisms with a common end result: alteration of availability of the drug at its primary site of absorption. The most common mechanisms include adsorption or complexation of the target drug by other drugs or by food, alterations in the ionization of the drug through pH changes, and perturbation of normal GI function (e.g., motility, bacterial colonization, mesenteric blood flow).

In the critical care setting, adsorption and complex formation are the most likely causes of decreased enteral drug absorption. Commonly prescribed drugs (e.g., sucralfate and kaolin pectin) are implicated in causing decreased absorption of other drugs by adsorbing target drugs and rendering them unavailable for absorption across the GI barrier.[29,35,95] Food, especially as enteral feeding products, is capable of causing adsorption of drugs. Considerable controversy surrounds the potential for this interaction in the case of phenytoin; the clinical importance of this interaction is still debatable.[11] Although less commonly prescribed in the pediatric setting, tetracyclines and quinolone antibiotics have long been known to cause drug complexes with metallic cations such as iron and calcium, resulting in a decreased effect of both the supplement and the antibiotic.[48,112]

Because only un-ionized drug is available for absorption through the intestinal (or gastric) mucosa, the pH at the site of GI absorption must be considered. In theory, absorption of weakly basic drugs such as penicillins or sulfonamides would be enhanced when given in the presence of concomitant H_2 antagonists or proton pump inhibitors for stress prophylaxis. However, most clinical investigations show this interaction is insignificant.[52,210,229] Logically, weakly acidic drugs such as phenobarbital would be expected to have reduced enteral absorption under the same circumstances; however, this has not been confirmed clinically.

Alterations in the structure or function of the GI tract are not often the cause for drug–drug interactions but nonetheless are important to consider. Drugs that affect gastric emptying or intestinal transit time can reduce or prolong the residence time of a drug at its site of absorption, potentially altering its systemic availability. Alterations in the normal bacterial flora of the gut can affect the absorption of drugs that are metabolized by these bacteria to active (or inactive) forms. Digoxin is the most common example of a drug whose absorption can be affected through this mechanism.[44,138,139] Alterations in mesenteric blood flow potentially could impact the absorption of any drugs administered enterally, but this has never been shown clinically. Although controversial, the ability of indomethacin to affect mesenteric blood flow has been cited as a theoretical reason to withhold feeds and enteral drugs in children being treated for patent ductus arteriosus.[69,252]

Alternative Sites of Absorption. Drug–drug interactions can occur when drugs are administered by nonenteral routes. A common concern in the intensive care unit setting is "compatibility" of drugs given by the IV route, whether the drugs are to be coadministered in the same IV bag or through common IV access lines. This concept is covered in greater detail in the section on pharmaceutical drug–drug interactions. Theoretically, intramuscular or subcutaneous absorption could be reduced when patients are receiving doses of vasopressor agents necessary to maintain blood pressure, secondary to reduced peripheral blood flow. Finally, it is common practice to instruct patients on combination therapy for asthma to administer β-agonist agents prior to controller medications (inhaled steroids, mast cell stabilizers) because their bronchodilatory effects may help to maximize absorption of the controller medication in the distal bronchial tree. However, an improvement in patient outcome secondary to this approach has never been proven.

Interactions Affecting Drug Distribution

Protein or Tissue Binding. Because the majority of drugs are bound to plasma proteins or tissue binding sites, the most commonly cited mechanisms for drug–drug interactions affecting distribution are those that involve protein or tissue binding. Several examples exist in which one drug displaces an object drug through competitive inhibition at a protein or tissue binding site. However, in most cases, the impact of the drug–drug interaction is minimal. The amount of free (active) drug may increase temporarily, but the free level falls back to its previous equilibrium as the clearance of drug subsequently increases. Most cases of increased free drug concentrations secondary to protein binding displacement occur when the displacing drug also inhibits the metabolism or excretion of the displaced drug. For example, probenecid not only displaces bound ceftriaxone from albumin binding sites but also inhibits the active secretion of the drug in the kidney, resulting in increased ceftriaxone concentrations.[235a] The clinical implications of this interaction are minimal because of the wide therapeutic index for ceftriaxone.

Alterations in Total Body Water. An important mechanism for drug–drug interactions affecting drug distribution that often is overlooked is alteration of body fluid composition. Severe dehydration can be caused iatrogenically, either through fluid restriction or overzealous diuretic use. In these cases, drug concentrations can be increased several-fold, resulting in untoward effects. Conversely, the volume of distribution of drugs can be increased significantly by increasing total body water. This can have the effect of decreasing drug concentrations to subtherapeutic levels. Drugs that distribute primarily in total body water, such as aminoglycosides, are particularly susceptible to these types of effects.[131]

Interactions Affecting Drug Metabolism

The majority of clinically relevant drug–drug interactions can be linked to an alteration in drug metabolism. The two major pathways for drug metabolism in humans are the phase I, oxidative pathway and the phase II, conjugation reactions.

Cytochrome P450 Interactions. Inhibition or induction of the phase I pathway is the most studied mechanism of drug–drug interactions, especially in relation to the cytochrome P450 system of enzymes. Table 112–3 lists the drugs that affect cytochrome P450 enzymes and those metabolized by the various, clinically relevant isoforms. Evaluation of a drug's potential to affect the P450 system is now an integral part of new drug development, and many of the older drugs have been studied extensively, such that these interactions often are predictable in adults. In fact, drug–drug interactions now are exploited clinically in human immunodeficiency virus (HIV) therapy through the use of low-dose ritonavir.[31a,33a,205a]

However, the relative lack of formal pediatric studies makes predicting the impact of a particular interaction difficult in a given child. Factors that must be considered include the state of maturation of the particular isoform and the presence of compensatory pathways. In general, it is reasonable to assume that a reaction that occurs in adults will also occur in children; proper action should be taken as necessary.

One important consideration is timing of drug–drug interactions secondary to P450 enzyme inhibition and/or induction. In general, enzyme inhibition results from competitive inhibition at the enzyme binding site and, therefore, becomes clinically relevant as soon as the offending drug reaches sufficient concentrations in the liver. Consequently, upon discontinuation of the offending drug, enzyme inhibition abates as the drug concentrations fall. Drugs with short half-lives have a relatively short offset of effect, whereas those with longer half-lives can cause significant effects for prolonged periods after discontinuation. In contrast, enzyme induction results from an increase in the amount of enzyme synthesized by hepatic cells. Thus there is a lag between the time an inducer is introduced and the onset of induction effect. As expected, the offset of effect also is somewhat prolonged.

Conjugative Enzyme Interactions. Because phase II reactions rarely are rate limiting, their potential to be the cause of clinically significant drug–drug interactions is low. However, the potential does exist for drugs to inhibit conjugation, thus impeding the conversion of object drugs to their inactive metabolites. A classic example is the interaction between high-dose ascorbic acid and acetaminophen. Ascorbic acid competitively inhibits the sulfation of acetaminophen, resulting in accumulation of the glucuronide metabolite.[98a]

Interactions Affecting Drug Excretion

The primary means for elimination of drugs or their metabolites is through renal excretion. The process of renal excretion involves three mechanisms: glomerular filtration rate (GFR), active tubular secretion, and tubular reabsorption. All three mechanisms can be affected by drug–drug interactions.

Glomerular Filtration Rate. Alterations in GFR secondary to drug–drug interactions most often result from alterations in renal blood flow. Drugs that act to reduce renal blood flow, such as cyclosporine or NSAIDs, can reduce GFR and thereby increase the blood concentration of drugs eliminated by this route.[40a,51a,83a,119a,263] Conversely, drugs that improve renal blood flow could increase GFR and decrease plasma concentrations of drugs eliminated through the kidneys. Use of low-dose dopamine to increase renal blood flow and GFR theoretically could cause a decrease in aminoglycoside concentrations; however, this has never been shown in humans.

Active Tubular Secretion. As its name implies, active tubular secretion is an active process whereby drugs bind to receptors and are transported across the tubular cells to be excreted. Drugs that compete for these bindings sites may inhibit the secretion of other drugs, causing increased concentrations. The two most commonly cited inhibitors of active tubular secretion are probenecid (inhibits the site for weak acids such as penicillin) and cimetidine (inhibits the site for weak bases such as procainamide). These reactions are rarely of clinical significance, although the probenecid–penicillin interaction has been used therapeutically to increase penicillin serum concentrations.[33b,44a,228a,259a]

Tubular Reabsorption. Tubular reabsorption is a passive process whereby drugs are reabsorbed into the systemic circulation from the lumen of the distal tubules. As with enteral absorption, only un-ionized molecules are available for reabsorption. Therefore drugs that alter the pH of the urine have the potential to cause increased tubular reabsorption of other drugs. A common example is phenobarbital, a weakly acidic drug. In overdose situations, sodium bicarbonate is administered to alkalinize the urine in the hopes that phenobarbital will become more ionized in urine, resulting in reduced tubular reabsorption and more rapid excretion. However, the effectiveness of this practice is not clear.[158a]

Interactions Affecting P-Glycoprotein Receptors

Research in the oncology field has led to the identification of an important drug transporter that is ubiquitous throughout the human body, namely, P-glycoprotein (PGP). PGP can be found in renal tubule cells, hepatic cells, in the blood-brain barrier, and in mucosal cells of the intestines, the pancreas, and adrenal glands. Table 112–3 lists drugs that are inhibitors and/or substrates for PGP. In general, PGP is believed to serve a protective function by transporting molecules out of the body or, in the case of the blood-brain barrier, out of the CNS. This is manifested in the gut by PGP-mediated secretion of molecules back into the intestinal lumen after absorption, in the kidney by active tubular secretion, in the liver by active secretion into the bile, and in the CNS by active removal of molecules out of the CNS. Thus those drugs that inhibit PGP are expected to increase the concentrations of substrates (either in plasma or the CNS). To date, few clinically relevant interactions have been identified because of the relatively low inhibitory activity of most known drugs. However, because of their ability to aid in the treatment of multiply drug-resistant carcinomas, potent PGP inhibitors are being developed and will be used therapeutically in the near future.[146,266]

Pharmacodynamic Drug–Drug Interactions

A pharmacodynamic drug–drug interaction can be defined as the combination of two or more drugs with additive, synergistic, or antagonistic pharmacodynamic effects. Additive pharmacodynamic interactions occur routinely when two or more drugs of the same class are given in combination, as in the case of antihypertensive medication or anticonvulsants. A synergistic interaction occurs when the combination of two drugs has an effect greater than the sum of their individual effects. One example of a clinically relevant synergistic interaction is the use of aminoglycosides in combination with β-lactam antibiotics. In theory, combining a cell-wall active agent (β-lactams) with an agent that inhibits bacterial protein synthesis (aminoglycosides) can achieve a greater antibiotic effect than the sum of the two individual effects.

TABLE 112–3

P-Glycoprotein and Cytochrome P450 Substrates, Inhibitors, and Inducers

	Substrates		Inhibitors		Inducers	
PGP*	Amiodarone	Itraconazole	Amiodarone	Midazolam	Amiodarone	Nicardipine
	Cimetidine	Levofloxacin	Carvedilol	Nicardipine	Cyclosporine	Nifedipine
	Ciprofloxacin	Methylprednisolone	Chlorpromazine	Nifedipine	Dexamethasone	Phenobarbital
	Cortisol	Morphine	Clarithromycin	Ofloxacin	Diltiazem	Phenytoin
	Cyclosporine	Nadolol	Cortisol	Prochlorperazine	Erythromycin	Probenecid
	Dexamethasone	Octreotide	Cyclosporine	Propranolol	Insulin	Rifampin
	Digoxin	Ondansetron	Desipramine	Quinidine	Midazolam	Tacrolimus
	Diltiazem	Phenytoin	Diltiazem	Quinine	Morphine	Verapamil
	Erythromycin	Ranitidine	Erythromycin	Sirolimus		
	Fentanyl	Sirolimus	Haloperidol	Spironolactone		
	Hydrocortisone	Verapamil	Imipramine	Tacrolimus		
		Itraconazole	Verapamil			
		Ketoconazole				
		Lidocaine				
CYP1A2	Acetaminophen	Nicardipine	Caffeine	Lidocaine	Carbamazepine	Pantoprazole
	Caffeine	Ondansetron	Cimetidine	Nifedipine	Insulin	Phenobarbital
	Carvedilol	Ranitidine	Ciprofloxacin	Omeprazole	Lansoprazole	Phenytoin
	Cisapride	R-warfarin	Clarithromycin	Ondansetron	Nafcillin	Rifampin
	Diazepam	Theophylline	Diltiazem	Propofol	Omeprazole	
	Haloperidol	Verapamil	Erythromycin	Propranolol		
	Lidocaine		Grapefruit juice	Ranitidine		
	Naproxen		Ketoconazole	Theophylline		
		Levofloxacin				
CYP1E2	Acetaminophen	Isoflurane		Isoniazid		
	Enflurane	Methoxyflurane				
	Halothane	Sevoflurane				
CYP2C9	Caffeine	Ondansetron	Chloramphenicol	Omeprazole	Carbamazepine	
	Carvedilol	Pantoprazole	Cimetidine	Phenobarbital	Phenobarbital	
	Cisapride	Phenobarbital	Diltiazem	Phenytoin	Phenytoin	
	Dextromethorphan	Phenytoin	Fluconazole	Probenecid	Rifampin	
	Diazepam	Propofol	Ibuprofen	Propofol		
	Diltiazem	Quinidine	Indomethacin	Propranolol		
	Fluconazole	S-warfarin	Itraconazole	Sulfonamides		
	Ibuprofen	Theophylline	Ketoconazole	Trimethoprim		
	Indomethacin	Valproic acid	Lansoprazole	Verapamil		

	Lansoprazole	Verapamil	Metronidazole	Voriconazole		
	Montelukast	Voriconazole	Nifedipine			
	Naproxen	Zafirlukast				
	Nicotine	Omeprazole				
CYP2C19	Cisapride	Phenobarbital	Cimetidine	Lansoprazole	Carbamazepine	
	Diazepam	Phenytoin	Diazepam	Omeprazole	Phenobarbital	
	Fluconazole	Propofol	Felbamate	Voriconazole	Phenytoin	
	Ibuprofen	Propranolol	Fluconazole		Prednisone	
	Indomethacin	Ranitidine	Indomethacin		Rifampin	
	Lansoprazole	R-warfarin	Ketoconazole			
	Metoprolol	Verapamil				
	Omeprazole	Voriconazole				
	Pantoprazole					
CYP2D6	Acetaminophen	Methadone	Amiodarone	Methylphenidate	Carbamazepine	Phenytoin
	Amphetamine	Methamphetamine	Chlorpheniramine	Metoprolol	Dexamethasone	Rifampin
	Caffeine	Metoprolol	Cimetidine	Nicardipine	Ethanol	
	Captopril	Morphine	Cisapride	Omeprazole	Phenobarbital	
	Carvedilol	Nelfinavir	Codeine	Ondansetron		
	Chlorpheniramine	Nevirapine	Dextromethorphan	Oxybutynin		
	Codeine	Omeprazole	Diltiazem	Propofol		
	Dextromethorphan	Ondansetron	Haloperidol	Propranolol		
	Diltiazem	Oxycodone	Ketoconazole	Quinidine		
	Fentanyl	Propofol	Lansoprazole	Ranitidine		
	Hydrocodone	Propranolol	Lidocaine	Verapamil		
	Lidocaine	Ranitidine	Methylamphetamine			
	Loratadine	Theophylline				
	Meperidine					
CYP3A4	Alfentanil	Losartan	Clarithromycin	Ketoconazole	Barbiturates	Phenytoin
	Alprazolam	Methadone	Cyclosporine	Methylprednisolone	Carbamazepine	Primidone
	Amiodarone	Methylprednisolone	Diltiazem	Metronidazole		
	Amlodipine	Miconazole	Erythromycin	Nefazodone		
	Atorvastatin	Midazolam	Ethinyl Estradiol	Norethindrone		
	Carbamazepine	Montelukast	Fluvoxamine	Prednisone	Dexamethasone	Rifabutin
	Clarithromycin	Nefazodone	Grapefruit juice	Verapamil	Griseofulvin	Rifampin
	Cisapride	Nimodipine	Isoniazid	Voriconazole		
	Citalopram	Nisoldipine	Itraconazole			
	Cyclophosphamide	Pioglitazone				
	Cyclosporine	Prednisolone				
	Dapsone	Quetiapine				

Continued

TABLE 112–3

P-Glycoprotein and Cytochrome P450 Substrates, Inhibitors, and Inducers—cont'd

Substrates		Inhibitors	Inducers
Dexamethasone	Rifabutin		
Diazepam	Sertraline		
Diltiazem	Sildenafil		
Dofetilide	Simvastatin		
Doxorubicin	Sirolimus		
Erythromycin	Tacrolimus		
Ethinyl Estradiol	Testosterone		
Etoposide	Theophylline		
Felodipine	Triazolam		
Fentanyl	Verapamil		
Fluconazole	Vinblastine		
Imatinib	Vincristine		
Ifosfamide	Voriconazole		
Itraconazole	R-warfarin		
Ketoconazole	Zolpidem		
Lidocaine			
Loratadine			

*Several drugs are listed as both P-glycoprotein (PGP) inhibitors and inducers because their effects on PGP expression can be concentration or duration related.

Although difficult to prove clinically, *in vitro* and animal studies have validated this theory.[17,222,238] Most antagonistic drug–drug interactions are more appropriately defined as pharmacokinetic interactions because they result from some alteration in drug concentrations, either in plasma or at the effect site. Antagonistic interactions that are truly pharmacodynamic in nature most often result from competitive inhibition at the receptor site for drug activity. Use of flumazenil to reverse benzodiazepine-induced sedation is an example of an antagonistic pharmacodynamic drug–drug interaction used clinically.[26,28,143]

Drug–Drug Interactions in Intravenous Admixtures

Parenteral administration of drug therapy poses a potential source of drug–drug interactions in the pediatric/neonatal intensive care unit. In this scenario, polypharmacy arising from an extensive problem list and limited IV access conspire to force the mixing of various drug solutions. However, disparate physicochemical properties and varying administration times preclude the indiscriminate admixing of numerous drugs into a single parenteral aliquot. In practice, both intermittently scheduled drugs and continuous infusions are often given concurrently by the Y-site of IV tubing, different lumens in the same IV line, or a different IV access altogether. This drug delivery strategy helps to reduce the contact time among different drug, electrolyte, and/or nutrient solutions. The majority of infusions require 15 to 60 minutes, a time frame in which most drugs will remain stable when they are infused with other drugs. Infusion of drugs with known incompatibilities could have serious consequences when administered to the patient. Introduction of a precipitate to venous circulation could produce adverse effects such as phlebitis and pulmonary embolism.[94] Admixing of IV drug solutions may lead to incompatibilities that could have serious consequences when administered to the patient. Factors influencing the coadministration of drugs include a limited number of IV access sites, an extensive drug therapy regimen, time constraints, and the need to administer other lengthy infusions (e.g., blood products).

Incompatibilities result from chemical reactions that may or may not be visible. Physical incompatibilities are easily identifiable because they illustrate any one of the following visual phenomena: precipitation, complexation, turbidity, color change, evolution of gas, or separation of the solution into distinct immiscible layers.[248] On the other hand, instability occurs when a mixture of drug solutions chemically react to yield a different species or degradation product, either of which could be pharmacologically inactive or even toxic. The rate at which these reactions occur adds another variable in determining whether or not two drug solutions can be coinfused and for what duration. Generally, incompatibility is defined as a 10% decomposition of one or more components in an admixture in less than 24 hours.[248] Drug solutions typically are pH buffered to optimize the solubility of the drug. Admixing solutions may alter the pH of the chemical environment and result in inactivation or visually ascertained incompatibilities such as precipitation. Reduction–oxidation reactions among incompatible drugs may lead to activation or generation of a toxic molecule. Salting out of drugs occurs when nonelectrolytes and weakly hydrated ions are exposed to strong electrolyte solutions. Chelation of drugs in incompatible admixtures can lead to inactivation or formation of insoluble complexes.

Drug–Drug Interactions by Therapeutic Class

Cardiovascular (see Chapter 23)

As opposed to many other classes of drugs, the most common mechanism of cardiovascular drug–drug interactions results through alterations in pharmacodynamics. The potential for two drugs to act upon the same receptor subtype sets the stage for pharmacodynamic interactions, which can be antagonistic, additive, or synergistic in nature. This section details some of potential interactions.

Sympathomimetic Amines. Sympathomimetic amines (epinephrine, norepinephrine, phenylephrine, dopamine, dobutamine, ephedrine, isoproterenol, metoproterenol, and isoetharine) are particularly susceptible to pharmacodynamic drug–drug interactions. The extent and significance of these interactions depend upon the selectivity of both the object drug and precipitant drug for adrenergic receptor types. β-Adrenergic blocking agents generally antagonize the cardiac and bronchodilating effects of the sympathomimetics.[149] However, propranolol and other nonspecific β-blockers (Table 112–4) may enhance the vasoconstriction produced with epinephrine. As a result, the patient may experience hypertension and bradycardia.[91,92] Labetalol possesses both α_1 and nonspecific β blocking activity, which produces an increase in diastolic blood pressure and a decrease in heart rate when given during an epinephrine infusion.[91,92] Metoprolol and possibly other β_1-cardioselective blockers have minimal effects on the pressor response when given concomitantly with epinephrine.[91,92]

Other classes of drugs can interact with the sympathomimetics. α-Adrenergic blocking agents (e.g., phentolamine), when added to a regimen containing a sympathomimetic, reduce vasoconstriction and attenuate the increase in blood pressure.[149] Tricyclic antidepressants (e.g., imipramine) tend to increase the pressor response to sympathomimetics such as epinephrine and norepinephrine and catecholamines such as phenylephrine. The effect has been shown to produce severe and persistent hypertension in patients receiving phenylephrine.[91,92,149] Ergot alkaloids may potentiate the pressor effects of sympathomimetics with pronounced α-adrenergic activity (e.g., epinephrine, norepinephrine, phenylephrine).[91,92,149] Antihistamines (diphenhydramine) and tricyclic antidepressants tend to inhibit tissue uptake of epinephrine and norepinephrine. They also can increase adrenoreceptor sensitivity to epinephrine.[149]

General anesthetics (e.g., cyclopropane) and halogenated hydrocarbons (e.g., halothane) tend to increase cardiac irritability and sensitize the myocardium to the effects of sympathomimetics. Tachycardia and arrhythmias (ventricular premature contractions and fibrillation) are reported with concurrent administrations.[149] Atropine also tends to block the reflex bradycardia produced by epinephrine, norepinephrine, and phenylephrine. This effect in turn augments the pressor response.[149] Finally, concurrent administration of dopamine and IV phenytoin (fosphenytoin) produces hypotension and bradycardia in case reports and animal studies. Cardiovascular status should be monitored closely when these medications are given concomitantly.[91, 92]

Vasodilators. The pharmacologic effect of vasodilators, such as nitroprusside, minoxidil, hydralazine, and diazoxide, are augmented by both β-blockers and diuretics. The decreased systemic vascular resistance and resultant reduction in arterial pressure provide stimuli for a compensatory increase in sympathetic nervous system impulses. Normalization of blood pressure to the set point then is mediated by an increase in cardiac contractility, increased heart rate, and stimulation of the renin-angiotensin-aldosterone (RAA) pathway. β-Blockers prevent this sympathetic outflow and thereby enhance the vasodilator response. Diuretics also block the compensatory sodium retention from the RAA pathway and thereby reduce the rise in arterial pressure that would have been produced from plasma volume expansion.[19] Caffeine, on the other hand, increases renin secretion.[245] Caffeine may attenuate the hypotensive response to vasodilators.

The combination of sodium nitroprusside and sildenafil may produce additive hypotensive effects. Although currently undergoing further evaluation, sildenafil holds some promise as a modality for treatment of pulmonary hypertension in pediatric and neonatal critical care. Thus the concomitant administration of nitroprusside and sildenafil is not outside the realm of possibility in the pediatric setting. Contact between sodium nitroprusside molecules and erythrocytes or the vascular wall results in generation of nitric oxide. Nitric oxide subsequently stimulates the cyclic guanosine monophosphate (cGMP) second messenger system in vascular smooth muscle upon activation of soluble guanylyl cyclase. The molecular process of increasing intracellular concentrations of cGMP translates to vasodilation and the resultant physiologic effect of reduced blood pressure. Sildenafil augments the response to cGMP through selective inhibition of type 5 phosphodiesterase, the enzyme that catalyzes degradation of cGMP. Therefore sildenafil can react similarly with other drugs (nitroglycerin, hydralazine) that promote the generation of a nitric oxide species. However, preliminary animal studies suggest that concomitant administration of sildenafil with nitroglycerin does not result in a dose-reducing effect for nitroglycerin.

Although the mechanism of action is unclear, concomitant administration of indomethacin with hydralazine may reduce the hypotensive effect of hydralazine.[41]

Approximately 90% of diazoxide is bound to plasma proteins, making protein binding displacement a likely scenario for drug–drug interactions. In vitro studies, for example, have illustrated the displacement of warfarin by diazoxide.[149] Children who have received both diazoxide and phenytoin experience difficulty in attaining therapeutic drug concentrations of phenytoin, which suggests that diazoxide may increase phenytoin metabolism.[149]

Antiarrhythmics. The antiarrhythmic drugs amiodarone, disopyramide, and quinidine are substrates for the CYP3A4 isoform of the P450 enzyme system. Plasma levels of these antiarrhythmics may increase and produce adverse effects when combined with CYP3A4 inhibitors such as the macrolide antibiotics (clarithromycin, erythromycin, troleandomycin), the azole antifungals (fluconazole, itraconazole, ketoconazole, voriconazole), and other miscellaneous inhibitors such as cyclosporine, the calcium channel blockers (diltiazem and verapamil), and grapefruit juice. Conversely, plasma levels decrease when therapy is combined with drugs that are known enzyme inducers, including phenobarbital, carbamazepine, phenytoin, oxcarbazepine, primidone, and rifampin. The antiarrhythmic drugs flecainide, mexiletine, and propafenone are substrates for CYP2D6. Concomitant therapy with enzyme inhibitors of CYP2D6, including amiodarone, cimetidine, diphenhydramine, fluoxetine, paroxetine, haloperidol, propafenone, and quinidine, could result in toxicity.[Hansten & Horn 2002]

As a substrate for PGP, digoxin exhibits reduced renal and nonrenal clearance when a PGP inhibitor is added to the drug regimen. The plasma levels of digoxin may double or quadruple, demanding close monitoring for digoxin toxicity. PGP inhibitors include amiodarone, clarithromycin, cyclosporine, diltiazem, erythromycin, ketoconazole, itraconazole, propafenone, quinidine, and verapamil.[91,92]

Pharmacodynamic interactions with drugs that modulate atrioventricular (AV) nodal conduction may produce clinically significant adverse effects, which include heart block, bradycardia, and other arrhythmias. Concurrent therapies with the antiarrhythmics, calcium channel blockers, and β-blockers should must be monitored closely or even reevaluated.[7] Patients with severe electrolyte imbalances may be susceptible to digoxin toxicities. Hypokalemia, hypomagnesemia, and hypercalcemia are all conditions that may be drug induced. Therefore drugs may interact with digoxin in an indirect manner through alteration of electrolyte homeostasis. The loop diuretics, thiazide diuretics, amphotericin B, corticosteroids, laxatives, and sodium polystyrene sulfonate may contribute to digoxin toxicity.[149]

Antihypertensives. Calcium channel blockers are implicated in several common pharmacokinetic drug–drug interactions involving the CYP3A substrates. In addition, inhibitors of CYP3A can cause significant interactions with calcium channel blockers. These interactions can lead to lower diastolic blood pressure, higher heart rates, and other vasodilation-related side effects.[104,169,170,171,255] Inducers of CYP3A4 are implicated in the reduced efficacy of calcium channel blockers.[7] Droperidol affects cardiac repolarization; it prolongs the QT/QTc interval and, when concurrently administered with calcium channel blockers, increases the risk of QT/QTc prolongation, torsades de pointes, and cardiac arrest.[192] Concomitant administration of fentanyl and nicardipine can result in severe hypotension.[189] Awareness of potential drug–drug interactions is necessary when administering calcium channel blockers.

β-Adrenergic antagonists are associated with a variety of pharmacodynamic and pharmacokinetic drug–drug interactions. Concomitant use of a β-blocker and verapamil or diltiazem can result in additive negative inotropic effects and can potentiate conduction abnormalities.[148,264]

Abrupt withdrawal of clonidine when concomitantly used with an β-adrenergic antagonist can exaggerate rebound hypertension symptoms associated with clonidine withdrawal.[16,137,236] The probable mechanism of this interaction is unopposed α-adrenergic agonism. Use of amiodarone with β-adrenergic antagonists potentates bradycardia, sinus arrest, and AV block.[189] Fentanyl anesthesia in combination with β-adrenergic antagonist and calcium channel antagonist reportedly causes hypotension.[189]

ACEIs have been implicated in a variety of drug–drug interactions. Electrolyte disturbances are a major source of complications with these drug–drug interactions. Potassium-sparing diuretics (spironolactone) in combination with ACEIs (e.g., enalaprilat) cause increases in potassium levels.[199]

Loop diuretics induce hypokalemia and hypomagnesemia and, when administered concomitantly with droperidol, may precipitate QT prolongation.[192] In addition, furosemide may produce digitalis toxicity when administered concurrently with digitalis therapy through this same mechanism.[121,231] There is increased risk for nephrotoxicity and ototoxicity when furosemide and aminoglycosides are administered concurrently.[109]

Antiepileptics (see Chapter 55)

The antiepileptics constitute a drug class that has the potential to be involved in a large array of drug–drug interactions. These interactions are mainly pharmacokinetic in nature and usually involve induction, inhibition, or competition among substrates for various isoforms of the cytochrome P450 enzyme system. Fortunately, these drugs typically are monitored using blood concentrations. Appropriate therapeutic drug monitoring can aid in the avoidance of adverse events secondary to drug–drug interactions. Table 112–3 lists the isoforms for which the various antiepileptics are substrates, inducers, or inhibitors.

Phenytoin. In the intensive care unit setting, phenytoin is generally administered intravenously in the form of the water-soluble prodrug fosphenytoin. Phosphatases in red blood cells and the liver catalyze the conversion of fosphenytoin to its active form phenytoin. Fosphenytoin generally has a serum half-life of 8 to 15 minutes.[152] Once fosphenytoin is converted to phenytoin, it is susceptible to all of the potential drug–drug interactions that affect orally administered phenytoin. Approximately 95% of phenytoin is metabolized in the liver by the CYP2C9/10 and CYP2C19 isoforms of the cytochrome P450 enzyme system to produce the inactive hydroxylated metabolite parahydroxyphenylhydantoin.[152] The CYP2C9/10 isoform is the main pathway of metabolism for this drug. Phenytoin metabolism is reduced and plasma levels increased via competition with other drugs that are substrates for CYP2C9 and CYP2C19, such as amiodarone, fluconazole, valproic acid, omeprazole, and fluoxetine. Conversely, phenytoin may competitively inhibit the metabolism of these drugs. Drugs that inhibit CYP2C9 reduce clearance of phenytoin and consequently increase plasma concentrations.[5] Examples include fluconazole, ketoconazole, cotrimoxazole, amiodarone, and valproate. Omeprazole, cimetidine, and fluoxetine are inhibitors of CYP2C19 and thus can increase phenytoin plasma concentrations.[5] In addition to serving as a substrate to CYP2C9/10 and CYP2C19, phenytoin can induce their activity. Moreover, phenytoin induces CYP3A4 and uridine diphosphate glucuronosyl transferase (UGT) activity.[152] It may take 1 to 2 weeks for maximum induction of these enzymes when phenytoin therapy is started and, conversely, the same amount of time for deinduction once the drug is discontinued.[5] Phenytoin exhibits a high degree of protein binding (≈90%) to serum proteins, mainly albumin, so displacement from its binding sites may produce clinically significant changes in free phenytoin concentration.[152] The free fraction is the pharmacologically active portion of the total phenytoin concentration in plasma. Populations in whom increased proportion of free drug may be found include neonates, patients with uremia, hyperbilirubinemia, or hypoalbuminemia, and/or patients taking concurrent anionic drugs and metabolites.[62,152,179] During the hospital course of critically ill children who experienced traumatic head injuries, protein binding and phenytoin metabolism are altered.[235] The free fraction of phenytoin may increase over time in patients with acute head injury.[87] Such a clinical condition makes this particular population of patients especially susceptible to potential protein displacement interactions with other highly protein-bound drugs, such as valproic acid. The potential clinical significance of this interaction is an increased risk for phenytoin toxicity.

Phenobarbital. Phenobarbital is a substrate for CYP2C9, CYP2C19, and CYP2E1. The CYP2C19 isoform serves as the primary pathway for metabolism.[152] Phenobarbital is converted to 5-p-hydroxyphenyl-5-ethyl-barbituric acid, an inactive species, and further conjugated with glucuronic acid or sulfuric acid for excretion in urine.[152] Phenobarbital has the potential to induce CYP2C9 and CYP3A4 enzymes.[272] The time frame for induction and deinduction of the P450 enzyme system depends upon phenobarbital's half-life, with induction beginning 1 week after initiating phenobarbital therapy and deinduction beginning 1 week after phenobarbital is discontinued. Maximum induction occurs in approximately 2 to 3 weeks. Phenobarbital also induces UGT.[5] Addition of phenobarbital or phenytoin to a regimen of methadone, which may be used in the intensive care unit for the purpose of weaning from long-term opiate sedation, may present a potential for significant drug–drug interaction. Induction of CYP2C9 and CYP3A4 leads to increased clearance of methadone. The reduced plasma concentration of methadone could result in signs of methadone withdrawal. In transplant patients, phenobarbital may reduce cyclosporine concentrations, which may lead to concerns regarding adequate immunosuppression. Another significant drug interaction involves the abrupt withdrawal of phenobarbital in a patient maintained on both phenobarbital and warfarin. In such a scenario, blood levels of warfarin may increase and lead to increased risk of bleeding. During maintenance of such a regimen, phenobarbital induces the same enzymes responsible for warfarin metabolism. As a result, warfarin dosing is adjusted based upon phenobarbital-mediated inhibition of the hypoprothrombinemia response.

Carbamazepine. The main pathway for metabolism of carbamazepine is through the CYP3A4 isoform. CYP1A2 and CYP2C8 also are sites for metabolism but are considered to play lesser roles. It is believed that carbamazepine may also be a substrate for CYP2C19.[5] Carbamazepine is metabolized to a 10,11-epoxide, which also possesses pharmacologic activity. Carbamazepine may undergo inactivation by hydroxylation and conjugation along another pathway. The 10,11-epoxide is further metabolized to inactive compounds for elimination. Carbamazepine induces CYP1A2, CYP2C9, CYP3A4, and UGT; therefore carbamazepine may reduce the plasma concentrations of drugs that are substrates for these isoforms. Carbamazepine illustrates autoinduction, the induction of its own metabolism through CYP3A4. Autoinduction is apparent in the initial weeks of carbamazepine therapy and doubles its rate of clearance within this time frame. Induction begins within the first week of therapy and maximizes at approximately 3 weeks.[5]

Concomitant therapy with drugs that are substrates, inducers, or inhibitors of the same isoforms involved in carbamazepine clearance changes its plasma concentration. Macrolide antibiotics (e.g., erythromycin, clarithromycin, troleandomycin) inhibit the CYP3A4 enzymes, which results in elevated carbamazepine plasma levels and a consequent decrease in 10,11-epoxide.[5] Calcium channel blockers (especially verapamil and diltiazem) also inhibit CYP3A4 and have similar effects on carbamazepine plasma levels.

Valproic Acid. The isoforms of the P450 enzyme system that metabolize valproic acid include CYP2C9 and CYP2C19, both of which represent minor pathways. The main route of metabolism for valproic acid involves glucuronidation by UGT and β-oxidation.[152] Valproate inhibits drugs that are metabolized by CYP2C9, such as phenytoin and phenobarbital. In addition to being a substrate for UGT, valproic acid inhibits drugs that are metabolized by this enzyme, such as lorazepam and lamotrigine. Felbamate, on the other hand, inhibits β-oxidation, resulting in reduced clearance of valproic acid.[5] Valproic acid also exhibits a high degree of protein binding to plasma albumin (90%), making protein displacement interactions likely with other highly protein-bound drugs.[152]

Lamotrigine. The main pathway for metabolism of lamotrigine is UGT-mediated glucuronidation. Lamotrigine is capable of inducing its own metabolism, with maximum autoinduction observed within 2 weeks. Autoinduction typically results in a 17% reduction in plasma blood levels.[101] Through their action on UGT, carbamazepine, phenytoin, and phenobarbital reduce plasma concentrations of lamotrigine when given concomitantly. Lamotrigine, on the other hand, reduces valproic acid plasma levels when added to a regimen containing valproic acid. Concentrations may be reduced by as much as 25% in the course of a few weeks.[152] When added to carbamazepine therapy, lamotrigine promotes increases in plasma levels of the 10,11-epoxide active metabolite of carbamazepine.[5]

Antiinfective/Antimicrobials (See Chapter 87)

Antimicrobial agents are commonly used in the intensive care unit to treat patients with serious infections. Some drug–drug interactions involve antimicrobial agents, but most are not clinically significant.[46] Some interactions involve complexation of the antimicrobial, such as quinolones (ciprofloxacin, levofloxacin) binding to multivalent cations (aluminum, calcium, magnesium, iron).[168,259] This interaction can be avoided by administering the drugs at separate times. Ciprofloxacin may interact with theophylline and caffeine, inhibiting their metabolism by the cytochrome P450 system. This interaction does not occur with third-generation (levofloxacin) and fourth-generation (gatifloxacin, moxifloxacin) quinolones.[259] Cyclosporine levels may be increased with concurrent use of ciprofloxacin. Monitoring of cyclosporine levels or changing to another antibiotic to which the pathogen is susceptible are ways to manage this interaction.

Many drug–drug interactions occur with macrolide antibiotics. Erythromycin may cause interactions through inhibition of the cytochrome P450 enzymes (1A,3A). Erythromycin may increase serum levels of theophylline, warfarin, carbamazepine, cyclosporine, midazolam, tacrolimus, and hydroxymethylglutaryl coenzyme A reductase inhibitors (e.g., lovastatin, simvastatin, atorvastatin).[3,75,178] Clarithromycin also inhibits cytochrome P450 enzymes and may increase the serum levels of carbamazepine, theophylline, caffeine, cyclosporine, warfarin, valproate, and midazolam.[3,178] Azithromycin is an azalide (macrolide subclass) that does not demonstrate cytochrome P450 complexation, so it has less drug interaction potential. No major drug–drug interactions have been shown with azithromycin and carbamazepine, theophylline, or midazolam.[3] Interactions with cyclosporine and warfarin are limited to case reports, so monitoring of serum levels and international normalized ratio (INR), respectively, is prudent when using this combination.[177]

Rifampin is a cytochrome P450 enzyme inducer that is involved in many drug–drug interactions. Rifampin may decrease serum concentrations of chloramphenicol, isoniazid, amiodarone, cyclosporine, prednisolone, and warfarin.[256,267] These interactions often complicate multidrug regimens for treatment of active tuberculosis.

Antifungal agents are used in the critical care setting for treatment and prophylaxis of systemic mycoses. The majority of drug–drug interactions with antifungals occur within the azole derivatives via inhibition of biotransformation. Azole derivatives inhibit sterol 14-α-demethylase, which is a hepatic microsomal cytochrome P450-dependent system. Unfortunately, this mechanism results in significant drug–drug interactions. Azole antifungals are known inhibitors of cytochrome P450 isoenzymes, although the specific CYP isoforms and potency of inhibition vary among agents.[240,255] Table 112–3 provides a description of cytochrome P450 isoforms inhibited by the azole antifungals.

Clinically significant interactions with azoles occur most frequently with agents that have narrow therapeutic windows and are metabolized by cytochrome P450 enzymes. Clinically significant interactions can occur when azole derivatives are administered with CYP3A substrates such as midazolam,[1,170] tacrolimus,[67] sirolimus,[201] cyclosporine,[66] nifedipine,[79] felodipine,[79,166] diltiazem,[201] and alfentanil.[180] Benzodiazepines that rely on the CYP3A4 enzyme for biotransformation are predisposed to drug–drug interactions with CYP3A inhibitors. The benzodiazepines most prone are alprazolam, diazepam, midazolam, and triazolam.[85,171,176] Ketoconazole, a potent inhibitor of CYP3A, increases the area under the concentration–time curve (AUC) of oral midazolam by 16-fold.[12-15,166,171] Whenever ketoconazole, itraconazole, voriconazole, or fluconazole is administered with midazolam, patients must be monitored for heightened response and altering the dosage or discontinuing therapy considered. Diazepam metabolism is mediated by CYP3A and CYP2C19 and is prone to interactions with azole derivatives.[175] Fluconazole and voriconazole have the potential to cause clinically significant drug–drug interactions with compounds that are metabolized via CYP3A, CYP2C9, and CYP2C19; therefore caution should be exercised when administering fluconazole or voriconazole with diazepam. Warfarin is a racemic mixture compound for which most pharmacodynamic activity occurs with the S-isomer, whose metabolism is dependent on CYP2C9, which is inhibited by fluconazole and voriconazole.[22,201] This interaction is significant, and appropriate dosage modifications or alteration of therapeutic agents must be considered. The calcium channel blocker class is metabolized by CYP3A isoenzymes and has the potential for interactions with azole derivatives.[166] Concomitant use of fluconazole and rifabutin has resulted in rifabutin toxicities from increased serum concentrations because of inhibition of cytochrome P450 isoenzymes.[247] Similar interactions are expected with voriconazole and itraconazole. Azole derivatives increase serum concentration of both phenytoin (after administration of fosphenytoin) and carbamazepine.[24,163] There is the potential for decreased efficacy of azole derivatives used in combination with rifampin, an inducer of the cytochrome P450 isoenzyme system.[9]

In addition to being CYP3A inhibitors, ketoconazole and itraconazole are substrates and inhibitors of PGP.[239,255] Drug–drug interactions mediated via PGP typically are important determinants of bioavailability, liver metabolism, and kidney excretion.[182,241] Thus ketoconazole and itraconazole with dual CYP3A and PGP inhibition could greatly impact the bioavailability of dual substrate drugs.[103,255] Diltiazem, verapamil, saquinavir, cyclosporine, and tacrolimus are dual CYP3A and PGP substrates.[40,270] Clearance of digoxin, a PGP substrate, is decreased with coadministration of itraconazole.[105] An increase in digoxin trough concentration is likely the result of impaired renal tubular secretion via inhibition of PGP.[105]

Concomitant administration of amphotericin B with cyclosporine, tacrolimus, or aminoglycosides results in increased nephrotoxicity.[33,217] Concomitant use of digoxin and amphotericin B products results in digitalis toxicities attributed to potassium depletion-mediated by amphotericin B.[187] Antifungal therapy is associated with a variety of potentially significant drug–drug interactions. Therapeutic drug monitoring is necessary in the critical care setting, but additional awareness is warranted when antifungal agents are being used (see Chapters 115 and 116).

Anesthetics and Sedatives

Several agents are used for anesthesia and sedation in the pediatric critical care setting. Many of these drugs have clinically significant drug–drug interactions. The ability to recognize potential drug–drug interactions related to the use of anesthetics or sedatives in the pediatric critical care setting requires a fundamental understanding of the agent's clinical pharmacology. Benzodiazepines are a class of anesthetics that are particularly susceptible to drug–drug interactions because of their route of biotransformation.[169,170,253] CYP3A4 plays a major role in the metabolism of midazolam, triazolam, and alprazolam, and caution should be exercised when combining these agents with CYP3A modulators.[190,200,202] As mentioned in the Antiinfective/Antimicrobials section, concomitant use of systemic antifungals and benzodiazepines results in a known clinically significant drug–drug interaction, caused by azole antifungals inhibiting the CYP3A isoenzyme.[169–171,253] Midazolam, a short-acting benzodiazepine used in the pediatric critical care setting, is almost exclusively metabolized via the CYP3A pathway. Interactions are most prominent with oral midazolam therapy because of the role of intestinal metabolism.[169–171] However, significantly increased plasma levels have been observed when IV midazolam therapy is administered with fluconazole.[Olkkola et al] Additionally, clarithromycin and erythromycin have been proven to significantly decrease systemic clearance of IV and oral midazolam.[82,83,171] Azithromycin, another macrolide, appears to not increase plasma concentrations of oral midazolam.[14] Propofol has been shown to decrease the clearance of midazolam by 37%, possibly by competitive inhibition of CYP3A4.[69] Concomitant administration of verapamil or diltiazem with oral midazolam is associated with dramatic increases in AUC and the maximum concentration (C_{max}).[13] Inducers of CYP3A can drastically decrease plasma concentrations of midazolam. Rifampin, a potent inducer of CYP3A and PGP expression in the gut mucosa, can cause dramatic decreases in plasma concentrations of oral midazolam.[13,83] Other inducers of CYP3A enzymes implicated in significant interactions with midazolam are carbamazepine and phenytoin.[3] Diazepam, a benzodiazepine with long-acting metabolites, is prone to drug–drug interactions with inhibitors or inducers of CYP2C19 or 3A4. Because the primary route of metabolism for lorazepam is through glucuronidation, this agent is associated with fewer potential pharmacokinetic drug–drug interactions.[85,86]

The potential for pharmacodynamic drug–drug interactions exists. Concomitant use of barbiturates and benzodiazepines causes additive respiratory and CNS depression. This additive mechanism is mediated via allosteric conformational changes with γ-aminobutyric acid (GABA), which regulates the opening of chloride channels, causing the neurons to become hyperpolarized and resistant to excitation.[250] The dosage of midazolam and other benzodiazepines often is reduced by 30% to 50% when they are administered concomitantly with opioid analgesics.[25] Flumazenil competitively inhibits the activity of benzodiazepines at its recognition site on the GABA–benzodiazepine receptor complex.[197] It does not reverse the CNS effects of GABA-mimetic agents such as barbiturates, propofol, and other general anesthetics.[197] The FDA has approved flumazenil for pediatric usage.[197] Clonidine, an α_2-adrenergic agonist agent with sedating properties, when used concomitantly with propofol, reduces the induction concentrations required for loss of consciousness.[93] Propofol can inhibit the clearance of alfentanil and act synergistically with opioids.[153,258] Caution should be exercised when using propofol in combination with drugs that lower seizure threshold, such as meperidine and enflurane.[162a] Neuromuscular blocking agents have some significant drug–drug interactions.[151] Concomitant use of IV antibiotics such as aminoglycosides or clindamycin has the potential to intensify the neuromuscular blockade produced by neuromuscular blocking agents.[151] Phenytoin has been shown to increase pancuronium requirements. Additionally, inhalation anesthetics can potentiate neuromuscular blockade.[151]

Analgesics (see Chapter 116)

A variety of agents are used for analgesia in pediatric critical care. Patients receiving opiate agonists are particularly susceptible to drug–drug interactions. Whenever an opiate agonist is administered with a CNS depressant, augmented effects or toxicity are possible. Therefore vigilance in monitoring for drug–drug interactions is necessary when administering these agents to help ensure that safe and effective analgesia is achieved.

Analgesic pharmacokinetic drug–drug interactions can mediate clinically relevant effects. CYP3A is involved in the metabolism of methadone and alfentanil.[117] Methadone metabolism is induced by rifampin and results in enhanced clearance of methadone.[18,42] One study of adults demonstrated an approximately fourfold increase in methadone clearance, with methadone clearance ranging from 0.538 L/hr/kg when administered with rifampin to 0.126 L/hr/kg when methadone was administered alone.[204] This effect could provoke withdrawal symptoms in patients receiving methadone.[18] In addition, phenobarbital, phenytoin, carbamazepine, nevirapine, and efavirenz have the potential to decrease methadone blood concentrations.[116,184] Rifampin significantly lowers alfentanil plasma concentrations by the same mechanism.[117]

Inhibition of CYP3A can result in increased plasma levels of methadone.[42] For example, fluconazole inhibits metabolism of methadone[42] and alfentanil.[180] Fluconazole decreased the clearance of alfentanil approximately 58% following IV fluconazole in healthy adults.[180]

Pharmacodynamic drug–drug interactions can result in synergic effects or antagonism. When a pure opiate agonist and a partial agonist/antagonist are used in combination, there is a risk for decreased clinical effects. For example, morphine (pure agonist) and nalbuphine (partial agonist/antagonist) used in combination can result in decreased opiate effect. This can have profound effects on analgesia and result in withdrawal symptoms for patients on long-term analgesia therapy.[185,195] Analgesic opioid therapy is associated with several side effects that can be heightened by drug–drug interactions, such as respiratory depression, hypotension, decreased GI motility, nausea, and vomiting. Use of a pure opioid antagonist, such as naloxone, is needed for reversal of undesirable effects. Most clinically significant drug–drug interactions associated with analgesics are pharmacodynamic in origin.

Anticoagulants

Warfarin is involved in a multitude of drug–drug interactions, including alterations in protein binding, hepatic metabolism by the cytochrome P450 system, in bacterial flora of the GI tract, and the clotting cascade. Aspirin, chloral hydrate, ibuprofen, and sulfamethoxazole can displace warfarin from protein binding sites, making more free fraction of warfarin available and hence augmenting anticoagulation. Warfarin metabolism may be inhibited by cimetidine, isoniazid, and erythromycin, resulting in decreased effect. Phenobarbital and rifampin can induce the metabolism of warfarin and decrease its effect. Several agents (e.g., amiodarone, erythromycin, and sulfamethoxazole) may decrease synthesis of vitamin K-dependent clotting factors and potentiate warfarin effect. Phytonadione (vitamin K) antagonizes the anticoagulation effect of warfarin.[272] Careful monitoring of bleeding and coagulation parameters (prothrombin time and INR) can help prevent serious adverse drug reactions. Many drug–drug interactions can occur when initiating warfarin therapy or when adding other medications to existing warfarin therapy.

Heparin may exhibit drug–drug interactions with oral anticoagulants (warfarin) and platelet inhibitors (e.g., aspirin, dextran, ibuprofen, and other agents that interfere with platelet aggregation). Other medications that may partially counteract the anticoagulant action of heparin include digitalis, the tetracyclines, nicotine, and antihistamines. Agents that may enhance the risk of hemorrhage with enoxaparin include anticoagulants and platelet inhibitors.[191,193]

Drotrecogin alfa (activated protein C) possesses anticoagulant activity, so potential interactions should be expected when it is administered with agents that have similar actions, depending on the drug and dosage.[172] Potential drug–drug interactions include those that may enhance anticoagulant activity (thrombolytic agents, other anticoagulants and antithrombotic agents, platelet aggregation inhibitors, glycoprotein IIb/IIIa inhibitors) and those that may interfere with anticoagulation activity of drotrecogin alfa (activated) (vitamin K, antihemophiliac factors, thrombin).[172]

Immunosuppressives (see Chapters 74, 77, 81, and 86)

Therapeutic agents that modulate the immune system frequently are involved in drug–drug interactions. Most immunosuppressive agents possess narrow therapeutic indexes and therefore require therapeutic drug monitoring.[51] As a result, a sophisticated knowledge of clinical pharmacology is required to evaluate the clinical relevance of potential drug–drug interactions involving these drugs.

Drug–drug interactions most commonly encountered with immunosuppressive drug therapy revolve around the inhibition or induction of the CYP3A enzymes. Cyclosporine, tacrolimus, prednisone, and sirolimus, all CYP3A substrates, are most prone to these types of pharmacokinetic drug–drug interactions.[127,213] Cyclosporine is extensively metabolized in the liver and GI tract, which explains its low bioavailability. Known CYP3A inhibitors have been used intentionally to maintain therapeutic levels in patients with high presystemic metabolism of cyclosporine.[20] Medications that inhibit CYP3A metabolism should be used with caution in patients taking cyclosporine, tacrolimus, or sirolimus because of the narrow therapeutic index of these agents; dosing adjustments of immunosuppressive therapy may be required. Erythromycin, clarithromycin, voriconazole, fluconazole, itraconazole, ketoconazole, diltiazem, verapamil, indinavir, and ritonavir inhibit CYP3A metabolism.[7,227,255] Several drugs can induce the metabolism of cyclosporine, tacrolimus, sirolimus, and prednisone. Rifampin causes induction of CYP3A and PGP,[65] leading to clinically significant decreases in cyclosporine and tacrolimus plasma concentrations.[65,71]

Potential pharmacodynamic drug–drug interactions must be considered. For example, cyclosporine and tacrolimus both are nephrotoxic agents and should be used with caution when they are administered with known nephrotoxins because of the heightened risk for nephrotoxicity. Patients on immunosuppressive therapy should not be administered live attenuated vaccines because such individuals lack the ability to mount a sufficient immune response.

Pulmonary Drugs

β_2-Adrenergic agonists (e.g., albuterol, levalbuterol, terbutaline) are useful agents for treatment of asthma. Drug–drug interactions can occur when β_2-adrenergic agonists are used in combination with β_1-adrenergic antagonists, especially the nonselective antagonists. A possible decreased β_2 effect could precipitate asthma symptoms. The nonselective antagonists include propranolol, nadolol, and labetalol (Table 112–4). Agents such as atenolol and metoprolol are selective for β_1 receptors at usual therapeutic doses and therefore are potentially safer to use in combination with β_2 agonists. However, these agents may lose their selectivity at higher doses. One potential side effect of the β_2 agonists is hypokalemia, which can be enhanced with concurrent use of loop and thiazide diuretics. Monitoring of potassium levels is recommended when these agents are used concurrently.[272]

TABLE 112–4

β-Blocker Receptor Selectivity

β-Blocker	Selectivity
Atenolol	β_1
Esmolol	β_1
Labetalol	None
Metoprolol	β_1
Nadolol	None
Pindolol	None
Propranolol	None
Sotalol	None
Timolol	None

Modified from Hoffman BB: Adrenoreceptor-activating and other sympathomimetic drugs. In Katzung BG, editor: Basic and clinical pharmacology. Stamford, Conn, 1998, Appleton & Lange.

Antineoplastics

Administration of a live vaccine (e.g., oral polio virus and measles, mumps, and rubella) should be avoided in patients receiving chemotherapeutic agents. Immunosuppression from chemotherapeutic regimens predisposes a patient to active infection when inoculated with a live vaccine. Severe and fatal infections from the combination are reported.[157] Administration of a live vaccine should not be attempted for at least 3 months after a chemotherapeutic agent is discontinued.[157]

Potential drug–drug interactions involving the cytochrome P450 enzyme system can be identified by pinpointing the substrates for the various isoenzymes of the mixed function oxidases among the antineoplastic agents. For example, the vinca alkaloids vincristine, vinorelbine, and vinblastine are substrates for CYP3A4. Known inhibitors and inducers of CYP3A4 increase and decrease plasma levels, respectively. Toxicities are more likely when vinca alkaloids are administered with classic CYP3A4 inhibitors such as the azole antifungals, macrolide antibiotics, calcium channel blockers (e.g., diltiazem and verapamil), quinupristin/dalfopristin, and cyclosporine. Antiepileptic drugs that are known inducers of the cytochrome P450 enzyme system may contribute to therapeutic failure with chemotherapeutic agents. In one study of pediatric patients with high-grade glioma, the presence of enzyme-inducing anticonvulsants increased irinotecan clearance.[45]

Multiple drug resistance in cancer cells has been attributed to the expression of a PGP efflux transmembrane transport protein.[266] This protein offers a potential target for future directed therapies in cancer treatment. Agents that modulate the activity of PGP currently are under development and may provide a drug interaction that favorably increases the efficacy of antineoplastic agents.[147] Coadministration of etoposide and cyclosporine, for example, results in elevation of the mean AUC of etoposide. Etoposide is a CYP3A4 substrate, whereas cyclosporine is both a CYP3A4 and PGP inhibitor.[128]

Inhibitors of the efflux pump, PGP, increase the cytotoxicity of the vinca alkaloids. Itraconazole, clarithromycin, and cyclosporine are known to inhibit PGP.[91,92] Colony-stimulating factors are often used to treat the ensuing neutropenia that accompanies cancer chemotherapy. Patients with lymphomas undergoing their first cycle of vincristine and receiving treatment with filgrastim or sargramostim are at risk for developing a severe atypical neuropathy. The neuropathy has been described as a severe, sharp, burning pain in the feet and appears to occur more commonly in lymphoma patients receiving this combination than in patients receiving vincristine alone.[261] The mechanism of action of this interaction is unclear.

Methotrexate elimination is governed by the kidneys; both filtration and active secretion are the main modes of methotrexate excretion. The process of tubular secretion requires both a carrier and energy, finite resources that create a saturable process. Competition among other drugs for secretion may lead to reduced clearance of methotrexate with consequent manifestations of toxicity. Concurrent administration of methotrexate with any of the penicillins (piperacillin, amoxicillin, etc.) have demonstrated this capacity.[49,50,211] The NSAIDs, aspirin, and other salicylates all increase the likelihood of methotrexate toxicity by this same mechanism.[36,47,56,72,73,232,233] Inhibition of renal prostaglandin synthesis and the resultant reduction in renal perfusion also are suggested to contribute to renal toxicities seen with methotrexate because this drug persists in renal tissue for weeks.[149] Omeprazole may exhibit another mode of interaction on the level of renal elimination. By inhibiting the transmembrane H^+/K^+-ATPase pump, omeprazole may decrease active secretion of methotrexate.[207] The antineoplastic activity of methotrexate stems from its inhibition of dihydrofolate reductase, the enzyme that catalyzes reduction of folic acid to tetrahydrofolic acid. In turn, tetrahydrofolic acid serves as a building block for purine and DNA synthesis. The clinician should be aware of other drugs that act along this pathway (e.g., ecotrimoxazole and pyrimethamine) because these agents may contribute to the toxicities associated with methotrexate therapy.[149,208]

REFERENCES

1. Ahonen J, Olkkola KT, Takala A: Interaction between fluconazole and midazolam in intensive care patients. *Acat Aaesthesiol Scand* 43:509-514, 1999.
2. Alldredge BK: Drug-induced seizures: controversies in their identification and management. *Pharmacotherapy* 17:857-860, 1997.
3. Alvarez-Elcoro S, Enzler MJ: The macrolides: erythromycin, clarithromycin and azithromycin: symposium on antimicrobial agents—part IX. *Mayo Clin Proc* 74:613-634, 1999.
4. American Society Health-System Pharmacists: ASHP guidelines on adverse drug reactions monitoring and reporting. *Am J Health Syst Pharm* 52:417-419, 1995.
5. Anderson GD: A mechanistic approach to antiepileptic drug interactions. *Ann Pharmacother* 32:554-563, 1998.
6. Anderson GD: Children verse adults: pharmacokinetics and adverse-effect differences. *Epilepsy* 43:53-59, 2002.
7. Anderson JR, Nawarskas JJ: Cardiovascular drug-drug interactions. *Cardiol Clin* 19:215-234, 2001.
8. Anonymous: Nitroprusside and cyanide toxicity. WHO Drug Information 4:176, 1990.
9. Apseloff G, Hilligoss DM, Gardner MJ, et al: Induction of fluconazole metabolism by rifampin: in vivo study in humans. *J Clin Pharmacol* 31:358-361, 1991.
10. Arslan E, Orzan E, Santarelli R: Global problem of drug-induced hearing loss. *Ann N Y Acad Sci* 884:1-14, 1999.
11. Au Yeung SC, Ensom MH: Phenytoin and enteral feedings: does evidence support an interaction? *Ann Pharmacother* 34:896-905, 2000.
12. Backman JT, Kivisto KT, Olkkola KT, et al: The area under the plasma concentration-time curve for oral midazolam is 400-fold larger during treatment with itraconazole than with rifampin. *Eur J Clin Pharmacol* 54:53-58, 1998.
13. Backman JT, Olkkola KT, Aranko K, et al: Dose of midazolam should be reduced during diltiazem and verapamil treatments. *Br J Clin Pharmacol* 37:221-225, 1994.
14. Backman JT, Olkkola KT, Neuvonen PJ: Azithromycin does not increase plasma concentrations of oral midazolam. *Int J Clin Pharmacol Ther* 33:356-359, 1995.
15. Backman JT, Olkkola KT, Ojala M, et al: Concentrations and effects of oral midazolam are greatly reduced in patients treated with carbamazepine or phenytoin. *Epilepsia* 37:253-257, 1996.
16. Bailey RR, Neale TJ: Rapid clonidine withdrawal with blood pressure overshoot exaggerated by beta-blockade. *Br Med J* 1:942-943, 1976.
17. Bayer AS, Chow AW, Morrison JO, et al: Bactericidal synergy between penicillin or ampicillin and aminoglycosides against antibiotic-tolerant lactobacilli. *Antimicrob Agents Chemother* 17:359-363, 1980.
18. Bending MR, Skacel PO: Rifampin-induced methadone withdrawal in AIDS. *J Clin Psychopharmacol* 10:443-444, 1990.
19. Benowitz NL: Antihypertensive agents. In Katzung BG, editor: *Basic and clinical pharmacology*, ed 7, Stamford, Conn, 1998, Appleton & Lange.
20. Berkovitch M, Bitzan M, Matsui D, et al: Pediatric clinical use of the ketoconazole/cyclosporine interaction. *Pediatr Nephrol* 8:492-493, 1994.
21. Bertino JS, Booker LA, Franck PA, et al: Incidence of significant risk factors for aminoglycoside-associated nephrotoxicity in patients dosed by using individualized pharmacokinetic monitoring. *J Infect Dis* 167:173-179, 1993.
22. Black D, Kunze K, Wienkers L, et al: Warfarin-fluconazole: a metabolically based drug interaction: in vivo studies. *Drug Metab Dispos* 24:422-428, 1996.
23. Blake PG, Ryan F: Rhabdomyolysis and acute renal failure after terbutaline overdose. *Nephron* 53:76-77, 1989.
24. Blum RA, Wilton JH, Hilligoss DM, et al: Effect of fluconazole on the disposition of phenytoin. *Clin Pharmacol Ther* 49:420-425, 1991.
25. Blumer JL: Critical analysis of deaths that occurred during a randomized clinical trial of sedation in pediatric intensive care unit. *Crit Care Med* 30(suppl):A95, 2003 (abstract).
26. Bonfiglio MF, Fisher-Katz LE, Saltis LM, et al: A pilot pharmacokinetic-pharmacodynamic study of benzodiazepine antagonism by flumazenil and aminophylline. *Pharmacotherapy* 16:1166-1172, 1996.
27. Brennan TA, Leape LL, Laird NM, et al: Incidence of adverse events and negligence in hospitalized patients: results of the Harvard medical practice study I. *N Engl J Med* 324:370-376, 1991.
28. Brogden RN, Goa KL: Flumazenil: a reappraisal of its pharmacological properties and therapeutic efficacy as a benzodiazepine antagonist. [published erratum appears in *Drugs* 43:442, 1992] *Drugs* 42:1061-1089, 1991.
29. Bucci AJ, Myre SA, Tan HS, et al: In vitro interaction of quinidine with kaolin and pectin. *J Pharm Sci* 70:999-1002, 1981.
30. Buratti S, Lavine JE: Drugs and the liver: advances in metabolism, toxicity, and therapeutics. *Curr Opin Pediatr* 14:601-607, 2002.
31. Burt M, Anderson DC, Kloss J, et al: Evidence-based implementation of free phenytoin therapeutic drug monitoring. *Clin Chem* 46:1132-1135, 2000.

31a. Buss N, Snell P, Bock J, et al: Saquinavir and ritonavir pharmacokinetics following combined ritonavir and saquinavir (soft gelatin capsules) administration. *British Journal of Clinical Pharmacology* 52:255-64, 2001.

32. Busto U, Naranjo CA, Sellers EM: Comparison of two recently published algorithms for assessing the probability of adverse drug reactions. *Br J Clin Pharmacol* 13:223-227,1982.
33. Campana C, Regazzi MB, Buggia I, et al: Clinically significant drug interactions with cyclosporin. *Clin Pharmacokinet* 30:141-179, 1996.

33a. Cardiello PG, van Heeswijk RP, Hassink EA, et al: Simplifying protease inhibitor therapy with once-daily dosing of saquinavir soft-gelatin capsules/ritonavir (1600/100 mg): HIVNAT 001.3 study. *JAIDS* 29:464-470, 2002.

33b. Carr RA, Pasutto FM, Foster RT: Influence of cimetidine coadministration on the pharmacokinetics of sotalol enantiomers in an anaesthetized rat model: evidence supporting active renal excretion of sotalol. *Biopharmaceutics & Drug Disposition* 17:55-69, 1996.

34. Carroll MC, Yueng-Yue KA, Esterly NB, et al: Drug-induced hypersensitivity syndrome in pediatric patients. *Pediatrics* 108:485-493, 2001.
35. Carver PL, Berardi RR, Knapp MJ, et al: In vivo interaction of ketoconazole and sucralfate in healthy volunteers. *Antimicrob Agents Chemother* 38:326-329, 1994.
36. Cassano WF: Serious methotrexate toxicity caused by interaction with ibuprofen. *Am J Pediatr Hematol Oncol* 11:481-482, 1989 (letter).
37. Chan JCN, Cockram CS, Critchley JAJH: Drug-induced disorders of glucose metabolism: mechanisms and management. *Drug Saf* 15:135-157, 1996.
38. Chan TYK. Drug-induced syndrome of inappropriate antidiuretic hormone secretion. *Drugs Aging* 11:27-44, 1997.
39. Christensen ML, Helms RA, Chesney RW: Is pediatric labeling really necessary? *Pediatrics* 104(3 pt 2):593-597, 1999.
40. Christians U, Jacobsen W, Benet LZ, et al: Mechanisms of clinically relevant drug interactions associated with tacrolimus. *Clin Pharmacokinet* 41:813-851, 2002.

40a. Christmann V, Liem KD, Semmekrot BA, van de Bor M: Changes in cerebral, renal and mesenteric blood flow velocity during continuous and bolus infusion of indomethacin. *Acta Paediatrica* 91:440-446, 2002.
41. Cinguegrani MP, Liang CS: Indomethacin attenuates the hypotensive action of hydralazine. *Clin Pharmacol Ther* 39:564-570, 1986.
42. Cobb MN, Desai J, Brown LS Jr, et al: The effect of fluconazole on the clinical pharmacokinetics of methadone. *Clin Pharmacol Ther* 63:655-662, 1998.
43. Cooper JAD: Drug-induced lung disease. *Adv Intern Med* 42: 231-268, 1997.
44. Corallo CE, Rogers IR: Roxithromycin-induced digoxin toxicity. *Med J Austr* 165:433-434, 1996.
44a. Corvaia L, Li SC, Ioannides-Demos LL, et al: A prospective study of the effects of oral probenecid on the pharmacokinetics of intravenous ticarcillin in patients with cystic fibrosis. *Journal of Antimicrobial Chemotherapy* 30:875-878, 1992.
45. Crews KR, Stewart CF, Jones-Wallace D, et al: Altered irinotecan pharmacokinetics in pediatric high-grade glioma patients receiving enzyme-inducing anticonvulsant therapy. *Clin Cancer Res* 8:2202-2209, 2002.
46. Cunha BA: Antibiotic side effects. *Med Clin North Am* 85: 149-185, 2001.
47. Daly H, Boyle J, Roberts C, et al: Interaction between methotrexate and non-steroidal anti-inflammatory drugs. *Lancet* 1:559, 1986.
48. D'amato RF, Thornsberry C, Baker CN, et al: Effect of calcium and magnesium ions on the susceptibility of Pseudomonas species to tetracycline, gentamicin, polymyxin B and carbenicillin. *Antimicrob Agents Chemother* 7:596-600, 1975.
49. Dawson JK, Abernathy VE, Lynch MP: Methotrexate and penicillin interaction. *Br J Rheumatol* 37:807, 1998 (letter).
50. Dean R, Nachman J, Lorenzana AN, et al: Possible methotrexate-mezlocillin interaction. *Am J Pediatr Hematol Oncol* 14:88-92, 1992.
51. del Mar Fernandez De Gatta M, Santos-Buelga D, Dominguez-Gil A, et al: Immunosuppressive therapy for paediatric transplant patients: pharmacokinetic considerations. *Clin Pharmacokinet* 41:115-135, 2002.
51a. Dello Strologo L, Massella L, Rizzoni G: Cyclosporine-induced transient renal hypoperfusion in adolescent transplant recipients. *Pediatric Nephrology* 10(1):81-83, 1996.
52. Deppermann KM, Lode H., Hoffken G, et al: Influence of ranitidine, pirenzepine, and aluminum magnesium hydroxide on the bioavailability of various antibiotics, including amoxicillin, cephalexin, doxycycline and amoxicillin-clavulanic acid. *Antimicrob Agents Chemother* 33:1901-1907, 1989.
53. Department of Health and Human Services, US FDA: The pediatric exclusivity provision: January 2001 Status Report to Congress, January 2001.
54. Diprivan (propofol). In: Medwatch 2001 Safety Information Summaries. Washington, DC, February 24, 2003, US Food and Drug Administration. Available at *www.fda.gov/medwatch/safety/2001/safety01.htm#dipriv*. Last accessed February 24, 2003.
55. Dubose TD Jr, Molony DA: Nephrotoxicity of non-steroidal anti-inflammatory drugs. *Lancet* 344:515-518, 1994.
56. Dupuis LL, Shore A, Silverman ED, et al: Methotrexate-nonsteroidal anti-inflammatory drug interaction in children with arthritis. *J Rheumatol* 17:1569-1473, 1990.
57. Duvoux C, Cherqui D, Dimartino V, et al: Nicardipine as antihypertensive therapy in liver transplant recipients: results of long term use. *Hepatology* 25:430-433, 1997.
58. Easton KL, Parsons BJ, Starr M, et al: The incidence of drug-related problems as a cause of hospital admissions in children. *Med J Austr* 169:356-359, 1998.
59. Eck P, Silver SM, Clark EC: Acute renal failure and coma after a high dose of acyclovir. *N Engl J Med* 325:1178, 1991.
60. Edwards IR, Aronson JK: Adverse drug reactions: definitions, diagnosis and management. *Lancet* 356:1255-1259, 2000.
61. Epstein M, Oster JR: Beta blockers and renal function: a reappraisal. *J Clin Hypertens* 1:85-99, 1985.
62. Evans WE, Schentag JJ, Jusko WJ, et al: Applied pharmacokinetics. Spokane, WA, 1986, Applied Therapeutics.
63. FDA issues warning on propofol (Diprivan). *CMAJ* 164:1608, 2001.
64. Feest TG: Low molecular weight dextran: a continuing cause of acute renal failure. *Br Med J* 2:1300, 1976.
65. Finch CK, Chrisman CR, Baciewicz AM, et al: Rifampin and rifabutin drug interactions. *Arch Intern Med* 162:985-992, 2002.
66. First MR, Schroeder TJ, Weiskittel P, et al: Concomitant administration of cyclosporine and ketoconazole in renal transplant recipients. *Lancet* II:1198-1201, 1989.
67. Floren LC, Bekersky I, Benet LZ, et al: Tacrolimus oral bioavailability doubles with coadministration of ketoconazole. *Clin Pharmacol Ther* 62:41-49, 1997.
68. Folb PI, Chalker J: Cytostatics and immunosuppressive drugs. In Dukes MNG, Aronson JK, editors: *Meyler's side effects of drugs: an encyclopedia of adverse reactions and interactions,* ed 14. New York, 2000, Elsevier.
69. Fowlie PW: Intravenous indomethacin for preventing mortality and morbidity in very low birth weight infants. *Cochrane Database Syst Rev*, 2002.
70. Frick PA, Cohen LG, Rovers JP: Algorithms used in adverse drug event reports: a comparative study. *Ann Pharmacother* 31: 164-167, 1997.
71. Furlan V, Perello L, Jacquemin E, et al: Interactions between FK506 and rifampicin or erythromycin in pediatric liver recipients. *Transplantation* 59:1217, 1995.
72. Furst DE, Herman RA, Koehnke R, et al: Effect of aspirin and sulindac on methotrexate clearance. *J Pharm Sci* 79:782-786, 1990.
73. Furst DE: Clinically important interactions of nonsteroidal anti-inflammatory drugs with other medications. *J Rheumatol Suppl* 17:58-62, 1988.
74. García, VP, Martínez FA, Augustí EB, et al: Drug-induced ototoxicity: current status. *Acta Otolaryngol* 121:569-572, 2001.
75. Garnett WR: Interactions with hydroxymethylglutaryl-coenzyme A reductase inhibitors. *Am J Health Syst Pharm* 52:1639-1645, 1995.
76. Gauthier PM, Szerlip HM: Metabolic acidosis in the intensive care unit. *Crit Care Med* 18:289-308, 2002.
77. Gibaldi M: Drug interactions: part I. *Ann Pharmacother* 26: 709-713, 1992.
78. Gilman AG, Rall TW, Nies AS, et al: *The Pharmacological Basis of Therapeutics*, ed 8, Elmsford, NY, 1990, Pergamon Press.
79. Gladtke E: Use of antipyretic analgesics in the pediatric patient. *Am J Med* 75:121-126, 1983.
80. Goetz MB, Sayers J: Nephrotoxicity of vancomycin and aminoglycoside therapy separately and in combination. *J Antimicrob Chemother* 32:325-334, 1993.
81. Goodman MS: Cancer: chemotherapy and care. Princeton, NJ, 1992, Bristol-Myers Squibb.
81a. Goodman ZD: Drug hepatotoxicity. *Clin Liver Dis* 6:381-397, 2002.
82. Gorski JC, Craven R, Haehner-Daniels B, et al: The effect of intestinal and hepatic CYP3A activity. *Clin Pharmacol Ther* 67:133, 2000.
83. Gorski JC, Jones DR, Haehner-Daniels BD, et al: The contribution of intestinal and hepatic CYP3A to the interaction between midazolam and clarithromycin. *Clin Pharmacol Ther* 64:133-143, 1998.
83a. Gossmann J, Radounikli A, Bernemann A, et al: Pathophysiology of cyclosporine-induced nephrotoxicity in humans: a role for nitric oxide? *Kidney & Blood Pressure Research* 24:111-115, 2001.
84. Grachalla RS: Clinical assessment of drug-induced disease. *Lancet* 356:1505-1511, 2000.
85. Greenblatt DJ, Ehrenberg BL, Gunderman J, et al: Kinetic and dynamic study of intravenous lorazepam: comparison with intravenous diazepam. *J Pharmacol Exp Ther* 250:134-139, 1989.
86. Greenblatt DJ, Wright CE, von Molkte LL, et al: Ketoconazole inhibition of triazolam and alprazolam clearance: differential kinetic and dynamic consequences. *Clin Pharmacol Ther* 64:237-247, 1998.
87. Griebel ML, Kearns GL, Fiser DH, et al: Phenytoin protein binding in pediatric patients with acute traumatic injury. *Crit Care Med* 18:385-391, 1990.
88. Hall AH, Rumack BH: Clinical toxicology of cyanide. *Ann Emerg Med* 15:1067-1074, 1986.
89. Hamaoka N, Oda Y, Hase I, et al: Propofol decreases the clearance of midazolam by inhibiting CYP3A4: an in vivo and in vitro study. *Clin Pharmacol Ther* 66:110-117, 1999.
90. Hansten PD, Horn JR: *Drug interactions and updates.* Philadelphia, 1990, Lea & Febiger: Drug Interactions Newsletter, Vancouver, 1990, Applied Therapeutics.
91. Hansten PD, Horn JR: *Managing clinically important drug interactions.* St. Louis, 2002, Facts and Comparisons.
92. Hansten PD, Horn JR: The top 100 drug interactions: a guide to patient management. Edmonds, WA, 2002, H&H Publications.

93. Higuchi H, Adachi Y, Dahan A, et al: The interaction between propofol and clonidine for loss of consciousness. *Anesth Analg* 94:886-891, 2002.
94. Hill SE, Heldman LD, Goo ED, et al: Fatal microvascular pulmonary emboli from precipitation of a total nutrient admixture solution. JPEN J Parenteral Enteral Nutr 20:81, 1996.
95. Hoeschele JD, Roy AK, Pecoraro VL, et al: In vitro analysis of the interaction between sucralfate and ketoconazole. Antimicrob Agents Chemother 38:319-325, 1994.
96. Hoffman BB, Lefkowitz RJ: Catecholamines, sympathomimetic drugs, and adrenergic receptor antagonist. In Gilman AG, editor: The pharmacological basis of therapeutics, ed 10, New York, 2001, Pergamon Press.
97. Holdsworth MT, Fichtl RE, Behta M, et al: Incidence and impact of adverse drug events in pediatric inpatients. Arch Pediatr Adolesc Med 157:60-65, 2003.
98. Hoogwerf B, Danese RD: Drug selection and the management of corticosteroid-related diabetes mellitus. Rheum Dis Clin North Am 25:489-505, 1999.
98a. Houston JB, Levy G: Drug biotransformation interactions in man VI: acetaminophen and ascorbic acid. *Journal of Pharmaceutical Sciences* 65:1218-1221, 1976.
99. Hricik DE, Browning PJ, Kopelman R, et al: Captopril induced function renal insufficiency in patients with bilateral renal artery stenosis, or stenosis in a solitary kidney. N Engl J Med 308: 377-381, 1983.
100. Hughes M, Binning A: Intravenous amiodarone in intensive care: time for reappraisal? *Intensive Care Med* 26:1730-1739, 2000.
101. Hussein Z, Posner J: Population pharmacokinetics of lamotrigine monotherapy in patients with epilepsy: retrospective analysis of routine monitoring data. *Br J Clin Pharmacol* 43:457-464, 1997.
102. Impicciatore P, Choonara I, Clarkson A, et al: Incidence of adverse drug reactions in paediatric in/out-patients: a systematic review and meta-analysis of prospective studies. *Br J Clin Pharmacol* 52:77-83, 2001.
103. Ito S, Woodland C, Harper PA, et al: P-glycoprotein-mediated renal tubular secretion of digoxin: the toxicological significance of the urine-blood barrier model. *Life Sci* 53: PL25-PL31, 1993.
104. Jalava KM, Olkkola KT, Neuvonen PJ: Itraconazole greatly increases plasma concentrations and effects of felodipine. *Clin Pharmacol Ther* 61:410-415, 1997.
105. Jalava KM, Partanen J, Neuvonen PJ: Itraconazole decreases renal clearance of digoxin. *Ther Drug Monit* 19:609-613, 1997.
106. Jick H: Drug-associated asymptomatic elevations of transaminase in drug safety assessments. *Pharmacotherapy* 15:23-25, 1995.
107. Joint Commission on Accreditation of Healthcare Organizations: Sentinel event glossary of terms. 2002. Available at *http:/www.jcaho.org*. Accessed July 6, 2002.
108. Jones JK: Adverse drug reactions in the community health setting: approaches to recognizing, counseling and reporting. *Fam Comm Health* 5:58-67, 1982.
109. Kaka JS, Lyman C, Kilarski DJ: Tobramycin-furosemide interaction. *Drug Intell Clin Pharm* 18:235-238, 1984.
110. Kaplowitz N: Drug-induced liver disorders: implications for drug development and regulations. *Drug Saf* 24:483-490, 2001.
111. Karch FE, Lasagna L: Toward the operational identification of adverse drug reactions. *Clin Pharmacol Ther* 21:247-254, 1977.
112. Kato R, Ueno K, Imano H, et al: Impairment of ciprofloxacin absorption by calcium polycarbophil. *J Clin Pharmacol* 42: 806-811, 2002.
113. Katoh M, Nakajima M, Shimada N, et al: Inhibition of human cytochrome P450 enzymes by 1,4-dihydropyridine calcium antagonists: prediction of in vivo drug-drug interactions. *Eur J Clin Pharmacol* 55:843-852, 2000.
114. Kaushal R, Bates DW, Landrigan C, et al: Medication errors and adverse drug events in pediatric inpatients. *JAMA* 285: 2114-2120, 2001.
115. Kessler DA: Introducing MedWatch, using FDA form 3500, a new approach to reporting medication and devise adverse effects and product problems. *JAMA* 269:2765-2768, 1993.
116. Ketter TA, Post RM, Worthington K: Principles of clinically important drug interactions with carbamazepine. Part I. *J Clin Psychopharmacol* 11:198-203, 1991.
117. Kharasch ED, Russell M, Mautz D, et al: The role of cytochrome P450 3A4 in alfentanil clearance. Implications for interindividual variability in disposition and perioperative drug interactions. *Anesthesiology* 87:36-50, 1997.
118. Kilpatrick CJ, Wanwimolruk S, Wing LMH: Plasma concentrations of unbound phenytoin in the management of epilepsy. *Br J Clin Pharmacol* 17:539-546, 1984.
119. Kirchain WR, Gill MA: Drug-induced liver disease. In Dipiro JT, editor: *Pharmacotherapy: a pathophysiologic approach*. Stamford, Conn, 1997, Appleton & Lange.
119a. Klein IH, Abrahams A, van Ede T, et al: Different effects of tacrolimus and cyclosporine on renal hemodynamics and blood pressure in healthy subjects. *Transplantation* 73:732-736, 2002.
120. Kleinknecht D, Vanhille P, Morel-Maroger L, et al: Acute Interstitial nephritis due to drug hypersensitivity. An up-to-date review of 19 cases. *Adv Nephrol* 12:277-308, 1983.
121. Knochel JP: Diuretic-induced hypokalemia. *Am J Med* 77:18-27, 1984.
122. Knowles S, Shapiro L, Shear NH: Serious dermatologic reactions in children. *Curr Opin Pediatr* 9:388-395, 1997.
123. Koselj M, Kveder R, Bren AF, et al: Acute renal failure in patients with drug-induced acute interstitial nephritis. *Ren Fail* 15:69-72, 1993.
124. Kramer MS, Leventhal JM, Hutchinson TA, et al: An algorithm for the operational assessment of adverse drug reactions, I. Background, description and instructions for use. *JAMA* 242:623-632, 1979.
125. Krasner AS: Glucorticoid-induced adrenal insufficiency. *JAMA* 282:671-676, 1999.
126. Krieble BF, Rudy DW, Glick MR, et al: Case report: acyclovir neurotoxicity and nephrotoxicity-the role for hemodialysis. *Am J Med Sci* 305:36-39, 1993.
127. Kronbach T, Fischer V, Meyer UA: Cyclosporine metabolism in human liver: identification of a cytochrome P-450III gene family as the major cyclosporine-metabolizing enzyme explains interactions of cyclosporine with other drugs. *Clin Pharmacol Ther* 43: 630-635, 1988.
128. Lacayo NJ, Lum BL, Becton DL: Pharmacokinetic interactions of cyclosporine with etoposide and mitoxantrone in children with acute myeloid leukemia. *Leukemia* 16:920-927, 2002.
129. Lam YWF, Arama CJ, Shikuma LR: The clinical utility of a published nomogram to predict aminoglycoside nephrotoxicity. *JAMA* 255:639-642, 1986.
130. Leape LL, Brennan TA, Laird N, et al: The nature of adverse events in hospitalized patients. Results of the Harvard medical practice study II. *N Engl J Med* 324:377-384, 1991.
131. Lecompte J, Dumont L, Hill J, et al: Effect of water deprivation and rehydration on gentamicin disposition in the rat. *J Pharmacol Exp Ther* 218:231-236, 1981.
132. Lenn NJ, Robertson M: Clinical utility of unbound antiepileptic drug blood levels in the management of epilepsy. *Neurology* 42:988-990, 1992.
133. Leuppi JD, Schnyder P, Hartmann K, et al: Drug-induced bronchospasms: analysis of spontaneously reported cases. *Respiration* 68:345-351, 2001.
134. Levin ML: The many causes of headache: migraine, vascular, drug-induced and more. *Postgrad Med* 112:67-68, 71-72, 75-76, 79-82, 2002.
135. Lewis JH: Drug-induced liver disease. *Med Clin North Am* 84:1275-1311, 2000.
136. Liano F, Pascual J: Epidemiology of acute renal failure: a prospective, multicenter, community-based study. Madrid Acute Renal Failure Study Group. *Kidney Int* 50:811-818, 1996.
137. Lilja M, Jounela AJ, Juustila HJ, et al: Abrupt and gradual change from clonidine to beta blockers in hypertension. *Acta Med Scand* 211:375-380, 1982.
138. Linday L, Dobkin JF, Wang TC, et al: Digoxin inactivation by the gut flora in infancy and childhood. *Pediatrics* 79:544-548, 1987.
139. Lindenbaum J, Rund DG, Butler VP Jr, et al: Inactivation of digoxin by the gut flora: reversal by antibiotic therapy. *N Engl J Med* 305:789-794, 1981.
140. Linton AL, Clark WF, Driedger AA, et al: Acute interstitial nephritis due to drugs. Review of the literature with a report of nine cases. *Ann Intern Med* 93:735-741, 1980.
141. Llanos A, Cieza J, Bernardo J, et al: Effect of salt supplementation on amphotericin B nephrotoxicity. *Kidney Int* 40:302-308, 1991.
142. Madias NE, Harrington JT: Platinum nephrotoxicity. *Am J Med* 65:307-314, 1978.

143. Mandema JW, Tukker E, Danhof M: In vivo characterization of the pharmacodynamic interaction of a benzodiazepine agonist and antagonist: midazolam and flumazenil. *J Pharmacol Exp Ther* 260:36-44, 1992.
144. Marcus FI: Drug interactions with amiodarone. *Am Heart J* 106: 924-930, 1983.
145. Marks V, Teale JD: Hypoglycemic disorders: drug-induced hypoglycemia. *Endocrinol Metab Clin North Am* 28:555-577, 1999.
146. Matheny CJ, Lamb MW, Brouwer KL, et al: Pharmacokinetic and pharmacodynamic implications of p-glycoprotein modulation. *Pharmacotherapy* 21:778-796, 2001.
147. Mayer KR: Multidrug resistance in cancer. Mechanisms, reversal using modulators of MDR and the role of MDR modulators in influencing the pharmacokinetics of anticancer drugs. *Eur J Pharm Sci* 11:265-283, 2000.
148. McCouty JC, Silas JH, Tucker GT, et al: The effect of combined therapy on the pharmacokinetics and pharmacodynamics of verapamil and propranolol in patients with angina pectoris. *Br J Clin Pharmacol* 25:349-357, 1988.
149. McEvoy GK, editor: *AHFS 2000 drug information*. Bethesda, Md, 2000, American Society of Health-System Pharmacists.
150. McInnes GT, Johnston GD: Positive inotropic drugs and drugs used in dysrhythmias. In Dukes MNG, Aronson JK, editors: *Meyler's side effects of drugs: an encyclopedia of adverse reactions and interactions,* ed 14, New York, 2000, Elsevier.
151. McManus CM: Neuromuscular blockers in surgery and intensive care, part 1. *Am J Health Syst Pharm* 58:2287-2299, 2001.
152. McNamara JO: Drugs effective in the therapy of epilepsies. In Gilman AG, editor: *The pharmacological basis of therapeutics,* ed 10. New York, 2001, Pergamon Press.
153. Mertens MJ, Vuyk J, Olofsen E, et al: Propofol alters the pharmacokinetics of alfentanil in healthy male volunteers. *Anesthesiology* 94:949-957, 2002.
154. Michel DJ, Knodel LC: Comparison of three algorithms used to evaluate adverse drug reactions. *Am J Hosp Pharm* 43:1709-1714, 1986.
155. Mignat C, Unger T: ACE inhibitors. Drug interactions of clinical significance. *Drug Saf* 12:334-347, 1995.
156. Miller M: Endocrine and metabolic dysfunction syndromes in the critically ill: syndromes of excess antidiuretic hormone release. *Crit Care Clin* 17:11-23, 2001.
156a. Mitra AG, Whitten MK, Laurent SL, et al: A randomized, prospective study comparing once-daily gentamicin versus thrice-daily gentamicin in the treatment of puerperal infection. *Am J Obstet Gynecol* 177:786-792, 1997.
157. MMWR: General recommendations on immunization. *MMWR* 38:205-214, 219-227, 1989.
158. Mockenhaupt M, Schöpf E: Epidemiology of drug-induced severe skin reactions. *Semin Cutan Med Surg* 15:236-243, 1996.
158a. Mohammed Ebid AH, Abdel-Rahman HM: Pharmacokinetics of phenobarbital during certain enhanced elimination modalities to evaluate their clinical efficacy in management of drug overdose. *Therapeutic Drug Monitoring* 23:209-216, 2001.
159. Mokhlesi B, Leiken JB, Murray P: Adult toxicology in critical care part I: general approach to the intoxicated patient. *Chest* 123:577-592, 2003.
160. Moore TJ, Weiss SR, Kaplan S, et al: Reported adverse drug events in infants and children under 2 years of age. *Pediatrics* 110:e53, 2002.
161. Morales-Olivas FJ, Martinez-Mir I, Ferrer JM, et al: Adverse drug reactions in children reported by means of the yellow card in Spain. *J Clin Epidemiol* 53:1076-1080, 2000.
162. Myers BD, Newton L: Cyclosporine-induced chronic nephropathy: an obliterative microvascular renal injury. *J Am Soc Nephrol* 2:S45-S52, 1991.
162a. Naguib M, Magboul MMA, Jaroudi R: Clinically significant drug interactions with general anaesthetics: incidence, mechanisms and management. *CNS Drugs* 8:51-78, 1997.
163. Nair DR, Morris HH: Potential fluconazole-induced carbamazepine toxicity. *Ann Pharmacother* 33:790-792, 1999.
164. Naranjo CA, Busto U, Sellers EM, et al: A method for estimating the probability of adverse drug reactions. *Clin Pharmacol Ther* 30:239-245, 1981.
165. Narins RG, Carley M, Bloom EJ, et al: The nephrotoxicity of chemotherapeutic agents. *Semin Nephrol* 10:556-564, 1990.
166. Neuvonen PJ, Suhonen R: Itraconazole interacts with felodipine. *J Am Acad Dermatol* 33:134-135, 1995.
167. Nies A, Spieldberg SP: Principles of therapeutics. In Hardman J, editor: *Goodman & Gilman's the pharmacological basis of therapeutics*. New York, 1996, McGraw-Hill.
168. Oliphant CM, Green GM: Quinolones: a comprehensive review. *Am Fam Physician* 34:455-464, 2002.
169. Olkkola KT, Ahonen J, Neuvonen PJ: The effect of the systemic antimycotics, itraconazole and fluconazole, on the pharmacokinetics and pharmacodynamics of intravenous and oral midazolam. *Anesth Analg* 82:511-516, 1996.
170. Olkkola KT, Aranko K, Luurila H, et al: A potentially hazardous interaction between erythromycin and midazolam. *Clin Pharmacol Ther* 53:298-305, 1993.
171. Olkkola KT, Backman JT, Neuvonen PJ: Midazolam should avoided in patients receiving the systemic antimycotics ketoconazole or itraconazole. *Clin Pharmacol Ther* 55:481-485, 1994.
172. Olsen KM, Martin SJ: Pharmacokinetics and clinical use of drotrecogin alfa (activated) in patients with severe sepsis. *Pharmacotherapy* 22(12 pt 2):196S-205S, 2002.
175. Ono S, Hatanaka T, Miyazawa S, et al: Human liver microsomal diazepam metabolism using cDNA-expressed cytochrome P450s: role of CYP2B6, 2C19 and the 3A subfamily. *Xenobiotica* 26:1155-1166, 1996.
176. Ozdemir M, Aktan Y, Boydag B, et al: Interaction between grapefruit juice and diazepam in humans. *Eur J Drug Metab Pharmacokinet* 23:55-59, 1998.
177. Page RL, Ruscin JM, Fish D, et al: Possible interaction between intravenous azithromycin and oral cyclosporine. *Pharmacotherapy* 21:1436-1443, 2001.
178. Pai MP, Graci DM, Amsden GW: Macrolide drug interactions: an update. *Ann Pharmacother* 34:495-513, 2000.
179. Painter MJ, Minnigh MB, Gaus L, et al: Neonatal phenobarbital and phenytoin binding profiles. *J Clin Pharmacol* 34:312-317, 1994.
180. Palkama VJ, Isohanni MH, Neuvonen PJ, et al: The effect of intravenous and oral fluconazole on the pharmacokinetics and pharmacodynamics of intravenous alfentanil. *Anesth Analg* 87:190-194, 1998.
181. Parke TJ, Stevens JE, Rice AS, et al: Metabolic acidosis and fatal myocardial failure after propofol infusion in children: five case reports. *BMJ* 305:613-616, 1992.
182. Pea F, Furlanut M: Pharmacokinetic aspects of treating infections in the intensive care unit: focus on drug interactions. *Clin Pharmacokinet* 40:833-868, 2001.
183. Piepho R, Whelton A, Mayor G, et al: Clinical therapeutic conference. *J Clin Pharmacol* 31:785-791, 1991.
184. Pinzani V, Faucherre V, Peyriere H: Methadone withdrawal symptoms with nevirapine and efavirenz. *Ann Pharmacother* 34:405-407, 2000.
185. Preston KL, Bigelow GE, Liebson IA: Antagonist effects of nalbuphine in opioid-dependent human volunteers. *J Pharmacol Exp Ther* 248:929-937, 1998.
186. Product Information: *Lanoxin®*. 2001, GlaxoSmithKline.
187. Product Information: *AmBisome(R), amphotericin B liposome for injection*. San Dimas, Calif, 2000, NeXstar Pharmaceutical.
188. Product Information: *Cardene(R), nicardipine hydrochloride*. Nutley, NJ, PI revised September 1999, reviewed July 2000, Roche Laboratories.
189. Product Information: *Cordarone(R) Intravenous, amiodarone*. Philadelphia, PI revised September 2001, reviewed March 2002, Wyeth-Ayerst Laboratories.
190. Product Information: *Halcion(R) triazolam*. Kalamazoo, Mich, 1994, Upjohn Laboratories.
191. Product Information: *Heparin Sodium Injection USP*. Los Angeles, 1999, American Pharmaceutical Partners.
192. Product Information: *Inapsine(R), droperidol*. Decatur, Ill, PI revised December 2001, reviewed April 2002, Akorn.
193. Product Information: *Lovenox®, Enoxaparin*. Bridgewater, NJ, 2001, Aventis Pharmaceutical Products.
194. Product Information: *Nitropress(R), sterile sodium nitroprusside, USP*. North Chicago, 1998, Abbott Laboratories.
195. Product Information: *Nubain(R), nalbuphine*. Manati, PR, PI revised December 1990, reviewed June 2002, Du Pont Pharmaceuticals.
196. Product Information: *Rapamune(R), sirolimus*. Philadelphia, PI revised January 2001, reviewed March 2001, Wyeth Laboratories, Division of Wyeth-Ayerst Pharmaceuticals.

197. Product Information: *Romazicon(R), flumazenil.* Nutley, NJ, 2002, Roche Laboratories.
198. Product Information: *Slo-Phyllin(R), theophylline tablets and syrup.* Collegeville, Penn, PI revised August 1996, reviewed May 2000, Rhone-Poulenc Rorer Pharmaceuticals.
199. Product Information: *Vasotec(R) I.V. injection, enalaprilat.* Whitehouse Station, NJ, PI revised October 2000, reviewed July 2001, Merck & Co.
200. Product Information: *Versed(R), midazolam.* Nutley, NJ, 1997, Roche Laboratories.
201. Product Information: *VFEND(R), voriconazole tablets and injection.* New York, PI issued May 2002, reviewed June 2002, Pfizer.
202. Product Information: *Xanax(R), alprazolam.* Kalamazoo, Mich, 1999, Pharmacia & Upjohn Company.
203. Pruchnicki MC, Dasta JF: Acute renal failure in hospitalized patients: part I. *Ann Pharmacother* 36:1261-1267, 2002.
204. Raistrick D, Hay A, Wolff K: Methadone maintenance and tuberculosis treatment. *BMJ* 313:925-926, 1996.
205. Rang HP, Dale MM: *Pharmacology,* ed 2, Edinburgh, 1991, Churchill-Livingstone.
205a. Rathbun RC, Rossi DR: Low-dose ritonavir for protease inhibitor pharmacokinetic enhancement. *Annals of Pharmacotherapy* 36:702-706, 2002.
206. Reed MD, Blumer JL: Propofol bashing. The time to stop is now! *Crit Care Med* 24:175-177, 1996.
207. Reid T, Yuen A, Catolico M, et al: Impact of omeprazole on the plasma clearance of methotrexate. *Cancer Chemother Pharmacol* 33:82-84, 1993.
208. Richmond R, McRorie ER, Ogden DA, et al: Methotrexate and triamterene: a potentially fatal combination? *Ann Rheum Dis* 56:209-210, 1997.
209. Rindone JP, Sloane EP: Cyanide toxicity from sodium nitroprusside: risks and management. *Ann Pharmacother* 26:515-520, 1992.
210. Rogers HJ, James CA, Morrison PJ, et al: Effect of cimetidine on oral absorption of ampicillin and cotrimoxazole. *J Antimicrob Chemother* 6:297-300, 1980.
211. Ronchera CL, Hernandex T, Peris JE, et al: Pharmacokinetic interaction between high-dose methotrexate and amoxicillin. *Ther Drug Monit* 15:375-379, 1993.
212. Roy LF, Villeneuve J-P, Dumont A, et al: Irreversible renal failure associated with triamterene. *Am J Nephrol* 11:486-488, 1991.
213. Sattler M, Guengerich FP, Yun CH, et al: Cytochrome P-450 3A enzymes are responsible for biotransformation of FK506 and rapamycin in man and rat. *Drug Metab Dispos* 20:753-761, 1992.
214. Schachter SC: Iatrogenic seizures. *Neurol Clin North Am* 16: 157-170, 1998.
215. Schlienger RG, Shear NH: Antiepileptic drug hypersensitivity syndrome. *Epilepsia* 39(suppl 7):53-57, 1998.
216. Schlondorff D: Renal complications of nonsteroidal anti-inflammatory drugs. *Kidney Int* 44:643-653, 1993.
217. Schutze GE: Antifungal agents for the treatment of systemic mycoses. *Semin Pediatr Infect Dis* 12:246-253, 2001.
218. Seeger JD, Kong SX, Schumock GT: Characteristics associated with ability to prevent adverse drug reactions in hospitalized patients. *Pharmacotherapy* 18;1284-1289, 1998.
219. Seelig CB, Maloley PA, Campbell JR: Nephrotoxicity associated with concomitant ACE inhibitor and NSAID therapy. *South Med J* 83:1144-1148, 1990.
220. Seligmann H, Podoshin L, Ben-David J, et al: Drug-induced tinnitus and other hearing disorders. *Drug Saf* 4:198-212, 1996.
221. Sens MA, Hazen-Martin DJ, Blackburn JG, et al: Growth characteristics of cultured human proximal tubule cells exposed to aminoglycoside antibiotics. *Ann Clin Lab Sci* 19:266-279, 1989.
222. Serra P, Brandimarte C, Martino P, et al: Synergistic treatment of enterococcal endocarditis: in vitro and in vivo studies. *Arch Intern Med* 137:1562-1567, 1977.
224. Silberstein, SD: Drug-induced headache. *Neurol Clin North Am* 16:107-123, 1998.
225. Simamora P, Pinsuwan S, Surakitbanharn Y, et al: Studies in phlebitis VIII: evaluations of pH solubilized intravenous dexverapamil formulations, PDA. *J Pharm Sci Technol* 50:123, 1996.
226. Simmons CF, Bogusky RT, Humes D: Inhibitory effects of gentamicin on renal cortical mitochondrial oxidative phosphorylation. *J Pharmacol Exp Ther* 12:17-22, 1980.
227. Slaughter RL, Edwards DJ: Recent advances: the cytochrome P450 enzymes. *Ann Pharmacother* 29:619-624, 1995.
228. Soldin S: Free drug measurements: when and why? An overview. *Arch Pathol Lab Med* 123:822-823, 1999.
228a. Somogyi A, McLean A, Heinzow B: Cimetidine-procainamide pharmacokinetic interaction in man: evidence of competition for tubular secretion of basic drugs. *European Journal of Clinical Pharmacology* 25:339-345, 1983.
229. Staniforth DH, Clarke HL, Horton R, et al: Augmentin bioavailability following cimetidine, aluminum hydroxide and milk. *Int J Clin Pharmacol Ther Toxicol* 23:154-157, 1985.
230. Steinbrook R: Testing medications in children. *N Engl J Med* 347:1462-1470, 2002.
231. Steiness E, Olesen KH: Cardiac arrhythmias induced by hypokalemia and potassium loss during maintenance digoxin therapy. *Br Heart J* 38:167-172, 1976.
232. Stewart CF, Fleming RA, Germain BF, et al: Aspirin alters methotrexate disposition in rheumatoid arthritis patients. *Arthritis Rheum* 34:1514-1520, 1991.
233. Stewart CL, Barnett R: Acute renal failure in infants, children and adults. *Crit Care Clin* 13:575-590, 1997.
234. Stillman MT, Napier J, Blackshear JL: Adverse effects of NSAIDs on the kidney. *Med Clin North Am* 68:371-385, 1984.
235. Stowe CD, Lee KR, Storgion SA, et al : Altered phenytoin pharmacokinetics in children with severe, acute traumatic brain injury. *J Clin Pharmacol* 40(12 pt 2):1452-1461, 2000.
235a. Stoeckel K, Trueb V, Dubach UC, McNamara PJ: Effect of probenecid on the elimination and protein binding of ceftriaxone. *European Journal of Clinical Pharmacology* 34:151-156, 1988.
236. Strauss FG, Franklin SS, Lewin AJ, et al: Withdrawal of antihypertensive therapy. *JAMA* 238:1734-1736, 1977.
237. Swan SK: Aminoglycosides nephrotoxicity. *Semin Nephrol* 17: 27-33, 1997.
238. Swingle HM, Bucciarelli RL, Ayoub EM: Synergy between penicillins and low concentrations of gentamicin in the killing of group B streptococci. *J Infect Dis* 152:515-520, 1985.
239. Takano M, Hasegawa R, Fukuda T, et al: Interaction with P-glycoprotein and transport of erythromycin, midazolam and ketoconazole in Caco-2 cells. *Eur J Pharmacol* 358:289-294, 1998.
240. Tan K: Clinical pharmacokinetics of a new azole—voriconazole. *Clin Microbiol Infect* 5:6, 1999.
241. Tanigawara Y: Role of P-glycoprotein in drug disposition. *Ther Drug Monit* 22:137-140, 2000.
242. Toto RD: Review: acute tubulointerstitial nephritis. *Am J Med Sci* 299:392-410, 1990.
243. Textor SC: Renal failure related to angiotensin-converting enzyme inhibitors. *Semin Nephrol* 17:67-76, 1997.
244. To err is human: building a safer health system. Washington, DC, 1999, National Academy Press.
245. Tofovic SP, Branch KR, Oliver RD, et al: Caffeine potentiates vasodilator-induced renin release. *J Pharmacol Exp Ther* 256:850-860, 1991.
246. Tong TG, Pond SM, Kreek MJ, et al: Phenytoin-induced methadone withdrawal. *Ann Intern Med* 94:349-351, 1981.
247. Trapnell CB, Narang PK, Li R, et al: Increased plasma rifabutin levels with concomitant fluconazole therapy in HIV-infected patients. *Ann Intern Med* 124:573-576, 1996.
248. Trissel LA: Drug stability and compatibility issues in drug delivery. *Cancer Bulletin* 42:393, 1990.
249. Tulkens PM: Nephrotoxicity of aminoglycoside antibiotics. *Toxicol Lett* 46:107-123, 1989.
250. Twyman RE, Rogers CJ, Macdonald RL: Differential regulation of gamma-aminobutyric acid receptor channels by diazepam and phenobarbital. *Ann Neurol* 25:213-220, 1989.
251. Upton RA: Pharmacokinetic interactions between theophylline and other medication (part I). *Clin Pharmacokinet* 20:66-80, 1991.
252. Van Bel F, Van Zoeren D, Schipper J, et al: Effect of indomethacin on superior mesenteric artery blood flow velocity in preterm infants. *J Pediatr* 116:965-970, 1990.
253. Varhe A, Olkkola KT, Neuvonen PJ: Oral triazolam is potentially hazardous to patients receiving systemic antimycotics ketoconazole or itraconazole. *Clin Pharmacol Ther* 56:601-607, 1994.
254. Vasa FR, Molitch ME: Prolonged critical illness management of long term acute care: endocrine problems in the chronically critically ill patient. *Clin Chest Med* 22:193-208, 2001.

255. Venkatakrishnan K, von Moktke LL, Greenblatt DJ: Effects of the antifungal agents on oxidative drug metabolism: clinical relevance. *Clin Pharmacokinet* 38:111-180, 2000.
256. Vesely JJK, Pien FD, Pien BCT: Rifampin, a useful drug for nonmycobacterial infections. *Pharmacotherapy* 18:345-357, 1998.
257. Vida JA: Anticonvulsants. In Foye WO, editor: *Principles of medicinal chemistry,* ed 3, Malvern, Penn, 1989, Lea & Febiger.
258. Vuyk J: Clinical interpretation of pharmacokinetic and pharmacodynamic propofol-opioid interactions. *Acta Anaesthesiol Belg* 52:445-451, 2001
259. Walker RC: The fluoroquinolones: symposium on antimicrobial agents—part XIII. *Mayo Clin Proc* 74:1030-1037, 1999.
259a. Waller ES, Sharanevych MA, Yakatan GJ: The effect of probenecid on nafcillin disposition. *Journal of Clinical Pharmacology* 22:482-489, 1982.
260. Wang E, Lew K, Casciano CN, et al: Interaction of common azole antifungals with P glycoprotein. *Antimicrob Agents Chemother* 46:160-165, 2002.
261. Weintraub M, Adde MA, Venzon DJ, et al: Severe atypical neuropathy associated with administration of hematopoietic colony-stimulating factors and vincristine. *J Clin Oncol* 14: 935-940, 1996.
262. Weiss J, Krebs S, Hoffmann C, et al: Survey of adverse drug reactions on a pediatric ward: a strategy for early and detailed detection. *Pediatrics* 110(2 pt 1):254-257, 2002.
263. Whelton A, Hamilton CW: Nonsteroidal anti-inflammatory drugs: effect on kidney function. *J Clin Pharmacol* 31:588-598, 1991.
264. Winniford MD, Fulton KL, Hillis LD: Symptomatic sinus bradycardia during concomitant propranolol-verapamil administration. *Am Heart J* 110:498, 1985.
265. World Health Organization: Requirements for adverse drug reactions. Genevea, Switzerland, 1975, World Health Organization.
266. Yu DK: The contribution of P-glycoprotein to pharmacokinetic drug-drug interactions. *J Clin Pharmacol* 39:1203-1211, 1999.
267. Zarembski DG, Fischer SA, Santucci PA, et al: Impact of rifampin on serum amiodarone concentrations in a patient with congenital heart disease. *Pharmacotherapy* 19:249-251, 1999.
268. Zenk KE: Y-site compatibility of drugs commonly used in the NICU. *Neonat Pharmacol Q* 1:13, 1992.
269. Zenk KE: Intravenous drug delivery in infants with limited IV access and fluid restriction. *Am J Hosp Pharm* 44:2542, 1987.
270. Zhang Y, Benet LZ: The gut as a barrier to drug absorption: combined role of cytochrome P450 3A and P-glycoprotein. *Clin Pharmacokinet* 40:159-168, 2001.
271. Zimmerman H: Hepatotoxicity: the adverse effects of drugs and other chemicals on the liver, ed 2, Philadelphia, 1999, Lippincott Williams & Wilkins.
272. Zucchero FJ, Hogan MJ, Sommer CD: Pocket guide to evaluations of drug interactions, ed 4, Washington DC, 2002, American Pharmaceutical Association.

PART

VI

Anesthesia and Analgesia Aspects of Pediatric Critical Care

CHAPTER

113

Organ System Considerations That Affect Anesthetic Management

Peter J. Davis and Joel B. Sarner

PEARLS

- The anesthetic care of intensive care unit (ICU) patients involves the extension of principles of medical management used in the operating room.
- The anesthesiologist caring for a critically ill child requires an understanding of the desired therapeutic endpoints and a knowledge of the patient's preexisting condition.
- For the intensivist, a patient returning to the ICU after surgery frequently requires an altered management plan. The physiologic perturbations of surgery and anesthesia frequently change the focus and direction of medical management. The intensivist must understand not only the events that occur in the operating room but also the rationale for using anesthetic agents and anesthetic techniques.

Cardiovascular Performance

For the anesthesiologist, knowledge of the hemodynamic characteristics that have ensured adequate organ perfusion in the pediatric intensive care unit (PICU) and the interventions that the intensivist has used to optimize the patient's cardiovascular function is essential to choosing the appropriate anesthetic.

Changes with Development

Cardiac assessment of the PICU patient requires a knowledge of normal cardiovascular growth and development and an understanding of the influence of disease and the effects of anesthesia on cardiovascular function (see Chapter 17). The myocardium of the neonate is less compliant than that of the adult, and the neonate's cardiac output depends primarily on the heart rate. Cardiac output increases substantially with age, whereas cardiac index (cardiac output divided by body surface area) ranges from 2.5 to 4.2 L/min/m^2 throughout life. Sympathetic innervation of the neonatal heart is not fully developed, and myocardial catecholamine stores are limited.[54] The response of the neonatal heart to vasoactive drugs is attenuated and the capacity for peripheral vasoconstriction during hypovolemia is reduced, probably because of the immature baroreceptor and α-adrenergic receptor systems.[81] Systemic vascular resistance is 800 to 1200 dyn·s·cm^5·m^2 at birth and reaches the adult value of 1600 by age 1 to 2 years. Systolic and diastolic blood pressures increase nonlinearly with age.

Pulmonary vascular resistance decreases dramatically after birth as hypoxemia-induced vasoconstriction is attenuated. During the first weeks of life, pulmonary vascular resistance continues to decrease, and by age 6 to 8 weeks pulmonary artery pressure and resistance have reached adult values. Mean right atrial (central venous) pressure normally is 1 to 5 mmHg. Mean left atrial pressure is

2 mmHg greater than mean right atrial pressure throughout life. Heart rate decreases markedly during the first few months of life and then decreases gradually until adulthood.

Oxygen consumption ($\dot{V}O_2$) increases from approximately 4.6 ml/kg/min in the term newborn infant to 7 ml/kg/min by age 10 days and 8 ml/kg/min by age 4 weeks. Oxygen consumption gradually decreases with age, reaching an adult value of 234 ml/min/1.7 m^2, or ≈140 ml/min/m^2, or 3.3 ml/kg/min.

Effects of Disease

Disease states can affect cardiovascular performance by their effects on the pulmonary and peripheral vasculatures and by their direct effects on the myocardium. Changes in myocardial compliance and filling pressures can profoundly influence myocardial performance. In addition, factors associated with disease states such as hypoxia, hypercarbia, acidosis, and hypothermia can affect pulmonary and systemic vascular resistances and thereby further modify myocardial function. The effects of changes in preload (i.e., the effects of fluid challenges) on the patient's blood pressure, cardiac output, and stroke volume and the clinical effects of changes in afterload heart rate, and myocardial contractility all influence the anesthesiologist's care of critically ill children.

Effects of Anesthetics

Anesthetic agents affect myocardial performance. During induction of anesthesia, potent inhaled agents such as halothane and isoflurane are associated with higher incidences of bradycardia, hypotension, and cardiac arrest in infants and children than in adults.[39] These cardiovascular depressant effects appear to be more pronounced in infants than in older children. Diaz and Lockard[27] found that more than 70% of healthy newborns had a greater than 30% decrease in systolic blood pressure during induction with halothane, whereas Friesen and Lichtor[39] noted that infants 1 to 6 months old had a 40% decrease in mean atrial pressure and a 30% decrease in heart rate when they received a halothane and nitrous oxide anesthetic. In a study of healthy children 1.5 to 12 years old undergoing halothane anesthesia, Barash et al.[3] noted that systolic blood pressure and heart rate decreased in a dose-dependent manner. Similar hemodynamic effects are noted in infants anesthetized with isoflurane.[40]

Because invasive monitors are difficult to insert in unsedated, awake children, much of the information about potent inhaled anesthetic agents and their effects on the determinants of cardiac output is derived from animal studies. In a neonatal piglet model, Boudreaux et al.[10] noted that the major adverse effect of halothane was its negative inotropic effect and not its negative chronotropic or unloading activity. In similarly designed studies, Schieber et al.[86] observed that, although isoflurane reduced contractility and decreased blood pressure and systemic vascular resistance more than did equipotent concentrations of halothane, cardiac index was better preserved in the isoflurane-anesthetized animals. Thus compared with halothane, the direct myocardial depressant effect of isoflurane is offset by its effect on the peripheral vasculature (afterload reduction).

Desflurane and sevoflurane are two new potent inhalational anesthetic agents. Because of their low blood solubility, they afford patients rapid induction and rapid awakening.[20,84,91,92,100,101] Desflurane has a blood gas solubility coefficient (0.42) that is similar to nitrous oxide in children. However, desflurane's pungent airway properties result in a high incidence of laryngospasm, coughing, and hypoxia that limit its utility as an induction agent in nonintubated children.[101]

The cardiovascular profile of desflurane is age dependent.[92] Compared with awake values, arterial blood pressure decreased in children anesthetized with 1 minimal alveolar concentration (MAC)* of desflurane by approximately 30%, whereas the heart rate decreased or remained the same. Thus at 1 MAC, desflurane, like isoflurane and halothane, appears to attenuate the baroresponse in children. Weiskopf et al.[95] demonstrated that rapid increases in desflurane from 0.55 to 1.66 MAC in adults can transiently increase arterial blood pressure and heart rate. This cardiovascular excitation is associated with an increase in sympathetic and renin-angiotensin system activity.

Information on the hemodynamics of sevoflurane in children suggests that sevoflurane (blood gas coefficient 0.68) appears to produce the same hemodynamic effects as isoflurane.[84] In adults anesthetized with sevoflurane or isoflurane, administration of exogenous epinephrine had similar dysrhythmogenic properties.[70]

In a study of children using echocardiograms in which sevoflurane and halothane were compared at equal MAC, Holzman et al.[53] noted sevoflurane had fewer myocardial depressant effects than sevoflurane.

The synthetic opioids may offer more hemodynamic stability than the inhaled anesthetics.[22,49,68] Robinson and Gregory[80] were the first to report the safety and efficacy of high-dose fentanyl anesthesia in children, in a study of premature infants undergoing patent ductus arteriosus ligation. In subsequent reports on pediatric patients, Hickey and Hansen[49] documented the safety of opioid anesthesia in children with complex congenital heart disease. Although these investigators noted that high doses of fentanyl (50 and 75 μg/kg) decreased heart rate and mean arterial pressure (MAP) 7% and 9%, respectively, in patients with bidirectional shunts, opioids had a salutary effect on pulmonary vascular resistance, increasing transcutaneous oxygenation by 45%.

Because of the prolonged respiratory and sedative effect associated with moderate- and high-dose administration of fentanyl and its congeners, shorter-acting opioids may offer the advantage of more predictable control with a similar cardiovascular profile than the longer-acting opioids. Remifentanil, a new μ opioid agonist with an ultrashort half-life, has been introduced into clinical practice. Remifentanil is metabolized by plasma and tissue esterases. It is independent of organ elimination. Consequently, its kinetic parameters do not change with the duration of infusion. This flat, context-sensitive half-time coupled with its ultrashort half-life (7–10 minutes) allow better drug effect predictability. Pharmacokinetic studies in children demonstrate faster clearances and larger volumes of distribution in neonates compared with older infants and children.[82] Comparative studies of remifentanil to inhaled anesthetic agents in children undergoing pyloromyotomy surgery suggest that the short half-life of remifentanil may be beneficial with regard to postoperative respiratory changes.[25,42] Because of remifentanil's ultrashort half-life and its nonaccumulation with prolonged infusion, it may be a beneficial agent for sedation of infants and children in the ICU setting.

Propofol is a sedative hypnotic agent frequently used for sedation and for induction of anesthesia. Propofol is hydrophobic and consequently is prepared in a lipid emulsion. It is irritating as an injection. In doses used for induction of anesthesia (2–3 mg/kg), propofol is associated with a 10% to 15% decrease in MAP. Its use in the PICU setting is controversial because of the report of five unexpected deaths in 1992 and because of other reports of its association with acidosis, rhabdomyolysis, and bradycardia[18,64,74] and with impaired fatty acid oxidation.[97] In a retrospective review of a case series involving 142 critically ill patients, Cornfield et al.[17] demonstrated that administration of continuous propofol was not associated with hemodynamic compromise or metabolic acidosis (see Chapter 116).

Developmental and disease-induced characteristics of cardiovascular performance are not readily predictable for individual infants and children. Therefore it is vital that the anesthesiologist glean as much as possible of the patient's cardiovascular behavior from the preanesthetic (PICU) experience.

Anemia and Transfusion

Concerns about transfusion-related disease transmission have forced clinicians to reassess transfusion criteria (see Chapter 75). Rothstein[83] previously recommended that in patients younger than 3 months, hemoglobin concentration should be greater than 10 g/dl, whereas in children older than 3 months a hemoglobin concentration of 9 g/dl was adequate. Slogoff[87] concluded that in normovolemic adults, a hematocrit of 20% (hemoglobin ≈7 g/dl) is adequate. Carson et al.[13] retrospectively reviewed mortality in 125 adult surgical patients who refused blood transfusion for religious reasons. Mortality correlated inversely with preoperative hemoglobin level and directly with operative blood loss. No operative deaths occurred among patients with a preoperative hemoglobin level above 8 g/dl and an operative blood loss of less than 500 ml.

Transfusion guidelines should anticipate age-related changes in the oxygen dissociation curve. P_{50} (partial pressure of oxygen at which hemoglobin is 50% saturated with oxygen) is lower in newborns than in adults. In a child age 1 year, P_{50} is higher than in normal adults; by age 9 to 12 years, P_{50} has decreased to adult values. These age-related changes in hemoglobin's affinity for oxygen alter oxygen unloading to the peripheral tissues.

Minimum acceptable hemoglobin (and approximate hematocrit) levels can be inferred from anticipated tissue oxygen delivery (Table 113–1). A hemoglobin concentration of 7 to 8 g/dl (hematocrit 21%–24%) is reasonable for adults and children based on the previous discussion. Minimum values chosen for infants should be more conservative (i.e., ensure greater oxygen delivery to tissues) than those for older patients. This takes into consideration the higher oxygen consumptions of infants and provides them with a larger margin of safety against hypoxic injury. Infants younger than 2 months probably require a hemoglobin level of 13 g/dl (hematocrit of 40%); infants older than 3 months require a hemoglobin level of 7 g/dl (hematocrit of 21%). Infants age 2 to 3 months are in a transitional phase, and minimum hemoglobin levels are more difficult to predict. These values are intended as guidelines only; each patient must be considered individually.

Patients with chronic anemia increase oxygen delivery by increasing cardiac output. Although potent inhaled anesthetic agents decrease myocardial function and cardiac output and thereby decrease oxygen delivery, these side effects are offset by the decrease in oxygen consumption that occurs in anesthetized patients.

The need to transfuse blood in the perioperative period frequently is determined by the patient's underlying hemodynamic stability, the type of surgery anticipated, and the known risks of administering blood products. In general, unless the procedure is minor, blood should be available for all ICU patients. Because ICU patients frequently are monitored with invasive catheters, serial measurements of hematocrit or hemoglobin usually can be obtained during the operative procedure to determine whether transfusion is warranted.

Respiratory Failure

When respiratory failure is present, the anesthesiologist must be aware of its precipitating factors. Acute respiratory distress syndrome (ARDS) is a clinical syndrome of respiratory distress, poor pulmonary compliance, and hypoxemia that usually occurs after a nonpulmonary condition such as shock, trauma, sepsis, or an unexplained condition leading to pulmonary parenchymal disease and respiratory failure. Direct mortality from respiratory failure is approximately 10% to 20%; overall mortality is as high as 65%. ARDS was first described as a clinical entity occurring in pediatric patients in 1980 (see Chapter 46).[75]

TABLE 113–1

Hemoglobin Requirement for Equivalent Tissue Oxygen Delivery

	P_{50} (mmHg)	Hb for Equivalent O_2 Delivery (g/dl)						
Adult	27	7	8	9	10	11	12	13
Infant >3 months	30	5.7	6.5	7.3	8.2	9.0	9.8	10.6
Neonate <2 months	24	10.3	11.7	13.2	14.7	16.1	17.6	19.1

Calculated from data of Motoyama EK, Zigas CJ, Troll G: *Am Soc Anesthiol* (abstratct), 1974.

Recognized factors predisposing pediatric patients to the development of ARDS include severe infection, cardiac arrest, shock, and aspiration. Although the cause of this condition is uncertain, the fundamental defect in the lung is injury to the pulmonary capillary endothelial cells leading to interstitial and, ultimately, alveolar pulmonary edema. This pulmonary vascular leakage results in hypoxemia, decreased pulmonary compliance, increased pulmonary vascular resistance, and venoarterial shunting.

The mainstays of treatment are endotracheal intubation, continuous positive-pressure ventilation with positive end-expiratory pressure (PEEP), and supplemental oxygen. Invasive monitoring by arterial, central venous, and pulmonary arterial cannulation may be necessary to optimize preload and cardiac output in the presence of high PEEP and high transpulmonary pressures. The patient's requirements for oxygen, PEEP, and pulmonary toilet must be understood preoperatively. Patients with poor pulmonary compliance challenge the ability to maintain adequate intraoperative ventilation. Preoperative knowledge of the interaction of PEEP with the adequacy of ventilation and cardiovascular function is an important concern of the anesthesiologist. Anesthetics can modify cardiovascular function, but anesthetics also can influence respiratory function by their effect on hypoxic pulmonary vasoconstriction.

Patients with ARDS may rely in part on regional hypoxic pulmonary vasoconstriction to minimize intrapulmonary shunting. Shifting of pulmonary blood flow away from atelectatic lung regions has been well described. The administration of vasoactive drugs and potent inhaled anesthetics has been shown in animal models to inhibit hypoxic pulmonary vasoconstriction and therefore may exacerbate hypoxemia by increasing intrapulmonary shunting.[30,61] However, the clinical relevance of the animal studies is not substantiated in human studies.[79,81] Nonetheless, the anesthesiologist must be aware that administration of potent inhaled anesthetics may increase the patient's shunt fraction.

Neurologic Injury

Head trauma is a major cause of pediatric mortality and morbidity. Trauma per se is the most common cause of death in patients age 1 to 38 years. Eighty percent of trauma patients have central nervous system (CNS) injury, and in 60% the CNS injury is the most severe. It is estimated that 185 of every 100,000 children experience head trauma requiring hospitalization (see Chapter 107).[58,59]

Neurologic injury may be the primary insult resulting from trauma. However, secondary cerebral injury may result from the development of intracranial hypertension and resultant cerebral ischemia. Recognition and control of elevated intracranial pressure (ICP) are key elements to preventing neurologic deterioration and patient morbidity.

Secondary traumatic brain injury can be characterized by an array of biochemical, cellular, and molecular events, which are associated with ischemia, excitotoxicity, energy failure, and cell death cascades, all of which result in cerebral swelling, axonal injury, inflammation, and regeneration.[56]

Intracranial Pressure

The signs of intracranial hypertension in infants and children are listed in Table 113–2. The presence of these signs and symptoms in conjunction with the baseline findings on neurologic examination may dramatically alter the patient's anesthetic care. The anesthesiologist must be aware of ongoing interventions to control ICP (see Chapter 52).

Control of cerebral perfusion is essential for maintaining neurologic function in pathologic states. Cerebral perfusion pressure is expressed as the difference between MAP and the larger of either central venous pressure or ICP. Thus in the presence of intracranial hypertension (ICP >15–20 mmHg), higher systemic blood pressures must be achieved to prevent cerebral ischemia.

Intracranial compliance depends on the volumes of the intracranial contents, cerebral tissue, blood, and extracellular fluid. The most dynamic of these is the blood compartment; changes in cerebral blood volume are mediated primarily through changes in cerebral vascular resistance. Cerebral vascular resistance is affected by both intracranial and extracerebral factors.

Regulation of Cerebral Blood Flow

Cerebral blood flow (CBF) regulation depends primarily on the local chemical and metabolic milieu, particularly on the concentrations of hydrogen ion, adenosine, and prostanoids. Production of these compounds correlates with normal cerebral activity and metabolic rate. Neurogenic and myogenic components also have minor roles in regulating cerebral vascular resistance.

Extracerebral factors that can change cerebral vascular resistance and CBF include arterial partial pressures of carbon dioxide ($Pa{CO_2}$) and oxygen ($Pa{O_2}$), MAP, and drugs (Figure 113–1). $Pa{CO_2}$ and CBF are directly related. As $Pa{CO_2}$ is rapidly lowered toward 20 mmHg, there is marked cerebral vasoconstriction and reduction in both CBF and ICP. Theoretically, an acute decrease in $Pa{CO_2}$ below 20 mmHg may be detrimental by reducing CBF enough to cause cerebral ischemia. The salutary effects of acute hyperventilation on ICP are diminished over time because acute changes in cerebrospinal fluid (CSF) pH are normalized in approximately 6 hours.

TABLE 113–2

Signs of Intracranial Hypertension in Infants and Children

Infants	Children	Infants and Children
Irritability	Headache	Decreased consciousness
Full fontanelle	Diplopia	Cranial nerve (III and VI) palsies
Widely separated cranial sutures	Papilledema	Loss of upward gaze (setting sun sign)
Cranial enlargement		Vomiting
		Signs of herniation, Cushing triad, papillary changes

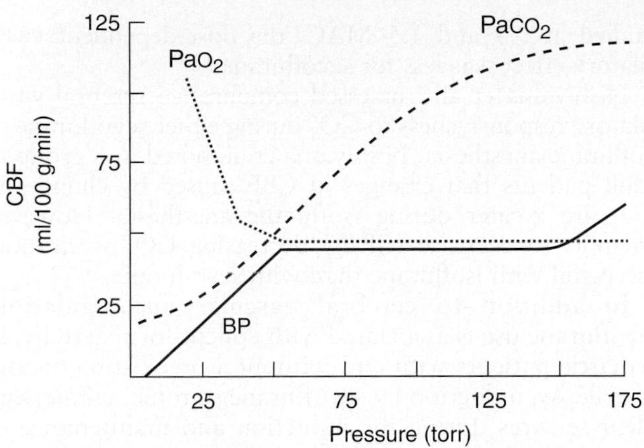

FIGURE 113–1 • Cerebral blood flow *(CBF)* changes resulting from alterations in $PaCO_2$, PaO_2, and blood pressure. The other two variables remain stable at normal values when the remaining variable is altered. (From Shapiro HM: *Anesthesiology* 43:445, 1975.)

Arterial oxygenation within the normal clinical range has little effect on cerebral vascular resistance. However, PaO_2 less than 50 mmHg results in cerebral vasodilation and increased CBF. Hyperoxia in excess of 300 mmHg may produce cerebral vasoconstriction.

Autoregulation, the ability of the brain to maintain constant CBF despite alterations in MAP, is functional over a MAP range from 50 to 150 mmHg in adults. At MAP less than 50 mmHg, symptoms of cerebral ischemia may appear. If the upper limit of MAP for autoregulation is exceeded, the resultant increase in CBF may cause cerebral edema. The autoregulatory curve may shift in the presence of chronic hypertension, intracranial tumors, head trauma, or shock states. This renders the brain more susceptible to ischemic effects.[27] The range of MAP over which autoregulation of CBF occurs in infants and children likely shifts in tandem with age-related changes in normal systemic blood pressures and cerebral perfusion pressures. Raju et al.[77] suggest that an infant's mean cerebral perfusion pressure is approximately equal to its gestational age in weeks and that this estimate holds true for growing preterm infants up to 5 weeks after birth.

Effects of Anesthetics on Cerebral Blood Flow

In general, potent inhaled anesthetics impair autoregulation and may cause hypotension and increased CBF (Figure 113–2). Consequently, they must be used cautiously, if at all, in patients with evidence of head trauma. Halothane and enflurane at 1 MAC abolish cerebral autoregulation. Isoflurane impairs autoregulation less than halothane does.[93] The effects of anesthetic agents on CBF and cerebral metabolism are summarized in Figure 113–3. In general, the preferred agents decrease both CBF and cerebral metabolic rate of oxygen ($CMRO_2$). The potent inhaled agents (halothane, enflurane, and isoflurane) "uncouple" the normal relationship between CBF and metabolism and cause marked cerebral vasodilation. Isoflurane is the only inhaled anesthetic with which CBF actually may decrease when concomitant hyperventilation to $PaCO_2$ of 20 to

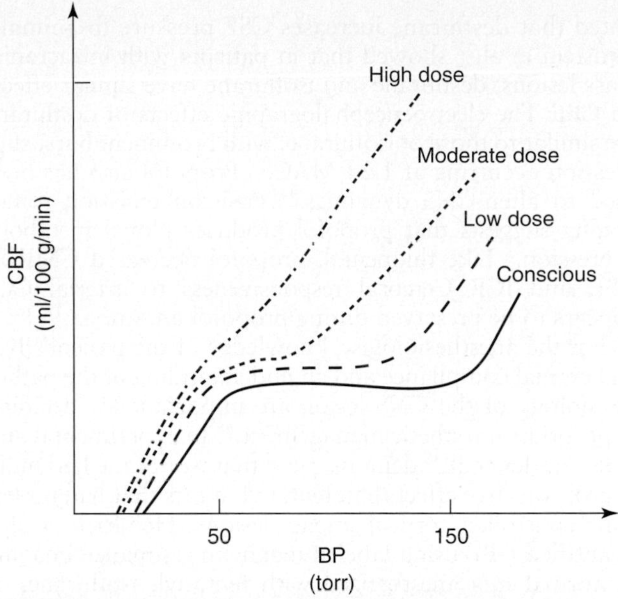

FIGURE 113–2 • Volatile anesthetics and autoregulation. Schematic representation of the effect of a progressively increased dose of a typical volatile anesthetic agent on cerebral blood flow *(CBF)* autoregulation. Both upper and lower thresholds are shifted to the left. (From Drummond K, Shapiro HM: Cerebral physiology. In Miller R, editor: *Anesthesia,* vol 2, ed 3, New York, 1990, Churchill Livingstone.)

25 mmHg[85] is used. Whereas nitrous oxide alone is known to cause mild cerebral vasodilation and to increase $CMRO_2$ (probably related to inadequate anesthetic depth), these effects are easily countered by the addition of intravenous sedatives, hypnotics, and narcotics.

Effects of desflurane on CBF have been demonstrated. Little information on the effects of sevoflurane on CNS physiology in human subjects is available. Artru et al.[2]

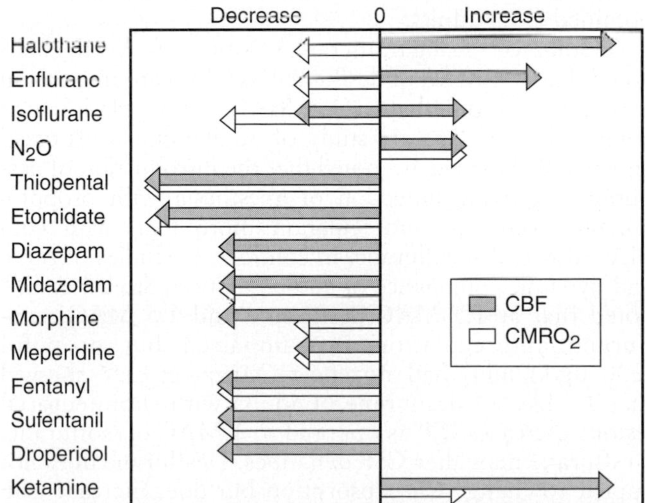

FIGURE 113–3 • Effects of anesthetic agents on cerebral blood flow *(CBF)* and cerebral metabolic rate of oxygen ($CMRO_2$). (From Cucchiara RF, Block S, Steinkeler JA: The effects of anesthetic agents on cerebral blood flow and cerebral metabolism: anesthesia for intracranial procedures. In Barash PG, Cullen BF, Stoelters SK, editors: *Clinical anesthesia.* Philadelphia, 1989, JB Lippincott.)

noted that desflurane increases CSF pressure in animals. Ornstein et al.[72] showed that in patients with intracranial mass lesions, desflurane and isoflurane have similar effects on CBF. The electroencephalographic effects of desflurane are similar to those of isoflurane, with prominent burst suppression occurring at 1.24 MAC.[78] Propofol also has been used to alter CNS dynamics.[94] Positron emission tomography suggests that propofol produces global metabolic depression.[1] Like thiopental, propofol decreased $CMRO_2$, CBF, and ICP. Cerebral responsiveness to arterial CO_2 appears to be preserved during propofol anesthesia.[19,76]

For the anesthesiologist, knowledge of the patient's ICP and cranial compliance and an understanding of the pathophysiology of the CNS lesion are important for deciding appropriate anesthetic management.[88] In experimental animals, Statler et al.[88] demonstrated that isoflurane had more neuroprotective effect than fentanyl in rats that had undergone controlled cortical impact lesions. Hendrich et al.[48] quantified CBF using labeled magnetic resonance imaging in normal rats anesthetized with fentanyl, isoflurane, or pentobarbital. In this study, CBF values were found to be approximately 2.5 to 3 times lower in most regions analyzed during anesthesia with either fentanyl (with N_2O/O_2) or pentobarbital versus isoflurane (with N_2O/O_2). In addition, these investigators noted that CBF was heterogeneous in rats anesthetized with isoflurane (with N_2O/O_2) but relatively homogenous in rats anesthetized with either fentanyl (with N_2O/O_2) or pentobarbital.

In previous human studies with opioids anesthesia, opioids maintained static cerebral autoregulation. Engelhard et al.[36] subsequently demonstrated that remifentanil, a μ opioid agonist with unique pharmacokinetic properties, when combined with low-dose propofol maintains both static and dynamic compliance of cerebrovascular autoregulation.

Most commonly, inhaled anesthetic agents are used in pediatric anesthesia. Most of the data on the effects of the inhaled anesthetic agents on cerebral autoregulation were obtained from adults.

In volunteers using transcranial Doppler, Bedforth et al.[6] noted that at 1 MAC of desflurane, cerebral autoregulation was impaired and that at 1.5 MAC autoregulation was abolished. In a separate study of adult nonneurosurgical patients, Bedforth et al.[5] noted that the introduction of desflurane following induction of anesthesia with propofol impaired cerebral autoregulation more than with equi MAC doses of sevoflurane. In contrast, in studies of static and dynamic compliance of autoregulation, Strebel et al.[89] noted that at 1.5 MAC desflurane and 1.5 MAC sevoflurane autoregulation was impaired but propofol (200 μg/kg/min) had no effect. Muzzi et al.[69] showed that 1 MAC of desflurane in adults with supratentorial lesions increases ICP as opposed to 1 MAC of isoflurane. Desflurane may alter CSF dynamics. Desflurane does not appear to change CSF absorption but does increase CSF production.[69]

In a study of patients undergoing nonintracranial neurosurgical procedures, Summors et al.[90] noted that dynamic cerebral autoregulation using transcranial Doppler ultrasonography is better preserved during 1.5 MAC sevoflurane than 1.5 MAC isoflurane anesthesia. Others noted similar findings with sevoflurane and isoflurane. In patients studied at 0.5 and 1.5 MAC, the dose-dependent vasodilatory effect was less for sevoflurane.[47,62]

Nishiyama et al.[71] assessed comparative cerebral vasodilatory responsiveness to CO_2 during either sevoflurane or isoflurane anesthesia. Nishiyama et al. noted in a group of adult patients that changes in CBF caused by changes in CO_2 are greater during isoflurane anesthesia. However, attempts to decrease ICP by decreasing CO_2 were more successful with isoflurane than with sevoflurane.[71]

In addition to cerebral vascular autoregulation, sevoflurane use is associated with epileptiform activity. In pediatric patients with and without a preexisting history of epilepsy, induction by sevoflurane of tonic, clonic, and silent seizures during the induction and maintenance of anesthesia is reported.[57,98,102]

Hepatic Dysfunction

Assessment of liver function is important for two aspects of anesthetic management. The liver is a major site of drug metabolism and is involved in homeostasis of the coagulation system. Anesthesia and surgery may exacerbate liver dysfunction in patients with preexisting liver disease and, in some instances, may cause life-threatening hepatic failure. Although the cause of hepatic dysfunction in surgical patients is unknown, it may be related to decreases in hepatic blood flow. Consequently, anesthetic drugs and techniques that may decrease hepatic blood flow should be avoided if possible.

Effects of Anesthetics on Hepatic Blood Flow

Blood flow in the splanchnic circulation can be altered by numerous factors. Mechanical ventilation, by altering the normal relationship between splanchnic venous outflow and venous outflow from the kidney and lower extremities, may affect splanchnic blood flow. The changes associated with mechanical ventilation can be further exacerbated by increasing tidal volume and applying PEEP.[63] Carbon dioxide concentration also influences splanchnic blood flow.[41]

Various anesthetic agents may have different effects on hepatic blood flow.[43] Gelman et al.[44] showed that hepatic oxygen supply is better maintained during isoflurane than during halothane anesthesia. In addition, in hypoxic rat models, the incidence of hepatic centrilobular necrosis was least with isoflurane compared with halothane, nitrous oxide, and fentanyl. Although anesthetic agents can decrease hepatic blood flow, Gelman et al. demonstrated that the decrease in hepatic blood flow is small compared with the decrease associated with the surgical stress of a laparotomy. Surgical procedures involving traction and manipulation of the abdominal viscera are associated with release of various vasoactive compounds that may further alter splanchnic blood flow. In sevoflurane-anesthetized dogs, Frank et al.[38] demonstrated that hepatic arterial blood flow was maintained, portal blood flow was decreased, and total hepatic blood flow was unchanged. In desflurane-anesthetized dogs, hepatic artery blood flow was maintained, portal blood flow was decreased, and total hepatic blood flow was reduced.[65]

Effects of Liver Disease on Pharmacokinetics

In addition to the effects of anesthetic agents on the liver, hepatic disease affects the pharmacology of anesthetic agents. Little is known about the pharmacologic properties of anesthetic agents in pediatric patients with liver disease.[21,24]

Although the liver is the major site of drug biotransformation, the effects of hepatic dysfunction on drug elimination and disposition are inconsistent.[96] The degree of liver dysfunction and a drug's ability to bind to plasma proteins are important variables in determining drug kinetics in patients with liver disease. For drugs with a high hepatic extraction ratio, hepatic clearance is sensitive to changes in hepatic blood flow, whereas for drugs with a low hepatic extraction ratio, hepatic drug clearance is a function of intrinsic hepatic enzyme activity and protein binding.[96] Thus the reported inconsistent effect of liver disease on drug pharmacology may be a function of the heterogeneous pathophysiology of liver disease with respect to hepatocellular function, protein binding, and hepatic blood flow.

Table 113–3 compares opioid pharmacokinetics in patients with and without liver disease. Note that the effects of hepatic disease are variable with respect to the pharmacokinetics of opioids.

Remifentanil, a μ opioid agonist that undergoes plasma and tissue esterase metabolism, is unaffected, with respect to its pharmacokinetic profile, by liver disease.[26,57] The pharmacokinetics of muscle relaxants in adults are well studied. Of the nondepolarizing muscle relaxants, pancuronium, vecuronium, and atracurium are significantly metabolized. Of these agents, only pancuronium and vecuronium pharmacokinetic profiles are altered by liver disease. In a study of children with moderate-to-severe liver dysfunction, Brandom et al.[12] showed that liver failure has no effect on atracurium pharmacokinetics.

Mivicurium is a benzylisoquinolium diester metabolized by plasma cholinesterase. It is a neuromuscular blocking agent of short duration. Greene et al.[46] noted that the severity of disease did not correlate with the duration of mivicurium block in pediatric patients with liver disease compared with controls. However, mivicurium's initial recovery and overall recovery from neuromuscular blockade did correlate inversely with the concentration of plasma cholinesterase.

Cisatracurium is a stereoisomer of atracurium. In patients with normal hepatic and renal function, the duration of action of cisatracurium is similar to that of atracurium. deWolf et al.[29] noted that although the kinetic profile of cisatracurium differed in patients with liver failure compared with control patients, the duration of clinical effectiveness was similar for the two groups of patients. In patients with hepatic failure, clearance of rocuronium is reduced, and the volume of distribution is increased. Consequently, the β elimination half-life is prolonged.

Role of Liver in Coagulation

The liver has a dual role in the coagulation system. It synthesizes proteins necessary for the coagulation cascade, and it functions as a clearing mechanism of the fibrinolytic system. Because coagulopathies are common in patients with liver disease and because hemostasis is paramount in any surgical procedure, coagulation monitoring and knowledge of the clinical effects of blood products on the coagulation system provide important information. Surgical procedures in which massive volumes of blood are expected to be transfused frequently result in dilutional thrombocytopenia. The need for platelet transfusions is a function of the amount of blood transfused and the initial platelet count. The appropriate use of blood products is discussed in Chapter 75. For patients with severe hepatic dysfunction undergoing surgical procedures, as well as for patients with

TABLE 113–3

Pharmacokinetics of Narcotics

Drug	Disease	V_d	$t_{1/2}\beta$	Clearance
Meperidine‡	Cirrhosis	263 ± 286	359 ± 77 min*	573 ± 158 ml/min*
	Control	232 ± 536	213 ± 25 min	900 ± 316 ml/min
Meperidine†	Acute hepatitis	5.56 ± 1.8 L/kg	6.94 ± 2.74 hr*	649 ± 228 ml/min*
	Control	5.94 ± 2.65 L/kg	3.37 ± 0.82 hr	1261 ± 527 ml/min
Morphine†	Cirrhosis	2.3 ± 1.3 L/kg	2.2 + 1.3 hr	1.15 ± 0.35 L/min
	Control	2.9 ± 2.4 L/kg	2.5 ± 1.5 hr	1.23 ± 0.43 L/min
Fentanyl†	Cirrhosis	4.27 ± 0.65 L/kg	304 ± 74 min	11.3 ± 1.6 ml/kg/min
	Control	3.44 ± 0.64 L/kg	263 ± 48 min	10.8 ± 1.2 ml/kg/min
Alfentanil†	Cirrhosis	351 ± 206 ml/kg	219 ± 128 min*	1.6 ± 1.0 ml/kg/min*
	Control	281 ± 97 ml/kg	90 ± 18 min	3.1 ± 1.6 ml/kg/min
Alfentanil‡	Cirrhosis§	0.46 ± 0.16 L/kg	45 ± 13 min	7.59 ± 3.6 ml/kg/min
	Control	0.40 ± 0.21 L/kg	41 ± 16 min	7.25 ± 4.3 ml/kg/min

From Davis PJ, Cook DR: *Transplant Proc* 21:3493, 1989.
$t_{1/2}\beta$-elimination half-life; V_d-volume of distribution.
* Significantly different from controls.
†Adults.
‡Children.
§Cirrhosis resulting from cholestatic liver disease.

normal coagulation profiles who are anticipated to need transfusion of more than one blood volume, an adequate supply of blood products must be available before surgery is started.

Renal Failure

One major function of the kidneys is the regulation of fluid and electrolyte balance. Hyponatremia and hyperkalemia, the electrolyte disorders seen most often in patients with renal failure, are discussed briefly. Management of fluid and electrolyte abnormalities associated with renal failure is reviewed in Chapters 60 and 62. However, some aspects of fluid and electrolyte disturbance have implications for anesthetic management.

Fluid and Electrolyte Disturbances

In clinical practice, it is desirable to maintain serum sodium concentrations greater than 125 mEq/L. At lower levels, symptoms including irritability, personality change, muscle weakness, and depressed deep tendon reflexes may occur. More severe hyponatremia (<120 mEq/L) may cause cerebral edema and may be associated with nausea, vomiting, confusion, convulsions, hypothermia, and even death. In addition, anesthetic requirements may decrease significantly in the presence of serum and CSF hyponatremia.

Hyperkalemia may produce well-recognized electrocardiographic changes, including symmetrical peaking of the T wave, ST-segment depression, and heart block. Ventricular fibrillation or asystole may result from extreme hyperkalemia. This has been observed after the use of depolarizing muscle relaxants, such as succinylcholine, which further increase plasma potassium concentrations by increasing muscle plasma membrane permeability.

The acidosis associated with renal failure would not be expected to interfere with reversal of neuromuscular blockade. Miller and Roderick[66] demonstrated that metabolic alkalosis, but not metabolic acidosis, may prevent neostigmine-induced antagonism of pancuronium. The mechanism proposed depends on simultaneous decreases in calcium and potassium levels. Whether the hypocalcemia associated with renal failure clinically affects reversal of neuromuscular relaxants remains to be demonstrated. In the event of prolonged neuromuscular blockade, dialysis should easily remove both muscle relaxants and anticholinesterase agents used for reversal of blockade. Both classes of drugs are highly ionized compounds.

Perioperative dialysis may be required to control hyponatremia, fluid overload, hyperkalemia, or severe acidosis in the surgical patient with renal failure. When possible dialysis should be accomplished shortly before surgery to optimize the patient's preoperative status (see Chapter 65). The goals of dialysis should not include dehydration. Patients who are dehydrated may become hypotensive during induction and maintenance of anesthesia.

Renal Drug Metabolism

The kidneys also function in drug elimination. The effects of renal failure on drug disposition and elimination are of particular interest to the anesthesiologist.

Nondepolarizing muscle relaxants are the major class of anesthetic drugs excreted primarily by the kidneys. Drugs that are almost exclusively eliminated by the kidney (e.g., gallamine and metocurine) should be avoided in the presence of renal failure. Pancuronium accumulates despite its hepatic metabolism and biliary excretion and may demonstrate as much as a fivefold increase in elimination half-life in anephric patients. Among the older, longer-duration muscle relaxants, D-tubocurarine is least affected by renal failure. Although the elimination half-life of D-tubocurarine is less prolonged in renal failure than that of gallamine, careful dosage titration and monitoring of neuromuscular blockade are essential when D-tubocurarine is used in this clinical setting.

The intermediate-duration relaxants vecuronium and atracurium are recommended for use in patients with renal failure.[8] Vecuronium depends primarily on hepatobiliary excretion; only 20% is excreted by the kidney. The pharmacokinetic and pharmacodynamic profiles of vecuronium in renal failure patients are similar to those in healthy patients.[7] Atracurium elimination occurs by Hoffmann elimination and ester hydrolysis in the plasma. Because these processes are independent of renal and hepatic function, the elimination half-life of atracurium is constant regardless of failure of these organs.[12,28] Atracurium metabolism produces laudanosine, which is associated with seizures in dogs at high plasma concentrations.[14] Data in human subjects indicate that the risk of such seizures probably is not clinically relevant. ICU patients receiving atracurium infusions for up to 219 hours had maximum plasma concentrations well below the threshold for canine seizures and showed no evidence of cerebral excitation.[99] The effects of renal failure on this scenario are not documented.

Mivicurium is a bisquarternary benzylisoquinolinium diester, nondepolarizing muscle relaxant metabolized by plasma cholinesterase. It is a mixture of three optical isomers. Mivicurium at a dose of 0.15 mg/kg prolonged neuromuscular blockade by a factor of 1.5 in patients with renal disease compared to patients with normal renal function.[103]

Cisatracurium is one of the stereoisomers of atracurium and is thought to be three times more potent than atracurium but with a similar duration of action. Like atracurium, cisatracurium is metabolized by Hoffmann elimination, and the drug does not accumulate. Its duration of action is not prolonged in patients with renal failure.[11]

Rocuronium is a monoquaternary steroidal muscle relaxant of rapid-to-intermediate onset of action and intermediate duration. The clinical duration of rocuronium is similar to that of vecuronium. It has a rapid onset of action, but in patients with renal disease clearance the onset of action is decreased by 30% to 40% and its duration of action is prolonged and variable.[60,67]

The anticholinesterases used to reverse neuromuscular blockade (neostigmine, pyridostigmine, and edrophonium) are eliminated primarily by the kidney, and renal failure markedly prolongs their duration of action. In the absence of renal function, the serum half-lives of neostigmine and D-tubocurarine were prolonged to similar degrees. Thus reversal of neuromuscular blockade induced by atracurium, vecuronium, and in many cases D-tubocurarine should not be complicated by recurrence of blockade.

Opioids are metabolized primarily by the liver. Thus renal failure should not have a major effect on narcotic administration. The pharmacokinetics of fentanyl, sufentanil, and alfentanil in children appear to be minimally affected by chronic renal failure.[23,24] However, morphine and meperidine are metabolized to active metabolites that are eliminated by the kidney. Morphine glucuronide accumulates at higher plasma concentration in patients with chronic renal failure.[15,73] Normeperidine, the major metabolite of meperidine, may accumulate and cause prolonged respiratory depression and seizures.

Of the inhaled anesthetics, isoflurane probably is the safest for patients with renal failure. It is not metabolized to fluoride ion or associated with potential renal toxicity, as are enflurane and methoxyflurane. It also is not associated with bromide ion production, as is halothane. Although bromide is not a renal toxin, it may account for persistent sedation.

The metabolic breakdown of desflurane is insignificant. Less than 1% of the absorbed dose is metabolized. Sevoflurane, however, undergoes metabolic breakdown into organic and inorganic compounds. Inorganic fluoride is a potential cause of nephrotoxicity. Studies with methoxyflurane show that plasma inorganic fluoride levels greater than 50 μM are associated with nephrotoxicity.

However, plasma levels may not accurately predict nephrotoxicity. Kharasch et al.[54] demonstrated that inhalational anesthetic agents are metabolized within the kidney by the cytochrome P-450 system and that various anesthetic agents are metabolized differently within the kidney. Consequently, it appears that intrarenally produced fluoride and not the plasma fluoride level may explain the relationship of nephrotoxicity to anesthetic metabolism.

The newer agents sevoflurane and desflurane have been studied in patients with and without renal disease. Desflurane is a polyfluorinated ethyl ether that does not undergo in vivo metabolism. Studies in both animals and humans suggest that desflurane has no hepatic or renal toxic effect; however, it does interact with dry carbon dioxide absorbants and produces carbon monoxide.[37]

Sevoflurane is a polyfluorinated methylisopropyl ether that undergoes in vivo degradation to difluorovinyl products and fluoride ion. In addition, sevoflurane undergoes degradation by the CO_2 absorber system to form fluoromethyl-1-1-difluoro-1-(trifluoromethyl) vinyl ether, also known as compound A. Both compound A and free fluoride ions have potential nephrotoxic effect. However, clinical studies in patients with normal renal function and those with abnormal renal function demonstrate that changes in kidney function following sevoflurane anesthesia are similar to changes that occur after desflurane, isoflurane, or enflurane anesthesia.[9,16,31,33,50,51,55]

Remifentanil is an opioid agonist that is metabolized by plasma and tissue esterases. The metabolic product of remifentanil metabolism has a potency of 1/3400 of its parent compound. It is independent of organ elimination, and its extremely rapid metabolism does not allow for drug accumulation. Ross et al.[82] reported the pharmacokinetic properties of remifentanil in children. Its ultrashort half-life (≈7 minutes) allows patients a rapid recovery from anesthesia. Because it is independent of organ elimination, the pharmacokinetic profile of remifentanil is unchanged in either renal or hepatic insufficiency.[52] Remifentanil also demonstrates a flat, context-sensitive half-time. Thus the length of time remifentanil is infused does not affect the time to patient recovery when infusion is discontinued.[32,45]

In addition to the fluid and electrolyte problems and pharmacologic concerns posed by renal failure, the presence or development of renal failure per se may affect perioperative outcome. In adults, perioperative renal failure is associated with mortality as high as 70%. Similar data from children are lacking. However, in a study of pediatric patients undergoing liver transplantation, the 1-year survival rate in patients with renal failure was 53% compared with 81% for patients in whom renal failure did not develop.[35]

Intravenous Alimentation

ICU patients frequently receive intravenous hyperalimentation for nutritional support. Intravenous hyperalimentation regimens should be adjusted in anticipation of surgery.

Surgical trauma results in accelerated protein catabolism. Administration of glucose to traumatized patients does not have the protein-sparing effect observed during starvation. The capacity of postoperative patients to handle exogenous glucose loads is impaired as a result of the neuroendocrine response to injury (see Chapter 68).[34] Hyperglycemic, hyperosmolar, nonketotic coma (HHNKC) is reported as a cause of delayed awakening after anesthesia. In two reports, the patients had diabetes mellitus, and they returned to the baseline level of consciousness within 1 to 3 postoperative days after appropriate therapy. Bedford[4] reported the fatal development of HHNKC postoperatively in a nondiabetic patient who received high-dose steroid therapy for thrombotic thrombocytopenic purpura.

Conversely, abrupt interruption of hyperalimentation containing high concentrations of dextrose may result in hypoglycemia, the signs and symptoms of which may be undetected in an anesthetized patient. Therefore optimal preoperative preparation should include weaning of glucose-containing solutions to concentrations less than or equal to 10% for a period of several hours before surgery. During this weaning period of dextrose, interval monitoring of serum glucose is mandatory. Such a practice should help prevent the problems of hyperglycemia and hypoglycemia. In addition, glucose concentrations less than or equal to 10% may be administered peripherally, thus facilitating central access for administration of fluid volume, vasopressors, and/or resuscitation medications. Glucose concentrations greater than 10% should be administered only through a central cannula; when administered peripherally, these solutions may result in intense thrombophlebitis associated with venous extravasation.

Although the perioperative administration of fat emulsions used for hyperalimentation has not been shown to increase anesthetic risk, the standard of anesthesia practice is to discontinue their use. Potential complications of intravenous lipids include hepatobiliary injury, pancreatitis, and hypoxemia resulting from interstitial lipoid pneumonitis with alveolar capillary block.

The pediatric intensivist must realize that concerns regarding caloric deprivation must be modified in the catabolic perioperative period. Nutritional supplementation should not be maintained at the expense of safe and effective intraoperative care.

REFERENCES

1. Alkire MT, Haier RJ, Barker SJ, et al: Cerebral metabolism during propofol anesthesia in humans studied with positron emission tomography. *Anesthesiology* 82:393, 1995.
2. Artru AA, Powers K, Doepfner P: CSF, sagittal sinus, and jugular venous pressures during desflurane or isoflurane anesthesia in dogs. *J Neurosurg Anesthesiol* 6:239, 1994.
3. Barash PG, Glanz S, Katz JD, et al: Ventricular function in children during halothane anesthesia: an echocardiographic evaluation. *Anesthesiology* 49:79, 1978.
4. Bedford RF: Hyperosmolar hyperglycemia nonketotic coma following general anesthesia: report of a case. *Anesthesiology* 35:652, 1971.
5. Bedforth NM, Hardman JG, Nathanson MH: Cerebral hemodynamic response to the introduction of desflurane: a comparison with sevoflurane. *Anesth Analg* 91:152-155, 2000.
6. Bedforth NM, Girling KJ, Skinner HJ, Mahajan RP: Effects of desflurane on cerebral autoregulation. *Br J Anaesth* 87:193-197, 2001.
7. Bell CF, Hunter JM, Jones RS, et al: Use of atracurium and vecuronium in patients with oesophageal varices. *Br J Anaesth* 57:160, 1985.
8. Bencini AF, Scaf AHJ, Sohn YJ, et al: Disposition and urinary excretion of vecuronium bromide in anesthetized patients with normal renal function or renal failure. *Anesth Analg* 65:245, 1986.
9. Bito H, Ikeuchi Y, Ikekda K: Effects of low flow sevoflurane anesthesia on renal function. *Anesthesiology* 86:1231-1237, 1997.
10. Boudreaux JP, Schieber RA, Cook DR: Hemodynamic effects of halothane in the newborn piglet. *Anesth Analg* 63:731, 1984.
11. Boyd AH, Eastwood NB, Parker CJR, Hunter JM: Pharmacodynamics of the 1R cis-1′R cis isomer of atracurium (51W89) in health and chronic renal failure. *Br J Anaesth* 174:400-404, 1995.
12. Brandom BW, Stiller RL, Cook DR, et al: Pharmacokinetics of atracurium in anaesthetized infants and children. *Br J Anaesth* 58: 1210, 1986.
13. Carson JL, Poses RM, Spence RK, et al: Severity of anaemia and operative mortality and morbidity. *Lancet* 1:727, 1988.
14. Chapple DJ, Miller AA, Ward JB, et al: Cardiovascular and neurological effects of laudanosine: studies in mice and rats, and in unconscious and anaesthetized dogs. *Br J Anesth* 59:218, 1987.
15. Chauvin M, Sandouk P, Schermann JM, et al: Morphine pharmacokinetics in renal failure. *Anesthesiology* 66:327, 1987.
16. Conzen PF, Nuscheler M, Melotte A, et al: Renal function and serum fluoride concentrations in patients with stable renal insufficiency after anesthesia with sevoflurane or enflurane. *Anesth Analg* 81:569-575, 1995.
17. Cornfield DN, Tegtmeyer K, Nelson MD, et al: Continuous propofol infusion in 142 critically ill children. *Pediatrics* 110:1177-1181, 2002.
18. Cray SH, Robinson BH, Cox PM: Lactic acidemia and bradyarrhythmia in a child sedated with propofol. *Crit Care Med* 26:2087-2092, 1998.
19. Dam M, Ori C, Pizzolato G, et al: The effects of propofol anesthesia on local cerebral glucose utilization in the rat. *Anesthesiology* 73:499, 1990.
20. Davis PJ, Cohen IT, McGowan FX Jr, et al: Recovery characteristics of desflurane vs. halothane for maintenance of anesthesia in pediatric ambulatory patients. *Anesthesiology* 80:298, 1994.
21. Davis PJ, Cook DR: Anesthetic problems in pediatric liver transplantation. *Transplant Proc* 21:3493, 1989.
22. Davis PJ, Cook DR, Stiller RL, et al: Pharmacodynamics and pharmacokinetics of high-dose sufentanil in infants and children undergoing cardiac surgery. *Anesth Analg* 66:203, 1987.
23. Davis PJ, Stiller RL, Cook DR, et al: Pharmacokinetics of sufentanil in adolescent patients with chronic renal failure. *Anesth Analg* 67:268, 1988.
24. Davis PJ, Stiller RL, Cook DR, et al: Effects of cholestatic hepatic disease and chronic renal failure on alfentanil pharmacokinetics in children. *Anesth Analg* 68:579, 1989.
25. Davis PJ, Galinkin J, McGowan FX, et al: A randomized multicenter study of remifentanil compared with halothane in neonates and infants undergoing pyloromyotomy. I. Emergence and recovery profiles. *Anesth Analg* 93:1380138-6, 2001.
26. Dershwitz M, Rosow CE: The pharmacokinetics and pharmacodynamics of remifentanil in volunteers with severe hepatic or renal dysfunction. *J Clin Anesth* 8:88S-90S, 1996.
27. Diaz JH, Lockard CH: Is halothane really safe in infancy? *Anesthesiology* 51:S313, 1979.
28. deBros FM, Lai A, Scott R, et al: Pharmacokinetics and pharmacodynamics of atracurium during isoflurane anesthesia in normal and anephric patients. *Anesth Analg* 65:743, 1986.
29. deWolf AM, Freeman JA, Scott VL, et al: Pharmacokinetics and pharmacodynamics of cisatracurium in patients with end-stage liver disease undergoing liver transplantation. *Br J Anaesth* 76: 624-628, 1996.
30. Domino KB, Borowec L, Alexander CM, et al: Influence of isoflurane on hypoxic pulmonary vasoconstriction in dogs. *Anesthesiology* 64:423, 1986.
31. Ebert TJ, Frink EJ, Kharasch ED: Absence of biochemical evidence for renal and hepatic dysfunction after 8 hours of 1.25 minimum alveolar concentration sevoflurane anesthesia in volunteers. *Anesthesiology* 88:601-610, 1998.
32. Egan TD, Lemmens HJ, Fiset P, et al: The pharmacokinetics of the new short-acting opioid remifentanil (GI87084B) in healthy adult male volunteers. *Anesthesiology* 79:881-892, 1993.
33. Eger EI 2nd, Koblin DD, Bowland T, et al: Nephrotoxicity of sevoflurane versus desflurane anesthesia in volunteers. *Anesth Analg* 84:160-168, 1997.
34. Elliott MJ, Alberti KGMM: Carbohydrate metabolism: effects of preoperative starvation and trauma. In Biebuyck JF, editor: *Nutritional aspects of anesthesia. Clinics in anesthesiology*, vol 1, Philadelphia, 1983, WB Saunders.
35. Ellis D, Avner ED, Starzl TE: Renal failure in children with hepatic failure undergoing liver transplantation. *J Pediatr* 108:393, 1986.
36. Engelhard K, Werner C, Mollenberg O, Kochs E: Effects of remifentanil/propofol in comparison with isoflurane on dynamic cerebrovascular autoregulation in humans. *Acta Anaesthesiol Scand* 45:971-976, 2001.
37. Fang ZX, Eger EI II, Laster MJ, et al: Carbon monoxide production from degradation of desflurane, enflurane, isoflurane, halothane, and sevoflurane by soda lime and Baralyme. *Anesth Analg* 89:1187-1193, 1995.
38. Frank EJ, Morgan SE, Coetzee A, et al: The effects of sevoflurane, halothane, enflurane, and isoflurane on hepatic blood flow and oxygenation in chronically instrumented greyhound dogs. *Anesthesiology* 76:85, 1992.
39. Friesen RH, Lichtor JL: Cardiovascular depression during halothane anesthesia in infants: a study of three induction techniques. *Anesth Analg* 61:42, 1982.
40. Friesen RH, Lichtor JL: Cardiovascular effects of inhalation induction with isoflurane in infants. *Anesth Analg* 62:411, 1983.
41. Fujita Y, Sakai T, Ohsumi A, et al: Effects of hypocapnia and hypercapnia on splanchnic circulation and hepatic function in the beagle. *Anesth Analg* 69:152, 1989.
42. Galinkin JL, Davis PJ, McGowan FX, et al: A randomized multicenter study of remifentanil compared with halothane in neonates and infants undergoing pyloromyotomy. II. Perioperative breathing patterns in neonates and infants with pyloric stenosis. *Anesth Analg* 93:1387-1392, 2001.
43. Gelman S: General anesthesia and hepatic circulation. *Can J Physiol Pharmacol* 65:1762, 1987.
44. Gelman S, Dillard E, Bradley EL Jr: Hepatic circulation during surgical stress and anesthesia with halothane, isoflurane, or fentanyl. *Anesth Analg* 66:936, 1987.
45. Glass P, Hardman D, Kamiyama Y: Preliminary pharmacokinetics and pharmacodynamics of an ultra-short-acting opioids: remifentanil (GI87084B). *Anesth Analg* 77:1031-1040, 1993.
46. Green DW, Fisher M, Sockalingham I: Mivacurium compared with succinylcholine in children with liver disease. *Br J Anaesth* 81: 463-465, 1998.
47. Gupta S, Heath K, Matta BF: Effect of incremental doses of sevoflurane on cerebral pressure autoregulation in humans. *Br J Anaesth* 79:469-472, 1997.

48. Hendrich KS, Kochanek PM, Melick JA, et al: Cerebral perfusion during anesthesia with fentanyl, isoflurane, or pentobarbital in normal rats studied by arterial spin-labeled MRI. *Magn Reson Med* 46:202-206, 2001.
49. Hickey PR, Hansen DD: Fentanyl- and sufentanil-oxygen-pancuronium anesthesia for cardiac surgery in infants. *Anesth Analg* 63:117, 1984.
50. Higuchi H, Adachi Y, Wada H, et al: The Effects of low-flow sevoflurane and isoflurane anesthesia on renal function in patients with stable moderate renal insufficiency. *Anesth Analg* 92:650, 2001.
51. Higuchi H, Sumita S, Wada H, et al: Effects of sevoflurane and isoflurane on renal function and on possible markers of nephrotoxicity. *Anesthesiology* 89:307-322, 1998.
52. Hoke JF, Shlugman D, Dershwitz M, et al: Pharmacokinetics and pharmacodynamics of remifentanil in persons with renal failure compared with healthy volunteers. *Anesthesiology* 87:531-541, 1997.
53. Holzman RS, van der Velde ME, Kaus SJ, et al: Sevoflurane depresses myocardial contractility less than halothane during induction of anesthesia in children. *Anesthesiology* 85:1260-1267, 1996.
54. Kharasch ED, Hankins DC, Thummel KE: Human kidney methoxyflurane and sevoflurane metabolism. *Anesthesiology* 82:689, 1995.
55. Kharasch ED, Frink EJ Jr, Zager R, et al: Assessment of low-flow sevoflurane and isoflurane effects on renal function using sensitive markers of tubular toxicity. *Anesthesiology* 86:1238-1253, 1997.
56. Kochanek PM, Clark R, Ruppel R, et al: Biochemical, cellular, and molecular mechanisms in the evolution of secondary damage after severe traumatic brain injury in infants and children: lesions learned from the bedside. *Pediatr Crit Care Med* 11:4-19, 2000.
57. Komatsu H, Taie S, Endo S, et al: Electrical seizures during sevoflurane anesthesia in two pediatric patients with epilepsy. *Anesthesiology* 81:1535, 1997.
58. Kraus JF, Fife D, Conroy C: Pediatric brain injuries: the nature, clinical course, and early outcomes in a defined United States' population. *Pediatrics* 79:501, 1987.
59. Kraus JF, Fife D, Cox P, et al. Incidence, severity, and external causes of pediatric brain injury. *Am J Dis Child* 140:687, 1986.
60. Magorian T, Wood P, Caldwell J, et al: The pharmacokinetics and neuromuscular effects of rocuronium bromide in patients with liver disease. *Anesth Analg* 80:754-759, 1995.
61. Marshall C, Lindgren L, Marshall BE: Effects of halothane, enflurane and isoflurane on hypoxic pulmonary vasoconstriction in rat lungs in vitro. *Anesthesiology* 60:304, 1984.
62. Matta BF, Heath KJ, Tipping K, et al: Direct cerebral vasodilatory effects of sevoflurane and isoflurane. *Anesthesiology* 91:677-680, 1999.
63. Matuschak GM, Pinsky MR, Rogers RM: Effects of positive end-expiratory pressure on hepatic blood flow and performance. *J Appl Physiol* 62:1377, 1987.
64. Mehta N, DeMunter C, Habibi P, et al: Short-term propofol infusions in children. *Lancet* 354:866-867, 1999.
65. Merin RG, Bernard JM, Doursout MF, et al: Comparison of the effects of isoflurane and desflurane on cardiovascular dynamics and regional blood flow in the chronically instrumented dog. *Anesthesiology* 74:568-574, 1991.
66. Miller RD, Roderick L: The influence of acid-base changes on neostigmine antagonism of a pancuronium neuromuscular blockade. *Br J Anaesth* 50:317, 1978.
67. Moore EW, Hunter JM: The new neuromuscular blocking agents: do they offer any advantages? *Br J Anaesth* 87:912-925, 2001.
68. Moore RA, Yang SS, McNicholas KW, et al: Hemodynamic and anesthetic effects of sufentanil as the sole anesthetic for pediatric cardiovascular surgery. *Anesthesiology* 62:725, 1985.
69. Muzzi DA, Losasso TJ, Dietz NM, et al: The effect of desflurane and isoflurane on cerebrospinal fluid pressure in humans with supratentorial mass lesions. *Anesthesiology* 76:720-724, 1992.
70. Navarro R, Weiskopf RB, Moore MA, et al: Humans anesthetized with sevoflurane or isoflurane have similar arrhythmic response to epinephrine. *Anesthesiology* 80:545, 1994.
71. Nishiyama T, Matsukawa T, Yokoyama T, Hanaoka K: Cerebrovascular carbon dioxide reactivity during general anesthesia: a comparison between sevoflurane and isoflurane. *Anesth Analg* 89:1437-1441, 1999.
72. Ornstein E, Young WL, Fleischer LH, et al: Desflurane and isoflurane have similar effects on cerebral blood flow in patients with intracranial mass lesions. *Anesthesiology* 79:498, 1993.
73. Osborne R, Joel S, Grebenik K: The pharmacokinetics of morphine and morphine glucuronides in kidney failure. *Clin Pharmacol Ther* 54:158, 1993.
74. Parke TJ, Stevens JE, Rice AS, et al: Metabolic acidosis and fatal myocardial failure after propofol infusion in children: five case reports. *BMJ* 305:613-616, 1992.
75. Pfennigner J, Gerber A, Tschappeler H, et al: Adult respiratory distress syndrome in children. *J Pediatr* 101:352, 1982.
76. Pinaud M, Lelausque J-N, Chetanneau A, et al: Effects of propofol on cerebral hemodynamics and metabolism in patients with brain trauma. *Anesthesiology* 73:404, 1990.
77. Raju TNK, Doshi UV, Vidyasagar D: Cerebral perfusion pressure studies in healthy preterm and term newborn infants. *J Pediatr* 100:139, 1982.
78. Rampil IJ, Lockhart SH, Eger EI, et al: The electroencephalographic effects of desflurane in humans. *Anesthesiology* 74:434, 1991.
79. Rees DI, Gaines GY III: One-lung anesthesia: a comparison of pulmonary gas exchange during anesthesia with ketamine or enflurane. *Anesth Analg* 63:521, 1984.
80. Robinson S, Gregory GA: Fentanyl-air-oxygen anesthesia for ligation of patent ductus arteriosus in preterm infants. *Anesth Analg* 60:331, 1981.
81. Rogers SN, Benumof JL: Halothane and isoflurane do not decrease PaO_2 during one-lung ventilation in intravenously anesthetized patients. *Anesth Analg* 64:946, 1985.
82. Ross AK, Davis PJ, Dear Gd GL, et al: Pharmacokinetics of remifentanil in anesthetized pediatric patients undergoing elective surgery or diagnostic procedures. *Anesth Analg* 93:1393-1401, 2001.
83. Rothstein P: What hemoglobin level is adequate in pediatric anesthesia? *Anesthesiol Update* 1:2, 1978.
84. Sarner JB, Levine M, Davis PJ, et al: Clinical characteristics of sevoflurane in children: a comparison with halothane. *Anesthesiology* 82: 38, 1995.
85. Scheller MS, Todd MM, Drummond JC: Isoflurane, halothane, and regional cerebral blood flow at various levels of $PaCO_2$ in rabbits. *Anesthesiology* 64:598, 1986.
86. Schieber RA, Namnoum A, Sugden A, et al: Hemodynamic effects of isoflurane in the newborn piglet: comparison with halothane. *Anesth Analg* 65:633, 1986.
87. Slogoff S: Anesthesia considerations in the anemic patient. *Anesthesiol Update* 2:7, 1979.
88. Statler KD, Kochanek PM, Dixon CE, et al: Isoflurane improves long-term neurologic outcome versus fentanyl after traumatic brain injury in rats. *J Neurotrauma* 12:1179-1189, 2000.
89. Strebel S, Lam AM, Matta B, et al: Dynamic and static cerebral autoregulation during isoflurane, desflurane, and propofol anesthesia. *Anesthesiology* 83:66-76, 1995.
90. Summors A, Gupta A, Matta B: Dynamic cerebral autoregulation during sevoflurane anesthesia: a comparison with isoflurane. *Anesth Analg* 88:341-345, 1999.
91. Taylor RH, Lerman J: Induction, maintenance, and recovery characteristics of desflurane in infants and children. *Can J Anaesth* 39:6, 1992.
92. Taylor RH, Lerman J: Minimum alveolar concentration of desflurane and hemodynamic responses in neonates, infants, and children. *Anesthesiology* 75:975, 1991.
93. Todd MM, Drummond JC: A comparison of the cerebrovascular and metabolic effects of halothane and isoflurane in the cat. *Anesthesiology* 60:276, 1984.
94. Van Hemelrijck J, Fitch W, Mattheuseen M, et al: Effect of propofol on cerebral circulation and autoregulation in the baboon. *Anesth Analg* 71:49, 1990.
95. Weiskopf RB, Moore MA, Eger EI II, et al: Rapid increase in desflurane concentration is associated with greater transient cardiovascular stimulation than with rapid increase in isoflurane concentration in humans. *Anesthesiology* 80:1035, 1994.
96. Williams RL: Drug administration in hepatic disease. *N Engl J Med* 309:1616, 1984.
97. Wolfe A, Weir P, Segar P, et al: Impaired fatty acid oxidation in propofol infusion syndrome. *Lancet* 357:606, 2001.
98. Woodforth IJ, Hicks RG, Crawford MR, et al: Electroencephalographic evidence of seizure activity under deep sevoflurane anesthesia in a nonepileptic patient. *Anesthesiology* 87:1579-1582, 1997.

99. Yate PM, Flynn PJ, Arnold RW, et al: Clinical experience and plasma laudanosine concentrations during the infusion of atracurium in the intensive therapy unit. Br J Anaesth 59:211, 1987.
100. Young WL: Effects of desflurane on the central nervous system. *Anesth Analg* 75:S32, 1992.
101. Zwass MS, Fisher DM, Welborn LG, et al: Induction and maintenance characteristics of anesthesia with desflurane and nitrous oxide in infants and children. *Anesthesiology* 76:373, 1992.
102. Bosenberg AT. Convulsions and sevoflurane. *Paediatr Anaesth* 7:477-478, 1997.
103. Cook DR, Freeman JA, Lai AA, et al: Pharmacokinetics of mivacurium in normal patients and in those with hepatic or renal failure. *Br J Anaesth* 69:580-585, 1992.

CHAPTER

114

Anesthetic Principles and Operating Room Anesthesia Regimens

James C. Fackler and John H. Arnold

PEARLS

- In the pediatric population, an understanding of the factors that alter the relationship between delivered anesthetic concentration and the concentration at the central nervous system site of action is important.
- Each inhaled agent has unique effects on the cardiovascular, respiratory, and central nervous systems.
  - All inhaled agents
  - Increase respiratory rate
  - Reduce tidal volume
  - Decrease ventilatory responses to hypoxemia and hypercapnia
  - Decrease bronchial smooth muscle tone
  - Decrease functional residual capacity
  - Produce dose-dependent increase in cerebral blood flow despite simultaneous depression of cerebral metabolic oxygen requirement
- Opioids can be administered intravenously, intramuscularly, subcutaneously, or neuraxially by intrathecal or epidural injection.
- No available pediatric data suggest that one class of anesthetic is safer than another in any particular situation.
- Many factors confound a safe anesthetic in a critically ill child. Airway considerations always take precedence. Most critically ill children who require general anesthesia are mechanically ventilated.
- Generally the transition of care between the providers in the operating room and the intensive care unit is an informal conversation at the bedside. Efforts to structure physician handoffs likely will reduce miscommunication errors.

Providing a safe anesthetic for a critically ill child is one of the most demanding challenges for an anesthesiologist. Children may require surgery with little advance warning. Cardiovascular and respiratory failure may be imminent or present. Even children who present with advance warning can present with multiorgan system failure. To provide optimal care in the postoperative period, the critical care specialist must develop an understanding of anesthetic techniques and alternatives. This chapter presents the anesthetic agents most commonly encountered in critical care practice and an overview of anesthetic techniques and alternatives. Specific conditions that demand unique anesthetic considerations are discussed. The reader is referred to a superb text of pediatric anesthesia for information beyond this overview.[15] An excellent short text also is recommended.[117]

Anesthetic Agents

Volatile Anesthetics

Although the precise mechanism of action of the inhalational agents remains incompletely understood,[39,77] the inhaled anesthetics are of major importance in modern anesthesia practice. The currently used agents include the an inorganic gas nitrous oxide and the volatile liquids isoflurane, desflurane, and sevoflurane. Until recently, halothane played an important role in pediatric anesthesia and is discussed in some detail. In children without overwhelming airway or respiratory disease, delivery of these potent inhaled agents by way of the respiratory system offers a reliable route of administration, a dependable mode of excretion, and the ability to quickly alter anesthetic concentrations in the central nervous system (CNS). For the initiation of anesthesia, halothane was used most often because of its relatively sweet (but strong) odor. In contrast, initiation of anesthesia with isoflurane is nearly impossible because of its pungent odor. High-concentration sevoflurane now is widely used for initiation of anesthesia in children.[21]

An understanding of the factors that alter the relationship between delivered anesthetic concentration and the concentration at the CNS site of action is important, particularly in the pediatric population. The inspired anesthetic concentration (usually represented in volume %) has a direct relationship with brain concentration. The gradient between inspired concentration (F_I) and alveolar concentration (F_A) determines the rapidity of anesthetic uptake and distribution to the CNS. When $F_A/F_I = 1$, equilibrium between inspired, alveolar, and brain anesthetic concentrations is achieved. The rate of rise of F_A/F_I is enhanced by increased alveolar ventilation. Increased cardiac output decreases the alveolar anesthetic concentration by removal of anesthetic from the alveolus. Although increased cardiac output enhances equilibration of tissue and arterial partial pressures, the net effect is lowering F_A and slowing the rise of brain anesthetic concentration. Further, the "blood solubility" of inhaled anesthetics is quantitatively described by the blood/gas partition coefficient. The higher the blood/gas partition coefficient, the more likely the anesthetic will be "partitioned" to the blood phase at the alveolar–capillary interface and the lower the F_A. Therefore the more "soluble" the agent, the slower the rise in F_A/F_I and thus brain anesthetic concentration.

The relative potencies of the inhaled anesthetics are quantitated by the minimum alveolar concentration (MAC) at equilibrium required to abolish purposeful movement in 50% of subjects exposed to a standardized noxious stimulus (expressed as a percentage at 1 atm). The greater the MAC, the higher the inspired anesthetic concentration needed to provide satisfactory surgical anesthesia (Table 114–1).

Each inhaled agent has unique effects on the cardiovascular, respiratory, and central nervous systems, which are not exhaustively reviewed here (Table 114–2). The volatile anesthetics produce dose-dependent decreases in mean arterial blood pressure as a result of direct myocardial depression and decreases in systemic vascular resistance. In contrast, nitrous oxide produces minimal alteration in either myocardial performance or systemic vascular resistance, and this may be partly accounted for by direct stimulation of the sympathetic nervous system.[28] However, when combined with a potent volatile agent or opioids, nitrous oxide is associated with significant depression of myocardial contractility. All inhaled agents increase the respiratory rate and decrease tidal volume, the ventilatory responses to hypoxemia and hypercapnia, bronchial smooth muscle tone, and functional residual capacity. All agents also produce a dose-dependent increase in cerebral blood flow despite simultaneous depression of cerebral metabolic oxygen requirement. In one clinical trial of children without CNS disease, sevoflurane did not affect cerebral blood flow velocity.[29] At concentrations above 2 MAC, isoflurane induces an isoelectric electroencephalogram (EEG), a property not shared by the other agents. There are a few case reports in children of poly spike-and-wave complexes appearing during sevoflurane anesthesia.[27]

Although halothane is most frequently cited as the agent responsible for perioperative hepatic dysfunction, multiple anesthetics have been examined in a hypoxic rat model and result in hepatic necrosis.[91] True halothane-induced hepatitis is a rare event, with an incidence of approximately 1:30,000,[99] and is seen most commonly after repeated administration. It most likely is mediated by an immune mechanism involving an intermediate oxidative metabolite.[50] Hepatotoxicity associated with desflurane and sevoflurane is exceptionally uncommon.[53]

TABLE 114–1

Solubilities and Potencies of Inhaled Anesthetics

	Blood/Gas Partition Coefficient	MAC (Vol %)
Nitrous oxide	0.47	105*
Isoflurane	1.4	1.15
Enflurane	1.8	1.68
Halothane	2.3	0.73
Desflurane	0.42	7.25
Sevoflurane	0.69	2.06

*Minimum alveolar concentration (MAC) of 105 is unachievable at atmospheric pressure.

TABLE 114–2

Cardiovascular and Cerebrovascular Effects of Inhaled Anesthetics

Myocardial Contractility	Heart Rate	Systemic Vascular Resistance	Cerebral Blood Flow
Halothane	—	–	±
Enflurane	–	+	–
Isoflurane	–	++	—
N_2O	±	±	±

++, greatly increased; +, moderately increased; ±, no consistent effect; –, moderately decreased; —, greatly decreased.
*In doses < 1.0 minimum alveolar concentration.

In every discipline of medicine, an understanding of genetic profiles will be increasingly important. Relevant to understanding responses to volatile anesthetics, in addition to the well-known variable of body temperature and age, a specific human genotype has been associated with an increased need for desflurane to achieve the same level of anesthesia.[57]

The inhaled agents produce dose-related decreases in renal blood flow and urine output as a result of effects on cardiac output and systemic vascular resistance. Fluoride-induced nephrotoxicity is a potential complication of prolonged exposure to the fluorinated hydrocarbons (halothane, enflurane, isoflurane, desflurane, sevoflurane), although it is of practical concern only during prolonged administration of enflurane.[53,66]

Opioid Anesthetics

The opiates (morphine) and synthetic opioids (meperidine, methadone, fentanyl, remifentanil) are used extensively in the intraoperative and postoperative care of children undergoing surgical procedures (Table 114–3). The virtues of opioids include minimal effects on myocardial performance and systemic vascular resistance, ablation of pulmonary vascular responsiveness to nociceptive stimuli, preservation of hypoxic pulmonary vasoconstriction, and analgesia for the immediate postoperative period.[6,47,48] Opioids can be administered intravenously, intramuscularly, subcutaneously, or neuraxially by intrathecal or epidural injection.

The opiates and synthetic opioids interact with stereospecific receptors in the CNS and peripheral tissues, which are identified as the site of action of the endogenous opioids (endorphins, enkephalins, dynorphins). Agonist–receptor interaction results in inhibition of adenylate cyclase and in alterations in the conductances of potassium and calcium channels.

The opioid receptors are classified according to clinical effect and anatomic site. The μ receptors mediate supraspinal (including brainstem) and spinal analgesia, respiratory depression, bradycardia, dependence, and euphoria. The predominant site of action of the opioids used in clinical practice is on the μ receptor. Neuraxially administered opioids have spinal and supraspinal effects.[92,109] At both spinal and supraspinal sites, opioids may act presynaptically and postsynaptically as inhibitory modulators of nociceptive transmission.[96] κ Receptor actions are associated with analgesia, sedation, and dysphoria.

TABLE 114–3

Relative Opioid Dosages

Agent	Relative Dose
Morphine	0.1 mg/kg
Meperidine	1.0 mg/kg
Methadone	0.1 mg/kg
Fentanyl 1	5 μg/kg
Sufentanil 0.2	1 μg/kg
Alfentanil 5	25 μg/kg

Dysphoria has been the major limitation to more widespread use of κ agents and mixed agonist-antagonists.

All currently available opioids, except meperidine, induce central parasympathetic stimulation and may directly depress the sinoatrial node, producing dose-related bradycardia. With the exception of meperidine, the opioids have negligible effects on myocardial performance. However, the combination of an opioid and potent volatile agents, nitrous oxide, or benzodiazepines may produce cardiovascular depression, which is not seen when these agents are administered alone.

All opioids produce dose-dependent respiratory depression by diminishing ventilatory response and the subjective distress produced by hypoxemia and hypercarbia. The CO_2 response curve is displaced to the right, and resting PCO_2 rises. Clinically, the respiratory rate decreases with an incomplete compensatory increase in tidal volume.

Although controversial, it has long been believed that infants and children are more prone than adults to respiratory depression after administration of opiates.[54] Unfortunately, no reliable pharmacodynamic information for infants younger than 3 months is available. However, clinical experience suggests that newborns, and particularly premature infants, have exaggerated respiratory depression after administration of opioids, possibly because of pharmacokinetic differences.[34,54,60]

Chest wall rigidity is a well-described complication of opioid administration in adults undergoing cardiac surgical procedures[7] and has been reported during use of morphine, meperidine, fentanyl, sufentanil, and alfentanil.[4,38] Most of the data derive from adult cardiac surgical patients receiving large doses of fentanyl or sufentanil,[13,52,59] but the condition definitely is seen in children.[37] Rigidity upon induction of anesthesia has been prevented by pretreatment with a "subrelaxant" dose of pancuronium (0.01–0.02 mg/kg)[2] and by slow intravenous infusion of opioid.[13,32] Rigidity also is reported in the postoperative period several hours after administration of opioid and in one report was severe enough to require reintubation.[38]

Morphine is generally the standard to which new opioids are compared. Peak analgesic effect after intravenous administration occurs at 20 minutes, reflecting delayed penetration of the blood-brain barrier. The relatively high pK_a, high degree of ionization at physiologic pH, and relatively low lipid solubility account for this delayed central effect. The lowest plasma concentration to provide effective analgesia intraoperatively is approximately 65 ng/ml; this value does not appear to vary with age.[19] Morphine undergoes extensive hepatic and extrahepatic glucuronidation, and metabolites are excreted principally in the urine. Prolonged respiratory depression has been observed in patients with renal failure receiving morphine.[44] This finding is attributed to accumulation of morphine-6-glucuronide, a secondary morphine metabolite previously thought to be inactive.[73,75,89] Newborns have demonstrated a wide variability in the clearance of morphine during the first 6 weeks of life.[83] Infants younger than 7 days have significantly lower clearance and greater elimination half-lives than older infants and tend to have a smaller volume of distribution.[60]

Morphine has cardiovascular effects that occasionally limit its usefulness in critically ill patients.

Morphine stimulates the release of significant amounts of histamine and inhibits compensatory sympathetic nervous system responses.[69] In supine, normovolemic patients, morphine causes little change in hemodynamics. However, rapid administration of intravenous morphine to hypovolemic or upright patients may provoke significant hypotension. Naloxone does not inhibit morphine-induced histamine release. Direct myocardial depression is not produced by morphine, even in large doses. However, the combination of morphine or any other opioid and potent volatile agents, nitrous oxide, or benzodiazepines may produce cardiovascular depression in critically ill patients, which is not seen when these agents are administered alone.

Fentanyl is a synthetic phenylpiperidine with approximately 100 times the analgesic potency of morphine. The pK_a of fentanyl is significantly lower than morphine, and its high lipid solubility provides a rapid onset of action and a short duration of effect by rapid redistribution. A second peak in plasma fentanyl concentration after intravenous bolus administration is reported by many authors[3,67,96] and may explain delayed respiratory depression seen after intraoperative use of fentanyl in adults.[65] This same phenomenon is described in neonates, and release of sequestered fentanyl from skeletal muscle or lung is proposed to explain this observation. Maximal analgesic effects are seen at plasma concentrations >25 to 30 ng/ml, and respiratory depression may be produced with plasma levels greater than 1 to 2 ng/ml.

Metabolism of fentanyl occurs almost exclusively in the liver, with very little unchanged drug excreted in the urine.[81] Clearance is profoundly affected by hepatic blood flow,[54] which may be significantly altered during intraabdominal procedures.[36,64,65] Halothane alters fentanyl pharmacokinetics,[7] presumably through changes in regional splanchnic blood flow.[62] In the neonatal population, the functional maturity of the cytochrome P-450 pathways may change significantly in the first few weeks of life.[55] These factors may explain the wide pharmacokinetic variability seen in infants and neonates. Calculated steady-state volumes of distribution may be larger in infants because of a greater percentage of body lipid composition or age-related changes in plasma protein binding. Increased clearance rates may reflect either increased hepatic extraction or increased hepatic blood flow in infants.[81] Elimination half-life appears to be prolonged in infants younger than 3 months, an important factor during repetitive dosing of fentanyl in neonates.

Fentanyl is widely used in neonatal and pediatric anesthesia because of its limited hemodynamic side effects, low cost, and intermediate duration of action. Fentanyl as a sole anesthetic in doses of 30 to 50 μg/kg produces minimal hemodynamic change even in critically ill premature infants[47,112,114] and may have beneficial effects in patients with pulmonary hypertension.[48,105] Even in such large doses, fentanyl does not release histamine. Bradycardia is more commonly seen with fentanyl anesthesia than with morphine at equipotent doses, although this rarely causes cardiovascular compromise.

Alfentanil is a fentanyl analogue with one fifth to one tenth the potency and approximately one third the duration of action of fentanyl. Alfentanil has a very low pK_a, with approximately 90% of the drug in the nonionized form at physiologic pH. The high degree of lipid solubility explains its short duration of action and rapid redistribution. The redistribution half-life of alfentanil is comparable to thiopental and fentanyl, but unlike those compounds a cumulative effect with prolonged administration is not seen.

Alfentanil is metabolized in the liver by pathways identical to those described for sufentanil. No active metabolites have been identified. The elimination half-life is significantly prolonged in patients with hepatic dysfunction,[30] and the plasma free-fraction also appears to be increased in these patients. These effects may account for the exaggerated and prolonged drug action seen in patients.

The alfentanil volume of distribution is small relative to fentanyl because of extensive protein binding. The elimination half-life is significantly shorter than any of the currently available opioids. A high degree of interpatient variability has, however, been seen in all pharmacokinetic studies of alfentanil.[64]

Remifentanil is a more recently introduced μ receptor agonist with pharmacologic effects similar to alfentanil.[76] However, remifentanil has a unique metabolism. Nonspecific plasma and tissue esterases hydrolyze remifentanil, and the drug has an extremely short duration. Also unique to remifentanil is its constant half-life from birth to adult, although the volume of distribution is larger in newborns.[84] As such, adverse reactions to remifentanil are brief (if the drug is stopped), but the analgesic effects also wane rapidly. Remifentanil has been studied specifically in neonates.[20] Given the short duration, careful attention must be paid (intraoperatively) to postoperative pain control.

Ketamine

Ketamine is a dissociative anesthetic that has been used as an induction agent for anesthesia, an analgesic for conscious sedation, a premedicant, and a sedative for critically ill patients (Table 114–4). There is a broad range of experience with this agent, as well as a host of opinions regarding its usefulness in the anesthetic armamentarium.[80]

Ketamine is chemically related to phencyclidine. It exists in two enantiomeric forms, which differ in their anesthetic potency and possibly in the incidence of emergence reactions.[110,111] Only the racemic mixture containing equal amounts of the (+) and (–) enantiomers is commercially available. The differing clinical effects of the enantiomeric forms suggest that ketamine interacts at a specific receptor site, although this site remains elusive. The precise CNS site of action of ketamine is inconclusive; however,

TABLE 114–4

Ketamine Dosages

Use	Doses
Induction	1–2 mg/kg IV 3–4 mg/kg IM 10–15 mg/kg PR
Analgesia	0.5 mg/kg IV 0.5 mg/kg PO

ketamine does interfere with excitatory transmission by way of N-methyl-D-aspartate receptor (NMDA) inhibiton.[8] Ketamine produces reliable serum levels when administered intravenously (within 1 minute) or intramuscularly (within 5 minutes). Ketamine is rapidly redistributed, with awakening occurring in 10 to 15 minutes. The redistribution half-life is approximately 5 minutes, and the elimination half-life is 130 minutes.[25,41] The most important metabolite is norketamine, which has approximately one third the anesthetic potency of ketamine.

Ketamine is a potent stimulator of the cardiovascular system, presumably by central sympathetic effects and by inhibiting catecholamine reuptake.[58] Heart rate, mean arterial pressure, and systemic vascular resistance all increase. Pulmonary vascular resistance does not appear to be altered in infants with or without preexisting pulmonary hypertension.[46] In an isolated heart preparation, ketamine inhibited contractile function.[85] Without compensatory sympathetic stimulation, therefore, ketamine may produce significant hypotension. Ketamine produces dose-related respiratory depression and shifts the CO_2 response curve to the right.[8] The bronchodilating properties of ketamine are well known and likely result from increased levels of endogenous catecholamines. Ketamine is as effective as halothane in preventing bronchoconstriction in dogs[49] and has been used successfully in therapy for life-threatening bronchospasm.[49,98] Oral and tracheal secretions are increased by ketamine, but this effect can be ameliorated by coadministration of an antisialagogue.

A number of animal studies demonstrate a significant increase in cerebral blood flow and intracranial pressure after ketamine administration.[70] Hypocapnia limits this response in animals[78] and in newborns.[33] Conventional wisdom suggests that ketamine should be avoided in patients with altered intracranial compliance. The theoretical benefit of NMDA antagonism in the amelioration of CNS ischemia is seen only in "heroic" ketamine doses.[56] However, maintenance of systemic blood pressure is so crucial in the setting of increased intracranial pressure that a role for ketamine should not be summarily dismissed.

Barbiturates

The barbiturates are all derivatives of the cyclic compound barbituric acid. Substitutions at the 2 and 5 carbon positions impart varying degrees of hypnotic, sedative, and anticonvulsant activity. These agents act by undetermined presynaptic actions and by γ-aminobutyric acid (GABA) potentiation at postsynaptic sites in the CNS. The rapid onset and prompt recovery are explained by the high degree of lipid solubility and rapid redistribution to peripheral sites. The oxybarbiturates (methohexital, pentobarbital) are metabolized only by the liver, whereas the thiobarbiturates (thiopental) also are metabolized at extrahepatic sites. Essentially, no unchanged drug is excreted in the urine, and elimination from the body depends primarily on hepatic oxidation, which explains the lengthy elimination half-lives of the barbiturates.

The clearance rate of thiopental in pediatric patients is approximately twice as great as in adults (6.6 vs. 3.1 ml/kg/min), accounting for the greatly reduced elimination half-life (6 vs. 12 hours).[93] Volumes of distribution or degree of protein binding do not appear to differ between pediatric and adult patients; however, minor but reproducible pharmacodynamic differences between adults and pediatric patients explain the increased induction doses of thiopental required in pediatric patients.[11,16]

Thiopental is frequently used for intravenous induction of anesthesia and is effective for use during endotracheal intubation. Methohexital administered either orally or rectally supports reliable and smooth induction. These agents produce direct and dose-related myocardial depression by calcium-contraction uncoupling. In the hemodynamically stable patient, this direct effect is offset by a baroreceptor-mediated increase in sympathetic activity, which produces a compensatory tachycardia and modest declines in blood pressure.[102,103] In patients with hypovolemia, hypotension, or myocardial dysfunction, the barbiturates may produce unacceptable decreases in blood pressure and coronary perfusion.

The barbiturates all share the potential for profound reduction in cerebral metabolic rate and cerebral blood flow[79,82] and frequently are used for this purpose in patients with altered intracranial compliance. Pentobarbital and thiopental in sufficient doses are capable of producing an isoelectric EEG and are potent anticonvulsants.[74] Methohexital, by virtue of a methylated *N*-1 carbon, has the potential to enhance seizure foci and has been used for this purpose during neurosurgical approaches to epilepsy with some success.[31]

Propofol

Propofol is widely used for intravenous induction and maintenance of anesthesia in children. Propofol is an intravenous agent that is structurally distinct from the barbiturates and other intravenous agents, with an undetermined site of action[90] (although the GABA receptor is implicated).[30] Its major advantages over other intravenous agents include the absence of active metabolites, rapid recovery time, and low incidence of nausea and vomiting when used for a variety of surgical procedures. Its disadvantages include pain upon injection and a number of apparent neurological sequelae when used for prolonged periods (primarily myoclonic activity and opisthotonic posturing).[104] Propofol is associated with an unusual and lethal syndrome in pediatric patients receiving the drug by continuous infusion in the critical care setting. The syndrome includes metabolic acidosis and refractory hypotension and has prompted the manufacturer to distribute a caution regarding its use for prolonged periods in the pediatric critical care setting.[10] Despite these adverse events, propofol (alone or in combination with ketamine or remifentanil) remains a popular agent among pediatric anesthetists.

Local Anesthetics

Local anesthetics act by interfering with impulse conduction within peripheral nerve fibers. Specifically, local anesthetics act at the sodium channel of nerve membranes. Lidocaine causes complete inhibition of sodium conductance but causes an only 5% decrease in potassium conductance. Thus the rate of neural depolarization is slowed, and action potential height is diminished.

Together, these effects produce complete conduction blockade. A review details the molecular mechanisms of local anesthetics.[12]

The local anesthetics are broadly classified into amide (e.g., lidocaine, bupivacaine) or ester (e.g., tetracaine, procaine) compounds, depending on the link between the aromatic portion and the intermediate chain of the molecules. The classes differ in their metabolism. The amide compounds are metabolized in the liver; the ester compounds are hydrolyzed in plasma by (hepatically produced) pseudocholinesterase. True allergies to local anesthetics are rare, although ester compounds are metabolized in part to paraaminobenzoic acid, which is allergenic.

Three specific chemical characteristics of the local anesthetics affect their action (Table 114–5).[97] The pK_a (pH when nonionized and ionized forms of the salt are present in equal concentrations) determines the speed of onset. The amount of protein binding determines the duration of action. The degree of lipid solubility correlates with potency. Because neonates, especially premature infants, have low concentrations of both albumin and α-lipoprotein, protein binding is diminished, which may result in increases in circulating free drug. Furthermore, because neonates and infants have low concentrations of plasma cholinesterase, clearance of the ester local anesthetics might be prolonged.

Local anesthetic toxicity is primarily manifested in the CNS. Circumoral numbness and dysgeusia are the first symptoms described by a verbal child or adult. Increasing toxicity produces visual disturbances, muscular fasciculations, convulsions, and coma, finally culminating in respiratory and circulatory failure. A 5 mg/kg dose of lidocaine is considered safe (7 mg/kg if lidocaine is administered with 1:200,000 epinephrine). Bupivacaine toxicity manifests as irreversible cardiovascular collapse more readily than does lidocaine toxicity. A safe bupivacaine dose is believed to be 3 mg/kg. A significant advantage of lidocaine is that lidocaine levels are easily measured.

Anesthetic Techniques

Options for providing safe and adequate surgical conditions are broadly classed into local, regional, or general anesthesia. No available pediatric data suggest that one class of anesthetic is safer than another in any particular situation. A few studies of adults report better outcomes after regional anesthesia.[88,116] No age limitations, including neonates, exist in the application of regional anesthetic techniques. Frequently, children receive a combination of regional and general anesthesia, the former often continued for postoperative analgesia. However, in part for historical and technical reasons, the vast majority of children requiring surgery, critically ill or otherwise, receive general anesthetics.

General Anesthesia

Induction of a "typical" anesthetic in a healthy adult is performed by intravenous administration of a short-acting barbiturate (sodium thiopental) or propofol. After the airway is found manageable with mask ventilation, neuromuscular blockade (with either succinylcholine or a nondepolarizing muscle relaxant) is followed by endotracheal intubation. Anesthesia is maintained with a combination of nitrous oxide and a potent volatile anesthetic. Narcotic is often added and provides postoperative analgesia.

There is no "typical" induction of anesthetic in a healthy child. Healthy newborns and young infants are most often taken to the operating room without premedication. Nitrous oxide and sevoflurane are delivered with a mask. When the appropriate depth of anesthesia is maintained, an intravenous catheter is placed. If necessary, neuromuscular blockade (usually with a nondepolarizing agent such as pancuronium) is followed by endotracheal intubation. Anxious older infants and toddlers can be sedated with oral midazolam approximately 30 minutes before the anesthetic induction. A less frequently used sedation technique is rectal methohexital; however, the necessary sedation dose of methohexital often leads to prolonged sedation. Most pediatric inductions of anesthesia occur in the presence of a parent.[42,43] When children are older than approximately 7 years, an intravenous catheter can be placed preoperatively, and a typical anesthetic used much like that outlined for the adult. Intravenous induction of anesthesia can be accomplished in infants and toddlers by deft placement of a 27-gauge "butterfly." Regardless, many older children and even adolescents prefer a mask induction. Mask inductions with a combination of nitrous oxide and halothane are problematic in older children and adolescents as they go through a sometimes prolonged, agitated phase. Nitrous oxide combined with sevoflurane works far better because the agitated phase is much shorter.

Many factors confound a safe anesthetic in a critically ill child. Airway considerations always take precedence. The compromised airway may present as single-system disease (e.g., epiglottitis or foreign body aspiration) or as a facet of multisystem disease (e.g., trauma). The primary anesthetic consideration in each case is establishment of a secure airway. Chapter 14 provides an expanded discussion of airway techniques, with specific discussion of the

TABLE 114–5

Chemical and Clinical Properties of Commonly Used Local Anesthetics

Agent	Class	Onset (min)	pK_a	Duration (hr)	Protein Binding	Relative Potency	Lipid Solubility
Procaine	Ester	14–18	8.9	1–1.5	5%	1	<1
Lidocaine	Amide	2–4	7.7	1–3	65%	2	4
Bupivacaine	Amide	5–8	8.1	3–10	95%	8	30
Tetracaine	Ester	10–15	8.6	3–10	85%	8	80

rapid-sequence induction of anesthesia (in situations of a full stomach).

Most critically ill children who require general anesthesia are mechanically ventilated. Most ventilators associated with anesthesia equipment are rather primitive volume ventilators. Although usually adequate, these "anesthesia" ventilators may contribute to postoperative pulmonary deteriorations, particularly in children with underlying lung pathology. All modalities of mechanical ventilation available in the intensive care unit also should be available in the operating room. If specifically modified ventilators (to deliver volatile anesthetics) are not available, narcotics can be used to maintain anesthesia, and standard pressure or volume ventilators can be used.

Regional Anesthesia

Although general anesthesia is chosen most frequently for pediatric surgical procedures, there is substantial use of regional anesthesia. Regional anesthesia often is preferred in premature infants undergoing lower abdominal or lower extremity operations (e.g., inguinal hernia repair) because neonates are at increased risk for apnea after general anesthesia. Other applications of regional anesthesia include children with a family history of malignant hyperthermia and children with chronic airway disease. Some suggest children with neuromuscular diseases associated with diminished pharyngeal or laryngeal reflexes and older children requiring emergency operations with a history of recent food intake also be considered for regional techniques. However, the latter conditions can present difficult airway problems if, during the operation, the regional anesthetic becomes unacceptable for surgery. Regional anesthesia is widely used in pediatric patients to provide postoperative analgesia.[5]

Spinal anesthesia consists of local injection of an anesthetic agent into the subarachnoid space (Table 114–6). The technique is easy to perform and is safe. The most frequent local anesthetic agents are lidocaine, tetracaine, and bupivacaine. Doses for infants and children are calculated on a body weight basis. When compared with older children and adults, infants and toddlers require more anesthetic per body weight, and the local anesthetic has a shorter duration of action. Complications are rare. Common side effects of spinal anesthesia in adults are dural puncture headaches and hemodynamic compromise. The latter results from both sympathectomy associated with the interruption of thoracic and lumbar nerve conduction and blockade of the cardiac accelerator function with high thoracic blockade. Surprisingly, neither complication is common in children. In fact, even a "total spinal" (if not associated with hypoxia) is not accompanied by profound blood pressure or heart rate changes in newborns.[23,61]

TABLE 114–6

Hyperbaric Tetracaine Doses for Spinal Anesthesia*

Age	Dose
Premature	0.8–1.0 mg/kg
Term neonate	0.6–0.8 mg/kg
1 to 3 mo	0.4–0.5 mg/kg
Older than 3 mo	0.3 mg/kg

*Generally for an anesthetic level to T_2–T_4.

Epidural anesthesia consists of injection of an anesthetic agent into the potential space between the dura mater and the ligamentum flavum. The medications can be administered by either a single injection or repeated injections through a catheter placed through a needle. Epidural analgesia probably is the most versatile regional analgesic technique.

Although the epidural space can be approached at any level, a lumbar or caudal epidural blockade is used for most children. The caudal epidural blockade with bupivacaine is used most frequently for postoperative pain relief after lower abdominal and lower extremity procedures. However, caudal anesthesia has been reported as sufficient for lower abdominal procedures (again, inguinal hernia repair) without the need for a general anesthetic.[94] Caudal epidural blockade also is used in combination with general anesthesia in children and infants during abdominal procedures. Complications are caused by improper placement of the needle, resulting in injection of the anesthetic agent into a vein, the dura, the subarachnoid space, or sacral marrow.

In pediatric patients, the most common peripheral nerve blockades are penile and ilioinguinal-iliohypogastric. These blocks are easy to perform, safe, and effective. Penile block is useful for circumcision and simple hypospadias repair. Bupivacaine is the preferred anesthetic agent; epinephrine must not be used because vasoconstriction of the blood supply to the penis may result in significant ischemia. Ilioinguinal and iliohypogastric nerve blocks are used for inguinal hernia repair, varicocele, and orchiopexy. The visceral pain produced from peritoneal traction and manipulation of the spermatic cord and testicles is not abolished.

Specific Anesthetic Considerations

Epiglottitis

Prototypical of the difficult airway is (was) epiglottitis. The past tense is mentioned because the incidence of epiglottitis has remarkably diminished[35,71] since the introduction of vaccinations for *Haemophilus influenzae* B in the early 1990s, but epiglottitis has not been eradicated.[68] The anesthetic regimen most commonly, but not exclusively,[24] chosen for epiglottitis is designed to maintain spontaneous ventilation until the upper airway obstruction is securely bypassed with an endotracheal tube. A surgeon should be scrubbed and poised to perform an emergency tracheostomy. To minimize (the child's) anxiety, a parent often is asked to accompany the child to the operating room. The sitting position optimizes the airway. Intravenous access is not obtained until the depth of anesthesia is sufficient to blunt pain responses. Noninvasive monitoring is placed only if leads, probes, and sensors can be attached without aggravating the child. Induction of anesthesia begins with 100% oxygen. In the event of complete airway obstruction, having denitrogenated the lungs allows a few extra moments of adequate oxygenation. Although nitrous oxide usually is blended with halothane to speed induction of anesthesia, 50% to 70% nitrous oxide is necessary. Also, 100% oxygen is far more important than a rapid induction; nitrous oxide should never be used in this setting. Therefore halothane is delivered in 100% oxygen. Because minute ventilation usually is impaired, halothane uptake is inhibited. As the level of anesthesia deepens, pharyngeal tone diminishes, further impairing the airway. Providing 10 to 12 cmH_2O positive end-expiratory pressure to the mask can partially alleviate the obstruction. The anesthesiologist may have to wait 30 to 40 minutes before the airway can be instrumented. At all times, spontaneous ventilation is maintained. When the anesthesiologist believes the child is sufficiently deep to tolerate laryngoscopy, it is wise to continue the induction another 5 minutes. An intravenous catheter then can be placed. Laryngoscopy is performed, and the airway is secured. Appropriate specimens should be obtained for cultures.

Many regimens for postoperative care of children with epiglottitis are available (see Chapter 39).[1,18,40] Options range from observation without endotracheal intubation to neuromuscular blockade and mechanical ventilation. A moderate course is 1 to 2 days of intubation in a sedated, but spontaneously breathing, child. Rarely, pulmonary edema develops after relief of the upper airway obstruction, and positive-end expiratory pressure is necessary.[51] Examination of the airway may be helpful before extubation. A fiberoptic nasopharyngoscopy works well. More simply, a short-acting barbiturate (sodium thiopental) and nondepolarizing muscle relaxant (atracurium) can provide safe conditions for a direct laryngoscopy in the intensive care unit.

Foreign Body Aspiration

Airway concerns similar to those described for epiglottitis arise during anesthesia for surgical recovery of an aspirated foreign body. Generally, an intravenous catheter can be placed preoperatively. Throughout the procedure, 100% oxygen is used. If the stomach is not empty, a rapid-sequence induction may be considered. However, spontaneous ventilation is theoretically preferred because positive-pressure ventilation (and particularly endotracheal intubation) risks forcing the foreign body more distal and makes recovery more difficult.[113] As with epiglottitis, close attention must be paid to the depth of anesthesia. Premature instrumentation of the airway may prompt coughing or laryngospasm. Unless significant airway manipulation raises concern of postoperative tracheal edema, early postoperative extubation is well tolerated.[63,106]

Blood Product Use and Conservation

Risks associated with transfusion of blood products have led to increased scrutiny of transfusion practices. Intraoperative administration of packed red blood cells is not recommended until the hematocrit falls below 23%.[14] Fresh-frozen plasma is indicated only for treatment of a documented coagulopathy. Major surgical procedures, during which significant blood loss can be anticipated, often are amenable to blood conservation techniques.[108] These techniques include autologous blood donation,[17,22] controlled hypotension,[115] and hemodilution.[86,87]

Multiple blood volumes can be lost, for example, during surgical correction of scoliosis, particularly when multiple vertebral laminectomies are necessary. Blood loss is diminished by lowering the mean systemic arterial blood pressure. Arterial pressure can be dropped to the limit of safe, autoregulated, cerebral perfusion (mean arterial pressure 50 mmHg). Many agents are effective. Nitroprusside, if coupled with a β-blocker to block reflex tachycardia, works well. If the nitroprusside dose is limited to 8 μg/kg/min, cyanide toxicity is of little concern. Labetolol, which provides both α-blockade and β-blockade, also is effective and is not associated with cyanide toxicity. Nitroglycerin is ineffective.[115] The short-acting β-blocker esmolol may play an important role in the future.

Hemodilution is nothing more than a short-term form of autologous transfusion and may be useful for reducing operative red blood cell loss. After induction of anesthesia and before the surgical procedure, maximally one third of the child's blood volume is removed and replaced normovolemically with crystalloid or colloid. The hematocrit should not be allowed to fall below 15%. In theory, surgical blood loss early in the procedure occurs with fewer red cells per volume. After the significant surgical bleeding is completed, the original blood can be reinfused as either whole blood or packed cells. Hypothermia (32°C) is useful as an adjunct to reduce metabolic demand. Hyperoxemia also is important because at a hematocrit of 15%, 100% oxygen significantly augments oxygen-carrying capacity in the form of dissolved oxygen.[87]

Handoff Between the Operating Room and the Intensive Care Unit

With strong justification, there is a focus on the identification and amelioration of medical errors in critical care.[9,26] Communication, or lack thereof, is a potent contributor, particularly to errors of omission.[100] Certainly the purpose of this chapter is to acquaint the critical care provider with sufficient anesthesia background so that communication can be facilitated. Generally the transition of care between the providers in the operating room and the intensive care unit is an informal conversation at the bedside. Typically nursing handoffs are structured. Efforts to structure physician handoffs likely will reduce miscommunication errors.[72]

REFERENCES

1. Arndal H, Andreassen UK: Acute epiglottitis in children and adults. Nasotracheal intubation, tracheostomy or careful observation? Current status in Scandinavia. *J Laryngol Otol* 102:1012, 1988.
2. Bailey PL, Wilbrink J, Zwanikken P, et al: Anesthetic induction with fentanyl. *Anesth Analg* 64:48, 1985.
3. Becker LD, Paulson BA, Miller RD, et al: Biphasic respiratory depression after fentanyl droperidol or fentanyl alone used to supplement nitrous oxide anesthesia. *Anesthesiology* 44:291, 1976.
4. Benthuysen JL, Smith NT, Sanford TJ, et al: Physiology of alfentanil-induced rigidity. *Anesthesiology* 64:440, 1986.
5. Berde CB: Pediatric postoperative pain management. *Pediatr Clin North Am* 36:921, 1989.
6. Bjertnaes L, Hauge A, Kriz M: Hypoxia-induced pulmonary vasoconstriction: effects of fentanyl following different routes of administration. *Acta Anaesthesiol Scand* 24:53, 1980.

7. Borel JD, Bentley JB, Nenad RE, et al: The influence of halothane on fentanyl pharmacokinetics. *Anesthesiology* 57:A239, 1982.
8. Bourke DL, Malit LA, Smith TC: Respiratory interactions of ketamine and morphine. *Anesthesiology* 66:153, 1987.
9. Bracco D, Favre JB, Bissonnette B, et al: Human errors in a multidisciplinary intensive care unit: a 1-year prospective study. *Intensive Care Med* 27:137-145, 2001.
10. Bray RJ: Propofol infusion syndrome in children. *Paediatr Anaesth* 8:491-499, 1998.
11. Brett CM, Fisher DM: Thiopental dose-response relations in unpremedicated infants, children, and adults. *Anesth Analg* 66:1024, 1987.
12. Butterworth JF, Strichartz GR: Molecular mechanisms of local anesthesia: a review. *Anesthesiology* 72:711, 1990.
13. Comstock MK, Carter JG, Moyers JR, et al: Rigidity and hypercarbia associated with high dose fentanyl induction of anesthesia. *Anesth Analg* 60:362, 1981
14. Consensus Conference: Perioperative red blood cell transfusion. *JAMA* 260:2700, 1988.
15. Cote CJ: *A practice of anesthesia for infants and children.* Baltimore, 2001, WB Saunders.
16. Cote CJ, Goudsouzian NG, Liu LM, et al: The dose response of intravenous thiopental for the induction of general anesthesia in unpremedicated children. *Anesthesiology* 55:703, 1981.
17. Council on Scientific Affairs: Autologous blood transfusions. *JAMA* 256:2378, 1986.
18. Crockett DM, Healy GB, McGill TJ, et al: Airway management of acute supraglottitis at the Children's Hospital, Boston: 1980-1985. *Ann Otol Rhinol Laryngol* 97:114, 1988.
19. Dahlstrom B, Bolme P, Feychting H, et al: Morphine kinetics in children. *Clin Pharmacol Ther* 26:354, 1979.
20. Davis PJ, Galinkin J, McGowan FX, et al: A randomized multicenter study of remifentanil compared with halothane in neonates and infants undergoing pyloromyotomy. I. Emergence and recovery profiles. *Anesth Analg* 93:1380-1386, 2001.
21. Delgado Herrera L, Ostroff RD, Rogers SA: Sevoflurane: approaching the ideal inhalational anesthetic a pharmacologic, pharmacoeconomic and clinical review. *CNS Drug Reviews* 7:48-120, 2001.
22. DePalma L, Luban NL: Autologous blood transfusion in pediatrics. *Pediatrics* 85:125, 1990.
23. Desparmet JF: Total spinal anesthesia after caudal anesthesia in an infant. *Anesth Analg* 70:665, 1990.
24. Diaz JH: Croup and epiglottitis in children: the anesthesiologist as diagnostician. *Anesth Analg* 64:621, 1985.
25. Domino EF, Domino SE, Smith RE, et al: Ketamine kinetics in unmedicated and diazepam-premedicated subjects. *Clin Pharmacol Ther* 36:645, 1984.
26. Donchin, YD, Gopher D, Donchin Y, et al: A look into the nature and causes of human errors in the intensive care unit. *Crit Care Med* 23:294-300, 1995.
27. Duffy CM, Matta BF: Sevoflurane and anesthesia for neurosurgery. *J Neurosurg Anesthesiol* 12:128-140, 2000.
28. Eisele JH, Smith NT: Cardiovascular effects of 40 percent nitrous oxide in man. *Anesth Analg* 51:956, 1972.
29. Fairgrieve R, Rowney DA, Karsli C, Bissonnette B: The effects of sevoflurane on cerebral blood flow velocity in children. *Acta Anaesthesiol Scand* 27:1226-1230, 2003.
30. Ferrier C, Marty J, Bouffard Y, et al: Alfentanil pharmacokinetics in patients with cirrhosis. *Anesthesiology* 62:480, 1985.
31. Fiset P: Functional brain imaging and propofol mechanisms of action. *Adv Exp Med Biol* 523:115-121, 2003.
32. Ford EW, Morrell F, Whisler WW: Methohexital anesthesia in the surgical treatment of uncontrollable epilepsy. *Anesth Analg* 61:997, 1982.
33. Freye E, Hartung E, Buhl R: Lung compliance in man is impaired by the rapid injection of alfentanyl. *Anaesthetist* 35:543, 1986.
34. Friesen RH, Thieme RE, Honda AT, et al: Changes in anterior fontanel pressure in preterm neonates receiving isoflurane, halothane, fentanyl, or ketamine. *Anesth Analg* 66:431, 1987.
35. Gauntlett IS, Fisher DM, Hertzka RE, et al: Pharmacokinetics of fentanyl in neonatal humans and lambs: effects of age. *Anesthesiology* 69:683, 1988.
36. Garpenholt O, Hugosson S, Fredlund H, et al: Epiglottitis in Sweden before and after introduction of vaccination against Haemophilus influenzae type B. *Pediatr Infect Dis J* 18:490-493, 1999.
37. Gelman S, Fowler KC, Smith LR: Liver circulation and function during isoflurane and halothane anesthesia. *Anesthesiology* 61:726, 1984.
38. Glick C, Evans OB, Parks BR: Muscle rigidity due to fentanyl infusion in the pediatric patient. *South Med J* 89:1119-1120, 1996.
39. Goldberg M, Ishak S, Garcia C, et al: Postoperative rigidity following sufentanil administration. *Anesthesiology* 63:199, 1985.
40. Gomez RS, Guatimosim C, Gomez MV: Mechanism of action of volatile anesthetics: role of protein kinase C. *Cell Mol Neurobiol* 23:877-885, 2003.
41. Gonzalez C, Reilly JS, Kenna MA, et al: Duration of intubation in children with acute epiglottitis. *Otolaryngol Head Neck Surg* 95:477, 1986.
42. Grant IS, Nimmo WS, McNicol LR, et al: Ketamine disposition in children and adults. *Br J Anaesth* 55:1107, 1983.
43. Hannallah RS, Abramowitz MD, Ot H, et al: Residents' attitudes toward parents' presence during anesthesia induction in children: does experience make a difference? *Anesthesiology* 60:598, 1984.
44. Hannallah RS, Rosales JK: Experience with parents' presence during anaesthesia induction in children. *Can Anaesth Soc J* 30: 286, 1983.
45. Hasselstrom J, Berg U, Lofgren A, et al: Long lasting respiratory depression induced by morphine-6-glucuronide. *Br J Clin Pharmacol* 27:515, 1989.
46. Hertzka RE, Gauntlett IS, Fisher DM, et al: Fentanyl-induced ventilatory depression: effects of age. *Anesthesiology* 70:213, 1989.
47. Hickey PR, Hansen DD, Cramolini GM, et al: Pulmonary and systemic hemodynamic responses to ketamine in infants with normal and elevated pulmonary vascular resistance. *Anesthesiology* 62:287, 1985.
48. Hickey PR, Hansen DD, Wessel DL, et al: Blunting of stress responses in the pulmonary circulation of infants by fentanyl. *Anesth Analg* 64:1137, 1985.
49. Hickey PR, Hansen DD, Wessel DL, et al: Pulmonary and systemic hemodynamic responses to fentanyl in infants. *Anesth Analg* 64:483, 1985.
50. Hirschman CA, Downes H, Farbood A, et al: Ketamine block of bronchospasm in experimental canine asthma. *Br J Anaesth* 51:713, 1979.
51. Hubbard AK, Roth TP, Gandolfi AJ, et al: Halothane hepatitis patients generate an antibody response toward a covalently bound metabolite of halothane. *Anesthesiology* 68:791, 1988.
52. Kanter RK, Watchko JF: Pulmonary edema associated with upper airway obstruction. *Am J Dis Child* 138:356, 1984.
53. Kentor ML, Schwalb AJ, Lieberman RW: Rapid high-dose fentanyl induction for CABG. *Anesthesiology* 53:393, 1980.
54. Kharasch ED: Metabolism and toxicity of the new anesthetic agents. *Acta Anaesthesiol Belg* 47:7-14, 1996.
55. Koehntop DE, Rodman JH, Brundage DM, et al: Pharmacokinetics of fentanyl in neonates. *Anesth Analg* 65:227, 1986.
56. Koren G, Goresky G, Crean P, et al: Pediatric fentanyl dosing based on pharmacokinetics during cardiac surgery. *Anesth Analg* 63:577, 1984.
57. Lees GJ: Influence of ketamine on the neuronal death caused by NMDA in the rat hippocampus. *Neuropharmacology* 34:411-417, 1995.
58. Liem EB, Lin CM, Suleman MI, et al: Anesthetic requirements is increased in redheads. *Anesthesiology* 101:279-283, 2004.
59. Lundy PM, Lockwood PA, Thompson G, et al: Differential effects of ketamine isomers on neuronal and extraneuronal catecholamine uptake mechanisms. *Anesthesiology* 64:359, 1986.
60. Lunn JK, Stanley TH, Eisele J, et al: High dose fentanyl anesthesia for coronary artery surgery: plasma fentanyl concentrations and influence of nitrous oxide on cardiovascular responses. *Anesth Analg* 58:390, 1979.
61. Lynn AM, Slattery JT: Morphine pharmacokinetics in early infancy. *Anesthesiology* 66:136, 1987.
62. Mahe V, Ecoffey C: Spinal anesthesia with isobaric bupivacaine in infants. *Anesthesiology* 68:601, 1988.
63. Mannering GJ: Drug metabolism in the newborn. *Fed Proc* 44:2302, 1985.
64. Mantel K, Butenandt I: Tracheobronchial foreign body aspiration in childhood. A report on 224 cases. *Eur J Pediatr* 145:211, 1986.

65. Masey SA, Koehler RC, Ruck JR, et al: Effect of abdominal distension on central and regional hemodynamics in neonatal lambs. *Pediatr Res* 19:1244, 1985.
66. Mather LE: Clinical pharmacokinetics of fentanyl and its newer derivatives. *Clin Pharmacokinet* 8:422, 1983.
67. Mazze RI, Calverley RK, Smith NT: Inorganic fluoride nephrotoxicity: prolonged enflurane and halothane anesthesia in volunteers. *Anesthesiology* 46:265, 1977.
68. McClain DA, Hug CC Jr: Intravenous fentanyl kinetics. *Clin Pharmacol Ther* 28:106, 1980.
69. McEwan J, Giridharan W, Clark RW, Spears P. Paediatric acute epiglottitis: not a disappearing entity. *Int J Pediatr Otorhinolaryngol* 67:317-221, 2003.
70. McQuay HJ, Moore RA, Paterson GM, et al: Plasma fentanyl concentrations and clinical observations during and after operation. *Br J Anaesth* 51:543, 1979.
71. Michenfelder JD: *Anesthesia and the brain.* New York, 1988, Churchill Livingstone.
72. Midwinter KI, Hodgson D, Yardley M: Paediatric epiglottitis: the influence of the Haemophilus influenzae B vaccine, a ten year review in the Sheffield region. *Clin Otolaryngol* 24:447-448, 1999.
73. Nearman HS, Popple CG: How to transfer a postoperative patient to the intensive care unit. Strategies for documentation, evaluation, and management. *J Crit Ill* 10:275-280, 1995.
74. Osborne RJ, Joel SP, Slevin ML: Morphine intoxication in renal failure: the role of morphine-6-glucuronide. *Br Med J [Clin Res]* 292:1548, 1986.
75. Partinen M, Kovanen J, Nilsson E: Status epilepticus treated by barbiturate anaesthesia with continuous monitoring of cerebral function. *Br Med J [Clin Res]* 282:520, 1981.
76. Pasternak GW, Bodnar RJ, Clark JA, et al: Morphine-6-glucuronide, a potent mu agonist. *Life Sci* 41:2845, 1987.
77. Patel SS, Spenscer CM: Remifentanil. *Drugs* 52:417-427, 1996.
78. Perouansky M, Pearce RA: Is anesthesia caused by potentiation of synaptic or intrinsic inhibition? Recent insights into the mechanism of volatile anesthetics. *J Basic Clin Physiol Pharmacol* 11:83-107, 2000
79. Pfenninger E, Dick W, Ahnefeld FW: The influence of ketamine on both normal and raised intracranial pressure of artificially ventilated animals. *Eur J Anaesthesiol* 2:297, 1985.
80. Pierce EC Jr, Lambertsen CJ, Deutsch S, et al: Cerebral circulation and metabolism during thiopental anesthesia and hyperventilation in man. *J Clin Invest* 41:1664, 1962.
81. Reich DL, Silvay G: Ketamine: an update on the first twenty-five years of clinical experience. *Can J Anaesth* 36:186, 1989.
82. Robinson S, Gregory GA: Fentanyl-air-oxygen anesthesia for ligation of patent ductus arteriosus in preterm infants. *Anesth Analg* 60:331, 1981.
83. Rockoff MA, Marshall LF, Shapiro HM: High-dose barbiturate therapy in humans: a clinical review of 60 patients. *Ann Neurol* 6:194, 1979.
84. Rosow CE, Moss J, Philbin DM, et al: Histamine release during morphine and fentanyl anesthesia. *Anesthesiology* 56:93, 1982.
85. Ross AK, Davis PJ, Dear DG, et al: Pharmacokinetics of remifentanil in anesthetized pediatric patients undergoing elective surgery or diagnostic procedures. *Anesth Analg* 93:1393-1401, 2001.
86. Saegusa K, Furukawa Y, Ogiwara Y, et al: Pharmacologic analysis of ketamine-induced cardiac actions in isolated, blood perfused canine atria. *J Cardiovasc Pharmacol* 8:414, 1986.
87. Schaller RT Jr, Schaller J, Furman EB: The advantages of hemodilution anesthesia for major liver resection in children. *J Pediatr Surg* 19:705, 1984.
88. Schaller RT Jr, Schaller J, Morgan A, et al: Hemodilution anesthesia: a valuable aid to major cancer surgery in children. *Am J Surg* 146:79, 1983.
89. Scott NB, Kehlet H: Regional anaesthesia and surgical morbidity. *Br J Surg* 75:299, 1988.
90. Sear JW, Hand CW, Moore RA, et al: Studies on morphine disposition: influence of renal failure on the kinetics of morphine and its metabolites. *Br J Anaesth* 62:28, 1989.
91. Sebel PS, Lowdon JD: Propofol: a new intravenous anesthetic. *Anesthesiology* 71:260, 1989.
92. Shingu K, Eger EI, Johnson BH, et al: Effect of oxygen concentration, hyperthermia, and choice of vendor on anesthetic-induced hepatic injury in rats. *Anesth Analg* 62:146, 1983.
93. Sjostrom S, Hartvig P, Persson MP, et al: Pharmacokinetics of epidural morphine and meperidine in humans. *Anesthesiology* 67:877, 1987.
94. Sorbo S, Hudson RJ, Loomis JC: The pharmacokinetics of thiopental in pediatric surgical patients. *Anesthesiology* 61:666, 1984.
95. Spear RM, Deshpande JK, Maxwell LG: Caudal anesthesia in the awake, high-risk infant. *Anesthesiology* 69:407, 1988.
96. Stoeckel H, Schuttler J, Magnussen H, et al: Plasma fentanyl concentrations and the occurrence of respiratory depression in volunteers. *Br J Anaesth* 54:1087, 1982.
97. Stoelting RK: *Pharmacology and physiology in anesthetic practice.* Philadelphia, 1987, JB Lippincott.
98. Strichartz GR, Sanchez V, Arthur R, et al: Fundamental properties of local anesthetics. II. Measured octanol: buffer partition coefficients and pka values of clinically used drugs. *Anesth Analg* 71:158, 1990.
99. Strube PJ, Hallam PL: Ketamine by continuous infusion in status asthmaticus. *Anaesthesia* 41:1017, 1986.
100. Summary of the National Halothane Study: Possible association between halothane anesthesia and postoperative hepatic necrosis. *JAMA* 197:775, 1966.
101. Thomas EJ, Sexton JB, Helmreich RL: Discrepant attitudes about teamwork among critical care nurses and physicians. *Crit Care Med* 31:956-959, 2003.
102. Thomson AM, West DC, Lodge D: An *N*-methylaspartate receptor-mediated synapse in rat cerebral cortex: a site of action of ketamine. *Nature* 313:479, 1985.
103. Todd MM, Drummond JC, U HS: The hemodynamic consequences of high-dose methohexital anesthesia in humans. *Anesthesiology* 61:495, 1984.
104. Todd MM, Drummond JC, U HS: The hemodynamic consequences of high-dose thiopental anesthesia. *Anesth Analg* 64:681, 1985.
105. Trotter C, Serpell MG: Neurologic sequelae in children after prolonged propofol infusion. *Anesthesia* 47:146, 199.
106. Vacanti JP, Crone RK, Murphy JD, et al: The pulmonary hemodynamic response to perioperative anesthesia in the treatment of high-risk infants with congenital diaphragmatic hernia. *J Pediatr Surg* 19:672, 1984.
107. Vane DW, Pritchard J, Colville CW, et al: Bronchoscopy for aspirated foreign bodies in children. Experience in 131 cases. *Arch Surg* 123:885, 1988.
108. Way WL, Costley EC, Way EL: Respiratory sensitivity of the newborn infant to meperidine and morphine. *Clin Pharmacol Ther* 6:454, 1965.
109. Weber TP, Grosse Hartlage MA, Van Aken H, Booke M. Anaesthetic strategies to reduce perioperative blood loss in paediatric surgery. *Eur J Anaesthesiol* 20:175-81, 2004.
110. Weddel SJ, Ritter RR: Serum levels following epidural administration of morphine and correlation with relief of postsurgical pain. *Anesthesiology* 54:210, 1981.
111. White PF, Ham J, Way WL, et al: Pharmacology of ketamine isomers in surgical patients. *Anesthesiology* 52:231, 1980.
112. White PF, Schuttler J, Shafer A, et al: Comparative pharmacology of the ketamine isomers. Studies in volunteers. *Br J Anaesth* 57:197, 1985.
113. Wiggum DC, Cork RC, Weldon ST, et al: Postoperative respiratory depression and elevated sufentanil levels in a patient with chronic renal failure. *Anesthesiology* 63:708, 1985.
114. Woods AM: Pediatric bronchoscopy, bronchography, and laryngoscopy. In Berry FA, editor: *Anesthetic management of difficult and routine pediatric patients.* New York, 1986, Churchill Livingstone.
115. Yaster M: The dose response of fentanyl in neonatal anesthesia. *Anesthesiology* 66:433, 1987.
116. Yaster M, Simmons RS, Tolo VT, et al: A comparison of nitroglycerin and nitroprusside for inducing hypotension in children: a double-blind study. *Anesthesiology* 65:175, 1986.
117. Yeager MP, Glass DD, Neff RK, Brinck-Johnsen T: Epidural anesthesia and analgesia in high-risk surgical patients. *Anesthesiology* 66:729, 1987.
118. Yemen TA: *Pediatric anesthesia handbook.* New York, 2002, McGraw-Hill Professional, New York.

CHAPTER

115

Neuromuscular Blocking Agents

D. Ryan Cook

PEARLS

- Although neuromuscular blocking agents are frequently used in the intensive care unit (ICU) as adjuncts to facilitate endotracheal intubation and controlled mechanical ventilation, they have no sedative, hypnotic, or analgesia side effects.
- The neuromuscular junctions mature, both physically and biochemically, throughout infancy, the contractile properties of skeletal muscle change; and the amount of muscle in proportion to body weight increases. Thus the neuromuscular junction is variably sensitive to relaxants.
- There are age-related changes in the apparent volume of distribution of relaxants, their redistribution and excretion (clearance), and possibly their rate of metabolism.
- Major organ failure, up-regulation of acetylcholine (ACh) receptors, poor nutrition, electrolyte and acid-base abnormalities, multiple drugs, and muscle atrophy can also have profound influences on the kinetics and dynamics of relaxants.
- Uncontrolled doses of relaxants for relatively long periods of time and limited monitoring of neuromuscular transmission may lead to prolonged muscle weakness or paralysis of patients in the ICU (i.e., critical illness polyneuropathy).

Neuromuscular blocking agents are frequently used in the intensive care unit (ICU) primarily to facilitate endotracheal intubation and controlled mechanical ventilation. Although intermittent mandatory ventilation is the usual method for providing ventilatory support of most patients in the ICU, those with serious head injury, tetanus, severe respiratory distress syndrome, or major organ failure may require and benefit from ventilatory support with partial or full neuromuscular blockade. Neuromuscular blocking agents have no sedative, hypnotic, or analgesic side effects, but they may indirectly decrease metabolic demand, prevent shivering, decrease nonsynchronous ventilation, decrease intracranial pressure (ICP), and improve chest wall compliance. Thus they may be useful adjuncts to other classes of drugs (e.g., sedative-hypnotics, narcotics, α_2 agonists).

The purposes of this chapter are to review the age-related pharmacologic characteristics of neuromuscular blocking agents and to define the clinical use of these drugs in the ICU. Throughout infancy the neuromuscular junction matures physically and biochemically, the contractile properties of skeletal muscle change, and the amount of muscle in proportion to body weight increases; as a result, the neuromuscular junction is variably sensitive to relaxants. In addition, there are changes in the apparent volume of distribution of relaxants, their redistribution and excretion (clearance), and possibly their rate of metabolism. These factors influence the dose-response relationship of relaxants and the duration of neuromuscular blockade.

Major organ failure, up-regulation of acetylcholine (ACh) receptors, poor nutrition, electrolyte and acid-base abnormalities, multiple drugs, and muscle atrophy can also have profound influences on the kinetics and dynamics of relaxants. In addition, uncontrolled doses of relaxants for relatively long periods of time and limited monitoring of neuromuscular transmission may lead to prolonged muscle weakness or paralysis of patients in the ICU. These issues have been the subject of many reviews and editorials.[1-12] Knowledge of neuromuscular pharmacology and its modification by age, concurrent medications, and concurrent disease processes will enhance the safe use of neuromuscular blocking agents in the ICU.

Neuromuscular Junction and Neuromuscular Transmission

The general anatomy, age-related physiology, and pharmacology of the neuromuscular junction have been well defined (see Chapter 48).[13-15] Advances in neuromuscular research have better defined the mechanisms of synaptic vesicular loading and exocytosis of ACh and further clarified the subtypes and functions of fetal and adult ACh receptors.

Anatomy

Single-cell motor neurons extend, uninterrupted, from the ventral horn of the spinal cord to the muscle. After entering a muscle, they branch and send unmyelinated axons to individual muscle fibers. The neuromuscular junction consists of a nerve terminal and a specialized area of the muscle fiber known as the *motor end-plate* (Fig. 115–1). This interface between motor neurons and their associated muscle fibers amplifies the electrical impulse from the nerve fibers to depolarize the relatively larger muscle fibers. The nerve terminal is an unmyelinated extension of the axon and has an abundance of mitochondria and vesicles containing ACh, adenosine triphosphate (ATP), calcium, choline, and a variety of lipids and proteins. The motor end-plate is contiguous with the muscle fiber membrane and features extensive infoldings that contain concentrated amounts of acetylcholinesterase. The nerve terminal and motor end-plate are separated by a distance of 500 Å. The motor end-plate is literally paved with ACh receptors at a density of 10,000 to 20,000/μm. Electron micrographs have shown specialized areas of the terminal axon membrane called *active zones,* which face invaginations of postsynaptic folds on the outside and feature a twin row of 20 to 30 synaptic vesicles on the inside. Each terminal has 500 to 1000 active zones.

There are three populations of cholinergic (nicotinic) ACh receptors involved with neuromuscular transmission: prejunctional, postjunctional, and extrajunctional. The classical ACh receptor contains the binding sites and the ion channel through which the ACh response occurs. This nicotinic, cholinergic, postjunctional receptor is a glycosylated polypeptide chain organized into five subprotein units forming a rosette with a central pit at the mouth of the ion channel, a so-called doughnut hole (Fig. 115–2). Each rosette is made up of two α1 units and a β1, γ, and δ unit. Although there are, in fact, nine different α-type subunits (α1 to α9) and four different β-type subunits, only α1 and β1 units are found in skeletal muscle. The brain contains receptors made up of all other subunits; α4 and β2 are the most common. Several proteins (e.g., agrin, rapsin) serve to aggregate and link the mature receptors in innervated muscle.

These subunits are arranged in a specific order (counterclockwise α1*–ε-α1–δ–β1). The α1* subunit has a higher affinity binding site for d-tubocurarine. The two Ach binding sites are at the α1*–ε (or δ) and the α1 δ interface. The α subunits contain the binding sites for both ACh and neuromuscular blocking drugs.[16-18] The other three subunits may alter the function of this receptor. Two molecules of Ach are needed to depolarize the Ach receptor, but only one molecule of nondepolarizing relaxant can block neuromuscular transmission. The fetal ACh receptor subtype differs in the structure of one subunit from the adult subtype (i.e., a γ subunit is present in the fetal ACh receptor instead of the ε subunit present in adult ACh receptors).

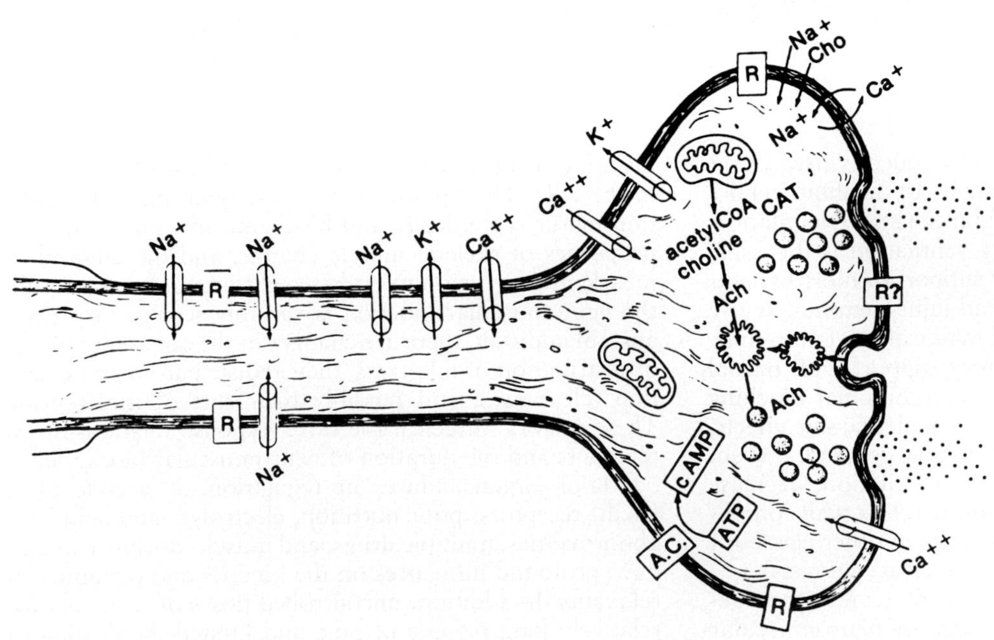

FIGURE 115–1 • Scheme of a motor nerve terminal. The proximal zone, immediately next to the last segment of myelin, is shown as rich in sodium channels (*Na+*) that may be activated by cholinergic receptors (*R*). A midzone contains enzyme systems related to metabolism and transmission (*CAT,* choline acetyl transferase; *A.C.*, adenylate cyclase). Some of these are dependent on the entry of sodium and choline (*Cho*), processes that are linked and may be modulated by a cholinergic receptor. Between the proximal and midzone, the terminal is shown as having a variety of ion channels, but to be rich in potassium channels. The final zone, that of release, is sketched as having calcium channels and perhaps having muscarinic or nicotinic receptors (*R?*) that can modulate the release of transmitter (*Ach*).

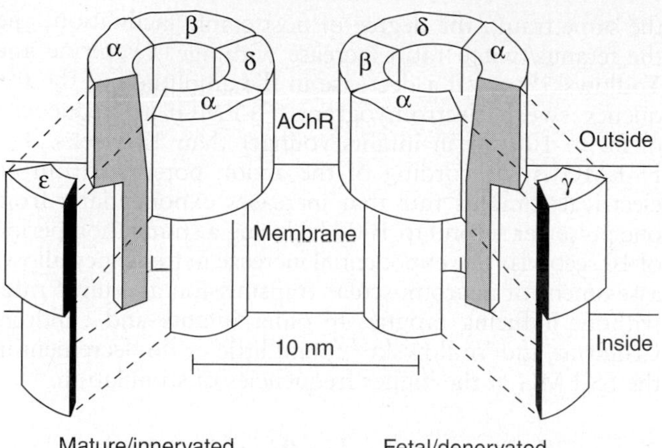

FIGURE 115–2 • AChR channels with the subunits (α, β, ε, and δ or α, β, γ, and δ) arranged around the central cation channel. Binding of acetylcholine to the two α-subunits induces the conformational change that converts the channel from closed to open, although the mean channel open times differ between the two types of AChRs depicted here. (Modified from Martyn JAJ et al: Up-and-down regulation of skeletal muscle acetylcholine receptors, *Anesthesiology* 76: 822, 1992.)

One presumes that neonates have a mix of both adult and fetal receptors. Functional differences exist between these two forms of ACh receptor. Immature ACh receptors vary markedly in many characteristics from more mature ones (Table 115–1 and Fig. 115–2). These differences appear to contribute to the sensitivity of fetal ACh muscle receptors to nondepolarizing and depolarizing neuromuscular blocking drugs. Some uncertainty exists, however, concerning these observations.[8,19-22] ACh receptors in mature animals are localized, and the binding sites are tightly packed (up to 20,000/μm^2) in the crests of the juxtaneural third of the folded postsynaptic surfaces just beneath the active zones. The deeper regions of the junctional cleft are practically devoid of receptors, and along the normal muscle fiber a 1000-fold decrease in receptor density occurs in the extrasynaptic membrane 200 μm from the end-plate.

Prejunctional autoreceptors (α3 subunits) are located in the membrane of the nerve terminal and function to modulate ACh mobilization and release. They have different binding characteristics and possibly different channel characteristics than the postjunctional receptors.[23] Antagonism of the prejunctional receptor results in diminished release of ACh from neurons stimulated at high frequency. These prejunctional nicotinic receptors increase ACh mobilization to readily releasable stores and provide feedback control during high-frequency stimulation. The ontogeny of α3 subunits is not known.

A limited number of extrajunctional ACh receptors are incorporated in the muscle plasma membrane of older infants, children, or adults. Extrajunctional receptors are more loosely attached to the cell membrane and can be located over the entire surface of the muscle membrane. Nerve activity serves as the regulatory stimulus inhibiting the biosynthesis of ACh receptors at extrajunctional sites. In the absence of nerve activity, this inhibition is less in evidence. Neurologic motor defects, direct muscle trauma, thermal injury, disease atrophy, sepsis, and prolonged use of relaxants can markedly increase the number of extrajunctional Ach receptors (i.e., up-regulation of receptors). Martyn et al[8] have reviewed these issues in great detail. Other studies provide further insights about these critical problems.[4, 24-26] For instance, months after the denervation of skeletal muscles, junctional receptors can be detected and extrajunctional receptors still recognized over much of the muscle membrane. Similarly, during periods of muscular inactivity the ACh-sensitive zone around the end-plates expands to several millimeters, and the sensitivity of the muscle to both natural and applied ACh increases.

TABLE 115–1

Distinguishing Features of Mature and Immature Junctional Receptors

Mature	Immature*
ε subunit	γ subunit
Localized to end-plate region	Junctional and extrajunctional sites
Metabolically stable (half-life 2 wk)	Metabolically unstable (half-life approximately 24 h)
Larger single-channel conductance	Smaller single-channel conductance
Shorter mean open time	Twofold to tenfold longer mean open time
Agonists depolarize less easily	Agonists depolarize more easily
Competitive agents block more easily	Competitive agents block less easily†

Data from Martyn JA, White DA, Gronert GA, et al: *Anesthesiology* 76:822, 1992.

*Immature junctional receptors have the same characteristics of up-regulated extrajunctional receptors.

†Recent data conflict with this statement.[20, 21]

Neuromuscular Transmission

Motor neurons synthesize ACh and store it in the nerve terminal that contains about half a million small vesicles, each containing about 12,000 molecules of Ach. Ach is loaded into the vesicles against a concentration gradient by an energy-dependent process. In the resting state ACh is spontaneously discharged in small amounts from the vesicles present in the presynaptic nerve ending, thus causing miniature end-plate potentials. Stimulation of the nerve produces the release of ACh molecules, which cross the synaptic cleft and bind to ACh receptors. Calcium promotes the release of ACh at the active zone and is required for quantal release of ACh. A nerve action potential usually releases about 200 to 500 quanta of ACh, each containing 2000 to 10,000 transmitter molecules. For release to occur, the vesicles must be appropriately docked at special release sites (active zones) that face the postjunctional Ach receptors. These vesicles form the immediately available store. Once the contents are discharged the vesicles are rapidly refilled. The immediately available store may be replenished from the reserve store of vesicles by the process of mobilization. Mobilization of Ach during tetanic stimulation may be limited in the neonate and particularly the premature infant. Docking of the vesicles to the release sites and subsequent exocytosis involves the interaction of a number of important proteins (e.g., synaptotagmin, synaptobrevin, VAMP, SNAP-25, and syntaxin). Vesamicol, botulinum toxins, and black widow spider venom (α-latrotoxin) can interfere with ACh transfer, release, or reformation, respectively.[27,28] Within microseconds a portion of released ACh binds to the receptors on the postsynaptic membrane, changing their conformational shape and inducing the opening of discrete sodium channels. Two ACh molecules must bind to the receptor before the ion channel can open. When the receptor and ACh interact, permeability of the membrane in the end-plate region increases, primarily to sodium but also to potassium. Sodium moves from outside to inside the cell, and the membrane depolarizes. This change in the end-plate potential is directly related to the amount of ACh released. If the end-plate potential is large, the muscle membrane is depolarized and the impulse is propagated along the entire muscle fiber, initiating muscle contraction. The released ACh diffuses from the end-plate region and is rapidly destroyed by acetylcholinesterase. The receptor thus acts as a powerful amplifier, converting the current carried by two ACh molecules to a current carried by thousands of cations. Furthermore, the receptor acts as a switch by opening and closing its ion channels, thereby switching the current on and off, as ACh molecules attach and detach.

Structural and Functional Development of the Neuromuscular System

The neuromuscular system is incompletely developed at birth. The conduction velocity of motor nerves increases throughout gestation as nerve fibers are myelinated. The myotubules connect to mature muscle fibers in the latter part of intrauterine life and in the first several weeks after birth. Some slow-contracting muscle (e.g., intrinsic muscles of the hand) is progressively converted to fast-contracting muscle, with a concomitant change in the force-velocity relationship. Both the diaphragm and the intercostal muscles increase their percentage of slow muscle fibers in the first months of life. Synaptic transmission is relatively slow at birth, but more important, the rate at which ACh is released during repeated nerve stimulation is limited in the infant.[29,30] Thus the margin of safety for neurotransmission is smaller in infants than in adults. Age-related changes in the ACh receptor may also contribute to the reduced margin of safety of neurotransmission.

Unanesthetized neonates appear to have less neuromuscular reserve during tetanic stimulation than adults. In neonates there is no fade of twitch height with repeated stimulation at rates of 1 to 2 Hz; at 20 Hz, however, there is significant fade. Premature infants may show posttetanic exhaustion for 15 to 20 minutes. Goudsouzian[31] noted slower contraction times of the thumb after slow and rapid rates of stimulation in term infants (1 to 10 days of age, anesthetized with halothane) than in older children. The percentage of fade at 20, 50, or 100 Hz did not differ between the infants and the older children, but the tetanic stimulus was applied for only 5 seconds. The train-of-four (TOF) ratio (the ratio of the amplitude of the fourth evoked response to the amplitude of the first response in the same train), the degree of posttetanic facilitation, and the tetanus/twitch ratio increase with age. Crumrine and Yodlowski[32] noted a decrease in the amplitude of the frequency sweep electromyogram (FS-EMG) at frequencies of 50 to 100 Hz in infants younger than 12 weeks. The FS-EMG is a recording of the action potential from an electrical stimulus rate that increases exponentially from one pulse per second to 100 Hz during a stimulation period of 10 seconds. The exponential increase in frequency allows assessment of neuromuscular transmission at tetanic rates without inducing fatigue. In older infants and children, Crumrine and Yodlowski[32] found little or no decrement in the FS-EMG at the higher frequencies of stimulation.

Types of Neuromuscular Blocking Agents

Neuromuscular blocking agents are described as being depolarizing or nondepolarizing, depending on their effect on the motor end-plate. Succinylcholine, the only commonly used depolarizing relaxant, produces two different types of blockade, phase 1 and phase 2 (Fig. 115–3). During phase 1, the binding of succinylcholine to ACh receptors causes membrane ionic channels to open in the same fashion as ACh does. The molecules remain bound to the receptor for an extended period and cause the membrane to remain depolarized and unable to trigger any further muscle action potentials. With prolonged exposure, a succinylcholine-induced blockade begins to assume the characteristics of a nondepolarizing blockade. This is referred to as phase 2, desensitization, or dual blockade.[33-36] The nondepolarizing agents bind to the α units of the ACh receptor and may also physically block the ion channel in the motor end-plate. When both α units are occupied by ACh, the channel opens and ions flow. Conversely, if one or both are occupied by a nondepolarizing agent, a competitive antagonism occurs, and ion flow is prevented. This competitive antagonism depends on the relative

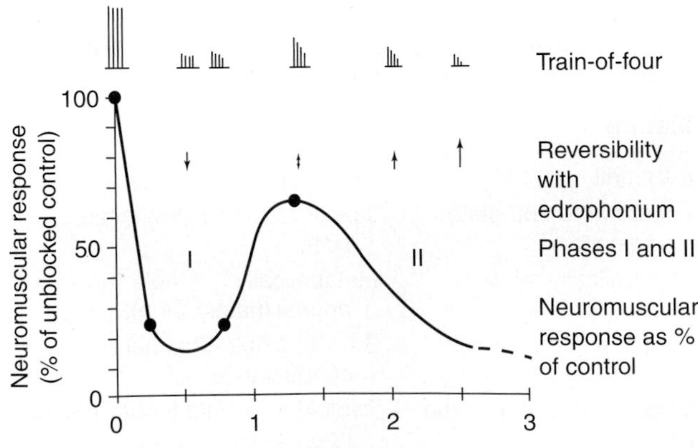

FIGURE 115–3 • During continuous infusion of succinylcholine chloride, a phase 1 block—characterized by reduced neuromuscular response, little fade of train-of-four (TOF), and increased blockade with edrophonium—is seen initially. During phase 2, there is a fade on TOF, increasing reversibility of the block by edrophonium, and accumulation of the slowly recovering residual block. (From Lee C: Succinylcholine: its past, present, and future, *Semin Anesth* 4:3, 1984, with permission.)

concentrations and the binding characteristics of the individual agent and is clearly the most important effect at the myoneural junction. Another mechanism by which such drugs affect neuromuscular transmission is channel blockade. Because the ion channel is much larger at its extracellular end than at its intracellular end, where it crosses the membrane, large molecules can enter the channel but fail to cross, thus acting as a plug preventing normal ion flow. This mechanism of action is not affected by increasing the concentration of ACh.

Dose-Response Relationships

The dose response to muscle relaxants is quantified by the degree of muscle twitch suppression (expressed as a percentage of baseline twitch [force], EMG height, or accelerometry height) observed after stimulation of a motor nerve (Fig. 115–4).[37,38] Although the dose-response curve is sigmoid, its midportion is relatively linear (Fig. 115–5). Dose-response relationships are therefore best defined in this 20% to 80% range of twitch suppression. Generally, doses producing 20%, 50%, and 80% inhibition define a line of best fit, which can be interpolated over the range studied to predict the response to any dose. Log-dose or log-dose probit transformations straighten the sigmoid curve and expand the range of linearity. The use of such curves permits determination of the mean dose that produces a maximal effect of 95% twitch suppression (ED_{95}) for a given drug (Table 115–2). The ED_{95} of a neuromuscular blocking agent can be viewed conceptually as proportional to both the volume of distribution (the bucket size) and the concentration of the blocker at its effect site. Although the concentration of drug at the neuromuscular junction in vivo is inaccessible, the drug concentration in plasma that produces, for example, 95% twitch suppression at steady-state conditions ($CP_{ss\,95}$), provides a means of comparing drug potencies and the factors that affect them. The volume of distribution of neuromuscular blocking agents is highly correlated with (but not equal to) the extracellular fluid (ECF) volume. The ECF of the volume of the

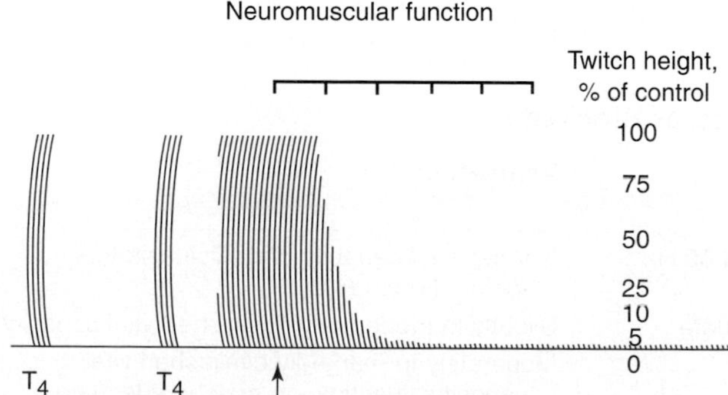

FIGURE 115–4 • Correlation of twitch height, clinical relaxation, and ventilation at increasing depths of neuromuscular blockade. A recording of evoked thumb adduction was made in a patient during nitrous oxide-narcotic-barbiturate anesthesia. The single twitch was evoked at 0.15 Hz. At T_4, train-of-four stimulation (2 Hz for 2 sec) was carried out. Time scale (minutes) at top. At the arrow, pancuronium, 0.1 mg/kg, was given intravenously, producing 99% twitch suppression.

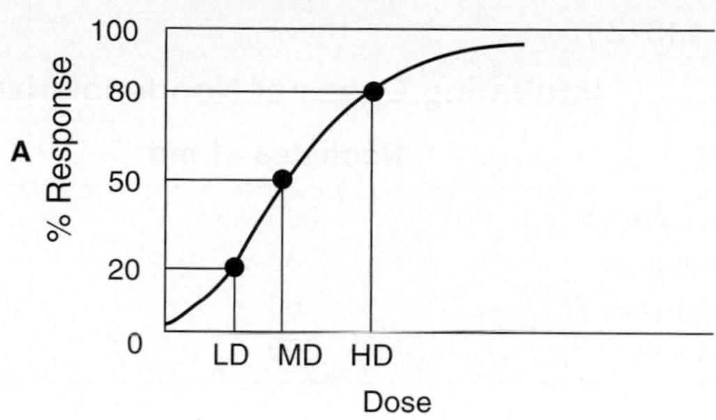

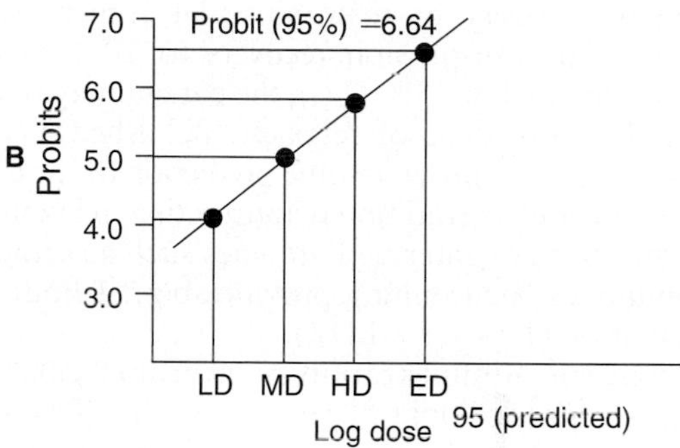

FIGURE 115–5 • **A,** Sigmoid dose-response relationship. The linear portion of the curve is defined by measuring the response of three doses of relaxant (*LD,* low dose; *MD,* middle dose; *HD,* high dose). These doses are best selected to cover a range encompassing 20% to 80% of the full measurable response. **B,** Creating a log-dose versus probit transformation extends the linearity to encompass 1% to 99% of the full measurable response. This allows extrapolation of the predicted ED_{95} from the straight line of best fit through three or more data points.

infant is significantly greater than that of the older child and adult on a weight basis. ECF volume and surface area, by contrast, bear a nearly constant relationship throughout life (6 to 8 L/m^2). The ED_{95} determined during the administration of so-called balanced anesthesia is more relevant to the patient in the ICU than that determined during the administration of a potent inhaled anesthetic. In clinical practice several multiples of the ED_{95} (e.g., $2 \times ED_{95}$)—the so-called intubating dose—are usually administered to ensure adequate neuromuscular blockade and to minimize the time to maximum neuromuscular blockade (the onset time).[39] Alternatively, small, priming doses of the nondepolarizing relaxant (less than $ED_{5\text{-}10}$) can be given to partially occupy the cholinergic receptor.[40] Larger, top-up doses (total dose $2 \times ED_{95}$) given several minutes later seem to accelerate the onset time. This approach avoids potential cardiovascular changes from even higher multiples of the ED_{95} (e.g., 6 to $8 \times ED_{95}$) and still provides rapid onset time of neuromuscular blockade.

If an endotracheal tube is already in place, smaller doses of neuromuscular blocking agents ($1 \times ED_{95}$) may suffice for controlled ventilation, depending on clinical needs. In general, with adequate sedation and analgesia *the clinician* should be able to achieve control of ventilation with ED_{75} to ED_{90} doses of relaxant unless the patient "fights" or "bucks" the ventilator because of hypoxia or hypercarbia (Table 115–3). Alternatively, an intubating dose of relaxant

TABLE 115–2

Intubating Doses of Nondepolarizing Muscle Relaxants in Pediatric Patients (μg/kg)

Agent	Neonates <1 mo	Infants <1 yr	Children 1-10 yr	Adolescents >12 yr
d-Tubocurarine	300	400	550	500-550
Pancuronium	80	80	100	80-100
Vecuronium	60	60	100	70-80
Atracurium	300	400	400	400

might be administered to achieve control of ventilation and then allow recovery of neuromuscular transmission. As neuromuscular transmission recovers to 10% of control twitch height (T_{10}) or 25% (T_{25}), the patient may require an additional top-up dose of relaxant. Published T_{10} or T_{25} indexes of recovery provide some prediction of the expected duration of effect. Traditional long-acting relaxants such as pancuronium or intermediate ones such as atracurium, vecuronium, or rocuronium, provide about 1 hour of clinical relaxation (1 to 1.5 × ED_{95}).

Intermittent administration of neuromuscular blocking agents for prolonged periods in the ICU may be inconvenient, and administration by infusion appears to be a practical alternative. The goal of such infusion techniques is to maintain a constant plasma concentration of relaxant and a constant degree of neuromuscular blockade. The steady-state infusion rate (I_{ss}) is proportional to the required plasma concentration (CP) and clearance rate and thus the removal rate (R_{ss}):

$$I_{ss} = R_{ss} = \text{clearance} \times CP_{ss\ 95}$$

Although traditional long-acting agents (e.g., pancuronium) have been used by infusion, there are drawbacks, such as recurrent cardiovascular effects and cumulation. Therefore it may be more prudent to infuse agents with an intermediate duration (e.g., atracurium, cisatracurium, rocuronium, or vecuronium) for prolonged periods. Short-acting agents (e.g., mivacurium) may be even more preferable. Shorter-acting agents may allow more rapid recovery of neuromuscular transmission and are more easily titrated but are clearly more expensive (Table 115–4). Monitoring of neuromuscular blockade with a nerve-muscle stimulator or clinical indicators diminishes the likelihood of prolonged neuromuscular blockade. Additional boluses of relaxant should not be administered until there is reappearance of a single twitch in the TOF-evoked response. Infusion rates can be adjusted to maintain a perceptible single twitch or a level that just abolishes the twitch. If complete neuromuscular blockade is deemed necessary, one would allow the patient to recover a single twitch every 24 hours.

Predictability of response is limited by electrolyte imbalances, drug interactions, and variable drug elimination. These issues have been well reviewed. Many drugs modify the action of muscle relaxants. Such substances may interfere directly with neuromuscular transmission, or they may influence the action of relaxants by extrajunctional mechanisms (Table 115–5). Knowledge of the interaction among muscle relaxants, drugs, and disease guides dosage adjustments.

Hypothermia may increase the intensity and duration of effect from neuromuscular blocking drugs. Decreasing ambient temperature from 37° to 27° C causes significant increases in the intensity of neuromuscular blockade by pancuronium and succinylcholine. The greater intensity of blockade at low temperatures may be related to possible retardation of metabolism and renal excretion of the drugs.

The short duration of action of succinylcholine and mivacurium are related to the hydrolysis of the drugs by butyrylcholinesterase (plasma or pseudocholinesterase), which is synthesized in the liver. There is wide variation in the time responses to succinylcholine in healthy patients

TABLE 115–3

Degrees of Neuromuscular Blockade

Neuromuscular Blockade (%)	Clinical Relaxation	Ventilation
0	None; train-of-four > 0.7; tetanus sustained at 50 Hz	Normal; vital capacity normal; inspiratory force > 50 cm H_2O
25	Poor; head lift inadequate; leg flexion inadequate	Slightly to moderately diminished vital capacity
50	Fair	Moderately to markedly diminished vital capacity; tidal volume may be adequate
75	Good	Tidal volume diminished
90	Good	Tidal volume inadequate
95	Very good; adequate for tracheal intubation under light anesthesia	Some diaphragmatic motion possible
100	Excellent; very good for tracheal intubation	Apnea

TABLE 115–4

Comparison of Neuromuscular Blocking Agents

	Loading Dose (μg/kg)	Infusion Rate (μg/kg/min)	Cost ($)* (24 hr)
Pancuronium	50-100	.5-1.0	10
Vecuronium	80-100	1.0-1.5	260
Pipecuronium	40-80	.2-.3	110
Atracurium	200-500	5-8	300
Doxacurium	25-50	.2-.35	190
Mivacurium	250-300	10-15	300

Modified from Fleming NW: *Semin Anesth* 13:255, 1994.
*Based on 70-kg adult.

because of considerable differences in butyrylcholinesterase activity. A prolonged response to succinylcholine and mivacurium may be expected in individuals whose butyrylcholinesterase activity is abnormally low because of congenital atypical enzyme, hepatic disease, or drugs that inhibit the enzyme.

Characteristics of Specific Agents

The sensitivity of the postjunctional cholinergic receptor to neuromuscular blocking agents may vary with age. When allowance is made for differences in the volume of distribution, infants appear as sensitive to succinylcholine

TABLE 115–5

Drug-Relaxant Interactions

Drug	Mechanism of Interaction	Clinical Implication
Magnesium	Blocks the release of acetylcholine at the neuromuscular junction, as well as accelerates the action of true cholinesterase	Potentiates the action of all relaxants when used in large amounts (e.g., eclampsia); this effect is reversed by calcium ions
Lithium	Increases transmitter release	Prolongs succinylcholine block; prolongs pancuronium block
Local anesthetics	Inhibit the release of acetylcholine	Potentiate nondepolarizing drugs and prolong the action of succinylcholine
Pitocin	Prolonged infusion alters the sensitivity of the end-plate to depolarization by succinylcholine	The duration of action of succinylcholine is prolonged, and increased dosage may be needed
Trimethaphan	Completes with acetylcholine at the neuromuscular junction	Potentiates nondepolarizing and antagonizes depolarizers; may potentiate succinylcholine
Quinidine	May diminish end-plate sensitivity to transmitter	May prolong the action of succinylcholine; potentiates nondepolarizing agents
Verapamil	Decreases sensitivity of end-plate at nonspecific sites	May potentiate nondepolarizing agents
Hydrocortisone	Unknown mechanism	Chronic administration inhibits nondepolarizing block; acute administration increases block
Dantrolene	Direct muscle effect diminishing excitation-contraction coupling	Can produce profound neuromuscular weakness
Cytotoxic drugs (alkylating agents): nitrogen mustard and related drugs	Inhibition of plasma cholinesterase by alkylating the enzyme	Prolong succinylcholine action
Echothiophate (eye drops)	A long-acting anticholinesterase; inhibits plasma cholinesterase	Prolonged response to succinylcholine
Antibiotics (streptomycin, neomycin, polymyxin, colimycin, kanamycin)	Reduce acetylcholine output by competing with calcium at presynaptic membrane binding sites (a "magnesium-like effect")	Increased sensitivity to curarelike drugs
Diuretics	Potassium loss	Hypokalemia may theoretically potentiate nondepolarizing block
Tricyclic antidepressant	Increased catecholamine levels	Cardiac dysrhythmias with pancuronium
Dilantin	Unknown mechanism	Resistance to nondepolarizing agents; increased clearance

Modified from Ali HH, Savarese JJ: *Anesthesiology* 45:216, 1976.

(the only depolarizing agent in use) as adults but more sensitive to nondepolarizing relaxants.

Succinylcholine

Succinylcholine, a rapid-acting and ultrashort-duration depolarizing muscle relaxant, is useful when given as a bolus to facilitate endotracheal intubation. The onset times (i.e., time to maximum neuromuscular blockade) at so-called intubating doses are listed in Table 115–6. Succinylcholine is metabolized by butyrylcholinesterase. Markedly prolonged neuromuscular blockade can result from atypical or abnormally low enzyme concentrations. When differences in volume of distribution and concentration of anesthesia are taken into account, infants and small children appear relatively resistant to succinylcholine, have a faster clearance, and have a shorter onset time (at equal multiples of the ED_{95}) than do older children and adults. Most of the side effects of succinylcholine were described within years of its introduction: dysrhythmias, increased intraocular pressure, prolonged apnea, injured muscle membranes with associated hyperkalemia, association with masseter spasm and malignant hyperthermia, and death. Infants and small children have a high incidence of such complications. Intractable, unexpected cardiac arrest (ventricular fibrillation or asystole) associated with a 40% to 50% death rate has been reported after the use of succinylcholine in children with undiagnosed Duchenne's muscular dystrophy. In these patients succinylcholine may cause rhabdomyolysis and massive hyperkalemia.[41-43] This series of case reports created a small firestorm that culminated in the Food and Drug Administration issuing a "box" warning against the elective use of succinylcholine.

Age-Related Responses

Neonates and infants require about twice as much succinylcholine on a weight basis as older children or adults to depress respiration or neuromuscular transmission or to produce apnea. In infants, 1 mg/kg succinylcholine has produced neuroblockade about equal to that produced by 0.5 mg/kg in children aged 6 to 8 years.[44] At these equipotent doses there is no statistically significant difference between the times to recover to 50% and 90% (T_{90}) neuromuscular transmission in the two groups. Complete neuromuscular blockade develops in children given 1 mg/kg of succinylcholine. Cook and Fischer[44] estimated the ED_{95} of succinylcholine to be 2.2 mg/kg. Better estimates of the ED_{95} of succinylcholine have been made more recently by others (Table 115–7; Fig. 115–6).[45] Neonates and infants may require 2 to 3 mg/kg and children 1 to 2 mg/kg of succinylcholine to achieve comparable intubation conditions seen in adults at 1 to 1.5 mg/kg of succinylcholine. In view of the marked variability in neuromuscular block produced by small doses of succinylcholine, it would seem advisable to select doses at the upper end of these ranges. Spontaneous recovery from succinylcholine-induced apnea may not occur sufficiently quickly to prevent hemoglobin desaturation in patients whose ventilation is not assisted.[46]

Goudsouzian and Liu[34] found that a threefold higher infusion rate of succinylcholine (mg/kg/hr) was needed to maintain a 90% twitch depression in young infants than in older infants or children. A slightly larger dose of succinylcholine was needed in infants than in the other age groups to achieve phase II block. Differences in butyrylcholinesterase activity, receptor sensitivity, or volume of distribution may explain these age-related differences in succinylcholine requirements. The neonate has about one half the butyrylcholinesterase activity of the older child or adult. Thus it is unlikely that augmented butyrylcholinesterase activity is responsible for the infant's resistance to succinylcholine. When succinylcholine was given on a surface area basis (40 mg/m^2), no difference existed between infants and adults in the times to recover to 10%, 50%, or 90% neuromuscular transmission; this dose of succinylcholine produced complete neuromuscular blockade in all patients. A linear relationship occurs between the log dose on a milligram per square meter basis and the maximum intensity of neuromuscular blockade for infants, children, and adults. They also observed a linear relationship between the logarithm of the dose on a milligram per square meter basis and either 50% or 90% recovery time for infants and children as a combined group. Similar findings have been noted by others (Table 115–7). Because of its small molecular size, succinylcholine is rapidly distributed throughout the extracellular fluid. The blood volume and ECF volume of the infant are significantly greater than those of the child and adult on a weight basis. Therefore on

TABLE 115–6

Variation in Onset Time at Different Epochs for Various Relaxants

	% Responders			
Onset Time (sec)	**Succinylcholine**	**Rapacuronium**	**Rocuronium**	**Mivacurium**
<30	0	0	0	0
31-60	90	62	50	27
61-90	10	19	25	45
91-120	0	14	17	9
121-150	0	0	0	9
151-180	0	0	8	9
>180	0	5	0	0

Data from various studies of the author.

TABLE 115–7

Calculated ED_{50} and ED_{95} for Succinylcholine as a Function of Age

Age Group	ED_{50} (µg/kg)	ED_{95} (µg/kg)	ED_{50} (µg/m^2)	ED_{95} (µg/m^2)
Neonates	250	625	3952	9881
Infants	317	729	6277	14,436
Children	184	423	4416	10,154
Adults	—	290	—	11,940

a weight basis (milligram per kilogram), twice as much succinylcholine is needed in infants as in adults to produce a given degree of neuromuscular blockade.

Because ECF volume and surface area bear a nearly constant relationship throughout life, it is not surprising that there is a good correlation between succinylcholine dose (µg/m^2) and response throughout life. The data of Goudsouzian and Liu[34] suggest that relative resistance to succinylcholine persists in some infants even when the dose is transformed to µg/m^2/min. These data suggest that the ACh receptor matures with age—or that pseudocholinesterase activity is high in infants. Indeed, butyrylcholinesterase activity is quite high in infants.

Side Effects

Succinylcholine can have profound cardiovascular effects; increase intraocular, intragastric, and ICPs; and be associated with hyperkalemia, myoglobinemia, and malignant hyperthermia.

Dysrhythmias. Succinylcholine exerts variable and seemingly paradoxical effects on the cardiovascular system. Typically, intravenous succinylcholine produces initial bradycardia and hypotension, followed after 15 to 30 seconds by tachycardia and hypertension. In the infant and small child, profound sustained sinus bradycardia (rates of 50 to 60 beats/min) is frequently observed; rarely, asystole occurs. Nodal rhythm and ventricular ectopic beats are seen in about 80% of children given a single intravenous injection of succinylcholine; such dysrhythmias are rarely seen after intramuscular injection of succinylcholine. The incidence of bradycardia and other dysrhythmias is higher after a second dose of succinylcholine.

Atropine (0.1 mg) appears to offer adequate protection against these bradyarrhythmias in all age groups of infants and children. (In infants vagolytic doses of 0.03 mg/kg are required for protection; in older children adequate protection is provided by doses of 0.005 mg/kg.)

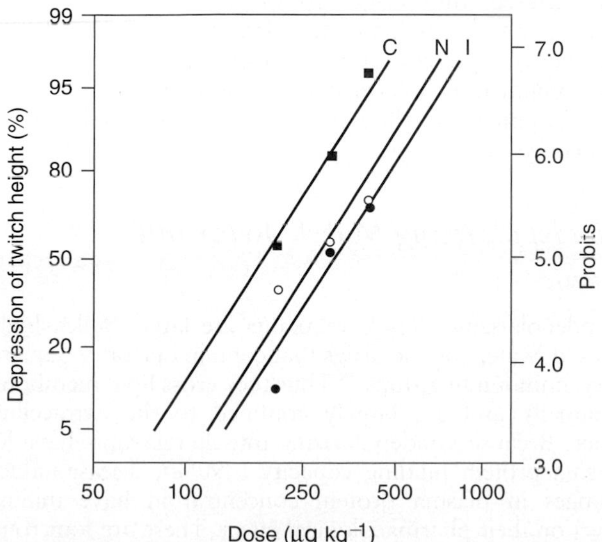

FIGURE 115–6 • Log dose-probit response regression lines for neonates (*N*), infants (*I*), and children (*C*). Points along the lines represent mean responses from subgroups of five patients.

Pulmonary Edema and Pulmonary Hemorrhage. Cook et al[47] have described several young infants in whom fulminant pulmonary edema developed only minutes after intramuscular injection of succinylcholine (4 mg/kg). The edema responded to ventilation with continuous positive airway pressure. Since that report I have seen additional cases of pulmonary edema and pulmonary hemorrhage after intravenous administration of succinylcholine. In each instance the patient was "lightly" anesthetized. I speculate that this complication represents a hemodynamic form of pulmonary edema caused by an acute increase in systemic vascular resistance and an acute decrease in pulmonary vascular resistance; in addition, "leaky" capillaries appear to be involved. Whether these cardiovascular changes are mediated by succinylcholine itself or by some other vasoactive substance (e.g., histamine) is not known.

Intragastric Pressure. Succinylcholine may increase intragastric pressure. The increase in intragastric pressure is directly related to the intensity of muscle fasciculations. In adults, pressures as high as 40 cm H_2O have been recorded after violent fasciculations. When the intragastric pressure exceeds 20 cm H_2O, the cardioesophageal valve ("sphincter") mechanism may become incompetent; regurgitation and aspiration may occur. Because of limited muscle mass, the infant or small child, in contrast to the adult, seldom has strong fasciculations. Salem and others observed an increase of only 4 cm H_2O in intragastric pressure after intravenous administration of succinylcholine in infants; in some patients the intragastric pressure decreased.

Intraocular Pressure. Intravenous or intramuscular administration of succinylcholine increases intraocular pressure in infants and adults. Although dilation of choroidal vessels by succinylcholine is a contributory factor, the increase in intraocular pressure is primarily the result of contraction of extraocular muscles. Typically after intravenous succinylcholine administration the intraocular pressure begins to increase within 60 seconds, peaks at 2 to 3 minutes, and then returns to control levels 5 to 7 minutes after injection.

A succinylcholine-induced increase in intraocular pressure in the presence of a penetrating wound of the eye can result in extrusion of vitreous humor through the site of injury and possibly loss of vision. The transient increase in intraocular pressure may be misinterpreted and lead to an unnecessary operation in a patient with glaucoma if tonometry is performed within 5 to 7 minutes of the injection of succinylcholine.

Increased Intracranial Pressure. Minton et al[48] suggested that succinylcholine per se may increase ICP. Increases in ICP after the administration of succinylcholine are produced by cerebral metabolic stimulation and increases in cerebral blood flow. These effects are attenuated by prior administration of a nondepolarizing agent and by treatment with thiopental or lidocaine.

Hyperkalemia and Myoglobinemia. In healthy patients, succinylcholine increases plasma levels of potassium by 0.3 to 0.5 mEq/L. Alarming concentrations of potassium, as high as 11 mEq/L, along with cardiovascular collapse, have been frequently reported with succinylcholine in a variety of conditions, including burns, massive trauma, stroke, spinal cord injury, and muscle diseases.[49-51] The common denominator appears to be either massive tissue destruction or central nervous system injury with muscle wasting. Strong fasciculations are not necessary to produce hyperkalemia in susceptible patients. There are no data to suggest that the infant is any less vulnerable than the adult to massive potassium flux from the listed conditions.[52,53] A high incidence of myoglobinemia occurs after succinylcholine (1 mg/kg) in prepubertal patients, especially those anesthetized with halothane. A much lower incidence was noted by Harrington et al.[54] Myoglobinemia rarely results from succinylcholine administration in adults. Plasma levels of creatine phosphokinase, an indicator of muscle injury, have been shown to be significantly increased after succinylcholine administration in children. Myoglobinemia and increased plasma levels of creatine phosphokinase occurred without strong fasciculations. The tendency of muscle in children to release myoglobin after depolarization with succinylcholine is not readily explained. Such changes seem rare in infants.

Masseter Spasm, Trismus, and Malignant Hyperthermia. Most clinicians are well aware of the association of succinylcholine with malignant hyperthermia. Typically malignant hyperthermia develops as a profound rigidity or violent fasciculations, a rapid increase in temperature, an increase in pulse rate, and an increase in end-tidal carbon dioxide tension. These are the classic signs, but occasionally the only manifestation of malignant hyperthermia is trismus.[55,56] The rigid jaw can be forced open but only with considerable difficulty. Only about half of the patients in whom trismus follows administration of succinylcholine have a predisposition to malignant hyperthermia.[55] Resting tension or stiffness in the masseter muscle increases in a dose-related manner as succinylcholine blocks neuromuscular function.[57-61] These changes can make laryngoscopy difficult. Perhaps masseter spasm is an extreme case of the apparently normal dose-related increase in resting tension observed in some studies. A more complete evaluation of the force required to open the mouth is necessary to clarify this issue. Perhaps masseter spasm is not only quantitatively different from the changes in resting tension but also qualitatively different. If so, the identifying features of masseter spasm have yet to be described in sufficient detail to allow differentiation of masseter spasm from an extreme instance of the normal increase in resting tension of the masseter after administration of succinylcholine. Therefore it is not possible to define susceptibility to malignant hyperthermia solely on the basis of trismus. Creatine phosphokinase measurement and muscle biopsy may be of some help, but most centers are reluctant to perform major muscle biopsies in children younger than 8 to 10 years. Thus the diagnosis is extraordinarily difficult to make on clinical grounds alone.

Decreasing Use

Rumors of the total withdrawal from use of succinylcholine have become more common in the past several years. Many have suggested that succinylcholine be eliminated from clinical use; others have demanded that succinylcholine be eliminated. Both the box warning against the elective use of succinylcholine and increased availability of alternative agents have contributed to the markedly diminished use of this agent.[62] Many of the profound cardiovascular complications of succinylcholine were described within 5 to 15 years of its introduction: the hazards of the use of succinylcholine in patients with neural injuries, neuromuscular disease, burns, and massive trauma were established, and the hazards of succinylcholine as a "triggering" agent for myotonia, masseter spasm, and malignant hyperthermia were established. Despite these hazards, succinylcholine remained popular to facilitate endotracheal intubation because there was no reasonable alternative. The clinical introduction of the new short-acting and intermediate-acting relaxants and the development of the so-called priming principle and other clinical strategies to minimize the onset time of relaxants have minimized the need for succinylcholine. Priming or administration of 8 to 10 times the ED_{95} of a relaxant can be used to accelerate the onset of neuromuscular blockade. Infants and small children rarely demonstrate histamine release after relaxants are administered; thus large top-up doses after the priming dose or initial megadoses of relaxants can be used. Such uses convert atracurium, cisatracurium, rocuronium, and vecuronium from intermediate-acting to long-acting relaxants. In patients in the ICU, however, this may be of little consequence.

Nondepolarizing Muscle Relaxants

Kinetics

Nondepolarizing muscle relaxants are large, bulky, highly ionized, water-soluble drugs that contain one or two quaternary ammonium groups.[28] Thus they cross lipid membranes minimally and are largely confined to the extracellular space. Because nondepolarizing muscle relaxants have low plasma protein binding capacity (<90%), disease-induced changes in plasma protein concentration have minimal effect on their pharmacological effect. There are four routes of elimination of nondepolarizing muscle relaxants: renal excretion, hepatic excretion, biotransformation (including Hofmann elimination), and tissue binding (Table 115–8).

TABLE 115–8

Elimination Routes of Muscle Relaxants

Agent	Metabolism in Plasma	Hepatobiliary Uptake and Metabolism	Renal Excretion
Mivacurium	XX		
Atracurium	XX		
Cisatracurium	XX		
Vecuronium		XX	X
Rocuronium		XX	X
Pancuronium		XX	X
Pipecuronium		XX	X
Doxacurium			XX

XX, Major route; *X*, Alternative route.

Nondepolarizing muscle relaxants filter freely through the glomerulus, and the renal clearance of these drugs does not exceed the glomerular filtration rate (1 to 2 ml/kg/min). Hepatic uptake and storage of steroidal nondepolarizing muscle relaxants (pancuronium and especially vecuronium) represent another aspect of drug distribution.[63] Bencini et al[63] estimated that 40% to 80% of an intravenous dose of vecuronium may be taken up by the liver within 30 minutes after its administration. The large hepatic uptake of vecuronium may be the cause of its short duration of action. The degree of metabolism that nondepolarizing muscle relaxants undergo varies widely. Hofmann elimination and ester hydrolysis are largely responsible for the breakdown of atracurium and cisatracurium. Hepatic biodegradation has been shown for steroidal relaxants.[64] A small fraction (20% to 30%) of pancuronium undergoes metabolism. The metabolism of vecuronium is significant.[64,65] Spontaneous deacetylation occurs in the liver, and the byproducts are 3-hydroxy and 17-hydroxy derivatives. The metabolism of steroidal relaxants is not mediated by cytochrome P450 systems (personal observations). The 3-OH metabolites of both vecuronium and pancuronium are roughly one half to equally potent at the neuromuscular junction as the parent compounds. The 17-OH and 3,17-OH metabolites are far less active.[65]

Long-Acting Agents

d-Tubocurarine. Although d-tubocurarine is no longer commercially available, studies of its dose-response relationships and kinetics were the prototypes for future studies with other nondepolarizing relaxants and have helped provide key concepts.[66-69] The volume of distribution for d-tubocurarine is high in the newborn infant compared with the older child or adult, but plasma clearance of d-tubocurarine does not differ with age. The volume of distribution for d-tubocurarine appears relatively constant on a liter per square meter basis (estimated by author). Adults and children require about 7 to 8 mg/m^2 of d-tubocurarine, 6- to 9-month-old infants require about 5 to 6 mg/m^2, and neonates only about 4 mg/m^2. These differences suggest that the neonate, and to a lesser degree the infant, is sensitive to d-tubocurarine if compensation is made for the wide variation in volumes of distribution. More important, the steady-state plasma concentration associated with 50% neuromuscular blockade ($Cp_{ss\,50}$) was age related; $Cp_{ss\,50}$ in neonates was about one third of that noted for adults. The largest variability in elimination half-lives and volumes of distribution was seen in the data from neonates.

Pancuronium. Pancuronium, a steroidal bisquaternary muscle relaxant, has been used frequently for infants and children in the ICU because of its rather predictable neuromuscular blocking action and associated cardiovascular stimulating properties. The dose-response relationships for pancuronium have been determined in infants and children by Goudsouzian, Liu, and Cote[66] and by Blinn et al.[70] Older children require a higher dose on a weight basis (μg/kg) than do infants and small children (Table 115–9).

Within 24 hours after administration of pancuronium, Duvaldestin et al[71] recovered 67% of the drug in the urine in the form of the parent compound and its metabolites. In other studies about 25% of the injected pancuronium appeared in the urine in the form of the 3-OH metabolite and less than 5% each in the form of the 17-OH and 3, 17-dehydroxy metabolites. Approximately 11% of the pancuronium was excreted in the bile as the parent compound and its metabolites.

Pancuronium has been studied extensively in patients with hepatic dysfunction or renal dysfunction (Table 115–10).[71,72] The studies indicate that different types of liver disease have different effects on the disposition of muscle relaxants. Studies show prolonged elimination half life and delayed recovery from pancuronium in patients with cholestasis. Duvaldestin et al[71] studied the pharmacokinetics of pancuronium in patients with cirrhosis and found a prolonged distribution half-life, an almost twofold increase in elimination half-life, and a 20% decrease in clearance. These effects are related primarily to an increase in ECF and therefore in volume of distribution (Table 115–10). On the basis of these observations, one would predict that, in patients with cirrhosis, resistance and increased sensitivity to pancuronium exist at the same time. On one hand, the onset time of pancuronium would be prolonged because of an increase in the volume of distribution, suggesting resistance to the drug; on the other hand, recovery would be delayed because of the prolonged elimination half-life, suggesting increased sensitivity.

TABLE 115–9

Cumulative Dose-Response Relationship of Pancuronium

	ED₅₀		*ED₉₅*	
Age	**(mg/kg)**	**(mg/m²)**	**(mg/kg)**	**(mg/m²)**
3-6 mo	24 ± 7	448 ± 136	45 ± 7	849 ± 151
7-12 mo	30 ± 5	602 ± 90	52 ± 9	1050 ± 175
1-3 yr	34 ± 9*	753 ± 198	62 ± 18*	1394 ± 401
4-6 yr	29 ± 8	1022 ± 524*	62 ± 13*	2136 ± 855*

Data from Brandom BW et al: Atracurium infusion in children during fentanyl, halothane, and isoflurane anesthesia, *Anesth Analg* 64:471, 1985.

*Statistically significant difference from the 3- to 6-month age group (analysis of variance).

TABLE 115–10

Pharmacokinetic Values in Healthy Patients and Patients with Organ Failure

	Healthy Patients			*Hepatic Patients*			*Renal Failure Patients*		
Drug	**Vd_{SS} (L/kg)**	**T 1/2β (hr)**	**Cl (ml/kg/min)**	**Vd_{SS} (L/kg)**	**T 1/2β (hr)**	**Cl (ml/kg/min)**	**Vd_{SS} (L/kg)**	**T 1/2β (hr)**	**Cl (ml/kg/min)**
d-Tubocurarine	0.3-0.5	2-5.8	1-2.7	NA	NA	NA	0.25	2.2	1.5
Pancuronium	0.14-0.4	1.7-2.4	1-2	0.21-0.42	3.4-5.1	0.6-1.5	0.29	4.3	0.9
Vecuronium	0.18-0.26	0.5-1.3	3	0.23	1.2	2.7	0.19	0.8	5.3
Atracurium	0.18	0.33	5-6	0.16	0.35	5.2	0.22	0.4	5.3

If given in renal failure, pancuronium may cause prolonged paralysis. The clearance of pancuronium is reduced by one half to two thirds, whereas the volume of distribution is only minimally affected (see Table 115–8). The metabolites accumulate in renal failure because they normally depend on renal excretion. The metabolites, especially 3-hydroxypancuronium, have some neuromuscular blocking activity, and they further prolong paralysis. A twofold to fourfold increase in elimination half-life results.

Pipecuronium. Pipecuronium, an analog of pancuronium, is free of cardiovascular side effects. It is a long-acting neuromuscular blocking drug with a duration of action similar to pancuronium. After administration of an ED_{95} dose, complete recovery of neuromuscular function occurs in approximately 1 hour in children. The ED_{95} of pipecuronium in children is 80 mg/kg during nitrous oxide-fentanyl anesthesia[115] and 50 mg/kg during nitrous oxide–halothane anesthesia.[74] The ED_{95} of pipecuronium in infants is only about 35 μg/kg during nitrous oxide–halothane anesthesia, but spontaneous recovery is not prolonged in infants relative to older patients after a dose titrated to produce close to maximal effect (i.e., not overdose).[73] Prolonged recovery is to be expected when multiples of the ED_{95} are administered.

Pipecuronium is largely excreted by the kidneys. In adults with renal failure, mean duration of neuromuscular blockade after one dose of 70 μg/kg was similar to that in patients with normal renal function, but there was more variability in duration of action in the renal failure group.[75] Prolonged neuromuscular blockade in an adult with renal failure has been reported.[76] It is to be expected that a dose of pipecuronium administered to facilitate rapid endotracheal intubation in children with no renal function will last at least several hours. Pipecuronium is not easily removed by peritoneal dialysis.

Doxacurium. Doxacurium has a duration of action similar to pancuronium. Unlike pancuronium, doxacurium has minimal cardiovascular side effects. In children, Sarner et al[77] have noted that the ED_{50} and ED_{95} of doxacurium in children during halothane-nitrous oxide-oxygen anesthesia are 14.8 μg/kg and 27.3 μg/kg, respectively. These values are comparable to the requirements seen in adults administered nitrous oxide–oxygen narcotic anesthesia. In addition, at equipotent doses of doxacurium the investigators noted age-related differences with respect to the time of recovery of neuromuscular transmission to T_{25} and time of onset to maximal blockade; the children anesthetized with halothane had shorter onset time to maximal block and shorter recovery times compared with adults anesthetized with nitrous oxide-oxygen and narcotic. Doxacurium is eliminated largely unchanged in the urine.[78] At equal doses of doxacurium patients with hepatic failure achieve a lesser and more variable degree of neuromuscular blockade than healthy patients; the onset time and clinical duration tended to be longer in patients with hepatic failure.[79]

Intermediate-Acting Agents

Atracurium. Atracurium, a muscle relaxant of intermediate duration, is metabolized by nonspecific esters and spontaneously decomposes by Hofmann degradation. Both processes are sensitive to pH and temperature. Under physiological conditions, the breakdown of atracurium is mainly by ester hydrolysis; Hofmann elimination plays a minor role. Deficient or abnormal butyrylcholinesterases have little or no effect on atracurium degradation. Other researchers and I have studied the effects of both age and potent inhaled anesthetics on the dose-response relationships of atracurium in infants, children, and adolescents.[80-84] On the basis of weight (μg/kg), the ED_{95} for atracurium was similar in infants aged 1 to 6 months and adolescents, whereas children had a higher dose requirement. On the basis of surface area (μg/m²), the ED_{95} for atracurium was similar in children and adolescents, and the ED_{95} (mg/m²) for atracurium in infants was much lower. At equipotent doses ($1 \times ED_{95}$) the duration of effect (time from injection to 95% recovery) was 23 minutes in infants and 29 minutes in children and adolescents, compared with 44 minutes in adults. The time from injection to T_{25} (i.e., 25% neuromuscular transmission) was 10 minutes in infants, 15 minutes in children and adolescents, and 16 minutes in adults. At T_{25}, supplemental doses are needed to maintain relaxation for surgery. At higher multiples of the ED_{95} the duration of effect is longer, but the times from T_5 to T_{25} are the same. The shorter duration of effect in the infant may represent a difference in pharmacokinetics. The pharmacokinetics of atracurium differs among infants, children, and adults. Volume of distribution is larger and the elimination half-life is seemingly shorter in infants than in children or adults. For these reasons clearance in infants is more rapid.

Brandom et al[80] have used a continuous infusion of dilute atracurium (200 μg/ml) after a bolus infusion to maintain neuromuscular blockade at 95% ± 5%. For this degree of steady-state blockade to be maintained, 8 to

10 μg/kg/min was required with nitrous oxide, thiopental, and narcotic anesthesia after an initial bolus. No accumulation was seen with prolonged infusion; recovery of neuromuscular transmission was prompt. The recovery of neuromuscular transmission from the same degree of blockade was similar with all three anesthetics. From these data the removal of atracurium can be estimated. At steady state the infusion rate (I_{ss}) equals the removal rate (R_{ss}) of atracurium. Removal is directly related to the clearance and the $CP_{ss\ 95}$. In children, during so-called balanced anesthesia, $CP_{ss\ 95}$ is about 2 μg/ml. Atracurium infusion requirements in children during nitrous oxide and narcotic anesthesia can be compared with those noted in several age groups of adults during similar anesthetic administrations. d'Hollander et al[85] noted that in patients aged 16 to 85 years, the steady-state atracurium infusion rate averaged 14.4 mg/m²/hr; this corresponds to 240 mg/m²/min. This value is similar to the 226 mg/m²/min I noted. Atracurium does not depend on the kidney or the liver for elimination because it is biodegraded by Hofmann elimination and ester hydrolysis. The parent compound and its metabolites, however, are normally found in bile and urine.[86] Because atracurium does not depend on the kidney for excretion, its elimination half-life and duration of action are not prolonged in patients with renal failure (see Table 115–10).[87-89] Fahey et al[87] found no change in the kinetics or the duration of action and rate of recovery from atracurium in these patients. Hunter, Jones, and Utting[88] also found no difference in duration of action.

Atracurium is a mixture of 10 optical and geometric isomers.[90] The R-R[91] optical isomer in the *cis-cis* configuration, cisatracurium, is about 1.5 times more potent than atracurium, and does not liberate histamine at high doses.[92] Cisatracurium is seemingly primarily degraded by Hofmann elimination, pH-dependent chemical degradation, with the initial formation of laudanosine and a monoquaternary acrylate. Plasma esterases hydrolyze the monoquaternary acrylate to a monoquaternary alcohol; further Hofmann elimination can form another molecule of laudanosine. Renal failure or liver disease has minimal effect on the pharmacodynamics of cisatracurium.[24,93] Because cisatracurium is more potent than atracurium, less laudanosine accumulates in patients after a bolus of prolonged infusion. Dhonneur et al[94] infused cisatracurium for one half to 8 days in patients with acute respiratory distress syndrome (ARDS). Clearance of cisatracurium differed little from that seen in healthy patients, and laudanosine plasma concentrations were less than 1200 ng/ml. Reich et al[95] infused cisatracurium in infants after congenital heart surgery. The clearance of cisatracurium was high, and the duration of residual blockade was low. Laudanosine plasma concentrations were less than 2000 ng/ml.

Laudanosine is the major end-product of atracurium degradation.[84,96] The byproducts of atracurium metabolism have no neuromuscular blocking effect, and they are excreted by the liver and the kidney.[86,97] Laudanosine accumulates in patients with liver or renal failure, and its serum concentration remains elevated for a prolonged period.[98] In large doses, laudanosine has been shown to cause central nervous system stimulation in dogs and rabbits[91] but not in cats.[99] It also increases the minimum alveolar concentration (MAC) of halothane in rabbits,[100] and in dogs it causes electroencephalographic changes of arousal during halothane anesthesia.[101] Adverse effects observed with laudanosine accumulation may be partially attributed to an interaction with neuronal nicotinic receptors (e.g., $\alpha4\beta2$ and $\alpha3\beta4$ receptors).[102] The clinical importance of laudanosine in patients with renal failure, particularly after repeated doses of atracurium, has not been determined. Atracurium has been infused in patients for 22 to 106 hours, however, without adverse effect.[97]

Vecuronium. The ED_{95} for vecuronium is somewhat higher in children than in infants and adults.[103,104] At equipotent doses ($2 \times ED_{95}$) of vecuronium, the duration of effect (time from injection to 90% recovery) was longest in infants (73 minutes) compared with that in children (35 minutes) and adults (53 minutes). Thus vecuronium does not have intermediate duration in infants. Other researchers and I have noted that a 2.4 μ/kg/min (60 μ/m²/min) infusion rate of vecuronium is required to maintain approximately 95% neuromuscular blockade in children during narcotic and nitrous oxide anesthesia. These infusion rates are several times higher than those noted by d'Hollander et al[103] in adults (aged 18 to 85 years). Young adults required 0.9 μg/kg/min (45 μg/m²/ min) to maintain 95% neuromuscular blockade. Children recover more rapidly from vecuronium infusion than do adults. Several groups have noted long-term vecuronium infusion requirements in adults with multiple organ failure in the ICU.[25] Infusion rates of about 1.6 μ/kg/min are required, and the degree of block may gradually increase—a sign of cumulation. Increasing vecuronium infusion requirements, by contrast, may be seen during prolonged infusions (i.e., 3 to 14 days). These increased requirements could not be clearly associated with various pathophysiological states, concurrent drug administration, or biochemical abnormalities. Proliferation of extrajunctional cholinergic receptors resulting from prolonged nondepolarizing blockade has also been offered as an explanation.

Fisher et al[105] determined the pharmacodynamics and pharmacokinetics of vecuronium in infants and children. The volume of distribution and mean residence time were greater in infants than in children. Clearance was similar in the two groups; the $CP_{ss\ 50}$ was lower in infants than in children. The combination of a large volume of distribution in infants and fixed clearance results in a longer mean residence time. After a single dose of relaxant, recovery of neuromuscular transmission depends on both distribution and elimination. The combination of a longer mean residence time and a lower sensitivity for vecuronium explains the prolongation of neuromuscular blockade in infants. Little or no 3-OH vecuronium is seemingly formed following a single dose of vecuronium (0.1 to 0.2 mg/kg).

Duvaldestin et al[106] studied the pharmacokinetics and pharmacodynamics of vecuronium in patients with cirrhosis compared with healthy subjects. The volume of distribution in patients with cirrhosis was normal, but the clearance was reduced by approximately 50%. The time interval between the administration of vecuronium and 50% recovery of twitch height was 130 minutes in patients with cirrhosis compared with 62 minutes in healthy subjects. The time to recovery from 25% to 75% of control twitch height was 68 minutes in patients with cirrhosis compared with 21 minutes in healthy subjects. Plasma concentration of vecuronium at 50% twitch recovery (CP_{50}) was similar in both groups. This similarity suggests that patients with cirrhosis have normal sensitivity to vecuronium. Despite the prolonged duration of action of vecuronium in patients with cirrhosis, it was still shorter than that of pancuronium in patients free of liver disease.

Vecuronium is only slightly dependent on renal elimination (10% to 30%), and therefore its elimination should be minimally affected by renal failure. Although some found no change in volume of distribution, clearance, elimination half-life, or recovery time with vecuronium in patients with renal failure, subsequent studies indicated that the duration of neuromuscular blockade was longer in patients with renal failure than in those with normal renal function.[107] This increased duration of effect may be related to both a decreased plasma clearance and a prolonged elimination half-life of vecuronium in the renal failure group. Similarly, Bencini et al[63] found a 50% decrease in clearance, an increase in volume of distribution, and a 50% increase in elimination half-life. The duration of action was not reported. Metabolites of vecuronium were not measured in these studies. Reich et al[95] infused vecuronium in infants following congenital heart surgery. The clearance of vecuronium was low, significant amounts of 3-OH vecuronium were noted, and return of neuromuscular transmission was slow.

Rocuronium. Rocuronium (ORG-9426) is a nondepolarizing, steroidal neuromuscular blocking drug similar to vecuronium, but with one eighth to one tenth of the potency. It is similar in many ways to vecuronium, but the lesser potency of rocuronium produces a more rapid onset of paralysis in comparison with equipotent doses of other drugs.[108] Bolus administration of 0.6 mg/kg of rocuronium, twice the ED_{95}, is associated with a transient increase in heart rate of about 15 beats/min.[109] Bolus intravenous administration of 0.6 mg/kg of rocuronium produces complete neuromuscular blockade (at the adductor pollicis) in infants and children in 50 and 80 seconds, respectively.[110] Increasing the dose to 0.8 mg/kg in children shortens this time to an average of 30 seconds.[109] The time to recovery of neuromuscular function to T_{25} after a dose of 0.6 mg/kg is almost twice as long in infants younger than 10 months compared with children aged 1 to 5 years (45.1 compared with 26.7 minutes, respectively). This age-related difference is similar to that observed with vecuronium.[111] Its rapid onset of action with minimal tachycardia and intermediate duration of action makes it an attractive neuromuscular blocking drug for use in pediatric patients. The role of rocuronium in patients in the ICU is unclear. Hepatic uptake and biliary excretion are the dominant mechanisms for its clearance; hepatobiliary clearance is about 75% and renal clearance is about 9%.[112] The effects of rocuronium are prolonged in patients with renal disease.[113] Little or no metabolism of rocuronium takes place (i.e., about 3%).

Short-Acting Relaxants

Mivacurium. Mivacurium, a short-duration of action nondepolarizing muscle relaxant, is metabolized by butyrylcholinesterase, which clearly influences the duration of action.[114-117] Mivacurium is a mixture of three optical isomers. The two active isomers of mivacurium (*trans*-trans and *cis*-trans) have a short half-life and rapid clearance because of rapid enzymatic hydrolysis. The *cis*-cis isomer has minimal neuromuscular blocking effects but is slowly hydrolyzed.[114,118-120] The ED_{95} of mivacurium during halothane anesthesia in infants and children is 85 μg/kg and 89 μg/kg.[121,122] Mivacurium is metabolized by butyrylcholinesterase more slowly than is succinylcholine. In infants, mivacurium produces complete neuromuscular blockade as quickly as succinylcholine, but at that time the intubating conditions were less desirable after mivacurium (i.e., a higher incidence of coughing and diaphragmatic movement).[123,124] In children, mivacurium produces complete neuromuscular blockade more slowly than does succinylcholine. During halothane anesthesia increasing the dose of mivacurium from 0.2 mg/kg to 0.3 mg/kg does not shorten the time to complete paralysis after mivacurium administration (1.5 minutes).[125] After administration of 0.3 mg/kg of mivacurium during halothane anesthesia, hypotension or cutaneous flushing was not observed in children. Mivacurium can induce histamine release when large bolus doses are administered rapidly. The most common manifestation of histamine release is cutaneous flushing as seen with d-tubocurarine. This is usually transient and associated with only mild decreases in blood pressure. Recovery to T_{25} was faster in infants (6.3 minutes) compared with children (10 minutes). Increasing the dose of mivacurium given to children from 0.2 to 0.3 mg/kg did not significantly prolong the time to spontaneous recovery of neuromuscular function to 25% of baseline.[123,124,126] Mivacurium (0.3 mg/kg) has little or no effect on lung mechanics (flow-volume loops).[127]

It is remarkable that the duration of action of mivacurium is so short in children. Mivacurium is one of the few neuromuscular blocking agents that are cleared in the plasma rather than by the kidneys or liver. This may be the reason why infants recover from this drug as least as rapidly as do children, and children recover more rapidly than do adults. There have been several studies of the kinetics of mivacurium in infants and children.[128,129] The volume of distribution of mivacurium is seemingly greater in the infant than in the child, and the clearance in infants and children is faster than that of the adult. These conclusions are indirectly supported by the observations that the infusion rate of mivacurium to maintain constant neuromuscular block (–95% twitch depression) is about twice as great in infants and children as in adults.[129] An advantage of mivacurium is that it can be given by infusion for hours without accumulation or prolongation of recovery once the infusion is stopped.[130,131]

In adults with renal or hepatic failure and subsequently reduced butyrylcholinesterase activity, the duration of mivacurium-induced neuromuscular blockade is increased by renal and hepatic failure. Similar studies in children have not been performed. In adults given 0.15 mg/kg the duration of block was approximately three times normal in those with liver failure.[118,119,132-134] There was a significant nonlinear, negative correlation between butyrylcholinesterase and time to spontaneous recovery of neuromuscular function to 25% of baseline in these patients.

Selection of Nondepolarizing Relaxant. At appropriate doses, all nondepolarizing relaxants produce neuromuscular blockade; at equipotent doses, each relaxant produces the same degree of relaxation as any other. Potency is important not only to the drug concentration in the vial but perhaps also to the disparity between neuromuscular blocking effects and autonomic side effects. In addition, onset time is markedly reduced with relaxants with high ED_{95}'s—a mass effect. In selecting one relaxant over another, one should consider its onset time, duration of effect, side effects, and routes of elimination (renal, liver, or spontaneous). In addition, one should consider how the age or the pathological condition of the patient may have an influence on the kinetics of the relaxant. The side effects of the nondepolarizing relaxants are primarily cardiovascular. These cardiovascular effects are related to the magnitude of histamine release, ganglionic blockade, and vagolysis. In addition, the cardiovascular effects appear to be age related. In infants and children minimal cardiovascular effects are seen after administration of atracurium or vecuronium at several multiples of the ED_{95}.[82,104,135,136] In adults, atracurium at three times the ED_{95} causes slightly less histamine release than two times the ED_{95} of metocurine and less than half as much histamine release as once the ED_{95} of d-tubocurarine.[137] Vecuronium (at any multiple of ED_{95}) is not associated with histamine release.[138] Infants and children appear to be less susceptible than adults to histamine release after administration of relaxants. In a small series of infants, five times the ED_{95} of atracurium did not elicit flushing or alter heart rate or blood pressure.[81,135] Local signs of histamine release after direct intravenous injection of atracurium in infants and children have been described, however[139]; rarely, flushing with or without mild hypotension is seen at high multiples of the ED_{95}. At high doses d-tubocurarine may cause hypotension and histamine release in children. The different pattern of tryptase release by the various types of relaxants suggests different mechanisms of mast cell activation.[140] Bronchospasm may be related to histamine release or release of leukotrienes. Some relaxants may block prejunctional muscarinic receptors in the airway.

At two times the ED_{95}, increases in heart rate are seen with pancuronium and rocuronium in children; in contrast, both have minimal effect on heart rate in infants. Because the infant responds with bradycardia to a variety of stimuli (hypoxia, tracheal intubation), the "potential" vagolytic effects of pancuronium or rocuronium may be desired side effects.

Modes of Evaluation of Neuromuscular Transmission

Restoration of complete skeletal muscle strength is essential to ensure that patients are able to sustain adequate ventilation, to cough, and to maintain a patent airway after chronic administration of relaxants. Peripheral nerve stimulation (usually the ulnar nerve) adequately measures recovery from nondepolarizing neuromuscular blockade. Peripheral nerve stimulation (e.g., TOF, double burst, or tetanic stimulation) is often used in preference to tests of ventilation. Nerve stimulators used for neuromuscular monitoring in the ICU may need to deliver at least 100 milliamps to generate supramaximal stimulation.[141] TOF stimulation has been established as the pattern of stimulation for clinical monitoring of neuromuscular blockade. This stimulation mode allows for convenient and reliable tactile evaluation of moderate degrees of nondepolarizing blockade without undue discomfort accompanying tetanic bursts (i.e., 50 to 100 Hz for 5 seconds). Several studies, however, suggest that these rigorous criteria for adequacy of neuromuscular transmission are indeed needed. The rationale for this approach is the following: first, the diaphragm recovers from the effects of nondepolarizing neuromuscular blocking drugs more rapidly than does the adductor pollicis; second, at a TOF ratio of 0.9, vital capacity returns to normal (>15 to 20 ml/kg), pharyngeal muscle strengthens with recovery of swallowing, diplopia disappears, and maximum inspiratory and expiratory force are only slightly depressed (−50 cm H_2O). Intense neuromuscular blockade of the peripheral muscles is indicated by disappearance of the response to TOF and single twitch stimulation.[142] It is possible, however, to quantify part of this period of no response by applying tetanic stimulation (50 Hz for 5 seconds), followed by 1-Hz stimulation and observing the posttetanic single twitch response (posttetanic count). The posttetanic count is highly correlated with recovery from intense blockade caused by relaxants and with antagonism less than or equal to the neuromuscular blockade.

During recovery of neuromuscular transmission it is difficult, however, to estimate the TOF ratio with sufficient certainty to exclude residual paralysis.[143] In this situation it may be more reliable to ascertain the ability to sustain tetanus (50 Hz) for 5 seconds or to evaluate double-burst stimulation (DBS). DBS is a new pattern of stimulation that was developed to reveal residual neuromuscular blockade.[144] DBS consists of two short tetanic bursts separated by 750 ms. A DBS with three impulses (200 μs square-wave impulses) in each of two tetanic bursts of 50 Hz (DBS 3.3) is most suitable for clinical work. Fade in the response results from residual neuromuscular blockade as is seen with TOF stimulation. DBS, however, is more sensitive than TOF in the manual detection of residual neuromuscular blockade. Absence of fade in response to DBS 3.3 normally excludes severe residual neuromuscular blockade but does not necessarily indicate adequate clinical recovery. Sustained tetanus (50 Hz) correlates with a TOF ratio of at least 0.85.[142]

Myoneuropathies (Critical Illness Polyneuropathy)

Unexpectedly prolonged duration of paralysis after administration of muscle relaxants to patients in the ICU has seemingly reached epidemic proportions.[25,26] Individual patients with so-called ICU neuromuscular syndrome have had a variety of relaxants administered for variable times, have had a variety of underlying critical diseases and coexisting conditions, and have had a spectrum of muscle weakness. Unfortunately, there is considerable overlap between this syndrome, disuse atrophy, polyneuropathy of critical illness, and steroid myopathy. Multiorgan dysfunction, corticosteroid administration, prolonged immobilization, and female sex have been suggested as key risk factors. Some cases appear to represent a pharmacological overdose (i.e., pharmacokinetic category), but other cases seemingly represent specific disease of the neuromuscular structures.[6,12,145] The disease includes marked atrophy of type I and type II muscle fibers, destruction of muscle, relatively little inflammation, and relatively intact motor and sensory nerves.[6] This syndrome may be related in part to synergistic dysfunctional up-regulation of ACh receptors from both a critical illness and the administration of muscle relaxants.[6] It has been suggested that reducing the amount of relaxants used (i.e., dose over time) by monitoring neuromuscular transmission may decrease the risk of prolonged paralysis.[146] Lee suggests that periodic interruption of relaxant administration, pharmacodynamic studies, and neurologic and electrophysiologic studies may be useful in the early detection of this complication. Prolonged neuromuscular blockade in infants and small children may interfere with normal growth and development of muscle and result in moderate to severe residual weakness for months. Immobilization-induced atrophy may not be reversible in developing muscle. Recovery of muscle function thus may be more likely in older infants and children, in whom neuromuscular development has already progressed to a fair degree, than in neonates and especially premature neonates immobilized shortly after birth.[147]

Reversal of Neuromuscular Blockade

Because of the increased potential for respiratory inadequacy from residual neuromuscular blockade in infants, most anesthesiologists routinely antagonize nondepolarizing relaxants. The rule has always been to reverse neuromuscular blockade. Large doses of neostigmine (70 μg/kg) are usually used. In infants, as in adults, neurotransmission returns promptly if few receptors are blocked at the time of reversal. Proper choice of relaxant and careful timing and titration of the dose of relaxant usually ensure that some motor tone is present by the time antagonism is attempted. Certain antibiotics, hypotension, hypothermia, acidosis, or hypocalcemia can prolong or potentiate neuromuscular blockade from nondepolarizing relaxants. Hypothermia, deep sedation, or narcosis per se can also lead to respiratory depression in infants.

The use of intermediate-acting relaxants forces one to reexamine the dictum always to reverse blockade. Clearly, the margin of safety of relaxants is increased with objective criteria to judge the adequacy of neuromuscular transmission. As stated in the preceding section, these criteria include a TOF ratio greater than 0.9, the ability to sustain tetanus at 50 Hz, a vital capacity of 15 to 20 ml/kg, the ability to flex the arms and legs, and an inspiratory force greater than 50 cm H_2O. If the infant or child can meet several of these criteria without reversal, no reversal is needed. When there is doubt, however, a drug should be given to reverse blockade.

Fisher et al[105,148] have examined the dose of neostigmine and edrophonium required in infants, children, and adults to reverse a 90% blockade from a continuous d-tubocurarine infusion. In infants and children 15 μg/kg of neostigmine produced a 50% antagonism of the d-tubocurarine blockade; in adults 23 μg/kg was required. It was claimed that the duration of antagonism was equal in all three groups, although the elimination half-life was clearly shorter in infants. A larger dose than that seemingly recommended would give a higher sustained blood concentration. Whether this is of pharmacological benefit in the absence of a continuous infusion or relaxant is doubtful. The dissociation between the elimination half-life and the duration of antagonism may result from the carbamylation of cholinesterase by neostigmine. In infants, 145 μg/kg of edrophonium produced a 50% antagonism of the d-tubocurarine blockade; in children, 233 μg/kg was required; and in adults, 128 μg/kg was required. The volume of distribution of edrophonium was similar in all age groups. The elimination half-life of edrophonium was shorter in infants than in children or adults; thus clearance was more rapid in infants. Because the molecular interaction between edrophonium and cholinesterase is readily reversible, Fisher et al[105,148] suggest that the shorter elimination half-life for edrophonium might limit its value in pediatric patients. This is doubtful.

Meakin et al[149] compared the rate of recovery from pancuronium-induced neuromuscular blockade after various doses of neostigmine (0.036 or 0.07 mg/kg) with edrophonium (0.7 or 1.43 mg/kg) in infants and children. In the first 5 minutes, recovery of neuromuscular transmission was more rapid after edrophonium than after neostigmine in all age groups; recovery was more rapid in infants and children than in adults. By 10 minutes there was no difference in neuromuscular transmission achieved in infants and children with either reversal agent (at either dose); adults had lower neuromuscular transmission at the lower dose (0.036 mg/kg) of neostigmine. Thus if speed of initial recovery is a critical issue, then edrophonium is better than neostigmine, and a high dose of neostigmine is better than a low dose. At 30 minutes after injection of either reversal agent (at any dose), there was no difference between neuromuscular transmission among age groups.

REFERENCES

1. Elliot JM, Bion JF: The use of neuromuscular blocking drugs in intensive care practice. *Acta Anaesthesiol Scand* 39:70, 1995.
2. Fiamengo SA, Savarese JJ: Use of muscle relaxants in intensive care units. *Crit Care Med* 19:1457, 1991.
3. Fleming NW: Neuromuscular blocking drugs in the intensive care unit: indications, protocols, and complications. *Semin Anesth* 13:255, 1994.
4. Kim C, Hirose M, Martyn JAJ: d-Tubocurarine accentuates the burn-induced upregulation of nicotinic acetylcholine receptors at the muscle membrane. *Anesthesiology* 83:309-315, 1995.
5. Klessig HT, Geiger HJ, Murray MJ, et al: A national survey on the practice patterns of anesthesiologist intensivists in the use of muscle relaxants. *Crit Care Med* 20:1341, 1992.
6. Lee C: Intensive care unit neuromuscular syndrome? *Anesthesiology* 83:237, 1995.
7. Magorian T, Lynam DP: Clinical use of muscle relaxants in patients with hepatic disease. In Rupp SM, editor: *Problems in anaesthesia: neuromuscular relaxants,* Philadelphia, 1992, JB Lippincott.
8. Martyn JAJ, White DA, Gronert GA, et al: Up-and-down regulation of skeletal muscle acetylcholine receptors. *Anesthesiology* 76: 822-843, 1992.
9. Miller RD: Use of neuromuscular blocking drugs in intensive care unit patients. *Anesth Analg* 81:1-2, 1995.
10. Rupp SM: Muscle relaxants and the patient with renal and/or hepatic failure. In Azar I, editor: *Muscle relaxants,* New York, 1993.
11. Viby-Mogensen J: Monitoring neuromuscular function in the intensive care unit. *Intensive Care Med* 19(suppl):S74, 1993.

12. Watling SM, Dasta JF: Prolonged paralysis in intensive care unit patients after the use of neuromuscular blocking agents: a review of the literature. *Crit Care Med* 22:884, 1994.
13. Calakos N, Scheller RH: Synaptic vesicle biogenesis, docking, and fusion: a molecular description. *Physiol Rev* 76:1-29, 1996.
14. Prince RJ, Since SM: The ligand binding domains of the nicotinic acetylcholine receptor. In Barrantes FJ, editor: The nicotinic acetylcholine receptor: current views and future trends, Berlin, New York,1998, Springer-Verlag.
15. Sanes JR, Lichtman JW: Development of vertebrate neuromuscular junction. *Ann Rev Neurosci* 22:389-442, 1999.
16 Blount P, Merlie JP: Molecular basis of the two nonequivalent ligand binding sites of the muscle nicotinic acetylcholine receptor. *Neuron* 3:349, 1989.
17. Gu Y, Franco A Jr, Gardner PD, et al: Properties of embryonic and adult muscle acetylcholine receptors transiently expressed in COS cells. *Neuron* 5:147, 1990.
18. Pedersen SE, Cohen JB: d-Tubocurarine binding sites are located at a-g and a-d subunit interfaces of the nicotinic acetylcholine receptor. *Proc Natl Acad Sci* 87:2785, 1990.
19.. Yost CS, Dodson BA: Inhibition of the nicotinic acetylcholine receptor by barbiturates and by procaine: do they act at different sites? *Cell Mol Neurobiol* 13:159, 1993.
20. Yost CS: Fetal-type acetylcholine receptors are more sensitive than adult-type to pancuronium blockade at equipotent agonist concentration. *Anesthesiology* 81:3A, 1994.
21. Paul M, Kindler CH, Fokt RM, et al: The potency of new muscle relaxants on recombinant muscle-type acetylcholine receptors. *Anesth Analg* 94:597-603, 2002.
22. Paul M, Fokt RM, Kindler CH, et al: Characterization of the interactions between volatile anesthetics and neuromuscular blockers at the muscle nicotinic acetylcholine receptor. *Anesth Analg* 95:362-367, 2002.
23. Bowman WC: Prejunctional and postjunctional cholinoreceptors at the neuromuscular junction. *Anesth Analg* 59:935, 1980.
24. Prielipp RC, Coursin DB, Scuderi PE, et al: Comparison of the infusion requirements and recovery profiles of vecuronium and cisatracurium 51W89 in intensive care unit patients. *Crit Care Trauma* 81:3, 1995.
25. Segredo V, Caldwell JE, Matthay MA, et al: Persistent paralysis in critically ill patients after long-term administration of vecuronium. *N Engl J Med* 327:524, 1992.
26. Tobias JD, Lynch A, McDuffee A, et al: Pancuronium infusion for neuromuscular block in children in the pediatric intensive care unit. *Anesth Analg* 81:13, 1995.
27. Naguib M, Flood P, McArdle JJ, et al: Advances in neurobiology of the neuromuscular junction. *Anesthesiology* 96:202-231, 2002.
28. Lee, C: Structure, conformation, and action of neuromuscular blocking drugs. *Br J Anaesth* 5:755-769, 1987.
29. Wareham AC, Morton RH, Meakin GH: Low quantal content of the endplate potential reduces safety factor for neuromuscular transmission in the diaphragm of the newborn rat. *Br J Anaesth* 72:205-209, 1994.
30. Meakin G, Morton RH, Wareham AC: Age-dependent variation in response to tubocurarine in the isolated rat diaphragm. *Br J Anaesth* 68:161-163, 1992.
31. Goudsouzian NG: Maturation of neuromuscular transmission in the infant. *Br J Anaesth* 52:205, 1980.
32. Crumrine RS, Yodlowski EH: Assessment of neuromuscular function in infants. *Anesthesiology* 54:29, 1981.
33. Donati F, Bevan DR: Long-term succinylcholine infusion during isoflurane. *Anesthesiology* 58:6, 1983.
34. Goudsouzian NG, Liu LMP: The neuromuscular response of infants to a continuous infusion of succinylcholine. *Anesthesiology* 60:97, 1984.
35. Lee C: Self antagonism: possible mechanism of tachyphylaxis in suxamethonium-induced neuromuscular block in man. *Br J Anaesth* 48:1097, 1986.
36. Sutherland GA, Bevan JC, Bevan DR: Neuromuscular blockade in infants following intramuscular succinylcholine in two or five percent solution. *Can J Anaesth* 30:342, 1980.
37. Dahaba AA, von Klobucar F, Rehak PH, et al: The neuromuscular transmission module versus the relaxometer mechanomyogaph for neuromuscular block monitoring. *Anesth Analg* 94:591-6, 2002.
38. Kopman AF, Kumar S, Klewicka MM, et al: The staircase phenomenon: Implications for monitoring of neuromuscular transmission. *Anesthesiology* 95:403-7, 2001.
39. Kopman AF, Klewicka MM, Neuman, GG: Reexamined: The recommended endotracheal intubating dose for nondepolarizing neuromuscular blockers of rapid onset. *Anesth Analg* 93:954-9, 2001.
40. Kopman AF, Khan NA, Neuman GG: Precurarization and priming: a theoretical analysis of safety and timing. *Anesth Analg* 93: 1253-1256, 2001.
41. Tang TT, Oechler HW, Siker D, et al: Anesthesia-induced rhabdomyolysis in infants with unsuspected Duchenne dystrophy. *Acta Paediatr* 81:716-719, 1992.
42. Gronert GA: Mortality greater with rhabdomyolysis than receptor upregulation, *Anesthesiology* 94:523-529, 2001.
43. Hopkins PM: Use of suxamethonium in children. *Br J Anaesth* 75:675-677, 1995.
44. Cook DR, Fischer CG. Neuromuscular blocking effects of succinylcholine in infants and children, *Anesthesiology* 42:662-665, 1975.
45. Meakin G, McKiernan EP, Morris P et al: Dose-response curves for suxamethonium in neonates, infants and children. *Br J Anaesth* 62:655, 1989.
46. Heir T, Feiner JR, Lin, J, et al: Hemoglobin desaturation after succinylcholine-induced apnea. *Anesthesia* 94:754-759, 2001.
47. Cook DR, Westman HR, Rosenfeld L, et al: Pulmonary edema in infants: possible association with intramuscular succinylcholine. *Anesth Analg* 60:220, 1981.
48. Minton MD, Grosslight K, Stirt JA, et al: Increases in intracranial pressure from succinylcholine: prevention by prior nondepolarizing blockade. *Anesthesiology* 65:165, 1986.
49. Delphin E, Jackson D, Rothstein P: Use of succinylcholine during elective pediatric anesthesia should be reevaluated. *Anesth Analg* 66:1190, 1987.
50. Rosenberg H, Gronert GA: Intractable cardiac arrest in children given succinylcholine, *Anesthesiology* 77:1054, 1992
51. Schow AJ, Lubarsky DA, Olson RP, et al: Can succinylcholine be used safely in hyperkalemic patients? *Anesth Analg* 95:119-22, 2002.
52. Dierdorf SF, McNiece WL, Wolfe TM, et al: Effect of thiopental and succinylcholine on serum potassium concentrations in children. *Anesth Analg* 63:1136, 1984.
53. Henning RD, Bush GH. Plasma potassium after halothanesuxamethonium induction in children. *Anaesthesia* 37:802, 1982.
54. Harrington JF, Ford DJ, Striker TW: Myoglobinemia and myoglobinuria after succinylcholine in children, *Anesthesiology* 59:A439, 1983.
55. Flewellen EH, Nelson TE: Halothane-succinylcholine induced masseter spasm: indicative of malignant hyperthermia susceptibility. *Anesth Analg* 63:693, 1984.
56. Schwartz L, Rockoff MA, Koka BV: Masseter spasm with anesthesia: incidence and implications. *Anesthesiology* 61:772, 1984.
57. DeCook TH, Goudsouzian NG: Tachyphylaxis and phase II block development during infusion of succinylcholine in children. *Anesth Analg* 59:639, 1980.
58. Plumley MH, Bevan JC, Saddler JM, et al: Dose-related effects of succinylcholine on the adductor pollicis and masseter muscles in children. *Can J Anaesth* 37:15, 1989.
59. Saddler JM, Bevan JC, Plumley MH, et al: Jaw tension after succinylcholine in children undergoing strabismus surgery. *Can J Anaesth* 37:21, 1989.
60. Van der Spek AF, Reynolds PI, Ashton-Miller JA, et al: Differing effect of agonist and antagonist muscle relaxants on cat jaw muscles. *Anesth Analg* 69:76, 1989.
61. Van der Spek AF, Fang WB, Ashton-Miller JA, et al: Increased masticatory muscle stiffness during limb muscle flaccidity associated with succinylcholine administration. *Anesthesiology* 69:11, 1988.
62. Cook DR: Can succinylcholine be abandoned? *Anesth Analg* 90:S24-S8, 2000.
63. Bencini A, et al: Clinical pharmacokinetics of vecuronium. In Agoston S et al, editors: *Clinical experiences with Norcuron (Org NC 45 vecuronium bromide)*, Amsterdam, 1983, Excerpta Medica.
64. Savage DS, Sleigh T, Carlyle I: The emergence of ORG NC 45 from the pancuronium series. *Br J Anaesth* 52:3S, 1980.
65. Marshall IG, Gibb AJ, Durant NN: Neuromuscular and vagal blocking actions of pancuronium bromide, its metabolites, and

vecuronium bromide (ORG NC 45) and its potential metabolites in the anesthetized cat. *Br J Anaesth* 55:703, 1983.
66. Goudsouzian NG, Liu LMP, Cote CJ: Comparison of equipotent doses of non-depolarizing muscle relaxants in children. *Anesth Analg* 60:862, 1981.
67. Goudsouzian NG, Martyn JJA, Liu LMP: The dose response effect of long-acting non-depolarizing neuromuscular blocking agents in children. *Can J Anaesth* 3:246, 1984.
68. Cook DR: Sensitivity of the newborn to tubocurarine. *Br J Anaesth* 53:320, 1981.
69. Fisher DM, O'Keeffe C, Stanski DR, et al: Pharmacokinetics and pharmacodynamics of d-tubocurarine in infants, children, and adults. *Anesthesiology* 57:203, 1982.
70. Blinn A, Woelfel SK, Cook DR, et al: Pancuronium dose-response revisited. *Paediatr Anesthe* 2:153, 1992.
71. Duvaldestin P, Saada J, Berger JL, et al: Pharmacokinetics, pharmacodynamics, and dose-response relationships of pancuronium in control and elderly subjects. *Anesthesiology* 56:36, 1982.
72. Lavine LM, Hindein BI: Hemodialysis as treatment for prolonged neuromuscular blockade in anephric patients. *Anesthesiology* 59:264, 1983.
73. Pittet JF, Tassonyi E, Morel DR, et al: Pipecuronium-induced neuromuscular blockade during nitrous oxide-fentanyl, isoflurane, and halothane anesthesia in adults and children. *Anesthesiology* 71:210, 1989.
74. Sarner JB, Brandom BW, Dong ML, et al: Clinical pharmacology of pipecuronium in infants and children during halothane anesthesia. *Anesth Analg* 71:362, 1990.
75. Caldwell JE, Canfell PC, Castagnoli KP, et al: The influence of renal failure on the pharmacokinetics and duration of action of pipecuronium bromide in patients anesthetized with halothane and nitrous oxide. *Anesthesiology* 70:7, 1989.
76. Caballero PA, Johnson RE: Long-lasting neuromuscular blockade from pipecuronium. *Anesthesiology* 76:154, 1992.
77. Sarner JB, Brandom BW, Cook DR, et al: Clinical pharmacology of doxacurium chloride (BW A938U) in children. *Anesth Analg* 67:303-306, 1988.
78. Dresner DL, Basta SJ, Ali HA, et al: Pharmacokinetics and pharmacodynamics of doxacurium in young and elderly patients during isoflurane anesthesia. *Anesth Analg* 71:498, 1990.
79. Cook DR, Freeman JA, Lai AA, et al: Pharmacokinetics and pharmacodynamics of doxacurium in normal patients and in those with hepatic or renal failure. *Anesth Analg* 72:145, 1991.
80. Brandom BW, Cook DR, Woelfel SK, et al: Atracurium infusion in children during fentanyl, halothane, and isoflurane anesthesia. *Anesth Anal*g 64:471, 1985.
81. Goudsouzian NG, et al: Neuromuscular effect of atracurium in infants and children. *Anesthesiology* 62:75, 1985.
82. Goudsouzian NG, Liu LM, Cote CJ, et al: Safety and efficacy of atracurium in adolescents and children anesthetized with halothane. *Anesthesiology* 59:459, 1983.
83. Stiller RL, Brandom BW, Cook DR: Determination of atracurium by high-performance liquid chromatography. *Anesth Analg* 64:58, 1985.
84. Stiller RL, Cook DR, Chakravorti S: In vitro degradation of atracurium in human plasma. *Br J Anaesth* 57:1085, 1985.
85. d'Hollander AA, Luyckx C, Barvais L, et al: Clinical evaluation of atracurium besylate requirement for a stable muscle relaxation during surgery: lack of age-related effects, Anesthesiology 59:237, 1983.
86. Neill EAM, Chapple DJ: Metabolic studies in the cat with atracurium: neuromuscular blocking agent designed for non-enzymatic inactivation at physiological pH. *Xenobiotica* 12:203, 1983.
87. Fahey MR, Rupp SM, Fisher DM, et al: The pharmacokinetics and pharmacodynamics of atracurium in patients with and without renal failure. *Anesthesiology* 61:699, 1984.
88. Hunter JM, Jones RS, Utting JE: Use of atracurium in patients with no renal function. *Br J Anaesth* 54:1251, 1982.
89. Ward S, Neil EAM: Pharmacokinetics of atracurium in acute hepatic failure (with acute renal failure). *Br J Anaesth* 55:1169, 1983.
90. Welch RM, Brown A, Ravitch J, et al: The in vitro degradation of cisatracurium, the R, cis-R'-isomer of atracurium, in human and rat plasma. *Clin Pharmacol Ther* 58:132, 1995.
91. Babel A: Etude comparative de la laudanosine et de la papaverine au point de vue pharmacodynamique. *Rev Med Suisse Romande* 19:657, 1989.
92. Tobias JD, Johnson JO, Sprague K, et al: Effects of rapacuronium on respiratory function during general anesthesia. *Anesthesiology* 95:908-912, 2001.
93. DeWolf AM, Freeman JA, Scott VL, et al: Pharmacokinetics and pharmacodynamics of cisatracurium in patients with end-stage liver disease undergoing liver transplantation. *Br J Anesth* 76: 624, 1996.
94. Dhonneur G, Cerf C, Lagneau F, et al: The pharmacokinetics of cisatracurium in patients with acute respiratory distress syndrome. *Anesth Analg* 93:400-404, 2001.
95. Reich DL, Hollinger I, Harrington DJ, et al: Pharmacokinetic comparison of cisatracurium and vecuronium infusions in neonates and infants following congenital heart surgery. *Anesthesiology*, October 2002.
96. Eddleston JM, Harper NJ, Pollard BJ, et al: Concentrations of atracurium and laudanosine in cerebrospinal fluid during intracranial surgery. *Br J Anaesth* 63:525, 1989.
97. Parker CJR, Jones JE, Hunter JM: Disposition of atracurium and its metabolite, laudanosine, in patients in renal and respiratory failure in an ITU. *Br J Anaesth* 61:531, 1988.
98. Fahey MR, Rupp SM, Canfell C, et al: The effect of renal failure on laudanosine excretion in man. *Br J Anaesth* 57:1049, 1985.
99. Ingram MD, Sclabassi RJ, Cook DR, et al: Cardiovascular and electroencephalographic effects of laudanosine in "nephrectomized" cats. *Br J Anaesth* 58:14S, 1986.
100. Shi WZ, Fahey MR, Fisher DM, et al: Laudanosine (a metabolite of atracurium) increases the minimum alveolar concentration of halothane in rabbits. *Anesthesiology* 63:584, 1985.
101. Lanier WL, Milde JH, Michenfelder JD: The cerebral effects of pancuronium and atracurium in halothane-anesthetized dogs. *Anesthesiology* 63:589, 1985.
102. Chiodini F, Charpantier E, Muller D, et al: Blockade and activation of the human neuronal nicotinic acetylcholine receptors by atracurium and laudanosine. *Anesthesiology* 94:643-651, 2001.
103. d'Hollander A, Massaux F, Nevelsteen M, et al: Age-dependent dose-response relationship of ORG NC45 in anesthetized patients. *Br J Anaesth* 54:653, 1982.
105. Fisher DM, Cronnelly R, Miller RD, et al: The neuromuscular pharmacology of neostigmine in infants and children, *Anesthesiology* 59:220, 1983.
110. Woelfel SK, Brandom BW, Cook DR, et al: Effects of bolus administration of ORG-9426 in children during nitrous oxide-halothane anesthesia. *Anesthesiology* 76:939, 1992.
115. Gatke MR, Ostergaard D, Bundgaard JR, et al: Response to mivacurium in a patient compound heterozygous for a novel and a known silent mutation in the butyrylcholinesterase gene: genotyping by sequencing. *Anesthesiology* 95:600-6, 2001.
140. Fisher DM, Miller RD: Neuromuscular effects of vecuronium (ORG NC45) in infants and children during N_2O-halothane anesthesia. *Anesthesiology* 58:519, 1983.
106. Duvaldestin P, et al: Pharmacokinetics and pharmacodynamics of ORG NC 45 in patients with cirrhosis. *Anesthesiology* 57:A238, 1982.
107. Lynam DP, Cronnelly R, Castagnoli KP, et al: The pharmacodynamics and pharmacokinetics of vecuronium in patients anesthetized with isoflurane with normal renal function or with renal failure. *Anesthesiology* 69:227, 1988.
108. Kopman A: Pancuronium, gallamine, and d-tubocurarine compared: Is speed of onset inversely related to drug potency? *Anesthesiology* 70:915, 1989.
109. O'Kelly B, Frossard J, Meistelman C, et al: Neuromuscular blockade following ORG 9426 in children during N_2O-halothane anesthesia. *Anesthesiology* 76:A787, 1991.
111. Meretoja OA: Is vecuronium a long-acting neuromuscular blocking agent in neonates and infants? *Br J Anaesth* 62:184, 1989.
112. Khuenl-Brady K, Castagnoli KP, Canfell C, et al: The neuromuscular blocking effects and pharmacokinetics of ORG 9426 and ORG 9616 in the cat. *Anesthesiology* 72:669-674, 1990.
113. Cooper RA, Maddineni VR, Mirakhur RK, et al: Time course of neuromuscular effects and pharmacokinetics of rocuronium bromide (ORG 9426) during isoflurane anesthesia in patients with and without renal failure. *Br J Anaesth* 71:222, 1993.

114 Cook DR, Chakravorti S, Brandom BW, et al: Effects of neostigmine, edrophonium and succinylcholine on the in vitro metabolism of mivacurium: clinical correlates. *Anesthesiology* 77:A948, 1992.
116. Ostergaard D, Rasmussen SN, Vib-Mogensen J, et al: The influence of drug-induced low plasma cholinesterase activity on the pharmacokinetics and pharmacodynamics of mivacurium. *Anesthesiology* 92:1581-1587, 2000.
117. Beaufort TM, Nigrovic V, Proost JH, et al: Inhibition of the enzymic degradation of suxamethonium and mivacurium increases the onset time of submaximal neuromuscular block. *Anesthesiology* 89:707-714, 1998.
118. Cook DR, Freeman JA, Lai AA, et al: Pharmacokinetics of mivacurium in normal patients and in those with hepatic or renal failure. *Br J Anaesth* 69:580, 1992.
119. Head-Rapson AG, Devlin JC, Parker CJR, et al: Pharmacokinetics of the three isomers of mivacurium and pharmacodynamics of the chiral mixture in hepatic cirrhosis. *Br J Anaesth* 73:613, 1994.
120. Lien CA, Schmith VD, Embree PB, et al: The pharmacokinetics and pharmacodynamics of the stereoisomers of mivacurium in patients receiving nitrous oxide/opioid/barbiturate anesthesia. *Anesthesiology* 80:1296, 1994.
121. Meretoja OA, Taivainen T, Wirtavuori K: Pharmacodynamics of mivacurium in infants. *Br J Anaesth* 73:490, 1994.
122. Woelfel SK, Brandom BW, McGowan FX, et al: Clinical pharmacology of mivacurium in pediatric patients less than two years old during nitrous oxide-halothane anesthesia. *Anesth Analg* 77:713, 1993.
123. Gronert BJ, Woelfel SK, Cook DR: Comparison of the neuromuscular effects of mivacurium and succinylcholine in infants and children. *Acta Anaesthesiol Scand* 39:35, 1995.
124. Gronert B, Woelfel S, Cook DR: Comparison of equipotent intubating doses of mivacurium and succinylcholine in infants 2-12 months old. *Anesthesiology* 79:A932, 1993.
125. Gronert BJ, Brandom: Neuromuscular blocking drugs in infants and children. *Pediatr Clin North Am* 41:73, 1994.
126. Gronert B, Woelfel S, Cook DR: Comparison of equipotent doses of mivacurium and succinylcholine in children 2-12 years old. *Anesthesiology* 79:A966, 1993.
127. Fine GF, Motoyama EK, Brandom BW, et al: The effect on lung mechanics in anesthetized children with rapacuronium: A comparative study with mivacurium. *Anesth Analg* 95:56-61, 2002.
128. Östergaard D, Gatke MR, Rasmussen BH, et al: The pharmacodynamics and pharmacokinetics of mivacurium in children. *Acta Anaesthesiol Scand* 46:512-518, 2002.
129. Markakis DA, Lau M, Brown R, et al: The pharmacokinetics and steady state pharmacodynamics of mivacurium in children. *Anesthesiology* 88:978-983, 1998.
130. Brandom BW, Sarner JB, Woelfel SK, et al: Mivacurium infusion requirements in pediatric surgical patients during nitrous oxide-halothane and during nitrous oxide-narcotic anesthesia. *Anesth Analg* 71:16, 1990.
131. Goudsouzian N, Chakravorti S, Denman W, et al: Lack of accumulation of the cis-cis isomer of mivacurium in patients with low plasma cholinesterase activity. *Anesthesiology* 81:1060, 1994.
132. Head-Rapson AG, Devlin JC, Parker CJ, et al: Pharmacokinetics and pharmacodynamics of the three isomers of mivacurium in health, in end-stage renal failure and in patients with impaired renal function. *Br J Anaesth* 75:31-36, 1995.
133. Head-Rapson AG, Devlin JC, Parker CJ, et al: Pharmacokinetics of the three isomers of mivacurium and pharmacodynamics of the chiral mixture in hepatic cirrhosis. *Br J Anaesth* 73:613-8, 1994.
134. Levy G: Effect of hepatic cirrhosis on the pharmacodynamics and pharmacokinetics of mivacurium in humans. *Pharm Res* 11: 772-773, 1994.
135. Brandom BW, Woelfel SK, Cook DR, et al: Clinical pharmacology of atracurium in infants. *Anesth Analg* 63:309, 1984.
136. Brandom BW, Rudd GD, Cook DR: Clinical pharmacology of atracurium in pediatric patients. *Br J Anaesth* 55:117S, 1983.
137. Basta SJ, Savarese JJ, Ali HH, et al: Histamine-releasing potencies of atracurium dimethyltubocurarine and tubocurarine. *Br J Anaesth* 55:105, 1983.
138. Basta SJ, Savareses JJ, Ali HH, et al: Vecuronium does not alter serum histamine within the clinical dose range. *Anesthesiology* 59:A273, 1983.
139. Nightingale DA, Bush GH: Atracurium in paediatric anesthesia. *Br J Anaesth* 55:115S, 1983.
140. Koppert W, Blunk JA, Petersen LJ: Different patterns of mast cel activation by muscle relaxants in human skin. *Anesthesiology* 95:659-667, 2001.
141. Harper NJ, Greer R, Conway D: Neuromuscular monitoring in intensive care patients: milliamperage requirements for supramaximal stimulation. *Br J Anaesth* 87:625-627, 2001.
142. Pavlin EG, Halle RH, Schaene R: Recovery of airway protection compared with ventilation in humans after paralysis with curare. *Anesthesiology* 70:381, 1989.
143. Viby-Mogensen J, Jensen NH, Engbaek J, et al: Tactile and visual evaluation of the response to train-of-four stimulation. *Anesthesiology* 63:440, 1985.
144. Drenck NE, Ueda N, Olsen NV, et al: Manual evaluation of residual curarization using double burst stimulation: a comparison with train of four. *Anesthesiology* 70:578, 1989.
145. De Jonghe B, Sharshar, T, Lefaucheur JP, et al: Paresis acquired in the intensive care unit. *JAMA* 288:2859-2867, 2002.
146. Fine GF, Brandom BW, Yellon RF: Unmasked residual neuromuscular block after administration of vecuronium for days. *Anesth Analg* 93:345-7, 2001.
147. Shear CR: Effects of disuse on growing and adult chick skeletal muscle. *J Cell Sci* 48:35, 1981.
148. Fisher DM, Cronnelly R, Sharma M, et al: Clinical pharmacology of edrophonium in infants. *Anesthesiology* 61:428, 1984.
149. Meakin G, Sweet PT, Bevan JC, et al: Neostigmine and edrophonium as antagonists of pancuronium in infants and children. *Anesthesiology* 59:316, 1983.

CHAPTER

116

Sedation and Analgesia

Christopher M.B. Heard and James E. Fletcher

PEARLS

- A wide selection of different sedation and analgesia options is available in the pediatric intensive care unit (PICU).
- There is no ideal sedative agent for all patients.
- Most children do well with a combination of opiates (fentanyl) and supplementation with benzodiazepines (BZDs) either by infusion (midazolam) or on an as required basis (PRN) (lorazepam) to provide adjunct anxiolysis and amnesia.
- Postoperatively, patients require adequate analgesia, which may include the use of epidural anesthesia or patient-controlled analgesia (PCA).
- In circumstances in which the ability to perform a rapid neurologic examination is required, use of short-acting agents such as remifentanil, propofol, or isoflurane may be warranted.
- All the sedative agents develop tolerance with prolonged use. The intensivist must be aware that, potentially, withdrawal can occur.
- A proactive treatment plan with methadone at the equivalent dose can effectively and safely prevent opiate withdrawal in the patient in the PICU.

Sedation is an integral part of patient management in the pediatric intensive care unit (PICU). It is necessary to minimize the perception and response to anxiety and pain. Children who are not adequately sedated or are experiencing pain may become tachycardic and hypertensive, and are at risk of losing their airway and central lines. Conversely, oversedation can cause cardiovascular depression and ileus and may interfere with a comprehensive neurologic examination. In patients who undergo prolonged sedation, tolerance and tachyphylaxis develop, and these lead to increasing sedative requirements.

Patients can recall their stay in the ICU. Many remember the tracheal tube or the ventilation of their lungs. Nightmares and hallucinations have also been reported.[1] Either single-drug therapy or inadequate dosing may be associated with a higher incidence of recall[2] in the patient with paralysis. In adults, delusional memories and an underlying anxiety state were predictors in the development of a posttraumatic stress disorder after sedation in the ICU.[3] Delusional memories were reported much more frequently than factual memory, probably because patients have difficulty correctly remembering the events that occur during their stay in the ICU. Taken together, the underlying illness, the multiplicity of different sedative agents, disorientation, and altered sleep patterns affect the ability of the patient to correctly remember. In the pediatric patient, recall of the PICU has also been reported.[4] More than 66% remembered their stay in the PICU. Eighteen percent had bad memories, 16% remembered ventilation and anxiety, and 29% remembered pain from a procedure or movement. Overall the recollections of patients in the PICU were only unpleasant in 15% of the patients. Sleep disturbance was also a problem.

Various scoring systems are often used to guide sedation. The most widely used is the Ramsay scale.[5] The patient's level of consciousness is classified as one of six scores (Table 116–1). The nurse at the bedside assesses the patient and then changes the sedation regimen as necessary to achieve the desired level of sedation. The ideal level of sedation varies from patient to patient, but in general,

TABLE 116–1

Ramsay Scale

Level	Description
1	Patient awake, anxious, and agitated or restless or both
2	Patient awake, cooperative, oriented, and tranquil
3	Patient awake, responds to command only
4	Patient asleep, brisk response to light glabellar tap or loud auditory stimulus
5	Patient asleep, sluggish response to light glabellar tap or loud auditory stimulus
6	Patient asleep, no response to light glabellar tap or loud auditory stimulus

most intensivists would seek to maintain a patient who is sleepy but easily awakened. A level of 2 or 3 seems to be ideal as the clinical endpoint for sedation in the Ramsay scale. Deeper sedation should be reserved for select patients who are often younger, are receiving muscle relaxants, or have a head injury. The use of a sedation scoring system to guide sedation of surgical critical care patients has been evaluated for cost-effectiveness. Scoring systems have proved to be cost saving for the ICU.[6] Because the patient can be more rapidly weaned from the ventilator through better control of the sedation level, the number of days a patient is connected to a ventilator is reduced.

The COMFORT score, composed of eight variables (each with five categories), has also been validated for use in the PICU to assess the sedation level in children. Use of this system, however, is more complicated and time-consuming.[7]

Many scoring systems are subjective and are limited by interobserver variability. The more objective methods may be too cumbersome for routine use. A simple scoring system has been devised, though, that is easy to use and minimizes subjectivity and observer variability.[8] This system is the Brussels sedation scale. It is similar to the Ramsay scale, but the Brussels scale levels that correspond to the Ramsay scale levels 4 and 5 are better differentiated (Table 116–2).

The Bispectral Index (BIS) is a processed electroencephalogram (EEG) monitor that measures the hypnotic effects of anesthetics and sedatives. The BIS is an empirical, statistically derived measurement. The BIS monitor reports a single number from 0 to 100 that represents an integrated measure of cerebral electrical activity. The BIS has been validated as a measure of hypnosis in adults in the operating room and ICU.[9] More recently it has been validated in the PICU.[10]

TABLE 116–2

Brussels Sedation Scale

Level	Description
1	Unable to be aroused
2	Responds to painful stimulation (trapezius muscle pinching) but not auditory stimulation
3	Responds to auditory stimulation
4	Awake and alert
5	Agitated

The BIS is an exciting new approach to EEG processing. It measures a state of the brain, representing the degree of alertness. It does not measure the concentration of a particular drug.[11] Although a number 100 on the BIS score indicates that the patient is fully awake, a number less than 40 is suggestive of a deep hypnotic effect. A BIS value of less than 60 in surgical patients was not associated with a recall.[12] The use of the BIS monitor in adult surgical patients and in older pediatric patients has shown a reduction in anesthesia requirements and a shorter recovery time.

The BIS monitor has been studied in several adult ICU populations. These studies have shown a correlation between the BIS score and a variety of sedation scores.[13] One of the main difficulties with clinical sedation scoring systems is their inability to assess depth of sedation in the patient with paralysis. Patients who require paralysis in the operating room are considered to be at increased risk of awareness during anesthesia.[14] This problem also exists for the sedated patient with paralysis in the PICU. It is well known that the clinical signs of inadequate anesthesia or sedation are not reliable,[15] and many other reasons account for alterations in the heart rate, blood pressure, perfusion, and pupillary responses in the patient in the PICU. In a study using the BIS in pediatric patients with paralysis,[16] researchers found that in more than 8% of the sedation assessments in which patients were thought to be adequately sedated by the bedside nurse, their BIS scores were greater than 80 (Fig. 116–1). This reflected a significant risk of awareness. The BIS correlates well with the Ramsay scale in the sedated child and may be a useful monitor to prevent inadequate sedation in a child with paralysis.

Opioids

Sedation in the PICU is most commonly achieved with a mixture of opioids and benzodiazepines (BZDs). Although many synthetic and naturally occurring opioids

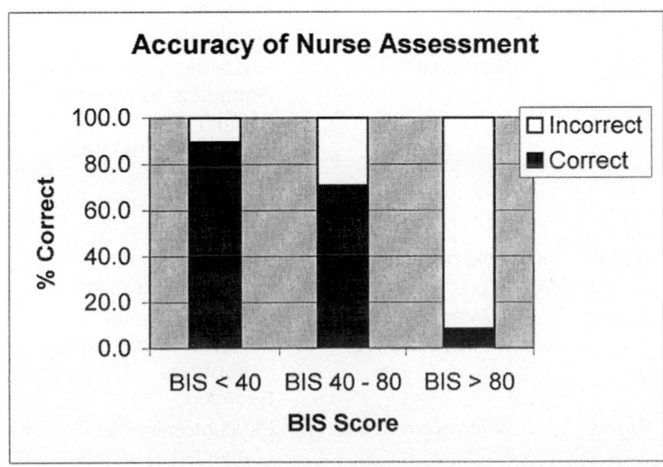

FIGURE 116–1 • Nurse sedation assessment of the paralyzed patient.

exist, morphine is considered the agent against which others are compared. The primary source of morphine is opium obtained from the opium poppy (*Papaver somniferum*), which also produces alkaloids such as codeine, thebaine, papaverine, and noscapine. *Opiates* are substances derived from opium; the term *opioid* also describes substances derived from opiates (e.g., oxycodone) but also includes substances that are created synthetically but have properties that are similar to those of opiates (e.g., fentanyl and methadone) and endogenous ligands. The terms are often used interchangeably because the pharmacological effects fall into the same category. Opioids are agonists at various opioid receptors, for which several endogenous ligands exist. There are three major classes of receptors: mu (μ), kappa (κ), and delta (δ). The opioid receptors possess the same general structure of an extracellular N-terminal region, seven transmembrane domains, and an intracellular C-terminal tail structure. Subtypes of each receptor (e.g., μ1, μ2) exist (Table 116–3), as does the possibility of less well-characterized opioid receptors ε, λ, ι, and ξ.

Most of the therapeutic and adverse effects can be accounted for by agonist activity at the μ receptor, which is responsible for analgesia, respiratory depression, pupillary constriction, and euphoria. At the cellular level, μ-receptor activation alters ionic permeability to K^+, causing hyperpolarization and depression of excitability in the neuronal system. There are associated effects on cholinergic, adrenergic, serotonergic, and dopaminergic neurotransmitter systems within the central nervous system (CNS). These receptors are found at multiple sites along pain pathways including the spinal cord, midbrain, thalamus, and the cortex. At the spinal cord level, pain reflexes (nociceptive) are depressed by receptors in the substantia gelatinosa that are mostly presynaptic and inhibit the release of substance P from C-fiber nerve terminals and account for the effectiveness of intrathecally and epidurally administered opioids. In the midbrain the analgesic effect is mediated in the periaqueductal gray matter (PAG) through ascending fibers and also descending fibers that modulate the function of the dorsal horn. Acetylcholine, γ-aminobutyric acid (GABA), norepinephrine, and serotonin are also involved in these pain-modulating pathways. Peripheral opioid receptors have also been shown and can be expressed in response to inflammation.[17] The intraarticular injection of morphine produces analgesia following arthroscopy through activation of opioid receptors located on white blood cells.[18] The endogenous ligands for the opioid receptors are the enkephalins, endorphins, and dynorphins. They have a morphine-like effect that can be specifically antagonized by the μ-receptor antagonist naloxone. The endomorphins have potent analgesic and gastrointestinal (GI) effects. At the cellular level, they activate G proteins ([35S] GTP gamma-S binding) and inhibit calcium currents.[19] Pro-opiomelanocortin is the precursor for β-endorphin (as well as adrenocorticotropic hormone [ACTH] and melanocyte-stimulating hormone [MSH]). β-Endorphin, itself very active, also includes the amino acid sequence for met-enkephalin, although the main precursor is proenkephalin A, which contains four copies of met-enkephalin and one copy of leu-enkephalin. The met-enkephalin sequence also gives opioid activity to a number of other larger peptides. Proenkephalin B (prodynorphin) gives rise to the dynorphin series and contains three leu-enkephalin sequences.

Local application of these endogenous substances to the brain provides effects that are similar to those of opiates. They do not function as analgesics because the administration of naloxone does not cause pain in the normal state. They are released during periods of sustained pain, stress, or activity to modulate physiologic pathways including those involved with pain. Therefore they are probably important to the physiologic condition of the patient in the ICU.

TABLE 116–3

Classification of Opiate Receptors and Subtypes

Subtype	Prototypic Drugs	Actions
Mu_1	Opiates and most opiate peptides	Supraspinal analgesia including periaqueductal gray matter, nucleus raphe magnus, and locus coeruleus Prolactin release Acetylcholine turnover in brain Catalepsy
Mu_2	Morphine	Respiratory depression Dopamine turnover in brain Gastrointestinal tract transit Most cardiovascular effects
Delta	Enkephalins	Spinal analgesia Dopamine turnover
Kappa	Dynorphin	Spinal analgesia Inhibition of antidiuretic hormone Sedation
Sigma	N-allynormetazocine	Psychotomimetic effects

Modified from Baresh PG, Cullen BF, Stoelting RK et al (editors): *Clinical anesthesia,* ed 2, Philadelphia, 1992, JB Lippincott.

Morphine

Morphine is an opiate, and its primary therapeutic actions are sedation and analgesia. Anxiolysis and euphoria may also occur, and these four therapeutic effects may be exploited to the benefit of the patient. These actions are mediated through the PAG, the ventromedial medulla, and the spinal cord. The reduction of nociceptive reflexes occurs all over the body, even below a completely transected spinal cord. In addition to increasing the sensory threshold for pain, morphine may decrease the hurting aspect (or unpleasantness) of pain; a patient given morphine may say something such as, "I have just as much pain, but it doesn't distress me as much." It blunts most types and intensities of pain, although some forms of neuropathic pain are relatively resistant. The resulting analgesia may be potent enough to abolish diagnostic symptoms and signs. The sedative effects reduce higher cortical function, cause difficulty in concentration, and cause a sense of drowsiness and dream-filled sleep. Higher doses will cause a state of unconsciousness or coma. The rate of respiration is reduced with a resultant fall in minute ventilation despite an accompanying increase in depth of breathing. This is associated with a decreased responsiveness to carbon dioxide (CO_2) and is an additive to the decreased CO_2 response seen during sleep. In some circumstances respiratory drive may be restricted to hypoxic stimulation of the carotid chemoreceptors. This is the most serious dose-related side effect of morphine. It can occur at doses used clinically for analgesia. In general all the opiates produce the same degree of respiratory depression for any given level of analgesia. Opioids are not anticonvulsants, and meperidine (and its metabolite normeperidine) may lower the seizure threshold.

Another CNS effect of morphine is pupillary constriction due to a central effect on the oculomotor nucleus. Nausea results from stimulation of the chemotrigger zone; however, opioids also depress the vomiting center, so the final effect is unpredictable. Nausea and vomiting are much more frequent in the ambulatory patient than in the patient confined to a hospital bed. Stress-related endocrine responses can be modified by morphine. It decreases the release of several hormones including ACTH, antidiuretic hormone (ADH), prolactin, growth hormone (GH), and epinephrine. The neuroendocrine stress response that is normally seen with trauma and surgery may be blunted. Itching may be caused by histamine release, but it may also be due to opiate receptor activation in the spinal cord.[20]

Morphine's effects on smooth muscle cause constipation. It reduces the intestinal propulsion activity through its central and peripheral effects. The central effects may be mediated by the vagus nerve. The direct smooth muscle relaxation and the increased local cholinergic transmission can be partly reversed by naloxone. This decreased motility is the basis of several over-the-counter antidiarrheal preparations including diphenoxylate, a μ agonist that does not cross the blood-brain barrier and thus acts as a peripheral opioid agonist. Morphine also causes an increase in biliary tract tone, which may cause biliary colic, as well as increased tone in the bladder detrusor muscle and vesical sphincter. Urinary retention is common with opioids and occurs in 55% of children receiving spinally administered opioid and 20% receiving intravenous (IV) opioid.[21]

Morphine has been studied extensively in term and preterm neonates. Glucuronidation is present in term babies and in many preterm ones. The half-life ($T_{1/2}$) of morphine, however, is 2 hours in children, 6.5 hours in term neonates, and 9 hours in the preterm child because of reduced clearance. Volume of distribution did not vary with age.[22]

Morphine causes histamine release and can cause peripheral vasodilatation. Infused at analgesic doses, it has little effect on the cardiovascular system, but skin flushing is not uncommon with rapid IV administration. The histamine-releasing potential should be considered in patients with asthma, especially during an acute exacerbation, and in patients with unstable cardiovascular systems for whom safer alternatives, such as fentanyl, exist.

Dosing recommendations in the ICU are the following: bolus, 0.05 to 0.1 mg/kg, and infusion, 10 to 30 μg/kg/hr (50% of this dose if patient is younger than 3 months). The pharmacokinetics of various opiates is shown in Table 116–4.

All opiates are weak bases and are moderately ionized at pH 7.4. Oral morphine is effective but is exposed to hepatic first-pass metabolism, which is variable among patients. The dose for acute pain is equivalent to 2 to 5 times the IV dose, and with long-term use the dose is 1.5 to 2.5 times the IV dose.

Morphine is metabolized to morphine-3-glucuronide (M3G) and M6G in the liver. M3G is the major metabolite and has little morphine-like activity, although some research has suggested that M3G may be associated with an antinociceptive effect, accounting for failure of analgesia during long-term use.[23] In contrast, M6G is many times more potent than morphine itself.

Morphine undergoes significant first-pass hepatic metabolism, whereby after a single parenteral dose, only morphine is initially active. After a single dose by mouth (PO), both morphine and M6G are active. With long-term oral use, M6G accumulates until its analgesic effect is greater than that of morphine. A similar effect can be anticipated with long-term morphine infusion in the patient in the PICU. The glucuronides are excreted by the kidney, together with only a small amount of free morphine. Ninety percent of total urinary excretion occurs within 24 hours.

Tolerance, defined as an increase in the dose required to create the same response, is a potential problem with all opiates. Tolerance is mainly limited to the depressant actions of morphine, including analgesia, respiratory depression, anxiolysis, and drowsiness. Tolerance of morphine's

TABLE 116–4

Opiate Pharmacokinetics

Drug	Elimination Half-life (hr)	Volume Distribution (SS) (L/kg)	Clearance (ml/kg/min)	Protein Binding
Morphine	2.2	3.3	15	30%
Meperidine	3.2	2.8	5	58%
Fentanyl	3.1	3.2	8	79%
Sufentanil	2.7	1.7	13	92%
Alfentanil	1.2	0.3	2.8	89%

Modified from Baresh PG, Cullen BF, Stoelting RK et al (editors): *Clinical anesthesia,* ed 2, Philadelphia, 1992, JB Lippincott.

is minimal. The mechanism of tolerance appears to involve the degree and duration of both μ and κ receptor occupancy. It appears more rapidly after continuous infusion, and cross-tolerance to other opiates is common, although anecdotal evidence suggests that when opioids are switched, a dose reduction may be possible because cross-tolerance sometimes appears incomplete.[24] Receptor down-regulation may also occur, as well as altered metabolism with an increased M3G/M6G ratio. Simultaneous blockade of N-methyl-D-aspartate (NMDA) receptors has been shown to be effective in reducing the development of tolerance.[25] Clinical tolerance appears uncommon with an exposure of less than 3 days, but after prolonged administration, doses 10 to 20 times that which would cause respiratory arrest in nontolerant patients may be tolerated.

Meperidine

Meperidine has one-tenth the potency of morphine. Compared with other common opioids, meperidine has more CNS excitatory effects including tremors, muscle spasm, myoclonus, psychiatric changes, and seizures. These may be due to a central serotoninergic effect.[26] It is metabolized by the liver to normeperidine, which is twice as toxic as meperidine and has a longer $T_{1/2}$ (15 hours). Normeperidine accumulation is enhanced in those patients with an induced cytochrome P450 system. Meperidine has a shorter duration of action (2 to 3 hours) and has a more rapid onset because of its increased lipid solubility, compared with morphine. Meperidine is unique among opioids because of its local anesthetic properties, which are capable of providing surgical spinal analgesia.[27] A small dose (0.125 to 0.25 mg/kg) of meperidine may be used to treat postoperative shivering.

Fentanyl

Fentanyl is one of the most commonly used opiates in the ICU. It is a synthetic derivative of meperidine without most of its unwanted side effects. It is a potent μ agonist and is 100 times more potent than morphine (100 μg fentanyl = 10 mg morphine at peak effect). It has a rapid onset and cessation because of its high lipid solubility (Fig. 116–2). Fentanyl may be administered by several routes, including IV, intramuscular (IM), transmucosal,[28] and subcutaneous (SC), when there is inadequate venous access.

Skeletal muscle rigidity (which can occur with all synthetic opiates) is well described in the literature. It is mediated through the CNS and is an idiopathic response usually associated with a large bolus dose (>5 μg/kg). It may improve with muscle relaxants and is reversible with naloxone. Fentanyl has little cardiovascular effect. Moderate bradycardia is the most common hemodynamic effect and is more likely when vecuronium is also administered. It does not cause histamine release. Dosing in the ICU is bolus, 1 μg/kg, and infusion, 1 to 4 μg/kg/hr (higher as tolerance develops). The short duration of effect of a single dose of fentanyl is not due to metabolism but rather to rapid redistribution. Maximum brain concentration after a bolus is achieved within 90 seconds. Then, because of rapid redistribution, the plasma level falls

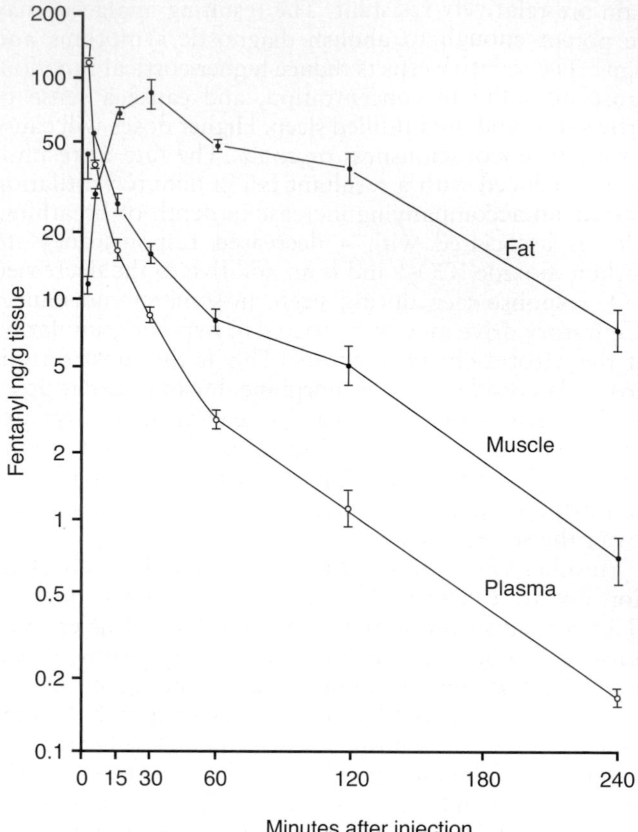

FIGURE 116–2 • Initial fentanyl redistribution.

by 50% in 30 minutes, and the result is a clinical duration of effect of a single dose of about 30 minutes. Fentanyl then accumulates in fat, where it is stored and slowly released with a longer elimination $T_{1/2}$ of about 4 hours (longer than morphine). Marked respiratory depression occurs within 120 seconds, and a single dose of 5 μg/kg will cause apnea in 50% of patients. Also, fentanyl is metabolized by the liver to nor-fentanyl and hydroxy fentanyl derivatives, both of which are thought to be inactive.

In the operating room, high-dose fentanyl is commonly used for cardiac anesthesia and for anesthetization of other unstable patients. A loading dose of 50 μg/kg, followed by 0.5 μg/kg/min, will occupy all opioid receptors and produce a state of anesthesia. Many cases of awareness with patients under anesthesia have been documented, however, even when these high doses of fentanyl were used.

Sufentanil

Sufentanil is another synthetic opiate that has actions and therapeutic effects that are similar to those of fentanyl. It is 5 to 10 times more potent than fentanyl and is the most potent opioid in clinical practice, posing a high risk of apnea with bolus administration. The following are the dosing recommendations:

- Bolus: 0.2 to 0.4 μg/kg
- Infusion: 0.2 to 1 μg/kg/hr

After a single bolus, sufentanil has kinetics similar to that of fentanyl with a short duration of clinical effect about 30 minutes. With prolonged use, however, sufentanil accumulates less and is associated with a more rapid recovery after infusion because of its smaller volume of distribution and similar clearance. When the patient is receiving high doses of fentanyl, sufentanil is useful to conserve infusion volume.

Alfentanil

Alfentanil is another synthetic opiate with a rapid onset. It is 5 times less potent than fentanyl. Although it is less lipid soluble than fentanyl because of its low pKa (negative logarithm of the acid ionization constant), there is a higher percentage of the drug in the active un-ionized form, and this results in a rapid onset. Because of its low volume of distribution, alfentanil has a short elimination $T_{1/2}$; this results in a short duration of action (5 to 10 minutes). Dosing bolus is 5 to 10 μg/kg if there is spontaneous respiration *or* 20 to 50 μg/kg if the patient's lungs are ventilated. Alfentanil is a useful agent for preventing the hypertensive or increased intracranial pressure (ICP) response to intubation. As with all synthetic opiates, there is a risk of muscle rigidity with the higher dosing. Infusion dose is 0.2 to 1 μg/kg/min for patients with ventilated lungs. Postinfusion recovery is quicker with alfentanil than with fentanyl. It is useful by infusion and safe in those patients with hepatic or renal failure.

Codeine

Codeine has a chemical structure and effects that are similar to those of morphine and is commonly used as an oral medication for cough suppression or mild to moderate pain relief. A large part of its effects are due to the metabolism of codeine to morphine. Ten to twenty percent of patients lack a metabolic pathway to convert codeine to morphine and this results an unpredictable effect. Dosing is 0.5 to 1 mg/kg. Constipation is a major side effect, and some patients complain of a vague peculiar or unpleasant feeling. Codeine can be habit-forming. It can be given orally, IM or rectally. Rapid IV use may result in cardiovascular collapse. Rectally administered codeine has been shown to have as rapid an onset as IM codeine, but it yields lower peak levels in children.[29] Codeine has been the analgesic of choice by neurosurgeons in the belief that pupillary signs are maintained. Morphine has been shown to be a more effective analgesic, however, in patients with head injuries.[30]

Remifentanil

Remifentanil is one of the newest synthetic opiates available. It was designed to be metabolized by plasma esterases to provide a short $T_{1/2}$. It is a potent μ agonist with mild K and Δ effects. It is substantially more potent than fentanyl. It is supplied as a white lyophilized powder that contains glycine (it should not be used for epidural or spinal analgesia). The metabolism is by nonspecific esterases not affected by pseudocholinesterase deficiency. The metabolite, a weak μ agonist, is excreted by the kidney.

The kinetics of remifentanil is different from those of most opiates used in the ICU. It has a short $T_{1/2}$, and this is due to metabolism rather than to redistribution. Therefore remifentanil has what is known as a *context-sensitive half-life*. The elimination $T_{1/2}$ for remifentanil is about 8 minutes. With an infusion of remifentanil, the $T_{1/2}$ does not increase but remains constant. With opiates such as fentanyl and alfentanil (Fig. 116–3), the clinical effect $T_{1/2}$ increases with time until it reflects the elimination $T_{1/2}$ of between 2 and 4 hours.

Kinetics reported for neonates is similar to adults. Continuous infusion rate depends on the degree of sedation/analgesia required (0.1 to 0.5 μg/kg/min for sedation; 0.75 to 2 μg/kg/min for balanced anesthesia; 4 μg/kg/min for loss of consciousness). Remifentanil has effects on the cardiovascular system that are similar to those of fentanyl. Remifentanil causes a mild bradycardia and a slight decrease in blood pressure,[31] which may be prevented with glycopyrrolate. There is no histamine release. Remifentanil is a potent respiratory depressant. For spontaneous respiration, a low continuous infusion dose (without a bolus) should be used (0.1 μg/kg/min). Sedation can be effectively managed by continuous infusion without the need for a bolus because of the short $T_{1/2}$. An increase or decrease of infusion rate is rapidly reflected by a change in the degree of sedation. This is important to note. Most other opiate sedatives require bolus dosing to achieve a rapid change in effect. This is neither appropriate nor needed for remifentanil.

Remifentanil has the usual opiate side effects; however, because of the short $T_{1/2}$, they will have only brief clinical effect. Remifentanil may prove to be a safe and effective choice for PICU sedation in those patients with severe renal or hepatic disease. It is an option only for those who require overnight ventilation or for those patients in whom a rapid awakening may be required for neurologic assessment. Remifentanil has been shown to reduce cerebral oxygen use and reduce cerebral blood flow if the CO_2 is maintained in a normal range.[32]

Remifentanil is currently an expensive option and should not be considered for every patient. Also, because of its short duration, the postoperative patient may need an alternative analgesic after extubation. Rapid development of opiate tolerance with remifentanil has been described in healthy volunteers[33]; however, this concern has not yet been reported in the literature on patients in the ICU.

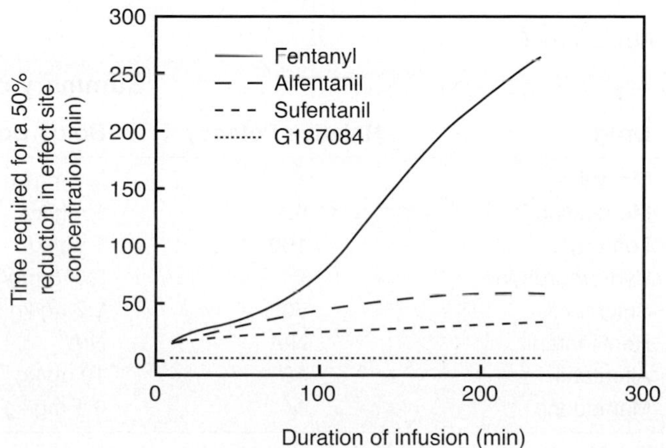

FIGURE 116–3 • Context-sensitive half-life.

TABLE 116–5

Dose Equivalents: Short Acting

	Oral	Parenteral
Morphine	0.5 mg/kg Q4	0.15 mg/kg Q3
Hydromorphone	0.1 mg/kg Q4	0.02 mg/kg Q4
Codeine	4 mg/kg Q3	
Hydrocodone	0.5 mg/kg Q3	
Oxycodone	0.5 mg/kg Q3	
Meperidine	5 μg/kg Q2	1.5 mg/kg Q2
Fentanyl		1.5 μg/kg Q2

Hydromorphone

Hydromorphone is a hydrogenated ketone of morphine. It is 7 times as potent as morphine with a similar onset and duration of action. It causes less histamine release than morphine.

Tramadol

This opiate analgesic relieves pain in two ways: by binding to opiate receptors and by inhibiting norepinephrine and serotonin, two pain-modifying neurotransmitters. It does not have antiinflammatory effects. Its use is indicated in cases of moderate to moderately severe pain.[34] Despite being a narcotic-like agent, the Food and Drug Administration (FDA) has not classified tramadol as a controlled substance. Dosage (not recommended for patients younger than 16 years) is an initial oral dose of 1 to 2 mg/kg every 6 hours and should not exceed 6 mg/kg/day (IV preparation is unavailable in the United States). Patients with a creatinine clearance less than 30 ml/min should not receive a dose more often than once every 12 hours with a maximum dose of 3 mg/kg/day; the dose for patients with cirrhosis is 1 mg/kg every 12 hours. Patients undergoing dialysis can receive their dose on the day of dialysis because only 7% of the drug is removed by the process. The adverse effects of tramadol most often involve the CNS and the GI tract. Patients may become dependent on tramadol. There is the possibility of abuse (little evidence so far of abuse), and it should not be given to opiate-dependent patients. Seizures have been seen in patients receiving high single oral doses of 10 mg/kg; this danger is even greater in patients with epilepsy and in anyone taking monoamine oxidase (MAO) inhibitors and neuroleptics (lower seizure threshold). Respiratory depression may occur if the recommended dosage is consistently exceeded or if another centrally acting depressant drug (e.g., alcohol) or an anesthetic is given concurrently. Because of the possibility of withdrawal symptoms, patients should not abruptly discontinue tramadol. Tramadol is not a useful drug for sedative action. Table 116–5 provides conversion doses for some commonly used oral opiates.

A summary of IV doses of different opiates is provided in Table 116–6.

Opiate Antagonists

Several opiate antagonists are available. The most commonly used is naloxone, which is a specific and sensitive receptor antagonist of all opiate receptors. Dosing can be either low dose (1 μg/kg) or high dose in an emergency situation (10 μg/kg). If the drug cannot be administered intravenously, then it can be given through an IM route or into the midventral surface of the tongue. When naloxone is being used for a long-acting agonist, an infusion may be necessary because its $T_{1/2}$ is only 30 to 81 minutes (mean, 64 ± 12 minutes). In neonates, the $T_{1/2}$ has been reported as 3.1 ± 0.5 hours; however, this prolonged effect is likely to be offset by a concomitant increase in the duration of action of the opioid for which the naloxone is given. No effect is seen in the healthy patient in the absence of administered opioids; however, in the setting of sepsis in the ICU, a vasopressor effect may occur, presumably because of an interaction with endogenous opioids released in response to stress. Nalmefene, a longer-acting antagonist, can be given through IV, IM, and SC routes. It has a redistribution $T_{1/2}$ of 41 minutes and a terminal $T_{1/2}$ of 10.8 hours in adults, and somewhat less in children. Thus reappearance of the antagonized opioid is unlikely if it is given in an adequate dose.[35]

TABLE 116–6

Summary of Opiate Dosing

Drug	Relative Potency	Bolus Dose	Initial Infusion Rate	Active Metabolites
Morphine	1	0.1 mg/kg	0.04 mg/kg/hr	M6G
Meperidine	0.1	1 mg/kg	N/A	Normeperidine
Fentanyl	100	1 μg/kg	1 μg/kg hr	None
Hydromorphone	7	0.015 mg/kg	0.005 mg/kg/hr	None
Sufentanil	500	0.2 μg/kg	0.2 μg/kg/hr	None
Remifentanil	N/A	N/A	0.1 μg/kg/min	None
Alfentanil	10	10 μg/kg	10 μg/kg/hr	None
Methadone	1	0.1 mg/kg	N/A	None

M6G, Morphine-6-glucuronide; *N/A*, not applicable.

BOX 116–1

Options for Controlling a Child's Pain

ANALGESICS

Opioids—weak, potent
NSAIDs
Nonopioids

ANESTHETICS

Regional block
Epidural anesthesia
Topical anesthesia

PHYSICAL

Thermal
Massage
Physical therapy
TENS

COGNITIVE

Imagery
Distraction
Hypnosis
Choices and control
Information
Role play

BEHAVIORAL

Biofeedback
Relaxation therapy

NSAID, Nonsteroidal antiinflammatory drug; *TENS,* transcutaneous electrical nerve stimulation.

Incidental Pain Syndromes in the Child in the Pediatric Intensive Care Unit

In addition to the techniques used to sedate children to facilitate their PICU management, many children will have pain related to their underlying condition.

There are many different options for controlling pain in the pediatric patient (Box 116–1). The pharmacological management of pain should follow the traditional World Health Organization (WHO) analgesic ladder, which begins with a nonopioid analgesic such as an NSAID or acetaminophen, followed by a weak opioid such as hydrocodone, added to the nonopioid, then moves on to a strong opioid as needed, such as morphine or hydromorphone. When taken orally, a sustained-release preparation is often useful once the dose requirement has been determined. The dose requirement of a strong opioid is variable in the patient taking opioids for a prolonged period of time, and failure to appreciate this is a common cause for therapeutic failure. In addition, once a dose requirement is known, the analgesic should be given to preempt pain rather than to relieve pain as required (PRN).

At each level of analgesic use, the addition of adjuvant medications should be considered. Adjuvant drugs fall into six groups: antidepressant, anticonvulsant, neuroleptic, steroid, stimulant, and local anesthetic. Of the tricyclic antidepressants, nortriptyline is available in a liquid form. The tricyclic antidepressants are indicated for neuropathic pain, particularly when the patient describes a burning pain. Also useful for neuropathic pain are the anticonvulsants gabapentin and carbamazepine. These often work best when the pain is described as shooting or lancinating. Neuropathic pain may result from tumor invasion, vincristine therapy, cytomegalovirus (CMV) infection, or human immunodeficiency (HIV) infection. The neuroleptics, including chlorpromazine and trimeprazine, may be useful in the management of nausea, anxiety, and pruritus. Steroids benefit mood, inflammation, nausea, appetite, nerve swelling/entrapment, and vasculitis. When opioid sedation is interfering with quality of life, a stimulant such as an amphetamine may restore energy and alertness while allowing ongoing analgesia from the opioid. Sometimes pain can be managed by local anesthetic, placed by peripheral nerve block, topically, or as a neuraxial block.

Sickle Cell Crisis

Sickle cell disease differs from cancer and acquired immune deficiency syndrome (AIDS) in that intermittent episodes of severe pain occur requiring urgent intensive treatment. A good review of this subject has been published.[36] Chronic pain may also be present because of long term tissue and bone damage from periods of ischemia during past crises, including persisting myocardial ischemia. Patients may be receiving long-acting opioids or may have had repeated exposure to opioids with past crises. Patients with a sickle crisis that involves the chest or brain are likely to be admitted to the PICU. Chest crises result from the sickling of erythrocytes in the pulmonary vasculature and result in hypoxia to the rest of the body and local lung damage. The systemic hypoxia worsens the crisis and is thus self-perpetuating. Chest radiograph changes may be late, and there may be an associated paralytic ileus. Poor pulmonary function may discourage the practitioner from using adequate opioid analgesics out of concern for worsening the hypoxia. It is important, however, not to underestimate the need for pain relief and to appreciate that past opioid exposure may have resulted in tolerance to opioids. If IV access is difficult to obtain, morphine may be given subcutaneously. Success has also been reported with nebulized morphine.[37]

Opiate Tolerance

The use of opiate infusions in the ICU is associated with the potential for the development of tolerance or dependence.[38] Iatrogenic withdrawal symptoms can occur if the opiates are discontinued abruptly. These effects have been shown to be related to the total dose and duration of fentanyl infusion. A fentanyl infusion of 5 days or a total cumulative dose of 1.6 mg/kg during the hospital stay was associated with 50% chance of the development of narcotic withdrawal, whereas a fentanyl infusion of 9 days or longer or a total cumulative fentanyl dose of 2.5 mg/kg or more during the hospital stay had an incidence of 100% withdrawal.[39] The rising plasma fentanyl levels caused by increased dosing suggested that increased metabolism or clearance was not responsible for the development of tolerance.

A study of patients in a PICU to determine the degree of opiate tolerance has shown a significant increase in opiate dosing required for adequate sedation.[40] The opiate infusion increased by about 80% per week for the first 3 weeks of opiate use. There was no difference in the rate of opiate increase with respect to age of the patient, postoperative status, mode of ventilation, and paralysis.

For those patients considered to be at risk of withdrawal, several options are available. If circumstances allow, it is better to start the treatment for withdrawal prevention before the patient has symptoms and signs of withdrawal. Opiate withdrawal is not usually a serious medical problem; it is rarely life threatening and is self limited. Treatment should be avoided, however, if possible for patient comfort. In a few circumstances, the associated hypersympathetic state may not be good for the patient. The signs and symptoms of withdrawal are nonspecific, and other causes, such as infection, hypoglycemia, hypocalcemia, hyperthyroidism, and hypoxia, should be excluded.

Because of the nonspecific nature of the symptoms of opiate withdrawal, several scoring systems have been described to aid with the diagnostic process. The Finnegan Score is based on 31 variables and is lengthy to use. The Lipsitz score is shorter and easier to use. Both of these scoring systems, however, were devised for use with neonates, and several of the measurements are not appropriate for patients in the PICU. Currently, there is no validated scoring system for assessing opiate withdrawal in the pediatric patient. In the limited number of articles in which opiate withdrawal in the PICU is evaluated, the authors have modified these scores (Table 116–7) in an attempt to provide an objective assessment of the patient.

The incidence of iatrogenic opiate withdrawal has also not been extensively studied in adult or pediatric ICUs. Many of the studies are retrospective with a varied description of opiate withdrawal symptoms and differences in drug dose comparisons. Although the pediatric data are even more limited, it appears that opiate withdrawal can complicate a patient's clinical course and that feeding difficulties are the main practical problems experienced.

TABLE 116–7

Signs and Symptoms of Opiate Withdrawal

	Examples
Neurologic excitability	Sleep disturbances Agitation Tremors Seizures Choreoathetoid movements
GI disturbances	Vomiting Diarrhea Autonomic dysfunction
Hypertension (>150 mmHg)	Tachycardia (>150) Tachypnea (>40) Fever (>38.5° C) Frequent yawning Sweating Goose flesh Mottling

GI, gastrointestinal.

Often the patients had already been transferred to the PICU before the onset of symptoms.

Several therapeutic options are available for the prevention and treatment of opiate withdrawal. Drugs from the same class are preferable. The FDA has approved methadone for opiate withdrawal. Other agents that may be useful include morphine, clonidine, phenobarbital, paregoric, chlorpromazine, transdermal clonidine patch,[41] and SC fentanyl. Paregoric contains morphine plus papaverine, noscapine, camphor (CNS stimulant), ethanol (45%), benzoic acid (which competes with bilirubin-binding sites), and glycerin (which causes diarrhea). Paregoric has been used for neonatal withdrawal, but because of its composition, it may cause side effects. Chlorpromazine may be useful for GI side effects, but hypothermia and hypotension may occur. Haloperidol may also be of use, having minimal respiratory depression and no active metabolites. It offers cardiovascular stability. Phenobarbital has been used for hyperactive behavior; however, it can cause significant CNS depression, it induces drug metabolism, and it is tolerance/dependence forming.

Methadone seems to be the most suitable agent. It has an oral bioavailability of 80% to 90% and an elimination $T_{1/2}$ of 12 to 24 hours. It is equipotent to morphine. Methadone has inactive metabolites and is less sedating than morphine while remaining an effective analgesic. Because of its higher bioavailability and reduced first-pass effect, it is more predictable orally than morphine. It has been extensively used in the outpatient management of opiate-addicted patients.

The convenience of oral route, the less-frequent dosing due to its longer $T_{1/2}$, and easy calculation because of its equal potency to morphine make methadone attractive for use in the management of opiate withdrawal in children. There is, however, a huge variability in recommendations regarding the methadone dose to prevent opiate withdrawal in children. In the dosing of methadone for conversion from fentanyl, several factors are important. Fentanyl, after prolonged IV administration, has a potency 100 times that of methadone; has a metabolic $T_{1/2}$ approximately one quarter that of methadone; and if given intravenously, has a bioavailability 20% greater than orally administered methadone. In a study in which the effectiveness of a fentanyl-methadone conversion protocol was assessed, researchers found that giving 2.4 times the daily fentanyl dose as methadone prevented withdrawal symptoms.[38] The methadone was given intravenously for 24 hours, and the fentanyl dose decreased by 50% on day 1 and then another 50% on day 2, and then discontinued. On day 3 the methadone was converted to oral dosing. The methadone was given intravenously initially. Because of its long $T_{1/2}$, oral dosing could take up to 5 days to reach a steady state. The duration of methadone requirement varied from 1 to 4 weeks, depending on the duration of opiate infusion. Methadone was being weaned by 3% to 15% per day when the patient exhibited no signs of withdrawal.

To date there have been no published cases of respiratory arrest when methadone has been used for opiate weaning. It would appear prudent, however, to initiate the conversion from fentanyl to methadone in the ICU environment in the event that problems arise and to ensure that an adequate dose is given. Once stabilized, the patient may be transferred to the floor and ultimately home, with a clearly described plan for decreasing the methadone dose over time. The weaning plan should also involve the home pediatrician so that patients have access to someone who is familiar with the process. In a follow-up of patients who had received methadone while in the ICU, 38% of patients were discharged home during the weaning process. No problems were associated with the weaning of methadone at home; a stigma regarding methadone use was not expressed by any of the parents.

The use of a clonidine patch has also been evaluated in the PICU. Clonidine has been shown to be effective in the management of nicotine, opiate, and alcohol withdrawal. It decreases sympathetic outflow from the CNS and has a synergistic effect for analgesia, both central and spinal. In one report, eight patients were described after tracheal reconstructive operations; they required postoperative sedation and ventilation for 7 days, which put them at high risk for withdrawal.[18] A clonidine patch was applied 12 hours before extubation, and the patients were weaned off the opiate. The dose used was approximately 6 μg/kg/day of clonidine, and the patch was left on for 7 days. One patch had to be removed because of hypotension. The patch seemed to be effective in preventing withdrawal. The patch is attractive because of its noninvasive approach, which is desired. The use of a transdermal patch prevents titration of effect, however, and problems with bradycardia, hypotension, hypothermia, sedation, and dysrhythmia may occur.

A confounding issue in many publications and in the clinical management of opiate withdrawal is the potential for simultaneous BZD withdrawal. Most researchers have not been able to separate these two issues. The symptoms of BZD withdrawal differ from those of opiate withdrawal; the BZD symptoms have less sympathetic activation. BZD withdrawal symptoms are characterized by agitation and a movement disorder. If it is a concern, low-dose lorazepam or diazepam may be added to the withdrawal management strategy (Table 116–8).

Rapid Opiate Detoxification

There have been reports of rapid opiate detoxification in the ICU. These procedures have used a form of deep sedation (often another propofol or other anesthetic agent) to facilitate opioid withdrawal in recreationally opiate-addicted patients.[42] The patients are given high doses of opiate antagonists to displace all opiates from the receptors and then heavy sedation to reduce the occurrence and effects of the sympathetic stimulation observed with short-term opiate withdrawal. These procedures have been safely performed in the ICU; however, there have been several reports of complications[43] when they were not performed with full ICU support. Currently, the effectiveness and safety of 1-day opiate detoxification is still an area of debate.[44] If used, however, it should be combined with an established long-term support plan to optimize long-term success.

In the PICU, deep sedation with propofol has been used to facilitate rapid opiate weaning of ventilator-dependent patients.[45] The use of propofol for up to 3 days allowed a reduction of fentanyl dosing from 24 to 9 μg/kg/hr (a 65% reduction). There were no signs or symptoms of opiate withdrawal noted and no development of metabolic acidosis. Opiate antagonists were not used for this rapid wean.

Benzodiazepines

Benzodiazepines (BZDs) are among the most commonly used agents for sedation in the ICU. They augment the function of the GABA type A GABA-A) receptor at the postsynaptic membrane. This pentameric protein controls a chloride channel, the opening of which leads to an inhibitory effect due to hyperpolarization of the cell membrane.[46, 47] They bind to BZD receptors, which in the CNS are usually found as part of the $GABA_A$ receptor, enhancing the effect of endogenous GABA.[48] Peripheral BZD receptors[49] are not usually associated with the GABA-A receptor but are a binding site for diazepam and midazolam. These 18-kDa proteins are associated with regulation of cellular proliferation, immunomodulation, porphyrin transport, heme biosynthesis, and anion transport. In particular they seem important in the regulation of steroid synthesis and apoptosis, and they have a significant effect on the hypothalamic-pituitary-adrenal axis.[50] These latter effects may be pertinent to the physiologic care of patients in the ICU.

BZD receptors are bound by a family of endogenous peptides called *endozepines,* which have similar effects to the BZDs.[51,52] The expression of this diazepam-binding inhibitor may be relevant to the development of dependence on not only BZDS, but also on alcohol and opioids,[53] and may therefore be relevant in the drug dependence commonly seen in patients in the PICU who are given these agents continuously. Naturally occurring BZDs have been detected with structures similar to those used clinically.[54] Subsets of alpha GABA-A receptors have been shown to have different effects. Type 1 receptors were responsible for sedation and anterograde amnesia, whereas type 2 mediated anxiolysis. It may be possible to develop selective subtype receptor agonists to provide anxiolysis without sedation, amnesia, or dependence.

The general pharmacological effects of BZDs are sedation, anxiolysis, euphoria (limbic system), reduced skeletal

TABLE 116–8

Pharmacokinetics of Benzodiazepines

Drug	Elimination Half-life (Hr)	Vol. Distribution (SS) (L/kg)	Clearance (ml/kg/min)	Protein Binding
Diazepam	46.6	1.13	0.4	97.8%
Midazolam	3.0	1.09	7.5	94%
Lorazepam	14.5	1.1	1.1	91%
Flumazenil	0.67	1.2	15.3	50%

muscle tone (through spinal BZD receptors), and anticonvulsant and neuroendocrine effects. They impair acquisition and encoding of new information, providing anterograde amnesia. They do not have any analgesic properties. They have little direct effect on ICP. Their effects are dose dependent. Patient cofactors influence response to BZDs. These include age, concurrent disease, and any cosedation therapy. Paradoxical reactions are reported in which agitation rather than calming is observed.[55] In healthy patients, BZDs have few cardiovascular side effects, but in a sick, intensive care population, profound cardiovascular depression may occasionally be observed. BZDs should be used judiciously until the patient response is known.[56] Midazolam has been most often associated with this effect,[57] and research in dogs has shown both negative inotropy and chronotropy, especially when the sympathetic response has been abolished.[58] Clinical use is largely encompassed by discussion of the pharmacologic properties of diazepam, midazolam, and lorazepam.

Diazepam

The first widely used BZD in the ICU was diazepam. Because of its low solubility in water, it is available in the IV or IM form dissolved in propylene glycol. This causes a significant amount of pain and thrombophlebitis with peripheral IV use. A lipid emulsion is available in the United Kingdom that has fewer side effects. Diazepam is inexpensive and is effective for short-term sedation, in which accumulation is less of a concern. It may be given orally because it has good absorption, but absorption tends to be erratic when it is given rectally or intramuscularly. It is highly lipid soluble with a long $T_{1/2}$ (24 hours). Metabolism by oxidative biotransformation generates several hypnotically active metabolites with elimination $T_{1/2}$s that may be longer than diazepam, including oxazepam ($T_{1/2}$, 10 hours) and n-dimethyldiazepam ($T_{1/2}$, 93 hours). Delayed recovery has been reported in neonates after they received diazepam, possibly because of the long $T_{1/2}$ of dimethyldiazepam.[59] Prolongation of effects occurs in patients when clearance is reduced because of hepatic dysfunction and when metabolism is inhibited by drugs such as cimetidine and omeprazole.

Midazolam

Midazolam is an imidazobenzodiazepine. It has a short elimination $T_{1/2}$ of 2 hours and is water soluble. This means that IV injection is nonirritating. Because of these factors, it has become popular in the ICUs for sedation by infusion. Intranasally (0.2 mg/kg), midazolam has proved as effective at controlling febrile seizures as IV diazepam (0.3 mg/kg).[60] It has extensive first-pass metabolism and provides less reliable results when given PO, although this route is often successfully used for premedication of children before general anesthesia in doses of 0.5 to 0.75 mg/kg (maximum, 20 mg). It is available in pleasant-tasting cherry syrup and is effective in 10 to 15 minutes, providing up to 1 hour of adequate anxiolysis, although residual hangover effects may persist.[61] Rectal and sublingual administration has been described.

Midazolam is about 8 times more potent than diazepam with a bolus dose of 0.05 to 0.1 mg/kg[62] and an infusion of 1 to 6 μg/kg/min. Midazolam is metabolized by the cytochrome P450 system subfamily IIIA (nifedipine oxidase), polypeptide 4 (CYP3A4),[63] to hydroxymidazolam (63% potency) and hydroxymidazolam glucuronide (9% potency). Because of the high degree of protein binding (94% protein bound), the free level can be significantly changed with interactions because of the protein binding, which may also occur with heparin. Hepatic or renal failure increases the free fraction by 2 to 3 times, and its effect can also be prolonged by the accumulation of active metabolites.[64] The $T_{1/2}$ of midazolam in patients in the ICU may be prolonged compared with that in healthy patients.[65] With short-term infusions (<12 hours), it retains a rapid recovery; however, with increased duration of use, the recovery becomes prolonged. Its clearance may be reduced by several commonly used ICU drugs, including calcium channel blockers, erythromycin, and triazole antifungals.[66]

Lorazepam

Lorazepam is an alternative water-soluble agent. It is well absorbed after both oral and IM administration.[67] It produces sedation for 4 to 8 hours after a single dose. It has a slower onset than midazolam. The elimination $T_{1/2}$ is about 14 hours. Metabolism is by glucuronyl transferase, not the cytochrome P450, and there are no active metabolites. This metabolism is unaffected by cimetidine or phenobarbitone, which only affects oxidative metabolic pathways. Sodium valproate may inhibit its metabolism, though.[68] In advanced liver disease, these phase II glucuronidation reactions are better preserved, and the increased T1/2 seen is due to increases in the volume of distribution rather than to reduced clearance. In patients with renal failure prolonged $T_{1/2}$ is also due to reduced protein binding because clearance is unchanged. There is no change in metabolism with aging or critical illness. In a comparison of infusions of midazolam and lorazepam, the recovery characteristics were found to be significantly different. In those patients receiving lorazepam it took an average of 260 minutes to return to baseline, whereas in those patients receiving midazolam, it took more than 6 times longer to return to baseline. Dosing may be by bolus (0.05 to 0.1 mg/kg every 2 to 4 hours) or by infusion (0.05 mg/kg/hr). Lorazepam was slightly less expensive than midazolam.[69] It has been recommended as the BZD of choice for long-term sedation because of its more predictable recovery profile in the sick patient in the ICU. Lorazepam for IV use has propylene glycol as a carrier. There is a risk of a metabolic lactic acidosis because of the metabolism of this carrier. Cases of fatal metabolic acidosis from propylene glycol have been reported in neonates taking a particular vitamin preparation. Several other potential ICU drugs may use propylene glycol as a carrier; these include some IV preparations of phenytoin and phenobarbitone, nitroglycerin, digoxin, and etomidate. There are reports of propylene glycol toxicity in adults who received multiple propylene glycol infusions.[70] Care should be taken when lorazepam is infused in patients who receive these other medications. In patients in the PICU, propylene glycol levels have been shown to correlate with the dose of lorazepam received; however, no metabolic abnormalities were detected.[71] Hemodialysis has been used successfully in the management of the lorazepam-associated propylene glycol toxicity.[72]

The metabolisms of different BZDs are intertwined with each other. Most of the agents require an oxidative process first with potentially active compounds before glucuronidation and excretion. The pharmacokinetics for different BZDs is shown in Table 116–8.

Tolerance and Dependence

Tolerance for and dependence on BZDs can occur as with opiates in the PICU.[73] This is not all due to receptor number down-regulation.[74] Withdrawal symptoms may be avoided with slow taper 10% per day or with a long-acting oral agent such as diazepam. Acute withdrawal symptoms may include anxiety, insomnia, nightmares, seizures, psychosis, and hyperpyrexia.

A postmidazolam infusion phenomenon has been described that includes poor social interaction, decreased eye contact, and a decreased interest in the surroundings. The patient may exhibit choreoathetotic movements with dystonic posturing. This can persist for 2 to 4 weeks but will resolve with no sequelae.

A single-dose abreaction to BZDs has also been described in children and in adults.[75] Some patients do not become sedated with normal doses and may even become agitated, and some patients may even worsen with increased dose. Postoperatively it has been described that up to 10% of patients who received a midazolam premedication were "squirrelly" for no apparent reason.

Flumazenil

Flumazenil is an imidazobenzodiazepine and is a specific competitive antagonist of the BZD receptor. It has no effect on other drugs such as barbiturates, ethanol, or other GABA-mimetic agents. It reverses the hypnotic and sedative effects of BZDs. It has a $T_{1/2}$ of about 1 hour after single IV bolus. In patients with hepatic impairment, its $T_{1/2}$ and clearance are prolonged, and there is a significant increase (>50%) of free drug because of reduced plasma protein binding. Renal failure has little effect on the pharmacokinetics. It is indicated for the complete or partial reversal of the central sedative effects of BZDs. Contraindications include patients who have a known hypersensitivity to BZDs, patients with epilepsy who are receiving BZD treatment, and those who have overdosed with a tricyclic antidepressant. Its use is often associated with mild to moderate tachycardia and hypertension.

In cases of multiple drug overdose, the use of flumazenil remains controversial. It is often overused in the emergency setting without due concern for potential adverse reactions[76] because of the potential toxic effects (cardiac arrhythmias or convulsions) of other psychotropic drugs ingested. The toxicity of tricyclic antidepressants becomes apparent as the effects of BZDs are antagonized. Patients should be evaluated for the signs and symptoms of a tricyclic antidepressant overdose, and an electrocardiogram (ECG) may be helpful in determining the risks involved.

The dosing information for pediatric patients is limited. The initial suggested dose used is 0.01 mg/kg (maximum, 0.2 mg) with incremental doses of 0.005 to 0.01 mg/kg (maximum, 0.2 mg) given every minute up to a maximum cumulative dose of 1 mg. The lower doses are suggested for sedation reversal and the higher doses for BZD overdose. Infusions at 0.05 to 0.01 mg/kg/hr have been used.[77]

The use of flumazenil in sedated patients in the ICU should be tempered by the potential for an unrecognized BZD dependence, which would increase the risks of side effects. If its use is required, then a carefully titrated dose would be appropriate. The $T_{1/2}$ of flumazenil is much shorter than some of the BZDs that it may be counteracting (see Table 116–8). The use of an infusion may be necessary because resedation has been reported after single-bolus use.[78] This should not, however, preclude the use of flumazenil in an intensive care setting.[79] Flumazenil has been used for reversal of conscious sedation. In the pediatric population, although it was well tolerated, it was not shown to significantly reduce recovery time.[80] Flumazenil has a limited duration with the potential for resedation after discharge from medical care, so an appropriate period of observation is required before discharge. A study in which researchers followed the effects of flumazenil after sedation indicated that some of the residual effects of midazolam were still present after reversal.[81] Flumazenil has also been used to treat a paradoxical midazolam reaction.

Chloral Hydrate

Chloral hydrate is a widely used oral hypnotic/sedative agent. It has been used for sedation for radiographic procedures, for EEGs, and in many different health care locations. It was first synthesized in 1832 and used in 1869 as a hypnotic agent. Shortly after, reports of acute and chronic toxicity were published.[82] In 1910 it was labeled as the most dangerous of hypnotics even though heroin and opium were in common use at that time. The addition of ethanol potentiates its effect (street name: Mickey Finn). It has been used to control agitation in the intensive care nursery (ICN) and to treat sleep difficulties in older patients.

It is rapidly and completely absorbed from the GI tract and is immediately converted into the active component trichloroethanol (TCE). The plasma levels peaks at 30 to 60 minutes TCE is 45% protein bound. It is metabolized by alcohol dehydrogenase, which converts the chloral hydrate to TCE.[83] This then undergoes glucuronidation with some oxidation to trichloroacetate (TCA). The $T_{1/2}$ of TCE is 8 to 12 hours (TCA, 67 hours). In infants and neonates this may be increased by 3 to 4 times. With multiple dosage regimens, there is a significant potential for accumulation. The metabolite TCA can displace bound bilirubin from albumin. Its actions include CNS depression with drowsiness and a sound sleep in less than an hour. With overdose the patient falls into a deep stupor or coma, and the pupils change from contracted to dilated. At therapeutic levels the blood pressure and respiratory rate are unaffected. It has little hangover effect. It has several effects on the cardiovascular system including decreased myocardial contractility, a shortened refractory period, and an increased sensitivity of the heart to catecholamines. It also has effects on mucous membranes.

Irritation can cause gastritis, nausea, and vomiting. With overdose a severe hemorrhagic gastritis with gastric necrosis and esophagitis has been described. Chloral hydrate and ethanol interfere with one another's metabolism through competition for alcohol dehydrogenase. Also, ethanol inhibits the conjugation of TCE, and TCE inhibits the oxidation of ethanol. Coumadin activity may be increased by chloral hydrate. Chloral hydrate is synergistic with other sedative agents. In children receiving amphetamine-based medication, chloral hydrate is contraindicated because there have been rare reports of arrhythmias. The reversal of chloral hydrate with flumazenil has been described; however, there has also been a report of ventricular tachycardia with this combination.

Dosing and Toxicity

Chloral hydrate is available as capsules, syrup (50 mg/ml), and suppositories. The sedative dose is 25 to 50 mg/kg (PO/PR [by way of the rectum]); up to 100 mg/kg can safely be used in children younger than 5 years with a maximum dose of 1 g. Because of an increased $T_{1/2}$, neonatal dosing should be lower (25 mg/kg). In preterm babies, toxicity resulted when chloral hydrate was used for 3 days; in term babies toxicity resulted when it was used for 7 days. The therapeutic level for TCE is 2 to 12 μg/L; toxicity occurs when the level is more than 25 μg/L. Chloral hydrate provides successful conscious sedation in about 90% of patients, but it appears to be less effective in those older than 2 years. A higher risk of failure with excessive effect can be seen in those patients with a history of obstructive sleep apnea or encephalopathy.

Signs of toxicity are usually noted within 3 hours of dosing. Paradoxical excitement has also been described in 6% of patients. There is some evidence that chloral hydrate may be genotoxic and carcinogenic. Mice studies have shown that a single-dose exposure can result in an increased risk of hepatic carcinomas and adenomas.[84] Chloral hydrate overdose produces a clinical picture that is similar to acute barbiturate poisoning. Ataxia, lethargy, and coma occur within 1 to 2 hours. Also, a pearlike odor may be noted. Cardiovascular instability poses the main threat to life. Severe arrhythmias including atrial fibrillation (AF), supraventricular tachyarrhythmia (SVT), ventricular tachyarrhythmia (VT), torsades de pointes, and ventricular fibrillation (VF) have been described.

Chronic use can cause a dependence syndrome. Also, chloral hydrate is not detectable in the blood. TCE levels are measurable, but they are not useful for clinical management, although they can be helpful for retrospective diagnosis.

The management of toxicity includes evaluation and monitoring at a medical facility if an amount greater than 50 mg/kg or unknown amount has been ingested. Two capsules may cause significant toxicity in a toddler, so there is little room for error in the history. Gastric lavage is not routine unless an hour has passed since ingestion of a large dose. Charcoal with intubation should be considered if significant toxicity is suspected. Standard antiarrhythmic management is often unsuccessful, although esmolol, overdrive pacing, and hemoperfusion have been tried.

Butyrophenones

Butyrophenones belong to the group of major tranquilizers.

Haloperidol is a potent antipsychotic agent with nonspecific dopamine antagonist action. It has little effect on the cardiovascular or respiratory systems. It produces the appearance of calm with minimal hypnotic effect and reduces operant behavior (purposeful movement). The patient appears tranquil and dissociated from surroundings but is readily accessible if spoken to. Haloperidol may mask actual feelings of mental restlessness. It is a potent antiemetic agent (action at the chemotrigger zone) and has no appreciable effect on the EEG. It potentiates analgesics and other sedative agents. Compared with less potent butyrophenones, it has fewer side effects. Neuroleptanalgesia, a dissociative form of anesthesia, can be induced when haloperidol is combined with high-dose opiates. This anesthetic state is useful for certain cardiac and neurosurgical procedures that require cardiovascular stability and a responsive patient. It is metabolized to inactive compounds with a $T_{1/2}$ of 15 to 25 hours. It is highly protein bound. Hepatic dysfunction increases the $T_{1/2}$ because of reduced clearance. Side effects include extrapyramidal signs, although acute dystonia is rare. Prolongation of QT interval is possible with the subsequent risk of ventricular tachycardia.[85] Hepatic toxicity can occur but is rare.

Haloperidol is indicated for the treatment of psychoses, Tourette's disorder, and severe behavioral problems in children. In the PICU it is used as a treatment for agitation in patients who are often unresponsive to other more commonly used agents. It has also proved to be effective as part of a sedative withdrawal strategy.

Haloperidol is available as syrup, tablets, and an IM preparation. The usual dosage for agitation in children younger than 3 years is 0.01 to 0.03 mg/kg every 4 hours. Maximum daily dose is 0.15 mg/kg/day. There are two IM preparations: the lactate is for repeated use, and the decanoate is a slow-release monthly formulation. Although not approved by the FDA, the IM lactate form has been given intravenously without problems.

Droperidol is faster acting with a shorter duration of action and a $T_{1/2}$ of 2 hours. It is available as an approved IV formulation. With an IV bolus, mild hypotension occurs because of mild α receptor blockade. Droperidol is more sedating than haloperidol and may be used as a sedation adjunct to general anesthesia. It is also used in low dose (0.05 mg/kg) as an antiemetic agent. There are concerns about the potential for droperidol also to cause prolongation of the QT interval and result in ventricular tachycardia.[86]

Phenothiazines

Chlorpromazine is a weaker antipsychotic agent with general CNS depressant activity. It has an antidopaminergic effect including extrapyramidal side effects, lethargy, and apathy with an EEG similar to normal sleep. It also causes a decrease in the body's ability to maintain temperature control, shivering is reduced, and it can be useful in hypothermic-induced states. Cardiovascular effects include α-adrenoreceptor blockade with hypotension and postural hypotension, but there is no effect on the ECG. Respiratory drive and depth are unaffected; however, there may be some dryness of the mucosa. On the GI tract its anticholinergic effect causes a decrease in secretions and motility. Liver effects include jaundice that occurs in 0.5% (recurrence rate, 40%), independent of dose or duration of therapy. This is associated with a rash, fever, and eosinophilia. This syndrome has a low death rate and usually resolves quickly on discontinuation of chlorpromazine.

Other effects include antihistamine-like action; local analgesia; a temporary leucopenia; and, rarely, agranulocytosis. It also has antiemetic properties. Indications include premedication, sedation as part of the lytic cocktail catheterization mixture number 3 (CM3),[87] intractable pain, antipsychosis, hiccups, prevention of succinylcholine pain, and induction of hypothermia (with other active measures). The dosage is a PO, an IM, an IV, or a rectal dose of 0.5 to 1 mg/kg every 6 hours.

Chlorpromazine is metabolized both in the gut wall and by the liver. It yields more than 50 metabolites, most of which are inactive.

Other phenothiazine derivatives include prochlorperazine, which has mainly antiemetic properties. Extrapyramidal side effects are more common in children younger than 5 years. Dosage is a PO or rectal dose of 0.1 mg/kg q8h and an IM or IV dose of 0.15 mg/kg.

Lytic Cocktail

The lytic cocktail (CM3) is a mixture of 25 mg/ml of meperidine, 6.5 mg/ml of promethazine, and 6.5 mg/ml of chlorpromazine. Its recommended dose is 0.1 ml/kg of body weight, but significant institutional variations exist. The CM3 was popular as sedation for cardiac catheterization. CM3 has been reported, however, to have a high failure rate and lacks several important characteristics of an ideal sedative for children. Dosing cannot be titrated easily and individually. Onset of action is delayed (30 minutes), and duration of effect is protracted (5 to 20 hours). CM3 has no anxiolytic or amnestic properties. Additional caution should also be exercised when this cocktail is used in children with seizure disorders. The metabolite of meperidine and the lowered seizure threshold from the chlorpromazine put the patient at risk. Patients with congenital heart disease with physiologic conditions such as a tetralogy of Fallot or left ventricular outflow obstruction may be put at risk because of systemic vasodilation that causes altered blood flow through shunts, a hypercyanotic spell, or decreased coronary blood flow due to diastolic hypotension.

Neuroleptic Malignant Syndrome

Both the butyrophenones and the phenothiazines have a rare but well-described side effect called the *neuroleptic malignant syndrome* (see Chapter 117). It is a cluster of adverse effects of antipsychotic medications first described in 1968. It involves the development of hypertonicity with autonomic instability, fever, and cognitive disturbance. The incidence is 0.5% to 1.4% of patients exposed to neuroleptics. The true incidence in children is unknown, however. Several different diagnostic criteria are available. Fever and rigidity present in all; others symptoms are shown in Box 116–2. A variety of therapies have been described (Table 116–9).

BOX 116–2

Signs and Symptoms of Neuroleptic Malignant Syndrome

Elevated creatine phosphokinase (97%)
Tachycardia (75%)
Altered consciousness (75%)
Tachypnea
Hypertension
Diaphoresis
Leucocytosis

Baclofen

Baclofen is a *p*-chlorophenol derivative of GABA analog. It has specific agonist activity at the $GABA_B$ receptor. It has a $T_{1/2}$ of 2 to 6 hours. It has inhibitory effects on the brain and spinal cord. At the spinal cord level it suppresses spinal reflexes to result in muscle relaxation. It is widely used as a skeletal muscle relaxant in patients with spasticity, such as cerebral palsy, spinal cord injury, and multiple sclerosis. It is most frequently given PO. Side effects include urinary retention, sedation, bradycardia, hypotension, respiratory depression, and apnea. Weakness may limit patient compliance. These "side effects" are sedative-like characteristics of the drug, which are not useful in clinical practice. Abrupt cessation of long-term baclofen therapy, therefore, resembles in part, short-term, sedative withdrawal.

Recently, intrathecal baclofen (ITB) was used with increasing frequency in children to treat spasticity. ITB was first introduced in 1984[88] with a pump delivery system that was available in 1992 for adults. This allows delivery of the drug to the spinal cord and reduces the dose significantly (1% of oral requirements), limiting systemic side effects.[89]

This GABA agonist inhibits the release of serotonin in the brainstem. After long-term use there is accommodation of the serotonin pathways to this long-term inhibition that is consistent with the usually observed increasing doses required for ITB over the first 12 to 18 months of treatment. When this inhibition is abruptly removed, sudden excess release of serotonin occurs. Acute overload of serotonin transmission, such as an overdose of serotonin reuptake inhibitors (SSRIs), can result in confusion, hyperthermia, myoclonus, and autonomic instability. It also has anticholinergic and antihistamine effects that may result in drowsiness; paradoxical excitation has been reported in children.

There have now been more than 25 case reports[90] of ITB withdrawal. ITB withdrawal seems to be more severe if the ITB treatment was for more than 1 year.

TABLE 116–9

Treatment Described in the Case Reports of Neuroleptic Malignant Syndrome

	Supportive Treatment	Neuroleptics DC'D	Anticholinergics/ Amantadine	Bromocriptine	Dantrolene	L-dopa	ECT
Frequency*	35	50	17	18	19	8	9
Total (*N*)†	55	55	48	57	58	58	59
Percent	63.6	90.9	35.4	31.6	32.8	13.8	15.3
Sequelae (*n*)	7	15	3	7	5	3	4
Deaths (*n*)	2	3	0	0	1	1	0
Duration of NMS‡							
Median	12	12.5	14	13	15	32	19.5
Mean	14.9	19.2	19.9	25.7	21.3	35	24.1
(SD)	(14.8)	(21.6)	(29.3)	(29.5)	(17.9)	(20.3)	(22.2)
NMS severity score							
Median	8	7	7.5	7	–	–	–
Mean	7.2	6.8	7.1	7.6	[illegible].6	7.4	5.6
(SD)	(2.1)	(2.1)	(2.5)	(1.3)	(1.4)	(2.1)	(2.1)

DC'D, discontinued; *ECT,* electroconvulsive therapy; *NMS,* neuroleptic malignant syndrome.
*Number of reports in which the treatment was administered.
†Number of reports in which the treatment was mentioned.
‡Duration in days.

A review of ITB pumps in 100 patients at a single center[91] has shown that problems with the delivery system are fairly common. Twenty-four percent of patients experienced a problem, with a follow-up period for a maximum of 5.6 years. There was an average of two problems per patient. Disconnection of the catheter from the implanted pump was the most common problem. Access ports on the pump seemed to increase the risk of problems (16% compared with a 2% disconnection rate); however, these ports do make troubleshooting easier. Causes of difficulty with ITB delivery are shown in Box 116–3.

The ITB withdrawal syndrome is interesting because it appears to have many similarities with the neuroleptic malignant syndrome. Prolonged muscle contraction caused by rebound spasticity results in thermogenesis, hyperthermia, and rhabdomyolysis.[92] Patients with ITB withdrawal are often managed initially as if they have sepsis and multisystem organ failure, with broad-spectrum antibiotics, and no improvement and delayed diagnosis.[93] The differential diagnosis of the hypermetabolic state is listed in Box 116–4.

The symptoms of ITB withdrawal can be classified into three categories (Table 116–10). Often the first clinical signs are the development of itching and some increase in spasticity. If replacement baclofen is not given, then the symptoms may progress to a severe hypermetabolic state that can be fatal if the cause is not recognized and treated. Of 27 patients reported to the FDA, six deaths were documented.[94]

The management of ITB withdrawal requires early diagnosis. It involves supportive ICU care and the onset of baclofen replacement therapy as soon as possible. Box 116–5 provides a guideline for the evaluation of the patient with suspected baclofen withdrawal. A definitive diagnosis may be obtained with measurement of cerebrospinal fluid (CSF) baclofen levels, but the results probably are not going to be available in the time course of treatment initiation.

Although the primary aim should be to replace baclofen, rapid replacement of ITB may not be possible. The required oral baclofen replacement dose may be

BOX 116–3

Causes of Interrupted Intrathecal Baclofen Delivery

Pump malfunction
Pump failure
Battery failure
Infections necessitating pump removal
Catheter problems (e.g., kinks, holes, tears, dislodgement, disconnection, migration)

BOX 116–4

Differential Diagnosis of Intrathecal Baclofen Withdrawal

Autonomic dysreflexia
NLMS
MH
Sepsis
Status epilepticus
Toxic
Metabolic
Immune-mediated disorders

TABLE 116–10

Severity of ITB Withdrawal

Designation	Description
Mild	Pruritic symptoms and increased spasticity
Moderate	High fever, altered mental status, seizures and profound rigidity, autonomic instability
Severe	Rhabdomyolysis, hepatic, renal failure, DIC brain injury, death

DIC, Disseminated intravascular coagulation; *ITB,* intrathecal baclofen.

50 to 100 times the intrathecal dose, and this is often not well tolerated by the patients because of side effects. An IV BZD should be the initial step in the treatment of baclofen withdrawal. Dantrolene has been used as an adjunct therapy for the increased spasticity.

The use of the potent serotonin antagonist cyproheptadine has been proposed as an alternative treatment adjunct.[95] It improved fever, spasticity, and itching in gout adult patients with ITB withdrawal. Dosages of cyproheptadine were in the range of 0.25 mg/kg/day every 6 hours, either PO or intramuscularly.

In some patients the ITB withdrawal is an elective management problem due to pump removal for infection. In these patients if a replacement pump cannot be placed, the patient needs to be observed and managed in the ICU to recognize and treat the withdrawal syndrome. The monitoring of creatine phosphokinase (CPK) levels may be helpful in managing withdrawal. In the reported cases of ITB withdrawal CPK levels have been in the range of 1800 to more than 40,000.[96] Mild elevations in CPK (300 t 500) may be an early marker of inadequate treatment.

BOX 116–5

Management of Suspected Baclofen Withdrawal

- Suspicion in at-risk patients
- Administer antipyretics and other cooling techniques for fever
- Administer benzodiazepines for seizures or spasticity
- Rule out medical causes
- Oral baclofen therapy
- Contact patient's ITB pump specialist to interrogate the pump and check the reservoir
- Abdominal radiographs (AP/lateral) to check for catheter integrity
- Neurosurgical consultation for possible surgical exploration and repair
- If catheter appears intact on plain radiographs, then consider performing a contrast catheter study to check for catheter integrity
- If problem is unresolved contact manufacturer (Medtronic 1-800-328-2518)

Modified from Kao LW, Amin Y, Kirk MA et al: Intrathecal baclofen withdrawal mimicking sepsis, *J Emerg Med* 24:423-427, 2003.
AP, Anteroposterior; *ITB,* intrathecal baclofen.

Dexmedetomidine

Dexmedetomidine (Precedex) is a selective α_2 agonist. It has an effect at receptors in the CNS and peripheral nervous system, as well as in autonomic ganglia. Stimulation of the α_2 receptor decreases the release of norepinephrine; inhibits sympathetic activity; and produces sedation, anxiolysis, and analgesia. It is 1600 times more active at the α_2 receptor than at the α_1 receptor and is thus 8 times more selective than clonidine. It is available as a white water-soluble powder in a 100-μg vial. In adults it has a redistribution phase of 6 minutes and an elimination $T_{1/2}$ of 2 hours. The pharmacokinetics appears to be similar in the pediatric patient, even after a 24-hour infusion.[97] It is almost completely metabolized in the liver by glucuronidation and P450 pathways to inactive metabolites. In patients with renal failure the pharmacokinetics did not show any prolongation of the terminal $T_{1/2}$; however, these patients were sedated for longer after the infusion was terminated compared with the control group.[98] This may be related to reduced protein binding of this normally highly protein bound drug (94%) and thus higher free drug levels in the patient with renal failure. In patients with hepatic dysfunction reduced clearance has been reported. With patients in severe hepatic failure a prolongation of the $T_{1/2}$ almost 3 times normal was reported.[99]

Dexmedetomidine has proved to be effective for sedation in the adult intensive care setting.[100] Currently, it is only licensed for 24 hours of sedation. The recommended dosage for dexmedetomidine is a loading dose of 1 μg/kg/min over 10 minutes followed by an infusion of 0.2 to 0.7 μg/kg/hr. It appears that in pediatric patients, the higher end of the dose range is required. Doses higher than 1.5 μg/kg/hr have not been shown to provide any further sedative action. Advantages of dexmedetomidine include minimal respiratory depression and predictable hemodynamic effects. Because of the reduced sympathetic activity, blood pressure and heart rate fall slightly. Clinical sedation trials have shown a decrease in heart rate of 7% and blood pressure by 10%. It has been infused before, during, and after the extubation process. Hypotension and bradycardia are more likely to occur during the loading phase, which may need to be prolonged or interrupted.

Dexmedetomidine cannot be given by rapid IV bolus because hypertension may occur due to direct stimulation of α_1 receptors. Mild transient hypertension is sometimes noted in adults during the loading phase, although this was not noticed in pediatric patients.

Long-term (160 hours) use of dexmedetomidine has also now been reported,[101] with no evidence of accumulation. The concern about rebound hypertension after long-term α_2 agonist treatment, such as that occurring with clonidine, has not been reported.

Sedation from dexmedetomidine often results in a patient who is tranquil yet easily aroused. Reduced analgesic requirements have been reported with its use. The easy arousal may make it a useful agent for when repeat neurologic examinations are required. Currently, pediatric experience in the ICU is limited. A small study of 16 patients (to date) in which dexmedetomidine was compared with midazolam in patients in the PICU showed equivalent sedation and only a slightly lower heart rate in the dexmedetomidine group. It has been safely used for a variety of noninvasive sedation procedures such as magnetic resonance imaging (MRI). There are also several case reports of its use as an adjunct to general anesthesia for the pediatric patient. It would appear to be a useful agent in the management of opiate withdrawal. Dexmedetomidine is useful for patients who are difficult to sedate, for treatment of postoperative shivering, and for postanesthesia agitation.

Dexmedetomidine is not without adverse effects. It is contraindicated in patients with heart block, and bradycardia has been reported in an infant treated with digoxin who received dexmedetomidine during the infusion phase.[102] It would also appear prudent to avoid its use with other drugs that can reduce arteriovenous (AV) node function such as beta-blockers and calcium channel blockers, and with patients with severe ventricular dysfunction or hypovolemia because reduction in sympathetic tone may cause a profound fall in blood pressure. There are little data on the use of dexmedetomidine in the PICU.

Propofol

Propofol (Diprivan) is a rapid-acting IV anesthetic agent. As a highly lipid-soluble 2,6 diisopropylphenol, it is an oil and insoluble in water. It is formulated as a 1% aqueous emulsion (1.2% egg phosphatide, 10% soyabean oil, 2.25% glycerol) with a propofol concentration of 10 mg/ml.

It has a rapid recovery because of its short redistribution $T_{1/2}$ (alpha) and is rapidly cleared by hepatic metabolism in healthy patients after short infusions, making it ideal for short procedures. The elimination $T_{1/2}$ is 2 hours (Table 116–11), but the $T_{1/2}$ is context sensitive and has been reported to be between 1 and 3 days after a 10-day infusion because of significant body accumulation. The kinetics follows a three-compartment model. The dose for induction of anesthesia in children is 2.5 mg/kg to 3.5 mg/kg; higher doses are required for infants and toddlers. Anesthesia can also be maintained by an infusion. The depth of sedation/anesthesia can be easily titrated, and an infusion rate of 25 to 150 μg/kg/min usually provides adequate sedation.

As with most sedative agents, propofol has side effects that may be a concern for the intensivist. It often causes hypotension in the sick child, and in those patients dependent on high sympathetic tone to maintain normal blood pressure, even small doses of propofol may result in a significant fall in the blood pressure. The hypotension is mainly caused by vasodilatation, and there is little direct myocardial depressant. Bradycardia can also occur on induction of anesthesia. Propofol increases atrial conduction time for neonatal rabbits and prolongs the refractory period. Propofol anesthesia can prevent the induction of known atrial tachycardias in the electrophysiology (EP) laboratory, and there are cases of conversion of atrial tachycardia to sinus rhythm on induction of propofol anesthesia. Propofol is a potent respiratory depressant, and it has a useful depressant effect on airway reflexes, which may facilitate endotracheal intubation. The injection of propofol often causes pain, and in the alert patient, strategies to minimize this are useful. Most commonly, lidocaine, either mixed with the propofol or injected before the injection of propofol, will markedly reduce the pain.

There are several advantages to propofol sedation in the ICU. It is rapidly acting and produces an easily controllable level of sedation. Unlike the barbiturates it provides rapid clinical recovery, even after prolonged infusion. It has antiemetic properties and can provide transient deep sedation if required for procedures. It has also been shown to facilitate sedative synergy with BZDs.[103]

In the adult ICU population, propofol has been compared with midazolam for long-term sedation. Both agents provide good sedation, but propofol has the advantage of being more titratable with a faster recovery.[104] Despite the increased drug cost, the use of propofol can reduce overall ICU costs because of a reduction in ventilator weaning time.[105]

Propofol has been used in the ICU as an anticonvulsant for refractory status epilepticus.[106] In a comparison with pentobarbital to provide burst suppression, both drugs were equally effective. Propofol was much more rapid in effect; there was no difference in outcome or ICU support measurements or length of stay.[107] In patients with raised ICP, propofol has the same effects on ICP and cerebral blood flow (CBF) and cerebral metabolic rate of oxygen ($CMRO_2$) as barbiturates. It also requires a similar level of hemodynamic support to maintain appropriate blood pressure and cerebral perfusion pressure (CPP). It can produce the same degree of burst suppression that may be required for uncontrolled intracranial hypertension. It also allows rapid changes in the level of sedation, to facilitate neurologic examination. In this regard it is a superior agent. As described later, however, the use of large doses of propofol in the ICU setting may be associated with worsened outcomes.

Special Issue Regarding Long-Term Infusion of Propofol

There are several important problems that may occur when propofol is used in the PICU. With long-term propofol

TABLE 116–11

Pharmacokinetics of Intravenous Anesthetic Agents

Drug	Elimination Half-life (Hr)	Volume Distribution (SS) (L/kg)	Clearance (ml/kg/min)	Protein Binding
Etomidate	2.9	2.52	17.9	76.9%
Ketamine	3.1	3.1	19.1	12%
Propofol	1.9	2.3	30	96.8%

infusions, a significant amount of lipid may be infused into the patient, with the same consequences as lipid infusions used for hyperalimentation. Hyperlipidemia and triglyceridemia have been reported in up to 10% of patients receiving propofol in the ICU. Pseudohyponatremia or the inability to do routine plasma electrolyte analysis has been described. It is important that the propofol calorie (20 mls/hr = 528 kcal/day)[108] and lipid load are included in the nutrition plan for the patient. It may be necessary to reduce enteral feeds or avoid intralipid in selected patients. With high propofol dosing, respiratory acidosis has been reported.[109]

The emulsion used for propofol administration is an excellent culture medium at room temperature. There have been cases of patients with systemic infection caused by propofol during operative procedures.[110] This is due to poor aseptic technique in the preparation and use of the propofol syringes and infusion lines. Unusual infective organisms were detected in several patients, and an epidemiological study by the Center for Disease Control (CDC) found propofol to be the common element.[111] Certain precautions should be followed when propofol is used in the PICU. The staff should be educated to the potential dangers of infection from propofol. The ampoule neck should be wiped with alcohol. There are no multidose vials of propofol. Syringes should be disposed when they are more than 6 hours old, and lines should be changed every 12 hours. Filters are available that can remove many of the potential pathogens and are compatible with the lipid-based propofol infusion.

There have been a few episodes of allergy to propofol; immune reactions are estimated at 1:45,000. These involve both anaphylactic and anaphylactoid types of reactions.[112] Although clinically indistinguishable, the anaphylactic response involves prior exposure to a component of the propofol suspension. Care should be taken when a history of allergy to soy or egg is found. Propofol does not release histamine and is an acceptable agent for use in patients with asthma.

A few patients who receive propofol may have dark-green urine. This is due to phenol metabolites and is not a clinical concern.[113]

Propofol Infusion Syndrome

One of the most important concerns is the development of a refractory metabolic acidosis in children who had received propofol sedation in the ICU. This was first described in 1992 as a series of five cases[114] with fatal myocardial failure in children with respiratory illnesses requiring ventilation and sedation. Five young patients from different ICUs had croup and went on to have a refractory cardiac failure, bradycardia, and acidosis. A lipemic serum had developed in all patients. They had all received propofol at an average rate of about 8 mg/kg/hr for more than 70 hours.

In review the case reports were not as simple or as complete in their reporting, with several published letters[115] from physicians involved with these patients showing incomplete data in the reporting. Several other case reports of an apparently similar clinical course were then subsequently described in the literature. This was enough evidence for the Committee on Safety of Medicines in the United Kingdom to issue a warning on propofol and its use in pediatric patients. At this time the FDA could not find a causal link between propofol and the deaths in children and did not issue a warning.

This reaction to propofol came to be known as the *propofol infusion syndrome*.[116] It is the sudden or relatively sudden onset of a marked bradycardia resistant to treatment with a least one of the following signs: lipemia, enlarged liver, severe metabolic acidosis, or rhabdomyolysis.

The syndrome is unlikely to be due to the carrier emulsion because intralipid has been used extensively in severely ill patients without problems. The propofol metabolites are acidic, highly water soluble, and have a short $T_{1/2}$.

A steady number of case reports of this syndrome have appeared in the literature since the initial description, as well as a couple of studies involving several hundred patients[117,118] who have not shown any problem with propofol in the PICU. In these studies, lower doses of propofol (4 mg/kg/hr) have been used, with regular monitoring of the acid base status and triglyceride levels. "Propofol bashing" became popular.[119] There are few drugs that are licensed specifically for the PICU, however, and there is a need for proper trials to avoid drugs being condemned as hearsay. Subsequently, a randomized, controlled trial of propofol was begun, and after its use in 327 patients, it was reviewed by the FDA.[120] The study was never published, but researchers found that, despite similar PRISM scores, patients who had received either 1% or 2% propofol preparations had a 2 to 3 times greater risk of death compared with the control sedative group. This led to a letter from AstraZeneca reminding health care workers that propofol was not approved for sedation of pediatric patients.[121]

There is still a lot of debate as to whether there is a safe infusion rate or duration of infusion for propofol in the PICU setting. It has been estimated that a study to show a significant increase in death would require 7000 patients, which would be difficult to accomplish.

The propofol infusion syndrome has also now been described in adult patients.[122] These patients had similar cardiac and metabolic findings, often associated with the management of intracranial hypertension. Propofol infusion syndrome appeared to be a higher risk if the 2% formulation was used. Patients with raised ICP require deeper levels of sedation; require higher doses of propofol; and also are receiving vasopressor support to maintain the CPP, which puts a further stress on a myocardium that is already failing.

The pathophysiologic cause of the syndrome is still poorly understood, but case reports have shown some metabolic abnormalities that may be the cause of the cardiac failure and acidosis. One report describes a 10-month-old child who had the syndrome and was successfully treated with hemofiltration and plasmapheresis.[123] Muscle and liver biopsy specimens showed changes consistent with a toxic insult. Analysis also showed a reduction in the cytochrome C oxidase activity in the muscle, with a normal activity in skin fibroblasts excluding an underlying respiratory chain defect. Profound acidosis with lactic acidosis is found in different types of genetically acquired cytochrome oxidase deficiency. It was postulated that the hemofiltration removed a water-soluble metabolite of propofol that had caused a reversible reduction in the oxidase activity. A second case report[124] also showed a metabolic abnormality. Elevated levels of malonylcarnitine and C5-acyl carnitine were found in a patient with propofol infusion syndrome. This patient was also treated successfully with hemofiltration. These findings are consistent with impaired fatty acid oxidation, with impaired entry of long chain fatty acids into the mitochondria and a failure of the respiratory chain. A review of the pathophysiologic function of the syndrome[125] suggested that propofol increases the activity of malonyl coenzyme A, which inhibits the carnitine palmityl transferase I, so long chain fatty acids cannot enter the mitochondria. Propofol also uncouples oxidation, so the short and medium chain fatty acids cannot be used, even though they have entered the mitochondria. Low energy production leads to cardiac and peripheral muscle necrosis.

In pediatric patients it has been suggested that an inadequate calorific intake coupled with a high metabolic demand requires a fully active fatty acid oxidation capacity. Propofol may inhibit this pathway and cause a cellular metabolic failure syndrome to develop. Children have lower glycogen stores and often require higher doses of sedative agents; thus the syndrome is more likely to occur in the pediatric patient. A carbohydrate intake of 6 to 8 mg/kg/min should be enough to suppress fat metabolism in the critically ill child. Also, there have been concerns raised about the influence of catecholamines and steroids in the development of the syndrome, especially in the adult population.

Propofol is still frequently used for procedural and short-term sedation,[126] but in a recent case report, researchers describe a patient who had a propofol infusion syndrome.[127] The patient had received a propofol infusion for 15 hours at 20 mg/kg/hr. After a 13-hour propofol-free period, an 8-hour infusion of propofol at 4 mg/kg/hr was given, after which the patient had intractable bradycardia and acidosis. This raises concerns about high-dose short-term propofol use in the PICU.

In a report on the use of propofol for two cases of refractory status epilepticus, patients aged 7 and 17 years had features similar to the propofol infusion syndrome.[128] Status epilepticus itself can result in neurologic deficit, hypoxia, rhabdomyolysis, cardiac arrhythmias, hyperthermia, metabolic acidosis, acute renal failure, and death. These patients, however, received high doses of propofol (18 to 27 mg/kg/hr) to achieve burst suppression for more than 48 hours, and both patients had rhabdomyolysis and cardiac failure. No monitoring of lipid status or acid base was performed, and propofol was used as the sole agent by practitioners with limited experience with this drug. In light of the reports now appearing in the adult neurointensive[129] care literature with the development of a propofol infusion-like syndrome in adult neurosurgical patients, it would appear that it is not the best choice for prolonged sedation for intracranial hypertension.[1]

Propofol remains a useful agent for procedural sedation in the PICU. When compared with midazolam and ketamine, propofol resulted in safe, effective sedation. The propofol-sedated patients awakened almost twice as fast; thus the efficiency of the sedation service was also improved.[130] It is also probably appropriate for overnight sedation, and higher doses should be avoided. It should probably not be used as a solo agent because tolerance appears to develop more rapidly. If its use is required for a prolonged period, then careful consideration should be given to its risks and benefits. A recent study showed that staff members of some PICUs are still using long-term high doses despite the potential risks involved.[131] Regular monitoring of the acid base status and triglycerides, as well as ensuring adequate calorific intake, should be maintained. If symptoms of the propofol infusion syndrome develop early, hemofiltration appears to be the current treatment of choice.

Sedation and Analgesia for Procedures

Many procedures performed on children involve pain and anxiety. In many hospitals the administration of sedation and analgesia falls to the pediatric intensivist.[132] The pediatric intensivist needs to be familiar with guidelines and protocols that are used for conscious sedation outside the ICU setting. Procedural pain accounts for most of the pain experienced by children with malignancies,[133] and many pediatric patients with trauma will require sedation for procedures such as correction in the emergency department of fractured limbs and lacerations.

Conscious sedation is a medically controlled state of depressed consciousness, whereby the patient remains responsive to verbal stimuli or, at most, a gentle shaking of the shoulder.[134] It anticipates that protective reflexes will be maintained and that the patient retains a patent airway independently. Neither airway patency nor airway protection should be taken for granted because patients with conditions such as obstructive sleep apnea may obstruct their airway with little sedation and aspiration of food can occur even without sedation.

Before conscious sedation is further explored, the insightful words spoken by Burton Epstein, in his "40th Rovenstine Lecture of the ASA" in the fall of 2002, should be considered: "The Myth . . . of the achievability of a state of conscious sedation in which pediatric patients are simultaneously responsive to voice stimulus while immobile in the face of pain is just that—a myth."[135]

A little consideration will reveal that for painless procedures, anxiolysis will most likely suffice, whereas for painful procedures, pharmacological elimination of the response to pain will result in a need for general anesthesia. Between these two extremes, the use of local anesthetics may modify the response so as to allow potentially

TABLE 116–12

States of Altered Consciousness

Designation	Description
1	Minimal sedation (anxiolysis)
2	Moderate sedation/analgesia ("conscious sedation")
3	Deep sedation/analgesia
4	General anesthesia

BOX 116–6

The Goals of Sedation

- Guard the patient's safety and welfare
- Minimize physical discomfort or pain
- Minimize negative psychological responses to treatment
- Control behavior
- Return patient to a state in which safe discharge is possible

BOX 116–7

Non-ICU Procedures Requiring Sedation

- Cardiac catheterization—diagnostic, angioplasty, stents, valvuloplasty, closure devices
- Neuroradiology—angiograms, stents, embolization
- Ultrasound—TEE, drainage procedures
- CT scan-guided abscess drainage

CT, Computed tomography; *ICU,* intensive care unit; *TEE,* transesophageal echocardiography.

painful procedures to be performed during conscious sedation. Another factor to consider is the effect of variation in the level of stimulation, whereby sedation titrated to effect during a painful stimulus becomes excessive once the stimulus is completed. Thus the practitioner treads on a narrow and sometimes impossible pathway when giving conscious sedation. The state of conscious sedation is part of a continuum (Table 116–12) defined by the working groups of the American Academy of Pediatrics (AAP) and the American Society of Anesthesiology (ASA),[136] which encompasses a range from anxiolysis to general anesthesia that is appropriate for surgery.

This continuum is difficult to control, and staff administering conscious sedation must be able to appropriately manage any patients who enter a deeper level of sedation than that planned. The goals of sedation are shown in Box 116-6.

It is helpful to think of conscious sedation as consisting of several components. A balanced sedation technique will involve amnesia, analgesia, relaxation, and inattention. Different procedures require different degrees of these components (Table 116–13).

Procedure

There are many instances when sedation may be beneficial in the PICU such as the placement of central lines, centesis tubes, and dressing changes. Sedation facilitates the procedure in the uncooperative patient and allows long or uncomfortable procedures to be performed. Outside the ICU, both noninvasive and invasive radiological examinations[137, 138] often require sedation (Box 116–7).

Safety with conscious sedation is largely determined by careful assessment and management of the airway, together with precautions to prevent aspiration of gastric contents. Adequacy of sedation largely depends on appropriate patient selection, the combination of the patients' known medical conditions, past sedation experience, and the nature (particularly pain) of the patients' procedures coupled with appropriate drug selection.

Conscious sedation may be better tolerated than deep sedation or general anesthesia when hemodynamic stability is compromised because many sedative and anesthesia agents induce cardiovascular instability such as vasodilation or myocardial depression. Furthermore, the ability to monitor the patient's neurologic status during the procedure through conversation or instruction may be helpful, especially during invasive neuroradiological procedures. Conscious sedation may allow an earlier discharge because less sedative is being used and may make the procedure, which would usually require the full operating room environment, possible outside of the operating room.

All patients should be assessed before conscious sedation. Box 116–8 lists the elements that should be included in the assessment.

The medical history should include evaluation of the cardiorespiratory system, any history of gastroesophageal reflux, and any previously failed or abnormal reaction to sedation. A recent asthmatic attack or respiratory tract infection, poorly controlled seizure disorder, or diabetes may require a change or postponement of the sedation plan. It is recommended that patients should be classified according to the ASA preoperative patient classification (Table 116–14). In most circumstances it is generally recommended that patients in ASA class VI and some in class III are not suitable for conscious sedation.

Fasting Recommendations

It is prudent to adopt the same guidelines as are used before general anesthesia is administered, in case sedation that is deeper than anticipated occurs. These are age dependent, and current recommendations are shown in Table 116–15.

TABLE 116–13

Suggested Sedation Quality for Different Procedures

	Amnesia	Analgesia	Relaxation	Inattention
MRI	0	0	1	4
Endoscopy	1	3	2	2
Paracentesis	1	3	0	2
Burn dressing	2	4	0	2
Local anesthesia	3	2	2	3

MRI, magnetic resonance imaging.

BOX 116–8

Presedation Assessment

History
- Medications
- Allergies
- Previous experience with sedation, anesthesia
- Alcohol, tobacco, illicit substance abuse

Fasting

Examination
- Head extension and neck flexion
- Mouth opening, jaw size
- Body habitus

Documentation
- Informed consent
- Instructions and information to responsible person

Despite this, less caution is often reported regarding fasting, without any apparent worsening of outcome. For example, in a survey of 450 radiology departments, 35% had no NPO (nothing by mouth) for neonates, and 17% used 2 hours NPO for infants. For oral contrast studies, most departments sedated the patient within 1 hour of the contrast being swallowed.[139] Consent should be obtained as with any medically indicated procedure or intervention. It should include discussion about the risks and benefits of the procedure and the sedation technique, as well as expectations of outcome and alternatives to the procedure and sedation.

The presedation interview for outpatients or non-ICU patients should also involve giving instructions and information to a responsible person, including postsedation instructions, a 24-hour phone contact phone number, guidelines concerning limitations of activity, and expected postsedation behavior. If conscious sedation is provided for nonscheduled patients, a review of several aspects is important (Box 116-9).

Sedation provided outside the ICU should be performed in a facility/area with the appropriately trained support staff. The staff should have had appropriate training with respect to pharmacology, monitoring, resuscitation (basic and advanced life support), emergency drugs, and cardiac arrest protocols and medications. Advanced cardiac life support (ACLS) and pediatric advanced life support (PALS) recommendations should be available to be followed.

TABLE 116–14

ASA Classification

Class	Description
I	A normally healthy patient
II	A patient with mild or well-controlled disease state
III	A patient with severe or poorly controlled disease state
IV	A patient with severe disease state that is a constant threat to life
V	A moribund patient who is not expected to survive without surgery

ASA, American Society of Anesthesiology.

TABLE 116–15

Presedation NPO Guidelines

	Solids/Nonclear Liquids*	Clear Liquids†
Adults	6 hr	3 hr
Children	6 hr	3 hr
Neonates (<3 mo)	4 hr	2 hr

NPO, Nothing by mouth.
*Milk, breast milk, pulp fruit juices.
†Clear fruit juices, water.

Monitoring of patients undergoing conscious sedation is an important component of safe, effective sedation. There are several different recommendations by the Joint Commission on Accreditation of Healthcare Organizations (JCAHO),[140] the American Board of Anesthesiology, and the American Academy of Pediatrics. These recommendations have not yet been fully followed by those providing sedation for children.[141] A study of pediatric dentists after publication by the AAP of its new recommendations found minimal monitoring and documentation of the sedation procedure. Baseline vital signs are important. Because of the possibility of oversedation, the level of consciousness should be assessed frequently, especially during titration of effect. This is best assessed with the Ramsay scale (see Table 116-1). A sedation record is important for documentation of the drugs used with times and doses and for the monitored measurements that are charted on a time-based record. Monitoring should include pulse oximetry for assessment of the degree of oxygenation and heart rate. The saturation should be maintained by supplemental oxygen. Breathing can be assessed either by monitoring the respiratory rate or by capnography. The blood pressure should be checked at regular intervals during the procedure. A study of 85 pediatric patients with complications after sedation showed that most severe complications resulted from a common pathway involving respiratory depression leading to respiratory arrest, cardiac arrest, and subsequent severe neurologic devastation. The most common causes for these complications are summarized in Box 116–10. There is no particular drug that is more

BOX 116–9

Preparing for Conscious Sedation

Consider airway
- Assess airway
- Preexisting risk factors
- Trauma-induced risk factors

Circulation
- Correct hypovolemia
- Hypovolemia is manifest when sympathetic tone is decreased

Fasting
- Time of last meal
- Trauma-induced delay in gastric emptying
- Drug-induced delay in gastric emptying

BOX 116–10

Causes of Sedation Complications

Drug overdose
Inadequate monitoring—during and after
Lack of appropriate skills by staff administering the sedation
Lack of appropriate pharmacology knowledge

likely to cause problems. Polypharmacy, especially with three or more drugs, has been shown to be a risk factor for pediatric sedation complications.[142] Dentists using nitrous oxide in combination with other agents appeared to have a higher incidence of problems. If long-acting drugs are used, the patient must be observed for an appropriate length of time. There were several reports of respiratory arrest occurring while the child was in the car seat on the way home. Any health care worker providing conscious sedation should be familiar with an emergency algorithm in case problems arise (Fig. 116–4).

There are many different pharmacological options for conscious sedation in children. The oral route is commonly used in children; it has a slow onset time that avoids a rapid peak effect, but also gives an unpredictable degree of sedation, which is not easy to titrate. IM administration is painful; however, it is useful in the uncooperative patient. The rectal route is nearly always available and has found favor in the past for barbiturate sedation. More contemporaneously, rectal diazepam at 0.2 to 0.5 mg/kg has proved useful in the control of seizures where IV access is not available.[143] Onset can be fairly slow and duration prolonged. The IV route offers a titratable effect but also adds the danger of acute uncontrolled overdose. Other routes include intranasal and transmucosal administration. Dosing recommendations are shown in Table 116–16.

Always keep in mind that BZD-opiate or barbiturate-opiate combinations are potent causes of respiratory depression, and extra monitoring and vigilance should be used. With IM and oral medications, adequate time should elapse to allow absorption before a further dose is given to avoid accidental overdose.

As noted in Table 116-13, different procedures require different qualities of sedation. These qualities are found in the array of drugs available to the intensivist (Table 116-17).

It may be useful to choose the sedative agent or agents that best fit the particular requirements for the procedure being performed.

Opiate and BZD antagonists should be readily available wherever conscious sedation is being performed. Staff caring for these patients should understand the drug indications and dosing of these medications to reduce any potential delay in their appropriate use. They can quickly

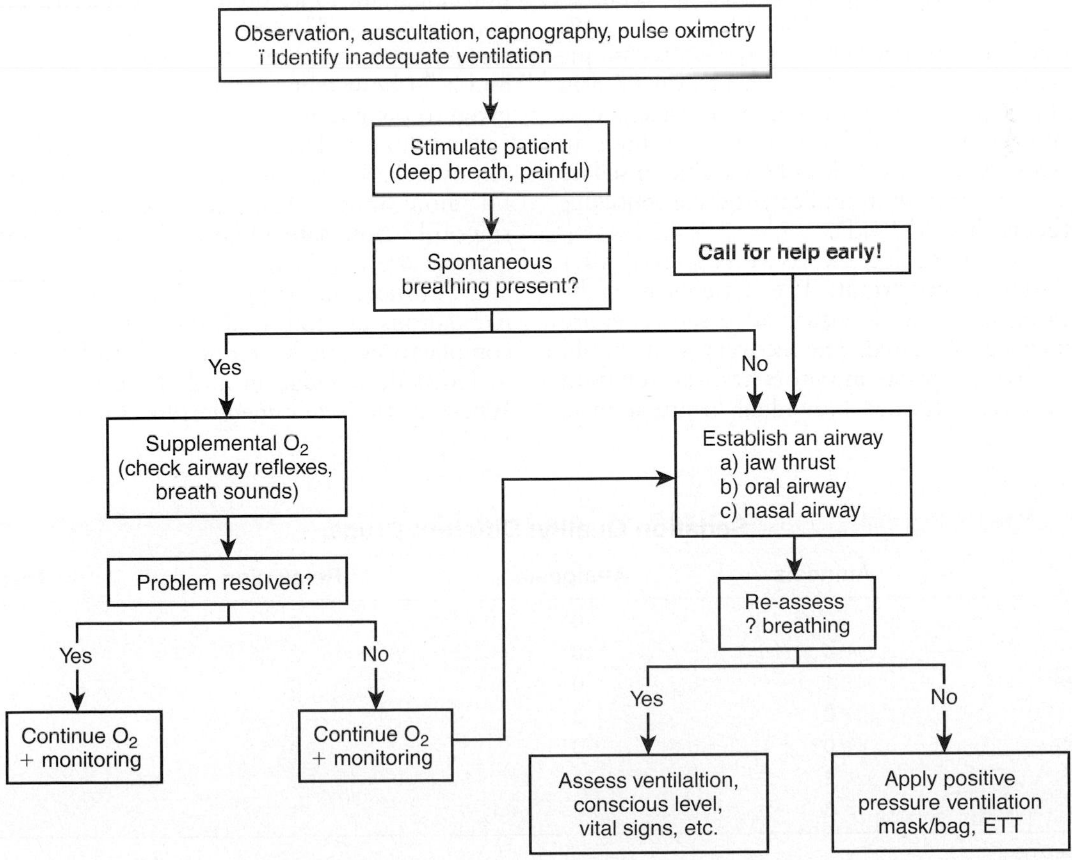

FIGURE 116–4 • Sedation emergency airway algorithm.

TABLE 116–16

Drug Dose Guidelines for Conscious Sedation

Route	Drug	Dose
PO	Chloral hydrate	50–75 mg/kg (repeat 25 mg/kg)
	Diazepam (Valium)	0.2–0.4 mg/kg (max, 20 mg)
	Midazolam (Versed)	0.5–0.75 mg/kg (max, 20 mg)
IM	Pentobarbital (Nembutal)	4–6 mg/kg (max, 100 mg)
	Fentanyl (Sublimaze)	1–3 μg/kg
	CM3	0.08–0.1 ml/kg (max, 2 ml)
IV	Morphine	0.1 mg/kg
	Meperidine (Demerol)	1–2 mg/kg (max, 75 mg)
	Fentanyl (Sublimaze)	1–2 μg/kg (max, 5 μg/kg)
	Midazolam (Versed)	0.05–0.1 mg/kg
	Diazepam (Valium)	0.05–0.1 mg/kg

CM3, Catheterization mixture number 3; *IM,* intramuscular; *IV,* intravenous; *PO,* by mouth.

and effectively reverse the respiratory depression from excessive doses of sedation.

In some circumstances the services of the anesthesia department may be useful. The anesthesia department has access to other pharmacological agents such as propofol and nitrous oxide, as well as the inhalational agents. The ability to use a deeper level of sedation if required is easily obtained with these rapidly acting, short-acting agents.

In emergency procedures where the patient's NPO status is unsafe or unknown, patients may need to undergo intubation to protect the airway. Anesthesiologists have the ability to perform a "needleless" sedation technique using a gas induction with anesthetic agents; an IV drip may be placed if required when the patient is asleep. This technique is especially useful for repeat procedures in oncology patients. Also, anesthesia is better able to sedate patients whose illness may contraindicate routine conscious sedation protocols (Box 116–11).

Care of the patient during the recovery period after conscious sedation is important. The patients must be monitored during recovery to ensure adverse events are rapidly recognized and treated. The recovery area should be equipped with appropriate monitors and resuscitation equipment and have a trained individual in attendance.

BOX 116–11

Patients Unsuitable for Conscious Sedation

- Premature (<60 weeks' gestation)
- Apnea, respiratory, or cardiac monitor at home
- Airway obstruction
- BPD, COPD, recent pneumonia, or croup
- Uncontrolled seizures or multiple medications
- Multiple psychotropic medications
- Poorly controlled asthma
- Vomiting
- GERD
- Raised ICP
- History of difficult sedation

BPD, Bronchopulmonary dysplasia; *COPD,* chronic obstructive pulmonary disease; *GERD,* gastroesophageal reflux disease; *ICP,* intracranial pressure.

The monitoring should be performed to the same degree as during the actual procedure. Level of consciousness and vital signs should be recorded at regular intervals. A physician who is responsible for the patient must be identifiable and must be easy to contact if required urgently. Patients may be discharged home when they are alert and orientated or when they have returned to baseline if baseline initial mental status was abnormal. Vital signs should be stable and within acceptable limits. A sufficient time should have elapsed if a reversal agent was used (2 hours). Patients should be discharged in the presence of a responsible adult to accompany them home and report any complications. Written instructions should be given to the parent concerning diet, medications, and activities, and a 24-hour contact telephone number should also be given to the parent.

Conscious sedation is safe and frequently used; unconscious sedation is potentially hazardous and needs careful monitoring. Hospital protocols are useful for a smoothly run, safe sedation policy.[144] Staff should be appropriately trained in sedation and resuscitation basic and advanced life support. When the ASA/AAP recommendations are followed, the risks of a sedation-related complication can be reduced.[145] Individual risk factors included deep sedation and the use of chloral hydrate. When all the recommendations for conscious sedation,

TABLE 116–17

Sedation Quality: Different Drugs

	Amnesia	Analgesia	Relaxation	Inattention
Barbiturates	0	0*	0	4
BZDs	4	0	2	4
Antihistamines	1	0	0	2
Opioids	0	2	0*	2
Chloral hydrate	0?	0	0	4
Ketamine	2	4	0*	4
Nitrous oxide	3	3	1	3

BZD, Benzodiazepine.
*May antagonize other drugs having this effect.

including NPO, ASA class, avoidance of deep sedation, sedation level monitoring, and drug use, were followed, the adverse event rate was zero.

Sedation for Magnetic Resonance Imaging

The PICU physician is often called on to provide sedation for the patient in the ICU undergoing MRI. Also, many institutions rely on the PICU team to provide a sedation service for other inpatients or outpatients undergoing MRI. The same standards should be adhered to as with any other child undergoing sedation[146] with respect to patient selection, monitoring, and postimaging care.

MRI is an imaging modality that is being increasingly used to aid in the diagnosis of neuroanatomic disorders. The patient is required to lie still within a small space while multiple images are obtained. MRI scanning is less rapid than computed tomography (CT) scanning. If the patient moves, this will cause degradation of the image quality, and a change in the patient's position may affect the homogeneity of the magnetic field, which is optimized at the beginning of the scan. Studies can take from 45 minutes to more than 2 hours, with individual sequences taking 3 to 10 minutes. The scanner is noisy and the restriction on space and movement can induce claustrophobia in some patients. The patient may also experience a slight increase in temperature. Most adults and older children (older than 6 years) are capable of lying still for the scan. With the use of earplugs and music it is well tolerated. There are several groups of patients, however, who may require sedation[147] for the scan to be performed (Box 116–12).

Because of the large magnetic field there are several unique problems[148] that can occur during a scan. These include the potential risk of the magnet causing a ferromagnetic object to move or heat up or the induction of an electric current from the radiofrequency (RF) pulses and switching magnetic gradients used in generating the images. This results in a significant list of contraindications to MRI (Box 116–13).

There are also several risk factors for sedating these patients. The patient is in a remote location, with limited access to and visibility of the airway. There are also several equipment issues (Box 116–14).

The monitors used must be suitable for use in the MRI suite.[149] They should be nonferromagnetic; the cables should be screened from electromagnetic interference (fiberoptic is ideal); and the signal should be filtered to avoid RF interference (interferes with image quality).

BOX 116–13

Contraindications to Magnetic Resonance Imaging (not a complete list)

Cardiac pacemaker
Aneurysm clips
Automatic implanted cardiac defibrillator
Neurostimulator
Pacing wires
Cochlear implant
Implanted insulin pump
Penile prosthesis
History of ocular injury involving metal object
History of vascular surgery < 3 months
History of soft tissue metal foreign body < 3 months
History of orthopedic hardware < 3 months

Despite the specialized technology that is available, several problems still remain. The ECG waveform is frequently altered, and analog information is often lacking during a scanning cycle. The ECG cables may cause burn injury, and special ECG electrodes are required to avoid burn injury. For pulse oximetry to be performed, a special probe is required. Heating of the usual probe may cause burn injury. Fiberoptic connection to the patient is best. Capnography requires long tubing, which results in a prolonged upsweep and delay in displaying real-time measurements. The respiratory rate and trends can still be useful. Any battery-powered monitor requires a nonmagnetic lithium battery. Exposure to the MRI shortens battery life. ICU ventilators are not MRI compatible. There are specialized MRI-safe anesthesia machines that have a ventilator; however, their use should be restricted to the anesthesia staff who are familiar with the equipment. The IV poles and the equipment carts should also be nonferromagnetic. Any equipment with a transformer (syringe pumps, IV pumps) must be kept out of the magnetic field. Gas cylinders *must* be aluminum. The area around any magnet that generates a magnetic field stronger than 5 G should not contain any ferromagnetic items.

Any staff entering the MRI suite should remember to remove any ferromagnetic objects. These include keys, watches, pens, and credit cards. Stethoscopes and laryngoscopes are also ferromagnetic. Infusion pumps should be outside the magnetic field, that is, outside the 5-G line. The electric motor in infusion pumps emits electromagnetic radiation and may run at an abnormal speed in the

BOX 116–12

Indications for Sedation for Magnetic Resonance Imaging (not a complete list)

Very young or agitated patient
A prolonged study (multiple scans)
Anxiety
Claustrophobia
Intensive care patient

BOX 116–14

Potential Difficulties in Magnetic Resonance Imaging

Malfunction of anesthesia or sedation equipment
Malfunction of monitoring
Anesthesia or sedation equipment causing interference with image quality
"High velocity ferromagnetic projectile" from loose object
Disruption of electronic devices

presence of a strong magnetic field. The pump is also a projectile risk. IV infusions through long tubing from outside the scanner can be useful so that the depth of anesthesia can be altered without having to enter the MRI suite.

The use of a cuffed endotracheal tube (ETT) may affect the quality of the MRI image because of metal in the valve of the pilot balloon and reinforcement of the mask airway. With the patient in the ICU, special care must be taken to ensure that all cables and transducers that may be carefully screened and all ferromagnetic objects are removed ("hiding in the sheets"). For invasive vascular pressure to be measured, the transducer should be as far from the patient as is practically possible and separated with a saline-filled pressure line. If cardiac arrest occurs, the patient should be removed from the magnetic field. The defibrillator should be kept outside the magnetic field and checked regularly. A nonferromagnetic code cart is also advisable. It is essential that the code team follow the rules about removing any loose magnetic items before entering the MRI suite or else a lethal projectile may be released. Ventilating the lungs of the ICU patient is often performed by hand ventilation by ICU staff in the MRI suite. The sedation technique is often a continuation of that used in the ICU, especially for a patient who undergoes intubation. In some children single doses of fentanyl or midazolam may be sufficient for a adequate sedation. If deeper sedation is required for patient comfort/cooperation, then IV sedation with supplemental oxygen with propofol is useful. A bolus of 2 mg/kg and an infusion of 100 μg/kg/min is a good method for patients with few medical problems and an easily maintained airway. It results in a rapid recovery with little nausea or vomiting.

Anesthesia Drugs

Ketamine

Ketamine is a phencyclidine derivative that provides sedation and analgesia. It results in a state of dissociative (trancelike) anesthesia. It is available in a variety of different dilutions, such as 10 mg, 50 mg, and 100 mg/ml; the latter is the most useful for IM use and the preparation of infusions. For a state of general anesthesia to be induced, a dose of 2 mg/kg IV is required. Onset takes 1 to 2 minutes with anesthesia lasting 10 to 15 minutes. Lower doses may be used for sedation. Anesthesia can also be induced by the IM route with a dose of 10 mg/kg, although onset is slower (5 to10 minutes) and duration of prolonged effect is 45 to 60 minutes. It is metabolized by the liver and excreted by the kidneys. The $T_{1/2}$ is 3.1 hours (see Table 116–11).

The side effects of ketamine include hypertension, tachycardia, increased intracranial pressure, and bronchodilation. The bronchodilation is probably due to its sympathomimetic action. It is a direct myocardial depressant, but blood pressure is usually maintained by the sympathetic stimulation that ketamine causes. In critically ill patients who already are using their maximum sympathetic drive, ketamine may cause a fall in cardiac output. Hallucinations and other psychiatric symptoms are often reported during and after its use in adults, but they occur less frequently in children. It is a potent sialogogue, and the use of an anticholinergic agent such as glycopyrrolate may be helpful. Its use is contraindicated in those patients who cannot tolerate hypertension,[150] have a history of cerebrovascular hemorrhage, have psychiatric disturbances, and have raised ICP. It is a useful agent for sedation for procedures, especially if there is no IV access. It has been used in patients with status asthmaticus as an adjunct bronchodilator both in intubated and nonintubated patients at an infusion rate of 0.5 to 2 mg/kg/hr. After discontinuing its use, the patient should receive BZDs to minimize the likelihood of hallucinations and be nursed in a quiet environment. Ketamine cannot be assumed to preserve pharyngeal reflexes any better than other sedatives agents, and apnea and airway obstruction can still occur.[151] NPO guidelines should still be observed.

Etomidate

Etomidate is a carboxylated imidazole, unrelated to other anesthetic agents. It is a rapidly acting IV anesthetic agent, which, like other rapid-onset anesthetic agents, partitions into the brain within one circulation time and redistributes out of the brain over the next few minutes. It is available dissolved in 30% propylene glycol, 2 mg/ml, and causes pain on injection. The anesthetic dose is 0.2 to 0.3 mg/kg. It has a favorable side effect profile with minimal cardiovascular and respiratory depression. Etomidate is associated with a high incidence of nausea and vomiting after emergence from anesthesia. Its pharmacokinetics is shown in Table 116–11.

The greatest disadvantage of etomidate in the intensive care setting is adrenocortical depression due to inhibition of adrenocortical mitochondrial 11-β-hydroxylase.[152] This effect is present in neonates and in adults.[153] The outcome of patients sedated with etomidate is worse than in those using alternative sedation, and steroid deficiency is thought to be the cause.[154]

In the CNS, etomidate suppresses seizure activity, although patients may show excitatory movements not associated with cortical EEG changes suggestive of seizures. The intracranial and intraocular pressures are lowered. It is the drug of choice for patients who are undergoing emergency intubation, those who have head injuries, and those who have a compromised cardiovascular system, and it is safe for use in patients with asthma because there is no histamine release. Etomidate has the highest therapeutic index of any anesthetic agent.

There have been several case reports of its satisfactory use for controlling refractory intracranial hypertension; it is associated with fewer cardiovascular problems than barbiturates are. Nevertheless, caution has to be taken concerning the development of a lactic acidosis due to the metabolism of propylene glycol.

Inhalational Agents

The inhalational agents remain the most widely used anesthetics in the operating room, although their mechanism of action is still poorly understood. The following are the five agents in clinical use: halothane, enflurane, isoflurane, sevoflurane, and desflurane. Sevoflurane and desflurane are newer agents that currently have limited use in the ICU.

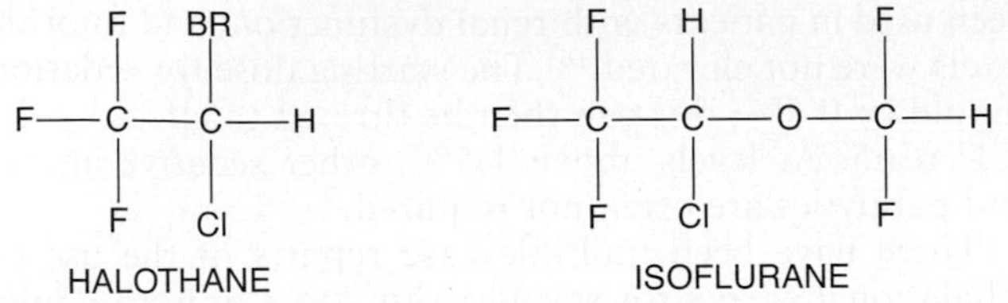

FIGURE 116–5 • Structures of inhalational agents.

Isoflurane remains the most logical choice of inhalational anesthetic in the ICU based on its cost/benefit ratio. As with any drug used in the ICU, it is important to understand the pharmacology; the side effect profile; and, in this case, the technical aspects of delivering these agents to the patient.

These agents are all fluorinated hydrocarbons (Fig. 116–5). Except for halothane they are ethyl-methyl esters. Each agent has different physicochemical properties that are important to its properties (Table 116–18).

The rate at which a change in inspired concentration is reflected in the brain is determined mainly by the blood/gas solubility. The more soluble the gas is in blood, the slower is the change due to the gas dissolving into the blood and reducing the partial pressure available to equilibrate with the brain. Sevoflurane and desflurane are the least soluble and therefore have the most rapid onset and offset; halothane has the slowest onset. The potency of the agents is represented by the minimal alveolar concentration (MAC). This is the percent of inhaled anesthesia agent that is required to prevent 50% of anesthetized patients from responding to a surgical incision. The lower the MAC, the more potent the agent is. Halothane is the most potent of the agents used and desflurane, the least. The MAC of anesthetic agents is not constant with age. For all the agents it is highest for those aged 1 to 12 months, and the MAC falls throughout childhood to reach adult levels. Neonates show a slightly reduced MAC compared with infants. The oil/water solubility determines the degree of accumulation of the agent within the body fat stores. A highly fat-soluble agent will have larger body stores; therefore recovery from the agent is delayed.

These agents all have significant effects on the cardiorespiratory systems. Although respiration can be controlled, the negative inotropic and vasodilator effects are pronounced and limit the concentrations that can be used. Halothane, the oldest of these agents still in use, has the greatest degree of cardiac depression. Sevoflurane and desflurane have a side effect profile similar to that of isoflurane, except that sevoflurane is partly metabolized to a potentially toxic metabolite, compound A, from a reaction with the soda lime used in anesthesia circle systems. For accumulation of compound A to be minimized in the circuit, a fresh gas flow of greater than 2 L/m should be used. Thus sevoflurane is currently not a good choice for prolonged ICU treatment with this type of circuit. Desflurane has some sympathomimetic effect, especially when the concentration is abruptly increased, and significant tachycardia and hypertension can occur.

Side effects of halothane include hypotension, which is due to direct myocardial depression. It also causes bradycardia because of effects on the sinoatrial node and vagal stimulation. Cardiac arrhythmias may occur, most commonly junctional rhythm. Halothane also sensitizes the myocardium to catecholamines, especially when the patient is hypercapnic or hypoxic. Because these physiologic changes are common in the intensive care patient, the potential for serious interactions with halothane abound. Halothane is metabolized approximately 20% by the liver, and a trifluoroacetic metabolite may cause an immune-mediated fatal hepatitis.[155]

Isoflurane causes hypotension mainly because of vasodilation, while maintaining cardiac output. There has been concern about a coronary steal phenomenon occurring in which blood is diverted from a partially obstructed coronary bed served by collateral arteries, due to vasodilation. The evidence for this is weak, however, and ischemia is probably due to hypotension rather than a true steal phenomena. Isoflurane vapor is pungent and may cause airway irritation, coughing, and laryngospasm if the patient is not adequately sedated before its use. It is only minimally metabolized (0.2%), and a hepatitis reaction is extremely unlikely.

Malignant hyperthermia is a rare reaction that may occur whenever the halogenated inhalational anesthetics or succinylcholine is given to a patient. It involves the unrestrained entry of calcium into myocytes and consequential consumption of adenosine triphosphate (ATP), resulting in metabolic failure. Hypermetabolism, manifested by increased CO_2 production, and acidosis occur. Later, the body temperature rises, and death from hyperkalemia occurs. Correction of blood chemistry, aggressive cooling, and the administration of dantrolene are urgently indicated (see Chapter 117).

The metabolism of all the anesthesia agents can result in the production of free fluoride ions. Concentrations of

TABLE 116–18

Vapor Characteristics

	Halothane	Isoflurane	Sevoflurane	Desflurane
MW	197.4	184.5	200	168
SVP (mmHg)	243	240	157	700
Boiling point ° C	50.2	48.5	58.5	22.8
MAC (%)	0.75–1.2	1.3–1.85	2.5–3.0	8.0–10
Blood/gas solubility	2.3	1.4	0.68	0.42
Oil/w% metabolized	20	0.2	3.3	0.02

MAC, Minimal alveolar concentration; *MW,* molecular weight; *SVP,* saturated vapor pressure.

fluoride greater than 50 μmol/L can cause renal dysfunction and a reduced concentrating capacity. This would appear to be a higher risk for both halothane and sevoflurane because of their more extensive metabolism. It may also be exaggerated by patients who are prescribed drugs that induce the cytochrome P450 enzyme complex.

Inhalational agents may cause hepatotoxicity in two ways: (1) by metabolism to reactive intermediates that are directly hepatotoxic or (2) through the intermediates that form adducts to hepatic proteins. These new proteins are then recognized as foreign, and an immune response that causes hepatic injury occurs. This is thought to be the mechanism of halothane hepatitis. This form of hepatitis is most common after halothane use; even then it is rare, occurring in 1 of 100,000 cases. It is less common with isoflurane, sevoflurane, or desflurane, which are much less metabolized. This fulminant hepatic failure, which may be fatal, is most common after repeated administrations of halothane in the older obese patient. The predominance of reductive halothane pathway metabolism results in a trifluoroacetic acid metabolite that forms a hapten. Halothane hepatitis is also less common in children.

All the inhalational agents cause cerebral vasodilation, which results in an increase in CBF (due to decoupling of the demand/flow ratio) and ICP. In pediatric patients with raised ICP, there was no difference among isoflurane, desflurane, and sevoflurane with respect to the increase in ICP and CBF.[156] In contrast, IV anesthetics maintain the demand/flow ratio, and CBF and ICP fall, with the exception of ketamine. In addition to an effect of CBF, the arterial blood pressure typically will decrease with anesthesia, and the effect of this on the CPP must be accounted for. In one study, the effect of the decrease in arterial pressure on CPP exceeded the effect of increasing ICP by a factor of 3.[157]

With these potential effects on CBF, the use of isoflurane should be carefully considered in those patients who have or are at risk of raised ICP. Nevertheless, isoflurane has been safely used in neuroanesthesia with controlled ventilation to a normal $PaCO_2$ and an inspired concentration not exceeding 1 MAC.[158]

Isoflurane has two main functions in the PICU: sedation and the management of refractory asthma. There are only a few reports of long-term sedative use of isoflurane in the ICU. In an adult study, 40 patients[159] who received an average of 96 MAC hours of isoflurane showed hemodynamic stability, less tachyphylaxis as compared with other sedative agents, and a more rapid wean from the ventilator. There was no evidence of renal or hepatic dysfunction with serum fluorides less than 50 μmol/L. In a pediatric study, 10 patients[160] who had been receiving large doses of opiates or BZDs received an average of 130 MAC hours of isoflurane. The range of use was from 1 to 30 days. Fifty percent of the patients experienced a withdrawal-like phenomenon, most commonly, those who had received more than 70 MAC hours of isoflurane. Fluoride levels were also measured, and although they were correlated with the duration of treatment, none was greater than 30 μmol/L. The highest levels were in a patient who was taking both phenytoin and phenobarbitone. Hypotension only occurred in one patient. There was no hepatic or renal dysfunction. The withdrawal was treated with a combination of BZDs and haloperidol with good effect. Isoflurane has also been used in patients with renal dysfunction, and fluoride levels were not elevated.[161] The starting dose for sedation should be 0.5%; this can then be titrated to effect by the ICU team. At levels above 1.5%, other sedative agents and paralytics are often not required.

There have been multiple case reports of the use of inhalational agents for status asthmaticus in both adults and children. Because of its speed of onset and its bronchodilation effects, isoflurane is a useful adjunct to β_2 agonists. If there is no improvement, or if unacceptable side effects occur, then its effects rapidly wane on discontinuation. Isoflurane is recommended for use because of its safer side effect profile. There have been no reports of renal or hepatic dysfunction despite use for often prolonged periods. Hypotension seems to be more common in these patients; it is possibly related to increased intrathoracic pressure and the potential for greater preload reduction with vasodilation. Fluid boluses and occasionally vasopressors are often required. Because isoflurane is not an analgesic agent, opiates may be needed for painful or uncomfortable procedures. Also, when the patient is weaned off the isoflurane, additional sedatives will be required. The isoflurane should be started at 0.5% and titrated for effect; doses of up to 2.5% have been reported as safely used.[162]

Delivery of Inhalation Agents

These gases are liquids at room temperature; a special delivery device called a *vaporizer* is required to deliver an accurate supply of the vapor. All vaporizers have several features in common. They provide a reservoir of the inhalational liquid with a level indicator and are capable of delivering a constant level of vaporization. Most newer vaporizers also have a color-coded keyed filler (e.g., purple, isoflurane; yellow, sevoflurane) that prevents the accidental filling of the vaporizer with the wrong agent. This could result in overdosing the patient because the vaporizer calibration is drug specific. If two vaporizers are accommodated in series on the anesthesia machine back bar, then an interlocking system should be used to prevent the accidental use of both vaporizers. Otherwise, the results would be contamination of the second vaporizer by gas from the first vaporizer and an uncontrolled excess delivery of gas to the patient.

One of the main problems with using these inhalational agents in the PICU is how to deliver them to the patient. One technique is to use an anesthesia machine to deliver the gas to an ICU ventilator with the correct oxygen percentage and inhalational agent. This mixture is delivered from the fresh gas outlet of the anesthesia machine. It is selected by adjustment of the flow rotameters on the anesthesia machine to give the desired oxygen concentration and then selection of the desired inspired concentration of inhalational agent on the vaporizer. Unfortunately, most ICU ventilators will not accept this low pressure gas supply as their driving gas. The Servo 900C is an exception because it has a low pressure inlet option for the driving gas. High flow rates are required to maintain filling the bellows of the ventilator; the flow rates must be higher than the minute ventilation. This sometimes results in a limitation of inspired oxygen because of the maximum flow of oxygen from the rotameters of the anesthesia machine being 10 to 12 L/m. Also, this consumes a lot of vapor.

Also available is another Servo ventilator, the 900D, that has a custom-fit vaporizer on the normal high pressure input. This machine is similar to the 900C, but it has been modified for anesthesia use and allows hand ventilation with inhalational agent also. Often the only alternative is to deliver anesthetic with an anesthesia machine. Anesthesia machine ventilators are not as sophisticated as ICU ventilators, may not be able to deliver appropriate volumes for pediatric patients, and often have limited positive end-expiratory pressure (PEEP) capabilities. The anesthesia machine needs to be checked before use and its correct function continually assessed during its use. This requires an understanding of the setup and alarms on the machine and an understanding of the procedures of the appropriate tests. This is usually not within the confines of a pediatric intensivist's scope of practice, and an anesthesiologist should be involved to ensure the safe and effective use of this apparatus.

Whenever inhalational agents are used, the waste gases from the expiratory limb of the ventilator should be scavenged to avoid prolonged exposure of the health care worker to these agents. The Occupational Safety and Health Administration (OSHA) limits occupational exposure to 2 ppm halothane for health care workers.[163] There are risks of the worker becoming sedated and also potential teratogenic effects. Several large studies about prolonged exposure to these agents have not shown any increase in risks for anesthesia personnel with respect to hepatic disease, teratogenesis, spontaneous abortions, psychological difficulties, infertility, neuropathy, or bone marrow depression.[164] Caution should also be taken when filling the vaporizer to avoid spilling the liquid during the process.[165] There are two forms of scavenging available. A passive system involves simply a tube connected to the expiratory limb connected to the outside. This system is at risk of occlusion because of kinking or someone standing inadvertently on the tubing; this will then occlude the expiratory limb of the ventilator. An active system involves an active suction to the expiratory limb, with a safety reservoir bag in series to prevent excess suction pressure being exposed to the patient.

In the operating room it is routine to monitor the levels of anesthesia agents given with a gas analyzer. This gives an inspired and expired inhalational agent concentration. This is helpful to ensure that the vaporizer is functioning correctly, that the vaporizer has not emptied without being detected, and that the concentration dialed on the vaporizer has reached its effect. When the end-tidal inhalational agent concentration equals the inspired agent, then steady state has been achieved. This normally occurs rapidly with isoflurane, but in a patient with severe asthma due to the severe limitation in airflow gas exchange, this may be delayed.

If the PICU staff is unfamiliar with the delivery system being used for the isoflurane, then it would be appropriate to have staff from the anesthesiology department set up the equipment and be sure that it functions correctly. Failure to configure the delivery system correctly has the potential to cause considerable harm or death. Once the situation has stabilized, an anesthesiologist may not be required at the bedside; however, an anesthesiologist should be available by pager to help troubleshoot any difficulties. The inspired agent should be monitored at least on a daily basis and ideally continually.

The use of inhalational agents in the PICU does involve the use of equipment that may be unfamiliar to pediatric intensivists. Isoflurane appears to be the best choice,[166] and it does offer several useful advantages, including the ability to deeply sedate patients (especially those difficult to sedate) without polypharmacy.[167] Although poorly defined currently,[168] tolerance and a withdrawal-like syndrome have been described, however, they appear to occur more slowly than with other sedative agents. It may be helpful to have a set of guidelines available for isoflurane use to facilitate its use in the PICU. These could include equipment use, monitoring requirements, dosing, and treatment of complications.[169] Caution should be used in patients who may have raised ICP because isoflurane may increase CBF. Isoflurane does allow, however, for a rapid wake-up if neurologic examinations are required.

Pharmacoeconomics

In today's economical climate it is important to consider the cost of the different sedation options available to the pediatric intensivist (Table 116–19). Most PICUs use a low-cost sedative regimen for the bulk of the sedations

TABLE 116–19

Relative Drug Costs of Different ICU Sedative Agents

Drug Class	Agent	Dose	Cost (cents /kg/hr)	Cost ($/kg/day)	Comments
Opiates	Fentanyl	4 μg/kg/hr	0.7	12	
	Morphine	50 μg/kg/hr	0.24	4	
	Sufentanil	0.8 μg/kg/hr	4.8	81	
	Remifentanil	0.4 μg/kg/min	21	353	
BZDs	Midazolam	0.1 mg/kg/hr	1.4	24	
	Lorazepam	0.1 mg/kg/hr	4.8	81	
Others	Dexmedetomidine	0.5 μg/kg/hr	38.5	643	
	Propofol	5 mg/kg/hr	18.9	318	
	Ketamine	2 mg/kg/hr	11.2	188	
	Isoflurane	0.5%	3.3	55	Servo 900D
	Sevoflurane	1%	59.8	1,005	Servo 900D

BZD, Benzodiazepine; *ICU,* intensive care unit.

required and keep the more expensive options for selected circumstances. Table 116–19 shows the different costs of some of the available agents in the PICU. They are presented as the cost per kilogram per hour of sedation at equipotent doses. The costs are the lowest hospital drug cost (Women's and Children's Hospital of Buffalo [WCHOB]) for each agent in its cheapest form and exclude preparation, delivery, and equipment issues related to each drug. Fentanyl is cheap, and for a 20-kg child, it costs $3.36 per day. Although morphine costs less, it has more potential side effects, which make the small extra cost of fentanyl warranted. Generic midazolam is now a cheaper option than lorazepam. The other synthetic opiates are expensive to use, and consideration should be given to appropriate indications for their use. A rapid recovery, however, with a quick extubation and early ICU discharge is also a considerable cost factor to be considered. Most of the nonopiate, non-BZD sedatives are expensive to use. The drug costs of isoflurane are comparable to those of the BZDs; however, it requires the availability of a specialized delivery system, which could increase the cost. If a device were available that could deliver isoflurane at low flows with most of the available ICU ventilators, then it would make isoflurane a more attractive option.

REFERENCES

1. Rundshagen I, Schnabel K, Wegner C, et al: Incidence of recall, nightmares, and hallucinations during analgosedation in intensive care, *Intensive Care Med* 28:38-43, 2002
2. Wagner BK, Zavotsky KE, Sweeney JB, et al: Patient recall of therapeutic paralysis in a surgical critical care unit, Pharmacotherapy 18:358-363, 1998.
3. Jones C, Griffiths RD, Humphris G, et al: Memory, delusions, and the development of acute posttraumatic stress disorder-related symptoms after intensive care, *Crit Care Med* 29:573-580, 2001.
4. Playfor S, Thomas D, Choonara I: Recollection of children following intensive care, *Arch Dis Child* 83:445-448, 2000.
5. Ramsay MA, Savege TM, Simpson BR, et al: Controlled sedation with aphaxalone-alphadone, *Br Med J* 2:656-659, 1974.
6. Brattebø G, Hofoss D, Flaatten H, et al: Effect of scoring system and protocol for sedation on duration of patients' need for ventilator support in a surgical intensive care unit, *BMJ* 324:1386-1389, 2002.
7. Ambuel B, Hamlett KW, Marx CM, et al: Assessing distress in pediatric intensive care environments: the COMFORT scale, J *Pediatr Psychol* 17:95-109, 1992.
8. Detriche O, Berre J, Massaut J, et al: The Brussels sedation scale: use of a simple clinical sedation scale can avoid excessive sedation in patients undergoing mechanical ventilation in the intensive care unit, *Br J Anaesth* 83:698-701, 1999.
9. Sebel PS, Lang E, Rampil IJ, et al: A multicenter study of bispectral electroencephalogram analysis for monitoring anesthetic effects, *Anesth Analg* 84:891-899, 1997.
10. Berkenbosch JW, Fichter CR, Tobias JD: The correlation of the bispectral index monitor with clinical sedation scores during mechanical ventilation in the pediatric intensive care unit, *Anesth Analg* 94:506-511, 2002.
11. Rosow C, Manberg PJ: Bispectral index monitoring, *Anesthesiol Clin North America* 2:89-107, 1998.
12. Struys M, Versichelen L, Byttebier G, et al: Clinical usefulness of the bispectral index for titrating target effect-site concentration, *Anesthesia* 53: 4-12, 1998.
13. Courtman SP, Wardurgh A, Petros AJ: Comparison of the bispectral index monitor with the comfort score in assessing level of sedation of critically ill children, *Intensive Care Med* 29:2239-2246, 2003.
14. Moerman N, Bonke B, Oosting J: Awareness and recall during general anesthesia, *Anesthesiology* 79:454-464, 1993.
15. Domino KB, Posner KL, Caplan RA, et al: Awareness during anesthesia. A closed claims analysis, *Anesthesiology* 90:1053-61, 1999.
16. Aneja R, Heard AM, Fletcher JE, et al: Sedation monitoring of children by the Bispectral Index in the pediatric intensive care unit, *Pediatr Crit Care Med* 4:60-64, 2003.
17. Zhou L, Zhang Q, Stein C, et al: Contribution of opioid receptors on primary afferent versus sympathetic neurons to peripheral opioid analgesia, *J Pharmacol Exp Ther* 286:1000-1006,1998.
18. Kalso E, Tramer MR, Carroll D, et al: Pain relief from intra-articular morphine after knee surgery: a qualitative systematic review, *Pain* 71:127-134, 1997.
19. Zadina JE, Martin-Schild S, Gerall AA, et al: Endomorphins: novel endogenous mu-opiate receptor agonists in regions of high mu-opiate receptor density, *Ann N Y Acad Sci* 897:136-144, 1999.
20. Slappendel R, Weber EW, Benraad B, et al: Itching after intrathecal morphine. Incidence and treatment, *Eur J Anaesthesiol* 17:616-621, 2000.
21. Sabbe MB, Yaksh TL: Pharmacology of spinal opioids, *J Pain Symptom Manage* 5:191-203, 1990.
22. Kart T, Christrup LL, Rasmussen M: Recommended use of morphine in neonates, infants and children based on a literature review: Part 1—Pharmacokinetics, *Paediatr Anaesth* 7:5-11, 1997.
23. Smith GD, Smith MT: Morphine-3-glucuronide: evidence to support its putative role in the development of tolerance to the antinociceptive effects of morphine in the rat, *Pain* 62:51-60, 1995.
24. Williams PI, Sarginson RE, Ratcliffe JM: Use of methadone in the morphine-tolerant burned paediatric patient, *Br J Anaesth* 80:92-95, 1998.
25. Laulin JP, Maurette P, Corcuff JB, et al: The role of ketamine in preventing fentanyl-induced hyperalgesia and subsequent acute morphine tolerance, *Anesth Analg* 94:1263-1269, 2002.
26. Latta KS, Ginsberg B, Barkin RL: Meperidine: a critical review, *Am J Ther* 9:53-68, 2002.
27. Kavuri S, Robalino J, Janardhan Y, et al: Low-dose intrathecal meperidine for lower limb orthopaedic surgery, *Can J Anaesth* 37:947-948, 1990.
28. Sharar SR, Bratton SL, Carrougher GJ, et al: A comparison of oral transmucosal fentanyl citrate and oral hydromorphone for inpatient pediatric burn wound care analgesia, J Burn Care Rehabil 19:521, 1998.
29. McEwan A, Sigston PE, Andrews KA, et al: A comparison of rectal and intramuscular codeine phosphate in children following neurosurgery, *Paediatr Anaesth* 10:189-193, 2000.
30. Goldsack C, Scuplak SM, Smith M: A double-blind comparison of codeine and morphine for postoperative analgesia following intracranial surgery, *Anaesthesia* 51:1029-1032, 1996.
31. Paris A, Scholz J, von Knobelsdorff G, et al: The effect of remifentanil on cerebral blood flow velocity, *Anesth Analg* 87:569-573, 1998.
32. Paris A, Scholz J, von Knobelsdorff G, et al: The effect of remifentanil on cerebral blood flow velocity, *Anesth Analg* 87:569-573, 1998.
33. Vinik RH, Kissin I: Rapid development of tolerance to analgesia during remifentanil infusion in humans, *Anesth Analg* 86:1307-1311, 1998.
34. Shipton EA: Tramadol—present and future, *Anaesth Intensive Care* 28:363-374, 2000.
35. Rosen DA, Morris JL, Rosen KR, et al: Nalmefene to prevent epidural narcotic side effects in pediatric patients: a pharmacokinetic and safety study, *Pharmacotherapy* 20:745-749, 2000.
36. Claster S, Vichinsky EP: Managing sickle cell disease, *BMJ* 327: 1151-1155, 2003.
37. Ballas SK, Viscusi ER, Epstein KR: Management of acute chest wall sickle cell pain with nebulized morphine, *Am J Hematol* 76: 190-191, 2004.
38. Siddappa R, Fletcher JE, Heard AM, et al: Methadone dosage for prevention of opioid withdrawal in children, *Paediatr Anaesth* 13:805-810, 2003.
39. Katz R, Kelly HW, His A: Prospective study on the occurrence of withdrawal in critically ill children who receive fentanyl by continuous infusion, *Crit Care Med* 22:763-767, 1994.
40. Joshi P et al: Opiate use and tolerance in the PICU, *Crit Care Med* A130:S526, 2003.
41. Deutsch ES, Nadkarni VM: Clonidine prophylaxis for narcotic and sedative withdrawal syndrome following laryngotracheal reconstruction, *Arch Otolaryngol Head Neck Surg* 122:1234-1238, 1996.
42. Kienbaum P, Scherbaum N, Thurauf N, et al: Acute detoxification of opioid-addicted patients with naloxone during propofol or methohexital anesthesia: a comparison of withdrawal symptoms,

neuroendocrine, metabolic, and cardiovascular patterns, *Crit Care Med* 28:969-976, 2000.

43. Pfab R, Hirtl C, Zilker T: Opiate detoxification under anesthesia: no apparent benefit but suppression of thyroid hormones and risk of pulmonary and renal failure, *J Toxicol Clin Toxicol* 37:43-50, 1999.
44. Stephenson J: Experts debate merits of 1-day opiate detoxification under anesthesia. *JAMA* 277:363-364, 1997.
45. Siddappa S et al: The use of propofol during rapid opiate weaning in the PICU, *Crit Care Med* A183:S606, 2002.
46. Sigel E: Mapping of the benzodiazepine recognition site on GABA(A) receptors, *Curr Top Med Chem* 2:833-839, 2002.
47. Ernst M, Brauchart D, Boresch S, et al Comparative modeling of GABA(A) receptors: limits, insights, future developments, *Neuroscience* 119:933-934, 2003.
48. Rudolph U: Identification of molecular substrate for the attenuation of anxiety: a step toward the development of better anti-anxiety drugs, *Sci World J* 1:192-193. 2001.
49. Beurdeley-Thomas A, Miccoli L, Oudard S, et al: The peripheral benzodiazepine receptors: a review, *J Neurooncol* 46:45-56, 2000
50. Casellas P, Galiegue S, Basile AS: Peripheral benzodiazepine receptors and mitochondrial function, *Neurochem Int* 40:475-486, 2002.
51. Arvat E, Giordano R, Grottoli S, et al: Benzodiazepines and anterior pituitary function, *J Endocrinol Invest* 25:735-747, 2002.
52. Kolmer M, Rovio A, Alho H: The characterization of two diazepam binding inhibitor (DBI) transcripts in humans, *Biochem J* 306(pt 2): 327 330, 1995.
53. Ohkuma S, Katsura M, Tsujimura A: Alterations in cerebral diazepam binding inhibitor expression in drug dependence: a possible biochemical alteration common to drug dependence, *Life Sci* 68:1215-1222, 2001.
54. Sand P, Kavvadias D, Feineis D, et al: Naturally occurring benzodiazepines: current status of research and clinical implications, *Eur Arch Psychiatry Clin Neurosci* 250:194-202, 2000.
55. Robin C, Trieger N: Paradoxical reactions to benzodiazepines in intravenous sedation: a report of 2 cases and review of the literature, *Anesth Prog* 49:128 132, 2002.
56. Jacqz-Aigrain E, Burtin P: Clinical pharmacokinetics of sedatives in neonates, *Clin Pharmacokinet* 31:423-443, 1996.
57. Langlois S, Kreeft JH, Chouinard G, et al: Midazolam: kinetics and effects on memory, sensorium, and haemodynamics, *Br J Clin Pharmacol* 23:273 278, 1987.
58. Saegusa K, Furukawa Y, Ogiwara Y, et al: Pharmacologic basis of responses to midazolam in the isolated, cross-perfused, canine right atrium, *Anesth Analg* 66:711-718, 1987.
59. Peinemann F, Daldrup T: Severe and prolonged sedation in five neonates due to persistence of active diazepam metabolites, *Eur J Pediatr* 160.378-381, 2001.
60. Lahat E, Goldman M, Barr J, et al: Comparison of intranasal midazolam with intravenous diazepam for treating febrile seizures in children: prospective randomised study, *BMJ* 321:83-86, 2000.
61. Cray SH, Dixon JL, Heard CM, et al: Oral midazolam premedication for paediatric day case patients, *Paediatr Anaesth* 6:265-270, 1996.
62. Blumer JL: Clinical pharmacology of midazolam in infants and children, *Clin Pharmacokinet* 35:37-47, 1998.
63. de Wildt SN, de Hoog M, Vinks AA, et al: Population pharmacokinetics and metabolism of midazolam in pediatric intensive care patients, *Crit Care Med* 31:1952-1958, 2003.
64. Bauer TM, Ritz R, Haberthur C, et al: Prolonged sedation due to accumulation of conjugated metabolites of midazolam, *Lancet* 346:145-147, 1995.
65. Malacrida R, Fritz ME, Suter PM, et al: Pharmacokinetics of midazolam administered by continuous intravenous infusion to intensive care patients, *Crit Care Med* 20:1123-1126, 1992.
66. Ahonen J, Olkkola KT, Takala A, et al: Interaction between fluconazole and midazolam in intensive care patients, *Acta Anaesthesiol Scand* 43:509-514, 1999.
67. Kyriakopoulos AA, Greenblatt DJ, Shader RI: Clinical pharmacokinetics of lorazepam: a review, *J Clin Psychiatry* 39(10 pt 2): 16-23, 1978.
68. Lee SA, Lee JK, Heo K: Coma probably induced by lorazepam-valproate interaction, *Seizure* 11:124-125, 2002.
69. Tobias JD, Rasmussen GE: Pain management and sedation in the pediatric intensive care unit, *Pediatr Clin North Am* 41:1269-1292, 1994.
70. Hayman M, Seidl EC, Ali M, et al: Acute tubular necrosis associated with propylene glycol from concomitant administration of intravenous lorazepam and trimethoprim-sulfamethoxazole, *Pharmacotherapy* 23:1190-1194, 2003.
71. Chicella M, Jansen P, Parthiban A, et al: Propylene glycol accumulation associated with continuous infusion of lorazepam in pediatric intensive care patients, *Crit Care Med* 30:2752-2756, 2002.
72. Parker MG, Fraser GL, Watson DM, et al: Removal of propylene glycol and correction of increased osmolar gap by hemodialysis in a patient on high dose lorazepam infusion therapy, *Intensive Care Med* 28:81-84, 2002.
73. Shafer A: Complications of sedation with midazolam in the intensive care unit and a comparison with other sedative regimens, *Crit Care Med* 26:947-956, 1998.
74. Bateson AN: Basic pharmacologic mechanisms involved in benzodiazepine tolerance and withdrawal, *Curr Pharm Des* 8:5-21, 2002.
75. Weinbroum AA, Szold O, Ogorek D, et al: The midazolam-induced paradox phenomenon is reversible by flumazenil. Epidemiology, patient characteristics and review of the literature, *Eur J Anaesthesiol* 18:789-797, 2001.
76. Mathieu-Nolf M, Babe MA, Coquelle-Couplet V, et al: Flumazenil use in an emergency department: a survey, *J Toxicol Clin Toxicol* 39:15-20, 2001.
77. Feld LG, Cimino M: *Pediatric dosing handbook,* Hudson, OH, 1997, Lexi-Comp.
78. Winkler E, Almog S, Kriger D, et al: Use of flumazenil in the diagnosis and treatment of patients with coma of unknown etiology, *Crit Care Med* 21:538-542, 1993.
79. Chern CH, Chern TL, Wang LM, et al: Continuous flumazenil infusion in preventing complications arising from severe benzodiazepine intoxication, *Am J Emerg Med* 16:238-241, 1998.
80. Peters JM, Tolia V, Simpson P, et al: Flumazenil in children after esophagogastroduodenoscopy, *Am J Gastroenterol* 94:1857-1861, 1999.
81. Girdler NM, Lyne JP, Wallace R, et al: A randomised, controlled trial of cognitive and psychomotor recovery from midazolam sedation following reversal with oral flumazenil, *Anaesthesia* 57: 868-876, 2002.
82. Pershad J, Palmisano P, Nichols M: Chloral hydrate: the good and the bad, *Pediatr Emerg Care* 15:432 433, 1999.
83. Lash LH, Fisher JW, Lipscomb JC, et al: Metabolism of trichloroethylene, *Environ Health Perspect* 108:177-200, 2000.
84. Salmon AG, Kizer KW, Zeise L, et al: Potential carcinogenicity of chloral hydrate—a review, *J Toxicol Clin Toxicol* 33:115-121, 1995.
85. Hassaballa HA, Balk RA: Torsade de pointes associated with the administration of intravenous haloperidol, *Am J Ther* 10:58-60, 2003.
86. Kao LW, Kirk MA, Evers SJ, et al: Droperidol, QT prolongation, and sudden death: what is the evidence? *Ann Emerg Med* 41: 559-560 2003 (comment).
87. Reappraisal of lytic cocktail/demerol, phenergan, and thorazine (DPT) for the sedation of children. American Academy of Pediatrics Committee on Drugs, *Pediatrics* 95:598-602, 1995.
88. Samson-Fang L, Gooch J, Norlin C: Intrathecal baclofen withdrawal simulating neuroleptic malignant syndrome in a child with cerebral palsy, *Dev Med Child Neurol* 42:561-565, 2000.
89. Kao LW, Amin Y, Kirk MA, et al: Intrathecal baclofen withdrawal mimicking sepsis, *J Emerg Med* 24:423-427, 2003.
90. Greenberg MI, Hendrickson RG: Baclofen withdrawal following removal of an intrathecal baclofen pump despite oral baclofen replacement, *J Toxicol Clin Toxicol* 41:83-85, 2003.
91. Gooch JL, Oberg WA, Grams B, et al: Complications of intrathecal baclofen pumps in children, *Pediatr Neurosurg* 39:1-6, 2003.
92. Reeves RK, Stolp-Smith KA, Christopherson MW: Hyperthermia, rhabdomyolysis, and disseminated intravascular coagulation associated with baclofen pump catheter failure, *Arch Phys Med Rehabil* 79:353-356, 1998.
93. Sampathkumar P, Scanlon P, Plevak D: Baclofen withdrawal presenting as multiorgan system failure, *Anesth Analg* 87:562 563, 1998.
94. Food and Drug Administration Safety Information and Adverse Event Reporting Program: 2002 safety alert - Lioresal (baclofen injection), Available at http://www.fda.gov/medwatch/SAFETY/2002/baclofen.htm. Accessed June 2004.
95. Meythaler JM, Roper JF, Brunner RC: Cyproheptadine for intrathecal baclofen withdrawal, *Arch Phys Med Rehabil* 84:638-642, 2003.

96. Colachis SC, Rea GL: Monitoring of creatinine kinase during weaning of intrathecal baclofen and with symptoms of early withdrawal, *Am J Phys Med Rehabil* 82:489-492, 2003.
97. Rodarte A, Diaz S, Foley J, et al: The pharmacokinetics of dexmedetomidine in post-surgical pediatric intensive care unit patients: a preliminary study, *Anesthesiology* 99:A423, 2003.
98. De Wolf AM, Fragen RJ, Avram MJ, et al: The pharmacokinetics of dexmedetomidine in volunteers with severe renal impairment, *Anesth Analg* 93:1205-1209, 2001.
99. Baughman VL, Cunningham F, Layden T, et al: Pharmacokinetic/pharmacodynamic effects of dexmedetomidine in patients with hepatic failure, *Anesth Analg* 90:S391,2000.
100. Venn RM, Bradshaw CJ, Spencer R, et al: Preliminary UK experience of dexmedetomidine, a novel agent for postoperative sedation in the intensive care unit, *Anaesthesia* 54:1136-1142, 1999.
101. Riker RR, Ramsay MAE, Prielipp RC, et al: Long-term dexmedetomidine infusions for ICU sedation: a pilot study, *Anesthesiology* 95:A383. 2001.
102. Berkenbosch JW, Tobias JD: Development of bradycardia during sedation with dexmedetomidine in an infant concurrently receiving digoxin, *Pediatr Crit Care Med* 4:203-205, 2003.
103. Short TG, Chui PT: Propofol and midazolam act synergistically in combination, *Br J Anaesth* 67:539-545, 1991.
104. Chamorro C, de Latorre FJ, Montero A, et al: Comparative study of propofol versus midazolam in the sedation of critically ill patients: results of a prospective, randomized, multicenter trial, *Crit Care Med* 24:932-939, 1996.
105. Barrientos-Vega R, Mar Sanchez-Soria M, Morales-Garcia C, et al: Prolonged sedation of critically ill patients with midazolam or propofol: impact on weaning and costs, *Crit Care Med* 25: 33-39, 1997.
106. Brown LA, Levin GM: Role of propofol in refractory status epilepticus, *Ann Pharmacother* 32:1053-1059, 1998.
107. Stecker MM, Kramer TH, Raps EC, et al: Treatment of refractory status epilepticus with propofol: clinical and pharmacokinetic findings, *Epilepsia* 39:18-26, 1998.
108. Platt M, White DC: Calories in sedation, *Anaesthesia* 42:322 AN2269, 1987.
109. Valente JF, Anderson GL, Branson RD, et al: Disadvantages of prolonged propofol sedation in the critical care unit, *Crit Care Med* 22:710-12, 1994.
110. Bach A, Geiss HK: Propofol and postoperative infections, *N Engl J Med* 30:1505-1506, 1995.
111. Bennett SN, McNeil MM, Bland LA, et al: Postoperative infections traced to contamination of an intravenous anesthetic, propofol, *N Engl J Med* 333:147-153, 1995.
112. Laxenaire MC, Mata-Bermejo E, Moneret-Vautrin DA, et al: Life-threatening anaphylactoid reactions to propofol (Diprivan), *Anesthesiology* 77:275-280, 1992.
113. Bodenham A, Culank LS, Park GR: Propofol infusion and green urine, *Lancet* 2:740, 1987 (letter).
114. Parke TJ, Stevens JE, Rice AS, et al: Metabolic acidosis and fatal myocardial failure after propofol infusion in children: five case reports, BMJ 305:613-616, 1992.
115. Propofol infusion in children, *BMJ* 305: 952-953, 1992 (letters to the editor).
116. Bray RJ: Propofol infusion syndrome in children, *Paediatr Anaesth* 8:491-499,1998.
117. Pepperman ML, Macrae D: A comparison of propofol and other sedative use in paediatric intensive care in the United Kingdom, *Paediatr Anaesth* 7:143-153, 1997.
118. Cornfield DN, Tegtmeyer K, Nelson MD, et al: Continuous propofol infusion in 142 critically ill children, *Pediatrics* 110: 1177-1181, 2002.
119. Reed MD, Blumer JL: Propofol bashing: the time to stop is now! *Crit Care Med* 24:175-176, 1996.
120. Felmet K, Nguyen T, Clark RS, et al: The FDA warning against prolonged sedation with propofol in children remains warranted, *Pediatrics* 112:1002-1003, 2003.
121. Dear health care provider letter, AstraZeneca, Newark, DE, March 26, 2001.
122. Kang TM: Propofol infusion syndrome in critically ill patients, *Ann Pharmacother* 36:1453-1456, 2002.
123. Cray SH, Robinson BH, Cox PN: Lactic academia and bradyarrhythmia in a child sedated with propofol, *Crit Care Med* 26:2087-2092, 1998.
124. Wolf A, Weir P, Segar P, et al: Impaired fatty acid oxidation in propofol infusion syndrome, *Lancet* 357:606-607, 2001.
125. Vasile B, Rasulo F, Candiani A, et al: The pathophysiology of propofol infusion syndrome: a simple name for a complex syndrome, *Intensive Care Med* 29:1417-1425, 2003.
126. Wheeler DS, Vaux KK, Ponaman ML, et al: The safe and effective use of propofol sedation in children undergoing diagnostic and therapeutic procedures: experience in a pediatric ICU and a review of the literature, *Pediatr Emerg Care* 19:385-392, 2003.
127. Hlozki J, Aring C, Gillor A: Death after re-exposure to propofol in a 3-year-old child: a case report, *Paediatric Anaesth* 14: 265-270, 2004.
128. Hanna JP, Ramundo ML: Rhabdomyolysis and hypoxia associated with prolonged propofol infusion in children, *Neurology* 50:301-303, 1998.
129. Cannon ML, Glazier SS, Bauman LA: Metabolic acidosis, rhabdomyolysis, and cardiovascular collapse after prolonged propofol infusion, *J Neurosurg* 95:1053-1056, 1995.
130. Seigler RS, Avant MG, Gwyn DR, et al: A comparison of propofol and ketamine/midazolam for intravenous sedation of children, *Pediatr Crit Care Med* 2:20-23, 2001.
131. Festa M, Bowra J, Schell D: Use of propofol infusion in Australian and New Zealand paediatric intensive care units, *Anaesth Intensive Care* 30:786-793, 2002.
132. Lowrie L, Weiss AH, Lacombe C: The pediatric sedation unit: a mechanism for pediatric sedation, *Pediatrics* 102:E30, 1998.
133. Friedman AG, Mulhern RK, Fairclough D, et al: Midazolam premedication for pediatric bone marrow aspiration and lumbar puncture, *Med Pediatr Oncol* 19:499-504, 1991.
134. American Academy of Pediatrics Committee on Drugs: Guidelines for monitoring management of pediatric patients during and after sedation for diagnostic and therapeutic procedures, *Pediatrics* 89:276-281, 1992.
135. Epstein BS: The American Society of Anesthesiologist's efforts in developing guidelines for sedation and analgesia for nonanesthesiologists: the 40th Rovenstine Lecture, *Anesthesiology* 98:1261-1268, 2003.
136. Practice guidelines for sedation and analgesia by non-anesthesiologists: American Society of Anesthesiologists Task Force on Sedation and Analgesia by Non-Anesthesiologists, *Anesthesiology* 84:459-471, 1996.
137. Dodson BA: Interventional neuroradiology and the anesthetic management of patients with arteriovenous malformations, In Cotrell JE, Smith DS, editors: *Anesthesia and neurosurgery,* St. Louis, 1994, Mosby.
138. Rheuban KS, Carpenter MA: Diagnostic cardiac catheterization, angiography, and interventional catheterization. In Lake CL (editor): *Pediatric cardiac anesthesia,* Norwalk, Conn, 1993, Appleton & Lange.
139. Keeter S, Benator RM, Weinberg SM, et al: Sedation in pediatric CT: national survey of current practice, *Radiology* 175:745-752, 1990.
140. Joint Commission on Accreditation of Healthcare Organizations: *Accreditation manual for hospitals,* St Louis, 1993, Mosby-Yearbook.
141. Wilson S: A survey of the American Academy of Pediatric Dentistry membership: nitrous oxide and sedation, *Pediatr Dent* 18:287-293,1996.
142. Cote CJ, Karl HW, Notterman DA, et al: Adverse sedation events in pediatrics: analysis of medications used for sedation, *Pediatrics* 106:633-644. 2000.
143. Dreifuss FE, Rosman NP, Cloyd JC, et al: A comparison of rectal diazepam gel and placebo for acute repetitive seizures, *N Engl J Med* 338:1869-1875, 1998.
144. Holzman RS, Cullen DJ, Eichhorn JH, et al: Guidelines for sedation by nonanesthesiologists during diagnostic and therapeutic procedures. The Risk Management Committee of the Department of Anaesthesia of Harvard Medical School, *J Clin Anesth* 6: 265-276, 1994.
145. Hoffman GM, Nowakowski R, Troshynski TJ, et al: Risk reduction in pediatric procedural sedation by application of an American Academy of Pediatrics/American Society of Anesthesiologists process model, *Pediatrics* 109:236-243, 2002.
146. Jorgensen NH, Messick JM Jr, Gray J, et al: ASA monitoring standards and magnetic resonance imaging, *Anesth Analg* 79: 1141-1147, 1994.

147. Heard CMB: Nuclear magnetic resonance Imaging. In Atlee JL, (editor): *Complications in anesthesia,* ed 1, Philadelphia, 1999, WB Saunders.
148. Menon DK, Peden CJ, Hall AS, et al: Magnetic resonance for the anaesthetist. Part 1: Physical principles, applications, and safety aspects, *Anaesthesia* 47:240-255, 1992.
149. Peden CJ, Menon DK, Hall AS, et al: Magnetic resonance for the anaesthetist. Part II. Anaesthesia and monitoring in MR units, *Anaesthesia* 47:508-516, 1992.
150. Roy TM, Pruitt VL, Garner PA, et al: The potential role of anesthesia in status asthmaticus, *J Asthma* 29:73-77, 1992.
151. Smith JA, Santer LJ: Respiratory arrest following intramuscular ketamine injection in a 4-year-old child, *Ann Emerg Med* 22: 613-615, 1993.
152. Kenyon CJ, McNeil LM, Fraser R: Comparison of the effects of etomidate, thiopentone and propofol on cortisol synthesis, *Br J Anaesth* 57:509-511, 1985.
153. Crozier TA, Flamm C, Speer CP, et al: Effects of etomidate on the adrenocortical and metabolic adaptation of the neonate, *Br J Anaesth* 70:47-53, 1993.
154. Watt I, Ledingham IM: Mortality amongst multiple trauma patients admitted to an intensive therapy unit, *Anaesthesia* 39: 973-978, 1984.
155. Clarke JB, Thomas C, Chen M, et al: Halogenated anesthetics form liver adducts and antigens that cross-react with halothane-induced antibodies, *Int Arch Allergy Immunol* 108:24-32, 1995.
156. Sponheim S, Skraastad O, Helseth E, et al: Effects of 0.5 and 1.0 MAC isoflurane, sevoflurane and desflurane on intracranial and cerebral perfusion pressures in children, *Acta Anaesthesiol Scand* 47:932-938, 2003.
157. Petersen KD, Landsfeldt U, Cold GE, et al: Intracranial pressure and cerebral hemodynamic in patients with cerebral tumors: a randomized prospective study of patients subjected to craniotomy in propofol-fentanyl, isoflurane-fentanyl, or sevoflurane-fentanyl anesthesia, *Anesthesiology* 98:329-336, 2003.
158. Fraga M, Rama-Maceiras P, Rodino S, et al: The effects of isoflurane and desflurane on intracranial pressure, cerebral perfusion pressure, and cerebral arteriovenous oxygen content difference in normocapnic patients with supratentorial brain tumors, *Anesthesiology* 98:1085-1090, 2003.
159. Tanigami H, Yahagi N, Kumon K, et al: Long-term sedation with isoflurane in postoperative intensive care in cardiac surgery, *Artif Organs* 21:21-23, 1997.
160. Arnold JH, Truog RD, Rice SA: Prolonged administration of isoflurane to pediatric patients during mechanical ventilation, *Anesth Analg* 76:520-526, 1993.
161. Fujino Y, Nishimura M, Nishimura S, et al: Prolonged administration of isoflurane to patients with severe renal dysfunction, *Anesth Analg* 86:440-441, 1998.
162. Johnston RG, Noseworthy TW, Friesen EG, et al: Isoflurane therapy for status asthmaticus in children and adults, *Chest* 97:698-701, 1990.
163. U.S. Department of Labor Occupational Safety and Health Administration: Waste anesthetic gases. OSHA Fact Sheet 91-38, Washington, DC, 1991.
164. U.S. Department of Labor Occupational Safety and Health Administration: Waste anesthetic gases. Available at http://www.osha.gov/SLTC/wasteanestheticgases. Accessed June 2004.
165. Curley MA, Molengraft JA: Providing comfort to critically ill pediatric patients, *Crit Care Nurs Clin North Am* 2:267-274, 1995.
166. Parnass SM, Feld JM, Chamberlin WH, et al: Status asthmaticus treated with isoflurane and enflurane, *Anesth Analg* 66:193-195, 1987.
167. Willatts SM, Spencer EM: Sedation for ventilation in the critically ill, *Anaesthesia* 49:422-428, 1994.
168. Kong KL, Willatts SM: Isoflurane sedation in pediatric intensive care, *Crit Care Med* 23:1308-1309, 1995.
169. Wheeler DS, Clapp CR, Ponaman ML, et al: Isoflurane therapy for status asthmaticus in children: a case series and protocol, *Pediatr Crit Care Med* 1:55-59, 2000.

CHAPTER

117

Malignant Hyperthermia

Barbara W. Brandom

PEARLS

- Malignant hyperthermia (MH) is a rare pharmacogenetic disorder that was first recognized as a complication of general anesthesia with potent inhaled gases.
- Initial signs of MH can occur postoperatively as fever with excessive metabolic rate and muscle injury.
- Myoglobinuria produces renal injury in about 10% of MH cases. Renal failure is more likely when treatment with dantrolene is delayed. Dantrolene will decrease the excessive metabolism in muscle that is the cause of MH. Mannitol, part of the formulation of dantrolene, is useful protection against myoglobin induced renal failure.
- Disseminated intravascular coagulation and cerebral edema are other frequent complications of MH.
- After initial treatment with 2.5 to 10 mg/kg of dantrolene, at least 1 mg/kg of dantrolene should be given every 6 hours for 4 doses because approximately 25% of patients experience an exacerbation or recrudescence of MH in the first 24 hours of an acute episode.
- Bolus administration of dantrolene may be associated with less phlebitis than is continuous infusion of dantrolene.

The physician in the intensive care unit (ICU) may first encounter a patient with malignant hyperthermia (MH) in transfer from the operating room or from an outpatient facility where general anesthesia was given and treatment for acute MH was begun. This patient may appear to be stable, but close observation for a relapse of MH is warranted. Approximately 25% of patients experience a recurrence of MH in the 24 hours after the initial episode. Administration of dantrolene for at least 24 hours after the initial episode is recommended. Alternatively, the ICU physician may be the first to entertain the diagnosis of MH in a patient admitted to the ICU for medical care or postoperative management. MH is clinically heterogeneous, and there are many causes of fever and muscle injury that are not MH. Regardless of the underlying cause, ICU management should avoid critical temperature and complications of rhabdomyolysis. The ICU physician should pursue common diagnoses while directing treatment for the rare syndrome of MH. Many months can be required to confirm a diagnosis of MH susceptibility.

Pathophysiology

MH is a clinically heterogeneous disorder in which a marked increase in the metabolic rate of genetically abnormal muscle can result in destruction of the muscle and multiorgan system failure. The underlying biochemical defect is a sudden increase in the concentration of calcium ion in the sarcoplasm.[1-3] An increased metabolic rate of muscle produces a load of acid sufficient to overwhelm the buffering capacity of the body and the ability of the lungs to excrete carbon dioxide (CO_2). Increased oxygen demand and the concomitant sympathetic response challenge the cardiovascular system. This syndrome can progress rapidly to severe acidosis, elevate temperature to levels consistent with heatstroke, and cause extensive rhabdomyolysis. This is fulminant MH, and without aggressive treatment death is likely. Before the introduction of dantrolene, the death rate of MH was 70%. Patients with the MH trait are often symptom free until exposed to the most common triggering agents, the anesthetic vapors such as sevoflurane, isoflurane, desflurane, and halothane and the depolarizing neuromuscular blocker succinylcholine.

As a result of inadequate oxygen delivery and high fever, multiorgan system failure may ensue. Organ systems affected are similar to those compromised by exertional heat stroke.[4] Renal failure, disseminated intravascular coagulation, cerebral edema, pulmonary edema, cardiac dysrhythmias, and decreased cardiac contractility are potential consequences of fulminant MH.[5]

The course of MH may often be less dramatic. People differ greatly in their rate of symptom development. Fulminant MH has been reported after many hours of inhalation anesthesia.[6] There are several different genetic abnormalities associated with MH.[7-10] Recently it has been suggested that two different genetic loci may be required to produce the MH phenotype in some families.[11,12] The factors that modify the expression of MH susceptibility are not completely determined.[13] A person may have fulminant MH during one anesthetic and no symptoms at all during other similar anesthetics.[14] If the pharmacological trigger agent is eliminated from the patient before the development of profoundly decreased pH in the muscle and shock, the metabolic abnormalities may resolve readily. This sequence of events could be termed *abortive MH.* The porcine model of MH can illustrate many of the features of MH in the human.[15]

Porcine Model

The pale, soft, exudative pork syndrome occurs when there is rapid postmortem glycolysis in muscle with a rapid fall in carcass muscle pH. This syndrome had been studied by the meat industry because the unfavorable meat qualities it produced made the susceptible breeds of pig less useful as sources of commercial pork. Exposure of animals of these breeds to halothane or succinylcholine produced the same biochemical changes in the muscle as did environmental, exercise, and anoxic stresses.[16,17]

In genetically susceptible pigs, the syndrome of MH is reproducible and follows a characteristic course. A rapidly developing sinus tachycardia, usually in excess of 200 beats/min, is often the earliest detectable sign. Tachycardia continues until shortly before death in the untreated animal. Open-mouthed breathing and hyperventilation proceed within minutes to apnea. There is blotchy cyanosis of the skin, most noticeably on the abdominal wall and the snout. Muscle tension increases. This is most evident in the hind legs, which become rigidly extended. There is a rapid and sustained rise in core temperature, which may reach 43° to 45° C before death (Fig. 117–1).[16,17]

The clinical signs of MH may appear in the pig within 5 to 15 minutes of the beginning of exposure to the pharmacological trigger. When halothane and succinylcholine are administered together to the genetically susceptible animal, MH is fulminant and usually fatal. If exposure to a trigger such as halothane is terminated within minutes of the first appearance of the major clinical signs of the syndrome, MH may resolve spontaneously.[16] There is a point, however, beyond which the pH of muscle falls rapidly, and the abnormal metabolic processes continue in the absence of the pharmacological trigger (Fig. 117–1).

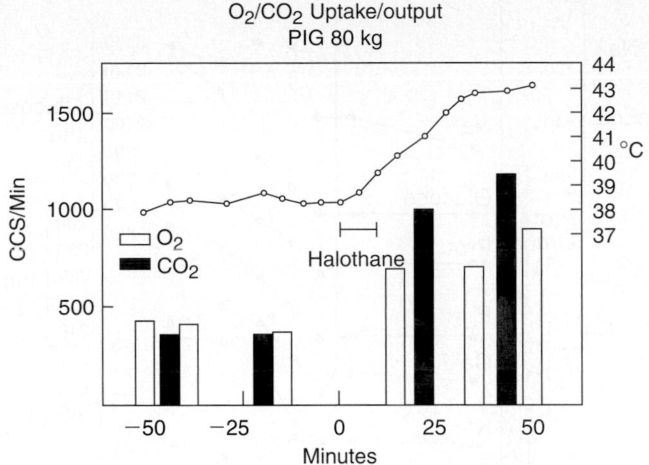

FIGURE 117–1 • Effect of halothane on O_2 consumption and CO_2 output. O_2/CO_2 exchange was measured over timed 4-minute periods. Halothane, 3% (v/v, in O_2), was given from 0 to 8 minutes. (Redrawn from Berman MC: *Nature,* 225:653, 1970.)

The biochemical changes that can be observed in the plasma of an MH-susceptible pig during an episode have been well documented (Figs. 117–2 and 117–3). The dramatic rise in Pa_{CO_2} is responsible for the observed hyperventilation followed by apnea, as CO_2 narcosis supervenes. Many of the other biochemical abnormalities are the result of a shift of water into the injured muscle cells and the concomitant leakage of intracellular ions into the plasma.[16,17]

An increase in myoplasmic calcium ion is the underlying biochemical event responsible for the manifestations of MH.

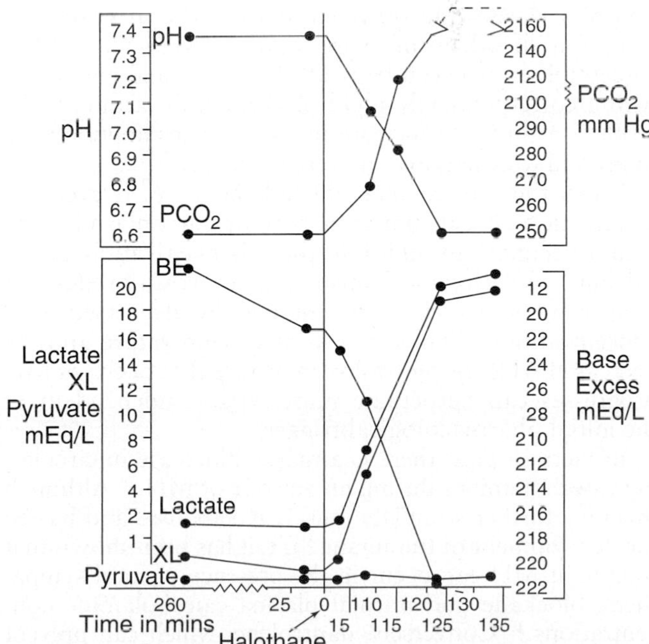

FIGURE 117–2 • Arterial blood acid-base changes recorded in an MHS Landrace pig during the course of an MH syndrome provoked by halothane after a control period of thiopentone and nitrous oxide anesthesia. (Redrawn from Harrison GG: *Int Anesthesiol Clin* 17: 25, 1979.)

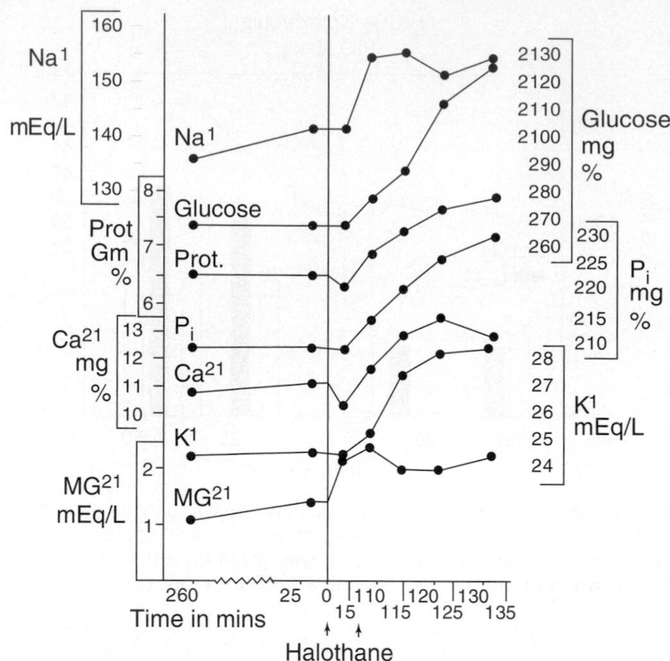

FIGURE 117–3 • Changes in serum biochemistry determinations during the course of an MH syndrome in the same animal as in Figure 119–2. (Redrawn from Harrison GG: *Int Anesthesiol Clin* 17: 25, 1979.)

A genetic defect in the ryanodine receptor (RYR),[18] through which calcium is released from the terminal cisternae of the sarcoplasmic reticulum, has been identified in many MH-susceptible pigs. Muscle rigor occurs as a result of calcium-induced inhibition of troponin and calcium-induced activation of adenosine triphosphatase. Metabolic rate is increased by calcium-induced activation of glycogen phosphorylase[16] and other enzymes.[19] The in vitro consumption of adenosine triphosphate (ATP) from MH-susceptible muscle can be twice that of normal muscle[19,20] with a correspondingly rapid production of lactate.[21] The result is a threefold increase in oxygen consumption with fifteenfold to twentyfold increase in lactate.[22,23]

When the intracellular pH falls below 6, irreversible inactivation of calcium transport by sarcoplasmic reticulum occurs.[24] In addition, there is inactivation of the calcium-regulating mechanism of actomyosin by elevated temperatures, which is potentiated by decreased ATP concentrations.[25] Thus the elevated temperature and the decreased ATP concentration in muscle that occur as MH progresses can perpetuate muscle rigor independent of the initial pharmacological trigger.

In Pietrain pigs, there is a marked increase in circulating catecholamines during an episode of MH.[26] Although this may further stimulate muscle metabolism and hasten the development of fulminant MH, it has been shown that fulminant MH can occur in the presence of total sympathetic blockade and normal plasma catecholamine concentrations.[27] Conversely, dantrolene, which can prevent the triggering of MH in the susceptible animal, has no effect on stress-induced increases in catecholamines.[27]

The susceptibility of the pig to the syndrome of MH was originally thought to be due to a single autosomal dominant gene; however, graded phenotypic variations[17] and failure to elicit MH in animals known to have genetically abnormal RYRs[13] suggest that the presence of one abnormal RYR gene is not a sufficient cause of MH. Studies of the effects of the most potent triggering agents in crossbred animals, normal pigs with MH-susceptible pigs, show that in a heterogeneous population, a relatively mild form of MH can be produced by the same triggers that would produce fulminant MH in the susceptible parent (Fig. 117–4).[28]

Trigger agents and therapeutic maneuvers have been examined in the porcine model of MH.[17] Symptomatic therapy including mechanical ventilation, aggressive administration of bicarbonate, expansion of the intravascular volume, treatment of dysrhythmias, and hyperkalemia can prolong the life of the animal during an episode of fulminant MH. The most effective therapy, however, is intravenous dantrolene (Fig. 117–5).[29] Also, a more water-soluble form of dantrolene, azumolene, has also been shown to be effective in the treatment of MH in the susceptible pig.[30]

Clinical Recognition of an Episode in Humans

The initial signs of an episode of MH are nonspecific. Hypercarbia is the earliest sign of MH. Tachycardia and dysrhythmias may also occur early in the course of an episode of MH. As in the porcine model of MH, there may be mottled cyanosis of the skin and generalized muscular rigidity. Masseter spasm, an extreme increase in tension of the masseter such that the mouth cannot be forced open, has been claimed to be an early sign of MH.[31] Later temperature elevation occurs. Because MH is a potentially fatal

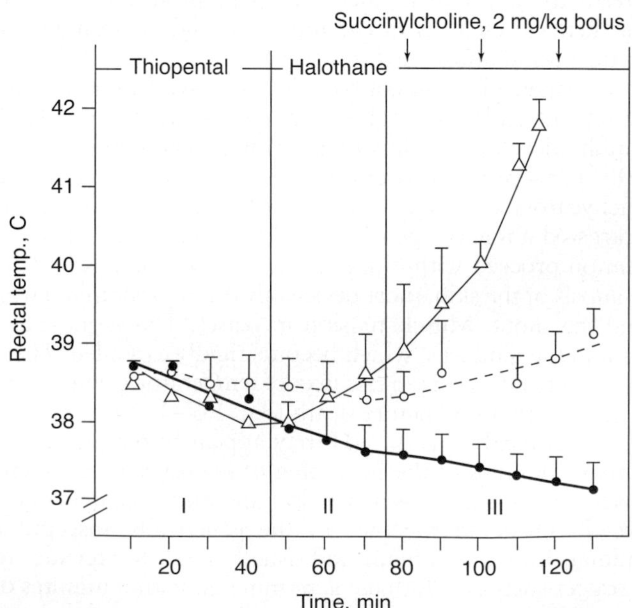

FIGURE 117–4 • Comparison of changes in rectal temperature during an anesthesia challenge for MH susceptibility among three different phenotype pig groups. (Redrawn from the International Anesthesia Research Society. Nelson TE, Flewellen EH, Gloyma DF: *Anesth Analg* 62:545, 1983.)

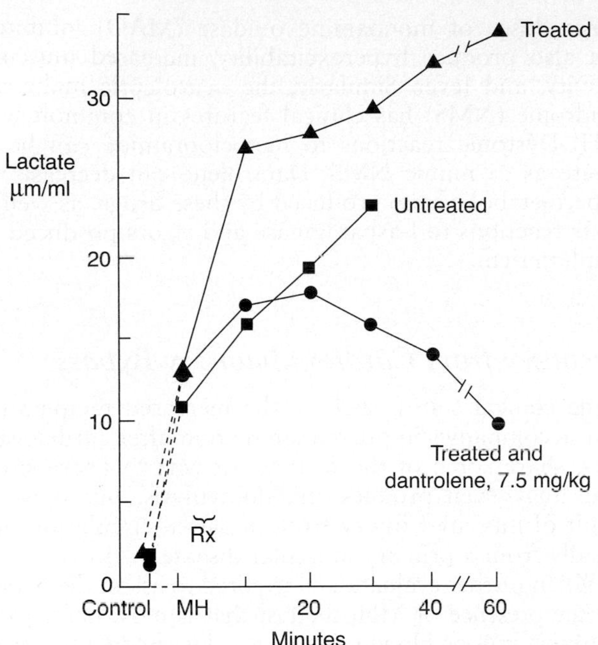

FIGURE 117–5 • Arterial blood lactate in MHS swine. During symptomatic treatment of MH, blood lactate continues to rise as a sign of unchecked fulminant metabolism (treated). When dantrolene is used in addition (treated and dantrolene), blood lactate decreases—a sign of dantrolene's specific inhibitory effect on muscle. (Redrawn from Gronert GA: *Anesthesioloy* 53:395, 1980.)

condition that may progress rapidly, anesthesiologists may be inclined to overdiagnose episodes of abortive MH. That is, when the nonspecific early signs of MH are noted during induction of anesthesia, anesthesia may be terminated, and the patient is considered MH-susceptible until proven otherwise. Alternatively, MH may develop insidiously during a long anesthetic.[6] There have been cases in which only mild signs of abortive MH occurred intraoperatively, but renal failure, hyperthermia, and death occurred postoperatively with no explanation other than MH.[32]

In a retrospective study of the Danish population, in which 386,250 anesthetics that occurred over 6.5 years in 87 hospitals were reviewed, the incidence of fulminant MH was 1 in 250,000 general anesthetics.[33] In this series, there were no cases of fulminant MH during regional anesthetics or "nontriggering" general anesthetics. When only anesthetics that included administration of succinylcholine and potent inhalation agents, such as halothane, isoflurane, and enflurane, were considered, the incidence of abortive MH was 1 in 4200 cases.[33] Abortive MH was defined as a masseter spasm or moderate changes in vital signs with slight metabolic or respiratory acidosis.

Two explanations can be proposed for the more than fiftyfold difference in incidence between fulminant and abortive MH. Early termination of the anesthetic in the presence of abortive MH may allow spontaneous resolution of the syndrome. No deaths occurred in the patients with abortive MH in this series. Alternatively, patients who received the diagnosis of abortive MH may not be susceptible to MH at all. The clinical signs of abortive MH, including masseter spasm, are not specific for MH.[34] In this retrospective series,[33] there was no information about further anesthetic experience or other evaluation of the potential for MH susceptibility, specifically the results of in vitro caffeine-halothane contracture testing, in those patients who had experienced abortive MH.

The sine qua non of MH is hypermetabolism. Rhabdomyolysis will occur when the energy supply of the muscle is exhausted. The physician who must evaluate a patient with abnormal vital signs and an increased expired CO_2 concentration should quickly rule out the most common causes of these abnormalities. If it is assumed that the findings are due to MH, dantrolene should be administered promptly. If sepsis, cardiovascular failure, central nervous system injury, or other conditions could have produced the abnormal vital signs, then these other diagnoses must be pursued and treated as well.

The following clinical scenarios frequently cause elevated expired and arterial CO^2 tension, tachycardia and other dysrhythmias, excessive jaw stiffness, and other nonspecific signs of MH in anesthetized children. A few causes of myoglobinuria, other than MH, are also listed here.

Elevated Inspired Carbon Dioxide

Inspiratory gas flow and minute ventilation must be documented to be adequate to preclude rebreathing of expired CO_2. Mapleson D type, nonvalved, gas delivery systems are frequently used in the operating room to supply anesthesia to pediatric patients. When the respiratory rate of a patient is increased without an increase in fresh gas flow through the Mapleson D type system, there is often an increase in inspired CO_2 tension.[35] Similarly, an undetected leak in the anesthesia circuit can produce an inadequate fresh gas flow, rebreathing of expired gas, and thus an elevated expired CO_2. Tachycardia and dysrhythmias may result from hypercarbia without an increase in metabolic rate.

Decreased Respiratory Drive

During induction of anesthesia with potent inhalation anesthetics, respiratory drive is depressed, upper airway obstruction may develop, and hypercarbia may result. This cause of hypercarbia is not related to increased metabolic rate. Indeed, during the first 5 to 15 minutes of anesthetic administration in a healthy pediatric patient, core body temperature decreases, while skin temperature increases.

Excitement

Although it is not the most desirable anesthetic situation, a pediatric patient may be subjected to an inhalation induction with sevoflurane or halothane while he or she is not cooperative. Induction of anesthesia may be prolonged in such a patient because of airway obstruction that results from excessive secretions. During induction of anesthesia with sevoflurane there may be transient stiffening of extremities and the torso. Hypercarbia may result. A child who underwent a prolonged, difficult induction of anesthesia may well demonstrate tachydysrhythmias. Inadequate depth of anesthesia may also result in increased resistance to opening of the mouth. During inhalation induction of anesthesia the use of a precordial stethoscope and capnography offers improved judgment of airway patency and adequacy of minute ventilation.

Other Causes of a Stiff Jaw

When difficulty opening the mouth is noted in the absence of obvious rigidity of the rest of the body, it may be due to previously unrecognized temporomandibular joint dysfunction, inadequate anesthesia, myotonia, or a normal response to succinylcholine.[36-38]

Muscular Disease

Myotonia congenita and myotonic dystrophy are two forms of primary muscular disease in which succinylcholine produces obvious rigidity rather than the anticipated flaccidity. The incidence of these disorders is similar to that of fulminant MH.[33,39] In a patient with dystrophinopathy (Duchenne's or Becker's muscular dystrophy), hyperkalemic cardiac arrest may occur after administration of succinylcholine during potent inhalation anesthesia.[40,41] During initial treatment, such cases have been difficult to differentiate clinically from MH. (see "Identification of Patients at Risk").

In the presence of neuromuscular disease, myoglobinuria may occur after exposure to potent inhalation anesthetics alone.[42,43] Myoglobinuria is to be expected after succinylcholine administration in patients with muscular dystrophy.[42] Even in healthy children, elevation of creatine phosphokinase (CPK) may be present more than 24 hours after exposure to succinylcholine in the presence of inhalation anesthesia.[44,45]

Fever

Temperature elevation is often the result of infection, traumatized tissues, or excessive environmental heat with inadequate opportunity for convective or evaporative heat loss. Inadequate fluid replacement predisposes to increased core temperature in children.[46] In these cases, there may be tachycardia and elevation in exhaled CO_2, which are consistent with the expected metabolic demands of fever. The systemic response to some viral infections, lymphomas, and leukemia[47-49] can be so extreme as to mimic MH.

Drug Interactions

Although pediatric surgical patients are less likely to be receiving medications that have potentially significant interactions with anesthetics than are older patients, some drug interactions in these children can produce dysrhythmias. Halothane is the cheapest inhalation induction agent for pediatric anesthetics. Halothane decreases the threshold for ventricular dysrhythmias. Other drugs with the same effect on ventricular conduction, such as aminophylline-containing compounds or β-stimulants, may produce multifocal premature ventricular contractions in the presence of halothane.

Ketamine, cocaine, and phencyclidine can produce tachycardia, muscle rigidity, and fever in humans. Large doses of monoamine oxidase (MAO) inhibitors can also produce hyperexcitability, increased muscular activity, and fever. Similarly, the neuroleptic malignant syndrome (NMS) has clinical features in common with MH. Dystonic reactions to metoclopramide can be so severe as to mimic NMS. Dantrolene can decrease the hypermetabolic state produced by these drugs, as well as toxic reactions to l-asparaginase and rigors produced by amphotericin.

Recovery from Cardiopulmonary Bypass

Some clinical states, such as the increased temperature that accompanies improved circulation after cardiac surgery, share some of the features of MH.[50] These situations may even produce rhabdomyolysis, but it is the result of muscular injury from impaired circulation, not usually from a primary muscular disease.

When further evaluation is required to assess the patient for the presence of MH, the test that is most likely to be helpful is venous blood gas analysis. Elevated CO_2 tension is apparent in mixed venous blood before it is abnormal in arterial blood during an episode of MH.[29] There is an increase in lactate release from muscle before a decrease in the partial pressure of oxygen in venous blood is observed during an episode of MH.[23] If venous blood indicates significant acidosis, partial pressure of CO_2 of greater than 60 torr, and bicarbonate less than 19 mEq/L[29] and the history of the patient is consistent with MH, the physician may assume that the patient is experiencing an episode of MH and treat accordingly. Further evidence of MH, evidence of rhabdomyolysis, may be available some hours or days after the episode has been treated.

Elevation of CPK or myoglobin in the plasma is evidence of rhabdomyolysis. There are many causes of rhabdomyolysis other than MH, though.[42] After administration of succinylcholine and halothane, moderate increases in these proteins in the plasma may be seen in healthy children.[51,52] Myoglobinemia occurs within minutes of exposure to succinylcholine in the presence of inhalation anesthetics in healthy children[53]; however, it is rare in healthy children to observe such an elevation in plasma myoglobin that myoglobinuria also occurs. The half-life of myoglobin in the plasma is approximately 12 hours. Therefore persistence of myoglobinuria for more than several days suggests that muscle cell integrity continues to be impaired. Renal injury is frequent when urine myoglobin is more than 1 μg/ml. CPK increases in the plasma with a slower time course than does myoglobin. After a major operation complicated by cardiopulmonary bypass and circulatory instability, CPK may be above 10,000 U/L.[50] Only when the CPK is greater than 20,000 U/L 24 hours after the anesthetic incident that elicited the suspicion of MH is the CPK elevation strongly suggestive that the patient would have a muscle contracture test consistent with susceptibility to MH.[34] Massive rhabdomyolysis, producing CPK of greater than 20,000 U/L, may occur in patients with underlying muscular disease not necessarily related to MH. Thus rhabdomyolysis in the absence of increased metabolic rate, increased production of CO_2, and metabolic acidosis should not be assumed to be MH.

Factors that "Trigger" Malignant Hyperthermia in Humans

MH is the result of acutely increased intracellular calcium concentrations in muscle. Excitation of the sarcolemma activates the voltage-sensitive dihydropyridine receptor that results in release of calcium through the RYR1[54] into the cytosol. The sarcoplasmic reticulum Ca^{2+}-ATPase pumps calcium back into the sarcoplasmic reticulum. Theoretically, any factors that increase calcium release or impair the removal of calcium out of the sarcoplasm could facilitate the appearance of MH. Because removal of calcium from the sarcoplasm requires ATP, any factor that impairs the formation of ATP could similarly facilitate the appearance of MH.

Potent inhalation anesthetics such as sevoflurane (Ultane, Sevorane), halothane (Fluothane), enflurane (Ethrane), isoflurane (Forane), and desflurane (Suprane) are acknowledged to be triggers of MH in humans. Depolarizing neuromuscular blocking drugs are also potent triggers of MH in humans. Succinylcholine (Anectine, Quelicin) is the only drug of this type currently in common use. The combination of succinylcholine and potent inhalation anesthetics produces more episodes of MH than do potent inhalation anesthetics administered without succinylcholine or succinylcholine administered in the presence of nitrous oxide and intravenous anesthetics.[33]

A number of drugs, such as amide local anesthetics, droperidol, ketamine, calcium, digitalis, methylxanthines, anticholinergics, anticholinesterases, and sympathomimetic drugs, had been considered to be potential triggers of MH in humans primarily on theoretical grounds. Review of clinical[55] and laboratory[56-58] experience suggests that these drugs are not triggers of MH, but, on rare occasions, MH may occur during an anesthetic in which no trigger agents were administered.[59]

Although myoglobinuria, heatstroke, and sudden cardiovascular collapse may be more common in families that contain known MH-susceptible persons, in general, MH in humans differs from porcine MH in that a pharmacological trigger is usually required for the syndrome to develop. There have been reports of MH[60] in humans, however, in the absence of anesthetic drugs. In a large, well-investigated kindred, two young patients who had the familial mutation associated with MH susceptibility died unexpectedly during febrile illnesses.[11] An athletic adolescent who had an RYR1 mutation associated with MH died after strenuous exercise.[61] Of 12 unrelated patients with exercise-induced rhabdomyolysis, 10 had in vitro contracture tests that were positive for MH and 3 of these had RYR1 mutations.[62] Others have also reported recurrent myoglobinuria associated with exercise in patients with MH-positive in vitro muscle contracture studies and mutation in the RYR1 gene.[63] Therefore the family members of a patient who experiences MH should be asked if they have voided "cola-colored" urine after exercise or experienced intolerance to heat. Individuals with such histories may be at increased risk of experiencing MH.

MH can occur during recovery from anesthesia.[64] The question of what triggers MH is complicated by the observation that a spectrum of susceptibility exists.[28] Current methods of evaluation are not sufficiently refined to differentiate perfectly between susceptibility and resistance to MH.[65,66]

The Course of a Clinical Episode of Malignant Hyperthermia in Humans

The initial clinical signs of an impending episode of MH are nonspecific. When MH is fulminant, metabolic and respiratory acidosis, tachycardia with dysrhythmias, a rapid increase in body temperature to 39.5° C or greater, hyperkalemia, myoglobinuria, and a marked increase in serum CPK are observed. The patient's medical history and clinical course usually help to differentiate fulminant MH from other metabolic or endocrinological crises such as sepsis, porphyria, thyroid storm,[67] and untreated pheochromocytoma.

If the patient is less susceptible or the trigger agent is removed before the syndrome becomes self-perpetuating (see "Porcine Model"), abortive MH could be said to have occurred. In this case, there are only mild signs suggestive of MH: moderate increases in heart rate, blood pressure, and temperature along with a slight respiratory acidosis. Mild metabolic acidosis and moderate increases in serum myoglobin and CPK may or may not be present. Masseter spasm may occur.[34] As previously suggested (see "Clinical Recognition of an Episode in Humans"), differentiating an abortive episode of MH from an anesthetic complicated by other factors can be difficult.

Treatment of an Episode of Malignant Hyperthermia

Remove Trigger Agents

When an episode of MH is suspected, it is prudent to alter, as soon as possible, the anesthetic technique to allow elimination of all trigger agents. A fresh gas flow of 10 L/min will eliminate residual potent inhalation anesthetic from some anesthesia machines and circuits within 15 minutes.[68,69] Other systems (Siemens KION) without the CO_2 absorber, however, require at least 25 minutes.[70] If sufficient clinical signs lead the physician to suspect the presence of MH and especially if blood gas analysis has proved the presence of significant metabolic and respiratory acidosis, dantrolene should be administered immediately and the operation should be terminated as soon as possible.

Administer Dantrolene

Dantrolene should be available in all locations where general anesthesia is administered—all anesthetic drug supply rooms. If dantrolene has to be obtained from a central location, such as the pharmacy, it must be stressed that the need for the initial and subsequent doses of drug is *urgent*. The initial dose of intravenous dantrolene for treatment of MH is 2.5[71] to 3 mg/kg. More than 10 mg/kg has sometimes been required to return metabolism to normal.[5]

Dantrolene has to be diluted with sterile, preservative-free, distilled water. Liter quantities of such water may be required. Note that 150 mg of mannitol accompanies each 60 mg of dantrolene in its current formulation.

Repeated dosing of dantrolene should be guided by clinical and laboratory signs. A flow sheet including heart rate and rhythm, arterial blood pressure, central venous pressure, minute ventilation, core temperature, urine output, mixed venous blood gas tensions, serum electrolytes, serum glucose, and total fluid intake is useful. Immediately after the administration of intravenous dantrolene, one may note a dramatic amelioration of the patient's tachycardia. If this is the result of an effect on the underlying hypermetabolic state, it is a "comforting sign." A modest decrease in heart rate after administration of intravenous dantrolene, however, could be caused by the increase in intravascular volume.

Intravenous dantrolene administration should be repeated until the clinical signs of MH and the metabolic and respiratory acidosis have resolved. The major side effect of dantrolene is muscle weakness.[72] Muscle weakness is noted in approximately 25% of patients after an acute episode of MH treated with dantrolene. The patient with MH is likely to require intubation and artificial ventilation anyway because of respiratory failure or pulmonary edema. Phlebitis is the other common side effect of dantrolene administration, noted in approximately 10% of patients.

After dantrolene has been effective in controlling an episode of fulminant MH, repeated intravenous administration of at least 1 mg/kg should be given every 6 hours after the initial dosing period. If no recurrences are noted after 24 hours, dantrolene administration could be withheld and weaning from supportive therapy begun. If weakness is marked and the patient is metabolically stable, dantrolene administration may be stopped. Weakness is expected when tissue levels of dantrolene are adequate to treat the syndrome.[72] The effects of dantrolene on strength may persist for more than 8 to 12 hours. Severe muscle weakness of variable duration can also be the result of an MH episode. Presumably this is due to muscle injury.

If dantrolene must be administered to a patient who is also receiving calcium channel blocking drugs, invasive hemodynamic monitoring is necessary. Serum potassium should be closely monitored. Patients receiving both verapamil and dantrolene have experienced severe hyperkalemia and myocardial depression.[73-75]

Symptomatic Treatment

Minute ventilation should be increased severalfold with supplemental oxygen. Sodium bicarbonate should be administered liberally, 2 to 4 mEq/kg, to treat metabolic acidosis. When repeated assessment of blood gases indicates resolution of acidosis, minute ventilation can be normalized.

If temperature is elevated, active measures should be taken to cool the patient. Drapes should be removed. A water mattress should be placed under the patient and turned to cooling temperatures. Cold intravenous saline can be administered through a peripheral vein, as indicated by central venous pressures. Hypovolemia should be avoided because even mild hypovolemia impairs dissipation of heat produced by increased metabolism.[46] The stomach can be lavaged with iced saline. Ice packs may be placed on the groin and the axillae. Wet cloths and a fan can be used to promote surface evaporation. Active cooling should be stopped when core temperature falls below 38.3° C to prevent inadvertent hypothermia.[76]

Cardiac dysrhythmias usually stop when the episode is adequately treated with dantrolene. Lidocaine may be administered with the usual precautions. Before lidocaine was accepted as a drug that was unlikely to trigger MH, procainamide was the antidysrhythmic of choice during an episode of MH. Procainamide must be administered slowly, starting at a dose of 15 mg/kg infused over 10 minutes, because it can be a potent myocardial depressant. Procainamide is no longer recommended for treatment of MH-susceptible patients. Calcium channel blockers are not indicated in MH because they may cause severe hyperkalemia and cardiovascular collapse in the presence of dantrolene.[75]

Hyperkalemia may require aggressive treatment, especially if myoglobinuria has compromised renal function. Calcium should be administered if necessary. Glucose and insulin (10 units regular insulin in 50 ml of 50% dextrose titrated to effect) can be administered as usually indicated, although if marked hyperglycemia exists, it may be advisable to reduce the dose of dextrose somewhat. β-Stimulants can be administered to reduce life-threatening hyperkalemia in the same doses used to treat bronchoconstriction or to support circulatory function.

Large losses of intravascular volume may occur because evaporative loss may be great, edema formation may occur in muscle and other tissues, and mannitol given as part of the formulation of dantrolene may induce significant diuresis. If diuresis is not occurring, additional mannitol should be administered to protect the kidneys from the effects of high concentrations of myoglobin in the urine.[77]

Cardiovascular support, in the form of fluid challenges, inotropic drugs, or both should be administered as guided by the customary monitoring.

Recrudescence

There are cases[59, 64] in which a patient was symptomatically treated for MH with dantrolene, appeared to recover, and then some hours later had another episode of increased metabolic rate. This second episode was sometimes accompanied by remarkable stiffness of the muscles. It is difficult to explain how these episodes occur in the apparent absence of a pharmacological trigger. Perhaps (as described under "Porcine Model") metabolic derangements in the muscle can become self-perpetuating. There is no definite or guaranteed time course for these events in the human. Some suggest observing a patient closely for 24 hours after the apparent end of an episode of fulminant MH to allow for the early recognition and treatment of recrudescence. Such patients should be monitored in an ICU because of the utility of invasive cardiovascular monitoring in documenting the course of an episode of MH. Recrudescence of MH can progress into fulminant MH and therefore warrants aggressive treatment with dantrolene and supportive therapy.

Potential Systemic Complications

During and after an episode of fulminant MH, several systemic complications may develop that require intensive care management. These complications are reminiscent of those occurring in heatstroke.[4]

Ventilatory failure may occur early in an episode of fulminant MH. The workload of the respiratory system may be further increased by the occurrence of pulmonary edema. Pulmonary edema may be the result of capillary leak. It may be worsened by impaired cardiac contractility in the presence of acidemia.

Cardiac dysrhythmias may occur in the presence of marked electrolyte abnormalities. In older patients, there may be foci of myocardial fibrosis as well. It has been hypothesized that such areas of fibrosis are the result of subclinical episodes of MH, which produced increased levels of circulating catecholamines.[78] Cardiac contractility can be impaired.

As a result of rhabdomyolysis, myoglobin appears in the plasma and may produce significant renal injury. Muscle damage sufficient to produce myoglobinuria and acute renal failure can occur in the absence of pigmenturia or dramatic elevation of CPK.[77] If myoglobin or hemoglobin is present, urine produces a positive reaction with orthotolidine (Hematest).

Cerebral edema and coma have been part of episodes of fulminant MH. Although it is thought that the metabolism of the brain is normal during an episode of MH,[3] oxygen supply to the central nervous system may be inadequate. Therefore supportive care to the patient during and after an episode of fulminant MH should include measures to document cerebral function and maximize cerebral perfusion.

Disseminated intravascular coagulation has also been part of episodes of fulminant MH. Presumably, this occurs as a result of tissue injury, either muscular injury or injury to other tissues as a result of hypoperfusion.

Treatment of any of these complications of MH is facilitated by the invasive monitoring used in the initial treatment of an episode of fulminant MH. Resolution of some of these complications may take longer than the adequate treatment of the acute episode of MH. Treatment of the life-threatening complications should not detract from the need to continue monitoring of metabolic status and continue administration of dantrolene, in increasing doses if necessary, until the metabolic state is normal.

Because pulmonary and cardiovascular compromise is a result of fulminant MH and because the major side effect of dantrolene is muscular weakness, mechanically controlled ventilation may be useful in the treatment of an episode of fulminant MH. When calculation of oxygen consumption and CO_2 production is simplified by the system of mechanical ventilation, these values serve as the most appropriate monitor of the adequacy of treatment of an episode of fulminant MH.

Identification of Patients at Risk

People who have survived an episode of fulminant MH are considered capable of having another episode, although they may have undergone many anesthetics uneventfully before their first episode of MH. The first-degree relatives (parents, siblings, children) of such individuals are generally considered potentially MH susceptible until they have been proved not to be susceptible by in vitro muscle contracture testing. MH was originally assumed to be an autosomal dominant genetic disorder with reduced penetrance. Multifactorial inheritance may be a more accurate description.[11,12,79,80] Multiple mutations associated with MH susceptibility are found throughout the RYR1 gene. Two mutations associated with MH susceptibility have been found in a subunit of the dihydropyridine receptor gene. Other loci associated with MH susceptibility have been identified in chromosomes 17q21-24, 1q32, 3q13, 7q21-24, and 5p. In families in which both muscle biopsy specimens for caffeine-halothane contracture testing have been strongly positive and a causative gene has been identified, genetic analysis is helpful in the diagnosis of MH susceptibility.[81,82]

The most efficient way to evaluate a family for MH susceptibility is to first evaluate the index patient with caffeine-halothane contracture tests of living muscle.[83] First-degree relatives of an individual with positive contracture results are assumed to have 50% probability of also being MH susceptible. This assumption improves the positive predictive value of the contracture test. Elements of the history and physical examination that could strengthen the suggestion that an individual may be susceptible to MH are a history of muscle cramping, heatstroke, hernias, clubfeet, scoliosis, spontaneous dislocation of the hip, eye muscle imbalance, or other minor muscular abnormalities.[84] It must be acknowledged that these findings are nonspecific, but they may occur with greater frequency in individuals susceptible to MH than in the population at large. Similarly, resting CPK concentrations may be elevated in MH-susceptible individuals. CPK levels, at rest, are of no predictive value in the general population.[85,86] In some populations, more than 25% of the patients with elevated CPK levels were not susceptible to MH on in vitro testing.[87] If a relative of a patient known to be susceptible to MH has an elevated CPK level, though, then that individual has an increased likelihood of being susceptible as well.[86,88]

There is some controversy about the evaluation of the individual who has experienced abortive MH or isolated masseter spasm. Abortive MH could be relatively slowly evolving MH or a group of signs produced by processes completely unrelated to MH. Increased stiffness of the masseter, even to the degree that endotracheal intubation is precluded, can be a normal response to succinylcholine.[37,38,44] Because MH could develop some minutes to hours after an occurrence of masseter spasm, some anesthesiologists recommend cancellation of an anesthetic after such an occurrence and evaluation of the CPK levels at 12 and 24 hours after the incident.[89,90] Neurological evaluation and muscle biopsy to rule out susceptibility to MH have also been recommended.[90] Neurological evaluation is relevant after abnormal intraoperative muscle tension because myotonia or an abnormality of ion channel may be present. Mutation in the muscle sodium channel has been noted in one family evaluated after severe rigidity followed succinylcholine administration.[91] Others recommend discontinuing the trigger agents of MH, careful evaluation of acid-base status, and continuation of the anesthetic and surgical procedure if no further problems are identified. Urine should be checked for the presence of myoglobin. If masseter spasm occurs without significant metabolic or cardiovascular changes, it is unlikely to be followed by fulminant MH.[45] Similarly, the low specificity of the contracture test for MH may produce many false-positive results in such patients.[92]

Some patients with muscular diseases have also been found to be susceptible to MH. This association was first described because episodes of MH, or exacerbations of rhabdomyolysis with cardiac arrest, occurred in individuals with myopathy. Later, individuals with myopathy and some of their relatives were found to have results indicative of susceptibility to MH by in vitro muscle contracture testing. Duchenne's muscular dystrophy,[93-95] Becker's muscular dystrophy, and central core disease[96,97] are the most common myopathies in which MH susceptibility has been described. MH has also been described in patients with the King-Denborough syndrome, myotonia congenita, hypokalemic periodic paralysis,[98,99] the Schwartz-Jampel syndrome, and several other conditions in which fever and muscle injury occur for unknown reason. In some of these conditions, such as the Schwartz-Jampel syndrome, there are some patients whose disease is related to neurologic abnormalities, not to muscle dysfunction. The genetic locus of central core disease has been found in the RYR1 gene,[100] and mutations in the dihydropyridine receptor gene have been associated with hypokalemic paralysis. If a coexisting myopathy is present in a patient who has experienced MH, it is important to confirm that diagnosis because the risk for other family members differs with different myopathies. Not all individuals with these muscle disorders, however, are susceptible to MH.[101] The anesthetic complications these patients are likely to develop may be difficult to differentiate from MH on the basis of clinical signs. For example, cardiac arrest resulting from marked hyperkalemia may occur several minutes after administration of succinylcholine to patients with dystrophinopathy (i.e., Duchenne's or Becker's muscular dystrophy).[40,41,102]

"The Safe Anesthetic"

An anesthetic designed for an individual who is or is suspected of being MH susceptible avoids drugs known to be triggers of MH; depolarizing neuromuscular blocking drugs, such as succinylcholine; and potent inhalation anesthetics (e.g., sevoflurane, halothane, enflurane, desflurane, and isoflurane). Anesthetic regimens considered to be "nontriggering" include any regional anesthetic, as well as intravenous drugs such as narcotics, barbiturates, benzodiazepines, and other sedatives (e.g., propofol); nitrous oxide; and nondepolarizing neuromuscular blocking drugs. Some intravenous anesthetics (e.g., thiopental and althesin) may attenuate or even prevent the initiation of MH in response to halothane.[17] Alternatively, etomidate may enhance the development of MH triggered by halothane.[17] In general, drugs should be selected that have the least potential to increase heart rate (because tachycardia is an early sign of MH) and the least need for pharmacological antagonism. Anticholinesterases can be administered, however, to patients with susceptibility to MH. It is advisable to avoid drugs that may affect temperature regulation and sympathetic tone to such an extent that it might be difficult to distinguish drug effects from early signs of MH.

No anesthetic regimen is guaranteed to preclude the development of MH in a susceptible individual. There have been case reports of MH in patients who received regional anesthesia or general anesthesia with nontriggering drugs.[59] It is to be expected, however, that the incidence of MH will be much lower during anesthetics that do not include the "trigger" agents of MH.[33]

Dantrolene

Dantrolene, a hydantoin with muscle relaxant properties, has greatly changed the treatment of and risk of death from MH.

Years ago it was thought that dantrolene decreases calcium release from the sarcoplasmic reticulum by decreasing the mobility of a calcium ionophore, which transports calcium across membranes.[103,104] Recently it was shown that dantrolene interacts with amino acids 590-609 in the N-terminal fragment of the RYR1.[105] By decreasing calcium release from the sarcoplasmic reticulum through RYR1, dantrolene decreases excitation-contraction coupling. It does not act on the neuromuscular junction or on the passive or active electrical properties of the surface membranes of muscle fibers. Therefore patients given effective doses of dantrolene have normal electromyograms and depressed force of muscle contraction.[72]

In children, intravenous infusion of dantrolene, 2.4 mg/kg over 10 to 12 minutes, produced stable blood levels of about 3.5 μg/ml for 4 hours, after which a slow decline in plasma concentration occurred (Fig. 117–6).[106] It appears that the half-life of dantrolene in the plasma of children is somewhat shorter than in adults: 7 to 10 hours

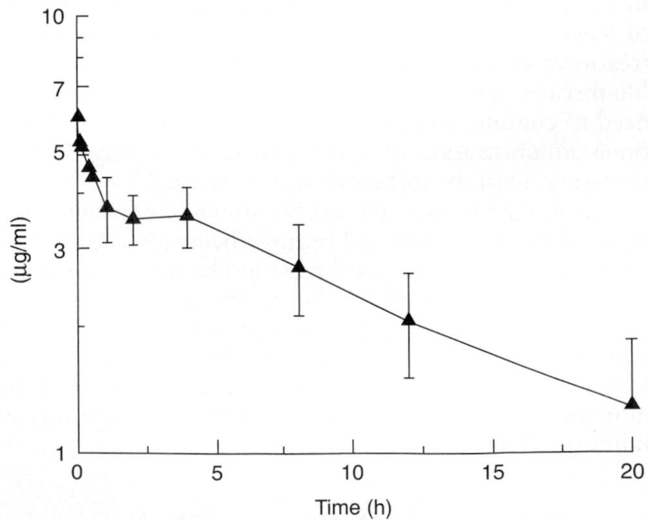

FIGURE 117–6 • Whole blood concentration of dantrolene vs. time for 10 children. (Redrawn from Lerman J, McLeod ME, Strong HA: *Anesthesiology* 70:625, 1989.)

compared with 12 hours, respectively.[72] This is consistent with the recommendation to repeat 1 mg/kg of dantrolene every 6 hours for prophylaxis against recurrence of MH in a child. Giving dantrolene by intermittent bolus rather than by continuous infusion may lessen the incidence of phlebitis noted after dantrolene administration. It is likely that when the plasma concentration of dantrolene is sufficient to inhibit an episode of MH, the patient will experience weakness and possibly disequilibrium. The ability to swallow could be compromised.

Dantrolene may be useful in the treatment of fever not associated with MH. Therefore if fever diminishes and abnormal vital signs associated with fever resolve after the administration of dantrolene, the patient did not necessarily have MH.

In Vitro Caffeine-Halothane Contracture Testing

In vitro caffeine-halothane contracture testing is the only specific test of MH susceptibility other than the occurrence of an episode of fulminant MH. At least 2 to 3 months should pass between an episode of suspected MH and the date of muscle biopsy.[65] This test has been described in detail, and the standards for its performance are now accepted by the specialized centers in North America and Europe that perform it.[66,107]

For the in vitro test to be performed according to the North American standards, a sample of skeletal muscle is obtained from the quadriceps. In a test chamber where pH, oxygen tension, and temperature are controlled, the muscle is exposed to 3% halothane for 10 minutes or to caffeine given incrementally to 32 mM. Muscle strips are stimulated supramaximally at 0.2 Hz, and tension is measured with a strain gauge.[107]

A positive halothane contracture test is defined as a contracture of any one of the four to eight muscle strips prepared, of greater than 0.2 to 0.7 g in the presence of 3% halothane. (The exact range of abnormal force is determined by each testing site after evaluation of at least 30 healthy controls.) A positive caffeine contracture test is defined as the observation of greater than 0.2 g tension in the presence of 2 mM caffeine, more than 1 g contracture at less than 4 mM caffeine, or an increase in maximal tension of more than 7% above baseline at 2 mM caffeine.[107]

Results may be reported in terms of the caffeine-specific concentration, the concentration of caffeine at which muscle produces a contracture equal to 1 g of tension. As noted, a caffeine-specific concentration of less than 4 mM caffeine is a positive caffeine contracture test.[107]

Reexamination of the results of the caffeine-halothane contracture test produced a statement of the operating characteristics of the test.[65] Its negative predictive value is high, but because the specificity of the in vitro test is only 85% at best, the positive predictive value of this test varies depending on the prior probability of the individual being susceptible to MH.[92] As much clinical and laboratory evidence as can be obtained should be used to interpret the results of the muscle biopsy specimen. Genetic analysis may be helpful if several generations of one family can be examined.

Less Invasive Tests of Malignant Hyperthermia Susceptibility

None of the relatively noninvasive tests of MH susceptibility have proved as sensitive and as specific as the in vitro caffeine-halothane contracture test. Tests that have been evaluated in the past include calcium uptake into frozen muscle, skinned fiber testing, platelet nucleotide depletion, ionized calcium concentration in lymphocytes, force of contracture, and phosphorus nuclear magnetic resonance spectroscopy.[108] Recently, other tests based on RYR1 function in β lymphocytes,[109,110] pharmacologic response in muscle cell cultures,[111-113] and microdialysis study of in situ muscle[55] have been proposed. Perhaps future studies will find abnormal genes or gene products that can identify the MH-susceptible individual without the need for a muscle biopsy and careful in vitro testing of muscle strips. In 2003 a diagnostic genetic test of MH susceptibility was available only through MH Diagnostic Centers in Europe[81] and New Zealand.[114] The sensitivity of a genetic test must be much less than that of the muscle contracture test, and its specificity has not been defined. Such tests were in the experimental phase in the United States in 2003.

Neuroleptic Malignant Syndrome and Serotonin Syndrome

NMS resembles MH in clinical findings with the exception that the time course of NMS is over hours to days rather than minutes to hours. NMS occurs only in association with a pharmacological trigger or potent neuroleptic agents, most frequently depot phenothiazines. NMS may occur in 1 of 200 patients treated with these drugs. Most of the patients are young men who received piperazine phenothiazines or haloperidol for the treatment of schizophrenia or mania.[53,115,116]

NMS can be fatal. Its initial signs are hypermetabolism, fever, tachycardia, muscle rigidity, and myoglobinuria. Acute renal failure and multiorgan failure such as observed in fulminant MH or heatstroke may occur in NMS. As is the case in patients who may have MH, the differential diagnosis must be carefully considered for the patient suspected of NMS. Rhabdomyolysis may occur from other causes. Severe dystonic reaction, catatonia, central nervous system infection or mass lesion, neuroleptic-related heatstroke, allergic drug reaction, toxic encephalopathy (caused by lithium, strychnine, or anticholinergic drugs), hyperthyroidism, and tetanus may present with symptoms similar to those of NMS.[117]

NMS is related to blockade of dopamine receptors. The dopamine antagonist, bromocriptine (2.5 to 20 mg q8h in the adult), has been used successfully to treat this disorder.[115] Dantrolene has also been used successfully to treat NMS.[118-120] Five of seven NMS patients who underwent muscle biopsy for in vitro halothane contracture testing had significantly abnormal results.[121] Therefore the recommendation has been made to treat NMS patients as MH susceptible until proved otherwise. Unfortunately, this can pose anesthetic difficulties because these psychiatric patients may receive electroconvulsive treatment (ECT). Succinylcholine, a potent trigger of MH, is a useful drug for lessening the force of the convulsions that accompany ECT. One patient who had experienced NMS did later receive succinylcholine repeatedly for ECT without complications.[122] Therefore it is unclear whether patients who have had NMS should be prevented from receiving anesthetic agents capable of triggering MH when these drugs are otherwise indicated.

The serotonin syndrome is caused by excessive serotoninergic activity at the 5-HT_{1A} receptors in the central nervous system.[123] Effects at dopamine receptors and 5-HT_2 receptors may also be important. Inhibitors of 5-HT (5-hydroxytryptamine) metabolism, 5-HT receptor antagonists and drugs such as cocaine that increase 5-HT release can all have similar effects. The symptoms of the serotonin syndrome include rapid onset of cognitive and behavioral changes, autonomic dysfunction, and neuromuscular abnormalities. Fever can be extreme.

Although there may be similarities in the presentation of MH, NMS, and the serotonin syndrome, they have pathophysiological differences. Nevertheless, there is experimental evidence in animals that stress-induced MH, more than anesthetic-induced MH, may be mediated in part by 5-HT.[123] Furthermore, there is evidence that patients with myotonic myopathies may be at increased risk of muscular complications during treatment with neuroleptic drugs.[124]

The Malignant Hyperthermia Association of the United States (MHAUS, 11 East State Street, Box 1069, Sherburne, NY, 13460-1069; fax, 607-674-7910) is a valuable resource for affected families and their physicians. This organization offers information, expert consultation, and referral. MHAUS maintains a 24-hour, professionally staffed telephone line to assist physicians and patients in dealing with MH, (1-800-644-9737) and NMS (1-888-667-8367). All cases of suspected MH and similar heat-related disorders should be reported to the North American MH Registry (telephone, 412-692-5464; website, www.mhreg.org) to support the continued epidemiologic study of MH.

REFERENCES

1. Britt BA: Aetiology and pathophysiology of malignant hyperthermia. In Britt BA, editor: *Malignant hyperthermia,* Norwell, Mass, 1987, Kluwer Academic.
2. Gommans IM, Vlak MH, de Haan A, et al: Calcium regulation and muscle disease, *J Muscle Res Cell Motil* 23:59, 2002.
3. Gronert GA, Mott J, Lee J: Aetiology of malignant hyperthermia, *Br J Anaesth* 60:253, 1988.
4. Bouchama A, Knochel JP: Heat Stroke, *N Engl J Med* 346:1978, 2002.
5. Nelson TE, Flewellen EH: Current concepts: the malignant hyperthermia syndrome, *N Engl J Med* 309:416, 1983.
6. Karan SM, Crowl F, Muldoon SM: Malignant hyperthermia masked by capnographic monitoring, *Anesth Analg* 78:590, 1994.
7. Fagerlund T, Ording H, Bendixen D, et al: Search for three known mutations in the RYR1 gene in 48 Danish families with malignant hyperthermia, *Clin Genet* 46:401, 1994.
8. Levitt RC, Nouri N, Jedlicka AE, et al: Evidence for genetic heterogeneity in malignant hyperthermia susceptibility, *Genomics* 11:543, 1991.
9. Levitt RC, Olckers A, Meyers S, et al: Evidence for the localization of a malignant hyperthermia susceptibility locus (MHS2) to human chromosome 17q, *Genomics* 14:562, 1992.
10. McCarthy TV, Healy JMS, Heffron JJA, et al: Localization of the malignant hyperthermia susceptibility locus to human chromosome 19q12-13.2, *Nature* 343:562, 1990.
11. Brown RL, Pollock AN, Couchman KG, et al: A novel ryanodine receptor mutation and genotype-phenotype correlation in a large malignant hyperthermia New Zealand Maori pedigree, *Hum Mol Genet* 9:1515, 2000.
12. Monnier N, Krivosic-Horber R, Payen JF, et al: Presence of two different genetic traits in malignant hyperthermia families: Implication for genetic analysis, diagnosis, and incidence of Malignant Hyperthermia Susceptibility, *Anesthesiology* 97:1067, 2002.
13. Fletcher JE, Calvo PA, Rosenberg H: Phenotypes associated with malignant hyperthermia susceptibility in swine genotyped as homozygous or heterozygous for the ryanodine receptor mutation, *Br J Anaesth* 71:410, 1993.
14. Claxton BA, Cross MH, Hopkins P: No response to trigger agents in a malignant hyperthermia susceptible patient, *Br J Anaesthesia* 88:870, 2002.
15. Iaizzo PA, Wedel DJ: Response to succinylcholine in porcine malignant hyperthermia, *Anesthesiology* 79:143, 1994.
16. Harrison GG: Porcine malignant hyperthermia, *Int Anesthesiol Clin* 17:25, 1979.
17. Harrison GG: Porcine malignant hyperthermia—the saga of the "hot" pig. In Britt BA, editor: *Malignant hyperthermia,* Norwell, Mass, 1987, Kluwer Academic.
18. MacLennan DH, Duff C, Zorzato F, et al: Ryanodine receptor gene is a candidate for predisposition to malignant hyperthermia, *Nature* 343:559, 1990.
19. Cheah KS: Mitochondria and malignant hyperthermia. In Britt BA, editor: *Malignant hyperthermia,* Norwell, Mass, 1987, Kluwer Academic.
20. Harrison GG, Saunders S, Biebuyck JF, et al: Anaesthetic induced malignant hyperpyrexia and a method for its prediction, *Br J Anaesth* 41:844, 1969.
21. Oka S, Igorashi Y, Takagi A, et al: Malignant hyperpyrexia and Duchenne muscular dystrophy: a case report, *Can Anaesth Soc J* 29:627, 1982.
22. Berman MC, Harrison GG, Bull AB, et al: Changes underlying halothane-induced malignant hyperpyrexia in Landrace pigs, *Nature* 225:653, 1970.
23. Gronert GA, Theye RA: Halothane-induced porcine malignant hyperthermia: metabolic and hemodynamic changes, *Anesthesiology* 44:36, 1976.
24. Berman MC, McIntosh DB, Kench JE: Proton inactivation of calcium transport by sarcoplasmic reticulum, *J Biol Chem* 256:994, 1977.
25. Fuchs F: Thermal inactivation of calcium regulating mechanism of human muscle actomyosin, *Anesthesiology* 42:584, 1975.
26. Hall GM, Lucke JN, Lister D: Porcine malignant hyperthermia. V: Fatal hyperthermia in the Pietrain pig associated with infusion of adrenergic agonists, *Br J Anaesth* 49:855, 1977.
27. Gronert GA, Milde JH, Theye RA: Role of sympathetic activity in porcine malignant hyperthermia, *Anesthesiology* 47:411, 1977.
28. Nelson TE, Flewellen EH, Gloyna DF: Spectrum of susceptibility to malignant hyperthermia-diagnostic dilemma, *Anesth Analg* 62:545, 1983.
29. Gronert GA: Malignant hyperthermia, *Anesthesiology* 53:395, 1980.
30. Dershwitz M, Sreter FA: Azumolene reverses episodes of malignant hyperthermia in susceptible swine, *Anesth Analg* 70:253, 1990.
31. Donlon JV, Newfield P, Sreter F et al: Implications of masseter spasm after succinylcholine, *Anesthesiology* 49:298, 1978.
32. Karger B, Tiege K: Fatal malignant hyperthermia-delayed onset and atypical course, *Forensic Sci Int* 129:187, 2002.
33. Ording H: Incidence of malignant hyperthermia in Denmark, *Anesth Analg* 64:700, 1985.
34. Larach MG, Rosenberg H, Larach DR, et al: Prediction of malignant hyperthermia susceptibility by clinical signs, *Anesthesiology* 66:547, 1987.
35. Rose DK, Froese AB: The regulation of $PaCO_2$ during controlled ventilation of children with a T-piece, *Can Anaesth Soc J* 26:104, 1979.
36. Hannallah RS, Kaplan RF: Jaw relaxation after a halothane/succinylcholine sequence in children, *Anesthesiology* 81:99, 1994.

37. Van der Spek AFL, Fang WB, Ashton-Miller JA, et al: The effects of succinylcholine on mouth opening, *Anesthesiology* 76:459, 1987.
38. Van der Spek AFL, Fang WB, Ashton-Miller JA, et al: Increased masticatory muscle stiffness during limb muscle flaccidity associated with succinylcholine administration, *Anesthesiology* 69:11, 1988.
39. Harper PS, Rudel R: Myotonic dystrophy. In Engel AG, Franzini-Armstrong C, editors: *Myology*, ed 2, New York, 1994, McGraw-Hill.
40. Delphin E, Jackson D, Rothstein P: Use of succinylcholine during elective pediatric anesthesia should be re-evaluated, *Anesth Analg* 66:1190, 1987.
41. Rosenberg H, Gronert GA: Intractable cardiac arrest in children given succinylcholine, *Anesthesiology* 77:1054, 1992.
42. Penn AS: Myoglobinuria. In Engel AG, Franzini-Armstrong C, editors: *Myology*, ed 2, New York, 1994, McGraw-Hill.
43. Rubiano R, Chang JL, Carroll J, et al: Acute rhabdomyolysis following halothane anesthesia without succinylcholine, *Anesthesiology* 67:856, 1987.
44. Kaplan RF, Rushing E: Isolated masseter muscle spasm and increased creatine kinase without malignant hyperthermia susceptibility or other myopathies, *Anesthesiology* 77:820, 1992.
45. Littleford JA, Patel LR, Bose D, et al: Masseter muscle spasm in children: implications of continuing the triggering anesthetic, *Anesth Analg* 72:151, 1991.
46. Ezri T, Szmuk P, Weisenberg M, et al: The effects of hydration on core temperature in pediatric surgical patients, *Anesthesiology* 98:838, 2003.
47. Lees DE, Gadde PL, Macnamara TE: Malignant hyperthermia in association with Burkitt's lymphoma: report of a third case, *Anesth Analg* 59:514, 1980.
48. Simmons PS, Smithson WA, Gronert GA, et al: Acute myelogenous leukemia and malignant hyperthermia in a patient with type 1b glycogen storage disease, *J Pediatr* 105:428, 1984.
49. Tsueda K, Dubick MN, Wright BD, et al: Intraoperative hyperthermic crisis in two children with undifferentiated lymphoma, *Anesth Analg* 57:511, 1978.
50. Casella ES, Soule LM, Blanck TJJ: Creatine kinase activity and temperature in children after cardiac surgery, *J Cardiothorac Anesth* 2:156, 1988.
51. Innes RKR, Stromme JH: Rise in serum creatine phosphokinase associated with agents used in anesthesia, *Br J Anaesth* 45:185, 1973.
52. Plotz J, Braun J: Failure of "self-taming" doses of succinylcholine to inhibit increases in post-operative serum creatine kinase activity in children, *Anesthesiology* 56:207, 1982.
53. Guze BH, Baxter LR: Neuroleptic malignant syndrome, *N Engl J Med* 313:163, 1985.
54. Ikemoto N, Yamamoto T: Regulation of calcium release by interdomain interaction within ryanodine receptors, *Front Biosci* 7:d671, 2002.
55. Anesteder M, Hager M, Muller CR, et al: Diagnosis of susceptibility to malignant hyperthermia by use of a metabolic test, *Lancet* 359:1579-1580, 2002.
56. Gronert GA, Ahern CP, Milde JH, et al: Effect of CO_2, calcium, digoxin, and potassium on cardiac and skeletal muscle metabolism in malignant hyperthermia susceptible swine, *Anesthesiology* 64:24, 1986.
57. Harrison GG, Morrell DF: Response of MHS swine to IV infusion of lignocaine and bupivacaine, *Br J Anaesth* 52:385, 1980.
58. Wingard DW, Bobko S: Failure of lidocaine to trigger porcine malignant hyperthermia, *Anesth Analg* 58:99, 1979.
59. Fitzgibbons DC: Malignant hyperthermia following preoperative oral administration of dantrolene, *Anesthesiology* 54:73, 1981.
60. Gronert GA, Thompson RL, Onofrio BM: Human malignant hyperthermia: awake episodes and correction by dantrolene, *Anesth Analg* 59:377, 1980.
61. Tobin JR, Jason DR, Challa VR, et al: Malignant hyperthermia and apparent heat stroke, *JAMA* 286:168, 2001.
62. Wappler F, Fiege M, Steinfath M, et al: Evidence for susceptibility to malignant hyperthermia in patients with exercise-induced rhabdomyolysis, *Anesthesiology* 96:941, 2001.
63. Davis M, Brown R, Dickson A, et al: Malignant hyperthermia associated with exercise-induced rhabdomyolysis or congenital abnormalities and a novel RYR1 mutation in new Zealand and Australian pedigrees, *Br J Anaesth* 88:508, 2002.
64. Mathieu A, Bogosian AJ, Ryan JF, et al: Recrudescence after survival of an initial episode of malignant hyperthermia, *Anesthesiology* 51:454, 1979.
65. Larach MG, Landis JR, Bunn JS, et al: The North American Malignant Hyperthermia Registry: Prediction of malignant hyperthermia susceptibility in low risk subjects, *Anesthesiology* 76:16, 1992.
66. Ording H, Bendixen D: Sources of variability in halothane and caffeine contracture tests for susceptibility to malignant hyperthermia, *Eur J Anaesthesiol* 9:367, 1992.
67. Shailesh Kumar MV, Carr RJ, Komanduri V, et al: Differential diagnosis of thyroid crisis and malignant hyperthermia in a porcine model, *Endocr Res* 25:87, 1999.
68. McGraw TT, Keon TP: Malignant hyperthermia and the clean machine, *Can Anaesth J* 36:530, 1989.
69. Ritchie PA, Cheshire MA, Pearce NH: Decontamination of halothane from anaesthesia machines achieved by continuous flushing with oxygen, *Br J Anaesth* 60:859, 1988.
70. Petroz GC, Lerman J: Preparation of the Siemens KION anesthetic machine for patients susceptible to malignant hyperthermia, *Anesthesiology* 96:941, 2002.
71. Koth MF, Horne ML, Martz R: Dantrolene in human hyperthermia: a multicenter study, *Anesthesiology* 56:254, 1982.
72. Flewellen EH, Nelson TE, Jones WP, et al: Dantrolene dose response in awake man: implications for management of malignant hyperthermia, *Anesthesiology* 59:275, 1983.
73. Lynch C, Durbin CG, Fisher NA, et al: Effects of dantrolene and verapamil on atrioventricular conduction and cardiovascular performance in dogs, *Anesth Analg* 65:252, 1986.
74. Rubin AS, Zablocki AD: Hyperkalemia, verapamil, and dantrolene, *Anesthesiology* 66:246, 1987.
75. Saltzman LS, Kates RA, Corke BC, et al: Hyperkalemia and cardiovascular collapse after verapamil and dantrolene administration in swine, *Anesth Analg* 63:473, 1984.
76. Jones DE, Ryan JF: Treatment of acute hyperthermia crises. In Britt BA, editor: *Malignant hyperthermia*, Norwell, Mass, 1987, Kluwer Academic.
77. Grossman RA, Hamilton RW, Morse BM, et al: Nontraumatic rhabdomyolysis and acute renal failure, *N Engl J Med* 291:807, 1974.
78. Huckell VF, Staniloff HM, Britt BA, et al: Cardiac manifestations of malignant hyperthermia susceptibility, *Circulation* 58:916, 1978.
79. Britt BA, Kalow W: Malignant hyperthermia: a statistical review, *Can Anaesth Soc J* 17:293, 1970.
80. Robinson R, Hopkins P, Carsana A, et al: Several interacting genes influence the malignant hyperthermia phenotype, *Hum Genetics* 112:217, 2003.
81. Girard T, Treves S, Voronkov E, et al: Molecular genetics of MH susceptibility, *Anesthesiology* 100:1076, 2004.
82. Urwyler A, Deufel T, McCarthy T, et al: Guidelines for molecular genetic detection of susceptibility to malignant hyperthermia, *Br J Anaesthesia* 86:283, 2001.
83. Loke JC, MacLennan D: Bayesian modeling of muscle biopsy contracture testing for malignant hyperthermia susceptibility, *Anesthesiology* 88:589, 1998.
84. Britt BA, Endrenyi L, Peters PL, et al: Screening of malignant hyperthermia susceptible families by creatine phosphokinase measurement and other clinical investigations, *Can Anaesth Soc J* 23:263, 1976.
85. Ellis FR, Clarke MC, Modgill M, et al: Evaluation of creatine phosphokinase in screening patients for malignant hyperthermia, *Br Med J* 3:511, 1975.
86. Paasuke RT, Brownell AKW: Serum creatine kinase level as a screening test for susceptibility to malignant hyperthermia, *JAMA* 255:769, 1986.
87. Moulds RFW, Denborough MA: Identification of susceptibility to malignant hyperthermia, *Br Med J* 2:245, 1974.
88. Allen GC, Rosenberg H: Malignant hyperthermia susceptibility in adult patients with masseter muscle rigidity, *Can J Anaesth* 37:31, 1990.
89. Gronert GA: Management of patients in whom trismus occurs following succinylcholine, *Anesthesiology* 68:653, 1988.
90. Rosenberg H: Trismus is not trivial, *Anesthesiology* 67:453, 1987.
91. Vita GM, Olckers A, Jedlicka AE, et al: Masseter muscle rigidity associated with glycine1306-to-alanine mutation in the adult muscle sodium channel *a*-subunit gene [see comments], *Anesthesiology* 82:1097, 1995.
92. Brandom BW, Gronert GA: Malignant hyperthermia. In Motoyama EK, Davis PJ, editors: *Smith's anesthesia for infants and children*, ed 6, Philadelphia, 1995, Mosby.

93. Brownell AKW, Paasuke RT, Elash A, et al: Malignant hyperthermia in Duchenne muscular dystrophy, *Anesthesiology* 58:180, 1983.
94. Heiman-Patterson TD, Martino S, Rosenberg H, et al: Malignant hyperthermia susceptibility in X-linked muscle dystrophies, *Pediatr Neurosci* 2:356, 1986.
95. Kelfer HM, Singer WD, Reynolds RN: Malignant hyperthermia in a child with Duchenne muscular dystrophy, *Pediatrics* 71:118, 1983.
96. Frank JP, Harati Y, Butler IJ, et al: Central core disease and malignant hyperthermia syndrome, *Ann Neurol* 7:11, 1980.
97. Robinson R, Brooks C, Brown SL, et al: RYR1 mutations causing central core disease are associated with more severe malignant hyperthermia in vitro contracture test phenotypes, *Hum Mutat* 20:88, 2002.
98. Lambert C, Blanloeil Y, Krivosic-Horber R, et al: Malignant hyperthermia in a patient with hypokalemic periodic paralysis, *Anesth Analg* 79:1012, 1994.
99. Rajabally YA, El Lahawi M: Hypokalemic periodic paralysis associated with malignant hyperthermia, *Muscle Nerve* 25:453, 2002.
100. Schwemmle S, Wolff K, Palmucci LM, et al: Multipoint mapping of the central core disease locus, *Genomics* 17:205, 1993.
101. Gronert GA, Fowler W, Cardinet GH, et al: Absence of malignant hyperthermia contractures in Becker-Duchenne dystrophy at age 2, *Muscle Nerve* 15:52, 1992.
102. Farrell PT: Anesthesia-induced rhabdomyolysis causing cardiac arrest, case report and review of anaesthesia and the dystrophinopathies, *Anaesth Int Care* 22:597, 1994.
103. Morgan KG, Bryant SH: The mechanism of action of dantrolene sodium, *J Pharmacol Exp Ther* 201:138, 1977.
104. Putney JW, Bianchi CP: Site of action of dantrolene in frog sartorius muscle, *J Pharmacol Exp Ther* 189:202, 1974.
105. Paul-Pletzer K, Yamamoto T, Bhat MB, et al: Identification of a dantrolene-binding sequence on the skeletal muscle ryanodine receptor, *J Biol Chem* 277(38):34918, 2002.
106. Lerman J, McLeod ME, Strong HA: Pharmacokinetics of intravenous dantrolene in children, *Anesthesiology* 70:625, 1989.
107. Larach MG: Standardization of the caffeine halothane muscle contracture test, *Anesth Analg* 69:511, 1989.
108. Olgin J, Rosenberg H, Allen G, et al: A blinded comparison of noninvasive, in vivo phosphorus nuclear magnetic resonance spectroscopy and the in vitro halothane/caffeine contracture test in the evaluation of malignant hyperthermia susceptibility, *Anesth Analg* 72:36, 1991.
109. Girard T, Cavagna D, Padovan E, et al: B-lymphocytes from malignant hyperthermia-susceptible patients have an increased sensitivity to skeletal muscle ryanodine receptor activators, *J Biol Chem* 276:48077, 2001.
110. Sei Y, Brandom BW, Bina S, et al: Patients with malignant hyperthermia demonstrate an altered calcium control mechanism in B lymphocytes, *Anesthesiology* 97:1052, 2002.
111. Girard T, Treves S, Censier K, et al: Phenotyping malignant hyperthermia susceptibility by measuring halothane-induced changes in myoplasmic calcium concentration in cultured human skeletal muscle cells, *Br J Anaesth* 89:571, 2002.
112. Klinger W, Baur C, Georgieff M, et al: Detection of proton release from cultured human myotubes to identify malignant hyperthermia susceptibility, *Anesthesiology* 97:1059, 2002.
113. Wehner M, Rueffert H, Koenig F, et al: Increased sensitivity to 4-chloro-m-cresol and caffeine in primary myotubes from malignant hyperthermia susceptible individuals carrying the ryanodine receptor 1 Thr2206Met (C6617T) mutation, *Clin Genet* 62:135, 2002.
114. Pollock AN, Langton EE, Couchman K, et al: Suspected malignant hyperthermia reactions in New Zealand. *Anaesth Intensive Care* 30:453, 2002.
115. Carroff SN: The neuroleptic malignant syndrome, *J Clin Psychol* 41:79, 1980.
116. Cohen BM, Baldessamini RJ, Pope HG, et al: Neuroleptic malignant syndrome, *N Engl J Med* 313:1293, 1985.
117. Levenson JL: Neuroleptic malignant syndrome, *Psychiatry* 142:1137, 1985.
118. Coons DJ, Hillman FJ, Marshall RW: Treatment of neuroleptic syndrome with dantrolene sodium: a case report, *Am J Psychiatry* 139:944, 1982.
119. Goulon M, de Rohan-Chabot P, Elkharrat D, et al: Beneficial effects of dantrolene in the treatment of neuroleptic malignant syndrome: a report of two cases, *Neurology* 33:516, 1983.
120. Granati JE, Stern BJ, Ringel A: Neuroleptic malignant syndrome: successful treatment with dantrolene and bromocriptine, *Ann Neurol* 14:89, 1983.
121. Carroff SN, Rosenberg H, Gerber JC: Neuroleptic malignant syndrome and malignant hyperthermia, *Lancet* 1:244, 1983.
122. Geiduschek J, Cohen SA, Khan A, et al: Repeated anesthesia for a patient with neuroleptic malignant syndrome, *Anesthesiology* 68:134, 1988.
123. Wappler F, Fiege M, Schulte am Esch J: Pathophysiological role of the serotonin system in malignant hyperthermia, *Brit J Anaesth* 87:794, 2001.

PART

VII

Cardiopulmonary Resuscitation

CHAPTER

118

Physiologic Foundations of Cardiopulmonary Resuscitation

Peter Trinkaus and Charles L. Schleien

PEARLS

- Both the cardiac and thoracic pump mechanisms play a role in infants and children during cardiopulmonary resuscitation (CPR), so attention to excellent chest compression technique is critical to attaining sufficient cardiac output to maintain coronary and cerebral blood flow.
- Use of high-dose epinephrine probably is not warranted during CPR given the results of large clinical trials in adults. However, use of any vasoconstrictor (including vasopressin) should be sufficient to raise aortic diastolic pressure during CPR above the critical level for resuscitation success (>15–20 mmHg).
- Amiodarone may be the most effective pharmacologic treatment for shock-resistant ventricular tachycardia or fibrillation.
- Use of the biphasic defibrillator is an important advance in the treatment of tachyarrhythmias.
- Mild to moderate hypothermia (33°–34° C) may improve survival and neurologic outcome following cardiac arrest.

With the development of basic cardiopulmonary resuscitation (CPR) in the early 1960s, skilled resuscitation teams both in and out of the hospital were developed. This development saved lives; previously every victim of cardiac arrest had died. Soon thereafter, successful resuscitation of patients by basic life support measures, defibrillation, and medications became common even as long as 5 hours after commencement of CPR. Data show that the success of CPR is dependent on many factors. Rapid institution of basic life support measures (bystander CPR for sudden out-of-hospital cardiac arrest [SOHCA]) and immediate electrical countershock for ventricular fibrillation (VF) improve the chances of survival for patients experiencing SOHCA.[175] These measures led to the growing deployment of automatic external defibrillators (AEDs) in public places. Although immediate defibrillation currently is the standard of care, accumulating evidence indicates that basic life support and other measures directed at restoring energy substrates to the myocardium before countershock in patients with prolonged VF may further improve outcome.[24,162,244] Other preexisting factors that play a role in successful resuscitation include the patient's age, prior medical condition, presenting cardiac rhythm, and the etiology of cardiac arrest. The low resuscitation rate in children, even when the patient does not suffer from preexisting disease, probably results from the high incidence of asystole as the presenting rhythm. Asystole is the most common presenting rhythm in both in-hospital and out-of-hospital arrests, noted in 55% to 70% of victims.[85,132,176,188,202] Bradycardia and pulseless electrical activity (PEA) are other common rhythms. The high incidence of asystole in pediatric arrest victims can be explained by systemic disturbances such as hypoxia, acidosis, sepsis, and hypovolemia that commonly precede the arrest. Although ventricular arrhythmias usually are reported as infrequent (range 1.3%–3.8%),[194] out-of-hospital series report VF in 10% to 19% of victims younger than 20 years.[155] These series, along with the observation that the frequency of witnessed arrest is much lower than in adults,[89] suggests that ventricular rhythms may be more common than usually estimated and that delay in resuscitation results in progression of nonperfusing rhythms to asystole. Increasing availability of AEDs may be contributing to the increased recognition of ventricular arrhythmias in out-of-hospital pediatric cardiac arrest. In specialized cardiac intensive care units (ICUs), ventricular arrhythmias account for as much as 30% of arrests.[172]

In their original work on CPR, Kouwenhoven et al.[130] proposed that blood flow during closed-chest compressions resulted from squeezing of the heart between the sternum and vertebral column, now termed the *cardiac blood flow mechanism*. In fact, the precise mechanism by which forward circulatory flow is generated during closed-chest cardiac massage has major implications for current approaches to CPR. Newer methods, such as vest CPR, simultaneous compression ventilation CPR (SCV-CPR), active compression-decompression CPR (ACD-CPR) both without and with an impedance threshold valve (ITV), and interposed abdominal compressions with CPR (IAC-CPR), take into account advances in our understanding of the mechanism of blood flow during resuscitation.

The pharmacology of resuscitation remains controversial, and these controversies have led to major changes in the guidelines for CPR. Use of sodium bicarbonate, calcium chloride, and glucose remains unresolved at this time. The role of epinephrine and especially high-dose epinephrine (HDE) is being readdressed because of concerns over postresuscitation deleterious effects on myocardial performance and poor outcomes. Evidence favoring a role for vasopressin, with a relatively pure vasoconstrictor effect, is accumulating. The role of lidocaine as the antiarrhythmic of choice for ventricular ectopy has been questioned as new data on the efficacy of amiodarone in arrest have been generated. Research is ongoing into alternative vasoconstrictors[224] and the use of "pharmacologic cocktails" that may include β-blockers, antiarrhythmics, antioxidants, nitroglycerin,[148,175,220] and a vasoconstrictor in attempts to improve the resuscitation outcome and postresuscitation cardiac function.

Developments in the use of direct current countershock have occurred. Biphasic defibrillators are now widely in use and appear to improve the success of defibrillation at lower delivered energies and, hopefully, decreased myocardial injury. As noted, the role of "shock first" is being reassessed as the success of electrical countershock in restoring spontaneous circulation declines rapidly after 3 to 4 minutes have elapsed.

Postresuscitation cerebral preservation has become an important area of focus, and mild therapeutic hypothermia has been found to improve neurologic outcome after adult cardiac arrest.

This chapter discusses the physiologic foundations of CPR. In the first section, the possible mechanisms of blood flow by the thoracic and cardiac pump mechanisms are discussed, including how the specific chest geometry of children and infants helps decide which of these mechanisms applies. Then, newer CPR techniques, which take into account the physiologic mechanisms discussed in the first section, are discussed. Controversies and advances in pharmacologic management during CPR and current guidelines for use of drugs for resuscitation are addressed. New developments in the use of countershock, including the timing of shocks, the energy used, and the type of current delivery system (biphasic or monophasic) are discussed. Finally, the role of therapeutic hypothermia is reviewed.

Mechanisms of Blood Flow

Cardiac Versus Thoracic Pump Mechanism

The cardiac pump hypothesis holds that blood flow is generated during closed-chest compressions when the heart is squeezed between the sternum and the vertebral column. This mechanism of flow implies that ventricular compression causes closure of the atrioventricular valves and that ejection of blood reduces ventricular volume. During chest relaxation, ventricular pressure falls below atrial pressure, allowing the atrioventricular valves to open and the ventricles to fill. This sequence of events resembles the normal cardiac cycle and occurs during cardiac compression when open-chest CPR is used.

Numerous clinical observations have conflicted with the cardiac pump hypothesis of blood flow. In 1964 MacKenzie[149] found that closed-chest CPR produced similar elevations in arterial and venous intravascular pressures, the result of a generalized increase in intrathoracic pressure. In 1976, Criley et al.[66] made the dramatic observation that several patients who developed VF during cardiac catheterization produced enough blood flow to maintain consciousness by repetitive coughing (Figure 118–1). The production of blood flow by increasing thoracic pressure without direct cardiac compression describes the thoracic pump mechanism of blood flow during CPR.

During normal cardiac function, the lowest pressure in the vascular circuit occurs on the atrial side of the atrioventricular valves. This low pressure compartment is the downstream pressure for the systemic circulation, which allows venous return to the heart. Angiographic studies

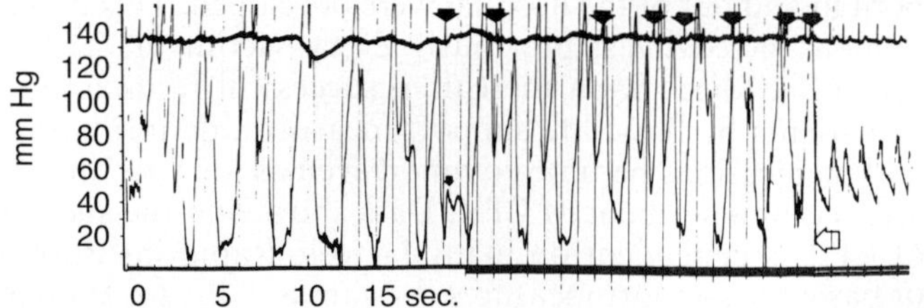

FIGURE 118–1 • Cough-CPR during prolonged ventricular asystole after coronary arteriographic injection. An 18-second period of asystole after right coronary arteriographic injection is depicted. During this period, the patient coughed every 2 seconds, generating peak aortic pressures > 140 mmHg. *Large arrows* mark the intrinsic QRS complexes after the 18-second period of asystole. *Small arrow* marks the resultant aortic pressure from the first intrinsic beat. The patient continued to cough until the cardiac rhythm stabilized 40 seconds later. (From Criley JM, Blaufuss AJ, Kissel G: *JAMA* 263:1246, 1976.)

show that blood passes from the venae cavae through the right heart into the pulmonary artery and from the pulmonary veins through the left heart into the aorta during a single chest compression. Echocardiographic studies show that, unlike normal cardiac activity or during open-chest CPR, during closed-chest CPR in both dogs[164] and humans[190] the atrioventricular valves are open during blood ejection and aortic diameter decreases rather than increases during blood ejection. These findings during closed-chest CPR support the thoracic pump theory and argue that the heart is a passive conduit for blood flow[203] (Figure 118–2).

Initial measurements of hemodynamic data during chest compression for CPR found the generation of almost equal pressures in the left ventricle, aorta, right atrium, pulmonary artery, and esophagus[128] (Figure 118–3). The finding that all intrathoracic vascular pressures are equal implies that suprathoracic arterial pressures must be higher than suprathoracic venous pressures. The unequal transmission of intrathoracic pressure to the suprathoracic vasculature establishes the gradient necessary for blood flow. The transmission of intrathoracic pressure to the suprathoracic veins may be modulated by venous valves. The presence of these jugular venous valves has been demonstrated in animals[104] and humans[54,170] undergoing CPR. An ultrasonography study of healthy children confirmed the presence of these valves in 84% of 239 jugular veins studied. The valves were bilateral in 74% of children.[71] Transmission of intrathoracic pressure to the intracranial vault during CPR indicates that any such valve function is partial. Pathologic studies have also identified valves in the subclavian vein in the large majority (87%) of cadavers studied. The absence of these valves in some patients is postulated to lead to failure of closed-chest CPR.[150]

Subsequent hemodynamic and echocardiographic studies found different results. Deshmukh et al.[76] demonstrated in a porcine model that mitral valve function persisted throughout resuscitation in 17 of 22 animals and that in successfully resuscitated animals maximal aortic pressure exceeded that in the right atrium throughout the resuscitation. In another porcine model of resuscitation, Hackl et al.[109] manipulated the compressive force and depth of resuscitation by using a mechanical resuscitator. The frequency of mitral valve closure during compressive systole was directly proportional to the force and depth of chest compression. When the depth of compression reached 25% of the AP diameter, valve closure occurred in 95% of cycles. They concluded that the mechanism of blood flow was dependent on force and depth of compression. In a study of CPR using transesophageal Doppler echocardiography in adults, Porter[181a] demonstrated mitral valve closure in compressive systole in the majority of (12/17) but not all patients. Peak mitral flow occurred in compressive diastole and was significantly higher in the group with mitral valve closure. Peak mitral flow occurred during compressive systole in those without valve closure. Left ventricular fractional shortening correlated with change in anteroposterior chest wall diameter and not mitral valve flow. These authors concluded that nonuniform increase in intrathoracic pressure plays a role in determining whether valve closure occurs during chest compressions. As noted, a decrease in aortic dimension during CPR has been demonstrated by echocardiography and taken as evidence for the thoracic pump mechanism of blood flow. Hwang[167] readdressed this issue using transesophageal echocardiography. He studied aortic dimension of the proximal and distal thoracic aorta and noted a decrease in aortic dimension in the distal aorta directly inferior to the zone of direct compression and an increase in dimension of the proximal aorta. He also noted mitral valve closure in all subjects

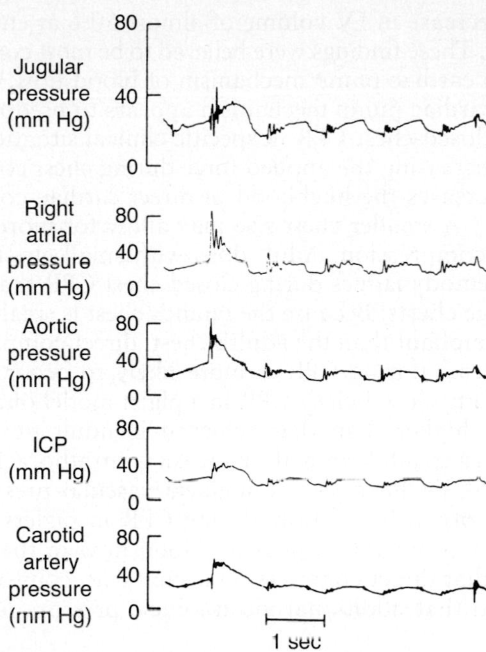

FIGURE 118–3 • Original record during conventional CPR. The first compression for conventional CPR follows the lung inflation that occurred during the previous release phase. Note increase in pressure on this compression. (From Koehler RC, Chandra N, Guerci AD, et al: *Circulation* 67:266, 1983.)

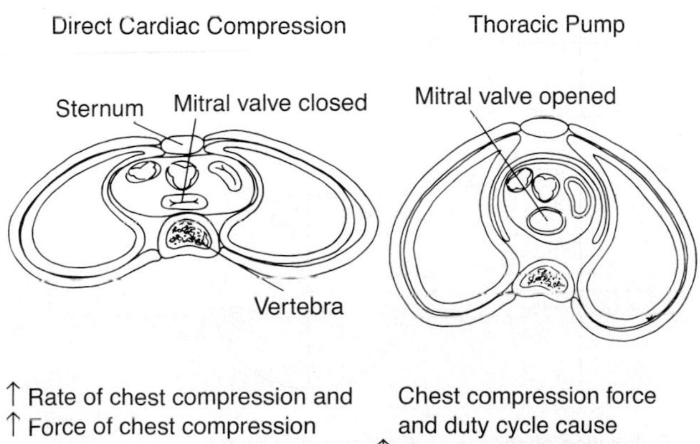

FIGURE 118–2 • Possible mechanisms for blood flow during CPR include direct cardiac compression **(left)** and the thoracic pump **(right).** With direct cardiac compression, an increase in chest compression rate causes an increase in blood flow by squeezing the heart between the vertebral column and sternum. With the thoracic pump mechanism, factors that increase pleural pressure cause an increase in pressure within the heart chambers and ultimately an increase in blood flow. (From Schleien CL: *Anesthesiology* 71:135, 1989.)

and a decrease in LV volume of almost 50% at end compression. These findings were believed to be most consistent with the cardiac pump mechanism of blood flow.[167]

The cardiac pump mechanism appears to predominate during closed-chest CPR in specific clinical situations. As noted, increasing the applied force during chest compressions increases the likelihood of direct cardiac compression.[78,109] A smaller chest size may allow for more direct cardiac compression. Adult dogs with small chests have better hemodynamics during closed-chest CPR than dogs with large chests. Because the infant's chest is smaller and more compliant than the adult's chest, direct compression of the heart during CPR is more likely to occur. Blood flow during closed-chest CPR in a piglet model of cardiac arrest is higher than that achieved in adult models.[154] In contrast to adult animals, increasing intrathoracic pressure by SCV-CPR does not augment vascular pressure or regional organ blood flow during CPR in piglets.[26] The failure of SCV-CPR to increase blood flow in the infant implies that direct compression occurs with conventional CPR and that additional intrathoracic pressure is of no benefit.

Rate and Duty Cycle

In 1986 the American Heart Association (AHA) increased the recommended rate of chest compressions from 60 to between 80 and 100 per minute. This change was a compromise between advocates of the thoracic pump mechanism and those of the cardiac pump mechanism. *Duty cycle* is defined as the ratio of the duration of the compression phase to the entire compression-relaxation cycle expressed as a percent. For example, at a rate of 30 compressions per minute, a 1.2-second compression time produces a 60% duty cycle. If blood flow is generated by direct cardiac compression, then the stroke volume is determined primarily by the force of compression. Prolonging the compression (increasing the duty cycle) beyond the time necessary for full ventricular ejection should have no additional effect on stroke volume. Increasing the rate of compressions should increase cardiac output because a fixed, relatively small volume of blood is ejected with each cardiac compression. In contrast, if blood flow is produced by the thoracic pump mechanism, the volume of blood to be ejected comes from a large reservoir of blood contained within the capacitance vessels in the chest. With the thoracic pump mechanism, flow is enhanced by increasing either the force of compression or the duty cycle but is not affected by changes in compression rate over a wide range of rates.[54] Mathematical models of the cardiovascular system confirm that blood flow is determined by both the applied force and the compression duration with the thoracic pump mechanism.[111] It appears from experimental animal data that both the thoracic pump and cardiac pump mechanisms can effectively generate blood flow during closed-chest CPR. Differences between various studies may be attributed to differences in animal models or compression techniques. Important differences in animal models include chest wall geometry, compliance and elastic recoil, compliance of the diaphragm, and intra-abdominal pressure. Differences in technique include the magnitude of sternal displacement, compression force, momentum of chest compression, compression rate, and duty cycle. Experimental and clinical data support both mechanisms of blood flow during CPR in human infants.

Results of several studies in dogs demonstrated a benefit of a compression rate of 120 per minute compared with slower rates during conventional CPR.[93,201] In studies of piglets,[74] puppies,[95] and humans,[54,169] no differences were found comparing different rates of compression during conventional CPR. In a study of piglet CPR, duty cycle was the major determinant of cerebral perfusion pressure. The duty cycle at which venous return became limited varied with age. A longer duty cycle was more effective in younger piglets.[74]

The discrepant importance of rate and duty cycle in various models (by different investigators) is confusing. However, increasing the rate of compressions during conventional CPR to 100 per minute satisfies both those who prefer the faster rates and those who support a longer duty cycle. This is true clinically because producing a longer duty cycle is easier when compressions are administered at a faster rate.

Chest Geometry

Chest geometry plays an important role in the ability of extrathoracic compressions to generate intrathoracic pressure. Shape, compliance, and deformability, which change greatly with age, are the chest characteristics that have the greatest impact during CPR.

The change in cross-sectional area of the chest during anterior to posterior delivered compressions is related to its shape[75] (Figure 118–4). The ratio of the chest anteroposterior diameter to the lateral diameter is referred to as the *thoracic index*. A keel-shaped chest, as seen in an adult dog, has a greater anteroposterior diameter and

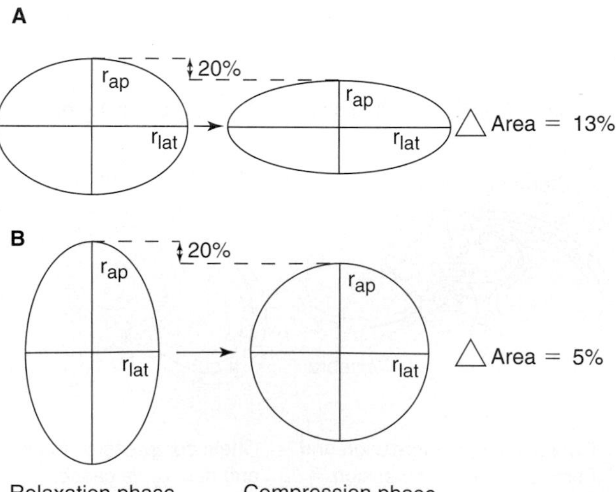

FIGURE 118–4 • Changes in area of ellipses with constant circumference. Each ellipse is labeled with the anteroposterior *(ap)* and lateral *(lat)* radii, and a 20% anteroposterior compression is applied. Indicated change in area equals relaxed area – compressed area. **A,** Initial anteroposterior/lateral ratio = 0.7, and compression leads to positive ejection because relaxed area – compressed area is negative. **B,** Initial anteroposterior/lateral ratio = 1.4, and compression toward a circular shape results in an increase in area. (From Dean JM, Koehler RC, Schleien CL, et al: *J Appl Physiol* 62:2212, 1987.)

thus a thoracic index greater than 1. A flat chest, as in a thin human, has a greater lateral diameter and thus a thoracic index less than 1. A circular chest has a thoracic index equal to 1. A circle has a larger cross-sectional area than either of these elliptical chests. As an anteroposterior compression flattens a circle, the cross-sectional area decreases and compresses its contents. In contrast, as an anteroposterior compression is applied to the keel-shaped chest, the cross-sectional area increases as a circular shape is approached. The cross-sectional area of the keel-shaped chest does not decrease until the chest compression continues past the circular shape to flatten the chest. This implies a threshold past which the compression must proceed before intrathoracic contents are decreased and squeezed.[75] Thus the rounder, flatter chests of small dogs and pigs may require less chest displacement than the keel-shaped chests of adult dogs to generate thoracic ejection of blood. This has been demonstrated in small dogs having round chests compared with adult dogs having keel-shaped chests.[13]

As humans age, the cartilage of the rib cage calcifies and chest wall compliance decreases. Older patients may require greater compression force to generate the same sternal displacement. A 3-month-old piglet requires a much greater compression force for anteroposterior displacement than its 1-month-old counterpart.[75] Direct cardiac compression is more likely to occur in the more compliant chest of younger animals. Cerebral and myocardial blood flow during closed-chest CPR was much higher in infant piglets than in adults[204] (Figures 118–5 and 118–6). This finding supports the cardiac pump mechanism of blood flow in infants because the level of organ blood flow achieved during closed-chest CPR in piglets approaches the level achieved during open-chest cardiac massage in adults.

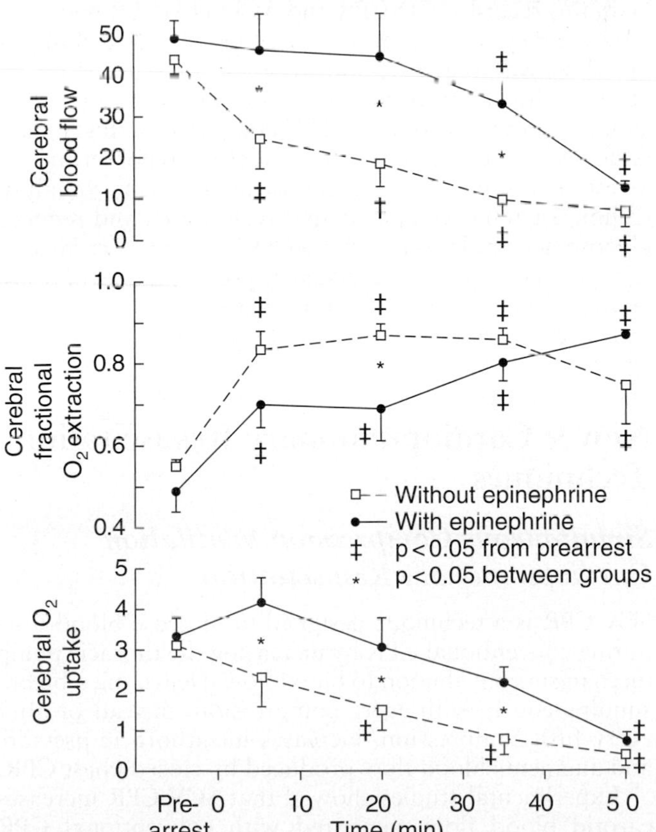

FIGURE 118–5 • Total cerebral blood flow, cerebral fractional O_2 extraction, and cerebral O_2 uptake before cardiac arrest and during 50 minutes of CPR in the groups with and without epinephrine.

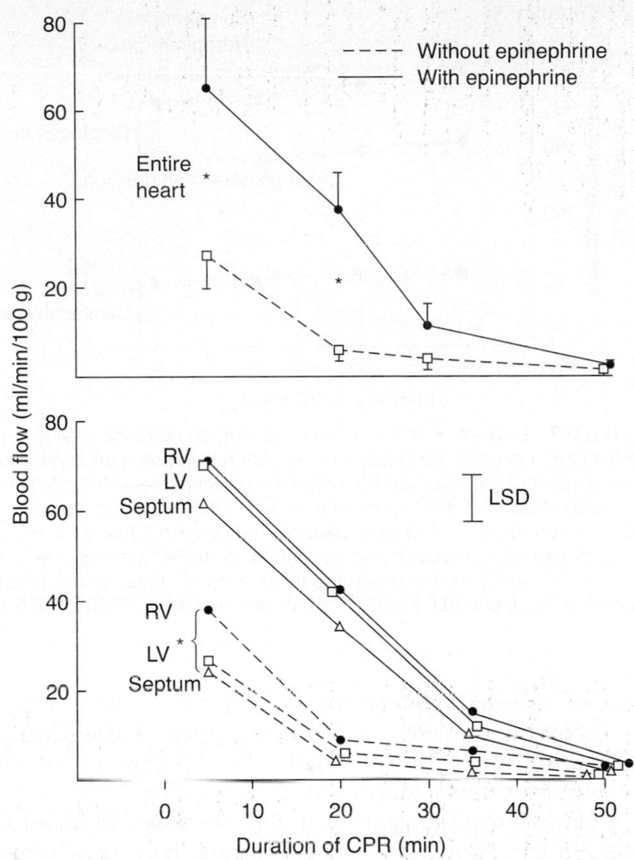

FIGURE 118–6 • **Top,** Total myocardial blood flow during CPR in piglets with and without epinephrine. *Asterisk* indicates significant difference between groups at 5 and 20 minutes. **Bottom,** Blood flow to right ventricular free wall *(RV, circle),* left ventricular free wall *(LV, squares),* and interventricular septum *(triangles)* in the groups with and without epinephrine. SE bars are omitted for clarity, but the least significant difference bar *(LSD,* derived from Duncan multiple-range test) is shown for comparisons among heart regions within an animal group. (Means must differ by height of bar for $p < 0.05$.) LSD for comparing means between groups is twice that shown for within-group LSD. *Asterisk* indicates that RV blood flow was greater than LV and septal blood flows at 5 minutes in the group without epinephrine. Flows in all three regions in the group with epinephrine were greater than those in the respective regions in the group without epinephrine at 5 and 20 minutes. (From Schleien CL, Dean MJ, Koehler RC, et al: *Circulation* 77:809, 1986.)

Marked deformation of the chest can occur during prolonged CPR and may alter the effectiveness of CPR[204] (Figure 118–7). Over time, the chest assumes a flatter shape, producing a larger percent decrease in cross-sectional area at the same absolute chest displacement. Progressive deformation may be beneficial if it leads to more direct cardiac compression. Unfortunately, too much deformation may decrease the recoil of the chest wall during the relaxation phase, leading to decreased cardiac filling. A progressive decrease in the effectiveness of chest compressions to produce blood flow is seen in piglets receiving conventional CPR.[204] Permanent deformation of the chest in this model approaches 30% of the original

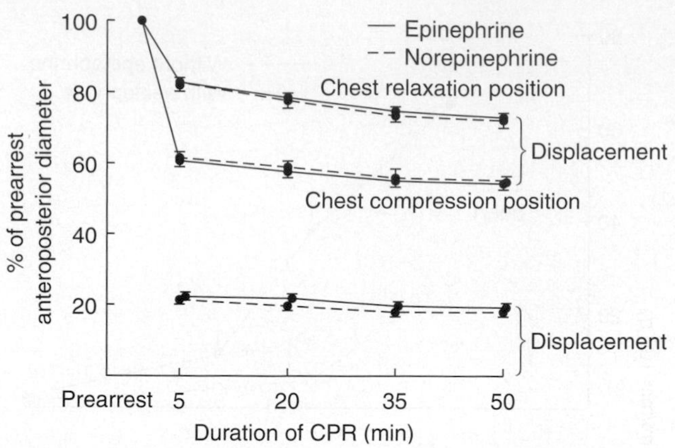

FIGURE 118–7 • Piston position during chest compression and relaxation phases of the cycle, and net piston displacement expressed as a percent of prearrest anteroposterior chest diameter (12.0 ± 0.3 cm) in piglets. Note that displacement was essentially unchanged over the 50-minute duration, but marked deformation occurred during the relaxation phase by 5 minutes and continued to further deform over the 50-minute period in the groups with or without epinephrine. (From Schleien CL, Dean MJ, Koehler RC, et al: *Circulation* 77:809, 1986.)

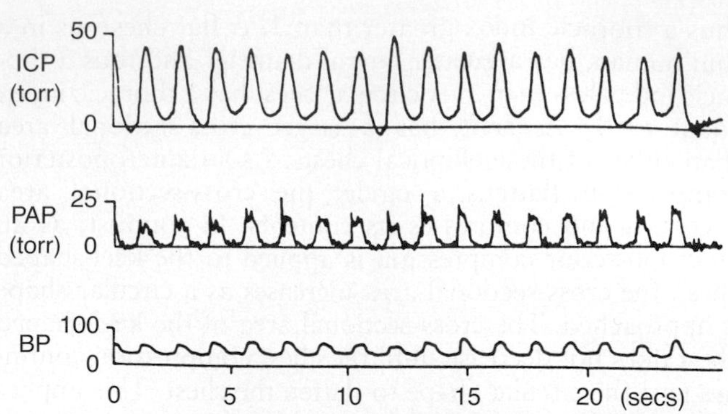

FIGURE 118–8 • Relationship of intracranial pressure, pulmonary artery pressure, and arterial blood pressure during closed-chest cardiac massage. Note that each chest compression is accompanied not only by a rise in arterial and pulmonary artery pressure but also by a sharp rise in intracranial pressure. (From Rogers MC, Nugent SK, Stidham GL: *Crit Care Med* 7:454, 1979.)

anteroposterior diameter. Attempting to limit deformation by increasing intrathoracic pressure from within during CPR with SCV-CPR was ineffective.[27] Using a thoracic vest to limit deformation when performing CPR greatly decreased the permanent chest deformation (3% vs. 30%) but did not attenuate the deterioration of vital organ blood flow with time.[211]

The characteristics of chest geometry of animals may relate to that in humans. Body weight, surface area, chest circumference, and diameter did not correlate with the magnitude of aortic pressure produced during CPR in a study of nine adults already declared dead.[211] A direct comparison of adult and pediatric human CPR has not been performed. The higher intravascular pressures and organ blood flow during CPR in infants compared with adults may result from more effective transmission of the force of chest compression because of the higher compliance and greater deformability of the infant chest.

Effects of Cardiopulmonary Resuscitation on Intracranial Pressure

When chest compressions are applied, the increase in intrathoracic pressure is transmitted through the venous system of the head and neck to the intracranial vault, resulting in an increased intracranial pressure (ICP). Pressure is transmitted via the paravertebral veins and the cerebrospinal fluid during CPR in dogs.[106] Large swings in ICP corresponding to chest compressions occur in children undergoing CPR[192] (Figure 118–8). This transmission of intrathoracic pressure to the intracranial contents accounts for the low cerebral perfusion pressure by increasing the downstream pressure and cerebral blood flow during closed-chest CPR.

The relationship of ICP to intrathoracic pressure during CPR is linear. In dogs receiving conventional CPR, ICP increased by one third of the rise of intrathoracic pressure in a range from 10 to 90 mmHg.[106] However, some modes of CPR change the intrathoracic to ICP relationship. In dogs, abdominal binding increases the transmission of pressure to the intracranial space to one half of the rise of intrathoracic pressure.[163] SCV-CPR, a mode of CPR designed to generate higher intrathoracic pressure, is similar to conventional CPR in its transmission of pressure to the cranium. Open-chest CPR decreases the transmission of pressure and improves cerebral perfusion pressure compared with conventional CPR. Thus increasing intrathoracic pressure may decrease cerebral blood flow because of the increase in downstream pressure, the ICP.

In this regard, ACD-CPR and ACD-ITV-CPR may have an advantage over conventional CPR. These techniques are designed to reduce intrathoracic pressure. Lindner et al.[139] showed in a porcine model that cerebral perfusion is increased with ACD-ITV compared with standard CPR. Using an adult porcine model of hypothermic VF arrest, the same group demonstrated by microdialysis techniques improved lactate/pyruvate ratios and reduced glucose accumulation in the ACD-ITV group compared with standard CPR.[16] In a pediatric porcine model of resuscitation, Voelckel et al.[234] found that ACD-CPR with ITV provided superior cerebral blood flow than standard CPR.

Newer Cardiopulmonary Resuscitation Techniques

Simultaneous Compression Ventilation Cardiopulmonary Resuscitation

SCV-CPR is a technique designed to increase blood flow during conventional CPR by increasing the thoracic pump mechanism contribution to blood flow. Delivering a breath simultaneously with every compression, instead of after every fifth compression, increases intrathoracic pressure and augments blood flow produced by closed-chest CPR.

Experimental studies showed that SCV-CPR increases carotid blood flow compared with conventional CPR alone.[52] Subsequent studies confirmed physiologic advantages of SCV-CPR in canine models.[128] However, in infant piglets[27] and small dogs,[13] SCV-CPR offered no advantage over conventional CPR. In these small animals, the compliance and geometry of the chest may allow more direct cardiac compression. Thus higher intrathoracic pressure may be achieved with conventional CPR alone.[74,204] Coronary perfusion pressure (CPP) was either only minimally increased or even decreased in humans during SCV-CPR compared with conventional CPR. Survival was significantly worse in both animals[198] and humans[131] who received SCV-CPR compared with conventional CPR. No study has shown an increased survival with this technique of CPR.

Interposed Abdominal Compression Cardiopulmonary Resuscitation

IAC-CPR is the delivery of an abdominal compression during the relaxation phase of chest compression. An extensive review by Babbs et al.[15] has been published. IAC-CPR may augment conventional CPR in several ways. First, IAC-CPR may return venous blood to the chest during chest relaxation.[97,145] Second, IAC-CPR increases intrathoracic pressure and augments the duty cycle of chest compression.[97,98] Third, IAC-CPR may compress the aorta and return blood retrograde to the carotid or coronary arteries.[145] IAC-CPR is an attractive alternative to some of the newer techniques of CPR because it requires no additional equipment for implementation; however, it does require training and manpower.

In animal experiments, cardiac output and cerebral and coronary blood flow were improved when comparing IAC-CPR with conventional CPR[84] but not in an infant model.[83] Initial human studies also demonstrated an increase in aortic pressure and CPP during IAC-CPR compared with conventional CPR.[120] Four randomized controlled trials have compared IAC-CPR with standard CPR. The first trial reported in 1985 by Mateer et al.[153] was the largest and included 291 patients. IAC-CPR was applied in the field by paramedics until ambulance transport. There were no differences in mortality. The later trials involved a total of 279 hospitalized patients.[195,196,239] The results from these trials are more positive, and a meta-analysis of these studies found an increased likelihood of return of spontaneous circulation (ROSC) and intact survival to discharge with IAC-CPR versus standard CPR.[14] No intraabdominal trauma was detected in any patient in these trials. Alternative techniques for abdominal hand position were studied in adult swine.[246] A stacked hand position similar to the usual position for chest compression over the abdominal aorta was compared with a diffuse hand position in which the hands were placed on the abdomen separately. This study demonstrated a significant increase in aortic diastolic pressure compared with standard CPR. However, CPP was not augmented as the right atrial diastolic pressure was also elevated. Stacked hand position was found to produce a CPP equivalent to standard CPR. Diffuse hand position, however, was associated with decreased CPP, so if the technique is applied this hand position should be avoided. Application of IAC-CPR is limited by the need for training and for the additional manpower. Although it has not been studied in a pediatric group, with skilled personnel available, IAC-CPR should be considered for use with inpatient arrests.

Active Compression-Decompression Cardiopulmonary Resuscitation and Impedance Threshold Valve Interposition

ACD-CPR uses a negative pressure "pull" on the thorax during the release phase of chest compression using a hand-held suction device[212] (Figure 118–9). This technique improves vascular pressures and minute ventilation during CPR in animals[61,141] and humans.[62,212] The mechanism of benefit of this technique is attributed to enhancement of venous return by the negative intrathoracic pressure generated during the decompression phase; in addition, it reverses the chest wall deformation that accompanies standard CPR.[96] Preliminary results in adults were promising,[60,61,147] and a large multi-institutional study of ACD-CPR completed in Europe found ACD-CPR was superior to standard CPR. In this study, a total of 750 patients were randomized to standard CPR or ACD-CPR. In the experimental group, 5% achieved 1 year (12 patients with intact neurologic status) versus 2% (three patients with intact neurologic status) in the standard group.[180] However, a number of other trials have not shown a difference between standard CPR and ACD-CPR. A Cochrane Database Systematic Review concluded there was no consistent benefit from this technique.[133] The effectiveness of ACD-CPR appears to be relatively site specific. Explanations for this variability have focused on the effectiveness of training for providers and intersite variation of on-scene advanced life support techniques.[96] Use of ACD-CPR requires significantly more physical effort

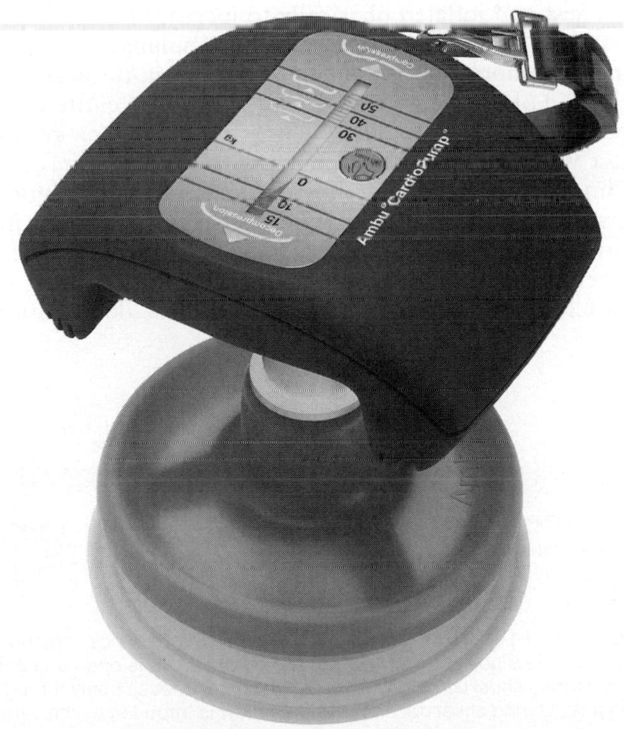

FIGURE 118–9 • Device for performing active compression-decompression CPR. The **upper part** is a hand and the **lower part** is a suction cup. (Courtesy AMBU Corporation. From Halperin H: *Curr Opin Crit Care* 10:188-192, 2004.)

than conventional CPR, and this requirement may have influenced outcome.[88]

Use of an inspiratory threshold valve has been evaluated in attempts to improve the outcome with ACD-CPR.[146,180] This technique involves the use of a valve placed between the ventilating bag and the airway, which is designed to close when the tracheal pressure falls below atmospheric pressure, enhancing the development of negative intrathoracic pressure during ACD-CPR (Figures 118–10 and 118–11). Animal studies,[185,235] including a young porcine model,[234] showed improved organ perfusion, and brain microdialysis studies demonstrated decreased lactate accumulation and improved glucose utilization.[16] In a small series of patients, diastolic pressure was raised along with CPP and end-tidal CO_2 release.[179] These studies led to an inclusion of the technique as an acceptable alternative to standard CPR in the 2000 AHA guidelines. Plaisance et al.[180] reported on a series of 400 patients randomized to ACD-CPR with ITV or sham-ITV. Survival at 24 hours was significantly improved. There was a nonsignificant trend toward improved neurologic survival with 6 of 10 discharged patients having intact survival compared with 1 of 8 discharged survivors in the sham-ITV group. The ultimate role of this technique, which requires specialized equipment and significant resuscitator training, remains to be determined.

Vest Cardiopulmonary Resuscitation

Vest CPR uses an inflatable bladder resembling a blood pressure cuff that is wrapped circumferentially around the chest and inflated phasically to increase intrathoracic pressure. Chest dimensions are changed minimally, so direct cardiac compression is unlikely. In addition, the even distribution of the force of compression over the entire chest wall decreases the likelihood of trauma to the skeletal chest wall and its thoracic contents.

Improvement of cerebral and myocardial blood flows[110,113] and survival[67,79] with vest CPR compared with conventional CPR was seen in dogs. In piglets, a 3% permanent chest deformation was seen after 50 minutes of vest CPR,[211] compared with an almost 30% deformation

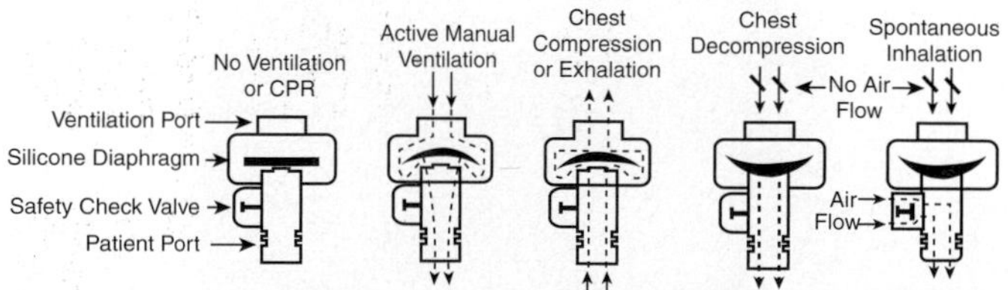

FIGURE 118–10 • Schematic diagram of impedance threshold valve. During a positive pressure ventilation the valve is open and gas flows. During chest compression or exhalation air moves freely through the valve. During chest decompression airflow is impeded by the valve decreasing intrathoracic pressure. During spontaneous ventilation the check valve opens allowing gas flow. Reproduced with permission from Lurie KG, Barnes TA, Zielinski TM, McKnite SH, Evaluation of a prototypic inspiratory impedance valve designed to enhance the efficiency of cardiopulmonary resuscitation. *Resp Care* 48(1):52-57, 2003.

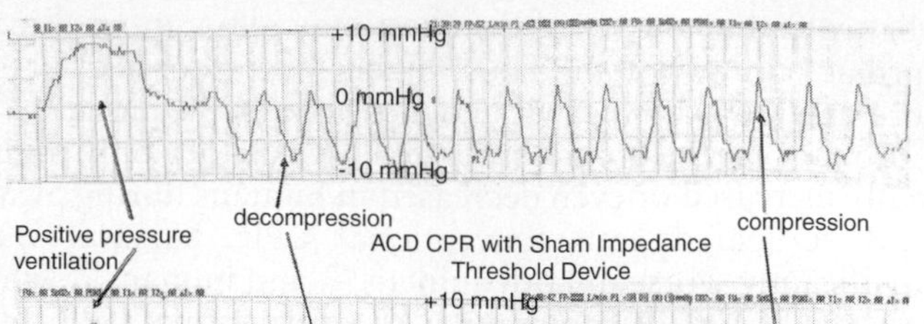

FIGURE 118–11 • Example of intratracheal pressures, a surrogate for intrathoracic pressures, in a patient undergoing cardiopulmonary resuscitation (CPR) with an automated compression device with and without an ITV (impedance threshold device) attached to a facemask. CPR was delivered at 100 compression/decompression cycles/min with a synchronized compression/ventilation ratio of 15:2. Note the absence of significant decreases in intratracheal pressures with a sham device. With the active ITD, wide fluctuations in intratracheal pressure are seen with each compression and decompression. Reproduced with permission. Courtesy of M. Lurie, MD and Advanced Circulatory Systems, Inc.

produced during an equivalent period of conventional CPR.[204] In a human study, vest CPR increased aortic systolic pressure but had little effect on aortic diastolic pressure compared with conventional CPR.[225] Despite its late application, vest CPR improved the hemodynamics and the rate of ROSC in adult patients in another study.[112] The lack of metallic parts has allowed vest CPR to be used experimentally during nuclear magnetic resonance spectroscopy to study brain intracellular pH.[86] The vest also has been used as an external cardiac assist device in nonarrested dogs with heart failure.[30] Clinically, the use of vest CPR depends on sophisticated equipment and remains experimental at this time.

Abdominal Binding

Abdominal binders and military antishock trousers (MAST) have been used to augment closed-chest CPR. Both methods apply continuous compression circumferentially below the diaphragm. Three mechanisms have been proposed for augmentation of CPR by these binders. First, binding the abdomen decreases the compliance of the diaphragm and raises intrathoracic pressure. Second, blood may be moved out of the intrathoracic structures to increase circulating blood volume. Third, applying pressure to the subdiaphragmatic vasculature and increasing its resistance may increase suprathoracic blood flow. These effects increase aortic pressure and carotid blood flow in both animals[128] and humans.[53] Unfortunately, as aortic pressure increases, the downstream component of CPP, namely, right atrial pressure, increases to an even greater extent, resulting in decreased CPP and myocardial blood flow.[164] These techniques also lower the cerebral perfusion pressure by enhanced transmission of intrathoracic pressure to the intracranial vault, which raises ICP (the downstream component of cerebral perfusion pressure). Clinical studies have failed to show an increased survival when an abdominal binder or MAST suit was used to augment CPR.

Open-Chest Cardiopulmonary Resuscitation

Use of open-chest cardiac massage has generally been replaced by closed-chest CPR. Compared with closed-chest CPR, open-chest CPR generates higher cardiac output and vital organ blood flow. During open-chest CPR there is less elevation of intrathoracic, right atrial, and intracranial pressure, resulting in higher coronary and cerebral perfusion pressure and higher myocardial and cerebral blood flow.[33]

Open-chest CPR is not a technique that can be applied by most health care personnel. It can be used in the operating room, ICU, or emergency department equipped with the necessary surgical and technical equipment and personnel. It is easily used in the operating room or ICU after cardiac surgery when the open chest can be easily accessed. Open-chest CPR is indicated for cardiac arrest secondary to cardiac tamponade, hypothermia, critical aortic stenosis, and ruptured aortic aneurysm. Other indications include cardiac arrest secondary to penetrating or crushed chest wall abnormalities that make closed-chest CPR impossible or ineffective.[4] Open-chest CPR is indicated for selected patients when closed-chest CPR has failed, although exactly which patients should receive this method of resuscitation under this condition is controversial. When initiated early after failure of closed-chest CPR, open-chest CPR may improve outcome.[127] When performed after 15 minutes of closed-chest CPR, open-chest CPR significantly improves CPP and the rate of successful resuscitation.[199]

Cardiopulmonary Bypass

Cardiopulmonary bypass (CPB) is one of the most effective ways to restore circulation after cardiac arrest. Animal studies show that CPB increases survival at 72 hours, increases recovery of consciousness, and preserves the myocardium better than conventional CPR.[138] In dogs, CPB resulted in better neurologic outcome than conventional CPR after a 4-minute ischemic period; however, neurologic outcome was dismal in both groups when the ischemic period lasted 12 minutes.[76] Some 90% of dogs survived 24 hours after 15 to 20 minutes of cardiac arrest, but only 10% survived when the arrest time was prolonged to 30 minutes when CPB was used for stabilization during defibrillation.[187] CPB decreased myocardial infarct size in a model involving coronary artery occlusion compared with conventional CPR.[1] In all animal models, CPB improves the success of resuscitation compared with conventional CPR.

Human experience with CPB for cardiac arrest outside the operating room is growing. Morris et al.[160] reviewed these data. Accumulated experience now includes seven pediatric series reporting on 127 cases and 10 adult series reporting on 331 cases. Overall survival is excellent compared with conventional CPR despite long arrest times. In both groups, survival to decannulation is approximately 60% despite average precannulation CPR times, where reported, ranging from 16 to 60 minutes for children and from 20 to 80 minutes for adults. Long-term survival is remarkable, with 47% of children and 31% of adults achieving long-term survival. In the largest series of children reported by Morris et al.,[160] between 1995 and 2002, 64 children underwent 66 extracorporeal membrane oxygenation (ECMO) runs initiated during active resuscitation with chest compressions or internal cardiac massage. Of these patients, 33 (50%) were decannulated and survived for more than 24 hours, 21 (33%) survived to hospital discharge, and 16 (26%) reportedly had no major changes in neurologic outcome. The average duration of CPR before cannulation in the survivors was 50 minutes. Of the six surviving children who required more than 60 minutes of CPR before ECMO, three had no apparent change in neurologic status. During the same period, 73 children underwent standard CPR; 10 received CPR for more than 30 minutes, with no survivors. Duncan et al.[82] reported a series of 18 pediatric cardiac surgical patients at the Boston Children's Hospital who received ECMO during active chest compressions. Of the first seven patients, only 29% survived. This led to the development of a rapid ECMO deployment strategy in which an ECMO pump is kept saline-primed in the ICU at all times, allowing initiation of extracorporeal support within 15 minutes. Precannulation support times dropped from an average of 90 minutes but still remained high at an average of 50 minutes. Of the remaining 11 patients, 10 were decannulated successfully, with 6 long-term survivors, 5 of whom were in New York Heart Association class I. This rapid deployment strategy likely will become more commonplace in large pediatric centers.

CPB requires a great deal of technical support and sophistication. In units with preprimed circuits on standby, CPB can be implemented quickly and with moderate success in a population of children who would otherwise almost certainly die. The success with some patients undergoing very long CPR times followed by ECMO use is encouraging and suggests the possibility of reversible myocardial injury as a cause of resuscitation failure in a subset of patients. Overall, ECMO is unlikely to have a major impact on pediatric outcome because of its limited availability.

Transcutaneous Cardiac Pacing

Transcutaneous cardiac pacing (TCP) is used as a method for noninvasive pacing of the ventricles for a relatively short period of time. Emergency cardiac pacing is successful in resuscitation only if it is initiated soon after the onset of arrest. In the absence of in situ pacing wires or an indwelling transvenous or esophageal pacing catheter, TCP is the preferred method for temporary electrical cardiac pacing. Since 1992, the AHA advanced cardiovascular life support (ACLS) guidelines have recommended the early use of an external pacemaker in patients with symptomatic bradycardia or asystole.[3]

Since Zoll[250] established TCP in 1952 as a clinically useful method of pacing adult patients during ventricular standstill (Stokes-Adams attacks) and bradycardia-associated hypotension, numerous anecdotal reports have supported its use for bradycardic or asystolic arrests.

Zoll et al.[251] reported successful in-hospital resuscitation of 12 of 16 patients with hypotensive bradycardia or asystole if TCP was initiated within 5 minutes of the arrest. In contrast, if TCP was started between 5 and 30 minutes after the arrest, only 8 of 44 patients with either of these rhythms could be resuscitated.[251] In two controlled clinical trials of prehospital TCP, no differences in the survival rate or success of resuscitation were observed in paced and nonpaced patients who had asystole or PEA.[18,115] In patients with symptomatic bradycardia, TCP improved resuscitation and the survival rate.[114]

To date the efficacy of TCP in pediatric resuscitation has not been studied. Beland et al.[20] showed that effective TCP could be achieved in hemodynamically stable children during induction of anesthesia for heart surgery. They were successful in 53 of 56 pacing trials, and the patients suffered no complications.[20]

TCP is indicated for patients whose primary problem is impulse formation or conduction, who have preserved myocardial function. TCP is most effective in patients with sinus bradycardia or high-grade atrioventricular block with slow ventricular response who also have a stroke volume sufficient to generate a pulse. TCP is not indicated for patients in prolonged arrest because in this situation TCP usually results in electrical but not mechanical cardiac capture, and its use may delay or interfere with other resuscitative efforts.

To set up pacing, one electrode is placed anteriorly at the left sternal border and the other posteriorly just below the left scapula. Smaller electrodes are available for infants and children; adult-sized electrodes can be used in children weighing more than 15 kg.[20] Electrocardiographic leads should be connected to the pacemaker, the demand or asynchronous mode selected, and an age-appropriate heart rate used. The stimulus output should be set at zero when the pacemaker is turned on and then increased gradually until electrical capture is seen on the monitor. The output required for a hemodynamically unstable rhythm is higher than that for a stable rhythm in children in whom the mean stimulus required for capture was between 52 and 65 mA. After electrical capture is achieved, one must ascertain whether an effective arterial pulse is generated. If pulses are not adequate, other resuscitative efforts should be used.

The most serious complication of TCP is induction of a ventricular arrhythmia.[21] Fortunately, this complication is rare and may be prevented by pacing only in the demand mode. Mild transient erythema beneath the electrodes is common. Skeletal muscle contraction can be minimized by using large electrodes, a 40-ms pulse duration, and the smallest stimulus required for capture. Sedatives or analgesics may be necessary in the awake patient. If defibrillation or cardioversion is necessary, one must allow a distance of 2 to 3 cm between the electrode and paddles to prevent arcing of the current.

Pharmacology

Adrenergic Agonists

In 1963, only 3 years after the original description of closed-chest CPR, Pearson and Redding[174] described the use of adrenergic agonists for resuscitation. They subsequently showed that early administration of epinephrine in a canine model of cardiac arrest improved the success rate of CPR. They also demonstrated that the increase in aortic diastolic pressure by administration of α-adrenergic agonists was responsible for the improved success of resuscitation. They theorized that vasopressors such as epinephrine were of value because the drug increased peripheral vascular tone, not by a direct effect on the heart.[186]

Yakaitis et al.[247] investigated the relative importance of α- and β-adrenergic agonist actions during resuscitation. Only 27% of dogs that received a pure β-adrenergic receptor agonist along with an α-adrenergic antagonist were resuscitated successfully, compared with all of the dogs that received a pure α-adrenergic agonist and a β-adrenergic antagonist (Figure 118–12). Later studies reconfirmed this finding. Michael et al.[154] demonstrated that the α-adrenergic effects of epinephrine result in intense vasoconstriction of the resistance vessels of all organs of the body, except those supplying the heart and brain. Because of the widespread vasoconstriction in nonvital organs, adequate perfusion pressure and thus blood flow to the heart and brain can be achieved despite the fact that cardiac output is very low during CPR[204] (Figure 118–13).

The increase in aortic diastolic pressure associated with epinephrine administration during CPR is critical for maintaining coronary blood flow and enhancing the success of resuscitation. Even though the contractile state of the myocardium is increased by use of β-adrenergic agonists in the spontaneously beating heart, during CPR, β-adrenergic agonists actually may decrease myocardial blood flow by increasing intramyocardial wall pressure and vascular resistance. This could redistribute intramyocardial blood flow away from the subendocardium, increasing the likelihood of ischemic injury to this region.[144] Moreover, evidence

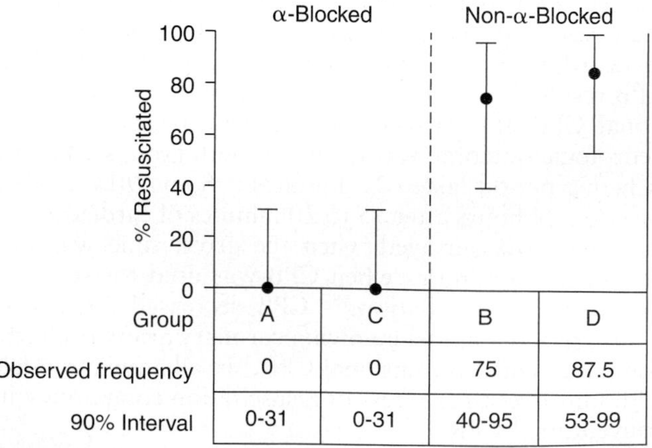

Group	A	C	B	D
Observed frequency	0	0	75	87.5
90% Interval	0-31	0-31	40-95	53-99

FIGURE 118–12 • Beneficial effect of α-adrenergic activity on resuscitation. Animals in group A received phenoxybenzamine; group B received propranolol; group C received phenoxybenzamine and propranolol; and group D received no drug. The 90% confidence intervals are reported for the sample size and observed resuscitation success. The lack of overlap between the α- and non–α-blocked groups indicates a significant benefit ($p \leq 0.01$) during resuscitation when α-adrenergic activity is intact. (From Yakaitis RW, Otto CW, Blitt CD: *Crit Care Med* 7:293, 1979.)

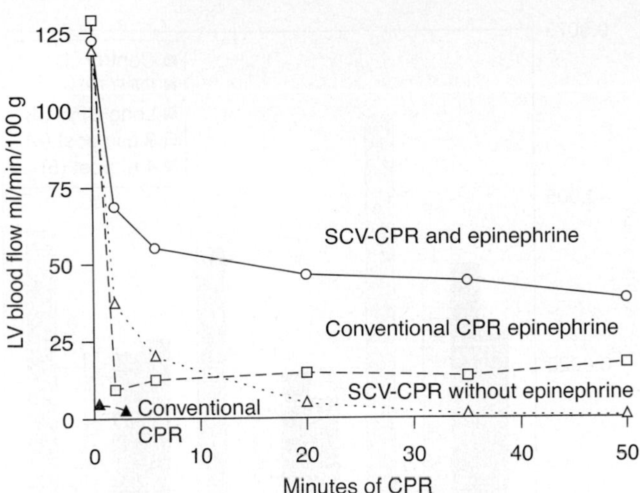

FIGURE 118–13 • Left ventricular (LV) blood flow before arrest and during four types of CPR. Note the rapid falloff of LV blood flow when epinephrine is not used. *SCV-CPR,* Simultaneous compression ventilation CPR. (From Michael JR, Guerci AD, Koehler RC, et al: *Circulation* 69:822, 1984.)

BOX 118–1

α-Adrenergic versus β-Adrenergic Agonist Effects

α-ADRENERGIC EFFECTS

Vasoconstrict peripheral vessels
Maintain aortic diastolic pressure
Improve coronary blood flow
No metabolic stimulatory effect

β-ADRENERGIC EFFECTS

Vasodilate peripheral vessels
Decrease aortic diastolic pressure
Increase cellular metabolic rate
Positive inotrope
Increase intensity of ventricular fibrillation
Increase heart rate and/or dysrhythmias following resuscitation

indicates that left ventricular end-diastolic pressure (LVEDP) rises with epinephrine use, reducing the overall impact of the vasoconstrictor effects of epinephrine on CPP. Tang et al.[229] showed elevated LVEDP and decreased measures of diastolic performance in epinephrine-resuscitated rats after induced VF compared with phenylephrine-resuscitated animals or epinephrine-resuscitated animals who also received a β-blocker. Similar data were found by McNamara, who used a rat pup model of asphyxial arrest. LVEDP was increased and diastolic function indices decreased with epinephrine compared with either saline alone or epinephrine combined with verapamil. These data imply that excessive β-adrenergic effects prevent the intracellular calcium reuptake during diastole that is required for myocardial relaxation. By its inotropic and chronotropic effects, β-adrenergic stimulation increases myocardial oxygen demand, which, when superimposed on low coronary blood flow, increases the risk of ischemic injury. This combination of increased oxygen demand by β-adrenergic agonists[77] and decreased oxygen supply may damage an already ischemic heart, raising the question of whether a pure α-adrenergic agonist would be better than epinephrine, which has significant β-adrenergic effects (Box 118–1). The effects on energy utilization and oxygen supply not only have implications for the success of the initial resuscitation but also for the postresuscitation function of the myocardium.

A number of studies have attempted to settle this controversy and actually have shown that pure α-adrenergic agonists can be used in place of epinephrine during CPR. Phenylephrine[186,204,247] and methoxamine are two pure α-adrenergic agonists that have been used in animal models of CPR with success equal to that of epinephrine. More recently vasopressin has been studied as a noncatecholamine vasoconstrictor in the management of cardiac arrest patients.[142] This agent is discussed in the section on vasopressin. These agents cause peripheral vasoconstriction and increase aortic diastolic pressure, resulting in improved myocardial and cerebral blood flow. This results in a higher oxygen supply/demand ratio in the ischemic heart and, at least, a theoretical advantage over the combined α- and β-adrenergic agonist effects of epinephrine. These agonists,[186,206] as well as vasopressors such as vasopressin,[142] have been used successfully for resuscitation. These drugs maintain blood flow to the heart during CPR as well as epinephrine. In an animal model of VF cardiac arrest, a resuscitation rate of 75% was reported for both epinephrine- and phenylephrine-treated groups. In this study, the ratio of endocardial to epicardial blood flow was lower in the epinephrine-treated group, suggesting the presence of subendocardial ischemia.[204] However, studies of this kind are difficult to interpret because of the inability to measure the degree of α-receptor activation by the different vasopressors. The higher subendocardial blood flow in the phenylephrine group may have been the result of less α-receptor activation.[36,41,42] Moreover, some investigators have questioned the merits of using a pure α-adrenergic agonist during CPR. Although the inotropic and chronotropic effects of β-adrenergic agonists may have deleterious hemodynamic effects during CPR administered for VF, increases in both heart rate and contractility increase cardiac output when spontaneous coordinated ventricular contractions are achieved.

Cerebral blood flow during CPR, like coronary blood flow, depends on peripheral vasoconstriction and is enhanced by use of α-adrenergic agonists. This action produces selective vasoconstriction of noncerebral peripheral vessels to areas of the head and scalp without causing cerebral vasoconstriction.[204] As with myocardial blood flow, pure α agents are as effective as epinephrine in generating and sustaining cerebral blood flow during CPR in adult animal models[206] and in infant models[204] (Figure 118–14). No difference in neurologic deficits 24 hours after cardiac arrest was found between animals receiving either epinephrine or phenylephrine during CPR.[35]

Analogous to the heart, β-adrenergic agonists could increase cerebral oxygen uptake if a sufficient amount of drug crosses the blood-brain barrier during or after resuscitation. In addition, adrenergic agonists may vasoconstrict

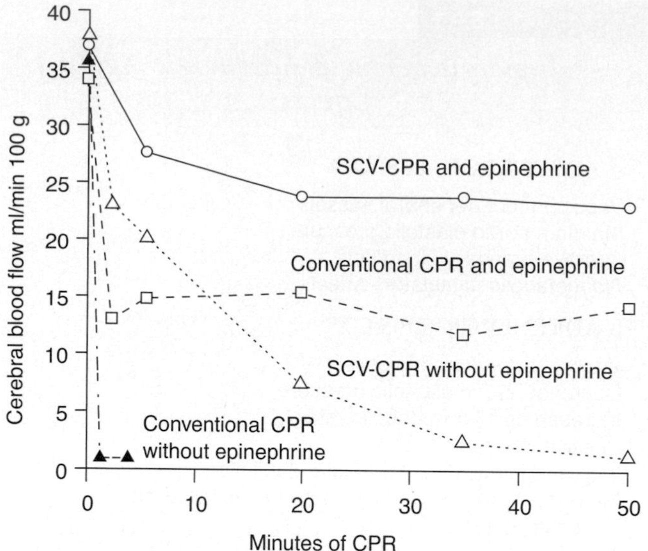

FIGURE 118–14 • Cerebral blood flow before arrest and during four types of 50 minutes of CPR. *SCV-CPR,* Simultaneous compression ventilation CPR. (From Michael JR, Guerci AD, Koehler RC, et al: *Circulation* 69:822, 1984.)

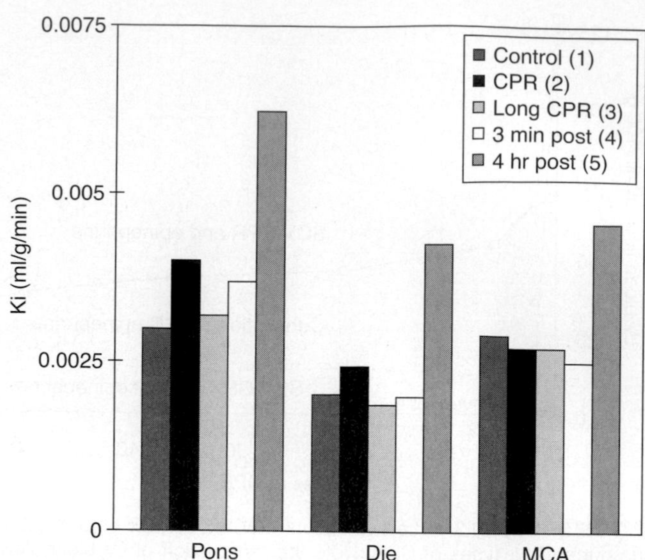

FIGURE 118–15 • Transfer coefficient (K_i) of α-aminoisobutyric acid for pons, diencephalon (DIE), and middle cerebral (MCA) artery regions. Control group; 8 minutes ischemia and 10 minutes cardiopulmonary resuscitation; 8 minutes ischemia and 40 minutes cardiopulmonary resuscitation; 3 minutes after resuscitation; 4 hours after resuscitation. Group 5 in each region $^*p < 0.05$, different from group 1 by one-way analysis of variance and Dunnett test for all three regions. (From Schleien CL, Koehler RC, Shaffner DH, et al: *Stroke* 22:477, 1991.)

or dilate cerebral vessels, depending on the balance between α- and β-adrenergic receptors. Epinephrine and phenylephrine had similar effects on cerebral blood flow and metabolism, maintaining normal cerebral oxygen uptake for 20 minutes of CPR in dogs. This implies that cerebral blood flow was high enough to maintain adequate cerebral metabolism and that β-receptor stimulation did not increase cerebral oxygen uptake, despite the fact that the combined effects of brain ischemia and CPR can increase the permeability of the blood-brain barrier to drugs used during CPR or when enzymatic barriers to vasopressors (e.g., by monoamine oxidase) are overwhelmed during tissue hypoxia. Mechanical disruption of the barrier could occur during chest compressions by large fluctuations in cerebral venous and arterial pressures. In addition, mechanical disruption could result from hyperemia, the large increase in cerebral blood flow that occurs during the early reperfusion period when the cerebral vascular bed is maximally dilated following resuscitation, particularly if systemic hypertension occurs.[208] We found no blood-brain barrier permeability changes during CPR immediately after or 4 hours after resuscitation in adult dogs.[208] However, after 8 minutes of cardiac arrest and 6 minutes of CPR in piglets, the blood-brain barrier was permeable to the small neutral amino acid α-aminoisobutyric acid, 4 hours after cardiac arrest[207] (Figure 118–15). We also found that this increase in permeability could be prevented by prearrest administration of conjugated superoxide dismutase and catalase,[205] indicating a role of oxygen free radicals in the pathogenesis of this injury to the blood-brain barrier (Figure 118–16). Using the same infant piglet model, we later found that these endothelial membrane changes frequently were associated with the presence of intravascular polymorphonuclear and monocytic leukocytes.[47] Whether leukocytes disrupt the blood-brain barrier by release of toxic substances, such as oxygen free radicals or proteases, or appear in the postischemic microvessels as an epiphenomenon of a more important derangement is unknown (Figure 118–17).

Vasopressin

The role of vasopressin as a noncatecholamine vasoconstrictor in the management of cardiac arrest patients has received a great deal of interest. Work by Lindner in Europe and Landry in the United States over the past 2 decades has established sufficient evidence of efficacy for its use to be included in the 2000 AHA Guidelines for Cardiopulmonary Resuscitation and Emergency Cardiovascular Care as an evidence class IIb alternate or adjunct to epinephrine for refractory VF in adults and as an option of indeterminate merit for children. Moreover, increasing evidence indicates that vasopressin is a useful agent in the management of shock of multiple etiologies and, therefore, may have a role in postresuscitation management of the arrest victim.

Arginine vasopressin is a short peptide hormone secreted by the posterior pituitary gland in response to changes in tonicity and changes in effective intravascular volume via baroreceptor unloading primarily in the aorta. Severe shock is the most potent stimulus to vasopressin secretion. Serum levels 20- to 200-fold higher than normal may be found immediately after cardiac arrest, as well as in other severe shock states. Despite these observations, lower than expected vasopressin levels have been found in some patients with profound shock,[117,118,135] and patients dying of cardiac arrest have been found to have significantly lower vasopressin levels than survivors.[143] The cause of lower than expected vasopressin levels in some patients is unclear. Observations in dogs suggest depletion of vasopressin stores as a potential mechanism. Dogs subjected to profound hemorrhagic shock have an early massive elevation

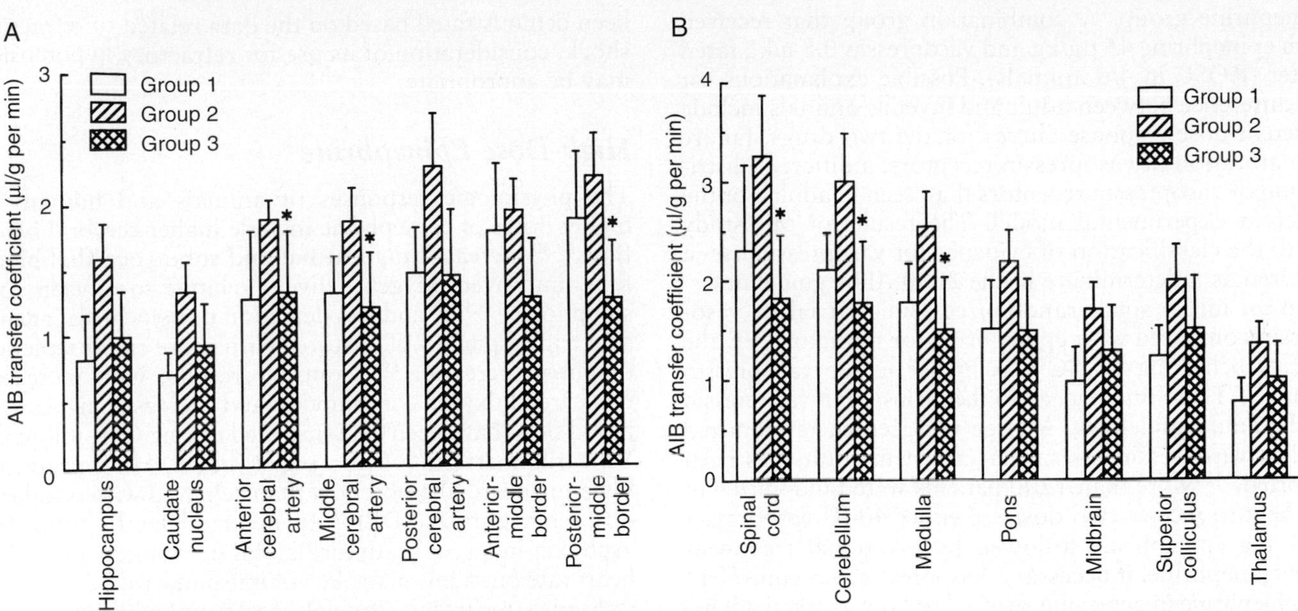

FIGURE 118–16 • **A,** Bar graph showing transfer coefficient of α-aminoisobutyric acid (AIB) from plasma to brain in hippocampus, caudate nucleus, and primary supply and border regions of cerebral arteries in nonischemic time controls (group 1; n = 5), ischemia group treated with polyethylene glycol (PEG) (group 2; n = 8), and ischemia group treated with PEG-superoxide dismutase and PEG-catalase (group 3; n = 8). Error bars represent SEM. $^*p < 0.05$ between groups 2 and 3 by Mann-Whitney U-test. **B,** Transfer coefficient of AIB from plasma to brain in caudal brain regions in nonischemic time controls (group 1; n = 5), ischemia group treated with polyethylene glycol (PEG) (group 2; n = 8), and ischemia group treated with PEG-superoxide dismutase and PEG-catalase (group 3; n = 8). Error bars represent SEM. $^*p < 0.05$ between groups 2 and 3 by Mann-Whitney U-test. (From Schleien CL, Eberle B, Schaffner DH, et al: *Stroke* 25:1830, 1994.)

of vasopressin levels immediately after the event, followed by a depression of levels below expected within 1 hour of the insult. Severe depletion of vasopressin stores from the posterior hypophysis was noted in these animals.[135] These animals developed a catecholamine-refractory, vasodilatory shock that responded dramatically to low doses of vasopressin.[157] These observations have led to an exploration

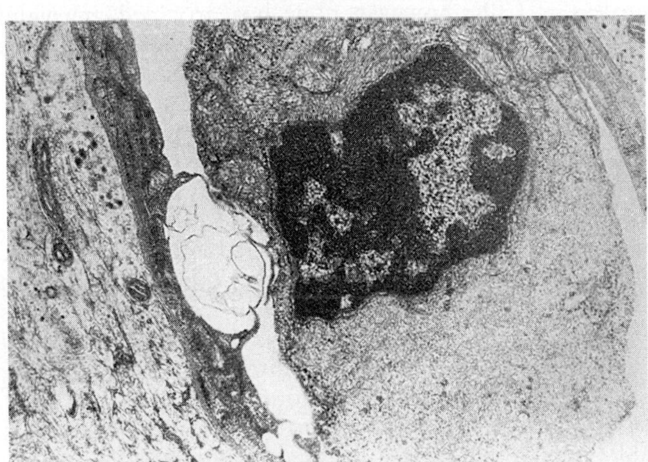

FIGURE 118–17 • Transmission electron micrograph of an infant piglet brain 4 hours after 8 minutes of cardiac arrest and 6 minutes of CPR (magnification ×5000). An intravascular leukocyte, which has the morphologic features of a monocyte, is adherent to the endothelial surface of a venule and appears to be occluding the lumen. The luminal surface of the endothelial cell contains membrane blebs and discontinuities. (From Caceres MJ, Schleien CL, Kuluz JW, et al: *Acta Neuropathol* 90:582, 1995.)

of the use of vasopressin in both cardiac arrest and shock states.

Vasopressin is an extremely potent vasoconstrictor. Its effects on vascular tone are primarily mediated through interaction with a specific G protein-coupled receptor referred to as the $V1_a$ receptor, which is distributed widely throughout vascular beds.[117] Of note, the $V1_a$ receptor is linked to the same second messenger system as the α-adrenergic receptor that mediates vasoconstriction through an alteration of intracellular calcium levels. Vasopressin also interacts with its V_2 receptor, which regulates aquaporin expression on the renal collecting duct epithelium. Stimulation of the V_2 receptor occurs at substantially lower levels than those required to activate the $V1_a$ receptor.

In the past decade, vasopressin use during resuscitation has been studied in animals and humans. In an adult porcine model of VF, vasopressin at a dose of 0.8 u/kg was found to be superior to the maximally effective dose of epinephrine 200 µg/kg in restoring left ventricular myocardial blood flow, increasing diastolic CPP and total cerebral blood flow, as well as rates of ROSC. Moreover, the duration of the effect was sustained for 4 minutes compared with 1.5 minutes for epinephrine.[139,142] Adverse effects noted in the postresuscitation phase included decreased renal and adrenal blood flow and reduced cardiac output.[183,184]

In a pediatric porcine model of cardiac arrest,[223] vasopressin at a dose of 0.8 u/kg was not as effective as epinephrine 200 µg/kg in restoring left ventricular myocardial blood flow or achieving ROSC. Only one of six animals achieved ROSC compared with six of six in the epinephrine group. A combination group that received both epinephrine 45 μg/kg and vasopressin 0.8 u/kg fared better (ROSC in 4/6 animals). Possible explanations for the difference between adult and juvenile animals include different dose-response curves for the two drugs, failure of maturation of vasopressin receptors, a different distribution of vasopressin receptors than seen in adults, or the different experimental model. The results of this study led to the classification of evidence for vasopressin use in children as indeterminate in the 2000 AHA guidelines.

In an initial small randomized clinical trial of vasopressin compared with epinephrine for refractory VF, the rate of achieving ROSC was higher in the vasopressin group.[140] These findings led to the inclusion of vasopressin in the adult guidelines. A large multicenter, randomized trial of vasopressin for cardiac arrest in adults has been reported.[242] More than 1200 patients were randomized in the field to receive two doses of either 40 IU vasopressin or 1 mg epinephrine followed by additional treatment with epinephrine, if necessary. Vasopressin was equivalent to epinephrine in achieving survival to both hospital admission and discharge in patients with either PEA or VF. In patients with asystole, vasopressin was superior to epinephrine in achieving both survival to admission and discharge, although intact neurologic outcome was not improved. In patients who failed to achieve ROSC after two doses of medication, a third dose of medication such as epinephrine could be added at the resuscitating physician's discretion. In the group receiving a third dose of medication such as epinephrine, survival was greater in the vasopressin group.

The published pediatric experience with vasopressin in cardiac arrest is limited to a case series. The outcome of four children with six prolonged refractory cardiac arrests unresponsive to standard resuscitation efforts was reported. Each child received one or more bolus doses of vasopressin (0.4 u/kg) as rescue therapy. In all children, the initial rhythm was a form of PEA that deteriorated to asystole in four of six events. Three children had ROSC for more than 60 minutes, including one child with asystole. Two children survived for more than 24 hours and one to hospital discharge. At this time, there is no clear role for vasopressin in pediatric resuscitation; however, its use as an adjunct for patients unresponsive to an initial dose of epinephrine may be appropriate.

The current recommended dose of vasopressin for adults in cardiac arrest is 40 IU. There are no data comparing this dose to other doses, and there is concern of postresuscitation complications related to this dose. At Morgan Stanley Children's Hospital, we have selected 0.5 u/kg as the standard for cardiac arrest. Further data are needed before more definitive dosing recommendations can be made.

Vasopressin use in postresuscitation management may be considered. A relative vasopressin deficiency has been noted in a number of shock states, including hemorrhage, sepsis, and post-CPB, as well as in patients who have unsuccessful resuscitations. In these settings, shock may be refractory to catecholamines (norepinephrine doses 2–4 μg/kg). These patients may respond to a vasopressin infusion, allowing the weaning of high-dose catecholamines. Although a role in the postresuscitation setting has not been demonstrated based on the data related to refractory shock, consideration of its use for refractory hypotension may be appropriate.

High-Dose Epinephrine

The physiologic responses of animals and humans to higher doses of epinephrine include higher cerebral blood flow,[28,40] increased myocardial and submyocardial blood flow, improved oxygen delivery relative to oxygen consumption,[38,39,41,55] and less depletion of myocardial adenosine triphosphate (ATP) stores with more rapid repletion of phosphocreatine.[116] Contrary results, with increased myocardial oxygen consumption and decreased myocardial blood flow, have been demonstrated during CPR following VF cardiac arrest.[26,78] In a piglet model, HDE produced lower myocardial blood flow than achieved with standard-dose epinephrine (SDE).[28] In neonatal lambs following asphyxia-induced bradycardia, HDE resulted in higher heart rate but a lower stroke volume and cardiac output.[44]

Studies regarding survival of patients who were given HDE have been contradictory. In out-of-hospital cardiac arrest patients, HDE produced higher aortic diastolic pressure during CPR and increased the rate of ROSC compared with standard doses of epinephrine. Gonzalez et al.[101,102] demonstrated a dose-dependent increase in aortic blood pressure by epinephrine in patients who failed to respond to prolonged resuscitative efforts. Paradis et al.[171] showed that HDE increased aortic diastolic pressure and improved the rate of successful resuscitation in patients who failed ACLS protocols. This group also reported on a series of 20 children treated with HDE and compared them with 20 historic controls of children with cardiac arrest treated with SDE.[100] They reported that 14 of the children in the HDE group had ROSC, 8 survived to hospital discharge, and 3 were neurologically intact. There were no survivors in the SDE comparison group. Other centers have claimed that higher-than-standard doses of epinephrine during CPR in children improve the hemodynamics and increase the success of CPR; however, none has provided any valid data that suggest that HDE improves survival beyond the immediate post resuscitation period.[57,151,171,181] Based on these studies, the 1992 AHA guidelines for pediatric advance life support recommended HDE if an initial SDE failed to resuscitate the child.

Three large multicenter studies subsequently were published that dampened the enthusiasm for the use of HDE. Stiell et al.[222] studied 650 adult patients after cardiac arrests who were randomly assigned to receive either an SDE or HDE (7 mg) epinephrine protocol. No differences were observed between the groups with regard to survival (23% vs. 18% 1-hour survival), rate of hospital discharge (5% vs. 3%), or neurologic outcome. Brown et al.[37] reported on 1280 adult patients who received either SDE (0.02 mg/kg) or HDE (0.2 mg/kg) after cardiac arrest. Again, no differences in ROSC, short-term survival, survival to hospital discharge, or neurologic outcome were observed between the two groups of patients. In a study of 816 adults, Callaham et al.[49] reported a higher ROSC in the HDE group. However, there were no differences in the rate of hospital discharge or ultimate survival of these patients.[49] In addition to these studies, a specific pediatric animal study was published that failed to demonstrate a clear survival benefit for HDE, although the occurrence of ROSC appeared to be greater.[26] The 2000 AHA guidelines changed the recommendation for HDE to an option for second and subsequent doses of epinephrine.

Most recently, a prospective, randomized, double-blind clinical trial of HDE in 68 pediatric in-patients was reported by Perondi et al.[176] ROSC for more than 20 minutes was achieved in 15 of 34 HDE patients but only 8 of 34 SDE patients ($p = 0.07$). However, survival to 24 hours occurred in only two of the HDE group versus seven of the SDE group ($p = 0.05$). In the group that suffered an asphyxial arrest, none of 12 treated with HDE group was alive at 24 hours, whereas as 7 of 18 patients in the SDE group survived. Four survived to hospital discharge, and two patients were neurologically normal.[176]

This trial reinforces concerns that HDE may account for some of the adverse effects that occur after resuscitation.[191,207] As discussed previously, epinephrine can worsen myocardial ischemic injury secondary to increased oxygen demand and result in tachyarrhythmias, hypertension, pulmonary edema, hypoxemia, and cardiac arrest.[2,207] Use of a β-adrenergic antagonist during or after ROSC has been suggested to attenuate the adverse effects of epinephrine.[79,80,98] Epinephrine causes hypoxemia and an increase in alveolar dead space ventilation by redistributing pulmonary blood flow.[226,238] In one study, HDE (>15 mg) given to adults during CPR resulted in a lower cardiac index, systemic oxygen consumption, and oxygen delivery immediately after resuscitation.[44] Prolonged peripheral vasoconstriction by excessive doses of epinephrine may delay or impair reperfusion of systemic organs, particularly the kidneys and gastrointestinal tract.

Given the accumulating evidence that subsequent deleterious effects may worsen outcome despite an improvement in ROSC, reassessment of HDE use seems appropriate.

Atropine

Atropine, a parasympatholytic agent, acts by blocking cholinergic stimulation of the muscarinic receptors of the heart. This usually results in an increase in the sinus rate and shortening of the atrioventricular node conduction time. Atropine may activate latent ectopic pacemakers. Atropine has little effect on systemic vascular resistance, myocardial perfusion pressure, or contractility.[99]

Atropine is indicated for treatment of asystole, PEA, bradycardia associated with hypotension, second- and third-degree heart block, and slow idioventricular rhythms. In children who present in cardiac arrest, sinus bradycardia and asystole are the most common initial rhythms, which makes atropine useful as a first-line drug. Atropine is particularly effective in clinical conditions associated with excessive parasympathetic tone.

The recommended dose of atropine is 0.02 mg/kg, with a minimum dose of 0.15 mg and a maximum dose of 2.0 mg. Smaller doses than 0.15 mg, even in small infants, may result paradoxically in bradycardia due to a central stimulatory effect on the medullary vagal nuclei by a dose that is too low to provide anticholinergic effects on the heart. Atropine may be given by any route, including intravenous (IV), endotracheal, intraosseous, intramuscular, and subcutaneous. Its onset of action occurs within 30 seconds, and its peak effect occurs between 1 and 2 minutes after an IV dose. The recommended adult dose is 0.5 mg every 5 minutes until the desired heart rate is obtained up to a maximum of 2 mg. For asystole, 1 mg is given intravenously and repeated every 5 minutes if asystole persists. Full vagal blockade usually is obtained with a dose of 2 mg in adults.

Because of its parasympatholytic effects, atropine should not be used in patients in whom tachycardia is undesirable. In patients after myocardial infarction or ischemia with persistent bradycardia, atropine should be used in the lowest dose possible to increase heart rate. This will limit tachycardia, a potent contributor to increased myocardial oxygen consumption, which could lead to VF. In addition, atropine should not be used in patients with pulmonary or systemic outflow tract obstruction or idiopathic hypertrophic subaortic stenosis because tachycardia decreases ventricular filling and lowers cardiac output in this setting.

Sodium Bicarbonate

The administration of sodium bicarbonate results in an acid-base reaction in which bicarbonate combines with hydrogen to form carbonic acid, which dissociates into water and carbon dioxide. Because of the generation of carbon dioxide, adequate alveolar ventilation must be present to achieve the normal buffering action of bicarbonate. Use of sodium bicarbonate during CPR remains controversial because of its potential side effects and the lack of evidence showing any benefit from its use during CPR.[105,215]

Sodium bicarbonate is indicated for correction of significant metabolic acidosis, especially when signs of cardiovascular compromise are present. Acidosis itself may have a number of negative effects on the circulation, including depression of myocardial function by prolonging diastolic depolarization, depressing spontaneous cardiac activity, decreasing the electrical threshold for VF, decreasing the inotropic state of the myocardium, and reducing the cardiac response to catecholamines. Acidosis also decreases systemic vascular resistance and attenuates the vasoconstrictive response of peripheral vessels to catecholamines. This is contrary to the desired effect during CPR. In addition, particularly in patients with a reactive pulmonary vascular bed, pulmonary vascular resistance is inversely related to pH. Rudolph and Yuan[193] observed a twofold increase in pulmonary vascular resistance in calves when pH was lowered from 7.4 to 7.2 under normoxic conditions. Therefore correction of even mild acidosis may be helpful in resuscitating patients who have the potential for increased right-to-left shunting through a cardiac septal defect, patent ductus arteriosus, or aortic-to-pulmonary shunt during periods of elevated pulmonary vascular resistance.

Multiple side effects of bicarbonate administration include metabolic alkalosis, hypercapnia, hypernatremia, and hyperosmolality. All of these side effects are associated with a high mortality rate. Alkalosis causes a leftward shift of the oxyhemoglobin dissociation curve, thus impairing release of oxygen from hemoglobin to tissues at a time when oxygen delivery already may be low. Alkalosis can result in hypokalemia, by enhancing potassium influx into cells, and ionic hypocalcemia, by increasing protein binding of ionized calcium. Hypernatremia and hyperosmolality may decrease tissue perfusion by increasing interstitial edema in microvascular beds. The marked hypercapnic acidosis that occurs during CPR on the venous side of the circulation, including the coronary sinus, may be worsened by administration of bicarbonate.[103,241] Myocardial acidosis during cardiac arrest is associated with decreased myocardial contractility. The mean venoarterial P_{CO_2} difference was 24 ± 15 mmHg in five patients during CPR and actually increased from 16 to 69 mmHg in one patient after administration of bicarbonate.[92] Another group showed a mean difference between Pv_{CO_2} and Pa_{CO_2} of 42 mmHg during CPR. Paradoxical intracellular acidosis after bicarbonate administration is possible because of rapid entry of carbon dioxide into cells with a slow egress of hydrogen ion out of cells. Paradoxical intracellular acidosis in the central nervous system after bicarbonate administration has been proposed but not definitively shown. In neonatal rabbits recovering from hypoxic acidosis, bicarbonate administration increased both arterial pH and intracellular brain pH as measured by nuclear magnetic resonance (NMR) spectroscopy.[210] In another study, intracellular brain ATP concentration in rats did not change during severe intracellular acidosis in the brain produced by extreme hypercapnia.[63] The rats who maintained ATP concentration even in the face of severe brain acidosis had no functional or histologic differences from normal controls. Using NMR spectroscopy of the brain in dogs during cardiac arrest and CPR, intracellular brain pH decreased to 6.29 with total depletion of brain ATP after 6 minutes of cardiac arrest. However, following effective CPR, ATP levels rose to 86% of prearrest levels and to normal by 35 minutes of CPR despite ongoing peripheral arterial acidosis[86] (Figure 118–18). However, cerebral pH decreased in parallel with blood pH when CPR was started immediately after arrest. Bicarbonate administration ameliorated and did not worsen the cerebral acidosis, indicating that the blood-brain pH gradient is maintained during CPR.[87]

When Pa_{CO_2} and pH are known, the dose of bicarbonate to correct the pH to 7.4 is calculated using the following equation:

$$0.3 \times \text{Weight M (kg M)} \times \text{Base deficit} = \text{mEq sodium bicarbonate.}$$

Because of its possible side effects and the large venous to arterial carbon dioxide gradient that develops during CPR, we recommend giving half the dose based on a volume distribution of 0.6. If blood gases are not available, the initial dose is 1 mEq/kg, followed by 0.5 mEq/kg every 10 minutes of ongoing arrest. Alveolar ventilation must be maintained because of the generation of carbon dioxide and can be assessed only by serial measurements of arterial blood gases and pH. Because of the potential side effects of bicarbonate, the indications for its use at this time are limited to cardiac arrest associated with hyperkalemia, patients with preexisting metabolic acidosis, and after approximately 10 minutes of CPR.

End-tidal CO_2 monitor is useful during CPR because it provides important information regarding both pulmonary and cardiac function. End-tidal CO_2 is measured

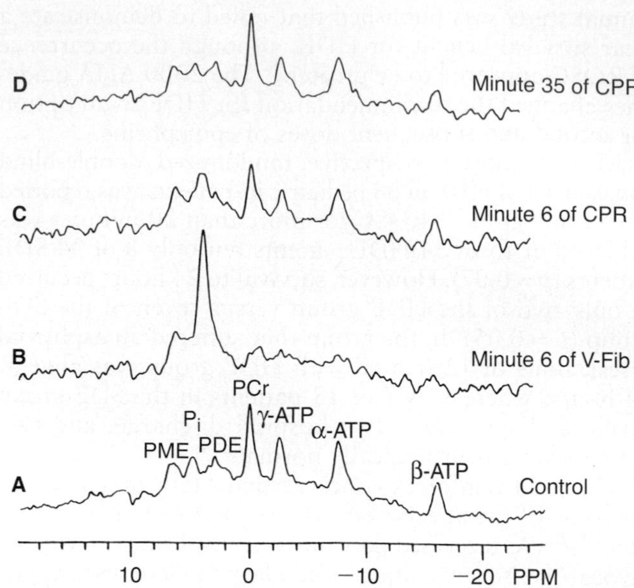

FIGURE 118–18 • ^{31}P magnetic resonance spectroscopy spectra from in situ dog brain during vest CPR after a 6-minute delay in the onset of CPR from time of arrest. Each spectrum was acquired in 1 minute. The frequency of the inorganic phosphate (P_i) peak is pH dependent. Note complete absence of adenosine triphosphate (ATP) and phosphocreatine (PCr), and pH_i = 6.28 in *trace B* after 6 minutes of ventricular fibrillation (v-fib) without CPR. After 6 minutes of CPR *(trace C),* ATP is more than 85% recovered, but pH is only 6.61. After 35 minutes of CPR *(trace D),* pH_i has returned to 7. (From Eleff SM, Schleien CL, Koehler RC, et al: *Anesthesiology* 76:77, 1992.)

instantaneously in the exhaled gas of every breath. In the absence of lung disease, end-tidal CO_2 correlates closely with Pa_{CO_2}, provided pulmonary blood flow is at least 20% to 25% of normal. As a respiratory monitor, end-tidal CO_2 analyzers accurately distinguish a tracheal (Et_{CO_2} >10) from an esophageal (Et_{CO_2} <5) intubation in infants and children.[31,32,168] Because measurements are made with every breath, dislodgment of the endotracheal tube from the trachea can be identified immediately. When cardiac output is extremely low, as occurs during ineffective CPR, delivery of carbon dioxide to the lungs is so limited that the total amount exchanged across the alveolar-capillary membrane is markedly reduced. In this situation, the measured end-tidal CO_2 is very low even when Pa_{CO_2} is elevated. As cardiac output increases, end-tidal CO_2 increases and the difference between end-tidal and arterial CO_2 becomes smaller.[200] End-tidal CO_2 has been correlated with CPP,[200] the critical parameter for resuscitation of the heart. However, a low end-tidal CO_2 may occur in the presence of adequate cardiac output during CPR after epinephrine because of its ability to increase intrapulmonary shunting.[50,152,226] In this case, a low end-tidal CO_2 underestimates cardiac output. Other causes of low end-tidal CO_2 include airway obstruction, tension pneumothorax, pericardial tamponade, pulmonary embolism, hypothermia, severe hypocapnia (which occurs commonly with overaggressive hand ventilation), and esophageal intubation.

Other Alkalinizing Agents

A number of other alkalinizing agents have been used experimentally in animals and humans. However, none has demonstrated any real advantages over sodium bicarbonate. Carbicarb, a solution of equimolar amounts of sodium bicarbonate and sodium carbonate, corrects metabolic acidosis without many of the side effects of sodium bicarbonate.[97] The buffering action of sodium carbonate occurs by consumption of carbon dioxide with generation of bicarbonate ion, as illustrated in the following equation:

$$Na_2CO_3 + CO_2 + H_2O \rightarrow HCO_3^- + 2Na^+.$$

During CPR, Carbicarb administration resulted in a greater increase in arterial pH and smaller increases in Pa_{CO_2}, lactate, and serum osmolality in animals.[29,97,223] However, Carbicarb was not superior to sodium bicarbonate when used for hypovolemic shock in rats.[19]

Dichloroacetate (DCA) increases the activity of pyruvate dehydrogenase, which facilitates the conversion of lactate to pyruvate.[216] When administered to patients with lactic acidosis, DCA decreased lactate concentration by half and increased bicarbonate concentration and pH.[218] In other studies, DCA improved cardiac output, possibly by increasing myocardial metabolism of lactate and carbohydrate.[217,240] In a multicenter trial of patients with lactic acidosis, DCA did not improve outcome when compared with sodium bicarbonate.[219]

Tromethamine (THAM; tris-hydroxymethyl-aminomethane) is an organic amine that attracts and combines with hydrogen ion, causing CO_2 and H_2O to combine to form bicarbonate and hydrogen ion. A dose of 3 ml/kg should raise the bicarbonate concentration by 3 mEq/L. Side effects of THAM include hyperkalemia, hypoglycemia, and acute hypocarbia resulting in apnea. In addition, peripheral vasodilation may occur after administration of THAM during CPR, an undesirable effect. THAM is contraindicated in patients with renal failure.

Calcium

Recommendations for use of calcium in CPR are restricted to a few specific situations, namely, hypocalcemia, hyperkalemia, hypermagnesemia, and calcium channel blocker overdose. These restrictions are based on the possibility that exogenously administered calcium may worsen ischemia/reperfusion injury. Intracellular calcium overload occurs during cerebral ischemia by the influx of calcium through voltage- and agonist-dependent (e.g., NMDA) calcium channels. Calcium plays an important role in the process of cell death in many organs, possibly by activating intracellular enzymes such as nitric oxide synthase, phospholipase A and C, and others.[158,243] Calcium channel blockers improve blood flow and function after ischemia to the heart,[59] kidney,[45] and brain.[119] Calcium channel blockers also raise the threshold of the ischemic heart to VF.[189] For these reasons, it appears that the recommended restrictions for use of calcium during CPR are well founded. On the other hand, no studies have shown that elevation of plasma calcium concentration, which occurs after calcium administration, worsens outcome of cardiac arrest. Because the normal ratio of extracellular to intracellular calcium is on the order of 1000:1 to 10,000:1, it seems unlikely that the rate of influx of calcium into cells would be influenced by a relatively small increase in its extracellular concentration.

The calcium ion is essential in myocardial excitation-contraction coupling, in increasing ventricular contractility, and in enhancing ventricular automaticity during asystole. Ionized hypocalcemia is associated with decreased ventricular performance and peripheral blunting of the hemodynamic response to catecholamines.[231,232] In addition, severe ionized hypocalcemia has been documented in adults suffering from out-of-hospital cardiac arrest (mean Ca 0.67 mmol/L),[231] during sepsis,[43] and in animals during prolonged CPR.[48] Thus patients at risk for ionized hypocalcemia should be identified and treated as expeditiously as possible. Both total and ionized hypocalcemia may occur in patients with chronic or acute disease. Total body calcium depletion leading to total serum hypocalcemia occurs in patients with hypoparathyroidism, DiGeorge syndrome, renal failure, pancreatitis, and long-term use of loop diuretics. Ionized hypocalcemia occurs after massive or rapid transfusion of blood products, a result of citrate and other preservatives in stored blood products that bind calcium. The magnitude of hypocalcemia in this setting depends on the rate of blood administration, the total dose, and the hepatic and renal function of the patient. Administration of 2 ml/kg/min of citrated whole blood causes a significant decrease in ionized calcium concentration in anesthetized patients.

The pediatric dose of calcium chloride for resuscitation is 20 mg/kg. The adult dose is 200 mg (2 ml of the 10% solution). Calcium gluconate is as effective as calcium chloride in raising ionized calcium concentration during CPR. Calcium gluconate is given at a dose of 30 to 100 mg/kg, with a maximum dose of 2 g in pediatric patients. Calcium should be given slowly through a large bore, free flowing IV line, preferably a central venous line. Severe tissue necrosis occurs when calcium infiltrates into subcutaneous tissue. When administered too rapidly, calcium may cause bradycardia, heart block, or ventricular standstill.

Glucose

Administration of glucose during CPR should be restricted to patients with documented hypoglycemia because of the possible detrimental effects of hyperglycemia on the brain during or following ischemia. Myers[161] found that infant monkeys that received glucose before cardiac arrest were more likely to develop seizures, prolonged coma, and brain death with cerebral necrosis than those that received saline. Siemkowicz and Hansen[213] confirmed this finding when they demonstrated that after 10 minutes of global brain ischemia, the neurologic recovery of hyperglycemic rats was worse than that of normoglycemic controls. The mechanism by which hyperglycemia exacerbates ischemic neurologic injury may be increased production of lactic acid in the brain by anaerobic metabolism. During ischemia under normoglycemic conditions, brain lactate concentration reaches a plateau. In a hyperglycemic milieu, however, brain lactate concentration continues to rise for the duration of the ischemic period. The severity of intracellular acidosis during ischemia is directly proportional to the preischemic glucose concentration.[56] The negative effect of hyperglycemia during brain ischemia is predicated on the presence of at least a small amount of blood flow to brain tissue. In one study, collaterally perfused but not end-arterial brain tissue had greater neuronal damage during hyperglycemic focal ischemia[182] (Figure 118–19).

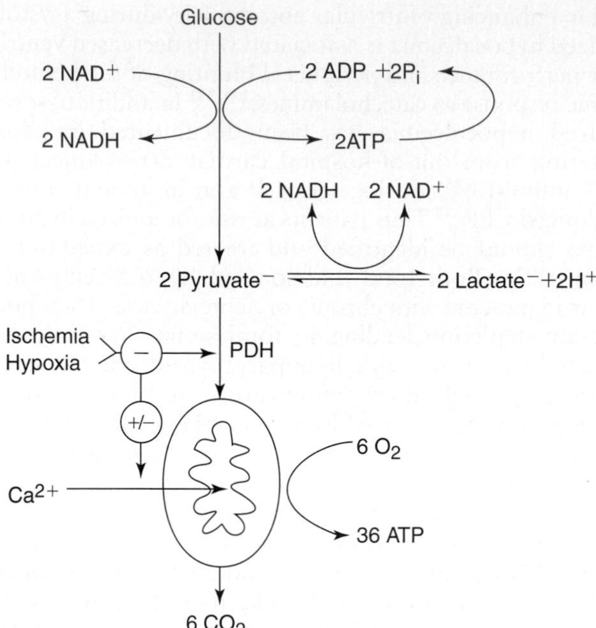

FIGURE 118–19 • Schematic diagram illustrating the aerobic/anaerobic metabolism of glucose. Oxidation of pyruvate to CO_2 (and H_2O) by pyruvate dehydrogenase and citric acid cycle enzymes is retarded to blocked by oxygen deficiency, causing a reduction of pyruvate to lactate. If the adenosine triphosphate *(ATP)* formed during glycolysis is hydrolyzed (that is, if the ATP concentration stays constant), one molecule of H^+ is released for each molecule of lactate formed. If the mitochondria retain a membrane potential, they will sequester excess calcium entering the cell; however, if they deenergized (with collapse of their membrane potential), they will release their calcium content. *ADP,* Adenosine diphosphate; *NAD,* nicotinamide adenine dinucleotide; *NADH,* reduced nicotinamide adenine dinucleotide; P_i, intracellular phosphorus; *PDH,* pyruvate dehydrogenase.

Clinical studies show a direct correlation between the initial postcardiac arrest serum glucose concentration and poor neurologic outcome.[9,45] However, a higher glucose concentration may just be an endogenous response to severe stress and thus a marker and not the cause of more severe brain injury.[145] In piglets, postischemic administration of glucose did not worsen neurologic outcome after global hypoxia-ischemia.[136] However, given the likelihood of additional ischemic and hypoxic events in the postresuscitation period, it seems prudent to maintain serum glucose in the normal range. Administration of insulin to hyperglycemic rats after global brain ischemia improved neurologic outcome.[236] The effect of insulin may be independent of its ability to lower blood glucose, as these investigators later showed that normoglycemic insulin-treated rats had a better outcome than normoglycemic placebo-treated controls.[237] Additional studies are needed to determine if the benefit from tight control of serum glucose following cardiac arrest or the use of insulin outweighs the risk of iatrogenic hypoglycemia.

Some groups of patients, including premature infants and debilitated patients with low endogenous glycogen stores, are more prone to developing hypoglycemia during and after a physiologic stress (e.g., surgery).[12] Bedside monitoring of serum glucose is critical during and after a cardiac arrest and allows for intervention before the critical point of low substrate delivery is reached. The dose of glucose needed to correct hypoglycemia is 0.5 to 1.0 g/kg given as 10% dextrose in infants. The osmolarity of 50% dextrose is approximately 2700 Osm/L and is associated with intraventricular hemorrhage in neonates and infants.

Management of Ventricular Fibrillation

The management of lethal ventricular arrhythmias traditionally has not played a major role in resuscitation teaching or management for children because of the low incidence of these arrhythmias. Newer evidence gathered in the environment of rapid access defibrillation suggests that as many as 19% of the presenting rhythms in pediatric arrests are ventricular in origin.[194] Moreover, the growing and aging population of children palliated for complex congenital heart disease in whom the occurrence of ventricular arrhythmias may be much higher than in the general pediatric population requires greater attention to ventricular arrhythmias than in the past. Other potential causes of ventricular arrhythmias include familial and acquired prolonged QT syndrome, other arrhythmogenic ventricular conditions,[137,166] cardiomyopathies, myocarditis, drug intoxications (illicit and accidental ingestion, therapeutic misadventures), electrolyte derangements (magnesium, calcium, potassium, glucose), and hypothermia.

Advances have been made in the management of ventricular arrhythmias. Rapid access to defibrillation has been shown to reduce mortality in adults, and the development of public access defibrillation (PAD) and AEDs has flowed from this knowledge. Initially AED devices had little utility for children, but the development of current-reducing electrodes and specific pediatric algorithms has made PAD a reality for children, and AEDs have been deployed in the many environments in which children would be the primary beneficiaries (e.g., schools, and public swimming pools). The technique of current delivery has undergone change with the development and deployment of biphasic defibrillators, which may offer increased efficacy with reduced risk of myocardial injury. Finally, amiodarone has started to replace lidocaine as the drug of choice for refractory ventricular arrhythmias and for atrial arrhythmias. The role of each of these factors in the resuscitation of pediatric arrest victims is discussed.

Defibrillation

VF is the chaotic electrical excitation of the ventricles. The electrical mechanism is usually explained as a reentrant depolarization of the myocardium, initially in waves that then take more circuitous routes and degenerate into smaller reentry circuits resulting in loss of the rhythmic contractile function of the ventricles.[230] This changing pattern of reentry circuits corresponds with the change from coarse to fine VF as the duration of fibrillation persists and may correlate with deterioration in energy stores associated with persistence of fibrillation.[23,126,165] Similarly, most cases of ventricular tachycardia are attributable to reentrant mechanisms, although increased automaticity is the likely mechanism in drug-induced torsades de pointes and electrolyte disturbances such as hypokalemia and hypomagnesemia.[11] Nonpulsatile ventricular tachycardia with loss of effective contractile function of the heart rapidly deteriorates into VF. Loss of effective ventricular function with these arrhythmias requires emergent management.

The standard for management of VF and pulseless ventricular tachycardia is immediate defibrillation. The standard voltage dose for pediatric defibrillation is 2 J/kg. If unsuccessful, the defibrillation is repeated at 4 J/kg twice before initiation of CPR and epinephrine.[4] This dosage is based on data reported by Gutgesell et al.[108] in 1976. They reported 71 defibrillation attempts in 27 children. Efficacy was 91% with 2 J/kg and 100% with 4 J/kg. Rhythms that fail to respond to three shocks are defined as "shock resistant." In this setting, the standard as defined in the AHA guidelines is epinephrine and CPR for a period of not more than 30 to 60 seconds, followed by a subsequent shock. If the rhythm remains refractory, amiodarone 5 mg/kg (or lidocaine, or magnesium for torsades de pointes) should be administered, followed by 30 to 60 seconds of CPR and then a repeat shock. An alternative to the pattern of CPR–drug–shock repeated twice is a pattern of CPR–drug–shock–shock–shock repeated twice.[4]

It is important to continue to deliver appropriate CPR while gathering defibrillation equipment.[25,249] Additional important considerations when delivering shocks include paddle size, position, contact pressure, and use of electrode paste. Large paddles reduce thoracic impedance, and infants older than 1 year or weighing more than 10 kg should be treated with adult paddles.[10] Adhesive patch electrodes are an acceptable alternative to paddles[73,124,125] and can be used when available if their use does not cause a delay in therapy. Paddles should be positioned to achieve current flow through the heart and an anterior–apex, posterior–apex, or anterior–posterior placement selected. Contact pressure has been demonstrated to reduce impedance. Firm pressure, commonly not properly applied, is required.[22] Proper electrode paste or gel is needed. Care is required to avoid smearing paste across the chest wall because this can lead to arcing of the circuit and a resultant short circuit. Bare paddles, ultrasound gel, saline-soaked pads, and alcohol pads are not acceptable alternatives to electrode cream or paste.[4]

The role of immediate defibrillation has come under question. The efficacy of defibrillation declines rapidly as fibrillation persists. When an arrest is witnessed and a defibrillator is immediately available, defibrillation likely will be successful. With any delay in resuscitation, the success of initial defibrillation declines at a rate estimated at between 7% and 10% per minute of continued fibrillation.[5] A number of studies have demonstrated in both animals and adults that if more than 3 to 5 minutes of fibrillation have occurred before institution of defibrillation, use of CPR for 90 to 180 seconds to restore myocardial energy stores will improve the likelihood of conversion to a perfusing rhythm with defibrillation.[24,68,129,244] Given the frequency of unwitnessed arrest in children and the relatively low frequency of ventricular arrhythmias, CPR first usually is the appropriate response in children.

Use of biphasic defibrillators is another important advance in the management of tachyarrhythmias. The optimal waveform—biphasic exponential truncated biphasic rectilinear (Figure 118–20), or other—and optimal energy dose are still being evaluated. Studies suggest that defibrillation can be achieved with lower energy and less myocardial injury than with a standard monophasic defibrillator current.[91,228] The first commercially available devices were approved by the Food and Drug Administration in 1996. An evidence based review was undertaken by the AHA and published in 1998.[69] The reviewers concluded that "Low-energy, non-progressive biphasic waveform defibrillators may be used for both out-of-hospital and in-hospital VF arrest, including persistent or recurrent VF that does not respond to the initial low-energy shock." These conclusions were based on observational studies and case reports. Subsequently, Schneider et al.[209] reported a randomized controlled trial of biphasic versus monophasic defibrillation for out-of-hospital cardiac arrest. Of 338 arrests, 115 patients had VF and were shocked with an AED. Defibrillation in the initial shock series was successful in 98% of patients receiving biphasic shocks but in only 69% of those receiving monophasic shocks ($p < 0.0001$), providing further evidence that biphasic waveforms are more efficacious than monophasic waveforms (Figure 118–21).

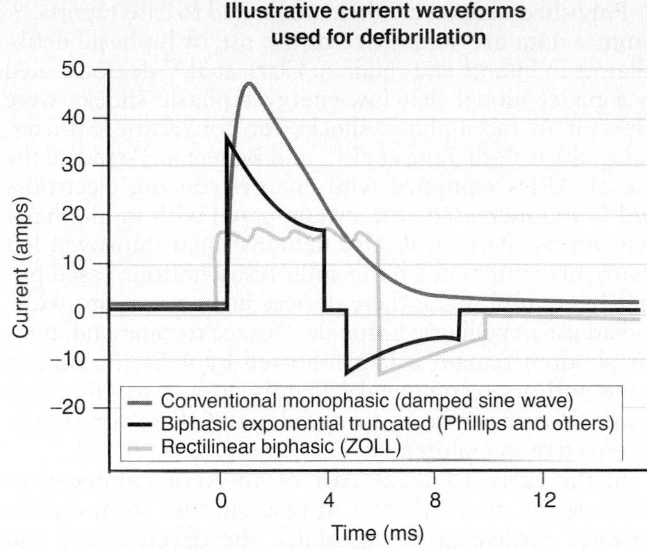

FIGURE 118–20 • Current flow for a conventional monophasic defibrillator, a biphasic truncated exponential waveform defibrillator, the Phillips HeartStart AED, and a rectilinear biphasic waveform defibrillator produced by Zoll. The Phillips waveform was produced with 150 J and 50-Ω impedance. Current will fall and duration will increase as impedance rises. The Zoll waveform was produced with 150 J and internally compensated impedance to maintain a stable current. (Waveforms courtesy Phillips and Zoll Corporations.)

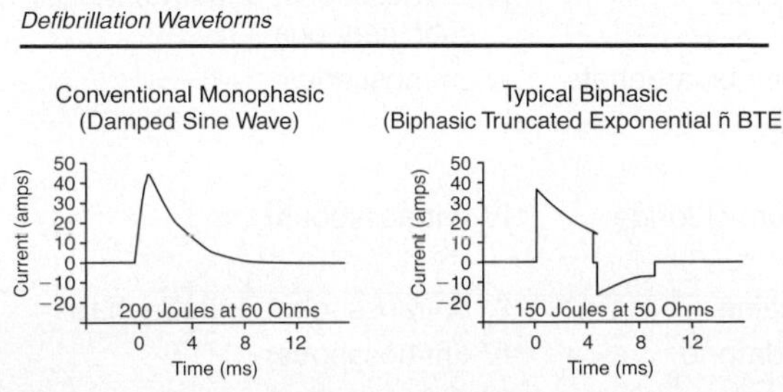

FIGURE 118–21 • Schematic patterns of current flow for conventional monophasic and typical biphasic defibrillator waveforms.

Published data on children are limited to case reports.[107] Animal data are supportive of the use of biphasic defibrillators in infants and children. Clark et al.[58] demonstrated in a piglet model that low-energy biphasic shocks were superior to monophasic shocks for converting catheter-induced VF. Both Tang et al.[227] and Berg et al.[23] studied the use of AEDs equipped with energy-reducing electrodes and found increased efficacy compared with monophasic waveforms. Berg et al. also demonstrated improved left ventricular function 5 hours after resuscitation. Based primarily on adult data, these devices have come into widespread use in pediatric hospitals. Dosage recommendations for children remain 2 J/kg followed by 4 J/kg, although some authors recommend half this dose, reasoning that lower doses are effective in adults and therefore should be effective in children.[121]

In the early 1990s as part of an AHA campaign to improve the abysmal rates of resuscitation from out-of-hospital cardiac arrest in adults, the development and deployment of AEDs was initiated. Both fixed and escalating dose devices were developed; however, the initial dose usually was at least 150 J. Because of the high fixed energy doses, the devices were not recommended for use in children younger than 9 years. Moreover, use of these devices for young children was questioned because the arrhythmia detection algorithms used in these devices were developed for adults. Cecchin et al.[51] used the Agilent Heartstream FR2 Patient Analysis System to analyze 696 five-second rhythms from 191 children younger than 12. Analysis revealed 100% accuracy for nonshockable rhythms and 96% accuracy for VF. This is similar to the accuracy reported for adults. In a more recent study, Atkinson et al.[11] tested the accuracy of the Lifepak 500 AED on 1561 fifteen-second rhythms from 203 children age 1 day to 7 years. The device correctly identified 99% of coarse VF as shockable and 99.1% of nonshockable rhythms. A number of manufacturers (Zoll and Agilent) have developed energy-reducing electrodes that should allow use of these devices in young children.

The International Liaison Committee on Resuscitation Task Force on Pediatric Advanced Life Support has issued a set of recommendations regarding the use of AEDs in young children to update the recommendations included in the 2000 AHA guidelines on resuscitation. They recommend use of an AED in children between the ages of 1 and 8 years who have no signs of circulation. The device should be adapted to deliver a pediatric dose. They found insufficient evidence to make a recommendation for infants younger than 1 year.[197] Despite these advances, given the epidemiology of pediatric cardiac arrest, the deployment of AEDs likely will not have a significant impact on the outcome of cardiac arrest in young children.[72]

Amiodarone

Amiodarone is an effective antiarrhythmic for both atrial and ventricular arrhythmias. The role of amiodarone in cardiac arrest was established after a series of studies demonstrated efficacy and superiority of amiodarone over lidocaine in the management of refractory VF and pulseless ventricular tachycardia in adults. Compared with lidocaine, amiodarone led to substantially higher rates of survival to hospital admission in patients with shock-resistant out-of-hospital VF.[81] These findings led to major changes in the AHA guidelines for management of ventricular arrhythmias (Table 118–1, and Figures 118–22 and 118–23).

Early reports on use of oral amiodarone in children were favorable.[64,65,178] Data on amiodarone use in children are limited to case reports and descriptive case series.[46,90,94,134,177] Nevertheless, it now is used widely for serious pediatric arrhythmias. It appears to be effective and have an acceptable short-term safety profile. The growing pediatric experience among experts and inference from adult studies led to inclusion of amiodarone in the 2000 AHA pediatric advanced life support guidelines as a drug of choice for pulseless ventricular tachycardia or VF, although the level of evidence was classified as indeterminate.[6] For hemodynamically stable ventricular tachycardia, it is also the drug of choice with the level of evidence classified as IIb. Procainamide and lidocaine remain alternative drug choices. Amiodarone is commonly

TABLE 118–1

DRUG THERAPY FOR PULSELESS ARREST

Drug	Route of Administration	Dosage	How Applied
Epinephrine	IV, intraosseous endotracheal	10 μg/kg	1:10,000 (0.1 ml/kg)
		100 μg/kg	1:1,000 should be used for ETT (0.1 ml/kg)
Atropine	IV, intraosseous, endotrachael, subcutaneous	0.02 mg/kg (minimum dose = 0.15 mg)	
Sodium bicarbonate	IV, intraosseous	1 mEq/kg/dose	1 mEq/ml
		or	0.5 mEq/ml
		0.3 × wgt (kg) × base deficit	
Calcium chloride	IV (intraosseous)	20 mg/kg	10% solution (100 mg/ml)
		0.2 ml/kg	
Lidocaine	IV (intraosseous) endotrachael	1 mg/kg	1%, 2%, 4% solution
Amiodarone	IV (intraosseous)	5 mg/kg	Dilute to 3 mg/ml
Magnesium	IV (intraosseous)	25–50 mg/kg for torsades de pointes or hypomagnesemia	50% solution

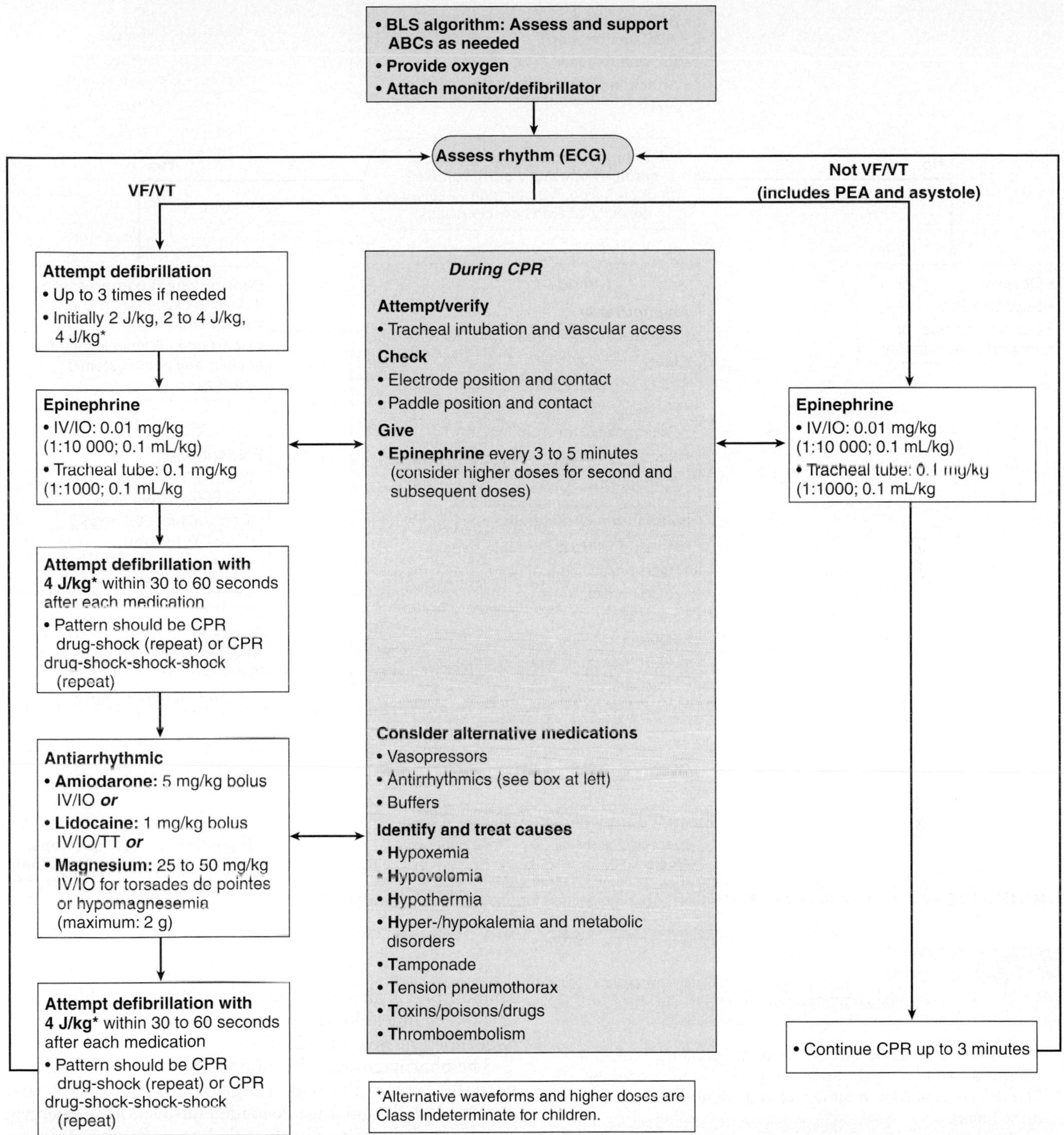

• BLS algorithm: Assess and support ABCs as needed
• Provide oxygen
• Attach monitor/defibrillator
Assess rhythm (ECG)
VF/VT
Not VF/VT (includes PEA and asystole)
Attempt defibrillation
• Up to 3 times if needed
• Initially 2 J/kg, 2 to 4 J/kg, 4 J/kg*
Epinephrine
• IV/IO: 0.01 mg/kg (1:10 000; 0.1 mL/kg)
• Tracheal tube: 0.1 mg/kg (1:1000; 0.1 mL/kg
Attempt defibrillation with 4 J/kg* within 30 to 60 seconds after each medication
• Pattern should be CPR drug-shock (repeat) or CPR drug-shock-shock-shock (repeat)
Antiarrhythmic
• Amiodarone: 5 mg/kg bolus IV/IO or
• Lidocaine: 1 mg/kg bolus IV/IO/TT or
• Magnesium: 25 to 50 mg/kg IV/IO for torsades de pointes or hypomagnesemia (maximum: 2 g)
Attempt defibrillation with 4 J/kg* within 30 to 60 seconds after each medication
• Pattern should be CPR drug-shock (repeat) or CPR drug-shock-shock-shock (repeat)
During CPR
Attempt/verify
• Tracheal intubation and vascular access
Check
• Electrode position and contact
• Paddle position and contact
Give
• Epinephrine every 3 to 5 minutes (consider higher doses for second and subsequent doses)
Consider alternative medications
• Vasopressors
• Antirrhythmics (see box at left)
• Buffers
Identify and treat causes
• Hypoxemia
• Hypovolemia
• Hypothermia
• Hyper-/hypokalemia and metabolic disorders
• Tamponade
• Tension pneumothorax
• Toxins/poisons/drugs
• Thromboembolism
Epinephrine
• IV/IO: 0.01 mg/kg (1:10 000; 0.1 mL/kg)
• Tracheal tube: 0.1 mg/kg (1:1000; 0.1 mL/kg
• Continue CPR up to 3 minutes
*Alternative waveforms and higher doses are Class Indeterminate for children.

FIGURE 118–22 • American Heart Association (AHA) guidelines for management of ventricular arrhythmias.

used for management of postoperative atrial and junctional ectopic tachycardia, especially in patients with ventricular pacing wires in place.

The wide range of effectiveness of amiodarone is demonstrated by the array of indications noted in the 2000 AHA guidelines for adults (Box 118–2).[7] Its role in the management of atrial arrhythmias in adults includes the following: as an adjunct to electrical cardioversion of refractory paroxysmal supraventricular tachycardia and atrial tachycardia, for rate control when digoxin has been ineffective, for pharmacologic conversion of atrial flutter, and for control of rapid ventricular response in preexcited atrial tachyarrhythmias. It is the drug of choice for junctional tachycardia with poor function. If function is preserved,

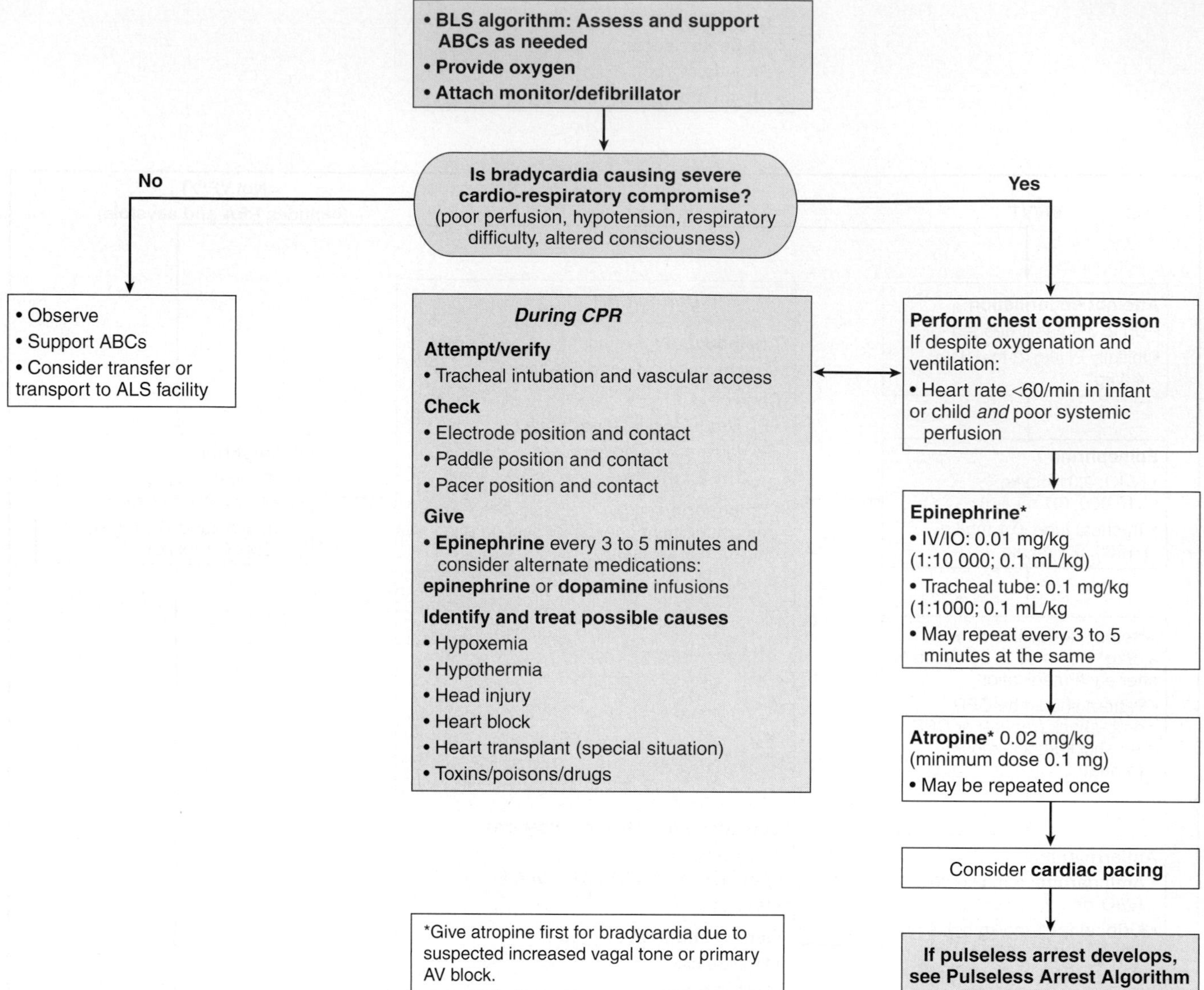

• BLS algorithm: Assess and support ABCs as needed
• Provide oxygen
• Attach monitor/defibrillator
Is bradycardia causing severe cardio-respiratory compromise? (poor perfusion, hypotension, respiratory difficulty, altered consciousness)
No
Yes
• Observe
• Support ABCs
• Consider transfer or transport to ALS facility
During CPR
Attempt/verify
• Tracheal intubation and vascular access
Check
• Electrode position and contact
• Paddle position and contact
• Pacer position and contact
Give
• Epinephrine every 3 to 5 minutes and consider alternate medications: epinephrine or dopamine infusions
Identify and treat possible causes
• Hypoxemia
• Hypothermia
• Head injury
• Heart block
• Heart transplant (special situation)
• Toxins/poisons/drugs
Perform chest compression
If despite oxygenation and ventilation:
• Heart rate <60/min in infant or child and poor systemic perfusion
Epinephrine*
• IV/IO: 0.01 mg/kg (1:10 000; 0.1 mL/kg)
• Tracheal tube: 0.1 mg/kg (1:1000; 0.1 mL/kg
• May repeat every 3 to 5 minutes at the same
Atropine* 0.02 mg/kg (minimum dose 0.1 mg)
• May be repeated once
Consider cardiac pacing
If pulseless arrest develops, see Pulseless Arrest Algorithm
*Give atropine first for bradycardia due to suspected increased vagal tone or primary AV block.

FIGURE 118–23 • American Heart Association (AHA) guidelines for management of bradycardia.

BOX 118–2

Amiodarone (IV)

Intravenous amiodarone affects sodium, calcium channels, and α- and β-adrenergic blocking properties. The drug is useful for treatment of both atrial and ventricular arrhythmias.

Amiodarone is also helpful for ventricular rate control of rapid atrial arrhythmias in patients with severely impaired LV function when digitalis has proved ineffective. Amiodarone is recommended after defibrillation and epinephrine in cardiac arrest with persistent VT or VF.

Amiodarone is effective for control of hemodynamically stable VT, polymorphic VT, and wide-complex tachycardia of uncertain origin.

Amiodarone is an adjunct to electrical cardioversion of refractory PSVTs, atrial tachycardia, and pharmacological cardioversion of AF.

Amiodarone can control rapid ventricular rate due to accessory pathway conduction in preexcited atrial arrhythmias.

Taken from Guidelines 2000 for CPR & ECCC.[5]

amiodarone is an acceptable alternative to a β-blocker or calcium channel blocker. Its role in ventricular arrhythmias is outlined in Box 118–2.

The pharmacology of amiodarone is complex and may partially explain the wide range of efficacy. It is poorly absorbed orally and must be loaded intravenously in urgent situations. It is primarily classified as a Vaughn-Williams class III agent that blocks the ATP-sensitive outward potassium channels, causing prolongation of the action potential and refractory period. However, this effect requires intracellular accumulation. Upon IV loading, the antiarrhythmic effects primarily result from noncompetitive α- and β-adrenergic receptor blockade, calcium channel blockade, and effects on inward sodium current causing a decrease in anterograde conduction across the atrioventricular node and an increase in the effective atrioventricular refractory period. The full antiarrhythmic impact requires a loading period for up to 1 to 3 weeks to achieve intracellular levels and full potassium channel blocking effects. Prolongation of the QT interval, an effect resulting from K-ATP channel blockade, is commonly described with amiodarone use; however, it does not manifest until several days into loading, underscoring its different effects during the acute period and after loading is accomplished. These effects are evident throughout all cardiac tissue, which may explain amiodarone's efficacy for so many arrhythmias, both atrial and ventricular. The α-adrenergic blockade leads to vasodilation, which may increase coronary blood flow.

Immediate hemodynamic effects are caused by the solubilizing agent Tween 80, which has both vasodilating and myocardial depressant effects.[173] Hypotension is commonly reported with IV administration and may limit the rate at which the drug can be given. The overall hemodynamic impact of IV administration depends on the balance of its effect on rate control, myocardial performance, and vasodilation. Cardiac output usually is unchanged or increases despite the decreased contractility because of both rate control and vasodilation. The effect on systemic vascular resistance and the limited impact on contractility make amiodarone the drug of choice for use in patients with impaired cardiac function.

The drug is highly lipid soluble, giving it a very large volume of distribution. This accounts for the need for loading over many days. Until all tissues are saturated, rapid redistribution out of the vascular compartment may lead to early recurrence of arrhythmias. Once tissue saturation has occurred, the half-life is estimated to be between 13 and 103 days.

Dosage recommendations for children are based on limited clinical studies and extrapolation of adult data. For life-threatening arrhythmias, the usual recommended dose is 5 mg/kg IV. This dose can be repeated if necessary to control the arrhythmia. IV loading doses are followed by a continuous infusion of 10 to 20 mg/kg/day if there is a risk for arrhythmia recurrence. The ideal rate of bolus administration is unclear, but once diluted the drug is given IV push in adults. The potential for profound vasodilation in children has led to concern by some pediatric intensivists and cardiologists, who recommend that amiodarone be given over 10 minutes as recommended in the package insert. This concern may not be valid in the pulseless arrest setting. Some delay always occurs with the current formulation of the IV drug because it must be diluted before it can be administered. Drug dilution should not delay administration of additional shocks. An average of five shocks are delivered to adults with refractory VF before amiodarone is administered. An alternative dosing regimen for children is administration of 1 mg/kg pushes every 5 minutes up to 5 mg/kg. This dose can be repeated up to 10 mg/kg if the arrhythmia is not controlled. Use of the small-aliquot bolus technique may be particularly appropriate for infants younger than 6 to 12 months.

Amiodarone IV leaches plasticizers, particularly DHEP, from polyvinyl chloride. This effect is enhanced at low infusion rates and at higher drug concentrations and may be minimized by frequent intermittent boluses. Whether these plasticizers have any significant toxicity at these doses is unknown, although evidence indicates testicular vacuolization in rodents. Additional caution is warranted in neonates because the solution contains benzyl alcohol, which is associated with metabolic acidosis and death in premature infants (gasping syndrome). Identification of the potential for these adverse events has led the manufacturer to issue a statement to health care professionals stating that use of IV amiodarone in pediatrics is not recommended. The AHA has responded with a reiteration of the recommendation for IV amiodarone use in the 2000 guidelines for emergency cardiac care. The statement concluded as follows, "In conclusion, the AHA Committee on Pediatric Resuscitation still considers amiodarone an acceptable option for acute management of pulseless arrest and ventricular tachyarrhythmias in pediatric patients. Practitioners who choose to administer amiodarone should be familiar with its safety profile and should seek to minimize toxicity from this agent."[8]

Adverse reactions to amiodarone can be life threatening. The drug prolongs the QT interval. In a series by et al.,[90] 29 of 50 infants and children experienced mild-to-moderate prolongation of the QTc. In the series by Burri et al.,[46] "most" infants experienced prolongation. Although none of the pediatric case series described patients developing drug-induced arrhythmias, amiodarone-induced torsades de pointes has been described in case reports,[214] and, although less common than in adults, caution is warranted. Use of amiodarone should be avoided in combination with other drugs that prolong the QT interval. In addition, caution should be exercised in the setting of hypomagnesemia and other electrolyte abnormalities that predispose to torsades de pointes. Severe bradycardia and heart block have been described, especially in the postoperative period, and ventricular pacing wires are recommended in this setting.

The manufacturer of the IV preparation (Wyeth) reports in the product literature a series of 61 children receiving amiodarone, of whom 36% had hypotension, 20% had bradycardia, and 15% developed AV block. These complications were severe or life threatening in some cases. In the published case series of children, the incidence of side effects appears to be much lower. In a series reported by Etheridge et al.,[90] two of six patients who received IV amiodarone experienced hypotension. In several other series, the incidence of hypotension ranged from zero of 15 to four of 40.[46,94,177] All patients who were believed to require treatment responded to a saline infusion or calcium. One patient with symptomatic bradycardia responded to temporary pacing. Two other patients required a reduction in the rate of drug infusion for mild bradycardia.

Noncardiac side effects are often seen, especially with chronic dosing.[122] The most serious side effect is development of interstitial pneumonitis, seen most often in patients with preexisting lung disease.[123] The incidence in children is unknown. Rarely an acute respiratory distress syndrome-like illness has been reported in both infants and adults at the initiation of treatment.[34,70] The lung disease may remit with early discontinuation of the drug. Thyroid disorders may occur with chronic use. Desethylamiodarone, the major metabolite of amiodarone, appears to have an antithyroid effect by noncompetitive binding to the nuclear receptors. Both hyperthyroidism with thyrotoxicosis and hypothyroidism have occurred. This may be of particular concern in the management of fetal tachycardias. Although amiodarone appears to be effective in controlling refractory life-threatening fetal tachycardias, evidence of fetal hypothyroidism was present in 19% of neonates based on cord blood TSH.[17] Other forms of toxicity include hepatotoxicity that may progress to cirrhosis, photosensitivity and skin discoloration, and local inflammation and cellulitis at the infusion site. Injection site reactions occurred in 5 of 20 patients who received amiodarone through a peripheral IV line. Corneal opacities are a common finding with chronic therapy but apparently do not affect vision.

Postresuscitation Care

Amelioration of neurologic injury after cardiac arrest has been a goal of many investigators over the last decades (Box 118–3). With the completion of two multicenter trials on mild hypothermia after cardiac arrest, one from Europe and the other from Australia, this goal appears to have been partially realized. In both studies, adult patients presenting with out-of-hospital VF who were resuscitated underwent rapid cooling to a target temperature between 32° C and 34° C. This temperature was maintained for 12 to 24 hours. Both neurologic outcome and mortality were improved compared with the control groups. The odds ratio for improved neurologic outcome were 1.4 in the European study, which included 275 patients, and was 5.25 in the Australian study, which included 77 randomized patients. The hypothermia groups had lower mean blood pressure, required more frequent use of epinephrine, and had higher systemic vascular resistance. Although these studies have a limited target population, data from animal studies[221] and other smaller case series[248] suggest that therapeutic hypothermia is a useful tool after cardiac arrest from all causes and its use appears warranted, especially because the incidence of serious attributable complications is low.

BOX 118–3

Experimental Cerebroprotective Therapy

- Calcium channel blockers
- Glutamate receptor antagonists
- Opiate receptor antagonists
- Central α_2-receptor antagonists
- β-Receptor antagonists
- Oxygen radical scavengers
- Iron chelators
- Xanthine oxidase inhibitors
- Inhibitors of arachidonic acid metabolism
- Thromobolytic agents
- Lazaroids
- Cerebral vasodilators
- Metabolic activators/inhibitors
- Hypothermia
- Nitric oxide synthase inhibitors
- Adenosine agonists
- Antiplatelet agents
- Antineutrophil strategies
- Protease inhibitors
- Growth factors

Future Directions

Despite the therapeutic advances highlighted, continued efforts to clarify the applicability to infants and children is important and ongoing. Actual clinical trials have been hampered by the federal regulation know as the "final rule" for resuscitation research.[156] In 1996, as part of a broad-ranging effort to protect patients rights as human subjects, the standard of community consent for research that required immediate intervention was developed. Since that time, resuscitation research in both adults and children has been limited, with most trials conducted in Europe, Australia, and other countries, often with US collaborators. The feasibility of obtaining a community standard to perform a hypothetical hypothermia after post cardiac arrest study in children was performed in 2004.[159] The relevant community was defined as hospital staff and the parents of ICU patients and parents of previously resuscitated children. They concluded that development of a study using an exemption from informed consent was feasible. However, in an accompanying editorial, Moler[156] reiterates that, despite feasibility, practicality is very different as evidenced by the complete lack of pediatric resuscitation trials since 1996. Whether revision of this rule will occur or techniques for acquiring community consent can be developed remains one of the major hurdles to future pediatric resuscitation research.

REFERENCES

1. Angelos MG, et al: Cardiopulmonary bypass in a model of acute myocardial infarction and cardiac arrest, Ann Emerg Med 19: 874-880, 1990.
2. Angelos MG, Ward KR, Beckley PD: Norepinephrine-induced hypertension following cardiac arrest: effects on myocardial oxygen use in a swine model, Ann Emerg Med 24:907-914, 1994.
3. Anonymous: Standards and guidelines for cardiopulmonary resuscitation (CPR) and emergency cardiac care (ECC), JAMA 268, 1992.
4. Anonymous: Guidelines 2000 for cardiopulmonary resuscitation and emergency cardiovascular care. Part 6: advanced cardiovascular life support: 7C: a guide to the international ACLS algorithms. The American Heart Association in collaboration with the International Liaison Committee on Resuscitation, Circulation 102(8 suppl):I291-I342, 2000.
5. Anonymous: Guidelines 2000 for cardiopulmonary resuscitation and emergency cardiovascular care. Part 6: advanced cardiovascular life support: 7C: a guide to the international ACLS algorithms. The American Heart Association in collaboration with the International Liaison Committee on Resuscitation, Circulation 102(8 Suppl):I86-I171, 2000.
6. Anonymous: Guidelines 2000 for cardiopulmonary resuscitation and emergency cardiovascular care. Part 6: advanced cardiovascular life support: section 1: introduction to ACLS 2000: overview of recommended changes in ACLS from the guidelines 2000 conference. The American Heart Association in collaboration with the International Liaison Committee on Resuscitation, Circulation 102(8 Suppl):I311-319, 2000.
7. Anonymous: Guidelines 2000 for cardiopulmonary resuscitation and emergency cardiovascular care. Part 6: advanced cardiovascular life support: section 1: introduction to ACLS 2000: overview of recommended changes in ACLS from the guidelines 2000 conference. The American Heart Association in collaboration with the International Liaison Committee on Resuscitation, Circulation 102(8 Suppl):I112-121, 2000.
8. Anonymous: Use of amiodarone in children. 2004, American Heart Association, Committee on Pediatric Resuscitation.
9. Ashwal S, et al: Prognostic implications of hyperglycemia and reduced cerebral blood flow in childhood near-drowning, Neurology 40:820-823, 1990.

10. Atkins DL, Kerber RE: Pediatric defibrillation: current flow is improved by using "adult" electrode paddles, *Pediatrics* 94:90-93, 1994.
11. Atkinson E, et al: Specificity and sensitivity of automated external defibrillator rhythm analysis in infants and children, *Ann Emerg Med* 42:185-196, 2003.
12. Auer R: Progress review: hypoglycemic brain damage, *Stroke* 17: 699-708, 1986.
13. Babbs CF, Tacker WA, Paris RL, et al: CPR with simultaneous compression and ventilation at high airway pressure in 4 animal models, *Crit Care Med* 10:501, 1982.
14. Babbs CF: Interposed abdominal compression CPR: a comprehensive evidence based review, *Resuscitation* 59:71-82, 2003.
15. Babbs CF: Simplified meta-analysis of clinical trials in resuscitation, *Resuscitation* 57:245-255, 2003.
16. Bahlmann L, et al: Brain metabolism during cardiopulmonary resuscitation assessed with microdialysis, *Resuscitation* 59:255-260, 2003.
17. Bartalena L, et al: Effects of amiodarone administration during pregnancy on neonatal thyroid function and subsequent neurodevelopment, *J Endocrinol Invest* 24:116-130, 2001.
18. Barthell E, et al: Prehospital external cardiac pacing: a prospective, controlled clinical trial, *Ann Emerg Med* 17:1221-1226, 1988.
19. Beech JS, et al: The effects of sodium bicarbonate and a mixture of sodium bicarbonate and carbonate ("Carbicarb") on skeletal muscle pH and hemodynamic status in rats with hypovolemic shock, *Metabolism* 43:518-522, 1994.
20. Beland MJ, et al: Noninvasive transcutaneous cardiac pacing in children, *Pacing Clin Electrophysiol* 10:1262-1270, 1987.
21. Beland MJ, et al: Ventricular tachycardia related to transcutaneous pacing, *Ann Emerg Med* 17:279-281, 1988.
22. Bennetts SH, et al: Is optimal paddle force applied during paediatric external defibrillation? *Resuscitation* 60:29-32, 2004.
23. Berg RA, et al: Attenuated adult biphasic shocks compared with weight-based monophasic shocks in a swine model of prolonged pediatric ventricular fibrillation, *Resuscitation* 61:189-197, 2004.
24. Berg RA, et al: Precountershock cardiopulmonary resuscitation improves ventricular fibrillation median frequency and myocardial readiness for successful defibrillation from prolonged ventricular fibrillation: a randomized, controlled swine study, *Ann Emerg Med* 40:563-570, 2004.
25. Berg RA, et al: Automated external defibrillation versus manual defibrillation for prolonged ventricular fibrillation: lethal delays of chest compressions before and after countershocks, *Ann Emerg Med* 42:458-467, 2003.
26. Berg RA, et al: High-dose epinephrine results in greater early mortality after resuscitation from prolonged cardiac arrest in pigs: a prospective, randomized study, *Crit Care Med* 22:282-290, 1994.
27. Berkowitz ID, et al: Blood flow during cardiopulmonary resuscitation with simultaneous compression and ventilation in infant pigs, *Pediatr Res* 26:558-564, 1989.
28. Berkowitz ID, et al: Epinephrine dosage effects on cerebral and myocardial blood flow in an infant swine model of cardiopulmonary resuscitation, *Anesthesiology* 75:1041-1050, 1991.
29. Bersin RM, Arieff AI: Improved hemodynamic function during hypoxia with Carbicarb, a new agent for the management of acidosis, *Circulation* 77:227-233, 1988.
30. Beyar R, et al: Circulatory assistance by intrathoracic pressure variations: optimization and mechanisms studied by a mathematical model in relation to experimental data, *Circ Res* 64:703-720, 1989.
31. Bhende MS, et al: Validity of a disposable end-tidal CO2 detector in verifying endotracheal tube placement in infants and children, *Ann Emerg Med* 21:142-5, 1992.
32. Bhende MS, Thompson AE, Orr RA: Utility of an end-tidal carbon dioxide detector during stabilization and transport of critically ill children, *Pediatrics* 89(6 pt 1):1042-1044, 1992.
33. Bircher N, Safar P, Stewart R: A comparison of standard, "MAST"-augmented, and open-chest CPR in dogs. A preliminary investigation, *Crit Care Med* 8:147-152, 1980.
34. Birmingham WP: More on an infant with acute pulmonary toxicity during amiodarone therapy, *Am J Cardiol* 81:1171, 1998.
35. Brillman JA, et al: Outcome of resuscitation from fibrillatory arrest using epinephrine and phenylephrine in dogs, *Crit Care Med* 13: 912-913, 1985.
36. Brown CG, et al: Methoxamine versus epinephrine on regional cerebral blood flow during cardiopulmonary resuscitation, *Crit Care Med* 15:682-686, 1987.
37. Brown CG, et al: A comparison of standard-dose and high-dose epinephrine in cardiac arrest outside the hospital. The Multicenter High-Dose Epinephrine Study Group, *N Engl J Med* 327:1051-1055, 1992.
38. Brown CG, et al: Myocardial oxygen delivery/consumption during cardiopulmonary resuscitation: a comparison of epinephrine and phenylephrine, *Ann Emerg Med* 17:302-308, 1988.
39. Brown CG, et al: Effect of standard doses of epinephrine on myocardial oxygen delivery and utilization during cardiopulmonary resuscitation, *Crit Care Med* 16:536-539, 1988.
40. Brown CG, et al: Comparative effect of graded doses of epinephrine on regional brain blood flow during CPR in a swine model, *Ann Emerg Med* 15:1138-1144, 1986.
41. Brown CG, et al: The effects of graded doses of epinephrine on regional myocardial blood flow during cardiopulmonary resuscitation in swine, *Circulation* 75:491-497, 1987.
42. Brown CG, et al: The effect of high-dose phenylephrine versus epinephrine on regional cerebral blood flow during CPR, *Ann Emerg Med* 16:743-748, 1987.
43. Burchard KW, et al: Hypocalcemia during sepsis. Relationship to resuscitation and hemodynamics, *Arch Surg* 127:265-272, 1992.
44. Burchfield DJ, et al: Effects of graded doses of epinephrine during asphxia-induced bradycardia in newborn lambs, *Resuscitation* 25: 235-244, 1993.
45. Burke TJ, et al: Protective effect of intrarenal calcium membrane blockers before or after renal ischemia. Functional, morphological, and mitochondrial studies, *J Clin Invest* 74:1830-1841, 1984.
46. Burri S, Hug MI, Bauersfeld U: Efficacy and safety of intravenous amiodarone for incessant tachycardias in infants, *Eur J Pediatr* 162:880-884, 2003.
47. Caceres MJ, et al: Early endothelial damage and leukocyte accumulation in piglet brains following cardiac arrest, *Acta Neuropathol (Berl)* 90:582-591, 1995.
48. Cairns CB, et al: Ionized hypocalcemia during prolonged cardiac arrest and closed chest CPR in a canine model, *Ann Emerg Med* 20:1178-1182, 1991.
49. Callaham M, et al: A randomized clinical trial of high-dose epinephrine and norepinephrine vs standard dose epinephrine in prehospital cardiac arrest, *JAMA* 268:2667-2672, 1992.
50. Cantineau JP, et al: Effect of epinephrine on end-tidal carbon dioxide pressure during prehospital cardiopulmonary resuscitation, *Am J Emerg Med* 12:267-270, 1994.
51. Cecchin F, et al: Is arrhythmia detection by automatic external defibrillator accurate for children?: sensitivity and specificity of an automatic external defibrillator algorithm in 696 pediatric arrhythmias, *Circulation* 103:2483-2488, 2001.
52. Chandra N, Rudikoff M, Weisfeldt ML: Simultaneous chest compression and ventilation at high airway pressure during cardiopulmonary resuscitation, *Lancet* 1:175-178, 1980.
53. Chandra N, Snyder LD, Weisfeldt ML: Abdominal binding during cardiopulmonary resuscitation in man, *JAMA* 246:351-353, 1981.
54. Chandra NC, et al: Observations of hemodynamics during human cardiopulmonary resuscitation, *Crit Care Med* 18:929-934, 1990.
55. Chase PB, et al: Effects of graded doses of epinephrine on both noninvasive and invasive measures of myocardial perfusion and blood flow during cardiopulmonary resuscitation, *Crit Care Med* 21:413-419, 1993.
56. Chopp M, et al: Global cerebral ischemia and intracellular pH during hyperglycemia and hypoglycemia in cats, *Stroke* 19:1383-1387, 1988.
57. Cipolotti G, Paccagnella A, Simini G: Successful cardiopulmonary resuscitation using high doses of epinephrine, *Int J Cardiol* 33: 430-431, 1991.
58. Clark CB, et al: Pediatric transthoracic defibrillation: biphasic versus monophasic waveforms in an experimental model, *Resuscitation* 51:159-163, 2001.
59. Clark RE, et al: Nifedipine: a myocardial protective agent, *Am J Cardiol* 44:825-831, 1979.
60. Cohen TJ, et al: A comparison of active compression-decompression cardiopulmonary resuscitation with standard cardiopulmonary resuscitation for cardiac arrests occurring in the hospital, *N Engl J Med* 329:1918-1921, 1993.
61. Cohen TJ, et al: Active compression-decompression. A new method of cardiopulmonary resuscitation. Cardiopulmonary Resuscitation Working Group, *JAMA* 267:2916-2923, 1992.

62. Cohen TJ, et al: Active compression-decompression resuscitation: a novel method of cardiopulmonary resuscitation, *Am Heart J* 124: 1145-1150, 1992.
63. Cohen Y, et al: Stability of brain intracellular lactate and 31P-metabolite levels at reduced intracellular pH during prolonged hypercapnia in rats, *J Cereb Blood Flow Metab* 10:277-284, 1990.
64. Coumel P, Fidelle J: Amiodarone in the treatment of cardiac arrhythmias in children: one hundred thirty-five cases, *Am Heart J* 100(6 pt 2):1063-1069, 1980.
65. Coumel P, Lucet V, Do Ngoc D: The use of amiodarone in children, *Pacing Clin Electrophysiol* 6(5 pt 1):930-939, 1983.
66. Criley JM, Blaufuss AH, Kissel GL: Cough-induced cardiac compression. Self-administered form of cardiopulmonary resuscitation, *JAMA* 236:1246-1250, 1976.
67. Criley JM, et al: Modifications of cardiopulmonary resuscitation based on the cough, *Circulation* 74(6 pt 2):IV42-IV50, 1986.
68. Cruz B, Niemann JT: Experimental studies on precordial compression or defibrillation as initial interventions for ventricular fibrillation, *Crit Care Med* 28(11 suppl):N225-N227, 2000.
69. Cummins RO, et al: Low-energy biphasic waveform defibrillation: evidence-based review applied to emergency cardiovascular care guidelines: a statement for healthcare professionals from the American Heart Association Committee on Emergency Cardiovascular Care and the Subcommittees on Basic Life Support, Advanced Cardiac Life Support, and Pediatric Resuscitation, *Circulation* 97:1654-1667, 1998.
70. Daniels CJ, et al: Acute pulmonary toxicity in an infant from intravenous amiodarone, *Am J Cardiol* 80:1113-1116, 1997.
71. Darge K, et al: Internal jugular venous valves in children: high-resolution US findings, *Eur Radiol* 11:655-658, 2001.
72. De Maio VJ, SI, Vaillancourt C, Wells GA, Spaite DW, Nesbitt L: Locations of pediatric cardiac arrest: implications for public access defibrillation, *Can J Emerg Med* 6:173, 2004.
73. Deakin CD, et al: A comparison of transthoracic impedance using standard defibrillation paddles and self-adhesive defibrillation pads, *Resuscitation* 39:43-46, 1998.
74. Dean JM, et al: Age-related effects of compression rate and duration in cardiopulmonary resuscitation, *J Appl Physiol* 68:554-560, 1990.
75. Dean JM, et al: Age-related changes in chest geometry during cardiopulmonary resuscitation, *J Appl Physiol* 62:2212-2219, 1987.
76. Deshmukh HG, et al: Mechanism of blood flow generated by precordial compression during CPR. I. Studies on closed chest precordial compression, *Chest* 95:1092-1099, 1989.
77. Ditchey RV, Goto Y, Lindenfeld J: Myocardial oxygen requirements during experimental cardiopulmonary resuscitation, *Cardiovasc Res* 26:791-797, 1992.
78. Ditchey RV, Lindenfeld J: Failure of epinephrine to improve the balance between myocardial oxygen supply and demand during closed-chest resuscitation in dogs, *Circulation* 78:382-389, 1988.
79. Ditchey RV, Rubio-Perez A, Slinker BK: Beta-adrenergic blockade reduces myocardial injury during experimental cardiopulmonary resuscitation, *J Am Coll Cardiol* 24:804-812, 1994.
80. Ditchey RV, Slinker BK: Phenylephrine plus propranolol improves the balance between myocardial oxygen supply and demand during experimental cardiopulmonary resuscitation, *Am Heart J* 127: 324-330, 1994.
81. Dorian P, et al: Amiodarone as compared with lidocaine for shock-resistant ventricular fibrillation, *N Engl J Med* 346:884-890, 2002.
82. Duncan BW, et al: Use of rapid-deployment extracorporeal membrane oxygenation for the resuscitation of pediatric patients with heart disease after cardiac arrest, *J Thorac Cardiovasc Surg* 116:305-311, 1998.
83. Eberle B, SC, Shaffner DH, et al: Effects of three models of abdominal compression on vital organ blood flow in piglet CPR model, *Anesthesiology* 73:A300, 1990.
84. Einagle V, et al: Interposed abdominal compressions and carotid blood flow during cardiopulmonary resuscitation. Support for a thoracoabdominal unit, *Chest* 93:1206-1212, 1988.
85. Eisenberg M, Bergner L, Hallstrom A: Epidemiology of cardiac arrest and resuscitation in children, *Ann Emerg Med* 12:672-674, 1983.
86. Eleff SM, et al: Brain bioenergetics during cardiopulmonary resuscitation in dogs, *Anesthesiology* 76:77-84, 1992.
87. Eleff SM, et al: Acidemia and brain pH during prolonged cardiopulmonary resuscitation in dogs, *Stroke* 26:1028-1034, 1995.
88. Elvira JC, et al: Active compression-decompression cardiopulmonary resuscitation in standing position over the patient (ACD-S), kneeling beside the patient (ACD-B), and standard CPR: comparison of physiological and efficacy parameters, Resuscitation 37:153-160, 1998.
89. Engdahl J, et al: The epidemiology of cardiac arrest in children and young adults, Resuscitation 58:131-138, 2003.
90. Etheridge SP, Craig JE, Compton SJ: Amiodarone is safe and highly effective therapy for supraventricular tachycardia in infants, Am Heart J 141:105-110, 2001.
91. Faddy SC, Powell J, Craig JC: Biphasic and monophasic shocks for transthoracic defibrillation: a meta analysis of randomised controlled trials, Resuscitation 58:9-16, 2003.
92. Falk JL, Rackow EC, Weil MH: End-tidal carbon dioxide concentration during cardiopulmonary resuscitation, N Engl J Med 318: 607-611, 1988.
93. Feneley MP, et al: Influence of compression rate on initial success of resuscitation and 24 hour survival after prolonged manual cardiopulmonary resuscitation in dogs, Circulation 77:240-250, 1988.
94. Figa FH, et al: Clinical efficacy and safety of intravenous amiodarone in infants and children, Am J Cardiol 74:573-577, 1994.
95. Fleisher G, Delgado-Paredes C, Heyman S: Slow versus rapid closed-chest cardiac compression during cardiopulmonary resuscitation in puppies, Crit Care Med 15:939-943, 1987.
96. Frascone RJ, Bitz D, Lurie K: Combination of active compression decompression cardiopulmonary resuscitation and the inspiratory impedance threshold device: state of the art, Curr Opin Crit Care 10:193-201, 2004.
97. Gazmuri RJ, et al: Cardiac effects of carbon dioxide-consuming and carbon dioxide-generating buffers during cardiopulmonary resuscitation, *J Am Coll Cardiol* 15:482-490, 1990.
98. Gervais HW, et al: Effect of adrenergic drugs on cerebral blood flow, metabolism, and evoked potentials after delayed cardiopulmonary resuscitation in dogs, *Stroke* 22:1554-1561, 1991.
99. Gilman AG, RT, Nies AS, et al: *Goodman and Gilman's the pharmacological basis of therapeutics*. New York, 1990, Pergamon Press.
100. Goetting MG, Paradis NA: High dose epinephrine in refractory pediatric cardiac arrest, *Crit Care Med* 17:1258-1262, 1989.
101. Gonzalez ER, et al: Dose-dependent vasopressor response to epinephrine during CPR in human beings, *Ann Emerg Med* 18:920-926, 1989.
102. Gonzalez ER, Ornato JP, Levine RL: Vasopressor effect of epinephrine with and without dopamine during cardiopulmonary resuscitation, *Drug Intell Clin Pharm* 22:868-872, 1988.
103. Grundler W, Weil MH, Rackow EC: Arteriovenous carbon dioxide and pH gradients during cardiac arrest, *Circulation* 74:1071-1074, 1986.
104. Gudipati CV, WM, Deshmukah HG, et al: Right atrial-jugular venous pressure gradients during experimental CPR, *Chest* 89:443S, 1986.
105. Guerci AD, Chandra N, Johnson E, et al: Failure of sodium bicarbonate to improve resuscitation from ventricular fibrillation in dogs, *Circulation* 74:IV75, 1986.
106. Guerci AD, et al: Transmission of intrathoracic pressure to the intracranial space during cardiopulmonary resuscitation in dogs, *Circ Res* 56:20-30, 1985.
107. Gurnett CA, Atkins DL: Successful use of a biphasic waveform automated external defibrillator in a high-risk child, *Am J Cardiol* 86:1051-1053, 2000.
108. Gutgesell HP, et al: Energy dose for ventricular defibrillation of children, *Pediatrics* 58:898-901, 1976.
109. Hackl W, et al: Echocardiographic assessment of mitral valve function during mechanical cardiopulmonary resuscitation in pigs, *Anesth Analg* 70:350-356, 1990.
110. Halperin HR, et al: Vest inflation without simultaneous ventilation during cardiac arrest in dogs: improved survival from prolonged cardiopulmonary resuscitation, *Circulation* 74:1407-1415, 1986.
111. Halperin HR, et al: Intrathoracic pressure fluctuations move blood during CPR: comparison of hemodynamic data with predictions from a mathematical model, *Ann Biomed Eng* 15:385-403, 1987.
112. Halperin HR, et al: A preliminary study of cardiopulmonary resuscitation by circumferential compression of the chest with use of a pneumatic vest, *N Engl J Med* 329:762-768, 1993.

113. Halperin HR, et al: Determinants of blood flow to vital organs during cardiopulmonary resuscitation in dogs, *Circulation* 73: 539-550, 1986.
114. Hedges JR, et al: Prehospital transcutaneous cardiac pacing for symptomatic bradycardia, *Pacing Clin Electrophysiol* 14: 1473-1478, 1991.
115. Hedges JR, et al: Prehospital trial of emergency transcutaneous cardiac pacing, *Circulation* 76:1337-1343, 1987.
116. Hoekstra JW, et al: Effect of standard-dose versus high-dose epinephrine on myocardial high-energy phosphates during ventricular fibrillation and closed-chest CPR, *Ann Emerg Med* 22:1385-1391, 1993.
117. Holmes CL, Landry DW, Granton JT: Science review: vasopressin and the cardiovascular system part 1—receptor physiology, *Crit Care* 7:427-434, 2003.
118. Holmes CL, Landry DW, Granton GT: Science review: vasopressin and the cardiovascular system part 2—clinical physiology, *Crit Care* 8:15-23, 2004.
119. Holthoff V, et al: Effect of nimodipine on glucose metabolism in the course of ischemic stroke, *Stroke* 21(12 suppl):IV95-IV97, 1990.
120. Howard M, et al: Interposed abdominal compression-CPR: its effects on parameters of coronary perfusion in human subjects, *Ann Emerg Med* 16:253-259, 1987.
121. Jacobs IG, et al: Energy levels for biphasic defibrillation, *Med J Aust* 179:451, 2003.
122. Jafari-Fesharaki M, Scheinman MM: Adverse effects of amiodarone, *Pacing Clin Electrophysiol* 21(1 pt 1):108-120, 1998.
123. Jessurun GA, Boersma WG, Crijns HJ: Amiodarone-induced pulmonary toxicity. Predisposing factors, clinical symptoms and treatment, *Drug Saf* 18:339-344, 1998.
124. Kerber RE, et al: Experimental evaluation and initial clinical application of new self-adhesive defibrillation electrodes, *Int J Cardiol* 8:57-66, 1985.
125. Kerber RE, et al: Self-adhesive preapplied electrode pads for defibrillation and cardioversion, *J Am Coll Cardiol* 3:815-820, 1984.
126. Kern KB, et al: Depletion of myocardial adenosine triphosphate during prolonged untreated ventricular fibrillation: effect on defibrillation success, *Resuscitation* 20:221-229, 1990.
127. Kern KB, Sanders AB, Ewy GA: Open-chest cardiac massage after closed-chest compression in a canine model: when to intervene, *Resuscitation* 15:51-57, 1987.
128. Koehler RC, et al: Augmentation of cerebral perfusion by simultaneous chest compression and lung inflation with abdominal binding after cardiac arrest in dogs, *Circulation* 67:266-275, 1983.
129. Kolarova J, et al: Optimal timing for electrical defibrillation after prolonged untreated ventricular fibrillation, *Crit Care Med* 31:2022-2028, 2003.
130. Kouwenhoven WB, Jude JR, Knickerbocker GG: Closed-chest cardiac massage, *JAMA* 173:1064-1067, 1960.
131. Krischer JP, et al: Comparison of prehospital conventional and simultaneous compression-ventilation cardiopulmonary resuscitation, *Crit Care Med* 17:1263-1269, 1989.
132. Kuisma M, Suominen P, Korpela R: Paediatric out-of-hospital cardiac arrests—epidemiology and outcome, *Resuscitation* 30: 141-150, 1995.
133. Lafuente-Lafuente C, Melero-Bascones M: Active chest compression-decompression for cardiopulmonary resuscitation, *Cochrane Database Syst Rev* CD002751, 2002.
134. Laird WP, et al: Use of intravenous amiodarone for postoperative junctional ectopic tachycardia in children, *Pediatr Cardiol* 24: 133-137, 2003.
135. Landry DW, Oliver JA: The pathogenesis of vasodilatory shock, *N Engl J Med* 345:588-595, 2001.
136. LeBlanc MH, et al: Glucose given after hypoxic ischemia does not affect brain injury in piglets, *Stroke* 25:1443-1447, 1994; discussion 1448.
137. Lehnart SE, et al: Sudden death in familial polymorphic ventricular tachycardia associated with calcium release channel (ryanodine receptor) leak, *Circulation* 109:3208-3214, 2004.
138. Levine R, et al: Cardiopulmonary bypass after cardiac arrest and prolonged closed-chest CPR in dogs, *Ann Emerg Med* 16:620-627, 1987.
139. Lindner KH, et al: Effect of vasopressin on hemodynamic variables, organ blood flow, and acid-base status in a pig model of cardiopulmonary resuscitation, *Anesth Analg* 77:427-435, 1993.
140. Lindner KH, et al: Randomised comparison of epinephrine and vasopressin in patients with out-of-hospital ventricular fibrillation, *Lancet* 349:535-537, 1997.
141. Lindner KH, et al: Effects of active compression-decompression resuscitation on myocardial and cerebral blood flow in pigs, *Circulation* 88:1254-1263, 1993.
142. Lindner KH, et al: Vasopressin improves vital organ blood flow during closed-chest cardiopulmonary resuscitation in pigs, *Circulation* 91:215-221, 1995.
143. Lindner KH, et al: Stress hormone response during and after cardiopulmonary resuscitation, *Anesthesiology* 77:662-668, 1992.
144. Livesay JJ, et al: Optimizing myocardial supply/demand balance with alpha-adrenergic drugs during cardiopulmonary resuscitation, *J Thorac Cardiovasc Surg* 76:244-251, 1978.
145. Longstreth WT Jr, et al: Neurologic outcome and blood glucose levels during out-of-hospital cardiopulmonary resuscitation, *Neurology* 36:1186-1191, 1986.
146. Lurie KG, et al: Improving active compression-decompression cardiopulmonary resuscitation with an inspiratory impedance valve, *Circulation* 91:1629-1632, 1995.
147. Lurie KG, et al: Evaluation of active compression-decompression CPR in victims of out-of-hospital cardiac arrest, *JAMA* 271: 1405-1411, 1994.
148. Lurie KG, et al: Combination drug therapy with vasopressin, adrenaline (epinephrine) and nitroglycerin improves vital organ blood flow in a porcine model of ventricular fibrillation, *Resuscitation* 54:187-194, 2002.
149. Mackenzie GJ, et al: Haemodynamic effects of external cardiac compression, *Lancet* 18:1342-1345, 1964.
150. Harmon JV Jr, Edwards WD: Venous valves in subclavian and jugular veins. Frequency, position and structure in 100 autopsy cases, *Am J Cardiovasc Pathol* 1:51-54, 1987.
151. Martin D, Werman HA, Brown CG: Four case studies: high-dose epinephrine in cardiac arrest, *Ann Emerg Med* 19:322-326, 1990.
152. Martin GB, et al: Effect of epinephrine on end-tidal carbon dioxide monitoring during CPR, *Ann Emerg Med* 19:396-398, 1990.
153. Mateer JR, et al: Pre-hospital IAC-CPR versus standard CPR: paramedic resuscitation of cardiac arrests, *Am J Emerg Med* 3: 143-146, 1985.
154. Michael JR, Guerci AD, Koehler RC: Mechanisms by which epinephrine augments cerebral and myocardial perfusion during cardiopulmonary resuscitation in dogs, *Circulation* 69:822-830, 1984.
155. Mogayzel C, et al: Out-of-hospital ventricular fibrillation in children and adolescents: causes and outcomes, *Ann Emerg Med* 25: 484-491, 1995.
156. Moler FW: Resuscitation research and the final rule: is there an impasse? *Pediatrics* 114:859-861, 2004.
157. Morales D, et al: Reversal by vasopressin of intractable hypotension in the late phase of hemorrhagic shock, *Circulation* 100: 226-229, 1999.
158. Morley P, Hogan MJ, Hakim AM: Calcium-mediated mechanisms of ischemic injury and protection, *Brain Pathol* 4:37-47, 1994.
159. Morris MC, et al: Exception from informed consent for pediatric resuscitation research: community consultation for a trial of brain cooling after in-hospital cardiac arrest, *Pediatrics* 114:776-781, 2004.
160. Morris MC, Wernovsky G, Nadkarni VM: Survival outcomes after extracorporeal cardiopulmonary resuscitation instituted during active chest compressions following refractory in-hospital pediatric cardiac arrest, *Pediatr Crit Care Med* 5:440-446, 2004.
161. Myers R:, Lactic acid accumulation as a cause of brain edema and cerebral necrosis resulting from oxygen deprivation. In GC Korbin R, editor: *Advances in perinatal neurology.* New York, 1979, Spectrum.
162. Niemann JT, et al: Immediate countershock versus cardiopulmonary resuscitation before countershock in a 5-minute swine model of ventricular fibrillation arrest, *Ann Emerg Med* 36:543-546, 2000.
163. Niemann JT, Rosborough JP, Pelikan PC: Hemodynamic determinants of subdiaphragmatic venous return during closed-chest CPR in a canine cardiac arrest model, *Ann Emerg Med* 19:1232-1237, 1990.
164. Niemann JT, et al: Hemodynamic effects of continuous abdominal binding during cardiac arrest and resuscitation, *Am J Cardiol* 53:269-274, 1984.

165. Noc M, et al: Ventricular fibrillation voltage as a monitor of the effectiveness of cardiopulmonary resuscitation, *J Lab Clin Med* 124:421-426, 1994.
166. Nof E, et al: A novel form of familial bidirectional ventricular tachycardia, *Am J Cardiol* 93:231-234, 2004.
167. Hwang SO, Lee KH, Cho JH, Yoon J, Choe KH: Changes of aortic dimension as evidence of cardiac pump mechanism during cardiopulmonary resuscitation in humans, *Resuscitation* 50:87-93, 2001.
168. O'Flaherty D, Adams AP: The end-tidal carbon dioxide detector. Assessment of a new method to distinguish oesophageal from tracheal intubation, *Anaesthesia* 45:653-655, 1990.
169. Ornato JP, et al: Effect of cardiopulmonary resuscitation compression rate on end-tidal carbon dioxide concentration and arterial pressure in man, *Crit Care Med* 16:241-245, 1988.
170. Paradis NA, et al: Simultaneous aortic, jugular bulb, and right atrial pressures during cardiopulmonary resuscitation in humans. Insights into mechanisms, *Circulation* 80:361-368, 1989.
171. Paradis NA, et al: Coronary perfusion pressure and the return of spontaneous circulation in human cardiopulmonary resuscitation, *JAMA* 263:1106-1113, 1990.
172. Parra DA, et al: Outcome of cardiopulmonary resuscitation in a pediatric cardiac intensive care unit, *Crit Care Med* 28:3296-3300, 2000.
173. Path GJ, et al: Effects of amiodarone with and without polysorbate 80 on myocardial oxygen consumption and coronary blood flow during treadmill exercise in the dog, *J Cardiovasc Pharmacol* 18:11-16, 1991.
174. Pearson JW, Redding JS: Epinephrine in cardiac resuscitation, *Am Heart J* 66:210-214, 1963.
175. Pepe PE, et al: Clinical review: reappraising the concept of immediate defibrillatory attempts for out-of-hospital ventricular fibrillation, *Crit Care* 8:41-45, 2004.
176. Perondi MB, et al: A comparison of high-dose and standard-dose epinephrine in children with cardiac arrest, *N Engl J Med* 350: 1722-1730, 2004.
177. Perry JC, et al: Pediatric use of intravenous amiodarone: efficacy and safety in critically ill patients from a multicenter protocol, *J Am Coll Cardiol* 27:1246-1250, 1996.
178. Pickoff AS, et al: Use of amiodarone in the therapy of primary ventricular arrhythmias in children, *Dev Pharmacol Ther* 6: 73-82, 1983.
179. Plaisance P, et al: A comparison of standard cardiopulmonary resuscitation and active compression-decompression resuscitation for out-of-hospital cardiac arrest. French Active Compression-Decompression Cardiopulmonary Resuscitation Study Group, *N Engl J Med* 341:569-575, 1999.
180. Plaisance P, et al: Evaluation of an impedance threshold device in patients receiving active compression-decompression cardiopulmonary resuscitation for out of hospital cardiac arrest, *Resuscitation* 61:265-271, 2004.
181. Polin K, Leikin JB: High-dose epinephrine in cardiopulmonary resuscitation. *JAMA* 269:1383, 1993; author reply 1383-1384.
182. Prado R, et al: Hyperglycemia increases infarct size in collaterally perfused but not end-arterial vascular territories, *J Cereb Blood Flow Metab* 8:186-192, 1988.
183. Prengel AW, et al: Cardiovascular function during the post-resuscitation phase after cardiac arrest in pigs: a comparison of epinephrine versus vasopressin, *Crit Care Med* 24:2014-2019, 1996.
184. Prengel AW, et al: Splanchnic and renal blood flow after cardiopulmonary resuscitation with epinephrine and vasopressin in pigs, *Resuscitation* 38:19-24, 1998.
185. Raedler C, et al: Vasopressor response in a porcine model of hypothermic cardiac arrest is improved with active compression-decompression cardiopulmonary resuscitation using the inspiratory impedance threshold valve, *Anesth Analg* 95:1496-502, 2002.
186. Redding JS, Pearson JW: Evaluation of drugs for cardiac resuscitation, *Anesthesiology* 24:203-207, 1963.
187. Reich H, et al: Cardiac resuscitability with cardiopulmonary bypass after increasing ventricular fibrillation times in dogs, *Ann Emerg Med* 19:887-890, 1990.
188. Reis AG, et al: A prospective investigation into the epidemiology of in-hospital pediatric cardiopulmonary resuscitation using the international Utstein reporting style, *Pediatrics* 109:200-209, 2002.
189. Resnekov L:, Calcium antagonist drugs—myocardial preservation and reduced vulnerability to ventricular fibrillation during CPR, *Crit Care Med* 9:360-361, 1981.
190. Rich S, Wix HL, Shapiro EP: Clinical assessment of heart chamber size and valve motion during cardiopulmonary resuscitation by two-dimensional echocardiography, *Am Heart J* 102(3 pt 1): 368-373, 1981.
191. Rivers EP, et al: The effect of the total cumulative epinephrine dose administered during human CPR on hemodynamic, oxygen transport, and utilization variables in the postresuscitation period, *Chest* 106:1499-1507, 1994.
192. Rogers MC, Nugent SK, Stidham GL: Effects of closed-chest cardiac massage on intracranial pressure, *Crit Care Med* 7: 454-456, 1979.
193. Rudolph AM, Yuan S: Response of the pulmonary vasculature to hypoxia and H+ ion concentration changes, *J Clin Invest* 45: 399-411, 1966.
194. Sacchetti A, et al: Primary cardiac arrhythmias in children, *Pediatr Emerg Care* 15:95-98, 1999.
195. Sack JB, Kesselbrenner MB, Bregman D: Survival from in-hospital cardiac arrest with interposed abdominal counterpulsation during cardiopulmonary resuscitation, *JAMA* 267:379-385, 1992.
196. Sack JB, Kesselbrenner MB, Jarrad A: Interposed abdominal compression-cardiopulmonary resuscitation and resuscitation outcome during asystole and electromechanical dissociation, *Circulation* 86:1692-1700, 1992.
197. Samson RA, Berg RA, Bingham R: Use of automated external defibrillators for children: an update—an advisory statement from the Pediatric Advanced Life Support Task Force, International Liaison Committee on Resuscitation, *Pediatrics* 112(1 pt 1): 163-168, 2003.
198. Sanders AB, et al: Failure of one method of simultaneous chest compression, ventilation, and abdominal binding during CPR, *Crit Care Med* 10:509-513, 1982.
199. Sanders AB, et al: Improved resuscitation from cardiac arrest with open-chest massage, *Ann Emerg Med* 13(9 pt 1):672-675, 1984.
200. Sanders AB, et al: End-tidal carbon dioxide monitoring during cardiopulmonary resuscitation. A prognostic indicator for survival, *JAMA* 262:1347-1351, 1989.
201. Sanders AB, Kern KB, Otto CW: The role of bicarbonate and fluid loading in improving resuscitation from prolonged cardiac arrest with rapid manual chest compression CPR, *Ann Emerg Med* 19: 1-8, 1990.
202. Schindler MB, et al: Outcome of out-of-hospital cardiac or respiratory arrest in children, *N Engl J Med* 335:1473-1479, 1996.
203. Schleien CL, et al: Controversial issues in cardiopulmonary resuscitation, *Anesthesiology* 71:133-149, 1989.
204. Schleien CL, et al: Effect of epinephrine on cerebral and myocardial perfusion in an infant animal preparation of cardiopulmonary resuscitation, *Circulation* 73:809-817, 1986.
205. Schleien CL, et al: Reduced blood-brain barrier permeability after cardiac arrest by conjugated superoxide dismutase and catalase in piglets, *Stroke* 25:1830-1834, 1994; discussion 1834-1835.
206. Schleien CL, et al: Organ blood flow and somatosensory-evoked potentials during and after cardiopulmonary resuscitation with epinephrine or phenylephrine, *Circulation* 79:1332-1342, 1989.
207. Schleien CL, et al: Blood-brain barrier disruption after cardiopulmonary resuscitation in immature swine, *Stroke* 22:477-483, 1991.
208. Schleien CL, et al: Blood-brain barrier integrity during cardiopulmonary resuscitation in dogs, *Stroke* 21:1185-1191, 1990.
209. Schneider T, et al: Multicenter, randomized, controlled trial of 150-J biphasic shocks compared with 200- to 360-J monophasic shocks in the resuscitation of out-of-hospital cardiac arrest victims. Optimized Response to Cardiac Arrest (ORCA) Investigators, *Circulation* 102:1780-1787, 2000.
210. Sessler D, et al: Effects of bicarbonate on arterial and brain intracellular pH in neonatal rabbits recovering from hypoxic lactic acidosis, *J Pediatr* 111(6 pt 1):817-823, 1987.
211. Shaffner DH, et al: Effect of vest cardiopulmonary resuscitation on cerebral and coronary perfusion in an infant porcine model, *Crit Care Med* 22:1817-1826, 1994.
212. Shultz JJ, et al: Evaluation of standard and active compression-decompression CPR in an acute human model of ventricular fibrillation, *Circulation* 89:684-693, 1994.
213. Siemkowicz E, Hansen AJ: Clinical restitution following cerebral ischemia in hypo-, normo- and hyperglycemic rats, *Acta Neurol Scand* 58:1-8, 1978.

214. Silvetti MS, et al: Amiodarone-induced torsade de pointes in a child with dilated cardiomyopathy, *Ital Heart J* 2:231-236, 2001.
215. Stacpoole PW: Lactic acidosis: the case against bicarbonate therapy, *Ann Intern Med* 105:276-279, 1986.
216. Stacpoole PW: The pharmacology of dichloroacetate, *Metabolism* 38:1124-1144, 1989.
217. Stacpoole PW, et al: Dichloroacetate derivatives. Metabolic effects and pharmacodynamics in normal rats, *Life Sci* 41:2167-2176, 1987.
218. Stacpoole PW, et al: Dichloroacetate in the treatment of lactic acidosis, *Ann Intern Med* 108:58-63, 1988.
219. Stacpoole PW, et al: A controlled clinical trial of dichloroacetate for treatment of lactic acidosis in adults. The Dichloroacetate-Lactic Acidosis Study Group, *N Engl J Med* 327:1564-1569, 1992.
220. Stadlbauer KH, et al: The effects of nifedipine on ventricular fibrillation mean frequency in a porcine model of prolonged cardiopulmonary resuscitation, *Anesth Analg* 97:226-230, 2003.
221. Sterz F, et al: Mild hypothermic cardiopulmonary resuscitation improves outcome after prolonged cardiac arrest in dogs, *Crit Care Med* 19:379-389, 1991.
222. Stiell IG, et al: High-dose epinephrine in adult cardiac arrest, *N Engl J Med* 327:1045-1050, 1992.
223. Sun JH, et al: Carbicarb: an effective substitute for NaHCO3 for the treatment of acidosis, *Surgery* 102:835-839, 1987.
224. Sun S, et al: alpha-Methylnorepinephrine, a selective alpha2-adrenergic agonist for cardiac resuscitation, *J Am Coll Cardiol* 37:951-956, 2001.
225. Swenson RD, et al: Hemodynamics in humans during conventional and experimental methods of cardiopulmonary resuscitation, *Circulation* 78:630-639, 1988.
226. Tang W, et al: Pulmonary ventilation/perfusion defects induced by epinephrine during cardiopulmonary resuscitation, *Circulation* 84:2101-2107, 1991.
227. Tang W, et al: Fixed-energy biphasic waveform defibrillation in a pediatric model of cardiac arrest and resuscitation, *Crit Care Med* 30:2736-2741, 2002.
228. Tang W, et al: The effects of biphasic waveform design on post-resuscitation myocardial function, *J Am Coll Cardiol* 43:1228-1235, 2004.
229. Tang W, et al: Epinephrine increases the severity of postresuscitation myocardial dysfunction, *Circulation* 92:3089-3093, 1995.
230. Topol EJ, CR, Isner J, et al., editors: *Textbook of cardiovascular medicine.* Baltimore, 2002, Lippincott, Williams & Wilkins.
231. Urban P, et al: Cardiac arrest and blood ionized calcium levels, *Ann Intern Med* 109:110-113, 1988.
232. Urban P, et al: The hemodynamic effects of heparin and their relation to ionized calcium levels, *J Thorac Cardiovasc Surg* 91:303-306, 1986.
233. Voelckel WG, et al: Effects of epinephrine and vasopressin in a piglet model of prolonged ventricular fibrillation and cardiopulmonary resuscitation, *Crit Care Med* 30:957-962, 2002.
234. Voelckel WG, et al: Effects of active compression-decompression cardiopulmonary resuscitation with the inspiratory threshold valve in a young porcine model of cardiac arrest, *Pediatr Res* 51:523-527, 2002.
235. Voelckel WG, et al: The effects of positive end-expiratory pressure during active compression decompression cardiopulmonary resuscitation with the inspiratory threshold valve, *Anesth Analg* 92:967-974, 2001.
236. Voll CL, Auer RN: The effect of postischemic blood glucose levels on ischemic brain damage in the rat, *Ann Neurol* 24:638-646, 1988.
237. Voll CL, Auer RN: Insulin attenuates ischemic brain damage independent of its hypoglycemic effect, *J Cereb Blood Flow Metab* 11:1006-1014, 1991.
238. von Planta I, et al: Coronary perfusion pressure, end-tidal CO2 and adrenergic agents in haemodynamic stable rats, *Resuscitation* 25:203-217, 1993.
239. Ward KR, et al: A comparison of interposed abdominal compression CPR and standard CPR by monitoring end-tidal PCO2, *Ann Emerg Med* 18:831-837, 1989.
240. Wargovich TJ, et al: Myocardial metabolic and hemodynamic effects of dichloroacetate in coronary artery disease, *Am J Cardiol* 61:65-70, 1988.
241. Weil MH, et al: Difference in acid-base state between venous and arterial blood during cardiopulmonary resuscitation, *N Engl J Med* 315:153-156, 1986.
242. Wenzel V, et al: A comparison of vasopressin and epinephrine for out-of-hospital cardiopulmonary resuscitation, *N Engl J Med* 350:105-113, 2004.
243. White BC, et al: Possible role of calcium blockers in cerebral resuscitation: a review of the literature and synthesis for future studies, *Crit Care Med* 11:202-207, 1983.
244. Wik L, et al: Delaying defibrillation to give basic cardiopulmonary resuscitation to patients with out-of-hospital ventricular fibrillation: a randomized trial, *JAMA* 289:1389-1395, 2003.
245. Woo E, et al: Admission glucose level in relation to mortality and morbidity outcome in 252 stroke patients, *Stroke* 19:185-191, 1988.
246. Xavier L, et al: Comparison of standard CPR versus diffuse and stacked hand position interposed abdominal compression-CPR in a swine model, *Resuscitation* 59:337-344, 2003.
247. Yakaitis RW, Otto CW, Blitt CD: Relative importance of alpha and beta adrenergic receptors during resuscitation, *Crit Care Med* 7:293-296, 1979.
248. Yanagawa Y, et al: Preliminary clinical outcome study of mild resuscitative hypothermia after out-of-hospital cardiopulmonary arrest, *Resuscitation* 39:61-66, 1998.
249. Yu T, et al: Adverse outcomes of interrupted precordial compression during automated defibrillation, *Circulation* 106:368-372, 2002.
250. Zoll PM: Resuscitation of the heart in ventricular standstill by external electric stimulation, *N Engl J Med* 247:768-771, 1952.
251. Zoll PM, et al: External noninvasive temporary cardiac pacing: clinical trials, *Circulation* 71:937-944, 1985.

CHAPTER

119

Pediatric Cardiopulmonary Resuscitation

Robert A. Berg, Arno Zaritsky, and Vinay Nadkarni

PEARLS

- Appropriate pediatric cardiopulmonary resuscitation (CPR) differs from that in adults because children are anatomically and physiologically different from adults.
- The four distinct phases of cardiac arrest and CPR are:
  Prearrest
  No flow
  Low flow
  Postresuscitation
- The most common precipitating event for cardiac arrests in children is respiratory insufficiency; adequate ventilation and oxygenation remain the first priority.
- Excellent standard closed-chest CPR generates cerebral blood flow that is approximately 50% of normal.
- Routine use of sodium bicarbonate for a child in cardiac arrest is not recommended.
- The attitude that ventricular fibrillation is rare in children can be a self-fulfilling prophecy with a uniformly fatal outcome.
- Strategically focused therapies to specific phases of cardiac arrest and resuscitation can lead to more successful CPR in children.

Cardiovascular disease remains the most common cause of disease-related death in the United States, resulting in approximately one million deaths per year. It is estimated that more than 400,000 Americans will suffer a cardiac arrest each year, nearly 90% in prehospital settings. Data regarding the incidence of childhood cardiopulmonary arrest is less robust, but the best data suggest that ≈16,000 American children suffer a cardiac arrest each year, with an annual incidence of ≈20/100,000 children. This chapter focuses on in-hospital pediatric cardiac arrest and cardiopulmonary resuscitation (CPR). Approximately 2% of children admitted to pediatric intensive care units have a cardiac arrest.[17]

Appropriate pediatric CPR differs from that in adults because children are anatomically and physiologically different from adults. In addition, the pathogenesis of cardiac arrests and the most common rhythm disturbances are different in children. In contrast to adults, children rarely suffer sudden ventricular fibrillation (VF) cardiac arrest from coronary artery disease. The causes of pediatric arrests are more diverse and usually are secondary to profound hypoxia or asphyxia resulting from respiratory failure or circulatory shock, which impair cardiac function and ultimately lead to cardiac arrest. By the time the arrest occurs, all organs of the body have generally suffered significant hypoxic-ischemic insults.

Importantly, children of various ages exhibit developmental changes that affect cardiac and respiratory physiology before, during, and after cardiac arrest. For example, newborns undergoing transitional physiologic changes during emergence from an environment of amniotic fluid to a gaseous environment certainly differ from adolescents.

Similarly, newborns and infants have much less cardiac and respiratory reserve and higher pulmonary vascular resistance than older children. Many children who experience in-hospital cardiac arrest have preexisting developmental challenges and other organ dysfunction.

Four Phases of Cardiac Arrest

The four distinct phases of cardiac arrest and CPR interventions (1) prearrest, (2) no flow (untreated cardiac arrest), (3) low flow (CPR), and (4) postresuscitation. Interventions to improve outcome of pediatric cardiac arrest should optimize therapies targeted to the time and phase of CPR, as suggested in Table 119–1.

The *prearrest* phase refers to relevant preexisting conditions (e.g., neurologic, cardiac, respiratory, or metabolic problems), developmental status, and precipitating events (e.g., respiratory failure or shock). It may represent a period of low, normal, or high blood flow. Interventions during the prearrest phase focus on preventing the cardiac arrest, with special attention to early recognition and treatment of respiratory failure and shock in children. In-hospital patients at high risk for a cardiac arrest generally should be in a monitored unit. Although data are limited in children, in-hospital medical emergency response teams have reduced the risk of cardiac arrest in hospitalized adult patients.[175,176]

Important factors in determining outcome from cardiac arrest are minimizing the *no-flow* phase of untreated cardiac arrest by monitoring high-risk patients, early recognition of the cardiac arrest, and prompt initiation of basic and advanced life support. Effective CPR optimizes coronary perfusion pressure and cardiac output to critical organs to support vital organ viability during the low flow phase. Important tenets of basic life support are *push hard, push fast,* and minimize interruptions of chest compression. Achieving optimal coronary perfusion pressure, exhaled carbon dioxide concentration, and cardiac output during the low-flow phase of CPR is consistently associated with an improved chance for return of spontaneous circulation (ROSC) and improved short- and long-term outcome. For VF and pulseless ventricular tachycardia (VT), rapid detection and prompt defibrillation are most important for successful resuscitation. For cardiac arrests resulting from asphyxia and/or ischemia, provision of adequate myocardial perfusion and myocardial oxygen delivery are most important.

The *postresuscitation* phase includes management of the *immediate postresuscitation* stage, the *next few hours to days,* and long-term *rehabilitation.* The immediate postresuscitation stage is a high-risk period for ventricular arrhythmias and other reperfusion injuries. Interventions during the immediate postresuscitation stage and the next few days include adequate tissue oxygen delivery, treatment of postresuscitation myocardial dysfunction, and minimizing postresuscitation tissue injury (e.g., preventing postresuscitation hyperthermia and hypoglycemia and perhaps providing postresuscitation hypothermia). Injured cells can hibernate, die, or partially or fully recover function. Cell death can occur as a result of necrosis or apoptosis (i.e., programmed cell death). This postarrest phase may have the greatest potential for innovative advances in the understanding of cell injury and death, inflammation, apoptosis, and hibernation, ultimately leading to novel interventions. The rehabilitation stage concentrates on salvage of injured cells, recruitment of hibernating cells, and reengineering of reflex and voluntary communications of these cell and organ systems to improve functional outcome.

The specific phase of resuscitation dictates the focus of care. Interventions that improve outcome during one phase may be deleterious during another. For instance, intense vasoconstriction during the *low-flow* phase of cardiac arrest improves coronary perfusion pressure and

TABLE 119–1

Phase	Interventions
Prearrest phase (protect)	Optimize community education regarding child safety Optimize patient monitoring Prioritize interventions to prevent progression of respiratory failure and/or shock to cardiac arrest Early recognition and activation of medical emergency response teams (or their equivalent)
Arrest (no-flow) phase (preserve)	Minimize interval to BLS and ACLS Organized 911/code blue response system Preserve cardiac and cerebral substrate Minimize interval to defibrillation, when indicated
Low-flow (CPR) phase (resuscitate)	Effective CPR to optimize myocardial blood flow and cardiac output (coronary and cerebral perfusion pressures and maximize exhaled CO_2 concentration) and avoid overventilation Consider adjuncts to improve vital organ perfusion during CPR Match oxygen delivery to oxygen demand (how?) Consider extracorporeal CPR if standard CPR/ALS are not promptly successful in patient with possibility of meaningful recovery
Postresuscitation phase, immediate (hours to days)	Optimize cardiac output and cerebral perfusion Treat arrhythmias, if indicated Prevent hyperglycemia, hyperthermia Consider mild resuscitative systemic hypothermia (for 24–48 hours following resuscitation) Possible future role for antioxidants, anti-inflammatory agents, thrombolytics, mediators of hibernation, and modulation of excitatory neurotransmitters
Postresuscitation phase, longer-term rehabilitation (regenerate)	Early intervention with occupational and physical therapy Bioengineering and technology interface Possible future role for stem cell transplantation

the probability of ROSC. The same intense vasoconstriction during the *postresuscitation* phase increases left ventricular afterload and may worsen myocardial strain and dysfunction. Current understanding of the physiology of cardiac arrest and recovery encourages us to crudely manipulate blood pressure, oxygen delivery and consumption, body temperature, inflammation, coagulation, and other physiologic parameters to optimize outcome. Future strategies likely will take advantage of increasing knowledge of cellular inflammation, thrombosis, reperfusion, mediator cascades, cellular markers of injury and recovery, and transplantation technology.

An overview of some of the pathophysiologic pathways perturbed by cardiac arrest and resuscitation, along with potential avenues for intervention, is shown in Figure 119–1.

Epidemiology of In-hospital Cardiac Arrest

The true incidence of pediatric pulseless arrest is difficult to estimate because of inconsistent terminology in the literature and the difficulty in assessing pulselessness in children. It is estimated that 5% of newborn infants require some degree of basic life support in the delivery room but that only 0.12% require chest compressions and/or administration of epinephrine.[14] Neonatal asphyxia accounts for one million deaths per year worldwide. Cardiac arrest occurred in 3% of children admitted to one children's hospital, in 1.8% of all children admitted to pediatric intensive care units,[17] and in 6% of children admitted to a pediatric cardiac intensive care unit.[177]

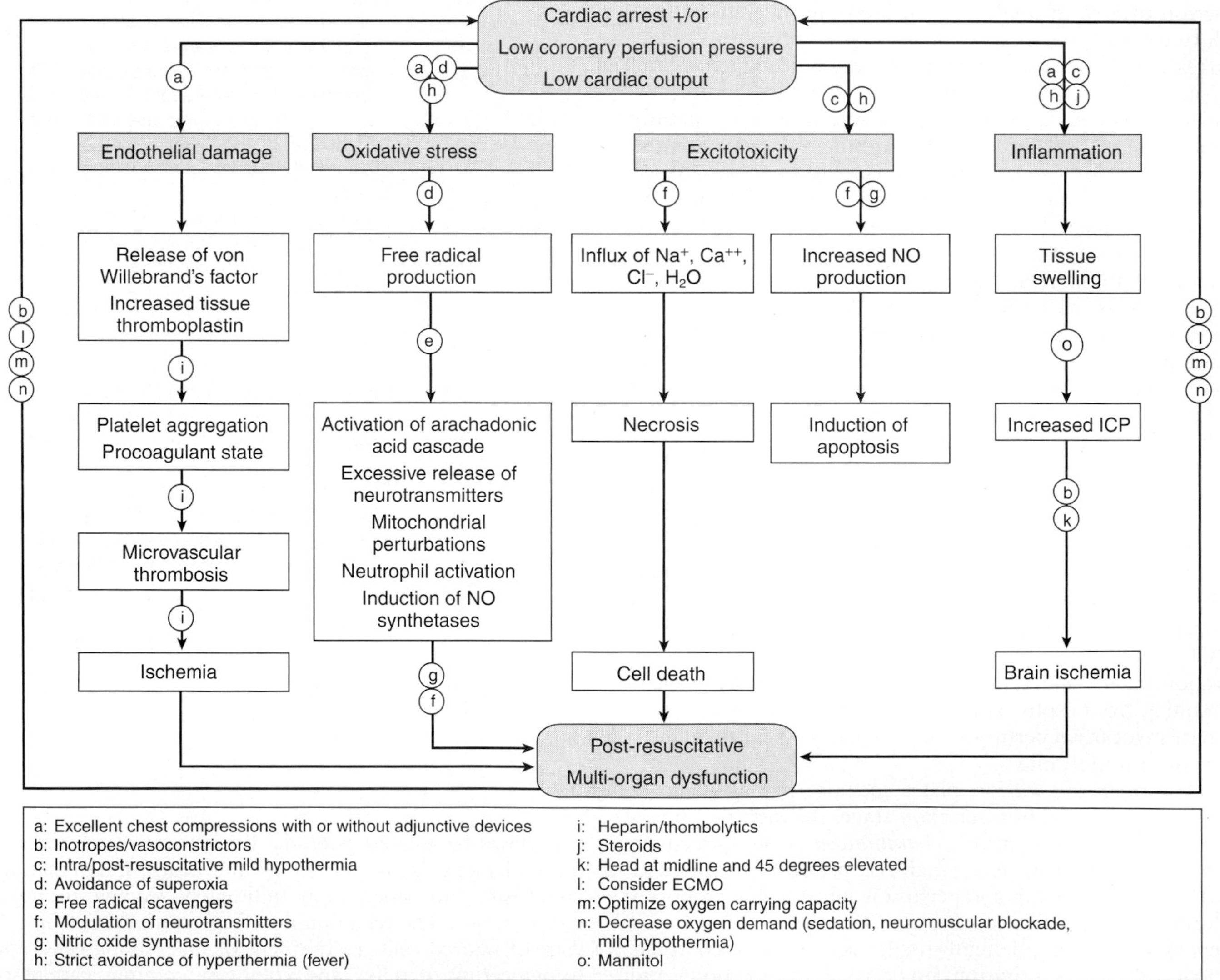

FIGURE 119–1 • Schematic of physiologic processes that result from cardiac arrest and initial resuscitation, with some promising interventions indicated by *lower case letters.* Many complex interconnections and feedback loops among these processes are omitted from the schematic in order to generate an overview of the processes and potential interventions. *a,* Excellent chest compressions with or without adjunctive devices; *b,* inotropes/vasoconstrictors; *c,* intra/postresuscitative mild hypothermia; *d,* avoidance of superoxia; *e,* free radical scavengers; *f,* modulation of neurotransmitters; *g,* nitric oxide (NO) synthase inhibitors; *h,* strict avoidance of hyperthermia (fever); *i,* heparin/thombolytics; *j,* steroids; *k,* head at midline and 45 degrees elevated; *l,* consider extracorporeal membrane oxygenation; *m,* optimize oxygen-carrying capacity; *n,* decrease oxygen demand (sedation, neuromuscular blockade, mild hypothermia); *o,* mannitol.

Several well-designed in-hospital pediatric CPR investigations with long-term follow-up have established that pediatric CPR and advanced life support can be remarkably effective (Table 119–2). Nearly two thirds of these patients initially were successfully resuscitated (i.e., attained sustained ROSC). Survival progressively decreased with time, in large part because of the underlying disease processes. Most of these arrests/events occurred in pediatric intensive care units as a result of progressive life-threatening illnesses that did not respond to treatment despite critical care monitoring and supportive care. The 1-year survival rates of 10% to 44% are superior to outcomes from out-of-hospital pediatric CPR and substantially superior to the certain 0% survival rate if CPR and advanced life support were not provided. The most recent data report 20% to 27% survival-to-hospital discharge rates, suggesting that outcomes improved compared with earlier studies with typically 5% to 15% survival-to-hospital discharge. Most importantly, the vast majority of survivors had good neurologic outcomes (i.e., normal or no demonstrable change in neurologic status compared with prearrest).

The National Registry of Cardiopulmonary Resuscitation (NRCPR) is an American Heart Association-sponsored, prospective, multisite, observational data collection instrument of in-hospital resuscitation, which currently is the largest registry of its kind in the world (*www.NRCPR.org*). Among the first 880 children in this registry, the initial electrocardiographic rhythm was VF/pulseless VT in 14%, asystole in 40%, and pulseless electrical activity in 24%; the initial rhythm was not reported in the remaining patients. Interestingly, another 200 children received CPR for severe bradycardia with

TABLE 119–2

Summary of Representative Studies of Outcome Following Pediatric Cardiac Arrest

Author, Year, Reference No.	Setting	No. of Patients	Return of Spontaneous Circulation (ROSC)	Survival to Discharge	Intact Neurologic Survival
Extracorporeal Life Support Organization, 2002[168]	In-hospital resuscitation from CA via ECMO	232	Included only patients successfully resuscitated via ECMO	88 (38%)	Not reported
NRCPR, 2002[169]	In-hospital CA	286	119 (42%)	65 (23%)	44 (15%)
Reis, 2002[16]	In-hospital CA	129	83 (64%)	21 (16%)	19 (15%)
Chamnanvanakij, 2000[167]	In-hospital intubated neonatal ICU patients who received chest compressions secondary to bradycardia	39	33/39 (85%)	20/39 (51%) overall; 9.5% of cardiac arrest patients	5 (13%) (6 additional patients lost to follow-up)
Gausche, 2000[21]	Out-of-hospital RA	820	N/A	233 (28%)	177 (22%)
Parra, 2000[18]	Pediatric cardiac ICU CA	32	24/38 arrests (63%)	14/32 patients (44%)	8/32 (25%)
Sirbaugh, 1999[19]	Out-of-hospital CA	300	33 (11%)	6 (2%)	1 (<1%)
Young, 1999[98]	Meta-analysis mixed in and out of hospital	Out-of-hospital CA: 1568 In-hospital CA: 544	Not reported	Out-of-hospital: 132 (8.4%) In-hospital: 129 (24%)	Not reported
Suominen, 1998[171]	Out-of-hospital CA in trauma patients	41	10 (24%)	3 (7%)	2 (5%)
Slonim, 1997[17]	In-hospital pediatric ICU CA	205	Not reported	28 (14%)	Not reported
Suominen, 1997[172]	Out-of-hospital CA	50	13 (26%)	8 (16%)	6 (12%)
Schindler, 1996[170]	Out-of-hospital RA or CA	101	64 (64%)	15 (15%)	0 (0%) of CA patients
Dieckmann, 1995[101]	Out-of-hospital CA	65	3 (5%)	2 (3%)	1 (1.5%)
Kuisma, 1995[8]	Out-of-hospital CA	34	10 (29%)	5 (15%)	4 (12%)
Tunstall-Pedoe, 1992[173]	In-hospital and out-of-hospital CA	3765	1411 (38%)	706 (19%)	Not reported
Zaritsky, 1987[174]	In-hospital RA or CA	CA 53 RA 40	Not reported	CA 5 (9%) RA 27 (68%)	Not reported

CA, cardiac arrest; *ECMO*, extracorporeal membrane oxygenation; *ICU*, intensive care unit; *NRCPR*, National Registry of Cardiopulmonary Resuscitation; *RA*, respiratory arrest.

pulses (i.e., at an earlier stage of the hypoxic-ischemic event). Sixty-five percent of the pulseless cardiac arrests occurred in an ICU, and 95% were witnessed and/or monitored. Twenty-seven percent survived to hospital discharge, and 81% had good neurologic outcomes or no deterioration from their neurologic baseline prior to hospital admission. In this large, multicenter in-hospital cardiac arrest database, children survived to hospital discharge more frequently following cardiac arrest than did adults (27% survival vs. 18% survival), predominantly because of better outcomes following asystole and pulseless electrical activity.

Interventions During the LOW-FLOW Phase: Cardiopulmonary Resuscitation

Airway and Breathing

The most common precipitating event for cardiac arrest in children is respiratory insufficiency. Therefore providing adequate ventilation and oxygenation remains the first priority. Effective ventilation does not necessarily require an endotracheal tube. One randomized, controlled study comparing outcomes of children with out-of-hospital respiratory arrest who received bag-mask ventilation compared with bag-mask ventilation followed by endotracheal intubation did not demonstrate that prehospital placement of a tracheal tube improves outcome.

Airway adjuncts such as pediatric laryngeal mask airways are available in most hospital settings. Their use may be considered for the patient in whom tracheal intubation is not immediately feasible. Pediatric emergency, critical care, and anesthesia physicians should be comfortable with their use. Emergency airway techniques such as transtracheal jet ventilation and emergency cricothyroidotomy are rarely, if ever, required during CPR. Effective bag-mask ventilation skills remain the cornerstone of providing effective emergency ventilation.

Provision of oxygen and adequate ventilation to normalize arterial oxygen content and remove carbon dioxide is the goal of initial assisted breathing. During CPR, cardiac output and pulmonary blood flow are approximately less than 33% of that during normal sinus rhythm. Consequently, much less ventilation is necessary for adequate gas exchange from the blood traversing the pulmonary circulation during CPR.

Cardiopulmonary interactions can have profound effects in the low-flow state of CPR. Animal and adult data indicate that a rapid rate of assisted ventilation (overexuberant rescue breathing) during CPR is common and can substantially compromise venous return and cardiac output. The adverse hemodynamic effects from ventilation during CPR plus the interruptions in chest compressions to open the airway and deliver rescue breathing can be a lethal combination.

End-Tidal Carbon Dioxide Monitoring During Cardiopulmonary Resuscitation

The magnitude of exhaled carbon dioxide (CO_2) during cardiac arrest depends largely upon pulmonary blood flow because the pulmonary artery blood typically has a high partial pressure of CO_2. Thus circulation generated by chest compressions can be assessed to an extent by measuring exhaled CO_2. Chest compressions can be titrated to exhaled CO_2 as an index of pulmonary perfusion and cardiac output. In adults with cardiac arrest, an end-tidal CO_2 >10 torr is associated with ROSC and with hospital survival. In an animal model, end-tidal CO_2 during CPR correlates with coronary perfusion pressure and with ROSC. If CPR does not produce adequate flow, the low-flow and consequent low end-tidal CO_2 during CPR can create a "false-negative" qualitative test for exhaled CO_2, a test often used for secondary confirmation of endotracheal tube placement during CPR.

In pediatric animal models of asphyxial cardiac arrest, end-tidal CO_2 is high at the initiation of CPR (representing exhalation of alveolar CO_2 that accumulated in the tissues and venous system and was delivered to the lungs while the animals were apneic but not yet pulseless) and then falls to levels similar to those seen during adult CPR. Although end-tidal CO_2 monitoring may be useful during pediatric CPR, pediatric-specific data are limited.

Circulation

Optimizing Cardiac Output and Coronary and Cerebral Perfusion Pressures During Cardiopulmonary Resuscitation

Blood is circulated during CPR by at least two different mechanisms: the cardiac pump (direct compression of the heart between the sternum and the spine) and the thoracic pump (increases in intrathoracic pressure generating a gradient for blood to flow from the pulmonary vasculature, through the heart, and into the peripheral circulation). Using special techniques, cardiac output can be supplemented by superimposing an abdominal pump (abdominal compression forces arterial blood from the abdomen to the periphery against a closed aortic valve and forces venous blood from the inferior vena cava back to the heart). The cardiac pump mechanism predominates in young children because of the relatively compliant thoracic wall. In children from infancy through adolescence, the heart is immediately posterior to the lower third of the sternum, suggesting that focusing compressions in this area may optimize the cardiac pump in pediatric CPR.

Compression/Ventilation Ratios

Current compression/ventilation ratios and tidal volumes recommended during CPR are based upon rational conjecture, tradition, and educational retention theory. Recent physiologic estimates suggest that the amount of ventilation provided should match, but not exceed, perfusion and should be titrated to the amount of circulation during a phase of resuscitation (no flow, low flow, high flow) and metabolic demand of the tissues. From 2000 to 2005, Pediatric Advanced Life Support (PALS) recommended a ratio of chest compressions to ventilations in a child younger than 8 years of five chest compressions to one ventilation, with a chest compression rate of 100/minute. In children older than 8 years, 15 chest compressions to two ventilations were recommended, with the chest compression rate remaining at 100/minute. Further studies suggest interruptions of chest compressions and overventilation are common, and laboratory and manikin studies suggest that more continuous chest compressions and fewer ventilations may be appropriate.

Although *A*irway and *B*reathing are prioritized in the *ABC* algorithm, that priority has been challenged in certain circumstances. Coronary perfusion pressure (which correlates with ROSC) rises during sequential chest compressions and falls during ventilation. In adult cardiac arrest, increasing the number of chest compressions between ventilations to as high as 50 or eliminating ventilation during bystander CPR may result in better hemodynamics and increased rates of ROSC. In animal models of sudden VF cardiac arrest, acceptable Pao_2 and $Paco_2$ persist with sudden cardiac arrest for 4 to 8 minutes in the absence of any rescue breathing. A randomized, controlled study of dispatcher-assisted bystander CPR in adults found a trend toward improved survival in the patients who received chest compressions alone compared with those who received dispatcher-instructed ventilation and chest compressions.

Oxygenation and ventilation clearly are important for survival from fibrillatory cardiac arrest, so why is rescue breathing not necessary for so long in VF yet quite important in asphyxia? Immediately after an acute fibrillatory cardiac arrest, aortic oxygen and carbon dioxide concentrations do not vary from the prearrest state because there is no blood flow and aortic oxygen consumption is minimal. Therefore when chest compressions are initiated, the blood flowing from the aorta to the coronary circulation provides adequate oxygenation at an acceptable pH. At that time, myocardial oxygen delivery is limited more by blood flow than by oxygen content. Over the next several minutes, arterial oxygenation and pH become increasingly important for effective resuscitation. Adequate oxygenation and ventilation can continue without rescue breathing because of chest compression-induced gas exchange and spontaneous gasping ventilation during CPR in victims of sudden cardiac arrest. Rescue breathing is not necessary in VF arrests for up to 12 minutes because arterial oxygenation and pH can be adequate with chest compressions alone. Most importantly, myocardial oxygen delivery does not differ whether or not rescue breathing is provided, in part because rescue breathing may have adverse effects on hemodynamics.

During asphyxia, as opposed to VF, blood continues to flow to tissues, and arterial and venous oxygen saturation decrease while carbon dioxide and lactate continue to increase for many minutes. In addition, continued pulmonary blood flow before the cardiac arrest depletes the pulmonary oxygen reservoir. Therefore asphyxia results in significant arterial hypoxemia and acidemia prior to resuscitation, in contrast to VF.

Consequently, children with asphyxial cardiac arrests typically have a significantly higher $Paco_2$ and lower Pao_2 at the onset of cardiac arrest and following tracheal intubation during resuscitation from cardiac arrest than do adults. Because respiratory failure and asphyxia generally precede pediatric cardiac arrest, foregoing ventilation in the pediatric cardiac arrest patient is not prudent.

A mathematical model of oxygen delivery during CPR performed with variable ratios of chest compressions to ventilations revealed that with correctly delivered chest compressions and appropriate tidal volumes, the optimal compression/ventilation ratio is 30:2 in adults. When the model was adjusted using chest compressions as generally delivered by a lay rescuer (i.e., compressions that were suboptimal), the optimal compression/ventilation ratio was 60:2. Mathematical models of compression/ventilation ratios suggest that matching the amount of ventilation to the amount of reduced pulmonary blood flow during closed-chest cardiac compressions should favor a very high compression/ventilation ratio.

Babbs and Kern[28] suggest that the best way to determine compression/ventilation ratios is to choose one that maximizes oxygen delivery to peripheral tissues (or perhaps a combination of oxygen delivery and blood flow). Maximizing oxygen delivery to peripheral tissues during single-rescuer CPR requires a tradeoff between time spent doing chest compressions and time spent doing mouth-to-mouth ventilations. Theoretically (ignoring the small amount of ventilation caused by chest compressions) neither compression only nor ventilation only CPR can sustain oxygen delivery to the periphery. Some intermediate value of the compression/ventilation ratio is needed. The best intermediate value depends upon many factors, including the compression rate, tidal volume, blood flow generated by compressions, and time interval that compressions are interrupted to perform ventilations. These factors can be related in a simple mathematical formula based upon classic physiology. These variables necessarily change as a function patient size. Such considerations may help refine the amount of ventilation recommended for both adults and children. Similar calculations in a pediatric mathematical model of CPR suggest that a variable compression/ventilation ratio for infants and children may be appropriate.

In a mannequin model of pediatric CPR, a chest compression/ventilation ratio of 15:2 delivered the same minute ventilation as CPR with a chest compression/ventilation ratio of 5:1, but the number of chest compressions delivered was 48% higher with the 15:2 ratio. This somewhat surprising observation was the result of the time interval of no compression or ventilation when the rescuer moved between delivering compressions and ventilation. The ratio of chest compressions to ventilations during "no flow" and "low flow" phases of CPR remains an area of high interest, controversy, and future research. Some have suggested the potential to simplify the algorithm to 15 chest compressions and 2 ventilations in all children.

Duty Cycle

In a model of human adult cardiac arrest, cardiac output and coronary blood flow are optimized when chest compressions last for 30% of the total cycle time (approximately 1:2 ratio of time in compression to time in relaxation). As the duration of CPR increases, the optimal duty cycle may increase to 50%. In a juvenile swine model, a relaxation period of at 250 to 300 ms (duty cycle of 40%–50% if 120 compressions are delivered per minute) correlates with improved cerebral perfusion pressure compared with shorter duty cycles of 30%.

Circumferential versus Focal Sternal Compressions

In adults and animal models of cardiac arrest, circumferential (vest) CPR has been demonstrated to improve CPR hemodynamics dramatically. In smaller infants, it often is possible to encircle the chest with both hands and depress the sternum with the thumbs, while compressing the thorax circumferentially (thoracic squeeze). In an infant animal model of CPR, this "two-thumb" method of compression with thoracic squeeze resulted in higher systolic and diastolic blood pressures and a higher pulse pressure than traditional two-finger compression of the sternum.

Open-Chest Cardiopulmonary Resuscitation

Excellent standard closed-chest CPR generates cerebral blood flow that is approximately 50% of normal. By contrast, open-chest CPR can generate cerebral blood flow that approaches normal. Whereas open-chest massage improves coronary perfusion pressure and increases the chance of successful defibrillation in animals and humans, performing a thoracotomy to allow open-chest CPR is impractical in many situations.

A retrospective review of 27 cases of CPR following pediatric blunt trauma (15 with open-chest CPR and 12 with closed-chest CPR) demonstrated that open-chest CPR increased hospital cost without altering rates of ROSC or survival to discharge. However, survival in both groups was 0%, indicating that the population may have been too severely injured or too late in the process to benefit from this aggressive therapy. Earlier institution of open-chest CPR may warrant reconsideration in selected special resuscitation circumstances.

Extracorporeal Membrane Oxygenation-Cardiopulmonary Resuscitation

Venoarterial extracorporeal membrane oxygenation (ECMO) has been increasingly used as a rescue therapy during CPR, especially for potentially reversible acute postoperative myocardial dysfunction or arrhythmias. In the largest published study, 33 (50%) of 66 events in 64 children resulted in decannulation, with the child surviving at least 24 hours; 21 (33%) of 64 children undergoing extracorporeal CPR survived to hospital discharge despite a median duration of chest compressions of approximately 50 minutes before ECMO.[178] The majority of survivors following prolonged CPR and ECMO had severe, but reversible, underlying cardiac disease. CPR and ECMO are not curative treatments. They are simply cardiopulmonary supportive measures that restore tissue perfusion until recovery from the precipitating disease process. As such, they can be powerful tools.

Intraosseous Vascular Access

In infants and children requiring emergent access for resuscitation from cardiac arrest, intraosseous vascular access should be established if reliable venous access cannot be achieved rapidly. Because of the difficulty establishing vascular access in pediatric cardiac arrest victims, it may be preferable to attempt intraosseous access immediately. A practical approach is to pursue intraosseous and peripheral or central venous access simultaneously.

Intraosseous vascular access provides access to a noncollapsible marrow venous plexus, which serves as a rapid, safe, and reliable route for administration of drugs, crystalloids, colloids, and blood during resuscitation. Intraosseous vascular access often can be achieved in 30 to 60 seconds. Although a styletted specially designed intraosseous or Jamshidi-type bone marrow needle is preferred to prevent obstruction of the needle with cortical bone, butterfly needles and standard hypodermic needles have been used successfully. The intraosseous needle typically is inserted into the anterior tibial bone marrow. Alternative sites are the distal femur, medial malleolus, anterior superior iliac spine, and distal tibia. In adults and older children, the medial malleolus, distal radius, distal ulna, and sternum are other options. The latter can be cannulated using a specifically designed device for this purpose.[179]

Intraosseous vascular access can be used in all age groups, from preterm neonates through adults. The needle should be twisted into, rather than shoved through, the bone marrow. Evidence for successful entry into the bone marrow includes (1) the sudden decrease in resistance after the needle passes through the bony cortex, (2) the needle remains upright without support, (3) aspiration of bone marrow into a syringe (this is not consistently achieved), and (4) the fluid infuses freely without evidence of subcutaneous infiltration.

Resuscitation drugs, fluids, and blood products can be safely administered by the intraosseous route. Continuous catecholamine infusions also can be provided by the intraosseous route. Onset of action and drug levels following intraosseous infusion during CPR are comparable to those achieved following vascular administration, including central venous administration. Intraosseous vascular access also can be used to obtain blood specimens for chemistry, blood gas analysis, and type and cross-match, although administration of sodium bicarbonate through the intraosseous cannula eliminates the close correlation with mixed venous blood gases.

Complications have been reported in less than 1% of patients following intraosseous infusion. Complications include tibial fracture, lower extremity compartment syndrome, extravasation of drugs, and osteomyelitis. Most of these complications may be prevented by careful technique. Although microscopic pulmonary fat and bone marrow emboli have been demonstrated in animal models, they have never been reported clinically and appear to occur just as frequently during cardiac arrest without intraosseous drug administration. Animal data and one human follow-up study indicate that local effects of intraosseous infusion on the bone marrow and bone growth are minimal.

Medications Used to Treat Cardiac Arrest

Vasopressors

Epinephrine (adrenaline) is an endogenous catecholamine with potent α- and β-adrenergic stimulating properties.

The α-adrenergic action (vasoconstriction) increases systemic and pulmonary vascular resistance. The resultant higher aortic diastolic blood pressure improves coronary perfusion pressure and myocardial blood flow even though it reduces global cardiac output during CPR. Adequacy of myocardial blood flow is a critical determinant of return of ROSC. Epinephrine also increases cerebral blood flow during CPR because peripheral vasoconstriction directs a greater proportion of flow to the cerebral circulation. The β-adrenergic effect increases myocardial contractility and heart rate and relaxes smooth muscle in the skeletal muscle vascular bed and bronchi; however, the β-adrenergic effects are not observed in the peripheral vascular beds secondary to the high dose used in cardiac arrest. Epinephrine also increases the vigor and intensity of VF, increasing the likelihood of successful defibrillation.

High-dose epinephrine (0.05–0.2 mg/kg) improves myocardial and cerebral blood flow during CPR more than standard-dose epinephrine (0.01–0.02 mg/kg) in animal models of cardiac arrest and may increase the incidence of initial ROSC. Administration of high-dose epinephrine, however, can worsen a patient's postresuscitation hemodynamic condition. Retrospective studies indicate that use of high-dose epinephrine in adults or children may be associated with a worse neurologic outcome. A randomized, controlled trial of rescue high-dose epinephrine versus standard-dose epinephrine following failed initial standard dose epinephrine in pediatric in-hospital cardiac arrest demonstrated a worse 24-hour survival in the high-dose epinephrine group (1/27 vs. 6/23, $p > 0.05$). Based on these clinical data, high-dose epinephrine cannot be recommended routinely for either initial or rescue therapy.

Wide variability in catecholamine pharmacokinetics and pharmacodynamics dictate individual titration of therapy in noncardiac arrest situations. Therefore a dose that is lifesaving during CPR for one patient may be life threatening to another. Perhaps, high-dose epinephrine should be considered an alternative to standard-dose epinephrine in special circumstances of refractory pediatric cardiac arrest (e.g., a patient on high-dose epinephrine infusion prior to cardiac arrest) and/or when continuous direct arterial blood pressure monitoring allows titration of the epinephrine dosage to diastolic (relaxation phase) arterial pressure during CPR. Nevertheless, high-dose epinephrine has never been demonstrated to improve outcome, so it should only be used with caution.

Vasopressin is a long-acting endogenous hormone that acts at specific receptors to mediate systemic vasoconstriction (V_1 receptor) and reabsorption of water in the renal tubule (V_2 receptor). The vasoconstriction is most intense in the skeletal muscle and skin vascular beds. Unlike epinephrine, vasopressin is not a pulmonary vasoconstrictor. In experimental models of cardiac arrest, vasopressin increases blood flow to the heart and brain and improves long-term survival compared with epinephrine. However, vasopressin can decrease splanchnic blood flow during and following CPR and can increase afterload in the postresuscitation period. Several adult randomized, controlled trials suggest that outcomes are similar after use of vasopressin or epinephrine during CPR. In an adult multicenter trial of out-of-hospital cardiac arrest assessing ROSC, vasopressin was equivalent to epinephrine. The combination of epinephrine following vasopressin in asystolic arrest improved the rate of ROSC.

In a pediatric porcine model of prolonged *VF*, use of vasopressin and epinephrine in combination resulted in higher left ventricular blood flow than either pressor alone, and both vasopressin alone and vasopressin plus epinephrine resulted in superior cerebral blood flow than epinephrine alone. In contrast, in a pediatric porcine model of *asphyxial* cardiac arrest, ROSC was more likely in piglets treated with epinephrine than in those treated with vasopressin. A case series of four children who received vasopressin during six prolonged cardiac arrest events suggests that use of bolus vasopressin may result in ROSC when standard medications have failed. Although vasopressin likely will not replace epinephrine as a first-line agent in pediatric cardiac arrest, preliminary data suggest that its use in conjunction with epinephrine in pediatric cardiac arrest deserves further investigation.

Antiarrhythmic Medications

(See section on ventricular fibrillation in children.)

Calcium

Calcium is used frequently in cases of cardiac arrest, despite the lack of evidence for efficacy when calcium is administered routinely in cardiac arrest. In the absence of hypocalcemia, administration of calcium does not improve outcome in cardiac arrest. Calcium administration is appropriate for the following known or suspected conditions: hypocalcemia, hyperkalemia, hypermagnesemia, and calcium channel blocker overdose.

Buffer Solutions

The routine use of sodium bicarbonate for a child in cardiac arrest is not recommended. Clinical trials involving critically ill adults with severe metabolic acidosis did not demonstrate a beneficial effect of sodium bicarbonate on hemodynamics despite correction of acidosis. However, the presence of severe acidosis may depress the action of catecholamines, so use of sodium bicarbonate may be considered in an acidemic child who is refractory to catecholamine administration. Acidosis may increase the threshold for myocardial stimulation in a patient with an artificial cardiac pacemaker; therefore, administration of bicarbonate or another buffer is appropriate for management of acidosis in these children. Administration of sodium bicarbonate also is indicated in the patient with a tricyclic antidepressant overdose, hyperkalemia, hypermagnesemia, or sodium channel blocker poisoning.

The buffering action of bicarbonate occurs when a hydrogen cation and a bicarbonate anion combine to form carbon dioxide and water. If carbon dioxide is not effectively cleared through ventilation, its buildup counterbalances the buffering effect of bicarbonate. Because carbon dioxide readily penetrates cell membranes, intracellular acidosis may increase without adequate ventilation. Therefore bicarbonate should not be used for management of respiratory acidosis.

Unlike sodium bicarbonate, tromethamine (THAM) buffers excess protons without generating carbon dioxide. Carbon dioxide is consumed following THAM administration. In a patient with limited ventilation, tromethamine may be preferable when buffering is necessary. Tromethamine undergoes renal elimination, and renal insufficiency may be a relative contraindication to its use.

Carbicarb, an equimolar combination of sodium bicarbonate and sodium carbonate, is another buffering solution that generates less carbon dioxide than sodium bicarbonate. In a canine model of cardiac arrest comparing animals given normal saline, sodium bicarbonate, THAM, or Carbicarb, the animals given any buffer solution had a higher rate of ROSC than the animals given normal saline. In the animals given sodium bicarbonate or Carbicarb, the interval to ROSC was significantly shorter than in animals given normal saline. However, at the end of the 6-hour study period, all resuscitated animals were in a deep coma, so no inferences regarding meaningful survival can be drawn. It is premature to recommend either THAM or Carbicarb during CPR at this time.

Ventricular Fibrillation in Children

VF has been an underappreciated pediatric problem. In the 1990s, two important studies demonstrated VF as the initial rhythm in 19% to 24% of out-of-hospital pediatric cardiac arrest victims. These studies excluded infants with sudden infant death syndrome (SIDS), who typically have been dead for some time, often with rigor mortis. In the NRCPR database, 18% of the children with a documented initial electrocardiogram had VF/pulseless VT. These arrhythmias also can occur during the reperfusion phase. In all, 27% of the children had VF/pulseless VT at some time during the resuscitation.

The incidence of VF varies by setting and age. In special circumstances, such as tricyclic antidepressant overdose, cardiomyopathy, postcardiac surgery, and prolonged QT syndromes, VF and pulseless VT are more likely. Furthermore, in one study, VF/VT occurred in only 3% of children ages 0 to 8 years in cardiac arrest but in 17% of cardiac arrest victims from age 8 to 30 years.

The treatment of choice for short-duration VF is prompt defibrillation. Because VF must be considered before defibrillation can be provided, early determination of the rhythm by electrocardiography is critical. An attitude that VF is rare in children can be a self-fulfilling prophecy with a uniformly fatal outcome.

The recommended defibrillation dose is 2 J/kg, but the data supporting this recommendation are not optimal and are based on old monophasic defibrillators. In the mid-1970s, authoritative sources recommended starting doses of 60 to 200 J for all children. Because of concerns for myocardial damage and animal data suggesting that shock doses ranging from 0.5 to 1 J/kg were adequate for defibrillation in a variety of species, Gutgesell et al.[90] evaluated the efficacy of their strategy to defibrillate with 2 J/kg monophasic shocks. Seventy-one transthoracic defibrillations in 27 children were evaluated. Shocks within 10 J of 2 J/kg resulted in successful defibrillation in 91% of defibrillation attempts.

The major determinant of successful defibrillation other than VF duration is countershock current. This current depends on the defibrillator energy and transthoracic impedance. Studies in children indicate that the transthoracic impedance of infants and children greatly overlap. Although there is a statistically significant correlation between size and transthoracic impedance, the correlation is weak. These studies provide only weak support for the present dogma that the defibrillator energy dose should vary directly with weight. Nevertheless, the present recommendation of 2 J/kg has stood the test of time.

Although the limited data regarding pediatric defibrillation used monophasic waveform shocks, most new defibrillators use biphasic waveform shocks. Defibrillation with these biphasic waveforms apparently is safer and more effective than monophasic waveform defibrillation. Therefore using 2 J/kg biphasic waveform shocks should be at least as effective as 2 J/kg monophasic shocks and possibly safer.

Antiarrhythmic Medications: Lidocaine and Amiodarone

Administration of antiarrhythmic medications should never delay administration of shocks to a patient with VF. However, after three unsuccessful attempts at electrical defibrillation, medications to increase the effectiveness of defibrillation should be considered. Epinephrine is the current first-line medication for both pediatric and adult patients in VF. If epinephrine with or without vasopressin and a subsequent repeat attempt to defibrillate are unsuccessful, lidocaine or amiodarone should be considered.

Lidocaine traditionally has been recommended for shock-resistant VF in adults and children. However, only amiodarone improved survival to hospital admission in the setting of shock-resistant VF compared with placebo. In another study of shock-resistant out-of-hospital VF, patients receiving amiodarone had a higher rate of survival to hospital admission than patients receiving lidocaine. Neither study included children. Because there is moderate experience with amiodarone use as an antiarrhythmic agent in children and because of the adult studies, it is rational to use amiodarone similarly in children with shock-resistant VF/VT. The recommended dosage is 5 mg/kg by rapid intravenous bolus. There are no published comparisons of antiarrhythmic medications for pediatric refractory VF. Although extrapolation of adult data and electrophysiologic mechanistic information suggest that amiodarone may be preferable for pediatric shock-resistant VF, the optimal choice is not clear.

Pediatric Automated External Defibrillators

Automated external defibrillators (AEDs) have improved adult survival from VF. AEDs are recommended for use in children 8 years or older with cardiac arrest. The available data suggest that some AEDs can accurately diagnose VF in children of all ages, but many AEDs are limited because the defibrillation pads and energy dosage are geared for adults. Adapters having smaller defibrillation pads that dampen the amount of energy delivered have been developed as attachments to adult AEDs, allowing their use in children.

Because lack of defibrillation clearly is lethal for pediatric VF, it is preferable to provide a shock with an appropriate pediatric dose or even a high-dose shock rather than no shock. However, it is important that the AED diagnostic algorithm is sensitive and specific for pediatric VF and VT. The diagnostic algorithms from several AED manufacturers have been tested for such sensitivity and specificity and therefore can be reasonably used in younger children.

Monophasic versus Biphasic Defibrillator Waveforms (and Beyond)

In a randomized, controlled trial comparing the efficacy of a biphasic (impedance-compensated biphasic truncated exponential) energy waveform with two different types of monophasic waveforms (monophasic truncated exponential and monophasic damped sine), defibrillation efficacy (i.e., termination of fibrillation) was superior with the biphasic waveform than for either of the two types of monophasic waveforms. AEDs currently use biphasic waveforms to deliver energy. Although internal (implantable) pediatric defibrillators are all biphasic waveform, no data on the safety and efficacy of biphasic transthoracic defibrillation in children are available, and a study in children is not feasible. Data suggest that doses greater than 2 J/kg and alternative waveforms may be safe and effective in small children.

Postresuscitation Myocardial Dysfunction

Postarrest myocardial stunning occurs commonly after successful resuscitation in animals.[36–42] In addition, most adults who survive to hospital admission after an out-of-hospital cardiac arrest die in the postresuscitation phase, many as a result of progressive myocardial dysfunction.[39,43,44] Animal studies demonstrate that postarrest myocardial stunning is a global phenomenon with biventricular systolic and diastolic dysfunction and typically resolves after 1 or 2 days. This postarrest myocardial stunning is pathophysiologically and physiologically similar to sepsis-related myocardial dysfunction[45] and postcardiopulmonary bypass myocardial dysfunction,[46,47] including increases in inflammatory mediator and nitric oxide production. Postarrest myocardial stunning is worse after a more prolonged untreated cardiac arrest,[36,48] after more prolonged CPR,[39,49] after defibrillation with higher-energy shocks,[50] and after a greater number of shocks.[39] Because cardiac function is essential to reperfusion following cardiac arrest, management of postarrest myocardial dysfunction may be important to improving survival.

Postresuscitation Interventions

Temperature Management

Hyperthermia following cardiac arrest is common in children, and fever following cardiac arrest is associated with poor neurologic outcome. Mild (32° C–34° C) resuscitative systemic hypothermia may improve neurologic outcome in adults after resuscitation from out-of-hospital VF arrest. Mild systemic hypothermia may benefit children resuscitated from cardiac arrest, but the question demands further study. At a minimum, it is advisable to strictly avoid even mild hyperthermia in children following CPR. Scheduled administration of antipyretic medications *and* use of external cooling devices often are necessary to prevent hyperthermia in this population.

Glucose Control

Hyperglycemia following adult cardiac arrest is associated with worse neurologic outcome after controlling for duration of arrest and presence of cardiogenic shock, but whether the hyperglycemia per se is harmful or is a marker of the severity of the stress hormone response and cellular injury from prolonged ischemia is not clear. In an animal model of asphyxial cardiac arrest, administration of insulin and glucose, but not administration of glucose alone, improved neurologic outcome compared with administration of normal saline. In critically ill adult patients, tight glucose control using an insulin infusion improved survival and reduced complications such as sepsis and renal failure.[180] Thus many critical care clinicians target tight glucose control with prevention of hyperglycemia and hypoglycemia following cardiac arrest, although the importance of this intervention remains to be determined.

Blood Pressure Management

Compared with healthy volunteers, adults resuscitated from cardiac arrest have impaired autoregulation of cerebral blood flow. Hence they may not maintain adequate cerebral blood flow in the context of low systemic pressure and likewise may not be able to protect the brain from excessive blood flow and microvascular perfusion pressure in the context of systemic hypertension. Therefore inasmuch as possible, blood pressure variability should be minimized following resuscitation from cardiac arrest.

A brief period of hypertension following resuscitation from cardiac arrest may diminish the no-reflow phenomenon. In animal models, brief induced hypertension following resuscitation results in improved neurologic outcome compared with normotensive reperfusion. In a retrospective human study, postresuscitative hypertension was associated with a better neurologic outcome after controlling for age, gender, duration of cardiac arrest, duration of CPR, and preexisting diseases.

Treatment of Postresuscitation Myocardial Dysfunction

Postresuscitation myocardial dysfunction is common. The classes of agents used to maintain circulatory function usually are characterized as inotropes, vasopressors, and vasodilators. Inotropes increase cardiac pumping function and often increase heart rate as well. Vasopressors increase systemic and often pulmonary vascular resistance; they are most commonly used in children with inappropriately low systemic vascular resistance. Vasodilators are designed to reduce systemic and pulmonary vascular resistance. Although they do not directly increase pumping function, vasodilators reduce ventricular afterload, which often improves stroke volume and therefore cardiac output. They are the only class of agents that can increase cardiac output and simultaneously reduce myocardial oxygen demand.

Optimal use of these agents involves titrating the medication to the patient's cardiovascular physiology. Invasive hemodynamic monitoring, including measurement of central venous pressure, pulmonary capillary wedge pressure, and cardiac output, may be appropriate. Furthermore, vasoactive agents have different hemodynamic effects at different infusion rates. For example, at low infusion rates, epinephrine is a potent inotrope and lowers systemic vascular resistance through a prominent action on vascular β-adrenergic receptors. At higher infusion rates, epinephrine remains a potent inotrope and increases systemic vascular resistance by activating vascular α-adrenergic receptors. Because pharmacokinetic and pharmacodynamic responses are not uniform across ages and across different diseases, careful monitoring of the patient's response to vasoactive agents is needed for optimal use.

Summary

Outcomes from pediatric cardiac arrest and CPR appear to be improving. Perhaps the evolving understanding of pathophysiologic events during and after pediatric cardiac arrest and the developing fields of pediatric critical care and pediatric emergency medicine have contributed to these apparent improvements. In addition, exciting breakthroughs in basic and applied science laboratories are on the immediate horizon for study in specific subpopulations of cardiac arrest victims. By strategically focusing therapies to specific phases of cardiac arrest and resuscitation and to the evolving pathophysiology, there is great promise that critical care interventions will lead the way to more successful cardiopulmonary and cerebral resuscitation in children.

REFERENCES

1. Cummins RO, Eisenberg MS, Hallstrom AP, Litwin PE: Survival of out-of-hospital cardiac arrest with early initiation of cardiopulmonary resuscitation. *Am J Emerg Med* 3:114-119, 1985.
2. Weaver WD, Cobb LA, Hallstrom AP, et al: Considerations for improving survival from out-of-hospital cardiac arrest. *Ann Emerg Med* 15:1181-1186, 1986.
3. Eisenberg MS, Copass MK, Hallstrom AP, et al: Treatment of out-of-hospital cardiac arrests with rapid defibrillation by emergency medical technicians. *N Engl J Med* 302:1379-1383, 1980.
4. Stults KR, Brown DD, Schug VL, Bean JA: Prehospital defibrillation performed by emergency medical technicians in rural communities. *N Engl J Med* 310:219-223, 1984.
5. Council ER: International guidelines 2000 for CPR and ECC—A consensus on science. *Resuscitation* 46:1-448, 2000.
6. Kern KB, Ewy GA, Voorhees WD, et al: Myocardial perfusion pressure: a predictor of 24-hour survival during prolonged cardiac arrest in dogs. *Resuscitation* 16:241-250, 1988.
7. Sanders AB, Kern KB, Atlas M, et al: Importance of the duration of inadequate coronary perfusion pressure on resuscitation from cardiac arrest. *J Am Coll Cardiol* 6:113-118, 1985.
8. Kuisma M, Suominen P, Korpela R: Paediatric out-of-hospital cardiac arrests—epidemiology and outcome. *Resuscitation* 30: 141-150, 1995.
9. Liberthson RR: Sudden death from cardiac causes in children and young adults. *N Engl J Med* 334:1039-1044, 1996.
10. Zaritsky A, Nadkarni V, Hazinski MF, et al: Recommended guidelines for uniform reporting of pediatric advanced life support. The Pediatric Utstein Style. *Pediatrics* 96:765-779, 1995.
11. Lee CJ, Bullock LJ: Determining the pulse for infant CPR: time for a change? *Mil Med* 156:190-193, 1991.
12. Whitelaw CC, Goldsmith LJ: Comparison of two techniques for determining the presence of a pulse in an infant. *Acad Emerg Med* 4:153-154, 1997.
13. Saugstad OD: Practical aspects of resuscitating asphyxiated newborn infants. *Eur J Pediatr* 157:S11-S15, 1998.
14. Perlman JM, Risser R: Cardiopulmonary resuscitation in the delivery room. Associated clinical events. *Arch Pediatr Adolesc Med* 149:20-25, 1995.
15. Saugstad OD, Rootwelt T, Aalen O: Resuscitation of asphyxiated newborn infants with room air or oxygen: an international controlled trial: the Resair 2 study. *Pediatrics* 102:e1, 1998.
16. Reis AG, Nadkarni V, Perondi MB, et al: A prospective investigation into the epidemiology of in-hospital pediatric cardiopulmonary resuscitation using the international Utstein reporting style. *Pediatrics* 109:200-209, 2002.
17. Slonim AD, PK, Ruttimann UE, Pollack MM: Cardiopulmonary resuscitation in pediatric intensive care units. *Crit Care Med* 25: 1951-1955, 1997.
18. Parra DA, Totapally BR, Zahn E, et al: Outcome of cardiopulmonary resuscitation in a pediatric cardiac intensive care unit. Critical Care Medicine 2000; 28:3296-3300.
19. Sirbaugh PE, Pepe PE, Shook JE, et al: A prospective, population-based study of the demographics, epidemiology, management, and outcome of out-of-hospital pediatric cardiopulmonary arrest. *Ann Emerg Med* 33:174-184, 1999.
20. Nadkarni V, Hazinski MF, Zideman D, et al: Pediatric resuscitation: an advisory statement from the Pediatric Working Group of the International Liaison Committee on Resuscitation. *Circulation* 95:2185-2195, 1997.
21. Gausche M, Lewis RJ, Stratton SJ, et al: Effect of out-of-hospital pediatric endotracheal intubation on survival and neurological outcome: a controlled clinical trial. *JAMA* 283:783-790, 2000.
22. Sanders AB, Ewy GA, Bragg S, et al: Expired PCO_2 as a prognostic indicator of successful resuscitation from cardiac arrest. *Ann Emerg Med* 14:948-952, 1985.
23. Cantineau JP, Lambert Y, Merckx P, et al: End-tidal carbon dioxide during cardiopulmonary resuscitation in humans presenting mostly with asystole: a predictor of outcome. *Crit Care Med* 24:791-796, 1996.
24. von Planta M, von Planta I, Weil MH, et al: End tidal carbon dioxide as an haemodynamic determinant of cardiopulmonary resuscitation in the rat. *Cardiovasc Res* 23:364-368, 1989.
25. Berg RA, Henry C, Otto CW, et al: Initial end-tidal CO_2 is markedly elevated during cardiopulmonary resuscitation after asphyxial cardiac arrest. *Pediatr Emerg Care* 12:245-248, 1996.
26. Bhende MS, Karasic DG, Karasic RB: End-tidal carbon dioxide changes during cardiopulmonary resuscitation after experimental asphyxial cardiac arrest. *Am J Emerg Med* 14:349-50, 1996.
27. Finholt DA, Kettrick RG, Wagner HR, Swedlow DB: The heart is under the lower third of the sternum. Implications for external cardiac massage. *Am J Dis Child* 140:646-649, 1986.
28. Babbs CF, Kern KB: Optimum compression to ventilation ratios in CPR under realistic, practical conditions: a physiological and mathematical analysis. *Resuscitation* 54:147-157, 2002.
29. MF H, editor: *American Heart Association: PALS provider manual.* Dallas, 2002, American Heart Association.
30. Berg RA, Sanders AB, Kern KB, et al: Adverse hemodynamic effects of interrupting chest compressions for rescue breathing during cardiopulmonary resuscitation for ventricular fibrillation cardiac arrest. *Circulation* 104:2465-2470, 2001.
31. Kern KB, Hilwig RW, Berg RA, et al: Importance of continuous chest compressions during cardiopulmonary resuscitation: improved outcome during a simulated single lay-rescuer scenario. *Circulation* 105:645-649, 2002.
32. Chamberlain D, Smith A, Colquhoun M, et al: Randomised controlled trials of staged teaching for basic life support: 2. Comparison of CPR performance and skill retention using either staged instruction or conventional training. *Resuscitation* 50:27-37, 2001.
33. Chandra NC, Gruben KG, Tsitlik JE, et al: Observations of ventilation during resuscitation in a canine model. *Circulation* 90: 3070-3075, 1994.
34. Noc M, Weil MH, Tang W, et al: Mechanical ventilation may not be essential for initial cardiopulmonary resuscitation. *Chest* 108:821-827, 1995.

35. Hallstrom AP: Dispatcher-assisted "phone" cardiopulmonary resuscitation by chest compression alone or with mouth-to-mouth ventilation. *Crit Care Med* 2000; 28:N190-N192.
36. Berg RA, Hilwig RW, Kern KB, Ewy GA: "Bystander" chest compressions and assisted ventilation independently improve outcome from piglet asphyxial pulseless "cardiac arrest." *Circulation* 101: 1743-1748, 2000.
37. Dorph E, Wik L, Steen PA: Effectiveness of ventilation-compression ratios 1:5 and 2:15 in simulated single rescuer paediatric resuscitation. *Resuscitation* 54:259-264, 2002.
38. Nadkarni V, GB, Tice L, Cox T, Rose MJ: Evaluation of a universal compression/ventilation ratio for one-rescuer CPR in infant, pediatric and adult manikins. *Crit Care Med* 25:A61, 1997 (abstract).
39. Kinney SB, Tibballs J: An analysis of the efficacy of bag-valve-mask ventilation and chest compression during different compression-ventilation ratios in manikin-simulated paediatric resuscitation. *Resuscitation* 43:115-120, 2000.
40. Babbs CF, Thelander K: Theoretically optimal duty cycles for chest and abdominal compression during external cardiopulmonary resuscitation. *Acad Emerg Med* 2:698-707, 1995.
41. Dean JM, Koehler RC, Schleien CL, et al: Age-related effects of compression rate and duration in cardiopulmonary resuscitation. *J Appl Physiol* 68:554-560, 1990.
42. Halperin HR, Tsitlik JE, Gelfand M, et al: A preliminary study of cardiopulmonary resuscitation by circumferential compression of the chest with use of a pneumatic vest. *N Engl J Med* 329:762-768, 1993.
43. Dorfsman ML, Menegazzi JJ, Wadas RJ, Auble TE: Two-thumb vs. two-finger chest compression in an infant model of prolonged cardiopulmonary resuscitation. *Acad Emerg Med* 7:1077-1082, 2000.
44. Bircher N, Safar P: Manual open-chest cardiopulmonary resuscitation. *Ann Emerg Med* 13:770-773, 1984.
45. Sanders AB, Kern KB, Ewy GA, et al: Improved resuscitation from cardiac arrest with open-chest massage. *Ann Emerg Med* 13: 672-675, 1984.
46. Boczar ME, Howard MA, Rivers EP, et al: A technique revisited: hemodynamic comparison of closed- and open-chest cardiac massage during human cardiopulmonary resuscitation. *Crit Care Med* 23:498-503, 1995.
47. Fleisher G, Sagy M, Swedlow DB, Belani K: Open- versus closed chest cardiac compressions in a canine model of pediatric cardiopulmonary resuscitation. *Am J Emerg Med* 3:305-310, 1985.
48. Sheikh A, Brogan T: Outcome and cost of open- and closed-chest cardiopulmonary resuscitation in pediatric cardiac arrests. *Pediatrics* 93:392-398, 1994.
49. Beattie C, Guerci AD, Hall T, et al: Mechanisms of blood flow during pneumatic vest cardiopulmonary resuscitation. *J Appl Physiol* 70:454-465, 1991.
50. Lafuente-Lafuente C, Melero-Bascones M: Active chest compression-decompression for cardiopulmonary resuscitation. *Cochrane Database Syst Rev* CD002751, 2001.
51. Kern KB, Figge G, Hilwig RW, et al: Active compression-decompression versus standard cardiopulmonary resuscitation in a porcine model: no improvement in outcome. *Am Heart J* 132:1156-1162, 1996.
52. Mauer DK, Nolan J, Plaisance P, et al: Effect of active compression-decompression resuscitation (ACD-CPR) on survival: a combined analysis using individual patient data. *Resuscitation* 41:249-256, 1999.
53. Plaisance P, Adnet F, Vicaut E, et al: Benefit of active compression-decompression cardiopulmonary resuscitation as a prehospital advanced cardiac life support. A randomized multicenter study. *Circulation* 95:955-961, 1997.
54. Skogvoll E, Wik L: Active compression-decompression cardiopulmonary resuscitation: a population-based, prospective randomised clinical trial in out-of-hospital cardiac arrest. *Resuscitation* 42: 163-172, 1999.
55. Arntz HR, Agrawal R, Richter H, et al: Phased chest and abdominal compression-decompression versus conventional cardiopulmonary resuscitation in out-of-hospital cardiac arrest. *Circulation* 104:768-772, 2001.
56. Babbs CF: Efficacy of interposed abdominal compression-cardiopulmonary resuscitation (CPR), active compression and decompression-CPR and Lifestick CPR: basic physiology in a spreadsheet model. *Crit Care Med* 28:N199-N202, 2000.
57. Paiva EF, Kern KB, Hilwig RW, et al: Minimally invasive direct cardiac massage versus closed-chest cardiopulmonary resuscitation in a porcine model of prolonged ventricular fibrillation cardiac arrest. *Resuscitation* 47:287-299, 2000.
58. Rozenberg A, Incagnoli P, Delpech P, et al: Prehospital use of minimally invasive direct cardiac massage (MID-CM): a pilot study. *Resuscitation* 50:257-262, 2001.
59. Langhelle A, Stromme T, Sunde K, et al: Inspiratory impedance threshold valve during CPR. *Resuscitation* 52:39-48, 2002.
60. Dalton HJ, Siewers RD, Fuhrman BP, et al: Extracorporeal membrane oxygenation for cardiac rescue in children with severe myocardial dysfunction. *Crit Care Med* 21:1020-1028, 1993.
61. Posner JC, Osterhoudt KC, Mollen CJ, et al: Extracorporeal membrane oxygenation as a resuscitative measure in the pediatric emergency department. *Pediatr Emerg Care* 16:413-415, 2000.
62. Duncan BW, Ibrahim AE, Hraska V, et al: Use of rapid-deployment extracorporeal membrane oxygenation for the resuscitation of pediatric patients with heart disease after cardiac arrest. *J Thorac Cardiovasc Surg* 116:305-311, 1998.
63. Holzer M, Sterz F, Schoerkhuber W, et al: Successful resuscitation of a verapamil-intoxicated patient with percutaneous cardiopulmonary bypass. *Crit Care Med* 27:2818-2823, 1999.
64. Younger JG, Schreiner RJ, Swaniker F, et al: Extracorporeal resuscitation of cardiac arrest. *Acad Emerg Med* 6:700-707, 1999.
65. Martin GB, Rivers EP, Paradis NA, et al: Emergency department cardiopulmonary bypass in the treatment of human cardiac arrest. *Chest* 113:743-751, 1998.
66. Kurose M, Okamoto K, Sato T, et al: The determinant of severe cerebral dysfunction in patients undergoing emergency extracorporeal life support following cardiopulmonary resuscitation. *Resuscitation* 30:15-20, 1995.
67. Mair P, Hoermann C, Moertl M, et al: Percutaneous venoarterial extracorporeal membrane oxygenation for emergency mechanical circulatory support. *Resuscitation* 33:29-34, 1996.
68. del Nido PJ, Dalton HJ, Thompson AE, Siewers RD: Extracorporeal membrane oxygenator rescue in children during cardiac arrest after cardiac surgery. *Circulation* 86:II300-II304, 1992.
69. Council ER. Part 4: the automated external defibrillator: key link in the chain of survival. European Resuscitation Council. *Resuscitation* 46:73-91, 2000.
70. Marenco JP, Wang PJ, Link MS, et al: Improving survival from sudden cardiac arrest: the role of the automated external defibrillator. *JAMA* 285:1193-1200, 2001.
71. Cecchin F, Jorgenson DB, Berul CI, et al: Is arrhythmia detection by automatic external defibrillator accurate for children?: sensitivity and specificity of an automatic external defibrillator algorithm in 696 pediatric arrhythmias. *Circulation* 103:2483-2488, 2001.
72. Atkins DL, Hartley LL, York DK: Accurate recognition and effective treatment of ventricular fibrillation by automated external defibrillators in adolescents. *Pediatrics* 101:393-397, 1998.
73. Jorgenson D, Morgan C, Snyder D, et al: Energy attenuator for pediatric application of an automated external defibrillator. *Crit Care Med* 30:S145-S147, 2002.
74. Tang W, Weil MH, Sun S, et al: The effects of biphasic and conventional monophasic defibrillation on postresuscitation myocardial function. *J Am Coll Cardiol* 34:815-822, 1999.
75. Martens PR, Russell JK, Wolcke B, et al: Optimal Response to Cardiac Arrest study: defibrillation waveform effects. *Resuscitation* 49:233-243, 2001.
76. Pellis T, Bisera J, Tang W, Weil MH: Expanding automatic external defibrillators to include automated detection of cardiac, respiratory, and cardiorespiratory arrest. *Crit Care Med* 30:S176-S178, 2002.
77. Marn-Pernat A, Weil MH, Tang W, et al: Optimizing timing of ventricular defibrillation. *Crit Care Med* 29:2360-2365, 2001.
78. Yu T, Weil MH, Tang W, et al: Adverse outcomes of interrupted precordial compression during automated defibrillation. *Circulation* 106:368-372, 2002.
79. Povoas HP, Bisera J: Electrocardiographic waveform analysis for predicting the success of defibrillation. *Crit Care Med* 28:N210-N211, 2000.
80. Noc M, Weil MH, Tang W, et al: Electrocardiographic prediction of the success of cardiac resuscitation. *Crit Care Med* 27:708-714, 1999.
81. Niemann JT, Criley JM, Rosborough JP, et al: Predictive indices of successful cardiac resuscitation after prolonged arrest and experimental cardiopulmonary resuscitation. *Ann Emerg Med* 14: 521-528, 1985.

82. Sanders AB, Ewy GA, Taft TV: Prognostic and therapeutic importance of the aortic diastolic pressure in resuscitation from cardiac arrest. *Crit Care Med* 12:871-873, 1984.
83. Otto CW, Yakaitis RW, Blitt CD: Mechanism of action of epinephrine in resuscitation from asphyxial arrest. *Crit Care Med* 9: 364-365, 1981.
84. Berg RA, Otto CW, Kern KB, et al: A randomized, blinded trial of high-dose epinephrine versus standard-dose epinephrine in a swine model of pediatric asphyxial cardiac arrest. *Crit Care Med* 24:1695-1700, 1996.
85. Stiell IG, Hebert PC, Weitzman BN, et al: High-dose epinephrine in adult cardiac arrest. *N Engl J Med* 327:1045-1050, 1992.
86. Brown CG, Martin DR, Pepe PE, et al: A comparison of standard-dose and high-dose epinephrine in cardiac arrest outside the hospital. The Multicenter High-Dose Epinephrine Study Group. *N Engl J Med* 327:1051-1055, 1992.
87. Callaham M, Madsen CD, Barton CW, et al: A randomized clinical trial of high-dose epinephrine and norepinephrine vs standard-dose epinephrine in prehospital cardiac arrest. *JAMA* 268:2667-2672, 1992.
88. Lipman J, Wilson W, Kobilski S, et al: High-dose adrenaline in adult in-hospital asystolic cardiopulmonary resuscitation: a double-blind randomised trial. *Anaesth Intensive Care* 21:192-196, 1993.
89. Lindner KH, Ahnefeld FW, Prengel AW: Comparison of standard and high-dose adrenaline in the resuscitation of asystole and electromechanical dissociation. *Acta Anaesthesiol Scand* 35:253-256, 1991.
90. Sherman BW, Munger MA, Foulke GE, et al: High-dose versus standard-dose epinephrine treatment of cardiac arrest after failure of standard therapy. *Pharmacotherapy* 17:242-247, 1997.
91. Choux C, Gueugniaud PY, Barbieux A, et al: Standard doses versus repeated high doses of epinephrine in cardiac arrest outside the hospital. *Resuscitation* 29:3-9, 1995.
92. Woodhouse SP, Cox S, Boyd P, et al: High dose and standard dose adrenaline do not alter survival, compared with placebo, in cardiac arrest. *Resuscitation* 30:243-249, 1995.
93. Gueugniaud PY, Mols P, Goldstein P, et al: A comparison of repeated high doses and repeated standard doses of epinephrine for cardiac arrest outside the hospital. European Epinephrine Study Group. *N Engl J Med* 339:1595-1601, 1998.
94. Berg RA, Otto CW, Kern KB, et al: High-dose epinephrine results in greater early mortality after resuscitation from prolonged cardiac arrest in pigs: a prospective, randomized study. *Crit Care Med* 22:282-290, 1994.
95. Hornchen U, Lussi C, Schuttler J: Potential risks of high-dose epinephrine for resuscitation from ventricular fibrillation in a porcine model. *J Cardiothorac Vasc Anesth* 7:184-187, 1993.
96. Tang W, Weil MH, Sun S, et al: Epinephrine increases the severity of postresuscitation myocardial dysfunction. *Circulation* 92: 3089-3093, 1995.
97. Rivers EP, Wortsman J, Rady MY, et al: The effect of the total cumulative epinephrine dose administered during human CPR on hemodynamic, oxygen transport, and utilization variables in the postresuscitation period. *Chest* 106:1499-1507, 1994.
98. Young KD, Seidel JS: Pediatric cardiopulmonary resuscitation: a collective review. *Ann Emerg Med* 33:195-205, 1999.
99. Behringer W, Kittler H, Sterz F, et al: Cumulative epinephrine dose during cardiopulmonary resuscitation and neurologic outcome. *Ann Intern Med* 129:450-456, 1998.
100. Gedeborg R, Silander HC, Ronne-Engstrom E, et al: Adverse effects of high-dose epinephrine on cerebral blood flow during experimental cardiopulmonary resuscitation. *Crit Care Med* 28:1423-1430, 2000.
101. Dieckmann RA, Vardis R: High-dose epinephrine in pediatric out-of-hospital cardiopulmonary arrest. *Pediatrics* 95:901-913, 1995.
102. Carpenter TC, Stenmark KR: High-dose epinephrine is not superior to standard-dose epinephrine in pediatric in-hospital cardiopulmonary arrest. *Pediatrics* 99:403-408, 1997.
103. Lindner KH, Prengel AW, Pfenninger EG, et al: Vasopressin improves vital organ blood flow during closed-chest cardiopulmonary resuscitation in pigs. *Circulation* 91:215-221, 1995.
104. Prengel AW, Lindner KH, Keller A: Cerebral oxygenation during cardiopulmonary resuscitation with epinephrine and vasopressin in pigs. *Stroke* 27:1241-1248, 1996.
105. Wenzel V, Lindner KH, Krismer AC, et al: Survival with full neurologic recovery and no cerebral pathology after prolonged cardiopulmonary resuscitation with vasopressin in pigs. *J Am Coll Cardiol* 35:527-533, 2000.
106. Prengel AW, Lindner KH, Wenzel V, et al: Splanchnic and renal blood flow after cardiopulmonary resuscitation with epinephrine and vasopressin in pigs. *Resuscitation* 38:19-24, 1998.
107. Voelckel WG, Lindner KH, Wenzel V, et al: Effects of vasopressin and epinephrine on splanchnic blood flow and renal function during and after cardiopulmonary resuscitation in pigs. *Crit Care Med* 28:1083-1088, 2000.
108. Lindner KH, Dirks B, Strohmenger HU, et al: Randomised comparison of epinephrine and vasopressin in patients with out-of-hospital ventricular fibrillation. *Lancet* 349:535-537, 1997.
109. Stiell IG, Hebert PC, Wells GA, et al: Vasopressin versus epinephrine for inhospital cardiac arrest: a randomised controlled trial. *Lancet* 358:105-109, 2001.
110. Voelckel WG, Lurie KG, McKnite S, et al: Effects of epinephrine and vasopressin in a piglet model of prolonged ventricular fibrillation and cardiopulmonary resuscitation. *Crit Care Med* 30: 957-962, 2002.
111. Voelckel WG, Lurie KG, McKnite S, et al: Comparison of epinephrine and vasopressin in a pediatric porcine model of asphyxial cardiac arrest. *Crit Care Med* 28:3777-3783, 2000.
112. Mann K, Berg RA, Nadkarni V: Beneficial effects of vasopressin in prolonged pediatric cardiac arrest: a case series. *Resuscitation* 52:149-156, 2002.
113. Dorian P, Cass D, Schwartz B, et al: Amiodarone as compared with lidocaine for shock-resistant ventricular fibrillation. *N Engl J Med* 346:884-890, 2002.
114. Kudenchuk PJ, Cobb LA, Copass MK, et al: Amiodarone for resuscitation after out-of-hospital cardiac arrest due to ventricular fibrillation. *N Engl J Med* 341:871-878, 1999.
115. Stueven HA, Thompson B, Aprahamian C, et al: Lack of effectiveness of calcium chloride in refractory asystole. *Ann Emerg Med* 14:630-632, 1985.
116. Stueven HA, Thompson B, Aprahamian C, et al: The effectiveness of calcium chloride in refractory electromechanical dissociation. *Ann Emerg Med* 14:626-629, 1985.
117. Cooper DJ, Walley KR, Wiggs BR, Russell JA: Bicarbonate does not improve hemodynamics in critically ill patients who have lactic acidosis. A prospective, controlled clinical study. *Ann Intern Med* 112:492-498, 1990.
118. Mathieu D, Neviere R, Billard V, et al: Effects of bicarbonate therapy on hemodynamics and tissue oxygenation in patients with lactic acidosis: a prospective, controlled clinical study. *Crit Care Med* 19:1352-1356, 1991.
119. Huang YG, Wong KC, Yip WH, et al: Cardiovascular responses to graded doses of three catecholamines during lactic and hydrochloric acidosis in dogs. *Br J Anaesth* 74:583-590, 1995.
120. Preziosi MP, Roig J, Hargrove N, Burchfield DJ: Metabolic acidemia with hypoxia attenuates the hemodynamic responses to epinephrine during resuscitation in lambs. *Crit Care Med* 21:1901, 1993.
121. Dohrmann ML, Goldschlager NF: Myocardial stimulation threshold in patients with cardiac pacemakers: effect of physiologic variables, pharmacologic agents, and lead electrodes. *Cardiol Clin* 3:527-537, 1985.
122. Bar-Joseph G, Weinberger T, Castel T, et al: Comparison of sodium bicarbonate, Carbicarb, and THAM during cardiopulmonary resuscitation in dogs. *Crit Care Med* 26:1397-1408, 1998.
123. Zeiner A, Holzer M, Sterz F, et al: Hyperthermia after cardiac arrest is associated with an unfavorable neurologic outcome. *Arch Intern Med* 161:2007-2012, 2001.
124. Hickey RW, Kochanek PM, Ferimer H, et al: Hypothermia and hyperthermia in children after resuscitation from cardiac arrest. *Pediatrics* 106:118-122, 2000.
125. Bernard SA, Gray TW, Buist MD, et al: Treatment of comatose survivors of out-of-hospital cardiac arrest with induced hypothermia. *N Engl J Med* 346:564-569, 2002.
126. The Hypothermia after Cardiac Arrest Study Group: Mild therapeutic hypothermia to improve the neurologic outcome after cardiac arrest. *N Engl J Med* 346:549-556, 2002.
127. Mullner M, Sterz F, Binder M, et al: Blood glucose concentration after cardiopulmonary resuscitation influences functional neurological recovery in human cardiac arrest survivors. *J Cereb Blood Flow Metab* 17:430-436, 1997.

128. Katz LM, Wang Y, Ebmeyer U, et al: Glucose plus insulin infusion improves cerebral outcome after asphyxial cardiac arrest. *Neuroreport* 9:3363-3367, 1998.
129. Sundgreen C, Larsen FS, Herzog TM, et al: Autoregulation of cerebral blood flow in patients resuscitated from cardiac arrest. *Stroke* 32:128-132, 2001.
130. Sterz F, Leonov Y, Safar P, et al: Hypertension with or without hemodilution after cardiac arrest in dogs. *Stroke* 21:1178-1184, 1990.
131. Safar P XF, Radovsky A, Tanigawa K, et al: Improved cerebral resuscitation from cardiac arrest in dogs with mild hypothermia plus blood flow promotion. *Stroke* 27:105-113, 1996.
132. Sasser HC, SP: Arterial hypertension after cardiac arrest is associated with good cerebral outcome in patients. *Crit Care Med* 27:A29, 1999 (abstract).
133. Sanders AB, Berg RA, Burress M, et al: The efficacy of an ACLS training program for resuscitation from cardiac arrest in a rural community. *Ann Emerg Med* 23:56-59, 1994.
134. Wik L, Thowsen J, Steen PA: An automated voice advisory manikin system for training in basic life support without an instructor. A novel approach to CPR training. *Resuscitation* 50:167-172, 2001.
135. Wik L, Myklebust H, Auestad BH, Steen PA: Retention of basic life support skills 6 months after training with an automated voice advisory manikin system without instructor involvement. *Resuscitation* 52:273-279, 2002.
136. Cappelle C, Paul RI: Educating residents: the effects of a mock code program. *Resuscitation* 31:107-111, 1996.
137. Madar J, Richmon S: Improving paediatric and newborn life support training by use of modified manikins allowing airway occlusion. *Resuscitation* 54:265-268, 2002.
138. Garden A, Robinson B, Weller J, et al: Education to address medical error—a role for high fidelity patient simulation. *N Z Med J* 115:133-134, 2002.
139. Kofranek J, Vu LD, Snaselova H, et al: GOLEM—multimedia simulator for medical education. *Medinfo* 10:1042-1046, 2001.
140. Milander MM, Hiscok PS, Sanders AB, et al: Chest compression and ventilation rates during cardiopulmonary resuscitation: the effects of audible tone guidance. *Acad Emerg Med* 2:708-713, 1995.
141. Berg RA, Sanders AB, Milander M, et al: Efficacy of audio prompted rate guidance in improving resuscitator performance of cardiopulmonary resuscitation on children. *Acad Emerg Med* 1:35-40, 1994.
142. Larsen PD Galletly PK: Patterns of external chest compression. *Resuscitation* 53:281-287, 2002.
143. Eisenburger P, Safar P: Life supporting first aid training of the public—review and recommendations. *Resuscitation* 41:3-18, 1999.
144. Klouche K, Weil MH, Tang W, et al: A selective alpha(2)-adrenergic agonist for cardiac resuscitation. *J Lab Clin Med* 140:27-34, 2002.
145. Bertsch T, Casarin W, Kretschmar M, et al: Protein S-100B: a serum marker for ischemic and infectious injury of cerebral tissue. *Clin Chem Lab Med* 39:319-323, 2001.
146. Horn M, Seger F, Schlote W: Neuron-specific enolase in gerbil brain and serum after transient cerebral ischemia. *Stroke* 26:290-297, 1995.
147. Rosen H, Sunnerhagen KS, Herlitz J, et al: Serum levels of the brain-derived proteins S-100 and NSE predict long-term outcome after cardiac arrest. *Resuscitation* 49:183-191, 2001.
148. Böttiger BW, Bode C, Kern S, et al: Efficacy and safety of thrombolytic therapy after initially unsuccessful cardiopulmonary resuscitation: a prospective clinical trial. *Lancet* 357:1583-1585, 2001.
149. Davies MJ, Bland JM, Hangartner JR, et al: Factors influencing the presence or absence of acute coronary artery thrombi in sudden ischaemic death. *Eur Heart J* 10:203-208, 1989.
150. Grieb P, Ryba MS, Debicki GS, et al: Changes in oxidative stress in the rat brain during post-cardiac arrest reperfusion, and the effect of treatment with the free radical scavenger idebenone. *Resuscitation* 39:107-113, 1998.
151. Ihnken K, Morita K, Buckberg GD, et al: Prevention of reoxygenation injury in hypoxaemic immature hearts by priming the extracorporeal circuit with antioxidants. *Cardiovasc Surg* 5:608-619, 1997.
152. Behringer W, Safar P, Kentner R, et al: Antioxidant Tempol enhances hypothermic cerebral preservation during prolonged cardiac arrest in dogs. *J Cereb Blood Flow Metabol* 22:105-117, 2002.
153. Liu Y, Rosenthal RE, Haywood Y, et al: Normoxic ventilation after cardiac arrest reduces oxidation of brain lipids and improves neurological outcome. *Stroke* 29:1679-1686, 1998.
154. Lipinski CA, Hicks SD, Callaway CW: Normoxic ventilation during resuscitation and outcome from asphyxial cardiac arrest in rats. *Resuscitation* 42:221-229, 1999.
155. Choi DW: Ischemia-induced neuronal apoptosis. *Curr Opin Neurobiol* 6:667-672, 1996.
156. Tseng EE, Brock MV, Lange MS, et al: Monosialoganglioside GM1 inhibits neurotoxicity after hypothermic circulatory arrest. *Surgery* 124:298-306, 1998.
157. Bolling SF, Tramontini NL, Kilgore KS, et al: Use of "natural" hibernation induction triggers for myocardial protection. *Ann Thorac Surg* 64:623-627, 1997.
158. Frerichs KU: Neuroprotective strategies in nature—novel clues for the treatment of stroke and trauma. *Acta Neurochir Suppl* 73:57-61, 1999.
159. Ortmann S, Heldmaier G: Regulation of body temperature and energy requirements of hibernating alpine marmots (Marmota marmota). *Am J Physiol Regul Integr Comp Physiol* 278: R698-R704, 2000.
160. Bottiger BW, Teschendorf P, Krumnikl JJ, et al: Global cerebral ischemia due to cardiocirculatory arrest in mice causes neuronal degeneration and early induction of transcription factor genes in the hippocampus. *Brain Res Mol Brain Res* 65:135-142, 1999.
161. Gourine A, Gonon A, Sjoquist PO, Pernow J: Short-acting calcium antagonist clevidipine protects against reperfusion injury via local nitric oxide-related mechanisms in the jeopardised myocardium. *Cardiovasc Res* 51:100-107, 2001.
162. Behringer W, Prueckner S, Safar P, et al: Rapid induction of mild cerebral hypothermia by cold aortic flush achieves normal recovery in a dog outcome model with 20-minute exsanguination cardiac arrest. *Acad Emerg Med* 7:1341-1348, 2000.
163. Paradis NA, Rose MI, Gawryl MS: Selective aortic perfusion and oxygenation: an effective adjunct to external chest compression-based cardiopulmonary resuscitation. *J Am Coll Cardiol* 23: 497-504, 1994.
164. Becker LB, Weisfeldt ML, Weil MH, et al: The PULSE initiative: scientific priorities and strategic planning for resuscitation research and life saving therapies. *Circulation* 105:2562-2570, 2002.
165. Affairs OoR: *Protection of human subjects*, vol. 2002. 1996, Food and Drug Administration.
166. Services DoHaH: *Informed consent requirements in emergency research*, vol. 2002. OPRR Reports, 1996.
167. Chamnanvanakij S, Perlman JM: Outcome following cardiopulmonary resuscitation in the neonate requiring ventilatory assistance. *Resuscitation* 45:173-180, 2000.
168. Organization ELS. *ECLS registry report*. Ann Arbor, Mich, 2002.
169. National Registry of Cardiopulmonary Resuscitation: National Registry of CPR SAB Participant Report: American Heart Association, 2002.
170. Schindler MB, Bohn D, Cox PN, et al: Outcome of out-of-hospital cardiac or respiratory arrest in children. *N Engl J Med* 335: 1473-1479, 1996.
171. Suominen P, Rasanen J, Kivioja A: Efficacy of cardiopulmonary resuscitation in pulseless paediatric trauma patients. *Resuscitation* 36:9-13, 1998.
172. Suominen P, Korpela R, Kuisma M, et al: Paediatric cardiac arrest and resuscitation provided by physician-staffed emergency care units. *Acta Anaesthesiol* Scand 41:260-265, 1997.
173. Tunstall-Pedoe H, Bailey L, Chamberlain DA, et al: Survey of 3765 cardiopulmonary resuscitations in British hospitals (the BRESUS Study): methods and overall results. *BMJ* 304:1347-1351, 1992.
174. Zaritsky A, Nadkarni V, Getson P, Kuehl K: CPR in children. *Ann Emerg Med* 16:1107-1111, 1987.
175. Bellomo R, Goldsmith D, Uchino S, et al: A prospective before-and-after trial of a medical emergency team. *Med J Aust* 179: 283-287, 2003.
176. DeVita MA, Braithwaite RS, Mahidhara R, et al: Use of medical emergency team responses to reduce hospital cardiopulmonary arrests. *Qual Saf Health Care* 13:251-254, 2004.
177. Rhodes JF, Blaufox AD, Seiden HS, et al: Cardiac arrest in infants after congenital heart surgery. *Circulation* 100:II194-II199, 1999.

178. Morris MC, Wernovsky G, Nadkarni VM: Survival outcomes following extracorporeal cardiopulmonary resuscitation instituted during active chest compressions following refractory in-hospital pediatric arrest. *Pediatr Crit Care Med* 5:440-446, 2004.

179. Dubick MA, Holcomb JB: A review of intraosseous vascular access: current status and military application. *Mil Med* 165: 552-559, 2000.

180. Van den Berghe G, Wouters P, Weekers F, et al: Intensive insulin therapy in critically ill patients. *N Engl J Med* 345:1359-1367, 2001.

Index

C

D

E

I

O

P

U

V

W

X

Y

Z